Medicine

Third Edition
Volume I

Edited by

James M. Rippe, M.D.
Associate Professor of Medicine, Tufts University
School of Medicine, Boston; Director, The Center for
Clinical and Lifestyle Research, Shrewsbury,
Massachusetts

Richard S. Irwin, M.D.
Professor of Medicine, University of Massachusetts
Medical School; Director, Division of Pulmonary,
Allergy, and Critical Care Medicine, University of
Massachusetts Medical Center, Worcester,
Massachusetts

Mitchell P. Fink, M.D.
Johnson & Johnson Professor of Surgery, Harvard
Medical School; Surgeon-in-Chief, Beth Israel Hospital,
Boston

Frank B. Cerra, M.D.
Dean of the Medical School and Professor of Surgery
and Clinical Pharmacy, University of Minnesota Medical
School—Minneapolis

Little, Brown and Company
Boston / New York / Toronto / London

Library of Congress Cataloging-in-Publication Data

Intensive care medicine / edited by James M. Rippe . . . [et al.] — 3rd ed.
  p.   cm.
Includes bibliographical references and index.
ISBN 0-316-74732-7 (vol. 1). — ISBN 0-316-74731-9 (vol. 2). — ISBN 0-316-74728-9 (set)
1. Critical care medicine.   I. Rippe, James M.
  [DNLM: 1. Critical Care. 2. Intensive Care Units.   WX 218 I60424 1996]
RC86.7.I555 1996
616′.028—dc20
DNLM/DLC
for Library of Congress   95-33188
                                                              CIP

Volume I ISBN 0-316-74732-7
Volume II ISBN: 0-316-74731-9
Set ISBN: 0-316-74728-9

Printed in the United States of America
MV-NY

Editorial: Nancy E. Chorpenning, Robert J. Stuart
Development Editor: Julie M. Jewell
Production Services: Ruttle, Shaw & Wetherill, Inc.
Copyeditors: Jane Grochowski, Julie Gillman, Peg
  Markow, Tina Rebane, Dana Singer
Cover Designer: Louis C. Bruno, Jr.

Intensive Care Medicine

Intensive Care

To our families
Stephanie, Diane, Rachel, Sara, Jamie, Rebecca,
Jan, Emily, Matthew, Kathie, Nicole, Christa, and Josh

Contents

XI. Surgical Problems in the Intensive Care Unit

XII. Shock and Trauma

XIII. Neurologic Problems in the Intensive Care Unit

XIV. Transplantation

XV. Metabolism and Nutrition

XVI. Pharmacokinetics and Pharmacodynamics

XVII. Dermatologic, Rheumatologic, and Immunologic Problems in the Intensive Care Unit

XVIII. Psychiatric Issues in Intensive Care

XIX. Moral, Ethical, Legal, and Public Policy Issues in the Intensive Care Unit

Preface

Publication of the third edition of *Intensive Care Medicine* marks a milestone in the history of the text. The first two editions established it as a leading source of information in the rapidly changing and complex field of critical care. The editorial challenge in assembling, writing, and editing the third edition was to ensure that the book changed and improved to meet the rigorous demands of clinicians of all specialties practicing in the adult intensive care environment without losing the fundamental strengths that have made it so popular. We hope and believe that the third edition of *Intensive Care Medicine* has risen to this challenge.

Since the publication of the first edition of *Intensive Care Medicine* over a decade ago, the field of intensive care has changed dramatically and so has the book. The first edition was edited by three cardiologists (James M. Rippe, Joseph S. Alpert, and James E. Dalen) and a pulmonologist/medical intensivist (Richard S. Irwin) and focused largely on medical intensive care. For the second edition we added as senior editor a surgical intensivist (Mitchell P. Fink) with a special interest in shock and trauma. With the third edition we added a second surgical intensivist (Frank B. Cerra) with special interests in nutrition and metabolism and their impact on disease processes. What started as a text focused largely on medical intensive care is now equally balanced between medical and surgical intensive care. This fact reflects our conviction concerning the increasingly unified and cooperative nature of the care of desperately sick individuals treated in modern intensive care units.

The third edition of *Intensive Care Medicine* is 25 percent larger than the second edition and over twice as long as the first. Every section has been fundamentally rewritten, expanded, and updated with major new sections in such crucial areas as transplantation, metabolism and nutrition, and pharmacokinetics. More than 40 new chapters have been added to keep pace with emerging knowledge and developing disciplines.

In medical intensive care important changes and advances have occurred since the publication of our second edition. The major advances have been in our better understanding of the pathophysiology of critical illness and increased knowledge of which therapeutic modalities are and are not likely to be efficacious. We also have acquired a better understanding of which therapies are likely to be harmful. Guided by results from an ever-increasing number of prospective, randomized, controlled studies, the care we now provide our critically ill patients is more scientifically based. For instance, as a reflection of our better understanding of the pathophysiology of respiratory failure, we now mechanically ventilate patients in different ways than we did 5 years ago; this is reflected in the totally rewritten chapter on initiation of mechanical ventilation. Moreover, given the results of randomized, controlled clinical trials, we have come to realize that prophylactic, selective digestive decontamination does not decrease mortality from pneumonia in the medically critically ill patient and that extracorporeal membrane oxygenation does not decrease mortality from the acute respiratory distress syndrome when it is compared with conventional mechanical ventilation.

Clinicians caring for critically ill surgical and medical patients encounter many of the same problems, including shock, acute lung injury, sepsis, and multiple organ system dysfunction. Nev-ertheless, certain issues (e.g., traumatic brain injury, burns, opportunistic infections in immunosuppressed solid organ transplant recipients) are peculiar to surgical patients. Progress in surgical critical care has been evolutionary rather than revolutionary. Many innovations (e.g., bioartificial liver, various substitutes for erythrocyte transition) are in the late stages of development but remain to be adopted as components of standard clinical practice. Even today, however, advances in such diverse areas as diagnostic and interventional radiology, antibiotics, and modes of mechanical ventilation have had major impacts on the care of critically ill surgical patients. Discussions of these and many other areas are incorporated into this edition of *Intensive Care Medicine*.

In coronary care, thrombolytic therapy has revolutionized the treatment of myocardial infarction and the other acute coronary syndromes. The entire coronary care section of the third edition has been rewritten and many new chapters added to emphasize new understandings and protocols based on the major advances in this area.

The complex nature of illnesses treated in the intensive care unit requires a sophisticated understanding of pharmacokinetics as well as nutrition and metabolic aspects of illness. Important new advances have emerged in both of these areas, which are covered in major new sections under the supervision of Frank Cerra.

The challenge we faced in producing the third edition of *Intensive Care Medicine* was broadening our scope to include major new sections in transplantation, coronary care, pharmacokinetics, and nutrition and metabolism without abandoning the practical, clinically oriented approach that many have come to expect from our first two editions. To accomplish this task our editorial approach and conceptual framework remained consistent with the first two editions.

We believe that intensive care is advanced medical and surgical care practiced by physicians possessing the specialized skills, clinical judgment, and knowledge required to treat the most complicated and desperately ill patients. The editorial approach to the book flows from this basic premise. Only conditions requiring the specialized resources of adult medical, surgical, and neurologic intensive care units are covered. Our focus remains on clinical management, while elements of basic history and physical examination, so critical for beginning physicians, are less emphasized.

As in previous editions the text opens with a detailed section on common techniques and procedures in the intensive care unit. This section, which so many have found so useful, has been reorganized and dramatically expanded. Every chapter has been updated with new references and figures. In addition, 13 new chapters have been added, covering such diverse procedures as temporary mechanical assistance of the failing left ventricle, peritoneal dialysis, extracorporeal membrane oxygenation, anesthesia for bedside procedures, and indirect calorimetry.

The next eight sections, which are arranged by organ system, explore major disease entities treated in the intensive care unit. Every chapter has been extensively rewritten and updated to reflect current understanding. Sections related to all aspects of surgical intensive care have been greatly expanded to underscore our balanced editorial approach equally emphasizing medical and surgical intensive care. The overdoses and poisonings section, often sadly lacking or underemphasized in other critical care texts, spans 30 chapters and almost constitutes an intensive care unit toxicology textbook imbedded in a larger book. The neurology, psychiatry, rheumatology, and immunology sections have all been fundamentally rewritten and updated. The moral, ethical, legal, and public policy section has been entirely reconfigured to reflect modern legal and financial realities now faced by intensivists on a daily basis.

As in previous editions, we have focused great attention on editorial consistency and writing clarity. Of course, in any effort of this magnitude certain editorial decisions must be made. Our emphasis remains, as it has been in previous editions, on clinical management. Discussions of pathophysiology are supplemented by extensive referencing to guide clinicians and researchers seeking more in-depth knowledge in this area. Where therapies reflect institutional bias or are considered controversial, we have attempted to indicate this.

Many fine individuals have made important contributions to the production of this book and deserve special recognition and thanks. First and foremost is our editorial coordinator, Elizabeth Porcaro. Beth's high energy, remarkable organizational skills, and unfailing good humor were critical to keeping this project moving forward. Our editorial assistants—Janet La-Bonte, Sherri Herland, Judith Camosse, Karol Lempicki, Joyce Speers, Janet Collins, and Kathy Anderson—have helped manage our busy professional lives while protecting the substantial amount of time required to write and edit. Our publisher and editors at Little, Brown and Company, including Tom Manning, Nancy Chorpenning, and Robert Stuart, have devoted great energy, constructive criticism, and sound guidance throughout the project. Peg Markow was invaluable during the final production process. Our families have provided unfailing love, support, and encouragement. To these individuals, and the many others who have helped in ways too numerous to recount, we are deeply grateful.

We hope that what has resulted from the arduous efforts of many people over the past 3 years is a useful and comprehensive text that will continue to inform, guide, and support intensive care practitioners in their daily efforts to relieve suffering and cure the complex diseases and conditions requiring intensive care management.

J. M. R.
R. S. I.
M. P. F.
F. B. C.

Section Editors

Cynthia K. Aaron, M.D.
Assistant Professor of Emergency Medicine, University of
Massachusetts Medical School; Director, Toxicology Services,
University of Massachusetts Medical Center, Worcester,
Massachusetts
Section X

Jack E. Ansell, M.D.
Professor of Medicine, Boston University School of Medicine;
Vice Chairman, Department of Medicine, Boston University
Medical Center, Boston
Section IX

Richard C. Becker, M.D.
Associate Professor of Internal Medicine, University of
Massachusetts Medical School; Director, Coronary Care Unit
and Thrombosis Research Center, University of Massachusetts
Medical Center, Worcester, Massachusetts
Section III

Lewis E. Braverman, M.D.
Professor of Medicine, Nuclear Medicine, and Physiology,
University of Massachusetts Medical School; Chairman,
Department of Nuclear Medicine, and Chief, Division of
Endocrinology, University of Massachusetts Medical Center,
Worcester, Massachusetts
Section VIII

Frank B. Cerra, M.D.
Dean of the Medical School and Professor of Surgery and
Clinical Pharmacy, University of Minnesota Medical School—
Minneapolis

Ray E. Clouse, M.D.
Professor of Medicine, Washington University School of
Medicine; Associate Physician, Department of Medicine,
Barnes Hospital, St. Louis
Section VII

Andrew J. Cohen, M.D.
Vice Dean of Medical Education, Department of Medicine
(Renal), University of Massachusetts Medical School;
Attending Physician, Department of Medicine, University of
Massachusetts Medical Center, Worcester, Massachusetts
Section V

Frederick J. Curley, M.D.
Associate Professor of Medicine, University of Massachusetts
Medical School; Director, Pulmonary Diagnostic Testing,
University of Massachusetts Medical Center, Worcester,
Massachusetts
Section I and Appendix

David A. Drachman, M.D.
Professor of Neurology and Chairman, Department of
Neurology, University of Massachusetts Medical School;
Chairman, Neurology Service, University of Massachusetts
Medical Center, Worcester, Massachusetts
Section XIII

David L. Dunn, M.D., Ph.D.
Professor of Surgery and Head, Surgical Infectious Diseases,
University of Minnesota—Minneapolis
Section XIV

Richard T. Ellison, M.D.
Associate Professor of Medicine, University of Massachusetts
Medical School; Clinical Director, Division of Infectious
Disease and Immunology, University of Massachusetts
Medical Center, Worcester, Massachusetts
Section VI

Mitchell P. Fink, M.D.
Johnson & Johnson Professor of Surgery, Harvard Medical
School; Surgeon-in-Chief, Beth Israel Hospital, Boston
Sections XI, XII

David F. Giansiracusa, M.D.
Professor of Medicine, University of Massachusetts Medical
School; Associate Chairman, Department of Medicine and
Division of Rheumatology, University of Massachusetts
Medical Center, Worcester, Massachusetts
Section XVII

Joel M. Gore, M.D.
Edward Budnitz Professor of Medicine and Vice Chairman of
Clinical Affairs, Department of Medicine, University of
Massachusetts Medical School; Worcester, Massachusetts
Section II

Stephen O. Heard, M.D.
Associate Professor of Anesthesiology and Surgery, University
of Massachusetts Medical School; Co-Director, Surgical
Intensive Care Unit, and Attending Anesthesiologist,
University of Massachusetts Medical Center, Worcester,
Massachusetts
Section I

Richard S. Irwin, M.D.
Professor of Medicine, University of Massachusetts Medical
School; Director, Division of Pulmonary, Allergy, and Critical
Care Medicine, University of Massachusetts Medical Center,
Worcester, Massachusetts
Section IV

Christopher H. Linden, M.D.
Associate Professor of Emergency Medicine, University of
Massachusetts Medical School; Director, Division of
Toxicology, University of Massachusetts Medical Center,
Worcester, Massachusetts
Section X

Aldo A. Rossini, M.D.
Professor of Medicine, University of Massachusetts Medical
School; Director, Division of Diabetes, University of
Massachusetts Medical Center, Worcester, Massachusetts
Section VIII

Theodore A. Stern, M.D.
Associate Professor of Psychiatry, Harvard Medical School;
Associate Psychiatrist and Director, Resident Psychiatric
Consultation Service, Massachusetts General Hospital, Boston
Section XVIII

Daniel Teres, M.D.
Associate Professor of Medicine and Surgery, Tufts University
School of Medicine, Boston; Director, Adult Critical Care
Division, Basystate Medical Center, Springfield, Massachusetts
Section XIX

Darwin E. Zaske, Pharm.D.
Professor of Pharmacy Practice, University of Minnesota
College of Pharmacy, Minneapolis; Director, Department of
Pharmaceutical Services, St. Paul-Ramsey Medical Center, St.
Paul, Minnesota
Section XVI

Contributing Authors

Cynthia K. Aaron, M.D.
Assistant Professor of Emergency Medicine, University of Massachusetts Medical School; Director, Toxicology Services, University of Massachusetts Medical Center, Worcester, Massachusetts

Tanyia L. Abel, Pharm.D.
Staff Pharmacist, Fairview-Riverside Medical Center, Minneapolis

Susan L. Abend, M.D.
Assistant Professor of Psychiatry, University of Massachusetts Medical School, Worcester, Massachusetts

William T. Adamson, M.D.
Research Fellow, Harrison Department of Surgical Research, University of Pennsylvania School of Medicine; Resident, Department of Surgery, Hospital of the University of Pennsylvania, Philadelphia

David H. Ahrenholz, M.D.
Associate Professor of Surgery, University of Minnesota Medical School—Minneapolis; Associate Director, The Burn Center, Ramsey Medical Center, St. Paul, Minnesota

Joseph S. Alpert, M.D.
Robert S. and Irene P. Flinn Professor of Medicine, University of Arizona College of Medicine; Chairman, Department of Medicine, University Medical Center, Tucson, Arizona

Neil M. Ampel, M.D.
Associate Professor of Medicine, University of Arizona College of Medicine; Staff Physician, Medical Service, Veterans Affairs Medical Center, Tucson, Arizona

Harry L. Anderson III, M.D.
Assistant Professor of Surgery, University of Pennsylvania School of Medicine; Attending Surgeon, Division of Trauma and Surgical Critical Care, Hospital of the University of Pennsylvania, Philadelphia

Jack E. Ansell, M.D.
Professor of Medicine, Boston University School of Medicine; Vice Chairman, Department of Medicine, Boston University Medical Center, Boston

Neil Aronin, M.D.
Professor of Medicine and Cell Biology, University of Massachusetts Medical School; Consultant Endocrinologist, University of Massachusetts Medical Center, Worcester, Massachusetts

Gerard P. Aurigemma, M.D.
Assistant Professor of Cardiovascular Medicine, University of Massachusetts Medical School; Director, Noninvasive Cardiology, University of Massachusetts Medical Center, Worcester, Massachusetts

Daniel T. Baran, M.D.
Professor of Orthopedics, University of Massachusetts Medical School, Worcester, Massachusetts

Robert H. Bartlett, M.D.
Professor of Surgery, University of Michigan Medical School; Director, Surgical Intensive Care Unit, and Chief, Division of Surgical Critical Care, University of Michigan Medical Center, Ann Arbor, Michigan

Steven P. Beaudette, M.D.
Instructor in Medicine, University of Massachusetts Medical School; Fellow, Division of Cardiovascular Medicine, University of Massachusetts Medical Center, Worcester, Massachusetts

Richard C. Becker, M.D.
Associate Professor of Internal Medicine, University of Massachusetts Medical School; Director, Coronary Care Unit and Thrombosis Research Center, University of Massachusetts Medical Center, Worcester, Massachusetts

Alexandra Beckett, M.D.
Assistant Professor of Psychiatry, Harvard Medical School; Director, HIV/AIDS Program, Department of Psychiatry, Beth Israel Hospital, Boston

Stanley B. Benjamin, M.D.
Chief, Division of Gastroenterology, Georgetown University Medical Center, Washington, DC

Joseph R. Benotti, M.D.
Associate Professor of Medicine, University of Massachusetts Medical School; Director, Invasive and Interventional Cardiology, St. Vincent Hospital, Worcester, Massachusetts

Laura Bilohrud, D.O.
Attending Physician, Kaiser Emergency Care Center, St. Joseph Hospital, Denver

Robert M. Black, M.D.
Associate Professor of Renal Medicine, University of Massachusetts Medical School; Director, Renal Division, St. Vincent Hospital, Worcester, Massachusetts

Neil R. Blacklow, M.D.
Richard M. Haidack Distinguished Professor of Medicine and Chairman, Department of Medicine, University of Massachusetts Medical School; Physician-in-Chief, Department of Medicine, University of Massachusetts Medical Center, Worcester, Massachusetts

Andrew M. Blumenfeld, M.D.
Instructor in Neurology, University of Massachusetts Medical School, Worcester, Massachusetts

Gregory J. Bonavita, M.D.
Electrophysiology and Pacing, Co-Director, Pacemaker Center, North Canton, Ohio

Frank V. McL. Booth, M.Sc., B.M.
Associate Professor of Surgery, State University of New York at Buffalo School of Medicine and Biomedical Studies; Chief, Division of Surgical Critical Care, The Buffalo General Hospital, Buffalo, New York

Pamela Borchardt-Phelps, M.D.

Steven Borzak, M.D.
Director, Cardiac Intensive Care Unit, Henry Ford Hospital, Detroit

Alfred A. Bove, M.D., Ph.D.
Bernheimer Professor of Medicine, Temple University School of Medicine; Chief, Department of Cardiology, Temple University Hospital, Philadelphia

Suzanne F. Bradley, M.D.
Assistant Professor of Internal Medicine, University of Michigan Medical School; Staff Physician, Department of Internal Medicine, Veterans Affairs Medical Center, Ann Arbor, Michigan

Lewis E. Braverman, M.D.
Professor of Medicine, Nuclear Medicine, and Physiology, University of Massachusetts Medical School; Chairman, Department of Nuclear Medicine, and Chief, Division of Endocrinology, University of Massachusetts Medical Center, Worcester, Massachusetts

Kenneth L. Brayman, M.D.
Assistant Professor of Surgery, University of Pennsylvania School of Medicine, Philadelphia

Patrick J. Brennan, M.D.

Doreen B. Brettler, M.D.
Professor of Medicine, University of Massachusetts Medical School; Director, New England Hemophilia Center, Medical Center of Central Massachusetts, Worcester, Massachusetts

Mary C. Burke, M.D.
Chief Resident, Division of Emergency Medicine, University of Massachusetts Medical Center, Worcester, Massachusetts

Gerard A. Burns, M.D.
Instructor, Division of Trauma and Critical Care, Yale University School of Medicine, New Haven, Connecticut

Paul E. Buse, M.D.
Fellow in Gastroenterology, Washington University School of Medicine, St. Louis

Michael D. Caldwell, M.D., Ph.D.
Professor of Surgery and Biochemistry, University of Minnesota Medical School—Minneapolis; Surgeon, University of Minnesota Hospital and Clinic of the University of Minnesota Health Sciences Center, Minneapolis

Daniel M. Canafax, Pharm.D.
Professor of Pharmacy Practice, Surgery, and Otolaryngology, University of Minnesota College of Pharmacy and University of Minnesota Medical School—Minneapolis

Christopher P. Cannon, M.D.
Assistant Professor of Medicine, Harvard Medical School, Boston

Ronald P. Caputo, M.D.
Clinical Instructor in Medicine, Harvard Medical School; Clinical Fellow, Division of Cardiology, Beth Israel Hospital, Boston

Ross S. Carol, M.D.
Resident, Division of Emergency Medicine, University of Massachusetts Medical Center, Worcester, Massachusetts

Karen Carroll, M.D.
Assistant Professor of Pathology and Adjunct Assistant Professor of Infectious Disease, University of Utah School of Medicine; Medical Director, Microbiology Laboratory, Associated Regional and University Pathologists, Salt Lake City

Philip F. Caushaj, M.D.
Associate Professor of Surgery, University of Massachusetts Medical School; Chairman, Department of Surgery, The Medical Center of Central Massachusetts, Worcester, Massachusetts

Frank B. Cerra, M.D.
Dean of the Medical School and Professor of Surgery and Clinical Pharmacy, University of Minnesota Medical School—Minneapolis

David A. Chad, M.D.
Professor of Neurology, University of Massachusetts Medical School; Attending Neurologist, University of Massachusetts Medical Center, Worcester, Massachusetts

Gary L. C. Chan, M.D.

Eugene B. Chang, M.D.
Associate Professor of Medicine, University of Chicago, Division of the Biological Sciences, Pritzker School of Medicine, Chicago

Sarah H. Cheeseman, M.D.
Professor of Medicine, Pediatrics, Molecular Genetics, and Microbiology, University of Massachusetts Medical School, Worcester, Massachusetts

Glenn M. Chertow, M.D.
Clinical Research Fellow, Division of Nephrology, Harvard Medical School; Amgen Clinical Scientist in Nephrology, American Kidney Fund, Boston

William K. Chiang, M.D.
Clinical Assistant Professor of Surgery/Emergency Medicine, New York University School of Medicine; Research Director, Department of Emergency Medicine, Bellevue Hospital Center, New York

Bernard D. Clifford, M.D.
Fellow, Division of Digestive Disease and Nutrition, University of Massachusetts Medical Center, Worcester, Massachusetts

David M. Clive, M.D.
Associate Professor of Medicine, University of Massachusetts Medical School; Residency Program Director, Department of Medicine, University of Massachusetts Medical Center, Worcester, Massachusetts

Christopher A. Clyne, M.D.
Director, Electrophysiology Laboratory, Community Medical Center, Scranton, Pennsylvania

Andrew J. Cohen, M.D.
Vice Dean of Medical Education, Department of Medicine (Renal), University of Massachusetts Medical School; Attending Physician, Department of Medicine, University of Massachusetts Medical Center, Worcester, Massachusetts

Stephen M. Cohn, M.D.
Associate Professor of Surgery, Yale University School of Medicine; Chief, Section of Trauma and Surgical Critical Care, Yale New Haven Hospital, New Haven, Connecticut

Jonathan F. Critchlow, M.D.
Assistant Professor of Surgery, Harvard Medical School; Co-Director, Respiratory-Surgical Intensive Care Unit, Beth Israel Hospital, Boston

Thomas G. Cropley, M.D.
Assistant Professor of Dermatology, University of Massachusetts Medical School; Dermatologist, University of Massachusetts Medical Center, Worcester, Massachusetts

Carlos Cuello, M.D.
Electrophysiology and Pacing, Director, Pacemaker Center, North Canton, Ohio

Frederick J. Curley, M.D.
Associate Professor of Medicine, University of Massachusetts Medical School; Director, Pulmonary Diagnostic Testing, University of Massachusetts Medical Center, Worcester, Massachusetts

Bruce S. Cutler, M.D.
Professor of Surgery, University of Massachusetts Medical School; Chairman, Division of Vascular Surgery, University of Massachusetts Medical Center, Worcester, Massachusetts

Seth T. Dahlberg, M.D.
Assistant Professor of Medicine, University of Massachusetts Medical Center; Physician, Division of Cardiology, University of Massachusetts Medical Center, Worcester, Massachusetts

James E. Dalen, M.D.
Vice Provost for Health Sciences, University of Arizona College of Medicine, Tucson, Arizona

Dimitar Danchev, M.D.
Assistant Professor of Medicine, Johns Hopkins Medical Center, Baltimore

Ashley Davidoff, M.D.
Associate Professor of Radiology, University of Massachusetts Medical School; Director, Abdominal Imaging, University of Massachusetts Medical Center, Worcester, Massachusetts

Robin I. Davidson, M.D.
Associate Professor of Surgery and Pediatrics, University of Massachusetts Medical School; Attending Neurosurgeon, University of Massachusetts Medical Center, Worcester, Massachusetts

John A. Dawson, M.D.
Associate Professor of Surgery, State University of New York Health Science Center at Syracuse College of Medicine; Director, Burn Unit and Surgical Critical Care Service, University Hospital, Syracuse, New York

Edwin A. Deitch, M.D.
Professor of Surgery and Chairman, Department of Surgery, UMDNJ-New Jersey Medical School; Surgeon and Chief, Department of Surgery, University Hospital, Newark, New Jersey

James Desemone, M.D.
Assistant Professor of Medicine, University of Massachusetts Medical School; Attending Physician, Division of Diabetes, University of Massachusetts Medical Center, Worcester, Massachusetts

Donald J. Deyo, D.V.M.
Assistant Professor of Anesthesiology, University of Texas Medical Branch, University of Texas Medical School at Galveston, Galveston, Texas

Sam T. Donta, M.D.
Professor and Associate Chairman of Medicine, University of Connecticut Health Center, Farmington, Connecticut

Robert P. Dowsett, B.M.
Fellow in Medical Toxicology, Department of Emergency Medicine, University of Massachusetts Medical Center, Worcester, Massachusetts

David A. Drachman, M.D.
Professor of Neurology and Chairman, Department of Neurology, University of Massachusetts Medical School; Chairman, Neurology Service, University of Massachusetts Medical Center, Worcester, Massachusetts

Thomas E. Ducker, M.D.

Gary L. Dudek, M.D.
Clinical Assistant Professor of Medicine, University of Rochester School of Medicine and Dentistry; Medical Director, Respiratory Therapy, The Genesee Hospital, Rochester, New York

David N. Dunbar, M.D.
Assistant Professor of Internal Medicine, University of Minnesota Medical School—Minneapolis; Director, Electrophysiology Laboratory, Hennepin County Medical Center, Minneapolis

David L. Dunn, M.D., Ph.D.
Professor of Surgery and Head, Surgical Infectious Diseases, University of Minnesota—Minneapolis

Philip A. Edelman, M.D.
Associate Professor of Medicine, Vanderbilt University School of Medicine; Chief, Section of Occupational and Environmental Medicine, Vanderbilt University Medical Center, Center for Clinical Toxicology, Nashville, Tennessee

Steven A. Edmundowicz, M.D.
Associate Professor of Medicine, Jefferson Medical College of Thomas Jefferson University; Chief of Endoscopy and Director of Clinical Gastrointestinal Services, Thomas Jefferson University Hospital, Philadelphia

William T. Edwards, M.D., Ph.D.
Associate Professor of Anesthesiology, University of Washington School of Medicine; Director, Pain Relief Service, Harborview Medical Center, Seattle

M. Francesca Egidi, M.D.

Richard S. Eisenstaedt, M.D.
Professor of Medicine, Temple University School of Medicine; Deputy Chair, Department of Medicine, Temple University Hospital, Philadelphia

Charles H. Emerson, M.D.
Professor of Medicine, University of Massachusetts Medical School, Worcester, Massachusetts

Nancy J. Evans, M.D.

Patrick G. Fairchild, M.D.
Associate Professor of Infectious Diseases and Immunology, University of Massachusetts Medical School; Director, HIV Clinical Center, University of Massachusetts Medical Center, Worcester, Massachusetts

Alan P. Farwell, M.D.
Assitant Professor of Medicine, University of Massachusetts Medical School; Attending Staff Physician, Department of Medicine, University of Massachusetts Medical Center, Worcester, Massachusetts

Alan M. Fein, M.D.
Professor of Medicine, State University of New York at Stony Brook, Health Sciences Center School of Medicine; Director, Division of Pulmonary and Critical Care Medicine, Winthrop-University Hospital, Mineola, New York

I. Alan Fein, M.D.
President, Critical Care Management Consultants, Inc., Albany, New York; Attending Physician, Department of Critical Care Medicine, Baptist Hospital of Miami, Miami

Kevin J. Felice, D.O.
Assistant Professor of Neurology, University of Connecticut School of Medicine; Attending Neurologist, University of Connecticut Health Center, Farmington, Connecticut

Robert P. Ferm, M.D.
Assistant Professor of Emergency Medicine, University of Massachusetts Medical School; Director, Medical Toxicology Fellowship, University of Massachusetts Medical Center, Worcester, Massachusetts

Massimo S. Fiandaca, M.D.
Clinical Assistant Professor of Neurological Surgery, Johns Hopkins University School of Medicine and University of Maryland School of Medicine, Baltimore

Mitchell P. Fink, M.D.
Johnson & Johnson Professor of Surgery, Harvard Medical School; Surgeon-in-Chief, Beth Israel Hospital, Boston

Judy Fish, M.M.Sc., R.D., C.N.S.D.
Nutrition Support Dietician, Geisinger Medical Center, Danville, Pennsylvania

Marc Fisher, M.D.
Professor of Neurology, University of Massachusetts Medical School; Chief, Department of Neurology, Medical Center of Central Massachusetts, Worcester, Massachusetts

Glenn Focht, M.D.
Instructor in Medicine, University of Massachusetts Medical School, Worcester, Massachusetts

Nancy M. Fontneau, M.D.
Instructor in Neurology, University of Massachusetts Medical School; Attending Neurologist, University of Massachusetts Medical Center, Worcester, Massachusetts

Marsha D. Ford, M.D.
Assistant Clinical Professor of Emergency Medicine, University of North Carolina at Chapel Hill School of Medicine, Chapel Hill; Director, Division of Medical Toxicology, and Assistant Chairman, Department of Emergency Medicine, Carolinas Medical Center, Charlotte, North Carolina

Cynthia T. French, M.S., R.N., C.S.
Coordinator of Division Clinical Programs, Division of Pulmonary, Allergy, and Critical Care Medicine, University of Massachusetts Medical Center, Worcester, Massachusetts

Gary M. Fudem, M.D.
Assistant Professor of Plastic Surgery, University of Massachusetts Medical School; Attending Surgeon, Division of Plastic Surgery, University of Massachusetts Medical Center, Worcester, Massachusetts

R. Brent Furbee, M.D.
Medical Director, Indiana Poison Center, Methodist Hospital of Indiana, Indianapolis

Nelson M. Gantz, M.D.
Clinical Professor of Medicine, Pennsylvania State University College of Medicine, Hershey; Chairman, Department of Medicine, and Chief, Division of Infectious Diseases, Polyclinic Medical Center, Harrisburg, Pennsylvania

Leonard I. Ganz, M.D.
Instructor in Medicine, Harvard Medical School, Boston

Marie J. George, M.D.
Assistant Professor of Infectious Disease and Immunology, University of Massachusetts Medical School, Worcester, Massachusetts

Edith S. Geringer, M.D.
Instructor in Psychiatry, Harvard Medical School; Co-Director, Primary Care Psychiatry Clinic, Massachusetts General Hospital, Boston

David F. Giansiracusa, M.D.
Professor of Medicine, University of Massachusetts Medical School; Associate Chairman, Department of Medicine and Division of Rheumatology, University of Massachusetts Medical Center, Worcester, Massachusetts

Richard H. Glew, M.D.
Professor of Medicine, Molecular Genetics, and Microbiology, University of Massachusetts Medical School; Academic Physician-in-Chief and Chairman, Department of Medicine, The Medical Center of Central Massachusetts, Worcester, Massachusetts

Junius J. Gonzales, M.D.
Assistant Professor of Psychiatry, Georgetown University School of Medicine; Director of Clinical Programs, Department of Psychiatry, Georgetown University Medical Center, Washington

Peter A. Gottlieb, M.D.
Assistant Professor of Pediatrics and Medicine, University of Colorado School of Medicine; Associate Physician, Barbara Davis Center for Childhood Diabetes, Young Adult Clinic, University of Colorado Health Sciences Center, Denver

Steven A. Gould, M.D.
Professor of Surgery, University of Illinois College of Medicine; Attending Surgeon, Michael Reese Hospital and Medical Center, Chicago

Donna B. Greenberg, M.D.
Assistant Professor of Psychiatry, Harvard Medical School; Associate Psychiatrist, Massachusetts General Hospital, Boston

Harry L. Greene, M.D.
Associate Professor of Internal Medicine, University of Arizona College of Medicine; Chief, Section of General Medicine, University of Arizona Health Sciences Center, Tucson, Arizona

Trevor O. Greene, M.D.
Assistant Professor of Medicine, University of Massachusetts Medical School; Director, Electrophysiology and Arrhythmia Service, St. Vincent Hospital, Worcester, Massachusetts

Donna R. Grogan, M.D.
Assistant Professor of Medicine, Department of Internal Medicine, University of Massachusetts Medical School, Worcester, Massachusetts

Ronald F. Grossman, M.D.
Associate Professor of Medicine, University of Toronto Faculty of Medicine; Head, Division of Respiratory Medicine, Mount Sinai Hospital, Toronto

Scott A. Gruber, M.D.

Ranier W. G. Gruessner, M.D.
Associate Professor of Surgery, University of Minnesota—Minneapolis

David R. P. Guay, Pharm.D.
Associate Professor, University of Minnesota College of Pharmacy, Minneapolis

Faustino Guinto, M.D.

Guillermo Gutierrez, M.D., Ph.D.
Professor of Pulmonary and Critical Care Medicine, University of Texas Medical School at Houston; Director, Medical Intensive Care Unit, Hermann Hospital, Houston

Nadim G. Haddad, M.D.
Assistant Professor of Medicine, Yale University School of Medicine, New Haven, Connecticut

Charles I. Haffajee, M.D.
Associate Professor of Medicine, Tufts University School of Medicine; Director, Cardiac Electrophysiology and Pacing Service, St. Elizabeth's Hospital, Boston

Alan H. Hall, M.D.
Clinical Assistant Professor of Preventive Medicine and Biometrics, University of Colorado School of Medicine; Editor-in-Chief, TOMES and TOMES Plus Information Systems, Micromedex, Inc., Denver

Ira M. Hanan, M.D.
Assistant Professor of Medicine, University of Chicago, Division of the Biological Sciences, Pritzker School of Medicine; Attending Physician, Section of Gastroenterology, University of Chicago Medical Center, Chicago

Stephen B. Hanauer, M.D.
Associate Professor of Medicine, University of Chicago, Division of the Biological Sciences, Pritzker School of Medicine; Attending Physician, Section of Gastroenterology, University of Chicago Medical Center, Chicago

Daniel Hanley, M.D.
Director, Neurosciences Critical Care Unit, Johns Hopkins Medical Center, Baltimore

Shawn Hansen, Pharm.D.
Clinical Specialist in Cardiology, Marshfield Clinic, Marshfield, Wisconsin

Robert A. Harrington, M.D.
Assistant Professor of Cardiology, Duke University School of Medicine; Interventional Cardiologist, Duke University Medical Center, Durham, North Carolina

Stephen O. Heard, M.D.
Associate Professor of Anesthesiology and Surgery, University of Massachusetts Medical School; Co-Director, Surgical Intensive Care Unit, and Attending Anesthesiologist, University of Massachusetts Medical Center, Worcester, Massachusetts

Robert C. Hendel, M.D.
Assistant Professor of Medicine, Northwestern University Medical School; Associate Director, Coronary Care Unit, Northwestern Memorial Hospital, Chicago

Robert J. Heyka, M.D.
Staff Physician, Nephrology/Hypertension, Cleveland Clinic Foundation, Cleveland

Lori L. Hoey, Pharm.D.
Assistant Professor, University of Minnesota College of Pharmacy, Minneapolis

Helen M. Hollingsworth, M.D.
Associate Professor of Medicine, Boston University School of Medicine; Director, Asthma and Allergy Services, Boston University Medical Center, Boston

Thomas A. Holly, M.D.
Fellow, Division of Cardiovascular Medicine, University of Massachusetts Medical School, Worcester, Massachusetts

Shoei K. S. Huang, M.D.
Professor of Medicine, University of Massachusetts Medical School; Director, Section of Cardiac Electrophysiology and Pacing, University of Massachusetts Medical Center, Worcester, Massachusetts

Rolf D. Hubmayr, M.D.
Professor of Pulmonary and Critical Care Medicine, Mayo
Medical School; Director, Pulmonary Research Unit, Mayo
Clinic, Rochester, Minnesota

James Hughes, M.D.
Assistant Professor of Surgery, University of Massachusetts
Medical School; Attending Otolaryngologist, University of
Massachusetts Medical Center, Worcester, Massachusetts

Richard S. Irwin, M.D.
Professor of Medicine, University of Massachusetts Medical
School; Director, Division of Pulmonary, Allergy, and Critical
Care Medicine, University of Massachusetts Medical Center,
Worcester, Massachusetts

J. Edward Jackson, M.D.
Associate Adjunct Professor of Medicine and Associate
Clinical Professor of Pharmacology, University of California,
San Diego, School of Medicine, La Jolla, California; Attending
Physician, Department of Medicine/Geriatrics, University of
California, San Diego, Medical Center, San Diego

Teresa E. Jacobs, M.D.
Clinical Instructor in Pulmonary and Critical Care Medicine,
University of Washington School of Medicine; Active Staff,
Department of Medicine, Swedish Medical Center, Providence
Medical Center, Seattle

Eric W. Jacobson, M.D.
Assistant Professor of Medicine, University of Massachusetts
Medical School, Worcester, Massachusetts

Connie A. Jastremski, M.S., R.N.
Adjunct Assistant Professor of Nursing, State University of
New York Health Science Center at Syracuse College of
Medicine; Director, Critical Care and Emergency Nursing,
University Hospital, Syracuse, New York

Michael S. Jastremski, M.D.
Director, Department of Critical Care, State University of New
York Health Sciences Center at Syracuse, Syracuse, New York

Peter J. Jederlinic, M.D.
Assistant Professor of Medicine, Columbia University College
of Physicians and Surgeons, New York; Director, Critical Care
Medicine, Mary Imogene Bassett Hospital, Cooperstown, New
York

Shailendra Joshi, M.D.

Wandana Joshi-Ryzewicz, D.O.
Assistant Professor of Anesthesiology, Tufts University School
of Medicine, Boston; Staff Anesthesiologist, Baystate Medical
Center, Springfield, Massachusetts

Carol A. Kauffman, M.D.
Professor of Internal Medicine, University of Michigan Medical
School; Chief, Infectious Diseases Section, Veterans Affairs
Medical Center, Ann Arbor, Michigan

Shubjeet Kaur, M.D.
Assistant Professor of Anesthesiology, University of
Massachusetts Medical School; Clinical Director, Department
of Anesthesiology, University of Massachusetts Medical
Center, Worcester, Massachusetts

Thomas E. Kearney, Pharm.D.
Clinical Professor of Pharmacy, University of California, San
Francisco, School of Pharmacy; Managing Director, San
Francisco Bay Area Regional Poison Control Center, San
Francisco General Hospital, San Francisco

Brian J. Kelly, M.D.
Head, Department of Critical Care Medicine, National Naval
Medical Center, Bethesda, Maryland

John G. Kelton, M.D.
Professor of Medicine and Pathology, McMaster University
School of Medicine; Chief, Department of Medicine, Chedoke-
McMaster Hospitals, Hamilton, Ontario, Canada

Mark A. Keroack, M.D.
Associate Professor of Infectious Diseases, University of
Massachusetts Medical School; Chief, Section of Infectious
Diseases, The Medical Center of Central Massachusetts,
Worcester, Massachusetts

Daniel Y. Kim, M.D.
Assistant Professor of Otolaryngology (Head and Neck
Surgery), University of Massachusetts Medical School; Chief,
Head and Neck Surgery, Division of Otolaryngology,
University of Massachusetts Medical Center, Worcester,
Massachusetts

Carey D. Kimmelstiel, M.D.
Assistant Professor of Medicine, Tufts University School of
Medicine; Assistant Director, Cardiac Catheterization
Laboratory, New England Medical Center Hospital, Boston

Mark A. Kirk, M.D.
Director, Medical Toxicology Fellowship, Indiana Poison
Center, Methodist Hospital, Indianapolis

Craig S. Kitchens, M.D.
Professor of Medicine and Vice Chairman, Department of
Medicine, University of Florida College of Medicine; Chief,
Medical Service, Veterans Affairs Medical Center, Gainesville,
Florida

Philip R. Kohls, Pharm.D.
Research Fellow, Department of Surgery, University of
Minnesota Medical School—Minneapolis; Clinical Pharmacist,
St. Paul-Ramsey Medical Center, St. Paul, Minnesota

Marin H. Kollef, M.D.
Assistant Professor of Internal Medicine, Washington
University School of Medicine; Medical Director, Respiratory
Therapy, and Assistant Director, Medical Intensive Care Unit,
Barnes Hospital, St. Louis

Peter E. Krims, M.D.
Assistant Professor of Medicine, University of Massachusetts
Medical School; Director, Endoscopic Services, University of
Massachusetts Medical Center, Worcester, Massachusetts

Ken Kulig, M.D.
Associate Clinical Professor of Trauma and Emergency
Medicine, University of Colorado School of Medicine;
Director, Porter Regional Toxicology Center, Porter Memorial
Hospital, Denver

Ajay Kumar, M.D.
Fellow in Gastroenterology, University of Tennessee College of Medicine, Memphis

Lawrence A. Labbate, M.D.

F. Marc LaForce, M.D.
Professor of Medicine, University of Rochester School of Medicine and Dentistry; Physician-in-Chief, Department of Medicine, The Genesee Hospital, Rochester, New York

Roger Laham, M.D.
Fellow in Cardiology, Beth Israel Hospital, Boston

Robert A. Lancey, M.D.
Assistant Professor of Surgery, University of Massachusetts Medical School; Attending Surgeon, Division of Thoracic and Cardiac Surgery, University of Massachusetts Medical Center, Worcester, Massachusetts

Laurence Landow, M.D.
Assistant Professor of Anesthesia and Surgery, University of Massachusetts Medical School, Worcester, Massachusetts

Stephen E. Lapinsky, M.D.
Assistant Professor of Medicine, University of Toronto; Staff Physician, Division of Respirology, Mt. Sinai Hospital, Toronto, Canada

John M. Lazarus, M.D.
Associate Professor of Medicine, Harvard Medical School; Director of Clinical Services, Division of Nephrology, Brigham and Women's Hospital, Boston

Stanley Lemeshow, Ph.D.
Professor of Biostatistics, University of Massachusetts School of Public Health and Health Sciences, Amherst, Massachusetts

Peter H. Levine, M.D.
Professor of Medicine, University of Massachusetts Medical School; Director, Blood Research Laboratory, and Physician-in-Chief, Medical Center of Central Massachusetts, Worcester, Massachusetts

William J. Lewander, M.D.
Associate Professor of Pediatrics, Brown University School of Medicine; Director, Pediatric Emergency Medicine, Hasbro Children's Hospital, Providence, Rhode Island

James G. Linakis, M.D., Ph.D.
Assistant Professor of Pediatrics, Brown University School of Medicine; Attending Physician, Emergency Department, Hasbro Children's Hospital/Rhode Island Hospital, Providence, Rhode Island

Christopher H. Linden, M.D.
Associate Professor of Emergency Medicine, University of Massachusetts Medical School; Director, Division of Toxicology, University of Massachusetts Medical Center, Worcester, Massachusetts

Carol F. Lippa, M.D.
Assistant Professor of Neurology, University of Massachusetts Medical School, Worcester, Massachusetts

Alan Lisbon, M.D.
Assistant Professor of Anesthesia, Harvard Medical School; Director, Division of Critical Care, Beth Israel Hospital, Boston

Nancy Y. N. Liu, M.D.
Assistant Professor of Medicine, University of Massachusetts Medical School, Worcester, Massachusetts

Bruce Lohr, Pharm.D.
Clinical Assistant Professor of Pharmacy, University of Minnesota College of Pharmacy; Clinical Specialist, Department of Pharmacy, University of Minnesota Hospital and Clinic of the University of Minnesota Health Sciences Center, Minneapolis

Randall R. Long, M.D., Ph.D.
Associate Professor of Neurology, University of Massachusetts Medical School; Vice-Chair, Department of Neurology, University of Massachusetts Medical Center, Worcester, Massachusetts

Christopher Longcope, M.D.
Professor of Medicine, University of Massachusetts Medical School; Attending Physician, Department of Obstetrics/Gynecology, University of Massachusetts Medical Center, Worcester, Massachusetts

Ana M. Lopez, M.D., M.P.H.
Research Fellow, Oncology Section, Department of Internal Medicine, University of Arizona, Tucson, Arizona

Donald G. Love, M.D.

John M. Luce, M.D.
Professor of Medicine and Anesthesia, University of California, San Francisco, School of Medicine; Associate Director, Medical Surgical Intensive Care Unit, San Francisco General Hospital, San Francisco

Margaret M. McCarron, M.D.
Professor of Internal Medicine and Emergency Medicine, University of Southern California School of Medicine; Associate Chief of Staff, Medical Administration, Los Angeles County/University of Southern California Medical Center, Los Angeles

George R. McKendall, M.D.
Assistant Professor of Medicine, Brown University School of Medicine; Director, Coronary Care Unit, Rhode Island Hospital, Providence, Rhode Island

Karl J. Madaras-Kelly, M.D.

J. Mark Madison, M.D.
Assistant Professor of Medicine, University of Massachusetts Medical School; Attending Physician, Division of Pulmonary, Allergy, and Critical Care Medicine, University of Massachusetts Medical Center, Worcester, Massachusetts

Henry J. Mann, Pharm.D.
Associate Professor of Pharmacy Practice, University of Minnesota College of Pharmacy; Critical Care Research Pharmacist, University of Minnesota Hospital and Clinic of the University of Minnesota Health Sciences Center, Minneapolis

Anthony S. Manoguerra, Pharm.D.
Professor of Clinical Pharmacy, University of California, San Francisco, School of Pharmacy; Director, San Diego Regional Poison Center, University of California, San Diego, Medical Center, San Diego

Susan J. Markowsky, Pharm.D.
Assistant Clinical Professor of Pharmacy Practice, University of Florida College of Pharmacy, Gainesville; Pharmacotherapy Specialist, Critical Care, Tampa General Hospital, Tampa, Florida

John R. Mathias, M.D.

Todd W. Mattox, Pharm.D.
Clinical Associate Professor, University of Florida College of Pharmacy; Nutrition Support Pharmacist, H. Lee Moffitt Cancer Center and Research Institute

Mani Menon, M.D.
Professor of Surgery and Physiology, University of Massachusetts Medical School; Chairman, Division of Urology and Transplantation Surgery, University of Massachusetts Medical Center, Worcester, Massachusetts

Ronald W. Mike, B.S., R.R.T.
Respiratory Therapist IV/Support Services, Division of Pulmonary, Allergy, and Critical Care Medicine, University of Massachusetts Medical Center, Worcester, Massachusetts

David I. Min, Pharm.D.
Assistant Professor of Pharmacy Practice, Northeastern University College of Pharmacy and Allied Health Professions; Clinical Pharmacist, Division of Organ Transplantation, New England Deaconess Hospital, Boston

Ann L. Mitchell, M.D.
Assistant Professor of Neurology, University of Massachusetts Medical School, Worcester, Massachusetts

Robert S. Mittleman, M.D.
Assistant Professor of Medicine, University of Massachusetts Medical School; Associate Director, Section of Cardiac Electrophysiology and Pacing, University of Massachusetts Medical Center, Worcester, Massachusetts

Michael G. Mooradd, M.D.
Assistant Professor of Medicine, University of Massachusetts Medical School, Worcester; Attending Cardiologist, Berkshire Medical Center, Pittsfield, Massachusetts

John P. Mordes, M.D.
Professor of Medicine, University of Massachusetts Medical School; Attending Physician, University of Massachusetts Medical Center, Worcester, Massachusetts

Gail Morrison, M.D.
Associate Dean for Clinical Curriculum, University of Pennsylvania School of Medicine; Associate Chairman, Department of Medicine, Hospital of the University of Pennsylvania, Philadelphia

Anne C. Mosenthal, M.D.
Assistant Professor of Surgery, UMDNJ-New Jersey Medical School, Newark; Chief, Laparoendoscopic Surgery, Veterans Affairs Medical Center, East Orange, New Jersey

Gerald S. Moss, M.D.
Dean, College of Medicine, University of Illinois at Chicago

Jonathan S. Moulton, M.D.

James B. Mowry, Pharm.D.
Affiliate Assistant Professor of Pharmacy Practice, Purdue University School of Pharmacy and Pharmacal Sciences, West Lafayette, Indiana; Director, Indiana Poison Center, Methodist Hospital of Indiana, Indianapolis

James L. Mullen, M.D.
Professor of Surgery and Director of Surgery Education, University of Pennsylvania School of Medicine, Philadelphia

Avi Nahum, M.D.
Assistant Professor of Medicine, University of Minnesota Medical School—Minneapolis; Director, Medical Intensive Care Unit, St. Paul-Ramsey Medical Center, St. Paul

Lena M. Napolitano, M.D.
Assistant Professor of Surgery, University of Massachusetts Medical School; Director, Surgical Critical Care, and Co-Director, Trauma Services, University of Massachusetts Medical Center, Worcester, Massachusetts

Gerald Nash, M.D.
Professor of Pathology, Tufts University School of Medicine, Boston; Chairman, Department of Pathology, Baystate Medical Center, Springfield, Massachusetts

Constance Nichols, M.D.

Michael S. Niederman, M.D.
Associate Professor of Medicine, State University of New York at Stony Brook Health Sciences Center School of Medicine, Stony Brook, New York; Director, Critical Care Subsection, Winthrop-University Hospital, Mineola, New York

Robert L. Norris, M.D.
Assistant Professor of Surgery, Stanford University School of Medicine; Associate Director, Division of Emergency Medicine, Stanford University Hospital, Stanford, California

Ira S. Ockene, M.D.
Professor of Cardiovascular Medicine, University of Massachusetts Medical School; Associate Director, Division of Cardiovascular Medicine, and Director, Preventive Cardiology Program, University of Massachusetts Medical Center, Worcester, Massachusetts

Timothy P. O'Connor, M.D.
Assistant Professor of Surgery, Southern Illinois University School of Medicine, Springfield, Illinois

Okike N. Okike, M.D.
Professor of Cardiothoracic Surgery, University of Massachusetts Medical School; Vice Chairman, Division of Cardiothoracic Surgery, University of Massachusetts Medical Center, Worcester, Massachusetts

Kent R. Olson, M.D.
Associate Clinical Professor of Medicine, University of California, San Francisco, School of Medicine; Medical Director, San Francisco Bay Area Regional Poison Control Center, San Francisco General Hospital, San Francisco

Steven M. Opal, M.D.
Associate Professor of Medicine, Brown University School of Medicine, Providence; Director, Infection Control Service, Memorial Hospital of Rhode Island, Pawtucket, Rhode Island

David A. Orsinelli, M.D.
Assistant Professor of Clinical Internal Medicine, Ohio State University College of Medicine; Attending Physician, Echocardiography Laboratory, The University Hospitals, Columbus, Ohio

Carlos R. Ortiz, M.D.
Associate Professor of Medicine and Anesthesiology, University of Rochester School of Medicine and Dentistry; Medical Director, Intensive Care Unit, The Genesee Hospital, Rochester, New York

William F. Owen, Jr., M.D.
Assistant Professor of Medicine, Harvard Medical School; Assistant Director of Dialysis, Brigham and Women's Hospital, Boston

Linda A. Pape, M.D.
Associate Professor of Cardiovascular Medicine and Pathology, University of Massachusetts Medical School; Attending Physician, Division of Cardiovascular Medicine, University of Massachusetts Medical Center, Worcester, Massachusetts

John A. Paraskos, M.D.
Professor of Medicine, University of Massachusetts Medical School; Director, Diagnostic Cardiology, University of Massachusetts Medical Center, Worcester, Massachusetts

John J. Paris, Ph.D.
Walsh Professor of Bioethics, Theology Department, Boston College; Clinical Professor of Community Health, Department of Community Health, Tufts University School of Medicine, Boston

Margaret M. Parker, M.D.
Associate Professor of Pediatrics, State University of New York at Stony Brook Health Sciences Center School of Medicine; Director, Pediatric Intensive Care Unit, University Medical Center, Stony Brook, New York

Liberto Pechet, M.D.
Professor Emeritus of Hematology/Oncology and Pathology, University of Massachusetts Medical School; Director, Hematology Laboratory, University of Massachusetts Medical Center, Worcester, Massachusetts

Paul R. Pentel, M.D.
Associate Professor of Medicine and Pharmacology, University of Minnesota Medical School—Minneapolis; Senior Physician, Division of Clinical Pharmacology and Toxicology, Hennepin County Medical Center, Minneapolis

Felix Perez-Villa, M.D.

A. Thomas Pezzella, M.D.
Associate Professor of Cardiothoracic Surgery, University of Massachusetts Medical School; Attending Cardiothoracic Surgeon, University of Massachusetts Medical Center, Worcester, Massachusetts

Catherine A. Phillips, M.D.
Assistant Professor of Neurology, University of Massachusetts Medical School; Director, EEG Laboratory, University of Massachusetts Medical Center, Worcester, Massachusetts

Daniel Picus, M.D.
Assistant Professor of Radiology, Washington University School of Medicine; Chief, Vascular Interventional Radiology, Mallinckrodt Institute of Radiology, Barnes Hospital, St. Louis

Mark H. Pollack, M.D.
Associate Professor of Psychiatry, Harvard Medical School; Director, Anxiety Disorders Program, Massachusetts General Hospital, Boston

Debra D. Poutsiaka, M.D.
Assistant Professor of Medicine, Division of Infectious Disease and Immunology, University of Massachusetts Medical School, Worcester, Massachusetts

Melvin R. Pratter, M.D.
Professor of Medicine, University of Medicine and Dentistry of New Jersey, Robert Wood Johnson Medical School at Camden; Head, Division of Pulmonary and Critical Care Medicine, Cooper Hospital/University Medical Center, Camden, New Jersey

Donald S. Prough, M.D.
Professor of Anesthesiology and Chairman, Department of Anesthesiology, University of Texas Medical Branch, University of Texas Medical School at Galveston; Medical Director, Surgical Intensive Care Unit, John Sealy Hospital, Galveston, Texas

Juan C. Puyana, M.D.
Assistant Professor of Surgery, University of Massachusetts Medical School, Worcester; Director, Surgical Intensive Care Unit, Brockton/West Roxbury Veterans Affairs Medical Center, West Roxbury, Massachusetts

G. Forrest Quimby, M.D.
Chief Resident, Department of Urology, University of Massachusetts Medical Center, Worcester, Massachusetts

Vassilios Raptopoulos, M.D.
Professor of Radiology, University of Massachusetts Medical School; Director, Abdominal Imaging, University of Massachusetts Medical Center, Worcester, Massachusetts

Paula Ravin, M.D.
Assistant Professor of Neurology, University of Massachusetts Medical School; Active Staff, Department of Neurology, University of Massachusetts Medical Center, Worcester, Massachusetts

Frank E. Reardon, J.D., M.S.
Attorney, Hassan and Reardon, Boston

Lawrence D. Recht, M.D.
Associate Professor of Neurology and Surgery, University of Massachusetts Medical School, Worcester, Massachusetts

Francis Renzi, M.D.
Assistant Professor of Emergency Medicine, University of Massachusetts Medical School, Worcester, Massachusetts

Marc Restuccia, M.D.
Resident, Division of Emergency Medicine, University of Massachusetts Medical Center, Worcester, Massachusetts

Randall R. Reves, M.D.
Associate Professor of Infectious Disease, University of Colorado School of Medicine; Director, Denver Metro Tuberculosis Clinic, Denver Disease Control Service, Denver

John R. Reynolds, Pharm.D.
Associate Professor of Clinical Pharmacy and Director, Division of Pharmacy Practice, Massachusetts College of Pharmacy and Allied Health Sciences, Boston

Peter E. Rice, M.D.
Clinical Assistant Professor of Surgery, State University of New York Health Science Center at Brooklyn, College of Medicine; Attending Surgeon, Brookdale Hospital Medical Center, Brooklyn, New York

Michael A. Rie, M.D.
Professor of Anesthesiology and Surgery, University of Kentucky College of Medicine; Director, Trauma Anesthesia Critical Care Service, University of Kentucky Medical Center, Lexington, Kentucky

Caroline A. Riely, M.D.
Professor of Medicine and Pediatrics, University of Tennessee College of Medicine, Memphis

James M. Rippe, M.D.
Associate Professor of Medicine, Tufts University School of Medicine, Boston; Director, The Center for Clinical and Lifestyle Research, Shrewsbury, Massachusetts

Michael J. Rohrer, M.D.
Assistant Professor of Surgery, University of Massachusetts Medical School; Co-Director, The Venous Clinic, University of Massachusetts Medical Center, Worcester, Massachusetts

John L. Rombeau, M.D.
Associate Professor of Surgery, Harrison Department of Surgical Research, University of Pennsylvania School of Medicine; Attending Surgeon, Hospital of the University of Pennsylvania, Philadelphia

Arthur L. Rosen, Ph.D.
Assistant Professor of Surgery, University of Chicago, Division of the Biological Sciences, Pritzker School of Medicine, Chicago

Barry Rosen, M.D.
Resident, Department of Surgery, Michael Reese Hospital and Medical Center, Chicago

Mark J. Rosen, M.D.
Associate Professor of Medicine, Albert Einstein College of Medicine of Yeshiva University; Chief, Division of Pulmonary and Critical Care Medicine, Department of Medicine, Beth Israel Medical Center, New York

Aldo A. Rossini, M.D.
Professor of Medicine, University of Massachusetts Medical School; Director, Division of Diabetes, University of Massachusetts Medical Center, Worcester, Massachusetts

Alan L. Rothman, M.D.
Assistant Professor of Medicine, University of Massachusetts Medical School, Worcester, Massachusetts

John C. Rotschafer, Pharm.D.
Professor of Pharmacy Practice, University of Minnesota College of Pharmacy, Minneapolis; Director, Antibiotic Pharmacokinetic Service, St. Paul Ramsey Medical Center, St. Paul, Minnesota

Lewis J. Rubin, M.D.
Professor of Medicine, University of Maryland School of Medicine; Head, Division of Pulmonary and Critical Care Medicine, University of Maryland Medical System, Baltimore

Steven A. Sahn, M.D.
Professor of Pulmonary-Critical Care Medicine, and Director, Division of Pulmonary-Critical Care Medicine, Medical University of South Carolina; Co-Director, Medical Intensive Care Unit, Medical University Hospital, Charleston, South Carolina

Diane Sauter, M.D.
Associate Professor of Emergency Medicine, New York Medical College, Valhalla, New York; Residency Director, Department of Emergency Medicine, Metropolitan Hospital Center, New York

Jay L. Schauben, Pharm.D.
Clinical Professor of Emergency Medicine and Pharmacy, University of Florida College of Medicine; Director, Florida Poison Information Center, University Medical Center, Jacksonville, Florida

Eric W. Schmidt, M.D.
Assistant Professor of Medicine, University of Massachusetts Medical School, Worcester, Massachusetts

Steven M. Schonholz, M.D.
Assistant Professor of Surgery, University of Massachusetts Medical School, Worcester, Massachusetts

Daniel P. Schuster, M.D.
Associate Professor of Internal Medicine and Radiology, Washington University School of Medicine; Director, Medical Intensive Care Unit, Barnes Hospital, St. Louis

William J. Schwartz, M.D.
Professor of Neurology, University of Massachusetts Medical School, Worcester, Massachusetts

Hansa L. Sehgal, B.S.
Research Associate, Department of Surgery, Michael Reese Hospital and Medical Center, Chicago

Lakshman R. Sehgal, Ph.D.
Research Assistant Professor of Surgery, University of Illinois College of Medicine; Research Associate, Michael Reese Hospital and Medical Center, Chicago

Frank W. Sellke, M.D.
Assistant Professor of Surgery, Harvard Medical School; Cardiothoracic Surgeon, Beth Israel Hospital, Boston

Michael G. Seneff, M.D.
Assistant Professor of Anesthesia and Medicine, George Washington University School of Medicine and Health Sciences; Director, Intensive Care Unit, George Washington University Medical Center, Washington

Michael W. Shannon, M.D.
Assistant Professor of Pediatrics, Harvard Medical School;
Associate Chief, Division of Emergency Medicine, Children's
Hospital, Boston

Thomas M. Sherman, M.D.
Fellow in Gastroenterology, Washington University School of
Medicine, St. Louis

Joan Mandt Shopbell, M.S.
Nutrition Support Dietitian, Methodist Hospital, St. Louis Park,
Minnesota

Eva P. Shronts, M.M.Sc., R.D., C.N.S.D.
Associate Director, Nutrition Support, Department of Surgery,
University of Minnesota Medical School—Minneapolis

Lawrence N. Shulman, M.D.
Assistant Professor of Medicine, Harvard Medical School;
Clinical Director, Division of Hematology-Oncology, Brigham
and Women's Hospital, Boston

Sara J. Shumway, M.D.
Associate Professor of Surgery, University of Minnesota
Medical School—Minneapolis

John L. Shuster, Jr., M.D.
Assistant Professor of Psychiatry and Director, Division of
Medical/Surgical Psychiatry, University of Alabama School of
Medicine, Birmingham, Alabama

Wayne E. Silva, M.D.
Professor of Surgery, University of Massachusetts Medical
School; Chairman, Division of General Surgery, and Director,
Trauma Center, University of Massachusetts Medical Center,
Worcester, Massachusetts

Dianne L. Silvestri, M.D.
Assistant Professor of Dermatology, University of
Massachusetts Medical School; Staff Physician, Division of
Dermatology, University of Massachusetts Medical Center,
Worcester, Massachusetts

Martin J. Smilkstein, M.D.
Assistant Professor of Emergency Medicine, Oregon Health
Sciences University School of Medicine; Medical Director,
Medical Toxicology Fellowship Program Director, Oregon
Poison Center, Portland, Oregon

Jeffrey R. Smith, M.D.
Fellow in Cardiology, Northwestern University Medical
School, Chicago

Nicholas A. Smyrnios, M.D.
Assistant Professor of Medicine, University of Massachusetts
Medical School; Director, Medical Intensive Care Unit,
University of Massachusetts Medical Center, Worcester,
Massachusetts

Joseph S. Solomkin, M.D.
Professor of Surgery, University of Cincinnati College of
Medicine, Cincinnati

David H. Spodick, M.D., D.Sc.
Professor of Medicine, University of Massachusetts Medical
School; Director, Clinical Cardiology and Cardiology Training,
St. Vincent Hospital, Worcester, Massachusetts

George Stathopoulos, M.D.
Gastroenterology Fellow, University of Chicago, Division of
the Biological Sciences, Pritzker School of Medicine, Chicago

Michael L. Steer, M.D.
Professor of Surgery, Harvard Medical School; Chief, Division
of General Surgery, Beth Israel Hospital, Boston

Theodore A. Stern, M.D.
Associate Professor of Psychiatry, Harvard Medical School;
Associate Psychiatrist and Director, Resident Psychiatric
Consultation Service, Massachusetts General Hospital, Boston

Donald S. Stevens, M.D.
Assistant Professor of Anesthesiology, University of
Massachusetts Medical School; Co-Director, Pain Treatment
Service, University of Massachusetts Medical Center,
Worcester, Massachusetts

F. Marc Stewart, M.D.
Associate Professor of Hematology/Oncology, and Chief,
Division of Hematology/Oncology, University of
Massachusetts Medical School, Worcester, Massachusetts

Robert J. Straka, Pharm.D.
Assistant Professor of Pharmacy Practice, University of
Minnesota College of Pharmacy, Minneapolis; Clinical
Pharmacy Specialist, St. Paul Ramsey Medical Center, St. Paul,
Minnesota

Martin A. Strosberg, Ph.D.
Associate Professor, Graduate Management Institute, Union
College, Schenectady, New York

Steven L. Strongwater, M.D.
Associate Professor of Medicine, University of Massachusetts
Medical School; Associate Chief of Staff, Department of
Quality Management Services, Office of the Chief of Staff,
University of Massachusetts Medical Center, Worcester,
Massachusetts

David E. R. Sutherland, M.D., Ph.D.
Professor of Surgery, University of Minnesota Medical
School—Minneapolis

Irma O. Szymanski, M.D.
Professor of Pathology, University of Massachusetts Medical
School; Director, Blood Bank, University of Massachusetts
Medical Center, Worcester, Massachusetts

Milton Tenenbein, M.D.
Professor of Pediatrics, Medicine, and Pharmacology,
University of Manitoba Faculty of Medicine; Director,
Emergency Services, Children's Hospital, Winnipeg, Manitoba,
Canada

Daniel Teres, M.D.
Associate Professor of Medicine and Surgery, Tufts University
School of Medicine, Boston; Director, Adult Critical Care
Division, Baystate Medical Center, Springfield, Massachusetts

George E. Tesar, M.D.
Chairman, Department of Psychiatry and Psychology,
Cleveland Clinic Foundation, Cleveland

Pierre Théroux, M.D.
Professor of Medicine, Université de Montréal Faculty of
Medicine; Director, Coronary Care Unit, Montreal Heart
Institute, Montreal

Christian Tomaszewski, M.D.
Assistant Clinical Professor of Emergency Medicine, University of North Carolina at Chapel Hill School of Medicine, Chapel Hill; Attending Physician, Department of Emergency Medicine, Carolinas Medical Center, Charlotte, North Carolina

John E. Tomaszewski, M.D.

Paula L. Townsend, Pharm.D.
TPN Inc., Reno, Nevada

Robert E. Tranquada, M.D.
Professor of Medicine, University of Southern California School of Medicine, Los Angeles

Arthur L. Trask, M.D.
Chief, Trauma Services, Fairfax Hospital, Falls Church, Virginia

Christoph Troppmann, M.D.

Sandra L. Turner, M.Ed., R.N., C.P.H.Q.
Manager, Medical Staff Services, Quality Assessment, Baystate Medical Center, Springfield, Massachusetts

Cynthia B. Umali, M.D.
Associate Professor of Radiology, University of Massachusetts Medical School; Thoracic Radiologist and Residency Program Director, Department of Radiology, University of Massachusetts Medical Center, Worcester, Massachusetts

Katherine S. Upchurch, M.D.
Associate Professor of Medicine, University of Massachusetts Medical School; Chief, Division of Rheumatology, Medical Center of Central Massachusetts, Worcester, Massachusetts

Kyle Vance-Bryan, Pharm.D.
Assistant Professor of Pharmacy, University of Minnesota College of Pharmacy, Minneapolis; Critical Care Specialist, Section of Clinical Pharmacology, St. Paul-Ramsey Medical Center, St. Paul, Minnesota

Thomas J. Vander Salm, M.D.
Professor of Surgery, University of Massachusetts Medical School; Chairman, Division of Cardiothoracic Surgery, University of Massachusetts Medical Center, Worcester, Massachusetts

Marc S. Visner, M.D.
Associate Professor of Surgery, University of Massachusetts Medical School; Attending Cardiothoracic Surgeon, University of Massachusetts Medical Center, Worcester, Massachusetts

Stephen J. Voyce, M.D.
Associate Clinical Professor of Medicine, Hahnemann University School of Medicine, Philadelphia; Attending Physician, Department of Cardiology, Community Medical Center, Scranton, Pennsylvania

Michael C. Vredenburg, D.O.
Cardiology Fellow, Henry Ford Heart and Vascular Institute, Henry Ford Hospital, Detroit

Alan B. Wagshal, M.D.
Assistant Professor of Medicine, University of Massachusetts Medical School, Worcester, MA

Karla J. Walker, Pharm.D.
Assistant Clinical Director, MedTox Laboratories, Inc., St. Paul

Andrea M. Sweeney Walsh, B.S., R.D.C.S.
Chief Cardiac Sonographer, University of Massachusetts Medical Center, Worcester, Massachusetts

Frank Walsh, M.D.

Robert L. Walton, Jr., M.D.
Professor of Surgery, University of Massachusetts Medical School; Chairman, Division of Plastic and Reconstructive Surgery, University of Massachusetts Medical Center, Worcester, Massachusetts

Rick Y. Wang, M.D.

Theodore E. Warkentin, M.D.
Assistant Professor of Pathology, McMaster University School of Medicine; Head, Transfusion Medicine and Hemostasis, Hamilton Civic Hospitals, Hamilton, Ontario, Canada

Paul M. Wax, M.D.
Assistant Professor of Emergency Medicine, University of Rochester School of Medicine and Dentistry; Attending Physician, Emergency Department, Strong Memorial Hospital, Rochester, New York

John P. Weaver, M.D.
Assistant Professor of Neurosurgery, University of Massachusetts Medical School, Worcester, Massachusetts

John G. Weg, M.D.
Professor of Pulmonary and Critical Care Medicine, University of Michigan Medical School, Ann Arbor, Michigan

Heather M. White, M.D.

Eric Wittbrodt, M.D.

Carol A. Wool, M.D.
Instructor in Psychiatry, Harvard Medical School; Assistant in Psychiatry (Primary Care), Massachusetts General Hospital, Boston

Jean-Dennis Yelle, M.D.
Clinical Associate Professor of Surgery, Georgetown University School of Medicine, Washington; Trauma Fellow, Fairfax Hospital, Falls Church, Virginia

Luke Yip, M.D.
Clinical Assistant Professor of Emergency Medicine, State University of New York Health Science Center at Syracuse College of Medicine; Attending Physician, Department of Emergency Medicine, University Health Science Center, Syracuse, New York

Darwin E. Zaske, Pharm.D.
Professor of Pharmacy Practice, University of Minnesota College of Pharmacy, Minneapolis; Director, Department of Pharmaceutical Services, St. Paul-Ramsey Medical Center, St. Paul, Minnesota

Gary R. Zuckerman, M.D.
Associate Professor of Medicine, Division of Gastroenterology, Washington University School of Medicine, St. Louis

I. Procedures and Techniques

Section Editors
Frederick J. Curley and Stephen O. Heard

Notice

1. Airway Management and Endotracheal Intubation

Shubjeet Kaur and Stephen O. Heard

In the emergency room and critical care environment, management of the airway to ensure optimal ventilation and oxygenation is of prime importance. Although initial efforts should be directed toward improving oxygenation and ventilation without intubating the patient, any prolonged efforts will eventually require the placement of an endotracheal tube. While endotracheal intubation is best left to the trained specialist, emergencies often require that the procedure be performed before a specialist arrives. Since intubated patients are common in the intensive care unit (ICU) and coronary care unit (CCU), all physicians working in these environments should be skilled in the techniques of airway management, endotracheal intubation, and management of intubated patients.

Historical Background

The earliest reported attempts at tracheal intubation occurred in the sixteenth and seventeenth centuries [1,2,3]. Vesalius reported sustaining respiration in a pig by blowing through a reed introduced into its trachea [2]. In 1667, Robert Hooke described an experiment in which he maintained ventilation in a dog by attaching its trachea to a bellows [1].

During the eighteenth century the idea of tracheal intubation must have occurred to a number of clinicians. Diphtheria and croup were common diseases (although not recognized as clinical entities and named until the early nineteenth century) and death often resulted from upper airway obstruction. In 1796, Herholdt and Rafu described mouth-to-mouth resuscitation, tracheal intubation, and tracheotomy as techniques to save drowning persons [4]. In the early nineteenth century the French surgeon P. J. Desault described successful tracheal intubation and outlined a technique of nasotracheal intubation.

During the 1870s, several investigators described successful anesthesia with chloroform delivered via tracheostomy [5,6]. In 1880, Macewen described successful intubation and survival of 2 patients who had been intubated for 35 and 36 hours [7]. In 1885, O'Dwyer described intubation employing a small metal tube [8]; 3 years later he published a series describing 50 patients with croup who had been treated with intubation, of whom 30 percent survived [9].

By the end of the nineteenth century a number of clinicians were experimenting with intubation and defining its clinical usefulness. Chevalier Jackson, one of the pioneers of otolaryngology, enthusiastically adopted the technique and in the early twentieth century (1907) published a guide to upper airway endoscopy that put tracheal intubation on firm clinical footing [10].

Anatomy

An understanding of the techniques of endotracheal intubation and potential complications is based on knowledge of the anatomy of the respiratory passages [11,12]. While a detailed anatomic description is beyond the scope of this book, an understanding of some features and relationships is essential to performing intubation.

NOSE. The roof of the nose is composed of the nasal and frontal bones, the cribriform plate, and the body of the sphenoid bone. The floor is formed by the palatine process of the maxillary bone and the horizontal plate of the palatine bone. The nasal septum (medial wall) contains septal cartilage, the vomer, and the perpendicular plate of the ethmoid. The lateral wall is formed by the superior and middle conchae of the ethmoid bone, pterygoid process of the sphenoid bone, perpendicular plate of the palatine bone, and the inferior concha. The orifices from the paranasal sinuses and nasolacrimal duct open onto the lateral wall. Blockage of these orifices by prolonged nasotracheal intubation may result in sinusitis [13]. The mucosa of the nose is provided with a rich blood supply from branches of the ophthalmic and maxillary arteries, which allow air to be warmed and humidified. Since the conchae provide an irregular, highly vascularized surface, they are particularly susceptible to trauma, with subsequent hemorrhage.

MOUTH AND JAW. The mouth is formed inferiorly by the tongue, alveolar ridge, and mandible. The hard and soft palate compose the superior surface and the oropharynx forms the posterior surface. Assessment of the anatomic features of the mouth and jaw is essential prior to orotracheal intubation.

NASOPHARYNX. The base of the skull forms the roof of the nasopharynx and the soft palate forms the floor. Both the roof and posterior walls of the nasopharynx contain lymphoid tissue (adenoids), which may become enlarged and compromise nasal airflow or become injured during nasal intubation, particularly in children. The eustachian tubes enter the nasopharynx on the lateral walls and may become blocked secondary to swelling during prolonged nasotracheal intubation.

OROPHARYNX. The soft palate defines the beginning of the oropharynx, which extends inferiorly to the epiglottis. The palatine tonsils protrude from the lateral walls and in children occasionally become so enlarged that exposure of the larynx for intubation becomes difficult. The oropharynx connects the posterior portion of the oral cavity to the hypopharynx.

HYPOPHARYNX. The epiglottis defines the superior border of the hypopharynx, and the beginning of the esophagus forms the inferior boundary. The larynx is anterior to the hypopharynx. The pyriform sinuses that extend around both sides of the larynx are part of the hypopharynx.

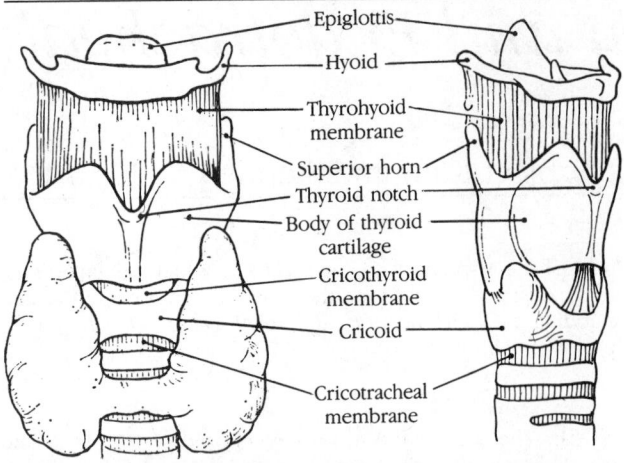

Fig. 1-1. Anatomy of the larynx, anterior and lateral aspects. Source: Ellis H: *Anatomy for Anaesthetists.* Oxford, UK, Blackwell Scientific, 1963. With permission.

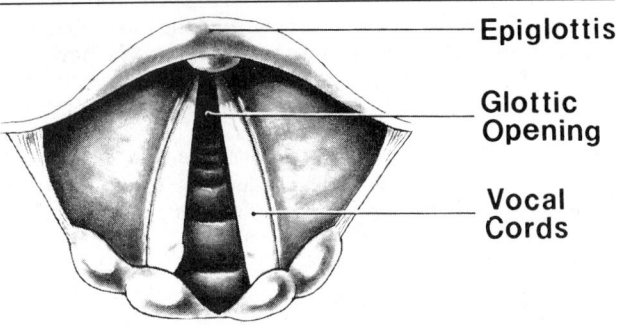

Fig. 1-2. Superior view of the larynx (inspiration). Source: Stoelting RK, Miller RD: *Basics of Anesthesia.* 2nd ed. Churchill Livingstone, New York, 1989. With permission.

LARYNX. The larynx (Fig. 1-1) is a complex, highly integrated area that houses the vocal cords. It allows the passage of air into the trachea, prevents aspiration, and provides support and protection to the apparatus of voice production. The larynx is bounded by the hypopharynx superiorly and is continuous with the trachea inferiorly. The thyroid, cricoid, epiglottic, cuneiform, corniculate, and arytenoid cartilages comprise the laryngeal skeleton. The thyroid and cricoid cartilages are readily palpated in the anterior neck. The cricoid cartilage articulates with the thyroid cartilage and is joined to it by the cricothyroid ligament. When the patient's head is extended, the cricothyroid ligament may be pierced with a scalpel or large needle to provide an emergency airway (Chap. 16). The cricoid cartilage completely encircles the airway. It is attached to the first cartilage ring of the trachea by the cricotracheal ligament. The anterior wall of the larynx is formed by the epiglottic cartilage, to which the arytenoid cartilages are attached. Fine muscles span the arytenoid and thyroid cartilages, as do the vocal cords. The true vocal cords and space between them are collectively termed the glottis (Fig. 1-2). The glottis is the narrowest space in the adult upper airway. In children, the cricoid cartilage defines the narrowest portion of the airway. Since normal voice production relies on the precise apposition of the true vocal cords, even a small lesion can cause hoarseness. The fact that lymphatic drainage to the true vocal cords is sparse indicates

that inflammation or swelling caused by tube irritation or trauma may take considerable time to resolve. The structures of the larynx are innervated by the superior and recurrent laryngeal nerve branches of the vagus nerve. The superior laryngeal nerve supplies sensory innervation from the inferior surface of the epiglottis to the superior surface of the vocal cords. From its takeoff from the vagus nerve, it passes deep to both branches of the carotid artery. A large internal branch pierces the thyrohyoid membrane just inferior to the greater cornu of the hyoid. This branch can be blocked with local anesthetics for oral or nasal intubations in awake patients. The recurrent laryngeal branch of the vagus nerve provides sensory innervation below the cords. It also supplies all the muscles of the larynx except the cricothyroid, which is innervated by the external branch of the superior laryngeal nerve.

TRACHEA. The adult trachea averages 15 cm long. Its external skeleton is comprised of a series of C-shaped cartilages. It is bounded in the rear by the esophagus and in front for the first few cartilage rings by the thyroid gland. The trachea is lined with ciliated cells that secrete mucus; through the beating action of the cilia, foreign substances are propelled toward the larynx. The carina is located at the fourth thoracic vertebral level (of relevance when judging proper endotracheal tube positioning on chest radiograph). The right main bronchus takes off at a less acute angle than the left, making right main bronchial intubation more common if the endotracheal tube is in too far.

Emergency Airway Management

In an emergency situation, establishing adequate ventilation and oxygenation assumes primary importance [14,15]. Too frequently, inexperienced personnel believe this requires immediate intubation; however, attempts at intubation may delay establishment of an adequate airway. Such efforts are time-consuming, can induce arrhythmias, and may induce bleeding and regurgitation, making subsequent attempts to intubate significantly more difficult. Some simple techniques and principles of emergency airway management can play an important role until the arrival of an individual skilled at intubation.

AIRWAY OBSTRUCTION. Compromised ventilation often results from upper airway obstruction by the tongue or substances retained in the mouth. If respiration is inadequate, the head-tilt-chin-lift or jaw-thrust maneuver should be performed. In patients with suspected cervical spine injuries, the jaw-thrust maneuver (without the head-tilt) is safest [16]. The head-tilt maneuver is accomplished by placing a palm on the patient's forehead and applying pressure to extend the head about the atlanto-occipital joint. The chin-lift is performed by placing several fingers of the other hand in the submental area and lifting the mandible. Care must be taken to avoid airway obstruction by pressing too firmly on the soft tissues in the submental area. The jaw-thrust is performed by lifting up on the angles of the mandible (Fig. 1-3) [14]. If the patient resumes spontaneous breathing, establishing this head position may constitute sufficient treatment. If obstruction persists, then abdominal thrusts and a check for foreign bodies, emesis, or secretions should be performed.

USE OF FACE MASK AND BAG VALVE DEVICE. If an adequate airway has been established and the patient is not breathing spontaneously, oxygen may be delivered via face

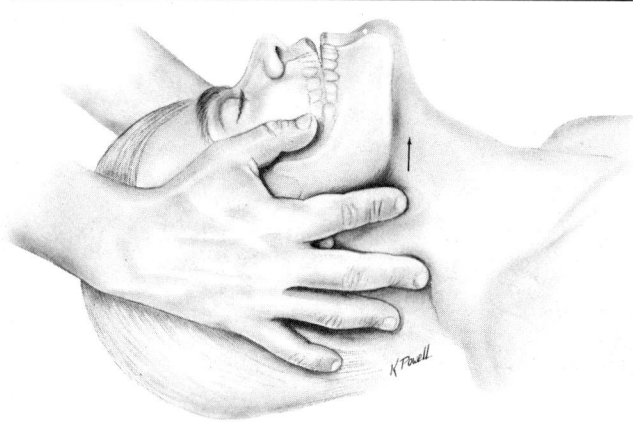

Fig. 1-3. In an obtunded or comatose patient, the soft tissues of the oropharynx become relaxed and may obstruct the upper airway. Obstruction can be alleviated by placing the thumbs on the maxilla with the index fingers under the ramus of the mandible and rotating the mandible forward with pressure from the index fingers (arrow). This maneuver will bring the soft tissues forward and therefore frequently reduce the airway obstruction.

mask and a bag valve device. It is important to establish a tight fit with the face mask, covering the patient's mouth and nose. This is accomplished by applying the mask initially to the bridge of the nose and drawing it downward toward the mouth, using both hands. The operator stands at the patient's head and presses the mask onto the patient's face with the left hand. The thumb should be on the nasal portion of the mask, the index finger near the oral portion, and the rest of the fingers spread on the left side of the patient's mandible so as to pull it slightly forward. The bag is then alternately compressed and released with the right hand. A good airway is indicated by the rise and fall of the chest; moreover, lung-chest wall compliance can be estimated from the amount of pressure required to compress the bag.

Fig. 1-4. Nasopharyngeal (A) or oropharyngeal (B) airways can be used to relieve soft tissue obstruction if elevating the mandible proves ineffective.

AIRWAY ADJUNCTS. If proper positioning of the head and neck or clearance of foreign bodies and secretions fails to establish an adequate airway, several airway adjuncts may be helpful if an individual skilled in intubation is not immediately available.

Oropharyngeal and Nasopharyngeal Airways. An oropharyngeal or nasopharyngeal airway occasionally helps to establish an adequate airway when proper head positioning alone is insufficient (Figs. 1-4 and 1-5) [16]. The oropharyngeal airway is semicircular and made of plastic or hard rubber. There are two types: the Guedel airway, with a hollow tubular design, and the Berman airway, with airway channels along the sides. Both types are most easily inserted by turning the curved portion toward the palate as it enters the mouth. It is then advanced beyond the posterior portion of the tongue and rotated downward into the proper position (Fig. 1-5). Often depressing the tongue or moving it laterally with a tongue blade helps to position the oropharyngeal airway. Care must be exercised not to push the tongue into the posterior pharynx, causing or exacerbating obstruction. Since insertion of the oropharyngeal airway can cause gagging and/or vomiting, it should be used only in unconscious patients.

The nasopharyngeal airway is a soft tube approximately 15 cm long made of rubber or plastic (Figs. 1-4 and 1-6). It is inserted via the nostril into the posterior pharynx. Prior to insertion, the airway should be lubricated with an anesthetic gel and, preferably, a vasoconstrictor should be administered into the nostril. The nasopharyngeal airway should not be used in patients with extensive facial trauma or cerebrospinal rhinorrhea, as it could be inserted through the cribriform plate into the brain.

Other Airway Adjuncts. The laryngeal mask airway, which has become available recently, can be positioned without direct visualization of the vocal cords and conforms to the shape of the laryngeal inlet (Fig. 1-7). Though a high rate of successful placement by inexperienced personnel has been touted [17,18], its use is limited mainly to anesthesiologists. A variety of other devices, including the esophageal obturator airway and transesophageal airway, have been developed to assist in maintaining a patent airway. These devices have virtually no role in the

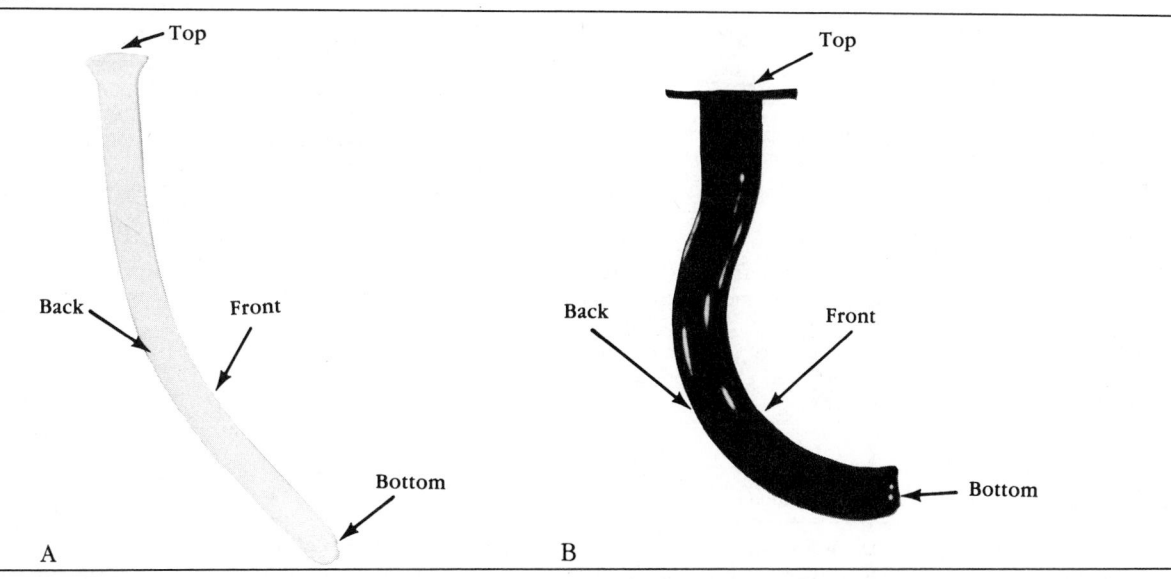

Top

Back   Front

Bottom

A

Top

Back   Front

Bottom

B

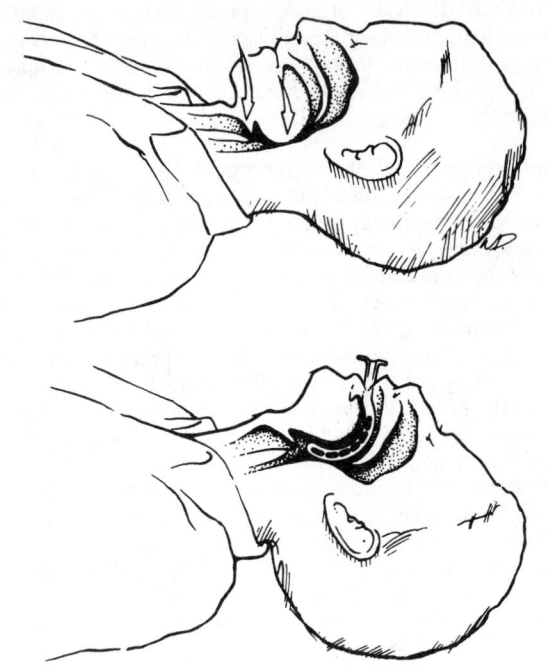

Fig. 1-5. The mechanism of upper airway obstruction and the proper position of the oropharygneal airway. With permission. *Textbook of Advanced Cardiac Life Support*, 1987, 1990. Copyright American Heart Association.

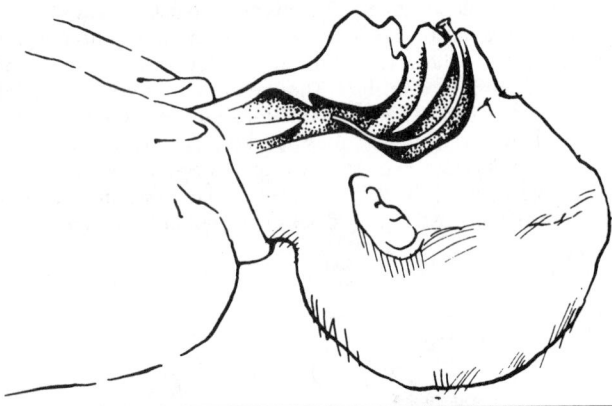

Fig. 1-6. The proper position of the nasopharygneal airway. With permission. *Textbook of Advanced Cardiac Life Support*, 1987, 1990. Copyright American Heart Association.

ICU; they are used only for out-of-hospital resuscitation by paramedical personnel. Furthermore, data from several recent studies suggest that these devices are no more effective than appropriately fitted masks with bag valve devices, and they subject patients to the risks of a variety of potentially serious complications [19]. The reader is referred elsewhere for information concerning their use [20].

Indications for Intubation

The indications for endotracheal intubation can be divided into four broad categories: (1) acute airway obstruction; (2) exces-

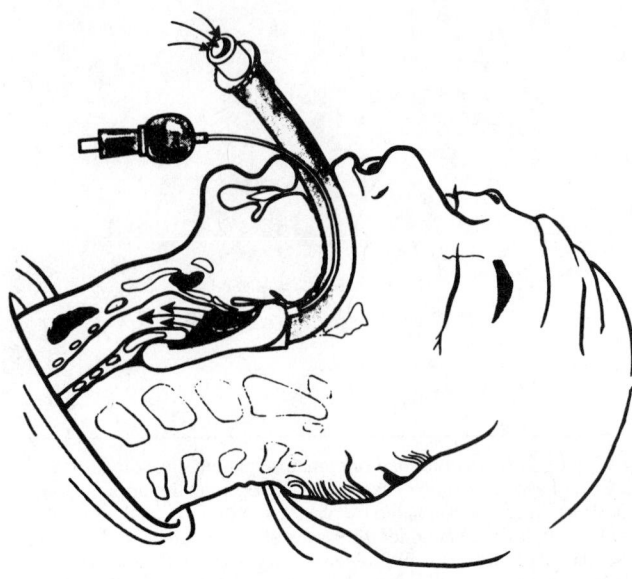

Fig. 1-7. Correct placement of the laryngeal mask airway. Source: Maltby JR, et al: The laryngeal mask airway: Clinical appraisal in 250 patients. *Can J Anaesth* 37:509-513, 1990. With permission.

sive pulmonary secretions or inability to clear secretions adequately; (3) loss of protective reflexes; and (4) respiratory failure (Table 1-1). Some conditions in each category require specific clinical measures or considerations and merit specific discussion.

ACUTE AIRWAY OBSTRUCTION. Acute upper airway obstruction is most often due to posterior displacement of the base of the tongue. Trauma can cause injury to the mandible, allowing posterior displacement of the tongue and other soft tissue structures that can lead to occlusion of the upper airway. Inhalation of smoke or noxious chemicals can result in acute laryngeal edema [21,22]. Aspiration of foreign bodies, particularly in children, can cause acute upper airway obstruction. Infections of the upper airway (epiglottitis, croup, diphtheria, retropharyngeal abscess) can lead to acute obstruction. Rapidly expanding hematomas can result from even minor trauma or coughing (particularly in patients with coagulopathies) and can obstruct the upper airway. Rapidly growing tracheal, paratracheal, laryngeal, or pharyngeal tumors can result in obstruction. Rare congenital conditions, such as laryngeal webs or supraglottic fusion, can cause obstruction in infants. Laryngeal edema or spasm caused by allergic reactions or anaphylaxis can result in acute airway obstruction (Chap. 183).

SECRETIONS. Patients with neuromuscular diseases or severe debilitation can experience problems in clearing their own secretions. Patients with chronic lung diseases (e.g., chronic obstructive pulmonary disease, cystic fibrosis) or acute lung pathology (e.g., pneumonia) sometimes produce copious secretions that overwhelm normal clearance mechanisms. Patients with these problems require frequent pulmonary suctioning, which is facilitated by placement of an endotracheal tube.

LOSS OF PROTECTIVE REFLEXES. Patients rendered unconscious by a head injury, drug overdose, or cerebrovascular

Table 1-1. Indications for Endotracheal Intubation

Acute airway obstruction
  Trauma
    Mandible
    Larynx (direct or indirect injury)
  Inhalation
    Smoke
    Noxious chemicals
    Foreign bodies
  Infection
    Acute epiglottitis
    Croup
    Retropharyngeal abscess
  Hematoma
  Tumor
  Congenital anomalies
    Laryngeal web
    Supraglottic fusion
  Laryngeal edema
  Laryngeal spasm (anaphylactic response)
Access for suctioning
  Debilitated patients
  Copious secretions
Loss of protective reflexes
  Head injury
  Drug overdose
  Cerebrovascular accident
Respiratory failure
  Hypoxemia
    Acute respiratory distress syndrome
    Hypoventilation
    Atelectasis
    Secretions
    Pulmonary edema
  Hypercapnia
    Hypoventilation
    Neuromuscular failure
    Drug overdose

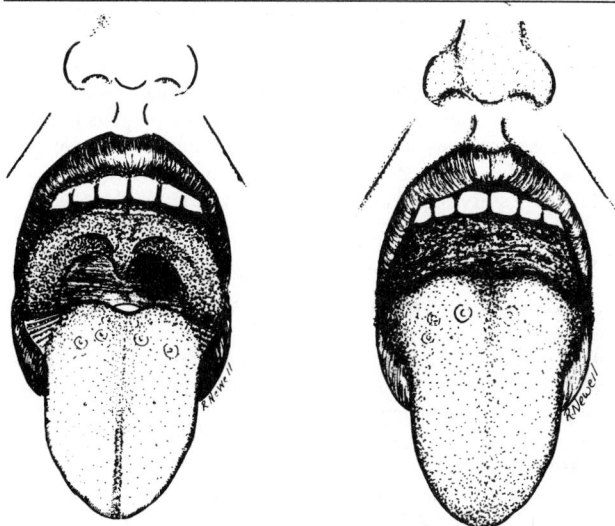

Fig. 1-8. The faucial pillars, soft palate, and uvula are not visible in the patient on the right. One should expect difficulty in orotracheal intubation. Source: Mallampati SR, Gatt SP, Gugino LD: A clinical sign to predict difficult tracheal intubation: A prospective study. *Can Anaesth Soc J* 32:429, 1985. With permission.

accident frequently lose their protective reflexes and are at high risk for regurgitation and aspiration of gastric contents. Endotracheal intubation can reduce the risk of aspiration.

RESPIRATORY FAILURE. A detailed discussion of the causes and treatment of respiratory failure is found in Chapters 42 to 47. The criteria for intubation of patients are similar to those for mechanical ventilation (Chap. 54).

Preintubation Evaluation

Even in the most urgent situation, a rapid assessment of the patient's airway anatomy can expedite the choice of the proper route for intubation, the appropriate equipment, and the most useful precautions to be taken. In the less emergent situation, several minutes of preintubation evaluation can decrease the likelihood of complications and increase the probability of successful intubation with minimal trauma.

Anatomic structures of the upper airway, head, and neck must be examined, with particular attention to abnormalities that might preclude a particular route of intubation. Evaluation of cervical spine mobility, temporomandibular joint function, and dentition is important. Any abnormalities that might prohibit alignment of the oral, pharyngeal, and laryngeal axes should be noted.

Cervical spine mobility is assessed by flexion and extension

of the neck (performed only after ascertaining that no cervical spine injury exists). The normal range of neck flexion-extension varies from 165 to 90 degrees, with the range decreasing approximately 20 percent by age 75. Conditions associated with decreased range of motion include any cause of degenerative disc disease (e.g., rheumatoid arthritis, osteoarthritis, ankylosing spondylitis), previous trauma, or age over 70 years.

Temporomandibular joint dysfunction can occur in any form of degenerative arthritis (particularly rheumatoid arthritis), any condition that causes a receding mandible, and in rare conditions such as acromegaly.

Examination of the oral cavity is mandatory. Loose, missing, or chipped teeth and permanent bridgework are noted, and removable bridgework and dentures should be taken out. Mallampati and associates [23] developed a clinical indicator based on the size of the posterior aspect of the tongue relative to the size of the oral pharynx (Fig. 1-8). The patient should be sitting and asked to protrude his or her tongue without phonating. When the faucial pillars, the uvula, the soft palate, and posterior pharyngeal wall are well visualized, the airway is classified as class I and a relatively easy intubation can be anticipated. When only the faucial pillars and soft palate are viable (class II), intubation may be difficult in up to 35 percent of patients. In a class III airway (only soft palate visualized), in most patients the glottis will not be exposed by direct laryngoscopy. Difficulties in orotracheal intubation can also be anticipated if (1) the patient is an adult and cannot open his or her mouth more than 40 mm (2 finger breadths), (2) the distance from the thyroid notch to the mandible is less than 3 finger breadths, (3) the patient has a high arched palate, (4) the normal range of flexion-extension of the neck is decreased [23,24].

Equipment for Intubation

Assembly of all appropriate equipment prior to attempted intubation can prevent potentially serious delays in the event of an unforeseen complication. Most equipment and supplies are readily available in the ICU but must be gathered so they are immediately at hand. A supply of 100% oxygen and a well-fitting mask with attached bag valve device are mandatory, as is suctioning equipment, including a large-bore tonsil suction attachment (Yankauer) and suction catheters. Adequate lighting facilitates airway visualization. The bed should be at the proper height, with the headboard removed and the wheels locked. Other necessary supplies include gloves, Magill forceps, oral and nasal airways, laryngoscope handle and blades (both straight and curved), endotracheal tubes of various sizes, stylet, tongue depressors, a syringe for cuff inflation, tape for securing the endotracheal tube in position, and tincture of benzoin. Table 1-2 is a checklist of supplies needed.

It is particularly important that an adequate number of personnel be available to assist the operator. Endotracheal intubation and emergency airway management are not one-person jobs. While the operator is performing a rapid preintubation assessment, ICU personnel should be gathering equipment. During and prior to intubation, a respiratory therapist should be present, whose sole concerns should be assisting in airway control prior to intubation and providing adequate oxygenation. It is helpful to have another assistant present who is familiar with the procedure and equipment and who should be ready to hand items to the operator on request.

LARYNGOSCOPES. The two-piece laryngoscope has a handle containing batteries that power the bulb in the blade. The blade snaps securely into the top of the handle, making the electrical connection. Failure of the bulb to illuminate suggests improper blade positioning, bulb failure, a loose bulb, or dead batteries. Modern laryngoscope blades with fiberoptic lights obviate the

Table 1-2. Equipment Needed for Intubation

Supply of 100% oxygen
Face mask
Bag valve device
Suction equipment
   Suction catheters
   Large-bore tonsil suction apparatus (Yankauer)
Stylet
Magill forceps
Oral airways
Nasal airways
Laryngoscope handle and blades (curved, straight; various sizes)
Endotracheal tubes (various sizes)
Tongue depressors
Syringe for cuff inflation
Head rest
Supplies for vasoconstriction and local anesthesia
Tape
Tincture of benzoin

problem of bulb failure. Many blade shapes and sizes are available. The two most commonly employed blades are the curved (MacIntosh) [25] and straight (Miller) [26] blades (Fig. 1-9). Although pediatric blades are available for use with the adult-sized handle, most anesthesiologists prefer a smaller handle for better control in the pediatric population. The choice of blade shape is a matter of personal preference and experience, although many inexperienced operators find the curved blade easier to use.

ENDOTRACHEAL TUBES. The internal diameter of the endotracheal tube is measured using both millimeters and French units (the former being most commonly used in the United States). This number is stamped on the tube. Tubes are available in 0.5-mm increments, starting at 2.5 mm. Lengthwise dimensions are also marked on the tube in centimeters, beginning at the distal tracheal end.

Selection of the proper tube diameter is of utmost importance

Fig. 1-9. The two basic types of laryngoscope blades, MacIntosh (left) and Miller (right). The MacIntosh blade is curved. The blade tip is placed in the vallecula and the handle of the laryngoscope pulled forward at a 45-degree angle. This allows visualization of the epiglottis. The Miller blade is straight. The tip is placed posterior to the epiglottis, pinning the epiglottis between the base of the tongue and the straight laryngoscope blade. The motion on the laryngoscope handle is the same as that used with the MacIntosh blade.

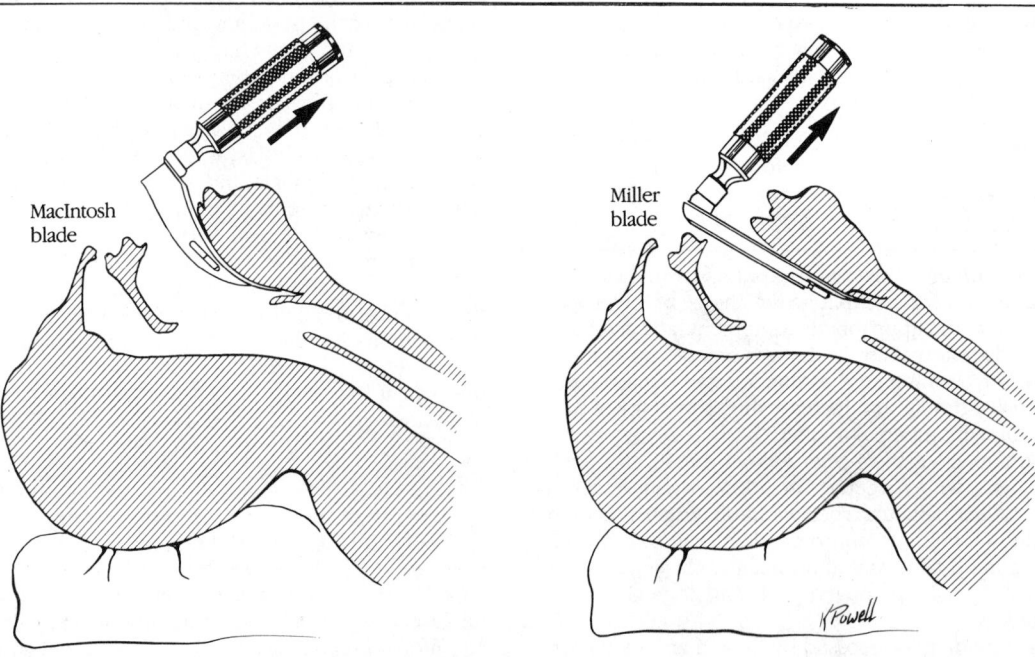

Table 1-3. Dimensions of
Endotracheal Tubes Based on Patient Age

Age	Internal diameter (mm)	French unit	Distance between lips and location in midtrachea of distal end (cm)*
Premature	2.5	10–12	10
Full term	3.0	12–14	11
1–6 mo	3.5	16	11
6–12 mo	4.0	18	12
2 yr	4.5	20	13
4 yr	5.0	22	14
6 yr	5.5	24	15–16
8 yr	6.5	26	16–17
10 yr	7.0	28	17–18
12 yr	7.5	30	18–20
≥14 yr	8.0–9.0	32–36	20–24

*Add 2 to 3 cm for nasal tubes.
Source: Stoelting RK: Endotracheal intubation, in Miller RD (ed): *Anesthesia,* 2nd ed. New York, Churchill Livingstone, 1986, p 531, with permission.

and is a frequently underemphasized consideration. The resistance to airflow varies with the fourth power of the radius of the endotracheal tube. Thus, selection of an inappropriately small tube can significantly increase the work of breathing [27]. Moreover, certain diagnostic procedures (e.g., bronchoscopy) done through endotracheal tubes require appropriately large tubes (Chap. 16).

In general, the larger the patient, the larger the endotracheal tube that should be used. Approximate guidelines for tube sizes and lengths by age are summarized in Table 1-3. Most adults should be intubated with an endotracheal tube with an inner diameter of at least 8.0 mm, although occasionally nasal intubation in a small adult requires a 7.0-mm tube.

ENDOTRACHEAL TUBE CUFF. Endotracheal tubes have low-pressure, high-volume cuffs to reduce the incidence of ischemia-related complications. Tracheal ischemia can occur any time cuff pressure exceeds capillary arteriolar pressure (approximately 32 mm Hg), causing inflammation, ulceration, infection, and dissolution of cartilaginous rings. Failure to recognize this progressive degeneration sometimes results in erosion through the tracheal wall (into the innominate artery if the erosion was anterior or the esophagus if the erosion was posterior) or long-term sequelae of tracheomalacia or tracheal stenosis [28,29,30]. With cuff pressures of 15 to 30 mm Hg, the low-pressure, high-volume cuffs conform well to the tracheal wall and provide an adequate seal during positive pressure ventilation. Although low cuff pressures can cause some damage (primarily ciliary denudation) [31], major complications are rare. Nevertheless, it is important to realize that a low-pressure, high-volume cuff can be converted to a high-pressure cuff if sufficient quantities of air are injected into the cuff. In addition, if lung-chest wall compliance is sufficiently low (and, hence, peak airway pressures are very high), high cuff pressures are required to maintain an adequate seal for mechanical ventilation [32].

Anesthesia prior to Intubation

Since patients requiring intubation often have a depressed level of consciousness, anesthesia is usually not required. If intubation must be performed on the alert, responsive patient, seda-

tion or general anesthesia exposes the patient to potential pulmonary aspiration of gastric contents because protective reflexes are lost. This is a particularly important consideration if the patient has recently eaten and must be weighed against the risk of various hemodynamic derangements that may occur secondary to tracheal intubation and initiation of positive-pressure ventilation. Laryngoscopy in an awake patient is a potent stimulus for sympathetic overflow and can result in tachycardia and an increase in blood pressure. This may be well tolerated in younger patients but may be detrimental in a patient with coronary artery disease or raised intracranial pressure. Sometimes laryngoscopy and intubation may result in a vasovagal response, leading to bradycardia and hypotension. Initiation of positive-pressure ventilation in a hypovolemic patient can lead to hypotension from diminished venous return.

Some of these responses may be attenuated by providing local anesthesia to the nares, mouth, and posterior pharynx prior to intubation. Lidocaine (1–4%) with phenylephrine (0.25%) or cocaine (4%, 200 mg total dose) can be used to anesthetize the nasal passages and provide local vasoconstriction. This allows the passage of a larger endotracheal tube with less likelihood of bleeding. Aqueous lidocaine-phenylephrine or cocaine can be administered via atomizer, nosedropper, or long cotton-tipped swabs inserted into the nares. Alternatively, viscous 2% lidocaine can be applied via a 3.5-mm endotracheal tube or small nasopharyngeal airway inserted into the nose. Anesthesia of the tongue and posterior pharynx can be accomplished with lidocaine spray (4–10%) administered via an atomizer. Alternatively, the glossopharyngeal nerve can be blocked with an injection of a local anesthetic, but this should be performed by experienced personnel.

Anesthetizing the larynx below the vocal cords prior to intubation is controversial. The cough reflex can be compromised, increasing the risk of aspiration. However, tracheal anesthesia may decrease the incidence of arrhythmias or untoward circulatory responses to intubation and improve patient tolerance of the endotracheal tube. Clinical judgment in this situation is necessary. Several methods can be used to anesthetize these structures. Transtracheal lidocaine (4%, 160 mg) is administered by cricothyroid membrane puncture with a small needle and anesthetizes the trachea and larynx below the vocal cords. Alternatively, after exposure of the vocal cords with the laryngoscope, the cords can be sprayed with lidocaine via an atomizer. Aerosolized lidocaine (4%, 6 ml) provides excellent anesthesia to the mouth, pharynx, larynx, and trachea [33,34]. The superior laryngeal nerve can be blocked with 2 ml of 1% to 1.5% lidocaine just inferior to the greater cornu of the hyoid bone. The rate of absorption of lidocaine differs by method, being greater with the aerosol and transtracheal techniques. The patient should be observed for signs of lidocaine toxicity (circumoral paresthesia, agitation, and seizures).

If general anesthesia is required for intubation, alternative means of airway control and oxygenation should be employed until an anesthesiologist arrives to administer the anesthetic and perform the intubation.

Techniques of Intubation [35]

In a true emergency, some of the preintubation evaluation is necessarily neglected in favor of rapid control of the airway. Attempts at tracheal intubation should not cause or exacerbate hypoxia. Whenever possible, an oxygen saturation monitor should be used. The risk of hypoxemia during intubation can be minimized with preoxygenation and by limiting the duration of the attempt to 30 seconds or less.

Preoxygenation (denitrogenation), which replaces the nitrogen in the patient's functional residual capacity with oxygen, can maximize the time available for intubation. During laryngoscopy, apneic oxygenation can occur from this reservoir. Preoxygenation is achieved by providing 100% oxygen at a high flow rate via a tight-fitting face mask for 3.5 to 4 minutes. Just prior to intubation, the physician should assess the likelihood of success of each route of intubation, the urgency of the clinical situation, the likelihood that intubation will be prolonged, and the prospect of whether diagnostic or therapeutic procedures such as bronchoscopy will eventually be required. Factors that will affect patient comfort should also be weighed. In the unconscious patient in whom a secure airway must be established immediately, orotracheal intubation with direct visualization of the vocal cords is generally the preferred technique. In the conscious patient, blind nasotracheal intubation is often preferred because it affords greater patient comfort. Nasotracheal intubation should be avoided in patients with coagulopathies or those anticoagulated for medical indications. In the accident victim with extensive maxillary and mandibular fractures and inadequate ventilation or oxygenation, cricothyrotomy may be mandatory (Chap. 16). In the patient with cervical spine injury or decreased neck mobility, intubation employing the fiberoptic bronchoscope may be necessary. Many of these techniques require considerable skill and should be performed only by those experienced in airway management [36].

Specific Techniques and Routes of Endotracheal Intubation

OROTRACHEAL INTUBATION. Orotracheal intubation is the technique most easily learned and most often employed for emergency intubations in the ICU. Perhaps the most important aspect of this technique is proper positioning of the patient. Successful orotracheal intubation requires alignment of the oral, pharyngeal, and laryngeal axes (Figs. 1-10 and 1-11). To facilitate this alignment, it is necessary to place the patient in the sniffing position (Fig. 1-11), in which the neck is flexed and the head is slightly extended. This can be accomplished by placing several bath towels under the occiput. In a patient with a full stomach, the esophagus can be occluded by compressing the cricoid cartilage posteriorly against the vertebral body. This technique, known as Sellick's maneuver, can prevent passive regurgitation of stomach contents into the trachea during intubation [37].

The laryngoscope handle is grasped in the left hand while the patient's mouth is opened with the gloved right hand. Often in the sniffing position, the unconscious patient's mouth will open; if not, the thumb and index finger of the right hand are placed on the lower and upper incisors, respectively, and moved past each other in a scissorlike motion. The laryngoscope blade is inserted on the right side of the mouth and advanced to the base of the tongue, pushing it toward the left. If the straight blade is used, it should be extended below the epiglottis. If the curved blade is used, it is inserted in the vallecula.

With the blade in place, the operator should lift forward in a plane 45 degrees from the horizontal to expose the vocal cords (Figs. 1-2 and 1-9). It is essential to keep the left wrist stiff and to do all lifting from the arm and shoulder, to avoid turning the patient's teeth into a fulcrum. The endotracheal tube is then held in the right hand and inserted at the right corner of the patient's mouth in a plane that intersects with the laryngoscope

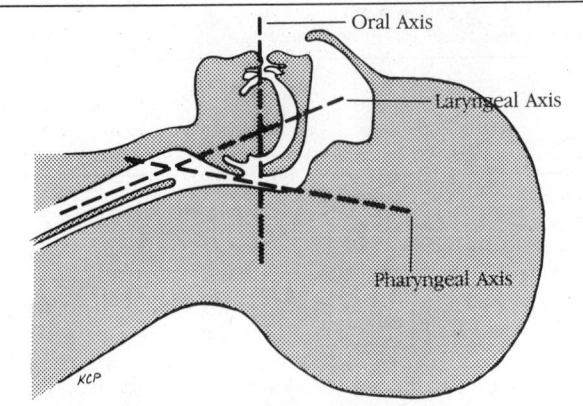

Fig. 1-10. In the supine patient, the axes of the mouth, pharynx, and larynx lie in divergent directions. To facilitate intubation, the axes of these three regions must be brought into close approximation.

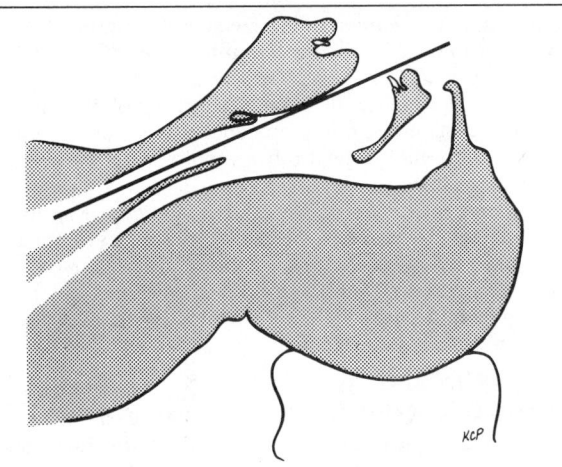

Fig. 1-11. With the patient's head in the proper position and with the use of the laryngoscope, the axes of the mouth, pharynx, and larynx can be brought into approximation, thus allowing easy visualization of the opening to the larynx.

blade at the level of the glottis. This prevents the endotracheal tube from obscuring the view of the vocal cords. The endotracheal tube is advanced through the vocal cords until the cuff just disappears from sight. The cuff is then inflated with enough air to prevent a leak during positive-pressure ventilation with a bag valve device.

Occasionally, the vocal cords cannot be seen entirely; only the corniculate and cuneiform tubercles, interarytenoid incisure, and posterior portion of the vocal cords are visualized (Fig. 1-2). In this situation it is helpful to insert the soft metal stylet into the endotracheal tube and bend it into a "hockey stick" configuration. The stylet should be bent or coiled at the proximal end to prevent the distal end from extending beyond the endotracheal tube and causing tissue damage. The stylet should be lubricated to ensure easy removal. Alternatively, a control-tip endotracheal tube may be used. This tube has a nylon cord running the length of the tube attached to a ring at the proximal end, which allows the operator to direct the tip of the tube anteriorly. A stylet with a maneuverable tip also has been described [38]. The tip is positioned through the glottic opening and the endotracheal tube passed into the trachea.

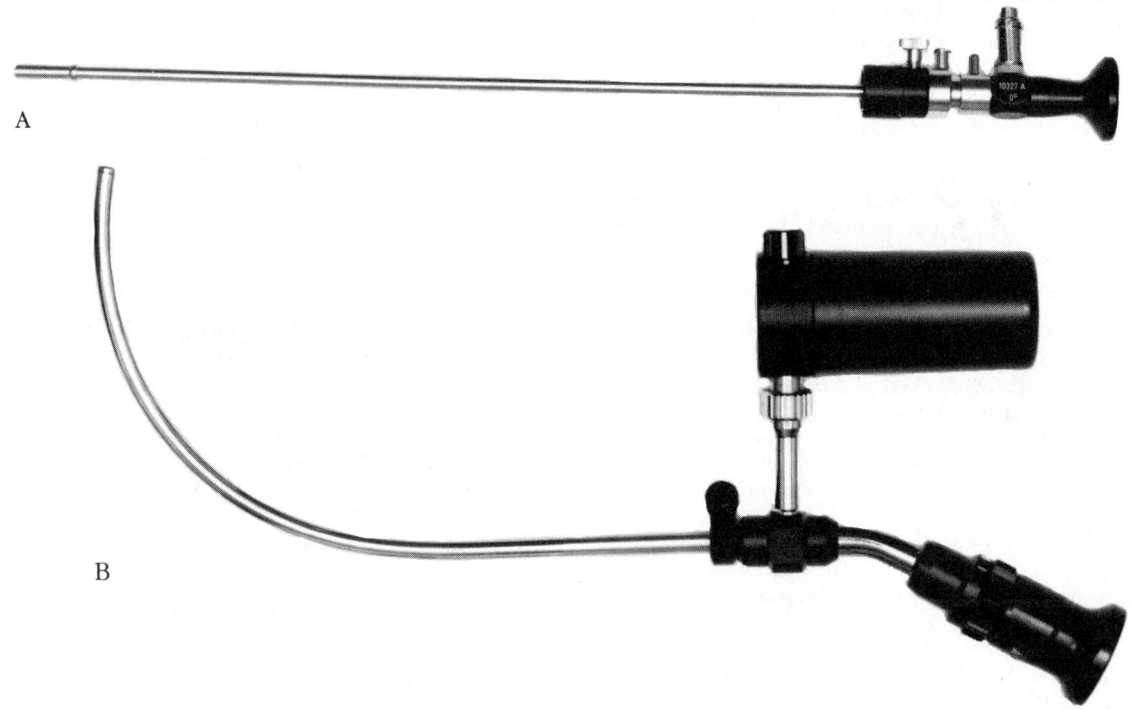

Fig. 1-12. Two rigid optical stylets are available for intubating the patient in whom such a procedure is expected to prove difficult: a straight optical stylet (A) and a curved stylet (B). Both require the use of a standard laryngoscope to move the soft tissue of the oropharynx out of the way to permit visualization of the upper part of the airway.

Another aid is a stylet with a light (light wand). With the room lights dimmed, the endotracheal tube containing the lighted stylet is inserted into the oropharynx and advanced in the midline. When it is just superior to the larynx, a glow is seen over the anterior neck. The stylet is advanced into the trachea and the tube is threaded over it. The light intensity is diminished if the wand enters the esophagus [39,40]. Curved or straight rigid optical stylets are also available for use in difficult intubations (Fig. 1-12). Both require the use of a standard laryngoscope to permit visualization of the upper airway.

Proper depth of tube placement is clinically ascertained by observing symmetric expansion of both sides of the chest and auscultating equal breath sounds in both lungs. A useful rule of thumb for tube placement in adults of "average" size is that the incisors shoud be at the 23-cm mark in men and the 21-cm mark in women [41]. Chander and Feldman advocate cuff palpation to ascertain correct tube position [42]. After intubation, the operator inflates the cuff to determine the amount of air necessary to prevent any leaks. The cuff is then deflated and a syringe with slightly more air (1–2 ml) than required to seal leaks is attached to the pilot line. The examiner then places his or her fingers just above the suprasternal notch and the cuff is rapidly inflated. The trachea is felt to expand at the level of the cuff. The process is repeated with the tube repositioned until the lower edge of the cuff is palpated just above the sternal notch. Auscultation of both lungs is then repeated to confirm equal breath sounds. The stomach should also be auscultated to ensure that the esophagus has not been entered. If the tube has been advanced too far, it will lodge in one of the main bronchi (particularly the right bronchus), and only one lung will be ventilated. If this error goes unnoticed, the nonventilated lung may collapse. Placement can also be confirmed by mea-

surement of end-tidal carbon dioxide if a capnograph is available [43]. Alternatively, a recently available chemical monitor of end-tidal carbon dioxide (FEF, Fenem) can be used to verify correct endotracheal tube placement or detect esophageal intubation. This device is attached to the proximal end of the endotracheal tube and changes color on exposure to carbon dioxide [44]. After estimating proper tube placement clinically, it should be confirmed by chest radiograph or (rarely) bronchoscopy. The tip of the endotracheal tube should be several centimeters above the carina (T_2 level). It must be remembered that flexion or extension of the head can advance or withdraw the tube 2 to 5 cm, respectively [45].

NASOTRACHEAL INTUBATION. Many of the considerations concerning patient preparation and positioning outlined for orotracheal intubation apply to nasal intubation as well. Blind nasal intubation is more difficult to perform than oral intubation because the tube cannot be observed directly as it passes between the vocal cords. However, nasal intubation is usually more comfortable for the patient and is generally preferable in the awake, conscious patient. Nasal intubation should not be attempted in patients with abnormal bleeding parameters, nasal polyps, extensive facial trauma, cerebrospinal rhinorrhea, sinusitis, or any anatomic abnormality that would inhibit atraumatic passage of the tube.

As discussed earlier, after the operator has alternately occluded each nostril to ascertain that both are patent, the nostril to be intubated is anesthetized. The patient should be monitored with a pulse oximeter and supplemental oxygen given as necessary. The patient may be either supine or sitting with the head extended in the sniffing position. The tube is guided slowly but firmly through the nostril to the posterior pharynx. Here the tube operator must continually monitor for the presence of air movement through the tube by listening for breath sounds with the ear near the open end of the tube. The tube must never be forced or pushed forward if breath sounds are lost, because damage to the retropharyngeal mucosa can result

[46]. If resistance is met, the tube should be withdrawn 1 to 2 cm and the patient's head repositioned (extended further or turned to either side). If the turn still cannot be negotiated, the other nostril or a smaller tube should be tried. Attempts at nasal intubation should be abandoned and oral intubation performed if these methods fail.

Once positioned in the oropharynx, the tube should be advanced to the glottis while listening for breath sounds through the tube. If breath sounds cease, the tube is withdrawn several centimeters until breath sounds resume, and the plane of entry is adjusted slightly. Passage through the vocal cords should be timed to coincide with inspiration. This is often signaled by a paroxysm of coughing and an inability to speak. The cuff should be inflated (as described for oral intubation) and proper positioning of the tube ascertained as previously outlined.

Occasionally, blind nasal intubation cannot be accomplished. In this case, after adequate topical anesthesia, a laryngoscope may be employed to visualize the vocal cords directly and Magill forceps used to grasp the distal end of the tube and guide it through the vocal cords (Fig. 1-13). Assistance in pushing the tube forward is essential during this maneuver, so that the operator merely guides the tube. The balloon on the tube should not be grasped with the Magill forceps.

FIBEROPTIC BRONCHOSCOPE INTUBATION. Fiberoptic bronchoscopy is an efficacious method of intubating the trachea in difficult cases [47,48,49] (Fig. 1-14). It may be particularly useful when the upper airway anatomy has been distorted by tumors, trauma, endocrinopathies [50,51,52], or congenital anomalies. This technique is sometimes valuable in accident victims where a question of cervical spine injury exists and the patient's neck cannot be manipulated. An analogous situation exists in patients with severe degenerative disc disease of the neck or rheumatoid arthritis with markedly impaired neck mobility. After obtaining adequate topical anesthesia, the bronchoscope can be used to intubate the trachea via either the nasal or oral route. An appropriately sized endotracheal tube is positioned over the bronchoscope, which is inserted into the mouth or nose and advanced through the vocal cords into the trachea. The endotracheal tube is moved over the bronchoscope and positioned above the carina under direct vision. The fiberoptic bronchoscope has also been used as a stent over which endotracheal tubes are exchanged and as a means to assess tracheal damage periodically during prolonged intubations. (A detailed discussion of bronchoscopy is found in Chap. 7.) Intubation by this technique requires skill and experience and is best performed by a fully trained operator.

CRICOTHYROTOMY. In a truly emergent situation, when intubation is unsuccessful, a cricothyrotomy may be required [53]. The technique is described in detail in Chapter 16. The quickest method, needle cricothyrotomy, is accomplished by introducing a large-bore (i.e., 14-gauge) catheter into the airway through the cricothyroid membrane while aspirating on a syringe attached to the needle of the catheter. When air is aspirated the needle is in the airway, and the catheter is passed over the needle into the trachea. A 3-ml syringe barrel is connected to the catheter. A 7-mm inside diameter endotracheal tube adapter fits into the syringe and can be connected to a high-pressure gas source or a high-frequency jet ventilator (Fig. 1-15). The patient can be adequately oxygenated for some time in this fashion [54]. A standard cricothyrotomy can be performed by making an incision through the skin and cricothyroid membrane and inserting a small (6.0–7.0 mm) endotracheal tube into the trachea (Chap. 16).

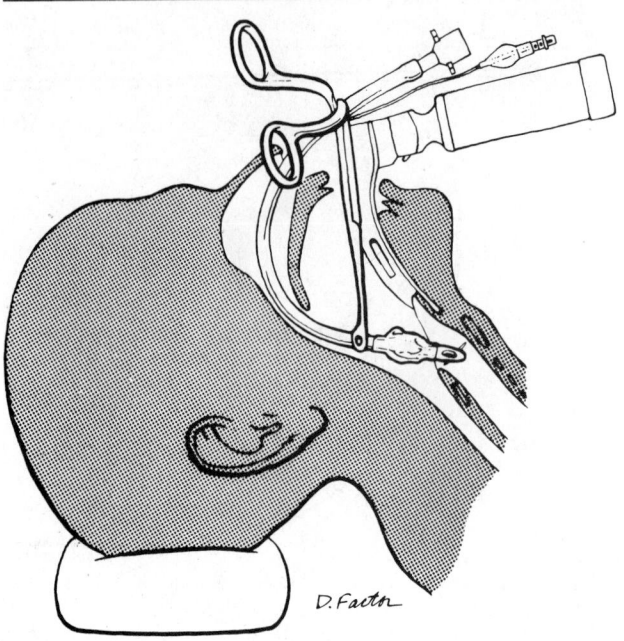

Fig. 1-13. McGill forceps may be required to guide the endotracheal tube into the larynx during nasotracheal intubation. Source: Barash PG, Cullen BF, Stoelting RK (eds): *Clinical Anesthesia.* 2nd ed. Philadelphia, JB Lippincott, 1992. With permission.

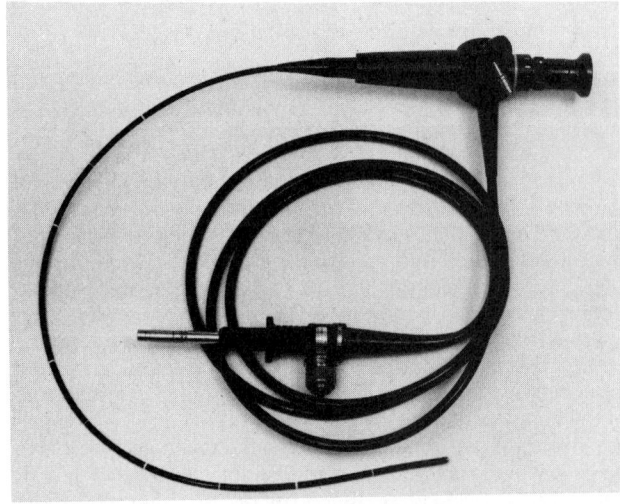

Fig. 1-14. The fiberoptic bronchoscope can be useful for intubating the trachea in the patient with a difficult airway or suspected cervical spine injury (see text for details).

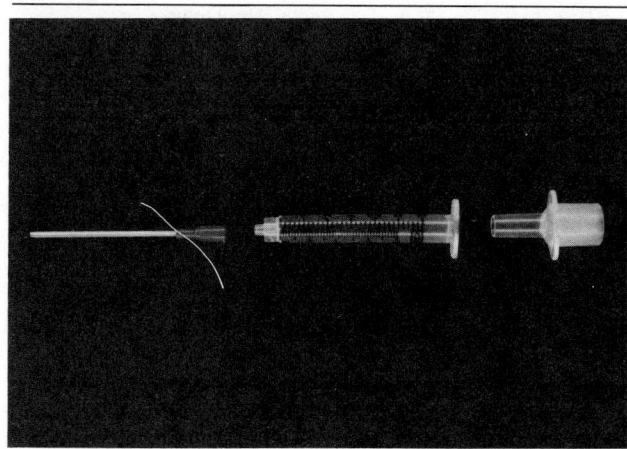

Fig. 1-15. A needle cricothyrotomy set. A large-bore (14-gauge) catheter is inserted through the cricothyroid membrane. The needle is removed and the catheter is attached to a 3-ml syringe barrel. A 7-mm endotracheal tube adapter is then attached to the syringe barrel. Alternatively, a 3-mm endotracheal tube adapter can be attached directly to the catheter.

Intubation of Difficult Airways [55,56]

Conditions that may predispose to difficulty in managing the airway can be classified as congenital or acquired lesions.

CONGENITAL ABNORMALITIES. Congenital hypoplasia or hyperplasia of the mandible makes it difficult to visualize the airway in the normal fashion [57]. Prominent incisors or maxillary hyperplasia can make placement of the laryngoscope in the oropharynx very difficult. Nasotracheal intubation or use of the fiberoptic bronchoscopy may be necessary.

ACQUIRED ABNORMALITIES. Acquired lesions that can lead to difficulties in airway management are those secondary to trauma or disease states. Massive injuries to the lower face following trauma can cause gross distortion of the mouth, and oral or nasal intubation may be impossible. Patients with acromegaly frequently have large tongues that can lead to difficulties in visualizing the airway [50]. Tumors of the neck can displace and distort the airway [51]. Prior operations such as radical neck dissection or hemimandibulectomy often result in distortion of the anatomy and make intubation difficult. Difficult laryngoscopy may also be anticipated in a subset of type I diabetic patients, secondary to the diabetic stiff joint syndrome with involvement of the atlanto-occipital joint [58]. Intubation with fiberoptic bronchoscopy can be particularly helpful in these situations.

SUSPECTED CERVICAL SPINE INJURY. Any patient with multiple trauma requiring intubation should be treated as if cervical spine injury is present [36,59,60]. In the absence of severe maxillofacial trauma or cerebrospinal rhinorrhea, nasal intubation is generally the preferred technique. However, in the profoundly hypoxemic or apneic patient, the orotracheal approach should be used [59]. If oral intubation is required, an assistant should maintain the neck in the neutral position by ensuring axial stabilization of the head and neck as the patient is intubated. A cervical collar also assists in immobilizing the cervical spine. In a patient with maxillofacial trauma and suspected cervical spine injury, retrograde intubation can be performed by puncturing the cricothyroid membrane with an 18-gauge catheter and threading a 125-cm Teflon-coated (0.025 cm diameter) guide wire through the catheter [61]. The wire is advanced into the oral cavity and the endotracheal tube is then advanced over the wire into the trachea. Alternatively, the wire can be threaded through the suction port of a 3.9-mm bronchoscope [62].

Airway Management in the Intubated Patient

Once the endotracheal tube is in position, proper management assumes utmost importance. From a pulmonary standpoint, an intubated patient is a "compromised host," robbed of normal upper airway defenses that protect the lungs from bacteria, other foreign bodies, and the aspiration of secretions. Some simple precautions and a careful approach to airway management will minimize complications.

SECURING THE TUBE. Properly securing the endotracheal tube in the desired position is important for three reasons: (1) to prevent accidental extubation; (2) to prevent advancement into one of the main bronchi; and (3) to minimize frictional damage to the upper airway, larynx, and trachea caused by patient motion. The endotracheal tube is usually secured in place with adhesive tape wrapped around the tube and applied to the patient's cheeks. Tincture of benzoin sprayed on the skin provides greater fixation. Alternatively, tape, intravenous (IV) tubing, or umbilical tape may be tied to the endotracheal tube and brought around the patient's neck to secure the tube. Care must be taken to prevent occlusion of neck veins. Other products (e.g., Velcro straps) to secure the tube are available. A bite block is positioned in the patient who is orally intubated to prevent the patient from biting down on the tube and occluding it. Once the tube has been secured and its proper position verified, it should be plainly marked on the portion protruding from the patient's mouth or nose so that advancement can be noted.

CUFF MANAGEMENT. Although low-pressure cuffs have markedly reduced the incidence of complications related to tracheal ischemia, monitoring cuff pressures remains important. The cuff should be inflated just beyond the point where an audible air leak occurs. Maintenance of intracuff pressures between 17 and 23 mm Hg should allow an adequate seal to permit mechanical ventilation under most circumstances while not compromising blood flow to the tracheal mucosa. The intracuff pressure should be checked periodically by attaching a pressure gauge and syringe to the cuff port via a three-way stopcock. The need to add air continually to the cuff to maintain its seal with the tracheal wall indicates that (1) the cuff or pilot tube has a hole in it, (2) the pilot tube valve is broken or cracked, or (3) the tube is positioned incorrectly and the cuff is between the vocal cords. The tube position should be re-evaluated to exclude the latter possibility. If the valve is broken, attaching a three-way stopcock to it will solve the problem. If the valve housing is cracked, cutting the pilot tube and inserting a blunt needle with a stopcock into the lumen of the pilot tube will maintain a competent system. Obviously, a hole in the cuff necessitates a change of tubes.

TUBE SUCTIONING. A complete discussion of tube suctioning can be found in Chapter 56. "Routine" suctioning should not be performed in patients in whom secretions are not a problem [63]. Suctioning can produce a variety of complications, including hypoxemia, elevations in intracranial pressure, and serious ventricular arrhythmias. Preoxygenation should reduce the likelihood of arrhythmias. Closed ventilation suction systems (Stericath) may reduce the risk of hypoxemia.

HUMIDIFICATION. Intubation of the trachea bypasses the normal upper airway structures responsible for heating and humidifying inspired air. It is thus essential that inspired air be heated and humidified (Chap. 54).

TUBE REPLACMENT. At times, endotracheal tubes may need to be replaced because of an air leak, obstruction, or other problem. Before attempting to change an endotracheal tube, one should assess how difficult it will be. After obtaining appropriate topical anesthesia or intravenous sedation and achieving muscle relaxation, direct laryngoscopy can be performed to ascertain whether there will be difficulties in visualizing the vocal cords. If the cords can be seen, the defective tube is removed under direct visualization and reintubation performed using the new tube. If the cords cannot be seen on direct laryngoscopy, then the tube can be changed over a long, plastic stylet (Eschmann stylet) or a fiberoptic bronchoscope. The disadvantage to using the bronchoscope is that the old tube must be cut away with a scalpel before the new tube can be advanced into the trachea. In a patient with a large intrapulmonary shunt, severe hypoxemia might develop while the old tube is being replaced. Alternatively, the bronchoscope (with the new tube on it) can be advanced into the trachea next to (rather than through) the old endotracheal tube after deflating the cuff. The old tube is then withdrawn and the new tube positioned over the bronchoscope [64].

Complications of Endotracheal Intubation

Complications associated with endotracheal intubation may occur: (1) during intubation, (2) while the endotracheal tube is in place, or (3) following extubation. Table 1-4 is a partial listing of these complications. The exact incidence of complications is difficult to determine, varying widely in published reports and depending to some extent on the vigor of efforts to identify them. Factors implicated in the etiology of complications include tube size, characteristics of the tube and cuff, trauma during intubation, duration and route of intubation, metabolic or nutritional status of the patient, tube motion, and laryngeal motor activity [65,66].

COMPLICATIONS DURING INTUBATION. During endotracheal intubation, traumatic injury can occur to any anatomic structure from the lips to the trachea. Possible complications include (1) aspiration, (2) damage to teeth and dental work, (3) corneal abrasions, (4) perforation or laceration of the pharynx,

Table 1-4. Complications of Endotracheal Intubation

Complications during intubation
  Spinal cord injury
  Excessive delay of CPR
  Aspiration
  Damage to teeth and dental work
  Corneal abrasions
  Perforation or laceration of:
    Pharynx
    Larynx
    Trachea
  Dislocation of an arytenoid cartilage
  Passage of endotracheal tube into cranial vault
  Epistaxis
  Cardiovascular problems
    Ventricular premature contractions
    Ventricular tachycardia
    Bradyarrhythmias
    Hypotension
    Hypertension
    Hypoxemia
Complications while tube is in place
  Blockage or kinking of tube
  Dislodgement of tube
  Advancement of tube into a bronchus
  Mechanical damage to any upper airway structure
  Problems related to mechanical ventilation (Chap. 54)
Complications following extubation
  Immediate complications
    Laryngospasm
    Aspiration
  Intermediate and long-term complications
    Sore throat
    Ulcerations of lips, mouth, pharynx, or vocal cords
    Tongue numbness (hypoglossal nerve compression)
    Laryngitis
    Vocal cord paralysis (unilateral or bilateral)
    Laryngeal edema
    Laryngeal ulcerations
    Laryngeal granuloma
    Vocal cord synechiae
    Tracheal stenosis

larynx, or trachea, (5) dislocation of an arytenoid cartilage [67], (6) retropharyngeal perforation [68,69], (7) epistaxis [46], (8) hypoxemia, (9) myocardial ischemia, and (10) laryngospasm with noncardiogenic pulmonary edema [70]. Many of these complications can be avoided by careful attention to technique. The eyes are vulnerable to damage from the operator's arms, sleeves, or instruments. Noncardiogenic pulmonary edema occurs during laryngospasm due to high negative intrapleural pressures causing a flux of fluid into the pulmonary interstitium [70].

A variety of cardiovascular complications can accompany intubation. Ventricular arrhythmias have been reported in 5 to 10 percent of intubations [71]. Ventricular tachycardia and ventricular fibrillation are uncommon but have been reported. Patients with myocardial ischemia are susceptible to ventricular arrhythmias, and lidocaine prophylaxis (100 mg IV bolus) prior to intubation may be warranted in such individuals. Bradyarrhythmias can also be observed and are probably caused by stimulation of the laryngeal branches of the vagus nerve [71]. They may not require therapy but usually respond to intravenous atropine (1 mg IV bolus). Both hypotension and hypertension during intubation have been reported [72]. The use of vasoactive medications for routine prophylaxis against hypotension or hypertension is unwarranted. However, in the patient with myocardial ischemia, short-acting agents to control blood pressure (nitroprusside) and heart rate (esmolol) during intubation may be needed.

COMPLICATIONS WHILE TUBE IS IN PLACE. Despite adherence to guidelines designed to minimize damage from endotracheal intubation, the tube can damage local structures. Microscopic alterations to the surface of the vocal cords can occur within 2 hours following intubation. Evidence of macroscopic damage can occur within 6 hours [73]. As might be expected, clinically significant damage typically occurs when intubation is prolonged [74]. The sudden appearance of blood in tracheal secretions suggests anterior erosion into overlying vascular structures, while the appearance of gastric contents suggests posterior erosion into the esophagus. Both situations require urgent bronchoscopy, and it is imperative that the mucosa underlying the cuff be examined. Other complications include tracheomalacia and stenosis, and damage to the larynx. Failure to secure the endotracheal tube properly or patient agitation can contribute to mechanical damage.

Another complication is blockage or kinking of the tube, resulting in compromised ventilation. Occlusion of the tube caused by the patient biting down on it can be minimized by placing a bite block in the patient's mouth. Blockage from secretions can usually be solved by suctioning, although changing the tube may be necessary.

Unplanned extubation and endobronchial intubation are potentially life-threatening. Appropriately securing and marking the tube should minimize these problems. Daily chest radiographs with the head always in the same position should be obtained on all intubated patients to assess the position of the tube [45].

Other complications occurring while the tube is in position relate to mechanical ventilation (e.g., pneumothorax) and are discussed in detail in Chapter 54.

COMPLICATIONS FOLLOWING EXTUBATION. Sore throat is so common following extubation that some authorities refuse to classify it as a complication [75]. It has been reported following 40 to 100 percent of intubations [76]. It probably results from mechanical irritation and usually resolves in 48 to 72 hours. The incidence of postextubation sore throat and hoarseness possibly can be decreased by using a smaller endotracheal tube [77]. Ulcerations of the lips, mouth, or pharynx can occur, being more common if the initial intubation was traumatic. Pressure from the endotracheal tube can traumatize the hypoglossal nerve, resulting in numbness of the tongue that can persist for 1 to 2 weeks [78,79]. Irritation of the larynx appears to be due to local mucosal damage and occurs in as many as 45 percent of individuals following extubation. Unilateral [80] or bilateral [81] vocal cord paralysis is an uncommon but serious complication following extubation. For reasons that are unclear, when unilateral vocal cord paralysis occurs, the left cord is involved twice as frequently as the right. Males are seven times more likely than females to experience cord paralysis [82]. Recurrent laryngeal nerve (RLN) damage can be caused by inflation of the cuff in the larynx, which compresses and damages the RLN as it passes between the arytenoid cartilage and thyroid lamina [83].

Some degree of laryngeal edema accompanies almost all endotracheal intubations. In adults, this is usually clinically insignificant. In children, however, even a small amount of edema can compromise the already small subglottic opening [84]. In a newborn, 1 mm of laryngeal edema results in a 65 percent narrowing of the airway. Laryngeal ulcerations are commonly observed following extubation. They are more commonly lo-

cated at the posterior portion of the vocal cords, where the endotracheal tube tends to rub [85]. Ulcerations become increasingly common the longer the tube is left in place. The incidence of ulceration is decreased by the use of endotracheal tubes that conform to the anatomical shape of the larynx [86]. Both laryngeal granulomata and synechiae of the vocal cords are extremely rare, but these complications can seriously compromise airway patency [87,88]. Surgical treatment is often required to treat these problems.

A feared late complication of endotracheal intubation is tracheal stenosis [88]. This occurs much less frequently now that high-volume, low-pressure cuffs are routinely used. Symptoms can occur weeks to months following extubation. In mild cases, the patient may experience dyspnea or ineffective cough. If the airway is narrowed to less than 5 mm, the patient presents with stridor. Dilation may provide effective treatment, but in some instances surgical intervention is necessary.

Extubation

The decision to extubate a patient is based on (1) a favorable clinical response to a carefully planned regimen of weaning from mechanical ventilation (Chap. 55), (2) recovery of consciousness following anesthesia, or (3) sufficient resolution of the initial indications for intubation.

TECHNIQUE OF EXTUBATION. The patient should be alert, lying with the head of the bed elevated to at least a 45-degree angle. The posterior pharynx must be thoroughly suctioned. In situations where postextubation difficulties are anticipated, equipment for emergency reintubation should be assembled at the bedside. The procedure is explained to the patient. The cuff is deflated and positive pressure is applied to expel any foreign material that has collected above the cuff as the tube is withdrawn. Supplemental oxygen is then provided.

The most serious complication of extubation is laryngospasm, which is much more likely to occur if the patient is not fully conscious. The application of positive pressure can sometimes relieve laryngospasm. If this maneuver is not successful, succinylcholine (by the intravenous or intramuscular route) can be administered. Succinylcholine can cause severe hyperkalemia in a variety of clinical settings, therefore only clinicians experienced with its use should administer it. Mechanical ventilation is needed until the patient has recovered from the succinylcholine.

TRACHEOSTOMY. In the past it was common to perform a tracheostomy to replace the endotracheal tube as soon as the need for prolonged airway control became apparent. Improvements in cuff design have permitted progressively longer periods of translaryngeal intubation. The optimal time of conversion from an endotracheal tube to a tracheostomy remains controversial [89,90,91]. The total complication rate of either procedure is reported to be similar (60%), but complications associated with tracheostomy are sometimes more serious. Tracheostomy has a reportedly higher mortality rate and incidence of secondary bacterial invasion and aspiration. Current data suggest that oral or nasal intubation is the method of choice when an artificial airway is required for less than 3 weeks. When airway protection or positive-pressure ventilation of longer duration is necessary, tracheostomy should be considered. Decisions regarding the timing of tracheostomy should be based on the overall clinical situation. The reader is referred to Chapter 16 for details on tracheostomy.

References

1. Hooke R: An account of an experiment made by R. Hooke on preserving animals alive by blowing through their lungs with bellows. *Philos Trans R Soc Lond [Biol]* 2:539, 1667.

2. Vesalius A: *Debumani corporis fabrica libri septem.* Basel, Oporinus, 1543, p 658.

3. Appelbaum EL, Bruce DL: A short history of tracheal intubation, in Appelbaum EL, Bruce DL (eds): *Tracheal Intubation.* Philadelphia, WB Saunders, 1976, p 1.

4. Herboldt JD, Rafu CG: An attempt at a historical survey of life saving measures for drowning persons and information on the best means by which they can again be brought back to life. Copenhagen, H Tikiobs, 1796. Reprinted in Denmark by Aarhuus Stiftsbogtrykkerie, 1960.

5. Snow J: *On Chloroform and Other Anaesthetics.* London, Churchill, 1858, p 117.

6. Trendelenberg F: Tamponade de trachea. *Arch Klin Chir* 12:121, 1871.

7. Macewen W: Clinical observations in the introduction of tracheal tubes by the mouth instead of performing tracheotomy or laryngotomy. *Br Med J Clin Res* 2:122, 163, 1880.

8. O'Dwyer J: Intubation of the larynx. *NY Med J* 42:145, 1885.

9. O'Dwyer J: Analysis of 50 cases of croup treated by intubation of the larynx. *NY Med J* 47:33, 1888.

10. Jackson C: *Tracheo-bronchoscopy, Esophagoscopy and Gastroscopy.* St. Louis, St. Louis Laryngoscope Co, 1907.

11. The respiratory system, in Goss CM (ed): *Gray's Anatomy of the Human Body.* 29th American ed. Philadelphia, Lea & Febiger, 1973, p 1120.

12. Ellis H, Feldman S: *Anatomy for Anaesthetists.* 4th ed. Oxford, UK, Blackwell Scientific, 1983, p 3.

13. Fassoulaki A, Pamouktsoglou P: Prolonged nasotracheal intubation and its association with inflammation of paranasal sinuses. *Anesth Analg* 69:50, 1989.

14. Natanson C, Shelhamer JH, Parrillo JE: Intubation of the trachea in the critical care setting. *JAMA* 253:1160, 1985.

15. Becker A: Airway management I: Indications for intubation and emergency airway management, in Rippe JM, Csete ME (eds): *Manual of Intensive Care Medicine.* 2nd ed. Boston, Little, Brown, 1989, p 3.

16. Standards and guidelines for cardiopulmonary resuscitation (CPR) and emergency cardiac care (ECC), II: Adult basic life support. *JAMA* 268:2184, 1992.

17. Benumof JL: Laryngeal mask airway: Indications and contraindications. *Anesthesiology* 77:843, 1992.

18. Pennant JH, White PF: Laryngeal mask airway: Its uses in anesthesiology. *Anesthesiology* 79:144, 1993.

19. Becker A: Airway management II: Techniques for intubation, in Rippe JM, Csete ME (eds): *Manual of Intensive Care Medicine.* 2nd ed. Boston, Little, Brown, 1989, p 8.

20. Standards and guidelines for cardiopulmonary resuscitation (CPR) and emergency cardiac care (ECC), III: Adult advanced cardiac life support. *JAMA* 268:2199, 1992.

21. Coleman DL: Smoke inhalation: Medical Staff Conference, University of California, San Francisco. *West J Med* 135:300, 1981.

22. Fein A, Leff A, Hopewell PC: Pathophysiology and management of the complications resulting from fire and inhaled products of combustion: Review of the literature. *Crit Care Med* 8:94, 1980.

23. Mallampati SR, Gatt SP, Gugino LD, et al: A clinical sign to predict difficult tracheal intubation: A prospective study. *Can Anaesth Soc J* 32:420, 1985.

24. Stone DJ, Gal TJ: Airway management, in Miller RD (ed): *Anesthesia.* 3rd ed. New York, Churchill Livingstone, 1990, p 1265.

25. MacIntosh RR: New laryngoscope. *Lancet* 1:205, 1943.

26. Miller RA: A new laryngoscope. *Anesthesiology* 2:317, 1941.

27. Wright PE, Marini JJ, Bernard GR: In vitro versus in vivo comparison of endotracheal tube airflow resistance. *Am Rev Respir Dis* 140:10, 1989.

28. Carroll R, Hedden M, Safar P: Intra-tracheal cuffs: Performance characteristics. *Anesthesiology* 31:275, 1969.

29. Knowlson GTG, Bassett HFM: The pressure exerted on the trachea by endotracheal inflatable cuffs. *Br J Anaesth* 42:824, 1970.

30. Andrews MJ, Pearson FG: Incidence and pathogenesis of tracheal injury following cuffed tube tracheostomy and assisted ventilation: Analysis of a two year perspective study. *Ann Surg* 173:249, 1971.

31. Klainer AS, Turndorf H, Wen-Hsien WU, et al: Surface alterations due to endotracheal intubation. *Am J Med* 58:674, 1975.

32. Guyton DC, Banner MJ, Kirby RR: High-volume, low pressure cuffs: Are they really low-pressure. *Crit Care Med* 17:S24, 1989.

33. Venus B, Polassani V, Pham CG: Effects of aerosolized lidocaine on circulatory responses to laryngoscopy and tracheal intubation. *Crit Care Med* 12:391, 1984.

34. Laurito CE, Baughman VL, Becker GL, et al: Effects of aerosolized and/or intravenous lidocaine on hemodynamic responses to laryngoscopy and intubation in outpatients. *Anesth Analg* 67:389, 1988.

35. Hee MKJ, Plevak DJ, Peters SG: Intubation of critically ill patients. *Mayo Clin Proc* 67:569, 1992.

36. Hastings RH, Marks JG: Airway management for trauma patients with potential cervical spine injuries. *Anesth Analg* 73:471, 1991.

37. Sellick BA: Cricoid pressure to control regurgitation of stomach contents during induction of anaesthesia. *Lancet* 2:404, 1961.

38. Rao TLK, Mathew M, Gorski EW, et al: Experience with a new intubation guide for difficult intubation. *Crit Care Med* 10:882, 1982.

39. Ellis DG, Jakymec A, Kaplan RM, et al: Guided orotracheal intubation in the operating room using a lighted stylet: A comparison with direct laryngoscopic technique. *Anesthesiology* 64:823, 1986.

40. Fox DJ, Castro T, Rastrelli AJ: Comparison of intubation techniques in the awake patient: The Flexi-lum Surgical light (lightwand) versus blind nasal approach. *Anesthesiology* 66:69, 1987.

41. Owen RL, Cheney FW: Endobronchial intubation: A preventable complication. *Anesthesiology* 67:255, 1987

42. Chander S, Feldman E: Correct placement of endotracheal tubes. *NY State J Med* 79:1843, 1979.

43. Gravenstein JS, Paulus DA, Hays TJ: *Capnography in Clinical Practice.* Stoneham, MA, Butterworths, 1989, p 43.

44. Winston RS, Layon AJ, Gravenstein N, et al: Detection of esophageal intubation with a new chemical monitor of end-tidal carbon dioxide. *Crit Care Med* 18:S216, 1990.

45. Conrardy PA, Goodman LR, Lainge F, et al: Alteration of endotracheal tube position: Flexion and extension of the neck. *Crit Care Med* 4:8, 1976.

46. Tintinall JE, Claffey J: Complications of nasotracheal intubation. *Ann Emerg Med* 10:142, 1981.

47. Taylor PA, Towey RM: The broncho-fiberscope as an aid to endotracheal intubation. *Br J Anaesth* 44:611, 1972.

48. Messeter KH, Pettersson KI: Endotracheal intubation with the fiberoptic bronchoscope. *Anaesthesia* 35:294, 1980.

49. Rosenbaum SH, Rosenbaum LM, Cole RP, et al: Use of the flexible fiberoptic bronchoscope to change endotracheal tubes in the critically ill patient. *Anesthesiology* 54:169, 1981.

50. Rees PJ, Webb JR, Hay JG: Acute exacerbation of upper airway obstruction in acromegaly. *Postgrad Med J* 58:429, 1982.

51. Hassard AD, Holland JG: Benign thyroid disease and upper airway obstruction. *J Otolaryngol* 11:77, 1982.

52. Ovassapian A, Doka JC, Romsa DE: Acromegaly: Use of fiberoptic laryngoscope to avoid tracheostomy. *Anesthesiology* 54:429, 1981.

53. Schecter WP, Wilson RS: Management of upper airway obstruction in the intensive care unit. *Crit Care Med* 9:577, 1981.

54. Koch E, Benumof JL: Percutaneous transtracheal jet ventilation: An important airway adjunct. *AANA J* 58:337, 1990.

55. Latto IP, Rosen M: *Difficulties in Tracheal Intubation.* London, Bailliere Tindall, 1987.

56. Shorten GD: Airway management. *Curr Opin Anesth* 5:772, 1992.

57. Payne KA: Difficult tracheal intubation. *Anaesth Intensive Care* 8:84, 1980.

58. Hogan K, Rusy D, Springman SR: Difficult laryngoscopy and diabetes mellitus. *Anesth Analg* 67:1162, 1988.

59. Shah JB, Skerman JH, Till WJ, et al: Appropriate techniques for airway management of emergency patients with suspected spinal cord injury. *Anesth Analg* 67:710, 1988.

60. Yealy DM, Cantees KK, Verdile VP, et al: Emergency airway management in trauma patients with a suspected cervical spine injury. *Anesth Analg* 68:413, 1989.

61. Barriot P, Riou B: Retrograde technique for tracheal intubation in trauma patients. *Crit Care Med* 16:712, 1988.

62. Stehling L: Evaluation of the airway, in *1989 Annual Refresher Course Lectures*. Chicago, American Society of Anesthesiologists, 1989, p 262/1.

63. Demers RR, Saklad M: Mechanical aspiration: A re-appraisal of its hazards. *Respir Care* 20:661, 1975.

64. Ovassapian A, Dykes MHM: The role of fiber-optic endoscopy in airway management. *Semin Anesth* 6:93, 1987.

65. Gaynor EB, Greenberg SB: Untoward sequelae of prolonged intubation. *Laryngoscope* 12:1461, 1985.

66. Kastanos N, Miro RE, Perez AM, et al: Laryngotracheal injury due to endotracheal intubation: Incidence, evolution, and predisposing factors—A prospective long-term study. *Crit Care Med* 11:362, 1983.

67. Quick C, Merwin G: Arytenoid dislocation. *Arch Otolaryngol* 104:267, 1978.

68. Levine PA: Hypopharyngeal perforation: An untoward complication of endotracheal intubation. *Arch Otolaryngol* 6:578, 1980.

69. Myers EM: Hypopharyngeal perforation: A complication of endotracheal intubation. *Laryngoscope* 92:583, 1982.

70. Willms D, Shure D: Pulmonary edema due to upper airway obstruction in adults. *Chest* 94:1090, 1988.

71. Gibbs JM: The effects of endotracheal intubation on cardiac rate and rhythm. *N Z Med J* 66:465, 1967.

72. Takeshima K, Noda K, Higaki M: Cardiovascular response to rapid anesthesia induction and endotracheal intubation. *Anesth Analg* 43:201, 1964.

73. Dubick MM, Wright BD: Problems of prolonged endotracheal intubations. *Chest* 74:479, 1978.

74. Vogelhut MM, Downs JB: Prolonged endotracheal intubation. *Chest* 76:110, 1979.

75. Baron SH, Kohlmoos HW: Laryngeal sequela of endotracheal anesthesia. *Ann Otol Rhinol Otolaryngol* 60:767, 1961.

76. Winkel E, Knudson J: Effect on the incidence of postoperative sore throat of one percent cinchocaine gel for endotracheal intubation. *Anesth Analg* 50:92, 1971.

77. Stout DM, Bishop MJ, Dwersteg JF, et al: Correlation of endotracheal tube size with sore throat and hoarseness following general anesthesia. *Anesthesiology* 67:419, 1987.

78. Teichner RL: Lingual nerve injury: A complication of lower tracheal anesthesia. *Br J Anaesth* 43:413, 1971.

79. Jones BC: Lingual nerve injury: A complication of intubation. *Br J Anaesth* 43:730, 1971.

80. Hahn SW, Martin JT, Lillie JC: Vocal cord paralysis of endotracheal intubation. *Arch Otolaryngol* 92:226, 1970.

81. Holley HS, Gildea JE: Vocal cord paralysis of endotracheal intubation. *JAMA* 215:281, 1971.

82. Cook WR: A comparison of idiopathic laryngeal paralysis in man and horse. *J Laryngol* 84:819, 1970.

83. Brandwein M, Abramson AL, Shikowitz MJ: Bilateral vocal cord paralysis following endotracheal intubation. *Arch Otolaryngol Head Neck Surg* 112:877, 1986.

84. Holinger P, Johnson K: Factors responsible for laryngeal obstruction in infants. *JAMA* 143:1229, 1950.

85. Jackson C: Contact ulcers, granuloma and other laryngeal complications of endotracheal anesthesia. *Anesthesiology* 14:425, 1953.

86. Eckerbom B, Lindholm CE, Alexopous C: Airway lesions caused by prolonged intubation with standard and with anatomically shaped tracheal tubes: A post-mortem study. *Acta Anaesthesiol Scand* 30:366, 1986.

87. Snow JC, Harano M, Balogy K: Post intubation granuloma of the larynx. *Anesth Analg* 45:425, 1966.

88. Bishop MJ, Weymuller EA, Fink BR: Laryngeal effects of prolonged intubation. *Anesth Analg* 63:335, 1984.

89. Berlauk JF: Prolonged endotracheal intubation vs. tracheostomy. *Crit Care Med* 14:742, 1986.

90. Stauffer JL, Olson DE, Petty TL: Complications and consequences of endotracheal intubation and tracheotomy. *Am J Med* 70:65, 1981.

91. Heffner JE, Miller S, Sahn SA: Tracheostomy in the intensive care unit, 1: Indications, technique, management. *Chest* 90:269, 1986.

2. Central Venous Catheters

Michael Seneff

Central venous catheterization remains an integral skill for the practice of critical care medicine. Continued technological advancements in catheter design and increased insight from animal and human research into the causes of catheter-related complications have made central venous catheterization easier and safer for physicians and patients. This chapter reviews the art and science of central venous catheterization, with special attention to the techniques and complications of the various routes of cannulation.

Historical Perspective

Although isolated experiments with central venous cannulation were performed in the early twentieth century [1], Aubaniac is credited with the first description of infraclavicular subclavian venipuncture in humans in 1952 [2]. A major advance in intravenous catheter technique came the following year, when Seldinger described the replacement of a catheter needle using a guidewire, a technique that now bears his name [3]. During the mid-1950s percutaneous catheterization of the inferior vena cava via a femoral vein approach became popular until reports of a high incidence of complications were published [4,5].

An important development occurred in 1959, when Hughes and Magovern described the clinical use of central venous pressure (CVP) measurements in humans undergoing thoracotomy [6]. In 1962, Wilson and associates extended the practicality of CVP monitoring by using percutaneous infraclavicular subclavian vein (SV) catheterization [7]. This technique achieved wide clinical acceptance, but enthusiasm was tempered when various, sometimes fatal, complications were reported. Subsequently, Yoffa reported his experience with supraclavicular subclavian venipuncture, claiming a lower incidence of complications, but his results were not uniformly reproduced [8].

Motivated by the search for a "golden route" [9], Nordlund and Thoren [10] and then Rams and associates [11] performed external jugular vein (EJV) catheterization and advocated a more extensive use of this approach. Although EJV catheterization met the goal of causing fewer complications during venipuncture, positioning of the catheter tip in a central venous location was sometimes impossible.

The first large series on internal jugular vein (IJV) catheterization appeared in 1969, when English et al. [12,13] reported their series of 500 percutaneous IJV catheterizations. Reports confirming this route's efficiency and low complication rate followed, and it has remained a popular site for central venous access.

The best route to establish central venous access remains controversial, and the search for the golden route continues. New techniques and concepts of central venous catheterization (CVC) are regularly introduced, but the four traditional routes are adequate to manage virtually all critically ill patients. Physicians must be aware of each route's advantages and disadvantages to be able to choose an appropriate site for the clinical situation.

Indications and Site Selection

Technical advances and a better understanding of anatomy have made insertion of central venous catheters easier and safer, but there still is an underappreciation of the inherent risks. Like any medical procedure, CVC has specific indications and should be reserved for the patient who has the potential truly to benefit from it (Table 2-1). After determining that CVC is necessary, inexperienced physicians often proceed with subclavian vein catheterization without a thoughtful consideration of the risk-benefit ratio for that route in that particular patient. The consequences of this cavalier approach can be disastrous [14]. It is the responsibility of all critical care physicians to conduct a scientific consideration of the risks and benefits of CVC for every patient who requires it. This will minimize the number of preventable complications and clinically justify those that do occur as a necessary risk of caring for the critically ill.

Volume resuscitation alone is not an indication for CVC. A 2.5-inch, 16-gauge catheter used to cannulate a peripheral vein can infuse two times the amount of fluid as an 8-inch, 16-gauge central venous catheter [15]. However, peripheral vein cannulation can be impossible in the hypovolemic, shocked individual. In this instance, the SV is the most reliable central site because it remains patent due to its fibrous attachments to the clavicle [16]. Depending on the clinical situation, the femoral vein (FV) is a reasonable alternative.

Central venous access is often required for the infusion of irritant medications (concentrated potassium chloride) or vasoactive agents, certain diagnostic or therapeutic radiologic procedures, and, obviously, in any patient in whom peripheral access is not possible. For these indications, the IJV is an ideal route because of its reliability and low rate of major complications with insertion. For experienced operators, the SV is an excellent alternative, as the risk of pneumothorax is low. The FV has many advantages as a primary alternative site but remains underutilized because of concern about the risk of complications from long-term (>72 hr) cannulation.

Long-term total parenteral nutrition with hyperosmolar solutions is best administered through SV catheters, which should be surgically implanted if appropriate. Acute hemodialysis is best accomplished with a subclavian catheter. Flow is more predictable, the catheter less prone to kinking, overall maintenance easier, and complications are rare [17,18]. There are increasing reports, however, of SV thrombosis and stenosis following temporary hemodialysis, causing some centers to switch to the IJV for temporary dialysis access in ambulatory patients [19,20]. The FV is also suitable for acute short-term hemodialysis or plasmapheresis in nonambulatory patients [21].

Table 2-1. Indication for CVC

	Site Selection		
	1st	2nd	3rd
Pulmonary artery catheterization	RIJV	LIJV	LSV
With coagulopathy	REJV	LEJV	RIJV
With pulmonary compromise or high-level PEEP	RIJV	LIJV	EJV
Total parenteral nutrition	SV	IJV	
Long-term	SV (surgically implanted)		
Acute hemodialysis/plasmapheresis	SV	FV	
		IJV (ambulatory)	
Cardiopulmonary arrest	FV	SV	IJV
Emergency transvenous pacemaker	RIJV	SV or LIJV	FV
Hypovolemia, inability to perform peripheral catheterization	SV or FV	IJV	
Preoperative preparation	IJV	EJV	SV
Neurosurgical procedure	AV	FV	SV
General-purpose venous access, vasoactive agents, caustic medications, radiological procedures	IJV	SV or FV	EJV
With coagulopathy	FV or EJV	IJV	AV
Emergency airway management	FV	SV	IJV
Inability to lie supine	FV	EJV	AV

SV, subclavian vein; IJV, internal jugular vein; EJV, external jugular vein; FV, femoral vein; R, right; L, left.

Emergency transvenous pacemakers are best inserted through the right IJV because of the direct path to the right ventricle. This route is associated with the fewest catheter tip malpositions. For the same reason, the right IJV is the primary route for insertion of flow-directed pulmonary artery catheters. In patients with coagulopathy, the EJV, if part of the surface anatomy, is a good alternative. When the SV is used for pulmonary artery catheterization, the left SV is the appropriate choice, for two reasons. First, in many patients, the tip of a standard introducer inserted into the right SV extends into the superior vena cava (SVC), requiring the pulmonary artery catheter to make a sharp bend when it exits the introducer. Malpositioning or kinking of the catheter may result [22]. This does not occur with left SV insertion because of the greater distance from the venipuncture site to the SVC. Second, catheters inserted from the left SV follow a natural curve, traversing the right ventricle into the right pulmonary artery. The reader is referred to Chapter 4 for additional information on the insertion and care of pulmonary artery catheters.

Preoperative CVC is desirable in a wide variety of clinical situations. If fluid status requires close monitoring, a pulmonary artery catheter should be inserted, since CVP is an unreliable predictor of left heart filling pressures [23–26]. In most preoperative patients, the IJV or EJV is the best route, since pneumothorax is very rare with these approaches and even a small pneumothorax is at risk of expanding under general anesthesia [27]. One specific indication for preoperative right ventricular catheterization is the patient undergoing a posterior craniotomy or cervical laminectomy in the sitting position. These patients are at risk for air embolism, and the catheter can be used to aspirate air from the right ventricle [28]. Neurosurgery is the only common indication for an antecubital approach, as IJV catheters can obstruct blood return from the cranial vault and increase intracranial pressure.

Venous access during cardiopulmonary resuscitation deserves special comment. Peripheral vein cannulation in circulatory arrest may prove impossible, and circulation times of drugs administered peripherally are prolonged when compared to central injection. Drugs injected through femoral catheters also have a prolonged circulation time unless the catheter tip is advanced beyond the diaphragm, although the clinical significance of this is controversial. Effective drug administration is an extremely important element of successful cardiopulmonary resuscitation, and all physicians should understand the appropriate techniques for establishing venous access. It is logical to establish venous access as quickly as possible, either peripherally or centrally if qualified personnel are present. Prolonged attempts at arm vein cannulation are not warranted, and under these circumstances the FV is a good alternative. If circulation is not restored after administration of appropriate drugs and defibrillation, then central access should be obtained by the most experienced operator available with a minimum interruption of cardiopulmonary resuscitation (CPR) [29,30,31]. Generally, SV cannulation can be achieved most rapidly during CPR, but IJV catheterization requires less interruption of external chest compressions and may be preferable if airway management is secured [30].

General Considerations and Complications

General considerations for CVC independent of the site of insertion are catheter tip location, vascular erosions, catheter-associated thrombosis, air and catheter embolism, and coagulopathy, which are discussed below. Catheter-associated infection is a complicated topic that is discussed separately.

CATHETER TIP LOCATION. Catheter tip location is a very important but often ignored consideration in CVC. The ideal location for the catheter tip is the distal innominate or proximal SVC, 3 to 5 cm proximal to the caval-atrial junction. Positioning of the catheter tip within the right atrium or right ventricle must be avoided. Cardiac tamponade secondary to catheter tip perforation of the cardiac wall is not rare, and two-thirds of patients suffering this complication die [32–35]. Perforation results from catheter tip migration that occurs from the motion of the beating heart as well as patient arm and neck movements. Migration of catheter tips can be impressive: 5 to 10 cm with antecubital catheters and 1 to 5 cm with IJV or SV catheters [36–39]. Other complications from intracardiac catheter tip position include provocation of arrhythmias from mechanical irritation or infusion of caustic medications or unwarmed blood [40].

Correct placement of the catheter tip is relatively simple, beginning with an appreciation of anatomy. The caval-atrial junction is approximately 13 to 16 cm from right-sided SV or IJV skin punctures and 15 to 20 cm from left-sided insertions. Insertion of a standard triple-lumen catheter to its full 20 cm almost always places the tip within the heart, especially with right-sided insertions. Catheters should therefore be secured at the 13- to 18-cm mark prior to obtaining a chest radiograph [41,42].

An accurate way to ensure proper catheter tip location is intravascular electrocardiography. Using an adapter, the catheter is inserted while monitoring lead II on a standard ECG. Advancement of the catheter tip into the right atrium is heralded by large P waves on the lead II tracing. Subsequent withdrawal of the catheter tip 3 to 5 cm usually ensures correct positioning [43]. Regardless of the technique used, a chest radiograph should be obtained following every initial central venous catheter insertion to ascertain catheter tip location and to detect complications. Although a cost-benefit analysis of this approach, especially with non-SV insertions, may not be favorable, the importance of correct placement of the catheter tip cannot be overstated.

VASCULAR EROSIONS. Large-vessel perforations secondary to central venous catheters are uncommon and often not immediately recognized. Vessel erosion typically occurs 1 to 7 days after catheter insertion. Patients usually present with sudden onset of dyspnea and often with new pleural effusions on chest radiograph [44]. Catheter stiffness, position of the tip within the vessel, and the site of insertion are probably important factors in causing vessel perforation. The relative importance of these variables is unknown. Repeated irritation of the vessel wall by a stiff catheter tip or infusion of hyperosmolar solutions may be the initiating event. Vascular erosions are more common with left IJV and EJV catheters, because for anatomic reasons the catheter tip is more likely to be positioned laterally under tension against the SVC wall [42,44–47]. Positioning of the catheter tip within the vein parallel to the vessel wall must be confirmed on chest radiograph. Free aspiration of blood from the catheter is not always sufficient to rule out a vascular perforation [44].

AIR AND CATHETER EMBOLISM. Significant air and catheter embolism are rare and preventable complications of CVC. Catheter embolism can occur at the time of insertion when a catheter-through- or over-needle technique is used and the operator withdraws the catheter without simultaneously retracting the needle. It more commonly occurs with antecubital or femoral catheters after insertion, because they cross joint lines and are prone to breakage when the agitated patient vigorously bends an arm or leg. Prevention, recognition, and management of catheter embolism are covered in detail elsewhere [48].

Air embolism is of greater clinical importance, often goes undiagnosed, and may prove fatal [49,50,51]. Theoretically, it is totally preventable with compulsive attention to proper catheter insertion and maintenance. Factors resulting in air embolism during insertion are well known, and methods to increase venous pressure, such as use of the Trendelenburg position, should not be forgotten. Catheter disconnect, typically occurring after insertion, is a more common cause. Air embolism should be suspected in any patient with an intrathoracic catheter tip who develops sudden unexplained hypoxemia or cardiovascular collapse, often after being moved between stretchers. A characteristic mill wheel sound may be auscultated over the precordium. Treatment involves placing the patient in the left lateral decubitus position and using the catheter to aspirate air from the right ventricle. Hyperbaric oxygen therapy to reduce bubble size has a controversial role in treatment [51]. The best treatment is prevention, including use of Luer-Lok equipment at all catheter connections [52].

COAGULOPATHY. Central venous access in the patient with a bleeding diathesis is problematic. The SV and IJV routes have increased risks in the presence of coagulopathy, but it is not known at what degree of abnormality the risk becomes unacceptable. A coagulopathy is generally defined as a prothrombin time greater than 15 seconds, platelet count less than 50,000, or bleeding time greater than 10 minutes. Although it is clear that safe venipuncture is possible with greater degrees of coagulopathy, the literature is fraught with case reports of serious hemorrhagic complications [53–56]. In patients with coagulopathy, the EJV is an excellent alternative for central venous access, especially pulmonary artery catheterization [57], while the FV offers a safe alternative for general-purpose venous access. If these sites cannot be used, the IJV is the best alternative, since it is a compressible site and there is positive experience with this route in patients with coagulopathy [58]. The SV is not a directly compressible site and is contraindicated except under unusual circumstances.

Although the antecubital veins can be safely cannulated in the presence of coagulopathy, this route is often not as practical as the alternatives. Triple-lumen catheters do not reach a central location when placed through antecubital veins, and the advantages of multilumen catheters in the patient at high risk for venipuncture are apparent; long single-lumen catheters are simply not as versatile. Consequently, antecubital vein CVC is a good option only in the patient with severe coagulopathy (i.e., disseminated intravascular coagulation with multiple sites of clinical bleeding).

THROMBOSIS. Catheter-related thrombosis is very common but usually of little clinical significance. The spectrum of thrombotic complications ranges from a sleeve of fibrin that surrounds the catheter from its point of entry into the vein distal to the tip, to mural thrombus, a clot that forms on the wall of the vein secondary to mechanical or chemical irritation, or occlusive thrombus, which occludes flow and may result in collateral formation [59]. All of these lesions are usually clinically silent, therefore studies that do not use venography to confirm the diagnosis are irrelevant. Using venography, fibrin sleeve formation can be documented in a majority of catheters, mural thrombi in 10 to 30 percent, and occlusive thrombi in 0 to 10 percent [59–65]. In contrast, clinical symptoms of thrombosis occur in only 0 to 3 percent of patients [59,63,66]. The incidence of thrombosis probably increases with duration of catheterization [62] but does not appear related to the site of insertion [59–65]. Recent studies have not confirmed the long-held impression that thrombosis is more common and/or more clinically relevant following FV catheterization than at other sites [67,68].

Catheter design and composition impact on the frequency of thrombotic complications. The ideal catheter material is nonthrombogenic and relatively stiff at room temperature to facilitate percutaneous insertion, yet soft and pliable at body temperature to minimize intravascular mechanical trauma. The catheter materials currently in use include polyethylene, polyvinylchloride, polyurethane, Teflon, and silicone elastomer (Silastic). All catheter materials are thrombogenic, but catheters with smooth surfaces are less prone to platelet aggregation [69]. Although not all studies are consistent, polyurethane, especially when coated with hydromer, appears to be the best material available for bedside catheter insertions. Silastic catheters have low thrombogenicity but must be surgically implanted, and pressure monitoring is usually not possible [38,70–73]. Heparin bonding of catheters decreases thrombogenecity, but the clinical importance of this remains uncertain [52,74,75,76]. Very-low-dose warfarin therapy also decreases the incidence of venogram-proved and clinically apparent thrombosis [77]. This approach holds promise, but since clinical sequelae from catheter-associated thrombosis are rare and warfarin has several relevant drug interactions in the critically ill patient, further study is needed.

Many physicians underappreciate the potential for catheter-associated thrombosis and are unaware of current catheter technology and research, but it is not a trivial issue. Physicians should be aware of the type of catheter in use in their hospital and be able to justify its use on a benefit-risk-cost basis.

Routes of Central Venous Cannulation

ANTECUBITAL APPROACH

Anatomic Considerations. Since the introduction of multilumen catheters and greater experience with the EJV and FV approaches, the antecubital veins are not commonly used for CVC. Advantages to this approach are a low incidence of major complications with insertion and the ability to use it in the presence of clotting abnormalities. Disadvantages include the fact that it is more time-consuming, the relative success rate is lower, the anatomy is less predictable, and catheters must be removed within 72 hours because of a high incidence of phlebitis and infection. These considerations have generally limited use of the antecubital veins to preoperative preparation of the neurosurgical patient at risk for intraoperative air embolism and as an alternative site in patients with severe coagulopathy.

The antecubital venous channels used for CVC are the basilic, cephalic, and brachial veins (Fig. 2-1). The basilic and cephalic veins are usually part of the surface anatomy and are cannulated percutaneously. A cutdown approach to the antecubital veins is not recommended because of a prohibitively high incidence of complications, especially infection. Although the brachial vein is occasionally cannulated percutaneously, it is rarely used for CVC.

Anatomy. The basilic vein is formed in the ulnar part of the dorsal venous network of the hand (Fig. 2-1). It may be found in the medial part of the antecubital fossa, where it is usually joined by the median basilic vein. It then ascends in the groove between the biceps brachii and pronator teres on the medial aspect of the arm to perforate the deep fascia distal to the midportion of the arm, where it joins the brachial vein to become the axillary vein. The basilic vein is almost always of substantial size and the anatomy is predictable; since the axillary vein is a direct continuation of it, the basilic vein provides an unimpeded path to the central venous circulation [78–81].

The cephalic vein begins in the radial part of the dorsal venous network of the hand and ascends around the radial border of the forearm (Fig. 2-1). In the lateral aspect of the antecubital fossa, it forms an anastomosis with the median basilic vein and then ascends the lateral part of the arm in the groove along the lateral border of the biceps brachii. It pierces the clavipectoral fascia in the deltopectoral triangle and empties into the proximal part of the axillary vein caudal to the clavicle. The variability of the cephalic vein anatomy renders it less suitable than the basilic vein for CVC. It joins the axillary vein at nearly a right angle, which can be difficult for a catheter to traverse. Instead of passing beneath the clavicle, the cephalic vein may pass through the clavicle, compressing the vein and making catheter passage impossible. Furthermore, in a significant percentage of cases, the cephalic does not empty into the axillary vein but divides into smaller branches or a venous plexus, which empties into the ipsilateral external jugular vein. The cephalic vein may also simply terminate or become attenuated just proximal to the antecubital fossa [78–81].

Technique of Cannulation. Several kits are available for antecubital CVC; the technique using a 24-inch, 16-gauge catheter-through-needle device is described here, but other devices have comparable efficacy [82].

The right basilic vein should be selected for the initial attempt at CVC because of anatomical considerations and clinical studies that confirm a higher success rate with the basilic than the cephalic vein [83,84,85]. The success rates from either arm are

If resistance to advancing the catheter is met, options are limited. Techniques such as abducting the arm are of limited value. With a catheter-through- or over-needle device, the catheter must never be withdrawn without simultaneously retracting the needle to avoid catheter embolism. If the catheter cannot be advanced easily, another site should be chosen.

Once the catheter has advanced the estimated distance, the stiff inner wire is removed and the catheter connected to an intravenous solution. Air embolism can occur with antecubital catheters; prophylactic measures are necessary. After the IV is infusing freely, the tubing should be placed in a dependent position to check for backflow of blood. The catheter is then sutured securely, the arm placed on an arm board to prevent bending at the elbow, and the insertion site bandaged in standard fashion. A chest radiograph is indicated to ascertain catheter tip position.

Success Rate and Complications. Using the above technique, a central venous catheter is placed successfully on the first attempt in approximately 70 percent of cases with the basilic vein and 40 to 50 percent with the cephalic vein [80–85,88,89,90]. In 5 percent or less, the failure is a result of an inability to perform venipuncture, but the major cause of failure is an inability to advance the catheter tip into the proper position. Several measures—abducting the arm to 90 degrees, turning the head to the ipsilateral side, and infusing intravenous solutions during cannulation—are advocated to improve the success rate; the efficacy of these measures is unproved.

Important complications resulting from antecubital CVC include sterile phlebitis, thrombosis (especially of the SV and IJV), infection, limb edema, and pericardial tamponade. Phlebitis is more common with antecubital central venous catheters, probably due to less blood flow in these veins as well as the proximity of the venipuncture site to the skin [91]. The risk of pericardial tamponade may also be increased because of greater catheter tip migration occurring with arm movements [38,92]. Complications are minimized by strict adherence to recommended techniques for catheter placement and care.

INTERNAL-EXTERNAL JUGULAR APPROACH. The IJV provides one of the most favorable sites for access to the great thoracic veins. Internal jugular vein cannulation offers a high success rate with few complications. Pediatricians used the IJV for venous access [93] long before Hermosura and colleagues described the technique and advocated its use in adults in 1966 [94]. In 1969, English et al. reported the first large series of IJV cannulations [12]; subsequently the procedure became commonplace, and in many centers the preferred method of CVC. In 1974, Blitt et al. described a technique of CVC via the EJV employing a J wire [95]. Although the success rate of this route is lower than with the IJV, a "central" venipuncture is avoided, and in selected cases catheterization via the EJV is an excellent alternative.

Anatomy. The IJV emerges from the base of the skull through the jugular foramen and enters the carotid sheath dorsally with the internal carotid artery (ICA) (Fig. 2-1). It then courses posterolaterally to the artery and runs beneath the sternocleidomastoid (SCM) muscle. The vein lies medial to the anterior portion of the SCM muscle in its upper part, then runs beneath the triangle formed by the two heads of the muscle in its medial portion before entering the SV near the medial border of the anterior scalene muscle beneath the sternal border of the clavicle. The junction of the right IJV (which averages 2–3 cm in diameter) with the right SV and then the innominate vein forms a straight path to the SVC. As a result, malpositions and looping

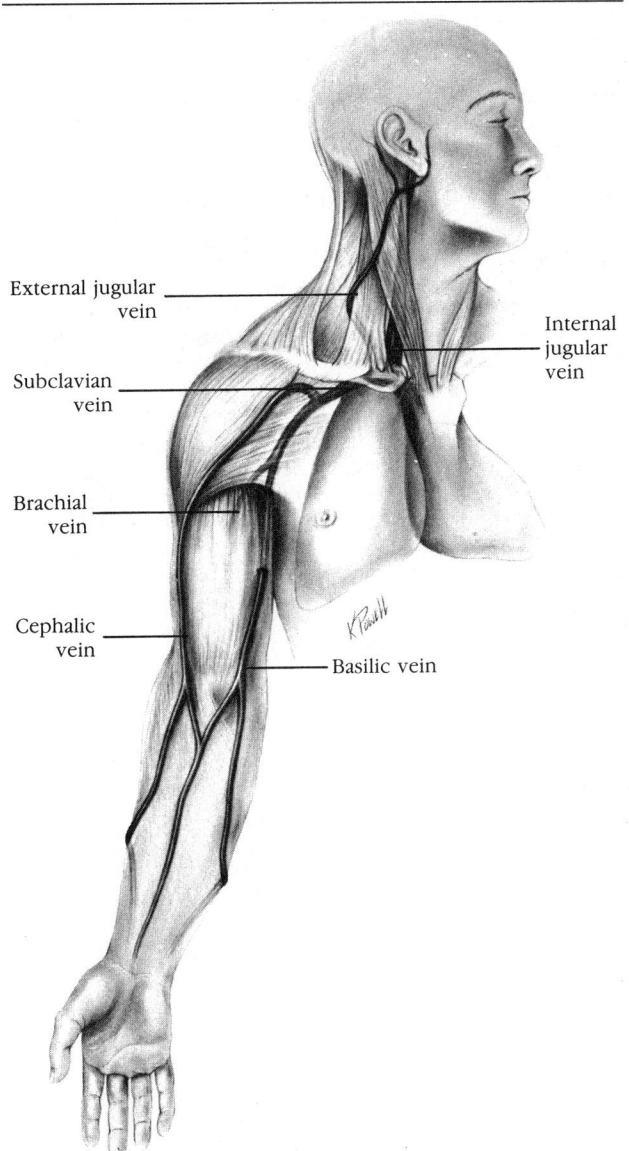

External jugular vein

Internal jugular vein

Subclavian vein

Brachial vein

Cephalic vein

Basilic vein

K. Powell

Fig. 2-1. Venous anatomy of the upper extremity. The internal jugular, external jugular, and subclavian veins are also shown.

comparable, although the catheter must traverse a greater distance when inserted via the left arm, which may result in a slightly higher rate of malposition [86].

With the patient's arm at his or her side, the antecubital fossa is prepared and draped, adhering to strict aseptic technique. A tourniquet is placed proximally to distend the vein, which is then entered at a 45-degree angle with the needle bevel pointing up and cephalad. When free backflow of blood is confirmed, the tourniquet is released and the catheter carefully threaded into the vein. The catheter should advance easily without undue resistance until the operator estimates the tip to be in the distal innominate or SVC. The length of insertion is estimated by measuring the distance from the venipuncture site to the manubriosternal junction; a more accurate method is intravascular electrocardiograhy (as discussed above) [87].

of a catheter inserted through the right IJV are unusual. In contrast, a catheter passed through the left IJV must negotiate a sharp turn at the left jugulosubclavian junction, which results in a greater percentage of catheter malpositions [96,97]. This sharp turn may also produce tension and torque at the catheter tip, resulting in a higher incidence of vessel erosion [44–47,98].

Knowledge of the structures neighboring the IJV is essential, because they may be invaded by a misdirected needle. The ICA runs medial to the IJV but, rarely, may lie directly posteriorly. Behind the ICA, just outside the sheath, lie the stellate ganglion and the cervical sympathetic trunk. The dome of the pleura, which is higher on the left, lies caudal to the junction of the IJV and SV. Posteriorly, at the root of the neck, course the phrenic and vagus nerves [78-81]. The thoracic duct lies behind the left IJV and enters the superior margin of the SV near the jugulo-subclavian junction. The right lymphatic duct has the same anatomical relationship but is much smaller, and chylous effusion occurs only with left-sided IJV cannulations [96,97].

Techniques of Cannulation. Internal jugular venipuncture may be accomplished by a variety of methods; as many as 14 variations have been described [99]. All methods use the same landmarks but differ in the site of venipuncture or orientation of the needle. Defalque grouped the methods into three general approaches: anterior, central, and posterior [100] (Fig. 2-2). I prefer the central approach for the initial attempt, but the method chosen varies with the institution and operator's experience. All approaches require identical equipment, and the operator may choose from many different catheters and pre-packaged kits. Multilumen catheters are now in common use, and the insertion of a triple-lumen catheter is described below. Insertion of an introducer for pulmonary artery catheterization follows the same basic technique and is described in detail in Chapter 4.

Standard triple-lumen catheter kits include a 7 Fr. triple-lumen catheter with 20 or 30 cm of usable length, a 0.035-inch diameter guidewire with straight and J tip, 18-gauge thin-wall needle, a 16-gauge catheter-over-needle, a 7 Fr. vein dilator, a 22-gauge "finder" needle, and appropriate syringes and suture material. Preparation of the guidewire and catheter prior to insertion is important; all lumens should be flushed with saline

Fig. 2-2. Surface anatomy and various approaches to cannulation of the internal jugular vein. A. Surface anatomy. B. Anterior approach. C. Central approach. D. Posterior approach.

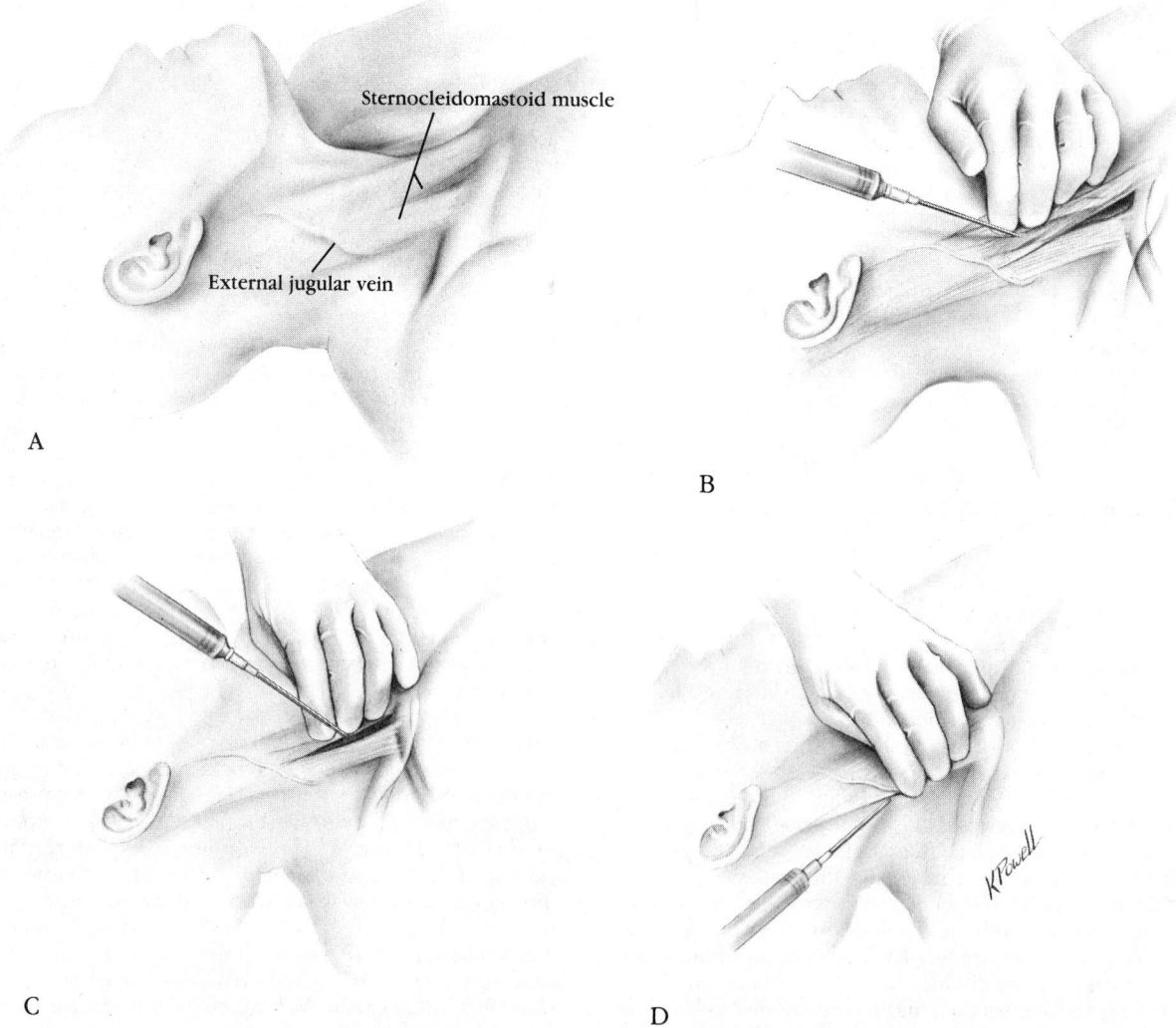

and the cap to the distal lumen removed. The patient is placed in a 15-degree Trendelenburg position to distend the vein and minimize the risk of air embolism, with the head turned gently to the contralateral side. The surface anatomy is identified, especially the angle of the mandible, the two heads of the SCM, the clavicle, the EJV, and the trachea (Fig. 2-2). The neck is then prepared with an iodine-containing solution, which is allowed to dry, and draped, with care to avoid covering the patient's eyes to minimize anxiety. For the central approach [13,100–103], skin puncture is at the apex of the triangle formed by the two muscle bellies of the SCM and the clavicle. The ICA pulsation is usually felt 1 to 2 cm medial to this point, beneath or just medial to the sternal head of the SCM. The skin at the apex of the triangle is infiltrated with 1% lidocaine using the 22-gauge needle, which is then used to locate the IJV. Use of a small-bore finder needle to locate the IJV should prevent inadvertent ICA puncture and unnecessary probing with a larger-bore needle. The operator should maintain slight or no pressure on the ICA with the left hand and insert the finder needle with the right hand at the apex of the triangle (or slightly more caudal) at a 30- to 45-degree angle with the frontal plane, directed at the ipsilateral nipple. After expulsion of any skin plug, the needle is advanced steadily with constant back pressure and venipuncture occurs within 3 to 5 cm. Deeper penetration is not recommended. If venipuncture does not occur on the initial thrust, back pressure should be maintained and the needle slowly withdrawn, as venipuncture frequently occurs on withdrawal. If the first attempt is unsuccessful, the operator should reassess patient position, landmarks, and techniques to ensure that he or she is not doing anything to decrease IJV lumen size (see below). Subsequent attempts may be directed slightly laterally or medially to the initial thrust, as long as the plane of the ICA is not violated. If venipuncture does not occur after three to five attempts, further attempts are likely to be unsuccessful and only increase complications [58,104,105]. When venipuncture has occurred with the finder needle, the operator can either withdraw the finder needle and introduce the large-bore needle in the identical plane or leave the finder needle in place and introduce the larger needle directly above it. If using the latter technique, the operator or assistant must be careful not to exert tension on the finder needle, as this may decrease the lumen size of the IJV and make catheterization more difficult. Many kits provide both an 18-gauge thin-wall needle through which a guidewire can be directly introduced and a 16-gauge catheter-over-needle device. With the latter apparatus, the catheter is threaded over the needle into the vein, the needle withdrawn, and the guidewire inserted through the catheter. Both techniques are effective; the choice is strictly a matter of operator preference. With the 18-gauge thin-wall needle, the operator must be sure to secure the needle in place with one hand while removing the syringe with the other, so that the needle does not migrate out of the vein prior to guidewire insertion. Many operators prefer the catheter-over-needle device for IJV catheterization because standard intravenous technique is used and the catheter is less likely to migrate from the vein before guidewire insertion. However, this technique requires that the catheter and needle be inserted and withdrawn simultaneously to avoid catheter embolism, and often the catheter does not pierce the tissue planes easily. Regardless of which large-bore needle is used, once venipuncture has occurred the syringe is removed during expiration or Valsalva maneuver and the hub occluded with a finger after ensuring that the backflow of blood is not pulsatile. The J tip of the guidewire is then inserted and should pass freely up to 20 cm, at which point the thin-wall needle or catheter is withdrawn. The tendency to insert the guidewire deeper than 15 to 20 cm should be avoided, as it is the most common cause of ventric-

ular arrhythmias during insertion and also poses a risk for cardiac perforation. Occasionally, the guidewire does not pass easily beyond the tip of the thin-wall needle (especially) or catheter. The guidewire should then be withdrawn, the syringe attached, and free backflow of blood reestablished and maintained while the syringe and needle are brought to a more parallel plane with the vein. The guidewire should then pass easily. If resistance is still encountered, rotation of the guidewire during insertion often allows passage, but extensive manipulation and force only lead to complications.

With the guidewire in place, a scalpel is used to make two generous 90-degree stab incisions at the skin entry site to facilitate passage of the 7 Fr. vein dilator. The dilator is inserted down the wire to the hub, ensuring that control and sterility of the guidewire is not compromised. The dilator is then withdrawn and gauze used at the puncture site to control oozing and prevent air embolism down the needle tract. The triple-lumen catheter is then inserted over the guidewire, ensuring that the guidewire protrudes from the distal lumen hub before the catheter tip penetrates the skin. The catheter is then advanced 15 to 17 cm (17–19 cm for left IJV) into the vein, the guidewire withdrawn, and the distal lumen capped. The catheter is sutured securely to limit tip migration and bandaged in a standard manner. A chest radiograph should be obtained to detect complications and tip location.

Alternative Approaches. The anterior and posterior approaches are identical in technique, differing only in venipuncture site and plane of insertion. For the anterior approach (Fig. 2-2) [99,100,106,107,108], the important landmark is the midpoint of the sternal head of the SCM, approximately 5 cm from both the angle of the mandible and the sternum. At this point, the carotid artery can be palpated 1 cm inside the lateral border of the sternal head. The index and middle fingers of the left hand gently palpate the artery, and the needle is introduced 0.5 to 1 cm lateral to the pulsation. The needle should form a 30- to 45-degree angle with the frontal plane and be directed caudally parallel to the carotid artery toward the ipsilateral nipple. Venipuncture occurs within 2 to 4 cm, sometimes only while the needle is slowly withdrawn. If the initial thrust is unsuccessful, the next attempt should be at a 5-degree lateral angle, followed by a cautious attempt more medially, never crossing the plane of the carotid artery.

The posterior approach (Fig. 2-2) [99,100,109,110,111] uses the EJV as a surface landmark. The needle is introduced 1 cm dorsally to the point where the EJV crosses the posterior border of the SCM or 5 cm cephalad from the clavicle along the clavicular head of the SCM. The needle is directed caudally and ventrally toward the suprasternal notch at an angle of 45 degrees to the sagittal plane, with a 15-degree upward angulation. Venipuncture occurs within 5 to 7 cm. If this attempt is unsuccessful, the needle should be aimed slightly more cephalad on the next attempt.

Success Rates and Complications.. Internal jugular vein catheterization is associated with a high rate of successful catheter placement regardless of the approach used. Elective procedures are successful more than 90 percent of the time, generally within the first three attempts, and catheter malposition is rare [96,97,100,101,102,104,106,107]. Operator experience does not appear to be as important a factor in altering the success rate of venipuncture as it is in increasing the number of complications [104,112]. Emergent IJV catheterization is less successful and is not the preferred technique during airway emergencies or other situations that may make it difficult to identify landmarks in the neck [104,112]. Some authors advocate the use of ultrasound localization to aid in IJV catheterization [113], but routine use of ultrasound is unnecessary for a procedure with such a high success rate. In special circumstances, ultrasound or Doppler localization is helpful in performing difficult or previously unsuccessful IJV catheterization [114,115].

Ultrasound studies have been useful in delineating factors that improve the efficiency of IJV cannulation. The ability to perform IJV venipuncture is directly proportional to its cross-sectional lumen area (CSLA), thus maneuvers that increase or decrease the veins' caliber impact on the success rate [41,113,115,116,117]. Maneuvers that decrease the CSLA include hypovolemia, carotid artery palpation, and excessive tension on a finder needle. Predictably, Valsalva maneuver and Trendelenburg position increase CSLA, as does high-level positive end-expiratory pressure (PEEP). There is also a progressive increase in CSLA as the IJV nears the SV. Overrotation of the neck may place the vein beneath the SCM muscle belly [115].

Often, a difficult IJV cannulation is successful on the first attempt by optimizing CLSA through attention to the above measures. If the IJV is still not punctured after one or two attempts, it is usually because of anatomical variation, not because of the absence of jugular flow [116,117]. In this situation, I use a Doppler device (Smart-Needle) to locate the IJV, because of its portability, overall convenience, and need for less operator expertise [118]. Others use ultrasound in an analogous fashion [119]. Whatever technique is employed, prolonged attempts at catheterization after optimization of IJV CSLA are only likely to increase complications.

Complications. The incidence and types of complications are similar regardless of the approach. Operator inexperience appears to increase the number of complications, but to an undefined extent, and probably does not have as great an impact as it does on the incidence of pneumothorax in subclavian venipuncture [100,120,121].

The overall incidence of complications in IJV catheterization is 0.1 to 4.2 percent [12,100,109,120,122], with a few studies reporting higher rates [58,104,123]. Important complications include ICA puncture, pneumothorax, vessel erosion, thrombosis, and infection. Vessel erosion, thrombosis, and infectious complications are common to all routes of CVC and are reviewed separately in this chapter.

By far the most common complication is ICA puncture, which constitutes 80 to 90 percent of all complications. In the absence of a bleeding diathesis, arterial punctures are benign and are managed conservatively without sequelae by applying local pressure for 10 minutes. Even in the absence of clotting abnormalities, a sizable hematoma may form, frequently preventing further catheterization attempts or, rarely, exerting pressure on vital neck structures [124–128]. Unrecognized arterial puncture can lead to catheterization of the ICA with a large-bore catheter or introducer and can have disastrous consequences, especially when heparin is administered [122]. Management of carotid cannulation with a large-bore catheter, such as a 7 Fr. introducer, is controversial. Some experts advise administration of anticoagulants to prevent thromboembolic complications, while others advise the opposite. My approach is to remove the catheter and avoid heparinization if possible, as hemorrhage appears to be a greater risk than thromboembolism [122].

Chronic complications that rarely complicate ICA puncture include hematomas requiring surgical excision [129], arteriovenous fistula [130], and pseudoaneurysm [131].

Coagulopathy is a relative contraindication to IJV catheterization, and the EJV or FV should be considered as primary alternatives. If these routes cannot be used, I proceed with the IJV approach. Under these circumstances, a finder needle technique is mandatory, because carotid puncture by a 22-gauge

needle is still unlikely to cause complications. Goldfarb and Lebrec [58] performed IJV cannulation in 1000 patients with liver disease and coagulopathy, defined as prothrombin activity less than 50 percent and/or bleeding time longer than 10 minutes and/or platelet count under 50,000. Despite a 7 percent incidence of arterial puncture, a clinically detectable hematoma formed in only 10 patients, one of whom required surgical drainage. The coagulopathy associated with liver disease cannot be equated to all coagulation abnormalities, but this experience suggests that the IJV can be used safely as an alternative to the EJV or FV in the presence of coagulopathy.

Pneumothorax is an unusual adverse consequence of IJV cannulation, with an average incidence of 0 to 0.2 percent [12,99,104,110,120]. It usually results from a skin puncture too close to the clavicle or, rarely, a guidewire inserted through a needle that has inadvertently migrated from the IJV lumen [58]. Pneumothorax may be complicated by heme, infusion of intravenous fluid, or tension [58,104,132,133].

An extraordinary number of case reports indicate that any complication from IJV catheterization is possible, even the intrathecal insertion of a Swan-Ganz catheter [134]. In reality, this route is reliable, with a low incidence of major complications. Operator experience is not as important a factor as in SV catheterization, the incidence of catheter tip malposition is low, and patient acceptance is high. It is best suited for elective catheterizations in volume-repleted patients, especially pulmonary artery catheterizations and insertion of temporary transvenous pacemakers. It is not the preferred site during airway emergencies, for administration of parenteral nutrition, or long-term catheterization. Anticoagulation is not an absolute contraindication, but EJV or FV catheterization may be more appropriate for initial attempts.

EXTERNAL JUGULAR VEIN APPROACH. The main advantages to the EJV route for CVC are that the EJV is part of the surface anatomy, it may be cannulated in the presence of clotting abnormalities, and the risk of pneumothorax is avoided. The main disadvantage is the unpredictability of passage of the catheter to the central compartment.

Anatomy. The EJV is formed anterior and caudal to the ear at the angle of the mandible by the union of the posterior auricular and retromandibular veins (Fig. 2-3). It courses obliquely across the anterior surface of the SCM, then pierces the deep fascia just posterior to the SCM and joins the SV behind the medial third of the clavicle. In 5 to 15 percent of patients, the EJV is not a distinct structure but a venous plexus, in which case it may receive the ipsilateral cephalic vein. The EJV varies in size and contains valves throughout its course. Its junction with the SV may be at a severe, narrow angle that can be difficult for a catheter to traverse.

Technique. The EJV should be cannulated using the 16-gauge catheter-over-needle, since guidewire manipulations are often necessary and secure venous access is preferable with a catheter. On occasion, especially after unsuccessful attempts and hematoma formation, an 18-gauge thin-wall needle must be used. The patient is placed in a slight Trendelenburg position, with arms to the side and head turned gently to the contralateral side. The right EJV should be chosen for the initial attempt and can be identified where it courses over the anterior portion of the clavicular belly of the SCM. The Valsalva maneuver may help identify the vein in the dehydrated patient, but because of venous valves, thoracic pressure is not consistently transmitted to the EJV. After sterile preparation, venipuncture is performed with the 16-gauge catheter-over-needle using the left index

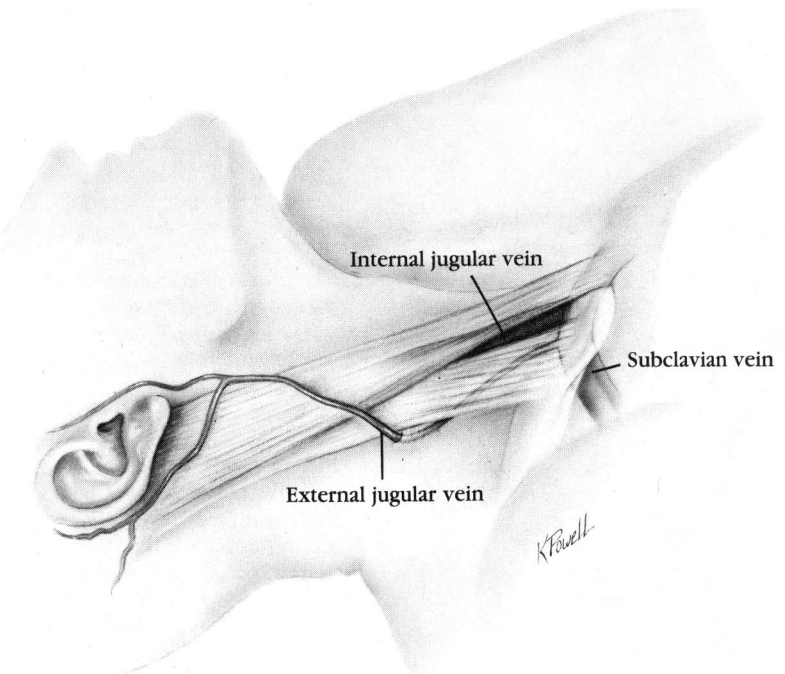

Fig. 2-3. External jugular vein.

finger and thumb to distend and anchor the vein. Skin puncture should be well above the clavicle and the needle advanced in the axis of the vein at 20 degrees to the frontal plane. The EJV may be more difficult to cannulate than expected because of its propensity to roll and displace rather than puncture in response to the advancing needle. A firm, quick thrust is often required to effect venipuncture. When free backflow of blood is established, the needle tip is advanced a few millimeters further into the vein and the catheter is threaded over the needle. The catheter may not thread its entire length because of valves, tortuosity, or the SV junction but should be advanced at least 3 to 5 cm to secure venous access. The syringe and needle can then be removed and the guidewire, J tip first, threaded up to 20 cm and the catheter removed. Manipulation and rotation of the guidewire, especially when it reaches the SV junction, may be necessary but should not be excessive. Various arm and head movements are advocated to facilitate guidewire passage. I have found abduction of the ipsilateral arm and anterior-posterior pressure exerted on the clavicle to be helpful. Once the guidewire has advanced 20 cm, two 90-degree skin stabs are made with a scalpel, and the vein dilator is inserted to its hub. Control of the guidewire should never be lost while the vein dilator is removed. The triple-lumen catheter is then inserted an appropriate length (16–17 cm on the right, 18 cm on the left). The guidewire is withdrawn, the catheter bandaged, and a chest radiograph obtained to screen for complications.

Success Rates and Complications. Central venous catheterization via the EJV is successful in 80 percent of patients (range 75–95%) [95,135,136,137]. Inability to perform venipuncture accounts for up to 10 percent of failures [96,135,138,139] and the remainder are a result of catheter tip malpositioning. Failure to position the catheter tip is a result of an inability to negotiate the EJV-SV junction, loop formation [96,139], or retrograde passage down the ipsilateral arm [112,135].

Serious complications arising from the EJV approach are rare and almost always associated with catheter maintenance rather than venipuncture. A local hematoma forms in 1 to 5 percent of patients at the time of venipuncture [96,135,139,140] but has little consequence unless it distorts the anatomy leading to catheterization failure. External jugular venipuncture is safe in the presence of coagulopathy. Infectious and thrombotic complications are no more frequent than with other central routes. Phlebitis is potentially more common because of lower blood flows, but this is unproved. Vascular erosions may occur more commonly with left-sided EJV catheters for the reasons discussed above [141]. A chest radiograph should be obtained to confirm catheter tip location within the SVC, parallel to the vessel wall.

There is considerable disagreement regarding the true usefulness of EJV catheterization in critical care practice. The reasons for the wide disparity in success rates reported in the literature are not apparent, but experience and enthusiasm for the route may play a role. My own experience with EJV catheterization is similar to the 80 percent success rate reported above, and I find it a valuable alternative to the IJV in anticoagulated patients or those with severe lung disease or on high-level PEEP. All critical care physicians should gain expertise with this route, as its success rate is at least comparable to that of the antecubital approach and major complications are rare.

FEMORAL VEIN APPROACH. The FV is an appealing site for CVC because it is directly compressible, it is remote from the airway and pleura, the technique is relatively simple, and the Trendelenburg position is not required during insertion. Femoral vein catheterization was a common site for CVC in the 1950s but was largely abandoned after 1959 when Moncrief [4]

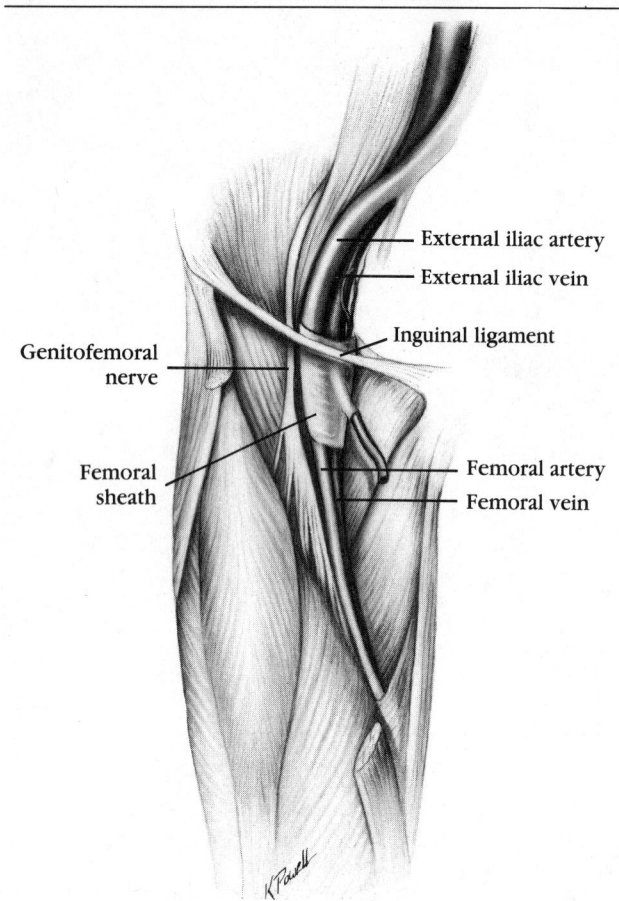

Fig. 2-4. Anatomy of the femoral vein.

and Bansmer et al. [5] reported a high incidence of complications, especially infection and thrombosis. In the subsequent two decades, FV cannulation was restricted to specialized clinical situations. Interest in short-term (<48 hr) FV catheterization was revived by positive experiences during the Vietnam conflict [142] and with patients in the emergency department [143,144]. More recent reports on long-term FV catheterization in children [145] and adults [67,68,146,147] suggest a complication rate no higher than that with other routes.

Anatomy. The FV (Fig. 2-4) is a direct continuation of the popliteal vein and becomes the external iliac vein at the inguinal ligament. At the inguinal ligament the FV lies within the femoral sheath a few centimeters from the skin surface. Within the intermediate compartment of the sheath, the FV lies medial to the femoral artery, which in turn lies medial to the femoral branch of the genitofemoral nerve. The medial compartment contains lymphatic channels and Cloquet's node. The external iliac vein courses cephalad from the inguinal ligament along the anterior surface of the iliopsoas muscle to join its counterpart from the other leg and form the interior vena cava (IVC) anterior to and to the right of the fifth lumbar vertebra [78–81].

Technique. Femoral vein cannulation is the easiest of all central venous procedures to learn and perform [143,148,149]. Either side is suitable, and the side chosen is based on operator convenience. The patient is placed in the supine position (if tolerated) with the leg extended and slightly abducted at the hip. Excessive hair should be clipped with scissors and the skin

prepped with an iodine-containing solution and wiped with alcohol or allowed to dry. The FV lies 1 to 1.5 cm medial to the arterial pulsation, and the skin should be infiltrated with 1% lidocaine at this point. In a patient without femoral artery pulsations, the FV can be located in the following manner [142]. The distance between the anterior superior iliac spine and the pubic tubercle is divided into three equal segments. The femoral artery is usually found where the medial segment meets the two lateral ones, and the FV lies 1 to 1.5 cm medial. An 18-gauge thin-wall needle is inserted at this point, 2 to 3 cm inferior to the inguinal ligament, so that venipuncture occurs caudal to the inguinal ligament and minimizes the risk of retroperitoneal hematoma in the event of arterial puncture. While maintaining constant back-pressure on the syringe, the needle, tip pointed cephalad, is advanced at a 45- to 60-degree angle to the frontal plane. Insertion of the needle almost to its hub is sometimes required in obese patients. Venipuncture may not occur until slow withdrawal. If the initial attempt is unsuccessful, landmarks should be reevaluated and subsequent thrusts oriented slightly more medial or lateral. A common error is to direct the needle tip medially, toward the umbilicus. The femoral vessels lie in the sagittal plane at the inguinal ligament (Fig. 2-4), and the needle should be directed accordingly. If inadvertent arterial puncture occurs, pressure is applied for 5 to 10 minutes.

When venous blood return is established, the syringe is depressed to skin level and free aspiration of blood reconfirmed. The syringe is removed, ensuring that blood return is not pulsatile. The guidewire should pass easily and never be forced, although rotation and minor manipulation are sometimes required. The needle is then withdrawn, two scalpel blade stab incisions made at 90 degrees above the guidewire insertion site, and the vein dilator inserted over the wire to the hub. The dilator is next withdrawn and a catheter appropriate to clinical requirements inserted, taking care never to lose control of the guidewire. The catheter is secured with a suture and antiseptic ointment and bandage applied.

Success Rate and Complications. Femoral vein catheterization is successful in 90 to 95 percent of patients, including those in shock or cardiopulmonary arrest [142,143,145,146,149,150]. Unsuccessful catheterizations are usually a result of venipuncture failure, hematoma formation, or inability to advance the guidewire into the vein. Operator inexperience may increase the number of attempts and complication rate but does not significantly decrease the overall success rate [146].

Only three complications occur regularly with FV catheterization: arterial puncture with or without local bleeding, infection, and thromboembolic events. Other reported complications are rare and include scrotal hemorrhage [151], right lower quadrant bowel perforation [152], retroperitoneal hemorrhage [153], puncture of the kidney [154], and perforation of IVC tributaries. These complications occur when skin puncture sites are cephalad to the inguinal ligament or when long catheters are threaded into the FV.

Femoral artery puncture occurs in 5 to 10 percent of adults [142,143,146,148,150], with a slightly higher incidence in children [145]. Most arterial punctures are uncomplicated, but major hematomas may form in 1 percent of patients [142,146]. Even in the presence of coagulopathy, arterial puncture with the 18-gauge thin-wall needle is usually of no consequence, with only rare reports of life-threatening thigh or retroperitoneal hemorrhage [149,155]. The long history of femoral vessel cannulation in the setting of renal failure attests to its safety in patients with bleeding tendencies [156]. Arteriovenous fistula and pseudoaneurysm are rare chronic complications of arterial puncture; the former is more likely to occur when both femoral vessels are cannulated concurrently [157].

Infectious complications from FV catheters are no more frequent than with other routes. The perception that FV catheters are more prone to infection derives from studies in the 1950s already cited, as well as the proximity of the site to the pubic area. All recent series involving both short- and long-term FV catheterization in adults and children have reported catheter-related infection rates of 5 percent or less [142,143,145,146,158]. Further evidence that the inguinal area is not an inherent "dirty" site is provided by experience with femoral artery catheters, which have an infection rate comparable to that with radial artery catheters [159,160].

The most feared complication of FV catheterization is deep venous thrombosis (DVT) of the lower extremity. Moncrief, in 1958, reported an incidence of autopsy-proven thrombosis of 13 percent with catheters left in place an average of 7 to 10 days in burn patients [4]. Bansmer and co-workers, also in 1958, reported a 29 percent incidence of IVC or ileofemoral thrombosis in patients with femoral catheters in place an average of 13 days [5]. These findings were largely responsible for the abandonment of FV catheters, but for several reasons these studies are probably not indicative of the true risk of thromboembolic complications from FV catheters. Both studies reported mainly autopsy findings from a small series of chronically ill patients, which is not a representative patient sample. Due to technological improvements in catheter design and material, catheters are not as thrombogenic as they were in the 1950s. Most important, these reports involved no comparative studies with catheters inserted at other central routes. Catheter-associated thrombosis is a risk of all central venous catheters, regardless of the site of insertion, and comparative studies using contrast venography are needed to better assess the relative risk of FV catheters. The available data suggest that FV catheters are no more prone to thrombosis than SV or IJV catheters [60,61,63,64,65,67,68]. However, thrombosis of the ileofemoral system is potentially more serious than upper extremity thrombosis, and the potential thromboembolic complications of FV catheters cannot be discounted [161,162]. Studies using serial impedance plethysmography or Doppler ultrasound to assess the incidence of DVT from FV catheters are in progress.

In summary, available evidence supports the view that the FV may be cannulated safely in critically ill adults. It is particularly useful for inexperienced operators because of the high rate of success and lower incidence of major complications. Femoral vein catheterizations may be performed during airway emergencies and cardiopulmonary arrest, in patients with coagulopathy, and in patients who are unable to lie flat. The only major complication during venipuncture is arterial puncture, which is usually easily managed. Infection is no more common than with other routes, and expanding clinical experience suggests that thromboembolism is not as clinically significant as once believed.

SUBCLAVIAN VEIN APPROACH. Since Aubaniac [2] described the use of subclavian venipuncture in humans, controversy has surrounded this route of access to the central circulation. Wilson et al.'s 1962 report [7] generated much enthusiasm for SV catheterization, but soon the large number of serious complications, some fatal, resulted in some investigators urging a moratorium on the procedure [163]. The controversy involving SV catheterization probably derives from the significant impact of operator experience on the incidence of complications. Experienced operators (see below) experience a pneumothorax rate of 1 percent or less and can justify use of the SV as primary central venous access in almost all patients. Inexperienced operators have a far greater rate of pneumothorax; therefore, in settings where relatively inexperienced

physicians perform the majority of CVC, the SV should be used more selectively [164,165]. The advantages of this route include consistent identifiable landmarks, easier long-term catheter maintenance, and relatively high patient comfort. The SV is the preferred site for CVC in patients with hypovolemia, for long-term total parenteral nutrition (TPN), for acute hemodialysis, and in patients with elevated intracranial pressure who require hemodynamic monitoring.

Anatomy. The SV is a direct continuation of the axillary vein, beginning at the lateral border of the first rib, extending 3 to 4 cm along the undersurface of the clavicle and becoming the brachiocephalic vein where it joins the ipsilateral IJV at Pirogoff's confluence behind the sternoclavicular articulation (Fig. 2-5) [78–81,166]. The vein is 1 to 2 cm in diameter, contains a single set of valves just distal to the EJV junction, and is fixed in position directly beneath the clavicle by its fibrous attachments. These attachments prevent collapse of the vein, even with severe volume depletion. Anterior to the vein throughout its course lies the subclavius muscle, clavicle, costoclavicular ligament, pectoralis muscles, and epidermis. Posteriorly, the SV is separated from the subclavian artery and brachial plexus by the anterior scalenus muscle, which is 10 to 15 mm thick in the adult. Posterior to the medial portion of the SV are the phrenic nerve and internal mammary artery as they pass into the thorax. Superiorly, the relationships are the skin, platysma, and superficial aponeurosis. Inferiorly, the vein rests on the first rib, Sibson's fascia, cupola of pleura (0.5 cm behind the vein), and pulmonary apex [19,42,167,168]. The thoracic duct on the left and right lymphatic duct cross the anterior scalene muscle to join the superior aspect of the SV near its union with the IJV.

Technique. Although there are countless variations, the SV may be cannulated by two basic techniques, the infraclavicular [2,7,9,16,99,166–172] or supraclavicular [16,99,166,167,173–177] approach (Fig. 2-6). The differences in success rate, catheter tip malposition, and complications between the two approaches are negligible, although catheter tip malposition and pneumothorax may be less likely with supraclavicular cannulation [178,179,180]. In general, when discussing the success rate and incidence of complications of SV catheterization, there is no need to specify the approach used. The 18-gauge thin-wall needle is preferable for SV cannulation. The catheter-over-needle device tends to be less effective for two reasons. First, the catheter often hangs up on the clavicle and does not advance easily over the needle. This may result in kinking or breakage of the catheter. Second, the catheter has a tendency to rebound out of the SV lumen after the needle is withdrawn because of tension exerted on it by the clavicle and tissue planes. Vascular access is then lost before insertion of the guidewire.

The patient is placed in a 15- to 30-degree Trendelenburg position, with a small bedroll between the shoulder blades. The head is turned gently to the contralateral side and the arms are kept to the side. The pertinent landmarks are the clavicle, the two muscle bellies of the SCM, the suprasternal notch, and the manubriosternal junction. For the infraclavicular approach (Fig. 2-6), the operator is positioned next to the patient's shoulder on the side to be cannulated. For reasons cited earlier, the left SV should be chosen for pulmonary artery catheterization; otherwise, the success rate appears to be equivalent regardless of the side chosen. Skin puncture is 2 to 3 cm caudal to the midpoint of the clavicle, corresponding to the area where the clavicle turns from the shoulder to the manubrium, and should be distant enough from the clavicle to avoid a downward angle of the needle in clearing the inferior surface of the clavicle, which also obviates the need to bend the needle. The path of

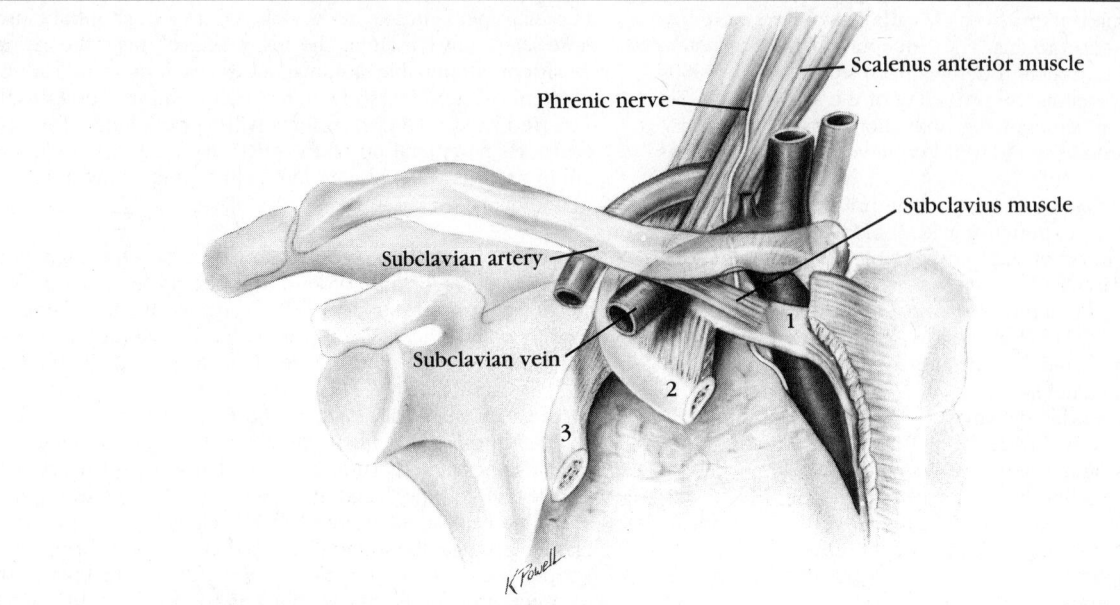

Fig. 2-5. Anatomy of the subclavian vein and adjacent structures.

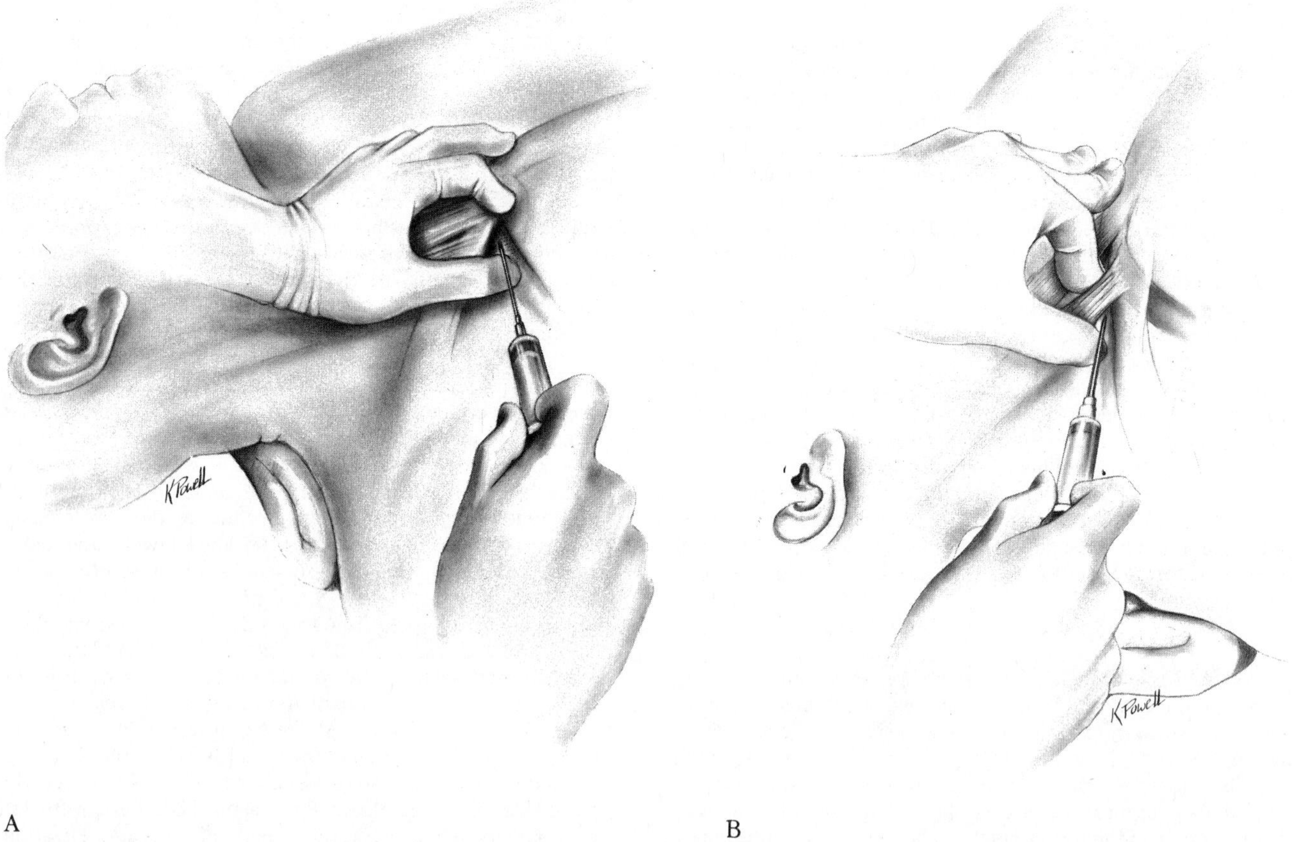

A   B

Fig. 2-6. A. Patient positioning for subclavian cannulation. B. Cannulation technique for supraclavicular approach.

the needle is toward the suprasternal notch or the medial end of the contralateral clavicle. After skin infiltration and liberal injection of the clavicular periosteum with 1% lidocaine, the 18-gauge thin-wall needle is mounted on a 10-ml syringe filled with saline. Skin puncture is accomplished with the needle bevel up, and a small amount of saline is expressed to eliminate any possible skin plug. The needle is advanced in the plane described above until the tip abuts the clavicle. The needle is then "walked" down the clavicle until the inferior edge is cleared. As the needle is advanced, the inferior surface of the clavicle should be felt hugging the needle. This ensures that the needle tip is as superior as possible to the dome of the pleura. The needle is advanced toward the suprasternal notch during breath holding or expiration, and venipuncture occurs when the needle tip lies beneath the medial end of the clavicle. This may require insertion of the needle to its hub. Venipuncture may not occur until slow withdrawal of the needle. If venipuncture is not accomplished on the initial thrust, the next attempt should be directed slightly more cephalad. If venipuncture does not occur by the third or fourth attempt, another site should be chosen, as additional attempts are unlikely to be successful and may result in complications [112,165]. When blood return is established, the bevel of the needle is rotated 90 degrees toward the heart. The needle is anchored firmly with the left hand while the syringe is detached with the right. Blood return should not be pulsatile, and air embolism prophylaxis is necessary at all times. The guidewire is then advanced through the needle to 15 cm and the needle withdrawn. The remainder of the procedure is as previously described. Triple-lumen catheters should be sutured at 13 to 15 cm on the right and 15 cm on the left to avoid intracardiac tip placement.

For the supraclavicular approach (Fig. 2-6), the important landmarks are the clavicular insertion of the SCM muscle and the sternoclavicular joint. The operator is positioned at the head of the patient on the side to be cannulated. The site of skin puncture is the claviculosternocleidomastoid angle, just above the clavicle and lateral to the insertion of the clavicular head of the SCM. The needle is advanced toward or just caudal to the contralateral nipple just under the clavicle. This corresponds to a 45-degree angle to the sagittal plane, bisecting a line between the sternoclavicular joint and clavicular insertion of the SCM [42,178]. The depth of insertion is from just beneath the SCM clavicular head at a 10- to 15-degree angle below the coronal plane. The needle should enter the jugulosubclavian venous bulb after 1 to 4 cm, and the operator may then proceed with catheterization.

Success and Complication Rates. Subclavian vein catheterization is successful in 90 to 95 percent of cases, generally on the first attempt [96,142,171,172,175,176,178,181]. The presence of shock does not alter the success rate as significantly as it does during IJV catheterization [142,181]. Unsuccessful catheterizations are a result of venipuncture failure or inability to advance the guidewire or catheter [96,171]. Catheter tip malposition occurs in 5 to 20 percent of cases [96,171,179,181] and tends to be more frequent with the infraclavicular approach [96,130,171,182]. Malposition occurs most commonly to the ipsilateral IJV and contralateral SV and is usually correctable without repeat venipuncture.

The overall incidence of complications varies depending on the operator's experience and the circumstances under which the catheter is inserted. Large series involving several thousand SV catheters have reported an incidence of major complications of 1 to 3 percent, with an overall rate of 5 percent [167–171]. In smaller, probably more clinically relevant studies, the major complication rate has ranged from 1 to 10 percent [96,142,178,181,183,184,185]. Factors resulting in a higher com-

plication rate are operator inexperience, multiple attempts at venipuncture, emergency conditions, and variance from standardized technique. Major complications include pneumothorax, arterial puncture, thromboembolism, and catheter-related infection. There are many case reports of isolated major complications involving neck structures or the brachial plexus; the reader is referred elsewhere for a complete listing of reported complications [99,167,186]. Infectious complications are reviewed later in this chapter; pneumothorax, arterial puncture, and thromboembolism are discussed in more detail below.

Pneumothorax accounts for one-fourth to one-half of reported complications, with an incidence of 1 to 5 percent [142,171,172,175,176,178,181,183,187–191]. The incidence varies inversely with the operator's experience and the number of "breaks" in technique [112,179,180,181,184,185]. There is no magic figure whereby an operator matures from inexperienced to experienced. Fifty catheterizations is cited frequently as a cutoff number, but it is reasonable to expect an operator to be satisfactorily experienced after having performed fewer [164]. For the experienced operator, a pneumothorax incidence < 0.5 percent is expected [7,142,167,171,176,178]. Most pneumothoraces are a result of lung puncture at the time of the procedure, but late-appearing pneumothoraces have been reported, and it is good practice to obtain a chest radiograph the day after the procedure.

One-fourth to one-half of pneumothoraces may be managed conservatively, without thoracostomy tube drainage [171, 181,183]. Rarely, a pneumothorax is complicated by tension [181,188], heme [175,192], infusion of intravenous fluid (immediately or days or weeks after catheter placement) [193–195], chyle, and massive subcutaneous emphysema [187]. Bilateral pneumothoraces can occur from unilateral attempts at venipuncture [196]. Pneumothorax can result in death, especially when it goes unrecognized [187,197,198].

Subclavian artery puncture occurs in 0.5 to 1.0 percent of cases, constituting one-fourth to one-third of all complications [96,142,171,175,176,185]. Arterial puncture is usually managed easily by applying pressure above and below the clavicle. Bleeding can be catastrophic in patients with coagulopathy. As with other routes, arterial puncture may result in arteriovenous fistula or pseudoaneurysm [199].

Clinical evidence of central venous thrombosis, including SVC syndrome, development of collaterals around the shoulder girdle, and pulmonary embolism, occurs in 0 to 3 percent of SV catheterizations [59,60,63,64,200], but routine phlebography performed at catheter removal reveals a much higher incidence of thrombotic phenomena. The importance of the discrepancy between clinical symptoms and radiologic findings is unknown, but it exists for all routes of CVC. Duration of catheterization, catheter material, and patient condition may have an impact on the frequency of thrombosis, but to an uncertain degree. Detection and treatment of catheter-associated thrombosis remains a controversial issue, discussed in detail elsewhere [38].

Infectious Complications

Infectious sequelae of central venous catheters include local phenomena, such as cellulitis, abscess formation, and suppurative thrombophlebitis, and systemic manifestations of bacteremia, septic shock, and metastatic infection. Catheter-related infection is a broad and complicated topic, and a review of the literature can be confusing. Many large series include peripheral intravenous catheters, peripheral arterial catheters, and central venous catheters of all types. Even in studies limited to central venous catheters, the duration of catheterization, site of venipuncture, condition of the patient, indication for placement, and medical decision-making about removal are uncontrolled or poorly recorded. Many frequently cited series are neither randomized nor prospective and include too small a patient sample to generate statistically significant results. The previous edition of this text identified several controversies surrounding infectious complications of central venous catheters. In the few years since publication of that text, human and animal research has provided considerable insight into many of these areas. This discussion will focus on much of these new data and how they impact on areas of particular interest to the critical care physician. Controversial topics that need clarification include the following: What type of site bandage is best? Do triple-lumen catheters have a higher rate of infection than conventional catheters? What is the role of new catheter technology? Are catheter changes over a guidewire an effective method of infection control? How long should catheters remain in place? Are there differences in infection rates among the different insertion sites? There are reasonably good answers to most of these questions, but controversy continues over others. Future prospective, randomized studies—utilizing standardized definitions of catheter-related infection—are needed to develop true consensus. The interested reader is referred to a recent excellent discussion of many of these topics [201].

Consensus regarding the definition and diagnosis of catheter-related infection is a necessary initial step in discussing catheter-related infectious complications [202,203]. The semiquantitative culture method described by Maki et al. [204] for culturing catheter segments is the most accepted technique for diagnosing catheter-related infection [205,206] and is one way to standardize results between institutions. Which catheter segment to culture routinely is controversial, and I do not believe available evidence strongly favors use of the intradermal segment over the catheter tip [201,202,205,206]; most centers routinely culture the catheter tip. Regardless of which segment is cultured, semiquantitative results are used to define catheter contamination as less than 15 colony-forming units (CFU) per culture plate. Catheter-related infection is defined as greater than 15 CFU and is identified as colonization (all other cultures negative); local or site infection (skin site with erythema, cellulitis, or purulence); catheter-related bacteremia (systemic blood cultures positive for identical organism on catheter segment and no other source); and catheter-related sepsis or septic shock.

PATHOPHYSIOLOGY OF CATHETER INFECTION.
Catheters can become infected from four potential sources: the skin insertion site; the catheter hub(s); hematogenous seeding; and infusate contamination, which generally results in epidemic nosocomial bacteremia, a distinct entity reviewed elsewhere [207]. Animal and human studies have shown that catheters are most commonly infected from bacteria colonizing the skin site, followed by invasion of the intradermal catheter tract. Once the external surface of the catheter in the tract is infected, bacteria can quickly traverse the entire length and infect the catheter tip, usually encasing the catheter in a slime layer known as a biofilm. From the catheter tip, bacteria may shed into the bloodstream, potentially creating metastatic foci of infection [201,208,209,210]. The pathophysiology of most catheter infections explains why guidewire changes are not effective in preventing or treating catheter-related infection: the colonized tract and, in many cases, biofilm remain intact and quickly reinfect the new catheter [211,212,213].

The catheter hub(s) also becomes colonized but contributes to catheter-related infectious complications less frequently than the insertion site [201,214–217]. Likewise, hematogenous seeding of catheters from bacteremia is an infrequent cause of catheter-related infection.

SITE PREPARATION AND CATHETER MAINTENANCE.
That the majority of catheter-related infections are caused by skin flora highlights the importance of site sterility during insertion and catheter maintenance. Organisms that colonize the insertion site originate from the patient's own skin flora or the hands of operators [210]. Iodine-containing disinfectants, such as 10% povidone-iodine, are the most commonly used skin disinfectants and provide a wide range of antibacterial activity. Proper application includes liberally scrubbing the site and allowing it to dry for 30 to 60 seconds before wiping with alcohol; defatting the skin with acetone is not necessary [210,218,219,220]. Excessive hair should be clipped with scissors prior to application of the antiseptic, as shaving can cause minor skin lacerations and disruption of the epidermal barrier to infection.

Iodine-containing solutions may not be the best antiseptic for site preparation. One recent study showed that when a 2% aqueous solution of chlorhexidine was used for site preparation and maintenance, the incidence of catheter-associated infection was reduced fourfold compared to povidone-iodine [221]. Chlorhexidine is a potent germicide, with a broad spectrum and longer duration of action. It is available in the United States primarily as a handwashing preparation. Further studies are needed before this agent can be recommended for site preparation and maintenance.

The hands of medical personnel are also a potential source of organisms for infecting intravascular devices [222,223]. Thorough handwashing and wearing sterile gloves are mandatory for persons involved in catheter insertion or care. Cap, masks, gowns, and a large drape (maximal sterile barriers) were shown to reduce the infection rate in one recent study [224]. If a break in sterile technique occurs during insertion, termination of the procedure and replacement of contaminated equipment is mandatory.

Care of the catheter after insertion is perhaps the single most important step in minimizing infection, and all medical personnel should follow standardized protocols [225,226]. The number of piggyback infusions and medical personnel handling tubing changes and manipulation of the catheter site should be minimized. Tubing changes every 48 to 72 hours are adequate; more frequent changes are unnecessary [227]. The use of transparent, semi-occlusive dressings is prevalent, but these may actually increase the risk of site colonization because of moisture trapping, and no dressing has been proved to be superior to gauze and tape [228,229,230]. Application of iodophor or polymicrobial ointment to the insertion site during dressing changes does not convincingly reduce the overall incidence of catheter infection, and certain polymicrobial ointments may increase the proportion of *Candida* infections [215,231].

FREQUENCY OF CATHETER-ASSOCIATED INFECTION.
Observing the above recommendations for catheter insertion and maintenance will minimize but not eliminate catheter-associated infection. Colonization of the insertion site can begin within 24 hours and increases with duration of catheterization; 20 to 40 percent of catheters eventually become colonized [214, 232–236]. Catheter-associated bacteremia and sepsis occurs in 2 to 8 percent of catheters [145,146,158,225,232,234–245], although some recent studies incorporating newer catheter technologies have demonstrated rates of catheter-associated bacteremia of 2 percent or less (see below) [214,246]. Bacteremia

is a significant complication, extending hospitalization and resulting in metastatic infection and death in a significant percentage of patients [207,210,228,244]. Gram-positive organisms, especially *Staphylococcus* species, are the most common infecting agents, but gram-negative enteric organisms are not rare. *Candida* species are less important today than in the past but still cause considerable morbidity, particularly in diabetic patients with prolonged catheterization and on broad-spectrum antibiotics.

TYPE OF CATHETER. The data presented above are derived from large studies and are not necessarily applicable to any given catheter because of variations in definitions, types of catheters, site of insertion, duration of catheterization, types of fluid infused, and policies regarding routine guidewire changes, all of which have been implicated at some point as important factors in the incidence of catheter-associated infection. The duration of catheterization in combination with the type of catheter are major factors; the site of insertion and type of fluid infused have a minor, if any, role. Guidewire changes have an important role in evaluation of the febrile catheterized patient, but routine guidewire changes do not prevent infection or extend the acceptable duration of catheterization at any given site (see below). Under ideal conditions, all of these factors are less important. Long-term TPN catheters can be maintained for months with low rates of infection, and there is no cutoff time at which colonization and clinical infection accelerate. Today, when the need for long-term catheterization is anticipated, surgically implanted silicone elastomer (Silastic) catheters are used. These catheters have low infection rates and are never changed routinely [247]. Catheters inserted percutaneously in the critical care unit, however, are not subject to ideal conditions and have a finite life span. For practical purposes, triple-lumen catheters have replaced single-lumen catheters for many indications for central venous access. Since catheter hubs are a potential source of infection and triple-lumen catheters can require three times the number of tubing changes, it was widely believed that they would have a higher infection rate. Studies have presented conflicting results, but overall the data support the view that triple-lumen catheters have a slightly higher rate of infection [234,238,242–245,248,249]. If used efficiently, however, they provide greater intravascular access per device and can decrease the total number of catheter days and exposure to central venipuncture. A slight increase in infection rate per catheter is therefore justifiable from an overall risk-benefit analysis, if triple-lumen catheters are used only when multiple infusion ports are truly indicated [244].

DURATION OF CATHETERIZATION. How long to leave a triple-lumen catheter in place is controversial and recommendations are changing. Based on older data, many institutions routinely move them to a new site or change over a guidewire every 72 to 96 hours. I have never recommended guidewire exchanges as an effective infection control measure, and two recently completed prospective controlled trials support this view [211,212]. Changing triple-lumen catheters to a new site every 72 to 96 hours minimizes infection but also increases mechanical complications associated with insertion. The intensivist is thus faced with balancing the risk of infection with the risks associated with insertion at a new site. Not surprisingly, the literature is interpreted differently and practices vary between and even within institutions; flexibility in management protocols is necessary. My approach is to leave triple-lumen catheters in place an average of 6 to 7 days before changing to

a new site, based on recent series and other data for daily risk of catheter colonization [211,236]. For selected patients, especially those at increased risk of complications from central venipuncture, I do not hesitate to leave triple-lumen catheters in place longer than a week.

The above recommendations do not necessarily apply to other special-use catheters, which can be exposed to different clinical situations and risk. Pulmonary artery catheters (PACs) should ideally be removed after 72 to 120 hours because of the increased risk of infection after this time. [234,239,250–255]. These catheters are at more risk for infection because patients are sicker, the introducer used for insertion is shorter, and catheter manipulations are frequent [256]. When PACs are removed to evaluate for infection, the introducer sheath must also be removed, as this, not the PAC, is in contact with the intradermal tract. Likewise, inserting a triple-lumen catheter through the introducer does not alter the risk of infection. Pulmonary artery catheter sheaths do not reduce the infection rate [257] but are clinically important because they allow frequent repositioning of the catheter if necessary. Catheters inserted for acute temporary hemodialysis historically have a risk of infection of approximately 3 percent per week [258,259]. Logically, patient factors influence the incidence of infection more than the type of catheter or site of insertion [21]. For acutely ill, hospitalized patients, these catheters should be managed similarly to other multiple-lumen catheters. For ambulatory outpatients, they can be left in place longer, akin to single-lumen catheters used for long-term parenteral nutrition.

New catheter technology (see below) is promising and may lead to changes in all of the above recommendations. For the present, every physician caring for the critically ill needs to be cognizant of existing data and infection rates in their own institution so that rational policies can be implemented.

SITE OF INSERTION. The condition of the site is more important than the location. Whenever possible, sites involved by infection, burns, or other dermatologic processes, or in close proximity to a heavily colonized area (e.g., tracheostomy) should not be used as primary access. The site of insertion is a relatively minor factor in infection rates, with the exception of antecubital fossa catheters. Catheters inserted through antecubital veins should be treated as peripheral catheters and removed at 72 hours, or a high incidence of phlebitis and infection results. [91,202,210,239]. Otherwise, there are relatively few and conflicting data demonstrating any difference between the EJV, IJV, FV, and SV. A few studies have reported a trend toward higher colonization rates with FV and IJV catheters and lower rates with SV catheters, but this has not convincingly translated into a higher incidence of clinical infection [236,240,241,254]. Once again, prospective, randomized studies are needed to clarify the issue.

GUIDEWIRE EXCHANGES. Guidewire exchanges have always been theoretically flawed as a form of infection control, because although a new catheter is placed, the site, specifically the intradermal tract, remains the same. Recent animal and human studies have shown that when the tract and old catheter are colonized, the new catheter invariably also becomes infected [213,260,261,262]. Alternatively, if the initial catheter is not colonized, there is no reason the new catheter will be more resistant to subsequent infection than the original one. In neither situation will a guidewire change prevent infection [211,212]. However, guidewire changes continue to have a valuable role for replacing defective catheters, exchanging one type of catheter for another, and in the evaluation of a febrile patient with an existing central catheter [211,263]. In the latter situation, the physician can assess the sterility of the catheter tract without subjecting the patient to a new venipuncture, as detailed below. However one decides to use guidewire exchanges, they must be performed properly. The catheter should be withdrawn until an intravascular segment is exposed, transected sterilely, and the guidewire inserted through the distal lumen. The catheter fragment can then be removed and a new catheter threaded over the guidewire. Insertion of the guidewire through the distal hub of the existing catheter is not appropriate.

New Catheter Technologies

Improvements in catheter technology continue to play an important role in minimizing catheter complications. Catheter material is an important factor in promoting thrombogenesis and adherence of organisms. Modern catheters are composed of flexible silicone (for surgical implantation) and polyurethane (for percutaneous insertion), because research has shown these materials are less thrombogenic [201]. Knowledge of the pathogenesis of most catheter-associated infection has stimulated improvements in catheter technology designed to interrupt bacterial colonization of the catheter and intradermal tract and subsequent migration to the tip. Two principle developments have resulted: the Vita-Cuff and antibiotic bonding of catheters. The Vita-Cuff is a silver-impregnated tissue-interface barrier that is attached to the catheter before insertion and then slipped into an intradermal position after placement. Subcutaneous tissue grows into the collagenous matrix of the cuff and acts as a mechanical, antibacterial barrier to invasion by skin flora [214]. The Vita-Cuff has been effective in clinical trials [214,264] but has not gained widespread acceptance; in my opinion, it is unlikely to in the future because of developments with catheter bonding.

Bonding drugs to catheter material is not new technology. Most PACs in use today are heparin-bonded to minimize thrombogenecity [74], but the effectiveness in preventing overall thrombotic phenomenon is minimized because the heparin rapidly disassociates from the catheter when it is exposed to serum. Interestingly, the heparin is bonded to the catheter with benzalkonium chloride, which has broad-spectrum antimicrobial properties and probably contributes to reducing PAC-associated infection [265].

Recently, antibiotic- and antiseptic-impregnated catheters have been studied in animals and humans [246,265-268]. Preliminary results with a commercially available catheter impregnated with silver sulfadiazine and chlorhexadine have been impressive, with a twofold reduction in colonization and fourfold reduction in bacteremia, to about 1 percent [246]. Small quantities of the silver sulfadiazine and chlorhexadine slowly disassociate from the catheter over a 15-day period, and toxicologic considerations are minimal, apparently even in patients allergic to sulfonamides [267]. The timed release of the three agents indicates a potential for substantially increasing the duration of catheterization, thus ensuring a favorable cost-benefit ratio. These catheters should have particular utility in patients who require prolonged percutaneous catheterization, such as those with acute renal failure; temporary dialysis catheters that have incorporated this technology are now available. Further studies are needed to delineate precisely all of the advantages of these catheters and the length of time they may safely remain in place.

Management of the Febrile Patient

Patients with a central venous catheter frequently develop fever. Removal of the catheter in every febrile patient is not feasible nor clinically indicated, because the fever is often unrelated to the catheter [269]. Management must be individualized and depends on type of catheter, duration of catheterization, anticipated need for continued central venous access, risk of establishing new central venous access, and underlying medical condition and prognosis. All critical care units have developed protocols for managing the febrile, catheterized patient. Decisions to withdraw, change over a guidewire, or leave catheters in place must be based on a fundamental knowledge of risks and benefits for catheters inserted at each site. Use of the new antibiotic/antiseptic-impregnated catheters will probably have an effect on the management algorithm (Fig. 2-7), but the full impact of these catheters will not be known for some time.

Catheter sites in the febrile patient should always be examined. Clinical infection of the site mandates removal of the catheter and institution of antibiotics. Surgically implanted catheters are not easily removed or replaced and can often be left in place while the infection is cleared with antibiotics, unless tunnel infection is present [247]. Percutaneously inserted central venous catheters are relatively easily removed, and the risks of leaving a catheter in place through an infected site outweighs the risk of replacement at a new site, except in very unusual circumstances.

In patients who develop septic shock, central venous catheters should be considered a possible source. If all catheter sites appear normal and a noncatheter site can be implicated as the source for infection, appropriate antibiotics are initiated and the catheters left in place. The usual guidelines for subsequent catheter management should be followed, and this rarely results in treatment failure. In contrast, if a noncatheter source cannot be identified, then central catheters in place more than a few days should be managed individually, with attention to duration of catheterization (Fig 2-7). For patients with excessive risks for new catheter placement (i.e., coagulopathy), guidewire exchange of the catheter is justifiable after obtaining two peripheral blood cultures and semiquantitative cultures of a catheter segment. If within the next 24 hours an alternative source for sepsis is found, or if the catheter segment culture is negative and the patient improves and stabilizes, the guidewire catheter can be left in place and a risky procedure avoided. Alternatively, if the catheter culture becomes positive, especially if the same organism is identified on peripheral blood cultures, the cutaneous tract is also infected and the guidewire catheter should be removed and alternative access achieved.

The most common situation is the stable febrile patient with a central venous catheter in place. As above, if a noncatheter source for fever is identified, appropriate antibiotics are given and the catheter left in place, assuming it is still needed and the site is clinically uninvolved. In the patient with no obvious source of fever, indications for the central venous catheters should be reviewed and the catheter withdrawn if it is no longer required. Also, if the catheter is within 24 hours of routine removal for infection control, it should be withdrawn and a new catheter inserted at an alternative site. Otherwise, the physician must decide between observation, potential premature withdrawal, or a guidewire change of the catheter. If the catheter is less than 72 to 96 hours old, observation is reasonable, as it is very unlikely that the catheter is already infected unless breaks in sterile technique occurred during insertion. For catheters more than 72 hours old but less than 120 hours old, guidewire exchanges are rational. Catheters inserted for this duration are still not likely to be the source of fever, but the risk cannot be ignored. Unfortunately, there is not a good way

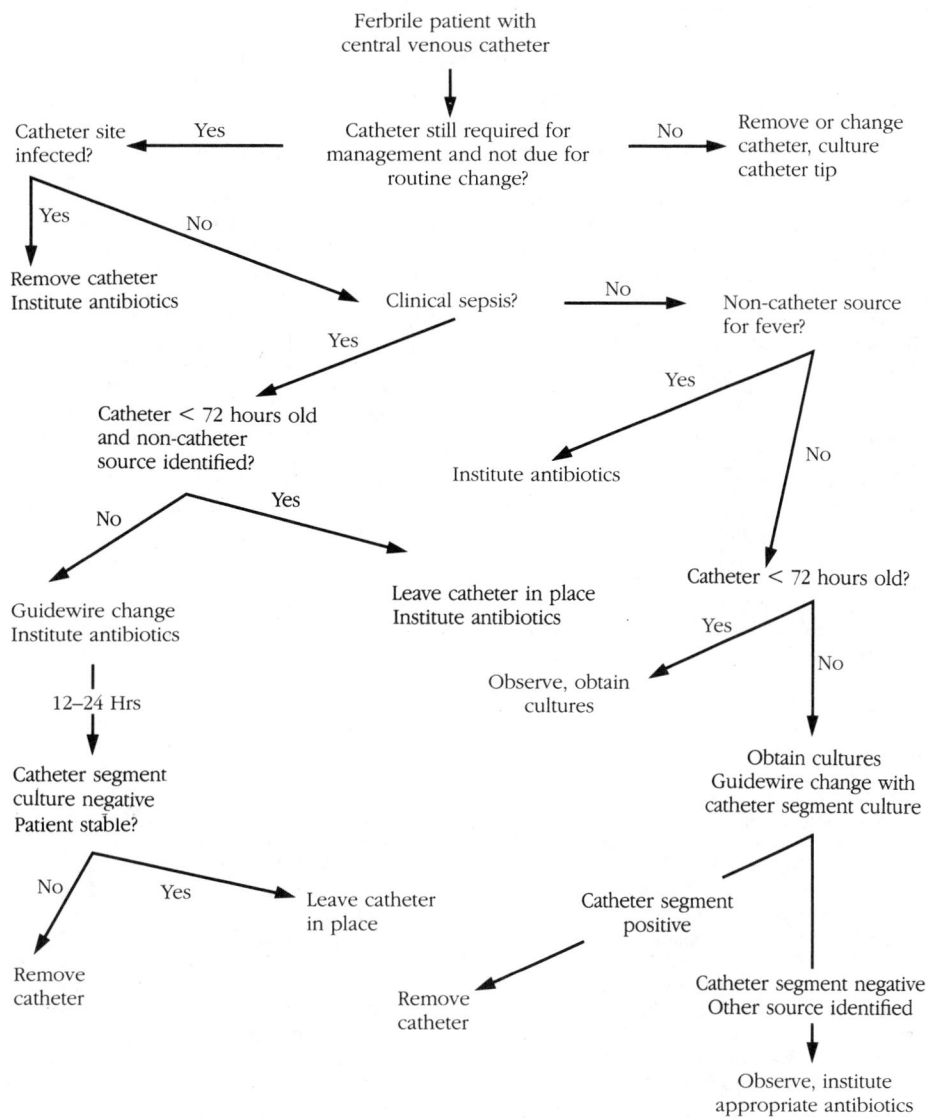

Fig. 2-7. Recommended approach to the catheterized patient with fever.

to assess the sterility of the catheter short of withdrawal and culture of a catheter segment. Drawback blood cultures obtained through the catheter may be positive for the same reason that peripheral blood cultures are positive, and isolated, positive drawback blood cultures are not necessarily indicative of catheter infection [202,206]. An appropriately performed guidewire change allows comparison of catheter segment cultures to other clinical cultures without subjecting the patient to repeat venipuncture. If within the next 24 hours an alternative source for fever is identified, and/or the initial catheter segment culture is negative, then the guidewire catheter can be left in place. Further management decisions regarding the catheter are complicated, but multiple guidewire changes of the same insertion site are probably not advisable.

When catheter-related bacteremia does develop, antibiotic therapy is necessary for a period of 7 to 14 days. Even in patients treated for 14 days, metastatic infection can develop [201, 270]. Catheter-related fever, infection, and septicemia is a complicated disease, and the expertise of an infectious disease

consultant may be required to assist with the decision on how long to continue antibiotic therapy.

References

1. Kalso E: A short history of central venous catheterization. *Acta Anaesth Scand* 81(suppl):7, 1985.
2. Aubaniac R: L'injection intraveneuse sousclaviculare advantage et technique. *Presse Med* 60:1456, 1952.
3. Seldinger SI: Catheter replacement of the needle in percutaneous arteriography: A new technique. *Acta Radiol* 39:368, 1953.
4. Moncrief JA: Femoral catheters. *Ann Surg* 147:166, 1958.
5. Bansmer G, Keith D, Tesluk H: Complications following use of indwelling catheters of inferior vena cava. *JAMA* 167:1606, 1958.
6. Hughes RE, Magovern GJ: The relationship between right atrial pressure and blood volume. *Arch Surg* 79:238, 1959.
7. Wilson JN, Grow JB, Demong CV, et al: Central venous pressure in optimal blood volume maintenance. *Arch Surg* 85:55, 1962.

8. Yoffa D: Supraclavicular subclavian venipuncture and catheterization. *Lancet* 2:614, 1965.

9. Linos DA, Mucha P, Van Heerden JA: Subclavian vein: A golden route. *Mayo Clin Proc* 55:315, 1980.

10. Nordlund S, Thoren L: Catheter in the superior vena cava for parenteral feeding. *Acta Chir Scand* 127:39, 1964.

11. Rams JJ, Dalcoff GR, Moulder PV: A simple method for central venous pressure measurements. *Arch Surg* 92:886, 1966.

12. English ICW, Frew RM, Pigott JF, et al: Percutaneous cannulation of the internal jugular vein. *Thorax* 24:496, 1969.

13. English ICW, Frew RM, Pigott JF, et al: Percutaneous catheterization of the internal jugular vein. *Anaesthesia* 24:521, 1969.

14. Hoshal VL Jr: The consequences of a cavalier approach to central venous catheterization. *Acta Anaesth Scand* 81(suppl):11, 1985.

15. Graber D, Dailey RH: Catheter flow rates updated. *JACEP* 6:518, 1977.

16. Novak RA, Venus B: Clavicular approaches for central vein cannulation, in Mallory DL, Venus B (eds): *Problems in Critical Care.* Philadelphia, JB Lippincott, 1987, p 246.

17. Fares LG, Hsu TC, Leva R, et al: Subclavian cannulation: A valuable dialysis access alternative. *Am Surg* 50:283, 1984.

18. Andersen JT, Gammelgoard J, Nielsen LM, et al: Subclavian vein catheterization for acute and chronic hemodialysis: A safe temporary vascular access. *Int Urol Nephrol* 18:327, 1986.

19. Schwab SJ, Quarles D, Middleton JP, et al. Hemodialysis-associated subclavian vein stenosis. *Kidney Int* 38:1156, 1988.

20. Cimochowski G, Sartain J, Worley E, et al: Clear superiority of internal jugular access over the subclavian vein for temporary dialysis. *Kidney Int* 33:230, 1987.

21. Firek AF, Cutler RE, St John Hammond PG: Reappraisal of femoral vein cannulation for temporary hemodialysis vascular access. *Nephron* 47:227, 1987.

22. Landow L: Complications of pulmonary artery catheter insertion. *Crit Care Med* 17:845, 1989.

23. Swan HJC: Central venous pressure monitoring is an outmoded procedure of limited practical value, in Ingelfinger FJ, Ebert RV, Finland MP, et al (eds): *Controversies in Internal Medicine.* vol 2. Philadelphia, WB Saunders, 1974, pp 185–193.

24. Forrester JS, Diamond G, McHugh TJ, et al: Filling pressures in the right and left sides of the heart in acute myocardial infarction: A reappraisal of central venous pressure monitoring. *N Engl J Med* 285:190, 1971.

25. Brisman R, Parks LC, Benson DW: Pitfalls in the clinical use of central venous pressure. *Arch Surg* 95:902, 1967.

26. Knobel E, Akamine N, Fernandes CJ Jr, et al: Reliability of right atrial pressure monitoring to assess left ventricular preload in critically ill septic patients. *Crit Care Med* 17:1344, 1989.

27. Martin JT, Patrick RT: Pneumothorax: Its significance to the anesthesiologist. *Anesth Analg* 39:420, 1960.

28. Dripps RD, Eckenhoff JE, Vandam LD: *Introduction to Anesthesia: The Principles of Safe Practice.* 6th ed. Philadelphia, WB Saunders, 1982, p 388.

29. Emerman CL, Pinchak AC, Hancock D, et al: Effect of injection site on circulation times during cardiac arrest. *Crit Care Med* 16:1138, 1988.

30. Kaye W, Bircher NG: Access for drug administration during cardiopulmonary resuscitation. *Crit Care Med* 16:179, 1988.

31. Emergency Cardiac Care Committee and Subcommittees, American Heart Association: Guidelines for cardiopulmonary resuscitation and emergency cardiac care . *JAMA* 268:2171, 1992.

32. Dane TEB, King EG: Fatal cardiac tamponade and other mechanical complications of central venous catheters. *Br J Surg* 62:6, 1975.

33. Brandt RL, Foley WJ, Fink GH, et al: Mechanism of perforation of the heart with production of hydropericardium by a venous catheter and its prevention. *Am J Surg* 119:311, 1970.

34. Defalque RJ, Campbell C: Cardiac tamponade from central venous catheters. *Anesthesiology* 50:249, 1979.

35. Long R, Kassum D, Donen N, et al: Cardiac tamponade complicating central venous catheterization for total parenteral nutrition: A review. *J Crit Care* 2:39, 1987.

36. Masachke SP, Rogove JH: Cardiac tamponade associated with a multilumen central venous catheter. *Crit Care Med* 12:611, 1984.

37. Curelaru I, Linder LE, Gustavsson B: Displacement of catheters inserted through internal jugular veins with neck flexion and extension. *Intensive Care Med* 6:179, 1980.

38. Wilson GL, McGregor PJ, Thompson GR: Long-term complications of intravascular cannulation, in Mallory DL, Venus B (eds): *Problems in Critical Care.* Philadelphia, JB Lippincott, 1987, p 309.

39. Wojciechowski J, Curelaru I, Gustavsson B, et al: "Half way" venous catheters, III: Tip displacements with upper extremity movements. *Acta Anesth Scand* 81:(suppl)36, 1985.

40. Marx GF: Clinical anesthesia conference: Hazards associated with venous pressure monitoring. *NY State J Med* 69:955, 1969.

41. McGee WT, Mallory DL: Cannulation of the internal and external jugular veins, in Mallory DL, Venus B (eds): *Problems in Critical Care.* Philadelphia, JB Lippincott, 1987, p 234.

42. Seneff MG: Central venous catheterization: A comprehensive review, part 1. *J Intensive Care Med* 2:163, 1987.

43. McGee WT, Mallory DL, Johans TG, et al: Safe placement of central venous catheters is facilitated using right atrial electrocardiography. *Crit Care Med* 4:S434, 1988.

44. Ellis LM, Vogel SB, Copeland EM: Central venous catheter vascular erosions: Diagnosis and clinical course. *Ann Surg* 209:475, 1989.

45. Ghani GA, Berry AJ: An unusual complication following cannulation of an external jugular vein. *Anesthesiology* 58:93, 1983.

46. Iberti TJ, Katz LB, Reiner MA, et al: Hydrothorax as a late complication of central venous indwelling catheters. *Surgery* 94:842, 1983.

47. Duntley P, Siever J, Korwes ML, et al: Vasular erosion by central venous catheters. *Chest* 101:1633, 1992.

48. Doering RB, Stemmer EA, Connolly JE: Complications of indwelling venous catheters with particular reference to catheter embolism. *Am J Surg* 114:259, 1967.

49. Campkin TV: Air embolism: Placement of central venous catheters. *Anesthesiology* 56:406, 1982.

50. Lambert MJ: Air embolism in central venous catheterization. *South Med J* 75:1189, 1982.

51. Orebaugh SL: Venous air embolism: Clinical and experimental considerations. *Crit Care Med* 20:1169, 1992.

52. Nichols PKT, Major E: Central venous cannulation. *Curr Anaesth Crit Care* 1:54, 1989.

53. Morgan RNW, Morrell DF: Internal jugular catheterization: A review of a potentially lethal hazard. *Anaesthesia* 36:512, 1981.

54. McEmany MT, Austen WG: Life-threatening hemorrhage from inadvertent cervical arteriotomy. *Ann Thorac Surg* 24:233, 1977.

55. Wisheart JD, Hasson MA, Jackson JW: A complication of internal jugular vein cannulation. *Anaesthesia* 34:1035, 1979.

56. Morrison SC, Jacobs P: Thrombocytopenia and subclavian cannulation. *Br Med J* 2:279, 1978.

57. Schwartz AJ, Jobes DR, Levy WJ, et al: Intrathoracic vascular catheterization via the external jugular vein. *Anesthesiology* 56:400, 1982.

58. Goldfarb G, Lebrec D: Percutaneous cannulation of the internal jugular vein in patients with coagulopathies: An experience based on 1000 attempts. *Anesthesiology* 56:321, 1982.

59. Ahmed N, Payne RF: Thrombosis after central venous cannulation. *Med J Aust* 1:217, 1976.

60. Brismar B, Hardstedt C, Jacobson S: Diagnosis of thrombosis by catheter phlebography after prolonged central venous catheterization. *Ann Surg* 194:729, 1981.

61. Chastre J, Cornud F, Bouchama A, et al: Thrombosis as a complication of pulmonary-artery catheterization via the internal jugular vein. *N Engl J Med* 306:278, 1982.

62. Wanscher M, Frifelt JJ, Smith-Sivertsen C, et al: Thrombosis caused by polyurethane double-lumen subclavian superior vena cava catheter and hemodialysis. *Crit Care Med* 16:624, 1988.

63. Efsing HO, Lindblad B, Mark J, et al: Thromboembolic complications from central venous catheters: A comparison of three catheter materials. *World J Surg* 7:419, 1983.

64. Axelsson K, Efsen F: Phlebography in long-term catheterization of the subclavian vein. *Scand J Gastroenterol* 13:933, 1978.

65. Bonnet F, Loriferne JG, Texier JP, et al: Evaluation of Doppler examination for diagnosis of catheter-related deep vein thrombosis. *Intensive Care Med* 15:238, 1989.

66. Bagwell CE, Marchildon MB: Mural thrombi in children: Potentially lethal complication of central venous hyperalimentation. *Crit Care Med* 17:295, 1989.

67. Durbec O, Albanese J, Rouzaud M, et al: Thrombotic risk of indwelling venous catheter in femoral position. *Anesthesiology* 75:A266, 1991.

68. Friedman B, Akers S, Gerber D, et al: The risk in ICU patients of deep venous thrombosis due to femoral vein catheterization. *Chest* 102:119S, 1992.
69. Hecker JF, Scandrett LA: Roughness and thrombogenicity of the outer surfaces of intravascular catheters. *J Biomed Mater Res* 19:381, 1985.
70. Linder LE, Curelaru I, Gustavsson B, et al: Material thrombogenicity in central venous catheterization: A comparison between soft, antebrachial catheters of silicone elastomer and polyurethane. *J Parenter Enter Nutr* 8:399, 1984.
71. StenQvist O, Curelaru I, Linder LE, et al: Stiffness of central venous catheters. *Acta Anaesthesiol Scand* 27:153, 1983.
72. Welch GW, McKeel DW, Silverstein P, et al: The role of catheter composition in the development of thrombophlebitis. *Surg Gynecol Obstet* 138:421, 1974.
73. Madan M, Alexander DJ, McMahon MJ: Influence of catheter type on occurrence of thrombophlebitis during peripheral intravenous nutrition. *Lancet* 339:101, 1992.
74. Hoar PF, Wilson RM, Mangano DT, et al: Heparin bonding reduces thrombogenecity of pulmonary artery catheters. *N Engl J Med* 305:992, 1981.
75. Mangano DT: Heparin bonding and long-term protection against thrombogenesis. *N Engl J Med* 307:894, 1982.
76. Kido DK, Poulin S, Algenghat JA, et al: Thrombogenicity of heparin and non-heparin coated catheters. *Am J Roentgenol* 139:957, 1982.
77. Bern MM, Lukich JJ, Wallach SR, et al: Very low doses of warfarin can prevent thrombosis in central venous catheters: A randomized prospective trial. *Ann Inter Med* 112:423, 1990.
78. Romanes GJ (ed): *Cunningham's Textbook of Anatomy*. London, Oxford University Press, 1972.
79. Williams PL, Warwick R (eds): *Gray's Anatomy*. Philadelphia, WB Saunders, 1980.
80. Hollinshead WH: *Textbook of Anatomy*. Hagerstown, MD, Harper & Row, 1974.
81. Anderson JE (ed): *Grant's Atlas of Anatomy*. 8th ed. Baltimore, Williams & Wilkins, 1983.
82. Lumley J, Russell WJ: Insertion of central venous catheters through arm veins. *Anesth Intensive Care* 3:101, 1975.
83. Holt MH: Central venous pressures via peripheral veins. *Anesthesiology* 28:1093, 1967.
84. Webre DR, Arens JF: Use of cephalic and basilic veins for introduction of central venous catheters. *Anesthesiology* 38:389, 1973.
85. Kellner GA, Smart JF: Percutaneous placement of catheters to monitor central venous pressure. *Anesthesiology* 36:515, 1972.
86. Kuramoto T, Sarabe T: Comparison of success in jugular versus basilic vein technique for central venous pressure catheter positioning. *Anesth Analg* 54:5, 1975.
87. Martin JT: Neuroanesthetic adjuncts for patients in the sitting position, III: Intravascular electrocardiography. *Anesth Analg Curr Res* 49:793, 1970.
88. Dietel M, McIntyre JA: Radiographic determination of site of central venous pressure catheters. *Can J Surg* 14:42, 1971.
89. Gilday DL, Downs AR: The value of chest radiography in the localization of central venous pressure catheters. *Can Med Assoc J* 101:363, 1969.
90. Bridges BB, Camden E, Takacs IA: Introduction of central venous pressure catheters through arm veins with a high success rate. *Can Anaesth Soc J* 26:128, 1979.
91. Giuffrida DJ, Bryan-Brown CW, Lumb PD, et al: Central vs peripheral venous catheters in critically ill patients. *Chest* 90:806, 1986.
92. Gustavsson B, Curelaru I, Hultman E, et al: Displacements of the soft, polyurethane central venous catheters inserted by basilic and cephalic veins with arm in maximal adduction and elevation. *Acta Anaesthesiol Scand* 27:102, 1983.
93. Silver HK, Kempe CH, Breyer HB: *Handbook of Pediatrics*. 5th ed. Los Altos, CA, Lange, 1963, p 37.
94. Hermosura B, Vanags L, Dickey NW: Measurement of pressure during intravenous therapy. *JAMA* 195:321, 1966.
95. Blitt CD, Wright WA, Petty WC, et al: Central venous catheterization via the external jugular vein: A technique employing the J-wire. *JAMA* 229:817, 1974.
96. Malatinsky J, Faybik M, Griffith M, et al: Venipuncture, catheterization, and failure to position correctly during central venous circulation. *Resuscitation* 10:259, 1983.

97. Fischer J, Lundstrom J, O'Hander HG: Central venous cannulation: A radiological determination of catheter positions and immediate intrathoracic complications. *Acta Anaesthesiol Scand* 21:45, 1977.
98. Criado A, Mena A, Figueredo R, et al: Late perforation of superior vena cava and effusion caused by central venous catheter. *Anesth Intensive Care* 9:286, 1981.
99. Rosen M, Latto IP, Ng WS: *Handbook of Percutaneous Central Venous Catheterization*. London, WB Saunders, 1981.
100. Defalque RJ: Percutaneous catheterization of the internal jugular vein. *Anesth Analg* 53:1, 1974.
101. McConnell RY, Fox RT: Experience with percutaneous internal jugular-innominate vein catheterizations. *Calif Med* 117:1, 1972.
102. Daily PO, Griepp RB, Shumway NE: Percutaneous internal jugular vein cannulation. *Arch Surg* 101:534, 1970.
103. Morgan RNW, Morrell DF: Internal jugular catheterization. *Anaesthesia* 36:512, 1981.
104. Johnson FE: Internal jugular vein catheterization. *NY State J Med* 78:2168, 1978.
105. Sznajder J, Zveibil FR, Bitterman H, et al: Central venous catheterization failure and complication rates by 3 percutaneous approaches. *Arch Intern Med* 146:259, 1986.
106. Mostert JW, Kenny GM, Murphy GP: Safe placement of central venous catheters into internal jugular veins. *Arch Surg* 101:431, 1970.
107. Civetta JM, Gabel JC, Geiner M: Internal jugular vein puncture with a margin of safety. *Anesthesiology* 36:622, 1972.
108. Petty C: An alternative method for internal jugular venipuncture for monitoring central venous pressure. *Anesth Analg* 54:157, 1975.
109. Jernigan WR, Gardner WC, Mahr NM, et al: Use of the internal jugular vein for placement of central venous catheter. *Surg Gynecol Obstet* 130:520, 1970.
110. Brinkman AJ, Costley DO: Internal jugular venipuncture. *JAMA* 223:182, 1973.
111. Kaiser CW, Koornick AR, Smith N, et al: Choice of route for central venous cannulation: Subclavian or internal jugular vein? A prospective randomized study. *J Surg Oncol* 17:345, 1981.
112. Bo-Linn GW, Anderson DJ, Anderson KC, et al: Percutaneous central venous catheterization performed by medical house officers. *Cathet Cardiovasc Diagn* 8:23, 1982.
113. Metz S, Horrow JC, Balcar I: A controlled comparison of techniques for locating the internal jugular vein using ultrasonography. *Anesth Analg* 63:673, 1984.
114. Legler D, Nugent M: Doppler localization of the internal jugular vein facilitates central venous cannulation. *Anesthesiology* 60:481, 1984.
115. Bazaral M, Harlan S: Ultrasonographic anatomy of the internal jugular vein relevant to percutaneous cannulation. *Crit Care Med* 9:307, 1981.
116. Mallory DL, Morrison GD, McGee WJ, et al: The effect of cannulation maneuvers and technique on internal jugular vein lumen cross-sectional area. *Crit Care Med* 16:447, 1988.
117. Denys BG, Uretsky BF: Anatomical variations of internal jugular vein location: Impact on central venous access. *Crit Care Med* 19:1516, 1991.
118. Gilbert TB, Señeff M: Facilitation of right internal jugular central venous cannulation using an audio-guided ultrasonic vascular access device. Presented at Annual Meeting of Society of Cardiovascular Anesthesiology, San Diego, April 1993.
119. Koski EMJ, Suhonen M, Mattila MAK: Ultrasound-facilitated central venous cannulation. *Crit Care Med* 20:424, 1992.
120. Tyden H: Cannulation of the internal jugular vein: 500 cases. *Acta Anaesthesiol Scand* 26:485, 1982.
121. Eisenhauer ED, Derveloy RJ, Hastings PR: Prospective evaluation of central venous pressure (CVP) catheters in a large city-county hospital. *Ann Surg* 196:560, 1982.
122. Schwartz AJ, Jobes CR, Greenhow DE, et al: Carotid artery puncture with internal jugular cannulation. *Anesthesiology* 51:S160, 1980.
123. Belani KG, Buckley JJ, Gordon JR, et al: Percutaneous cervical central venous line placement: A comparison of the internal and external jugular vein routes. *Anesth Analg* 59:40, 1980.
124. Butsch JL, Butsch WL, Darosa JF: Bilateral vocal cord paralysis. *Arch Surg* 111:828, 1976.

125. Knoblanche GE: Respiratory obstruction due to hematoma following internal jugular vein cannulation. *Anesth Intensive Care* 7:286, 1979.

126. Klineberg PL, Greenhow DE, Ellison N: Hematoma following internal jugular vein cannulation. *Anesth Intensive Care* 8:94, 1980.

127. Parikh RK: Horner's syndrome: A complication of percutaneous catheterization of the internal jugular vein. *Anaesthesia* 27:327, 1972.

128. Briscoe CE, Brishman JA, McDonald WI: Extensive neurological damage after cannulation of internal jugular vein. *Br Med J* 1:314, 1974.

129. Brown CS, Wallace CT: Chronic hematoma: A complication of percutaneous catheterization of the internal jugular vein. *Anesthesiology* 45:368, 1976.

130. Hansbrough JF, Narrod JA, Rutherford R: Arteriovenous fistulas following central venous catheterization. *Intensive Care Med* 9:287, 1983.

131. Shield CF, Richardson JD, Buckley CJ, et al: Pseudoaneurysm of the brachiocephalic arteries: A complication of percutaneous internal jugular vein catheterization. *Surgery* 78:190, 1975.

132. Cook TL, Dueker CW: Tension pneumothorax following internal jugular cannulation and general anesthesia. *Anesthesiology* 45:554, 1976.

133. Koch MJ: Bilateral IV hydrothorax. *N Engl J Med* 286:218, 1972.

134. Nagai K, Kemmotsu O: An inadvertent insertion of a Swanz-Ganz catheter into the intrathecal space. *Anesthesiology* 62:848, 1985.

135. Schwartz AJ, Jobes DR, Levy WJ, et al: Intrathoracic vascular catheterization via the external jugular vein. *Anesthesiology* 56:400, 1982.

136. Blitt CD, Carlson GL, Wright WA, et al: J-wire versus straight wire for central venous system cannulation via the external jugular vein. *Anesth Analg* 61:536, 1982.

137. Abadir AR, Ung KA, Chaudhry R: Evaluation of external jugular vein for Swanz-Ganz catheter insertion. *Anesthesiology* 51:S159, 1979.

138. Giesy J: External jugular vein access to central venous system. *JAMA* 219:216, 1972.

139. Riddell GS, Latto IP, Ng WS: External jugular vein access to the central venous system: A trial of two types of catheters. *Br J Anaesth* 54:535, 1982.

140. Jobes DR, Schwartz AJ, Greenhow DE: Safer jugular vein cannulation. Recognition of arterial puncture and preferential use of the external jugular route. *Anesthesiology* 59:353, 1983.

141. Ghani GA, Berry AJ: Right hydrothorax after left external jugular vein catheterization. *Anesthesiology* 53:93, 1983.

142. Getzen LC, Pollak EW: Short-term femoral vein catheterization. *Am J Surg* 138:875, 1979.

143. Swanson RS: Emergency intravenous access through the femoral vein. *Ann Emerg Med* 13:244, 1984.

144. Dailey RH: "Code red" protocol for resuscitation of the exsanguinated patient. *J Emerg Med* 2:373, 1985.

145. Kanter RK, Zimmerman JJ, Strauss RH, et al: Central venous catheter insertion by femoral vein: Safety and effectiveness for the pediatric patient. *Pediatrics* 77:842, 1986.

146. Williams JF, Friedman BC, McGrath BJ, et al: The use of femoral venous catheters in critically ill adults: A prospective study. *Crit Care Med* 17:584, 1989.

147. Kruse JA, Carlson RW: Infectious complications of femoral vs internal jugular and subclavian vein central venous catheterization. *Crit Care Med* 19:843, 1991.

148. Dailey RH: Femoral vein cannulation: A review. *J Emerg Med* 2:367, 1985.

149. Gilston A: Cannulation of the femoral vessels. *Br J Anaesth* 48:500, 1976.

150. Bozzetti F: Percutaneous femoral vein catheterization. *Anaesthesia* 33:761, 1978.

151. Sung JP, Bikangaga AW, Abbott JA: Massive hemorrhage to scrotum from laceration of inferior epigastric artery following percutaneous femoral vein catheterization: Case report. *Mil Med* 146:362, 1981.

152. Nidus BD, Neusy AJ: Chronic hemodialysis by repeated femoral vein cannulation. *Nephron* 29:195, 1981.

153. Kjellstrand CM, Merino GE, Mauer SM, et al: Complications of percutaneous femoral vein catheterizations for hemodialysis. *Clin Nephrol* 4:37, 1975.

154. Kalzsa SA, Cohen EL: Urologic complication associated with Swanz-Ganz catheter. *Urology* 6:716, 1975.

155. Sharp KW, Spees EK, Selby LR, et al: Diagnosis and management of retroperitoneal hematomas after femoral vein cannulation for hemodialysis. *Surgery* 95:90, 1984.

156. Shaldon S, Chiandussi L, Higgs B: Hemodialysis by percutaneous catheterization of the femoral artery and vein with regional heparinization. *Lancet* 2:857, 1961.

157. Fuller TJ, Mahoney JJ, Juncos LI, et al: Arteriovenous fistula after femoral vein catheterization. *JAMA* 236:2943, 1976.

158. Stenzel JP, Green TP, Fuhrman BP, et al: Percutaneous femoral venous catheterizations: A prospective study of complications. *J Pediatr* 114:411, 1989.

159. Russell JA, Joel M, Hudson RJ, et al: Prospective evaluation of radial and femoral artery catheterization sites in critically ill adults. *Crit Care Med* 11:936, 1983.

160. Graves PW, Davis AL, Maggi C, et al: Femoral artery cannulation for monitoring in critically ill children: Prospective study. *Crit Care Med* 18:1363, 1990.

161. Lynn KL, Maling TMJ: A major pulmonary embolus as a complication of femoral vein catheterization. *Br J Radiol* 50:667, 1977.

162. Nolewajika AJ, Goddard MD, Brown TC: Temporary pacing and femoral vein thrombosis. *Circulation* 62:646, 1980.

163. Shapira M, Stern WZ: Hazards of subclavian vein cannulation for central venous pressure monitoring. *JAMA* 201:327, 1967.

164. Tremper KK: Central venous catheterization: A perspective. *J Intensive Care Med* 2:121, 1987.

165. Sznadjer JI, Zveibil FR, Bitterman H, et al: Central vein catheterization: Failure and complication rates by three percutaneous approaches. *Arch Intern Med* 146:259, 1986.

166. Schechter, DC, Acinapura AJ: Subclavian vein catheterization, part 1. *NY State J Med* 79:346, 1979.

167. Grant JP: Subclavian catheter insertion and complications, in Grant JP (ed): *Handbook of Total Parenteral Nutrition*. Philadelphia, WB Saunders, 1980, p 47.

168. Moosman DA: The anatomy of infraclavicular subclavian vein catheterization and its complications. *Surg Gynecol Obstet* 136:71, 1973.

169. Keeri-Szanto M: The subclavian vein: A constant and convenient intravenous injection site. *Arch Surg* 72:179, 1956.

170. Voegele LD: Subclavian venipuncture for vascular access. *South Med J* 73:1288, 1980.

171. Eerola R, Kaukinen L, Kaukinen S: Analysis of 13,800 subclavian catheterizations. *Acta Anaesthesiol Scand* 29:293, 1985.

172. Mogil RA, Delaurentis DA, Rosemond GP: The infraclavicular venipuncture. *Arch Surg* 95:320, 1967.

173. James PM, Myers RT: Central venous pressure monitoring: Misinterpretation, abuses, indications, and a new technique. *Ann Surg* 175:693, 1972.

174. Brahos GJ: Central venous catheterization via the supraclavicular approach. *J Trauma* 17:872, 1977.

175. Yoffa D: Supraclavicular subclavian venipuncture and catheterization. *Lancet* 2:614, 1965.

176. Haapaniemi L, Slatis P: Supraclavicular catheterization of the superior vena cava. *Acta Anaesthesiol Scand* 18:12, 1974.

177. MacDonnell JE, Perez H, Pitts SR, et al: Supraclavicular subclavian vein catheterization: Modified landmarks for needle insertion. *Ann Emerg Med* 21:421, 1992.

178. James PM, Myers R: Central venous pressure monitoring: Complications and a new technique. *Am Surg* 39:75, 1981.

179. Dronen S, Thompson B, Nowak R, et al: Subclavian vein catheterization during cardiopulmonary resuscitation: Comparison of supra- and infraclavicular percutaneous approaches. *JAMA* 247:3227, 1982.

180. Sterner S: A comparison of the supraclavicular approach and the infraclavicular approach for subclavian vein catheterization. *Ann Emerg Med* 15:421, 1986.

181. Simpson ET, Aitchison JM: Percutaneous infraclavicular subclavian vein catheterization in shocked patients: A prospective study in 172 patients. *J Trauma* 22:781, 1982.

182. Malatinsky J, Kadlic T, Majek M, et al: Misplacement and loop formation of central venous catheters. *Acta Anaesthesiol Scand* 20:237, 1976.

183. McCormack T, Lane BE, Tanner WA, et al: Complications of subclavian vein cannulation. *Ir Med J* 74:373, 1981.

184. Herbst CA Jr: Indications, management, and complications of percutaneous subclavian catheters: An audit. *Arch Surg* 113:1421, 1978.

185. Bernard RW, Stahl WM: Subclavian vein catheterization: A prospective study, 1—Non-infectious complications. *Ann Surg* 173:184, 1971.

186. McGoon MD, Benedetto PW, Greene BM: Complications of percutaneous central venous catheterization: A report of two cases and review of the literature. *John Hopkins Med J* 145:1, 1979.

187. Smith BE, Modell JH, Graub ML, et al: Complications of subclavian vein catheterization. *Arch Surg* 90:228, 1965.

188. Christensen KH, Nerstrom B, Baden H: Complications of percutaneous catheterization of the subclavian vein in 129 cases. *Acta Chir Scand* 133:615, 1967.

189. Defalque RJ: Subclavian venipuncture: A review. *Anesth Analg* 47:677, 1968.

190. Ryan JA, Abel RM, Abbott WM, et al: Catheter complications in total parenteral nutrition: A prospective study of 200 consecutive patients. *N Engl J Med* 270:757, 1974.

191. Feiler EM, de Alva WE: Infraclavicular percutaneous subclavian vein puncture: A safe technique. *Am J Surg* 118:906, 1969.

192. Host S, Kiriham N, Myerscough E: Haemothorax after subclavian vein cannulation. *Thorax* 32:101, 1977.

193. Allsop JRM, Askew AR: Subclavian vein cannulation: A new complication. *Br Med J* 4:262, 1975.

194. La Penna R, Whinnery C: An unusual complication of subclavian vein catheterization for total parenteral nutrition. *Postgrad Med J* 64:171, 1978.

195. Reilly JJ, Cosini AB, Russell PS: Delayed perforation of the innominate vein during hyperalimentation. *Arch Surg* 112:96, 1977.

196. Weiner P, Sznajder I, Plavnick L, et al: Unusual complications of subclavian vein catheterization. *Crit Care Med* 12:538, 1984.

197. Adar R, Mozes M: Fatal complication of central venous catheter. *Br Med J* 3:746, 1971.

198. Matz R: Complications of determining the central venous pressure. *N Engl J Med* 273:703, 1965.

199. Hagley SR: Subclavian arteriovenous fistula from central venous catheterization. *Anesth Intensive Care* 13:103, 1985.

200. Warden GD, Wilmore DW, Pruitt BA: Central venous thrombosis: A hazard of medical progress. *J Trauma* 13:620, 1973.

201. Raad II, Bodey GP: Infectious complications of indwelling vascular catheters. *Clin Infect Dis* 15:197, 1992.

202. Plit ML, Lipman J, Eidelman J, et al: Catheter related infection: A plea for consensus with review and guidelines. *Intensive Care Med* 14:503, 1988.

203. Corona ML, Peters SG, Narr BJ, et al: Infections related to central venous catheters. *Mayo Clin Proc* 65:979, 1990.

204. Maki DG, Weise CE, Sarafin HW: A semiquantitative culture method for identifying intravenous catheter related infection. *N Engl J Med* 296:1305, 1977.

205. Collignon PJ, Soni N, Pearson IY, et al: Is semiquantitative culture of central vein catheter tips useful in the diagnosis of catheter associated bacteremia. *J Clin Microbiol* 24:532, 1986.

206. Rello J, Coll P, Prats G: Laboratory diagnosis of catheter-related bacteremia. *Scand J Infect Dis* 23:583, 1991.

207. Maki DG: Noscomial bacteremia: An epidemiologic overview. *Am J Med* 70:719, 1981.

208. Passerini L, Lam K, Costerton JW, et al: Biofilms on indwelling vascular catheters. *Crit Care Med* 20:665, 1992.

209. Cooper GL, Schiller AL, Hopkins CC: Possible role of capillary action in pathogenesis of experimental catheter-associated dermal tunnel infections. *J Clin Microbiol* 26:8, 1988.

210. Maki DG: Pathogenesis, prevention, and management of infections due to intravascular devices used for infusion therapy, in Bisno A, Waldvogel F (eds): *Infections associated with Indwelling Medical Devices*. Washington, DC, American Society for Microbiology, 1989, pp 161–177.

211. Eyer S, Brummitt C, Crossley K, et al: Catheter-related sepsis: Prospective, randomized study of three methods of long-term catheter maintenance. *Crit Care Med* 18:1073, 1990.

212. Cobb DK, High KP, Sawyer RG, et al: A controlled trial of scheduled replacement of central venous and pulmonary artery catheters. *N Engl J Med* 327:1062, 1992.

213. Olson ME, Lam K, Bodey GP, et al: Evaluation of strategies for central venous catheter replacement. *Crit Care Med* 20:797, 1992.

214. Maki DG, Cobb L, Garman JK, et al: An attachable silver-impregnated cuff for prevention of infection with central venous catheters: A prospective randomized multi-center trial. *Am J Med* 85:307, 1988.

215. Beam TR, Goodman EL, Maki DG, et al: Preventing central venous catheter-related complications: A roundtable discussion. *Inf Surg* 12:1, 1990.

216. Sitges-Serra A, Linares J, Garau J, et al: Catheter sepsis: The clue is the hub. *Surgery* 97:355, 1985.

217. Cooper GL, Hopkins CC: Rapid diagnosis of intravascular catheter-associated infection by direct gram staining of catheter segments. *N Engl J Med* 312:1142, 1985.

218. King, TC, Price PB: An evaluation of iodophors as skin antiseptics. *Surg Gynecol Obstet* 105:361, 1963.

219. White JJ, Wallace CK, Burnett LS: Drug letter: Skin disinfections. *Johns Hopkins Med J* 126:169, 1970.

220. Maki DG, McCormack KN: Defatting catheter insertion sites in total parenteral nutrition is of no value as an infection control measure. *Am J Med* 83:833, 1987.

221. Maki DG, Ringer M, Alvarado CJ: Prospective randomized trial of povidone-iodine, alcohol, and chlorhexadine for prevention of infection associated with central venous and arterial catheters. *Lancet* 338:339, 1991.

222. Roberts FJ, Cockroft WH: Infection associated with intravenous catheters. *Can Med Assoc J* 102:89, 1970.

223. Morse LJ, Williams HL, Grenn FP Jr, et al: Septicemia due to *Klebsiella pneumoniae* originating from a handcream dispenser. *N Engl J Med* 277:472, 1967.

224. McCormick R, Maki DG: The importance of maximal sterile barriers during insertion of central venous catheters: A prospective study, abstract no. 1077 in *Program and Abstracts of the 29th Interscience Conference on Antimicrobial Agents and Chemotherapy*. Washington, DC, American Society for Microbiology, 1989.

225. Nehme AE: Nutritional support of the hospitalized patient: The team concept. *JAMA* 243:1906, 1980.

226. Freeman JB, Lemire A, MacLean LD: Intravenous alimentation and septicemia. *Surg Gynecol Obstet* 135:708, 1972.

227. Maki DG, Ringer M: Evaluation of dressing regimens for prevention of infection with peripheral intravenous catheters. *JAMA* 258:2396, 1987.

228. Conly JM, Grieves K, Peters B: A prospective randomized study comparing transparent and dry gauze dressings for central venous catheters. *J Infect Dis* 159:310, 1989.

229. Masur H: Central venous catheters: Dry gauze dressings versus clear plastic dressings. *Update Crit Care* 4:5, 1989.

230. Hoffman KK, Weber DJ, Samsa GP, et al: Transparent polyurethane film as an intravenous catheter dressing. *JAMA* 267:2072, 1992.

231. Maki DG, Band JD: A comparative study of polyantibiotic and iodophor ointments in prevention of vascular catheter-related infection. *Am J Med* 70:739, 1981.

232. Mogensen JV, Frederiksen W, Jensen JK: Subclavian vein catheterization infection: A bacteriological study of 130 catheter insertions. *Scand J Infect Dis* 4:31, 1972.

233. Bernard RW, Stahl WM, Chase RM: Subclavian vein catheterizations: A prospective study—Infectious complications. *Ann Surg* 173:191, 1971.

234. Miller JJ, Venus B, Mathru M: Comparison of the sterility of long term central venous catheterization using single lumen, triple lumen, and pulmonary artery catheters. *Crit Care Med* 2:634, 1984.

235. Bozzetti F, Terno G, Bonfanti G, et al: Prevention and treatment of central venous catheter sepsis by exchange via a guidewire. *Ann Surg* 198:48, 1983.

236. Gil RT, Krause JA, Thill-Baharozian MC, et al: Triple vs single lumen central venous catheters. *Arch Intern Med* 149:1139, 1989.

237. Prager RL, Silva J: Colonization of central venous catheters. *South Med J* 77:458, 1984.

238. Voegele LD: Routine subclavian vein catheterization in abdominal surgical practice. *Am J Surg* 131:178, 1976.

239. Pinilla JC, Ross DF, Martin T, et al: Study of the incidence of intravascular catheter infection and associated septicemia in critically ill patients. *Crit Care Med* 11:21, 1983.

240. Collignon P, Suni N, Pearson I, et al: Sepsis associated with central vein catheters in critically ill patients. *Intensive Care Med* 14:227, 1988.

241. Sitzmann JV, Townsend TR, Siler MC, et al: Septic and technical complications of central venous catheterizations: A prospective study of 200 consecutive patients. *Ann Surg* 202:766, 1985.

242. Pemberton LB, Lyman B, Lander V, et al: Sepsis from triple vs single-lumen catheters during total parenteral nutrition in surgical or critically ill patients. *Arch Surg* 121:591, 1986.

243. Kelly CS, Ligas JR, Smith CA, et al: Sepsis due to triple lumen central venous catheters. *Surg Gynecol Obstet* 163:14, 1986.

244. Hilton E, Haslett TM, Borenstein MT, et al: Central catheter infections: Single- versus triple-lumen catheters. *Am J Med* 84:667, 1988.

245. McCarthy MC, Shives JK, Robison RJ, et al: Prospective evaluation of single and triple lumen catheters in total parenteral nutrition. *J Parenteral Nutr* 11:259, 1987.

246. Maki DG, Wheller SJ, Stolz SM, et al: Clinical trial of a novel antiseptic-coated central venous catheter, abstract no. 461 in *Program and Abstracts of the 31st Interscience Conference on Antimicrobial Agents and Chemotherapy*. Washington, DC, American Society for Microbiology, 1991.

247. Clarke DE, Raffin TA: Infectious complications of indwelling long-term central venous catheters. *Chest* 97:966, 1990.

248. Appelgran KN: Triple-lumen catheters: Technological advances or setbacks. *Arch Surg* 53:113, 1987.

249. Christoff-Clark N, Watters VA, Sparks W, et al: Use of triple-lumen subclavian catheters for administration of total parenteral nutrition. *J Parenter Enter Nutr* 16:403, 1992.

250. Myers ML, Austin TW, Sibbald WJ: Pulmonary artery catheter infections: A prospective study. *Ann Surg* 201:237, 1985.

251. Hudson-Civetta JA, Civetta JM, Martinez OV, et al: Risk and detection of pulmonary artery catheter-related infection in septic surgical patients. *Crit Care Med* 15:29, 1987.

252. Michel L, Marsh HM, McMichan JC, et al: Infection of pulmonary artery catheters in critically ill patients. *JAMA* 245:1032, 1981.

253. Applefeld JJ, Caruthers TE, Reno DJ, et al: Assessment of the sterility of long term cardiac catheterization using the thermodilution Swanz-Ganz catheter. *Chest* 74:377, 1978.

254. Sise MJ, Hollingsworth P, Brimm JE, et al: Complications of the flow-directed pulmonary artery catheter. *Crit Care Med* 9:315, 1981.

255. Senagore A, Waller JD, Bonnell BW, et al: Pulmonary artery catheterization: A prospective study of internal jugular and subclavian approaches. *Crit Care Med* 15:35, 1987.

256. Hampton AA, Sheretz RJ: Vascular access infections in hospitalized patients. *Surg Clin North Am* 68:57, 1988.

257. Heard SO, Davis RF, Sheretz RJ, et al: Influence of sterile protective sleeves on the sterility of pulmonary artery catheters. *Crit Care Med* 15:499, 1987.

258. Sheretz RJ, Falk RJ, Huffman KA, et al: Infections asociated with subclavian Uldall catheters. *Arch Intern Med* 143:52, 1983.

259. Dahlberg PJ, Yutuc WR, Newcomer KL: Subclavian hemodialysis catheter infections. *Am J Kidney Dis* 7:421, 1986.

260. Mermel LA, McCormick RD, Springman SR, et al: The pathogenesis and epidemiology of catheter-related infection with pulmonary artery Swan-Ganz catheters: A prospective study utilizing molecular subtyping. *Am J Med* 91 (suppl B): 197S, 1991.

261. Pettigrew RA, Lang SDR, Haydock DA, et al: Catheter-related sepsis in patients on intravenous nutrition: A prospective study of quantitative catheter cultures and guidewire changes for suspected sepsis. *Br J Surg* 72:52, 1985.

262. Graeve AH, Carpenter CM, Schiller WR: Management of central venous catheters using a wire introducer. *Am J Surg* 142:752, 1981.

263. Hagley MT, Martin B, Gast P, et al: Infectious and mechanical complications of central venous catheters placed by percutaneous venipuncture and over guidewires. *Crit Care Med* 20:1426, 1992.

264. Flowers RH III, Schwenzer KJ, Kopel RF, et al: Efficacy of an attachable subcutaneous cuff for the prevention of intravascular catheter-related infection. *JAMA* 261:878, 1989.

265. Mermel LA, Stolz SM, Maki DG: Surface antimicrobial activity of heparin-bonded and antiseptic-impregnated vascular catheters. *J Infect Dis* 167:920, 1993.

266. Sheretz RJ, Carruth WA, Hampton AA, et al: Efficacy of antibiotic-coated catheters in preventing subcutaneous staphylococcal aureus infections in rabbits. *J Infect Dis* 167:98, 1993.

267. Modak SM, Samputh L: Development and evaluation of a new polyurethane central venous antiseptic catheter: Reducing central venous catheter infections. *Infect Med* 10:23, 1992.

268. Kamal GD, Pfaller MA, Rempe LE, et al: Reduced intravascular catheter infection by antibiotic bonding: A prospective, randomized controlled trial. *JAMA* 265:2364, 1991.

269. Davis S, Raad I, Umphrey J, et al: Low infection rate and high durability of central venous catheters (CVC) in cancer patients, abstract L-41 in *Proceedings of the Annual Meeting of the American Society for Microbiology*. Washington, DC, American Society for Microbiology, 1991.

270. Rahal JJ: Preventing second-generation complications due to *Staphylococcus aureus*. *Arch Intern Med* 149:503, 1989.

3. *Arterial Line Placement and Care*

Michael Seneff

Arterial catheterization is performed in 50 to 75 percent of all patients admitted to intensive care units, making it the second most frequent invasive procedure, surpassed only by venous catheterization. Arterial cannulation is well tolerated, and technological improvements and a better understanding of risk factors have minimized complications. In many centers critical care technicians routinely insert, maintain, calibrate, and troubleshoot arterial catheters and pressure-monitoring equipment. While this has standardized care, many physicians no longer possess an adequate working knowledge of these important systems. This chapter presents a scientific review of the indications, techniques, equipment, and complications of arterial cannulation. An overview of physical principles governing pressure monitoring and equipment calibration is also presented, with the intent that every physician caring for critically

ill patients be able to troubleshoot measurement errors when they arise.

Historical Perspective

Physicians have achieved access to the arterial circulation for many years, but early methods were comparatively crude and accompanied by a substantial risk of morbidity. The modern age of arterial monitoring was initiated by Farinas in 1941, when he described cannulation of the aorta with a urethral catheter introduced through a surgically exposed femoral artery [1]. Cannulation technique, catheters, and monitoring equipment have since improved. The strain gauge manometer, introduced in

1947, consisted of a wheatstone bridge with four-strain sensitive wire elements [2]. Displacement of a bellows attached to the bridge caused a change in resistance of the wires, altering current output and converting a mechanical stimulus into a proportional electrical signal. Peterson et al. described on-line arterial monitoring in 1949 [3], using specially adapted intraarterial plastic cannulas, a capacitance manometer, amplifier, and ink recorder. These authors were among the first to appreciate and describe the various factors that can result in over- or under-damping of pressure tracings.

Two important advances in arterial cannulation technique followed. In 1950, Massa and associates reported the development of a cannula through which a needle protruded at the tip [4]. This allowed simultaneous insertion of both needle and catheter into a vein, with the catheter being advanced over the needle into the vessel. Barr described use of this device for radial artery cannulation in 1961 [5]. In 1953, Seldinger described percutaneous placement of a catheter using a guidewire [6], a technique now used extensively for central venous and large artery cannulation.

The technological explosion of the last 20 years has resulted in improvements to each component of the monitoring system. Catheters are more uniform and less thrombogenic. Transparent and disposable solid-state systems have replaced troublesome wire elements in transducers. Monitors are more user-friendly, with internal calibration, better filtering capabilities, and pleasing color visual displays. Additional technological improvements will undoubtedly follow, but it is likely that future systems will continue to be plagued by certain physical and man-made restraints.

Indications for Arterial Cannulation

The indications for arterial cannulation can be grouped into four broad categories (Table 3-1): (1) hemodynamic monitoring, (2) frequent arterial blood gas sampling, (3) arterial administration of drugs, and (4) intraaortic balloon pump use. In critical care units, continuous arterial access is usually established for the first two indications, although infusion of thrombolytic drugs is increasingly more common.

Noninvasive, indirect blood pressure measurements determined by auscultation of Korotkoff sounds distal to an occluding cuff (Riva-Rocci method) are generally accurate, although readings consistently average 10 to 20 mm Hg lower than a simultaneous direct measurement [7]. In hemodynamically unstable patients, however, indirect techniques may significantly underestimate blood pressure, especially in patients with shock and on vasoconstrictor agents [8]. Automatic oscillometric devices (i.e., Dinamap) can also be inaccurate, particularly in rapidly changing situations, at the extremes of blood pressure, and in patients with dysrhythmias [9,10]. For these reasons, direct

Table 3-1. Indications for Arterial Cannulation

Hemodynamic monitoring
   Acutely hypertensive or hypotensive patients
   With use of vasoactive drugs
Multiple blood sampling
   Ventilated patients
   Limited venous access
Arterial administration of drugs
Intraaortic balloon pump use

blood pressure monitoring is mandatory for unstable patients. Rapid beat-to-beat changes can easily be monitored and appropriate therapeutic modalities initiated, and variations in individual pressure waveforms may prove diagnostic. Waveform inspection can rapidly diagnose ECG lead disconnect, indicate the presence of aortic valve disease, help determine the effect of dysrhythmias on perfusion, and reveal the impact of the respiratory cycle on blood pressure (pulsus paradoxus) [11].

Management of patients in critical care units typically requires multiple laboratory determinations. Patients on mechanical ventilators or in whom intubation is contemplated need frequent monitoring of arterial blood gases. In these situations, arterial cannulation prevents repeated trauma by frequent arterial punctures and permits routine laboratory tests without multiple needle sticks. Typically, an arterial line for blood gas determination should be placed when a patient will require three or more measurements daily.

Arterial catheters should be removed when no longer needed. Too often, they are left in place for convenience and to prevent late-night "nuisance" calls to house officers to perform venipuncture. This cannot be justified on a risk-benefit basis. Pulse oximeters can accurately monitor arterial hemoglobin saturation, and in selected patients end-tidal carbon dioxide monitors are a noninvasive alternative to direct arterial measurement. In many cases these monitors can limit or eliminate the need for routine blood gas determinations, even for patients on ventilators.

Equipment, Monitoring Techniques, and Sources of Error

The equipment necessary to display and measure an arterial waveform includes: (1) an appropriate intravascular catheter, (2) fluid-filled noncompliant tubing with stopcocks, (3) a transducer and dome, (4) a constant flush device, and (5) electronic monitoring equipment, consisting of a connecting cable, monitor with amplifier, oscilloscope display screen, and recorder. Using this equipment, intravascular pressure changes are transmitted through the hydraulic (fluid-filled) elements to the transducer, which converts mechanical displacement into a proportional electrical signal. The signal is amplified and processed by the monitor and the waveform is displayed on the oscilloscope screen, accompanied by a digital readout [12]. Undistorted presentation of the arterial waveform is dependent on the performance of each component. A detailed discussion of relevant pressure monitoring principles is beyond the scope of this chapter, but consideration of a few basic concepts is adequate to understand the genesis of most monitoring inaccuracies.

The major problems inherent to pressure monitoring with a catheter system are inadequate dynamic response, improper zeroing and zero drift, and improper transducer/monitor calibration [12–15]. Most physicians are aware of zeroing and calibration techniques but underappreciate the importance of dynamic response in ensuring system fidelity. Catheter-tubing-transducer systems used for pressure monitoring can best be characterized as underdamped second-order dynamic systems with mechanical parameters of elasticity, mass, and friction [12]. Overall, the dynamic response of such a system is determined by its resonant frequency and damping coefficient (zeta). The resonant or natural frequency of a system is the frequency at which it oscillates when stimulated. When the frequency content of an input signal (i.e., pressure waveform) approaches the resonant frequency of a system, progressive amplification of the output signal occurs, a phenomenon known as ringing [16]. To ensure a flat frequency response (accurate recording across a spectrum of frequencies), the resonant frequency of a monitoring system should be at least five times higher than the highest frequency in the input signal [12]. Physiological peripheral arterial waveforms have a fundamental frequency of 3 to 5 Hz, although they have been shown to have components that range up to 20 Hz [13]. It follows, then, that the resonant frequency of a system used to monitor arterial pressure should ideally be greater than 20 Hz to avoid ringing and systolic overshoot. This same system may be inadequate to display a left ventricular pressure wave, which has a fundamental frequency of greater than 20 Hz [17].

The system component most likely to cause amplification of a pressure waveform is the hydraulic elements. A good hydraulic system will have a resonant frequency between 10 and 20 Hz, which may overlap with arterial pressure frequencies. Thus amplification can occur, which may require damping to reproduce the waveform faithfully [17].

The damping coefficient is a measure of how quickly an oscillating system comes to rest [16]. A system with a high damping coefficient absorbs mechanical energy well (i.e., compliant tubing), causing a diminution in the transmitted waveform. Conversely, a system with a low damping coefficient results in underdamping and systolic overshoot. Damping coefficient and resonant frequency together determine the dynamic response of a recording system. If the system's resonant frequency is less than 7.5 Hz, the pressure waveform will be distorted no matter what the damping coefficient. On the other hand, a resonant frequency of 24 Hz allows a range in the damping coefficient of 0.15 to 1.1 without resultant distortion of the pressure waveform [12,13,15].

The damping coefficient and resonant frequency of a monitoring system can be assessed at the bedside by the fast-flush test, performed by briefly opening and closing the valve in the continuous flush device, producing a square wave displacement on the oscilloscope followed by a return to baseline, usually after a few smaller oscillations (Fig. 3-1). Values for the damping coefficient and resonant frequency can be computed by printing the wave on graph paper [12], but visual inspection is usually adequate to ensure a proper frequency response. An optimum fast-flush test results in one undershoot followed by small overshoot, then settles to the patient's waveform (Fig. 3-1) [13].

For peripheral pulse pressure monitoring, an adequate fast-flush test usually corresponds to a resonant frequency of 10 to 20 Hz coupled with a damping coefficient of 0.5 to 0.7 [13]. To

ensure the continuing fidelity of a monitoring system, dynamic response validation by fast-flush test should be performed frequently: with every significant change in patient hemodynamic status, after each opening of the system (zeroing, blood sampling, tubing change), whenever the waveform appears dampened, and at least every 8 hours [12].

With consideration of the above concepts, components of the monitoring system are designed to optimize the frequency response of the entire system. The 18- and 20-gauge catheters used to gain vascular access are not a major source of distortion but can become kinked or occluded by thrombus, resulting in overdamping of the system. Connecting tubing with stopcocks are the major source of underdamped tracings. Standard, noncompliant tubing is provided with most disposable transducer kits and should be as short as possible to minimize signal amplification [16]. Air bubbles in the tubing are a notorious source of overdamping of the tracing and can be cleared by flushing through a stopcock. Currently available disposable transducers incorporate microchip technology, are very reliable, and have relatively high resonant frequencies (>40 Hz) [18]. Transducer domes are small and transparent to disclose air bubbles. The transducer assembly has an orifice to which a stopcock is attached, allowing the system to be zeroed but also providing a source for air bubble accumulation [19]. The transducer is attached to the electronic monitoring equipment by a cable. Modern monitors have internal calibration and filter artifacts and print the oscilloscope display on request. Many monitors can freeze a display and provide on-screen calibration with a cursor to measure beat-to-beat differences in amplitude precisely. This allows measurement of the effect of ectopic beats on blood pressure or assessment of the severity of pulsus paradoxus. The digital readout display is an average of values over time and may not be an accurate representation of beat-to-beat variability.

When presented with pressure data or readings believed to be inaccurate, or which are significantly different from indirect readings (>20 mm Hg difference), a few quick checks can ensure system accuracy. Improper zeroing of the system is the single most important source of error. Zeroing can be checked by opening the transducer stopcock to air and aligning with the midaxillary line, confirming that the monitor displays zero. Zeroing should be repeated with patient position changes, when significant changes in blood pressure occur, and routinely every 6 to 8 hours because of zero drift [15]. Calibration of the system is usually not necessary, due to standardization of current disposable transducers [18,20,21]. Transducers are faulty on occasion, however, and calibration can be checked by attaching a mercury manometer to the stopcock and applying 100, 150, and/or 200 mm Hg pressure. If the monitor does not display the pressure within an acceptable range (±5 mm Hg), most

Fig. 3-1. Fast-flush test. A. Overdamped system. B. Underdamped system. C. Optimal damping.

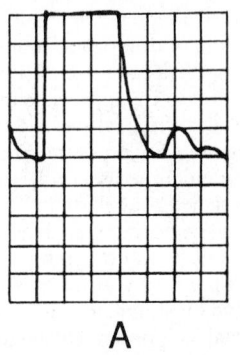
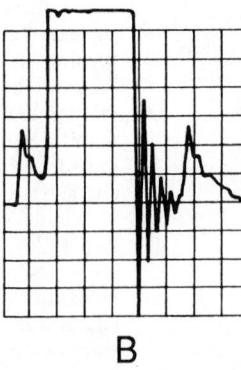
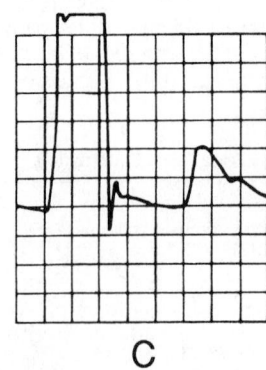

A   B   C

are equipped with a calibration device or gauge factor knob that allows for linear calibration.

If zero referencing and calibration are correct, a fast-flush test will assess the system's dynamic response. Overdamped tracings are usually caused by air bubbles, kinks, clot formation, compliant tubing, loose connections, a deflated pressure bag, or anatomical factors affecting the catheter. All of these are usually correctable. An underdamped tracing results in systolic overshoot and can be secondary to excessive tubing length or patient factors such as increased inotropic or chronotropic state. Many monitors can be adjusted to filter out frequencies above a certain limit, which can eliminate frequencies in the input signal causing ringing. However, this may also cause inaccurate readings if important frequencies are excluded. Rarely, when an underdamped tracing cannot be corrected by tubing changes or other manipulations, a disposable damping device (e.g., Accudynamic or Rose) can be attached to the transducer and adjusted to achieve optimal damping [12,13].

Technique of Arterial Cannulation

SITE SELECTION. Several factors are important in selecting the site for arterial cannulation. The ideal artery has extensive collateral circulation that will maintain the viability of distal tissues if thrombosis occurs. The site should be comfortable for the patient, accessible for nursing care, and close to the monitoring equipment. Sites involved by infection or disruption in the epidermal barrier should be avoided. Certain procedures, such as coronary artery bypass grafting, may dictate preference for one site over another [22,23]. Larger arteries and catheters provide more accurate (central aortic) pressure measurements. Though not usually clinically relevant, physicians should also be cognizant of differences in pulse contour recorded at different sites. As the pressure pulse wave travels outward from the aorta, it encounters arteries that are smaller and less elastic, with multiple branch points, causing reflections of the pressure wave. This results in a peripheral pulse contour with increased slope and amplitude, causing recorded values to be artificially elevated. As a result, femoral artery recordings yield higher systolic values than central aortic recordings, and lower extremity arteries have higher systolic pressures than upper extremity arteries. Diastolic pressures tend to be less affected, and mean arterial pressures measured at the different sites are similar [24,25].

The most commonly used sites for arterial cannulation are the radial, femoral, axillary, dorsalis pedis, brachial, and, in children, temporal arteries. All sites are cannulated percutaneously—peripheral sites with a 2-inch, 20-gauge, nontapered Teflon catheter-over-needle and larger arteries using the Seldinger technique with a prepackaged kit, typically containing a 6-inch, 18-gauge Teflon catheter and appropriate introducer needles and guidewire. Surgical cutdown at any site is no longer recommended due to increased risk of complications, especially infection and thrombosis, and is almost never required when adequate attention is given to alternative arterial sites.

Critical care physicians should be facile with arterial cannulation at all sites, but at most centers radial and femoral artery catheters constitute more than 90 percent of all arterial catheterizations. Although each site has unique complications, available data do not indicate a preference for any one site [26].

Radial artery cannulation is usually attempted initially unless the patient is in shock and/or pulses are not palpable. If this fails, femoral artery cannulation should be performed rather than attempting radial artery cannulation at another peripheral site. A traditional bias against femoral artery cannulation has

been disproven by multiple studies demonstrating a complication rate no higher, and sometimes lower, than radial artery cannulation [27–32]. In some centers, the femoral artery is the preferred site, especially when long-term cannulation is anticipated [19].

The dorsalis pedis artery is absent in 3 to 14 percent of patients and may be more difficult to catheterize than other sites [33,34,35]. The brachial artery is not commonly used because it does not possess good collateral circulation and there is theoretically an increased risk for distal ischemia, but centers that routinely employ brachial artery catheters do not report a higher complication rate [32,36,37]. Finally, the axillary artery has many attractive features for direct pressure monitoring, including its rich collateral circulation and central location [28,32,38,39].

RADIAL ARTERY CANNULATION. A thorough understanding of normal arterial anatomy and common anatomic variants greatly facilitates insertion of catheters and management of unexpected findings at all sites. The reader is referred elsewhere for a comprehensive review of arterial anatomy [40]; only relevant anatomic considerations are presented here. The radial artery is one of two final branches of the brachial artery (the ulnar being the other). It courses over the flexor digitorum sublimis, flexor pollicis longus, and pronator quadratus muscles and lies just lateral to the flexor carpi radialis in the forearm (Fig. 3-2). As the artery enters the floor of the palm, it ends in the deep volar arterial arch at the level of the metacarpal bones and communicates with the ulnar artery. A second site of collateral flow for the radial artery occurs via the dorsal arch running in the dorsum of the hand.

The ulnar artery runs between the flexor carpi ulnaris and flexor digitorum sublimis in the forearm, with a short course over the ulnar nerve. In the hand the artery runs over the transverse carpal ligament and becomes the superficial volar arch, which forms an anastomosis with a small branch of the radial artery. These three anastomoses provide excellent collateral flow to the hand. Not all individuals, however, are born with three patent arches, and disease processes such as atherosclerosis and scleroderma may compromise previously existing channels. A competent superficial or deep palmar arch must be present to ensure adequate collateral flow. At least one of these arches may be absent in up to 20 percent of individuals.

Modified Allen's Test. Prior to placement of a radial or ulnar arterial line, it must be demonstrated that the blood supply to the hand would not be eliminated by a catheter-induced thrombus. In 1929, Allen described a technique of diagnosing occlusive arterial disease [41]. His technique has been modified and serves as the most common screening test prior to radial artery cannulation. The examiner compresses both radial and ulnar arteries and asks the patient to clinch and unclinch the fist repeatedly until pallor of the palm is produced. Hyperextension of the hand is avoided, as it may cause a false negative result, suggesting inadequate collateral flow [42]. One artery is then released and the time to blushing of the palm noted. The procedure is repeated with the other artery. Normal palmar blushing is complete before 7 seconds (positive test); 8 to 14 seconds is considered equivocal; and 15 or more seconds abnormal (negative test).

Allen's test is not an ideal screening procedure. In one study, a normal Allen's test was confirmed using Doppler study in only 86 percent of patients [43]. In another study comparing Allen's test to Doppler examination, Allen's test had a sensitivity of 87 percent (i.e., it detected ulnar collateral flow in 87% of cases in which Doppler study confirmed its presence) and a

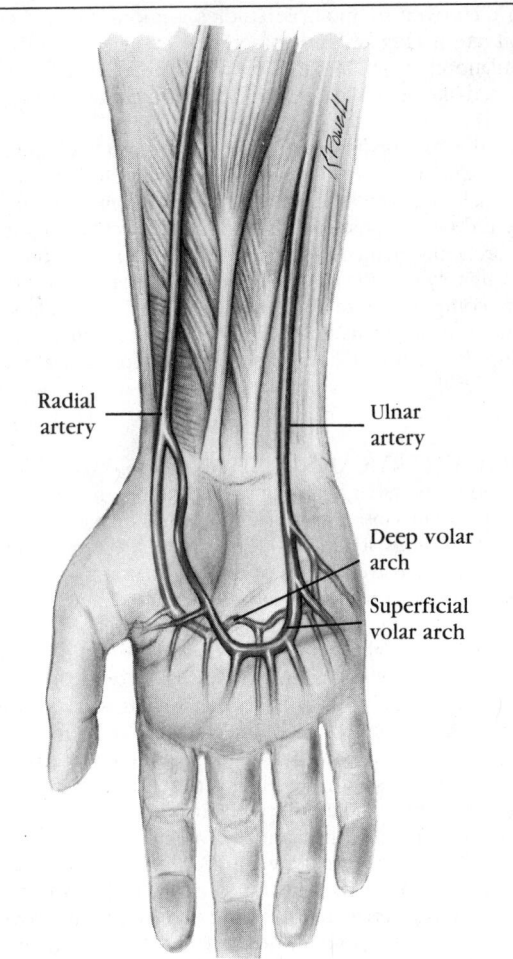

Radial artery

Ulnar artery

Deep volar arch

Superficial volar arch

Fig. 3-2. Anatomy of the radial artery. Note the collateral circulation to the ulnar artery through the deep volar arterial arch and dorsal arch.

negative predictive value of only 0.18 (i.e., only 18% of patients with no collateral flow by Allen's test had this confirmed by Doppler study) [44]. Other studies have compared Allen's test to plethysmography, with similiar results [45]. Thus, the modified Allen's test does not necessarily predict the presence of collateral circulation [46,47]; as a result, some centers have abandoned its use as a routine screening procedure [48]. Each institution should establish its own guidelines regarding routine Allen's testing and the evaluation and management of negative results. If a lack of collateral circulation is verified by confirmatory testing, I believe it is advisable to avoid arterial cannulation on that hand.

Percutaneous Insertion. Following a normal modified Allen's test, the hand is placed in 30 to 60 degrees of dorsiflexion with the aid of a roll of gauze and armband, with care not to hyperabduct the thumb, which may obliterate the pulse. The volar aspect of the wrist is prepared and draped using sterile technique, and approximately 0.5 ml of lidocaine is infiltrated on both sides of the artery through a 25-gauge needle. Lidocaine serves to decrease patient discomfort and the likelihood of arterial vasospasm. If the pulse is obscured following lidocaine infiltration, massaging the wheal should quickly restore pulsation.

A 20-gauge, nontapered, Teflon 1¼- or 2-inch catheter-over-needle apparatus is used for the puncture. Entry is made at a 30- to 60-degree angle to the skin approximately 2 to 3 inches proximal to the distal wrist crease. The needle and cannula are advanced until blood return is noted in the hub, signifying intraarterial placement of the tip of the needle (Fig. 3-3). A small amount of further advancement is necessary for the cannula to enter the artery as well. With this accomplished, needle and cannula are brought flat to the skin and the cannula advanced to its hub with a firm, steady rotary action. Correct positioning is confirmed by pulsatile blood return on removal of the needle. If the initial attempt is unsuccessful, anatomic considerations indicate that subsequent attempts should be more proximal, rather than closer to the wrist crease [40].

Not uncommonly, difficulty is encountered when attempting to pass the catheter. Carefully replacing the needle and slightly advancing the whole apparatus occasionally remedies the problem. Alternately, a fixation technique can be attempted (Fig. 3-3). The artery is purposely transfixed by advancing the needle and catheter through the far wall of the vessel. The needle is then removed and the cannula pulled back until vigorous arterial blood return is noted. The catheter can then be advanced into the arterial lumen, although occasionally the needle must be carefully partially reinserted (never forced, to avoid shearing the catheter) to serve as a rigid stent. Return of pulsatile blood flow confirms proper placement.

Catheters with self-contained guidewires to facilitate passage of the cannula into the artery are available. Percutaneous puncture is made in the same manner, but when blood return is noted in the catheter hub the guidewire is passed through the needle into the artery, serving as a stent for subsequent catheter advancement. The guidewire and needle are then removed and placement confirmed by pulsatile blood return. The cannula is then attached to transducer tubing and secured by suturing, antiseptic ointment is applied, and the site is bandaged.

DORSALIS PEDIS ARTERY CANNULATION. Dorsalis pedis artery catheterization is uncommon in most critical care units; compared to the radial artery, the anatomy is less predictable and the success rate lower [35]. The dorsalis pedis artery is the main blood supply of the dorsum of the foot. The artery runs from the level of the ankle to the great toe. It lies very superficial and just lateral to the tendon of the extensor hallucis longus (Fig. 3-4). The dorsalis pedis anastomoses with branches from the posterior tibial (lateral plantar artery) and, to a lesser extent, peroneal arteries, creating an arterial arch network analogous to that in the hand. Collateral circulation is assessed by occluding the dorsalis pedis and posterior tibial pulses and blanching the great toe by repeated flexion. Release of the posterior tibial artery should result in blushing of the toe within 10 seconds; longer blushing times may represent poor collateral circulation. Tests using Doppler probes or pneumatic cuffs around the great toe have also been proposed [33,34,35].

The foot is placed in plantar flexion and prepared in the usual fashion. Vessel entry is obtained approximately halfway up the dorsum of the foot; advancement is the same as with cannulation of the radial artery. Patients usually find insertion here more painful but less physically limiting. Systolic pressure readings are usually 5 to 20 mm Hg higher with dorsalis pedis catheters than radial artery catheters, but mean pressure values are generally unchanged.

BRACHIAL ARTERY CANNULATION. Cannulation of the brachial artery is infrequently performed because of concern regarding the lack of effective collateral circulation. Centers

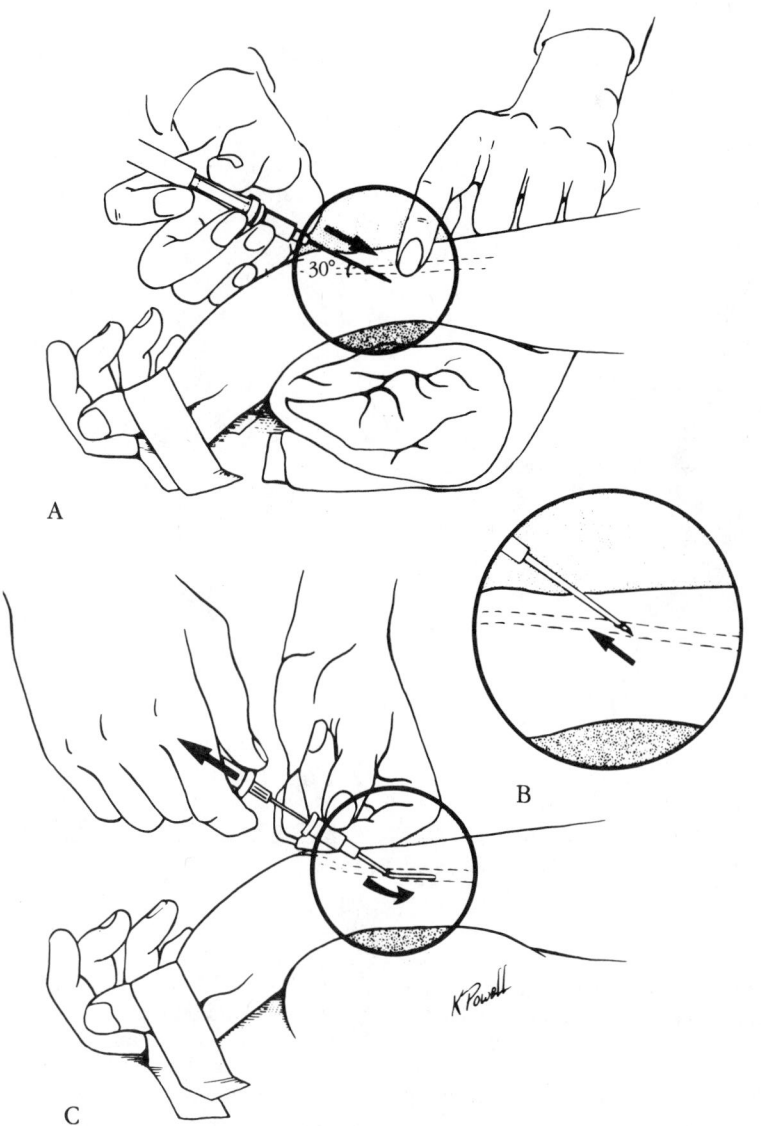

Fig. 3-3. Cannulation of the radial artery. A. A towel is placed behind the wrist, and the hand is immobilized with tape. The radial artery is fixated with a 20-gauge angiocath connected to a 5-ml syringe (optional). B. The angiocath is withdrawn until pulsatile blood return is noted. C. The trocar is withdrawn as the Teflon catheter is simultaneously advanced.

experienced in the use of brachial artery catheters, however, have reported complication rates no higher than with other routes [30,36,37]. Even when diminution of distal pulses occurs, either because of proximal obstruction or distal embolization, clinical ischemia is unlikely [36]. An additional anatomic consideration is the median nerve, which lies in close proximity to the brachial artery in the antecubital fossa and may be punctured by a misdirected needle in 1 to 2 percent of cases [37]. This usually causes only transient paresthesias, but median nerve palsy has been reported [49]. Median nerve palsy is a particular risk in patients with coagulopathy because even minor bleeding into the fascial planes can produce compression of the median nerve [50]. Coagulopathy should be considered a contraindication to brachial artery cannulation.

It is good practice to perform a modified Allen's test or Doppler studies of the ulnar and radial arteries prior to brachial artery cannulation. An alternative site should be selected if one is missing or collateral circulation is inadequate. Clinical examination of the hand, and Doppler studies if indicated, should be repeated daily while the brachial catheter is in place. The catheter should be promptly removed if diminution of any pulse occurs.

Cannulation of the brachial artery can be performed with a 2-inch catheter-over-needle as described for the radial artery, but most centers use the Seldinger technique as described in the section on femoral artery cannulation. Inserting a 6-inch catheter into the brachial artery places the catheter tip in the axillary artery, and pressures obtained are more representative of aortic pressures. The brachial artery is punctured by extending the arm at the elbow and locating the pulsation in or slightly proximal to the antecubital fossa, just medial to the bicipital tendon (Fig. 3-5). Once the catheter is established, the elbow must be kept in full extension to avoid kinking or breaking the catheter.

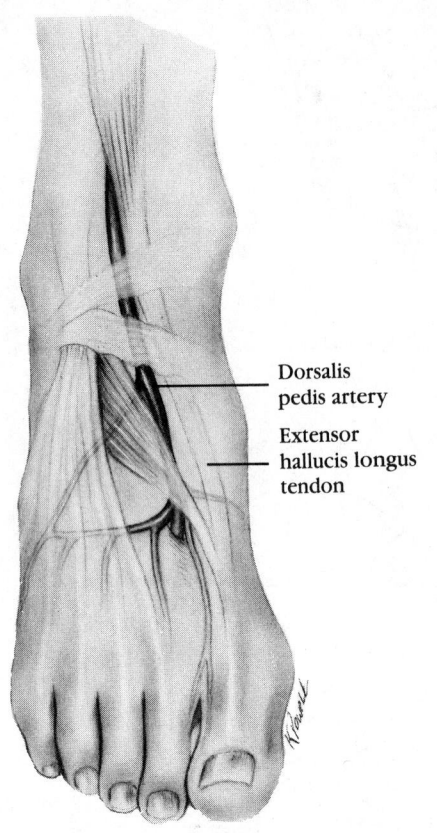

Fig. 3-4. Anatomy of dorsalis pedis artery and adjacent structures.

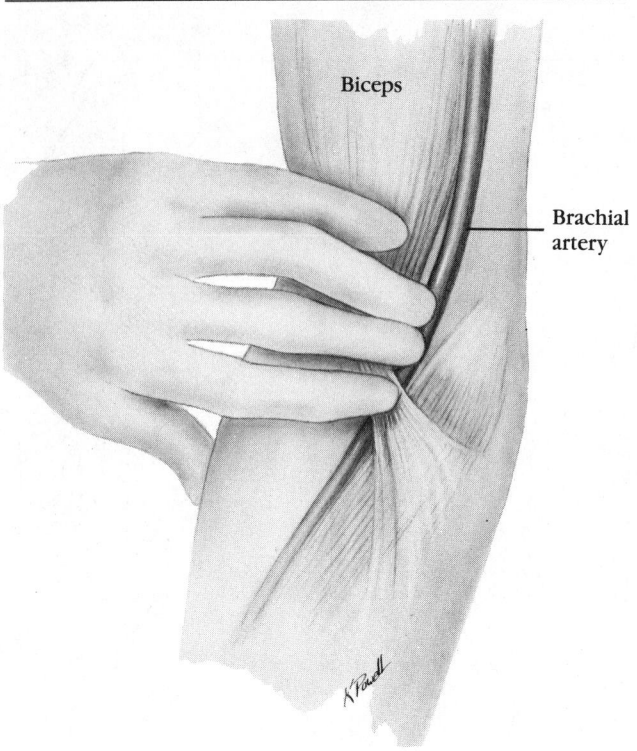

Fig. 3-5. Palpation of the brachial artery. The arm is fully extended at the elbow and the artery palpated in the antecubital fossa as indicated. The brachial artery is then cannulated at this site.

FEMORAL ARTERY CANNULATION. Femoral artery catheters are gaining wider clinical use. The once held belief that they were associated with a higher risk for complications has been disproved by multiple studies [27–32,51]. In practice, the femoral artery is usually the next alternative when radial artery cannulation fails or is inappropriate. The femoral artery is large and often palpable when other sites are not, and the technique of cannulation is easy to learn. The most common cause for failure to cannulate is severe atherosclerosis or prior vascular procedures involving both femoral arteries, in which case axillary or brachial artery cannulation is appropriate. Complications unique to this site are rare but include retroperitoneal hemorrhage and intraabdominal viscus perforation. These complications only occur because of poor technique or in the presence of a large hernia. Ischemic complications from femoral artery catheters are rare.

The external iliac artery becomes the common femoral artery at the inguinal ligament (Fig. 3-6). The artery courses under the inguinal ligament near the junction of the medial and the middle third of a straight line drawn between the pubis and the anterior superior iliac spine. The artery is cannulated using the Seldinger technique and any one of several available prepackaged kits. Kits contain the equivalent of a 19-gauge thin-wall needle, appropriate guidewire, and a 6-inch, 18-gauge Teflon catheter. The patient lies supine with the leg extended and slightly abducted. Site preparation includes clipping of pubic hair if necessary. Skin puncture should be a few centimeters caudal to the inguinal ligament to minimize the risk of retroperitoneal hematoma or bowel perforation, which can occur when the needle is cephalad to the inguinal ligament. The thin-wall needle is directed, bevel up, cephalad at a 45-degree angle. When arterial blood return is confirmed, the needle and syringe are brought down against the skin to facilitate guidewire passage. The guidewire should advance smoothly, but minor manipulation and rotation is sometimes required if the wire meets resistance at the needle tip or after it has advanced into the vessel. Inability to pass the guidewire may be due to an intimal flap over the needle bevel or atherosclerotic plaques in the vessel. In the latter instance, cannulation of that femoral artery might not be possible. When the guidewire will not pass beyond the needle tip it should be withdrawn and blood return reestablished by advancing the needle or repeat vascular puncture. The guidewire is then inserted, the needle withdrawn, and a stab incision made with a scalpel at the skin puncture site. The catheter is next threaded over the guidewire to its hub and the guidewire withdrawn. The catheter is then sutured securely and connected to the transducer tubing.

AXILLARY ARTERY CANNULATION. Axillary artery catheterization is often the next alternative after radial or femoral artery cannulation. Again, considerable bias exists against use of this vessel, but centers experienced with axillary artery monitoring report a low rate of complications [38,39,52]. The axillary artery is large and frequently palpable when all other sites are not and has a rich collateral circulation. The tip of a 6-inch catheter inserted through an axillary approach lies in the subclavian artery, and thus accurate central pressures are obtained. The central location of the tip makes cerebral air embolism a greater risk, therefore left axillary catheters are preferred for the initial attempt, since air bubbles passing into the right subclavian artery are more likely to traverse the aortic arch [39].

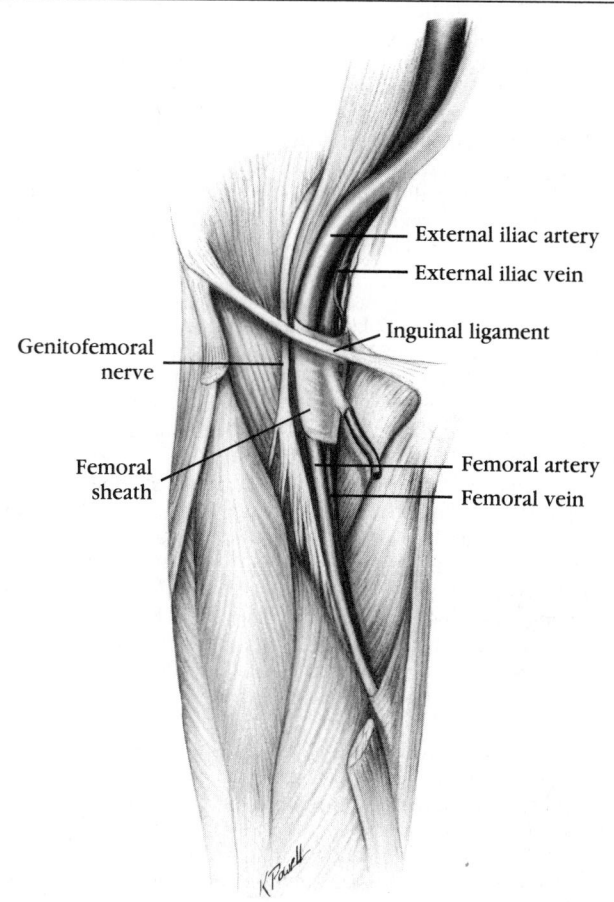

Fig. 3-6. Anatomy of the femoral artery and adjacent structures. The artery is cannulated below the inguinal ligament.

Caution should be exercised in flushing axillary catheters, and some experts recommend hand flushing with small volumes [11].

The axillary artery begins at the lateral border of the first rib as a continuation of the subclavian artery and ends at the inferior margin of the teres major muscle, where it becomes the brachial artery. The optimal site for catheterization is the junction of the middle and lower third of the vessel, which usually corresponds to its highest palpable point in the axilla. At this point the artery is superficial and is located at the inferior border of the pectoralis major muscle. The artery is enclosed in a neurovascular bundle, the axillary sheath, with the medial, posterior, and lateral cords of the brachial plexus. Medial to the medial cord is the axillary vein [11,19,53]. Not surprisingly, brachial plexus neuropathies have been reported from axillary artery cannulation. Coagulopathy is a relative contraindication, as the axillary sheath can rapidly fill with blood from an uncontrolled arterial puncture, resulting in a compressive neuropathy.

The axillary artery is cannulated using the Seldinger technique and kit as described in the section on femoral artery cannulation. The arm is abducted, externally rotated, and flexed at the elbow by having the patient place his or her hand under his or her head. Axillary hair should be clipped and the site prepared in standard fashion. The artery is palpated at the lower border of the pectoralis major muscle and fixed against the shaft of the humerus. After local infiltration with lidocaine, the thin-wall needle is introduced at a 30- to 45-degree angle to the

vertical plane until return of arterial blood. The remainder of the catheterization proceeds as described for femoral artery cannulation.

Complications of Arterial Cannulation

Arterial cannulation is a relatively safe invasive precedure. Although estimates of the total complication rate range from 15 to 40 percent, clinically relevant complications occur in 5 percent or less (Table 3-2). Risk factors for infectious and noninfectious complications have been identified [11,26,47,54–57] (Table 3-3), but the clinical impact of most of these factors is minimal, given the overall low incidence of complications [46].

THROMBOSIS. Thrombosis is the single most common complication of intraarterial lines. The incidence of thrombosis varies with the site, method of detection, size of the cannula, and

Table 3-2. Complications Associated with Arterial Cannulation

Site	Complication
All sites	Pain and swelling
	Thrombosis
	Asymptomatic
	Symptomatic
	Embolization
	Hematoma
	Hemorrhage
	Limb ischemia
	Catheter-related infection
	Local
	Systemic
	Diagnostic blood loss
	Pseudoaneurysm
	Heparin-associated thrombocytopenia
Radial artery	Cerebral embolization
	Peripheral neuropathy
Femoral artery	Retroperitoneal hemorrhage
	Bowel perforation
	Arteriovenous fistula
Axillary artery	Cerebral embolization
	Brachial plexopathy
Brachial artery	Median nerve damage
	Cerebral embolization

Table 3-3. Factors Predisposing to Complications with Arterial Cannulation

Large tapered cannulas (>20 gauge except at the large artery sites)
Hypotension
Coagulopathy
Low cardiac output
Multiple puncture attempts
Use of vasopressors
Altherosclerosis
Hypercoagulable state
Placement by surgical cutdown
Site inflammation
Intermittent flushing system
Bacteremia

duration of cannulation. Thrombosis is common with radial and dorsalis pedis catheters, but very rare with femoral or axillary catheters. The incidence of radial artery thrombosis following cannulation has progressively declined due to recognition of the importance of catheter size and composition and the use of continuous versus intermittent heparin flush systems [19,54,56,58–64]. The incidence probably increases significantly with duration of cannulation [65]. When a 20-gauge nontapered Teflon catheter with a continuous 3 ml per hour heparinized saline flush is used to cannulate the radial artery for 3 to 4 days, thrombosis of the vessel can be detected by Doppler study in 5 to 25 percent of cases [46,60,63,64]. Use of a flush solution containing heparin is standard and may reduce the incidence of thrombosis [66], but in patients with relative or absolute contraindications to heparin use, sodium citrate [67] or saline alone may be substituted [68].

Thrombosis often occurs after decannulation. Women represent a preponderance of patients who experience flow abnormalities following radial artery cannulation, probably because of smaller arteries and a greater tendency to exhibit vasospasm [46]. All patients eventually recanalize, generally by 3 weeks after removal of the catheter. Despite the high incidence of Doppler-detected thrombosis, clinical ischemia of the hand is rare and usually resolves following catheter removal. Symptomatic occlusion requiring surgical intervention occurs in less than 1 percent of cases. Most patients who develop clinical ischemia have an associated contributory cause, such as prolonged circulatory failure with high-dose vasopressor therapy [46].

The lack of association between a high incidence of thrombosis as detected by Doppler study and subsequent clinical ischemia is intriguing. The traditional explanation is that radial artery cannulation is performed in patients only after a normal modified Allen's test, thus adequate ulnar collateral flow is assured. However, most cases of clinically significant ischemia occur in patients with an antecedent normal Allen's test [47] and, as previously discussed, the modified Allen's test is not ideal for predicting the presence of adequate ulnar collateral flow. Thrombosis is frequent enough, and Allen's test imprecise enough, that more clinical episodes of ischemia should be expected. Based on military and civilian trauma experience, Slogoff et al. [46] postulated that radial artery thrombosis is more likely to occur only when there is adequate collateral circulation, a kind of self-protective mechanism. Whatever the reasons, the incidence of permanent sequelae resulting from arterial catheter-related thrombosis is exceedingly low.

Significant ischemic complications are minimized by regular inspection of the extremity for unexplained pain, blanching, or other signs of ischemia and immediate withdrawal of the catheter when they appear. If evidence of ischemia persists after catheter removal, thrombolytic therapy, radiologic or surgical embolectomy, or cervical sympathetic blockade are treatment options [47].

CEREBRAL EMBOLIZATION. Continuous flush devices used with arterial catheters are designed to deliver 3 ml per hour of heparinized saline (generally 1–5 units heparin/ml saline) from an infusion bag pressurized to 300 mm Hg. Commercially available systems are not necessarily uniform in performance [69]. When the flush valve is opened, a bolus of fluid is administered directly upstream. Lowenstein and associates [70] demonstrated that with rapid flushing of radial artery lines with relatively small volumes of radiolabeled solution, traces of the solution could be detected in the central arterial circulation in a time frame representative of retrograde flow. Chang and associates [71] demonstrated that injection of greater than 2 ml of air into the

radial artery of small primates resulted in retrograde passage of air into the vertebral circulation. Factors that increase the risk for retrograde passage of air are patient size and position (air travels up in a sitting patient), injection site, and flush rate. Air embolism has been cited as a risk mainly for radial arterial catheters [71] but logically could occur with all arterial catheters, especially axillary and brachial artery catheters. The risk is minimized by clearing all air from tubing before flushing, opening the flush valve for no more than 2 to 3 seconds, and avoiding overaggressive manual flushing of the line with small syringes.

DIAGNOSTIC BLOOD LOSS. Diagnostic blood loss (DBL) is patient blood loss that occurs due to frequent blood sampling obtained for laboratory testing. The significance of DBL is underappreciated. It is a particular problem in patients with standard arterial catheter setups that are used as the site for sampling, because 3 to 5 ml of blood is typically wasted (to avoid heparin/saline contamination) every time a sample is obtained. In patients with frequent arterial blood gas determinations, DBL can be substantial and result in a transfusion requirement [72,73]. There are several ways to minimize DBL. Tubing systems employing two stopcocks or a distal stopcock with a proximal sampling port (VAMP and others) allow for heparin-free blood to be sampled without wastage. Intraarterial blood gas monitoring is a new technology that essentially allows continuous sampling of arterial blood gas values; preliminary results have been promising [74,75]. Other techniques that minimize DBL include blood microchemistry analysis [76] and the use of pediatric collection tubes [77]. Given the expense and risks of blood component therapy, any or all of the above techniques should be routinely implemented in every intensive care unit. The added expense of closed sampling tubing systems is probably justified on a cost-risk-benefit analysis. It is simply good medicine always to minimize tests to those that are truly indicated and to discontinue the arterial catheter as soon as it is no longer required.

HEPARIN-ASSOCIATED THROMBOCYTOPENIA. Thrombocytopenia is very common in critically ill adults and is usually not due to heparin [78]. However, when the platelet count falls below 80,000 to 100,000 per milliliter, it is advisable to discontinue all heparin, even the small amount contained in continuous flush devices, because of the possibility of heparin-associated thrombocytopenia (HAT) [79]. Although the data are conflicting, heparin probably is beneficial in minimizing the risk of thrombosis with arterial catheters, and its routine use should be continued. In the presence of thrombocytopenia, however, sodium citrate, saline, and lactated Ringer's solution are suitable replacements. The need for increased flushing requirements to prevent more complications with nonheparin solutions requires further study in a large number of patients [68].

OTHER MECHANICAL AND TECHNICAL COMPLICATIONS. Other noninfectious complications reported with arterial lines are pseudoaneurysm formation [80,81], hematoma, local tenderness, hemorrhage, neuropathies [50,82], and embolization.

INFECTION. Infectious sequelae are the most important clinical complications occurring because of arterial cannulation. In a 1979 study, 12 percent of nosocomial bacteremias were related to direct arterial pressure-monitoring systems [57], but improvements in equipment and system design have resulted in a decreased rate of infection. Many concepts and definitions applied to central venous catheter-related infection (Chap. 2) are also relevant to arterial catheters.

Catheter-associated infection is usually initiated by skin flora that invade the intracutaneous tract, causing colonization of the catheters and, ultimately, bacteremia. An additional source of infection from pressure-monitoring systems is contaminated infusate or equipment, which generally causes epidemic nosocomial bacteremia [83]. Arterial pressure-monitoring systems have been the cause of a number of epidemics in the past [84] and are at greater risk for this type of infection than central venous catheters for several reasons: (1) the transducer can become colonized because of inadequate sterilization or stagnant flow; (2) the flush solution is infused at a slow rate (3 ml/hr) and may hang for several hours; and (3) multiple blood samples are obtained by several different personnel from stopcocks in the system, which can serve as entry sites for bacteria [85,86].

Appreciation of the mechanisms responsible for initiating arterial catheter-related infection is important in understanding how to minimize infection. Thorough operator and site preparation is paramount. Iodine-containing solutions are the most commonly used skin disinfectants. Proper application involves scrubbing the area and allowing it to dry or stand for 30 to 60 seconds before wiping with alcohol [87]. Chlorhexadine as a topical agent has a broader antibacterial spectrum and longer duration of action than 10% povidone-iodine solution, and recent experience has demonstrated an impressive reduction in catheter-related infection [88]; more studies are needed. Skin flora introduced from the hands of medical personnel are an important source of infection. Operators must wash their hands and wear sterile gloves during insertion and care of the catheter. Breaks in sterile technique during insertion mandate termination of the procedure and replacement of the compromised equipment. Nursing personnel should follow strict guidelines when drawing blood samples or manipulating tubing. Ideally, stopcocks are covered with diaphragms instead of caps. Blood withdrawn to clear the tubing prior to drawing samples should not be reinjected unless a specially designed system is in use. In many hospitals, critical care technicians perform daily maintenance checks; regardless of who is responsible, standardized techniques should be observed. Flush solutions should not contain glucose and should be changed every 24 hours. Daily inspection of the site is mandatory, and the catheter should be removed promptly if abnormalities are noted. Dressings are changed at least every 48 hours. Expensive transparent dressings have not been shown to be superior to gauze and tape in preventing infection [89,90]. Application of a polymicrobial ointment to the insertion site during dressing changes is standard but may not reduce the incidence of clinically important infection [87].

Improvements in equipment have also removed potential sources of contamination. One-piece, disposable transducers alleviate the problem of inadequate sterilization of reusable transducer domes. Flush systems are designed to minimize stagnant flow in the transducer [85]. Finally, most centers change the entire monitoring setup every 48 hours.

These measures have contributed to an impressive decrease in arterial catheter-related infection. Older studies and those that did not observe a standardized maintenance protocol should be interpreted with caution. Recent prospective data demonstrate that catheter-related infection, defined as 15 or more colonies on semiquantitative culture of a catheter segment [92], occurs in 4 to 20 percent of catheters but contributes to bacteremia or septicemia in only 0 to 3 percent of cases [27,28,29,57,88,93,94]. The site of insertion does not appear to be an important factor impacting on the incidence of infection [28,29,95]; duration of catheterization continues to be important, but recommendations are changing. In 1979, Maki and Band [57] reported an increase in arterial catheter-related infection and bacteremia after 96 hours of catheterization. This figure was widely accepted, and most centers adopted a policy of changing arterial catheters after 72 to 96 hours. This is no longer necessary, however, as recent studies of catheters remaining in place a week or longer have not demonstrated a higher rate of clinically important infection [28,29,93,94,95].

Recent data also demonstrate the futility of guidewire changes in preventing infection [94]. Whether or not advancements that appear promising in reducing central venous catheter-associated infection, such as antibiotic-impregnated catheters, will be available or equally effective for arterial catheters is speculative at present. Currently, at my institution arterial catheters remain in place for 7 days and sometimes longer, unless site inspection is abnormal; an increased catheter infection rate has not been detected. Although not all centers are willing to adopt a policy of prolonged or indefinite catheterization, each center should determine its own catheter-associated infection rate so that rational policies can be formulated based on existing infection rates.

When arterial catheter infection does occur, *Staphylococcus* species, especially *S. epidermidis,* are most commonly isolated [88]. Gram-negative organisms are less frequent, but predominate in contaminated infusate or equipment-related infection [83,96]. *Candida* species are a greater risk in prolonged catheterization of the glucose-intolerant patient on multiple systemic broad-spectrum antibiotics. Catheter-associated bacteremia should be treated with a 7- to 14-day course of appropriate antibiotics. In complicated cases, longer courses are sometimes necessary [87].

The optimal evaluation of febrile catheterized patients is a challenging problem. The decision to discontinue or change an arterial catheter differs from the approach with central venous catheters discussed in Chapter 2 in some fundamental ways. Arterial catheters are less likely to be the source of fever than central venous catheters, and changing of arterial lines is frequently not indicated. I have never recommended guidewire changes of arterial catheters to evaluate for infection because of pathophysiological considerations and because arterial catheters may be inserted at alternative sites at low risk to the patient. Obviously, if the site is abnormal, the catheter should be removed regardless of the duration of catheterization. More specific guidelines are difficult to recommend, and individual factors should always be considered. In general, arterial catheters in place less than 3 days will not be the source of fever unless insertion was contaminated. Catheters in place 7 days or longer should be changed to a different site because of the small but measurable chance of infection.

Recommendations

Either the radial or femoral artery is an appropriate initial site for percutaneous arterial cannulation. Most centers have more experience with radial artery cannulation, but femoral artery catheters are reliable and have a comparable incidence of complication. In more than 95 percent of patients, one of these two sites is adequate to achieve arterial pressure monitoring. When these sites are not appropriate, the dorsalis pedis artery is a good alternative, but cannulation is frequently not possible, especially if radial artery cannulation failed because of poor perfusion. Under these circumstances, the axillary or brachial artery can be safely cannulated unless a coagulopathy is present. The site selected for any given patient may not be of prime importance, as centers experienced in the use of alternative sites report excellent results with low rates of complication. Recent experience indicates that arterial catheters can be left in place longer than 4 days without significantly increasing infection, but each institution needs to conduct its own studies to standardize policies and document catheter-associated infection rates. Arterial catheters should be discontinued promptly when they are no longer required for patient management.

References

1. Farinas PL: A new technique for arteriographic examination of the abdominal aorta and its branches. *Am J Roentgenol* 46:641, 1941.

2. Lambert E, Wood E: The use of a resistance wire strain gauge manometer to measure intra-arterial pressure. *Proc Soc Exp Biol Med* 64:186, 1947.

3. Peterson LH, Dripps RD, Risman GC: A method for recording the arterial pressure pulse and blood pressure in man. *Am Heart J* 37:771, 1949.

4. Massa DJ, Lundy JS, Faulconer A Jr, et al: A plastic needle. *Mayo Clin Proc* 25:413, 1950.

5. Barr PO: Percutaneous puncture of the radial artery with a multi-purpose Teflon catheter for intravenous use. *Acta Physiol Scand* 51:353, 1961.

6. Seldinger SI: Catheter replacement of the needle in percutaneous arteriography. *Acta Radiol* 39:368, 1953.

7. Finnie KJC, Watts DG, Armstrong PW: Biases in the measurement of arterial pressure. *Crit Care Med* 12:965, 1984.

8. Cohn JN: Blood pressure measurement in shock: Mechanism of inaccuracy in ausculatory and palpatory methods. *JAMA* 199:972, 1967.

9. Hutton P, Dye J, Prys-Roberts C: An assessment of the Dinamap 845. *Anaesthesia* 39:261, 1984.

10. Johnson CJ, Kerr JH: Automated blood pressure monitors: A clinical evaluation of 5 models in adults. *Anesthesiology* 40:471, 1985.

11. Harman EM: Arterial cannulation, in Mallory DL, Venus B (eds): *Problems in Critical Care.* Philadelphia, JB Lippincott, 1988, p 286.

12. Gardner RM: Direct arterial pressure monitoring. *Curr Anaesth Crit Care* 1:239, 1990.

13. Gardner RM: Direct blood pressure measurement: Dynamic response requirements. *Anesthesiology* 54:227, 1981.

14. Veremakis C, Halloran TH: The technique of monitoring arterial blood pressure. *J Crit Illness* 4:82, 1989.

15. Gardner RM, Hollingsworth KW: Optimizing the electrocardiogram and pressure monitoring. *Crit Care Med* 14:651, 1986.

16. Boutros A, Albert S: Effect of the dynamic response of transducer-tubing system on accuracy of direct-blood pressure measurement in patients. *Crit Care Med* 11:124, 1983.

17. Rothe CF, Kim KC: Measuring systolic arterial blood pressure. Possible errors from extension tubes or disposable transducer domes. *Crit Care Med* 8:683, 1980.

18. Cliffe P: Transducers for the measurement of pressure, in Scurr C, Feldman S (eds): *Scientific Foundations of Anaesthesia.* Chicago, Yearbook, 1982, p 40.

19. Sladen A: Arterial pressure monitoring, in *Invasive Monitoring and Its Complications in the Intensive Care Unit.* St. Louis, CV Mosby, 1990, p 47.

20. Disposable pressure transducers. *Health Devices* 13:268, 1984.

21. Gardner RM, Kutik M (co-chairs): *American National Standard for Interchangeability and Performance of Resistive Type Blood Pressure Transducers.* Arlington, VA, Association for the Advancement of Medical Instrumentation (AAMI/ANSI), 1986.

22. Bazaral MG, Nacht A, Petre J, et al: Radial artery pressure compared with subclavian artery pressure during coronary artery surgery. *Cleve Clin J Med* 55:448, 1988.

23. Lamantia KR, Barash PG: Arterial pressure monitoring: What are we really monitoring? *Cleve Clin J Med* 55:415, 1988.

24. Pauca AL, Wallenhaupt SL, Kon ND, et al: Does radial artery pressure accurately reflect aorta pressure? *Chest* 102:1193, 1992.

25. O'Rourke MF, Yaginuma T: Wave reflections and the arterial pulse. *Arch Intern Med* 144:366, 1984.

26. Veremakis C, Halloran TH: The technique of arterial cannulation. *J Crit Illness* 4:63, 1989.

27. Soderstrom CA, Wasserman DH, Dunham CM, et al: Superiority of the femoral artery for monitoring: A prospective study. *Am J Surg* 44:309, 1982.

28. Gurman GM, Kriemerman S: Cannulation of big arteries in critically ill patients. *Crit Care Med* 13:217, 1985.

29. Russell JA, Joel M, Hudson RJ, et al: Prospective evaluation of radial and femoral artery catheterization sites in critically ill adults. *Crit Care Med* 11:936, 1983.

30. Norwood SH, Cormier B, McMahon NG, et al: Prospective study of catheter-related infection during prolonged arterial catheterization. *Crit Care Med* 16:836, 1988.

31. Pinilla JC, Ross DF, Martin T, et al: Study of the incidence of intravascular catheter infection and associated septicemia in critically ill patients. *Crit Care Med* 11:21, 1983.

32. Gordon LH, Brown M, Brown OW, et al: Alternative sites for continuous arterial monitoring. *South Med J* 77:1498, 1984.

33. Husum B, Palm T, Eriksen J: Percutaneous cannulation of the dorsalis pedis artery: A prospective study. *Br J Anaesth* 51:1055, 1979.

34. Youngberg JA, Miller ED: Evaluation of percutaneous cannulations of the dorsalis pedis artery. *Anesthesiology* 44:80, 1976.

35. Johnson RE, Greenhow DE: Catheterization of the dorsalis pedis artery. *Anesthesiology* 39:654, 1973.

36. Barnes RW, Foster EJ, Janssen GA, et al: Safety of brachial arterial catheters as monitors in the intensive care unit: A prospective evaluation with the Doppler ultrasonic velocity detector. *Anesthesiology* 44:260, 1976.

37. Mann S, Jones RI, Miller-Craig MW, et al: The safety of ambulatory intra-arterial pressure monitoring: A clinical audit of 1000 studies. *Int J Cardiol* 5:585, 1984.

38. DeAngelis J: Axillary artery monitoring. *Crit Care Med* 4:205, 1976.

39. Bryan-Brown CW, Kwun KB, Lumb PD, et al: The axillary artery catheter. *Heart Lung* 12:492, 1983.

40. Mathers LH Jr: Anatomical considerations in obtaining arterial access. *J Intensive Care Med* 5:110, 1990.

41. Allen EV: Thromboangiitis obliterans: Method of diagnosis of chronic occlusive arterial lesions distal to the wrist with illustrative cases. *Am J Med Sci* 178:237, 1929.

42. Ejrup B, Fischer B, Wright IS: Clinical evaluation of blood flow to the hand: The false-positive Allen test. *Circulation* 33:778, 1966.

43. Clarke W, Freund PR, Wasse L, et al: Assessment of adequacy of ulnar arterial flow prior to radial artery catheterization. *Anesthesiology* 55:A38, 1981.

44. Glavin, RJ, Jones HM: Assessing collateral circulation in the hand: Four methods compared. *Anaesthesia* 44:594, 1989.

45. Fuhrman TM, Reilley TE, Pippin WD: Comparison of digital blood pressure, plethysmography, and the modified Allen's test as means of evaluating the collateral circulation of the hand. *Anaesthesia* 47:959, 1992.

46. Slogoff S, Keats AS, Arlund C: On the safety of radial artery cannulation. *Anesthesiology* 59:42, 1983.

47. Wilkins RG: Radial artery cannulation and ischemic damage: A review. *Anaesthesia* 40:896, 1985.

48. Vaghadia H, Schechter MT, Sheps SB, et al: Evaluation of a postocclusive reactive circulatory hyperaemia (PORCH) test for the assessment of ulnar collateral circulation. *Can J Anaesth* 35:591, 1988.

49. Littler WA: Median nerve palsy: A complication of brachial artery cannulation. *Postgrad Med J* 52(suppl):110, 1976.

50. Macon WL, Futrell JW: Median nerve neuropathy after percutaneous puncture of the brachial artery in patients receiving anticoagulants. *N Engl J Med* 288:1396, 1973.

51. Ersoz CJ, Hedden M, Lain L: Prolonged femoral arterial catheterization for intensive care. *Anesth Analg* 49:160, 1970.

52. Brown M, Gordon LH, Brown OW, et al: Intravascular monitoring via the axillary artery. *Anesth Intensive Care* 13:38, 1984.

53. Lipchik EO, Sugimoto H: Percutaneous brachial artery catheterization. *Radiology* 160:842, 1986.

54. Bedford RF, Wollman H: Complications of percutaneous radial artery monitoring. *Anesthesiology* 38:228, 1973.

55. Puri UK, Carlson RW, Bander JJ, et al: Complications of vascular catheterization in the critically ill. *Crit Care Med* 8:495, 1980.

56. Gardner RM, Schwartz R, Wong HC, et al: Percutaneous indwelling radial artery catheterization for monitoring cardiovascular function. *N Engl J Med* 290:1227, 1974.

57. Band JD, Maki DG: Infections caused by arterial catheters used for hemodynamic monitoring. *Am J Med* 67:735, 1979.

58. Downs JB, Rackstein AD, Klein EF, et al: Hazards of radial artery catheterization. *Anesthesiology* 38:283, 1973.

59. Davis FM: Radial artery cannulation: Influence of catheter size and material on arterial occlusion. *Anesth Intensive Care* 6:49, 1978.

60. Bedford RF: Radial arterial function following percutaneous cannulation with 18- and 20-gauge catheters. *Anesthesiology* 47:37, 1977.

61. Downs JB, Chapman RL, Hawkins IF: Prolonged radial-artery catheterization: An evaluation of heparinized catheters and continuous irrigation. *Arch Surg* 108:671, 1974.

62. Oh T, Opie NJ, Davis NJ: Continuous flush system for radial artery cannulation. *Anesth Intensive Care* 4:29, 1976.

63. Weiss BM, Galtiker RI: Complications during and following radial artery cannulation: A prospective study. *Intensive Care Med* 14:424, 1986.

64. Jones RM, Hill AB, Nahrwold MC, et al: The effect of method of radial artery cannulation on post-cannulation blood flow and thrombus formation. *Anesthesiology* 55:76, 1981.

65. Bedford RF: Long-term radial artery cannulation: Effects on subsequent vessel function. *Crit Care Med* 6:64, 1978.

66. Clifton GD, Branson P, Kelly HJ, et al: Comparison of normal saline and heparin solutions for maintenance of arterial catheter patency. *Heart Lung* 20:115, 1990.

67. Herrera N, Kaiser MB, Dovidas B: Sodium cittrae solution: Alternative to heparin flushes. *Int Pharm Abstr* 26:519, 1989.

68. Hook ML, Reuling J, Luettgen ML, et al: Comparison of the patency of arterial lines maintained with heparinized and nonheparinized infusions. *Heart Lung* 16:693, 1987.

69. Rithalia SVS, Tinker J: Continuous flush devices for vascular pressure monitoring. *Intensive Care Med* 9:295, 1983.

70. Lowenstein E, Little JW, Lo HH: Prevention of cerebral embolization from flushing radial artery cannulas. *N Engl J Med* 285:414, 1971.

71. Chang C, Dughi J, Shitabata P, et al: Air embolism and the radial arterial line. *Crit Care Med* 16:141, 1988.

72. Peruzzi WT, Parker MA, Lichtenthal PR, et al: A clinical evaluation of a blood conservation device in medical intensive care unit patients. *Crit Care Med* 21:501, 1993.

73. Silver MJ, Jubran H, Stein S, et al: Evaluation of a new blood-conserving arterial line system for patients in intensive care units. *Crit Care Med* 21:507, 1993.

74. Shapiro BA, Mahutte K, Cane RD, et al: Clinical performance of a blood gas monitor: A prospective, multicenter trial. *Crit Care Med* 21:487, 1993.

75. Zimmerman JL, Dellinger RP: Initial evaluation of a new intraarterial blood gas system in humans. *Crit Care Med* 21:495, 1993.

76. Chernow B, Salem M, Stacey J: Blood conservation: A critical care imperative. *Crit Care Med* 19:313, 1991.

77. Mann MC, Votto J, Kambe J, et al: Management of the severely anemic patient who refuses transfusion: Lessons learned during the care of a Jehovah's witness. *Ann Intern Med* 117:1042, 1992.

78. Wittels EG, Siegel RD, Mazur EM: Thrombocytopenia in the intensive care unit setting. *J Intensive Care Med* 5:224, 1990.

79. Warkentin TE, Kelton JG: Heaparin-induced thrombocytopenia. *Ann Rev Med* 40:31, 1989.

80. Wolf S, Mangano DT: Pseudoaneurysm, a late complication of radial artery catheterization. *Anesthesiology* 52:80, 1980.

81. Altin RS, Flicker S, Naidech HJ: Pseudoaneurysm and arteriovenous fistula after femoral artery catheterization: Associated with low femoral punctures. *Am J Roentgenol* 152:629, 1989.

82. Marshall G, Edelstein G, Hirshman CA: Median nerve compression following radial artery puncture. *Anesth Analg* 59:953, 1980.

83. Maki D: Nosocomial bacteremia: An epidemiologic overview. *Am J Med* 70:719, 1981.

84. Mermel LA, Maki DG: Epidemic bloodstream infections from hemodynamic pressure monitoring: Signs of the times. *Infect Control Hosp Epidemiol* 10:47, 1989.

85. Shinozaki T, Deane RS, Mazuzan JE, et al: Bacterial contamination of arterial lines: A prospective study. *JAMA* 249:223, 1983.

86. Stamm WE, Colella JJ, Anderson RL, et al: Indwelling arterial catheters as a source of nosocomial bacteremia. *N Engl J Med* 292:1099, 1975.

87. Maki DG: Pathogenesis, prevention, and management of infections due to intravascular devices used for infusion therapy, in Bisno A, Waldvogel F (eds): *Infections Associated with Indwelling Medical Devices.* Washington, DC, American Society for Microbiology, 1989, p 166.

88. Maki DG, Ringer M, Alvarado CJ: Prospective, randomised trial of povidone-iodine, alcohol, and chlorhexadine for prevention of infection associated with central venous and arterial catheters. *Lancet* 338:339, 1991.

89. Conly JM, Grieves K, Peters B: A prospective, randomized study comparing transparent and dry gauze dressings for central venous catheters. *J Infect Dis* 159:310, 1989.

90. Hoffmann KK, Weber DJ, Samsa GP, et al: Transparent polyurethane film as an intravenous catheter dressing: A meta analysis of the infection risks. *JAMA* 267:2072, 1992.

91. Maki DG, Band JD: A comparative study of polyantibiotic and iodophor ointments in prevention of vascular catheter-related infection. *Am J Med* 70:739, 1981.

92. Maki DG, Weise CE, Sarafin HW: A semiquantitative culture method for identifying intravenous-catheter related infection. *N Engl J Med* 296:1305, 1977.

93. Leroy O, Billiau V, Beuscart C, et al: Nosocomial infections associated with long-term radial artery cannulation. *Intensive Care Med* 15:241, 1989.

94. Eyer S, Brummitt C, Crossley K, et al: Catheter-related sepsis: Prospective randomized study of three methods of long-term catheter maintenance. *Crit Care Med* 18:1073, 1990.

95. Thomas F, Parker J, Burke J, et al: Prospective randomized evaluation of indwelling radial vs. femoral arterial catheters in high risk critically ill patients. *Crit Care Med* 10:226, 1982.

96. Ransjo V, Good Z: An outbreak of *Klebsiella oxytoca* septicemia associated with the use of invasive blood pressure monitoring. *Acta Anaesthesiol Scand* 36:289, 1992.

4. Pulmonary Artery Catheters

Stephen J. Voyce and James M. Rippe

Since their introduction in 1970 by Swan and associates, balloon-tipped, flow-directed pulmonary artery (PA) catheters have found widespread use in the clinical management of critically ill patients [1]. In unstable situations, during which hemodynamic changes often occur rapidly, clinical evaluation may be misleading [2–6]. Pulmonary artery catheters allow direct measurement of several major determinates and consequences of cardiac performance (preload, afterload, cardiac output), thereby supplying additional data to aid clinical decision-making [7–10].

Indications

The wide potential of the PA catheter should not preclude a careful clinical assessment, since hemodynamic monitoring entails a risk, albeit small, for the patient. Clinicians who employ hemodynamic monitoring should understand the fundamentals of insertion technique, the equipment used, and the data that can be generated [9].

Hemodynamic monitoring has four central objectives: (1) to assess left and/or right ventricular function; (2) to monitor changes in hemodynamic status; (3) to guide treatment with pharmacologic and nonpharmacologic agents; and (4) to provide prognostic information. The conditions in which PA catheterization may be useful are characterized by a clinically unclear and/or rapidly changing hemodynamic status. Numerous sources review the indications for placement of PA catheters [9,11,12,13]. Table 4-1 is a partial listing of these indications. Use of PA catheters in specific disease entities is discussed in other chapters.

In addition to the classic indications for PA catheterization detailed in Table 4-1, three reports describe novel uses of PA catheters in the intensive care unit (ICU). Scalea and colleagues describe using mixed venous and/or central venous oxygen saturation as an early accurate measurement of occult blood loss in trauma victims [14]. Two studies describe using cytologic examination of an aspirate of pulmonary capillary blood (withdrawn with the catheter in the wedge position) as a means of antemortem diagnosis of pulmonary lymphangitic carcinoma [15,16].

Other uses of PA catheters outside the ICU include applications in the anesthesia suite and cardiac catheterization laboratory [17–20]. These are not discussed further here.

Basic Catheter Features and Construction

The basic catheter is constructed from polyvinylchloride and has a pliable shaft that softens further at body temperature. Because polyvinylchloride has a high thrombogenicity, the catheters are generally coated with heparin. Heparin bonding of catheters, introduced in 1981, has been shown effective in reducing cather thrombogenicity [21,22]. The standard catheter length is 110 cm and the most commonly used external diameter is 5 or 7 Fr. (one Fr. = 0.0335 mm). A balloon is fastened 1 to 2 mm from the tip (Fig. 4-1); when inflated, it guides the catheter (by virtue of fluid dynamic drag) from the greater intrathoracic veins through the right heart chambers into the pulmonary artery. When fully inflated in a vessel of sufficiently large caliber, the balloon protrudes above the catheter tip, thus distributing tip forces over a large area and minimizing the chances for endocardial damage or arrhythmia induction during catheter insertion (Fig. 4-2). Progression of the catheter is stopped when it impacts in a PA slightly smaller in diameter than the fully inflated balloon. From this position the pulmonary artery wedge pressure (PAWP) is obtained. Balloon capacity varies according to catheter size, and the operator must be aware of the individual balloon's maximal inflation volume as recommended by the manufacturer. The balloon is usually inflated with air, but filtered carbon dioxide should be used in any situation in which balloon rupture might result in access of the inflation medium to the arterial system (e.g., if a right-to-left intracardiac shunt or a pulmonary arteriovenous fistula is suspected). If carbon dioxide is used, periodic deflation and reinflation may be necessary, since carbon dioxide diffuses through the latex balloon at a rate of approximately 0.5 ml per minute. Liquids should never be used as the inflation medium.

A variety of catheter constructions are available, each designed for particular clinical applications. Double-lumen catheters allow balloon inflation through one lumen, and a distal opening at the tip of the catheter is used to measure intravascular pressures and sample blood. Triple-lumen catheters have a proximal port terminating 30 cm from the tip of the catheter, allowing simultaneous measurement of right atrial and PA or wedge pressures. The most commonly employed PA catheter in the ICU setting is a quadruple-lumen catheter, which has a lumen containing electrical leads for a thermistor positioned at the catheter surface 4 cm proximal to its tip (Fig. 4-1) [23]. The thermistor measures PA blood temperature and allows thermodilution cardiac output measurements. A five-lumen catheter is also available, with the fifth lumen opening 40 cm from the tip of the catheter. The fifth lumen provides additional central venous access for fluid or medication infusions when peripheral access is limited or when drugs requiring infusion into a large vein (e.g., dopamine, epinephrine) are used.

Several special-purpose PA catheter designs are available. Pacing PA catheters incorporate two groups of electrodes on the catheter surface, enabling intracardiac electrocardiographic (ECG) recording or temporary cardiac pacing [24]. These catheters are used for emergency cardiac pacing, although it is often difficult to position the catheter for reliable simultaneous cardiac pacing and PA pressure measurements. A new five-lumen catheter (Paceport right ventricular catheter; C.R. Bard, Billerica, MA) allows passage of a specially designed 2.4 Fr. bipolar pacing electrode (probe) through the additional lumen, located 19 cm from the catheter tip (Figs. 4-3 and 4-4). This allows emergency temporary intracardiac pacing without the need for a separate central venous puncture. The pacing probe is Teflon-coated to allow easy introduction through the paceport lumen; the intracavitary part of the probe is heparin-impregnated to reduce the risk of thrombus formation. A recent report demonstrated satisfactory ventricular pacing in 19 of 23 patients using this catheter design (83% success rate) [25]. When a pacing probe is not in use, the fifth lumen may be used for addi-

Table 4-1. General Indications
for Pulmonary Artery Catheterization

1. Management of complicated myocardial infarction
   a. Hypovolemia vs. cardiogenic shock
   b. Ventricular septal rupture vs. acute mitral regurgitation
   c. Severe left ventricular failure
   d. Right ventricular infarction
   e. Unstable angina
   f. Refractory ventricular tachycardia
2. Assessment of respiratory distress
   a. Cardiogenic vs. noncardiogenic (e.g., ARDS) pulmonary edema
   b. Primary vs. secondary pulmonary hypertension
3. Assessment of shock
   a. Cardiogenic
   b. Hypovolemic
   c. Septic
   d. Pulmonary embolism
4. Assessment of therapy in selected individuals
   a. Afterload reduction in patients with severe left ventricular function
   b. Inotropic agent
   c. Vasopressors
   d. Beta-blockers
   e. Temporary pacing (ventricular vs. atrioventricular)
   f. Intraaortic balloon counterpulsation
   g. Mechanical ventilation (e.g., with PEEP)
5. Management of postoperative open heart surgical patients
6. Assessment of cardiac tamponade/constriction
7. Assessment of valvular heart disease
8. Perioperative monitoring of patients with unstable cardiac status during noncardiac surgery
9. Assessment of fluid requirements in critically ill patients
   a. Gastrointestinal hemorrhage
   b. Sepsis
   c. Acute renal failure
   d. Burns
   e. Decompensated cirrhosis
   f. Advanced peritonitis
10. Management of severe preeclampsia [198]

ARDS = adult respiratory distress syndrome; PEEP = positive end-expiratory pressure.
Adapted from Gore, et al: *Handbook of Hemodynamic Monitoring.* Boston, Little, Brown, 1985, with permission.

tional central venous access or continuous right ventricular pressure monitoring. This is the preferred PA catheter at our institution.

Continuous mixed venous oxygen saturation measurement is clinically available using a fiberoptic five-lumen PA catheter [26]. Segal and colleagues described a catheter that incorporates Doppler technology for continuous cardiac output determinations [27]. Catheters equipped with a fast-response (95 msec) thermistor and intracardiac ECG monitoring electrodes are also available. These catheters allow determination of right ventricular ejection fraction (RVEF) and right ventricular systolic time intervals in critically ill patients [28–31]. The calculated RVEF has correlated well with simultaneous radionuclide first-pass studies [28]. The clinical utility of these and other catheter modifications is under investigation [27,32–35].

PRESSURE TRANSDUCERS. Hemodynamic monitoring requires a system able to convert changes in intravascular pressure into an electrical signal suitable for interpretation. The most commonly employed hemodynamic monitoring system is a catheter-tubing-transducer system. A fluid-filled intravascular

catheter is connected to a transducer by a fluid-filled tubing system. The transducer (Fig. 4-5) has a fluid-filled chamber (dome) that is connected to the fluid-filled catheter. The system transmits pressure changes from the intravascular space through the catheter to the dome. A diaphragm connected to the transducer is displaced by the transmitted pressure changes. The diaphragm deforms a series of resistance wires that are connected to form a Wheatstone bridge (which allows changes in resistance to induce an electrical current). The current produced is proportional to the displacement of the diaphragm and after amplificaiton is displayed as a waveform on a cathode-ray tube. Digital pressure meters display these changes numerically, allowing continuous monitoring of intravascular pressure changes.

Insertion Techniques

GENERAL CONSIDERATIONS. Techniques for insertion of Swan-Ganz catheters and handling of the monitoring equipment are described in many sources [36–40]. Manufacturers' recommendations should be carefully followed, as should the individual institution's uniform procedure techniques and equipment preferences.

Pulmonary artery catheterization can be performed in any hospital location where continuous ECG and hemodynamic monitoring is possible and where equipment and supplies needed for cardiopulmonary resuscitation are readily available. Fluoroscopy is not essential, but it can facilitate difficult placements. Properly constructed beds and protective aprons are mandatory for safe use of fluoroscopic equipment. Meticulous attention to sterile technique is of obvious importance; all involved personnel must wear sterile caps, gowns, masks, and gloves.

The catheter may be inserted percutaneously or via cutdown into the basilic, brachial, femoral, subclavian, or internal jugular veins using techniques described in Chapter 2. For the following reasons, many clinicians prefer the percutaneous internal jugular approach: (1) patient arm movements are not encumbered and are unlikely to alter catheter tip position; (2) it can be used in patients undergoing intrathoracic surgery; and (3) fewer thrombotic and septic complications may occur. We often use a prepackaged catheter introducer kit (including a sheath vessel dilator, guidewire, sterile sleeve adapter, and related supplies) (Fig. 4-6), which is reflected in our recommended procedure (described below).

EQUIPMENT PREPARATION. Gathering the equipment, setup, and calibration are usually accomplished by the nursing staff, but all personnel participating in Swan-Ganz placements should be aware of the procedure.

1. Gather the equipment needed for pressure monitoring.
   a. IV pole with attached manifold
   b. One 250-ml bag of normal saline with 500 units of heparin added
   c. One pressure bag
   d. One clysis (bifurcated) IV tubing and two pressure tubings
   e. One disposable transducer dome
   f. Two fast-flush devices (Sorenson Intraflows)
   g. Three 3-way stopcocks
2. Set up the pressure lines and transducer.
   a. Connect the clysis tubing to the bag of heparinized saline and purge air from the tubing.

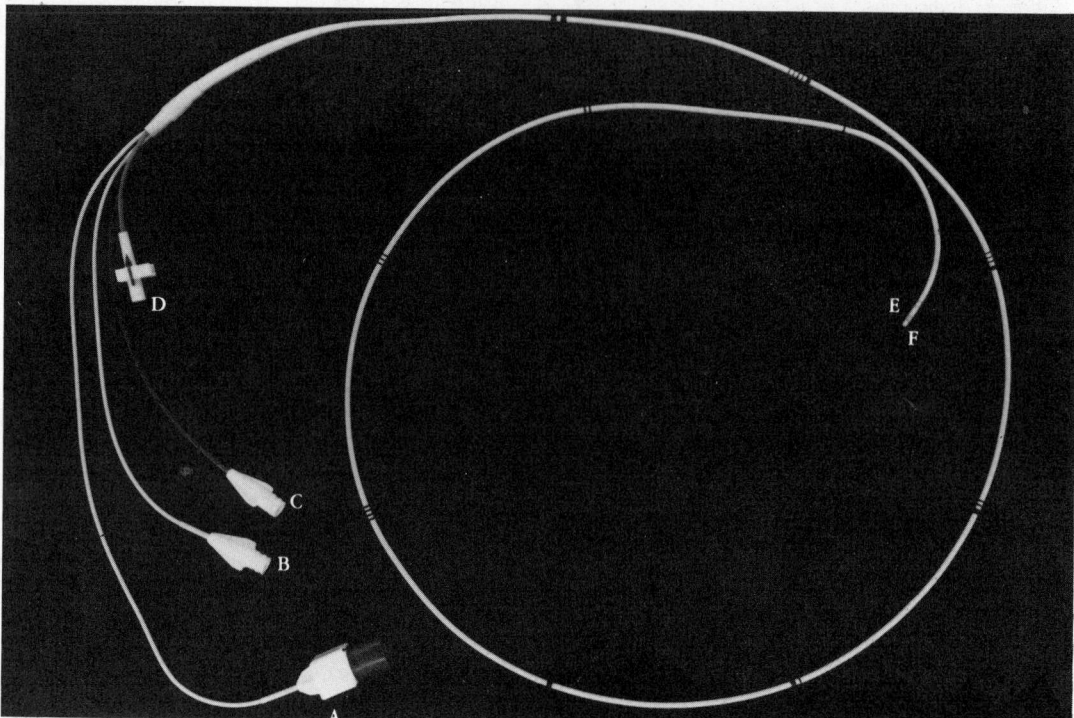

Fig. 4-1. Quadruple-lumen pulmonary artery catheter. A. Connection to thermodilution cardiac output computer. B. Connection to distal lumen. C. Connection to proximal lumen. D. Stopcock connected to balloon at the catheter tip for balloon inflation. E. Thermistor. F. Balloon. Note that the catheter is marked in 10-cm increments.

b. Cap all unused ports on the manifold.
c. Connect the male end of intraflow to the manifold and the clysis tubing to the IV tubing on the intraflow.
d. Connect the pressure tubing to the remaining female port on the intraflow and place a three-way stopcock on the distal end of the pressure tubing.
e. Place the saline bag into the pressure bag and inflate pressure to approximately 150 mm Hg.
f. Turn the stopcocks on the manifold to the off position, open the clamps on the IV tubing, and pull the red tail of the intraflow to flush the system of air.
g. Clear both ports of the distal stopcock and then close the system to air.
h. Inflate the pressure bag to 300 mm Hg.
i. Place 2 ml of normal saline on top of the disposable dome, attach the dome to the transducer, and attach the transducer to the manifold.
j. Turn the stopcocks on the manifold such that the flush system is open to the transducer.
k. Place a stopcock on the remaining port of the disposable dome and open the transducer to air.
l. Flush the transducer until all air is eliminated, then close the system to air.
3. Zero-balance the transducer.
 a. Attach the appropriate end of the transducer to the monitor and allow the transducer to warm up for about 15 minutes.
 b. Turn the stopcocks on the manifold off to the pressure lines and open the transducer stopcock to air.
 c. Zero-balance the transducer following the manufacturer's instructions.

4. Calibrate the transducer against mercury.
 a. Open the transducer stopcock to air and turn the manifold stopcocks off to the lines.
 b. Connect a clean filter and a three-way stopcock to a mercury manometer. Connect the male end of the filter to the stopcock on the transducer.
 c. Use a large syringe or bulb to apply pressure to the transducer through the manometer (200 mm Hg is recommended).
 d. The monitor readout and manometer reading should agree to ±5 percent.
 e. If the pressures do not correlate, adjust the monitor following the manufacturer's instructions or replace the transducer.
 f. Release the pressure and close the stockcock on the transducer.
 Note: A detailed description of the pressure monitoring system setup and troubleshooting are available elsewhere [9].
5. Gather the equipment needed for catheter insertion.
 a. Bedside table
 b. Cutdown trays for peripheral placements
 c. Catheter and vein introducer kits
 d. Sterile gowns, masks, gloves, and drapes
 e. 1% lidocaine HCl
 f. 1-ml and 5-ml syringes
 g. Small cup of sterile saline or water to test balloon integrity
 h. Suture and dressing materials
 i. Arrange the instruments and kits on a sterile field.

CATHETER INSERTION PROCEDURE

1. Position the patient, providing as much patient comfort and operator ease of access as possible. Scrub insertion area with povidone-iodine or other antibacterial solution and drape the area appropriately.
2. Anesthetize the skin using a 1% lidocaine HCl (Fig. 4-7).

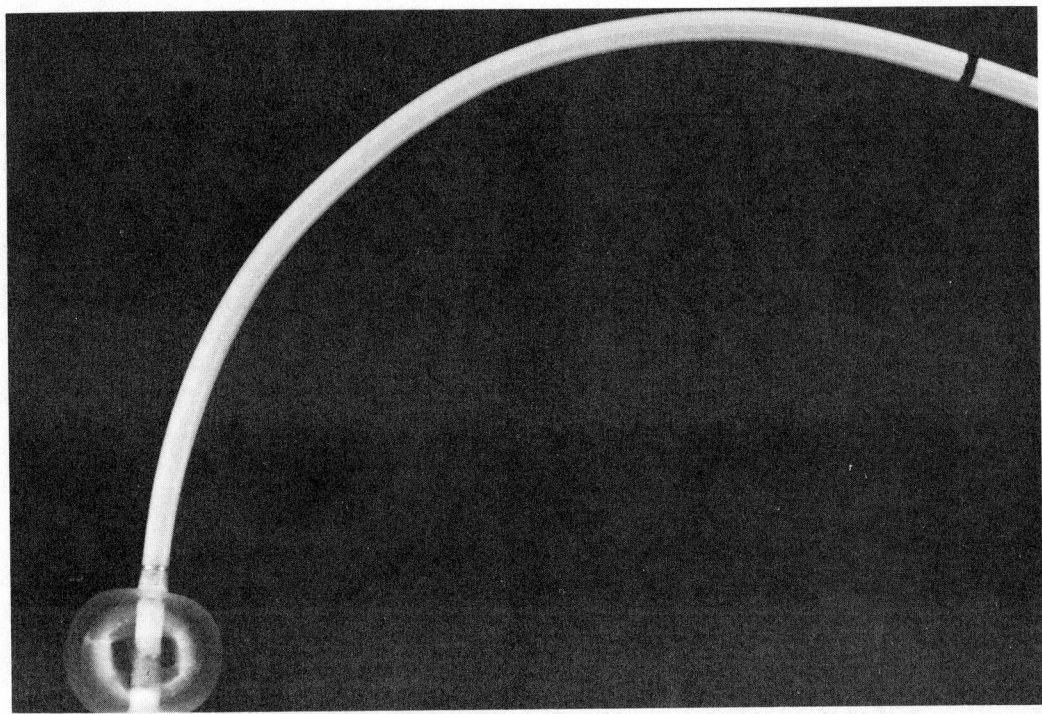

Fig. 4-2. Balloon properly inflated at the tip of a pulmonary artery catheter. Note that the balloon shields the catheter tip and prevents it from irritating cardiac chambers on its passage to the pulmonary artery.

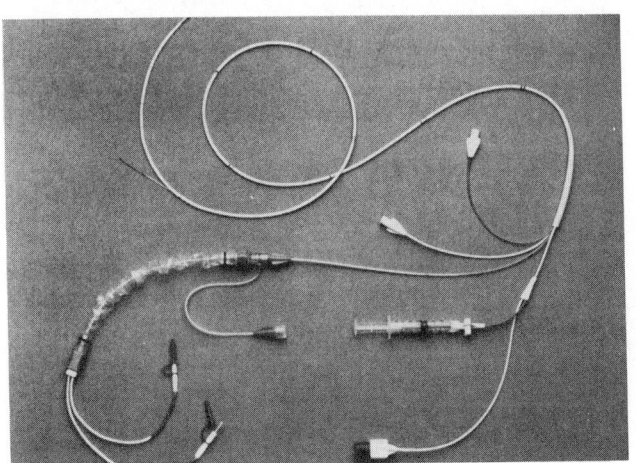

Fig. 4-3. Pacing port pulmonary artery catheter. Note additional lumen with pacing probe and protective sheath attached *(arrow)*.

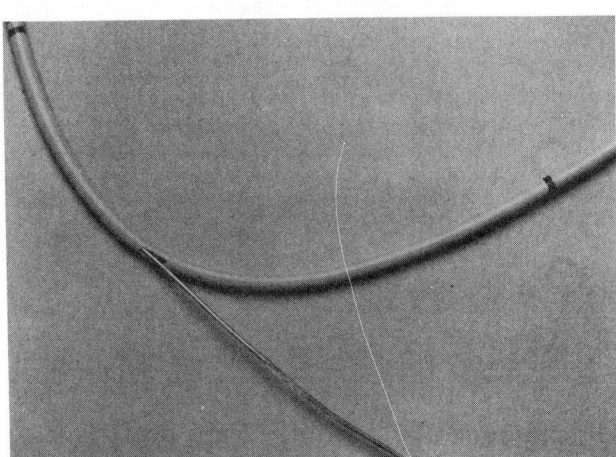

Fig. 4-4. Close-up view of the pacing port catheter with the pacing electrode extending out the additional lumen.

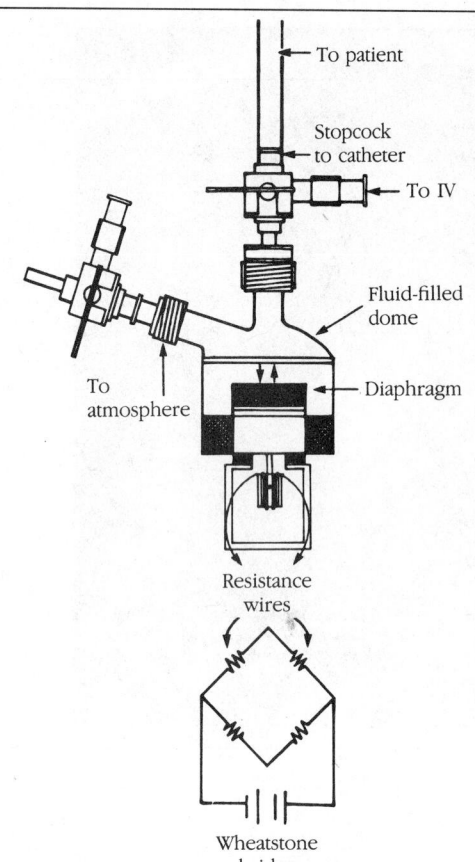

Fig. 4-5. Transducer/Wheatstone bridge. (From Gore JM, Zwerner PL: Hemodynamic monitoring in acute myocardial infarction, in Alpert JS, Francis GS (eds): *Modern Coronary Care,* Boston, Little, Brown, 1990. With permission.)

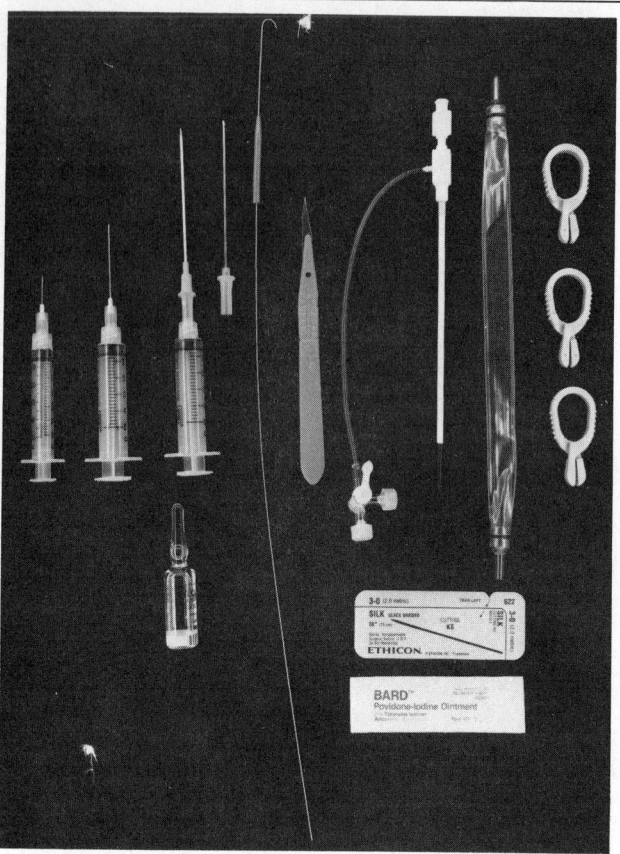

Fig. 4-6. Equipment available in a commercially supplied kit for pulmonary artery catheter introduction. Supplies shown include (clockwise from left: 3-ml syringe with 25-gauge needle for anesthetizing the skin, 5-ml syringe with 1½-inch, 21-gauge needle for anesthetizing superficial tissues and locating the vein to be cannulated, 5-ml syringe with catheter-over-needle to cannulate vein, needle to cannulate vein (alternative to cannula-over-needle), 25-cm guidewire, scalpel, introducer, and sheath, sterile sheath for catheter, towel clips, 3-0 suture for fixing catheter in place, iodine ointment, and 1% lidocaine. The technique for catheter introduction using this equipment is outlined in the text.

3. Remove the sterile balloon-tipped catheter from its container and wipe the outside with gauze soaked in sterile water or saline. Test for balloon integrity by submerging it in a small amount of fluid and checking for air leaks as the balloon is inflated (using the amount of air recommended by the manufacturer). Deflate the balloon.

4. Locate the vessel to be cannulated using a 21-gauge, 1 1/2-inch needle attached to a 5-ml syringe (see Chap. 2 for cannulization techniques). Leave this locator needle and syringe in place once free blood has been aspirated (Fig. 4-8).

5. Next to the locator needle insert an 18-gauge guidewire introducer needle-cannula into the vessel (Fig. 4-9). When blood is easily aspirated into a syringe attached to the guidewire introducer needles (Fig. 4-10A), remove the locator needle.

6. Advance the Teflon cannula over the inner needle of the introducer assembly into the vessel and remove the inner needle (Fig. 4-10B). Thread a spring guidewire through the cannula into the vessel, making certain to advance the soft end of the guidewire first (Fig. 4-10C). Holding the guidewire in place, withdraw the cannula from the vessel by pulling it over and off the length of the guidewire (Fig. 4-10). This technique leaves the guidewire located in the vessel as indicated (Fig. 4-11).

7. Make a small incision with a scalpel to enlarge the puncture site (Fig. 4-12).

8. Thread a vessel dilator sheath apparatus (size 8 Fr. if a 7 Fr. catheter is to be used) over the guidewire and advance it into the vessel using a twisting motion to get through the puncture site (Fig. 4-13).

9. Remove the guidewire and vessel dilator, leaving the introducer sheath in the vessel (Fig. 4-14).

10. Attach stockcocks to the right atrium and PA ports of the PA catheter and fill the proximal and distal catheter lumens with flush solution. Close the stopcocks (to keep flush solution within the lumens and avoid introduction of air into the circulation).

11. If a sterile sleeve adapter is to be used, insert the catheter through it and pull the adapter proximally over the catheter to keep it out of the way. Once the catheter is advanced to its desired intravascular location, attach the distal end of the sleeve adapter to the introducer sheath hub.

12. Pass the catheter through the introducer sheath into the vein (Fig. 4-15). Advance it, using the marks on the catheter shaft indicating 10-cm distances from the tip, until the tip is in the right atrium. This requires advancement of approximately 35 to 40 cm from the left antecubital fossa, 10

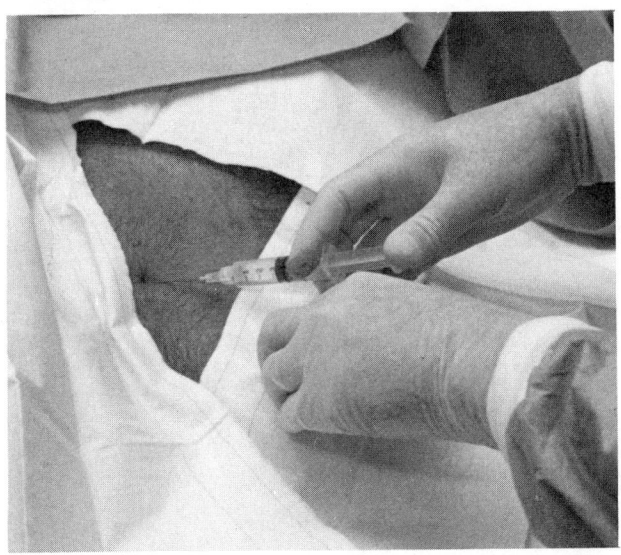

Fig. 4-7. The skin is anesthetized with 1% lidocaine HCl. (In this situation the left subclavian approach was chosen.)

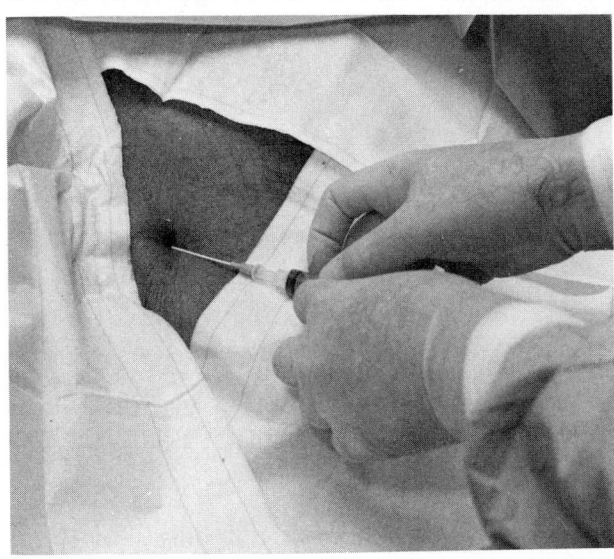

Fig. 4-9. Once the subclavian vein has been located, an 18-gauge guidewire introducer needle-cannula is introduced into the vessel.

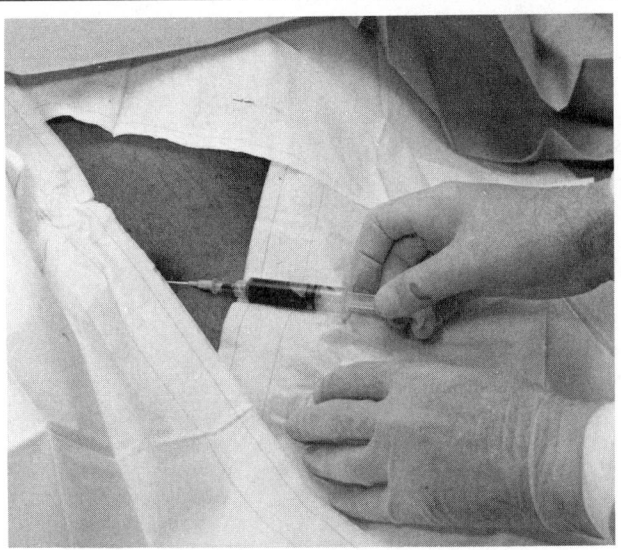

Fig. 4-8. The subclavian vein has been located with a 21-gauge, 1½-inch needle, and free blood aspiration has been demonstrated.

to 15 cm from the internal jugular vein, 10 cm from the subclavian vein, and 35 to 40 cm from the femoral vein. A right atrial waveform on the monitor with appropriate fluctuations accompanying respiratory changes or cough confirms proper intrathoracic location (Fig. 4-16 center). Obtain right atrial blood for oxygen saturation from the distal port. Flush the distal lumen with heparinized saline and record the right atrial pressures. (Occasionally, it is necessary to inflate the balloon to keep the tip from adhering to the atrial wall during blood aspiration.)

13. With the catheter tip in the right atrium, inflate the balloon with the recommended amount of air or carbon dioxide (Fig. 4-16A). Inflation of the balloon should be associated with a slight feeling of resistance—if it is not, suspect bal-

loon rupture and do not attempt further inflation or advancement of the catheter until properly reevaluating balloon integrity. If significant resistance to balloon inflation is encountered, suspect malposition of the catheter in a small vessel; withdraw the catheter and readvance it to a new position. Do not use liquids to inflate the balloon, since they might be irretrievable and could prevent balloon deflation.

14. With the balloon inflated, advance the catheter until a right ventricle pressure tracing is seen on the monitor (Fig. 4-16 center). Obtain and record right ventricular pressures. Catheter passage into and through the right ventricle is an especially risky time in terms of arrhythmias. Maintaining the balloon inflated in the right ventricle minimizes ventricular irritation (Fig. 4-16B), but it is important to monitor vital signs and ECG throughout the entire insertion procedure.

15. Continue advancing the catheter until the diastolic pressure tracing rises above that in the right ventricle (Fig. 4-16 center), indicating PA placement (Fig. 4-16C). If a right ventricular trace still appears after the catheter has been advanced 15 cm beyond the original distance needed to reach the right atrium, suspect curling in the ventricle; deflate the balloon, withdraw it to the right atrium, then reinflate it and try again. Advancement beyond the PA position results in a fall on the pressure tracing from the levels of systolic pressure noted in the right ventricle and PA. When this is noted, record the PAWP (Fig. 4-16 center and D) and deflate the balloon. Phasic PA pressure should reappear on the pressure tracing when the balloon is deflated. If it does not, pull back the catheter with the deflated balloon until the PA tracing appears. With the balloon deflated, blood may be aspirated for oxygen saturation measurement. Watch for intermittent right ventricular tracings indicating slippage of the catheter backwards into the ventricle.

16. Carefully record the balloon inflation volume needed to change the PA pressure tracing to the PAWP tracing. If PAWP is recorded with an inflation volume significantly lower than the manufacturer's recommended volume, or if subsequent PAWP determinations require lessening

Text continues on page 57.

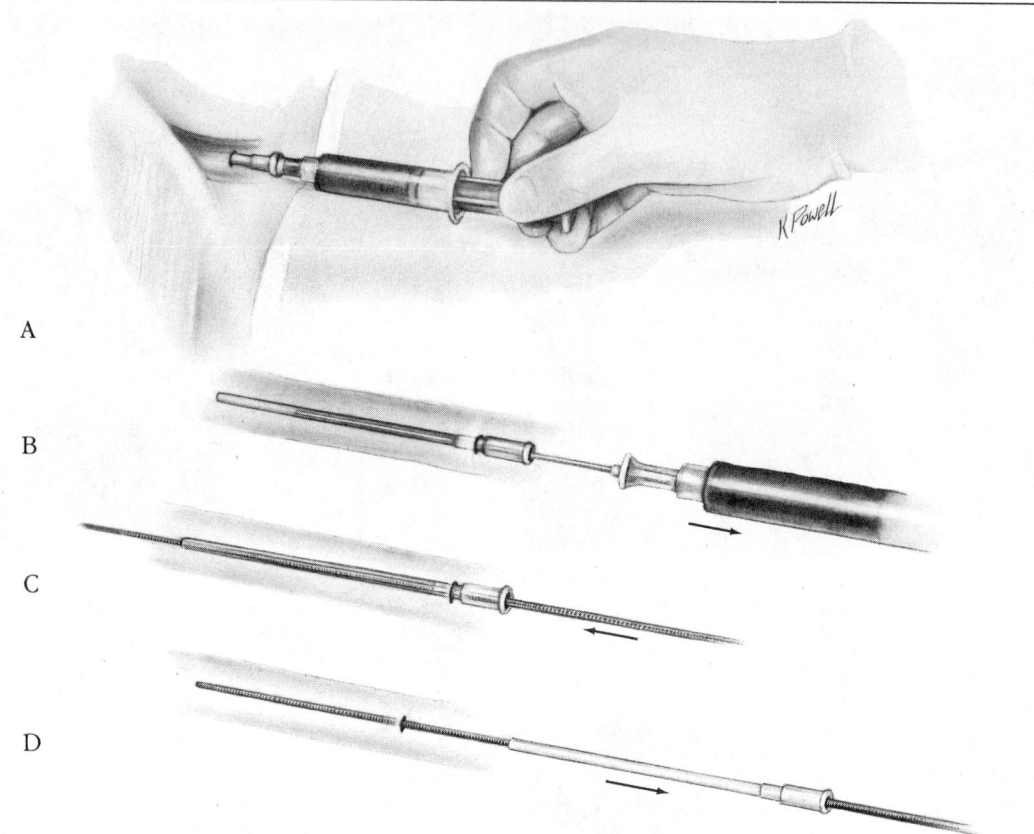

Fig. 4-10. A. Easy blood aspiration has been demonstrated using the guidewire introducer needle. B. The inner needle is removed. C. The spring guidewire is advanced, soft end first, through the cannula into the vessel. D. With the guidewire held in place, the cannula is withdrawn from the vessel by being pulled over and off the length of the guidewire.

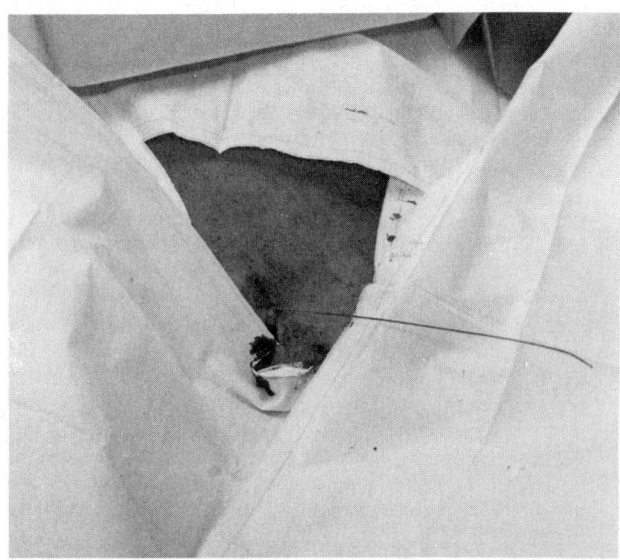

Fig. 4-11. The spring guidewire, stiff end protruding, is now located in the subclavian vein.

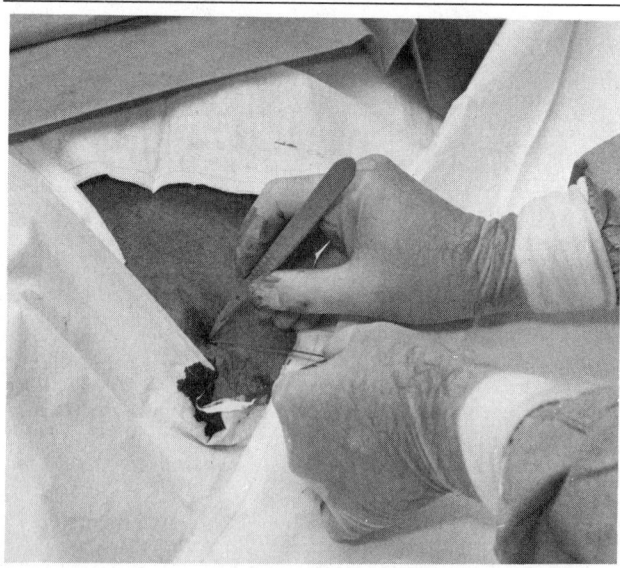

Fig. 4-12. A small incision is made with a scalpel to enlarge the puncture site.

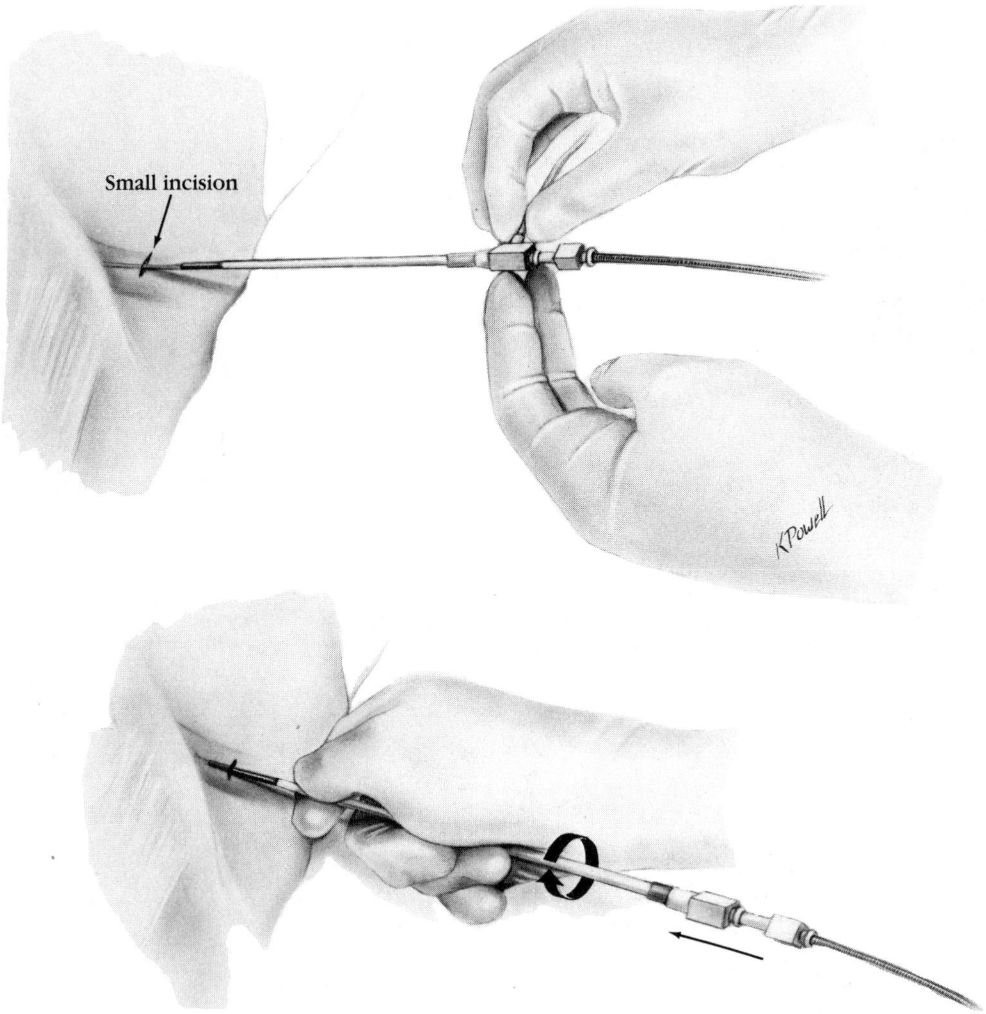

Small incision

A

B

Fig. 4-13. A. The vessel dilator-sheath apparatus is threaded over the guidewire and advanced into the vessel. B. A twisting motion is used to thread the apparatus into the vessel.

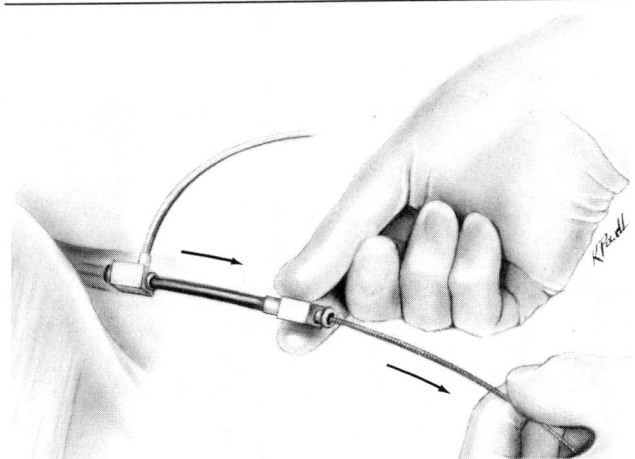

Fig. 4-14. The guidewire and vessel dilator are removed, leaving the introducer sheath in the vessel.

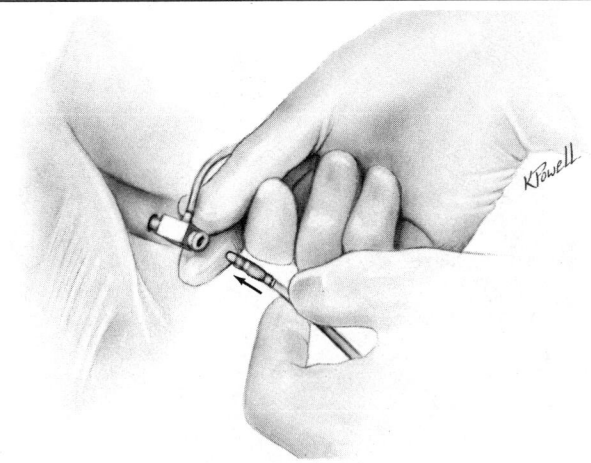

Fig. 4-15. The catheter is passed through the introducer sheath into the vein.

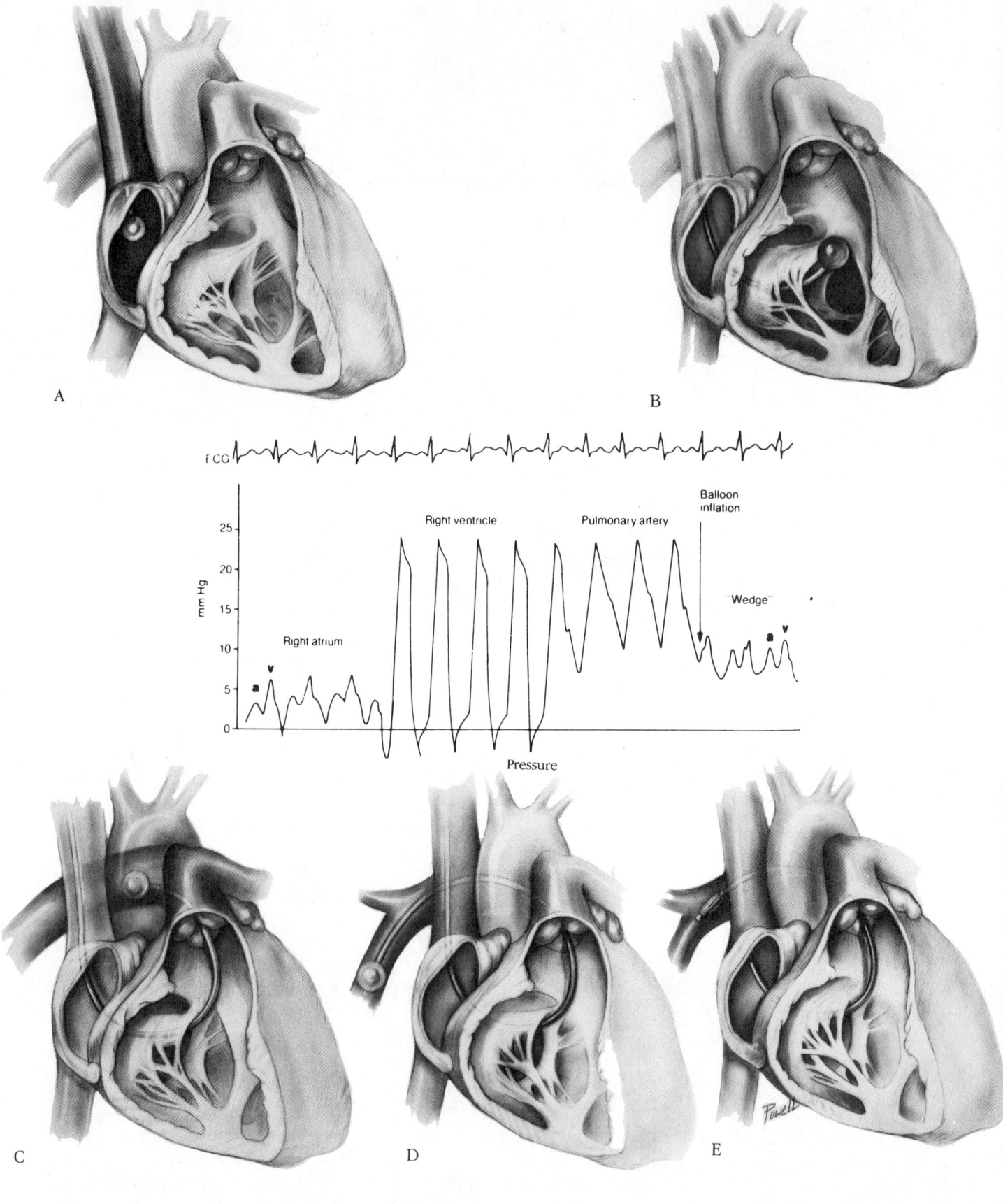

Fig. 4-16. Center. Waveform tracings generated as the balloon-tipped catheter is advanced through the right heart chambers into the pulmonary artery. RA = right atrium; RV = right ventricle; PA = pulmonary artery; PAWP = pulmonary artery wedge pressure. A. With the catheter tip in the RA, the balloon is inflated. B. The catheter is advanced into the RV with the baloon inflated and RV pressure tracings are obtained. C. The catheter is advanced through the pulmonary valve into the pulmonary artery. A rise in diastolic pressure will be noted. D. The catheter is advanced to the PAWP position. A typical PAWP tracing will be noted with A and V waves. E. The balloon is deflated. Phasic PA pressure should reappear on the monitor. (See text for details.) (Center figure adapted from Wiedmann HP: Cardiovascular-pulmonary monitoring in the intensive care unit, I. *Chest* 85:540, 1984. With permission.)

amounts of balloon inflation volume as compared to an initial appropriate amount, the catheter tip has migrated too far peripherally and should be pulled back immediately.

17. Secure the catheter in the correct PA position by suturing and/or taping it to the skin to prevent inadvertent advancement. Apply a germicidal agent and dress appropriately.

18. Order a chest radiograph to confirm catheter position; the catheter tip should appear no more than 3 to 5 cm from the midline. To assess whether peripheral catheter migration has occurred, daily chest radiographs are recommended to supplement pressure monitoring and checks on balloon inflation volumes. An initial cross-table lateral radiograph should be obtained in patients on positive end-expiratory pressure (PEEP) to rule out superior placements.

PACEPORT CATHETER INSERTION TECHNIQUE. The Paceport catheter has an additional lumen 19 cm from the catheter tip (the right ventricular port), which allows passage of a specially designed 2.4 Fr. pacemaker wire (probe). These catheters are used in patients who require hemodynamic monitoring and temporary ventricular pacing. When the probe is not in use, the right ventricular port may be used to infuse fluid or medication. The catheter is inserted as described for a standard PA catheter. The pacemaker is introduced as follows.

1. Connect the right ventricular port to a pressure transducer to verify the location of the opening in the RV. Ideally, the right ventricular port opening is positioned 1 to 2 cm distal to the tricuspid valve [25]. To achieve this after initial placement, pull the catheter back until a right atrial pressure tracing is recorded from the right ventricular port. Advance the catheter (with balloon inflated) until a right ventricular pressure tracing is first obtained. At this point the opening of the right ventricular port is at the level of the tricuspid valve; simply advancing the catheter an additional 1 to 2 cm will place the opening in the desired position. The pacemaker probe can be introduced now or at a later stage.

2. A special package (Fig. 4-17) enables sterile introduction of the pacemaker probe. Mark the external part of the right ventricle lumen to indicate how far the probe extends from the right ventricular lumen opening into the right ventricle.

3. Attach the tip of the pacemaker probe introducer package to the hub of the right ventricular port. Advance the 2.4 Fr. pacing probe gently through the Paceport lumen. Passage of the probe is facilitated by keeping the extravascular portion of the PA catheter as straight as possible and keeping the probe on its packaging spool during insertion. Allow the spool to spin slowly as the probe is advanced.

4. When the marker on the probe reaches the 0 marking on the external part of the right ventricular lumen, the tip of the probe is at the lumen opening.

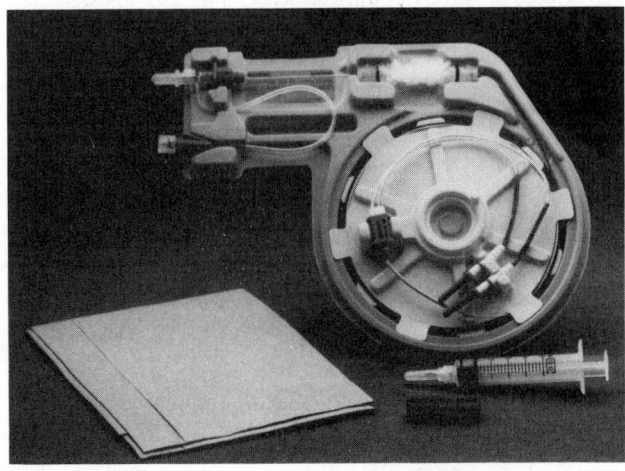

Fig. 4-17. Commercially available special packaging for pacing probe.

5. Connect the distal electrode of the probe to an ECG recorder (see Chap. 8 on pacemaker insertion) and advance it until the intracardiac electrogram demonstrates S–T segment elevation, indicating contact with the endocardium.

6. Connect the probe to a pacemaker generator and check the thresholds.

7. Obtain a chest radiograph to ensure proper pacemaker probe placement at the RV apex.

SPECIAL CONSIDERATIONS. Generally, patients should have normal coagulation parameters before central venous access is attempted. However, patients on anticoagulant medications or those receiving thrombolytic therapy are frequently encountered in the ICU setting. Special attention to central venous cannulation is necessary to minimize the risk of serious hemorrhagic complications in this patient population. The anticoagulant (intravenous heparin or oral warfarin) should be discontinued and sufficient time allowed to pass before the procedure is undertaken. Intravenous heparin should be discontinued 3 to 4 hours prior to the procedure to allow the partial thromboplastin time to normalize. Heparin may be restarted on completion of the procedure. Protamine may also be used to antagonize the effect of heparin acutely. Discontinuation of oral warfarin has little acute effect on the prothrombin time, due to the drug's protracted half-life. The prothrombin time can be acutely normalized by infusion of fresh frozen plasma. Vitamin K can be administered, but it may take several days to reverse the anticoagulant effect of warfarin and makes reanticoagulation with warfarin more difficult.

Although anticoagulation is a relative contraindication for hemodynamic monitoring, it may be imprudent or impossible to correct a patient's coagulation profile prior to pulmonary artery catheterization. In these cases a number of techniques may be used to minimize hemorrhagic risks. Cannulation of the basilic vein by a cutdown approach is recommended. This allows the operator direct access to the point of catheter insertion. The internal and external jugular veins are secondary approaches in this patient population. These vessels are anatomically accessible to direct compression of potential bleeding sites. Extreme care to avoid inadvertent carotid artery puncture is mandatory. If carotid artery puncture does occur, bleeding is usually controlled with direct pressure. The subclavian approach should be avoided in patients with coagulopathies, since this site is inaccessible to direct pressure.

If a patient receiving thrombolytic therapy requires hemodynamic monitoring, the medication infusion must be discontinued immediately. Approaches to central venous access are similar to those discussed in anticoagulated patients. The half-life of tissue plasminogen ativator is 8 to 9 minutes, allowing rapid reversal of the drug's thrombolytic effects. Streptokinase has a half-life of approximately 20 minutes but also induces a systemic fibrinolytic state that may last 24 hours. Fresh frozen plasma and discontinuation of the streptokinase are required to normalize bleeding parameters.

In certain disease states (right atrial or right ventricular dilatation, severe pulmonary hypertension, severe tricuspid insufficiency, low cardiac output syndromes), it may be difficult to position a flow-directed catheter properly. These settings may require fluoroscopic guidance to aid in catheter positioning. Infusion of 5 to 10 ml of cold saline through the distal lumen may stiffen the catheter and aid in positioning. Alternatively, a 0.025-cm guidewire (length 145 cm) may be used to stiffen the catheter when placed through the distal lumen of a 7 Fr. PA catheter. This manipulation should be performed only under fluoroscopic guidance by an experienced operator. Rarely, non-flow-directed PA catheters (e.g., Cournand catheters) may be required. Because of their rigidity, these catheters have a potential for perforating the right heart and must be placed only under fluoroscopy by a physician experienced in cardiac catheterization techniques.

Physiologic Data

Measurement of a variety of hemodynamic parameters and oxygen saturations is possible using the PA catheter. A summary of normal values for these parameters is found in Tables 4-2 and 4-3.

PRESSURES

Right Atrium. With the tip of the PA catheter in the right atrium (Fig. 4-16A), the balloon is deflated and a right atrial waveform recorded (Fig. 4-18). Normal resting right atrial pressure is 0 to 6 mm Hg. Two major positive atrial pressure waves, the A wave and V wave, can usually be recorded. The A wave is due to atrial contraction and follows the simultaneosly recorded electrocardiographic P wave [11,41]. The A wave peak generally follows the peak of the electrical P wave by approximately 80 msec [42]. The V wave represents the pressure generated by venous filling of the right atrium while the tricuspid valve is closed. The peak of the V wave occurs at the end of ventricular systole when the atrium is maximally filled. This occurs near the end of the electrocardiographic T wave. A third minor positive wave, the C wave, is due to the sudden motion of the atrioventricular valve ring toward the right atrium at the onset of ventricular systole. The C wave follows the A wave by a time period equal to the electrocardiographic P–R interval. The C wave is more readily visible in cases of P–R prolongation [42]. The x descent follows the A wave and reflects atrial relaxation. The y descent is due to rapid emptying of the atrium following opening of the tricuspid valve. The mean right atrial pressure decreases during inspiration (secondary to a decrease in intrathoracic pressure), whereas the A and V waves and the x and y descents become more prominent. Once a multilumen PA catheter is in position, right atrial blood can be sampled and pressure monitored using the proximal lumen. It should be noted that the pressures obtained via the proximal lumen may not accurately reflect right atrial pressure, due to positioning of the lumen against the atrial wall or within the introducer sheath.

Table 4-2. Normal Resting Pressures Obtained During Right Heart Catheterization

Cardiac chamber	Pressure (mm Hg)
Right atrium	
Range	0–6
Mean	3
Right ventricle	
Systolic	17–30
Diastolic	0–6
Pulmonary artery	
Systolic	15–30
Diastolic	5–13
Mean	10–18
Pulmonary artery wedge	
(mean)	2–12

Adapted from Gore JM, Alpert JS: *Handbook of Hemodynamic Monitoring.* Boston, Little, Brown, 1984, with permission.

Table 4-3. Approximate Normal Oxygen Saturation and Content Values

Chamber sampled	Oxygen content (vol%)	Oxygen saturation (%)
Superior vena cava	14	70
Inferior vena cava	16	80
Right atrium	15	75
Right ventricle	15	75
Pulmonary artery	15	75
Pulmonary vein	20	98
Femoral artery	19	96
A–V oxygen content difference	3.5–5.5	

Adapted from Gore JM, Alpert JS: *Handbook of Hemodynamic Monitoring.* Boston, Little, Brown, 1984, with permission.

The latter problem is more frequently encountered in shorter patients [43].

Right Ventricle. The normal resting right ventricular pressure is 17 to 30/0 to 6 mm Hg recorded when the PA catheter crosses the tricuspid valve (Fig. 4-16B). The right ventricular systolic pressure should equal the PA systolic pressure (except in cases of pulmonic stenosis or right ventricular outflow tract obstruction). The right ventricular pressure should equal the mean right atrial pressure during diastole when the tricuspid valve is open. Introduction of the right ventricular Paceport catheter allows continuous monitoring of right ventricular hemodynamics when the pacer probe is not in place. Right ventricular monitoring is increasingly used in the surgical critical care setting [44]. Right ventricular end-diastolic volume index (RVEDVI) and RVEF can now be accurately measured. A number of studies [45,46,47] have suggested that RVEDVI may be a more accurate measure of ventricular preload and correlates better with cardiac index than does the PAWP. It is important to note that these studies did not include patients with underlying left ventricular dysfunction or arrhythmia, therefore the conclusions may not apply to these latter groups. The role of right ventricular monitoring in critically ill patients requires further investigation.

Pulmonary Artery. With the catheter in proper position and the balloon deflated, the distal lumen transmits PA pressure

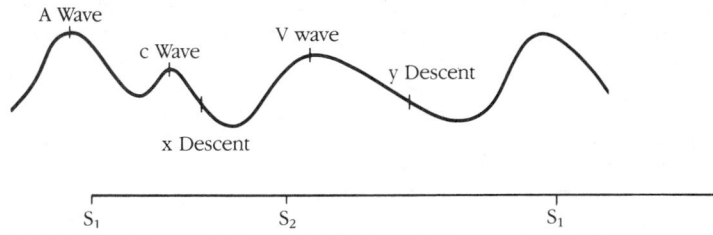

Fig. 4-18. Stylized representation of a right atrial waveform in relation to heart sounds. See text for discussion of A, C, and V waves and *x* and *y* descents. (Adapted from Gore JM, Zwerner PL: Hemodynamic monitoring in acute myocardial infarction, in Alpert JS, Francis GS (eds): *Modern Coronary Care.* Boston, Little, Brown, 1990. With permission.)

(Fig. 4-16E). Normal resting PA pressure is 15 to 30/5 to 13 mm Hg, with a normal mean pressure of 10 to 18 mm Hg. The PA waveform is characterized by a systolic peak and diastolic trough with a dicrotic notch due to closure of the pulmonic valve. The peak PA systolic pressure occurs in the T wave of a simultaneously recorded ECG.

Since the pulmonary vasculature is normally a low-resistance circuit, PA diastolic pressure (PADP) is closely related to mean PAWP (PADP is usually 1 to 3 mm Hg higher than mean PAWP) and thus can be used as an index of left ventricle filling pressure in patients in whom a wedge pressure is unobtainable or in whom PADP and PAWP have been shown to correlate closely. However, if pulmonary vascular resistance is increased, as in pulmonary embolic disease, pulmonary fibrosis, or "reactive" pulmonary hypertension (Chap. 64), PADP may markedly exceed mean PAWP and thus become an unreliable index of left heart function [36,48]. Similar provisos apply when using PA mean pressure as an index of left ventricular function [2].

Pulmonary Artery Wedge Pressure. An important application of the balloon flotation catheter is the recording of PAWP. This measurement is obtained when the inflated balloon impacts into a slightly smaller branch of the PA (Fig. 4-16D). In this position, the balloon stops the flow, and the catheter tip senses pressure transmitted backward through the static column of blood from the next active circulatory bed—the pulmonary veins. Pulmonary venous pressure is a prime determinant of pulmonary congestion and thus of the tendency for fluid to shift from the pulmonary capillaries into the interstitial tissue and alveoli [37]. Also, pulmonary venous pressure and PAWP closely reflect left atrial pressure (except in rare instances, such as pulmonary venocclusive disease, in which there is obstruction in the small pulmonary veins), and serve as indices of left ventricular filling pressure [48,49,50]. The PAWP is required to assess left ventricular filling pressure, since multiple studies have demonstrated that right atrial (e.g., central venous) pressure correlates poorly with the PAWP [51,52,53].

The PAWP is a phase-delayed, amplitude-dampened version of the left atrial pressure. The normal resting PAWP is 2 to 12 mm Hg and averages 2 to 7 mm Hg below the mean PA pressure. The PAWP waveform is similar to that of the right atrium with A, C, and V waves and *x* and *y* descents (Fig. 4-18). However, in contradistinctino to the right atrial waveform, the PAWP waveform demonstrates a V wave that is slightly larger than the A wave [11]. Due to the time required for left atrial mechanical events to be transmitted through the pulmonary vasculature, PAWP waveforms are further delayed when recorded with a simultaneous ECG. The peak of the A wave follows the peak of the electrocardiographic P wave by approximately 240 msec and the peak of the V wave occurs after the electrocardio-

graphic T wave has been inscribed. Wedge position is confirmed by withdrawing a blood specimen from the distal lumen and measuring oxygen saturation. Measured oxyen saturation of 95 percent or more is satisfactory [50]. The lung segment from which the sample is obtained will be well ventilated if the patient breathes slowly and deeply.

A valid PAWP measurement requires a patent vascular channel between the left atrium and catheter tip. Thus, the PAWP approximates pulmonary venous pressure (and therefore left atrial pressure) only if the catheter tip lies in zone 3 of the lungs [13,54,55]. (The lung is divided into three physiologic zones, dependent on the relationship of PA, pulmonary venous, and alvolar pressures. In zone 3, the PA and pulmonary venous pressure exceed the alveolar pressure, ensuring an uninterrupted column of blood between the catheter tip and the pulmonary veins.) If, on portable lateral chest radiograph, the catheter tip is below the level of the left atrium (posterior position in supine patients), it can be assumed to be in zone 3. This assumption holds if applied PEEP is less than 15 cm H_2O and the patient is not markedly volume-depleted. Position of the catheter in zone 3 may also be determined by certain physiologic characteristics (Table 4-4). A catheter wedged outside zone 3 will show marked respiratory variation, an unnaturally smooth vascular waveform, and misleading high pressures.

With a few exceptions [56], estimates of capillary hydrostatic filtration pressure from PAWP are acceptable [55]. It should be noted that measurement of PAWP does not take into account capillary permeability, serum colloid osmotic pressure, interstitial pressure, or actual pulmonary capillary resistance [57,58]. These factors all play a role in the formaiton of pulmonary edema, and the PAWP should be interpreted in the context of the specific clinical situation.

Mean PAWP correlates well with left ventricular end diastolic pressure (LVEDP), provided the patient has a normal mitral valve and normal left ventricular function. In myocardial infarction, conditions with decreased left ventricular compliance (e.g., ischemia, left ventricular hypertrophy), and conditions

Table 4-4. Checklist for Verifying Position of Pulmonary Artery Catheter

	Zone 3	Zone 1 or 2
PAWP contour	Cardiac ripple (A + V waves)	Unnaturally smooth
PAD vs PAWP	PAD > PAWP	PAD < PAWP
PEEP Trial	$\Delta PAWP < 1/2 \Delta PEEP$	$\Delta PAWP > 1/2 \Delta PEEP$
Respiratory variation of PAWP	$< 1/2 \Delta P_{ALV}$	$\geq 1/2 \Delta P_{ALV}$
Catheter tip location	LA level or below	Above LA level

PAWP = pulmonary artery wedge pressure; PAD = pulmonary artery diastolic pressure; P_{ALV} = alveolar pressure; PEEP = positive end-expiratory pressure; LA = left atrium.
Adapted from Marini JJ: Hemodynamic monitoring with the pulmonary artery catheter. *Critical Care Clinics* 2:3, 1986, with permission.

with markedly increased left ventricular filling pressure (e.g., dilated cardiomyopathy), the contribution of atrial contraction to left ventricular filling is increased. Thus, the LVEDP may be significantly higher than mean left atrial pressure or PAWP [13,55].

End expiration provides a readily identifiable reference point for PAWP interpretation because pleural pressure returns to baseline at the end of passive deflation (approximately equal to atmospheric pressure). Pleural pressure can exceed the normal resting value with active expiratory muscle contraction or use of PEEP. How much PEEP is transmitted to the pleural space cannot be estimated easily, since it varies depending on lung compliance and other factors. When normal lungs deflate passively, end-expiratory pleural pressure increases by approximately one-half the applied PEEP. In patients with reduced lung compliance (e.g., adult respiratory distress syndrome [ARDS]), the "transmitted" fraction may be one-fourth or less of the PEEP value. In the past, PEEP levels greater than 10 mm Hg were thought to interrupt the column of blood between the left atrium and PA catheter tip, causing the PAWP to reflect alveolar pressure more accurately than left atrial pressure. However, two recent studies suggest that this may not hold true in all cases. Hasan and colleagues concluded that the PAWP-left atrial fluid column was protected by lung injury [59], and Teboul and coworkers could find no significant discrepancy between PAWP and simultaneosly measured LVEDP at PEEP levels of 0, 10, and 16 to 20 cm H_2O in patients with ARDS [60]. They hypothesize that (1) a large intrapulmonary right-to-left shunt may provide a number of microvessels shielded from alveolar pressure, allowing free communication from PA to pulmonary veins; or (2) in ARDS, both vascular and lung compliance may decrease, reducing transmission of alveolar pressure to the pulmonary microvasculature, maintaining an uninterrupted blood column from the catheter tip to the left atrium.

Although it is difficult to estimate precisely the true transmural vascular pressure in a patient on PEEP, temporarily disconnecting PEEP to measure PAWP is not recommended. Since the hemodynamics have been destabilized, these measurements will be of questionable value. Venous return increases acutely after discontinuation of PEEP [61,62,63], and abrupt removal of PEEP will cause hypoxia, which may not reverse quickly on reinstitution of PEEP [63,64,65]. A more in-depth discussion of measurement and interpretation of pulmonary vascular pressures on PEEP is found in Chapter 66.

CARDIAC OUTPUT

Thermodilution Technique. A catheter equipped with a thermistor 4 cm from its tip allows calculation of cardiac output using the thermodilution principle [23,66]. Correlation with the Fick technique as applied in the cardiac catheterization laboratory is excellent [67]. The thermodilution principle holds that if a known quantity of cold solution is introduced into the circulation and adequately mixed (passage through two valves and a ventricle is adequate), the resultant cooling curve recorded at a downstream site allows calculation of net bloodflow. Cardiac output is inversely proportional to the integral of the time-versus-temperature curve.

In practice, a known amount of cold solution (typically 10 ml of D_5W in adults and 5 ml of D_5W in children) is injected into the right atrium via the catheter's proximal port. The thermistor allows recording of the baseline PA blood temperature and subsequent temperature change. The resulting curve is usually analyzed by computer, although it can be analyzed manually by simple planimetric methods. Correction factors are

added by catheter manufacturers to account for the mixture of cold indicator with warm residual fluid in the catheter injection lumen and the heat transfer from the catheter walls to the cold indicator.

Reported coefficients of variation using triplicate determinations, using 10 ml of cold injectate and a bedside computer, are approximately 4 percent or less [36,37]. Use of room-temperature injectate causes a slightly greater variability and is not recommended in states in which variations in PA blood temperature are expected (patients with severe shortness of breath, on mechanical ventilators, or in very-high-output states). Attempts to repeat the injection of cold solution during the same point in the respiratory cycle should be made in these patients [27]. Variations in the rate of injection can also introduce error into cardiac output determinations, and it is thus important that the solution be injected as rapidly as possible. Careful attention must be paid to the details of this procedure; even then, changes of less than 10 to 15 percent above or below an initial value may not truly establish directional validity [38]. Thermodilution cardiac output is inaccurate in low-output states, tricuspid regurgitation, and atrial or ventricular septal defects [68].

Fick Technique. When thermodilution technology is unavailable, cardiac output can be estimated using the Fick principle. This principle states that the total release or uptake of a substance by an organ equals the product of bloodflow through that organ times the difference of arteriovenous concentrations of the substance. Oxygen is the substance most conveniently used, and pulmonary bloodflow is in practice assumed to be equal to cardiac output. The formula employed is:

$$\text{Cardiac output} = \frac{\text{oxygen consumption (ml/min)}}{\text{arterial } O_2 \text{ content} - \text{venous } O_2 \text{ content}}$$

Oxygen consumption (VO_2) varies according to individual as well as by age and sex; accurate measurement in the cardiac catheterization laboratory involves collection of expired oxygen in a Douglas bag over a specified time period. Oxygen consumption is estimated in the ICU setting, for practical reasons, as being 250 ml per minute for a 70-kg man. It can be more generally estimated as 130 ml times body surface area if body weight consists of 15 percent or more of fat, or 140 ml times body surface area if fat content is estimated at 5 percent or less. Body surface area can be estimated using the patient's height and weight (Fig. 4-19).

Blood oxygen content is calculated by accounting for the patient's hemoglobin content and the theoretic oxygen-carrying capacity of hemoglobin as follows:

$$\text{Oxygen content} = \% \text{ saturation} \times \text{Hgb (gm/dl)} \\ \times 1.39 \text{ (ml } O_2/\text{gm Hgb)} \times 10$$

This equation to determine mixed venous oxygen content in the PA cannot be employed when any right-to-left, left-to-right, or bidirectional intracardiac shunt exists, since these situations violate the fundamental assumption that pulmonary bloodflow equals cardiac output. Also, since both oxygen consumption and blood oxygen content are estimated in the ICU setting, absolute values for cardiac output using this technique should be treated with caution. The utility of the Fick technique lies in its convenience and ability to provide an accurate sense of trends in cardiac output changes. Normal values for arterial-venous oxygen content difference, mixed venous oxygen saturation, and cardiac output can be found in Table 4-5.

A sample calculation of cardiac output for a 70-kg man on room air with a hemoglobin of 14 gm per deciliter, an arterial

BSA

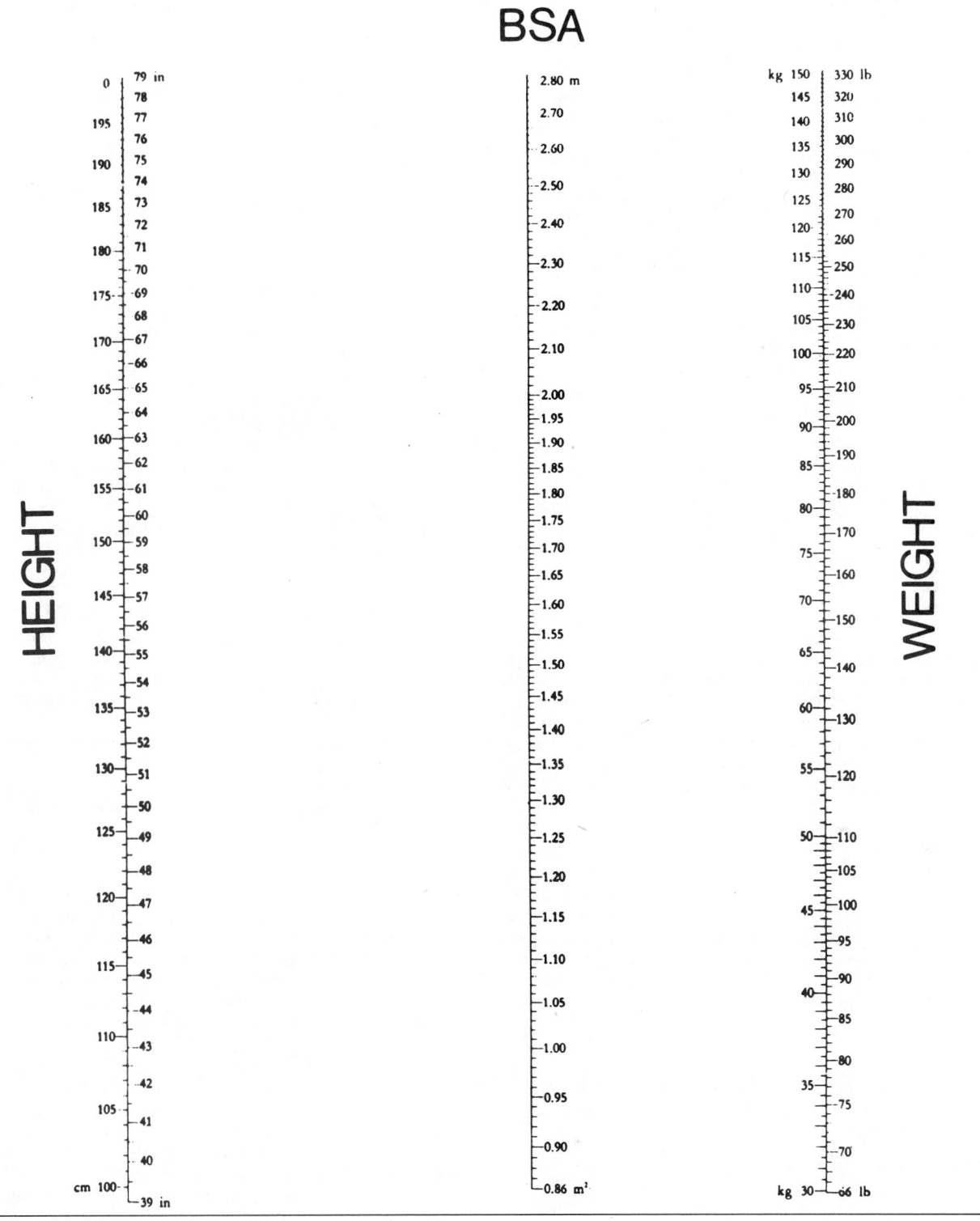

Fig. 4-19. Nomogram for calculating body surface area of adults from height and weight (in m²). (From Gore JM, Alpert JS: *Handbook of Hemodynamic Monitoring.* Boston, Little, Brown, 1984. With permission.)

Table 4-5. Selected Hemodynamic
Variables Derived from Right Heart Catheterization

Hemodynamic variable	Normal range
Arterial venous content difference	3.5–5.5 ml/100 ml
Cardiac index	2.5–4.5 L/min/m²
Cardiac output	3.0–7.0 L/min
Left ventricular stroke work index	45–60 gm/beat/m²
Mixed venous oxygen content	18.0 ml/100 ml
Mixed venous saturation	75% (approx.)
Oxygen consumption	200–250 ml/min
Pulmonary vascular resistance	120–250 dyne/sec/cm⁻⁵
Stroke volume	70–130 ml/contraction
Stroke volume index	40–50 ml/contraction/m²
Systemic vascular resistance	1100–1500 dyne/sec/cm²

Adapted from Gore JM, Alpert JS: *Handbook of Hemodynamic Monitoring.* Boston, Little, Brown, 1984, with permission.

oxygen saturation of 95 percent, and a mixed venous oxygen saturation of 70 percent, follows:

$$\text{Cardiac output} = \frac{250 \text{ ml/min}}{(0.95)(14)(1.39)(10) - (0.70)(14)(1.39)(10)}$$

$$= \frac{250 \text{ ml/min}}{181 - 136 \text{ ml/L}}$$

$$= 5.55 \text{ L/min}$$

ANALYSIS OF MIXED VENOUS BLOOD. Cardiac output can be approximated merely by examining mixed venous (pulmonary artery) oxygen saturation. If cardiac output rises, then the mixed venous oxygen partial pressure will rise, since peripheral tissues need to exact less oxygen per unit of blood. Conversely, if cardiac output falls, peripheral extraction from each unit will increase to meet the needs of metabolizing tissues. Thus there is a direct proportionality, and serial determinations of mixed venous oxygen saturation can display trends in cardiac output. Normal mixed venous oxygen saturation is 70 to 75 percent; values less than 60 percent are associated with heart failure and values less than 40 percent with shock [69]. Potential sources of error in this determination include extreme low flow states where poor mixing may occur and contamination of desaturated mixed venous blood by saturated pulmonary capillary blood when the sample is aspirated too quickly through the nonwedged catheter [17]. Fiberoptic reflectance oximetry pulmonary artery catheters can continuously measure and record mixed venous oxygen saturations in appropriate clinical situations [26,33].

DERIVED PARAMETERS. Useful hemodynamic parameters that can be derived using data with PA catheters include:

1. Cardiac index = $\dfrac{\text{cardiac output (CO) in L/min}}{\text{body surface area (BSA) in m}^2}$

2. Stroke Volume = $\dfrac{\text{cardiac output (L/min)}}{\text{heart rate (beats/min)}}$

3. Stroke index = $\dfrac{\text{CO (L/min)}}{\text{heart rate (beats/min)} \times \text{BSA (m}^2)}$

4. Mean arterial pressure (mm Hg) = $\dfrac{(2 \times \text{diastolic}) + \text{systolic}}{3}$

5. Systemic vascular resistance (dyne/sec/cm⁻⁵) =

$$\frac{\text{mean arterial pressure} - \text{mean right atrial pressure (mm Hg)}}{\text{cardiac output (L/Min)}} \times 80$$

6. Pulmonary arteriolar resistance (dyne/sec/cm⁻⁵) =

$$\frac{\text{mean PA pressure} - \text{mean PCW pressure (mm Hg)}}{\text{CO (L/min)}} \times 80$$

7. Total pulmonary resistance (dyne/sec/cm⁻⁵) =

$$\frac{\text{mean PA pressure (mm Hg)}}{\text{CO (L/min)}} \times 80$$

8. Left ventricular stroke work index =

$$\frac{1.36 \, (\text{MAP} - \text{PAWP}) \times \text{SI}}{100}$$

9. Oxygen delivery (DO₂) (ml/min/M²) =

Cardiac index × arterial O₂ content

Normal values are listed in Table 4-5.

Clinical Applications

Table 4-6 summarizes specific hemodynamic patterns for a variety of disease entities in which PA catheters are indicated. (See Chaps. 37, 38, 42, 60, 171, and 173 for more detailed discussion.) The examples given here illustrate the type of data generated and how they influence clinical decisions.

NORMAL RESTING HEMODYNAMIC PROFILE. The finding of normal cardiac output associated with normal left and right heart filling pressures is useful in establishing a noncardiovascular basis to explain abnormal symptoms or signs and as a baseline to gauge a patient's disease progression or response to therapy. Right atrial pressures of 0 to 6 mm Hg, PA systolic pressures of 15 to 30 mm Hg, PA diastolic pressures of 5 to 12 mm Hg, PA mean (PAM) pressures of 9 to 18 mm Hg, PAWP of 5 to 12 mm Hg, and a cardiac index exceeding 2.5 liters per minute per M² characterize a normal cardiovascular state at rest.

HYPOVOLEMIA. Decreases in cardiac index, right atrial pressure, and PAWP (with or without an accompanying fall in systemic blood pressure and the clinical picture of shock) are consistent with hypovolemia. Overvigorous diuretic therapy, hemorrhage, and "third space" fluid losses are common etiologies. At a PAWP less than 15 to 18 mm Hg, particularly in patients with acute myocardial infarction and decreased left ventricular compliance, small increases in PAWP/LVEDP resulting from volume replacement therapy may cause marked increases in stroke volume as ventricular function moves along the steep portion of the Starling curve. Attainment of slightly higher left heart filling pressures (18–24 mm Hg) may prove optimal for improving cardiac index in patients in whom "relative" hypovolemia complicates acute myocardial infarction. Right ventricular failure (as manifested by elevated right atrial and right ventricular end-diastolic pressures) may complicate hypovolemia and should not preclude volume loading in patients whose PAWP levels and other clinical signs indicate its requirement. Septic shock may cause the coexistence of a high cardiac index, a low PAWP, and a markedly low peripheral vascular resistance. Vasoconstricting agents and volume repletion may be helpful in such patients.

PULMONARY CONGESTION. Pulmonary congestion resulting from fluid overload or left ventricular failure is characterized

Table 4-6. Hemodynamic Parameters in Commonly Encountered Clinical Situations (Idealized)

	RA	RV	PA	PAWP	AO	CI	SVR	PVR
Normal	0–6	25/0–6	25/6–12	6–12	130/80	≥2.5	1500	≤250
Hypovolemic shock	0–2	15–20/0–2	15–20/2–6	2–6	≤90/60	<2.0	>1500	≤250
Cardiogenic shock	8	50/8	50/35	35	≤90/60	<2.0	>1500	≤250
Septic shock								
Early	0–2	20–25/0–2	20–25/0–6	0–6	≤90/60	≥2.5	<1500	<250
Late[a]	0–4	25/4–10	25/4–10	4–10	≤90/60	<2.0	>1500	>250
Acute massive pulmonary embolism	8–12	50/12	50/12–15	≤12	≤90/60	<2.0	>1500	>450
Cardiac tamponade	12–18	25/12–18	25/12–18	12–18	≤90/60	<2.0	>1500	≤250
AMI without LVF	0–6	25/0–6	25/12–18	≤18	140/90	≤2.5	1500	≤250
AMI with LVF	0–6	30–40/0–6	30–40/18–25	>18	140/90	>2.0	>1500	>250
Biventricular failure 2° to LVF	>6	50–60/>6	50–60/25	18–25	120/80	~2.0	>1500	>250
RVF 2° to RVI	12–20	30/12–20	30/12	<12	≤90/60	<2.0	>1500	>250
COR pulmonale	>6	80/>6	80/35	<12	120/80	~2.0	>1500	>400
Idiopathic pulmonary hypertension	0–6	80–100/0–6	80–100/40	<12	100/60	<2.0	>1500	>500
Acute VSR[b]	6	60/6–8	60/35	30	≤90/60	<2.0	>1500	>250

RA = right atrium; RV = right ventricle; PA = pulmonary artery; PAWP = pulmonary artery wedge pressure; AO = aortic; SVR = systemic vascular resistance; PVR = pulmonary vascular resistance; AMI = acute myocardial infarction; LVF = left ventricular failure; RVI = right ventricular infarction; RVF = right ventricular failure; VSR = ventricular septal rupture; CI = cardiac index
[a]Hemodynamic profile seen in approximately $\frac{1}{3}$ of patients in late septic shock.
[b]Confirmed by appropriate RA–PA oxygen saturation step-up. See text for discussion.
Adapted from Gore JM, Alpert JS: *Handbook of Hemodynamic Monitoring*. Boston, Little, Brown, 1984, with permission.

by a PAWP in excess of 18 mm Hg or as high as 30 mm Hg or more in pulmonary edema. Diuretics in such circumstances tend to relieve congestion without alteration in cardiac output, since changes occur on the flat portion of the Starling curve. Inotropic drugs and/or vasodilator agents are added as indicated to attempt further preload or afterload reduction in cases of severe pump failure (Chap. 42).

Pulmonary edema can occur at PAWP levels considerably lower than those listed above when the primary problem involves either a decrease in plasma colloid oncotic pressure or changes in the pulmonary capillary membranes. Examples include ARDS (with "capillary leakage"), severe hypoproteinemia, and overzealous administration of crystalloid solutions. Clinical evidence of respiratory distress and radiographic suggestion of pulmonary edema with normal left heart filling pressures and function suggest the presence of noncardiac pulmonary edema (Chap. 54).

HEART FAILURE. Cardiogenic shock is characterized by signs of peripheral hypoperfusion and shock in conjunction with hemodynamic data evidencing a markedly diminished cardiac index and markedly elevated PAWP. Milder degrees of left ventricular failure show correspondingly less depression in cardiac output (diminished stroke volumes often compensated by increases in heart rate) but are still characterized by elevated PAWP and varying degrees of pulmonary congestion (Chap. 42).

Right ventricular failure is suggested by increases in right ventricular end-diastolic and mean right atrial pressures. If it is caused by left ventricular failure, these increases will be accompanied by an increased PAWP and a decreased cardiac output. If caused by pulmonary vascular disease or occlusion, or in the setting of an isolated RV infarction, indices of left heart filling and function may be normal (Chaps. 45, 64, 171) [70].

TRICUSPID INSUFFICIENCY. Tricuspid insufficiency generally occurs in the setting of pulmonary hypertension and right ventricular dilatation and usually presents as a chronic condition [71]. It causes accentuation of the right atrial V wave with a steep *y* descent and attendant elevation of the mean right atrial pressure. Tricuspid insufficiency interferes with measurement of thermodilution cardiac output because of the back-and-forth flow of the indicator between the right atrium and right ventricle.

ACUTE MITRAL REGURGITATION. Acute mitral regurgitation should be considered when a systolic murmur develops in the setting of acute ischemia or severe left ventricular failure of any origin. Left ventricular blood floods a normal-sized, noncompliant left atrium during ventricular systole, causing giant V waves in the wedge pressure tracing (Fig. 4-20). The giant V wave of acute mitral regurgitation may be transmitted to the PA tracing, yielding a bifed PA waveform composed of the PA systolic wave and the V wave. As the catheter is wedged, the PA systolic wave is lost but the V wave remains. It is important to note that the PA systolic wave occurs earlier in relation to the QRS of a simultaneously recorded ECG (between the QRS and T waves) than does the V wave (after the T wave).

Although a large V wave is not diagnostic of acute mitral regurgitation and is not always present in this circumstance, acute mitral regurgitation remains the most common cause of giant V waves in the PAWP tracing (Chap. 30). Prominent V waves may occur whenever the left atrium is distended and noncompliant due to left ventricular failure from any cause (e.g., ischemic heart disease, dilated cardiomyopathy) [72,73] or secondary to the increased pulmonary bloodflow in acute ventricular septal defect [74]. Acute mitral regurgitation is the rare instance when the PA end-diastolic pressure may be lower than the computer-measured mean wedge pressure [42].

ACUTE VENTRICULAR SEPTAL RUPTURE. Acute ventricular septal perforation often occurs in the same clinical settings as and produces physical findings similar to those of acute mitral regurgitation. Ventricular septal rupture can be rapidly demonstrated by documenting a marked oxygen saturation step-up in the PA or right ventricle as compared to the right atrium [75]. An oxygen step-up greater than 1.0 volume percent (10% oxygen saturation step-up) between the right atrium and right ventricle indicates a significant left-to-right shunt at the ventricular level (Chap. 40).

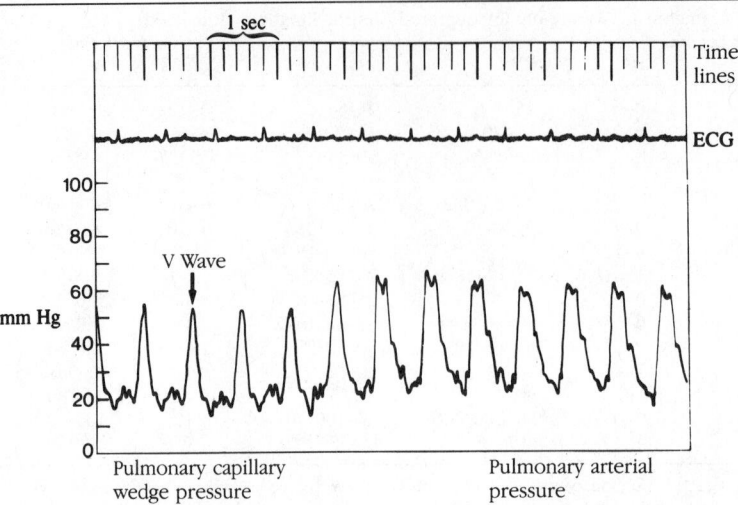

Fig. 4-20. Pulmonary artery and pulmonary artery wedge tracings with giant V waves distorting with PA recording. (Adapted from Gore JM, Zwerner PL: Hemodynamic monitoring in acute myocardial infarction, in Alpert JS, Francis GS (eds): *Modern Coronary Care.* Boston, Little, Brown, 1990. With permission.)

Care must be taken when interpreting oxygen saturations obtained in acute ventricular septal rupture. Right atrial venous blood is from three sources: the inferior vena cava, the superior vena cava, and the coronary sinus. Right atrial oxygen saturation is misleadingly low if sampled adjacent to the coronary sinus. However, if significant tricuspid insufficiency is present in addition to acute ventricular septal rupture, the right atrial saturation will be misleadingly increased, since arterial blood will cross the ventricular septum and then regurgitate into the right atrium. In patients with an acute ventricular septal rupture, mixed venous blood should be sampled from the inferior and superior vena cavae [11]. As previously noted, a prominent V wave may be present in the PAWP tracing. Unusual causes of an oxygen step-up in the right ventricle are coronary fistula to the right ventricle, atrial septal defect primum, and patent ductus arteriosus with pulmonic regurgitation.

RIGHT VENTRICULAR INFARCTION. Right ventricular infarction typically occurs in the setting of inferior myocardial infarction. The signs and symptoms of right ventricular infarction are discussed in Chapter 45. The hemodynamic findings are characteristic, although they may be confused with cardiac tamponade or constrictive pericarditis. The right atrial pressure is elevated (frequently >10 mm Hg) and often disproportionately increased relative to the PAWP [76]. Right atrial waveform reveals prominent x and y descents, with the y descent occasionally exceeding the x descent due to a dilated noncompliant right ventricle confined by a nondistensible pericardium [77,78]. These abnormalities may become exaggerated as right atrial pressure increases during volume expansion therapy. The right atrial pressure does not decline with inspiration and may actually increase (Kussmaul's sign). Right ventricular end-diastolic pressure and volume are elevated and right ventricular stroke volume is decreased, resulting in a narrowed pulmonary artery pulse pressure. Tricuspid regurgitation may complicate right ventricular infarction if right ventricular dilatation or papillary muscle dysfunction occurs [79].

CARDIAC TAMPONADE. Cardiac tamponade constitutes a medical emergency, since rising intrapericardial pressure inter-feres with diastolic filling of the heart. The hemodynamic hallmarks of cardiac tamponade are elevation and equalization of the right atrial, right ventricular diastolic, pulmonary artery diastolic, and mean pulmonary artery wedge pressures. Examination of the right atrial pressure tracing reveals a dominant x descent due to the diminished cardiac volume during ventricular systole. The y descent is frequently absent, resulting in a unimodal right atrial pressure recording. Even in severe cardiac tamponade, the mean right atrial pressure declines with inspiration. This fact can be helpful for distinguishing cardiac tamponade from other conditions that result in elevated right-sided diastolic pressures, such as right ventricular infarction and pericardial constriction. Hypovolemia and severe underlying left ventricular dysfunction may modify the hemodynamics of cardiac tamponade. The venous pressures are only modestly elevated in the former situation, while the PAWP may be significantly higher than the right atrial pressure in the latter [80,81].

PULMONARY HYPERTENSION. A mean PA pressure greater than 20 mm Hg defines pulmonary hypertension (Chap. 51). Pulmonary hypertension can be classified as passive (increases in left atrial or left ventricular end-diastolic pressure lead to increased pulmonary pressures), active, or reactive. For a comprehensive discussion of pulmonary hypertension and how to distinguish these three types, see Chapter 64.

PULMONARY EMBOLISM. Approximately 70 percent of patients with acute pulmonary embolism demonstrate some degree of pulmonary hypertension. Generally, 25 to 30 percent of a previously normal pulmonary vascular bed becomes obstructed [82]. The mean PA pressure is typically in the range of 20 to 40 mm Hg, with right ventricular and PA systolic pressure rarely exceeding 50 mm Hg. Higher PA systolic pressures suggest a chronic component of pulmonary hypertension, since a previously normal right ventricle lacks hypertrophy and cannot generate higher PA pressures acutely. The right ventricle generally dilates and fails once right ventricular systolic pressure reaches 50 to 60 mm Hg. Pulmonary vascular resistance is elevated in pulmonary embolism, with the PA diastolic pressure remaining significantly higher (>5 mm Hg) than the mean PAWP. The PAWP is usually low or normal. The A and V waves of the PAWP tracing may disappear because the abnormal pulmonary vasculature may not allow retrograde transmission of these pressure waves from left atrium to catheter tip [42].

In patients with pulmonary emboli and/or respiratory distress of any cause, wide swings in intrathoracic pressure may be transmitted to the PAWP tracing and reduce the accuracy of the measurement. The true left ventricular filling pressure is usually overestimated in this setting. As previously mentioned, measurements should be made at end expiration [83].

Massive pulmonary embolism presenting as acute cor pulmonale with cardiogenic shock occurs when the pulmonary cross-sectional area is acutely obstructed by more than 60 percent [9]. In this setting right atrial pressure is elevated (often >10 mm Hg), right ventricular and PA systolic pressures are increased, PAWP is usually low, pulmonary vascular resistance is significantly elevated (usually greater than two times normal), and cardiac output is markedly decreased (Table 4-6).

ARRHYTHMIA DIAGNOSIS. The right atrial pressure tracing can be used both to diagnose arrhythmias and to aid in understanding their hemodynamic consequences. In atrial fibrillation, atrial systole is lost. This is reflected in the right atrial pressure tracing by disappearance of the A wave. Atrial flutter can be diagnosed by the presence of mechanical flutter waves in the right atrial pressure recording at a rate of approximately 300 per minute. During atrioventricular nodal reentrant tachycardia, the retrograde P wave is often hidden in the QRS complex on the ECG, however atrial mechanical activity can be demonstrated by the presence of regular cannon A waves in the right atrial pressure tracing [42]. Cannon A waves are the result of atrial contraction at a time when the atrioventricular valves are closed during ventricular systole. The sequence of atrial and ventricular contraction is reversed, but the two events remain associated, causing the cannon A waves to be regular. Cannon A waves are also commonly encountered during ventricular arrhythmias. The presence of irregular cannon A waves during a wide-complex tachycardia suggests ventricular tachycardia.

Pulmonary artery catheters incorporating atrial and ventricular sensing electrodes on the catheter surface help in diagnosing complex cardiac arrhythmias by allowing recording of the intracardiac electrogram. The pacing PA catheter and Paceport catheter also allow selective pacing and establishment of an optimal heart rate. The pacing PA catheter allows for atrioventricular synchronous pacing, while the Paceport allows only ventricular pacing. A Paceport catheter with separate atrial and ventricular probes is in design [25].

Complications

Minor and major complications associated with bedside balloon flotation pulmonary artery catheterization have been reported (Table 4-7). During the first 10 years the catheters were used clinically (in the 1970s), a number of studies reported a relatively high incidence of certain complications. Consequent revision of guidelines for PA catheter use and improved insertion and maintenance techniques resulted in a decreased incidence of these complications in the 1980s [84]. The majority of complications are avoidable by scrupulous attention to detail in catheter placement and maintenance [85,86].

COMPLICATIONS ASSOCIATED WITH CENTRAL VENOUS ACCESS. The insertion techniques and complications of central venous cannulation are discussed in Chapter 2. Reported local vascular complications include local arterial or venous hematomas, inadvertent entry into the carotid system, atrioventricular fistulas, and pseudoaneurysm formation [87,

Table 4-7. Complications of Pulmonary Artery Catheterization

1. Associated with central venous access
2. Balloon rupture
3. Knotting
4. Pulmonary infarction
5. Pulmonary artery perforation
6. Thrombosis, embolism
7. Arrhythmias
8. Intracardiac damage
9. Infections
10. Miscellaneous complications

88,89]. Adjacent structures, such as the thoracic duct, can be damaged, with resultant chylothorax formation. Pneumothorax can be a serious complication of insertion, although the incidence is relatively low (1–2%) [40,90,91]. The incidence of pneumothorax is higher with the subclavian approach than the internal jugular approach in some reports [92], but other studies demonstrate no difference between the two sites [93,94]. The incidence of complications associated with catheter insertion is generally considered to be inversely proportional to the operator's experience.

Some complications may be avoided by inserting the catheter from an arm vein under direct vision. Such placements, however, may be associated with a higher rate of thrombosis and make catheter manipulation more difficult; fluoroscopic guidance is generally required. To minimize the risk of mediastinal bleeding, peripheral placement should be considered in patients with abnormal hemostatic parameters and those with severe pulmonary hypertension.

BALLOON RUPTURE. This complication occurred more frequently in the early 1970s and was generally related to exceeding recommended inflation volumes. The main problems posed by balloon rupture are air emboli gaining access to the arterial circulation and/or balloon fragments embolizing to the distal pulmonary circulation. If rupture occurs during catheter insertion, the loss of the balloon's protective cushioning function can predispose to endocardial damage and attendant thrombotic and arrhythmic complications.

KNOTTING. Knotting of a catheter around itself is most likely to occur when loops form in the cardiac chambers and the catheter is repeatedly withdrawn and readvanced [95]. Knotting is avoided if care is taken not to advance the catheter significantly beyond the distances at which entrance to the ventricle or PA would ordinarily be anticipated. Knotted catheters can usually be extricated transvenously; guidewire placement [96], venotomy, or more extensive surgical procedures are occasionally necessary.

Knotting of PA catheters around intracardiac structures [97] or other intravascular catheters [98] has been reported. Rarely, entrapment of a PA catheter in cardiac sutures following open heart surgery has been reported, requiring varying approaches for removal [99].

PULMONARY INFARCTION. Peripheral migration of the catheter tip (caused by catheter softening and loop tightening with time) with persistent, undetected wedging in small branches of the PA is the most common mechanism underlying pulmonary ischemic lesions attributable to Swan-Ganz catheters [100]. These lesions are usually small and asymptomatic, often diagnosed solely on the basis of changes in the chest radiograph demonstrating a wedge-shaped pleural based density with a convex proximal contour [101].

Severe infarctions are produced if the balloon is left inflated in the wedge position for an extended period of time, thus obstructing more central branches of the PA, or if solutions are injected at relatively high pressure through the catheter lumen in an attempt to restore an apparently damped pressure trace. Pulmonary embolic phenomena resulting from thrombus formation around the catheter or over areas of endothelial damage can also result in pulmonary infarction.

The reported incidence of pulmonary infarction secondary to PA catheters in 1974 was 7.2 percent [100], but recently reported rates of pulmonary infarction are much lower. Boyd and colleagues [102] found a 1.3 percent incidence of pulmonary infarction in a prospective study of 528 PA catheterizations. Sise and co-workers [103] reported no pulmonary infarctions in a prospective study of 319 PA catheter insertions. Use of continuous heparin flush solution and careful monitoring of PA waveforms are important reasons for the decreased incidence of this complication.

PULMONARY ARTERY PERFORATION. A serious and feared complication of PA catheterization is rupture of the PA leading to hemorrhage, which can be massive and sometimes fatal [104–112]. Rupture may occur during insertion or may be delayed a number of days [112]. Pulmonary artery rupture or perforation has been reported in approximately 0.1 to 0.2 percent of patients [102,113,114], although recent pathologic data suggest the true incidence of PA perforation is somewhat higher [115]. Proposed mechanisms by which PA rupture can occur include an increased pressure gradient between PAWP and PA pressure brought about by balloon inflation and favoring distal catheter migration where perforation is more likely to occur; a wedged catheter tip position favoring eccentric or distended balloon inflation with a spearing of the tip laterally and through the vessel; cardiac pulsation causing shearing forces and damage as the catheter tip repeatedly contacts the vessel wall; presence of the catheter tip near a distal arterial bifurcation where vessel wall integrity against which the balloon is inflated may be compromised; and simple lateral pressure on vessel walls caused by balloon inflation (this tends to be greater if the catheter tip was wedged before inflation began). Patient risk factors for PA perforation include pulmonary hypertension, mitral valve disease, advanced age, hypothermia, and anticoagulant therapy. (In patients with these risk factors and in whom PADP reflects PAWP reasonably well, avoidance of subsequent balloon inflation altogether constitutes prudent prophylaxis.)

Another infrequent but life-threatening complication is false aneurysm formation associated with rupture or dissection of the PA [116]. Technique factors related to PA hemorrhage are distal placement or migration of the catheter; failure to remove large catheter loops placed in the cardiac chambers during insertion; excessive catheter manipulation; use of stiffer catheter designs; and multiple overzealous, or prolonged balloon inflations. Adherence to strict technique may decrease the incidence of this complication. In a prospective study reported in 1986, no cases of PA rupture occurred in 1400 patients undergoing PA catheterization for cardiac surgery [92].

Pulmonary artery perforation typically presents with massive hemoptysis. Emergency management includes immediate wedge arteriogram and bronchoscopy, intubation of the unaffected lung, and consideration of emergency lobectomy or pneumonectomy. Pulmonary artery catheter balloon tamponade resulted in rapid control of bleeding in one case report [117]. Application of PEEP to intubated patients may also tamponade hemorrhage caused by a PA catheter [118,119].

THROMBOEMBOLIC COMPLICATIONS. Since PA catheters constitute foreign bodies in the cardiovascular system and can potentially damage the endocardium, they are associated with an increased incidence of thrombosis. Thrombi encasing the catheter tip and aseptic thrombotic vegetations forming at endocardial sites in contact with the catheter have been reported [100,120,121,122]. Extensive clotting around the catheter tip can occlude the pulmonary vasculature distal to the catheter, and thrombi anywhere in the venous system or right heart can serve as a source of pulmonary emboli. Subclavian venous thrombosis, presenting with unilateral neck vein distention and upper extremity edema, may occur in up to 2 percent of subclavian placements [123,124]. Venous thrombosis complicating percutaneous internal jugular vein catheterization is fairly commonly reported, although its clinical importance remains uncertain [125]. Consistently damped pressure tracings without evidence of peripheral catheter placement or pulmonary vascular occlusion should arouse suspicion of thrombi at the catheter tip. A changing relationship of PADP to PAWP over time should raise concern about possible pulmonary emboli.

If an underlying hypercoagulable state is known to exist, if catheter insertion was particularly traumatic, or if prolonged monitoring becomes necessary, one should consider cautiously anticoagulating the patient.

Heparin-bonded catheters reduce thrombogenicity [21] and have become the most commonly employed PA catheters. An important complication of heparin-bonded catheters is heparin-induced thrombocytopenia [126,127]. Routine platelet counts are recommended for patients with heparin-bonded catheters in place.

RHYTHM DISTURBANCES. Atrial and ventricular arrhythmias occur commonly during insertion of PA catheters [128]. Premature ventricular contractions occurred during 11 percent of the catheter insertions originally reported by Swan and co-workers [1].

Recent studies have reported advanced ventricular arrhythmias (three or more consecutive ventricular premature beats) approximately 30 to 60 percent of patients undergoing right heart catheterization [92,129–132]. Most arrhythmias are self-limited and do not require treatment, but sustained ventricular arrhythmias requiring treatment occur in 0 to 3 percent of patients [102,131,133]. Risk factors associated with increased incidence of advanced ventricular arrhythmias are acute myocardial ischemia or infarction, hypoxia, acidosis, hypocalcemia, and hypokalemia [131,132]. Prophylactic use of lidocaine in these higher-risk patients may reduce the incidence of this complication [134]. A recent study [135] suggests that a right lateral tilt position (5-degree angle) during PA catheter insertion is associated with a lower incidence of malignant ventricular arrhythmias than the Trendelenburg position.

Although the majority of arrhythmias occur during catheter insertion, arrhythmias may develop at any time after the catheter has been correctly positioned. These arrhythmias are due to mechanical irritation of the conducting system and may be persistent. Ventricular ectopy may also occur if the catheter tip falls back into the right ventricular outflow tract. Evaluation of catheter-induced ectopy should include assessment of the distal lumen pressure tracing to ensure the catheter has not slipped into the right ventricle and portable chest radiograph to evaluate catheter position. Lidocaine may be used but is unlikely to ablate the ectopy because the irritant is not removed. If the arrhythmia persists after lidocaine therapy or is associated with hemodynamic compromise, the catheter should be removed. Catheter removal should be performed by physicians under continuous ECG monitoring, since the ectopy occurs almost as frequently during catheter removal as during insertion [136,137].

Right bundle branch block (usually transient) can also complicate catheter insertion [138–141]. Patients undergoing anesthesia induction, those in the early stages of acute anteroseptal myocardial infarction, and those with acute pericarditis appear particularly susceptible to this complication. Patients with preexisting left bundle branch block are at risk for developing complete heart block during catheter insertion [142,143,144].

The frequency of catheter-induced right bundle branch block may be low, but the results may be disastrous. We suggest that these patients not be catheterized unless a temporary pacemaker can be inserted quickly or even prophylactically [142,143,144]. If a prophylactic temporary pacemaker is not selected, alternative considerations include use of an external transthoracic pacing device, a PA catheter with a specially designed Paceport, or a pacing PA catheter (electrodes mounted on catheter surface). The operator should be familiar with the various limitations on these methods.

INTRACARDIAC DAMAGE. Damage to the right heart chambers, tricuspid valve, pulmonic valve, and their supporting structures as a consequence of PA catheterization has been reported [124,145–152]. The incidence of catheter-induced endocardial disruption detected by pathologic examination varies from 3.4 [153] to 75 percent [148], but most studies suggest a range of 20 to 30 percent [124,149,150]. These lesions consist of hemorrhage, sterile thrombus, intimal fibrin deposition, and nonbacterial thrombotic endocarditis. The clinical significance is not clear, but there is concern that they may serve as a nidus for infectious endocarditis. Garrison and Freedman [154] demonstrated this theory in 1970. They produced infective endocarditis in rabbit hearts after induction of platelet-fibrin thromb (created by intracardiac manipulation of polyethylene catheters) and subsequent catheter contamination with *Staphylococcus aureus*.

Direct damage to the cardiac valves and supporting chordae occurs primarily by withdrawal of the catheters while the balloon is inflated [1]. However, chordal rupture has been reported despite balloon deflation [118]. The incidence of intracardiac and valvular damage discovered on postmorten examination is considerably higher than that of clinically significant valvular dysfunction.

INFECTIONS. Catheter-related septicemia (same pathogen growing from blood and catheter tip) was reported in up to 2 percent of patients undergoing bedside catheterization in the 1970s [129,155]. However, the incidence of septicemia related to the catheter appears to have declined in recent years, with a number of recent studies suggesting a rate of 0 to 1 percent [92,156,157]. In situ time of more than 72 to 96 hours significantly increases the risk of catheter-related sepsis. Right-sided septic endocarditis has been reported [151,158], but the true incidence of this complication is unknown. Becker and colleagues noted two cases of left ventricular abscess formation in patients with PA catheters and *S. aureus* septicemia [147]. Incidence of catheter colonization or contamination varies from 5 to 20 percent, depending on the duration of catheter placement and criteria used to define colonization [157,159]. Currently, it appears that there is no method to assess in situ bacterial colonization of PA catheters accurately and that there is no correlation between positive and negative blood cultures and catheter-related infection [118].

Pressure transducers have also been identified as an occasional source of infection [160]. The chance of introducing infection into a previously sterile system is increased during injections for cardiac output determinations and during blood withdrawal. Approaches to reduce the risk of catheter-related infection include use of a sterile protective sleeve, antibiotic bonding to the catheter, and empiric changing of catheters over a guidewire [93,161–164].

OTHER COMPLICATIONS. Rare miscellaneous complications that have been reported include (1) hemodynamically significant decreases in pulmonary bloodflow caused by balloon inflation in the central PA in postpneumonectomy patients with pulmonary hypertension in the remaining lung [165]; (2) disruption of the catheter's intraluminal septum as a result of injecting contrast medium under pressure [166]; (3) artifactual production of a midsystolic click caused by a slapping motion of the catheter against the interventricular septum in a patient with right ventricular strain and paradoxical septal motion [167]; (4) thrombocytopenia secondary to heparin-bonded catheters [126,127]; and (5) dislodgment of pacing electrodes [168]. Multiple unusual placements of PA catheters have also been reported, including in the left pericardiophrenic vein, via the left superior intercostal vein into the abdominal vasculature, and from the superior vena cava through the left atrium and left ventricle into the aorta after open heart surgery [169,170,171].

Guidelines for Safe Use of Pulmonary Artery Catheters

As experience with PA catheters and understanding of their potential complications increase, multiple revisions and changes of emphasis in the original recommended techniques and guidelines have emerged [37,39,55,84,85,100,105,108,120,144,172]. These precautions are summarized and outlined below:

A. Avoid complications associated with catheter insertion.
1. Inexperienced personnel performing insertions must be supervised. Many hospitals require that PA catheters be inserted by a fully trained cardiologist.
2. Keep the patient as still as possible. Restraints and/or sedation may be required.
3. Strict sterile technique is mandatory.
4. Avoid vein irritation by wetting the catheter and inserting it quickly without undue manipulation.
5. Examine the postprocedure chest radiograph for pneumothorax (especially after subclavian or internal jugular venipuncture) and for catheter tip position.

B. Avoid balloon rupture.
1. Always inflate the balloon gradually. Stop inflation if no resistance is felt.
2. Do not exceed recommended inflation volume. At the recommended volume, excess air will automatically be expelled from a syringe with holes bored in it that is constantly attached to the balloon port. Maintaining recommended volume also helps prevent the inadvertent injection of liquids.
3. Keep the number of inflation-deflation cycles to a minimum.
4. Do not reuse catheters designed for single usage, and do not leave catheters in place for prolonged periods of time.
5. Use carbon dioxide as the inflation medium if communication between the right and left sides of the circulation is suspected.

C. Avoid knotting. Discontinue advancement of the catheter if entrance to right atrium, right ventricle, or PA has not been achieved at distances normally anticipated from a given insertion site. If these distances have already been significantly exceeded, or if the catheter does not withdraw easily, use fluoroscopy before attempting catheter withdrawal. Never pull forcefully on a catheter that does not withdraw easily.

D. Avoid damage to pulmonary vasculature and parenchyma.
1. Keep recording time of PAWP to a minimum, particularly in patients with pulmonary hypertension and other risk factors for PA rupture. Be sure the balloon is deflated after each PAWP recording. There is never an indication for continuous PAWP monitoring.
2. Constant pressure monitoring is required each time the balloon is inflated. It should be inflated slowly, in small increments, and must be stopped as soon as the pressure tracing changes to PAWP or damped.
3. If a wedge is recorded with balloon volumes significantly less than the inflation volume recommended on the catheter shaft, withdraw the catheter to a position where full (or near full) inflation volume produces the desired trace.
4. Anticipate catheter tip migration. Softening of the catheter material with time, repeated manipulations, and cardiac motion make distal catheter migration almost inevitable.
   a. Continuous tip pressure monitoring is recommended, and the trace must be closely watched for changes from characteristic PA pressures to those indicating a PAWP or damped tip position.
   b. Decreases in balloon inflation volumes necessary to attain wedge tracings over time should raise suspicion regarding catheter migration.
   c. Confirm satisfactory tip position with chest radiographs immediately after insertion, at the 6- to 12-hour mark, and then at least daily.
5. Do not use liquids to inflate the balloon. They may prevent deflation, and their relative incompressibility may increase lateral forces and stress on the walls of pulmonary vessels.
6. Hemoptysis is an ominous sign and should prompt an urgent diagnostic evaluation and rapid institution of appropriate therapy.
7. Avoid injecting solutions at high pressure through the catheter lumen on the assumption that clotting is the cause of the damped pressure trace. First, aspirate from the catheter. Then consider problems related to catheter position, stopcock position, transducer dome, transducers, pressure bag, flush system, or trapped air bubbles. Never flush the catheter in the wedge position.

E. Avoid thromboembolic complications.
1. Minimize trauma induced during insertion.
2. Use heparin-bonded catheters if there are no clinical contraindications.
3. Consider the judicious use of anticoagulants in patients with hypercoagulable states or other risk factors.
4. Avoid flushing the catheter under high pressure.
5. Watch for a changing PADP-PAWP relationship along with other clinical indicators of pulmonary embolism.

F. Avoid arrhythmias.
1. Constant ECG monitoring during insertion and maintenance as well as ready accessibility of all supplies for performing cardiopulmonary resuscitation, defibrillation, and temporary pacing are mandatory.
2. Use caution when catheterizing patients with an acutely ischemic myocardium or preexisting left bundle branch block. Use prophylactic antiarrhythmic drugs and/or a temporary pacemaker as indicated.
3. When the balloon is deflated, do not advance the catheter beyond the right atrium.
4. Avoid overmanipulation of the catheter.
5. Secure the catheter in place at the insertion site.
6. Watch for intermittent right ventricular pressure tracings when the catheter is thought to be in the PA position. An unexplained ventricular arrhythmia in a patient with a PA catheter in place indicates the possibility of catheter-provoked ectopy.

G. Avoid valvular damage.
1. Avoid prolonged catheterization and excessive manipulation.
2. Do not withdraw the catheter when the balloon is inflated.

H. Avoid infections.
1. Use meticulously sterile technique on insertion.
2. Avoid excessive cardiac output determinations and blood withdrawals.
3. Avoid prolonged catheterization.
4. Remove the catheter if signs of phlebitis develop. Culture the tip and use antibiotics as indicated.

Controversies

Clinical use of PA catheters has increased in recent years [173]. Although it is generally agreed that hemodynamic monitoring enhances the understanding of cardiopulmonary pathophysiology in critically ill patients, it is important to remember that the catheter itself has no direct therapeutic benefit. There is increasing concern that bedside PA catheterization may be overused [174] and the data obtained not be optimally used.

OPTIMAL HEMODYNAMIC PARAMETERS. The normal resting hemodynamic parameters listed in Table 4-2 and 4-5 are appropriate physiologic goals in normal unstressed patients. Shoemaker and colleagues [175,176,177] have proposed that patients with greater degrees of illness (e.g., postsurgery, trauma, burns, sepsis) require "supranormal" physiologic parameters to improve outcome. Using data derived from PA catheterization, these investigators retrospectively described the hemodynamic and oxygen transport variables of critically ill postoperative survivors versus nonsurvivors [178,179]. Subsequent application of these supranormal physiologic goals in prospective studies [175,177] has demonstrated favorable results. High-risk surgical patients maintained with supranormal parameters (cardiac index >4.5 L/min/m², oxygen delivery >600 ml/min/m², oxygen consumption >170 ml/min/m²) had a significantly lower mortality and fewer medical complications than patients maintained with normal hemodynamic values. It is important to recognize that patients with left ventricular dysfunction or acute myocardial infarction were not included in these studies. Attempts to maintain supranormal physiologic parameters in the latter patient groups may, in fact, be detrimental [177,180]. Further study is required to determine the applicability of this strategy in critically ill medical patients.

APPROPRIATE USE OF PULMONARY ARTERY CATHETERS. In 1987, a retrospective study by Gore and colleagues [173] showed that PA catheterization in patients with acute myocardial infarction complicated by heart failure, hypotension, or shock was associated with a higher mortality than in patients with similar complications of myocardial infarction who were not catheterized. The difference in mortality rates persisted despite multivariate analysis of the data to adjust for infarct size. The authors acknowledged the difficulty in assessing whether the patients who received a PA catheter were actually "sicker" than those who did not, given the study's retrospective nature. No specific complication of PA catheterization could be related to the increased short-term mortality, and the authors were careful not to suggest that the increased mortality was due to the use of the PA catheter [181].

Two additional studies reported similar results [182,183]. Zion and colleagues [182] reported a retrospective study of PA catheters in patients with acute myocardial infarction; survival was not improved in patients receiving a PA catheter. In a unique prospective study, Guyatt et al. [183] demonstrated a mortality benefit of PA catheterization in a diverse critically ill patient population.

Varying interpretations of these reports have spurred a spirited debate in the medical literature. Certain authorities believe the risk-benefit ratio for PA catheterization is far too great to continue use of this technique [184,185,186]. Others contend that the limitations of the previously mentioned studies do not allow such a definitive conclusion and therefore do not support such a moratorium [84,180,187–193]. They suggest that a prospective, randomized trial of the efficacy of PA catheters be undertaken, first called for as far back as 1980 [194]. The recent controversy regarding the PA catheter has added fuel to the fire [189,195]. Such a study would require strict treatment protocols and standardization of physician skills [180]. This fact was underscored by a 1990 multicenter study that reported physicians' abilities to interpret and apply data obtained from PA catheterization to be extremely variable (mean test score 67% correct) and stressed that such deficiencies may lead to "inappropriate therapeutic decisions and increased patient morbidity" [196]. Until the results of future studies are available, clinicians employing hemodynamic monitoring should carefully assess the risk-benefit ratio on an individual patient basis. The physician should understand the indications, insertion techniques, equipment, and data that can be generated prior to undertaking PA catheter insertion [197]. Pulmonary artery catheterization must not delay or replace bedside clinical evaluation and treatment.

References

1. Swan HJC, Ganz W, Forrester J, et al: Catheterization of the heart in man with use of a flow-directed balloon-tipped catheter. *N Engl J Med* 283:447, 1970.
2. Rutherford BD, McCann WD, O'Donovan TPB: The value of monitoring pulmonary artery pressure for early detection of left ventricular failure following myocardial infarction. *Circulation* 43:655, 1971.
3. Carabello B, Cohn PF, Alpert JS: Hemodynamic monitoring in patients with hypotension after myocardial infarction. *Chest* 74:5, 1978.
4. Connors AF, McCaffree DR, Gray BA: Evaluation of right heart catheterization in the critically ill patient without acute myocardial infarction. *N Engl J Med* 308:263, 1983.
5. Waller J, Johnson SP, Kaplan JA: Usefulness of pulmonary artery catheters during aortocoronary bypass surgery. *Anesth Analg* 61:221, 1982.
6. Iberti TJ, Fisher CJ: A prospective study on the use of the pulmonary artery catheter in a medical intensive care unit: Its effects on diagnosis and therapy. *Crit Care Med* 11:238, 1983.
7. Gorlin R: Current concepts in cardiology: Practical cardiac hemodynamics. *N Engl J Med* 296:203, 1977.
8. Dalen JE: Bedside hemodynamic monitoring. *N Engl J Med* 301:1176, 1979.
9. Gore JM, Alpert JS, Benotti JR, et al: *Handbook of Hemodynamic Monitoring.* Boston, Little, Brown, 1984.
10. Keefer FR, Barash PG: Pulmonary artery catheterization: A decade of clinical progress? *Chest* 84:241, 1984.
11. Gore JM, Zwerner PL: Hemodynamic monitoring of acute myocardial infarction, in Alpert JS, Francis GS (eds): *Modern Coronary Care.* Boston, Little, Brown, 1990, p 139.
12. Wiedermann HP, Matthay MA, Matthay RA: Cardiovascular-pulmonary monitoring in the intensive care unit, 2. *Chest* 85:656, 1984.
13. Marini JJ: Hemodynamic monitoring with the pulmonary artery catheter. *Crit Care Clin* 2:551, 1986.
14. Scalea TM, Holman M, Fuortes M, et al: Central venous blood oxygen saturation: An early, accurate measurement of volume during hemorrhage. *J Trauma* 28:725, 1988.
15. Safian RD, Come SE, Kadin M, et al: Use of pulmonary capillary wedge aspirates for the antemortum diagnosis of pulmonary microvascular tumor. *Cathet Cardiovasc Diagn* 17:112, 1989.
16. Masson RG, Krikorian J, Kukl P, et al: Pulmonary microvascular cytology in the diagnosis of lymphocytic carcinomas. *N Engl J Med* 321:71, 1989.
17. Pace NL: A critique of flow-directed pulmonary artery catheterization. *Anesthesiology* 47:455, 1977.
18. Steele P, Davies H: The Swan-Ganz catheter in the cardiac laboratory. *Br Heart J* 35:647, 1973.
19. Hesdorffer CS, Milne JF, Meyers AM, et al: The value of Swan-Ganz catheterization and volume loading in preventing renal failure in patients undergoing abdominal aneurysmectomy. *Clin Nephrol* 28:372, 1987.
20. Tuman KJ, McCarthy RJ, Spiess BD, et al: Effect of plmonary artery catheterization on outcome in patients undergoing coronary artery surgery. *Anesthesiology* 70:199, 1989.
21. Hoar PF, Wilson RM, Mangano DT, et al: Heparin bonding reduces thrombogenicity of pulmonary-artery catheter. *N Engl J Med* 305:993, 1981.
22. Mangano DT: Heparin bonding long term protection against thrombosis. *N Engl J Med* 307:894, 1982.
23. Forrester JS, Ganz W, Diamond G, et al: Thermodilution cardiac output determination with a single flow-directed catheter. *Am Heart J* 83:306, 1972.
24. Chatterjee K, Swan JHC, Ganz W, et al: Use of a balloon-tipped flotation electrode catheter for cardiac monitoring. *Am J Cardiol* 36:56, 1975.
25. Simoons ML, Demey HE, Bossaert LL, et al: The Paceport catheter: A new pacemaker system introduced through a Swan-Ganz catheter. *Cathet Cardiovasc Diagn* 15:66, 1988.
26. Baele PL, McMechan JC, Marsh HM, et al: Continuous monitoring of mixed venous oxygen saturation in critically ill patients. *Anesth Analg* 61:513, 1982.
27. Segal J, Pearl RG, Ford AJ, et al: Instantaneous and continuous cardiac output obtained with a Doppler pulmonary artery catheter. *J Am Coll Cardiol* 13:1382, 1989.
28. Vincent JL, Thirion M, Bumioulle S, et al: Thermodilution measurement of right ventricular ejection fraction with a modified pulmonary artery catheter. *Intensive Care Med* 12:33, 1986.
29. Guerrero JE, Munoz J, De Lacalle B, et al: Right ventricular systolic time intervals determined by means of a pulmonary artery catheter. *Crit Care Med* 20:1529, 1992.
30. Dhainaut JF, Brunet F, Monsallier JF, et al: Bedside evaluation of right ventricular performance using a rapid computerized thermodilution mode. *Crit. Care Med* 15:148, 1987.
31. Vincent JL: Measurement of right ventricular ejection fraction. *Intensive Care World* 7:133, 1990.
32. Nishimura RA: Another measurement of cardiac output: Is it truly needed? *J Am Coll Cardiol* 13:1393, 1989.
33. Rayput MA, Rickey HM, Bush BA, et al: A comparison between a fiberoptic flow-directed thermal dilution pulmonary artery catheter in critically ill patients. *Arch Intern Med* 149:83, 1989.
34. Hankeln K, Michelsen H, Kubeak V, et al: Continuous, on-line, real-time measurement of cardiac output and derived cardiorespiratory variables in the critically ill. *Crit Care Med* 13:1071, 1985.
35. Normann RA, Johnson RW, Messinger JE, et al: A continuous cardiac output computer based on thermodilution principles. *Ann Biomed Eng* 17:61, 1989.

36. Buchbinder N, Ganz W: Hemodynamic monitoring: Invasive techniques. *Anesthesiology* 45:146, 1976.

37. Swan HJC, Ganz W: Use of balloon flotation catheters in critically ill patients. *Surg Clin North Am* 55:501, 1975.

38. Hurst, JW, Logue RB, Rackley CE, et al: *The Heart*. New York, McGraw-Hill, 1982.

39. Russel RO, Rackley CE: *Hemodynamic Monitoring in a Coronary Intensive Care Unit*. Mount Kisco, NY, Futura, 1981.

40. Ganz W, Swan HJC: Balloon-tipped flow-directed catheters, in Grossman W (ed): *Cardiac Catheterization and Angiography*, 2nd ed. Philadelphia, Lea & Febiger, 1980, pp 78–85.

41. Barry WA, Grossman W: Cardiac catheterization, in Braunwald E (ed): *Heart Disease: A Textbook of Cardiovascular Medicine*, vol 1. Philadelphia, WB Saunders, 1988, p 287.

42. Sharkey SW: Beyond the wedge: Clinical physiology and the Swan-Ganz catheter. *Am J Med* 83:111, 1987.

43. Bohrer H, Fleischer F: Errors in biochemical and haemodynamic data obtained using introducer lumen and proximal port of Swan-Ganz catheter. *Int Care Med* 15:330, 1989.

44. Huford WE, Zapol WM: The right ventricle and critical illness: A review of anatomy, physiology, and clinical evaluation of its function. *Intensive Care Med* 14:448, 1988.

45. Diebel LN, Wilson RF, Tagett MG, et al: End diastolic volume: A better indicator of preload in the critically ill. *Arch Surg* 127:817, 1992.

46. Martyn JA, Snider MT, Farago LF, et al: Thermodilution right ventricular volume: A novel and better predictor of volume replacement in acute thermal injury. *J Trauma* 21:619, 1981.

47. Reuse C, Vincent JL, Pinsky MR, et al: Measurement of right ventricular volume during fluid challenge. *Chest* 98:14050, 1990.

48. Walston A, Kendall ME: Comparison of pulmonary wedge and left atrial pressure in man. *Am Heart J* 86:159, 1973.

49. Lange RA, Moore DM, Cigarroa RG, et al: Use of pulmonary capillary wedge pressure to assess severity of mitral stenosis: Is true left atrial pressure needed in this condition? *J Am Coll Cardiol* 13:825, 1989.

50. Alpert JS: The lessons of history as reflected in the pulmonary capillary wedge pressure. *J Am Coll Cardiol* 13:830, 1989.

51. Mond HG, Hunt D, Sloman G: Hemodynamic monitoring in the coronary care unit using the Swan-Ganz right heart catheter. *Br Heart J* 35:635, 1973.

52. Scheinman MM, Aggott JA, Rapaport E: Clinical uses of a flow-directed right heart catheter. *Arch Intern Med* 124:19, 1969.

53. Forrester JS, Diamond G, McHugh TJ, et al: Filling pressures in the right and left sides of the heart in acute myocardial infarction. *N Engl J Med* 285:190, 1971.

54. O'Quin R, Marini JJ: Pulmonary artery occlusion pressure: Clinical physiology, measurement, and interpretation. *Am Rev Respir Dis* 128:319, 1983.

55. Wiedermann HP, Matthay MA, Matthay RA: Cardiovascular-pulmonary monitoring in the intensive care unit, 1. *Chest* 85:537, 1984.

56. Timmis AD, Fowler MB, Burwood RJ, et al: Pulmonary edema without critical increase in left atrial pressure in acute myocardial infarction. *Br Med J* 283:636, 1981.

57. Holloway H, Perry M, Downey J, et al: Estimation of effective pulmonary capillary pressure in intact lungs. *J Appl Physiol* 54:846, 1983.

58. Dawson CA, Linehan JH, Rickaby DA: Pulmonary microcirculatory hemodynamics. *Ann NY Acad Sci* 384:90, 1982.

59. Hasan FM, Weiss WB, Braman SS, et al: Influence of lung injury on pulmonary wedge-left atrial pressure correlation during positive and expiratory pressure ventilation. *Ann Rev Respir Dis* 131:246, 1985.

60. Teboul JL, Zapol WM, Brun-Buisson C, et al: A comparison of pulmonary artery occlusion pressure and left ventricular end diastolic pressure during mechanical ventilation with PEEP in patients with severe ARDS. *Anesthesiology* 70:261, 1989.

61. Quist J, Pontoppridan H, Wilson R, et al: Hemodynamic responses to mechanical ventilation with PEEP: The effect of hypervolemia. *Anesthesiology* 42:45, 1975.

62. Zarins CK, Virgilio RW, Smith DE, et al: The effect of vascular volume on positive end-expiratory pressure induced cardiac output depression and wedge-left atrial pressure discrepancy. *J Surg Res* 23:348, 1977.

63. Downs JB, Douglas ME: Assessment of cardiac filling pressure occurring in continuous positive-pressure ventilation. *Crit Care Med* 8:285, 1980.

64. DeCampo T, Civetta JM: The effect of short-term discontinuation of high-level PEEP in patients with acute respiratory failure. *Crit Care Med* 7:47, 1979.

65. Luterman A, Horovitz JH, Carrico CJ, et al: Withdrawal from positive end-expiratory pressure. *Surgery* 83:328, 1978.

66. Ganz W, Swan HJC: Measurement of blood flow by thermodilution. *Am J Cardiol* 29:241, 1972.

67. Branthwaite MA, Bradley RD: Measurement of cardiac output by thermal dilution in man. *J Appl Physiol* 24:434, 1968.

68. Grossman W: Blood flow measurement: The cardiac output, in Grossman W (ed): *Cardiac Catheterization and Angiography*. Philadelphia, Lea & Febiger, 1985, p 116.

69. Goldman RH, Klughaupt M, Metcalf T, et al: Measurement of central venous oxygen saturation in patients with myocardial infarction. *Circulation* 38:941, 1968.

70. Cohn JN, Guiha NH, Broder MI, et al: Right ventricular infarction: Clinical and hemodynamic features. *Am J Cardiol* 33:209, 1974.

71. Ockene IS: Tricuspid valve disease, in Dalen JE, Alpert JS (eds): *Valvular Heart Disease*. Boston, Little, Brown, 1981, p 281.

72. Pichard AD, Kay R, Smith H, et al: Large V waves in the pulmonary wedge pressure tracing in the absence of mitral regurgitation. *Am J Cardiol* 50:1044, 1982.

73. Ruchs RM, Heuser RR, Yin FU, et al: Limitations of pulmonary wedge V waves in diagnosing mitral regurgitation. *Am J Cardiol* 49:849, 1982.

74. Bethen CF, Peter RH, Behar VS, et al: The hemodynamic simulation of mitral regurgitation in ventricular septal defect after myocardial infarction. *Cathet Cardiovasc Diagn* 2:97, 1976.

75. Meister SG, Helfant RH: Rapid bedside differentiation of ruptured interventricular septum from acute mitral insufficiency. *N Engl J Med* 287:1024, 1972.

76. Lopez-Senden J, Coma-Corella I, Gamallo C: Sensitivity and specificity of hemodynamic criteria in the diagnosis of acute right ventricular infarction. *Circulation* 64:515, 1981.

77. Arma-Canella I, Lopez-Sendon J: Ventricular compliance in ischemic right ventricular dysfunction. *Am J. Cardiol* 45:555, 1980.

78. Lorell B, Leinback RC, Pohost GM, et al: Right ventricular infarction: Clinical diagnosis and differentiation from cardiac tamponade and pericardial constriction. *Am J Cardiol* 43:465, 1979.

79. MacAllister RG, Friesinger GG, Sinclair Smith BC: Tricuspid regurgitation following inferior myocardial infarction. *Arch Intern Med* 136:95, 1976.

80. Reddy PS, Antiss EL, O'Toole JD, et al: Cardiac tamponade: Hemodynamic observations in man. *Circulation* 58:265, 1978.

81. Antman EM, Cargill V, Grossman W: Low pressure cardiac tamponade. *Ann Intern Med* 91:403, 1979.

82. McIntyre KM, Sasahara AA: The hemodynamic response to pulmonary embolism in patients without prior cardiopulmonary disease. *Am J Cardiol* 28:288, 1971.

83. Rice DL, Gaasch WH, Alexander JK, et al: Wedge pressure measurements in obstructive pulmonary disease. *Chest* 66:628, 1974.

84. Matthay MA, Chatterjee K: Bedside catheterization of the pulmonary artery: Risks compared with benefits. *Ann Intern Med* 109:826, 1988.

85. Swan HJC, Ganz W: Complications with flow-directed balloon-tipped catheters. *Ann Intern Med* 91:494, 1979.

86. Swan HJC, Ganz W: Hemodynamic measurements in clinical practice: A decade in review. *J Am Cardiol* 1:103, 1983.

87. McNabb TG, Green CH, Parket FL: A potentially serious complication with Swan-Ganz catheter placement by the percutaneous internal jugular route. *Br J Anaesth* 47:895, 1975.

88. Hansbroyh JF, Narrod JA, Rutherford R: Arteriovenous fistulas following central venous catheterization. *Intensive Care Med* 9:287, 1983.

89. Shield CF, Richardson JD, Buckley CJ, et al: Pseudoaneurysm of the brachiocephalic arteries: A complication of percutaneous internal jugular vein catheterization. *Surgery* 78:190, 1975.

90. Patel C, LaBoy V, Venus B, et al: Acute complications of pulmonary artery catheter insertion in critically ill patients. *Crit Care Med* 14:195, 1986.

91. McNabb TG, Green LH, Parker FL: A potentially serious compli-

cation with Swan-Ganz catheter placement by the percutaneous internal jugular route. *Br J Anaesth* 47:895, 1975.

92. Danen J, Bolton D: A prospective analysis of 1400 pulmonary artery catheterizations in patients undergoing cardiac surgery. *Acta Anaesthesiol Scand* 14:1957, 1986.
93. Senagere A, Waller JD, Bonnell BW, et al: Pulmonary artery catheterization: A prospective study of internal jugular and subclavian approaches. *Crit Care Med* 15:35, 1987.
94. Nembre AE: Swan-Ganz catheter. *Arch Surg* 115:1194, 1980.
95. Lipp H, O'Donoghue K, Resnekov L: Intracardiac knotting of a flow-directed balloon catheter. *N Engl J Med* 284:220, 1971.
96. Mond HG, Clark DW, Nesbitt SJ, et al: A technique for unknotting an intracardiac flow-directed balloon catheter. *Chest* 67:731, 1975.
97. Meister SG, Furr CM, Engel TR, et al: Knotting of a flow-directed catheter about a cardiac structure. *Cathet Cardiovasc Diagn* 3:171, 1977.
98. Swaroop S: Knotting of two central venous monitoring catheters. *Am J Med* 53:386, 1972.
99. Loggam C, Sanborn TA, Christian F: Ventricular entrapment of a Swan-Ganz catheter: A technique for nonsurgical removal. *J Am Coll Cardiol* 13:1422, 1989.
100. Foote GA, Schabel SI, Hodges M: Pulmonary complications of the flow-directed balloon-tipped catheter. *N Engl J Med* 290:927, 1974.
101. Wechsler RJ, Steiner RM, Kinori F: Monitoring the monitors: The radiology of thoracic catheters, wires and tubes. *Semin Roentgenol* 23:61, 1988.
102. Boyd KD. Thomas SJ, Gold J, et al: A prospective study of complications of pulmonary artery catheterizations in 500 consecutive patients. *Chest* 84:245, 1983.
103. Sise MJ, Hollingsworth P, Bumm JE, et al: Complications of the flow directed pulmonary artery catheter: A prospective analysis of 219 patients. *Crit Care Med* 9:315, 1981.
104. Barash PG, Nardi D, Hammond G, et al: Catheter-induced pulmonary artery perforation: Mechanisms, management and modifications. *J Thorac Cardiovasc Surg* 82:5, 1981.
105. Pape LA, Haffajee CI, Markis JE, et al: Fatal pulmonary hemorrhage after use of the flow-directed balloon-tipped catheter. *Ann Intern Med* 90:344, 1979.
106. Lapin ES, Murray JA: Hemoptysis with flow-directed cardiac catheterization. *JAMA* 220:1246, 1972.
107. Haapaniemi J, Gadowski R, Naini M, et al: Massive hemoptysis secondary to flow-directed thermodilution catheters. *Cathet Cardiovasc Diagn* 5:151, 1979.
108. Golden MS, Pinder T, Anderson WT, et al: Fatal pulmonary hemorrhage complicating use of a flow-directed balloon-tipped catheter in a patient receiving anticoagulant therapy. *Am J Cardiol* 32:865, 1973.
109. Page DW, Teres D, Hartshorn JW: Fatal hemorrhage from Swan-Ganz catheter. *N Engl J Med* 291:260, 1974.
110. Chun GMH, Ellestad MH: Perforation of the pulmonary artery by a Swan-Ganz catheter. *N Engl J Med* 284:1041, 1971.
111. Fleischer AG, Tyers FO, Manning GT, et al: Management of massive hemoptysis secondary to catheter-induced perforation of the pulmonary artery during cardiopulmonary bypass. *Chest* 95:1340, 1989.
112. Carlson TA, Goldenberg IF, Murray PD, et al: Catheter-induced delayed recurrent pulmonary artery hemorrhage. *JAMA* 261:1943, 1989.
113. McDaniel DD, Stone JG, Faltas AN, et al: Catheter induced pulmonary artery hemorrhage: Diagnosis and management in cardiac operations. *J Thorac Cardiovasc Surg* 82:1, 1981.
114. Shah KB, Rao TL, Laughlin S, et al: A review of pulmonary artery catheterization in 6245 patients. *Anesthesiology* 61:271, 1984.
115. Fraser RS: Catheter-induced pulmonary artery perforation: Pathologic and pathogenic features. *Hum Pathol* 18:1246, 1987.
116. Declen JD, Friloux LA, Renner JW: Pulmonary artery false-aneurysms secondary to Swan-Ganz pulmonary artery catheters. *Am J Roentgenol* 149:901, 1987.
117. Thoms R, Siproudhis L, Laurent JF, et al: Massive hemoptysis from iatrogenic balloon catheter rupture of pulmonary artery: Successful early management by balloon tamponade. *Crit Care Med* 15:272, 1987.
118. Slacken A: Complications of invasive hemodynamic monitoring in the intensive care unit. *Curr Probl Surg* 25:69, 1988.
119. Scuderi PE, Prough DS, Price JD, et al: Cessation of pulmonary artery catheter-induced endobronchial hemorrhage associated with the use of PEEP. *Anesth Analg* 62:236, 1983.
120. Yorra FH, Oblath R, Jaffe H, et al: Massive thrombosis associated with use of a Swan-Ganz catheter. *Chest* 65:682, 1974.
121. Pace NL, Horton W: Indwelling pulmonary artery catheters: Their relationship to aseptic thrombotic endocardial vegetations. *JAMA* 233:893, 1975.
122. Greene JF, Cummings KC: Aseptic thrombotic endocardial vegetations: A complication of indwelling pulmonary artery catheters. *JAMA* 225:1525, 1973.
123. Dye LE, Segall PH, Russell RO, et al: Deep venous thrombosis of the upper extremity associated with use of the Swan-Ganz catheter. *Chest* 73:673, 1978.
124. Elliot CG, Zimmerman GA, Clemmer TP: Complications of pulmonary artery catheterization in the care of critically ill patients: A prospective study. *Chest* 76:647, 1979.
125. Chastre J, et al: Thrombosis as a complication of pulmonary artery catheterization via the internal jugular vein. *N Engl J Med* 306:278, 1982.
126. Laster JL, Nichols WK, Silver D: Thrombocytopenia associated with heparin-coated catheters in patients with heparin-associated antiplatelet antibodies. *Arch Intern Med* 149:2285, 1989.
127. Laster JL, Silver D: Heparin coated catheters and heparin-induced thrombocytopenia. *J Vasc Surg* 7:667, 1988.
128. Geha DG, Davis NJ, Lappas DG: Persistent atrial arrhythmias associated with placement of a Swan-Ganz catheter. *Anesthesiology* 39:651, 1973.
129. Elliot CG, Zimmerman GA, Clemmer TP: Complications of pulmonary artery catheterization in the care of critically ill patients. *Chest* 76:647, 1979.
130. Spring CL, Jacobs JL, Caralis PV, et al: Ventricular arrhythmias during Swan-Ganz catheterization of the critically ill. *Chest* 79:413, 1981.
131. Spring CL, Pozen PG, Rozanski JJ, et al: Advanced ventricular arrhythmias during bedside pulmonary artery catheterization. *Am J Med* 72:203, 1982.
132. Patel C, Laboy V, Venus B, et al: Acute complications of pulmonary artery catheter insertion in critically ill patients. *Crit Care Med* 14:195, 1986.
133. Iberti TJ, Benjamin E, Grupzi L, et al: Ventricular arrhythmias during pulmonary artery catheterization in the intensive care unit. *Am J Med* 78:451, 1985.
134. Spring CL, Marical EH, Garcia AA, et al: Prophylactic use of lidocaine to prevent advanced ventricular arrhythmias during pulmonary artery catheterization: Prospective, double blind study. *Am J Med* 75:906, 1983.
135. Keusch DJ, Winters S, Thys DM: The patient's position influences the incidence of dysrhythmias during pulmonary artery catheterization. *Anesthesiology* 70:582, 1989.
136. Johnston W, Royster R, Beamer W, et al: Arrhythmias during removal of pulmonary artery catheters. *Chest* 85:296, 1984.
137. Damen J: Ventricular arrhythmia during insertion and removal of pulmonary artery catheters. *Chest* 88:190, 1985.
138. Luck JC, Engel TR: Transient right bundle branch block with "Swan-Ganz" catheterization. *Am Heart J* 92:263, 1976.
139. Thomson IR, Dalton BC, Lappas DG, et al: Right bundle branch block and complete heart block caused by the Swan-Ganz catheter. *Anesthesiology* 51:359, 1979.
140. Abernathy WS: Complete heart block caused by the Swan-Ganz catheter. *Chest* 65:349, 1974.
141. Morris D, Mulvihill D, Lew WY: Risk of developing complete heart block during bedside pulmonary artery catheterization in patients with left bundle branch block. *Arch Intern Med* 147:2005, 1987.
142. Lavie CJ, Gersh BJ: Pacing in left bundle branch block during Swan-Ganz catheterization (letter). *Arch Intern Med* 148:981, 1988.
143. Kaye W: Invasive monitoring techniques, in McIntyre KM, Lewis AJ (eds): *Textbook of Advanced Cardiac Life Support*, Dallas, American Heart Association, 1983, p 165.
144. Moser KM, Spragg RG: Use of the balloon tipped pulmonary artery catheter in pulmonary disease. *Ann Intern Med* 98:53, 1983.
145. Smith WR, Glauser FL, Jenison P: Ruptured chordae of the tricuspid valve: The consequence of flow-directed Swan-Ganz catheterization. *Chest* 70:790, 1976.

146. O'Toole JD, Wurtzbacher JJ, Wearner NE, et al: Pulmonary valve injury and insufficiency during pulmonary artery catheterization. *N Engl J Med* 301:1167, 1979.

147. Becker RC, Martin RG, Underwood DA: Right sided endocardial lesions and flow directed pulmonary artery catheters. *Cleve Clin J Med* 54:384, 1987.

148. Ford SE, Manley PN: Indwelling cardiac catheters: An autopsy study of associated endocardial lesions. *Arch Pathol Lab Med* 106:314, 1982.

149. Lange HW, Galliani CA, Edwards JE: Local complications associated with indwelling Swan-Ganz catheters. *Am J Cardiol* 52:1108, 1983.

150. Sage MD, Koelmeyer TD, Smeeton WMI: Evolution of Swan-Ganz catheter related pulmonary valve nonbacterial endocarditis. *Am J Forensic Med Pathol* 9:112, 1988.

151. Rowley KM, Clubb KS, Smith GJW, et al: Right sided infective endocarditis as a consequence of flow directed pulmonary artery catheterization. *N Engl J Med* 311:1152, 1984.

152. Van der Belkahn J, Fowler NO, Doerger P: Right heart catheter lesions: Any significance? *Am J Clin Pathol* 82:137, 1984.

153. Pace NL, Horton W: Indwelling pulmonary artery catheters: Their relationship to aseptic thrombotic endocardial vegetations. *JAMA* 233:893, 1975.

154. Garrison PK, Freedman LR: Experimental endocarditis. I. Staphylococcal endocarditis in rabbit hearts resulting from placement of a polyethylene catheter in the right side of the heart. *Yale J Biol Med* 42:394, 1970.

155. Prochan H, Dittei ᴍ, Jobst C, et al: Bacterial contamination of pulmonary artery catheters. *Intensive Care Med* 4:79, 1978.

156. Pinella JC, Ross DF, Martin T, et al: Study of the incidence of intravascular catheter infection and associated septicemia in critically ill patients. *Crit Care Med* 11:21, 1983.

157. Michel L, Marsh HM, McMichan JC, et al: Infection of pulmonary artery catheters in critically ill patients. *JAMA* 245: 1032, 1981.

158. Greene JF, Fitzwater JE, Clemmer TP: Septic endocarditis and indwelling pulmonary artery catheters. *JAMA* 233:891, 1975.

159. Myers ML, Austin TW, Sibbald WJ: Pulmonary artery catheter infections: A prospective study. *Ann Surg* 201:237, 1985.

160. Weinstein RA, Stamm WE, Kramer L: Pressure monitoring devices: Overlooked source of nosocomial infection. *JAMA* 236:936, 1976.

161. Singh SJ, Puri VK: Prevention of bacterial colonization of pulmonary artery catheters. *Infect Surg* 853, 1984.

162. Kopman EA, Sandza JG Jr: Manipulation of the pulmonary artery catheter after placement: Maintenance of sterility. *Anesthesiology* 48:373, 1978.

163. Heard SO, Davis RF, Skeretz RJ, et al: Influence of sterile protective sleeves on the sterility of pulmonary artery catheters. *Crit Care Med* 15:499, 1987.

164. Cobb DK, High KP, Sawyer RG, et al: A controlled trial of scheduled replacement of central venous and pulmonary artery catheters. *N Engl J Med* 327:1062, 1992.

165. Berry AJ, Geer RT, Marshall BE: Alteration of pulmonary blood flow by pulmonary artery occluded pressure measurement. *Anesthesiology* 51:164, 1979.

166. Schluger J, Green J, Giustra FX, et al: Complication with use of flow-directed catheter. *Am J Cardiol* 32:125, 1973.

167. Isner JM, Horton J, Ronan JAS: Systolic click from a Swan-Ganz catheter: Phonoechocardiographic depiction of the underlying mechanism. *Am J Cardiol* 42:1046, 1979.

168. Lawson D, Kushkins LG: A complication of multipurpose pacing pulmonary artery catheterization via the external jugular vein approach (letter). *Anesthesiology* 62:377, 1985.

169. McLellan BA, Jerman MR, French WJ, et al: Inadvertent Swan-Ganz catheter placement in the left pericardiophrenic vein. *Cathet Cardiovasc Diagn* 16:173, 1989.

170. Allyn J, Lichtenstein A, Koski EG, et al: Inadvertent passage of a pulmonary artery catheter from the superior vena cava through the left atrium and left ventricle into the aorta. *Anesthesiology* 70:1019, 1989.

171. Lazzam C, Sanborn TA, Christian F: Ventricular entrapment of a Swan-Ganz catheter: A technique for nonsurgical removal. *J Am Coll Cardiol* 13:1422, 1989.

172. Swan HJC, Ganz W: Guidelines for use of balloon-tipped catheter. *Am J Cardiol* 34:119, 1974.

173. Gore JM, Goldberg RJ, Spodick DH, et al: A community wide assessment of the use of pulmonary artery catheters in patients with acute myocardial infarction. *Chest* 92:721, 1987.

174. Robin ED: The cult of the Swan-Ganz catheter. *Ann Intern Med* 103:445, 1985.

175. Shoemaker WC, Appel PL, Dram HB, et al: Prospective trial of supranormal values of survivors as therapeutic goals in high risk surgical patients. *Chest* 94:1176, 1988.

176. Shoemaker WC, Appel PC, Kram HB: Oxygen transport measurement to evaluate tissue perfusion and titrate therapy: Dobutamine and dopamine effcts. *Crit Care Med* 19:672, 1991.

177. Shoemaker WC, Kram HB, Appel PL: Therapy of shock based on pathophysiology, monitoring, and outcome prediction. *Crit Care Med* 18:S19, 1990.

178. Bland RD, Shoemaker WC, Abraham E, et al: Hemodynamic and oxygen transport patterns in surviving and nonsurviving patients. *Crit Care Med* 13:85, 1985.

179. Bland R, Shoemaker WC, Shabot MM: Physiologic monitoring goals for the critically ill patient. *Surg Gynecol Obstet* 147:833, 1978.

180. Voyce SJ, Goldberg RJ, Gore JM: Evaluation of right heart catherization: Where do we go from here? *J Intensive Care Med* 6:98, 1991.

181. Gore JM, Dalen JE: Pulmonary artery catheters (letter). *Chest* 93:1115, 1988.

182. Zion MM, Balkin J, Rosenmann D, et al: Use of pulmonary artery catheters in patients with acute myocardial infarction: Analysis of experience in 5841 patients in the SPRINT registry. *Chest* 98:1331, 1990.

183. Guyatt G: A randomized control trial of right heart catheterization in critically ill patients. *J Intensive Care Med* 6:91, 1991.

184. Robin ED: Death by pulmonary artery flow-directed catheter. Time for a moratorium? (editorial). *Chest* 92:727, 1987.

185. Robin ED: Hazards of the Swan-Ganz catheter (letter). *Ann Intern Med* 108:151, 1988.

186. Russel RO Jr: Swan-Ganz (commentary). *Patient Care* 22:39, 1988.

187. Robin ED: Defenders of the pulmonary artery catheter (letters and reply). *Chest* 93:1059, 1988.

188. Scanlon PD: The pulmonary artery catheter dilemma (letter). *Am Rev Respir Dis* 138:491, 1988.

189. Spodick DH: Flow directed pulmonary artery catheterization: Moratorium vs clinical trial (editorial). *Chest* 95:489, 1989.

190. Sibbald WJ, Spring CL; The pulmonary artery catheter: The debate continues (editorial). *Chest* 94:899, 1988.

191. Chatterjee K, Matthay M: Right heart catheterization is a diagnostic procedure not a therapeutic intervention. *J Intensive Care Med* 6:101, 1991.

192. Goldberg RJ: Risk and benefit of pulmonary artery catheterization. *J Intensive Care Med* 3:69, 1988.

193. Dalen JE: Does pulmonary artery catheterization benefit patients with acute myocardial infarction? *Chest* 98:1313, 1990.

194. Spodick DH: Physiologic and prognostic complications of invasive monitoring: Undetermined risk/benefit ratios in patients with heart disease. *Am J Cardiol* 46:173, 1980.

195. Spodick DH: Analysis of flow-directed pulmonary artery catheterization (editorial). *JAMA* 261:1946, 1989.

196. Ibetri TJ, Fischer EP, Leibowitz AB, et al: A multicenter study of physicians' knowledge of the pulmonary artery catheter. *JAMA* 264:2928, 1990.

197. Friesinger GC, Williams SV: Clinical competence in hemodynamic monitoring: A statement for physicians from the ACP/ACC/AHA task force on clinical privileges in cardiology. *J Am Coll Cardiol* 7:1460, 1990.

198. Clark SL, Cotton DB: Clinical indications for pulmonary artery catheterization in the patient with severe preeclampsia. *Am J Obstet Gynecol* 158:453, 1988.

199. Shoemaker WC, Montgomery ES, Kaplan E, et al: Physiologic patterns in surviving and nonsurviving shock patients. *Arch Surg* 106:630, 1973.

200. Vincent JL, Reuse C, Frank N, et al: Right ventricular dysfunction in septic shock: Assessment by measurements of right ventricular ejection fraction using the thermodilution technique. *Acta Anesthesiol Scand* 33:34, 1989.

5. Temporary Cardiac Pacing

Michael G. Mooradd and
Seth T. Dahlberg

Temporary cardiac pacing may be lifesaving in a number of disease states commonly treated in the intensive care unit (ICU). The indications as well as techniques for initiating and maintaining temporary cardiac pacing should be familiar to ICU personnel.

Indications for Temporary Cardiac Pacing

As outlined in Table 5-1, temporary pacing is indicated in the management of a number of serious rhythm and conduction disturbances [1,2]. Temporary pacing catheters may also be important tools for the diagnosis of rapid heart rhythms.

BRADYARRHYTHMIAS. Rate disturbances that respond to temporary cardiac pacing include sinus bradycardia and high-grade atrioventricular (A-V) block, as well as ventricular tachycardia precipitated by episodic bradycardia [1].

Sinus bradycardia may occur in any critically ill patient; it is commonly seen in patients with myocardial infarction, hyperkalemia, antiarrhythmic medication intoxication, myxedema, and increased intracranial pressure. Bradyarrhythmias also commonly result from exaggerated vasovagal reactions to procedures routinely performed in the ICU, such as suctioning of the tracheobronchial tree in the intubated patient. High-grade A-V block with secondary inadequate cardiac output may result from digitalis toxicity, hyperkalemia, or any other infectious, inflammatory, or metabolic process predisposing to the emergence of a junctional pacer. Bradycardia-dependent ventricular tachycardia often occurs in association with ischemic heart disease and acute coronary insufficiency.

TACHYARRHYTHMIAS. Temporary cardiac pacing has been used in both prevention and termination of supraventricular and ventricular tachyarrhythmias [3–7].

Atrial pacing is often effective in terminating atrial flutter and paroxysmal nodal supraventricular tachycardia [8]. A critical pacing rate (usually 125–135% of the flutter rate) and pacing duration (usually about 10 seconds) are important in the successful conversion of atrial flutter to sinus rhythm [9,10]. This method is nearly always effective in patients with classic atrial flutter; however, it is typically ineffective for atypical or type II atrial flutter (rate 400 beats/min, P waves upright in the inferior leads). Although pacing termination of atrial flutter may be more successful from sites in the low right atrium, this requires great care to avoid rapid ventricular stimulation, which may precipitate ventricular fibrillation with hemodynamic collapse.

In many clinical situations pacing termination of atrial flutter may be more attractive than synchronized cardioversion, which requires anesthesia with its attendant risks. Pacing termination is the treatment of choice for atrial flutter in patients with epicardial atrial wires in place after cardiac surgery. It may be preferred as the means to convert atrial flutter in patients on digoxin and those with sick sinus syndrome, as these groups often demonstrate prolonged sinus pauses after DC cardioversion [11,12].

Rapid atrial pacing (at rates of 400–700 beats/min) has also been used to prevent recurrent supraventricular tachycardias by inducing atrial fibrillation. This technique may be useful in situations in which the ventricular rate cannot be adequately controlled in response to an automatic or reentrant supraventricular tachycardia [13].

Regarding ventricular arrhythmias, temporary pacing has proved lifesaving in preventing paroxysmal ventricular tachycardia in patients with prolonged Q–T intervals (*Torsades de pointes*), particularly when secondary to drugs. Temporary cardiac pacing is the treatment of choice to stabilize the patient while a type I antiarrhythmic agent exacerbating ventricular irritability is metabolized [14]. In this situation, the pacing rate is set to provide a mild tachycardia. The effectiveness of cardiac pacing probably relates to decreasing the dispersion of refractoriness of the ventricular myocardium (shortening the Q–T interval).

Temporary ventricular pacing is also frequently successful in terminating ventricular tachycardia [15,16,17]. If ventricular tachycardia must be terminated urgently, cardioversion is mandated (Chap. 10). However, in less urgent situations, conversion of ventricular tachycardia via rapid ventricular pacing may be useful. The success of this technique depends on the setting in which ventricular tachycardia occurs as well as the type of pacing used (rapid overdrive pacing or programmed extrastimulation). Programmed stimulation techniques are usually effective in terminating ventricular tachycardia in a patient with remote myocardial infarction or in the absence of heart disease. This technique is less effective when ventricular tachycardia complicates acute myocardial infarction or cardiomyopathy. Rapid ventricular pacing is most successful in terminating ventricular tachycardia when the ventricle can be "captured" (asynchronous pacing for 5–10 beats at a rate of 50 beats/min greater than that of the underlying tachycardia). Extreme caution is advised, as it may be accompanied by acceleration of ventricular tachycardias in more than 40 percent of patients; a cardiac defibrillator should be available at the bedside.

DIAGNOSIS OF RAPID RHYTHMS. Temporary atrial pacing electrodes allow accurate diagnosis of tachyarrhythmias when the morphology of the P wave and its relation to the QRS complexes cannot be elucidated from the surface electrocardiogram (ECG) [18,19]. The ability to record an intraatrial electrogram is particularly helpful in a rapid, regular, narrow-complex tachycardia in which the differential diagnosis includes atrial flutter with rapid ventricular response, reentry-type or other supraventricular tachycardia. This technique is also useful to distinguish wide-complex tachycardias in which the differential diagnosis includes supraventricular tachycardia with aberrant conduction, sinus tachycardia with bundle branch block, and ventricular tachycardia.

To record an intraatrial ECG, the limb leads are connected in the standard fashion and a precordial lead (usually V_1) is connected to the proximal electrode of the atrial pacing catheter.

A rhythm strip is run at a rapid paper speed, simultaneously demonstrating two limb leads as well as the atrial electrogram obtained via lead V_1. The rhythm strip should reveal the conduction pattern between atria and ventricle as antegrade, simultaneous, retrograde, or dissociated.

ACUTE MYOCARDIAL INFARCTION. Temporary pacing may be used therapeutically or prophylactically in acute myocardial infarction. Recommendations for temporary cardiac pacing have been provided by a Task Force of the American College of Cardiology and the American Heart Association (Table 5-2) [20]. Bradyarrhythmias unresponsive to medical treatment that result in hemodynamic compromise require urgent treatment. Patients with anterior infarction and bifascicular block or type II second-degree A-V block, while hemodynamically stable, may require a temporary pacemaker, as they are at risk for sudden development of complete heart block with an unstable escape rhythm.

Because coordinated atrial transport may be essential for preservation and maintenance of effective stroke volume, A-V sequential pacing is frequently the pacing modality of choice [21,22,23]. For example, when right ventricular involvement complicates inferoposterior infarction, transvenous A-V sequential pacing may be necessary to ensure adequate cardiac output [24,25].

Prophylactic temporary cardiac pacing has aroused considerable debate for the role it may play in complicated anterior wall myocardial infarction [26,27]. Thrombolytic therapy, when indicated, should take precedence over placement of prophylactic cardiac pacing, as prophylactic pacing has not been shown to improve mortality. Transthoracic (transcutaneous) cardiac pacing is safe and usually effective [28–31] and would be a reasonable alternative to prophylactic transvenous cardiac pacing, particularly soon after thrombolytic therapy has been administered.

Equipment Available for Temporary Pacing

Several methods of temporary pacing are currently available for use in the ICU. Transvenous pacing of the right ventricle or right atrium with a pacing catheter or modified pulmonary artery catheter is the most widely used technique; intraesophageal, transcutaneous, and epicardial pacing are also available.

TRANSVENOUS PACING CATHETERS. Some of the many transvenous pacing catheters available for use in the critical care setting are illustrated in Figure 5-1. Pacing catheters range in size from 4 Fr. (1.2 mm) to 7 Fr. (2.1 mm). Stiff catheters (Fig. 5-1, middle) can be inserted under fluoroscopic guidance using standard central venous cannulation techniques. In more urgent situations, or where fluoroscopy is unavailable, a flow-directed flexible balloon-tipped catheter (Fig. 5-1, left) may be placed in the right ventricle using ECG guidance. The stiff catheter is easier to manipulate than the balloon-tipped catheter.

A flexible J-shaped catheter (Fig. 5-1, right) is available specifically for temporary atrial pacing [32]. This lead is positioned by "hooking" it in the right atrial appendage, providing stable contact with the atrial endocardium (Fig. 5-2). Either the subclavian or internal jugular venous approach may be used. Fluoroscopic guidance is needed to achieve the proper pacing position.

Table 5-1. Indications for Acute (Temporary) Cardiac Pacing

A. Conduction disturbances
  1. Symptomactic persistent complete heart block with inferior myocardial infarction
  2. Complete heart block, Mobitz type II A-V block, new bifascicular block (e.g., right bundle branch block and left anterior hemiblock, left bundle branch block, first-degree heart block), or alternating left and right bundle branch block complicating acute anterior myocardial infarction
  3. Symptomatic idiopathic complete heart block, or high-degree A-V block
  4. Asystole
B. Rate disturbances
  1. Hemodynamically significant or symptomatic sinus bradycardia
  2. Bradycardia-dependent ventricular tachycardia
  3. A-V dissociation with inadequate cardiac output
  4. Polymorphic ventricular tachycardia with long Q–T interval (*Torsades de pointes*)
  5. Recurrent ventricular tachycardia unresponsive to medical therapy
  6. Evaluation and treatment of supraventricular arrhythmias, including atrial flutter, A-V nodal tachycardia, and Wolff-Parkinson-White syndrome
C. During electrophysiologic studies
  1. Evaluation of sinus node, A-V node, and His bundle function
  2. Evaluation of wide QRS tachycardias
  3. Evaluation of therapeutic modalities for inducible ventricular and supraventricular tachycardia

Table 5-2. Recommendations for Temporary Pacemaker in Acute Myocardial Infarction

A. Class I (indicated)
  1. Asystole
  2. Complete heart block
  3. Right bundle branch with left anterior or posterior hemiblock developing in acute myocardial infarction
  4. Type II second-degree A-V block
  5. Symptomatic bradycardia unresponsive to atropine
B. Class IIa (probably indicated)
  1. Type I second-degree heart block with hypotension unresponsive to atropine
  2. Sinus bradycardia with hypotension unresponsive to atropine
  3. Recurrent sinus pauses unresponsive to atropine
  4. Atrial or ventricular overdrive pacing for incessant ventricular tachycardia
C. Class IIb (possibly indicated)
  1. Left bundle branch block with first-degree heart block of unknown duration
  2. Bifascicular block of unknown duration

Source: ACC/AHA Task Force Report

A multilumen pulmonary artery catheter with a small (2.4 Fr.) bipolar pacing lead through a right ventricular lumen allows intracardiac pressure monitoring and pacing through a single catheter [33]. Details on its use and insertion are described in Chapter 4.

ESOPHAGEAL ELECTRODE. Esophageal "pill" electrode allows atrial pacing and recording of atrial depolarizations without requiring central venous cannulation. As mentioned, detecting atrial depolarization aids in the diagnosis of tachyarrhythmias. Esophageal pacing has also been used to terminate supraventricular tachycardia and atrial flutter [34].

TRANSCUTANEOUS EXTERNAL PACEMAKERS. Transcutaneous external pacemakers have external patch electrodes

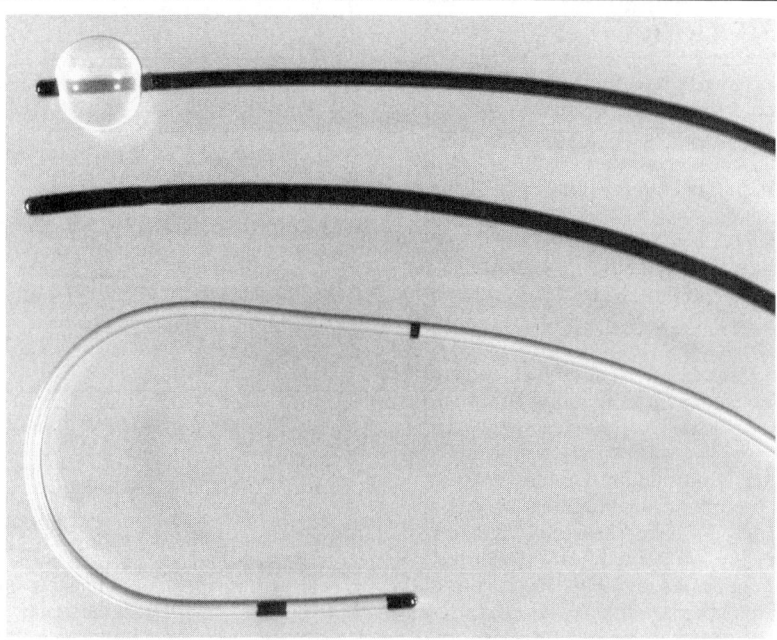

Fig. 5-1. Cardiac pacing catheters. Several designs are available for temporary pacing in the critical care unit. Bottom. Atrial J-shaped wire. Middle. Standard 5 Fr. pacing wire. Top. Balloon-tipped, flow-directed pacing wire.

Fig. 5-2. Temporary atrioventricular (A-V) demand pulse generators, older (left) and recent (right) models. Adjustable parameters on the older model include pacing mode (synchronous or asynchronous), ventricular rate, ventricular current output (mA), atrial output (mA), and A-V interval (msec). The updated model, in addition, allows atrial sensing.

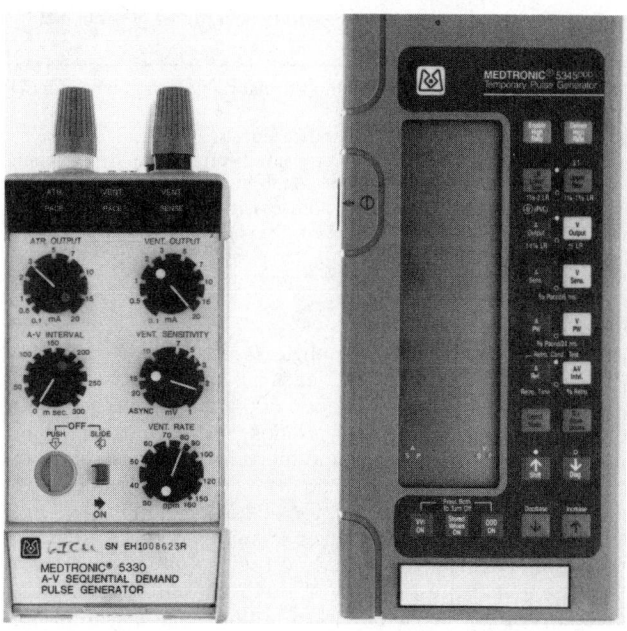

that deliver a higher current (up to 200 mA) and longer pulse duration (20–40 msec) than transvenous pacemakers. External pacing can be implemented immediately and the risks of central venous access avoided. Some patients may require sedation for the discomfort of skeletal muscle stimulation. Transcutaneous external pacemakers have been used to treat bradyasystolic cardiac arrest, symptomatic bradyarrhythmias, and overdrive pacing of tachyarrhythmias and prophylactically for conduction abnormalities during myocardial infarction. They may be particularly useful when transvenous pacing is unavailable, as in the prehospital setting, or relatively contraindicated, as during thrombolytic therapy for acute myocardial infarction [28,29, 30,3536,37].

EPICARDIAL PACING. The placement of epicardial electrodes requires open thoracotomy. These electrodes are routinely placed electively during cardiac surgical procedures for use during the postoperative period [18,19].

PULSE GENERATORS FOR TEMPORARY PACING. Temporary pulse generators are capable of ventricular, atrial, and A-V sequential pacing. Figure 5-2 is an illustration of two temporary atrioventricular pulse generators. Adjustable ventricular and atrial parameters in these generators include pacing modes (synchronous or asynchronous), rates, current outputs (mA), sensing thresholds (mV), and A-V pacing interval/delay (msec). The earlier model (Fig. 5-2, left) is limited in that it senses only ventricular depolarization; without atrial sensing, atrial pacing may occur when the atrium is refractory (due to a recent intrinsic depolarization). Consequently, with this model the atrial pacing rate must be set continuously to exceed the intrinsic atrial rate to maintain A-V sequential pacing.

The more recent model (Fig. 5-2, right) has atrial sensing/inhibiting capability in addition to the capabilities of the earlier model. This pacemaker also may be set with an upper rate limit (to avoid rapid ventricular pacing while "tracking" an atrial tachycardia); in addition, an atrial pacing refractory period may be programmed (to avoid pacemaker-mediated/endless loop tachyarrhythmias).

Choice of Pacing Mode

A pacing mode must be selected when temporary cardiac pacing is initiated. Common modes for cardiac pacing are outlined in Table 5-3. The mode most likely to provide the greatest hemodynamic benefit should be selected. In patients with hemodynamic instability, establishing ventricular pacing is of paramount importance prior to attempts at A-V sequential pacing.

Although ventricular pacing effectively counteracts bradycardia, it cannot restore normal cardiac hemodynamics because it disrupts the synchronous relationship between atrial and ventricular contraction [38–56]. The result of asynchronous contraction of the atria and ventricles (via random dissociation or retrograde/V-A conduction) is increased left atrial pressure and reduced cardiac output. The undesirable hemodynamic and arrhythmic consequences of A-V dyssynchrony are outlined in Tables 5-4 and 5-5.

The importance of the atrial contribution to total ventricular stroke volume has recently become well recognized. With A-V dissociation, the normal atrial "kick" is lost. Previously, this was considered unimportant, since in the normal heart, under resting conditions, the atrium contributes less than 15 percent to ventricular filling; however, in patients with diseases characterized by noncompliant ventricles (ischemic heart disease, hypertrophic cardiomyopathy, aortic stenosis, and congestive cardiomyopathy), the atrial contribution to ventricular stroke volume may be quite substantial. In one study, loss of a properly timed atrial contraction in patients following inferior or anterior myocardial infarction was associated with a 25 percent decrease in systolic blood pressure and cardiac output [23]. Figure 5-3 illustrates the drop in systolic blood pressure observed as the pacing mode is changed from A-V sequential to ventricular in a patient with hypertrophic cardiomyopathy.

In addition to the hemodynamic benefit of atrial or A-V sequential pacing, the risk of atrial fibrillation or flutter may be reduced because of decreased atrial size and/or atrial pressure. This suggests that patients with intermittent atrial fibrillation may be better maintained in normal sinus rhythm with atrial or A-V sequential pacing, rather than ventricular demand pacing. Table 5-6 lists subsets of patients who are particularly likely to benefit from A-V sequential pacing [57,58].

Procedure to Establish Temporary Pacing

After achieving venous access (Chap. 2), the pacing catheter is advanced to the central venous circulation. Under fluoroscopic guidance, the tip is advanced across the tricuspid valve to the right ventricular apex (Fig. 5-4). If fluoroscopy is not available, a flexible balloon-tipped pacing catheter may be positioned using ECG guidance [59,60]. The patient is connected to the limb leads of the ECG machine, and the distal (negative) electrode of the pacing catheter is connected to lead V with an alligator clip or a special adaptor supplied with the lead. Lead V is then used to monitor continuously a unipolar intracardiac electrogram. The morphology of the recorded electrogram indicates the position of the catheter tip (Fig. 5-5). The balloon is inflated in the superior vena cava, and the catheter is advanced while observing the recorded intracardiac electrogram. When the tip of the catheter is in the right ventricle, the balloon is deflated and the catheter advanced to the right ventricular apex. The S–T segment of the intracardiac electrogram is elevated due to a current of injury when the catheter tip contacts the ventricular endocardium.

Table 5-3. Common Pacemaker Modes for Temporary Cardiac Pacing

AOO Atrial pacing: pacing is asynchronous
AAI Atrial pacing, atrial sensing: pacing is on demand to provide a minimum programmed rate
VOO Ventricular pacing: pacing is asynchronous
VVI Ventricular pacing, ventricular sensing: pacing is on demand to provide a minimum programmed rate
DVI Dual-chamber pacing, ventricular sensing: atrial pacing is asynchronous, ventricular pacing is on demand following a programmed A-V delay
DDD Dual-chamber pacing and sensing: atrial and ventricular pacing is on demand to provide a minimum rate, ventricular pacing follows a programmed A-V delay, and upper-rate pacing limit should be programmed

Table 5-4. Adverse Effects of Ventricular Pacing

1. Loss of atrial kick
2. Intermittent mitral and tricuspid regurgitation
3. V–A conduction in some patients
4. Potential arrhythmia indication (AF, SVT)
5. Hypotension, especially orthostatic

AF = atrial fibrillation; SVT = supraventricular tahycardia

Table 5-5. Hemodynamic Consequences of Ventriculoatrial Conduction

1. Increased left and right atrial pressure
2. Decreased left ventricular stroke volume
3. Mitral and tricuspid insufficiency
4. Vasodepressor reflexes with resultant vasodilatation and hypotension
5. Cannon A waves

Table 5-6. Patients Most Likely to Benefit from A-V Sequential Temporary Pacing

1. Acute myocardial infarction, in particular right ventricular (inferior) infarction
2. Stiff, noncompliant ventricle: aortic stenosis, idiopathic hypertrophic subaortic stenosis, hypertensive heart disease, hypertrophic cardiomyopathy (obstructive or nonobstructive)
3. Low cardiac output states (cardiomyopathy)
4. Recurrent atrial arrhythmias (overdrive pacing of the atria)
5. Postcardiac surgery

After the tip of the pacing catheter is satisfactorily inserted in the right ventricular apex, the leads are connected to the ventricular output positions at the top of the pulse generator, with the pacemaker box in the off position. The pacemaker is then put on asynchronous mode and the ventricular rate set to exceed the patient's intrinsic ventricular rate by 10 to 20 beats per minute. The threshold current for ventricular pacing is set at 5 to 10 mA. Then the pacemaker is switched on. Satisfactory ventricular pacing is evidenced by a wide QRS complex, with S–T segment depression and T wave inversion immediately preceded by a pacemaker depolarization (spike). With pacing from the apex of the right ventricle, the paced rhythm usually demonstrates a pattern of left bundle branch block on the surface ECG [61].

Ventricular pacing is maintained as the output current for ventricular pacing is slowly reduced. The pacing threshold is

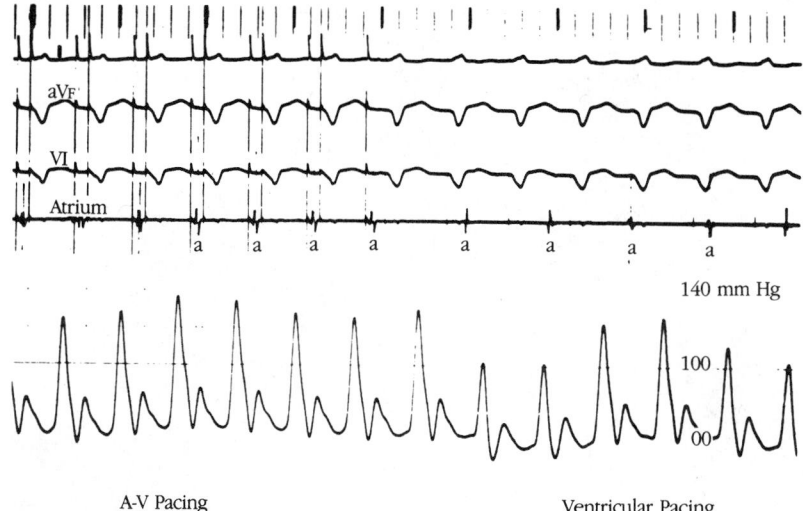

aVF

VI

Atrium

140 mm Hg

100

00

A-V Pacing   Ventricular Pacing

Fig. 5-3. Effects of atrioventricular (A-V) sequential and ventricular pacing at identical rates on systolic blood pressure in a patient with hypertrophic cardiomyopathy and a noncompliant left ventricle. Note the decline in systolic and mean arterial (a) pressures with ventricular pacing. The phasic blood pressure increase on the right is due to the coincident association of properly timed P waves with the ventricularly paced rhythm, the result of A-V dissociation characteristic of ventricular pacing in this patient.

Fig. 5-4. Appropriate fluoroscopic lead position of atrial and ventricular leads. SVC = superior vena cava; Ao = aorta; RV = right ventricle. (From Harthorne JW, et al: Cardiac pacing, in Eagle KA, Haber E, DeSanctis RW, et al (eds): *The Practice of Cardiology: The Medical and Surgical Units at Massachusetts General Hospital.* Boston, Little, Brown, 1989. With permission.)

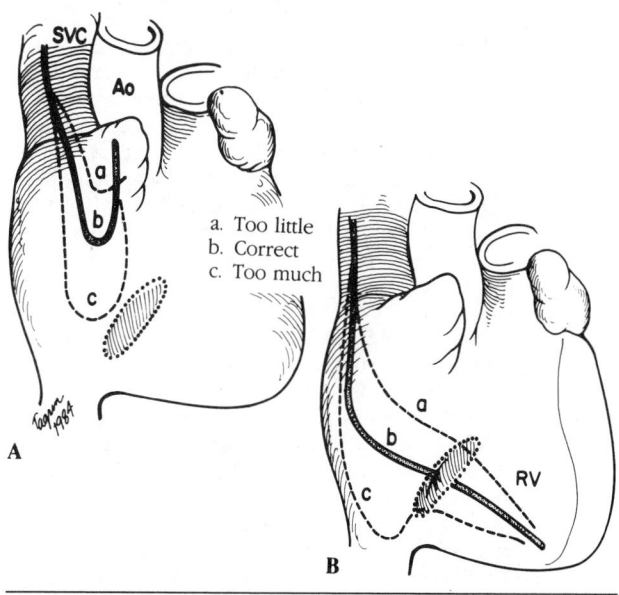

a. Too little
b. Correct
c. Too much

defined as the lowest current at which consistent ventricular capture occurs. With the ventricular electrode appropriately positioned at or near the apex of the right ventricle, a pacing threshold of less than 0.5 to 1.0 mA should be achieved. If the output current for continuous ventricular pacing is consistently greater than 1 to 1.5 mA, the pacing threshold is too high. Possible causes of a high pacing threshold include relatively refractory endomyocardial tissue (fibrosis) or, most commonly, unsatisfactory positioning of the pacing electrode. The tip of the pacing electrode should be repositioned in the region of the ventricular apex until satisfactory ventricular capture at a current of less than 1.0 mA is consistently maintained. After the threshold current for ventricular pacing has been established at a satisfactory level, the ventricular output is set to exceed the threshold current at least threefold. This guarantees uninterrupted ventricular capture despite any modest increase in the pacing threshold.

The pacemaker is now set in a VOO mode. However, the pacing generator generally should be set in the VVI ("demand") mode, as this prevents pacemaker discharge soon after an intrinsic or spontaneous premature depolarization, while the heart lies in the electrically vulnerable period for induction of sustained ventricular arrhythmias [62]. To set the pacemaker in VVI mode, the pacing rate is set at 10 beats per minute less than the intrinsic rate and the sensitivity control is moved from asynchronous to the minimum sensitivity level. The sensitivity is gradually increased until pacing spikes appear. This level is the sensing threshold. The sensitivity is then set at a level slightly below the determined threshold and the pacing rate reset to the minimum desired ventricular rate.

If A-V sequential pacing is desired, the atrial J-shaped pacing catheter should be advanced into the right atrium. Using fluoroscopic guidance, the catheter is rotated anteromedially to achieve a stable position in the right atrial appendage (Fig. 5-4) [60,63]. The leads are connected to the atrial output of the pulse generator. The atrial current is set to 20 mA and the atrial pacing rate adjusted to at least 10 beats per minute greater than the intrinsic atrial rate. The A-V interval is adjusted at 100 to 200 msec (shorter intervals usually provide better hemodynamics), and the surface ECG is inspected for evidence of atrial pacing (electrode depolarization and capture of the atrium at the pacing rate).

The manifestation of atrial capture on ECG is atrial depolarization immediately following the atrial pacing spike. In patients with intact A-V conduction, satisfactory atrial capture can be

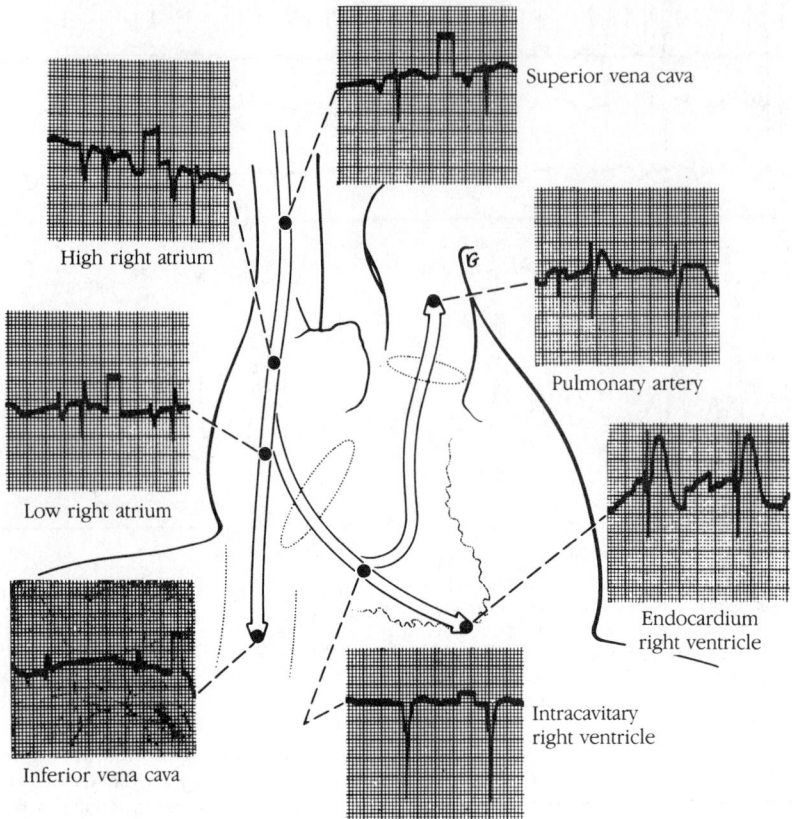

High right atrium

Superior vena cava

Low right atrium

Pulmonary artery

Endocardium
right ventricle

Inferior vena cava

Intracavitary
right ventricle

Fig. 5-5. Pattern of recorded electrogram at various locations in the venous circulation.(From Harthorne JW, et al: Cardiac pacing, in Eagle KA, Haber E, DeSanctis RW, et al (eds): *The Practice of Cardiology: The Medical and Surgical Units at Massachusetts General Hospital.* Boston, Little, Brown, 1989. With permission.)

verified by shutting off the ventricular portion of the pacemaker and demonstrating A-V synchrony during atrial pacing. As long as the atrial pacing rate continually exceeds the intrinsic sinus rate, the atrial P wave activity should track with the atrial pacing spike.

The dual-chamber temporary pacemaker may not have atrial sensing capability. If not, the pacemaker will function in a DVI mode (Table 5-3). Should the intrinsic atrial rate equal or exceed the atrial pacing rate, the atrial stimulus will fail to capture and A-V sequential pacing will be lost. If the pacemaker has atrial sensing capability, the atrial sensing threshold should be determined and an appropriate level set. The pacer will then function in the DDD mode. The DDD mode is usually preferred, as it provides optimum cardiac hemodynamics through a range of intrinsic atrial rates. In this mode an upper-rate limit must be set to prevent rapid ventricular pacing in response to a paroxysmal supraventricular tachycardia.

Complications of Temporary Pacing

Although temporary endocardial pacing can be accomplished from several alternate venous access sites, rational selection of the optimal route requires understanding of the results and complications of each. A 43 percent incidence of pacemaker malfunction (i.e., failure to sense or capture the R wave properly) and a 16.9 percent incidence of pacemaker-related complications were reported in 142 episodes of temporary pacemaker insertion by the brachial (61 cases) or femoral (81 cases) approach [64]. Austin and associates reported pacemaker malfunction in 37 percent and complications in 20 percent of 100 patients requiring pacemaker insertion by the antecubital or femoral route [65]. The Mayo Clinic's early experience with temporary cardiac pacing in the coronary care unit revealed a 17.9 percent incidence of malfunction of the temporary pacemaker and a 13.7 percent incidence of complications [64]. Over the 4-year interval from 1976 to 1980, there was a decline in use of the basilic vein surgical approach (the initially preferred method for temporary pacemaker insertion) from 95.6 percent to 22.8 percent. As use of the antecubital route declined, so did the rate of complications (pacemaker malfunction, infection) when compared to the subclavian or internal jugular venous approaches. Using predominantly the subclavian or internal jugular approaches, Donovan and Lee reported a 7 percent rate of serious complications related to temporary cardiac pacing [66]. Complications of temporary pacing from any venous access route include pericardial friction rub, arrhythmia, right ventricular perforation, cardiac tamponade, infection, inadvertent arterial injury, diaphragmatic stimulation, phlebitis, and pneumothorax. The Mayo Clinic experience revealed that percutaneous cannulation of the right internal jugular vein has provided the simplest, most direct route to the right-sided cardiac chambers. In addition, for selected patients placement of the catheter in the coronary sinus provides the benefit of stable atrial stimulation. Temporary endocardial pacing via this route is convenient and may be associated with a lower rate of pacemaker complications [67].

Although insertion via direct cutdown of the brachial vein

may be satisfactory for short-term pacing, percutaneous vascular access by the subclavian or internal jugular vein provides more stable long-term vascular access for temporary pacing (Chap. 2). Insertion from the brachial vein reduces the risk of arterial injury, hematoma formation, and pneumothorax, but the motion of the patient's arm relative to the torso increases the risk of dislodgement of the pacing electrode from a stable ventricular or atrial position [67]. The risk of infection may also be increased with this approach. The brachial approach is still preferred for the patient receiving thrombolytic therapy or full-dose anticoagulation.

Complications of internal jugular venous cannulation may include pneumothorax, carotid arterial injury, and pulmonary embolism (Chap. 2). These risks are minimized by knowledge of anatomic landmarks, adherence to proved techniques, and use of a small-caliber needle to localize the vein before insertion of the large-caliber needle (for full discussion see Chap. 2). Full-dose systemic anticoagulation, thrombolytic therapy, and prior neck surgical procedures are relative contraindications to routine internal jugular vein cannulation [65,68]. The risk of venous thrombosis following temporary cardiac pacemaker insertion using the internal jugular or subclavian venous approach has not been prospectively studied [69].

Percutaneous subclavian venipuncture is also frequently used for insertion of temporary pacemakers [62,70,71]. When the operator has a good understanding of the subclavian anatomy, the latter procedure is relatively simple and safe (Chap. 2). This approach should be avoided in patients with severe obstructive lung disease or a bleeding diathesis (including thrombolytic therapy), in whom the risk of pneumothorax or bleeding is increased.

The femoral venous approach is used for electrophysiologic studies when the catheter is left in place for only a few hours. Although temporary cardiac pacing can be established through the percutaneous femoral approach, this approach is less desirable when long-term cardiac pacing is required, since there is a risk of deep venous thrombosis around the catheter. In one study, venographic or autopsy evidence of deep venous thrombosis was present in 34 percent and pulmonary embolism in 50 percent of patients in whom a temporary pacing catheter had been inserted by the femoral venous approach [72]. The occurrence of deep venous thrombosis has been documented by objective criteria (impedance plethysmography, measurement of fibrin degradation products, and/or ^{125}I-fibrinogen scanning) in 25 percent of patients prospectively studied after insertion of a temporary cardiac pacemaker via the femoral approach [73,74].

References

1. Wiener I: Pacing techniques in the treatment of tachycardias. *Ann Intern Med* 93:326, 1980.
2. Silver MD, Goldschlager NG: Temporary transvenous cardiac pacing in the critical care setting. *Chest* 93:607, 1988.
3. Wellens HJJ, Bar F, Gorges AP, et al: Electrical management of arrhythmias with emphasis on the tachycardia. *Am J Cardiol* 41:1025, 1978.
4. Haft J: Treatment of arrhythmias by intracardiac electrical stimulation. *Prog Cardiovasc Dis* 16:539, 1974.
5. Batchelder JL, Zipes DP: Treatment of tachyarrhythmias by pacing. *Arch Intern Med* 135:1115, 1975.
6. Harold SS: Therapeutic uses of cardiac pacing in tachyarrhythmias, in Naruba O (ed): *His Bundle Electrocardiography and Clinical Electrophysiology.* Philadelphia, F.A. Davis, 1975.
7. Spurrell RAJ: Artificial cardiac pacemakers, in Kribler DC, Goodwin JF (ed): *Cardiac Arrhythmias.* London, WB Saunders, 1975, p 238.
8. Wellens HJJ: Value and limitations of programmed electrical stimulation of the heart in the study and treatment of tachycardias. *Circulation* 57:845, 1978.
9. Wills JI Jr, MacLean WAH, James TN, et al: Characterization of atrial flutter studies in man after open heart surgery using fixed atrial electrodes. *Circulation* 60:665, 1979.
10. Waldo AL, MacLean WAH, Karp RB, et al: Entrainment and interruption of atrial flutter with atrial pacing studies in man following open heart surgery. *Circulation* 56:737, 1977.
11. Das G, Anand K, Ankinfedu K, et al: Atrial pacing for cardioversion of atrial flutter in digitalized patients. *Am J Cardiol* 41:308, 1978.
12. Radford DJ, Julian DG: Sick sinus syndrome: Experience of a cardiac pacemaker clinic. *Br Med J* 3:504, 1974.
13. Waldo AL, MacLean WAH, Karp RB, et al: Continuous rapid atrial pacing to control recurrent or sustained supraventricular tachycardias following open heart surgery. *Circulation* 54:245, 1976.
14. Scarovsky S, Strasberg B, Lewin RF, et al: Polymorphous ventricular tachycardia: Clinical features and treatment. *Am J Cardiol* 44:339, 1979.
15. Wellens HJJ, Schuilenburg RM, Durrer DL: Electrical stimulation of the heart in patients with ventricular tachycardia. *Circulation* 46:216, 1972.
16. Wellens HJJ, Duren DR, Lie KI: Observations on mechanisms of ventricular tachycardia in man. *Circulation* 54:237, 1976.
17. Josephson ME, Horowitz LN, Farshidi A, et al: Recurrent sustained ventricular tachycardia, 1: Mechanisms. *Circulation* 57:431, 1978.
18. Waldo AL, MacLean WAH, Cooper TB, et al: Use of temporarily placed epicardial atrial wire electrodes for the diagnosis and treatment of cardiac arrhythmias following open-heart surgery. *J Thorac Cardiovasc Surg* 76:500, 1978.
19. Waldo AL: *Cardiac Arrhythmias: Their Mechanisms, Diagnosis, and Management.* Philadelphia, JB Lippincott, 1987.
20. Gunnar RM, Bourdillon PDV, Dixon DW, et al: Guidelines for the early management of patients with acute myocardial infarction: ACC/AHA Task Force Report. *J Am Coll Cardiol* 16:249, 1990.
21. Nimetz AA, Shubrooks SJ Jr, Hunter AM, et al: The significance of bundle branch block during acute myocardial infarction. *Am Heart J* 90:439, 1975.
22. Mullins CB, Atkins JM: Prognosis and management of ventricular conduction blocks in acute myocardial infarction. *Mod Concepts Cardiovasc Dis* 45:129, 1976.
23. Chamberlain DA, Leinbach RC, Vassau CE, et al: Sequential atrioventricular pacing in heart block complicating acute myocardial infarction. *N Engl J Med* 282:577, 1970.
24. Love JC, Haffajee CI, Gore JM, et al: Reversibility of hypotension and shock by atrial or atrioventricular sequential pacing in patients with right ventricular infarction. *Am Heart J* 108:5, 1984.
25. Topol EJ, Goldschlager N, Ports TA, et al: Hemodynamic benefit of atrial pacing in right ventricular myocardial infarction. *Ann Intern Med* 96:594, 1982.
26. Resnekov L, Lipp H: Pacemaking and acute myocardial infarction. *Prog Cardiovasc Dis* 14:475, 1972.
27. Lamas GA, Muller JE, Zoltan GT, et al: A simplified method to predict occurrence of complete heart block during acute myocardial infarction. *Am J Cardiol* 57:1213, 1986.
28. Falk RH, Ngai STA: External cardiac pacing: Influence of electrode placement on pacing threshold. *Crit Care Med* 14:931, 1986.
29. Hedges JR, Syverud SA, Dalsey WC, et al: Prehospital trial of emergency transcutaneous cardiac pacing. *Circulation* 76:1337, 1987.
30. Madsen JK, Meibom J, Videbak R, et al: Transcutaneous pacing: Experience with the Zoll noninvasive temporary pacemaker. *Am Heart J* 116:7, 1988.
31. Dunn DL, Gregory JJ: Noninvasive temporary pacing: Experience in a community hospital. *Heart Lung* 1:23, 1989.
32. Littleford PO, Curry RC Jr, Schwartz KM, et al: Clinical evaluation of a new temporary atrial pacing catheter: Results in 100 patients. *Am Heart J* 107:237, 1984.
33. Simoons ML, Demey HE, Bossaert LL, et al: The Paceport catheter: A new pacemaker system introduced through a Swan-Ganz catheter. *Cathet Cardiovasc Diagn* 15:66, 1988.
34. Benson DW: Transesophageal electrocardiography and cardiac pacing: The state of the art. *Circulation* 75:86, 1987.
35. Luck JC, Grubb BP, Artman SE, et al: Termination of sustained ventricular tachycardia by external noninvasive pacing. *Am J Cardiol* 61:574, 1988.

36. Kelly JS, Royster RL, Angert KC, et al: Efficacy of noninvasive transcutaneous cardiac pacing in patients undergoing cardiac surgery. *Anesthesiology* 70:747, 1989.

37. Blocka JJ: External transcutaneous pacemakers. *Ann Emerg Med* 18:1280, 1989.

38. Yashar JJ, Kitzes DL, Araf M, et al: Atrioventricular sequential pacemakers: Indications, complications and long-term follow-up. *Ann Thorac Surg* 29:91, 1980.

39. Samet P, Bernstein W, Natha DA, et al: Atrial contribution to cardiac output in complete heart block. *Am J Cardiol* 16:1, 1965.

40. Carleton PA, Passovoy M, Graettinger JS: The importance of the contribution and timing of left atrial systole. *Clin Sci* 30:151, 1966.

41. Romero LR, Haffajee CI, Doherty P, et al: Comparison of ventricular function and volume with A-V sequential and ventricular pacing. *Chest* 80:346, 1981.

42. Knuse I, Arnman K, Conradson TB, et al: A comparison of the acute and long-term hemodynamic effects of ventricular inhibited and atrial synchronous ventricular inhibited pacing. *Circulation* 65:846, 1982.

43. Judge RD, Wilson WJ, Siegel JH: Hemodynamic studies in patients with implanted cardiac pacemakers. *N Engl J Med* 270:1391, 1961.

44. Escher DJW, Schwedel JB, Schwartz LS, et al: Transvenous electrical stimulation of the heart, II. *Ann N Y Acad Sci* 111:981, 1964.

45. Samet P, Bernstein WH, Levin S: Significance of atrial contribution to ventricular filling. *Am J Cardiol* 15:195, 1965.

46. Benchimol A, Ellis JG, Dimond EG: Hemodynamic consequences of atrial and ventricular pacing in patients with normal and abnormal hearts: Effects of exercise at a fixed atrial and ventricular rate. *Am J Med* 39:911, 1965.

47. Benchimol A, Dimond EG: Cardiac function in man during artificial stimulation of the left ventricle, right ventricle and right atrium. *Am J Cardiol* 17:118, 1966.

48. Humphries JO, Hinman EJ, Bernstein L, et al: Effect of artificial pacing of the heart on cardiac and renal function. *Circulation* 36:717, 1967.

49. Leinbach RC, Chamberlain DC, Kastor JA, et al: A comparison of the hemodynamic effects of ventricular and sequential A-V pacing in patients with heart block. *Am Heart J* 78:502, 1969.

50. Bashour T, Naughton JP, Cheng TO: Systolic time intervals in patients with artificial pacemakers. *Am J Cardiol* 32:287, 1973.

51. van Hemel NM, Schapekens van Riemptst ALE, Bakema H, et al: Long-term follow-up after pacemaker implantation in sick sinus syndrome. *PACE* 4:8, 1981.

52. DeSanctis RW: Diagnostic and therapeutic uses of atrial pacing. *Circulation* 43:748, 1971.

53. Haas JM, Strait GB: Pacemaker induced cardiovascular failure. *Am J Cardiol* 33:295, 1974.

54. Patel AK, Yap VM, Thomsen JH: Adverse effects of right ventricular pacing in a patient with aortic stenosis. *Chest* 72:103, 1977.

55. Segel N, Samet P: Physiologic aspects of cardiac pacing, in Samet P (ed): *Cardiac Pacing,* 2nd ed. New York, Grune & Stratton, 1980, p 111.

56. Murphy P, Morton P, Murtaugh G, et al: Hemodynamic effects of different temporary pacing modes for the management of bradycardias complicating acute myocardial infarction. *PACE* 15:391, 1992.

57. Stone JM, Bhakta RD, Lutgen J: Dual chamber sequential pacing management of sinus node dysfunction: Advantages over single-chamber pacing. *Am Heart J* 104:1319, 1982.

58. Fields J, Berkovitz B, Matloff JM: Surgical experience with temporary and permanent AV sequential demand pacing. *J Thorac Cardiovasc Surg* 66:865, 1973.

59. Bing OHL, McDowell JW, Hantman J, et al: Pacemaker placement by electrocardiographic monitoring. *N Engl J Med* 287:651, 1972.

60. Harthorne JW, Eisenhauer AC, Steinhaus DM: Cardiac pacing, in Eagle KA, Haber E, De Sanctis RW (ed): *The Practice of Cardiology: The Medical and Surgical Cardiac Units at the Massachusetts General Hospital.* Boston, Little, Brown, 1989.

61. Morelli RL, Goldschlager N: Temporary transvenous pacing: Resolving postinsertion problems. *J Crit Illness* 2:73, 1987.

62. Donovan KD: Cardiac pacing in intensive care. *Anaesth Intensive Care* 13:41, 1984.

63. Holmes DR Jr: Temporary cardiac pacing, in Furman S, Hayes DL, Holmes DR Jr (ed): *A Practice of Cardiac Pacing.* Mount Kisco, NY, Futura, 1989.

64. Lumia FJ, Rios JC: Temporary transvenous pacemaker therapy: An analysis of complications. *Chest* 64:604, 1973.

65. Austin JL, Preis LK, Crampton RS, et al: Analysis of pacemaker malfunction and complications of temporary pacing in the coronary care unit. *Am J Cardiol* 49:301, 1982.

66. Donovan KD, Lee KY: Indications for and complications of temporary transvenous cardiac pacing. *Anaesth Intensive Care* 13:63, 1984.

67. Hynes JK, Holmes DR, Harrison CE: Five year experience with temporary pacemaker therapy in the coronary care unit. Mayo *Clin Proc* 58:122, 1983.

68. Civetta JM, Gabel JC, Gemer M: Internal-jugular-vein puncture with a margin of safety. *Anesthesiology* 36:622, 1972.

69. Chastre J, Cornud F, Bouchama A, et al: Thrombosis as a complication of pulmonary-artery catheterization via the internal jugular vein: Prospective evaluation by phlebography. *N Engl J Med* 306:278, 1982.

70. Davidson JT, Ben-Hur N, Nathen H: Subclavian venepuncture. *Lancet* 2:1139, 1963.

71. Linos DA, Mucha P Jr, van Heerden JA: Subclavian vein: A golden route. *Mayo Clin Proc* 55:315, 1980.

72. Nolewajka AJ, Goddard MD, Brown TC: Temporary transvenous pacing and femoral vein thrombosis. *Circulation* 62:646, 1980.

73. Pandian NG, Kosowaky BD, Gurewich V: Transfemoral temporary pacing and deep vein thrombosis. *Am Heart J* 100:847, 1980.

74. Kakkar VV, Corrigan TP: Detection of deep vein thrombosis: Survey and current status. *Prog Cardiovasc Dis* 17:207, 1974.

6. *Cardioversion and Defibrillation*

Trevor O. Greene and
Robert S. Mittleman

The use of electric countershock to restore a normal cardiac rhythm is an essential part of modern arrhythmia management, particularly in the intensive care setting. In the 200 years since it was originally described, this technique has proved valuable due to its simplicity, effectiveness, and rapid action.

Synchronized cardioversion is frequently performed on an elective basis; under these circumstances the utmost care must be taken to reduce the risk and discomfort for the patient. It is often preferable to attempt to convert to normal sinus rhythm by other means, so that electrical cardioversion is not necessary. At the other end of the spectrum is the need for emergent defibrillation for ventricular fibrillation. Under these circumstances, other priorities must be subsidiary to the goal of restoring a stable rhythm as rapidly as possible. In the intensive care setting, there is very frequently an intermediate priority for restoring a normal rhythm, and the risks and benefits of a variety of management options must be weighed carefully.

The initial experience with electrical therapy for arrhythmias was apparently that of Abildgaard, who recorded experiments in 1775 in which a shock delivered to hens rendered them lifeless, while subsequent shocks were successful in resuscitating them [1].

During the twentieth century, prior to the use of direct current shocks, alternating current was initially used by Zoll and colleagues [2] and others [3] to restore normal sinus rhythm. However, it was not until the pioneering work of Lown and associates in the 1960s that direct current was used routinely in treating a variety of arrhythmias and therefore became an essential part of modern arrhythmia management [4–8].

Cardioversion

The term *cardioversion* describes the means by which electrical countershock is used to terminate cardiac arrhythmias other than ventricular fibrillation. *Defibrillation,* on the other hand, is the process of electrically depolarizing a critical mass of myocardium in an effort to terminate ventricular fibrillation [8,9,10]. Cardioversion differs from defibrillation in that in the former the electric shock is synchronized. *Synchronization* is the process whereby the electric unit recognizes the R or S wave to avoid discharge of energy during the vulnerable period of the ventricle.

Early investigators noted a 5 percent incidence of ventricular fibrillation following cardioversion and postulated the existence of a vulnerable phase of ventricular excitability [11]. Wiggers and Wegria demonstrated that such a vulnerable period does indeed occur [12]. In mammalian ventricles it measures approximately 27 to 30 msec before the end of ventricular systole, or just before inscription of the apex of the T wave on the surface electrocardiogram (ECG). Synchronization of the electrical discharge to occur outside of the vulnerable period prevents ventricular fibrillation. Most cardioversion equipment is designed to trigger on the R or S wave of the ECG. It is therefore important to remember that when a defibrillator is in the synchronized mode it will usually not discharge if the rhythm is ventricular fibrillation. The operator, having synchronized for cardiover-sion, must remember that the device must be desynchronized to deliver electrical therapy for defibrillation.

PHYSIOLOGY OF CARDIOVERSION. The physiologic basis for electrical cardioversion is linked to the pathogenesis of cardiac arrhythmias. The mechanisms of cardiac arrhythmias can be classified into three categories: disorders of impulse formation (automaticity and triggered activity due to after depolarizations), disorders of impulse conduction (reentry), and a combination of the two.

Cardioversion is effective in terminating tachycardias perpetuated on the basis of reentry. Reentrant tachycardias require at least two functionally distinct pathways that have initial and final common pathways. Once unidirectional block develops in one pathway, and if conduction delay and tissue refractoriness permit, a propagated circulating electrical wavefront can exist. The advancing wavefront of depolarization is separated from its "tail" by fully recovered tissue, referred to as the excitable gap. Depolarization of the excitable tissue in the reentry circuit essentially closes the gap, thereby preventing perpetuation of the tachycardia. That such depolarization of the excitable gap is the basis for the effectiveness of cardioversion is supported by the observation that this technique is equally effective irrespective of where in the cycle the discharge is delivered: Invasive electrophysiologic evaluation supports reentrant mechanisms for many arrhythmias commonly seen in the intensive care setting, which are consequently, under normal circumstances, effectively terminated by a synchronized shock (Table 6-1).

In contrast, tachycardias that result from enhanced automaticity rather than reentrant mechanisms do not respond to cardioversion (Table 6-1).

INDICATIONS FOR CARDIOVERSION. Electrical therapy for cardiac arrhythmias may be elective or urgent. The procedure is performed on an urgent basis if a rhythm results in hemodynamic instability or is associated with severe symptoms. For elective cardioversion, the likelihood of obtaining and maintaining normal sinus rhythm must be weighed against the potential risks of the procedure.

Indications for electrical cardioversion can be grouped according to the following classifications (Table 6-2):

1. Class I—Conditions for which there is general agreement that cardioversion should be performed.
2. Class II—Conditions for which controversy exists with respect to the necessity of the procedure.
3. CLASS III—Conditions for which there is general agreement that the procedure is unnecessary or may incur undue risk and therefore is contraindicated.

Class I. Hemodynamically decompensating tachyarrhythmias are almost always an indication for urgent cardioversion. Occasionally, the patient will tolerate the rhythm for brief or intermediate periods of time. If the arrhythmia is known to be ventricular in origin, it may be possible to administer lidocaine in an attempt to convert it to sinus rhythm. If the rhythm has a

Table 6-1. Classification of Tachyarrhythmias based on Predicted Responses to External Cardioversion/Defibrillation

Responsive (reentrant)
    Atrial fibrillation
    Atrial flutter
    Sinoatrial nodal tachycardia
    A-V nodal tachycardia
    Intraatrial tachycardia
    A-V reciprocating tachycardia
    Ventricular tachycardia
    Ventricular flutter
    Ventricular fibrillation
Nonresponsive (automatic)
    Automatic atrial tachycardias
    A-V junctional tachycardias
    Accelerated idioventricular tachycardia
    Parasystole

A-V = atrioventricular.

Table 6-2. Indications and Contraindications for Elective and Emergency Cardioversion

A. Class I
  1. Emergency cardioversion—situations caused by reentrant arrhythmias resulting in:
    a. Hemodynamic instability
    b. Ischemia
    c. Congestive heart failure
  2. Ventricular tachycardia
  3. Atrial fibrillation or atrial flutter in the following situations:
    a. Hemodynamic compromise
    b. Difficulty in controlling ventricular rate
    c. After removal of inciting cause
    d. Idiopathic atrial fibrillation < 1 year's duration
    e. Embolic episodes
  4. Supraventricular tachycardia (wide or narrow complex) with resulting hemodynamic instability
B. Class II
  1. *Torsades de pointes*
  2. Ventricular flutter
  3. Atrial fibrillation
    a. Longstanding atrial fibrillation >1 year's duration
    b. Markedly enlarged left atrium >45 mm diameter
    c. Intolerance of antiarrhythmic medications
    d. Revision of atrial fibrillation after previous cardioversion
    e. Failure of mechanical atrial systole to follow electrical systole
    f. Stable atrial fibrillation and sick sinus syndrome
C. Class III
  1. Atrial fibrillation with slow ventricular response in the absence of digitalis or beta-blockade
  2. Digitalis toxicity
  3. Infrequent atrial fibrillation with spontaneous conversion
  4. Chaotic atrial tachycardia
  5. Severe conduction system disease

wide QRS complex and its origin (supraventricular or ventricular) is unknown after analysis by Wellens's or other criteria [13,14] intravenous procainamide is the preferred medication.

Under other circumstances the patient may be very stable hemodynamically, and a more cautious approach to management is reasonable. After weighing the risks and benefits, it may still be appropriate to proceed. Factors to consider include the patient's cardiac status and overall condition (which may affect their ability to tolerate an arrhythmia over a prolonged period of time), the risk of thromboembolic events (in the case of atrial fibrillation), and the value of other measures to increase the likelihood of correcting the arrhythmia without cardioversion

and of maintaining sinus rhythm once achieved. This could indicate treatment of contributing factors or the use of oral or intravenous antiarrhythmic agents, such as procainamide. If the patient has a supraventricular tachyarrhythmia, an alternative approach is to administer medications such as verapamil or digoxin to slow the ventricular rate and improve the hemodynamic condition, with plans to convert the patient to normal sinus rhythm later, when the risk is lower.

Class II. A particular form of ventricular tachycardia, *Torsades de pointes,* may occur in patients taking class IA antiarrhythmic agents (quinidine and procainamide). This is a distinct form of polymorphic ventricular tachycardia first described by Dessertenne in 1966 [15]. It is frequently associated with a long Q–T interval, and although it may be temporarily terminated by cardioversion it usually requires atrial and ventricular pacing at rates greater than 110 beats per minute to prevent a recurrence [16].

Extremely rapid ventricular tachycardia (>200 beats/min), or ventricular flutter, may display a sawtooth configuration with tall, peaked T waves. Under these circumstances synchronization for cardioversion is virtually impossible. The synchronizing circuit may mistake the T wave for the QRS spike, thus markedly increasing the likelihood of provoking ventricular fibrillation. In this setting, nonsynchronized electrical countershock (defibrillation) is preferable to synchronized therapy (cardioversion).

Class III. In some individuals, particularly those with extremely unstable atrial tachyarrhythmias and those with conduction system disease, atrial fibrillation may be the most stable rhythm attainable and attempts at cardioversion may be contraindicated. Individuals with infrequent episodes of atrial fibrillation who convert spontaneously to sinus rhythm would not benefit from cardioversion, therefore it is deemed unnecessary. In addition, digitalis intoxication increases the risk of direct current countershock. The procedure can be performed safely when digoxin levels are maintained in the therapeutic range (0.8–2.0 mg/ml) [17].

METHOD OF CARDIOVERSION

Preparation. In extreme emergencies, such as impending hemodynamic collapse or ischemia, many of the steps in the following description must be shortened or eliminated to facilitate prompt termination of dangerous rhythms.

Under elective circumstances, the procedure should be fully explained to the patient to allay fear and anxiety. The medical history should be reviewed and a brief physical examination performed, focusing on the heart and peripheral pulses. The procedure should be performed following an overnight fast in elective cases or after skipping a meal in more urgent cases. Intubation is usually not necessary. An ECG should be obtained both before and after the procedure and continuous monitoring performed throughout. If the patient is on digitalis, it need not be withheld. Serum digoxin level and electrolytes should generally be obtained on the day prior to the procedure (see below). Prothrombin time (INR) is also obtained if anticoagulation is in progress.

Elective cardioversion is preferably performed in the morning to allow for an adequate duration of monitoring prior to discharge. The patient should be comfortable and lying on a hard surface in case cardiopulmonary resuscitation (CPR) is required. The procedure should be performed only in an area fully equipped for CPR. An intravenous catheter should be placed and an intravenous infusion started for drug administration. Blood pressure, heart rate, and respiratory rate should be monitored prior to, during, and after administration of anesthesia. The patient's ECG and vital signs should be monitored for at least 4 hours after the procedure.

Anesthesia. Ideally, an anesthesiologist or respiratory technician should manage the airway and sedation. Initial sedation can be accomplished with a variety of medications, including short-acting barbiturates or benzodiazepines such as diazepam, the latter group also being amnestic agents. Blood pressure is monitored throughout anesthesia and 100% oxygen is administered via Ambu-bag or face mask. Just prior to cardioversion, an intravenous agent is given for final sedation and amnesia. Although there has been extensive experience with intravenous diazepam, the recent trend has been to use medications with a shorter half-life, such as midazolam, sodium methohexital, or propofol. Normally at the time of cardioversion, the patient should not be responsive to simple verbal stimuli (e.g., calling their name), to assure that he or she will have no recollection of the shock after recovery.

Technique. The principal danger in transthoracic elective cardioversion is the provocation of ventricular fibrillation. To avoid this complication, the cardioversion equipment is set on the

synchronous mode and adequate synchronization of the R wave must be demonstrated. The ECG lead that shows the largest R wave amplitude should be selected.

Electrode size and placement have been the subject of some controversy [18]. Both anterolateral and anteroposterior paddle placement have been employed [18]. Placement of the electrodes determines the transthoracic current pathway; incorrect placement has been considered the most common cause of unsuccessful cardioversion or defibrillation [19]. The most important factor to ensure success of a pathway is to locate the maximum area of myocardium in the pathway. When the anterolateral configuration is used, the anterior paddle is positioned just to the left of the sternum and below the sternomanubrial joint, while the lateral paddle is placed at the cardiac apex (Fig. 6-1A). In the anteroposterior configuration, the anterior paddle is in the same position used in the anterolateral configuration, while the patient lies on the posterior paddle, which is centered at the tip of the left scapula (Fig. 6-1B). The anteroposterior configuration reduces cardioversion energy requirements up to 50 percent and should be employed in all cardioversion [20]. The anterolateral position has the virtue of rapid application in the emergency setting.

The size of the electrodes alters the transthoracic impedance and intracardiac current density. For adults, the optimal paddle size appears to be 8 to 10 cm in diameter [18–21]. Although smaller paddles have been manufactured for children, adult-size paddles should be used for children who weigh more than 10 kg (approximately 1 year old) to minimize transthoracic impedance [18]. As is true for defibrillation, the presence of epicardial patch electrodes from implantable defibrillators may affect optimal paddle orientation (see below).

Fig. 6-1. Paddle position for cardioversion. The paddles are coated with conductive gel and pressed firmly against the chest wall. A. Anterolateral configuration. The anterior paddle is positioned just to the left of the sternum below the sternomanubrial joint while the lateral paddle is placed at the cardiac apex. B. Anteroposterior position. The anterior paddle is in the same location noted for the anterolateral position while the patient lies on the posterior paddle, which is centered at the tip of the left scapula.

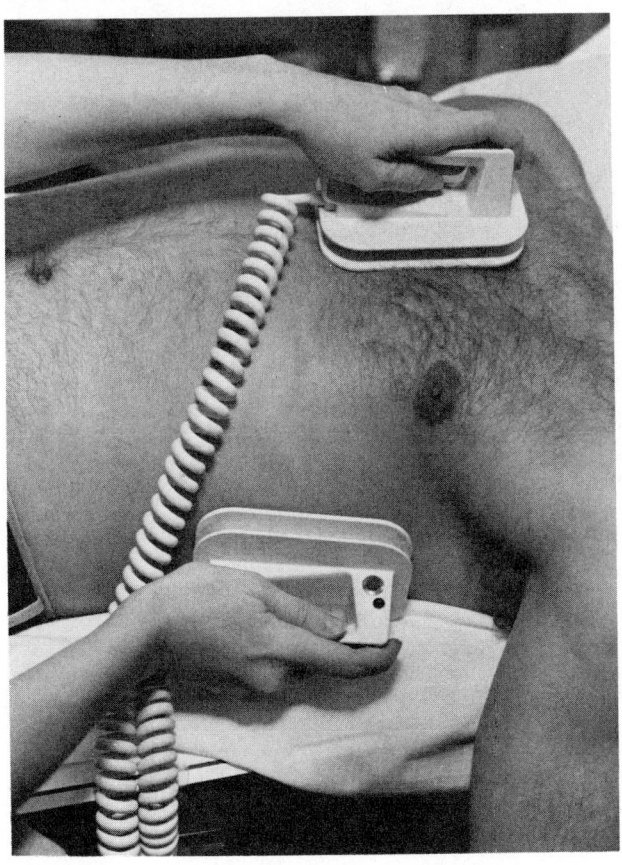

A

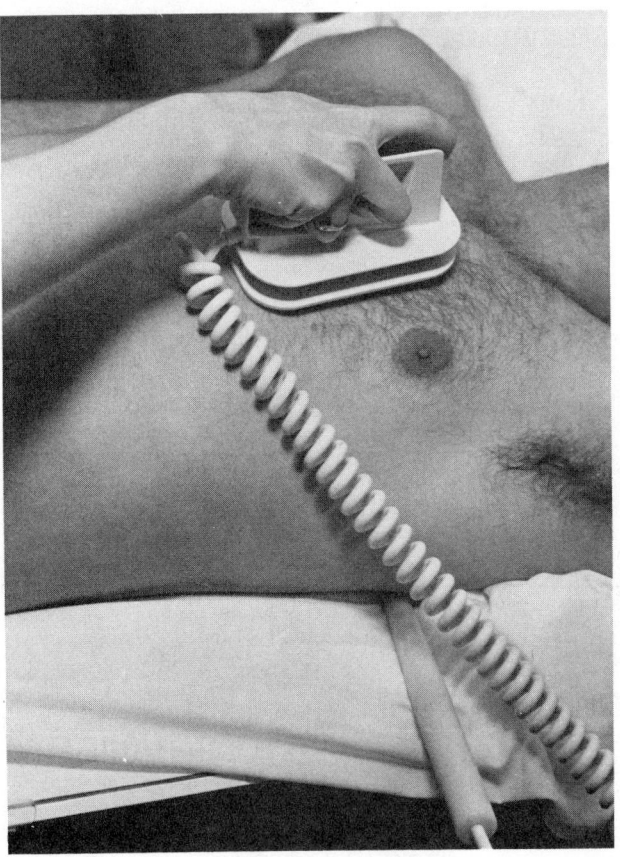

B

Both electrodes should be completely covered with conductive gel to prevent skin burns (Fig. 6-2). Alcohol swabs are contraindicated because of the potential fire hazard. The electrodes should be applied firmly to the chest wall. The monitor should be checked to ensure that proper synchronization is occurring immediately prior to discharge. The shock is delivered only after the operator is certain that no assisting personnel are in contact with the patient or the bed.

Energy Level. The amount of energy used for cardioversion should be titrated starting with the lowest dose thought most likely to revert the rhythm. The amount necessary varies with the specific arrhythmia (Table 6-3). In urgent situations with hemodynamic instability every effort should be made to terminate the tachyarrhythmia as promptly as possible, usually with a single shock.

Atrial flutter and most supraventricular tachycardia require lower energies, 30 to 50 joules being an appropriate starting level. Atrial fibrillation requires higher energy, an optimal starting point being 100 joules. Each successive dose should be doubled, to a maximum of 400 joules, if reversion does not occur. In stable ventricular tachycardia a minimum of 100 joules should be used, as this is most often successful with a single effort.

CARDIOVERSION OF SPECIFIC ARRHYTHMIAS

Atrial Fibrillation. In the general population, the most common indication for cardioversion is atrial fibrillation. On ECG, atrial fibrillation is characterized by low-amplitude, irregular undulations of the baseline with a variable morphologic configuration reflecting atrial activity. The decision to perform cardioversion depends on multiple factors, including symptomatic and clinic benefits seen in hypertrophic hearts once sinus rhythm is achieved; the reported 20 to 30 percent increase in

Table 6-3. Suggested Initial Energy Levels for External Cardioversion or Defibrillation of Common Arrhythmias

Rhythm	Energy (joules)
Atrial flutter	50
Supraventricular tachycardias	50
Atrial fibrillation	100
Monomorphic ventricular tachycardia	100
Polymorphic ventricular tachycardia and ventricular fibrillation	200 (asynchronous)

cardiac output from coordinated atrial contraction in congestive heart failure; and associated increase in the incidence of strokes in atrial fibrillation [22,23]. This is particularly important when there is a relative or absolute contraindication to anticoagulation.

Elective electrical cardioversion has offered a reliable alternative to chemical cardioversion. Early series demonstrated an initial success rate greater than 85 percent [8], but most investigators have found that less than 50 percent of patients remain in this rhythm longer than 1 year without maintenance therapy. The energy required for reversion is a function of the duration of the disorder. Patients with atrial fibrillation of greater than 6 months' duration require, on average, 150 joules for cardioversion; those with atrial fibrillation of less than 3 months duration require 100 joules [8]. The energy required for successful cardioversion may also depend on transthoracic impedance [24]. Some investigators have found that 24 to 48 hours of pretreatment with quinidine diminishes the energy required for cardioversion and confers the additional benefit of chemical cardioversion in 15 to 25 percent of patients. Another option is the use of intravenous procainamide. Prior to cardioversion, a total of 1000 mg of procainamide may be given intravenously over 30 minutes, with frequent monitoring of blood pressure. Up to 25 percent of patients will revert to sinus rhythm during administration and will not require electrical cardioversion.

Electrocardiographic patterns following reversion may be quite variable. In atrial fibrillation of recent onset, P waves will return in 1.0 to 3.0 seconds following the delivery of shock. In chronic atrial fibrillation, long periods of asystole with junctional escape beats and subsequent sinus bradycardia may oc-

---

Fig. 6-2. A. Self-adhesive pads, used increasingly in the intensive care setting. The adhesive backing is removed and the pads are applied in the position shown in B. As with paddles, the rhythm can be monitored directly. Some models also provide external pacing capability. Note that an adapter is included for connection to the defibrillator, so that the defibrillator can be connected either to the pads or to the paddles, but not to both simultaneously.

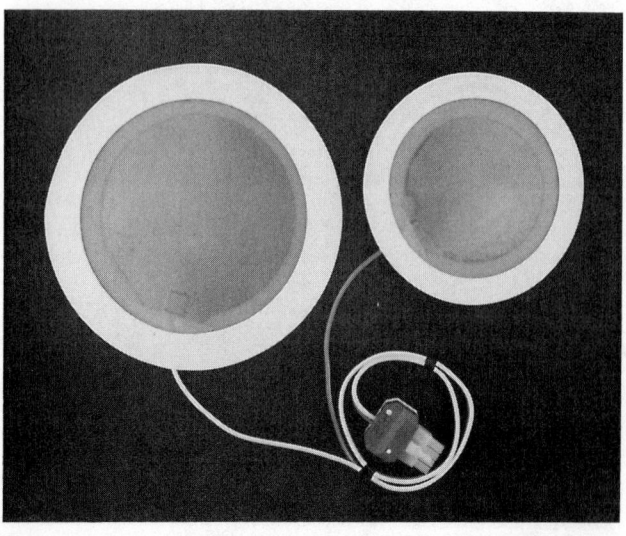

A

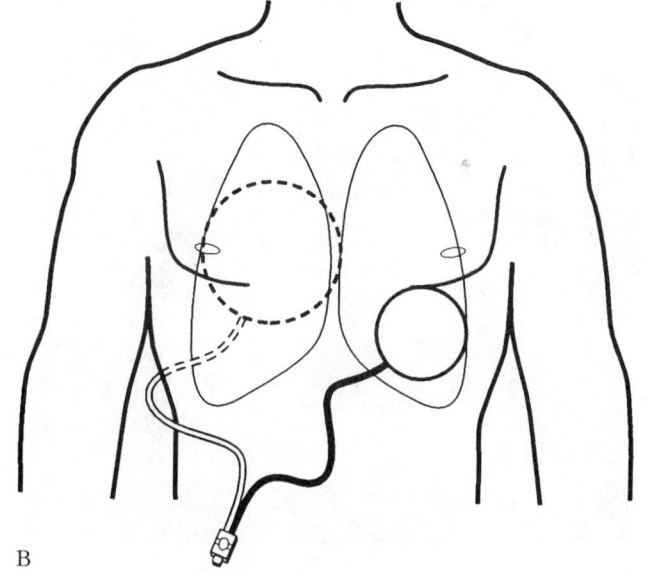

B

cur. The chances of maintaining long-term sinus rhythm are higher in patients maintained on quinidine [25–29].

Favorable candidates for cardioversion include patients (1) who display hemodynamic compromise in atrial fibrillation and who would benefit from normal sinus rhythm; (2) whose ventricular rate is difficult to control; (3) who remain in atrial fibrillation after the underlying or inciting cause has been removed; (4) with idiopathic atrial fibrillation of less than 1 year's duration; and (5) who suffer embolic episodes.

Patients in atrial fibrillation who present a relatively unfavorable subset for cardioversion include patients (1) with long-standing atrial fibrillation (>1 year's duration); (2) with an enlarged left atrium; (3) with stable atrial function and sick sinus syndrome; (4) who cannot tolerate antiarrhythmic medications; and (5) who have had previous cardioversion and subsequently reverted to atrial fibrillation.

An enlarged left atrium correlates with failure to remain in sinus rhythm. Patients with left atrial dimensions of more than 45 mm rarely remain in sinus rhythm for 6 months [30]. In general, large left atrial size and longstanding atrial fibrillation are considered unfavorable conditions for successful cardioversion. Nonetheless, every case of atrial fibrillation should be considered for one attempt at cardioversion, especially with the adjunct of the newer antiarrhythmic agents such as sotalol and propafenone.

Reversion of atrial electrical activity without return of mechanical activity is not uncommon [31]. Once atrial electrical activity has resumed, mechanical activity may lag for as long as 4 to 6 weeks [32]. This may occasionally be a contributing factor in pulmonary edema following cardioversion [33]. These patients are likely to revert to atrial fibrillation.

Atrial Flutter. This is a regular atrial rhythm that is usually most evident on the surface ECG as a characteristic saw tooth appearance in the inferior leads. Atrial flutter has been divided into type I (classic), in which the atrial rate is in the range of 240 to 340 complexes per minute, and type II, in which the rate is 340 to 430 complexes per minute [34]. Type I atrial flutter can occasionally be converted to normal sinus rhythm with rapid atrial pacing, whereas type II cannot. Occasionally, patients may have flutter in one atrium and fibrillation in another [35]. Cardioversion is the treatment of choice for terminating type II atrial flutter. Success rates in the range of 72 to 100 percent have been reported [36,37,38]. The electrical energy required to convert atrial flutter is low, usually of the order of 25 to 50 joules. Anticoagulation prior to elective cardioversion of atrial flutter is not currently recommended, although there is persistent controversy.

Supraventricular Tachycardias. While the success rate for electrical cardioversion of supraventricular tachycardias is high, approximately 75 to 80 percent, it is not the first line of treatment, since medications can generally be used effectively [39]. In instances where these rhythms are induced by digitalis toxicity, cardioversion may represent a real danger because of the likelihood of precipitating ventricular fibrillation. If digitalis toxicity is suspected, attempted cardioversion should begin at low electrical energies. This may provide both diagnostic information and therapeutic benefit. Increasing ventricular ectopy following low-dose shocks suggests that digitalis toxicity is contributing to the arrhythmia and further attempts at cardioversion should be abandoned [40].

Wolff-Parkinson-White Syndrome. Reciprocating tachycardias may occur in 40 to 80 percent of patients with Wolff-Parkinson-White syndrome and atrial fibrillation in 14 to 20 percent (Chapter 41) [41]. Atrial fibrillation in these patients can be associated with 1:1 conduction over the accessory pathway, leading to a ventricular response that may be extremely rapid (occasionally > 300 beats/min) [42,43]. Atrial fibrillation with preexcited R–R intervals of less than 250 msec suggests that the rhythm may degenerate to ventricular fibrillation. Digoxin and verapamil may exacerbate the condition by blocking normal conduction via the atrioventricular (A-V) node while providing even more rapid conduction down the accessory pathway. If there is hemodynamic instability, prompt electrical cardioversion is the treatment of choice. If the patient remains hemodynamically stable, intravenous procainamide is the drug of choice for rate control and chemical cardioversion.

Ventricular Tachycardia. Cardioversion is one of the leading therapeutic options for monomorphic paroxysmal ventricular tachycardia [44]. The energy required to revert ventricular tachycardia is typically 100 joules, and the success rate is approximately 95 to 100 percent [45]. Even lower energy levels are occasionally effective, most often in the hemodynamically stable patient in a controlled environment; however, even if synchronized to the QRS complex, lower energies have the potential to convert the rhythm to ventricular fibrillation. It is almost always preferable to employ a countershock in the synchronous mode to terminate ventricular tachycardia, with three exceptions: (1) in an extreme emergency with rapid hemodynamic compromise with insufficient time for synchronization; (2) in digitalis intoxication-provoked ventricular tachycardia (where the increased risk of ventricular fibrillation makes overdrive pacing preferable); and (3) in ventricular flutter. In the latter instance, the presence of tall T waves may occasionally cause inadvertent synchronization and provoke an episode of ventricular fibrillation. Under these circumstances, nonsynchronized electrical shock is preferable. Polymorphic ventricular tachycardia should be treated as ventricular fibrillation.

CARDIOVERSION IN SPECIAL CIRCUMSTANCES

Cardioversion and Digitalis Preparation. Cardioversion of patients on digitalis remains a dilemma. Early studies in dogs demonstrated that a toxic dose of ouabain resulted in an 8000-fold increase in sensitivity of the myocardium to electrical shock [46]. Patients reported to suffer ventricular fibrillation and die following cardioversion were those who received high electrical doses in the setting of digitalis toxicity [47]. Patients on digitalis have also been observed to display increased ventricular ectopic activity during cardioversion [48].

Cardioversion can be safely undertaken in patients receiving digitalis preparations as long as there is no clinical evidence of digitalis toxicity. When cardioversion must be performed in a patient with a question of toxicity, most investigators recommend titration beginning with low-energy shocks. One approach recommended an initial dose of 5 joules, followed by 10, 25, 50, 100, 200, 300, and 400 joules, until reversion occurs [8]. Increased ectopy at any energy level should prompt administration of lidocaine. Atrial overdrive pacing should be considered as an alternative cardioversion technique in patients with atrial flutter who are on digitalis preparations and as the treatment of choice in digitalis toxicity. In one series, 23 of 25 patients in atrial flutter and on digitalis were successfully reverted to sinus rhythm with atrial pacing [49].

Many investigators routinely withhold digitalis preparations on the day of cardioversion. Others advocate prophylactic use of lidocaine. A normal serum potassium level is particularly important before cardioversion is attempted in patients on digitalis preparations. In life-threatening arrhythmias that warrant emergency cardioversion in the setting of digitalis toxicity, it may be prudent to administer antidigoxin antibodies (Digibind) along with intravenous lidocaine.

Cardioversion and Amiodarone. Amiodarone has enjoyed increasing use for supraventricular and ventricular arrhythmia, with widespread use limited mainly by its side effects and organ toxicity. It is often used as a third-line drug in atrial fibrillation, prescribed only after the patient becomes refractory to alternative antiarrhythmic therapy. There is controversy as to the effect of amiodarone on energy requirements for cardioversion and defibrillation. Some investigators have not observed any effect [50], whereas others have noted impeded cardioversion [51]. Our center has not identified any change in cardioversion or defibrillation thresholds during chronic amiodarone therapy [52]. No increased hazards appear to accompany cardioversion in patients being treated with amiodarone. The medication appears to have some stabilizing properties in the atrium, which help to maintain sinus rhythm.

Cardioversion During Pregnancy. Synchronized, direct current cardioversion has been performed successfully in all trimesters of pregnancy without apparent adverse fetal effects [53,54]. Arrhythmias are not uncommon during pregnancy. The approach to therapy does not change, with the obvious exception that known or potentially teratogenic antiarrhythmic medications should be avoided.

Cardioversion of paroxysmal supraventricular tachycardia with 100 joules and atrial fibrillation with as great as 300 joules has been reported to be effective and without substantial risk to the fetus or the woman [55,56,57]. A number of studies have shown that electrical countershock does not induce premature labor [58,59], although in one instance cesarean section was performed for fetal distress [56]. Fetal rhythm should be monitored during cardioversion [58]. Defibrillation of unstable tachyarrhythmias in a pregnant woman poses no ethical dilemma, since it may be lifesaving to both woman and fetus [60].

It is currently recommended that if the maternal arrhythmia is serious and refractory to other treatments, synchronized direct current cardioversion should be performed. The fetus should be monitored immediately after the procedure for signs of fetal distress if age of fetal viability has been reached and if maternal status permits operative delivery should fetal compromise ensue.

Cardioversion in Children. In general, the energy level to revert any arrhythmia should be reduced in the pediatric population. Cardioversion has been successful in treating atrial tachyarrhythmias in children [61]. With ventricular fibrillation, a success rate of 91 percent has been reported in children weighing 2.1 to 5.0 kg with energy levels of 1 to 2 joules/kg [62,63,64]. The American Heart Association has published guidelines for paddle size, location, and energy levels for defibrillation in children (Chap. 19) [65].

COMPLICATIONS OF CARDIOVERSION

Embolization and Anticoagulation. The risk of embolism and the value of anticoagulation in cardioversion have been reviewed in a number of studies [66–71]. The high risk of arterial embolization complicating atrial fibrillation in both rheumatic and nonrheumatic heart disease has been well documented. Approximately 30 percent of patients with chronic atrial fibrillation suffer at least one episode of embolism if not anticoagulated, and 10 to 20 percent of all deaths from rheumatic heart disease are embolic in origin [72]. This high incidence of embolism is the major rationale for cardioverting patients with atrial fibrillation. A number of studies have shown an appreciable incidence of embolism (1–3%) after cardioversion [67–71]. The risk of embolism prompted a number of trials of anticoagulation around the time of cardioversion. At least one series documented that anticoagulation lowers the risk of embolism associated with cardioversion to between zero and 0.8 percent [73].

Certain guidelines have emerged with respect to anticoagulation around the time of cardioversion. The American College of Chest Physicians–National Heart, Lung and Blood Institute's national conference on antithrombotic therapy recommended at least 3 weeks of anticoagulation prior to cardioversion of atrial fibrillation present for more than 2 days, followed by an additional 4 weeks after the procedure [74]. This approach is based on the theory that clot formation may take up to 2 weeks to develop and atrial mechanical function can require 3 to 4 weeks to return after cardioversion [32]. Current recommendations do not call for anticoagulation prior to cardioversion of atrial flutter [74].

Atrial thrombi are poorly detected by conventional noninvasive techniques, such as transthoracic electrocardiography. Transesophageal echocardiography is a highly accurate tool for detecting atrial thrombi [75–78], in large measure because of its ability to visualize thrombi in the left atrial appendage. If atrial thrombi can be excluded by the technique, early cardioversion can be performed safely without the need for prolonged oral anticoagulation before the procedure [79].

Myocardial Injury during Cardioversion. Myocardial injury following cardioversion is a common clinical dilemma, especially in patients with underlying myocardial ischemia. Interpretation of the creatinine kinase (CK) levels becomes difficult. A number of studies have demonstrated that electrical shock can cause both functional and morphologic changes in the myocardium [80,81]. Direct current has been shown to cause less damage than alternating current [5]. Myocardial damage appears to be greatest when shocks are repetitive and closely spaced [82]. However, measurable myocardial damage rarely occurs following cardioversion at currently recommended energy levels (Table 6-3). Elevations in CK-MB are extremely rare and when they do occur are usually small [83,84,85].

Pulmonary Edema following Cardioversion. In older studies, pulmonary edema following cardioversion was reported to occur in as many as 2 to 3 percent of patients within 3 hours after the procedure [86,87]. In our personal experience, this has occurred much less commonly. When it does occur, it may be related to failure of the left atrial systole to begin promptly following cardioversion or to left ventricular dysfunction caused by the electrical shock. Return of left atrial systole may contribute to volume overload in a compromised left ventricle [88,89].

Prophylactic Temporary Pacemaker Insertion prior to Cardioversion. There is general agreement that patients with proven or strongly suspected sinus node dysfunction should have a temporary transvenous pacemaker placed prior to cardioversion [90]. Such patients would include those in atrial fibrillation with a slow ventricular response in the absence of medication with a blocking effect on the A-V node and those in atrial fibrillation with a history of sick sinus syndrome. Permanent pacing should also be considered for these patients.

Although a conduction disturbance (right or left bundle branch block or nonspecific intraventricular conduction delay) portends a high risk, it has not been noted to increase the complication rate of cardioversion [91]. Consequently, cardioversion can be performed safely in these patients without prophylactic temporary pacing.

Defibrillation

Defibrillation is the process of electrically depolarizing a critical mass of myocardium to terminate ventricular fibrillation and reestablish normal sinus rhythm. It differs from cardioversion in that the latter involves synchronization to avoid accidental delivery during the vulnerable ventricular period. Higher energies are generally required for defibrillation than for cardioversion.

Although practical considerations in defibrillation have changed very little over the last 25 years, insight into the mechanism has grown tremendously. This has been an area of intense study, spurred in part by the explosive growth in the use of implantable defibrillators. Although many issues remain unresolved, it is generally accepted that during fibrillation there is continuous reentrant excitation of the ventricle and that when defibrillation is successful it can extinguish these depolarizing wavelets without precipitating new activation waves [92,93].

Our concept of the method by which defibrillation restores normal depolarization has evolved. The total extinction hypothesis, developed by Wiggers in 1940, suggested that to terminate ventricular fibrillation it was necessary simultaneously to terminate all activation fronts in the ventricles [94]. This approach was subsequently supplanted by the critical mass hypothesis of Zipes and associates, which suggested that if fibrillation could be terminated in the vast majority of the ventricular myocardium, the remaining mass was insufficient to perpetuate the arrhythmia [95].

Current concepts of defibrillation have tried to reconcile the complex effects of defibrillation shocks on myocardial cells depending on their refractory state, the apparent potential for defibrillation shocks to terminate and reinitiate ventricular fibrillation, and the improved efficacy of biphasic shocks over monophasic shocks. It is generally accepted that below a certain energy level, a direct current shock has only a certain probability of terminating ventricular fibrillation, but when a certain threshold is reached it will always be effective [93]. The upper limit of vulnerability hypothesis suggests that subthreshold shocks may terminate the reentrant fronts that perpetuate ventricular fibrillation but often will reinitiate new reentrant fronts elsewhere in the ventricle [93,96]. Shocks above a certain energy level will prevent new activation fronts from reinducing fibrillation. The extension of refractoriness hypothesis suggests that a direct current shock will depolarize all excitable cells, but for cells that are partly refractory (which appears to be most cells in the fibrillating ventricle), it will produce a considerable prolongation of the refractory period, such that the perpetuation of reentrant wavefronts is impaired [93,97,98]. Reconciliation of these competing hypotheses may ultimately lead to more effective means of external defibrillation.

COMPONENTS OF DEFIBRILLATORS AND ELECTRICAL CONCEPTS. Early work by Lown et al. showed that direct current was superior to alternating current because it is safer and causes less myocardial damage [5]. The direct current defibrillator contains a high-voltage power source that charges an energy storage capacitor, which in turn is connected to the paddles or adhesive shocking electrodes. Several thousand volts are delivered over 4 to 12 msec. In most commercially available defibrillators, the defibrillation waveform has a dampened sinusoidal morphology, which differs from the truncated exponential or biphasic truncated exponential waveform that is currently used for implanted defibrillators but nonetheless has proved to be highly effective [99].

Although the energy used in essentially all marketed defibrillators is expressed in joules, it has become clear that the transcardiac current density (i.e., the current that passes directly through the heart) is the critical factor in defibrillation [100,101,102]. Under most circumstances, only a small percentage (approximately 4%) of the transthoracic energy (the energy delivered directly through the defibrillation electrodes) is actually delivered to the heart [103,104]. With any particular energy delivery, the transthoracic impedance ultimately determines the current delivered; a low impedance results in a higher energy delivery and a high impedance results in low current. It therefore could be anticipated that a low impedance would facilitate effective defibrillation.

There are multiple factors involved in determining the impedance, which can roughly be grouped into patient-specific factors and equipment-specific factors, the former including factors affecting the skin-electrode interface. Equipment-specific factors include the amount of energy discharged from the defibrillator as well as the size, type, and location of the defibrillation electrodes. All of the considerations for cardioversion discussed earlier in this chapter also apply to defibrillation. As for cardioversion, skin contact is important; adequate contact should be maintained and a generous amount of conductive gel used. The transthoracic impedance decreases immediately after the first shock; consequently, a second shock may be effective even when an initial shock at the same energy was not [105].

Self-adhesive electrode patches are used increasingly as an alternative to paddles [106]. They provide impedances comparable to those of paddles and offer a stable reliable option for situations in which shocks may be necessary over a prolonged period of time.

There appear to be a multitude of patient-specific factors, which have not been completely characterized. For example, defibrillation during expiration appears to be preferable to that during inspiration [107]. It has been calculated that a pleural effusion would reduce the percentage of transthoracic current delivered to the heart from 4 to 2 percent, which evidently could have a major impact on success [103,104]. It has also been reported that transthoracic impedance decreases following surgery requiring median sternotomy [108]. Further study may allow development of more effective strategies for patient defibrillation; for the present, the usual anteroposterior or anterolateral electrode placement appears to be desirable for defibrillation as well as for cardioversion. A number of studies have demonstrated that the longer ventricular fibrillation persists, the more difficult it becomes to defibrillate the patient successfully [101,109]. Metabolic factors may also contribute to refractory ventricular fibrillation, and vigorous attempts should be made to correct acidosis, electrolyte imbalance, hypoglycemia, and hypoxia during cardiopulmonary resuscitation.

LOGISTICS AND EQUIPMENT FOR DEFIBRILLATION

Testing Defibrillators. Every intensive and coronary care unit should develop protocols for ensuring that defibrillators are in proper working order. The following guidelines for defibrillator testing are recommended by the American Heart Association (AHA) [65].

LINE-POWERED DEFIBRILLATORS. Engineering personnel should perform a maintenance inspection every 3 months. Each day clinical personnel should perform a visual inspection and charge-discharge test at 50 joules. A full energy charge-discharge test should be done weekly.

BATTERY-POWERED DEFIBRILLATORS. Engineering personnel should perform a maintenance inspection every 3 months. Clinical personnel should perform tests at the same energy levels

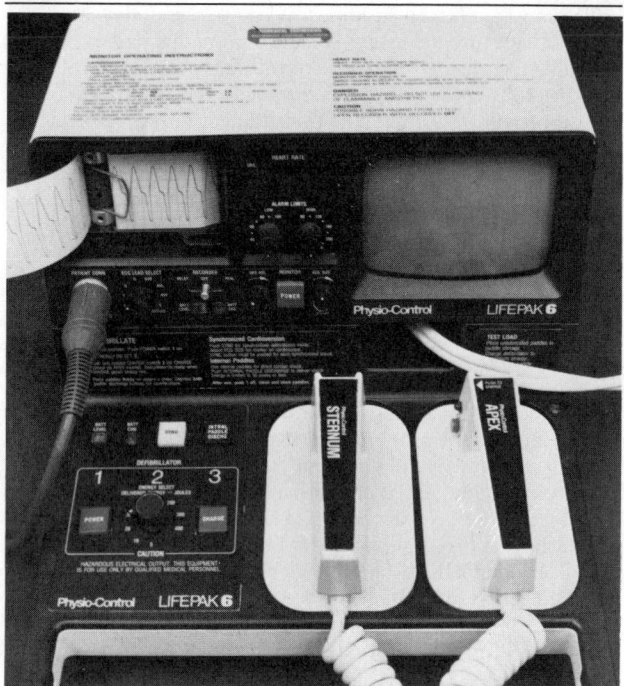

Fig. 6-3. Standard equipment used in cardioversion and defibrillation. Note the synchronization circuit. This circuit must be activated to sense the QRS spike for cardioversion and must be deactivated to allow unsynchronized defibrillation.

and frequency as for line-powered defibrillators. Battery maintenance should be performed as outlined in the manufacturer's operating instructions.

Operating a Defibrillator. Successful use of defibrillation equipment requires an understanding of the electronic controls and settings on both the defibrillator and monitor (Fig. 6-3). The monitor and defibrillator both have power on-off switches, either separate or combined in one unit. In addition, many defibrillators have a synchronizer circuit to allow cardioversion. If the synchronizer circuit is activated, a shock can be delivered only when the monitor recognizes a QRS spike, thus the synchronizer circuit must be shut off during attempted conversion of ventricular fibrillation.

Most defibrillators are now equipped with "quick-look" paddles that allow ECG monitoring from the paddles. The paddles will not function simultaneously with patient leads, so one or the other must be activated. Once the main power source to the circuit is switched on, the amount of energy must be selected and a separate switch engaged to charge the capacitor. An indicator light or gauge indicates when the desired charge has been stored, with the charge time dependent on the amount of energy selected. The stored charge can then be delivered through the paddles. There are several systems for discharging the paddles, but the safest system involves simultaneously depressing discharge buttons on each paddle.

TECHNIQUE OF DEFIBRILLATION. Adherence to a standard protocol for defibrillation will ensure optimal safety and the highest possible success rate. The following protocol is recommended by the AHA for defibrillation in cardiac arrest [65,110].

1. *Begin basic cardiac life support and call for defibrillation equipment and assistance.* Recent trends in emergency defibrillation emphasize the importance of rapid defibrillation as the major determinant of survival in cardiac arrest due to ventricular defibrillation. Call for assistance and perform basic life support until a defibrillator is available. Do not allow other subsidiary measures to delay the delivery of therapy. A precordial thump, sometimes of value in terminating ventricular tachycardia and in a small number of cases for ventricular fibrillation, is now considered an optional, possibly effective (class IIb) technique. Blind defibrillation, previously considered an important first step, is now rarely necessary because most defibrillators allow quick-look rapid monitoring of the heart rhythm.

2. *Delegate basic cardiac life support duties to qualified assistants.* It is essential that basic cardiac life support not be unduly interrupted by repeated attempts at defibrillation. At least a peripheral and, in some instances, a central venous catheter, control of the airway, and adequate oxygenation must be established as early as possible.

3. *Evaluate cardiac rhythm.* Continuous rhythm monitoring is essential throughout the resuscitation effort.

4. *Treat ventricular fibrillation.* If ventricular fibrillation is present and a defibrillator is available, accomplish the following steps rapidly and with minimum interruption of basic cardiac life support (BCLS) and advanced cardiac life support (ACLS) measures.

a. Apply conductive gel to the defibrillator paddles.
b. Turn on the main power supply to the defibrillator.
c. Ensure that the defibrillator is not in synchronous mode.
d. Select the energy level (typically 200 joules).
e. Charge the capacitor.
f. Place the paddles on the patient's chest and press firmly.
g. Recheck the monitor rhythm.
h. Clear the area, being certain that no personnel are in contact with the patient or the bed.
i. Deliver the countershock by depressing the buttons on both defibrillator paddles.

5. *Check the ECG and pulse.* If ventricular fibrillation persists after the first countershock, recharge the capacitor and rapidly deliver a second countershock at 200 to 300 joules. If ventricular fibrillation still persists, increase the energy to 360 joules for the third shock. Subsequent shocks should not exceed 360 joules. If the third shock fails to convert the rhythm, continue CPR, including ventilation, administer epinephrine, and repeat shocks. Epinephrine may be of value in converting fine to coarse ventricular fibrillation. It is important to remember that organized electrical activity can resume without mechanical activity (electromechanical dissociation), so the carotid or femoral pulse as well as the ECG must be checked. If no pulse returns, immediately resume basic cardiac life support.

6. *Apply ACLS procedures.* If ventricular fibrillation persists after two countershocks, turn attention toward factors that may explain defibrillation failure (electrode size, placement, and interface as well as a clinical picture of pneumothorax, acidosis, or hypoxemia). Consider administering intravenous lidocaine, followed by bretylium, magnesium sulfate, or procainamide, to aid in defibrillation.

PEDIATRIC DEFIBRILLATION. Defibrillation in children differs from that in adults in several important respects. The following considerations are based on AHA guidelines for pediatric defibrillation [110].

1. Blind countershock is not recommended in infants and children. Ventricular fibrillation is very uncommon in this pop-

ulation; heart block or bradyarrhythmias are much more likely to have led to cardiac arrest. If ventricular fibrillation is demonstrated by monitor, defibrillation should be attempted only after a minimum of 2 minutes of basic cardiac life support.

2. The energy levels used to defibrillate ventricular fibrillation in children are considerably lower than those required for adults. The recommended energy level for the first countershock is 2 joules per kilogram (1 joule/pound), which is doubled on the second countershock if the first is unsuccessful. Failure of the second countershock to convert ventricular fibrillation should prompt vigorous correction of acidosis and hypoxia.

If the infant or child who suffers ventricular fibrillation has been treated with digitalis preparations, defibrillation should be undertaken with great caution, since it can lead to irreversible cardiac arrest. The initial countershock should be performed with the lowest energy level available on the defibrillator, with a slow, cautious progression toward higher energy levels if the first countershock is unsuccessful.

CONTROVERSIES IN DEFIBRILLATION

Amount of Electric Energy Used. There is considerable debate concerning the appropriate amount of electrical energy to employ in defibrillation [111–114]. In the past, many clinicians advocated use of 400 joules of stored energy in the initial attempt to defibrillate ventricular fibrillation in adults.

Most defibrillators that store 400 joules of energy deliver 270 to 330 joules across a 50-ohm resistance (a typical resistance across an adult chest wall with adequately prepared and applied paddles). In 1974, Tacker et al. suggested that this amount of energy is insufficient to defibrillate 35 percent of individuals weighing more than 50 kg and 60 percent of individuals weighing 90 to 100 kg [111]. This was based on a retrospective analysis of data in children and some animal experiments. Several subsequent large, prospective studies have established that 95 to 98 percent of patients with ventricular fibrillation can be successfully cardioverted using an average of 200 joules of stored energy [105,115]. Ninety percent of patients studied by Pantridge et al. had ischemic heart disease and 74 percent had an acute myocardial infarction [115]. No failure to defibrillate successfully was recorded when 400 joules of stored energy was applied. Other case reports show the efficacy of defibrillation using 400 joules of stored energy in even extremely obese individuals [116,117]. Several studies have demonstrated that failure to defibrillate ventricular fibrillation successfully does not directly correlate with body size but is related to factors such as metabolic abnormalities and transthoracic impedance [101,105,118]. Furthermore, several investigators have emphasized the potential for increased myocardial damage following higher-energy countershocks [113]. While some uncertainty remains, the guidelines established by the AHA appear prudent [110]. An initial countershock of 200 joules of *delivered* energy is recommended, followed immediately by another countershock of 200 to 300 joules. A subsequent shock at 360 joules can be instituted if ventricular fibrillation persists. Countershocks should not exceed 360 joules of delivered energy. Open heart defibrillation can typically be accomplished with energies of 5 to 40 joules.

Chest Thump. Pennington and colleagues were the first to recommend "thumpversion" for reversion of ventricular tachycardia [119]. They reported 12 instances in 5 patients in whom a blow with the fist to the precordium successfully reverted ventricular tachycardia. The exact mechanism by which the chest thump works is not well understood. Early in the course

of ventricular tachycardia, the rhythm may be reverted with small amounts of electrical energy (<1 joule), and the thump may supply this. The thump may also work in some mechanical way. A hazard associated with the chest thump includes inadvertently administering it during the ventricular vulnerable period and causing ventricular fibrillation [120]. The AHA considers chest thump a class IIB (possibly effective, probably not harmful) therapy for pulseless cardiac arrest when a defibrillator is not available. It should never be used in ventricular tachycardia with a pulse unless a defibrillator and pacemaker are immediately available [110]. Chest thump is not recommended in children.

Effect of Medication on Defibrillation Thresholds. Despite the extensive use of antiarrhythmic medications, there is extremely limited information on their effects on defibrillation thresholds in humans [121]. While the chronic use of cardiac defibrillation was limited to transthoracic (external) high-energy shocks, little attention was paid to the effects of exogenous factors. Early studies, which were technically excellent even by today's most critical criteria, showed convincingly that quinidine, lidocaine, and phenytoin resulted in an increase in cardiac defibrillation energy requirements [122,123]. More recently, however, the negative effect of quinidine on the ability to defibrillate the heart was not confirmed in a dog model of internal defibrillation [124]. This discrepancy may be attributable to the high doses of quinidine used in previous studies.

With the advent of low-energy internal, implantable defibrillators, many studies have described the effects of various pharmacologic interventions on cardiac defibrillation [52,125,126]. The results are conflicting, unsettled, or lacking confirmation, thus no firm conclusion of clinical pertinence can be drawn from available data [121].

CURRENT-BASED DEFIBRILLATION. Most currently available defibrillators deliver a constant energy output regardless of the transthoracic impedance. However, since it is the transcardiac current delivery that ultimately determines the success of defibrillation, external defibrillators have been developed that are capable of measuring the transthoracic impedance [100,101,102]. This allows control of the current delivered to the patient so that a shock of sufficient energy to terminate the arrhythmia but not so high as to cause adverse effects can be delivered. This has been done manually, but a device that automatically adjusts the energy output based on the transthoracic impedance has been developed [100]. It was able to achieve success comparable to that of a standard protocol while delivering significantly less energy (145 joules vs. 200 joules), which in principle would minimize the adverse effects produced by defibrillation. It is unclear at this time when or whether such a device will become widely available.

IMPLANTABLE DEFIBRILLATORS AND PACEMAKERS. Permanent pacemakers have long been known to be susceptible to temporary or permanent effects on their performance as a result of electrical countershock [127,128]. Potential problems include lead dislodgement (generally only early after implantation), acute and/or chronic impairment of pacing and sensing parameters, reprogramming of pacing mode, and damage to the electric circuitry, which can have unpredictable effects [128]. Essentially all pacemakers have protective circuitry to prevent damage to their components. Prominent effects can nonetheless occur at the electrode-tissue interface, which under the worst of circumstances can result in electrical burns. The most common abnormality is a transient rise in pacing and sensing thresholds, which can result in temporary failure to pace and/or inhibit appropriately. Bipolar pacemakers are less susceptible to problems than unipolar pacemakers.

For cardioversion or defibrillation of patients with permanent pacemakers, it is recommended to (1) use the lowest possible defibrillator energy; (2) place defibrillation paddles as far as possible (at least 10 cm) from the pulse generator; (3) use a vector of defibrillation as close as possible to perpendicular to the tip of the ventricular pacing lead; (4) be prepared to reprogram the pacemaker or to use an alternate means of pacing; (5) monitor patients carefully following therapy for evidence of pacemaker malfunction [128].

There has been explosive growth in the use of implantable cardioverter defibrillators (ICDs) worldwide, and this growth is likely to continue [125,129]. Patients with these devices will be seen in increasing numbers in the intensive care setting. To manage such patients appropriately, it is important to understand their function and interaction with external defibrillators and other influences in the intensive care environment.

Unless the ICD is programmed to an inactive state, it will continue to work as originally programmed, independent of treatments such as external defibrillation. As mentioned above, when an external defibrillation is delivered, commonly the pacing and sensing parameters of a permanent pacemaker are temporarily impaired (generally for less than 24 hours), due to a complex set of factors acting at the electrode-tissue interface [128]. It is likely that the same effects could be seen in implantable defibrillators, but we are unaware of any such reports. There is also the possibility of dislodgement of any recently implanted transvenous pacing or shocking lead; the chance of this is markedly reduced for a chronic implant.

Implantable defibrillators can sometimes respond to nonphysiologic influences in the environment, such as electromagnetic interference [127]. For example, the use of electrocautery for surgery very commonly causes a defibrillator discharge, and an ICD must be inactivated if electrocautery is being considered. For any operation not involving the use of electrocautery, the risks and benefits of inactivating the device should be weighed before preceding. Magnetic resonance imaging studies are contraindicated.

As for pacemakers, there is a potential to damage an ICD from an external defibrillation. Similar to pacemakers, all ICDs come with protective circuitry to reduce the potential damage of such a shock, but because of the uncertainty of the effectiveness of such circuitry it is best to inactivate the device and to take the same precautions as for pacemakers if an elective external cardioversion is planned.

The traditional standard configuration of defibrillation electrodes has been two or three patches placed on the epicardial surface of the heart for delivery of the defibrillation shock. There has been justifiable concern that the ICD patches themselves may impede the delivery of an external defibrillation shock because material used in the patches may act as an insulator, altering or blocking the current flow through the heart.

One study examined this issue in detail and determined that epicardial ICD patches in dogs produced a significant elevation in the threshold for external defibrillation regardless of the orientation of the patches with respect to the defibrillation shock [130]. The effect was even greater when the axis of the defibrillation shock was the same as the axis for the ICD patches.

Thus it seems reasonable to use a higher defibrillation energy for a patient with epicardial ICD patches, and it is preferable to orient the external defibrillation electrodes perpendicular to the plane of the ICD patches (i.e., along the anteroposterior axis if the patches are along the lateral surface of the heart and with the anterolateral paddle location if the patches are oriented

more along the anteroposterior plane). The patch position can be readily determined on a chest radiograph. In any case, since time is critical in defibrillation, delivery of a shock should never be delayed because of uncertainty about epicardial patch position. It should also be remembered that newer, recently released, and investigational lead placements use transvenous defibrillation electrodes instead of epicardial patches. These will undoubtedly come into common clinical practice in the next few years and would seem less likely to interfere with an external shock, although definitive information is lacking at this point.

References

1. Driscol TE, Ratnoff OR, Nygaard OF: The remarkable Dr. Abildgaard and countershock. *Ann Intern Med* 83:878, 1975.
2. Zoll PM, Linethal AJ, Gibson W, et al: Termination of ventricular fibrillation in man by externally applied countershock. *N Engl J Med* 25:727, 1956.
3. Beck CS, Pritchard WH, Feil SA: Ventricular fibrillation of long duration abolished by electric shock. *JAMA* 135:985, 1947.
4. Lown B, Amarasingham R., Newman J: New method for terminating cardiac arrhythmias: Use of synchronized capacitor discharge. *JAMA* 182:548, 1962.
5. Lown B, Bey SK, Perlroth MG, et al: Comparison of alternating current with direct current countershock across the chest. *Am J Cardiol* 10:223, 1963.
6. Alexander S, Kleiger R, Lown B: Use of external electric countershock in the treatment of ventricular tachycardia. *JAMA* 177:916, 1961.
7. Lown B, Bey SK, Perlroth MG, et al: Comparative studies of ventricular fibrillation. *J Clin Invest* 42:953, 1963.
8. Lown B, Perlroth MG, Bey SK, et al: "Cardioverson" of atrial fibrillation: A report on the treatment of 65 episodes in 50 patients. *N Engl J Med* 269:325, 1963.
9. DeSilva RA, Graboys DB, Podrid PJ, et al: Cardioversion and defibrillation. *Am Heart J* 100:881, 1980.
10. Lown B, Wolf M: Approaches to sudden cardiac death from coronary artery disease. *Circulation* 44:130, 1981.
11. King BG: *Effect of Electric Shock on Heart Action with Special Reference to Varying Susceptibility in Different Parts of the Cardiac Cycle.* Ph.D. dissertation, New York, Columbia University Press, 1934.
12. Wiggers CJ, Wegria R: Ventricular fibrillation due to single localized induction and condenser shocks applied during the vulnerable phase of ventricular systole. *Am J Physiol* 128:500, 1921.
13. Wellens HJ, Brugada P: Diagnosis of ventricular tachycardia from the 12-lead electrocardiogram. *Cardiol Clin* 5:511, 1987.
14. Brugada P, Brugada J, Mont L, et al: A new approach to the differential diagnosis of a regular tachycardia with a wide QRS complex. *Circulation* 83:1644, 1991.
15. Dessertenne F: La tachycardia ventriculaire à deux foyes oposes variables. *Arch Mal Coeur* 59:263, 1966.
16. Greene TO, Spodick DH: Recognition and management of *Torsades de pointes. Heart Dis Stroke* 1:383, 1992.
17. Mann DL, Maisel AS, Atwood JE, et al: Absence of cardioversion-induced ventricular arrhythmias in patients with therapeutic digoxin levels. *J Am Coll Cardiol* 5:882, 1985.
18. Kerber RE, Jensen SR, Grayzel J, et al: Elective cardioversion: Influence of paddle electrode location and size on success rates and energy requirements. *N Engl J Med* 305:658, 1981.
19. Crampton RA: Accepted, controversial and speculative aspects of ventricular defibrillation. *Prog Cardiovasc Dis* 23:167, 1980.
20. Lown B, Kleiger R, Wolff G: Technique of cardioversion. *Am Heart J* 67:282, 1964.
21. Thomas ED, Ewy GA, Dahl CF, et al: Effectiveness of direct current defibrillation: Role of paddle electrode size. *Am Heart J* 93:463, 1967.
22. Wolf PA, Kannel WB, McGee DL, et al: Duration of atrial fibrillation

and the imminence of stroke: The Framingham study. *Stroke* 14:664, 1983.

23. Wolf PA, Abbott RD, Kannel WB: Atrial fibrillation: A major contributor to stroke in the elderly—The Framingham study. *Arch Intern Med* 147:1561, 1987.

24. Kerber RE, Martins JB, Kienzie MG, et al: Energy current and success in defibrillation and cardioversion: Clinical studies using an automated impedance-based method of energy adjustment. *Circulation* 77:1038, 1988.

25. Hartel G, Louhija A, Konttinen A, et al: Value of quinidine in maintenance of sinus rhythm after electrical conversion of atrial fibrillation. *Br Heart J* 33:518, 1971.

26. Hilestead L, Bjerkelund C, Dale J, et al: Quinidine and maintenance of sinus rhythm after electrical conversion of chronic atrial fibrillation. *Br Heart J* 33:518, 1971.

27. Sodermark T, Johnsson B, Olsson A, et al: Effect of quinidine on maintaining sinus rhythm after conversion of atrial fibrillation or flutter: A multi-center study from Stockholm. *Br Heart J* 37:486, 1975.

28. Normand JP, Legendre M, Kahn JC, et al: Comparative efficacy of short acting and long acting quinidine for maintenance of sinus rhythm after electrical conversion of atrial fibrillation. *Br Heart J* 38:381, 1976.

29. Boissel JP, Wolff E, Gillete J, et al: Controlled trial of a long acting quinidine for maintenance of sinus rhythm after conversion of sustained atrial fibrillation. *Eur Heart J* 2:49, 1981.

30. Henry WL, Morganroth J, Pearlman AS, et al: Relation between echocardiographically determined left atrial size and atrial fibrillation. *Circulation* 53:273, 1976.

31. Logan WSWE, Rowlands DJ, Howitt G, et al: Left atrial activity following cardioversion. *Lancet* 1:472, 1965.

32. Manning WJ, Leeman DE, Gorch PJ, et al: Pulse Doppler evaluation of atrial mechanical function after electrical cardioversion of atrial fibrillation. *J Am Coll Cardiol* 13:617, 1989.

33. Budo WJ, Natarajan P, Kroop IG: Pulmonary edema following direct current cardioversion for atrial arrhythmias. *JAMA* 218:1803, 1971.

34. Wells JL Jr, Maclean WAH, James TN, et al: Characterization of atrial flutter: Studies in man after open heart surgery using fixed atrial electrodes. *Circulation* 60:665, 1975.

35. Genetos BC, Gaum WE, Elharrar V, et al: Dissimilar atrial rhythms in a patient with Wolff-Parkinson-White syndrome. *Chest* 72:663, 1977.

36. Szekely P, Batson G, Stock DC: Direct current shock treatment of cardiac arrhythmias. *Br Heart J* 28:366, 1966.

37. Bjerkelund C, Orning M: Evaluation of direct current shock therapy of atrial arrhythmias. *Acta Med Scand* 184:481, 1968.

38. Frithz G, Aberg H: Direct current conversion of atrial flutter. *Acta Med Scand* 187:271, 1970.

39. Vassaux C, Lown B: Cardioversion of supraventricular tachycardia. *Circulation* 39:791, 1969.

40. Katz MJ, Zitnik RJ: Direct current shock and lidocaine in the treatment of digitalis induced ventricular tachycardia. *Am J Cardiol* 18:552, 1966.

41. Newman BJ, Donoso E, Friedbert CK: Arrhythmias in the Wolff-Parkinson-White syndrome. *Prog Cardiovasc Dis* 9:147, 1966.

42. Wellens HJD: Wolff-Parkinson-White syndrome and atrial fibrillation. *Am J Cardiol* 34:777, 1974.

43. Alimurung BN, Robinson TH, Clements SD Jr: Atrial fibrillation and the Wolff-Parkinson-White syndrome. *South Med J* 73:806, 1980.

44. Brusca A, DeFrancheschi A, DiLeo M, et al: Electrical treatment of paroxysmal ventricular tachycardia. *Acta Cardiol* 23:169, 1968.

45. Lown B, Bey SK, Perlroth MG, et al: Cardioversion of ectopic tachyarrhythmias. *Am J Med Sci* 246:257, 1963.

46. Lown B, Kleiger R, Williams BJ: Cardioversion and digitalis drugs: Changed threshold of electric shock in digitalized animals. *Circ Res* 17:519, 1965.

47. Rabbino MD, Likoff W, Dreifus LS: Complications and limitations of direct current countershock. *JAMA* 190:147, 1964.

48. Kleiger R, Lown B: Cardioversion and digitalis, II: Clinical studies. *Circulation* 33:878, 1966.

49. Das G, Anand KM, Ankinedu K, et al: Atrial pacing for cardioversion of atrial flutter in digitalized patients. *Am J Cardiol* 41:301, 1978.

50. Varna MPS, Geddes JS, Pantridge JF: DC cardioversion in patients on amiodarone. *Eur J Cardiol* 12:371, 1981.

51. Fogoros RN: Amiodarone-induced refractoriness to cardioversion. *Ann Intern Med* 100:699, 1984.

52. Huang SK, Tan de Guzman WL, Chenarides JG, et al: Effects of long-term amiodarone therapy on the defibrillation threshold and the rate of shocks of the implantable cardioverter defibrillator. *Am Heart J* 122:720, 1991.

53. Robards GJ, Saunders PM: Refractory supraventricular tachycardia complicating pregnancy. *Med J Aust* 2:278, 1973.

54. Vogel JH, Pryor K, Blound SG: Direct current defibrillation during pregnancy. *JAMA* 193:970, 1965.

55. Schroeder JS, Harrison DC: Repeated cardioversion during pregnancy. *Am J Cardiol* 27:445, 1971.

56. Grand A, Bernard J: Cardioversion et grossesse. *Nouv Presse Med* 2:2327, 1973.

57. Sanchez Diaz CJ, Gonzalez Carmona VM, Ruesga Zamora E, Monteverda Grether CA: Electrical cardioversion in the emergency service. *Arch Inst Cardiol Mex* 57:387, 1987.

58. Meitus ML: Fetal electrocardiography and cardioversion with direct current countershock. *Dis Chest* 48:324, 1965.

59. Sussman HI, Duque D, Lesser ME: Atrial flutter with one to one conduction: Report of a case in a pregnant women successfully treated with DC countershock. *Dis Chest* 49:99, 1966.

60. Curry JJ, Quintana F: Myocardial infarction with ventricular fibrillation during pregnancy treated by direct current defibrillation with fetal survival. *Chest* 58:82, 1970.

61. Radford DJ, Izukawa T: Atrial fibrillation in children. *Pediatrics* 59:250, 1977.

62. Gutgesell HP, Tacker WA, Geddes LA, et al: Energy dose for ventricular defibrillation of children. *Pediatrics* 58:898, 1976.

63. Ewy GA: Electrical therapy of cardiovascular emergency. *Circulation* (suppl 4):111, 1974.

64. Kerber RE: Energy requirements for defibrillation. *Circulation* (suppl 4):117, 1974.

65. Shade BR, et al: *Advanced Cardiac Life Support*. Englewood Cliffs, NJ, American Heart Association, 1986.

66. Dunn M, Alexander J, DeSilva R, Hildner F: Antithrombolytic therapy in atrial fibrillation. *Chest* 89:685, 1986.

67. Bjerkelund CJ, Orning OM: Efficacy of anticoagulant therapy in preventing embolism related to DC electrical conversion of atrial fibrillation. *Am J Cardiol* 23:208, 1969.

68. Freeman I, Wexler J, Howard F: Anticoagulants for treatment of atrial fibrillation. *JAMA* 184:73, 1963.

69. Morris JJ Jr, Kong Y, Norse WC, et al: Experience with "cardioversion" of atrial fibrillation and flutter. *Am J Cardiol* 14:94, 1964.

70. Hearst JW, Paulk EA Jr, Proctor HD, et al: Management of patients with atrial fibrillation. *Am J Med* 37:728, 1964.

71. Morris JJ Jr, Peter RH, McIntosh HD: Electrical conversion of atrial fibrillation: Immediate and long term results and selection of patients. *Ann Intern Med* 65:216, 1966.

72. Goldman MJ: Management of chronic atrial fibrillation: Indications for a method of conversion to sinus rhythm. *Prog Cardiovasc Dis* 2:465, 1960.

73. Bjerkelund CJ, Orning OM: Evaluation of DC shock treatment of atrial arrhythmias: Immediate results and complications in 437 patients with long term results in the first 290 of these. *Acta Med Scand* 184:481, 1978.

74. Laupacus A, Allers G, Dunn M, et al: Antithrombotic therapy in atrial fibrillation. *Chest* 102:4265, 1992.

75. Daniel WG, Freedberg RS, Grote J, et al: Incidence of left atrial thrombi in patients with nonvalvular atrial fibrillation: A multicenter study using trans-esophageal echocardiography. *Circulation* 86:1396, 1992.

76. Aschenberg L, Scheuster M, Kremer P, et al: Transesophageal two-dimensional echocardiography for the detection of left atrial appendage thrombus. *J Am Coll Cardiol* 7:163, 1986.

77. Mugge A, Daniel WG, Hawsmann D, et al: Diagnosis of left atrial appendage thrombi by transesophageal echocardiography: Clinical implications and follow-up. *Am J Cardiac Imaging* 4:173, 1990.

78. Manning WJ, Reis GJ, Douglas PS: Use of transesophageal echocardiography to detect left atrial thrombi before percutaneous balloon dilatation of the mitral valve: A prospective study. *Br Heart J* 67:170, 1992.

79. Manning WJ, Silverman DI, Gordon SP, et al: Cardioversion from atrial fibrillation without prolonged anticoagulation with use of transesophageal echocardiography to exclude the presence of atrial thrombi. *N Engl J Med* 328:750, 1993.
80. Tedeschi CG, White CW Jr: Morphologic study of canine heart subjected to defibrillation, electrical defibrillation and manual compression. *Circulation* 9:916, 1954.
81. Rivkin LM: Defibrillation and cardiac burns. *J Thorac Cardiovasc Surg* 46:755, 1963.
82. Dahl CF, Ewy GA, Warner ED, et al: Myocardial necrosis from direct current discharge: Effect of paddle electrode size and time interval between discharges. *Circulation* 50:596, 1974.
83. Ehsani A, Ewy GA, Sobel BE: Effects of electrical countershock on serum creatine phosphokinase (CPK) isoenzyme activity. *Am J Cardiol* 37:12, 1976.
84. Reiffel JA, Gambino R, McCarthy DM, et al: Direct current cardioversion: Effect of creatine kinase, lactic dehydrogenase, myocardial isoenzymes. *JAMA* 239:122, 1978.
85. Chun PKC, Davia JE, Donohue DJ: ST segment evaluation with elective DC cardioversion. *Circulation* 63:220, 1981.
86. Sutton RB, Tsataris TO: Pulmonary edema following direct current cardioversion. *Chest* 57:191, 1970.
87. Lindsey J Jr: Pulmonary edema following cardioversion. *Am Heart J* 74:434, 1967.
88. Ikram H, Nixon PGP, Arcan T: Left atrial function after electrical conversion to sinus rhythm. *Br Heart J* 30:80, 1968.
89. Rowlands DJ, Logan WSWE, Howart E: Atrial function after conversion. *Am Heart J* 74:149, 1967.
90. Mancini GBJ, Goldberger AL: Cardioversion of atrial fibrillation: Consideration of embolism, anticoagulation, prophylactic pacemaker and long term success. *Am Heart J* 104:617, 1982.
91. Cascio WE, Foster JR, Sheps DS: Elective cardioversion in the presence of conduction disturbance. *J Electrocardiol* 17:63, 1984.
92. Kerber RE: External direct current defibrillation and cardioversion, in Zipes DP, Jalife J (eds): *Cardiac Electrophysiology: From Cell to Bedside.* Philadelphia, WB Saunders, 1990, pp 954–962.
93. Ideker RE, Tang AS, Frazier DW, et al: Ventricular defibrillation: Basic concepts, in El-Sherif N, Samet P (eds): *Cardiac Pacing and Electrophysiology.* Philadelphia, WB Saunders, 1991.
94. Wiggers CJ: The mechanism and nature of ventricular defibrillation. *Am Heart J* 20:399, 1940.
95. Zipes DP, Fisher J, King RM, et al: Termination of ventricular fibrillation in dogs by depolarizing a critical amount of myocardium. *Am J Cardiol* 36:37, 1975.
96. Chen P-S, Shibata N, Dixon EG, et al: Comparison of the defibrillation threshold and the upper limit of vulnerability. *Circulation* 73:1022, 1986.
97. Sweeney RJ, Gill RM, Steinberg MI, Reid PR: Ventricular refractory period extension caused by defibrillation shocks. *Circulation* 82:965, 1990.
98. Swartz JF, Jones JL, Fletcher RD: Characterization of ventricular fibrillation based on monophasic action potential morphology in the human heart. *Circulation* 87:1907, 1993.
99. Miles WM, Zipes DP: Cardioversion and defibrillation: clinical aspects, in El-Sherif N, Samet P (eds): *Cardiac Pacing and Electrophysiology.* Philadelphia, WB Saunders, 1991.
100. Dalzell DW, Cunningham SR, Anderson J, Adgey AA: Initial experience with microprocessor controlled current based defibrillator. *Br Heart J* 61:502, 1989.
101. Dalzell GW, Adgey AA: Determinants of successful transthoracic defibrillation and outcome in ventricular fibrillation. *Br Heart J* 65:311, 1991.
102. Dalzell GW, Cunningham SR, Anderson J, Adgey AA: Electrode pad size, transthoracic impedance and successful external defibrillation. *Am J Cardiol* 64:741, 1989.
103. Deale OC, Lerman BB: Intrathoracic current flow during transthoracic current fraction. *Circ Res* 67:1405, 1990.
104. Lerman BB, Deale OC: Relation between transcardiac and transthoracic current during defibrillation in humans. *Circ Res* 67:1420, 1990.
105. Kerber RE, Grayzel J, Hoyt R, et al: Transthoracic resistance in human defibrillation: Influence of body weight, chest size, serial shocks, paddle size, and paddle contact pressure. *Circulation* 63:676, 1981.
106. Kerber RE, Martins KB, Kelly KJ, et al: Self-adhesive preapplied electrode pads for defibrillation and cardioversion. *J Am Coll Cardiol* 3:815, 1984.
107. Ewy GA, Hellman DAM, McClung S, et al: Influence of ventilation phase on transthoracic impedance and defibrillation effectiveness. *Crit Care Med* 8:164, 1980.
108. Kerber RE, Vance S, Schomer SJ, et al: Transthoracic defibrillation: Effect of sternotomy on chest impedance. *J Am Coll Cardiol* 20:94, 1992.
109. Bardy GH, Ivey TD, Allen M, Johnson GA: Prospective, randomized evaluation of effect of ventricular fibrillation duration on defibrillation thresholds in humans. *J Am Coll Cardiol* 13:1362, 1989.
110. Emergency Cardiac Care Committee and Subcommittees, American Heart Association: Guidelines for cardiopulmonary resuscitation and emergency cardiac care. *JAMA* 268:2171, 1992.
111. Tacker WA Jr, Galioto FM Jr, Giuliana E, et al: Energy dosage of human transchest electrical ventricular defibrillation. *N Engl J Med* 290:214, 1974.
112. Lown B, Crampton RS, DeSilva RA, et al: The energy for ventricular defibrillation: Too little to too much? *N Engl J Med* 298:1252, 1978.
113. Adgey AAJ, Patton JN, Campbell NPS, et al: Ventricular defibrillation: Appropriate energy levels. *Circulation* 60:219, 1979.
114. Tacker WA Jr, Ewy GA: Emergency defibrillation dose: Recommendations and rationale. *Circulation* 60:223, 1979.
115. Pantridge JF, Adgey AAJ, Webb SW, et al: Electrical requirements for ventricular defibrillation. *Br Med J* 2:313, 1975.
116. DeSilva RA, Lown B: Energy requirement for the markedly overweight patient. *Circulation* 57:827, 1978.
117. Lappin HA: Ventricular defibrillators in heavy patients. *N Engl J Med* 291:153, 1974.
118. Gascho JA, Crampton RS, Cherwek ML, et al: Determinance of ventricular defibrillation in adults. *Circulation* 60:231, 1979.
119. Pennington JE, Taylor J, Lown B: Chest thump for reverting ventricular tachycardia. *N Engl J Med* 283:1192, 1970.
120. Yakaitis RW, Redding JS: Precordial thumping during cardiac resuscitation. *Crit Care Med* 1:22, 1973.
121. Ruffy R: Pharmacological modulation of ventricular defibrillation, in Zipes DP, Jaliffe J (eds): *Cardiac Electrophysiology from Cell to Bedside.* Philadelphia, WB Saunders, 1990, pp 959–962.
122. Woodfolk DI, Craffee WR, Cohen W, et al: The effect of quinidine on electrical energy required for ventricular fibrillation. *Am Heart J* 72:659, 1966.
123. Babbs CF, Yim GKW, Whistler SJ, et al: Elevation of ventricular defibrillation threshold in dogs by antiarrhythmic drugs. *Am Heart J* 98:345, 1979.
124. Dorian P, Fair ES, Davy JM, et al: Effect of quinidine and bretylium on defibrillation energy requirements. *Am Heart J* 112:19, 1986.
125. Troup PJ, Chapman PD, Olinger GN, et al: The implanted defibrillator: Relation of defibrillating lead configuration and clinical variables to defibrillation threshold. *J Am Coll Cardiol* 6:1315, 1985.
126. Guarnieri T, Levine JH, Veltri EP, et al: Success of chronic defibrillation and the role of antiarrhythmic drugs with the automatic implantable cardioverter/defibrillator. *Am J Cardiol* 60:1061, 1987.
127. Furman S, Hayes DL, Holmes DR: *A Practice of Cardiac Pacing.* 2nd ed. Mount Kisko, NY, Futura, 1989.
128. Barold SS, Falkoff MD, Ong LS, Heinle RA: Interference in cardiac pacemakers: Exogenous sources, in El-Sherif N, Samet P (eds): *Cardiac Pacing and Electrophysiology.* Philadelphia, WB Saunders, 1991.
129. Manolis AS, Rastegar H, Estes NAM III: Automatic implantable cardioverter defibrillator: Current status. *JAMA* 262:1362, 1989.
130. Lerman BB, Deale OC: Effect of epicardial patch electrodes on transthoracic defibrillation. *Circulation* 81:1409, 1990.

7. Echocardiography in the Intensive Care Unit

Gerard P. Aurigemma, David A. Orsinelli, and Andrea M. Sweeney Walsh

Echocardiography has proven to be an invaluable tool for evaluation of the critically ill patient in the intensive care unit (ICU) because of the wealth of information it can provide rapidly and because studies can be performed at the patient's bedside. At our institution approximately 30 percent of all echocardiographic studies are performed emergently in the ICU or emergency room, principally to diagnose life-threatening conditions such as aortic dissection or cardiac tamponade or to evaluate left ventricular function in patients with hypotension or congestive heart failure. In these and other clinical situations, echocardiography provides diagnostic information with excellent sensitivity and specificity and is frequently the only cardiac diagnostic test necessary.

Echocardiography may be performed either with the transducer placed directly on the patient's chest (transthoracic echocardiography [TTE]) or mounted on a gastroscope that is passed into the patient's esophagus and stomach (transesophageal echocardiography [TEE]). In the past the major limitation of TTE in the ICU setting was that many studies were technically inadequate for a variety of reasons: mechanical ventilation, chronic obstructive lung disease, and the presence of incisions/bandages in the postoperative patient. However, the advent and widespread use of TEE has extended the capabilities of echocardiography in the ICU by providing high-quality, diagnostic images in situations where TTE is technically limited. Thus at present, with very few exceptions, echocardiography provides the answer to the major clinical question, rapidly, in the ICU patient.

Ultrasound Principles

Echocardiography uses ultrasonic energy to create real-time, two-dimensional (2-D) images of the beating heart. In this chapter we use the term *echocardiography* to refer to ultrasound examination of the heart; a routine echocardiographic study consists of M-mode, 2-D, and Doppler echocardiographic examinations (discussed below). Details about ultrasound physics may be found elsewhere [1,2]. The echocardiography machine consists of a device that transmits and receives ultrasound (transducer), a central processor that converts the received ultrasound into a 2-D image, and a video display. The echocardiographic examination is recorded by the operator on videotape and chart paper and reviewed, off-line, either on the machine or at a separate VCR/television viewing station. It is likely that in the future routine echocardiographic examination will be recorded and displayed using digital technology, which promises enhanced resolution and streamlined study storage, retrieval, and playback. Digital technology is already used extensively in stress echocardiography.

Transthoracic Echocardiographic Imaging

A 2-D echocardiogram depicts the beating heart on a video display, from a series of viewpoints or "windows." The operator performs the examination using a standard routine and sequentially images the heart from each of these windows (see below and Figs. 7-1 and 7-2). The standard echocardiographic examination utilizes three separate ultrasound technologies: M-mode echo, 2-D echo, and Doppler flow analysis. The M-mode echocardiogram displays the motion of cardiac structures with respect to time, along a single "icepick" view (Fig. 7-3); this examination is recorded on strip-chart paper. At present, M-mode recordings are used principally for measurements of cardiac chamber sizes and to time events precisely in the cardiac cycle, since the temporal resolution of M-mode technique is superior to that of 2-D echo. This means, for example, that the M-mode recording may be used to detect diastolic collapse of the right ventricle in patients with cardiac tamponade or early closure of the mitral valve in patients with acute, severe aortic regurgitation due to bacterial endocarditis. In most other respects, however, M-mode echo has been supplanted by 2-D echo, which images much more of the cardiac volume than M-mode echo and therefore permits a better spatial appreciation of cardiac structures (Fig. 7-2); however the M-mode examination is still a vital part of the routine echocardiographic study in our laboratory for the analysis of dimensions and in situations that call for precise timing of cardiac events.

The third ultrasound technology used in routine echocardiographic studies is Doppler echocardiography. A detailed discussion of the physics of Doppler ultrasound is provided elsewhere [3,4]. In brief, Doppler ultrasound provides a measure of the velocity of flowing blood in the heart and great vessels. The techniques of pulsed and continuous-wave Doppler (Fig. 7-4) display the flow velocity recording, or spectrum, alongside a 2-D echocardiographic image. By use of the Bernoulli equation, which relates the peak velocity of flow across valves or septal defects to the associated pressure drop, a pressure gradient may be estimated from the Doppler recording of peak velocity [3,4]. The Doppler technique is therefore used to estimate, from the velocity profile, the peak and mean pressure gradients associated with aortic and mitral stenosis [4,5]. The same principle is used to estimate the right ventricular (RV) systolic pressure from the peak velocity associated with tricuspid regurgitation (TR) [6]. The difference between RV and right atrial (RA) pressure can be derived from the TR velocity profile; this number is added to an estimate of RA pressure to derive the RV systolic pressure. In the absence of pulmonic stenosis, the RV pressure is equal to the pulmonary artery pressure.

A recent addition to the routine transthoracic echocardiographic examination is Doppler color flow mapping [7,8,9]. The principles underlying color flow mapping are the same as

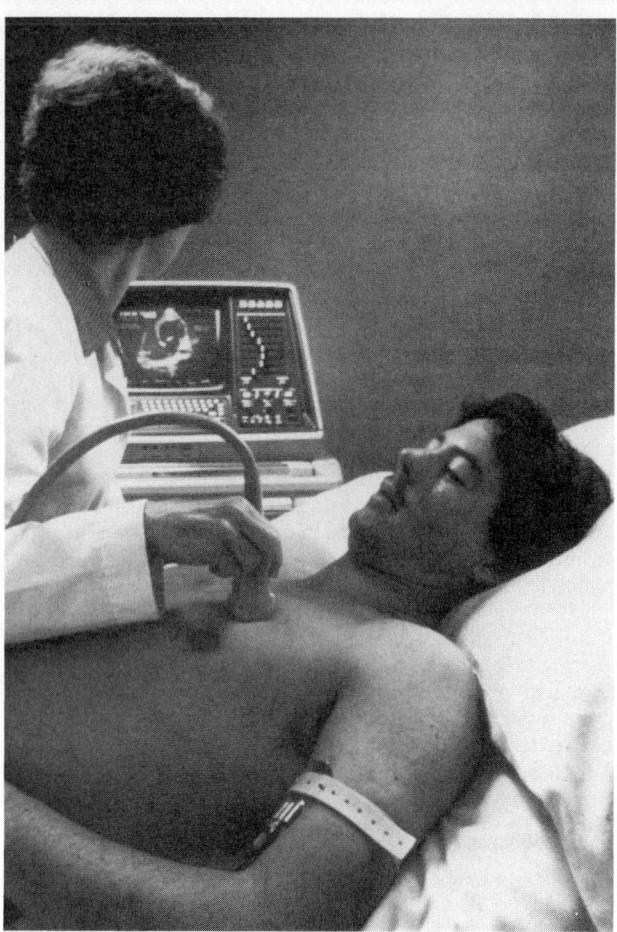

Fig. 7-1. 2-D echo performed with the probe in the parasternal position. The patient is either supine or in the left decubitus position, with electrocardiographic leads placed on the arms, shoulders, or chest. The ultrasonographer sits on the examination bed or stands at the bedside and continuously views the video display. The controls on the echocardiographic machine are set to optimize image quality. (Courtesy of Hewlett-Packard)

those used in pulsed and continuous-wave Doppler. However, instead of a display of Doppler velocities with respect to time, as is used in pulsed and continuous-wave Doppler, color flow mapping provides a color-coded display of velocities superimposed on the 2-D echocardiographic image. In this manner, the spatial extent of disturbed flow may be appreciated in the context of the 2-D image. Color flow Doppler therefore provides an immediate assessment of disturbed flow in valvular regurgitation, intracardiac shunts, and hypertrophic cardiomyopathy [10]. Moreover, color flow Doppler is the most widely used noninvasive technique to quantitate valvular regurgitation, providing results that are similar to semiquantitative angiographic grading of regurgitation [8,9].

TRANSTHORACIC IMAGING TECHNIQUE. Echocardiographic imaging requires that the ultrasound transducer be placed in certain specific locations on the chest wall ("acoustic windows"); placement of the transducer in these locations permits the ultrasound beam to avoid interference by the lungs and ribs as it travels to and from the cardiac structures (see Fig. 7-2). Routine echo is performed using several acoustic win-

dows, as described below. Transmission gel applied to the transducer serves as an interface between the transducer and the chest wall, since air transmits ultrasound poorly.

An ECG signal recorded and displayed simultaneously with the echocardiographic examination; ECG timing is crucial for analysis of the motion of cardiac structures throughout the cardiac cycle. The ECG electrodes are usually placed on the patient's shoulders and lower part of the abdomen. Imaging is performed with the patient supine or in left lateral decubitus position, with the upper body lifted 30 to 40 degrees. This position is useful during imaging from the apical and parasternal windows (see below).

In our laboratory, a routine examination comprises M-mode, 2-D, and Doppler echo; the examination is problem-oriented, however, and is tailored to answer the major clinical questions. Routine examination includes imaging from four major acoustic windows, to view the heart from different angles. Additional images may be required to answer certain clinical questions; these images are obtained from any standard location by rotating and tilting the transducer. A complete examination generally takes 30 to 50 minutes but may be much longer in instances when precise Doppler quantitation of disturbed flow is required.

Parasternal Views (Figs. 7-1 and 7-2). The transducer is first positioned at the second or third intercostal space just left of sternum, with the patient in left lateral decubitus position; this positioning acts to shift the left lung to allow better visualization of the heart. The reference point of the transducer is positioned toward the patient's right shoulder so that the plane of the image transects the heart along its long axis from apex to base. The resulting image, the parasternal long-axis view (Fig. 7-2a), displays the heart sagittally, with the LV at the center of the screen. The M-mode recording is made from this view.

A short-axis, or transverse, view of the heart is obtained by rotating the transducer 90 degrees from the long-axis view so the reference point is directed toward the patient's left shoulder (Fig. 7-2b,c). The resulting images depict the right side of the heart, including the tricuspid valve, on the left of the screen, the pulmonic valve on right side of screen, and the three cusps of the aortic valve in the center of screen. The transducer is tilted or rocked to a position that is more perpendicular to the chest wall so the ultrasound beam intersects the heart at the mitral valve level. Finally, the transducer is tilted inferiorly and toward the apex of the heart so the ultrasound beam bisects the midportion of the LV chamber and depicts the LV at the level of the papillary muscles. This view permits a comprehensive evaluation of LV function, since segmental wall motion abnormalities in all three coronary perfusion beds may be visualized at once.

Apical Views. The transducer is moved to the apical window, with the patient remaining in left lateral decubitus position, and placed at or near the cardiac apex and angled superiorly. The apical long-axis view is obtained by orienting the reference point on the transducer superiorly toward the patient's right shoulder. The resulting image displays the heart upside-down, with the apex of the heart displayed at the top of the monitor and the base displayed at the bottom. The apical four-chamber view is obtained by orienting the reference point on the transducer toward the patient's left shoulder. All four cardiac chambers (ventricles and atria) are seen simultaneously. This view is useful for evaluations of the LV lateral and septal walls, RV anterior wall, and mitral and tricuspid valves. The apical five-chamber view is obtained by tilting the transducer more anteriorly so the beam travels through the LV outflow tract and aortic valve.

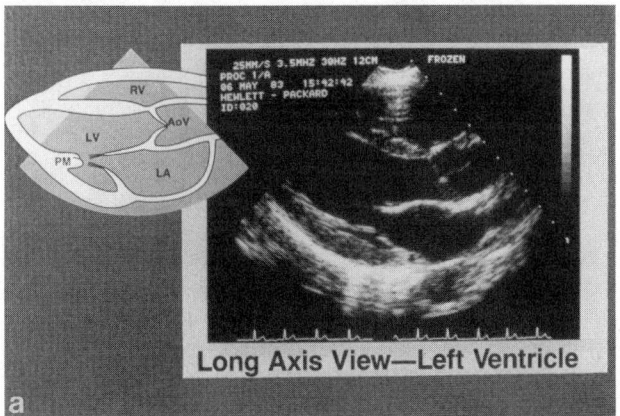

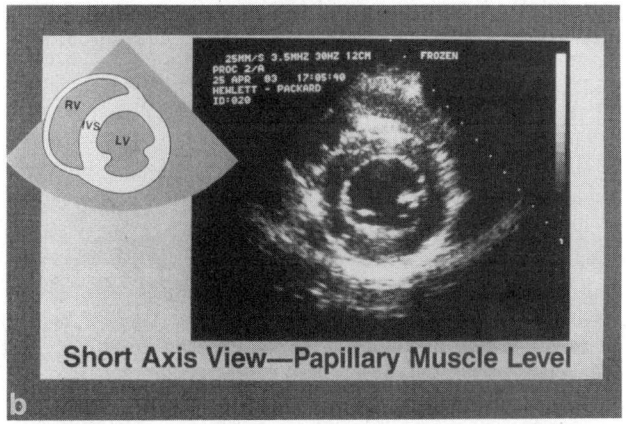

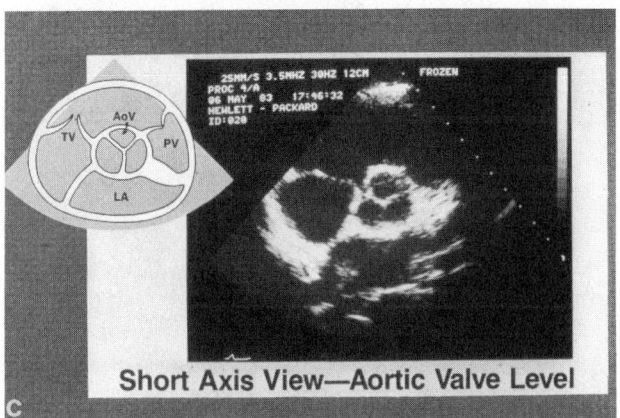

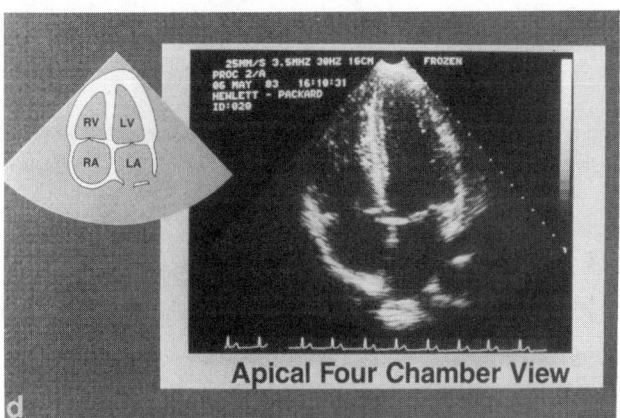

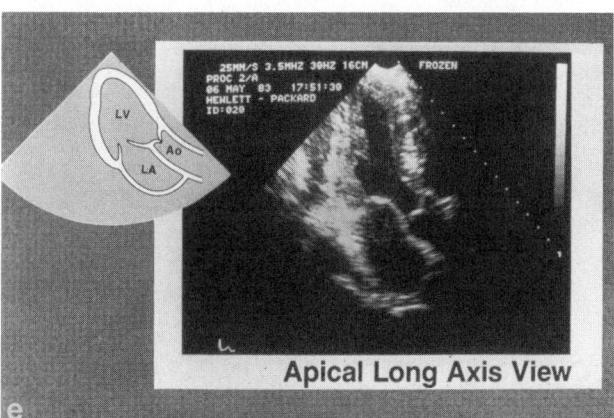

Fig. 7-2. Standard 2-D echo views with corresponding schematic diagrams to demonstrate cardiac anatomy. a. Parasternal long-axis view. b. Parasternal short-axis view at the level of the papillary muscle. c. Parasternal short-axis view at the level of the aortic valve. d. Apical four-chamber view. e. Apical long-axis view. The operator obtains sequential images from parasternal and apical windows. Thus, after a comprehensive examination all four cardiac valves and all four cardiac chambers are completely examined. The combination of the parasternal short-axis view and the apical views permit a comprehensive examination of wall motion of the left ventricular myocardium in all three coronary perfusion beds. (Courtesy of Hewlett-Packard)

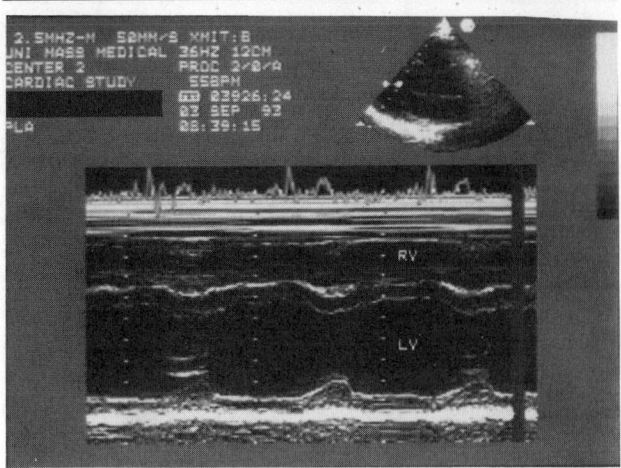

Fig. 7-3. 2-D-directed M-mode examination. The inserted 2-D image is used to target the single icepick view through the midportion of both ventricles (dotted vertical line). The motion of cardiac structures along this view is displayed with respect to the ECG, which is above the M-mode display. The right ventricular (RV) and left ventricular (LV) cavities are labeled; the intervening structure is the interventricular septum, which thickens and moves posteriorly in systole.

Rotating the transducer so the reference point is directed toward the left side of the patient's neck causes the beam to bisect the chambers of the left side only. This positioning produces the apical two-chamber view, which displays the inferior and anterior walls of the LV.

Subcostal View. The transducer is positioned over the lower section of the chest just below the xyphoid. The ultrasound beam travels through the abdominal wall, liver, and diaphragm before reaching the heart. The reference point on the transducer is directed toward the right shoulder, with anterior and superior angulation of the transducer. The resulting image displays the base of the heart on the left and the apex on the right of the monitor. The anatomic relation of the plane of the interatrial septum to the path of the ultrasound beam is particularly important in evaluation of patients with suspected atrial septal defect. This view provides images that may supplement suboptimal images obtained from the parasternal or apical windows.

LIMITATIONS OF TRANSTHORACIC ECHOCARDIOGRAPHY. Several important limitations of TTE should be noted. Imaging from the chest wall requires the use of relatively low-frequency transducers (usually 2.5 or 3.5 mHz for adults), which provides poor resolution of cardiac structures. Since both air and the chest wall impede ultrasound transmission, high-quality TTE requires optimal acoustical windows. Consequently, patients who are obese, have obstructive lung disease, or have suffered chest wall injury or undergone sternotomy may not be suitable ultrasound subjects; similarly, patients who hyperventilate because of pain, anxiety, or poor gas exchange may be expected to have suboptimal studies. Prosthetic aortic and mitral valves present obstacles to the ultrasound beam transmission and result in acoustic "shadowing." Such shadowing will, for example, prevent the Doppler beam from reaching the left atrium on apical views and therefore prevent complete color Doppler mapping of mitral regurgitation in most instances.

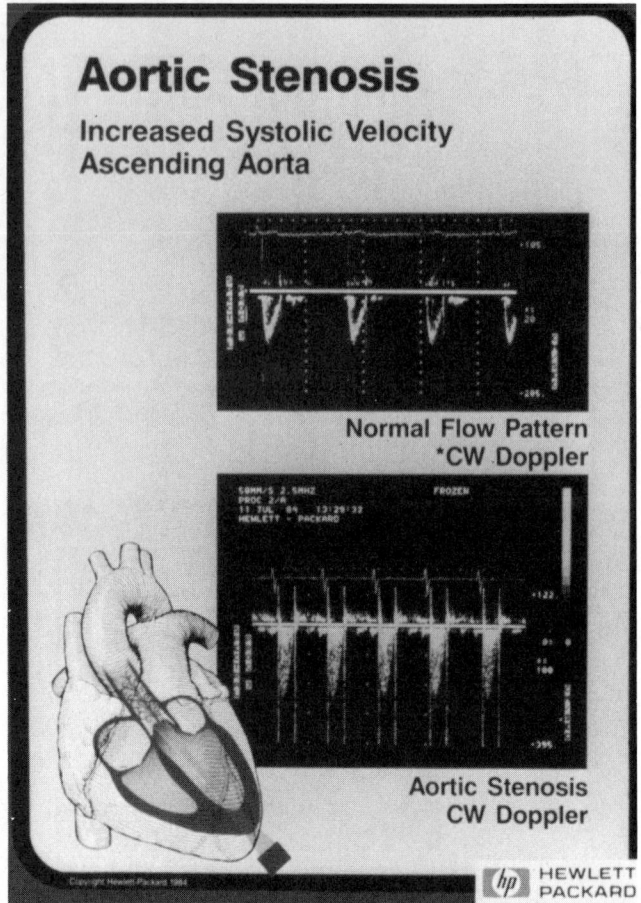

Fig. 7-4. Schematic and spectral flow recordings from a patient with aortic stenosis illustrates the relationship between Doppler velocity and pressure gradients. The upper panel demonstrates a normal flow pattern by continuous-wave Doppler in the ascending aorta. In contrast, the patient with aortic stenosis (lower panel) has an increase in peak systolic velocity, indicative of pressure differential across the aortic valve. The corresponding pressure gradient can be estimated from the peak velocity recording using the Bernouilli equation, where the pressure gradient is $4 \times$ peak velocity^2. (Courtesy of Hewlett-Packard)

Transesophageal Echocardiographic Imaging

Transesophageal echo overcomes many of the technical limitations of TTE by imaging via the esophagus and avoiding the interference of the intervening chest wall structures and the lungs. In addition to providing a novel set of imaging windows, the proximity of the esophagus to the heart and great vessels permits the use of higher-frequency transducers, providing better image resolution. For these reasons TEE images are, with few exceptions, of very high quality. Thus the advantages of TEE (compared to TTE) include improved image quality and expanded diagnostic capabilities.

EQUIPMENT. The TEE probe consists of an ultrasound transducer mounted on the tip of a modified flexible gastroscope

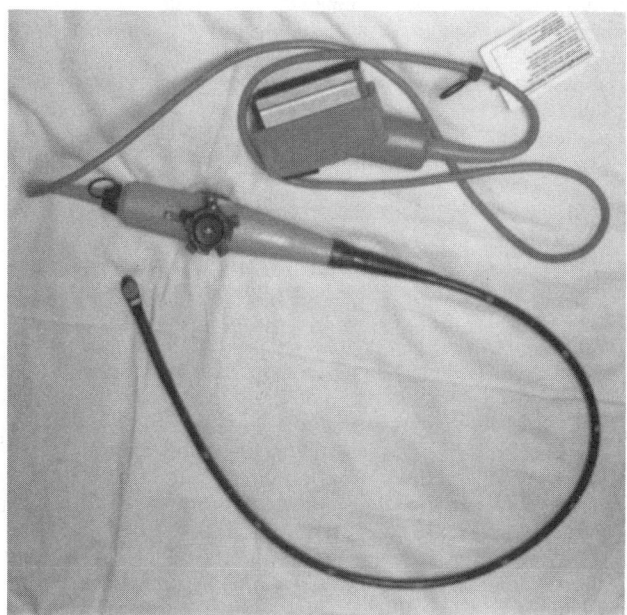

A

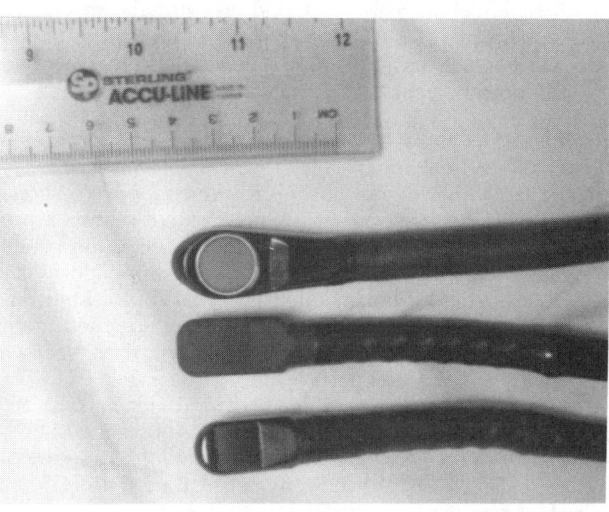

B

Fig. 7-5. Transesophageal echo probes. A. Hewlett-Packard OmniPlane probe, showing the flexible probe, handle with control wheels, connecting cable, and electrical transducer connector. B. Distal tip of three probes. From left to right, an OmniPlane probe (Hewlett-Packard), a Hewlett-Packard single-plane probe, and an Advanced Technology Laboratories single-plane probe.

Table 7-1. Clinical Situations in which Transesophageal Echo Is Superior to Transthoracic Echo

1. Assessment of patients with suspected endocarditis, both native and prosthetic valve, and complications of endocarditis
2. Assessment of suspected prosthetic valve dysfunction, especially mitral prostheses
3. Evaluation of suspected thoracic aortic pathology, including aortic dissection
4. Evaluation of suspected intracardiac masses, especially in the atria (e.g., atrial myxoma, atrial thrombi)
5. Evaluation of patients with a suspected cardiac source of systemic emboli
6. Assessment of the interatrial septum (e.g., atrial septal defect, patent foramenovale)
7. Diagnosis of central pulmonary emboli

The current generation of TEE transducers have biplane or multiplane imaging capabilities, often with multiple imaging frequencies, and full Doppler capabilities.

INDICATIONS. Transesophageal echo is indicated in the assessment of cardiac structure and function in patients in whom TTE images are inadequate to answer the clinical question. In addition, TEE has been shown to be superior to TTE for a variety of specific indications and is usually indicated as an adjunctive test to TTE. Table 7-1 lists indications for which TEE has been shown to be superior to TTE [11–31]. Transesophageal echo may also provide diagnostic information beyond that derived from a good-quality TTE in patients with native valve dysfunction, congenital heart disease, and complications of acute myocardial infarction. The precise role of TEE in many of these situations is rapidly evolving.

EXAMINATION. The TEE procedure has been described by several authors [32,33,34]. Our approach is described below, with mention of special considerations when performing TEE in the critical care setting (Table 7-2).

Personnel. While TTE is routinely performed by nonphysician sonographers, TEE is always performed by a physician who has extensive training in echocardiography and who has completed appropriate training in both esophageal intubation and interpretation of TEE images [34].

For optimal patient safety, TEE requires the presence of one or two ancillary personnel to assist the physician operator and monitor the patient. A nurse or physician should be present to help position the patient, administer medications, monitor the patient's vital signs and respiratory status, and operate the suction device. It is helpful to have a second assistant present to adjust the image settings on the echocardiography machine and to assist with videotaping; this is generally performed by an ultrasonographer or cardiology fellow.

Preparation. An appropriate patient history should be obtained to confirm the need for the study, screen for contraindications to the procedure, determine the need for endocarditis prophylaxis (see below), determine any drug allergies, and assess the patient's respiratory and hemodynamic status. Patients with compromised respiratory status should be stabilized prior to TEE, since sedation and/or esophageal intubation may result in further respiratory compromise. In such patients, the

that is approximately 100 cm long (Fig. 7-5A). The distal flexible tip of the scope houses the ultrasound transducer (Fig. 7-5B). The controls for manipulating the tip of the probe are located on the handle of the probe. Two lockable wheels on the handle control motion of the tip of the probe. A large outer wheel controls probe flexion (anteroposterior motion) while a smaller inner wheel controls lateral (right-left) motion. A cable connects the probe handle to an electrical transducer connector, which is inserted into the ultrasound imaging system. Controls for adjusting the echocardiographic image (e.g., sector size, depth, gain) and Doppler modalities are located on the echocardiographic machine.

Table 7-2. Procedure for Transesophageal Echo

1. Patient preparation
   a. Screen for appropriate indications/contraindications
   b. Hemodynamic/respiratory status assessment
   c. Patient consent
   d. NPO (NG tube in selected patients)
   e. IV access
2. Pharyngeal anesthesia
3. Sedation (midazolam and/or meperidine)
4. Monitor vital signs during and after procedure
5. Esophageal intubation
   a. Manual guidance or blind intubation
6. Image acquisition (goal-directed examination)
7. Equipment care

procedure should be delayed until the patient is stabilized; on occasion, intubation and controlled ventilation is required for airway protection and adequate oxygenation.

It is mandatory to review prior TTE studies; a careful review of the findings may sometimes obviate the need for TEE. In our experience this is often the case when intracardiac masses are suspected: the TTE may demonstrate that the suspected mass is a Chiari network, prominent eustachian valve, or imaging artifact.

The TEE probe should be inspected for damage to the probe and to ensure that the controls of the scope are operational, and it should be confirmed that the echocardiography machine is operating properly. An appropriate suction device, supplemental oxygen, resuscitation equipment, and appropriate medications must be readily available during the procedure.

Patient Preparation and Monitoring. The procedure should be explained to the patient and consent obtained from the patient or surrogate. Dentures and other dental prostheses should be removed. To avoid the potential complication of aspiration of gastric contents, except in truly emergent situations, patients should fast a minimum of 4 hours prior to TEE and preferably take nothing orally (except medications) overnight prior to the study. Critically ill patients often develop a paralytic ileus and even with an adequate overnight fast may have retained gastric contents. If there is any question as to the presence of gastric contents, a nasogastric (NG) tube should be passed prior to TEE to decompress the stomach. The NG tube may remain in place during TEE if no difficulty is encountered in passing the probe; if there is difficulty in passing the TEE probe or if suboptimal images are obtained, the NG tube should be removed. For patients with an NG or feeding tube in place, the position of the tube should be confirmed after TEE, as it may be displaced during the procedure. Many patients in the ICU have central venous access present, which can be used to administer medications. If access is not present, a stable peripheral intravenous catheter (preferably located in an antecubital vein if a saline contrast study is to be performed) is needed to administer medications.

During the procedure, the patient's respiratory status, vital signs, and ECG should be continuously monitored. Continuous monitoring of the arterial oxygen saturation with pulse oximetry is helpful, especially in the unstable patient with compromised respiratory status. Following the procedure, the patient must be observed to ensure that he or she has recovered from the effects of sedation and is stable. Food should be withheld until the effects of pharyngeal anesthesia have resolved, usually 1 to 2 hours.

Local Anesthesia. Local pharyngeal anesthesia is used to suppress the gag reflex, even in the intubated patient. For the paralyzed or unconscious patient, local anesthesia is not necessary. Patients who are able to swallow are asked to gargle then swallow 15 to 30 ml of viscous lidocaine. Following this, the pharynx is sprayed with a topical anesthetic, such as Cetacaine (Cetylite Industries, Pennsauken, N.J.). The adequacy of the anesthesia is tested using a gloved finger to confirm that the gag reflex has been suppressed.

Sedation. Intravenous sedation is not mandatory [36], but we believe the procedure is much better tolerated with judicious use of conscious sedation [32,33]. We prefer a short-acting benzodiazepine, such as midazolam, given in 0.5- to 1-mg increments (to an average total dose of 4 mg). In addition, we frequently use meperidine in doses of 12.5 to 25 mg intravenously (average total dose 25–50 mg). In patients with renal failure we use morphine sulfate in doses of 1 mg (to a total of 1–4 mg) in place of meperidine to avoid the accumulation of a major metabolite of meperidine that undergoes renal excretion. These drugs must be used with caution in critically ill patients who may have altered metabolism due to underlying disease (e.g., cardiac, renal, or hepatic failure), which may result in oversedation and respiratory depression. Hemodynamically unstable patients also may be more vulnerable to the potential hypotensive effects of these drugs.

Adequate sedation is imperative in patients with suspected aortic dissection or acute myocardial infarction to avoid potentially deleterious increases in blood pressure and myocardial oxygen demand. This may be especially important in the patient with aortic dissection, in whom increases in blood pressure may lead to propagation of dissection.

Endocarditis Prophylaxis. The need for endocarditis prophylaxis for TEE is controversial [32–38]. The incidence of bacteremia related to TEE and thus the risk of endocarditis should be similar to that of upper endoscopy without biopsy, a procedure thought to be low-risk [38,39]. However, the patient population evaluated by TEE is at greater risk for endocarditis, since many patients have underlying valvular and/or congenital heart disease. While there have been reports of endocarditis apparently related to TEE [39,40], most prospective studies have found a low incidence of positive blood cultures related to TEE, most if not all of which were thought to represent contaminants [40–47]. Khandheria summarized the results of several of these studies [39] and concluded that the incidence of positive blood cultures related to TEE is no different than the rate of blood culture contamination; therefore, with the possible exception of patients with poor dentition and a history of endocarditis, antibiotic prophylaxis for TEE is not warranted. Patients at high risk (e.g., prosthetic heart valves, prior endocarditis, surgically constructed systemic-pulmonary shunts) may be considered for prophylaxis. Our current practice is to administer prophylactic antibiotics only to patients with prosthetic valves, unless there is a clinical question of endocarditis, in which case such treatment could render diagnostic blood cultures negative. The most appropriate role for prophylactic antibiotics remains to be determined, and some authorities recommend no such routine prophylaxis [44–47].

Esophageal Intubation. The technique of inserting the probe (esophageal intubation) and performing the TEE procedure has been described in detail [31,32]. We will describe our approach. The nonintubated patient is positioned in the left lateral decubitus position; the intubated patient (see below) is usually studied in the supine position. Both the operator and assistant wear disposable gloves. In patients with teeth, a bite guard is placed around the probe. The distal 10 to 15 cm of the probe is lubricated with a combination of a water-soluble lubricating gel and

2% lidocaine gel. The lock on the wheel controlling flexion/anteflexion is released while the medial/lateral control wheel is kept locked in the neutral position. Once the probe is inserted, this lock is released. After adequate conscious sedation and pharyngeal anesthesia, one or two fingers of one hand is placed in the posterior pharynx to guide the probe. Since fiberoptic guidance is not available for TEE, the probe is inserted with manual guidance, with care to keep the probe in the midline. Once the probe has been advanced to the posterior pharynx, the patient is asked to swallow to help advance the probe through the upper esophageal sphincter and into the distal esophagus (a depth of 25–35 cm as measured from the incisors), where the aortic valve and left atrium are visualized. The patient's neck may need to be flexed to facilitate probe placement. Gentle pressure may be used to pass the probe, but it should never be forcefully advanced. Once the probe is placed, the bite guard is positioned and images obtained. An alternative method of esophageal intubation is to place the bite guard in the patient's mouth and insert the probe blindly.

Intubated Patients. Probe insertion in the intubated patient is similar to that described above. Because the airway is protected, patients are routinely studied in the supine position. Since respiration is supported, sedatives and analgesics may be used somewhat more generously, though hypotension should be avoided. For awake patients, the posterior pharynx may be anesthetized with a topical anesthetic spray. If difficulty is encountered with esophageal intubation, the cuff of the endotracheal tube may be temporarily deflated to facilitate probe passage. The cuff is reinflated once the probe has been placed. A laryngoscope may be used to facilitate esophageal intubation in the intubated patient where there is extreme difficulty passing the probe blindly. We occasionally use vecuronium (Norcuron), a short-acting nondepolarizing neuromuscular blocking agent, when the patient is extremely uncooperative despite maximal amounts of intravenous sedation; the usual dose of vecuronium is 0.05 to 0.1 mg/kg, given as an intravenous bolus.

Image Acquisition. Image acquisition commences with probe passage. Figures 7-6 to 7-9 show the standard TEE images recorded in a routine study. In the critical care setting, a brief, directed examination must sometimes suffice. On completion of the procedure, the probe is cleaned and disinfected with a 2% glutaraldehyde solution in accordance with the manufacturer's recommendations.

CONTRAINDICATIONS. The contraindications to TEE in the ICU patient are similar to those in the ambulatory patient [33,48]. A history of dysphagia should be elicited and if present evaluated to confirm that no significant esophageal disease is present. Esophageal pathology, such as strictures, varices, diverticuli, scleroderma, prior surgery, or radiation is an absolute contraindication to TEE, as are gastric volvulus, perforation, and active upper gastrointestinal bleeding. If there are questions concerning the safety of TEE in a patient with known or suspected esophageal pathology, a gastroenterologist should be consulted.

While the patient with a coagulopathy may be at increased risk of complications, therapeutic anticoagulation is not a contraindication to TEE. Relative contraindications to TEE include inability of the patient to cooperate, oropharyngeal distortion, and cervical spondylosis, which may make probe passing difficult. A hiatal hernia may interfere with image acquisition. Patients with head and neck trauma must be evaluated carefully to ensure that no oral/pharyngeal trauma exists that could interfere with safe passage of the probe. In patients with sus-

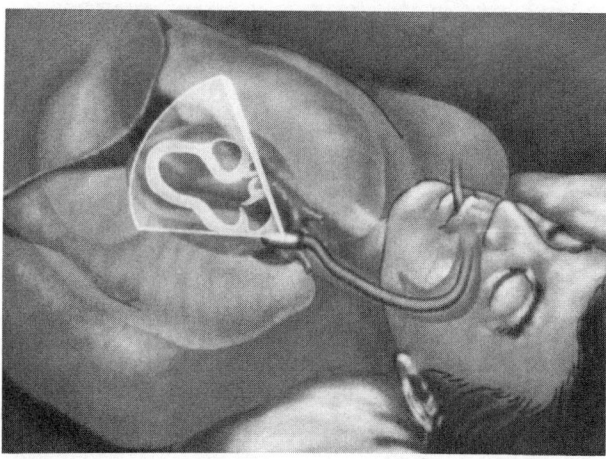

Fig. 7-6. Schematic drawing of a transesophageal echo probe in relationship to mediastinal structures. The probe is positioned in the esophageal imaging plane, providing a sagittal view of the heart. The probe may be further advanced into the stomach and retroflexed to image the heart in cross-section. (Courtesy of Hewlett-Packard)

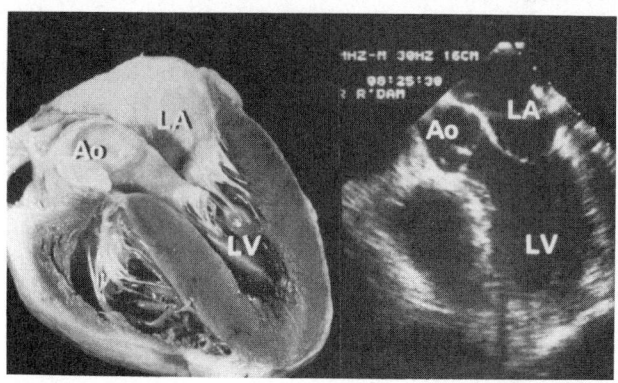

Fig. 7-7. Anatomic specimen and corresponding transesophageal echo image, illustrating the plane of the section when the probe is in the esophagus. Cardiac structures are labeled. This view provides a coronal image of the left ventricle with an excellent view of the mitral apparatus, aortic valve, aortic outflow tract, and left atrium. (Courtesy of Hewlett-Packard)

pected cervical spine injury, cervical spine radiographs should be reviewed by a radiologist to exclude cervical spine fractures or dislocations prior to any attempt at probe passage or head positioning.

COMPLICATIONS. Transesophageal echo has proven to be an extremely safe procedure, even in the critically ill patient [36,48–53]. The potential complications are similar to those encountered in the ambulatory patient and include pharyngeal and esophageal injury, aspiration, laryngospasm, tracheal intubation, respiratory depression, hypotension, and arrhythmias. Critically ill patients may be more susceptible to the untoward effects of intravenous sedation, and unconscious or heavily sedated patients may be at an increased risk of esophageal injury due to their inability to inform the operator of discomfort. In the largest series to date, Daniel et al. [36] reported that the

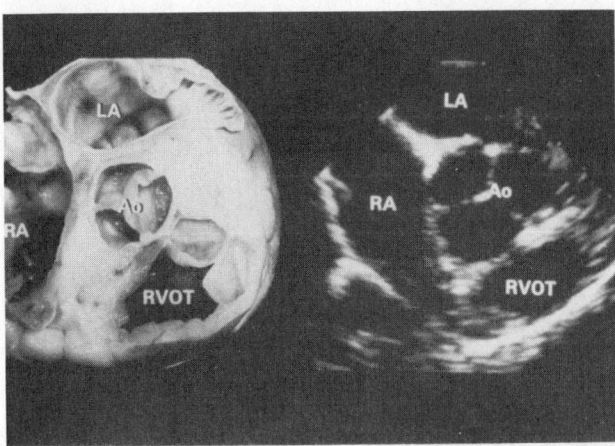

Fig. 7-8. Transesophageal view of the base of heart, with the probe in the esophagus. Cardiac structures are labeled. Note the excellent detail of the aortic valve leaflets (Courtesy of Hewlett-Packard)

most common complication was failure to intubate the esophagus, which occurred in 201 (1.9%) of 10,419 procedures. The procedure was prematurely aborted in 90 (0.88%), in most cases due to patient intolerance (n = 65) or complications (n = 18). The complications included bronchospasm (n = 6), hypoxia (n = 2), arrhythmia (n = 7), severe angina (n = 1), pharyngeal bleeding (n = 1) and severe hematemesis resulting in death (n = 1). Thus the mortality rate in this series was 0.0098 percent. The patient who died had a lung tumor that eroded into the esophagus, resulting in uncontrollable bleeding. The Mayo Clinic recently reported their experience in 3827 TEE studies performed over four years [50]. They reported complications in 2.9 percent of studies and death in 1 patient. The mortality rate was 0.026 percent (ventricular fibrillation in a patient with congestive heart failure. Several studies have shown that TEE is safe in the critical care setting [51,52,53].

Fig. 7-9. The transesophageal echo probe has been advanced into the stomach and retroflexed, to provide a short-axis image of the left ventricle similar to that obtained from transthoracic echo windows. From this transgastric window, wall motion of the myocardium in all three coronary perfusion beds may be visualized. The corresponding anatomy is labeled at left. (Courtesy of Hewlett-Packard)

Clinical Applications of Echocardiography in the Intensive Care Unit

We will now review the application of echocardiography in ICU patients. The application of echocardiography in specific cardiovascular disorders is also discussed in Chapters 33 to 38, 40, and 42.

In our experience, echocardiography is most commonly indicated in the ICU setting for the evaluation of LV function. Echocardiographic data is most helpful in guiding management in unexplained hypotension, congestive heart failure, and suspected mechanical complications following acute myocardial infarction. This experience is similar to that reported by other centers: in a recent study hemodynamic instability was the indication for TEE in approximately one-half of ICU patients [53]. In these instances a bedside echocardiogram (TTE, TEE, or both) rapidly furnishes information concerning LV size and systolic performance and LV diastolic filling and can depict disturbed flow resulting from valvular regurgitation or acquired ventricular septal defects.

LEFT VENTRICULAR STRUCTURE AND FUNCTION

Hypotension. Comprehensive 2-D echo, using TEE where TTE is inadequate, rapidly provides an estimate of the ejection fraction (EF), the most widely used clinical index of LV systolic function. The EF may be estimated by visual inspection of the 2-D echo images or by computing LV end-diastolic and end-systolic volumes [54,55,56]. Most commercially available echocardiographic machines are equipped with software that allows for off-line computation of EF; these methods require that endocardial edges of the LV cavity be traced manually in both systole and diastole. The EF is then calculated from the resulting cavity areas, using geometric assumptions about LV shape [54]. However, a recent study suggests that visual estimate of EF by an experienced physician compares favorably with results of the more labor-intensive, off-line computer computation of EF from the same images [57]. There is much current interest in the use of semiautomated border detection algorithms, which permit rapid determination of LV volumes and ejection fraction without the need for off-line, manual tracing of echocardiographic images. This technique appears to hold promise for the rapid quantitation of LV volumes and function in clinical practice (Fig. 7-10).

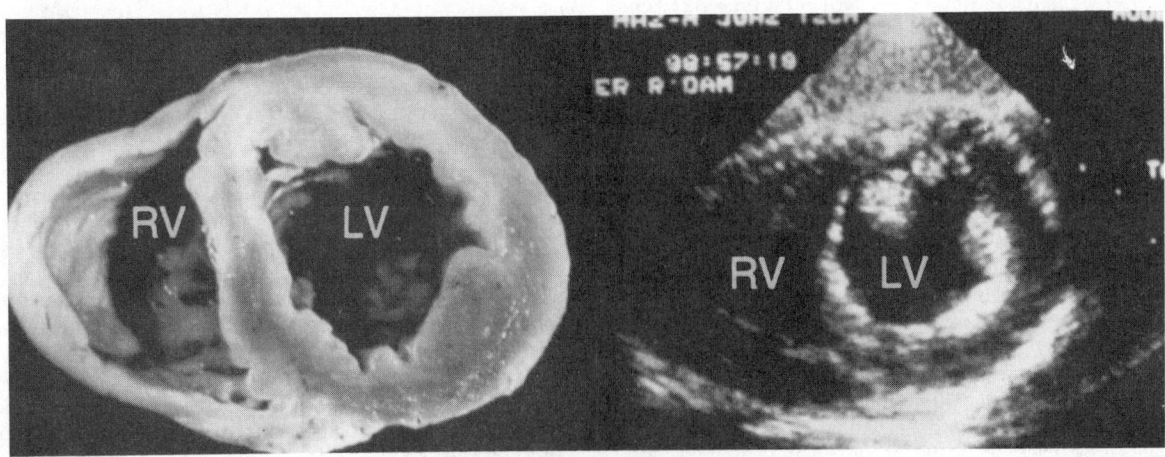

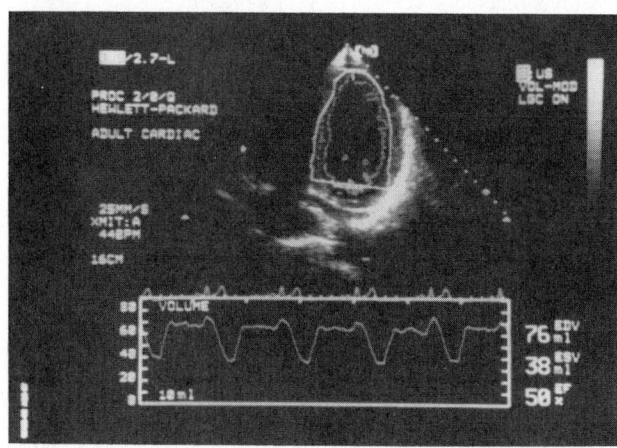

Fig. 7-10. The technique of automated boundary detection and its application to the study of cardiac volumes and ejection fraction. Top. Apical four-chamber view. Bottom. Corresponding beat-to-beat volume display. This technique may be used for on-line, rapid quantitation of end-diastolic and end-systolic volumes and ejection fraction. (Courtesy of Hewlett-Packard)

Since LV chamber dimensions and volumes may be estimated either visually or by quantitative analysis, echocardiography can be used to diagnose hypovolemia. The echocardiogram demonstrates small end-diastolic and end-systolic LV volumes and normal or supranormal ejection fraction (Fig. 7-11). In our experience, hypovolemia is an important cause of hypotension in the postoperative patient, particularly within the first 24 to 48 hours.

Fig. 7-11. A patient evaluated for hypotension following aortic valve replacement for aortic stenosis. Though systolic dysfunction was the suspected cause of hypotension, the study reveals that the ejection performance is supranormal and there is very small end-systolic volume. A. Diminished left ventricular cavity size on this diastolic frame. Posteromedial and anterolateral papillary muscles are shown at 1 and 5 o'clock, respectively. B. End-systolic frame, demonstrating almost total cavity obliteration and small end-systolic volume. These findings led to discontinuation of intravenous pressor support and substitution of fluid resuscitation with subsequent hemodynamic improvement.

Echocardiography is an essential part of the evaluation and postoperative management of elderly patients following aortic valve replacement for aortic stenosis [58–61]. In a subset of these patients (generally older women) who had echocardiography to investigate hypotension, we have noted marked hypertrophy, hyperdynamic systolic function with an EF greater than 70 percent, small chamber volumes, and Doppler evidence consistent with outflow tract obstruction [58]. Often, these findings were completely unexpected and led to dramatic changes in postoperative management, such as discontinuation of positive inotropic agents and institution of fluid resuscitation; in some instances, institution of beta-blockers and/or calcium channel blockers was required. In our experience, these changes are often associated with a restoration of adequate blood pressure, probably due to improved LV filling. Since proper management is predicated on correct diagnosis, we have a low threshold for performing an echocardiogram on postoperative aortic valve disease patients, since routine clinical, radiographic, and even Swan-Ganz catheter data may be misleading [58].

Congestive Heart Failure. Up to 40 percent of patients presenting with congestive heart failure have an EF of 45 percent or greater [62,63]. When the EF is normal, cardiac causes for congestive heart failure may include acute, severe mitral, or aortic regurgitation or impairment of LV filling (diastolic dysfunction) caused by myocardial ischemia and/or hypertensive heart disease. In fact, most patients with congestive heart failure and a normal EF have an antecedent history of hypertension [62,63]. In longstanding hypertension with or without myocardial ischemia, the LV loses its ability to fill completely at normal diastolic pressure [64]. Adequate filling of the LV is then associated with a rise in LV diastolic pressure, resulting in pulmonary congestion [64].

The Doppler mitral inflow velocity pattern has been used to identify abnormalities in diastolic function [65,66]. A pattern of "abnormal relaxation" (Fig. 7-12) generally accompanies patients with longstanding hypertension. However, a shift in the Doppler inflow pattern to a "restrictive" pattern generally indicates high LV filling pressures associated with abnormal LV compliance [67,68,69]. These diastolic filling profiles may be dynamic, as indicated by the fact that treatment with agents such as nitroglycerin or diuretics, which reduce filling pressures, results in a reversion of this restrictive pattern to the

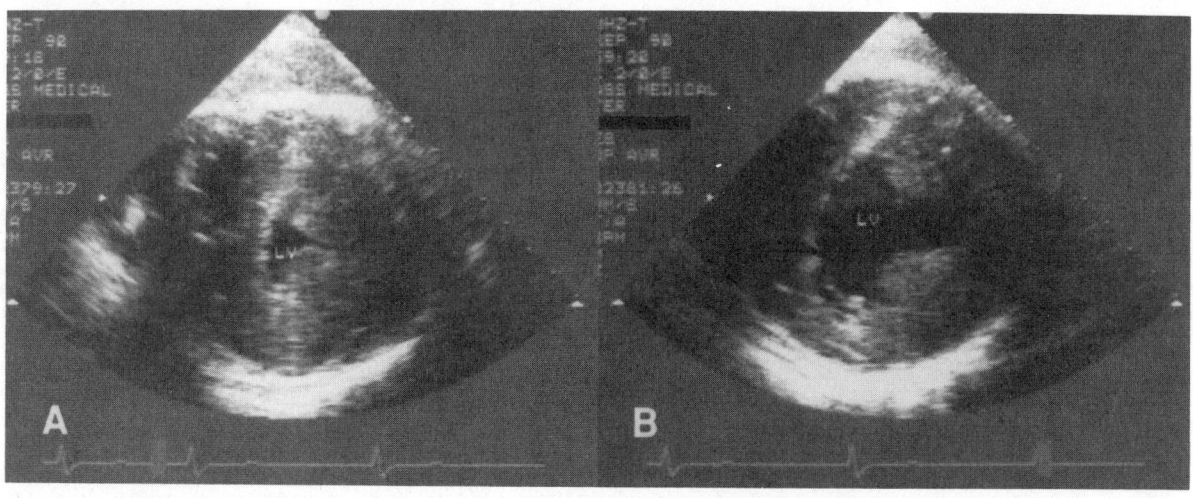

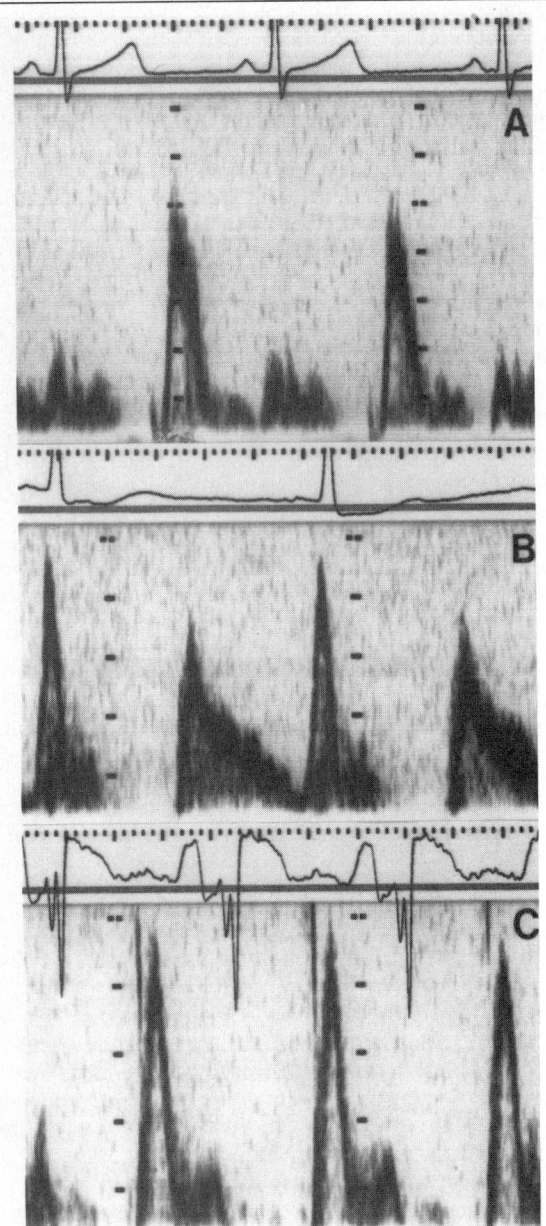

Fig. 7-12. Doppler mitral inflow patterns: strip chart recordings of mitral inflow velocities showing three commonly encountered patterns. Velocity is on the vertical axis and ECG on the horizontal axis. A. A normal individual. In each cardiac cycle, denoted by the R wave, the first velocity profile is associated with passive filling of the left ventricle (LV) (E wave, occurring at the time of the T wave of the ECG) and the second profile is associated with atrial systole (A wave, occurring shortly after the p wave on the ECG). In normals, peak E exceeds peak A velocity. B. A patient with hypertensive LVH, showing reduced E velocity and enhanced A velocity. This pattern is consistent with abnormal LV relaxation. C. A patient with clinical congestive heart failure. This pattern (E velocity exceeding A velocity) is similar to normal, but the rapid deceleration of the E velocity profile reflects abnormal LV compliance and abnormal elevation in diastolic filling pressures.

abnormal relaxation pattern [70]. The presence of an abnormal relaxation or restrictive filling pattern in the face of a normal LV ejection fraction signifies diastolic dysfunction as a possible etiology for congestive heart failure. Thus 2-D echo coupled with Doppler mitral inflow analysis supports the diagnosis of diastolic dysfunction as a cause for congestive heart failure by demonstrating normal ejection fraction and an abnormal LV filling pattern.

Echeverria and co-workers [71] demonstrated the clinical utility of echocardiography in evaluation of patients with congestive heart failure in a study performed prior to the widespread use of Doppler mitral inflow analysis. These investigators reported on 50 consecutive patients referred for echocardiography; in patients with ejection fractions less than 50 percent, echocardiography revealed findings that were worse than clinically expected in 12 (40%). In this group of patients with reduced ejection fraction, echocardiography led to changes in clinical management in 37 percent. The clinical impact of echocardiography, however, was greater in the 40 percent of patients with congestive heart failure and normal ejection fraction (mean EF 70 ± 9%). These patients generally suffered from hypertensive heart disease; interestingly, a normal EF was unexpected by the clinician in 18 of these 20 patients (90%). The echocardiographic findings led to changes in clinical management in 12 (90%) of these patients.

A similar study by Aguirre and co-workers is noteworthy because the investigators used Doppler echocardiography to characterize diastolic function [73]. The combination of 2-D echo and Doppler techniques delineated a mechanism for congestive heart failure in approximately two-thirds of the study population.

Oh and co-workers demonstrated that the Doppler transmitral flow profile correlates with the presence of clinical heart failure in patients suffering an acute myocrdial infarction [73]. This is presumably because the restrictive mitral inflow pattern is indicative of abnormally elevated LV diastolic pressures. Therefore, in patients with congestive heart failure, diastolic filling variables complement the assessment of systolic function and permit a comprehensive assessment of ventricular function.

Myocardial Infarction. At our institution, echocardiography is the principal method used to investigate suspected mechanical complications following myocardial infarction (Chap. 45). Echocardiography can rapidly estimate LV ejection fraction and therefore determine whether hypotension in the patient following myocardial infarction is due to depressed pump function, RV infarction, hypovolemia, or a mechanical complication such as ventriculoseptal rupture.

The ability of echocardiography to detect wall motion abnormalities in myocardial infarction is well established [74,75,76]; in general, reduction in coronary flow of 20 percent or more is required to produce an abnormality in wall motion detectable by echocardiography [77]. The hallmark of such flow reduction is systolic thinning of the myocardium and an apparent outward motion of the endocardium. Coronary flow reductions of 50 percent or greater are reliably associated with a wall motion abnormality on the echocardiogram.

An extensive literature has also documented that 2-D echo accurately diagnoses acute myocardial infarction. Stamm and co-workers correlated location of regional wall motion abnormality with coronary anatomy in patients with their first acute myocardial infarction [75]. These investigators also established that in patients with single-vessel disease there is an excellent correspondence between the echocardiographic site of infarction and coronary anatomy, with the exception of some circumflex coronary occlusions, which tend to be less specifically localized. As is to be expected, patients with multivessel disease present more problems with precise localization of wall motion abnormality.

Echocardiography is also used to estimate the amount of myocardial damage by acute infarction. Though there has been an excellent correlation between echocardiographic and autopsy estimates of the extent of myocardial infarction in both experimental and human studies [78,79,80], echocardiography tends to overestimate the anatomic extent of infarction [81,82,83]. This phenomenon is most likely due to the fact that echocardiography depicts the abnormal function of anatomically normal myocardium that is "tethered" to the infarcted myocardium [77]. Despite this limitation, echocardiography is useful in estimating the extent of myocardial damage following infarction.

In addition to diagnosing myocardial infarction and stratifying risk in patients presenting with chest pain syndromes, 2-D echo sensitively and accurately depicts mechanical complications of myocardial infarction [84–88]. These complications include aneurysm formation, infarct expansion, pseudoaneurysm formation, development of right ventricular infarction [84], and development of mural thrombus (Figs. 7-13 to 7-17). These complications are discussed in detail in Chapter 45.

Doppler color flow mapping enables the clinican rapidly to visualize flow disturbances complicating acute myocardial infarction. The echocardiographic examination can sensitively detect acute ventricular septal rupture as well as papillary muscle dysfunction or ruptured chordae tendineae complicating acute myocardial infarction [87]. Thus 2-D echo and color flow mapping are invaluable adjuncts to clinical examination in the postmyocardial infarction patient with a new holosystolic murmur. Transesophageal echocardiography supplements the transthoracic examination and in our experience has been particularly useful in diagnosing severe mitral regurgitation or ventricular septal rupture in patients with inadequate TTE studies.

CARDIAC VALVES

Stenosis and Regurgitation. Echocardiographic assessment of heart valve disease requires a combination of M-mode, 2-D, and Doppler techniques and a skilled and conscientious ultrasonographer. For regurgitant lesions, the anatomic defect (e.g., flail mitral leaflet) is depicted by 2-D echo, and the location and spatial extent of the flow disturbances is semiquantitated by color flow mapping [7,8,9]. A combination of 2-D echo and M-mode echo is used to assess LV size and function, to help determine the impact on LV performance of the valvular regurgitation. Echocardiographic parameters of size and function are increasingly used to help guide the timing of mitral and aortic valve replacement [89].

Echocardiographic techniques are likewise used extensively in valvular stenosis. Pulsed and continuous-wave Doppler study is used to measure the peak velocity associated with valvular stenosis and, using the Bernoulli principle, estimated peak and mean pressure gradients [5,90]. These velocity measurements may also be used to estimate the stenotic valve area in mitral and aortic stenosis [5]. Doppler-derived gradients correlate closely with invasive determinations. In addition, TEE allows for the investigation of mitral and aortic prosthetic valves, which are incompletely examined by TTE.

Suspected Endocarditis. Echocardiography is commonly requested in the ICU to evaluate patients with suspected bacterial endocarditis. The reported sensitivity of TTE ranges from 44 to 80 percent in patients with clinically suspected endocarditis [91–96]; it has been shown to have excellent specificity and

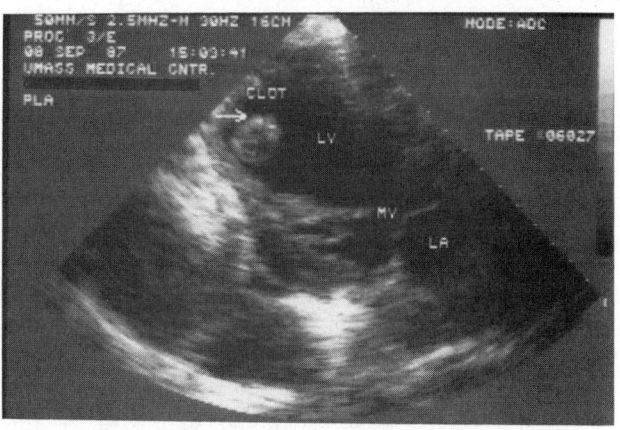

Fig. 7-13. A patient with a large apical myocardial infarction, apical long-axis orientation. The left ventricular cavity is enlarged and there is a pedunculated, large freely mobile clot (*arrow*) attached to the inferoapical portion of the left ventricle.

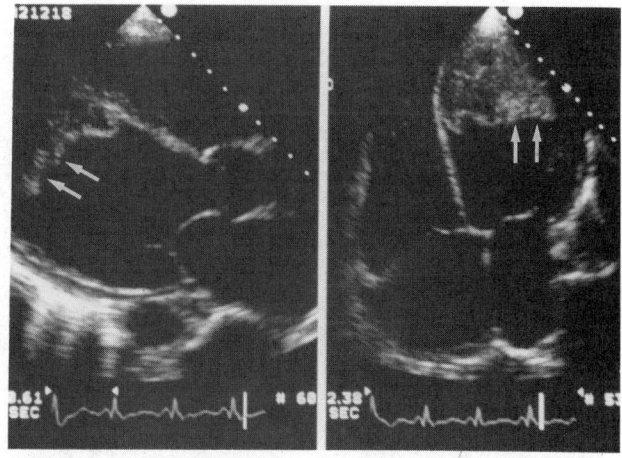

Fig. 7-14. Left. Transthoracic echo, parasternal long-axis view. The left ventricle (LV) is markedly dilated; 2-D echo revealed marked decrease in systolic function. There is a large echo-dense region (*arrows*) (apical four-chamber view). This region indicates a large apical thrombus in this patient with dilated cardiomyopathy and depressed LV systolic function. (Courtesy of Hewlett-Packard)

negative predictive value and can demonstrate abscess formation complicating endocarditis [31,97,98]. However, false positive results may be caused by nonspecific valve thickening, degenerative or rheumatic leaflet sclerosis, ruptured chordae tendineae, or severe myxomatous degeneration of valve leaflets. Pulsed and color flow Doppler imaging supplement TTE in bacterial endocarditis by enabling the clinician to assess the site and severity of associated valvular regurgitation [95]. Jaffe et al. recently demonstrated that when bacterial endocarditis is associated with minimal valvular regurgitation, the risk of in-hospital mortality is low and progression to valve replacement is unlikely [99].

Considering the high-quality images routinely obtained with

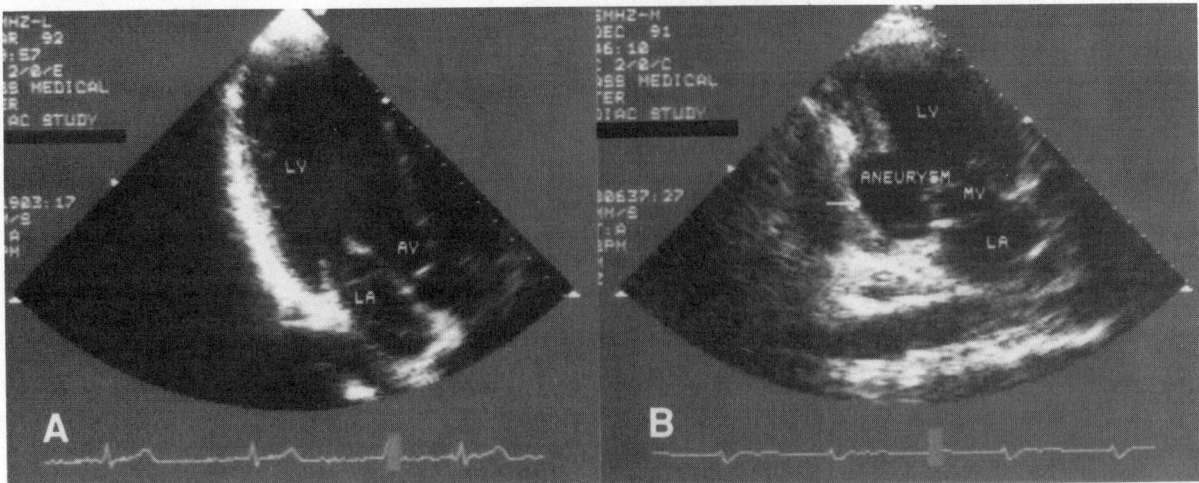

Fig. 7-15. Aneurysm of the inferoposterior wall of the left ventricle (LV). A. Normal LV inferoposterior wall. B. A patient with an inferior myocardial infarction. Large outpouching of the LV wall in the vicinity of papillary muscle (*arrow*), which represents an aneurysm of the inferior wall.

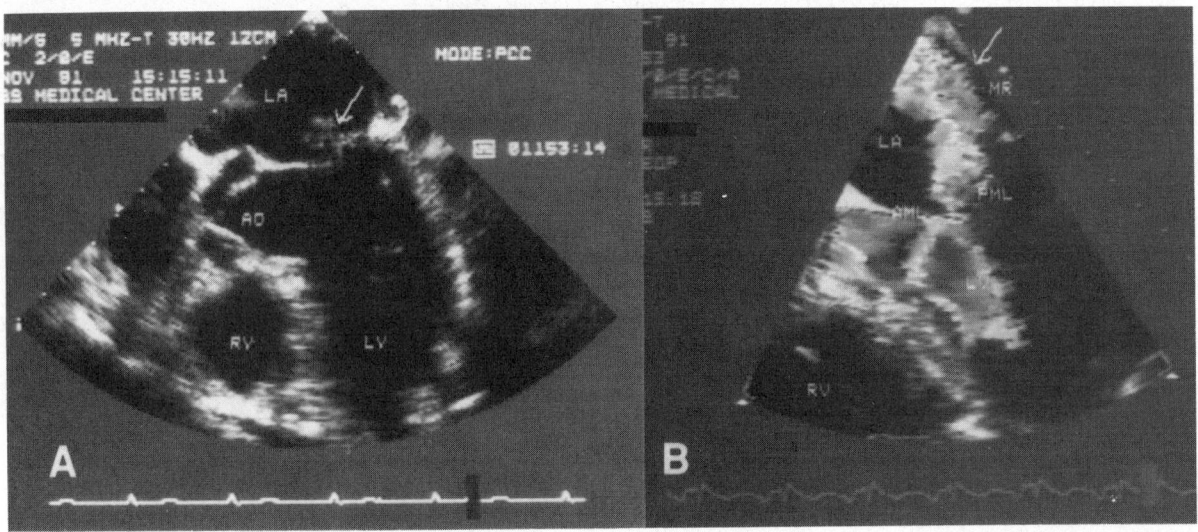

Fig. 7-16. Transesophageal study of a patient with holosystolic murmur. The cardiac structures are labeled. The large mobile mass attached to the posterior leaflet of the mitral valve is consistent with chordal rupture and flail mitral leaflet. Right. The associated jet of mitral regurgitation, which is eccentric (adheres to the lateral wall of the left ventricle). It can be difficult to distinguish among severe, myxomatous degeneration of the mitral valve, vegetation, and flail mitral leaflet.

TEE, it is not surprising that this procedure has an impressive incremental yield in sensitivity and specificity in patients with suspected endocarditis compared with TTE. Shively et al. recently showed that the sensitivity of TEE was much greater than that of TTE (94% vs. 44%, p<0.01) when echocardiographic studies were considered "almost certainly" to demonstrate endocarditis [96]. At lesser levels of diagnostic certainty, TEE was still associated with a much higher sensitivity than TTE (94% vs. 69%) with no sacrifice in specificity. In our experience, TEE

is particularly helpful when TTE is suggestive but not diagnostic of a vegetation (Fig. 7-18).

Transesophageal echo may also demonstrate clinically unsuspected intracardiac abscesses (Fig. 7-19). Daniel and coworkers [31] recently reported the findings of TEE examination in 118 consecutive patients with infective endocarditis of both native and prosthetic valves. Forty-four of their patients had one or more areas of an intracardiac abscess, typically the result of *Staphylococcus aureus* infection of the aortic valve. Transesophageal echo successfully demonstrated 40 to 46 areas of abscess, compared with only 13 of 46 identified by TTE (sensitivity 87% for TEE vs. 28% for TTE).

Transthoracic echo also appears to identify endocarditis patients at increased risk of complications. Stafford and Buda [100,101] observed more complicated clinical courses in endocarditis patients whose TTE studies demonstrated vegetations. In Buda's series, patients with maximal vegetation diameter

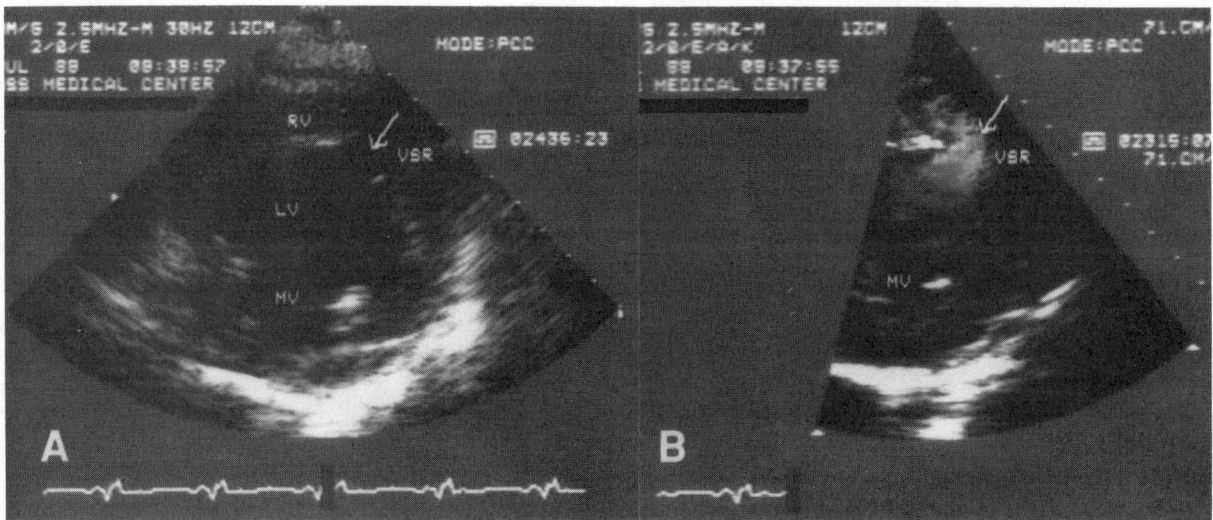

Fig. 7-17. A patient with a myocardial infarction and holosystolic murmur. A. Short-axis view, demonstrating discontinuity in the anteroseptal region (*arrow*). B. Turbulent flow, diagnostic of left ventricle to right ventricle septal rupture flow, is demonstrated (*arrow*).

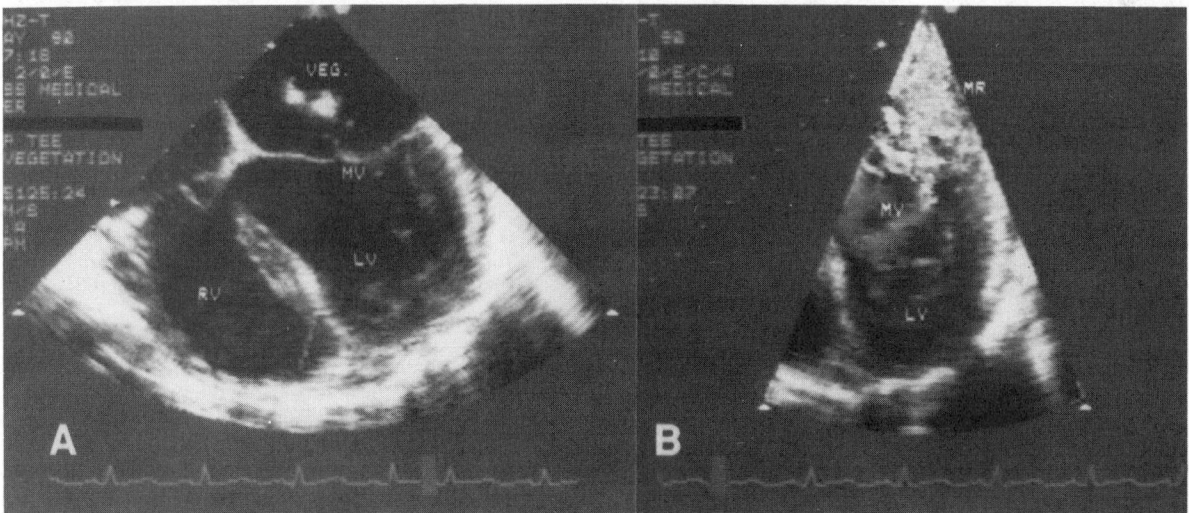

Fig. 7-18. Patient with clinical evidence of bacterial endocarditis. A. Transesophageal view, showing all four cardiac chambers. There is a large, freely mobile vegetation attached to the posterior mitral valve leaflet. B. Associated severe mitral regurgitation, denoted by mosaic color flow pattern that completely fills the left atrium. This patient was taken to the operating room for mitral valve replacement.

exceeding 10 mm were at higher risk for the development of emboli, congestive heart failure, need for surgical intervention, and death than those with smaller vegetations [100]. Mugge and co-workers showed that 22 to 47 patients with a vegetation greater than 10 mm suffered embolic events, in comparison to 11 of 58 patients with a vegetation diameter of 10 mm or less [103]. Sanfilippo and co-workers retrospectively reviewed medical records and 2-D echo in 204 consecutive patients with a clinical diagnosis of endocarditis [102]. These investigators demonstrated that the probability of complications (antibiotic fail-

ure, congestive heart failure, embolization, need for surgery, in-hospital mortality) was related to vegetation size as a continuous variable. Moreover, echocardiographic descriptions of the vegetation (i.e., consistency, mobility, and extent) were predictors of complications [103]. Jaffee and co-workers also demonstrated that in patients with vegetations greater than 10 mm as depicted by 2-D echo the risk of subsequent embolism significantly exceeded that in patients with smaller vegetations [99].

In summary, TTE and TEE are complementary diagnostic techniques in infective endocarditis. A negative, high-quality TTE provides strong evidence against the diagnosis of bacterial endocarditis, particularly when valvular regurgitation is minimal. Transesophageal echo offers an important increase in diagnostic sensitivity when the TTE is of poor quality or when the TTE is negative or equivocal in high clinical suspicion of

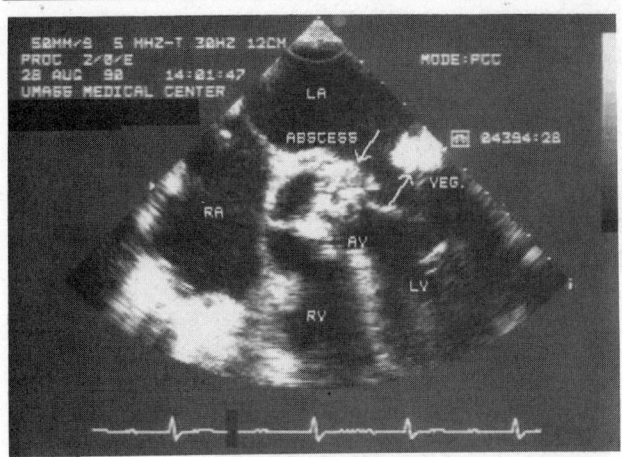

Fig. 7-19. Transesophageal image of a patient who had aortic valve surgery and subsequently developed bacterial endocarditis. The cardiac structures are labeled. The large mobile mass attached to the mitral valve represents a vegetation (*arrow*). There is also an aortic root abscess (*arrows*).

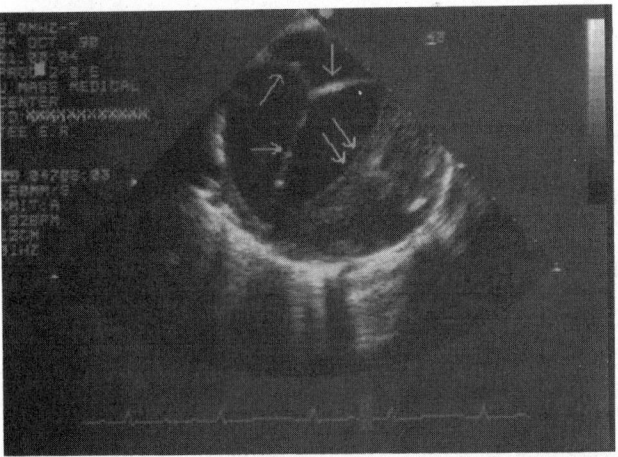

Fig. 7-20. Transesophageal study of a patient with Marfan syndrome. Transverse view of the descending aorta, demonstrating a complex intimal flap (*single arrows*) with thrombus in a false lumen (*double arrows*).

endocarditis. Certain TTE findings appear to identify IE patients at high risk for embolic and other complications.

AORTA/GREAT VESSELS

Thoracic Aortic Dissection. Thoracic aortic dissection is a catastrophic event in which a rapid, accurate diagnosis can be lifesaving. Until recently, the evaluation of aortic dissection relied on aortography or contrast-enhanced computed tomography. Recently, TEE and magnetic resonance imaging (MRI) have been introduced into use for diagnosis of aortic dissection. A complete discussion of aortic dissection is found in Chapter 36. Transesophageal echo has greatly expanded the role of echocardiography in the evaluation of aortic dissection [14–17,104–109] and is also useful in detecting pulmonary embolism [23,25,110], conditions that often enter the differential diagnosis of the patient presenting with acute chest pain and/or dyspnea.

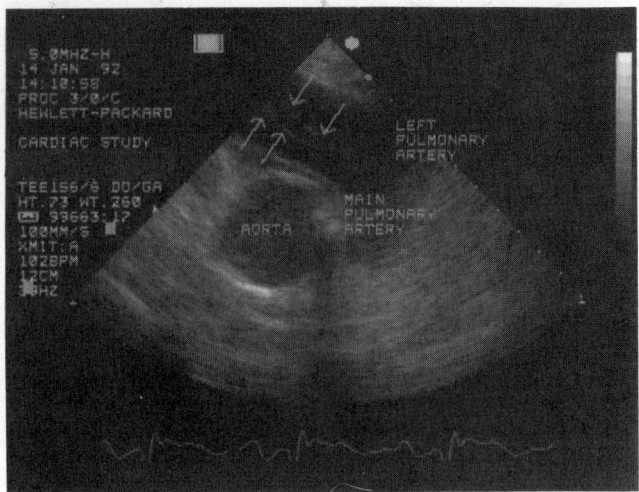

Fig. 7-21. Transverse view of the pulmonary artery bifurcation, demonstrating a large central pulmonary embolus (*arrows*). This patient presented with dyspnea and chest pain. Transesophageal echo was requested following inadequate transthoracic echo, to evaluate left ventricular function.

Transthoracic echo has been used to evaluate patients with suspected aortic dissection [111,112], but its inadequate sensitivity, especially for descending aortic dissection, has until recently precluded the use of echocardiography as a definitive diagnostic test for aortic dissection [109,111,112]. The diagnosis of aortic dissection by echocardiography depends on the identification of an intimal flap, an abnormal linear echo in the aortic lumen, which may be undulating or stationary [104,109]. If the false lumen is thrombosed, the presence of central displacement of intimal calcification may be used to diagnose aortic dissection [105].

Transthoracic echo is hampered by its inability to image the entire thoracic aorta, especially the descending aorta, as well as in obtaining adequate acoustic windows in critically ill patients. The reported sensitivity and specificity of TTE for diagnosing aortic dissection range from 59 to 100 percent and 63 to 96 percent, respectively [108,109,113,114]. Transesophageal echo overcomes many of the limitations of TTE in assessment of the aorta. Due to the close proximity of the esophagus to the aorta, the entire thoracic aorta is well visualized by TEE, with the exception of a small blind spot in the distal ascending aorta that is obscured from view due to the interposition of the trachea between the esophagus and the aorta. Figure 7-20 demonstrates the appearance of aortic dissection on TEE.

Several studies comparing multiple imaging modalities have demonstrated that TEE is, with the possible exception of MRI, most accurate in the diagnosis of aortic dissection [105]. Two recent studies showed a lower specificity than originally reported, due to a significant number of false positive findings in the ascending aorta [107,108]. False positive studies are often due to the presence of imaging artifacts resulting from reverberations from vessel or aortic root calcification or atherosclerotic disease that mimics an intimal flap as well as multiple path artifacts from ultrasound reflection in the left atrium [108,115]. The aorta-lung interface may cause mirror image artifacts in the arch and descending aorta, giving the appearance of a double-lumen aorta [115,116]. Thus, accurate evaluation of the aorta using TEE requires considerable operator experience and knowledge of the potential pitfalls.

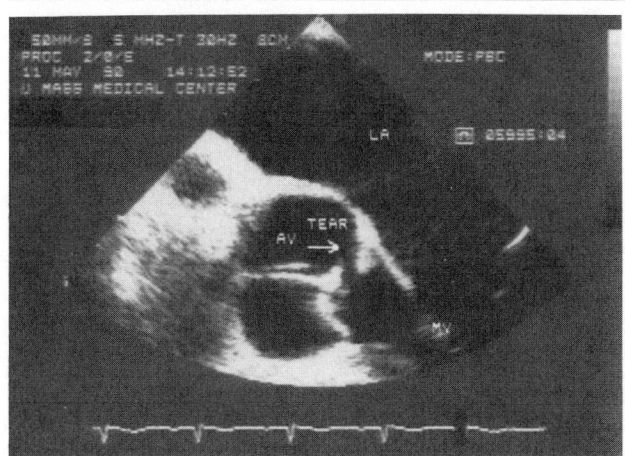

Fig. 7-22. A patient who developed acute, severe aortic regurgitation following blunt chest trauma during a motor vehicle accident. A tear in commissure between the noncoronary and left cusp is clearly demonstrated. Color flow Doppler examination demonstrated severe aortic regurgitation. Based on this study, the patient was sent for semiurgent aortic valve replacement.

Transesophageal echo has several advantages over other imaging modalities: it is portable, thus allowing bedside diagnosis as well as ongoing treatment and monitoring of the patient's hemodynamic status; it is readily available; it allows rapid diagnosis (dissection can be excluded in minutes after the probe is placed); it is minimally invasive; it does not require the use of intravenous contrast material or ionizing radiation; and it is relatively inexpensive [109]. It can also assess LV function, the status of the aortic valve, degree of aortic regurgitation, and the presence of a pericardial effusion that may cause cardiac tamponade. With the possible exception of MRI, no other imaging

modality shares all of these advantages, and MRI is hampered by the need for long scan times, which limits its applicability in acutely ill patients with hemodynamic compromise. Thus, in many institutions, including ours, TEE has become the imaging modality of choice in the initial evaluation of aortic dissection and in many circumstances has obviated the need for further diagnostic imaging, including aortography [109].

Acute Pulmonary Embolism. Transthoracic echo may demonstrate suggestive evidence of pulmonary embolus, such as right ventricular enlargement or evidence of pulmonary hypertension. While it is not a primary imaging modality for the diagnosis of pulmonary embolus, TEE can detect central pulmonary embolus [23,25,110]. In patients undergoing TEE for chest pain syndromes and/or unexplained dyspnea or hypoxemia, careful scanning of the pulmonary arteries is warranted, especially if no other findings that may explain the patient's symptoms are detected (Fig. 7-21).

Trauma. Traumatic injury to the aorta commonly accompanies serious, nonpenetrating injury to the thorax. Several recent preliminary studies have demonstrated the superiority of TEE in the evaluation of patients with thoracic trauma, compared with angiography and CT scanning.

Traumatic valve injuries may result clinically in aortic regurgitation. Most commonly traumatic injury involves the aortic valve. The 2-D echo, either TTE or TEE, usually visualizes aortic valve rupture and aortic regurgitation. Echocardiography and color flow Doppler mapping are also useful in penetrating chest injuries (Fig. 7-22).

PERICARDIAL DISEASE. Echocardiography is the principal method used in the ICU setting to evaluate the patient with suspected cardiac tamponade. M-mode and 2-D echo readily detect pericardial effusions and can help distinguish loculated from free-flowing collections (Figs. 7-23 and 7-24). Echocardiography may also be used at the bedside to guide pericardiocentesis and to help the clinician decide when an operative approach is advisable, in the case of localized collection of fluid.

In patients with sizable pericardial effusions, several echocardiographic signs indicate increased intrapericardial pressure, including early diastolic collapse of the RV free wall and diastolic collapse of the right atrial free wall. However, these are

Fig. 7-23. A patient with hypotension. A. From the parasternal window, showing all four cardiac chambers. PE = pericardial effusion. B. From the apical window. There is a very large pericardial effusion and clear-cut compromise of right ventricular filling. Note the compression of the right ventricle in this diastolic frame (*arrow*).

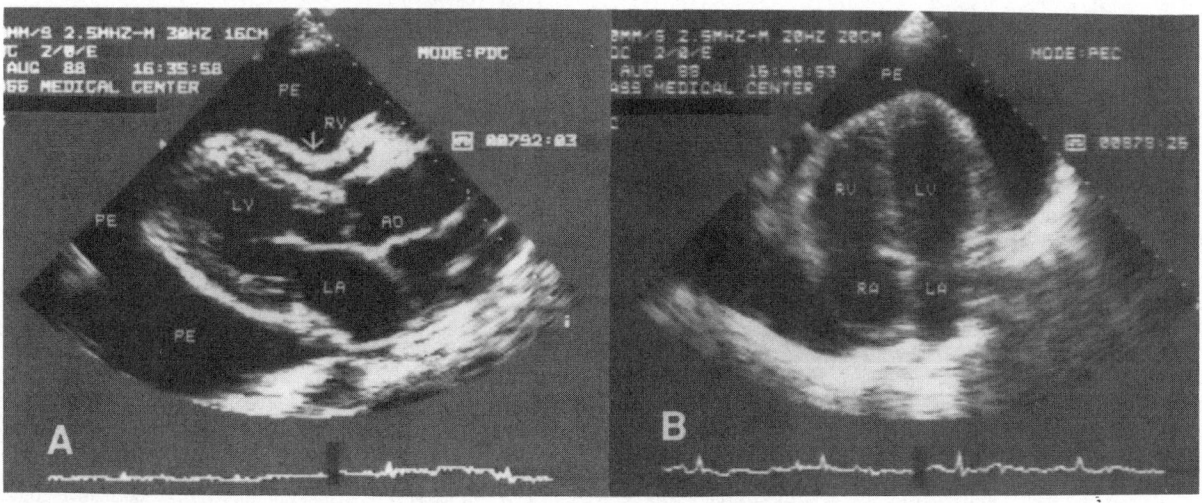

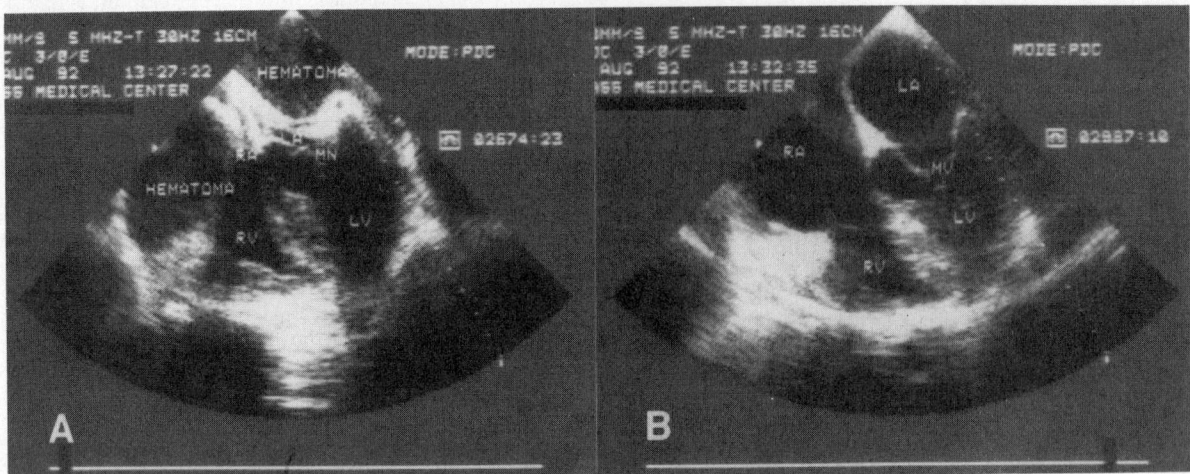

Fig. 7-24. A. Postoperative transesophageal study of a patient with profound hemodynamic compromise following cardiac surgery, demonstrating a large hematoma compressing the right atrium and left atrium, limiting ventricular filling. B. Obtained approximately 5 minutes later after drainage of large sanguineous pericardial effusion. Note the restoration of normal-sized right atrium and left atrium and increase in size of the right ventricle. Pericardiocentesis was associated with dramatic increase in systolic pressure.

both sensitive signs of increases in intrapericardial pressure and do not necessarily diagnose cardiac tamponade, which is a clinical diagnosis made at the bedside. Additional signs of increased intrapericardial pressure include exaggerated respiratory variation in the Doppler mitral inflow and hepatic vein flow profiles.

References

1. Feigenbaum H: *Echocardiography.* 4th ed. Philadelphia, Lea & Febiger, 1986.
2. Geiser EA: Echocardiography: Physics and instrumentation, in Marcus et al (eds) *Cardiac Imaging.* Philadelphia, WB Saunders, 1991.
3. Hatle L, Angelsen B: *Doppler Ultrasound in Cardiology: Physical Principles and Clinical Applications.* 4th ed. Philadelphia, Lea & Febiger, 1984.
4. Cannon SR, Richards KL: Principles and physics of Doppler, in Marcus et al, (eds) *Cardiac Imaging.* Philadelphia: WB Saunders, 1991.
5. Currie RJ, Seward JB, Reeder GS, et al: Continuous wave Doppler echocardiographic assessment of severity of calcific aortic stenosis. *Circulation* 79:1165, 1985.
6. Yock PG and Popp RL: Non-invasive estimation of right ventricular systolic pressure by Doppler ultrasound in patients with tricuspid regurgitation. *Circulation* 70:657, 1984.
7. Miyatako K, Izumo S, Okamoto M, et al: Semiquantitative grading of severity of mitral regurgitation by real-time two-dimensional Doppler flow imaging technique. *J Am Coll Cardiol* 7:82, 1986.
8. Spain MG, Smith MD, Grayburn PA, et al: Quantitative assessment of mitral regurgitation by Doppler color flow imaging: Angiographic and hemodynamic correlations. *J Am Coll Cardiol* 13:585, 1989.
9. Perry GJ, Helmcke F, Nanda NC, et al: Evaluation of aortic insufficiency by Doppler color flow mapping. *J Am Coll Cardiol* 9:952, 1987.
10. Hoit BD, Penonen E, Dalton N, et al: Doppler color flow mapping studies of jet formation and spatial orientation in obstructive hypertrophic cardiomyopathy. *Am Heart J* 117:1119, 1989.
11. Alton ME, Pasierski TJ, Orsinelli DA, et al: Comparison of transthoracic and transesophageal echocardiography in evaluation of 47 Starr-Edwards prosthetic valves. *J Am Coll Cordiol* 20:1503, 1992.
12. Gussenhoven EJ, Taams MA, Roelandt JRTC, et al: Transesophageal two-dimensional echocardiography: Its role in solving clinical problems. *J Am Coll Cardiol* 8:975, 1986.
13. Erbel R, Schweizer P, Besdos P, et al: Two-dimensional echocardiographic diagnosis of papillary muscle rupture. *Chest* 79:595, 1981.
14. Erbel R, Bornor N, Steller D, et al: Detection of aortic dissection by transesophageal echocardiography. *Br Heart J* 58:45, 1987.
15. Erbel R, Engberding R, Daniel W, et al: Echocardiography in diagnosis of aortic dissection, *Lancet* 1:457, 1989.
16. Nienaber C, Spielmann R, Kodolitsch Y, et al: Diagnosis of thoracic aortic dissection: Magnetic resonance imaging versus transesophageal echocardiography. *Circulation* 85:434, 1992.
17. Nienaber CA, von Kodolitsch Y, Nicolas V, et al: The diagnosis of thoracic aortic dissection by noninvasive imaging procedures. *N Engl J Med* 328:1, 1993.
18. Pearson AC, Labovitz A., Tatineni S, Gomez CR: Superiority of transesophageal echocardiography in detecting cardiac source of embolism in patients with cerebral ischemia of uncertain etiology. *J Am Coll Cardiol* 17:66, 1991.
19. Pearson AC, Nagelhout D, Castello R, et al: Atrial septal aneurysm and stroke: A transesophageal echocardiographic study. *J Am Coll Cardiol* 18:1223, 1991.
20. Schneider B, Hanrath P, Vogel P, Meinertz T: Improved morphologic characterization of atrial septal aneurysm by transesophageal echocardiography: Relation to cerebrovascular events. *J Am Coll Cardiol* 16:1000, 1990.
21. Khandheria BK, Takik AJ, Taylor CL, et al: Aortic dissection: Review of value and limitations of two-dimensional echocardiography in a six-year experience. *J Am Soc Echocardiogr* 2:17, 1989.
22. van den Brink RBA, Visser CA, Basart DCG, et al: Comparison of transthoracic and transesophageal color Doppler flow imaging in patients with mechanical prostheses in the mitral valve position. *Am J Cardiol* 63:1471, 1989.
23. Nixdorff U, Erbal R, Drexler M, Meyers J: Detection of thromboembolus of the right pulmonary artery by transesophageal two-dimensional echocardiogapy. *Am J Cardiol* 61:488, 1988.
24. Reeder GS, Khandheria BK, Seward JB, Tajik AJ: Transesophageal echocardiography and cardiac masses. *Mayo Clin Proc* 66:1101, 1991.
25. Wittlich N, Erbal R, Eichler A, et al: Detection of central pulmonary artery thromboemboli by transesophageal echocardiography in patients with severe pulmonary embolism. *J Am Soc Echocardiogr* 5:515, 1992.
26. Taams MA, Gussenhoven EJ, Calahan MK, et al: Transesophageal Doppler color-flow imaging in the detection of native and Bjork-Shiley mitral valve regurgitation. *J Am Coll Cardiol* 13:95, 1989.

27. Karolis DG, Chandrasekaran K, Victor MF, et al: Recognition and embolic potential of intraortic athrosclerotic debris. *J Am Coll Cardiol* 17:73, 1991.

28. Tunick PA, Kronzon I: Protruding atherosclerotic plaque in the aortic arch of patients with systemic embolization: A new finding seen by transesophageal echocardiography. *Am Heart J* 120:658, 1990.

29. Tunick PA, Culliford AT, Lamparello PJ, Kronzon I: Brief report: Antheromatosis of the aortic arch as an occult source of multiple systemic emboli. *Ann Intern Med* 114:391, 1991.

30. Chen C, Koschyk D, Hamm C, et al: Usefulness of transesophageal echocardiography in identifying small left ventricular apical thrombus. *J Am Coll Cardiol* 21:208, 1993.

31. Daniel WG, Mugge A, Martin RP, et al: Improvement in the diagnosis of abscesses associated with endocarditis by transesophageal echocardiography. *N Engl J Med* 324:795, 1991.

32. Seward JB, Khandheria BK, Oh JK, et al: Transesophageal echocardiography: Technique, anatomic correlation, implementation, and clinical applications. *Mayo Clin Proc* 63:649, 1988.

33. Labovitz AJ, Pearson AC: *Transesophageal Echocardiography: Basic Principles and Clinical Applications*. Philadelphia, Lea & Febiger, 1992.

34. Ansari A: Transesophageal two-dimensional echocardiography: Current perspectives. *Prog Cardiovasc Dis* 35:349, 1993.

35. Pearlman AS, Gardin JM, Martin RP: Guidelines for physician training in transesophageal echocardiography: Recommendations of the American Society of Echocardiography Committee for physician training in echocardiography. *J Am Soc Echocardiogr* 5:187, 1992.

36. Daniel WG, Erbel R, Kasper W, et al: Safety of transesophageal echocardiography. A multicenter survey of 10,419 examinations. *Circulation* 83:817, 1991.

37. Fisher EA, Stahl JA, Budd JH, Goldman ME: Transesophageal echocardiography: Procedures and clinical applications. *J Am Coll Cardiol* 18:1333, 1991.

38. Khandheria BK: Prophylaxis or no prophylaxis before transesophageal echocardiography? *J Am Soc Echocardiogr* 5:285, 1992.

39. Dajani AS, Bisno AL, Chung KJ, et al: Prevention of bacterial endocarditis. A statement for health professionals from the Committee on Rheumatic Fever, Endocarditis, and Kawasaki Disease of the Council of Cardiovascular Disease in the Young, the American Heart Association. *Circulation* 82:1170, 1991.

40. Foster E, Kusumoro FM, Sobol SM, Schiller NB: Streptococcal endocarditis temporally related to transesophageal echocardiography. *J Am Soc Echocardiogr* 3:424, 1990.

41. Read RC, Finch RG, Donald FE, et al: Infective endocarditis after transesophageal echocardiography. *Circulation* 87:1426, 1993.

42. Steckelberg JM, Khandheria BK, Anhalt JP, et al: Prospective evaluation of the risk of bacteremia associated with transesophageal echocardiography. *Circulation* 84:177, 1991.

43. Voller H, Spielberg C, Schroder K, et al: Frequency of positive blood cultures during transesophageal echocardiography. *Am J Cardiol* 68:1538, 1991.

44. Nikutta P, Mantev-Stiers F, Becht I, et al: Risk of bacteremia induced by transesophageal echocardiography: Analysis of 100 consecutive procedures. *J Am Soc Echocardiogr* 5:168, 1992.

45. Melendez LJ, Chan K, Cheung PK, et al: Incidence of bacteremia in transesophageal echocardiography: A prospective study of 140 consecutive patients. *J Am Coll Cardiol* 18:1650, 1991.

46. Shyu K, Hwang J, Lin S, et al: Prospective study of blood culture during transesophageal echocardiography. *Am Heart J* 124:1541, 1992.

47. Gal RA, Gaeckle TC, Gadasalli S: Chemoprophylaxis before transesophageal echocardiography in patients with prosthetic or bioprosthetic cardiac valves. *Am J Cardiol* 72:115, 1993.

48. Schiller NB, Maurer G, Ritter SB, et al: Transesophageal echocardiography. *J Am Soc Echocardiogr* 2:354, 1989.

49. Chan K, Cohen GI, Sochowski RA, Baird MG: Complications of transesophageal echocardiography in ambulatory adult patients: Analysis of 1500 consecutive examinations. *J Am Soc Echocardiogr* 4:577, 1991.

50. Seward JB, Khandheria BK, Oh JK, et al.: Critical appraisal of transesophageal echocardiography: Limitations, pitfalls, and complications. *J Am Soc Echocardiogr* 5:288, 1992.

51. Pearson AC, Castello R, Labovitz AJ: Safety and utility of transesophageal echocardiography in the critically ill patient, *Am Heart J* 119:1083, 1990.

52. Foster E, Schiller NB: The role of transesophageal echocardiography in critical care: UCSF experience. *J Am Soc Echocardiogr* 5:368, 1992.

53. Oh JK, Seward JB, Khandheria BK, et al: Transesophageal echocardiography in critically ill patients. *Am J Cardiol* 66:1492, 1990.

54. Folland ED, Parisi AF, Moynihan PF, et al: Assessment of left ventricular ejection fraction and volumes by real-time, two-dimensional echocardiography. A comparison of cineangiographic and radionuclide techniques. *Circulation* 60:760, 1979.

55. Schiller NB, Acquatella H, Ports TA, et al: Left ventricular volume from paired biplane two-dimensional echocardiography. *Circulation* 60:547, 1979.

56. Quinones MA, Waggoner AD, Reduto LA, et al: A new, simplified and accurate method for determining ejection fraction with two-dimensional echocardiography. *Circulation* 64:744, 1981.

57. Amico AF, Lichtenberg GS, Reisner SA, et al: Superiority of visual versus computerized echocardiographic estimation of radionuclide left ventricular ejection fraction. *Am Heart J* 118:1259, 1989.

58. Aurigemma G, Battista S, Orsinelli D, et al: Abnormal LV intracavity flow acceleration in patients undergoing aortic valve replacement for aortic stenosis: A marker for high post-operative morbidity and mortality. *Circulation* 86:926, 1992.

59. Cutrone F, Coyle JP, Novoa R, et al: Severe dynamic left ventricular outflow tract obstruction following aortic valve replacement diagnosed by intraoperative echocardiography. *Anesthesiology* 72:563, 1990.

60. Laurent M, Leborgne O, Clement C, et al: Systolic intra-cavitary gradients following aortic valve replacement: An echo-Doppler study. *Eur Heart J* 12:1098, 1991.

61. Schwinger ME, O'Brien F, Freedberg RS, Kronzon I:' Dynamic outflow obstruction after aortic valve replacement: A Doppler echocardiographic study. *J Am Soc Echocardiogr* 3:205, 1990.

62. Soufer R, Wohlgelernter D, Vita NA, et al: Intact systolic LV function in clinical congestive heart failure. *Am J Cardiol* 55:1032, 1985.

63. Dougherty AH, Naccarelli GV, Gray EL, et al: Congestive heart failure with normal systolic function. *Am J Cardiol* 54:778, 1984.

64. Bonow RO, Udelson JE: LV diastolic dysfunction as a cause of congestive heart failure. *Ann Intern Med* 117:502, 1992.

65. Pearson AC, Labovitz AJ, Mrosek D, et al: Assessment of diastolic function in normal and hypertrophied hearts: Comparison of Doppler echocardiography and M-mode echocardiography. *Am Heart J* 113:1417, 1987.

66. Choong CY, Abascal VM, Weyman J, et al: Prevalence of valvular regurgitation by Doppler echocardiography in patients with structurally normal hearts by two-dimensional echocardiography. *Am Heart J* 117:636, 1989.

67. Stoddard MF, Pearson AC, Kern MJ, et al: Left ventricular diastolic function: Comparison of pulsed Doppler echocardiographic and hemodynamic indexes in subjects with and without coronary artery disease. *J Am Coll Cardiol* 13:327, 1989.

68. Appleton CP, Hatle LK, Popp RL: Cardiac tamponade and pericardial effusion: Respiratory variation in transvalvular flow velocities studied by Doppler echocardiography. *J Am Coll Cardiol* 11:1020, 1988.

69. Appleton CP, Hatle LK, Popp RL: Demonstration of restrictive ventricular physiology by Doppler echocardiography. *J Am Coll Cardiol* 11:757, 1988.

70. Choong CY, Abascal VM, Thomas JD, et al: Combined influence of ventricular loading and relaxation of the transmitral flow velocity profile in dogs measured by Doppler echocardiography. *Circulation* 78:672, 1988.

71. Echeverria HH, Bilsker MS, Myerburg RJ, Kessler KM: Congestive heart failure: Echocardiographic insights. *Am J Med* 75:750, 1983.

72. Aguirre FV, Pearson AC, Lewen MK, et al: Usefulness of Doppler echocardiography in the diagnosis of congestive heart failure. *Am J Cardiol* 63:1098, 1989.

73. Oh JK, Ding ZP, Gersh BJ, et al: Restrictive left ventricular diastolic filling identifies patients with heart failure after acute myocardial infarction. *J Am Soc Echocardiogr* 5:497, 1992.

74. Stamm RB, Gibson RS, Bishop HL, et al: Echocardiographic detection of infarct-localized asynergy and remote asynergy during

acute myocardial infarction: Correlation with the extent of angiographic coronary disease. *Circulation* 67:233, 1983.

75. Heger JJ, Weyman AE, Wann LS, et al: Cross-sectional echocardiography in acute myocardial infarction: Detection and localization of regional left ventricular asynergy. *Circulation* 60:531, 1979.

76. Heger JJ, Weyman AE, Wann LS, et al: Cross-sectional echocardiographic analysis of the extent of left ventricular asynergy in acute myocardial infarction. *Circulation* 61:1113, 1980.

77. Armstrong WM, Francis GS (ed), *Modern Coronary Care*. Boston, Little, Brown & Co., 1990, pp 455-494.

78. Pandian NG, Koyanagi S, Skorton DJ, et al: Relations between 2-dimensional echocardiographic wall thickening abnormalities, myocardial infarct size and coronary risk area in normal and hypertrophied myocardium in dogs. *Am J Cardiol* 52:1318, 1983.

79. Kerber RE, Marcus ML, Ehrhardt J, et al: Correlation between echocardiographically demonstrated segmental dyskinesis and regional myocardial perfusion. *Circulation* 52:1097, 1975.

80. Buda AL, Zotz RJ, LeMire MS, et al: Comparison of two-dimensional echocardiographic wall motion and wall thickening abnormalities in relation to the myocardium at risk. *Am Heart J* 111:587, 1986.

81. Guth BD, White FC, Gallagher KP, Bloor CM: Decreased systolic wall thickening in myocardium adjacent to ischemic zones in conscious swine during brief coronary artery occlusion. *Am Heart J* 107:458, 1984.

82. Force T, Kemper A, Perkins L, et al: Overestimation of infarct size by quantitative two-dimensional echocardiography: The role of tethering and of analytic procedures. *Circulation* 73:1360, 1986.

83. Hecht HS, Taylor R, Wong M, Shah PM: Comparative evaluation of segmental asynergy in remote myocardial infarction by radionuclide angiography, two-dimensional echocardiography, and contrast ventriculography. *Am Heart J* 101:740, 1981.

84. Lopez-Sendon J, Garcia-Fernandez A, Coma-Conella I, et al: Segmental right ventricular function after acute myocardial infarction: Two-dimensional echocardiographic study in 63 patients. *Am J Cardiol* 51:390, 1983.

85. Come PC, Riley MF, Weintraub R: Echocardiographic detection of complete and partial papillary muscle rupture during acute myocardial infarction. *Am J Cardiol* 56:787, 1985.

86. Come PA: Doppler detection of acquired ventricular septal defect. *Am J Cardiol* 55:586, 1985.

87. Miyatake K, Okamoto M, Kinoshita N, et al: Doppler echocardiographic features of ventricular septal rupture in myocardial infarction. *J Am Coll Cardiol* 5:182, 1985.

88. Mintz GS, Victor MF, Kotler MN, et al: Two-dimensional echocardiographic identification of surgically correctable complications of acute myocardial infarction. *Circulation* 64:91, 1981.

89. Ross J Jr: Afterload mismatch in aortic and mitral valve disease: Implications for surgical therapy. *J Am Coll Cardiol* 5:811, 1985.

90. Stamm RB, Martie RP: Quantification of pressure gradients across stenotic valves by Doppler ultrasound. *J Am Coll Cardiol* 2:707, 1983.

91. Gilbert BW, Haney RS, Crawford F, et al: Two-dimensional echocardiographic assessment of vegetative endocarditis. *Circulation* 55:346, 1977.

92. Stewart JA, Silimperi D, Harris P, et al: Echocardiographic documentation of vegetative lesions in infective endocarditis. *Circulation* 62:374, 1980.

93. Wann LS, Hallam CC, Dillon JC, et al: Comparison of M-mode and cross-sectional echocardiography in infective endocarditis. *Circulation* 60:728, 1979.

94. O'Brien JT, Geiser E: Infective endocarditis and echocardiography. *Am Heart J* 104:386, 1984.

95. Stafford WJ, Petch J, Radford DJ: Vegetations in infective endocarditis: Clinical relevance and diagnosis by cross-sectional echocardiography. *Br Heart J* 53:301, 1985.

96. Shively BK, Gurule FT, Roldan CA, et al: Diagnostic value of transesophageal compared with transthoracic echocardiography in infective endocarditis. *J Am Coll Cardiol* 18:391, 1991.

97. Enzler MJ, Wilson WR, Giuliani ER: Noninvasive detection of cardiac abscesses complicating infective endocarditis. *Am J Noninvas Cardiol* 1:109, 1987.

98. Zeineddin M, Stewart JA: Echocardiographic detection of nonvalve-ring abscess complicating aortic valve endocarditis. *Am J Med* 85:97, 1988.

99. Jaffe WM, Morgan ED, Pearlman AS, Otto CM: Infective endocarditis, 1983–1988: Echocardiographic findings and factors influencing morbidity and mortality. *J Am Coll Cardiol* 15:1227, 1990.

100. Buda AJ, Zotz RJ, LeMire MS, Bach DS: Prognostic significance of vegetations detected by two-dimensional echocardiography in infective endocarditis. *Am Heart J* 112:1291, 1986.

101. Stafford WJ, Petch J, Radford DJ: Vegetations in infective endocarditis: Clinical relevance and diagnosis by cross-sectional echocardiography. *Br Heart J* 53:301, 1985.

102. Mugge A, Daniel WG, Frank G, Lichtlen PR: Echocardiography in infective endocarditis: Reassessment of prognostic implications of vegetation size determined by the transthoracic and the transesophageal approach. *J Am Coll Cardiol* 14:631, 1989.

103. Sanfilippo AJ, Picard MH, Newell JB, et al: Echocardiographic assessment of patients with infectious endocarditis: Prediction of risk for complications. *J Am Coll Cardiol* 18:1191, 1991.

104. Erbel R, Bornor N, Steller D, et al: Detection of aortic dissection by transesophageal echocardiography. *Br Heart J* 58:45, 1987.

105. Erbel R, Engberding R, Daniel W, et al: Echocardiography in diagnosis of aortic dissection. *Lancet* 1:457, 1989.

106. Ballal RS, Nanda NC, Gatewood R, et al: Usefulness of transesophageal echocardiography in assessment of aortic dissection. *Circulation* 84:1903, 1991.

107. Nienaber C, Spielmann R, Kodolitsch Y, et al: Diagnosis of thoracic aortic dissection: Magnetic resonance imaging versus transesophageal echocardiography. *Circulation* 85:434, 1992.

108. Nicnaber CA, von Kodolitsch Y, Nicolas V, et al: The diagnosis of thoracic aortic dissection by noninvasive imaging procedures. *N Engl J Med* 328:1, 1993.

109. Cigarroa JE, Isselbacher EM, DeSanctis RW, Eagle KA: Diagnostic imaging in the evaluation of suspected aortic dissection. *N Engl J Med* 328:35, 1991.

110. Rittoo D, Sutherland GR, Flapan SL: Role of transesophageal echocardiography in diagnosis and management of central pulmonary artery thromboembolism. *Am J Cardiol* 71:1115, 1993.

111. Victor MF, Mintz GS, Kotler MN, et al: Two dimensional echocardiographic diagnosis of aortic dissection. *Am J Cardiol* 48:1155, 1981.

112. Granato JE, Dee P, Gibson RS: Utility of two-dimensional echocardiography in suspected ascending aortic dissection. *Am J Cardiol* 56:123, 1985.

113. Khandheria BK, Takik AJ, Taylor CL, et al: Aortic dissection: Review of value and limitations of two-dimensional echocardiography in a six-year experience. *J Am Soc Echocardiogr* 2:17, 1989.

114. Kotler M: Is transesophageal echocardiography the new standard for diagnosing dissecting aortic aneurysms? *J Am Coll Cardiol* 14:1263, 1989.

115. Khandheria BK, Seward JB, Oh JK, et al: Valve and limitations of transesophageal echocardiography in the assessment of mitral valve prothesis. *Circulation* 83:1956, 1993.

116. Appelbe AF, Walker PG, Ycoh JK, et al: Clinical significance and origin of artifacts in transesophageal echocardiography of the thoracic aorta. *J Am Coll Cardiol* 21:754, 1993.

8. Pericardiocentesis

Glenn Focht and Richard C. Becker

Pericardiocentesis is an important and sometimes lifesaving procedure performed in the critical care setting. It is not performed with enough frequency to allow most physicians to master the procedure. This chapter reviews the indications for pericardiocentesis, summarizes the pathophysiology of pericardial effusions, and provides a step-by-step approach to pericardiocentesis, including management of patients following the procedure.

Indications for Pericardiocentesis

The initial management of a patient with known or suspected pericardial effusion is largely determined by overall clinical status. In the absence of hemodynamic instability (or in rare cases of suspected purulent bacterial pericarditis) there is no need for emergent or urgent pericardiocentesis, but it may be performed for diagnostic purposes. A thorough noninvasive work-up should be completed prior to consideration of an invasive diagnostic procedure [1]. Whenever possible, elective pericardiocentesis should be performed using ultrasound or fluoroscopic guidance.

In contrast, the management of hemodynamically compromised patients requires emergent removal of pericardial fluid to restore adequate ventricular filling and hasten clinical stabilization. The exact method and timing of pericardiocentesis is ultimately dictated by the patient's overall degree of instability. Patients with profound hypotension unresponsive to fluid resuscitation require immediate, often unguided (blind), pericardiocentesis. In this setting, there are no absolute contraindications to the procedure, and it should therefore be performed without delay at the patient's bedside.

Urgent pericardiocentesis is indicated for patients who are initially hypotensive but respond quickly to aggressive fluid resuscitation. The procedure should be performed within several hours of presentation while careful monitoring and hemodynamic support continue. As in elective circumstances, pericardiocentesis in these patients should be undertaken with appropriate visual guidance, the method of which depends on the physician's experience and resources. The modalities used most commonly are ultrasonography, echocardiography, and fluoroscopy.

Three additional points must be stressed regarding patients undergoing expedited pericardiocentesis. First, coagulation parameters (PT, PTT, platelet count) should be checked and, when possible, quickly normalized prior to the procedure. Second, some critical care authorities advocate performance of all pericardiocentesis procedures in the catheterization laboratory with concomitant right heart pressure monitoring to document efficacy of the procedure and to exclude a constrictive element of pericardial disease (Chapter 34) [2]. We support this approach; however, excessive delays because of scheduling difficulties must be avoided. Finally, efforts to assure a cooperative and stationary patient during the procedure will greatly facilitate the performance, safety, and success of pericardiocentesis.

The clinical presentation of hemodynamically significant pericardial effusions varies widely among patients. A comprehensive understanding requires knowledge of normal pericardial anatomy and physiology.

Anatomy

The pericardium is a membranous structure with two layers separated by a small potential space. The visceral pericardium is closely but loosely adherent to the epicardial surface. It is a monolayer of mesothelial cells and attaches to the epicardium by a loose collection of small blood vessels, lymphatics, and connective tissue. The parietal pericardium is a fibrous structure that defines the outer membrane. Its inner surface is also composed of a monolayer of mesothelial cells. The remainder of the parietal pericardium consists of a dense network of connective tissue that is relatively nondistensible; therefore, it defines the dimensions and shape of the pericardium [3].

Further anatomic definition of the pericardium is derived from multiple attachments of the parietal pericardium in the thorax. Superiorly, the fibrous parietal pericardium attaches to the ascending aorta just below the arch. The inferior portion adheres strongly to the fibrous center of the diaphragm on which it rests. Anteriorly, the outer membrane is anchored to the sternum and costal cartilages by ligaments, as well as by a less organized collection of connective tissue. The posterior margin of the parietal pericardium abuts the esophagus and pleural sacs; here, the visceral pericardium is absent and the parietal pericardium attaches directly to the epicardium at the borders of the entrance of the inferior and superior vena cavae and pulmonary veins [4]. Beyond providing stability, these multiple attachments also limit the inherent elasticity and distensibility of the pericardium.

This complex anatomic arrangement provides an anchor for the contracting myocardium and results in a small space between the visceral and parietal layers (pericardial space). The pericardial space or sac usually contains a small volume (15–50 ml) of clear serous fluid that is chemically similar to a plasma ultrafiltrate [5,6]. The mechanism responsible for the production of pericardial fluid is not well understood. A homeostasis usually exists between new production of pericardial fluid and its drainage into the venous circulation via lymphatics.

The major determinant of when and how pericardial effusions come to clinical attention is directly related to the speed at which they develop. Effusions that collect rapidly (over minutes to hours) may cause hemodynamic compromise with volumes of 250 ml or less. These effusions are usually located posteriorly and are often difficult to detect without echocardiography. In contrast, effusions developing slowly (over days to weeks) allow for hypertrophy and distention (stretch) of the fibrous parietal membrane. Volumes of 2000 ml or greater may accumulate without significant hemodynamic compromise. These patients may present with symptoms due to compression of adjacent thoracic structures, such as cough, dyspnea, dysphagia, or early satiety. Three other clinical conditions will promote hemodynamic compromise, even in the absence of large pericardial effusions: intravascular hypovolemia, impaired ventricular systolic function, and ventricular hypertrophy with decreased elasticity of the myocardium.

Pericardiocentesis: Procedure

Since the first blind or "closed" pericardiocentesis in 1840 [7], several different approaches have been described [8]. These approaches have varied considerably, particularly in the needle apparatus entry site. Marfan described the subcostal approach in 1911 [9], which then became the standard approach for unguided pericardiocentesis.

The advent of clinically applicable ultrasonography has opened a new chapter in diagnostic and therapeutic approaches to pericardial disease, allowing clinicians to quantitate and localize pericardial effusions quickly and noninvasively [10,11]. Work by Callahan et al. at the Mayo Clinic established the increased efficacy and safety of two-dimensional (2-D) echocardiography to guide pericardiocentesis [12,13]. This has resulted in two major trends in clinical practice. First, 2-D echocardiography is commonly used to guide pericardiocentesis. Second, approaches other than the subxyphoid method have been investigated due to the ability to clearly define the anatomy (location and volume) of each patient's effusion [8,12,13]. Typically, a four-chamber view of the heart is obtained by positioning the transducer at the apex. After insertion of the pericardiocentesis needle (described below), appropriate positioning in the pericardial space can be confirmed by injecting 5 ml of agitated saline (contrast). Echocardiography can also be used to reposition the needle safely if fluid return is suboptimal. Standard fluoroscopy can be used to confirm needle and catheter positioning within the pericardial space.

Formulas for quantitating the amount of pericardial fluid by echocardiographic or fluoroscopic means have not been established. As a rule, however, an effusion of moderate size (>250 ml) is required for a pericardiocentesis.

Regardless of whether echocardiography or another guidance method is used, the subxyphoid approach remains the standard of practice. The materials required for bedside pericardiocentesis are listed in Table 8-1 (Fig. 8-1). Table 8-2 (Fig. 8-2) lists the materials required for simultaneous placement of an intrapericardial drainage catheter. The materials are available in prepackaged kits or individually. We do not have a preference; the key to success is immediate availability of the necessary materials.

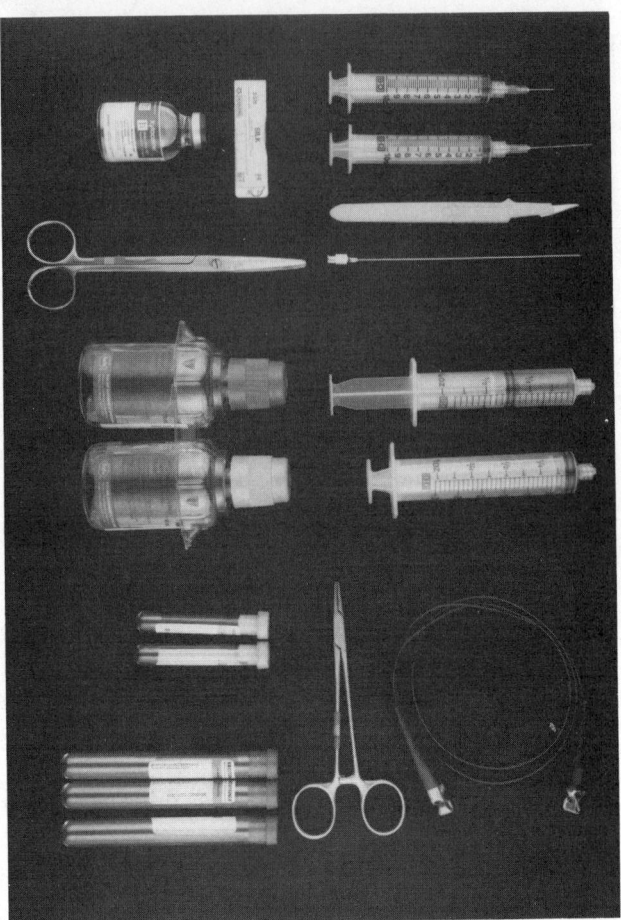

Fig. 8-1. Materials required for pericardiocentesis (clockwise from upper left): 10-ml syringe with 25-gauge needle, 10-ml syringe with 22-gauge needle, no. 11 blade, 18-gauge 8-cm thin-walled needle, 20-ml syringe, 30-ml syringe, alligator clip, hemostat, three red-top tubes, two purple-top tubes, culture bottles, scissors, 1% lidocaine solution, suture material.

Table 8-1. Materials for Pericardiocentesis

1. Site preparation
   a. Antiseptic
   b. Gauze
   c. Sterile drapes and towels
   d. Sterile gloves, masks, gowns, caps
   e. 5-ml or 10-ml syringe with 25-gauge needle
   f. 1% lidocaine (without epinephrine)
   g. Code cart
   h. Atropine (1-mg dose vial)
2. Procedure
   a. No. 11 blade
   b. 20-ml syringe with 10 ml of 1% lidocaine (without epinephrine)
   c. 18-gauge, 8-cm, thin-walled needle with blunt tip
   d. Multiple 20- and 40-ml syringes
   e. Hemostat
   f. Sterile alligator clip
   g. ECG machine
   h. 3 red-top tubes
   i. 2 purple-top (heparinized) tubes
   j. Culture bottles
3. Postprocedure
   a. Suture material
   b. Scissors
   c. Sterile gauze and bandage

Table 8-2. Materials for Intrapericardial Catheter

1. Catheter placement
   a. Teflon-coated flexible J-curved guidewire
   b. 6 Fr. dilator
   c. 8 Fr. dilator
   d. 8 Fr., 35-cm flexible pigtail catheter with multiple fenestrations (end and side holes)
2. Drainage system*
   a. Three-way stopcock
   b. Sterile IV tubing
   c. 500-ml sterile collecting bag (or bottle)
   d. Sterile gauze and adhesive bag (or bottle)
   e. Suture material

*System described allows continuous drainage.

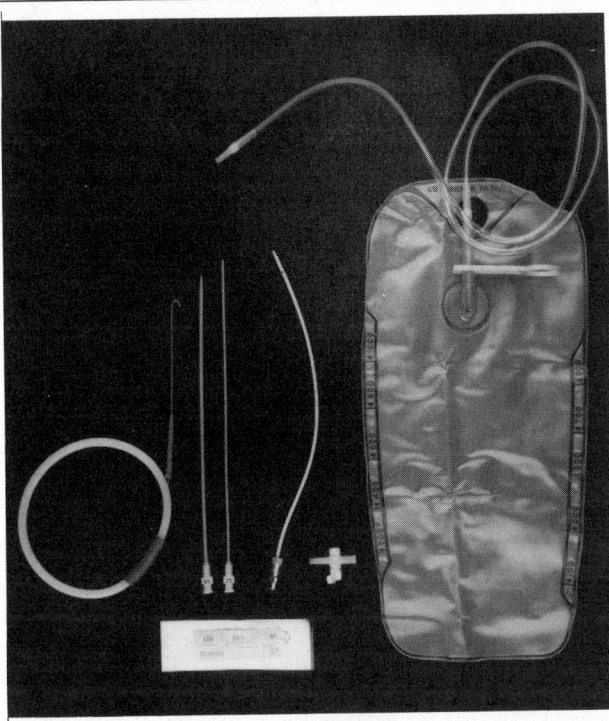

Fig. 8-2. Materials required for intrapericardial catheter placement and drainage (clockwise from lower left): Teflon-coated flexible 0.035-inch J-curved guidewire, 8 Fr. dilator, 6.3 Fr. dilator, 8 Fr. catheter with end and side holes (35-cm flexible pigtail catheter not shown), three-way stopcock, 500-ml sterile collecting bag and tubing, suture material.

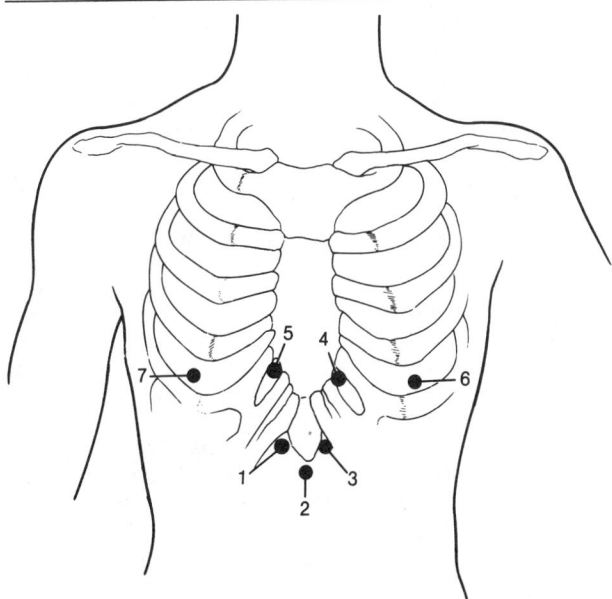

Fig. 8-3. Selected locations for pericardiocentesis. In most cases, the subxiphoid approach (1–3) is preferred. (From Spodick DH: *Acute Pericarditis,* New York, Grune & Stratton, 1959. With permission.)

While the patient is being prepared for emergent or urgent pericardiocentesis, it is imperative that aggressive resuscitation measures are undertaken. Several large-bore peripheral IV lines should be placed for infusion of isotonic saline or colloid solutions. The use of inotropic agents and other vasoactive drugs remains controversial [14,15,16], but when fluid resuscitation alone is inadequate their use should be strongly considered.

The subxyphoid approach for pericardiocentesis is as follows.

1. *Patient Preparation.* Assist the patient in assuming a comfortable supine position with the head of the bed elevated to approximately 45 degrees from the horizontal plane. It is important for the patient to maintain this position during the procedure. Extremely dyspneic patients may need to be positioned fully upright. Elevation of the thorax will allow free-flowing effusions to collect inferiorly and anteriorly, sites that are safest and easiest to access using the subxyphoid approach. The patient's bed should be placed at a comfortable height for the physician performing the procedure.

2. *Needle Entry Site Selection.* Locate the patient's xyphoid process and the border of the left costal margin using both inspection and careful palpation. The needle entry site should be 0.5 cm to the (patient's) left of the xyphoid process and 0.5 to 1.0 cm inferior to the costal margin (Fig. 8-3). It is essential that the surface anatomy be accurately defined before proceeding further. It is helpful to estimate (by palpation) the distance between the skin surface and the posterior margin of the bony thorax. This will help guide subsequent needle insertion. The usual distance is 1.0 to 2.5 cm, increasing with obesity or protuberance of the abdomen.

3. *Site Preparation.* Strict sterile techniques must be maintained at all times in preparation of the needle entry site. Prepare a wide area in the subxyphoid region and lower thorax with a povidone-iodine solution and drape the field with sterile towels, leaving exposed the subxyphoid region. Raise a 1- to 2-cm subcutaneous wheal by infiltrating the needle entry site with 1% lidocaine solution (without epinephrine). Incise the skin with a no. 11 blade at the selected site after achieving adequate local anesthesia. This facilitates needle entry, which is at times difficult because of the absence of a bevel on the Teflon needle apparatus.

4. *Insertion of the Needle Apparatus.* Place the needle apparatus in the dominant hand (right-handed operators should stand to the patient's right and left-handed operators to the left) and insert it in the subxyphoid incision. The angle of entry (with the skin) should be approximately 45 degrees. Direct the needle tip superiorly, aiming for the patient's left shoulder. Continue to advance the needle posteriorly while alternating between aspiration and injection of lidocaine, until the tip has passed just beyond the posterior border of the bony thorax (Fig. 8-4). The posterior border usually lies within 2.5 cm of the skin surface. If the needle tip contacts the bony thorax, inject lidocaine after aspirating to clear the needle tip and anesthetize the periosteum. Then "walk" the needle behind the posterior (costal) margin.

5. *Needle Direction.* Reduce the angle of contact between the needle and skin to 15 degrees once the tip has passed the posterior margin of the bony thorax. This will be the angle of approach to the pericardium; the needle tip, however, should still be directed toward the patient's left shoulder. A 15-degree angle is used regardless of the height of the patient's thorax (whether at 45 degrees or sitting upright) (Fig. 8-5).

6. *Needle Advancement.* Advance the needle slowly while alternating between aspiration of the syringe and injection of 1% lidocaine solution. If ECG guidance is employed, apply the sterile alligator clip to the needle hub, being certain not to

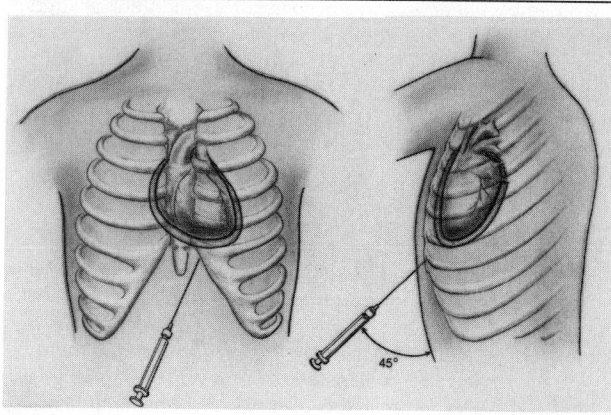

Fig. 8-4. Insertion of the needle apparatus. After the subxiphoid region and lower thorax are prepared and adequate local anesthesia is given, the pericardiocentesis needle is inserted in the subxiphoid incision. The angle of entry (with the skin) should be approximately 45 degrees. The needle tip should be directed superiorly, toward the patient's left shoulder.

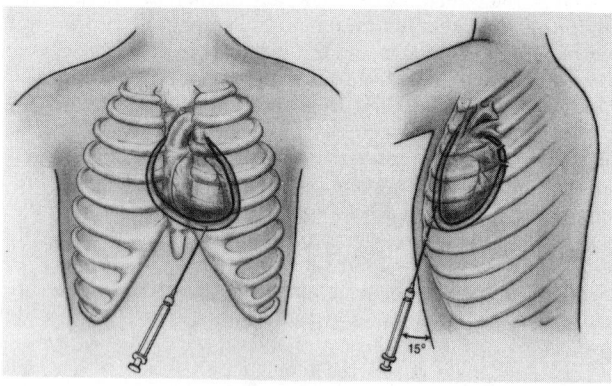

Fig. 8-5. Needle direction. The needle tip should be reduced to 15 degrees once the posterior margin of the bony thorax has been passed. Needle advancement. The needle is advanced toward the left shoulder slowly while alternating between aspiration and injection. A "give" is felt and fluid is aspirated when the pericardial space is entered.

occlude the needle's lumen. Obtain a baseline lead V tracing and monitor a continuous tracing for the presence of ST segment elevation or premature ventricular contractions (evidence of epicardial contact) as the needle is advanced. Advance the needle along this extrapleural path until either:

a. A "give" is felt and fluid is aspirated from the pericardial space (usually 6.0–7.5 cm from the skin) (Fig. 8-6). Some patients may experience a vasovagal response at this point and require atropine intravenously to increase their blood pressure and heart rate.

b. ST segment elevation or premature ventricular contractions are observed on the ECG lead V tracing when the needle tip contacts the epicardium. If ST segment elevation or premature ventricular complexes occur, immediately (and carefully) withdraw the needle toward the skin surface while aspirating. Avoid any lateral motion, which could damage the epicardial vessels. Completely withdraw the needle if no fluid is obtained during the initial repositioning.

The patient's hemodynamic status should improve promptly

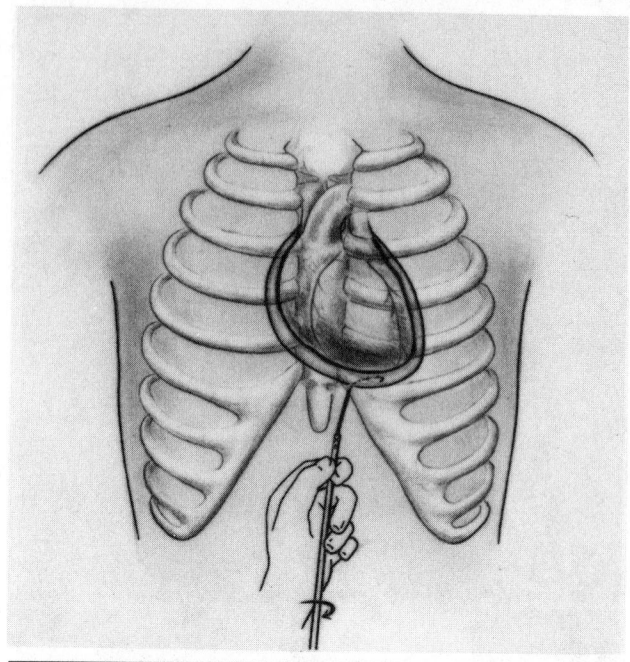

Fig. 8-6. Placement technique. Holding the needle in place, a Teflon-coated, 0.035-inch guidewire is advanced into the pericardial space. The needle is then removed. Following a series of skin dilations, an 8 Fr., 35-cm flexible pigtail catheter is placed over the guidewire into the pericardial space. Passage of dilators and the pigtail catheter is facilitated by a gentle clockwise/counterclockwise motion.

with removal of sufficient fluid. Successful relief of tamponade is supported by (a) a fall of intrapericardial pressure to levels between -3 and $+3$ mm Hg; (b) a fall in right atrial pressure and a separation between right and left ventricular diastolic pressures; (c) augmentation of cardiac output; (d) increased systemic blood pressure; and (e) reduced pulsus paradoxus to physiologic levels. An improvement may be observed after removal of the first 50 to 100 ml of fluid. If the right atrial pressure remains elevated after fluid removal an effusive-constrictive process should be considered. The diagnostic studies performed on pericardial fluid are outlined in Table 8-3. Several options exist for continued drainage of the pericardial space. The simplest approach is to use large-volume syringes and aspirate the fluid by hand. This approach is not always practical (i.e., in large-volume effusions), however, and manipulation of the needle apparatus may cause myocardial trauma. Alternatively, some pericardiocentesis kits include materials and instructions for a catheter-over-needle technique for inserting a pericardial drain. Finally, the Seldinger technique may be used to place an indwelling pericardial drain.

7. *Placement Technique.* Create a track for the catheter by passing a 6 Fr. dilator over a firmly held guidewire. After removing the dilator, use the same technique to pass an 8 Fr. dilator. Then advance an 8 Fr. flexible pigtail catheter over the guidewire into the pericardial space. Remove the guidewire. Passage of the dilators is facilitated by use of a torquing (clockwise/counter clockwise) motion. A wider incision at the base of the guidewire may be required to pass the dilators. Proper positioning of the catheter using radiography, fluoroscopy, or bedside echocardiography facilitates fluid drainage.

8. *Drainage System* [17–20]. Attach a three-way stopcock to the intrapericardial catheter and close the system by attaching the stopcock to the sterile collecting bag with the connecting tubing. The catheter may also be connected to a transducer,

Table 8-3. Diagnostic Studies Performed on Pericardial Fluid

1. Hematocrit
2. White count with differential
3. Glucose
4. Protein
5. Gram stain
6. Routine aerobic and anaerobic cultures
7. Smear and culture for acid-fast bacilli
8. Cytology
9. Other studies as indicated
   a. Cholesterol
   b. Amylase
   c. Lactate dehydrogenase
   d. Special cultures (viral, parasite studies)
   e. Antinuclear antibody
   f. Rheumatoid factor
   g. Total complement, C_3

Table 8-4. Complications of Pericardiocentesis

1. Cardiac puncture
   a. Uncomplicated
   b. Secondary hemopericardium, myocardial infarction
2. Pneumothorax
3. Arrhythmias
   a. Bradycardia
   b. Ventricular tachycardia
4. Trauma to abdominal organs (liver, gastrointestinal tract)
5. Cardiac arrest (predominantly electromechanical dissociation from myocardial perforation, but occasionally tachyarrhythmia or bradyarrhythmia)*
6. Rare
   a. Coronary artery laceration (left anterior descending coronary artery, right coronary artery)
   b. Infection
   c. Fistula formation
   d. Pulmonary edema

*Incidence has varied from 0 to 5% in studies and was less common in guided procedures, more common in "blind" procedures [1,21,22].

allowing intrapericardial pressure monitoring. The system may be secured as follows:

   a. Suture the pigtail catheter to the skin, making sure the lumen is not compressed. Cover the entry site with a sterile gauze and dressing.
   b. Secure the drainage bag (or bottle) using tape at a level approximately 35 to 50 cm below the level of the heart. This system may be left in place for 48 to 72 hours. Echocardiography or fluoroscopic guidance may be used to reposition the pigtail catheter, facilitating complete drainage of existing pericardial fluid.

Short-Term and Long-Term Management

Following pericardiocentesis, close monitoring is required to detect evidence of recurrent tamponade and procedure-related complications. Table 8-4 lists the most common serious complications associated with pericardiocentesis [1,21,22]. Factors associated with an increased risk of complications include (1) small effusion (< 250 ml), (2) posterior effusion, (3) localized effusion, (4) maximum anterior clear space (by echocardiography) less than 10 mm, and (5) unguided approach. All patients undergoing pericardiocentesis should have a portable chest radiograph performed immediately after the procedure to exclude the presence of pneumothorax. In addition, a transthoracic 2-D echocardiogram should be obtained within several hours to evaluate the adequacy of pericardial drainage. Echocardiography can also be used to confirm catheter placement.

Finally, careful technique is required to maintain the sterility of the pericardial catheter drainage system. With meticulous local care, the complication rate is exceptionally low, even when the catheter is left in place for 36 to 48 hours [12,18].

The long-term management of patients with significant pericardial fluid collections is beyond the scope of this chapter (see Chap. 34); however, the role of surgical intervention is reviewed briefly. The indications for surgical intervention are controversial and vary widely (Table 8-5) [2,23–28]. Several indications that have been established include (1) pericardial disease with concomitant constrictive physiology, (2) known loculated or posteriorly located effusions not amenable to pericardiocentesis, (3) suspected purulent pericarditis, and (4) effusions not successfully drained by pericardiocentesis [2, 29]. The etiology of the effusion (Table 8-6) and the patient's functional status are of central importance in determining the pre-

Table 8-5. Major Surgical Options for the Management of Pericardial Effusions

Procedure	Approach	Resection Margins
Pericardial Window		
Subxyphoid	Subxyphoid	<9cm² block
Pleural	Thoracotomy	<9cm² block
Partial pericardiectomy	Thoracotomy	Right phrenic nerve; great vessels to diaphragmatic reflection
Complete pericardiectomy	Thoracotomy or sternotomy	Right phrenic nerve to left pulmonary vein; great vessels to midportion of diaphragmatic pericardium

Table 8-6. Common Causes of Pericardial Effusion

1. Idiopathic
2. Malignancy
3. Uremia
4. Postpericardiotomy syndrome
5. Connective tissue disease
6. Trauma
   a. Blunt
   b. Penetrating
7. Infection
   a. Viral
   b. Bacterial
   c. Fungal
   d. Tuberculosis
8. Aortic dissection
9. Complication of cardiac catheterization or pacemaker insertion
10. Myxedema
11. Postirradiation

ferred treatment. Aggressive attempts at nonsurgical management of chronically debilitated patients or those with metastatic disease of the pericardium may be in order [25,30,31]. Pericardial sclerosis with tetracycline or other agents has shown promise in carefully selected patients with malignant pericardial disease [30,32,33]. Patients with a guarded prognosis who fail aggressive medical therapy should be offered the least invasive procedure.

References

1. Permayer-Miulda G, Sagrista-Savleda J, Soler-Soler J: Primary acute pericardial disease: A prospective study of 231 consecutive patients. *Am J Cardiol* 56:623, 1985.
2. Lovell BH, Braunwald E: Pericardial disease, in Braunwald E (ed): *Heart Disease: A Textbook of Cardiovascular Medicine.* Philadelphia, WB Saunders, 1988, pp 1484–1501.
3. Tandler J: Anatomie des Harsens. Jeng, Fischer, 1913. Quoted by Elias H, Boyd LJ: Notes on the anatomy, embryology and histology of the pericardium. *J NY Med Coll* 2:50, 1960.
4. Roberts WC, Spray TL: Pericardial heart disease: A study of its causes, consequences, and morphologic features, in Spodick D (ed): *Pericardial Diseases.* Philadelphia, FA Davis, 1976, p 17.
5. Shabatai R: Function of the pericardium, in Fowler NO (ed): *The Pericardium in Health and Disease.* Mount Kisco, NY: Futura, 1985, pp 19–46.
6. Shabetai R: *The Pericardium.* New York, Grune & Stratton, 1981, pp 1–33.
7. Schuh R: Erfahrungen uber de Paracentese der Brust und des Herz Beutels. *Med Jahrb d KK Osterr Staates Wien* 33: 388, 1841.
8. Tilkian AG, Daily EK: Pericardiocentesis and drainage, in Tilkian AG, Daily EK (eds): *Cardiovascular Procedures: Diagnostic Techniques and Therapeutic Approaches.* St. Louis, CV Mosby, 1986, pp 231–254.
9. Marfan AB: Poncitian du pericarde par l'espigahe. *Ann Med Chir Infarct* 15:529, 1911.
10. Pandian NG, Brockway B, et al: Pericardiocentesis under 2-dimensional echocardiographic guidance in loculated pericardial effusion. *Ann Thorac Surg* 45:99, 1988.
11. Anthony D, Chandraratna N, et al: Application of 2-dimensional contrast studies during pericardiocentesis. *Am J Cardiol* 52:1120, 1983.
12. Callahan JA, Seward JB, et al: 2-dimensional echocardiography-guided pericardiocentesis: Experience in 117 consecutive patients. *Am J Cardiol* 55:476, 1985.
13. Callahan, JA, Seward JB, et al: Pericardiocentesis assisted by 2-dimensional echocardiography. *J Thorac Cardiovasc Surg* 85:877, 1983.
14. Callahan M: Pericardiocentesis in traumatic and non-traumatic cardiac tamponade. *Ann Emerg Med* 13:924, 1984.
15. Fowler NO, Guberman BA, Gueron M: Cardiac tamponade, in Eliot RS (ed): *Cardiac Emergencies.* 2nd ed. Mount Kisco, NY, Futura, 1982, pp 415–427.
16. Sedlinger S: Catheter replacement of the needle in percutaneous angiography. *Acta Radiol Diagn (Stock)* 39, 368.
17. Kapoor AS: Technique of pericardiocentesis and intrapericardial drainage, in Kapoor AS (ed): *International Cardiology.* New York, Springer-Verlag, 1989, pp 146–153.
18. Kopecky SL, Callahan JA, et al: Percutaneous pericardial catheter drainage: Report of 42 consecutive cases. *Am J Cardiol* 58:633, 1986.
19. Massumi RA, Rios JC, Ewy GA: Technique for insertion of an indwelling pericardial catheter. *Br Heart J* 30:333, 1960.
20. Patel AK, Kogol Charoen PK, et al. Catheter drainage of the pericardium: Practical method to maintain long-term patency. *Chest* 92:1018, 1987.
21. Wong B, Chandraratha M, et al: The risk of pericardiocentesis. *Am J Cardiol* 44:1110, 1979.
22. Krikorian JG, Hancock EW: Pericardiocentesis. *Am J Med* 65:808, 1978.
23. Piehler JM, et al: Surgical management of effusive pericardial disease: Influence of extent of pericardial resection on clinical cause. *J Thorac Cardiovasc Surg* 90:506, 1985.
24. Little AG, Kremser PC, Wade JL, et al: Operation for diagnosis and treatment of pericardial effusions. *Surgery* 96:738, 1984.
25. Palatianos GM, Thuer RJ, Karser GA: Comparison of effectiveness and safety of operations on the pericardium. *Chest* 88:30, 1985.
26. Little AG, Fergusen MK. Pericardioscopy as adjunct to pericardial window. *Chest* 89:53, 1986.
27. Prager RL, Wilson CH, Border WH Jr: The subxiphoid approach to pericardial disease. *Ann Thorac Surg* 34:6, 1982.
28. Spodick DH: Pericardial windows are suboptimal. *Am J Cardiol* 51:607, 1983.
29. Rub RH, Moelleering RC: Clinical microbiologic and therapeutic aspects of purulent pericarditis. *Am J Med* 59:68, 1975.
30. Shepher FA, Christopher M, et al: Medical management of malignant pericardial effusion by tetracycline sclerosis. *Am J Cardiol* 60:1161, 1987.
31. Morm JE, Hallonby D, Gonda A, et al: Management of uremia pericarditis: A report of 11 patients with cardiac tamponade and a review of the literature. *Ann Thorac Surg* 22:588, 1976.
32. Reit Knecht F, Regal AM, et al: Management of cardiac tamponade in patients with malignancy. *J Surg Oncol* 30:19, 1985.
33. Biran S, Bruinian G, et al: The management of pericardial effusion in cancer patients. *Chest* 71:182, 1977.

9. *The Intraaortic Balloon and Counterpulsation*

Bruce S. Cutler

Cardiogenic shock is still a highly lethal complication of acute myocardial infarction, despite modern pharmocologic support [1,2,3]. Left ventricular assist devices (LVAD) are of two types. First are those that reduce left ventricular work by functioning as a pump in a parallel circuit with the heart. They withdraw venous blood from the circulation and then return it under pressure to a peripheral artery. The second group of devices are not pumps in the conventional sense of the word: they assist the ischemic ventricle through improvement in coronary artery perfusion and reduction in systemic afterload by counterpulsation. The intraaortic balloon pump (IAB), which falls into this second group, is by far the most widely used LVAD because of its effectiveness, ease of application, and relative safety.

Equipment

The balloon is made from a thin film of polyurethane because of its strength and antithrombotic properties. Mechanical failures, including leaks, are rare [4–7]. Intraaortic balloons are available in 30-ml and 40-ml volumes. The 40-ml IAB measures 15 × 280 mm and is mounted on the end of a plastic catheter with two concentric lumens. The central lumen is used to pass a guidewire during insertion and to monitor central aortic pressure. The outer lumen is the passageway for gas exchange and is connected to a console that synchronizes inflation and deflation with the cardiac cycle and makes automatic adjustments for changes in heart rate and rhythm. Circuitry in the console detects arrhythmias, gas leaks, and internal malfunctions. Helium is used as the driving gas because its low molecular weight allows the high gas velocities necessary at elevated heart rates without excessive generation of heat [8]. For optimal unloading, the balloon should inflate just after the dicrotic notch of the arterial pulse wave and deflate just prior to left ventricular ejection. If inflation occurs prematurely, or if deflation is delayed at a time when the aortic valve is open, the left ventricle is forced to contract against an inflated balloon. In a patient with a recent myocardial infarction, this could potentially result in ventricular rupture. Conversely, if inflation is delayed, or deflation occurs too early, maximal reduction in afterload is not achieved. Although the IAB can cycle as rapidly as 150 to 160 times per minute, the efficiency of counterpulsation is reduced at heart rates over 130. Pharmacologic control of tachycardias or other arrhythmias may be necessary for optimal IAB function.

Physiology

Counterpulsation improves left ventricular performance [9] through an increase in coronary perfusion and a decrease in myocardial oxygen consumption [10,11]. In contrast to other types of circulatory assist devices, the IAB requires a minimum cardiac index of 1.2 to 1.4 L/min/m² to be effective [12]. Because of the requirement for minimum intrinsic left ventricular ejection, the IAB cannot assist the patient who is asystolic or in ventricular fibrillation. Counterpulsation causes an increase in cerebral and peripheral blood flow [13] but no significant alteration of renal perfusion, unless the renal orifices are occluded by the balloon [14,15].

Indications

CARDIOGENIC SHOCK. The IAB was developed with the hope of reversing cardiogenic shock after myocardial infarction. Clinical studies from a number of institutions have confirmed that counterpulsation is successful in reversing the shock state, at least temporarily, in 80 to 85 percent of patients [3,16,17]. Postmortem studies of those who are refractory show extensive infarction of 40 percent or more of the left ventricle [18,19]. Such patients are salvageable only by cardiac transplantation. Although counterpulsation is initially effective in reversing shock following myocardial infarction, a disappointingly high percentage of such patients become dependent on the IAB, as demonstrated by a fall in systemic arterial pressure and cardiac output and a rise in left atrial filling pressures when circulatory support is temporarily discontinued. Under these circumstances there is relatively little potential for spontaneous improvement in left ventricular function following myocardial infarction, and counterpulsation by itself simply postpones the inevitable outcome. When the IAB is used alone in the treatment of cardiogenic shock following myocardial infarction, the 1-year survival rate is only 9 to 22 percent [19–22]. Since counterpulsation is of limited effectiveness in patients with very low cardiac output, combining IAB with other methods of cardiac support is potentially attractive. Early studies have reported greater hemodynamic support and improved survival rates when counterpulsation is combined with percutaneous cardiopulmonary bypass in the treatment of patients in refractory cardiogenic shock [23].

It is important that the anatomic and functional derangements responsible for cardiogenic shock be corrected if the high rate of IAB dependence is to be reduced. Animal [24–27] and clinical [10] studies suggest that infarcted myocardium is surrounded by a zone of ischemic tissue that may redevelop effective contractility if satisfactory coronary perfusion can be restored through thrombolytic therapy, angioplasty, or aortocoronary surgery. Counterpulsation should be initiated as soon as it is determined that the shock state is not responsive to volume expansion and drug therapy. Once stabilized, as judged by improvement in the cardiac index, peripheral perfusion, and urinary output, the patient should undergo cardiac catheterization and, if feasible, revascularization. The IAB is usually removed a day or two later. Only about 40 percent of patients with cardiogenic shock after myocardial infarction are suitable candidates for revascularization. Although the overall mortality rate for early revascularization after myocardial infarction is 50 percent this represents a clear improvement when compared with medical therapy alone [28–31].

REVERSIBLE MECHANICAL DEFECTS. Counterpulsation is very effective in the initial stabilization of patients with mechanical intracardiac defects complicating infarction such as acute mitral regurgitation and ventricular septal perforation. Counterpulsation reduces pulmonary artery pressure and increases cardiac output for both of these lesions, and it also decreases the regurgitant V wave seen in mitral insufficiency.

Mitral valve replacement with concomitant coronary revascularization is the usual treatment for rupture of a papillary muscle. Acute ventricular septal defects are usually caused by infarction of the septum due to occlusion of the left anterior or posterior descending artery or both. The timing of surgical repair of an acute ventricular septal defect remains controversial. Some have advocated early repair, before the development of multiple organ failure. Early operation poses the technical difficulty of suturing recently infarcted tissue and is associated with a surgical mortality of 36 percent [32]. With the delayed approach the mortality is only 24 percent, but some patients succumb before operation [33]. Both methods of treatment rely on counterpulsation to maintain pre- and postoperative hemodynamic stability.

UNSTABLE ANGINA. Counterpulsation is effective in the treatment of unstable angina. The use of the IAB before irreversible myocardial injury and cardiogenic shock have supervened would seem to be theoretically sound, were the method without serious potential complications. Some institutions use counterpulsation very liberally for the treatment of unstable angina and report surgical mortality rates approaching those for chronic stable angina, in the range of 2.0 to 5.5 percent [34,35]. Such statistics are difficult to evaluate since the majority of patients with unstable angina also do well with aggressive medical therapy, and other centers have reported that counterpulsation is rarely necessary [36,37]. Until more exact guidelines are developed and randomized comparative trials performed, treatment of patients with unstable angina rests on clinical judgment. Counterpulsation should not be used as a substitute for vigorous pharmacologic therapy; however, counterpulsation is indicated when the angina is persistent and when there is ongoing electrocardiographic evidence of ischemia, despite maximal pharmacologic therapy.

WEANING FROM CARDIOPULMONARY BYPASS. One of the most useful indications for IAB is to aid in weaning patients from cardiopulmonary bypass who have suffered perioperative myocardial injury. Myocardial dysfunction following surgery is often reversible if the patient's circulation can be assisted for

24 to 48 hours [21,38,39]. The best results are achieved when counterpulsation is used in conjunction with optimal preloading with volume expansion, reduction of afterload with vasodilators, and positive inotropic agents to increase cardiac output [40]. When used in this setting, approximately 75 percent of bypass-dependent patients can be successfully weaned, with a 42 to 56 percent 2-year survival rate [12,40–44]. The best results are reported for patients with pure coronary disease, rather than those requiring valve replacement.

PREOPERATIVE USE. Routine preoperative use of IAB has been advocated by some groups for certain high-risk patients, including those with hemodynamically significant stenosis of the left main coronary artery and those with marked impairment of left ventricular function, as indicated by an ejection fraction less than 0.35 [45,46]. Operative mortality rates as high as 40 percent seemed to justify this approach; however, with improvements in anesthetic techniques and more sophisticated monitoring, many institutions now report surgical mortality rates for left main coronary artery disease equivalent to those for other types of coronary surgery without preoperative counterpulsation [47,48]. Since the incidence of peripheral vascular complications associated with the use of IAB is significant, this risk must be weighed against the potential benefits when counterpulsation is routinely applied to a large class of patients. Most centers use counterpulsation selectively rather than routinely for patients with left ostial coronary stenosis or diminished ejection fraction.

BRIDGE TO TRANSPLANTATION. Counterpulsation has been used to provide mechanical support for patients in failure while awaiting cardiac transplantation. The IAB may be used alone or in combination with other assist devices, such as extracorporeal membrane oxygenator (ECMO), LVAD, or an implantable artificial heart. Not surprisingly, the incidence of bacteremia is somewhat higher and the survival rate reduced for bridged patients compared to those not requiring preoperative assistance [49,50,51].

PERCUTANEOUS CORONARY ANGIOPLASTY. The indications and experience with percutaneous coronary angioplasty have expanded to include patients with multiple coronary lesions and those with impaired left ventricular function. Many centers now use counterpulsation to control unstable angina prior to and during coronary angioplasty [45,52,53]. The IAB is also recommended for prophylactic use in patients with severe left ventricular dysfunction or wall abnormalities and during dilatation of an unprotected left main coronary stenosis or a protected stenosis with reduced left ventricular function [30]. Counterpulsation has been reported to increase peak coronary blood flow velocity and may be a promising method to prevent coronary reocclusion following angioplasty for acute myocardial infarction [54]. Counterpulsation may be lifesaving following a failed angioplasty to support the myocardium until emergency aortocoronary revascularization can be performed [55,56,57].

LESS FREQUENT INDICATIONS. Counterpulsation is occasionally employed in a variety of other clinical situations. The IAB has been used to control pharmacologically refractory ventricular irritability after myocardial infarction [58,59]. Counterpulsation effectively diminishes ventricular irritability in as many as 90 percent of patients, apparently through a favorable influence on the myocardial oxygen supply-demand ratio. The best long-term survival rate has been for patients who subsequently undergo surgical revascularization before being weaned from IAB. With the advent of more potent antiarrhythmic drugs, the use of IAB to control ventricular arrhythmia will probably be less frequent.

Counterpulsation is also employed to stabilize patients in cardiogenic shock or with refractory angina during transit from a community hospital to a tertiary care facility, where more definitive treatment, including cardiac catheterization and revascularization, is available [60,61]. With the development of smaller portable consoles, counterpulsation will probably be used more frequently for transportation of patients with cardiac dysfunction. Successful use of IAB for treatment of heart failure following myocardial trauma has been reported [62,63,64]. Counterpulsation has also been used for perioperative support for high-risk noncardiac surgery, such as aortic aneurysm resection [65,66] or general surgical procedures [67]. Under most circumstances, it is preferable to improve the cardiac status of such patients with preliminary aortocoronary surgery. In some instances, however, coronary revascularization is not feasible because of diffuse disease or limited ventricular function, yet the patient requires a major surgical procedure. Preliminary results from counterpulsation for noncardiac operations are encouraging, but the experience is still too limited to recommend its widespread use in this setting.

Counterpulsation has been proposed as a method of limiting infarct size. Experimental evidence from canine studies supports this application [25,27]; however, data from other animal models, such as swine [24,26] and baboons [68] (which have a coronary circulation similar to that of humans), have not shown a benefit from counterpulsation. Moreover, the incidence and magnitude of potential complications remains sufficiently great to preclude recommending routine use of IAB in this application [17,69].

Contraindications

Aortic valvular insufficiency, aortic dissection, and severe aortoiliac disease are absolute contraindications to counterpulsation. In the presence of significant aortic regurgitation, the augmented diastolic pressure is transmitted directly to the left ventricle, compounding the deleterious effects of valvular insufficiency. Because of the need for anticoagulation during counterpulsation, gastrointestinal bleeding, thrombocytopenia, and other bleeding diatheses are relative contraindications to counterpulsation.

Technique of Insertion

The technique of IAB insertion described here, while generally applicable to all guidewire-directed IABs, is not intended to be a substitute for thorough familiarity with the manufacturer's instructions. New IAB devices are frequently introduced, each with its own variations in technique and list of precautions.

The following equipment is needed.

1. Manufacturer-supplied sterile insertion kit, including IAB, Potts-Cournand needle, guidewires, dilators, sheaths, connector tubing, one-way valve, syringe, stopcock
2. Portable fluoroscope
3. Povidone-iodine prep solution, sterile drapes, towel clips

4. 1% lidocaine with syringe and 22-gauge, 1 1/2-inch needle
5. Sterile gauze pads
6. No. 11 scalpel blade and handle
7. Dilute heparin solution (10,000 units in 500 ml of normal saline)
8. Two 0 silk sutures on curved cutting needles
9. Needleholder
10. 5000 units of heparin and a 10-ml syringe

Prior to insertion, the reasons for recommending counterpulsation therapy and potential complications should be fully explained to the patient and family and informed consent obtained. Since the IAB should be inserted in the side with the best circulation, any history suggesting vascular insufficiency, such as intermittent claudication, should be ascertained. Femoral and pedal pulses in both lower extremities should be palpated. If pedal pulses are absent, the ankle pressure may be measured using a portable Doppler ultrasonic flow detector [70].

An indwelling cannula in the radial artery is very helpful to monitor arterial pressure and time counterpulsation; it may be placed prior to insertion of the IAB (Chap. 3). In an emergency, the IAB may be placed first and the central lumen of the balloon used to measure arterial pressure.

The procedure should be performed with the patient supine. Cannulation of the femoral artery is very difficult if the patient cannot lie perfectly flat. In the severely orthopneic patient, controlled respiration with a mechanical ventilator may be required. Insertion of the IAB should be carried out on a radiolucent bed, operating table, or cardiac catheterization table to permit the use of fluoroscopy. An assistant should be available to prepare a sterile table on which supplies can be arranged.

Both inguinal areas are shaved and cleansed with povidone soap and water, followed by povidone-iodine solution. Sterile towels and sheets are used as drapes, leaving exposed a wide area over both femoral arteries. The contents of the insertion kit should be opened and arranged in order of usage. The balloon should be handled very carefully to avoid damage to the delicate membrane. The instructions for preparing the IAB should be followed closely, since the technique varies with the manufacturer. The most common method involves placement of a sterile one-way valve on the IAB male Luer fitting. A 60-ml syringe is connected to the valve and a 30-ml vacuum is applied. The syringe is then removed, leaving the valve in place and the IAB fully collapsed. The balloon should be left in its protective sleeve until the femoral artery is cannulated. The central lumen of the balloon and the Potts-Cournand needle should be flushed with dilute heparin saline.

Next, 10 ml of 1% lidocaine is instilled subdermally and subcutaneously over the femoral artery pulse. The puncture site should be 1 cm below the inguinal crease directly over the femoral pulsation. The femoral artery can be immobilized between the third and fourth fingers of the left hand while the Potts-Cournand needle is inserted at a 45-degree angle with the bevel pointing cephalad. The needle is passed through *both* walls of the artery. The central stylet is removed and the needle is slowly withdrawn until a strong, pulsatile jet of blood returns (Fig. 9-1). A weak jet of blood indicates that the needle is not properly located in the center of the arterial lumen; it should be withdrawn and replaced. When the outer cannula is properly placed in the artery, a J guidewire, 145 çm long and 0.030 inches in diameter, is passed through the cannula and advanced under fluoroscopic control until the tip is in the thoracic aorta (Fig. 9-2). The guidewire should pass *very easily* through the cannula. Even minimal resistance indicates that the guidewire is coiling. Under these circumstances, the guidewire is removed, the cannula repositioned for a brisk jet of blood, and another attempt

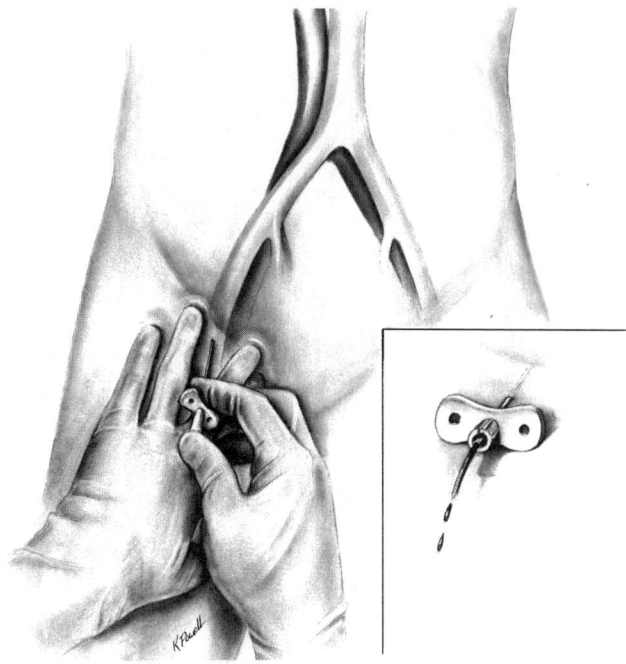

Fig. 9-1. The Potts-Cournand needle is inserted at a 45-degree angle into the common femoral artery. *Inset:* Pulsatile jet of blood indicates that the needle is properly located in the center of the arterial lumen.

made with a new wire. When the tip of the guidewire is satisfactorily positioned in the thoracic aorta, the patient should be intravenously anticoagulated with 5000 units of heparin. The Potts-Cournand needle is withdrawn, leaving the guidewire in place. To facilitate passage of the dilators and sheaths, a 4-mm incision is made at the puncture site, using a no. 11 scalpel blade. An 8 Fr. dilator is passed over the guidewire and, with a rotating motion, passed through the skin and subcutaneous tissue into the femoral artery (Fig. 9-3). This dilator is removed and exchanged for a 9.5 Fr. dilator with overlying Teflon sheath. Pressure is maintained over the puncture site to control bleeding during the exchange. About 4 cm of the sheath is left exposed caudal to the puncture site. The IAB is removed from the protective sleeve with care not to touch the balloon surface with metal instruments, which can damage the polyurethane membrane. The dilator is removed, leaving the sheath and guidewire in the artery. The sheath contains a valve to prevent back-bleeding during this maneuver. The free end of the guidewire is passed through the central lumen of the IAB. The IAB is advanced over the guidewire and through the sheath into the descending aorta, under fluoroscopic guidance (Fig. 9-4). As the IAB is advanced, a slight "give" or decrease in resistance is detected as the IAB exits from the distal end of the sheath. The tip of the balloon is radiopaque and should be positioned 2 cm distal to the orifice of the left subclavian artery. The IAB must be inserted to the level of the manufacturer's mark (usually a double line) on the IAB catheter to ensure that the entire membrane has emerged from the sheath to permit complete balloon opening; failure to exit the sheath completely will reduce diastolic augmentation, cause high balloon filling pressures, and lead to balloon fatigue and eventually balloon rupture with gas embolization. When the IAB is properly positioned, the sheath seal is pushed over the hub of the sheath to control bleeding (Fig. 9-5). Return of blood through the central lumen of the IAB provides reassurance that the device

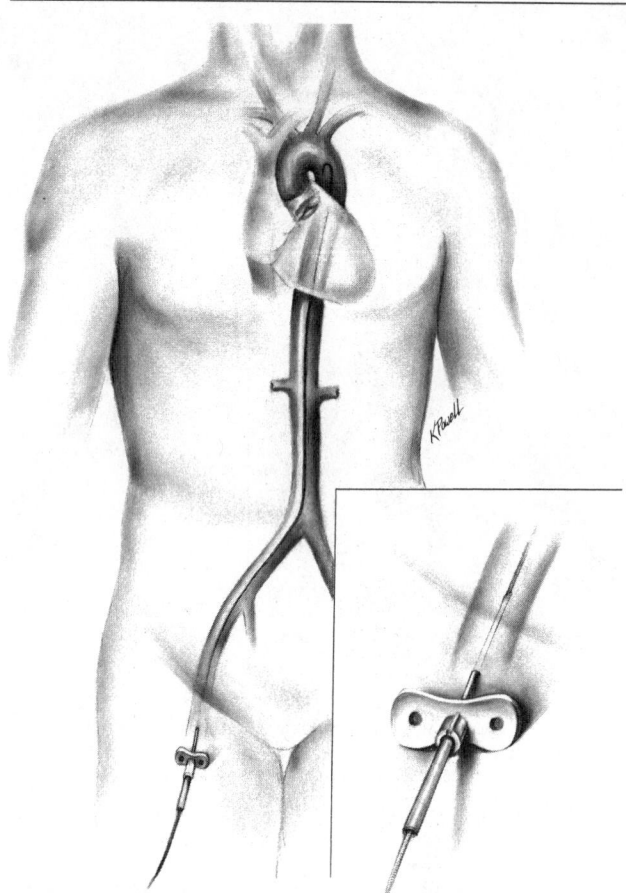

Fig. 9-2. When the Potts-Cournand needle is properly placed in the artery, the guidewire is advanced under fluoroscopic control until the tip is in the thoracic aorta.

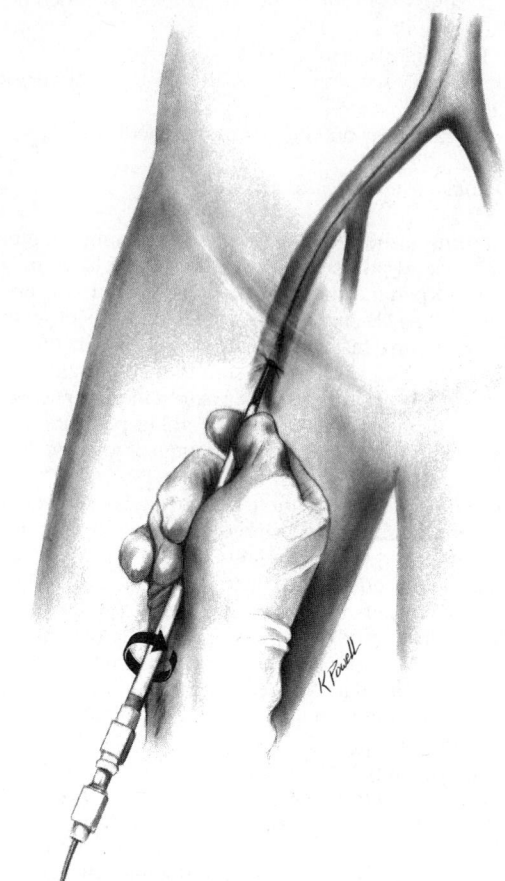

Fig. 9-3. A 9.5 Fr. dilator with overlying Teflon sheath is passed over the guidewire. A rotary motion and firm pressure are necessary to enter the lumen of the femoral artery.

has not caused a dissection. When in doubt, a small quantity of angiographic dye may be injected to confirm the final position of the IAB; thereafter, the central lumen should be carefully aspirated and then flushed with heparinized saline and used to monitor intraaortic pressure and to time counterpulsation. The one-way valve is removed and the male Luer fitting connected to the pressure line from the IAB console. The IAB and sheath should be secured to the inner thigh with heavy silk sutures. Antibiotic ointment should be applied to the puncture site, followed by a sterile gauze dressing.

Alternatively, the IAB may be inserted without the use of the sheath, which reduces the intraluminal arterial obstruction from 12 Fr. to 9.5 Fr. and may decrease the risk of ischemic complications to the lower limb. The sheathless technique is identical to that described above to the point where a 0.030 guidewire is positioned in the descending thoracic aorta. Passage of the IAB without a sheath requires a more spacious subcutaneous tunnel, which can be produced by gently spreading a hemostat along the tract of the guidewire. The IAB should be moistened with sterile saline. The inner stylet is removed by rotating the Luer lock fitting one-half turn counterclockwise. The free end of the guidewire is inserted into the tip of the IAB until it exits from the female Luer fitting of the hub. The IAB is advanced over the guidewire through the skin and subcutaneous tissue, holding the IAB close to the insertion point to prevent kinking. As the IAB enters the artery, blood under arterial pressure will run back along the folds of the balloon but will stop once the

IAB is completely inserted. The balloon is advanced to the proper position in the descending thoracic aorta. Sterility of the exposed catheter is maintained until its position has been confirmed by fluoroscopy or chest radiograph, since it cannot be repositioned once it has been contaminated. The guidewire is removed and the central lumen flushed with heparin saline. When the final position of IAB has been verified, the hub is secured to the inner thigh with heavy silk sutures and covered with a sterile occlusive dressing. Counterpulsation is initiated as described earlier [71,72].

Insertion of the IAB is most safely performed under fluoroscopic control. Under emergency conditions, however, the position of the IAB may be approximated by laying the device on the patient's chest so that the tip lies at the level of the third intercostal space and then marking the site on the catheter with a silk tie where it will pass through the introducer. The final position of the IAB may then be verified with a portable chest radiograph and adjusted as necessary. Transesophageal echocardiography is used increasingly to evaluate left ventricular function before and even during cardiac operations. It also shows promise as a relatively noninvasive means of evaluating the position of the IAB in the thoracic aorta and can be used to monitor coronary blood flow velocity during counterpulsation [73].

Anticoagulation with a heparin infusion to maintain the partial thromboplastin time at twice the control value is recommended to reduce the risk of embolism from the surface of the

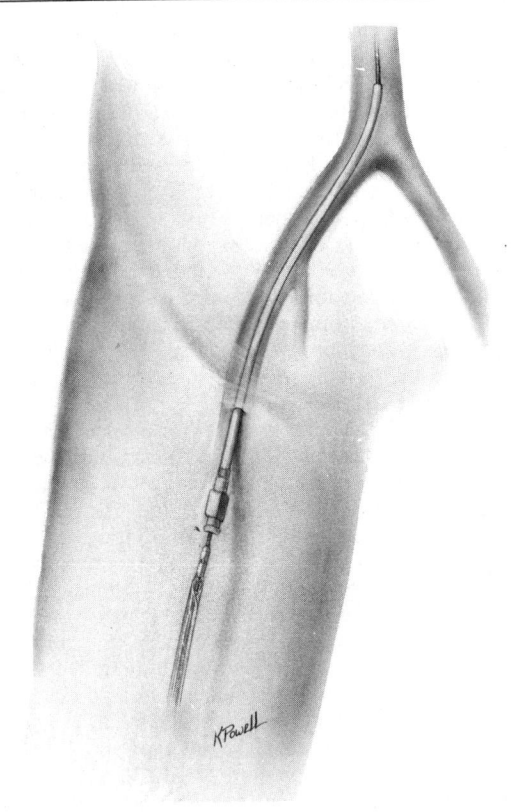

Fig. 9-4. The intraaortic balloon is advanced over the guidewire into the descending thoracic aorta under fluoroscopic guidance.

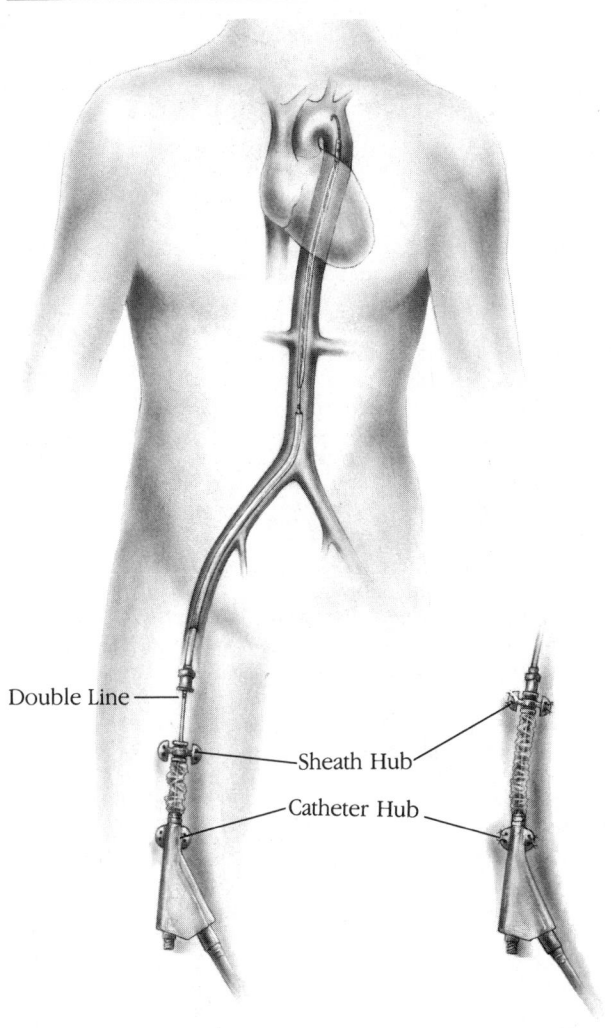

Fig. 9-5. The tip of the intraaortic balloon is positioned 2 cm distal to the orifice of the left subclavian artery. The IAB must be inserted to the level of the *double line* to be sure the entire membrane has emerged from the sheath. *Inset:* The sheath seal is pushed over the sheath hub to control bleeding. The sheath and catheter hubs are sutured in place.

balloon and thrombosis of the femoral artery at the puncture site. When anticoagulation is contraindicated because of thrombocytopenia, gastrointestinal bleeding, or recent surgery, an infusion of low-molecular-weight dextran at 20 ml per hour may be used. Prophylactic antibiotics effective against *Staphylococcus aureus* are recommended because of the potential threat of bacterial seeding of the IAB. We typically use intravenous cephalothin or oxacillin.

As soon as the IAB is in position, the circulatory status of the limb should be checked. Due to obstruction of blood flow in the iliac and femoral arteries, it is not unusual for the IAB to cause previously palpable pedal pulses to decrease or even to become absent. Usually, there is sufficient collateral flow to prevent severe ischemia. Adequacy of circulation is indicated by the preservation of sensation, motion, and normal color and the absence of pain. Measurement of Doppler ankle pressures provides an objective evaluation of the circulation. The ankle arm index may be compared with the preinsertion value. A Doppler ankle pressure less than 40 mm Hg or ankle arm index less than 0.25 indicates severe circulatory impairment. While the IAB is in position, it is imperative that the circulatory status be monitored every 2 to 4 hours. It is a common error to concentrate on the patient's cardiac problems on counterpulsation and to overlook progressive limb ischemia.

Acute limb ischemia may occur any time after initiation of counterpulsation but is most likely to occur immediately after IAB placement; following a decrease in cardiac output, especially if accompanied by an increase in inotropic support; or immediately after surgery. Some degree of ischemia occurs in many patients and is usually well tolerated and reversible when the IAB is removed. Consequently, initial management, partic-

ularly if the ischemia is mild, is conservative. Improvement in cardiac output, increase in systemic blood pressure, and weaning from alpha-adrenergic agents often improves peripheral perfusion. Sliding the insertion sheath back until the distal end just emerges from the femoral artery may allow enough increased blood flow past the catheter to relieve limb ischemia [74].

Severe ischemia, as indicated by the absence of an arterial Doppler signal over the dorsalis pedis or posterior tibial arteries at the ankle, requires prompt treatment. If the patient is not balloon-dependent, the easiest solution is to wean rapidly and remove the IAB. If the patient is balloon-dependent and the indication for counterpulsation was unstable or postinfarction angina, urgent cardiac catheterization and emergency coronary revascularization, followed by prompt removal of the IAB, should be considered. If coronary angiography and revascularization are not feasible or if the ischemia is sufficiently severe that the circulation must be improved promptly to prevent tissue necrosis, transfer of the IAB to the opposite limb is most expeditious. Even if the ischemia recurs on the second side, it may allow enough time to establish adequate pharmacologic support of the myocardium to proceed with cardiac catheterization and revascularization. Alternatively, a vascular bypass from the opposite common femoral artery to the superficial femoral artery distal to the IAB can effectively restore nearly normal circulation [75]. Although it may require transporting the patient to the operating room, the procedure is relatively minor and can be performed under local anesthesia. The procedure is highly successful in relieving limb ischemia, and the graft may be left in place when the IAB is removed. The final option for the IAB-dependent patient is to accept the possibility of future amputation and leave the device in place. Usually, this choice is made only in the patient whose chances for survival are considered extremely poor.

Triggering and Timing of Intraaortic Balloon Pump

The most important prerequisites for effective counterpulsation are the means of triggering inflation and timing the inflation-deflation cycle [76]. The R wave of the patient's ECG is the most common means for triggering balloon inflation. The IAB console is designed to detect the R wave of the ECG and is initially set so that inflation occurs at the peak of the T wave, which corresponds approximately with closure of the aortic valve. Deflation is then timed to occur just prior to the next QRS, which correlates with ventricular systole. It is important to select the ECG lead with the most pronounced R wave. Most triggering problems are due to an ECG with an R wave of low amplitude, dislodged electrodes, or electrical interference. If the patient has an implanted or external pacemaker, the pacing artifact may cause false triggering. In this setting, the lead in which the artifact has minimum amplitude or is of a negative sign is selected. Most IAB consoles have circuitry designed to reject the pacing artifact. In addition, intermittent right bundle branch block in which the R wave is of varying magnitude, or atrial fibrillation in which the R–R interval is variable, may interfere with effective ECG triggering.

The arterial waveform may also be used to trigger the IAB. In this mode, the upstroke of the arterial wave is sensed by the console. A fairly sharp upstroke with a pulse pressure of at least 40 mm Hg is necessary for reliable arterial triggering. This mode is useful when ECG triggering is not feasible because of the lack of a consistently good R wave or when there is electrical interference, such as intraoperative use of electrocautery.

The IAB may be triggered by an external pacemaker. In this mode the pacing artifact, rather than the patient's R wave, is used to trigger inflation. This mode is very useful when the ECG is of poor electrical quality or when pacing is necessary for bradycardia, complete heart block, or overdriving ventricular ectopy; however, it must be emphasized that this is a potentially lethal means of triggering. If pacing capture is lost, the timing of inflation and deflation will follow the pacemaker rather than the cardiac ejection pattern. Consequently, it is possible for the IAB to inflate during systole. Because of the potential hazards of the pacemaker triggering of the IAB, we recommend use of this mode only in an emergency when triggering cannot be effected by ECG or arterial waveform, and then only with an IAB technician in constant attendance. Finally, counterpulsation can be triggered by an internally generated signal from the IAB console at a fixed rate of 80 per minute. This triggering mode is used only to generate a pulse during cardiopulmonary bypass.

When initiating counterpulsation, the console should be set to a 1:2 assist ratio so the effects of augmentation on every other beat can be analyzed. The IAB should be inflated initially to one-half the operating volume until proper timing is effected. Slide switches on the console permit adjustment of the timing of both inflation and deflation during the cardiac cycle (Fig. 9-6). If the IAB is inflated too early when the aortic valve is still open, left ventricular workload is increased rather than reduced. If inflation occurs too late, diastolic aortic root pressure fails to rise significantly, and there is no improvement in coronary perfusion. Deflation should occur just prior to systole; consequently, it should be timed so the intraaortic pressure is at a minimum when the aortic valve opens. If deflation occurs too early, the benefit of improved coronary filling in late diastole is lost. When deflation is too late, the left ventricle must contract against the residual pressure caused by a partially inflated IAB.

A good arterial waveform is essential for proper IAB timing. Since a finite time is necessary for transmission of the pulse pressure from the aortic root to the periphery, IAB timing varies, depending on the location of the arterial line. The pulse wave requires about 50 msec to be transmitted from the aortic root to the radial artery and about 120 msec to be transmitted from the aortic root to the femoral artery. Ideally, IAB inflation should occur just after closure of the aortic valve, which corresponds with the dicrotic notch of the aortic root pulse when measured through the lumen of the IAB. Therefore, if the radial artery is used to monitor arterial pressure, inflation should occur midway between the peak of the waveform and the dicrotic notch. If the femoral artery line is employed, inflation should occur at the time of the peak arterial pressure (Fig. 9-7).

When the IAB technician and physician are satisfied with both triggering and timing, the IAB may be fully inflated and set to a 1:1 ratio to assist each cardiac cycle. The IAB inflation will result in a diastolic pressure that exceeds the systolic pressure. Conversely, deflation of the balloon will reduce end-diastolic pressure by 15 to 20 mm Hg and systolic pressure by 5 to 10 mm Hg [76]. Timing should be rechecked every 1 to 2 hours and whenever there is a significant change in heart rate or cardiac output, development of arrhythmia, or change in triggering mode. When retiming, it is helpful to return to the 1:2 assist ratio.

Finally, the console should be switched from manual to automatic operation. This activates internal monitoring circuits that will stop the IAB and sound an alarm when certain malfunctions are detected. Some of the monitored functions are volume and pressure in the IAB, the presence of leaks causing loss of driving gas, loss of ECG or arterial trigger signal, and improper deflation of the IAB. Since many patients are adversely affected by even a brief loss of counterpulsation, it is important that physicians and intensive care unit nurses be completely familiar with the detection and prompt correction of common problems associated with the use of counterpulsation. An experienced IAB technician must be available on a 24-hour basis to manage the more complicated, but fortunately unusual, equipment malfunctions.

Weaning from Counterpulsation

Cessation of counterpulsation involves two steps: weaning and IAB removal. The IAB console can provide counterpulsation ratios of 1:1, 1:2, and 1:3. In addition, some consoles permit weaning by a gradual reduction in balloon volume. The patient may be progressively weaned by reducing the assist ratio or IAB volume and checking the cardiac index and filling pres-

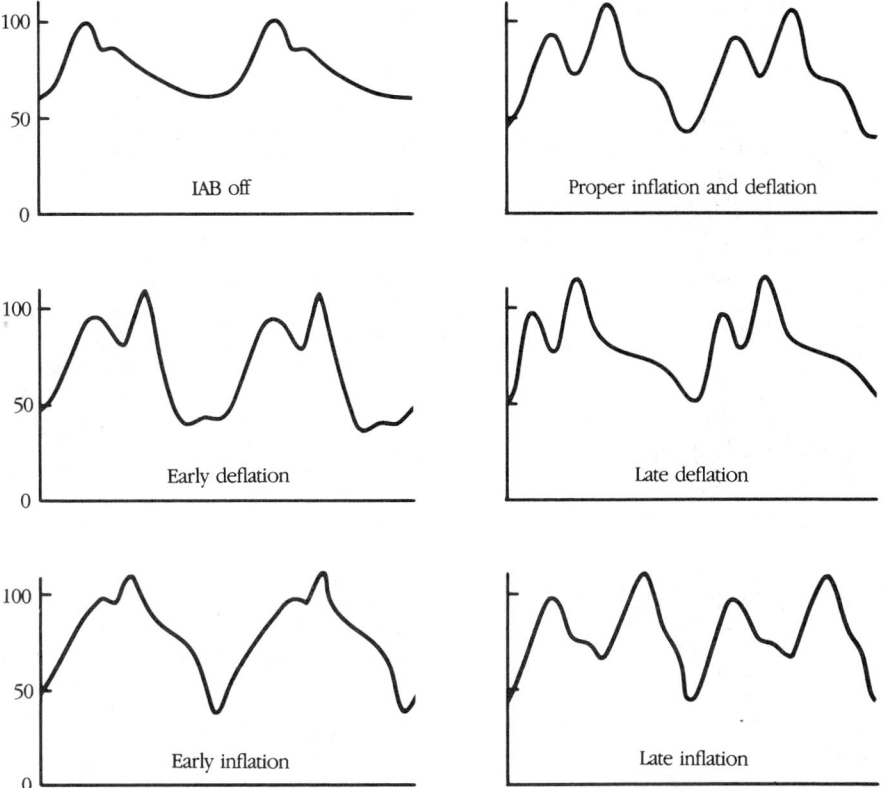

Fig. 9-6. Slide switches on the intraaortic balloon (IAB) console permit proper timing of inflation and deflation during the cardiac cycle.

sures at each level. Usually, at least 2 hours is required to establish stability at each new assist level. When the patient has been weaned to 1:3 and has been stable for a few hours, the IAB may be removed.

The heparin infusion should be stopped 2 hours before removing the percutaneous IAB. The prothrombin and partial thromboplastin times should be near normal and the platelet count greater than 75,000 before removal of a percutaneous IAB. The IAB console should be put on standby or off. The dressing and securing sutures should be removed. The IAB catheter should be removed from the back of the console, and an assistant should use a 50-ml syringe to apply continuous negative pressure. The gasket is then removed from the sheath connector and the IAB is withdrawn until it abuts the sheath. The operator should not attempt to withdraw the balloon into the sheath. The IAB and sheath are then removed as a unit. Arterial bleeding is allowed for 1 or 2 seconds to "flush" any residual thrombus. Sufficient pressure to obliterate the femoral pulse is applied for 45 minutes before the operator checks for bleeding. If there is any evidence of hematoma formation, pressure should be applied for an additional 15 minutes. The use of sandbags is not recommended, since they do not apply sufficient localized pressure over the puncture site and can conceal a developing hematoma. Occasionally, particularly in obese or hypertensive patients, local pressure, even for an hour or more, will not control bleeding from the puncture site and a hematoma forms. This is best managed with early surgical exploration, evacuation of the hematoma, and direct surgical repair of the puncture site.

Complications of Counterpulsation

Complications of counterpulsation may be grouped into three categories: (1) those that occur during the insertion procedure, (2) those that develop while the IAB is in place, and (3) those that are consequences of IAB removal. The overall complication rate for percutaneous IAB ranges from 17 to 28 percent [43,77–85].

COMPLICATIONS DURING INSERTION. The most common complication related to insertion is failure of the IAB to pass the iliofemoral system because of atherosclerotic occlusive disease. With the currently available 9.5 Fr. percutaneous IAB, the reported failure rate ranges from 5 to 7 percent [77–80] and may be slightly higher with the sheathless technique [72]. If severe peripheral vascular disease precludes IAB implantation, the IAB may be inserted via the ascending aorta at the time of cardiac surgery [86,87]. The transthoracic route permits expiditious placement under direct vision and avoids potential ischemic complications to the lower extremities. The disadvantages of this approach are the risk of cerebral embolism during insertion, increased rate of balloon rupture, risk of mediastinal bleeding and infectious complications, and the need for a second operative procedure for its removal [88]. Clearly, transthoracic placement of IAB is not available to the nonsurgical patient. There have been case reports of successful IAB placement via the right subclavian artery, but the experience is so limited that this must be considered experimental [89]. Under emergency circumstances, an IAB may be inserted through the femoral limb of an aortobifemoral graft, with a reported infection rate of 12 percent [90]. Because of the risk of introducing infection into a prosthetic graft, with its associated high morbidity and

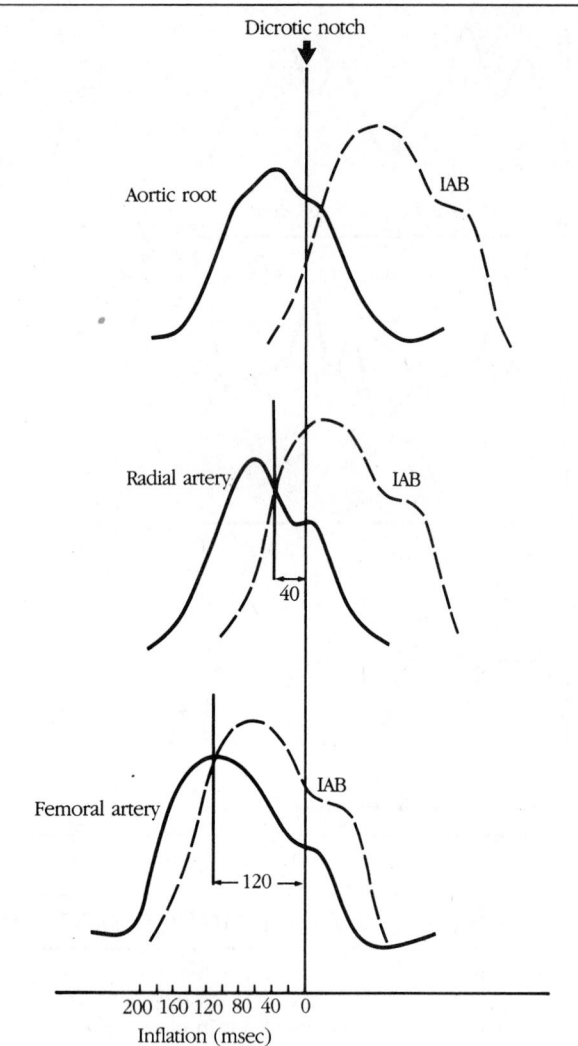

Dicrotic notch

Aortic root   IAB

Radial artery   IAB

40

Femoral artery   IAB

120

200 160 120 80 40 0
Inflation (msec)

Fig. 9-7. Proper timing of intraaortic balloon (IAB) inflation depends on the artery from which the arterial pressure is measured.

mortality, the duration of counterpulsation should be minimized when this method of access is employed.

Other complications of IAB insertion include aortic dissection and arterial perforation [43,77–81,91]. Although both are serious complications, there are many reports of successful counterpulsation with an IAB in a subintimal location [90,91]. Perforation usually occurs in the common iliac artery because of difficulty in negotiating a tortuous vessel or angulation at the aortic bifurcation. Arterial perforation is an acute emergency requiring urgent surgical intervention. The reported incidence of aortic dissection or arterial perforation is 1 to 2 percent [82,92,93]. These types of arterial injuries can be minimized by the use of wire-guided IAB and continuous fluoroscopy during the insertion procedure.

COMPLICATIONS WHILE INTRAAORTIC BALLOON IS IN PLACE. Limb ischemia is the most common complication of counterpulsation and is sufficiently severe to require removal of the IAB in 11 to 27 percent of patients [44,76–81,94,95]. Early intraaortic balloon pumps used a 12 Fr. catheter placed through a surgical cutdown over the common femoral artery. Smaller

catheters (8.0 to 9.5 Fr.) and sheathless insertion technique may reduce the incidence of ischemic complications [71,72].

A large review of the complications of counterpulsation found that limb ischemia sufficiently severe to require cessation of IAB therapy occurred in 32 percent of women, 34 percent of insulin-dependent diabetics, and 75 percent of patients with significant peripheral vascular occlusive disease as indicated by a preinsertion ankle arm index less than 0.6 [81]. The caliber of the IAB, duration of counterpulsation, and use of anticoagulation were not shown to be significant risk factors for ischemia. Although the physician does not have the luxury of selecting patients who are free of risk factors, earlier catheterization and revascularization can be considered in patients in whom they are present.

Since the IAB is a foreign body in continuous contact with the circulation, there is justifiable concern about infection. Surprisingly, septic complications are relatively unusual, even with prolonged periods of counterpulsation [96]. In one study of more than 700 patients, only 1.4 percent developed septicemia [81]. However, when sepsis does occur in the presence of IAB, the mortality rate is high. Positive blood cultures in a patient on counterpulsation require prompt removal and culture of the IAB and treatment with the appropriate intravenous antibiotic.

Some degree of thrombocytopenia is observed in most patients with an IAB. Platelet counts should be performed daily. Since heparin has been associated with thrombocytopenia, the patient should be changed to an infusion of low-molecular-weight dextran if the platelet count falls below 100,000 per cubic millimeter. There is usually no need to transfuse platelets unless the patient develops overt bleeding. The platelet count usually returns to normal soon after the IAB is removed.

There have been case reports of embolization of platelet aggregates from the surface of the balloon or dislodgement of atherosclerotic debris from the aortic wall to the mesenteric [97,98], renal [99], spinal [100,101], cerebral, and peripheral arteries [77]. Such complications are unpredictable and not preventable with the use of anticoagulation or antiplatelet drugs. Rupture of the IAB occurs in 2 to 4 percent of patients and may cause embolization of the helium driving gas, resulting in a cerebrovascular accident [6] or death [5]. Balloon rupture is probably not due to fatigue of the polyurethane membrane, since one IAB was used for nearly a year (30 million inflations) in a single patient without leaking [7]. Microscopic analysis of a failed IAB usually shows abrasions, presumably from contact with atherosclerotic plaques. Balloon rupture seems to be most frequent in patients with a small-caliber aorta, where there is intimate contact between the IAB and the wall of the aorta with each inflation. In this situation, a sharp plaque can abrade the balloon membrane, causing gas to escape into the circulation. Further evidence for this theory is the observation that patients with IAB rupture often have unusually high diastolic augmentation pressures. An IAB rupture, therefore, may be heralded by console alarms detecting high balloon-filling pressures [4]. Blood in the connecting tubing is a hallmark of rupture and requires immediate cessation of counterpulsation, placement of the patient in the Trendelenburg position, and IAB removal. Antibiotic coverage should be broadened, since the gas chamber of the IAB is not sterile. If the patient is dependent on counterpulsation, the IAB may be replaced over a guidewire. A related, recently recognized serious complication, is IAB entrapment. A small perforation in the balloon membrane permits a slow leak of blood into the balloon lumen. The leak is sufficiently small that the loss of driving gas is not detected by the IAB console. The dry helium desiccates the collected blood, forming a rock-hard pellet, which impinges against the orifice of the common iliac artery during attempted removal. The entrapped balloon can be removed only by surgical aortotomy.

Since entrapment can occur only if there is a balloon perforation, even a trace of blood in the tubing is an indication to remove or exchange the IAB. Furthermore, resistance during removal may indicate entrapment, which should be confirmed radiologically to determine the safest means of removal [100,101].

COMPLICATIONS DURING OR FOLLOWING REMOVAL.

As noted above, the IAB may be removed percutaneously by withdrawing the balloon and sheath together, after which the puncture site is compressed for 45 to 60 minutes. A randomized prospective study showed that the incidence of vascular complications for IABs removed with this technique was 4 percent, which was the same as with an open surgical procedure [104]. Although the majority of percutaneously placed IABs may be safely removed "percutaneously," surgical removal is still recommended for patients who are anticoagulated, who have a coagulopathy, or in whom the IAB was placed with an operative procedure. Arterial perfusion of the limb should be checked soon after removal of the IAB by palpation of pulses and measurement of the ankle-arm index. The puncture site should be examined for hematoma, false aneurysm formation, and arteriovenous fistula. In obese patients, ultrasound is a useful objective means to distinguish a hematoma from a false aneurysm. A characteristic continuous bruit heard over the puncture site indicates an arteriovenous fistula. The diagnosis may be confirmed by duplex scan or arteriography.

Conclusions

The IAB is the most widely used LVAD currently available. Its major value lies in its ability to "buy time" for the medical patient so that cardiac catheterization can be performed to look for a surgically correctable mechanical defect or remediable coronary artery disease. In addition, it can often permit weaning from cardiopulmonary bypass of the cardiac surgical patient with depressed left ventricular function. The ease with which the IAB can be inserted has aroused speculation that the indications for its use will broaden and that it may be implanted by less experienced physicians, thus increasing the possibility of more frequent and more severe complications. Even in the most capable hands, there is probably an irreducible incidence of complications due to associated severe peripheral vascular disease and diminished cardiac output. The incidence of complications can be minimized by limiting the use of the IAB to well-accepted indications, using meticulous insertion technique, and careful monitoring of limb circulation after implantation.

References

1. Forsell G, Nordlander R, Nyquist O, et al: Intraaortic balloon pumping in the treatment of cardiogenic shock complicating acute myocardial infarction. Acta Med Scand 206:189, 1979.
2. Lorente P, Gourgon R, Beaufils P, et al: Multivariate statistical evaluation of intraaortic counterpulsation in pump failure complicating acute myocardial infarction. Am J Cardiol 46:124, 1980.
3. Moulopoulos S, Stamatelopoulos S, Petrou P: Intraaortic balloon assistance in intractable cardiogenic shock. Eur Heart J 7:396, 1986.
4. Stahl KD, Tortolani AJ, Nelson RL, et al: Intraaortic balloon rupture. Trans Am Soc Artif Intern Organs 34:496, 1988.
5. Haykal HA, Wang AM: CT diagnosis of delayed cerebral air embolism following intraaortic balloon pump catheter insertion. Comput Radiol 10:307, 1986.
6. Frederiksen JW, Smith J, Brown P, et al: Arterial helium embolism from a ruptured intraaortic balloon. Ann Thorac Surg 46:690, 1988.
7. Freed PS, Wasfie T, Zado B, et al: Intraaortic balloon pumping for prolonged circulatory support. Am J Cardiol 61:554, 1988.
8. Kayser KL, Johnson WD, Shore RT: Comparison of driving gases for IABPs. Med Instrum 15:51, 1981.
9. Akyurekli Y, Taichman GC, Keon WJ: Effectiveness of intra-aortic balloon counterpulsation on systolic unloading. Can J Surg 23:122, 1980.
10. Williams DO, Korr KS, Gewirtz H, et al: The effect of intraaortic balloon counterpulsation on regional myocardial blood flow and oxygen consumption in the presence of coronary artery stenosis in patients with unstable angina. Circulation 66:593, 1982.
11. Gewirtz H, Ohley W, Williams DO, et al: Effect of intraaortic balloon counterpulsation on regional myocardial blood flow and oxygen consumption in the presence of coronary artery stenosis: Observations in an awake animal model. Am J Cardiol 50:829, 1982.
12. Sturm JT, McGee MG, Fuhrman TM, et al: Treatment of postoperative low output syndrome with intraaortic balloon pumping: Experience with 419 patients. Am J Cardiol 45:1033, 1980.
13. Juhlin-Dannfelt A, Nordlander R, Nyquist O: Peripheral hemodynamics in assisted circulation with intra-aortic balloon pumping in patients with cardiogenic shock. Acta Med Scand 205:505, 1979.
14. Bhayana JN, Scott SM, Sethi GK, et al: Effects of intraaortic balloon pumping on organ perfusion in cardiogenic shock. J Surg Res 26:108, 1979.
15. Swartz MT, Sakamoto T, Arai H, et al: Effects of intraaortic balloon position on renal artery blood flow. Ann Thorac Surg 53:604, 1992.
16. Scheidt S, Wilner G, Mueller H, et al: Intra-aortic balloon counterpulsation in cardiogenic shock: Report of a cooperative clinical trial. N Engl J Med 288:979, 1973.
17. O'Rourke MF, Norris RM, Campbell TJ, et al: Randomized controlled trial of intraaortic balloon counterpulsation in early myocardial infarction with acute heart failure. Am J Cardiol 47:815, 1981.
18. Bourdarias JP, Gourgon R, Bardet J: Mechanical circulatory assistance by intraaortic balloon pumping for the treatment of cardiogenic shock. Intensive Care Med 4:29, 1978.
19. Sturm JT, Fuhrman TM, Igo SR, et al: Quantitative indices of intraaortic balloon pump (IABP) dependence during post-infarction cardiogenic shock. Artif Organs 4:8, 1980.
20. Johnson SA, Scanlon PJ, Loeb HS, et al: Treatment of cardiogenic shock in myocardial infarction by intraaortic balloon counterpulsation and surgery. Am J Med 62:687, 1977.
21. Jackson G, Cullum P, Pastellopoulos A, et al: Intra-aortic balloon assistance in cardiogenic shock after myocardial infarction or cardiac surgery. Br Heart J 39:598, 1977.
22. Kuhn LA: Management of shock following acute myocardial infarction; II: Mechanical circulatory assistance. Am Heart J 95:789, 1978.
23. Phillips SJ, Zeff RH, Kongtahworn C, et al: Benefits of combined balloon pumping and percutaneous cardiopulmonary bypass. Ann Thorac Surg 54:908, 1992.
24. Laas J, Campbell CD, Takanashi Y, et al: Failure of intra-aortic balloon pumping to reduce experimental myocardial infarct size in swine. J Thorac Cardiovasc Surg 80:85, 1980.
25. Jett GK, Dengle SK, Barnett PA, et al: Intraaortic balloon counterpulsation: Its influence alone and combined with various pharmacological agents on regional myocardial blood flow during experimental acute coronary occlusion. Ann Thorac Surg 32:144, 1981.
26. Takanashi Y, Campbell CD, Laas J, et al: Reduction of myocardial infarct size in swine: A comparative study of intraaortic balloon pumping and transapical left ventricular bypass. Ann Thorac Surg 32:475, 1981.
27. Muller KD, Lubbecke F, Schaper W, et al: Effect of intraaortic balloon counterpulsation (IABP) on myocardial infarct size and collateral flow in an experimental dog model. Intensive Care Med 8:131, 1982.
28. McEnany MT, Kay HR, Buckley MJ, et al: Clinical experience with intraaortic balloon pump support in 728 patients. Circulation 58(suppl I):I124, 1978.
29. DeWood MA, Notske RN, Hensley GR, et al: Intraaortic balloon

counterpulsation with and without reperfusion for myocardial infarction shock. *Circulation* 61:1105, 1980.

30. Hartzler GO, Rutherford BD, McConahay DR, et al: "High-risk" percutaneous transluminal coronary angioplasty. *Am J Cardiol* 61:33G, 1988.

31. Kuhn LA: External pressure circulatory assistance: No light on the shadow. *Am J Cardiol* 46:1069, 1980.

32. Blanche C, Khan SS, Matloff JM, et al: Results of early repair of ventricular septal defect after an acute myocardial infarction. *J Thorac Cardiovasc Surg* 104:961, 1992.

33. Muehrcke DD, Daggett WM Jr, Buckley MJ, et al: Postinfarct ventricular septal defect repair: Effect of coronary artery bypass grafting. *Ann Thorac Surg* 54:876, 1992.

34. Bardet J, Rigaud M, Kahn JC, et al: Treatment of post-myocardial infarction angina by intra-aortic balloon pumping and emergency revascularization. *J Thorac Cardiovasc Surg* 74:299, 1977.

35. Harris PL, Woollard K, Bartoli A, et al: The management of impending myocardial infarction using coronary artery bypass grafting and an intra-aortic balloon pump. *J Cardiovasc Surg* 21:405, 1980.

36. Craver JM, Kaplan JA, Jones EL: What role should the intraaortic balloon have in cardiac surgery. *Ann Surg* 189:769, 1979.

37. Brundage BH, Ullyot DJ, Winokur S, et al: The role of aortic balloon pumping in postinfarction angina: A different perspective. *Circulation* 62(suppl I):I119, 1980.

38. Buckley MJ, Craver JM, Gould HK, et al: Intra-aortic balloon pump assist for cardiogenic shock after cardiopulmonary bypass. *Circulation* 48(suppl III):90, 1973.

39. Lund O, Johansen G, Allermand H, et al: Intraaortic balloon pumping in the treatment of low cardiac output following open heart surgery: Immediate results and long-term prognosis. *Thorac Cardiovasc Surg* 36:332, 1988.

40. Macoviak J, Stephenson LW, Edmunds LH Jr, et al: The intraaortic balloon pump: An analysis of five years' experience. *Ann Thorac Surg* 29:451, 1980.

41. Sturm JT, Fuhrman TM, Sterling R, et al: Combined use of dopamine and nitroprusside therapy in conjunction with intra-aortic balloon pumping for the treatment of post-cardiotomy low-output syndrome. *J Thorac Cardiovasc Surg* 82:13, 1981.

42. Golding LAR, Loop FD, Peter M, et al: Late survival following use of intraaortic balloon pump in revascularization operations. *Ann Thorac Surg* 30:48, 1980.

43. Di Lello F, Mullen DC, Flemma RJ, et al: Results of intraaortic balloon pumping after cardiac surgery: Experience with the Percor balloon catheter. *Ann Thorac Surg* 46:442, 1988.

44. Naunheim KS, Swartz MT, Pennington DG, et al: Intraaortic balloon pumping in patients requiring cardiac operations: Risk analysis and long-term follow-up. *J Thorac Cardiovasc Surg* 104:1654, 1992.

45. Tommaso CL: Management of high-risk coronary angioplasty. *Am J Cardiol* 64:33E, 1989.

46. Tahan SR, Geha AS, Hammond GL: Bypass surgery for left main coronary artery disease: Reduced perioperative myocardial infarction with preoperative intraaortic balloon counterpulsation. *Br Heart J* 43:191, 1980.

47. Brandt B III, Wright CB, Doty DB, et al: Surgical treatment of left main coronary artery disease: Operative risk. *Surgery* 87:436, 1980.

48. Vijayanager R, Bognolo DA, Eckstein PF, et al: The role of intraaortic balloon pump in the management of patients with main left coronary artery disease. *Cathet Cardiovasc Diagn* 7:397, 1981.

49. Maccioli GA, Lucas WJ, Norfleet EA: The intra-aortic balloon pump: A review. *J Cardiothorac Anesth* 2:365, 1988.

50. Bolman RM III, Spray TL, Cox JL, et al: Heart transplantation in patients requiring preoperative mechanical support. *J Heart Transplan* 6:273, 1987.

51. Oaks TE, Wisman CB, Pae WE, et al: Results of mechanical circulatory assistance before heart transplantation. *J Heart Transplan* 8:113, 1989.

52. Voudris V, Marco J, Morice MC, et al: "High-risk" percutaneous transluminal coronary angioplasty with preventive intra-aortic balloon counterpulsation. *Cathet Cardiovasc Diagn* 19:160, 1990.

53. Kahn JK, Rutherford BD, McConahay DR, et al: Supported "high risk" coronary angioplasty using intraaortic balloon pump counterpulsation. *J Am Coll Cardiol* 15:1151, 1990.

54. Ishihara M, Sato H, Tateishi H, et al: Effects of intraaortic balloon pumping on coronary hemodynamics after coronary angioplasty in patients with acute myocardial infarction. *Am Heart J* 124:1133, 1992.

55. Ferguson TB Jr, Mulhbaier LH, Salai DL, et al: Coronary artery bypass grafting after failed elective and failed emergent percutaneous angioplasty: Relative risks of emergent surgical intervention. *J Thorac Cardiovasc Surg* 95:761, 1988.

56. Akins CW, Block PC: Surgical intervention for failed percutaneous transluminal coronary angioplasty. *Am J Cardiol* 53:108C, 1984.

57. Talley JD, Jones EL, Weintraub WS, et al: Coronary artery bypass surgery after failed elective percutaneous transluminal coronary angioplasty: A status report. *Circulation* 79:I126, 1989.

58. Willerson JT, Curry GC, Watson JT, et al: Intraaortic balloon counterpulsation in patients in cardiogenic shock, medically refractory left ventricular failure and/or recurrent ventricular tachycardia. *Am J Med* 58:183, 1975.

59. Hanson EC, Levine FH, Kay HR, et al: Control of postinfarction ventricular irritability with the intraaortic balloon pump. *Circulation* 63(suppl I):I130, 1980.

60. Gottlieb SO, Chew PH, Chandra N, et al: Portable intraaortic balloon counterpulsation: Clinical experience and guidelines for use. *Cathet Cardiovasc Diagn* 12:18, 1986.

61. Singh JB, Connelly RN, Kocot S, et al: Intraaortic balloon counterpulsation in a community hospital. *Chest* 79:58, 1981.

62. Fallahnejad M, Kutty ACK, Menut H: The importance of intraaortic balloon pumping in the management of coronary artery laceration. *J Cardiovasc Surg* (Torino) 23:426, 1982.

63. Snow N, Lucas AE, Richardson JD: Intra-aortic balloon counterpulsation for cardiogenic shock from cardiac contusion. *J Trauma* 23:426, 1982.

64. Jacobs JP, Horowitz MD, Ladden DA, et al: Case report: Intra-aortic balloon counterpulsation in penetrating cardiac trauma. *J Cardiovasc Surg* 33:38, 1992.

65. Bonchek LI, Olinger GN: Intra-aortic balloon counterpulsation for cardiac support during noncardiac operations. *J Thorac Cardiovasc Surg* 78:147, 1979.

66. Hollier LH, Spitell JA Jr, Puga FJ: Intra-aortic balloon counterpulsation as adjunct to aneurysmectomy in high-risk patients. *Mayo Clin Proc* 56:565, 1981.

67. Siu SC, Kowalchuk GJ, Welty FK, et al: Intra-aortic balloon counterpulsation support in the high-risk cardiac patient undergoing urgent noncardiac surgery. *Chest* 99:1342, 1991.

68. Haston HH, McNamara JJ: The effects of intraaortic balloon counterpulsation on myocardial infarct size. *Ann Thorac Surg* 28:335, 1979.

69. Amsterdam EA, Awan NA, Lee G, et al: Intra-aortic balloon counterpulsation: Rationale, application and results. *Cardiovasc Clin* 11:179, 1980.

70. Loebl EC, Pomajzl MJ, Platt MR, et al: Noninvasive assessment of limb ischemia associated with intraaortic balloon pumping, in Diethrich EB (ed): *Noninvasive Cardiovascular Diagnosis*. 2nd ed. Littleton, MA, PSG, 1981.

71. Nash IS, Lorell BH, Fishman RF, et al: A new technique for sheathless percutaneous intraaortic balloon catheter insertion. *Cathet Cardiovasc Diagn* 23:57, 1991.

72. Phillips SJ, Tannenbaum M, Zeff RH, et al: Sheathless insertion of the percutaneous intraaortic balloon pump: An alternative method. *Ann Thorac Surg* 53:162, 1992.

73. Katz ES, Tunick PA, Kronzon I: Observations of coronary flow augmentation and balloon function during intraaortic balloon counterpulsation using transesophageal echocardiography. *Am J Cardiol* 69:1635, 1992.

74. Cutler BS: Acute leg ischemia secondary to intraaortic balloon pump insertion, in Brewster DC (ed): *Common Problems in Vascular Surgery*. Chicago, Year Book, 1989, pp 325–529.

75. Alpert J, Parsonnet V, Goldenkranz RJ, et al: Limb ischemia during intra-aortic balloon pumping: Indication for femorofemoral crossover graft. *J Thorac Cardiovasc Surg* 79:729, 1980.

76. Weber KT, Janicki JS: Intraaortic balloon counterpulsation: A review of physiologic principles, clinical results, and device safety. *Ann Thorac Surg* 17:602, 1974.

77. Grayzel J: Clinical evaluation of the Percor percutaneous intraaortic balloon: Cooperative study of 722 cases. *Circulation* 66(suppl I):I223, 1982.

78. Bregman D, Nichols AB, Weiss MB, et al: Percutaneous intraaortic balloon insertion. *Am J Cardiol* 46:261, 1980.

79. Alderman JD, Gabliani GI, McCabe CH, et al: Incidence and management of limb ischemia with percutaneous wire-guided intraaortic balloon catheters. *J Am Coll Cardiol* 9:524, 1987.

80. Goldberg M, Kantrowitz A, Rubenfire M, et al: Intraaortic balloon pump insertion: A randomized study comparing percutaneous and surgical techniques. *J Am Coll Cardiol* 9:515, 1987.

81. Kantrowitz A, Wasfie T, Freed PS, et al: Intraaortic balloon pumping 1967 through 1982: Analysis of complications in 733 patients. *Am J Cardiol* 57:976, 1986.

82. Inverson LIG, Herfindahl G, Ecker RR, et al: Vascular complications of intraaortic balloon counterpulsation. *Am J Surg* 154:99, 1987.

83. Wasfie T, Freed PS, Rubenfire M, et al: Risks associated with intraaortic balloon pumping in patients with and without diabetes mellitus. *Am J Cardiol* 61:558, 1988.

84. Leinbach RC, Goldstein J, Gold HK, et al: Percutaneous wire-guided balloon pumping. *Am J Cardiol* 49:1707, 1982.

85. Sanfelippo PM, Baker NH, Ewy HG, et al: Experience with intraaortic balloon counterpulsation. *Ann Thorac Surg* 41:36, 1986.

86. McGeehin W, Sheikh F, Donahoo JS, et al: Transthoracic intraaortic balloon pump support: Experience in 39 patients. *Ann Thorac Surg* 44:26, 1987.

87. Meldrum-Hanna WG, Deal CW, Ross DE: Complications of ascending aortic intraaortic balloon pump cannulation. *Ann Thorac Surg* 40:241, 1985.

88. Hazelrigg SR, Auer JE, Seifert PE: Experience in 100 transthoracic balloon pumps. *Ann Thorac Surg* 54:528, 1992.

89. Mayer JH: Subclavian artery approach for insertion of intraaortic balloon. *J Thorac Cardiovasc Surg* 76:61, 1978.

90. LaMuraglia GM, Vlahakes GJ, Moncure AC, et al: The safety of intraaortic balloon pump catheter insertion through suprainguinal prosthetic vascular bypass grafts. *J Vasc Surg* 13:830, 1991.

91. Jacobs LE, Fraifeld M, Kotler MN, et al: Aortic dissection following intraaortic balloon insertion: Recognition by transesophageal echocardiography. *Am Heart J* 124:536, 1992.

92. Biddle TL, Stewart S, Stuard ID: Dissection of the aorta complicating aortic balloon counterpulsation. *Am Heart J* 92:781, 1976.

93. Isner JM, Cohen SR, Virmani R, et al: Complications of the intraaortic balloon counterpulsation device: Clinical and morphologic observations in 54 necropsy patients. *Am J Cardiol* 45:260, 1980.

94. Goldman BS, Hill TJ, Rosenthal GA, et al: Complications associated with use of the intra-aortic balloon pump. *Can J Surg* 25:153, 1982.

95. Felix WR Jr, Barsamian E, Silverman AB: Long-term follow-up of limbs after use of intraaortic balloon counterpulsation device. *Surgery* 91:183, 1982.

96. Karlson KB, Martin EC, Bregman D, et al: Superior mesenteric artery obstruction by intraaortic counterpulsation balloon simulating embolism: A case report. *Cardiovasc Intervent Radiol* 4:236, 1981.

97. Lazar JM, Ziady GM, Dummer SJ, et al: Outcome and complications of prolonged intraaortic balloon counterpulsation in cardiac patients. *Am J Cardiol* 69:955, 1992.

98. Jarmolowski CR, Poirier RL: Small bowel infarction complicating intra-aortic balloon counterpulsation via the ascending aorta. *J Thorac Cardiovasc Surg* 79:735, 1980.

99. Baciewicz FA Jr, Kaplan BM, Murphy TE, et al: Bilateral renal artery thrombotic occlusion: A unique complication following removal of a transthoracic intraaortic balloon. *Ann Thorac Surg* 33:631, 1982.

100. Harris RE, Reimer KA, Crain BJ, et al: Spinal cord infarction following intraaortic balloon support. *Ann Thorac Surg* 42:206, 1986.

101. Scott IR, Goiti JJ: Late paraplegia as a consequence of intraaortic balloon pump support: A case report. *Ann Thorac Surg* 40:300, 1985.

102. Millham FH, Hudson HM, Woodson J, et al: Intraaortic balloon pump entrapment. *Ann Vasc Surg* 5:381, 1991.

103. Schechter D, Murali S, Uretsky BF, et al: Case reports: Vascular entrapment of intra-aortic balloon after short-term balloon counterpulsation. *Cathet Cardiovasc Diagn* 22:174, 1991.

104. Rohrer MJ, Sullivan CA, McLaughlin DJ, et al: A prospective randomized comparison of surgical and percutaneous intraaortic balloon pump removal. *J Thorac Cardiovasc Surg* 103:569, 1992.

Acknowledgment: Thanks to Kevin Cotter, C.C.P., for assistance with the technical aspects of the manuscript.

10. Temporary Mechanical Assistance of the Failing Left Ventricle

Robert A. Lancey and Okike N. Okike

Cardiovascular disease continues to be the leading cause of death in the United States, with approximately two-thirds of these fatalities attributed to left ventricular failure. Cardiogenic shock occurs in 15 percent of patients who reach the hospital after an acute myocardial infarction. Despite maximum medical support and use of an intraaortic balloon pump (IABP), only 15 percent of these patients will survive [1]. Likewise, of approximately 250,000 cardiac surgical procedures performed each year in the United States, 1 to 7 percent require placement of an IABP. Of these, only 65 percent will survive [2]. It is further estimated that 1 to 2 percent of patients undergoing cardiac surgery will fail attempts at weaning from cardiopulmonary bypass, even with IABP support.

The patient populations identified above, and those with progressive cardiac failure awaiting transplantation, constitute a population in whom placement of a ventricular assist device (VAD) is potentially lifesaving. These devices provide an improved means of support for a failing left ventricle and are often the only means of support to prevent progression to complete cardiac decompensation and death.

Pathophysiology of Left Ventricular Failure

To manage a patient with ventricular failure, a thorough understanding of cardiac physiology and pathophysiology is essential. Cardiac function in both the normal and failing states is best described by Starling's law, which identifies cardiac performance as directly proportional to ventricular preload in a pressure-volume relationship. As ventricular volume is increased (producing a concomitant rise in end-diastolic filling pressure) the resultant stroke volume also increases within a normal physiologic range. The ability of the ventricle to respond with an increase in stroke volume (and thus an increase in cardiac output) depends on the ability of the myocardial fibril to respond to stretching with an increased force of contraction.

When the myocardial fibril stretches beyond twice its normal length there is progressive loss of active tension and an increase in resting tension. This point is marked by a shift to the descending limb of Starling's curve. Progressive cardiac failure and a decline in cardiac output ensues, as further volume loading simply produces a greater rise in left ventricular end-diastolic pressure and a decline in stroke volume. With profound myocardial ischemia or frank myocardial infarction, Starling's curve shifts downward and to the right, representing a progressive decline in myocardial contractility.

This model of progressive loss of ventricular power may begin with an imbalance between myocardial oxygen supply and demand. A reduction in high-energy phosphate stores in the myocardium results in a decline in velocity and extent of myocardial fibril shortening (depressed contractility) as well as an increase in ventricular wall tension. With rising wall tension, oxygen demand is increased, while at the same time supply is decreased to the subendocardium. Progressive deterioration of left ventricular performance ultimately results in inadequate body tissue perfusion, accompanying acidosis, and eventual end-organ dysfunction. Left ventricular failure specifically results in pulmonary congestion and hypoxemia, compounding the insult to tissue perfusion.

Treatment of this progressive loss of ventricular power is aimed at reducing myocardial oxygen demand, augmenting myocardial oxygen supply, and improving ventricular performance. Inotropic agents can increase cardiac contractile function; however, this therapy is at the expense of an increase in myocardial oxygen demand and may hasten the progression of ischemia. Better treatment is provided by an IABP, which not only increases myocardial perfusion but also reduces left ventricular afterload and left ventricular wall tension [3]. For patients with postcardiotomy cardiogenic shock (2–6% of those undergoing coronary revascularization or valvular heart operations) [4], a similar pattern may ensue. Aggressive pharmacologic support with inotropic agents and prompt use of an IABP can lead to successful weaning from cardiopulmonary bypass in 75 to 85 percent of these patients, but in 1 percent of patients undergoing cardiac operation a mechanical VAD may be indicated [4].

In experimental studies, left heart bypass has been shown to reduce infarct size [5–9] and decrease myocardial oxygen consumption and ventricular workload [8,9]. Left ventricular bypass devices have also been found to be more effective than IABP in reducing myocardial oxygen consumption [10] and more effective than a combination of IABP and pharmacologic inotropic support in preserving myocardial structure and function in an experimental model [11].

Left VADs function by diverting blood flow away from the left ventricle (usually with a cannula placed in the left atrium or left ventricle) and pumping blood back beyond the left ventricle (most commonly into the aorta). By reducing the workload of the heart, the VAD allows a period of recuperation and metabolic recovery for ischemic myocytes. "Resting" the ventricle allows high-energy phosphate stores to be repleted in the setting of profound ischemia and promotes salvage of myocardium bordering the infarct zone during infarction.

An equally important goal in the use of assist devices is to attain a level of perfusion pressure and cardiac output necessary for adequate end-organ perfusion. Thus, tissue perfusion is maintained while myocardial reparative processes occur as myocardial work is minimized.

Historical Perspective

All types of cardiopulmonary bypass are based on the pioneering work of Gibbon, who developed extracorporeal circulation and was the first to apply it clinically, in 1953. With the growth of cardiac surgery, the concept of prolonged ventricular assistance for postcardiac surgical ventricular failure arose. Liotta was the first to use a left VAD clinically [12]. Roller pumps were used initially [13,14] but were replaced over time by centrifugal pumps, which provided longer periods of support without the embolic and hemolytic consequences of roller pumps. Before 1985, most assist devices were used for postcardiotomy cardiogenic shock. Since then, attention has also focused on those with acute myocardial infarction and cardiogenic shock and as a means for bridging to cardiac transplantation [15].

Recent years have been characterized by tremendous growth in research and technological development in the field of cardiac assist devices. Nonpulsatile devices used as a part of cardiopulmonary bypass circuits in the operating room have been modified and have found widespread application in the postoperative setting. Pulsatile devices with valves and pneumatic or electrical power sources have been designed and used under guidelines established by the Food and Drug Administration (FDA). As long-term support is becoming more widespread (with an increased emphasis on bridging to transplantation) devices capable of implantation have gained popularity.

The future will likely see expansion of the use of VADs. Improvements in management and understanding of their role following cardiac surgery along with success in bridging patients to transplantation may make these devices valuable not only clinically but also economically [16]. The expanding use of percutaneous transluminal coronary angioplasty (PTCA) and improvements in emergency medical service systems provide settings in which greater use of assist devices may be necessary for acute myocardial infarction and cardiogenic shock.

Features of Ventricular Assist Devices

A wide range of VADs and systems has been developed, some more compatible in certain clinical situations than in others (Table 10-1). Ventricular assist devices may vary in location in relation to the patient, pumping mechanism used, and expected time course of support and may be classified as short-term, intermediate-term, or long-term. Short-term VADS are used to allow for tissue perfusion in a setting of acute myocardial infarction or cardiogenic shock. Intermediate-term VADS are used most commonly following cardiac surgery, either in the operating room for a patient who cannot be separated from cardiopulmonary bypass or in the intensive care unit for progressive low cardiac output syndrome in the first 24 to 48 hours after surgery. Long-term VADS are primarily for bridging to transplantation.

Most VADS are tethered, requiring the patient to be connected to an external component at all times by wires or tubes through the skin. These devices are either extracorporeal, with the pumping mechanism set apart from the body, or paracorporeal, in which the pumping mechanism is in contact with the

Table 10-1. Spectrum of Mechanical Ventricular Assistance

Intraaortic balloon pump (IABP)
Extracorporeal membrane oxygenators (ECMO)
Ventricular assist devices (VAD)
Ventricular assist systems (VAS)
Total artificial hearts (TAH)

Table 10-2. Ventricular Assist Device Pumping Mechanisms

Roller pump
Centrifugal pump
Rotary pump
Pneumatic pulsatile pump
Electrical pulsatile pump

Table 10-3. Ventricular Assist Devices

Short-term	Intermediate-term	Long-term
Bard ECMO	Centrifugal pumps	Novacor LVAS
Datascope ECMO	Bio-medicus	TCI Heart-mate
Hemopump	Sarns	
Roller pumps	Pierce-Donachy Thoratec*	
	Symbion AVAD*	
	Abiomed BVS System 5000*	

*May also be used long-term.

patient. With implantable VADs, the patient is able to ambulate. Power is provided by a battery pack with wires connected to the pumping mechanism or is transduced using a transcutaneous energy transmission system (TETS). Implantable devices are more common in the setting of bridging to transplantation.

A variety of pumps can be used for VADs (Table 10-2). Roller pumps were initially used, and recent data demonstrate acceptable patient survival rates when they are used for up to 48 hours [7]. Besides being associated with hemolysis and embolization during prolonged use, these pumps are able to provide only a limited amount of flow (no greater than 3 liters/min) [17]. Centrifugal pumps are more common. Originally there was concern about pump-induced damage to blood components, but animal studies on long-term use have not supported this concern [18]. These pumps provide nonpulsatile flow and are available in two types: Biopumps (Bio-medicus, Eden Prairie, MT), which use a vortex mechanism to provide flow [19–23], and Sarns pumps (Sarns/3M, Ann Arbor, MI), which use impeller blades [24]. Devices using other means of pumping have been designed specifically for ventricular assistance. The Hemopump (Johnson & Johnson, Warren, NJ) uses a rotary pump and others use pneumatic or electrical mechanisms. The latter two methods provide pulsatile blood flow from the VAD. Retrospective analysis comparing nonpulsatile and pulsatile modes in terms of ability to wean from VADs and survival rates has shown no significant statistical difference [25]. This may be due, in part, to the fact that nonpulsatile VADs are used almost exclusively with an IABP, thereby providing some degree of pulsatile flow to the system.

Pulsatile flow systems vary in their mode of function. Asynchronous systems pump at a fixed rate whereas synchronous systems pump in coordination with native ventricular contraction. Although synchronous pumping theoretically results in better decompression of the native ventricle, the intrinsic heart rate is often too fast and irregular for optimal filling [26].

Types of Ventricular Assist Devices

There is a wide variety of VADs, each with specific design features. A thorough discussion of the specifications of each device (e.g., maximal flow rate, cannulation technique, complications) is well beyond the scope of this chapter. The general features of the devices currently in use are outlined below (Table 10-3).

The Hemopump, developed in the late 1980s, is for short-term use. It consists of a rotary pump contained in a narrow 7-mm chamber on the end of a catheter [27,28,29]. This high-speed pump provides for axial flow up to 3.5 to 4.0 liters per minute. It is inserted through a graft sewn onto the common femoral artery and is placed with its tip in the left ventricle. Blood is drawn from the ventricle and ejected into the aorta. This provides nonpulsatile flow over a short period of time and is perhaps most useful in a setting of acute hemodynamic deterioration from cardiogenic shock.

Nonpulsatile flow using a centrifugal pump is a common form of ventricular assistance [20–25,30]. This device is tethered to the patient and placed in an extracorporeal position. Vortex pumps (Biomedicus) and impeller pumps (Sarns) have been used and may provide assistance for the left ventricle, the right ventricle, or both. When used as a left VAD, blood is pumped from the left atrium to the aorta. Standard cardiopulmonary bypass cannulas are often used. Although they were originally used for intermediate-term assistance, Bolman et al. described use of the Biopump as a bridge to transplantation [19]. Ambulation is impractical, as the cannulas are held in place by purse string sutures and could become dislodged.

The Abiomed B.V.S. System 5000 (Abiomed Cardiovascular, Danvers, MA) is another extracorporeal assist device that may function for left, right, or biventricular assistance. This is a polyurethane, pneumatically driven pump with trileaflet valves. The atrial chambers are gravity-filled from the patient's atrium, and blood is pumped back into the aorta through a Dacron graft for left ventricular assistance. Good results have been obtained with this device after cardiotomy [12], and it has been used successfully as a bridge to cardiac transplantation [31].

Another device designed for intermediate-term use that has subsequently found more widespread use than the Biopump and the Abiomed as a bridge to transplantation is the Pierce-Donachy Thoratec VAD (Thoratec Laboratories, Berkeley, CA) [32,33]. It is a pneumatically driven polyurethane pump with mechanical valves for pulsatile flow and is tethered in a paracorporeal position on the abdominal wall. Cannulas penetrate the chest wall and connect to the left atrium or left ventricle and to the aorta, the latter via a Dacron graft. These devices may also be used for right ventricular or biventricular assistance. The flow is timed either synchronously or asynchronously.

The Symbion Acute Ventricular Assist Device (AVAD) (Symbion, Tempe, AZ) is a pneumatically driven paracorporeal assist device that may be used for either or both ventricles. It uses mechanical valves and by virtue of its design allows patient ambulation. It, too, has seen use in bridging to transplantation [26].

Left ventricular assist systems (LVAS) are fully implantable devices used almost exclusively long-term as a bridge to transplantation. The Novacor LVAS (Baxter Healthcare, Oakland, CA) has an electrically driven pulsatile device that uses biologic valves. Power is provided via wires from a battery belt worn on the outside to the device, which is placed in the abdominal cavity. Dacron grafts are used to connect the system to the aorta and left ventricle. This device serves only for left ventricular support [34]. The TCI Heart-mate (Thermo Cardiosystems, Woburn, MA) is an implantable pulsatile pump that is positioned in the abdomen or within the abdominal wall and is connected to an external power source through a percutaneous lead [35,36]. It uses porcine xenograft valves and is connected to the left ventricular apex via a Dacron graft sewing ring. Minimal antithrombotic therapy is needed, as contact surfaces are impregnated with microspheres to promote formation of a biologic lining.

Table 10-4. Criteria for Left Ventricular Assist Device Insertion

Hemodynamic parameters
    Cardiac index < 1.8 L/m^2/min
    Mean arterial pressure < 60 mm Hg
    Left atrial pressure > 20 mm Hg
    Urine output < 20 ml/hr
    Systemic vascular resistance > 2100 dyne/sec/cm^{-5}
No correctable surgical lesions
Metabolic abnormalities absent
Maximal inotropic support
Optimal preload
Use of intraaortic balloon pump

Indications for Use

Left ventricular assistance may be necessary either acutely or chronically. In an acute setting the device is often used to assist a patient failing to wean from cardiopulmonary bypass after cardiac surgery. Patients may acutely develop left ventricular failure with cardiogenic shock secondary to myocardial ischemia or infarction in the cardiac catherization laboratory, coronary care unit, or emergency room [37,38,39]. Criteria have evolved for patient selection (Table 10-4). Norman et al. defined cardiogenic shock in terms of hemodynamic parameters [40], which have since been modified and adapted for defining patients requiring mechanical VAD support. The accepted criteria include a cardiac index of less than 1.8 L/m^2/min, mean arterial pressure of less than 60 mm Hg, left atrial pressure or right atrial pressure greater than 20 mm Hg, urine output less than 20 ml/hr, and systemic vascular resistance greater than 2100 dyne/sec/cm^{-5} [15,21,41]. When these conditions exist for more than a few hours, there is less than a 15 percent chance of survival [40]. In addition to the hemodynamic criteria, neither surgically correctable lesions nor metabolic abnormalities should be present. Preload must be maximized and an IABP placed. Maximal inotropic support should be provided, although the degree and nature of this has not been standardized. In fact, the attempt to produce "adequate" blood pressure, systemic vascular resistance, and cardiac index with the use of inotropes may inflict harm on the already ischemic myocardium.

Numerous studies have emphasized the need for early decision making in VAD placement, and early institution of ventricular support has been identified as an important prognostic factor for success in weaning from ventricular assistance [42]. McGovern noted no survivors if the device was placed after four or more attempts at weaning from cardiopulmonary bypass following unsuccessful cardiac surgery [43]. In general, it is thought that ventricular assistance should be instituted within 1 hour of conclusion of the cardiac surgical procedure [1].

When a VAD is inserted, it is assumed that the heart will recover to a degree that will allow removal of the device. During unsuccessful attempts at weaning from cardiopulmonary bypass, it is often quite difficult to determine whether frank infarction has occurred or myocardial stunning is present. Ventricular assist devices will not rescue infarcted myocardium but may provide optimal conditions in which stunned myocardium may recover. Perioperative infarct is thus a poor prognostic factor for survival, as most patients with extensive myocardial necrosis do not survive even with VAD support [15].

Stunning as a state of reversal of myocardial dysfunction secondary to a postischemic period was first proposed by Braunwald and Kloner [44]. During initial perfusion of ischemic myocardium, cellular and metabolic abnormalities may exist which produce impaired left ventricular function [45,46]. Such stunned myocardium often requires several days before base-

line function is regained. Ellis et al. have shown that acute coronary artery occlusion for just 15 minutes can lead to detectable functional and metabolic derangements lasting up to a week [46]. Unfortunately, no definitive method of determining the presence and degree of myocardial infarction in the immediate postcardiotomy setting has been developed. Transesophageal echocardiography may assist in identifying wall motion abnormalities, but they may occur transiently as a result of ischemia. Myocardial biopsy is obviously more definitive but is neither feasible nor practical in the acute setting.

The use of VADs, and more specifically left ventricular assist systems, as bridges to transplantation is growing rapidly. They are meant to provide essentially "permanent" support until a donor heart is available.

Contraindications to Use

Whereas indications for placement of a VAD are clearly defined, contraindications are still evolving. Massive myocardial infarction is obviously a contraindication, but this condition may not be obvious in the immediate postoperative period. Most published contraindications [15,41] are relative (Table 10-5).

Sepsis may be an appropriate reason to avoid VAD placement, yet infections responding to antibiotic therapy should not absolutely preclude mechanical ventricular support. Because of the need to anticoagulate patients with VADs, those with bleeding disorders or active bleeding (as from the gastrointestinal tract or in the central nervous system) should be excluded as candidates for support. Bleeding remains the most common complication and is a poor prognostic factor for survival.

The presence of a chronic debilitating disease would also serve as a contraindication to VAD placement. Metastatic cancer should preclude VAD insertion, and severe pulmonary hypertension secondary to underlying pulmonary disease, severe peripheral vascular disease, and neurologic impairment are all relative contraindications. The presence of chronic renal failure has served as a deterrent to VAD placement in the past, as has severe hepatic failure, because of the potential for significant bleeding.

Single-organ dysfunction should not preclude placement of a VAD. If organ dysfunction, rather than irreversible failure, is present, VAD support can ultimately improve organ function [47].

Advanced age is felt by many to represent a relative contraindication to VAD placement. The exact age above which VAD placement is absolutely contraindicated has not been generally accepted, as the patient's general condition prior to left ventric-

Table 10-5. Contraindications to Left Ventricular Assist
Device Use

Massive myocardial infarction
Sepsis
Metastatic malignancy
Bleeding disorder
Active bleeding (gastrointestinal, central nervous system)
Severe pulmonary hypertension
Severe hepatic failure
Chronic renal failure
Severe peripheral vascular disease
Neurologic impairment

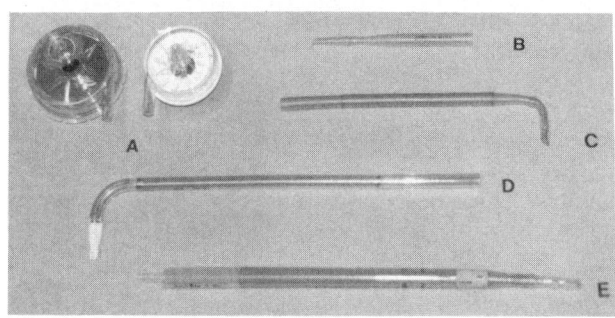

Fig. 10-1. Equipment for ventricular assist devices. A. Centrifugal
pumps. B. Cannula for main pulmonary artery (RVAD inflow). C.
Cannula for aorta (LVAD inflow). D. Cannula for left atrium (LVAD
outflow). E. Cannula for right atrium (RVAD outflow).

ular failure must also be considered. Retrospective analysis of
prognostic factors has shown poor survival (13%) in patients
older than 70 years of age [48]. Others have identified age
greater than 65 as a poor prognostic factor for VAD placement
[41,42]. At the other end of the age spectrum, survival rates in
children supported with VADs after cardiac surgery have been
greater than in adults [49].

Techniques of Placement
(Figures 10-1 and 10-2)

For most types of mechanical ventricular assistance, cannulation is performed through a median sternotomy. The Hemopump, a short-term assist device, is placed in the common
femoral artery through a graft sewn onto the artery. Technical
difficulties with this device have centered on problems with
insertion and kinking of the catheter at the insertion site [29].

In the common setting for VAD placement (in the operating
room after unsuccessful attempts to wean from cardiopulmonary bypass), placement of an intermediate-term VAD may be
performed expeditiously. A patent foramen ovale should be
sought and closed, since unloading the left atrium with the VAD
may result in shunting across the patent foramen ovale and
subsequent cyanosis. Centrifugal pumping systems generally
use standard cardiopulmonary bypass cannulas for both inflow
and outflow. Purse string sutures with Teflon pledgets passed
through rubber tourniquets help secure cannulas in the left
atrium and aorta [20]. Left atrial drainage is performed with a
cannula placed through the right superior pulmonary vein, roof
of the atrium, or left atrial appendage. Restriction of venous
return at the time of cannulation helps raise the left atrial pressure and prevents air embolization. These cannulation sites
serve as sources of troublesome bleeding in the postoperative
period; therefore care should be taken to protect against and
identify bleeding from around the cannulas. Whereas centrifugal and roller pumps use standard cardiopulmonary bypass
cannulas and tubing, paracorporeal and implantable VADs are
often connected to the aorta with a Dacron graft and to the left
ventricular apex with similar material using a sewing ring.

Controversy exists as to the efficacy of left ventricular unloading using left atrial cannulation versus left ventricular cannulation. The advantages of left atrial cannulation include relative technical simplicity as well as a notable reduction in inflow
obstruction [1]. In clinical settings, left atrial cannulation has
been shown to be associated with better survival rates than left
ventricular cannulation [15]. Left ventricular function is preserved by avoiding injury to the apex, whereas potential loss
of future function may accompany left ventricular cannulation
[1].

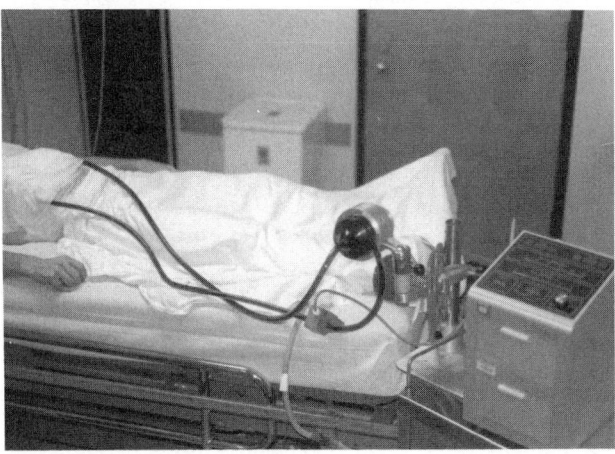

Fig. 10-2. Left ventricular assist device with console, centrifugal
pumps, and tubing.

Left ventricular cannulation, however, provides greater flow
rates (in the range of 5.5–6.5 liters/min) than does left atrial
cannulation (4.0–4.5 liters/min) [32]. Animal studies have demonstrated better decompression of the left ventricle and greater
reduction in myocardial infarct size with left ventricular cannulation compared with left atrial cannulation [9,15,50]. Pulsatile pumps seem to fill better with left ventricular cannulation
than with left atrial cannulation, probably due to the difference
between active filling (from left ventricular contraction) versus
passive filling from the left atrium [15]. In a nondilated heart
following cardiac surgery, left ventricular cannulation may be
more difficult. In addition, the goal in this setting is maximal
recovery of left ventricular function. Thus, left atrial cannulation
seems a logical choice for assisting the postcardiotomy stunned
myocardium. In the setting of bridging to transplantation with
a possibly dilated left ventricle, since the left ventricle will be
sacrificed when a transplant is available, left ventricular cannulation appears to be a more logical choice.

One further technical point involves positioning of the cannulas in relation to the chest wall. Although compression of
bypass grafts is a concern, it is rarely a problem. To minimize
infection, the cannulas should penetrate through the chest wall
and not out the sternotomy wound. Every attempt should be
made to approximate the skin over the mediastinum and to

close the sternum itself. Care should be taken to avoid compromising flow within the cannulas to achieve this goal.

Management of Assist Devices

Once a VAD has been inserted, careful surveillance in the intensive care unit is required. Close monitoring of hemodynamic parameters, fluid and blood product intake, and urine output and blood loss is mandatory. Hemodynamic parameters to maintain include a mean arterial blood pressure of between 65 to 80 mm Hg, right and left atrial pressures in the range of 5 to 15 mm Hg (often by adjustments in volume), a cardiac index of 2.2 to 3.0 L/m²/min, and mixed venous saturation of 65 to 70 percent [15] (Table 10-6). If biventricular assistance is used, left ventricular flow should exceed right ventricular flow by 500 to 1000 ml because of return of bronchial flow to the left ventricle [15].

Pharmacologic inotropic support should be minimized as much as possible. In a setting of left ventricular assistance, its major purpose would be to support function of the right ventricle. Usually only dopamine (1–3 μg/kg/min) is necessary, primarily to improve renal flow. Often peripheral vasomotor tone must be controlled, using vasodilators (e.g., sodium nitroprusside) or vasopressors (e.g., phenylephrine, norepinephrine). Drugs that vasodilate the pulmonary vasculature (isoproterenol, prostaglandin E₁) may also be necessary, should signs of right ventricular failure develop.

Given the thrombogenicity of device contact surfaces, anticoagulation is often necessary during mechanical ventricular assistance. The necessity for and degree of anticoagulation depends on the device used. For short-term control, heparin and dextran are commonly chosen. Aspirin, dipyridamole and warfarin are used for longer-term placement, in particular for ventricular assist systems. Frequent monitoring of the activated clotting time (ACT) is required immediately after placement, and the degree of anticoagulation must be strictly controlled, as bleeding remains one of the most common complications and worse prognostic factors for survival in VAD use.

The VAD apparatus itself must be secured next to or on the patient (extracorporeal or paracorporeal). The tubings and their connections must remain secured tightly to each other and to the patient and remain without kinks.

Dressings must be changed under sterile conditions at least twice daily at the sites where the cannulas enter the body. Nutritional needs must be addressed early in the postoperative course. Special attention must be paid to skin care, especially for patients with extracorporeal devices who are limited in movement. Decubitus ulcers may develop rapidly; therefore, frequent turning or use of specialized support beds is essential. In addition, psychological needs of the patient and family involving anxiety about the device and fear of death must be addressed.

Adequate care of a patient with a VAD requires a team of physicians, nurses, and perfusionists familiar with the device and the possible complications.

Table 10-6. Left Ventricular Assist Device Maintenance Parameters

Mean arterial pressure	65–80 mm Hg
Left and right arterial pressure	5–15 mm Hg
Cardiac index	2.2–3.0 L/m²/min
Mixed venous oxygen saturation	65–70%

Weaning

The ultimate goal of ventricular assistance is removal of the device after ventricular recovery. Hemodynamic parameters are assessed and used in the decision-making process. Transesophageal echocardiography and radionuclide angiography have also been used to assist in weaning.

Timing of VAD removal is critical. In the postcardiotomy setting, the device is placed to allow time for replenishment of high-energy phosphates and adenine nucleotides and resolution of myocardial edema that accompanies cardiopulmonary bypass [1]. Attempts to wean from mechanical ventricular support in less than 24 hours usually fail [43]. In 90 percent of survivors, ventricular support is discontinued within a week [25]. If failure to wean persists beyond 10 days, transplantation should be considered [15]. Retrospective analyses of large groups of patients on ventricular assistance postcardiotomy show that an average of 4 days of support is necessary [25]. If no significant improvement in left ventricular function can be identified within 72 hours as assessed by transesophageal echocardiography, the chances of weaning are severely reduced [51].

Initial assessment of suitability for VAD removal usually begins 24 hours after insertion. Hemodynamic parameters are measured with the VAD on and repeated with the flow turned down. Flow is decreased (to no less than 1 liter/min) until the left atrial pressure rises to 20 to 25 mm Hg while monitoring the arterial pressure waveform for evidence of left ventricular ejection. If none is present, full support is reinstituted. If there is evidence of recovery, transesophageal echocardiography is performed to evaluate left ventricular function more precisely. Along with monitoring left atrial pressure as the flow is decreased, the change in right atrial pressure, pulmonary arterial pressures, mean arterial blood pressure, and cardiac index is observed. Removal of the device is frequently successful when (at low flow) right and left atrial pressures are less than 20 mm Hg, mean arterial blood pressure is maintained at greater than 70 mm Hg, and the cardiac index is greater than 2.2 liters/min/m².

It should be emphasized that during weaning, ventricular support must never be discontinued totally. When flow is reduced it should be to a minimum of 1 liter/min. With reduction of flow during weaning efforts, anticoagulation must be increased. It is recommended that at 1 liter/min the ACT should be maintained at greater than 180 seconds, and the flow rate at this level should not be maintained for more than 2 minutes [20].

In recent years, transesophageal echocardiography (TEE) has been used more frequently to assess the feasibility of VAD removal. An ejection fraction greater then 30 percent has been found to be a reliable indicator of successful weaning [15]. Transesophageal echocardiography has also been useful in identifying intrapericardial clots compromising left ventricular function and intracavitary thrombi [51]. At times, TEE is performed with injections of epinephrine or dobutamine to assess myocardial viability in severely hypokinetic segments [51]. In addition to assessing ejection fraction and identifying evidence of tamponade, TEE may help to locate cannula position in the left atrium to maximize unloading of the left ventricle [52]. Radionuclide angiography has also been used to determine ejection fraction as an adjunct to hemodynamic parameters to assess ability to wean [15,53].

The most significant predictors of successful weaning are adequate mean arterial pressure and cardiac index, acceptable mixed venous oxygen saturation, improved ejection fraction, and normal left atrial pressure [54]. Early signs of patients who will be weaned successfully include those requiring less than

75 hours of ventricular support, some degree of left ventricular recovery within 24 hours, mild or absent right ventricular failure, and no evidence of postoperative myocardial infarction by ECG [43] (Table 10-7). Patients who are weaned at the appropriate time and who attain adequate hemodynamic parameters have a 70 percent chance of survival [54].

Complications

Despite appropriate placement of VADs and meticulous management, numerous complications may occur. These are classified into patient-related and device-related complications (Table 10-8).

Bleeding is the most common patient-related complication, occurring in up to 83 percent of those requiring ventricular assistance [20,33], and is especially common following reoperative cardiac procedures [22]. Causes include thrombocytopenia, which occurs primarily in the first several days [15], platelet dysfunction, and hypofibrinogenemia. During VAD use, there appears to be increased fibrin degradation for the first 3 days [15]. Anticoagluation, both at the time of surgery and during ventricular assistance, contributes to excessive bleeding. Surgical bleeding is common and requires aggressive repair. Early institution of ventricular support has been found to carry fewer subsequent bleeding problems [15]. Heparin administered during cardiopulmonary bypass should be reversed with protamine and clotting allowed to normalize before institution of a heparin infusion in the intensive care unit. An adequate hemoglobin level must be maintained to optimize oxygen delivery, and transfusion of platelets is indicated if the platelet count is less than 100,000 [55]. If surgical bleeding is suspected, early exploration is mandatory. The application of fibrin glue at the site of cannulation at the time of cannula insertion or during subsequent exploration may prove useful. Failure to control bleeding within the first 24 hours or the presence of bleeding at the time of weaning portends a poor chance of survival [41]. In addition to the hemodynamic compromise and potential deleterious effects on oxygen delivery that accompany massive bleeding, multiple transfusions in these patients are associated with adult respiratory distress syndrome (ARDS) and multiple organ failure [15,56].

Infection is also a frequent patient-related complication and portends poor survival. The incidence is often related to the duration of support, occurring infrequently if support lasts less than a week [15] but in as many as 70 percent of patients who are supported for up to 3 weeks [56]. Contributing causes include multiple blood transfusions, the presence of numerous invasive catheters, including pulmonary artery catheters and IABPs, tissue edema, and exploration for bleeding. Device-related infection must be aggressively treated but does not require removal of the device. Appropriate antibiotic therapy is undertaken, and patients with this problem have been weaned or bridged to transplantation successfully. Prevention of infection entails control of bleeding and removal of invasive catheters as expeditiously as possible. Frequent dressing changes at cannulation sites as well as routine surveillance cultures, including fungal titers [56], may also help prevent serious infections. Prophylactic antibiotics are administered, most commonly a cephalosporin for the first 3 days the device is in place, along with an aminoglycoside if the patient has been in the hospital more than 5 days before insertion [56].

Patients on VADs are prone to strokes, from both inadequate cerebral blood flow and thromboemboli. Pulmonary insufficiency may occur in up to 60 percent [57], usually related to volume overload, pulmonary edema secondary to multiple

Table 10-7. Left Ventricular Assist Device Weaning: Early Signs of Potential Success

< 75 hours of pump support
No evidence of postoperative myocardial infarction by ECG
Some left ventricular recovery by 24 hours
Right ventricular failure mild or absent
Control of bleeding
Maintenance of renal function

Table 10-8. Complications of Ventricular Assist Devices

Patient-related	Device-related
Bleeding	Thromboembolism
Infection	Hemolysis
Ventricular arrhythmias	Device failure
Stroke	Device infection
Respiratory failure	Right ventricular failure
Renal failure	

blood transfusions, or a prolonged period of cardiopulmonary bypass, pneumonia, or ARDS. Renal failure likewise may occur in up to 60 percent [57], caused by low flow before and after insertion of the device, extended time on cardiopulmonary bypass, and multiple blood transfusions [15]. Renal failure is an important prognostic factor [56], usually associated with a poor outcome. It may be progressive and unresponsive to therapy [15] and is perhaps best treated by continuous arterial-venous hemofiltration (CAVH), with or without dialysis, at the time the device is inserted. CAVH is effective in treating hypervolemia and acute renal failure in this patient population [56,58].

Ventricular arrhythmias may complicate therapy in the VAD patient. Often transient, there is no significant difference in their occurrence before or during support with a VAD between survivors and nonsurvivors [59]. If severe and potentially lethal arrhythmias are present and persistent, bilateral ventricular assistance may be required [32].

Device-related complications are also numerous. Thromboembolism is inherent to the use of mechanical ventricular assistance, as the foreign surfaces all possess some degree of thrombogenicity [21,48,60,61,62]. The incidence has been found to be related to the length of support, usually not occurring before day 4 [63]. Anticoagulation should be instituted when coagulation parameters have returned to normal following cardiopulmonary bypass and bleeding has been brought under control (less than 100 ml/min) [55]. Attempts to lower the incidence of thromboembolism have centered on the contact surfaces themselves. Textured surfaces have been developed (e.g., lining tubes with microspheres) to enhance the formation of a neointimal lining [64]. The use of heparin-coated tubing has been studied but results have been mixed [65,66]. Thromboembolism must also raise suspicion of a patent foramen ovale with a paradoxical embolus.

Hemolysis occurs to a certain degree with most VADS but is rarely a major problem. Device failure also may occur but is quite rare. Failure may be due to fractured valves, split tubings, or drive unit failures. Cannula obstruction may present as low cardiac output.

Right ventricular failure occurring after placement of a left VAD is common, with an incidence of up to 50 percent [15]. It is a common cause of mortality in patients originally requiring only a left VAD [67,68], but the etiology is unclear. Possible mechanisms include impairment of interventricular septal function [69] due to septal ischemia [70] and progressive elevation of pulmonary vascular resistance due to complement-mediated polymorphonuclear leukocyte activation and stasis in pulmonary capillaries [56,71,72]. However, not all investigators have found evidence for left VAD-induced right ventricular failure [73]. Although some surgeons routinely employ biventricular assistance to avoid right heart failure [26], this practice is not universally adopted.

Prognostic Factors

A number of prognostic factors have been identified during use of VADs. Improved survival is associated with operator experience, use of biventricular assist devices, early institution of ventricular assistance, absence of perioperative myocardial infarction and/or right ventricular failure, and evidence of left ventricular recovery within 24 hours [20,60]. Conversely, factors associated with a poor outcome include patients who arrived in the operating room in full cardiac arrest or cardiogenic shock, cardiopulmonary bypass of greater than 7 hours' duration, biventricular failure, excessive bleeding during cardiopulmonary bypass, age greater than 65 years, and an unsuccessful or incomplete operation [41,42].

Overall Results

The American Society for Artificial and Internal Organs (ASAIO) and the International Society for Heart Transplantation (ISHT) developed a database on the clinical application of VADs in 1985. The most recent report from this voluntary registry presents data from contributing centers up to December 31, 1990 [25]. Data were collected on 965 patients supported with a VAD for postcardiotomy cardiogenic shock and 544 patients who were bridged to transplantation. In the postcardiotomy group, 45 percent were weaned successfully from their VAD and 25 percent were discharged from the hospital. Of those bridged to transplantation, 70 percent eventually underwent transplantation and 66 percent of those initially supported with a VAD or ventricular assist system were eventually discharged from the hospital.

Certain trends were identified in the postcardiotomy patients in cardiogenic shock. Although twice as many were supported with nonpulsatile centrifugal pumps versus pulsatile pumps, weaning and survival rates were equal for the two groups. Support times averaged 3 days for those on centrifugal pumps and 6 days for those on pneumatic pumps. Those requiring only univentricular support had better weaning and survival rates, but this is likely due to the severity of the underlying pathology compared to those requiring biventricular support. Of the 25 percent who were eventually discharged from the hospital (survivors), 86 percent were New York Heart Association functional class I or II [25]. Another study supports these data: two-thirds of survivors of VAD support felt they had returned to a normal life-style after discharge [74].

Although complications of mechanical ventricular systems were numerous and frequently multiple for each patient, patient characteristics (e.g., age greater than 70 years) had a greater effect on overall outcome. Complications associated with an inability to wean from VAD support included bleeding, disseminated intravascular coagulation, renal failure, biventricular failure, cyanosis secondary to a patent foramen ovale, inadequate cardiac output, and inlet cannulation obstruction pro-

ducing a low cardiac output. Once weaned from ventricular support, factors associated with lower survival included renal failure, perioperative myocardial infarction, and infection [25].

Patient dependence on the left VAD was rare, indicating improved patient selection. Insufficient ventricular recovery, while an identifiable cause of death, was not the cause of the majority of eventual mortalities. Multiple factors, such as stroke, multiple organ dysfunction syndrome, sepsis, or a combination of these, were implicated as causes of death [60].

Overall, results from the combined registry reflect not only acceptable rates of weaning and survival, but a gradual improvement in these numbers over time. Continued improvements in patient selection, technical expertise in placing VADs, and improved management of those with VADs will continue to make them viable, if not preferred, options for those with acute or progressive left ventricular decompensation.

References

1. Jorge E, Pae WE, Pierce WS: Left heart and biventricular bypass. *Crit Care Clin* 2:267, 1986.
2. Pennington DG, Swartz MT: Temporary circulatory support in patients with post-cardiotomy cardiogenic shock, in Spence PA, Chitwood WR (eds): *Cardiac Surgery: State of the Art Reviews.* Philadelphia, Hanley & Belfus, 1991, pp 373–392.
3. Mundth ED: Assisted circulation, in Sabiston DC, Spencer FC (eds): *Surgery of the Chest.* Philadelphia, WB Saunders, 1990, pp 1777–1799.
4. Pae WE, Miller CA, Matthews Y, et al: Ventricular assist devices for post-cardiotomy cardiogenic shock. *J Thorac Cardiovasc Surg* 104:541, 1992.
5. Catinella FP, Cunningham JN, Glassman E, et al: Left atrium-to-femoral artery bypass: Effectiveness in reduction of acute experimental myocardial infarction. *J Thorac Cardiovasc Surg* 86:887, 1983.
6. Laschinger JC, Cunningham JN, Catinella FP, et al: "Pulsatile" left atrial-femoral artery bypass. *Arch Surg* 118:965, 1983.
7. Rose DM, Grossi E, Laschinger JC, et al: Strategy for treatment of acute evolving myocardial infarction with pulsatile left heart assist device. *Crit Care Clin* 2:251, 1986.
8. Grossi EA, Laschinger JC, Cunningham IN, et al: Time course of myocardial salvage with left heart assist in evolving myocardial infarction. *Surg Forum* 35:322, 1984.
9. Pennock JL, Pae WE, Pierce WS, et al: Reduction of myocardial infarct size: Comparison between left atrial and left ventricular bypass. *Circulation* 59:275, 1979.
10. McDonnell MA, Kralior AC, Tsagarir TJ, et al: Comparative effect of counterpulsation and bypass on left ventricular myocardial oxygen consumption and dynamics before and after coronary occlusion. *Am Heart J* 97:78, 1979.
11. Mickleborough LL, Rebeyka I, Wilson GJ, et al: Comparison of left ventricular assist and intra-aortic balloon counterpulsation during early reperfusion after ischemic arrest of the heart. *J Thorac Cardiovasc Surg* 93:597, 1987.
12. Champseur G, Ninet J, Vigneron M, et al: Use of the Abiomed BVS System 5000 as a bridge to cardiac transplantation. *J Thorac Cardiovasc Surg* 100:122, 1990.
13. Spencer FC, Eisenman NG, Trinkle JK, et al: Assisted circulation for cardiac failure following intracardiac support with cardiopulmonary bypass. *J Thorac Cardiovasc Surg* 49:56, 1965.
14. DeBakey ME: Left ventricular bypass for cardiac assistance: Clinical experience. *Am J Cardiol* 27:3, 1971.
15. Pennington DG, Swartz MT: Current status of temporary circulatory support, in Karp RB, Kouchoukos N, Laks H, et al (eds): *Advances in Cardiac Surgery.* Chicago, Year Book, 1990, pp 177–197.
16. Poirier VL: Can our society afford mechanical hearts? *ASAIO Trans* 37:540, 1991.
17. Rose DM, Connolly M, Cunningham JN, et al: Technique and results with a roller pump left and right heart assist device. *Ann Thorac Surg* 47:124, 1989.

18. Taenaka Y, Inoue K, Masuzawa T, et al: Influence of an impeller centrifugal pump on blood components in chronic animal experiments. *ASAIO Journal* 38:M577, 1992.
19. Bolman RM, Cox JL, Marshall W, et al: Circulatory support with centrifugal pump as a bridge to cardiac transplantation. *Ann Thorac Surg* 47:108, 1989.
20. McGovern GJ: The Biopump and postoperative circulatory support. *Ann Thorac Surg* 54:245, 1993.
21. Hoy FB, Stables C, Gomez RC, et al: Prolonged ventricular support using a centrifugal pump. *Can J Surg* 32:342, 1989.
22. Killen DA, Piehler JM, Borkon AM, et al: Bio-Medicus ventricular assist device for salvage of cardiac surgical patients. *Ann Thorac Surg* 52:230, 1991.
23. Parks B, Liebler GA, Burkholder JA, et al: Mechanical support of the failing heart. *Ann Thorac Surg* 42:627, 1986.
24. Curtis JJ, Walls JT, Schmaltz R, et al: Experience with the Sarns centrifugal pump in postcardiotomy ventricular failure. *J Thorac Cardiovasc Surg* 104:554, 1992.
25. Pae WE: Ventricular assist devices and total artificial hearts: A combined registry experience. *Ann Thorac Surg* 55:295, 1993.
26. Lick SL, Copeland JG, Smith RG, et al: Use of the Symbion biventricular assist device in bridging to transplantation. *Ann Thorac Surg* 55:283, 1993.
27. Scholz KH, Tebbe U, Chemnitius M, et al: Transfemoral placement of the left ventricular assist device "Hemopump" during mechanical resuscitation. *J Thorac Cardiovasc Surg* 38:69, 1990.
28. Frazier OH, Wampler RK, Duncan JM, et al: First human use of the Hemopump, a catheter-mounted ventricular assist device. *Ann Thorac Surg* 49:299, 1990.
29. Frazier OH, Nakatani T, Duncan JM, et al: Clinical experience with the Hemopump. *ASAIO Trans* 35:604, 1989.
30. Drinkwater DC, Laks H: Clinical experience with centrifugal pump ventricular support at UCLA Medical Center. *ASAIO Trans* 34:505, 1988.
31. Kaan GL, Noyez L, Vincent JG, et al: Management of postcardiotomy cardiogenic shock with a new pulsatile ventricular assist device. *ASAIO Trans* 37:559, 1991.
32. Farrar DJ, Hill JD: Univentricular and biventricular Thoratec VAD support as a bridge to transplantation. *Ann Thorac Surg* 55:276, 1993.
33. Pennington DG, McBride LR, Swartz MT, et al: Use of the Pierce-Donachy ventricular assist device in patients with cardiogenic shock after cardiac operations. *Ann Thorac Surg* 47:130, 1989.
34. Portner PM, Oyer PE, Pennington DG, et al: Implantable electrical left ventricular assist system: Bridge to transplantation and the future. *Ann Thorac Surg* 47:142, 1989.
35. Frazier OH: Chronic left ventricular support with a vented electric assist device. *Ann Thorac Surg* 55:273, 1993.
36. McGee MG, Paynis SM, Nakatani T, et al: Extended clinical support with an implantable left ventricular assist device. *ASAIO Trans* 35:614, 1989.
37. Phillips SJ: Percutaneous cardiopulmonary bypass and innovations in clinical counterpulsation. *Crit Care Clin* 2:297, 1986.
38. Dembitsky WP, Moreno-Cabral RJ, Adamson RM, et al: Emergency resuscitation using portable extracorporeal membrane oxygenation. *Ann Thorac Surg* 55:304, 1993.
39. Moritz A, Wolner E: Circulatory support with shock due to acute myocardial infarction. *Ann Thorac Surg* 55:238, 1993.
40. Norman JC, Cooley DA, Igo SR, et al: Prognostic indices for survival during postcardiotomy intra-aortic balloon pumping. *J Thorac Cardiovasc Surg* 74:709, 1977.
41. Pennington DG: Circulatory support symposium: Patient selection. *Ann Thorac Surg* 47:77, 1989.
42. Emery RW, Joyce LD: Direction in cardiac assistance. *J Cardiovasc Surg* 6:400, 1991.
43. McGovern GJ: Circulatory support symposium: Weaning and bridging. *Ann Thorac Surg* 47:102, 1989.
44. Braunwald E, Kloner RA: The stunned myocardium: Prolonged, post-ischemic ventricular dysfunction. *Circulation* 66:1146, 1982.
45. Kloner RA, Ellis ST, Lange R, et al: Studies of experimental coronary artery reperfusion: effects on infarct size, myocardial function, biochemistry, ustrastructure and microvasculature damage. *Circulation* 68 (suppl 1):8, 1983.
46. Ellis SB, Henschke CI, Sandor T, et al: Time course of functional

and biochemical recovery of myocardium salvaged by reperfusion. *J Am Coll Cardiol* 11:1047, 1983.
47. Burnett CM, Duncan JM, Frazier OH, et al: Improved multiorgan function after prolonged univentricular support. *Ann Thorac Surg* 55:65, 1993.
48. Miller CA, Pae WE, Pierce WS: Combined registry for the clinical use of mechanical ventricular assist devices: Postcardiotomy cardiogenic shock. *Trans Am Soc Artif Intern Organs* 36:43, 1990.
49. Pennington DG, Swartz MT: Circulatory support in infants and children. *Ann Thorac Surg* 55:233, 1993.
50. Laks H, Hahn IW, Blair O, et al: Cardiac assistance and infarct size: Left atrial-to-aortic vs. left ventricular-to-aortic bypass. *Surg Forum* 27:226, 1976.
51. Barzilai B, Davila-Roman VG, Eaton MH, et al: Transesophageal echocardiography predicts successful withdrawal of ventricular assist devices. *J Thorac Cardiovasc Surg* 104:1410, 1992.
52. Nasu M, Okada Y, Fujiwara H, et al: Transesophageal echocardiography findings of intracardiac events during cardiac assist. *Artif Organs* 14:377, 1990.
53. Verani MS, Sekela ME, Mahmarian JJ, et al: Left ventricular function in patients with centrifugal left ventricular assist device. *ASAIO Trans* 35:544, 1989.
54. Termuhlen DF, Swartz MT, Ruzevich SA, et al: Hemodynamic predictors for weaning patients from ventricular assist devices (VADS). *J Biomater Appl* 4:374, 1990.
55. Copeland JG: Circulatory support symposium: Bleeding and anticoagulation. *Ann Thorac Surg* 47:88, 1989.
56. Pierce WS: Circulatory support symposium: Other postoperative complications. *Ann Thorac Surg* 47:96, 1989.
57. Zumbro GL, Kitchens WR, Shearer G, et al: Mechanical assistance for cardiogenic shock following cardiac surgery, myocardial infarction, and cardiac transplantation. *Ann Thorac Surg* 44:11, 1987.
58. Macris MP, Barcenas CG, Parnis SM, et al: Simplified method of hemofiltration in ventricular assist device patients. *ASAIO Trans* 34:708, 1988.
59. Moroney DA, Swartz MT, Reedy JE, et al: Importance of ventricular arrhythmias in recovery patients with ventricular assist devices. *ASAIO Trans* 37:M516, 1991.
60. Adamson RM, Dembitsky WP, Reichman RT, et al: Mechanical support: Assist or nemesis? *J Thorac Cardiovasc Surg* 98:915, 1989.
61. Kanter KR, Ruzevich SA, Pennington DG, et al: Follow-up of survivors of mechanical circulatory support. *J Thorac Cardiovasc Surg* 96:72, 1988.
62. Icenogle TB, Smith RG, Cleavinger M, et al: Thromboembolic complications of the Symbion AVAD system. *Artif Organs* 13:532, 1989.
63. Termuhlen DF, Swartz MT, Pennington DG, et al: Thromboembolic complications with the Pierce-Donachy ventricular assist device. *ASAIO Trans* 35:616, 1989.
64. Graham TR, Dasse K, Coumbe A, et al: Neo-intimal development on textured biomaterial surfaces during clinical use of an implantable left ventricular assist device. *Eur J Cardiothorac Surg* 4:182, 1990.
65. Von Segesser LK, Weiss BM, Bisang B, et al: Ventricular assist with heparin surface coated devices. *ASAIO Trans* 37:M278, 1991.
66. Bianchi JJ, Swartz MT, Raithel SC, et al: Initial clinical experience with centrifugal pumps coated with the carmeda process. *ASAIO Trans* 38:M143, 1992.
67. Pennington DG, Reedy JE, Swartz MT, et al: Univentricular versus biventricular assist device support. *J Heart Lung Transplant* 10:258, 1991.
68. Elbeery JR, Owen CH, Savitt MA, et al: Effects of left ventricular assist device on right ventricular function. *J Thorac Cardiovasc Surg* 99:809, 1990.
69. Nishigaki K, Matsuda H, Hirose H, et al: The effect of left ventricular bypass on the right ventricular function: Experimental analysis of the effects of ischemic injuries to the right ventricular free wall and interventricular septum. *Artif Organs* 14:218, 1990.
70. Daly RC, Chandrasekaran K, Cavarocchi NC, et al: Ischemia of the interventricular septum: A mechanism of right ventricular failure during mechanical left ventricular assist. *J Thorac Cardiovasc Surg* 103:1186, 1992.
71. Pennington DG, Merjavy JP, Swartz MT, et al: The importance of biventricular failure in patients with postoperative cardiogenic shock. *Ann Thorac Surg* 39:16, 1985.

72. Hammerschmidt DE, Stroncek DF, Bowers TK, et al: Complement activation and neutropenia occuring during cardiopulmonary bypass. *J Thorac Cardiovasc Surg* 81:370, 1981.
73. Farrar DJ, Compton PG, Hershon JJ, et al: Right ventricular function in an operating room model of mechanical left ventricular assistance

and its effects in patients with depressed left ventricular function. *Circulation* 72:1279, 1985.
74. Ruzevich SA, Swartz MT, Reedy JE, et al: Retrospective analysis of the psychologic effects of mechanical circulatory support. *J Heart Transplant* 9:209, 1990.

11. Chest Tube Insertion and Care

Robert A. Lancey and
A. Thomas Pezzella

Chest tube insertion, or tube thoracostomy, involves placement of a sterile tube into the pleural space for evacuation of air and/or fluid, often into a closed collection system. The purpose of this procedure (also known as closed intercostal drainage) is to promote lung expansion and prevent potentially lethal levels of pressure from developing in the thorax. Less acutely, tube thoracostomy allows drainage of blood or infected collections that could organize and prevent full expansion of the lung.

Although tube thoracostomy is not complex in the scope of all surgical procedures, it may result in serious and life-threatening complications if performed by a novice or hastily without proper preparation. Insertion and care of chest tubes are common issues not only in the intensive care unit (ICU) but throughout the hospital. In addition, chest tube insertion has become a component of the training for certification in Advanced Trauma Life Support [1].

This chapter will familiarize ICU personnel with the indications and the contraindications for chest tube insertion. Potential complications, technique of insertion, and subsequent management principles are discussed.

History

Hippocrates was the first to describe drainage of the pleural space, proposing the insertion of metal tubes to relieve empyema [2]. Playfair introduced the concept of underwater seal drainage in 1872 [3], and Hewitt, 4 years later, was the first to describe a method of closed tube drainage of the pleural space as treatment for empyema [4]. However, it was not until the 1917 influenza epidemic, which was associated with high mortality due to open chest drainage of empyemas, that Graham and Bell reintroduced closed chest aspiration and drainage [5]. With the use of postthoracotomy closed chest drainage in World War II and closed drainage of traumatic hemothorax in the Korean conflict, closed chest tube insertion and drainage became widespread.

Pleural Anatomy and Physiology

Since the primary goal of chest tube placement is drainage of pathologic processes of the pleural space, a basic knowledge of the anatomy and physiology is essential. The lung fills all but approximately 10 ml of the hemithorax in the normal physiologic state. This pleural space is a closed, serous sac surrounded by two layers, the parietal pleura and the visceral pleura, which are contiguous at the pulmonary hilum and the inferior pulmonary ligament. During development in utero, the lungs are enveloped by the visceral pleura, which is formed from splanchnic mesenchyme. The parietal pleura is derived from somatic mesoderm and lines the inner thoracic wall [6].

The parietal pleura may be subdivided into four anatomic sections: the costal pleura (lining the ribs, costal cartilages, and intercostal spaces), the cervical pleura (lining the most superior aspect of the pleural space), the mediastinal pleura (lining the medial aspect of the pleural space), and the diaphragmatic pleura (overlying the diaphragm). The visceral pleura covers completely and is adherent to the pulmonary parenchyma, following the indentations and lining the interlobar spaces to varying degrees. Lined by mesothelial cells, the pleural layers are in close approximation to each other and under normal physiologic conditions allow free expansion of the lung in a lubricated environment. In some areas, true potential spaces exist where parietal pleural surfaces are in contact during expiration, most notably inferoposteriorly in the costodiaphragmatic sinus and retrosternally in the costomediastinal sinus [7].

Drainage of the pleural space is necessary when the normal physiologic processes of this space are disrupted. Violation of the visceral pleura allows accumulation of air (pneumothorax) and possibly blood (hemopneumothorax). Disruption of the parietal pleura may result in hemothorax if an underlying vascular structure is disrupted, or pneumothorax if the defect communicates to the environment. In addition, derangements of the normal fluid dynamics in the pleural space may result in the accumulation of clinically significant effusions.

Fluid enters the pleural space from the parietal pleura and is reabsorbed through stomata in the parietal pleura and into the lymphatics, which drain regionally into the mediastinal, intercostal, phrenic, and substernal lymph nodes. Although up to 500 ml per day may enter the pleural space, normally less than 3 ml of fluid is present at any given time [8]. This normal equilibrium may be disrupted by increased fluid entry into the space due to alterations in hydrostatic (e.g., congestive heart failure) or oncotic pressures or by changes in the parietal pleura itself (e.g., inflammatory diseases). A derangement in lymphatic drainage, such as that seen with lymphatic obstruction by malignancy, may also result in fluid accumulation.

Chest Tube Placement

INDICATIONS. Numerous conditions indicate the need for drainage of the pleural space. The procedure may be performed to palliate a chronic disease process, as with drainage of malignant pleural effusions, or to relieve an acute, life-threatening process, as with decompression of a tension pneumothorax. Additional therapeutic maneuvers may be enhanced by placement of a chest tube, as when used with antibiotic therapy for treatment of an empyema or to instill sclerosing agents to prevent recurrence of malignant pleural effusions. The indications for closed intercostal drainage encompass a variety of disease processes in the hospital setting (Table 11-1).

Pneumothorax. Accumulation of air in the pleural space (pneumothorax) is the most common indication for chest tube placement. Although in many cases the diagnosis is made by physical examination and chest radiograph, in others it is not so obvious and may be accompanied by acute hemodynamic decompensation if a tension pneumothorax develops. Common symptoms include tachypnea, shortness of breath, and pleuritic-type chest pain, although some patients (in particular those with a small spontaneous pneumothorax) may be asymptomatic. Pneumothorax in a mechanically ventilated patient often presents acutely with deteriorating oxygenation and an increase in airway pressures.

Diagnosis is often confirmed by chest radiograph, demonstrating a thin opaque line beyond which exists a hyperlucent area in which lung markings are absent. The size of the pneumothorax may be estimated, but this is at best a rough estimation of a three-dimensional process based on two-dimensional information. No single grading system is yet universally accepted. Inspiratory and expiratory films may be helpful in equivocal situations, and a lateral decubitus film with the affected side up may yield further diagnostic information. Associated abnormalities, such as hemothorax, should be sought.

The decision to insert a chest tube for pneumothorax is based on the patient's overall clinical status and/or serial chest radiographs. Patients who are symptomatic, are receiving positive pressure ventilation, or have an enlarging pneumothorax should undergo tube decompression.

A spontaneous pneumothorax occurs most commonly in tall, young, slender males secondary to rupture of apical alveoli with subsequent formation of subpleural blebs, which then rupture into the pleural space. Patients may present with pleuritic pain, tachypnea, and coughing but also may be asymptomatic. Physical findings include diminished breath sounds and hyperresonance to percussion on the affected side. An associated hemothorax secondary to torn adhesions may occur in up to 5 percent of cases [9].

Small, stable, asymptomatic pneumothoraces may be observed with serial chest radiographs, with the rate of reexpansion being approximately 1.25 percent of lung volume per day [10]. Needle aspiration and nonoperative therapy have been attempted but result in longer hospitalization and higher recurrence rates. Definitive operative intervention involving resections of apical blebs, pleurodesis, and/or pleurectomy via open thoracotomy or thoracoscopy is often reserved for those with recurrence or persistent air leak. The risk of a recurrent ipsilateral pneumothorax is as high as 50 percent, and of a third episode up to 60 to 80 percent [11].

Pneumothorax in trauma patients is often accompanied by bleeding (hemopneumothorax) and almost invariably requires tube decompression, especially if mechanical ventilation is planned. Rib fractures are often present and may cause a life-threatening tension pneumothorax. Air continuously leaking

Table 11-1. Indications for Chest Tube Insertion

A. Pneumothorax
 1. Spontaneous
 2. Traumatic
 3. Necrotizing pneumonia
 4. Interstitial fibrosis
 5. Malignancy
  a. Primary
  b. Metastatic
 6. Bullous emphysema
 7. Pulmonary infarction
 8. Iatrogenic
  a. Central line placement
  b. Positive-pressure ventilation
  c. Thoracentesis
B. Hemothorax
 1. Traumatic
  a. Blunt
  b. Penetrating
 2. Iatrogenic
 3. Malignancy
  a. Primary
  b. Metastatic
 4. Infectious
 5. Pulmonary AV malformation
 6. Spontaneous pneumothorax
 7. Blood dyscrasias
 8. Ruptured thoracic aortic aneurysm
C. Empyema
 1. Parapneumonic
 2. Posttraumatic
 3. Postoperative
 4. Septic emboli
 5. Intraabdominal infection
D. Chylothorax
 1. Traumatic
  a. Blunt
  b. Penetrating
  c. Surgical
 2. Congenital
 3. Malignancy
 4. Miscellaneous
  a. Filariasis
  b. Tuberculosis
  c. Subclavian vein obstruction
E. Pleural effusion
 1. Transudate
 2. Exudate
  a. Malignancy
  b. Postoperative
  c. Iatrogenic
  d. Immunologic
  e. Inflammatory

into the pleural space with no route of escape will collapse the affected lung, flatten the diaphragm, and eventually cause contralateral shift of the mediastinum. Compression of the contralateral lung and of venous return results in hypoxemia and hypotension, respectively. Emergency decompression with a 14- or 16-gauge catheter in the second intercostal space in the midclavicular line may be lifesaving while preparations for chest tube insertion are being made. In fact, in a hypotensive trauma patient, pleural space decompression may be required before the diagnosis of tension pneumothorax is confirmed.

Bullous disease, malignancies (particularly metastatic disease from soft tissue sarcomas), and necrotizing pneumonia are potential sources of a persistent pneumothorax. Iatrogenic causes of pneumothorax, such as thoracentesis and attempted insertion of central venous catheters, are not uncommon. The incidence of pneumothorax associated with attempts at subclavian vein access has been reported to be as high as 6 percent [12]. The incidence is lower with an internal jugular approach, but pneumothorax still may result, since the lung apices rise above the clavicles. Patients on mechanical ventilation, especially with elevated levels of positive end-expiratory pressure (PEEP), are also at risk. In this setting, a tension pneumothorax may rapidly develop and require emergency measures as described above. Although prophylactic insertion of bilateral pleural tubes has been reported for patients on extremely high levels of PEEP (greater than 40 cm H_2O) [13], no controlled study has yet documented its benefit.

Hemothorax. Accumulation of blood in the pleural space (hemothorax) may be classified as spontaneous or traumatic. A hemothorax may also occur secondary to attempted thoracentesis or tube placement from injury to the intercostal or internal mammary arteries or to the pulmonary parenchyma. In trauma, a pulmonary source of hemorrhage is often self-limiting due to the low pressure of the pulmonary vascular system. However, if the source is systemic (intercostal, internal mammary or subclavian arteries, aorta, or heart), bleeding is often persistent and potentially life-threatening.

Different guidelines have been proposed to determine timing of operation for a traumatic hemothorax. In general, indications for open thoracotomy are initial blood loss greater than 1000 to 1500 ml, or continued blood loss greater than 500 ml over the first hour, greater than 200 ml per hour after 2 to 4 hours, or greater than 100 ml per hour after 6 to 8 hours, or in an unstable patient not responding to volume resuscitation [14,15,16]. Placement of a large bore (36–40 Fr.) drainage tube not only assists in ventilation but also helps assess the need for immediate thoracotomy.

Incomplete drainage of a traumatic hemothorax due to poor positioning of the tube or clotting in the tube may result in a fibrothorax when the intrapleural blood clots and organizes. Subsequent significant reduction of pulmonary reserve may occur as a result of lung trapped by this process, and an empyema may develop. Early removal of this collection via open thoracotomy enables full reexpansion of the lung and prevents empyema formation in those able to tolerate the procedure [17,18]. If the patient's condition mandates nonoperative management, a waiting period of several weeks will allow an organized peel to form, facilitating its removal during decortication.

Common causes of nontraumatic hemothoraces include spontaneous pneumothorax (from tearing of adhesions between the lung and the parietal pleura), pulmonary arteriovenous malformations, and malignancies of the lung and pleura, both primary and metastatic. In addition, necrotizing pulmonary infections and pulmonary infarctions may result in a secondary hemothorax.

Empyema. Empyemas are pyogenic infections of the pleural space. They are seen most commonly in association with a necrotizing pneumonia, from septic pulmonary emboli or secondary spread of intraabdominal infections, and after trauma to the chest requiring a chest tube (especially in the setting of an inadequately drained hemothorax).

Definitive management of an empyema requires both drainage and antibiotic therapy. Pyothorax was a more common complication of pneumonia in the preantibiotic area; since then, in addition to a decline in incidence, the microbial spectrum has changed. The most common organisms now isolated are no longer *Streptococcus* species but rather *Staphylococcus aureus* and anaerobic and gram-negative organisms. Chest tube drainage is indicated for pleural collections with any of the following characteristics: pH less than 7.0, glucose less than 40 mg/dl, lactate dehydrogenase greater than 1000 u/dl, frank purulence, or gram-positive or culture-positive specimens [19].

Large-bore drainage tubes (36–40 Fr.) are used, and success is evidenced by resolving fever and leukocytosis, improving clinical status, and eventual resolution of tube drainage. The tube is removed slowly over several days, allowing a fibrous tract to form. If no improvement is seen, rib resection and open drainage may be indicated. Chronic empyema may require decortication or, in more debilitated patients, open flap drainage (Eloesser procedure). Bergh and associates described the instillation of fibrinolytic enzymes (streptokinase) through the tube to break up persistent purulent collections and loculations [20].

Chylothorax. Chylothorax is lymphatic leakage into the pleural space with subsequent accumulation. This fluid is almost always sterile, due to the immunologic properties of lymph, and may accumulate at a rate of up to 1500 ml per day, causing hemodynamic compromise and metabolic sequelae due to loss of protein, fat, and fat-soluble vitamins. Fluid triglyceride level greater than 110 mg/dl [21] or a cholesterol-to-triglyceride ratio of less than 1 [22] confirms the diagnosis.

The primary causes of chylothorax are trauma (including surgery), malignancy, congenital, and miscellaneous, such as filariasis invasion or subclavian vein obstruction. Surgical procedures most often implicated include those involving mobilization of the aortic arch (e.g., repair of aortic coarctation, patent ductus arteriosus, or vascular rings) or esophageal resection [23]. The appearance of chyle in the pleural space may be delayed for 7 to 10 days after injury, especially if there are dietary restrictions after surgery. The fluid may collect in the posterior mediastinum before rupturing into the pleural space (often on the right side) [22]. Nonsurgical trauma, such as crush or blast injuries or those causing sudden hyperextension of the spine or neck, may result in chylothorax, as may a violent bout of vomiting or coughing.

In nontraumatic settings, malignancy must always be suspected. Leak occurs secondary to direct invasion of the thoracic duct or from obstruction by external compression or tumor embolus. Lymphosarcoma, lymphoma, and primary lung carcinomas are those most frequently implicated [22].

Treatment consists of tube drainage and aggressive maintenance of fluid and nutritional status. Hyperalimentation and intestinal rest are recommended to limit flow through the duct. Approximately 50 percent will resolve spontaneously [24], and while no consensus exists as to the optimal time to intervene surgically, a minimum of 2 weeks of observation is usually appropriate [25,26] unless the patient is already in a malnourished state. Open thoracotomy is recommended to ligate the duct and close the fistula. Identification of the site is aided by preoperative oral administration of cream or olive oil or injection of Evans blue dye into the leg [22].

Pleural Effusion. Management of a pleural effusion begins with thoracentesis to differentiate the nature of the fluid collection as transudative or exudative. Treatment of transudative pleural effusions is aimed at controlling the underlying cause, such as congestive heart failure, the nephrotic syndrome, or cirrhosis. Only rarely is tube thoracostomy indicated. Exudative effusions, however, often require tube drainage.

Prior to drainage it is essential to identify the fluid as free-flowing or loculated, using decubitus chest films. If the latter is suspected, localization of the collection and proper tube placement may require use of ultrasound or computed tomographic (CT) scanning. For malignant pleural effusions, chest tube insertion may serve not only to relieve symptoms and enable lung expansion but also to allow instillation of sclerosing agents to facilitate pleural symphysis. Once the pleural space has been evacuated of fluid and air and apposition of the pleural surfaces is present, a chemical pleurodesis may be performed with one of a number of agents, thereby obliterating the pleural space and preventing further fluid accumulation. Bleomycin, doxycycline, and talc are among the more commonly used agents [27].

CONTRAINDICATIONS. The most obvious contraindication to chest tube insertion seems straightforward—lack of a pneumothorax or of a fluid collection in the pleural space—yet this distinction is not always clear. What may appear at first to be a pneumothorax may instead be a skinfold, the medial border of the scapula, or even the tract of a recently removed chest tube. A large bulla may also be mistaken for a pneumothorax, a circumstance in which attempted pleural tube placement may result in significant morbidity. An expiration chest film, which highlights the pulmonary parenchyma by increasing its density, or a decubitus view with the suspected side up may help confirm the diagnosis, as may CT scanning. Likewise, an apparent pleural effusion may be a lung abscess or consolidated pulmonary parenchyma. Again, CT scanning or ultrasonography may prove helpful in delineating the pathology prior to tube placement.

Past history of a process that would promote pleural symphysis, such as a sclerosing procedure, pleurodesis, pleurectomy, or even previous thoracotomy on the affected side, should raise caution and prompt evaluation with CT scanning. This will help identify the exact area of pathology and direct tube placement away from areas where the lung is adherent to the chest wall. In a postpneumonectomy patient, the pleural tube should be placed above the original incision, as the diaphragm frequently rises to this height.

The possibility of herniation of abdominal contents through the diaphragm in patients with severe blunt abdominal trauma or stab wounds in the vicinity of the diaphragm requires more extensive evaluation prior to tube placement. In addition, coagulopathies should be corrected prior to tube insertion in a nonemergency setting.

TECHNIQUE. Chest tube insertion requires knowledge not only of the anatomy of the chest wall and intrathoracic and intraabdominal structures but also of general aseptic technique. The procedure should be performed or supervised only by experienced surgeons, since the complications of an improperly placed tube may have immediate life-threatening results. Prior to tube placement, the patient must be evaluated thoroughly by physical examination and chest films to avoid insertion of the tube into a bulla or lung abscess, into the abdomen, or even into the wrong side. Particular care must be taken before and during the procedure to avoid intubation of the pulmonary parenchyma.

The equipment necessary is listed in Table 11-2. Sterile technique is mandatory whether the procedure is performed in the operating room, ICU, emergency room or on the ward. Detailed informed consent is obtained as conditions dictate and contributes to alleviating patient anxiety during the procedure. Administration of parenteral narcotics or benzodiazepines as well as careful and generous administration of local anesthetic will provide a relatively painless procedure.

Drainage tubes are made from either silastic or rubber. The older, right-angled rubber tubes elicit more pleural inflammation, have fewer drainage holes, and are not easily identified on chest radiograph. Silastic tubes are either right-angled or straight, have multiple drainage holes, and contain a radio-

Table 11-2. Chest Tube Insertion Equipment

1. Povidone-iodine solution
2. Sterile towels and drapes
3. Sterile sponges
4. 1% xylocaine without epinephrine (40 ml)
5. 10-ml syringe
6. 18, 21, and 25-gauge needles
7. 2 Kelly clamps
8. Mayo scissors
9. Standard tissue forceps
10. Towel forceps
11. Needle holder
12. 0-Silk suture with cutting needle
13. Scalpel handle and no. 10 blade
14. Chest tubes (24, 28, 32, and 36 Fr.)
15. Chest tube drainage system (filled appropriately)
16. Petrolatum gauze
17. 2-inch adhesive tape
18. Sterile gowns and gloves, masks, caps

paque stripe with a gap to mark the most proximal drainage hole. They are available in sizes ranging from 6 to 40 Fr.; the type selected depends on the patient population (sizes 6–24 Fr. for infants and children) and the collection being drained (sizes 24–28 Fr. for air, 32–36 Fr. for pleural effusions, and 36–40 Fr. for blood or pus).

Before performing the procedure, it is important to review the steps that will be taken, ensuring that all necessary equipment is available. Patient comfort and safety are paramount.

1. The patient is placed supine with the head of the bed adjusted for comfort. The involved side is elevated slightly and the arm on that side brought up over the head (Fig. 11-1). Supplemental oxygen is administered as needed.
2. In most instances, the tube is inserted into the fourth or fifth intercostal space in the anterior axillary line, to avoid intraabdominal structures and the pectoral muscles. An alternative entry site is the second intercostal space anteriorly in the midclavicular line for decompression of a pneumothorax only, but based on cosmetic considerations and to avoid the thick pectoral muscles, the former site is preferred in adults.
3. Under sterile conditions, the area is prepared with 10% povidone-iodine solution and draped to include the nipple, which serves as a landmark. A 2- to 3-cm area is infiltrated with 1% lidocaine to raise a wheal in the anterior axillary line located two finger-breadths below the intercostal space that will be penetrated. This allows for a subcutaneous tunnel to develop, through which the tube will travel, and discourages air entry into the chest following removal of the tube.
4. To confirm location of air or fluid, a thoracentesis is first performed at the proposed site of tube insertion. If air or fluid is not aspirated, the anatomy should be reassessed and chest radiographs and CT scans reexamined before proceeding.
5. A 2-cm transverse incision is made with a scalpel and additional lidocaine administered to infiltrate the tissues through which the tube will pass as well as a generous area in the intercostal space, including the periosteum of the ribs above and below. Care should be taken to fully anesthetize the parietal pleura, as it (unlike the visceral pleura) contains pain fibers. Each injection of lidocaine should be preceded by aspiration on the syringe to prevent injection into the intercostal vessels. Up to 30 to 40 ml of lidocaine may be needed to achieve adequate local anesthesia (Fig. 11-1).
6. A short tunnel is created to the chosen intercostal space,

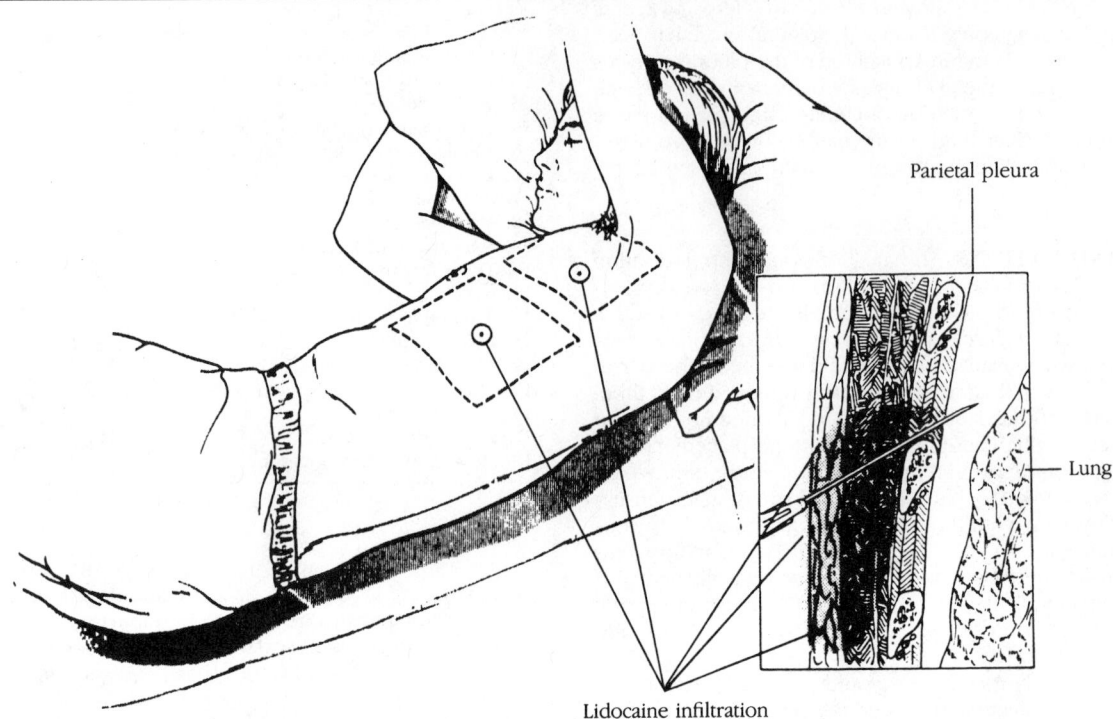

Parietal pleura

Lung

Lidocaine infiltration

Fig. 11-1. Proper patient positioning for chest tube insertion. Note that the involved side is slightly elevated and the arm is flexed over the head. Lidocine infiltrates progressively through the tissue. (From Vander Salm TJ, Cutler BS, Wheeler HB (eds): *Atlas of Bedside Procedures.* Boston, Little, Brown, 1989, p 186)

using Kelly clamps. The intercostal muscles are then bluntly divided and the closed Kelly clamp carefully inserted through the parietal pleura, hugging the superior portion of the lower rib to prevent injury to the intercostal bundle of the rib above. The Kelly clamp is inserted less than 1 cm to prevent injury to the intrathoracic structures and is spread open approximately 2 cm (Fig. 11-2).

7. A finger is inserted into the pleural space to explore the anatomy and confirm proper location and lack of pleural symphysis. Only easily disrupted adhesions should be broken. Bluntly dissecting strong adhesions will tear the lung and potentially initiate troublesome bleeding from the systemic circulation.

8. The chest tube is inserted into the pleural space and positioned appropriately (apically for a pneumothorax and dependently for fluid removal). All holes must be confirmed to be within the pleural space by palpation. The use of undue pressure or force to insert the tube should be avoided. Tube placement may be guided by Kelly clamping the tip to direct it apically or posteriorly (Fig. 11-3).

9. The location of the tube should be confirmed by flow of air (seen as condensation) or fluid from the tube. The tube is

Table 11-3. Complications of Chest Tube Insertion

1. Unintentional tube placement into vital structures (lung, liver, spleen, etc.)
2. Bleeding
3. Reexpansion pulmonary edema
4. Residual pneumothorax
5. Residual hemothorax
6. Empyema

then sutured to the skin securely to prevent slippage (Fig. 11-4). A horizontal mattress suture may be used to allow the hole to be tied closed when the tube is removed. A petrolatum gauze dressing is applied and the tube connected to a drainage apparatus and securely taped to both the dressing and the patient. All connections between the patient and the drainage apparatus must be tight and securely taped also.

COMPLICATIONS. Chest tube insertion may be accompanied by signficant complications. In one series, insertion and management of pleural tubes in patients with blunt chest trauma carried a 9 percent incidence of complications [28]. Insertion alone is usually accompanied by a 1 to 2 percent incidence of complications even when performed by experienced personnel (Table 11-3) [28,29].

Unintentional placement of the tube through intercostal vessels or into the lung, heart, liver, or spleen can result in considerable morbidity and possible mortality. Adequate knowledge of the anatomy in general and of the pathologic process in particular should prevent such occurences. Reexpansion pulmonary edema on the affected side in the setting of a large, chronic, pleural effusion may be avoided by incremental removal of the fluid, limiting initial removal to no more than 1 liter over the first 30 minutes. Factors that contribute to this process include a trapped lung and placement of negative pressure on the tube via the drainage system at the time of initial tube placement [30,31].

Residual pneumothorax may follow removal of the tube and may be due to a persistent air leak or entry of air through the tube site during or after removal. The two causes may be differentiated based on serial chest films, with a persistent pulmonary leak showing an increasing pneumothorax and requiring replacement of the tube. A small stable pneumothorax may be treated by sealing the wound securely and with observation. If the pneumothorax is large or symptomatic, tube decompression is indicated.

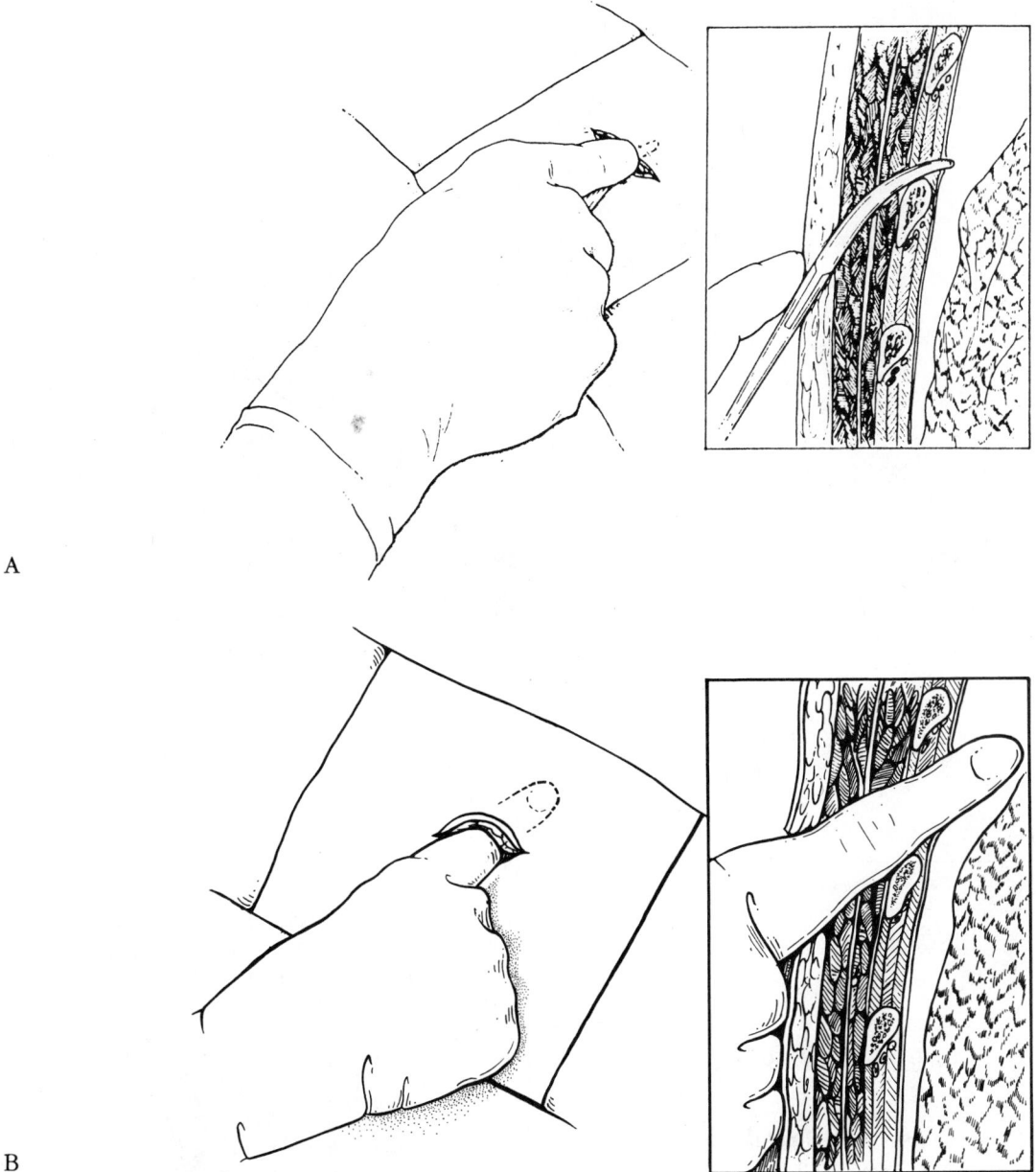

A

B

Fig. 11-2. A. The clamp penetrates the intercostal muscle. B. The index finger is gently inserted to explore the immediate area around the incision. No instruments are inserted into the pleural space at this time.

Secondary infection of the pleural space may occur after chest tube insertion, forming an empyema. Although this is rare, it is more common following treatment for a traumatic hemothorax. Numerous studies have examined the utility of prophylactic antibiotics for tube thoracostomy. It is generally accepted that antibiotics are not indicated for drainage of a spontaneous pneumothorax, as there is no proved benefit for their use [32], but controversy exists as to their benefit in trauma patients. Some studies have shown advantages in antibiotic therapy while others have found no significant difference [33,34,35]. It is perhaps prudent to administer prophylactic antibiotics for those with a traumatic hemothorax, especially when other injuries are present.

Chest Tube Management and Care

While a chest tube is in place, the tube and drainage system must be checked daily for adequate functioning. In the past, drainage systems employed one to three bottles, closed to the environment, serving as a one-way valve to allow egress of air and fluid while preventing their return back into the pleural space. This enabled the development of a negative-pressure environment in the pleural space. Today most institutions employ a one-piece three-chambered system that contains a calibrated collection trap for fluid, an underwater seal unit to allow escape of air while maintaining negative pleural pressure, and a suction regulator (Fig. 11-5). Suction is routinely established at 15 to 20 cm, controlled by the height of the column in the suction regulator unit, and maintained as long as an air leak is present. The drainage system is examined daily to ensure that

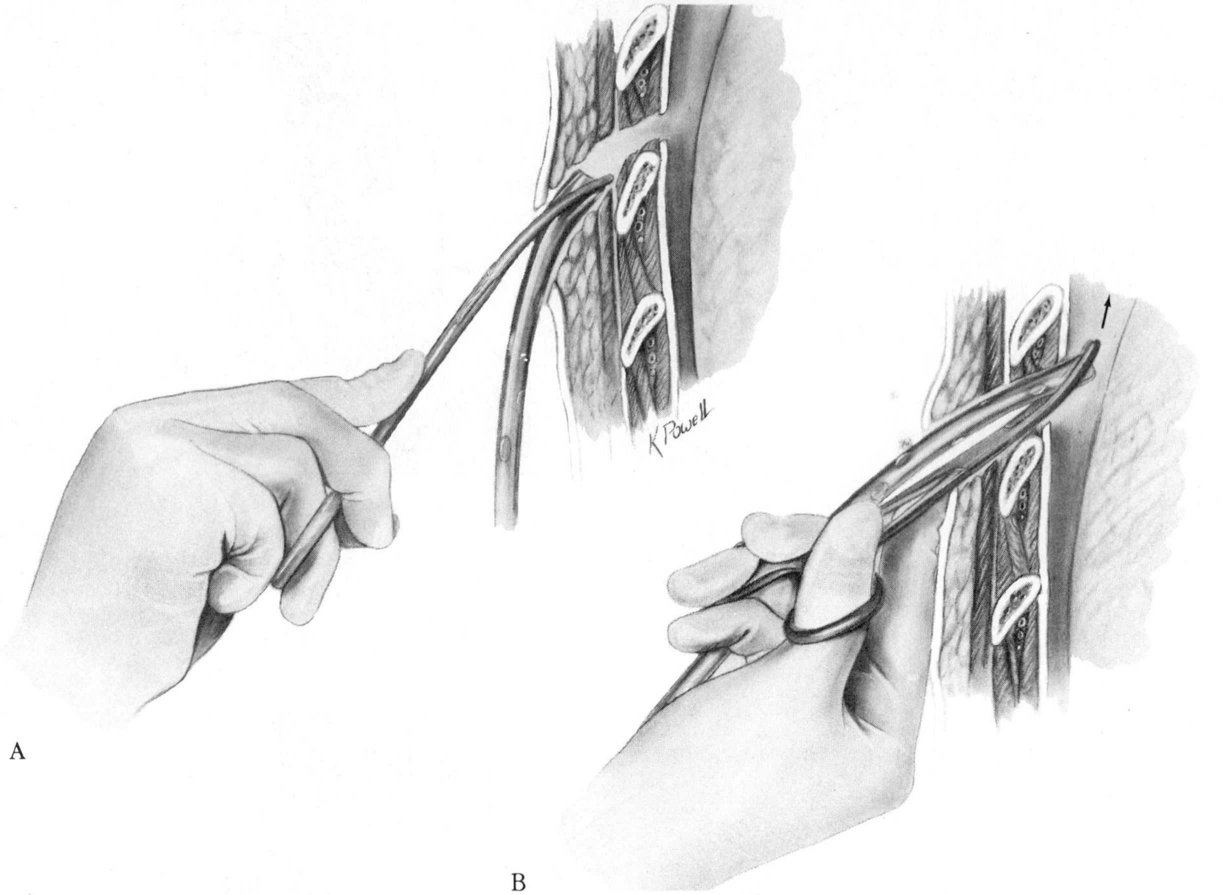

Fig. 11-3. A. The end of the chest tube is grasped with a Kelly clamp and guided with a finger through the chest incision. B. The clamp is rotated 180 degrees to direct the tube toward the apex.

Fig. 11-4. The tube is securely sutured to the skin with a 1–0 or 2–0 silk suture. This suture is left long, wrapped around the tube, and secured with tape. To seal the tunnel, this suture is tied when the tube is pulled out.

appropriate levels are maintained in the underwater seal and suction regulator chambers. If suction is desired, bubbling should be noted in the suction regulator unit. Connections between the chest tube and the drainage system should be tightly fitted and securely taped. For continuous drainage, the chest tube and the tubing to the drainage system should remain free of kinks and should not be left in a dependent position or clamped (which may result in life-threatening tension pneumothorax). The tube may be "milked" and gently stripped, but irrigation of the tube is discouraged. Dressing changes should be performed every 2 or 3 days and as needed, and adequate pain control is mandatory to encourage coughing and ambulation (which serve to reexpand the lung).

Serial chest films should be obtained routinely to follow the response to closed intercostal drainage and ensure that the most proximal drainage hole has not migrated from the pleural space. This situation may result in a pneumothorax or produce subcutaneous emphysema. If this occurs and the *pathologic* process is not corrected, replacement of the tube is usually indicated, especially if subcutaneous emphysema is developing. A tube should never be readvanced into the pleural space, and if a tube is to be replaced it should always be at a different site rather than through the same hole. If a pneumothorax persists, increasing the suction level may be benecial, but an additional tube may be required if no improvement results.

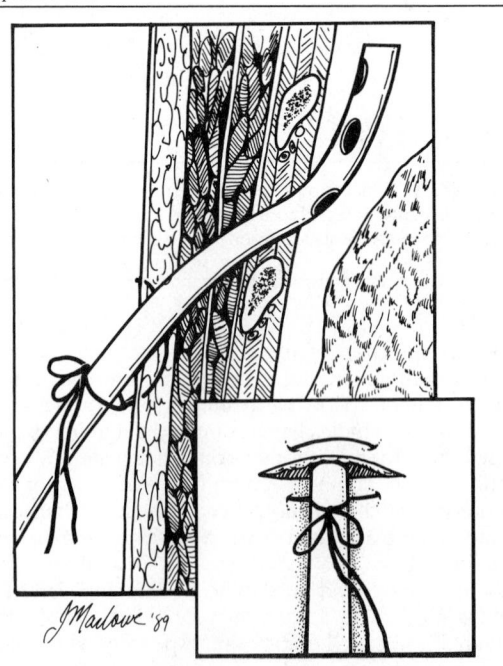

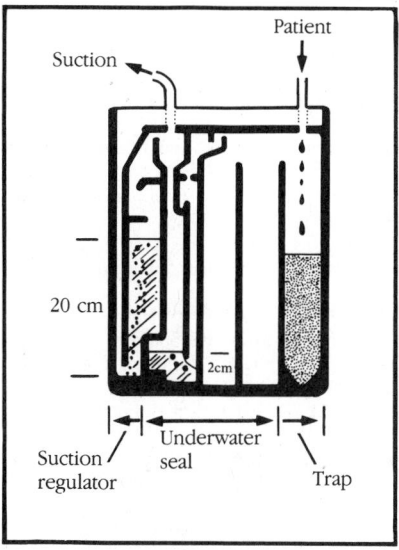

Contained single plastic unit

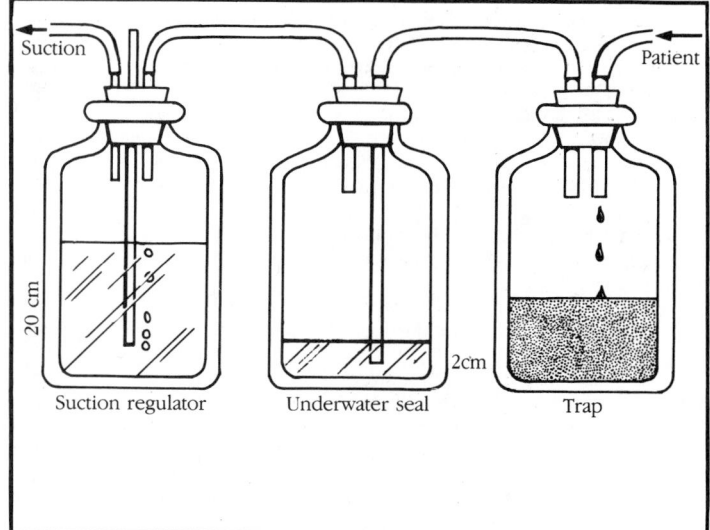

3 bottle system

Fig. 11-5. Three bottle drainage system in contrast with contained single plastic unit.

Chest Tube Removal

Indications for removal of chest tubes include resolution of the pneumothorax and/or fluid accumulation in the pleural space. For a pneumothorax, the drainage system is left on suction until the air leak stops. If an air leak persists, brief clamping of the chest tube is performed to be sure the leak is indeed from the patient and not the system. If an air leak persists from the lung, another tube may be indicated. When the leak has ceased for more than 24 to 48 hours (or if no fluctuation is seen in the underwater seal chamber), the drainage system is placed on water seal by disconnecting the wall suction. A chest film is obtained several hours later. If no reaccumulation of air is identified and no air leak appears in the system with coughing, deep breathing, and reestablishment of suction, the tube may be removed. For fluid collections, the tube may be removed when drainage has become minimal, unless sclerotherapy is planned.

Tube removal is often preceded by oral or parenteral analgesia at an appropriate time interval. A petrolatum gauze dressing and tape are readied and the patient instructed to take maximal deep breaths slowly and successively. The suture holding the tube to the skin is cut and the tube removed while the hole is simultaneously covered with the petrolatum gauze dressing at the peak of inspiration. At this point, the patient can generate only positive pressure in the pleural space, minimizing the possibility of drawing air back into the pleural space. Some prefer placing a horizontal mattress suture at the time of tube insertion, left untied, to be secured at the time of tube removal, especially for individuals with thin chest walls and for children and infants. A chest radiograph is performed immediately to confirm lack of recurrence of the pneumothorax and is repeated 24 hours later to check for reaccumulation of air or fluid.

Related Systems

A brief mention is made here of related systems that supplement the ability to drain the pleural space. Percutaneous aspiration of the pleural space to relieve a pneumothorax with no active air leak has been attempted in a number of settings. Although successful in up to 75 percent of cases of needle-induced or traumatic pneumothoraces, the success rate falls to about 50 percent for those with spontaneous pneumothoraces [36]. Small percutaneous catheters placed via Seldinger technique or using a trocar have gained attention recently for treatment of simple pneumothoraces and loculated pleural fluid collections (the latter via CT scan guidance). These may be especially helpful for collections not easily accessible by tube thoracostomy.

Heimlich valves, which are one-way flutter valves that allow egress of air from pleural tubes or catheters, have also gained greater attention over the past several years. They facilitate ambulation in patients with persistent air leaks and allow outpatient therapy for such patients. In fact, in one study, almost 75 percent of patients with spontaneous pneumothoraces treated as outpatients with Heimlich valves required no further therapy [37].

References

1. *Advanced Trauma Life Support Instructor Manual.* Chicago, American College of Surgeons, 1989, p 105–110.
2. Hippocrates: Writings, in Hutchins RA (ed): *Great Books of the Western World.* vol. 29. Chicago, Encyclopedia Britannica, 1952, p 142.
3. Playfair GE: Case of empyema treated by aspiration and subsequently by drainage: Recovery. *Br Med J* 1:45, 1875.
4. Mead RH: *A History of Thoracic Surgery.* Springfield, IL, Charles C. Thomas, 1961, p 238–256.
5. Graham EA, Bell RD: Open pneumothorax: Its relation to the treatment of empyema. *Am J Med Sci* 156:839, 1918.
6. Moore KL: *The Developing Human.* Philadelphia, WB Saunders, 1977, pp 190–192.
7. DeMeester TR, Lafontaine E: The pleura, in Sabiston DC, Spencer FC (eds): *Surgery of the Chest.* Philadelphia, WB Saunders, 1990, pp 444–497.
8. Sahn SA: Benign and malignant pleural effusions, in Shields TW (ed): *General Thoracic Surgery.* Philadelphia, Lea & Febiger, 1989, pp 613–624.

9. Deslauriers J, LeBlanc P, McClish A: Bullous and bleb diseases of the lung, in Shields TW (ed): *General Thoracic Surgery*. Philadelphia, Lea & Febiger, 1989, pp 727–749.

10. Kircher LT Jr, Swartzel RL: Spontaneous pneumothorax and its treatment. *JAMA* 155:24, 1954.

11. Gobbel WG, Rhea WG, Nelson IA, et al: Spontaneous pneumothorax. *J Thorac Cardiovasc Surg* 46:331, 1963.

12. Bernard RW, Stahl WM: Subclavian vein catheterization: A prospective study, I.—Non-infectious complications. *Ann Surg* 173:184, 1971.

13. Hayes DF, Lucas CE: Bilateral tube thoracostomy to preclude tension pneumothorax in patients with acute respiratory insufficiency. *Am Surg* 42:330, 1976.

14. Sandrasagra FA: Management of penetrating stab wounds of the chest: Assessment of the indications for early operation. *Thorax* 33:474, 1978.

15. McNamara JJ, Messersmith JK, Dunn RA, et al: Thoracic injuries in combat casualties in Vietnam. *Ann Thorac Surg* 10:389, 1970.

16. Boyd AD: Pneumothorax and hemothorax, in Hood RM, Boyd AD, Culliford AT (eds): *Thoracic Trauma*. Philadelphia, WB Saunders, 1989, pp 133–148.

17. Collins MP, Shuck JM, Wachtel TL, et al: Early decortication after thoracic trauma. *Arch Surg* 113:440, 1978.

18. Beall AC, Crawford HW, DeBakey NE: Considerations in the management of acute traumatic hemothorax. *J Thorac Cardiovasc Surg* 52:351, 1966.

19. Miller JI Jr: Infections of the pleura, in Shields TW (ed): *General Thoracic Surgery*. Philadelphia, Lea & Febiger, 1989, pp 633–649.

20. Bergh NP, Ekroth R, Larsson S, et al: Intrapleural streptokinase in the treatment of hemothorax and empyema. *Scand J Thorac Cardiovasc Surg* 11:265, 1977.

21. Staats RA, Ellefson RD, Budahn LL, et al: The lipoprotein profile of chylous and unchylous pleural effusions. *Mayo Clin Proc* 55:700, 1980.

22. Miller JI Jr: Chylothorax and anatomy of the thoracic duct, in Shields TW (ed): *General Thoracic Surgery*. Philadelphia, Lea & Febiger, 1989, pp 625–632.

23. Bessone LN, Ferguson TB, Burford TH: Chylothorax. *Ann Thorac Surg* 12:527, 1971.

24. Ross JK: A review of the surgery of the thoracic duct. *Thorax* 16:12, 1961.

25. Williams KR, Burford TH: The management of chylothorax. *Ann Surg* 160:131, 1964.

26. Selle JG, Snyder WA, Schreiber JT: Chylothorax. *Ann Surg* 177:245, 1977.

27. Hausheer FH, Yarbro JW: Diagnosis and treatment of malignant pleural effusions. *Semin Oncol* 12:54, 1985.

28. Daly RC, Mucha P, Pairolero PC, et al: The risk of percutaneous chest tube thoracostomy for blunt thoracic trauma. *Ann Emerg Med* 14:865, 1985.

29. Millikan JS, Moore EE, Steiner E, et al: Complications of tube thoracostomy for acute trauma. *Am J Surg* 140:738, 1980.

30. Trapneel DH, Thurston JGB: Unilateral pulmonary edema after pleural aspiration. *Lancet* 1:1367, 1970.

31. Waqaruddin M, Bernstein A: Re-expansion pulmonary oedema. *Thorax* 30:54, 1975.

32. Neugebauer MK, Fosburg RG, Trummer MJ: Routine antibiotic therapy following pleural space intubation: A reappraisal. *J Thorac Cardiovasc Surg* 61:882, 1971.

33. Stone HH, Symbas PN, Hooper CA: Cefamandole for prophylaxis against infection in closed tube thoracostomy. *J Trauma* 21:975, 1981.

34. Mandal AK, Montaño J, Thadepaldi H: Prophylactic antibiotics and no antibiotics compared in penetrating chest trauma. *J Trauma* 25:639, 1985.

35. LoCurto JJ, Tischler CD, Swank G, et al: Tube thoracostomy and trauma: Antibiotics or not? *J Trauma* 26:1067, 1986.

36. Delius RE, Obeid FN, Horst HM, et al: Catheter aspiration for simple pneumothorax. *Arch Surg* 124:883, 1989.

37. Mercier C, Page A, Verdant A, et al: Outpatient management of intercostal tube drainage in spontaneous pneumothorax. *Ann Thorac Surg* 22:163, 1976.

12. Bronchoscopy

Richard S. Irwin

Bronchoscopy is the endoscopic examination of the tracheobronchial tree. Whether performed with a flexible or rigid instrument (Fig. 12-1), it is a procedure of the trained specialist familiar with all of its potential indications, complications, and contraindications. Unless otherwise stated, this chapter will focus on the flexible instrument.

Since its commercial introduction for clinical use in 1968, flexible fiberoptic bronchoscopy has had a dramatic impact on the approach and management of patients with a wide variety of respiratory problems [1]. The procedure has revolutionized the practice of clinical chest medicine. It offers a variety of features and capabilities that have fostered its widespread use: (1) it is easily performed; (2) it is associated with few complications [2]; (3) it is much more comfortable [3] and safer [4] for the patient than rigid bronchoscopy; (4) it exposes a far greater proportion of the tracheobronchial tree (especially the upper lobes) to direct visualization than does rigid bronchoscopy [5]; (5) it does not require general anesthesia or the use of an operating room [3]; and (6) it may be performed at the bedside [3]. For all of these reasons, flexible fiberoptic bronchoscopy has largely replaced rigid bronchoscopy as the procedure of choice for most endoscopic evaluations of the airway. On the other hand, rigid bronchoscopy may be the procedure of choice [1,6] for (1) brisk hemoptysis (>200 ml/24 hr), (2) extraction of foreign bodies, (3) endobronchial resection of granulation tissue that might occur after traumatic and/or prolonged intubation, (4) biopsy of vascular tumors (e.g., bronchial adenoma) in which brisk and excessive bleeding can be controlled by packing, (5) endoscopic laser surgery, and (6) dilation of tracheobronchial strictures and placement of airway stents.

Diagnostic Indications

GENERAL CONSIDERATIONS. Since flexible fiberoptic bronchoscopy can be performed easily even in intubated patients, the same general indications apply to critically ill patients on ventilators and to noncritically ill patients; however, only the indications most commonly encountered in critically ill patients are discussed here. A complete list of indications for bronchoscopy appears in Table 12-1.

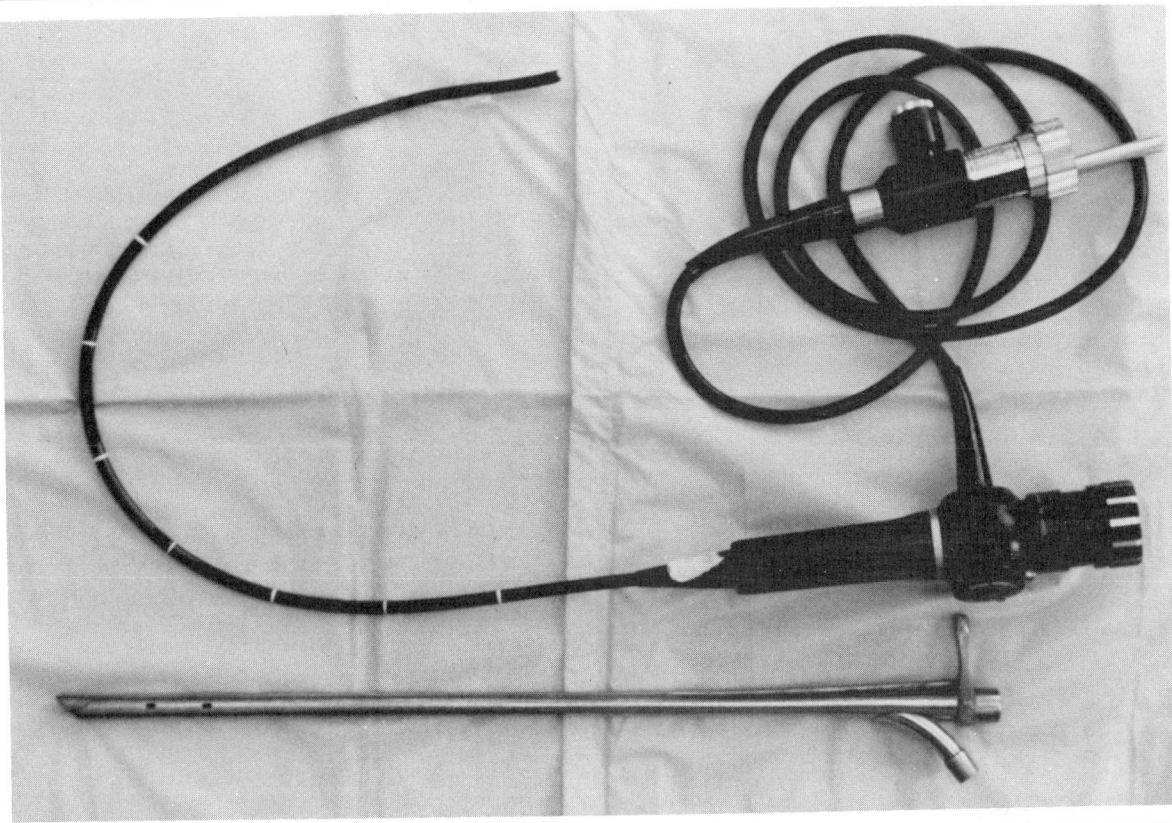

Fig. 12-1. Rigid (*bottom*) and flexible (*top*) fiberoptic broncho-
scopes. The standard rigid bronchoscope is a hollow tube, 40 cm
long, with a blunted, beveled tip and a 7-mm lumen. A light source
can be introduced into the channel that begins at the top of the
scope's proximal end. The side arm at the proximal end can be used
for oxygen administration. A standard flexible fiberoptic bronchoscope consists of a control section with a light source attachment connected to a flexible insertion tube, 4.8–5.9 mm in outer diameter, with
a distal bending section. The control section has an eyepiece at its
most proximal end as well as an angle lever that allows rotation of
the distal end up and down and an inner channel for instillation or
aspiration of liquids and/or insertion of cytology brushes or biopsy
forceps.

COMMON INDICATIONS

Hemoptysis. This is one of the most common clinical problems
for which bronchoscopy is indicated [16,40] (see Chap. 61 for
a detailed discussion). Whether the patient complains of blood
streaking or massive hemoptysis (expectoration of >600 ml in
48 hr) [61], bronchoscopy should be considered to localize the
site of bleeding and to diagnose the cause. Localization of the
site of bleeding is crucial if definitive therapy such as surgery
becomes necessary. If flexible fiberoptic bronchoscopy is performed before hemoptysis ceases entirely, the site and etiology
of the bleeding will be determined in approximately 90 percent
of patients [40]. If it is performed after bleeding ceases entirely,
the etiology will be determined in no more than 50 percent of
patients [40]. Since hemoptysis can be caused by tracheobronchial tree disorders, cardiovascular diseases, hematologic conditions, and localized and diffuse pulmonary parenchymal disorders, clinical judgment must dictate whether and when
bronchoscopy is indicated [38]. For instance, it is not indicated
in patients with obvious pulmonary embolism with infarction.
In intubated or tracheotomized patients, hemoptysis should always be evaluated, since it may indicate potentially life-threatening tracheal damage. Unless the bleeding is massive, a flexible fiberoptic bronchoscope, rather than a rigid bronchoscope,
is the instrument of choice for evaluating hemoptysis.

Atelectasis. Although atelectasis may be due to mucus plugging, fiberoptic bronchoscopy should be performed to rule out
endobronchial obstruction by carcinoma or foreign body. When
atelectasis occurs in critically ill patients who had a normal chest
film on admission, mucus plugging is the most likely cause [10].
In intubated patients, the position of the endotracheal tube,
which may have slipped down the right mainstem bronchus
and obstructed the right upper lobe, should be determined on
a chest radiograph [62].

Diffuse Parenchymal Disease. Bronchoscopy can be used to
assess both airways and lung parenchyma by visualization and
transbronchoscopic lung biopsy, respectively. Because bronchoalveolar lavage specimens yield representative cellular material of simultaneously obtained lung biopsy specimens, it is
not surprising that bronchoalveolar lavage is useful in diagnosing opportunistic infections in immunocompromised hosts
(e.g., in acquired immunodeficiency syndrome [AIDS]). Transbronchial lung biopsy is performed under fluoroscopic guidance to minimize the chance of pneumothorax from inadvertent
biopsy of the visceral pleura. The reader is referred to Chapter
77 for an in-depth discussion of lung biopsy procedures.

Three factors should be considered in choosing the bronchoscopy procedure in critically ill patients with diffuse parenchymal infiltrates: (1) local expertise, (2) the patient's condition,
and (3) the potential yield of the particular procedure.

LOCAL EXPERTISE. This factor refers to the availability of individuals skilled in performing the procedure and laboratory per-

Table 12-1. Indications for Bronchoscopy

Diagnostic indications	Therapeutic indications
Acute inhalation injury [7,8]	Brachytherapy for central airway neoplasms [47]
Assessment of intubation damage [9]	Closure of bronchopleural fistula [48]
Atelectasis [10–14]	Endotracheal intubation [29,49]
Blunt chest trauma [15]	Excessive secretions and atelectasis [10–14,29]
Chest radiograph consistent with neoplasia [16,17,18]	Foreign bodies [50,51]
Cough [19,20]	Hemoptysis [52–55]
Cultures [21–28]	Laser resection for central airway neoplasms [56]
Diaphragmatic paralysis [29]	Lung abscess [1,57]
Diffuse parenchymal disease and/or bilateral hilar adenopathy [30–38]	Preoperative assessment of resectability [58,59]
Hemoptysis [39,40]	Pulmonary alveolar proteinosis lavage [60]
Local recurrence [29]	
Localized wheeze [29]	
Lung abscess [41]	
Metastatic disease with unknown primary [42]	
Pleural effusion of unknown etiology [3]	
Positive cytology and normal chest radiograph [43]	
Recurrent laryngeal nerve paralysis [29]	
Recurrent pneumonia [44]	
Segmental bronchography [45]	
Symptoms after resectional surgery [46]	
Unresolving infiltrate [3]	

sonnel skilled in specimen processing and analysis. If local expertise is limited (e.g., a skilled cytopathologist is not available to read bronchial brush or percutaneous needle aspiration specimens, or the microbiology laboratory is not equipped reliably to process specimens for the variety of organisms seen in immunocompromised hosts), the patient should be transferred to another institution with expanded resources.

PATIENT'S CONDITION. Once it has been decided that the patient's prognosis is potentially good enough to justify a lung biopsy technique, the next decision involves choosing the biopsy procedure. If it is determined that the patient could not tolerate any complication, no matter how minor, or that the patient's condition allows time for only one diagnostic procedure (i.e., the patient is rapidly deteriorating), then an open lung biopsy should be performed. Immediate morbidity and mortality from open lung biopsy in the critically ill, immunocompromised patient on a ventilator appear to be minimal, except in patients with a poor prognosis from the underlying disease. Useful information with acceptable morbidity (e.g., pneumothorax, hemorrhage) can also be obtained in hemodynamically stable patients on mechanical ventilation with transbronchial lung biopsy [63,64]. If there are no contraindications to bronchoalveolar lavage or transbronchoscopic lung biopsy and the patient's condition is such that there will be time for another diagnostic procedure if necessary, then one of these procedures may be preferable.

POTENTIAL YIELD OF PROCEDURE. In patients with diffuse pulmonary disease, the clinical setting influences the choice of procedure. When a biopsy is performed to document the presence and type of inorganic pneumoconiosis, open lung biopsy

is the only procedure that will yield a sufficient amount of tissue for all of the requisite analyses (chemical analysis must be included). When diffuse pulmonary infiltrates suggest sarcoidosis and carcinomatosis, transbronchoscopic lung forceps biopsy should be considered initially because it has an extremely high yield in these situations (Chap. 77).

In the non-AIDS immunocompromised host, transbronchoscopic lung biopsy and bronchoalveolar lavage have high yields for identifying *Pneumocystis carinii, Legionella* species, and cytomegalovirus (CMV) infections [31,34]. In patients with AIDS, transbronchial lung biopsy and lavage have been shown to have a 94 to 100 percent sensitivity for the diagnosis of *P. carinii* pneumonia [65]. Lavage alone may have a sensitivity of up to 97 percent [65]. In AIDS patients, the sensitivity of lavage or transbronchial lung biopsy for identifying all opportunistic organisms (*Pneumocystis,* CMV, *Mycobacterium avium-intracellulare, Cryptococcus neoformans, Coccidioides immitis,* and *Histoplasma capsulatum*) can be as high as 86 percent and 87 percent, respectively [66,67]. However, since sputum samples can also be positive for *Pneumocystis* in up to 79 percent of cases [65], expectorated sputum, when available, should be evaluated first for this organism before resorting to bronchoscopy. The highest yields of identifying CMV infections have been obtained on lavage fluid examined by immunofluorescence with CMV-specific monoclonal antibodies [66]. On the other hand, transbronchoscopic lung biopsy and lavage are not the best procedures to evaluate whether lung changes are drug-induced.

Acute Inhalation Injury. In patients exposed to smoke inhalation, fiberoptic laryngoscopy and bronchoscopy are indicated to identify the anatomic level and severity of injury [7,8]. Prophylactic intubation should be considered if considerable upper airway mucosal injury is noted early; acute respiratory failure is more likely in patients with mucosal changes seen at segmental or lower levels [68].

Blunt Chest Trauma. Patients who present with an atelectatic lung, lobar atelectasis, pneumomediastinum, and/or pneumothorax after blunt chest trauma may have sustained a fractured airway [15]. Since this requires surgical intervention, bronchoscopy should be performed immediately. The fiberoptic instrument allows an initial quick, thorough examination without general anesthesia.

Postresectional Surgery. Flexible fiberoptic bronchoscopy can identify a disrupted suture line causing bleeding and pneumothorax [29] following surgery and an exposed endobronchial suture causing cough [46].

Assessment of Intubation Damage. Although laryngeal and tracheal complications have been markedly reduced with soft, low-pressure balloons on the new nonirritating endotracheal tubes, damage still occurs. In these cases, to determine when a tracheostomy should be performed, flexible fiberoptic bronchoscopy with an average adult-sized instrument (outside diameter of scope 4.8–5.9 mm) can be easily performed in a ventilated patient if the patient has an endotracheal tube in place that is 8 mm or larger in internal diameter. A tube 8 mm in internal diameter usually allows rapid, intermittent insertions of a standard, adult bronchoscope, but this is the minimal size that can be used without risking complications [69,70,71]. For this reason, adult patients should always be intubated with an endotracheal tube at least 8 mm in internal diameter, if possible. If the endotracheal tube is smaller, it will not be possible to ventilate and bronchoscope the patient simultaneously, unless a pediatric bronchoscope (outside diameter 3.5 mm) or intubation endoscope (outside diameter 3.8 mm) is used or a special low-resistance endotracheal tube is already in place [72].

When a nasotracheal or orotracheal tube of the proper size is in place, the balloon can be routinely deflated and the tube withdrawn over the bronchoscope to look for subglottic damage. The tube is withdrawn up through the vocal cords and over the fiberoptic bronchoscope and glottic and supraglottic damage sought. We recommend that this procedure be performed at least weekly; however, available data demonstrate no clear-cut observations that assist in determining the ideal timing of tracheostomy in patients previously intubated. Nevertheless, if subglottic ulcers or necrosis or glottic edema or ulcers occur, tracheostomy is indicated to avoid the serious sequelae of tracheomalacia, tracheostenosis, and laryngostenosis. In patients with no obvious lesions and no reasonable chance of immediately being weaned from the ventilator, tracheostomy should be considered after 11 days of intubation when severe laryngeal injury becomes a very real potential concern [73]. In patients on long-term ventilatory assistance with cuffed tracheostomy tubes, fiberoptic bronchoscopy can help differentiate aspiration from tracheoesophageal fistula. With the bronchoscope in the distal trachea, the patient is asked to swallow a dilute solution of methylene blue. The absence of methylene blue in the trachea and its presence leaking around and out of the tracheostomy stoma provide accurate evidence of a swallowing abnormality and the absence of a tracheoesophageal fistula.

Cultures. Transnasal or transoral fiberoptic bronchoscopy aspirates from a nonintubated patient [23,25] are no more reliable than nasotracheal suction aspirates or expectorated sputum specimens for culture of routine aerobic and anaerobic organisms [21]. All of these methods generate excessive false positive and false negative bacteriologic data. Fiberoptic bronchoscopy aspirates may, however, be extremely useful in identifying *Mycobacterium tuberculosis* [28], *Nocardia* species [27], pathogenic fungi [27], and *Legionella* species [74] when patients are unable to expectorate adequate quantities of sputum. A new sampling device (a retractable sterile wire brush within two telescoped catheters plugged at the distal end) improves routine bronchoscopy culture, but only when the brush specimen is quantitatively cultured [75,76]. See Chapter 13 for an indepth discussion of methods of obtaining lower respiratory tract secretions in pneumonia.

Therapeutic Indications

EXCESSIVE SECRETIONS AND ATELECTASIS. When chest physiotherapy, incentive spirometry, and sustained maximum inspiration with cough fail to clear the airways of excessive secretions and reexpand lobar atelectasis [77], flexible fiberoptic bronchoscopy may be successful. Occasionally, the direct instillation of acetylcysteine (Mucomyst) through the bronchoscope may be necessary to liquify the thick, tenacious inspissated mucus [78]. Since acetylcysteine may induce bronchospasm in asthmatics, these patients must be pretreated with a bronchodilator. Flexible fiberoptic bronchoscopy effectively clears excessive secretions and is more comfortable for the patient than rigid bronchoscopy and therefore appears to be the procedure of choice [10].

FOREIGN BODIES. Although the rigid bronchoscope is considered by many to be the instrument of choice for removing foreign bodies, devices with which to grasp objects are available for use with the flexible fiberoptic bronchoscope [51].

ENDOTRACHEAL INTUBATION. In patients with ankylosing spondylitis and other mechanical problems of the neck, the flexible fiberoptic bronchoscope may be used as an obturator for endotracheal intubation [29]. The bronchoscope with an endotracheal tube passed over it can be passed transnasally (after proper local anesthesia) through the vocal cords into the trachea. Then the tube can be passed over the scope. This same technique can be used in patients with tetanus complicated by trismus and in patients with acute epiglottitis [49]. In the latter two instances, the procedure should preferably be done in the operating room with an anesthesiologist and otolaryngologist present.

HEMOPTYSIS. On rare occasions where brisk bleeding threatens asphyxiation, endobronchial tamponade may stabilize the patient before definitive therapy is performed (Chap. 61) [53]. With the use of the flexible bronchoscope, usually passed through a rigid bronchoscope, a Fogarty catheter with balloon is passed into the bleeding lobar orifice. When the balloon is inflated and wedged tightly, the patient may be transferred to surgery or angiography for bronchial arteriography and bronchial artery embolization [52,54,55].

CENTRAL OBSTRUCTING AIRWAY LESIONS. Some patients with cancer and others with benign lesions that obstruct the larynx, trachea, and major bronchi can be treated by photoresection using a laser through a bronchoscope. It is not unusual for patients to be transferred to an ICU for a life-threatening airway obstruction that could be relieved by laser resection [79].

CLOSURE OF BRONCHOPLEURAL FISTULA. Bronchopleural fistula (BPF) is an acquired pathway between the bronchial tree and pleural space. After placement of a chest tube, drainage of the pleural space, and stabilization of the patient (e.g., infection, cardiovascular and respiratory systems), bronchoscopy can be used to visualize a proximal BPF or localize a distal BPF; it can also be used in attempts to close the BPF [80,81]. Although the published experience on bronchoscopically sealing BPFs is limited, a number of case reports have suggested that a variety of materials, injected through the bronchoscope, may successfully seal BPFs [80–83]. These materials have included doxycycline and tetracycline followed by autologous blood instillation to form an obstructive blood clot, lead fishing weights or shot, tissue adhesive, fibrin glue, absorbable gelatin sponge, angiographic occlusion coils, silver nitrate, and balloon occlusion. For an in-depth discussion of BPF and its management, see Chapter 65.

Complications

When performed by a trained specialist, routine flexible fiberoptic bronchoscopy is extremely safe. Mortality should not exceed 0.1 percent [2] and overall complications should not exceed 8.1 percent [2]. The rare deaths have been due to excessive premedication or topical anesthesia, respiratory arrest from hemorrhage, laryngospasm, or bronchospasm, and cardiac arrest from acute myocardial infarction [84,85]. Nonfatal complications occurring within 24 hours of the procedure include fever (1.2–16%) [2,86], pneumonia (0.6–6%) [2,86], vasovagal reactions (2.4%) [2], laryngospasm and bronchospasm (0.1–

0.4%) [2,84], hypotension and cardiac arrhythmias (0.9%) [2], pneumothorax (0.2%) [2], anesthesia-related problems (0.1%) [2,84], and aphonia (0.1%) [2]. Although transient bacteremias occur (15.4–33%) after rigid bronchoscopy [87,88], probably due to trauma to the teeth and airways, they do not predictably occur after transnasal flexible fiberoptic bronchoscopy [89]. The incidence of bacteremia after transoral fiberoptic bronchoscopy has not been studied.

The patients in whom complications are likely to occur are asthmatics, who are prone to develop laryngospasm and bronchospasm; patients with cardiovascular problems (e.g., angina, arrhythmias), who are prone to develop cardiovascular problems; and immunoincompetent hosts, who are at increased risk for developing infection [2]. Patients with hemoptysis are more likely to bleed, whereas patients with partially obstructing endobronchial lesions are more likely to develop pneumonia.

Contraindications

Bronchoscopy should not be performed: (1) when an experienced bronchoscopist is not available; (2) when the patient will not or cannot cooperate and cooperation is needed; (3) when adequate oxygenation cannot be given during and for approximately 4 hours after the procedure (arterial oxygen tension will drop an average of 20 mm Hg during a routine diagnostic bronchoscopy) [90]; (4) when coagulation studies cannot be normalized in patients in whom biopsies, brush or forceps, will be taken; (5) in unstable cardiac patients [91,92,93]; and (6) in untreated symptomatic asthmatics [94]. Although patients with stable carbon dioxide retention can be safely bronchoscoped with a flexible instrument [95], premedication, sedation during the procedure, and supplemental oxygen must be used with caution.

Procedure

PREPROCEDURAL CONSIDERATIONS. The following is a checklist for use before performing the procedure:

1. Does the patient have asthma?
2. Does the patient have cardiovascular disease?
3. Is the patient uremic?
4. Is the patient immunoincompetent?
5. Does the patient have drug allergies?
6. Have the chest film and ECG been ordered?
7. Have arterial blood gas analysis, platelet count, prothrombin time, and partial thromboplastin time been ordered?
8. Has the patient recently taken any medication that will interfere with platelet function? If so, has a bleeding time been ordered?
9. Has the patient fasted for 3 to 4 hours before the procedure?
10. Has a procedure consent form been signed?
11. Has premedication been ordered (e.g.,1 mg intramuscular atropine and 50 mg intramuscular meperidine [Demerol])?
12. Has an angiocath been placed in an arm vein?

PROCEDURAL CONSIDERATIONS. In nonintubated patients, flexible fiberoptic bronchoscopy can be performed by the transnasal route (Fig. 12-2) or transoral route with a bite block through an endotracheal tube or through a rigid bronchoscope [1]. The overwhelming majority of bronchoscopists in the United States prefer the transnasal route in a patient who

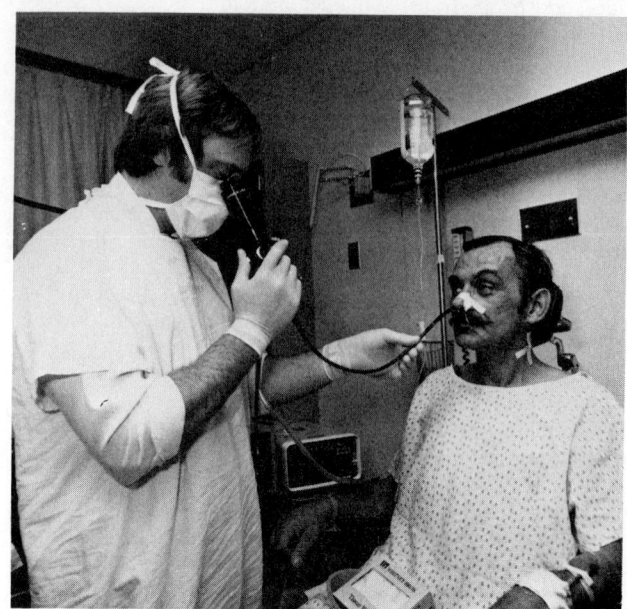

Fig. 12-2. Transnasal flexible fiberoptic bronchoscopy. This procedure can be easily and safely performed with topical anesthesia with minimal patient discomfort. An operating room is not required.

has been previously anesthetized by hand-nebulized lidocaine and lidocaine jelly as a lubricant [1]. Since lidocaine is absorbed through the mucus membranes, significant blood levels may be reached after topical administration; however, if a total of less than 200 mg is used during the procedure, only levels in the low therapeutic range will be obtained [96,97]. In patients on a lidocaine drip, another anesthetic, such as topical cocaine, should be given. A sudden change in mental status, tremulousness, hallucinations, increased sedation, or a hypotensive reaction should suggest lidocaine toxicity [96,97].

In intubated and mechanically ventilated patients, the flexible fiberoptic bronchoscope can be passed through a swivel adapter with a rubber diaphragm (Fig. 12-3), which will prevent loss of the delivered respiratory gases [98]. In this setting, the following points are important: (1) Never use a tracheal tube smaller than 8 mm in internal diameter with a bronchoscope with the standard external diameter, because (a) it will not be possible to deliver an adequate tidal volume, owing to increased airway resistance [69], and (b) positive end-expiratory pressure (PEEP) caused by standard scopes and tube will approach 20 cm H_2O with the potential for barotrauma [69]. (2) PEEP, if already being delivered, must be discontinued [69]. (3) The inspired oxygen concentration (FIO_2) must be temporarily increased to 100 percent [69]. (4) With the help of a respiratory therapist, expired volumes should be constantly measured to ensure that they are adequate (tidal volumes usually have to be increased 40–50%) [69]. (5) As little as possible should be suctioned, and for short periods of time, because suctioning will decrease the tidal volumes being delivered [69]. During bronchoscopy, continuous oxygen therapy and ECG monitoring are necessary.

POSTPROCEDURAL CONSIDERATIONS. The following is a checklist for use after performing the procedure:

1. After performing a transbronchoscopic lung biopsy in the nonintubated patient or routine bronchoscopy in the intu-

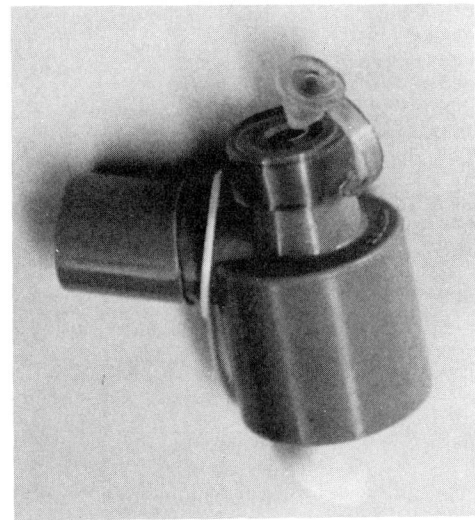
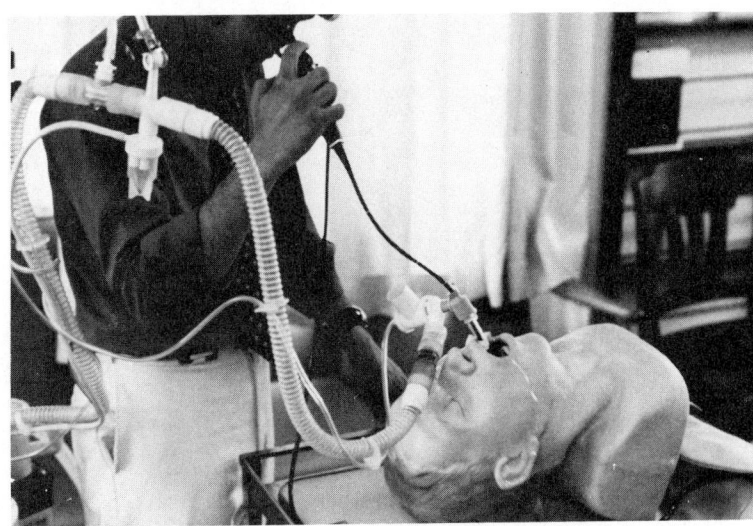

A   B

Fig. 12-3. Flexible fiberoptic bronchoscopy in intubated and mechanically ventilated patients. With the use of a swivel adapter with a rubber diaphragm (A), flexible fiberoptic bronchoscopy can be easily and safely performed in mechanically ventilated patients without losing the delivered respiratory gases (B).

bated, mechanically ventilated patient, obtain a chest radiograph to look for a pneumothorax.

2. In the ventilated patient, return the ventilator settings back to the preprocedure settings.

3. In the nonintubated patient, continue supplemental oxygen for 4 hours following the procedure [90].

4. Obtain frequent vital signs until the patient has been stable for 2 hours.

5. Do not allow the nonintubated patient to eat or drink until the local anesthesia has worn off. Approximately 1 to 2 hours after the procedure, allow the patient to sip some water [97]. If the patient does not cough and sputter, allow the patient to resume a regular diet.

6. Although postbronchoscopy fever ($\geq$ 101°F) will develop in up to 16 percent of patients, it usually lasts 24 hours or less [86]. If it lasts longer, evaluate the patient for a postbronchoscopy pneumonia; this complication is most likely to occur in patients older than 60 years who have endoscopic lesions that are brushed [86].

References

1. Sackner MA: Bronchofiberscopy. *Am Rev Respir Dis* 111:62, 1975.

2. Pereira W Jr, Kovnat DM, Snider GL: A prospective cooperative study of complications following flexible fiberoptic bronchoscopy. *Chest* 73:813, 1978.

3. Rath GS, Schaff JT, Snider GL: Flexible fiberoptic bronchoscopy: Techniques and review of 100 bronchoscopies. *Chest* 63:689, 1973.

4. Lukomsky GI, Ovchinnikov AA, Bilal A: Complications of bronchoscopy: Comparison of rigid bronchoscopy under general anesthesia and flexible fiberoptic bronchoscopy under topical anesthesia. *Chest* 79:316, 1981.

5. Kovnat DM, Rath GS, Anderson WM, et al: Maximal extent of visualization of bronchial tree by flexible fiberoptic bronchoscopy. *Am Rev Respir Dis* 110:88, 1974.

6. Prakash UBS, Stuffs SE: The bronchoscopy survey: Some reflections. *Chest* 100:1660, 1991.

7. Wanner A, Cutchavaree A: Early recognition of upper airway obstruction following smoke inhalation. *Am Rev Respir Dis* 108:1421, 1973.

8. Hunt JL, Agree RN, Pruitt BA Jr: Fiberoptic bronchoscopy in acute inhalation injury. *J Trauma* 15:641, 1975.

9. Amikam B, Landa J, West J, et al: Bronchofiberscopic observations of the tracheobronchial tree during intubation. *Am Rev Respir Dis* 105:747, 1972.

10. Mahajan VK, Catron PW, Huber GL: The value of fiberoptic bronchoscopy in the management of pulmonary collapse. *Chest* 73:817, 1978.

11. Lindholm CE, Ollman B, Snyder J, et al: Flexible fiberoptic bronchoscopy in critical care medicine: Diagnosis, therapy and complications. *Crit Care Med* 2:250, 1974.

12. Bartlett CR Jr, Vecchione JJ, Bell ALL Jr: Flexible fiberoptic bronchoscopy for airway management during acute respiratory failure. *Am Rev Respir Dis* 109:429, 1974.

13. Feldman NT, Huber GL: Fiberoptic bronchoscopy in the intensive care unit. *Int Anesthesiol Clin* 14:31, 1976.

14. Barrett CR Jr: Flexible fiberoptic bronchoscopy in the critically ill patient: Methodology and indications. *Chest* 73 (suppl):746, 1978.

15. Fraser RG, Pare JAP: Diseases of the thorax caused by external physical agents, in Fraser RG, Pare JA (eds): *Diagnosis of Diseases of the Chest.* 2nd ed. Philadelphia, WB Saunders, 1979, p 1577.

16. Khan MA, Whitcomb ME, Snider GL: Flexible fiberoptic bronchoscopy. *Am J Med* 61:151, 1976.

17. Richardson RH, Zavala DC, Mukerjee PK, et al: The use of fiberoptic bronchoscopy and brush biopsy in the diagnosis of suspected pulmonary malignancy. *Am Rev Respir Dis* 109:63, 1974.

18. Zavala DC: Diagnostic fiberoptic bronchoscopy: Techniques and results of biopsy in 600 patients. *Chest* 68:12, 1975.

19. Irwin RS, Corrao WM, Pratter MR: Chronic persistent cough in the adult: The spectrum and frequency of causes and successful outcome of specific therapy. *Am Rev Respir Dis* 123:413, 1981.

20. Poe RH, Israel RH, Utell MJ, et al: Chronic cough: Bronchoscopy or pulmonary function testing? *Am Rev Respir Dis* 126:160, 1982.

21. Irwin RS, Corrao WM: A perspective on sputum analyses in pneumonia. *Respir Care* 24:328, 1979.

22. Irwin RS, Garrity FL, Erickson AD, et al: Sampling lower respiratory tract secretions in primary lung abscess: A comparison of the accuracy of four methods. *Chest* 79:559, 1981.

23. Bartlett JG, Alexander J, Mayhew J, et al: Should fiberoptic bronchoscopy aspirates be cultured? *Am Rev Respir Dis* 114:73, 1976.

24. Halperin SA, Suratt PM, Gwaltney JM Jr, et al: Bacterial cultures of the lower respiratory tract in normal volunteers with and without experimental rhinovirus infection using a plugged double catheter system. *Am Rev Respir Dis* 125:678, 1982.

25. Fossieck BE Jr, Parker RH, Cohen MH, et al: Fiberoptic bronchoscopy and culture of bacteria from the lower respiratory tract. *Chest* 72:5, 1977.

26. Higuchi JH, Coalson JJ, Johanson WG Jr: Bacteriologic diagnosis of nosocomial pneumonia in primates: Usefulness of the protected specimen brush. *Am Rev Respir Dis* 125:53, 1982.

27. George RB, Jenkinson SG, Light RW: Fiberoptic bronchoscopy in the diagnosis of pulmonary fungal and nocardial infections. *Chest* 73:33, 1978.

28. Jett Jr, Cortese DA, Dines DE: The value of bronchoscopy in the diagnosis of mycobacterial disease: A five-year experience. *Chest* 80:575, 1981.

29. Landa JF: Indications for bronchoscopy. *Chest* 73 (suppl):686, 1978.

30. Andersen HA: Transbronchoscopic lung biopsy for diffuse pulmonary diseases: Results in 939 patients. *Chest* 73 (suppl):734, 1978.

31. Ellis JH Jr: Transbronchial lung biopsy via the bronchoscope: Experience with 107 consecutive cases and comparison with bronchial brushing. *Chest* 68:524, 1975.

32. Zavala DC: Transbronchial biopsy in diffuse lung disease. *Chest* 73 (suppl):727, 1978.

33. Feldman NT, Pennington JE, Ehrie MG: Transbronchial lung biopsy in the compromised host. *JAMA* 238:1377, 1977.

34. Springmeyer SC, Silvestri RC, Sale GE, et al: The role of transbronchial biopsy for the diagnosis of diffuse pneumonias in immunocompromised marrow transplant recipients. *Am Rev Respir Dis* 126:763, 1982.

35. Poe RH, Utell MJ, Hall WJ, et al: Sensitivity and specificity of the nonspecific transbronchial lung biopsy. *Am Rev Respir Dis* 119:25, 1979.

36. Wilson RK, Fechner RE, Greenberg SD, et al: Clinical implications of a "non-specific" transbronchial biopsy. *Am J Med* 65:252, 1978.

37. Toledo-Pereyra LH, DeMeester TR, Kinealey A, et al: The benefits of open lung biopsy in patients with previous non-diagnostic transbronchial lung biopsy: A guide to appropriate therapy. *Chest* 77:647, 1980.

38. Koerner SK, Sakowitz AJ, Appelman RI, et al: Transbronchial lung biopsy for the diagnosis of sarcoidosis. *N Engl J Med* 293:268, 1975.

39. Braman SS, Irwin RS, Constantine H: Hemoptysis, in Conn HF, Conn RB (eds): *Current Diagnosis.* 5th ed. Philadelphia, WB Saunders, 1977, p 15.

40. Selecky PA: Evaluation of hemoptysis through the bronchoscope. *Chest* 73 (suppl):741, 1978.

41. Petty TL, Mitchell RS: Suppurative lung diseases. *Med Clin North Am* 51:529, 1967.

42. Mohsenifar Z, Chopra SK, Simmons DH: Diagnostic value of fiberoptic bronchoscopy in metastatic pulmonary tumors. *Chest* 74:369, 1978.

43. Sanderson DR, Fontana RS, Wollner LB, et al: Bronchoscopic localization of radiographically occult lung cancer. *Chest* 65:608, 1974.

44. Winterbauer RH, Bedon GA, Ball WCJ: Recurrent pneumonia: Predisposing illness and clinical patterns in 158 patients. *Ann Intern Med* 70:689, 1969.

45. Lutch JS, Ryan KG: Bronchography combined with bronchoscopy: A new method. *Chest* 75:108, 1979.

46. Albertini RE: Cough caused by exposed endobronchial sutures. *Ann Intern Med* 94:205, 1981.

47. Schray MF, McDougall JC, Martinez A, et al: Management of malignant airway compromise with laser and low dose rate brachytherapy: The Mayo Clinic experience. *Chest* 93:265, 1988.

48. Powner DJ: Pulmonary barotrauma in the intensive care unit. *J Intensive Care Med* 3:224, 1988.

49. Giudice JC, Komansky HJ: Acute epiglottitis: The use of a fiberoptic bronchoscope in diagnosis and therapy. *Chest* 75:211, 1979.

50. Holinger PH, Holinger LD: Use of the open tube bronchoscope in the extraction of foreign bodies. *Chest* 73 (suppl):721, 1978.

51. Cunanan OS: The flexible fiberoptic bronchoscope in foreign body removal: Experience in 300 cases. *Chest* 73:725, 1978.

52. Bredin CP, Richardson PR, King TKC: Treatment of massive hemoptysis by combined occlusion of pulmonary and bronchial arteries. *Am Rev Respir Dis* 117:969, 1978.

53. Saw EC, Gottlieb LS, Yokoyama T, et al: Flexible fiberoptic bronchoscopy and endobronchial tamponade in the management of massive hemoptysis. *Chest* 70:589, 1976.

54. Remy J, Arnaud A, Fardou H, et al: Treatment of hemoptysis by embolization of bronchial arteries. *Radiology* 122:33, 1977.

55. White RI, Kaufman SL, Barth KH: Therapeutic embolization with detachable silicone balloons: Early clinical experience. *JAMA* 241:1257, 1979.

56. Cavaliere S, Foccoli P, Farina PL: Nd: Yag laser bronchoscopy: A five-year experience with 1,396 applications in 1,000 patients. *Chest* 94:15, 1988.

57. Safdar F, Draman SS: Fiberoptic bronchoscopy in pulmonary abscess. *Chest* 77:707, 1980.

58. Robbins HM, Morrison DA, Sweet ME, et al: Biopsy of the main carina: Staging lung cancer with the fiberoptic bronchoscope. *Chest* 75:484, 1979.

59. Robbins HM, Sweet ME, Jefferson SE, et al: The determination of resectability of lung cancer by fiberoptic bronchoscopy. *Arch Intern Med* 141:649, 1981.

60. Brach BB, Harrell JH, Moser KM: Alveolar proteinosis: Lobar lavage by fiberoptic bronchoscopic technique. *Chest* 69:224, 1976.

61. Crocco JA, Rooney JJ, Fankushen DS, et al: Massive hemoptysis. *Arch Intern Med* 121:495, 1968.

62. Goodman LR, Putnam CE: Radiological evaluation of patients receiving assisted ventilation. *JAMA* 245:858, 1981.

63. Papin TA, Grum CM, Weg JG: Transbronchial biopsy during mechanical ventilation. *Chest* 89:168, 1986.

64. Pincus PS, Kallenbach JM, Hurwitz MD, et al: Transbronchial biopsy during mechanical ventilation. *Crit Care Med* 15:1136, 1987.

65. Hopewell PC: *Pneumocystis carinii* pneumonia: Diagnosis. *J Infect Dis* 157:1115, 1988.

66. Emanuel D, Peppard J, Stover D, et al: Rapid immunodiagnosis of cytomegalovirus pneumonia by bronchoalveolar lavage using human and murine monoclonal antibodies. *Ann Intern Med* 104:476, 1986.

67. Broaddus C, Dake MD, Stulbarg MS, et al: Bronchoalveolar lavage and transbronchial biopsy for the diagnosis of pulmonary infections in the acquired immunodeficiency syndrome. *Ann Intern Med* 102:747, 1985.

68. Brandstetter RD: Flexible fiberoptic bronchoscopy in the intensive care unit. *J Intensive Care Med* 4:248, 1989.

69. Lindholm C-E, Ollman B, Snyder JV, et al: Cardiorespiratory effects of flexible fiberoptic bronchoscopy in critically ill patients. *Chest* 74:362, 1978.

70. Shinnick JP, Johnston RF, Oslick T: Bronchoscopy during mechanical ventilation using fiberscope. *Chest* 65:613, 1974.

71. Feldman NT, Sanders J: An alternate method for fiberoptic bronchoscopic examination of the intubated patient. *Am Rev Respir Dis* 111:562, 1975.

72. Carden E: Recent improvements in technique for general anesthesia for bronchoscopy. *Chest* 73 (suppl):697, 1978.

73. Heffner JE: Medical indications for tracheotomy. *Chest* 96:186, 1989.

74. Saravolatz LD, Russell G, Cvitkovich D: Direct immunofluorescence in the diagnosis of Legionnaire's disease. *Chest* 79:566, 1981.

75. Wimberly NW, Bass JB, Boyd BW, et al: Use of a bronchoscopic protected catheter brush for the diagnosis of pulmonary infections. *Chest* 81:556, 1982.

76. Torres A, Bellacasa JP, Xaubert A, et al: Diagnostic value of quantitative cultures of bronchoalveolar lavage and telescoping plugged catheters in mechanically ventilated patients with bacterial pneumonia. *Am Rev Respir Dis* 140:306, 1989.

77. Marini JJ, Pierson DJ, Hudson LD: Acute lobar atelectasis: A prospective comparison of fiberoptic bronchoscopy and respiratory therapy. *Am Rev Respir Dis* 119:971, 1979.

78. Lieberman J: The appropriate use of mucolytic agents. *Am J Med* 49:1, 1970.

79. Dedhia HV, Lapp NL, Jain RR, et al: Endoscopic laser therapy for respiratory distress due to obstructive airway tumors. *Crit Care Med* 13:464, 1985.

80. Powner DJ, Bierman MI: Thoracic and extrathoracic bronchial fistulas. *Chest* 100:480, 1991.

81. Baumann MH, Sahn SA: Medical management and therapy of bronchopleural fistulas in the mechanically ventilated patient. *Chest* 97:721, 1990.

82. Salmon CJ, Ponn RB, Westcott JL: Endobronchial vascular occlusion coils for control of a large parenchymal bronchopleural fistula. *Chest* 98:233, 1990.
83. Martin WR, Siefkin AD, Allen R: Closure of a bronchopleural fistula with bronchoscopic instillation of tetracycline. *Chest* 99:1040, 1991.
84. Credle WF, Smiddy JF, Elliott RC: Complications of fiberoptic bronchoscopy. *Am Rev Respir Dis* 109:67, 1974.
85. Suratt PM, Smiddy JF, Gruber B: Deaths and complications associated with fiberoptic bronchoscopy. *Chest* 69:747, 1976.
86. Pereira W, Kovnat DM, Khan MA, et al: Fever and pneumonia after flexible fiberoptic bronchoscopy. *Am Rev Respir Dis* 112:59, 1975.
87. Burman SO: Bronchoscopy and bacteremia. *J Thorac Cardiovasc Surg* 40:635, 1960.
88. Everett ED, Hirschmann JV: Transient bacteremia and endocarditis prophylaxis: A review. *Medicine* 56:61, 1977.
89. Kane RC, Cohen MH, Fossieck BE Jr, et al: Absence of bacteremia after fiberoptic bronchoscopy. *Am Rev Respir Dis* 111:102, 1975.
90. Albertini RE, Harrell JH, Kurihara N, et al: Arterial hypoxemia induced by fiberoptic bronchoscopy. *Chest* 65:117, 1974.
91. Shrader DL, Lakshminarayan S: The effect of fiberoptic bronchoscopy on cardiac rhythm. *Chest* 73:821, 1978.
92. Lundgren R, Haggmark S, Reiz S: Hemodynamic effects of flexible fiberoptic bronchoscopy performed under topical anesthesia. *Chest* 82:295, 1982.
93. Luck JC, Messeder OH, Rubenstein MJ, et al: Arrhythmias from fiberoptic bronchoscopy. *Chest* 74:139, 1978.
94. Sahn SA, Scoggin C: Fiberoptic bronchoscopy in bronchial asthma: A word of caution. *Chest* 69:39, 1976.
95. Salisbury BG, Metzger LF, Altose MD, et al: Effect of fiberoptic bronchoscopy on respiratory performance in patients with chronic airways obstruction. *Thorax* 30:441, 1975.
96. Perry LB: Topical anesthesia for bronchoscopy. *Chest* 73 (suppl):691, 1978.
97. Chinn WM, Zavala DC, Ambre J: Plasma levels of lidocaine following nebulized aerosol administration. *Chest* 71:346, 1977.
98. Reichert WW, Hall WJ, Hyde RW: A simple disposable device for performing fiberoptic bronchoscopy on patients requiring continuous artificial ventilation. *Am Rev Respir Dis* 109:394, 1974.

13. Methods of Obtaining Lower Respiratory Tract Secretions in Pneumonia

Richard S. Irwin

Ideally, patients with bacterial pneumonia should be treated with an effective, narrow-spectrum antibiotic. The drug should be selected based on identification of the causative organism. Although blood, pleural fluid, open thoracotomy, and percutaneous needle lung aspiration cultures are all generally accepted as standards that yield accurate diagnostic information, physicians must frequently rely on the results of analyses of lower respiratory tract secretions (sputum). Sputum may be obtained by indirect and direct approaches. The indirect approach, exemplified by expectorated sputum, tracheal suction, wire brushing under direct vision through a flexible fiberoptic bronchoscope (WBB), and bronchoalveolar lavage (BAL), samples sputum that passes through the upper airway (larynx and above). The direct approach, exemplified by transtracheal aspiration (TTA) and percutaneous needle aspiration, samples sputum that does not pass through the upper airway. While percutaneous needle aspiration cultures are referred to throughout this chapter, this technique is not discussed in great detail because it is not commonly employed for cultures in adults.

Indirect Methods

EXPECTORATED SPUTUM. Although many physicians reflexively order and make therapeutic decisions on the basis of routine expectorated sputum analysis, data on its reliability are conflicting and confusing. A routine sputum culture is one in which a specimen has been expectorated into a container, transported to the laboratory after a variable period of time, and then plated on culture media without undergoing dilution or homogenization. The portion to be cultured is chosen in the laboratory. It is uniformly agreed that expectorated sputum should not be routinely cultured in anaerobic pulmonary infections, since it invariably is contaminated by indigenous anaerobic mouth and oropharyngeal flora [1]. There is uncertainty about the accuracy of expectorated sputum analysis in aerobic pulmonary infections, also. Pecora and Yegian [2] compared cultures of expectorated sputum with those obtained at thoracotomy; Lees and McNaught [3] and Laurenzi et al. compared expectorated sputum cultures with direct bronchoscopy cultures [4]. All concluded that contamination of expectorated sputum by aerobic pharyngeal organisms occurs readily, and that the bacteriologic flora of the expectorated sputum may not reflect the nature of the bronchial flora. In patients with bacteremic pneumococcal pneumonia, correlation between expectorated sputum and blood cultures has varied from poor to excellent. In three representative articles showing poor correlation, pneumococci were not found in routine expectorated sputum cultures an average of 45 percent of the time [5,6,7]. In addition, another potential pathogen was found 27 percent of the time [7]. On the other hand, in 13 patients with pneumococcal pneumonia diagnosed by TTA, Thorsteinsson et al. grew the pneumococcus as the predominant organism in all routine expectorated sputum cultures [8]. They grew other potential pathogens also in 33 percent of the same patients. Thorsteinsson et al. concluded that their routine expectorated sputum specimens were accurate because they personally collected, streaked, and read their own cultures.

To improve the results of routinely processed expectorated sputum, special manipulations and techniques have been tried. By using special culture techniques (mouse inoculation and anaerobic incubation for pneumococci), several workers have improved correlation between expectorated sputum and blood cultures, identifying the pneumococcus in 83 to 97 percent of cultures [5,9,10]; however, expectorated sputum cultures still grew a significant number of other pathogens. Homogenization of sputum has been advocated to overcome the problem of missing the causative organism because of its uneven distribution in the specimen. To assess the usefulness of homogenized expectorated sputum specimens quantitatively cultured in acute pneumonia after initiation of therapy, serial expectorated sputum and TTA cultures were compared [11]. While the lower respiratory tract became sterile after initiation of antibiotic therapy as assessed by serial TTA cultures, expectorated sputum cultures continuously grew large concentrations of *Staphylococcus aureus* and various facultative gram-negative bacilli. Using quantitative bacteriology, Hahn and Beaty compared homogenized expectorated sputum and TTA cultures and concluded that the cause of pneumonia could not be predicted based on the colony counts of potential pathogens isolated from expectorated sputum [12]. Only 45 percent of their patients with pneumococcal pneumonia, diagnosed by TTA and clinical data, had pneumococci in their expectorated sputum. On the other hand, by washing macroscopically purulent or mucoid expectorated sputum in addition to culturing it quantitatively, Bartlett and Finegold found an excellent correlation between expectorated sputum and TTA cultures [13].

Data on the usefulness of the expectorated sputum Gram smear are also conflicting. Hahn and Beaty found that the Gram smear was not a reliable predictor of the cause of pneumonia [12]. Shulman et al. showed that even competent, conscientious physicians may miss the causative agent on routine expectorated sputum Gram smears [14]. Lepow et al. showed a poor correlation between expectorated sputum Gram smears and cultures [15]. For example, when gram-positive diplococci were seen, pneumococci grew only 50 percent of the time; when *Haemophilus influenzae* was not seen, it grew 65 percent of the time. On the other hand, when gram-positive, lancet-shaped diplococci were seen, Rein et al. were able to grow pneumococci 90 percent of the time [16]. In this study, a positive Gram stain was defined as one in which 10 or more gram-positive diplococci were seen in an oil immersion field in which squamous epithelial cells were absent. Geckler et al. recently reported that in approximately 50 percent of cases of pneumonia, Gram stain smear analyses of both TTA and expectorated sputum were inaccurate and led to the initial selection of inappropriate antibiotic therapy [17]. While interpretation of TTA data in this study is not possible because of methodologic inadequacies, expectorated sputum data revealed that Gram smear analysis of expectorated sputum is frequently inaccurate, even when interpreted by infectious disease specialists, and therefore may be unreliable in predicting the cause of lower respiratory tract infection [18].

To improve on the variable accuracy of routine expectorated sputum analysis without imposing on the clinical microbiology laboratory the time-consuming and cumbersome special techniques mentioned earlier, attempts have been made to define "good" expectorated sputum microscopically. Murray and Washington concluded retrospectively that when a purulent portion of expectorated sputum had less than 10 squamous epithelial cells per low-power field, it was as accurate as TTA cultures performed in their institution, since the average number of organisms isolated was similar for both methods (2.4 for TTA, 2.7 for expectorated sputum) [19]. Since their results also showed that the best expectorated sputum specimen was not necessarily the one with the greatest number of white blood cells but the one with the fewest squamous epithelial cells, VanScoy reanalyzed the same data [20]. After eliminating organisms that he considered unlikely to cause pneumonia in adults, VanScoy concluded that a "good" expectorated sputum sample had greater than 25 white blood cells per low-power field even if there were greater than 25 squamous epithelial

cells per low-power field. Geckler et al. prospectively compared TTA and "good" expectorated sputum in the same patients [21]. They defined a "good" expectorated sputum specimen as one with greater than 25 leukocytes and fewer than 10 squamous epithelial cells per low-power field. The results showed that a potential pathogen growing in one of these good specimens was predictive of the same growth in 94 percent of companion TTAs. If a potential pathogen did not grow in one of these specimens, expectorated sputum was false negative 45 percent of the time. Overall, the good expectorated sputum was not a reliable predictor 23 percent of the time. If the specimen was not good, its accuracy dropped dramatically.

Difficulties in diagnosing bacterial pneumonia by expectorated sputum culture have led to development of immunologic detection methods. Only a few studies have assessed the diagnostic reliability of the Quellung reaction of sputum or the detection of pneumococcal polysaccharide in sputum by counterimmunoelectrophoresis (CIE). In 21 cases of definite pneumococcal pneumonia (positive blood and pleural fluid cultures in 19 and 2, respectively) [22], CIE was positive in 81 percent and Quellung reaction in 86 percent. While these results are promising for diagnosing pneumococcal pneumonia, the specificity of these tests in patients merely colonized with pneumococci in the oropharynx is not known.

TRACHEAL SUCTION. Tracheal suction is another indirect means of sampling sputum. When orotracheal cultures in children were compared with direct lung aspirates, the orotracheal aspirate grew the causative organism 20 percent of the time [23]. Using cultures aspirated through a fiberoptic bronchoscope as an example of tracheal suction, Bartlett et al. found that specimens were uniformly contaminated by oropharyngeal organisms [24]. The bronchoscope had been passed through an endotracheal tube. In 16 patients without infection, 85 aerobes and anaerobes were isolated, an average of greater than 5 bacterial species per aspirate. In 7 additional patients with suspected lower respiratory tract infection who had companion TTAs, bronchoscopy aspirates yielded 7 of the 8 organisms present in the TTAs; however, they grew 23 other organisms also, many of which were potential pathogens. The authors concluded that fiberoptic bronchoscopy aspirates do not accurately reflect lower respiratory tract bacteriology.

In 31 clinically uninfected patients with lung cancer, Fossieck et al. compared fiberoptic bronchoscopy and TTA cultures [25]. In this study, the bronchoscope was passed transnasally. Potential pathogens were present in 87 percent of bronchoscopy aspirates but only 31 percent of companion TTAs. The results of cultures agreed completely in only one instance. These data led the authors to state that cultures of washings or secretions obtained by routine fiberoptic bronchoscopy provide inaccurate and clinically confusing information about the presence and types of bacteria in the lower respiratory tract.

Although the detection of antibody-coated bacteria in lower respiratory tract secretions obtained by tracheal suction has been used to distinguish pneumonia from colonization, this test cannot identify specific organisms [26].

WIRE BRUSHING AT TIME OF BRONCHOSCOPY. Over the past 21 years, a variety of wire brushing methods have been studied. The earlier brushes were passed within open-ended catheters; those being used and studied today are passed in telescoping plugged catheters. Wanner et al. were among the first to evaluate lower respiratory tract secretions obtained by wire sampling through a fiberoptic bronchoscope [27]. The instrument was passed through a nasopharyngeal airway, however secretions were not suctioned but obtained under direct vision by passing a wire loop contained in a sterile polyethylene catheter. In vitro experiments designed to mimic passage through the upper respiratory tract failed to demonstrate contamination of the catheter—wire loop system. Consequently, wire loop cultures were compared with expectorated sputum and nasopharyngeal cultures in 38 patients with respiratory tract infections and in 41 with noninfectious lung disorders. On the basis of isolating fewer organisms from bronchi compared with tracheae and upper respiratory tracts, Wanner et al. concluded that the bronchoscope-catheter-wire loop system prevents contamination from regions through which the bronchoscope has previously passed. Pecora also compared the results of bronchoscopy and TTA cultures in 44 patients with infectious and noninfectious pulmonary disorders [28]. Bronchoscopy cultures were obtained with the use of a rigid bronchoscope and a catheter arrangement similar to that of Wanner. Specimens were handled only aerobically. The TTA cultures were rarely contaminated and correlated well with the diagnoses, whereas bronchoscopy cultures were more frequently contaminated.

Irwin et al. evaluated the relative sensitivity of cultures obtained by TTA, WBB, and expectorated sputum in localized pulmonary infections by comparing each method with percutaneous lung aspiration (PLA) cultures, an accepted standard, in patients with peripheral lung abscesses [29]. Lung abscess (the end result of a necrotizing pneumonia) abutting the chest wall was used as an example of a localized pulmonary infection, since gross pus could be aspirated safely and easily through the chest wall. This experimental design theoretically eliminated the possibility of the causative organism(s) being unevenly distributed in the localized infections. Wire brush cultures were obtained under direct vision through a fiberoptic bronchoscope with a sterile, open-ended polyethylene catheter with retracted wire brush. Only macroscopically mucopurulent expectorated sputum was homogenized and then semiquantitatively cultured. Of the 27 organisms that PLA cultures isolated from 10 lung abscesses (8 aerobic, 2 anaerobic), TTA identified 81 percent plus an additional 5 and WBB identified 68 percent plus 16. Of the 14 organisms that PLA cultures isolated from 8 aerobic abscesses, TTA identified 93 percent plus an additional 2, WBB identified 83 percent plus 12, and expectorated sputum identified 71 percent plus 19. From a laboratory standpoint, the authors concluded the following: (1) when PLA cultures cannot be obtained, the most accurate method for determining the cause of a localized pulmonary infection is TTA, followed by WBB and then expectorated sputum; and (2) since TTA generates false negative and false positive information, it may not be an appropriate standard by which to evaluate other methods, such as expectorated sputum.

Wimberly et al. developed another WBB method, which employed a wire brush retracted in telescoping cannulas with a distal occlusion [30]. This has become known as the protected brush catheter (PBC) method of sampling lower respiratory tract secretions. Although this closed-end brush-in catheter system appeared to be superior to the open-end brush-in catheter systems in minimizing contamination from upper airway secretions in the inner channel of the bronchoscope [31,32], false positive information was still generated [33]. Presumably, the contaminating bacteria were aspirated into the lower respiratory tract during anesthesia or bronchoscopy or were brought to the lower respiratory tract by the bronchoscope or outer wall of the catheter. Bass and Pollock believed that careful quantitative bacteriology could distinguish contamination from infection in the closed-end catheter system [34]. Following the publication of their article, a number of studies have been published assessing the role of PBC quantitative cultures in diagnosing

the etiology of acute bacterial pneumonia in immunocompetent, spontaneously breathing and mechanically ventilated patients. In these studies, more than 10^3 colony-forming units (cfu) per milliliter was defined as significant (causative) bacterial growth.

In multiple studies published on spontaneously breathing humans with acute bacterial pneumonia using PBC quantitative cultures, the etiologic diagnosis of pneumonia has been from 50 to 96 percent, with the majority in the 70- to 90-percent range [35].

In diagnosing nosocomial pneumonia in mechanically ventilated patients [36], sensitivity and specificity of PBC quantitative cultures have ranged from 60 to 100 percent. A study in a primate model of pneumonia showed that cultures using the PBC system with quantitative bacteriology identified the causative pathogen in 70 percent of animals and generated 10 percent false positives [37].

While the PBC quantitative culture method has achieved popularity, especially in diagnosing pneumonia in patients on mechanical ventilation, it has important limitations that should preclude its uniform and reflex acceptance as a consistently accurate method. It can generate false positive results in 32 to 58 percent of cases and false negative information from 16 to 33 percent [38]. Since it can provide only cultural, not direct smear, data, it can yield results only after a delay of 24 to 48 hours. It involves bronchoscopy, an invasive procedure, with its attendant costs and complications (e.g., hypoxemia, arrhythmias, transient worsening of pulmonary infiltrates) [36]. Finally, a recent study revealed that the diagnostic threshold of greater than 10^3 cfu per milliliter that has been recommended to diagnose the presence of bacterial pneumonia may not be as reliable as was previously thought. Its repeatability can vary in 59 percent of patients by more than $1 \log_{10}$ [38]. In this study, 25 pecent of isolates had results on each side of the 10^3 cfu per milliliter threshold point. This variability was probably due to inhomogeneity of bacterial concentrations in lower respiratory tract secretions and/or variability in the volume of secretions sampled.

BRONCHOALVEOLAR LAVAGE. Since BAL theoretically samples a larger and more representative amount of lower respiratory tract secretions than PBC and provides a sufficient sample to do smears for rapid identification as well as culture, it has been evaluated as an alternative or complementary method to PBC with quantitative cultures. However, the role of BAL with quantitative bacteriology in diagnosing the etiology of pneumonia has not yet been clearly defined. While some studies have shown results similar to PBC with quantitative bacteriology [38,39,40], others have revealed poor correlation [41]. Differences in these studies probably relate to technical issues concerning the BAL procedure, sample processing, and use of different diagnostic thresholds of bacterial growth that have varied from greater than 10^3 to 10^5 cfu per milliliter [36,39]. Investigators have also begun to evaluate the usefulness of Gram stain analysis of BAL fluid. Limited data show that with a cutoff of greater than 7 percent of BAL cells containing intracellular bacteria to identify patients with pneumonia, Gram smear had a sensitivity of 86 percent and a specificity of 96 percent [42].

In a few studies, when expectorated sputum culture has been negative, BAL has been useful in diagnosing *Legionella pneumophila* by culture and direct fluorescent antibody examination and *Mycobacterium tuberculosis* [36]. In diagnosing *Mycobacterium tuberculosis* by bronchoscopy, BAL has a higher yield than bronchial washing and postbronchoscopy sputum cultures

[36]. In patients with miliary tuberculosis, BAL cultures were positive in 100 percent while sputum cultures were positive in 25 percent [36].

While quantitative cultures of transbronchial needle aspirates, another method, offer no advantage to PBC quantitative cultures in diagnosing pneumonia [35], it is too soon to assess the role of three newer methods (e.g., nonbronchoscopic BAL, nonbronchoscopic protected BAL, and bronchoscopic protected BAL) [36]. The ongoing search for an accurate and safe method of sampling lower respiratory tract secretions attests to the fact that such a method has yet to be identified.

Direct Methods

TRANSTRACHEAL ASPIRATION. There are a number of different ways to sample directly lower respiratory tract secretions (transthoracic needle aspiration, lung biopsy, and TTA). Pecora first described TTA, in 1959 [43]. The technique has since been modified slightly and performed by piercing the cricothyroid membrane rather than the membranous trachea below the cricoid cartilage; consequently, it may be more accurate to call the procedure translaryngeal aspiration rather than transtracheal aspiration.

In general, the literature concerning the accuracy of TTA sputum analysis in characterizing lower respiratory tract bacteriology is less conflicting than that on expectorated sputum and tracheal suction. Using transthoracic needle aspiration culture as a standard for comparison in 16 patients with pneumococcal pneumonia, Tempest et al. found that the homologous-type pneumococcus was present in 94 percent of companion TTAs [10]. Other potential pathogens were isolated in 6 instances. Although Davidson et al. found that TTA did not reflect the bacteriology of the transthoracic aspiration standard any better than did special expectorated sputum cultures, TTA gave false positive results much less frequently [44]. By comparing TTA with blood culture data in 23 patients with bacteremic pneumonia, Bartlett isolated the same bacterial species in 100 percent of TTAs [45]. In addition, 7 TTAs grew other potential pathogens. Correlation of TTA cultures in clinical diagnoses in 488 instances in this retrospective study showed that the incidence of false positives was 21 percent. In patients receiving no prior antibiotic, the incidence of false negatives was 1 percent. Using PLA cultures as a standard for comparison in 10 patients with peripheral lung abscesses, Irwin et al. prospectively determined the relative accuracy of TTA compared with WBB and expectorated sputum cultures [29]. Of these, TTA was found to be the most accurate sampling method (see above). This study was remarkable for controlling TTA against oropharyngeal contamination that might occur during the procedure.

Other studies have been used to support the accuracy of TTA analysis. Patients with bacterial pneumonia who have been treated solely on the basis of TTA culture results have uniformly done well [11,12,46,47]. Since anaerobes, with few exceptions, are not present in TTA specimens in normal subjects and in patients with chronic bronchitis [1], TTA has been found to be very useful in diagnosing anaerobic bronchopulmonary infection [47]. In normal subjects and in patients with nonbacterial pulmonary disease, TTA cultures have been sterile [46]. Although normal individuals have been shown to aspirate pharyngeal secretions during sleep [48], this sterility has been explained by the fact that pulmonary defense mechanisms efficiently clear and detoxify inhaled bacteria [49].

Limited data concerning TTA Gram smears show them to be accurate in predicting bacteriologic diagnoses in greater than 90 percent of instances [47].

Though TTA in large series of patients has been associated with low morbidity and no mortality [12,28,46,50,51,52], isolated case reports have described life-threatening complications and death [53,54,55]. Partly because of these reports and the development of the PBC quantitative culture method, TTA is infrequently performed today. An in-depth discussion of the complications and contraindications of TTA and a detailed description of the procedure is found in Irwin [56].

PERCUTANEOUS NEEDLE ASPIRATION AND OPEN LUNG BIOPSY. Unless gross fluid is obtained by percutaneous needle aspiration (e.g., sampling a lung abscess [29]), the causative organisms of an infiltrate may not be obtained because they are unevenly distributed in the infectious process. Because of this limitation and the more than modest complication rate (Chap. 77), percutaneous needle aspiration should be used only in carefully selected patients. Though open lung biopsy is the most definitive method of identifying the cause(s) of a pulmonary infection, it is associated with modest morbidity and rare mortality. Moreover, the additional information gained over less invasive procedures, primarily in immunocompromised hosts, frequently makes no difference in patient outcome (Chap. 77). Consequently, open lung biopsy also should be used only in carefully selected patients.

Conclusions

FROM A LABORATORY STANDPOINT. Controversy and conflict surround methods of sampling sputum. Routine expectorated sputum analysis is generally reliable in lower respiratory tract infections when the isolated organism cannot be considered an oropharyngeal contaminant (e.g., *Mycobacterium tuberculosis*). In other instances, routinely handled expectorated sputum is frequently inaccurate. By microscopically screening expectorated sputum and processing only "good" specimens, the inaccuracy of routine cultures may possibly be minimized. The accuracy of expectorated sputum cultures can be improved by using special techniques, but false positive information is still frequently generated. Expectorated sputum must be swarming with a morphologically distinct organism for Gram smears to be predictive of subsequent cultures. These comments also apply to tracheal suction and WBB analyses with an open-end catheter system. The use of TTA diminishes the deficiencies of expectorated sputum, tracheal suction, and WBB analyses with an open-end catheter system. In the nonintubated and nontracheotomized patient, TTA and bronchoscopy using PBC with quantitative bacteriology are the most accurate methods; by extrapolation of data, they appear to give similar results. In the intubated and mechanically ventilated patient, bronchoscopy using PBC with quantitative bacteriology using the greater than 10^3 cfu per milliliter [38] threshold and bronchoscopy BAL with quantitative culture (using the greater than 10^5 cfu/ml threshold [38]) are most accurate. Although TTA and bronchoscopy PBC and BAL using quantitative bacteriology generate the least false positive and false negative information, they still have these shortcomings and should not be used as standards for comparing other methods.

FROM A CLINICAL STANDPOINT. While the more invasive procedures are more likely to yield more accurate bacteriologic results, the most important issues are when and in whom are the costs of TTA, PBC, and BAL procedures worth the benefit. Are they, or any sampling method, significantly better from clinical standpoints than empiric antibiotic therapy? Until a prospective study designed to evaluate cost-benefit endpoints in a large group of patients with pneumonia is undertaken, the role of the more invasive methods in the evaluation of lower respiratory tract infections will remain controversial.

References

1. Bartlett JG, Rosenblatt JE, Finegold SM: Percutaneous transtracheal aspiration in the diagnosis of anaerobic pulmonary infection. *Ann Intern Med* 79:535, 1973.
2. Pecora DV, Yegian D: Bacteriology of the lower respiratory tract in health and chronic diseases. *N Engl J Med* 258:71, 1958.
3. Lees AW, McNaught W: Bacteriology of lower respiratory tract secretions, sputum and upper respiratory tract secretions in "normals" and chronic bronchitis. *Lancet* 2:1112, 1959.
4. Laurenzi GA, Potter RT, Kass EH: Bacteriologic flora of the lower respiratory tract. *N Engl J Med* 265:1273, 1961.
5. Rathbun HK, Govani I: Mouse inoculation as a means of identifying pneumococci in the sputum. *Johns Hopkins Med J* 120:46, 1967.
6. Fiala M: A study of the combined role of viruses, mycoplasmas and bacteria in adult pneumonia. *Am J Med Sci* 257:44, 1969.
7. Barrett-Connor E: The nonvalue of sputum culture in the diagnosis of pneumococcal pneumonia. *Am Rev Respir Dis* 103:845, 1971.
8. Thorsteinsson SB, Musher DM, Fagan T: The diagnostic value of sputum culture in acute pneumonia. *JAMA* 233:894, 1975.
9. Drew WL: Value of sputum culture in diagnosis of pneumococcal pneumonia. *J Clin Microbiol* 6:62, 1977.
10. Tempest B, Morgan R, Davidson M, et al: The value of respiratory tract bacteriology in pneumococcal pneumonia among Navajo Indians. *Am Rev Respir Dis* 109:577, 1974.
11. Benner EJ, Munzinger JP, Chan R: Superinfections of the lung: An evaluation by serial transtracheal aspirations. *West J Med* 121:173, 1974.
12. Hahn HH, Beaty HN: Transtracheal aspiration in the evaluation of patients with pneumonia. *Ann Intern Med* 72:183, 1970.
13. Bartlett JG, Finegold SM: Bacteriology of expectorated sputum with quantitative culture and wash technique compared to transtracheal aspirates. *Am Rev Respir Dis* 117:1019, 1978.
14. Shulman JA, Phillips IA, Petersdorf RG: Errors and hazards in the diagnosis and treatment of bacterial pneumonias. *Ann Intern Med* 62:41, 1965.
15. Lepow ML, Balassanian N, Emmerich J, et al: Interrelationships of viral, mycoplasmal and bacterial agents in uncomplicated pneumonia. *Ann Rev Respir Dis* 97:533, 1968.
16. Rein MF, Gwaltney JM, O'Brien WM, et al: Accuracy of Gram's stain in identifying pneumococci in sputum. *JAMA* 239:2671, 1978.
17. Geckler RW, McAllister CK, Gremillion DH, et al: Clinical value of paired sputum and transtracheal aspirates in the initial management of pneumonia. *Chest* 87:631, 1985.
18. Pratter MR, Irwin RS: Clinical value of the Gram-stain smear of respiratory secretions. *Chest* 88:163, 1985.
19. Murray PR, Washington JA: Microscopic and bacteriologic analysis of expectorated sputum. *Mayo Clin Proc* 50:339, 1975.
20. VanScoy RE: Bacterial sputum cultures: A clinician's viewpoint. *Mayo Clin Proc* 52:39, 1977.
21. Geckler RW, Gremillion DH, McAllister CK, et al: Microscopic and bacteriological comparison of paired sputa and transtracheal aspirates. *J Clin Microbiol* 6:396, 1977.
22. Perlino CA: Laboratory diagnosis of pneumonia due to *Streptococcus pneumoniae*. *J Infect Dis* 150:139, 1984.
23. Mimica I, Donoso E, Howard JE, et al: Lung puncture in the etiological diagnosis of pneumonia: A study of 543 infants and children. *Am J Dis Child* 122:278, 1971.
24. Bartlett JG, Alexander J, Mayhew J, et al: Should fiberoptic bronchoscopy aspirates be cultured? *Am Rev Respir Dis* 114:73, 1976.
25. Fossieck BE Jr, Parker RH, Cohen MH, et al: Fiberoptic bronchoscopy and culture of bacteria from the lower respiratory tract. *Chest* 72:5, 1977.
26. Wunderink RG, Russell GB, Mezgar E, et al: The diagnostic utility of the antibody-coated bacteria test in intubated patients. *Chest* 99:84-88, 1991.
27. Wanner A, Amikam B, Robinson MJ, et al: Comparison between the bacteriologic flora of different segments of the airways: Examination by bedside bronchofiberscopy. *Respiration* 30:561, 1973.
28. Pecora DV: A comparison of transtracheal aspiration with other methods of determining the bacterial flora of the lower respiratory tract. *N Engl J Med* 269:664, 1963.
29. Irwin RS, Garrity FL, Erickson AD, et al: Sampling lower respiratory tract secretions in primary lung abscess: A comparison of the accuracy of four methods. *Chest* 79:559, 1981.
30. Wimberly N, Faling LJ, Bartlett JG: A fiberoptic bronchoscopy technique to obtain uncontaminated lower airway secretions for bacterial culture. *Am Rev Respir Dis* 119:337, 1979.
31. Hayes DA, McCarthy LC, Friedman M: Evaluation of two bronchofiberscopic methods of culturing the lower respiratory tract. *Am Rev Respir Dis* 122:319, 1980.
32. Joshi JH, Wang K-P, DeJongh CA, et al: A comparative evaluation of two fiberoptic bronchoscopy catheters: The plugged telescoping catheter versus the single sheathed nonplugged catheter. *Am Rev Respir Dis* 126:860, 1982.
33. Halperin SA, Suratt PM, Gwaltney JM Jr, et al: Bacterial cultures of the lower respiratory tract in normal volunteers with and without experimental rhinovirus infection using a plugged double catheter system. *Am Rev Respir Dis* 125:678, 1982.
34. Bass JB Jr, Pollock HM: Use of the plugged double catheter system for obtaining bacterial cultures of the lower respiratory tract. *Am Rev Respir Dis* 126:939, 1982.
35. Lorch DG Jr, John JF Jr, Tomlinson JR, et al: Protected transbronchial needle aspiration and protected specimen brush in the diagnosis of pneumonia. *Am Rev Respir Dis* 136:565, 1987.
36. Meduri GU, Baselski V: The role of bronchoalveolar lavage in diagnosing nonopportunistic bacterial pneumonia. *Chest* 100:179, 1991.
37. Higuchi JH, Coalson JJ, Johanson WG Jr: Bacteriologic diagnosis of nosocomial pneumonia in primates: Usefulness of the protected brush specimen brush. *Am Rev Respir Dis* 125:53, 1982.
38. Marquette CH, Herengt F, Mathieu D, et al: Diagnosis of pneumonia in mechanically ventilated patients:repeatability of the protected specimen brush. *Am Rev Respir Dis* 147:211, 1993.
39. Rankin JA: Getting the bugs out of BAL. *Chest* 100:1, 1991.
40. Torres A, De La Bellacasa JP, Xaubert A, et al: Diagnostic value of quantitative cultures of bronchoalveolar lavage and telescoping plugged catheters in mechanically ventilated patients with bacterial pneumonia. *Am Rev Respir Dis* 140:306, 1989.
41. Chastre J, Fagon J-Y, Soler P, et al: Diagnosis of nosocomial bacterial pneumonia in intubated patients undergoing ventilation: Comparison of the usefulness of bronchoalveolar lavage, and the protected specimen brush. *Am J Med* 85:499, 1988.
42. Chastre J, Fagon J-Y, Soler P, et al: Quantification of BAL cells containing intracellular bacteria rapidly identifies ventilated patients with nosocomial pneumonia. *Chest* 95 (suppl):191S, 1989.
43. Pecora DV: A method of securing uncontaminated tracheal secretions for bacterial examination. *J Thorac Surg* 37:653, 1959.
44. Davidson M, Tempest B, Palmer DL: Bacteriologic diagnosis of acute pneumonia: Comparison of sputum, transtracheal aspirates and lung aspirates. *JAMA* 235:158, 1976.
45. Bartlett JG: Diagnostic accuracy of transtracheal aspiration bacteriologic studies. *Am Rev Respir Dis* 115:777, 1977.
46. Kalinske RW, Parker RH, Brandt D, et al: Diagnostic usefulness and safety of transtracheal aspiration. *N Engl J Med* 276:604, 1967.
47. Reis K, Levison ME, Kaye D: Transtracheal aspiration in pulmonary infection. *Arch Intern Med* 133:453, 1974.
48. Huxley EJ, Viroslav J, Gray WR, et al: Pharyngeal aspiration in normal adults and patients with depressed consciousness. *Am J Med* 64:564, 1978.
49. Green GM, Jakab GJ, Low RB, et al: Defense mechanisms of the respiratory membrane. *Am Rev Respir Dis* 115:479, 1977.

50. Pratter MR, Irwin RS: Transtracheal aspiration: Guidelines for safety. *Chest* 76:518, 1979.
51. Pratter MR, Pape LA, Irwin RS: The effect of transtracheal aspiration on cardiac rate and rhythm: A prospective study. *Chest* 80:439, 1981.
52. Pecora DV: Bronchofiberscopy. *Am Rev Respir Dis* 111:887, 1975.
53. Schillaci RF, Iacovoni VE, Conte RS: Transtracheal aspiration complicated by fatal endotracheal hemorrhage. *N Engl J Med* 295:488, 1976.
54. Unger KM, Moser KM: Fatal complication of transtracheal aspiration. *Arch Intern Med* 132:437, 1973.
55. Parsons GH, Price JE, Auston PW: Bilateral pneumothorax complicating transtracheal aspiration. *West J Med* 125:73, 1976.
56. Irwin RS: Methods of sampling lower respiratory tract secretions in pneumonia, in Rippe JM, Irwin RS, Alpert JS, Fink MP (eds). *Intensive Care Medicine*. 2nd ed. Boston, Little, Brown, 1991, pp 140–148.

14. Thoracentesis

Donna R. Grogan and Richard S. Irwin

Thoracentesis is an invasive procedure that involves the introduction of a trocar, needle, or cannula into the pleural space for the removal of accumulated fluid or air. Since it was first described in 1852 [1], thoracentesis, which does not involve thoracotomy, has been frequently performed by physicians at all levels of training. Despite approximately 130 years of combined medical and surgical experience with the procedure, not until recently have a few prospective studies critically evaluated the clinical value and complications associated with it [2,3,4]. Most studies concerning thoracentesis have dealt with the interpretation of the pleural fluid analyses [5].

Indications

Thoracentesis may be performed for diagnostic and/or therapeutic reasons. Diagnostic thoracentesis should be performed to obtain a sample of pleural fluid for gross, microscopic, and laboratory analysis whenever a pleural effusion of unknown etiology is recognized. Analysis of pleural fluid has been shown to yield clinically useful information in greater than 90 percent of cases [3]. To avoid confusion in interpreting laboratory results, the procedure should be performed, whenever possible, before any treatment has been given. The four most common diagnoses for symptomatic (cough, dyspnea, or chest pain) and asymptomatic pleural effusions are malignancy, congestive heart failure, parapneumonia, and postoperative sympathetic effusions [6]. A recommended diagnostic algorithm for evaluation of a pleural effusion of unknown etiology is presented in Figure 14-1 [6]. In patients whose pleural effusion remains undiagnosed after thoracentesis and closed pleural biopsy, thoracoscopy should be considered for visualization of the pleura and directed biopsy. Thoracoscopy has provided a positive diagnosis in 80.3 pecent of patients with recurrent pleural effusions not diagnosed by repeated thoracentesis, pleural biopsy, or bronchoscopy [7].

Therapeutic thoracentesis is indicated to remove fluid or air that is causing cardiopulmonary embarrassment. When performed for recurrent malignant pleural effusion, it should be followed by chest tube drainage with instillation of a sclerosing agent (Table 14-1) [8]; when performed for a tension pneumothorax or a pneumothorax that is slowly enlarging, it must be followed by chest tube placement (see Chap. 11).

Thoracentesis should not be performed to determine whether fluid is present; that must be known before performing the procedure. Although history (pleuritic pain) and physical findings (dullness to percussion, decreased breath sounds, and decreased vocal fremitus) suggest that an effusion is present, chest radiograph or ultrasonic examination is essential to confirm the clinical suspicion (Chap. 70).

Contraindications

Absolute contraindications to performing a thoracentesis include (1) an uncooperative patient, (2) inability to clearly identify the top of the rib under the percutaneous puncture site, (3) lack of expertise in performing the procedure, and (4) presence of a coagulation abnormality that cannot be corrected. Relative contraindications to a thoracentesis include all clinical settings in which a risk of a complication from the procedure may be potentially catastrophic for the patient, which might include (1) an area where known bullous lung disease exists, (2) a patient on positive end-expiratory pressure (PEEP), (3) a patient who has only one lung (the other having been surgically removed), and (4) a patient with a markedly elevated left hemidiaphragm, splenomegaly, and pleural effusion on the left. In these settings, it may be safer to perform the thoracentesis under ultrasonic guidance.

Table 14-1. Sclerosing Technique for Managing Malignant Pleural Effusions*

1. Completely drain the pleural space with a chest tube; connect the tube to water-sealed drainage with a pressure of −15 to −20 cm water for 24 hours or until drainage is complete.
2. Once drainage is complete, instill a solution of doxycycline (1 gram) or bleomycin (60 units) through the tube into the pleural space.
3. To facilitate the contact of the sclerosing agent with all pleural surfaces, instill 200 ml of air, clamp the tube, and rotate the patient in right and left lateral decubitis, prone, and supine positions for intervals of 3 minutes each.
4. With the tube clamped, rotate the patient again in the same four positions, but for 30-min intervals.
5. At the end of 2 hours, reconnect the chest tube to water-sealed drainage with negative pressure.
6. Remove the tube when drainage is <150 ml/24 hr; it may need to remain in place for 48–72 hr after instillation.

*This technique is a modification of that reported by Good and Sahn [8] in which they achieved an 80% success rate in preventing the reaccumulation of a malignant effusion. Doxycycline or bleomycin or another sclerosing agent (e.g., talc) must be used rather than tetracycline since injectable tetracycline is no longer available in the U.S.

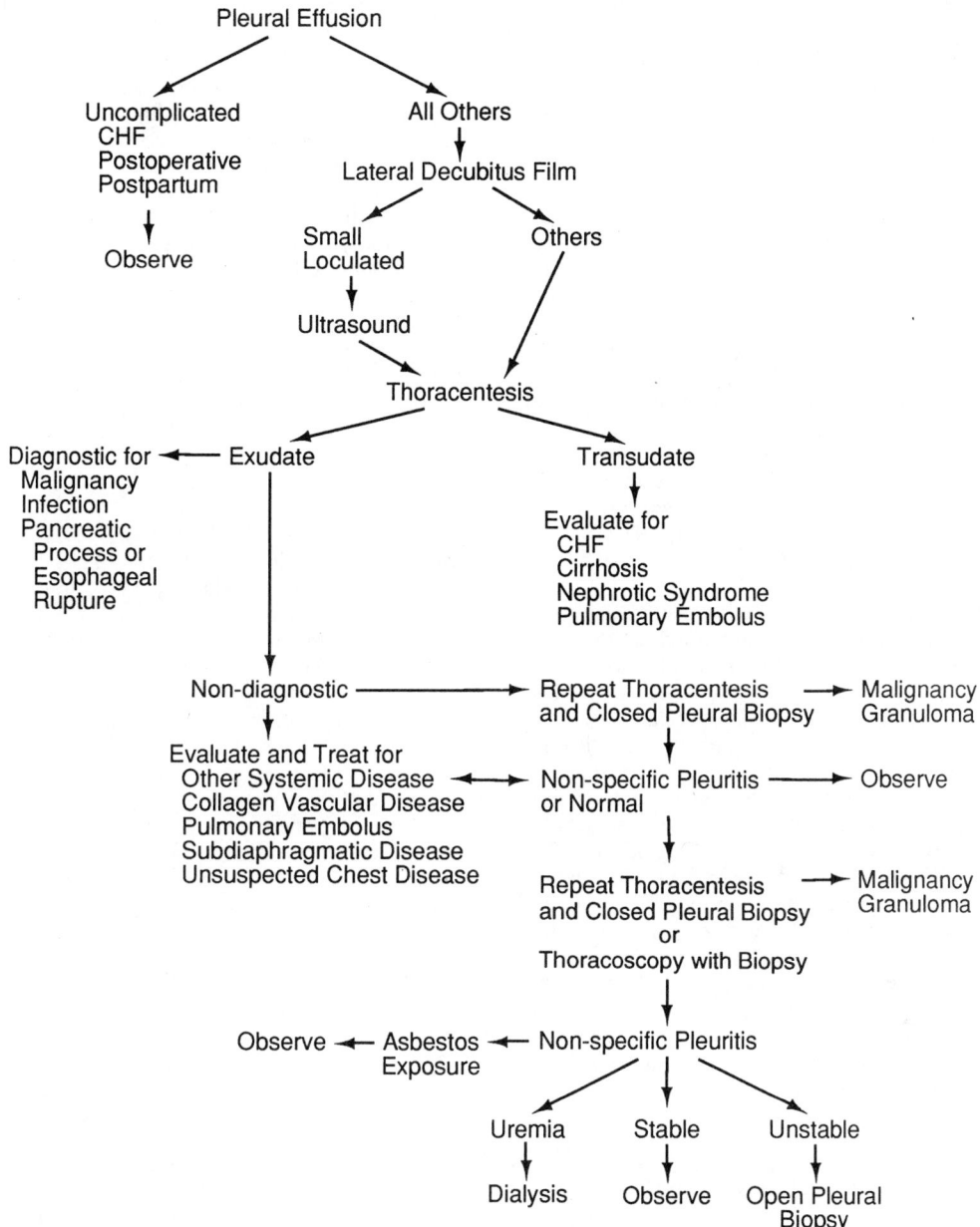

Fig. 14-1. Diagnostic algorithm for evaluation of pleural effusion. (Adapted from Smyrnios NA, Jederlinic PJ, Irwin RS: Pleural effusion in an asymptomatic patient: Spectrum and frequency of causes and management considerations. *Chest* 97:192, 1990.)

Complications

It has been assumed that thoracentesis is a relatively uncomplicated, low-risk procedure that is well tolerated [9]. However, a number of recent prospective studies have documented that complications associated with the procedure are not infrequent [2,3] and that the method by which thoracentesis is performed can significantly influence the spectrum and frequency of these complications [4]. The overall complication rate has been reported to be as high as 50 to 78 percent and can be further categorized as major (15–19%) or minor (31–63%) [3,4]. Although death due to the procedure is infrequently reported, complications may often be life-threatening [2,10].

Major complications include pneumothorax, hemopneumothorax, hemorrhage, hypotension, and reexpansion pulmonary edema. The rate of pneumothorax varies depending on the method used, ranging from 0 to 3 percent for sonographically localized and performed procedures and 19 to 39 percent for clinically localized and performed procedures [4,11]. There is no difference in pneumothorax rate for clinically localized and performed procedures as compared with sonographically localized but clinically performed taps [11,12]. However, the pneumothorax rate of clinically localized and performed procedures differs depending on the type of equipment used (20% for needle only, 20-gauge, 1.5 inches; and 39% for needle catheter, 16-gauge catheter inserted through a 14-gauge needle) [4]. Although pneumothorax is most commonly due to laceration of lung parenchyma, room air may enter the pleural space if the thoracentesis needle is open to room air when the patient takes a deep breath (intrapleural pressure will be subatmospheric). The pneumothorax may be small and asymptomatic, resolving spontaneously, or large and associated with respiratory compromise, requiring chest tube drainage. Hemorrhage can occur from laceration of an intercostal artery or inadvertent puncture of the liver or spleen, even if coagulation studies are normal. The risk of intercostal artery laceration is greatest in the elderly because of increased tortuosity of the vessels [13]. This complication is potentially lethal, and open thoracotomy may be required to control the bleeding.

Hypotension may occur during the procedure (as part of a vasovagal reaction) or hours after the procedure (most likely due to reaccumulation of fluid from intravascular space). Hypotension in the latter setting responds to volume expansion. It can usually be prevented by limiting pleural fluid drainage to 1 liter or less. High-protein, noncardiogenic, unilateral pulmonary edema may also occur due to lung reexpansion [14]. Although its frequency is not known, it is more likely to occur the longer an effusion has been present before evacuation and when larger amounts of fluid are removed [15].

Other major complications are rare and include implantation of tumor along the needle tract of a previously performed thoracentesis [16], venous and cerebral air embolism [17,18], and inadvertent placement of a sheared catheter into the pleural space [2].

Minor complications include dry tap or insufficient fluid, pain, subcutaneous hematoma or seroma, anxiety, dyspnea, and cough. Reported rates for these minor complications range from 16 to 63 percent and depend on the method used to perform the procedure, with higher rates associated with the needle-catheter technique [3,4]. Dry tap and insufficient fluid are technical problems and expose the patient to increased risk of morbidity related to the need to perform a repeat thoracentesis. Under these circumstances, it is recommended that the procedure be repeated under direct sonographic guidance. Pain may originate from parietal pleural nerve endings from inadequate local anesthesia [19], inadvertent scraping of rib periosteum, or piercing an intercostal nerve during a misdirected needle thrust. Anxiety is commonly associated with thoracentesis (up to 21% of procedures [3]) and can be minimized by proper patient positioning, description of the procedure to the patient, and proper technique. Coughing may occur when a large effusion is evacuated, perhaps due to stimulation of pleural and/or airway cough receptors [20].

Procedure

GENERAL CONSIDERATIONS. The most common techniques for performing thoracentesis are catheter-through-needle, needle only, and needle under direct sonographic guidance. Theoretically, the catheter-through-needle technique has been thought to be safest, for a number of reasons: (1) the risk of pneumothorax should be minimized since a needle is in the pleural space for an extremely short period of time; (2) laceration of subdiaphragmatic structures should be totally avoided by introducing a catheter through a needle well above the diaphragm and by directing the catheter downward; (3) as long as freely moving fluid or air is present, the catheter procedure should be 100 percent successful since the patient can be easily and safely maneuvered, with no discomfort, into a position that will allow the catheter to assume an optimal sampling location; and (4) removal of large effusions should be easy for the operator [21].

However, a recent prospective randomized study comparing these three techniques revealed that the risk of pneumothorax is significantly greater with the catheter-through-needle tech-

nique compared with the needle only or sonography guided needle. The procedures were performed by house officers in training on cooperative patients with free-flowing effusions, predominantly for diagnostic reasons [4]. Based on this information, we recommend the following. (1) All physicians-in-training who perform the procedure should attend a lecture stressing normal chest landmarks and observe a movie demonstrating the proper techniques on performing a thoracentesis. (2) When the procedure is indicated for diagnosis, the procedure should be performed by direct sonographic guidance or needle-only methods, and the catheter-through-needle method should be avoided. (3) When a dry tap or inadequate fluid has complicated a procedure performed by needle only, the procedure should be repeated with direct sonographic guidance. (4) The catheter-through-needle method can be used for procedures performed for therapeutic reasons until future studies better evaluate its relative risk for this indication. Protocols for each procedure are outlined below.

CATHETER-THROUGH-NEEDLE TECHNIQUE FOR RE-MOVAL OF FREELY FLOWING FLUID

1. Describe the procedure to the patient and obtain written informed consent.
2. Although premedication for pain is rarely needed, a narcotic may be occasionally needed for spasmodic or uncontrollable cough, and 1 mg of subcutaneous atropine may be given to prevent a vasovagal episode.
3. Collect all items that will be needed for the thoracentesis (Table 14-2). Most commercially available kits contain many of these items.
4. With the patient sitting, arms at side, mark the tip of the scapula on the side to be tapped. This should define the eighth intercostal space and should be the lowest interspace that is punctured, unless it has been previously de-

Table 14-2. Thoracentesis Equipment

Purpose	Equipment
Skin preparation and local anesthesia	Sterile gloves
	Sterile drape
	Iodophor solution
	Sterile sponges
	Local anesthetic (2% lidocaine)
	Small needle (25-gauge)
	Large needle (18–22-gauge, 2 in. long)
	5-ml syringe for anesthesia
Thoracentesis	20-ml (2) or 50-ml (1) Luer-Lok syringes
	14-gauge needle with 16-gauge catheter (12 in. long) (American Pharmoseal Laboratories, Glendale, CA) or 20-gauge, 1.5-inch needle
	Three-way stopcock (1), 1-liter sterile container, connecting tubing
	Sterile clamp
	Adhesive tape
	Bandaid
Collection	15-ml red-top tubes (2)
	7-ml purple-top tubes containing EDTA (2)
	5-ml heparinized glass syringe (1) with iced-slush bag for transportation
	Sterile anaerobic transport media bottle (1)
	Heparin solution (1:1000) for cytology and cell block specimens
	Sterile tubes for routine aerobic, fungal, and TB cultures

EDTA = ethylenediaminotetraacetate.

termined by sonography that a lower interspace can be safely entered.

5. Whenever possible, position the patient in a comfortable position (Fig. 14-2), such as sitting and leaning forward over a pillow-draped, height-adjusted bedside table. The patient's arms should be crossed in front to elevate and spread the scapulae. An assistant should stand in front of the patient to prevent any unexpected movements.

6. Percuss the posterior chest to determine the highest point of the effusion. The interspace below this point should be entered in the posterior axillary line, unless it is below the eighth intercostal space. If it is, sonography should be performed to mark the fluid level and level of the diaphragm.

7. With a fingernail, gently mark the superior aspect of the rib in the posterior axillary line of the chosen interspace. (The inferior portion of each rib contains an intercostal artery and should be avoided.)

8. Cleanse the area with an iodophor and allow it to dry.

9. Wear sterile gloves and sterilely drape the area surrounding the puncture site. Handle all syringes with sterile technique.

10. Except for the instillation of local anesthesia (2% lidocaine) with a 25-gauge needle, the procedure should cause the patient little discomfort. After the superficial skin has been anesthetized, aim for the top of the rib with an 18- to 22-gauge needle, 2 inches long, and generously anesthetize the deeper soft tissues. Always aspirate through the syringe before instilling to ensure that the needle is not in a vessel or the pleural space. On reaching the rib, infiltrate along the superior and lateral aspects of the rib. Carefully aspirate through the syringe as the pleura is approached. (The rib is 1–2 cm wide.) Fluid will enter the syringe if the height of the fluid and the needle are at the same level.

11. Be careful not to instill anesthetic into the pleural space; it is bactericidal for most organisms, including *Mycobacterium tuberculosis* [22,23].

12. To prevent room air from entering the pleural space during the procedure, place the three-way stopcock on the 16-gauge catheter with the valve closed to the needle.

13. Insert the 14-gauge needle into the anesthetic tract with the bevel of the needle down. (A 14-gauge needle allows passage of a 16-gauge catheter; a smaller catheter might get kinked and bend on itself.) Put the catheter into the needle; the catheter should be several millimeters proximal to the end of the needle (Fig. 14-3A). After the needle is just past the superior surface of the rib, gently try to advance the catheter (Fig. 14-3B). It will not advance unless the parietal pleura has been punctured. Continue to advance the needle a few millimeters at a time, pausing only to try to advance the catheter gently. At the precise moment when the catheter begins to pass freely through the needle, the pleural space has been entered (Fig. 14-3C). At this juncture, direct the needle downward to ensure that the catheter descends to the most dependent area of the pleural space (Fig. 14-3D).

14. As the catheter is advanced forward in a single smooth motion, the needle is simultaneously pulled back out of the chest (Fig. 14-4).

15. Never pull the catheter back through the needle, since it may be sheared off by the needle.

16. Attach a 20- or 50-ml Luer-Lok syringe to the three-way stopcock, open the stopcock to the syringe, and aspirate. If fluid does not appear in the syringe, continue to reposition the patient, not the catheter, until the optimum fluid-catheter position is achieved.

17. Once fluid can easily be obtained, fill a heparinized glass syringe from the other side of the three-way stopcock and handle the specimen as an arterial blood gas sample; that

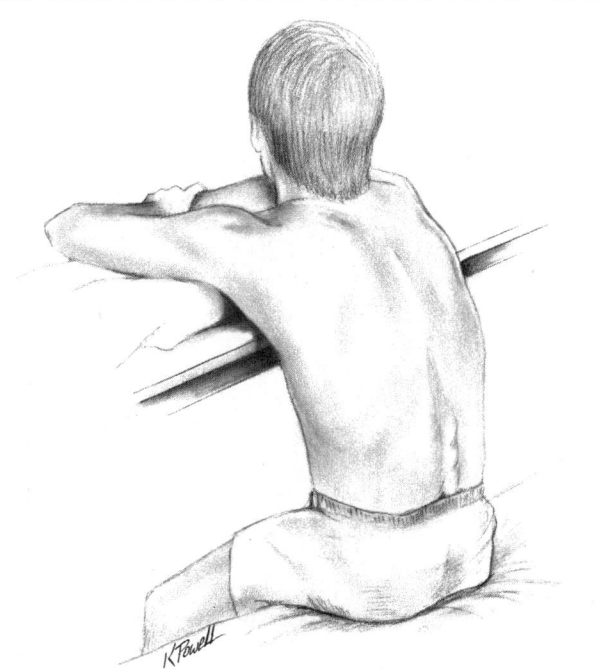

Fig. 14-2. Standard position for patient undergoing thoracentesis. The patient is comfortably positioned, sitting up and leaning forward over a pillow-draped, height-adjusted bedside table. The arms are crossed in front of the patient to elevate and spread the scapulae.

is, express all of the air bubbles and cork and place it in an iced-slush bag for immediate transportation.

18. Continue to refill the 20- or 50-ml syringe and transfer its contents into the appropriate collection tubes and containers.

19. To collect large amounts of fluid for cytology, cell block, or estrogen receptor analysis, add 10,000 units of heparin to the collection bag; attach the bag to the three-way stopcock with connecting tubing.

20. Fluid can be quickly aspirated and transferred into the bag by turning the three-way stopcock into appropriate positions.

21. After the thoracentesis has been completed, remove the catheter from the chest. Apply pressure to the wound for several minutes, then apply a sterile bandage.

22. Obtain a postprocedure expiratory chest radiograph to look for a pneumothorax.

23. Immediately after the procedure, draw venous blood for total protein, lactate dehydrogenase (LDH), and glucose determinations; draw arterial blood for pH study. These studies are necessary to interpret pleural fluid values (see the section on interpretation of pleural fluid analysis).

NEEDLE-ONLY TECHNIQUE FOR REMOVAL OF FREELY FLOWING FLUID

1. Follow steps 1 to 11 as described in the catheter-through-needle technique.

2. Once pleural fluid is aspirated through the needle used to anesthetize the tissue, and with the needle left in place, place a gloved finger at the point on the needle where it exits the skin, then remove the needle. This will estimate the required depth of insertion for the thoracentesis needle.

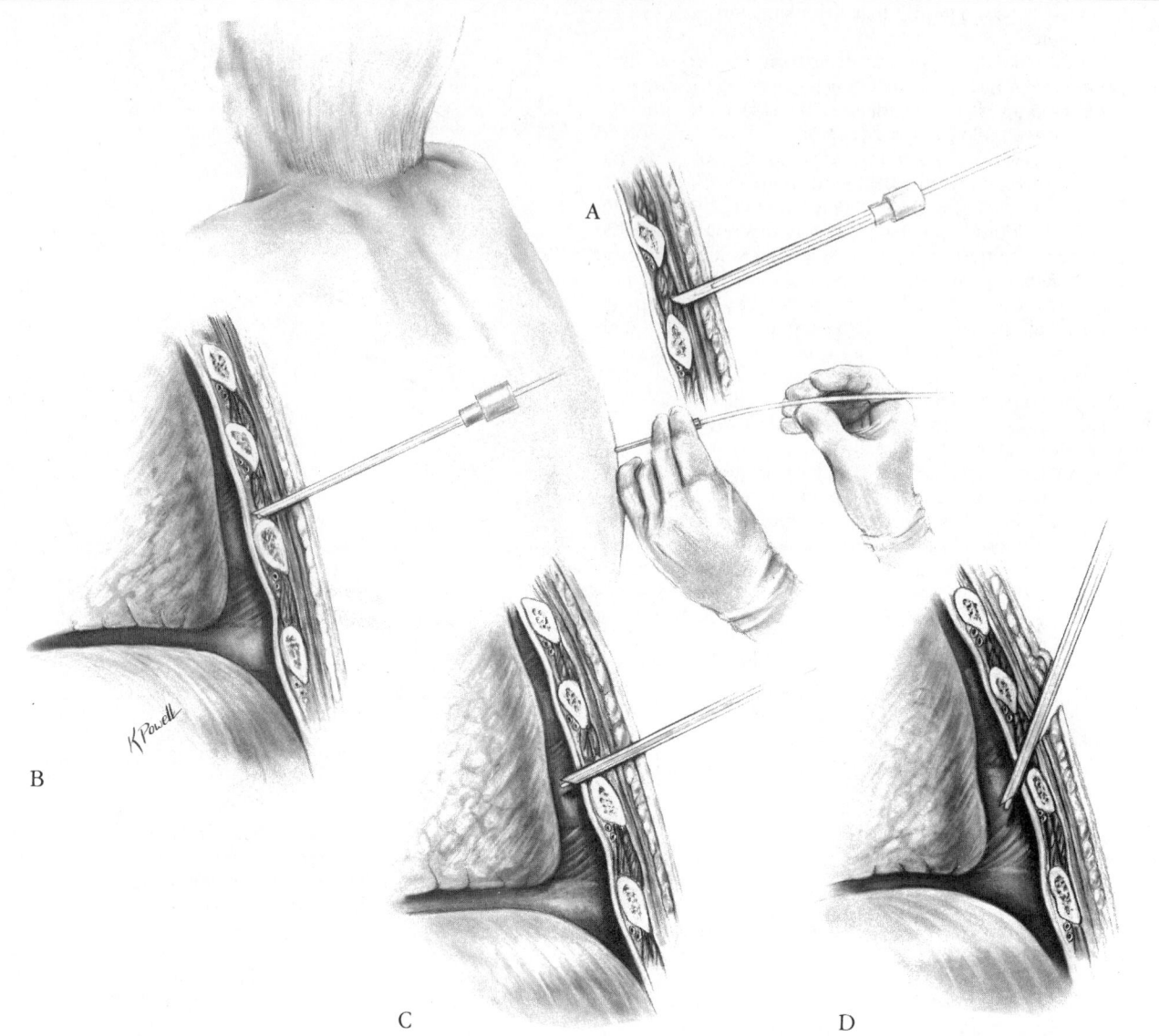

Fig. 14-3. Catheter technique for thoracentesis of freely flowing pleural field. A. A standard 14-gauge needle with 16-gauge catheter and three-way stopcock are used. After the needle has been inserted into the skin and soft tissue just above the rib, the catheter is placed into the needle several millimeters proximal to the tip of the needle. B. The catheter is gently advanced after the needle has crossed the surface of the rib. It will not advance if it meets the resistance of soft tissue. (The catheter is not forced into the soft tissue.) C. The needle is advanced several millimeters at a time only after attempts at passing the catheter have met with resistance. As soon as the parietal pleura has been punctured, the catheter will begin to advance easily. D. Before advancing the catheter any farther, the needle is directed downward.

3. Attach a three-way stopcock to a 20 gauge, 1.5-inch needle and attach a 50-ml syringe to the stopcock. The valve on the stopcock should be open to the needle to allow aspiration of fluid during needle insertion.

4. Insert the 20-gauge needle along the anesthetic tract. Slowly advance the needle through the subcutaneous tissue toward the pleura, always aspirating through the syringe. When pleural fluid is obtained in the syringe, stabilize the needle by attaching a clamp to the part of the needle that exits the skin. This will prevent further advancement of the needle into the pleural space.

5. When fluid can easily be obtained, fill a heparinized glass syringe from the other side of the three-way stopcock and handle the specimen as an arterial blood gas sample; that is, express all of the air bubbles and cork and place it in an iced-slush bag for immediate transportation.

6. Fill the 50-ml syringe, transferring its contents into the appropriate collection tubes and containers. One hundred milliliters should be ample fluid for diagnostic studies.

7. When the thoracentesis is complete, remove the needle from the chest. Apply pressure to the wound for several minutes, then apply a sterile bandage.

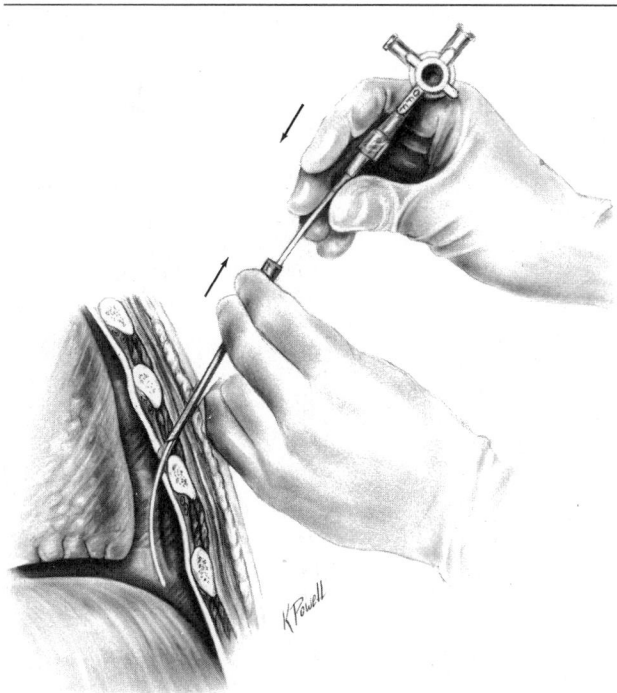

Fig. 14-4. The final step in removal of freely flowing pleural fluid. In rapid sequence, the catheter is advanced and the needle withdrawn from the chest.

8. Obtain a postprocedure expiratory chest radiograph to look for a pneumothorax.
9. Immediately after the procedure, draw venous blood for total protein, LDH, and glucose determinations; draw arterial blood for pH study. These studies are necessary to interpret pleural fluid values (see the section on interpretation of pleural fluid analysis).

NEEDLE WITH DIRECT SONOGRAPHIC GUIDANCE FOR REMOVAL OF FREELY FLOWING FLUID. A dynamic (real-time) sonographic scanner is used to document the pleural effusion fluid level as well as the depth of needle insertion necessary to enter the pleural space. The protocol is similar to that described above for the needle-only technique, but that the needle is inserted under direct sonographic guidance.

REMOVAL OF LOCULATED FLUID. To obtain pleural fluid successfully and minimize complications when the fluid is loculated, we believe the procedure should be performed with computerized tomography (CT) or under sonographic guidance or that the percutaneous insertion site should have been previously determined and marked during a CT scan or ultrasound examination. Although skin preparation, local anesthesia, and the procedure are generally carried out as enumerated above, the use of a catheter is optional in this setting.

REMOVAL OF FREELY MOVING PNEUMOTHORAX
1. Follow the same catheter protocol described above for removing freely moving fluid, but position the patient supine with the head of the bed elevated 30 to 45 degrees.
2. Prepare the second or third intercostal space in the anterior, midclavicular line (this will avoid hitting the more medial

internal mammary artery) for the needle and catheter insertion.
3. Have the bevel of the 14-gauge needle facing up and direct the needle upward so that the catheter can be guided toward the superior aspect of the hemithorax.
4. Air may be actively withdrawn by syringe or pushed out when intrapleural pressure is supraatmospheric (e.g., during a cough), as long as the catheter is intermittently open to the atmosphere. In the latter setting, air can leave but not reenter if the catheter is attached to a one-way valve apparatus (Heimlich valve) or if it is put to underwater seal (see Chap. 11).
5. When local anesthesia and skin cleansing are not possible because a tension pneumothorax is life-threatening, perform the procedure without them. If a tension pneumothorax is known to be present and a chest tube is not readily available, quickly insert a 14-gauge needle into the second anterior intercostal space. If a tension pneumothorax is suspected and a 14-gauge needle and 16-gauge catheter are handy, place the catheter according to the above technique to avoid puncturing the lung. If a tension pneumothorax is present, air will escape under pressure. When the situation has stabilized and the tension pneumothorax has been diagnosed, leave the needle or catheter in place until a sterile chest tube can be inserted.

Interpretation of Pleural Fluid Analysis

To determine the etiology of a pleural effusion, a number of tests on pleural fluid have been found to be helpful (Table 14-3). A two-stage laboratory approach to the evaluation of pleural effusion should be used [24]. The initial determination should be to classify the effusion as a transudate or an exudate using the following criteria.

Table 14-3. Helpful Tests in Determining Etiology of a Pleural Effusion

1. Biochemistry*
   a. LDH
   b. Total protein
   c. pH
   d. Amylase
   e. Glucose
   f. ± Triglyceride
   g. ± Cholesterol
2. Hematology
   a. Cell counts
   b. Differential
3. Microbiology
   a. Anaerobic and aerobic cultures
   b. Fungal and AFB cultures
   c. Gram and AFB stain
   d. ± Direct fluorescent antibody for *Legionella* species
4. Serology
   a. ± Cryptococcal antigen
   b. ± Rheumatoid factor
   c. ± Complement determinations
5. Pathology
   a. Cytology
   b. Cell block
   c. ± Estrogen receptors

*To interpret these pleural fluid tests, simultaneous blood values must also be obtained.
LDH = lactate dehydrogenase; AFB = acid-fast bacteria.

TRANSUDATE. A transudate is biochemically defined by meeting all of the following criteria: pleural fluid-to-serum total protein ratio less than 0.5; pleural fluid-to-serum lactate dehydrogenase (LDH) ratio less than 0.6; and absolute pleural fluid LDH less than 200 IU [25]. The former diagnostic criteria of pleural fluid specific gravity less than 1.015 or total protein less than 3.0 gm per deciliter are no longer used.

EXUDATE. An exudate is also biochemically defined by the following criteria [25]: protein ratio greater than 0.5, LDH ratio greater than 0.6, or pleural fluid LDH value greater than 200 IU. Only if all three biochemical criteria have not been met is it nearly 100 percent certain that one is dealing with a transudate (Table 14-4). If a transudate is present, then no further tests on pleural fluid are indicated [24] (Table 14-4). If an exudate is present, then further laboratory evaluation is warranted (Fig. 14-1). If the tests listed in Table 14-3 do not narrow the differential diagnosis, a percutaneous pleural biopsy should be performed [26,27]. Thoracoscopy-guided pleural biopsy should be considered in those patients with pleural effusion of unknown etiology despite the above-listed procedures [7].

pH. Pleural fluid pH determinations are diagnostically and therapeutically useful [28,29,30]. For instance, the differential diagnosis associated with a pleural fluid pH less than 7.2 is consistent with systemic acidemia, bacterially infected effusion (empyema), malignant effusion, rheumatoid or lupus effusion, tuberculous effusion, ruptured esophagus, noninfected parapneumonic effusion that needs drainage, and urinothorax [31,32]. Parapneumonic effusions with a pH less than 7.2 act similar to infected empyemas and require chest tube drainage for adequate resolution.

AMYLASE. A pleural fluid amylase level twice the serum level or an absolute value greater than 160 Somogyi units has been reported [33,34,35] with acute and chronic pancreatitis, pancreatic pseudocyst that has dissected or ruptured into the pleural space, primary and metastatic cancer, and esophageal rupture.

GLUCOSE. A low pleural fluid glucose value is defined as less than 50 percent of the serum value [5]. In this situation, the differential diagnosis includes rheumatoid and lupus effusion, infected nontuberculous bacterial empyema, malignancy, tuberculosis, and esophageal rupture [5, 36–40].

TRIGLYCERIDE AND CHOLESTEROL. Chylous pleural effusions are chemically defined by a triglyceride level greater than 110 mg per deciliter and the presence of chylomicrons on a pleural fluid lipoprotein electrophoresis [41]. The usual appearance of a chylous effusion is milky, but an effusion with elevated triglycerides may also appear serous [41]. The measurement of a triglyceride level is therefore important. Chylous effusions occur when the thoracic duct has been disrupted somewhere along its course. The most common causes are trauma and malignancy (e.g., lymphoma) [41]. A pseudochylous effusion appears grossly milky due to an elevated cholesterol level; the triglyceride level is normal [41]. Chronic effusions, especially those associated with rheumatoid and tuberculous pleuritis, are characteristically pseudochylous [41].

Table 14-4. Causes of Pleural Effusions

Transudates	Exudates
Congestive heart failure	Parapneumonic effusion (bacterial pneumonia)
Cirrhosis with ascites	Pulmonary infarction
Nephrotic syndrome	Malignancy (direct pleural involvement, late mediastinal involvement)
Hypoalbuminemia	Viral pneumonia
Peritoneal dialysis	Connective tissue disease (lupus, rheumatoid, mixed)
Atelectasis (acute)	Tuberculosis
Superior vena cava obstruction	Fungal disease
Subclavian catheter misplacement	Parasitic disease (*Entamoeba histolytica, Paragonimus westermani*)
Early mediastinal malignancy	Gastrointestinal disease (pancreatitis, esophageal rupture, subphrenic abscess)
Meigs syndrome	Drug reaction (nitrofurantoin, methysergide)
Urinothorax	Asbestos
	Meigs syndrome
	Postmyocardial infarction and postcardiac surgical operation
	Trapped lung
	Lymphatic abnormality
	Uremic pleurisy
	Atelectasis (chronic)
	Chylothorax
	Sarcoidosis
	Longstanding congestive heart failure
	Congestive heart failure after vigorous diuresis
	Hepatitis

Adapted from Sahn SA: The pleura. *Am Rev Respir Dis* 134:184, 1988. With permission [51].

CELL COUNTS AND DIFFERENTIAL. Although pleural fluid white blood cell count and differential are never diagnostic of any disease, it would be distinctly unusual for an effusion other than one associated with bacterial pneumonia to have a white blood cell count exceeding 50,000 per cubic millimeter [42]. In an exudative pleural effusion of acute origin, polymorphonuclear leukocytes predominate early, while mononuclear cells predominate in chronic exudative effusions. Although pleural fluid lymphocytosis is nonspecific, severe lymphocytosis (>80% of cells) plus less than 1 percent mesothelial cells is suggestive of tuberculosis [42,43]. Finally, pleural fluid eosinophilia is nonspecific [44,45,46].

Grossly bloody effusions (red blood count 5,000–10,000 cells/mm³ must be present for fluid to appear pinkish) containing greater than 100,000 red blood cells per cubic millimeter are most consistent with trauma, malignancy, or pulmonary infarction [42]. To distinguish a traumatic thoracentesis from a preexisting hemothorax, several observations are helpful [5]. First, because a preexisting hemothorax has been defibrinated, it will not form a clot on standing. Second, a traumatic thoracentesis is suggested when pleural fluid and blood hematocrit values match.

CULTURES AND STAINS. To maximize the yield from pleural fluid cultures, anaerobic as well as aerobic cultures should be obtained. If the sample of pleural fluid sent for culture is transported in an oxygen-free atmosphere (a capped glass syringe that has had all bubbles squirted out is all that is necessary), the microbiology laboratory can perform all necessary anaerobic, aerobic, fungal, and mycobacterial cultures and smears. Since acid-fast stains may be positive in 20 percent of tuberculous effusions [5], they should always be performed in addition to Gram smears. By submitting pleural biopsy pieces to both the pathology and microbiology laboratories, it is possible to diagnose up to 90 percent of tuberculous effusions percutaneously [25]. The value and yield of direct fluorescent antibody staining for *Legionella* species in pleural fluid is currently unknown.

SEROLOGY. Serologic tests on pleural fluid are of some diagnostic value. Positive cryptococcal antigen is consistent with cryptococcal pulmonary infection [47]. Since positive rheumatoid factors can be found in rheumatoid as well as nonrheumatoid effusions, a positive test should be interpreted only as being consistent with, not diagnostic of, a rheumatoid pleural effusion [37]. Since low pleural fluid complement levels can be seen in rheumatoid arthritis, systemic lupus erythematosus, malignancy, and infected pleural effusions, they are of limited value [48].

CYTOLOGY. Malignancies can produce pleural effusions by implantation of malignant cells on the pleura or impairment of lymphatic drainage secondary to tumor obstruction [49]. The tumors that most commonly cause pleural effusions are lung, breast, and lymphoma. Pleural fluid cytology should be performed for an exudative effusion of unknown etiology, using 100 to 200 ml of fluid. If initial cytology results are negative and strong clinical suspicion exists, additional samples of fluid can increase the chance of a positive result. In patients who are ultimately proved to have a malignancy as an etiology of their effusion, 59 percent have positive cytology on a single sample, 65 percent on the second sample, and 70 percent on the third sample. The addition of a pleural biopsy increases the positive results to 81 percent [50]. Heparin should be added to the container to prevent clotting of fluid. In addition to malignancy, cytologic examination can definitively diagnose rheumatoid pleuritis [52]. The pathognomonic picture [52] consists of slender, elongated macrophages and giant, round, multinucleated macrophages, accompanied by amorphous granular background material.

References

1. Bowditch HI: Paracentesis thoracis. *Am J Med Sci* 23:105, 1852.
2. Seneff MG, Corwin RW, Gold LH, et al: Complications associated with thoracentesis. *Chest* 89:97, 1986.
3. Collins TR, Sahn SA: Thoracentesis: Clinical value, complications, technical problems, and patient experience. *Chest* 91:817, 1987.
4. Grogan D, Irwin RS, Channick R, et al: Complications associated with thoracentesis: A prospective randomized study comparing three different methods. *Arch Intern Med* 150:873, 1990.
5. Sahn SA: The differential diagnosis of pleural effusions. *West J Med* 137:99, 1982.
6. Smyrnios NA, Jederlinic PJ, Irwin RS: Pleural effusion in an asymptomatic patient. Spectrum and frequency of causes and management considerations. *Chest* 97:192, 1990.
7. Kendall SWH, Bryan AJ, Large SR, Wells FC: Pleural effusions: Is thoracoscopy a reliable investigation? A retrospective review. *Respir Med* 86:437, 1992.
8. Good JT, Sahn SA: Intrapleural therapy with tetracycline in malignant pleural effusions. *Chest* 74:602, 1978.
9. Hall WJ, Mayerski RJ: Diagnostic thoracentesis and pleural biopsy in pleural effusions: Position paper. *Ann Intern Med* 103:799, 1985.
10. Capps JA: Air embolism versus pleural reflex as the cause of pleural shock. *JAMA* 109:852, 1937.
11. Raptopoulos V, Davis LM, Lee G, et al: Factors affecting the development of pneumothorax associated with thoracentesis. *Am J Roentgenol* 156:917, 1991.
12. Kohan JM, Poe RH, Isreal RH, et al: Value of chest ultrasonography versus decubitus roentgenography for thoracentesis. *Am Rev Respir Dis* 133:1124, 1986.
13. Carney PA, Ravin CE: Intercostal artery laceration during thoracentesis. *Chest* 75:520, 1979.
14. Marland AM, Glauser FL: Hemodynamic and pulmonary edema protein measurements in a case of re-expansion pulmonary edema. *Chest* 81:250, 1982.
15. Trapnell DH, Thurston JGB: Unilateral pulmonary edema after pleural aspiration. *Lancet* 1:1367, 1970.
16. Stewart BN, Block AJ: Subcutaneous implantation of cancer following thoracentesis. *Chest* 66:456, 1974.
17. O'Quinn JR, Lakshminarayan S: Venous air embolism. *Arch Intern Med* 142:2173, 1982.
18. Diamond S, Kaplitz S, Novick O: Cerebral air embolism as a complication of thoracentesis. *GP* 30:87, 1964.
19. Capps JA, Coleman GH: *An Experimental and Clinical Study of Pain in the Pleura, Pericardium and Peritoneum.* New York, MacMillan, 1932.
20. Irwin RS, Rosen MJ: Cough: A comprehensive review. *Arch Intern Med* 137:1186, 1977.
21. Gott PH: A simplified method for thoracentesis and pleural fluid drainage. *Am Rev Respir Dis* 92:295, 1965.
22. Kleinfeld J, Ellis PP: Inhibition of microorganisms by topical anesthetics. *Appl Microbiol* 15:1296, 1967.
23. Schmidt RM, Rosenkranz HS: Antimicrobial activity of local anesthetics: Lidocaine and procaine. *J Infect Dis* 121:597, 1970.
24. Peterman TA, Speicher CE: Evaluating pleural effusions: A two stage laboratory approach. *JAMA* 252:1051, 1984.
25. Light RW, MacGregor MI, Luchsinger PC, et al: Pleural effusions: The diagnostic separation of transudates and exudates. *Ann Intern Med* 77:507, 1972.
26. Levine H, Meteger W, Lacera D, et al: Diagnosis of tuberculous pleurisy by culture of pleural biopsy specimen. *Arch Intern Med* 126:269, 1970.
27. Salyer WR, Eggleston JC, Erozan YS: Efficacy of pleural needle biopsy and pleural fluid cytopathology in the diagnosis of malignant neoplasm involving the pleura. *Chest* 67:536, 1975.
28. Potts DE, Levin DC, Sahn SA: Pleural fluid pH in parapneumonic effusions. *Chest* 70:328, 1976.
29. Light R, Girard WM, Jenkinson SG, et al: Parapneumonic effusions. *Am J Med* 69:507, 1980.
30. Good JT, Taryle DA, Maulitz RM, et al: The diagnostic value of pleural fluid pH. *Chest* 78:55, 1980.
31. Stark DD, Shanes JG, Baron RL, et al: Biochemical features of urinothorax. *Arch Intern Med* 142:1509, 1982.
32. Sahn SA, Miller RS: Obscure pleural effusion: Look to the kidney. *Chest* 90:31, 1986.
33. Enide N: Studies of amylase activity in pleural fluid and ascites. *Cancer* 13:283, 1960.
34. Sherr HP, Light RW, Merson MH, et al: Origin of pleural fluid amylase in esophageal rupture. *Ann Intern Med* 76:985, 1972.
35. Light RW, Ball WC: Glucose and amylase in pleural effusions. *JAMA* 225:257, 1973.
36. Carr DT, Power MH: Pleural fluid glucose with special reference to its concentration in rheumatoid pleurisy with effusion. *Dis Chest* 37:321, 1960.
37. Good JT Jr, King TE, Sahn SE: Natural and drug-induced lupus pleuritis: A cause of low glucose-low pH pleural effusion. *Chest* 78:518, 1980.
38. Potts DE, Taryle DA, Sahn SA: The glucose-pH relationship in parapneumonic effusions. *Arch Intern Med* 138:1378, 1978.
39. Clarkson B: Relationship between cell type, glucose concentrations, and response to treatment in neoplastic effusions. *Cancer* 17:914, 1964.

40. Maulitz RM, Good JT Jr, Kaplan RL, et al: The pleuropulmonary consequences of esophageal rupture: An experimental model. *Am Rev Respir Dis* 120:363, 1979.
41. Staats BA, Ellefson RD, Budahn LL, et al: The lipoprotein profile of chylous and nonchylous pleural effusions. *Mayo Clin Proc* 55:700, 1980.
42. Light RS, Erozan YS, Ball WC: Cells in pleural fluid. *Arch Intern Med* 132:854, 1973.
43. Spriggs AI, Boddington MM: Absence of mesothelial cells from tuberculous pleural effusions. *Thorax* 15:169, 1960.
44. Campbell GD, Webb WR: Eosinophilic pleural effusion. *Am Rev Respir Dis* 90:194, 1964.
45. Bower G: Eosinophilic pleural effusion. *Am Rev Respir Dis* 95:746, 1967.
46. Deresinski SC, Leff A, Hopewell PC: Eosinophils, pleural effusions, and malignancy. *Ann Intern Med* 89:424, 1978.

47. Young EJ, Hirsh DD, Fainstein V, et al: Pleural effusions due to *Cryptococcus neoformans:* A review of the literature and report of two cases with cryptococcal antigen determinations. *Am Rev Respir Dis* 121:743, 1980.
48. Hunder GG, McDuffie FC, Hepper NGG: Pleural fluid complement in systemic lupus erythematosus and rheumatoid arthritis. *Ann Intern Med* 76:357, 1972.
49. Hausheer FH, Yarbro IW: Diagnosis and treatment of malignant pleural effusion. *Semin Oncol* 12:54, 1985.
50. Winkelman M, Pfitzer P: Blind pleural biopsy in combination with cytology of pleural effusions. *Acta Cytol* 25:373, 1981.
51. Sahn SA: The pleura. *Am Rev Respir Dis* 138:184, 1988.
52. Naylor B: The pathognomic cytologic picture of rheumatoid pleuritis. *J Clin Cytol Cytopathol* 34:465, 1990.

15. Arterial Puncture for Blood Gas Analysis

Richard S. Irwin

Analysis of a sample of arterial blood for pH_a carbon dioxide tension ($PaCO_2$), oxygen tension (PaO_2), bicarbonate, and percent oxyhemoglobin saturation is performed with a single laboratory test, arterial blood gas analysis (ABG). Since an ABG can be safely and easily obtained and furnishes rapid and accurate information on how well the lungs and kidneys are working [1,2,3], it is the single most useful laboratory test in managing patients with respiratory and metabolic disorders; moreover, since it is not possible to predict the level of PaO_2 and $PaCO_2$ reliably using physical signs of cyanosis [4] and depth of breathing [5], the ABG provides the most important way of making a diagnostic assessment of the nature, progression, and severity of a respiratory disturbance. Though the clinical evaluation will not be as reliable and accurate as an ABG in uncovering unsuspected hypoxemia and/or hypercapnia (acidemia), these blood gas derangements may cause a constellation of central nervous system and cardiovascular signs and symptoms (Table 15-1) that should provoke one to obtain an ABG. In other words, the clinician should have a high index of suspicion that a respiratory and/or metabolic disorder is present in patients with a wide variety of central nervous system and/or cardiovascular signs and symptoms. While acute hypercapnia to 70 mm Hg (pH 7.16) and acute hypoxemia to less than 30 mm Hg may lead to circulatory collapse and coma, chronic exposures permit adaptation with more subtle effects [7].

Normal values are as follows [6]: for pH_a the accepted range of two standard deviations is 7.35 to 7.45; for $PaCO_2$ the accepted range of two standard deviations is 35 to 45 mm Hg; for PaO_2 the accepted predictive regression equation in nonsmoking, upright normal individuals is $PaO_2 = 109 - (0.43 \times \text{age in years})$.

Historical Perspective

The ABG is a relatively recent addition to the diagnostic armamentarium. In 1947, Comroe and Botelho demonstrated that the clinical estimation of hypoxemia by observing cyanosis was unreliable [4]. In 1956, Clark invented the modern oxygen partial pressure tension (PO_2) electrode [8]. Sanz, in 1957, reintroduced [9] the modern capillary glass pH electrode invented in 1933 by McInnes and Belcher. That same year, Stow et al. invented the modern carbon dioxide partial pressure tension (PCO_2) electrode [10]. In 1962, Severinghaus discussed the state of the art of the electrodes for pH, PCO_2, and PO_2 and began clinical studies [11]. In 1966, Petty et al. demonstrated the simplicity and safety of arterial puncture performed by physicians [2]. In 1968, Mithoefer et al. reconfirmed by systematic demonstration that the clinical estimation of alveolar ventilation was unreliable [5]. In 1971, Sackner et al. demonstrated the simplicity and safety of arterial puncture performed by nurses [3].

Indications

An ABG analysis is indicated whenever there is a reason to rule in or out the presence of a respiratory or metabolic disturbance, and to assess the nature, progression, or severity of a respiratory or metabolic disorder.

Drawing the ABG Specimen

PERCUTANEOUS ARTERIAL PUNCTURE. The conventional technique of sampling arterial blood using a glass syringe is described in detail, since it is the standard to which all other methods are compared. Drawing arterial blood should be no more difficult than drawing venous blood. The vessel is easily palpated in most cases and entry is easily noted if a large enough needle is used, since the syringe is filled by the pressurized, pulsatile flow of blood. It is logical preferentially to enter arterial vessels that have the best collateral circulation, so that if spasm or clotting occurs the distal tissue will not be deprived of perfusion. Logic also dictates that puncture of a site

Table 15-1. Common Signs and Symptoms of Hypoxemia and Hypercapnia

Hypoxemia	Hypercapnia (acidemia)
Judgment and personality changes	Headache, confusion
	Dizziness
Confusion, stupor, coma	Somnolence to coma
Insomnia, restlessness, seizures	Papilledema, increased CSF pressure
Headache	
Tachycardia, bradycardia	Focal twitching, asterixis
Cardiac arrhythmias	Diaphoresis
Hypertension (systemic or pulmonary)	Systemic hypertension, pulmonary vascular hypertension
Hypotension	Hypotension (late)
Tachypnea, dyspnea	Cardiac failure

CSF = cerebrospinal fluid.
Source: Weiss EB, Faling LJ, Mintz S, et al: Acute respiratory failure in chronic obstructive pulmonary disease: I. Pathophysiology. *Disease-a-Month*, October 1969. Copyright © 1969 by Year Book Medical Publishers, Inc., Chicago. With permission.

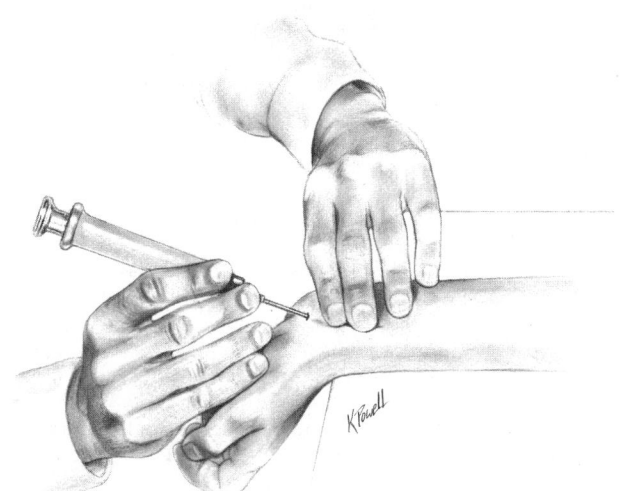

Fig. 15-1. Arterial puncture procedure. See text for description.

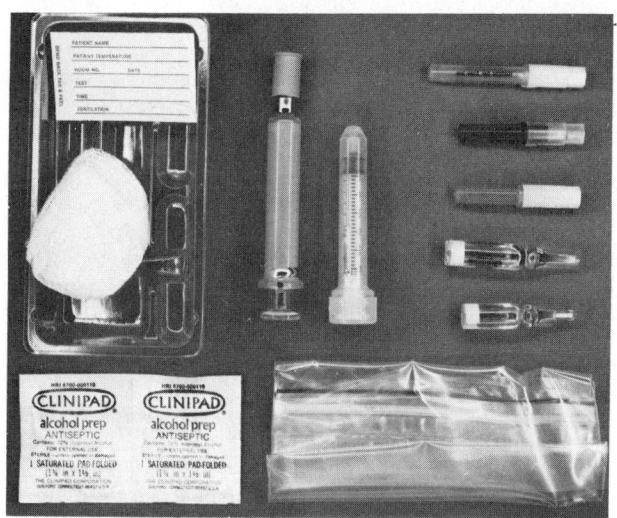

Fig. 15-2. A representative ABG kit. It should include 1% lidocaine, sodium heparin solution (1000 units/ml), 2 syringes (1 for lidocaine injection, 1 for blood sample), 22- and 25-gauge needles, alcohol wipes, sterile gauze, a bag of slush for transportation of the syringe with the blood sample, and a gummed information label.

where the artery is superficial is preferable, since that is where entry is easiest. This will also minimize pain. The radial artery best fulfills the above criteria; it is very superficial at the wrist, and the collateral circulation to the hand by the ulnar artery provides adequate blood flow in approximately 92 percent of normal adults in case of total occlusion of the radial artery [12]. The absence of a report of total occlusion of the radial artery following puncture for ABG in an adult with normal hemostasis not only attests to the safety of the percutaneous arterial puncture, but also suggests that it is probably not necessary routinely to check, prior to puncture, for the adequacy of the superficial palmar arch by Allen's test [13], a modification of Allen's test (Chap. 3) [14], or Doppler ultrasound [12]. If radial artery sites are not accessible, dorsalis pedis, posterior tibial, superficial temporal (in infants), brachial, and femoral arteries are alternatives (Chap. 3). Brachial and especially femoral artery punctures are contraindicated in patients with abnormal hemostatic mechanisms, because adequate vessel tamponade may not be possible, since these vessels are not located superficially. Moreover, any vessel that has been reconstructed surgically should not be punctured.

The syringe material may influence the results of PaO_2 [15,16,17]. The most accurate results have been consistently obtained using a glass syringe. Falsely low PaO_2 values may be obtained with plastic syringes, due to the diffusion of PaO_2 through plastic. This may become a significant problem only when blood specimens have PaO_2 values greater than 221 mm Hg. Because of their lower cost, many hospitals now predominantly use plastic syringes.

The conventional, recommended radial artery technique is as follows (Fig. 15-1).

1. Put protective gloves on and seat yourself in a comfortable position facing the patient. Open an ABG kit (Fig. 15-2).
2. With the patient's palm up, slightly hyperextend the wrist and palpate the radial artery. Severe hyperextension may obliterate the pulse.
3. Cleanse the skin with an alcohol swab.
4. With a 25-gauge needle, inject enough 1% lidocaine intradermally to raise a small wheal at the point where the skin puncture will be made. Although many physicians eliminate this step, I believe the local anesthetic makes subsequent needle puncture with a 22-gauge needle less painful and often painless. If local anesthesia is not given, however,

the potential pain and anxiety with concomitant hyperventilation and breath holding that might be associated with a percutaneous arterial puncture have not been shown to be real concerns. In 100 patients with an intraarterial catheter in place who had simultaneous sampling of arterial blood from the catheter and a percutaneous puncture without local anesthesia, there was no significant difference in blood gas values [18].

5. Attach a needle no smaller than a 22-gauge to a glass syringe that will accept 5 ml of blood.
6. Wet the needle and syringe with a sodium heparin solution (1000 units/ml). Express all of the excess.
7. With the needle, enter the artery at an angle of approximately 30 degrees to the long axis of the vessel. This insertion angle minimizes the pain due to inadvertently scraping the periosteum below the artery.

8. As soon as the artery is entered, blood will appear in the syringe. Allow the arterial pressure to fill the syringe with at least 3 ml of blood [19]. Do not apply suction by pulling on the syringe plunger.

9. Immediately after obtaining the specimen, squirt out any tiny air bubbles. To ensure that the specimen will be anaerobic when transported, cap the syringe by first removing the needle and then plugging the syringe with the rubber stopper found in most commercial blood gas kits. (By removing the needle, the blood gas technician will avoid the risk of inadvertently being stuck by it.) To avoid being stuck by the needle or being exposed to expelled blood, one of several ABG kits can be purchased that provide safeguards against these potential hazards.

10. Roll the blood sample between both palms for 5 to 15 seconds to mix the heparin and blood. Apply pressure to the puncture site for 5 minutes. If the arterial sample was obtained from the brachial artery, compress this vessel so that the radial pulse cannot be palpated.

11. Immerse the capped sample in a bag of ice and water (slush) and immediately transport it to the blood gas laboratory.

12. Write on the ABG slip the time of the drawing and the conditions under which it was drawn (e.g., fraction of inspired oxygen, ventilator settings, position of the patient).

Deviations from the recommended technique enumerated above may introduce errors as follows.

1. Plastic, not glass, syringes will allow oxygen to diffuse to the atmosphere from a sample with a high PO_2. In addition, plastic syringes tenaciously retain air bubbles unless extra effort is used to remove them [16]. Because these syringes may impede smooth filling, they usually require plunger assistance in collecting specimens. Consequently, there is not the reassurance that an artery, rather than a vein, has been sampled.

2. If suction is applied for plunger assistance, gas bubbles may be pulled out of solution. If they are expelled, measured tensions may be falsely lowered [20].

3. Dilution of blood by heparin solution does not affect the pH, but it does reduce the measured PCO_2 and calculated bicarbonate, in direct proportion to the amount of dilution [19,21]. The dilution error will be no greater than 4 percent if a glass syringe is only wetted with a 22-gauge needle and 3 to 5 ml of blood collected; the amount of heparin in this setting is approximately 0.2 ml. Although a new device avoids the dilutional heparin problem by employing crystalline heparin, clinical experience is insufficient to recommend it over the conventional technique [22,23].

4. If an ABG specimen is not analyzed within 1 minute of being drawn, or if it is not immediately cooled to 2°C, the PO_2 and pH will fall and PCO_2 will rise due to oxygen use by leukocytes, platelets, and reticulocytes. This can be troublesome in patients with leukemia and/or thrombocytosis [24].

5. Inadvertent sampling of a vein causes a falsely low PaO_2. Even a PO_2 greater than 50 mm Hg can be obtained from a vein. For example, arm vein PO_2 can approximate arterial PO_2 if flow is greatly increased by warming. Since oxygen consumption of the arm in this situation will not appreciably change, according to the Fick principle (Chap. 4), flow must increase by venous oxygen concentration approaching arterial. Using a large enough needle to allow the arterial pulse to fill the syringe provides reassurance that an artery, not a vein, has been sampled.

COMPLICATIONS. Using the conventional radial artery technique described above, complications are unusual. They include a rare vasovagal episode, local pain, and limited hematomas, occurring no more frequently than 0.58 percent of the time [1,2,3]. An expanding aneurysm of the radial artery has been reported even more rarely after frequent punctures [25].

CONTRAINDICATIONS. In patients with abnormal hemostasis, percutaneous puncture of any artery that is not superficial is contraindicated, due to the theoretically greater chance of complications [26]. If frequent sampling of superficial arteries in the same situation becomes necessary, arterial cannulation is advised (Chap. 3).

Measuring the ABG Specimen

Although most blood gas laboratories include pH, PCO_2, PO_2, bicarbonate, and percent oxyhemoglobin saturation values on their ABG reporting slip, it is important to know which values are actually measured. Those laboratories using Radiometer, Instrumentation Laboratory, and Corning machines actually measure pH, PCO_2, and PO_2. The bicarbonate and percent oxyhemoglobin saturation values are calculated. While the calculated bicarbonate value is as reliable as the pH and PCO_2 values, the calculated percent oxyhemoglobin saturation value is often inaccurate, due to the many unknown variables that cannot be corrected for (e.g., 2,3-DPG [diphosphoglycerate], binding characteristics of hemoglobin). By convention, arterial blood gas specimens are analyzed at 37°C.

Should blood gas measurements be corrected for the patient's temperature? Although no studies have demonstrated that this is clinically necessary, blood gases drawn at temperatures greater than 39°C should probably be corrected for temperature [27]. Because the solubility of oxygen and carbon dioxide increases as blood is cooled to 37°C, the hyperthermic patient is more acidotic and less hypoxemic than uncorrected values indicate. Therefore, for each 1°C that the patient's temperature is greater than 37°C, PaO_2 should be increased 7.2 percent, $PaCO_2$ increased by 4.4 percent, and pH decreased by 0.015. It is not necessary to correct the $PaCO_2$ and pH in the hypothermic patient [28], since acid-base changes in vivo parallel the changes of blood in vitro. However, PaO_2 values must be corrected for temperature or significant hypoxemia may be overlooked. The PaO_2 at 37°C is decreased by 7.2 percent for each degree that the patient's temperature is less than 37°C.

Physician Responsibility

Even when a laboratory has a good quality control program and the ABG values of pH, PCO_2, PO_2, and bicarbonate are reliable, the clinician should check the accuracy of the laboratory by periodically sending aliquots of arterial blood from the same specimen to the chemistry laboratory for a total CO_2 content and to the blood gas laboratory. The blood gas laboratory's values can be checked using Henderson's simple mathematical equation, which is a rearrangement of the Henderson-Hasselbalch equation [29]:

$$[H^+] = 25 \times PaCO_2/TCO_2$$

The accuracy of $PaCO_2$ is solved for by using the $[H^+]$ measured in the blood gas laboratory (Table 15-2) and the TCO_2 measured in the chemistry laboratory. The value solved for should be

Table 15-2. Relation Between pH and [H$^+$] Shown over a Small Range of Values*

pH	[H$^+$](nM/L)
7.36	44
7.37	43
7.38	42
7.39	41
7.40	40
—	—
7.41	39
7.42	38
7.43	37
7.44	36

*Note that pH 7.40 corresponds to hydrogen ion concentration of 40 nM/L and that each deviation in pH of 0.01 unit corresponds to opposite deviation in [H$^+$] of 1 nM/L. For pH values between 7.28 and 7.45, [H$^+$] calculated empirically in this fashion agrees with the actual value obtained by means of logarithms to the nearest nM/L (nearest 0.01 pH unit). Below pH 7.28 and above pH 7.45, the estimated [H$^+$] is always lower than the actual value, the discrepancy reaching 11 percent at pH 7.10 and 5 percent at pH 7.50.
Source: Kassirer JP, Bleich HL: Rapid estimation of plasma carbon dioxide tension from pH and total carbon dioxide content. Reprinted by permission of the *New England Journal of Medicine* 272:1067–1068, 1965.

close to that measured. Venous TCO$_2$ should not be used in this exercise, since it is often greater than arterial TCO$_2$.

Alternatives

Although little progress has been made in noninvasive pH measurement, there have been four important areas of technologic development: oximetry, transcutaneous PO$_2$ and PCO$_2$ gas measurements, expired PCO$_2$, and indwelling intravascular electrode systems. See Chapter 29 for further discussion.

References

1. Fleming WH, Bowen JC: Complications of arterial puncture. *Milit Med* 139:307, 1974.
2. Petty TL, Bigelow B, Levine BE: The simplicity and safety of arterial puncture. *JAMA* 195:181, 1966.
3. Sackner MA, Avery WG, Sokolowski J: Arterial punctures by nurses. *Chest* 59:97, 1971.
4. Comroe JH, Botelho S: The unreliability of cyanosis in the recognition of arterial anoxemia. *Am J Med Sci* 214:1, 1947.
5. Mithoefer JC, Bossman OG, Thibeault DW, et al: The clinical estimation of alveolar ventilation. *Am Rev Respir Dis* 98:868, 1968.
6. Raffin TA: Indications for arterial blood gas analysis. *Ann Intern Med* 105:390, 1986.
7. Weiss EB, Faling LJ, Mintz S, et al: Acute respiratory failure in chronic obstructive pulmonary disease, I: Pathophysiology. *Disease-a-Month* October 1969, 1.
8. Clark LC Jr: Monitor and control of blood and tissue oxygen tensions. *Trans Am Soc Artif Intern Organs* 2:41, 1956.
9. Sanz MC: Ultramicro methods and standardization of equipment. *Clin Chem* 3:406, 1957.
10. Stow RW, Baer RF, Randall BF: Rapid measurement of the tension of carbon dioxide in blood. *Arch Phys Med Rehabil* 38:646, 1957.
11. Severinghaus JW: Electrodes for blood and gas PCO$_2$, PO$_2$ and blood pH. *Acta Anaesth Scand* 11(suppl):207, 1962.
12. Felix WR Jr, Sigel B, Popky GL: Doppler ultrasound in the diagnosis of peripheral vascular disease. *Semin Roentgenol* 4:315, 1975.
13. Allen EV: Thromboangiitis obliterans: Methods of diagnosis of chronic occlusive arterial lesions distal to the wrist, with illustrative cases. *Am J Med Sci* 178:237, 1929.
14. Bedford RF: Radial arterial function following percutaneous cannulation with 18- and 20-gauge catheters. *Anesthesiology* 47:37, 1977.
15. Janis KM, Fletcher G: Oxygen tension measurements in small samples: Sampling errors. *Am Rev Respir Dis* 106:914, 1972.
16. Winkler JB, Huntington CG, Wells DE, et al: Influence of syringe material on arterial blood gas determinations. *Chest* 66:518, 1974.
17. Ansel GM, Douce FH: Effects of syringe material and needle size on the minimum plunger-displacement pressure of arterial blood gas syringes. *Respir Care* 27:147, 1982.
18. Glauser FL, Morris JF: Accuracy of routine arterial puncture for the determination of oxygen and carbon dioxide tensions. *Am Rev Respir Dis* 106:776, 1972.
19. Bloom SA, Canzanello VJ, Strom JA, et al: Spurious assessment of acid-base status due to dilutional effect of heparin. *Am J Med* 79:528, 1985.
20. Adams AP, Morgan-Hughes JO, Sykes MK: pH and blood gas analysis: Methods of measurement and sources of error using electrode systems. *Anaesthesia* 22:575, 1967.
21. Hansen JE, Simmons DH: A systematic error in the determination of blood PCO$_2$. *Am Rev Respir Dis* 115:1061, 1977.
22. Petty TL, Bailey D, Best C: A new device for arterial blood gas sampling. *JAMA* 239:2016, 1978.
23. Gayed AM, Marino ME, Dolanski EA: Comparison of the effects of dry and liquid heparin on neonatal arterial blood gases. *Am J Perinatol* 9:159, 1992.
24. Hess CE, Nichols AB, Hunt WB, et al: Pseudohypoxemia secondary to leukemia and thrombocytosis. *N Engl J Med* 301:361, 1979.
25. Mathieu A, Dalton B, Fischer JE, et al: Expanding aneurysm of the radial artery after frequent puncture. *Anesthesiology* 38:401, 1973.
26. Macon WL IV, Futrell JW: Median-nerve neuropathy after percutaneous puncture of the brachial artery in patients receiving anticoagulants. *N Engl J Med* 288:1396, 1973.
27. Curley FJ, Irwin RS: Disorders of temperature control, I: Hyperthermia. *J Intensive Care Med* 1:5, 1986.
28. Curley FJ, Irwin RS: Disorders of temperature control, III: Hypothermia. *J Intensive Care Med* 1:270, 1986.
29. Kassirer JP, Bleich HL: Rapid estimation of plasma carbon dioxide tension from pH and total carbon dioxide content. *N Engl J Med* 272:1067, 1965.

16. Tracheotomy

Wayne E. Silva and James Hughes

The term *tracheotomy*, derived from the Greek words *tracheia arteria* (rough artery) and *tome* (incision), refers to the operation that opens the trachea, resulting in the formation of a tracheostoma, or the opening itself. Tracheotomy was referred to by Galen in the second century and is reputed to have first been performed by Asclepiades in the first century B.C., but there is some evidence that it was practiced by the ancient Egyptians more than 3500 years ago [1,2]. The first surgical description of tracheotomy was that of the Italian physician Antonio Musa Brasavola, in approximately 1540. The procedure was done for an abscess of the windpipe, from which the patient recovered, following drainage. For the next 300 years tracheotomy fell into disfavor; Goodall could find detailed reports of only 28 successful tracheotomies over that period [3]. Tracheotomy regained approval in the early 1800s when used by Trousseau and Bretonneau in the management of diphtheria. In the early 1900s, Chevalier Jackson described refinements to the operation, particularly warning against high tracheotomy involving the cricothyroid membrane or the first tracheal ring because of the risk of injury to the cricoid cartilage and subsequent subglottic stenosis [4]. During this period, the procedure was used to treat difficult cases of respiratory paralysis from poliomyelitis. Largely because of improvements in tubes and advances in clinical care, endotracheal intubation gradually has become the treatment of choice for airway management [3,5]. Subglottic stenosis, caused by excessive pressure from the cuffs of endotracheal tubes, is relatively rare; nevertheless, other laryngeal problems, including permanent voice change, are recognized as potential sequelae of intubation. In view of these problems, and because patients increasingly require extended periods of airway management at many institutions, tracheotomy is performed more frequently today than just a few years ago. Since tracheotomy and other emergency surgical airways are occasionally required in critically ill and injured patients who cannot be intubated for various reasons (e.g., cervical spine injury, upper airway obstruction, laryngeal injury, anatomic considerations), the indications, contraindications, complications, and techniques associated with tracheotomy and other surgical airways should be familiar to all physicians involved in intensive care.

Indications

The indications for tracheotomy can be divided into three general categories: (1) to bypass obstruction of the upper airway, (2) to provide an avenue for tracheal toilet and removal of retained secretions, and (3) to provide a means for ventilatory support (Table 16-1).

TRACHEOTOMY TO BYPASS AIRWAY OBSTRUCTION

Laryngeal Dysfunction. Varying degrees of upper airway obstruction can result from vocal cord paralysis, particularly abductor paralysis from recurrent laryngeal nerve injury. Although cord paralysis (even if bilateral) may be tolerated at rest, increased activity or laryngeal edema from an upper respiratory tract infection can result in stridor or even complete obstruction [6].

Trauma. In the management of trauma, tracheotomy or cricothyrotomy may be necessary as an elective or emergent procedure. Oral or nasotracheal intubation may be impossible because of upper airway obstruction due to hemorrhage or edema or direct crush or transection injury to the larynx, or because mandibular fractures may result in lack of support for the glossal musculature. Cervical spine injury may preclude manipulation of the neck for orotracheal intubation. A fractured skull with cribriform plate involvement dictates against the use of nasotracheal intubation.

Burns and Corrosives. Inhalation of hot smoke, caustic gas, or corrosives may result in significant edema in the supraglottic larynx.

Foreign Bodies. Although most commonly seen in the pediatric age group, foreign body aspiration occasionally occurs in adults. Attempts to dislodge the bolus may be unsuccessful, necessitating bypass of the obstruction through tracheotomy.

Congenital Anomalies. Stenosis of the glottic or subglottic area is a well-recognized entity in the newborn. If the stenosis is significant, emergency tracheotomy may be required.

Infections. Bacterial or viral inflammation of the larynx may result in significant upper airway compromise. Croup, a laryngotracheitis of viral origin, presents in the pediatric age group. Epiglottitis, also primarily a childhood disease, is occasionally seen in adults, manifesting as increasing shortness of breath and stridor associated with severe sore throat and odynophagia (painful swallowing) [7,8]. Ludwig's angina and deep neck space infections can compromise the upper airway, necessitating tracheotomy.

Neoplasms. Neglected malignancies of the larynx may present with progressive upper airway obstruction. Such tumors are usually associated with a history of smoking and/or alcohol use. Although emergency tracheotomy should be avoided, it is occasionally necessitated by this type of obstruction.

Postoperative Airway Obstruction. Certain surgical procedures, such as surgery of the base of the tongue or hypopharynx, may require prophylactic tracheotomy in anticipation of progressive postoperative upper airway obstruction secondary to edema.

Obstructive Sleep Apnea. Patients with this syndrome present with daytime hypersomnolence and nocturnal insomnia. They are often obese and snore, usually loudly. Tracheotomy is curative because it bypasses the upper airway obstruction due to adipose tissue and/or pharyngeal and tongue muscle dysfunction [9,10,11]. Hypertrophied tonsils, nasopharyngeal tissues, and pharyngeal mucosa may cause a similar type of upper airway obstruction [6]. Tracheotomy may be used alone or in combination with other surgical procedures (nasal sep-

Table 16-1. Indications for Tracheotomy

1. Upper airway obstruction
   a. Laryngeal dysfunction
   b. Trauma
   c. Burns and corrosives
   d. Foreign bodies
   e. Congenital anomalies
   f. Infections
   g. Neoplasms
   h. Postoperative
   i. Obstructive sleep apnea
2. Tracheal toilet
   a. Old age
   b. Weakness
   c. Neuromuscular disease
3. Ventilatory support

toplasty, tonsillectomy, adenoidectomy, uvulopalatoplasty) to relieve the peripheral obstruction. See Chapter 58 for a comprehensive discussion of this disorder.

TRACHEOTOMY FOR TRACHEAL TOILET. Due to age, weakness, or neuromuscular disease, many patients are unable to clear secretions effectively and therefore require frequent suctioning. Tracheotomy provides an easy access to the lower airway. (See Chap. 69 for a complete discussion on augmentation of mucociliary clearance.)

TRACHEOTOMY FOR VENTILATORY SUPPORT. Ventilatory support is sometimes required for patients who cannot maintain adequate oxygen saturation or who have progressive carbon dioxide retention. While endotracheal intubation is usually the initial method of providing ventilatory support (see Chap. 1), tracheotomy is generally preferred for long-term management. Tracheotomy in chronic lung disease patients allows bypass of the non-gas-exchanging upper airway, reducing dead space ventilation [6]. Also, ventilator-dependent patients tolerate weaning from a tracheotomy tube better than from an endotracheal tube [12]. Tracheotomy is typically more comfortable than endotracheal intubation. Patients with a tracheotomy can eat normally (if they are awake and alert and have a functioning gastrointestinal tract), whereas endotracheal intubation precludes eating. Other advantages to tracheotomy over orotracheal intubation are that it facilitates safe patient mobility because it has a more secure tube and allows transfer of the patient from the intensive care unit (ICU) [13,14,15].

Special Considerations

PSYCHOLOGICAL FACILITATED CARE. A tracheotomy helps improve patients' psychoemotional state, as they are able to communicate their level of comfort. Tracheotomy also facilitates nursing care [13,16]. These factors should be considered when deciding whether to perform tracheotomy.

PREVENTION OF ASPIRATION. Though some physicians perform tracheotomy to prevent aspiration, it may actually cause aspiration [6] (see the section on dysphagia and aspiration). In general, tracheotomy to prevent aspiration is not recommended.

Contraindications

There are no absolute contraindications to tracheotomy, but certain conditions, such as anticoagulation and significant medical problems, warrant special attention prior to anesthesia and surgery.

Timing of Tracheotomy

When to convert from endotracheal tube to tracheotomy has been a matter of great controversy, with a range of 3 days to 3 weeks advised [13,17,18]. Eleven days seems to be an optimal time for conversion, but the decision is to be based on anticipated length of need for the mechanical airway [13,19]. Some reports have suggested that early tracheotomy (as early as within 72 hours of injury) is associated with a reduced incidence of pneumonia and should be performed in conjunction with percutaneous endoscopic gastrostomy (PEG) [20,21].

EMERGENCY TRACHEOTOMY. Emergency tracheotomy is a moderately difficult procedure, requiring training and skill; experience; adequate assistance, time, and lighting; and proper equipment and instrumentation [22]. When time is short, the patient uncooperative, the anatomy distorted, and the aforementioned requirements not met, tracheotomy can be very hazardous. Emergency tracheotomy can pose significant risk to nearby neurovascular structures, particularly in small children in whom the trachea is small and not well defined. The risk of complications for emergency tracheotomy is 2 to 5 times higher than for elective tracheotomy [23,24]. Nonetheless, there are occasional indications for emergency tracheotomy [25], including transected trachea; anterior neck trauma with crushed larynx [26]; and pediatric (younger than 12 years) patients requiring an emergency surgical airway, in whom cricothyrotomy is generally not advised.

TRACHEOTOMY IN THE INTENSIVE CARE UNIT. As many as 33 percent of critically ill ICU patients moved to other areas of the hospital for tests or procedures have significant and potentially dangerous physiologic changes [14,15,23]. While tracheotomy is best performed in the operating room, bedside tracheotomy can be performed safely [14,15,21] (complication rate 5–6%) under certain conditions (i.e., the patient is in the ICU; the patient is properly monitored and already intubated; the procedure is performed by an experienced surgeon with proper assistance, lighting, and equipment) [1].

Techniques

After an endotracheal intubation, the patient is properly positioned, with a large roll supporting the shoulders and the head and neck extended (Fig. 16-1). The area from the mandible to below the clavicles is prepared with an antiseptic solution, and the patient is sterilely draped. A local anesthetic, usually with epinephrine, is injected at the site of the anticipated incision. A 4- to 5-cm transverse incision is made approximately 1 fingerbreadth above the jugular notch of the sternum (Fig. 16-2). After the subcutaneous tissues have been transected and the bleeding is controlled, dissection is continued in the midline.

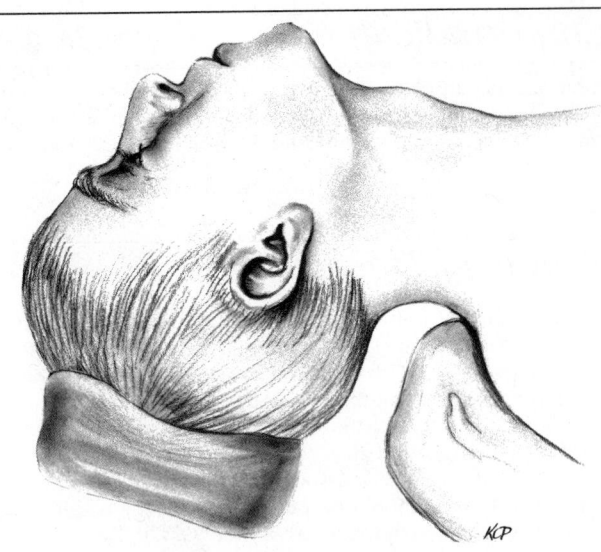

Fig. 16-1. Proper positioning for elective tracheotomy.

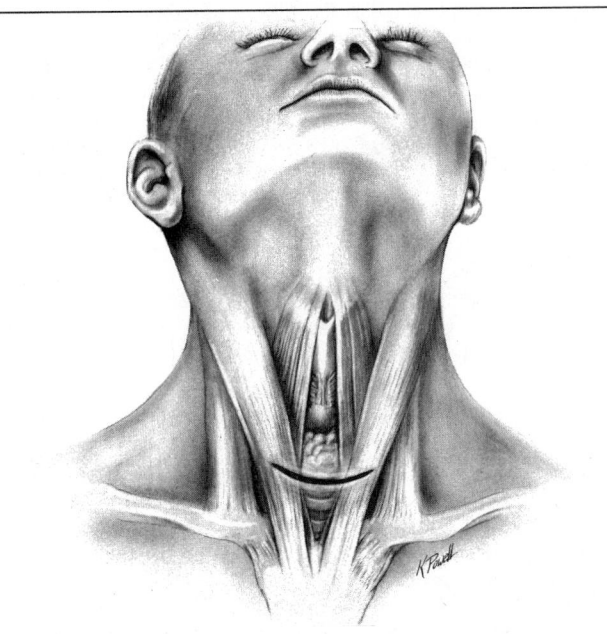

Fig. 16-2. Standard transverse incision for elective tracheotomy.

The strap muscles are identified and retracted. The thyroid isthmus, which overlies the second to fourth tracheal rings, usually must be retracted or transected and ligated. When the trachea has been identified and the pretracheal fascia cleared from its anterior wall, lidocaine is injected directly into the trachea to suppress the cough reflex. Several methods have been described to fenestrate the trachea [27]. We prefer making a cruciate incision in the anterior wall of the trachea. Care must be taken not to injure the posterior tracheal wall or esophagus (Fig. 16-3). Next, a window is created in the anterior wall of the trachea. It is sometimes preferable to create a superiorly or inferiorly based (Bjork) flap, which is sutured to the skin to provide ready access for recannulation should the tracheotomy

tube be dislodged [27]. In infants and young children, no tracheal wall is removed; the trachea is entered by a vertical midline incision. Sutures are placed laterally in the pretracheal fascia and taped to the neck so the trachea can be identified and recannulated should the tube become displaced. After hemostasis is achieved, the tube is inserted through the fenestration and is secured in position by cloth tapes tied around the neck with several square knots. In young children and neurosurgical patients, it is frequently preferable to suture the tracheotomy tube to the skin. If the tracheotomy wound is gaping, partial closure may be indicated. A tight closure should be avoided, since it can lead to dissection of air into the subcutaneous tissues. Finally, a tracheotomy dressing is applied [28–31]. In emergency tracheotomy the technique is modified by making a vertical incision and doing all dissection in the midline until the anterior tracheal wall is identified, then entering the trachea (Fig. 16-4A).

Tubes and Cannulas

From the sixteenth century, when Fabricius described the first tracheotomy tube, until synthetic materials were developed virtually all tubes were made of metal (generally silver or stainless steel) and contained an inner cannula that could be removed for cleaning. Characteristics of a good tracheotomy tube are flexibility to accommodate varying patient anatomies, inert material, wide internal diameter, the smallest external diameter possible, a smooth surface to allow easy insertion and removal, and sufficient length to be secure once placed but not so long as to impinge the carina or other tracheal parts [13]. In the late 1960s, surgeons began to experiment with silicone and other synthetic materials for tracheotomy tubes. At present, almost all tracheotomy tubes are made of synthetic material. One disadvantage of the silicone tube is the increased thickness of the tube wall, necessitating a larger outer diameter to obtain the same inner diameter. Silicone tubes are available with or without a cuff. The cuff allows occlusion of the airway around the tube, which is necessary for positive-pressure ventilation. It also minimizes aspiration. In the past, cuffs were associated with a fairly high incidence of tracheal stenosis caused by ischemia and necrosis of the mucous membrane and subsequent cicatricial contracture at the cuff site [32,33,34]. The high-volume, low-pressure cuffs now used diminish the pressure on the wall of the trachea, thereby minimizing (but not eliminating) problems due to focal areas of pressure necrosis [35]. If the only purpose of the tube is to secure the airway (sleep apnea) or to provide access for suctioning secretions, a tube without a cuff can be placed.

If the patient does not require constant ventilatory support, a fenestrated or valved tube can be used (Fig. 16-5). A fenestrated tube has a hole on the superior wall through which air can escape, allowing phonation. The valved fenestrated tube has a one-way flap that directs the expired air through the valve where it escapes (Fig. 16-6). The Kistner button (Fig. 16-7A) developed approximately 20 years ago, is a short cannula that extends from the skin to the anterior tracheal wall and permits immediate access to the airway as needed [36]. The Montgomery tracheal cannula (Fig. 16-7B) has an external collar that fixes the tube in place, preventing it from becoming displaced in the trachea [37]. One major advantage of a button or cannula is that they cause less irritation of the tracheal wall, thereby decreasing the production of secretions. They are particularly useful in patients who require intermittent access to the airway (myasthenia gravis, sleep apnea syndrome), because the tubes

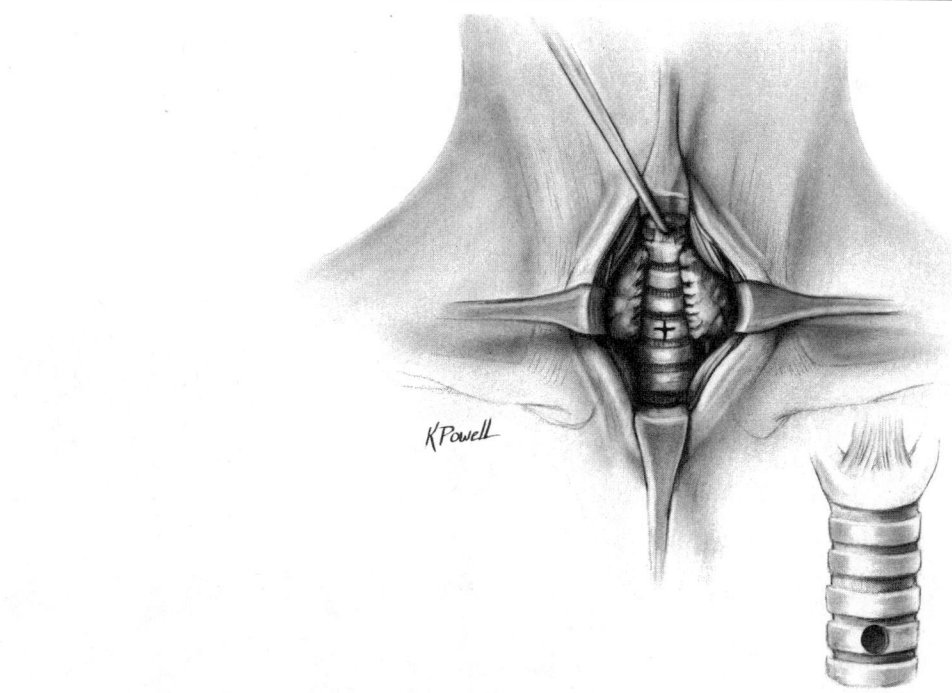

Fig. 16-3. Location of the cruciate incision in the anterior tracheal wall.

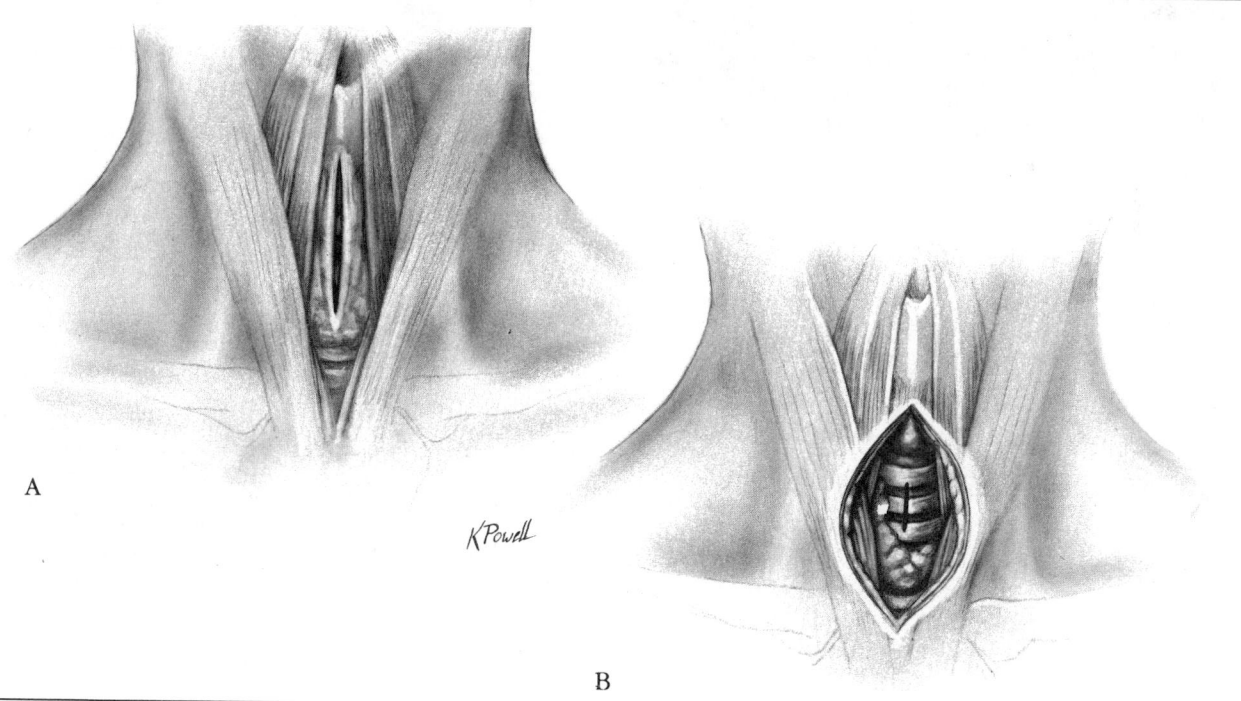

A

B

Fig. 16-4. Technique for emergency tracheotomy. A. A vertical incision is made and dissection to the anterior tracheal wall performed. B. Entrance is made into the trachea.

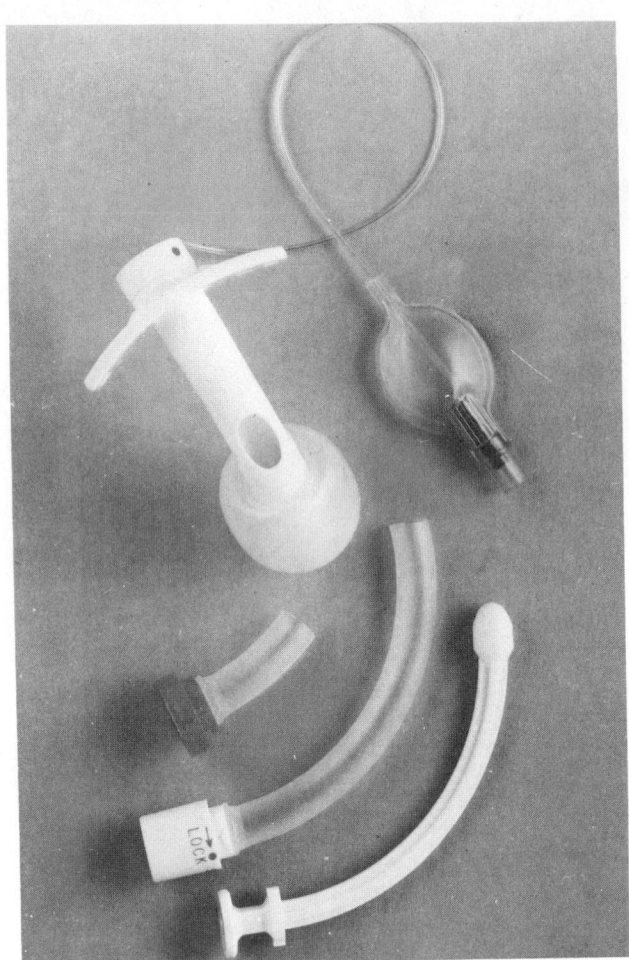

Fig. 16-5. Fenestrated Silastic tracheotomy tube.

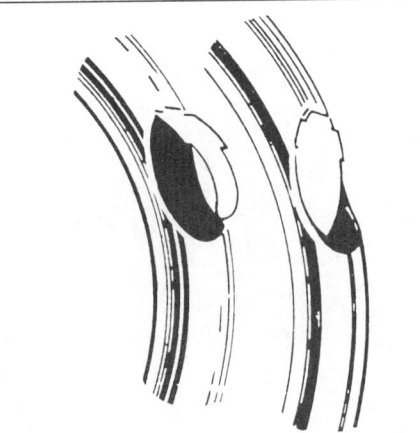

Fig. 16-6. Valved fenestrated tracheotomy tube. The Tucker valve shown is open on the left and closed on the right.

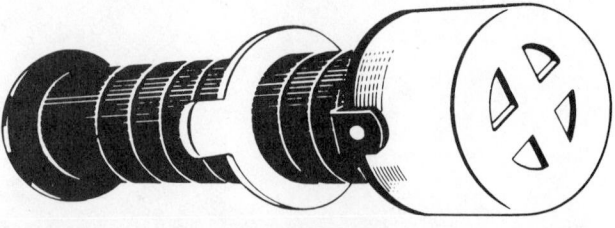

A

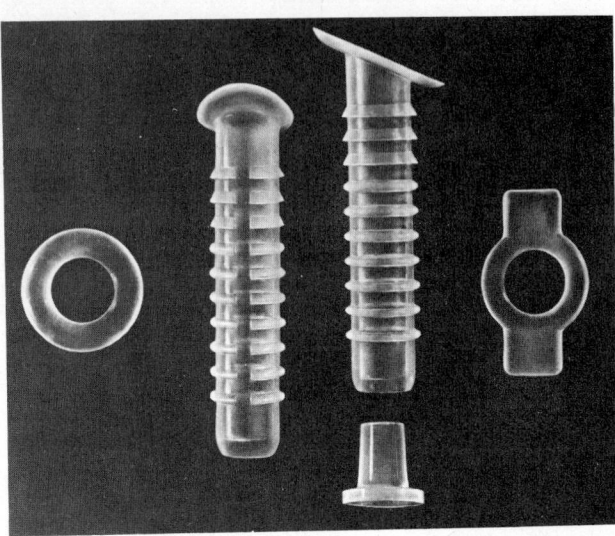

B

Fig. 16-7. A. Kistner button. B. Montgomery tracheal cannula.

can be opened at night and plugged during the day. This sort of tube is also cosmetically more acceptable.

Occasionally, a patient requires more distal cannulation of the trachea because of extensive stenosis or tracheomalacia. Jackson's extra-long tracheotomy tubes and cane-shaped tracheotomy tubes are available for that purpose (Fig. 16-8A).

Patients who have had laryngectomy and require splinting of the tracheostoma to prevent stenosis are typically cannulated with a laryngectomy tube, which is somewhat shorter and of different design than the standard tracheotomy tube (Fig. 16-8B). The shorter length is required because the trachea is sutured to the skin and the tube need not extend through a variable distance of soft tissue. Patients who have reconstruction of the trachea or subglottic larynx may require placement of a T tube (Fig. 16-8C), which is generally left in place for several months following the operation, until the cicatrix has matured. The vertical portion of the tube extends from the subglottic region to the proximal trachea. It has a horizontal limb that extends to the anterior neck. T tubes are generally used to support the trachea, to provide access for suctioning, and to maintain an opening for respiration and phonation until healing is complete.

Postoperative Care

The care of a tracheotomy tube after surgery is of paramount importance. Until the first tracheotomy tube change, the tapes should not be changed or disturbed by anyone other than the

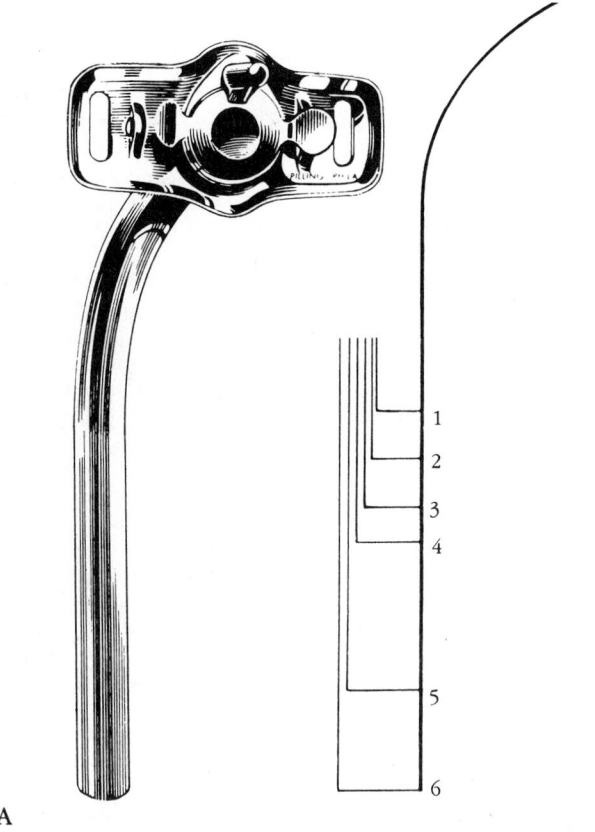

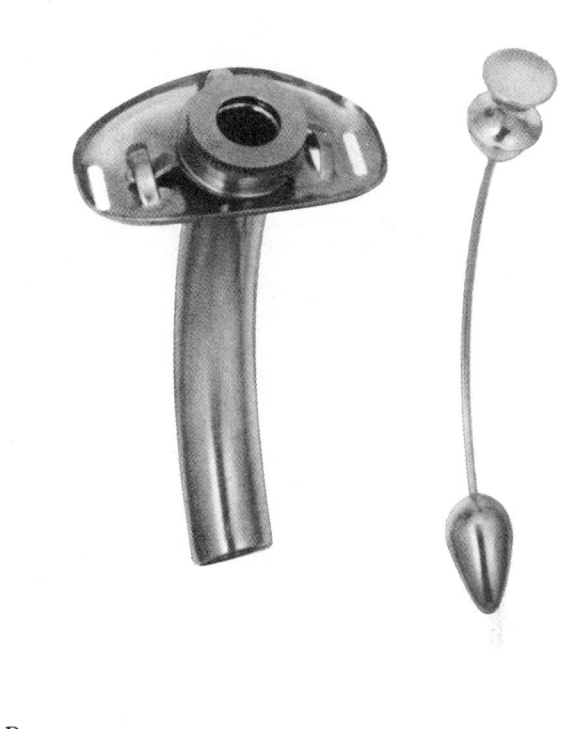

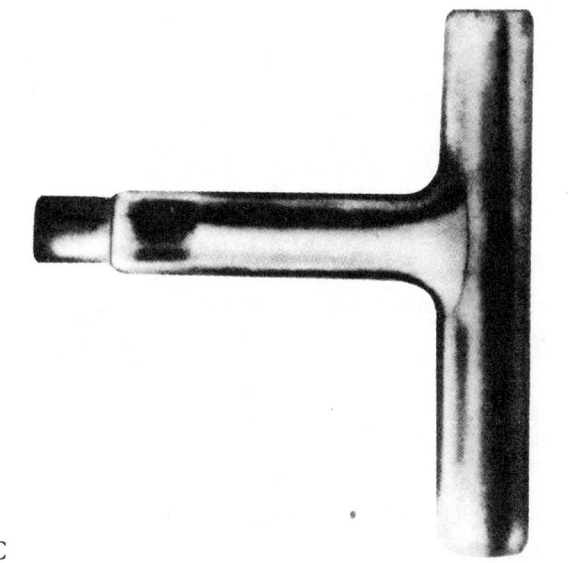

Fig. 16-8. A. Jackson cane-shaped tracheotomy tube. B. Laryngectomy tube. C. Montgomery tube.

surgeon or his or her representative. Ideally, the first tube change should not be attempted until the tract has matured, which requires at least 7 to 10 days. Silicone tubes do not require changing as frequently as metal tubes and generally can be left for periods of several months. If the tube has been sutured into position, the sutures should be left in place until the first tube change. The frequency of posttracheotomy suctioning is dictated by the volume of secretions produced. Excessive bronchorrhea or atelectasis may require suctioning as often as every 5 to 10 minutes. The inner cannula of the tube should be removed regularly under sterile conditions for inspection and cleaning. Humidification is very important in preventing obstruction of the tube by inspissated secretions and crusting (see Chap. 69). The obturator should be kept at the bedside at all times. Prior to discharge from the hospital, patients with permanent tracheotomies (and their families) must be fully instructed in care and cleaning of the tube and techniques for replacing it should it become dislodged.

Complications

A variety of complications (Table 16-2) are associated with tracheotomy [38–58]. The reported incidence of complications varies from 6.0 to 50 percent [23,39] and mortality from 0.9 to 4.5 percent [1,23,39,40]. Posttracheotomy mortality is caused by hemorrhage, tube dislodgment, infection, and obstruction. Neurosurgical patients have a higher posttracheotomy complication rate than do other patients [17,30,41].

Table 16-2. Complications of Tracheotomy

Complication	Etiology	Treatment
Tube obstruction	Inspissated secretions	Remove tube and clean tube
Tube dislodgment	Loose ties Patient movement Anatomic considerations	Replace tube or intubate orally
Hemorrhage Minor (early)	Small skin, subcutaneous tissue, and muscle bleeding	Packing/hemostatics Elevate head of bed
Moderate (late)	Thyroid isthmus Anterior/transverse Jugular veins Granulation tissue	Laser/cautery Return to OR Elevate head of bed
Major (late)	Tracheoarterial fistula	Inflate cuff Surgery
Tube misplacement	See text	Reintubate orally
Bronchorrhea	Tracheal irritation	Increased suctioning
Stomal infection	Tracheal irritation	Antibiotics Stoma care
Subcutaneous emphysema	Tight wound closure	May resolve Open wound
Recurrent laryngeal nerve injury	Iatrogenic	Delayed repair
Pneumothorax	Misplaced tube Tight wound closure Dissection of air into pleural space	Chest tube
Atelectasis	Inadequate ventilation or bleeding into trachea	Suctioning
Tracheoesophageal fistula	Iatrogenic Tube movement or angulation	Surgical repair
Aerophagia	Tube stimulates swallowing	Nasogastric tube Deflate cuff
Subglottic edema and stenosis	High tracheotomy Laryngeal inflammation	Surgical correction
Dysphagia	Pressure of tracheotomy tube and cuff	Decannulate Deflate cuff
Aspiration	Limited movement of larynx	Decannulate Deflate cuff
Tracheocutaneous fistula	Epithelialization of tracheotomy tract	Surgical closure
Difficult decannulation	Granuloma, stenosis, psychological dependence	Laser surgery Decrease tube sizes gradually

OBSTRUCTION. Occasionally, a tube becomes plugged with clotted blood or inspissated secretions. In this case the inner cannula should be removed immediately and the patient suctioned. Should that fail, it may be necessary to remove the outer cannula also, a decision that must take into consideration the reason the tube was placed and the length of time it has been in place. Obstruction also may be due to angulation of the distal end of the tube against the anterior or posterior tracheal wall. An undivided thyroid isthmus pressing against the angled tracheotomy tube can force the tip against the anterior tracheal wall, while a low superior transverse skin edge can force the tip of the tracheotomy tube against the posterior tracheal wall. An indication of this type of obstruction is an expiratory wheeze. Division of the thyroid isthmus and proper placement of transverse skin incisions help prevent anterior or posterior tube angulation and obstruction [42].

TUBE DISPLACEMENT/DISLODGMENT. Dislodgment of a tracheotomy tube that has been in place 2 weeks or longer is managed simply by replacing the tube. If it cannot be immediately replaced or if it is replaced and the patient cannot be ventilated (indicating that the tube is not in the trachea), orotracheal intubation should be performed. Immediate postoperative displacement can be fatal if the tube cannot be promptly replaced and the patient cannot be reintubated. Dislodgment in the early postoperative period is usually caused by one of several technical problems. Failure to divide the thyroid isthmus may permit the intact isthmus to ride up against the tracheotomy tube and thus displace it [42]. Excessively low placement of the stoma (i.e., below the second and third rings) can occur when the thoracic trachea is brought into the neck by overextending the neck or by excessive traction on the trachea. When the normal anatomic relationships are restored, the trachea recedes below the suprasternal notch, causing the tube to be dislodged from the trachea [42,43]. The risk of dislodgment of the tracheotomy tube, a potentially lethal complication, can be minimized by: (1) transection of the thyroid isthmus at surgery, if indicated; (2) proper placement of the stoma; (3) avoidance of excessive neck hyperextension and/or tracheal traction; (4) application of sufficiently tight tracheotomy tube retention tapes; and (5) suture of the tracheotomy tube flange to the skin in patients with short, stocky necks. Some surgeons apply retaining sutures to the trachea for use in the early postoperative period in case the tube should become dislodged, allowing the trachea to be pulled into the wound for reintubation. Reintubation of a tracheostomy can be accomplished using a smaller, beveled endotracheal tube and then applying a tracheotomy tube over the smaller tube, using Seldinger technique [44]. Making a Bjork flap involves suturing the inferior edge of the trachea stoma to the skin, thus allowing a "sure" pathway for tube placement. Bjork flaps, however, tend to interfere with swallowing and to promote aspiration [6].

EARLY HEMORRHAGE

Minor. Postoperative fresh tracheotomy bleeding occurs in up to 37 percent of cases [1]. Postoperative coughing and straining can cause venous bleeding by dislodging a clot or ligature. Elevating the head of the bed, packing the wound, and/or using hemostatic materials usually controls minor bleeding. Major bleeding occurs in 5 percent of tracheotomies and is due to hemorrhage from the isthmus of the thyroid gland, loss of a ligature from one of the anterior jugular veins, or injury to the transverse jugular vein that crosses the midline just above the jugular notch. Persistent bleeding may require a return to the operating room for management. Techniques to decrease the likelihood of early posttracheotomy hemorrhage include: (1) use of a vertical incision; (2) careful dissection in the midline, with care to pick up each layer of tissue with instruments rather than simply spreading tissues apart; (3) liberal use of ligatures rather than electrocautery; and (4) careful division and suture ligation of the thyroid isthmus [1,13,24,28,29,31,40,42,43].

Delayed. Late hemorrhage after tracheotomy is usually due to bleeding granulation tissue or another relatively minor cause. However, it previously was reported that 50 percent of all tracheotomy bleeding occurring more than 48 hours after the procedure is due to an often fatal complication of rupture of the innominate artery caused by erosion of the tracheotomy tube at its tip or cuff into the vessel [44,45]. Since the advent of the low-pressure cuff, the incidence of this complication has decreased considerably.

Eighty-five percent of tracheal-innominate fistulas occur within the first month after tracheotomy [46], although it has been reported as late as 7 months after operation. Other sites of delayed exsanguinating posttracheotomy hemorrhage include the common carotid artery, superior and inferior thyroid arteries, aortic arch, and innominate vein [46]. Rupture and fistula formation is caused by erosion through the trachea into the artery due to excessive cuff pressure, or angulation of the tube tip against the anterior trachea. Infection and other factors that weaken local tissues, such as malnourishment and steroids, also seem to play a role [39]. The innominate artery rises to about the level of the sixth ring anterior to the trachea, so low placement of the stoma can also create close proximity of the tube tip or cuff to the innominate artery. Rarely, an anomaly of the innominate, occurring with an incidence of 1 to 2 percent [18,46], is responsible for this disastrous complication. There have been fewer reports of tracheal-innominate fistulas recently, perhaps due to the use of low-pressure cuffs [46]. Pulsation of the tracheotomy tube is an indication of potentially fatal positioning [46]. Initially, hemorrhage from a tracheal-innominate fistula is usually not exsanguinating. "Herald" bleeds must be sought promptly using fiberoptic tracheoscopy. If a tracheal-innominate fistula seems probable (minimal tracheitis, anterior pulsating erosions), then the patient should be taken to the operating room for evaluation. Definitive management involves resection of the artery. The mortality rate is greater than 50 percent. Sudden exsanguinating hemorrhage may be managed by hyperinflation of the tracheotomy cuff tube or reintubation with an endotracheal tube through the stoma, attempting to place the cuff at the level of the fistula. A lower neck incision with blind digital compression on the artery may be part of a critical resuscitative effort [47].

MISPLACEMENT OF TUBE. This technical error occurs at the time of surgery or when the tube is changed or replaced through a fresh stoma. If not recognized, associated mediastinal emphysema and tension pneumothorax can occur, along with alveolar hypoventilation. Injury to neurovascular structures, including the recurrent laryngeal nerve, is possible [40,43]. The patient must be orally intubated or the tracheostoma recannulated. Some advise placing retaining sutures in the trachea at the time of surgery. The availability of a tracheotomy set at the bedside following tracheotomy facilitates emergency reintubation.

BRONCHORREA. Tracheotomy tubes virtually always irritate the trachea, resulting in an increase in normal secretions. This can generally be managed by frequent suctioning.

STOMAL INFECTIONS. An 8 to 12 percent incidence of cellulitis or purulent exudate is reported [1,16,38,48]. Attention to the details of good stoma care and early use of antibiotics are advised.

SUBCUTANEOUS EMPHYSEMA. Approximately 5 percent of patients develop subcutaneous emphysema following tracheotomy [44]. It is most likely to occur when dissection is exten-

sive and/or the wound is closed tightly. Partial closure of the skin wound is appropriate, but the underlying tissues should be allowed to approximate naturally. Subcutaneous emphysema generally resolves over the 48 hours following tracheotomy, but when the wound is closed tightly and the patient is coughing or on positive-pressure ventilation, pneumomediastinum, pneumopericardium, and/or tension pneumothorax may occur [4,42].

RECURRENT LARYNGEAL NERVE INJURY. Injury to the recurrent laryngeal nerve with resultant vocal cord paralysis is a rare complication of tracheotomy. It is more likely if the tracheotomy was done under emergency conditions. Recurrent laryngeal nerve injury leads to a hoarse, breathy voice. Diagnosis is made by indirect examination of the larynx. Surgical exploration and repair may be necessary.

PNEUMOTHORAX AND PNEUMOMEDIASTINUM. The cupola of the pleura extends well into the neck, especially in patients with emphysema; thus, the pleura can be damaged during tracheotomy. This complication is more common in the pediatric age group because the pleural dome extends more cephalad in children [1]. The incidence of pneumothorax following tracheotomy is about 5 percent [1,44]. Many surgeons routinely obtain a postoperative chest radiograph.

ATELECTASIS. Atelectasis following tracheotomy is due to hypoventilation, excessive blood entering the trachea at the time of surgery, or placement of a tube that is too long or too low, which leads to occlusion of one of the main bronchi. Treatment is increased suctioning and/or placement of a tube of a more appropriate length.

TRACHEOESOPHAGEAL FISTULA. Tracheoesophageal fistula caused by injury to the posterior tracheal wall and cervical esophagus occurs in less than 1 percent of patients, more commonly in the pediatric age group. Early postoperative fistula is a result of iatrogenic injury during the procedure [18,44,47]. The chances of creating a fistula can be minimized by entering the trachea initially with a horizontal incision between two tracheal rings (the second and third), thereby eliminating the initial cut into a hard cartilaginous ring [42]. A late tracheoesophageal fistula may be due to tracheal necrosis caused by tube movement or angulation, as in neck hyperflexion, or excessive cuff pressure [24,44,47]. A tracheoesophageal fistula should be suspected in patients with cuff leaks, abdominal distention, recurrent aspiration pneumonia, and reflux of gastric fluids through the tracheotomy site. It may be demonstrated on endoscopy and contrast studies. Tracheoesophageal fistulas require surgical repair.

AEROPHAGIA. The tracheotomy tube may stimulate repeated swallowing by the patient, who attempts to clear the sensation of a lump in his or her throat. This can lead to gastric distention, which should be treated by insertion of a nasogastric tube. If the condition persists, the patient should be decannulated as soon as possible.

SUBGLOTTIC EDEMA AND STENOSIS. Placement of the tracheotomy tube in close proximity to the glottic area (cricothyrotomy or first tracheal ring tracheotomy) may lead to edema and eventual subglottic stenosis. This is more likely to occur if there is mucosal injury from a previous endotracheal intubation and/or infection at the stoma site [19,48]. Meticulous care of tracheotomy stomas and prompt treatment of upper airway infections can help prevent this complication. Removal of a button of cartilage during tracheotomy in adults is acceptable, but in an infant or young child this maneuver may result in tracheal stenosis. Subglottic edema is a significant cause of decannulation problems. (See the section on cricothyrotomy for a more complete discussion.)

DYSPHAGIA AND ASPIRATION. Some patients with tracheotomy tubes complain of the sensation of a mass in the lower neck. This may lead to dysphagia, particularly if the cuff is left inflated while the patient is eating [49]. As discussed above, although some physicians perform tracheotomy to prevent aspiration [6], the major swallowing disorder associated with tracheotomy is aspiration. Even the presence of a gag reflex does not confer protection against aspiration of pharyngeal contents. The defects reported are delayed triggering of the swallow response and pharyngeal pooling of contrast materials [50]. The causes include (1) decreased laryngeal elevation and anterior movement during deglutition, because the tube itself or a Bjork flap fixes the trachea to the skin; (2) esophageal compression by an inflated cuff; and (3) desensitization of the larynx, leading to loss of protective reflexes and uncoordinated laryngeal closure. If dysphagia is a problem, simple measures (e.g., deflation of the cuff during eating or use of a nasogastric tube for enteral nutrition) should be attempted. Following extubation the deficits usually improve with time [50]. If the problem is severe and/or chronic, further evaluation and even surgery may be indicated [6].

TRACHEOCUTANEOUS FISTULA. Although the tracheostoma generally closes rapidly following decannulation, a persistent fistula occasionally remains, particularly when the tracheotomy tube was present for a prolonged period. If this occurs, the fistula tract can be excised and the wound closed primarily, under local anesthesia [51].

DIFFICULTY IN DECANNULATION. The usual causes of difficulty with decannulation are the presence of a granuloma or edema at the stoma site or indentation and collapse of the anterior tracheal wall above the stoma site. Some granulomas are pedunculated and easily removed [1], but others may require endoscopic laser treatment. Subglottic stenosis, another cause of decannulation problems, may require surgical management. At times, particularly in children, patients are reluctant to allow removal of tracheotomy tubes. This can generally be managed by changing the tube to progressively smaller sizes until it can be plugged for 24 hours and then removed. Occasionally, in the infant and newborn, the tube must be left in place until the trachea has had a chance to grow [52,53,54].

Cricothyrotomy

Cricothyrotomy, also known as laryngostomy, laryngotomy, cricothyroidotomy, and coniotomy [59], was condemned in Jackson's 1921 paper on high tracheotomies because of excessive complications, particularly subglottic stenoses [4,60,61]. He em-

phasized the importance of the cricoid cartilage as an encircling support for the larynx and trachea. However, Brantigan and Grow's favorable report evaluating 655 cricothyrotomies, with a complication rate of only 6.1 percent and no cases of subglottic stenosis, prompted reevaluation of cricothyrotomy for elective and emergency airway access [62]. Further reports emphasized the advantages of cricothyrotomy over tracheotomy, which included technical simplicity, speed of performance, low complication rate [61,63–66], suitability as a bedside procedure, usefulness for isolation of the airway from median sternotomy [65,67] and radical neck dissection incisions [68], lack of need to hyperextend the neck, and formation of a smaller scar. Also, because cricothyrotomy results in less encroachment on the mediastinum, there is less chance of esophageal injury and virtually no chance of pneumothorax or tracheoarterial fistula [61].

Despite these considerations, many authorities currently recommend that cricothyrotomy be used as an elective long-term method of airway access only in highly selected patients [60,61,69]. Use of cricothyrotomy in the emergency setting, particularly for managing trauma, is not controversial [26,59,70,71]. Described in 1984 as a method of managing retained secretions in the intensive care setting [72], cricothyrotomy is in fairly wide use in Great Britain.

ELECTIVE CRICOTHYROTOMY. Indications for elective cricothyrotomy include (1) need for a surgical airway in patients after median sternotomy or neck reconstruction [60,65,67]; (2) presence of (rare) anatomic variations that preclude tracheotomy or make it dangerous to perform or manage (e.g., in severe cervical kyphosis); (3) need for airway management in terminally ill patients [60]; and (4) need for short-term (less than 5 days) surgical airway following facial reconstruction. Recommended precautions are: (1) to avoid cricothyrotomy following long periods of endotracheal intubation, particularly in diabetics and the elderly; (2) to assess the airway endoscopically prior to cricothyrotomy, particularly following endotracheal intubation, to rule out the presence of antecedent laryngeal inflammation; (3) to provide antibiotic coverage for airway infections and stoma inflammation; and (4) to convert to tracheotomy should inflammation or infection occur [69].

EMERGENCY CRICOTHYROTOMY. Because cricothyrotomy requires a small number of instruments and less training than tracheotomy and can be performed quickly, it is indicated as a means for controlling the airway in an emergency when oral or nasotracheal intubation is unsuccessful or contraindicated. In emergency situations, translaryngeal intubations fail because of massive oronasal hemorrhage or regurgitation, structural deformities of the upper airway, muscle spasm and clenched teeth, and obstruction by foreign bodies of the upper airway [26,59]. Cricothyrotomy finds its greatest use in trauma management. Actual or suspected cervical spine injury, alone or in combination with severe facial trauma, makes nasotracheal and orotracheal intubation both difficult and hazardous. Thus, cricothyrotomy has an important role in emergency airway management [70] (see Fig. 16-9).

CONTRAINDICATIONS. Cricothyrotomy should not be used to manage airway obstruction occurring immediately following endotracheal extubation, because the obstruction may be found below the larynx [4,61,70]. Likewise, with primary laryngeal trauma or disease such as tumor and infection, cricothyrotomy may prove useless. It is contraindicated in infants and children

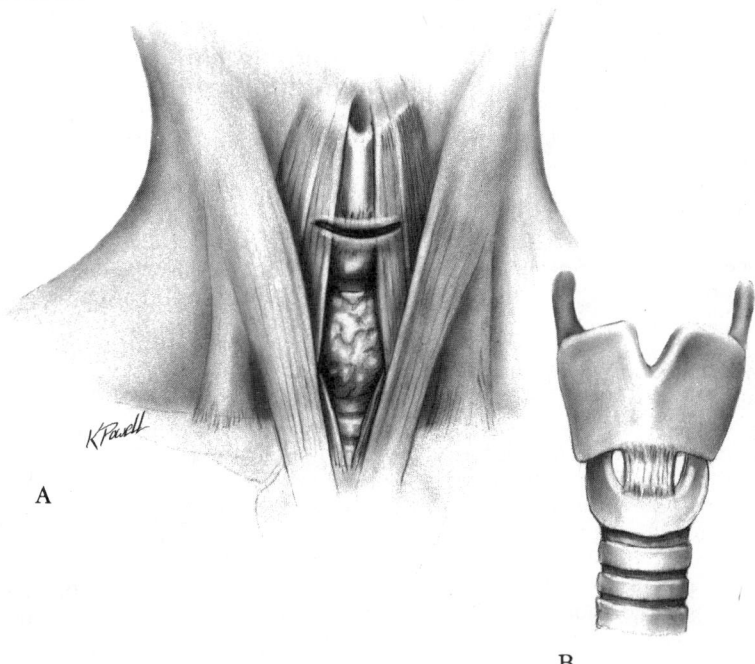

A

B

Fig. 16-9. Emergency cricothyrotomy.

younger than 10 to 12 years under all circumstances [70]. In this age group, percutaneous transtracheal jet ventilation may be a temporizing procedure until tracheotomy can be performed.

ANATOMY. The cricothyroid space is no larger than 7 to 9 mm in its vertical dimension, smaller than the outside diameter of most tracheotomy tubes (no. 6 Shiley outside diameter is 10.0 mm). The cricothyroid artery runs across the midline in the upper portion and the membrane fuses vertically in the midline. The anterosuperior edge of the thyroid cartilage is the laryngeal prominence. The cricothyroid membrane is approximately 2 to 3 cm below this laryngeal prominence and can be identified as an indentation immediately below the thyroid cartilage. The lower border of the cricothyroid membrane is the cricoid cartilage [26,59,69,73,74].

PROCEDURE

1. After palpating for location of the cricothyroid membrane, clean the area over the membrane with antiseptic solution and anesthetize, using a local anesthetic. Make a 3-cm skin incision in the vertical direction, thereby avoiding some cutaneous and subcutaneous bleeding.
2. Palpate the cricothyroid membrane through the open incision. Stabilize the larynx by grasping it between the thumb and index finger or using a tracheal hook.
3. Create a short transverse incision directly through the membrane in its lower third. A no. 11 blade is best used, as only the tip of the blade will go through the membrane. Spread the membrane horizontally, using a hemostat or scissors. Leave this "dilator" in place and insert a no. 4 Shiley tracheotomy tube or an appropriately tailored endotracheal tube.
4. Secure the tube in place and inflate the cuff.
5. The cricothyrotomy may remain in place for up to 5 days if extubation is feasible within that time. Otherwise, it should

be converted to a standard tracheotomy under controlled operative conditions [26,74].

COMPLICATIONS. The reported incidence of short- and long-term complications of cricothyrotomy ranges from 6.1 percent [62] for procedures performed in elective, well-controlled, carefully selected cases to greater than 50 percent [59,60,69,71,75] for procedures performed under emergency or other suboptimal conditions.

Subglottic Stenosis. The incidence of subglottic stenosis following cricothyrotomy is 2 to 3 percent [60,61]. This major complication occurs at the tracheotomy or cricothyrotomy site but not at the cuff site [18,76]. Necrosis of cartilage due to iatrogenic injury to the cricoid cartilage or pressure from the tube on the cartilage may play a role [70]. Possible reasons that subglottic stenosis may occur more commonly with cricothyrotomy than with tracheotomy include: (1) the larynx is the narrowest part of the laryngotracheal airway; (2) subglottic tissues, especially in children, are intolerant of contact; and (3) division of the cricothyroid membrane and the cricoid cartilage destroy the only complete ring supporting the airway [3,60]. Prior laryngotracheal injury, as with prolonged translaryngeal intubation, is a major risk factor for the development of subglottic stenosis following cricothyrotomy [60,61,69].

Decannulation Difficulties. Subglottic stenosis and growth of granulation tissue are the causes of difficulties with decannulation in 50 percent of cases [60,69]. The granulation tissue may sometimes be managed endoscopically using a laser, but conversion to tracheotomy may be necessary.

Voice Change (Hoarseness). The most frequent complication, occurring in up to 50 percent of patients, is hoarseness due to vocal cord paresis [60,69].

Persistent Laryngotracheal Cutaneous Fistula. This problem is caused by damage to the cricoid cartilage, either at the time of the operation or later, due to pressure from a tube too large for the relatively small cricothyroid space. The maximum tube size for the cricothyroid space is a no. 4 Shiley.

Hemorrhage. Early bleeding is a frequent complication of emergency cricothyrotomy [73,77]. Significant arterial hemorrhage is usually due to laceration of the cricothyroid artery that courses across the upper portion of the cricothyroid membrane. A vertical incision may transect the artery, whereas a lower transverse membrane incision avoids the artery and does not disrupt the membrane's midline fusion. Such disruption is thought to be another potential source of subglottic stenosis [73]. Late hemorrhage from cricothyrotomy is rare.

Tube Misplacement. Tube misplacement is a common and potentially disastrous complication of cricothyrotomy. Cricothyrotomy is performed in a relatively blind fashion, and the usual methods of confirming correct placement of a tracheotomy tube are not as effective with cricothyrotomy. In one study, tube misplacement occurred in 36 percent of cases [71]. In 22 percent of cases, the tube was placed either through the pharyngeal membrane or outside the trachea altogether. Pneumothorax, subcutaneous emphysema, and neurovascular injury are associated with misplacement of tubes outside the trachea [78].

Percutaneous Airway Technique

The concept of a tracheotomy by percutaneous dilatation was described by Toye and Weinstein in 1969 and again in 1986 [79]. Seldinger's wire-guided insertion technique for intravascular catheters has been adapted to many tube and catheter placement procedures [80]. Several modifications and variations of the Seldinger technique have resulted in development of percutaneous techniques for tracheotomy and cricothyrotomy, as well as commercially available kits for performing these procedures. Percutaneous methods of creating a surgical airway can be used wherever elective or emergency tracheotomy or cricothyrotomy is indicated. This "mini-tracheostomy" through the cricothyroid membrane has found particular favor in Great Britain, where it is used as suction access to the trachea [81,82]. Strong advocates now recommend some percutaneous (dilatational) method as the method of choice for creating a surgical airway.

ADVANTAGES

1. In experienced hands, some percutaneous techniques frequently can be performed in only 30 seconds, and usually in less than 2 minutes [79]. Compared to the 10 to 20 minutes required for standard operative tracheotomy, this represents a substantial saving of time, particularly with upper airway emergencies

2. Because there is less dissection and the tube fits snugly in the hole created, there is less immediate bleeding with the percutaneous technique [83]. Even penetration of the thyroid isthmus with this technique apparently does not result in a significant incidence of pretracheal hematoma [79].

3. Because the direction of the tube is controlled by a preplaced wire and entry into the trachea is confirmed before the tube is placed, the risk of perforation of the posterior trachea and esophagus is lessened [84].

4. The small skin incision required for the percutaneous technique and the smaller size of the stoma result in a more cosmetically acceptable scar [79,83].

5. Stomal infection or stenosis is very rare [79,80,83].

6. The procedure can be performed by nonsurgeons.

7. The procedure can be performed at the bedside.

8. Lighting is not critical.

9. The procedure can be done without an assistant.

TECHNIQUES AND INSTRUMENTS. There are several percutaneous tracheotomy and cricothyrotomy techniques and commercially available instruments and kits [85-89]. All use some form of the Seldinger artery cannulation technique with various adaptations for cutting (using a tracheostome [Nu-Trake, Pediatrake]) or dilating the pretracheal tissues and trachea (vide infra) (Figs. 16-10 and 16-11). Percutaneous airways are performed at the cricothyroid membrane, subcricoid space (between the cricoid and the first tracheal ring) [83], or the level of the second to fourth tracheal rings. The cricothyroid membrane is more difficult to puncture and dilate than the trachea; considerable force must be used. All of the techniques require a skin incision, but it should be no larger than the tracheotomy tube that is to be placed [79]. Although lower complication rates are cited for the dilatational technique, methods using a cutting instrument (tracheostome) have their advocates. Advantages of tracheostome techniques are that they can be used in emergencies, tracheostomy tubes with balloon cuffs are more easily advanced, and larger tubes can be inserted than with techniques that use sequential dilators [82,88,89]. Except under emergency conditions, percutaneous airway procedures should be done with an endotracheal tube in place. Despite their attractiveness as methods for the "unskilled," considerable training and practice are necessary for both techniques, if significant, even lethal, complications are to be avoided [90,91,92].

COMPLICATIONS. Several percutaneous methods are associated with a significant complication rate in the hands of those who have had little or no training or experience with the procedure, particularly when used under emergency conditions. In an evaluation of one percutaneous cricothyrotomy instrument, 5 of 15 physicians failed to cannulate the trachea [93]. Under emergency conditions, percutaneous cricothyrotomy often results in placement in the airway but above or below the expected position, with the potential for significant complications, such as injury to vocal cords or transection of the larynx [93]. However, in some studies the complication rates for percutaneous tracheotomy (11–14%) are lower than those for some major series of operative tracheotomies [79,80]. Nevertheless, paratracheal insertion occurred in 6 percent of cases even when percutaneous tracheotomy was performed by experienced operators under elective conditions [79]. This complication is avoided when intratracheal placement of the needle is proved by aspiration of air before proceeding further. Endoscopic confirmation of accurate needle placement ensures correct placement of the tracheostomy tube and prevents paratracheal placement [94,95,96]. The importance of proper training and practice with the percutaneous technique cannot be overemphasized [85]. Training videos are available with some of the commercially available percutaneous airway kits.

PERCUTANEOUS DILATATIONAL TRACHEOTOMY. Ciaglia and Graniero reported on percutaneous dilatational subcricoid tracheotomy from 1985 to 1992 [97], prior to which percutaneous techniques involved instruments with sharp cut-

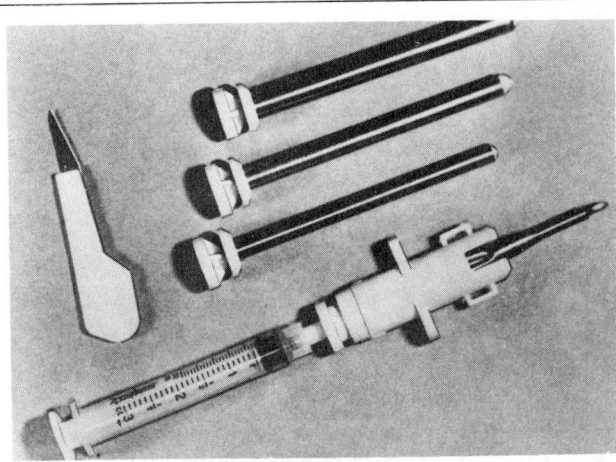

Fig. 16-10. "Nu-Trake" cricothyrotomy instrument.

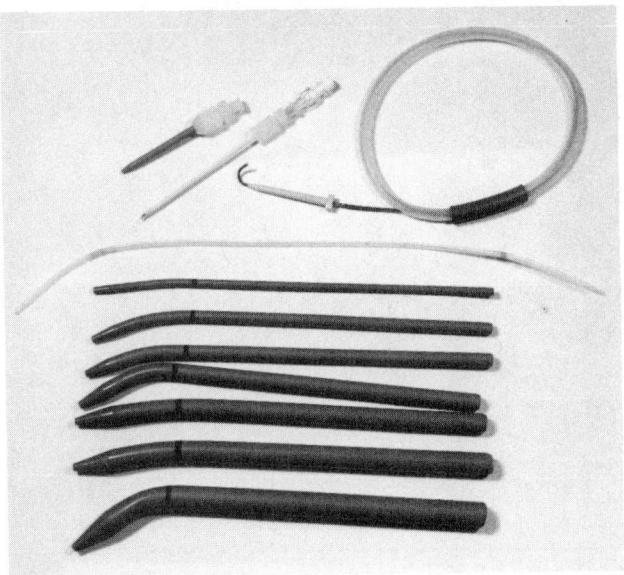

Fig. 16-11. Cook Percutaneous Tracheostomy Introducer Set.

ting blades. Since then, Ciaglia and others [21,98] have reported significant success rates and fewer complications than with other percutaneous techniques and even than standard tracheotomy [98,99]. Wang et al. [92] reported significant, even disastrous, complications from the technique and emphasize performance of the procedure by a trained surgeon capable of conventional tracheotomy. This technique should not be used for emergency cricothyroidotomy [98].

Advantages of the percutaneous (guidewire) dilatational elective tracheotomy technique cited by investigators are that (1) no operating room is necessary; (2) it is faster than standard conventional tracheotomy; (3) it is inexpensive; (4) dissection is decreased, therefore there is less risk of infection. One difficulty is that it is basically a "blind" procedure, but upper airway endoscopy may help identify intratracheal placement of the needle and J guidewire and with the selection of the exact intratracheal ring membrane to puncture [94,95,96].

The technique of percutaneous dilatational guidewire elective tracheotomy and tips of numerous operators are described in the literature [15,21,87,97,98,99]. Briefly, the procedure is as follows.

1. Intubate the trachea and monitor oxygen saturation. Adjust FIO_2, tidal volume, respiratory rate, and positive end-expiratory pressure as needed to compensate for necessary air leak during the procedure.
2. Loosen the tapes fixing the endotracheal tube in place and secure the tube by hand throughout the procedure. Identify neck landmarks (Fig. 16-12A).
3. Under local anesthesia and intravenous sedation, insert a needle and cannula between the first and second tracheal rings. Obtain free aspiration of air (Fig. 16-12B). If the needle impales the endotracheal tube, withdraw the tube a bit further. Some use a laryngoscope while removing the endotracheal tube to identify the correct position.
4. Remove the needle, insert a J guidewire through the cannula, and then remove the cannula (Fig. 16-12C). Make an incision about the guidewire (Fig. 16-12D).
5. Place a silicone guiding catheter over the guidewire and perform all dilations over this "double guide" (wire and silicone catheter) to prevent any kinking (Fig. 16-12E).
6. Insert and remove dilators of increasing size, up to a 36 Fr. for an 8-mm internal diameter cannula tracheotomy tube. Slightly overdilate the tracheotomy (Fig. 16-12F,G).
7. Lubricate a proper size dilator and preload it with the tracheostomy tube (Fig. 16-12H).
8. Thread the dilator carrying the tracheotomy tube over the silicone guide and insert it into the trachea. Positioning marks on the silicone guide and dilators assist in positioning (Fig. 16-12I).
9. Remove the dilator, silicone guide, and J guidewire. Fix the tracheotomy tube in place and remove the endotracheal tube. Dilatation of some tracheas can be extremely difficult; numerous tips and techniques are reported.

Reported complications include many of the same complications of standard tracheotomy, as well as placement of the dilators extratracheally, perforation of the esophagus, and development of a mucosal endobronchial flap [98]. However, early and late complications, including tracheal stenosis, have been few. The technique described here compares favorably with standard tracheotomy and has some advantages [98–101]. It has clearly been shown to be safe and valuable for ICU use [102]. Intraoperative and early complications seem to be related to lack of experience with the technique, therefore the procedure should be performed only by those capable of performing conventional tracheotomy.

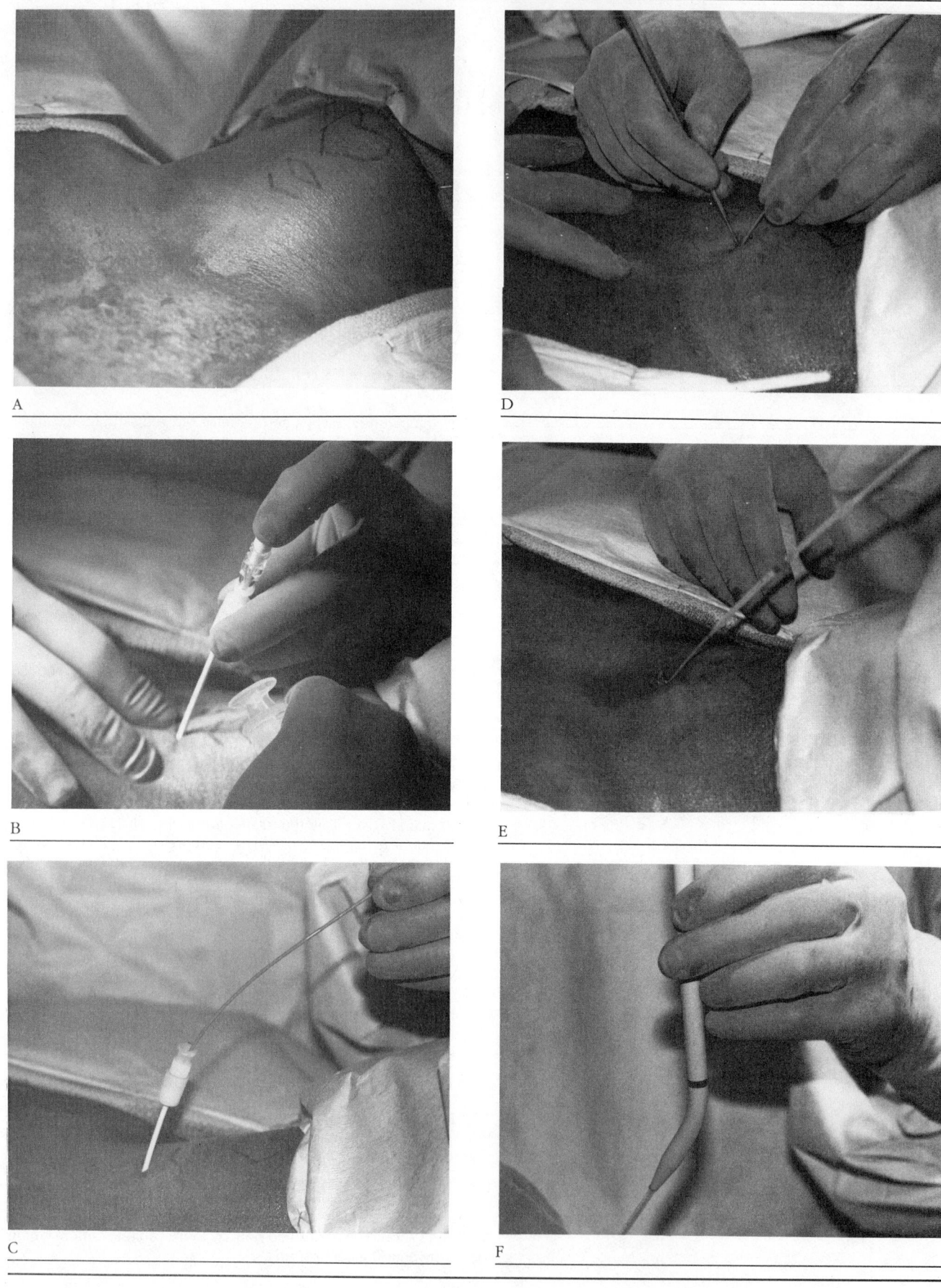

A

B

C

D

E

F

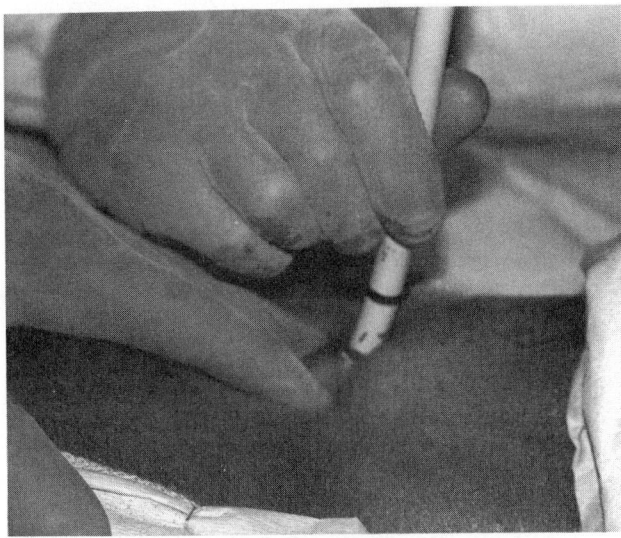

G

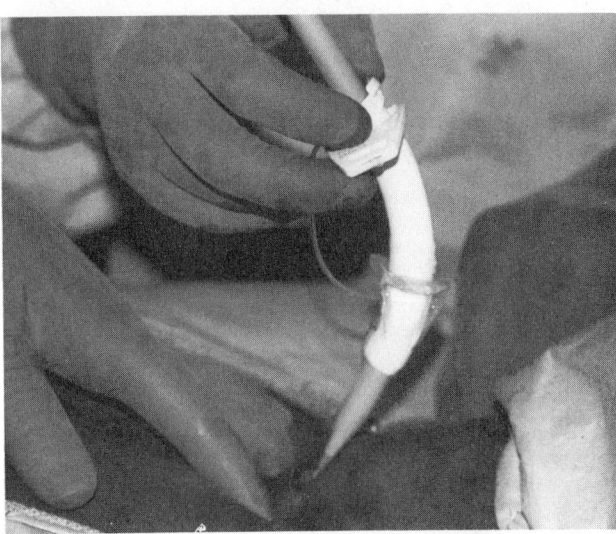

H

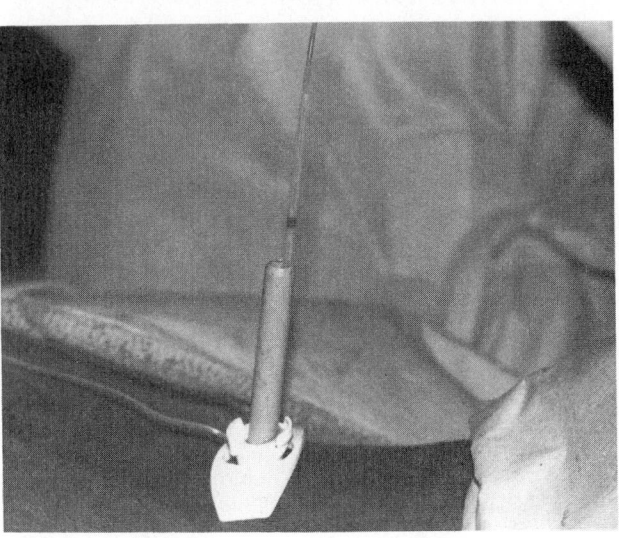

I

Fig. 16-12. A–I. Percutaneous dilatational tracheotomy technique. (See text for details.)

References

1. Goldstein SI, Breda SD, Schneider KL: Surgical complications of bedside tracheotomy in an otolaryngology residency program. *Laryngoscope* 97:1407, 1987.
2. Heffner JE, Miller KS, Sahn SA: Tracheostomy in the intensive care unit, 1: Indication, techniques, management. *Chest* 90:269, 1986.
3. Goodall EW: The story of tracheotomy. *Br J Child Dis* 31:167, 1934.
4. Jackson C: High tracheotomy and other errors: The chief causes of chronic laryngeal stenosis. *Surg Gynecol Obstet* 32:392, 1921.
5. McClelland RMA: Tracheostomy: Its management and alternatives. *Proc R Soc Med* 65:401, 1972.
6. Nash M: Swallowing problems in the tracheotomized patient. *Surg Clin North Am* 21:701, 1988.
7. Bjure J: Tracheotomy: A satisfactory method in the treatment of acute epiglottis—A clinical and functional follow-up study. *Int J Pediatr Otorhinolaryngol* 3:37, 1981.
8. Hanline MH Jr: Tracheotomy in upper airway obstruction. *South Med J* 74:899, 1981.
9. Guilleminault C, Simmons FB, Motta J, et al: Obstructive sleep apnea syndrome and tracheostomy. *Arch Intern Med* 141:985, 1981.
10. Burwell C, Robin E, Whaley R, et al: Extreme obesity associated with alveolar hypoventilation. *Am J Med* 141:985, 1981.
11. Tilkian A, Guilleminault C, Schroeder JS, et al: Sleep induced apnea syndrome. *Am J Med* 63:348, 1977.
12. Yung MW, Snowdon SL: Respiratory resistance of tracheostomy tubes. *Arch Otolaryngol* 110:591, 1984.
13. Lewis RJ: Tracheostomies: Indications, timing, and complications. *Clin Chest Med* 13:137, 1992.
14. Indeck M, Peterson S, Brotman S: Risk, cost and benefit of transporting patients from the ICU for special studies. *Crit Care Med* 15:350, 1987.
15. Hawkins ML, Burrus EP, Treat RC, et al: Tracheostomy in the intensive care unit: A safe alternative to the operating room. *South Med J* 82:1096, 1989.
16. Astrachan DI, Kirchner JC, Goodwin JW Jr: Prolonged intubation vs tracheotomy: Complications, practical and psychological considerations. *Laryngoscope* 98:1165, 1988.
17. Dunham CM, LaMonica C: Prolonged tracheal intubation in the trauma patient. *J Trauma* 24:120, 1984.
18. Stauffer JL, Olson DE, Petty TL: Complications and consequences of endotracheal intubation and tracheostomy: A prospective study of 150 critically ill adult patients. *Am J Med* 70:65, 1981.
19. El-Naggar M, Sadogopan S, Levine H, et al: Factors influencing choice between tracheostomy and prolonged translaryngeal intubation in acute respiratory failure: A prospective study. *Anesth Analg* 55:195, 1976.
20. Rodriques JL, Steinberg SM, Luchetti FA, et al: Early tracheostomy for primary airway management in the surgical critical care setting. *Surgery* 108:655, 1990.
21. Moore FA, Haenel JB, Moore EE, Read RA: Percutaneous tracheostomy/gastrostomy in brain-injured patients: A minimally invasive alternative. *J Trauma* 33:435, 1992.
22. Thomas GK: Tracheostomy, in Paparella MM, Shumrick DA (eds): *Otolaryngology.* vol. 3. Philadelphia, WB Saunders, 1973.
23. Stock CM, Woodward CG, Shapiro BA, et al: Perioperative complications of elective tracheostomy in critically ill patients. *Crit Care Med* 14:861, 1986.
24. Skaggs JA, Cogbill CL: Tracheostomy: Management, mortality, complications. *Am Surg* 35:393, 1969.
25. American College of Surgeons Committee on Trauma: *Advanced Trauma Life Support Course for Physicians, Instructor Manual.* Chicago, American College of Surgeons, 1985, p 159.
26. Kline SN: Maxillofacial trauma, in Kreis DJ, Gomez GA (eds): *Trauma Management.* Boston, Little, Brown, 1989.
27. Eliachar I, Goldsher M, Joachims HZ, et al: Superiorly based tra-

cheostomal flap to counteract tracheal stenosis: Experimental study. *Laryngoscope* 91:976, 1981.
28. Orringer MB: Endotracheal intubation and tracheostomy: Indications, techniques, and complications. *Surg Clin North Am* 60:1447, 1980.
29. Montgomery WW: Surgery of the trachea, in Montgomery WW (ed): *Surgery of the Upper Respiratory Tract.* 2nd ed., vol. 2. Philadelphia, Lea & Febiger, 1979, p 365.
30. Seid AB, Thomas GK: Tracheostomy, in Paparela MM, Shumrick DA (eds): *Otolaryngology.* vol. 3. Philadelphia, WB Saunders, 1980, p 3004.
31. Dugan DJ, Samson PC: Tracheostomy: Present day indications and techniques. *Am J Surg* 106:290, 1963.
32. Cooper JD, Grillo HC: The evolution of tracheal injury due to ventilatory assistance through cuffed tubes: A pathologic study. *Ann Surg* 169:334, 1969.
33. Lomholt N: A new tracheostomy tube. *Acta Anaesthesiol Scand* 11:311, 1967.
34. Stool SE, Campbell JR, Johnson DG: Tracheostomy in children: The use of plastic tubes. *J Pediatr Surg* 3:402, 1968.
35. Grillo HZ, Cooper JD, Geffin B, et al: A low pressured cuff for tracheostomy tubes to minimize tracheal inner injury. *J Thorac Cardiovasc Surg* 62:898, 1971.
36. Venus B: Five year experience with Kistner tracheostomy tube. *Crit Care Med* 8:106, 1980.
37. Montgomery WW: Silicone tracheal cannula. *Ann Otol Rhinol Laryngol* 89:521, 1980.
38. Dayal VS, ElMasri W: Tracheostomy in intensive care settings. *Laryngoscope* 96:58, 1986.
39. Oshinsky AE, Rubin JS, Gwozdz CS: The anatomical basis for post-tracheotomy innominate artery rupture. *Laryngoscope* 98:1061, 1988.
40. Meade JW: Tracheotomy: Its complications and their management. *N Engl J Med* 264:519, 587, 1961.
41. Miller JD, Kapp JP: Complications of tracheostomies in neurosurgical patients. *Surg Neurol* 22:186, 1984.
42. Kirchner JA: Avoiding problems in tracheotomy. *Laryngoscope* 96:55, 1986.
43. Kenan PD: Complications associated with tracheotomy: Prevention and treatment. *Otolaryngol Clin North Am* 12:807, 1979.
44. Heffner JE, Miller KS, Sahn SA: Tracheostomy in the intensive care unit: 2: Complications. *Chest* 90:430, 1986.
45. Mathog RH, Denan PD, Hudson WR: Delayed massive hemorrhage following tracheostomy. *Laryngoscope* 81:107, 1971.
46. Mamikunian C: Prevention of delayed hemorrhage after tracheotomy. *Ear Nose Throat J* 67:881, 1988.
47. Thomas AN: The diagnosis and treatment of tracheoesophageal fistula caused by cuffed tracheal tubes. *J Thorac Cardiovasc Surg* 65:612, 1973.
48. Burns HP, Dayar VS, Scott A, et al: Laryngotracheal trauma: Observations on its pathogenesis and its prevention following prolonged orotracheal intubation in the adult. *Laryngoscope* 89:1316, 1979.
49. Bonanno PC: Swallowing dysfunction after tracheotomy. *Ann Surg* 174:29, 1971.
50. DeVita MA, Spierer-Rundback L: Swallowing disorders in patients with prolonged orotracheal intubation or tracheostomy tubes. *Crit Care Med* 18:1328, 1990.
51. Hughes M, Kirchner JA, Branson RJ: A skin-lined tube as a complication of tracheostomy. *Arch Otolaryngol* 94:568, 1971.
52. Louis R: Decannulation after tracheostomy in infants and children. *J Laryngol Otol* 79:435, 1965.
53. Tepas JJ III, Herog JH, Shermeta DW, et al: Tracheostomy in neonates and small infants. Problems and pitfalls. *Surgery* 89:635, 1981.
54. Gaudet PT, Peerless A, Sosaki CT, et al: Pediatric tracheostomy and associated complications. *Laryngoscope* 81:107, 1071.
55. Chew JY, Cantrell RW: Tracheostomy: Complications and their management. *Arch Otolaryngol* 96:538, 1972.
56. Kirchner JA: Tracheostomy and its problems. *Surg Clin North Am* 60:1093, 1980.
57. Harrington CT: Complications of tracheostomy. *Arch Surg* 91:652, 1965.
58. Grillo HC: Surgery of the trachea, in *Current Problems in Surgery.* Chicago, Year Book, 1970.
59. Mace SE: Cricothyrotomy. *Emerg Med* 6:309, 1988.
60. Esses BA, Jafek BW: Cricothyroidotomy: A decade of experience in Denver. *Ann Otol Rhinol Laryngol* 96:519, 1987.
61. Cole RR, Aguilar EA: Cricothyroidotomy versus tracheotomy: An otolaryngologist's perspective. *Laryngoscope* 98:131, 1988.
62. Brantigan CO, Grow JB: Cricothyroidotomy: Elective use in respiratory problems requiring tracheotomy. *J Thorac Cardiovasc Surg* 71:72, 1976.
63. Boyd AD, Romita MC, Conlan AA, et al: A clinical evaluation of cricothyroidotomy. *Surg Gynecol Obstet* 149:365, 1979.
64. Sise MJ, Shacksord SR, Cruickshank JC, et al: Cricothyroidotomy for long term tracheal access. *Ann Surg* 200:13, 1984.
65. O'Connor JV, Reddy K, Ergin MA, et al: Cricothyroidotomy for prolonged ventilatory support after cardiac operations. *Ann Thorac Surg* 39:353, 1985.
66. Lewis GA, Hopkinson RB, Matthews HR: Minitracheotomy: A report of its use in intensive therapy. *Anesthesia* 41:931, 1986.
67. Pierce WS, Tyers FO, Waldhausen JA: Effective isolation of a tracheostomy from a median sternotomy wound. *J Thorac Cardiovasc Surg* 66:841, 1973.
68. Morain WD: Cricothyroidotomy in head and neck surgery. *Plast Reconstr Surg* 65:424, 1980.
69. Kuriloff DB, Setzen M, Portnoy W, et al: Laryngotracheal injury following cricothyroidotomy. *Laryngoscope* 99:125, 1989.
70. Jorden RC, Rosen P: Airway management in the acutely injured, in Moore EE, Eiseman B, Van Way CW (eds): *Critical Decisions in Trauma.* St. Louis, Mosby, 1984.
71. McGill J, Clinton JE, Ruiz E: Cricothyrotomy in the emergency department. *Ann Emerg Med* 11:361, 1982.
72. Matthews HR, Hopkinson RB: Treatment of sputum retention by minitracheotomy. *Br J Surg* 71:147, 1984.
73. Terry RM, Cook P: Hemorrhage during minitracheostomy: Reduction of risk by altered incision. *J Laryngol Otol* 103:207, 1989.
74. Cutler BS: Cricothyroidotomy for emergency airway, in Vander Salm TJ, Cutler BS, Wheeler HB (eds): *Atlas of Bedside Procedures.* Boston, Little, Brown, 1988.
75. Erlandson MJ, Clinton JE, Ruiz E, et al: Cricothyrotomy in the emergency department revisited. *J Emerg Med* 7:115, 1989.
76. Brantigan CO, Grow JB: Subglottic stenosis after cricothyroidotomy. *Surgery* 91:217, 1982.
77. Little CM, Parker MG, Tanopolsky R: The incidence of vasculature at risk during cricothyroidotomy. *Ann Emerg Med* 15:805, 1986.
78. Silk JM, Marsh AM: Pneumothorax caused by minitracheostomy. *Anesthesia* 44:663, 1989.
79. Toye FJ, Weinstein JD: Clinical experience with percutaneous tracheostomy and cricothyroidotomy in 100 patients. *J Trauma* 26:1034, 1986.
80. Hazard PB, Garrett HE Jr, Adams JW, et al: Bedside percutaneous tracheostomy: Experience with 55 elective procedures. *Ann Thorac Surg* 46:63, 1988.
81. Av J, Walker WS, Inglis D, et al: Percutaneous cricothyroidostomy (minitracheostomy) for bronchial toilet: Results of therapeutic and prophylactic use. *Ann Thorac Surg* 48:850, 1989.
82. Fisher EW, Howard DJ: Percutaneous tracheostomy in a head and neck unit. *J Laryngol Otol* 106:625, 1992.
83. Ciaglia P, Firsching R, Suniec C: Elective percutaneous dilatational tracheostomy: A new simple bedside procedure—Preliminary report. *Chest* 6:715, 1985.
84. Helms U, Heilman K: Ein neues Krikothyreoidotomie-Besteck für den Nontfall. *Anaesthetist* 34:47, 1985.
85. Wain JC, Wilson DJ, Mathisen DJ: Clinical experience with minitracheotomy. *Ann Thorac Surg* 49:881, 1990.
86. Weiss S: A new instrument for pediatric emergency cricothyrotomy. *National Pediatric Trade Journal,* Winter 1987, pp 9–11.
87. Weiss S: A new emergency cricothyroidotomy instrument. *J Trauma* 23:155, 1983.
88. Schachner A, Ovil J, Sidi J, et al: Rapid percutaneous tracheostomy. *Chest* 98:1266, 1990.
89. Ivatury R, Siegel JH, Stahl WM, et al: Percutaneous tracheostomy after trauma and critical illness. *J Trauma* 32:133, 1992.
90. Ravlo O, Bach V, Lybecker H, et al: A comparison between two emergency cricothyroidotomy instruments. *Acta Anaesthesiol Scand* 31:317, 1987.
91. Bjoraker DG, Kumar NB, Brown ACD: Evaluation of an emergency cricothyrotomy instrument. *Crit Care Med* 15:157, 1987.

92. Wang MB, Berke GS, Ward PH, et al: Early experience with percutaneous tracheotomy. *Laparoscope* 102:157, 1992.

93. Clancy MJ: A study of the performance of cricothyroidotomy on cadavers using the Minitrach II. *Arch Emerg Med* 6:143, 1989.

94. Paul A, Marelli D, Chiu RC-J, et al: Percutaneous endoscopic tracheotomy. *Ann Thorac Surg* 47:314, 1989.

95. Friedman Y, Franklin C: Endoscopic guided percutaneous tracheotomy: Early results of a consecutive trial. *JOTRA* 31:303, 1991.

96. Marelli D, Paul A, Manolidis S, et al: Endoscopic guided percutaneous tracheotomy: Early results of a consecutive trial. *J Trauma* 30:433, 1990.

97. Ciaglia P, Graniero KD: Percutaneous dilatational tracheostomy: Results and long-term follow-up. *Chest* 101:464, 1992.

98. Anderson HL, Bartlett RH: Elective tracheotomy for mechanical ventilation by the percutaneous technique. *Clin Chest Med* 12:555, 1991.

99. Hazard P, Jones C, Benitone J: Comparative clinical trial of standard operative tracheostomy with percutaneous tracheostomy. *Crit Care Med* 19:1018, 1991.

100. Leinhardt DJ, Mughal M, Bowles B, et al: Appraisal of percutaneous tracheostomy. *Br J Surg* 79:255, 1992.

101. Bodenham A, Diament R, Cohen A, et al: Percutaneous dilational tracheostomy. *Anaesthesia* 46:570, 1991.

102. Friedman Y, Mayer A: Bedside percutaneous tracheotomy in critically ill patients. *Chest* 104:532, 1993.

17. Extracorporeal Membrane Oxygenation and Carbon Dioxide Elimination

Harry L. Anderson III and
Robert H. Bartlett

Extracorporeal membrane oxygenation (ECMO), or extracorporeal life support (ECLS) as it is called today, is a modification of cardiopulmonary bypass (usually reserved for the operating room during open heart surgery) for prolonged use at the bedside. Extracorporeal life support became standard therapy for neonatal respiratory failure in 1986; its routine use in pediatric and adult patients has been more controversial. There were several anecdotal reports of success with the use of ECMO for treatment of respiratory failure in the early 1970s, until Zapol et al. reported the results of a National Institutes of Health (NIH)-sponsored multicenter trial of ECMO in adults with respiratory failure [1]. In this study, conventional mechanical ventilation was compared against ECMO as therapy for patients with adult respiratory distress syndrome (ARDS). Survival in each group was 10 percent, and thereafter the use of ECMO for adults was essentially abandoned.

Gattinoni et al., in 1986, reported a technique of low-flow extracorporeal perfusion using percutaneous vascular access, which emphasized carbon dioxide removal [2]. Using this technique of extracorporeal carbon dioxide removal (ECCO$_2$R), they reported an initial experience of 43 patients with 21 survivors. Based on this experience, several centers returned to the use of ECLS for the treatment of adult respiratory failure. Increasingly over the last few years, ECLS has been used to treat respiratory and cardiac failure in the pediatric patient, for what would seemingly be a logical jump from the treatment of neonates to smaller pediatric patients.

In this chapter, the technique of ECLS and indications and contraindications for the procedure in children and adults are described. Future directions for extracorporeal technology, particularly with regard to the intravascular oxygenator (IVOX), are discussed.

Background

The concept of cardiopulmonary bypass was introduced by Gibbon in 1937, when he described a system for cardiopulmonary support after operation on the heart [3]. His system consisted of a roller pump for perfusion of the blood through the system and a vertically mounted cylinder over which blood flowed, allowing exchange of carbon dioxide and oxygen between the thin film of blood and ambient air. Blood was then returned to the aorta.

The technology of cardiopulmonary bypass advanced, particularly with the refinement of the oxygenator. Various configurations have since evolved, particularly the bubble oxygenator, the disc oxygenator, the membrane oxygenator, and the hollow fiber oxygenator. In 1972, Hill et al. reported the first adult patient with respiratory failure treated with prolonged extracorporeal support [4]. Several other anecdotal reports of successes followed. In 1979, Zapol and collaborators reported the results of the NIH-sponsored multicenter comparison of ECMO versus conventional mechanical ventilation in adult patients with respiratory failure due to ARDS [1]. The patients were entered into the study based on having severe respiratory failure as predicted by strict entry criteria (mortality greater than 80%) and randomized to either continuing mechanical ventilation or ECMO. Although it was anticipated that 300 patients would be entered into the study, the study was terminated after 92 patients, due to a meager 10 percent survival in each group.

Bartlett et al., in 1976, described the first newborn with neonatal respiratory distress syndrome successfully treated with ECMO [5]. Several other centers reported the use of ECMO for treatment of persistent fetal circulation. Not until neonatal series from three centers were reported was ECMO considered standard therapy [6]. Randomized trials testing a new and very effective therapy against another, much less effective therapy resulting in almost certain mortality are difficult to perform, particularly when the endpoint is death. Randomization to the conventional therapy group is essentially randomization to death. Several randomized studies of ECMO in the neonate were stopped prematurely because of this ethical and moral dilemma. In one controversial randomized study of ECMO versus conventional management for newborns, Bartlett and colleagues achieved statistical significance, with 13 patients treated with ECMO (who survived) and 1 patient in the control group (who died), a statistical technique aptly named "randomized play-the-winner" [7,8].

As ECMO remained standard therapy for neonatal respiratory failure, several encouraging reports described its use for pediatric and adult respiratory failure [2,9–15]. In 1985, Gattinoni and colleagues reported 48.8 percent survival in 43 adult patients with respiratory failure treated by $ECCO_2R$ [2]. They used entry criteria similar to those in the 1977 NIH-sponsored adult ECMO trial (entry threshold with predicted mortality of 80%). Their technique incorporated percutaneous vascular access and a low-flow extracorporeal system that was particularly efficient at carbon dioxide removal. Oxygen transfer was accomplished with low-pressure, low-rate "apneic oxygenation" across the patient's lungs. Several other European and U.S. centers reported similar successes with varying techniques of extracorporeal circulation. As the technology of perfusion and understanding of the pathophysiology and treatment of cardiac and pulmonary failure have improved in recent years (compared to the 1970s), the term *ECMO* has been replaced by *ECLS* to acknowledge this modern approach to cardiopulmonary failure.

Technique of ECLS Perfusion

As ECLS also has its origin in cardiothoracic perfusion, the ECLS circuit has many similarities to the bypass perfusion equipment found in the operating room. The two most common modes of perfusion, venoarterial bypass and venovenous bypass, are depicted in Figures 17-1 and 17-2. Venoarterial perfusion is similar to heart-lung bypass—blood is drained from the right atrium (usually via a catheter placed in the right internal jugular vein) and pumped through a roller pump to a device designed for gas exchange (an oxygenator). Blood is returned to the aorta, usually via the common carotid artery or femoral artery, after warming by passage through a water-jacketed heat exchanger. This mode of perfusion is suitable for providing *both* cardiac and respiratory support. With venovenous bypass, on the other hand, blood is returned to a major vein (usually the femoral vein), raising the oxygen content of venous blood before it enters the heart. Venovenous perfusion provides *only* respiratory support—cardiac function must be intact, since no blood pressure or cardiac support is provided by venovenous ECLS. Table 17-1 compares venoarterial and venovenous perfusion.

CANNULATION. Cannulation can be performed by surgical exposure and direct cannulation of vessels or by the percutaneous method described by Pesenti and colleagues [16]. Percutaneous cannulation is usually reserved for access of veins, and not arteries; arterial cannulation usually requires direct vascular repair of the artery at the time of decannulation.

Once a mode of perfusion has been selected, the patient is anticoagulated (heparin, 100 units/kg body weight). Catheters

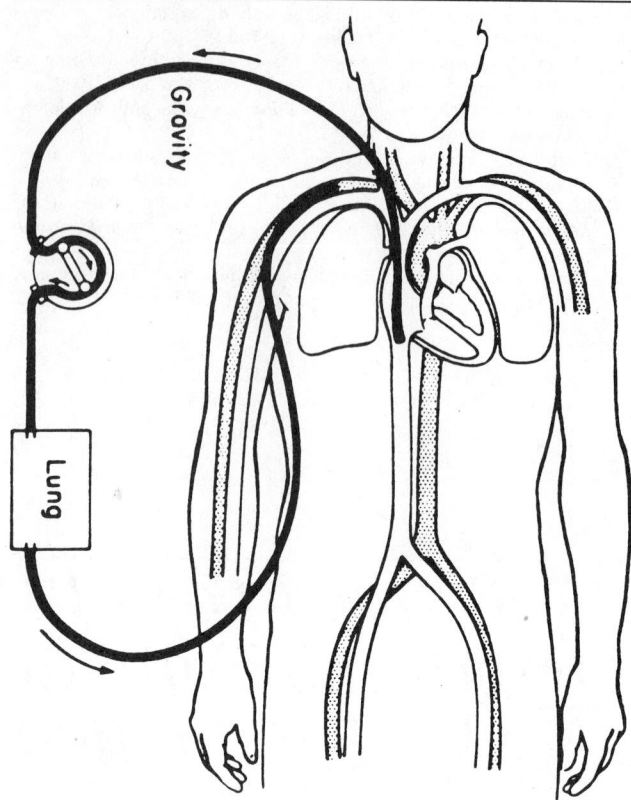

Fig. 17-1. Venoarterial extracorporeal life support perfusion. Blood is typically drained by a right internal jugular catheter with the tip near the right atrium and returned to the aorta (by a catheter in the axillary, carotid, or femoral artery or by direct cannulation of the aorta through the chest). (From Bartlett RH: Extracorporeal life support for cardiopulmonary failure. *Curr Prob Surg* 27:635, 1990. With permission.)

are usually chosen on the basis of the vessel size(s), and the expected or required blood flow through the catheter. Montoya et al. described an indexing system describing the resistance to flow in various catheters, based on a single number (the M number) [17]. Sinard et al. tested and categorized various cannulas used today for extrathoracic cannulation [18]. Thin-wall, wire-reinforced catheters manufactured by Bio-Medicus (Minneapolis, MN) typically provide low-resistance, high-flow access and are ideally suited for percutaneous access.

As the limiting factor for bypass flow is the rate at which venous blood can be drained from the patient, usually the largest possible catheter is selected for venous drainage and usually the internal jugular vein is used as it is the largest extrathoracic vein leading to the right atrium of the heart. Additional catheters may be placed in the femoral veins or the right atrium by thoracotomy, should additional venous drainage be necessary. Oxygenated, warmed blood is typically returned to the femoral vein with venovenous perfusion, and with this configuration percutaneous cannulation can be considered.

For venoarterial perfusion, oxygenated blood is returned to the carotid, femoral, or axillary arteries by direct surgical cutdown and exposure of the vessels. Surgical exposure is performed at the right neck so the internal jugular vein and common carotid artery each can be ligated distally and cannulas placed in each vessel proximally after a venotomy and arteriotomy, respectively, are created. During operation in the

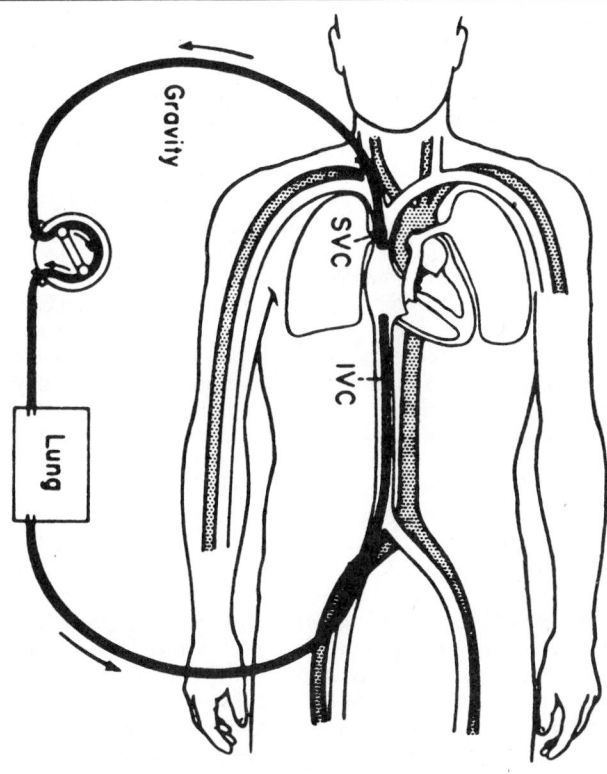

Fig. 17-2. Venovenous extracorporeal life support perfusion. Blood is typically drained by a right internal jugular catheter with the tip near the right atrium and returned to the vena cava by a catheter in the femoral vein. (From Bartlett RH: Extracorporeal life support for cardiopulmonary failure. *Curr Prob Surg* 27:635, 1990. With permission.)

Table 17-1. Comparison of Venoarterial and Venovenous Extracorporeal Life Support

	Venoarterial	Venovenous
Type of support	Cardiac and/or respiratory failure	Respiratory failure only
Vascular access	Vein to artery	Vein to vein
Decannulation	Requires arterial ligation or repair	No repair needed
Arterial access	Yes	No
Typical pump flow rate	80–100 ml/kg/min	100–120 ml/kg/min
Systemic oxygen delivery	Cardiac output + pump flow	Cardiac output only
Inotrope requirements	None	Usually required
Weaning of ventilator on initiation of bypass	Rapid	Gradual
Arterial waveform	Flattened pulse contour	Normal pulse contour
Central venous pressure	Inconsistent; depends on pump flow	Accurate indicator of volume status
Pulmonary artery pressure	Low; depends on pump flow	Accurate
Arterial oxygen saturation	95–100%; proportional to pump flow rates	80–95% common at maximum flow
Mixed venous oxygen saturation	Accurate	Artificially high due to recirculation

thorax, particularly that involving cardiopulmonary bypass, direct cannulation of the aortic arch is accomplished using an aortic perfusion cannula, and this cannula is connected to the ECLS circuit. A separate operation is necessary for decannulation, at which time the sternum and chest wall are closed. As the femoral and axillary arteries are considered "end arteries," with minimal collateral supply of the distal limb, distal perfusion must be provided when using these vessels for return of oxygenated blood. Usually a small perfusion catheter is placed opposite the perfusion cannula (through the same arteriotomy) to perfuse the limb distally.

Unilateral ligation and cannulation of the common carotid artery is the usual method of cannulation in the neonate and is typically used for cannulation of pediatric and adult patients. Neurologic sequelae of occlusion of the common carotid artery are infrequent, owing to the generous collateral circulation from the external carotid artery and the circle of Willis to the ipsilateral hemisphere of the brain. Unilateral ligation of the common carotid artery is usually performed after removal of a carotid catheter; attempts at repair of the arteriotomy can be complicated by distal thromboembolization, carotid stenosis at the site of repair, and pseudoaneurysm formation. Several centers have attempted repair of the carotid artery in pediatric and neonatal patients, with satisfactory results [19,20].

PUMPING SYSTEMS. There are two types of pumps used for perfusion: the servo-controlled roller pump and the centrifugal pump. The roller pump has behind it many years of laboratory and clinical use in the operating room. It is inexpensive and has no moving parts that contact the blood, but pump rotation speed must be regulated in response to changes in venous blood drainage from the patient. The centrifugal pump, of which the Bio-Medicus Bio-Pump is most commonly used, is a more expensive device that uses a spinning impeller which contacts and propels blood through the system. Although the centrifugal pump has no absolute requirement for servoregulation of the pump head rotational speed based on venous drainage, periods of occlusion at the inlet can result in cavitation of blood (gas bubble formation) in the pumping chamber. This results in hemolysis of blood and potential for air embolism. The centrifugal pump head must also be replaced every few days, due to wear of the impeller bearing, necessitating cessation of ECLS for a short period during the exchange. A pumping system incorporating advantages of both systems is currently in use in Europe [21] and under development in our laboratory for manufacture [22].

GAS EXCHANGE DEVICES (OXYGENATORS). The oxygenator is the key component to the ECLS system and probably the component of the circuit most prone to failure. In contrast to the drum-type oxygenator used by Gibbon and the disc or older plate-type oxygenators, modern oxygenators are of the spiral sandwich membrane (Kolobow membrane lung) or hollow fiber type. Both membrane types are used in the operating room for cardiac perfusion. The spiral wrapped membrane oxygenator consists of a single, long envelope constructed of silicone, with gas ports at either end. This envelope is spirally wound into a cylindrical shape, which is housed in a molded plastic container. Deoxygenated blood flows from one end of the device to the other, and thus through and around the wound membrane envelope. Oxygen gas is supplied to the inlet port of the oxygenator and passes through the envelope in countercurrent fashion, allowing oxygen and carbon dioxide gas exchange with blood. Gas exchange capability of oxygenators is rated in terms of square meters of surface area available for gas exchange. This design has had decades of satisfactory clinical use. For extended periods of use, however, the membrane lung is limited by the higher resistance to flow in the blood path and areas of stagnant flow leading to clot formation. Effort is currently underway to provide a thromboresistant heparin-bonded surface to the blood path.

The hollow fiber-type oxygenator is best typified by the Medtronic Maxima (Medtronic, Minneapolis, MN) oxygenator. This device has hollow microporous fibers through which the oxygen sweep gas flows and around which blood passes, an arrangement that allows gas exchange between blood and the gas phase. This design offers relatively small size and low resistance to blood flow, but the priming volume is much higher than with the membrane-type oxygenator. This oxygenator is available with a heparin-bonded coating that is Food and Drug Administration (FDA)-approved for *short-term* perfusion (in the operating room). It has been used extensively in Europe and in some U.S. centers for prolonged $ECCO_2R$ or ECLS [14,23,24]. In theory, the level of anticoagulation can be reduced with heparin-bonded components, but in practice "wetting" of the microporous membrane in these particular oxygenators leads to leakage of plasma to the gas phase, resulting in sudden profuse outpouring of serum containing foam 1 to 7 days after beginning ECLS. The oxygenator must be quickly replaced when plasma leak degrades oxygenating efficiency.

HEAT EXCHANGER. The heat exchanger in the blood path channels blood and warms it with a surrounding jacket of water supplied by a constant-temperature water bath. The heat exchanger is placed at the end (reinfusion) side of the circuit, warming the blood back to physiologic temperature just prior to its return to the patient. Several available devices involve long cylindrical chambers in which the blood enters the top and exits the bottom. Water warmed to just above physiologic temperature (38°C) is ported to the bottom of the same device, exiting the top and warming the blood in countercurrent fashion. There is a small visible reservoir of blood at the top of the heat exchanger, which doubles as a trap for bubbles that may make their way beyond the oxygenator, preventing passage to the patient.

PATIENT SELECTION. One of the more difficult aspects of this technology is deciding which patients in the intensive care unit, with early reversible cardiac and/or respiratory failure, might benefit from ECLS. The key terms here are *early* and *reversible:* our experience has shown that early intervention, particularly after the initiation of mechanical ventilation in patients with respiratory failure, is important for a successful outcome [15]. For patients with primary cardiac dysfunction, ECLS intervention must begin early enough to avoid the likely and inevitable deterioration of other organ systems (kidney, brain, etc.) when systemic perfusion is low.

Entry criteria for the neonate with persistent fetal circulation from primary pulmonary hypertension are well described. Entry is based on the patient attaining 50 to 80 percent or greater mortality with continued conventional management. Each neonatal ECLS center defines its mortality rate for any given patient with given physiologic parameters. For example, the alveolar-arterial oxygen gradient [$P(A-a)O_2$] can be used, or more commonly, oxygenation index (OI), defined as:

$$OI = \frac{[FIO_2] \times [MAP \ (cm \ H_2O)]}{[PaO_2 \ (mm \ Hg)]} \times 100$$

where FIO_2 is the inspired oxygen fraction, MAP is the mean airway pressure, and PaO_2 is the arterial partial pressure of oxygen [25]. In our institution, three successive calculations at 2-hour intervals resulting in OI values of 25 or greater predict at least 50 percent mortality, and OI values greater than 40 predict 80 percent mortality. A neonate consistently at the 50 percent mortality threshold for several hours, or one who reaches the 80 percent mortality threshold, is placed on ECLS, should no contraindication to anticoagulation exist.

Selection of the pediatric or adult (cardiac or respiratory failure) patient is more involved, as the many disease processes that result in cardiac or respiratory failure in these age groups do not result in the common pathophysiology of cardiorespiratory failure in the newborn. During the NIH-sponsored ECMO trial of the 1970s, criteria were developed to predict mortality at the 80 percent level or greater. Most centers still use these physiologic criteria for the selection of pediatric and adult patients. A more complete summary of indications and contraindications for pediatric and adult patients can be found in Table 17-2.

Extracorporeal life support is designed to allow "lung rest," and when instituted for severe respiratory failure has the primary purpose of providing sufficient oxygen transfer and carbon dioxide removal so that ventilator settings (inspired oxygen concentration, peak inflating pressures) may be decreased to less injurious levels. This is predicated on the expectation of lung recovery, which often is based on an educated guess. Sudden onset and deterioration in previously healthy lungs is more likely to reverse with ECLS than would an acute process superimposed on some other chronic pulmonary condition (e.g., pulmonary fibrosis, pulmonary hypertension), when initially presenting with identical degrees of respiratory dysfunction.

Pure capillary leak syndromes, bronchoreactive disease (asthma), and nonnecrotizing pneumonia (some viral pneumonias, *Legionella* infection) are typically treated with ECLS, and these diseases are expected to reverse within 1 to 2 weeks of ECLS.

For primary cardiac failure, ECLS has been used extensively by some centers, particularly in pediatric cardiac patients [9–13] (see Chap. 10). Venoarterial perfusion is the mainstay of cardiac support for patients with right and/or left ventricular failure. As with patients with respiratory failure, reversibility of the cardiac insult is a prerequisite to instituting ECLS for cardiac failure, and near full recovery should be expected after a *few days* of ECLS support.

Typical medical cardiac conditions treated by ECLS are myocarditis and cardiomyopathy resulting in a cardiac index less than 2 $L/min/m^2$ and mixed venous oxygen saturation of 50 percent or less for 2 hours or more, despite optimal pharmacologic and mechanical intervention. The capability for ECLS

Table 17-2. Indications and Contraindications for Extracorporeal Life Support for Pediatric and Adult Patients

Indications
  Total static lung compliance < 0.5 ml/cm H_2O/kg
  Transpulmonary shunt > 30% on inspired oxygen fraction of 0.6 or greater
  Reversible respiratory failure
  Time on mechanical ventilation ≤ 5 days (10 days absolute maximum)
Contraindications
  Potential for severe bleeding
  Time on mechanical ventilation ≥ 11 days
  Necrotizing pneumonia
  Poor quality of life (metastatic malignancy, major central nervous system injury, quadriplegia)
  Age > 60 years

cardiac support has been a useful addition to medical centers with active pediatric cardiothoracic and cardiac transplantation programs [12,26,27]. In such cases, ECLS provides short-term support prior to cardiac operation or transplantation (i.e., bridge to transplant). After cardiac operation, ECLS provides support while depressive effects of myocardial preservation or "myocardial stun" reverse. In the postoperative patient requiring ECLS, the potential for severe bleeding might at first seem to be a contraindication; special consideration and techniques are used under these circumstances (see below).

Management of Patients Undergoing ECLS

Once the patient has undergone cannulation and initiation of bypass, several considerations are necessary to minimize the likelihood of complication and to optimize the benefit derived from ECLS. This technology is expensive in both hospital resources and the combined effort of medical personnel in hour-to-hour management. Attention to certain details with regard to management improves the likelihood of more rapid success.

ANTICOAGULATION. After the initial loading dose of heparin at the time of cannulation, the patient is started on a continuous systemic heparin infusion. The activated clotting time (ACT) is checked hourly and the rate of heparin administration modified, if necessary, to maintain the ACT within desired limits. The ACT is a measure of heparin activity on *whole blood* (involving coagulation factors, platelets, etc.) and is preferred over individual assays of partial thromboplastin time (PTT) or thrombin clotting time, which are isolated measurements of heparin activity in *plasma*. Usually the target ACT is 180 to 200 seconds (normal 90–120 seconds). The desired ACT range is selected as a balance between too much anticoagulation (and higher ACT), which would result in bleeding, and inadequate anticoagulation, which results in circuit component clotting, particularly in the oxygenator. For patients at risk for bleeding, a lower ACT range (150–170 seconds) is usually selected. For patients actively bleeding while on ECLS, we sometimes stop administration of heparin for several hours (up to 1–2 days), with the expectation of the eventual need to change a membrane oxygenator (because of thrombosis in the blood path and deterioration of gas transfer). In such cases, an additional circuit is primed and kept ready nearby to swap should complete circuit failure by thrombosis occur. Whittlesey et al. described ECLS conducted without systemic heparin for several days [28].

To assure sufficient anticoagulation as well as prothrombosis when using systemic heparinization, antithrombin III activity and fibrinogen levels can be monitored with some regularity and increased by transfusion with fresh frozen plasma or cryoprecipitate. When heparin-bonded surfaces are perfected and suitable for long-term perfusion, full systemic heparinization will become unnecessary.

BLOOD PRODUCT MANAGEMENT. The most common complication of ECLS is bleeding, which occurred in up to 80 percent of cases in some series. The pediatric and adult patient are most prone to bleeding, given the propensity for other severe and unrelated illnesses (i.e., gastric ulcer) or even conditions specific to the disease being treated (fractures, chest tubes, recent operation and bleeding from a surgical site). Blood loss during the NIH-sponsored ECMO trial in the 1970s routinely exceeded 2 liters per day. Blood products (red blood cells, platelets, clotting factors) must be administered as part of the ECLS routine, due to bulk loss (bleeding and laboratory sampling), consumption (platelet activation and aggregation in the membrane oxygenator) and sequestration (usually noted as an increase in liver and spleen size in patients undergoing ECLS).

Packed red blood cells are transfused to maintain a hematocrit of 40 to 45 percent, to maximize the amount of oxygen delivered to the patient per liter of perfused blood. The small but possible risk of transfusion-associated disease must be understood by all parties involved, as by necessity blood products are required during some phase of the patient's ECLS course, beginning with priming of the circuit. Concentrated platelets are administered to keep platelet counts greater than 100,000/mm^3, and if ongoing bleeding is present a higher target platelet level of 150,000/mm^3 or greater is used. Although platelet *numbers* may appear adequate during ECLS, platelet *function* is usually less than normal due to platelet activation with the foreign surface of the ECLS circuit and the ongoing addition of older, more senescent platelets found in exogenous blood sources.

FLUID MANAGEMENT. Most critically ill patients, particularly those requiring resuscitation to maintain adequate blood pressure in the presence of higher airway pressures or additional preload to compensate for diminished cardiac contractility, are usually several kilograms (more correctly measured in *liters*) above dry weight. One goal early in ECLS is to augment net fluid loss, with the intention of achieving near dry weight at the time of decannulation. Fluid balance is carefully monitored during ECLS, and fluids are usually administered in an amount approximately 80 percent of maintenance. In addition, diuretics (furosemide [Lasix], ethacrynic acid [Edecrine], and mannitol) are added to the daily medication regimen to force diuresis. Should rapid fluid removal be necessary, a dialyzer/hemofilter membrane can be placed in the circuit and filtration driven by the higher pressure of the preoxygenator portion of the circuit. Slow continuous ultrafiltration (SCUF) or conventional continuous arteriovenous hemofiltration (CAVH) without or with dialysis (CAVH-D), in the case of renal failure, can be performed [29]. Parenteral nutrition is typically employed, since full enteral feeding using a nasoduodenal tube often proves unsatisfactory due to adynamic ileus.

VENTILATOR MANAGEMENT. Patients with respiratory failure who have failed conventional management usually require high peak and mean ventilatory pressures and high inspired oxygen fraction. The primary goal of ECLS for respiratory failure is to allow lung rest, by taking over a majority of oxygenation and ventilation, so ventilatory parameters can be decreased to more moderate settings. For cardiac and respiratory failure patients, a modification of the approach used by Gattinoni has been adopted: limited pressure (peak pressures no higher than 30–40 cm H$_2$O), low inspired fraction (FIO$_2$ ≤ 0.5), low respiratory rate (10 breaths/min) ventilation, using modest levels of positive end-expiratory pressure (PEEP, to 5–15 cm H$_2$O) [2]. Inspiratory time is prolonged to augment alveolar recruitment and expansion. For longer ECLS runs, percutaneous tracheostomy using the Ciaglia method is usually performed [30]. Standard and routine tracheal suctioning is continued, as are other standard respiratory care and nursing maneuvers.

WEANING FROM ECLS. During ECLS, improvement in pulmonary function or cardiac function is usually obvious, as blood gases improve and pump flow is decreased over time. When extracorporeal support is weaned to about 10 percent of metabolic requirement or cardiac output, a "trial off" ECLS is performed, with the anticipation of eventual decannulation. For patients on venoarterial bypass, moderate ventilatory settings are chosen (e.g., FIO_2 of 0.5) and any inotropes adjusted to modest rates of infusion. The catheters connecting the patient to the ECLS circuit are clamped and the bridge opened to allow idling of the blood to prevent thrombosis in the circuit. The trial off is continued until the patient shows signs of deterioration (decreasing blood pressure, cardiac output, arterial or mixed venous saturation), in which case the patient is placed back on ECLS, or until it is clear the patient is ready for decannulation. A modest trial off bypass of 2 to 4 hours without deterioration usually indicates that the patient is ready to be decannulated. Failure during a trial off simply means the patient is not yet ready, and another trial off is attempted 1 to 2 days later. The trial off during venovenous bypass is much simpler, because only the oxygen supply needs to be removed from the oxygenator and the bypass circuit allowed to circulate mixed venous blood away from and back to the patient (essentially providing a vena cava-to-vena cava shunt). The ECLS circuit, with blood oxygen saturation monitoring capability in the drainage limb of the circuit, acts to give the same information a fiberoptic oxygen saturation catheter would give if left in the central venous position. This information is invaluable when the progress of a trial off is followed noninvasively.

Results

To date more than 10,000 patients have been treated with ECLS at more than 90 centers worldwide [31]. A current summary of the use of ECLS for cardiorespiratory failure, as compiled by the Extracorporeal Life Support Organization (ELSO) Registry, is listed in Table 17-3. ELSO is an organization of health care professionals involved with ECLS from centers around the world, which was founded in 1989. The Registry is maintained for and is useful to member centers by offering data analysis of the accumulated ECLS patient database, and under the direction of ELSO several multicenter trials have been conducted. ELSO and the ELSO Registry have provided answers regarding ECLS issues of more than just the anecdotal experience of one or two investigators.

The ECLS experience is greatest in neonates, and this group of patients also has the highest survival rate. Survival for meconium aspiration syndrome is highest (93%); that for congenital diaphragmatic hernias is much lower (58%) due to the complex surgical nature of this disease [31]. Survival is higher in the more experienced centers, and survival rates increase over time at any new center beginning an ECLS program, lending support to the concept of a learning curve with this technology.

For pediatric patients, experience with cardiac and respiratory failure has grown as the number of centers has grown, and there is a natural tendency of neonatal centers to "move up" to ECLS support of larger pediatric cardiorespiratory failure patients in the pediatric critical care unit. This growth has been most notable for the treatment of pediatric patients after cardiac operation for congenital anomaly and transplantation.

After Gattinoni's report of improved survival with $ECCO_2R$ for adults with respiratory failure, several centers returned to this technology as an additional technique used in the critical care unit (Table 17-4). For patients with primary illness resulting in a survival of only 10 percent (by entry criteria), the 50 percent survival offered by ECLS, though not at the level for newborns (85–95%), is an improvement. We are now completing a phase I trial of ECLS for adults.

Morris et al reported a unique approach to the treatment of ARDS using a computer-driven algorithm, in an attempt to standardize ventilatory manipulations and changes during the testing of a new technology [32]. Comparing conventional mechanical ventilation to pressure-controlled, inverse-ratio ventilation and $ECCO_2R$, they found no difference in survival of the two treatment groups [33]. They did, however, note an improvement in survival of patients with respiratory failure using this computer-driven algorithm. A definitive test of any advantage of ECLS over conventional therapy still needs to be performed in centers experienced with prolonged perfusion and this new technology. We have yet to answer fully the question, "Is ECLS better than conventional management?"

Advances in ECLS

The development and testing of several new technologies related to ECLS deserve special mention, as these innovations will simplify ECLS and automate the process to the point where minute-by-minute attendance by an ECLS specialist will not be necessary. ECLS will be maintained and monitored by the critical care nurse already at the bedside.

First and foremost on the horizon is the development of a suitable thromboresistant surface coating for perfusion components. Although success has been achieved with heparin coating of short-term cardioperfusion components used in the operating room, currently two processes are under development for coating the oxygenators for long-term use: Carmeda Bio-Active Surface (Medtronic/Carmeda, Stockholm, Sweden) and DuraFlo II (Baxter-Bentley Laboratories, Irvine, CA) [14,34,35]. Leakage of plasma from the blood phase to the gas phase (as previously described) is inconsistent in its timing of appearance during ECLs, but this peculiar event has been reported in European centers where hollow fiber oxygenators with the Carmeda coating are routinely used and in our center and other U.S. centers [36]. Plasma leakage from the oxygenator has been duplicated in the laboratory and work toward refinement in the physical interaction of blood with the heparin-coated membrane may yet yield satisfactory results.

The roller pump and centrifugal pump have remained the only options for perfusion in the United States. A third system, previously marketed in Europe by Rhone-Poulenc (Collin-Cardio, Paris, France) combines the low cost and durability of these two systems and has safety features to prevent cavitation during periods of decreased venous return and overpressurization with subsequent tubing rupture during accidental occlusion of higher-pressure outlet lines. This system uses ovoid, distensible tubing, which collapses flat during inlet occlusion (preventing further blood flow and thus cavitation) and becomes round during outlet occlusion (overcoming the occlusion of the rollers, thus preventing high pressures). This system has been used

Table 17-3. Results of Extracorporeal Life Support in Neonatal and Pediatric Patients*

Group	Patients reported	Number survived	Percent survival
Neonatal respiratory	8913	7213	81%
Pediatric respiratory	672	336	50%
Pediatric cardiac	1109	493	44%
Total	10694	8042	75%

*Compiled by the ELSO Registry as of April 1994 [31].

Table 17-4. International and U.S. Centers Performing Extracorporeal Life Support for Adult Patients

Center	Number of Patients	Number survived	Percent survival
Armand-Trousseau Children's Hospital (Paris, France)	64	27	42%
Free University of Berlin (Berlin, Germany)	41	22	55%
Albert-Ludwigs University (Freiburg, Germany)	19	11	58%
Klinikum Mannheim, University of Heidelberg (Mannheim, Germany)	7	2	29%
Hospital Phillips University (Marburg, Germany)	150	86	57%
Ludwig-Maximilians University (Munich, Germany)	9	7	78%
Ospedale S. Gerardo/University of Milan (Monza/Milan, Italy)	93	41	44%
Karolinska Hospital/St. Goran's Hospital (Stockholm, Sweden)	26	9	35%
Groby Road Hospital (Leicester, United Kingdom)	18	12	67%
Sharpe Memorial Hospital (San Diego, CA)	9	3	33%
University of Michigan (Ann Arbor, MI)	46	25	54%
Hershey Medical Center (Hershey, PA)*	–	–	–
University of Pittsburgh (Pittsburgh, PA)	11	7	64%
LDS Hospital, University of Utah (Salt Lake City, UT)	21	7	33%
Total	514	259	50%

*Not available.

successfully by Durandy and colleagues in Paris [21]. A prototype is under development for FDA approval and manufacture in the United States [22].

Advances in catheter technology have been driven primarily by the needs of cardiothoracic perfusion. The thin-walled, low-resistance catheters manufactured by Bio-Medicus are ideal for percutaneous insertion and allow relatively high flow. A double-lumen catheter has been designed for single-site cannulation and venovenous perfusion in the newborn [37]. This design allows both drainage and return of blood through a single catheter barrel. A larger design for percutaneous placement in pediatric and adult patients is under development.

The existing ECLS perfusion system requires a specialist at the bedside full time for routine monitoring of the circuit, assessment of the level of anticoagulation, and modification of the rate of heparin administration and someone knowledgeable about the circuit to intervene effectively and quickly with circuit emergencies (raceway tubing rupture, oxygenator failure) or patient emergencies (e.g., bleeding, tension pneumothorax, hypotension). Our team of ECLS specialists is comprised of nurses, respiratory care personnel, perfusionists, and physicians who are specially trained to assemble, prime, monitor, and troubleshoot the ECLS circuit. The ECLS specialist remains at the bedside along with the critical care nurse. One objective has been to add sufficient automation and servoregulation to the system such that once cannulation and initial operation of the circuit have been completed and confirmed, the critical care nurse can both continue critical care duties and monitor the ECLS circuit.

This servoregulated ECLS circuit would automatically wean the system based on data input of mixed venous oxygen saturation, arterial oxygen saturation (by pulse oximetry), pulmo-

nary mechanics (from the ventilator), and assay of blood gases. Pump flow and oxygenator sweep gas composition and flow would be modulated based on feedback from these physiologic parameters. Safety mechanisms would be built in to detect the presence of air bubbles in the arterial return side or high pressures within the system. Merz et al. have designed a system for ECLS perfusion that incorporates some of these features [38].

The intravascular oxygenator (IVOX, CardioPulmonics, Salt Lake City, UT) is a gas exchange device that accomplishes what would be more correctly called intracorporeal respiratory support. The device, introduced in 1987, somewhat resembles a balloon pump in configuration and method of insertion; it is surgically placed into the vena cava via the right internal jugular vein or the right femoral vein (Fig. 17-3) [39]. Gas transfer of oxygen and carbon dioxide occur in *venous blood*, somewhat mimicking the process of venovenous perfusion.

The device is constructed of thin fibers of siloxane-coated microporous polypropylene suspended from either end by a central gas tube "stalk." The device is wound spirally to decrease its insertion diameter (similar to a balloon pump catheter). After surgical exposure of the right internal jugular vein or right femoral vein, it is inserted, under fluoroscopic guidance, through a venotomy into the vena cava. When in place, the fibers are unwound, or "unfurled," and allowed to spread out to occupy the lumen of the vena cava. Oxygen is supplied to the distal ends of the fibers via the central gas tube. Subatmospheric pressure (vacuum) is applied to the proximal ends of

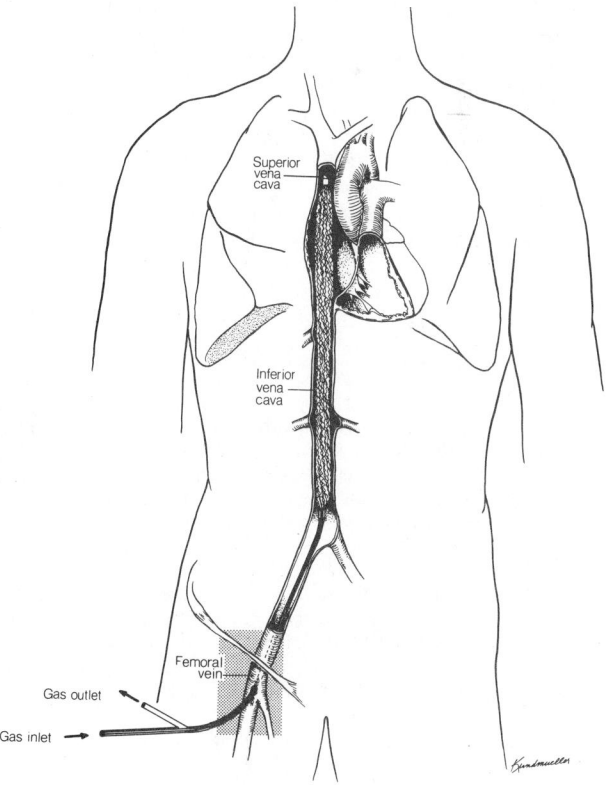

Fig. 17-3. Intravascular Oxygenator (IVOX). The device is inserted into the vena cava through a venotomy after surgical exposure of the right femoral or right internal jugular vein. Oxygen sweep gas is drawn through the hollow fibers (by negative pressure at the gas outlet), allowing diffusion of oxygen to venous blood and carbon dioxide from venous blood to the sweep gas. (From CardioPulmonics, Inc., Salt Lake City, Utah. With permission.)

the fibers, drawing the oxygen sweep gas through the fibers. As subatmospheric pressures are used, gas embolism is prevented after breakage of a fiber, since blood will enter the fiber and clot, occluding it. Thrombus formation is minimized by a thromboresistant coating on the fibers of the device and the concomitant use of systemic anticoagulation. Oxygen gas is transferred from the sweep gas by diffusion across the fiber membrane into the venous blood, and carbon dioxide similarly diffuses from venous blood into the sweep gas. As the carbon dioxide concentration in the exhaust gas can be measured, carbon dioxide excretion can be calculated by multiplying by the sweep gas flow rate.

Several centers have reported safety and efficacy of the IVOX device, but because of the limited surface area available for gas exchange in the blood path, maximal removal of carbon dioxide is limited to about one-third of metabolically produced carbon dioxide [40,41]. Oxygen transfer to venous blood is less efficient. Cox and co-workers developed a mathematical model describing gas transfer across the IVOX, and showed that an arterial pCO_2 of 75 to 80 mm Hg was necessary to achieve carbon dioxide removal rates of 90 to 100 ml per minute [42]. These observations confirm the earlier work of Hickling et al. on enhanced augmentation of carbon dioxide excretion using permissive hypercapnia [43]. A phase I study of the IVOX is nearing completion at 30 centers worldwide. The gas-exchanging capabilities of the IVOX are limited and certainly less than those afforded by ECLS or $ECCO_2R$. The IVOX does, however, represent a novel approach to augmentation of gas exchange by a route other than the native lungs.

Conclusion

Extracorporeal life support has made significant technologic advance in recent years. It is standard therapy for neonatal respiratory failure and is used in pediatric and adult cardiorespiratory failure. A key factor to success with ECLS is early intervention in the disease process, prior to irreversible organ damage. Proper application of this technology requires an organized and experienced team of surgeons, intensivists, ECLS specialists, and nurses. Recent improved success with ECLS can be attributed to improved perfusion technology and better patient selection. As understanding of the pathophysiology of cardiac and respiratory failure continues to advance, ECLS may well find a more important role in the critical care unit.

References

1. Zapol WM, Snider MT, Hill JD, et al: Extracorporeal membrane oxygenation in severe acute respiratory failure: A randomized prospective study. *JAMA* 242:2193, 1979.
2. Gattinoni L, Pesenti A, Mascheroni D, et al: Low-frequency positive-pressure ventilation with extracorporeal CO_2 removal in severe acute respiratory failure. *JAMA* 256:881, 1986.
3. Gibbon JH Jr: Artificial maintenance circulation during experimental occlusion of the pulmonary artery. *Arch Surg* 34:1105, 1937.
4. Hill JD, O'Brien TG, Murray JJ, et al: Extracorporeal oxygenation for acute post-traumatic respiratory failure (shock-lung syndrome): Use of the Bramson membrane lung. *N Engl J Med* 286:629, 1972.
5. Bartlett RH, Gazzaniga AB, Jefferies R, et al: Extracorporeal membrane oxygenation (ECMO) cardiopulmonary support in infancy. *ASAIO Trans* 22:80, 1976.
6. Short BL, Pearson GD: Neonatal extracorporeal membrane oxygenation: A review. *J Intensive Care Med* 1:47, 1986.
7. Bartlett RH, Roloff DW, Cornell RG, et al: Extracorporeal circulation

in neonatal respiratory failure: A prospective randomized study. *Pediatrics* 4:479, 1985.
8. Cornell RG, Landenberger BD, Bartlett RH: Randomized play-the-winner clinical trials. *Communicat Stat Theory Methods* 1:159, 1986.
9. Anderson HL III, Attorri RJ, Custer JR, et al: Extracorporeal membrane oxygenation (ECMO) for pediatric cardiopulmonary failure. *J Thorac Cardiovasc Surg* 99:1011, 1990.
10. Adolph V, Heaton J, Steiner R, et al: Extracorporeal membrane oxygenation for nonneonatal respiratory failure. *J Pediatr Surg* 26:326, 1991.
11. Redmond CR, Graves ED, Falterman KW, et al: Extracorporeal membrane oxygenation for respiratory and cardiac failure in infants and children. *J Thorac Cardiovasc Surg* 93:199, 1987.
12. Pennington GD, Swartz MT: Circulatory support in infants and children. *Ann Thorac Surg* 55:233, 1993.
13. O'Rourke PP, Stolar CJH, Zwischenberger JB, et al: Extracorporeal membrane oxygenation: Support for overwhelming pulmonary failure in the pediatric population—Collective experience from the Extracorporeal Life Support Organization. *J Pediatr Surg* 28:523, 1993.
14. Bindslev L: Adult ECMO performed with surface-heparinized equipment. *ASAIO Trans* 34:1009, 1988.
15. Anderson HL III, Steimle CN, Shapiro MB, et al: Extracorporeal life support for adult cardiorespiratory failure. *Surgery* 114:161, 1993.
16. Pesenti A, Gattinoni L, Kolobow T, et al: Extracorporeal circulation in adult respiratory failure. *ASAIO Trans* 34:43, 1988.
17. Montoya JP, Merz SI, Bartlett RH: A standardized system for describing flow/pressure relationships in vascular access devices. *ASAIO Trans* 37:4, 1991.
18. Sinard JM, Merz SI, Hatcher MD, et al: Evaluation of extracorporeal perfusion catheters using a standardized measurement technique: The M-number. *ASAIO Trans* 37:60, 1991.
19. Spector ML, Wiznitzer M, Walsh-Sukys MC, et al: Carotid reconstruction in the neonate following ECMO. *J Pediatr Surg* 26:357, 1991.
20. Taylor BJ, Seibert JJ, Glasier CM, et al: Evaluation of the reconstructed carotid artery following extracorporeal membrane oxygenation. *Pediatrics* 90:568, 1992.
21. Durandy Y, Chevalier JY, Lecompte Y: Single cannula venovenous bypass for respiratory membrane lung support. *J Thorac Cardiovasc Surg* 99:404, 1990.
22. Montoya JP, Merz SI, Bartlett RH: Laboratory experience with a novel, non-occlusive, pressure-regulated peristaltic pump. *ASAIO J* 38:M406, 1992.
23. Anderson HL III, Delius RE, Sinard JM, et al: Early experience with adult extracorporeal membrane oxygenation in the modern era. *Ann Thorac Surg* 53:553, 1992.
24. Pesenti A, Gattinoni L, Bombino M: Long term extracorporeal respiratory support: 20 years of progress. *Intensive Crit Care Dig* 12:15, 1993.
25. Bartlett RH: Extracorporeal life support for cardiopulmonary failure. *Curr Prob Surg* 10:627, 1990.
26. Delius RE, Bove EL, Meliones JN, et al: Use of extracorporeal life support in patients with congenital heart disease. *Crit Care Med* 20:1216, 1992.
27. Klein MD, Shaheen KW, Whittlesey GC, et al: Extracorporeal membrane oxygenation for the circulatory support of children after repair of congenital heart disease. *J Thorac Cardiovasc Surg* 100:498, 1990.
28. Whittlesey GC, Kundu SY, Salley SO, et al: Is heparin necessary for extracorporeal circulation? *ASAIO Trans* 34:823, 1988.
29. Heiss KF, Petit B, Hirschl RB, et al: Renal insufficiency and volume overload in neonatal ECMO managed by continuous ultrafiltration. *ASAIO Trans* 10:557, 1987.
30. Ciaglia P, Firsching R, Syniec C: Elective percutaneous dilatational tracheostomy—A new simple bedside procedure—Preliminary report. *Chest* 87:715, 1985.
31. ECMO Quarterly Report. Ann Arbor, MI. ECMO Registry of the Extracorporeal Life Support Organization, April 1994.
32. Morris AH, Menlove RL, Rollins RJ, et al: A controlled clinical trial of a new 3-step therapy that includes extracorporeal CO_2 removal for ARDS. *ASAIO Trans* 34:48, 1988.
33. Clemmer T, Morris A, Suchyta M, et al: Extracorporeal support does not improve ARDS survival (abstract). *Crit Care Med* 20:S61, 1992.
34. Shanley CJ, Hultquist KA, Rosenberg DM, et al: Prolonged extra-

corporeal circulation without heparin: Evaluation of the Medtronic Minimax oxygenator. *ASAIO Trans* 38:M311, 1992.

35. Toomasian JM, Hsu L-C, Hirschl RB, et al: Evaluation of Duraflo II heparin coating in prolonged extracorporeal membrane oxygenation. *ASAIO Trans* 34:410, 1988.
36. Mottaghy K, Oedekoven B, Starmans H, et al: Technical aspects of plasma leakage prevention in microporous capillary membrane oxygenators. *ASAIO Trans* 35:640, 1989.
37. Anderson HL III, Otsu T, Chapman RA, et al: Venovenous extracorporeal life support in neonates using a double lumen catheter. *ASAIO Trans* 35:650, 1989.
38. Merz S, Montoya PJ, Shanley CJ, et al: Implementation of a controller for extracorporeal life support (abstract). *ASAIO Trans* 22:69, 1993.
39. Mortensen JD: An intravenacaval blood gas exchange (IVCBGE) device: Preliminary report. *ASAIO Trans* 33:570, 1987.
40. Jurmann JM, Demertzis S, Schaefers H-J, et al: Intravascular oxygenation for advanced respiratory failure. *ASAIO J* 38:120, 1992.
41. Conrad SA, Eggerstedt JM, Morris VF, et al: Prolonged intracorporeal support of gas exchange with an intravenacaval oxygenator. *Chest* 103:158, 1993.
42. Cox CS Jr, Zwischenberger JB, Grave DF, et al: Intracorporeal CO_2 removal and permissive hypercapnia to reduce airway pressure in acute respiratory failure: The theoretical basis for permissive hypercapnia with IVOX. *ASAIO J* 39:97, 1993.
43. Hickling KG, Henderson SJ, Jackson R: Low mortality associated with low volume pressure limited ventilation with permissive hypercapnia in severe adult respiratory distress syndrome. *Intensive Care Med* 16:372, 1990.

18. Peritoneal Dialysis, Hemodialysis, and Hemofiltration Techniques in the Intensive Care Unit

Glenn M. Chertow and J. Michael Lazarus

Dialytic techniques were first used in clinical practice in 1946, when Kolff successfully dialyzed a 45-year-old woman with drug-induced oliguric acute renal failure and uremic encephalopathy [1]. For many years thereafter, acute dialysis was considered both cumbersome and experimental. Over the past 20 years, however, refinements in techniques and technology have made dialysis precise, reliable, and extremely effective. This chapter describes currently available dialytic procedures and their indications, potential benefits, and risks in the management of critically ill patients.

Indications for Acute Dialysis

Management of critically ill patients is often complicated by derangements in fluid and electrolyte balance as well as impaired renal function. Renal function is typically gauged by an assay of serum creatinine, a molecule whose clearance approximates glomerular filtration [2]. Some define acute renal failure as a finite rise or percent elevation in the serum creatinine; others use the term more loosely. Table 18-1 lists several common causes of acute renal failure in critically ill patients. Renal failure is often the result of two or more factors, such as nephrotoxin exposure and hypoperfusion, that alone might be insufficient to induce significant injury.

Evaluation of the patient with acute renal failure in the intensive care unit (ICU) must include careful investigation into possible causes of reversible disease. Many ICU patients suffer from renal hypoperfusion, due to volume depletion from gastrointestinal bleeding or vigorous diuretic therapy, low cardiac output states, such as cardiogenic shock or severe congestive heart failure, or vascular shunting, as in sepsis or hepatic cirrhosis.

These patients characteristically have reduced urine output, and, in the absence of diuretic therapy or underlying renal disease, low fractional excretion of sodium [3]. Volume expansion may augment renal blood flow and urine output but may complicate cardiac and pulmonary function, particularly in the setting of congestive heart failure. A pulmonary artery catheter may be required in some cases to guide therapy.

Complete or partial urinary tract obstruction can lead to acute renal failure in critically ill patients, either in association with their primary disease or as a result of therapy. For instance, retroperitoneal lymphadenopathy in a patient with lymphoma or metastatic cervical or colonic carcinoma may cause ureteral obstruction, leading to bilateral hydronephrosis and acute renal failure [4]. More subtle presentations of urinary tract obstruction may develop in the ICU as well; for example, an elderly man with prostatic hypertrophy may have mild urethral obstruction with relatively normal renal function at baseline but develop urinary retention and obstruction after surgery, which can be exacerbated by the anticholinergic side effects of commonly used sedatives and analgesics, such as diphenhydramine, hydroxyzine, thioridazine, morphine, and meperidine [5]. Bedside ultrasound study of the kidneys is reliable and relatively inexpensive; we recommend that all patients with acute renal failure be screened for urinary tract obstruction before dialysis is initiated.

If acute renal failure is due to intrinsic renal disease or injury, it is useful to consider it as an entity of two major subtypes: oliguric and nonoliguric acute renal failure. In nonoliguric renal failure, the patient has a diminished ability to clear by-products of metabolism, such as urea nitrogen and drugs, but maintains a urine output (with or without diuretics) sufficient to avoid the sequelae of volume overload. Typically, preserved urine output protects the patient from the development of severe hyperka-

Table 18-1. Common Causes of Acute Renal Failure in the Intensive Care Unit

Intraoperative hypotension
Acute blood loss
Prolonged volume depletion
Cardiogenic shock
Sepsis syndrome
Nephrotoxicity
    Intravenous contrast
    Nonsteroidal antiinflammatory drugs
    Aminoglycosides
    Amphotericin B
    Cyclosporin A
    Angiotensin-converting enzyme inhibitors
Prolonged aortic or renal artery cross-clamping
Atheroemboli
Acute parenchymal renal disease
Urinary tract obstruction
Hepatorenal syndrome
Trauma (rhabdomyolysis)

Table 18-2. Indications for Dialysis in the Intensive Care Unit

Absolute
    Volume overload refractory to diuretic therapy
    Hyperkalemia poorly responsive to conservative therapy
    Uremic complications
        Pericarditis or serositis
        Severe bleeding diathesis
        Encephalopathy
    Specific drug overdose
Relative
    Failing nutritional status with need for hyperalimentation
    Obligate excess fluid intake (e.g., antibiotics)
    Metabolic derangements
        Acidemia
        Hyperphosphatemia
        Hypermagnesemia
        Hyperuricemia

lemia as well, as renal potassium excretion is in part flow-dependent [6]. In contrast, oliguric renal failure portends a poorer renal prognosis, as there is often insufficient time for renal recovery before dialysis is required. Unfortunately, a reliable laboratory surrogate for uremia is not available. The blood urea nitrogen is frequently considered an adequate gauge of the presence of uremia, although its level may be affected by several factors that are independent of renal function. These include comorbid illnesses, such as gastrointestinal bleeding or hypercatabolism, as well as drug therapy with glucocorticoids or tetracyclines [7]. Serum creatinine generally serves as a more reliable marker of impaired glomerular filtration, although it too is subject to error, as creatinine generation is dependent on body muscle mass, a widely variable factor [8].

ABSOLUTE INDICATIONS. Table 18-2 lists the usual indications for dialysis in the ICU. Volume overload with pulmonary edema is the most common reason for initiating dialysis in the ICU. Acute renal failure may result in extravascular (peripheral edema, ascites, pleural effusions) as well as intravascular (hypertension, pulmonary congestion) volume expansion. Although the extravascular manifestations of volume overload can be dramatic, they are rarely of sufficient morbidity to warrant dialytic intervention. On the other hand, pulmonary congestion mandates acute intervention if it cannot be controlled with diuretic agents alone. Individuals with left ventricular dysfunction, whether due to intrinsic heart disease or secondary to the effects of sepsis, acidemia, or hypoxia, suffer the greatest morbidity from volume excess. Volume overload may occur even in individuals with nonoliguric renal failure, if diuresis is insufficient in the face of large amounts of fluid administered with antibiotics, hyperalimentation, and the like.

Even in patients with oliguric acute renal failure, diuretic challenge should be undertaken before ultrafiltration or dialysis is initiated. A loop diuretic, such as furosemide (200–400 mg) or bumetanide (5–10 mg) can be administered intravenously in combination with a thiazide agent, such as chlorthiazide (250–500 mg) or oral metolazone (5–10 mg). If there is no response to a diuretic challenge and no major change in the patient's hemodynamics, repeated large doses of diuretics should be avoided to reduce the risk of ototoxicity. Low-dose dopamine (1–2 μg/kg/min) may be added to the diuretic regimen to augment renal perfusion and enhance natriuresis [9].

Hyperkalemia that is sufficient to cause disturbances of cardiac conduction can complicate some cases of acute renal fail-

ure. Typically, individuals with primary disorders associated with hypercatabolism and tissue breakdown are at highest risk; these include rhabdomyolysis, gastrointestinal bleeding, hemolytic anemia, disseminated intravascular coagulation, and tumor lysis syndrome. An orally administered cation exchange resin (sodium polystyrene sulfonate) may efficiently bind intestinal potassium [10], but its use is limited in many critically ill patients with ileus or gastrointestinal bleeding. Efforts to direct extracellular potassium excess into the intracellular compartment with glucose with or without insulin, beta-adrenergic agonists (e.g., albuterol) [11], and sodium bicarbonate are effective but will not reduce potassium burden over the long term. When conservative measures are insufficient to control potassium excess, dialysis should be initiated.

Unlike pulmonary edema or hyperkalemia, which are readily diagnosed, the clinical consequences of uremia may be difficult to detect in the ICU. For instance, encephalopathy, a clinical hallmark of uremia, is common among seriously ill patients and may be the result of medication, pain, sleep disturbance, and/or underlying disease (e.g., liver or central nervous system). Another complication of uremia, pericarditis, may be seen following cardiac surgery, after myocardial infarction, or as a complication of infectious (e.g. pneumonia), neoplastic (e.g., breast or lung carcinoma), or autoimmune (e.g., systemic lupus erythematosus) disease. Uremia can lead to bleeding due to platelet malfunction, although underlying coagulopathy, stress gastritis, and anticoagulant and antiplatelet drugs are more common causes of bleeding in ICU patients. When uremia can be implicated as a likely additive cause of encephalopathy, serositis, or a bleeding diathesis, dialysis should be initiated.

RELATIVE INDICATIONS. Metabolic acidosis invariably accompanies acute renal failure, as endogenously generated organic acids are retained and the kidney suffers from a diminished ability to retain bicarbonate and maximally to acidify the urine [13]. In ICU patients, acidosis can be worsened by hypoventilation, severe diarrhea, or the composition of intravenous fluids and hyperalimentation. Usually, metabolic acidosis can be controlled conservatively, but dialysis may be required in selected settings. For instance, an individual with acidosis and compensatory tachypnea may experience respiratory fatigue and require intubation, particularly if pulmonary edema and hypoxia are present. Others may not tolerate the administration of sodium bicarbonate for treatment of acidosis because of preexistent volume overload. An arterial pH of 7.20 or less should heighten concern; although acidosis itself may not be directly deleterious, when severe it is often a marker of advanced underlying disease. The management of patients with lactic acidosis due to low cardiac output or hypoxic states is especially challenging, as the administration of sodium bicarbonate to this subgroup may paradoxically worsen acidosis [14]. Unfortunately, concurrent hemodynamic instability frequently complicates dialysis in these patients.

Metabolic alkalosis due to nasogastric suction or prolonged diuretic therapy is common among ICU patients but is nearly always treated conservatively, predominantly with the administration of chloride salts or agents that reduce gastric acid production (e.g., cimetidine, omeprazole). Hypocalcemia typically accompanies acute renal failure and can be treated effectively with intravenous or oral calcium supplementation. Severe hypercalcemia due to malignancy, vitamin D intoxication, or milk-alkali syndrome only rarely requires dialysis, with a modified low-calcium dialysate (0–1 mEq/L) [15]. Saline diuresis, biphosphanates, corticosteroids, and/or mithramycin are effective and safer for most patients than dialysis. Similarly, hypermagnesemia, due to cathartic abuse, for example, and hyperuricemia, as might be encountered in tumor lysis syndrome, can be rapidly corrected with dialysis, although conservative measures usually suffice.

Most drugs of abuse, such as barbiturates, tricyclic antidepressants, and benzodiazepines, are highly protein-bound [16], and only limited fractions of free drug are cleared by dialysis. In contrast, acute intoxication with water-soluble drugs of relatively low molecular weight, such as aspirin or methanol, is effectively managed with hemodialysis or charcoal hemoperfusion [17]. Acute peritoneal dialysis is much less efficient than hemodialysis for clearance of small solutes and should not be used for acute intoxications.

Some investigators have advocated hemofiltration in the treatment of adult respiratory distress syndrome (ARDS) [18]. The rationale for hemofiltration is twofold: in addition to its ability to reduce total body water and sodium, hemofiltration may result in the clearance of "culprit" cytokines, such as tumor necrosis factor (TNF) [19], which may be of critical importance in the pathobiology of ARDS. However, hemofiltration in this setting may be hazardous. For instance, volume depletion secondary to overzealous ultrafiltration may reduce ventricular filling and impair oxygen delivery, thereby worsening existent hypoxemia. In addition, the hemofilter itself may induce cytokine activation and counterbalance the clearance achieved. Until more definitive evidence is available, hemofiltration or dialysis should not be performed routinely for patients with ARDS.

Contraindications

The only absolute contraindication to hemodialysis is the inability to establish vascular access, which is rarely problematic in the acute setting. Bleeding can usually be controlled, even in uremic patients, with careful technique, and if necessary, with dDAVP and blood product support [20]. Peritoneal dialysis is contraindicated in individuals with peritonitis or a history of extensive abdominal surgery. Individuals with reduced lung volumes may also fare poorly with peritoneal dialysis, as the abdominal distention required may impair diaphragmatic excursion. Arterial access for continuous hemofiltration and related techniques is contraindicated in individuals with severe peripheral vascular disease or a history of femoral artery bypass grafting because of the potential for atheroembolic or ischemic sequelae.

Although lifesaving in many circumstances, dialysis is not without substantial risk. Table 18-3 lists the complications common to all forms of renal replacement therapy and those that

Table 18-3. Complications of Renal Replacement Therapy in the Intensive Care Unit

General
Hypotension from volume depletion
Electrolyte disturbances
Acid-base disturbances
Infection
Peritoneal dialysis
Peritonitis
Hyperglycemia
Impaired ventilation
Protein loss
Conventional hemodialysis
Hemorrhage
Thromboembolism
Leukopenia*
Hypoxemia*
Continuous hemofiltration techniques
Hemorrhage
Arterial insufficiency
Cholesterol embolization
Arteriovenous shunting

*Seen most commonly with nonbiocompatible hemodialysis membranes (e.g. cuprophane).

could be considered modality-specific. An important underrecognized risk of dialysis is the delay in recovery of renal function that may occur after dialysis for acute renal failure [21]. After an ischemic or toxic insult, tissue repair and recovery of function may require days to weeks [22]. Hemodynamic or immunologic factors related to dialysis can delay these processes. For example, repeated bouts of hypotension during dialysis may aggravate renal ischemia. In addition, complement-mediated injury sustained by blood dialyzer contact with nonbiocompatible membranes (see below) may delay or prevent renal recovery.

General Principles of Dialysis

ULTRAFILTRATION. Ultrafiltration in its simplest form is the removal of protein-free plasma water as a result of an osmotic gradient across a semipermeable membrane. For instance, ultrafiltration during peritoneal dialysis is driven by the instillation in the peritoneal cavity of an osmotically active solute, typically dextrose. The uptake of dextrose from the peritoneum is time- and concentration-dependent, such that the rate of ultrafiltration (milliliters per minute) decreases with extended dwell time and lower dextrose (1.5%) concentration. Maximal ultrafiltration can be achieved with shortened dwell times (20–30 minutes) and increased volume and tonicity (2.5% or 4.25% dextrose) of dialysate [23].

In contrast, ultrafiltration during conventional hemodialysis depends on the permeability characteristics of the dialyzer (artificial kidney) and the transmembrane pressure (TMP) gradient [24]. The permeability of the dialyzer is a function of pore size (ultrafiltration coefficient) and surface area. In general, dialyzers manufactured from synthetic plastics, such as polysulfone, polymethylmethacrylate (PMMA), and polyacrilonitrile (PAN), offer higher ultrafiltration rates than those comprised of cellulose, cuprophane, or related materials. The TMP gradient necessary for ultrafiltration can be applied as positive pressure along the blood path or as negative pressure along the dialysate side of the membrane. In the past, the transmembrane pressure necessary to ultrafilter a desired volume was calculated at the bed-

Table 18-4. Performance Characteristics of Available Hemodialyzers

Fiber	Surface area (m²)	Ultrafiltration coefficient (ml/hr/mm Hg)	Urea clearance (ml/min)	Vitamin B$_{12}$ clearance (ml/min)	Cost ($)	Biocompatability
Cuprophan	0.2–2.0	0.9–9.0	51–190	8–63	+	0
Cellulose Ace.	0.5–2.1	2.4–10	128–198	26–77	+	+
Hemophan	0.7–1.6	2.0–7.6	160–194	43–91	+ +	+ +
Polyacrilonitrile	0.5–2.0	14–62	118–195	37–112	+ + +	+ + +
Polysulfone	0.4–1.8	20–60	125-192	20–139	+ + + +	+ + +

*Clearance values at blood flow rate 200 ml/minute.

side, based on the patient's blood flow and the ultrafiltration coefficient of the dialyzer. This practice has been largely supplanted recently by the use of ultrafiltration control systems, which automatically calculate and modify transmembrane pressure to achieve precisely desired ultrafiltration rates [25]. This precision is critical in ICU patients who may be hemodynamically unstable. In fact, ultrafiltration control is necessary to use the newer, more powerful synthetic membranes with high ultrafiltration capacity (Table 18-4).

Hemofiltration and related continuous techniques are particularly well suited to ICU patients who require ultrafiltration, because ultrafiltration can be monitored and modified on nearly a minute-to-minute basis. During hemofiltration, the formation of ultrafiltrate depends on the cardiac output and blood flow into the hemofilter, as well as the negative pressure generated by the height of the ultrafiltrate collection system [26]. If the ultrafiltrate collection system is located substantially below the hemofilter, ultrafiltration rates as high as 10 to 15 liters per day can be achieved, even in the presence of low arterial blood pressure [27]. An alternative approach is the use of a negative-pressure pump or suction device, which can dramatically increase ultrafiltration rates [28]. Of course, caution must be exercised to avoid excessive ultrafiltration under these circumstances.

CLEARANCE. The movement of solute from blood to dialysate can be accomplished by diffusive or convective transport. Diffusive clearance is achieved by the concentration-dependent movement of solute across a semipermeable membrane. In contrast, convective transport is ultrafiltration- or flow-dependent. Substances of variable molecular weight (e.g., urea, vitamin B$_{12}$) have been used as markers to characterize the contributions of diffusive and convective clearance among available dialytic modalities [29]. It is known that smaller-molecular-weight solutes, such as urea and potassium, have high diffusive clearances, whereas larger molecules, such as vitamin B$_{12}$ and beta$_2$-microglobulin, depend predominantly on ultrafiltration for clearance.

During peritoneal dialysis, diffusive clearance of small solutes is accomplished by the presence of concentration gradients between the peritoneal capillary bed and the dialysate, which is free of urea and potassium, for example (Table 18-5). Small solute clearance can increase by as much as 25 percent with more rapid exchanges, as the patient (peritoneum) and dialysate are not given time to reach equilibrium. The use of hypertonic dialysate (2.5% or 4.25% dextrose) can also improve small solute clearance via convective transport and will enhance the clearance of medium-sized and large molecules, which depends on ultrafiltration [30].

During conventional hemodialysis, the majority of small solute clearance is accomplished by diffusion. In a hollow fiber dialyzer, blood flows in each fiber, which is itself a semiperme-

able membrane, while dialysate bathes the outer surface of each fiber (Fig. 18-1). This results in mass transfer of small solutes from the blood to the dialysate. Clearance is maximized when blood and dialysate flow at rapid rates in a countercurrent direction; this situation maintains a maximal concentration gradient throughout blood-dialysate contact. A double-lumen, semisoft dialysis catheter is most often used in the ICU and blood flow rates of 250 to 350 ml per minute through these catheters can usually be achieved. Dialysate flow is standardized on many hemodialysis machines to either 500 or 800 ml per minute. Near-maximal solute clearance with conventional hemodialysis can be achieved with a large hemodialyzer, a blood flow rate of 400 ml per minute, a dialysate flow rate of 800 ml per minute, and 4 or more hours of treatment. Medium-sized and large molecule clearance is augmented with increased ultrafiltration.

In contrast, continuous arteriovenous hemofiltration (CAVH) and continuous venovenous hemofiltration (CVVH) depend on ultrafiltration alone for small and large solute clearance (i.e., convective clearance). With these techniques, whole blood enters the hemofilter, which is a dialyzer selected for its high permeability and capacity to retain cellular elements (Fig. 18-2). As ultrafiltration proceeds, the patient "excretes" fluid with a composition similar to that of plasma. A physiologic replacement fluid is administered intravenously, diluting the plasma of urea and other metabolic by-products. Judiciously selected replacement fluid (Table 18-6) can compensate for specific metabolic disturbances (e.g., base-containing fluid for patients with acidosis) and allows for individualization of care among critically ill patients with different underlying diseases.

Table 18-5. Dialysate Formulation for Peritoneal Dialysis and Conventional Hemodialysis

Peritoneal dialysis	
Na$^+$	132 mEq/L
K$^+$	0
Cl$^-$	96 mEq/L
Lactate	40 mEq/L
Ca$^+$	2.5 or 3.5 mEq/L
Mg$^+$	0.5 or 1.5 mEq/L
Glucose	347 (1.5%), 398 (2.5%), or 486 (4.25%) mOsm/L

Conventional hemodialysis		Range
Na$^+$	140 mEq/L	138–145
K$^+$	2.0 mEq/L	0–4
Cl$^-$	106 mEq/L	100–110
HCO$_3$$^-$	38 mEq/L	35–45
Ca$^+$	2.5 mEq/L	1.0–3.5
Mg$^+$	1.5 mEq/L	1.5
Dextrose	2.0 g/L	1.0–2.5

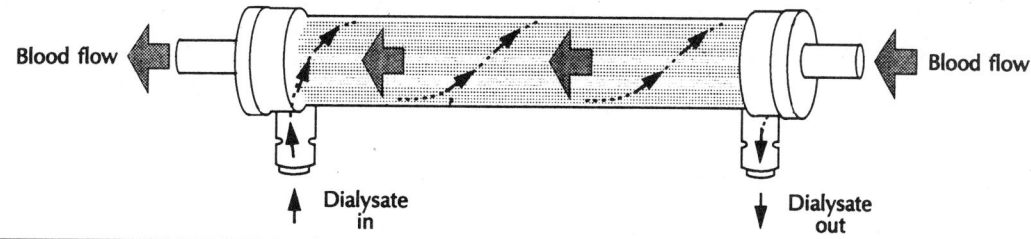

Fig. 18-1. Hollow fiber dialyzer.

Continuous arteriovenous hemodialysis (CAVHD) and continuous venovenous hemodialysis (CVVHD) differ from hemofiltration in the addition of diffusive dialysis. A sterile dialysate (typically peritoneal dialysate, although custom solutions may be formulated) is infused countercurrent to blood flow via side ports in the hemofilter (Fig. 18-2). The dialysate contacts the hollow fibers in the hemofilter, as in conventional hemodialysis, resulting in additional diffusion of small solutes. While far less efficient per unit time than conventional hemodialysis, CAVHD or CVVHD can provide time-averaged clearances with continuous therapy that exceed those of all other modalities [31].

Vascular Access Procedures

PERITONEAL CAVITY ACCESS. In acute renal failure, access to the peritoneal cavity can be achieved with a rigid temporary stylet catheter or a chronic soft catheter with a protective Dacron cuff. Use of a temporary peritoneal dialysis catheter is most appropriate if the anticipated duration of peritoneal dialysis is less than 48 to 72 hours, as in the treatment of hypothermia, or if a soft silicone catheter and surgical personnel are not available. A rigid catheter can be placed at the bedside by ICU personnel.

Table 18-6. Physiologic Intravenous Infusion Fluids for Replacement in Hemofiltration

1. Hyperalimentation
2. Lactated Ringer's solution

Na$^+$	130 mEq/L
Cl$^-$	110 mEq/L
Lactate	28 mEq/L
K$^+$	4 mEq/L
Ca$^+$	3 mEq/L

3. Alternative solution
1 liter IV D 10 0.9% normal saline with 5 mEq calcium gluconate and 0–4 mEq magnesium sulfate, followed by
1 liter IV D 10 0.45% normal saline with 44 mEq (1 amp) NaHCO$_3$, followed by
1 liter IV D 10 0.9% normal saline with 5 mEq calcium gluconate and 0–4 mEq magnesium sulfate, followed by
1 liter IV D 10 W with 132 mEq (3 amp) NaHCO$_3$
Cycle can then be repeated

Net:	
Na$^+$	140 mEq/L
Cl$^-$	96 mEq/L
HCO$_3$$^-$	44 mEq/L
K$^+$	0 mEq/L
Ca$^+$	2.5 mEq/L
Mg$^+$	0–2 mEq/L

The procedure for placement of a temporary peritoneal dialysis catheter is as follows. The urinary bladder is emptied to prevent inadvertent perforation. The abdomen is prepared with povidone-iodine solution and draped, as it would be for an abdominal paracentesis. A point one-third the distance between the umbilicus and symphysis pubis is infiltrated with local anesthetic to the peritoneum. To distend the peritoneum, 1 to 2 liters of 1.5% dextrose peritoneal dialysate is introduced into the peritoneal cavity via a 16-gauge spinal needle or angiocath. A small puncture is made at the same site with a scalpel blade. The stylet-catheter is inserted into the skin puncture site and passed through the skin, underlying fascia, and linea alba. Entrance of the catheter tip into the peritoneum is evidenced by a sudden reduction in resistance and dialysis fluid in the transparent catheter. If cloudy or feculent fluid is withdrawn, the bowel has been punctured [32]. The catheter should be left in place until a decision is made regarding the need for a diagnostic procedure (e.g., contrast computed tomography). Intravenous antibiotics to cover bowel flora (e.g., gentamicin and metronidazole, or ampicillin-sulbactam) should be started. If peritoneal dialysis is to be continued, another access site should be chosen and the above process repeated.

If the peritoneal drainage is clear, the stylet is withdrawn until the obturator point meets the catheter tip. The catheter is then advanced into the posteroinferior area of the peritoneal cavity and connected to a closed-gravity manual instillation drainage system or an automatic cycler. The catheter can then be secured to the skin by a superficial purse-string suture.

Unfortunately, peritoneal access with a rigid catheter is frequently complicated by peritonitis. If dialysis is required for more than 48 to 72 hours, a new site should be selected and the original catheter removed. Otherwise, a catheter designed for chronic use with Dacron cuffing, such as the Tenckoff catheter, should be inserted. Although a chronic dialysis catheter can be placed in the ICU by experienced skilled personnel using a percutaneous technique, the preferred method in most hospitals is surgical placement under sterile conditions in the operating suite. Surgical catheter placement is not addressed in this chapter.

HEMODIALYSIS ANGIOACCESS. Conventional hemodialysis requires access to the circulation at a site large enough to provide blood flow rates of 250 to 400 ml per minute. For patients with chronic renal failure, an endogenous upper extremity arteriovenous fistula or synthetic arteriovenous graft is usually placed to allow repeated hemodialysis treatments via percutaneous needle puncture. Such a procedure is not warranted for potentially reversible acute renal failure. In the acute setting, angioaccess typically requires cannulation of the femoral, subclavian, or internal jugular vein. In critically ill patients, the choice of site for angioaccess may be dictated by the underlying disease, such as respiratory failure or coagulopathy (Table 18-7). Although of historical importance, external shunts, such as the Quinton-Scribner shunt, are no longer used for temporary hemodialysis access.

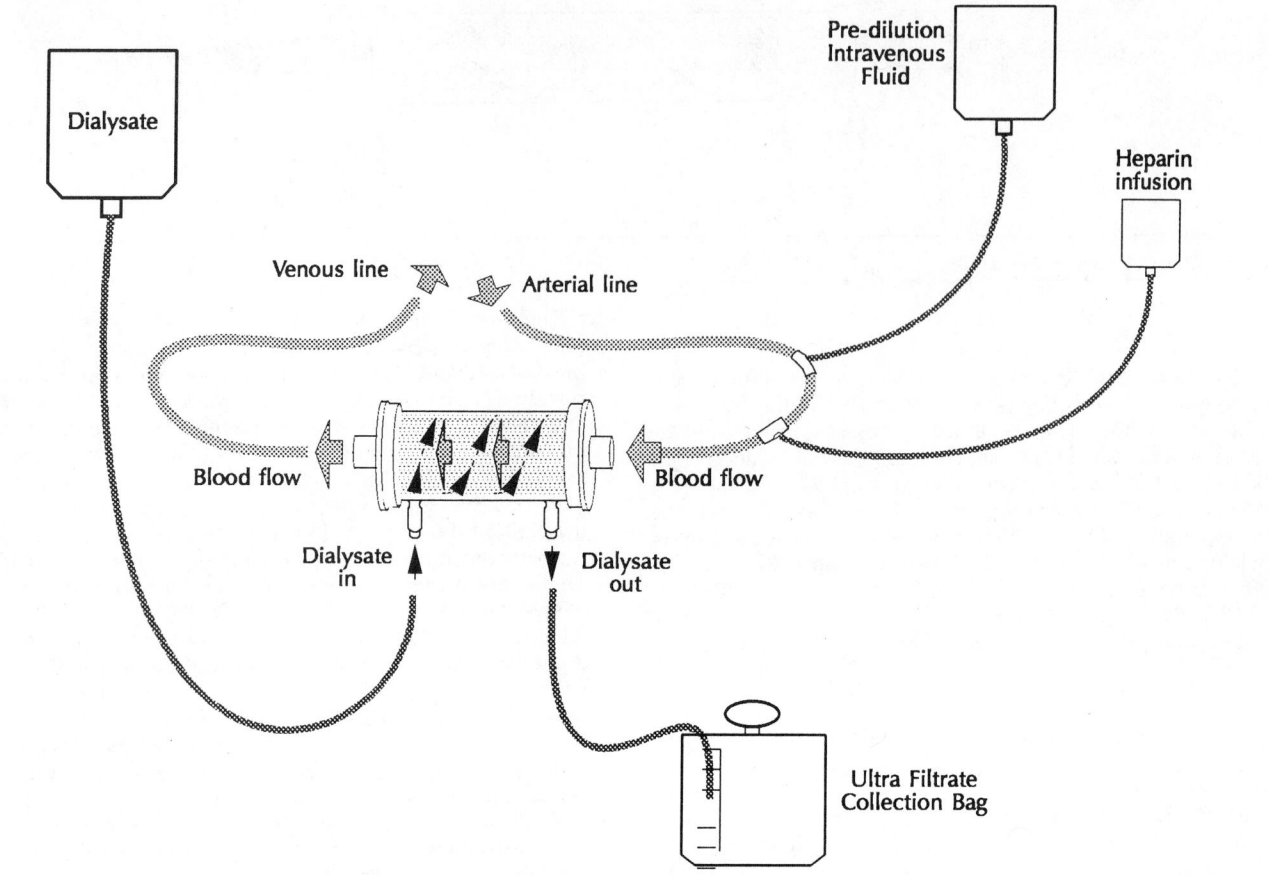

Fig. 18-2. Continuous arteriovenous hemodialysis.

Femoral Vein. The procedure for placement of a femoral venous catheter for conventional hemodialysis is similar to that described in Chapter 2 for placement of a femoral cannula. Once the vein is cannulated with a needle, a flexible wire is passed through the needle. If any obstruction is encountered, the wire is removed and the needle and syringe repositioned. The needle is then removed, leaving only the wire entering the skin. A small nick is made at the wire entrance site and a dilator is placed over the wire and twisted gently at the entrance site. A double-lumen catheter, 13.5 cm long, is passed over the wire and into the femoral vein. The wire is removed and blood is drawn back through the catheter lumen and flushed to confirm accurate catheter placement.

A temporary catheter at the femoral site is prone to thrombosis, particularly in an ambulatory patient whose catheter may kink with bending at the hips. Catheter patency is usually maintained by continuous infusion of a heparinized saline solution (2000 units heparin per 500 ml 0.9% saline, at 10 ml per hour through each catheter port). If heparin is contraindicated, catheter patency can usually be maintained with low-flow saline infusion alone. Should the catheter become occluded with thrombus, we recommend placement of a new catheter over a guidewire or at a more proximal or distal site along the vein. The femoral site is also prone to infection, particularly in obese patients. Meticulous local care is required to limit infection risk. The use of prophylactic antibiotics is not advocated. Under optimal conditions, a femoral dialysis catheter may remain in place up to 2 to 3 weeks. A patient with an indwelling femoral dialysis catheter should remain supine as much as possible to limit bending and kinking of the catheter. Unfortunately, this may delay rehabilitation and recovery. It is reasonable to perform same-day femoral vein catheterizations with dialysis if the anticipated duration of therapy is limited, thereby reducing the risks of thromboembolism, infection, and catheter malfunction.

Femoral venous access is preferable in patients with coagulopathy. If the artery is inadvertently punctured, the site is easily compressible; in contrast, puncture of the subclavian or carotid artery (located beside the internal jugular vein) may result in hemothorax or stroke, respectively, among other complications [33]. Patients critically ill, on mechanical ventilation, and at increased risk of pneumothorax should have femoral catheterization when temporary hemodialysis is required.

Subclavian Vein. Subclavian vein catheterization is described in detail in chapter 2. After the vein is cannulated, the syringe is removed and a flexible wire passed through the needle into the subclavian vein. The needle hub is covered by the thumb to reduce the risk of air embolism. It is advisable to rotate the needle 90 degrees clockwise so the wire exits in the caudal direction. The needle is then removed. A scalpel blade is used to nick the skin at the wire entrance site. After dilation, the 13.5-cm double-lumen dialysis catheter is passed into the subclavian vein. Mild resistance may be experienced as the catheter travels below the clavicle. As with femoral cannulation, if substantial resistance is encountered the catheter should be removed and repositioned. When the procedure is complete, the patient may be taken out of the Trendelenburg position. The catheter is then secured to the skin with several sutures.

A chest radiograph should be obtained after all attempts at subclavian access to rule out pneumothorax and confirm placement of the catheter in the subclavian vein or superior vena

Table 18-7. Comparison of Vascular Access Sites for Conventional Hemodialysis or Venovenous Hemofiltration Hemodialysis

Femoral vein	Advantages
	Easily accessible
	Companion artery compressible
	Disadvantages
	Infection risk
	Impaired patient mobility
	Indications
	Inability to tolerate Trendelenburg position
	Inability to tolerate pneumothorax (e.g., pneumonia, emphysema)
	Coagulopathy
	Poorly defined anatomic landmarks (e.g., morbid obesity)
Subclavian vein	Advantages
	Patient comfort and mobility
	Extended duration of access
	Disadvantages
	Requires skilled operator
	Risk of pneumothorax
	Inability to compress companion artery if punctured
	Long-term adverse sequelae (subclavian vein thrombosis)
	Indications
	Anticipated need for dialysis greater than 1 week
	Need for mobility and rehabilitation
Internal jugular vein	Advantages
	Patient comfort and mobility
	Extended duration of access
	Disadvantages
	Requires surgical placement
	Risk of pneumothorax
	Contraindicated with tracheostomy
	Indications
	Ability to tolerate minor surgical procedure
	Anticipate dialysis requirement for extended period
	Need for mobility and rehabilitation

cava. Occasionally, the catheter may travel cephalad, into the internal jugular vein. If this occurs, the catheter should be repositioned, preferably under fluoroscopy. In the event of subclavian arterial puncture, topical pressure should be applied for at least 15 minutes and the femoral site used. Rarely, the superior vena cava or right atrium can be perforated, especially if the catheter is long and has been advanced to the hub in a person of short stature. This constitutes a surgical emergency.

Catheter patency in the subclavian vein is more easily maintained than for the femoral vein, so continuous heparinized saline solutions are not necessary. Our practice is to instill 7500 units of heparin into each catheter lumen after placement and to withdraw the heparin from the catheter before dialysis. This procedure is repeated after each treatment. If the catheter does become occluded with thrombus, it can usually be successfully changed over a guidewire.

Subclavian vein catheterization offers the advantages of increased patient comfort and mobility and lower risk of local infection. For the patient with acute renal failure, the subclavian vein is a useful angioaccess site, particularly if the patient is too unstable to undergo surgical placement of a tunneled internal jugular vein dialysis catheter. Unfortunately, subclavian vein stenosis is a frequent complication of long-term subclavian vein cannulation and may seriously impair venous drainage of any

permanent ipsilateral hemodialysis access that might be used if renal function does not recover [34].

Internal Jugular Vein. Placement of temporary or semipermanent hemodialysis catheters in the internal jugular vein has emerged in recent years as the optimal angioaccess for patients with end-stage renal disease, although relatively few patients with acute renal failure have undergone this procedure [35]. Percutaneous internal jugular venous cannulation can be performed, although a tunneled technique is more often used. Percutaneous cannulation of the internal jugular vein (described in detail in Chap. 2) is usually accomplished at the neck via the anterior approach, puncturing the skin approximately 2 cm above the clavicle between the bellies of the sternocleidomastoid muscle. Caution must be exercised to avoid inadvertent puncture of the common carotid artery. The right internal jugular vein is more commonly used and is recommended, as its passage into the superior vena cava is more direct and reliably performed. However, a large dialysis catheter can be easily manipulated or displaced at this awkward location. Therefore, most internal jugular catheters are surgically placed and tunneled beneath the skin under fluoroscopic guidance. A tunneled catheter in the internal jugular vein offers several distinct advantages over a percutaneous temporary dialysis catheter, even for patients with acute renal failure in the ICU. The internal jugular catheters are comfortable, do not require immobility or the supine position, and include a Dacron cuff, which may reduce the risk of line infection. Unfortunately, the internal jugular site may be prone to bacterial contamination in ICU patients with a tracheostomy and copious secretions. Therefore, we have avoided placement of internal jugular catheters in patients with tracheostomies.

Tunneled internal jugular catheters have been used in some patients for months to years and are optimal for those with acute renal failure whose renal recovery is unlikely. Local management of the catheter is similar to management at the subclavian site. Heparin (7500 units) is routinely instilled into each catheter lumen after dialysis. If in spite of heparin the catheter becomes occluded with thrombus or fibrin, 5000 units of urokinase may be instilled for 20 to 30 minutes, achieving thrombolysis with negligible systemic absorption. Fortunately, the internal jugular veins are less prone to stenosis than the subclavian veins, even after long-term cannulation, so compromised permanent angioaccess is less of a concern.

HEMOFILTRATION ANGIOACCESS. The techniques used to establish venous access for CVVH or CVVHD are exactly as described above. On the other hand, CAVH and related arteriovenous techniques, such as slow continuous ultrafiltration (SCUF) by definition require access to both arterial and venous limbs of the circulation. Vascular access is usually achieved by percutaneous cannulation of the common femoral artery and vein. Alternative sites, including the axillary artery and vein, and external shunts have been attempted but do not provide adequate blood flow for effective hemofiltration. Patients with femoral artery bypass grafts and those with severe atherosclerotic vascular disease are extremely poor candidates for arteriovenous techniques. Before femoral artery cannulation, dorsalis pedis pulses should be examined by Doppler study. If pulses are inaudible or a bruit is present over the femoral artery, an alternative dialytic modality, such as conventional hemodialysis or continuous venovenous hemofiltration or hemodialysis via the femoral, subclavian, or internal jugular vein, should be used.

Femoral Artery. The common femoral artery is palpated beneath the inguinal ligament. Cannulation of the femoral artery is described in detail in Chapter 2. The artery should be punctured no more than 2 cm below the ligament to avoid the superficial femoral artery. The surrounding skin and subcutaneous tissue are infiltrated with local anesthetic. A 14-gauge needle attached to a non-Luer lock 10-ml syringe is slowly advanced at a 45-degree angle until the artery is punctured. The needle is steadied with the left hand and the syringe removed while the operator's left thumb covers the needle aperture to limit blood loss from the pulsatile arterial flow. A flexible wire is passed through the needle. The needle is then removed, after which a nick is made in the skin at the needle entrance site. A dilator that fills the lumen of the 0.317-cm diameter (Vygon) catheter is gradually passed into the artery, followed by the catheter itself. The wire and dilator are then removed in succession. Again, the thumb must cover the catheter outflow site. After the catheter is capped, it may be sutured in place. The corresponding vein is then cannulated as described above with the same single-lumen catheter. The arterial and venous limbs of the system may originate from either side (e.g., a patient with an arterial pressure monitor in the left femoral artery and a central venous triple-lumen catheter in the left femoral vein may undergo right femoral artery and left femoral vein cannulation for arteriovenous hemofiltration). Catheter patency is usually maintained by the systemic anticoagulation required to prevent clotting of the hemofilter.

Specific Dialytic Modalities

ACUTE PERITONEAL DIALYSIS

Intermittent Peritoneal Dialysis. Intermittent peritoneal dialysis (e.g., 8–12 hours of hourly to half-hourly exchanges on alternate days) rarely provides sufficient clearance or ultrafiltration for patients with acute renal failure. In the ICU, acute peritoneal dialysis should be continuous, to optimize solute clearance and provide hour-to-hour volume control.

Continuous Peritoneal Dialysis. Peritoneal dialysis is in many ways simpler than hemodialysis to perform, and despite its limitations it enjoys a following among nephrologists who care for critically ill patients. Because direct access to the circulation is not required, attention need only be given to sterility as well as intake and output measures, techniques familiar to all ICU nursing personnel, even those with limited experience in critical care nephrology. In general, 1 to 3 liters of peritoneal dialysate (Table 18-5) is instilled every 1 to 2 hours to achieve maximal solute clearance. As described above, the dextrose concentration can be modified as ultrafiltration needs are assessed; often insulin is needed (or increased) as the dextrose concentration is increased to prevent significant hyperglycemia. When performed intensively, peritoneal dialysis may achieve urea clearances comparable to those with hemofiltration or hemodialysis.

Peritoneal dialysis may be inadequate for some ICU patients, especially those who are hypercatabolic. As exchanges become more frequent, a larger proportion of total dialysis time is spent on instillation and drainage, with increasingly less time available for contact between the dialysate and the peritoneal membrane, which is necessary for effective diffusive clearance. Rapid exchange may also increase infection risk and is labor-intensive. In addition, ultrafiltration and clearance can be reduced in the setting of hypotension or shock with reduced mesenteric blood flow. Individuals with a wide variety of vascular disorders, including diabetes mellitus, chronic systemic hypertension, and vasculitis, are prone to this complication [36]. A subset of ICU patients who require renal replacement therapy but who are less catabolic may be successfully managed with less frequent peritoneal dialysis treatments. Four to 12 exchanges daily (every 2, 4 or 6 hours) can provide satisfactory ultrafiltration and clearance for patients of small to modest body size, assuming proper technique and good peritoneal membrane function. A blood urea nitrogen of approximately 60 mg per 100 ml or lower in this setting is usually indicative of adequate dialysis, assuming adequate nitrogen intake.

CONVENTIONAL HEMODIALYSIS. Conventional hemodialysis is the most common mode of dialysis employed for patients with acute renal failure in the ICU. Per unit time, it is by far the most efficient in terms of both ultrafiltration and clearance. Patients who undergo conventional hemodialysis for acute renal failure typically are dialyzed for 3 to 5 hours, every other day or 3 times weekly.

A conventional hemodialysis machine consists of a blood pump, a dialysate delivery system, and numerous safety control devices (Fig. 18-3). The usual dialysis membrane is comprised of thousands of hollow fibers made of modified cellophane or cellulose, such as cuprophane or cellulose acetate, or synthetic plastics, such as polysulfone, PAN, or PMMA (Figure 18-1). Whole blood traverses these fibers and is bathed by dialysate, which can be formulated to regulate plasma electrolytes and pH optimally. As dialysis proceeds, equilibrium between the contents of plasma and dialysate is approached. Blood flow rates of 250 to 400 ml per minute can be maintained with successful vascular access and a volumetric pump. Dialysate flow rates range from 500 to 800 ml per minute. With larger membranes and high flows (high-flux dialysis), a urea reduction ratio (URR) or percent reduction of urea (PRU) on the order of 60 to 80 percent or more can be achieved with a single 4-hour dialysis treatment.

Selection of the hemodialysis membrane is usually based on the performance characteristics of the dialyzer (Table 18-4), issues of biocompatibility and potential membrane-related side effects, and cost. Most currently available membranes can achieve satisfactory urea clearances, although the clearance of larger molecules may be substantially greater with the more porous synthetic membranes [37]. Ultrafiltration rates differ among the traditional cellulosic and newer noncellulosic membranes. For a patient with marked volume overload, a synthetic membrane with a large ultrafiltration coefficient should be used if a dialysis machine with ultrafiltration control is available.

The contact of blood with cuprophane fibers frequently results in activation of the alternate complement pathway as well as pulmonary leukosequestration [38], peripheral leukopenia [39], transient hypoxemia, and stimulation of other cytokines, such as interleukin-1 and TNF [40]. These effects are less marked with synthetic noncellulosic "biocompatible" membranes and therefore may influence the choice of hemodialyzer for certain ICU patients with acute renal failure. For instance, a patient with ARDS or severe pneumonia may be unable to tolerate further hypoxia, so a biocompatible membrane would be indicated. A single study recently demonstrated improved survival and rate of renal recovery in a small cohort of patients dialyzed with PMMA versus cuprophane [41]. We use biocompatible membranes exclusively for patients with acute renal failure, although definitive evidence for their superiority from a large randomized trial is currently lacking.

Systemic anticoagulation is routinely administered during conventional hemodialysis, although it may be limited in some high-risk patients to low-dose continuous, fractional, or regional heparinization. The high blood flow rates during con-

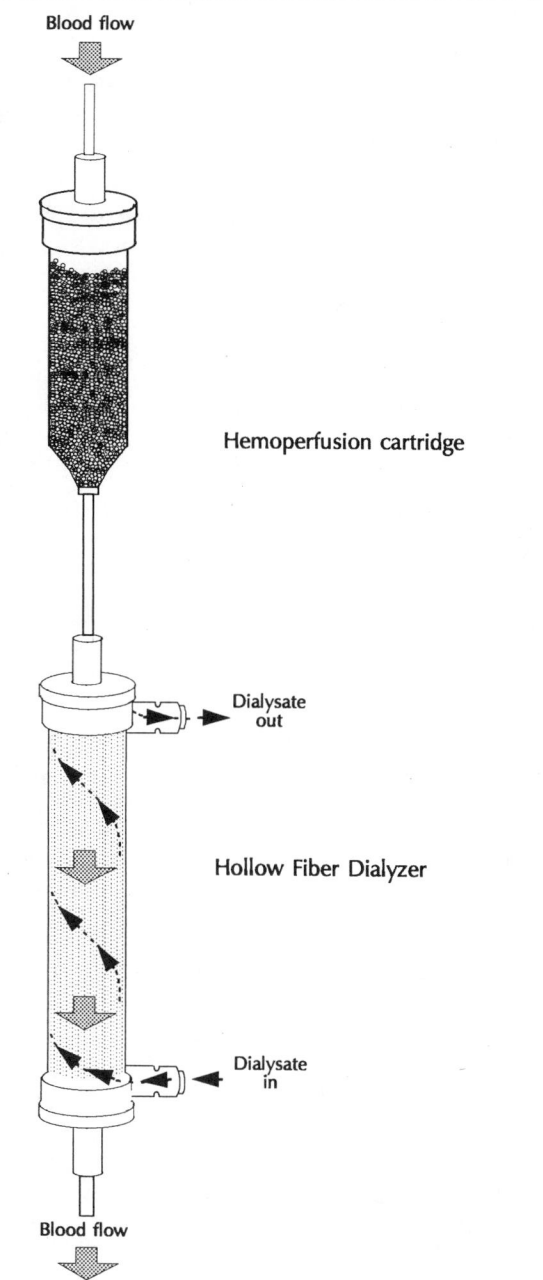

Blood flow

Hemoperfusion cartridge

Dialysate out

Hollow Fiber Dialyzer

Dialysate in

Blood flow

Fig. 18-3. Activated charcoal hemoperfusion.

ventional hemodialysis may permit successful treatment without anticoagulation, particularly in the patient with liver disease or a bleeding diathesis. Careful visual inspection of the dialyzer and blood lines is necessary to detect dialyzer clotting, which will impair dialysis efficiency and risk systemwide clotting and substantial blood loss. Monitoring the venous pressure in the system is also important, as a sudden decrease often suggests dialyzer clotting. Fractional heparinization requires frequent monitoring of the activated clotting time (ACT) to limit systemic heparin exposure to a minimum [42]. Regional (i.e., nonsystemic) heparinization can be performed by adding heparin to the blood before it enters the dialyzer, followed by protamine

(a heparin antagonist) to the blood after it exits. This technique requires highly skilled nursing personnel but can be extremely useful in selected settings. The use of regional citrate, which binds ionized calcium, a cofactor in hemostasis, is another alternative to systemic heparinization in high-risk patients [43]. Unfortunately, the use of citrate carries the additional risk of worsening renal failure-induced hypocalcemia if strict attention to electrolytes and intravenous replacement of calcium is not maintained.

Although patients often do well with a standard hemodialysis regimen, it may be difficult to tolerate because of hypotension in some critically ill patients, particularly those with cardiovascular disease. Many factors can influence intradialytic hemodynamics. In the past, acetate served as the buffer base for hemodialysate and frequently led to hypotension and reduced cardiac output by virtue of its direct vasodilatory and myocardial depressant properties [44]. In recent years, acetate has been replaced by bicarbonate dialysis, which less commonly exacerbates vasodilatation and systemic hypotension during treatment. The dialysis sodium concentration can also have profound effects on blood pressure during treatment. A high sodium concentration (e.g., 145 mEql) during hemodialysis results in maintenance of blood pressure despite fluid removal [45], but often leads to excessive thirst and a tendency to increased interdialytic weight gain. Reducing dialysate sodium concentration in regular decrements (sodium modeling) during treatment can often achieve volume removal without hypotension [46]. Ultrafiltration control devices have also been helpful in avoiding rapid volume fluxes. Unfortunately, hypotension and cardiovascular instability may still be seen among ICU patients who receive conventional hemodialysis, beyond that expected by virtue of volume removal alone. Osmotic factors resulting from rapid diffusion of small solutes such as urea may be in part responsible for these effects, although the exact mechanism for this phenomenon is unknown.

SEQUENTIAL ULTRAFILTRATION HEMODIALYSIS. A particularly useful modification of conventional hemodialysis for acute renal failure is sequential ultrafiltration hemodialysis. Ultrafiltration of large volumes of fluid over brief time periods (e.g., >1–2 L/hour) during conventional hemodialysis may be poorly tolerated, especially in critically ill patients. In the past, it was thought that this hypotension resulted from the rapid depletion of intravascular volume during ultrafiltration and that insufficient time was given to allow for equilibration of extravascular fluid into the intravascular "available" space. However, if ultrafiltration is performed without concurrent diffusive dialysis, volume removal is more often tolerated without hypotension [47]. During sequential ultrafiltration hemodialysis, a patient typically undergoes ultrafiltration for 1 to 2 hours to achieve desired volume removal, followed by 3 to 4 hours of diffusive dialysis without any further ultrafiltration. With this technique, up to 4 liters per hour can be removed initially, and solute clearance can often proceed without major hemodynamic instability. It is important to recognize that clearance is limited during ultrafiltration, and to achieve adequate control of azotemia the usual duration of conventional hemodialysis should be prescribed during the diffusive phase.

SLOW CONTINUOUS ULTRAFILTRATION. Slow continuous ultrafiltration (SCUF) is a closed pump-free system that uses indwelling single-lumen catheters in the femoral artery and vein, a shortened tubing apparatus, and a porous hollow fiber membrane, from which plasma water is extracted by hydrostatic and oncotic pressure gradients (Fig. 18-2). Using a small hollow fiber filter made from polysulfone (Amicon D-20) or a parallel-plate polyacrilonitrile filter (Hospal Biospal), up to 10 liters per day of plasma water can be removed. The ultrafiltration rate can be increased further by use of negative-pressure devices. The major advantages of SCUF are the continuous nature of volume removal and the ability to perform the technique without a dialysis machine, blood pump, or specialized nursing personnel. Slow continuous ultrafiltration may be the treatment of choice for ICU patients with life-threatening volume overload, but unlike hemofiltration or hemofiltration hemodialysis techniques, SCUF alone rarely provides adequate control of azotemia in the critically ill patient with renal dysfunction.

Anticoagulation is almost always required with continuous renal replacement therapies. The relatively low blood flows and increased blood viscosity as a result of ultrafiltration make blood within the hollow fibers susceptible to clotting. Anticoagulation is usually achieved with low-dose heparin administered into a sleeve of the arterial catheter tubing. In general, we administer a 2000-unit bolus followed by a continuous infusion of approximately 10 units/kg/hour; partial thromboplastin time should be monitored routinely. Regional heparinization or regional citrate anticoagulation can also be employed. In patients with adequate blood pressure and a bleeding diathesis, the continuous techniques can often be performed successfully without anticoagulation if ultrashort lines are used.

One of two methods of regulating ultrafiltration-induced volume loss may be employed. In the first, the ultrafiltrate drainage bag is raised relative to the patient and hemofilter, so reducing the negative pressure exerted on the filter; this results in a decrease in the ultrafiltration rate. Alternatively, ultrafiltration is allowed to continue at a high rate, with gravity alone or assisted by a suction device, while a physiologic replacement fluid is administered intravenously to achieve the desired net rate of ultrafiltration. When replacement fluid is given, by definition, the process is known as hemofiltration.

CONTINUOUS ARTERIOVENOUS HEMOFILTRATION AND CONTINUOUS VENOVENOUS HEMOFILTRATION.
Continuous arteriovenous hemofiltration was first described in 1977 [48] and quickly became an important mode of acute renal replacement therapy. Hemofiltration is a practical and effective means of controlling volume overload with partial control of azotemia in critically ill patients with acute renal failure. It is particularly well-suited when hour-to-hour volume control is necessary or when conventional hemodialysis might be complicated by severe hemodynamic instability. Hemofiltration also enables provision of nutritional support to patients without concern for excessive volume administration, because high ultrafiltration rates are feasible. In fact, hyperalimentation may be the replacement fluid of choice in most cases (Table 18-6).

In addition to achieving ultrafiltration, hemofiltration results in convective solute clearance. For example, as plasma water containing a high concentration of urea and other "toxins" is lost in the ultrafiltrate, a replacement fluid containing no urea or "toxins" is administered intravenously to the patient, thereby diluting the concentration of unwanted compounds. With time, the nitrogenous by-products of metabolism are eliminated. Although clearance of small solutes, such as urea or potassium, can be achieved more efficiently by diffusion, convection results in some small solute clearance and is the main mode of clearance for medium-sized and larger molecules. These molecules may play an important role in uremia and in critical illness, although to date specific uremic toxins have not been identified. Diluting the plasma before the site of entry at the hemofilter with physiologic intravenous fluids (predilution) reduces the risk of fiber thrombosis by limiting the ultrafiltration-induced increase in plasma viscosity and also results in improved solute clearance [49]. We recommend the use of predilution fluids with these techniques.

Continuous arteriovenous hemofiltration (CAVH) and CVVH are equally useful techniques for patients in the ICU with acute renal failure. The advantages and disadvantages of each are given in Table 18-8.

CONTINUOUS ARTERIOVENOUS HEMODIALYSIS AND CONTINUOUS VENOVENOUS HEMODIALYSIS.
The addition of diffusive dialysis to continuous hemofiltration is easily accomplished. Each hemofilter is equipped with two side ports, which can be used to instill dialysate (Fig. 18-2). Typically, dialysate is instilled countercurrent to blood flow at a rate of 900 ml per hour, or 15 ml per minute. Net ultrafiltration is calculated by measuring the total volume in the collection bag and subtracting the dialysate volume along with any administered replacement fluid. Higher rates of dialysate flow may provide a marginal increase in small solute clearance when blood flow is brisk, but this is costly and generally not required [50]. Peritoneal dialysate is most commonly used for this technique. Satisfactory control of volume and azotemia can almost always be achieved, even in hypercatabolic patients, with the combination of continuous hemofiltration and hemodialysis.

When the use of peritoneal dialysate as the dialysate source is contraindicated, such as with severe lactic acidosis, a customized dialysate that contains sodium, chloride, glucose, and bicarbonate can be prepared. Calcium and magnesium cannot be added to bicarbonate-containing solutions, as calcium- and magnesium-carbonate will precipitate. Therefore, they must be given through alternative intravenous sites. The inadvertent use of saline or other non-base-containing intravenous fluids as the dialysate will lead to severe metabolic acidosis and should be avoided under all circumstances. Anticoagulation is usually required.

Complications are not uncommon (Table 18-3) but in many cases reflect the severity of underlying disease, rather than complications of the technique per se. At present, no randomized controlled clinical trials have proved continuous hemofiltration hemodialysis superior to conventional hemodialysis, although the continuous therapies have gained widespread acceptance in many centers.

Table 18-8. Comparison of Continuous Arteriovenous Hemofiltration/Hemodialysis (CAVH/CAVHD) and Continuous Venovenous Hemofiltration/Hemodialysis (CVVH/CVVHD)

CAVH/CAVHD	Advantages
	Can be performed without mechanical blood pump
	No dialysis nursing staff required
	Less costly
	Disadvantages
	Requires arterial access
	Erratic blood flow depending on arterial pressure
	Patients with femoral bypass grafts or severe atherosclerosis ineligible
CVVH/CVVHD	Advantages
	Venous access only
	Precise control of blood flow and clearance rate
	Easy crossover to conventional dialysis treatment
	Disadvantages
	More costly
	Skilled dialysis nursing staff often required

HEMOPERFUSION. Acute drug intoxication is a relatively common reason for admission to medical ICUs. The nephrologist is often consulted regarding the potential benefit of dialysis or activated charcoal hemoperfusion for rapid drug removal in cases of life-threatening intoxications. In fact, most patients do well with respiratory support and conservative measures, including volume expansion, oral charcoal administration, and the like, but occasionally do benefit from dialytic management.

Peritoneal dialysis should not be used for acute intoxications, as the drug clearance rate is much slower than that of hemodialysis or hemoperfusion. Hemodialysis and hemoperfusion are generally limited to intoxications due to small, water-soluble, and non-protein-bound drugs, such as lithium, methanol, and aspirin. During charcoal hemoperfusion, blood is passed through a column of activated charcoal resin along with a standard hemodialyzer (Fig. 18-4). Charcoal hemoperfusion may be somewhat more effective for lipid-soluble drugs. Table 18-9 lists drugs whose intoxication may be amenable to dialytic therapy.

PLASMAPHERESIS. Membrane plasmapheresis (fully discussed in Chap. 23) entails the use of a special separator membrane that is extremely porous, so plasma proteins, including immunoglobulins as large as IgM, may be removed. The procedure is similar to CVVH but the replacement fluid is typically a combination of albumin and crystalloid or plasma (Table 18-

Table 18-9. Intoxications Amenable to Treatment with Hemodialysis or Hemoperfusion

Methanol
Lithium
Aspirin
Ethylene glycol
Theophylline

10) and the procedure lasts only 2 to 4 hours. The nephrologist may perform plasmapheresis in ICU patients with acute renal failure due to anti-glomerular basement membrane antibody disease, renal vasculitis, or multiple myeloma or patients with intact renal function but life-threatening thrombotic thrombocytopenic purpura (TTP), hemolytic uremic syndrome (HUS), or Guillain-Barré syndrome. Plasma removal is measured by a bedside collection bag or cylinder and is generally replaced milliliter for milliliter.

Plasmapheresis may also be performed with a centrifugation device rather than a porous membrane. As with all forms of extracorporeal therapy, caution must be exercised to avoid volume depletion.

Nutrition

The importance of adequate nutrition in patients with chronic renal failure has been definitively demonstrated [51]. Critically

Fig. 18-4. Delivery system for conventional hemodialysis.

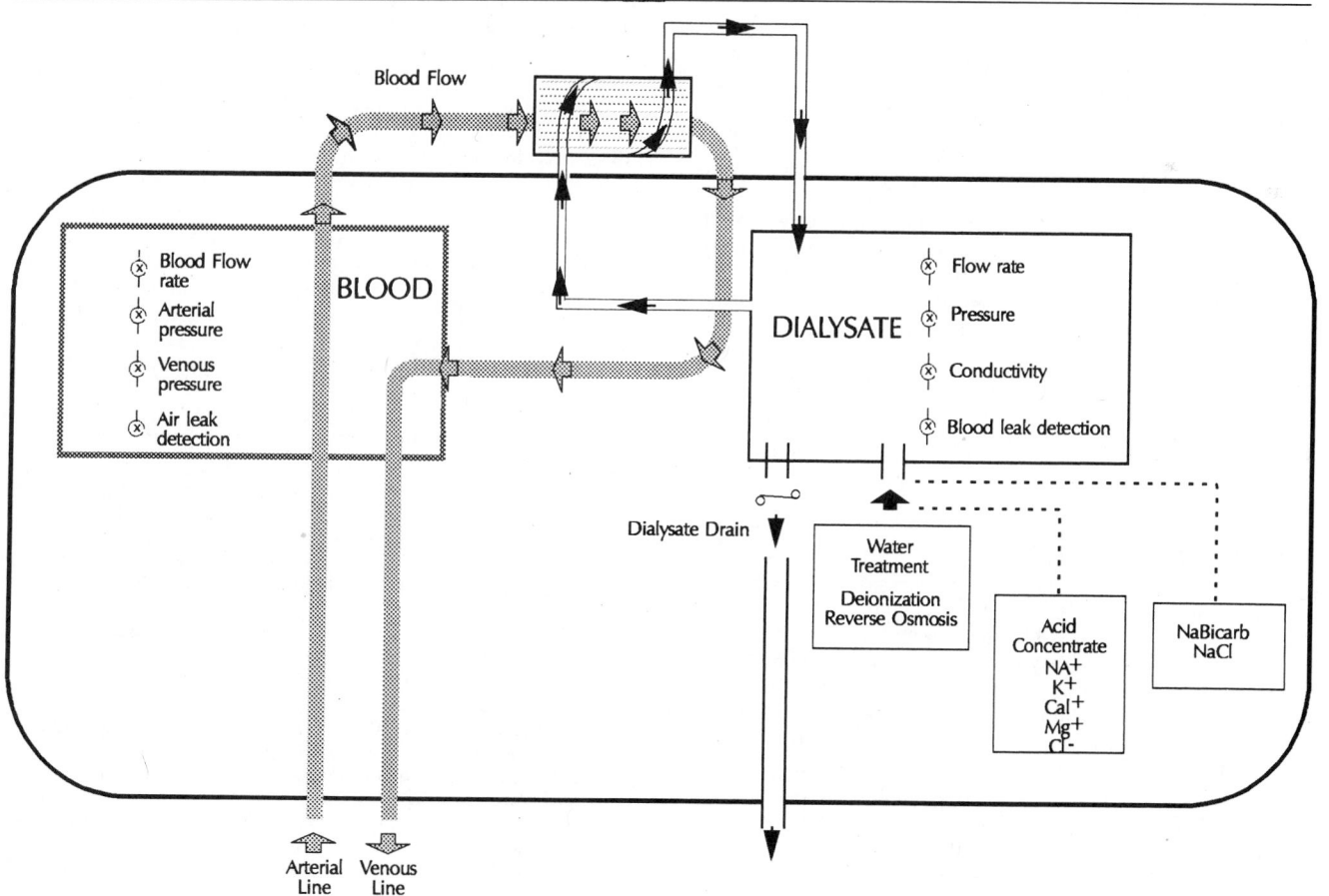

Table 18-10. Plasmapheresis Protocol

Phase I
  5 treatments within first week
  40 ml/kg/day of plasma removal
  Low-dose systemic heparin
  Replacement fluid
    2/3 5% albumin
    1/3 crystalloid
    1 unit fresh frozen plasma (FFP) with fifth treatment
    (All FFP with TTP or HUS)
Phase II
  3 treatments during weeks 2 and 3, if indicated

Table 18-11. Factors Associated with Functional Renal Recovery

Increase in urine output
Increase in urine osmolality or specific gravity
Improvement in metabolic acidosis
Decrease in serum creatinine or decreased rate of rise

ill patients with acute renal failure are at high risk for malnutrition, in part because of reduced nutritional intake (supply) and in part because of hypercatabolic processes (demand) such as sepsis, glucocorticoid therapy, surgical trauma, and, especially, multiple organ failure [52]. Inadequate nutrition in this population can lead to endogenous protein breakdown, worsening catabolism, and delayed postoperative healing and impaired host defenses. Intensive nutritional support may be important in improving outcome.

In past years, protein intake was severely restricted in patients with acute renal failure in an effort to reduce uremic symptomatology. Recently, however, early and aggressive institution of nutritional support has become standard practice in many centers. We advocate that dialysis be initiated to allow nutritional support, especially in catabolic patients, even when traditional absolute indications for dialysis (Table 18-1) are absent. Accordingly, dialysis must be more intensive, so that resultant nitrogenous waste products can be sufficiently cleared.

Several factors related to dialysis itself may affect nutritional status. For example, amino acids and water-soluble vitamins are readily removed with all types of dialysis and must be repleted daily. Peritoneal dialysis results in substantial protein loss, far more so than conventional hemodialysis or continuous renal replacement therapy. On the other hand, hemodialysis with bioincompatible membranes (see above) may worsen catabolism.

Our current recommendations for nutrition in patients with acute renal failure include enteral or parenteral administration of at least 35 kcal per kilogram per day, including 1.2 to 1.4 gm of protein per kilogram. Dialysis should be prescribed to maintain control of azotemia without compromising nutrition, even if treatments are prolonged (5–6 hours) or more frequent (4–5 per week). For critically ill patients who require large volumes of hyperalimentation, CAVHD and CVVHD may be especially practical and effective.

Stopping Therapy

Patients usually recover from acute renal failure within 4 weeks but may take 6 to 8 weeks or longer. It is imperative periodically to examine factors that may be associated with functional recovery (Table 18-11). Generally, urine output of less than 0.5 liter per day is insufficient to provide clearance of obligate solute. However, even brisk urine output is not sufficient to withhold dialysis, particularly in critically ill patients, if clearance remains poor. Care must be individualized, balancing the risks of holding renal replacement therapy against the risks associated with dialysis, including the reduced chance for recovery with continued therapy.

Several laboratory parameters may provide indications that function is returning. A urine osmolality dissimilar to plasma or a specific gravity of greater than 1.020 or less than 1.010 indicates the kidney's ability to concentrate or dilute the urine, a capacity lost when function is severely impaired. Paradoxically, urea nitrogen may increase during recovery because of improved tubular reabsorptive capacity. The creatinine typically plateaus or slowly decreases over time as function improves.

It is reasonable to monitor intradialytic serum creatinine and urea nitrogen in patients with acute renal failure. If the intradialytic rate of rise of creatinine is progressively less with time, it most likely indicates improving renal function. If the creatinine decreases between treatments and the patient is not threatened by volume overload or other complications, dialysis can be withheld and the patient followed carefully.

Stopping therapy in the face of declining clinical status is far more challenging. In most critically ill patients who develop acute renal failure, the extent of comorbid disease (e.g., sepsis, cardiac failure, surgical trauma) determines clinical outcome. The decision to withdraw dialysis may be appropriate when further aggressive care is futile but will almost certainly hasten death. As with most dilemmas encountered by ICU staff, the clinical and ethical care of the dying patient with acute renal failure must be individualized. It is vital fully to inform the patient and his or her representatives of the potential risks and benefits of dialysis before it is begun. As with other interventions, such as the use of an intraaortic balloon pump or mechanical ventilation, it is often helpful to recommend a trial period of 1 to 2 weeks, after which the patient's clinical condition can be reassessed and the decision to proceed with dialysis readdressed. The institution of dialysis should not mandate that treatment be continued indefinitely; in fact, many patients agree to short-term therapy but elect a priori to decline chronic dialysis should it be deemed necessary, based on quality-of-life considerations. A thoughtful, realistic, and compassionate approach to the patient with acute renal failure should allow the patient and his or her family and primary physician to participate in decision-making.

References

1. Kolff WJ: The artificial kidney. M.D. thesis, University of Groningen, Kampen, The Netherlands, 1946.
2. Bauer JH, Brooks CS, Burch RN: Clinical appraisal of creatinine clearance as a measurement of glomerular filtration rate. *Am J Kidney Dis* 2:337, 1982.
3. Miller T, Anderson R, Linas S: Urinary diagnostic indices in acute renal failure. *Ann Intern Med* 89:47, 1978.
4. Fer MF, McKinney TD, Richardson RL, et al: Cancer and the kidney: Complications of neoplasms. *Am J Med* 71:704, 1981.
5. Novicki DE, Willscher MK: Case-profile, anticholinergic-induced hydronephrosis. *Urology* 13:324, 1979.
6. Van Ypersele De Strihou C: Potassium hemostasis in renal failure. *Kidney Int* 11:491, 1977.
7. Edwards OM, Huskisson EC, Taylor R: Azotemia aggravated by tetracycline. *Br J Med* 1:26, 1970.
8. Hunter A: The physiology of creatine and creatinine. *Physiol Rev* 2:586, 1922.

9. Parker S, Carlon GC, Isaacs M, et al: Dopamine administration in oliguric and non-oliguric renal failure. *Crit Care Med* 9:630, 1981.

10. Flinn RB, Merrill JP, Wlezant WR: Treatment of the oliguric patient with a new sodium-exchange resin and sorbitol. *N Engl J Med* 264:111, 1961.

12. Montoliu J, Lens XM, Revert L: Potassium-lowering effect of albuterol for hyperkalemia in renal failure. *Arch Intern Med* 147:713, 1987.

13. Rose BD: *Clinical Physiology of Acid-Base and Electrolyte Disorders.* New York, McGraw-Hill, 1989.

14. Androgue HJ, Rashad MN, Gorin AB, et al: Assessing acid-base status in circulatory failure: Differences between arterial and central venous blood. *N Engl J Med* 320:1312, 1989.

15. Cardella CJ, Birkin BL, Roscoe M, et al: Role of dialysis in the treatment of severe hypercalcemia: Report of two cases successfully treated with hemodialysis and review of the literature. *Clin Nephrol* 12:285, 1979.

16. Harvey SC: Hypnotics and sedatives, in Gilman AG, Goodman LS, Rall TW, Murad F (eds): *The Pharmacologic Basis of Therapeutics.* New York, MacMillan, 1985.

17. Garella S: Extracorporeal techniques in the treatment of exogenous intoxication. *Kidney Int* 33:735, 1988.

18. Cosentino F, Paganini E, Lockrem J, et al: Continuous arteriovenous hemofiltration in the adult respiratory distress syndrome: A randomized trial. *Contrib Nephrol* 93:94, 1991.

19. Bellomo R, Tipping P, Boyce N: Tumor necrosis factor clearance during veno-venous hemodiafiltration in the critically ill. *Trans Am Soc Artif Int Organs* 37:M322, 1991.

20. Vigan G, Remuzzi G: Prevention and therapeutic management of bleeding in dialysis patients, in Nissenson AR, Fine RN (eds): *Dialysis Therapy.* Philadelphia, Hanley & Belfus, 1992.

21. Schulman G, Fogo A, Gung A, et al: Complement activation retards resolution of acute ischemic renal failure in the rat. *Kidney Int* 40:1069, 1991.

22. Serdengecti K, Onen K: Renal recovery patterns in acute renal failure. *Cerrahpassa Med Rev* 2:25, 1983.

23. Bomar JB, Dechard JF, Hlavinka D, et al: The elucidation of maximum efficiency minimum costs peritoneal dialysis protocols. *Trans Am Soc Artif Int Organs* 20:120, 1974.

24. Henderson LW: Biophysics of ultrafiltration and hemofiltration, in Maher JF (ed): *Replacement of Renal Function by Dialysis.* Dordrecht, The Netherlands, Kluwer, 1989.

25. Keshaviah PR, Shaldon S: Hemodialysis monitors and monitoring, in Maher JF (ed): *Replacement of Renal Function by Dialysis.* Dordrecht, The Netherlands, Kluwer, 1989.

26. Lauer A, Saccaggi A, Ronco C, et al: Continuous arteriovenous hemofiltration in the critically ill patient. *Ann Intern Med* 99:455, 1983.

27. Golper TA: Continuous arteriovenous hemofiltation in acute renal failure. *Am J Kidney Dis* 6:373, 1985.

28. Chanard J, Milcent T, Toupance O, et al: Ultrafiltration-pump assisted continuous arteriovenous hemofiltration. *Kidney Int* 33 (suppl 24): S157, 1988.

29. Sargent JA, Gotch FA: Principals and biophysics of dialysis, in Maher JF (ed): *Replacement of Renal Function by Dialysis.* Dordrecht, The Netherlands, Kluwer, 1989.

30. Henderson LW: Peritoneal ultrafiltration dialysis: Enhanced urea transfer using hypertonic peritoneal dialysis fluid. *J Clin Invest* 45:950, 1966.

31. Sigler MH, Teehan BP, Van Valkenburgh D: Solute transport in continuous hemodialysis: A new treatment for acute renal failure. *Kidney Int* 32:562, 1987.

32. Similin EP, Wright FH: Perforating injuries of the bowel complicating peritoneal catheter insertion. *Lancet* 1:64, 1968.

33. Vanholder R, Lameire N, Verbank J, et al: Complications of subclavian catheter hemodialysis: A 5-year prospective study in 257 consecutive patients. *Int J Artif Organs* 5:297, 1982.

34. Cimochowski GE, Worley E, Rutherford WE, et al: Superiority of internal jugular over the subclavian access for temporary dialysis. *Nephron* 54:154, 1990.

35. Uldall R, DeBruyne M, Besley M, et al: A new vascular access catheter for hemodialysis. *Am J Kidney Dis* 21:270, 1993.

36. Nolph KD, Stoltz M, Maher JF: Altered peritoneal permeability in patients with systemic vasculitis. *Ann Intern Med* 78:891, 1973.

37. Salem M, Mujais SK: Technical and functional considerations in choosing hollow-fiber dialyzers, in Nissenson AR, Fine RN (eds): *Dialysis Therapy.* Philadelphia, Hanley & Belfus, 1992.

38. Craddock PR, Fehr J, Brigham KL: Complement and leukocyte-mediated pulmonary dysfunction in hemodialysis. *N Engl J Med* 296:769, 1977.

39. Craddock PR, Fehr J, Delmasso AP, et al: Hemodialysis leukopenia: Pulmonary vascular leukostasis resulting from complement activation by dialyzer cellophane membranes. *J Clin Invest* 59:879, 1977.

40. Yamagami S, Yoshihara H, Kishimoto T, et al: Cuprophan membrane induces interleukin-1 activity. *Trans Am Soc Artif Organs* 32:98, 1986.

41. Hakim RM, Wingard RL, Lawrence P, et al: Use of biocompatible membranes improves outcome and recovery from acute renal failure (abstract). *Am Soc Nephrol* 367, 1992.

42. Gotch F, Keen M: Precise control of minimal heparinization for high bleeding risk hemodialysis. *Trans Am Soc Artif Int Organs* 234:168, 1977.

43. von Brecht J, Flanagan M, Freeman R, Lim V: Regional anticoagulation: Hemodialysis with hypertonic trisodium citrate. *Am J Kidney Dis* 8:196, 1986.

44. Wolff J, Pedersen T, Rossen M, Cleeman-Rasmussen K: Effects of acetate and bicarbonate dialysis on cardiac performance, transmural myocardial perfusion, and acid-base balance. *Int J Artif Organs* 9:105, 1986.

45. Van Stone JC, Bauer J, Carey J: The effect of dialysate sodium concentration on body fluid distribution during hemodialysis. *Trans Am Soc Artif Intern Organs* 26:383, 1980.

46. Raja R, Kramer M, Barber K, Chin S: Sequential changes in dialysate sodium during dialysis. *Trans Am Soc Artif Organs* 29:649, 1983.

47. Shinaberger JH, Brautbar N, Miller JH, Gardner PW: Successful application of sequential hemofiltration followed by diffusion dialysis with standard dialysis equipment. *Trans Am Soc Artif Int Organs* 24:677, 1978.

48. Kramer P, Wigger W, Rieger J, et al: Arteriovenous hemofiltration: A new and simple method for treatment of overhydrated patients resistant to diuretics. *Klin Wochenschr* 55:1121, 1977.

49. Geronemus R, von Albertini B, Glabman S, et al: Enhanced molecular clearance in hemofiltration. *Proc Clin Dial Transplant Forum* 8:147, 1978.

50. Bonnardeaux A, Pichette V, Quimet D, et al: Solute clearances with high dialysate flow rates and glucose absorption from the dialysate in continuous arteriovenous hemodialysis. *Am J Kidney Dis* 19:31, 1992.

51. Lowrie EG, Lew NL: Death risk in hemodialysis patients: The predictive value of commonly measured variables and an evaluation of death risk differences between facilities. *Am J Kidney Dis* 15:458, 1990

52. Chima CS, Meyer L, Hummell AC, et al: Protein catabolic rate in patients with acute renal failure on continuous arteriovenous hemofiltration and total parenteral nutrition. *J Am Soc Nephrol* 3:1516, 1993.

19. Gastrointestinal Endoscopy

Peter Krims and Bernard Clifford

Over the past 30 years, quantum leaps in endoscope technology have led to dramatic changes in gastrointestinal endoscopy practice in critically ill patients. From the development of the first widely used semiflexible gastroscope popularized by Schindler in the 1940s, to the current generation of video endoscope technology, gastrointestinal endoscopy has moved from an esoteric elective diagnostic procedure to a commonly performed therapeutic procedure in intensive care units (ICUs) worldwide [1]. This chapter reviews the indications, contraindications, techniques, and complications of gastrointestinal endoscopy in critically ill patients.

Endoscopes

Current fiberoptic gastrointestinal endoscopes are slim, flexible, and capable of visualizing more than 90 percent of the upper gastrointestinal tract (esophagus, stomach, duodenum) and colon. The areas most commonly not visualized in the gastrointestinal tract on endoscopic examination are the fundus or body of the stomach when there is an inherent blood clot and the colon when colonic preparation is poor. Newer endoscopes can visualize portions of the small bowel, and the terminal ileum can be examined with a standard colonscope [2]. Charged couple device (CCD) chip technology and video monitors have replaced fiberoptic bundles on newer instruments, allowing for digital storage of images and greater teamwork during difficult therapeutic procedures. The endoscopes are equipped with a fiberoptic bundle for light delivery; a CCD chip (video endoscope) or a fiberoptic bundle (fiberscope) for image delivery; operating channels for suctioning, biopsies, and various therapies; and a separate channel for insufflation of air and water. Wheels and buttons on the handle of the instrument control tip deflection, suction, and air/water insufflation (Fig. 19-1).

Indications

The indications for elective gastrointestinal endoscopy in the ICU are similar to those for other hospitalized patients. (Table 19-1); however, it is usually delayed until the patient's cardiopulmonary status has been stabilized. Although cardiopulmonary complications of gastrointestinal endoscopy are infrequent, it should be performed only when the tangible benefits clearly outweigh the risks. Gastrointestinal endoscopy in patients with clinically insignificant bleeding or minimally troublesome gastrointestinal complaints should be postponed until their medical-surgical illnesses improve. Endoscopy is sometimes indicated in patients with occult blood loss, when anticoagulation or thrombolytic therapy is contemplated. Generally it should be performed only when the results will alter plans for therapy.

Some authors have distinguished between indications for diagnostic and therapeutic endoscopic procedures. However, it cannot always be predicted when therapy may be needed during a procedure anticipated to be diagnostic. Therefore, all endoscopists performing diagnostic gastrointestinal procedures

should be competent in endoscopic therapy. This recommendation is bolstered by recent randomized trials in upper gastrointestinal bleeding showing that patient outcome is improved only if endoscopic therapy is provided [3,4].

UPPER GASTROINTESTINAL ENDOSCOPY. The indications for upper gastrointestinal endoscopy, listed in Table 19-1, include upper gastrointestinal bleeding, caustic ingestion, and foreign body ingestion. In patients with upper gastrointestinal bleeding, those with severe or recurrent bleeding and those with significant underlying cardiopulmonary disease have the highest morbidity and mortality and may benefit most from therapeutic endoscopy directed towards hemostasis [5]. Therefore, patients with upper gastrointestinal bleeding, evidence of hemodynamic instability, and continuing need for transfusions should undergo urgent upper endoscopy with plans for appropriate endoscopic therapy (see below).

Endoscopically placed gastrostomy feeding tubes are increasingly used in ICUs for enteral nutrition. Percutaneous endoscopic gastrostomy (PEG) tubes can be placed at the beside under intravenous and local sedation (see Chap. 22). They are less easily dislodged than nasogastric tubes, but severe, life-threatening complications are rarely associated with PEG placement [6].

ENDOSCOPIC RETROGRADE CHOLANGIOPANCREATOGRAPHY (ERCP). Endoscopic retrograde cholangiopancreatography is used only occasionally in the ICU and is therefore discussed only briefly here. It is indicated in ICU patients with severe gallstone pancreatitits and those with cholangitis unresponsive to medical therapy (Table 19-1). A number of retrospective and prospective controlled trials have shown that ERCP combined with sphincterotomy and stone extraction reduces complications in patients with severe gallstone pancreatitis and cholangitis [7,8,9]. Emergent ERCP can be performed safely on the day of admission without increased risk of complications, and it reduces the incidence of biliary sepsis.

LOWER GASTROINTESTINAL ENDOSCOPY. Lower gastrointestinal endoscopy can be performed for acute lower gastrointestinal bleeding (Table 19-1), but it is technically difficult in this setting and the diagnostic accuracy may therefore be lower. In addition, there are no randomized trials demonstrating improvement in patient outcome in patients undergoing urgent lower gastrointestinal endoscopy for acute lower gastrointestinal bleeding. Techetium-labeled erythrocyte scanning and/or angiography are the methods of choice for localizing a bleeding site. Elective endoscopic evaluation after a complete colonic cleansing preparation generally yields more satisfactory results.

Endoscopic colonic decompression has been advised in critically ill patients with acute adynamic ileus. Anecdotal reports and small uncontrolled series suggest that when the diameter of the right colon exceeds 12 cm perforation is imminent and decompression is necessary [10,11]. Other studies suggest that the colonic dilation may not progress to life-threatening complications and that decompression is unnecessary [12].

A trial of nasogastric suction, rectal tube placement, and frequent position changes should be initiated before attempts at

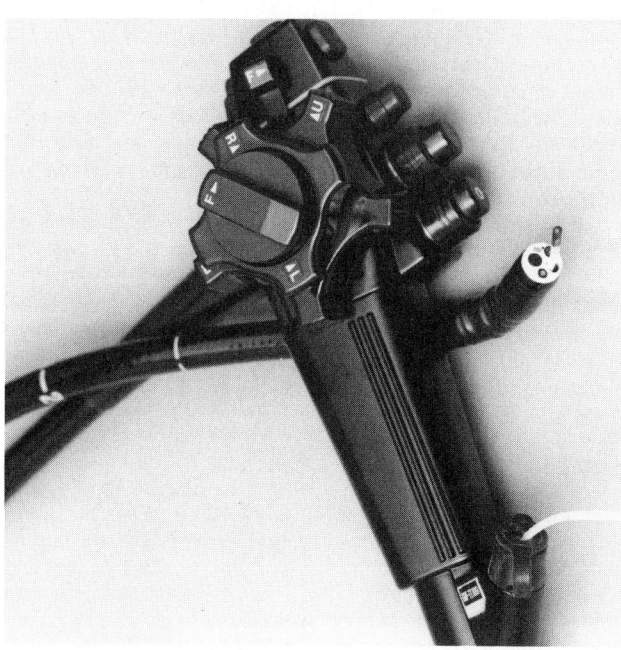

Fig. 19-1. Video upper endoscope. Note the control knobs controlling tip deflection, buttons controlling suction, air and water insufflation, and the tip of the insertion tube with a heater probe catheter protruding through the operating channel.

endoscopic decompression. Placement of a decompression tube into the colon is recommended, since relapse is common [13,14].

Contraindications

Table 19-2 lists contraindications to endoscopy. In general, endoscopy (and the associated air insufflation) should be avoided in patients with known or suspected gastrointestinal perforation and those known to be at high risk for perforation. Hemodynamic instability is a relative contraindication for endoscopy, but the benefit of therapeutic endoscopy may outweight the risks in some critically ill patients. For example, patients with severe cholangitis are likely to benefit from therapeutic ERCP, even in the presence of refractory hypotension or hypoxemia. The risk of a bleeding complication from endoscopic sphincterotomy is higher in patients with a gross coagulopathy, and ERCP may be delayed while the coagulopathy is corrected. Patients who are unable to cooperate should have endoscopy

Table 19-1. Indications for Gastrointestinal (GI) Endoscopy

Upper GI endoscopy
  GI bleeding
  Caustic ingestion
  Foreign body ingestion
Endoscopic retrograde cholangiopancreatography
  Severe gallstone parcreatitis
  Severe cholangitis
Lower GI endoscopy
  GI bleeding
  Acute adynamic ileus

Table 19-2. Contraindications to Endoscopy

1. Suspected/impending perforated viscus
2. Severe diverticulitis or severe inflammatory bowel disease
3. Refractory hypotension or hypoxemia (unstable patient)
4. Uncooperative patient
5. Unprotected airway in a confused or stuporous patient with acute upper gastrointestinal bleeding

Table 19-3. Complications of Endoscopy

1. Bleeding
2. Perforation of the gastrointestinal tract lumen by endoscope, catheters, or guidewires
3. Aspiration
4. Reaction to sedative medication

delayed; otherwise, endotracheal intubation and heavy sedation or general anesthesia may be necessary to facilitate the procedure. Finally, patients with acute upper gastrointestinal bleeding who are confused or stuporous should have their airway protected with an endotracheal tube prior to endoscopy. This is especially applicable to patients with variceal hemorrhage.

Complications

The principal risks of any endoscopic procedure are bleeding and perforation. These and other complications are outlined in Table 19-3. Bleeding can occur after biopsy, polypectomy, endoscopic sphincterotomy and therapeutic treatment of bleeding sites (varices, ulcers, AVMs). Most bleeding is minimal and self-limited, but repeat endoscopy and surgery may be necessary to control recurrent bleeding. Angiography can assist in localizing the bleeding source in postendoscopy bleeding. Perforation of the lumen may result from direct pressure of the endoscope, catheters, or guidewires on the wall or insufflation of air and resultant rupture of a severely inflamed and weakened gut wall, as in severe infectious or inflammatory colitis. Antibiotics and intravenous fluids should be given, and surgery may be required. If duodenal perforation is encountered following endoscopic sphincterotomy, early medical therapy and stabilization of the patient may preclude the need for surgery [15]. Aspiration of stomach contents and blood in acute upper gastrointestinal bleeding can be mimimized by protecting the airway with endotracheal intubation in patients with severe bleeding or altered mental state. A history of medication allergies and reactions should be obtained prior to administering sedative drugs. Patients with a history of alcohol abuse can have paradoxical reactions to benzodiazepine medications; caution should be used in sedating these patients. In our experience, sedation with relatively high-dose narcotics has been successful for patients who abuse alcohol.

Techniques

UPPER GASTROINTESTINAL ENDOSCOPY. Proper patient preparation is crucial to a safe and complete endoscopic examination. The patient should understand the nature of the examination, indications, and complications. Fluid resuscitation and optimal treatment of hypoxemia should precede all endoscopic examinations. Obtunded patients with gastrointestinal bleeding should be intubated to prevent aspiration, and intubation should be considered in nonobtunded patients with severe bleeding and those undergoing foreign body removal. Nasogastric or orogastric lavage with a large-bore tube (greater than 40 Fr.) should be performed to evacuate blood and clots from the stomach prior to endoscopy in acute gastrointestinal bleeding.

Proper patient selection will optimize outcome and minimize risk. Upper gastrointestinal bleeding is the most common indication for upper endoscopy in the ICU. Patients with continued or recurrent upper gastrointestinal bleeding as evidenced by red blood in the nasogastric aspirate should have urgent uper endoscopy as early as possible, certainly within 6 to 8 hours after presentation. In patients with massive hemorrhage endoscopy may be performed in the operating room in anticipation of surgical therapy.

A team approach is required to perform endoscopy in critically ill patients. The team consists of an experienced endoscopist, a specially trained endoscopy assistant, and a nurse skilled in monitoring patients undergoing endoscopy. For complex procedures, the nurse is situated at the patient's head, ensuring airway patency and administering intravenous sedation as needed, while the assistant provides technical help to the endoscopist. The procedure is generally performed under local and intravenous (conscious) sedation. A topical anesthetic is applied to the pharynx to reduce the gag reflex. Intravenous anxiolytics (diazepam, midazolam) and/or narcotics (meperidine, fentanyl) are commonly used. We prefer midazolam and fentanyl becuse of their amnestic effect and short half-life, respectively. Proper patient monitoring is needed, with frequent (every 5 minutes) blood pressure and pulse measurements and continuous measurement of oxygen saturation via pulse oximetry.

Endoscopy is performed with a "therapeutic" instrument, equipped with a large operating channel to allow suctioning of blood, and hemostatic therapy. The endoscope is passed into the patient's mouth to the posterior pharynx under direct visualization. Gentle pressure on the upper esophageal sphincter allows passage of the instrument into the esophagus. If the patient is awake, voluntary swallow may facilitate passage of the endoscope into the esophagus. The upper gastrointestinal tract is rapidly surveyed to locate the site of bleeding to facilitate surgical therapy should endoscopic therapy fail. If an active bleeding site is found, hemostatic therapy may be attempted immediately. Otherwise, the esophagus, stomach, and duodenum should be rapidly examined. Frequently, a large clot remains in the fundus or the body of the stomach, obscuring the mucosa in this area. In this case, the remainder of the upper gastrointestinal tract should be examined for a bleeding site and clot removal momentarily deferred. If no other bleeding lesion is located the clot should be removed, if possible, and the underlying mucosa examined. In patients with significant recent bleeding and endoscopic evidence of recent hemorrhage (a visible vessel or adherent clot on an ulcer), hemostatic therapy to prevent rebleeding should be strongly considered [16].

HEMOSTATIC THERAPY IN UPPER GASTROINTESTINAL ENDOSCOPY.
Actively bleeding lesions in the upper gastrointestinal tract can be treated with laser photocoagulation, heater probe therapy, mono- and bipolar electrocoagulation, or injection therapy. Preliminary data suggest that all forms of hemostatic therapy are effective. However, laser photocoagulation is expensive and cumbersome and has fallen out of favor. Injection therapy is simple and inexpensive, requiring only a needle catheter and various liquid media to effect hemostasis, including absolute ethanol, sclerosants (sodium morrhuate), or vasoconstrictors (epinephrine). Injection therapy may be less effective in briskly bleeding ulcers [17]. Injection sclerotherapy is most commonly used to treat bleeding esophageal varices. A newer method of banding esophageal varices may be associated with fewer complications than sclerotherapy [18,19,20]. Further trials are needed to determine the best method of treating bleeding varices.

The precise technique of hemostasis of bleeding lesions of the gastrointestinal tract varies depending on the hemostatic method employed. The most commonly used methods are the heater probe, bipolar electrocautery needle, and injection therapy. Heater probes generate heat using electrical current delivered to the tip of the catheter, while bipolar electrocautery delivers electrical current directly to the tissue, causing coagulation necrosis. Therapy using heater probes or bipolar electrocoagulation probes is most effective when coaptive coagulation is applied. With this method, the actively bleeding vein or artery is compressed using stiff probes until hemostasis is effected. Continuous pressure is applied as the bleeding ceases, and then the bipolar coagulation or heat is applied, "welding" the vessel shut. Because hemostatic therapy with the heater probe or bicap equipment requires an en-face view, lesions seen tangentially may be difficult to treat with these methods. Injection therapy using epinephrine, absolute alcohol, or sclerosants (sodium morruhate, ethanolamine) allows treatment of lesions even when seen tangentially. Injection therapy generally begins on the periphery of the lesion, with four injections in all four quadrants. Sclerotherapy is performed for active or recent bleeding in esophageal varices. It is currently the most widely used treatment in the United States for esophageal variceal bleeding. Direct intravariceal injection and/or perivariceal injection is performed. One to 4 ml is injected in each varix, starting in the distal esophagus just above the gastroesophageal junction. The addition of methylene blue to the sclerosant may help identify previously injected varices [21].

LOWER GASTROINTESTINAL ENDOSCOPY.
Lower gastrointestinal endoscopy is infrequently performed in the ICU because it is relatively insensitive at localizing the source of colonic bleeding. The procedure, which is technically difficult at times in well-prepared, healthy outpatients, can be extremely hard to perform in critically ill patients with colonic hemorrhage. Also, the colon tends to act as a reservoir for blood, making even the relative source of hemorrhage (left versus right colon), which is most useful to the surgeon, almost impossible to identify.

Instruments available for the examination of the lower gastrointestinal tract include the anoscope, which is useful mainly to evaluate for hemorrhoids or fissures, sigmoidoscopes, and colonoscopes. Rigid sigmoidoscopes are rarely used in the ICU and cannot be inserted as far as the standard 65-cm flexible sigmoidoscope. Colonoscopes are generally 140 to 180 cm long and are necessary to reach colonic lesions situated proximal to the splenic flexure.

Patient preparation for colonoscopy is more intensive than for upper gastrointestinal endoscopy. Usually, a gallon of nonabsorbed polyethylene glycol is given by mouth over 4 to 6 hours or by nasogastric tube 12 hours prior to examination. Magnesium citrate may be used over 24 to 48 hours in patients who have been taking clear liquids. Any oral iron preparations should be discontinued several days prior to examination. The examination is similar to gastrointestinal endoscopy with respect to support staff, sedation, and monitoring of the patient (see above). Abdominal pressure applied by an assistant during colonoscopy may assist in advancing the colonoscope.

Colonoscopy has been reported as therapy for pseudoobstruction [10–14]. Decompression by colonoscopy should not be first-line therapy for pseudoobstruction. Nasogastric and rectal tube placement, discontinuation of offending medications (narcotics and phenothiazines), treatment of underlying illness, and frequent repositioning (every 2 hours) of debilitated ICU patients often allows for resolution of pseudoobstruction.

References

1. Hirschowitz BI: Development and application of endoscopy. *Gastroenterology* 104:337, 1993.
2. Barkin JS, Reiner DK, Lewis BS, et al: Diagnostic and therapeutic jejunoscopy with the SIF 10L enteroscope: Longer really is better (abstract). *Gastrointest Endosc* 36:214, 1990.
3. Peterson WL, Barnett CC, Smith HJ, et al: Routine early endoscopy in upper gastrointestinal tract bleeding. *N Engl J Med* 304:925, 1981.
4. Laine L: Multipolar electrocoagulation in the treatment of active upper gastrointestinal tract hemorrhage: A prospective controlled trial. *N Engl J Med* 316:1613, 1987.
5. NIH Consensus Conference: Therapeutic endoscopy and bleeding ulcers. *JAMA* 262:1369, 1989.
6. Larson DE, Burton DD, Schroeder KW, et al: Percutaneous endoscopic gastrostomy: Indication, success, complications and mortality in 314 consecutive patients. *Gastroenterology* 93:48, 1987.
7. Neoptolemos JP, Carr-Locke DL, London NJ, et al: Controlled trial of urgent ERCP and endoscopic sphincterotomy versus conservative treatment for acute pancreatitis due to gallstones. *Lancet* 2:979, 1988.
8. Fan S, Lai E, Mok F, et al: Early treatment of acute biliary pancreatitis by endoscopic papillotomy. *N Engl J Med* 328:228, 1993.
9. Leese T, Neoptolemos JP, Baker AR, et al: Management of acute cholangitis and the impact of endoscopic sphincterotomy. *Br J Surg* 73:988, 1986.
10. Dorudi S, Berry AR, Kerrlewell MGW: Acute colonic pseudoobstruction. *Br J Surg* 79:99, 1992.
11. Strodel WE, Nostrant TT, Eckhauser FE, et al: Therapeutic and diagnostic colonoscopy in non-obstructive colonic dilation. *Ann Surg* 197:416, 1983.
12. Sloyer AF, Panella VS, Demas BE, at al: Olgivie's syndrome: Successful management without colonoscopy. *Dig Dis Sci* 33:1391, 1988.
13. Harig JM, Fumo DE, Loo FD, et al: Treatment of acute nontoxic megacolon during colonoscopy: Tube placement versus simple decompression. *Gastrointest Endosc* 34:23, 1988.
14. Burke G, Shellito PC: Treatment of recurrent colonic pseudoobstruction by endoscopic placement of a fenestrated overtube. *Dis Colon Rectum* 30:615, 1987.
15. Chung RS, Sviak MV, Ferguson DR: Surgical decisions in the management of duodenal perforation complicating endoscopic sphincterotomy. *Am J Surg* 165:700, 1993.
16. Laine L: Refining the prognostic value of endoscopy in patients presenting with bleeding ulcers. *Gastrointest Endosc* 39:461, 1993.
17. Lin H, Perng C, Lee F, et al: Endoscopic injection for the arrest of peptic ulcer hemorrhage: Final results of a prospective, randomized, comparative trial. *Gastrointest Endosc* 39:15, 1993.
18. Steigmann GV, Goff JS, Michaletz-Onody PA, et al: Endoscopic sclerotherapy as compared with endoscopic ligation for bleeding esophageal varices. *N Engl J Med* 326:1527, 1992.
19. Laine L, El-Newihi HM, Migikovsky B, et al: Endoscopic ligation compared with sclerotherapy for the treatment of bleeding esophageal varices. *Ann Intern Med* 119:1, 1993.
20. Saltzman JR, Aurora S: Complications of esophageal variceal band ligation. *Gastrointest Endosc* 39:185, 1993.
21. Planas R, Boiz J, Broggi M, et al: Portacable shunt vs. endoscopic sclerotherapy in the elective treatment of variceal hemorrhage. *Gastroenterology* 100:1078, 1991.

20. Paracentesis and Diagnostic Peritoneal Lavage

Lena M. Napolitano

I. Abdominal Paracentesis

INDICATIONS. Abdominal paracentesis is a simple procedure that can be easily performed at the bedside in the intensive care unit (ICU) and may provide important diagnostic information or therapy in critically ill patients with ascites. Diagnostic abdominal paracentesis is usually performed to determine the exact etiology of the ascites that has accumulated or to determine whether infection is present, as in spontaneous bacterial peritonitis. It can also be used in any clinical situation where the analysis of a sample of peritoneal fluid might be useful in ascertaining a diagnosis and guiding therapy [1].

As a therapeutic intervention, abdominal paracentesis is usually performed to drain large volumes of abdominal ascites. This role is becoming less prevalent, however, as chronic diuretic therapy becomes more successful. Therapeutic abdominal paracentesis can be palliative by diminishing abdominal pain from abdominal distention or improve pulmonary function by allowing better diaphragmatic excursion in patients who have chronic ascites refractory to aggressive medical management.

TECHNIQUES. Prior to initiating abdominal paracentesis, a catheter must be inserted to drain the urinary bladder (see Chap. 26) and any underlying coagulopathy or thrombocytopenia corrected. The patient must be positioned correctly. If the patient is critically ill, the procedure is performed in the supine position. If the patient is clinically stable and abdominal paracentesis is being performed for therapeutic volume removal of ascites, the patient can be placed in the sitting position, leaning slightly forward, to increase the total volume of ascites removed.

The site for paracentesis on the anterior abdominal wall is then chosen (Fig. 20-1). The preferred site is in the lower abdomen, just lateral to the rectus abdominis muscle and inferior to the umbilicus. It is important to stay lateral to the rectus

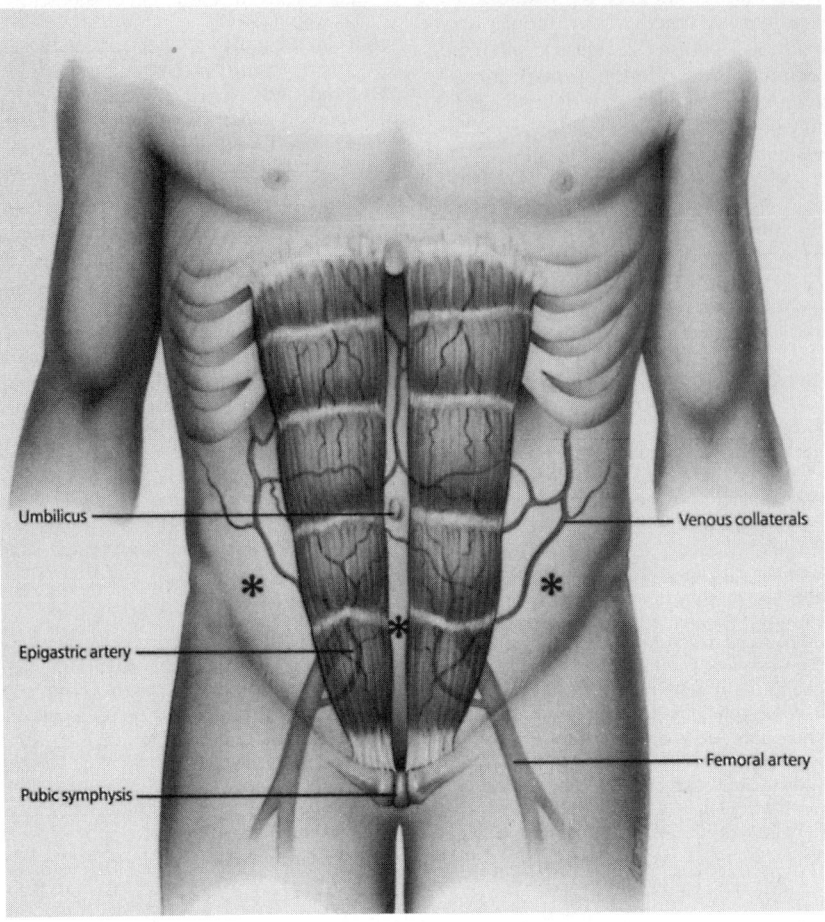

Fig. 20-1. Suggested sites for paracentesis.

abdominal muscle to avoid injury to the inferior epigastric artery and vein. In patients with chronic cirrhosis and caput medusae (engorged anterior abdominal wall veins), these visible vascular structures must be avoided. Injury to these veins can cause significant bleeding due to underlying portal hypertension and may result in hemoperitoneum. The left lower quadrant of the abdominal wall is preferred over the right lower quadrant for abdominal paracentesis because critically ill patients often have cecal distention. The ideal site is therefore in the left lower quadrant of the abdomen, lateral to the rectus abdominis muscle in the midclavicular line, and inferior to the umbilicus. If the patient has had previous abdominal surgery limited to the lower abdomen, it may be difficult to perform a paracentesis in the lower abdomen and the upper abdomen may be chosen. The point of entry, however, remains lateral to the rectus abdominis muscle in the midclavicular line. If there is concern that the ascites is loculated due to previous abdominal surgery or peritonitis, then abdominal paracentesis should be performed under ultrasound guidance to prevent iatrogenic complications.

Abdominal paracentesis can be performed by the needle technique, the catheter technique, or with ultrasound guidance. Diagnostic paracentesis usually requires 20 to 50 ml of peritoneal fluid and is commonly performed using the needle technique. However, if large volumes of peritoneal fluid are required (i.e., for cytologic examination) the catheter technique is used, as it is associated with a lower incidence of complica-

tions. Therapeutic paracentesis, as in the removal of large volumes of ascites, should always be performed with the catheter technique. Ultrasound guidance can be helpful in diagnostic paracentesis using the needle technique or in therapeutic paracentesis with large volume removal using the catheter technique.

Needle Technique. With the patient in the appropriate position and the access site for paracentesis determined, the patient's abdomen is prepared with 10% povidone-iodine solution and sterile drapes are applied. If necessary, intravenous sedation is administered to prevent the patient from moving excessively during the procedure (see Chap. 28). Local anesthesia, using 1% or 2% lidocaine with 1:200,000 epinephrine, is infiltrated into the site. A skin wheal is created with the local anesthetic, using a short 25- or 27-gauge needle. Then, using a 22-gauge 1 1/2-inch needle, the local anesthetic is infiltrated into the subcutaneous tissues and anterior abdominal wall, with the needle perpendicular to the skin. Before infiltrating the anterior abdominal wall and peritoneum, the skin is pulled taut inferiorly, allowing the peritoneal cavity to be entered at a different location than the skin entrance site, thereby decreasing the chance of ascitic leak. This is known as the Z-track technique. While maintaining tension inferiorly on the abdominal skin, the needle is advanced through the abdominal wall fascia and peritoneum, and local anesthetic is injected. Intermittent aspiration identifies when the peritoneal cavity is entered, with return of ascitic fluid into the syringe. The needle is held securely in this position with the left hand, and the right hand is used to withdraw approximately 20 to 50 ml of ascitic fluid into the syringe for a diagnostic paracentesis. Once adequate fluid is withdrawn, the needle and syringe are withdrawn from the anterior abdominal wall and the paracentesis site is covered with a sterile dressing. The needle is removed from the syringe, since this may be contaminated with skin organisms. A small amount of peritoneal fluid is sent in a sterile container for Gram stain and culture and sensitivity test. The remainder of the fluid is sent for appropriate studies, which may include cytology, cell count and differential, protein, specific gravity, amylase, pH, lactate dehydrogenase, bilirubin, triglycerides, and albumin. Peritoneal fluid may be sent for smear and culture for acid-fast bacilli, if tuberculous peritonitis is in the differential diagnosis for that particular patient.

Catheter Technique. The patient is placed in the proper position, and the anterior abdominal wall site for paracentesis is prepared and draped in the usual sterile fashion. Aseptic technique is used throughout the procedure. The site is anesthetized with local anesthetic as described for the needle technique. A 22-gauge, 1 1/2-inch needle attached to a 10-ml syringe is used to document the free return of peritoneal fluid into the syringe at the chosen site. This needle is removed from the peritoneal cavity and a catheter-over-needle assembly is used to gain access to the peritoneal cavity. If the anterior abdominal wall is thin, an 18- or 20-gauge angiocath may be used as the catheter-over-needle assembly. If the anterior abdominal wall is quite thick, as in obese patients, it may be necessary to use a long (5 1/4-inch) catheter-over-needle assembly (18- or 20-gauge) or a percutaneous single-lumen central venous catheter (18- or 20-gauge) and gain access to the peritoneal cavity using the Seldinger technique. The peritoneal cavity is entered as for the needle technique. The catheter-over-needle assembly is inserted perpendicular to the anterior abdominal wall using the Z-track technique; once peritoneal fluid returns into the syringe barrel, the catheter is advanced over the needle, the needle is removed, and a 20- or 50-ml syringe is connected to the catheter. The tip of the catheter is now in the peritoneal cavity and can be left in place until the appropriate amount of peritoneal fluid is removed. This technique, rather than the needle technique, should be employed when large volumes of peritoneal fluid must be removed, since complications (e.g., intestinal perforation) may occur if a needle is left in the peritoneal space for an extended period.

When the Seldinger technique is used in patients with a large anterior abdominal wall, access to the peritoneal cavity is initially gained with a needle or catheter-over-needle assembly. A guidewire is then inserted through the needle and an 18- or 20-gauge single-lumen central venous catheter threaded over the guidewire. It is very important to use the Z-track method for the catheter technique, to prevent development of an ascitic leak, which may be difficult to control and may predispose the patient to peritoneal infection.

Ultrasound Guidance Technique. Patients who have had previous abdominal surgery or peritonitis are predisposed to abdominal adhesions, and it may be quite difficult to gain free access into the peritoneal cavity for diagnostic or therapeutic paracentesis. Ultrasound-guided paracentesis can be very helpful in this population by providing accurate localization of the peritoneal fluid collection and determining the best abdominal access site. This procedure can be performed using the needle or catheter technique as described above, depending on the volume of peritoneal fluid to be drained. Once the fluid collection is localized by the ultrasound probe, the abdomen is prepared and draped in the usual sterile fashion. A sterile sleeve can be placed over the ultrasound probe so there is direct ultrasound visualization of the needle or catheter as it enters the peritoneal cavity. The needle or catheter is thus directed to the area to be drained and the appropriate amount of peritoneal or ascitic fluid is removed. If continued drainage of a loculated peritoneal fluid collection is desired, the radiologist can place a chronic indwelling peritoneal catheter, using a guidewire technique (see Chap. 31).

The use of ultrasound guidance for drainage of loculated peritoneal fluid collections has markedly decreased the incidence of iatrogenic complications related to abdominal paracentesis. If the radiologist does not identify loculated ascites on the initial ultrasound evaluation and documents that there is a large amount of peritoneal fluid which is free in the abdominal cavity, he or she can then indicate the best access site by marking the anterior abdominal wall with an indelible marker. The paracentesis can then be performed by the clinician and repeated whenever necessary. This study can be performed at the bedside in the ICU with a portable ultrasound unit.

COMPLICATIONS. The most common complications related to abdominal paracentesis are bleeding and persistent ascitic leak. Since most patients who have developed ascites also have some component of chronic liver disease with associated coagulopathies, it is very important to correct any underlying coagulopathy before proceeding with abdominal paracentesis. In addition, it is very important to select an avascular access site on the anterior abdominal wall. The Z-track technique is very helpful in minimizing persistent ascitic leak and should always be used. Other complications associated with abdominal paracentesis include intestinal or urinary bladder perforation, with associated peritonitis and infection. Intestinal injury is more common when the needle technique is used. Since the needle is free in the peritoneal cavity, iatrogenic intestinal perforation may occur if the patient moves or if intraabdominal pressure increases with Valsalva maneuver or coughing. Urinary bladder injury is less common and underscores the importance of draining the urinary bladder with a catheter before the procedure. This injury is more common when the abdominal access site is in the suprapubic location; therefore, this access site is not recommended.

Patients who have large-volume chronic abdominal ascites, such as that secondary to hepatic cirrhosis or ovarian carcinoma, frequently develop transient hypotension when a considerable amount of ascitic fluid is removed during therapeutic abdominal paracentesis. It is therefore very important to obtain reliable peripheral or central venous access in these patients so fluid resuscitation can be performed should transient hypotension develop during the procedure. Large-volume ascites removal in such patients is only transiently therapeutic; the underlying chronic disease will induce reaccumulation of the ascites. Careful adherence to proper technique will minimize complications.

Diagnostic Peritoneal Lavage

Prior to the introduction of diagnostic peritoneal lavage by Root and colleagues in 1965 [2], nonoperative evaluation of the injured abdomen was limited to standard four-quadrant abdominal paracentesis. Abdominal paracentesis for evaluation of hemoperitoneum was associated with a high false negative rate. This clinical suspicion was confirmed by Giacobine and Siler in an experimental animal model of hemoperitoneum documenting that a 500 ml blood volume in the peritoneal cavity yielded a positive paracentesis rate of only 78 percent [3]. The initial study by Root and co-workers reported 100 percent accuracy in identification of hemoperitoneum using 1 liter of peritoneal lavage fluid. Many subsequent clinical studies have confirmed these findings, with the largest series reported by Fischer and colleagues in 1978 [4]. They reviewed 2586 cases of diagnostic peritoneal lavage and reported a false positive rate of 0.2 percent, false negative rate of 1.2 percent, and overall accuracy of 98.5 percent. Since its introduction in 1965, diagnostic peritoneal lavage has become a cornerstone in the evaluation of blunt and penetrating abdominal injuries.

INDICATIONS. The primary indication for diagnostic peritoneal lavage is evaluation of blunt abdominal trauma in patients with associated hypotension or altered level of consciousness. Altered neurologic status in trauma patients may be secondary to drug or alcohol ingestion or due to traumatic brain injury. Such findings make abdominal physical examination unreliable, necessitating definitive evaluation for traumatic abdominal injury. If the patient is hemodynamically stable and can be transported safely, the clinician may consider obtaining an abdominal computed tomography (CT) scan. If the patient is hemodynamically unstable or requires emergent surgical intervention for a craniotomy, thoracotomy, or vascular procedure, it is imperative to determine whether there is a coexisting intraperitoneal source of hemorrhage, to prioritize treatment of life-threatening injuries. Peritoneal lavage is therefore used to diagnose the extent of abdominal trauma in patients with multisystem injury or those requiring general anesthesia for treatment of associated traumatic injuries. Patients with associated thoracic or pelvic injuries should also have definitive evaluation for abdominal trauma, and diagnostic peritoneal lavage can be used in these patients.

Diagnostic peritoneal lavage can be used to evaluate penetrating abdominal trauma [5,6]. Thal [7,8] evaluated the utility of diagnostic peritoneal lavage in patients with stab wounds to the lower thorax and abdomen. Diagnostic peritoneal lavage had a false positive rate of 2.4 percent and a false negative rate of 4.9 percent, defining a positive lavage as a red blood cell count greater than 100,000 cells per milliliter of lavage fluid. Diagnostic peritoneal lavage has also been evaluated as a tool for determining intraabdominal injury in patients with gunshot wounds to the lower thorax and abdomen. These clinical studies [5,9] have documented high false positive and false negative rates; therefore, diagnostic peritoneal lavage is not recommended in patients with gunshot wounds to the thorax or abdomen, and mandatory exploratory laparotomy or thoracotomy is indicated.

Diagnostic peritoneal lavage may prove useful in evaluation for possible peritonitis or ruptured viscus in patients with an altered level of consciousness but no evidence of traumatic injury. Diagnostic peritoneal lavage can be considered in critically ill patients with sepsis to determine whether intraabdominal infection is the underlying source. When diagnostic peritoneal lavage is used to evaluate intraabdominal infection, a white blood cell count greater than 500 cells per milliliter of lavage fluid is considered positive. Diagnostic peritoneal lavage can also serve a therapeutic role. It is very effective in rewarming patients with significant hypothermia. It may potentially be used therapeutically in pancreatitis, fecal peritonitis, and bile pancreatitis, but multiple clinical studies have not documented its efficacy in these cases.

Diagnostic peritoneal lavage should not be performed in patients with clear signs of significant abdominal trauma and hemoperitoneum associated with hemodynamic instability. These patients should be transported to the operating room immediately and undergo emergent celiotomy. Pregnancy is a relative contraindication to diagnostic peritoneal lavage; it may be technically difficult to perform due to the gravid uterus and is associated with a higher risk of complications. Bedside ultrasound evaluation of the abdomen in the pregnant trauma patient is associated with least risk to both woman and fetus. An additional relative contraindication to diagnostic peritoneal lavage is multiple previous abdominal surgeries. These patients commonly have multiple abdominal adhesions, and it may be very difficult to gain access to the free peritoneal cavity. If diagnostic peritoneal lavage is indicated, it must be performed by the open technique to prevent iatrogenic complications such as intestinal injury.

TECHNIQUES. There are three techniques of diagnostic peritoneal lavage: closed percutaneous technique, semiclosed technique, and open technique. The closed percutaneous technique, introduced by Lazarus and Nelson in 1979 [10], is easy to perform, can be done rapidly, is associated with a low complication rate, and is as accurate as the open technique. It should not be used in patients who have had previous abdominal surgery or a history of abdominal adhesions. The open technique entails the placement of the peritoneal lavage catheter into the peritoneal cavity under direct visualization. It is more time-consuming than the closed percutaneous technique. It is recommended by the American College of Surgeons Committee on Trauma and in the Advanced Trauma Life Support Course. The semiclosed technique requires a smaller incision than the open technique and uses a peritoneal lavage catheter with a metal stylet to gain entrance into the peritoneal cavity. It has become less popular as clinicians have become more familiar and skilled with the Lazarus-Nelson closed technique.

The patient must be placed in the supine position for all three techniques. A catheter is placed into the urinary bladder and a nasogastric tube inserted into the stomach to prevent iatrogenic bladder or gastric injury. The nasogastric tube is placed on continuous suction for gastric decompression. The skin of the anterior abdominal wall is prepared with 10% povidone-iodine solution and sterile drapes are applied, leaving the periumbilical area exposed. Standard aseptic technique is used throughout the procedure. Local anesthesia with 1% or 2% lidocaine with 1:200,000 epinephrine is used as necessary throughout the procedure.

Closed Percutaneous Technique (Fig. 20-2). Local anesthesia is infiltrated inferior to the umbilicus and a 5-mm skin incision is made just at the inferior umbilical edge. An 18-gauge needle is inserted through this incision and into the peritoneal cavity, angled toward the pelvis at approximately a 45-degree angle with the skin. The penetration through the linea alba and then through the peritoneum will be felt as two separate "pops." A J-tipped guidewire is passed through the needle and into the peritoneal cavity, again directing the wire toward the pelvis by maintaining the needle at a 45-degree angle to the skin. The 18-gauge needle is then removed and the peritoneal lavage catheter inserted over the guidewire into the peritoneal cavity, using a twisting motion and guiding it inferiorly toward the pelvis. The guidewire is then removed, and a 10-ml syringe is attached to the catheter for aspiration. If free blood returns from the peritoneal catheter before the syringe is attached or if gross blood returns in the syringe barrel, then hemoperitoneum has been documented; the catheter is removed and the patient transported quickly to the operating room for emergent celiotomy. If no gross blood returns on aspiration through the catheter, then peritoneal lavage is performed using 1 liter of Ringer's lactate solution or normal saline previously warmed to prevent hypothermia. The fluid is instilled into the peritoneal

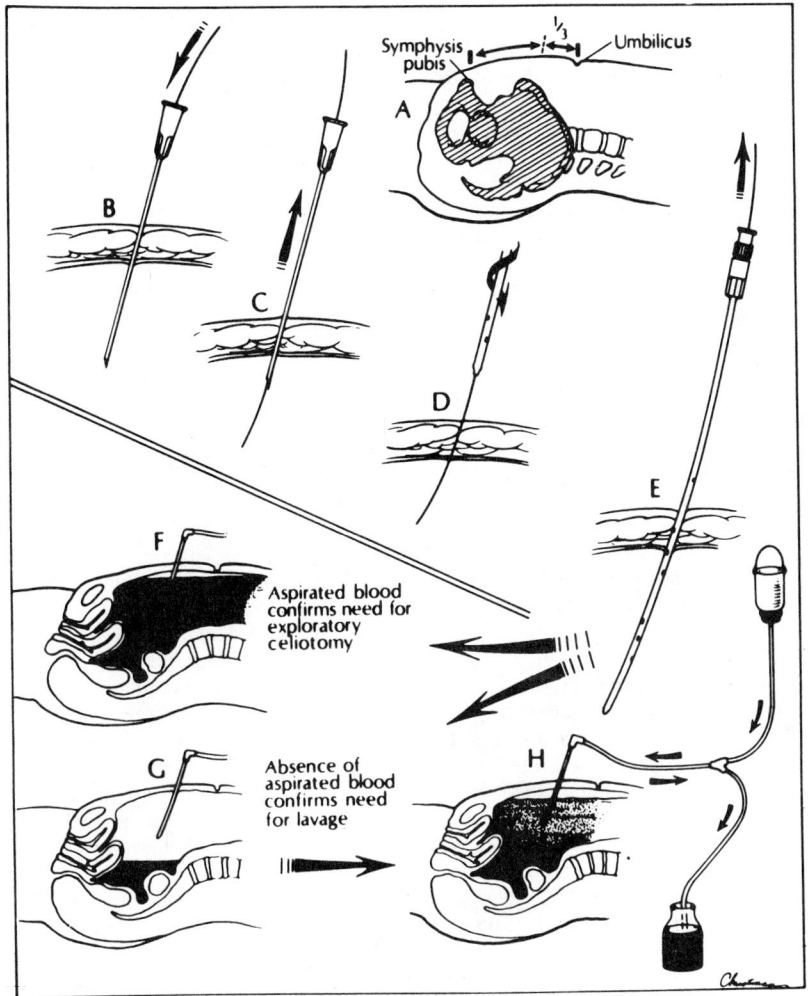

Fig. 20-2. The closed percutaneous technique for diagnostic peritoneal lavage, using a Seldinger guidewire method.

cavity through the peritoneal lavage catheter; afterward, the peritoneal fluid is allowed to drain out of the peritoneal cavity by gravity until the fluid return slows. A minimum of 300 ml of lavage fluid is considered a representative sample of the peritoneal fluid. A sample is sent to the laboratory for determination of red blood cell count, white blood cell count, amylase concentration, and presence of bile, bacteria, or particulate matter. When the lavage is completed, the catheter is removed and a sterile dressing applied over the site. Suture approximation of the skin edges is not necessary when the closed technique is employed for diagnostic peritoneal lavage.

Semiclosed Technique. Local anesthetic is infiltrated in the area of the planned incision and a 2- to 3-cm vertical incision made in the infraumbilical or supraumbilical area. The incision is continued sharply down through the subcutaneous tissue and linea alba, and the peritoneum is then visualized. Forceps, hemostats, or Allis clamps are used to grasp the edges of the linea alba and elevate the fascial edges, to prevent injury to underlying abdominal structures. The peritoneal lavage catheter with a metal inner stylet is inserted through the closed peritoneum into the peritoneal cavity at a 45-degree angle to the anterior abdominal wall, directed toward the pelvis. When the catheter-

metal stylet assembly is in the peritoneal cavity, the peritoneal lavage catheter is advanced into the pelvis and the metal stylet removed. A 10-ml syringe is attached to the catheter, and aspiration is conducted as previously described. When the lavage is completed, the fascia must be reapproximated with sutures, the skin closed, and a sterile dressing applied.

Open Technique. After the administration of appropriate local anesthetic, a vertical midline incision approximately 3 to 5 cm long is made. This incision is commonly made in the infraumbilical location, but in patients with presumed pelvic fractures or retroperitoneal hematomas or in pregnant patients, a supraumbilical location is preferred. The vertical midline incision is carried down through the skin, subcutaneous tissue, and linea alba, under direct vision. The linea alba is grasped on either side using forceps, hemostats, or Allis clamps and the fascia elevated to prevent injury to the underlying abdominal structures. The peritoneum is identified, and a small vertical peritoneal incision is made to gain entrance into the peritoneal cavity. The peritoneal lavage catheter is then inserted into the peritoneal cavity under direct visualization and advanced inferiorly toward the pelvis. It is inserted without the stylet or metal trocar. When in position, a 10-ml syringe is attached for aspiration. If aspiration of the peritoneal cavity is negative (i.e., no gross blood returns), then peritoneal lavage is performed as described above. As in the semiclosed technique, the fascia and skin must be reapproximated to prevent dehiscence and/or evisceration.

A recent prospective randomized study documented that the Lazarus-Nelson technique of closed percutaneous diagnostic peritoneal lavage can be performed faster than the open procedure [11]. The procedure times with the closed technique varied from 1 to 3 minutes, compared with 5 to 24 minutes for the open technique. In addition, it was documented that the closed percutaneous technique is as accurate as the open procedure and was associated with a lower incidence of wound infections and complications. This study concluded that the closed percutaneous technique, using the Seldinger technique, should be used initially in all patients except those who have had previous abdominal surgery or pregnant patients.

Cotter and colleagues recently reported a modification of diagnostic peritoneal lavage that allows for more rapid infusion and drainage of lavage fluid [12]. This modification uses cystoscopy irrigation tubing for instillation and drainage of the peritoneal lavage fluid. The cystoscopy irrigation system dramatically reduced both influx and efflux times, saving an average of 19 minutes per patient for the completion of peritoneal lavage. This modification can be applied to the closed percutaneous or open technique for diagnostic peritoneal lavage to decrease the procedure time in critically ill patients.

INTERPRETATION OF RESULTS. The current guidelines for interpretation of positive and negative results of diagnostic peritoneal lavage are listed in Table 20-1. A positive result can be estimated by the inability to read newsprint or typewritten print through the lavage fluid as it returns through clear plastic tubing. This test is not reliable, however, and a quantitative red blood cell count in a sample of the peritoneal lavage fluid must be performed. For patients with nonpenetrating abdominal trauma, a red blood cell count greater than 100,000 cells per milliliter of lavage fluid is considered positive and requires emergent celiotomy, and less than 50,000 cells per milliliter is

considered negative. Red blood cell counts in the range of 50,000 to 100,000 red blood cells per milliliter are considered indeterminate.

The guidelines for patients with penetrating abdominal trauma are much less clear. Feliciano and colleagues support the use of the same criteria established for blunt abdominal trauma and reported an overall accuracy of 91.2 percent using these guidelines in penetrating abdominal trauma [13]. Thal reported a false positive rate of 2.4 pecent, and false negative rate of 4.9 percent in patients who had diagnostic peritoneal lavage using the standard guidelines for blunt abdominal trauma in patients with thoracoabdominal stab wounds [7]. Other clinical studies have used a red blood cell count of greater than 2000 cells per milliliter or greater than 10,000 cells per milliliter as the criterion for a positive diagnostic peritoneal lavage in patients with penetrating thoracic or abdominal trauma [5,6]. This leads to a higher false positive rate and a lower false negative rate and improves the overall accuracy of the procedure. Future clinical studies with a large trauma patient population will be required to establish clearly the guidelines for positive and negative diagnostic peritoneal lavage results in patients with penetrating thoracoabdominal injury.

Determination of hollow viscus injury by diagnostic peritoneal lavage is much more difficult. A white blood cell count greater than 500 cells per milliliter of lavage fluid or an amylase concentration greater than 175 U per 100 ml of lavage fluid is usually considered positive. These studies, however, are not as accurate as the use of red blood cell count in the lavage fluid to determine presence of hemoperitoneum. A recent study in blunt abdominal trauma patients determined that the white blood cell count in lavage fluid has a positive predictive value of only 23 percent and probably should not be used as an indicator of a positive diagnostic peritoneal lavage [14]. Other studies have recently analyzed alkaline phosphatase levels in diagnostic peritoneal lavage fluid to determine whether this assay is helpful in diagnosis of hollow viscus injuries [15,16]. The results have been variable. One study of 545 patients who sustained blunt or penetrating abdominal injury determined that alkaline phosphatase levels greater than 10 in the diagnostic peritoneal lavage effluent was predictive of hollow visceral injury with a specificity of 99.4 percent and a sensitivity of 93.3 percent [16]. Additional studies will be required to confirm these results and establish the use of alkaline phosphatase levels as a positive indicator of significant intraabdominal injury.

It must be stressed that diagnostic peritoneal lavage is not accurate for determination of retroperitoneal visceral injuries or diaphragmatic injuries [17]. The incidence of false negative diagnostic peritoneal lavage results is approximately 30 percent in patients who sustained traumatic diaphragmatic rupture. In addition, diagnostic peritoneal lavage is insensitive in detecting subcapsular hematomas of the spleen or liver that are contained, with no evidence of hemoperitoneum. Although diagnostic peritoneal lavage is now used in the evaluation of nontraumatic intraabdominal pathology, the criteria for positive lavage in these patients have not yet been established. Additional clinical studies are needed.

Table 20-1. Interpretation of Diagnostic Peritoneal Lavage Results

Positive
  Nonpenetrating abdominal trauma
    Immediate gross blood return via catheter
    Immediate return of intestinal contents or food particles
    Aspiration of 10 ml of blood via catheter
    Return of lavage fluid via chest tube or urinary catheter
    RBC count > 100,000/ml
    WBC count > 500/ml
    Amylase > 175 units/100 ml
  Penetrating abdominal trauma
    Immediate gross blood return via catheter
    Immediate return of intestinal contents or food particles
    Aspiration of 10 ml of blood via catheter
    Return of lavage fluid via chest tube or Foley catheter
    RBC count used is variable, from > 10,000/ml to > 100,000/ml
    WBC count > 500/ml
    Amylase > 175 units/100 ml
Negative
  Nonpenetrating abdominal trauma
    RBC count < 50,000/ml
    WBC count < 100/ml
    Amylase < 75 units/100 ml
  Penetrating abdominal trauma
    RBC count used is variable, from < 2000/ml to < 50,000/ml
    WBC count < 100/ml
    Amylase < 75 units/100 ml

RBC = red blood cell; WBC = white blood cell.

COMPLICATIONS. Complications of diagnostic peritoneal lavage by either of the techniques described here include malposition of the lavage catheter, injury to the intraabdominal organs or vessels, iatrogenic hemoperitoneum, wound infection or dehiscence, evisceration, and possible unnecessary laparotomy. Diagnostic peritoneal lavage is a very valuable technique, however, and if it is performed carefully, with attention to detail, these complications will be minimized. Wound infection, dehiscence, and evisceration are more common with the open technique, therefore the closed percutaneous technique is recommended in all patients who do not have a contraindication to this technique. Knowledge of both techniques is necessary, however, since the choice of technique should be based on the individual patient's presentation.

References

1. Gerber DR, Bekes CE: Peritoneal catheterization. *Crit Care Clin* 8:727, 1992.
2. Root H, Hauser C, McKinley C, et al: Diagnostic peritoneal lavage. *Surgery* 57:633, 1965.
3. Giacobine JW, Siler VE: Evaluation of diagnostic abdominal paracentesis with experimental and clinical studies. *Eur Gynaecol Obstet* 110:676, 1960.
4. Fischer R, Beverlin B, Engrav L, et al: Diagnostic peritoneal lavage 14 years and 2586 patients later. *Am J Surg* 136:701, 1978.
5. Merlotti GJ, Marcet E, Sheaff CM, et al: Use of peritoneal lavage to evaluate abdominal penetration. *J Trauma* 25:228, 1985.
6. Gruenberg JC, Brown RS, Talbert JG, et al: The diagnostic usefulness of peritoneal lavage in penetrating trauma. *Am Surg* 48:402, 1982.
7. Thal ER: Evaluation of peritoneal lavage and local exploration in lower chest and abdominal stab wounds. *J Trauma* 17:642, 1977.
8. Thal ER: Peritoneal lavage: Reliability of RBC count in patients with stab wounds to chest and abdomen. *Arch Surg* 119:579, 1984.
9. Thal ER, May RA, Beesinger D: Peritoneal lavage: Its unreliability in gunshot wounds of the lower chest and abdomen. *Arch Surg* 115:430, 1980.
10. Lazarus HM, Nelson JA: A technique for peritoneal lavage without risk or complication. *Surg Gynecol Obstet* 149:889, 1979.
11. Howdieshell TR, Osler RM, Demarest GB: Open versus closed peritoneal lavage with particular attention to time, accuracy and cost. *Am J Emerg Med* 7:367, 1989.
12. Cotter CP, Hawkins ML, Kent RB, et al: Ultrarapid diagnostic peritoneal lavage. *J Trauma* 29:615, 1989.
13. Feliciano D, Bitondo C, Steed G, et al: Five hundred open taps or lavages in patients with abdominal stab wounds. *Am J Surg* 148:772, 1984.
14. Soyka J, Martin M, Sloan E, et al: Diagnostic peritoneal lavage: Is an isolated WBC count greater than or equal to 500/mm^3 predictive of intra-abdominal trauma requiring celiotomy in blunt trauma patients? *J Trauma* 30:874, 1990.
15. Megison SM, Weigelt JA: The value of alkaline phosphatase in peritoneal lavage. *Ann Emerg Med* 19:5, 1990.
16. Jaffin JH, Ochsner G, Cole FJ, et al: Alkaline phosphatase levels in diagnostic peritoneal lavage as a predictor of hollow visceral injury. *J Trauma* 34:829, 1993.
17. Fischer RP, Freeman T: The inadequacy of peritoneal lavage in diagnosing acute diaphragmatic rupture. *J Trauma* 16:538, 1976.

21. Management of Acute Esophageal Variceal Hemorrhage with Gastroesophageal Balloon Tamponade

Juan Carlos Puyana

Esophageal variceal hemorrhage is an acute, severe, dramatic complication of the patient with portal hypertension that carries a high mortality and significant incidence of recurrence [1]. Until recently, balloon tamponade of the esophagus was considered the first line of treatment to control variceal hemorrhage; however, management of this entity has changed during the last decade, mainly due to the results obtained with urgent diagnostic and therapeutic endoscopy and sclerotherapy [2–5]. This chapter describes the use of devices designed for gastric and esophageal balloon tamponade, summarizes the experience with these tubes, and describes the current role of balloon tamponade in the overall management of bleeding esophageal varices.

Indications and Contraindications

A Sengstaken-Blakemore tube is indicated in patients with a diagnosis of esophageal variceal hemorrhage in which sclerotherapy is not technically possible or readily available or has failed [6]. An adequate anatomic diagnosis is imperative before any of these balloon tubes are inserted. Severe upper gastrointestinal bleeding attributed to esophageal varices in patients with clinical evidence of chronic liver disease results from other causes in 40 percent of cases [7]. The tube is contraindicated in patients with recent esophageal surgery or esophageal stricture [8]. Some authors do not recommend balloon tamponade when a hiatal hernia is present, but, there are reports of successful hemorrhage control in some of these patients [9].

Technical and Practical Considerations

AIRWAY CONTROL. Endotracheal intubation is imperative in patients with hemodynamic compromise and/or encephalopathy. The incidence of aspiration pneumonia is directly related to the presence of encephalopathy or impaired mental status [10,11]. Suctioning of pulmonary secretions and blood accumulated in the hypopharynx is facilitated in patients with endotracheal intubation. Sedatives and analgesics are more readily administered in intubated patients and may be required often, since these tubes are poorly tolerated in most patients. Sedatives must be used cautiously, however, since a number of these patients have impaired liver metabolism. I recommend inserting an endotracheal tube in any patient who will have balloon tamponade. The incidence of pulmonary complications is significantly lower when endotracheal intubation is routinely used [10].

HYPOVOLEMIA, SHOCK, AND COAGULOPATHY.

Adequate intravenous access should be obtained with large-bore venous catheters and aggressive fluid resuscitation undertaken with crystalloids and colloids. A central venous catheter or pulmonary artery catheter may be required to monitor intravascular filling pressures, especially in patients with severe cirrhosis, advanced age, or underlying cardiac and pulmonary disease. The hematocrit should be maintained above 28 percent and coagulopathy should be treated with fresh frozen plasma and platelets. Four to 6 units of packed red cells should always be available in case of severe recurrent bleeding, which commonly occurs in these patients [12].

CLOTS AND GASTRIC DECOMPRESSION.

Placement of an Ewald tube and aggressive lavage and suctioning of the stomach and duodenum facilitate endoscopy and diminish the risk of aspiration and may help control hemorrhage from causes other than esophageal varices.

The diagnostic endoscopic procedure should be done as soon as the patient is stabilized following basic resuscitation. Endoscopy is performed in the intensive care unit (ICU) or operating room under controlled monitoring and with adequate equipment and personnel. An endoscope with a large suction channel should be used.

TUBE, PORTS, AND BALLOONS.

Minnesota (Fig. 21-1) and Sengstaken-Blakemore (Fig. 21-2) tubes are most commonly used. Other tubes have been described for balloon tamponade (Table 21-1). Several studies have published combined experience with tubes such as the Linton and Nachlas tube [12,13]. The techniques described here are limited to the use of the Minnesota and Sengstaken-Blakemore tubes. All lumens should be patent and balloons should be inflated and checked for leaks. The Minnesota tube has a fourth lumen that allows intermittent suctioning above the esophageal balloon, facilitating suctioning of saliva, blood, and pulmonary secretions in the hypopharynx [11,14] (Fig. 21-3). When using a standard Sengstaken-Blakemore tube, a no. 18 Salem sump with surgical ties is attached above the esophageal balloon as originally described by Boyce [15] and inserted through the mouth. Suctioning above the esophageal balloon and hypopharynx diminishes but does not eliminate the risk of aspiration pneumonia.

INSERTION AND PLACEMENT OF THE TUBE.

The tube should be generously lubricated with lidocaine jelly. It can be inserted through the nose or mouth, but the nasal route is not recommended in patients with coagulopathy. The tube is passed into the stomach. Auscultation in the epigastrium while a flush of air is injected through the gastric lumen verifies the position of the tube, but the position of the gastric balloon must be confirmed radiologically at this time. The gastric balloon is inflated with no more than 80 ml of air and a (portable) radiograph obtained that includes the upper abdomen and lower chest (Fig. 21-4). When it is documented that the gastric balloon is below the diaphragm, it should be further inflated with air, slowly, to a volume of 250 to 300 ml [16]. The

Fig. 21-1. Minnesota tube.

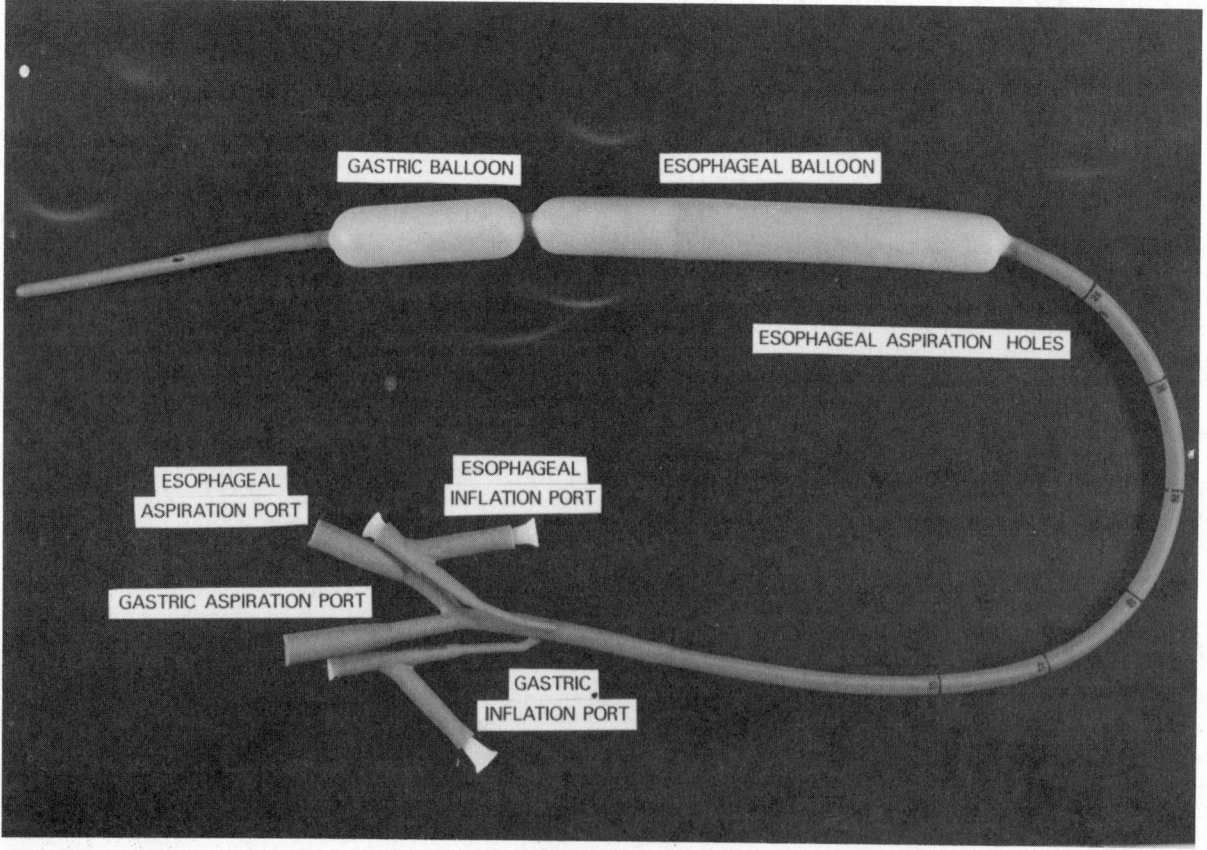

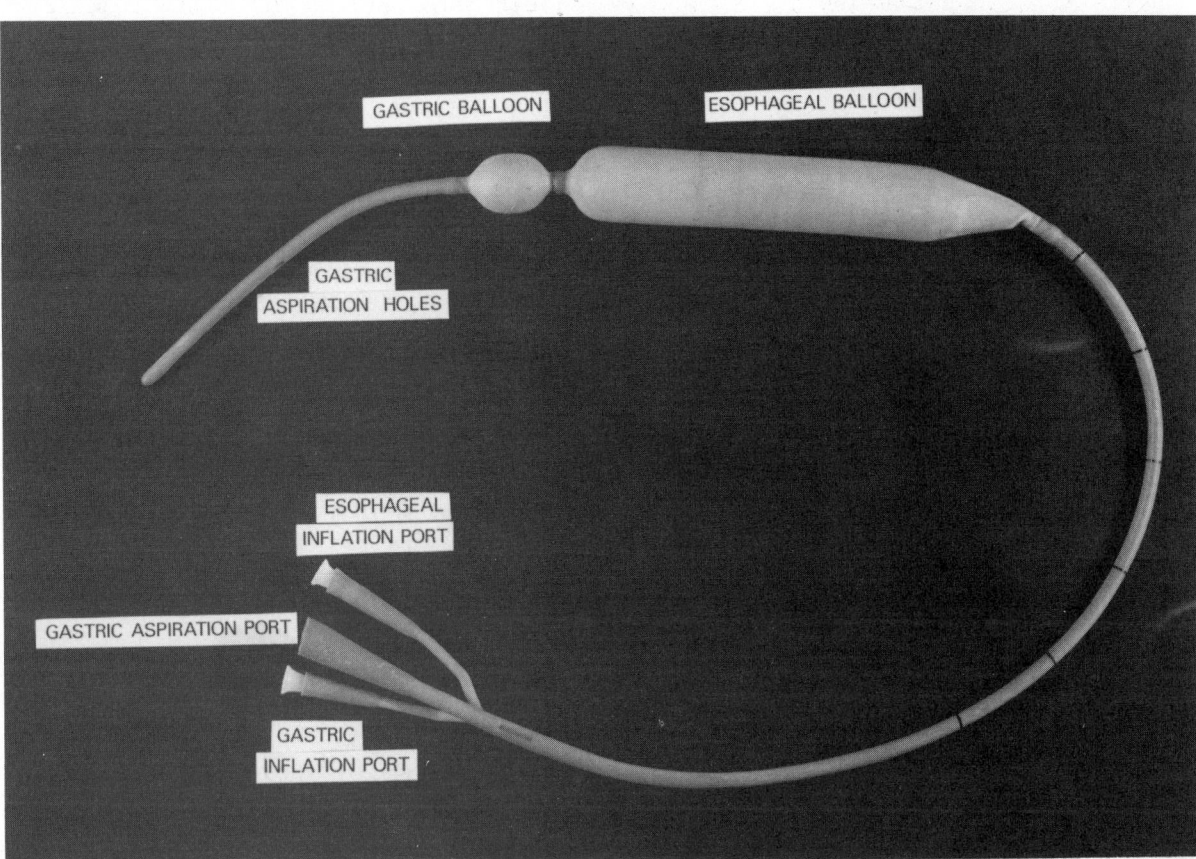

Fig. 21-2. Sengstaken-Blakemore tube.

gastric balloon of the Minnesota tube can be inflated to 450 ml. Tube balloon inlets should be clamped with rubber shod hemostats after insufflation. Hemorrhage is frequently controlled with insufflation of the gastric balloon alone without applying traction [17], but in patients with torrential hemorrhage it is necessary to apply traction (vide infra). If the bleeding continues, the esophageal balloon should be inflated with a bedside manometer to about 45 mm Hg and this pressure monitored and maintained. Some authors [12] inflate the esophageal balloon in all patients immediately after it is inserted.

FIXATION AND TRACTION TECHNIQUES. Fixation and traction on the tube depend on the route of insertion. When the nasal route is used, traction should not be applied against the nostril, since this can easily cause skin and cartilage necrosis. When traction is required, the tube should be attached to a cord that is passed over a pulley in a bed with an overhead orthopedic frame and aligned directly as it comes out of the nose to avoid contact with the nostril. This system allows maintenance of traction with a known weight (500–1500 gm) that is easily measured and constant. When the tube is inserted through the mouth, traction is better applied by placing a football helmet on the patient and attaching the tube to the bar of the helmet after a similar weight is applied for tension [18]. Pressure sores can occur in the head and forehead when the helmet does not fit properly or when it is used for a prolonged period of time. Several authors recommend overhead traction for both oral and nasal insertion [19].

Table 21-1. Tubes Available for Balloon Tamponade

Tube	Manufacturer	Description
Minnesota four-lumen tube	Davol	18 Fr., 42-in.-long tube, 1 1/2-in. gastric balloon, 8-in. esophageal balloon; rubber, non-sterile, single use
Blakemore tube	Davol, Rush	12, 16, and 20 Fr., child, medium, and adult sizes (adult = 39 in. long); rubber, nonsterile, single use
Nachlas gastrointestinal tube	Davol	20 Fr., 52-in., triple-lumen, gastric balloon only; 2 suction ports (above and below balloon); rubber, nonsterile, single use
Linton esophageal tube	Davol	20 Fr., 42-in., 3 1/2-in. gastric balloon, 800 ml air; 2 suction ports (above and below balloon); rubber, nonsterile, single use
Idezuki tube	See Idezuki et al. [28]	Gastric and esophageal balloon; transparent tube with significantly larger inner diameter that allows passage of bronchoscope for direct visualization of bleeding varices, permitting "titration" of balloon pressure; polyurethane and polyvinyl chloride

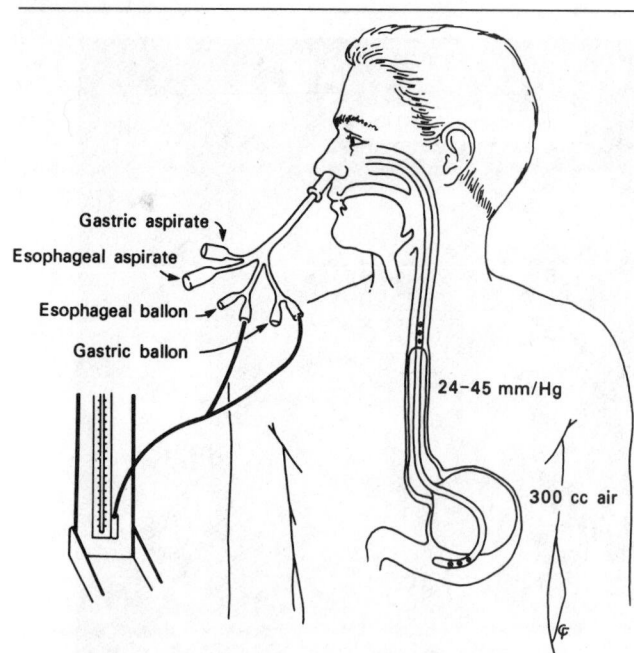

Gastric aspirate
Esophageal aspirate
Esophageal ballon
Gastric ballon

24-45 mm/Hg

300 cc air

Fig. 21-3. Proper positioning of the Minnesota tube.

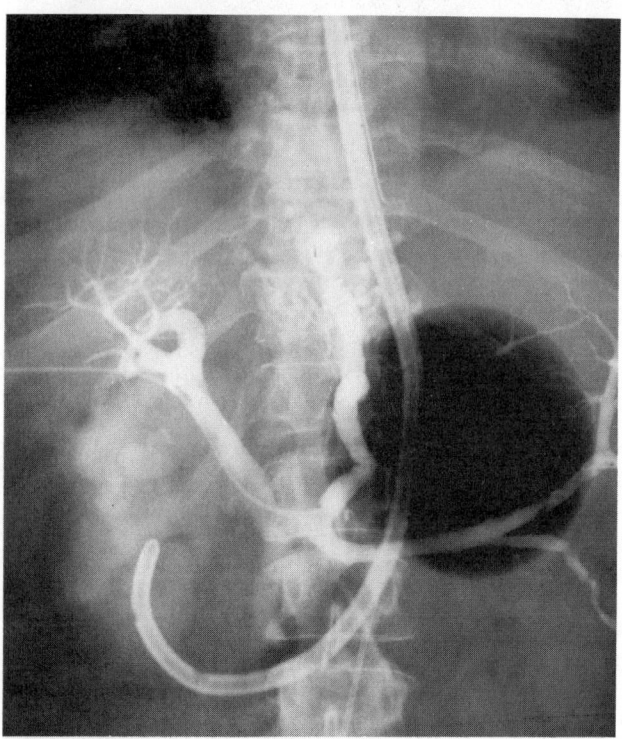

Fig. 21-4. Radiograph showing correct position of the tube; the gastric balloon is seen below the diaphragm. Note the Salem sump above the gastric balloon and adjacent to the tube. (Courtesy of Ashley Davidoff, M.D.)

MAINTENANCE AND MONITORING. The gastric lumen is placed to intermittent suction. The Minnesota tube has an esophageal lumen that can also be placed to low intermittent suction. If the Salem sump has been used as previously described, then continuous suction can be used on the sump tube. The tautness and inflation of balloons should be checked an hour after insertion and periodically by experienced personnel. The tube should be left in place a minimum of 24 hours. The gastric balloon tamponade can be maintained continuously up to 48 hours. The esophageal balloon, however, must be deflated for 30 minutes every 8 hours [10]. The position of the tube should be monitored radiologically every 24 hours or sooner if there is any indication of tube displacement. A pair of scissors should be at the bedside in case the balloon ports need to be cut for rapid decompression, since the balloon can migrate and acutely obstruct the airway [20].

REMOVAL OF THE TUBE. Once hemorrhage is controlled, the esophageal balloon is deflated first; the gastric balloon is left inflated for an additional 24 to 48 hours. If there is no evidence of bleeding, the gastric balloon is deflated and the tube is left in place 24 hours longer. If bleeding recurs, the appropriate balloon is reinflated. The tube is removed if no further bleeding occurs.

Role of Balloon Tamponade in the Management of Bleeding Esophageal Varices

Extensive clinical experience on the use of balloon tamponade has been accumulated since 1950, when it was described by Sengstaken and Blakemore. However, some controversy remains regarding the safety and effectiveness of these techniques [20,21,22]. Early series were characterized by a high incidence of rebleeding and lethal complications directly related to the tubes. Table 21-2 summarizes results from several studies since 1967 [23,24]. There is a wide range in the incidence of rebleeding and mortality, with the discrepancy explained in part by the diversity of techniques employed. In some instances the tube was used after prolonged unsuccessful pharmacologic therapy, usually in patients with severe hemodynamic compromise. More recent studies stratified patients according to Child's classification, using transfusion requirements, hypotension, and response to treatment [25]. Independent predictors of mortality in ICU patients with bleeding esophageal varices were recently described by Lee et al [26]. These predictors are total volume of sclerosing agent (ethanolamine), blood transfusion greater

Table 21-2. Efficacy and Mortality of Balloon Tamponade for Bleeding Esophageal Varices

Author, date	n	% hemostasis	% rebleed	% mortality
Pitcher (1967)	50	92	16	36
Novis (1976)	41	85	60	60
Chojkier (1980)	39	41	20	90
Hunt (1982)	103	94	29	28
Barsoum (1982)	50	42	58	60
Correia (1984)	17	70	15	24
Paquet (1985)	21	73	44	27
Panes (1988)	151	91	47	34
Teres (1990)	52	87	20	30

than 10 units of red cells, Glasgow Coma Scale, coagulopathy reflected by an average 2.6±1.6 INR (international normalized ratio for prothrombin test), and presence of shock. The objective of treatment of acute esophageal bleeding is to arrest the hemorrhage and allow time for patient stabilization for elective treatment. During the last 10 years, a number of studies comparing the efficacy of balloon tamponade against sclerotherapy have shown that the incidence and severity of complications as well as the results in controlling bleeding favor the use of sclerotherapy as the first line of treatment [27–31]. However, balloon tamponade continues to have an important place in the management of patients with acute esophageal variceal hemorrhage (Fig. 21-5). The decision to use other therapeutic alternatives depends on the initial response to sclerotherapy, the severity of the hemorrhage, and the patient's underlying condition. Combined pharmacologic therapy with vasoactive drugs and balloon tamponade can control the hemorrhage in 90 percent of cases [12]. Terblanche et al. advocate vasopressin and nitroglycerin infusion to diminish portal vein pressure while emergency endoscopy is performed to confirm the diagnosis [31]. Other alternatives include percutaneous transhepatic embolization, which is recommended in poor-risk patients who do not stop bleeding despite other measures [32]. Recent preliminary reports described endoscopic band ligation of the bleeding vessel [33,34], which seems to have lower morbidity than sclerotherapy [35,36], and is better tolerated by patients. However, a larger experience is required before definite recommendations are made.

HISTORICAL DEVELOPMENT. Westphal, in 1930, described the use of an esophageal sound as a means of controlling var-

iceal hemorrhage [37]. In 1947, successful control of hemorrhage by balloon tamponade was achieved by attaching an inflatable latex bag to the end of a Miller-Abbot tube [38]. In 1949, a two-balloon tube was described by Patton and Johnson [39]. A triple-lumen tube with a gastric and an esophageal balloon (one lumen for gastric aspiration and the other two for balloon inflation) was described by Sengstaken and Blakemore in 1950 [40]. Linton, in 1953, proposed a single gastric balloon tube with a suction lumen below the balloon as a diagnostic tool to differentiate between gastric and esophageal bleed and a larger balloon (800 ml) capable of compressing the submucosal veins in the cardia, thereby minimizing flow to the esophageal veins [41,42]. An additional suction port above Linton's gastric balloon was introduced by Nachlas in 1955 [43]. The Minnesota tube was described in 1968 as a modification of the Sengstaken-Blakemore tube, incorporating the esophageal suction port described above [14].

COMPLICATIONS. Aspiration pneumonia is the most common complication of balloon tamponade. The severity and fatality rate is related to the presence of impaired mental status and encephalopathy in patients with poor control of the airway. The incidence ranges from 0 to 12 percent. Acute laryngeal obstruction is the most severe of all complications and the worst example of tube migration. Migration of the tube occurs when the gastric balloon is not inflated properly after adequate positioning in the stomach or when excessive traction (greater than 1.5 kg) is used. Aspiration pneumonia and esophageal perforation can both occur when the balloon migrates into the esophagus or hypopharynx [44,45]. Mucosal ulceration of the gastroesophageal junction is common and is directly related to prolonged traction time (greater than 36 hours). Perforation of the esophagus is reported as a result of misplacing the gastric

Fig. 21-5. Management of esophageal variceal hemorrhage.

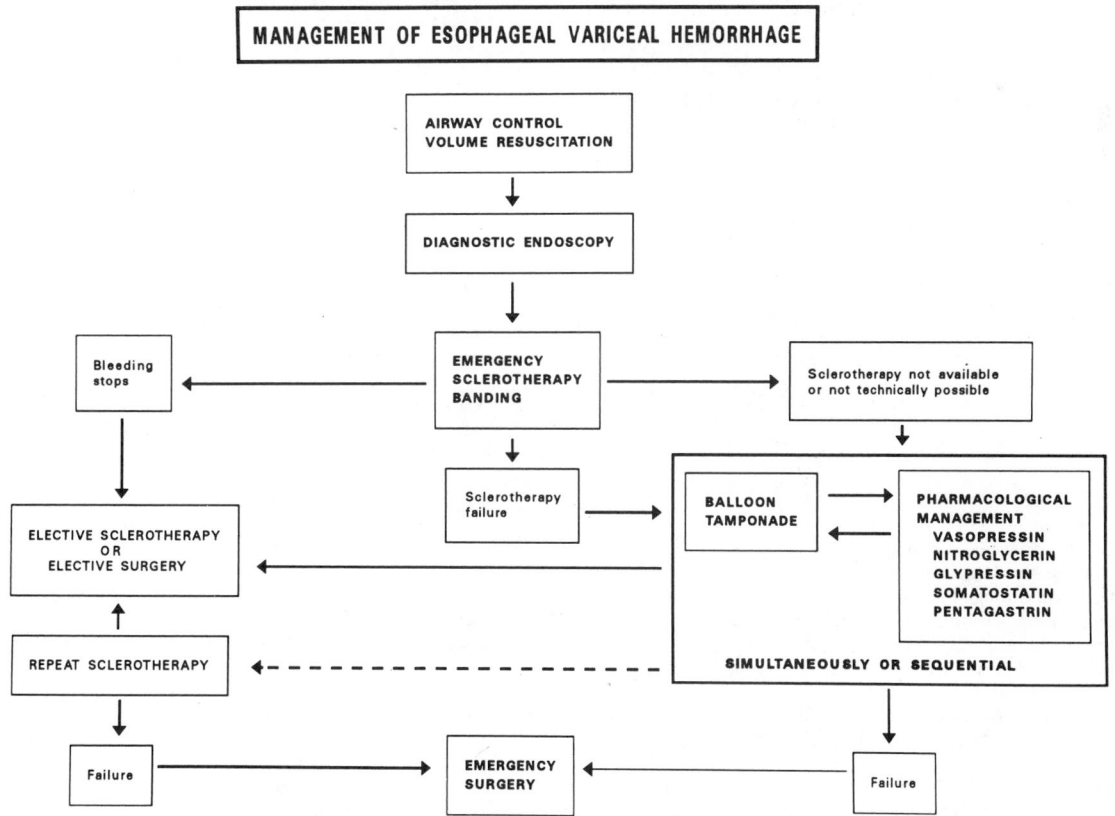

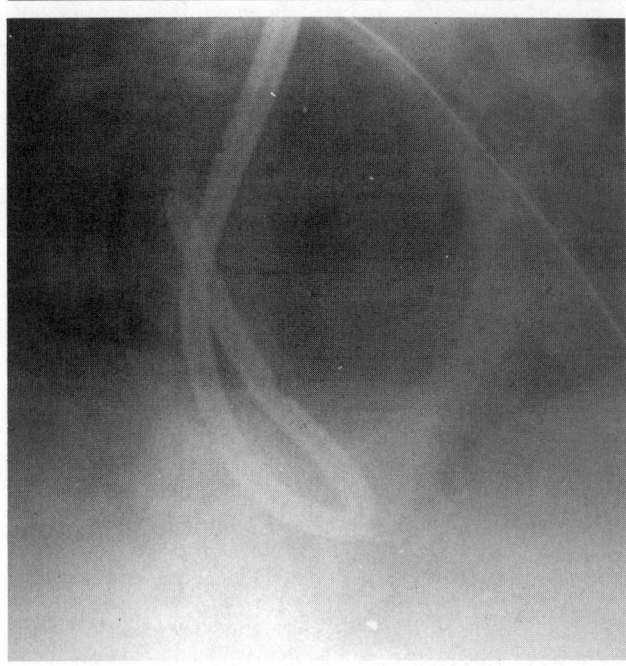

Fig. 21-6. Chest radiograph, showing distal segment of the tube coiled in the chest and the gastric balloon inflated above the diaphragm in the esophagus. (Courtesy of Ashley Davidoff, M.D.)

balloon above the diaphragm (Fig. 21-6). It is imperative that the position be confirmed radiologically immediately after passing the tube and before the gastric balloon is inflated with more than 80 ml of air. Rupture of the esophagus carries a high mortality, especially in patients with severe hemorrhage who already have serious physiologic impairment. The incidence of complications that are a direct cause of death ranges from 0 to 20 percent. Unusual complications, such as impaction, result from obstruction of the balloon ports making it impossible to deflate the balloon. Occasionally surgery is required to remove the tube [46]. Other complications include necrosis of the nostrils and nasopharyngeal bleeding.

Acknowledgments

The author thanks Charles F. Foltz and Susan A. Bright, Medical Media Service, West Roxbury VA Medical Center.

References

1. Terblanche J, Krige JE, Bornman PC: The treatment of esophageal varices. *Annu Rev Med* 43:69, 1992.
2. Westaby D, MacDougall BRD, Williams R: Improved survival following injection sclerotherapy for esophageal varices: Final analysis of a controlled trial. *Hepatology* 5:827, 1985.
3. Terblanche J, Krige JE, Bornman PC: Endoscopic sclerotherapy. *Surg Clin North Am* 70:341, 1990.
4. Barsoum MS, Ibrahim AS, Bolous FI, et al: Tamponade and injection sclerotherapy in the management of bleeding oesophageal varices. *Br J Surg* 69:76, 1982.
5. Paquet KJ, Feussner H: Endoscopic sclerosis and esophageal balloon tamponade in acute hemorrhage from esophagogastric var-

ices: A prospective controlled randomized trial. *Hepatology* 5:580, 1985.
6. Burnett DA, Rikkers LF: Nonoperative emergency treatment of variceal hemorrhage. *Surg Clin North Am* 70:291,1990.
7. Fleisher D: Etiology and prevalence of severe persistent upper gastrointestinal bleeding. *Gastroenterology* 80:800, 1983
8. McCormick PA, Burroughs AK, McIntyre N: How to insert a Sengstaken-Blakemore tube. *Br J Hosp Med* 43:274, 1990.
9. Minocha A, Richards RJ: Sengstaken-Blakemore tube for control of massive bleeding from gastric varices in hiatal hernia. *J Clin Gastroenterol* 14:36, 1992.
10. Cello JP, Crass RA, Grendell JH, et al: Management of the patient with hemorrhaging esophageal varices. *JAMA* 256:1480, 1986.
11. Pasquale MD, Cerra FB: Sengstaken-Blakemore tube placement. *Crit Care Clin* 8:743, 1992.
12. Panes J, Teres J, Bosch J: Efficacy of balloon tamponade in treatment of bleeding gastric and esophageal varices: Results in 151 consecutive episodes. *Dig Dis Sci* 33:454, 1988.
13. Teres J, Cecilia A, Bordas JM, et al: Esophageal tamponade for bleeding varices: Controlled trial between the Sengstaken-Blakemore tube and the Linton-Nachlas tube. *Gastroenterology* 75:566, 1978.
14. Edlich RF, Lande AJ, Goodale RL, Wangensteen OH: Prevention of aspiration pneumonia by continuous esophageal aspiration during esophagogastric tamponade and gastric cooling. *Surgery* 64:405, 1968.
15. Boyce HW: Modification of the Sengstaken-Blakemore balloon tube. *N Engl J Med* 267:195, 1962.
16. Duarte B. Technique for the placement of the Sengstaken-Blakemore tube. *Surg Gynecol Obstet* 168:449, 1989.
17. Pinto Correia J, Martins Alves M, Alexandrino P, et al: Controlled trial of vasopressin and balloon tamponade in bleeding esophageal varices. *Hepatology* 4:885, 1984.
18. Head HB, Kukral JC, Preston FW: Helmet-mounted constant traction spring for maintenance of position of Sengstaken tube. *Am J Surg* 112:465, 1966.
19. Hunt PS, Korman MG, Hansky J, et al: An 8-year prospective experience with balloon tamponade in emergency control of bleeding esophageal varices. *Dig Dis Sci* 27:413, 1982.
20. Chojkier M, Conn HO: Esophageal tamponade in the treatment of bleeding varices: A decadal progress report. *Dig Dis Sci* 25:267, 1980.
21. Conn HO, Simpson JA: Excessive mortality associated with balloon tamponade of bleeding varices: A critical reappraisal. *JAMA* 202:587, 1967.
22. Orloff MJ: Emergency treatment of variceal hemorrhage. *Can J Surg* 22:550, 1979.
23. Pitcher JL: Safety and effectiveness of the modified Sengstaken-Blakemore tube: A prospective study. *Gastroenterology* 61:291, 1967.
24. Novis BH, Duys P, Terblanche J: Fiberoptic endoscopy and the use of the Sengstaken tube in acute gastrointestinal hemorrhage in patients with portal hypertension and varices. *Gut* 17:258, 1976.
25. Teres J, Planas R, Panes J, et al: Vasopressin/nitroglycerin infusion versus esophageal tamponade in the treatment of acute variceal bleeding: A randomized controlled trial. *Hepatology* 11:964, 1990.
26. Lee H, Hawker FH, Selby W, et al: Intensive care treatment of patients with bleeding esophageal varices: Results, predictors of mortality, and predictors of the adult respiratory distress syndrome. *Crit Care Med* 20:1555, 1992.
27. Fleig WE, Stange EF, Ruettenauer K, et al: Emergency endoscopic sclerotherapy for bleeding esophageal varices: A prospective study in patients not responding to balloon tamponade. *Gastrointest Endosc* 29:8, 1983.
28. Idezuki Y, Sanjo K, Bandai Y, et al: Current strategy for esophageal varices in Japan. *Am J Surg* 160:98, 1990.
29. Lewis J, Chung RS, Allison J: Sclerotherapy of esophageal varices. *Arch Surg* 115:476, 1980.
30. Moreto M, Zaballa M, Bernal A, et al: A randomized trial of tamponade or sclerotherapy as immediate treatment for bleeding esophageal varices. *Surg Gynecol Obstet* 167:331, 1988.
31. Terblanche J, Yakoob HI, Bornman PC, et al: Acute bleeding varices: A five-year prospective evaluation of tamponade and sclerotherapy. *Ann Surg* 194:521, 1981.

32. Bengmark S, Borjesson B, Hoevels J, et al: Obliteration of esophageal varices by PTP: A follow-up of 43 patients. *Ann Surg* 190:549, 1979.
33. Stiegman GV, Goff JS, Sun JH, et al: Endoscopic variceal ligation: An alternative to sclerotherapy. *Gastrointest Endosc* 35:431, 1989.
34. Saeed ZA, Michaletz PA, Winchester CB, et al: Endoscopic variceal ligation in patients who have failed endoscopic sclerotherapy. *Gastrointest Endosc* 36:572, 1990.
35. Mal F, Labadie H, Meicler C, et al: Acute pericarditis with tamponade after endoscopic sclerosis of esophageal varices. *Gastroenterol Clin Biol* 11:910, 1987.
36. Brown DL, Luchi RJ: Cardiac tamponade and constrictive pericarditis complicating endoscopic sclerotherapy. *Arch Intern Med* 147:2169, 1987.
37. Westphal K: Uber eine Kompressions Behandlun der Blutungen aus Oesophagusvarizen. *Dtsch Med Wochenschr* 56:1135, 1930.
38. Rowentree LG, Zimmerman EF, Todd MH, et al: Intraesophageal venous tamponade: Its use in case of variceal hemorrhage from the esophagus. *JAMA* 13:630, 1947.
39. Patton TB, Johnson CG: Method for control of bleeding from esophageal varices. *Arch Surg* 59:502, 1949.
40. Sengstaken RW, Blakemore AH: Balloon tamponage for the control of hemorrhage from esophageal varices. *Ann Surg* 131:781, 1950.
41. Linton RR: The emergency and definitive treatment of bleeding esophageal varices. *Gastroenterology* 21:1, 1953.
42. Linton RR: The treatment of esophageal varices. *Surg Clin North Am* 46:485, 1966.
43. Nachlas MN: A new triple-lumen tube for diagnosis and treatment of upper gastrointestinal hemorrhage. *N Engl J Med* 252:720, 1955.
44. Vlavianos P, Gimson AES, Westaby D, Williams R: Balloon tamponade in variceal bleeding: Use and misuse. *Br Med J* 298:29, 1989.
45. McGrath RB: Inadvertent gastric balloon inflation within the chest in the management of esophageal varices. *Crit Care Med* 14:580, 1986.
46. Gossat D, Bolin TD: An unusual complication of balloon tamponade in the treatment of esophageal varices: A case report and brief review of the literature. *Am J Gastroenterol* 80:600, 1985.

22. Endoscopic Placement of Feeding Tubes

Lena M. Napolitano, Steven Schonholz, and Philip Caushaj

Indications for Enteral Feeding

Nutritional support is an essential component of intensive care medicine (see Chaps. 200 and 201) [1–5]. It has become increasingly evident that nutritional support administered via the enteral route is far superior to total parenteral nutrition [6,7]. Although there are absolute or relative contraindications to enteral feeding in selected cases, most critically ill patients can receive some or all of their nutritional requirements via the gastrointestinal tract. Even when some component of nutritional support must be provided intravenously, feeding via the gut is desirable.

Provision of nutrition through the enteral route aids in prevention of gastrointestinal mucosal atrophy, thereby maintaining the integrity of the gastrointestinal mucosal barrier [8,9]. Derangements in the barrier function of the gastrointestinal tract may permit the systemic absorption of gut-derived microbes and microbial products (bacterial translocation), which has been implicated as important in the pathophysiology of syndromes of sepsis and multiple organ system failure (see Chap. 199) [10]. Other advantages of enteral nutrition are preservation of immunologic gut function and normal gut flora, improved utilization of nutrients, and reduced cost. Recent studies suggest that clinical outcome is improved and infectious complications are decreased in patients who receive enteral nutrition compared with parenteral nutrition [11,12].

Several developments, including new techniques for placement of feeding tubes, availability of smaller-caliber, minimally reactive tubes, and an increasing range of enteral formulas, have expanded the ability to provide enteral nutritional support to critically ill patients. Enteral feeding at a site proximal to the pylorus may be absolutely or relatively contraindicated in patients with increased risk of pulmonary aspiration, but feeding more distally (particularly distal to the ligament of Treitz) decreases the likelihood of aspiration. Other relative or absolute contraindications to enteral feeding include fistulas, intestinal obstruction, upper gastrointestinal hemorrhage, and severe inflammatory bowel disease [13]. Enteral feeding is not recommended in patients with severe malabsorption or early in the course of severe short gut syndrome [14,15].

Access to the Gastrointestinal Tract

After deciding to provide enteral nutrition, the clinician must decide whether to deliver the formula into the stomach, duodenum, or jejunum and determine the optimal method for accessing the site, based on the function of the patient's gastrointesinal tract, duration of enteral nutritional support required, and risk of pulmonary aspiration. Gastric feeding provides the most normal route for enteral nutrition, but it is commonly poorly tolerated in the critically ill patient due to gastric dysmotility with delayed emptying. Enteral nutrition infusion into the duodenum or jejunum may decrease the incidence of aspiration because of the protection afforded by a competent pyloric sphincter; however, the risk of aspiration is not completely eliminated by feeding distal to the pylorus [16]. Infusion into the jejunum is associated with the lowest risk of pulmonary aspiration. An advantage of this site of administration is that enteral feeding can be initiated early in the postoperative period, because postoperative ileus primarily affects the colon and stomach and only rarely involves the small intestine [17,18,19].

Techniques

Enteral feeding tubes can be placed via the transnasal, transoral or percutaneous transgastric routes. If these procedures are contraindicated or unsuccessful, the tube may be placed by endoscopy using endoscopic and laparoscopic technique or surgically via a laparotomy [20,21].

NASOENTERIC ROUTE. Nasoenteric tubes are the most commonly used means of providing enteral nutritional support in critically ill patients. This route is preferred for short- to intermediate-term enteral support when eventual resumption of oral feeding is anticipated. It is possible to infuse enteral formulas into the stomach using a conventional 16 or 18 Fr. polyvinyl-chloride nasogastric tube, but patients are usually much more comfortable if a small-diameter silicone or polyurethane feeding tube is used. Nasoenteric tubes vary in luminal diameter (6–14 Fr.) and length, depending on the desired location of the distal orifice: stomach, 30 to 36 inches; duodenum, 43 inches; jejunum, at least 48 inches [22]. Some tubes have tungsten-weighted tips designed to facilitate passage into the duodenum via normal peristalsis; others have a stylet. Most are radiopaque. Newer tubes permit gastric decompression while delivering formula into the jejunum [23].

Nasoenteric feeding tubes should be placed with the patient in a semi-Fowler's or sitting position. The tip of the tube should be lubricated, placed in the patient's nose, and advanced to the posterior pharynx. If possible, the patient should be permitted to sip water as the tube is slowly advanced into the stomach. Once in position, air should be insufflated through the tube while auscultating over the stomach with a stethoscope. The presence of a gurgling sound suggests, but does not prove, that the tube is in the gastric lumen. A chest radiograph should be obtained to confirm the position of the tube prior to initiating feeding. The tube should be securely taped to the forehead or cheek without tension. If the tube is placed for duodenal or jejunal feeding, a loop 6 to 8 inches long may be left extending from the nose and the tube advanced 1 to 2 inches every hour. Placing the patient in a right lateral decubitus position may facilitate passage through the pylorus.

Spontaneous transpyloric passage of enteral feeding tubes in critically ill patients is commonly unsuccessful secondary to the preponderance of gastric atony in these patients. The addition of a tungsten weight to the end of enteral feeding tubes and the development of wire or metal stylets in enteral feeding tubes are aimed at improving the success rate for spontaneous transpyloric passage. The administration of intravenous metoclopramide has also been recommended to improve spontaneous transpyloric placement of enteral feeding tubes. A recent randomized prospective trial in critically ill patients compared the success rate of transpyloric passage of weighted versus unweighted enteral feeding tubes, both with inner stylets. This study demonstrated that the combination of preinsertion metoclopramide and a tapered, unweighted feeding tube with inner stylet achieved transpyloric position in 84 percent of patients at 4 hours after placement, compared to 36 percent with the weighted enteral feeding tubes (p < .002) [24]. Nasoenteral feeding tubes with inner stylets are therefore recommended for use in critically ill patients. However, these tubes must be inserted by skilled practitioners.

If the tube does not migrate into the duodenum over several hours, placement can be attempted under endoscopic assistance or fluoroscopic guidance. Endoscopic placement of nasoenteral feeding tubes is easily accomplished in the critically ill patient and can be performed at the bedside using portable equipment. The patient is sedated appropriately, and topical anesthetic is applied to the posterior pharynx with lidocaine or benzocaine spray. A nasoenteric feeding tube 43 to 48 inches long with an inner wire stylet is passed transnasally into the stomach. The endoscope is inserted and advanced through the esophagus into the gastric lumen. An endoscopy forceps is passed through the biopsy channel of the endoscope and used to grasp the tip of the enteral feeding tube. The endoscope, along with the enteral feeding tube, is advanced distally into the duodenum as far as possible (Fig. 22-1). The endoscopy forceps and feeding tube remain in position in the distal duodenum as the endoscope is withdrawn back into the gastric lumen. The endoscopy forceps is opened, the feeding tube released, and the endoscopy forceps withdrawn carefully back into the stomach. On first pass, the feeding tube is usually lodged in the second portion of the duodenum. The portion of the feeding tube that is redundant in the stomach is advanced slowly into the duodenum using the endoscopy forceps, aiming to achieve a final position distal to the ligment of Treitz (Fig. 22-2). An abdominal radiograph is obtained at the completion of the procedure to document the final position of the nasoenteral feeding tube. Endoscopic placement of postpyloric enteral feeding tubes is highly successful, eliminates the risk of transporting the patient to radiology for fluoroscopic placement, and allows for prompt achievement of nutritional goals, since enteral feeding can be initiated immediately following the procedure.

PERCUTANEOUS ROUTE. Percutaneous endoscopic gastrostomy (PEG) tube placement has become the procedure of choice for patients requiring prolonged enteral nutritional support [20,21,25,26,27]. Tubes range in size from 20 to 28 Fr. Unlike surgical gastrostomy, PEG does not require general anesthesia and laparotomy, and it eliminates the discomfort associated with chronic nasoenteric tubes. This procedure can be considered in patients who have normal gastric emptying and low risk for pulmonary aspiration and can be performed in the operating room, an endoscopy unit, or at the bedside in the intensive care unit (ICU) with portable endoscopy equipment.

Percutaneous endoscopic gastrostomy should not be performed in patients with near or total obstruction of the pharynx or esophagus, in the presence of coagulopathy, or when trans-

Fig. 22-1. Endoscopic placement of nasoenteral feeding tube. Endoscopy forceps and gastroscope advancing the feeding tube in the duodenum.

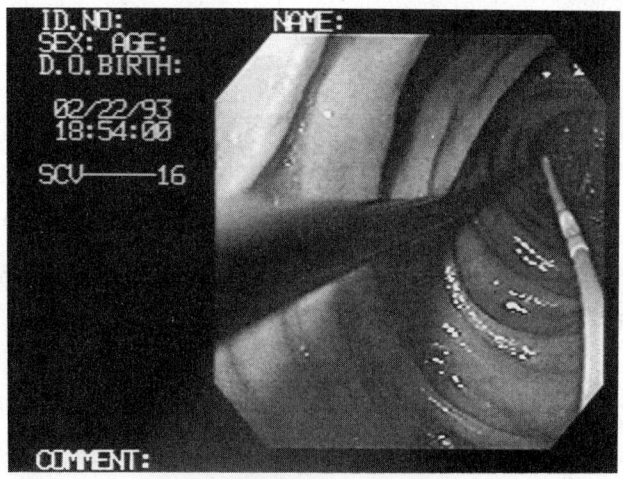

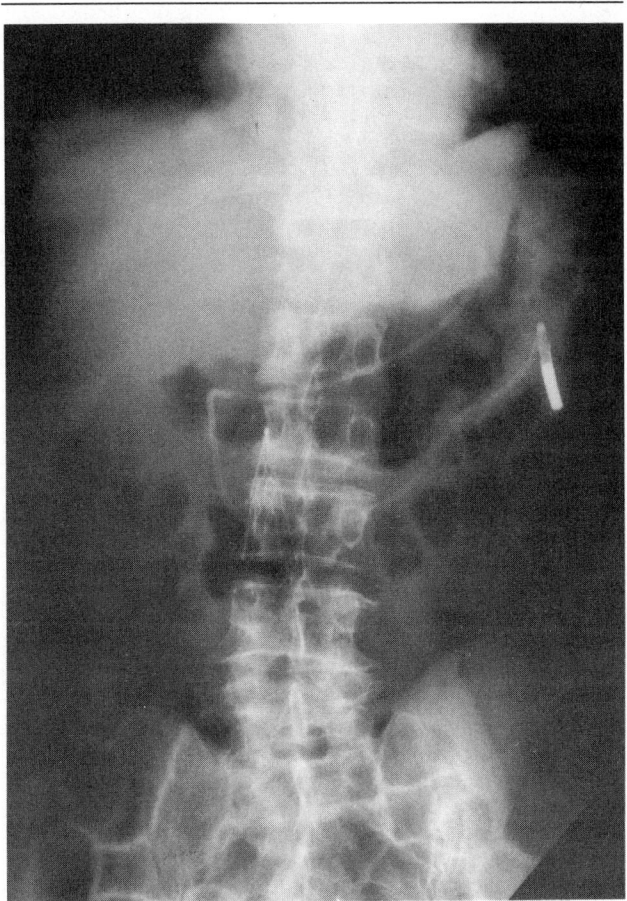

Fig. 22-2. Abdominal radiograph, documenting the optimal position of an endoscopically placed nasoenteral feeding tube, past the ligament of Treitz.

illumination is inadequate. Relative contraindications are ascites, gastric cancer, and gastric ulcer. Previous abdominal surgery is not a contraindication. The original method for PEG was the "pull" technique. More recent modifications are the "push" and "introducer" techniques.

Pull Technique. The procedure is performed with the patient in the supine position. The abdomen is prepared and draped. The posterior pharynx is anesthetized with a topical spray or solution (e.g., benzocaine spray or viscous lidocaine) and intravenous sedation (e.g., 1–2 mg of midazolam) is administered. A prophylactic antibiotic, usually a first-generation cephalosporin, is administered prior to the procedure. The fiberoptic gastroscope is inserted into the stomach, which is then insufflated with air. The lights are dimmed and the assistant applies digital pressure to the anterior abdominal wall in the left subcostal area approximately 2 cm below the costal margin, looking for the brightest transillumination. The endoscopist should be able to identify clearly the indentation in the stomach created by the assistant's digital pressure on the anterior abdominal wall; otherwise, another site should be chosen. When the correct spot has been identified, the assistant anesthetizes the anterior abdominal wall. The endoscopist then introduces a polypectomy snare through the endoscope. A small incision is made in the skin and the assistant introduces a large-bore catheter-needle stylet assembly into the stomach and through the

snare. The snare is then tightened securely around the catheter. The inner stylet is removed and a looped insertion wire is introduced through the catheter and into the stomach. The cannula is slowly withdrawn so the snare grasps the wire. The gastroscope is then pulled out of the patient's mouth with the wire firmly grasped by the snare. The end of the transgastric wire exiting the patient's mouth is then tied to a prepared gastrostomy tube. The assistant pulls on the end of the wire exiting from the abdominal wall while the endoscopist guides the lubricated gastrostomy tube into the posterior pharynx and the esophagus. With continued traction, the gastrostomy tube is pulled into the stomach so that it exits on the anterior abdominal wall. The gastroscope is reinserted into the stomach to confirm adequate placement of the gastrostomy tube against the gastric mucosa and to document that no bleeding has occurred. The intraluminal portion of the tube should contact the mucosa, but excessive tension on the tube should be avoided, since this can lead to ischemic necrosis of the gastric wall. The tube is secured to the abdominal wall using sutures. Feedings may be initiated immediately following the procedure or 24 hours later.

Push Technique. This method is very similar to the pull technique. The gastroscope is inserted and a point on the anterior abdominal wall localized as for the pull technique. Rather than introducing a looped insertion wire, however, a straight guidewire is snared and brought out through the patient's mouth by withdrawing the endoscope and snare together. A commercially developed gastrostomy tube (Sachs-Vine) with a tapered end is then passed in an aboral direction over the wire, which is held taut. The tube is grasped and pulled the rest of the way out. The gastroscope is reinserted to check the position and tension on the tube.

Introducer Technique. This method uses a peel-away introducer technique originally developed for the placement of cardiac pacemakers and central venous catheters. The gastroscope is inserted into the stomach and an appropriate position for placement of the tube is identified. After infiltration of the skin with local anesthetic, a 16- or 18-gauge needle is introduced into the stomach. A J-tipped guidewire is inserted through the needle into the stomach and the needle is withdrawn. Using a twisting motion, a 16 Fr. introducer with a peel-away sheath is passed over the guidewire into the gastric lumen [28,29]. The guidewire and introducer are removed, leaving in place the sheath that allows placement of a 14 Fr. Foley catheter. The sheath is peeled away after the balloon is inflated with 10 ml of normal saline.

Percutaneous Endoscopic Jejunostomy. If postpyloric feeding is desired (especially in patients at high risk for pulmonary aspiration), a percutaneous endoscopic jejunostomy (PEJ) may be performed. The PEJ tube allows for simultaneous gastric decompression and duodenal/jejunal enteral feeding. A second smaller feeding tube can be attached and passed through the gastrostomy tube and advanced endoscopically into the duodenum or jejunum. When the PEG is in position, a guidewire is passed through the PEG and grasped using endoscopy forceps. The guidewire and endoscope are passed into the duodenum as distally as possible. The jejunal tube is then passed over the guidewire through the PEG into the distal duodenum and advanced into the jejunum, and the endoscope is withdrawn [30]. An alternative method is to grasp a suture at the tip of the feeding tube or the distal tip of the tube itself and pass the tube into the duodenum using forceps advanced through the biopsy channel of the endoscope. This obviates the need to pass the gastroscope into the duodenum, which may result in dislodgment of the tube when the endoscope is withdrawn [20,27,31].

Fluoroscopic Technique. Percutaneous gastrostomy can also be performed using fluoroscopy [32]. The stomach is insufflated with air using a nasogastric tube or a skinny needle if the patient is obstructed proximally. Once the stomach is distended and position is checked again with fluoroscopy, the stomach is punctured with an 18-gauge needle. A heavy-duty wire is passed and the tract is dilated to 7 Fr. A gastrostomy tube may then be inserted into the stomach. An angiographic catheter is introduced and manipulated through the pylorus. The percutaneous tract is then further dilated and the gastrojejunostomy tube is advanced as far as possible.

Complications. The most common complication following percutaneous placement of enteral feeding tubes is infection, usually involving the cutaneous exit site and surrounding tissue. Gastrointestinal hemorrhage has been reported but is usually due to excessive tension on the tube, leading to necrosis of the stomach wall. Gastrocolic fistulas, which develop if the colon is interposed between the anterior abdominal wall and stomach when the needle is introduced, have been reported [33]. Adequate transillumination aids in avoiding this complication. Separation of the stomach from the anterior abdominal wall can occur, resulting in peritonitis when enteral feeding is initiated. In most instances, this complication is caused by excessive tension on the gastrostomy tube. Another potential complication is pneumoperitoneum, secondary to air escaping following puncture of the stomach during the procedure [20,34]. This is usually clinically insignificant. If the patient develops fevers and abdominal tenderness, a Gastrografin study should be obtained to exclude the presence of a leak.

All of the percutaneous gastrostomy and jejunostomy procedures described above have been established as safe and effective. The method is selected based on the endoscopist's experience and training and the patient's nutritional needs.

SURGICAL PROCEDURES. Since the advent of PEG, surgical placement of enteral feeding tubes is usually performed as a concomitant procedure as the last phase of a laparotomy performed for another indication. Occasionally an operation solely for tube placement is performed in patients requiring permanent tube feedings when a percutaneous approach is contraindicated or unsuccessful.

Gastrostomy. This is a simple procedure when performed as part of another intraabdominal operation. It should be considered when prolonged enteral nutritional support is anticipated after surgery.

Complications are quite common after surgical gastrostomy. This may reflect the poor nutritional status and associated medical problems in many of the patients who undergo this procedure [35]. Potential complications include wound infection, dehiscence, gastrostomy disruption, internal or external leakage, gastric hemorrhage, and tube migration.

Needle-Catheter Jejunostomy. This procedure consists of the insertion of a small (5 Fr.) polyethylene catheter into the small intestine at the time of laparotomy for another indication [36]. Kits containing the necessary equipment for the procedure are available from commercial suppliers (e.g., Vivonex). A needle is used to create a submucosal tunnel from the serosa to the mucosa on the antimesenteric border of the jejunum. A catheter is inserted through the needle and then the needle is removed. The catheter is brought out through the anterior abdominal wall and the limb of jejunum is secured to the anterior abdominal

wall with sutures. The tube can be used for feeding immediately after the operation [37]. The potential complications are similar to those associated with gastrostomy, but patients may have a higher incidence of diarrhea. Occlusion of the needle-catheter jejunostomy is common due to its small luminal diameter, and elemental nutritional formulas are preferentially used.

Transgastric Jejunostomy. Critically ill patients who undergo laparotomy commonly require gastric decompression and a surgically placed tube for enteral nutritional support. Routine placement of separate gastrostomy and jejunostomy tubes is very common in this patient population and achieves the objective of chronic gastric decompression and early initiation of enteral nutritional support through the jejunostomy. Technical advances in surgically placed enteral feeding tubes led to the development of transgastric jejunostomy and duodenostomy tubes, which allow simultaneous decompression of the stomach and distal feeding into the duodenum or jejunum. The advantage of these tubes is that only one enterotomy into the stomach is needed, eliminating the possible complications associated with open jejunostomy tube placement. In addition, only one tube is necessary for gastric decompression and jejunal feeding, eliminating the potential complications of two separate tubes for this purpose. The transgastric jejunostomy tube is placed surgically in the same manner as a gastrostomy tube, and the distal portion of the tube is advanced manually through the pylorus, into the duodenum, with its final tip resting as far distally as possible in the duodenum or jejunum (Fig. 22-3). The transgastric jejunostomy tube is preferred to transgastric duodenostomy tubes because it is associated with less reflux of feedings into the stomach and a decreased risk of aspiration pneumonia. Surgical placement of transgastric jejunostomy tubes at the time of laparotomy is recommended for patients who will likely require prolonged gastric decompression and enteral feeding.

Delivering the Tube Feeding Formula

The enteral formula can be delivered by intermittent bolus feeding, gravity infusion, or continuous pump infusion.

Fig. 22-3. Transgastric duodenal feeding tube, which allows simultaneous gastric decompression and duodenal feeding, can be placed percutaneously (with endoscopic or fluoroscopic assistance) or surgically.

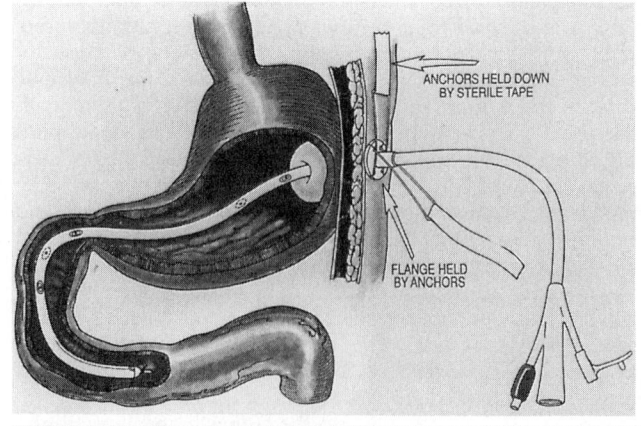

In the intermittent bolus method, the patient receives 300 to 400 ml of formula every 4 to 6 hours. The bolus is usually delivered with the aid of a catheter-tipped, large-volume (60-ml) syringe. The main advantage of bolus feeding is simplicity. This approach is often used for patients requiring prolonged supplemental enteral nutritional support after discharge from the hospital. Unfortunately, bolus feeding can be associated with serious side effects. Bolus enteral feeding into the stomach can cause gastric distention, nausea, cramping, and aspiration. The intermittent bolus method should not be used when feeding into the duodenum or jejunum, since boluses of formula can cause distention, cramping, and diarrhea.

Gravity infusion systems allow the formula to drip continuously over 16 to 24 hours or intermittently over 20 to 30 minutes four to six times per day. This method requires constant monitoring, as the flow rate can be extremely irregular. The main advantages of this approach are simplicity, low cost, and close simulation of a normal feeding pattern [38].

Continuous pump infusion is the preferred method for the delivery of enteral nutrition in the critically ill patient. A peristaltic pump can be used to provide a continuous infusion of formula at a precisely controlled flow rate. This decreases problems with distention and diarrhea. Gastric residuals tend to be smaller with continuous pump-fed infusions and the risk of aspiration may be decreased [39,40]. In adult burn patients, continuous feedings are associated with less stool frequency and shorter time to achieve nutritional goals [41].

Medications

When medications are administered via an enteric feeding tube, it is important to be certain the drugs are compatible with each other and with the enteral formula. In general, medications should be delivered separately, rather than as a combined bolus. For medications that are better absorbed in an empty stomach, tube feedings should be suspended for 30 to 60 minutes prior to administration [42].

Medications should be administered in an elixir formulation via enteral feeding tubes whenever possible to prevent occlusion of the tube. Enteral tubes should always be flushed with 20 ml of saline after medications are administered. To use an enteral feeding tube to administer medications dispensed in tablet form, often the pills must be crushed and delivered as a slurry mixed with water. This is inappropriate for some medications, however, such as those absorbed sublingually or formulated as a sustained-released tablet or capsule.

Complications

Enteral tube placement is associated with few complications, if physicians adhere to appropriate protocols and pay close attention to the details of the procedures.

NASOPULMONARY INTUBATION. Passage of an enteral feeding tube into the tracheobronchial tree most commonly occurs in patients with diminished cough or gag reflexes due to obtundation, altered mental status, or other causes. The presence of a tracheostomy or endotracheal tube does not guarantee proper placement. A chest (or upper abdominal) radiograph should always be obtained prior to initiating tube feedings with a new tube, to ensure that the tube is properly positioned. Endotracheal or transpulmonary placement of a feeding tube can be associated with pneumothorax, hydrothorax, pneumonia, and abscess formation [43–46].

ASPIRATION. Pulmonary aspiration is a serious and potentially fatal complication of enteral nutritional support [47–50]. The incidence of this complication is variable and depends on the patient population studied.

Major risk factors for aspiration include obtundation or altered mental status, absence of cough or gag reflexes, delayed gastric emptying, gastroesophageal reflux, and feeding in the supine position. The risk of pulmonary aspiration is minimized when the enteral feeding tube is positioned in the jejunum past the ligament of Treitz.

GASTROINTESTINAL INTOLERANCE. Delayed gastric emptying is sometimes improved by administering the prokinetic agent metoclopramide (10–20 mg IV) [51]. Dumping syndrome (diarrhea, distention, and abdominal cramping) can limit the use of enteral feeding. Dumping may be caused by delivering a hyperosmotic load into the small intestine.

Diarrhea in critically ill patients should not be attributed to intolerance of enteral feeding until other causes are excluded. Other possible etiologies for diarrhea include medications (e.g., magnesium-containing antacids, quinidine), alterations in gut microflora due to prolonged antibiotic therapy, antibiotic-associated colitis, ischemic colitis, viral or bacterial enteric infection, electrolyte abnormalities, and excessive delivery of bile salts into the colon. Diarrhea can also be a manifestation of intestinal malabsorption due to enzyme deficiencies or villous atrophy [52,53,54].

Even if diarrhea is due to enteral feeding, it can be controlled in nearly 50 percent of cases by instituting a continuous infusion of formula (if bolus feedings are used), slowing the rate of infusion, changing the formula, adding fiber to the enteral formula, or adding antidiarrheal agents (e.g., deodorized tincture of opium) [55].

METABOLIC COMPLICATIONS. Prerenal azotemia and hypernatremia can develop in patients fed with hyperosmolar solutions [52,56–59]. The administration of free water, either added to the formula or as separate boluses, to replace obligatory losses can avert this situation. Deficiencies of essential fatty acids and fat-soluble vitamins can develop after prolonged support with enteral solutions that contain minimal amounts of fat. Periodic enteral supplementation with linoleic acid or intravenous supplementation with emulsified fat (Intralipid) can prevent this [60]. The amount of linoleic acid necessary to prevent chemical and clinical fatty acid deficiency has been estimated to be 2.5 to 20 gm per day [61].

BACTERIAL CONTAMINATION. Bacterial contamination with enteral solutions [62,63] occurs when commercial packages are opened and mixed with other substances [64]. The risk of contamination depends on the duration of feeding [65,66]. Tube feeding formulas have been implicated in causing *Pseudomonas* and *Enterobacter* sepsis [67,68]. The presence of gram-negative bacilli in enteral formulas has been associated with abdominal distention, presumably secondary to an ileus [69].

OCCLUDED FEEDING TUBES. Precipitation of certain proteins when exposed to an acid pH may be an important factor leading to the solidifying of formulas [70]. Most premixed intact protein formulas solidify when acidified to a pH less than 5. To prevent occlusion of feeding tubes, the tube should be flushed with saline before and after checking residuals. Small-caliber nasoenteric feeding tubes should be flushed with 20 ml of saline every 4 to 6 hours to prevent tube occlusion, even when enteral feedings are administered by continuous infusion.

Medications are a frequent cause of clogging. When administering medications enterally, liquid elixirs should be used if available, since even tiny particles of crushed tablets can occlude the distal orifice of small-caliber feeding tubes. If tablets are used, it is important to crush them to a fine powder and solubilize in liquid prior to administration. In addition, tubes should be flushed with saline before and after the administration of any medications.

Several maneuvers are useful for clearing a clogged feeding tube. The tube can be irrigated with warm saline, a carbonated liquid, cranberry juice, or an enzyme solution (e.g., Viokase). Commonly, a mixture of lipase, amylase, and protease (Pancrease) dissolved in sodium bicarbonate solution is instilled into the tube with a syringe and the tube clamped for approximately 30 minutes to allow enzymatic degradation of precipitated enteral feedings. The tube is then vigorously flushed with saline. A catheter can be inserted into the enteral tube through the area of occlusion [70]. The catheter itself may break up the precipitate; warm saline with or without an enzyme preparation may facilitate this process.

References

1. Apelgren KN, Rombeau JL: Comparison of nutritional indices and outcome in critically ill patients. *Crit Care Med* 10:305, 1982.
2. McCarthy MC: Nutritional support in the critically ill surgical patient. *Surg Clin North Am* 71:831, 1991.
3. Warnold I, Lundholm K: Clinical significance of preoperative nutritional status in 215 non-cancer patients. *Ann Surg* 199:299, 1984.
4. Mullen JL, Buzby GP, Matthews DC, et al: Reduction of operative morbidity and mortality by combined preoperative and postoperative nutritional support. *Ann Surg* 192:604, 1980.
5. Blackburn GL: Hyperalimentation in the critically ill patient. *Heart Lung* 8:67, 1979.
6. Koruda MJ, Guenter P, Rombeau JL: Enteral nutrition in the critically ill. *Crit Care Clin* 3:133, 1987.
7. Saito H, Trocki O, Alexander JW, et al: The effect of nutrient administration on nutritional state, catabolic hormone secretion, and gut mucosal integrity after burn injury. *J Parenter Enter Nutr* 11:1, 1987.
8. Levine GM, Deren JJ, Steiger E, et al: Role of oral intake in maintenance of gut mass and disaccharidase activity. *Gastroenterology* 67:975, 1974.
9. Raul F, Noriegar R, Duffeol M, et al: Modifications of brush border enzyme activities during starvation in the jejunum and ileum of adult rats. *Enzyme* 28:328, 1982.
10. Napolitano LM, Baker CC: Bacterial translocation: Fact or fancy. *Adv Trauma Crit Care*, 7:79, 1992.
11. Daly JM, Lieberman MD, Goldfine J, et al: Enteral nutrition with supplemental arginine, RNA, and omega-3 fatty acids in patients after operation: Immunologic, metabolic, and clinical outcome. *Surgery* 112:56, 1992.
12. Moore FA, Feliciano DV, Andrassy RJ, et al: Early enteral feeding, compared with parenteral, reduces postoperative septic complications: The results of a meta-analysis. *Ann Surg* 216:172, 1992.
13. Hemysfield SB, Bethel RA, Ansley JD, et al: Enteral hyperalimentation: An alternative to central venous hyperalimentation. *Ann Intern Med* 90:6371, 1979.
14. Bury KD: Elemental diets, in Ficher JE (ed): *Total Parenteral Nutrition*. Boston, Little, Brown, 1976, p 395.
15. Shils ME, Randall HT: Diet and nutrition in the care of the surgical patient, in Goodhart RS, Shils ME (eds): *Modern Nutrition in Health and Disease*. 6th ed. Philadelphia, Lea & Febiger, 1980, p 1082.
16. Strong R, Condon S, Solinger M, et al: Equal aspiration rates from postpylorus and intragastric-placed small-bore nasoenteric feeding tubes: A randomized, prospective study. *J Parenter Enter Nutr* 16:59, 1992.
17. Dunn EL, Moore EE, Bohus RW: Immediate postoperative feeding following massive abdominal trauma: The catheter jejunostomy. *J Parenter Enter Nutr* 4:393, 1989.
18. Hoover HC Jr, Ryan JA, Anderson EJ, et al: Nutritional benefits of immediate postoperative jejunal feeding of an elemental diet. *Am J Surg* 139:153, 1980.
19. Smith RC, Hartemink RJ, Holinshead JW, et al: Fine bore jejunostomy feeding following major abdominal surgery: A controlled randomized clinical trial. *Br J Surg* 72:458, 1985.
20. Ponsky JL: Evolving trends in enteral alimentation. *Ann Surg* 18:327, 1986.
21. Gauderer MWL, Stellato TA: Gastrostomies: Evolution techniques, indications and complications. *Curr Probl Surg* 23:657, 1986.
22. Chernoff R: *Directory of Penn Products and Services*. Silver Spring, MD, American Society for Parenteral and Enteral Nutrition, 1985.
23. Rombeau JL, Twomey PL, McLean GK, et al: Experience with a new gastrostomy: Jejunal feeding tube. *Surgery* 93:574, 1983.
24. Lord LM, Weiser-Maimone A, Pulhamus M, et al: Comparison of weighted vs unweighted enteral feeding tubes for efficacy of transpyloric intubation. *J Parenter Enter Nutr* 17:271, 1993.
25. Larson DE, Fleming CR, Ott BJ, et al: Percutaneous endoscopic gastrostomy: Simplified access for enteral nutrition. *Mayo Clin Proc* 58:103, 1983.
26. Ponsky JL, Gauderer MWL, Stellato TA, et al: Percutaneous approaches to enteral alimentation. *Am J Surg* 149:102, 1985.
27. Kozarek RA, Ball TJ, Ryan JA: When push comes to shove: A comparison between two methods of percutaneous endoscopic gastrostomy. *Am J Gastroenterol* 81:642, 1986.
28. Russell TR, Brotman M, Norris F: Percutaneous gastrostomy: A new simplified and cost effective technique. *Am J Surg* 148:132, 1984.
29. Miller RE, Kummer BA, Tiszenkel HI, et al: Percutaneous endoscopic gastrostomy: Procedure of choice. *Ann Surg* 204:543, 1986.
30. Duckworth PF Jr, Kirby DF, McHenry L: Percutaneous endoscopic gastrojejunostomy made easy: A simplified endoscopic technique. *Gastrointest Endosc* 37:241, 1991.
31. Gottfried EB, Plumser AB: Endoscopic gastrojejunostomy: A technique to establish small bowel feeding without laparotomy. *Gastrointest Endosc* 30:355, 1984.
32. Gray RR, St. Louis EL, Grosman H: Modified catheter for percutaneous gastrojejunostomy. *Radiology* 173:275, 1989.
33. Nghiem CH, Bui HD, Dang CV, et al: A new complication of percutaneous endoscopic gastrostomy. *Am J Gastroenterol* 83:448, 1988.
34. Gottfried EB, Plumser, AB, Clair MR: Pneumoperitoneum following percutaneous endoscopic gastrostomy: A prospective study. *Gastrointest Endosc* 32:397, 1986.
35. Strodel WE, Ponsky JL: Complications of percutaneous gastrostomy, in Ponsky JL (ed): *Techniques of Percutaneous Gastrostomy*. New York, Igaku-Shoin, 1988.
36. Sagar S, Harland P, Shields R: Early postoperative feeding with elemental diet. *Br Med J* 1:293, 1979.
37. Dunn EL, Moore EE, Bohus RW: Immediate postoperative feeding following massive abdominal trauma: The catheter jejunostomy. *J Parenter Enter Nutr* 4:393, 1980.
38. Hansen BC: Feeding methods and gastointestinal function, in Rombeau JL, Caldwell MD (eds): *Clinical Nutrition: Enteral and Tube Feeding*. vol. 1. Philadelphia, WB Saunders, 1985.
39. Askanazi J, Elwyn DH, Silverberg PA, et al: Respiratory distress secondary to a high carbohydrate load: A case report. *Surgery* 87:596, 1980.
40. Orr G, Wade J, Bothe A, et al: Alternatives to total parenteral nutrition in the criticaly ill patient. *Crit Care Med* 8:29, 1980.
41. Hiebert J, Brown A, Anderson R, et al: Comparison of continuous vs intermittent tube feedings in adult burn patients. *J Parenter Enter Nutr* 5:73, 1981.
42. Visconti JA, Gora ML, Tschampel MM: Considerations of drug therapy in patients receiving enteral nutrition. *Nutr Clin Pract* 4:105, 1989.
43. Woodall BH, Winfield DF, Bisset GS III: Inadvertent tracheobronchial placement of feeding tubes. *Radiology* 165:727, 1987.
44. Lipman TO, Kessler T, Arabian A: Nasopulmonary intubation with

feeding tubes: Case reports and a review of the literature. *J Parenter Enter Nutr* 9:618, 1985.

45. Scholten DJ, Wood TL, Thompson DR: Pneumothorax from nasoenteric feeding tube insertion. *Am Surg* 52:381, 1985.
46. Toews A, DeLaRocha, AG: Oropharyngeal sepsis with endothoracic spread. *Can J Surg* 23:265, 1980.
47. Cataldi-Betcher EL, Seltzer MH, Slocum BA, et al: Complications occurring during enteral nutritional support: A prospective study. *J Parenter Enter Nutr* 7:546, 1983.
48. Olivares L, Segovia A, Revuelta R: Tube feeding and lethal aspiration in neurological patients: A review of 720 autopsy cases. *Stroke* 5:654, 1974.
49. Winterbauer RH, Durning RB, Barron E, et al: Aspirated nasogastric feeding solution detected by glucose strips. *Ann Intern Med* 95:67, 1981.
50. Metheny NA, Eisenberg D, Spies M: Aspiration pneumonia in patients fed through nasoenteral tubes. *Heart Lung* 15:256, 1986.
51. McCallum RW, Albibi R: Metoclopramide: Pharmacology and clinical application. *Ann Intern Med* 98:86, 1983.
52. Silk DBA: *Nutritional Support in Hospital Practice*. Oxford, UK, Blackwell, 1983.
53. Heymsfield SB, Erbland M, Casper K, et al: Enteral nutritional support: Metabolic, cardiovascular, and pulmonary interrelations. *Clin Chest Med* 7:41, 1986.
54. Zagoren AJ, Water DW, Beck S, et al: Colloid osmotic pressure: Sensitive predictor of enteral feeding intolerance. *J Am Coll Nutr* 3:260, 1964.
55. Niemiec PN, Vanderveen TW, Morrison JT, et al: Gastrointestinal disorders caused by medication and electrolytes solution osmolarity during enteral nutrition. *J Parenter Enter Nutr* 7:387, 1983.
56. Kaminski MV: Enteral hyperalimentation. *Surg Gynecol Obstet* 143:12, 1976.
57. Bernard M, Forlaw L: Complications and their prevention, in Rombeau JL, Caldwell MD (eds): *Clinical Nutrition: Enteral and Tube Feeding*. vol. 1. Philadelphia, WB Saunders, 1984.
58. Gault MH, Dixon ME, Doyle M, et al: Hypernatremia, azotemia, and dehydration due to high protein tube feeding. *Ann Intern Med* 68:778, 1968.
59. Telfer N: The effect of tube feeding on the hydration of elderly patients. *J Gerontol* 20:536, 1965.
60. Dodge JA, Yassa JG: Essential fatty acids deficiency after prolonged treatment with elemental diet. *Lancet* 2:192, 1975.
61. Holman RT: Function and biologic activities of essential fatty acids in man, in Meng HC, Wilmore DW (eds): *Fat Emulsions in Parenteral Nutrition*. Chicago, American Medical Association, 1976, p 5.
62. Flynn NM, Freeland CP, Roller RD, et al: Microbial contamination of continuous drip feedings. *J Parenter Enter Nutr* 13:18, 1989.
63. Schreiner R, Eitzen H, Gfell M, et al: Environmental contamination of continuous drip feedings. *Pediatrics* 63:232, 1979.
64. Anderson KR, Norris DJ, Godfrey LB, et al: Bacterial contamination of tube feeding formulas. *J Parenter Enter Nutr* 8:673, 1984.
65. Paauw JD, Fagerman KE, McCamish MA, et al: Enteral nutrient solutions: Limiting bacterial growth. *Am Surg* 50:312, 1984.
66. Anderson A: Growth of bacteria in enteral feeding solutions. *J Med Microbiol* 20:63, 1985.
67. Casewell M, Cooper J, Webster M: Enteral feeds contamination with *Enterobacter cloacae* as a cause of septicema. *Br Med J* 282:973, 1981.
68. Devries E, Mulder N, Houwen B, et al: Enteral nutrition by nasogastric tube in adult patients treated with intensive chemotherapy for acute leukemia. *Am J Clin Nutr* 35:1490, 1982.
69. Perkins AM, Marcuard SP: Clogging of feeding tubes. *J Parenter Enter Nutr* 12:403, 1988.
70. Boysen D, Heinzelmann MJ, Bommarito AA: A new approach to the management of obstructed enteral feeding tubes. *Clin Pract* 4:111, 1989.

23. Therapeutic Hemapheresis

Irma O. Szymanski

The art of blood letting was rediscovered during the twentieth century after Abel et al., in 1914, demonstrated in a dog model that a large amount of a single blood component, plasma, could be removed safely [1]. They called this procedure *plasmapheresis*, from the Greek word *aphaeresis*, meaning "removal." The clinical usefulness of this approach became apparent in the 1960s, when it was demonstrated that the hyperviscosity syndrome of Waldenström's macroglobulinemia could be treated effectively with manual plasmapheresis [2]. Currently, hemapheresis (removal of a blood component) is useful in the treatment of many diseases. Modern techniques are available for harvesting platelets (plateletpheresis, thrombocytapheresis), white cells (leukapheresis, leukocytapheresis), red cells (erythrocytapheresis), and plasma (plasmapheresis, plasma exchange). This chapter focuses on the technical aspects, effectiveness, adverse effects, and indications for therapeutic hemapheresis.

Techniques

Hemapheresis involves separation of whole blood into blood components, removal of a selective component, and reinfusion of the remaining blood. Blood components of different specific gravities are usually separated by centrifugation, but plasma can also be separated from whole blood by filtration. The latter method is not used commonly in the United States, although they are popular in Western Europe and Japan [3]. The centrifugal separation of blood components can be done using manual or automated methods.

MANUAL HEMAPHERESIS. Manual hemapheresis requires a minimum of technology. Four hundred fifty milliliters of the patient's whole blood is collected into a bag, which is disconnected from the patient for centrifugation and harvesting of the desired component. This is a time-consuming process and only rarely used. Physical separation of the bag of blood from the patient is potentially dangerous, as any error in identification of patient or component could lead to hemolytic transfusion reaction.

AUTOMATED HEMAPHERESIS

Discontinuous Flow. Haemonetics (Braintree, MA) pioneered hemapheresis technology, in which aliquots (about 500 ml) of whole blood are collected and separated into blood components using a sterile, disposable collection apparatus that remains connected to the patient throughout the procedure. Whole blood drawn from the patient is anticoagulated with acid-citrate-dextrose (ACD) in an ACD-to-whole blood ratio of approximately 1:8 and flows at a rate of up to 60 ml per minute into a spinning centrifuge bowl. As the bowl fills, blood components settle into different layers on the basis of specific gravity. An exit port at the top of the bowl is connected by integrally attached tubing to collection bags. When the bowl is filled, plasma, the lightest component, exits first, followed by platelets and white cells. When plasma exchange is performed, the collection cycle may be terminated any time before the platelet layer emerges from the bowl. In platelet collection, the platelet layer together with some plasma is diverted into a collection bag. In leukapheresis, white cells, which are located just under the platelet band, may be harvested together with some red cells. After removing the desired component, red cells and the remaining components are pumped into a transfusion bag and reinfused to the patient. Erythrocytapheresis differs slightly in that the patient's red cells are discarded, and plasma and platelets are returned together with donor red cells. In any of these apheresis methods, the reconstituted blood can be infused to the same vein from which it was collected (single-needle procedure) or to the vein in the opposite arm (dual-needle procedure). If two needles are used, blood collection and reinfusion can be simultaneous. To collect enough of the desired component, several aliquots of blood must be processed. Replacement fluid must also be administered if more than 10 percent of blood volume is removed.

The extracorporeal blood volume (EV) varies during the collection and return cycle in the one-needle procedure and is greatest at the end of the collection cycle. If two needles are used, EV remains relatively constant after completion of the first collection cycle. Extracorporeal blood volume should never exceed 15 percent of the patient's total blood volume. The EV is calculated as follows. At the end of a collection cycle for plateletpheresis the bowl is full of a red cell-plasma mixture with a hematocrit (Hct) of approximately 80 percent. Hence EV is calculated by the formula:

$$EV = (BV \times 0.8)/Hct$$

where BV is the bowl volume. Bowls with 375-, 225-, and 125-ml volumes are available to control EV in different-sized individuals. Although the Haemonetics Blood Processor is still used, procedures employing continuous flow are now generally preferred.

Continuous Flow. Hemapheresis can be done in continuous fashion using blood processors manufactured by Baxter Healthcare (Deerfield, IL) and Cobe BCT (Lakewood, CO). Of the two systems, the Cobe Spectra is ideal for therapeutic hemapheresis. It uses a separation channel that, when inserted into the Cobe centrifuge, resembles a hollow belt, with a volume of about 180 ml. As the belt turns in the centrifuge, anticoagulated whole blood flows into one end. During the centrifugal journey the blood components settle into layers, according to specific gravity. Red cells, being the most dense, sediment next to the outer wall of the belt, with white cells, platelets, and plasma forming the other successive layers toward the center. As the layers are established, the components are harvested through segments of tubing that join the belt at right angles to the inner wall, resembling the spokes of a wheel. The segments of tubing extend into the hollow belt to depths appropriate for harvesting the desired components. Sets of different designs are used to collect plasma, white cells, platelets, and red cells. Each procedure is automated and individualized according to the pa-

tient's size, blood and plasma volume, quantity of the blood component to be removed, and type of replacement fluid used. Because the extracorporeal volume is small, this machine allows for hemapheresis to be done safely in children and small adults and is generally preferred for less stable intensive care unit (ICU) patients. The procedure can also be performed more quickly with this machine than with any other blood processor.

REMOVAL OF A SPECIFIC PLASMA CONSTITUENT. Removal of only the pathologic plasma constituent, rather than whole plasma, would be the most efficient way of performing therapeutic plasma exchange. Devices to be incorporated into plasmapheresis sets are available for removal of circulating immune complexes, immunoglobulins, or low-density lipoprotein (LDL). In this type of plasmapheresis it is not necessary to administer replacement fluids.

The Prosorba column (Imre, Seattle, WA), designed to remove circulating immune complexes and IgG from plasma, has been approved by the Food and Drug Administration (FDA) for treatment of certain immune disorders (e.g., intractable idiopathic thrombocytopenic purpura and HIV-ITP) [4]. Each column has 200 mg of purified staphylococcal protein A covalently coupled to an inert silica matrix. Protein A has a high avidity for the Fc portion of IgG, particularly when it is immune-complexed. It is believed that circulating immune complexes suppress the development of anti-idiotypes, which blunt the formation of harmful autoantibodies. Data show that after Prosorba treatment, titers of autoantibody (idiotype) decreased and those of anti-idiotype increased in patient's plasma [4]. Therefore, this treatment is thought to modulate and normalize the immune response.

Excorim (Lund, Sweden) has manufactured a device that removes large amounts of circulating immune complexes and IgG from plasma. It consists of a set of two small columns that can be regenerated after use. While the patient's plasma is passed through one column to absorb immunoglobulins, the other is regenerated with special elution procedure. The two-column sets have not yet been licensed in the United States.

Low-molecular-weight dextran sulfate, covalently bound to cellulose, may be used to remove LDL from the plasma of patients with familial hypercholesterolemia. Low-density lipoprotein can also be removed by columns containing anti-LDL or modified macroporous cellulose [5].

VASCULAR ACCESS. Good vascular access is essential for hemapheresis. At least one good antecubital vein is required to draw whole blood from the patient; the processed blood can be returned to a smaller vein through an indwelling catheter. Hemapheresis cannot be reliably performed via a peripheral vein unless at least a 17-gauge cannula can be inserted; if this is impossible, a femoral or subclavian catheter must be used. The selection of an appropriate catheter is important to permit rapid, continuous blood flow, as thin, pliable catheters tend to collapse during blood withdrawal. In my experience, Acu Flex-FSN (Cobe, Lakewood, CO), a 5.5-inch double-lumen catheter, is excellent for femoral vein blood access, whereas I have had good experience with the Mahurkar dual-lumen catheter (11.5 Fr., 13.5 cm in length; Quinton, Seattle, WA) inserted into the subclavian vein. Femoral catheters can be left in place for 3 to 4 days and subclavian catheters for 2 to 3 weeks. Infusion of donor plasma, which contains citrate, via the subclavian catheter may cause cardiac arrhythmias due to the calcium-lowering effects of citrate.

Effectiveness of Therapeutic Hemapheresis

Degree of dilution of blood cells or plasma constituents in the patient's blood immediately after hemapheresis depends on the distribution of the component between extra- and intravascular space and the percentage of component removed. Assuming that plasma analytes do not equilibrate between intra- and extravascular spaces during the procedure, the expected concentration immediately after plasma exchange can be estimated on the basis of percentage of plasma volume removed (Table 23-1). Unfortunately, the effectiveness of the removal decreases as more plasma is harvested, because the patient's plasma becomes increasingly diluted during the procedure. Subsequently, the concentration of the specific component depends on the rate of production. To maintain a low or normal concentration of blood cells or plasma constituents, a course of hemapheresis to supplement other therapy is usually prescribed. Recommended schedules for treating a number of diseases exist but are individualized, if possible, according to the patient's response. The efficacy of hemapheresis in treating various diseases may be demonstrated by means of randomized, controlled clinical trials or by showing that the pathogenesis of the disease or its manifestations involves a blood component or plasma constituent that can be removed during the procedure and that removal is associated with improvement in the patient's condition [6]. Unfortunately, reduction in the concentration of a pathogenic protein is not always associated with clinical improvement. This could have many explanations; for example, the damage done by an antibody could have been irreversible, or the avidity of an antibody to its target tissue may be high even when plasma concentration is low.

The level of normal plasma constituents also decreases following plasma exchange, each being diluted to a different degree. A study involving 10 patients who had a total of 30 plasma exchange procedures with 5 percent albumin as replacement fluid revealed that IgG, IgM, cholesterol, alkaline phosphatase, and SGPT were removed as expected, but the concentrations of glucose and HCO_3 did not change [7]. The concentrations of fibrinogen and C3 decreased more than expected, suggesting consumption of these proteins during the procedure. Uric acid, calcium, potassium, SGOT, LDH, amylase, and CPK decreased less than expected, suggesting that they equilibrated rapidly between intra- and extravascular spaces. Most plasma constituents returned to baseline levels within 24 to 72 hours, but normalization of fibrinogen, C3, cholesterol, IgG, and IgM concentrations required 1 to 2 weeks [7]. Normalization of plasma constituents in critically ill patients after plasma exchange using albumin as replacement fluid has not been studied but could require a longer time because of decreased protein synthesis. As a rule, I do not order any laboratory assays immediately after the procedure because the results can be misleading unless analytes that equilibrate quickly between intra- and extravas-

cular spaces are tested. Usually I obtain Ig levels before each procedure (unless fresh frozen plasma is used as a replacement fluid) and infuse Ig if the level decreases to less than 200 mg per deciliter.

Adverse Effects

HYPOTENSIVE EPISODES. Patients undergoing hemapheresis may experience vasovagal reactions or hypotensive episodes due to procedure-induced fluctuations in the blood volume. Hypotensive episodes respond readily to crystalloids or colloid infusion.

DONOR PLASMA-INDUCED REACTIONS. Infusion of cold plasma can cause chills, and allergic or anaphylactic reactions may occur in a sensitized patient. To prevent allergic reactions, I usually premedicate patients with diphenhydramine hydrochloride (Benadryl) about 30 minutes before giving plasma. Anaphylactic reactions are rare, occurring in IgA-deficient patients who have formed anti-IgA antibodies. These reactions must be treated with epinephrine and intravenous fluids.

The citrate in donor plasma may lower ionized calcium levels, causing cardiac arrhythmias, particularly when plasma is infused through the subclavian catheter to the superior vena cava [8].

EFFECTS DUE TO DECREASE OF PLASMA ANALYTES. The concentration of antithrombin III decreases in patients whose plasma is replaced with albumin, and thrombotic phenomena have been suspected to occur in such patients [9]. Similarly, plasma cholinesterase, necessary for degradation of suxamethonium anesthetic, is reduced by extensive plasma removal [10]. To avoid prolonged apnea after suxamethonium anesthesia, it is prudent to allow at least 72 hours between plasma exchange and anesthesia. As a less desirable alternative, fresh frozen plasma infusions may be given.

REBOUND PHENOMENON. Decrease in the concentration of specific antibodies by plasma removal is thought to cause a rebound phenomenon in antibody synthesis [11]. Orlin & Berkman showed, that although the concentration of immunoglobulins was 40 percent of the initial value on the tenth day after plasmapheresis, anti-A at that time had 100 percent agglutinating activity, indicating either enhanced synthesis of these antibodies or production of antibodies with high avidity [7].

ADVERSE REACTIONS DUE TO MEDICATIONS. Removal of large volumes of plasma may lower the concentration of medications. It may be advisable to administer medications after the procedure has been completed.

Therapeutic hemapheresis is not recommended in patients who are receiving intravenous heparin, because removal of large amounts of heparin might compromise the anticoagulant therapy.

Patients on ACE inhibitors may have life-threatening anaphylactoid reactions when undergoing hemodialysis, LDL removal from plasma using dextran sulfate columns, or treatment of plasma with Prosorba columns [12,13,14]. Seven fatalities have been reported, thought to be caused by generation of bradykinin, induced by certain membranes, accompanied by a de-

Table 23-1. Expected Removal of Plasma Constituents*

% Plasma volume removed	% Plasma constituent removed
50	40
100	65
150	80
200	88

* As a function of the amount of diluted and undiluted plasma volume removed.

crease in the availability of kininase II, identical to angiotensin I-converting enzyme, which normally contributes to the inactivation of bradykinin. In this setting, bradykinin may reach toxic levels and the patient may experience severe flushing, dyspnea, hypotension, and bradycardia. In such cases the procedure must be discontinued immediately and the patient treated with intravenous fluids and epinephrine.

ADVERSE REACTIONS DUE TO PROSORBA COLUMN. Passage of plasma through the Prosorba column initiates complement activation. A variety of flulike symptoms, including chills, fever, muscle and joint pain, nausea, respiratory difficulties, and hypo- or hypertension, have been noted in about 35 percent of procedures performed [4]. Since the usual course of therapy consists of several procedures, about 70 percent of patients experienced some of these symptoms. To reduce complications, I medicate the patient with Tylenol and Benadryl before giving the treated plasma. It has also been reported that patients on small doses of prednisone during treatment have a lower incidence of adverse reactions [4].

ADVERSE EFFECTS DUE TO CATHETERS. When catheters are used, they may become clotted or infected, requiring removal to avoid systemic complications. Apheresis via central venous catheters, particularly, requires strict adherence to protocols to maintain patency and sterility.

Indications

Therapeutic hemapheresis is employed to remove excessive or abnormally functioning cells (cytapheresis) and plasma or its constituents (plasma exchange). Because it is relatively expensive, invasive, and time-consuming, it should be used discriminately in conditions for which it has been shown clearly to be beneficial. Indications for therapeutic cytapheresis are listed in Table 23-2 [15]. These procedures should be repeated only as necessary to reach or maintain the target cell value. Diseases in which plasma exchange is considered standard, primary therapy or supplemental but possibly effective therapy are shown in Table 23-3. Note that data have shown plasma exchange not be effective in treating chronic ITP, lupus nephritis, polymyositis/dermatomyositis, or renal transplant rejection.

In severe, intractable systemic lupus erythematosus, pemphigus vulgaris, and hemolytic anemia, a combination of plasma exchange with pulse cyclophosphamide therapy has shown good results in several case reports [16,17,18]. The concept behind this approach is that lowering of plasma antibody levels by plasmapheresis induces, by a negative feedback mechanism, proliferation of B cells, thought at that stage to be vulnerable to chemotherapy.

Contraindications

Except for inappropriate indications, there are only relative contraindications for performance of therapeutic hemapheresis. Patients with severe cardiac failure or who are otherwise hemodynamically unstable might not tolerate the blood volume changes during the procedure. Patients receiving intravenous heparin therapy are not recommended for plasma exchange

Table 23-2. Indications for Therapeutic Cytapheresis

Procedure	Disease	Indications
Erythrocytapheresis	Sickle cell disease	Unrelenting crises, pregnancy, acute pulmonary syndromes, retinal artery occlusion, intrahepatic cholestasis, priapism
Leukapheresis	AML	To relieve leukostasis when blast count > 100,000/μl
	CML	To relieve leukostasis when WBC count > 200,000/μl
Plateletpheresis	Thrombocytosis	To prevent thrombosis or hemorrhage when platelet count > 1,000,000/μl

Table 23-3. Diseases in Which Plasma Exchange Therapy Is Effective

Standard, primary therapy
  Hyperviscosity syndrome
  Cryoglobulinemia
  Thrombotic thrombocytopenic purpura
  Hemolytic uremic syndrome
  Posttransfusion purpura
  Acute Guillain-Barré syndrome
  Chronic idiopathic demyelinating polyradiculopathy
  Myasthenia gravis
  Refsum's disease
  Goodpasture syndrome
  Familial hyperlipoproteinemia
Adjunctive therapy
  Cold agglutinin disease
  Circulating anticoagulants, refractory to other therapy
  HELLP syndrome, postpartum
  Renal failure with myeloma
  Systemic vasculitis due to systemic lupus erythematosus or RA
  Pemphigus vulgaris
  Poisonings and drug overdose (protein-bound)

Based in part on *Guidelines for Therapeutic Hemapheresis.* American Association of Blood Banks, May 1993.

due to adverse effects of heparin removal. Patients with thrombotic events should not undergo treatment with Prosorba columns because the complement activation can aggravate thrombotic tendencies. Patients on ACE inhibitors should not undergo treatment with Prosorba columns because of possible anaphylactoid reactions.

Therapeutic Plasma Exchange in the Intensive Care Unit

Some ICU patients may need therapeutic cytapheresis or plasma exchange. The recommended schedules and therapeutic endpoints for plasma exchange treatment in some situations are shown in Table 23-4.

Table 23-4. Treatment Schedules and Therapeutic Endpoints of Diseases Treated with Plasma Exchange in the Intensive Care Unit

Disease	Total amount of plasma removed	Replacement fluid	Therapeutic endpoints
Acute Guillain-Barré syndrome	200–250 ml/kg within 2 weeks	Albumin	Not applicable
Acute myasthenia gravis	150 ml/kg within 3 exchanges or until therapeutic endpoint	Albumin	Amelioration of symptoms
Thrombotic thrombocytopenic purpura	1.5 plasma volume removal daily for 3 days, then 1 plasma volume removal until therapeutic endpoint	Fresh frozen or cryo-poor plasma	Normal platelet count for 2–3 days, normal LDH
Severe autoimmune hemolytic anemia, (cold antibody)	1–1.5 plasma volume removal daily or every other day until therapeutic endpoint	Albumin	Decrease in hemolysis
Goodpasture syndrome	1 plasma volume daily or every other day until therapeutic endpoint	Albumin, IVIG supplementation when IgG < 200 mg/dl	Control of pulmonary hemorrhage, stabilization of renal disease

ACUTE GUILLAIN-BARRÉ SYNDROME. A controlled clinical trial comparing plasma exchange to standard therapy for Guillain-Barré syndrome appeared in 1985 [19]. This study of 245 patients found statistically significant differences favoring plasma exchange in the following recovery parameters: improvement at 4 weeks, time to improve one clinical grade, time to independent walking, and outcome at 6 months. In general, patients treated with plasma exchange spent less time in the ICU and hospital. Patients who were treated within 7 days of onset of the symptoms fared better than patients whose treatment was started later. The replacement fluid in most cases was 5 percent albumin. A French study published in 1987 confirmed the beneficial effects of plasma exchange, although the volume of plasma exchanged was slightly greater and the composition of the replacement solution was different (including IVIG) [20]. In some patients, fresh frozen plasma was used as replacement solution, and this was associated with more complications (fever, skin rash, hepatitis) [20]. A recent report from the Netherlands indicates that IVIG is as effective as plasma exchange in the treatment of Guillain-Barré syndrome [21]. In contrast, reports from the United States show worsening of some patients' symptoms following IG infusions [22]. According to the literature and in my experience, plasma exchange is also effective in ameliorating symptoms of Miller Fisher syndrome, an unusual variant of Guillain-Barré syndrome [23].

MYASTHENIA GRAVIS. Plasma exchange therapy is indicated in myasthenia gravis only in the following situations: myasthenic crisis; rapidly progressive disease, especially with uncontrolled bulbar or respiratory muscle compromise; preparation of some patients for thymectomy or a worsening condition after thymectomy; to avoid the use of corticosteroids in patients with contraindications to these drugs; to decrease the dose of corticosteroids in patients with unacceptable side effects; and in patients who are refractory to other treatment modalities [24]. When plasma exchange is used for these indications, improvement is usually rapid.

THROMBOTIC THROMBOCYTOPENIC PURPURA. A recent Canadian multicenter controlled trial compared plasma exchange to plasma infusion in 102 patients with thrombotic thrombocytopenic purpura (TTP). The results, published in 1991, showed plasma exchange to be the more effective treatment, with a mortality rate of 21.5 percent compared to 37.2 percent in the plasma infusion group [25]. My protocol for treatment of TTP involves daily plasma exchanges with removal of 1.5 plasma volumes per procedure. The replacement fluid is a combination of 5 percent albumin (during the first half of the procedure) and fresh frozen plasma (during the latter half). Daily plasma exchange sessions are continued until platelet count and LDH level normalize and may be followed with one or two further procedures. If the patient does not respond adequately, other treatment modalities (prednisone, antiplatelet drugs, or vincristine) are added. It has been stated that cryopoor plasma might be a more desirable replacement fluid than fresh frozen plasma (because it lacks large-molecular-weight forms of the von Willebrand factor), but there are no definitive studies comparing these two replacement fluids. It has been reported that resistant cases have responded when plasma exchange was combined with Prosorba column treatment [26].

SEVERE AUTOIMMUNE HEMOLYTIC ANEMIA (COLD-REACTING ANTIBODY). Removal of cold agglutinins, such as anti-I, by plasma exchange may relieve severe hemolysis in some cases of severe autoimmune hemolytic anemia [27]. The patient's blood and other intravenous fluids must be warmed before they are returned to the patient. This method of antibody removal, unfortunately, may not prevent fatal outcome.

RAPIDLY PROGRESSIVE GLOMERULONEPHRITIS. Therapeutic plasma exchange is currently the primary line of therapy for only one type of rapidly progressive glomerulonephritis (RPGN), the antiglomerular basement membrane-positive Goodpasture syndrome, particularly when there is moderate or severe renal disease with pulmonary hemorrhage. Since pulmonary hemorrhage can be fatal, it constitutes a medical emergency and plasma exchange must be done immediately. The role of plasma exchange is only secondary in patients who have RPGN associated with antineutrophil cytoplasm antibodies (i.e., systemic vasculitis due to Wegener's granulomatosis or polyarteritis nodosa) [28,29,30]. Plasma exchange is not thought to be beneficial in patients with immune complex-mediated RPGN [31].

DRUG OVERDOSE AND POISONING. Theoretically, plasma exchange is effective in removing protein-bound toxins and drugs that have been given in overdose. Case reports have confirmed the beneficial effect of this approach when treating patients poisoned with the mushroom toxin amanitin [32], the nephrotoxic herbicide paraquat [33], and the organophosphate insecticide methylparathion [34]. In the treatment of the latter poisoning, which is mediated by anticholinesterase activity, plasma might be useful as a replacement fluid.

Summary

Techniques of performing hemapheresis have changed since the times of Abel, even outpaced our understanding of its proper clinical use. Therapeutic hemapheresis is useful in ameliorating acute symptoms by virtue of decreasing the concentration of pathologic cells or plasma constituents. It is quite effective, even lifesaving, in certain disease processes that are of limited duration. The role of plasma exchange in the treatment of chronic disease is less clear-cut, but it is considered useful in the management of acute crises and as a method to decrease the concentration of pathologic antibodies for which no other therapy is effective. Development and licensing of newer devices capable of selectively removing specific abnormal plasma proteins will add to the sophistication of hemapheresis therapy.

References

1. Abel JJ, Rowntree LG, Turner BB: Plasma removal with return of corpuscles (plasmapheresis). *J Pharmacol Exp Ther* 5:625, 1914.
2. Solomon A, Fahey JL: Plasmapheresis therapy in macroglobulinemia. *Ann Intern Med* 58:789, 1963.
3. Gurland HJ: Therapeutic apheresis update. *Adv Exp Med Biol* 260:193, 1989.
4. Snyder HW Jr, Cochran SK, Balint JP Jr, et al: Experience with protein A-immunoadsorption in treatment-resistant adult immune thrombocytopenic purpura. *Blood* 79:2237, 1992.
5. Mimori A, Takahashi K, Mitamura T, et al: Clinical evaluatin of three types of plasmapheresis in a patient with type IIa familial hypercholesterolemia. *J Clin Apheresis* 3:209, 1987.
6. Shumak KH, Rock GA: Therapeutic plasma exchange. *N Engl J Med* 310:762, 1984.
7. Orlin JB, Berkman EM: Partial plasma exchange using albumin replacement: Removal and recovery of normal plasma constituents. *Blood* 56:1055, 1980.
8. Sutton DMC, Cardella CJ, Uldall PR, et al: Complications of intensive plasma exchange. *Plasma Ther* 2:19, 1981.
9. Sultan Y, Bussel A, Maisonneuve P, et al: Potential danger of thrombosis after plasma exchange in the treatment of patients with immune disease. *Transfusion* 19:588, 1979.
10. Evans RT, Macdonald R, Robinson A: Suxamethonium apnoea associated with plasmaphoresis. *Anaesthesia* 35:198, 1980.
11. Schlansky R, DeHoratius RJ, Pincus T, et al: Plasmapheresis in systemic lupus erythematosus: A cautionary note. *Arthritis Rheum* 24:49, 1981.
12. Tielemans C, Madhoun P, Lenaers M, et al: Anaphylactoid reactions during hemodialysis on AN69 membranes in patients receiving ACE inhibitors. *Kidney Int* 38:982, 1990.
13. Siami G, Morrow J, James L, et al: Anaphylactoid reactions associated with eval hollow fiber plasma filter pheresis and ACE-inhibitors. Presented at the American Society for Apheresis 14th Annual Meeting, April 1993, Boston, abstract 89.
14. Keller C, Grutzmacher P, Bahr F, et al: LDL-apheresis with dextran sulphate and anaphylactoid reactions to ACE inhibitors. *Lancet* 341:60, 1993.
15. Berkman EM: Therapeutic apheresis: What it can and can't do. *Diagn Med* 7:55, 1984.
16. Schroeder JO, Euler HH, Löffler H: Synchronization of plasmapheresis and pulse cyclophosphamide in severe systemic lupus erythematosus. *Ann Intern Med* 107:344, 1987.
17. Euler HH, Löffler H, Christophers E: Synchronization of plasmapheresis and pulse cyclophosphamide therapy in pemphigus vulgaris. *Arch Dermatol* 123:1205, 1987.
18. Lupus Plasmapheresis Study Group: Plasmapheresis and subsequent pulse cyclophosphamide versus pulse cyclophosphamide alone in severe lupus: Design of the LPSG trial. *J Clin Apheresis* 6:40, 1991.
19. The Guillain-Barré Syndrome Study Group: Plasmapheresis and acute Guillain-Barré syndrome. *Neurology* 35:1096, 1985.
20. French Gooperative Group on Plasma Exchange in Guillain-Barré Syndrome: Efficiency of plasma exchange in Guillain-Barré syndrome: Role of replacement fluids. *Ann Neurol* 22:753, 1987.
21. van der Meché FGA, Schmitz PIM, the Dutch Guillain Barré Study Group: A randomized trial comparing intravenous immune globulin and plasma exchange in Guillain-Barré syndrome. *N Engl J Med* 326:1123, 1992.
22. Stricker RB, Kwiatkowska BJ, Habis JA et al: Response to plasmapheresis following failure of intravenous gammaglobulin in patients with myasthenia gravis and Guillain-Barré syndrome. Presented at the American Society for Apheresis 14th Annual Meeting, April 1993, Boston, abstract 98.
23. Littlewood R, Bajada S: Successful plasmapheresis in the Miller-Fisher syndrome. *Br Med J* 282:778, 1981.
24. Lisak RP: Plasma exchange in neurologic diseases. *Arch Neurol* 41:654, 1984.
25. Rock GA, Shumak KH, Buskard NA, et al: Comparison of plasma exchange with plasma infusion in the treatment of thrombotic thrombocytopenic purpura. *N Engl J Med* 325:393, 1991.
26. Gaddis T, Guthrie T, Mittleman A, et al: Protein A immunoadsorption (PAI) in classical thrombotic thrombocytopenic purpura (TTP) refractory to plasma exchange report of eleven patients. Presented at the American Society of Hematology meeting, December 1992.
27. Silberstein LE, Berkman EM: Plasma exchange in autoimmune hemolytic anemia (AIHA). *J Clin Apheresis* 1:238, 1983.
28. Lockwood CM, Boulton-Jones JM, Lowenthal RM, et al: Recovery from Goodpasture's syndrome after immunosuppressive treatment and plasmapheresis. *Br Med J* 2:252, 1975.
29. Johnson JP, Whitman W, Briggs WA, et al: Plasmapheresis and immunosuppressive agents in antibasement membrane antibody induced Goodpasture's syndrome. *Am J Med* 64:354, 1978.
30. Erickson SB, Kurtz SB, Donadio JV Jr, et al: Use of combined plasmapheresis and immunosuppression in the treatment of Goodpasture's syndrome. *Mayo Clin Proc* 54:714, 1979.
31. Glöckner WM, Sieberth HG, Wichmann HE, et al: Plasma exchange and immunosuppression in rapidly progressive glomerulonephritis: A controlled, multicenter study. *Clin Nephrol* 29:1, 1988.
32. Mercuriali F, Sirchia G: Plasma exchange for mushroom poisoning. *Transfusion* 17:644, 1977.
33. Miller J, Sanders E, Webb D: Plasmapheresis for paraquat poisoning. *Lancet* 1:875, 1978.
34. Luznikov EA, Yaroslavsky AA, Molodenkov MN, et al: Plasma perfusion through charcoal in methylparathion poisoning. *Lancet* 1:38, 1977.

24. Aspiration of Cerebrospinal Fluid

John P. Weaver and Robin I. Davidson

This chapter presents guidelines for safe cerebrospinal fluid (CSF) aspiration for the emergency room (ER) or intensive care unit (ICU) physician and provides a basic understanding of the indications, techniques, and potential complications for these procedures.

Most procedures to aspirate CSF require readily accessible equipment and sterile supplies located on most hospital patient care units, and certainly in the ER or ICU. Radiographic imaging is required for procedures in which the external anatomic landmarks provide inadequate guidance for safe needle placement, or when needle placement by external landmarks alone has proved unsuccessful due to anatomic variations caused by trauma, operative scar, congenital defects, or degenerative changes. Fluoroscopy is typically the most useful radiographic tool for C1–2 puncture, failed lumbar puncture, and myelography. Computed tomography (CT) is used for stereotactic placement of ventricular catheters.

The clinician should recognize the relative expertise required to perform these procedures and when other assistance is necessary. Some procedures are relatively safe and routinely performed, but others require equipment that may be available only in a radiology department or operating room. Many procedures can be done by a primary care physician or intensivist, but some require the assistance of a radiologist, neurologist, or neurosurgeon.

A radiologist may be needed for fluoroscopy. Other procedures require other expertise, such as for a shunt or CSF reservoir tap. It would be prudent to seek a neurosurgeon's counsel prior to performing such a procedure regarding the indications and potential risks of violating an implanted system, since the central nervous system (CNS) is an immunologically privileged system and the consequences of infection are significant, often resulting in multiple subsequent operative procedures.

Most procedures require only local anesthesia, and lidocaine is most commonly used. General anesthesia or sedation is uncommonly required but is sometimes helpful for toddlers, anxious patients, or those who are confused, combative, or otherwise uncooperative (see Chap. 28). Chloral hydrate is often used for children; morphine, haloperidol, or midazolam may be used in adult and pediatric populations. Midazolam can reduce anxiety-related behaviors before and after the procedure and has an amnestic effect, but during the procedure it may not provide adequate sedation [1].

Indications

CEREBROSPINAL FLUID ASPIRATION OR PRESSURE MEASUREMENT FOR DIAGNOSIS.
There are many indications for CSF sampling, including suspicion of CNS bacterial, fungal, or viral infections or subarachnoid hemorrhage (SAH). Headache can be a prominent symptom of cerebrovascular disease. The headache of SAH may be similar to migraine, and headache may accompany or precede cerebral thrombosis and embolism as a forerunner to stroke [2]. Cerebrospinal fluid pressure recording is important in the diagnosis and treatment of normal pressure hydrocephalus, benign intracranial hyperten-

sion, and severe head injury. Cytologic study enables identification of cells from CNS primary or metastatic tumors and differentiation from inflammatory disorders [3]. Neuroradiographic procedures, including myelography, cisternography, pneumoencephalography, and ventriculography or therapeutic intervention for intrathecal chemotherapy or antibiotic administration, require access to the CSF compartment.

The fluid analysis performed depends on the patient's age, history, and differential diagnosis. Information such as the presence of meningeal irritative signs or symptoms, history of systemic or intracranial neoplasm, and radiographic evidence of an abnormality guides the choice of diagnostic tests. Cerebrospinal fluid composition also depends on cerebral metabolism, blood-brain barrier function, systemic or CNS disease, and drug therapies, among other factors. Normal values for CSF solute, amino acid, protein, neurotransmitter, and metabolite compositions are available from the hospital clinical chemistry laboratory.

The CSF glucose depends on the blood glucose level and is usually two-thirds of serum glucose. Because glucose depends on carrier-facilitated diffusion, CSF glucose levels lag behind changes in the serum glucose. Simultaneous levels, preferably fasting levels, should be compared. Low CSF glucose in inflammatory or infectious meningeal disorders reflects increased glucose utilization by the CNS or leukocytes and inhibited transport mechanisms. The increased glucose metabolism is usually accompanied by increased CSF lactate, reflecting increased anaerobic glycolysis.

Cerebrospinal fluid protein content is normally low and less than 0.5 percent of that in plasma. Immunoglobulin G (IgG) is the major gamma-globulin and is increased in response to inflammation and demyelination. Protein electrophoresis to measure the relative amount of protein fractions is useful for diagnosis in a number of diseases. The protein also varies in different CSF spaces. The total protein in the ventricles is 6 to 12 mg per deciliter, in the cisterna magna 15 to 25 mg per deciliter, and in the lumbar subarachnoid space 20 to 50 mg per deciliter. Increased protein is a nonspecific indicator of CNS disease. Elevation greater than 500 mg per deciliter is consistent with meningitis, intraspinal tumor with CSF block, and bloody CSF. Low protein can be demonstrated in children younger than 2 years, some patients with pseudotumor cerebri, acute water intoxication, and hyperthyroid or leukemic patients.

Hemorrhage. Lumbar puncture is indicated following SAH if the head CT is nondiagnostic or unavailable and if the clinical history and presentation are not convincing of SAH. Lumbar puncture should not be performed without prior CT scan if the patient has any focal neurologic deficits, because an intracranial hematoma may be present, which would increase the risk of transtentorial herniation with lumbar puncture. Ventriculomegaly due to acute obstructive hydrocephalus following subarachnoid hemorrhage may also be demonstrated by CT. In this case a ventriculostomy catheter for ventricular CSF diversion would better benefit the patient, and lumbar puncture is not needed. One of the biggest problems with CSF examination is a traumatic lumbar puncture yielding bloody fluid that makes the determination of SAH difficult. All specimens should be spun down and examined carefully against white paper in comparison to a tube of water. If a lumbar puncture is performed and the CSF examined at least 2 hours after the initial hemorrhage, it will be xanthochromic. The protein may be elevated and glucose very slightly depressed, and the opening pressure at the time of lumbar puncture may reflect the elevation of intracranial pressure. Another method to differentiate between blood in CSF due to intracranial hemorrhage and that due to a traumatic spinal tap has been demonstrated in neonates [4]. The mean corpuscular volume (MCV) of erythrocytes in the CSF can be compared with that from peripheral blood. The MCV of CSF is lower than that of peripheral blood following intracranial hemorrhage, but in patients with a traumatic tap the values are similar.

Infection

Cerebrospinal fluid evaluation is the single most important aspect of the laboratory diagnosis of meningitis. However, a cautious approach to CSF aspiration is prudent in patients with brain abscess or suspected intracranial hypertension to avoid brain herniation and a potentially fatal outcome [5]. Basic CSF examination usually includes a Gram stain, cell count with white cell differential, protein and glucose levels, and aerobic culture with antibiotic sensitivities. With suspicion of tuberculosis or fungal meningitis the fluid can be analyzed by acid-fast stain, India ink preparation, and cryptococcal antigen. Tests to identify bacterial antigens for *Streptococcus pneumoniae*, *Streptococcus* group B, *Hemophilus influenzae*, and *Neisseria meningitides* (meningococcus) groups allow rapid diagnosis and early treatment. In cases in which the patient presents with a rapidly deteriorating clinical course, however, antibiotic therapy should not be delayed for diagnostic imaging or reduction of intracranial pressure by other therapeutic measures [6].

Rodewald et al. reported an argument to perform only limited CSF analysis in a pediatric population [7]. In their study, the decision to analyze CSF for protein or glucose was based on initial analysis of the nucleated blood cell count (NucBC). A negative screening test was defined as a CSF NucBC less than 6 per cubic millimeter. The results demonstrated that the screening test was much more sensitive and specific than other routine tests in predicting the presence of infection. These results provided a basis of a strategy for sequential testing of CSF. First submitting the specimen for NucBC and culture limited the samples that required further testing, with a potential savings of time, effort, and healthcare dollars. In a neonatal population, Schwersenski et al. reported that lumbar puncture and CSF analysis may be more useful after 1 week of age than during the first week of life. This prospective study assessed the frequency and diagnostic utility of lumbar punctures as part of evaluation for suspected congenital or postnatal infection in neonates. It showed rare positive CSF cultures during the first week of life. Of these, only one had a simultaneous positive blood culture and clinically evident meningitis. The yield after the first week of life was approximately 5 times higher [8].

Shunt System Failure. Aspiration from the valves and reservoirs of shunt systems is performed to determine patency and collect CSF to rule out an infectious process. Instrumenting a shunt can potentially contaminate a clean functioning system with skin flora, so the shunts should be tapped selectively and perhaps a neurosurgeon should be consulted prior to doing this. Indications for shunt tap include clinical presentation of an infectious process after all reasonable and common sources have been evaluated and excluded. An invasive test for patency should follow a head CT scan that shows ventriculomegaly. If possible, this should be compared to a previous study, because in some cases the ventricles remain enlarged despite adequate drainage. Clinical presentation of shunt obstruction is highly variable; it may be slowly progressive, intermittent, or stuttering or there may be a rapid decline in mentation and progression into coma. If the proximal catheter is patent, then aspiration may temper the neurologic impairment or even be lifesaving until formal shunt revision can be performed.

Normal Pressure Hydrocephalus. Serial lumbar punctures or continuous CSF drainage via a lumbar catheter can be used as a provocative diagnostic test to select patients who would benefit from a shunt for CSF diversion. They are most useful and have a positive predictive value if the patient improves. The CSF access can also be used for infusion tests and measurement of CSF production rate, pressure-volume index, and outflow resistance or absorption. Some studies suggest that these values are also predictive of therapeutic CSF diversion [9,10,11].

Benign Intracranial Hypertension (Pseudotumor Cerebri). Benign intracranial hypertension, or pseudotumor cerebri, occurs in young persons, often obese young women. Intracranial pressure (ICP) is elevated without ventriculomegaly, perhaps from a disturbance in CSF circulation. Etiologic factors for childhood presentation include chronic middle ear infection, dural sinus thrombosis, head injury, vitamin A overdosage, tetracycline exposure, internal jugular venous thrombosis, and idiopathic causes [12]. There may actually be a broader group of closely associated syndromes with a single underlying pathophysiologic mechanism [13]. Intracranial hypertension develops and becomes symptomatic over several months. Headache is the earliest and most common presenting symptom, but blurred vision, dizziness, diplopia, transient visual obscurations, and abnormal facial sensations can also occur [14]. Objective findings of papilledema, abducens palsy, and visual impairment are common sequelae of the intracranial hypertension. When lumbar puncture is performed as part of the evaluation, the CSF pressure is usually elevated to 25 to 40 cm H_2O, and CSF dynamics demonstrate an increase in CSF outflow resistance. Serial lumbar punctures can be therapeutic with daily taps performed and CSF withdrawn until the closing pressure is normal. In some cases, this can restore the balance between CSF formation and absorption. Other patients may need shunting after other medical therapies, including weight loss, steroids, acetazolamide, diuretics, and glycerol, have failed. A lumboperitoneal shunt is commonly used, but ventricular shunt systems also work well.

Lymphoma and Leukemia. Lymphoma and leukemia frequently infiltrate the subarachnoid space, with little brain involvement. Cerebrospinal fluid sampling may provide a diagnosis or be done periodically to screen neurologically asymptomatic patients who have a type of leukemia with a tendency to recur. Cerebrosinal fluid for cytologic study can be collected through routine or serial lumbar punctures; cisternal CSF examination will enhance the diagnosis if the lumbar CSF is nondiagnostic [15]. Acute varieties that involve CNS include acute lymphocytic leukemia (ALL), acute nonlymphocytic leukemia (ANLL), acute myelogenous leukemia (AMoL), acute myelomonocytic leukemia (AMMoL), and acute undifferentiated leukemia (AUL) [16]. Nuclear morphology is often distorted, and blast forms in these disorders have high nuclear to cytoplasmic ratios, smooth chromatin, and prominent nucleoli. Individual proliferating T and B lymphocytes can be detected in the CSF in patients with inflammatory and neoplastic diseases and may aid in the differentiation of opportunistic infection from leukemic infiltration [17].

Meningeal Carcinomatosis and Subarachnoid Spread of Primary CNS Tumors. Some systemic neoplasms have a high propensity for CNS metastases (e.g., malignant melanoma). In patients with a known history of systemic neoplasm who develop signs and symptoms of meningeal irritation, CSF cytologic study can determine whether there are tumor cells present. Sometimes a generous volume of CSF or serial sampling is needed for cytologic diagnosis. Metastatic tumors have meningeal dissemination far more frequently than primary brain tumors, and in some cases their intracranial extension may be the initial clinical presentation. Of the primary brain tumors, high-grade gliomas most commonly disseminate in the subarachnoid space, but it is difficult to differentiate between tumor types [18]. Childhood brain tumors also disseminate in the subarachnoid space with some frequency, depending on tumor type.

Myelography. Access to the CSF space is required to perform myelography. Lumbar puncture is the most common means of access for lumbar and cervical myelography because the contrast agent is denser than CSF and may be directed by gravity to the area of interest. Cervical C1–2 puncture may be the usual access for cervical myelography at some centers, but for many the technique is reserved for patients in whom a successful lumbar puncture is not possible due to extensive arachnoiditis, epidural tumor, severe spinal stenosis, or CSF block.

Other Neurologic Disorders. There is an extensive literature of the CSF changes in multiple sclerosis. Usually the ICP is normal and the CSF composition shows normal glucose, mononuclear pleocytosis, an increase in protein level due to increased endothelial cell permeability associated with demyelinating lesions, and an increase in immunoglobulins (IgG) preferentially in CSF relative to serum [19]. Oligoclonal bands are useful in the diagnosis of multiple sclerosis and other inflammatory diseases, and electrophoretic separation of inflammatory proteins can increase specificity of diagnosis. A very elevated CSF protein with relative absence of pleocytosis is characteristic of acute idiopathic polyneuritis or Guillain-Barré syndrome, and normal CSF is more common in the Miller Fisher variant of this disease. Elevated CSF protein is found in diabetic neuropathy, although the elevation and clinical disease are not well correlated.

CEREBROSPINAL FLUID ACCESS FOR THERAPEUTIC INTERVENTION

Fistulas. Cerebrospinal fluid leaks occur for a variety of reasons, including nontraumatic and traumatic etiologies. Traumatic etiologies, including accidental injury and iatrogenic causes, are considered here because there is a therapeutic role for CSF access.

Postoperative CSF fistulas may occur following tumor resections located at the skull base and are a result of dura and skull defects and the pressure effects of gravity. For example, patients who have lesions, such as an olfactory groove meningioma or a pituitary tumor resected from the frontal fossa, may develop a CSF fistula despite intraoperative measures to provide a watertight dural closure. Orthostatic headaches are a characteristic symptom and the leak is clinically evident as CSF rhinorrhea. Cerebrospinal fluid fistulas following skull base lesions from the middle cranial fossa and cerebellar-pontine angle occur infrequently, and usually the CSF leaks through the auditory tube to the nasopharynx [20]. Closure of the dura in the posterior fossa following suboccipital craniectomy may be difficult and often is not watertight. A CSF fistula in this region leads to a CSF pseudomeningocele and potential subsequent wound breakdown. Cerebrospinal fluid leak following lumbar surgery is unusual but may occur due to recent myelography, a dural tear, postlaminectomy bone spikes, or inadequate dural closure [21,22].

The most common presentation of a CSF fistula is following trauma. Basilar skull fractures that cross the ethmoid or frontal sinus can lead to CSF rhinorrhea. Another relatively common fracture follows the long axis of the petrous bone and usually involves the middle ear. Hemotympanum may be noted on examination or, if the tympanic membrane is ruptured, the patient will demonstrate CSF otorrhea. Delayed leaks are not uncommon because the fistula can become occluded with adhesions or herniated brain tissue, which temporarily tamponades the defect until brain swelling resolves. In fact, leaks sometimes provide CSF decompression from posttraumatic intracranial hypertension, which must be treated prior to or concurrently with repairing the leak.

Placement of a lumbar drainage catheter or daily lumbar punctures can be useful nonoperative approaches to treating a CSF fistula. The use of continuous drainage by a lumbar catheter is somewhat controversial because of the potential for intracranial contamination from the sinuses if the intracranial pressure is lowered. Such intervention should follow several days of postural drainage, achieved by keeping the patient sitting upright. If a lumbar drainage catheter is used, the collection bag should be maintained no lower than the patient's shoulder level to prevent complications of low intracranial pressure, and duration of continuous drainage should be limited to about 5 days to reduce the risk of infection.

Intracranial Hypertension. Intracranial hypertension (see Chaps. 25 and 175) can cause significant neurologic injury and even death. The CSF serves to protect brain tissue against various mechanisms of cerebral injury, so access to the intracranial CSF space is useful in diagnosis and treatment [23]. A ventriculostomy is commonly used both as an ICP monitor and a means to treat intracranial hypertension by CSF drainage. An ICP measuring device is often placed following traumatic brain injury for patients who suffer from deterioration of mental status to a Glasgow Coma Score (GCS) less than 8 or 9 or a motor score less than 6 (not aphasic), diffuse brain edema, hematoma (epidural, subdural, intraparenchymal), cortical contusions, or absent or compressed basal cisterns on initial CT. ICP monitoring can be indicated in cerebrovascular diseases, including aneurysmal subarachnoid hemorrhage, spontaneous intracerebral hematoma, ischemic and hypoxic cerebral insults, intraventricular hemorrhage, and clinical or radiographic indication of elevated ICP. It is sometimes required in patients treated with paralytics, sedatives, or barbiturates that may mask the neurological examination. Obstructive hydrocephalus is caused by mechanical mechanisms that may raise ICP acutely with dilatation of the ventricles and resultant compression of surrounding brain. Disease processes that can cause hydrocephalus are aneurysmal subarachnoid hemorrhage, third-ventricular tumors, intraventricular hemorrhage, intraventricular cysticercosis, and colloid cysts. Brain edema often surrounds tumors, intracranial hemorrhage, infarcted brain, and traumatic brain contusions and can occur after operation. Diffuse brain swelling more often occurs in the setting of inflammatory and infectious disorders such as Reye syndrome or meningitis or as a result of hyperthermia, carbon dioxide retention, or intravascular congestion.

Drug therapy. The CSF can be a route to administer medications such as chemotherapeutic agents and antibiotics. Treatment of CNS lymphoma or leukemia is accomplished in part by intrathecal injections of various agents that may be infused through a lumbar injection or by intraventricular injection through an Ommaya reservoir. Serial small doses of these agents, such as methotrexate, are recommended for intrathecal chemotherapy of meningeal carcinomatosis to prevent neurotoxicity [24]. Meningitis and ventriculitis are treated with systemic intravenous administration of antibiotics that may be supplemented by direct injection into the CSF through a ventriculostomy or lumbar puncture. Again, small doses are recommended to prevent neurotoxicity, especially when the ventricular route is used.

Techniques

There are several techniques for CSF aspiration. All procedures should be performed using sterile technique with adequate hand washing, masks, sterile gloves, towels, and instruments. The skin is prepared with an antiseptic solution and draped with sterile towels.

LUMBAR PUNCTURE. Lumbar puncture (LP) is a common procedure readily performed by the general practitioner and uncommonly requiring the assistance of radiology. It can be performed in nearly any hospital or outpatient setting where commercially prepared lumbar puncture trays are available. In patients with advanced degenerative changes or extensive previous lumbar surgery or congenital defects the use of fluoroscopy for needle placement may be required. C1–2 or cisternal punctures are seldom required for CSF collection but are occasionally used. Premedication is typically not required, as local anesthesia is quite effective. It has even been demonstrated in a controlled clinical trial that in the neonatal population, injection with a local anesthetic for lumbar puncture is probably not required and does not reduce perceived stress or discomfort [25].

Figures 24-1 and 24-2 depict some of the steps for lumbar puncture [26]. The patient is placed in the lateral knee-chest position or sitting while leaning forward over a table or tray at bedside (Fig. 24-1). The sitting position is sometimes preferred in obese patients, in whom adipose tissue can obscure the midline, or in elderly patients with significant lumbar spinal degenerative disease (Fig. 24-2). Local anesthetic (usually lidocaine) is injected using a 25- or 27-gauge needle to form a skin wheal. A 1.5-inch needle is used to inject anesthetic along the midline to anesthetize the intraspinous ligament and muscles. This usually provides adequate anesthesia, but if not, more extensive regional anesthesia can be given. A field block is accomplished by additional injections on each side of the interspinous space near the lamina [27].

A 18- to 20-gauge spinal needle is used for pressure measurement. Needles as small as 27-gauge can be used for aspiration or therapeutic infusion [28]. The smaller needles decrease the risk of CSF leak, consequent headache, and backache and should be used if intracranial hypertension is suspected. The point of skin entry is midline between the spinous processes of L3–4, at the level of the superior iliac crests. Lower needle placement, at L4–5 or L5–S1, is required in children and neonates to avoid injury to the conus medullaris, which lies more caudal than in adults. The needle is advanced with the stylet or obturator in place to maintain needle patency and prevent iatrogenic intraspinal epidermoid tumors [5]. With proper needle orientation, the bevel will be parallel to the spinal column and the longitudinal fibers of the dura. The needle will pass through the following structures before entering the subarachnoid space: skin, superficial fascia, supraspinous ligament, interspi-

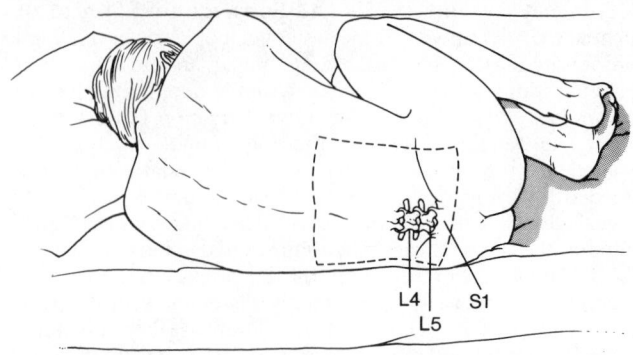

Fig. 24-1. Patient in the lateral decubitis position with back at edge of bed and knees, hips, back and neck flexed. (From Davidson RI: Lumbar puncture, in VanderSalm TJ (ed): *Atlas of Bedside Procedures.* Boston, Little Brown, 1988. With permission.)

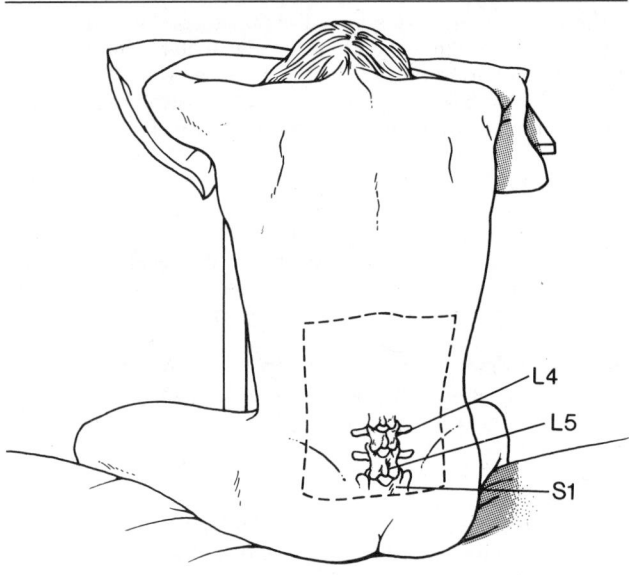

Fig. 24-2. Patient sitting on the edge of the bed leaning on bedside stand. (From Davidson RI: Lumbar puncture, in VanderSalm TJ (ed): *Atlas of Bedside Procedures.* Boston, Little Brown, 1988. With permission.)

nous ligament, ligamentum flavum, epidural space with fatty areolar tissue and internal vertebral venous plexus, dura mater, and arachnoid mater (Fig. 24-3). The depth will vary from 1 inch or less in a child to as much as 4 inches in an obese adult. The tactile sensations of passing through the intraspinous ligaments into the epidural space followed by dural puncture are consistent and are recognized with practice. Once intradural, the bevel of the needle is redirected to point cephalad to improve CSF flow.

The opening CSF pressure is measured with the patient's legs relaxed and extended partly from the knee-chest position. Because it is often difficult to measure CSF pressure in children, a technique that measures CSF flow rate can be used to estimate it [29]. After CSF is collected for diagnostic studies, the closing pressure can be measured prior to needle withdrawal. The CSF opening and closing pressures are more difficult to measure with the patient in the sitting position because the static pres-

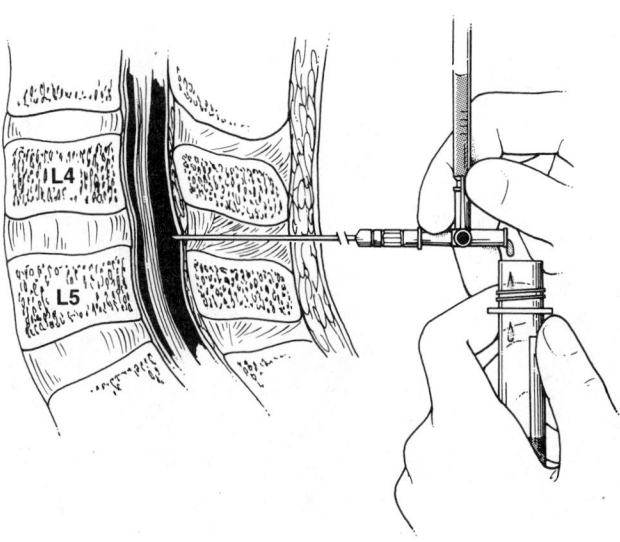

Fig. 24-3. The spinal needle is advanced to the spinal subarachnoid space and cerebrospinal fluid samples collected after opening pressure is measured. (From Davidson RI: Lumbar puncture, in VanderSalm TJ (ed): *Atlas of Bedside Procedures.* Boston, Little Brown, 1988. With permission.)

sure of the column of fluid is higher and CSF may be lost when the needle stylet is first withdrawn. The pressure may be measured by attaching plastic tubing and holding it up to the level of the foramen magnum, or by reclining the patient in the lateral position and proceeding as already described.

Although lumbar puncture is typically safe, there are a number of significant complications and potential risks involved. Hemorrhage is uncommon but can be seen in association with a bleeding disorder or anticoagulation. Spinal subarachnoid hemorrhage is rare but can occur in the face of anticoagulation or thrombocytopenia resulting in a blockage of CSF flow and causing back and radicular pain with sphincter disturbances and even paraparesis [30]. Spinal subdural hematoma is rare but is associated with a high morbidity and mortality; surgical intervention for clot evacuation must be prompt. Infection by the introduction of skin flora into the subarachnoid space can cause meningitis, but this is uncommon if aseptic technique is used. Lumbar drainage for the treatment of cranial base CSF leak fistulas, whether by serial taps or continuous drainage by an implanted catheter, increases the risk of infection by reducing the pressure gradient and potentially introducing flora intracranially from the paranasal or mastoid sinuses. Another complication is the inability to access CSF, or "dry tap," which may be caused by excessively deep needle penetration.

Headache is the most renowned side effect of lumbar puncture. It may be due to a reduced CSF pressure causing the stretching of pain-sensitive intracranial structures. Magnetic resonance imaging (MRI) can be used to measure intracranial CSF volume and demonstrate reduced CSF volume following lumbar puncture, but most of the CSF is lost from cortical structures and the brain is not measurably changed in position [31]. Postlumbar puncture headaches are not significantly related to a change in MRI-demonstrated CSF volume. The use of a fine-gauge needle significantly decreases the pain associated with needle placements and the severity of the postural headaches following lumbar puncture [32]. The shape of the needle point seems to play a significant role in subsequent CSF leakage and headache; new needle designs, many with smaller diameters,

are being evaluated for routine clinical use [33]. A coaxial needle is sometimes helpful when the patient is morbidly obese [34]. Several studies have demonstrated that psychologic factors strongly influence patient tolerance to the procedure [32,35]. Treatment of postural headaches following lumbar puncture includes initially keeping the patient recumbent to reduce the hydrostatic fluid pressure at the puncture site. The patient should take fluids generously and avoid activities that cause stress or strain. Caffeine products and intravenous lidocaine may be beneficial. If noninvasive therapies such as these have failed after several days, an epidural blood patch or even epidural injection of dextran may be applied at the puncture site and can provide a lasting cure of CSF fistula [36].

A very uncommon sequela of lumbar puncture or continuous CSF drainage is hearing loss. Drainage of CSF decreases intracranial pressure, which is transmitted to the perilymph via the cochlea aqueduct and in some patients causes a temporary but perceptive partial hearing loss. Transient hearing loss is apparently not uncommon, but irreversible losses can be significant [37,38]. Transient sixth nerve palsy can also occur, due to traction from excessive CSF removal.

Neurovascular injury is also uncommon but can occur, particularly in the setting of complete subarachnoid block due to a spinal cord tumor located cephalad to the level of the aspiration. Traction of the spinal cord can produce neurologic deterioration (spinal coning) from CSF drainage [39,40].

C1–2 PUNCTURE. The C1–2 or lateral cervical puncture was originally developed for percutaneous cordotomy. It does not require fluoroscopic control but is most safely performed by a radiologist with fluoroscopy. It is occasionally used for myelography and CSF collection when aspiration from the lumbar space is impossible.

The puncture is performed with the patient supine, the head and neck flexed, and the lateral neck washed and draped. The skin puncture site is localized 1 cm caudal and 1 cm dorsal to the tip of the mastoid process. After the skin is prepared and infiltrated with lidocaine, a spinal needle under fluoroscopic control is directed toward the junction of the middle and posterior thirds of the bony canal to avoid an anomalous vertebral or posterior inferior cerebellar artery that may lie in the anterior half of the canal. If performed without fluoroscopy, the stilette should be removed frequently to check for CSF. When performed under fluoroscopic guidance, the needle is seen to be directed perpendicular to the neck and just under the posterior ring of C1. The same "pop" is felt piercing the dura as in the lumbar puncture, and the bevel is then directed cephalad in a similar fashion.

Complications of lateral cervical puncture include injury to the spinal cord or the vertebral artery. Irritation of a nerve root, causing local pain and headache, is not uncommon.

CISTERNAL PUNCTURE. Cisternal puncture provides another source of access to the CSF space, via the cisterna magna, when lumbar puncture is technically impossible or contraindicated.

A preoperative lateral flexed skull radiograph should be performed to ensure normal anatomy. The patient is placed in the sitting position with the head slightly flexed. The hair is shaved in the occipital region and the skin prepared and infiltrated with lidocaine. The point of entry is on the midline between the external occipital pertuberance in the upper margin of the spinous process of C2 or through an imaginary line through both external auditory meati [5]. The spinal needle is directed in a slightly cephalad direction and usually strikes the occipital bone. The needle can be partially withdrawn and redirected more caudally in a stepwise fashion until it passes through the atlantooccipital membrane and dura, producing the familiar "popping" sensation. The cisterna magna usually lies at a depth of 4 to 6 cm from the skin surface; certainly the needle should not be advanced more than 7.5 cm, to prevent injury to the medulla.

Complications can include injury to the medulla or a vertebral artery. With a cooperative patient this is usually a reasonably safe procedure, since the cisterna magna is a relatively large CSF space. However, it is still not commonly practiced because it is potentially more hazardous than a C1-2 puncture under fluoroscopic control.

ASPIRATION OF SHUNTS AND RESERVOIRS

Shunt Reservoir Aspiration. In-line subcutaneous reservoirs in ventriculoatrial (VA) or ventriculoperitoneal (VP) shunting systems are located proximal to the unidirectional valve and can be accessed percutaneously. The reservoirs are usually button-sized, measuring approximately 1 cm in diameter and 2 mm high and either are in the burr hole, directly affixed to the ventricular catheter (Fig. 24-4) or are an integral part of the valve system (Fig. 24-5).

Shunt reservoirs may be tapped to remove CSF to diagnose infection (ventriculitis) or to assess shunt patency. Absence of flow indicates obstruction of the ventricular catheter, a common cause of shunt failure. With flow present, a radionuclide can be injected to perform a "shunt flow study" to diagnose a complete or partial distal blockade.

Gloves, masks, antiseptic solution, razor, no. 23 and no. 25 needle (short hub or butterfly), tuberculin syringe, drapes, and sterile collecting tubes are readied. The procedure may be performed in the ER, ICU, treatment room, at bedside or in the nuclear medicine department. No special position is required as long as the reservoir is readily accessible. Sedation may be required for toddlers. Infants can be swaddled, and older children are usually cooperative. The reservoir is palpated and the overlying hair shaved to a diameter of approximately 25 mm. Reference to a skull radiograph may be needed to determine the appropriate location. Mask and gloves are donned and the skin cleansed with the antiseptic solution. No local anesthesia is used. The use of topical EMLA Cream (lidocaine 2.5% and prilocaine 2.5%, Astra Pharmaceutical) may require removal of an excessive amount of hair but may be considered. The needle is inserted perpendicular to the reservoir and through the scalp, usually no more than 2 to 3 mm. Cerebrospinal fluid is then collected if needed or the antibiotics or isotope injected. Aspiration should not be done routinely and should be done only under the supervision or with the approval of a neurosurgeon. After the needle is removed, the area should be gently digitally massaged for a minute.

Risks and complications of shunt reservoir aspiration include improper insertion, induction of infection, introduction of blood into the CSF, and bleeding from choroid plexus through too vigorous aspiration. Older shunting systems may not have reservoirs. When aspiration is indicated, the neurosurgeon may be able to aspirate the pumping segment of a cylindric valve or the shunt tubing itself.

Lumboperitoneal Shunt Aspiration. Lumboperitoneal shunts are placed via percutaneous insertion of the lumbar subarachnoid catheter or through a small superficial incision. Typically the shunt is tunneled in the subcutaneous tissue around the patient's flank to the abdomen, where another incision and dissection is performed to place the distal catheter into the peritoneal cavity. A reservoir or valve may be used and

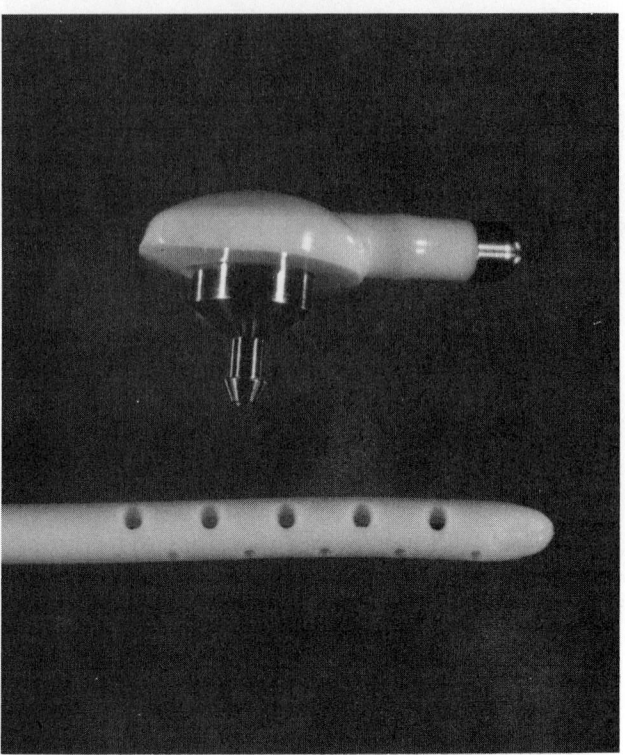

Fig. 24-4. Close-up view of Rickham reservoir in the calvarial opening, the funneled base connected directly to the proximal end of the ventricular catheter. The distal perforated end is shown.

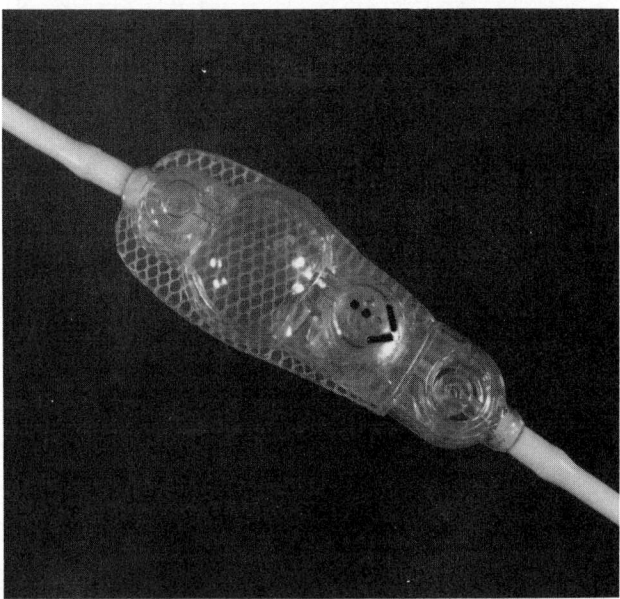

Fig. 24-5. A domed reservoir in series in one type of shunt valve. The large clear-domed area for puncture lies immediately proximal to the one-way valve.

is usually located on the lateral aspect of the flank. With careful palpation and recognition of the location of the two incisions, this portion of the tubing can usually be found, although it can be a difficult endeavor in an obese patient.

Aspiration is simple following positioning of the patient in the lateral decubitus position. A pillow resting under the dependent flank may be helpful. The skin is prepared using the antiseptic solution and a small needle is used without local anesthesia to perforate the reservoir and aspirate the CSF. Aspiration should be gentle, since aside from infection the most significant complication is nerve root irritation.

Ommaya and Other Reservoir Aspiration. Blind reservoirs are those that do not have a distal "runoff" system and consist only of a catheter located in a CSF-containing space (usually a ventricle) secured to a subcutaneous aspirating chamber or reservoir. They are placed only to access CSF and have no other transmitting function. In premature infants who weigh 800 to 2000 gm, reservoirs without shunts are frequently used to control hydrocephalus secondary to intraventricular hemorrhage prior to the insertion of a formal shunting system. They are tapped daily to attempt to maintain a stable ventricular size. Ommaya reservoirs are dome-shaped structures (Fig. 24-6), approximately 1 to 2 cm in diameter, with an access port coming from the base or side, placed subcutaneously, and connected to a ventricular catheter (Fig. 24-7) or, rarely, to a catheter that enters the lumbar thecal sac. These reservoirs are used to instill antibiotics in the treatment of bacterial ventriculomeningitis or chemotherapeutic agents for neoplasms of the CSF and for CSF analysis to monitor treatment.

To perform reservoir apiration, razor, gloves, mask, antiseptic solution, no. 23 or 25 butterfly needle, tuberculin and 3-ml syringes, appropriate sterile agents for instillation, drapes, and sterile collecting tubes are readied. A lumbar puncture set provides most of the needed materials. Reservoir aspiration may be performed in the ER, ICU, or treatment room or at the patient's bedside. The patient is positioned to expose the cranial or spinal reservoir. Sedation may be required for toddlers but is otherwise unnecessary. The reservoir is palpated (usually frontal scalp) and overlying hair generously shaved. Mask and gloves are donned and the area thoroughly prepared with an antiseptic solution. Sterile drapes are secured and the reservoir entered with a vertically oriented puncture. Cerebrospinal fluid is removed by gravity (aspiration is avoided, if possible) and can be sent for analysis or reinjection. A volume equal to that to be instilled should be removed. The antibiotic or chemotherapeutic agent is injected; 1 ml of CSF or sterile saline can be used to flush the dose into the ventricle, or the reservoir may be gently barbotaged to accomplish the same end—diffusion of the agent from the reservoir into the CSF spaces.

Risks and complications of reservoir aspiration include improper insertion, inability to obtain CSF, induction of infection, introduction of blood into the CSF, choroid plexus bleeding into the ventricle or (in the case of a lumbar reservoir) root symptoms with too vigorous aspiration, and chemical ependymitis or arachnoiditis.

VENTRICULOSTOMY. Ventricular catheterization is performed for diagnosis (e.g., cytology and neuroradiographic procedures, such as pneumoencephalography and ventriculography) and therapy, such as CSF drainage, treatment of intracranial hypertension, and administration of intrathecal chemotherapy or antibiotics.

Ventricular catheterization is performed by a neurosurgeon at the bedside in the ICU or in the operating room. The entry sites most commonly used are the coronal entry (Kocher's

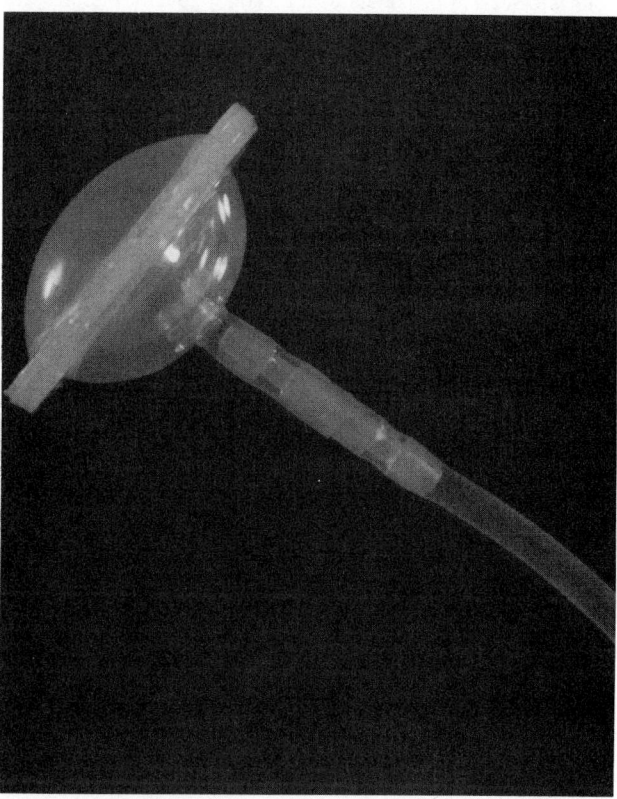

Fig. 24-6. Close-up view of a Ommaya double-domed reservoir, the caudal half of which is designed to lie within the burr hole.

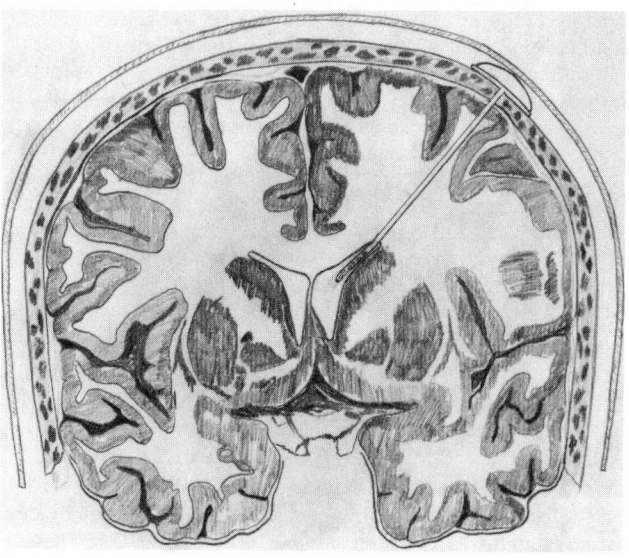

Fig. 24-7. Coronal section through the brain at the level of the frontal horns, illustrating the subgaleal/epicalvarial location at the Ommaya reservoir, with the distal ostia of the catheter lying within the ventricle.

point), located approximately at the midpupillary line just anterior to the coronal suture, and the occipital parietal approach, which is 4 cm from the midline and 6 cm above the inion. The frontal and occipital horns of the lateral ventricle are cannulated by these two approaches, respectively.

For the coronal approach, the patient is positioned supine with the head midline. For the occipital parietal approach the patient is positioned so the head is in the full lateral position. Premedication is usually not needed but may be helpful in the patient who is combative, extremely apprehensive, or unable to cooperate. Radiographic guidance is typically not required unless the ventricular catheter is placed using a stereotactic technique. Computed tomography stereotaxis is used to place ventricular catheters in patients whose ventricles are normally small or pathologically small (e.g., diffuse brain swelling, slit ventricle syndrome). This is common in patients with myeloproliferative disorders who require access for CSF surveillance or chemotherapeutic administration. Details regarding the techniques of placement are beyond the scope of this chapter.

Complications of ventriculostomy placement include meningitis or ventriculitis, scalp wound infection, intracranial hematoma, and failure to cannulate the ventricle.

LUMBAR DRAINAGE. Continuous CSF drainage via a lumbar catheter is useful in the treatment of CSF fistulas and as a provocative test to demonstrate the potential therapeutic effect of CSF shunting in patients with normal-pressure hydrocephalus, intracranial hypertension, or ventriculomegaly due to a failure in CSF absorption (e.g., SAH, infection).

Commercially available lumbar drainage kits, which are closed sterile systems that drain into a replaceable collection bag, are most convenient. Catheter placement is performed just as in lumbar puncture, but a large-bore Touhy needle is used, through which the proximal catheter is passed after CSF return is noted. Needle orientation is the same as in lumbar puncture and is probably more important, due to the size of the Touhy needle. Epidural catheter kits can also be used, though they tend to be slightly stiffer and have a narrower inner diameter.

Complications can include hemorrhage in the epidural space, introduction of infectious agents, inability to aspirate CSF, headache, persistent CSF leak, lumbosacral nerve root irritation, and, probably most serious, subdural hematoma due to CSF overdrainage. The potential for overdrainage is significant because the catheter has a relatively large caliber and because the amount of drainage depends on the cooperation of the nursing staff and patient: the drainage bag must not be lowered past a predetermined level (e.g., external auditory meatus to shoulder height). Subdural hematoma more commonly occurs in the elderly.

Summary

Of the various techniques for CSF aspiration, lumbar puncture is by far the most commonly performed by the general practitioner or intensivist. Other techniques may require the expertise or assistance of radiologic, neurologic, and neurosurgical colleagues.

References

1. Friedman AG, Mulhern RK, Fairclough D, et al: Midazolam premedication for pediatric bone marrow aspiration and lumbar puncture. *Med Pediatr Oncol* 19:499, 1991.

2. Edmeads J: Headache as a symptom of cerebrovascular disease. *Clin J Pain* 5:89, 1989.

3. Bigner SH: Cerebrospinal fluid (CSF) cytology: Current status and diagnostic applications. *J Neuropathol Exp Neurol* 51:235, 1992.

4. Yurdakok M, Kocabas CN: CSF erythrocyte volume analysis: A simple method for the diagnosis of traumatic tap in newborn infants. *Pediatr Neurosurg* 17:199, 1991–92.

5. Wood JH: Cerebrospinal fluid: Techniques of access and analytical interpretation, in Wilkins RH, Rengacharg SS (eds): *Neurosurgery.* New York, McGraw-Hill, 1985.

6. Greenlee JE: Approach to diagnosis of meningitis: Cerebrospinal fluid evaluation. *Infect Dis Clin North Am* 4:583, 1990.

7. Rodewald LE, Woodin KA, Szilagyi PG, et al: Relevance of common tests of cerebrospinal fluid in screening for bacterial meningitis. *J Pediatr* 119:363, 1991.

8. Schwersenski J, McIntyre L, Bauer CR: Lumbar puncture frequency and cerebrospinal fluid analysis in the neonate. *Am J Dis Child* 145:54, 1991.

9. Albeck MJ, Borgesen SE, Gjerris F, et al: Intracranial pressure and cerebrospinal fluid outflow conductance in healthy subjects. *J Neurosurg* 74:597, 1991.

10. Lundar T, Nornes H: Determination of ventricular fluid outflow resistance in patients with ventriculomegaly. *J Neurol Neurosurg Psychiatry* 53:896, 1990.

11. Tans JT, Poortvliet DC: Reduction of ventricular size after shunting for normal pressure hydrocephalus related to CSF dynamics before shunting. *J Neurol Neurosurg Psychiatry* 51:521, 1988.

12. Dhiravibulya K, Ouvrier R, Johnston I, et al: Benign intracranial hypertension in childhood: A review of 23 patients. *J Paediatr Child Health* 27:304, 1991.

13. Johnston I, Hawke S, Halmagyi J, et al: The pseudotumor syndrome: Disorders of cerebrospinal fluid circulation causing intracranial hypertension without ventriculomegaly. *Arch Neurol* 48:740, 1991.

14. Adams RD, Victor M: *Principles of Neurology.* 3rd ed., New York, McGraw-Hill, 1985.

15. Rogers LR, Duchesneau PM, Nunez C, et al: Comparison of cisternal and lumbar CSF examination in leptomeningeal metastasis. *J Neurol* 42:1239, 1992.

16. Bigner SH, Johnston WWW: The cytopathology of cerebrospinal fluid, I: Non-neoplastic condition, lymphoma and leukemia. *Acta Cytol* 25:335, 1981.

17. Thomas RS, Beuche W, Felgenhauer K: The proliferation rate of T and B lymphocytes in cerebrospinal fluid. *J Neurol* 238:27, 1991.

18. Onda K, Tanaka R, Takahashi H, et al: Cerebral glioblastoma with cerebrospinal fluid dissemination: A clinicopathological study of 14 cases examined by complete autopsy. *J Neurosurg* 25:533, 1989.

19. Fishman RA: *Cerebrospinal Fluid in Diseases of the Nervous System.* 2nd ed. Philadelphia, WB Saunders, 1992.

20. Bryce GE, Nedzelski JM, Rowed DW, et al: Cerebrospinal fluid leaks and meningitis in acoustic neuroma surgery. *Otolaryngol Head Neck Surg* 104:81, 1991.

21. Waisman M, Schweppe Y: Postoperative cerebrospinal fluid leakage after lumbar spine operations: Conservative treatment. *Spine* 16:52, 1991.

22. Agrillo U, Simonetti G, Martino V: Postoperative CSF problems after spinal and lumbar surgery: General review. *J Neurosurg Sci* 35:93, 1991.

23. Lyons MK, Meyer FB: Cerebrospinal fluid physiology and the management of increased intracranial pressure. *Mayo Clin Proc* 65:684, 1990.

24. Nakagawa H, Murasawa A, Kubo S, et al: Diagnosis and treatment of patients with meningeal carcinomatosis. *J Neurooncol* 13:81, 1992.

25. Porter FL, Miller JP, Cole FS, et al: A controlled clinical trial of local anesthesia for lumbar punctures in newborns [see comments]. *Pediatrics* 88:663, 1991.

26. Davidson RI: Lumbar puncture, in VanderSalm TJ (ed): *Atlas of Bedside Procedures.* 2nd ed. Boston, Little Brown, 1988.

27. Wilkinson HA: Technical note: Anesthesia for lumbar puncture. *JAMA* 249:2177, 1983.

28. van DeKelft E, Bosmans J, Parizel P, et al: Intracerebral hemorrhage after lumbar myelography with iohexol: Report of a case and review of the literature. *Neurosurgery* 28:570, 1991.

29. Ellis RW III, Strauss LC, Wiley JM, et al: A simple method of esti-

mating cerebrospinal fluid pressure during lumbar puncture. *Pediatrics* 89:895, 1992.

30. Scott EW, Cazenave CR, Virapongse C: Spinal subarachnoid hematoma complicating lumbar puncture: Diagnosis and management. *Neurosurgery* 25:287, 1989.
31. Grant R, Condon B, Hart I, et al: Changes in intracranial CSF volume after lumbar puncture and their relationship to post-LP headache. *J Neurol Neurosurg Psychiatry* 54:440, 1991.
32. Wilkinson AG, Sellar RJ: The influence of needle size and other factors on the incidence of adverse effects caused by myelography. *Clin Radiol* 44:338, 1991.
33. A prospective double-blind clinical trial, comparing the sharp Quincke needle (22G) with an "atraumatic" needle (22G) in the induction of post-lumbar puncture headache. *Acta Neurol Scand* 86:50, 1992.
34. Johnson JC, Deeb ZL: Coaxial needle technique for lumbar puncture in the morbidly obese patient. *Radiology* 179:874, 1991.

35. Lee T, Maynard N, Anslow P, et al: Post-myelogram headache: Physiological or psychological? *Neuroradiology* 33:155, 1991.
36. Barrios-Alarcon J, Aldrete JA, Paragas-Tapia D: Relief of post-lumbar puncture headache with epidural dextran 40: A preliminary report. *Regional Anesth* 14:78, 1989.
37. Walsted A, Salomon G, Thomsen J: Hearing decrease after loss of cerebrospinal fluid: A new hydrops model? *Acta Otolaryngol* 111:468, 1991.
38. Michel O, Brusis T: Hearing loss as a sequel of lumbar puncture. *Ann Otol Rhinol Laryngol* 101:390, 1992.
39. Wong MC, Krol G, Rosenblum MK: Occult epidural chloroma complicated by acute paraplegia following lumbar puncture. *Ann Neurol* 31:110, 1992.
40. Mutoh S, Aikou I, Ueda S: Spinal coning after lumbar puncture in prostate cancer with asymptomatic vertebral metastasis: A case report. *J Urol* 145:834, 1991.

25. Neurologic and Intracranial Pressure Monitoring

Donald S. Prough and Donald Deyo

Central nervous system (CNS) disease is common in neurologic and neurosurgical as well as general medical-surgical intensive care units (ICUs). Despite the large number of patients with such diverse diseases as traumatic brain injury, subarachnoid hemorrhage, stroke, and postischemic encephalopathy, clinical neurologic monitoring remains as rudimentary as systemic hemodynamic monitoring was two decades ago. Most clinical management protocols rely on inferences from normal physiology supplemented by fragmentary brain-specific data, usually nothing more than intracranial pressure (ICP) and systemic blood pressure. Although clinical experience suggests that morbidity and mortality can be altered by therapeutic alteration of cerebral blood flow (CBF) and cerebral metabolism in some neurologically injured patients, no data confirm the general clinical utility of neurologic monitoring. Intuitively, monitoring of systemic hemodynamics and gas exchange would seem to be more important than brain-specific monitoring, because of the exquisite sensitivity of the injured brain to decreases in cerebral oxygen delivery.

Current neurologic monitoring equipment is often costly, cumbersome, and dependent on highly skilled technicians; many techniques are applied primarily as research tools rather than routine clinical monitors. An impressive array of devices is currently available or under development. Some offer an unprecedented opportunity to recognize impending neurologic injury and, ideally, to reduce morbidity and mortality. However, technologic developments in the 1990s require demanding evaluation, incorporating traditional methods, such as the randomized clinical trial, but adding broader and more complex assessments of effectiveness, quality of life, patient preferences, and costs and benefits [1].

This chapter reviews the techniques currently available for neurologic monitoring and summarizes their use in several common neurologic and neurosurgical diseases. Throughout the chapter, three questions should be constantly in mind:

1. Under what circumstances do blood pressure, arterial carbon dioxide tension ($PaCO_2$), arterial oxygen tension (PaO_2), and body temperature provide insufficient information about the adequacy of cerebral oxygen delivery ($CBF \times CaO_2$)?
2. Under what circumstances does more precise information about the adequacy of cerebral oxygen delivery permit therapeutic interventions that improve outcome?
3. Is the proportion of patients in a specific diagnostic category who will develop avoidable injury sufficiently large to justify extensive (and potentially expensive) application of neurologic monitoring devices?

Goals of Brain Monitoring

Monitoring devices cannot independently improve outcome—they can only contribute to decreased morbidity and mortality by providing physiologic data that can be integrated into a more effective therapeutic plan (Fig. 25-1). Neurologic monitoring falls into two distinct categories. The first category, which includes electroencephalography and evoked potential monitoring, defines a qualitative threshold beyond which additional morbidity becomes likely. The second category, which includes monitors of ICP, CBF, and cerebral metabolism, provides quantitative physiologic information. Such devices can potentially define a threshold for intervention that provides a margin of safety between the level at which neurologic injury might occur and the level at which treatment can be implemented. For instance, pulse oximeters, which monitor a critical aspect of brain oxygenation, are widely applied in critically ill patients. The threshold of hemoglobin (Hgb) saturation below which tissue hypoxia becomes likely varies among individuals but is less than 75 percent (equivalent to $PaO_2 < 40$ mm Hg) in otherwise

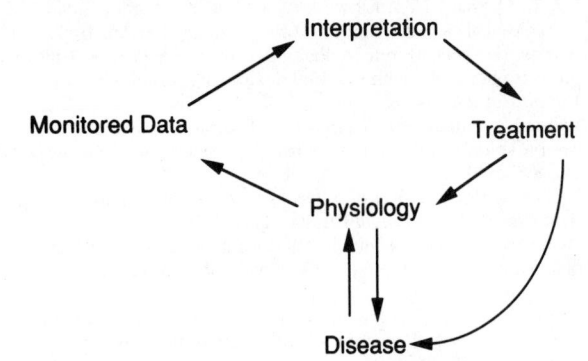

Fig. 25-1. Monitored data are dynamically integrated into the management of critical neurologic illness. Acute neurologic disease produces alterations in physiology that are detected by monitors. The monitored data are then interpreted and, based on that interpretation, incorporated into a treatment plan. Treatment may alter the disease process or physiologic expression of the disease process. In turn, monitored data will change as a consequence of therapy. (From Prough DS: Neurologic monitoring, in Carlson RW, Geheb MA (eds): *Principles & Practices of Medical Intensive Care.* Philadelphia, WB Saunders, 1993, p 222. With permission.)

healthy persons. However, the threshold for intervention, the Hgb saturation below which most clinicians usually change treatment, is 90 percent.

Quantitative physiologic monitors may therefore be used to develop and test therapeutic goals that substantially exceed minimally acceptable levels. For instance, Bland and colleagues defined a threshold for systemic oxygen delivery (cardiac output × CaO$_2$) at 600 ml O$_2$/min/m^2, below which mortality and morbidity increase in high-risk surgical patients [2,3]. Subsequently, by using that value as a threshold above which systemic oxygen delivery was maintained by hemodynamic support, Shoemaker et al. demonstrated a decline in mortality and morbidity in comparison to patients managed without reference to the threshold [4]. That strategy provides a model for the definition of critical and interventional thresholds. Nevertheless, few data define thresholds for intervention for neurologic monitoring devices or even quantify the relationship between monitored variables and the risk of preventable neurologic injury.

Cerebral Ischemia

Virtually all neurologic monitors are intended to detect actual or possible cerebral ischemia. Cerebral ischemia, defined as cerebral oxygen delivery (CDO$_2$) insufficient to meet metabolic needs, can result from a critical reduction of any of the components of CDO$_2$, including CBF, Hgb concentration, and arterial Hgb saturation (SaO$_2$). The brain constitutes only 2 percent of total body weight but receives 15 percent of cardiac output and accounts for 15 to 20 percent of total oxygen consumption (Table 25-1). Certain regions of the brain, such as the cerebellum, the basal ganglia, the CA-1 layer of the hippocampus, and the arterial boundary zones between major branches of the intracranial vessels, appear to be selectively vulnerable to ischemic injury [5].

The severity of ischemic brain damage is proportional to the magnitude and duration of the lowering of CDO$_2$. In monkeys, paralysis develops if regional CBF declines below about 23 ml/

Table 25-1. Comparison of Systemic and Cerebral Oxygenation Variables

Variable	Systemic	Cerebral
Blood flow (ml/100 gm/min)	7.0	50
Oxygen consumption (ml/100 gm/min)	0.3	3.4
Oxygen delivery (ml/100 gm/min)	1.4	10
AVDO$_2$ (ml O$_2$/100 ml)	5.0	7.0
Venous saturation (%)	75	65

100 gm/min [6]. Infarction of brain tissue, however, requires that CBF remain below 18 ml/100 gm/min [6]. Therefore, prolonged paralysis is potentially reversible if the paralysis is associated with CBF values of 18 to 23 ml/100 gm/min. The tolerable duration of more profound ischemia is inversely proportional to the severity of CBF reduction; that is, CBF less than 10 ml/100 gm/min for 2 hours results in infarction (Fig. 25-2).

Cerebral ischemia is traditionally characterized as focal or global and complete or incomplete (Table 25-2). From a practical standpoint, a clinically useful brain monitor should detect focal cerebral ischemia. Most global cerebral insults, such as hypotension, hypoxemia, and cardiac arrest, are readily detected by systemic monitors. Therefore, brain-specific monitors can provide additional information primarily in situations in which regional cerebral oxygenation may be impaired despite adequate systemic oxygenation and perfusion, such as stroke, subarachnoid hemorrhage (SAH) with vasospasm, and cerebral trauma.

Fig. 25-2. Schematic representation of ischemic thresholds in awake monkeys. The threshold for reversible paralysis occurs at a local cerebral blood flow (l CBF) of approximately 23 ml/100 gm/min. Irreversible injury (infarction) is a function of the magnitude of blood flow reduction and the duration of that reduction. Relatively severe ischemia is potentially reversible if the duration is sufficiently short. (From Jones TH, Morawetz RB, Crowell RM, et al: Thresholds of focal cerebral ischemia in awake monkeys. *J Neurosurg* 54:773, 1981. With permission.)

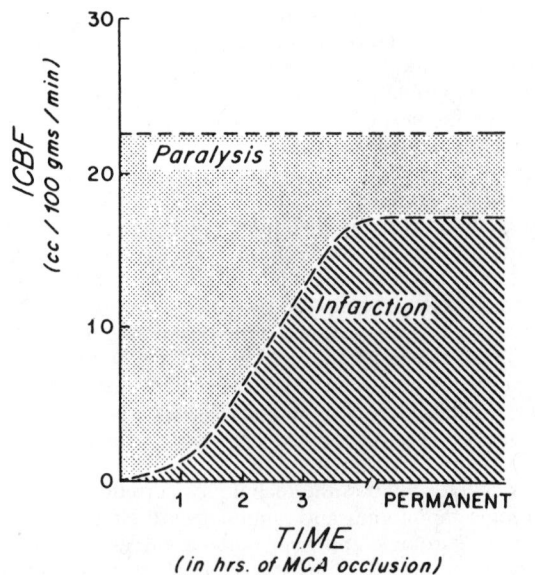

Table 25-2. Characteristics of Cerebral Ischemic Insults

Characteristics	Examples
Global, incomplete	Hypotension, hypoxemia, cardiopulmonary resuscitation
Global, complete	Cardiac arrest
Focal, incomplete	Stroke, subarachnoid hemorrhage with vasospasm

Table 25-3. Neurologic Monitoring Approaches

Cerebral perfusion	Cerebral oxygen extraction	Cerebral function
Cerebral blood flow	Jugular bulb saturation	EEG
Cerebral blood flow velocity	Near-infrared spectroscopy	Raw
Intracranial pressure		Processed
		Evoked potentials

Cerebral ischemia may necessitate ICU admission or may develop during the course of hospitalization. Nevertheless, the value of brain monitoring has been poorly defined in most critical neurologic and neurosurgical illness. Many clinicians assume that ischemic damage (e.g., that associated with stroke or cardiac arrest) is irreversible by the time patients are first seen by a physician. In addition, many brain monitors, such as those that record CBF, ICP, and computer-processed electroencephalograms (EEG), require specifically trained technicians. Therefore, no generally accepted protocols have been developed that establish clinically important thresholds for intervention, that define appropriate therapeutic interventions, and that have been demonstrated to improve outcome. In the absence of such protocols, highly individualized approaches have arisen.

Techniques of Neurologic Monitoring

Brain monitors directly or indirectly assess cerebral perfusion, cerebral oxygen extraction, or cerebral function (Table 25-3). Brain monitors can be classified in terms of the validity of the measurements performed and in terms of the ease with which monitored information can be incorporated into the clinical reasoning process (Table 25-4). The design and use of monitoring devices necessitate trade-offs among various performance characteristics. For instance, a monitor with high positive predictive value (i.e., that falls outside threshold values only when cerebral ischemia is unequivocally present) is unlikely to detect less profound ischemia. A monitor that is highly sensitive to changes in cerebral oxygenation will frequently warn of small changes that are unlikely to produce brain injury. For example, pulse oximetry frequently demonstrates transient declines in SaO_2 that would result in no adverse sequelae were no action taken. Presumably, prompt correction of episodes of desaturation that would result in no harm in most patients will avoid unexpected injury in an occasional patient.

Practical use of brain monitors requires definition of critical thresholds at which therapeutic interventions should be undertaken. Thresholds of CBF that correlate with various clinical outcomes, physiologic changes, and changes in monitored variables have been defined based upon animal experiments [6–9] and to a lesser extent on clinical data [10] (Table 25-5). If a monitor of brain function detects cerebral ischemia, the actual severity is not established. All that is known is that cerebral oxygenation in a region of brain that contributes to that function has fallen below a critical threshold. The shortfall could be slight or severe. Because more severe ischemia will produce neurologic injury in less time, it is impossible to predict with certainty whether changes in function will be followed by cerebral infarction. In addition, if regional ischemia involves structures that do not participate in the monitored function, infarction could develop without warning. This predictable relationship no doubt explains the failure of monitors to detect cerebral ische-

Table 25-4. Glossary of Neurologic Monitor Characteristics

Term	Definition
Bias	Average difference (positive or negative) between monitored values and "gold standard" values
Precision	Standard deviation of the differences (bias) between measurements
Sensitivity	Probability that the monitor will demonstrate cerebral ischemia when cerebral ischemia is present
Positive predictive value	Probability that cerebral ischemia is present when the monitor suggests cerebral ischemia
Specificity	Probability that the monitor will not demonstrate cerebral ischemia when cerebral ischemia is not present
Negative predictive value	Probability that cerebral ischemia is not present when the monitor reflects no cerebral ischemia
Threshold value	The value used to separate acceptable (i.e., no ischemia present) from unacceptable (i.e., ischemia present)
Speed	The time elapsed from the onset of actual ischemia or the risk of ischemia until the monitor provides evidence

Source: Prough DS: Brain monitoring. In Shoemaker W, Taylor R (eds): *Critical Care: State of the Art*. vol. 12. Fullerton, CA, Society of Critical Care Medicine, 1991.

Table 25-5. Clinical, Pathophysiologic, and Monitoring Thresholds in Cerebral Ischemia

CBF ($ml \cdot 100g^{-1} \cdot min^{-1}$)	Clinical	Pathophysiologic Changes	Monitored Changes
50	Normal		
23	Reversible paralysis		EEG slowing, EP change
20		Na^+/K^+ pump dysfunction	
18	Infarction		EEG flat
15			EP absent
10		K^+ efflux, Ca^{++} influx	

Source: Prough DS: Brain monitoring. In Shoemaker W, Taylor R (eds): *Critical Care: State of the Art*. vol. 12. Fullerton, CA, Society of Critical Care Medicine, 1991.

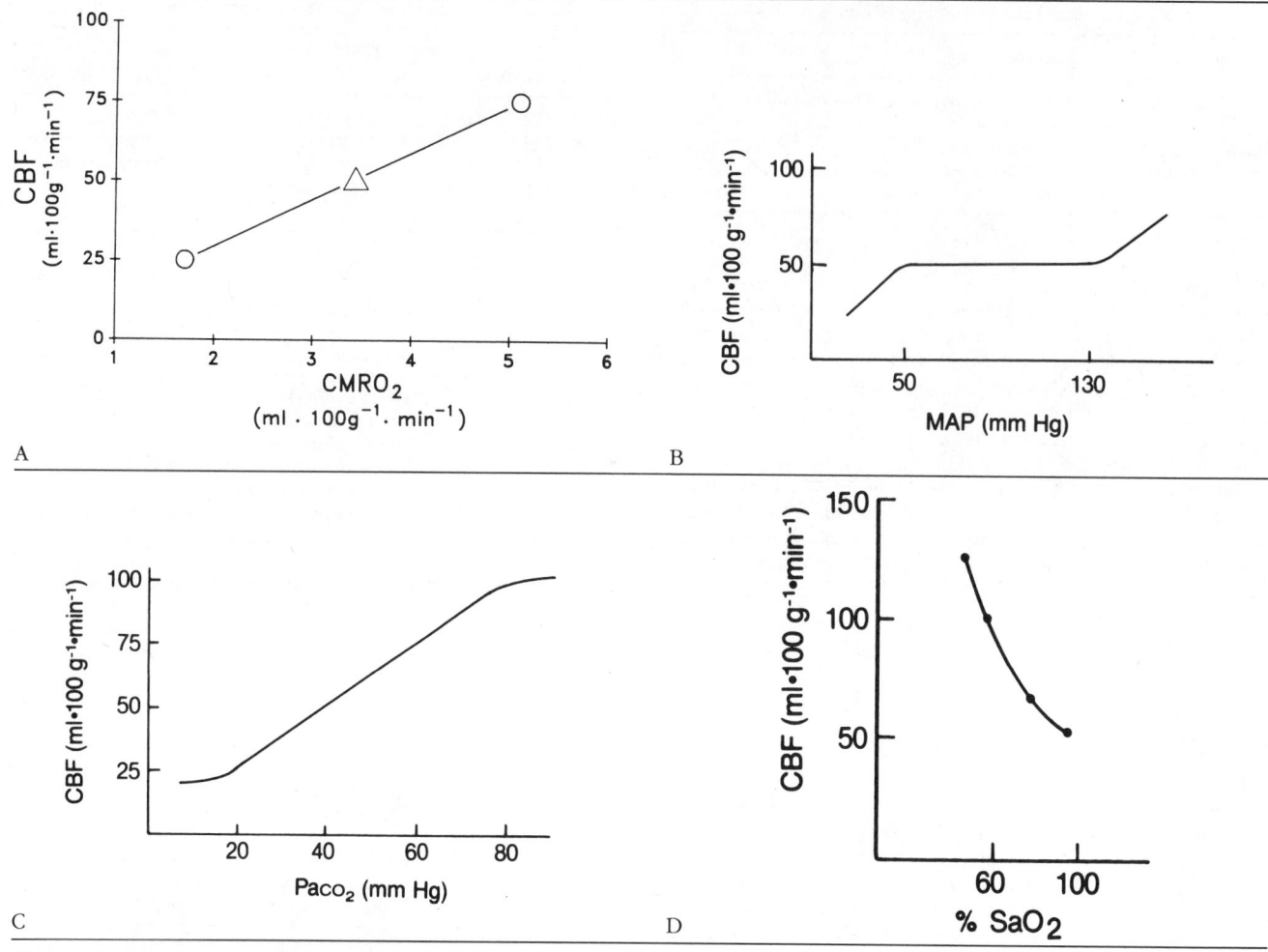

Fig. 25-3. **A.** The normal relationship between the cerebral metabolic rate of oxygen consumption (CMRO$_2$) and cerebral blood flow (CBF) is characterized by closely coupled changes in both variables. Normally, CBF is 50 ml/100 gm/min at a CMRO$_2$ of 3.4 ml/100 gm/min in adults (open triangle). As CMRO$_2$ increases or decreases, CBF changes in a parallel fashion (solid line). (From Butterworth JF IV, Prough DS, Head trauma, in Rippe JR, Irwin RS, Alpert JS, et al (eds): *Intensive Care Medicine,* 2nd ed. Boston, Little, Brown, 1991. With permission.) **B.** Effect of mean arterial pressure (MAP) on cerebral blood flow (CBF). Note that changes in MAP produce little change in CBF over a broad range of pressures. If intracranial pressure (ICP) exceeds normal limits, substitute cerebral perfusion pressure (CPP) on the horizontal axis. **C.** Effect of PaCO$_2$ on cerebral blood flow (CBF). Changes in PaCO$_2$ exert powerful effects on cerebral vascular resistance across the entire clinically applicable range of values. **D.** Effect of arterial oxygen saturation (SaO$_2$) on cerebral blood flow (CBF). Extreme changes in SaO$_2$ cause reciprocal changes in CBF.

mia in patients who subsequently develop clinical evidence of brain infarction as well as reports of profound changes in monitored variables that are followed by no apparent change in clinical condition. The complexity and heterogeneity of brain tissue virtually preclude development of a single, perfectly predictive brain monitor.

CARDIORESPIRATORY MONITORING. Neurologic function is easily disrupted by alterations of nutrient supply or biochemical milieu. In critically ill neurologic patients, routine

monitoring, including arterial blood gases, blood pressure, and electrolytes, permits early detection and treatment. Blood pressure monitoring and pulse oximetry provide important clues about the adequacy of global brain oxygenation. Cerebral blood flow is controlled in normal persons by metabolic demand, pressure autoregulation, PaCO$_2$, and CaO$_2$. Figure 25-3A depicts the normal "coupled" relationship in which CBF is dependent on the cerebral metabolic rate for oxygen (CMRO$_2$). Metabolic demand varies directly with body temperature and the level of brain activation, examples being increases in CMRO$_2$ produced by fever, seizures, or pain. Changes in cerebral perfusion pressure (CPP) (or mean arterial pressure [MAP] if ICP is normal) do not alter CBF over a range of pressures of about 50 to 130 mm Hg (Fig. 25-3B) [11,12]. Normally, PaCO$_2$ powerfully regulates cerebral vascular resistance over a range of PaCO$_2$ of 20 to 80 mm Hg (Fig. 25-3C). Cerebral blood flow is acutely halved if PaCO$_2$ is halved and doubles if PaCO$_2$ doubles. Pulse oximetry monitors arterial oxygen saturation SaO$_2$, a primary determinant of CaO$_2$ and therefore CDO$_2$. The brain normally increases CBF in response to decreasing CaO$_2$, whether the reduction is secondary to a decrease in Hgb or in SaO$_2$ (Fig. 25-3D) [13–16]. Consequently, brain-specific monitors are of greatest value in patients in whom global or regional CBF cannot increase in response to either decreasing oxygen supply or increasing metabolic requirements.

Rising blood pressure, bradycardia, and respiratory irregularities constitute Cushing's triad, a manifestation of rising ICP.

However, many patients who have acute brain disease have elevated circulating levels of catecholamines, which may cause hypertension independent of ICP. Heart rate, a variable component of the triad, often fails to show the expected vagally induced decrease, despite intracranial hypertension. Respiratory irregularities will not be apparent in patients who receive neuromuscular blockers or mechanical ventilation.

NEUROLOGIC EXAMINATION. Frequent, accurately recorded neurologic examinations are an essential aspect of neurologic monitoring. Ideally, any neurologic examination will include a meaningful, easily interpreted description of the patient's ability to interact with the environment. Neurologic examination quantifies two key characteristics: changes in consciousness and focal brain dysfunction. The state of consciousness and the trend in neurologic function are the most important indications of the severity of neurologic disease and the most important predictors of survival. Comparable levels of consciousness imply different prognoses in patients who are improving versus those who are deteriorating.

The Glasgow Coma Scale (GCS), originally developed as a prognostic tool and a way to compare series of patients in different institutions [17], has become popular as a quick, reproducible estimate of level of consciousness in critically ill patients (Table 25-6). The scale, which includes observations regarding eye opening, motor response in the "best" limb, and verbal responses, is less useful in intubated patients who cannot make verbal responses. At a minimum, the GCS score should be supplemented by recording pupillary size and reactivity and the status of focal neurologic findings.

Impaired consciousness is nonspecific; however, recognition of changing consciousness may warn of a variety of treatable conditions, including progression of intracranial hypertension, developing vasospasm in patients after SAH, delayed posttraumatic intracranial hematomas, and systemic complications of intracranial pathology, such as hyponatremia, hypoxemia, and hypercarbia. Focal neurologic findings often suggest a specific lesion; that is, unilateral weakness or reflex changes developing after carotid endarterectomy suggest the possibility of ipsilateral carotid occlusion.

Table 25-6. Glasgow Coma Scale

Component	Response	Score
Eye opening	Spontaneously	4
	To verbal command	3
	To pain	2
	None	1
		Subtotal: 1–4
Motor response (best extremity)	Obeys verbal command	6
	Localizes pain	5
	Flexion—withdrawal	4
	Flexor (decorticate posturing)	3
	Extensor (decerebrate posturing)	2
	No response (flaccid)	1
		Subtotal: 1–6
Best verbal response	Oriented and converses	5
	Disoriented and converses	4
	Inappropriate words	3
	Incomprehensible sounds	2
	No verbal response	1
		Subtotal: 1–5
		Total: 3–15

NEUROIMAGING. Although the explosive growth of sophisticated neuroimaging techniques has revolutionized the initial evaluation of patients who have life-threatening neurologic and neurosurgical conditions, these devices do not function as monitors per se. Rather, they provide a rapid means of diagnosing sudden deteriorations in neurologic status, whether evident on neurologic examination or changes in a monitored physiologic variable. Examples of acute pathology evident on computed tomography (CT) and magnetic resonance imaging (MRI) are presented in Chapter 175.

Cerebral CT and MRI scans are indicated in response to reasonable suspicion that a new or progressive anatomic lesion will be evident and that recognition of that change is likely to alter treatment. Examples include new or expanded subdural hematomas and intracerebral hemorrhage. However, CT scanning has several limitations. First, CT scans provide information about brain structure, not function; important, treatable conditions may not be evident. Second, unlike physiologic monitors, CT scans provide static, infrequent data. Third, moving a critically ill patient to a CT scanner necessitates considerable investment of personnel and substantial risk to the patient. Often, MRI scans provide better resolution than CT scans. However, utility in critically ill patients is impaired by the incompatibility of MRI with ferrous metals, a ubiquitous component of ventilators, monitors, and infusion pumps. Both CT and MRI scans require an extended interval in which the ability of personnel to observe and treat patients is limited.

In patients with clinical evidence of brain death, confirmatory studies should be rapidly available, portable, and specific for irreversible brain damage. Cerebral flow studies (the initial component of radionuclide brain scans) can document cessation of CBF and have generally replaced repeated electroencephalography for confirmation of brain death [18].

CEREBRAL BLOOD FLOW MONITORING

Xenon[133] Clearance. The first quantitative method for the measurement of human CBF was the Kety-Schmidt technique [19,20], in which global CBF was calculated from the difference between the arterial and jugular bulb saturation curves of an inhaled, inert gas. Shortly thereafter, techniques were developed that measured regional cortical CBF using an intraarterially injected radioisotope such as Xenon[133] (^{133}Xe) [21,22]. The washout curves are determined by placing one or multiple collimated scintillation counters or gamma detectors close to the scalp and measuring the counts for each detector over time, usually 11 to 15 minutes. The biological half-life of the gas in brain tissue is proportional to blood flow. Clearance from extracranial tissues is considered insignificant in proportion to cortical flow. Concerns regarding the risk of carotid puncture prompted the development of techniques that measured cortical CBF after inhaled [23,24] or intravenous administration of ^{133}Xe, using gamma counting of exhaled gas to correct clearance curves for recirculation of [133]Xe (Figs. 25-4 and 25-5). Currently, the inhalation and intravenous techniques are most commonly employed, because neither requires placement of arterial catheters or jugular venous bulb catheters.

[133]Xe clearance estimates of regional cortical CBF represent a powerful research technique. Nevertheless, few clinicians have used the technique for primary diagnosis, surveillance, or goal-directed management. Among the obstacles to wider use of ^{133}Xe clearance are the cumbersome regulations governing the administration of radionuclides, the technically demanding nature of the measurements, and the sustained stable conditions (5–15 minutes) required to perform a single measurement.

Transcranial Doppler Flow Velocity. Arterial flow velocity can be readily measured in intracranial vessels, especially the

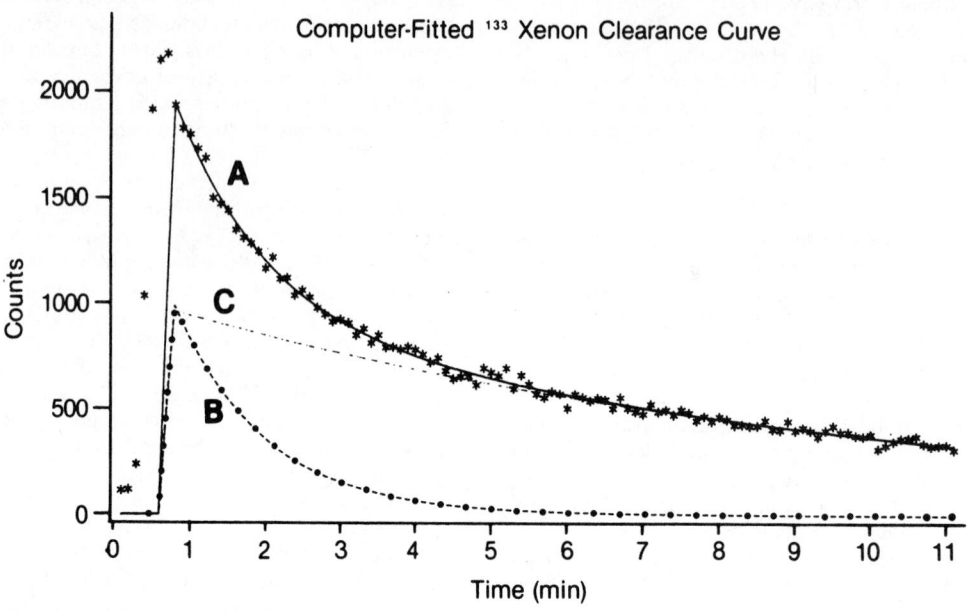

Fig. 25-4. ^{133}Xe clearance curve after intraarterial injection. After rapid bolus arrival in the cerebral circulation, clearance of the radioisotope usually is biexponential. The asterisks represent actual counted gamma emissions with the computer-fitted, computer-smoothed curve (A) superimposed. The rapidly clearing compartment (predominantly gray matter flow) is represented by curve B. The slowly clearing compartment is designated C. (From Prough DS, Michenfelder JD: Cerebral blood flows and metabolism, in Cerra FB, Shoemaker WC (eds): *Critical Care: State of the Art.* vol. 8. Fullerton, CA, Society of Critical Care Medicine, 1987, pp 43–70. With permission.)

middle cerebral artery (MCA), in most patients using transcranial Doppler (TCD) equipment. Transcranial Doppler measurements initially appeared to offer useful diagnostic information in a variety of acute and chronic cerebrovascular problems.

Doppler flow velocity utilizes the shift in frequency observed when a sound wave is reflected by a moving substance, in this case red blood cells. The frequency shift is higher for high flow velocities and low for low velocities. Blood moving toward the transducer shifts the transmitted frequency to higher frequencies and blood moving away to lower frequencies.

Usually the middle cerebral artery or the retinal artery is insonated. The resultant velocity waveform appears similar to the pulsatile arterial waveform. Transcranial Doppler assesses blood flow *velocity* rather than blood flow per se. Velocity is a function not only of blood flow rate but also of vessel diameter. If the arterial diameter changes, changes in velocity will not correlate with changes in flow. If the diameter of the middle cerebral artery remains constant, changes in velocity are proportional to changes in CBF measured using ^{133}Xe clearance; however, intersubject differences in flow velocity correlate poorly with intersubject differences in CBF measured using ^{133}Xe clearance (Fig. 25-6) [25].

As a monitor for patients at risk for ischemic cerebral complications, TCD appears promising. Entirely noninvasive, TCD measurements can be repeated at frequent intervals or even applied continuously. Therefore, TCD could potentially be used not only as a diagnostic and prognostic tool, but as a surveillance monitor and an essential component of goal-directed therapy. However, further work is necessary to define those situations in which the excellent capacity for rapid trend monitoring should be exploited. One possible approach is to combine intermittent ^{133}Xe clearance measurements with continuous TCD monitoring. In effect, ^{133}Xe clearance measurements could be used to "calibrate" the TCD, improving its quantitative value in individual patients.

Thermal Diffusion. The loss of thermal energy from heated tissue is proportional to the blood flow (assuming the blood is cooler than the tissue) adjacent to a thermal detector [26,27,28]. In this technique, a thermal transducer is placed in contact with the brain surface. The device heats the brain surface very slightly; circulating blood carries away the added thermal energy. Because the device determines CBF in one small region of cortex, the technique provides potentially important monitoring information in states in which global CBF would be expected to change in parallel with monitored flow or in which a specific region at risk for ischemia can be identified. The necessity of surgical placement and maintenance of an invasive intracranial device carries a risk of infection.

Intracranial Pressure Monitoring. Because of the spatial constraints imposed by the rigid skull, the brain, cerebrospinal fluid, and cerebral blood volume have little room to expand without increasing ICP. Although intracranial hypertension contributes to morbidity and mortality in such diverse diseases as traumatic brain injury, SAH, stroke, and postischemic encephalopathy, clinical estimates of ICP cannot provide accurate information. The symptoms and signs of raised ICP are neither sensitive nor specific. However, certain findings suggest evidence of intracranial hypertension. Cushing's triad (hypertension, bradycardia, and respiratory irregularity) suggests the possibility of severely increased ICP, although its absence does not exclude intracranial hypertension. Neither does hypertension in patients with acute brain disease necessarily imply increased ICP. In patients with traumatic coma, a GCS score of 4 to 6 suggests a high probability of increased ICP. Patients at risk for intracranial hypertension who have a decreasing level of consciousness probably have increased ICP. In the final stages of intracranial hypertension, patients typically progess through stages of progressively poorer responsiveness; if this is not interrupted it usually culminates in pupillary dilation and brain

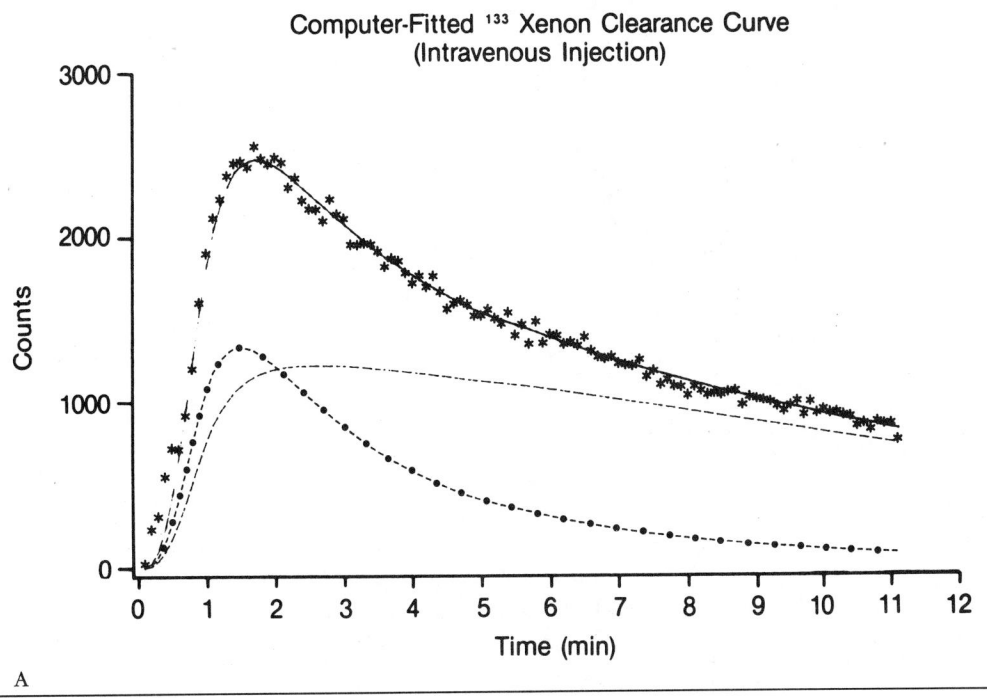

Computer-Fitted ¹³³ **Xenon Clearance Curve**
(Intravenous Injection)

A

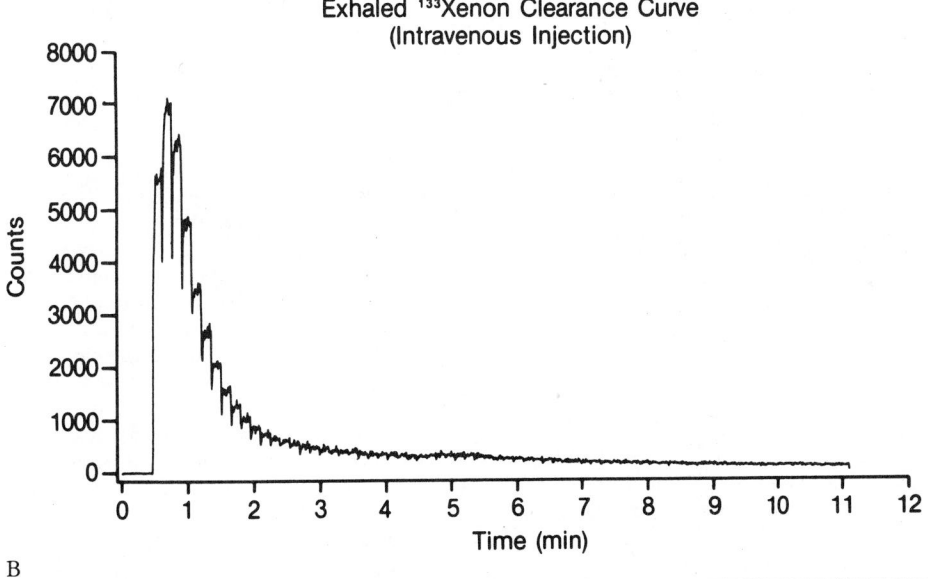

Exhaled ¹³³**Xenon Clearance Curve**
(Intravenous Injection)

B

Fig. 25-5. **A.** In contrast to the ¹³³Xe clearance curve generated by intraarterial injection, an intravenous injection produces a later, broader peak in the gamma emission rate. Because larger doses are necessary for intravenous studies, recirculation of ¹³³Xe slows the clearance rate. **B.** Correction of the ¹³³Xe clearance curve for recirculation requires estimation of the decline in arterial ¹³³Xe clearance by counting the rate of gamma emissions in end-tidal exhaled gas. (From Prough DS, Michenfelder JD: Cerebral blood flows and metabolism: Implications for clinical monitoring, in Cerra FB, Shoemaker WC (eds): *Critical Care: State of the Art*. vol. 8. Fullerton, CA, Society of Critical Care Medicine, 1987, pp 43–70. With permission.)

death. In effect, the physical findings associated with increasing ICP become apparent only when intracranial hypertension is sufficiently severe to injure the brain. The probability of increased ICP is less if patients moan, grimace, or withdraw to painful stimuli. Patients able to follow simple commands rarely have clinically important intracranial hypertension.

Because ICP cannot be adequately assessed by physical examination or intermittent neurologic imaging techniques, direct measurement and monitoring of ICP has become a common intervention. During the development of ICP monitoring, multiple sites and technologies have been employed. Short-term and long-term measurement and monitoring have been performed in the lumbar or cervical subarachnoid space, lateral cerebral ventricles, subdural (subarachnoid) space, epidural

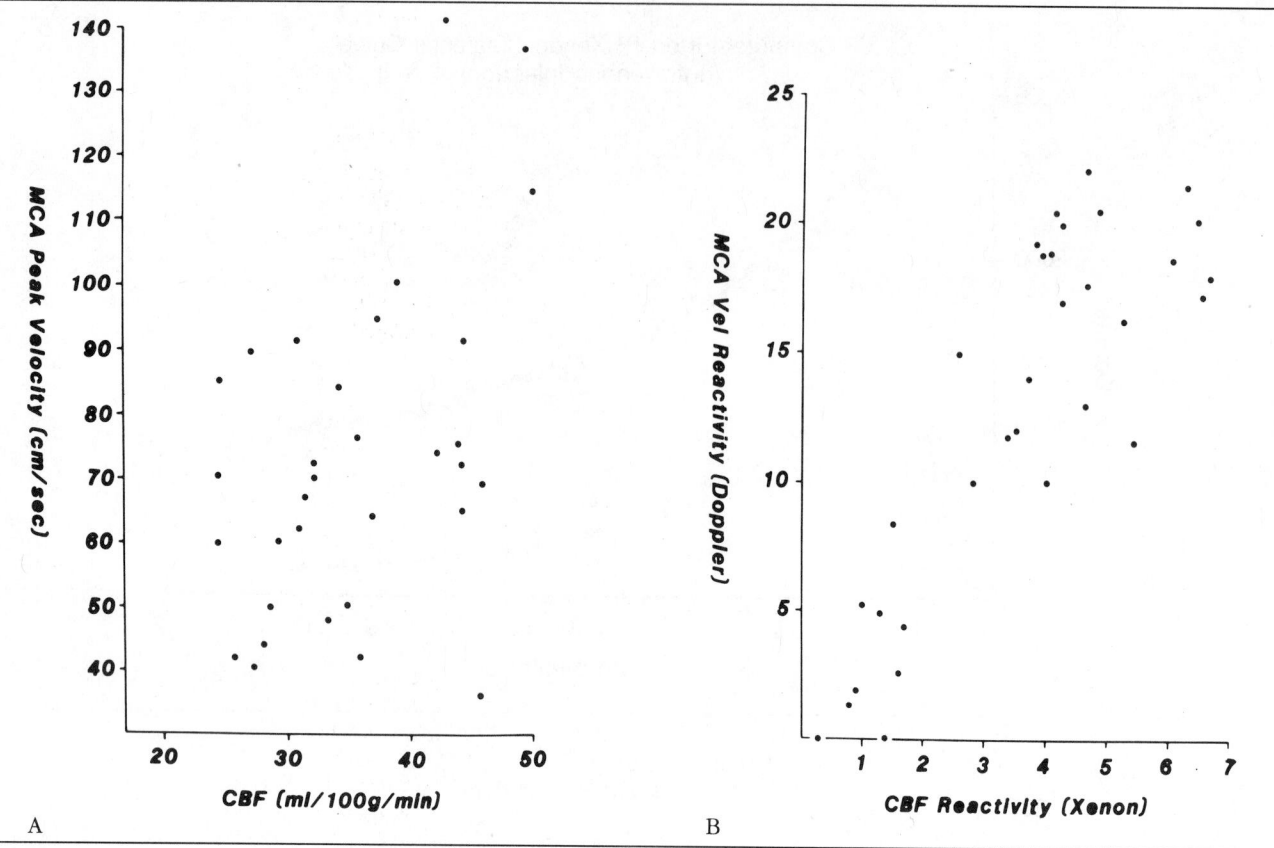

Fig. 25-6. **A.** Relationship between cerebral blood flow (CBF), measured using ^{133}Xe, and peak flow velocity in the middle cerebral artery (MCA), measured using the transcranial Doppler. The intersubject correlation is poor (r = 0.0424). **B.** Reactivity to changes in $PaCO_2$ demonstrates that intrasubject changes in CBF, measured using ^{133}Xe, correlate better with changes in MCA peak velocity (r = 0.489). (Reproduced with permission. Bishop CCR, Powell S, Rutt D, et al: Transcranial Doppler measurement of middle cerebral artery blood flow velocity: A validation study. *Stroke* 17:913, 1986. Copyright 1986 American Heart Association.)

space, transcutaneously over open fontanels in infants [29], and in the brain parenchyma. Measurement or monitoring from the spinal subarachnoid space can release cerebrospinal fluid distal to the site of impending herniation, thereby precipitating brain herniation. Herniation may cause misleadingly low spinal subarachnoid pressures because of compartmentalization of fluid on either side of an obstructed foramen magnum or tentorium. Currently one of three sites—one of the lateral ventricles, the subdural space, or the brain parenchyma—is most often used. Monitoring ICP from each of these sites usually provides equivalent data, but because pressure gradients may exist among various sites, it may be advantageous to monitor in or adjacent to the most severely damaged hemisphere.

Lundberg et al. first proposed that cerebral ventricular pressure monitoring could be used to improve management of patients with closed head trauma [30]. Ventricular catheterization for ICP monitoring and CSF drainage, ideally inserted under strict aseptic technique, is the method of choice in patients in whom clinical outcome is dependent on hydrocephalus and CSF excess. In contrast, intraventricular catheters may be quite difficult to place if cerebral edema or brain swelling has com-

pressed the cerebral ventricular system. Two types of transducers can be used in the lateral ventricles—ventricular catheters that are fluid-coupled to external pressure transducers or transducer-tipped catheters (Camino Laboratories, San Diego, CA). All fluid-coupled systems that passively connect to external transducers must be zeroed at the level of the external auditory meatus. The transducer-tipped catheters measure either the amount or change in wavelength of reflected light, either of which is proportional to changes in pressure at the transducer tip. Although they gradually lose calibration ("drift") and must be removed for recalibration, fiberoptic catheters are less susceptible to short-term malfunction than the previous generation of fluid-filled, subdural catheters [31,32].

Intracranial pressure monitoring from the subdural space is usually performed with commercially available monitors of three basic designs: fluid-coupled bolts, fluid-coupled subdural catheters, and fiberoptic transducer-tipped catheters. Intracranial pressure monitoring became commonplace in tertiary care centers after the development of the subarachnoid bolt by Vries et al. [33]. Though generally accurate, subdural bolts may generate erroneous information [34,35]. Subdural bolts are open tubes facing end-on against the brain surface, and brain tissue may herniate into the system at high pressures, both damaging the brain cortex and obstructing the device. Plastic catheters designed for ventricular drainage or other purposes can be placed in the subdural space for ICP monitoring but usually suffer from severe artifacts of transmitted pressures. A version of the fiberoptic system described above is also used for subdural pressure monitoring [36] and appears to demonstrate acceptably low drift over periods of up to 5 days [31].

Intracranial pressure functions as the outflow pressure for

the cerebral circulation (assuming jugular venous pressure is lower), according to the equation:

$$CPP = MAP - ICP$$

where CPP is cerebral perfusion pressure, MAP is mean arterial pressure, and ICP exceeds jugular venous pressure. Although CBF cannot be directly inferred from knowledge of MAP and ICP, severe increases in ICP reduce both CPP and CBF.

Because intracranial hypertension can produce global cerebral ischemia or herniation, an increasing ICP merits concern. However, other information available from an ICP monitor also may prompt concern. This includes widening of the intracranial pulse pressure, diminution of the ability to compensate for increasing intracranial volume, and pathologic waveforms. Pathologic waveforms can best be appreciated by reviewing a printed record of trends. B waves, cycling at a rate of 2 to 4 per minute with an amplitude of 10 mm Hg or greater warn of possible decompensation of reserve but are not pathognomic [37]. Plateau, or A waves, which have long been recognized as a sign of impending catastrophe, consist of cyclic increases in ICP, often 50 mm Hg or greater and lasting as long as 15 to 30 minutes [30].

Numerous authors have investigated ways to enhance the value of ICP monitoring. Brain compliance can be assessed by calculating the pressure volume index (PVI). This requires the addition of volume to CSF or withdrawal of CSF through a ventricular cannula, then substituting measured values in the equation:

$$PVI = \frac{V}{\log P_0/P_{m \text{ or } p}}$$

where V is the volume withdrawn or injected, P_0 is the pressure before withdrawing or injecting fluid, P_m is the minimum pressure following fluid withdrawal, and P_p is the peak pressure following volume addition [38]. Based on the PVI, Tans and Poortvliet determined that the critical PVI was less than 13 ml, at which level treatment was likely to be necessary by either reducing ventricular fluid pressure or improving compliance [39]. Calculations based on changes in ICP in response to withdrawal or addition of fluid through a ventricular cannula indicate that reduction of ICP is nearly always required if PVI is less than 10 ml. Robertson et al. correlated PVI with a computerized frequency analysis of the ICP waveform in 55 severely head-injured patients and determined that this continuous technique provided information that correlated very highly with PVI, provided earlier evidence of changes in intracranial compliance than ICP alone, and did not require manipulation of intracranial fluid volume [40]. Marmarou et al. determined that changes in cerebrospinal fluid dynamics contributed much less to increases in ICP following severe head injury than did vascular mechanisms [41].

The problems associated with ICP monitoring generally fall into three categories: risks to patients, inaccurate data, and inappropriate use or misinterpretation of data. Patient risks include aggravation of cerebral edema, intracranial hemorrhage, cortical damage, and infection [42,43,44]. Most clinicians agree that intraventricular catheters carry a greater risk of infection than subdural monitors. Inaccurate data may result from complexity of equipment, improper maintenance, and unfamiliarity with equipment. Inappropriate use or misinterpretation of data usually results from improper choice of techniques or unwarranted decisions to initiate therapy or to withhold indicated therapy. In a recent series of 46 patients monitored with fiberoptic catheters in the intraparenchymal (n = 43) or intraven-

tricular (n = 3) positions, 12 percent developed broken components, 8.6 percent required repositioning for erroneous readings, and epidural hematomas complicated 3.4 percent [45].

CEREBRAL OXYGEN EXTRACTION

Jugular Venous Saturation. Measurements of oxygen in blood obtained from the jugular venous bulb provide information about the adequacy of CBF that is equivalent to the type of reasoning applied to the relationship between systemic "mixed venous" blood and the adequacy of cardiac output. Cerebral blood flow, $CMRO_2$, CaO_2, and jugular venous oxygen content ($CjvO_2$) are related according to the following equation:

$$CMRO_2 = CBF \times (CaO_2 - CjvO_2)$$

Rearranged, the equation becomes:

$$CjvO_2 = CaO_2 - \frac{CMRO_2}{CBF}$$

By inference, jugular venous oxygen saturation ($SjvO_2$), a major determinant of $CjvO_2$, represents a monitor of the adequacy of CBF. Mixed cerebral venous blood, like mixed systemic blood, is a global average of effluent from a variety of brain regions and may not reflect marked regional hypoperfusion. Therefore, abnormally low jugular venous saturation suggests the possibility of cerebral ischemia, but normal or elevated jugular venous saturation, while reassuring, is not adequate evidence of satisfactory cerebral perfusion. If, in addition to the cerebral arteriovenous oxygen content difference ($AVDO_2$), CBF is simultaneously measured, $CMRO_2$ can be calculated. Jugular venous blood gas sampling or continuous monitoring in clinical use has demonstrated excessive hyperventilation and unexpected cerebral desaturation and has been used in clinical investigation to guide therapy for head-injured patients.

The jugular venous bulb was first used as a sampling site more than 60 years ago [46]. Today, retrograde cannulation of the jugular bulb is a low-risk, technically simple procedure [47]. The internal jugular vein can be located by external anatomic landmarks and a "seeker" needle as it is for antegrade passage of central venous catheters or pulmonary artery catheters; however, the catheter is directed toward the mastoid process, below which lies the jugular venous bulb. A skull radiograph can confirm the position. An alternative method of placement uses Doppler ultrasound to identify and guide cannulation of the vein. Continuous monitoring of $SjvO_2$ is feasible using commercially available oximetry catheters. However, because of the configuration of the jugular bulb, continuous monitoring requires frequent repositioning and recalibration.

Near-Infrared Spectroscopy. Near-infrared spectroscopy may eventually offer the opportunity to assess the adequacy of brain oxygenation continuously, thereby facilitating either surveillance or goal-directed therapy. Near-infrared light penetrates the skull and, during transmission through or reflection from brain tissue, undergoes changes in wavelength that are proportional to the relative concentrations of oxygenated and deoxygenated Hgb in the tissue beneath the field [48]. Reflectance spectroscopy is technically easier because the high absorption by cranial tissue normally prevents transmittance of sufficient light unless a high-intensity laser light source is used.

The basic physical theories underlying near-infrared spectroscopy have been developed over the past 30 years. Cerebral near-infrared spectroscopy takes advantage of the different wavelengths of light absorbed by saturated versus desaturated hemoglobin. The absorption (A) of light by a chromophore (i.e., hemoglobin) is defined by the equation (known as Beer's law):

$$A = abc$$

where a is the absorption constant, b is the path length of the light, and c is the concentration of the chromophore.

Extensive preclinical and clinical data demonstrate the sensitivity of the technique for the detection of qualitative changes in brain oxygenation [48–53] (Fig. 25-7). Technical challenges to quantification of the signal include difficulty in determining the path lengths of reflected lights of different wavelengths and estimating the relative proportions of arterial, venous, and capillary blood in the field. For practical purposes, 75 percent of the blood is assumed to be venous and 25 percent arterial for calculation of mixed brain oxygen saturation. Recent data suggest that quantification of the signal may be practical [54,55,56]. If subsequent clinical validation of one or more of the current variety of approaches is satisfactory, a noninvasive, continuous monitor of cerebral circulatory adequacy will be possible. The availability of an inexpensive, simple-to-operate surveillance monitor as well as a monitor that could be used for goal-directed therapy would provide an unprecedented opportunity to manage the cerebral circulation as comprehensively as the systemic circulation can now be managed. The challenge then

Fig. 25-7. Electroencephalogram ([EEG] DSA display), analog EEG, blood pressure, and near-infrared spectroscopic estimation of hemoglobin saturation in brain and muscle (O.D., for optical density in brain and muscle) during an episode of ventricular fibrillation in a patient undergoing implantation of an automatic implantable defibrillator. With abrupt cessation of cerebral circulation, O.D. in brain and muscle declined abruptly. After an interval of absent circulation, defibrillation resulted in restoration of perfusion. The postdefibrillation increase in O.D. brain may represent transient postischemic hyperemia. (From Smith DS, Levy W, Maris M, et al: Reperfusion hyperoxia in brain after circulatory arrest in humans. *Anesthesiology* 73:12, 1990. With permission.)

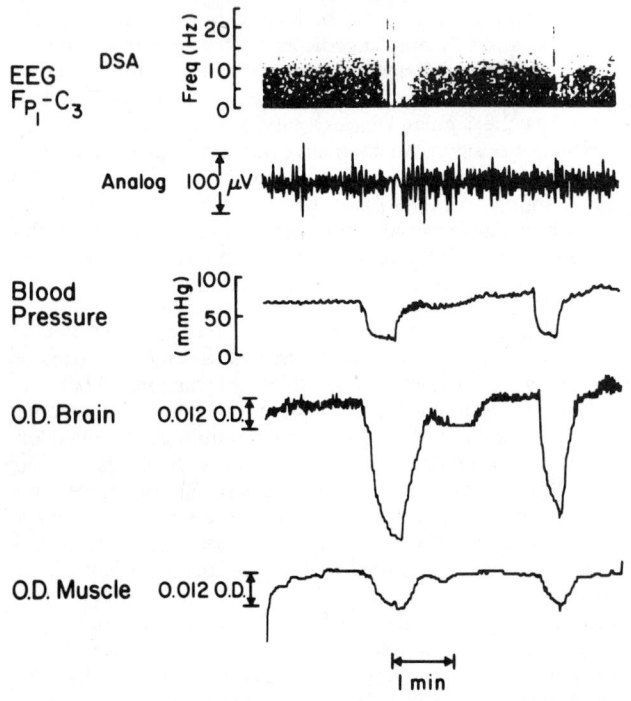

will be to demonstrate that improved therapy based on enhanced monitoring will improve outcome.

ELECTROPHYSIOLOGIC MONITORING

Electroencephalographic Monitoring. The cortical EEG, altered by mild cerebral ischemia and abolished by profound cerebral ischemia, can be used to indicate potentially damaging hypoperfusion. Traditionally used in some centers during carotid endarterectomy to detect cerebral ischemia after carotid cross-clamping and in neurologically devastated patients to document brain death, the EEG has not been used extensively in critically ill patients. Nonetheless, intermittent monitoring may be useful in patients suspected of isolated seizures or status epilepticus. Also helpful in defining the depth or the type of coma, the EEG may document focal or lateral intracranial abnormalities, but it has limited value as an anatomically or etiologically precise diagnostic tool. However, improved computer processing may improve the practicality of day-to-day monitoring of high-risk patients.

The EEG detects brain electrical activity as recorded at the scalp. In the ICU environment, technically adequate EEGs are often difficult to obtain because of electrical noise from electronic equipment such as monitors and nearby computers. Usually the EEG electrodes are placed in the 10–20 electrode configuration (Fig. 25-8) and the leads are connected to a 16-channel amplifier. The amplifier increases the intensity of the tiny potentials and filters noise by excluding signals outside a defined frequency window. The amplifier also has a high common-mode rejection ratio (i.e., changes in potential that are seen equally in all leads are rejected).

The unprocessed EEG is a complex waveform that consists of components of different frequencies and amplitudes. The spectrum of EEG frequencies is divided into delta (<4 Hz), theta (4–8 Hz), alpha (8–13 Hz), and beta (>13 Hz). Monitoring the unprocessed EEG requires the presence of an expert technician or physician who can rapidly recognize changes in the pattern of the waveform.

Continuous EEG recording is cumbersome due to the sheer volume of data (300 pages per hour of hard copy). Therefore, various methods have been designed to compress the data and still give meaningful information. If the complex waveform is filtered and digitized, a computer-driven rapid Fourier analysis can determine the relative amplitude in each frequency band. In the most commonly employed software programs, the data are then displayed as a compressed spectral array (CSA), a three-dimensional method of plotting the frequency of the EEG waveforms versus power time. Another method of processing, density spectral array (DSA), has the advantage of being able to detect small peaks that might be hidden in the CSA [57]. Computerized compression of the data permits frequent, repetitive assessment of the EEG with a minimum of specific training.

Extensive development and marketing of hardware and software suitable for EEG monitoring in critically ill patients has not appreciably increased its use. The equipment is relatively expensive, depends for successful use on the ready availability of dedicated technicians, and requires a modest level of sophistication for interpretation of changes. Also, EEG monitoring in critically ill patients appears to have little value for either surveillance or goal-directed therapy.

Evoked Potential Monitoring. Sensory evoked potentials (EPs), which include somatosensory evoked potentials (SSEPs), brainstem auditory evoked potentials (BAEPs), and visual evoked potentials (VEPs), can be used as qualitative threshold

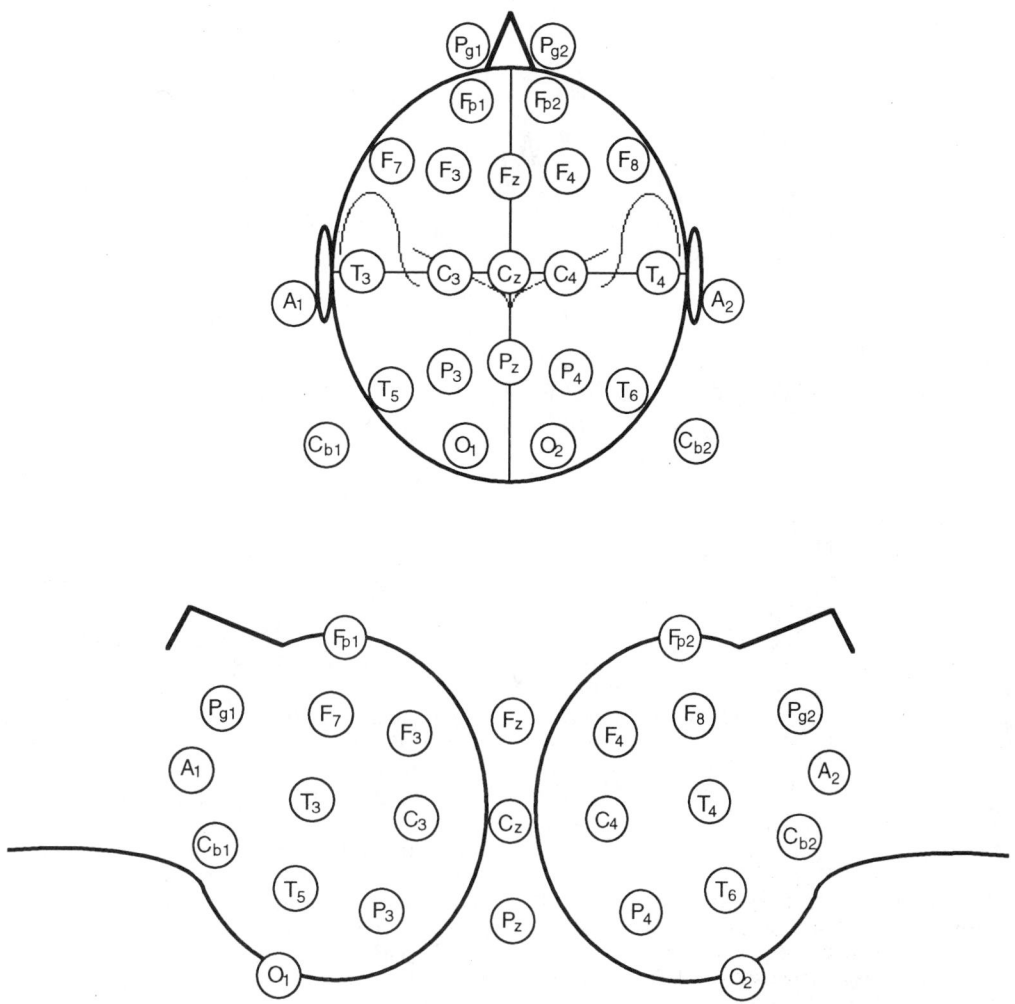

Fig. 25-8. Electrode placement using the 10–20 configuration.

monitors to detect severe neural ischemia. Whereas the EEG records the continuous, spontaneous activity of the brain, EPs evaluate the responses of the brain to specific stimuli. In the unprocessed EEG, the change in potential in response to a single stimulus cannot be detected. To quantify the BAEP, repeated identical stimuli are applied and signal averaging is used to visualize the reproducible evoked responses while removing the inconsistent background EEG (Fig. 25-9). High-quality amplifiers are necessary because the evoked response is approximately one-tenth the amplitude of the EEG. The resulting signal, displayed as voltage (in microvolts or nanovolts) on the vertical axis and time (in milliseconds) on the horizontal axis, is described in terms of the amplitude of individual peaks and the delay (latency) from stimulus administration until the appearance of specific portions of the waveform.

The sensitivity of EP monitoring is similar to that of EEG monitoring. Evoked potentials are generated by integrated neural networks, including the initial sensory structure, the transmitting pathways, and cortical and subcortical stimulus-processing centers. As the response to a stimulus is transmitted centrally, characteristic waveforms are generated that correspond to electrophysiologic activity in structures through which the stimulus passes. Evoked potentials, especially BAEPs, are

relatively robust, although they are modified by sedatives, narcotics, and anesthetics as well as trauma, hypoxia, or ischemia. Because obliteration of EPs occurs only under conditions of profound cerebral ischemia or mechanical trauma, EP monitoring is one of the most specific ways in which to assess neurologic integrity. However, EPs are insensitive to less severe deterioration of cerebral or spinal cord oxygen availability.

To record BAEPs, the A_1–C_z and A_2–C_z montages (Fig. 25-8) are commonly used. To elicit BAEPs, stimuli, usually clicks of 90 dB, are broadcast through a small speaker earphone. Each stimulus generates electrical activity in the cochlear nerve and its associated ipsilateral pathways.

The SSEP is similar to the BAEP, but usually the stimulus is applied to a peripheral nerve, usually the median nerve at the wrist, by a low-amplitude current of approximately 20 msec in duration. The resultant sensory (afferent) nerve stimulation is sufficient to provoke a slight thumb twitch. Because peripheral nerve stimulation can be uncomfortable, SSEPs are usually obtained on comatose patients. Somatosensory evoked potentials are unaffected by neuromuscular blocking agents. The C_3–C_z or C_4–C_z and C_3–C_4 montages (Fig. 25-8) are commonly used. The montage is intended to record from the contralateral brain. Erb's point (F_z–EP) and the cervical spinal cord (F_z–C_{11}) (Fig. 25-10) may also be recorded to check the conduction of the afferent nerves.

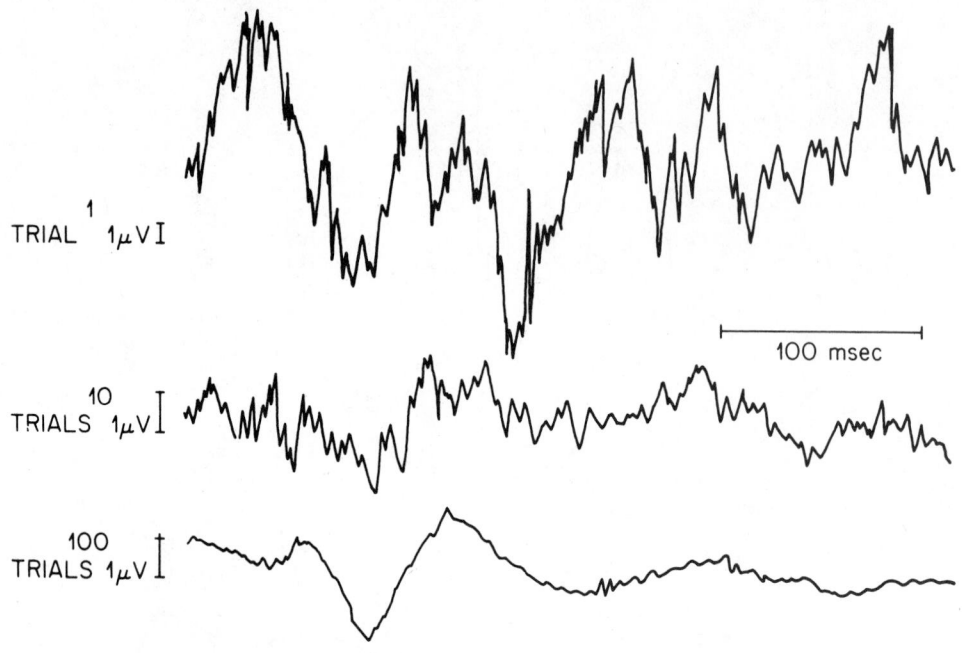

TRIAL ^{1} $1\mu V$ I

TRILS ^{10} $1\mu V$ I

$\overline{100\ msec}$

^{100}
TRIALS $1\mu V$ I

Fig. 25-9. Averaging reduces background noise. After 100 trials, this visual evoked potential (EP) is relatively noise-free. The same EP is hard to distinguish after only 10 trials and would be impossible to find in the original unaveraged data. (From Nuwer MR: *Evoked Potential Monitoring in the Operating Room.* New York, Raven, 1986, p 29. With permission.)

As with EEG monitoring, despite extensive development of hardware and software to support clinical EP monitoring, a variety of factors have limited extensive use of these techniques. First, the equipment is expensive, although less costly devices have recently been introduced. Second, highly trained technicians are essential for recording accurate data and for frequent observation of ongoing monitoring. Third, interpretation of changes requires considerable clinical sophistication in the art of pattern recognition. Perhaps most important, EP monitoring appears to have little value for either surveillance or goal-directed therapy in critically ill patients, in contrast to its possible value for intraoperative monitoring.

Specific Neurologic and Neurosurgical Diseases

MONITORING IN CENTRAL NERVOUS SYSTEM TRAUMA. Cerebral blood flow measurements have never become a routine part of management of head-injured patients, although considerable quantities of descriptive data have been generated. Lower CBF correlates with poorer outcome, after adjustment for confounding variables, in head-injured patients [58].

Human acute head injury sufficiently severe to produce coma (GCS score $\leq$ 8) is associated with decreased $CMRO_2$, moderately decreased CBF, and highly variable autoregulation. In the majority of comatose, head-injured patients, CBF is less than the normal value of 50 ml/100 gm/min and $CMRO_2$ is well below the normal value of 3.5 ml/100 gm/min [59]. Many older patients demonstrate persistently subnormal CBF of 15 to 20

ml/100 gm/min [60]. In some patients with head injury, $CMRO_2$ and CBF are proportionately reduced (i.e., coupling is preserved); in others CBF substantially exceeds that necessary to meet $CMRO_2$ [61]. Ninety percent of patients younger than 18 years demonstrate cerebral hyperemia (CBF exceeding metabolic demand) at some point during intensive monitoring [62]. Patients who demonstrate appropriate coupling between low $CMRO_2$ and low CBF may be vulnerable to excessive vasoconstriction during acute hyperventilation. Nearly 20 percent of patients develop a wide cerebral $AVDO_2$ during hyperventilation (Table 25-7), suggesting that hyperventilation therapy should be accompanied by an estimate of the adequacy of cerebral perfusion [61]. In some patients with severely reduced $CMRO_2$, acute hyperventilation actually increases $CMRO_2$ [63].

Cerebral blood flow after head trauma is pressure-dependent in approximately one-third of patients; two-thirds demonstrate intact pressure autoregulation. However, even in patients with impaired pressure autoregulation and high CPP, CBF may not increase to normal levels. Neither ICP, neurologic status, nor baseline CBF predicts the status of autoregulation [59]. Most patients with mass lesions demonstrate defective autoregulation, while autoregulation remains intact in many patients without intracranial mass lesions [59]. In children, either abnormally high or abnormally low CBF is associated with impaired autoregulation [64]. In head-injured patients in whom autoregulation is intact, mannitol reduces ICP and does not change CBF; if autoregulation is defective, ICP changes little and CBF increases [65].

The regional distribution of CBF is more variable in head-injured patients than in normal individuals [66,67]. Patients who do not survive and those who survive in a persistent vegetative state frequently demonstrate regional CBF values less than 20 ml/100 gm/min, especially in the frontal and parietal lobes [66]. Low flow in arterial boundary regions in the frontoparietal cortex, often secondary to high ICP, contributes to poor neurologic outcome [67]. However, even in patients who ultimately progress to good recovery, CBF may be less than 20 ml/100 gm/min in some brain regions. Recently, transcranial Doppler flow velocity measurements have been used to identify moderate and severe cerebral vasospasm after head injury [68]; all patients

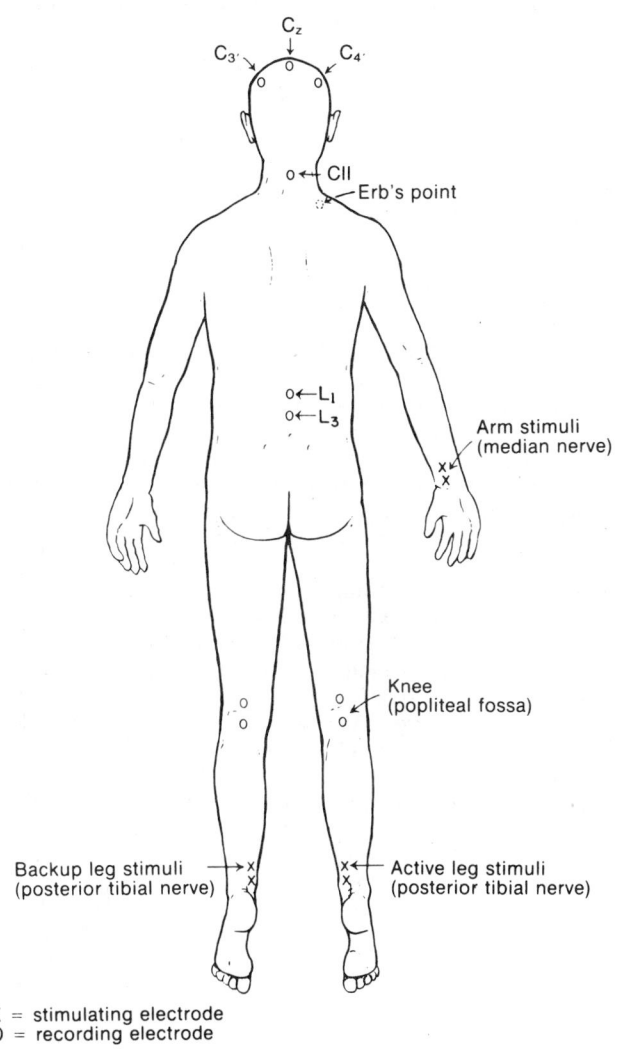

X = stimulating electrode
O = recording electrode

Prone Patient

Fig. 25-10. Sites used commonly for stimulating and recording electrodes for somatosensory evoked potentials from median and posterior tibial nerves. (From Gravenstein JS, Paulus DA: *Clinical Monitoring Practice.* 2nd ed. Philadelphia, JB Lippincott, 1987, p 270. With permission.)

Table 25-7. Cerebral Oxygenation in 10 Patients with Widely Increased Cerebral Oxygen Extraction

Hemodynamic variable	Hyperventilated patients	Normal value
CMRO$_2$ (ml/100 gm/ min)	1.9 ± 0.5	3.3 ± 0.4
CBF$_{15}$ (ml/100 gm/ min)	18.6 ± 4.4	53.3 ± 6.8
AVDO$_2$ (ml/100 ml)	10.5 ± 0.7	6.3 ± 1.2
VpO$_2$ (mm Hg)	22.3 ± 1.8	37.5 ± 5.6

Of 31 patients who were acutely hyperventilated (PaCO$_2$ 18–26 mm Hg) after severe head injury, 10 demonstrated increased oxygen extraction.

CMRO$_2$ = cerebral metabolic rate for oxygen consumption; CBF$_{15}$ refers to the specific formula used to calculate cerebral blood flow; AVDO$_2$ = cerebral arteriovenous oxygen content difference; and VpO$_2$ = jugular venous oxygen tension.

(Modified from Obrist WD, Langfitt TW, Jaggi JL, et al: Cerebral blood flow and metabolism in comatose patients with acute head injury. *J Neurosurg* 61:241, 1984, with permission of the publisher)

creases in cerebral hemispheric blood volume accompanied by a decline in CBF [71].

Intracranial pressure monitors are usually considered a fundamental part of the care of patients with severe closed head injury (i.e., GCS score ≤ 8) [72]. In more than one-third of patients with severe brain trauma, ICP exceeds 20 mm Hg. Severe intracranial hypertension is the primary cause of death in more than 10 percent of severely injured patients, and ICP greater than 20 mm Hg increases morbidity in those who survive [73]. Marshall et al. reported that consistent ICP monitoring was associated with more favorable outcome than had previously been achieved in patients with severe head injury [74]. Saul and Ducker compared the results in two sequential series, the first consisting of 127 patients managed in 1977 and 1978 and the second consisting of 106 patients managed in 1979 and 1980 [75]. In the first group, management was initiated when ICP rose to 20 to 25 mm Hg; in the second, ICP was managed earlier and more aggressively. The overall mortality in the second group was 28 percent compared to 46 percent in the first group [75]. Therefore, many neurosurgeons consider that aggressive monitoring and control of ICP improves outcome in severe head injury. Although ICP monitoring has been credited by some investigators with improving prognosis in acute closed head injury [73–77], others question whether concurrent improvements in management, rather than ICP monitoring, explain the improvement [78].

Unlike the modalities previously discussed, ICP monitoring has been used for surveillance and goal-directed therapy. In head-injured patients, clinicians have applied systematic, though institutionally specific, protocols for avoidance of intracranial hypertension and reduction of increased ICP when a threshold of 15 or 20 mm Hg is exceeded. In particular, decisions about diuretics, hyperventilation, position changes, and additional diagnostic procedures may be made using ICP data. The information is considered necessary in patients in whom neuromuscular blocking agents are administered as part of treatment to reduce ICP, because of the inability to perform a comprehensive neurologic examination. If intracranial hypertension is refractory to conventional therapy, ICP monitoring is one of the alternative techniques used to titrate barbiturate coma [79], although prophylactic barbiturate coma has failed to improve neurologic outcome after head injury [80].

Intracranial hypertension or reduced intracranial compliance can be managed using a variety of strategies, all of them based on the central concept that reduction of ICP or improvement

with severe vasospasm (5 of 8 patients with vasospasm in a group of 30 head-injured patients) had traumatic SAH [68].

Conceptually, much of the management of acute head injury patients is intended to maintain adequate CBF. However, CBF is not routinely measured. Most cerebral circulatory information is inferred from knowledge of MAP, PaCO$_2$ and ICP. Langfitt and Obrist originally described the brain elastance curve produced by gradually adding volume to the intracranial space [69]. Lundberg first proposed that changes in therapy based on ICP monitoring could improve outcome [70], based on the underlying assumption that intracranial hypertension, if untreated, may cause herniation or cerebral hypoperfusion. Through extensive monitoring of ventricular fluid pressure in patients with brain tumors, he demonstrated that ICP is subject to periodic wave phenomena, of which the most dangerous is the plateau wave. Plateau waves, the occurrence of which often precipitates acute neurologic deterioration, appear to result from in-of intracranial compliance can be accomplished only by reducing brain blood volume, brain tissue volume, or cerebrospinal fluid volume.

Robertson et al. recently reported extensive experience with monitoring the cerebral arteriovenous oxygen content difference [81]. In a series of 100 patients, they accumulated evidence that measurements of the cerebral arteriovenous differences of lactate and oxygen content could be used to predict CBF and to differentiate patients with patterns consistent with ischemia or infarction, normal CBF, cerebral hyperemia, and compensated hypoperfusion (Fig. 25-11) [81]. Near-infrared spectroscopy also has been used to localize posttraumatic intracranial hematomas [82].

Occasionally, hyperventilation may result in local, paradoxic increases in CBF (so-called "inverse steal") [83]. If increased ICP develops in patients with a wide cerebral AVDO$_2$, mannitol may be more appropriate than further hyperventilation [84]. Excessive regional vasoconstriction is a possible mechanism for the reported worsening of outcome in patients hyperventilated after head trauma in comparison to those maintained at a higher level of PaCO$_2$ [85].

After traumatic brain injury, the brain is even more dependent on aerobic and anaerobic metabolism of glucose [86]; head-injured patients appear to use other cerebral metabolic substrates, such as acetoacetate and beta-hydroxybutyrate, poorly.

In head-injured [87–96] and spinal cord-injured [97–102] patients, EP monitoring has been employed as a diagnostic and prognostic aid. After head injury, BAEPs correlate less well with clinical outcome than cortical SSEPs [87–90], the disappearance of which is a particularly ominous prognostic sign [88]. Multimodality EPs improve the prognostic accuracy of clinical examination and measurement of ICP in head-injured patients [89,92,94,95,96]. After acute spinal cord injury, SSEPs differentiate complete from incomplete transection but do not accu-

rately predict recovery of function [97–101]. Li et al. reported that a combination of quantitative SSEP assessment in the ulnar and posterior tibial regions, motor index score, and pinprick sensory score provided a strong prognostic battery in patients with cervical spinal cord injury [102].

MONITORING IN ISCHEMIC NEUROLOGIC DISEASE.

Neurologic monitoring in patients with nontraumatic, ischemic neurologic and neurosurgical conditions has been less extensive than in patients with traumatic coma. However, some data are available.

Cerebral blood flow has been investigated in patients who have suffered cardiac arrest, because of the well-documented experimental phenomenon of postischemic hypoperfusion (PIH) [103,104]. Clinical data support the concept that some patients develop PIH after cardiac arrest [105,106], but CMRO$_2$ tends to be proportionally reduced [105]. Because the cerebral vasodilator nimodipine increased CBF and improved neurologic outcome in animals after complete cerebral ischemia [107,108], immediate postresuscitation administration of nimodipine was investigated in patients [109,110]. However, neurologic outcome was not improved. In some patients, CBF actually increased markedly within 24 to 48 hours after cardiac arrest, and this was associated with a poor prognosis [106].

Neurologic deterioration after SAH often represents cerebral vasospasm. Although CBF decreases, vasospasm reduces blood vessel diameter, thereby increasing flow velocity in the middle cerebral artery [111,112,113]. As vasospasm resolves (and CBF increases), velocity decreases [47]. The value of TCD evaluation appears to be established in noninvasively "detecting severe stenosis (>65%) in the major basal intracranial arteries; assessing patterns and extent of collateral circulation . . . ; evaluating and following vasoconstriction . . . , especially after SAH . . . "[114]. In patients randomized to receive nicardipine (a calcium entry blocker) or placebo after SAH, the incidence of vasospasm, as reflected in mean middle cerebral artery flow velocities exceeding 120 cm per second, was 23 percent in the nicardipine versus 49 percent in the placebo group [115]. Elevated middle cerebral artery velocity has also been used to determine the success of angioplasty to treat intracranial vasospasm [116]. Nevertheless, some investigators find TCD to be of questionable value, failing to predict delayed ischemic deficits [117] even if pulsatility indices are used [118].

Intracranial pressure monitoring has been applied by a limited number of investigators in diverse acute ischemic and nonischemic neurologic conditions, including SAH and anoxic cerebral insults [119-125]. When ICP monitoring is used in nontraumatic brain disease, the rationale and strategies are similar to those used in head trauma. However, data defining the impact of ICP monitoring on outcome are more fragmentary and less convincing than those available for traumatized patients.

Cant and Shaw monitored 51 patients using a CSA device [126] and reported that persistence or return of a peak of activity in the theta or alpha frequency bands within 10 days of the onset of coma was associated with a favorable recovery. In contrast, patients in whom such a peak was lost were likely to die or suffer residual neurologic damage. In patients comatose from a mixture of traumatic and ischemic injuries, an alternating pattern of CSA activity was associated with a more favorable outcome [127]. Alpha-coma, unconsciousness associated with an EEG pattern resembling normal wakefulness occurring after brainstem stroke or hypoxic/anoxic cerebral injury, suggests a poor prognosis for survival [128]. Serial EEGs have been used to improve prognostication in children with nontraumatic coma; the worst prognostic findings were low-amplitude activ-

Fig. 25-11. Conceptual model of the relationship between cerebral blood flow (CBF) and cerebral metabolism in comatose, head-injured patients. In nonischemic brain, the arteriovenous oxygen difference (AVDO$_2$) and CBF vary reciprocally, as illustrated by the solid curve, representing a cerebral metabolic rate of oxygen (CMRO$_2$) averaging 0.9 μmol/gm/min (substantially less than 1.5 μmol/gm/min in normal individuals; 1.5 μmol/gm/min = 3.4 ml O$_2$/100 gm/min). In the presence of cerebral ischemia/infarction (*open arrows*), AVDO$_2$ and CBF have an unpredictable relationship. (From Robertson C, Narayan RK, Gokaslan ZI, et al: Cerebral arteriovenous oxygen difference as an estimate of cerebral blood flow in comatose patients. *J Neurosurg* 70:222, 1989. With permission.)

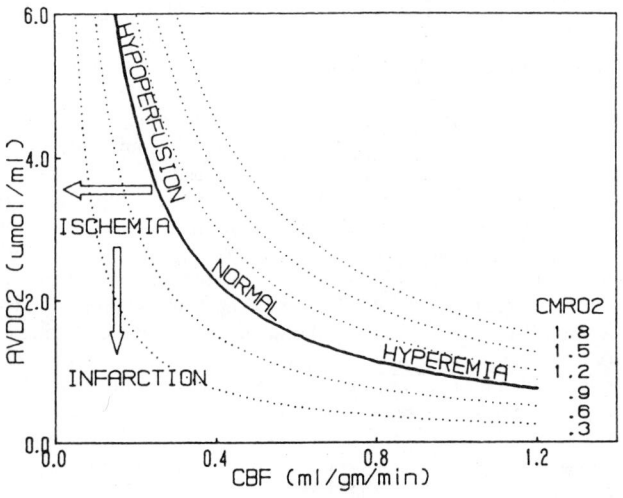

Table 25-8. Techniques for Assessing Cerebral Circulation

Characteristic	MODALITY						
	Evoked potentials	EEG	CBF (^{133}Xe clearance)	CBF (transcranial Doppler flow velocity)	ICP monitoring	Brain metabolic monitoring (jugular venous saturation)	Brain metabolic monitoring (near-infrared spectroscopy)
Bias	N/A	N/A	±5%	N/A	Excellent	Gold standard	Not established
Precision	N/A	N/A	±5%	N/A	Excellent	Gold standard	Not established
Sensitivity	High for ischemia	Good for ischemia; sensitive to drug effects	Good for 5% change	Good for CBF change (relative)	Good for ICP change; poor for ischemia	Good for global; poor for regional	Good for severe global desaturation
Positive predictive value	Good for ischemia	Poor for ischemia	Good for CBF decrease	Good for CBF change	Good for ICP change; poor for ischemia	Good for global; poor for regional	Not established
Specificity	High for ischemia	Poor for ischemia	Poor for ischemia; good for CBF decrease	Good for CBF change	Good for ICP change; poor for ischemia	Good	Not established
Negative predictive value	Good for ischemia	Fair for ischemia	Poor for ischemia	Poor for ischemia; good for vasospasm	Good for ICP change; poor for ischemia	Good	Not established
Threshold definition	Ischemia (CBF 15–23 ml/ 100 gm/min)	Ischemia (CBF 18–23 ml/ 100 gm/min)	Can be set at desired level	Interpatient variability	15–20 mm Hg or <50 mm Hg CPP	Saturation <50	Probably similar to jugular saturation
Speed	Good	Good	Poor	Poor	Good (once inserted)	Fair (good if continuous)	Excellent
Utility in clinical:							
Diagnosis	Good	Good	Poor	Good	Poor	Poor	Untested
Surveillance	Poor	Fair	Poor	Fair in SAH	Good (CHI)	Poor (good if continuous)	Should be excellent
Prognosis	Good	Fair	Fair	Fair in SAH	Good (CHI)	Fair	Untested
Goal-directed therapy	Poor	Poor	Poor	Untested	Fair (CHI); Reye syndrome	Untested	Potentially valuable but untested

NA = not applicable; EEG = electroencephalography; CBF = cerebral blood flow; ICP = intracranial pressure; SAH = subarachnoid hemorrhage; CPP = cerebral perfusion pressure; CHI = closed head injury.

ity or electrocerebral silence [128]. Quantitative EEG monitoring has been used to identify delayed ischemic deficits after SAH, occasionally before clinical deterioration [129].

Because of the sensitivity of the EEG to drug effects, either unprocessed or processed EEG monitoring can be used to assess sedation in critically ill patients. It can also be used to provide early evidence of seizure activity or cerebral ischemia [130]. However, despite considerable interest in the intraoperative use of computer-processed EEG monitoring [130–135], particularly in patients undergoing carotid endarterectomy and cardiac surgery, few centers have extensively used EEG monitoring techniques in the ICU.

When used for brain and spinal cord monitoring, EPs are intended to detect deterioration in neurologic function at a time when corrective action may still reverse changes. Thus, they have been used most extensively for monitoring during neurosurgical procedures and for diagnosis in such diseases as multiple sclerosis [136,137]. However, neurologic deficits occur that have not been predicted by changes in EPs [138], and apparently severe changes in EPs may not be followed by neurologic deficits. The former probably represents damage to tissue that has not been part of the conducting pathway for the monitored response; the latter presumably reflects either ischemia of insufficient duration to produce irreversible injury or ischemia of insufficient magnitude to produce cell death.

To a limited extent, EPs have been used to facilitate diagnosis and prognostication in ischemic and hypoxic brain injury. Central conduction time is prolonged by ischemia in primates [139] and in humans who have ischemic complications of SAH [140]. With impending brain death, cortical SSEPs disappear first; BAEPs disappear only when brain death is imminent [141,142]. Persistence of the medullary components of the SSEP at a time when the cortical components are no longer present confirms brain death [141]. In children, absence of the cortical components of SSEPs with preserved brainstem function suggests the likelihood of a chronic vegetative state [143].

Somatosensory evoked potentials persist, though in altered form, during barbiturate administration; BAEPs are resistant to the effects of barbiturates [144]. Central conduction time, a measure of the time required to transmit the response to a stimulus from the periphery to the cortex, appears to be unaffected even by high levels of barbiturates [145]. Therefore, EPs assist in assessing neurologic status even in patients in barbiturate coma.

Summary

A variety of powerful techniques, all of which can be performed at the bedside of the critically ill patient, are available for assessing the cerebral circulation (Table 25-8). The next step in the evolution of neurologic monitoring necessitates the development of physiologically and pharmacologically sound protocols for goal-directed therapy. These must then be carefully tested to determine whether they can reduce morbidity and mortality in patients with critical neurologic illness.

References

1. Fuchs VR, Garber AM: What is new about the new technology assessment? *N Engl J Med* 323:673, 1990.
2. Bland RD, Shoemaker WC, Abraham E, et al: Hemodynamic and oxygen transport patterns in surviving and nonsurviving patients. *Crit Care Med* 13:85, 1985.
3. Bland RD, Shoemaker WC: Probability of survival as a prognostic and severity illness score in critically ill surgical patients. *Crit Care Med* 13:91, 1985.
4. Shoemaker WC, Appel PL, Kram HB, et al: Prospective trial of supranormal values of survivors as therapeutic goals in high-risk surgical patients. *Chest* 94:1176, 1988.
5. Graham DI: The pathology of brain ischaemia and possibilities for therapeutic intervention. *Br J Anaesth* 57:3, 1985.
6. Jones TH, Morawetz RB, Crowell RM, et al: Thresholds of focal cerebral ischemia in awake monkeys. *J Neurosurg* 54:773, 1981.
7. Symon L: Flow thresholds in brain ischaemia and the effects of drugs. *Br J Anaesth* 57:34, 1985.
8. Holbach K-H, Wassmann HW, Hohelüchter KL: Reversibility of the chronic post-stroke state. *Stroke* 7:296, 1976.
9. Hossmann K-A, Olsson Y: Suppression and recovery of neuronal function in transient cerebral ischemia. *Brain Res* 22:313, 1970.
10. Sharbrough FW, Messick JM Jr, Sundt TM Jr: Correlation of continuous electroencephalograms with cerebral blood flow measurements during carotid endarterectomy. *Stroke* 4:674, 1973.
11. Strandgaard S, Paulson OB: Cerebral autoregulation. *Stroke* 15:413, 1984.
12. Strandgaard S: Cerebral blood flow in hypertension. *Acta Med Scand* [Suppl] 678:11, 1983.
13. Tommasino C, Moore S, Todd MM: Cerebral effects of isovolemic hemodilution with crystalloid or colloid solutions. *Crit Care Med* 16:862, 1988.
14. Todd MM, Tommasino C, Moore S: Cerebral effects of isovolemic hemodilution with a hypertonic saline solution. *J Neurosurg* 63:944, 1985.
15. Phillis JW, Preston G, DeLong RE: Effects of anoxia on cerebral blood flow in the rat brain: Evidence for a role of adenosine in autoregulation. *J Cereb Blood Flow Metab* 4:586, 1984.
16. Hoffman WE, Albrecht RF, Miletich DJ: The role of adenosine in CBF increases during hypoxia in young vs. aged rats. *Stroke* 15:124, 1984.
17. Teasdale G, Jennett B: Assessment of coma and impaired consciousness: A practical scale. *Lancet* 2:81, 1974.
18. Korein J, Braunstein P, Kercheff I, et al: Radioisotope bolus technique as a test to detect circulatory deficit associated with cerebral death. *Circulation* 51:924, 1975.
19. Kety SS, Schmidt CF: The determination of cerebral blood flow in man by the use of nitrous oxide in low concentrations. *Am J Physiol* 143:53, 1945.
20. Kety SS, Schmidt CF: The nitrous oxide method for the quantitative determination of cerebral blood flow in man: Theory, procedure and normal values. *J Clin Invest* 27:476, 1948.
21. Hoedt-Rasmussen K, Sveinsdottir E, Lassen NA: Regional cerebral blood flow in man determined by intra-arterial injection of radioactive inert gas. *Circ Res* 18:237, 1966.
22. Olesen J, Paulson OB, Lassen NA: Regional cerebral blood flow in man determined by the initial slope of the clearance of intra-arterially injected ^{133}Xe. *Stroke* 2:519, 1971.
23. Obrist WD, Thompson HK Jr, Wang HS, et al: Regional cerebral blood flow estimated by ^{133}Xenon inhalation. *Stroke* 6:245, 1975.
24. Risberg J, Ali Z, Wilson EM, et al: Regional cerebral blood flow by ^{133}Xenon inhalation. *Stroke* 6:142, 1975.
25. Bishop CCR, Powell S, Rutt D, et al: Transcranial Doppler measurement of middle cerebral artery blood flow velocity: A validation study. *Stroke* 17:913, 1986.
26. Tenjin H, Yamaki T, Nakagawa, et al: Impairment of CO_2 reactivity in severe head injury patients: An investigation using thermal diffusion method. *Acta Neurochir* 104:121, 1990.
27. Kuwayama N, Takaku A, Harada J, et al: Modified thermal diffusion flow probe for the continous monitoring of cortical blood flow. *Neurosurgery* 29:583, 1991.
28. Dickman CA, Carter LP, Baldwin HZ: Continuous regional cerebral blood flow monitoring in acute craniocerebral trauma. *Neurosurgery* 28:467, 1991.
29. Salmon JH, Hajjar W, Bada HS: The fontogram: A noninvasive pressure monitor. *Pediatrics* 60:721, 1977.
30. Lundberg N, Troupp H, Lorin H: Continuous recording of the ventricular-fluid pressure in patients with severe acute traumatic brain injury. *J Neurosurg* 22:581, 1965.
31. Crutchfield JS, Narayan RK, Robertson CS, et al: Evaluation of a fiberoptic intracranial pressure monitor. *J Neurosurg* 72:482, 1990.
32. Chambers IR, Mendelow AD, Sinar EJ, et al: A clinical evaluation of the Camino subdural screw and ventricular monitoring kits. *Neurosurgery* 26:421, 1990.
33. Vries JK, Becker DP, Young HF: A subarachnoid screw for monitoring intracranial pressure. *J Neurosurg* 100:1117, 1973.
34. Miller JD, Bobo H, Kapp JP: Inaccurate pressure readings for subarachnoid bolts: Case report. *Neurosurgery* 19:253, 1986.
35. Allen R: Intracranial pressure: A review of clinical problems, measurement techniques and monitoring methods. *J Med Eng Technol* 10:299, 1986.
36. Ostrup RC, Luerssen TG, Marshall LF, Zornow MH: Continuous monitoring of intracranial pressure with a miniaturized fiberoptic device. *J Neurosurg* 67:206, 1987.
37. Wilkinson HA, Schuman N, Ruggiero J: Nonvolumetric methods of detecting impaired intracranial compliance or reactivity: Pulse width and waveform analysis. *J Neurosurg* 50:758, 1979.
38. Maset AL, Marmarou A, Ward JD, et al: Pressure-volume index in head injury. *J Neurosurg* 67:832, 1987.
39. Tans JT, Poortvliet DC: Intracranial volume-pressure relationship in man, II: Clinical significance of the pressure volume index. *J Neurosurg* 59:810, 1983.
40. Robertson CS, Narayan RK, Contant CF, et al: Clinical experience with a continuous monitor of intracranial compliance. *J Neurosurg* 71:673, 1989.
41. Marmarou A, Maset AL, Ward JD, et al: Contribution of CSF and vascular factors to elevation of ICP in severely head-injured patients. *J Neurosurg* 66:883, 1987.
42. Kanter RK, Weiner LB, Patti AM, et al: Infectious complications and duration of intracranial pressure monitoring. *Crit Care Med* 13:837, 1985.
43. Aucoin PJ, Kotilainen HR, Gantz NM, et al: Intracranial pressure monitors: Epidemiologic study of risk factors and infections. *Am J Med* 80:369, 1986.
44. Clark WC, Muhlbauer MS, Lowrey R, et al: Complications of intracranial pressure monitoring in trauma patients. *Neurosurgery* 25:20, 1989.
45. Yablon JS, Lantner HJ, McCormack TM, et al: Clinical experience with a fiberoptic intracranial pressure monitor. *J Clin Monit* 9:171, 1993.
46. Myerson A, Halloran RD, Hirsch HL: Technic for obtaining blood from the internal jugular vein and internal carotid artery. *Arch Neurol Psychiatry* 17:807, 1927.
47. Goetting MG, Preston G: Jugular bulb catheterization: Experience with 123 patients. *Crit Care Med* 18:1220, 1990.
48. Jobsis-Vandervliet FF, Fox E, Sugioka K: Monitoring of cerebral oxygenation and cytochrome aa3 redox state, in Tremper KK, Barker SJ (eds): *Advances in Oxygen Monitoring: International Anesthesiology Clinics.* Boston, Little, Brown, 1987, pp 209–230.
49. Proctor HJ, Cairns C, Fillipo D, et al: Brain metabolism during increased intracranial pressure as assessed by niroscopy. *Surgery* 96:273, 1984.
50. Brazy JE, Lewis DV, Mitnick MH: Noninvasive monitoring of cerebral oxygenation in preterm infants: Preliminary observations. *Pediatrics* 75:217, 1985.
51. Smith DS, Levy W, Maris M, et al: Reperfusion hyperoxia in brain after circulatory arrest in humans. *Anesthesiology* 73:12, 1990.

52. Delpy DT, Arridge SR, Cope M, et al: Quantitation of pathlength in optical spectroscopy. *Adv Exp Med Biol* 248:41, 1989.
53. Delpy DT, Cope M, van der Zee P, et al: Estimation of optical pathlength through tissue from direct time of flight measurement. *Phys Med Biol* 33:1433, 1988.
54. Ferrari M, Wilson DA, Hanley DF, et al: Noninvasive determination of hemoglobin saturation in dogs by derivative near-infrared spectroscopy. *Am J Physiol* 256:H1493, 1989.
55. Prough DS, Scuderi PE, Lewis G, et al: Initial clinical experience using in vivo optical spectroscopy to quantify brain oxygen saturation. *Anesthesiology* 73:A424, 1990.
56. McCormick PW, Stewart M, Dujovny M, et al: Clinical application of diffuse near-infrared transmission spectroscopy to measure cerebral oxygen metabolism. *Hospimedica* 8:39, 1990.
57. Levy WJ, Shapiro HM, Maruchak G, et al: Automated EEG processing for intraoperative monitoring: A comparison of techniques. *Anesthesiology* 53:223, 1980.
58. Robertson CS, Contant CF, Gokaslan ZL, et al: Cerebral blood flow, arteriovenous oxygen difference, and outcome in head injured patients. *J Neurol Neurosurg Psychiatry* 55:594, 1992.
59. Bruce DA, Langfitt TW, Miller JD, et al: Regional cerebral blood flow, intracranial pressure, and brain metabolism in comatose patients. *J Neurosurg* 38:131, 1973.
60. Cold GE, Jensen FT: Cerebral blood flow in the acute phase after head injury, 1: Correlation to age of the patients, clinical outcome and localization of the injured region. *Acta Anaesthesiol Scand* 24:245, 1980.
61. Obrist WD, Langfitt TW, Jaggi JL, et al: Cerebral blood flow and metabolism in comatose patients with acute head injury: Relationship to intracranial hypertension. *J Neurosurg* 61:241, 1984.
62. Muizelaar JP, Marmarou A, DeSalles AA, et al: Cerebral blood flow and metabolism in severely head-injured children, 1: Relationship with GCS score, outcome, ICP, and PVI. *J Neurosurg* 71:63, 1989.
63. Obrist WD, Clifton GL, Robertson CS, et al: Cerebral metabolic changes induced by hyperventilation in acute head injury, in Meyer JS, Lechner H, Reivich M (eds): *Cerebral Vascular Disease.* vol. 6. New York, Elsevier, 1977, pp 251–255.
64. Muizelaar JP, Ward JD, Marmarou A, et al: Cerebral blood flow and metabolism in severely head-injured children, 2: Autoregulation. *J Neurosurg* 71:72, 1989.
65. Muizelaar JP, Lutz HA III, Becker DP: Effect of mannitol on ICP and CBF and correlation with pressure autoregulation in severely head-injured patients. *J Neurosurg* 61:700, 1984.
66. Overgaard J, Mosdal C, Tweed WA: Cerebral circulation after head injury, 3: Does reduced regional cerebral blood flow determine recovery of brain function after blunt head injury? *J Neurosurg* 55:63, 1981.
67. Overgaard J, Tweed WA: Cerebral circulation after head injury, 4: Functional anatomy and boundary-zone flow deprivation in the first week of traumatic coma. *J Neurosurg* 59:439, 1983.
68. Martin NA, Doberstein C, Zane C, et al: Posttraumatic cerebral arterial spasm: Transcranial Doppler ultrasound, cerebral blood flow, and angiographic findings. *J Neurosurg* 77:575, 1992.
69. Langfitt TW, Obrist WD: Cerebral blood flow and metabolism after intracranial trauma. *Prog Neurol Surg* 10:14, 1981.
70. Lundberg N: Continuous recording and control of ventricular fluid pressure in neurosurgical practice. *Acta Psychiatr Scand* 36(Suppl 149):1, 1960.
71. Hayashi M, Kobayashi H, Handa Y, et al: Brain blood volume and blood flow in patients with plateau waves. *J Neurosurg* 63:556, 1985.
72. Ward JD: Intracranial pressure monitoring, in Society of Critical Care Medicine: *Critical Care: State of the Art.* Fullerton, CA, 1989, pp 173–185.
73. Miller JD, Becker DP, Ward JD, et al: Significance of intracranial hypertension in severe head injury. *J Neurosurg* 47:503, 1977.
74. Marshall LF, Smith RW, Shapiro HM: The outcome with aggressive treatment in severe head injuries, I: The significance of intracranial pressure monitoring. *J Neurosurg* 50:20, 1979.
75. Saul TG, Ducker TB: Effect of intracranial pressure monitoring and aggressive treatment on mortality in severe head injury. *J Neurosurg* 56:498, 1982.
76. Miller JD, Butterworth JF IV, Gudeman SK, et al: Further experi-
77. Becker DP, Miller JD, Ward JD, et al: The outcome from severe head injury with early diagnosis and intensive management. *J Neurosurg* 47:491, 1977.
78. Colohan AR, Alves WM, Gross CR, et al: Head injury mortality in two centers with different emergency medical services and intensive care. *J Neurosurg* 71:202, 1989.
79. Eisenberg HM, Frankowski RF, Contant CF, et al: High-dose barbiturate control of elevated intracranial pressure in patients with severe head injury. *J Neurosurg* 69:15, 1988.
80. Ward JD, Becker DP, Miller JD, et al: Failure of prophylactic barbiturate coma in the treatment of severe head injury. *J Neurosurg* 62:383, 1985.
81. Robertson CS, Narayan RK, Gokaslan ZL: Cerebral arteriovenous oxygen difference as an estimate of cerebral blood flow in comatose patients. *J Neurosurg* 70:222, 1989.
82. Gopinath SP, Robertson CS, Grossman RG, Chance B: Near-infrared spectroscopic localization of intracranial hematomas. *J Neurosurg* 79:43, 1993.
83. Darby JM, Yonas H, Marion DW, et al: Local "inverse steal" induced by hyperventilation in head injury. *Neurosurgery* 23:84, 1988.
84. Cruz J, Miner ME, Allen SJ, et al: Continuous monitoring of cerebral oxygenation in acute brain injury: Injection of mannitol during hyperventilation. *J Neurosurg* 73:725, 1990.
85. Muizelaar JP, Marmarou A, Ward JD, et al: Adverse effects of prolonged hyperventilation in patients with severe head injury: A randomized clinical trial. *J Neurosurg* 75:731, 1991.
86. Robertson CS, Clifton GL, Grossman RG, et al: Alterations in cerebral availability of metabolic substrates after severe head injury. *J Trauma* 28:1523, 1988.
87. Seales DM, Rossiter VS, Weinstein ME: Brainstem auditory evoked responses in patients comatose as a result of blunt head trauma. *J Trauma* 19:347, 1979.
88. Ganes T, Lundar T: EEG and evoked potentials in comatose patients with severe brain damage. *Electroencephalogr Clin Neurophysiol* 69:6, 1988.
89. Greenberg RP, Newlon PG, Hyatt MS, et al: Prognostic implications of early multimodality evoked potentials in severely head-injured patients. *J Neurosurg* 55:227, 1981.
90. Hume AL, Cant BR: Central somatosensory conduction after head injury. *Ann Neurol* 10:411, 1981.
91. Cant BR, Hume AL, Judson JA, et al: The assessment of severe head injury by short-latency somatosensory and brain-stem auditory evoked potentials. *Electroencephalogr Clin Neurophysiol* 65:188, 1986.
92. Anderson DC, Bundlie S, Rockswold GL: Multimodality evoked potentials in closed head trauma. *Arch Neurol* 41:369, 1984.
93. Newlon PG, Greenberg RP, Hyatt MS, et al: The dynamics of neuronal dysfunction and recovery following severe head injury assessed with serial multimodality evoked potentials. *J Neurosurg* 57:168, 1982.
94. Greenberg RP, Mayer DJ, Becker DP, et al: Evaluation of brain function in severe human head trauma with multimodality evoked potentials, 1: Evoked brain-injury potentials, methods, and analysis. *J Neurosurg* 47:150, 1977.
95. Greenberg RP, Becker DP, Miller JD, et al: Evaluation of brain function in severe head trauma with multimodality evoked potentials, 2: Localization of brain dysfunction and correlation with posttraumatic neurological conditions. *J Neurosurg* 47:163, 1977.
96. Narayan RK, Greenberg RP, Miller JD, et al: Improved confidence of outcome prediction in severe head injury. *J Neurosurg* 54:751, 1981.
97. Rowed DW, McLean JAG, Tator CH: Somatosensory evoked potentials in acute spinal cord injury: Prognostic value. *Surg Neurol* 9:203, 1976.
98. Powers SK, Bolger CA, Edwards MSB: Spinal cord pathways mediating somatosensory evoked potentials. *J Neurosurg* 57:472, 1982.
99. McGarry J, Friedgood DL, Woolsey R, et al: Somatosensory-evoked potentials in spinal cord injuries. *Surg Neurol* 22:341, 1984.
100. Dorfman LJ, Perkash I, Bosley TM, et al: Use of cerebral evoked potentials to evaluate spinal somatosensory function in patients

with traumatic and surgical myelopathies. *J Neurosurg* 52:654, 1980.

101. Chabot R, York DH, Watts C, et al: Somatosensory evoked potentials evaluated in normal subjects and spinal cord-injured patients. *J Neurosurg* 63:544, 1985.

102. Li C, Houlden DA, Rowed DW: Somatosensory evoked potentials and neurological grades as predictors of outcome in acute spinal cord injury. *J Neurosurg* 72:600, 1990.

103. Snyder JV, Nemoto EM, Carroll RG, et al: Global ischemia in dogs: Intracranial pressures, brain blood flow and metabolism. *Stroke* 6:21, 1975.

104. Steen PA, Michenfelder JD, Milde JH: Incomplete versus complete cerebral ischemia: Improved outcome with a minimal blood flow. *Ann Neurol* 6:389, 1979.

105. Beckstead JE, Tweed WA, Lee J, et al: Cerebral blood flow and metabolism in man following cardiac arrest. *Stroke* 9:569, 1978.

106. Cohan SL, Mun SK, Petite J, et al: Cerebral blood flow in humans following resuscitation from cardiac arrest. *Stroke* 20:761, 1989.

107. Steen PA, Newberg LA, Milde JH, et al: Nimodipine improves cerebral blood flow and neurologic recovery after complete cerebral ischemia in the dog. *J Cereb Blood Flow Metab* 3:38, 1983.

108. Steen PA, Gisvold SE, Milde JH, et al: Nimodipine improves outcome when given after complete cerebral ischemia in primates. *Anesthesiology* 62:406, 1985.

109. Forsman M, Aarseth HP, Nordby HK, et al: Effects of nimodipine on cerebral blood flow and cerebrospinal fluid pressure after cardiac arrest: Correlation with neurologic outcome. *Anesth Analg* 68:436, 1989.

110. Roine RO, Kaste M, Kinnunen A, et al: Nimodipine after resuscitation from out-of-hospital ventricular fibrillation: A placebo-controlled, double-blind, randomized trial. *JAMA* 264:3171, 1990.

111. Seiler RW, Grolimund P, Aaslid R: Cerebral vasospasm evaluated by transcranial ultrasound correlated with clinical grade and CT-visualized subarachnoid hemorrhage. *J Neurosurg* 64:594, 1986.

112. Aaslid R, Huber P, Nornes H: Evaluation of cerebrovascular spasm with transcranial Doppler ultrasound. *J Neurosurg* 60:37, 1984.

113. Sekhar LN, Wechsler LR, Yonas H, et al: Value of transcranial Doppler examination in the diagnosis of cerebral vasospasm after subarachnoid hemorrhage. *Neurosurgery* 22:813, 1988.

114. American Academy of Neurology: Assessment: Transcranial Doppler. *Neurology* 40:680, 1990.

115. Haley EC, Kassell NF, Torner JC: A randomized trial of nicardipine in subarachnoid hemorrhage: Angiographic and transcranial Doppler ultrasound results. *J Neurosurg* 78:548, 1993.

116. Hurst RW, Schnee C, Raps EC, et al: Role of transcranial Doppler in neuroradiological treatment of intracranial vasospasm. *Stroke* 24:299, 1993.

117. Laumer R, Steinmeier R, Gönner F, et al: Cerebral hemodynamics in subarachnoid hemorrhage evaluated by transcranial Doppler sonography, 1: Reliability of flow velocities in clinical management. *Neurosurgery* 33:1, 1993.

118. Steinmeier R, Laumer R, Bondár I, et al: Cerebral hemodynamics in subarachnoid hemorrhage evaluated by transcranial Doppler sonography, 2: Pulsatility indices—Normal reference values and characteristics in subarachnoid hemorrhage. *Neurosurgery* 33:10, 1993.

119. Tasker RC, Matthew DJ, Helms P, et al: Monitoring in non-traumatic coma, I: Invasive intracranial measurements. *Arch Dis Child* 63:888, 1988.

120. Barnett GH, Ropper AH, Romeo J: Intracranial pressure and outcome in adult encephalitis. *J Neurosurg* 68:585, 1988.

121. Hanid MA, Davies M, Mellon PJ, et al: Clinical monitoring of intracranial pressure in fulminant hepatic failure. *Gut* 21:866, 1980.

122. Bailes JE, Spetzler RF, Hadley MN, et al: Management morbidity and mortality of poor-grade aneurysm patients. *J Neurosurg* 72:559, 1990.

123. Sarnaik AP, Preston G, Lieh-Lai M, et al: Intracranial pressure and cerebral perfusion pressure in near-drowning. *Crit Care Med* 13:224, 1985.

124. Nussbaum E, Galant SP: Intracranial pressure monitoring as a guide to prognosis in the nearly drowned, severely comatose child. *J Pediatr* 102:215, 1983.

125. Griswold WR, Viney J, Mendoza SA, et al: Intracranial pressure monitoring in severe hypertensive encephalopathy. *Crit Care Med* 9:573, 1981.

126. Cant BR, Shaw NA: Monitoring by compressed spectral array in prolonged coma. *Neurology* 34:35, 1984.

127. Karnaze DS, Marshall LF, Bickford RG: EEG monitoring of clinical coma: The compressed spectral array. *Neurology* 32:289, 1982.

128. Westmoreland BF, Klass DW, Sharbrough FW, et al: Alpha-coma: Electroencephalographic, clinical, pathologic, and etiologic correlations. *Arch Neurol* 32:713, 1975.

129. Labar DR, Fisch BJ, Pedley TA, et al: Quantitative EEG monitoring for patients with subarachnoid hemorrhage. *Electroencephalogr Clin Neurophysiol* 78:325, 1991.

130. Tasker RC, Boyd S, Harden A, et al: Monitoring in non-traumatic coma, II: Electroencephalography. *Arch Dis Child* 63:895, 1988.

131. Cant BR, Shaw NA: Electroencephalography and compressed spectral array in severe intracranial disease. *Int Anesthesiol Clin* 17:343, 1979.

132. Rampil IJ, Matteo RS: Changes in EEG spectral edge frequency correlate with the hemodynamic response to laryngoscopy and intubation. *Anesthesiology* 67:139, 1987.

133. Algotsson L, Messeter K, Rehncrona S, et al: Cerebral hemodynamic changes and electroencephalography during carotid endarterectomy. *J Clin Anesth* 2:143, 1990.

134. Silbert BS, Kluger R, Cronin KD, et al: The processed electroencephalogram may not detect neurologic ischemia during carotid endarterectomy. *Anesthesiology* 70:356, 1989.

135. Muizelaar JP: The use of electroencephalography and brain protection during operation for basilar aneurysms. *Neurosurgery* 25:899, 1989.

136. Chiappa KH, Ropper AH: Evoked potentials in clinical medicine (first of two parts). *N Engl J Med* 306:1140, 1982.

137. Chiappa KH, Ropper AH: Evoked potentials in clinical medicine (second of two parts). *N Engl J Med* 306:1205, 1982.

138. Lesser RP, Raudzens P, Lüders H, et al: Postoperative neurological deficits may occur despite unchanged intraoperative somatosensory evoked potentials. *Ann Neurol* 19:22, 1986.

139. Hargadine JR, Branston NM, Symon L: Central conduction time in primate brain ischemia: A study in baboons. *Stroke* 11:637, 1980.

140. Symon L, Hargadine J, Zawirski M, et al: Central conduction time as an index of ischaemia in subarachnoid hemorrhage. *J Neurol Sci* 44:95, 1979.

141. Goldie WD, Chiappa KH, Young RR, et al: Brainstem auditory and short-latency somatosensory evoked responses in brain death. *Neurology* 31:248, 1981.

142. Garcia-Larrea L, Bertrand O, Artru F, et al: Brain-stem monitoring, II: Preterminal BAEP changes observed until brain death in deeply comatose patients. *Electroencephalogr Clin Neurophysiol* 68:446, 1987.

143. Frank LM, Furgiuele TL, Etheridge JE Jr: Prediction of chronic vegetative state in children using evoked potentials. *Neurology* 35:931, 1985.

144. de Weerd AW, Groeneveld C: The use of evoked potentials in the management of patients with severe cerebral trauma. *Acta Neurol Scand* 72:489, 1985.

145. Hume AL, Cant BR, Shaw NA: Central somatosensory conduction time in comatose patients. *Ann Neurol* 5:379, 1979.

26. Percutaneous Cystostomy

G. Forrest Quimby and Mani Menon

Percutaneous suprapubic cystostomy is a proved method of treatment of acute urinary retention when standard urethral catheterization of the bladder is impossible or contraindicated [1–6]. The placement of a small-diameter trocar suprapubic tube is rapid, safe, and easily accomplished at the bedside, requiring only local anesthesia.

Indications

The indications for percutaneous suprapubic cystostomy in the intensive care unit (ICU) are restricted (Table 26-1). Inability to place a urethral catheter in the setting of acute urinary retention is undoubtedly the most common indication for percutaneous suprapubic urinary diversion. Rarely, urethral disruption or infection is an indication. Before attempting suprapubic tube placement, one should be familiar with the various methods of urethral catheterization.

Urethral Catheterization

Typically, urethral catheters are used in the ICU to drain urine and monitor urinary output. Catheters differ in size (outside diameter, in French size) and shape, type of material, number of lumens, and type of retaining mechanism. The catheter selected depends on a thorough history and physical examination, as well as the indication for the catheter.

Prior to catheterization, it is important to note the patient's urinary history and history of previous prostate or urethral surgery. Male patients with a typical history of obstructive voiding symptoms such as decreased stream, intermittency, hesitation, nocturia, and dribbling may present difficulties with catheterization. In these patients, the standard 16 or 18 Fr. catheter may be deflected by large lateral lobe hypertrophy of the prostate and coil or create a false passage in the urethra. If an attempt at passing a small catheter is unsuccessful, often a 20 or 22 Fr. catheter is large enough to "push" its way through the hypertrophied prostate. Adequate lubrication, as described below, is essential. In patients with a history of previous open prostatectomy, radical prostatectomy, or transurethral resection of the prostate (TURP), catheterization may be difficult. The use of a Coudé-tip catheter may aid in negotiating a high bladder neck as a result of contracture after surgery.

Routine examination of the patient, including digital rectal examination, is necessary prior to catheterization. It is important to note the presence of blood at the urethral meatus or a high-riding prostate in a trauma patient, as urethral disruption may have occurred. In this situation, a retrograde urethrogram demonstrating lack of contrast extravasation is necessary prior to the procedure. In the patient with a large prostate, one might consider starting with a large urethral catheter.

The indication for catheter drainage may determine the type of catheter employed. Drainage in the setting of gross hematuria may necessitate a 22 or 24 Fr. catheter that has larger holes for the irrigation and removal of clots. Occasionally, continuous bladder irrigation is necessary via a three-way urethral catheter to prevent reclotting. Typically in men, larger indwelling catheters cause retention of urethral secretions and subsequent urethritis. Epididymitis may follow if large catheters are used over prolonged periods. Therefore, unless otherwise indicated, a 16 or 18 Fr. Foley catheter should be used.

TECHNIQUE OF URETHRAL CATHETERIZATION. After the patient is prepared and draped, 10 ml of local anesthetic in lubricant (2% lidocaine hydrochloride jelly) may be injected retrograde into the urethra in males. Anesthesia to the urethral mucosa requires 5 to 10 minutes, accomplished by a penile clamp or manually occluding the urethral meatus. Prior to introducing the catheter, the balloon must be tested to be sure it will deflate. Following generous lubrication with a water-soluble lubricant, the catheter is grasped near the tip with sterile gloves and is inserted into the external meatus while the penis is stretched with the other hand. The catheter is advanced gently; if there is resistance to advancement the location is determined by palpating of the catheter tip. The membranous urethra in males is a normal site of resistance, usually due to involuntary constriction of the external sphincter. This can be overcome by gentle, constant pressure applied to the catheter. In patients who have had a radical retropubic prostatectomy, the lack of support of the membranous urethra after surgery may increase the angulation between the bulbous and membranous urethra, obstructing catheter passage. This may be solved by having an assistant elevate the urethra by placing a finger in the rectum during catheter passage. Bladder neck stricture may be a barrier that cannot be bypassed, although a Coudé catheter might be successful where a straight catheter will fail. If urethral catheter drainage is expected to be necessary for more than a few days, the catheter is secured to the abdomen instead of the leg, to avoid a potential stricture at the penoscrotal junction.

In females, short, straight catheters are preferred. Due to the shorter urethra, only 5 ml of local anesthetic in lubricant is necessary. Rarely, due to vulvectomy secondary to vulvar cancer, vaginal atrophy, or morbid obesity, the urethral meatus will not be visible. In this case, blind catheter placement over a finger located in the vagina at the palpated site of the urethral meatus may be successful.

Contraindications to Suprapubic Cystostomy

The contraindications to percutaneous suprapubic cystostomy are listed in Table 26-2. The bladder may not be palpable if the patient is in acute renal failure and oliguric or anuric, has a small contracted neurogenic bladder, or is incontinent. In males with a nonpalpable bladder a 14 Fr. urethral catheter may be placed into the fossa navicularis and the balloon inflated with

Table 26-1. Indications for Percutaneous Cystostomy

1. Acute urinary retention when urethral catheterization is unsuccessful
2. Urethral disruption due to pelvic trauma
3. Bladder drainage required in the presence of severe urethral, prostatic, or epididymal infection

Table 26-2. Contraindications to Percutaneous Cystostomy

1. Nonpalpable bladder
2. Previous lower abdominal surgery
3. Coagulopathy
4. Known bladder tumor
5. Clot retention

2 to 3 ml of sterile saline to occlude the urethra. Saline can then be slowly injected in a retrograde fashion into the bladder to distend it, using a catheter-tip syringe. Once the bladder is easily palpable, a suprapubic tube may be placed. In the patient with a small contracted neurogenic bladder, it may be impossible to distend the bladder adequately and perform suprapubic urinary diversion safely with this method. Ultrasound guidance can be used to locate the bladder and a 22-gauge spinal needle then used to enter it. Saline is instilled into the bladder via the needle to distend it enough for easy suprapubic tube placement.

In patients with previous lower abdominal surgery, ultrasound evaluation may be necessary before a cystostomy catheter can be placed safely, because adhesions from previous surgery may hold a loop of bowel in the area of insertion. Coagulopathy is an obvious relative contraindication to suprapubic cystostomy. In patients with known bladder tumor, percutaneous bladder access should be avoided since tumor cell seeding of the percutaneous tract can occur. Finally, percutaneous suprapubic catheters are generally ineffective for draining bladders in patients with retained clots because of the small caliber of the catheters. Open surgical placement of a large-caliber tube is necessary if urethral catheterization is impossible.

Technique

There are several kits available for percutaneous suprapubic cystostomy, differing principally in how the catheter is retained in the bladder (Fig. 26-1). The Stamey unit (Cook Urological, Spencer, IN) uses a polyethylene Malecot catheter and the Bonanno catheter (Beckton Dickinson and Co., Franklin Lakes, NJ) uses a flexible Teflon tube inserted over a trocar that pigtails in the bladder after the trocar is withdrawn. We prefer the Stamey catheter because it appears to provide the most secure retention and the best drainage.

The patient is placed in the supine position; a roll may be placed under the hips to extend the pelvis. The distended bladder is confirmed by palpation and the suprapubic area is shaved, prepared with povidone-iodine or equivalent, and draped to include an area around the midline from the pubis to midway between the pubis and umbilicus. Then 1% lidocaine is infiltrated in the midline, approximately 4 cm above the pubis (Fig. 26-2). Lidocaine is injected to anesthetize the skin down to and including the anterior bladder wall. A 22-gauge spinal needle is used to find the bladder. If the bladder is distended adequately the needle can be directed vertically. If the bladder is smaller, however, a 60-degree caudal angle can be used (Fig. 26-2). The bladder is punctured by the spinal needle and confirmed by aspirating urine with a 3-ml syringe. At this point, both the angle and depth of puncture can be noted by placing the fingers on the spinal needle at the junction of the skin and withdrawing the needle. The fingers are placed at an equivalent depth on the cystostomy trocar to determine where bladder puncture should be obtained. At the site of spinal needle puncture, a 2-mm stab wound is then made with a no. 11 blade in preparation for trocar puncture. Using the trocar apparatus provided in the kit, the trocar is advanced into the bladder, duplicating the angle and depth used on the successful spinal needle puncture. Urine is aspirated again to ascertain that the trocar tip is in the bladder and the trocar is removed, leaving the suprapubic tube in the bladder. In a patient with urinary retention, urine should flow freely through the suprapubic catheter. The catheter (if it is a Stamey catheter) may then be pulled back gently until the resistance of the flange of the catheter is full against the anterior bladder wall and then advanced approximately 2 cm back into the bladder to allow for movement. This maneuver pulls the catheter away from the trigone and helps reduce bladder spasms.

Fig. 26-1. Stamey Suprapubic Cystostomy trochar set.

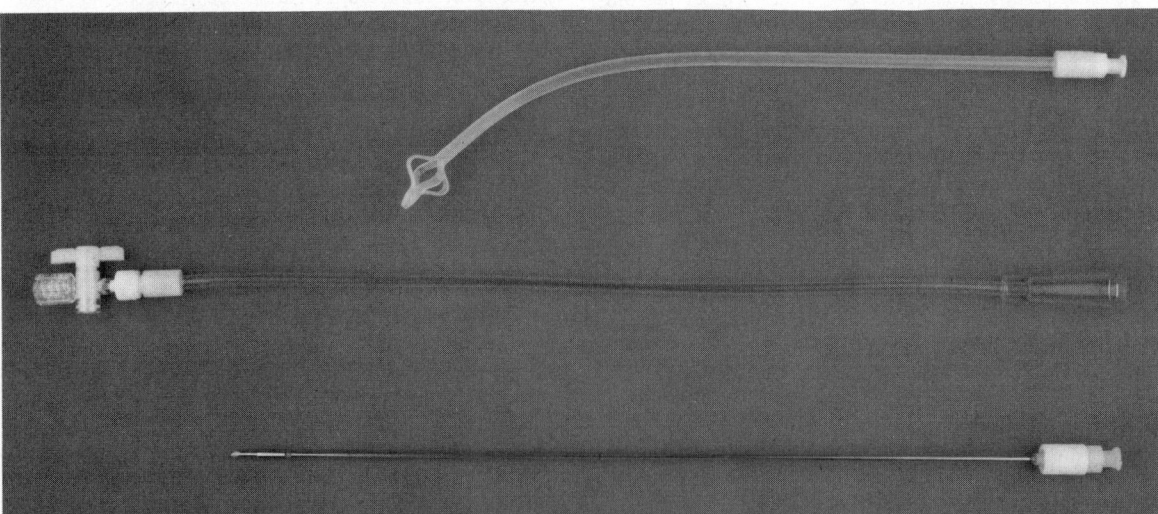

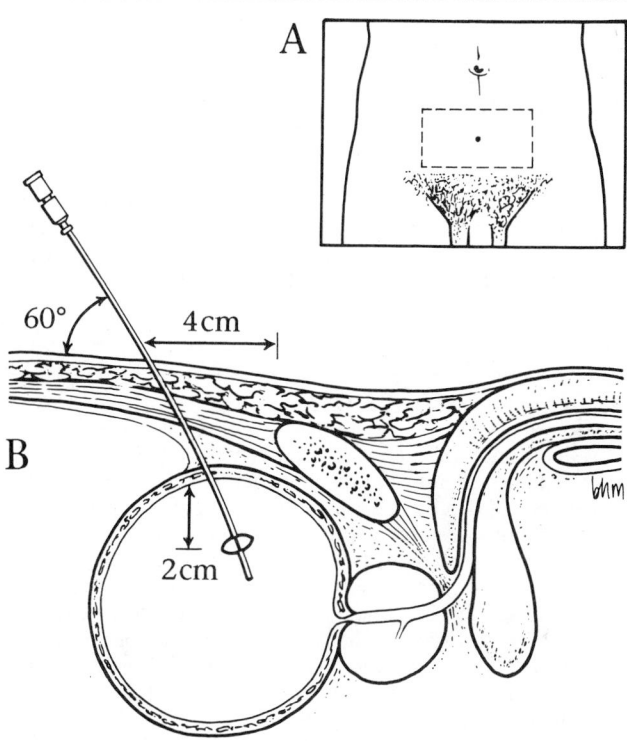

Fig. 26-2. Technique of suprapubic trochar placement. A. Area to be shaved, prepared and draped prior to trochar placement. B. Position of the Stamey trochar in the bladder. The angle, distance from the pubis, and position of the catheter in relation to the bladder wall are demonstrated.

Table 26-3. Complications of Percutaneous Cystostomy

1. Bladder spasms
2. Hematuria
3. Bowel perforation
4. Hypotension
5. Postobstructive diuresis
6. Loss of a portion of the catheter in the bladder

the procedure only on well-distended bladders and taking a midline approach no more than 4 cm above the pubis. In patients who have had previous lower abdominal or pelvic surgery, an ultrasound examination should be performed before the procedure to rule out entrapped bowel.

Hypotension rarely occurs following suprapubic tube placement. It may be secondary to a vasovagal response or be caused by relief of pelvic venous compression from bladder distention. It is easily treated with fluid resuscitation. If urinary obstruction is prolonged and the blood urea nitrogen is significantly elevated, then the patient is at risk for postobstructive diuresis after suprapubic tube placement. Patients at highest risk include those with azotemia, peripheral edema, congestive heart failure, and mental status changes [8]. If urine output continues at greater than 200 ml per hour the patient needs aggressive monitoring of vital signs and intake and output and may require intravenous fluid replacement (replace half of urine output with normal saline). The mechanisms of this diuresis include urea-mediated solute diuresis and natriuresis secondary to the enormous increase in distal tubule solute delivery, which overwhelms the distal reabsorption mechanism [9].

Other rare but possible complications include through-and-through perforation of the bladder and loss of a portion of the catheter in the bladder [10].

Complications

The complications that can occur following percutaneous suprapubic cystostomy are listed in Table 26-3. Bladder spasms, the most common complication, can be avoided using the technique described previously. Severe bladder spasms can be treated with 5 mg oxybutynin chloride two times per day, to a maximal dosage of 5 mg four times per day. This medication must be withdrawn prior to suprapubic tube removal, since its anticholinergic activity may aggravate urinary retention in patients with underlying obstructive uropathy.

Hematuria is probably the second most common complication following suprapubic tube placement. It is rarely severe enough to necessitate open cystostomy for placement of a large-bore tube for irrigation. The etiology is varied but usually secondary to laceration of a submucosal vessel or rapid decompression of a chronically distended bladder. It can be avoided by gradually decompressing a chronically distended bladder.

Bowel perforation, a well-known complication of percutaneous suprapubic cystostomy [7], can be avoided by attempting

References

1. Hodgkinson CP, Hodari AA: Trocar suprapubic cystostomy for postoperative bladder drainage in the female. *Am J Obstet Gynecol* 96:773, 1966.
2. Cook JB, Smith PH: Percutaneous suprapubic cystostomy after spinal cord injury. *Br J Urol* 48:119, 1976.
3. Morehouse DD: Emergency management of urethral trauma. *Urol Clin North Am* 9:251, 1982.
4. Walsh PC, Retik AB, Stamey TA, Vaughan ED (eds): *Campbell's Urology.* 6th ed. Philadelphia, WB Saunders, 1992.
5. Bonanno PJ, Landers DE, Rock DE: Bladder drainage with the suprapubic catheter needle. *Obstet Gynecol* 35:807, 1970.
6. Stamey TA: Suprapubic cystostomy. *Monogr Urol* 1:1 editorial, 1980.
7. Noller KL, Pratt JH, Symmonds RE: Bowel perforation with suprapubic cystostomy: Report of two cases. *Obstet Gynecol* 48(suppl 1):67s, 1976.
8. Vaughan ED, Gillenwater JY: Diagnosis, characterization and management of post-obstructive diuresis. *J Urol* 109:286, 1973.
9. Howards SS: Post-obstructive diuresis: A misunderstood phenomenon. *J Urol* 110:537, 1973.
10. McGruder CJ: Suprapubic bladder drainage following gynecologic operations. *Am J Obstet Gynecol* 113:267, 1972.

27. Aspiration of Joints

Eric W. Jacobson

Arthrocentesis is a safe and relatively simple procedure that involves the introduction of a needle into the joint space to remove synovial fluid. It constitutes an essential part of the evaluation of any arthritis of unknown cause, frequently with the intent to rule out a septic process [1,2,3].

Ropes and Bauer first categorized synovial fluid as inflammatory or noninflammatory in 1953 [4], terms that are still used today. Hollander et al. coined the term *synovianalysis* to describe the process of joint fluid analysis in 1961 [5]. He and others [6,7] were instrumental in establishing the critical role of synovial fluid analysis to diagnose certain forms of arthritis. Septic arthritis and crystalline arthritis can be diagnosed by synovial fluid analysis alone. They may present similarly but require markedly different treatments, thus necessitating early arthrocentesis and prompt synovial fluid analysis.

Indications

Arthrocentesis is performed for both diagnostic and therapeutic purposes [8,9]. The main indication for arthrocentesis is to assist in the evaluation of arthritis of unknown cause. In the intensive care unit (ICU) it is most commonly performed in the setting of acute monoarthritis or oligoarthritis (presenting with one to three inflamed joints) to rule out septic arthritis. Many types of inflammatory arthritis mimic septic arthritis. Synovial fluid analysis is useful in differentiating the various causes of inflammatory arthritis [4,10] (Table 27-1). Therefore, patients presenting with mono- or oligoarthritis of recent onset require prompt arthrocentesis with subsequent synovial fluid analysis, preferably before initiation of treatment.

Before performing arthrocentesis, it must be ascertained that the true joint is inflamed and an effusion is present. This requires a meticulous physical examination to differentiate arthritis from periarticular inflammation. Bursitis, tendinitis, and cellulitis all may mimic arthritis. In the knee, the examination begins with assessment of swelling. A true effusion may cause bulging of the parapatellar gutters and the suprapatellar pouch [11]. The swelling should be confined to the joint space. To check for small effusions, the bulge test is performed [12]. Fluid is stroked from the medial joint line into the suprapatellar pouch and then from the suprapatellar pouch down along the lateral joint line. If a bulge of fluid is noted at the medial joint line, then a small effusion is present (Fig. 27-1). If a large effusion is suspected a patellar tap is performed [13]. The left hand is used to apply pressure to the suprapatellar pouch while the right hand taps the patella against the femur with sharp downward pressure. If the patella is ballottable, then an effusion is probably present. Comparison with the opposite joint is helpful. Many texts describe joint examination and assessment for fluid in the knee and other joints [11–14].

Arthrocentesis is also used for therapeutic purposes. In a septic joint, serial joint aspirations are required to remove accumulated inflammatory or purulent fluid. This allows serial monitoring of the total white blood cell count, Gram stain, and culture to assess response to treatment and accomplishes complete drainage of a "closed space." Inflammatory fluid contains many destructive enzymes that contribute to cartilage and bony degradation; removal of the fluid may slow this destructive process [15,16]. Finally, arthrocentesis allows for injection of long-acting corticosteroid preparations into the joint space, which may be a useful treatment for various inflammatory and noninflammatory forms of arthritis [17,18,19].

Contraindications

Absolute contraindications to arthrocentesis include local infection of the overlying skin or other periarticular structures and severe coagulopathy [1,2,3,20]. If coagulopathy is present and septic arthritis is suspected, every effort should be made to correct the coagulopathy (with fresh frozen plasma or alternate factors) prior to joint aspiration. Therapeutic anticoagulation is not an absolute contraindication, but every effort should be made to avoid excessive trauma during aspiration in this circumstance. Known bacteremia is a contraindication because inserting a needle into the joint space disrupts capillary integrity and thus allows joint space seeding [21]. If septic arthritis is strongly suspected, however, joint aspiration is indicated. The presence of articular instability (e.g., that seen with badly damaged joints) is a relative contraindication, though the presence of a large presumed inflammatory fluid may still warrant joint aspiration.

Complications

The major complications of arthrocentesis are iatrogenically induced infection and bleeding, both of which are extremely rare [1]. The risk of infection after arthrocentesis has been estimated to be less than 1 in 10,000 [22]. Hollander reported an incidence of less than 0.005 percent in 400,000 injections [23]. Owen reported an incidence of 0.002 to 0.004 percent in more

Table 27-1. Common Causes of Inflammatory Arthritis

Rheumatoid arthritis
Spondyloarthropathies
   Psoriatic arthritis
   Reiter's syndrome/reactive arthritis
   Ankylosing spondylitis
   Ulcerative colitis/regional enteritis
Crystal-induced arthritis
   Monosodium urate (gout)
   Calcium pyrophosphate dihydrate (pseudogout)
   Hydroxyapatite
Infectious arthritis
   Bacterial
   Mycobacterial
   Fungal
Connective tissue diseases
   Systemic lupus erythematosus
   Vasculitis
   Scleroderma
   Polymyositis
Hypersensitivity
   Serum sickness

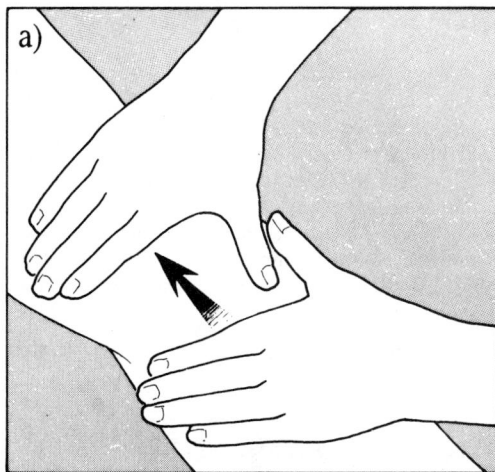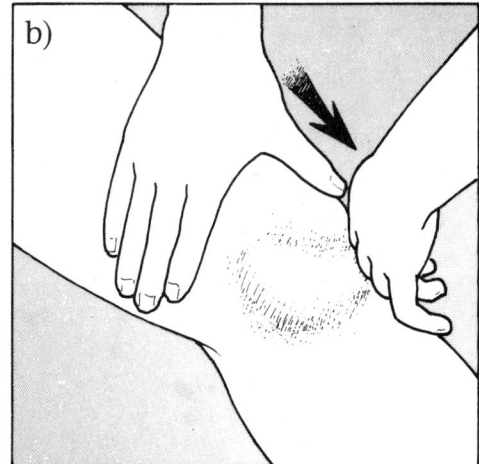

Fig. 27-1. The bulge test. A. Milk fluid from the suprapatellar pouch into the joint. B. Slide hand down the lateral aspect of the joint line and watch for a bulge medial to the joint.

than 50,000 injections [24]. Strict adherence to aseptic technique will reduce the risk of postarthrocentesis infection. Significant hemorrhage is also extremely rare. Correction of prominent coagulopathy prior to arthrocentesis will reduce this risk.

Another potential complication of arthrocentesis is direct injury to the articular cartilage by the needle. This is not quantifiable, but any injury to cartilage could be associated with degenerative change over time. To avoid cartilaginous damage the needle should be pushed in only as far as necessary to obtain fluid; excessive movement of the needle during the procedure and aggressive complete drainage should be avoided.

A rare complication is separation of the hypodermic needle from its hub during arthrocentesis [25]. A hemostat should be available to remove a separated needle from the soft tissue if necessary.

Technique

Joint aspiration is easily learned. A sound knowledge of the joint anatomy, including the bony and soft tissue landmarks used for joint entry, is needed. Strict aseptic technique must be followed to minimize risk of infection, and relaxation of the muscles surrounding the joint should be encouraged, since muscular contraction can impede the needle's entry into the joint.

Most physicians in the ICU can aspirate the knee, as it is one of the most accessible joints. Other joints should probably be aspirated by an appropriate specialist, such as a rheumatologist or orthopedic surgeon. Certain joints are quite difficult to enter blindly and are more appropriately entered using radiologic guidance, such as with fluoroscopy or computed tomography (CT). These include the hip, sacroiliac, and temporomandibular joints. Here we describe the technique for knee aspiration. Many texts describe in detail the aspiration technique of other joints [3,7,23,24].

1. Describe the procedure to the patient, including the possible complications, and obtain written informed consent.
2. Collect all items needed for the procedure (Table 27-2).
3. With the patient supine and the knee fully extended, ex-

amine the knee to confirm the presence of an effusion, as described earlier.
4. Identify landmarks for needle entry. The knee may be aspirated from a medial or lateral approach. The medial approach is more commonly used and is preferred when small effusions are present. Identify the superior and inferior borders of the patella. Entry should be halfway between those borders just inferior to the undersurface of the patella (Fig. 27-2). The entry site may be marked with pressure from the end of a ballpoint pen with the writing tip retracted. An indentation mark should be visible.
5. Cleanse the area with an iodine-based antiseptic solution, such as Betadine. Allow the area to dry, then wipe once with an alcohol swab. Practice universal precautions: wear gloves at all times while handling any body fluid, though they need not be sterile for routine knee aspiration. Do not touch the targeted area once it has been cleaned.
6. Apply local anesthesia. We prefer ethyl chloride, which is sterile and provides superficial anesthesia. Spray ethyl chloride directly onto the designated area; stop when the first signs of freezing are evident so as not to cause any skin damage. Alternatively a local anesthetic (1% lidocaine) may be instilled with a 25-gauge needle into the subcutaneous skin. Once numbing has occurred, deeper instillation of the

Table 27-2. Arthrocentesis Equipment

Skin preparation and local anesthesia	Idophor solution
	Alcohol swab
	Ethyl chloride spray
	For local anesthesia—1% lidocaine, 25-gauge, 1-inch needle, 22-gauge, 1.5-inch needle, 5-ml syringe
	Sterile sponge/cloth
Arthrocentesis	Gloves
	10–60-ml syringe (depending on size of effusion)
	18–20-gauge, 1.5-inch-needle
	Sterile sponge/cloth
	Sterile clamp
	Bandaid
Collection	15-ml anticoagulated tube (with sodium heparin or EDTA)
	Sterile tubes for routine cultures
	Slide, cover slip

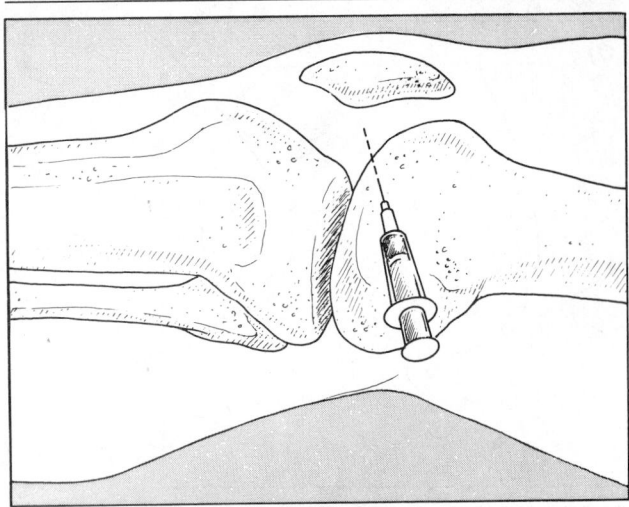

Fig. 27-2. Technique of aspirating the knee joint. The needle enters halfway between the superior and inferior borders of the patella and is directed just inferior to the patella.

local anesthetic (to the joint capsule) can be performed using a 22-gauge, 1.5-inch needle.

7. To enter the knee joint, use an 18-gauge, 1.5-inch needle with a 20- to 60-ml syringe, depending on the size of the effusion. Use a quick thrust through the skin and on through the capsule to minimize pain. Avoid hitting periosteal bone, which causes significant pain, or cartilage, which causes cartilaginous damage. Aspirate fluid to fill the syringe. If the fluid appears purulent or hemorrhagic, try to tap the joint "dry," which will remove mediators of inflammation that may perpetuate an inflammatory or destructive process. If the syringe is full and further fluid remains, the sterile hemostat may be used to clamp the needle, thus stabilizing it, while switching syringes. When the syringes have been switched, more fluid can be withdrawn. The syringes must be sterile.

8. When the fluid has been obtained, quickly remove the needle and apply pressure to the needle site with a piece of sterile gauze. When bleeding has stopped, remove the gauze, clean the area with alcohol, and apply an adhesive bandage. If the patient is anticoagulated or has a bleeding diathesis, apply prolonged pressure.

9. Document the amount of fluid obtained. Perform gross examination, noting the color and clarity. A "string sign" may be performed at the bedside to assess fluid viscosity (see

below). Send fluid for cell count with differential, Gram stain, routine culture, specialized cultures for *Gonococcus, Mycobacterium,* and fungus, if indicated, and polarized microscopic examination for crystal analysis. Other tests, such as glucose and complement determinations, are generally not helpful. Use an anticoagulated tube to send fluid for cell count and crystal analysis. Sodium heparin and EDTA are appropriate anticoagulants. Lithium heparin and calcium oxalate should be avoided because they can precipitate out of solution to form crystals, thus potentially giving a false positive assessment for crystals [6,26]. Fluid may be sent for Gram stain and culture in the syringe itself or in a sterile red-top tube.

Synovial Fluid Analysis

Synovial fluid analysis is identical for all joints and begins with bedside observation of the fluid. The color, clarity, and viscosity of the fluid are characterized. Synovial fluid is divided into noninflammatory versus inflammatory types based on the total nucleated cell count. A white blood cell count less than or equal to 2000 per cubic millimeter is defined as a noninflammatory fluid and greater than 2000 per cubic millimeter is defined as an inflammatory fluid. Table 27-3 shows how fluid is divided into major categories based on appearance and cell count.

GROSS EXAMINATION

Color. Color and clarity should be tested using a clear glass tube. Translucent plastic, as used in most disposable syringes, interferes with proper assessment [1].

Normal synovial fluid is colorless. Both noninflammatory and inflammatory synovial fluid appear yellow or straw-colored. Septic effusions frequently appear purulent and whitish. Depending on the number of white blood cells present, pure pus may be extracted from a septic joint. Hemorrhagic effusions appear red or brown. If the fluid looks like pure blood, the tap may have aspirated venous blood. The needle is removed, pressure applied, and the joint reentered from an alternate site. If the same bloody appearance is noted, the fluid is a hemorrhagic effusion probably not related to the trauma of the aspiration. If any question remains, the hematocrit of the effusion is compared to that of peripheral blood. The hematocrit in a hemorrhagic effusion is typically lower than that of peripheral blood. In the case of a traumatic tap, the hematocrit of the "fluid" should be equal to that of peripheral blood.

Table 27-3. Joint Fluid Characteristics

	Normal	Group I (noninflammatory)	Group II (inflammatory)	Group III (septic)
Color	Clear	Yellow	Yellow or opalescent	Variable—may be purulent
Clarity	Transparent	Transparent	Translucent	Opaque
Viscosity	Very high	High	Low	Typically low
Mucin clot	Firm	Firm	Friable	Friable
WBC/mm³	200	200–2000	2000–100,000	>50,000, usually >100,000
PMN (%)	<25	<25	>50	>75
Culture	Negative	Negative	Negative	Usually positive

PMN = polymorphonuclear cells.

Clarity. The clarity of synovial fluid depends on the number and types of cells or particles present. Clarity is tested by reading black print on a white background through a glass tube filled with the synovial fluid. If the print is easily read, the fluid is transparent. This is typical of normal and noninflammatory synovial fluid. If the black print can be distinguished from the white background but is not clear, the fluid is translucent. This is typical of inflammatory effusions. If nothing can be seen through the fluid, it is opaque. This occurs with grossly inflammatory, septic, and hemorrhagic fluids (Table 27-3).

Viscosity. The viscosity of synovial fluid is a measure of the hyaluronic acid content. Hyaluronic acid is one of the major substances in synovial fluid that gives it a viscous quality. Degradative enzymes such as hyaluronidase are released in inflammatory conditions, thus destroying hyaluronic acid and other proteinaceous material, resulting in a thinner, less viscous fluid.

Viscosity can be assessed at the bedside using the string sign [1]. A drop of fluid is allowed to fall from the end of the needle or syringe and the length of the continuous "string" that forms estimated. Normal fluid typically forms at least a 6-cm continuous string. Inflammatory fluid will not form a string; instead, it drops off the end of the needle or syringe like water dropping from a faucet. Again, universal precautions should always be used when handling synovial fluid.

The mucin clot, another measure of viscosity, estimates the presence of intact hyaluronic acid and hyaluronic acid-protein interactions. This test is performed by placing several drops of synovial fluid in 5% acetic acid and then mixing with a stirring stick. A "good" mucin clot forms in normal and noninflammatory fluid. The fluid remains condensed in a clot resembling chewed gum. A "poor" mucin clot is seen with inflammatory fluid; the fluid disperses diffusely within the acetic acid.

CELL COUNT AND DIFFERENTIAL. The cell count should be done as soon as possible after arthrocentesis, as a delay of even several hours may cause an artificially low white blood cell count [27]. The total white blood cell count of synovial fluid differentiates noninflammatory from inflammatory fluid, as noted above. The technique for the cell count is identical to that used with peripheral blood. The fluid may be diluted with normal saline for a manual count, or an automated counter may be used. Viscous fluid with excessive debris may clog a counter or give falsely elevated results, thus making the manual procedure somewhat more accurate.

The differential white blood cell count is also performed using the technique used for peripheral blood, typically using Wright's stain. The differential is calculated based on direct visualization. The differential count includes cells typically seen in peripheral blood, such as polymorphonuclear cells, monocytes, and lymphocytes, as well as cells localized to the synovial space. In general, the total white blood cell count and the polymorphonuclear cell count increase with inflammation and infection [28]. Septic fluid typically has a differential of greater than 75 percent polymorphonuclear cells (Table 27-3).

CRYSTALS. All fluid should be assessed for the presence of crystals. As with cell count, crystal analysis should be performed as soon as possible after arthrocentesis. A delay is associated with a decreased yield [27]. One drop of fluid is placed on a slide and covered with a cover slip; this is examined for crystals using a compensated polarized light microscope. The presence of *intracellular* monosodium urate or calcium pyrophosphate dihydrate (CPPD) crystals confirms a diagnosis of gout or pseudogout, respectively. Even in the presence of crystals, infection must be considered since crystals can occur concomitantly with a septic joint. Monosodium urate crystals are typically long and needle-shaped. They may appear to pierce through a white blood cell. They are negatively birefringent, appearing yellow when parallel with the plane of reference. Typically, CPPD crystals are small and rhomboid. They are weakly positively birefringent, appearing blue when oriented parallel to the plane of reference. Rotating the stage of the microscopic and thereby the orientation of the crystals 90 degrees changes their color: monosodium urate crystals will turn blue and CPPD crystals yellow. The yield for crystals can be increased by spinning the specimen and examining the sediment. If the fluid cannot be examined immediately, it should be refrigerated to preserve the crystals.

GRAM STAIN AND CULTURE. The Gram stain is done as with other body fluids. It should be performed as soon as possible to screen for the presence of bacteria. Synovial fluid in general should be cultured routinely for aerobic and anaerobic bacterial organisms. In certain circumstances (e.g., in *chronic* monoarticular arthritis), fluid may be cultured for the presence of mycobacteria and fungus. If disseminated gonorrhea is suspected, fluid should be plated directly onto chocolate agar or Thayer-Martin media. A positive culture confirms septic arthritis.

Other studies on synovial fluid (glucose, protein, complement, immune complexes) generally are not helpful.

References

1. Gatter RA: *A Practical Handbook of Joint Fluid Analysis.* Philadelphia, Lea & Febiger, 1984.
2. Stein R: *Manual of Rheumatology and Outpatient Orthopedic Disorders.* Boston, Little Brown, 1981.
3. Krey PR, Lazaro DM: *Analysis of Synovial Fluid.* Summit, NJ, CIBA-GEIGY, 1992.
4. Ropes MW, Bauer W: *Synovial Fluid Changes in Joint Disease.* Cambridge, MA, Harvard University Press, 1953.
5. Hollander JL, Jessar RA, McCarty DJ: Synovianalysis: An aid in arthritis diagnosis. *Bull Rheum Dis* 12:263, 1961.
6. Gatter RA, McCarty DJ: Synovianalysis: A rapid clinical diagnostic procedure. *Rheumatism* 20:2, 1964.
7. Coggeshell HC: *Arthritis and Allied Conditions.* 6th ed. Philadelphia, Lea & Febiger, 1960.
8. Hasselbacher P: *Primer on the Rheumatic Diseases,* 9th ed. Atlanta, Arthritis Foundation, 1988.
9. Eisenberg JM, Schumacher JM, Davidson PK, et al: Usefulness of synovial fluid analysis in the evaluation of joint effusions: Use of threshold analysis and likelihood ratios to assess a diagnostic test. *Arch Intern Med* 144:715, 1984.
10. Schumacher HR: Synovial fluid analysis. *Orthop Rev* 13:85, 1984.
11. Polley HF, Hunder GG: *Rheumatolic Interviewing and Physical Examination of the Joints.* 2nd ed. Philadelphia, WB Saunders, 1978.
12. Doherty M, Hazelman BL, Hutton CW, et al: *Rheumatology Examination and Injection Techniques.* London, WB Saunders, 1992.
13. Hoppenfeld S: *Physical Examination of the Spine and Extremities.* Norwalk, CT, Appleton-Century-Crofts, 1976.
14. Kelley WN, Harris ED, Ruddy S, et al: *Textbook of Rheumatology.* 2nd ed. Philadelphia, WB Saunders, 1985.
15. Greenwald RA: Oxygen radicals inflammation and arthritis: Pathophysiological considerations and implications for treatment. *Semin Arthritis Rheum* 20:219, 1991.
16. Robinson DR, Tashjian AH, Levine L: Prostaglandin E2 induced bone resorption by rheumatoid synovia: A model for bone destruction in RA. *J Clin Invest* 56:1181, 1975.

17. Hollander JL, et al: Hydrocortisone and cortisone injected into arthritic joints. *JAMA* 147:1629, 1951.
18. Hollander JL: Intrasynovial corticosteroid therapy in arthritis. *Maryland State Med J* 19:62, 1970.
19. Steinbrocker P, Neustadt DH: *Aspiration and Injection Therapy in Arthritis and Musculoskeletal Diseases*. Hagerstown, MD, Harper & Row, 1972.
20. Gray RG, Tenenbaum J, Gottlieb NL: Local corticosteroid injection treatment in rheumatic disorders. *Semin Arthritis Rheum* 10:231, 1981.
21. McCarthy DJ Jr: A basic guide to arthrocentesis. *Hosp Med* 4:77, 1968.
22. Gottlieb NL, Riskin WG: Complications of local corticosteroid injections. *JAMA* 243:1547, 1980.
23. Hollander JL: Intrasynovial corticosteroid therapy. *Arthritis and Allied Conditions*. 8th ed. Philadelphia, Lea & Febiger, 1972.

24. Owen DS Jr: Aspiration and injection of joints and soft tissues, in Kelly WN, Harris ED, Ruddy S, et al (eds): *Textbook of Rheumatology*. 3rd ed. Philadelphia, WB Saunders, 1989.
25. Gottlieb NL: Hypodermic needle separation during arthrocentesis. *Arthritis Rheum* 24:1593, 1981.
26. Tanphaichitr K, Spilberg I, Hahn B: Lithium heparin crystals simulating calcium pyrophosphate dihydrate crystals in synovial fluid (letter). *Arthritis Rheum* 9:966, 1976.
27. Kerolus G, Clayburne G, Schumacher HR Jr: Is it mandatory to examine synovial fluids promptly after arthrocentesis? *Arthritis Rheum* 32:271, 1989.
28. Krey PR, Bailen DA: Synovial fluid leukocytosis: A study of extremes. *Am J Med* 67:436, 1979.

28. Anesthesia for Bedside Procedures

Laurence Landow and
Wandana Joshi-Ryzewicz

High on the list of contributions by anesthesiologists to the practice of critical care medicine is the introduction of intravenous (IV) anesthetics. Intravenous anesthesia as we know it today dates from the administration of thiopental (sodium pentothal) by John S. Lundy at the Mayo Clinic in 1935 [1]. Ironically, in a landmark issue of the journal *Anesthesiology* 8 years later, thiopental was branded "the ideal method of euthanasia in war surgery" because of the large number of fatalities that arose from its use in sailors injured during the attack on Pearl Harbor in 1941 [2]. Had there not been a companion article and accompanying editorial in the same issue detailing the safety of thiopental in a patient with a severe gunshot wound [3], many patients might have been denied access to the innovative surgical techniques (e.g., cardiopulmonary bypass) that emerged after World War II.

Formation of intensive care units (ICUs) in this country was fueled by the recognition that a specialized team of physicians and nurses was needed for postoperative care of patients undergoing open heart surgery. Until the 1970s, only a handful of IV anesthetic drugs (e.g., morphine, meperidine, diazepam) was available for these and other high-risk patients. Since that time, the pharmaceutical industry has produced opioids that are more potent than morphine by several orders of magnitude and sedatives that induce loss of consciousness within seconds. By allowing us to model different dose regimens, computers have been instrumental in increasing understanding of the pharmacokinetics of these drugs and their implications in critically ill patients. No less important has been the introduction of computer-driven programmable infusion pumps and continuous IV infusion technique. Continuous IV drug administration is superior to the repeated bolus method because it (1) provides relatively constant blood and central nervous system (CNS) levels of drugs, thereby avoiding the peaks and valleys incurred with intermittent dosing; (2) decreases drug accumulation; and (3) permits changes in the infusion rate to meet individual patient requirements. Anesthesiologists use this technique in the operating room in total IV anesthesia (TIVA). Acclaim for TIVA

is growing because analgesia and hypnosis (lack of awareness) can be managed separately, without polluting the environment with nitrous oxide and other inhalation agents that are potential ozone depleters.

Surveys of hospitalized patients leave little doubt that pain has been, and continues to be, underrated and undertreated by the medical profession. To deal with this issue effectively, intensivists have a responsibility to familiarize themselves with anesthetic agents currently available. In this chapter we examine various aspects of delivering anesthesia to patients in the ICU. We begin with a discussion of pain management problems encountered in the critically ill, then describe the properties of various analgesics and hypnotics (commonly referred to as sedatives) and the pitfalls to avoid when using them, and finally offer practical suggestions for using TIVA in the ICU.

Benefits of Pain Relief

While a causal relationship between pain and outcome of critical illness might appear unlikely at first glance, increasing evidence suggests the opposite. Studies show that effective pain control (1) decreases the incidence of pulmonary complications in patients with abdominal or thoracic injury and long bone fractures [4]; (2) promotes patient mobilization and attendant reductions in deep venous thrombosis [5]; (3) attenuates the stress response to injury (i.e., catecholamine-associated hypertension, tachycardia, and increased oxygen consumption) [6] (4) improves nitrogen balance [7]; (5) improves the metabolic and immune responses to injury (i.e., stimulation of the complement, arachidonic acid, cytokine, and hypothalamic-pituitary-adrenal cascades) [8,9]; (6) blunts the stimulatory effects of pain on cerebral blood flow and metabolic rate in closed-head injury patients [10]; and (7) decreases the severity of ischemic episodes in the first 18 hours following coronary artery bypass surgery [11].

Common Pain Management Problems in ICU Patients

INAPPROPRIATE DOSING. Selecting the proper dose of an analgesic to administer to a patient in the ICU is problematic due to difficulty in assessing the effectiveness of pain relief, pharmacokinetic differences between the critically ill and other patients, and normal physiologic changes associated with aging.

Assessing the Effectiveness of Pain Relief. Often, ICU patients are incapable of communicating their feelings because of delirium, obtundation, or endotracheal intubation. As a result, medical staff must rely on autonomic hyperactivity (e.g., tachycardia, hypertension, lacrimation, diaphoresis) to assess pain intensity and the effectiveness of drug therapy, a task made nearly impossible by confounding variables inherent in the host response to critical illness.

Pharmacokinetic Considerations. The aim of administering a drug intravenously is to achieve and maintain occupancy of tissue receptors in sufficient numbers to obtain the desired effect, minimize side effects, and facilitate quick recovery. The manner in which the body distributes a drug from the plasma (central compartment) into the tissues (peripheral compartments) and back again into the plasma, ultimately eliminating it from the body, defines its pharmacokinetic profile. Traditionally, serum drug levels have been believed to decrease over time following a bolus injection (elimination half-life [T1/2]) in proportion to the volume of the compartments in which the drug is distributed (volume of distribution at steady state [VdSS]), divided by its rate of elimination from the body (clearance [Cl]):

$$T1/2 = VdSS/Cl$$

Elimination half-lives in critically ill patients are unlike those in normal subjects for several reasons [12]. Because ICU patients frequently have renal and/or hepatic dysfunction, drug elimination is significantly impaired. Hypoalbuminemia, common in critical illness, decreases protein binding and increases free drug concentration [13]. Since free drug is the only moiety that occupies tissue receptors, decreased protein binding increases VdSS. Capillary permeability is often altered during critical illnes. Drugs ordinarily restricted to the intravascular compartment because of their large diameter or molecular weight are free to enter peripheral tissues (i.e., fat, muscle, skin), effectively decreasing the concentration of drug delivered to the CNS. This, in turn, necessitates larger loading doses to achieve the desired response and correspondingly longer periods of time to clear the drug from the body.

With increasing use of continuous IV drug infusions, the notion that elimination half-life predicts serum drug concentrations and, by implication, treatment-effect, has undergone major revision. For example, investigators have noticed that return of consciousness following an 8-hour propofol infusion takes only 5 to 10 minutes, even though the elimination half-life of propofol approaches 5 hours. This suggests that the initial fall in drug concentration following termination of an infusion is more a function of redistribution from the plasma and other highly perfused tissues to less-well perfused peripheral compartments than it is a function of drug elimination rate from the body. In this light, intercompartmental clearances, volumes, and rate constants take on primary importance, whereas elimination half-lives, in and of themselves, provide virtually no insight about the rate of decline of drug concentrations [14].

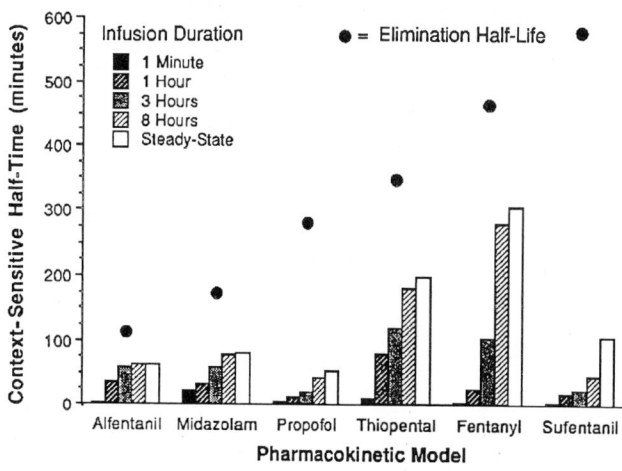

Fig. 28-1. Elimination half-lives and context-sensitive half-times from computer simulation models for several anesthetic drugs. (From Hughes MA, Glass PSA, Jacobs JR: Context-sensitive half-time in multicompartment pharmacokinetic models for intravenous anesthetic drugs. *Anesthesiology* 76:336, 1992. With permission.)

Hughes et al. coined the term *context-sensitive half-time,* or the time required for serum drug concentrations to decrease 50 percent after an infusion is stopped, as a more realistic measure of its duration of action [15]. *Context* in this sense is the duration of the infusion prior to switching it off. Figure 28-1 provides elimination half-lives and context-sensitive half-times from computer simulation models for several commonly used anesthetic drugs.

Physiologic Changes Associated with Aging. People 65 years of age and older comprise the fastest growing segment of the population and constitute the majority of patients in many ICUs. Aging inevitably leads to (1) a decrease in total body water and lean body mass; (2) an increase in body fat and, hence, an increase in the VdSS for lipid-soluble drugs; and (3) a decrease in drug clearance rates, due to reductions in plasma protein binding, liver mass, hepatic enzyme activity, liver blood flow, and renal excretory function. Double-blind studies indicate a progressive, age-related increase in pain relief [16] and electroencephalographic suppression [17] among elderly patients receiving the same dose of narcotic as younger patients. Corresponding studies show an increase in CNS depression [18,19] following administration of identical doses of benzodiazepines.

IMPROPER SELECTION OF AGENT. Procedures performed in ICUs today (Table 28-1) span a spectrum that extends from those associated with minimal pain but considerable discomfort (e.g., esophagogastroscopy) to those that are very painful without adequate analgesia (e.g., orthopedic manipulations, dressing changes). Depending on technical difficulty, the duration of these procedures can range from minutes to hours. To provide an acceptable level of anesthesia, IV anesthetics should be selected according to the nature of the procedure and titrated according to the patient's response to surgical stimulus. Choice of anesthetic agents also should be guided by the following to maximize clinical effectiveness.

Head Trauma. Head-injured patients require a technique that provides effective yet brief analgesia and sedation so the ca-

Table 28-1. Bedside Procedures and Associated Levels of Discomfort

Level of Discomfort	Procedure
Irritating and/or mildly to moderately painful; necessitates a modest degree of sedation and analgesia	Esophagogastroscopy Transesophogeal echocardiography Transtracheal aspiration Thoracocentesis Paracentesis
Considerably more irritating and/or painful; necessitates considerably more sedation and analgesia	Thoracostomy Endotracheal intubation Pericardiocentesis/pericardial window Bronchoscopy Colonoscopy Peritoneal dialysis catheter insertion Peritoneal lavage
Extremely painful; necessitates profound sedation and analgesia	Debridement of open wounds Dressing changes Orthopedic manipulations Percutaneous intra-aortic balloon insertion Tracheostomy Bone marrow biopsy Percutaneous gastrostomy Open lung biopsy Ventriculostomy

pability to assess neurologic status is not lost for extended periods of time. In addition, the technique must not adversely affect cerebral perfusion pressure (mean arterial pressure minus intracranial pressure [ICP]). Drugs eliminated too rapidly can lead to episodes of agitation and ICP surges during the procedure, thereby jeopardizing cerebral perfusion. Longer-acting drugs lead to oversedation and difficulty in making an adequate neurologic examination following the procedure.

Coronary Artery Disease. Despite improved medical management, the prevalence of coronary artery disease will continue to rise as life span increases. In patients younger than 65 years, ischemic heart disease should be suspected in those with (1) diabetes mellitus; (2) hypertension, especially if they are cigarette smokers or are hyperlipidemic [20]; (3) left ventricular hypertrophy on electrocardiogram (ECG) [21]; (4) peripheral vascular disease [22]; or (5) carotid bruits [23]. Recent data confirm the findings of earlier studies that suggest that postoperative myocardial ischemia following cardiac and noncardiac surgery strongly predicts adverse outcome [24]. Accordingly, sufficient anesthesia should be provided during *and* after invasive procedures to reduce plasma catecholamine and stress hormone levels. The IV anesthetics and techniques that are used should cause tachycardia and/or significant hypotension.

Renal and/or Hepatic Failure. The association between sepsis and postoperative acute renal failure has been recognized for many years [25]. The risk of an adverse drug reaction is at least three times higher in azotemic patients than in those with normal renal function [26]. This risk is magnified by excessive circulating drug (or drug metabolite) levels and/or physiologic changes in target tissues induced by the uremic state.

Adverse drug reactions are no less common in patients with hepatic dysfunction. Liver failure increases VdSS by impairing synthesis of two plasma-binding proteins, albumin and alpha$_1$-acid glycoprotein. In addition, reductions in hepatic blood flow and hepatic enzymatic activity (e.g., cytochrome P-450) decrease rates of drug clearance.

Advantages and Disadvantages of Specific Drugs Used for Bedside Procedures (Table 28-2)

MORPHINE, FENTANYL, SUFENTANIL, ALFENTANIL (OPIOIDS)

Classification: Analgesic

Dose: See Table 28-3.

Elimination: Hepatic and renal

Summary. Newer opioids (e.g., alfentanil) have very short half-lives. When administered as a loading dose and continuous infusion, they are rapid in onset, easily titratable, and ideal for alleviating pain associated with brief bedside procedures. They should be used in conjunction with a short-acting sedative administered as a bolus (e.g., midazolam) or as a continuous infusion (e.g., propofol).

Pitfalls. Alfentanil quickly disappears from CNS receptors. Thus, longer-acting opioids must be added to the analgesic regimen toward the end of the procedure if pain is expected to persist for some time afterward.

Description. Opium, the source of all natural opioids, has been used (and abused) for more than 4000 years. It is composed of over 20 distinct alkaloids, including morphine, codeine, and papaverine. Although morphine can be synthesized in the laboratory, it is still obtained from the poppy, *Papaver somniferum.*

Pain relief by morphine and its surrogates is relatively selective, in that other sensory modalities (touch, vibration, vision, hearing) are not obtunded. Moreover, continuous dull pain is relieved more effectively than sharp intermittent pain, but in sufficient amounts morphine relieves even severe pain (e.g., renal or biliary colic). Opioids blunt pain by (1) inhibiting pain processing by the dorsal horn of the spinal cord; (2) decreasing transmission of pain by activating descending inhibitory pathways in the brainstem; and (3) altering the emotional response to pain by actions on the limbic cortex.

Various types of opioid receptors (denoted by Greek letters) have been discovered in the spinal cord, brainstem, thalamus, limbic system, and cerebral cortex [27]. Their stimulation causes the subject to experience emotions that can be described as pleasant (analgesia [μ_1] and sedation [κ]), or unpleasant (hallucinations [σ]) [28,29]. Transmission of impulses from these receptors to other centers is facilitated or inhibited by many substances, including substance P, neurotensin, vasoactive intestinal peptide, serotonin, cholecystokinin, gamma aminobutyric acid (GABA), and noradrenalin [30,31].

Pharmacokinetic data reveal that morphine and the newer opioids are similar except for their lipid solubility. Differences in lipid solubility affect the ease with which these drugs cross the blood-brain barrier. Morphine enters the CNS with difficulty, and peak analgesic effects may not occur for 15 to 30 minutes after IV injection. Hence, the plasma profile of morphine does not parallel its clinical effects. In contrast, fentanyl, sufentanil, and alfentanil enter and leave the brain and spinal cord easily, permitting easier titration, more effective attenuation of the stress response, and earlier return of spontaneous ventilation and extubation [32,33].

In view of their marked advantages, it is our bias that newer opioids have supplanted morphine for analgesia during bedside procedures. This line of reasoning applies less to fentanyl

Table 28-2. Characteristics of Intravenous Anesthetics (Bolus)

Properties	Thiopental	Etomidate	Midazolam	Ketamine	Propofol
Dose (mg/kg)	4	0.5	0.1	2	2
Onset	Rapid	Rapid	**Intermediate**	Rapid	Rapid
Duration (min)	5–10	5–10	**15–30**	10–15	5–10
Cardiovascular effects	↓	**0**	Minimal	↑	↓
Respiratory effects	↓	Minimal	↓	Minimal	↓
Analgesia	0	0	0	**Potent**	0
Amnesia	0	0	**Potent**	**Potent**	0
CNS effects	Drowsiness	Minimal	Drowsiness	**± Dysphoria**	Minimal

Dose indicated should be reduced 50% in elderly patients. Entries in bold type indicate noticeable differences among drugs.

Table 28-3. Analgesic-Sedative Combinations for Use at the Bedside

Component	Loading Dose (μg/kg)	Maintenance Infusion (μg/kg/min)
Analgesic		
Alfentanil	10–50	0.5–2.0
Sufentanil	0.25–0.75	0.005–0.020
Ketamine	500–1000	20–100
Sedative		
Propofol	1000–2000	100–200
Midazolam	100–250	0.5–2.0

Loading doses should be reduced 25–50% in the elderly and hemodynamically compromised. Titrate maintenance infusion doses to the level of stimulus.

and more to sufentanil and alfentanil, as illustrated by several clinical studies. For example, following injection of equivalent analgesic dosages of alfentanil or fentanyl and production of apnea, return of spontaneous ventilation was achieved within 10 to 20 minutes with alfentanil versus more than 2 hours with fentanyl [34]. However, the newer opioids are more expensive than morphine or fentanyl and should be reserved for those patients in whom faster recovery is desired.

Side Effects

GASTROINTESTINAL. Constipation, nausea, and/or vomiting are well-described side effects of opioid administration. Reduced gastric emptying and bowel motility (both small and large intestine), often leading to adynamic ileus, appear to be both peripherally (by opioid receptors located in the gut) and centrally (by the vagus nerve) mediated [35].

CARDIOVASCULAR. Hypotension is not unusual following morphine administration (5–10 mg IV) [36], especially if it is given rapidly (i.e., >5–10 mg/min). Several mechanisms have been proposed to explain this effect, including vagal-induced bradycardia, venous and arterial vasodilation, splanchnic sequestration of blood, and histamine release [37–41]. In patients pretreated with both H_1- and H_2-antagonists, the hypotensive response following morphine administration is significantly attenuated despite comparable increases in plasma histamine concentrations. These data strongly implicate histamine as the cause of these changes [42].

Although fentanyl, sufentanil, and alfentanil do not affect plasma histamine concentrations [43], bolus doses can be associated with hypotension, especially when infused rapidly (i.e., <1 minute). This action is related to medullary vasomotor center depression and vagal nucleus stimulation.

RESPIRATORY. A dose-dependent reduction in responsiveness of brainstem respiratory centers to carbon dioxide follows opioid administration. Key features of opioid-induced respiratory depression are a reduction in the slope of the ventilatory and occlusion pressure responses to carbon dioxide, a rightward shift of the minute ventilatory response to hypercarbia [44], and an increase in the apneic threshold (i.e., the $PaCO_2$ below which spontaneous ventilation is not initiated without hypoxia) and resting end-tidal carbon dioxide. Perhaps most important, opioids decrease hypoxic ventilatory drive [45]. Often overlooked is the observation that the onset and duration of respiratory depression may exceed the time course of analgesia [46,47]. However, it has not been proved that an equianalgesic dose of one narcotic (or agonist-antagonist) produces more or less respiratory depression than any other opiate. It is worth emphasizing that morphine administration in patients with renal failure has been associated with prolonged respiratory depression secondary to circulating active metabolites [48].

The practice of administering small doses of naloxone (0.04 mg) to patients to reverse the respiratory depression of iatrogenic narcotic overdose is risky and inadvisable for a number of reasons. Although in the past naloxone was thought to have little intrinsic agonist activity, this view is no longer tenable. Many reports indicate that naloxone has significant effects on cardiovascular function with or without prior narcotic administration. Recent anecdotal reports describe the precipitation of vomiting, delirium, arrhythmias, pulmonary edema, cardiac arrest, and sudden death subsequent to the sudden withdrawal of analgesia by naloxone administration, even in otherwise healthy postoperative patients [49–52]. Furthermore, naloxone levels decline rapidly, whereas narcotic levels may remain elevated for quite some time. Intramuscular or subcutaneous injections provide increased protection against delayed effects of opioids but are not foolproof. Recurring respiratory depression, therefore, remains a distinct possibility and in the unintubated patient is a source of potential morbidity.

Some recent data [53] suggest that reversal with an opioid agonist-antagonist such as nalbuphine may be safer than with naloxone. Antagonists with some intrinsic analgesic properties produce a more gradual reversal than naloxone. However, it is important to note that a mixed agonist-antagonist can either increase or decrease the opioid effect, depending on the dose administered, the particular agonist already in the bloodstream, and the amount of drug to be reversed [54].

For bedside procedures in the ICU, many of these problems can be obviated by using a short-acting opioid, such as alfentanil.

NEUROLOGICAL. Opioids have little effect on cerebral metabolic rate or cerebral blood flow when ventilation is controlled. Most reports suggest that narcotics do not increase intracranial pressure. However, fentanyl and sufentanil have been reported to increase ICP in patients following head trauma [55], and other opioids may affect cerebral perfusion pressure adversely by lowering mean arterial pressure [56–59].

THIOPENTAL, METHOHEXITAL (BARBITURATES)

Classification: Sedative-hypnotic

Dose: Thiopental: 3 to 4 mg per kilogram IV; Methohexital: 1 to 2 mg per kilogram

Elimination: Hepatic

Summary. Barbiturates have a long record of safety and are renowned for their beneficial effect on cerebral oxygen kinetics.

Pitfalls. Barbiturate administration can lead to significant hypotension and tachycardia.

Description. Sodium thiopental and methohexital, which act by suppressing the reticular activating system, are the barbiturates most often used for brief periods of sedation and hypnosis. Thiopental has a context-sensitive half-time (i.e., duration) of 5 to 10 minutes, despite a long elimination half-life (10–12 hours), due to redistribution from the plasma to the peripheral compartment (muscle, skin, to a lesser extent fat) [60]. Methohexital, which is two to three times more potent than thiopental, has a slightly shorter duration of action.

For the purposes of this discussion, barbiturates are used primarily to facilitate endotracheal intubation. The ideal candidate for a barbiturate induction is the euvolemic head-injured patient with normal cardiovascular function. Following induction doses, ICP decreases to a greater extent than arterial pressure; hence, cerebral perfusion pressure usually increases. Furthermore, barbiturates reduce cerebral oxygen utilization (CMRO$_2$) more than they reduce cerebral blood flow, favorably affecting the cerebral oxygen demand-delivery ratio.

Side Effects

CARDIOVASCULAR. Profound hypotension, occasionally leading to cardiac arrest, may occur with thiopental administration in critically ill patients. Since thiopental is highly bound (72–86%) to albumin [61], increased plasma levels of the free drug can result in patients with hypoalbuminemia due to critical illness, renal failure, or hepatic dysfunction [62,63]. Myocardial depression and an increase in venous capacitance [64] are responsible for the hypotension.

RESPIRATORY. Thiopental (but not methohexital) causes histamine release [65]. Though anecdotal evidence suggests this is not a significant clinical problem, some anesthesiologists avoid thiopental in patients with a history of bronchospastic disease. Thiopental depresses respiration and carbon dioxide responsiveness in a dose-related manner [66]. It also decreases the ventilatory response to hypoxia [67].

NEUROLOGIC. The one absolute contraindication to the use of barbiturates is a history of variegate or acute intermittent porphyria. Induction of liver cytochrome P-450 enzymes by barbiturates depletes the free heme pool and results in decreased synthesis of tryptophan pyrrolate, the enzyme responsible for tryptophan metabolism. The tryptophan that accumulates is diverted to serotonin synthesis, which may be responsible for the gastrointestinal and CNS symptoms of an acute attack of porphyria [68]. Thiopental administration has been associated with severe demyelination syndromes, leading to death in some cases.

ETOMIDATE

Classification: Sedative-hypnotic

Dose: 0.2 to 0.5 mg per kilogram

Elimination: Hepatic and plasma esterases

Summary. Etomidate has the same beneficial effect on cerebral oxygen kinetics as the barbiturates yet is virtually devoid of cardiovascular side effects.

Pitfalls. The clinical implications of adrenocortical suppression must be appreciated when selecting this agent.

Description. Etomidate is an intravenous anesthetic with a rapid onset and recovery [69] and a cardiovascular profile that is unrivaled, even in the setting of cardiomyopathy [70–73]. Not only does etomidate lack significant effects on myocardial contractility, but baseline sympathetic output and baroreflex regulation of sympathetic activity are well preserved [74]. Similar to the barbiturates, etomidate causes a dose-related depression of cerebral oxygen metabolism and blood flow [75,76] without changing the intracranial volume-pressure relationship [77]. Unlike thiopental, etomidate does not cause histamine release [78].

Etomidate was used extensively in Europe during the late 1970s. Reports appeared shortly thereafter describing excess mortality associated with low plasma cortisol levels in patients receiving prolonged sedation with etomidate [79,80]. Additional anecdotes confirmed an association between etomidate administration and decreased plasma cortisol levels [81]. It is now recognized that even single doses of etomidate can produce adrenal cortical suppression lasting 24 hours or more in normal patients undergoing elective surgery [82]. These effects are more pronounced as the dose is increased or if continuous infusions are used for sedation [83,84]. Etomidate-induced adrenocortical suppression occurs because the drug blocks a key step in the metabolic pathway, leading to adrenal steroidogenesis [85]. Since the drug does not affect the response of tissue cortisol receptors, supplementation with exogenous steroids should prevent the adverse effects of adrenal cortical suppression and allow clinical use of etomidate for brain protection or anesthetic induction.

We routinely use etomidate (rather than thiopental) in certain patient subgroups: hypovolemic patients, multitrauma patients with closed-head injury, and patients with low ejection fraction, severe aortic stenosis, left main coronary artery disease, or severe cerebral vascular disease. Etomidate should be used with the understanding that adrenocortical suppression may last 24 hours or longer.

DIAZEPAM, LORAZEPAM, MIDAZOLAM (BENZODIAZEPINES)

Classification: Sedative-hypnotic

Dose: See Table 28-3.

Elimination: Hepatic

Summary. Midazolam, the most appropriate benzodiazepine for short-term use in the ICU, provides effective sedation and amnesia during endoscopy and other relatively painless procedures.

Pitfalls. Because recovery of cognitive function following midazolam is more prolonged than with other sedatives (e.g., propofol), it may not be appropriate in situations where rapid return of consciousness is a priority.

Description. Benzodiazepine receptors in the cerebral cortex, limbic system, and cerebellar cortex lie in close proximity to receptors for GABA, the most important inhibitory neurotransmitter in the brain. Benzodiazepine receptor activation induces conformational changes in GABA receptors, potentiating the inhibitory action of GABA and mediating clinical effects such as sedation and anticonvulsion. Benzodiazepines also have an affinity for glycine receptors, another CNS inhibitory neurotransmitter. Interaction with glycine receptors inhibits afferent conduction to motor neurons in the spinal cord and higher anxiety centers, accounting for muscle relaxation and anxiolysis [86].

Midazolam provides more complete anterograde amnesia [87] and, due to its water solubility, produces less pain on IV injection than diazepam and lorazepam [88]. Anterograde amnesia following midazolam (5 mg IV) peaks 2 to 5 minutes after injection and lasts 20 to 40 minutes [89]. Plasma levels of midazolam and clinical endpoints have been correlated [90]. Amnesia occurs at concentrations greater than 100 ng per milliliter, whereas concentrations greater than 250 to 300 ng per milliliter are necessary for hypnosis (unconsciousness). Since midazolam is highly (95%) protein-bound to albumin, drug effect is likely to be exaggerated in ICU patients. Likewise, though the elimination half-life of midazolam is comparatively short (2 hours, versus 36 hours for diazepam and 12 hours for lorazepam) [91], it is noticeably prolonged in obese and elderly patients, in about 6 percent of normal patients [92,93], and following prolonged infusions [94].

Similar to the barbiturates, benzodiazepines cause dose-dependent reductions in $CMRO_2$ and cerebral blood flow, suggesting that these agents may be beneficial in patients with cerebral ischemia.

All benzodiazepines attenuate the tachycardia and hypertension induced by ketamine administration. The psychotic sequelae of ketamine, however, are more effectively eliminated with midazolam than with diazepam (see below).

Midazolam does not suppress adrenal steroidogenesis [95].

Side Effects

RESPIRATORY. The respiratory effects of the various benzodiazepines are qualitatively similar. Diazepam (0.4 mg/kg IV) depresses the slope of the carbon dioxide response minute-ventilation curve in normal volunteers [96] and increases the dead space-tidal volume ratio and arterial PCO_2 [97]. Respiratory depression is even more marked and prolonged in patients with chronic obstructive pulmonary disease (COPD) [98]. This effect begins 1 minute after injection, peaks at 3 minutes, and lasts longer than 30 minutes after injection. The level and time course of depression after 0.15 mg per kilogram of midazolam is similar to that seen after 0.3 mg per kilogram of diazepam in healthy patients and in those with COPD [99]. Midazolam blunts the ventilatory response to hypoxia [100].

CARDIOVASCULAR. Small (< 10%) increases in heart rate and small decreases in systemic vascular resistance are frequently observed after administration of these agents [101,102]. Midazolam (0.2 mg/kg) has no significant effects on coronary vascular resistance or autoregulation [103].

KETAMINE

Classification: Sedative-hypnotic, analgesic

Dose: Sedation-hypnosis, mild analgesia: 10 to 20 mg IV as needed; TIVA: see Table 28-3.

Elimination: Primarily hepatic, but extrahepatic as well (sites to be determined)

Summary. Ketamine is one of the most useful IV drugs available. Combined with propofol or midazolam to minimize dysphoria, ketamine is a superlative sedative, analgesic, and amnestic agent.

Pitfalls. Tachycardia associated with repeated bolus doses can be reduced by administering ketamine as a constant infusion and by adding propofol or midazolam to the regimen.

Description. Ketamine is a safe, rapidly acting agent that induces a state of sedation, amnesia, and marked analgesia known as dissociative analgesia. This term describes a functional dissociation between the thalamocortical and limbic systems, which is derived from the strong feeling of dissociation from the environment experienced by subjects anesthetized with the drug [104]. Administered orally, intramuscularly, or rectally, ketamine can provide excellent analgesia and sedation for patients with limited intravenous access (e.g., patients with extensive burns) or for procedures near the airway, where physical access and ability to secure an airway is limited (e.g., gunshot wounds to the face).

Following IV administration, ketamine is rapidly distributed to highly perfused tissues and subsequently redistributed to lean muscle and fat in a manner similar to that for thiopental. It is rapidly metabolized by the liver to norketamine, which is also pharmacologically active. Though the elimination half-life is 2 to 3 hours, the context-sensitive half-time is similar to that of propofol.

Many consider ketamine to be the analgesic of choice in patients with a history of bronchospasm. In the usual dosage, it decreases airway resistance, probably by blocking norepinephrine uptake, which, in turn, stimulates beta-adrenergic receptors in the lungs. In contrast to many beta-agonist bronchodilators, ketamine is not arrhythmogenic when given to asthmatic patients receiving aminophylline [105,106].

Ketamine is often used in unintubated patients because it ordinarily permits retention of airway reflexes. Unlike other intravenous induction agents, ketamine (1–2 mg/kg IV) is only a mild respiratory depressant, causing the carbon dioxide-response curve to shift to the right without affecting the slope of the curve [107]. Because salivary and tracheobronchial secretions are increased by ketamine, 0.2 mg of glycopyrrolate should be administered 5 minutes prior to injecting the anesthetic. In patients with borderline hypoxemia despite maximal therapy, ketamine may be the drug of choice, since there is evidence to suggest that ketamine does not inhibit hypoxic pulmonary vasoconstriction [108].

A major feature that distinguishes ketamine from most other intravenous anesthetics is that it stimulates the cardiovascular system (i.e., raises heart rate and blood pressure). Cardiovascular stimulation appears to result from direct stimulation of the CNS with increased sympathetic nervous system outflow and blockade of norepinephrine reuptake in adrenergic nerves [109–112]. Ketamine, however, causes direct myocardial depression [113-118]. While significant systolic dysfunction is distinctly unusual in the clinical setting, hypotension has been reported following ketamine administration in hemodynamically compromised patients with chronic catecholamine depletion [119].

Because pulmonary hypertension is a characteristic feature of the adult respiratory distress syndrome, drugs that increase right ventricular afterload should be avoided. Earlier investigations suggested that ketamine increases pulmonary vascular resistance [120,121,122]. More recent data obtained by studying infants with either normal or elevated pulmonary vascular resistance reveal that ketamine does not affect pulmonary vascular resistance as long as ventilation is maintained at a constant rate [123]. These findings have been confirmed in adults [124].

Earlier reports also suggested that ketamine increases ICP in vivo [125,126], an effect attributed to increased cerebral blood flow. However, these data were obtained in spontaneously breathing subjects and did not control for changes in ICP due to hypercarbia. Although a recent in vitro study found that ketamine directly dilates cerebral arteries (by acting as a calcium channel antagonist) [127], blood flow does not change when ketamine is injected directly into cerebral vessels [128]. Furthermore, in mechanically ventilated pigs with artificially produced intracranial hypertension (in which ICP is on the "shoulder" of the compliance curve), 0.5 to 2.0 mg per kilogram of ketamine IV does not raise ICP [129], and in mechanically ventilated preterm infants, 2 mg per kilogram of ketamine IV does not increase anterior fontanelle pressure, an indirect monitor of ICP [130]. Nevertheless, until additional data are available, ketamine should be used with caution in patients with raised intracranial pressure.

Side Effects

PSYCHOLOGICAL. The psychic emergence phenomena of ketamine have been described as floating sensations, vivid dreams (pleasant or unpleasant), hallucinations, and delirium. These effects are more common in patients older than 16 years, in females, after short operative procedures, after large doses (>2 mg/kg IV), and after rapid administration (>40 mg/min) [131]. Pretreatment with benzodiazepines prevents these phenomena [132,133,134]. In a study comparing ketamine-midazolam with ketamine-diazepam, the former resulted in fewer emergence reactions and a shorter time to complete recovery [135].

CARDIOVASCULAR. As of this writing, the effect of ketamine on myocardial contractile performance in humans remains to be demonstrated. Nonetheless, since ketamine increases myocardial oxygen consumption (Table 28-2) [136], there is a risk of precipitating myocardial ischemia in patients with coronary artery disease if ketamine is used alone. Surprisingly, ketamine-diazepam, ketamine-midazolam, and ketamine-sufentanil combinations are well tolerated by patients undergoing coronary artery bypass surgery [137,138].

The effect of ketamine on cardiac rhythm is another controversial topic. In some experiments, ketamine abolishes epinephrine-induced arrhythmias by prolonging the relative refractory period; in others, it sensitizes the myocardium to catecholamines and enhances the arrhythmogenicity of epinephrine [139,140].

NEUROLOGIC. Ketamine does not lower the minimal electroshock seizure threshold in mice. When administered with aminophylline, however, a clinically apparent reduction in seizure threshold is observed [141].

HEMATOLOGIC. Ketamine irreversibly inhibits platelet aggregation in baboons [142]; however, no significant hemostatic changes have been observed in humans undergoing ketamine-midazolam anesthesia [143].

PROPOFOL

Classification: Sedative-hypnotic

Dose: See Table 28-3.

Elimination: Hepatic, extrahepatic

Summary. Propofol is extremely popular because it is easily titratable and reaches equilibration across the blood-brain barrier far more rapidly than midazolam. Thus, patients return to a lighter level of sedation more quickly with propofol than with midazolam, a factor that probably makes propofol the preferred agent for sedation in general and in patients with altered level of consciousness in particular.

Pitfalls. The effect of propofol on level of consciousness will dissipate faster than the effects from concomitantly administered alfentanil and sufentanil, especially as the duration of anesthesia increases.

Description. Propofol is a sedative drug *without* amnestic properties that can be given as a bolus or continuous infusion.

Propofol, thiopental, and methohexital cross the blood-brain barrier at roughly equivalent rates, but the extensive tissue distribution and high metabolic clearance of propofol make awakening and "clear-headed" emergence significantly faster than with the barbiturates. Even after a 10-hour infusion of propofol, only 10 to 15 minutes is required for a 50 percent decrease in concentration, whereas methohexital necessitates approximately 90 minutes and thiopental several hours. At the higher end of a recommended bolus dose (2 mg/kg), propofol is approximately twice as potent in reducing blood pressure as thiopental when used for induction of anesthesia.

Despite having similar elimination half-lives (2 hours), propofol has a far more evanescent duration of action than midazolam when given as a single dose or as a short-term infusion [144]. Similarly, recovery following long-term sedation (>7 days) is significantly faster in ICU patients receiving propofol than in those receiving midazolam [145]. As discussed earlier, these phenomena occur because during continuous infusions context-sensitive half-time increases very slightly, whereas elimination half-life is prolonged (Fig. 28-1) [146]. Elimination half-life is also prolonged in elderly patients [147] and those with liver dysfunction [148]. There are no known active metabolites of propofol [149].

In patients sedated with propofol in the absence of muscle relaxant drugs, respiratory rate appears to be a more predictable sign of inadequate sedation than hemodynamic changes (i.e., propofol is a potent respiratory depressant). The ventilatory response to rebreathing carbon dioxide during a maintenance infusion of propofol is similar to that induced by other sedative drugs: propofol significantly decreases the slope of the carbon dioxide-response curve by 40 to 60 percent [150]. Nevertheless, in one study, spontaneously breathing propofol-anesthetized patients were able to maintain normal end-tidal carbon dioxide values during minor outpatient surgical procedures [151].

Bolus doses of propofol in the range of 1 to 2 mg per kilogram induce hypnosis within 30 seconds. Maintenance infusion doses of 100 to 200 µg/kg/min are adequate in younger subjects, whereas doses should be reduced by 20 to 50 percent in the elderly [152]. Unlike etomidate, propofol does not inhibit adrenal steroidogenesis [153]. Because sedation can be induced and deepened so rapidly, propofol is ideal for extremely irritating procedures, such as endotracheal tube suctioning and positioning. Equally important, rapid recovery of neurologic status makes propofol the paradigm for ICU patients in general and those with head trauma in particular who cannot tolerate mechanical ventilation without pharmacologic sedation. Unfortunately, the cost of propofol is substantial; thus, it should not be used for sedation for prolonged periods of time.

Side Effects

CARDIOVASCULAR. Propofol depresses ventricular systolic function and lowers afterload [154,155,156] but has no effect on diastolic function [157]. Vasodilation with propofol results from calcium channel blockade [158]. In patients undergoing coronary artery bypass surgery, propofol (2 mg/kg IV bolus) produces a 23 percent fall in mean arterial blood pressure, a 20 percent increase in heart rate, and a 26 percent decrease in stroke volume [159]. Other studies show that propofol administration in patients with coronary artery disease can be associated with increased myocardial lactate production, a sign of myocardial ischemia [160,161]. In a study of 10 patients 50 to 75 years old without known coronary artery disease who were undergoing total hip replacement, propofol (2 mg/kg bolus plus 6 mg/kg/hr infusion) did not affect heart rate, cardiac output, central venous pressure, or pulmonary artery pressures, but systemic arterial pressure and systemic vascular resistance decreased 25 percent [162].

NEUROLOGIC. Propofol may improve neurologic outcome and reduce neuronal damage by depressing cerebral metabolism. Propofol decreases cerebral oxygen consumption, cerebral blood flow, and cerebral glucose utilization in humans and animals to the same degree as reported for thiopental and etomidate [163–166].

Practical Considerations for Total Intravenous Anesthesia

We and others have observed that propofol and sufentanil-alfentanil-ketamine combinations are the drugs most suited for TIVA. Each drug is delivered as a bolus plus infusion, as indicated in Table 28-3, using a programmable infusion pump. Bolus doses should not be used in hemodynamically unstable patients and the elderly. For *light* sedation, we start an infusion of propofol (no bolus) and titrate to level of wakefulness, respiratory rate, and so on. In most other situations, patients should be paralyzed during the procedure, preferably with a short-acting muscle relaxant (e.g., vecuronium, atracurium, mivacurium) and monitored with a nerve stimulator. The reader is referred to anesthesia textbooks for additional information regarding pharmacologic muscle paralysis.

Several other points deserve consideration in this context:

1. It is clear from carefully controlled clinical investigations and individual case reports that some patients may be completely aware of intraoperative events at times when there is absolutely no change in hemodynamics or any manifestation of increased sympathetic activity [167–171]. Hence, administering sufentanil or alfentanil to blunt incisional pain without inducing lack of awareness with a sedative-hypnotic is inappropriate [172].

2. Propofol is not amnesic, so patients must receive adequate sedation to prevent recall. Clinical experience suggests that usually several minutes of light anesthesia is required before patient recall is possible. Prompt treatment of unexplained tachycardia or hypertension with a propofol bolus of 1 to 4 ml (10–40 mg) usually prevents this problem, except as indicated previously.

3. It is our practice never to infuse medications directly without the use of a carrier IV fluid running continuously at a rate of approximately 50 ml per hour. This method not only helps deliver medication into the circulation, it also serves as a further monitor against occlusion of the drug delivery system. Occlusion of the infusion line for more than a few minutes may lead to patient awareness.

4. Because of their pharmacologic properties, alfentanil and sufentanil infusions are stopped 15 to 30 minutes prior to the end of the procedure, whereas propofol and ketamine infusions may be continued until the last 5 to 10 minutes. Continual communication with the surgeon during the procedure may be necessary to meet these endpoint criteria.

5. To maintain reasonably constant propofol blood concentrations, the maintenance infusion rate should be decreased during the procedure, because rapid distributional volumes saturate over time.

6. Strict aseptic technique is especially important during the handling of propofol, because the vehicle in which the drug is dispersed, a mixture of soybean oil and egg lecithin, supports the rapid growth of microorganisms. Recent reports highlight the consequences of bacterial contamination, including fever and infection, which can lead to or aggravate life-threatening illness.

References

1. Lundy JS: Intravenous anesthesia: Preliminary report of the use of two new thiobarbiturates. *Proc Mayo Clin* 10:536, 1935.
2. Halford FJ: A critique of intravenous anesthesia in war surgery. *Anesthesiology* 4:67, 1943.
3. Adams RC, Gray HK: Intravenous anesthesia with pentothal sodium in the case of a gunshot wound associated with accompanying severe traumatic shock and loss of blood: Report of a case. *Anesthesiology* 4:70, 1943.
4. Trinkle JK, Richardson JD, Franz JL, et al: Management of flail chest without mechanical ventilation. *Ann Thorac Surg* 19:355, 1975.
5. Modig J, Borg T, Karistrom G, et al: Thromboembolism after total hip replacement: Role of epidural and general anesthesia. *Anesth Analg* 62:174, 1983.
6. Jorgensen BC, Anderson HB, Engquist A: Influence of epidural morphine on postoperative pain, endocrine, metabolic, and renal responses to surgery: A controlled study. *Acta Anaesthesiol Scand* 26:63, 1982.
7. Brandt MR, Fernandes A, Mordhurst R, et al: Epidural analgesia improves postoperative nitrogen balance. *Br Med J* 1:1106, 1978.
8. Kehlet H: Modification of responses to surgery by neural blockade: Clinical implications, in Cousins MJ, Brindenbaugh PO (eds): *Neural Blockade in Clinical Anesthesia and Management of Pain.* 2nd ed. Philadelphia, JB Lippincott, 1988, pp 145–188.
9. Rem J, Brandt MR, Kehlet H: Prevention of postoperative lymphopenia and granulocytosis by epidural analgesia. *Lancet* 1:283, 1980.
10. Buchweitz E, Grandison L, Weiss HR: Effect of morphine on regional cerebral oxygen consumption and supply. *Brain Res* 291:301, 1984.
11. Mangano DT, Siliciano D, Hollenberg M, et al: Postoperative myocardial ischemia: Therapeutic trials using intensive analgesia following surgery. *Anesthesiology* 76:342, 1992.
12. Townsend PO, Fink MP, Stein KL: Aminoglycoside pharmacokinetics: Dosage requirement and nephrotoxicity in trauma patients. *Crit Care Med* 17:154, 1989.
13. Koch-Weser J, Sellers EM: Binding of drugs to serum albumin. *N Engl J Med* 294:311, 1976.
14. Shafer SL, Stanski DR: Improving the clinical utility of anesthetic drug pharmacokinetics (editorial). *Anesthesiology* 176:327, 1992.
15. Hughes MA, Glass PSA, Jacobs JR: Context-sensitive half-time in multicompartment pharmacokinetic models for intravenous anesthetic drugs. *Anesthesiology* 76:334, 1992.
16. Bellvile JW, Forrest W, Miller E: A study of postoperative patients. *JAMA* 217:1835, 1971.
17. Scott JC, Stanski DR: Decreased fentanyl and alfentanil dose requirements with age: A simultaneous pharmacokinetic and pharmacodynamic evaluation. *J Pharmacol Exp Ther* 240:160, 1987.
18. Greenblatt DJ, Locniskar AA, Shader RI: Lorazepam kinetics in the elderly. *Clin Pharmacol Ther* 26:103, 1979.
19. Reidenberg MM, Levy M, Warner H: Relationship between diazepam dose, plasma level, age, and CNS depression. *Clin Pharmacol Ther* 23:371, 1978.
20. Gordon T, Kannel WB: The Framingham, Massachusetts study twenty years later, in Kessler II, Levin ML (eds): *Community as an*

Epidemiologic Laboratory: A Case-Book of Community Studies. Baltimore, Johns Hopkins University Press, 1970, pp 123–146.

21. Benchimol A, Harris CL, Desser KB, et al: Resting electrocardiogram in major coronary artery disease. *JAMA* 224:1489, 1973.

22. Hertzer NR, Beven EG, Young JR, et al: Coronary artery disease in peripheral vascular patients: A classification of 1000 angiograms and results of surgical management. *Ann Surg* 199:223, 1984.

23. Barnes RW, Marzalek PB: Asymptomatic carotid disease in the cardiovascular surgical patient: Is prophylactic endarterectomy necessary? *Stroke* 12:497, 1981.

24. Mangano DT, Browner WS, Hollenberg M: Association of perioperative myocardial ischemia with cardiac morbidity and mortality in men undergoing noncardiac surgery. *N Engl J Med* 323:1781, 1990.

25. Fischer RP, Polk HC Jr: Changing etiologic patterns of renal insufficiency in surgical patients (editorial). *Surg Gynecol Obstet* 140:85, 1975.

26. Rubin AL, Stenzel KH, Reidenberg MM: Symposium on drug action and metabolism in renal failure. *Am J Med* 62:459, 1977.

27. Boukoms AJ: Pain relief in the intensive care unit. *J Intensive Care Med* 3:32, 1988.

28. Pleuvry BJ: An update on opioid receptors. *Br J Anaesth* 55:1435, 1983.

29. Rosow C: Newer opioid analgesics and antagonists. *Anesthesiol Clin North Am* 6:319, 1988.

30. Watkins LR, Mayer DJ: Multiple endogenous opiate and nonopiate analgesia systems: Evidence for their existence and clinical implication. *Ann NY Acad Sci* 467:273, 1986.

31. Cousins MJ, Mather LE: Intrathecal and epidural administration of opioids. *Anesthesiology* 61:276, 1984.

32. Yate PM, Thomas D, Sebel PS: Alfentanil infusion for sedation and analgesia in intensive care. *Lancet* 2:396, 1984.

33. Van Peer A, Vercauteren M, Noorduin R, et al: Alfentanil kinetics in renal insufficiency. *Eur J Clin Pharmacol* 30:245, 1986.

34. Stanski DR, Hug CC Jr: Alfentanil: A kinetically predictable narcotic analgesic. *Anesthesiology* 57:435,1982.

35. Steward JJ, Weisbrodt NW, Burks TF: Central and peripheral actions of morphine on intestinal transit. *J Pharmacol Exp Ther* 205:547, 1978.

36. Drew JH, Dripps RD, Comroe JH: Clinical studies on morphine, II: The effect of morphine upon the circulation of man and upon the circulatory and respiratory responses to tilting. *Anesthesiology* 7:44, 1946.

37. Greene JF, Jackman AP, Parsons G: The effects of morphine on the mechanical properties of the systemic circulation in the dog. *Circ Res* 42:474, 1978.

38. Lowenstein E, Whiting RB, Bittar DA, et al: Local and neurally mediated effects of morphine on skeletal muscle vascular resistance. *J Pharmacol Exp Ther* 180:359, 1972.

39. Henney RP, Vasko JS, Brawley RK, et al: The effects of morphine on the resistance and capacitance vessels of the peripheral circulation. *Am Heart J* 72:242, 1966.

40. Hsu HO, Hickey RF, Forbes AR: Morphine decreases peripheral vascular resistance and increases capacitance in man. *Anesthesiology* 50:98, 1979.

41. Green JF, Jackman AP, Krohn KA: Mechanisms of morphine induced shifts in blood volume between extracorporeal reservoir and the systemic circulation of the dog under conditions of constant blood flow and vena caval pressures. *Circ Res* 42:479, 1978.

42. Moss J, Rosow CE: Histamine release by narcotics and muscle relaxants in humans. *Anesthesiology* 59:330, 1983.

43. Rosow CE, Moss J, Philbin DM, et al: Histamine release during morphine and fentanyl anesthesia. *Anesthesiology* 56:93, 1982.

44. Ngai SH: Effects of morphine and meperidine on the central respiratory mechanisms in the cat: The action of levallorphan in antagonizing these effects. *J Pharmacol Exp Ther* 131:91, 1961.

45. Weil JV, McCullough RE, Kline JS, et al: Diminished ventilatory response to hypoxia and hypercapnia after morphine in normal man. *N Engl J Med* 292:1103, 1975.

46. Nielslen CH, Camporesi EM, Bromage PR, et al: CO_2 sensitivity after epidural and IV morphine. *Anesthesiology* 55:A372, 1981.

47. Downes JJ, Kemp RA, Lambertsen CJ: The magnitude and duration of respiratory depression due to fentanyl and meperidine in man. *J Pharmacol Exp Ther* 158:416, 1967.

48. Aitkenhead AR, Vater M, Achola K, et al: Pharmacokinetics of single-dose intravenous morphine in normal volunteers and patients with end-stage renal failure. *Br J Anaesth* 56:813, 1984.

49. Azar I, Turndorf H: Severe hypertension and multiple atrial premature contractions following naloxone administration. *Anesth Analg* 58:524, 1979.

50. Michaelis LL, Hickey PR, Clark TA, et al: Ventricular irritability associated with the use of naloxone hydrochloride. *Ann Thorac Surg* 18:608, 1974.

51. Taff RH: Pulmonary edema following naloxone administration in a patient without heart disease. *Anesthesiology* 59:576, 1983.

52. Azar I, Patel AK, Phau CQ: Cardiovascular responses following naloxone administration during enflurane anesthesia. *Anesth Analg* 60:237, 1981.

53. Moldenhauer CC, Roach GW, Finlayson DC, et al: Nalbuphine antagonism of ventilatory depression following high-dose fentanyl anesthesia. *Anesthesiology* 62:647, 1985.

54. Bailey PL, Clark NJ, Pace NL, et al: Failure of nalbuphine to antagonize morphine: A double-blind comparison with naloxone. *Anesth Analg* 65:605, 1986.

55. Sperry RJ, Bailey PL, Reichman MV, et al: Fentanyl and sufentanil increase intracranial pressure in head trauma patients. *Anesth Analg* 77:416, 1992.

56. Markovitz BP, Duhaime A-C, Sutton L, et al: Effects of alfentanil on intracranial pressure in children undergoing ventriculoperitoneal shunt revision. *Anesthesiology* 76:71, 1992.

57. Lutz LJ, Milde JH, Milde LN: Cerebral effects of alfentanil in dogs with reduced intracranial compliance. *J Neurosurg Anesth* 1:169, 1989.

58. McPherson RW, Krempansanka E, Eimerl D, et al: Effects of alfentanil on cerebral vascular reactivity in dogs. *Br J Anaesth* 57:1232, 1985.

59. Herrick IA, Gelb AW, Manninen PH, et al: Effects of fentanyl, sufentanil, and alfentanil on brain retractor pressure. *Anesth Analg* 72:359, 1991.

60. Price HL: A dynamic concept of the distribution of thiopental in the human body. *Anesthesiology* 21:40, 1960.

61. Ghoneim MM, Pandya HB: Plasma protein binding of thiopental in patients with impaired renal or hepatic function. *Anesthesiology* 42:545, 1975.

62. Burch PG, Stanski DR: Thiopental pharmacokinetics in renal failure. *Anesthesiology* 55:A7176, 1981.

63. Shideman FE, Kelley AR, Lee LE, et al: The role of the liver in the detoxification of thiopental (pentothal) by man. *Anesthesiology* 10:421, 1949.

64. Sonntag H, Hellborg K, Schenk HD, et al: Effects of thiopental on coronary blood flow and myocardial metabolism in man. *Acta Anaesthesiol Scand* 19:69, 1975.

65. Hirshman CA, Edelstein RA, Eastman CL, et al: Histamine release by barbiturates in human mast cells. *Anesthesiology* 61:A352, 1984.

66. Bellville JW, Seed JC: The effect of drugs on the respiratory response to carbon dioxide. *Anesthesiology* 21:727, 1960.

67. Hirshman CH, McCullough RE, Cohen JP, et al: Hypoxic ventilatory drive in dogs during thiopental, ketamine or pentobarbital anesthesia. *Anesthesiology* 43:628, 1975.

68. Litman DA, Correia MA: L-tryptophan: A common derivative of biochemical and neurological events of acute hepatic porphyria. *Science* 222:1031, 1983.

69. Kay B: A dose-response relationship for etomidate with some observations on accumulation. *Br J Anaesth* 48:213, 1976.

70. Goading JM, Wang JT, Smith RA, et al: Cardiovascular and pulmonary responses following etomidate induction of anesthesia in patients with demonstrated cardiac disease. *Anesth Analg* 58:40, 1979.

71. Criado A, Maseda J, Navarro E, et al: Induction of anesthesia with etomidate: Hemodynamic study of 36 patients. *Br J Anaesth* 52:803, 1980.

72. Riou B, Lecarpentier Y, Chemia D, et al: In vitro effects of etomidate on intrinsic myocardial contractility in the rat. *Anesthesiology* 72:330, 1990.

73. Riou B, Lecarpentier Y, Viars P: Effects of etomidate on the cardiac papillary muscle of normal hamsters and those with cardiomyopathy. *Anesthesiology* 78:83, 1993.

74. Ebert TJ, Muzi M, Berens R, et al: Sympathetic responses to induc-

tion of anesthesia in humans with propofol or etomidate. *Anesthesiology* 76:725, 1992.

75. Renou AM, Vernhiet J, Macrez P, et al: Cerebral blood flow and metabolism during etomidate anaesthesia in man. *Br J Anaesth* 50:1047, 1978.

76. Milde LN, Milde JH, Michenfelder JD: Cerebral functional, metabolic, and hemodynamic effects of etomidate in dogs. *Anesthesiology* 63:371, 1985.

77. Artru AA: Intracranial volume-pressure relationship following thiopental or etomidate. *Anesthesiology* 71:763, 1989.

78. Doenicke A, Lorenz W, Beigl R, et al: Histamine release after intravenous application of short-acting hypnotics: A comparison of etomidate, althesin (CT1341) and propranidid. *Br J Anaesth* 45:1097, 1973.

79. Ledingham IM, Watt I: Influence of sedation on mortality in critically ill multiple trauma patients. *Lancet* 1:1270, 1983.

80. Ledingham IM, Finlay WEI, Watt I, et al: Etomidate and adrenocortical function. *Lancet* 1:1434, 1983.

81. Fragen RJ, Shanks CA, Molteni A: Effect on plasma cortisol concentrations of a single induction dose of etomidate or thiopentone. *Lancet* 2:625, 1983.

82. Fragen RJ, Shanks CA, Molteni A, et al: Effects of etomidate on hormonal responses to surgical stress. *Anesthesiology* 61:652, 1984.

83. Wagner RL, White PF, Kan PB, et al: Inhibition of adrenal steroidogenesis by the anesthetic etomidate. *N Engl J Med* 310:1415, 1984.

84. Wagner RL, White PF: Etomidate inhibits adrenocortical function in surgical patients. *Anesthesiology* 61:647, 1984.

85. Wagner RL, White PF, Kan PB, et al: Inhibition of adrenal steroidogenesis by the anesthetic etomidate. *N Engl J Med* 310:1415, 1984.

86. Richter JJ: Current theories about the mechanisms of benzodiazepines and neuroleptic drugs. *Anesthesiology* 54:66, 1981.

87. Aun C, Flynn PJ, Richards J, et al: A comparison of midazolam and diazepam for intravenous sedation in dentistry. *Anesthesiology* 39:589, 1984.

88. Reves JG, Fragen RJ, Vinik HR, et al: Midazolam: Pharmacology and uses. *Anesthesiology* 62:310, 1985.

89. Dundee JW, Samuel IO, Toner W, et al: Midazolam: A water-soluble benzodiazepine. *Anaesthesia* 35:454, 1980.

90. Persson MP, Nilsson A, Hartvig P: Relation of sedation and amnesia to plasma concentrations of midazolam in surgical patients. *Clin Pharmacol Ther* 43:324, 1988.

91. Greenblatt DJ, Abernathy DR, Locknixkar A, et al: Effect of age, gender and obesity on midazolam kinetics. *Anesthesiology* 61:27, 1984.

92. Dundee JW, Collier PS, Carlisle RJT, et al: Prolonged midazolam elimination half-life. *Br J Clin Pharmacol* 21:425, 1986.

93. Dirksen MSC, Vree TB, Driessen JJ: Midazolam in the intensive care unit. *Drug Intell Clin Pharm* 20:805, 1986.

94. Brown CR, Sarnquist FH, Canup CA, et al: Clinical, electroencephalographic and pharmacokinetic studies of a water-soluble benzodiazepine, midazolam maleate. *Anesthesiology* 50:467, 1979.

95. Shapiro JM, Westphal LM, White PF, et al: Midazolam infusion for sedation in the intensive care unit: Effect on adrenal function. *Anesthesiology* 64:394, 1986.

96. Catchlove RFH, Kafer ER: The effects of diazepam on the ventilatory response to carbon dioxide and on steady-state gas exchange. *Anesthesiology* 34:9, 1971.

97. Gross JB, Smith L, Smith TC: Time course of ventilatory response to carbon dioxide after intravenous diazepam. *Anesthesiology* 57:18, 1982

98. Forster A, Gardaz JP, Suter PM, et al: Respiratory depression by midazolam and diazepam. *Anesthesiology* 53:494, 1980.

99. Gross JB, Zebrowski ME, Carel WD, et al: Time course of ventilatory depression after thiopental and midazolam in normal subjects and in patients with chronic obstructive pulmonary disease. *Anesthesiology* 58:540, 1983.

100. Alexander CM, Gross JB: Sedative doses of midazolam depress hypoxic ventilatory responses in humans. *Anesth Analg* 67:377, 1988.

101. Massant J, d'Hollander A, Barvais L, et al: Haemodynamic effects of midazolam in the anaesthetized patient with coronary artery disease. *Acta Anaesthesiol Scand* 27:299, 1983.

102. Rao S, Sherbaniuk RW, Prasad K, et al: Cardiopulmonary effects of diazepam. *Clin Pharmacol Ther* 14:182, 1973.

103. Marty J, Nitenberg A, Blanchet F, et al: Effects of midazolam on the coronary circulation in patients with coronary artery disease. *Anesthesiology* 64:206, 1986.

104. Winters WD, Ferrer-Allado T, Guzman-Flores C: The cataleptic state induced by ketamine: A review of the neuropharmacology of anesthesia. *Neuropharmacology* 11:303, 1972.

105. Stirt JA, Berger JM, Roe SD, et al: Cardiovascular effects of ketamine following administration of aminophylline in dogs. *Anesth Analg* 61:685, 1982.

106. Hirschman CA, Downes H, Farbood A, et al: Ketamine block of bronchospasm in experimental canine asthma. *Br J Anaesth* 51:713, 1979.

107. Bourke DL, Malit LA, Smith TC: Respiratory interactions of ketamine and morphine. *Anesthesiology* 66:153, 1987.

108. Lumb PD, Silvay G, Weinreich AI, et al: A comparison of the effects of continuous ketamine infusion and halothane on oxygenation during one-lung anaesthesia in dogs. *Can Anaesth Soc J* 26:394, 1979.

109. Chodoff P: Evidence for central adrenergic action of ketamine. *Anesth Analg* 51:247, 1972.

110. Lundy PM, Gverzdys S, Frew R: Ketamine: Evidence of tissue specific inhibition of neuronal and extraneuronal catecholamine uptake processes. *Can J Physiol Pharmacol* 63:298, 1985.

111. Salt PJ, Barnes PK, Beswick FJ: Inhibition of neuronal and extraneuronal uptake of noradrenaline by ketamine in the isolated perfused rat heart. *Br J Anaesth* 51:835, 1979.

112. Wong DHW, Jenkins LC: The cardiovascular effects of ketamine in hypotensive states. *Can Anaesth Soc J* 22:339, 1975.

113. Pagel PS, Kampine JP, Schmeling WT, et al: Ketamine depresses myocardial contractility as evaluated by the preload recruitable stroke work relationship in chronically instrumented dogs with autonomic nervous system blockade. *Anesthesiology* 76:564, 1992.

114. Dowdy EG, Kaya K: Studies of the mechanism of cardiovascular responses to CI-581. *Anesthesiology* 29:931, 1968.

115. Adams HR, Parker JL, Mathew BP: The influence of ketamine on inotropic and chronotropic responsiveness of heart muscle. *J Pharmacol Exp Ther* 201:171, 1977.

116. Saegusa K, Furukawa Y, Ogiwara Y, et al: Pharmacologic analysis of ketamine-induced cardiac actions in isolated, blood-perfused canine atria. *J Cardiovasc Pharmacol* 8:414, 1986.

117. Urthaler F, Walter AA, James TN: Comparison of the inotropic action of morphine and ketamine studied in canine cardiac muscle. *J Thorac Cardiovasc Surg* 72:142, 1976.

118. Barrigon S, De Miguel B, Tamargo J, et al: The mechanism of the positive inotropic action of ketamine on isolated atria of the rat. *Br J Pharmacol* 76:85, 1982.

119. Waxman K, Shoemaker WC, Lippmann M: Cardiovascular effects of anesthetic induction with ketamine. *Anesth Analg* 59:335, 1980.

120. Tarnaw J, Hess W, Schmidt D, et al: Narkoseeinleitung bei Patienten mit Koronarer Herzkrankheit: Flunitrazepam, Diazepam, Ketamin, Fentanyl. *Anaesthesist* 28:9, 1979.

121. Goading JM, Dimick AR, Tavakili M: A physiologic analysis of cardiopulmonary responses to ketamine anesthesia in non-cardiac patients. *Anesth Analg* 56:813, 1977.

122. Takahashi K, Shima T, Koga Y, et al: Effects of ketamine hydrochloride on the pulmonary hemodynamics. *Jpn J Anaesth* 20:842, 1971.

123. Hickey PR, Hansen DD, Cramolini GM: Pulmonary and systemic hemodynamic responses to ketamine in infants with normal and elevated pulmonary vascular resistance. *Anesthesiology* 61:A438, 1984.

124. Balfors E, Haggmark S, Nyhman H, et al: Droperidol inhibits the effects of intravenous ketamine on central hemodynamics and myocardial oxygen consumption in patients with generalized atherosclerotic disease. *Anesth Analg* 62:193, 1983.

125. Shapiro HM, Wyte SR, Harris AB: Ketamine anaesthesia in patients with intracranial pathology. *Br J Anaesth* 44:1200, 1972.

126. Takeshita H, Okuda Y, Sari A: The effects of ketamine on cerebral circulation and metabolism in man. *Anesthesiology* 36:69, 1972.

127. Wendling WW, Daniels FB, Harakal C, et al: Ketamine directly dilates cerebral arteries by acting as a calcium antagonist. *Anesthesiology* 77:A772, 1992.

128. Schwedler M, Miletich DJ, Albrecht RF: Cerebral blood flow and metabolism following ketamine administration. *Can Anaesth Soc J* 29:222, 1982.

129. Pfenninger E, Dick W, Ahnefeld FW: The influence of ketamine on both normal and raised intracranial pressure of artificially ventilated animals. *Eur J Anaesthesiol* 2:297, 1985.

130. Friesen RH, Thieme RE, Honda AT, et al: Changes in anterior fontanel pressure in preterm neonates receiving isoflurane, halothane, fentanyl, or ketamine. *Anesth Analg* 66:431, 1987.

131. White PF, Way WL, Trevor AJ: Ketamine: Its pharmacology and therapeutic uses. *Anesthesiology* 56:119, 1982.

132. White PF: Pharmacologic interactions of midazolam and ketamine in surgical patients. *Clin Pharmacol Ther* 31:280, 1982.

133. Mattila MAK, Larni HM, Nummi SE, et al: Effect of diazepam on emergence from ketamine anaesthesia: A double-blind study. *Anaesthesist* 28:20, 1979.

134. Cartwright PD, Pingel SM: Midazolam and diazepam in ketamine anaesthesia. *Anaesthesia* 39:439, 1984.

135. Toft P, Romer U: Comparison of midazolam and diazepam to supplement total intravenous anaesthesia with ketamine for endoscopy. *Can J Anaesth* 34:466, 1987.

136. Smith G, Thorburn J, Vance JP, et al: The effects of ketamine on the canine coronary circulation. *Anaesthesia* 34:555, 1979.

137. Kumar SM, Kothary SP, Zsigmond EK: Lack of cardiovascular stimulation during endotracheal intubation in cardiac surgical patients anaesthetized with diazepam-ketamine-pancuronium. *Clin Ther* 3:43, 1980.

138. Sperring SJ, Sinisi NJ, Robson NJ, et al: Sufentanil plus low-dose ketamine, the ideal induction mixture? *Anesth Analg* 67:S215, 1988.

139. Dowdy EG, Kaya K: Studies of the mechanism of cardiovascular responses to CI-581. *Anesthesiology* 29:931, 1968.

140. Koehntop DE, Liao JC, Van Bergen FH: Effects of pharmacologic alterations of adrenergic mechanisms by cocaine, aminophylline and ketamine on epinephrine-induced arrhythmias during halothane-nitrous oxide anesthesia. *Anesthesiology* 46:83, 1977.

141. Hirshman CA, Krieger W, Littlejohn G, et al: Ketamine-aminophylline-induced decrease in seizure threshold. *Anesthesiology* 56:464, 1982.

142. Atkinson PM, Taylor DI, Chetty N: Inhibition of platelet aggregation by ketamine hydrochloride. *Thromb Res* 40:227, 1985.

143. Heller W, Fuhrer G, Juhner M, et al: Haemostaseologische Untersuchungen unter der Anwendung von Midazolam/Ketamin. *Anaesthesist* 35:419, 1986.

144. Roekaerts PMHJ, Huygen FJPM, de Lange S: Infusion of propofol versus midazolam for sedation in the intensive care unit following coronary artery surgery. *J Cardiothorac Vasc Anesth* 7:142, 1993.

145. Carrasco G, Molina R, Costa J, et al: Propofol vs midazolam in short-, medium-, and long-term sedation of critically ill patients: A cost-benefit analysis. *Chest* 103:557, 1993.

146. Albanese J, Martin C, Lacarelle B, et al: Pharmacokinetics of long-term propofol infusion used for sedation in ICU patients. *Anesthesiology* 73:214, 1990.

147. Dundee JW, Robinson FP, McCollum JSC, et al: Sensitivity to propofol in the elderly. *Anaesthesia* 41:482, 1986.

148. Servin F, Desmonts JM, Haberer JP, et al: Pharmacokinetics and protein binding of propofol in patients with cirrhosis. *Anesthesiology* 69:887,1988.

149. Cockshott ID: Propofol ("Diprivan") pharmacokinetics and metabolism: An overview. *Postgrad Med J* 61(suppl 3):45, 1985.

150. Goodman NW, Black AMS, Carter JA: Some ventilatory effects of propofol as a sole anaesthetic agent. *Br J Anaesth* 59:1497, 1987.

151. Doze VA, Westphal LM, White PF: Comparison of propofol with methohexital for outpatient anesthesia. *Anesth Analg* 65:1189, 1986.

152. Cummings GC, Dixon J, Kay NH, et al: Dose requirements of ICI 35 868 (propofol, "Diprivan") in a new formulation for induction of anaesthesia. *Anaesthesia* 39:1168, 1984.

153. Fragen RJ, Weiss HW, Molteni A: The effect of propofol on adrenocortical steroidogenesis: A comparative study with etomidate and thiopental. *Anesthesiology* 66:839, 1987.

154. Pagel PS, Warltier DC: Negative inotropic effects of propofol as evaluated by the regional preload recruitable stroke work relationship in chronically instrumented dogs. *Anesthesiology* 78:100, 1993.

155. Coates DP, Monk CR, Prys-Roberts C, et al: Haemodynamic effects of infusions of the emulsion formulation of propofol during nitrous oxide anesthesia in humans. *Anesth Analg* 66:64, 1987.

156. Mulier JP, Wouters PF, Van Aken H, et al: Cardiodynamic effects of propofol in comparison with thiopental: Assessment with a transesophageal echocardiographic approach. *Anesth Analg* 72:28, 1991.

157. Pagel PS, Schmeling WT, Kampine JP, et al: Alteration of canine left ventricular diastolic function by intravenous anesthetics *in vivo*: Ketamine and propofol. *Anesthesiology* 76:419,1992.

158. Chang KSK, Davis RF: Propofol produces endothelium-independent vasodilation and may act as a Ca^{2+} channel blocker. *Anesth Analg* 76:24, 1993.

159. Al-Khudhairi D, Gordon G, Morgan M, et al: Acute cardiovascular changes following propofol. *Anaesthesia* 37:1007, 1982.

160. Mayer N, Legat K, Weinstabl C, et al: Effects of propofol on the function of normal, collateral-dependent, and ischemic myocardium. *Anesth Analg* 76:33, 1993.

161. Stephan H, Sonntag H, Schenk HD, et al: Effects of propofol on cardiovascular dynamics, myocardial blood flow and myocardial metabolism in patients with coronary artery disease. *Br J Anaesth* 58:969, 1986.

162. Claeys MA, Gepts E, Camu F: Haemodynamic changes during anaesthesia induced and maintained with propofol. *Br J Anaesth* 60:3, 1988.

163. Werner c, Hoffman WE, Kochs E, et al: The effects of propofol on cerebral blood flow in correlation to cerebral blood flow velocity in dogs. *Anesthesiology* 73:A556, 1990.

164. Vandesteene A, Trempont V, Engelman E, et al: Effect of propofol on cerebral blood flow and metabolism in man. *Anesthesia* 43(suppl):42, 1988.

165. Van Hemelrijck J, Fitch W, Mattheussen M, et al: Effect of propofol on cerebral circulation and autoregulation in baboons. *Anesth Analg* 71:49, 1990.

166. Dam M, Ori C, Pizzolato G, et al: The effects of propofol anesthesia on local cerebral glucose utilization in the rat. *Anesthesiology* 73:499, 1990.

167. Ausems ME, Hug CC Jr, Stanski DR, et al: Plasma concentrations of alfentanil required to supplement nitrous oxide anesthesia for general surgery. *Anesthesiology* 65:362, 1986.

168. Hug CC Jr, Hall RI, Angert KC, et al: Alfentanil plasma concentrations v. effect relationships in cardiac surgical patients. *Br J Anaesth* 61:435, 1988.

169. Mummaneni N, Rao TLK, Montoya A: Awareness and recall with high-dose fentanyl-oxygen anesthesia. *Anesth Analg* 59:948, 1980.

170. Hilgenberg JC: Intraoperative awareness during high-dose fentanyl-oxygen anesthesia. *Anesthesiology* 54:341, 1981.

171. Philbin DM, Rosow CE, Schneider RC, et al: Fentanyl and sufentanil anesthesia revisited: How much is enough? *Anesthesiology* 73:5, 1990.

172. Shafer SL, Varvel JR: Pharmacokinetics, pharmacodynamics, and rational opioid selection. *Anesthesiology* 74:53, 1991.

29. Routine Monitoring of Critically Ill Patients

Frederick J. Curley and
Nicholas A. Smyrnios

When intensive care units (ICUs) came into being 30 years ago, most vital signs were monitored intermittently by a nurse and continuous measurement either was unavailable or necessitated invasive procedures. The explosion in the use of computers and other technology over the past few decades has significantly changed critical care. In no part of the hospital is the patient more intensively and continuously monitored, with the possible exception of the operating room, than in the ICU. All vital signs can now be monitored accurately, noninvasively, and continuously.

This chapter deals with the routine, predominantly noninvasive monitoring that should be done for most patients in critical care units. It also examines the indications for, the fundamental technology of, and the problems encountered in the routine monitoring of temperature, blood pressure, pulse and electrocardiographic rhythm, respiratory rate and pattern, oxygenation, and carbon dioxide levels, and gastric intramucosal pH. Since the intent of most monitoring is to warn the supervising staff of impending danger or to alert them to present danger in the patient's condition, our discussion focuses on those uses of the monitors that are clearly established with regard to patient safety.

Temperature Monitoring

Abnormal temperature is common in critically ill patients. In the surgical ICU in one study, rectal temperatures on admission were normal in only 30 percent of patients, were above 37.6°C in 37.6 percent, and were below 36.8°C in 32.3 percent [1]. Recognition of abnormal temperature is clinically important. Abnormal temperature is frequently the earliest clinical sign of infection, inflammation, central nervous system (CNS) dysfunction, or drug toxicity. Both hypo- and hyperthermia have a significant morbidity and mortality (see Chaps. 72 and 73). Accurate measurement of temperature depends on the type of thermometer used and the site of temperature measurement.

TYPES OF THERMOMETERS. A mercury in glass thermometer is the type in most common clinical use. Falsely low measurements may result from failure to leave the thermometer in place for a minimum of 3 minutes equilibration time. Falsely high temperatures result from failure to shake the mercury down. Due to practical limitations in length, different models of mercury thermometers are used for the hypothermic temperature range.

Liquid crystal display (LCD) thermometers usually involve liquid crystals embedded in thin adhesive strips that are directly attached to the patient's skin. The crystals may be sensitive to temperature changes as small as 0.2°C, but the displays usually limit discrimination of temperature changes to no more than 0.5°C. Liquid crystal display thermometers can be applied to any area of the skin but are most commonly applied to the

forehead for ease of use and steady perfusion. Like all skin temperature measurements, they poorly reflect core temperature when the skin is hypoperfused. Forehead skin temperature is typically lower than core temperatures by 2.2°C [2], and changes in LCD forehead temperature lag behind changes in core temperature by more than 12 minutes [3]. The LCD strip may be left in place for several hours without skin irritation but must be discarded after use [4]. Liquid crystal display skin thermometry is probably best used in patients with stable, normal hemodynamics who are not anticipated to experience major temperature shifts and in whom the trend of temperature change is more important than the accuracy of the measurement.

Thermocouples and thermistors are frequently used as probes in electric thermometers that convert the electrical temperature signal into analog or digital displays. Thermocouples consist of a tight junction of two dissimilar metals. The voltage change across the junction can be precisely related to temperature. The measuring thermocouple must be calibrated against a second constant temperature junction for absolute temperature measurements. The measured voltage changes are of the order of 50 μV per degree Celsius and must be amplified to generate a usable temperature display. In the range of 20 to 50°C, thermocouples may have a linearity error of less than 0.1° [4]. Thermocouples are faster and cheaper but less sensitive than thermistors and semiconductors.

Thermistors consist of semiconductor metal oxides in which the electrical resistance changes inversely with temperature. A linearity error of up to 4°C may occur over the temperature range of 20 to 50°, but this can be substantially reduced by making mathematical adjustments or placing a fixed resistance in parallel with the thermistor, which decreases its sensitivity and usable temperature range [4]. Thermistors are more sensitive, faster responding, and less linear and costly than thermocouples or semiconductors [4,5]. Semiconductors measure temperature by taking advantage of the fact that the base to emitter voltage change is temperature-dependent, while the collector current of the silicon resistor is constant. Both thermocouples and thermistors can be fashioned into thin wires embedded in flexible probes that are suitable for placing in body cavities to measure deep temperature.

Zero heat flow thermometry involves placing a thermistor, a heat flow sensor, and a heater immediately adjacent to the skin. Heat loss from the skin is detected by the flow sensor and is compensated by the heater. In this manner, the skin beneath the probe is isolated from ambient temperature changes and more directly reflects deep body temperature or core temperature [6,7]. Response time to changes in core temperature is generally about 10 minutes [7] but may be substantially longer in obese patients [5]. Inaccuracies during hypoperfusion have been reported [5]. Despite its convenience, this type of thermometer remains infrequently used in the clinical setting due to its cost, 30-minute warm-up time, and inadequate data on local variation of deep body temperature at different sites.

Radiotelemetry thermometers have been made in the form of ingestible pills. The temperature sensor in the pill is an inductor and functions in such a way that temperature-dependent changes in inductance result in changes in radiofrequency. Changes in radiofrequency can then be detected by a remote unit and translated electronically into a digital display of temperature. These thermometers have little application in the ICU, as temperature differences of up to 2°C may occur just by transit of the pill in the intestine [8].

Infrared emission detection tympanic thermometers [9] are probably now most commonly used in the hospital setting. These thermometers employ an infrared sensor that detects infrared energy emitted by the core temperature tissues behind the tympanic membrane. The infrared emissions through the tympanic membrane vary linearly with core temperature. The thermometer's sensor sends a signal to a microprocessor, which converts the signal into a digitally displayed temperature. Measurements are most accurate when the measuring probe blocks the entrance of ambient air into the ear canal and when the midposterior external ear is tugged posterosuperiorly so as to direct the probe to the anterior, inferior third of the tympanic membrane. Operator error due to improper calibration, setup, or poor probe positioning can significantly alter temperatures [10]. Mathematical corrections are available so tympanic temperature may be compared with that at other sites.

SITES OF MEASUREMENT.

Core temperature refers to the deep body temperature that is carefully regulated by the hypothalamus so as to be independent of transient small changes in ambient temperature. Core temperature exists more as a physiologic concept than as the temperature of an anatomic location. Ideal sites of temperature measurement would be protected from heat loss, painless, and convenient to use and would not interfere with the patient's ability to move and communicate. No one location provides an accurate measurement of core temperature in all clinical circumstances. Rectal, bladder, and tympanic temperatures are in general the most reliable sites for measuring approximate core temperatures.

Sublingual temperature measurement is convenient but suffers numerous limitations. Although open versus closed mouth breathing [11] and use of nasogastric tubes do not alter temperature measurement [12], oral temperature is obviously altered if measured during or immediately after the patient has consumed hot or cold drinks. Falsely low oral temperatures may occur due to cooling from tachypnea [13]. Sixty percent of sublingual temperatures are more than 1°F lower than simultaneously measured rectal temperatures; 53 percent differ by 1 to 2°F and 6 percent differ by more than 2°F. Continuous sublingual measurement interferes with the patient's ability to eat and speak, and it is difficult to maintain a good probe position. Sublingual measurement is best suited for intermittent monitoring when highly accurate measurement of core temperature is unnecessary.

Axillary temperatures have been used as an index of core temperature and may be taken with a mercury in glass thermometer or a flexible probe. Temperatures average 1.5 to 1.9°C lower than tympanic temperatures [14]. Positioning the sensor over the axillary artery is thought to improve accuracy. The accuracy and precision of axillary temperature measurement are less than at other sites [14], perhaps due in part to the difficulty of maintaining a good probe position.

Rectal temperature is conveniently measured with a mercury in glass thermometer or a flexible temperature sensor. It is clearly the most accepted standard of measuring core temperature in clinical use. Prior to inserting a rectal thermometer, a digital rectal examination should be performed, as feces can blunt temperature measurement. Readings are more accurate when the sensor is passed more than 10 cm (4 inches) into the rectum [5]. Rectal temperature correlates well in most patients with distal esophageal, bladder, and tympanic temperatures [14,15]. Due to thermal inertia in the rectum, it is typically the slowest of the central measurement sites to respond to induced changes in temperature [16,17].

Esophageal temperature is usually measured with an electric, flexible temperature sensor and varies greatly with the position of the sensor in the esophagus. In the proximal esophagus, as well as in the midportion near the trachea and bronchi, temperature is influenced by that of the ambient air [18]. During hypothermia, temperatures in different portions of the esophagus may differ by up to 6°C [18]. Stable, more accurate temperatures are reached when the sensor is 45 cm from the nose [18,19]. Esophageal temperatures on average are 0.6°C lower than rectal temperatures [20]. Due to the proximity of the distal esophagus to the great vessels and heart, distal esophageal temperature responds rapidly to changes in core temperature [5]. Changes in esophageal temperature may inaccurately reflect changes in core temperature when induced temperature change occurs due to the inspiration of heated air, warm or cold gastric lavage, or cardiac bypass or assist [5]. Complications apart from mild discomfort and epistaxis are rare.

Tympanic temperature must be measured with a specifically designed thermometer and correlates well with rectal and distal esophageal temperature [5]. During induced hypothermia in animals, tympanic temperature better approximates brain temperature than distal esophageal temperature [21]. Perforation of the tympanic membrane [22] and bleeding from the external canal [23] due to trauma from the probe have been reported. One series had a 1.25 percent complication rate [17]. Tympanic temperature measurement should always be preceded and followed by an otoscopic examination. Current thermometers do not permit continuous measurement, which limits their utility in the ICU.

Urinary bladder temperature can be easily measured with a specially designed temperature probe embedded in a Foley catheter [14–17]. In patients undergoing induced hypothermia and rewarming, bladder temperatures correlate well with great vessel and rectal temperatures and less well with esophageal temperatures [15,16,17]. Bladder temperature under steady-state conditions is more reproducible than that taken at other sites [15].

Central venous temperature may be easily measured with a thermistor-equipped pulmonary artery catheter. The temperature sensor is located at the distal tip and can record accurate great vessel temperatures when the tip of the catheter is in the distal vena cava. Temperatures would, of course, differ from core temperatures when heated air was breathed or warm or cold intravenous fluids infused.

Temperature measured on the medial aspect of the great toe varies with core temperature and toe perfusion [1]. The gradient between toe and core temperature is therefore an index of perfusion. A normal rectal-to-toe temperature difference of 3 to 7°C occurs once patient hemodynamics have been optimized. Abnormal toe-to-rectal temperature gradients occur during hypovolemia, low cardiac output, pain, and hypoxemia acidosis [1,24]. The absolute value of great toe temperature has been predictive of mortality in some populations. Great toe temperature less than 27°C persisting more than 3 hours after admission is associated with death in 67 percent of adults [24], and temperatures less than 32°C lasting 4 hours after cardiac surgery predicted significantly increased mortality in children [25]. Toe temperature is an unreliable indicator of core temperature because it is so greatly affected by perfusion. It should be used only to assess peripheral circulatory flow in comparison with other measurements of core temperature.

The choice of site used to monitor temperature must be

individualized, but certain generalizations can be made. Tympanic, bladder, and esophageal temperatures in general appear to be most accurate and reproducibile [26]. In a study of 56 patients undergoing general anesthesia, esophageal, bladder, and rectal temperatures were more accurate than forehead and axillary measurements and esophageal and bladder temperatures were more precise than rectal, axillary, and forehead temperatures when compared to tympanic temperature [15,27]. As bladder, esophageal, tympanic, and rectal sites appear comparable, convenience may help dictate appropriate site selection. Routine measurement of esophageal temperatures would necessitate insertion of a nasal probe in all patients. In addition, accuracy varies greatly with small changes in position. Therefore, routine esophageal temperature measurement is probably of benefit only in patients undergoing treatment for hyper- or hypothermia. Tympanic temperature measurement requires physician involvement for otoscopy and decreases the patient's ability to hear. Placement of probes may also be traumatic. Rectal probes are frequently extruded and may be refused by patients. Reusable electronic sheath-covered rectal thermometers have been associated with the transmission of *Clostridium difficile* and vancomycin-resistant *Enterococcus* [28,29]. Due to the risk of infecting other patients, all rectal thermometers should be used only once. Patients with a thermistor-tipped pulmonary artery catheter already in place require no additional monitoring, but insertion of a central venous thermistor to monitor temperature is probably warranted only in hyper- or hypothermia. As most critically ill patients have an indwelling Foley catheter, bladder temperature could be easily measured at a cost of less than $10 per thermistor-equipped catheter. Continuous temperature monitoring is in general probably best accomplished by measurement of bladder, great vessel, or rectal temperature. Intermittent measurements for reasons of accuracy should probably be rectal rather than sublingual.

INDICATIONS FOR TEMPERATURE MONITORING. Temperature monitoring was identified as an essential service for critical care units by the Task Force on Guidelines of the Society of Critical Care Medicine recommendations for services and personnel for delivery of care in a critical care setting [30]. Critically ill patients are at high risk for temperature disorders due to debility, impaired voluntary control of temperature, frequent use of sedative drugs, and high predisposition to infection. All critically ill patients should have core temperature measured at least every 4 hours. As the morbidity and mortality of hypo- and hyperthermia vary with the severity and duration of the abnormality, patients with temperatures above 39°C or below 36°C should have their temperature continuously monitored. Patients who are undergoing active interventions to alter temperature, for example breathing heated air or using a cooling-warming blanket, should have continuous monitoring to prevent over- or undertreatment of temperature disorders.

Arterial Pressure Monitoring

Arterial pressure has traditionally been measured with a mercury sphygmomanometer and a stethoscope. Techniques of direct blood pressure measurement via intraarterial catheter were initially developed in the 1930s and popularized in the 1950s [31,32]. These measurements were soon accepted as representing "true" systolic and diastolic pressures.

Since that time a variety of alternative indirect methods have been developed that equal and even surpass auscultation in reproducibility and ease of measurement. However, the accuracy of even direct blood pressure measurements in certain situations has been questioned [33,34]. What represents "true" blood pressure has been reevaluated in an attempt to find a method that accurately describes the patient's condition and is reproducible enough to allow comparison between groups for research purposes. This section examines the advantages and disadvantages of the various methods of arterial pressure monitoring and provides recommendations for their use in the ICU.

INDIRECT BLOOD PRESSURE MEASUREMENT. There are several methods of indirect blood pressure monitoring [35–38], most of which describe the external pressure applied when flow is observed in an artery distal to the occlusion. Therefore, what is actually detected is blood flow, not intraarterial pressure [35]. One method describes the pressure required to maintain a distal artery with a transmural pressure of zero. These differences in what is actually measured are the major points of discrepancy between direct and indirect measurements and are discussed further below.

Indirectly measured pressures vary depending on the size of the cuff used. Cuffs of inadequate width and length can provide falsely elevated readings. Bladder width should equal 40 percent and bladder length at least 60 percent of the circumference of the extremity measured [39]. Anyone making indirect pressure measurements must be aware of these factors and carefully select the cuff to be used.

Manual Methods

AUSCULTATORY (RIVA-ROCCI) PRESSURES. The traditional method of blood pressure measurement involves inflating a sphygmomanometer cuff around an extremity and auscultating over an artery distal to the occlusion. Sounds from the vibrations of the artery under pressure (Korotkoff sounds) indicate systolic and diastolic pressures [38]. The level at which the sound first becomes audible is taken as the systolic pressure. The point where there is an abrupt diminution or disappearance of sounds is used as diastolic pressure [35]. This remains the most commonly used method of blood pressure monitoring in the ICU and yields an acceptable value in most situations. Its advantages include low cost, time-honored reliability, and simplicity. Disadvantages include operator variability and the absence of Korotkoff sounds when pressures are very low. Auscultatory pressures also correlate poorly with directly measured pressures at the extremes of pressure [35,40]. There is a tendency for pressures obtained by auscultation to fall increasingly below those measured directly as the pressure increases. However, the difference between these values is unpredictable and at times the indirectly measured value can exceed its direct counterpart by as much as 20 mm Hg [35]. Therefore, auscultatory pressures must be interpreted with full knowledge of their limitations in the critically ill.

OSCILLATION METHOD. The oscillation method has served as the basis for the development of several automated blood pressure monitoring devices. The first discontinuity in the needle movement of an aneroid manometer indicates the presence of blood flow in the distal artery and is taken as systolic pressure [35]. This oscillation is caused by vibration of the walls of the artery when blood begins to flow through it. Diastolic pressure is not measured by this technique. The advantages of the oscillation method are low cost and simplicity. The disadvantages include the inability to measure diastolic pressure, poor correlation with directly measured pressures [35], and lack of utility in situations where Riva-Rocci measurements are also unobtainable. In one study, 34 percent of all aneroid manometers in use in one large medical system demonstrated inaccurate measurements, even when more lenient standards were used than those advocated by the National Bureau of Standards and the Association for the Advancement of Medical Instrumentation [41]. In the same survey, 36 percent of the devices were found to be mechanically defective. This points out the need for regular maintenance of these devices. While the manometers themselves may also be used for auscultatory measurements, oscillometric readings probably provide no advantage over auscultation in the ICU.

PALPATION METHOD. Palpatory systolic pressures are obtained by detecting the pulse in the radial artery as the cuff is slowly deflated. This resembles the oscillation method because it does not measure diastolic pressure. Palpation is most useful in emergency situations where Korotkoff sounds cannot be heard and an arterial line is not in place. The inability to measure diastolic pressure makes the palpation method less valuable for continuous monitoring. In addition, palpation obtains no better correlation with direct measurements than the previously described techniques. In one study, variation from simultaneously obtained direct pressure measurements was as high as 60 mm Hg [40]. Like other indirect methods, palpation tends to underestimate actual values to greater degrees at higher levels of arterial pressure.

Automated Methods.

Automated indirect blood pressure devices provide measurements of arterial blood pressure without manual inflation and deflation of the sphygmomanometer cuff. They operate on one of six principles: Doppler flow, infrasound, oscillometry, photoplethysmography, arterial tonometry, and Doppler echocardiography.

DOPPLER FLOW. Doppler systems operate on the Doppler principle, which takes advantage of the change in frequency of an echo signal when there is movement between two objects. These devices emit brief pulses of sound at a high frequency that is reflected back to the transducer [42]. The compressed artery exhibits a large amount of wall motion when flow first appears in the vessel distal to the inflated cuff. This causes a change in frequency of the echo signal, called a Doppler shift. The first appearance of flow in the distal artery represents systolic pressure. In an uncompressed artery the small amount of motion does not cause a change in frequency of the reflected signal. Therefore, the disappearance of the Doppler shift in the echo signal represents diastolic pressure [43,44].

INFRASOUND. Infrasound devices use a microphone to detect low-frequency (20–30 Hz) sound waves associated with the oscillation of the arterial wall [37,45]. These sounds are processed by a minicomputer and the processed signals usually displayed in digital form [46].

OSCILLOMETRY. Oscillometric devices operate on the same principle as manual oscillometric measurements. The cuff senses pressure fluctuations caused by vessel wall oscillations in the presence of pulsatile blood flow [37,47]. Maximum oscillation is seen at mean pressure, while wall movement greatly decreases below diastolic pressure [48]. As with the other automated methods described, the signals produced by the system are processed electronically and displayed in digital form.

PHOTOPLETHYSMOGRAPHY. The photoplethysmographic method avoids the use of an arm cuff. A finger cuff is applied to the proximal or middle phalanx, to keep the artery at a constant size [49]. The pressure in the cuff is changed as necessary by a servocontrol unit strapped to the wrist. The feedback in this system is provided by a light source and detector that measure absorption at a frequency specific for arterial blood. The pressure needed to keep the artery at a constant size is always equal to the intraarterial pressure, thereby creating a transmural pressure of zero [50]. Advocates of photoplethysmography claim it

is the only noninvasive method that actually measures pressure and the only one that gives a truly continuous reading.

ARTERIAL TONOMETRY. Arterial tonometry provides continuous noninvasive measurement of arterial pressure, including pressure waveforms. Essentially, it involves flattening a superficial artery against a bone to remove any force due to wall tension and then placing a pressure transducer on the skin over the flattened artery. The resultant force sensed by the pressure transducer is thought to measure intraarterial pressure only [51]. Preliminary studies indicate a high degree of accuracy and reproducibility of measurements, although more definitive studies are needed [51,52].

ECHOCARDIOGRAPHY. The Doppler echocardiogram has been used occasionally to estimate aortic pressures. This is primarily of value for the rare patient in whom peripheral pressures cannot be obtained. This measurement takes advantage of the Bernoulli equation, which describes the relationship between pressure gradient and flow (V). In its modified form, this relationship is [53]:

Pressure gradient = $4V^2$

In patients who demonstrate regurgitation across the aortic valve, the pressure gradient measured is that seen across the valve. This can give an estimation of systolic pressure which is accurate only to within the wide range of variation of the left ventricular diastolic pressure. Therefore, this method should be used only when all other methods have failed.

Utility of Noninvasive Blood Pressure Measurements.

All four of the methods described for which there are adequate data on which to base an analysis (Doppler flow, infrasound, oscillometry, photoplethysmography) yield only marginally acceptable correlation with direct blood pressure measurement [36,37,45,47,54–60]. The group average values obtained by oscillometric methods can correlate to within 1 mm Hg of the directly measured average values [37,55], but they vary greatly from predicting intraarterial pressures in individual subjects. Methods employing infrasound technology correlate least well with direct measures [36,37], obtaining correlation coefficients of 0.58 to 0.84 in comparison with arterial lines. Doppler sensing devices offer a slightly better correlation but still vary sufficiently to be clinically inadequate. Correlation coefficients range from 0.83 to 0.99 for systolic pressures and 0.71 for diastolic pressures [36]. These highly positive correlations coincide with individual variations of as much as 30 mm Hg. Oscillometric monitors have shown varying degrees of argeement in different studies [47,48,54,55,61]. Correlation coefficients of 0.739 to 0.99 and 0.52 to 0.82 are seen for systolic and diastolic pressures, respectively. The reasons for these differences are uncertain but may be related to the setting in which the trial was carried out or the specifics of the populations studied. In many cases a difference of more than 20 mm Hg was seen in individual readings, when compared to directly measured pressures [37,47,62]. Photoplethysmography using a finger cuff has been compared to standard methods in multiple studies [56–60]. While these devices respond rapidly to changes in blood pressure and give excellent correlation in group averages, they suffer from the same lack of precise correlation to individual values that the other methods do.

While they have not been consistently accurate, automated methods do have the potential to yield as accurate a value as pressures derived by auscultation [61,62,63]. One study revealed as good a correlation with directly measured pressures as Riva-Rocci pressures have traditionally obtained [37]. A study by Aitken et al. demonstrated acceptable correlation of photoplethysmography with systolic pressures measured directly [57]. Another study demonstrated that mean arterial pressures determined by auscultation were extremely close to those measured by automated devices [62].

One of the proposed advantages of automated noninvasive monitoring is patient safety [64]. The incidence of vessel occlusion and hemorrhage is thought to be reduced when arterial lines are avoided. Automated methods have complications of their own, however. Ulnar nerve palsies have been reported with frequent inflation and deflation of a cuff [65]. Decreased venous return from the limb and eventually reduced perfusion to that extremity can also be seen when the cuff is set to inflate and deflate every minute [64,66].

In summary, automated noninvasive blood pressure monitors may have a role in following trends of pressure change [67]. They are probably adequate for frequent blood pressure checks in essentially stable patients. They are also of some use when arterial lines cannot be easily used, such as in patient transport. Automated blood pressure monitors may be particularly helpful in the severely burned patient, where direct arterial pressure measurement may lead to an unacceptably high risk of infection [68]. They are useful when measurement of group averages rather than of individual patients are of concern. They are of little value in situations where blood pressure is likely to fluctuate rapidly. Also, they exhibit such divergence from directly obtained values that critical patient management decisions should not be made based on information derived from automated monitors unless confirmation using a more reliable method is possible.

DIRECT INVASIVE BLOOD PRESSURE MEASUREMENT.
Direct blood pressure measurement is performed with an intraarterial catheter. The techniques of insertion and care of arterial lines are covered thoroughly in Chapter 3. Here, we discuss the advantages and disadvantages of invasive monitoring compared to noninvasive means.

In theory, intraarterial pressure can be measured in two ways. Pressure can be detected by a wire transducer at the tip of an indwelling catheter. Electrical impulses can then be conducted back along the wire to the processor for display. Alternatively, the catheter can contain a fluid column that transmits the pressure back through the tubing to the transducer. In practice, only the second system is used. A low-compliance diaphragm in the transducer creates a reproducible volume change in response to the applied pressure change. The volume change alters the resistance of a Wheatstone bridge and is thus converted into an electrical signal [69]. The pressure is displayed both in waveform and digitally in most systems.

Problems in Direct Pressure Monitoring
PATIENT-RELATED PROBLEMS. Several technical problems can affect the measurement of arterial pressure via the arterial line. Transducers must be calibrated to zero at the level of the heart. Improper zeroing can lead to erroneous interpretation of essentially accurate measurements. Thrombus formation at the catheter tip can cause occlusion of the catheter, making accurate measurement impossible. This problem can be essentially eliminated by using a 20-gauge Teflon catheter, rather than a smaller one, with a slow, continuous heparin flush [70,71]. Because movement of the limb may interrupt the column of fluid and prevent accurate measurement, it should be immobile during readings.

SYSTEM-RELATED PROBLEMS. Direct pressure values are also affected by several factors specific to the measurement system itself. For example, effective transducer design must take into

account the natural frequency of the transducer system. The natural frequency is the frequency at which the system oscillates independent of changes in the measured variable. Signals that approach the natural frequency in wavelength become amplified and may result in an exaggerated reported pressure [72]. This phenomenon is referred to as overshoot. Above the natural frequency, the signal is attenuated and an erroneously low pressure can be reported. Accurate recording systems require a natural frequency at least five times greater than the fundamental frequency (i.e., the range of expected heart rates) [34,73]. This is necessary to account for the multiple harmonic frequencies produced along with the main (fundamental) frequency.

The frequency response of the system is a phenomenon not only of transducer design but also of the tubing and the fluid within it. The length, width, and compliance of the tubing all affect the system's response to change. Tubing shorter than 60 cm should be used [74]. Small-bore catheters are preferable to minimize the mass of fluid that can oscillate and amplify the pressure [73]. The compliance of the system (change in volume of the tubing and the transducer for a given change in pressure) should be low [73]. In addition, bubbles in the tubing can affect measurements in two ways. Large amounts of air in the measurement system damp the system response and cause underestimation of pressure [75]. This is usually easily detectable. Small air bubbles cause an increase in the compliance of the system and can lead to significant amplification of the reported pressure [73,74,75].

SITE-RELATED PROBLEMS. Other problems arise in relation to the location of catheter placement. The radial artery is the most common site of arterial cannulation for pressure measurement. This site is accessible and easily immobilized for protection of the catheter and the patient. The major alternative site is the femoral artery. Both sites are relatively safe for insertion [70,76,77]. Other available sites include the brachial, dorsalis pedis, and axillary arteries [77,78]. Site-specific problems with arterial lines center on whether pressures measured directly at one site can be compared to pressures measured at another site. Although it was thought that upper extremity pressures were different from those measured in the leg, this probably reflects the location of measurement rather than the extremity. Systolic pressure is augmented toward the periphery by reflection of the pressure from the distal vessels due to impedance discontinuity [33], the abrupt increase in resistance due to the narrowing of peripheral vessels. Changes in the pressure-pulse contour as it approaches the periphery are manifestations of this. This waveform becomes narrower and more peaked as it proceeds distally [66]. In practice, this means systolic pressures measured in the radial artery are, on average, 6 mm Hg higher than those in the brachial artery [33]. Similarly, in the absence of a significant arterial obstruction, dorsalis pedis pressures are higher than femoral pressures. These differences are less significant in older patients and those with noncompliant vessels. The elevation of central systolic pressures in these situations eliminates the increase seen along the course of the vessels in young, healthy persons. Pressures should be measured from a single site whenever possible, and comparisons should not be made between values obtained at different sites.

Advantages. Despite technical problems, direct arterial pressure measurement offers several advantages. Arterial lines actually measure the end-on pressure propagated by the arterial pulse. This is in contrast to indirect methods, which report the external pressure necessary either to obstruct flow or to maintain a constant transmural vessel pressure. Arterial lines can also detect pressures at which Korotkoff sounds are either absent or inaccurate [40]. Arterial lines provide a continuous measurement. They provide an immediate report of changes in blood pressure without the need for repeated inflation and deflation of a cuff. In situations where frequent blood drawing is necessary, indwelling arterial lines eliminate the need for multiple percutaneous punctures.

CONCLUSIONS. Arterial blood pressure can be monitored indirectly or directly. Most indirect methods detect flow, while direct methods measure intraarterial pressure. Indirect techniques can be manual or automated. Manual methods have the advantages of being inexpensive and easy to perform. Auscultation sphygmomanometry is the standard by which most correlations of blood pressure to pathology in humans have been made. It continues to be the most commonly used and valuable method of blood pressure monitoring. Other manual methods offer no advantage over auscultation. Automated indirect methods are more complicated and expensive, while offering no improvement in accuracy over auscultation. Direct measurements via arterial lines have the advantage of actually measuring the parameter in question. They are accurate to greater extremes of pressure than indirect methods and allow rapid recognition of changes in pressure and heart rate. They should be used whenever auscultation is considered inadequate to meet the needs of blood pressure monitoring in an intensive care setting.

Electrocardiographic Monitoring

Continuous electrocardiographic (ECG) monitoring is performed routinely in almost all ICUs in the United States. It combines the principles of electrocardiography, which have been known since 1903, with the principles of biotelemetry, first put into practical application in 1921 [79,80]. Here we review the principles of arrhythmia monitoring and the problems associated with it. We also discuss the automatic detection of arrhythmias and the role of automated S–T segment analysis. Although telemetry is not usually used in ICUs, it is a useful adjunct in the advancement of recuperating patients to more routine levels of care and is briefly discussed here.

JUSTIFICATION FOR ARRHYTHMIA MONITORING IN THE INTENSIVE CARE UNIT. Electrocardiographic monitoring in most ICUs is done over hard-wired apparatus. Skin electrodes detect cardiac impulses and transform them into an electrical signal, which is transmitted over wires directly to the signal converter and display unit. This removes the problems of interference and frequency restrictions seen in telemetry systems at the cost of reduced mobility for the patient. Most often, mobility is not an immediate concern for this group of patients.

Arrhythmia monitoring has clearly improved the prognosis of patients admitted to the ICU for acute myocardial infarction (AMI) [81,82,83]. In coronary care, arrhythmia monitoring is necessary for the following reasons. (1) Up to 95 percent of patients with AMI have some disturbance of their rate or rhythm within 48 hours of admission [84]. Ventricular premature beats (VPBs) are the most common arrhythmia, present in up to 100 percent of patients [83,84,85]. Monitoring allows the recognition and treatment of minor arrhythmias such as frequent VPBs, which may be entirely asymptomatic but also may predict sudden death [86]. (2) Ventricular tachycardia (VT) occurs in approximately one-third of patients with AMI. Other serious arrhythmias are seen less frequently. Monitoring enables the rapid detection of ventricular fibrillation or VT, increasing the likelihood of successful resuscitation. Arrhythmia monitoring has been shown to improve prognosis in the postmyocardial infarction period when combined with an aggressive, formalized approach to the treatment of arrhythmias [83]. It also can demonstrate the response to therapy so alternative treatments can be begun, if necessary. (3) Thrombolytic therapy for AMI may lead to a slight increase in arrhythmias within 8 to 12 hours after successful reperfusion [87]. Frequent premature ventricular contractions and accelerated idioventricular rhythm are the most common of these and rarely cause clinical compromise [87,88,89]. Monitoring allows the detection of these arrhythmias as one indicator of successful reperfusion.

The effect of monitoring in a noncardiac ICU is less certain. One study demonstrated a 23.9 percent incidence of atrial fibrillation and a 17.4 percent incidence of VT in a medical ICU [90]. Twenty-five percent of the episodes of VT were not detected by an experienced ICU staff. Computerized detection of arrhythmias altered therapy in 43 to 62 percent of cases, depending on the abnormality detected. The effect of monitoring on the prognosis of these patients has not been investigated.

EVOLUTION OF ARRHYTHMIA MONITORING SYSTEMS FOR CLINICAL USE. After the continuous ECG monitoring in ICUs was begun, some deficiencies with the systems were recognized. Initially, the responsibility for arrhythmia detection was assigned to specially trained coronary care nurses, occupying a great deal of their time and efforts. Despite this, several studies documented that manual methods of arrhythmia detection failed to identify arrhythmias in up to 77 percent of cases [85,91,92]. Salvos of ventricular tachycardia were among the undetected arrhythmias. This failure was probably due to an inadequate number of staff nurses to watch the monitors for the appearance of arrhythmias. Other possibilities included inadequate staff education and faulty monitors [91].

The next generation of monitors was equipped with built-in rate alarms that sounded whenever a preset maximum or minimum rate was detected. These proved inadequate because many runs of VT are too brief to exceed the rate limit for a given time interval [85,92]. Subsequently, computerized arrhythmia detection systems were incorporated into the monitors. The computer software in these systems is capable of diagnosing arrhythmias based on recognition of heart rate, variability, rhythm, intervals, segment lengths, complex width, and morphology [93,94]. These systems have been validated in both coronary care and general medical ICUs [92,95]. While they are susceptible to some error due to movement, artifact, and signal noise, they generally perform very well [95]. A quick look at the patient and review of the tracing is adequate to detect most errors [93]. Computerized arrhythmia detection systems are well accepted by nursing personnel, who must work most closely with them [96].

TECHNICAL CONSIDERATIONS. As with any other biomedical measurement, technical problems can arise in the monitoring of cardiac rhythm. Arrhythmia monitoring is fairly simple, and modern systems have removed much of what previously caused difficulty. Standards have been devised to guide manufacturers and purchasers of ECG monitoring systems [97,98].

Whenever a patient is directly connected to an electrically operated piece of equipment by a low-resistance path, the possibility of electrical shock exists. This would most commonly occur with improper grounding of equipment when a device such as a pacemaker is in place. Precautions necessary to avoid this potential catastrophe include (1) periodic checks to ensure that all equipment in contact with the patient is at the same ground potential as the power ground line; (2) insulation of exposed lead connections; and (3) use of appropriately wired three-prong plugs [99,100].

The size of the ECG signal is important for accurate recognition of cardiac rate and rhythm. Several factors may affect signal size. The amplitude can be affected by mismatching between skin-electrode and preamplifier impedance. The combination of a high skin-electrode impedance, generally the result of poor contact between the skin and electrode, with low-input impedance of the preamplifier can result in a decrease in the size of the ECG signal [101]. Skin-electrode impedance should be less than 3500 ohm [98]. This can be promoted by good skin preparation, site selection, and conducting gels. A high preamplifier input impedance or the use of buffer amplifiers can also improve impedance matching and thereby improve the signal obtained.

Another factor that affects complex size is critical damping, the system's ability to respond to changes in the input signal. An underdamped system will respond to changes in input with displays that exaggerate the signal, called overshoot. An overdamped system will respond slowly to a given change and may exhibit a complex that underestimates the actual amplitude. The accepted guidelines followed by most manufacturers state that a system should be able to respond to 1 mV peak voltage variation up to 300 Hz, with a response equal to input [101].

The ECG signal can also be affected by the presence of inherent, unwanted voltages at the point of input into the ECG. These include the common mode signal, a response to surrounding electromagnetic forces; the direct current (DC) skin potential produced by contact between the skin and the electrode; and a potential caused by internal body resistance. These can disrupt the signal and affect interpretation. They can be reduced by the use of a negative feedback circuit that deamplifies these voltages to allow clean signal reception [101].

Finally, the ECG system must have a frequency response that is accurate for the signals being monitored. A range of 0.05 to 100 Hz has generally been accepted as adequate to represent signal amplitudes accurately.

PERSONNEL. The staff's ability to interpret the information received is crucial to the effectiveness of arrhythmia monitoring [98]. Primary interpretation may be by nurses or technicians under the supervision of a physician. All personnel responsible for interpreting rhythm strips must have formal training developed cooperatively by the hospital's medical and nursing staffs. At a minimum, this training should include basic ECG interpretation skills and arrhythmia recognition. Formal protocols for responding to and verifying alarms should be established and adhered to. Finally, a physician should be available in the hospital to assist with interpretation and made decisions regarding therapy.

ISCHEMIA MONITORING. Just as episodes of VT and ventricular fibrillation are missed with simple monitoring systems, significant episodes of myocardial ischemia often go undetected [102]. This is either because the episode is asymptomatic or because the patient's ability to communicate is impaired due to intubation or altered mental status. Electrocardiographic monitoring systems with automated S–T segment analysis exist to attempt to deal with this problem.

In most S–T segment monitoring systems, the computer initially creates a template of the patient's "normal" QRS complexes. It then recognizes the QRS complexes and the J points

of subsequent beats and compares an isoelectric point just prior to the QRS with a portion of the S–T segment 60 to 80 msec after the J point [103]. It compares this relationship to that of the same points in the QRS complex template. The system must decide whether the QRS complex in question was generated and conducted in standard fashion or whether the beats are aberrant, which negates the validity of comparison. Therefore, an arrhythmia detection system must be included in all ischemia monitoring systems designed for use in the ICU. In standard systems, three leads can be monitored simultaneously. These leads are usually chosen to represent the three major axes (anteroposterior, left-right, and craniocaudal). They can be displayed individually, or the S–T segment deviations can be summed up and displayed in a graph over time [103].

Automated S–T segment analysis has gained widespread popularity among cardiologists; in fact, an American Heart Association Task Force recommended that ischemia monitoring be included in new monitoring systems developed for use in the coronary care unit [98]. However, the impact of automated S–T segment analysis on patient outcomes has not been determined. While the early detection of ischemic episodes could lead to early interventions, such as rate control or thrombolysis, to prevent further damage, studies are needed to assess the effect of this, especially during the postmyocardial infarction period.

PRINCIPLES OF TELEMETRY. Intensive care patients frequently continue to require ECG monitoring after they are released from the ICU. At this point, increased mobility is important to allow physical and occupational therapy as well as other rehabilitation services. Telemetry systems can facilitate this.

Telemetry means measurement at a distance [104]. Biomedical telemetry consists of measuring various vital signs, including heart rhythm, and transmitting them to a distant terminal [105]. Telemetry systems in the hospital consist of four major components [105]. (1) A signal transducer detects heart activity via skin electrodes and converts it into electrical signals. (2) A radio transmitter broadcasts the electrical signal over ultrahigh frequencies (UHF) or very high frequencies (VHF). (3) The radio receiver detects the transmission and converts it back into an electrical signal. (4) The signal converter and display unit presents the signal in its most familiar format.

Telemetry can be continuous or intermittent. Post-ICU patients, when monitored, are almost always followed continuously. Continuous telemetry requires an exclusive frequency so the signal can be transmitted without interruption from other signals [106], which means the hospital system must have multiple frequencies available to allow monitoring of several patients simultaneously. The telemetry signal may be received in one location or simultaneously in multiple locations, depending on staffing practices. The signal transducer and display unit should also be equipped with an automatic arrhythmia detection and alarm system to allow rapid detection and treatment of arrhythmias.

SUMMARY. Continuous ECG monitoring for the detection of arrhythmias is and should be ubiquitous in the ICU, as it has been shown to improve the prognosis in post-AMI patients. Because a large percentage of arrhythmias can be missed by ICU staff when monitors without computerized arrhythmia detection systems are used, these computerized systems should be standard equipment in ICUs that care for AMI patients.

A survival benefit has not been clearly demonstrated in other populations of critically ill patients, due to a lack of studies addressing this issue. It appears that computerized monitoring devices can detect a significant number of arrhythmias not noted manually in these patients also. A large percentage of these lead to an alteration in patient care. Therefore, it seems wise to include them as standard equipment in all medical and surgical ICUs.

Monitoring systems currently used to detect arrhythmias include detection electrodes, transmission wires, and signal converter and display units. Despite the variety of potential technical problems discussed above, modern arrhythmia detection systems are extremely sensitive and usually very accurate. Simple measures, such as a rapid glance at the printed tracing and the patient, are usually sufficient to explain their errors. Automated S–T segment analysis may facilitate the early detection of ischemic episodes. Telemetry provides close monitoring of recuperating patients while allowing them increased mobility. Since most sophisticated monitoring systems are extremely expensive, further studies are needed to clarify their role in the noncardiac patient.

Respiratory Monitoring

The primary respiratory parameters that must be monitored in critically ill patients include respiratory rate, tidal volume or minute ventilation, and oxygenation. Routine monitoring of carbon dioxide levels and pH would be desirable, but the technology for monitoring these parameters is not yet developed enough to consider continuous monitoring mandatory. In mechanically ventilated patients, many physiologic functions can be monitored routinely and continuously by the ventilator. This section does not discuss monitoring by the mechanical ventilator but examines those devices that might be routinely used to monitor continuously and noninvasively the parameters mentioned above.

RESPIRATORY RATE, TIDAL VOLUME, AND MINUTE VENTILATION. Clinical suspicion of a new respiratory problem in a critically ill patient may lead to further evaluation with arterial blood gases (ABG), a chest radiograph, or other testing. Visual inspection of the patient frequently is inadequate to detect changes in respiratory rate or tidal volume. Physicians, nurses, and hospital staff frequently report inaccurate respiratory rates, possibly because they underestimate the importance of the measurement [107]. Two studies in which physicians and staff were asked to assess tidal volume and minute ventilation indicate that tidal volume is (1) assessed poorly, (2) frequently overestimated, and (3) not reproducible on repeat assessment [108,109]. In another study, ICU staff had a greater than 20 percent error more than one-third of the time when the recorded respiratory rate was compared to objective tracings [110]. Objective monitoring must be employed because clinical evaluation is inaccurate.

Impedance Monitors. Impedance monitors are commonly used to measure respiratory rates and approximate tidal volume in ICUs and home apnea alarms. These devices typically employ ECG leads and measure changes in impedance generated by the change in distance between leads as a result of the thoracoabdominal motions of breathing. To obtain a quality signal, leads must be placed at points of maximal change in thoracoabdominal contour and/or sophisticated computerized algorithms must be used. Alarms can then be set for a high and low rate or for a percentage drop in the signal thought to correlate with a decrease in tidal volume.

In clinical use, impedance monitors suffer confounding problems. They have failed to detect obstructive apnea when it has occurred and falsely detected apnea when it has not [90,111,112]. Although computerized impedance monitors may falsely report bradypnea in up to 17 percent of patients, they detect tachypnea more accurately [90]. Detection of obstructive apnea by impedance monitors is poor because chest wall motion may persist and be counted as breaths by these monitors as the apneic patient struggles to overcome airway obstruction [111,112]. Tidal volume estimates may be artifactually affected by changes in patient position or patient movement. Impedance monitors offer the advantage of being very inexpensive when ECG is already in use but lack accuracy when precise measurements of tidal volume, change in tidal volume, or bradypnea-apnea are required.

Respiratory Inductive Plethysmography. The most commonly used respiratory inductive plethysmograph (RIP) measures changes in the cross-sectonal area of the chest and abdomen that occur with respiration and processes these signals into respiratory rate and tidal volume. Two 3- to 10-cm-wide bands consisting of elastic fabric containing a wire sewn in a zigzag fashion are placed around the patient's upper chest and around the abdomen below the ribs. As the cross-sectional area of the bands changes with respiration, the self-inductance of the coils changes the frequency of attached oscillators. The signals from the oscillator pass through a demodulator, yielding a voltage signal. The voltage signals may be calibrated by numerous methods to within 10 percent of spirometry or may be internally calibrated so that further measurements reflect a percentage change from baseline. Respiratory inductive plethysmography can accurately measure respiratory rate and the percent of change in tidal volume, as well as detect obstructive apnea [113,114,115]. These measurements are more accurate than impedance measurements [112].

In addition to displaying respiratory rate and percent of change in tidal volume, RIP can provide continuous measurement of asynchronous and paradoxical breathing and signal an alarm for predetermined changes in these values. Studies of patients during weaning have demonstrated that asynchronous and paradoxical movements are common during early weaning and may be helpful in predicting respiratory failure [116,117] (Fig.29-1). However, as a single parameter, an increase in respiratory rate is more predictive of imminent failure to wean [118]. The noninvasive nature of the tidal volume measurement may be extremely helpful in patients in whom direct measurement of expired volume is confounded due to technical problems or leaks (e.g., patients with bronchopleural fistulas, undergoing ventilation with nasal ventilators, or on nasal constant positive airway pressure). In addition, RIP can display changes in functional residual capacity (FRC), which permits rapid assessment of the effect of changing positive end-expiratory pressure (PEEP). Determinations of the presence and estimation of the amount of auto (intrinsic) PEEP can be made by observing the effect of applied (extrinsic) PEEP on FRC [119].

Respiratory inductive plethysmography systems are available with central station configurations designed specifically for ICU use. Routine use of RIP has resulted in decreased ICU length of stay and reduced hospital cost [102]. Compared to inductance methods, RIP is more accurate and offers a variety of other useful measurements but is slightly less convenient and more expensive. It is useful for the careful monitoring of patients with obstructive apnea.

Other Methods. Although respiratory rate can be measured accurately with a pneumotachometer, capnographs, or electromyography, none of these methods has achieved a level of

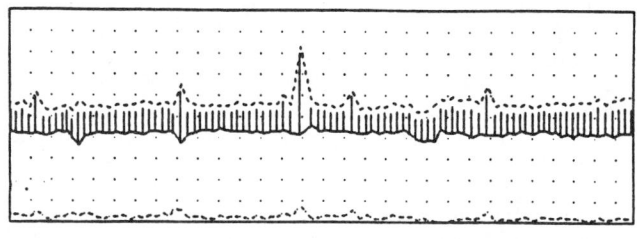

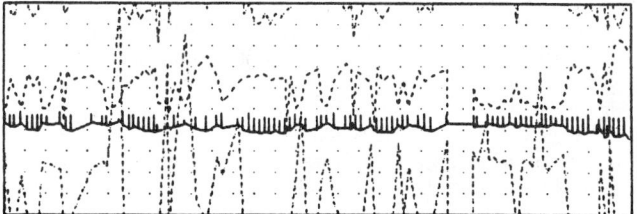

Fig. 29-1. Respiratory inductive plethysmography (RIP) tracing demonstrating impending respiratory failure during weaning from mechanical ventilation. Each panel is a 15-minute recording in which the height of the vertical lines represents the tidal volume of individual breaths. The spacing between lines varies with the respiratory rate. The solid horizontal line represents functional residual capacity. The height of the dotted line above the tidal volume bars increases with asynchronous or paradoxical breathing. Percent of tidal volume generated by the rib cage is indicated by the dotted line at the bottom of each panel. In panel A, ventilated breaths are regular and tidal volume is generated mostly by the abdominal compartment. In panel B, taken during impending respiratory failure, there are periods of apnea, tidal volume is decreased, asynchrony is increased, and there is alternation of motion (respiratory alternans) between rib cage and abdomen, as seen by the variation in the percentage of tidal volume generated by the rib cage. (Courtesy of Non Invasive Monitoring Systems, Inc., Miami Beach, FL.)

popular usage in the ICU. A pneumotachometer requires complete collection of exhaled gas and therefore requires either intubation or use of a tight-fitting face mask. Due to this inconvenience and difficulties with calibration and maintenance, pneumotachometers are infrequently used routinely in the ICU. Surface electromyography of respiratory muscles can be used to calculate respiratory rate accurately [121] but cannot detect obstructive apnea or provide a measure of tidal volume. Electromyography works well in infants but has difficulties in adults, especially in obese adults and those with edema. Capnography works exceedingly well as a respiratory rate monitor, does not require intubation or a face mask, and is a useful tool in many circumstances. Capnography is discussed in more detail below.

A pneumotachometer can assess tidal volume but suffers from the same limitations as those discussed for respiratory rate.

Measurements of Gas Exchange

PULSE OXIMETRY. Oximeters offer a noninvasive method of determining whether oxygen supplementation is needed and, once delivered, whether supplementation is adequate. Co-oximeters perform measurements on whole blood obtained from an artery or a vein. They frequently measure absorbance at multiple wavelengths and compute the percentage of oxyhemoglobin, deoxyhemoglobin, methemoglobin, and carboxyhemoglobin in total hemoglobin. They are mostly free of the artifacts that limit the accuracy of tissue oximeters and

are regarded as the gold standard by which other methods of assessing saturation are measured. Noninvasive tissue oximeters usually measure only the percentage of oxyhemoglobin of total hemoglobin. Early oximeters tended to be bulky and inconvenient, in that they required exposed vessels, heat, or histamine to induce vasodilation, arterial occlusion to render a tissue bloodless for calibration, or multistep calibration procedures [122]. As pulse oximeters circumvent most of these problems with no significant loss of accuracy, they have supplanted virtually all older types of oximeters in clinical use. Pulse oximeters measure the saturation of hemoglobin in the tissue during the arterial and venous phases of pulsation and mathematically derive arterial saturation. This section reviews the fundamental technology involved in pulse oximetry, practical problems that limit its use, and indications for the use of oximeters in critically ill patients.

More than 20 manufacturers now market pulse oximeters. Due to the variety of manufacturers, the numerous algorithms used, and the diverse patient populations studied, it is difficult to generalize the studies performed with one particular instrument, with its specific version of software, in one defined group of patients to critically ill patients in general. The reader should always check with an oximeter's manufacturer before generalizing the discussion below to his or her oximeter and patient population.

Technology. Oximeters distinguish between oxy- and reduced hemoglobin on the basis of their different absorption of light. Oxyhemoglobin absorbs much less red ($\pm$ 660 nm) and slightly more infrared ($\pm$ 910–940 nm) light than reduced hemoglobin. Oxygen saturation thereby determines the ratio of red to infrared absorption. When red and infrared light are directed from light-emitting diodes (LEDs) to a photodetector across a pulsatile tissue bed, the absorption of each wavelength by the tissue bed varies cyclically with pulse. During diastole, absorption is due to the nonvascular tissue components (e.g., bone, muscle, and interstitium) and venous blood. During systole, absorption is determined by all of these components and arterialized blood. The pulse amplitude accounts for only 1 to 5 percent of the total signal [123]. Thus, the difference between absorption in systole and diastole is theoretically due to the presence of arterialized blood. The change in ratio of absorption between systole and diastole can then be used to calculate an estimate of arterial saturation (SaO_2). Absorption is typically measured hundreds of times per second. Signals are generally averaged over several seconds and then displayed digitally. The algorithm used for each oximeter is determined by calibration on human volunteers. Most oximeters under ideal circumstances measure the saturation indicated by the pulse oximeter (SpO_2) to within 2 percent of SaO_2 [124].

Oximeters are typically equipped to display the measured SpO_2 and pulse and to sound alarms for high and low values of each. Most employ software algorithms to send warning messages or stop display analysis when signal quality deteriorates.

Problems Encountered in Use. Any process that affects or interferes with the absorption of light between the LEDs and photodetector or alters the quality of pulsatile flow has the potential for artifactually distorting the oximeter's calculations. Pulse oximeters should be able to obtain valid readings in 98 percent of patients in an operating room or postanesthesia care unit [125]. Table 29-1 lists the problems that must be considered in clinical use.

CALIBRATION. Since early attempts to calibrate pulse oximeters in accord with the principles of Beer's law of absorbance proved unsuccessful, manufacturers now use normal individ-

Table 29-1. Conditions Adversely Affecting
Accuracy of Oximetry

May result in poor signal detection	
Probe malposition	No pulse
Motion	Vasoconstriction
Hypothermia	Hypotension

Fasely lowers SpO₂	Falsely raises SpO₂
Nail polish	Elevated carboxyhemoglobin
Dark skin	Elevated methemoglobin
Ambient light	Ambient light
Elevated serum lipids	Hypothermia
Methylene blue	
Indigo carmine	
Indocyanine green	

uals to derive calibration algorithms. This results in three problems. First, manufacturers use different calibration algorithms, which results in a difference in SpO₂ of up to 2.7 percent between oximeters of different manufacturers when used to measure the same patient [126]. Second, manufacturers define SpO₂ differently for calibration purposes. Calibration may or may not account for the interference of small amounts of dyshemoglobinemia (e.g., methemoglobin or carboxyhemoglobin). For example, if an oximeter is calibrated on the basis of a study of nonsmokers with a 2 percent carboxyhemoglobin (COHB) level, the measured SpO₂ percentage would differ depending on whether the value used to calibrate SpO₂ included or excluded the 2 percent COHB [126]. Third, it is difficult for ethical reasons for manufacturers to obtain an adequate number of validated readings in people with SpO₂ less than 70 percent to develop accurate calibration algorithms in this saturation range. Most oximeters give less precise readings and underestimate saturation in this saturation range [127]. Until better calibration algorithms are available, oximeters should be considered unreliable when SpO₂ is less than 70 percent. The accuracy of a unit can be checked by sytematically comparing the oximetry values of the oximeter with simultaneous co-oximeter values measured from arterial blood. An in vitro system to evaluate oximeter performance has been designed but is too complex for routine validation of individual oximetry devices [128].

SITE OF MEASUREMENT. Accurate measurements may be obtained from fingers, foreheads, and earlobes [129,130]. The response time from a change in PaO₂ to a change in displayed SpO₂ is delayed in finger and toe probes as compared to ear, cheek, or glossal probes [129,131]. Forehead edema, wetness, and head motion have resulted in inaccurate forehead SpO₂ values [132]. Motion and perfusion artifacts are the greatest problems with digital measurements. Glossal pulse oximetry has been useful in some patients where no other measuring site was available [133], and specific glossal probes may be developed soon. The earlobe is believed to be the site least affected by vasoconstriction artifact [134].

FINGER NAILS. Long finger nails may prevent correct positioning of the finger pulp over the diodes used in inflexible probes and therefore produce inaccurate SpO₂ readings without affecting the pulse rate [135]. Synthetic nails have produced erroneous results [124]. Nail polish of several colors has been shown to lower SpO₂ falsely [136]. Not surprisingly, those colors with the greatest difference in absorption between 660 and 940 nm produced the greatest artifact. While thickness of applied polish may also be a factor, adhesive tape, even when placed over both sides of a finger, did not affect measured SpO₂ [137].

SKIN COLOR. The effect of skin color on SpO₂ was assessed in a study of 655 patients [138]. Although patients with the darkest skin had significantly less accurate SpO₂ readings, the mean difference in SpO₂ between subjects with light skin and those with the darkest skin compared to control co-oximeter readings was only 0.5 percent, a clinically insignificant difference. Pulse oximeters, however, encountered major difficulties in obtaining readings in darker-skinned patients; 18 percent of patients with darker skin triggered warning lights or messages versus 1 percent of lighter-skinned patients. Thus, dark skin may prevent a measurement from being obtained, but when the oximeter reports an error-free value the value is accurate enough for clinical use.

AMBIENT LIGHT. Ambient light that affects absorption in the 660- or 910-nm wavelengths or both may affect calculations of saturation and pulse. Xenon arc surgical lights [139], fluorescent lights [140], and fiberoptic light sources [140] have caused falsely elevated saturation but typically obvious dramatic elevations in pulse. An infrared heating lamp [142] has produced falsely low saturations and a falsely low pulse, and a standard 15-watt fluorescent bulb resulted in falsely low saturation without a change in heart rate [143]. Interference from surrounding lights should be suspected by the presence of pulse values discordant from the palpable pulse or ECG and/or changes in the pulse-saturation display when the probe is transiently shielded from ambient light with an opaque object. Most manufacturers have now modified their probes to minimize this problem.

HYPERBILIRUBINEMIA. Bilirubin's absorbance peak is maximal in the 450-nm range but has tails extending in either direction [144]. Bilirubin therefore does not typically affect pulse oximeters that use the standard two-diode system [144,145]. However, it may greatly interfere with the measurement of saturation by co-oximeters. Co-oximeters typically employ four to six wavelengths of light and measure absolute absorbance to quantify the percentage of all major hemoglobin variants. Serum bilirubin values as high as 44 mg per 100 ml produced no effect on the accuracy of pulse oximeters but produced falsely low levels of oxyhemoglobin measured by co-oximetry [144].

DYSHEMOGLOBINEMIAS. Conventional two-diode oximeters cannot detect the presence of fetal hemoglobin, methemoglobin, or COHB. Fetal hemoglobin may confound readings in neonates but is rarely a problem in adults. As methemoglobin absorbs more light at 660 nm than at 990 nm, oxygen saturation is falsely elevated whenever methemoglobin levels exceed 6 percent [146]. Moreover, higher levels of methemoglobin tend to bias the reading toward 85 to 90 percent [147]. Carboxyhemoglobin is typically read by a two-diode oximeter as 90 percent oxyhemoglobin and 10 percent reduced hemoglobin [148], resulting in false elevations of SpO₂. As COHB may be 10 percent in smokers, pulse oximetry may fail to detect significant desaturation in this group of patients. Hemolytic anemia may also elevate COHB up to 2.6 percent [149]. As other etiologies of COHB are rare in the hospital and the half-life of COHB is short, this problem is unusual in the critical care setting except in new admissions or patients with active hemolysis.

ANEMIA. There are few clear data on the effect of anemia on pulse oximetry. In dogs, there was no significant degradation in accuracy until the hematocrit was less than 10 percent [150].

LIPIDS. Patients with elevated chylomicrons and those receiving lipid infusions may have falsely low SpO₂ due to interference in absorption by the lipid [151].

HYPOTHERMIA. Quality signals may be unobtainable in 10 percent of hypothermic (< 35°C) patients [152] and signal detection fails at temperatures less than 26.5°C [153]. The decrease in signal quality probably results from hypothermia-induced vasoconstriction. When quality signals could be obtained, SpO₂ differed from co-oximetry measured saturation by only 0.6 percent [152] in one series and tended to be falsely elevated by 0.9 to 3.0 percent SpO₂ in another [153].

INTRAVASCULAR DYES. Methylene blue, used to treat methemoglobinemia, has a maximal absorption at 670 nm and therefore falsely lowers measured SpO_2 [154]. Indocyanine green and indigo carmine also lower SpO_2, but the changes are minor and brief [155]. Fluorescein has no effect on SpO_2 [155]. Due to the rapid vascular redistribution of injected dyes, the effect on oximetry readings typically lasts only 5 to 10 minutes [156].

MOTION ARTIFACT. Shivering and other motions that change the distance from diode to receiver may result in artifact. Oximeters account for motion by different algorithms. Some oximeters display a warning sign, others stop reporting data, and others display erroneous values. The display of a pulsatile waveform rather than a signal strength bar helps to indicate that artifact has distorted the pulse signal and lowered the quality of the subsequent SpO_2 analysis [157].

HYPOPERFUSION. During a blood pressure cuff inflation model of hypoperfusion, most oximeters remained within 2 percent of control readings [158]. Increasing systemic vascular resistance (SVR) and decreasing cardiac output can also increase the inability to obtain a quality signal. In one series the lowest cardiac index and highest SVR at which a signal could be detected were 2.4 L/min/m² and 2930 dyne sec/cm⁵/m² [153]. Warming the finger [159], sympathetic digital block [160], or applying a vasodilating cream [153] tended to extend the range of signal detection in individual patients. The oximeter's ability to display a waveform and detect perfusion degradation of the signal were crucial in determining when the readings obtained were valid [158].

PULSATILE VENOUS FLOW. In physiologic states where venous and capillary flows become pulsatile, the systolic pulse detected by the oximeter may no longer reflect the presence of just arterial well-saturated blood. In patients with severe tricuspid regurgitation or hyperperfusion the measured saturation may be falsely low [161,162].

Indications. Unsuspected hypoxemia is common in critically ill patients. Sixteen percent of patients not receiving supplemental oxygen in the recovery room have saturations less than 90 percent [163]. Thirty-five percent of patients develop saturations less than 90 percent during transfer out of the operating room [164]. Due to the high frequency of hypoxemia in critically ill patients, the frequent need to adjust oxygen flow to avoid toxicity and insufficiency, and the unreliability of visual inspection to detect mild desaturation, oximeters should be useful in most critically ill patients for routine, continuous monitoring. In one study that randomized more than 20,000 operative and perioperative patients to continuous or no oximetric monitoring, the authors concluded that oximetry permitted detection of more hypoxemic events, prompted increases in the fraction of oxygen in inspired air (FiO_2), and significantly decreased the incidence of myocardial ischemia but did not significantly decrease mortality or complication rates [165]. In the ICU, continuous oximetric monitoring may spare patients oxygen toxicity by facilitating the rapid tapering of FiO_2 [166].

Oximeters have been employed in the ICU for reasons other than continuous monitoring. They can be useful in locating an artery that is difficult to palpate. When the oximeter is placed distal to the artery, the signal strength will decrease and the saturation may decrease when the more proximal vessel is compressed [167,168]. Oximeters may be helpful during difficult intubations. Once desaturation occurs, attempts to intubate should be postponed until manual ventilation restores saturation. Oximetry is not helpful in promptly detecting inadvertent esophageal intubation, in that desaturation may lag behind apnea by more than 30 seconds [169] in this setting. Oximeters can be useful in detecting systolic blood pressure. In one study where the blood pressure cuff was inflated proximal to the

oximeter, the point at which the pulse signal was lost was within 2 mm Hg of Doppler measurements of systolic pressure [170]. In trauma patients an abrupt, sustained 10 percent drop in saturation in the presence of a stable chest radiograph and static compliance was highly predictive of pulmonary embolism [171].

TRANSCUTANEOUS OXYGEN AND CARBON DIOXIDE MEASUREMENT. Transcutaneous systems measure partial pressures of oxygen ($P_{tc}O_2$) and carbon dioxide ($P_{tc}CO_2$) that diffuse out of the vasculature and through the skin. This section examines the technology most commonly used to measure transcutaneous partial pressures, the differences between the values obtained by cutaneous measurement and arterial measurement, and the indications for use of transcutaneous gas measurement.

Technology. The technology used to obtain transcutaneous gas measurements varies slightly between manufacturers but generally employs similar techniques. Typically, a unit less than 1 inch in diameter is attached to the skin with an adhesive. An electrode is used to heat the skin that promotes arterialization of capillaries and improves diffusion of gases through the skin's lipid layers. A temperature sensor measures skin temperature at the skin surface and adjusts the heater to provide a constant temperature. In adults, temperatures of 43.5 to 44.5°C produce the most satisfactory results. Some systems do not rely on heating to improve diffusion of gas. Similar results may be produced by stripping off the stratum corneum with adhesive tape or measuring from a site with a thinner layer of skin, such as the conjunctiva.

Oxygen and carbon dioxide diffuse out of the capillaries into the interstitium and through the skin to measuring electrodes. The diffusing distance from capillary to sensor may be as small as 0.3 mm. Precalibrated Clarke and Severinghaus-type electrodes, similar to those used in blood gas machines, then measure the partial pressure of oxygen and carbon dioxide. The temperature at which partial pressure is measured and reported can be adjusted on some units. These signals are then electronically averaged and converted into a continuous digital display. Alarms may be set for high and low values of both gases measured. Many units also display trend signals to indicate whether and in which direction a change occurs.

Since units do use electrodes for partial pressure measurement, problems with calibration and electrode drift during prolonged monitoring can clearly alter measurements. Drift may alter readings by up to 12 percent over a 2-hour period [172].

Differences between Arterial and Transcutaneous Measurements. Numerous factors may cause $P_{tc}O_2$ and $P_{tc}CO_2$ to differ from partial pressures of arterial oxygen (PaO_2) and partial pressures of arterial carbon dioxide ($PaCO_2$). Most differences can be traced to factors involving probe temperature, blood flow, local metabolism, or skin thickness.

The increased temperature of the heating probe shifts the oxygen dissociation curve to the right and promotes off-loading of bound oxygen, which increases the PO_2 in the surrounding interstitium. Different temperature settings will alter this effect to varying degrees and may directly influence the final value measured at the skin surface. Heat-induced artifacts may be avoided by using a measurement site that does not require heating, such as a conjunctival probe site [173].

Blood flow is a critical determinant of the value measured at the skin. If there is no flow to the region below the sensor there is no delivery of oxygen and no elimination of CO_2 by the vasculature, resulting in lower PO_2 and higher PCO_2 than in an adjacent artery. Some units provide an index of cutaneous blood flow by displaying changes in the amount of heat necessary to keep the probe at a constant temperature. As perfusion increases, heat is carried away from the probe faster and more heat must be applied to maintain a constant temperature. As perfusion decreases, the opposite occurs. Thus, a decrease in probe heat output may reflect a fall in perfusion.

Local metabolism alters values from arterial levels, in that gases diffusing from the capillaries may be consumed or added to by local metabolism. Local oxygen consumption by the tissues between capillary and skin surface can reduce $P_{tc}O_2$ by 20 to 40 mm Hg during hypoperfused states [174]. The $P_{tc}CO_2$ in hypoxemic or underperfused regions may also be dramatically increased, in some cases more than 30 mm Hg higher than in arterial samples.

Thick or edematous skin provides a diffusion barrier that amplifies all of the above effects. The longer the distance the gases must diffuse to be measured, the more important are the effects of temperature, perfusion, and local metabolism. This appears to be the fundamental reason why transcutaneous measurements are generally more accurate in neonates than in adults. Edema, burns, abrasions, or scleroderma would all alter transcutaneous values.

Clinical Correlations and Utility. In healthy adults, $P_{tc}O_2$ and $P_{tc}CO_2$ accurately reflect PaO_2 and $PaCO_2$ [172,175]. The measured transcutaneous values of oxygen and carbon dioxide are typically 10 mm Hg lower [176] and 5 to 23 mm Hg higher [177,178] than arterial values, respectively. Fever and tissue edema alter the correlation between arterial and transcutaneous values. Systemic hypoperfusion due to low cardiac output, regional hypoperfusion due to sepsis or shock, and local hypoperfusion due to cutaneous vasoconstriction to medication or cold produce discrepancies. In these cases transcutaneous measurements cease to reflect arterial values and better track oxygen delivery and tissue metabolism [174,179].

Several studies have demonstrated the value of transcutaneous oxygen measurements as indices of perfusion or oxygen delivery. When PaO_2 remains constant, a decrease in $P_{tc}O_2$ is probably due to changes in perfusion. Changes in local perfusion and metabolism may cause $P_{tc}O_2$ values to fall to zero and $P_{tc}CO_2$ values to climb to more than 30 mm Hg above arterial values [177]. When the cardiac index is less than 2 liters per minute, $P_{tc}O_2$ correlates best with PaO_2 [174]. In hemorrhagic shock, the ratio of $P_{tc}O_2$ to PaO_2 decreases, even though PaO_2 may remain normal [180,181]. Values are more sensitive to changes in flow than in pressure, but flow is always compromised at a blood pressure less than 50 mm Hg. Deterioration of $P_{tc}O_2$ values may occur up to 4 minutes before a decrease in blood pressure [181]. Improvements in flow were detected within 1 minute by a rise in $P_{tc}O_2$ [174]. As the measurements are very sensitive to changes in flow, they can be useful in predicting or warning of imminent change before a blood pressure response is seen. In perioperative patients, declines in the $P_{tc}O_2$-to-PaO_2 ratio to less than 0.77 were predictive of hemodynamic collapse within the next 50 minutes [182]. In cardiogenic shock, $P_{tc}O_2$ values of 25 mm Hg or less have been predictive of death [174].

In other circumstances, transcutaneous measurements may be helpful in assessing a complex interaction between perfusion and oxygenation factors. During the titration of PEEP in critically ill patients, $P_{tc}O_2$ correlates well and directly with PaO_2 and pulmonary artery PO_2 and correlates inversely with a shunt fraction [178]. In this setting, where the clinical goal is to optimize oxygen delivery, the single noninvasive measurement of $P_{tc}O_2$ might replace more invasive blood measurements.

Partial pressures of carbon dioxide measurements are af-

fected in virtually all situations that alter $P_{tc}O_2$. In most cases, the variations have been less sensitive predictors of changes in perfusion [174]. Studies in hemodynamically stable patients have shown that $P_{tc}O_2$ reliably tracks arterial PCO_2 values in patients being weaned from mechanical ventilation. Partial pressures of carbon dioxide remained within 5.2 ± 1.5 mm Hg of $PaCO_2$ [177]. In cases where $P_{tc}O_2$ remains near constant, changes in $P_{tc}O_2$ would be expected to track changes in minute ventilation or dead space.

Transcutaneous equipment also requires meticulous attention to provide quality readings. Probes must be firmly attached to the skin, or leaks from the surrounding atmosphere will lower $P_{tc}CO_2$ and alter $P_{tc}O_2$ values. Adhesion is a problem in diaphoretic patients. Patient motion may produce tension on the cable connecting the sensor to the processing unit, causing leaks or disconnection. Probe sites must be changed at least every 4 to 6 hours to prevent burns. Units must be recalibrated whenever the probe temperature is changed and every 4 to 6 hours to prevent artifact from electrode drift. Many units take 15 to 60 minutes to warm the skin and establish stable readings. These factors can combine in many patients to make transcutaneous measurements very inconvenient.

Indications. Transcutaneous monitors have little role in the ICU as simple tools to replace other means of measuring arterial gas. Their application in practice is not complex but is far from simple. They predictably reflect arterial values only in hemodynamically stable patients, who are least likely to demand intensive care or to benefit from ICU monitoring. As monitors of trends in PCO_2 and PO_2, they can be regarded as effective only in the sense that they typically do not produce false negative alarms—that is, if the arterial values change, the transcutaneous values reflect the change. So many other factors, such as changes in tissue edema and perfusion, may result in alterations in transcutaneous trends that the supervising staff can initially determine only that something has changed. An accurate interpretation of the clinical event usually requires reassessment of either cardiac status or arterial gases.

Therefore, transcutaneous monitors are inadequate cardiac monitors and inadequate pulmonary monitors but are quality cardiopulmonary monitors. Transcutaneous monitoring is currently most useful in patients in whom changes in either perfusion or gas exchange are likely, but not both. When perfusion is stable, values will reflect gas exchange. When gas exchange is stable, values will reflect perfusion. When both are unstable, the results cannot be interpreted without additional information. In the future, transcutaneous measurements could be combined with noninvasive monitors of cardiac output or with results from indwelling arterial monitors of blood gases to provide continuous analysis of perfusion, gas exchange, and local metabolism. Until such time, this complex assessment must be provided by the supervising staff.

CAPNOGRAPHY. Capnography involves the measurement and display of expired PCO_2 concentrations. This section reviews the technology, the sources of difference between end-tidal PCO_2 and arterial PCO_2, and the indications for capnography in the ICU.

Technology. Expired PCO_2 concentration is usually determined by infrared absorbance or mass spectrometry. The infrared technique relies on the fact that CO_2 has a characteristic absorbance of infrared light with maximal absorbance near a wavelength of 4.28 mm. A heated wire with optical filters is used to generate an infrared light of appropriate wavelength. When CO_2 passes between a focused beam of light and a semiconductor photodetector, an electronic signal can be generated, which, when calibrated, accurately reflects the PCO_2 of the tested gas. A mass spectrometer bombards gas with an electron stream. The ion fragments that are generated can be deflected by a magnetic field to detector plates located in precise positions to detect ions characteristic of the molecule being evaluated. The current generated at the detector can be calibrated to be proportional to the partial pressure of the molecule being evaluated.

The two techniques have different strengths. Mass spectrometers can detect the partial pressures of several gases simultaneously and can monitor several patients at once. Infrared techniques measure only PCO_2 and are usually employed on only one patient at a time. The calibration and analysis time required for mass spectrometry is significantly longer than with infrared techniques. Infrared systems respond to changes in approximately 100 msec, whereas mass spectrometers take 45 seconds to 5 minutes to respond [183]. Although costs vary widely, mass spectrometers are generally far more expensive and are most frequently purchased to be the central component of a CO_2 monitoring system. In the operating room, mass spectrometry has the advantage of being able to measure the partial pressure of anesthetic gases, and the need for a technical specialist to oversee its operation can be more easily justified. For these reasons, mass spectrometry has achieved much more popularity in the operating room than in the ICU.

Gases may be sampled by mainstream or sidestream techniques. Mainstream sampling involves placing the capnometer directly in line in the patient's respiratory circuit. All air leaving the patient passes through the capnometer. The sidestream sampling techniques pump 100 to 300 ml of expired air per minute through thin tubing to an adjacent analyzing chamber. The mainstream method can be used only on patients who are intubated or wearing a tight-fitting face or nose mask. Due to the size of mass spectrometer equipment, mainstream sampling is applicable only to infrared analysis. Mainstream sampling offers the advantage of almost instantaneous analysis of sampled air, but it increases the patient's dead space and adds uncomfortable weight to the endotracheal tube. Sidestream sampling removes air from the expiratory circuit, confounding measurement of tidal volume. The aspirating flow rate and tubing length significantly affect the ability to detect a rapid rise in CO_2 and the delay between physiologic change in the patient and display of the change at the monitor [184]. When the delay exceeds the respiratory cycle time, the generated data are inaccurate [184]. The sidestream sampling line is also prone to clogging with pulmonary secretions, saliva, or water condensation. Clogging affects accuracy and delay time. Sidestream sampling can detect cyclic changes in CO_2 concentration easily in the unintubated patient if the sampling tube is located near the mouth or nose. Because of all of these issues, accurate sidestream sampling requires short tubes and constant attention to the possibility of clogged sample lines.

Differences between End-Tidal and Arterial Carbon Dioxide. The PCO_2 in exhaled air measured at the mouth changes in a characteristic pattern in normal individuals that reflects the underlying physiologic changes in the lung (Fig. 29-2). During inspiration, the PCO_2 is negligible and rises abruptly with expiration. The rate of rise reflects the washout of dead space air with air from perfused alveoli. A plateau concentration is reached after dead space air has been exhaled. The plateau level is determined by the mean alveolar PCO_2, which is in equilibration with pulmonary artery PCO_2 (P_vCO_2). The end alveolear plateau level of PCO_2 measured during the last 20 percent of exhalation is the end-tidal PCO_2 [183]. In normal individuals at rest, the difference between end-tidal PCO_2 and

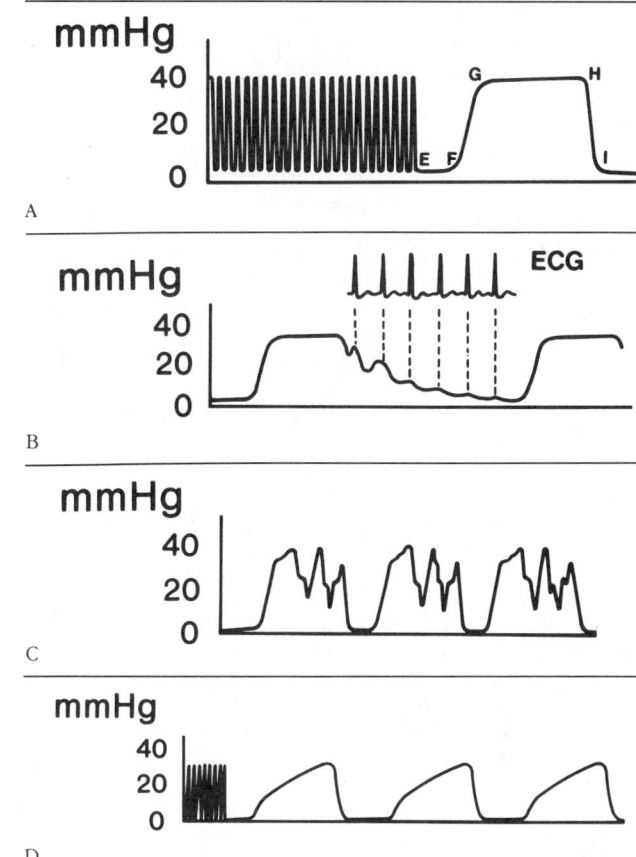

Fig. 29-2. Normal and abnormal capnograms. Panel A shows a normal capnogram; on the right of the trace the paper speed has been increased. The EF segment is inspiration. The FG segment reflects the start of expiration with exhalation of dead space gas. The GH segment is the alveolar plateau. End-tidal values are taken at point H. HI is the beginning of inspiration. The alveolar plateau is distorted and the end-tidal point cannot be clearly determined in panel B due to cardiac oscillations, in panel C due to erratic breathing, and in panel D due to obstructive airways disease. (Modified from Stock MC: Noninvasive carbon dioxide monitoring. *Crit Care Clin* 4:511, 1988. With permission.)

arterial PCO_2 is ± 1.5 mm Hg. A difference exists due to the presence of dead space (i.e., ventilation without perfusion) and a physiologic shunt (i.e., perfusion without ventilation). Any change in anatomic dead space or pulmonary perfusion alters ventilation perfusion mismatch so as to increase the difference between end-tidal and arterial PCO_2 values. As dead space increases, the end-tidal PCO_2 represents more the PCO_2 of nonperfused alveoli, thereby diverging from the arterial PCO_2 value. As perfusion decreases, less alveoli are perfused, creating a similar effect.

In most equipment, the end-tidal PCO_2 level is determined by a computerized algorithm. As algorithms are imperfect, a waveform display is considered essential for accurate interpretation of derived values [185]. In slowly breathing patients, cardiac pulsations may cause the intermittent exhalation of small amounts of air at the end of the lungs' expiratory effort. This results in oscillations that may obscure the plateau phase. An irregular respiratory pattern or large increases in dead space can also distort the plateau phase. Visual inspection of traces can detect situations where algorithms are prone to produce errors [183].

Indications. In the ICU, capnography is most useful for determining the presence or absence of respiration. Such determinations do not require that end-tidal PCO_2 be measured accurately, only that changes be detected reliably. Apnea can be defined as an absence of variation in PCO_2 levels. Alarms for apnea and tachypnea can be set and relied on. However, capnography cannot discriminate between obstructive and central apnea, as it cannot reliably detect muscular efforts of the thorax or abdomen.

For similar reasons, capnography is a useful adjunct for detecting unintentional extubation, malposition of the endotracheal tube, or absence of perfusion. Cyclic variation of end-tidal PCO_2 is absent in esophageal intubation or disconnection from the ventilator [186]. Pharyngeal intubation with adequate ventilation may, however, produce a normal capnogram. Capnography can demonstrate the return of circulation after cardiopulmonary arrest or bypass [187].

Due to changes in dead space and perfusion, end-tidal PCO_2 measurements are unreliable indicators of arterial PCO_2 in critically ill patients. In one study of anesthetized, stable, generally healthy adults $PaCO_2$ could not be reliably determined from end-tidal values [188]. In patients undergoing weaning from mechanical ventilation, end-tidal PCO_2 was also shown to have no predictable relationship to $PaCO_2$ [189,190]. Although end-tidal and arterial values correlated well ($R = 0.78$) and rarely differed by more than 4 mm HG, changes in end-tidal PCO_2 correlated poorly with changes in arterial PCO_2 ($R^2 = 0.58$). Due to changes in dead space and perfusion, arterial and end-tidal measurements at times moved unpredictably in opposite directions.

If arterial PCO_2 is followed, the difference between end-tidal PCO_2 and $PaCO_2$ can be used as an index of the severity of ventilation perfusion mismatch. The alveolar-arterial gradient of oxygen [$P(A-a)O_2$] is more easily calculated and in most clinical settings provides similar information. Although theoretically attractive, use of end-tidal CO_2 measurements to evaluate changes in ventilation perfusion mismatch has failed to yield clinical benefits [191].

Capnography has been helpful in the operating room in detecting air and pulmonary embolism as well as malignant hyperthermia [183,187]. In these situations, the capnograph does not provide a diagnosis; it records a change, which, if limits are exceeded, will signal an alarm. The responsibility for accurately interpreting the subtleties of changes in the capnogram remains the task of an experienced physician.

Conclusion. Capnography is of very limited use in the critically ill patient. It cannot reliably replace arterial PCO_2 monitoring. Although it monitors respiratory rate accurately, it is far more expensive and inconvenient than other types of respiratory rate monitors. Capnography is better suited to the operating room, where its value is increased due to its ability to help detect endotracheal tube malposition, air embolism, pulmonary embolism, and malignant hyperthermia, and the immediate availability of a highly skilled anesthesiologist to interpret subtle changes in the capnogram.

CONTINUOUS INVASIVE INTRAARTERIAL OXYGEN AND CARBON DIOXIDE MONITORS. Devices specifically designed to measure intraarterial pH, PCO_2, and PO_2 continuously are now commercially available [192]. Arterial blood may be continuously monitored by the placement of a fiberoptic sensor catheter into a 20-gauge radial artery catheter or intermittently monitored by creating a flow of blood from a radial artery catheter past an external fiberoptic sensor. Sensors are designed so that chemical indicators responsive to pH, PCO_2, and PO_2 are exposed to blood at the distal tip of the sensor. Light in the fiber may be reflected, absorbed, or otherwise altered when the indicator reacts with the analyte of interest. The change in the light is measured at the other end of the fiber and converted via a microprocessor into a digital readout. Systems that employ optical detection of altered light have been named optodes. Fluorescence and transmission optodes are the primary technologies now employed. Transmission optodes carry light to the indicator via one fiber path and measure attenuation of the light by the indicator in another fiber path. Fluoresence optodes have a dye at the tip of the sensor, which increases or decreases fluoresence as the concentration of the analyte changes in the dye. These systems require an in vitro calibration against known standards prior to use and intermittent in vivo calibration against arterial samples processed on a traditional ABG analyzer.

Initial studies have shown such monitoring systems to be safe, reliable, and accurate [193,194]. The optode catheters have a tremendous potential to improve quality of care by more rapidly and reliably detecting adverse events than trancutaneous, capnographic, or oximetric monitors. When coupled with these other monitors or with intramucosal monitors, they should be able to enhance our knowledge regarding regional organ perfusion and lung ventilation. In addition, changes in these parameters could be measured quickly in response to a therapeutic intervention. The technology has not been available long enough to assess its impact on clinical outcome or any measure of cost-effectiveness. Further studies are needed to evaluate the clinical impact of these devices before they can be recommended for routine use in the ICU.

Gastric Intramucosal pH Monitoring

Intramucosal pH monitoring is used to monitor trends in tissue pH in response to changes in local oxygen delivery and metabolism. The trends can be used to identify impending distress and predict survival. The technique measures PCO_2 and pH in saline in a gas-permeable balloon placed in the lumen of a viscus. The pH and PCO_2 of the adjacent mucosa equilibrates with the saline. The pH and PCO_2 of the saline can be measured by withdrawing it from the balloon and analyzing it with a blood gas machine. Although several sites can be used to monitor intramucosal values, the stomach is most frequently monitored in the ICU setting.

BACKGROUND AND THEORY. Most authors define *shock* as a state of inadequate perfusion that leads to diffuse cellular hypoxia and organ dysfunction. Many parameters have been considered in an attempt to detect early changes in tissue oxygenation, including arterial oxygen saturation, pH, and serum lactate levels; subcutaneous and transcutaneous PO_2; arterial blood pressure, cardiac output, urine output, and mixed venous oxyhemoglobin saturation. None of these can accurately and noninvasively predict the development of shock (or other common complications) in a broad range of ICU patients.

Recently, investigators have studied regional tissue perfusion as an indicator of shock. In healthy animals, oxygen consumption is independent of delivery except below a critical minimum level [195]. In dogs that critical level has been found to be approximately 50 to 60 percent of the resting DO_2. Below that level oxygen uptake depends on the supply of oxygen delivered; anaerobic metabolism takes place; and acid is produced.

However, in shock states there may be a defect in tissue utilization of oxygen that changes the critical level of oxygen delivery at which oxygen consumption is dependent on its supply [196]. (See Chapters 171 and 173 for a discussion of supply dependency of oxygen consumption.) In that setting, oxygen delivery to an organ may be inadequate for that organ's needs despite a systemic level of oxygen delivery that is considered adequate. Tissue hypoxia can develop and local anaerobic metabolism may result.

Anaerobic metabolism causes acidosis because the hydrolysis of adenosine triphosphate (ATP) produces protons that cannot be used up by simultaneous oxidative phosphorylation of adenosine 5′-diphosphate (ADP) to ATP. The presence of these protons drives the carbonic anhydrase reaction to produce more CO_2, which subsequently diffuses into and develops an equilibrium with any adjacent intraluminal fluid. Thus the measurement of an intraluminal PCO_2 and the capillary HCO_3^- (estimated as equivalent to the arterial HCO_3^-) allows calculation of the intramucosal pH (pHi) by the modified Henderson-Hasselbalch equation:

$$pH = pK + \log (HCO_3^-)/(f \times PaCO_2)$$

where f is a correction factor used to account for differing periods of measurement.

Intramucosal acidosis is therefore a marker of local hypoperfusion. Several factors other than acidosis may alter cellular metabolism and intramucosal values; (1) loss of adenine nucleotides; (2) formation of oxygen-free radicals; (3) increases in intracellular calcium; (4) degradation of membrane phopholipids; and (5) mechanical alterations due to cellular edema [197]. However, an accurate, noninvasive way of measuring tissue acidosis could be beneficial if it allows detection of hypoperfusion of vital organs before systemic signs can be detected.

TECHNICAL CONSIDERATIONS

Procedure. The technique of pHi monitoring has evolved steadily over the past 30 years. Measurement of pHi in the gallbladder and urinary bladder was initially described by Bergofsky [198]. Subsequently it was shown that the intramucosal pH of the small intestine could also be determined [199]. Early intramucosal pH monitors consisted of glass or wire electrodes that were surgically implanted in the wall of the organ being studied. These devices were limited to research applications because an operation was required to place them and their presence in the mucosa of the organ caused tissue damage, therefore altering the conditions being measured. This prompted investigators to search for a less invasive, equally accurate way to obtain this measurement.

In 1973, an implantable catheter made of silicone impregnated with silver was described [200]. This material is extremely permeable to oxygen and carbon dioxide and allowed rapid equilibration between the tensions of these gases in the tissues and the saline that filled the catheter. Because this catheter, too, required surgical implantation and caused injury to the tissue surrounding it, it was limited to research applications. However, it was confirmed that the gases in tissue will equilibrate rapidly with saline in close proximity to it; it was subsequently confirmed that this principle would hold for the fluid in the lumen of a hollow viscus [201].

The current gastrointestinal tonometry catheter consists of a saline-filled silicone balloon attached near the end of a nasogastric or sigmoid tube. Before insertion, the balloon is repeatedly infused with normal saline until all air is eliminated. The upper gastrointestinal catheter is inserted with standard technique for nasogastric tube placement and placement confirmed radiographically. The stopcock is flushed with saline to eliminate any trapped air and the balloon is filled to the manufacturer's specifications with saline and the tonometer lumen closed to the outside environment. The saline is allowed to equilibrate with the fluid in the lumen of the organ being monitored. It is believed that the saline in the balloon requires approximately 90 minutes to equilibrate with the saline in the lumen, although there are mathematical formulas available to correct the values obtained with 30 to 90 minutes of equilibration [202]. After adequate time for equilibration, the dead space (usually 1.0 ml) is aspirated and discarded, and the saline in the balloon is completely aspirated under anaerobic conditions. The tonometer lumen is closed until a decision is made to refill it for subsequent measurement. An ABG sample is taken simultaneously, and both samples are sent for analysis. The PCO_2 of the tonometer sample and the HCO_3^- of the arterial blood are used in the modified Henderson-Hasselbalch equation to calculate pHi.

Measurements of gastric PCO_2 for determination of pHi have been validated on a limited number of blood gas analyzers. Machines other than those previously validated may show errors in the measurement of gastric PCO_2 despite the ability to measure systemic arterial PCO_2 accurately. To our knowledge, all such errors identified to date have been systematic in nature, and therefore could be adjusted with appropriate correction factors. Before making clinical decisions based on the information derived, the clinician should determine whether the blood gas analyzer in use has been validated and, if a systematic error has been found, that correction factors are available.

Sites of Measurement. As described above, original descriptions of viscus tonometry used the gallbladder and urinary bladder as primary sites of monitoring [198]. Tonometry of the gastrointestinal tract was described soon thereafter and currently is by far the preferred site for monitoring tissue metabolism. This site is preferred because the intestine is easily accessible and can be cannulated from above or below, is sensitive to decreases in perfusion, and may be involved in initiating sepsis. The intestinal mucosa is thought to be affected early during circulatory insufficiency because blood is shunted away from it to preserve the function of the brain and heart. Ironically, because of the unique countercurrent microcirculation in the walls of the intestine, it may be particularly vulnerable to reductions in blood flow and may demonstrate conversion to anaerobic metabolism and tissue acidosis before other tissues. Finally, many have postulated that the intestine has a role in propagation of sepsis. Ischemia of the intestinal mucosa may damage the mucosal barrier and allow bacteria and toxins from the lumen to enter the bloodstream and exacerbate an early shock state.

Several sites in the intestinal tract can serve as sites for pHi monitoring. The most easily accessible is the stomach. In many cases the patient requires nasogastric tube placement independent of the placement of the tonometer, so no additional procedures are necessary. Tubes that serve for both nasogastric drainage and tonometry are commercially available. In animals, gastric pHi moves in parallel with changes in small intestinal and sigmoid pHi, although both alternative sites appear more sensitive to changes in intravascular volume and oxygen delivery induced by experimental bleeding [203]. Gastric pHi has been shown to have significant correlations with important measures of pathology, although measurement in the small bowel or sigmoid may be more effective in specific situations.

Tonometrically derived gastric pHi can be affected by the acid secretory status of the stomach. In one study, mean gastric pHi was 7.30 in untreated normal volunteers but 7.39 in a similar group treated with ranitidine [204]. This was because the PCO_2 in the gastric fluid of the treated patients was 42 ± 4 mm Hg, compared to 52 ± 14 mm Hg in the untreated group. The difference in CO_2 content of the fluid is thought to be due to production of CO_2 by the conversion of secreted H^+ and HCO_3^- into water and CO_2. The CO_2 produced can then back-diffuse into the mucosa and cause it to be more acidotic and theoretically less accurate in its representation of the state of tissue perfusion. Reduction of hydrogen ion secretion prevents the reaction from being driven in that direction. This observation leaves unresolved the question of whether the secretion of acid needs to be controlled or whether the limits of normalcy can be adjusted to compensate for acid secretion. This is particularly important since some have suggested that inhibition of gastric acid secretion predisposes to nosocomial pneumonia [205]. Another issue is how, if acid is to be controlled, can it be controlled in consistent fashion. Further investigation is needed to answer these questions.

INDICATIONS FOR USE. In general, the goals of monitoring in the ICU are to (1) measure key indices of underlying pathology; (2) aid with diagnosis; (3) alert the healthcare team to changes in the patient's condition; (4) guide therapy; and (5) track trends and assess prognosis [206]. Due to its ability to detect early changes in intestinal perfusion and the potential for therapeutic actions to improve ICU survival based on this information, pHi monitoring satisfies many of those goals. In addition, since it is relatively noninvasive, it can be performed rapidly and by anyone with the ability to place a nasogastric tube. However, while proponents advocate its use in all seriously ill hospitalized patients, no clear survival or cost savings advantage has been demonstrated [207]. Therefore, an attempt should be made to identify patients most likely to benefit from this form of monitoring.

Intramucosal pH monitoring has been better studied in postoperative ICU patients than in other critically ill patients. In particular, intra- and postoperative cardiac surgery patients have been well studied, and in that group gastric pHi appears to predict complications well [208,209]. Patients who have had abdominal aortic surgery and are at risk for postoperative intestinal ischemia may benefit from a tonometer placed in their sigmoid colon [210]. Based on studies performed on mixed medical-surgical populations, any critically ill patient with a high likelihood of developing hemodynamic instability may be considered for pHi monitoring, including those with myocardial infarction and pulmonary edema or high CPK elevations; fever, leukocytosis, and tachycardia; positive blood cultures; APACHE II score greater than 18; overdoses of potentially vasoactive drugs; overt gastrointestinal bleeding and orthostatic hypotension; unexplained respiratory failure; and postoperative patients with histories of cardiac disease or intraoperative hemodynamic instability. Other patients may also benefit from pHi monitoring, but more definite recommendations await more extensive experience.

The level of gastric pHi has been correlated with survival. In a study by Gutierrez et al., gastric pHi less than 7.32 was associated with increased mortality [211]. However, in another study the level of gastric pHi correlated only with short-term (72-hour) survival and failed to predict long-term outcome [212]. Gastric pHi is also useful in predicting complications after cardiac surgery [208] and has been used to predict the development of gastrointestinal bleeding and mesenteric ischemia, although small intestinal pHi appears to be a more sensitive indicator of the latter [213].

Therapeutic interventions based on gastric pHi have been reported to improve survival in critically ill patients who pre-sented with initially normal pHi values [214]. Infusions of dobutamine and saline given in response to changes in gastric pHi improved survival in patients who presented with initial pHi levels greater than 7.35. No difference was seen in the survival rates of patients whose initial gastric pHi levels were less than 7.35.

Gastric pHi has often failed to correlate with more conventional measures of tissue perfusion. In one animal study using experimental bleeding, gastric pHi failed to change significantly until systolic blood pressure of 45 mm Hg was reached [203]. In another study, DO_2 correlated with VO_2 and oxygen extraction ratio but not with gastric pHi [214]. It has been postulated that the reason is the insensitivity of global measures of oxygen delivery and consumption to reflect localized hypoperfusion to the intestine. Alternatively, our understanding of the significance of pHi values may be incomplete and our interpretation therefore mistaken. Only further investigation will answer this question.

Complications of gastric pHi monitoring are limited to those associated with nasogastric tube use and arterial blood gas measurement. These include discomfort, gastroesophageal reflux, pulmonary aspiration, and aggravation of bleeding from esophageal or gastric lesions from tube placement and vasovagal episodes, pain, and hematomas from blood gas measurement.

CONCLUSIONS. Conventional methods of determining the adequacy of tissue oxygenation may be insensitive to the localized changes that may precede systemic hemodynamic collapse. Inadequate tissue oxygenation causes tissue acidosis because of the shift to anaerobic metabolism. Because the carbon dioxide present in the tissue is in equilibrium with that in the intraluminal fluid of a viscus, the intramucosal pH of that organ can be determined by measuring intraluminal PCO_2 and arterial HCO_3^-. The stomach, small intestine, or sigmoid colon can be used, with the stomach being most popular because of the ease of cannulation. The results of these tests may be helpful in determining prognosis in critically ill patients, and therapy based on these findings may improve survival. Definite indications for use have not been clearly established, but the procedure may be beneficial to any critically ill patient at risk of local ischemia or the systemic hypoperfusion state of shock.

References

1. Kholoussy AM, Sufian S, Pavlides C, et al: Central peripheral temperature gradient: Its value and limitations in the management of critically ill surgical patients. *Am J Surg* 140:609, 1980.
2. Burgess GE III, Cooper JR, Marino RJ: Continuous monitoring of skin temperature using a liquid-crystal thermometer during anesthesia. *South Med J* 71:516, 1978.
3. Roberts NH: The comparison of surface and core temperature devices. *J Am Assoc Nurse Anesth* 48:53, 1980.
4. Silverman RW, Lomax P: The measurement of temperature for thermoregulatory studies. *Pharmacol Ther* 27:233, 1985.
5. Vale RJ: Monitoring of temperature during anesthesia. *Int Anesthesiol Clin* 19:61, 1981.
6. Fukuoka M, Yamori Y, Toyoshima T: Twenty-four hour monitoring of deep body temperature with a novel flexible probe. *J Biomed Eng* 9:173, 1987.
7. Lees DE, Kim YD, MacNamara TE: Noninvasive determination of core temperature during anesthesia. *South Med J* 73:1322, 1980.
8. Watson BW: Clinical uses of radio pills. *Br J Hosp Med* 25:618, 1981.
9. Terndrup TE: An appraisal of temperature assessment by infrared emission detection tympanic thermometry. *Ann Emerg Med* 21:1483, 1992.

10. Terndrup TE, Rajk J: Impact of operator technique and device on infrared emission detection tympanic thermometry. *J Emerg Med* 10:683, 1992.

11. Erickson R: Thermometer placement for oral temperature measurement in febrile adults. *Int J Nurs Stud* 13:199, 1976.

12. Heinz J: Validation of sublingual temperatures in patients with nasogastric tubes. *Heart Lung* 14:128, 1985.

13. Tandberg D, Sklar D: Effect of tachypnea on the estimation of body temperature by an oral thermometer. *N Engl J Med* 313:945, 1985.

14. Cork RC, Vaughan RW, Humphrey LS: Precision and accuracy of intraoperative temperature monitoring. *Anesth Analg* 62:211, 1983.

15. Bone ME, Feneck RO: Bladder temperature as an estimate of body temperature during cardiopulmonary bypass. *Anaesthesia* 43:181, 1988.

16. Ramsay JG, Ralley FE, Whalley DG, et al: Site of temperature monitoring and prediction of afterdrop after open heart surgery. *Can Anaesth Soc J* 32:607, 1985.

17. Moorthy SS, Winn BA, Jallard MS, et al: Monitoring urinary bladder temperature. *Heart Lung* 14:90, 1985.

18. Severinghaus JW: Temperature gradients during hypothermia. *Ann NY Acad Sci* 80:515, 1962.

19. Webb GE: Comparison of esophageal and tympanic temperature monitoring during cardiopulmonary bypass. *Anesth Analg* 52:729, 1973.

20. Crocker BD, Okumura F, McCuaig, et al: Temperature monitoring during general anaesthesia. *Br J Anaesth* 52:1223, 1980.

21. Davis FM, Barnes PK, Bailey JS: Aural thermometry during profound hypothermia. *Anaesth Intensive Care* 9:124, 1981.

22. Wallace CT, Marks WE, Adkins WY, et al: Perforation of the tympanic membrane: A complication of tympanic thermometry during anesthesia. *Anesthesiology* 41:290, 1974.

23. Benzinger M: Tympanic thermometry in surgery and anesthesia. *JAMA* 209:1207, 1969.

24. Joly HR, Weil MH: Temperature of the great toe as an indication of the severity of shock. *Circulation* 39:131, 1969.

25. Knight RW, Opie JC: The big toe in the recovery room: Peripheral warm-up patterns in children after open-heart surgery. *Can J Surg* 24:239, 1981.

26. Nierman DM: Core temperature measurement in the intensive care unit. *Crit Care Med* 19:818, 1991.

27. Heidenreich T, Giuffre M, Doorley J: Temperature and temperature measurement after induced hypothermia. *Nurs Res* 41:296, 1992.

28. Brooks SE, Veal RO, Kramer M, et al: Reduction in the incidence of *Clostridium difficile* associated diarrhea in an acute care hospital and a skilled nursing facility following replacement of electronic thermometers with single-use disposables. *Infect Control Hosp Epidemiol* 13:98, 1992.

29. Livnorese LL, Dias S, Samel C, et al: Hospital-acquired infection with vancomycin-resistant *Enterococcus faecium* transmitted by electronic thermometers. *Ann Intern Med* 117:112, 1992.

30. Task Force on Guidelines: Recommendations for services and personnel for delivery of care in a critical care setting. *Crit Care Med* 16:809, 1988.

31. Pierce EC: Percutaneous arterial catheterization in man with special reference to aortography. *Surg Gynecol Obstet* 93:56, 1951.

32. Donald DC Jr, Kesmodel KF Jr, Rollins SL Jr, et al: An improved technique for percutaneous cerebral angiography. *Arch Neurol Psychiatry* 65:500, 1951.

33. Bruner JMR, Krenis LJ, Kunsman JM, et al: Comparison of direct and indirect methods of measuring arterial blood pressure, part I. *Med Instrum* 15:11, 1981.

34. Bruner JMR, Krenis LJ, Kunsman JM, et al: Comparison of direct and indirect methods of measuring arterial blood pressure, part II. *Med Instrum* 15:97, 1981.

35. Bruner JMR, Krenis LJ, Kunsman JM, et al: Comparison of direct and indirect methods of measuring arterial blood pressure, part III. *Med Instrum* 15:182, 1981.

36. Reder RF, Dimich I, Cohen ML, el al: Evaluating indirect blood pressure measurement techniques: A comparison of three systems in infants and children. *Pediatrics* 62:326, 1978.

37. Nystrom E, Reid KH, Bennett R, et al: A comparison of two automated indirect arterial blood pressure meters: With recordings from a radial arterial catheter in anesthetized surgical patients. *Anesthesiology* 62:526, 1985.

38. DeGowin EL, DeGowin RL: The thorax and cardiovascular system, in DeGowin EL, DeGowin RL (eds): *Bedside Diagnostic Examination.* New York, Macmillan, 1981, p 229.

39. Carrol GC: Blood pressure monitoring. *Crit Care Clin* 4:411, 1988.

40. Van Bergen FH, Weatherhead S, Treloar AE, et al: Comparison of direct and indirect methods of measuring arterial blood pressure. *Circulation* 10:481, 1954.

41. Bailey RH, Knaus VL, Bauer JH: Aneroid sphygmomanometers: An assessment of accuracy at a university hospital and clinics. *Arch Intern Med* 151:1409, 1991.

42. Zagzebski JA: Physics and instrumentation in Doppler and B-mode ultrasonography, in Zwiebel WJ (ed): *Introduction to Vascular Ultrasonography.* Orlando, Grune & Stratton, 1986, p 21.

43. Kirby RR, Kemmerer WT, Morgan JL: Transcutaneous Doppler measurement of blood pressure. *Anesthesiology* 31:86, 1969.

44. Hochberg HM, Salomon H: Accuracy of automated ultrasound blood pressure monitor. *Curr Ther Res* 13:129, 1971.

45. Chastonay P, Morel D, Forster A, et al: Evaluation of a new monitoring device for arterial blood pressure and heart rate measurement by automatic sphygmomanometry. *Anaesth Intensivther Notfallmed* 17:348, 1982.

46. Puritan Bennett Corporation: *Infrasonde Model D4000 Electronic Blood Pressure Monitor Operating Manual.* Los Angeles, Puritan Bennett Corporation.

47. Cullen PM, Dye J, Hughes DG: Clinical assessment of the neonatal Dinamap 847 during anesthesia in neonates and infants. *J Clin Monit* 3:229, 1987.

48. Borow KM, Newberger JW: Non-invasive estimation of central aortic pressure using the oscillometric method for analyzing systemic artery pulsatile blood flow: Comparative study of indirect systolic, diastolic, and mean brachial artery pressure with simultaneous direct ascending aortic pressure measurements. *Am Heart J* 103:879, 1982.

49. Van Egmond J, Hasenbros M, Crul JF: Invasive v non-invasive measurement of arterial pressure. *Br J Anaesth* 57:434, 1985.

50. Boehmer RD: Continuous, real-time, noninvasive monitor of blood pressure: Penaz methodology applied to the finger. *J Clin Monit* 3:282, 1987.

51. Kemmotsu O, Ueda M, Otsuka H, et al: Arterial tonometry for non-invasive, continuous blood pressure monitoring during anesthesia. *Anesthesiology* 75:333, 1991.

52. Kemmotsu O, Ueda M, Otsuka H, et al: Blood pressure measurement by arterial tonometry in controlled hypotension. *Anesth Analg* 73:54, 1991.

53. Jawad IA: Quantitative applications of Doppler ultrasonography, in Jawad IA (ed): *A Practical Guide to Echocardiography and Cardiac Doppler Ultrasound.* Boston, Little Brown, 1993.

54. Casadei R, Parati G, Pomidossi G, et al: 24-hour blood pressure monitoring: Evaluation of Spacelabs 5300 monitor by comparison with intra-arterial blood pressure recording in ambulant subjects. *J Hypertens* 6:797, 1988.

55. Baker LK: Dinamap monitor versus direct blood pressure measurements. *Dimensions Crit Care Nurs* 5:228, 1986.

56. Latman NS: Evaluation of finger blood pressure monitoring instruments. *Biomed Instrum Technol* 26:52, 1992.

57. Aitken HA, Todd JG, Kenny GNC: Comparison of the Finapres and direct arterial pressure monitoring during profound hypotensive anesthesia. *Br J Anaesth* 67:36, 1991.

58. Kermode JL, Davis NJ, Thompson WR: Comparison of the Finapres blood pressure monitor with intra-arterial manometry during induction of anaesthesia. *Anaesth Intensive Care* 17:470, 1989.

59. Farquhar IK: Continuous direct and indirect blood pressure measurement (Finapres) in the critically ill. *Anaesthesia* 46:1050, 1991.

60. Bos WJW, Imholz BPM, van Goudoever J, et al: The reliability of non-invasive continuous finger blood pressure measurement in patients with both hypertension and vascular disease. *Am J Hypertens* 5:529, 1992.

61. Yelderman M, Ream AK: Indirect measurement of mean blood pressure in the anesthetized patient. *Anesthesiology* 50:253, 1979.

62. Rutten AJ, Isley AH, Skowronski GA, et al: A comparative study of the measurement of mean arterial blood pressure using automatic

oscillometers, arterial cannulation and auscultation. *Anaesth Intensive Care* 14:58, 1986.

63. Modesti PA, Gensini GF, Conti C, et al: Clinical evaluation of an automatic blood-pressure monitoring device. *J Clin Hypertens* 3:631, 1987.

64. Paulus DA: Noninvasive blood pressure measurement. *Med Instrum* 15:91, 1981.

65. Sy WP: Ulnar nerve palsy possibly related to use of automatically cycled blood pressure cuff. *Anesth Analg* 60:687, 1981.

66. Betts EK: Hazard of automated noninvasive blood pressure monitoring. *Anesthesiology* 55:717, 1981.

67. Hutton P, Prys-Roberts C: An assessment of the Dinamap 845. *Anaesthesia* 39:261, 1984.

68. Bainbridge LC, Simmons HM, Elliot D: The use of automatic blood pressure monitors in the burned patient. *Br J Plastic Surg* 43:322, 1990.

69. Sladen A: Complications of invasive hemodynamic monitoring in the intensive care unit. *Curr Probl Surg* 25:69, 1988.

70. Davis FM, Stewart JM: Radial artery cannulation. *Br J Anaesth* 52:41, 1980.

71. Gardner RM, Schwarz R, Wong HC, et al: Percutaneous indwelling radial-artery catheters for monitoring cardiovascular function. *N Engl J Med* 290:1227, 1974.

72. Schwid HA: Frequency response evaluation of radial artery catheter-manometer systems: Sinusoidal frequency analysis versus flush method. *J Clin Monit* 4:181, 1988.

73. Rothe CF, Kim KC: Measuring systolic arterial blood pressure: Possible errors from extension tubes or disposable transducer domes. *Crit Care Med* 8:683, 1980.

74. Hughes VG, Prys-Roberts C: Intra-arterial pressure measurements: A review and analysis of methods relevant to anaesthesia and intensive care. *Anaesthesia* 26:511, 1971.

75. Shinozaki T, Deane RS, Mazuzan JE: The dynamic responses of liquid filled catheter systems for direct measurements of blood pressure. *Anesthesiology* 53:498, 1980.

76. Russell JA, Joel M, Hudson RJ, et al: Prospective evaluation of radial and femoral artery catheterization sites in critically ill adults. *Crit Care Med* 11:936, 1983.

77. Colvin MP, Curran JP, Jarvis D, et al: Femoral artery pressure monitoring. *Anaesthesia* 32:451, 1977.

78. Bryan-Brown CW, Kwun KB, Lumb PD, et al: The axillary artery catheter. *Heart Lung* 12:492, 1983.

79. Thys DM: The normal ECG, in Thys DM, Kaplan JA (eds): *The ECG in Anesthesia and Critical Care*. New York, Churchill Livingstone, 1987, p 1.

80. Winters SR: Diagnosis by wireless. *Sci Am* 124:465, 1921.

81. Lown B, Klein MD: Coronary and precoronary care. *Am J Med* 46:705, 1969.

82. Yu PN, Fox SM, Imboden CA, et al: A specialized intensive care unit for acute myocardial infarction. *Mod Concepts Cardiovasc Dis* 34:23, 1965.

83. Kimball JT, Killip T: Aggressive treatment of arrhythmias in acute myocardial infarction: Procedures and results. *Prog Cardiovasc Dis* 10:483, 1968.

84. Julian DG, Valentine PA, Miller GG: Disturbances of rate, rhythm, and conduction in acute myocardial infarction. *Am J Med* 37:915, 1964.

85. Romhilt DW, Bloomfield SS, Chou T, et al: Unrealiability of conventional electrocardiographic monitoring for arrhythmia detection in coronary care units. *Am J Cardiol* 31:457, 1973.

86. American Heart Association: Myocardial infarction, in *Textbook of Advanced Cardiac Life Support*. Dallas, American Heart Association, 1987, p 11.

87. Cercek B, Lew AS, Laramee P, et al: Time course and characteristics of ventricular arrhythmias after reperfusion in acute myocardial infarction. *Am J Cardiol* 60:214, 1987.

88. Buckingham TA, Devine JE, Redd RM, et al: Reperfusion arrhythmias during coronary reperfusion therapy in man: Clinical and angiographic correlations. *Chest* 90:346, 1986.

89. Linnik W, Tintinalli JE, Ramos R: Associated reactions during and immediately after rtPA infusion. *Ann Emerg Med* 18:234, 1989.

90. Bartter T, Curley FJ, Larrivee G, et al: The value of arrhythmia monitoring in medical intensive care units. *Am Rev Respir Dis* 139:A152, 1989.

91. Holmberg S, Ryden L, Waldenstrom A: Efficiency of arrhythmia detection by nurses in a coronary care unit using a decentralized monitoring system. *Br Heart J* 39:1019, 1977.

92. Vetter NJ, Julian DG: Comparison of arrhythmia computer and conventional monitoring in coronary-care unit. *Lancet* 1:1151, 1975.

93. Pierpoint GL: Pitfalls of computer use in acute care medicine. *Heart Lung* 16:207, 1987.

94. Watkinson WP, Brice MA, Robinson KS: A computer-assisted electrocardiographic analysis system: Methodology and potential application to cardiovascular toxicology. *J Toxicol Environ Health* 15:713, 1985.

95. Alcover IA, Henning RJ, Jackson DL: A computer-assisted monitoring system for arrhythmia detection in a medical intensive care unit. *Crit Care Med* 12:888, 1984.

96. Badura FK: Nurse acceptance of a computerized arrhythmia monitoring system. *Heart Lung* 9:1044, 1980.

97. Association for the Advancement of Medical Instrumentation: American National Standard for Cardiac Monitors, Heart Rate Meters, and Alarms (EC 13-1983). Arlington, VA, ANSI/AAMI, 1984.

98. Mirvis DM, Berson AS, Goldberger AL, et al: Instrumentation and practice standards for electrocardiographic monitoring in special care units. *Circulation* 79:464, 1989.

99. Starmer CF, Whalen RE, McIntosh HD: Hazards of electric shock in cardiology. *Am J Cardiol* 14:537, 1964.

100. Bruner JMR: Hazards of electrical apparatus. *Anesthesiology* 28:396, 1967.

101. Hewlitt-Packard Corporation. *ECG Measurement-Application Note* AN711. Waltham, MA, Hewlitt Packard.

102. Cecchi AC, Dovellini EV, Marchi F, et al: Silent myocardial ischemic during ambulatory electrocardiographic monitoring in patients with effort angina. *J Am Coll Cardiol* 1:934, 1983.

103. Clements FM, Bruijn NP: Noninvasive cardiac monitoring. *Crit Care Clin* 4:435, 1988.

104. Hanley J: Telemetry in health care. *Biomed Eng* 11:269, 1976.

105. Pittman JV, Blum MS, Leonard MS: *Telemetry Utilization for Emergency Medical Services Systems*. Atlanta, Health Systems Research Center, Georgia Institute of Technology, 1974.

106. Anderson GJ, Knoebel SB, Fisch C: Continuous prehospitalization monitoring of cardiac rhythm. *Am Heart J* 82:642, 1971.

107. McFadden JP, Price RC, Eastwood HD, et al: Raised respiratory rate in elderly patients: A valuable physical sign. *Br J Med* 284:626, 1982.

108. Mithoefer JC, Bossman OG, Thibeault DW, et al: The clinical estimation of alveolar ventilation. *Am Rev Respir Dis* 98:868, 1968.

109. Semmes BJ, Tobin MJ, Snyder JV, et al: Subjective and objective measurement of tidal volume in critically ill patients. *Chest* 87:577, 1985.

110. Krieger B, Feinerman D, Zaron A, et al: Continuous noninvasive monitoring of respiratory rate in critically ill patients. *Chest* 90:632, 1986.

111. Shelly MP, Park GR: Failure of a respiratory monitor to detect obstructive apnea. *Crit Care Med* 14:836, 1986.

112. Sackner MA, Bizousky F, Krieger BP: Performance of impedance pneumograph and respiratory inductive plethysmograph as monitors of respiratory frequency and apnea. *Am Rev Respir Dis* 135:A41, 1987.

113. Chadha TS, Watson H, Birch S, et al: Validation of respiratory inductive plethysmography using different calibration procedures. *Am Rev Respir Dis* 125:644, 1982.

114. Sackner MA, Watson H, Belsito AS, et al: Calibration of respiratory inductive plethysmograph during natural breathing. *J Appl Physiol* 66:410, 1989.

115. Tobin MJ, Jenouri G, Lind B, et al: Validation of respiratory inductive plethysmography in patients with pulmonary disease. *Chest* 83:615, 1983.

116. Tobin MJ, Jenouri G, Birch S, et al: Effect of positive end-expiratory pressure on breathing patterns of normal subjects and intubated patients with respiratory failure. *Crit Care Med* 11:859, 1983.

117. Tobin MJ, Guenther SM, Perez W, et al: Konno-Mead analysis of ribcage-abdominal motion during successful and unsuccessful trials of weaning from mechanical ventilation. *Am Rev Respir Dis* 135:1320, 1987.

118. Krieger BP, Chediak A, Gazeroglu HB, et al: Variability of breathing pattern before and after extubation. *Chest* 93:767, 1988.

119. Hoffman RA, Ershowsky P, Krieger BP: Determination of auto-

PEEP during spontaneous and controlled ventilation by monitoring changes in end-expiratory thoracic gas volume. *Chest* 96:613, 1989.

120. Krieger BP, Ershowsky P, Spivack D, et al: Initial experience with a central respiratory monitoring unit as a cost-saving alternative to the intensive care unit for medicare patients who require long-term ventilator support. *Chest* 93:395, 1988.

121. O'Brien MJ, Van Eykern LA, Oetomo SB, et al: Transcutaneous respiratory electromyographic monitoring. *Crit Care Med* 15:394, 1987.

122. Chapman KR, Rebuck AS: Oximetry, in Nochomovitz ML, Cherniak NS (eds): *Noninvasive Respiratory Monitoring.* New York, Churchill Livingstone, 1986, p 803.

123. Huch A, Huch R, Konig V, et al: Limitations of pulse oximetry. *Lancet* 1:357, 1988.

124. New W: Pulse oximetry. *J Clin Monit* 1:126, 1985.

125. Moller JT, Pederen T, Rasmussen LS, et al: Randomized evaluation of pulse oximetry in 20,802 patients, I: Design, demography, pulse oximeter failure rate, and overall complications rate. *Anesthesiology* 78:436, 1993.

126. Choe H, Tashiro C, Fukumitsu K, et al: Comparison of recorded values from six pulse oximeters. *Crit Care Med* 17:678, 1989.

127. Severinghaus JW, Naifeh KH, Koh SO: Errors in 14 pulse oximeters during profound hypoxia. *J Clin Monit* 5:72, 1989.

128. Reynolds KJ, Moyle JTB, Gale LB, et al: In vitro performance test system for pulse oximeters. *Med Biol Eng Comput* 30:629, 1992.

129. Severinghaus JW, Naifeh KH: Accuracy of responses of six pulse oximeters to profound hypoxia. *Anesthesiology* 67:551, 1987.

130. Cheng EY, Stommel KA: Quantitative evaluation of a combined pulse oximetry and end-tidal CO_2 monitor. *Biomed Instrum Tech* 23:216, 1989.

131. Reynolds LM, Nicolson SC, Steven JM, et al: Influence of sensor site location on pulse oximetry kinetics in children. *Anesth Analg* 76:751, 1993.

132. Cheng EY, Hopwood MB, Kay J: Forehead pulse oximetry compared with finger pulse oximetry and arterial blood gas measurement. *J Clin Monit* 4:223, 1988.

133. Hickerson W, Morrell M, Cicala RS: Glossal pulse oximetry. *Anesth Analg* 69:72, 1989.

134. Evans ML, Geddes LA: An assessment of blood vessel vasoactivity using photoplethysmography. *Med Instrum* 22:29, 1988.

135. Tweedie IE: Pulse oximeters and finger nails. *Anaesthesia* 44:268, 1989.

136. Cote CJ, Goldstein EA, Fuchsman WH, et al: The effect of nail polish on pulse oximetry. *Anesth Analg* 67:683, 1988.

137. Read MS: Effect of transparent adhesive tape on pulse oximetry. *Anesth Analg* 68:701, 1989.

138. Ries AL, Prewitt LM, Johnson JJ: Skin color and ear oximetry. *Chest* 96:287, 1989.

139. Costarino AT, Davis DA, Keon TP: Falsely normal saturation reading with the pulse oximeter. *Anesthesiology* 67:830, 1987.

140. Hanowell L, Eisele JH Jr, Downs D: Ambient light affects pulse oximeters. *Anesthesiology* 67:864, 1987.

141. Block FE Jr: Interference in a pulse oximeter from a fiberoptic light source. *J Clin Monit* 3:210, 1987.

142. Brooks TD, Paulus DA, Winkle WE: Infrared heat lamps interfere with pulse oximeters. *Anesthesiology* 61:630, 1984.

143. Amar D, Neidzwski J, Wald A, et al: Fluorescent light interferes with pulse oximetry. *J Clin Monit* 5:135, 1989.

144. Beall SN, Moorthy SS: Jaundice, oximetry, and spurious hemoglobin desaturation. *Anesth Analg* 68:806, 1989.

145. Veyckemans F, Baele P, Guillaume JE, et al: Hyperbilirubinemia does not interfere with hemoglobin saturation measured by pulse oximetry. *Anesthesiology* 70:118, 1989.

146. Watcha MF, Connor MT, Hing AV: Pulse oximetry in methemoglobinemia. *Am J Dis Child* 143:845, 1989.

147. Reynolds KJ, Palayiwa E, Moyle JTB, et al: The effect of dyshemoglobins on pulse oximetry, I: Theoretical approach. II: experimental results using an in vitro system. *J Clin Monitor* 9:81, 1993.

148. Barker SJ, Tremper KK: The effect of carbon monoxide inhalation on pulse oximetry and transcutaneous PO_2. *Anesthesiology* 66:677, 1987.

149. Coburn RF, Williams WJ, Kahn SB: Endogenous carbon monoxide production in patients with hemolytic anemia. *J Clin Invest* 45:460, 1966.

150. Lee SE, Tremper KK, Barker SJ: Effects of anemia on pulse oximetry and continuous mixed venous oxygen saturation monitoring in dogs. *Anesth Analg* 67:S130, 1988.

151. Cane RD, Harrison RA, Shapiro BA, et al: The spectrophotometric absorbance of intralipid. *Anesthesiology* 53:53, 1980.

152. Gabrielczyk MR, Buist RJ: Pulse oximetry and postoperative hypothermia: An evaluation of the Nellcor N-100 in a cardiac surgical intensive care unit. *Anaesthesia* 43:402, 1988.

153. Palve H, Vuori A: Pulse oximetry during low cardiac output and hypothermia states immediately after open heart surgery. *Crit Care Med* 17:66, 1989.

154. Rieder HU, Frei FJ, Zbinden AM, et al: Pulse oximetry in methemoglobinemia: Failure to detect low oxygen saturation. *Anaesthesia* 44:326, 1989.

155. Scheller MS, Unger RJ, Kelner MJ: Effects of intravenously administered dyes on pulse oximetry readings. *Anesthesiology* 65:550, 1986.

156. Unger R, Scheller MS: More on dyes and pulse oximeters. *Anesthesiology* 67:148, 1987.

157. Taylor MB: Erroneous actuation of the pulse oximeter. *Anaesthesia* 42:1116, 1987.

158. Morris RW, Nairn M, Torda TA: A comparison of fifteen pulse oximeters, I: A clinical comparison. II: A test of performance under conditions of poor perfusion. *Anaesth Intensive Care* 17:62, 1989.

159. Paulus DA: Cool fingers and pulse oximetry. *Anesthesiology* 71:168, 1989.

160. Mineo R, Sharrock NE: Pulse oximeter waveforms from the finger and the toe during lumbar epidural anesthesia. *Regional Anesth* 18:106, 1993.

161. Broome IJ, Mills GH, Spiers P, et al: An evaluation of the effect of vasodilatation on oxygen saturations measured by pulse oximetry and venous blood gas analysis. *Anaesthesia* 48:415, 1993.

162. Stewart KG, Rowbottam SJ: Inaccuracy of pulse oximetry in patients with severe tricuspid regurgitation. *Anaesthesia* 46:668, 1991.

163. Smith DC, Canning JJ, Crul JF: Pulse oximetry in the recovery room. *Anaesthesia* 44:345, 1989.

164. Tyler IL, Tantisera B, Winter PM: Continuous monitoring of arterial oxygen saturation with pulse oximetry during transfer to the recovery room. *Anesth Analg* 64:1108, 1985.

165. Moller JT, Johannenssen NW, Espersen K, et al: Randomized evaluation of pulse oximetry in 20,802 patients, II: Perioperative events and postoperative complications. *Anesthesiology* 78:423, 1993.

166. Rotello LC, Warren J, Jastremski MS, et al: A nurse directed protocol using pulse oximetry to wean mechanically ventilated patients from toxic oxygen concentrations. *Chest* 102:1833, 1992.

167. Introna RPS, Silverstein PI: A new use for the pulse oximeter. *Anesthesiology* 65:342, 1986.

168. Katz Y, Lee ME: Pulse oximetry for localization of the dorsalis pedis artery. *Anaesth Intensive Care* 17:114, 1989.

169. Guggenberger H, Lenz G, Federle R: Early detection of inadvertent esophageal intubation: Pulse oximetry vs. capnography. *Acta Anaesthesiol Scand* 33:112, 1989.

170. Korbon GA, Wills MH, D'Lauro F, et al: Systolic blood pressure measurement: Doppler vs. pulse oximeter. *Anesthesiology* 67:A188, 1987.

171. Brathwaite CEM, O'Malley KF, Ross SE, et al: Continuous pulse oximtery and the diagnosis of pulmonary embolism in critically ill trauma patients. *J Trauma* 33:528, 1992.

172. Wimberley PD, Pedersen KG, Thode J, et al: Transcutaneous and capillary pCO_2 and pO_2 measurements in healthy adults. *Clin Chem* 29:1471, 1983.

173. Abraham E, Smith M, Silver L: Continuous monitoring of critically ill patients with transcutaneous oxygen and carbon dioxide and conjunctival oxygen sensors. *Ann Emerg Med* 13:1021, 1984.

174. Tremper KK, Keenan B, Applebaum R, et al: Clinical and experimental monitoring with transcutaneous PO_2 during hypoxia, shock, cardiac arrest, and CPR. *J Clin Eng* 6:149, 1981.

175. Rooth G, Hedstrand U, Tyden H, et al: The validity of the transcutaneous oxygen tension method in adults. *Crit Care Med* 4:162, 1976.

176. Gothgen I, Jacobsen E: Transcutaneous oxygen tension measurement, I: Age variation and reproducibility. *Acta Anaesthesiol Scand* 67:66, 1978.

177. Eletr S, Jimison H, Ream AK, et al: Cutaneous monitoring of sys-

temic PCO$_2$ on patients in the respiratory intensive care unit being weaned from the ventilator. *Acta Anaesthesiol Scand* 68:123, 1978.

178. Tremper KK, Waxman K, Shoemaker WC: Use of transcutaneous oxygen sensors to titrate PEEP. *Ann Surg* 193:206, 1981.

179. Tremper KK, Shoemaker WC: Transcutaneous oxygen monitoring of critically ill adults, with and without low flow shock. *Crit Care Med* 9:706, 1981

180. Shoemaker WC, Fink S, Ray CW, et al: Effect of hemorrhagic shock on conjunctival and transcutaneous oxygen tensions in relation to hemodynamic and oxygen transport changes. *Crit Care Med* 12:949, 1984.

181. Abraham E, Oye R, Smith M: Detection of blood volume deficits through conjunctival oxygen tension monitoring. *Crit Care Med* 12:931, 1984.

182. Nolan LS, Shoemaker WC: Transcutaneous O$_2$ and CO$_2$ monitoring of high risk surgical patients during the perioperative period. *Crit Care Med* 10:762, 1982.

183. Stock MC: Noninvasive carbon dioxide monitoring. *Crit Care Clin* 4:511, 1988.

184. Schena J, Thomspon J, Crone R: Mechanical influences on the capnogram. *Crit Care Med* 12:672, 1984.

185. Paulus DA: Capnography. *Int Anesthesiol Clin* 27:167, 1989.

186. Murray IP, Modell JM: Early detection of endotracheal tube accidents by monitoring of carbon dioxide concentration in respiratory gas. *Anesthesiology* 59:344, 1983.

187. Falk JL, Rackow EC, Weil MH: End tidal carbon dioxide concentration during cardiopulmonary resuscitation. *N Engl J Med* 318:607, 1988.

188. Raemer DB, Francis D, Philip JH, et al: Variation in PCO$_2$ between arterial blood and peak expired gas during anesthesia. *Anesth Analg* 62:1065, 1983.

189. Hoffman RA, Krieger BP, Kramer MR, et al: End-tidal carbon dioxide in critically ill patients during changes in mechanical ventilation. *Am Rev Respir Dis* 140:1265, 1989.

190. Morley TF, Giaimo J, Maroszan E, et al: Use of capnography for assessment of the adequacy of alveolar ventilation during weaning from mechanical ventilation. *Am Rev Respir Dis* 148:339, 1993.

191. Jardin F, Genevray B, Pazin M, et al: Inability to titrate PEEP in patients with acute respiratory failure using end tidal carbon dioxide measurements. *Anesthesiology* 62:530, 1985.

192. Shapiro BA: In-vivo monitoring of arterial blood gases and pH. *Resp Care* 37:165, 1992.

193. Shapiro BA, Mahutte CK, Cane RD, et al: Clinical performance of a blood gas monitor: A prospective, multicenter trial. *Crit Care Med* 21:487, 1993.

194. Zimmerman JI, Dellinger RP: Initial evaluation of a new intraarterial blood gas system in humans. *Crit Care Med* 4:495, 1993.

195. Grum CM, Fiddian-Green RG, Pittenger GL, et al: Adequacy of tissue oxygenation in intact dog intestine. *J Appl Physiol* 55:1065, 1984.

196. Nelson DP, Samsel RW, Wood LDH, et al: Pathologic supply dependence of systemic and intestinal O$_2$ uptake during endotoxemia. *J Appl Physiol* 64:2410, 1988.

197. Gutierrez G: Cellular energy metabolism during hypoxia. *Crit Care Med* 19:619, 1991.

198. Bergofsky EM: Determination of tissue O$_2$ tensions by hollow visceral tonometers: Effects of breathing enriched O$_2$ mixtures. *J Clin Invest* 43:193, 1964.

199. Dawson AM, Trenchard D, Guz A: Small bowel tonometry: Assessment of small gut mucosal oxygen tension in dog and man. *Nature* 206:943, 1965.

200. Kivisaari J, Niinikoski J: Use of silastic tube and capillary sampling technic in the measurement of tissue pO$_2$ and pCO$_2$. *Am J Surg* 125:623, 1973.

201. Fiddian-Green RG, Pittenger G, Whitehouse WM: Back-diffusion of CO$_2$ and its influence on the intramural pH in gastric mucosa. *J Surg Res* 33:39, 1982.

202. Fiddian-Green RG: Tonometry: Theory and applications. *Intensive Care World* 9:1, 1992.

203. Hartmann M, Montgomery A, Jonsson K, Haglund U: Tissue oxygenation in hemorrhagic shock measured as transcutaneous oxygen tension, subcutaneous oxygen tension, and gastric intramucosal pH in pigs. *Crit Care Med* 19:205, 1991.

204. Heard SO, Helsmoortel CM, Kent JC, et al: Gastric tonometry in healthy volunteers: Effect of ranitidine on calculated intramural pH. *Crit Care Med* 19:271, 1991.

205 Eddleston JM, Vohra A, Scott P, et al: A comparison of stress ulceration and secondary pneumonia in sucralfate or ranitidine treated intensive care unit patients. *Crit Care Med* 19:1491, 1991.

206. Gutierrez G: Advances in ICU monitoring. Presented at the Annual Meeting of the American College of Chest Physicians, Chicago, October 1992.

207. Fiddian-Green RG: Should the measurements of tissue pH and pO$_2$ be included in the routine monitoring of intensive care unit patient? *Crit Care Med* 19:141, 1991.

208. Fiddian-Green RG, Baker S: Predictive value of the stomach wall pH for complications after cardiac operations: Comparison with other monitoring. *Crit Care Med* 15:153, 1987.

209. Landow L, Phillips DA, Heard SO, et al: Gastric tonometry and venous oximetry in cardiac surgery patients. *Crit Care Med* 19:1226, 1991.

210. Shiedler MG, Cutler BS, Fiddian-Green RG: Sigmoid intramural pH for prediction of ischemic colitis during aortic surgery. *Arch Surg* 122:881, 1987.

211. Gutierrez G, Bismar H, Dantzker DR, et al: Comparison of gastric intramucosal pH with measures of oxygen transport and consumption in critically ill patients. *Crit Care Med* 20:451, 1992.

212. Gys T, Hubens A, Neels H, et al: Prognostic value of gastric intramucosal pH in surgical intensive care patients. *Crit Care Med* 16:1222, 1988.

213. Fiddian-Green RG, McGough E, Pittenger G: Predictive value of intramural pH and other risk factors for massive bleeding from stress ulceration. *Gastroenterology* 85:613, 1983.

214. Gutierrez G, Palizas F, Doglio G, et al: Gastric intramucosal pH as a therapeutic index of tissue oxygenation in critically ill patients. *Lancet* 339:195, 1992.

30. Indirect Calorimetry

Nicholas A. Smyrnios and
Frederick J. Curley

Indirect calorimetry is a technique that uses measurements of inspired and expired gas flows, volumes, and concentrations to calculate oxygen consumption and carbon dioxide production. Energy expenditure, respiratory quotient, and other values may then be derived from the measured values.

Numerous studies over the past 25 years indicate that the outcome of intensive care unit (ICU) patients improves when their nutritional needs are optimized. Over the past decade several studies have suggested that measurement of oxygen delivery and oxygen consumption in septic or hypotensive patients may be helpful in improving outcome. Indirect calorimetry provides a noninvasive, accurate method of measuring both caloric requirements and oxygen consumption. This chapter focuses on the technique of performing indirect calorimetry in the ICU setting. Chapters 200 and 201 more fully discuss the use of the estimates of energy expenditure to determine caloric requirements in the critically ill, and Chapters 171, 173, and 181 address the use of these values in understanding the pathophysiology and management of sepsis and shock.

Prediction equations, the Fick equation, and direct calorimetry have been used to estimate caloric requirements and oxygen consumption in the critically ill. Prediction equations usually offer an estimate based on data derived from calorimetric studies performed on groups of similar patients. This provides a guideline for individual patients but lacks specificity and accuracy. The Fick equation calculates oxygen consumption by multiplying cardiac output by the difference in arterial and venous oxygen content. This technique is usually limited to patients with pulmonary artery catheters in place to provide measurements of cardiac output and mixed venous saturation. In addition, it relies on the incorrect assumption that the subject's respiratory quotient can be accurately estimated [1]. Direct calorimetry measures energy by quantitating the subject's heat production. Because it requires placing the subject in a thermically isolated whole-body enclosure for more than an hour [2], it is virtually impossible to use in a critical care setting. Indirect calorimetry provides estimates of caloric expenditure and oxygen consumption by direct measurement of inhaled and exhaled gases and subsequent analysis by a computerized metabolic cart system. Indirect calorimetry is noninvasive and relatively convenient and has a solid scientific basis. Indirect calorimetry should be the preferred technique for these measurements in the modern ICU.

Theoretical Basis of Indirect Calorimetry

An understanding of the uses and limitations of indirect calorimetry requires an understanding of the theoretical basis of the procedure. All indirect calorimetry systems rely on measures of inhaled and exhaled air flow, volume, and concentrations of oxygen and carbon dioxide. Indirect calorimetry systems can be classified as open-circuit systems, which measure minute ventilation and the difference between inspired and expired gas concentrations, or closed-circuit systems, which measure changes in the amount of gases in a fixed reservoir over time [3]. This chapter reviews only open-circuit systems, as most ICUs use this technique.

DEFINITIONS. Chemical energy used to fuel the human body is stored primarily in the form of adenosine triphosphate (ATP), which is formed by the oxidation of glucose, protein, and lipid. Indirect calorimetry measures the oxygen used and carbon dioxide produced during oxidation. Therefore it is the *production* of chemical energy that is indirectly measured by the gas exchange parameters. Despite this, it is the convention to describe this quantity as energy expended. Therefore, we use the term *energy expenditure* to describe the amount of energy measured by indirect calorimetry.

In any discussion of energy expenditure it is important to define what level of energy expenditure is being considered. Basal metabolic rate or basal energy expenditure (BEE) is the energy used by the body at complete rest and in the postabsorptive state (absence of active nutritional intake for at least 4–6 hours). This measurement can be obtained reliably only in deep sleep. Basal energy expenditure does take into account the effects of illness and stress. Resting energy expenditure (REE) is obtained from an awake subject at rest, also in the postabsorptive state. It is usually expected to be approximately 10 percent greater than BEE [4,5,6]. Total energy expenditure (TEE) is REE plus the energy used during activity plus the energy used to metabolize foodstuffs, also called diet-induced thermogenesis (DIT). It is important to remember that these levels describe only the number of calories being used. Determining the appropriate number of calories to feed a patient is much more complicated and depends on overall nutritional status. For most ICU patients we wish to know 24-hour TEE, rather than BEE or REE.

CALCULATION OF ENERGY EXPENDITURE. Most indirect calorimetry systems use the modified Weir equation to calculate energy expenditure. In its more complete form, this equation uses oxygen consumption ($\dot{V}O_2$), carbon dioxide production ($\dot{V}CO_2$), and nonprotein urinary nitrogen (UN):

$$\text{Energy expenditure} = 3.9\ \dot{V}O_2\ \text{ml/min} + 1.1\ \dot{V}CO_2\ \text{ml/min} - 2.2\ \text{UN gm/day}$$

The Weir equation is not experimentally derived from measurements on humans but is mathematically derived based on physiologic facts. The derivation relies on the knowledge that: (1) TEE is equal to the sum of the energy expended from the combustion of carbohydrate, fat, and protein; (2) the caloric equivalents of each of glucose (3.7 kcal/gm), fat (9.5 kcal/gm), and protein (4.1 kcal/gm) are known; (3) the oxygen consumed and carbon dioxide produced in burning each of these fuels is known; and (4) therefore the equation for energy expenditure can be expressed in terms of oxygen consumption and carbon dioxide production by solving the system of equations that describe the stoichiometry of fuel combustion. The reader is referred to other sources for a complete derivation of the equation [7]. In practice, the amount of urea nitrogen in the urine is often not measured because of the inconvenience of measurement and the fact that its contribution to TEE is considered minimal.

CALCULATION OF OXYGEN CONSUMPTION. The essential measurements of indirect calorimetry are the inspired and expired oxygen fractions, carbon dioxide fractions, and minute ventilations. Oxygen consumption and carbon dioxide production can be calculated using similar equations, which compute the difference between inspired (I) and expired (E) volumes:

Oxygen consumption = $\dot{V}O_2 = \dot{V}_I(FIO_2) - \dot{V}_E(FEO_2)$
Carbon dioxide production = $\dot{V}CO_2 = V_E(FECO_2) - V_I(FICO_2)$

To avoid the need to measure the concentrations and volumes of both expiratory and inspiratory gases, techniques that preferentially measure the expiratory gases only have been developed. Most systems measure only exhaled volumes and mathematically derive an estimate of inhaled volume. Any assumption that the volume exhaled is equal to the volume inhaled is erroneous whenever $\dot{V}CO_2$ and $\dot{V}O_2$ are not equal (i.e., respiratory quotient [RQ] is not equal to 1) and becomes more erroneous as FIO_2 increases. A mathematical relationship of $\dot{V}_E$ to $\dot{V}_I$, also called the Haldane transformation, can be used to explain this phenomenon. It takes advantage of the fact that nitrogen is an essentially inert gas. Therefore:

Volume inspired $(\dot{V}_I)$ x FIN_2 = Volume expired $(\dot{V}_E) \times FEN_2$

Rearranged, this reads:

$\dot{V}_I = \dot{V}_E \times FEN_2/FIN_2.$

Since

$FIO_2 + FIN_2 = 1$

and

$FEO_2 + FECO_2 + FEN_2 = 1$

then

$FIN_2 = 1 - FIO_2$

and

$FEN_2 = 1 - FECO_2 - FEO_2.$

If we substitute back into the previous equation:

$\dot{V}_I = \dot{V}_E \times (1 - FECO_2 - FEO_2)/1 - FIO_2.$

As the inspired oxygen concentration increases, the denominator decreases and the difference between inspired and expired gas volume becomes greater. Therefore, the calculation of oxygen consumption becomes progressively more erroneous. The Haldane equation can therefore be used to determine the value of $\dot{V}_I$ without measuring inspired volume. The accuracy of the Haldane equation in estimating inspired volume, and thereby oxygen consumption and energy expenditure, then depends greatly on the accuracy of measurement of FIO_2 and $\dot{V}_E$. Accuracy increases with more frequent and precise measurement of FIO_2 and/or delivery of a fixed oxygen concentration.

It is important to emphasize that any error in measuring exhaled volumes or gas concentration directly produces an error of a greater magnitude in the calculation of oxygen consumption, carbon dioxide production, or energy expenditure. At a minute ventilation of 10 liters per minute and an inspired-to-expired oxygen concentration difference of 0.03, the oxygen consumption would be 300 ml per minute. If the FIO_2 was measured to be 0.46 instead or 0.45 and the FEO_2 remained at 0.42, the oxygen consumption would be 400 ml per minute, a 33 percent change. If the measured minute ventilation was 10.1 liters per minute and the actual value was 10 liters per minute, there would be an error in the oxygen consumption of 30 ml per minute, or 10 percent. The analysis system must be free of leaks, and extremely accurate sensors must be used. Most oxygen sensors are less accurate at higher FIO_2. Due to the difficulty in obtaining accurate measures at higher FIO_2 most indirect calorimetry studies are usually limited to patients on 60% oxygen or less.

CALCULATION OF SUBSTRATE UTILIZATION. Indirect calorimetry may be used to determine what percentage of energy expenditure comes from each of the major foodstuffs. Once carbon dioxide production and oxygen consumption have been measured, their ratio, the respiratory quotient, and a measure of protein metabolism can be used to solve mathematically for the percentage of calories burned derived from fat or carbohydrate. The amount of protein catabolized in a day may be estimated to be the sum of urine urea nitrogen (measured in grams) and daily losses from skin and in stool, usually assumed to be approximately 4 gm. The value calculated is multiplied by 6.25 to describe grams of protein metabolized per day.

The respiratory exchange ratio, or respiratory quotient, is the ratio of carbon dioxide produced to oxygen consumed. The primary foodstuffs have established RQs: fat, 0.7; protein, 0.8; carbohydrate, 1.0. Using the amount of protein catabolized (and therefore the amount of energy derived from protein), the RQs of fat and carbohydrate, the REE, the RQ of the patient's metabolism as a whole, and the proportion of energy derived from fat, carbohydrate, and protein can be calculated [8]. The normal range of RQ is from 0.7, for pure fat metabolism, to 1.0, for pure carbohydrate metabolism. Almost always a combination of processes is occurring. Respiratory quotients greater than 1.0 indicate that the sum of all the reactions occurring is the synthesis of fat (lipogenesis). Values less than 0.7 may be noted when ketones are the primary fuel. These calculations yield only an estimate of substrate utilization, because (1) the mathematics make assumptions regarding the average RQ of foods and (2) protein metabolism is only estimated.

Equipment and Technique

Open-circuit indirect calorimetry systems all involve certain basic components, typically an oxygen analyzer, carbon dioxide analyzer, and a flow meter (usually a pneumotach). Various systems include masks, canopies, mixing chambers, tubing, desiccants, and pumps, and most have a personal computer with a monitor for graphic displays. We describe only the equipment necessary for the techniques discussed here.

METHODS OF MEASUREMENT. Oxygen sensors in commercially available systems are either zirconium or differential paramagnetic sensors. The zirconium oxide sensor is coated with an oxygen-permeable substance. At temperatures of approximately 800°C, oxygen diffuses across this outer layer and an electrical signal that is proportional to the partial pressure of oxygen is created [3,9]. Differential paramagnetic analyzers measure the difference in concentration of the gas between the inspiratory and expiratory lines. These analyzers typically have an accuracy of ±0.02 percent and a response time of 130 msec or less. Essentially all available carbon dioxide analyzers are nondispersed infrared devices. A gas sample in the path of infrared energy creates an alteration in an electrical signal that is proportional to the concentration of carbon dioxide. These analyzers have an accuracy of ±0.02 percent with a response time of 110 msec. Some systems measure both inspired and expired carbon dioxide and some measure only expired, assuming the inspired value to be negligible. Volume is measured by measuring flow and integrating the result over time to obtain volume. Flow is usually determined with a pneumotach, which calculates flow for a measured pressure drop across a known resistance. An alternative is the mass flow sensor, which actually measures the number of gas molecules that flow by two heated wires. Both methods are extremely accurate, although the mass flow meter is reported to be accurate at slightly lower tidal volumes.

Gas concentrations are measured using one of three techniques: mixing chamber, breath by breath, and dilution. All of these have several steps in common. All tests must begin with calibration of the essential components. Gas analyzer calibrations usually involve measurement of at least two known concentrations of the gas to create a calibration line. Calibration of the flow meter involves measurement of a known volume passing through the sensor at varying flow rates. Some machines have automated much of this process.

Mixing Chamber Method. The mixing chamber is the most well-established method and has been considered the gold standard. A mixing chamber is an automated Douglas bag that mixes expired gases over a predetermined interval and provides the material to be sampled [9]. Expired gas is passed from a mouthpiece or the ventilator exhalation port into a collection chamber, which is in series with the flow meter and gas analyzers. Inside the chamber, flow is interrupted by baffles to allow more even mixing of gases. A sample of mixed gas is withdrawn from the chamber, the gas concentrations analyzed, and the sample returned to the chamber. Depending on the design, the gas is either vented or passed through the flow meter. The concentrations (but not flows or volumes) of inspiratory gas are sampled from the inspiratory side of a mouthpiece or a ventilator circuit. Inspiratory volumes are calculated from expiratory volumes, as explained above. A computer compares mixed expired versus inspired concentrations and multiplies by volume to yield a measure of consumption or production. The results reflect the values of gases mixed over time and are usually reported as values per time interval of measurement (e.g., oxygen consumption per 5 minutes).

Breath-by-Breath Method. The collection and analysis of gases in the breath-by-breath method is similar to that in the mixing chamber technique, but each breath is analyzed. A sample of gases is taken for analysis from each inspiration and expiration. These samples are coupled with flow measurements for each breath to calculate $\dot{V}O_2$, $\dot{V}CO_2$, and REE. The concentrations of expiratory gases are measured directly from samples drawn from the expiratory side of the mouthpiece or ventilator circuit prior to entering a mixing chamber. Inspired concentrations are measured from samples drawn from the inspiratory side of a mouthpiece or ventilator circuit. Oxygen consumption

and carbon dioxide production values are usually expressed as millimeters per minute and energy expenditure as kilocalories per day for each breath and can be averaged or summed over varying periods, depending on the clinician's needs. The crucial component in these measurements is the alignment of various signals. If the time needed for the gases to reach the analyzer and the expiratory flow to reach the flow meter is known, the $\dot{V}O_2$, $\dot{V}CO_2$, and $\dot{V}_E$ signals can be precisely aligned and accurate measurements made. Instruments that use breath-by-breath analysis align the signals automatically by computer. Improper alignment can render the measurements useless. Both oxygen and carbon dioxide sensors must have a very rapid response time. The placement of the gas analysis line just distal to the endotracheal tube can standardize transit time and eliminate artifact, which assists in this process. The counterpoint to this is that proximal placement of the gas analysis line may predispose it to obstruction by bronchial secretions emanating from the endotracheal tube.

Dilution Method. The dilution method is the only technique that can be used in nonintubated patients who cannot use a mouthpiece. It is used most often in nonintubated patients, but some systems have adopted it for use with mechanical ventilation. A predetermined flow of gas of known oxygen and carbon dioxide concentration passes through a face shield mask or a hoodlike canopy past the subject's mouth. The exhaled gases are diluted into the passing stream of known gas. The amount of gas the machine puts into the stream is adjusted to keep the flow constant as the patient alters his or her own ventilation. Samples of the diluted gases are removed for analysis and the values obtained multiplied by the flow rate to yield a measure of volume. Oxygen consumption and carbon dioxide production are calculated by comparing concentrations in and out of the system. As volume is not directly measured with this method, measurement of minute ventilation and respiratory rate are not typically reported.

FACTORS AFFECTING ACCURACY. Accurate measurements require close attention to technique. Several problems are frequently encountered in the ICU setting. In the mixing chamber or breath-by-breath method, even a small error in measuring volume can produce a large error in calculated values. All connections to the metabolic cart and in the ventilator circuit must be checked for leaks. In intubated patients, it may be necessary to eliminate the small leak at the endotracheal tube cuff by overdistending the cuff for the brief duration of the study. It may be impossible to eliminate this leak in patients with high peak pressures. In all techniques, an error in measuring oxygen or carbon dioxide concentrations leads to larger errors in the subsequently calculated values. If the patient's oxygen source produces any variation in FIO_2, inspiratory concentrations of oxygen must be continuously measured. If the equipment is not capable of this, a high-quality blender or tank of oxygen of known concentration can be used for the testing period. Many ventilators and virtually all oxygen standard flow meters do not provide a steady enough concentration of oxygen to permit a single measurement of FIO_2. Any change in inspired oxygen concentration during the study will render the measurements invalid until the inspired oxygen concentration is remeasured.

Inspired and expired gas concentrations are typically sampled with long, narrow tubes leading from taps into the respiratory circuit. Tubing can easily clog with patient secretions and invalidate collected data. Most systems also somehow condition the gas from these sample tubings to standardize for temperature and water vapor. Failure to follow the manufacturer's advice on desiccant change or timing of tubing change alters the accuracy of the data.

Care must also be taken to interface the metabolic cart with the ventilator and associated equipment carefully. Disruption of the normal ventilator circuit with inappropriately placed sampling devices may lead to ventilator malfunction or trigger alarms. All connections to ventilators must be according to manufacturer's specifications. Inappropriate location of sampling tubes may also lead to artifacts in flow or concentration measurements. The use of positive end-expiratory pressure (PEEP) may variably alter the ventilator circuit compressible volume, leading to errors in volume and concentration measurements. Techniques to isolate sensors from the effects of PEEP have been incorporated into the latest generation of equipment. No equipment has yet been validated with high frequency or oscillator ventilation.

Few measures can be used to determine whether the data obtained are reliable. The RQ can act as a quality control in that values outside the physiologic range (approximately 0.65–1.3 in the ICU) indicate that the measurement needs correction before any of the data can be used [3]. Data averaged over 30 to 60 seconds can be used to determine whether the degree of variability is physiologic. If possible, inspiratory values, which should be stable, should be frequently measured and displayed during the test. When inspiratory values are not frequently monitored, leaks in the inspiratory circuit lower FiO_2 values, falsely lower oxygen consumption and energy expenditure measurements, and falsely elevate RQ. Leaks in the expiratory circuit falsely decrease volume measurements. Leaks in the breath-by-breath sampling line produce marked variability in the derived values.

Uses of Indirect Calorimetry in the Intensive Care Unit

The primary role of indirect calorimetry in the ICU to date has been to assess energy expenditure and nutritional requirements. Recently, there has been increasing interest in using metabolic carts to assist in the management of septic or hypotensive patients. There has always been interest in using indirect calorimetry in research into the pathophysiology of critical illness.

NUTRITIONAL ASSESSMENT. Accurate determination of daily caloric needs is important because inappropriate feeding causes problems in the critically ill. Malnutrition is associated with an increased mortality [10,11]. Inadequate caloric intake can cause muscle weakness, impaired immunity, and delayed wound healing [12,13]. Excess alimentation can lead to hyperglycemia, hepatic dysfunction, increased carbon dioxide production [14,15], increased minute ventilation (V_E), respiratory distress, and respiratory failure [16].

In most ICUs the patient's caloric intake is determined by estimating a daily TEE. Basal energy expenditure is calculated from a standard equation and adjusted for level of illness, diet-induced thermogenesis, and amount of activity. Studies comparing this practice with measurement of energy expenditure by indirect calorimetry have inconclusive results. Some conclude that estimates of energy expenditure routinely overestimate caloric need [1–20]; others conclude that estimates of energy expenditure are inaccurate but in no consistent direction [21,22,23] and still others conclude that clinical estimates are as accurate as measured values [24–27]. The results may differ due

to the different techniques and patient populations in each study.

There is no standard as to length and frequency of studies needed to estimate accurately 24-hour caloric needs. Studies from 5 minutes to 24 hours in duration have been used [20,28,29]. The cost of technicians and equipment and the demands for other interventions in the ICU that would confound calorimetry necessitate that the study be brief. The more unstable the patient, the more inaccurate will be the prediction of that day's 24-hour caloric need. Even if the test accurately predicts that day's energy expenditure, it is unclear whether it can predict caloric need for subsequent days. Weissman et al. found day-to-day changes of 12 to 46 percent, depending on the patient's clinical condition [30]. Testing conditions must be developed that make it practical to repeat the test multiple times if the patient remains in the ICU for an extended period and to determine the appropriate frequency of remeasurement.

Even if energy expenditure can be measured more accurately than it can be estimated, does it alter clinical outcome? Some investigators believe providing an average energy requirement suffices for most patients and that indirect calorimetry can be reserved for the 10 to 20 percent with more complex cases [31]. Others believe accurate determination of energy requirements is crucial [32]. This question could be answered by a randomized study comparing outcomes of large numbers of patients who have their caloric intake determined by traditional or indirect calorimetric methods.

SUBSTRATE UTILIZATION. Substrate utilization analysis is probably not necessary for the average patient. An elevated RQ may indicate excessive levels of carbohydrate metabolism and with it elevated levels of carbon dioxide production. It has been suggested that this may precipitate or perpetuate respiratory failure [15,16,33,34]. Indirect calorimetry can be used to help detect elevated carbohydrate metabolism and follow the response of carbon dioxide production and RQ to a change in diet. In more complicated cases of hepatic or renal failure an analysis of substrate utilization may be used to assess quickly the efficacy of a change in diet.

OXYGEN CONSUMPTION. Oxygen consumption data can assist in the management of hemodynamic status. Proponents believe oxygen consumption varies linearly with oxygen delivery over a broad range in patients with septic shock. They propose that increases in oxygen delivery to levels above the normal physiologic range can increase oxygen consumption in this serious condition. In several studies that support this theory, $\dot{V}O_2$ has usually been calculated from the same variables used to calculate DO_2 [35,36,37]. This "mathematic coupling" of data may introduce a systematic error, making the correlation of DO_2 and $\dot{V}O_2$ more likely [38,39]. A way to negate this error is to measure $\dot{V}O_2$ through the analysis of respiratory gases. A metabolic cart can be used to monitor $\dot{V}O_2$ while oxygen delivery is measured using hemodynamic variables. One study that used this method failed to show significant changes in $\dot{V}O_2$ despite large increases in DO_2 induced by dobutamine infusion [40]. When the breath-by-breath method of calorimetry is employed, changes in oxygen consumption in response to a therapeutic intervention should be readily apparent.

RESEARCH AND FUTURE APPLICATIONS. Although this discussion has focused primarily on the indirect calorimeter as a monitor of oxygen consumption and energy expenditure, other values measured by the calorimeter have potential value in the ICU. Many computerized indirect calorimetry systems permit analog or digital inputs from other monitoring equipment into the system's computer. Many values derived from the combination of device inputs have not been adequately studied to recommend routine clinical use. If the oxygen consumption measurement is combined with data from an arterial and mixed venous oximeter (an oximetric pulmonary artery catheter), continuous measurements of cardiac output may be displayed. The values of oxygen pulse, measured as oxygen consumption divided by heart rate, correlate well as an index of left ventricular stroke volume. The ventilatory equivalences of oxygen and carbon dioxide, calculated by dividing minute ventilation by oxygen consumption or carbon dioxide production, respectively, can serve as an index of ventilation perfusion mismatch. As technology improves and equipment cost declines, the use of indirect calorimeters as short-term monitors of complex physiologic changes resulting from disease and treatment may markedly increase.

References

1. Ligett SB, St. John RE, Lefrak SS: Determination of resting energy expenditure utilizing the thermodilution pulmonary artery catheter. *Chest* 91:562, 1987.
2. McManus C, Newhouse H, Seitz S, et al: Human gradient-layer calorimeter: Development of an accurate and practical instrument for clinical studies. *J Parenter Enter Nutr* 8:317, 1984.
3. Branson RD: The measurement of energy expenditure: Instrumentation, practical considerations, and clinical application. *Respir Care* 35:640, 1990.
4. Feurer ID, Crosby LO, Mullen JL: Measured and predicted resting energy expenditure in clinically stable patients. *Clin Nutr* 3:27, 1984.
5. Owen OE: Resting metabolic requirements of men and women. *Mayo Clin Proc* 63:503, 1988.
6. Weissman C, Kemper M, Elwyn EH, et al: The energy expenditure of the mechanically ventilated critically ill patient: An analysis. *Chest* 89:254, 1986.
7. Ferrannini E: The theoretical bases of indirect calorimetry: A review. *Metabolism* 37:287, 1988.
8. Bursztein S, Elwyn DH, Askanazi J, et al: *Energy Metabolism, Indirect Calorimetry, and Nutrition.* Baltimore, Williams & Wilkins, 1989.
9. Teirlinck HC: Sensormedics 2900 metabolic measurement cart: Technical and fundamental considerations in gas exchange measurements. *Cardiopulm Rev* 1991. (Sensormedics Corporation publication)
10. Apelgren KN, Rombeau JL, Twomey P, et al: Comparison of nutritional indices and outcome in critically ill patients. *Crit Care Med* 10:305, 1982.
11. Murray MJ, Marsh HM, Wochos DN, et al: Nutritional assessment of intensive care unit patients. *Mayo Clin Proc* 63:1106, 1988.
12. Arora NS, Rochester DF: Respiratory muscle strength and maximal voluntary ventilation in undernourished patients. *Am Rev Respir Dis* 126:5, 1982.
13. Kahan BD: Nutrition and host defense mechanisms. *Surg Clin North Am* 61:557, 1981.
14. Askanazi J, Rosenbaum SH, Hyman AI, et al: Respiratory changes induced by the large glucose loads of total parenteral nutrition. *JAMA* 243:1444, 1980.
15. Gieske T, Gurushanthaiah G, Glauser FL: Effects of carbohydrates on carbon dioxide excretion in patients with airway disease. *Chest* 71:55, 1977.
16. Covelli HD, Black JW, Olsen MS, et al: Respiratory failure precipitated by high carbohydrate loads. *Ann Intern Med* 95:579, 1981.
17. Daly JM, Heymsfield SB, Head CA, et al: Human energy requirements: Overestimation by widely used prediction equation. *Am J Clin Nutr* 42:1170, 1985.
18. Cortes V, Nelson LD: Errors in estimating energy expenditure in critically ill surgical patients. *Arch Surg* 124:287, 1989.
19. Mann S, Westenkow DR, Houtchens BA: Measured and predicted caloric expenditure in the acutely ill. *Crit Care Med* 13:173, 1985.
20. Makk LJK, McClave SA, Creech PW, et al: Clinical application of the metabolic cart to the delivery of total parenteral nutrition. *Crit Care Med* 18:1320, 1990.
21. Saffle JR, Medina E, Raymond J, et al: Use of indirect calorimetry in the nutritional management of burned patients. *J Trauma* 25:32, 1985.
22. Weissman C, Kemper M, Askanazi J, et al: Resting metabolic rate of the critically ill patient: Measured versus predicted. *Anesthesiology* 64:673, 1986.
23. Smyrnios NA, Curley FJ, Jederlinic PJ, et al: Indirect calorimetry in the medical ICU: Comparison with traditional practice and effect on cost of care. *Am Rev Respir Dis* 141:A581, 1990.
24. Hunter DC, Jaksic T, Lewis D, et al: Resting energy expenditure in the critically ill: Estimations versus measurement. *Br J Surg* 75:875, 1988.
25. Van Lanschot JB, Feenstra BWA, Vermeij CG, et al: Calculation versus measurement of total energy expenditure. *Crit Care Med* 14:981, 1986.
26. Saffle JR, Larson CM, Sullivan J: A randomized trial of indirect calorimetry-based feedings in thermal injury. *J Trauma* 30:776, 1990.
27. Liggett SB, Renfro AD: Energy expenditures of mechanically ventilated nonsurgical patients. *Chest* 98:682, 1990.
28. Vermeij CG, Feenstra BW, Van Lanschot JB, et al: Day-to-day variability of energy expenditure in critically ill surgical patients. *Crit Care Med* 17:623, 1989.
29. Rumpler WV, Seale JL, Conway JM, et al: Repeatability of 24-h energy expenditure measurements in humans by indirect calorimetry. *Am J Clin Nutr* 51:147, 1990.
30. Weissman C, Kemper M, Hyman AI: Variation in the resting metabolic rate of mechanically ventilated critically ill patients. *Anesth Analg* 68:457, 1989.
31. Bursztein S, Elwyn DH: Measured and predicted energy expenditure in critically ill patients. *Crit Care Med* 21:312, 1993.
32. Mullen JL: Indirect calorimetry in critical care. *Proc Nutr Soc* 50:239, 1991.
33. Herve P, Simmonneau G, Girard P, et al: Hypercapneic acidosis induced by nutrition in mechanically ventilated patients: Glucose versus fat. *Crit Care Med* 13:537, 1985.
34. Sherman BW, Hamilton C, Panacek EA: Adequacy of early enteral nutrition support by the enteral route in patients with acute respiratory failure. *Chest* 98:104S, 1990.
35. Bihari D, Smithies M, Gimson A, et al: The effects of vasodilation with prostacyclin on oxygen delivery and uptake in critically ill patients. *N Engl J Med* 317:397, 1987.
36. Kaufman BS, Rackow EC, Falk JL: The relationship between oxygen delivery and consumption during fluid resuscitation of hypovolemic and septic shock. *Chest* 85:336, 1984.
37. Astiz ME, Rackow EC, Falk JL, et al: Oxygen delivery and consumption in patients with hyperdynamic septic shock. *Crit Care Med* 15:26, 1987.
38. Archie JP Jr: Mathematic coupling of data: A common source of error. *Ann Surg* 193:296, 1981.
39. Stratton HH, Feustel PJ, Newell JC: Regression of calculated variables in the presence of shared measurement error. *J Appl Physiol* 62:2083, 1987.
40. Ronco JJ, Fenwick JC, Wiggs BR, et al: Oxygen consumption is independent of increases in oxygen delivery by dobutamine in septic patients who have normal or increased plasma lactate. *Am Rev Respir Dis* 147:25, 1993.

31. Interventional Radiology: Drainage Techniques

Ashley Davidoff

The intensive care unit (ICU) patient manifests unique problems, most commonly presenting to the radiologist with problems of sepsis. Often the role of the radiologist is to identify the source of sepsis and to characterize and drain problematic collections. When the source of sepsis is visualized, imaging modalities can contribute to diagnosis and therapy. Plain film, ultrasound, computed tomography (CT), and nuclear medicine are the tools at hand.

General Aims

Abnormal fluid collections may be a result of physiologic stasis (e.g., cholestasis) or pathologic accumulation (hematoma, urinoma, lymphocele, seroma), which may be complicated by secondary infection and abscess formation. The aim, therefore, is to characterize the abnormal fluid collection and drain infected collections in a safe manner.

Indications

The indications for imaging and intervention may be diagnostic or therapeutic. Accumulation of fluid may occur in normal (pleural space, peritoneal space) or abnormal (interloop collections [Fig. 31-1], dissecting pseudocysts [Fig. 31-2], anastamotic leakages) spaces. Normal fluid may accumulate in abnormal places (biloma, hematoma, urinoma). These collections are all within the capability of percutaneous drainage. Detection of these accumulations usually requires imaging, because clinical examination lacks sensitivity, and characterization of the fluid usually requires needle aspiration, because imaging modalities lack specificity. The presence of infection in any fluid accumulation in the abdomen is almost always an absolute indication for drainage. The most common indications for bedside imaging, aspiration, and drainage are presented in Table 31-1.

Contraindications

The contraindications to intervention mostly reflect risks that may supersede the advantages of the procedure. Contraindications that relate to patient safety include perforation of organs and bleeding, specifically of lung (with resultant pneumothorax), blood vessels, large bowel, pancreas, spleen, and small bowel (Fig. 31-1). Perforations by small-gauge needles (except of the lung) commonly have a benign course, but morbidity increases significantly when these organs are traversed with a drainage catheter. An important consideration when draining fluid accumulations in the abdominal cavity is the position of the pleural space, situated at the twelfth rib anteriorly and posteriorly and at the tenth rib along the midaxillary line. The pleural space is normally not visualized. Subacute or chronic secondary infection of the pleural space is usual when this space is traversed during catheter passage to the abdomen; therefore, drainage of an abdominal collection through the pleural space is contraindicated.

Attention to clotting factors is important before embarking on an invasive procedure. When the prothrombin time is 3 seconds longer than control, the partial thromboplastin time measures 50 seconds or more, the platelet count is less than 70,000, or the bleeding time is greater than 8 minutes, a procedure is relatively contraindicated [1,2]. Each case is weighed on its own merit, however, and more "liberal" allowance is often made for small-gauge needle procedures and superficial collections.

A second set of relative contraindications stems from limitations of the drainage procedure related to features of the disease process. Collections surrounded by bowel or bone cannot be safely accessed (Fig. 31-1). In the past, multilocular collections were considered a contraindication because of inability to drain all but the first abscess entered. It has been recently suggested that drainage of multilocular collections should be attempted because the loculations may communicate, may be mechanically broken by the catheter [3], or may be lysed chemically with urokinase [4,5].

Presence of more than three abscess cavities, fistulous tracts, and fungi, were previously considered contraindications to drainage, but some of these have become only relative contraindications. Many patients with these conditions are given a trial of percutaneous therapy if they can tolerate the time necessary to show a therapeutic response.

There are many circumstances in which patients are not candidates for curative surgery or curative percutaneous drainage. Temporary drainage may allow partial recovery and make subsequent surgical treatment more feasible [6].

Risks

The risk of complication is low, with minor complications reported in 9.8 percent [7] and serious complications in 5 percent [8] of procedures. Risks include bleeding, perforation, and secondary infection. Death as a result of the procedure is rare, but

Table 31-1. Indications for Imaging, Aspiration, and Drainage

Imaging
1. Evaluation of the gallbladder for cholecystitis
2. Evaluation of the pleural space for pleural fluid
3. Evaluation of the peritoneal cavity for peritoneal fluid

Aspiration
1. Thoracentesis for characterization of pleural fluid
2. Paracentesis for characterization of peritoneal fluid
3. Characterization of an intraabdominal fluid collection

Drainage
1. Abscess drainage
2. Cholecystostomy for acalculous cholecystitis

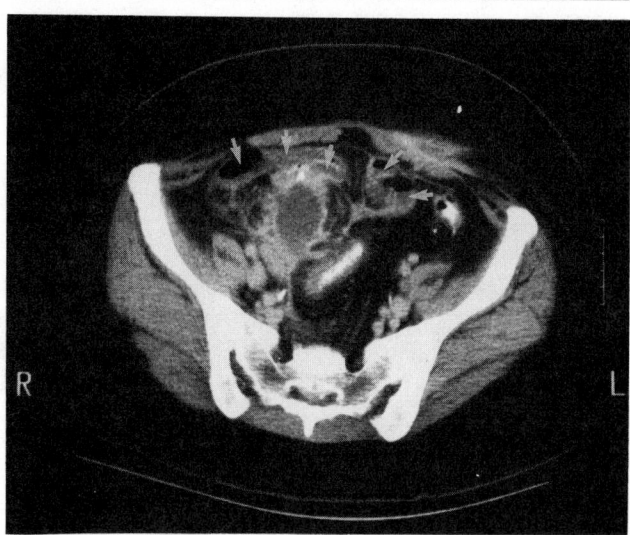

Fig. 31-1. Computed tomography scan demonstrating an inter-loop collection characterized by an enhancing rim and low-density center. Access to the collection via a drainage catheter is prohibited anteriorly by surrounding bowel loops (*arrows*) and posteriorly and laterally by the bony pelvis.

mortality following the maneuver can be as high as 14.2 percent, with the cause of death attributed to "sepsis" and underlying multisystem disease rather than the procedure itself [7].

Benefits

The benefits of drainage include avoidance of surgery and anesthesia and the ability to mobilize immediately after the procedure. Drainage has a cure rate of 60 to 85 percent [1,7,9,10,11].

Method

PATIENT PREPARATION. Informed consent is imperative. Although most procedures are relatively safe, it is important that the patient and family understand the risks.

Prothrombin time and partial thromboplastin time are essential tests; platelet count and bleeding time are requested only if there are clinical concerns. For ultrasound, enteric nutrition should be discontinued 4 hours prior to the procedure, since the introduction of air into the gastrointestinal tract or added peristalsis limits visualization. For CT, oral contrast is given 4 to 8 hours prior to the procedure. The contrast is a 2% solution, close to water; unless there are contraindications to drinking water, there are no contraindications to the use of oral contrast. Water-soluble contrast media (as opposed to barium-based solutions) are used in patients with suspected gastrointestinal leakage.

Broad-spectrum antibiotic coverage is essential prior to procedures that involve infected collections and should be continued as dictated by the sensitivities of the bacteria.

EQUIPMENT AND SPECIAL NEEDS. Portable ultrasound is now well established as the workhorse for diagnostic and in-

terventional procedures at the bedside. The overall strength of ultrasound in this setting is its portability and ability to identify and characterize fluid collections. It can provide very specific information in the ICU setting. Ultrasound is best used when the collection is superficial (pleural, peritoneal, or gall bladder [Fig. 31-3]); CT is best used when the fluid is thought to be deeper in the peritoneal cavity or in the retroperitoneum (Fig. 31-2).

When the questions are of a global nature, such as ruling out abdominal abscess, when they relate to the retroperitoneum, or if the disease lies beyond bowel (Fig. 31-1), CT is the diagnostic and therapeutic tool of choice. Although ultrasound can portray needles and catheters as they pass through the tissues to the final target, CT is far more consistent in this regard. When a "treacherous" path has to be taken and bowel, spleen and pleural space have to be avoided, CT is preferred (Fig. 31-2).

Procedures done in the ICU require the assistance of an ultrasound technologist and ICU nursing staff. Since sterile method is used, the ultrasound technologist is needed to operate the equipment. The nursing staff assists in monitoring the patient during the procedure, administers required analgesic and anxiolytic medication (see Chap. 28), maintains optimal patient positioning, and provides additional equipment needed.

Kits for aspiration and drainage containing lidocaine, needles, syringes, test tubes, gloves and vacutainers should be readily available. Needles, catheters, and guidewires should be selected in the radiology department, as they are not usually available in the ICU.

Standard sterile precautions are used including hand washing and patient skin preparation using 10% povidone-iodine, sterile drapes, and sterile surgical gloves. If the Seldinger technique, in which guidewire exchange is usually cumbersome, is contemplated, gown, mask, and cap should be worn to prevent unintentional contamination.

A spinal needle is used for the initial aspiration. A conventional 22-gauge "spinal" needle with 0.7 mm outside diameter does not accept the skinny guidewire (0.018 inch). Thus, if the Seldinger technique is contemplated the small-gauge needle used initially is of the manufacture that will accept the skinny wire. If the collection cannot be aspirated, then a 20-gauge or 18-gauge needle is used.

Appropriate tests are ordered on the aspirated fluid, depending on the indications for the procedure. A vacuum-protected culture medium is used for culture of fungi and aerobic and anaerobic bacteria.

There is a wide selection of guidewires available. We routinely use the 15-cm Bentson guidewire (Cook, Bloomington, IN) with a flexible straight tip. When the Seldinger technique is used, a small-gauge stainless steel wire is used initially. A series of dilators should be available so the Seldinger tract can be progressively dilated to 1 French larger than the catheter to be inserted.

Many types of catheters are available. In general, we use 5 to 10 Fr. catheters, depending on the character of the fluid aspirated. When the fluid is thin and not obviously infected, the 5 Fr. catheter is adequate; the thicker the fluid the larger the catheter used. The Luer lock at the end of the catheter is usually only 5 or 6 Fr., thus limiting the ability of even a 14 Fr. catheter. There is a tendency to think the largest catheter with a sump yields the best results, but we have found this not to be the case. We tend to place 7 to 9 Fr. catheters without a sump, with comparable success.

TECHNIQUES

Diagnostic Aspirates. The key to successful diagnostic aspiration is a well-planned needle path. The site of insertion, angle

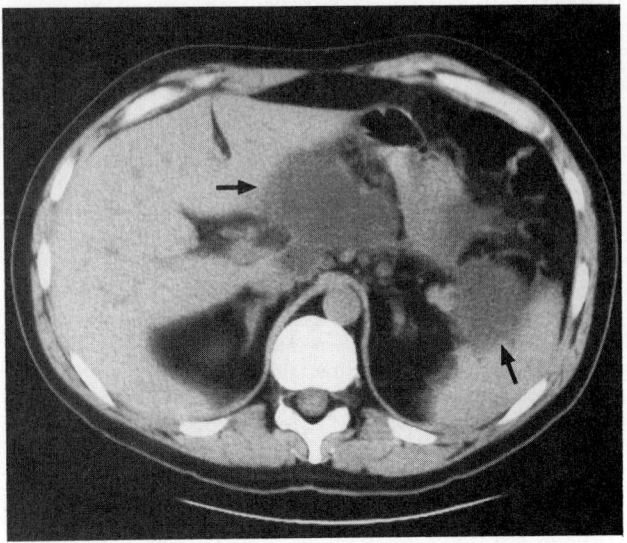

A

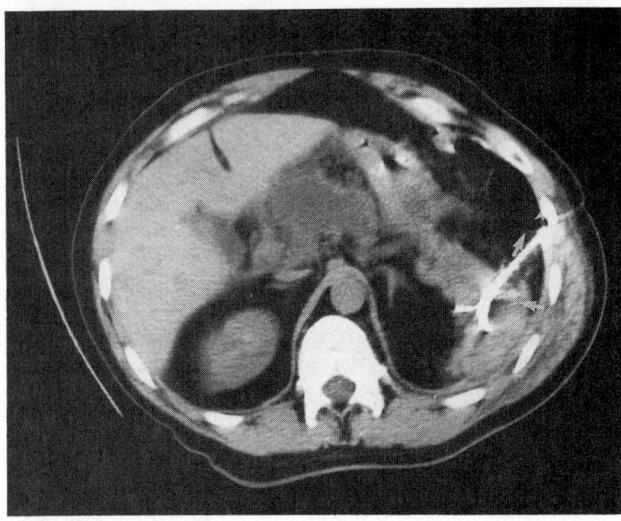

B

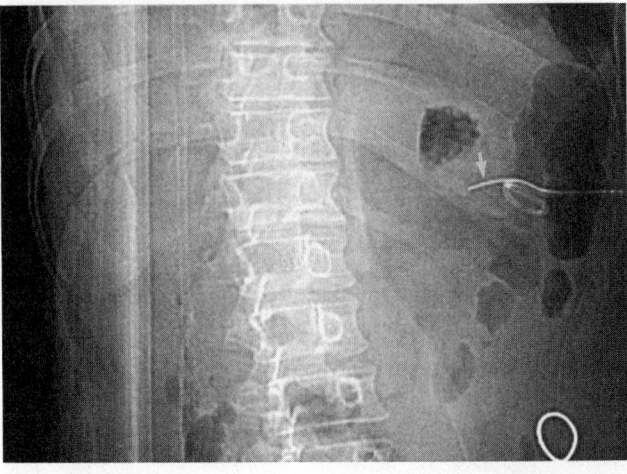

C

Fig. 31-2. A. Two pseudocysts superior to the pancreas, the first in the lesser sac and the second near the hilum of the spleen. B. Drainage of the latter was accomplished via an angled approach to avoid the spleen (*arrow*) and colon (*arrow*). Access to the first was accomplished using an unimpeded inferior approach. C. The scout film, performed after the first drainage, shows the catheter coiled and fixed in shape. The arrow indicates the safety guidewire that is left in place until the position of the catheter is deemed satisfactory.

of introduction, and depth of the needle are the three important factors to consider. A right angle entry (needle to skin) and the shortest path to the collection are optimal but not always possible (Fig. 31-2). Real-time guided ultrasonography allows one to trace the path of the needle as it passes along the planned course. This technique is sometimes cumbersome, particularly when the puncture is between the ribs, where visualization of the needle is inconsistent. Others find the guide indispensable. Many attempts have been made to improve visualization, in both needle design (Teflon-coated, side holes) and technique (introduction of air through the needle, mechanical shaking of the needle). If aspiration is unsuccessful after the needle has been introduced, either the needle is placed incorrectly or the fluid is too thick to be aspirated through a small-gauge needle. The collection is imaged to identify the needle position; a larger-bore needle is usually attempted if the fluid is too thick for the small-gauge needle.

Drainage

INTRODUCTION OF THE CATHETER. The catheter is introduced by using either the trocar technique or the Seldinger technique.

When the fluid collection appears to be easily accessible, the trocar technique is preferred. This technique is easier to perform but does carry the risk of more severe complications if a viscus is perforated, since the hole produced by a catheter is larger than that from the first step in the Seldinger technique. Usually a guiding small-gauge needle is used to "sound out" the direction and course of the final catheter path. Once the needle is placed, it is imaged and its placement revised until an optimal course has been accomplished. An attempt is made to aspirate the fluid to confirm appropriate placement and to evaluate the character and thickness. The aspirated fluid is evaluated to determine whether drainage is needed. Macroscopic evaluation of the aspirate is sometimes confusing. The supernatant (which is the usual initial aspirate) may appear clear, serous, and noninfected, while the sediment obviously contains more complex material. One is cautioned not to make the decision of "noncomplex" or "sterile" collection based on the initial aspirate. Often the referring physician's instructions are to drain if infected, leave if not. In practice, waiting 10 minutes for this decision is impractical, and late growth on a previously negative Gram stain is common. We have adopted a policy of liberal placement of catheters, particularly if clinical suspicion is high and the fluid appears complex. If on subsequent culture there is no growth of organisms, the catheter is removed. Secondary infection of a previously sterile collection is possible, but we have found that cautious and judicious use of this policy has been effective and uncomplicated, particularly when decisions are made in conjunction with the referring clinician. The choice of catheter size and type depends mostly on thickness of the fluid. If the fluid is too thick to be aspirated through the small-gauge needle, we usually opt for a 9 or 10 Fr. catheter and use Seldinger technique.

The catheter is inserted alongside the guiding needle. Attention to depth of the collection, position of the sideholes in relation to this depth, and the final position and shape of the catheter are considerations at this stage.

In the Seldinger technique, needle, guidewire, and dilators

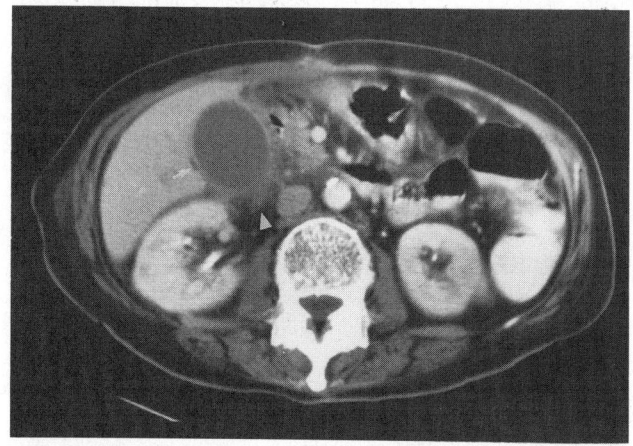

A

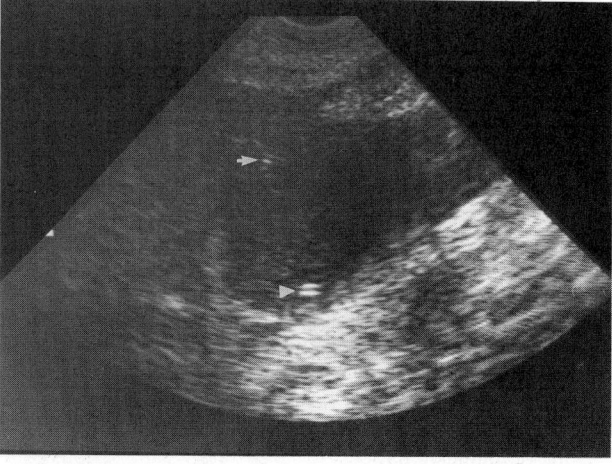

C

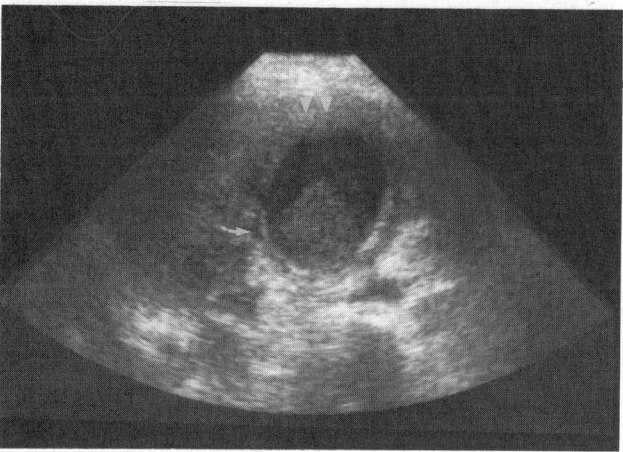

B

Fig. 31-3. A. Computed tomography scan demonstrating a distended gallbladder with a small amount of pericholecystic fluid (*arrow*) and induration of the surrounding fat (*closed arrow*) suggesting cholecystitis with extension of the inflammatory process or early perforation. B. Transverse ultrasound image of the gallbladder, confirming the presence of pericholecystic fluid (*arrow*), the rounded and distended shape of the gallbladder, and tumefactive bile in the lumen. A small amount of liver tissue anterior to the gallbladder (*closed arrows*) is the planned path to the gallbladder. C. Transverse ultrasound image of the gallbladder showing two echogenic foci. The first reflects the path of the catheter through the liver (*arrow*) and bare area of the gallbladder; the second (*closed arrow*) reflects the satisfactory intracystic position of the catheter.

are progressively introduced until an appropriate tract has been formed to allow for the final introduction of the catheter. Theoretically, it is the safer of the two procedures. However, when the procedure is performed under CT or ultrasound guidance, the real-time visualization of needles, guidewires, dilators, and catheter cannot be appreciated and the technique loses some of its advantage. It is the better method when the path to the collection is hazardous, the catheter size required is large, or fluoroscopic guidance is needed.

The considerations of catheter choice are similar to those outlined for the trocar technique. Once the collection has been entered and there is free drainage of fluid, careful manipulation is suggested. At this point, with free drainage of fluid from the catheter, it is useful to document the satisfactory position of the catheter (Figs. 31-2C and 31-3C). Distention of the abscess cavity by contrast, air, or aggressive manipulation is discouraged, to prevent bacteremia or septicemia that may originate from the inflamed and bleeding surface of the cavity. It is reasonable, however, to aspirate obviously purulent material, with the aim of evacuating the contents as completely as possible. The sudden appearance of blood tinged material is usually an indication to discontinue aspiration and to rely on left gravity drainage.

FIXING THE CATHETER. Anchoring the catheter with self-retaining locks is essential to prevent the catheter from being accidently pulled out. These locks consist of a string that threads through the catheter to its tip. When the string is pulled and fixed in position, the tension retains the pigtail in a fixed, rounded, more stable position. In addition, the catheter is fixed to the skin using a disk or belt. It is important to anchor the bag to the patient's clothing so it does not put tension on the catheter.

AFTERCARE AND FOLLOW-UP. Frequent flushing of the catheter is necessary starting a few hours after insertion. Normal saline is injected initially in small amounts (5–10 ml) every 4 hours to flush the catheter and prevent clogging of the sideholes. After 24 hours, the aim of flushing is to agitate the dependent debris of the collection, so that the sediment can eventually work its way into the catheter. Larger volumes, approximating the size of the cavity, are used to prevent the development of adhesions and loculation. We recommend 4-hourly flushing until the drainage fluid clears. When the fluid is too viscous to permit drainage, it may be liquefied with N-acetyl cysteine [12]; loculations may be loosened by mechanical [3] or chemical means with urokinase [4,5].

Follow-up study of the abscess should be performed using CT or fluoroscopy 3 to 4 days after catheter insertion to evaluate the extent of the abscess and identify undrained collections and fistulous tracts. This is an important and often ignored procedure. Frequently the findings drastically alter management when unsuspected fistulous tracts are revealed, indicating the need for surgery.

Kinking, blockage by debris, and dislodgement of the catheter are common causes of failed drainage. The interventional team should evaluate daily for these problems.

WHEN TO REMOVE THE CATHETER. Once the patient has defervesced (usually within 24 hours), the cavity has decompressed (5–10 days), antibiotics are discontinued, and drainage has ceased or is minimal, it is recommended that the three-way stopcock of the catheter be turned off to the patient and a trial of 24 hours with the patient off antibiotics be performed. If fever, leukocytosis, or reaccumulation of fluid occurs, then the catheter should be left in. Otherwise, it can be withdrawn.

Expected Results

Defervescence usually occurs within 24 hours but may take up to 4 to 5 days. Successful drainage may take 2 weeks or even longer.

Successful drainage and cure is usually accomplished in 60 to 85 percent of patients [1,7,9,13,14], with partial success attained in 7 to 18 percent [10,11]. The procedure fails in 8 to 20 percent of patients [7,8,10,11] and must be repeated in 2.1 percent [7].

Minor complications occur in 9.8 percent [7] and serious complications in 5 percent [8]. Mortality after the procedure ranges from 1.4 to 14.2 percent [3,8,13], though most groups who report mortality following the procedure suggest that death was due not to the technique but to the patient's severely compromised condition.

Special Circumstances

CHOLECYSTOSTOMY. A cholestatic situation exists in most ICU patients, and distention of the gallbladder is common. Cholecystostomy is indicated in the patient with a distended gallbladder and sepsis of unknown origin (Fig. 31-3). This relatively simple procedure is safe when performed by an experienced physician and can be performed at the bedside. The trocar technique, using the liver as a window to the gallbladder fossa, is our method of choice. Special attention should be paid to the exact depth of the gallbladder since there is little room for error. If the catheter is advanced too far, it may perforate the wall, with resultant bile peritonitis. The bile in acalculous cholecystitis is black (like crank case oil) and does not appear grossly purulent. Frequently, neither organisms nor white cells are present, and the real test of successful drainage is the patient's subsequent clinical course.

EMPYEMA. The percutaneous insertion of large chest tubes by a thoracic surgeon is the procedure of choice for empyemas in our institution (see Chap. 11). Occasionaly, small inaccessible empyemas require imaging guidance. Special considerations for this procedure include the use of a large-bore catheter and underwater seal and care to prevent introduction of air through the needles and catheters into the pleural space, as inspiratory effort by the patient causes a negative intrathoracic pressure. Urokinase has been used in the pleural space to lyse loculated collections [4,5].

PSEUDOCYSTS. Percutaneous drainage has an 80 percent cure rate and is an effective front-line treatment for most pancreatic pseudocysts, whether the collection is sterile or infected. It is particularly suitable for the ICU patient. Cure is likely if sufficient time is allowed for closure of fistulas from the pancreatic duct [6]. Because low-output fistulas are present in 44 percent of patients [2], it is recommended that the catheter be maintained for an average of 7 weeks, sometimes longer. Paradoxically, infected pseudocysts require a shorter period. Duvnjak et al. [14] suggest that the amylase concentration in the pseudocyst allows one to predict to some degree the potential for cure and recommend that this level be evaluated during the course of drainage.

References

1. Ferrucci JT, Wittenberg J, Mueller PR, Simeone JF (eds): *Interventional Radiology of the Abdomen*. 2nd ed. Baltimore, Williams & Wilkins, 1985.
2. Kandarpa K: *Handbook of Cardiovascular and Interventional Radiologic Procedures*. Boston, Little, Brown, 1989.
3. Lang EK, Springer RM, Glorioso LW, Cammarata CA: Abdominal abscess drainage under radiologic guidance: Causes of failure. *Radiology* 159:329, 1986.
4. Couser JI Jr, Berley J, Timm EG: Intrapleural urokinase for loculated effusion. *Chest* 101:1467, 1992.
5. Lieberman RP, Hahn FJ, Imray TJ, Phalen JT: Loculated abscesses: Management by percutaneous fracture of septations. *Radiology* 161:827, 1986.
6. van Sonnenberg E, Mueller PR, Ferrucci JT Jr: Percutaneous drainage of 250 abdominal abscesses and fluid collections, I: Results, failures, and complications. *Radiology* 151:337, 1984.
7. Kerlan RK Jr, Jeffrey RB Jr, Pogany AC, Ring EJ: Abdominal abscess with low-output fistula: Successful percutaneous drainage. *Radiology* 155:73 1985.
8. Lambiase RE, Deyoe L, Cronan JJ, Dorfman GS: Percutaneous drainage of 335 consecutive abscesses: Results of primary drainage with 1-year follow-up. *Radiology* 184:167, 1992.
9. Brolin RE, Flancbaum L, Ercoli FR, et al: Limitations of percutaneous catheter drainage of abdominal abscesses. *Surg Gynecol Obstet* 173:203, 1991.
10. Gerzof SG, Johnson WC: Radiographic aspects of diagnosis and treatment of abdominal abscesses. *Surg Clin North Am* 64:53, 1984.
11. Moulton JS, Moore PT, Mencini RA: Treatment of loculated pleural effusions with transcatheter intracavitary urokinase. *Am J Roentgenol* 153:941, 1989.
12. van Sonnenberg E, Wittich GR, Casola G, et al: Percutaneous drainage of infected and noninfected pancreatic pseudocysts: Experience in 101 cases. *Radiology* 170:757, 1989.
13. Dahnert W, Gunther R, Klose K, Gamstatter G: Results of percutaneous abscess drainage. *ROFO Fortschr Geb Nuklearmed* 139:400, 1983.
14. Duvnjak M, Vucelic B, Rotkvic I, et al: Assessment of value of pancreatic pseudocyst amylase concentration in the treatment of pancreatic pseudocysts by percutaneous evacuation. *J Clin Ultrasound* 20:183, 1992.
15. Jacques P, Mauro M, Safrit H, et al: CT features of intraabdominal abscesses: Prediction of successful percutaneous drainage. *Am J Roentgenol* 146:1041, 1986.
16. van Waes PF, Feldberg MA, Mali WP, et al: Management of loculated abscesses that are difficult to drain: A new approach. *Radiology* 147:57, 1983.

II. Cardiovascular Problems in the Intensive Care Unit

Section Editor
Joel M. Gore

32. Cardiopulmonary Resuscitation

John A. Paraskos

History

Since the introduction of cardiopulmonary resuscitation (CPR), we have been forced to rethink our definitions of life and death. Although sporadic accounts of attempted resuscitations are recorded from antiquity [1,2,3], until recently no rational quarrel could be found with the sixth century B.C. poetic fragment of Ibycus, "You cannot find a medicine for life once a man is dead" [4]. Until 1960, successful resuscitation was largely limited to artificial ventilation for victims of respiratory arrest, such as near drowning, smoke inhalation, and aspiration. Such attempts were likely to succeed if performed before cardiac arrest had resulted from hypoxia and acidosis. Emergency thoracotomy with "open heart massage" was rarely employed and was occasionally successful if definitive therapy was readily available [5]. Electrical reversal of ventricular fibrillation by externally applied electrodes was described in 1956 by Zoll et al. [6]. This ability to reverse a fatal arrhythmia without opening the chest challenged the medical community to develop a method of sustaining adequate ventilation and circulation long enough to bring the electrical defibrillator to the patient's aid. By 1958, adequate rescue ventilation became possible with the development of the mouth-to-mouth technique by Safar et al. [7,8] and Elam et al. [9]. In 1960, Kouwenhoven et al. [10] described closed chest cardiac massage, thus introducing the modern era of cardiopulmonary resuscitation. The simplicity of this technique—". . . all that is needed are two hands"—has led to its widespread dissemination. The interaction of this technique of sternal compression with mouth-to-mouth ventilation was developed as basic CPR. The first national conference on CPR was sponsored by the National Academy of Sciences in 1966 [11]. Instruction in CPR for both professionals and the public soon followed through community programs in basic life support (BLS) and advanced cardiac life support (ACLS). Standards for both BLS and ACLS were set in 1973 [12] and were updated in 1979 [13], 1985 [14], and 1992 [15].

For some individuals with adequately preserved cardiopulmonary and neurologic systems, the cessation of breathing and cardiac contraction may be reversed if CPR and definitive care are quickly available. If other systems are also spared, prolonged and vigorous life may ensue. The short period during which loss of vital signs may be reversed is often referred to as "clinical death." For clinical death to be reversed, however, ventilation and circulation must be restored before irreversible damage to vital structures occurs. The state of irreversible death is referred to as "biologic death." In difficult circumstances, the best single criterion (medical and legal) for the ultimate death of the functioning integrated human individual (i.e., the person) is brain death [16–20]. By this criterion, we can make decisions as to the appropriateness of continuing "life-sustaining" techniques.

Efficacy

The value of standardized CPR continues to undergo considerable scrutiny. Unfortunately, it appears that its efficacy is limited. Cardiopulmonary resuscitation does not seem to go be-yond the short-term sustaining of viability until definitive therapy can be administered. This was Kouwenhoven's stated goal. The benefit of rapid initiation of CPR has been demonstrated in numerous studies [21–24]. Data from prehospital care systems in Seattle showed that 43 percent of patients found in ventricular fibrillation were discharged from the hospital if CPR (i.e., BLS) was applied within 4 minutes and defibrillation (i.e., ACLS) within 8 minutes. If either was delayed, survival rates were much lower. Survival rates for patients in asystole or with pulseless electrical activity were much lower [25,26]. In a Miami study, none of the patients found in bradyarrhythmia or asystole survived, whereas 23 percent of those in ventricular fibrillation were eventually discharged [27,28]. Perhaps one of the benefits of the early initiation of CPR is the prolongation of ventricular fibrillation, thereby increasing the likelihood that ACLS with attempts at defibrillation will be successful. If the onset of CPR is delayed or if the time to defibrillation is greater than 10 minutes, the probability is greater that the victim will be in asystole or in "fine" ventricular fibrillation and will convert to asystole. Even though patients suffering cardiac arrest in the hospital can be expected to receive CPR and definitive therapy well within the 4- and 8-minute time frames, their chances of being discharged alive are generally worse than for out-of-hospital victims. This seems to be due to serious underlying medical problems [29–33].

Almost three decades ago, Pantridge and Geddes [34] introduced the "mobile intensive care unit" in Belfast, Ireland. Since then, emergency medical transport programs have spread throughout the world. In recent years there has been a move to add the capability of defibrillation to the emergency medical services system [35–38]. This is already in place in some metropolitan areas that use full paramedics. Recognizing the importance of early defibrillation, it is imperative that all first-response systems provide this necessary service, either by using emergency medical technicians capable of performing defibrillation (EMT-Ds) or by equipping and training EMTs with automatic or semiautomatic defibrillators [39–42].

Although the present approach is modestly successful for ventricular fibrillation, CPR techniques have most likely not yet been optimized, and further improvement is greatly needed [43]. Cardiac output has been measured at no better than 25 percent of normal during conventional CPR in humans [44–47]. In animal models, myocardial perfusion and coronary flow have been measured at 1 to 5 percent of normal [48–51]. Cerebral blood flow has been estimated to be 3 to 15 percent of normal when CPR is begun immediately [50,52,53], but it decreases progressively as CPR continues [54,55] and intracranial pressures rise [56,57]. Despite these pessimistic findings, complete neurologic recovery has been reported in humans even after prolonged administration of CPR [58].

Researchers continue to evaluate new approaches and techniques, and further refinements in the delivery of CPR can be expected. Although research in this area must be enthusiastically encouraged, assiduous attention to research methods and their applicability to humans is required to prevent an overly hasty and potentially injurious change in the present guidelines. The wide variety of experimental methods and models makes evaluation of apparently contradictory research results difficult. Animal preparations for research in resuscitative techniques have limited applicability to humans, largely because of differences in size and configuration of the thoracic cage. Before new CPR techniques can be reasonably endorsed, they must have been demonstrated to improve either survival or neurologic outcome. In addition, they must be simple to apply in an arrest, and, optimally, they should be simple to teach and be applicable by one rescuer without undue effort.

Mechanisms of Blood Flow during Resuscitation

Any significant improvement in CPR technique would seem to require an understanding of the mechanism by which blood flows during CPR. However, there is currently no unanimity among researchers in this area. It is of interest that significant advances seem to have been made by research groups holding very different ideas concerning the basic mechanism of blood flow during CPR. Indeed, it is possible that several mechanisms are operative; one or the other may be more important in individuals of different size and chest configuration.

CARDIAC COMPRESSION THEORY. In 1960, when Kouwenhoven et al. reported on the efficacy of closed chest cardiac massage, most accepted the theory that blood is propelled by compressing the heart "trapped between the sternum and the vertebral column" [10]. According to this theory, during sternal compression the intraventricular pressures would be expected to rise higher than the pressures elsewhere in the chest. With each sternal compression, the semilunar valves would be expected to open and the atrioventricular valves to close. With sternal release, the pressure in the ventricles would be expected to fall and the atrioventricular valves to open, allowing the heart to fill from the lungs and systemic veins. Indeed, an echocardiographic study using minipigs has shown such valve motion [59]. Although some animal studies have demonstrated pressure changes consistent with this theory [60], most have not [61]. If the cardiac compression mechanism were operative, ventilation would best be interposed between sternal compressions so as not to interfere with cardiac compression. Also, the faster the sternal compression, the higher the volume of blood flow, assuming the ventricles could fill adequately. The theory of cardiac compression was first brought into question in 1962, when Weale and Rothwell-Jackson demonstrated that during chest compression there was a rise in the venous pressure almost equal to that in the arterial pressure [62]. The following year, Wilder et al. showed that ventilating synchronously with chest compression produced higher arterial pressures than alternating ventilation and compression [63]. It was more than a decade, however, before more data confirmed these initial findings.

THORACIC PUMP THEORY. In 1976, Criley et al. [64] reported that during cardiac arrest, repeated forceful coughing was capable of generating systolic pressures comparable to those of normal cardiac activity. This finding strongly suggested that high intrathoracic pressures were capable of sustaining blood flow, independent of sternal compression. Subsequently, Niemann et al. proposed that the propulsion of blood during sternal compression was due to the same mechanism of increased intrathoracic pressure [65]. Studies using pressure measurements [66,67], angiography [68], and echocardiography [69,70] support this hypothesis. According to this theory, during CPR the heart serves only as a conduit. Forward flow is generated by a pressure gradient between intrathoracic and extrathoracic vascular structures. Flow to the arterial side is favored

by functional venous valves and greater compressibility of veins as compared to arteries at their exit points from the thorax [61,68,71,72]. The thoracic pump theory provides the rationale for experimental attempts at augmenting forward flow by increasing intrathoracic pressure.

Experimental and Alternate Techniques of Cardiopulmonary Resuscitation

Several experimental and alternate techniques of CPR are presented in Table 32-1.

OPEN CHEST CARDIOPULMONARY RESUSCITATION. One of the first forms of successful CPR was open chest CPR [92,93,94]. It was shown to be effective when definitive care was rapidly available, with survival rates, largely in operating room arrests, ranging from 16 to 37 percent [5,95,96]. Mechanistically, open chest CPR clearly involves cardiac compression without the use of a thoracic gradient. Weale and Rothwell-Jackson demonstrated lower venous pressures and higher arterial pressures than with closed chest compression [62]. There is considerable evidence that open chest CPR may be more efficacious than closed chest CPR in terms of cardiac output as well as cerebral and myocardial preservation [97,98]. Clearly, some patients with penetrating chest trauma are unlikely to respond to chest compression and are candidates for open chest CPR [46,99,100]. Several studies suggest a benefit from thoracotomy in these patients [101,102,103]. If open chest CPR is to be used, it should be used early in the sequence [104,105]. Patients with blunt chest and abdominal trauma may also be considered candidates for open chest CPR. Obviously, this technique should not be attempted unless adequate facilities and trained personnel are available.

CARDIOPULMONARY BYPASS FOR UNRESPONSIVE ARREST. Cardiopulmonary bypass is certainly not a form of routine life support; however, it has been considered a possible adjunct to artificial circulation. It is an indispensable adjunct to cardiac surgery and is being used more frequently for invasive procedures as a standby for sudden cardiac collapse. Cardiopulmonary bypass has been used in arrests unresponsive to standard CPR methods [106]. In dog models bypass has been shown capable of providing near normal end-organ blood flow with improved resuscibility and neurologic status [107–111]. Emergency bypass can be instituted with femoral artery and vein access, without thoracotomy [112]. Further study of its use in humans is necessary before it can be recommended for wider use in cardiac arrest. Obviously, its potential use is restricted to centers capable of providing this technological level of treatment. The cost necessitates careful consideration of the potential to save the patient.

Infectious Diseases and Cardiopulmonary Resuscitation

The fear provoked by the spread of human immunodeficiency virus (HIV) may lead to excessive caution when dealing with strangers; it has clearly decreased the willingness of the lay

Table 32-1. Experimental and Alternate Techniques of Cardiopulmonary Resuscitation

Reseacher	Technique	Notes
Taylor et al. (1977) [73]	Longer compression duration	Proposed use of longer duration to 40–50% of the compression-relaxation cycle.
Chandra et al. (1980) [51,74]	Simultaneous chest compression and lung inflation	High airway pressures of 60–110 mm Hg are used to augment carotid flow, requiring intubation and a mechanical ventilator. This would be an advanced life support method needing sophisticated skills and equipment; its use has not met with universal success [75,76].
Harris et al. (1967) [77,78] Redding (1971) [79] Chandra et al. (1981) [80] Koehler et al. (1983) [53]	Abdominal binding	Abdominal binding increases intrathoracic pressure by redistributing blood into the thorax during CPR. Studies have demonstrated adverse effects on coronary perfusion [81], diminished cerebral oxygenation [82], and less successful canine resuscitation [76].
Ralston et al. (1982) [83]	Interposed abdominal compression	A variation of the abdominal binding technique. The abdominal compression is released when the sternum is compressed. Higher oxygen delivery and higher cerebral and myocardial blood flows have been reported [84,85]. There is less potential for liver and gastric injury than with continuous abdominal binding [86]. A second or third rescuer is needed, the instructions are complex, and one study did not show an improvement in outcome [87]. A recent study suggested an improvement in survival and neurologic outcome [88]. Simultaneous abdominal and chest compression provided higher thoracic pressures in humans [89].
Maier et al. (1984) [60]	High-impulse cardio-pulmonary resuscitation	In dogs, peak cardiac and vascular pressures were 2–4 times greater than the corresponding intrathoracic pressures. Stroke volume and coronary blood flow were maximized with chest compression of moderate force and brief duration. At compression rates of 150 per minute, cardiac output increased as the coronary flow remained as high as 75% of prearrest values. High impulse and high compression rates can result in rescuer fatigue and increased injury.
Crul et al. (1985) [90]	Compression-ventilation sequence	Crul et al. argued that the standard sequence causes an unnecessary delay in brain perfusion and that early sternal compression might trigger heart contraction similar to a sternal thump. Lesser et al. countered that no data exist to support the clinical value of the compression-ventilation sequence [91].

public as well as health professionals to learn and perform CPR. The effect of this fear with regard to CPR is serious and must be addressed at some length [113].

The lay public's concern about infectiousness of HIV has been blamed on ignorance or mass hysteria. However, it is worth trying to place the issue in perspective. It is not unreasonable for the lay public to maintain a respectful distrust of scientific authorities when dealing with a public health issue whose existence was not even suspected 15 years ago. In the public's view, it was these same authorities who gave the blood transfusions and factor VIII infusions during the late 1970s and early 1980s that caused a significant number of HIV infections. The public's fear can be counteracted only by continued education and by stressing the facts. Health care professionals have less of an excuse to be unnecessarily frightened, but their opportunity for exposure to patients with HIV is considerable and must be adequately addressed [114].

Historically, the wide dissemination of CPR coincided with a unique period of relative freedom from fear of severe respiratory contagion. The CPR effort would have been unthinkable during earlier decades. Bacterial pneumonia, influenza, diphtheria, syphilis, tuberculosis, and poliomyelitis are a few of the deadly diseases that caused great fear and countless deaths and could easily have been spread by mouth-to-mouth ventilation. The age of powerful antibiotics and immunizations allowed us to exchange saliva with strangers in CPR classes and with victims of sudden death, with no greater concern than catching a cold or the flu. It is ironic that this freedom from fear has been dispelled by a disease that has not been shown to be transmitted by either respiratory aerosol or saliva.

Saliva has not been implicated in the transmission of HIV even after bites, percutaneous inoculation, or contamination of open wounds with saliva from HIV-infected patients [115–120]. Hepatitis B-positive saliva also has not been demonstrated to be infectious when applied to oral mucous membranes or through contamination by shared musical instruments or CPR training manikins used by hepatitis B carriers. However, it is not impossible that the mouth-to-mouth technique might result in the exchange of blood between victim and rescuer if there were open lesions or trauma to the buccal mucosa or lips. Diseases such as tuberculosis, herpes, or respiratory viral infections are potentially spread during mouth-to-mouth ventilation. The impact of these facts is different for lay people and health care professionals and different for those carrying infection and those at risk of infection [121].

IMPLICATIONS FOR RESCUERS WITH KNOWN OR POTENTIAL INFECTION. Potential rescuers who know or highly suspect they are infected with a serious pathogenic organism should not perform mouth-to-mouth ventilation if there is another rescuer who is less likely to be infectious or another immediate and effective method of ventilation, such as mechanical ventilation devices.

IMPLICATIONS FOR HEALTH CARE PROFESSIONALS. Though the probability of a rescuer becoming infected with HIV during CPR seems to be minimal, all those called on to provide CPR in the course of their employment should have ready access to mechanical ventilation devices. Bag-valve mask devices should be available as initial ventilation equipment, and early endotracheal intubation should be encouraged when equipment and trained professionals are available. Masks with one-way valves and plastic mouth and nose covers with filtered openings provide some protection from transfer of oral fluids and aerosols. S-shaped mouthpieces, masks without one-way valves, and handkerchiefs provide little if any barrier protection and should not be considered for routine use. With these guidelines in mind, health care professionals are reminded that they have a special moral and ethical obligation, and in some instances a legal obligation, to provide CPR, especially in the setting of their occupational duties.

IMPLICATIONS FOR LAY RESCUERS. There is no legal obligation for a trained lay person to provide CPR. The obligation is a moral and ethical one. The informed lay person should be motivated to perform CPR by the knowledge that a delay in initiating ventilation could result in death or disablement for an otherwise salvageable person. The potential rescuer should also recognize that the risk, even with a known HIV-positive victim, is considered very low. Lay persons should also be motivated to be trained in CPR by the knowledge that they will most often be called on to provide CPR to members of their own family or close acquaintances. A useful strategy would be to target family members of patients at increased risk of sudden cardiac death for CPR training [122,123].

IMPLICATIONS FOR MANIKIN TRAINING IN CARDIO-PULMONARY RESUSCITATION. The American Heart Association (AHA) guidelines specify that students or instructors should not actively participate in CPR training sessions with manikins if they have dermatologic lesions on their hands or in oral or circumoral areas, if they are known to be infected with hepatitis or HIV, or if they have reason to believe they are in the active stage of any infectious process. In routine ventilation training, instructors should not allow participants to exchange saliva by performing mouth-to-mouth ventilation in sequence without barrier mouth pieces. Special plastic mouth pieces and specialized manikins protect against such interchange of mucus.

TRAINING IN CARDIOPULMONARY RESUSCITATION FOR PERSONS WITH CHRONIC INFECTIONS. If a potentially infectious person is to be trained in CPR, common sense precautions should be taken to protect other participants from any risk of infection. The chronically infected individual should be given a separate manikin for practice that is adequately disinfected before anyone else uses it. The chronically infected trainee should be made aware of the preceding guidelines for potential rescuers with infections. In addition, the potential risk of infection for the immunocompromised rescuer should not be ignored.

An agency that requires successful completion of a CPR course as a prerequisite for employment must decide whether or not to waive its requirement for an employee who is unable to complete a CPR course for whatever reason. That agency also must determine whether a chronically infected individual should continue to work in a situation in which CPR administration is a duty of employment.

Standard Procedures and Team Effort

The distinctive function of the intensive care unit (ICU) is to serve as a locus of concentrated expertise in medical and nursing care, life-sustaining technologies, and treatment of complex multiorgan system derangement. Historically, it was the development of effective treatment for otherwise rapidly fatal arrhythmias during acute myocardial infarction that impelled the medical community to establish ICUs [124]. Rapid response by medical personnel has been facilitated by constant professional attendance and the development of uniform standards of resuscitation. Each member of the professional team is expected to respond according to the same standards.

The skills necessary to perform adequately during a cardiac or respiratory arrest and to interface smoothly with advanced cardiac life support techniques cannot be learned from reading texts and manuals. Cardiopulmonary resuscitation courses taught according to AHA guidelines allow hands-on experience that approximates the real situation and tests the psychomotor skills needed in an emergency. All those who engage in patient care should be trained in BLS. Those whose duties require a higher level of performance should be trained in ACLS as well. As these skills deteriorate with disuse, they need to be updated. It is worth noting that there is no "certification" in BLS or ACLS. Issuance of a "card" is neither a license to perform these techniques nor a guarantee of skill but simply an acknowledgment that an individual attended a specific course and passed the required tests. If employers or government agencies require such a card of their health workers, it is by their own mandate.

The ensuing discussion of BLS and ACLS techniques follows the recommendations and guidelines established by the AHA and presented in the 1992 Journal of the American Medical Association supplement [15]. The scientific basis and rationale behind the recommendations and guidelines are discussed in greater depth in the "Proceedings of the 1992 National Conference on Cardiopulmonary Resuscitation and Emergency Cardiac Care" [125].

Basic Life Support for Adults with an Unobstructed Airway

Basic life support is meant to support the circulation and respiration of a victim of cardiac or respiratory arrest. After recognizing and ascertaining the need, definitive help is summoned without delay and CPR is initiated.

RESPIRATORY ARREST. This may result from airway obstruction, drowning, stroke, smoke inhalation, drug overdose, electrocution, or physical trauma. In the ICU, pulmonary congestion, respiratory distress syndrome, and mucous plugs are frequent causes of primary respiratory arrests. The heart usually continues to circulate blood for several minutes, and residual oxygen in the lungs and blood may keep the brain viable. Early intervention by opening the airway and providing ventilation may prevent cardiac arrest and may be all that is required to restore spontaneous respiration. In the intubated patient, careful suctioning of the airway and attention to the ventilator settings are required.

CARDIAC ARREST. This results in rapid depletion of oxygen in vital organs. After 6 minutes brain damage is expected to occur, except in hypothermia (e.g., near drowning in cold water). Therefore, early bystander CPR (within 4 minutes) and rapid ACLS with attempted defibrillation (within 8 minutes) are essential to improve survival and neurologic recovery rates [42,126].

The sequence of steps in CPR may be summarized as the ABCs of CPR: airway, breathing, and circulation. This mnemonic device is useful in teaching the public, but it should be remembered that each step is preceded by *assessment* of the need for intervention: before opening the airway the rescuer determines unresponsiveness; before breathing the rescuer determines breathlessness; before circulation the rescuer determines pulselessness.

ASSESSMENT, DETERMINATION OF UNRESPONSIVENESS, AND ALERTING OF EMERGENCY MEDICAL SERVICES. The victim of a cardiac arrest may be found in an apparently unconscious state (i.e., an unwitnessed arrest) or may be observed to lapse suddenly into apparent unconsciousness (i.e., a witnessed arrest). In either case, the rescuer must promptly assess the victim's responsiveness by attempting to wake and communicate with the victim by tapping or gently shaking and shouting. The rescuer should summon nearby persons for help. If no other person is immediately available, the rescuer should call for emergency medical services immediately (dial 911 in most localities) and identify the location and nature of the emergency. This "phone first" dictum assumes that telephone services are reasonably close by and that emergency medical services are available (Fig. 32-1). Obviously, defibrillators and other emergency equipment should be immediately available in an ICU. More than one person should always be present so that CPR can be initiated promptly and the resuscitation team can be alerted within the first few seconds after an arrest has been recognized.

In an optimally functioning ICU, nearly all arrests should be witnessed. Early recognition of cardiac and respiratory arrests is facilitated by electronic monitoring of cardiac rhythm and often of respiratory rate and hemodynamic measurements. Video monitors often extend visual monitoring. Unfortunately, it is quite possible for a patient to become lost behind this profusion of electronic signals, the dependability of which varies widely. For several precious minutes, a heart with pulseless electrical activity will continue to provide a comforting electronic signal, while the brain suffers hypoxic damage. A high frequency of false alarms due to loose electrodes or other artifacts may dangerously raise the threshold of awareness and prolong the response time of the ICU team. The overall efficacy of monitoring devices, therefore, is highly dependent on meticulous skin preparation, care of electrodes, transducers, pressure cables, and the like.

Sudden apparent loss of consciousness, occasionally with seizures, may be the first signal of arrest and requires prompt reaction. After determining unresponsiveness, the pulse may be assessed as the next step. If the carotid pulse cannot be palpated in a 5- to 10-second period and a monitor-defibrillator is not immediately available, a precordial thump may be performed by striking the lower third of the sternum with the fist, from a height of approximately 8 inches (or the span of the stretched fingers of one hand). If the pulse does not return and a monitor defibrillator is not immediately available, the rescuer should proceed with establishing the airway (see below). If a defibrillator is immediately available, it should be used in preference to a precordial thump; this is expected to be the case in a monitored arrest in an ICU.

OPENING THE AIRWAY AND DETERMINING BREATHLESSNESS. After establishing unresponsiveness and positioning the victim on his or her back (Fig. 32-2), the next step is to open the airway and check for spontaneous breathing. In a monitored arrest with ventricular fibrillation or tachycardia this step is often taken after initial attempts to defibrillate. Meticulous attention to establishing an airway and supplying adequate ventilation is essential to any further resuscitative effort. The team leader must carefully monitor the adequacy of ventilation.

The head tilt-chin lift maneuver (Figs. 32-3 and 32-4) is usually successful in opening the airway. The head is tilted backward by a hand placed on the forehead. The fingers of the other hand are positioned under the mandible and the chin is lifted upward. The teeth are almost approximated but the mouth is not allowed to close. Because considerable cervical hyperextension occurs, this method should be avoided in patients with cervical injuries or suspected cervical injuries. The jaw thrust maneuver (Fig. 32-5) provides the safest initial approach to opening the airway of a patient with a cervical spine injury; it usually allows excellent airway opening with a minimum of cervical extension. The angles of the mandible are

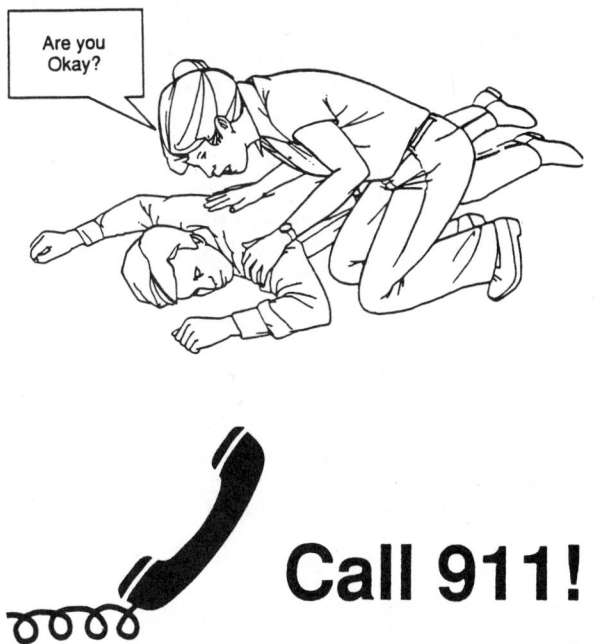

Fig. 32-1. Initial steps of cardiopulmonary resuscitation. Top. Determine unresponsiveness. Bottom. Activate the emergency medical services system. (From *Guidelines for Cardiopulmonary Resuscitation and Emergency Cardiac Care,* 1992, copyright American Medical Association. With permission.)

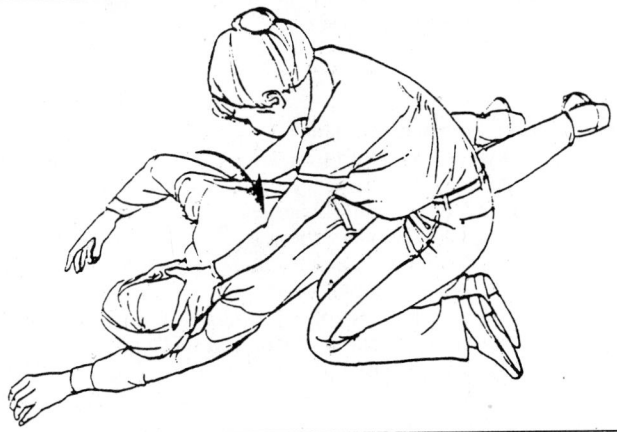

Fig. 32-2. The victim must be supine on a firm flat surface. (From *Guidelines for Cardiopulmonary Resuscitation and Emergency Cardiac Care,* 1992, copyright American Medical Association. With permission.)

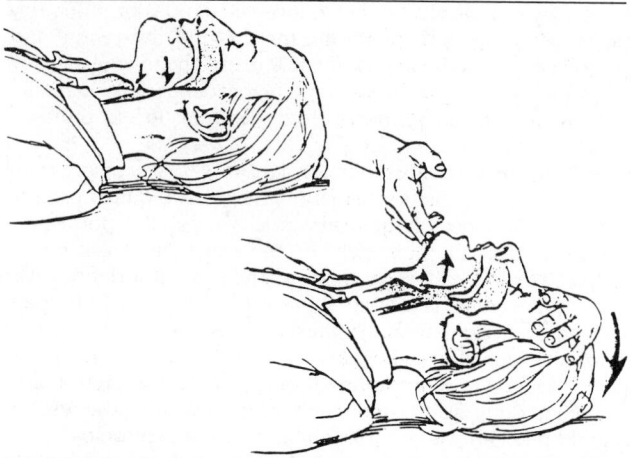

Fig. 32-3. Opening the airway. Top. Airway obstruction caused by tongue and epiglottis. Bottom. Opening the airway with the head tilt-chin lift maneuver. (From *Guidelines for Cardiopulmonary Resuscitation and Emergency Cardiac Care*, 1992, copyright American Medical Association. With permission.)

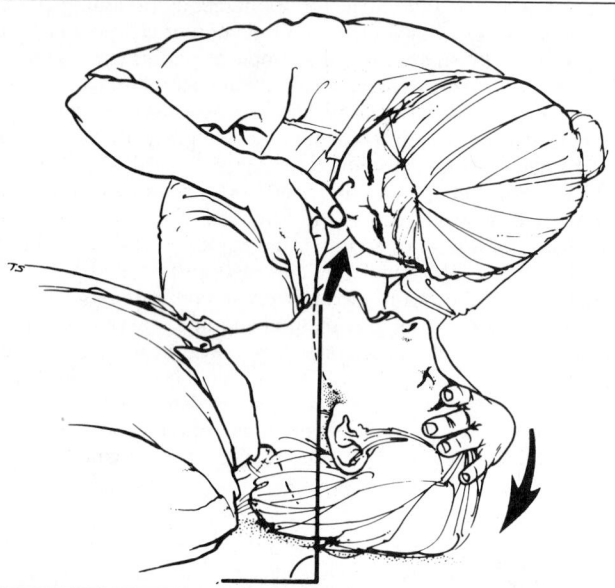

Fig. 32-4. Determining breathlessness. Open the airway and "look, listen, and feel." (From *Guidelines for Cardiopulmonary Resuscitation and Emergency Cardiac Care*, 1992, copyright American Medical Association. With permission.)

grasped with both hands and lifted upward, thus tilting the head gently backward. If mouth-to-mouth ventilation is required while the jaw thrust is being performed, the victim's nostrils must be occluded by the fleshy aspect of the rescuer's cheek.

After opening the airway, the rescuer should take 3 to 5 seconds to determine whether there is spontaneous air exchange. This is accomplished by placing an ear over the patient's mouth and nose while watching to see if the chest and abdomen rise and fall ("look, listen, and feel") (Fig. 32-4). If the rescuer fails to see movement, hear respiration, and feel the rush of air against the ear and cheek, rescue breathing should be initiated.

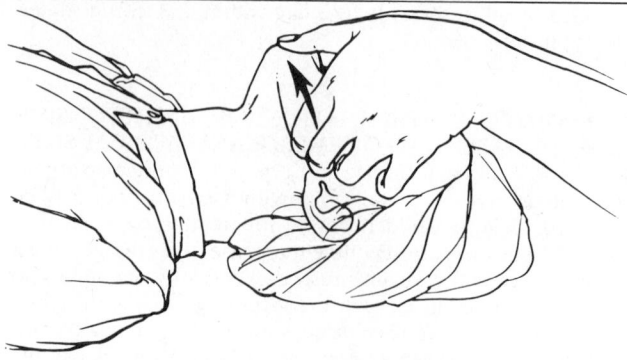

Fig. 32-5. Jaw thrust maneuver. Opening the airway with minimum extension of the neck. (From Standards and guidelines for CPR and ECC. *JAMA* 255:2843, 1986. With permission.)

RESCUE BREATHING. If spontaneous breathing is absent, rescue breathing must be initiated (Fig. 32-6). If equipment is immediately available and the rescuer is trained, intubation and ventilatory adjuncts should be used initially; otherwise, the victim's nostrils are pinched with thumb and forefinger and mouth-to-mouth ventilation is begun. The rescuer takes a deep breath and makes a tight seal over the victim's mouth. The rescuer breathes into the victim's mouth twice, completely refilling his or her lungs after each breath. Each breath should be delivered over 1.5 to 2 seconds, allowing the victim's lungs to deflate between breaths. Thereafter, the rate of 12 breaths per minute is maintained for as long as necessary, with tidal volumes of 800 to 1200 cc. Delivering the breath over 1.5 second or more prevents gastric insufflation. Melker et al. [127,128,129] demonstrated airway pressures well in excess of those required to open the lower esophageal sphincter when quick breaths are used to ventilate patients. If the victim wears dentures, they are usually best left in place to assist in forming an adequate seal. As soon as possible, airway adjuncts with 100 percent delivered oxygen are substituted for mouth-to-mouth ventilation.

If air cannot be passed into the victim's lungs, another attempt at opening the airway should be made. The jaw thrust maneuver may be necessary. If subsequent attempts at ventilation are still unsuccessful, the victim should be considered to have an obstructed airway and attempts should be made to dislodge a potential foreign body obstruction.

Mouth-to-nose ventilation may be necessary in cases of severe facial trauma or trismus (Fig. 32-6 center). The head tilt-chin lift maneuver is used to open the airway while the rescuer's mouth forms a seal over the victim's nose. During delivery of air, the victim's mouth is occluded, using the palm of the hand if necessary. During exhalation, the mouth is allowed to reopen so that the soft palate does not obstruct the airflow through the nasopharynx.

If a tracheostomy tube is in place, direct application of mouth-to-stoma ventilation is necessary until ventilatory adjuncts are available (Fig. 32-6 bottom). Unless there is a cuff on the tracheostomy tube that can be inflated, the victim's mouth must be occluded with one hand throughout the ventilatory cycle. Mouth-to-stoma ventilation is also preferable if the victim has an established tracheostomy stoma.

DETERMINING PULSELESSNESS. In the adult, the absence of a central pulse is best determined by palpating the carotid

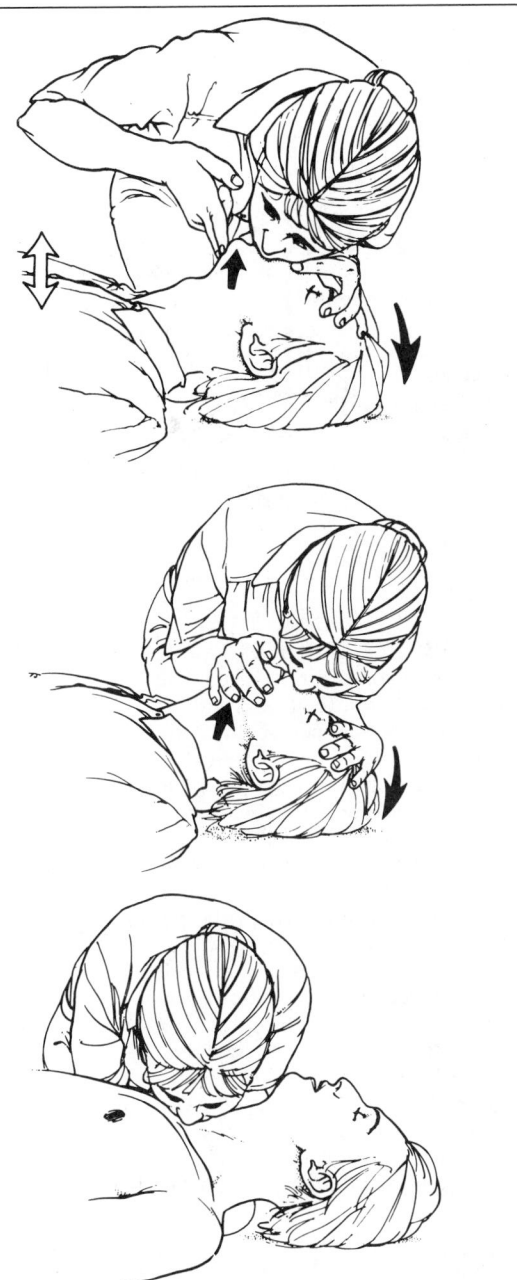

Fig. 32-6. Rescue breathing. Top. Mouth-to-mouth. Center. Mouth-to-nose. Bottom. Mouth-to-stoma. (From *Cardiopulmonary Resuscitation*. Washington, DC, American Red Cross, 1981. Courtesy of the American Red Cross. All rights reserved in all countries.)

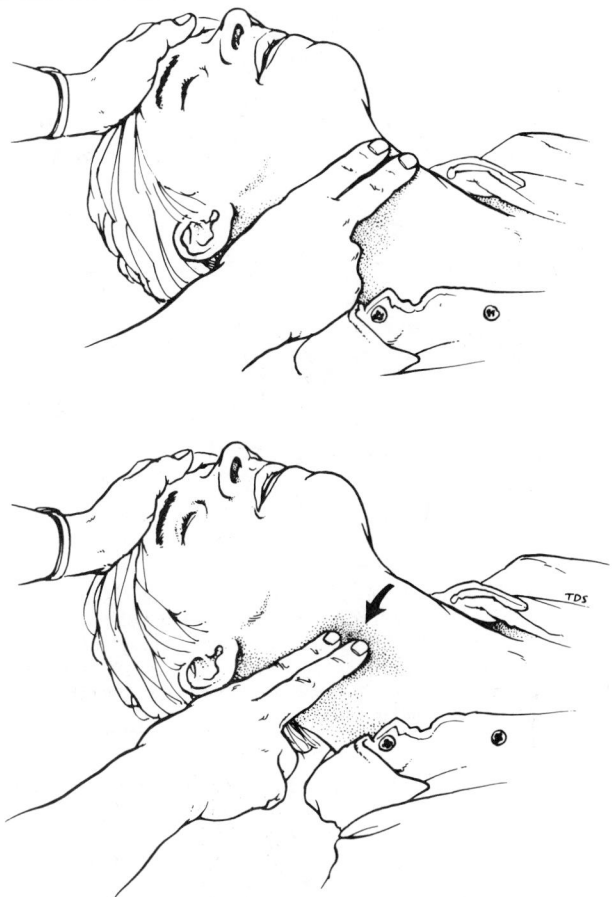

Fig. 32-7. Determining pulselessness. Top. Feeling the laryngeal cartilage. Bottom. Fingers slide into groove between treachea and sternomastoid muscle, searching for carotid pulse. (From Standards and guidelines for CPR and ECC. *JAMA* 255:2843, 1986. With permission.)

artery (Fig. 32-7), although rarely the carotid artery may be absent because of localized obstruction. If a pulse is not felt after 10 seconds of careful searching, chest compression is initiated, unless electrical countershock for ventricular arrhythmia or artificial pacing for asystole is immediately available.

CHEST COMPRESSION. Artificial circulation depends on adequate chest compression through sternal depression. The safest manner of depressing the sternum is with the heel of the rescuer's hand on the lower half of the sternum, with the fingers

kept off the rib cage (Fig. 32-8). It is usually most effective to cover the heel of one hand with the heel of the other, the heel being parallel to the long axis of the sternum. If the rescuer's hands are placed either too high or too low on the sternum, or if the fingers are allowed to lie flat against the rib cage, broken ribs and organ laceration can result.

The rescuer's elbows should be kept locked and the arms straight, with the shoulders directly over the patient's sternum (Fig. 32-9). This position allows the rescuer's upper body to provide a perpendicularly directed force for sternal depression. The sternum is depressed 1.5 to 2 inches (3.9–3.75 cm) at a rate of 80 to 100 per minute. At the end of each compression, pressure is released and the sternum is allowed to return to its normal position, without removing the hand from the sternum. Equal time should be allotted to compression and relaxation with smooth movements, avoiding jerking or bouncing the sternum. Manual and automatic chest compressors for fatigue-free sternal compression are used by some emergency medical services crews and emergency room and ICU personnel. Whether using hinged manually operated devices or compressed air-powered plungers, the rescuer must be constantly vigilant about proper placement and adequacy of sternal compression. An experimental device using a suction plunger-like device may improve flows by facilitating sternal rebound and thoracic

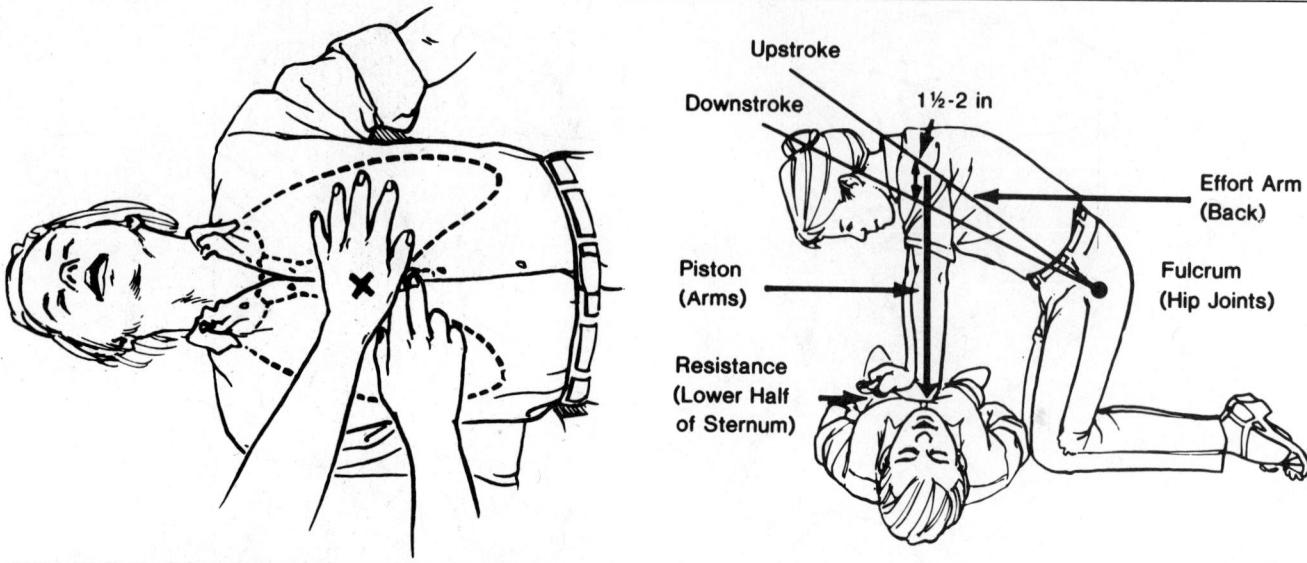

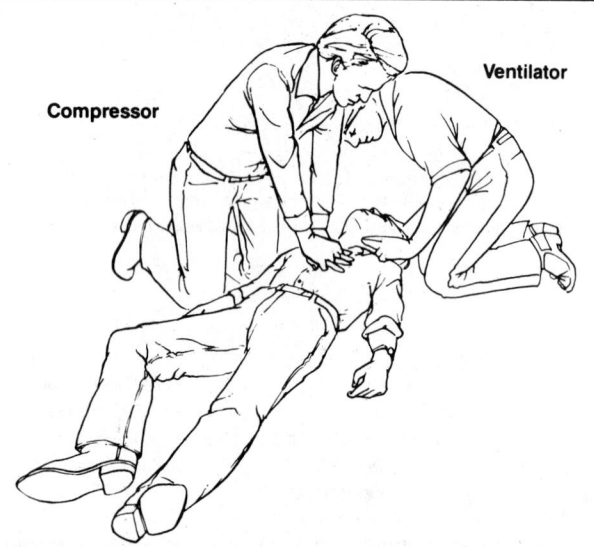

Fig. 32-8. External chest compression. Left. Locating the proper hand position on the lower half of the sternum. Right. Proper position of the rescuer, with shoulders directly over the victim's sternum and elbows locked. (From *Cardiopulmonary Resuscitation*. Washington, DC, American Red Cross, 1987, p. 95. Courtesy of the American Red Cross. All rights reserved in all countries.)

Fig. 32-9. Two-rescuer CPR. The ventilator assesses the victim while the compressor assumes the proper position for external chest compressions. (Reproduced with permission. *Healthcare Provider's Manual for Basic Life Support*. 1988. Copyright American Heart Association.)

vascular filling; this has been referred to as "active compression–decompression CPR" [130,130a,130b].

Ventilation and sternal compression should not be interrupted for longer than 7 seconds to check on the return of a pulse, except under special circumstances. Warranted interruptions include execution of ACLS procedures (e.g., endotracheal intubation, placement of central venous lines) or an absolute need to move the patient. Even in these limited circumstances, CPR should not be interrupted longer than 30 seconds.

TWO-RESCUER CARDIOPULMONARY RESUSCITATION.
The combination of artificial ventilation and circulation can be delivered more efficiently and with less fatigue by two rescuers. One rescuer, positioned at the victim's side, performs sternal compressions while the other, positioned at the victim's head, maintains an open airway and performs ventilation (Fig. 32-10). This technique should be mastered by all health care workers called on to perform CPR. Lay persons have not been routinely taught this method, in the interest of improving retention of basic skills. The compression rate for two-rescuer CPR, as for one-rescuer CPR, is 80 to 100 per minute. To ensure adequate time (1.5–2 seconds) for filling the lungs, a pause for a breath should be allowed after each fifth compression [129]. Exhalation occurs during chest compressions. When the rescuer performing compressions is tired, the two rescuers should switch responsibilities, with the minimal possible delay.

The effectiveness of chest compressions should be monitored by the ventilating rescuer feeling the carotid pulse. Chest compressions should be stopped for 5 seconds after the first minute and every few minutes thereafter to determine whether spontaneous breathing and circulation have resumed.

COMPLICATIONS OF BASIC LIFE SUPPORT PROCEDURES. Proper application of CPR should minimize serious complications, but serious risks are inherent in BLS procedures and should be accepted in the context of cardiac arrest. Awareness of these potential complications is important in the post-resuscitative care of the arrest victim.

Gastric distention and regurgitation are common complications of artificial ventilation without endotracheal intubation. These complications are more likely to occur when ventilation pressures exceed the opening pressure of the lower esophageal sphincter [131,132]. In mouth-to-mouth ventilation, 1.5 to 2 seconds should be allowed for air delivery to the lungs to prevent airway pressures from exceeding 20 to 25 cm H_2O. "Staircase ventilation," or breathing rapidly without allowing full exhalation, should be avoided for the same reason. To avoid causing regurgitation and aspiration no attempts should be made to relieve gastric distention unless it is so severe that it interferes with adequate ventilation. If ventilation appears to be severely compromised, BLS should be interrupted briefly while the victim is rolled on the side and moderate pressure is applied over

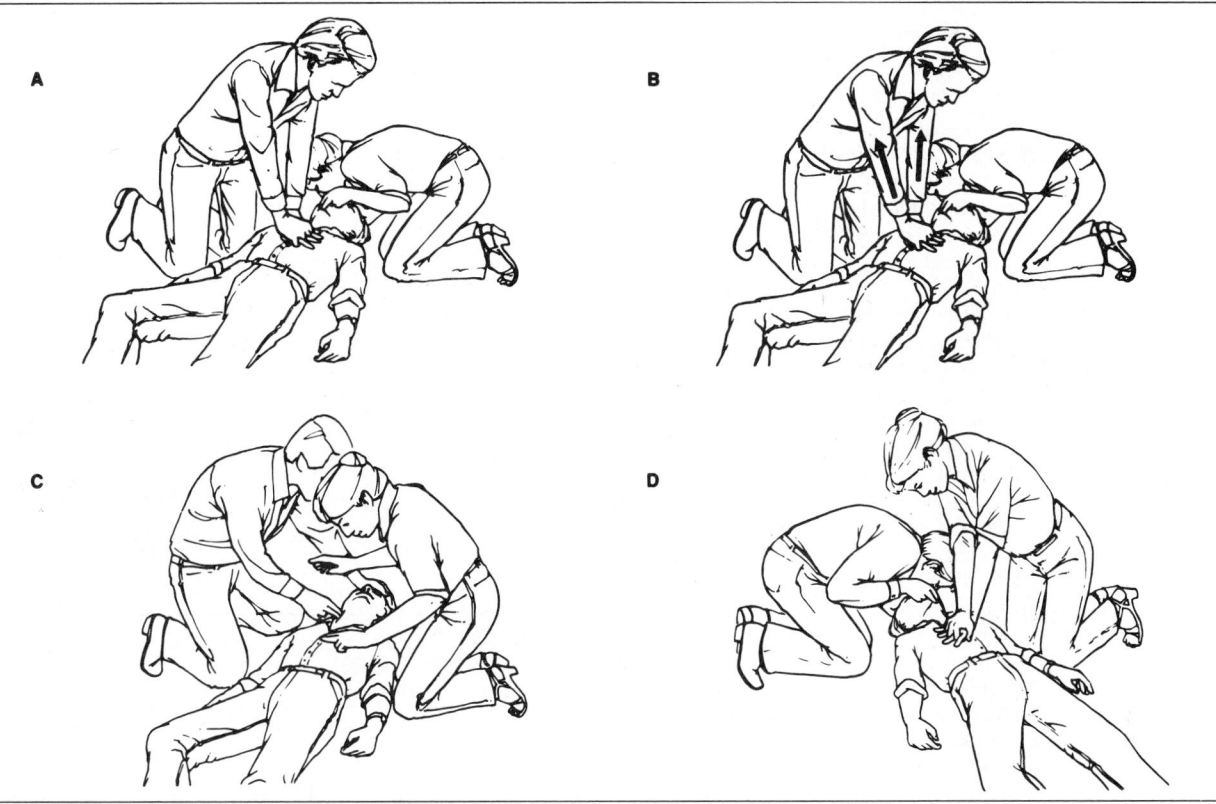

Fig. 32-10. Switching responsibilities in two-rescuer CPR. A. Compressor indicates desire to switch, "Change and two, and three and, four and, five." B. Ventilator delivers a rescue breath after the fifth compression. C. Ventilator moves to the victim's chest and finds proper position while the compressor moves to the victim's head and checks for spontaneous breathing and pulse. D. The new ventilator delivers a breath, signaling need for a new cycle of compressions and ventilations in a 5:1 ratio. (Reproduced with permission. *Healthcare Provider's Manual for Basic Life Support.* 1988. Copyright American Heart Association.)

the epigastrium to expel some of the accumulated air. If regurgitation occurs, the vomitus should be allowed to drain from the mouth while the victim is lying on the side. After removing residual vomitus and clearing the mouth, the victim is repositioned and CPR is reinstituted immediately. While an esophageal obturator airway may decrease the threat of distention and regurgitation during its use, the risk is increased at the time of its removal. To obviate this risk, the trachea should be intubated and protected with an inflated cuff before the esophageal cuff is deflated and the esophageal obturator removed.

Complications of sternal compression and manual thrusts include rib and sternal fractures, costochondral separation, flail chest, pneumothorax, hemothorax, hemopericardium, subcutaneous emphysema, mediastinal emphysema, pulmonary contusions, bone marrow and fat embolism, as well as lacerations of esophagus, stomach, inferior vena cava, liver, or spleen [133,134,135]. While rib fractures are common during CPR, especially in the elderly, no serious sequelae are likely unless tension pneumothorax occurs and is ignored. The more serious complications are unlikely to occur in CPR if proper hand position is maintained and exaggerated depth of sternal compression is avoided. Overzealous or repeated abdominal or chest thrusts for relief of airway obstruction are more likely to cause

fractures or lacerations. For this reason, abdominal thrust is not recommended for infants less than 1 year of age.

MONITORING THE EFFECTIVENESS OF BASIC LIFE SUPPORT. The victim should be monitored for resumption of spontaneous breathing and circulation after the first minute and every few minutes thereafter. Chest compression must be stopped for 5 seconds and breathlessness and pulselessness rechecked as noted previously.

The effectiveness of the rescue effort is assessed regularly by the ventilating rescuer, who notes the chest motion and escape of expired air. Adequacy of circulation is assessed by noting an adequate carotid pulse with sternal compressions.

Animal studies suggest that the best guidelines to the efficacy of ongoing CPR efforts are aortic diastolic pressure and myocardial perfusion pressure (aortic diastolic minus right atrial diastolic) [48,79,136–140]. In instrumented patients for whom systemic arterial pressure (with or without central venous pressure) is available, attempts should be made to optimize myocardial perfusion pressure during CPR.

Pupillary response, if present, is a good indicator of cerebral circulation. However, fixed and dilated pupils should not be accepted as evidence for irreversible or biologic death. Ocular pathology, such as cataracts, and a variety of drugs (e.g., atropine and ganglion-blocking agents) interfere with the pupillary light reflex. The decision to cease BLS should be made only by the physician in charge of the resuscitation effort; this decision should not be made until it is obvious that the victim's cardiovascular system will not respond with return of spontaneous circulation to adequate administration of ACLS, including electrical and pharmacologic interventions. Remediable problems, such as airway obstruction, severe hypovolemia, and pericardial tamponade, should also have been reasonably excluded by careful attention to ACLS protocols.

Pediatric Resuscitation

The majority of infants and children who require resuscitation have had a primary respiratory arrest. Cardiac arrest results from the ensuing hypoxia and acidosis; therefore, the focus of pediatric resuscitation is airway maintenance and ventilation. The outcomes for CPR in children with cardiac arrest are poor because the cessation of cardiac activity is usually the manifestation of prolonged hypoxia. Brain damage is, therefore, all too common. Respiratory arrest, if treated before cessation of cardiac activity has supervened, carries a much better prognosis [141,142]. It is for this reason that it is recommended to provide the initial steps of CPR for infants and children before taking time to telephone for emergency assistance. The first minute of CPR will allow opening of the airway and beginning of artificial ventilation. If an obstructed airway is found, attempts at dislodging a foreign body will not be delayed.

Effective techniques for ventilation and chest compression vary with the child's size. Infant procedures are applicable to patients who appear to be younger than 1 year of age. Child techniques are applicable to patients who appear to be 1 to 8 years of age. Adult techniques are appropriate for patients who appear older than 8 years of age.

If the child is found to be apneic, the patient is placed in the supine position and the head tilt-chin lift maneuver is used to open the airway (Fig. 32-11). Overextension of the neck is unnecessary and best avoided. Some believe overextension of the child's flexible neck may obstruct the trachea; however, there are no data to support this. The jaw thrust should be used if an adequate airway is not obtained with the head tilt-chin lift maneuver or if neck injury is suspected.

Artificial ventilation of the infant requires the rescuer's mouth

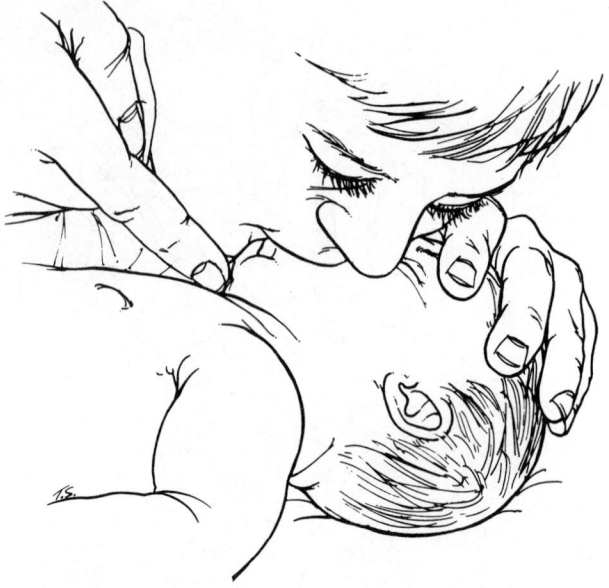

Fig. 32-12. Rescue breathing in infant: mouth-to-mouth and nose seal. (From Standards and guidelines for CPR and ECC. *JAMA* 255:2843, 1986. With permission.)

to cover both the mouth and nose to make an effective seal (Fig. 32-12). If the child's face is too large to form a tight seal over both nose and mouth, the mouth alone is covered, as for the adult.

The lung volume of the infant or small child is small enough that a "puff" of air from the rescuer's mouth might be adequate to inflate the lungs. However, the smaller diameter of the tracheobronchial tree and any pulmonary disease that may be contributing to the arrest usually provides considerable resistance to airflow. Therefore, a surprising amount of inspiratory pressure may be needed to move adequate air into the lungs. This is especially true for the child who may have edematous respiratory passages. Accordingly, adequacy of ventilation must be monitored by observing the rise and fall of the chest and by feeling and listening for exhaled air from the mouth and nose. Excessive ventilatory volumes may exceed esophageal opening pressure and cause gastric distention.

Gastric decompression is dangerous and should be avoided until the patient has been intubated and the cuff inflated to protect the respiratory tract from aspiration. If gastric distention is so severe that ventilation is greatly compromised, the child's body should be turned to one side before pressure on the abdomen is applied. It is preferable to use a gastric tube with suction whenever possible.

The ventilation rate for infants is 20 per minute (once every 3 seconds) and for children is 15 per minute (once every 4 seconds). Adolescents are ventilated at the adult rate of 12 per minute (once every 5 seconds). If artificial circulation is not necessary, more rapid ventilatory rates are acceptable. However, if the airway is unprotected, 1 to 1.5 seconds should be taken to fill the lungs of the infant or child. This is faster than in adults or adolescents because less volume is required.

Artificial circulation is instituted in the absence of a palpable pulse. The pulse of the larger child or adolescent can easily be detected at the carotid artery, as in the adult. The neck of the infant, however, is too short and fat for reliable palpation of the carotid artery. Palpation of the precordium is also unreliable; some infants have no precordial impulse in spite of ade-

Fig. 32-11. Head tilt-chin lift in infant: opening the airway. (From Standards and guidelines for CPR and ECC. *JAMA* 255:2843, 1986. With permission.)

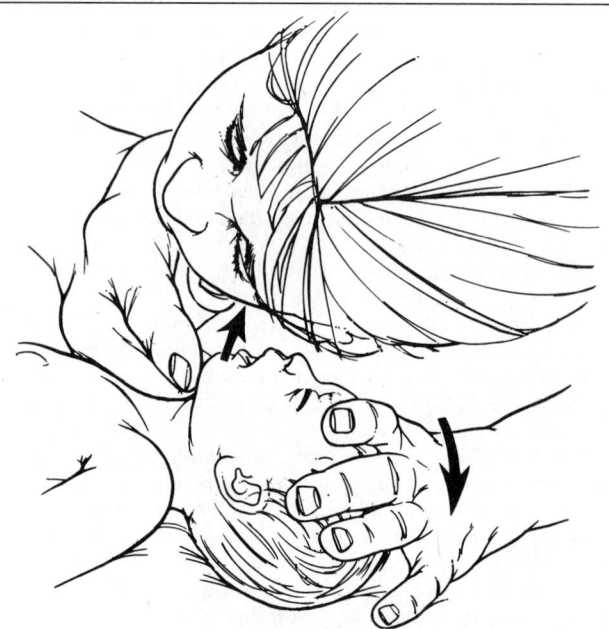

quate cardiac output. It is recommended, therefore, that the presence of an infant's pulse be determined by palpating the brachial artery between the elbow and shoulder.

To apply chest compression in an infant, the rescuer's index finger is placed on the sternum, just below the intermammary line. The proper area for compression is one finger's breadth below the intermammary line on the lower sternum, at the location of the middle and ring fingers (Fig. 32-13). Using two or three fingers, the sternum is compressed 0.5 to 1 inch (1.25–2.5 cm). For the child, the heel of one hand is positioned on the lower third of the sternum (Fig. 32-14). The sternum is compressed 1 to 1.5 inches (2.5–3.75 cm). The frequency of sternal compressions for infants and children is 100 per minute. The ratio of compressions to ventilations is 5:1 for all ages (except adults and larger children, when a single rescuer will follow a 15:2 ratio).

Fig. 32-13. Locating finger position for sternal compression in infant, using an imaginary line between the nipples. (From Standards and guidelines for CPR and ECC. *JAMA* 255:2843, 1986. With permission.)

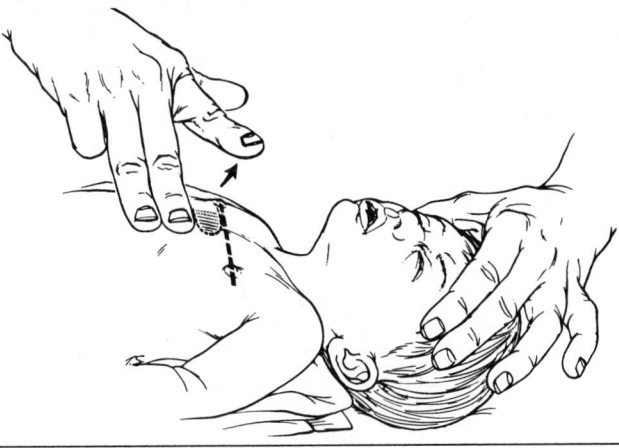

Fig. 32-14. Locating hand position for sternal compression in child: using heel of one hand. (From Standards and guidelines for CPR and ECC. *JAMA* 255:2843, 1986. With permission.)

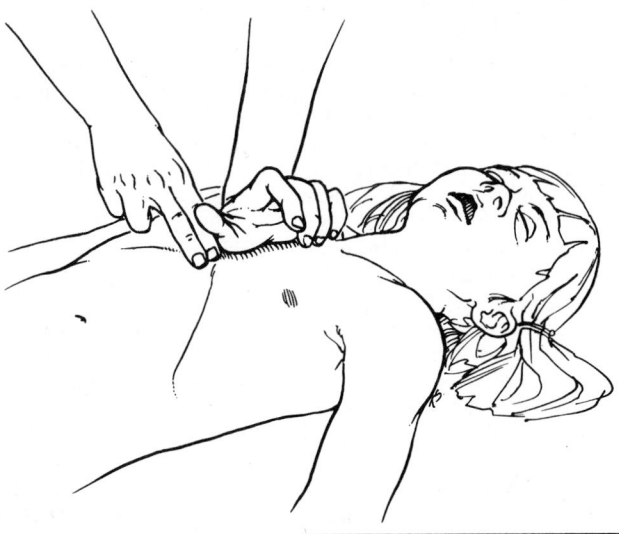

Obstructed Airway

An unconscious patient can develop airway obstruction when the tongue falls backward into the pharynx. Alternatively, the epiglottis may block the airway when pharyngeal muscles are lax. In the sedated or ill patient, regurgitation of stomach contents into the pharynx is a frequent cause of respiratory arrest. Blood clots from head and facial injuries are another source of pharyngeal and upper airway obstruction. Even otherwise healthy individuals may develop foreign body obstruction from poorly chewed food, large wads of gum, and so forth. The combination of attempting to swallow unchewed food, drinking alcohol, and laughing is particularly conducive to pharyngeal obstruction. Children's smaller airways are likely to obstruct with small nuts or candies. Children are also prone to obstruct their airways by placing toys or objects such as marbles or beads in their mouths.

Victims of partial obstruction with reasonable gas exchange should be encouraged to continue breathing efforts with attempts at coughing. The emergency medical services system should be called and the patient monitored until the obstruction can be properly visualized. This is best performed in a facility in which suction, intubation, and possible tracheostomy can be performed. A patient whose obstruction is so severe that air exchange is obviously markedly impaired (cyanosis with lapsing consciousness) should be treated as having complete obstruction.

Victims of complete obstruction may still be conscious. They are unable to cough or vocalize. A subdiaphragmatic abdominal thrust (Heimlich maneuver) may force air from the lungs in sufficient quantity to expel a foreign body from the airway [143,144].

If the victim is still standing, the rescuer stands behind the victim and wraps his or her arms around the victim's waist. The fist of one hand is placed with the thumb side against the victim's abdomen in the midline slightly above the navel and well below the xiphoid process (Fig. 32-15). The fist is grasped with the other hand and quickly thrust inward and upward. It may be necessary to repeat the thrust 6 to 10 times to clear the airway. Each thrust should be a separate and distinct movement.

If the patient is unconscious or lying down, he or she should be positioned in the supine position with the face up (Fig. 32-16). The rescuer kneels astride the victim's thighs and places the heel of one hand against the victim's abdomen, slightly above the navel and well below the xiphoid process. The other hand is placed directly on top of the first and pressed inward and upward with separate quick forceful thrusts.

In the unconscious patient a finger sweep should be used to attempt to dislodge the foreign body if it remains lodged after multiple subdiaphragmatic abdominal thrusts. With the face up, the victim's mouth is opened by grasping the lower jaw and tongue with the thumb and fingers. The jaw is lifted upward (tongue-jaw lift). The index finger of the other hand is inserted down along the inside of the cheek, deeply to the base of the tongue. A hooking action is used to maneuver the foreign body into the mouth, where it can be removed. Blind finger sweeps should be avoided in infants and children because it is more likely that a foreign object or swollen epiglottis will be pushed further into the airway. The tongue-jaw lift should be used and may in itself partially relieve the obstruction. If a foreign body is visualized, however, it should be grasped and removed.

If attempted rescue breathing in an arrested patient fails to move air into the lungs, an obstructed airway must be presumed to be present. It may simply be due to the tongue or epiglottis, rather than a foreign body. If the airway remains closed after repositioning the head, other maneuvers to open the airway,

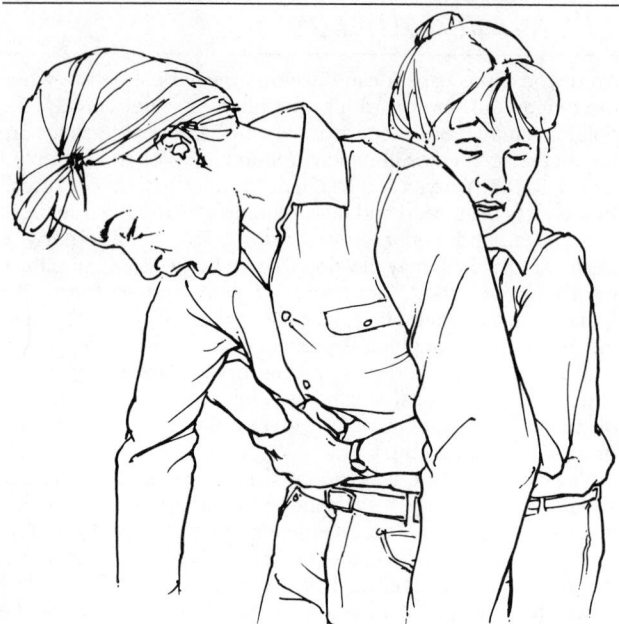

Fig. 32-15. Abdominal thrust with conscious victim standing: rescuer standing behind victim of foreign body airway obstruction. From Standards and guidelines for CPR and ECC. *JAMA* 255:2843, 1986. With permission.)

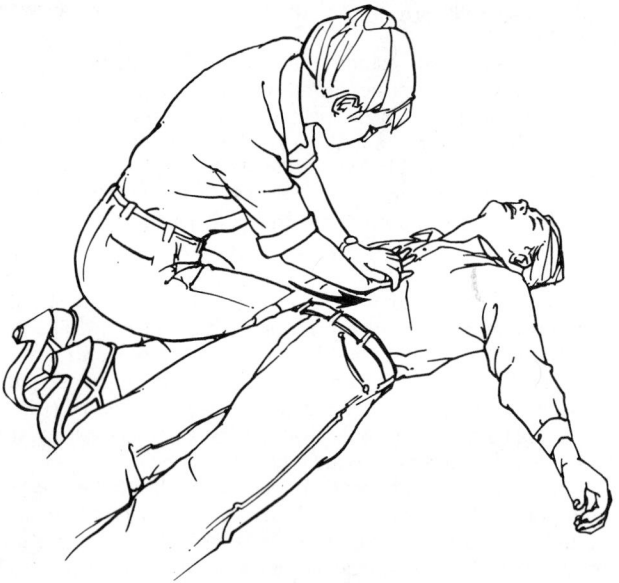

Fig. 32-16. Abdominal thrust with unconscious victim: victim of foreign body airway obstruction lying supine. (From Standards and guidelines for CPR and ECC. *JAMA* 255:2843, 1986. With permission.)

including the jaw thrust and tongue-jaw lift, must be used. If the airway remains obstructed, subdiaphragmatic abdominal thrusts are used, as described previously. Careful suction and direct visualization are also used when available.

Chest thrusts may be substituted for abdominal thrusts in women in advanced stages of pregnancy, in patients with severe ascites, or in the markedly obese. The fist is placed in the midsternum for the erect and conscious patient. For the supine victim, the hand is positioned on the lower sternum, as for

external cardiac compression. Each thrust is delivered slowly and distinctly.

If attempts at dislodging a foreign body or relieving airway obstruction fail, advanced procedures are necessary to provide oxygenation until direct visualization, intubation, or tracheostomy is accomplished.

Advanced Cardiac Life Support in Adults

The use of adjunctive equipment, more specialized techniques, and pharmacologic and electrical therapy in the treatment of cardiac or respiratory arrest victims is generally referred to as ACLS. These techniques and their interface with BLS and the emergency medical services system are considered in the AHA's ACLS teaching program [145]. An improvement in survival after in-hospital cardiac arrest was demonstrated after medical house officers were trained in ACLS [146]. An in-depth discussion is available in the ACLS text published by the American Heart Association.

The focus of the following sections is on the techniques and medications used in initial resuscitative efforts. The demarcation from therapies more commonly reserved for the ICU is often indistinct; indeed, it is expected to vary with the experience of the prehospital team and the degree of physician supervision. In general, most ACLS measures should be applied by trained individuals operating within an emergency medical services system in the community, in transport, as well as in the hospital setting.

AIRWAY AND VENTILATORY SUPPORT. Oxygenation and optimal ventilation are prerequisites of successful resuscitation. Ventilation with the rescuer's exhaled breath, which provides 16 to 17 percent oxygen, may produce an alveolar partial pressure of oxygen (PaO_2) of 80 mm Hg. Arterial hypoxemia is inevitable because of diminished cardiac output (including pulmonary blood flow), intrapulmonary shunting, and ventilation-perfusion (V/Q) mismatch. Therefore, supplemental oxygen should be administered as soon as it becomes available, beginning with 100 percent. In the period following a successful resuscitation, the amount of administered oxygen may be decreased as guided by the arterial blood partial pressure of oxygen (PaO_2).

Emergency ventilation performed in the hospital or by emergency medical services personnel commonly begins with the combined use of a mask and oral airway. Mouth-to-mask ventilation is very effective, as long as an adequate seal is maintained between the mask and face. Most masks are best fitted by flaring the top and molding it over the bridge of the nose. The inflated rim is then carefully molded to the cheeks as the mask is allowed to recoil. Relatively firm pressure is required to maintain the seal. Masks with one-way valves also provide a measure of isolation from the victim's saliva and breath aerosol. Bag-valve-mask ventilation requires strong hands and a self-inflating bag. The bag should be connected to a gas reservoir and oxygen so that 100 percent oxygen delivery can be approximated. It cannot be overemphasized that the success of this method depends on airway patency and an adequate seal between the mask and face. Equally important is adequate compression of the bag to deliver the required tidal volume. It is advisable that everyone who uses this technique practice on a recording ventilating manikin to assess the adequacy of the method in their hands. Many people discover that their hands are not large enough or strong enough to deliver 800 to 1200 cc of air. Some may have to squeeze the bag between their elbow and chest wall to supply adequate ventilation. If two people are available to ventilate, one should secure the mask while the other uses both hands to attend to the bag.

The mask design should include the following features:

The use of transparent material, which allows the rescuer to assess lip color and to observe vomitus, mucus, or other obstructing material in the patient's airway

A cushioned rim around the mask's perimeter to conform to the patient's face and to facilitate a tight seal

A standard 15- to 22-mm connector, which allows the use of additional airway equipment

A comfortable fit to the rescuer's hand

An oxygen insufflation inlet, which allows oxygen supplementation during mouth-to-mask ventilation

A one-way valve, which allows some protection from the patient's breath and aerosol during mouth-to-mask ventilation

Availability in appropriate sizes and shapes, for various sized faces. Most adults are accommodated by a standard medium-sized (no. 4) oval-shaped mask.

Ventilating bags must be designed to include the following features:

A self-refilling bag, which allows operation independent of a fresh gas source (often called Ambu bags)

A fresh gas inlet, which allows ambient air or supplemental oxygen to flow into the reservoir bag through a valve inlet

A nipple for oxygen connection, located near the gas inlet valve

A reservoir bag that is easy to clean and sterilize without damaging it

Availability in pediatric and adult sizes

A non-rebreathing valve, directing flow to the patient during inhalation and to the atmosphere during exhalation. The valve casing should be transparent to allow visual inspection of its function. It should be easy to clean and assemble. A pop-off feature is often present to prevent inadvertently high airway pressures; however, such valves should have provision to override the pop-off feature because higher airway pressures are sometimes required to ventilate lungs with unusually high resistances, especially in children.

Reservoir tubing that can be attached to the fresh gas inlet valve, which allows an accumulation of oxygen to refill the reservoir bag during the refill cycle. Such a reservoir allows delivered oxygen to approach 100 percent; without it the self-refilling bag can deliver only 40 to 50 percent oxygen.

Oxygen-powered resuscitators allow the pressure of compressed oxygen tanks at 50 psi to drive lung inflation. They are usually triggered by a manual control button, and the oxygen can be delivered through a mask or tube for ease of ventilation. These devices deliver oxygen at a flow rate of 100 liters per minute and allow airway pressures of 60 cm H_2O. However, when used with masks and unprotected airways (not separated from the esophagus by an inflated cuff), these devices are likely to cause gastric distention and poor ventilation. They are not as reliable as mouth-to-mask or bag-valve-mask ventilation. When used in adults, they should be recalibrated to deliver flows of no more than 40 liters per minute, to avoid opening the lower esophageal sphincter. A relief valve that opens at approximately 60 cm H_2O and vents any excess volume into the atmosphere should be present. In addition, an audible alarm

that sounds whenever the relief valve pressure is exceeded should be present. This alarm warns the rescuer that the victim requires higher inspiratory pressures and may not be adequately ventilated. Barotrauma is likely to occur in infants and children. Children often have high airway resistances and are difficult to ventilate with these resuscitators. These devices should be avoided in general and should not be used with infants or children.

Endotracheal intubation is required if the patient cannot be rapidly resuscitated or when adequate spontaneous ventilation does not resume quickly. Experienced personnel should attempt intubation. The patient should be hyperventilated before each attempt, and resuscitative efforts should not be interrupted by more than 30 seconds with each attempt. Cricoid pressure should be applied, when possible, by a second person during endotracheal intubation to protect against regurgitation of gastric contents. The prominence inferior to that of the thyroid cartilage is the cricoid cartilage. Downward pressure should be applied with the thumb and index finger (Fig. 32-17) until the cuff of the endotracheal tube is inflated [131,147].

Once the victim is intubated and the trachea is protected from regurgitation, faster inspiratory flow rates are possible and ventilations may be more frequent and asynchronous with the compressions. Under these circumstances, ventilations more rapid than 12 to 15 per minute are advisable in an attempt to hyperventilate and improve carbon dioxide removal.

Some prehospital emergency medical services use esophageal obturator airways, designed to be inserted blindly through the victim's mouth into the esophagus. Once the device has been positioned in the esophagus, the distal balloon is inflated, occluding the esophagus. The lungs are ventilated through proximal holes in the pharynx. Several modifications are available. The esophageal gastric tube airway allows decompression of the stomach through a gastric lumen. Should a patient arrive in the emergency room with either of these devices in place, endotracheal intubation should be performed and the cuff inflated before the esophageal obturator is removed. Vomiting is common after removal of such a device. The data regarding the adequacy of oxygenation with these devices compared to endotracheal intubation are conflicting [148–151]. Endotracheal intubation is the much preferred technique, and time should be taken to teach it well to paramedics and emergency personnel who are called upon to ventilate patients.

Fig. 32-17. Cricoid pressure: application of downward pressure over the cricoid with neck extended. (From Sellick BA: Cricoid pressure to control regurgitation of stomach contents during induction of anesthesia. *Lancet* 2:404, 1961. With permission.)

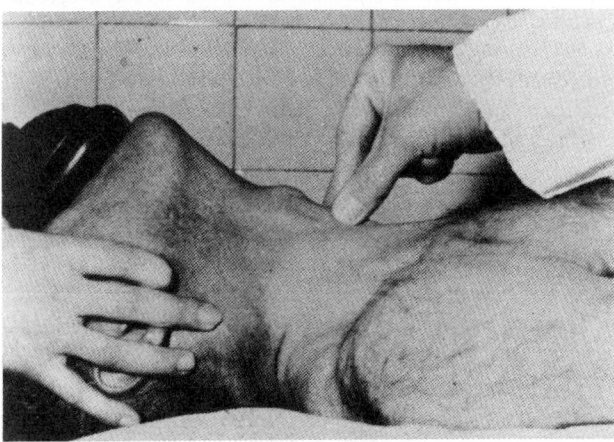

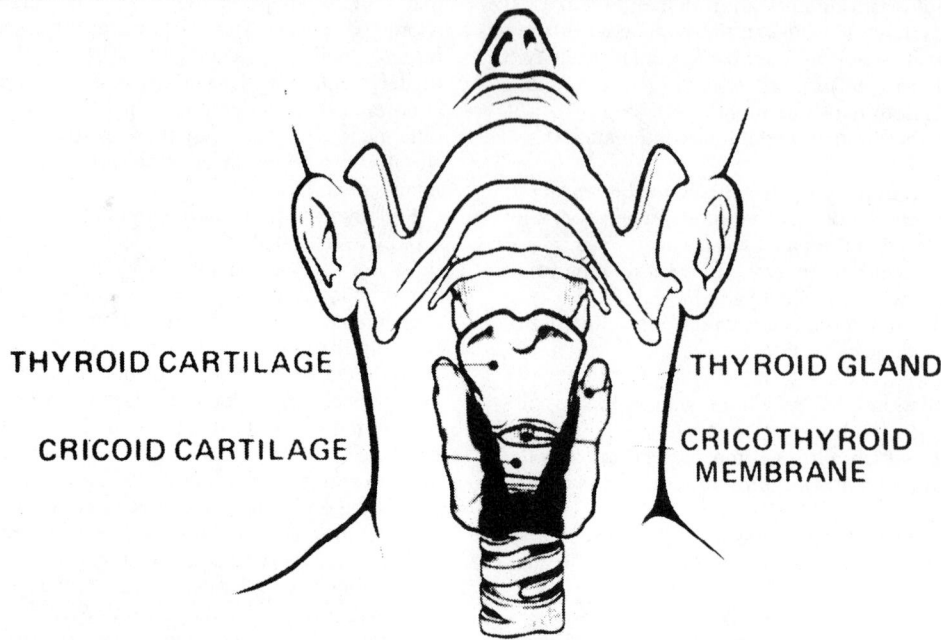

THYROID CARTILAGE

CRICOID CARTILAGE

THYROID GLAND

CRICOTHYROID MEMBRANE

Fig. 32-18. Landmarks for locating the cricothyroid membrane for use of transtracheal catheter ventilation or cricothyrotomy. (Reproduced with permission. *Textbook of Advanced Cardiac Life Support,* 1987. Copyright American Heart Association.)

If attempts at relieving an obstructed airway have failed, several advanced techniques may be used to secure the airway until intubation or tracheostomy is successfully performed. In transtracheal catheter ventilation, a catheter is inserted over a needle through the cricothyroid membrane (Fig. 32-18). The needle is removed and intermittent jet ventilation initiated [152]. In cricothyrotomy, an opening is made in the cricothyroid membrane with a knife [153,154,155]. Tracheostomy, if still necessary, is best performed in the operating room by a skilled surgeon after the airway has been secured by one of the aforementioned techniques.

CIRCULATORY SUPPORT. Chest compression should not be unduly interrupted while adjunctive procedures are instituted. The rescuer coordinating the resuscitative effort must ensure that adequate pulses are generated by the compressor. The carotid or femoral pulse should be evaluated every few minutes.

Mechanical chest compressors seem useful in the hands of experienced resuscitators. It is important that such devices be correctly calibrated to provide a stroke of 1.5 to 2 inches. The position of the press on the sternum must be checked frequently to ensure adequate compression with a minimum of damage. The press may be a manually operated hinged device or powered by compressed gas (usually 100% O_2). The plunger is mounted on a backboard and is associated with a time-pressure cycled ventilator. This device is programmed to deliver CPR in a 5:1 compression ventilation ratio using a compression duration that is 50 percent of the cycle length. Such units allow the patient to be harnessed to the backboard, fixing the location of the plunger. When used properly, with careful monitoring of patient position, this device facilitates CPR during transport. An acceptable electrocardiogram (ECG) can often be recorded with the compressor in operation, and defibrillation can be delivered during the downstroke of chest compression, without delays in CPR.

Electrocardiographic monitoring is necessary during resuscitation to guide appropriate electrical and pharmacologic therapy. Until ECG monitoring allows diagnosis of the rhythm, the patient should be assumed to be in ventricular fibrillation (vide infra).

Most defibrillators currently marketed have built-in monitoring circuitry in the paddles ("quick-look" paddles). On application of the defibrillator paddles, the patient's ECG is displayed on the monitor screen. This facilitates appropriate initial therapy. For continuous monitoring beyond the first few minutes, a standard ECG monitoring unit should be employed.

Electrocardiographic monitoring must never be relied on without frequent reference to the patient's pulse and clinical condition. What appears on the monitor screen to be ventricular fibrillation or asystole must not be treated as such unless the patient is found to be without a pulse. An apparently satisfactory rhythm on the monitor must be accompanied by an adequate pulse and blood pressure.

Defibrillation is the definitive treatment for the vast majority of cardiac arrests. It should be delivered as early as possible and repeated frequently until ventricular fibrillation or pulseless ventricular tachycardia has been terminated.

If an electrical defibrillator is not immediately available, a precordial thump may be employed. Conversion of ventricular tachycardia and ventricular fibrillation by a precordial thump (and even with a cough) has been well documented [156, 157,158]. A solitary precordial thump, therefore, is warranted in monitored ventricular fibrillation or pulseless ventricular tachycardia in the absence of a defibrillator. If the thump leads to a rhythm with a pulse, a bolus of lidocaine should be given. In patients with ventricular tachycardia who have a pulse, a precordial thump should not be used unless an electric defibrillator is available, because a thump can induce ventricular fibrillation [159].

Electrical defibrillation involves passing an electric current through the heart and causing synchronous depolarization of the myofibrils. As the myofibrils repolarize, the opportunity arises for the emergence of organized pacemaker activity.

Proper use of the defibrillator requires special attention to the following.

1. *Selection of proper energy levels.* This lessens myocardial damage and arrhythmias occasioned by unnecessarily high energies. Inadequate energies will not terminate the arrhythmia. An initial energy of 200 joules appears to be safer than higher energies [160] and equally effective [160,161]. If the patient remains pulseless after the initial shock, the next defibrillation attempt should be at 200 to 300 joules. The third and subsequent attempts should be at no higher than 360 joules. If ventricular fibrillation recurs after successful defibrillation, the prior successful energy level should be tried again.

2. *Proper asynchronous mode.* The proper mode must be selected if the rhythm is ventricular fibrillation. The synchronizing switch must be deactivated or the defibrillator will dutifully await the nonforthcoming R wave. For rapid pulseless ventricular tachycardia (approximately 150–200 beats/min) it is best not to attempt synchronization with the R wave, since this increases the likelihood of delivering the shock on the T wave. If the countershock should fall on the T wave and induce ventricular fibrillation, another unsynchronized countershock must be delivered promptly after confirming pulselessness.

3. *Proper position of the paddles.* This allows the major energy of the electric arc to traverse the myocardium. The anterolateral position requires that one paddle be placed to the right of the upper sternum, just below the clavicle. The other paddle is positioned to the left of the nipple in the left midaxillary line. In the anteroposterior position, one paddle is positioned under the left scapula with the patient lying on it. The anterior paddle is positioned just to the left of the lower sternal border.

4. *Adequate contact between paddles and skin.* This should be assured, using just enough electrode paste to cover the paddle face, without spilling over the surrounding skin. The rescuer should hold the paddles with firm (approximately 25 pounds) pressure. The pressure should be delivered using the forearms; leaning into the paddles should be avoided for fear that the rescuer may slip. If defibrillator electrode paddles are used, the skin must be carefully prepared according to the manufacturer's directions.

5. *No contact with anyone other than the victim.* The rescuer must be sturdily balanced on both feet and not standing on a wet floor. Cardiopulmonary resuscitation must be discontinued with no one remaining in contact with the patient. It is the responsibility of the person holding the paddles to check the patient's surroundings, ensure the safety of all participants, loudly announce the intention to countershock, and depress both buttons. The use of an automatic or semiautomatic defibrillator does not decrease the operator's need for diligence.

6. *If no skeletal muscle twitch or spasm has occurred.* The equipment, contacts, and synchronizer switch used for elective cardioversions should be rechecked.

7. *The rhythm should be assessed after each countershock and the patient should be checked for a pulse at appropriate times.* This must be done before proceeding with therapeutic interventions. After the first and second defibrillation attempt, the rhythm is assessed by the monitor screen; the next defibrillation attempt is performed if the rhythm has clearly not changed on the monitor. If there is a question, the pulse should be checked. After the third defibrillation attempt, a pulse check is in order. After apparently successful defibrillation, the pulse should be checked before it is assumed that spontaneous circulation has resumed. If the patient remains pulseless, CPR should be resumed, an intravenous line placed, epinephrine administered, and reshock performed at 360 joules, or three sequential shocks should be used, as in the first attempt.

Pacemaker therapy requiring positioning of transvenous or transthoracic electrodes is time-consuming and technically demanding and usually interferes with adequate performance of CPR. External pacing equipment often allows myocardial capture with some discomfort and skeletal muscle contraction [162]. Obviously, this is unimportant during asystole or bradycardic cardiac arrest. Unfortunately, pacing does not produce a perfusing rhythm in most cases of cardiac arrest [163,164,165]. Patients who respond to emergency pacing are those with severe bradycardias or conduction block who have reasonably well-preserved myocardial function [166].

Venous access with a reliable intravenous route must be established early in the course of the resuscitative effort to allow administration of necessary drugs and fluids. However, initial defibrillation attempts and CPR should not be delayed for the placement of an intravenous line. Peripheral venous access through antecubital veins is often more convenient because it is less likely to interfere with other rescue procedures. Cannulation of such veins may be difficult, however, because of venous collapse or constriction. A large-bore catheter system should be used, because needles in the vein are apt to become dislodged during CPR. A long catheter may be threaded into the central circulation. Alternatively, the extremity may be elevated and a large volume of flush solution used to help entry of the drug into the central circulation. Lower extremity peripheral veins should be avoided, because entry of drugs into the central circulation from such veins during CPR is questionable [68,167].

Central venous access offers a more secure route for drug administration and should be attempted if initial resuscitative efforts are not successful. Femoral vein cannulation is difficult to achieve during CPR [168] and flow into the thorax is slower than with upper torso access. If the femoral vein is successfully cannulated, a long line should be placed into the vena cava above the level of the diaphragm. Internal jugular or subclavian routes are preferable, but their placement should not be allowed to delay defibrillation attempts or interfere with CPR. They should be placed by experienced operators. In infants and children up to 6 years of age, the intraosseous route is easy to achieve and is very effective for venous access.

Drugs such as epinephrine, atropine, and lidocaine can be administered via the endotracheal tube if there is delay in achieving venous access. However, this route requires a higher dose to achieve an equivalent blood level [169,170,171], and a sustained duration of action (a "depot effect") can be expected if there is a return in spontaneous circulation [170,171]. It is suggested that 2.5 times the intravenous dose be administered when using the endotracheal route. Delivery of the drug to the circulation is facilitated by diluting the drug to a 10 ml volume and delivering it through a catheter positioned to the tip of the endotracheal tube. Intracardiac injection of epinephrine should be avoided and is indicated only if intravenous and endotracheal routes are not available.

Drug Therapy

CORRECTION OF HYPOXIA. Hypoxemia should be corrected early during CPR with administration of the highest possible oxygen concentration. Inadequate perfusion, decreased pulmonary blood flow, pulmonary edema, atelectasis, and ventilation-perfusion mismatch all contribute to the difficulty in maintaining adequate tissue oxygenation. Inadequate tissue oxygenation results in anaerobic metabolism, generation of lactic acid, and development of metabolic acidosis.

CORRECTION OF ACIDOSIS. Correction of acidosis must be considered when the arrest has lasted more than several minutes. *Metabolic acidosis* develops because of tissue hypoxia and conversion to anaerobic metabolism. *Respiratory acidosis* occurs because of the apnea or hypoventilation with intrapulmonary ventilation-perfusion abnormalities; the marked decrease in pulmonary blood flow that exists even with well-performed CPR also contributes. Exhaled carbon dioxide during CPR is markedly diminished [172–175] and cannot be adequately increased even with endotracheal intubation and increased volume of moved air, as a result the $PaCO_2$ rises. Hyperventilation should be attempted to remove as much carbon dioxide as possible. Early intubation is an important goal so that larger volumes of gas can be moved in and out of the lung, without causing gastric insufflation. Once the airway is protected, ventilation can proceed asynchronously with sternal compression and at a faster rate than the 5:1 ratio would allow.

Sodium bicarbonate reacts with hydrogen ions to buffer metabolic acidosis by forming carbonic acid and then carbon dioxide and water. Each 50 mEq of sodium bicarbonate will generate 260 to 280 mm Hg of carbon dioxide, which can be eliminated only through expired air. As carbon dioxide of exhaled gas during CPR is markedly decreased, the carbonic acid generated by sodium bicarbonate cannot be eliminated. Paradoxical intracellular acidosis is likely to result, and arterial blood gases may not correctly reflect the state of tissue acidosis [176,177]. The sodium and osmolar load of bicarbonate is high; excessive administration will result in hyperosmolarity, hypernatremia, and worsened cellular acidosis. With these concerns in mind, the AHA guidelines suggest that sodium bicarbonate be avoided until successful resuscitation has reestablished a perfusing rhythm [178]. In the postresuscitative state, the degree of acidosis can be better estimated from blood gases and the acidemia corrected with hyperventilation and possibly bicarbonate administration. Sodium bicarbonate is of questionable value in treating metabolic acidosis during cardiac arrest; it has not been shown to facilitate ventricular defibrillation or survival in cardiac arrest [179]. In any case, bicarbonate should not be used during cardiac arrest until at least 10 minutes have passed, the patient is intubated, and the patient has not responded to initial defibrillatory attempts and drug intervention. An exception is the patient who has known preexisting hyperkalemia in whom the administration of bicarbonate is recommended. The use of bicarbonate may also be of value in patients who have a known preexisting bicarbonate-responsive acidosis or a tricyclic antidepressant overdosage or to alkalinize the urine in drug overdosage.

VOLUME REPLACEMENT. Increased central volume is often required during CPR, especially if the initial attempts at defibrillation have failed. Pulseless electrical activity is particularly likely to be caused either by acute severe hypovolemia (e.g., exsanguination) or by a cardiovascular process for which volume expansion may be a lifesaving temporizing measure (e.g., pericardial tamponade, pulmonary embolism, and septic shock). The usual clues for hypovolemia, such as collapsed jugular and peripheral veins and evidence of peripheral vasoconstriction, are unavailable during cardiac arrest; furthermore, dry mucous membranes and absence of normal secretions (tears, saliva) are unreliable in acute hypovolemia. Most physical findings of tamponade, pulmonary embolism, or septic shock are absent during arrest. Therefore, one must be guided by an appropriate clinical history and have a low threshold to administer volume during CPR.

Simple crystalloids, such as 5% dextrose in water, are inappropriate for rapid expansion of the circulatory blood volume. Isotonic crystalloids (0.9% saline, Ringer's lactate), colloids, or blood are necessary for satisfactory volume expansion. Crystalloids are more readily available, easier to administer, and less expensive than colloids. They are also free of the potential to cause allergic reactions or infections. Colloids are more likely to sustain intravascular volume and oncotic pressure. Some studies have suggested shorter resuscitation times and better survival with colloids as opposed to crystalloids [180].

If the patient has a weak pulse, simple elevation of the legs may help by promoting venous return to the central circulation. In profound hypovolemia with subsequent arrest, medical antishock garments (MAST suits) may ameliorate the hypovolemia until fluid administration or surgical intervention can supervene. Volume challenges should be given as needed until pulse and blood pressure have been restored or until there is evidence of volume overload. In the postresuscitative phase, pulmonary artery and central venous catheterization are usually needed to monitor volume replacement adequately. Fluid replacement is guided by the patient's clinical course, urine output, and catheterization data. The goal is to achieve optimal cardiac output and perfusion pressure without excessive fluid expansion or pulmonary congestion.

SYMPATHOMIMETIC DRUGS AND VASOPRESSORS. Sympathomimetic drugs either act directly on adrenergic receptors or act indirectly by releasing catecholamines from nerve endings. Most useful during cardiac emergencies are the adrenergic agents, which include the endogenous biogenic amines epinephrine, norepinephrine, and dopamine and the synthetic agents isoproterenol and its derivative dobutamine [181, 182,183]. The effects of these adrenergic agents can be divided into several broad categories: stimulation of certain peripheral smooth muscles, inhibition of other peripheral smooth muscles, cardiac stimulation, metabolic effects, and central nervous system effects. The variable effects of different agents appear to be caused by the presence of several species of adrenergic receptor. The classification of adrenergic receptors into alpha- and beta-receptors was first proposed by Ahlquist in 1948 [184]. The concept was based on the variable activity of a series of sympathomimetic agents at effector sites. Alpha-receptors are associated with vasoconstriction, mydriasis, and intestinal relaxation. Beta-receptors are associated with vasodilatation, cardioacceleration, positive inotropism, bronchial relaxation, and intestinal relaxation. Metabolic effects of adrenergic agents are largely beta effects, including glycogenolysis and fatty acid release. Insulin release is increased by beta-receptors and inhibited by alpha-receptors.

Beta-receptors are of two types: beta$_1$ and beta$_2$. Beta$_1$-receptors are responsible for cardiac stimulation and lipolysis. Beta$_2$-receptors are responsible for vasodilatation and bronchodilatation. Alpha$_1$- and alpha$_2$-receptors are found at postsynaptic and presynaptic locations, respectively.

Norepinephrine acts on both alpha- and beta$_1$-receptors, but its alpha effects predominate. Epinephrine also acts on both receptors, with its *alpha and beta effects more balanced*. The synthetic agent isoproterenol is a pure beta-agonist, and its actions are blocked by beta-blockers such as propranolol. The synthetic agents methoxamine and phenylephrine are pure alpha-agonists, and their effects are blocked by phenoxybenzamine or phentolamine.

Dopamine has beta activity and (at higher doses) alpha activity. At all doses, it has vasodilator activity on renal, mesenteric, coronary, and intracerebral arteries that cannot be blocked by beta-blockers. This effect can be attenuated by haloperidol and phenothiazines. This suggests the presence of specific dopaminergic receptors in these vascular beds.

Epinephrine. This is the pressor agent used most frequently during cardiopulmonary resuscitation. Epinephrine is a naturally occurring catecholamine with both alpha and beta activity.

Indications for the use of epinephrine include all forms of cardiac arrest, because its alpha-vasoconstrictive activity is important in raising the perfusion pressure of myocardium and brain. The importance of alpha-adrenergic activity during resuscitation has been noted in several studies [185,186,187], whereas administration of pure beta-agonists (e.g., isoproterenol or dobutamine) has been shown to be ineffective [188,189]. The beta action of epinephrine is theoretically useful in asystole and bradycardic arrests by increasing heart rate. The beta effect has also been touted to convert asystole to ventricular fibrillation or to convert "fine" ventricular fibrillation to "coarse." Coarse or wide-amplitude ventricular fibrillation is easier to convert to a perfusing rhythm than is fine or small-amplitude ventricular fibrillation. However, this may be due primarily to the shorter time course of the arrest in patients still manifesting wide-amplitude rather than small-amplitude ventricular fibrillation.

Epinephrine is best administered intravenously. As soon as possible after failed ventricular defibrillation attempts (or if de-

fibrillation is not an option), an adult in cardiac arrest should be given a 1-mg dose at a 1:10,000 dilution (10 ml). It should be given in the upper extremity or centrally (vide supra) and may be repeated every 5 minutes. If a peripheral line is used, the drug should be administered rapidly and should be followed by a 20-ml bolus of intravenous fluid and elevation of the extremity. It should not be administered in the same intravenous line as an alkaline solution. If an intravenous line has not been established the endotracheal route may be used, but the intracardiac route should be avoided, as it is prone to serious complications such as intramyocardial injection, coronary laceration, and pneumothorax. An intravenous titration of 1 to 4 µg per minute can also be given for inotropic and pressor support. Brown et al. published data using a swine model which strongly suggest that doses of epinephrine 10 times those prescribed previously may be more advantageous during arrest [190,191]. Martin et al. demonstrated a drop in end-tidal PCO_2 during CPR in a dog model with high-dose epinephrine [192]. This occurred despite a rise in coronary perfusion pressure and may be due to pulmonary vascular shunting or a further diminution of cardiac output. Early results with the use of high-dose epinephrine in humans were encouraging [193,194,195], but two multicenter trials have failed to demonstrate an improvement in survival or neurological outcome [196,197]. Intermediate- or high-dose epinephrine is therefore considered an option mode to the standard dose (Fig. 32-19).

Precautions in the use of epinephrine and other alpha-agonists include tissue necrosis from extravasation and inactivation from admixture with bicarbonate.

Norepinephrine. This is a potent alpha-agonist with beta activity. Its salutary alpha effects during CPR are similar to those of epinephrine [198,199]. However, there are no data to support the belief that it is superior to epinephrine during an arrest.

The major effect of norepinephrine is on the blood vessels.

Fig. 32-19. Ventricular fibrillation and pulseless ventricular tachycardia (VF/VT). (From *Guidelines for Cardiopulmonary Resuscitation and Emergency Cardiac Care,* 1992, copyright American Medical Association. With permission.)

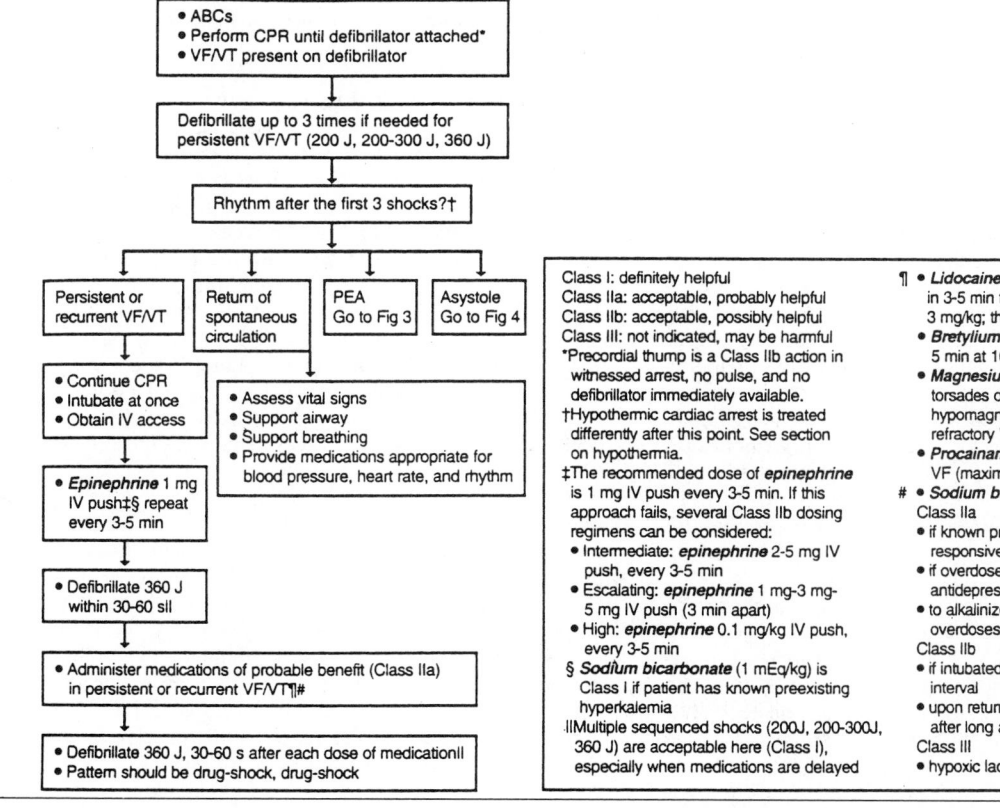

Initial coronary vasoconstriction usually gives way to coronary vasodilatation, probably as a result of increased myocardial metabolic activity. In a heart with compromised coronary reserve, this may cause further ischemia. During cardiac arrest, its usefulness, like that of epinephrine, is most likely due to peripheral vasoconstriction with an increase in perfusion pressure. In patients with spontaneous circulation who are in cardiogenic shock (when peripheral vasoconstriction is often already extreme) its effect is more difficult to predict. Norepinephrine also causes considerable renal and mesenteric vasoconstriction, whereas dopamine at low infusion rates causes vasodilatation in these vascular beds.

Indications for the use of norepinephrine during cardiac arrest are similar to those for epinephrine, although there does not appear to be any reason to prefer it to epinephrine. Norepinephrine appears to be most useful in the treatment of shock caused by inappropriate decline in peripheral vascular resistance, such as septic shock and neurogenic shock.

It is administered by intravenous infusion, titrated to an adequate perfusion pressure. Four to 8 mg of the bitartrate (2–4 mg of the base) should be diluted in 500 ml of D5W or 5% dextrose in normal saline. If 8 mg of the bitartrate is diluted in 500 ml, 1 ml will contain 16 μg per milliliter; a microdrip administration set may be used to deliver 1 ml in 60 drops. After observing the response to an initial dose of 2 μg/kg/min, the dose is adjusted to maintain a low normal blood pressure (85–90 mm Hg systolic or somewhat higher in a previously hypertensive individual). An average effective adult dose is 2 to 12 μg/kg/min. Higher doses are needed in some individuals. Norepinephrine should not be administered in the same intravenous line as an alkaline solution. After the patient has been transferred to a critical care unit, the drug may be continued for several days but should be gradually tapered when possible. Abrupt termination of the infusion (as may occur in transport) may lead to sudden severe hypotension.

Precautions to the use of norepinephrine include its inappropriate use in hypovolemic shock and in patients with already severe vasoconstriction. Intraarterial pressure monitoring is strongly recommended when using norepinephrine, because indirect blood pressure measurement is often incorrect in patients with severe vasoconstriction. In patients with myocardial ischemia or infarction, myocardial oxygen requirements are increased by all catecholamines, but especially by norepinephrine, due to its marked afterload increasing properties. Unless the increased oxygen delivery occasioned by the rise in perfusion pressure outweighs the increase in myocardial oxygen requirement caused by the afterload increase, norepinephrine is likely to have deleterious effects. Heart rate, rhythm, electrocardiographic evidence for ischemia, direct systemic and pulmonary pressures, urine output, as well as cardiac output should be closely monitored when using this drug in patients with myocardial ischemia or infarction. Extravasation of norepinephrine in superficial tissues is apt to result in ischemic necrosis and sloughing. Therefore, norepinephrine should be administered through a catheter well advanced into the vein. If extravasation does occur, 5 to 10 mg of phentolamine in 10 to 15 ml of saline should be infiltrated as soon as possible into the area of extravasation.

Isoproterenol. This synthetic catecholamine has almost pure beta-adrenergic activity. Its cardiac activity includes potent inotropic and chronotropic effects, both of which increase myocardial oxygen demand. In addition to bronchodilatation, the arterial beds of skeletal muscle, kidneys, and gut dilate, resulting in a marked drop in systemic vascular resistance. Cardiac output can be expected to increase markedly unless the increased myocardial oxygen demand results in sufficient myocardial ischemia. Systolic blood pressure is usually maintained because of the rise in cardiac output, but the diastolic and mean pressures usually decrease. As a result, coronary perfusion pressure drops at a time when myocardial oxygen requirement is increased. This combination can be expected to have deleterious effects in patients with ischemic heart disease, especially during cardiac arrest. The main clinical usefulness of isoproterenol is in its ability to stimulate pacemakers within the heart.

Indications for isoproterenol are primarily in the setting of atropine-resistant, hemodynamically significant bradyarrhythmias, including profound sinus and junctional bradycardia as well as various forms of high-degree atrioventricular block. It should be used only as an interim measure, until a temporary pacemaker can be inserted. If the aortic diastolic pressure is already low, epinephrine is likely to be better tolerated as a stimulus to pacemakers. *Under no circumstances should isoproterenol be used during cardiac arrest* [183].

Isoproterenol is administered by titration of an intravenous solution. One milligram of isoproterenol (Isuprel) is diluted with either 250 ml D5W (4 μg/ml) or 500 ml D5W (2 μg/ml). The infusion rate should be only rapid enough to effect an adequate perfusing heart rate (2–20 μg/per min, or 0.05–0.5 μg/kg/min). Depending on the adequacy of cardiac reserve, a target heart rate as low as 50 to 55 beats per minute may be satisfactory. Occasionally more rapid rates are necessary.

Precautions in the use of isoproterenol are largely due to the increase in myocardial oxygen requirement, with its potential to provoke ischemia; *this effect, coupled with the possibility of dropping the coronary perfusion pressure, makes isoproterenol a dangerous selection in the coronary patient.* The marked chronotropic effects may cause tachycardia and may provoke serious ventricular arrhythmias, including ventricular fibrillation. Isoproterenol is generally contraindicated if tachycardia is already present, especially if the arrhythmia may be secondary to digitalis toxicity. If significant hypotension develops with its use, it may be combined with another beta-agonist with alpha activity. However, switching to dopamine or epinephrine is usually preferable; better yet is the use of another modality for rate control, such as pacing.

Dopamine Hydrochloride. This naturally occurring precursor of norepinephrine has alpha-, beta-, and dopamine-receptor stimulating activity. The dopamine-receptor activity dilates renal and mesenteric arterial beds at low doses (1–2 μg/kg/min), which may not produce an increase in heart rate or blood pressure. These effects cannot be blocked with either beta- or alpha-blocking agents. At doses from 2 to 10 μg/kg/min, dopamine exerts primarily beta-adrenergic activity, with an increase in contractile force and heart rate. At doses of 10 μg/kg/min and greater, the alpha-adrenergic activity becomes more and more prominent, causing peripheral vasoconstriction and constriction of renal and splanchnic arterial beds. At doses greater than 20 μg/kg/min, alpha activity is likely to overcome dopaminergic effects and lower renal and mesenteric blood flow.

Indications for the use of dopamine are primarily significant hypotension and cardiogenic shock. Its dopaminergic effects may be useful in early shock, with decreasing urine output; it may be started at low doses along with volume expansion.

Dopamine is administered by intravenous titration. A 200-mg ampule is diluted to 250 or 500 ml in D5W or D5NS, for a concentration of 800 or 400 μg per milliliter. Dopamine should not be administered in the same intravenous line as an alkaline solution. For hypotension, the initial infusion rate is usually 2 to 5 μg/kg/min, which is increased until a satisfactory response is achieved in blood pressure and urine output. As with all catecholamine infusions, the lowest infusion rate that results in satisfactory perfusion should be the goal of therapy. Rarely, a patient may need in excess of 20 μg/kg/min. Urine output, cardiac output, systemic vascular resistance, and left ventricular filling pressure monitoring is necessary for optimal control of the hemodynamic response.

Precautions for dopamine use are similar to those for other catecholamines. Tachycardia or ventricular arrhythmias may require reduction in dosage or discontinuation of the drug. If significant hypotension occurs from the dilating activity of dopaminergic or beta-active doses, small amounts of an alpha-active drug may be added. Dopamine may increase myocardial ischemia. Sloughing may occur if dopamine extravasates into subcutaneous tissues. If this occurs, phentolamine should be infiltrated into the area of extravasation, as for norepinephrine extravasation.

Dobutamine. This is a potent synthetic beta-adrenergic agent that differs from isoproterenol in that tachycardia is less problematic. Unless ischemia supervenes, cardiac output will increase, as will renal and mesenteric blood flow.

Dobutamine is indicated primarily for the short-term enhancement of ventricular contractility in the heart failure patient. It may be used for postresuscitative stabilization of the arrest victim or the patient with heart failure refractory to other drugs. It may also be used in combination with intravenous nitroprusside, which lowers peripheral vascular resistance and thereby left ventricular afterload. Whereas nitroprusside lowers peripheral resistance, dobutamine maintains the perfusion pressure by augmenting cardiac output.

Dobutamine is administered by slow titrated intravenous infusion. A dose as low as 0.5 μg/kg/min may be effective, but the usual dose range is 2.5 to 10.0 μg/kg/min. A 250-mg vial is dissolved in 10 ml of sterile water and then to 250 or 500 ml of D_5W, for a concentration of 1 or 0.5 mg per milliliter. Dobutamine should not be administered in the same intravenous line as alkaline solutions.

Precautions for dobutamine use are similar to those for other beta-agonists. Dobutamine may cause tachycardia, ventricular arrhythmias, myocardial ischemia, and extension of infarction. It must be used with caution in patients with coronary artery disease.

ANTIARRHYTHMIC AGENTS. Antiarrhythmics play an important role in stabilizing rhythm in many resuscitation situations. Lidocaine has proved the most useful in counteracting the tendency to ventricular arrhythmias. Bretylium has a similar use. Procainamide is occasionally used in postresuscitative care.

Lidocaine. This antiarrhythmic agent often proves effective against ventricular arrhythmias, such as premature ventricular complexes and ventricular tachycardia. Premature ventricular complexes are not unusual in apparently healthy people and most often are benign. Even in the patient with chronic heart disease, premature ventricular complexes and nonsustained ventricular tachycardia are usually asymptomatic, and controversy exists concerning the need to treat under these circumstances. The situation is very different for patients with myocardial ischemia or recent myocardial infarction, who are much more likely to progress from premature ventricular complexes to sustained ventricular tachycardia or fibrillation. Such patients should be treated promptly with antiarrhythmic agents such as lidocaine (Figs. 32-20 and 32-21). The efficacy of prophylactic lidocaine in reducing primary ventricular fibrillation in patients with acute myocardial infarction has been established [200,201]. However, the toxic-to-therapeutic ratio is not favorable enough to warrant its routine use in patients suspected of acute myocardial infarction [202–206].

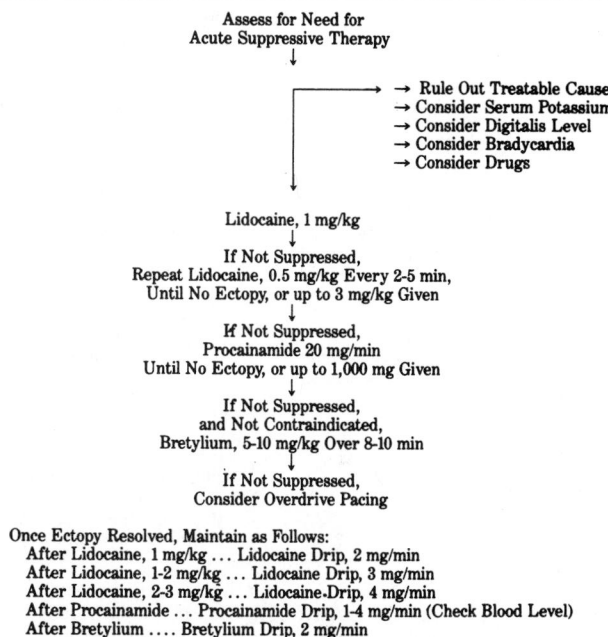

Fig. 32-20. Ventricular ectopy: acute suppressive therapy according to a sequence developed to assist in teaching how to treat a broad range of patients with ventricular ectopy. Some patients may require therapy not specified herein. This algorithm should not be construed as prohibiting such flexibility. (From Standards and guidelines for CPR and ECC. *JAMA* 255:2843, 1986. With permission.)

Lidocaine is indicated primarily to suppress ventricular arrhythmias in patients with myocardial ischemia and recent myocardial infarction. While its routine prophylactic use is not recommended for patients with suspected myocardial infarction, it is recommended in ventricular tachycardia and fibrillation, for control of premature ventricular complexes, and for wide-complex tachycardia of uncertain type. It is used after successful conversion of ventricular tachycardia or fibrillation to protect against recurrence. Correction of the underlying cause of the ventricular irritability (myocardial ischemia, hypoxemia, hypercarbia, electrolyte imbalance, digitalis excess, etc.) must also be addressed for successful management of the arrhythmia.

Administration of lidocaine begins with an intravenous bolus. The onset of action is rapid. Its duration of action is brief but may be prolonged by continuous infusion. A solution of lidocaine, typically 20 mg per milliliter (2%), should be prepared for intravenous administration. Prefilled syringes are available for bolus injection. Several dosage schedules are in use, but most common is to give a bolus of 1 mg per kilogram, followed by a continuous infusion of 2 to 4 mg per minute (15–50 μg/kg/min). If the patient has suffered an acute myocardial infarction *and has had ventricular arrhythmias,* the infusion is continued for hours to days and tapered slowly. If the cause of the arrhythmia has been corrected, the infusion may be tapered more rapidly.

Precautions should be taken against excessive accumulation of lidocaine. The dosage should be reduced in patients with low cardiac output, congestive failure, hepatic failure, and age greater than 70 years, because of decreased liver metabolism of the drug. Toxic manifestations are usually neurologic and can vary from slurred speech, tinnitus, sleepiness, and dysphoria to localizing neurologic symptoms. Frank seizures may occur with

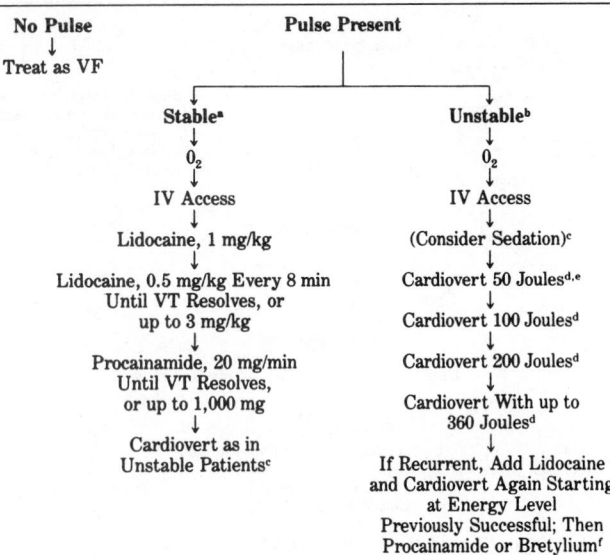

No Pulse
↓
Treat as VF

Pulse Present

Stable^a
↓
O₂
↓
IV Access
↓
Lidocaine, 1 mg/kg
↓
Lidocaine, 0.5 mg/kg Every 8 min
Until VT Resolves, or
up to 3 mg/kg
↓
Procainamide, 20 mg/min
Until VT Resolves,
or up to 1,000 mg
↓
Cardiovert as in
Unstable Patients^c

Unstable^b
↓
O₂
↓
IV Access
↓
(Consider Sedation)^c
↓
Cardiovert 50 Joules^d,e
↓
Cardiovert 100 Joules^d
↓
Cardiovert 200 Joules^d
↓
Cardiovert With up to
360 Joules^d
↓
If Recurrent, Add Lidocaine
and Cardiovert Again Starting
at Energy Level
Previously Successful; Then
Procainamide or Bretylium^f

Fig. 32-21. Sustained ventricular tachycardia. This sequence was developed to assist in teaching how to respond to a broad range of patients with sustained ventricular tachycardia. Some patients may require therapy not specified herein. This algorithm should not be construed as prohibiting such flexibility. a. If a patient becomes unstable (see footnote b) at any time, move to "unstable" arm of the algorithm. b. "Unstable" indicates symptoms (e.g., chest pain, dyspnea), hypotension, congestive heart failure, ischemia, or infarction. c. Sedation should be considered for all patients except those who are unconscious or who cannot wait because of severe hemodynamic instability. d. For patients in shock or marked pulmonary edema, unsynchronized cardioversion should be performed if synchronization would cause a delay; for patients with rapid ventricular tachycardia greater than 150 beats/min, unsynchronized cardioversion is preferable to avoid synchronizing on the T wave. If ventricular fibrillation appears to result on the monitor and the patient is pulseless, countershock immediately without synchronization. e. A precordial thump may be employed prior to cardioversion. f. If ventricular tachycardia resolves, begin IV infusion of antiarrhythmic drug that aided resolution; if cardioversion is unsuccessful, use IV lidocaine, followed by bretylium. Procainamide may also be considered. (From Standards and guidelines for CPR and ECC. *JAMA* 255:2843, 1986. With permission.)

or without preceding neurologic symptoms and may be controlled with short-acting barbiturates or diazepam. Conscious patients should be warned about the possible symptoms of neurologic toxicity and asked to report them immediately if they occur. Enlisting the patient's aid also allays the fear that would otherwise develop from unexpected neurologic symptoms. Excessive blood levels can significantly depress myocardial contractility.

Bretylium Tosylate. Bretylium is an adrenergic-blocking agent that initially causes a release of norepinephrine from peripheral adrenergic nerve terminals. It subsequently prevents further release of norepinephrine from these same terminals or their uptake of norepinephrine. The latter effect potentiates the actions of circulating catecholamines. Bretylium is effective in suppressing ventricular arrhythmias in a variety of conditions, including acute myocardial infarction and ischemia. It has been demonstrated in animal studies to have a primary antifibrillatory effect [207,208]. Clinically, it has been found effective in the treatment of ventricular tachycardia and ventricular fibrillation. It has not been found to be more effective than lidocaine in

direct comparisons. Based on animal work [209], higher doses than those currently recommended may be needed for improved efficacy, but data in humans are not yet available.

Bretylium causes an initial release of norepinephrine from nerve endings that results in an increase in cardiac output and mean systemic pressure which lasts 10 to 20 minutes after parenteral administration. This is followed by a delayed hypotensive effect secondary to peripheral adrenergic blockade. In fact, hypotension is the most common side effect of bretylium, but it is generally mild and usually does not require discontinuation of the drug. Hypotension is most marked in patients with volume depletion or limited myocardial reserve. Paradoxically, hypotension is more often produced by low doses (<5 mg/kg), which are apt to cause peripheral dilatation without augmentation of cardiac output.

Bretylium is indicated for ventricular tachycardia and fibrillation, especially if they prove refractory to lidocaine and electrical countershocks. It may also be used to suppress recurrent ventricular tachycardia or fibrillation and has been used for arrhythmia prophylaxis in acute myocardial infarction.

Bretylium is administered by intravenous bolus. It is available in 10-ml ampules containing 500 mg. For unresponsive ventricular fibrillation, 5 mg per kilogram undiluted is given in a rapid bolus, followed by additional attempts at electrical defibrillation. If this dose fails, a 10 mg per kilogram bolus is administered, repeated if necessary every 15 to 30 minutes, up to a maximum total initial dose of 30 mg per kilogram. Each bolus should be followed by an attempt at electrical defibrillation at maximum delivered energy (or at previously successful energy level). For slow drips, 500 mg should be diluted to 50 ml with saline. An intravenous drip of 5 to 10 mg per kilogram over 10 to 20 minutes may be given for recurrent or refractory ventricular tachycardia; this may be repeated as needed every 6 to 8 hours. Alternatively, a 1 to 2 mg per minute drip may be administered.

Precautions for bretylium include the production of nausea and vomiting, especially by rapid infusions. There is a high incidence of mild orthostatic hypotension. More severe hypotension may occur, requiring that the patient be placed in the Trendelenburg position and that fluids be administered. Rarely, low dosages of pressor agents may be required. Digitalis toxic ventricular arrhythmias are likely to be worsened during early transient norepinephrine release. Bretylium is relatively contraindicated in patients with a marked restriction in ability to increase their stroke volume; these patients include those with severe aortic or pulmonic stenosis and those with severe pulmonary hypertension.

Procainamide Hydrochloride. Procainamide is an antiarrhythmic agent, with quinidinelike activity. Like quinidine, it is useful in suppressing a wide variety of both ventricular and supraventricular arrhythmias. It is effective against reentrant as well as ectopic arrhythmogenic mechanisms. It has somewhat less vagolytic effect than quinidine and does not cause the rise in digoxin level seen with quinidine. Procainamide is sometimes used in the critical care setting for the suppression of ventricular arrhythmias not effectively treated by lidocaine or bretylium or in patients who cannot be treated with either of these agents. Procainamide is indicated for the suppression of ventricular arrhythmias refractory to lidocaine or both lidocaine and bretylium. It may also be used in patients with supraventricular arrhythmias causing hemodynamic compromise or worsening ischemia.

Procainamide is administered either orally or by intravenous injection. For serious arrhythmias in the critical care setting, intravenous injection is preferable. An infusion of 20 mg per minute (0.3 mg/kg/min) is given up to a loading dose of 1 gm

(15 mg/kg) or until the arrhythmia is suppressed, hypotension develops, or the QRS interval widens by 50 percent of its original width. A maintenance infusion may then be started at 1 to 4 mg per minute. The dosage should be lowered in the presence of renal failure. Blood levels of procainamide and its metabolite *N*-acetylprocainamide should be monitored in patients with renal failure or those receiving more than 3 mg per minute for more than 24 hours. Infusions as low as 1.4 mg/kg/hr may be needed in patients with renal insufficiency.

Precautions in the use of procainamide include its production of systemic hypotension, disturbance in atrioventricular conduction, and decreased ventricular contractility. Intravenous infusion must be carefully monitored, with frequent blood pressure determinations and measurement of ECG intervals P–R, QRS, and Q–T. Hypotension usually responds to slowing the infusion rate. If the QRS interval increases by more than 50 percent of its initial width, procainamide infusion should be discontinued. Widened QRS signifies toxic blood levels and may herald serious atrioventricular conduction abnormalities and asystole. This is particularly true of patients with digitalis intoxication and those with antecedent atrioventricular conduction abnormalities. A marked decrease in Q–T interval may predispose a patient to *Torsades de pointes* ventricular arrhythmias. Patients who have ventricular arrhythmias of the *Torsades* variety or ventricular arrhythmias associated with bradycardias should not be treated with procainamide.

Adenosine. Adenosine is an endogenous purine nucleoside that depresses atrioventricular (AV) nodal conduction and sinoatrial (SA) nodal activity. Because of the delay in A-V nodal conduction, adenosine is effective in terminating arrhythmias that use the A-V node in a reentrant circuit (e.g., paroxysmal supraventricular tachycardia [PSVT]) [210]. In supraventricular tachycardias such as atrial flutter, atrial fibrillation, or atrial or ventricular tachycardia that do not use the A-V node in a reentrant circuit, blocking transmission through the A-V node may prove helpful in clarifying the diagnosis [211]. The half-life of adenosine is less than 5 seconds, as it is rapidly metabolized.

Administration is by intravenous bolus of 6 mg given over 1 to 3 seconds, followed by a 20-ml saline flush. An additional dose of 12 mg may be given if no effect is seen within 1 to 2 minutes. Patients on theophylline may need higher doses [212].

Side effects caused by adenosine are transient and may include flushing, dyspnea, and anginalike chest pain (even in the absence of coronary disease). Sinus bradycardia and ventricular ectopy are common after terminating PSVT with adenosine, but the arrhythmias are typically so short-lived as to be clinically unimportant. The reentrant tachycardia may recur after the effect of adenosine has dissipated and may require additional doses of adenosine or a longer-acting drug, such as verapamil or diltiazem.

Theophylline and other methylxanthines, such as theobromine and caffeine, block the receptor responsible for adenosine's electrophysiologic effect; therefore, higher doses may be required in their presence. Dipyridamole and carbamazepine, on the other hand, potentiate and may prolong the effect of adenosine; therefore, other forms of therapy may be advisable [212].

Verapamil and Diltiazem. Unlike other calcium channel-blocking agents, verapamil and diltiazem increase refractoriness in the A-V node and significantly slow conduction. This action may terminate reentrant tachycardias that use the A-V node in the reentrant circuit (e.g., PSVT). These drugs may also slow the ventricular response in patients with atrial flutter or fibrillation and even in patients with multifocal atrial tachycar-

dia. They should be used only in patients in whom the tachycardia is known to be supraventricular in origin.

Administration of verapamil is by intravenous bolus of 2.5 to 5 mg over 2 minutes. Additional doses of 5 to 10 mg may be given at 15- to 30-minute intervals in the absence of a response. The maximum cumulative dose is 20 mg. Diltiazem may be given as an initial dose of 0.25 mg per kilogram with a follow-up dose of 0.35 mg per kilogram, if needed [213,214]. A maintenance infusion of 5 to 15 mg per hour may be used to control the rate of ventricular response in atrial fibrillation.

Both verapamil and diltiazem may decrease myocardial contractility and may worsen congestive heart failure or even provoke cardiogenic shock in patients with significant left ventricular dysfunction. They should be used with caution, therefore, in patients with known cardiac failure or suspected diminished cardiac reserve and in the elderly. If a patient develops worsened failure or hypotension after the use of these agents, calcium should be administered as described previously.

Magnesium. Cardiac arrhythmias and even sudden death have been associated with magnesium deficiency [215]. Hypomagnesemia decreases the uptake of intracellular potassium and may precipitate ventricular tachycardia or fibrillation. Magnesium supplementation may reduce the incidence of ventricular arrhythmias following myocardial infarction [215,216,217]. Magnesium is the treatment of choice for patients with *Torsades de pointes*.

Magnesium is administered intravenously. For rapid administration during ventricular tachycardia or ventricular fibrillation with suspected or documented hypomagnesemia, 1 to 2 gm may be diluted in 100 ml of D_5W and given over 1 to 2 minutes. A 24–hour infusion of magnesium may be used for peri-infarction patients with documented hypomagnesemia. A loading dose of 1 to 2 gm is diluted in 100 ml D_5W and slowly given over 5 minutes to 1 hour, followed by an infusion of 0.5 to 1.0 gm per hour over the ensuing 24 hours. Clinical circumstances and the serum magnesium level dictate the rate and duration of the infusion. Hypotension or asystole may occur with rapid administration.

Amiodarone. Amiodarone is a benzofurane derivative that is structurally similar to thyroxine and contains a considerable level of iodine. Gastrointestinal absorption is slow, therefore when given orally the onset of action is delayed while the drug slowly accumulates in adipose tissue. The mean elimination half-life is 64 days (24–160 days). Intravenous administration allows rapid onset of action, with therapeutic blood levels achieved with 600 mg given over 24 hours.

Amiodarone decreases myocardial contractility and may provoke congestive heart failure. It also causes vasodilation, however, which may counterbalance the decrease in contractility. In general, therefore, it is well tolerated even by those with myocardial dysfunction.

Amiodarone given intravenously has been found successful in terminating a variety of reentrant and non-reentrant supraventricular and ventricular rhythms [218,219]. It may be considered especially if other agents have failed.

Administration is by an intravenous infusion of 5 mg per kilogram over 2 to 5 minutes. If significant hypotension supervenes, the infusion must be discontinued.

OTHER AGENTS. Additional drugs occasionally found useful or necessary during resuscitation or in the immediate postresuscitation period include atropine, calcium, nitroprusside, and nitroglycerine. These agents are discussed below. Many other drugs may be required in particular emergencies and are discussed in other parts of this text. An incomplete list of these drugs includes digoxin, antibiotics, thiamine, thyroxin, morphine, naloxone, adrenocorticoids, fibrinolytic agents, anticoagulants, and dextrose.

Atropine Sulfate. Atropine is a vagolytic drug of use in increasing heart rate by stimulating pacers and facilitating atrioventricular conduction suppressed by excessive vagal tone.

Atropine is indicated primarily in bradycardias causing hemodynamic difficulty or associated with ventricular arrhythmias (Fig. 32-22). Atropine may be useful in atrioventricular block at the nodal level. It is also used in asystole and bradycardic arrests in the hope that decreased vagal tone will allow the emergence of an effective pacemaker [220].

Atropine is administered by intravenous bolus. If a rapid full vagolytic response is desired, as in asystole or bradycardic ar-

rest, 1 mg should be administered intravenously at once. If a satisfactory response has not occurred within several minutes (2–5 minutes) additional 1-mg doses should be given in a bolus, to a maximum dose of 3 mg (0.04 mg/kg) [221]. For bradycardia with a pulse, the initial dose should be 0.5 mg, repeated every 5 minutes until the desired effect is obtained, to a maximum dose of 3 mg (0.04 mg/kg). Atropine may be given by the endotracheal route at doses 2.5 times the intravenous dose.

Precautions for atropine include the concern that an inordinately rapid heart rate not be produced. Patients with ischemic heart disease are likely to have worsened ischemia or ventricular arrhythmias if the rate is too rapid. Uncommonly, a patient will have a paradoxical slowing of rate with atropine; this is more likely with smaller first doses and is caused by a central vagal effect. This effect is rapidly counteracted by additional atropine. In this situation, the next dose of atropine should be given immediately. If additional atropine does not correct the problem, the patient may require judicious use of isoproterenol and/or pacemaker therapy.

Calcium. Calcium's positive inotropic effect has led to its use in cardiac arrest. The contractile state of the myocardium depends in part on the intracellular concentration of the calcium ion. Transmembrane calcium flux serves an important regulatory function in both active contraction and active relaxation. The use of calcium in cardiac arrest is based on an early report by Kay and Blalock in which several pediatric cardiac surgical patients were successfully resuscitated, apparently with the aid of calcium [222]. However, several field studies have failed to demonstrate an improvement in survival or neurologic outcome with the use of calcium versus a control [223,224,225]. In addition, many patients during arrest are found to have severely hypercalcemic blood levels after usual doses of calcium [226,227]. This is apparently due to the markedly contracted volume of distribution of the ion in the arrested organism. In addition, calcium has the theoretical disadvantage of facilitating postanoxic tissue damage, especially in brain and heart. Digitalis toxicity may be exacerbated by the administration of calcium.

Calcium is indicated only in those circumstances in which it has been shown to be of benefit [220,228]: calcium channel blocker toxicity, severe hyperkalemia, severe hypocalcemia, arrest after multiple transfusions with citrated blood, fluoride toxicity, and coming off heart-lung bypass after cardioplegic arrest.

Calcium is available as calcium chloride, calcium glucceptate, or calcium gluconate. The gluconate salt is unstable and less frequently available. The chloride salt provides the most direct source of calcium ion and produces the most rapid effect. The glucceptate and gluconate salts require hepatic degradation to release the free calcium ion. Calcium chloride is, therefore, the best choice. It is highly irritating to tissues and must be injected into a large vein with precautions to avoid extravasation. Calcium chloride is available in a 10% solution. An initial dose of 250 to 500 mg may be administered slowly over several minutes. It may be repeated as necessary at 10-minute intervals, if strong indications exist.

Precautions for calcium use include the need for slow injection without extravasation. If bicarbonate has been administered through the same line, it must be cleared before introducing the calcium. If the patient has a rhythm, rapid injection may result in bradycardia. Calcium salts must be used with caution in patients receiving digitalis.

Sodium Nitroprusside. This is a rapidly acting dilator of both arteries and veins. Systemic arterial dilatation decreases impedance to left ventricular outflow (afterload reduction), thereby

Fig. 32-22. Bradycardia with a pulse. (From *Guidelines for Cardiopulmonary Resuscitation and Emergency Cardiac Care,* 1992, copyright American Medical Association. With permission.)

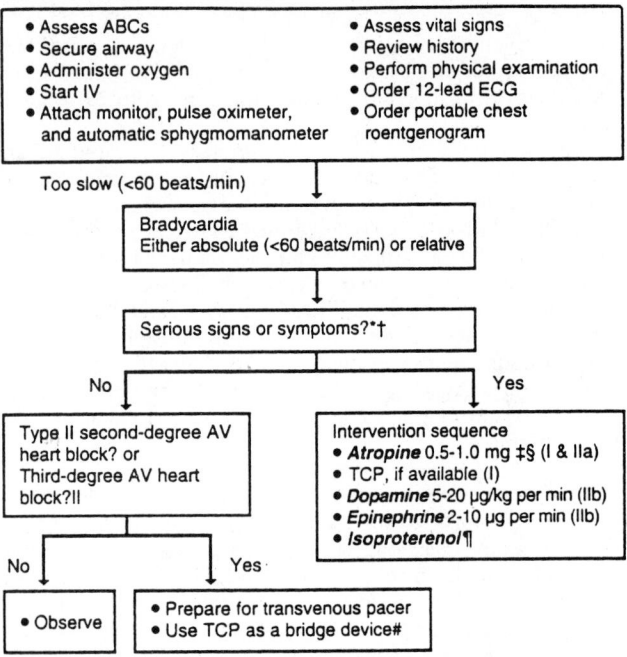

- Assess ABCs
- Secure airway
- Administer oxygen
- Start IV
- Attach monitor, pulse oximeter, and automatic sphygmomanometer
- Assess vital signs
- Review history
- Perform physical examination
- Order 12-lead ECG
- Order portable chest roentgenogram

Too slow (<60 beats/min)

Bradycardia
Either absolute (<60 beats/min) or relative

Serious signs or symptoms?*†

No   Yes

Type II second-degree AV heart block? or Third-degree AV heart block?||

Intervention sequence
- *Atropine* 0.5-1.0 mg ‡§ (I & IIa)
- TCP, if available (I)
- *Dopamine* 5-20 µg/kg per min (IIb)
- *Epinephrine* 2-10 µg per min (IIb)
- *Isoproterenol*¶

No   Yes

- Observe

- Prepare for transvenous pacer
- Use TCP as a bridge device#

*Serious signs or symptoms must be related to the slow rate.
  Clinical manifestations include:
  symptoms (chest pain, shortness of breath, decreased level of conciousness) and
  signs (low BP, shock, pulmonary congestion, CHF, acute MI).
†Do not delay TCP while awaiting IV access or for *atropine* to take effect if patient is symptomatic.
‡Denervated transplanted hearts will not respond to *atropine*. Go at once to pacing, *catecholamine* infusion, or both.
§*Atropine* should be given in repeat doses in 3-5 min up to total of 0.04 mg/kg. Consider shorter dosing intervals in severe clinical conditions. It has been suggested that atropine should be used with caution in atrioventricular (AV) block at the His-Purkinje level (type II AV block and new third-degree block with wide QRS complexes) (Class IIb).
||Never treat third-degree heart block plus ventricular escape beats with *lidocaine.*
¶*Isoproterenol* should be used, if at all, with exteme caution. At low doses it is Class IIb (possibly helpful); at higher doses it is Class III (harmful).
#Verify patient tolerance and mechanical capture. Use analgesia and sedation as needed.

diminishing resistance to left ventricular ejection and improving cardiac output. Venous dilatation simultaneously provides preload reduction by withholding blood from the central circulation and reducing left ventricular filling pressure and volume. Myocardial oxygen consumption drops and subendocardial blood flow may rise as ventricular wall stress is lowered. In addition, the lowered left ventricular filling pressures cause a decrease in pulmonary capillary pressure and pulmonary congestion. Although vasodilators are most commonly used in the critical care unit, they are occasionally needed in the emergency room to aid in stabilizing the resuscitated patient with severe left ventricular dysfunction.

Nitroprusside is indicated in any situation in which cardiac output is severely reduced, causing either cardiogenic shock with elevated systemic vascular resistance or pulmonary congestion from elevated left ventricular filling pressure. Patients with aortic or mitral regurgitation or a left-to-right shunt from a ventricular septal rupture are apt to respond especially well to nitroprusside infusion. Nitroprusside has also become a preferred treatment for patients in hypertensive crisis.

Nitroprusside is administered by intravenous infusion. The onset of action is rapid, so that the effects of dose change become apparent within several minutes. For patients with severe left ventricular failure, infusion should begin at 10 μg per minute, with increments of 5 to 10 μg per minute at 5-minute intervals. Most patients will respond to a total dose of 50 to 100 μg per minute, although an occasional patient will require a significantly higher dose. Patients in hypertensive crisis may be started at 50 μg per minute and may require as much as 400 to 1000 μg per minute. Nitroprusside is available in 50-mg vials of dihydrate. The drug should be dissolved in 5 ml of D$_5$W and diluted to a volume of 250 to 1000 ml of D$_5$W. Because of the instability of the reconstituted solution, it is recommended that it be used within 4 hours. The solution should be wrapped in opaque material because nitroprusside deteriorates more rapidly with exposure to light.

Precautions for nitroprusside include hypotension, generally secondary to excessive dosage. While most patients with hypotension cannot tolerate nitroprusside, others can be given nitroprusside with volume repletion. Nitroprusside is converted to thiocyanate by a hepatic enzyme, and the thiocyanate is cleared by the kidneys. Signs and symptoms of thiocyanate toxicity include nausea, tinnitus, blurred vision, and delirium. Thiocyanate blood levels should be measured in patients with renal dysfunction and those on high doses for a prolonged period.

Nitroglycerine. Like nitroprusside, nitroglycerine is a vasodilator that may prove useful in the emergency treatment of the postresuscitation patient. It may be given sublingually, transdermally, or intravenously, depending on the situation and desired dose. Unlike nitroprusside, nitroglycerine is a more potent dilator of venous capacitance vessels than of arterioles; therefore, it is more a preload reducer than an afterload reducer. Coronary dilatation does occur and may be particularly beneficial in patients with coronary spasm and acute ischemia. Myocardial ischemia is reversed through the lowering of preload and myocardial oxygen consumption as well as by coronary dilatation.

Sublingual or transdermal nitroglycerine is indicated for angina. The sublingual route is preferable. For persistent or frequently recurring ischemia unrelieved by other routes of administration, an infusion of nitroglycerine is often effective. It is useful for suspected coronary spasm. An infusion of nitroglycerine may also be used for preload reduction in patients with left ventricular failure. It may be given together with an infusion of nitroprusside, especially if ischemia has not been reversed by the hemodynamic effects of nitroprusside alone.

Nitroglycerine is administered by a sublingual tablet or spray (0.3–0.4 mg) or by transdermal patch or ointment. For rapid effect the sublingual route should be used. It may be repeated every 3 to 5 minutes, if pain relief or return of S–T segments to baseline has not yet occurred. If ischemia persists, an infusion should be started and titrated to achieve the desired result. A 50-μg bolus of nitroglycerine may be given before the initiation of an intravenous drip. Two 20-mg vials may be diluted in 250 ml of D$_5$W for a concentration of 160 μg per milliliter. The infusion is started at 10 to 20 μg per minute and increased by 5 to 10 μg every 5 to 10 minutes until the desired effect is achieved (e.g., fall in left ventricular pressure to 15 to 18 mm Hg or relief of chest pain and return of ST segments to baseline). While most patients respond to 50 to 200 μg per minute, an occasional patient will require 500 μg per minute or more; however, the maintenance of high plasma levels of nitroglycerine may induce tolerance. *Whenever possible, intermittent dosing with nitrate-free periods is recommended, and the use of the lowest effective dose is advised.*

Precautions for nitroglycerine use include hypotension and syncope, especially if the patient has had an acute myocardial infarction, is volume-depleted, or has restriction to either left ventricular filling (e.g., pericardial constriction or tamponade, hypertrophic disease, mitral stenosis, pulmonic stenosis, or pulmonary hypertension) or restriction in left ventricular outflow (e.g., aortic stenosis or hypertrophic obstructive cardiomyopathy). Rapid titration of intravenous nitroglycerine in patients with left ventricular failure requires careful hemodynamic monitoring to ensure efficacy and safety. The hypotensive patient may be placed in the Trendelenburg position and given volume replacement. Rarely, a patient with severe obstructive coronary disease develops worsened ischemia with nitroglycerine through a coronary steal mechanism. If ischemia is persistent in spite of maximum tolerated nitroglycerine dose, attempts should be made to decrease the dose and other modalities of therapy, including heparin or cardiac catheterization, considered, with a view to early revascularization.

Clinical Settings

The procedures involved in resuscitation of a victim of cardiovascular or respiratory collapse are part of a continuum progressing from initial recognition of the problem and institution of CPR to intervention with defibrillators, drugs, pacemakers, transport, and postresuscitative evaluation and care. The following sections focus on the pharmacologic and electrical intervention appropriate to various clinical settings common in cardiac arrest.

VENTRICULAR FIBRILLATION. Ventricular fibrillation is the initial rhythm encountered in 50 to 70 percent of prehospital cardiac arrests and 30 to 40 percent of hospital cardiac arrests. In a significant percentage of hospital cardiac arrests and in a smaller number of prehospital arrests, pulseless ventricular tachycardia is the first rhythm encountered by rescue personnel. Electrical defibrillation is the most important intervention in treating these arrhythmias (Fig. 32-19). The sooner it is administered, the more likely it is to succeed. If a defibrillator is not immediately available and an adult cardiac arrest is witnessed, a precordial thump should be delivered after determining pulselessness [156,157]. Many witnessed arrests in the emergency room will be in monitored patients; the rescuer, however, must not initially rely solely on the monitored signal but must confirm the need for CPR by determining the absence of a pulse. If after the precordial thump a pulse has not returned, CPR is continued. In unmonitored cases in which a defibrillator is readily available, quick-look paddles should confirm the diagnosis of ventricular fibrillation or ventricular tachycardia and countershock should be attempted at an energy level of 200 joules without delay. If the patient remains in ventricular fibrillation or pulseless tachycardia, a second shock at 200 to 300 joules should be delivered immediately. A third countershock at 360 joules should be given if the ventricular arrhythmia persists. Between the second and third shocks, the rhythm is determined by assessing the monitor. If the arrhythmia has not demonstrated a change, the subsequent shock is delivered. Pulse need not be checked at those times unless the monitored rhythm shows a possible change. If ventricular fibrillation or tachycardia recurs after transiently converting (rather than persisting without converting), the previously successful energy level should be used in the next attempt to defibrillate.

In cases that persist in pulseless ventricular tachycardia or fibrillation despite three attempts at countershock, CPR is initiated, supplemental oxygen added when available, intravenous access established, and epinephrine (10 ml of a 1:10,000 dilution) administered as a bolus. It is best to administer the drug into the central circulation. If the antecubital vein is used, the arm should be elevated and the drug flushed with 20 ml of intravenous fluid to facilitate access to the central circulation. During CPR, drugs should not be given into more peripheral veins or below the level of the diaphragm, as access into the thoracic circulation is sluggish [229,230]. Early intubation is preferable if it can be performed without delaying defibrillation attempts and administration of epinephrine. Within 30 to 60 seconds of epinephrine administration, defibrillation should again be attempted at 360 joules. Three sequential shocks are also acceptable at this point if the monitor fails to display a change in the rhythm. If ventricular fibrillation or tachycardia has not responded or has responded only transiently, lidocaine

hydrochloride, 1 mg per kilogram, should be administered as an intravenous push. Large clinical studies of refractory ventricular fibrillation have failed to demonstrate any differential advantage between bretylium and lidocaine [231,232], therefore either repeated doses of lidocaine (0.5 mg/kg boluses every 8 minutes for a total of 3 mg/kg) or bretylium (initially 5 mg/kg, then 10 mg/kg) may be used. Repeated doses of epinephrine (10 ml of a 1:10,000 dilution or higher doses, if selected) should also be administered at 3- to 5-minute intervals in an attempt to maintain an adequate coronary perfusion pressure during CPR.

Adequacy of ventilation should be assessed with an arterial blood gas determination, if possible. Sodium bicarbonate is of questionable value during most cardiac arrests but should be administered if the patient has known preexisting hyperkalemia. Otherwise, it is probably effective and may be considered if the patient is intubated and has known preexisting bicarbonate-responsive acidosis or tricyclic antidepressant overdose or to alkalinize the urine in drug overdose. It is possibly useful and may be considered in an intubated patient with a long arrest interval. When used, it is administered at 1 mEq per kilogram.

Repeated countershocks at 360 joules (or three sequential shocks) should be administered after each major drug intervention. If a perfusing supraventricular rhythm develops, a lidocaine bolus should be administered, if one has not yet been given during the sequence of interventions. In addition, blood gas determination and sodium bicarbonate administration may be of use once a perfusing rhythm has been restored and the PCO_2 of expired air has presumably risen.

ASYSTOLE. Asystole (Fig. 32-23) is the first rhythm encountered in 30 to 40 percent of prehospital as well as hospital cardiac arrests. Asystole is obviously the end result of any pulseless rhythm, and as such, when it is the presenting rhythm it is often the termination of untreated ventricular fibrillation. In the prehospital setting, many cases of asystole are related to delayed initiation of BLS and/or ACLS. Primary asystole associated with increased parasympathetic tone is less common but does occur. Whether this rhythm occurs as the initial rhythm or fol-

Fig. 32-23. Asystole. (From *Guidelines for Cardiopulmonary Resuscitation and Emergency Cardiac Care,* 1992, copyright American Medical Association. With permission.)

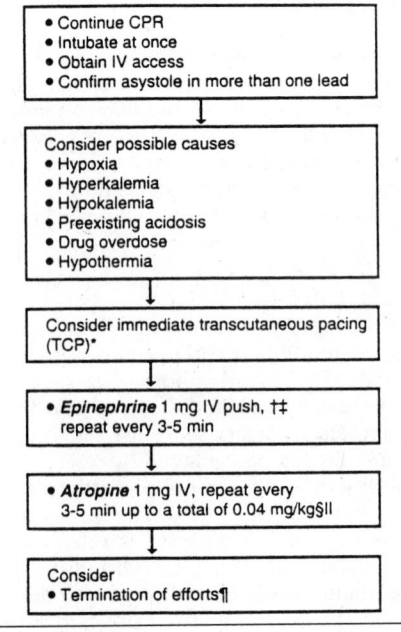

Class I: definitely helpful
Class IIa: acceptable, probably helpful
Class IIb: acceptable, possibly helpful
Class III: not indicated, may be harmful
*TCP is a Class IIb intervention. Lack of success may be due to delays in pacing. To be effective TCP must be performed early, simultaneously with drugs. Evidence does not support routine use of TCP for asystole.
†The recommended dose of *epinephrine* is 1 mg IV push every 3-5 min. If this approach fails, several Class IIb dosing regimens can be considered:
• Intermediate: *epinephrine* 2-5 mg IV push, every 3-5 min
• Escalating: *epinephrine* 1 mg-3 mg-5 mg IV push (3 min apart)
• High: *epinephrine* 0.1 mg/kg IV push, every 3-5 min
‡*Sodium bicarbonate* 1 mEq/kg is Class I if patient has known preexisting hyperkalemia.

§Shorter *atropine* dosing intervals are Class IIb in asystolic arrest.
‖*Sodium bicarbonate* 1 mEq/kg:
Class IIa
• if known preexisting bicarbonate-responsive acidosis
• if overdose with tricyclic antidepressants
• to alkalinize the urine in drug overdoses
Class IIb
• if intubated and continued long arrest interval
• upon return of spontaneous circulation after long arrest interval
Class III
• hypoxic lactic acidosis
¶If patient remains in asystole or other agonal rhythms after successful intubation and initial medications and no reversible causes are identified, consider termination of resuscitative efforts by a physician. Consider interval since arrest.

lows on ventricular tachycardia or fibrillation, it carries a very poor prognosis: Fewer than 1 to 2 percent of patients can be expected to revert successfully to a perfusing rhythm. Even more rarely will such a patient leave the hospital with reasonable neurologic integrity or significantly long-term survival. Such a patient's best hope lies in the early discovery and treatment of a reversible cause for cardiovascular collapse, such as hypovolemia. Occasionally, asystole develops due to excessive vagal tone, such as that seen with induction of anesthesia during surgical procedures, or stimulation of carotid body, bladder, biliary, or gastrointestinal tract. Unfortunately, most patients with asystole suffer from severe coronary artery disease and are unlikely to be salvageable.

In patients with apparent asystole, CPR is initiated; as soon as possible an intravenous line should be established and epinephrine administered, as in pulseless ventricular tachycardia or fibrillation. Transcutaneous pacing, if available, may be considered. While evidence does not support the routine use of transcutaneous pacing in asystole, lack of success is likely to be due to delays in its use [233]. If used, it should be used early along with drug administration. If a perfusing rhythm is not promptly restored, a full vagolytic dose of atropine should be given, with 1 mg initially and every 3 to 5 minutes, to a total dose of 3 mg (0.04 mg/kg). Additional doses of epinephrine should be given at 3- to 5-minute intervals if a favorable response has not occurred.

It has been demonstrated that ventricular fibrillation may masquerade as asystole in several leads and for minutes at a time [234]. It is therefore important to check at least two different lead configurations at 90-degree orientation to confirm the diagnosis of asystole. Routine shocking of asystole, however, is discouraged because of the possibility of increasing parasympathetic tone [235,236] and thus decreasing further any chance of return of spontaneous rhythm. No improvement in survival has been demonstrated with the use of shocks for presumed asystole [237,238,239].

As in other forms of arrest, neither sodium bicarbonate nor calcium has been shown to be of benefit; these agents should be considered only under specific circumstances (see above).

Temporary artificial pacing is of no likely benefit in primary or postcountershock asystole. Pacing with endocardial electrodes, percutaneous transthoracic electrodes, or external transcutaneous electrodes has led to pitifully few long-term survivals in these cases [163,164,165].

The use of isoproterenol in an attempt to stimulate pacemakers through its beta-adrenergic agonist effects has not proved beneficial. Indeed, its peripheral beta-stimulation produces a decrease in arterial resistance and perfusion pressure that is detrimental, whereas alpha-agonists seem to increase myocardial and cerebral perfusion [185–188,240,241].

PULSELESS ELECTRICAL ACTIVITY. Pulseless electrical activity (PEA) is present when an arrest victim is found to have organized electrocardiographic ventricular complexes (QRS) unassociated with a palpable pulse. Pulseless ventricular tachycardia is not considered a form of PEA. Electromechanical dissociation (EMD) is a form of PEA in which the QRS is unaccompanied by any evidence of ventricular contraction and the emergency response is the same (Fig. 32-24). Along with PEA and EMD may be considered bradyasystolic rhythms and severe wide-complex bradycardias. These arrhythmias may be associated with specific clinical states that, if reversed early, may lead to the return of a pulse. It is best, therefore, to consider them together. When PEA is encountered, severe hypovolemia, cardiac tamponade, massive pulmonary embolism, tension

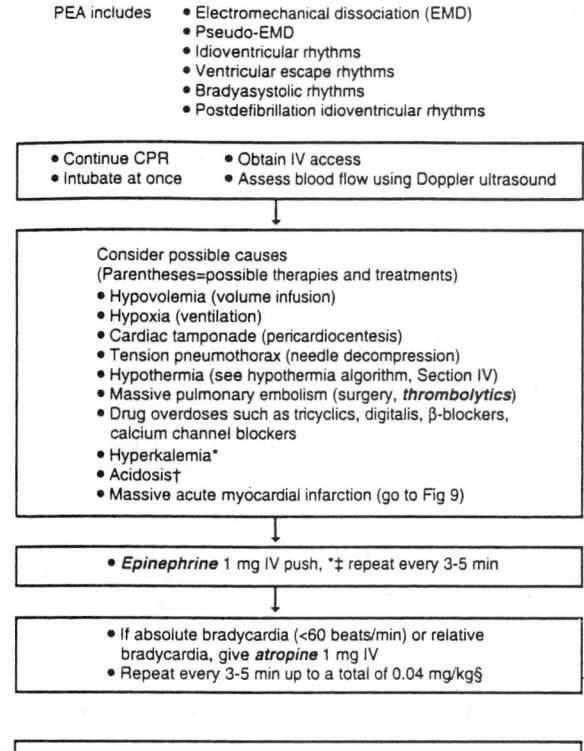

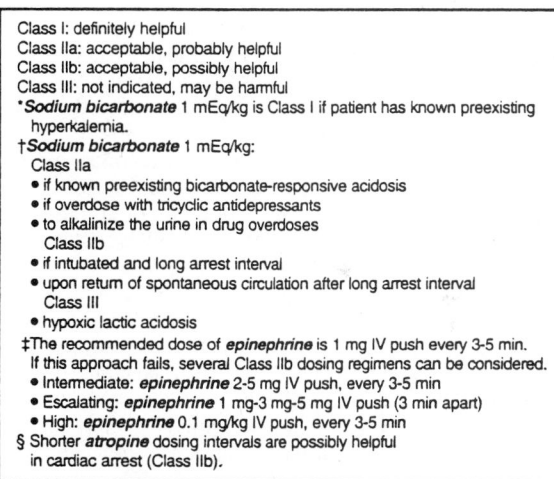

Fig. 32-24. Pulseless electrical activity (PEA) and electromechanical dissociation (EMD). (From *Guidelines for Cardiopulmonary Resuscitation and Emergency Cardiac Care,* 1992, copyright American Medical Association. With permission.)

pneumothorax, and severe myocardial contractile dysfunction should be considered.

With the diagnosis of PEA, CPR is initiated and, as soon as possible, volume is administered in the form of intravenous crystalloid or colloid. If PEA is indeed caused by intravascular volume depletion, a fluid challenge may return a pulse. Epinephrine should be administered as in other forms of arrest and doses repeated at 3- to 5-minute intervals if a pulse has not returned. In patients at high risk for pericardial effusions (i.e., patients hospitalized with known malignancy, severe renal failure, recent myocardial infarction, or cardiac catheterization) pericardiocentesis should be attempted early in the course of

CPR if the patient is not responding to volume and alpha-agonists. In prehospital arrests pericardial tamponade is rare, but an attempt at pericardiocentesis is warranted if there is no favorable response to volume or alpha-agonists. Echocardiography, when available, will almost always confirm or rule out the possibility of tamponade and may be useful in delineating the volume status as well as the function of the ventricles.

SPECIAL SITUATIONS. Near drowning victims in cold water may recover after prolonged periods of submersion. Apparently, the hypothermia coupled with the bradycardia of the diving reflex may serve to protect against organ damage [242,243]. Successful resuscitation has been described after considerable periods of submersion [243,244]. Since it is often difficult for bystanders and rescuers to estimate the duration of submersion, in most cases it is warranted to initiate CPR at the scene, unless there exists physical evidence of irreversible death, such as putrefaction or dependent rubor (see Chap. 63).

Hypothermia may occur with environmental exposures other than cold water drowning. The body's ability to maintain temperature is diminished by alcohol, sedation, antidepressants, neurologic problems, and advanced age. Because of the associated bradycardia and oxygen-sparing effects, prolonged hypothermia and arrest may be tolerated with complete recovery. A longer period may be needed to establish breathlessness and pulselessness because of the profound bradycardia and slowed respiratory rate. Resuscitative efforts should not be abandoned until near normal temperature has been reestablished [245].

Electric shock and lightning strike may lead to tetanic spasm of respiratory muscles or convulsion causing respiratory arrest. Ventricular fibrillation or asystole may occur from the electric shock or after prolonged respiratory arrest. Before initiating assessment and CPR, the potential rescuer must ascertain whether the victim is still in contact with the electrical energy and that "live wires" are not in dangerous proximity. If the victim is located at the top of a utility pole, CPR is best instituted after the victim is lowered to the ground [246].

Open chest CPR with thoracotomy should be applied early in cases of penetrating chest trauma associated with cardiac arrest (see preceding). In such patients, thoracotomy by trained personnel will allow for the relief of pericardial tamponade and possible control of exsanguinating hemorrhage. Well-equipped trauma centers should have multidisciplinary teams that can provide early definitive surgical treatment. The unanswered question is whether another subgroup of patients who have not responded to conventional ACLS techniques (including defibrillation attempts and drugs) would benefit by thoracotomy and open chest CPR. Animal studies suggest that survival may be improved over closed chest compression if open chest CPR is used within the first 15 minutes of arrest [247,248,249]. If open chest CPR is delayed until 20 minutes or more of closed chest CPR, there is no improvement in outcome despite improved hemodynamics [233,234]. In patients with out-of-hospital arrest in whom open chest CPR was attempted after 30 minutes of conventional CPR, survival did not improve [250].

Other instances in which open chest CPR may be considered include cardiac arrest in patients with chest deformity in which closed chest CPR is not providing a pulse; penetrating abdominal trauma with deterioration and cardiac arrest in which aortic cross-clamping may provide temporary control of abdominal hemorrhage; blunt trauma with cardiac arrest; and cardiac arrest due to hypothermia, pulmonary embolism, pericardial tamponade, or abdominal hemorrhage in which initiation of conventional therapy and closed chest CPR is not proving effective. In the aforementioned cases, the decision to use open chest CPR presupposes quick availability of definitive surgical intervention.

References

1. Paraskos JA: Biblical accounts of resuscitation. *J Hist Med Allied Sci* 47:310, 1992.
2. Paraskos JA: History of CPR and the role of the national conference. *Ann Emerg Med* 22:275, 1993.
3. Safar P: History of cardiopulmonary-cerebral resuscitation, in Kaye W, Bircher N (eds): *Cardiopulmonary Resuscitation*. New York, Churchill Livingstone, 1989.
4. Ibycus: Chrysippus, quoted in Strauss MB (ed): *Familiar Medical Quotations*. Boston, Little Brown, 1968.
5. Stephenson HE Jr: *Cardiac Arrest and Resuscitation*. St. Louis, Mosby, 1958.
6. Zoll PM, Linenthal AJ, Gibson W, et al: Termination of ventricular fibrillation in man by externally applied electrical countershock. *N Engl J Med* 254:727, 1956.
7. Safar P: Mouth to mouth airway. *Anesthesiology* 18:904, 1957.
8. Safar P, Escarraga L, Elam JO: A comparison of the mouth to mouth and mouth to airway methods of artificial respiration with the chest pressure arm-lift method. *N Engl J Med* 258:671, 1958.
9. Elam JO, Green DG, Brown ES, et al: Oxygen and carbon dioxide exchange and energy cost of expired air resuscitation. *JAMA* 167:328, 1958.
10. Kouwenhoven WB, Jude JR, Knickerbocker GG: Closed chest cardiac massage. *JAMA* 173:1064, 1960.
11. Cardiopulmonary resuscitation: Statement by the Ad Hoc Committee on Cardiopulmonary Resuscitation of the Division of Medical Sciences, National Academy of Sciences, National Research Council. *JAMA* 178:372, 1966.
12. Standards for cardiopulmonary resuscitation (CPR) and emergency cardiac care (ECC). *JAMA* 227(suppl):833, 1974.
13. Standards and guidelines for cardiopulmonary resuscitation (CPR) and emergency cardiac care (ECC). *JAMA* 244:453, 1980.
14. Standards and guidelines for cardiopulmonary resuscitation (CPR) and emergency cardiac care (ECC). *JAMA* 255:2843, 1986.
15. Guidelines for cardiopulmonary resuscitation and emergency cardiac care. *JAMA* 268:2171, 1992.
16. A definition of irreversible coma: Report of the Ad Hoc Committee of the Harvard Medical School to Examine the Definition of Brain Death. *JAMA* 205:337, 1968.
17. An appraisal of the criteria of cerebral death—A summary statement: A collaborative study. *JAMA* 237:982, 1976.
18. Guidelines for the determination of death: Report of the medical consultants on the diagnosis of death to the President's Commission for the Study of Ethical Problems in Medicine and Biomedical and Behavioral Research. *JAMA* 246:2184, 1981.
19. Kansas Session Laws of 1970, chap 378.
20. *Commonwealth v. Golston*, 366 NE 2d 744, 1977.
21. Lund I, Skulberg A: Resuscitation of cardiac arrest outside hospitals: Experience with a mobile intensive care unit in Oslo. *Acta Anesthesiol Scand* 53(suppl):13, 1973.
22. Copley DP, Mantle JA, Roger WJ, et al: Improved outcome for prehospital cardiopulmonary collapse with resuscitation by bystanders. *Circulation* 56:902, 1977.
23. Cummins RO, Eisenberg MS, Hallstrom AP, et al: Survival of out-of-hospital cardiac arrest with early initiation of cardiopulmonary resuscitation. *Am J Emerg Med* 3:114, 1985.
24. Weaver WD, Cobb LA, Hallstrom AP, et al: Considerations for improving survival from out-of-hospital cardiac arrest. *Ann Emerg Med* 15:1181, 1986.
25. Eisenberg MS, Bergner L, Hallstrom A: Cardiac resuscitation in the community: Importance of rapid provision and implications for program planning. *JAMA* 241:1905, 1979.
26. Weaver WD, Copass MK, Bufi D, et al: Improved neurologic recovery and survival after early defibrillation. *Circulation* 69:943, 1984.
27. Myerburg RJ, Conde CA, Sung RJ, et al: Clinical electrophysiologic and hemodynamic profile of patients resuscitated from prehospital cardiac arrest. *Am J Med* 68:568, 1980.
28. Myerburg RJ, Kessler KM, Zaman L, et al: Survivors of prehospital cardiac arrest. *JAMA* 247:1485, 1982.
29. Camarata SJ, Weil MH, Hanashiro PK, et al: Cardiac arrest in the critically ill. 1. A study of predisposing causes in 132 patients. *Circulation* 44:688, 1971.

30. Hahn RG, Hutchinson JC, Conte JE: Cardiopulmonary resuscitation in a university hospital, an analysis of survival and cost. *West J Med* 131:344, 1979.

31. DeBard ML: Cardiopulmonary resuscitation: Analysis of six years' experience and review of the literature. *Ann Emerg Med* 10:408, 1981.

32. Bedell SE, Delbanco TL, Cook EF, et al: Survival after cardiopulmonary resuscitation in the hospital. *N Engl J Med* 309:569, 1983.

33. Lemire JG, Johnson AL: Is cardiac resuscitation worthwhile? A decade of experience. *N Engl J Med* 286:970, 1972.

34. Pantridge JF, Geddes JS: A mobile intensive care unit in the management of myocardial infarction. *Lancet* 2:271, 1967.

35. Tweed WA, Bristow G, Donen N: Resuscitation from cardiac arrest: Assessment of a system providing only basic life support outside of hospital. *Can Med Assoc J* 122:297, 1980.

36. Vertesi L, Wilson L, Glick N: Cardiac arrest: Comparison of paramedic and conventional ambulance services. *Can Med Assoc J* 128:809, 1983.

37. Stults KR, Brown DD, Schug VL, et al: Prehospital defibrillation performed by emergency medical technicians in rural communities. *N Engl J Med* 310:219, 1984.

38. Smith JP, Bodai BI: The urban paramedic's scope of practice. *JAMA* 253:544, 1985.

39. Stults KR, Brown DD, Kerber RE: Efficacy of an automated external defibrillator in the management of out-of-hospital cardiac arrest: Validation of the diagnostic algorithm and initial clinical experience in a rural environment. *Circulation* 73:701, 1986.

40. Weaver WD, Hill D, Fahrenbruch CE, et al: Use of the automatic external defibrillator in the management of out-of-hospital cardiac arrest. *N Engl J Med* 319:661, 1988.

41. Eisenberg MS, Copass MK, Hallstrom AP, et al: Treatment of out-of-hospital cardiac arrest with rapid defibrillation by emergency medical technicians. *N Engl J Med* 302:1379, 1980.

42. Emergency Cardiac Care Committee: Automated external defibrillators and advanced cardiac life support: A new initiative from the American Heart Association. *Am J Emerg Med* 9:91, 1991.

43. Paraskos JA: External compression without adjuncts. *Circulation* 74(suppl):IV-33, 1986.

44. MacKenzie GJ, Taylor SH, McDonald AH, et al: Haemodynamic effects of external cardiac compression. *Lancet* 1:1342, 1964.

45. DelGuercio LRM, Coomaraswamy RP, State D: Cardiac output and other hemodynamic variables during external cardiac massage in man. *N Engl J Med* 269:1398, 1963.

46. DelGuercio LRM, Feind NR, Cohn JD, et al: Comparison of blood flow during external and internal cardiac massage in man. *Circulation* 31(suppl 1):171, 1965.

47. Oriol A, Smith HJ: Hemodynamic observations during closed-chest cardiac massage. *Can Med Assoc J* 98:841, 1968.

48. Ditchey RV, Winkler JV, Rhodes CA: Relative lack of coronary blood flow during closed-chest resuscitation in dogs. *Circulation* 66:297, 1982.

49. Niemann JT, Rosborough JP, Ung S, et al: Coronary perfusion pressure during experimental cardiopulmonary resuscitation. *Ann Emerg Med* 11:127, 1982.

50. Luce JM, Ross BK, O'Quin RJ, et al: Regional blood flow during cardiopulmonary resuscitation in dogs using simultaneous and nonsimultaneous compression and ventilation. *Circulation* 67:258, 1983.

51. Chandra N, Weisfeldt ML, Tsitlik J, et al: Augmentation of carotid flow during cardiopulmonary resuscitation by ventilation at high airway pressure simultaneous with chest compression. *Am J Cardiol* 48:1053, 1981.

52. Jackson RE, Joyce K, Danosi SF, et al: Blood flow in the cerebral cortex during cardiopulmonary resuscitation in dogs. *Ann Emerg Med* 13:657, 1984.

53. Koehler RC, Chandra N, Guerci AD, et al: Augmentation of cerebral perfusion by simultaneous chest compression and lung inflation with abdominal binding after cardiac arrest in dogs. *Circulation* 67:266, 1983.

54. Stajduhar K, Steinberg R, Sotosky M, et al: Cerebral blood flow and common carotid artery blood flow during open-heart CPR in dogs. *Ann Emerg Med* 13:385, 1984.

55. Sharff JA, Pantley G, Noel E: Effect of time on regional organ perfusion during two methods of cardiopulmonary resuscitation. *Ann Emerg Med* 13649, 1984.

56. Guerci A, Chandra N, Levin H, et al: Hemodynamic determinants of intracranial pressure during resuscitation. *Circulation* 64:IV-304, 1981.

57. Bircher N, Safar P: Open-chest CPR: An old method whose time has returned. *Am J Emerg Med* 2:568, 1984.

58. Krug JJ: Cardiac arrest secondary to Addison's disease. *Ann Emerg Med* 15:735, 1986.

59. Deshmukh HG, Weil MH, Rackow EC, et al: Echocardiographic observations during cardiopulmonary resuscitation: A preliminary report. *Crit Care Med* 13:904, 1985.

60. Maier GW, Tyson GS Jr, Olsen CO, et al: The physiology of external cardiac massage: High-impulse cardiopulmonary resuscitation. *Circulation* 70:86, 1984.

61. Weisfeldt ML, Chandra N: Physiology of cardiopulmonary resuscitation, in Creger WP (ed): *Annual Review of Medicine: Selected Topics in Clinical Sciences.* Palo Alto, CA, Annual Reviews, 1981, vol 32, p 437.

62. Weale FE, Rothwell-Jackson RL: The efficiency of cardiac massage. *Lancet* 1:990, 1962.

63. Wilder RJ, Weir D, Rush BF, et al: Methods of coordinating ventilation and closed chest cardiac massage in the dog. *Surgery* 53:186, 1963.

64. Criley JM, Blaufuss AJ, Kissel GL: Cough induced cardiac compression. *JAMA* 236:1246, 1976.

65. Niemann JT, Rosborough JP, Brown D, et al: Cough-CPR: Documentation of systemic perfusion in man and in an experimental model—A "window" to the mechanism of blood flow in external CPR. *Crit Care Med* 8:141, 1980.

66. Rudikoff MT, Maughan WL, Effron M, et al: Mechanisms of blood flow during cardiopulmonary resuscitation. *Circulation* 61:345, 1980.

67. Weisfeldt ML, Chandra N, Tsitlik J: Increased intrathoracic pressure—not direct heart compression—causes the rise in intrathoracic vascular pressures during CPR in dogs and pigs. *Crit Care Med* 9:377, 1981.

68. Niemann JT, Rosborough JP, Hausknecht M, et al: Pressure-synchronized cineangiography during experimental cardiopulmonary resuscitation. *Circulation* 64:985, 1981.

69. Rich S, Wix HL, Shapiro EP: Clinical assessment of heart chamber size and valve motion during cardiopulmonary resuscitation by two dimensional echocardiography. *Am Heart J* 102:368, 1981.

70. Werner JA, Greene HL, Janko CL, et al: Visualization of cardiac valve motion in man during external chest compression using two-dimensional echocardiography: Implications regarding the mechanism of blood flow. *Circulation* 63:1417, 1981.

71. Babbs CF: New versus old theories of blood flow during CPR. *Crit Care Med* 8:191, 1980.

72. Fisher J, Vaghaiwalla F, Tsitlik J, et al: Determinants and clinical significance of jugular venous valve competence. *Circulation* 65:188, 1982.

73. Taylor GJ, Tucker WM, Greene HL, et al: Importance of prolonged compression during cardiopulmonary resuscitation in man. *N Engl J Med* 296:1515, 1977.

74. Chandra N, Rudikoff M, Weisfeldt ML: Simultaneous chest compression and ventilation at high airway pressure during cardiopulmonary resuscitation. *Lancet* 1:175, 1980.

75. Bircher N, Safar P: Comparison of standard and "new" closed-chest CPR and open-chest CPR in dogs. *Crit Care Med* 9:384, 1981.

76. Sanders AB, Ewy GA, Alferness CA, et al: Failure of one method of simultaneous chest compression, ventilation, and abdominal binding during CPR. *Crit Care Med* 10:509, 1982.

77. Harris LC Jr, Kirimli B, Safar P: Augmentation of artificial circulation during cardiopulmonary resuscitation. *Anesthesiology* 28:730, 1967.

78. Harris LC Jr, Kirimli B, Safar P: Ventilation-cardiac compression ratios in CPR. *Anesthesiology* 28:806, 1967.

79. Redding JS: Abdominal compression in cardiopulmonary resuscitation. *Anesth Analg* 50:668, 1971.

80. Chandra N, Snyder LD, Weisfeldt ML: Abdominal binding during cardiopulmonary resuscitation in man. *JAMA* 246:351, 1981.

81. Niemann JT, Rosborough JP, Ung S, et al: Hemodynamic effects of continuous abdominal binding during cardiac arrest and resuscitation. *Am J Cardiol* 53:269, 1984.

82. Bircher N, Safar P: Cerebral preservation during cardiopulmonary resuscitation. *Crit Care Med* 13:185, 1985.

83. Ralston SH, Babbs CF, Niebauer MJ: Cardiopulmonary resuscitation with interposed abdominal compression in dogs. *Anesth Analg* 61:645, 1982.

84. Voorhees WD, Babbs CF, Niebauer MJ: Improved oxygen delivery during cardiopulmonary resuscitation with interposed abdominal compressions. *Ann Emerg Med* 12:128, 1983.

85. Voorhees WD, Ralston SH, Babbs CF: Regional blood flow during cardiopulmonary resuscitation with abdominal counterpulsation in dogs. *Am J Emerg Med* 2:123, 1984.

86. Babbs CF, Schoenlein WE, Lowe MW: Gastric insufflation during IAC-CPR and standard CPR in a canine model. *Am J Emerg Med* 3:99, 1985.

87. Mateer JR, Stueven HA, Thompson BM, et al: Prehospital IAC-CPR versus standard CPR: Paramedic resuscitation of cardiac arrests. *Am J Emerg Med* 3:143, 1985.

88. Sack JB, Kesselbrenner MB, Bregman D: Survival from in-hospital cardiac arrest with interposed abdominal counterpulsation during cardiopulmonary resuscitation. *JAMA* 267:379, 1992.

89. Barranco F, Lesmes A, Irles JA, et al: Cardiopulmonary resuscitation with simultaneous chest and abdominal compression: Comparative study in humans. *Resuscitation* 20:67, 1990.

90. Crul JF, Neursing BTJ, Zimmerman AHE: The ABC sequence of cardiopulmonary resuscitation (CPR). *J World Assoc Emerg Disaster Med* 1(suppl):236, 1985.

91. Lesser R, Bircher N, Safar P, et al: Sternal compression before ventilation in cardiopulmonary resuscitation (CPR). *J World Assoc Emerg Disaster Med* 1(suppl):239, 1985.

92. Hake TG: Studies on ether and chloroform from Professor Schiff's physiological laboratory. *Practitioner* 12:241, 1874.

93. Boehm R: Ueber Wiederbelebung nach Vergiftungen und Asphyxie. *Arch Exp Pathol Pharmacol* 8:68, 1878.

94. Pike FH, Guthrie CC, Stewart GN: Studies in resuscitation. I. The general conditions affecting resuscitation, and the resuscitation of blood and the heart. *J Exp Med* 10:371, 1908.

95. Stephenson HE Jr, Reid C, Hinton JW: Some common denominators in 1200 cases of cardiac arrest. *Ann Surg* 137:731, 1953.

96. Turk LN, Glenn WW: Cardiac arrest: Results of attempted resuscitation in 42 cases. *N Engl J Med* 251:795, 1954.

97. Bartlett RL, Stewart NJ, Raymond J, et al: Comparative study of three methods of resuscitation: Closed-chest, open-chest manual, and direct mechanical ventricular assistance. *Ann Emerg Med* 13:773, 1984.

98. Bircher N, Safar P: Manual open-chest cardiopulmonary resuscitation. *Ann Emerg Med* 13:770, 1984.

99. Shocket E, Rosenblum R: Successful open cardiac massage after 75 minutes of closed chest massage. *JAMA* 200:157, 1967.

100. Sykes MK, Ahmed N: Emergency treatment of cardiac arrest. *Lancet* 2:347, 1963.

101. Bodai BI, Smith JP, Ward RE, et al: Emergency thoracotomy in the management of trauma: A review. *JAMA* 249:1891, 1983.

102. Cogbill TH, Moore EE, Milikan JS, et al: Rationale for selective application of emergency department thoracotomy in trauma. *J Trauma* 23:453, 1983.

103. Danne PD, Finelli F, Champion HR: Emergency bay thoracotomy. *J Trauma* 24:796, 1984.

104. Kern KB, Sanders AB, Badylak SF, et al: Long-term survival with open-chest cardiac massage after ineffective closed-chest compression in a canine model. *Circulation* 75:498, 1987.

105. Kern KB, Sanders AB, Janas W, et al: Limitations of open-chest cardiac massage after prolonged, untreated cardiac arrest in dogs. *Ann Emerg Med* 20:761, 1991.

106. Long WB, Rosenblum S, Grady IP: Successful resuscitation of bupivacaine-induced cardiac arrest using cardiopulmonary bypass. *Anesth Analg* 69:403, 1989.

107. Pretto E, Safar P, Saito R, et al: Cardiopulmonary bypass after prolonged cardiac arrest in dogs. *Ann Emerg Med* 16:611, 1987.

108. Levine R, Gorayeb M, Safar P, et al: Emergency cardiopulmonary bypass after cardiac arrest and prolonged closed-chest CPR in dogs. *Ann Emerg Med* 16:620, 1987.

109. Martin GB, Nowak RM, Carden DL, et al: Cardiopulmonary bypass vs CPR as treatment for prolonged canine cardiopulmonary arrest. *Ann Emerg Med* 16:628, 1987.

110. Carden DL, Martin GB, Nowak RM, et al: The effect of cardiopulmonary bypass resuscitation on cardiac arrest induced lactic acidosis in dogs. *Resuscitation* 17:153, 1989.

111. Beyersdorf F, Acar C, Buckberg GD, et al: Studies on prolonged acute regional ischemia. IV. Aggressive surgical treatment for intractable ventricular fibrillation after myocardial infarction. *J Thorac Cardiovasc Surg* 98:557, 1989.

112. Hartz R, LoCicero J III, Sanders JH Jr, et al: Clinical experience with portable cardiopulmonary bypass in cardiac arrest patients. *Ann Thorac Surg* 50:437, 1990.

113. Ornato JP, Hallagan LF, McMahon SB, et al: Attitudes of BCLS instructors about mouth-to-mouth resuscitation during the AIDS epidemic. *Ann Emerg Med* 19:151, 1990.

114. Block AJ: The physician's responsibility for the care of AIDS patients: An opinion. *Chest* 94:1283, 1988.

115. Fox PC, Wolff A, Yeh CK, et al: Saliva inhibits HIV-1 infectivity. *J Am Dent Assoc* 116:635, 1988.

116. Freidland GH, Saltzman BR, Rogers MF, et al: Lack of transmission of HTLV III/LAV infection to household contacts of patients with AIDS or AIDS-related complex with oral candidiasis. *N Engl J Med* 314:344, 1986.

117. Marcus R, CDC Cooperative Needlestick Surveillance Group: Surveillance of health care workers exposed to blood from patients infected with the human immunodeficiency virus. *N Engl J Med* 319:1118, 1988.

118. Sande MH: Transmission of AIDS: The case against casual contagion. *N Engl J Med* 314:380, 1986.

119. Recommendations for prevention of HIV transmission in health care settings. *MMWR* 36(2S):3S, 1987.

120. Update: Universal precautions for prevention of transmission of human immunodeficiency virus, hepatitis B virus, and other bloodborne pathogens in health care settings. *MMWR* 37(24):377, 1988.

121. Risk of infection during CPR training and rescue: Supplemental guidelines. *JAMA* 262:2714, 1989.

122. Dracup K, Heaney DM, Taylor SE, et al: Can family members of high risk cardiac patients learn cardiopulmonary resuscitation? *Arch Intern Med* 149:61, 1989.

123. Goldberg RJ: Training of family members of high-risk cardiac patients in cardiopulmonary resuscitation: Skills performance and need for physician recommendations. *Arch Intern Med* 149:25, 1989.

124. Adgey AAJ, Geddes JS, Webb SW, et al: Acute phase of myocardial infarction. *Lancet* 2:501, 1971.

125. Proceedings of the 1992 National Conference on Cardiopulmonary Resuscitation and Emergency Cardiac Care. *Ann Emerg Med* 22:275, 1993.

126. Thompson RG, Hallstrom AP, Cobb LA: Bystander-initiated cardiopulmonary resuscitation in the management of ventricular fibrillation. *Ann Intern Med* 90:737, 1979.

127. Melker R, Cavallaro D, Krischer J: One-rescuer CPR: A reappraisal of present recommendations for ventilation. *Crit Care Med* 9:423, 1981.

128. Melker RJ: Asynchronous and other alternative methods of ventilation during CPR. *Ann Emerg Med* 13:758, 1984.

129. Melker RJ, Banner MJ: Ventilation during CPR: Two-rescuer standards reappraised. *Ann Emerg Med* 14:397, 1985.

130. Cohen TJ, Tucker KJ, Lurie KG, et al: Active compression-decompression: A new method of cardiopulmonary resuscitation. *JAMA* 267:2916, 1992.

130a. Shultz JJ, Coffeen P, Sweeney M, et al: Evaluation of standard and active compression-decompression CPR in an acute human model of ventricular fibrillation. *Circulation* 89:684, 1994.

130b. Tucker KJ, Galli F, Savitt MA, et al: Active compression-decompression resuscitation: Effect on resuscitation success after in-hospital cardiac arrest. *J Am Coll Cardiol* 24:201, 1994.

131. Salem MR, Wong AY, Mani M, et al: Efficacy of cricoid pressure in preventing gastric inflation during bag-mask ventilation in pediatric patients. *Anesthesiology* 40:96, 1974.

132. Melker RJ: Alternative methods of ventilation during respiratory and cardiac arrest. *Circulation* 74(suppl): IV-63, 1986.

133. Krischer JP, Fine EG, Davis JH, et al: Complications of cardiac resuscitation. *Chest* 92:287, 1987.

134. Nagel EL, Fine EG, Krischer JP, et al: Complications of CPR. *Crit Care Med* 9:424, 1981.

135. Powner DJ, Holcombe PA, Mello LA: Cardiopulmonary resuscitation-related injuries. *Crit Care Med* 12:54, 1984.

136. Crile G, Dolley DH: Experimental resuscitation of dogs killed by anesthetics and asphyxia. *J Exp Med* 6:713, 1906.

137. Sanders AB, Ewy GA, Taft TV: Prognostic and therapeutic importance of the aortic diastolic pressure in resuscitation from cardiac arrest. *Crit Care Med* 12:871, 1984.

138. Michael JR, Guerci AD, Koehler RC, et al: Mechanisms by which epinephrine augments cerebral and myocardial perfusion during cardiopulmonary resuscitation in dogs. *Circulation* 69:822, 1984.

139. Ralston SH, Voorhees WD, Babbs CF: Intrapulmonary epinephrine during prolonged cardiopulmonary resuscitation: Improved regional blood flow and resuscitation in dogs. *Ann Emerg Med* 13:79, 1984.

140. Paradis NA, Martin GB, Rivers EP, et al: Coronary perfusion pressure and the return of spontaneous circulation in cardiopulmonary resuscitation in humans. *JAMA* 263:1106, 1990.

141. Ludwig S, Kettrick RG, Parker M: Pediatric cardiopulmonary resuscitation. *Clin Pediatr* 23:71, 1984.

142. Torphy DE, Minter MG, Thompson BM: Cardiorespiratory arrest and resuscitation of children. *Am J Dis Child* 138:1099, 1984.

143. Heimlich HJ, Hoffman KA, Canestri FR: Food-choking and drowning deaths prevented by external subdiaphragmatic compression: Physiologic basis. *Ann Thorac Surg* 20:188, 1975.

144. Heimlich HJ, Uhtley MH: The Heimlich maneuver. *Clin Symp* 31:22, 1979.

145. Carveth SW, Burnap TK, Bechtel J, et al: Training in advanced cardiac life support. *JAMA* 235:2311, 1976.

146. Lowenstein SR, Sabyan EM, Lassen CF, et al: Benefits of training physicians in advanced cardiac life support. *Chest* 89:512, 1986.

147. Sellick BA: Cricoid pressure to control regurgitation of stomach contents during induction of anaesthesia. *Lancet* 2:404, 1961.

148. Meislin H: The esophageal obturator airway: A study of respiratory effectiveness. *Ann Emerg Med* 9:54, 1980.

149. Hammargren Y, Clinton JE, Ruiz E: A standard comparison of esophageal obturator airway and endotracheal tube ventilation in cardiac arrest. *Ann Emerg Med* 14:953, 1985.

150. Auerbach PS, Geehr EC: Inadequate oxygenation and ventilation using the esophageal gastric tube airway in the prehospital setting. *JAMA* 250:3067, 1983.

151. Smith JP, Bodai BI, Aubourg R, et al: A field evaluation of the esophageal obturator airway. *J Trauma* 23:317, 1983.

152. Smith RB, Babinski M, Klain M, et al: Percutaneous transtracheal ventilation. *J Am Coll Emerg Phys* 5:765, 1976.

153. McGill J, Clinton JE, Ruiz E: Cricothyrotomy in the emergency department. *Ann Emerg Med* 11:361, 1982.

154. Simon RR, Brenner BE: Emergency cricothyroidotomy in the patient with massive neck swelling. 1. Anatomical aspects. *Crit Care Med* 11:114, 1983.

155. Simon RR, Brenner BE, Rosen MA: Emergency cricothyroidotomy in the patient with massive neck swelling. 2. Clinical aspects. *Crit Care Med* 11:119, 1983.

156. Caldwell G, Millar G, Quinn E, et al: Simple mechanical methods of cardioversion: A defense of the precordial thump and cough version. *Br Med J* 291:627, 1985.

157. Pennington JE, Taylor J, Lown B: Chest thump for reverting ventricular tachycardia. *N Engl J Med* 283:1192, 1970.

158. Wei JY, Green HL, Weisgeldt ML: Cough facilitated cardioversion of ventricular tachycardia. *Am J Cardiol* 45:174, 1980.

159. Yakaitis RW, Redding JS: Precordial thumping during cardiac resuscitation. *Crit Care Med* 1:22, 1973.

160. Weaver WD, Cobb LA, Copass MK, et al: Ventricular defibrillation: A comparative trial using 175–J and 320–J shocks. *N Engl J Med* 207:1101, 1982.

161. Kerber RE, Jensen SR, Gascho JA, et al: Determinants of defibrillation: Prospective analysis of 183 patients. *Am J Cardiol* 52:739, 1983.

162. Zoll PM, Zoll RH, Falk RH, et al: External noninvasive temporary cardiac pacing: Clinical trials. *Circulation* 71:937, 1985.

163. Falk RH, Jacobs L, Sinclair A, et al: External non-invasive cardiac pacing in out-of-hospital cardiac arrest. *Crit Care Med* 11:779, 1983.

164. Hedges JR, Syverud SA, Dalsey WC: Developments in transcutaneous and transthoracic pacing during bradyasystolic arrest. *Ann Emerg Med* 13:822, 1984.

165. Hedges JR, Syverud SA, Dalsey WC, et al: Prehospital trial of emergency transcutaneous cardiac pacing. *Circulation* 76:1337, 1987.

166. Clinton JE, Zoll PM, Zoll RH, et al: Emergency noninvasive external pacing. *J Emerg Med* 2:155, 1985.

167. Kuhn GJ, White BC, Swetnam RE, et al: Peripheral vs central circulation times during CPR: A pilot study. *Ann Emerg Med* 10:417, 1981.

168. Jastremski MS, Matthias HD, Randell PA: Femoral venous catheterization during cardiopulmonary resuscitation: A critical appraisal. *J Emerg Med* 1:387, 1984.

169. Ralston SH, Tacker WA, Showen L, et al: Endotracheal versus intravenous epinephrine during electromechanical dissociation with CPR in dogs. *Ann Emerg Med* 14:1044, 1985.

170. Hoernchen U, Schuettler J, Stoeckel H, et al: Endobronchial instillation of epinephrine during cardiopulmonary resuscitation. *Crit Care Med* 15:1037, 1987.

171. Haehnel J, Lindner KH, Ahnefeld FW: Endobronchial administration of emergency drugs. *Resuscitation* 17:261, 1989.

172. Falk JL, Rackow EC, Weil MH: End-tidal carbon dioxide concentration during cardiopulmonary resuscitation. *N Engl J Med* 318:607, 1988.

173. Garnett AR, Ornato JP, Gonzalez ER, et al: End-tidal carbon dioxide monitoring during cardiopulmonary resuscitation. *JAMA* 257:512, 1987.

174. Trevino RP, Bisera J, Weil MH, et al: End-tidal CO_2 as a guide to successful cardiopulmonary resuscitation: A preliminary report. *Crit Care Med* 13:910, 1985.

175. Weil MH, Bisera J, Trevino RP, et al: Cardiac output and end-tidal carbon dioxide. *Crit Care Med* 13:907, 1985.

176. Weil MH, Grundler W, Yamaguchi M, et al: Arterial blood gases fail to reflect acid-base status during cardiopulmonary resuscitation: A preliminary report. *Crit Care Med* 13:884, 1985.

177. Weil MH, Ruiz CE, Michaels S, et al: Acid-base determinants of survival after cardiopulmonary resuscitation. *Crit Care Med* 13:888, 1985.

178. Jaffe A: Cardiovascular pharmacology I. *Circulation* 74(suppl IV):IV-70, 1986.

179. Guerci AD, Chandra N, Johnson E, et al: Failure of sodium bicarbonate to improve resuscitation from ventricular fibrillation in dogs. *Circulation* 74(suppl IV):IV-75, 1986.

180. Shoemaker WC, Schluchter M, Hopkins JA, et al: Fluid therapy in emergency resuscitation: Clinical evaluation of colloid and crystalloid regimens. *Crit Care Med* 9:367, 1981.

181. Otto CW, Yakaitis RW, Blitt CD: Mechanism of action of epinephrine in resuscitation from asphyxial arrest. *Crit Care Med* 9:364, 1981.

182. Otto CW, Yakaitis RW, Redding JS, et al: Comparison of dopamine, dobutamine, and epinephrine in cardiopulmonary resuscitation. *Crit Care Med* 9:366, 1981.

183. Otto CW: Cardiovascular pharmacology II. The use of catecholamines, pressor agents, digitalis, and corticosteroids in CPR and emergency cardiac care. *Circulation* 74(suppl IV):IV-80, 1986.

184. Ahlquist RP: A study of the adrenotropic receptors. *Am J Physiol* 153:586, 1948.

185. Redding JS, Pearson JW: Evaluation of drugs for cardiac resuscitation. *Anesthesiology* 24:203, 1963.

186. Redding JS, Pearson JW: Resuscitation from ventricular fibrillation: Drug therapy. *JAMA* 203:255, 1968.

187. Otto CW, Yakaitis RW, Redding JS, et al: Comparison of dopamine, dobutamine, and epinephrine in CPR. *Crit Care Med* 9:640, 1981.

188. Otto CW, Yakaitis RW, Ewy GA: Effects of epinephrine on defibrillation in ischemic ventricular fibrillation. *Am J Emerg Med* 3:285, 1985.

189. Niemann JT, Haynes KS, Garner D, et al: Postcountershock pulseless rhythms: Response to CPR, artificial cardiac pacing, and adrenergic agonists. *Ann Emerg Med* 15:112, 1986.

190. Brown CG, Katz SE, Werman HA, et al: The effect of epinephrine versus methoxamine on regional myocardial blood flow and defibrillation rates following a prolonged cardiorespiratory arrest in a swine model. *Am J Emerg Med* 5:362, 1987.

191. Brown CG, Taylor RB, Werman HA, et al: Myocardial oxygen delivery/consumption during cardiopulmonary resuscitation: A

comparison of epinephrine and phenylephrine. *Ann Emerg Med* 17:302, 1988.

192. Martin GB, Gentile NT, Paradis NA, et al: Effect of epinephrine on end-tidal carbon dioxide monitoring during CPR. *Ann Emerg Med* 19:396, 1990.

193. Koscove EM, Paradis NA: Resuscitation from cardiac arrest using high-dose epinephrine therapy. *JAMA* 259:3031, 1988.

194. Gonzalez ER, Ornato JP, Garnett AR, et al: Dose-dependent vasopressor response to epinephrine during CPR in human beings. *Ann Emerg Med* 18:920, 1989.

195. Martin D, Werman HA, Brown CG: Four case studies: High-dose epinephrine in cardiac arrest. *Ann Emerg Med* 19:322, 1990.

196. Stiell IG, Hebert PC, Weitzman BN, et al: High-dose epinephrine in adult cardiac arrest. *N Engl J Med* 327:1045, 1992.

197. Brown CG, Martin DR, Pepe PE, et al: A comparison of standard-dose and high-dose epinephrine in cardiac arrest outside the hospital. *N Engl J Med* 327:1051, 1992.

198. Robinson LA, Brown CG, Jenkins J, et al: The effects of norepinephrine versus epinephrine on myocardial hemodynamics during CPR. *Ann Emerg Med* 18:336, 1989.

199. Brown CG, Robinson LA, Jenkins J, et al: The effect of norepinephrine versus epinephrine on regional cerebral blood flow during cardiopulmonary resuscitation. *Am J Emerg Med* 7:278, 1989.

200. DeSilva RA, Hennekens CH, Lown B, Casscells W: Lignocaine prophylaxis in acute myocardial infarction: An evaluation of randomised trials. *Lancet* 2:855, 1981.

201. Koster RW, Dunning AJ: Intramuscular lidocaine for prevention of lethal arrhythmias in the prehospital phase of acute myocardial infarction. *N Engl J Med* 313:1105, 1985.

202. Carruth JE, Silverman ME: Ventricular fibrillation complicating acute myocardial infarction: Reasons against the routine use of lidocaine. *Am Heart J* 104:545, 1982.

203. Dunn HM, McComb JM, Kinney CD, et al: Prophylactic lidocaine in the early phase of suspected myocardial infarction. *Am Heart J* 110:353, 1985.

204. MacMahon S, Collins R, Peto R, et al: Effects of prophylactic lidocaine in suspected acute myocardial infarction: An overview of results from the randomized controlled trials. *JAMA* 260:1910, 1988.

205. American College of Cardiology/American Heart Association Task Force on Assessment of Diagnostic and Therapeutic Cardiovascular Procedures: Guidelines for the early management of patients with acute myocardial infarction. *Circulation* 82:664, 1990.

206. Gunnar RM, Passamani ER, Bourdillon PD, et al: Guidelines for the early management of patients with acute myocardial infarction: A report of the American College of Cardiology/American Heart Association Task Force on Assessment of Diagnostic and Therapeutic Cardiovascular Procedures. *J Am Coll Cardiol* 16:249, 1990.

207. Anderson JL, Patterson E, Conlon M, et al: Kinetics of antifibrillatory effects of bretylium: Correlation with myocardial drug concentration. *Am J Cardiol* 46:583, 1980.

208. Babbs CF, Yim GKW, Whistler SJ, et al: Elevation of ventricular defibrillation threshold in dogs by antiarrhythmic drugs. *Am Heart J* 98:345, 1979.

209. Bacaner MB: Treatment of ventricular fibrillation and other acute arrhythmias with bretylium tosylate. *Am J Cardiol* 21:530, 1968.

210. DiMarco JP, Sellers TD, Berne RM, et al: Adenosine: Electrophysiologic effects and therapeutic use for terminating paroxysmal supraventricular tachycardia. *Circulation* 68:1254, 1983.

211. DiMarco JP, Sellers TD, Lerman BB, et al: Diagnostic and therapeutic use of adenosine in patients with supraventricular tachyarrhythmias. *J Am Coll Cardiol* 6:417, 1985.

212. Parker RB, McCollam PL: Adenosine in the episodic treatment of paroxysmal supraventricular tachycardia. *Clin Pharm* 9:261, 1990.

213. Salerno DM, Dias VC, Kleiger RE, et al: Efficacy and safety of intravenous diltiazem for treatment of atrial fibrillation and atrial flutter. *Am J Cardiol* 63:1046, 1989.

214. Ellenbogen KA, Dias VC, Plumb VJ, et al: A placebo-controlled trial of continuous intravenous diltiazem infusion for 24-hour heart rate control during atrial fibrillation and atrial flutter: A multicenter study. *J Am Coll Cardiol* 18:891, 1991.

215. Teo KK, Yusuf S, Collins R, et al: Effects of intravenous magnesium in suspected acute myocardial infarction: Overview of randomised trials. *Br Med J* 303:1499, 1991.

216. Woods KL, Fletcher S, Roffe C, Haider Y: Intravenous magnesium sulphate in suspected acute myocardial infarction: Results of the second Leicester Intravenous Magnesium Intravention Trial (LIMIT-2). *Lancet* 339:1553, 1992.

217. Ceremzynski L, Jurgiel R, Kulakowski P, Gübalska J: Threatening arrhythmias in acute myocardial infarction are prevented by intravenous magnesium sulfate. *Am Heart J* 118:1333, 1989.

218. Waxman HL, Groh WC, Marchlinski FE, et al: Amiodarone for control of sustained ventricular tachyarrhythmias: Clinical and electrophysiologic effects in 51 patients. *Am J Cardiol* 50:1066, 1982.

219. McGovern B, Ruskin JN: The efficacy of amiodarone for ventricular arrhythmias can be predicted with clinical electrophysiological studies. *Int J Cardiol* 3:71, 1983.

220. Paraskos JA: Cardiovascular pharmacology. III. Atropine, calcium, calcium blockers, and beta blockers. *Circulation* 74(suppl IV):IV-86, 1986.

221. Chamberlain DA, Turner P, Sneddon JM: Effects of atropine on heart rate in healthy man. *Lancet* 2:12, 1967.

222. Kay JH, Blalock A: The use of calcium chloride in the treatment of cardiac arrest in patients. *Surg Gynecol Obstet* 93:97, 1951.

223. Stueven HA, Thompson BM, Aprahamian C, et al: Use of calcium in prehospital cardiac arrest. *Ann Emerg Med* 12:136, 1983.

224. Stueven HA, Thompson BM, Aprahamian C, et al: Calcium chloride: Reassessment of use in asystole. *Ann Emerg Med* 13:820, 1984.

225. Harrison EE, Amey BD: The use of calcium in electromechanical dissociation. *Ann Emerg Med* 13:844, 1984.

226. Carlon GC, Howland WS, Kahn RC, et al: Calcium chloride administration in normocalcemic critically ill patients. *Crit Care Med* 8:209, 1980.

227. Dembo DH: Calcium in advanced life support. *Crit Care Med* 9:358, 1981.

228. Thompson BM, Stueven HA, Tonsfeldt DJ: Calcium: Limited indications, some danger. *Circulation* 74(suppl IV):IV-90, 1986.

229. Barsan WG, Levy RC, Weir H: Lidocaine levels during CPR: Differences after peripheral venous, central venous, and intracardiac injections. *Ann Emerg Med* 10:73, 1981.

230. Hedges JR, Barsan WB, Doan LA, et al: Central versus peripheral intravenous routes in cardiopulmonary resuscitation. *Am J Emerg Med* 2:385, 1984.

231. Haynes RE, Chinn TL, Copass MK, et al: Comparison of bretylium tosylate and lidocaine in management of out of hospital ventricular fibrillation: A randomized clinical trial. *Am J Cardiol* 48:353, 1981.

232. Olson DW, Thompson BM, Darin JL, et al: A randomized comparison study of bretylium tosylate and lidocaine in resuscitation of patients from out-of-hospital ventricular fibrillation in a paramedic system. *Ann Emerg Med* 13:807, 1984.

233. Bocka JJ: External transcutaneous pacemakers. *Ann Emerg Med* 18:1280, 1989.

234. Ewy GA, Dahl CF, Zimmerman M, et al: Ventricular fibrillation masquerading as ventricular standstill. *Crit Care Med* 9:841, 1981.

235. Brown DC, Lewis AJ, Criley JM: Asystole and its treatment: The possible role of the parasympathetic nervous system in cardiac arrest. *J Am Coll Emerg Phys* 8:448, 1979.

236. Vassale M: On the mechanisms underlying cardiac standstill: Factors determining success or failure of escape pacemakers in the heart. *J Am Coll Cardiol* 5:35B, 1985.

237. Thompson BM, Brooks RC, Pionkowski RS, et al: Immediate countershock treatment of asystole. *Ann Emerg Med* 13:827, 1984.

238. Stults K, Brown D, Kerber R: Should ventricular asystole be cardioverted? (abstract) *Circulation* 76:IV-12, 1987.

239. Stults K, Brown D: Converting asystole. *J Emerg Med Serv* 9:38, 1984.

240. Michael JR, Guerci AD, Koehler RC, et al: Mechanisms by which epinephrine augments cerebral and myocardial perfusion during cardiopulmonary resuscitation in dogs. *Circulation* 69:822, 1984.

241. Sanders AB: The roles of methoxamine and norepinephrine in electromechanical dissociation. *Ann Emerg Med* 13:835, 1984.

242. Scholander PF: The master switch of life. *Sci Am* 209:92, 1963.

243. Siebke H, Rod T, Breivik H, et al: Survival after 40 minutes submersion without cerebral sequelae. *Lancet* 1:1275, 1975.

244. Southwick FS, Dalgish PH: Recovery after prolonged asystolic cardiac arrest in profound hypothermia: A case report and literature review. *JAMA* 243:1250, 1980.

245. Steinman AM: The hypothermic code: CPR controversy revisited. *J Emerg Med Serv* 10:32, 1983.

246. Gordon AS, Ridolpho PF, Cole JE: *Definitive Studies on Pole-top Resuscitation.* Camarillo, CA, Research Resuscitation Laboratories, Electric Power Research Institute, 1983.

247. Sanders AB, Kern KB, Ewy GA, et al: Improved resuscitation from cardiac arrest with open-chest CPR in dogs. *Crit Care Med* 9:384, 1981.

248. Sanders AB, Kern KB, Atlas M, et al: Importance of the duration of inadequate coronary perfusion pressure in resuscitation from cardiac arrest. *J Am Coll Cardiol* 6:113, 1985.

249. Safar P, Abramson NS, Angelos M, et al: Emergency cardiopulmonary bypass for resuscitation from prolonged cardiac arrest. *Am J Emerg Med* 8:55, 1990.

250. Geehr EC, Lewis FR, Auerbach PS: Failure of open-heart massage to improve survival after prehospital non-traumatic cardiac arrest (letter). *N Engl J Med* 314:1189, 1986.

33. Critical Aortic Stenosis and Hypertrophic Cardiomyopathy

Gerard P. Aurigemma and
John A. Paraskos

Obstruction to left ventricular outflow, due to either valvular aortic stenosis or hypertrophic obstructive cardiomyopathy, may lead to syncope, congestive heart failure, or sudden cardiac death. In addition, supraventricular tachyarrhythmias in patients with marked ventricular hypertrophy, due to either aortic stenosis or hypertrophic cardiomyopathy, may be met with dire hemodynamic consequences. Recent work suggests that the management of elderly patients with aortic stenosis following valve replacement may be complicated by a low-output state despite normal ejection fraction. For these and other reasons, patients with aortic stenosis or hypertrophic cardiomyopathy will come to the attention of the intensive care unit (ICU) physician. In most instances, proper management requires, in addition to a working knowledge of the pathophysiology of these disorders, access to two-dimensional (2-D) and Doppler echocardiography (see Chap. 7). These techniques permit a comprehensive, noninvasive assessment of left ventricular systolic and diastolic function, as well as the disturbed flow resulting from left ventricular outflow obstruction.

Table 33-1 lists the variety of lesions that may cause left ventricular outflow obstruction. In general, left ventricular outflow obstruction is either fixed (valvular, subvalvular, or supra-

valvular) or dynamic (hypertrophic cardiomyopathy with obstruction). The discussion in this chapter is limited to valvular aortic stenosis and hypertrophic cardiomyopathy.

Aortic Stenosis

ETIOLOGY. Stenosis of the aortic valve is by far the most common cause of obstruction to left ventricular outflow; valvular lesions may develop in a previously normal or a congenitally deformed valve. While the vast majority of patients who have acquired stenosis of both the aortic and mitral valves have rheumatic heart disease [1,2], isolated disease of the aortic valve is rarely due to rheumatic heart disease [3,4,5]. The age at which the hemodynamic obstruction develops is highly dependent on the etiology of the stenosis (Table 33-2). The bicuspid aortic valve is the most common congenital heart defect, excluding mitral valve prolapse, occurring in as many as 2 percent of live births. The bicuspid valve is not stenotic at birth; however, degenerative changes eventually cause significant stenosis or regurgitation in the majority of patients [6,7].

While degeneration of congenitally malformed valves accounts for most cases of isolated aortic stenosis in patients younger than 65 years of age, beyond that age the most common cause of severe aortic stenosis is degenerative change of a previously normal three-cusped aortic valve [8]. This degenerative process is very common, causing some degree of aortic valvular calcification in as many as 30 percent [9] and a systolic ejection murmur in 69 percent of the population over age 80 [10]; however, only a small fraction of these people develop hemodynamically significant aortic stenosis [11].

Table 33-1. Causes of Left Ventricular Outflow Obstruction

A. Congenital lesions
  1. Valvular
    a. Unicuspid
    b. Bicuspid with degeneration
    c. Deformed 3- or 4-cusped valves with degeneration (rare)
  2. Subvalvular
    a. Discrete fibromembranous
    b. Tunnel lesion (diffuse fibromuscular)
    c. Hypertrophic cardiomyopathy
  3. Supravalvular
    a. Hourglass deformity
    b. Hypoplastic
    c. Membranous
B. Acquired lesions
  1. Degenerative changes (fibrocalcific deformity)
    a. Of congenitally abnormal valve
    b. Of normal 3-cusped valve
  2. Rheumatic heart disease

Table 33-2. Symptoms of Discrete Aortic Stenosis: Age of Onset and Likely Etiology

Childhood: Nonvalvular and unicuspid valvular
Adolescence: Nonvalvular, unicuspid, or bicuspid valvular
Young adult: Bicuspid valvular and rheumatic
Middle age: Bicuspid valvular, rheumatic, occasionally degenerative
Above age 65: Degenerative change of previously normal valve

PATHOPHYSIOLOGY. In valvular aortic stenosis, increased impedance to left ventricular ejection is the primary hemodynamic disturbance; the severity of the obstruction determines the hemodynamic consequences for the left ventricle. In fixed valvular stenoses, a cross-sectional area as small as 1.0 cm² (compared with the normal 3.0–3.5 cm²) causes a significant rise in left ventricular outflow impedance and results in a pressure gradient across the valve, even at rest [12]; with further reduction of the orifice size to 0.6 to 0.8 cm², outflow impedance increases. As intraventricular pressure rises, afterload (as determined by wall stress, from the Laplace relationship) increases. Though the rise in afterload may be expected to reduce ejection performance (since afterload and ejection fraction are inversely related) the left ventricle maintains a normal stroke volume through the development of compensatory hypertrophy (see Fig. 33-1). In this manner, the development of concentric hypertrophy (an increase in the ratio of wall thickness to left ventricular cavity dimension) offsets the increase in intraventricular pressure and maintains normal wall stress until late in the course of the disease [13,14].

As long as compensatory left ventricular hypertrophy allows for normalization of afterload, ejection performance remains normal. Stroke volume therefore remains normal, and the patient may remain free of symptoms of low cardiac output. However, total myocardial oxygen demand increases due to the increase in myocardial mass, and even unobstructed coronary arteries may fail to provide adequate blood flow, especially with exertion. The adverse consequences of a mismatch between myocardial oxygen demand and supply include angina pectoris, myocardial infarction, and even lethal arrhythmias.

Both myocardial hypertrophy and ischemia may lead to increased left ventricular chamber stiffness or reduced diastolic compliance. This reduction in compliance is manifested as an elevation in left ventricular diastolic pressures, especially at end diastole, when there may be a significant increment in left ventricular diastolic pressure produced by atrial contraction. A forceful atrial contraction is therefore necessary to provide an elevation in end-diastolic pressure to provide for adequate filling. The physical findings associated with this reduction in left ventricular compliance include a fourth heart sound and even a palpable presystolic apical impulse. For this reason, the loss of a normally synchronized atrial contraction may seriously compromise left ventricular stroke volume by decreasing late diastolic filling. Likewise, excessive preload reduction by any mechanism (i.e., volume depletion or administration of vasodilators) may seriously decrease the ability of the left ventricle to deliver an adequate stroke volume. With progressive reductions in left ventricular compliance, the mean left ventricular diastolic pressure may rise to a level (approximately 25 mm Hg) that can provoke pulmonary congestion. Thus, pulmonary congestion signifies heart failure due to an inability of the left ventricle to fill normally at low pressure ("diastolic dysfunction") and may occur in the face of a normal ejection fraction, as has been demonstrated in patients with hypertensive disease [15,16,17].

While left ventricular size and systolic function are preserved in most patients with aortic stenosis without coronary heart disease, some patients develop contractile dysfunction. This may be manifested on 2-D echocardiography (or other imaging techniques) as a reduction in ejection fraction. With reduced systolic function, the systolic gradient falls along with the stroke volume. The systolic murmur tends to lessen in both intensity and duration, since these features are dependent, in part, on the magnitude of the gradient. As the mean left ventricular diastolic pressure rises further, pulmonary congestion and passive pulmonary hypertension may develop [18]. In turn, some patients may develop right ventricular failure; thus, it is possible for a patient with longstanding aortic stenosis to have a clinical presentation dominated by signs and symptoms of right ventricular failure.

The rate of progression of valvular aortic stenosis is highly variable but may be more rapid in patients with degenerative calcific than congenital or rheumatic disease. The peak systolic gradient across the valve has been observed to proceed at rates of 0.8 to 1.3 mm Hg per month [19]; however, an individual patient with initially mild stenosis may develop severe stenosis as quickly as 2 years [20]. Doppler echocardiography permits serial noninvasive monitoring of the progression of stenosis [21,22].

In summary, the clinical presentation, physical findings, and hemodynamic assessment of patients with valvular aortic stenosis depend not only on the severity of the obstruction, but also on left ventricular systolic and diastolic function .

Fig. 33-1. Inverse relationship between wall stress and ejection fraction [13]. Wall stress is shown on the x-axis and ejection fraction on the y-axis. As wall stress (estimate of afterload on the left ventricle) increases, ejection fraction may be expected to fall. However, most patients' stress-ejection fraction coordinates fall along the regression line; depressed ejection fraction in these patients is due to afterload excess and may increase following aortic valve replacement. In contrast, individuals whose stress-ejection fraction coordinates fall below the regression line are likely to have suffered irreversible fibrotic changes. Left ventricular function in these individuals is unlikely to improve substantially following valve replacement.

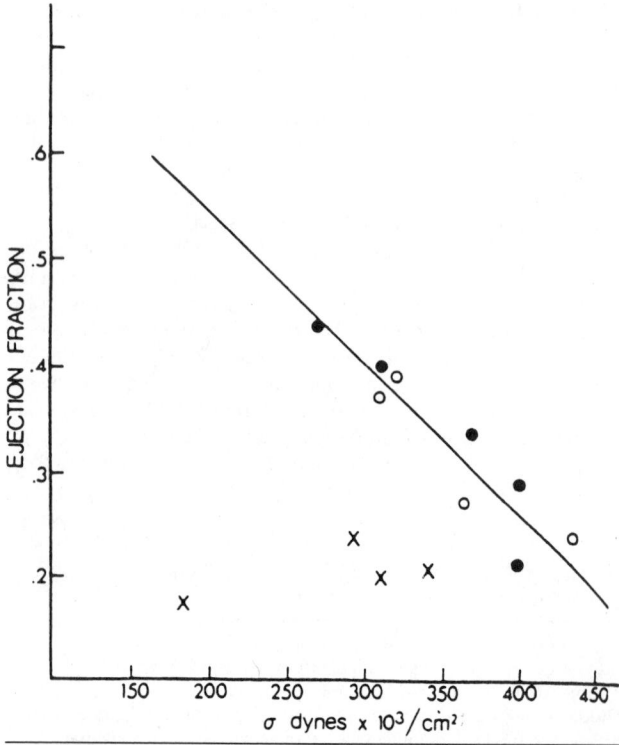

HISTORY. The cardinal symptoms associated with outflow obstruction include angina pectoris, dizziness, syncope, and dyspnea (Table 33-3). Characteristically, these symptoms are effort-induced. However, it is also possible that patients with significant outflow obstruction of the left ventricle may remain free of symptoms for many years.

Angina pectoris is the most commonly encountered symptom, occurring in more than half of patients with symptomatic

Table 33-3. Features Common to All Forms
of Severe Left Ventricular Outflow Obstruction

Angina, syncope, dyspnea
Systolic ejection murmur
Paradoxically split second sound
Fourth sound
Sustained apical impulse
Left ventricular hypertrophy

aortic stenosis [23,24]. In the absence of epicardial coronary disease, myocardial ischemia is presumed to be due to the exaggerated oxygen requirements caused by left ventricular hypertrophy [25,26]. In older patients, associated coronary atherosclerosis is common, occurring in two-thirds of patients with aortic stenosis over the age of 60 years and in one-third of those aged 40 to 60 years [25]; in older individuals this incidence is much higher [26,27,28].

Syncope occurring with or immediately after physical exertion is the next most common symptom, elicited from approximately a third of symptomatic patients [23,24,29,30]. More frequently, however, patients complain of effort-induced dizziness or lightheadedness. The usual explanation of syncope in patients with aortic stenosis is a sudden drop in peripheral vascular resistance, caused by exercise, in the face of a fixed cardiac output [31,32]. Alternatively, syncope may be caused by an abrupt fall in cardiac output without a compensatory rise in peripheral resistance, or by an arrhythmia [30]. There is also evidence that excessive stimulation of cardiac mechanoreceptors may play a role in syncope in patients with significant aortic stenosis [31].

Patients presenting with left ventricular systolic failure due to unrelieved aortic stenosis may complain of progressive dyspnea on exertion, paroxysmal nocturnal dyspnea, orthopnea, cough, or generalized fatigue. Rarely, a patient presents with predominantly right-sided findings: peripheral edema or right upper quadrant discomfort due to hepatic congestion. In these instances the left ventricle may show dilation in addition to a reduction in ejection fraction. A small percentage (perhaps 5%) of adults with unrecognized aortic valvular stenosis may suffer sudden death without premonitory symptoms.

Once the symptoms of angina pectoris, syncope, or dyspnea develop, mean life expectancy is several years, and prompt measures should be taken to define the severity of the lesion and determine the need for surgical intervention. An analysis of survival curves of unoperated patients with aortic stenosis indicates that median survival following onset of heart failure is 2 years, 3 years for syncope, and 5 years for angina [5,22,33].

PHYSICAL EXAMINATION. In aortic stenosis, blood pressure is usually normal, although pulse pressure tends to be restricted; significant hypertension is not rare, especially in the elderly. Experienced clinicians are aided in assessing the carotid by simultaneously listening over the precordium. The normal carotid pulse is perceived as coincident with the first heart sound. If the carotid pulse follows the first heart sound by an appreciable time delay, significant obstruction can be presumed to exist. Systolic vibrations or "shudders" of the carotid pulse correlate with the presence of a transmitted murmur but not with the severity of the stenosis (Fig. 33-2) [34]. Careful palpation of the carotid artery may reveal a delayed upstroke, following the slow rise in the aortic pressure curve ("pulsus parvus et tardus"), a finding that identifies hemodynamically severe aortic stenosis with great specificity.

In all forms of significant outflow obstruction, the apical im-

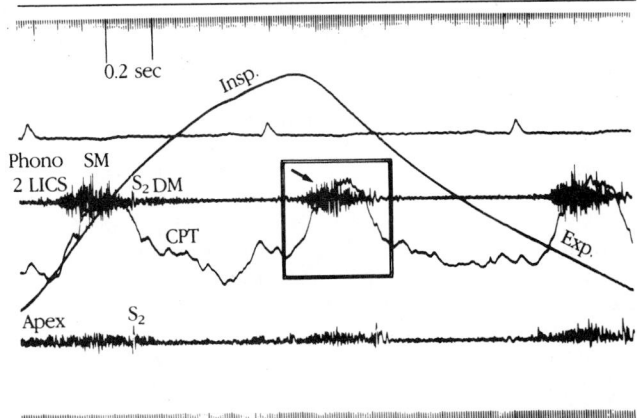

Fig. 33-2. Carotid pulse tracing (CPT) and phonocardiogram (Phono) of a patient with severe aortic stenosis. Note the delay in carotid upstroke. The prominent shudder on the carotid upstroke (*arrow*) is a manifestation of the transmission of the prolonged systolic murmur (SM) into the carotid vessels. A higher-pitched diastolic murmur (DM) is not well recorded. The intensity of the S₂ is diminished. 2 LICS = second left intercostal space.

pulse tends to be forceful and sustained because of protracted emptying of the hypertrophied left ventricle. The impulse is usually medial to or at the left midclavicular line, unless there is insignificant left ventricular dilatation, in which case the apical impulse is displaced laterally. Occasionally, a presystolic thrust is noted, due to a forceful atrial contraction.

An aortic ejection click may be audible at the onset of the murmur (Table 33-4). This click is perceived as an explosive high-pitched beginning to the murmur; however, this sound is not appreciated in the majority of adult patients with calcified and relatively immobile aortic valves [35]. In severe aortic stenosis, the second heart sound is expected to be paradoxically split due to the prolongation of left ventricular ejection time. However, in adult patients with critical aortic stenosis, the aortic closure sound is considerably diminished in intensity, so that paradoxical splitting cannot usually be appreciated. A fourth heart sound should be audible in all forms of severe left ventricular outflow obstruction, unless atrial fibrillation has supervened.

An auscultatory finding common to all forms of left ventricular outflow obstruction is the systolic ejection (crescendo-decrescendo) murmur (Tables 33-3 and 33-4). This murmur is often accompanied by a palpable thrill. It is important to note, however, that the intensity of the murmur is related poorly to the severity of the stenosis; duration of the murmur is a better index of the severity of obstruction. A late-peaking, prolonged murmur is suggestive of severe stenosis. A valvular aortic ste-

Table 33-4. Differentiating Features among Etiologies
for Left Ventricular Outflow Obstruction

Age at onset of symptoms
Years symptoms have been present
Maximal location of systolic murmur
Systolic ejection click
Dilatation of ascending aorta
Differential carotid delay and brachial pressures
Presence of aortic regurgitation
Presence of mitral disease
Decreased aortic closure sound

notic murmur is low-pitched and often described as "rough" or "harsh"; it tends to be loudest at the aortic area and is usually well transmitted to the apex. In the elderly, the murmur often has a musical or "cooing" quality at the apex and is often mistaken as an independent murmur of mitral regurgitation (Fig. 33-2).

An aortic regurgitation murmur is common in valvular as well as discrete subvalvular aortic stenosis. This murmur may be very faint and may require maneuvers that raise peripheral vascular resistance to become audible; such maneuvers include isometric contraction (hand grip) or squatting. Aortic regurgitation is much less common in association with supravalvular stenosis or hypertrophic obstructive cardiomyopathy (Table 33-5).

LABORATORY STUDIES

Electrocardiogram. With severe aortic stenosis, evidence for left ventricular hypertrophy is present in the majority of patients. Increased R wave voltage over left precordial leads is expected with associated S–T segment sagging and T wave inversion ("strain pattern") typical of pressure overload left ventricular hypertrophy. Left bundle branch block may also occur.

The P wave is usually normal, although with left ventricular failure a prominent terminal negative deflection in leads V_1 and V_2 is not uncommon. Severe left atrial abnormality or atrial fibrillation is uncommon and should raise the suspicion of associated mitral valve disease.

Chest Radiograph. In most patients, the heart is not dilated and the cardiothoracic ratio is normal on a posteroanterior chest film. However, the left lower border of the heart shadow is often rounded or convex as a result of left ventricular hypertrophy. With systolic failure of the left ventricle, the chest film shows cardiac enlargement, as well as evidence for pulmonary venous engorgement or congestion.

Calcification of the aortic valve is expected in adults with valvular aortic stenosis. If valvular calcium cannot be observed with careful fluoroscopy, critical aortic stenosis is unlikely. Poststenotic dilatation of the proximal aorta is usual in severe valvular stenosis. The dilatation should cause a bulge to the right side of the mediastinum on the chest film (Fig. 33-3).

Echocardiogram. In patients with critical aortic stenosis, the echocardiogram is expected to demonstrate concentric left ventricular hypertrophy, as well as thickened aortic valve cusps with diminished mobility (Figs. 33-4 and 33-5).

The majority of bicuspid aortic valves are identified by 2-D echocardiography (Fig. 33-6). When the bicuspid valve has become calcified and stenotic, the leaflet echoes become dense and reduplicated, with a restriction in systolic excursion similar to that seen in three-cusped stenotic valves; with heavy calcification it may be difficult to distinguish bicuspid from trileaflet aortic valves by echocardiography.

Sclerotic trileaflet valves exhibit multiple dense echoes with diminished systolic excursion and separation. If cusp echoes are normal in intensity and thickness and their separation is greater than 12 mm, hemodynamically significant aortic stenosis is essentially excluded in the adult. Multiple dense echoes with a separation of less than 8 mm are correlated with at least moderate stenosis [36,37].

Recent work by Carroll and co-workers [38] suggests that there is a gender association to the pattern of left ventricular hypertrophy in aortic stenosis, at least in elderly individuals. Women tend to display a more marked concentric response, with smaller left ventricular cavities and higher ejection fractions; conversely, men with equivalent degrees of valvular stenosis are more likely to have larger left ventricular cavities and depressed ejection fraction.

Doppler Echocardiogram. Echocardiographic investigation of the aortic valve for stenosis requires careful Doppler analysis and a skilled and meticulous ultrasonographer. The velocity of the jet of blood traversing the stenotic valve correlates with the transvalvular gradient (Fig. 33-7) [39–42]. Continuous-wave Doppler study is necessary to record the extremely high velocities (2–6 m/sec) that accompany valvular aortic stenosis. Proper angling of the Doppler beam parallel to the orientation of the systolic jet is critical to obtain a reliable estimate of the velocity. It is important to note that the failure to record a high velocity jet of aortic stenosis by Doppler echocardiography does not necessarily exclude critical aortic stenosis, but may result from the inability to align the Doppler beam parallel to an eccentric systolic jet. Thus, if the clinical suspicion of critical aortic stenosis is high, invasive hemodynamic measurements

Table 33-5. Aortic Stenosis: Physical Findings

Lesion	Murmur	Ejection click	Aortic closure sound	Aortic regurgitation	Carotid pulse
Congenital					
Unicuspid valvular	Aortic area to neck and apex	Common	Normal or loud in children	Uncommon in children	Delayed
Bicuspid valvular	Aortic area to neck and apex	Common in young adults	Decreased in adults	Common	Delayed
Discrete subvalvular	Left sternal border	Rare	Normal or decreased	Very common	Delayed
Hypertrophic	Left sternal border and apex	Rare	Normal or decreased	Uncommon	Brisk
Supravalvular	Aortic area to neck	Rare	Normal or decreased	Uncommon	Rapid right; delayed left
Acquired					
Degenerative	Aortic area to neck and apex	Uncommon	Decreased	Common	Delayed
Rheumatic	Aortic area to neck and apex with mitral murmurs	Uncommon	Decreased	Very common	Delayed

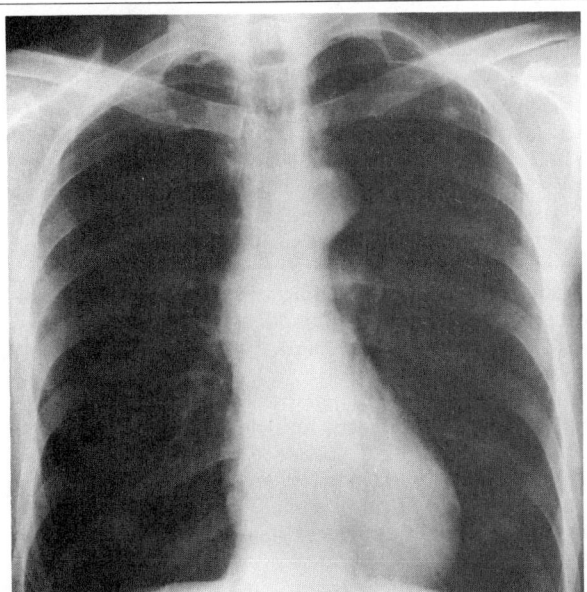

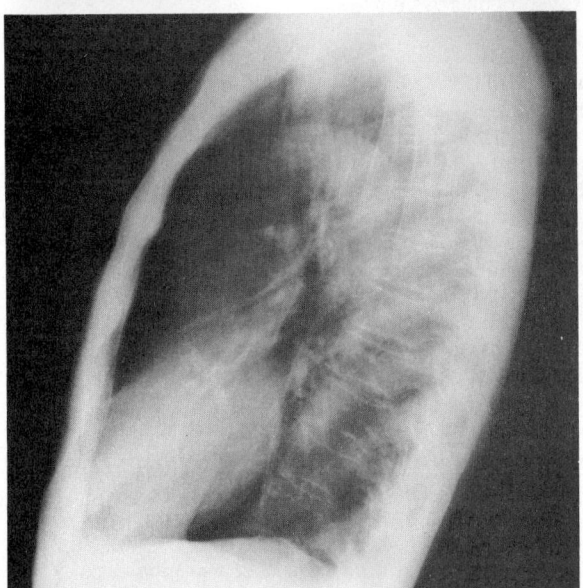

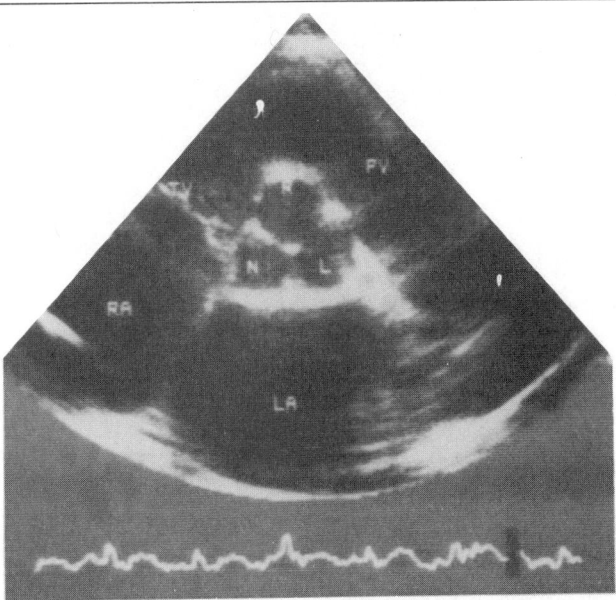

Fig. 33-4. Two-dimensional echocardiogram of normal aortic valve in cross-section. Three aortic valve leaflets can be seen in the closed position. The commissures form a Y shape and the three sinuses of Valsalva form a trifoil. N = noncoronary cusp; L = left coronary cusp; R = right coronary cusp; LA = left atrium; RA = right atrium; TV = tricuspid valve; PV = pulmonic valve.

Fig. 33-3. Chest roentgenograms in a patient with valvular aortic stenosis. Top. The posteroanterior film shows rounding of the left ventricular shadow consistent with concentric hypertrophy, a dilated ascending aorta, and calcium flecks in a position consistent with the aortic cusps. There is no cardiomegaly. Bottom. The lateral view is consistent with poststenotic dilatation of the ascending aorta and the aortic valvular location of the calcification. (From Dalen JE, Alpert JS (eds): *Valvular Heart Disease*. Boston, Little, Brown, 1981. With permission.)

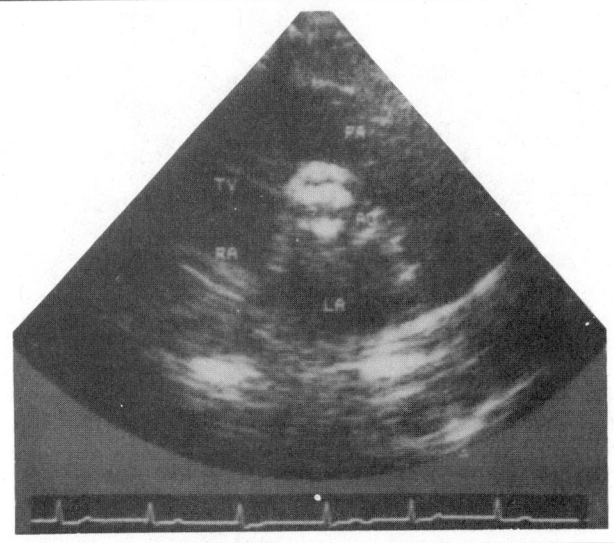

Fig.33-5. Echocardiogram in calcific valvular aortic stenosis. Thickened immobile valve cusps are seen to fill the aortic valve area in the cross-sectional view in diastole. Systolic views failed to demonstrate significant opening. AO = aortic valve; LA = left atrium; RA = right atrium; TV = tricuspid valve.

may be necessary despite an unimpressive Doppler transvalvular gradient.

The use of the continuity equation permits estimation of the stenotic aortic valve area. This calculation requires Doppler meaurement of the peak flow velocity both immediately proximal and distal to the stenotic valve and an estimate, from 2-D echocardiography, of the cross-sectional area of the left ventricular outflow tract. Continuity equation estimates correlate well with the Gorlin equation estimates at cardiac catheterization [43–49].

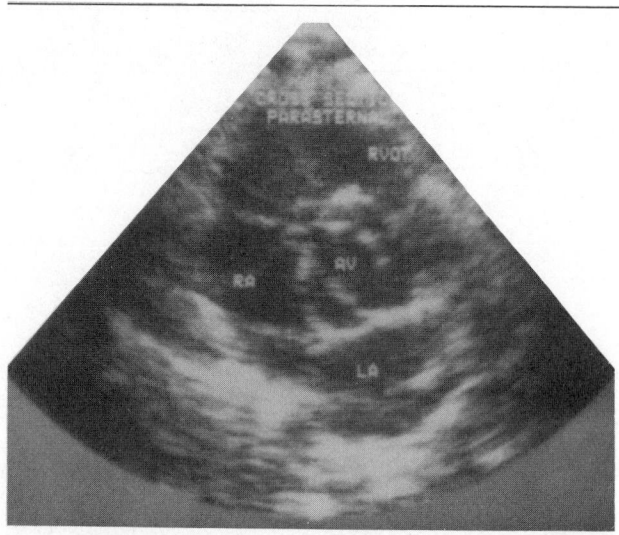

Fig. 33-6. Echocardiogram of a bicuspid aortic valve (AV) in systole. Note the two abnormally positioned valve leaflets with a single commissure running from right and superior to left and inferior. The systolic opening appears adequate. LA = left atrium; RA = right atrium; RVOT = right ventricular outflow tract.

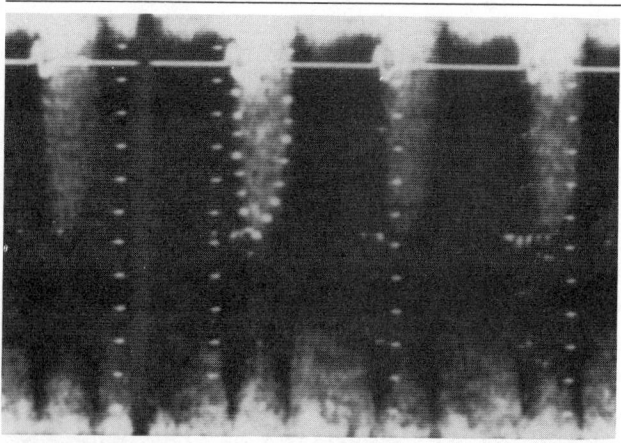

Fig. 33-7. Continuous-wave Doppler recording across the left ventricular outflow tract and aortic valve. The maximum velocity is almost 7 m per second, giving a peak gradient of 189 mm Hg and a mean gradient of 118 mm Hg. The mean gradient at catheterization was 100 mm Hg.

CARDIAC CATHETERIZATION. Cardiac catheterization is warranted in any patient with suspected severe symptomatic aortic stenosis. Catheterization has two principal objectives: to corroborate Doppler findings and to delineate important coronary artery stenosis. While it is feasible to proceed to valve replacement without catheterization in younger individuals with rheumatic disease, the older age and associated high incidence of coronary artery disease in patients with degenerative calcific aortic stenosis make coronary arteriography mandatory prior to surgery.

The pressure gradient across the aortic obstruction is usually

measured by passing a catheter across the aortic valve retrograde into the left ventricle. An accurate measure of cardiac output by either the Fick method or the dye dilution technique should be performed as close as possible to the measurement of the gradient (Figs. 33-8 and 33-9). The cross-sectional valve area can then be estimated using the hydraulic formula of Gorlin and Gorlin [50]. Occasionally, a catheter cannot be passed across a deformed and stenotic aortic valve and must instead be passed into the left ventricle by puncturing the interatrial septum (transseptal technique) or, rarely, by directly puncturing the left ventricular apex transcutaneously.

With a normal cardiac output, a mean systolic gradient of 50 mm Hg or more is usually found with severe aortic stenosis. In such severe cases, the calculated valve area is usually less than 0.8 cm²; however, as cardiac output drops due to systolic pump dysfunction, mean systolic gradients less than 50 mm Hg are often recorded. The calculated valve area, however, should faithfully estimate the severity of stenosis in these cases.

Right heart catheterization is of limited value in the evaluation of most patients with aortic stenosis, unless associated pulmonary or right-sided lesions are suspected. Monitoring pulmonary capillary, pulmonary arterial, and right atrial pressures is most useful, however, in managing critically ill patients with left ventricular dysfunction.

MANAGEMENT. In general, asymptomatic individuals with aortic stenosis do not require surgical intervention. This conclusion is based on a review of recent Doppler echocardiographic studies performed by Kelly and associates [51] and Pellikka and co-workers [52]. Kelly and associates followed 51 asymptomatic patients with significant aortic stenosis by Doppler for an average of 17 months (range 1–45 months). Forty-one percent of these initially asymptomatic patients developed symptoms and two patients (4%) died. Sudden death did not occur in any patient [51]. Pellikka et al. [52] reported similar findings in a larger cohort of patients who did not undergo valve replacement and were followed for an average of 20

Fig. 33-8. Simultaneous left ventricular and left brachial artery pressures in a patient with aortic stenosis. The mean systolic gradient across the aortic valve was 50 mm Hg, with a cardiac output of 5.1 liters per minute by the Fick method. An aortic valve area was calculated at 0.7 cm². This patient had an abnormal upstroke time (*arrow*). The widening of the pulse pressure after a premature beat (*bracket*) is to be expected in valvular aortic stenosis, in contrast to hypertrophic obstructive cardiomyopathy (see Fig. 33-2).

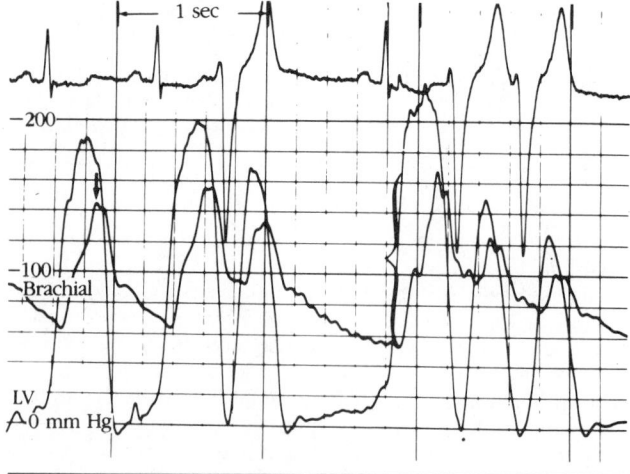

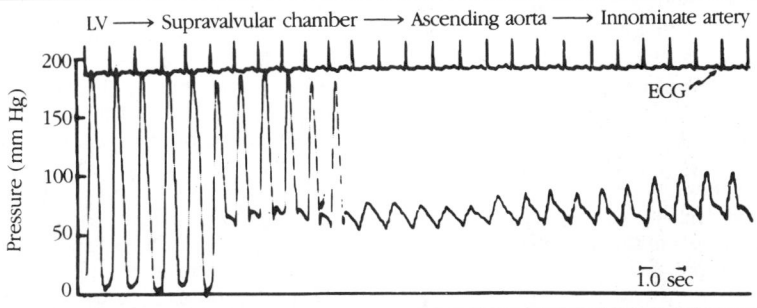

Fig. 33-9. Pressures recorded as a catheter is pulled back from the left ventricle (LV) to the innominate artery in a patient with supravalvular aortic stenosis. There is a gradient between the proximal and distal ascending aorta. (From Glancey DL, Epstein SE: Differential diagnosis of type and severity of obstruction to left ventricular outflow. *Prog Cardiovasc Dis* 14:153, 1971. With permission.)

months. These investigators found that 3 of the 113 asymptomatic patients not undergoing surgery suffered cardiac death during follow-up; however, all three developed cardiac symptoms prior to death [52]. Thus, none of the patients who remained asymptomatic died during the follow-up period.

In view of these studies, we believe it is reasonable to delay aortic valve replacement until symptoms attributable to aortic stenosis develop. Clearly, the risk of death, sudden or otherwise, in asymptomatic individuals with severe aortic stenosis must be weighed against the risk of death attributable to "prophylactic" valve replacement. Of 30 asymptomatic patients at the same institution who underwent aortic valve replacement, 2 died suddenly within 2 weeks of operation [52]. Braunwald, in an editorial accompanying this study, argued that "operative treatment is the most common cause of sudden death in asymptomatic patients with aortic stenosis" [53]. Moreover, in many instances, symptoms develop during close follow-up. In Kelly's series [51], approximately 40 percent of initially asymptomatic patients developed symptoms within 45 months; in Pellikka's series, 38 percent developed symptoms with 2 years. Asymptomatic individuals with evidence for significant aortic stenosis should be cautioned against strenuous physical exertion and should be followed closely for the development of symptoms. Valve replacement is recommended if the valve area is found to be less than 0.8 cm² in the symptomatic patient. Once angina, syncope, or left ventricular failure occurs urgent cardiac catheterization is necessary, and early surgical correction is warranted if catheterization corroborates the presence of severe stenosis.

INTENSIVE CARE UNIT MANAGEMENT. Medical therapy of symptomatic aortic stenosis in the ICU is at best a temporizing measure until definitive diagnosis and surgical correction can be undertaken. Surgery for severe fixed stenosis should not be delayed until cardiac therapy is "optimized," except for the rapid correction of volume and pressure abnormalities. On the other hand, if serious noncardiac medical or medication problems exist, surgery should indeed be delayed if the hemodynamic situation permits.

In the ICU, a high suspicion for aortic stenosis should lead to prompt noninvasive evaluation. If severe fixed stenosis is demonstrated by Doppler study, prompt left-sided catheterization should be performed to corroborate findings and evaluate the need for myocardial revascularization. With the exception of some patients with severe left ventricular systolic

dysfunction (manifested by mean transvalvular gradient below 30 mm Hg) surgery should be performed if the valve area is less than 0.8 cm².

If the echocardiogram reveals features of hypertrophic cardiomyopathy without significant valvular stenosis, catheterization is rarely needed, and a change in medical management often leads to gratifying results. While awaiting surgical correction, the patient with both fixed aortic stenosis and myocardial ischemia may be treated with judicious use of nitrates. Nitrates decrease preload and effectively reduce both end-diastolic and end-systolic volumes. This may be achieved with either nitroglycerin ointment (½ to 1 inch applied topically every 4 to 6 hours) or intravenous nitroglycerin (titrated to systolic blood pressure). Both systolic and diastolic aortic pressures tend to drop so that overall wall stress and myocardial oxygen requirements may be lessened dramatically. Excessive nitrate effect, however, is potentially deleterious, because preload reduction may drop the stroke volume and precipitously lower the blood pressure.

Patients with left ventricular failure and pulmonary congestion may be cautiously treated with diuretics. Careful monitoring of the pulmonary capillary wedge pressure is recommended to prevent excessive reduction in preload and subsequent hypotension. A pulmonary capillary pressure of 16 to 18 mm Hg usually averts pulmonary congestion while permitting an adequate stroke volume. However, in the postoperative patient (see below) the compliance characteristics of the left ventricle may be such that an adequate stroke volume may come at the expense of higher filling pressures.

In spite of the fixed orifice in valvular aortic stenosis, afterload reduction has also met with some success in the treatment of left ventricular failure in these patients [51,55]. Arterial vasodilators must be employed, however, with even more caution than in other patients with left ventricular failure. In this setting, captopril 6.25 to 25 mg orally, three times per day, might be considered. Care must be taken to avoid pharmacologic agents with a significant myocardial depressant effect. Beta-blockers, calcium channel blockers, and most antiarrhythmics (especially disopyramide, procainamide, quinidine, flecainide, encainide, and amiodarone) should therefore be used with caution.

SURGICAL THERAPY. As noted above, a symptomatic patient with valvular stenosis and a valve area of less than 0.8 cm² should be offered aortic valve replacement. If left ventricular systolic function is preserved, the mean gradient usually exceeds 50 mm Hg in these individuals.

In adults, the absolute mean gradient is not used as an indication for surgery, since individuals with significant left ventricular systolic dysfunction may have low transvalvular gradients, even with critical stenosis [13]. The presence of a mean transvalvular gradient below 30 mm Hg appears to identify a subgroup of patients in whom valve replacement is associated with poor outcome [13]. It is of interest that preoperative ejection fraction alone does not correlate well with surgical risk or postoperative morbidity; in fact, ejection fraction may improve dramatically following valvular replacement. This point is illustrated in Figure 33-1, which shows the known relationship between afterload (wall stress) and ejection fraction. As afterload increases, because of either increased intraventricular pressure or left ventricular cavity dilatation, there is an obligatory decrease in ejection fraction, even if there is no change in contractile state. Thus, as mentioned above, a depressed ejection fraction may belie normal intrinsic contractile function if afterload is abnormally high ("afterload excess").

Work by Carabello and co-workers and by others has shown that an increase in ejection fraction may be expected following aortic valve replacement if the preoperative depression in ejection fraction was the result of afterload excess rather than irreversible myocardial damage [13,56]. Thus, it is not uncommon for patients with congestive heart failure and depressed ejection fraction due to aortic stenosis to experience a marked functional recovery following aortic valve replacement. Conversely, in patients with critical aortic stenosis a transvalvular gradient of less than 30 mm Hg, as shown by Carabello et al., usually reflects irreversible myopathic changes in the left ventricle. Since in this subset of patients reduced ejection is not due to afterload excess, valve replacement is not usually met with functional recovery [13]. Brogan and co-workers recently showed that despite refinement in the surgical approach to patients in the decade since Carabello's study, the prognosis for these patients remains grim: of 13 patients undergoing valve replacement for severe aortic stenosis, 6 died in the perioperative period [57].

For the vast majority of patients with valvular stenosis, the native valve must be excised and replaced with a prosthetic device. If coronary artery bypass grafting is necessary, it is routinely performed at the time of valve replacement [57,58]. Replacement of the aortic valve with a bioprosthesis is theoretically more advantageous if lifelong anticoagulation can be avoided. Calcific degeneration of porcine prostheses is common and is more likely to progress in children and young adults, at a rate as high as 10 percent per year [59,60,61]. Dysfunction of the bioprosthesis is usually caused by stenosis, although significant regurgitation may also develop [60]. Premature dysfunction also is found in patients undergoing long-term renal dialysis. Other prosthetic valves require lifelong anticoagulation.

The long-term survival of patients with aortic stenosis is greatly improved with surgical correction, with associated coronary artery disease as the leading cause of death after successful aortic valve replacement [62,63].

POSTOPERATIVE HYPOTENSION. Numerous reports have described the coexistence of aortic stenosis and hypertrophic cardiomyopathy. The coexistence of these lesions is likely to come to attention in the patient who undergoes initially successful aortic valvular surgery but develops a low-output state, with or without pulmonary congestion, in the early postoperative period [27]. In the patient with these coexistent lesions the sudden afterload reduction afforded by aortic valve replacement leads to a small left ventricular cavity and evidence on Doppler study of outflow obstruction. Either transthoracic or transesophageal echocardiographic evaluation is critical for optimal management of this life-threatening condition and should be performed to exclude potentially reversible problems such as early valve dysfunction or cardiac tamponade.

If the echocardiogram reveals poor systolic function, continued diuretics and inotropic agents are warranted; aortic balloon

pump assistance may also be necessary. In our experience, however, the echocardiogram often reveals excellent systolic function without significant valve dysfunction. This scenario is especially common in elderly patients, usually women, with marked left ventricular hypertrophy [27]. While in some patients, the pathophysiology of the low-output state may involve left ventricular outflow tract obstruction caused by coexistent, unrecognized hypertrophic cardiomyopathy [64–70], it is our impression that the low-output syndrome results from the sudden unloading of a heart with marked secondary hypertrophy (due to valvular stenosis, hypertension, or both) [27,68,69,70]. This sudden unloading, we hypothesize, leads to a small left ventricular cavity and is exacerbated by diastolic dysfunction. This situation is further aggravated by preload or afterload reducing agents and by positive inotropic agents; tachycardia may further exacerbate the situation by interfering with left ventricular filling.

Treatment of this potentially catastrophic situation is best dictated by the echocardiographic findings, including transesophageal echocardiography (TEE) if necessary. Optimal treatment usually involves fluid administration, discontinuation of intravenous positive inotropic and chronotropic support, and administration of calcium channel blockers and/or beta-blockers. We have used metoprolol intravenously (in 5 mg doses to a total dose of 15 mg) to achieve adequate beta blockade. Similar effects can be achieved with oral metoprolol (25–100 mg two times per day), titrated to heart rate, or verapamil, 40 to 80 mg orally three times per day, titrated to heart rate or blood pressure. Atrial fibrillation should be treated immediately, since atrial booster function may be especially important for optimal left ventricular systolic performance in this situation.

PERCUTANEOUS VALVULOPLASTY. Percutaneous balloon aortic valvuloplasty has been used to increase the orifice size of a stenotic aortic valve [71–74]. This technique has been applied successfully in children and young patients to cure the stenosis or to improve hemodynamics enough to allow for valve replacement [75,76]. While some success has been described in adults in lowering transaortic gradients and improving symptoms, it appears that the benefits, in most cases, are not long-standing [77–83], with restenosis occurring within 6 months of the procedure in roughly half of patients. Many patients experience no benefit [78]. Risks include worsening of aortic regurgitation, death, systemic embolization, vascular damage, and endocarditis [84–87]. In our institution this procedure is reserved as a palliative measure for those who cannot undergo surgery and those who do not have significant aortic regurgitation. It has been used with apparent success in elderly patients with critical aortic stenosis in an attempt to reduce the risk of general anesthesia for major noncardiac surgery [88].

Hypertrophic Cardiomyopathy

ETIOLOGY. Hypertrophic cardiomyopathy comprises a wide spectrum of structural abnormalities resulting in a variety of clinical syndromes. Marked degrees of hypertrophy may accompany hypertension and aortic stenosis ("secondary hypertrophy"); however, *hypertrophic cardiomyopathy* refers to a disorder whose structural features include marked left ventricular wall thickness, asymmetric hypertrophy of the interventricular septum, narrowed outflow tract, and systolic anterior motion of the mitral valve [89–92]. Functionally this hypertrophy is inappropriate, that is, it is unexplained by the degree of afterload, which is low or normal. Systolic function is hyperdynamic and left ventricular emptying is virtually complete, at least early in the course of the disorder. Obstruction of left ventricular outflow, related to asymmetric septal hypertrophy and systolic anterior motion of the mitral valve, occurs in approximately 25 percent of patients [91–95].

Hypertrophic cardiomyopathy appears to be inherited in an autosomally dominant manner in most individuals, with a slight male preponderance [96,97]. Phenotypic expression, however, is quite variable, ranging from asymptomatic hypertrophy identified on an echocardiogram ordered for other reasons to marked hypertrophy, outflow obstruction, and sudden death. Hypertrophic cardiomyopathy is found in a disproportionately large percentage of young individuals who suffer sudden death during athletic competion [91,92].

The discovery of large kindreds with familial hypertrophic cardiomyopathy has helped elucidate the variable phenotypic expression of this disorder and provided insight into the inheritance of hypertrophy. Recent analysis has identified abnormalities in genes coding for myosin heavy chain [98,99].

PATHOPHYSIOLOGY. The ventricle of patients with hypertrophic obstructive cardiomyopathy is found to be massively hypertrophied in an asymmetric fashion, with disordered histologic architecture. Most often the interventricular septum is both disproportionately hypertrophied [93] and hypokinetic [94]. In some patients, the hypertrophied ventricle displays evidence of an apparent obstruction to outflow, denoted by associated systolic apposition of the mitral valve apparatus and the interventricular septum on M-mode or 2-D echocardiography [95] or the appearance of a systolic intracavitary gradient in association with systolic anterior motion. Controversy still exists concerning the role of systolic anterior motion in the pathophysiology of this disorder [89–92,95,100,101,102]. Some have hypothesized that the gradient and systolic anterior motion of the mitral valve are consequences of hyperdynamic systolic function and rapid, near-complete emptying of the cavity and the creation of Venturi forces in the left ventricular outflow tract [91,92,100,101,102]. Alternatively, it has been argued that the systolic anterior motion of the mitral valve, resulting from abnormal position of the mitral apparatus, causes true obstruction to outflow. A recent study using TEE provided insight into the pathophysiology of this disorder [103]. Griggs and co-workers demonstrated that initial coaptation occurs abnormally in the midportion of both leaflets [103]. In addition, this study documented that leaflet length was abnormally increased in patients in the series. Thus, it is possible that abnormal structural features of the mitral valve apparatus contribute to the pathophysiology of hypertrophic, obstructive cardiomyopathy.

However, it should be kept clearly in mind that in both fixed and dynamic obstruction, the consequences of progressive hypertrophy (with or without ischemia) include abnormalities in left ventricular filling, which may lead to pulmonary congestion, low cardiac output, or both. Marked decrease in diastolic compliance of the left ventricle leads to an elevation of left atrial and pulmonary venous pressures with resulting pulmonary congestion and dyspnea [15]. In some individuals this diastolic dysfunction is associated with a reduced stroke volume, a direct consequence of the small left ventricular end-diastolic volume. This diminution in volume may have consequences during or immediately following exercise, when the drop in peripheral vascular resistance may cause an exaggerated fall in blood pressure, resulting in dizziness or even syncope. In addition, it is hypothesized that the left ventricle is "underfilled" at a time when the septum is thickening, leading to abutment of the mitral apparatus against the septum (cavity obliteration).

It is not yet clear how many patients with hypertrophic obstructive cardiomyopathy actually have symptoms caused by a significant obstruction to left ventricular emptying. Symptoms specifically caused by reduced stroke volume due to blood "entrapment" below the muscular obstruction may indeed be unusual [89]; nevertheless, some patients demonstrate obstructive features, with a subaortic systolic pressure gradient and a systolic murmur [91,92]. Reduction in preload exaggerates these obstructive features by causing a decrease in diastolic filling. Afterload reduction also accentuates the obstructive phenomena by bringing about earlier systolic emptying. However, this finding of early systolic emptying has not been universal; continued low-grade ventricular emptying has been documented in many subjects [100,101]. In the dynamic obstruction hypothesized to occur in hypertrophic cardiomyopathy, as well as in fixed outflow obstruction, the contribution of atrial contraction to diastolic filling may be much greater than usual. In both instances, the onset of atrial fibrillation may cause a serious reduction in stroke volume and lead to profound hypotension [104].

HISTORY. Recent work by Spirito and co-workers [105] highlights the fact that most patients with hypertrophic cardiomyopathy have only mild symptoms. The diagnosis is often made in adulthood, with patients usually in their fourth or fifth decade of life. Clinical manifestations vary widely; many patients are asymptomatic, while the first presentation in some affected individuals may be sudden cardiac death. There appears to be a male preponderance [91,92,105].

Common symptoms include dyspnea, which is the result of abnormal diastolic filling, angina, and syncope [91,92]. As in aortic stenosis, it is common for typical angina pectoris (and even myocardial infarction) to occur despite normal epicardial coronary arteries. Near syncope and syncope are also common symptoms and may indicate a predisposition to serious ventricular arrhythmias.

PHYSICAL EXAMINATION. Some of the physical findings in patients with hypertrophic cardiomyopathy are similar to those of other patients with pressure overload hypertrophy. The apical impulse may be laterally displaced and a presystolic impulse may be palpable. In hypertrophic cardiomyopathy with obstruction, the carotid pulse has a "bisfieriens" quality, characterized by an abrupt decline in midsystole.

The murmur of hypertrophic obstructive cardiomyopathy is usually best heard between the apex and the left sternal border and is usually made louder by the Valsalva maneuver and by standing. This murmur is therefore distinguished from all other outflow murmurs, which tend to decrease in intensity with these maneuvers [105].

LABORATORY STUDIES

Electrocardiogram. In hypertrophic cardiomyopathy, the asymmetric nature of the septal hypertrophy may cause deep Q waves in inferior and lateral leads, mimicking a prior infarction (Fig. 33-10).

Chest Radiograph. Enlargement of the overall cardiac silhouette is seen in approximately one-half of patients with hypertrophic cardiomyopathy.

Echocardiogram. Echocardiography is the most important diagnostic test for patients with suspected hypertrophic cardiomyopathy and, it may be argued, has been responsible for

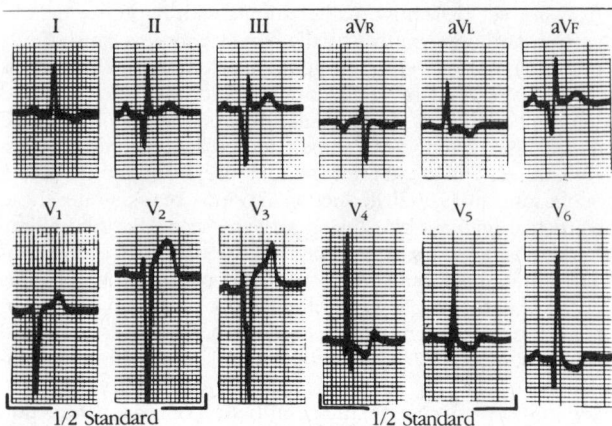

Fig. 33-10. Electrocardiogram of a patient with asymmetric septal hypertrophy. Q waves in leads II, III, aVF, V₅, and V₆. Precordial leads exhibit voltage criteria for left ventricular hypertrophy with S–T segment and T wave abnormalities suggestive of "strain." (From Braunwald E, Lambrew CT, Rockoff SD, et al: Idiopathic hypertrophic subaortic stenosis: Description of the disease based upon an analysis of 64 patients. *Circulation* 29(suppl IV):1, 1964. With permission.)

delineating most of the clinical and morphologic features of this disorder. A universal echocardiographic feature of hypertrophic cardiomyopathy is marked left ventricular hypertrophy, which often predominantly involves the interventricular septum. The left ventricular cavity is diminished in both systole and diastole. In patients with systolic gradients, there is systolic anterior motion of the mitral valve apparatus (Figs. 33-11 to 33-14), prolonged contact of the anterior mitral leaflet with the septum, and early closure of the aortic valve. These features are usually best appreciated on M-mode echocardiography (Figs. 33-13 and 33-14). The usual criterion for the diagnosis of hypertrophic cardiomyopathy by echocardiography is a ratio of septal to posterior wall thickness of 1.3 to 1.5:1 (assuming that the posterior wall has not been thinned by prior infarction). This excessive hypertrophy is associated with hyperdynamic left ventricular systolic function, perhaps as a consequence of systolic unloading. In certain patients there is a characteristic appearance of the left ventricular myocardium on M-mode echo ("ground glass" appearance). It is possible that this appearance is related to abnormal tissue, produced by fibrosis.

Doppler Echocardiogram. Doppler echocardiography has also been successfully used to record the subaortic gradient of hypertrophic obstructive cardiomyopathy (Figs. 33-15 and 33-16) [106,107,108]. In general, the Doppler gradient correlates

Fig. 33-11. Echocardiogram in the parasternal long axis in hypertrophic obstructive cardiomyopathy, during diastole. Note the marked hypertrophy of the interventricular septum (IVS) in comparison to the posterior wall of the left ventricle (LVPW). LV = left ventricle; LA = left atrium; RV = right ventricle.

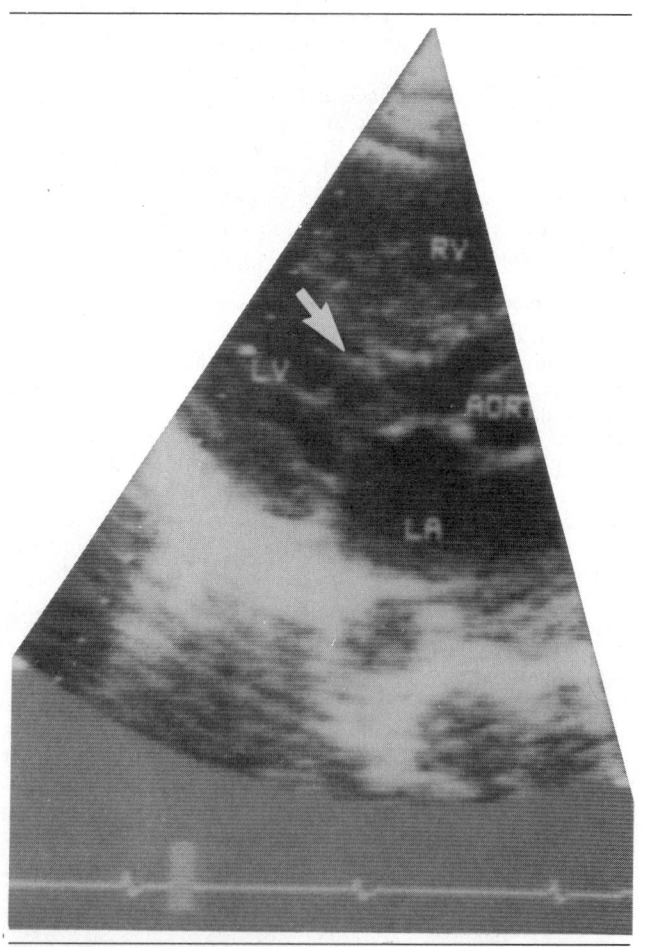

Fig. 33-12. Echocardiogram in the parasternal long axis in hypertrophic obstructive cardiomyopathy, during systole. Note the systolic anterior position of mitral valve structures (*arrow*). LV = left ventricle; LA = left atrium; RV = right ventricle.

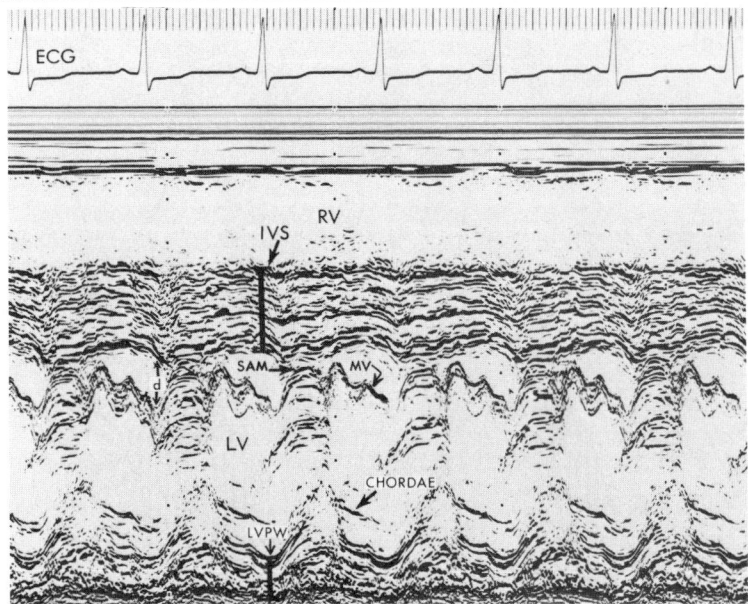

Fig. 33-13. Echocardiogram (time-motion study) in hypertrophic obstructive cardiomyopathy. Note the systolic anterior motion (SAM) of the mitral valve, which here results in sustained abutment of the anterior leaflet against the interventricular septum (IVS) during systole. RV = right ventricle; LV = left ventricle; MV = mitral valve. (From Dalen JE, Alpert JS (eds): *Valvular Heart Disease.* Boston, Little, Brown, 1981. With permission.)

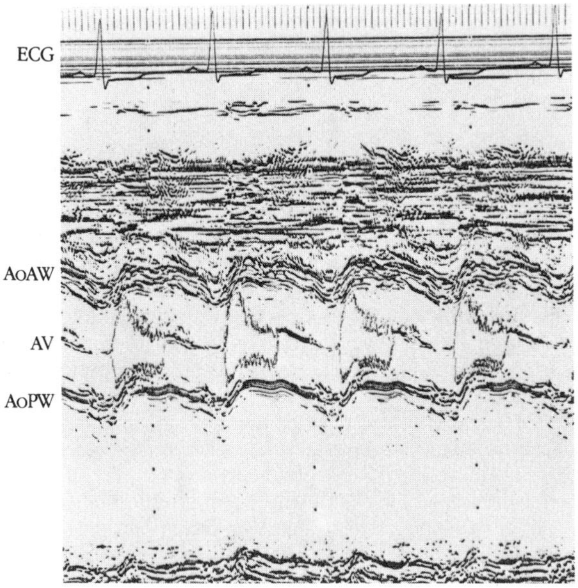

Fig. 33-14. Echocardiogram (time-motion study) in hypertrophic obstructive cardiomyopathy. After the aortic valve (AV) opens, the leaflets are seen to move away from the anterior and posterior aortic walls (AoAW and AoPW) to a position of partial systolic closure. Note also the fine fluttering of the leaflets, which occurs commonly in normal valves and in all varieties of subvalvular obstruction but is rare in valvular aortic stenosis. (From Dalen JE, Alpert JS (eds): *Valvular Heart Disease.* Boston, Little, Brown, 1981. With permission.)

well with invasive gradient estimates. In addition, abnormalities in diastolic function are observed by Doppler analysis of the left ventricular filling velocities [79].

CARDIAC CATHETERIZATION. In nonvalvular obstructions, the cardiac catheterization allows localization of the site of obstruction by recording, on careful retrograde pullback of the catheter, the pressure gradient either above or below the aortic valve (Fig. 33-17). Hypertrophic obstructive cardiomyopathy is characterized by a variable gradient below the aortic valve. This gradient is dynamic in that it is markedly affected by physiologic or pharmacologic interventions. Any decrease in left ventricular size or increase in contractility raises the gradient. Premature ventricular beats are particularly useful in assessing patients with suspected obstruction due to hypertrophic cardiomyopathy: the obstruction is exaggerated during the postextrasystolic beat because of a marked increase in contractility (Fig. 33-17). Characteristically, the pulse pressure of the postextrasystolic beat is diminished in this disorder, whereas it is likely to rise in fixed forms of left ventricular outflow obstruction.

MEDICAL THERAPY. The medical treatment of hypertrophic cardiomyopathy is aimed at providing symptomatic relief and preventing sudden death. Digitalis (digoxin, 0.125–0.25 mg orally per day) should be reserved for rate control in patients with atrial fibrillation, in view of the potential for adverse consequences of positive inotropism. Diuretics may be used cautiously in patients with pulmonary congestion; care must be taken not to reduce preload excessively.

Beta-blockers have salutary effects for patients with hypertrophic cardiomyopathy and symptoms: They decrease both contractility and heart rate and therefore lessen myocardial oxygen demand. The usual doses of metroprolol are 50 to 200 mg per day; for atenolol, 50 to 100 mg by mouth daily. Calcium channel blockers may also have salutary effects on left ventricular diastolic function by relieving ischemia, lowering blood pressure, or reducing asynchrony of relaxation. Verapamil appears to be the most widely used agent (usual dose 240–360 mg/day), though nifedipine (30–90 mg per day in divided doses) and

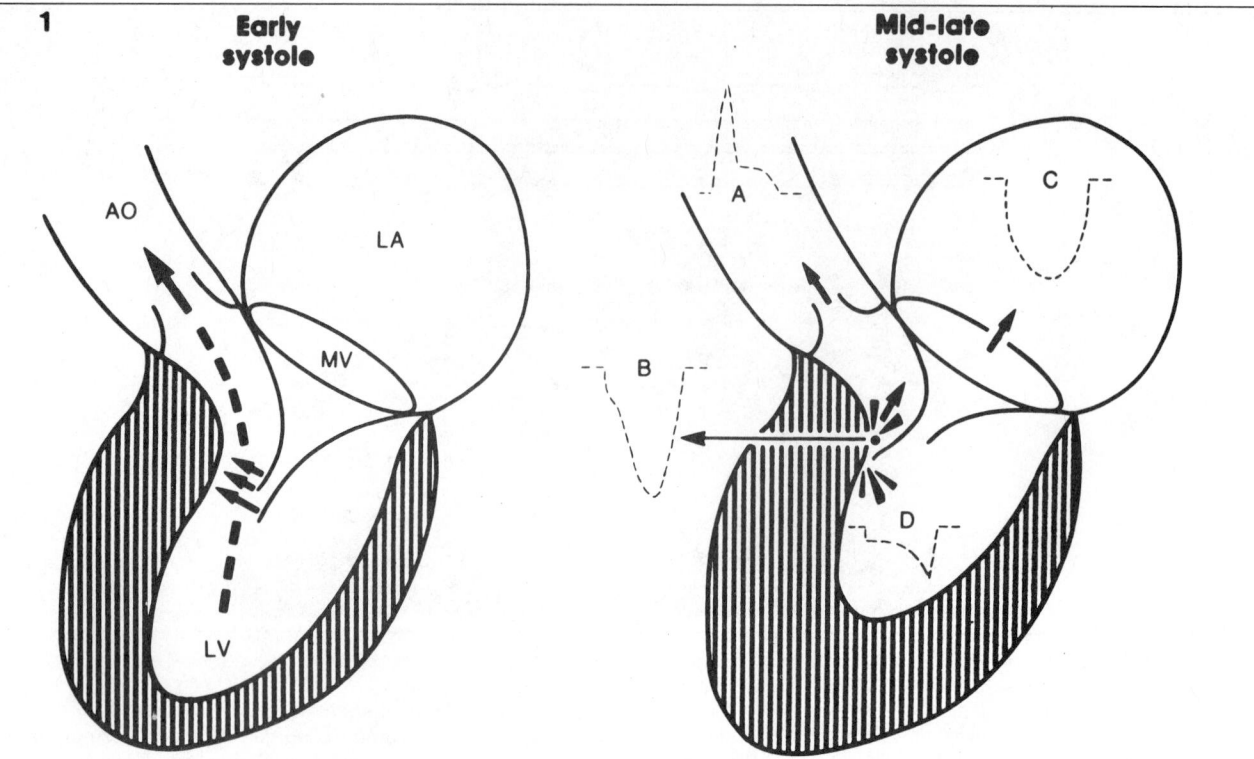

Fig. 33-15. Left. Proposed mechanism of mitral leaflet systolic anterior motion in early systole in obstructive hypertrophic cardiomyopathy. The ventricular septal hypertrophy and narrow outflow tract are associated with rapid and complete ejection (dashed line), thus the path of ejection is closer to the mitral leaflets than is normal. In patients with obstruction, these are thought to result in Venturi forces (*short arrows*), which may draw the mitral leaflet(s) toward the septum (systolic anterior motion), with the subsequent development of mitral leaflet-septal contact as seen on the right panel. AO = aorta; LA = left atrium; MV = mitral valve; LV = left ventricle. Right. According to Wigle [90], by midsystole, anterior mitral-leaflet septal contact causes obstruction to left ventricular outflow (converging and diverging lines at this site) and a diminution in forward aortic flow (*short aortic arrows*) as well as mitral regurgitation (*arrow* arising from mitral orifice). Letters indicate Doppler velocity recordings throughout systole in the ascending aorta (A); at the level of mitral leaflet-septal contact (B); in the left atrium (C); and near the apex of the left ventricle (D). In B,C, and D, flow is away from the transducer. (From Wigle ED: Hypertrophic cardiomyopathy: A 1987 viewpoint. *Circulation* 75: 311, 1987. With permission).

diltiazem (90–270 mg orally per day in divided doses) have also been reported to have beneficial effects.

Nitrates have proved helpful in treating angina in patients with hypertrophic cardiomyopathy and coronary artery disease, but, as in valvular stenosis, they must be used with caution because of the potentially deleterious effects of preload reduction. At present there does not appear to be a role for direct arterial vasodilators (hydrazine) or angiotensin-converting enzyme inhibitors in patients with hypertrophic cardiomyopathy, since a drop in arterial pressure can be expected to result in an undesired increase in left ventricular emptying. Disopyramide, an antiarrhythmic drug, has been shown to effect symptomatic improvement; this may be due to its negative inotropic properties. The usual daily dose is 400 to 1600 mg.

It is not unusual for patients with hypertrophic cardiomyopathy to suffer from incapacitating and life-threatening ar-

rhythmias. Recurrent syncope or symptomatic palpitations require investigation into possible arrhythmias and may require antiarrhythmic therapy [109,110]. Amiodarone (total daily dose: 200–600 mg) appears to be efficacious in the treatment of both supraventricular and ventricular arrhythmias [110]. There are also reports that it improves prognosis [110].

SURGICAL THERAPY. Surgery is rarely indicated for hypertrophic cardiomyopathy. If symptoms persist despite treatment with beta-blockers, calcium channel blockers, or disopyramide, surgical removal of ventricular muscle may be attempted. Surgery for hypertrophic cardiomyopathy generally involves a septal myomectomy to remove a portion of proximal interventricular septum to widen the left ventricular outflow tract. Occasionally, mitral valve replacement may be performed to relieve mitral regurgitation [111,112]. Intraoperative TEE appears to be helpful in intraoperative decision making. In successful cases, TEE demonstrates that following myectomy there is dramatic thinning of the septum and resolution of the systolic anterior motion of the mitral valve. Mitral regurgitation is usually either reduced or abolished [103]. Symptomatic and hemodynamic improvement has been noted in most series [113–118]. Whether survival is actually improved by surgery, however, is unknown.

Recently, Fananapazir and co-workers described dramatic symptomatic improvement in a group of hypertrophic cardiomyopathy patients in response to dual chamber pacing [119]. The rationale for pacemaker implantation was that preexcitation of the interventricular septum by right ventricular pacing would lead to motion of the septum away from the posterior wall in systole and widening of the left ventricular outflow tract. This widening, it was hypothesized, would lead to lesser degrees of systolic anterior motion of the mitral valve, a diminution in the left ventricular outflow tract pressure gradient, and

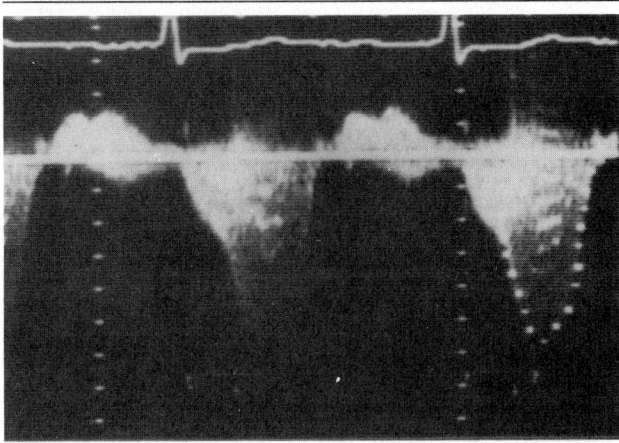

Fig. 33-16. Continuous-wave Doppler recording across the left ventricular outflow tract in a patient with hypertrophic obstructive cardiomyopathy. The maximum gradient was 138 mm Hg with a mean gradient of 70 mm Hg. Note the typical shoulder on the gradient, with the highest velocities achieved in late systole (dagger-shaped).

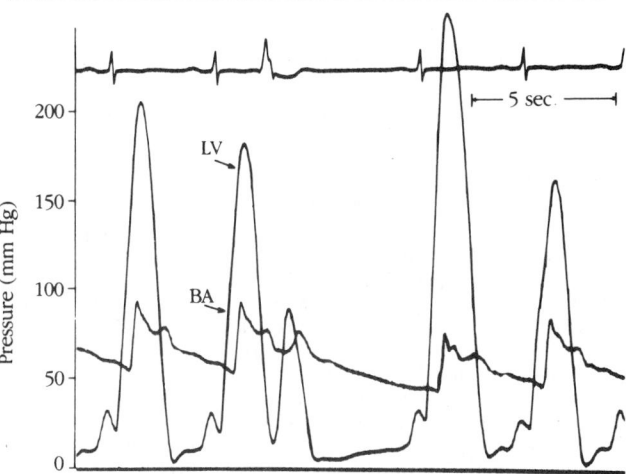

Fig. 33-17. Simultaneous pressures recorded in the left ventricle (LV) and brachial artery (BA) in a patient with hypertrophic obstructive cardiomyopathy. During the postpremature contraction beat, the pulse pressure in the brachial artery is less than it is during the control beats. (From Braunwald E, Lambrew CT, Rockoff SD, et al: Idiopathic hypertrophic subaortic stenosis: Description of the disease based upon an analysis of 64 patients. *Circulation* 29(suppl IV):1, 1964. With permission.)

reduction in the severity of mitral regurgitation. The patients in this series were elected based on their failure to respond to medical therapy with beta- and calcium channel blockers and disopyramide; all were in New York Heart Association's functional class III or IV. According to the authors, DDD pacing led to either abolition or significant improvement in symptoms in virtually all patients. All 15 class IV patients improved two functional grades by the time of follow-up evaluation (1.5–3 months after initiation of DDD pacing). The functional improvement paralleled a 57 percent reduction in the peak left ventricular outflow tract gradient (from 64 ± 7 to 27 ± 5 mm Hg). Sur-

prisingly, at the time of follow-up study, the gradient was reduced significantly even when the patients were studied in normal sinus rhythm (i.e., when not paced).

This study suggests that DDD pacing is an attractive alternative to myomyectomy, which, as noted above, has a relatively high associated mortality in severely symptomatic patients. The widespread use of this modality awaits confirmation of the authors' findings by investigators in other referral centers with large populations of patients with hypertrophic cardiomyopathy.

References

1. Levinson GE: Valvular heart disease, in Gordon BL (ed): *Clinical Cardiopulmonary Physiology,* 3rd ed. New York, Grune & Stratton, 1969, p 245.
2. Roberts WC, Virmani R: Aschoff bodies at necropsy in valvular heart disease: Evidence from an analysis of 543 patients over 14 years of age that rheumatic heart disease, at least anatomically, is a disease of the mitral valve. *Circulation* 57:803, 1978.
3. Bacon APC, Mathews MB: Congenital bicuspid aortic valves and the aetiology of isolated aortic valvular stenosis. *Q J Med* 28:545, 1959.
4. Roberts WC: The structure of the aortic valve in clinically isolated aortic stenosis: An autopsy study of 162 patients over 15 years of age. *Circulation* 42:91, 1970.
5. Selzer A: Changing aspects of the natural history of valvular aortic stenosis. *N Engl J Med* 317:91, 1987.
6. Fenoglio JJ Jr, McAllister HA, DeCastro CM, et al: Congenital bicuspid aortic valve after age 20. *Am J Cardiol* 39:164, 1977.
7. Roberts WC: The congenitally bicuspid aortic valve: A study of 85 autopsy cases. *Am J Cardiol* 26:72, 1970.
8. Roberts WC, Perloff JK, Constantino T: Severe valvular aortic stenosis in patients over 65 years of age: A clinicopathologic study. *Am J Cardiol* 27:497, 1971.
9. Campbell M: Calcific aortic stenosis and congenital bicuspid aortic valve. *Br Heart J* 30:606, 1968.
10. Burns DL, Van der Hauwaert LG: Aortic systolic murmur developing with increasing age. *Br Heart J* 20:370, 1958.
11. Davidson ET, Friedman SA: Significance of systolic murmurs in the aged. *N Engl J Med* 279:225, 1968.
12. Dexter L, Harken DE, Cobb LA Jr, et al: Aortic stenosis. *Arch Intern Med* 101:754, 1958.
13. Carabello BA, Green LH, Grossman W, et al: Hemodynamic determination of prognosis of aortic valve replacement in critical aortic stenosis and advanced congestive heart failure. *Circulation* 62:42, 1980.
14. Ross J Jr: Afterload mismatch in aortic and mitral valve disease: Implications for surgical therapy. *J Am Coll Cardiol* 5:811, 1985.
15. Bonow RO, Udelson JE: LV diastolic dysfunction as a cause of congestive heart failure. *Ann Intern Med* 117:502, 1992.
16. Soufer R, Wohlgelernter D, Vita NA, et al: Intact systolic LV function in clinical congestive heart failure. *Am J Cardiol* 55:1032, 1985.
17. Dougherty AH, Naccarelli GV, Gray EL, et al: Congestive heart failure with normal systolic function. *Am J Cardiol* 54:778, 1984.
18. Silver K, Aurigemma G, Krendel S, et al: Pulmonary artery hypertension in severe aortic stenosis: Incidence and mechanism. *Am Heart J* 125:146, 1993.
19. Cheitlin MD, Gertz EW, Brundage BH, et al: Rate of progression of valvular aortic stenosis in the adult. *Am Heart J* 98:689, 1979.
20. Bogart D, Murphy BL, Wond BYS, et al: Progression of aortic stenosis. *Chest* 76:391, 1979.
21. Currie RJ, Seward J, Reeder GS, et al: Continuous wave Doppler echocardiographic assessment of severity of calcific aortic stenosis. *Circulation* 79:1165, 1985.
22. Lombard JT, Selzer A: Valvular aortic stenosis: A clinical and hemodynamic profile of patients. *Ann Intern Med* 106:292, 1987.
23. Wood P: Aortic stenosis. *Am J Cardiol* 1:553, 1958.
24. Mitchell AM, Sackett CH, Hunzicker WJ, et al: The clinical features of aortic stenosis. *Am Heart J* 48:694, 1954.
25. Hakki AH, Kimbiris D, Iskandrian AS, et al: Angina pectoris and

coronary artery disease in patients with severe aortic valvular disease. *Am Heart J* 100:441, 1980.

26. Hancock EW: Aortic stenosis, angina pectoris, and coronary artery disease. *Am Heart J* 93:382, 1977.

27. Aurigemma GP, Battista S, Orsinelli D, et al: Abnormal left ventricular intracavitary flow acceleration in patients undergoing aortic valve replacement for aortic stenosis: A marker for high postoperative morbidity and mortality. *Circulation* 86:926, 1992.

28. Orsinelli D, Aurigemma GP, Battista S, et al: Left ventricular hypertrophy and mortality following aortic valve replacement for aortic stenosis. *J Am Coll Cardiol* 22:1679, 1993.

29. Hammersten JG: Syncope and aortic stenosis. *Arch Intern Med* 87:274, 1951.

30. Flamm MD, Braniff BA, Kimball R, et al: Mechanism of effort syncope and aortic stenosis. *Circulation* 36(suppl 2):109, 1967.

31. Johnson AM: Aortic stenosis, sudden death and left ventricular baroreceptors. *Br Heart J* 33:1, 1971.

32. Mark AL, Kioschos JM, Abboud FM, et al: Abnormal vascular response to exercise in patients with aortic stenosis. *J Clin Invest* 52:1138, 1973.

33. Ross J Jr, Braunwald E: Aortic stenosis. *Circulation* 38(suppl 5):61, 1968.

34. Alpert JS, Vieweg WVR, Hagan AD: Incidence and morphology of carotid shudders in aortic valve disease. *Am Heart J* 92:435, 1976.

35. Aronow WS, Kronzon I: Correlation of prevalence and severity of valvular aortic stenosis determined by continuous-wave Doppler echocardiography with physical signs of aortic stenosis in patients aged 62 to 100 years with aortic systolic ejection murmurs. *Am J Cardiol* 60:399, 1987.

36. Godley RW, Green D, Dillon JC, et al: Reliability of two-dimensional echocardiography in assessing the severity of valvular aortic stenosis. *Chest* 79:657, 1981.

37. Parisi AF, Folland ED: Are non-invasive tests sufficient for preoperative evaluation of aortic stenosis? *J Am Coll Cardiol* 3:1092, 1984.

38. Carroll JD, Carroll EP, Feldman T, et al: Sex-associated differences in left ventricular function in aortic stenosis of the elderly. *Circulation* 86:1099, 1992.

39. Schwartz A, Vignola PA, Walker JH, et al: Echocardiographic estimation of aortic-valve gradient in aortic stenosis. *Ann Intern Med* 89:329, 1978.

40. Hatle L, Angelsen BA, Tromsdal A: Non-invasive assessment of aortic stenosis by Doppler ultrasound. *Br Heart J* 43:284, 1980.

41. Hatle L: Noninvasive assessment and differentiation of left ventricular outflow obstruction with Doppler ultrasound. *Circulation* 64:381, 1981.

42. Hegrenaes L, Hatle L: Aortic stenosis in adults: Noninvasive estimation of pressure differences by continuous wave Doppler echocardiography. *Br Heart J* 54:396, 1985.

43. Kosturakis D, Allen HD, Goldberg SJ, et al: Noninvasive quantification of stenotic semilunar valve areas by Doppler echocardiography. *J Am Coll Cardiol* 3:1256, 1984.

44. Warth DC, Stewart WJ, Block PC, et al: A new method to calculate aortic valve area without left heart catheterization. *Circulation* 70:978, 1984.

45. Richards KL, Cannon SR, Miller JF, et al: Calculation of aortic valve area by Doppler echocardiography: A direct application of the continuity equation. *Circulation* 73:964, 1986.

46. Teirstein P, Yeager M, Yock PG, et al: Doppler echocardiographic measurement of aortic valve area in aortic stenosis: A noninvasive application of the Gorlin formula. *J Am Coll Cardiol* 8:1059, 1986.

47. Oh JK, Taliercio CP, Holmes DR, et al: Prediction of the severity of aortic stenosis by Doppler aortic valve area determination: Prospective Doppler-catheterization correlation in 100 patients. *J Am Coll Cardiol* 11:1227, 1988.

48. Jaffe WM, Roche AHG, Coverdale HA, et al: Clinical evaluation versus Doppler echocardiography in the quantitative assessment of valvular heart disease. *Circulation* 78:267, 1988.

49. Miller FA: Aortic stenosis: Most cases no longer require invasive hemodynamic study. *J Am Coll Cardiol* 13:551, 1989.

50. Gorlin R, Gorlin SG: Hydraulic formula for calculating the area of the stenotic mitral valve, other cardiac valves, and central circulatory shunts. *Am Heart J* 41:1, 1951.

51. Kelly TA, Rothbart RM, Cooper CM, et al: Comparison of outcome of asymptomatic to symptomatic patients older than 20 years of age with valvular aortic stenosis. *Am J Cardiol* 61:123, 1988.

52. Pellikka PA, Nishimura RA, Bailey KR, et al: The natural history of adults with asymptomatic, hemodynamically significant aortic stenosis. *J Am Coll Cardiol* 15:1012, 1990.

53. Braunwald E: On the natural history of severe aortic stenosis. *J Am Coll Cardiol* 15:1018, 1990.

54. Greenberg BH, Massie BM: Beneficial effects of afterload reduction therapy in patients with congestive failure and moderate aortic stenosis. *Circulation* 61:1212, 1980.

55. Awan NA, DeMaria AN, Miller RR, et al: Beneficial effects of nitroprusside administration on left ventricular dysfunction and myocardial ischemia in severe aortic stenosis. *Am Heart J* 101:386, 1981.

56. St. John Sutton M, Plappert T, Spiegel A, et al: Early post-operative changes in left ventricular chamber size, architecture, and function in aortic stenosis and aortic regurgitation and their relation to intraoperative changes in afterload: A prospective two-dimensional echocardiographic study. *Circulation* 76:77, 1987.

57. Brogan W, Grayburn P, Lange R, Hillis L: Prognosis after valve replacement in patients with severe aortic stenosis and a low transvalvular pressure gradient. *J Am Coll Cardiol* 21:1657, 1993.

58. Richardson JV, Kouchoukos NT, Wright JO III, et al: Combined aortic valve replacement and myocardial revascularization: Results in 220 patients. *Circulation* 59:75, 1979.

59. Ferrans VJ, Boyce SW, Billingham ME, et al: Calcific deposits in porcine bioprostheses: Structure and pathogenesis. *Am J Cardiol* 46:721, 1980.

60. Oyer PE, Miller DC, Stinson EB, et al: Clinical durability of the Hancock porcine bioprosthetic valve. *J Thorac Cardiovasc Surg* 80:824, 1980.

61. Curcio CA, Commerford PJ, Rose AG, et al: Calcifications of glutaraldehyde-preserved porcine xenografts in young patients. *J Thorac Cardiovasc Surg* 81:621, 1981.

62. Rahimtoola SH: Valve replacement: A perspective. *Am J Cardiol* 35:711, 1975.

63. Roberts DL, DeWeese JA, Mahoney EB, et al: Long-term survival following aortic valve replacement. *Am Heart J* 91:311, 1976.

64. Parker DP, Kaplan MA, Connolly JE, et al: Co-existent aortic valvular and functional subaortic stenosis: Clinical, physiologic and angiographic aspects. *Am J Cardiol* 24:307, 1969.

65. Nanda NC, Gramiak R, Shah PM, et al: Echocardiography in the diagnosis of idiopathic hypertrophic subaortic stenosis co-existing with aortic valve disease. *Circulation* 50:752, 1974.

66. Stewart S, Nanda NC, DeWeese JA: Simultaneous operative correction of aortic valve stenosis and idiopathic hypertrophic subaortic stenosis. *Circulation* 51(suppl I):I-34, 1975.

67. Feizi O, Farrer-Brown G, Emanuel R: Familial study of hypertrophic cardiomyopathy and congenital aortic valve disease. *Am J Cardiol* 41:956, 1978.

68. Hess OM, Schneider J, Turina M, et al: Asymmetric septal hypertrophy in patients with aortic stenosis: An adaptive mechanism or a coexistence of hypertrophic cardiomyopathy? *J Am Coll Cardiol* 1:783, 1983.

69. Schwinger ME, O'Brien F, Freedberg RS, et al: Dynamic outflow obstruction after aortic valve replacement: A Doppler echocardiographic study. *J Am Soc Echocardiogr* 3:205, 1990.

70. Cutrone F, Coyle JP, Novoa R, et al: Severe dynamic left ventricular outflow tract obstruction following aortic valve replacement diagnosed by intraoperative echocardiography. *Anesthesiology* 72:563, 1990.

71. Lababidi Z, Wu RJ, Walls JT: Percutaneous balloon aortic valvuloplasty: Results in 23 patients. *Am J Cardiol* 53:194, 1984.

72. Cribier A, Saoudi N, Berland J, et al: Percutaneous transluminal valvuloplasty of acquired aortic stenosis in elderly patients: An alternative to valve replacement? *Lancet* 1:63, 1986.

73. McKay RG, Safian RD, Lock JE, et al: Balloon dilatation of calcific aortic stenosis in elderly patients: Postmortem, intraoperative, and percutaneous valvuloplasty studies. *Circulation* 74:119, 1986.

74. Isner JM, Samuels DA, Slovenkai GA, et al: Mechanism of aortic balloon valvuloplasty: Fracture of valvular calcific deposits. *Ann Intern Med* 108:377, 1988.

75. Lababidi Z, Weinhaus L: Successful balloon valvuloplasty for neonatal critical aortic stenosis. *Am Heart J* 112:913, 1986.

76. Desnoyers MR, Slem DN, Rosenfield K, et al: Treatment of cardiogenic shock by emergency aortic balloon valvuloplasty. *Ann Intern Med* 108:833, 1988.

77. Safian RD, Berman AD, Diver DJ, et al: Balloon aortic valvuloplasty in 170 consecutive patients. *N Engl J Med* 319:125, 1988.

78. Brady ST, Davis CA, Kussmaul WG, et al: Percutaneous aortic balloon valvuloplasty in octogenarians: Morbidity and mortality. *Ann Intern Med* 110:761, 1989.

79. Berland J, Cribier A, Savin T, et al: Percutaneous balloon valvuloplasty in patients with severe aortic stenosis and low ejection fraction: Immediate results and 1-year follow-up. *Circulation* 79:1189, 1989.

80. Holmes DR, Nishimura RA, Reeder GS, et al: Clinical follow-up after percutaneous aortic balloon valvuloplasty. *Arch Intern Med* 148:1405, 1989.

81. Lewin RF, Dorros G, King JF, et al: Percutaneous transluminal aortic valvuloplasty: Acute outcome and follow-up of 125 patients. *J Am Coll Cardiol* 14:1210, 1989.

82. Sherman W, Hershman R, Lazzam C, et al: Balloon valvuloplasty in adult aortic stenosis: Determinants of clinical outcome. *Ann Intern Med* 110:421, 1989.

83. Davidson CJ, Harrison JK, Leithe ME, et al: Failure of balloon aortic valvuloplasty to result in sustained clinical improvement in patients with depressed left ventricular function. *Am J Cardiol* 65:72, 1990.

84. Cujec B, McMeekin J, Lopez J: Bacterial endocarditis after percutaneous aortic valvuloplasty. *Am Heart J* 115:178, 1988.

85. Cribier A, Berland J, Koning R, et al: Percutaneous transluminal aortic valvuloplasty: Indications and results in adult aortic stenosis. *Eur Heart J* 9:149, 1988.

86. Acar J, Vahanian A, Slama M, et al: Treatment of calcified aortic stenosis: Surgery or percutaneous transluminal aortic valvuloplasty? *Eur Heart J* 9:163, 1988.

87. Davidson CJ, Skelton TN, Kisslo KB, et al: The risk for systemic embolization associated with percutaneous balloon valvuloplasty in adults. *Ann Intern Med* 108:557, 1988.

88. Roth RB, Palacios IF, Block PC, et al: Percutaneous aortic balloon valvuloplasty: Its role in the management of patients with aortic stenosis requiring major noncardiac surgery. *J Am Coll Cardiol* 13:1039, 1989.

89. Criley JM, Siegel RJ: Has "obstruction" hindered our understanding of hypertrophic cardiomyopathy? *Circulation* 72:1148, 1985.

90. Wigle ED: Hypertrophic cardiomyopathy: A 1987 viewpoint. *Circulation* 75:311, 1987.

91. Maron BJ, Bonow RO, Cannon RO III, et al: Hypertrophic cardiomyopathy: Interrelations of clinical manifestations, pathophysiology, and therapy. 1. *N Engl J Med* 316:780, 1987.

92. Maron BJ, Bonow RO, Cannon RO III, et al: Hypertrophic cardiomyopathy: Interrelations of clinical manifestations, pathophysiology, and therapy. 2. *N Engl J Med* 316:844, 1987.

93. Henry WI, Clark CE, Epstein SE: Asymmetric septal hypertrophy (ASH): Echocardiographic identification of the pathognomonic anatomic abnormality of IHSS. *Circulation* 47:225, 1973.

94. Rossen RM, Goodman DJ, Ingham RE, et al: Ventricular systolic septal thickening and excursion in idiopathic hypertrophic subaortic stenosis. *N Engl J Med* 291:1317, 1974.

95. Henry WL, Clark CE, Griffith JM: Mechanism of left ventricular outflow obstruction in patients with obstructive asymmetric septal hypertrophy (idiopathic hypertrophic subaortic stenosis). *Am J Cardiol* 35:337, 1975.

96. Clark CE, Henry WL, Epstein SE: Familial prevalence and genetic transmission of idiopathic hypertrophic subaortic stenosis. *N Engl J Med* 289:709, 1973.

97. Maron BJ: The genetics of hypertrophic cardiomyopathy. *Ann Intern Med* 105:610, 1986.

98. Jarcho JA, McKenna W, Pare JAP, et al: Mapping a gene for familial hypertrophic cardiomyopathy to chromosome. *N Engl J Med* 321:1372, 1989.

99. Tanigawa G, Jarcho JA, Kass S, et al: A molecular basis for familial hypertrophic cardiomyopathy: An α/β cardiac myosin heavy chain hybrid gene. *Cell* 62:991, 1990.

100. Bonow RO: Left ventricular ejection dynamics and outflow obstruction in hypertrophic cardiomyopathy. *J Am Coll Cardiol* 13:1280, 1989.

101. Sasson Z, Henderson M, Wilansky S, et al: Causal relation between the pressure gradient and left ventricular ejection time in hypertrophic cardiomyopthy. *J Am Coll Cardiol* 13:1275, 1989.

102. Murgo JP, Alter BR, Dorethy JF, et al: Dynamics of left ventricular ejection in obstructive and nonobstructive hypertrophied cardiomyopathy. *J Clin Invest* 66:1369, 1980.

103. Griggs LE, Wiggle ED, Williams WG, et al: Transesophageal Doppler echocardiography in obstructive hypertrophic cardiomyopathy: Clarification of pathophysiology and importance in intraoperative decision making. *J Am Coll Cardiol* 20: 42, 1992.

104. Savage DD, Seides SF, Maron BJ, et al: Prevalence of arrhythmias during 24-hour electrocardiographic monitoring and exercise testing in patients with obstructive and nonobstructive hypertrophic cardiomyopathy. *Circulation* 59:866, 1979.

105. Spirito P, Chiarella F, Carratino L, et al: Clinical course and prognosis of hypertrophic cardiomyopathy in an outpatient population. *N Eng J Med* 320: 749, 1989.

106. Maron BJ, Gottdiener JS, Arce J, et al: Dynamic subaortic obstruction in hypertrophic cardiomyopathy: Analysis by pulsed Doppler echocardiography. *J Am Coll Cardiol* 6:1, 1985.

107. Yock PG, Hatle L, Popp RL: Patterns and timing of Doppler-detected intracavitary and aortic flow in hypertrophic cardiomyopathy. *J Am Coll Cardiol* 8:1047, 1986.

108. Bryg RJ, Pearson AC, Williams GA, et al: Left ventricular systolic and diastolic flow abnormalities determined by Doppler echocardiography in obstructive hypertrophic cardiomyopathy. *Am J Cardiol* 59:925, 1987.

109. Maron BJ, Savage DD, Wolfson JK, et al: Prognostic significance of 24 hour ambulatory electrocardiographic monitoring in patients with hypertrophic cardiomyopathy: A prospective study. *Am J Cardiol* 48:252, 1981.

110. McKenna WJ, Harris L, Rowland E, et al: Amiodarone for long-term management of patients with hypertrophic cardiomyopathy. *Am J Cardiol* 54:802, 1984.

111. Cooley DA, Leachman RD, Wukasch DC: Diffuse muscular subaortic stenosis: Surgical treatment. *Am J Cardiol* 31:1, 1973.

112. Fighali S, Krajcer Z, Leachman RD: Septal myomectomy and mitral valve replacement for idiopathic hypertrophic subaortic stenosis: Short- and long-term follow-up. *J Am Coll Cardiol* 3:1127, 1984.

113. Morrow AG, Reitz BA, Epstein SE, et al: Operative treatment in hypertrophic subaortic stenosis: Techniques, and the results of pre- and postoperative assessments in 83 patients. *Circulation* 52:88, 1975.

114. Shah PM, Adelman AG, Wigle ED, et al: The natural (and unnatural) history of hypertrophic obstructive cardiomyopathy. *Circ Res* 35(suppl II):II-179, 1974.

115. Wigle ED, Adelman AG, Felderhof CH: Medical and surgical treatment of the cardiomyopathies. *Circ Res* 35(suppl II):II-196, 1974.

116. Maron BJ, Merrill WH, Freier PA, et al: Long-term clinical course and symptomatic status of patients after operation for hypertrophic subaortic stenosis. *Circulation* 57:1205, 1978.

117. Redwood DR, Goldstein RE, Hirshfeld J, et al: Exercise performance after septal myotomy and myectomy in patients with obstructive hypertrophic cardiomyopathy. *Am J Cardiol* 44:215, 1979.

118. Beahrs MM, Tajik AJ, Seward JB, et al: Hypertrophic obstructive cardiomyopathy: Ten- to 21-year follow-up after partial septal myectomy. *Am J Cardiol* 51:1160, 1983.

119. Fananapazir L, Cannon III R, Tripodi D, et al: Impact of dual-chamber permanent pacing in patients with obstructive hypertrophic cardiomyopathy with symptoms refractory to verapamil and β-adrenergic blocker therapy. *Circulation* 85:2149, 1992.

34. Critical Care of Pericardial Disease

David H. Spodick

General Considerations

The pericardium surrounds the heart by a double envelopment of its one-celled mesothelial serous sac (*serosa*), clasped externally by a fibrous coat of varying thickness (*fibrosa*). The portion of the serous sac covering the cardiac surface is the visceral pericardium; the rest of the sac's monolayer, sandwiched with the fibrosa, forms the parietal pericardium. The many functions and physiology of the normal pericardium beyond the scope of this chapter are adequately covered in other reviews [1].

Pericardial diseases cover a very wide etiopathogenetic spectrum, including every kind of medical and surgical disease (condensed in Table 34-1; detailed in reference 2). For a pericardial syndrome to require critical care, it must impose on the patient very unpleasant symptoms, hemodynamic embarrassment, or urgent differential diagnosis from other syndromes. For practical purposes, there are three pericardial conditions to be considered: (1) acute pericarditis with or without pericardial effusion, (2) cardiac tamponade, and (3) constrictive pericarditis, including effusive-constrictive pericarditis.

Acute Pericarditis

Acute pericarditis most often presents as a strictly inflammatory fibrinous lesion without clinically recognizable pericardial fluid. Radiographs and echocardiograms frequently show small or moderate effusions, but most do not progress to significant cardiac compression (tamponade).

ETIOLOGY. A burgeoning list of diseases, syndromes, and agents has been shown to produce pericarditis [2]. The etiology in any given case can be found in nine major categories (see Table 34-1). Category 9 in Table 34-1 includes a vast array of unusual diseases, some fairly reliably associated with a remarkable prevalence of pericarditis, such as thalassemia, the (probably immunopathic) postmyocardial and pericardial injury syndromes, inflammatory bowel disease, and so on.

Etiology is important to critical care in the sense that certain forms (e.g., certain infections and neoplasms) are amenable to

Table 34-1. Major Etiologic Categories of Acute Pericarditis and Myopericarditis Overlapping Pathogenesis

1. Idiopathic pericarditis (syndrome)
2. Pericarditis due to living agents
3. Pericarditis in the vasculitis-connective tissue disease group
4. Immunopathic pericarditis; pericarditis in "hypersensitivity" states
5. Pericarditis in diseases of contiguous structures
6. Pericarditis in disorders of metabolism
7. Neoplastic pericarditis
8. Traumatic pericarditis
9. Pericarditis of uncertain origin or in association with syndromes of uncertain cause

specific therapy. A careful medication history may disclose agents that cause or aggravate pericarditis, such as lupus-producing drugs and anticoagulants. Certain etiologies are also more prone to induce tamponade and various forms of constriction that require critical care.

SYMPTOMS. Acute pericarditis may be asymptomatic, but more often there is central chest pain, usually very sharp and with a pleuritic component and sometimes with only vague precordial distress [3,4]. Precordial distress may closely mimic angina, including a predominant pressure sensation. The onset is frequently perceived as sudden, particularly when it interrupts sleep; the pain is frequently reduced by sitting up. It may radiate in an anginal distribution, remain precordial, or migrate to one side of the chest. A quasi-specific feature is its frequent radiation to the trapezius ridge; pain may also be confined to one or both *trapezius ridges* [3]. (While radiation to the shoulder also is frequent, when the patient describes "shoulder pain" it is important to ask him or her to point to the area, since little else causes trapezius ridge pain.) Patients describe breathing difficulty, but not true dyspnea. The difficulty described tends to be shallow, "splinted" breathing or tachypnea and is due to trying to avoid pain with deeper respiratory movements. If a pleural, bronchial, pulmonary, or cardiac disorder coexists, true dyspnea may precede or accompany the pericardial syndrome. Odynophagia (pain on swallowing) occasionally occurs and can be the only symptom. (It also occurs in esophageal disorders that cause pain resembling that of pericarditis and, in the case of esophageal ulcer, can involve the pericardium [4].) Patients with myopericarditis, notably Coxsackie virus-induced, may also have considerable skeletal muscle pain. Fever varies, depending on etiology. Anorexia and anxiety are common. Etiologic or associated diseases (e.g., acute myocardial infarction, tuberculosis, rheumatic fever) may produce signs that can coexist or even dominate the clinical tableau [4].

SIGNS. The *pericardial rub* (friction sound) is pathognomonic of pericarditis and remains common with pericardial effusions [5]. Rubs are sometimes faint and nearly always wax and wane, even to the point of disappearing and reappearing within the same hour. Yet they are often unmistakable due to their unusual superficiality and peculiar scratchy, grating, creaking, or shuffling character; the most intense rubs produce thrills (very common in uremic pericarditis). Because of their changeable qualities, rubs must be sought diligently from the time pericardial disease is first suspected. A fully developed rub has three components, usually distinguishable by careful auscultation even at rather rapid heart rates: a ventricular systolic rub, preceded by an atrial rub, and followed by an early diastolic rub. The latter follows the second heart sound and is usually the faintest of the three components [5]. Its weakness or absence accounts for the traditional "to-and-fro" description of pericardial friction. At very rapid heart rates the diastolic rub and atrial rub summate, again giving the impression of two components [5]. With pleuropericarditis, a pleuropericardial rub is heard with the pericardial component when the patient holds his or her breath [6].

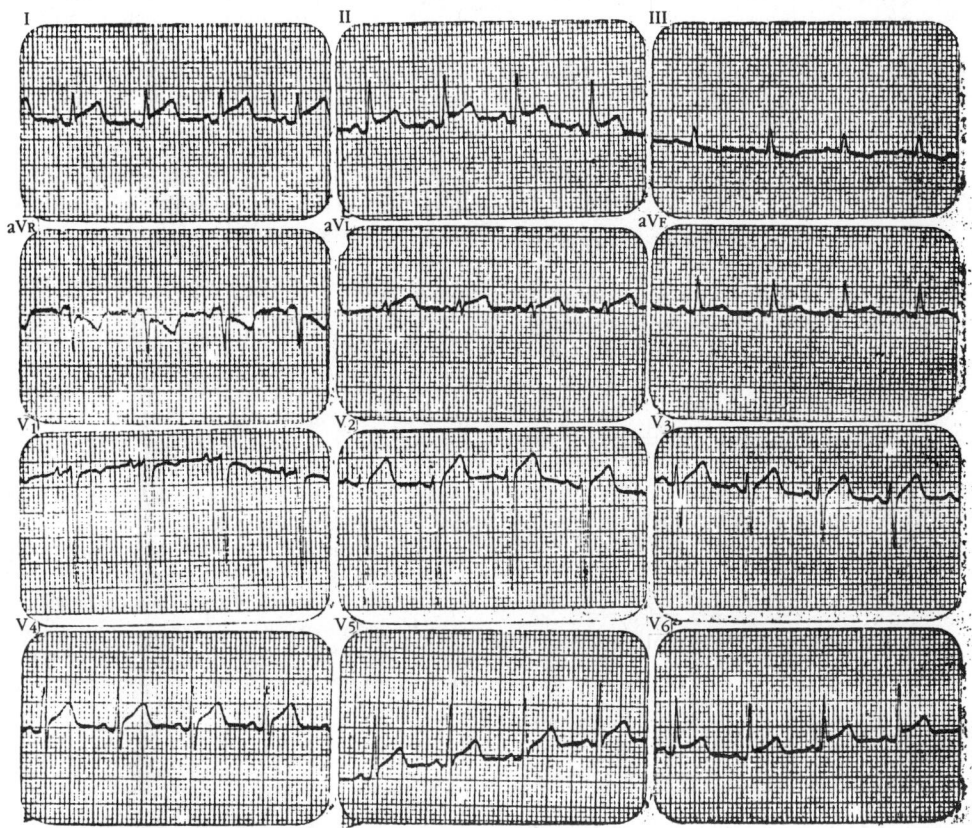

Fig. 34-1. Acute pericarditis. Typical stage I electrocardiogram showing J–ST elevations in most leads (I, II, aVL, aVF, and V₃ to V₆) and J–ST depressions in leads aVR and V₁. P–R segments are depressed below the T–P baseline in leads I, II, aVL, aVF, and V₃ to V₆.

LABORATORY INVESTIGATIONS. Except in the presence of significant accompanying myocarditis or other heart disease, true cardiomegaly does not occur with pure pericarditis. About 250 ml of pericardial fluid is needed to begin to enlarge the roentgenographic cardiac silhouette. The white blood cell count, sedimentation rate, and other acute phase reactants vary according to the etiologic agent or primary illness. Serum levels of cardiac enzymes vary widely from no change to rather major increases.

Electrocardiogram. Electrographic changes (Fig. 34-1) are of three types: typical [7,8], typical variants [9], and atypical (the last including no change) (10). Of four potential ECG stages, an entirely typical stage I ECG is virtually diagnostic. Stage I produces concave S–T elevation in most ECG leads, particularly those of "left ventricular epicardial" deviation (i.e., mainly leads I, II, aVL, aVF, and V₃ to V₆. Lead aVR consistently shows S–T depression. V₁ usually shows S–T depression; less often shows isoelectric S–T; and occasionally shows S–T elevation [8].

During the evolutionary phase (stage II), all S–T junctions return to baseline more or less "in phase," with little change in T waves. In most patients, P–R segments may be depressed in stage I or, more commonly, stage II. Rarely, P–R depression occurs in stage III. The T waves progressively flatten and invert in all or most of the leads that showed S–T elevations [7,8]. Widespread T wave inversions appear in stage III and are not distinguishable from those of diffuse myocardial injury, myocarditis, or "biventricular injury." Indeed, stage III is quite consistent with myocarditis because all ST–T changes are due to involvement of the myocardium immediately underlying the inflamed visceral pericardium. In stage IV, the T waves return to their prepericarditic condition. The entire electrocardiographic evolution occurs in a matter of days or weeks. Usually, transition from stage III and stage IV is relatively slow, while stage II may evolve rapidly. Some patients are left with some degree of T wave inversion for an indefinite period.

TYPICAL ELECTROCARDIOGRAPHIC VARIANTS. Common ECG variants include (1) progression directly from stage I to stage IV (i.e., restitution without going through stages II and III; more frequent in recent years); (2) nonresolution after stage III (no stage IV); (3) depressed S–T junction in lead III in hearts with a horizontal QRS axis; and (4) depressed S–T in lead aVL in hearts with a vertical axis [9]. Depending on the frequency of ECG monitoring, one or another stage may be missed, although a single daily ECG usually registers all. *Yet, appearance of a typical stage I at any time makes the ECG virtually diagnostic of acute pericarditis.*

ATYPICAL ELECTROCARDIOGRAPHIC VARIANTS. Atypical ECGs occur in more than 40 percent of cases of mixed etiologies [10]. These are particularly disturbing when only a few leads are affected, since they may suggest a local rather than general injury, specifically myocardial infarction (by definition a "local" lesion). Yet, unlike infarction, "reciprocal" S–T deviations are quite rare, and their absence should raise the possibility of pericarditis in the appropriate clinical setting. Other atypical variants occur in the presence of other diseases that have already modified the ECG.

An important ECG variant that can be quasi-diagnostic is P–R segment (not P–R interval) depression in the absence of true S–T segment elevation, although this often gives the illusion of S–T elevation. This is sometimes the only sign of pericarditis [10]. It should be emphasized that this highly sensitive sign of unknown specificity may be missed unless it is remembered that the appropriate baseline for the ECG is the succeeding T–P interval (7).

DIAGNOSIS. While pericarditis may be either an "isolated" lesion or part of a more generalized disease or a disorder affecting a neighboring organ (especially the heart or lungs), it must be recognized and differentiated from syndromes causing similar symptoms and signs. Central chest pain should always raise a question of pericarditis, while radiation or referral of pain to the trapezius ridge makes it mandatory to rule pericarditis in or out. Most pericardial rubs are easily distinguished from murmurs because of their apparent superficiality and because rubs are often clearly triphasic. Even biphasic rubs may be distinguished from continuous murmurs. In contrast, monophasic rubs, particularly ventricular systolic rubs, can mimic murmurs of tricuspid regurgitation and ventricular septal defect, principally because all rubs (not only monophasic rubs) tend to be most intense, or heard only at the left mid- to lower sternal border, where they are also most likely to be palpable [5]. Here, the frequent association of a pericarditic syndrome, short-term changeable nature, and unpredictable precordial extent of rubs as well as the frequent absence of associated heart disease are all distinguishing features.

Multiple-observer studies employing blinded auscultation and phonocardiography show generally about 40 percent of rubs to be louder in inspiratory, 15 percent in expiration, and 25 percent of equal intensity of both phases; thus, respiratory behavior of many rubs is not sufficiently specific to help make a differential diagnosis [5].

The electrocardiographic stages are almost always diagnostic when they evolve typically. Typical stage I alone is virtually diagnostic, although it can be confused with early repolarization, a normal ECG variant. The latter does not evolve, although it often occurs in nervous young males—and the pain of acute pericarditis could make anyone nervous—and is corrected by exercise, as is acute pericarditis [11].

Elevation of the J point above the level of the P–R segment is likely to be more than one-fourth the height of the T wave in pericarditis and less than that in early repolarization, but this is not "100 percent specific" [12].

The pain of angina pectoris and myocardial infarction may be like that of acute pericarditis; however, pericarditic pain usually lasts much longer and is usually sharper. Anginal and infarctional pains do not have the pleuritic qualities most common in pericarditis.

The ECG in angina pectoris is nearly always marked by depressed, rather than elevated, S–T segments, except for variant (Prinzmetal) angina, yet an atypical ECG evolution in acute pericarditis may be confused with the latter in as many as one-third of patients [10]. P–R segment depressions in such cases favor pericarditis.

Without associated or preexisting coronary disease, Q waves do not occur in pericarditis (save for some cases associated with myocarditis) [8]. However, if a patient with pericarditis first presents with stage III changes (all T waves inverted), a primarily myocardial versus pericardial disorder must be distinguished on clinical grounds.

MANAGEMENT. The treatment of clinically noneffusive pericarditis or pericarditis without overtly compressing effusion is symptomatic (i.e., aimed at pain, malaise, and fever). In my experience, the optimal treatment is to begin with ibuprofen (Motrin) 600 mg every 6 hours, which often relieves pain within 15 minutes to 2 hours. Depending on patient tolerance and therapeutic response, the individual dose can be reduced to 400 mg or raised to 800 mg or greater with continued observation for side effects. Should this fail, aspirin up to 900 mg four times per day may be given. Indomethacin may be used, always given on a full stomach and in divided doses from 100 to 200 mg per day, beginning with 25 mg every 6 hours. In patients with myocardial infarction ("epistenocardiac") pericarditis, indomethacin perhaps should not be used because of experimental work showing that it reduces coronary flow, increases experimental infarction, and increases blood pressure.

Intractably symptomatic pericarditis occasionally calls for alternative, even more drastic, treatment, such as phenylbutazone over 2 or 3 days or even azathioprine (Imuran), beginning with very small doses and with constant vigilance for side effects. Corticosteroid therapy may be employed at the lowest effective dose with appropriate tapering but should be avoided if at all possible because patients may become addicted, with consequent extreme difficulty in weaning. Although pericardiectomy may be resorted to in extreme cases of treatment failure, it may not be successful in relieving pain and must be considered as a last-ditch measure. Any known etiologic disease process or agent should be treated specifically when specific treatment (e.g., appropriate antibiotics) is available.

Noncompressing ("Lax") Pericardial Effusion

Most cases of acute pericarditis without tamponade probably involve some excess fluid due to intrapericardial exudation, with those amounting to 250 ml or more becoming clinically obvious either on physical examination or (more likely) chest radiograph. Yet even rather large effusions may not clinically embarrass the heart as long as the rate of exudation is slow enough to permit the pericardium to stretch. (Studies of systolic time intervals show that even small lax effusions, without any significant blood pressure drop during inspiration, are not physiologically inert, although they have no apparent clinical significance [3].

The configuration of the cardiac silhouette cannot be used to distinguish between cardiomegaly, large pericardial cysts, and pericardial effusions; this must be done by contrast radiography, radioisotope scanning, computed tomography, or, perhaps optimally, echocardiography. Lacking these, a "water bottle" silhouette or unusually wide mediastinal shadow is highly suggestive, particularly when lung fields are not congested. The appearance of a unilateral left pleural effusion in addition to these findings points also to pericardial disease without being specific [4]. Well-penetrated lateral films may show *pericardial fat lines* well within the cardiopericardial outline [3].

Noncompressing effusions may produce no clinical manifestations and may be the only sign of pericardial disease, so that any symptoms or signs are those of pericarditis itself, either occurring with or preceding the effusion. If a systemic or extrapericardial disease is responsible for the pericarditis, signs and symptoms of that condition may dominate the picture. Very large, though noncompressing, effusions may produce precordial discomfort and symptoms due to pressure on adjacent structures, such as dyspnea (from reduced lung capacity), cough, hoarseness, dysphagia, and hiccoughs. Heart sounds may be reduced with massive effusions, and percussion of the precordium may give a dull (classically, "flat") note.

In up to 70 percent of patients in whom pericardial fluid is an inflammatory exudate, a pericardial rub is audible. With very large effusions, the Bamberger-Pins-Ewart sign—dullness and bronchial breathing between the tip of the left (rarely the right) scapula and the vertebral column—is common [4].

LABORATORY INVESTIGATIONS. Radiography shows an increased cardiac silhouette and, in the absence of cardiac and pulmonary disease, clear lung fields, and often left pleural effusion [13]. The ECG may show low-voltage QRS and T waves (nearly always with normal P wave voltage). Low voltage is nonspecific and not very sensitive.

Echocardiograms at first show small amounts of fluid posteriorly at the left ventricular level in systole only (Table 34-2). Progressive accumulation extends the posterior fluid into both systole and diastole; with larger effusions, fluid appears anteriorly [3]. Occasionally, fluid can be found behind the left atrium (i.e., in the oblique sinus of the pericardium), exposing the atrial contraction pattern, but only with rather large effusions. Tumors can simulate this finding. It is important to adjust echo gain, reject, and damping controls and, with M-mode echo, to scan extensively.

Anterior pericardial fluid tends to reveal brisk pulsations of the right ventricular wall. Large amounts of posterior fluid are associated with decreased amplitude of movement in the parietal pericardium-lung interface. Only occasionally, with large posterior effusions, is anterior fluid absent, usually due to anterior adhesions (especially after cardiac surgery). When fluid appears to be only anterior, it is possible that posterior adhesions may be present, yet an anterior echo-free space alone should not be considered pericardial effusion unless this is demonstrated. Epicardial fat, pericardial cysts, and tumors can simulate anterior pericardial fluid. If echocardiograms are technically poor or equivocal in the face of strong evidence of effusion, computed tomography or a right atriogram can be done to show a wide band between that structure and the lung.

With echocardiography, the heart may be seen to "swing" within the pericardium in large effusions; that is, the left ventricular posterior wall echo and right ventricular anterior wall echo seem to move synchronously along with the intervening structures (Fig. 34-2). Swinging movements are distinct from contraction and relaxation. Occasionally (and usually with some degree of cardiac tamponade), the swinging reverses direction on alternate beats instead of every beat. Often, some degree of swinging produces pseudoprolapse of the mitral and tricuspid valves. (At heart rates >120 beats/min pansystolic "prolapse" may be present, whereas at <120 beats/min there is early or late prolapse.)

Swinging on alternate beats may also produce electric alternation, owing to repetitive change of the heart position with respect to the fixed positions of the ECG electrodes. This is a helpful ancillary diagnostic sign when there is clinical cardiac tamponade (pathognomonic when P waves, as well as QRS and T, alternate). Rarely, swinging also produces a small mechanical pulsus alternans.

With any amount of pericardial fluid (with or without cardiac tamponade) systolic time intervals show remarkably exaggerated respiratory changes—much greater than normal prolongation of the preejection period and shortening of the ejection time during inspiration (14).

Patients with noncompressing pericardial effusions may not need critical care, although removal of fluid for diagnostic purposes may sometimes be required to be rule out or in specific etiologies. Therapeutic agents used for clinically "dry" pericarditis sometimes help resolve noncompressing effusions.

Table 34-2. Echocardiogram in Pericardial Effusion and Cardiac Tamponade[a]

I. Pericardial effusion: M-mode and 2-D
  A. Echo-free space
    1. Posterior to LV (small to moderate effusions)
    2. Posterior and anterior (moderate to large effusions)
    3. Behind left atrium in some large to very large effusions
  B. Decreased movement of posterior pericardium-lung interface
  C. RV pulsations brisk (with anterior fluid)
  D. Aortic root movement abnormal or attenuated
  E. "Swinging heart" (large effusions)
    1. Periodicity 1:1 or 2:1 (rarely 3:1)
    2. RV and LV walls move synchronously
    3. Mitral-tricuspid pseudoprolapse (pansystolic at HR>120 beats/min)
  F. 2-D only
    1. Loculated fluid
    2. Adhesions (fibrinous and fibrous)
II. Cardiac tamponade: M-mode and 2-D
  Evidence of effusion plus
  A. Cardiac compression
    1. Decreased total transverse dimension (RV epicardium to LV epicardium at end diastole: may be apparent only after tap)
    2. RV diameters decreased (may be apparent only after tap), unless previous RV enlargement
    3. Early diastolic collapse of RV outflow tract with continued diastolic inward wall motion (≥50 msec after mitral D point)
  B. Inspiratory effects (with pulsus paradoxus)
    1. RV expands from greatly reduced expiratory end-diastolic size
    2. IV septum shifts to left
    3. LV compressed
    4. Mitral excursion-D/E amplitude and open valve area decreased
      a. E/F slope decreased or rounded
      b. Open time[b] decreased
    5. Aortic valve[b] opening decreased; premature closure
    6. Reduced increase in inferior vena cava diameter (<25%)
    7. Echocardiographic stroke volume decreased
    8. Decreased fractional shortening (short axis)
    9. Doppler: Right-sided transvalvular flows greatly exaggerated; left-sided flows greatly reduced (reversed during expiration)
  C. Notch in RV epicardium during isovolumic contraction (M-mode)
  D. Coarse oscillations of LV posterior wall (2-D echocardiography only)
  E. RA free wall indentation (buckling) during late diastole or isovolumic contraction
  F. RV indentation (buckling) during early diastole
  G. LA free wall indentation (cases with fluid behind LA)
  H. SVC and IVC dilation (unless volume depletion) and relatively fixed diameter during respiration
  I. Presystolic reflux or contrast media into IVC

[a] Sensitivities and specificities vary for each item.
[b] Often difficult to define during pericardial effusion; mitral valve may open with atrial systole only during inspiration.
IV = interventricular; IVC = inferior vena cava; LA = left atrium; LV = left ventricle; RA = right atrium; RV = right ventricle; SVC = superior vena cava; 2-D = two dimensional.

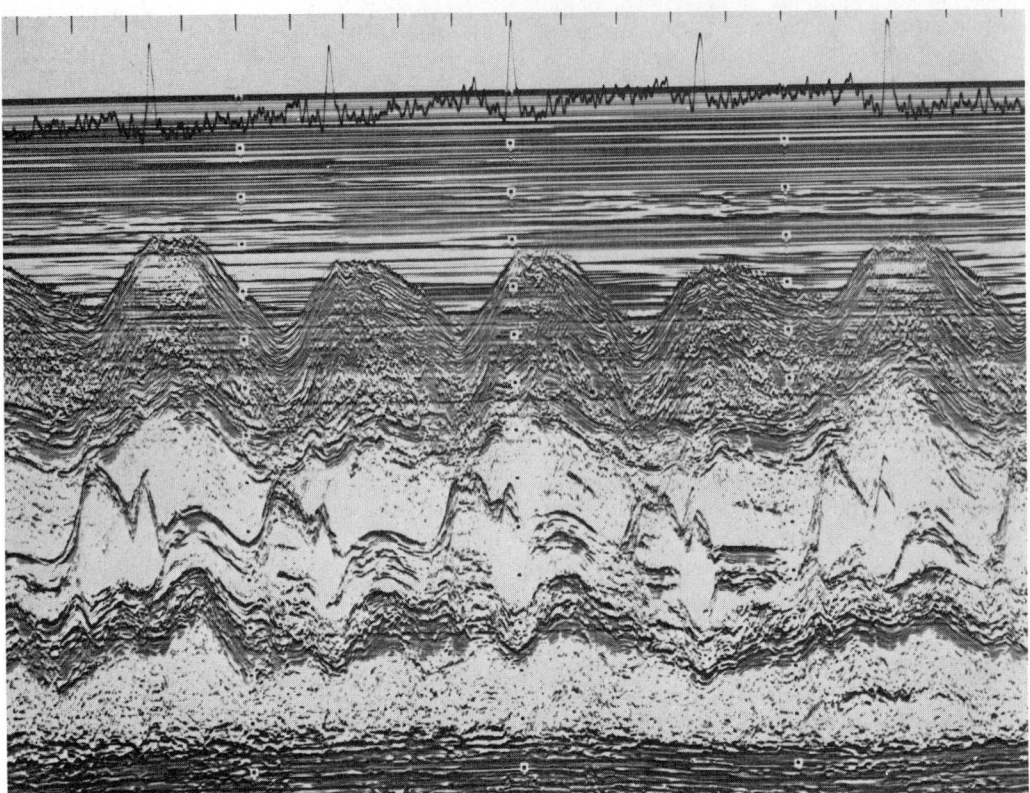

Fig. 34-2. Pericardial effusion with cardiac tamponade. M-mode echocardiogram and electrocardiogram showing features of tamponade. Pericardial fluid is seen anterior and posterior to the left ventricle. 2:1 "swinging" of the heart is seen best in the anterior right ventricular echo with larger excursions on alternate beats, producing in the electrocardiogram (*top*) electric alternation. The right ventricle is greatly compressed. There is pseudoprolapse of the mitral valve, confined to late systole because of the only mildly accelerated heart rate (90 beats/min).

Although computed tomographic scans and magnetic resonance images are more sensitive and specific, echocardiography is the mainstay for diagnosis of pericardial effusion. Echocardiography can be done more rapidly (including portable bedside studies) and provides "instant" functional data.

Cardiac Tamponade

Cardiac tamponade is defined as hemodynamically significant cardiac compression due to accumulated pericardial contents that evoke and defeat compensatory mechanisms (Fig. 34-3) [1]. A relatively wide range of severity of cardiac compression may be encountered. The pericardial contents may be effusion fluid, blood, pus, or gas (including air), singly or in combinations, occasionally with underlying constrictive epicarditis. Tamponade must be considered in any patient with cardiogenic shock and systemic congestion.

PHYSIOLOGY. For significant cardiac compression, the pericardial contents must increase at a rate exceeding the rate of stretch of the parietal pericardium and, to some degree, the rate at which venous blood volume expands to maintain the small filling gradient to the right heart [1]. In uncomplicated tamponade, central venous pressure rises in parallel with intrapericardial pressures to 12 to 25 mm Hg; mean atrial and ventricular diastolic pressures equilibrate within 4 mm Hg of this level. In exceptional cases, these pressures may exceed 30 mm Hg; in "low-pressure tamponade" (see below) they may be less than 10 mm Hg.

Relentlessly increasing intrapericardial pressure progressively reduces ventricular volume, producing rising diastolic pressures that resist filling to the point that even a normal ejection fraction cannot avert critical reduction of stroke volume at any heart rate. Both ventricles fill against a common stiffness (pericardium plus fluid), evoking corresponding increases in left and right atrial pressures. Cardiac transmural pressures are progressively reduced by rising intrapericardial pressure and in extreme tamponade may become negative so that the ventricles probably fill by diastolic suction and during atrial contraction [1]. Transmural pressure equals cavity pressure minus pericardial pressure; therefore, normally negative pericardial pressure sums with cavity pressure (minus minus = plus), whereas positive (i.e., tamponading) pericardial pressure reduces transmural pressure (minus plus = minus) [1]. (Transmural pressure is a true "filling pressure," although net chamber distending forces must represent total distending minus total compressing forces.)

The course of ventricular filling is incompletely understood, but it is slow, and ultimately the ventricles may fill only during atrial systole (particularly at rapid heart rates). Pericardial pressure quickly exceeds early diastolic pressure in the atria and right ventricle and rises further during ventricular diastolic expansion with transient early diastolic right ventricular collapse, so that atrial emptying is impeded; moreover, the thin right atrium, exposed to pericardial pressure, collapses in diastole,

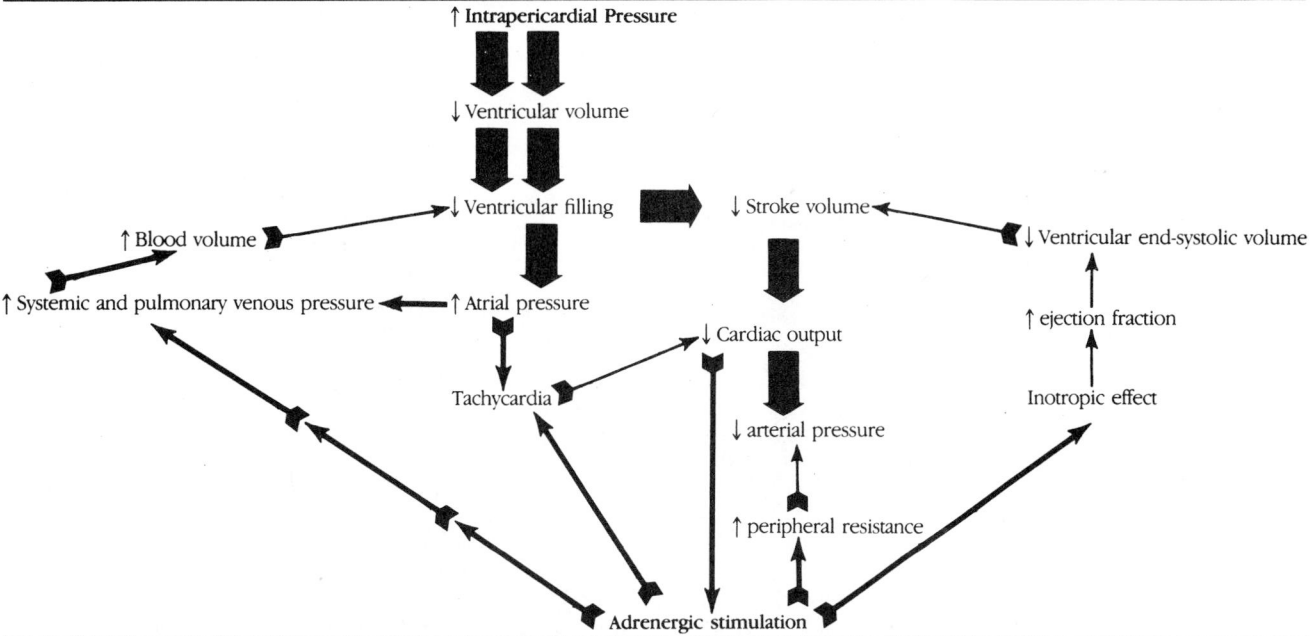

Fig. 34-3. Cardiac tamponade (*heavy arrows without tails*) and compensatory mechanisms (*arrows with tails*). Thin tailed arrows represent immediate mechanisms directed against tamponade changes; intermediate mechanisms are represented by heavier tailed arrows. For example, decreased ventricular filling due to decreased ventricular volume is immediately supported by increased blood volume. Development of the latter is stimulated by the intermediate mechanism, increased venous pressures (see text).

both phenomena leading to amputation of the normal y descent. The x descent remains, owing to active movement of the atrial "floor" toward the ventricular apices during ventricular ejection. Characteristic pressure curves in cardiac tamponade thus show absence or amputation of the atrial y descent and rising ventricular diastolic pressures with a high end-diastolic pressure.

Considering the diastolic pressure "clamp" on the myocardium, disturbances of coronary flow are not surprising. Whether significant ischemia occurs is unknown, except in severe experimental tamponade, which produces subendocardial hypoperfusion and hemorrhage [15]. With less severe tamponade, decreased flow tends to remain proportional to the reduced work of the heart [1].

Elevated end-diastolic pressure is reflected in atrial mean pressure elevation and systemic and pulmonary venous hypertension. As long as venous pressure is maintained sufficiently to support atrial pressures, ventricular inflow can be maintained. Due mainly to reduced filling, ventricular systolic pressure ultimately falls, along with stroke volume, so that cardiac output is principally maintained by tachycardia [3].

COMPENSATION. Beyond pericardial stretch, compensatory mechanisms for tamponade are mainly adrenergically mediated, including tachycardia, peripheral vasoconstriction, and maintained ejection fraction (in pure tamponade without heart disease, the ejection fraction is normal or increased) [1]. The success of compensation is reflected clinically in reasonably good and occasionally even elevated systemic systolic and pulse pressures, until a life-and-death crisis is precipitated by

relentlessly increasing pericardial contents. Except in rapid traumatic tamponade, increased blood volume helps maintain cardiac output and systemic blood pressure. Compensation involves a complex set of interactions, condensed in Figure 34-3. The myocardium itself is also important, so that an additionally diseased or injured heart may not maintain circulatory pressures as well as a normal heart.

PULSUS PARADOXUS. Excessive fluid in the pericardium increases the normal pericardial effect on ventricular interaction and exaggerates the normal inspiratory decrease in systemic blood pressure, thus leading to pulsus paradoxus. The latter is always the net effect of several mechanisms of individually varying contribution in any given case. The appearance in the systemic circulation of clinically measurable pulsus paradoxus (a systolic pressure drop ≥ 10 mm Hg) depends primarily on an increase in right heart filling (as in normal circumstances) during inspiration, which produces a further increase in pericardial pressure, i.e., exaggerating the effects of tamponade during inspiration [16]. The complex chain of events is summarized in Figure 34-4. Although pulsus paradoxus is the hallmark of tamponade, at the bedside it must be borne in mind that pulsus is common to other disorders: obstructive lung disease (including severe asthma), pulmonary embolism, tense ascites, obesity, mitral stenosis with right heart failure, right ventricular infarction, and hypovolemic and cardiogenic shock. In occasional cases of restrictive cardiomyopathy and constrictive pericarditis with some pericardial effusion, a relatively small pulsus may be present as well.

CLINICAL MANIFESTATIONS. Tamponade may appear insidiously as the first sign of pericardial injury or intrapericardial bleeding, especially in conditions such as neoplasia, trauma, and connective tissue disorders. Commonly, however, it follows clinical acute pericarditis. The symptoms of tamponade are not specific, and patients may have symptoms and signs of

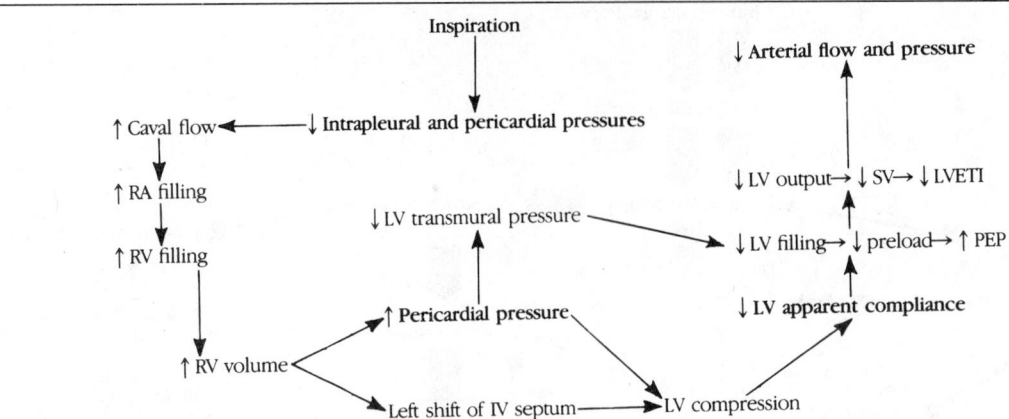

Fig. 34-4. Mechanisms of pulsus paradoxus. RA = right atrial; RV = right ventricular; LV = left ventricular; IV = interventricular; SV = stroke volume; PEP = preejection period.

an associated disease. Usually they progressively feel "sicker" and with advanced cardiac compression have pallor, tachycardia, cyanosis, impaired cerebral function, sweating, and cold acral points. Most patients (clearly not all until quite late) are relatively or absolutely hypotensive. The clinical tableau tends to resemble congestive heart failure. The lungs, however, are nearly always clear, possibly because despite high left heart filling pressures, the right ventricle cannot receive and eject enough blood to cause pulmonary engorgement or edema, but this remains speculative. Since atrial natriuretic factor increases only after relief of tamponade (and constriction), it may be a "permissive" factor when it rises in myocardial failure.

In patients with rapid tamponade due to hemorrhage, as in wounds and cardiac or aortic rupture, the dominant picture is one of shock. If unchecked, shock leads to electromechanical dissociation. Lack of time for blood volume expansion often permits tamponade to occur with relatively low central venous pressures, without jugular distention (although jugular pulsations may be seen) [4].

Hemothorax, rather than hemopericardium, is more common with wounds of the left atrium because of the special clasp of its overlying pericardium and because high-velocity cardiac wounds produce large pericardial lacerations through which blood can exit [4]. In traumatized patients, it is well to remember that multiple wounds may be present and that abdominal wounds often penetrate the thorax.

PHYSICAL EXAMINATION. When tamponade is due to inflammatory or neoplastic lesions, pericardial rubs frequently are present and can be quite loud, although the heart sounds themselves may be distant due to insulation by the surrounding fluid and feeble heart action. Heart sounds are usually better heard over the base of the heart, sometimes with relative accentuation of the pulmonic second sound (P_2). The precordium may be quiet and the apex beat not palpable, but there are many exceptions in which sounds and apex beat seem normal. Neck veins are usually engorged, even with the patient at 90 degrees, and sometimes there are prominent forehead, scalp, and retinal veins. If the venous level can be accurately discerned, the single negative systolic phase in midsystole (x trough) is a valuable finding that may be timed while listening to the heart sounds as one watches a rapid inward darting of the neck veins between S_1 and S_2. Neck veins should also show normal reduction in size during inspiration. Kussmaul's sign (inspiratory expan-

sion of neck veins) is evidence *against* uncomplicated cardiac tamponade; thus, if there is fluid, even under pressure, Kussmaul's sign should be absent unless there is epicardial constrictive pericarditis as well as fluid. The possibility of the latter should also be suspected if a third heart sound is found before or after drainage. Like Kussmaul's sign, a third heart sound in adults virtually rules out uncomplicated cardiac tamponade. Kussmaul's sign is always difficult to authenticate, even with constriction.

Clinically significant tamponade without extreme hypotension usually yields a palpable pulsus paradoxus at any available artery. This should be quantitated by sphygmomanometer; if the systolic pressure equals or exceeds 100 mm Hg, a clinically significant inspiratory drop should exceed 10 mm Hg. With lower systolic pressures a small pulsus can be considered significant as long as it occupies over half the pulse pressure. (During hypotensive and shocklike states, intraarterial measurements generally give higher values for blood pressure than a cuff.) Serial sphygmomanometer measurements of pulsus can be used for noninvasive monitoring of the progress of tamponade and its management.

Absence of Pulsus Paradoxus. Pulsus occurs when both ventricles are filling against a common pericardial stiffness and respiratory changes alternately favor right and left heart filling [1]. It is absent or minimal with any significant degree of constriction. On the other hand, advanced left ventricular hypertrophy or severe left heart failure (i.e., greatly reduced left ventricular chamber compliance) complicating tamponade may maintain left-sided filling pressures well above right ventricular and pericardial pressures (and may produce an S_3).

Here, pericardial pressure matches only right ventricular filling pressure, because both are determined by compliance of the tense pericardial sac, while filling pressure in the left ventricle is determined by its greatly reduced compliance, so that pulsus paradoxus will not be present in systemic arteries.

In atrial septal defect, pulsus paradoxus is absent because increased systemic venous return is balanced by shunting to the left atrium. Left ventricular filling during severe aortic regurgitation can damp respiratory fluctuations and eliminate pulsus. Finally, severe tamponade with extreme hypotension may not show measurable respiratory changes. Right heart tamponade also nullifies pulsus paradoxus, often due to loculated pericardial fluid after cardiac surgery. In some patients, low-pressure tamponade associated with hypovolemia produces only slight elevation of right-sided pressures. Further reduction in blood volume can precipitate florid tamponade.

GRAPHIC FINDINGS. Echocardiographic and radiographic signs of tamponade (see Fig. 34-2) are basically the same as for noncompressing pericardial effusion with certain physiologic changes superimposed. Ultrasound and Doppler findings are summarized in Table 34-2.

With strong clinical evidence for tamponade, an equivocal or technically poor echocardiogram, or uncertainty as to the type of pericardial disease, a right atriogram may be performed through a flow-directed catheter (which can monitor pressures). It clearly shows the right atrial border to be straight in mild tamponade and buckled, especially at end-atrial systole, along with dilation of the superior vena cava and compression (tapering and/or abrupt narrowing) of its intrapericardial segments. Cardioangiography also shows small atria and ventricles, increased transcardiac circulation time, increased distance between right atrium and lung, and inferior vena cava reflux. Some or all of these, however, can also be seen in constrictive pericarditis and restrictive cardiomyopathies.

The ECG usually is not specific, although S–T and P–R deviations may persist. Frequently, there is some decrease in voltage of the QRS and T waves (the P wave nearly always being spared), reflecting not only insulation by fluid but also the effects of cardiac compression [17]. Low voltage is not a reliable finding. Electric alternation is strong evidence of some degree of tamponade and is virtually pathognomonic when it affects the P waves as well as QRS–T (simultaneous alternation) [18]. Systolic time intervals show exaggeration of respiratory changes [3] (much as in lax pericardial effusion) [13].

SUSPECTED TAMPONADE. Effusions with elevated venous pressure with or without hypotension or pulsus paradoxus that do not resolve rapidly should be drained and the effects on heart rate and arterial and venous pressures observed. When the diagnosis of tamponade cannot be made noninvasively, right cardiac catheterization should be performed; if necessary, angiography of the right atrium or superior vena cava should be performed (see above).

CRITICAL CARE. Removal of pericardial fluid as soon as possible by paracentesis or surgical drainage is the definitive treatment, indeed the only rational treatment. Surgical drainage is favored for either traumatic tamponade or tamponade due to pericarditis caused by pyogenic organisms. Otherwise, needle aspiration can be used with the introduction of a pericardial catheter with minimal trauma to permit optimal drainage and protection against refilling. The pericardium can be tapped from almost any reasonable place on the chest wall, and it is desirable to use two-dimensional echocardiography as a guide. The subxiphoid approach is preferred for the usual blind pericardiocentesis. A complete description of pericardiocentesis appears in Chapter 8. The optimal and safest approach is through a thoracoscope inserted in the subxiphoid zone.

Failure of paracentesis to deliver fluid does not rule out pericardial effusion or hemorrhage. When brisk intrapericardial bleeding overwhelms fibrinolytic activity of the pericardium and the defibrinating effect of cardiac movement, the resulting intrapericardial clot cannot be aspirated and can seriously compress the heart. In this circumstance, rebleeding along with the clot produces especially severe tamponade. If diagnostic suspicion is strong and aspiration is unsuccessful, surgical intervention becomes mandatory. Subxiphoid surgical drainage can be performed, with the following advantages: (1) it is extrapleural and extraperitoneal; (2) it permits digital exploration of the pericardium; (3) it permits visual inspection with an endoscope; (4) a generous biopsy can be resected; and (5) it permits a "window" into the adjacent pleural cavity [19,20]. The subxi-

poid approach may be technically difficult in obese patients and in those with a very narrow costal arch. Recently, balloon catheter pericardiostomy by experienced operators has been successful both for external drainage and to create a pericardiopleural "window."

The physiology of tamponade (Fig. 34-3) provides a theoretic basis for medical management: attacks on key points in the tamponade sequence, support for the compensation sequence, or both. These methods include (1) inotropic agents that increase stroke volume or support systemic resistance or both, (2) blood volume expansion to maintain the venoatrial gradients, (3) afterload-reducing agents in patients with adequate blood pressure, and (4) combined therapy (e.g., afterload reduction plus blood volume expansion). Despite the success of these agents in experimental tamponade, some clinical trials demonstrate disappointing results in patients who are not hypovolemic [21].

Anticoagulant therapy should be withheld or discontinued. This consideration becomes especially important in ruling in or out pulmonary embolism, which can produce chest pain, high central venous pressure, and pulsus paradoxus. Finally, positive-pressure ventilation should be avoided, as it tends to reduce cardiac output in tamponade.

Pericarditis versus Myocardial Infarction

Special consideration must be given to differentiating acute pericarditis, with or without effusion or tamponade, from both acute myocardial infarction and acute pericarditis in the setting of (and presumably due to) myocardial infarction. Because pericarditic pain may occasionally masquerade as ischemic pain, it sometimes becomes critical, particularly in older patients, to distinguish between the two. This is also the case when the ECG either is nonspecific or evolves in an atypical manner [10]. Although the clinical course ultimately settles most diagnoses, at onset it is crucial to narrow the odds. The differentiation is most critical because thrombolytic therapy for coronary thrombosis is a cause of hemotamponade in some patients with pericarditis. An outline of the differential diagnosis is given in Table 34-3.

Myocardial infarction produces two forms of pericarditis: a common one in which pericardial involvement results directly from myocardial injury ("epistenocardiac" pericarditis) and the relatively uncommon post-myocardial infarction syndrome, an indirect, probably immunopathic result of infarction. The latter can appear from the first few days to several weeks or even longer after myocardial infarction, may be associated with arthralgias, pleuritis, and pneumonitis, and has a tendency to recur. The former appears on the second to fifth day after clinical onset in up to 20 percent of cases and is the form most likely to be met in the critical care setting. (At postmortem, epistenocardiac pericarditis is associated only with anatomically transmural infarctions, occurring in almost 40% of these [22]. This form of pericarditis may be heralded by new and severe pain, different from and often worse than that of the infarct—the pain is often specifically pleuritic and frequently involves the trapezius ridge—with secondary fever rise and only rarely with general S–T junction elevation on the ECG (Figs. 34-5A and 34-5B). In most cases there are no reciprocal S–T deviations—indeed, the original S–T depressions reciprocal to the infarct are often obliterated or converted to S–T elevations by the generalized pericarditis—while infarct T wave inversions per se may be reversed or may remain. As a rule, however, the ECG does not

Table 34-3. Differential Diagnosis of Acute Pericarditis

Finding	Acute pericarditis	Acute ischemia
Pain		
Onset	More often sudden	Usually gradual, crescendo
Main location	Substernal or left precordial	Same or confined to zones of radiation
Radiation	May be same as ischemic, also trapezius ridge(s)	Shoulders, arms, neck back; not trapezius ridge(s)
Quality	Usually sharp; stabbing, "background" ache	Usually "heavy" or "burning"
Inspiration	Worse	No effect unless with infarct in pericarditis
Duration	Persistent; may wax and wane	Usually intermittent
Electrocardiogram		
J–ST	Diffuse elevation usually concave, without reciprocal depressions	Localized deviation usually convex (with reciprocal infarction)
P–R segment depressions	Frequent	Almost never
Abnormal Q waves	None unless with infarction	Common with infarction ("Q wave" infarcts)
T waves	Inverted after J points return to baseline	Inverted while S–T still elevated (infarct)
Myocardial enzymes	Normal or elevated	Elevated (infarct)
Pericardial friction	Rub (most cases)	Rub only if with pericarditis
Abnormal S_3	Absent unless preexisting	May be present
Abnormal S_4	Absent unless preexisting	Nearly always present
S_1	Intact	Often dull, mushy after first day
Pulmonary congestion	Absent	May be present
Arrhythmia	None (in absence of heart disease)	Frequent
Conduction abnormalities (A-V and IV)	None (in absence of heart disease)	Frequent

AP = angina pectoris; MI = myocardial infarction; IV = interventricular; A-V = atrioventricular.

change sufficiently and a pericardial rub is needed for diagnosis. Yet, the condition is well tolerated by most patients and can be handled with the addition of 1 to 3 days of pain-relieving and antiinflammatory agents on the schedule previously noted. These may resolve the pain in as little as 20 minutes. Rarely, tamponade develops, precipitating a crisis that may resemble congestive heart failure, shock, right ventricular infarction, or acute cor pulmonale and requiring rapid drainage. The intrapericardial effect of anticoagulants remains controversial, but it is prudent to withhold them in most cases of pericarditis complicating myocardial infarction. On the other hand, thrombolytics have definitely caused pericardial hemorrhage in a few (strangely not all) patients with pericarditis.

Constrictive Pericarditis

Constrictive pericarditis is seen less in its traditional chronic form and more in subacute and acute forms, following relatively soon after a detectable bout of acute pericarditis with or without effusion. The etiologies are essentially the same as for acute pericarditis (Table 34-1), although acute rheumatic fever with pericarditis, even when severe, does not produce constriction. Certain etiologic factors, however, are especially likely to lead to constriction, sometimes without evidence of antecedent acute pericarditis. These include tuberculosis, therapeutic irradiation of the chest, trauma, and a "new" form during uremia under dialysis [1]. Purified protein derivative (tuberculin) (PPD) skin tests are nearly always positive in cases with tuberculosis but may be falsely negative in constriction with protein-losing enteropathy due to high venous pressure that results in intestinal loss of lymphocytes.

Like tamponade, constriction severely limits ventricular filling, with equalization of left and right heart filling pressures. Systolic right ventricular pressure rises, but usually to less than 50 mm Hg, and the right ventricular end-diastolic pressure to systolic pressure ratio is usually greater than 0.3. Unlike the situation with tamponade, the heart is encased in a quasi-yield-

ing shell that does not transmit fluctuating pleural pressure. Consequently, respiratory changes in cardiac pressures are minimal and jugular venous pressure increases during inspiration (Kussmaul's sign; also seen in right ventricular infarction, acute cor pulmonale, and tricuspid stenosis). Inspiratory decrease in arterial pressure in pure constriction is slight, nearly always less than 10 mm Hg. The exception is constriction with additional pericardial fluid that is itself under pressure.

Many early reports that alleged pulsus paradoxus to be present in constriction did not exclude concomitant tamponade or pleuropulmonary disease that could produce pulsus. True pulsus paradoxus ($\geq$ 10 mm Hg) during constrictive pericarditis thus implies the diagnosis of effusive-constrictive disease or some other causative factor.

Unlike cardiac tamponade, the heart is not compressed in early diastole and relaxes normally or quite abruptly (rubber bulb effect) as filling proceeds until it reaches its pericardial limit. There is, therefore, a "square root" configuration to the diastolic pressure (not seen in tamponade, particularly when measured by manometer tip catheters). Early diastolic pressure drops to, or near, 0 mm Hg, unless there is concomitant myocardial disease, and then rises rapidly to its plateau, the point at which the constricting scar stops it. Unlike the situation in tamponade, venous and atrial pressures show prominent y as well as x troughs. The y descent tends to be deeper and quite precipitous as it corresponds to the ventricular pressure dip when the atrioventricular valves are open (Fig. 34-6). This brief filling period begins with torrential early diastolic ventricular filling and ends abruptly as the ventricles reach their constricted limit. At this point there is usually an intense third heart sound (S_3). A few patients with some "give" in the constricting tissue retain the end-diastolic "atrial kick" in ventricular pressure with a corresponding fourth heart sound (S_4) [6]. An S_4 may also occur in an ill-defined group with "elastic constriction," in whom there may be enough give in the constricting tissue to extend early ventricular filling and minimize or make undetectable the S_3. In the absence of myocardial disease, inotropic function of the heart is well preserved.

The clinical picture of constrictive pericarditis depends on the tempo of onset. A history of acute pericarditis is frequent

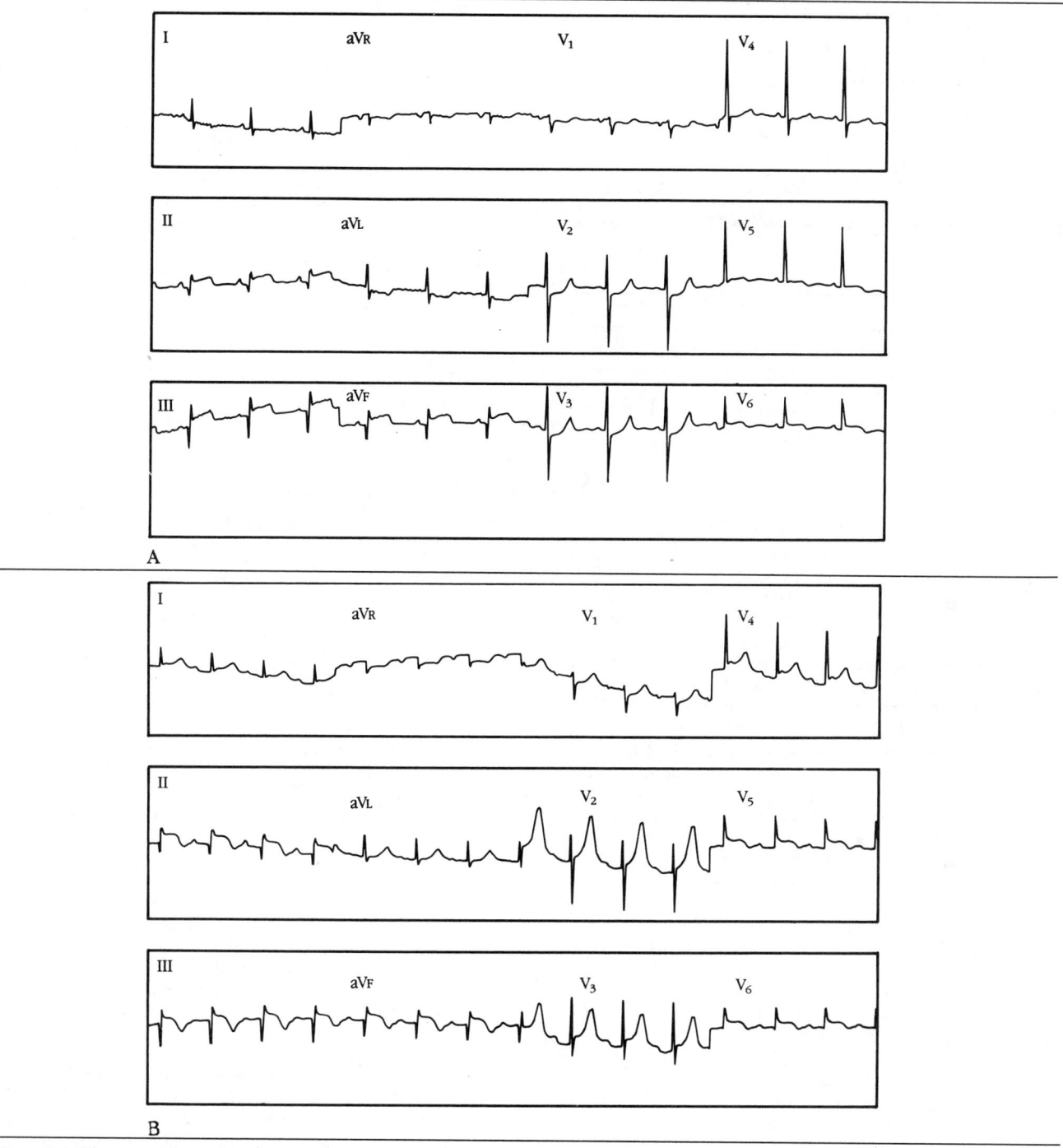

Fig. 34-5. A. Acute inferolateral myocardial infarction. Note the associated S–T depressions in leads V_1 to V_3 and reciprocal J–ST depression in lead aVL. B. Acute "epistenocardiac" pericarditis during acute infarction (same patient as shown in A). J points are elevated in leads I, II, III, aVF, and V_2 to V_6. J–ST depressions occur in leads aVR and V_1. Formerly inverted T waves in leads I and aVL are now upright, although evolutionary T wave inversions proceed in II, III, aVF, V_5, and V_6 (compare with A). The P–R interval is 0.24 seconds and due primarily to consequences of inferior infarction.

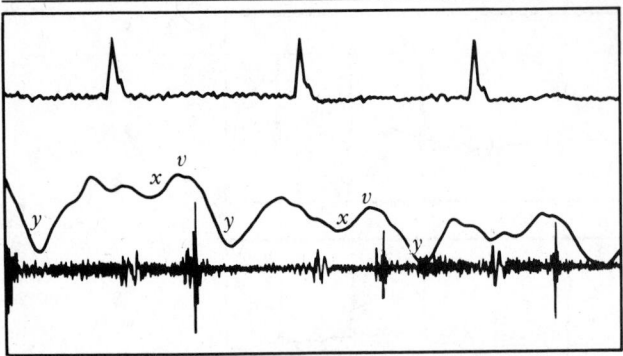

Fig. 34-6. Constrictive pericarditis. Jugular venous pulse tracing taken 2.5 months after successful coronary bypass surgery. The patient developed systemic congestion and distention of neck veins with prominent *x* and *y* descents. The *x* trough falls between the first and second heart sounds, and the *y* trough follows the second heart sound on the phonocardiogram.

Table 34-4. Echocardiography of Pericardial Scarring and Constriction

A. Pericardial thickening
   1. Condensed parietal pericardial echo
   2. Doubled parietal pericardial echo
B. Adhesions (fibrous or fibrinous)
   1. Adhesive strands seen (2-D) between LVPW and parietal pericardial echo (fluid present)
   2. Parietal pericardium moves with LVPW
      a. Without intervening space
      b. With intervening space = residual pericardial fluid ("halo sign")
C. Constrictive pericarditis
   1. Reduced ventricular size
   2. Atrial dilated
   3. Flat LVPW motion in mid- to late diastole
   4. Usually no posterior "depression" after atrial systole (post-P wave endocardial echo moves <1 mm posteriorly)
   5. Mitral E/F slope sharp
   6. Early A-V valve closure
   7. IVS notchings: sharp posterior, then anterior motion (septal "flip-flop")
      a. During atrial systole
      b. During early diastole
   8. Inspiratory effects
      a. Interatrial and interventricular septa bulge to left
      b. Premature (pre-P wave) pulmonary valve opening (at very high RVDP)
      c. Marked inspiratory post-P wave deepening of pulmonary valve A wave
D. 2-D only (most of A, B, and C on both M-mode and 2-D)
   1. Pericardium forms immobile single or double "shell"
   2. Ventricular expansion ends abruptly
   3. A-V valves hyperactive
   4. SVC, IVC, and hepatic veins dilated and lack normal inspiratory narrowing

*Most signs are relatively nonspecific.
LVPW = left ventricular posterior wall; IVS = interventricular septum; RVDP = right ventricular diastolic pressure; SVC = superior vena cava; IVC = inferior vena cava.

but by no means uniform. The pericardium may show calcification, its prevalence increasing with chronicity. Patients have mainly the signs and symptoms of systemic congestion, usually with clear lung fields and a normal or slightly enlarged (almost never small) cardiac size; easy fatigability; dyspnea on exertion, usually without orthopnea; pedal edema, ascites, or both; hepatomegaly (and, in some chronic cases, splenomegaly); and, above all, distention of the neck veins in which the x and y descents are easily seen unless the heart rate is very fast. Timing with the heart sounds, therefore, discloses a prominent systolic collapse, the x descent, and a prominent and often larger early diastolic collapse, the y descent, both collapses departing from a high standing level of pressure. *In pericardial disease, it is important to inspect the neck veins for brisk inward motion, rather than outward pulsations.* These may be difficult to elicit if there is atrial fibrillation, seen in chronic constriction and in patients with preexisting cardiac disease. In the critical care setting or catheterization laboratory, the pressure relations and morphology of the pressure curves are easily demonstrated. Noninvasive jugular pulse tracings nearly always clearly show the typical morphology and are very useful for differentiating pure constriction (Fig. 34-6). Computed tomography in constriction demonstrates tubelike ventricles, atrial enlargement, septal changes, and enlargement of the inferior vena cava as well as pericardial thickening. Magnetic resonance imaging (MRI) is comparable (and clearer).

It is not difficult to differentiate between constrictive pericarditis and congestive heart failure. Sometimes important diagnostic problems remain, however, particularly with regard to restrictive cardiomyopathies such as amyloidosis, which are not common lesions but entities that sometimes require biopsy or diagnostic thoracotomy as a last resort. Restrictive cardiomyopathies tend to have higher left-sided than right-sided pressures and show greater inequalities during exercise and slower early- to midsystolic filling. The echocardiographic diagnosis of constrictive pericarditis is not specific, although the echocardiogram may be very helpful in conjunction with the clinical picture. Echocardiographic findings in constriction are summarized in Table 34-4.

In the absence of associated heart disease, an important hallmark of the constricted patient is a normally functioning myocardium that is prevented from doing its job by external restraint, thus being underloaded and underworked. Functional indices of contraction, such as ejection fraction, are normal. This can be determined from echocardiographic data quite easily, and noninvasively from systolic time intervals, which show a normal preejection period, virtually excluding cardiomyopathies. In postradiation therapy constriction, restrictive cardiomyopathies due to myocardial fibrosis may coexist.

MANAGEMENT. Medical management of constrictive pericarditis resembles that of congestive heart failure, since most signs and symptoms are related to systemic congestion. Digitalis, therefore, has been used, although its effect in the absence of complicating heart disease is uncertain. It is, however, useful in the presence of certain arrhythmias. Antiarrhythmic agents other than digitalis can also be used for particular arrhythmias; however, in the usual subacute or acute constriction they are generally not needed (acute pericarditis, in the absence of heart disease, does not produce arrhythmias) [10,23]. Tuberculous pericarditis, usually a chronic lesion, can be associated with arrhythmias and atrioventricular blocks, but probably because of involvement of the myocardium and conducting tissues [24]. Diuretics have long been a mainstay to relieve systemic congestion and its symptoms. The definitive treatment of constrictive pericarditis is always surgical removal of as much of the pericardium as possible [1].

Cardiac Compression after Cardiac Surgery

The rapidly increasing number of patients undergoing cardiac surgery is producing significant increases in postsurgical cardiac compression from four major causes: bleeding, pericardial effusion, postpericardiotomy syndrome, and constrictive pericarditis (Fig. 34-6).

Cardiac compression by these mechanisms (and combinations of them, e.g., bleeding with effusion or effusion with constriction) may easily be confused with other causes of postoperative low cardiac output, such as myocardial failure and prosthetic valve dysfunction. Shortly after operation, mediastinal bleeding is usually detected by monitoring drainage, but after the drains are removed hemorrhage and effusion can be concealed, particularly if they develop slowly. It should be noted that leaving the pericardium open or suturing it loosely does not necessarily permit adequate drainage; indeed, many authorities anticipate less trouble from completely closing the pericardium. Postoperative surveillance should include regular searches for pulsus paradoxus and increasing central venous pressure. Localized cardiac compression by local constriction, hematoma, or loculated effusion compressing the right or left heart may result in a shocklike picture without pulsus paradoxus (see "Absence of Pulsus Paradoxus," above) (1). Echocardiography may help but is technically difficult after thoracic surgery; computed tomography and magnetic resonance imaging are superior; moreover, cardiac compression—constrictive as well as effusive—may develop insidiously days to months after discharge. In the absence of a typical clinical picture, right heart pressures should be measured when tamponade is suspected; pericardiocentesis can be tried, although if there is a "dry tap" surgical pericardiotomy may be more productive. Pericardiotomy is particularly desirable when pericardial hematomas clot and acutely compress the heart or organize and form potentially constrictive adhesions.

References

1. Spodick DH: The normal and diseased pericardium: Current concepts of pericardial physiology, diagnosis and treatment. *J Am Coll Cardiol* 1:240, 1983.
2. Spodick DH: The pericardium: Structure, function and disease spectrum, in Spodick DH (ed): *Pericardial Diseases.* Philadelphia, FA Davis, 1976, pp 1–10.
3. Spodick DH: Acute pericardial disease: Pericarditis, effusion, and tamponade. *JCE Cardiol* 14:9, 1979.
4. Spodick DH: *Acute Pericarditis.* New York, Grune & Stratton, 1959.
5. Spodick DH: The pericardial rub: A prospective, multiple observer investigation of pericardial friction in 100 patients. *Am J Cardiol* 35:357, 1975.
6. Spodick DH: Acoustic phenomena in pericardial disease. *Am Heart J* 81:114, 1971.
7. Spodick DH: Diagnostic electrocardiographic sequences in acute pericarditis: Significance of PR segment and PR vector changes. *Circulation* 48:575, 1973.
8. Spodick DH: The electrocardiogram in acute pericarditis: Distributions of morphologic and axial changes by stages. *Am J Cardiol* 33:470, 1974.
9. Spodick DH: Differentiatial diagnosis of acute pericarditis. *Prog Cardiovasc Dis* 14:192, 1972.
10. Bruce MA, Spodick DH: Atypical electrocardiogram in acute pericarditis: Characteristics and prevalence. *J Electrocardiol* 13:61, 1980.
11. Spodick DH: Differential characteristics of the electrocardiogram in early repolarization and acute pericarditis. *N Engl J Med* 295:523, 1976.
12. Ginzton LE, Laks MM: The differential diagnosis of acute pericarditis from the normal variant: New electrocardiographic criteria. *Circulation* 65:1004, 1982.
13. Weiss JM, Spodick DH: Association of left pleural effusion with pericardial disease. *N Engl J Med* 303:696, 1983.
14. Spodick DH, Paladino D, Flessas AP: Respiratory effects on systolic time intervals during pericardial effusion. *Am J Cardiol* (in press).
15. Wechsler AS, Auerback BJ, Graham TC, et al: Distribution of intramyocardial blood flow during pericardial tamponade. *J Thorac Cardiovasc Surg* 68:847, 1974.
16. Shabetai R, Fowler NO, Fenton JC, et al: Pulsus paradoxus. *J Clin Invest* 44:1882, 1965.
17. Toney JC, Kolmen SN: Cardiac tamponade: Fluid and pressure effects on electrocardiographic changes. *Proc Soc Exp Biol Med* 121:642, 1966.
18. Spodick DH: Electric alternation of the heart: Its relation to the kinetics and physiology of the heart during cardiac tamponade. *Am J Cardiol* 10:155, 1962.
19. Prager RL, Wilson CH, Bender HW: The subxiphoid approach to pericardial disease. *Ann Thorac Surg* 34:6, 1982.
20. Spodick DH: Pericardial windows are suboptimal. *Am J Cardiol* 51:607, 1983.
21. Kerber RE, Jascho JA, Litchfield R, et al: Hemodynamic effects of volume expansion and nitroprusside compared with the pericardiocentesis in patients with acute cardiac tamponade. *N Engl J Med* 307:929, 1982.
22. Erhardt KR: Clinical and pathologic observations in different types of myocardial infarction. *Acta Med Scand* 560 (suppl):1, 1974.
23. Spodick DH: Arrhythmias during acute pericarditis: A prospective study of one hundred consecutive cases. *JAMA* 235:39, 1976.
24. Spodick DH: Tuberculous pericarditis. *Arch Intern Med* 98:737, 1956.

35. Sudden Cardiac Death

Charles I. Haffajee

History

Sudden cardiac death occurs in approximately 400,000 patients per year in the United States, accounting for approximately 50 percent of all cardiovascular mortality. Sudden cardiac death is defined in this chapter as loss of consciousness within 1 hour of the onset in symptoms in an individual with or without known preexisting heart disease. It does not spare any age, gender, or socioeconomic group and is much more common in patients with underlying coronary artery disease.

Sudden cardiac death is the leading cause of death in the 20- to 64-year-old age group and affects men twice as often as women. This results in disruption of families and incalculable human suffering and has a profound economic impact; thus, sudden cardiac death is one of the major public health challenges at this time.

Each year 1.5 million Americans experience myocardial infarction, from which about 40 percent die. Of these patients roughly two-thirds die before they reach a hospital or receive medical attention. Of the remaining one-third, about half die after reaching the hospital, and the remaining deaths occur in the first year after discharge [1].

Most advances in treatment and a better understanding of the mechanisms leading to sudden cardiac death have resulted from monitoring during the process of sudden cardiac death. Specifically, ambulatory monitoring, cardiac catheterization, and electrophysiologic findings during programmed ventricular stimulation in survivors of sudden cardiac death have led to a better pathogenetic understanding of it [2,3]. Substudies have suggested that the vast majority of patients die either from primary ventricular fibrillation (40%) or rapid ventricular tachycardia leading to ventricular fibrillation (60%) [4,5].

It appears that the expression of myocardial infarction frequently follows a circadian variation: Myocardial infarction occurs much more commonly in the early hours of the morning. This is presumably associated with increased catecholamine release. Table 35-1 and Figure 35-1 list the causes of cardiac death and of ventricular fibrillation and ventricular tachycardia.

Causes

Coronary artery disease is the major cause of sudden cardiac death. Acute myocardial infarction causes only about 20 percent of these deaths and global ischemia (left main, triple-vessel atherosclerotic coronary artery disease or coronary artery spasm) accounts for another 15 to 20 percent [6,7]. The remaining 50 to 60 percent of sudden cardiac deaths appear to result from ventricular tachycardia or ventricular fibrillation associated with prior myocardial infarction. This is particularly true in patients with either left ventricular aneurysms or markedly lowered ejection fractions (< 30%).

A smaller percentage of sudden cardiac death is due to cardiac diseases other than coronary artery disease, such as cardiomyopathies (congestive, hypertrophic, infiltrative, and right ventricular dysplasia) [8], primary electrical disease (primary ventricular fibrillation, long Q–T syndrome, and Wolff-Parkinson-White syndrome), end-stage valvular heart disease, con-

genital heart disease, acute massive pulmonary embolism, and rupture and/or dissection of the aorta. Bradyarrhythmia leading to cardiac standstill occasionally causes sudden cardiac death, more often in the setting of end-stage congestive heart failure.

Clearly, identification of patients at high risk for sudden cardiac death should be a prime responsibility. The major impact will be in prevention of coronary artery disease, such as coronary risk factor modification, from an early age. Factors identified as increasing the risk for the development of coronary artery disease are cigarette smoking, hypertension, particularly associated with left ventricular hypertrophy, low high-density lipoproteins with hyperlipidemia, and diabetes mellitus (Table 35-2).

Diagnosis of Arrhythmias (VT/VF) Leading to Sudden Cardiac Death

Arrhythmias observed in the immediate postresuscitation period are frequently different from those responsible for the ventricular tachycardia or ventricular fibrillation initiating death in sudden cardiac death victims. Following resuscitation, once hemodynamic stability has been achieved, only a minority of patients exhibit spontaneous arrhythmias that may have resulted in sudden cardiac death [9,10]. The arrhythmias leading to sudden cardiac death may be identified in these patients by extensive Holter monitoring and/or exercise testing [11] or, more reliably, by electrophysiologic testing. Approximately 25 percent of resuscitated sudden cardiac death patients do not exhibit ambient significant arrhythmias during Holter monitoring or exercise testing even though their sudden cardiac death resulted from ventricular tachycardia or ventricular fibrillation. On the other hand, routine electrophysiologic testing using programmed ventricular stimulation in these patients has a higher probability of exposing arrhythmia leading to sudden cardiac death [12,13]. As is often the case in diagnostic tests, the more stringent and more severe the protocol for programmed ventricular stimulation in an attempt to induce ventricular tachycardia and ventricular fibrillation, the lesser the specificity and

Table 35-1. Cardiac Causes of VT/VF in Absence of Acute Myocardial Infarction

1. Prior myocardial infarction
2. Cardiomyopathies
   Idiopathic dilated
   Valvular heart disease
   Hypertrophic myopathies
   Arrhythmogenic right ventricular dysplasia
   Congenital heart disease
   Infiltrative disease (sarcoid, collagen, vascular, malignancy)
3. Electrical disorders
   Long Q–T syndrome
   Preexcitation syndromes (e.g., Wolff-Parkinson-White)
   Conduction disorders
   Primary idiopathic VF

VT = ventricular tachycardia; VF = ventricular fibrillation.

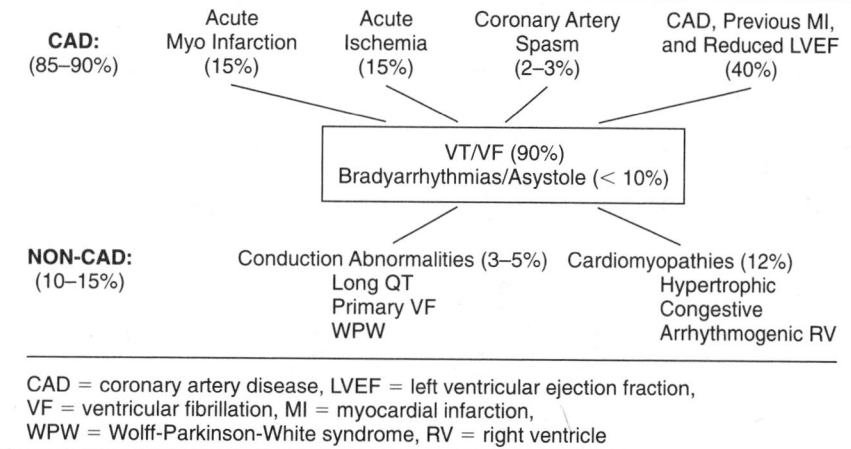

Fig. 35-1. Mechanisms of sudden cardiac death. CAD = coronary artery disease; LVEF = left ventricular ejection fraction; MI = myocardial infarction; VF = ventricular fibrillation; VT = ventricular tachycardia; RV = right ventricle; WPW = Wolff-Parkinson-White syndrome.

the higher the sensitivity. However, a variety of protocols have been used and it appears that programmed stimulation with two extra stimuli is highly specific, though not very sensitive. If using two or three extra stimuli and pacing at fast rates induces monomorphic ventricular tachycardia with a cycle length less than 220 msec (slower than 280 beats/min), then it appears that such an arrhythmia has high specificity and can be used as an endpoint for therapy in survivors of arrhythmic sudden cardiac death [11,12,13]. Unfortunately, a significant percentage of patients can have polymorphic ventricular tachycardia or ventricular fibrillation inducible only during electrophysiologic study, and this may be the only arrhythmia seen during resuscitation. However, polymorphic ventricular tachycardia or ventricular fibrillation lacks specificity, since it can be induced in patients not at risk of sudden death by similar protocols of programmed ventricular stimulation [21]. Thus, it is very important to try to obtain the patient's initial arrhythmia at the time of the cardiac arrest. Several studies [18,21] have addressed this issue, since polymorphic ventricular tachycardia or ventricular fibrillation may be the only arrhythmia inducible during electrophysiologic studies in patients experiencing sudden cardiac death. Most often the initial arrhythmia at the time of cardiac arrest is not available for comparison with the arrhythmia initiated in the laboratory, and the laboratory findings must be extended to that leading to sudden cardiac death. It appears from several studies that the initiation of monomorphic ventricular tachycardia can be considered a positive endpoint in survivors of sudden death [13,15]. However, if polymorphic ventricular tachycardia or ventricular fibrillation is inducible, especially with two extra stimuli, this finding may be considered specific in such patients, though its specificity is less so than that of monomorphic ventricular tachycardia. A significant number of patients, when undergoing programmed ventricular stimulation, have inducible monomorphic ventricular tachycardia (Table 35-3). A smaller percentage have inducible polymorphic ventricular tachycardia, especially with two extra stimuli. It is important that one-third of patients may have no arrhythmia initiated during electrophysiologic study; this can pose a problem in terms of preventive therapy [17,19,21]. In some patients who experienced ventricular tachycardia or ventricular fibrillation while taking antiarrhythmic therapy no arrhythmia is inducible. Drug-induced proarrhythmia has to be considered in such patients. Quinidine or quinidinelike drugs (procainamide, disopyramide), certain antihistamines (hismanal), and erythromycin or its analogs can cause polymorphic ventricular tachycardia or ventricular fibrillation in association with increased Q–T interval, especially with a low serum potassium. Other antiarrhythmics, such as flecainide, encainide, ethmozin, and propafenone (class IC), may cause incessant monomorphic ventricular tachycardia that can be provoked by exercise testing in some patients.

About 30 to 40 percent of patients surviving sudden cardiac death may have no inducible arrhythmia during programmed ventricular stimulation, Holter monitoring, and exercise testing, and other diagnostic tests may not yield an underlying significant cardiac abnormality or cause sudden cardiac death [13–17,20,21,22]. Subtle abnormalities, such as long Q–T syndrome, may be sought in these patients and may involve repetitive monitoring and/or exercise testing.

Table 35-2. Causes of Sudden Cardiac Death

1. CAD (> 90%)
   a. Primary ventricular electrical instability (VT/VF) in patients with CAD and previous myocardial infarction (60%)
   b. Acute myocardial infarction (15%)
   c. Acute myocardial ischemia (10%)
   d. Coronary artery spasm (2–5%)
2. Non-CAD (5–10%)
   a. Congenital QT syndrome
   b. Preexcitation disorders (e.g., W-P-W syndrome)
   c. Primary ventricular fibrillation
   d. Drug-induced polymorphous ventricular tachycardia (*Torsades de pointes*)
   e. Bradyarrhythmic conditions (complete heart block, sinus arrest)
   f. Cardiomyopathies (congestive, hypertrophic)
   g. Severe valvular heart disease (aortic stenosis)
   h. Pulmonary embolism
   i. Aortic rupture or dissection

CAD = coronary artery disease; VT = ventricular tachycardia; VF = ventricular fibrillation; W-P-W = Wolff-Parkinson-White.

Management (Table 35-4)

Prevention rather than treatment should be the goal for sudden cardiac death. Despite better understanding of the mechanisms

Table 35-3. Electrophysiologic Findings in Survivors of Out-of-Hospital Cardiac Arrest

Authors	No. of patients	Sustained VT	Polymorphic VT/VF	NSVT	Total % of patients inducible	Noninducible
Eldar et al. [12]	108	41	11	23	69%	33
Freedman et al. [13]	150	82	23	8	25%	371
Hays et al. [14]	100	40	29	—	69%	31
Kehoe et al. [15]	38	18	4	—	58%	16
Knilans et al. [16]	57	24	8	—	54%	25
Roy et al. [17]	119	63	9	11	70%	36
Stevenson et al. [18]	15	7	4	—	73%	4
Swerdlow et al. [19]	140	56	27	16	71%	41
Wilbur et al. [20]	166	61	25	45	79%	35

VT = ventricular tachycardia; VF = ventricular fibrillation, NSVT = nonsustained ventricular tachycardia (≤ 30 sec duration).

leading to sudden cardiac death, the identification of patients at risk continues to be a challenge.

Preventing or delaying expression of coronary artery disease should make a major impact on sudden cardiac death. This involves counseling patients with a family history of coronary artery disease; identification and aggressive treatment of risk factors, such as smoking, diet, and use of antihyperlipidemic agents, especially with drugs that affect the metabolism of cholesterol, such as Lovastatin; attempts to increase the high-density lipoprotein fraction of cholesterol (exercise program and/or alcohol); aggressive treatment of hypertension and prevention of left ventricular hypertrophy; and control of diabetes mellitus. In relatives of patients with known coronary artery disease, risk factors should be assessed and treadmill exercise testing considered when they reach the age of 40.

Patients with known coronary artery disease and previous myocardial infarction should be assessed for risk of sudden cardiac death. Unless there is a contraindication, these patients should receive beta-blockers and aspirin. Both therapies have been shown to decrease the risk of infarction and sudden death in patients who have previously experienced a myocardial infarction [18]. Coronary artery bypass graft surgery should be considered in patients with multivessel disease and angina with reduced left ventricular ejection fractions, as revascularization has been shown to decrease myocardial reinfarction and sudden cardiac death [23].

Patients who have experienced a life-threatening arrhythmia or have been resuscitated from arrhythmic sudden cardiac death should be considered for aggressive individualized therapy for the prevention of recurrence [21,22]. If ventricular

Table 35-4. Approaches to Management and Prevention of Sudden Cardiac Death

1. Coronary risk factor modification
   a. Cessation of cigarette smoking
   b. Blood pressure control
   c. Diet
   d. Antihyperlipidemic agents (e.g., Lovastatin)
   e. Exercise program
2. General treatment of at-risk patients
   a. β-blockers in post-myocardial infarction patients
   b. Revascularization or angioplasty in patients with severe coronary artery disease
   c. "Prophylactic" ICD or amiodarone in high-risk patients
3. Aggressive individualized therapy of survivors
   a. ICD
   b. Sotalol or amiodarone
   c. CABG ± ICD

ICD = implantable defibrillator; CABG = coronary artery bypass graft.

tachycardia or ventricular fibrillation occurred in these patients in the setting of a reversible factor, such as hypokalemia, drug-induced *Torsades de pointes,* or global ischemia, corrective steps should be taken to prevent their recurrence.

Resuscitated sudden cardiac death victims in whom ventricular tachycardia or ventricular fibrillation occurred in the absence of a reversible factor or acute myocardial infarction should be stabilized. Once neurologic status returns to normal electrophysiologic evaluation and cardiac catheterization should be considered (Fig. 35-2).

Cardiac catheterization allows assessment of the extent of coronary artery disease and degree of left ventricular dyfunction. This information should be interpreted together with the history and perhaps objective ischemic tests, such as exercise or persantine thallium imaging. Programmed ventricular stimulation during electrophysiologic studies for induction of ventricular tachycardia or ventricular fibrillation after normalization of electrolytes and elimination of all antiarrhythmics should then be performed [21,22]. The induction of sustained monomorphic ventricular tachycardia, polymorphic ventricular tachycardia or ventricular fibrillation with single or double extra stimuli or hemodynamically embarrassing, nonsustained monomorphic ventricular tachycardia should be considered a significant response. Several studies have identified these endpoints as predictive of future events and they should serve as a guide for therapeutic intervention. Antiarrhythmic therapy can be used to determine whether they will prevent reinduction of sustained baseline arrhythmias leading to sudden cardiac death [20]. However, these results have been disappointing with standard antiarrhythmic agents such as quinidine or quinidinelike agents (procainamide, disopyramide), newer, more toxic antiarrhythmic agents, such as flecainide, encainide, and ethmozine, and the lidocaine derivatives (mexilitene and tocainide).

Recent data with sotalol (ESVEM Trial) [24] and amiodarone [25] suggest that these drugs may prevent future arrhythmic events leading to sudden cardiac death. A 2-year follow-up study of sotalol showed that this agent may confer protection against sudden cardiac death by suppressing inducible ventricular tachycardia or ventricular fibrillation during programmed ventricular stimulation or suppressing significant baseline ventricular arrhythmias (by Holter monitoring or exercise testing). Empiric amiodarone has been shown to confer protection against sudden cardiac death in relatively noncontrolled, nonrandomized trials [25,26]. Ongoing prospective controlled trials with amiodarone are addressing this issue and in patients with congestive cardiomyopathy and ventricular arrhythmias. Several trials are comparing amiodarone and the implantable cardioverter-defibrillator (ICD) for protection against sudden cardiac death in survivors and in patients at risk.

In general, as Table 35-4 demonstrates, an organized ap-

1. Sudden cardiac death survivor

    ↓

2. Stabilize
   —Treat complications of resuscitation
   —Assess neurological status
   —Extubate

    ↓

3. Identify reversible causes
   —Acute myocardial infarction
   —Hypokalemia
   —Drug-induced torsades de pointes

    ↓

4. Define cardiac status and anatomy
   —Exercise/persantine thallium scan
   —Echocardiography (LVEF, valvular status,
     four chamber size)
   —Nuclear (MUGA) scan
   —Cardiac catheterization

    ↓

5. Define VT/VF; conduction abnormalities
   —EP study
   —Holter
   —Exercise testing

    ↓

6. Select therapy
   —Implantable defibrillator
   —CABG ± defibrillator
   —Empiric amiodarone
   —Possibly sotalol

Fig. 35-2. Management of patients with sudden cardiac death.

proach should be made to management of sudden cardiac death survivors. Individualized therapy has been shown to decrease the recurrence of death from 30 percent per year to less than 10 percent per year. In particular, use of the ICD for arrhythmic sudden death survivors appears to reduce the incidence of recurrent sudden death to 1 to 2 percent per year.

Several noncontrolled, nonrandomized studies appear to demonstrate that the ICD can decrease the recurrence of sudden cardiac death to 1 percent or less per year [28]. However, in follow-up of patients who have received the ICD, the mortality in years 3 to 5 following ICD implantation remains high (20–35%) and may be more dependent on left ventricular dysfunction and/or coronary artery disease [28]. Definitive trials addressing these issues (AVID, SIDS, CASCADE [27], and CASH trials) have not been completed. One of the major challenges is the prevention of primary sudden cardiac death in high-risk patients such as those with low ejection fraction (< 40%) following myocardial infarction with asymptomatic nonsustained ventricular tachycardia, and positive signal-averaged ECGs; patients with advanced congestive and other forms of cardiomyopathies; and patients with primary electrical disease.

More problematic is the appropriate preventive therapy for patients with coronary artery disease and depressed left ventricular function and no inducible arrhythmias by programmed ventricular stimulation, exercise testing, and/or prolonged Holter monitoring and for patients with other types of structural heart disease and no inducible or documented arrhythmias. It appears that the incidence of recurrent sudden death is high in these patients, and they are at high risk for recurrent ventricular tachycardia or ventricular fibrillation. Unless some obvious, correctable, reversible factor for sudden cardiac death can be identified in these patients, ICD implantation is recommended at

this time; it may even be recommended as a prophylactic therapy in such high-risk patients.

Due to the difficulty in assessing the effectiveness and safety of antiarrhythmic therapy and the risk of proarrhythmia, the need for preventive therapy continues to be a major challenge. The technologic advances of implantable ICDs allow for total transvenous implants [29] with smaller devices placed pectorally, with minimal risk to the patient. There is therefore increasing pressure to consider prophylactic ICDs in high-risk patients.

One hopes that data emanating from trials being implemented will allow for better management of patients at high risk of sudden cardiac death.

References

1. Greene HL: Sudden arrhythmic cardiac death: Mechanisms, resuscitation and classification: The Seattle perspective. *Am J Cardiol* 65:4B, 1990.
2. Liberthson RR, Nagel EL, Hirschman JC, et al: Prehospital ventricular defibrillation: Prognosis and follow-up course. *N Engl J Med* 291:317, 1974.
3. Hosenpud JF, McAnulty JH, Niles NR: Unexpected myocardial disease in patients with life threatening arrhythmias. *Br Heart J* 56:55, 1986.
4. Weaver WD, Cobb LA, Hallstrom AP: Ambulatory arrhythmias in resuscitated victims of cardiac arrest. *Circulation* 66:212, 1982.
5. deLuna AB, Coumel P, LeClercq JF: Ambulatory sudden cardiac death: Mechanisms of production of fatal arrhythmias on the basis of data from 157 cases. *Am Heart J* 117:151, 1989.
6. Stevenson WG, Wiener I, Yeatman L, et al: Complicated atherosclerotic lesions: A potential cause of ischemic ventricular arrhythmias in cardiac arrest survivors who do not have inducible ventricular tachycardia? *Am Heart J* 116:1, 1988.
7. Fellows CL, Weaver WD, Greene HL: Cardiac arrest associated with coronary artery spasm. *Am J Cardiol* 60:1397, 1987.
8. Thiene G, Nava A, Corrado D, et al: Right ventricular cardiomyopathy and sudden death in young people. *N Engl J Med* 318:129, 1988.
9. Weaver WD, Cobb LA, Hallstrom AP, et al: Factors influencing survival after out-of-hospital cardiac arrest. *J Am Coll Cardiol* 7:752, 1986.
10. Lionkowski RS, Thompson DM, Gruschow AW: Resuscitation time in ventricular fibrillation: A prognostic indicator. *Ann Emerg Med* 12:733, 1983.
11. Weaver WD, Cobb LA, Hallstrom AP, et al: Considerations for improving survival from out-of-hospital cardiac arrest. *Ann Emerg Med* 15:1181, 1986.
12. Eldar M, Sauve MJ, Scheinman MM: Electrophysiologic testing and follow-up of patients with aborted sudden death. *J Am Coll Cardiol* 10:291, 1987.
13. Freedman RA, Swerdlow CD, Soderholm-Difatte V, et al: Prognostic significance of arrhythmia inducibility or non-inducibility at initial electrophysiologic study in survivors of cardiac arrest. *Am J Cardiol* 61:578, 1988.
14. Hays, LJ, Lerman BB, DiMarco JP: Non-ventricular arrhythmias as precursors of ventricular fibrillation in patients with out-of-hospital cardiac arrest. *Am Heart J* 118:53, 1989.
15. Kehoe R, Tommaso C, Zhentlin T, et al: Factors determining programmed stimulation responses and long term arrhythmic outcome in survivors of ventricular fibrillation with ischemic heart disease. *Am Heart J* 116:355, 1988.
16. Knilans TK, Prystowsky EN: Antiarrhythmic drug therapy in management of cardiac arrest survivors. *Circulaton* 85(suppl I):118, 1992.
17. Roy D, Waxman HL, Kienzle MG, et al: Clinical characteristics and long-term follow-up in 119 survivors of cardiac arrest: Relation to inducibility at electrophysiologic testing. *Am J Cardiol* 52:969, 1983.
18. Stevenson WG, Brugada P, Waldecker B, et al: Clinical, angiographic, and electrophysiologic findings in patients with aborted sudden death as compared with patients with sustained ventricular tachycardia after myocardial infarction. *Circulation* 71:1146, 1985.

19. Swerdlow CD, Bardy GH, McAnulty J, et al: Determinants of induced sustained arrhythmias in survivors of out-of-hospital ventricular fibrillation. *Circulation* 76:1053, 1987.
20. Morady P, DiCarlo L, Winston S, et al: Clinical features and prognosis of patients with out-of-hospital cardiac arrest and a normal electrophysiologic study. *J. Am Coll Cardiol* 4:39, 1984.
21. Wilber DJ, Garan H, Finkelstein D, et al: Out-of-hospital cardiac arrest: Use of electrophysiologic testing in the prediction of long-term outcome. *N Engl J Med* 318:19, 1988.
22. Waller TJ, Kay HR, Spielman SR, et al: Reduction in sudden death and total mortality by antiarrhythmic therapy evaluated by electrophysiologic drug testing: Criteria of efficacy in patients with sustained ventricular tachyarrhythmia. *J Am Coll Cardiol* 10:83, 1987.
23. Kelly P, Ruskin JN, Vlahakes G: Surgical coronary revascularization in survivors of prehospital cardiac arrest: Its effect on inducible ventricular arrhythmias and long-term survival. *J Am Coll Cardiol* 15:267, 1990.
24. ESVEM Investigators: The ESVEM trial: Electrophysiologic study versus electrocardiographic monitoring for selection of antiarrhythmic therapy of ventricular tachyarrhythmias. *Circulation* 79:1354, 1989.
25. Kay GN, Pryor DB, Lee KL, et al: Comparison of survival of amiodarone-treated patients with coronary artery disease and malignant ventricular arrhythmias with that of a control group with coronary artery disease. *J Am Coll Cardiol* 9:877, 1987.
26. Ceremuzynski L, Kleczar E, Krzeminska-Pakula M, et al: Effect of amiodarone on mortality after myocardial infarction: A double-blind, placebo-controlled, pilot study. *J Am Coll Cardiol* 20:1056, 1992.
27. Greene HL, Poole JE, Fellows CL, et al: Cardiac arrest in Seattle: Conventional versus amiodarone drug evaluation (CASCADE): Mortality results (abstract). *Circulation* 86:(Suppl I):1-656, 1992.
28. Winkle RA, Mead RH, Ruder MA, et al: Long-term outcome with the automatic implantable cardioverter-defibrillator. *J Am Coll Cardiol* 13:1353, 1989.
29. Yee R, Klein G, Leitch J, et al: A permanent transvenous lead system for an implantable pacemaker cardioverter-defibrillator. *Circulation* 85:196, 1992.

36. *Dissection of the Aorta*

Linda A. Pape

Aortic dissection occurs when a hematoma develops within the wall of the aorta and advances, sometimes along the entire length of the aorta. The clinical presentation is quite varied, and the condition is life-threatening [1–8]. The hematoma may rupture into the pericardial sac or the pleural space, causing cardiac tamponade or massive hemothorax. It often disrupts the aortic valve, causing acute aortic insufficiency and left ventricular failure. Compromise of branch vessels may lead to stroke or limb ischemia.

Death due to aortic dissection may occur within 24 hours, and the majority of patients die within days of the onset of symptoms unless definitive medical and surgical therapy is instituted [1]. Without treatment, 90 percent of patients die within a year. [1]

Because it progresses so rapidly and has such diverse clinical manifestations, acute aortic dissection is one of the greatest challenges in cardiovascular medicine. Over the past 20 years faster and more accurate diagnosis, advances in surgical technique, and more rapidly instituted medical and surgical treatment have transformed aortic dissection from an almost uniformly fatal process to one with a 5-year survival rate up to 75 percent [1,9–13].

The severe chest pain associated with aortic dissection usually leads to a mistaken initial diagnosis of acute myocardial infarction [7]; however, acute aortic dissection is much less common than acute myocardial infarction. Estimates indicate that 1 in 10,000 patients admitted to the hospital or 1 in 205 patients at autopsy have aortic dissection [1] [14].

The most common underlying etiologies of aortic dissection are hypertension and connective tissue disorders. In Marfan's syndrome, aortic dissection is one of the most frequent causes of death [15]. Definitive diagnosis is made by cineangiography or cut-film aortography, echocardiography, contrast computerized tomography, or magnetic resonance imaging (MRI).

Initial medical therapy in all cases is directed toward limiting the spread of the dissection. This is best accomplished by decreasing the force of left ventricular contractility and lowering systolic blood pressure. Surgery is the treatment of choice in virtually all cases of acute dissection involving the ascending aorta. Surgery for dissection confined to the descending aorta is usually limited to patients with actual or impending complications: expansion or rupture.

Etiology

ANATOMY. The thoracic aorta includes the aortic valve and sinuses of Valsalva, from which originate the coronary arteries, the ascending aorta, the aortic arch, and the descending aorta. Two-thirds of all dissections originate in the ascending aorta, the 5-cm segment above the aortic valve. The aortic arch (also approximately 5 cm long) gives rise to the brachiocephalic, left common carotid, and left subclavian arteries. After the takeoff of the left subclavian artery, the descending aorta courses along in the posterior mediastinum for approximately 20 cm until it reaches the diaphragm. Important branches in this segment include the intercostal and spinal cord arteries.

HISTOLOGY. The normal aorta is composed of three distinct layers. The thin innermost layer, the intima, consists of smooth muscle cells, elastic fibers, and fibroblasts. The intima is lined by endothelial cells, which border the aortic lumen. Adjacent to the intima is the media, the layer most important for the aorta's structural integrity. The media consists of multiple layers of fenestrated elastic tissue, with collagen fibers and smooth muscle cells between. These elements are embedded in ground substance composed primarily of acid mucopolysaccharides. The third, outermost layer of the aorta is the adventitia, which is relatively thin but also structurally important. The adventitia is composed of collagen and elastin and contains the vasa vasorum.

In nearly all cases aortic dissection begins when an intimal tear permits blood to enter the aortic media and advance along a plane within the outer third of the aortic wall. The transversely oriented intimal tear most commonly occurs in the proximal ascending aorta (61%). The next most common sites are the proximal descending aorta between the origin of the left subclavian artery and the ligamentum arteriosum (16%), the remainder of the descending aorta (10%), the aortic arch (9%), and the abdominal aorta (3%) [1].

Although it is generally accepted that the process of aortic dissection begins with an intimal tear, this has not been proved conclusively. In fact, most reported series include a few cases, usually less than 5 percent, in which an intimal tear or entry site cannot be demonstrated [1]. In a review of 204 autopsied patients, Wilson and Hutchins reported 21 (13%) cases without intimal tears [16]; however, all of those without a demonstrable entry site had dissection confined to the descending thoracic or abdominal aorta. The alternative explanation to the primary intimal tear is that dissection begins with hemorrhage of the vasa vasorum within the media and subsequent rupture into the intima [17,18].

The cause of the break in the intima that allows dissection to occur is unknown. Numerous studies have failed to identify any consistent pathology sufficient to explain the tears. Atherosclerosis does not seem to be an etiologic factor; intimal tears were found to originate in an atherosclerotic plaque in only 5 percent of cases in two series [1,19]. Furthermore, the distribution of atherosclerosis in the aorta is nearly the reverse of the distribution of intimal tears. The abdominal aorta, the site of the most severe atherosclerosis, is rarely the site of an intimal tear.

Still, there is some disagreement regarding the role of atherosclerosis in the pathogenesis of dissection. Braunstein found, in his 1963 histologic study of 35 cases of aortic dissection, that in 50 percent an atherosclerotic plaque penetrated deeply into the media at the site of the intimal tear [20]. He commented on the frequent finding of histologically apparent atherosclerosis in the absence of grossly evident disease. Murray and Edwards, in their series of 56 cases, found atherosclerosis to be uncommon in areas of intimal laceration [19]. In a more recently published series, Wilson and Hutchins found that atherosclerosis was slightly but significantly more prevalent in the dissection group than in an age-, race-, and sex-matched control group; they concluded that atherosclerosis may therefore have an etiologic role [16]. The question remains unresolved. More recently, Larson and Edwards found severe atherosclerosis involving the intimal tear in only 9 percent of 121 cases of type I or II dissection but in 80 percent of 40 type III dissections [21].

Another important consideration in the pathogenesis of aortic dissection is what abnormality of the aortic media allows dissection to occur. Extensive histologic studies of normal, aging aortas and aortas from patients with aortic stenosis, Marfan's syndrome, and aortic dissection do not show a specific defect responsible for dissection [17,22]. Medionecrosis, elastin fragmentation, and fibrosis all occur in the "normal," aging aorta but are present in greater severity in patients with dissection [22,23]. Cystic medionecrosis, seen in Marfan's syndrome (3% of all dissections) and in patients younger than 40 years of age with dissection, is the one finding that does not increase with age [23]. Even here, however, controversy exists, with some studies showing an increase with age and hypertension [17,24].

Cystic medionecrosis is associated with defects in elastic tissue and collagen organization. In Marfan's syndrome a deficiency in the formation of collagen cross-links was reported in 1981 [25]. Although *cystic medionecrosis* has become almost synonymous with *Marfan's syndrome,* some patients with Marfan's syndrome with dissection do not have cystic medionecrosis [26]. Observations of the biochemical composition of the aorta in patients with dissections compared with controls have shown localized increased collagen, which effectively dilutes

the matrix components important for mechanical integrity [27]. Other recent studies have shifted attention from collagen to elastic architecture [28,29], suggesting defects in elastin production. There may be a varying combination of defects in collagen, elastin, and the interconnections between laminae, fibers, and smooth muscle cells, which depends in turn on underlying genetic defects (Marfan's) and acute and chronic vascular stresses (hypertension). The vast majority of non-Marfan's patients with dissection have degenerative changes, including elastin fragmentation, medionecrosis, and fibrosis, not cystic medionecrosis [18].

ETIOLOGIC FACTORS (Table 36-1). Hypertension is by far the most important disease associated with the development of aortic dissection. Clinical evidence or a history of hypertension was present in 92 percent of 463 autopsied cases reviewed in Hirst and co-workers' classic article [1]. Clinical series likewise record a prevalence of 52 to 82 percent [5–8,10,16,30,31]. Although a recent autopsy study from Italy reported an apparent increasing prevalence of dissection [32], a more recent study from Japan over the years 1975 to 1985 showed an incidence of 1 in 205, similar to that of older studies [14].

After hypertension, congenitally malformed aortic valves are the most common factor predisposing to aortic dissection [33]. Bicuspid valves accounted for 11.4 percent of aortic dissections in a recent clinical series from the Mayo Clinic [34]. All were associated with ascending aortic dissection, as were those reported by Roberts and Roberts [33]. Other conditions associated with aortic dissection include Marfan's syndrome, Ehlers-Danlos syndrome, pregnancy, coarctation of the aorta, aortic stenosis, Turner's syndrome, and relapsing polychondritis [16,26,35,36,37]. In coarctation and Turner's syndrome, hypertension is probably a significant contributing factor in the development of dissection. Rare associations also include giant cell aortitis and syphilitic aortitis and cocaine use [38]. Iatrogenic causes include cardiac catheterization, femoral artery insertion of an intraaortic balloon catheter, and balloon angioplasty of aortic coarctation [39]. Cardiovascular surgery [40] is a rare cause of acute aortic dissection, with a recently reported incidence of 24 of 14,877 surgical procedures at Massachusetts General Hospital (0.16%) [41]. Nevertheless, in the Mayo Clinic series of 236 cases of dissection, an additional 31 cases were iatrogenic (11.6% of total) [34]. In Roberts and Roberts' series, 6.5 percent of cases were iatrogenic [33]. Thus, after hypertension and bicuspid aortic valve, cardiac procedures appear to be the next most common cause of aortic dissection.

Table 36-1. Etiologies and Associations of Aortic Dissection

Hypertension
Congenital aortic valve disease
    Bicuspid
    Unicuspid
Coarctation of aorta
Marfan's syndrome
Cystic medionecrosis
Pregnancy
Ehlers-Danlos syndrome
Turner's syndrome
Relapsing polychondritis
Giant cell arteritis
Cocaine use
Iatrogenic
    Cardiac catheterization
    Intraaortic balloon insertion
    Cardiac surgery

Classification

The original classification of DeBakey still in use divides aortic dissection into three types. Type I dissection begins in the ascending aorta and extends distally to the arch and descending aorta. Type II dissection begins in and is limited to the ascending aorta. Type II is more likely in patients with the Marfan's syndrome [42]. Type III begins in and is limited to the descending aorta. The most useful classification of aortic dissections was proposed by Daily et al. in 1970 [43]. Recognizing the distinct difference in clinical course and prognosis, they divided dissection patients into two groups: those with involvement of the ascending aorta (type A) and those in whom the dissection was limited to the descending aorta (type B). Thus Daily type A includes DeBakey types I and II, and type B is equivalent to DeBakey type III. Dissection is considered acute if it is of less than 2 weeks' duration and chronic if evidence of dissection had been present for more than 2 weeks. This system has gained wide acceptance because of its clinical relevance as well as simplicity [5,7,10,44].

Pathophysiology

Most intimal tears occur in those portions of the aorta that are attached to relatively fixed structures and are therefore subject to the greatest mechanical stress. These two areas are the ascending aorta immediately above the aortic valve and the proximal descending aorta just beyond the origin of the left subclavian artery [1].

As blood enters the intima and media, it usually tracks along in a plane between the inner two-thirds and outer one-third of the media. As it pulses along this plane, the blood creates a double-lumened aorta. Usually the blood reenters from the false channel into the true lumen at some distal site. The false lumen may remain patent, become dominant, and compress the true lumen. Both true and false lumen may remain patent indefinitely. The false lumen may in time thrombose spontaneously. This "healing" occurs primarily in cases with descending aortic dissection and may account for the survival of some untreated patients [45,46].

The most important factors influencing the spread of aortic dissection, aside from the tissue characteristics of the aorta itself, are left ventricular contractility, aortic compliance, and stroke volume. Left ventricular contractility determines the rate of rise of the aortic pressure pulse and is thought to be the most important single factor. In vitro studies in a Tygon tubing model and in the dog aorta by Prokop and co-workers showed that the rate of change of pressure (dp/dt) in pulsatile flow is more important than the absolute level of blood pressure [47]; however, since absolute pressure increases wall tension, both rate of rise and absolute pressure play a role in the spread of dissection [48].

The consequences of dissection may be divided into three main groups: arterial compromise, aortic insufficiency, and external rupture. In general, dissection tends to propagate distally from the intimal tear. Some degree of retrograde dissection is common, however, especially in dissection of the ascending aorta [49]. As the dissection spreads, it may compromise any of the aortic branch vessels by compression. The dissection may extend into the walls of the branch vessels themselves or spiral around and skip branches. The result of arterial compression may be myocardial, limb, cerebral, or visceral ischemia or infarction [50,51]. Absent or diminished pulse is a frequent finding in patients with type A dissection and is often asymptomatic.

Dissection of the ascending aorta in 50 to 60 percent of cases results in aortic insufficiency [2,5,44]. The intramural hematoma may either undermine support of one or more aortic cusps or commissures or actually disrupt the valve itself. Dilation or distortion of the root likewise may prevent normal coaptation of the cusps and result in valvular incompetence. Another common mechanism is prolapse of the intimal flap across the valve. The normal or concentrically hypertrophied left ventricle (50% of these patients have hypertension) does not accommodate a sudden diastolic overload well. When severe aortic insufficiency occurs acutely, left ventricular diastolic pressure is abruptly elevated, resulting in left ventricular failure and pulmonary venous congestion. The wide pulse pressure usually seen in compensated chronic aortic insufficiency is usually not seen in acute aortic insufficiency associated with dissection.

In as many as 25 percent of cases of ascending aortic dissection, there is a history of an aortic insufficiency murmur [44]. These murmurs may be due to root dilation secondary to hypertension or to medial degeneration, both common in ascending aorta dissections. Some may be due to primary valvular disease. Rarely, prior dissection is the apparent cause of the murmur.

External rupture constitutes the third important aspect of the pathophysiology of aortic dissection. External rupture through the thoracic aortic adventitia most frequently causes hemorrhage into the pericardium or left pleural space. The site of rupture was correlated to the site of the intimal tear by Gore and Hirst (Table 36-2) [52]. Dissection of the descending thoracic aorta and abdominal aorta (the latter is rare) may also rupture into the retroperitoneum.

Diagnosis

HISTORY. The predominant symptom in approximately 90 percent of patients with acute aortic dissection is the very abrupt onset of very severe chest pain [1,5,44]. Anterior chest pain is most common, with frequent radiation to the interscapular region of the back. If pain is limited to the anterior chest, ascending aortic dissection is more likely. If pain is limited to the back, the dissection is more likely due to dissection of the descending aorta; however, pain in both anterior chest and back is common enough in either type of dissection that pain location alone, though suggestive, is not sufficiently specific to diagnose the site of dissection.

Although the admitting diagnosis in patients with dissection is most frequently given as "rule out myocardial infarction," the pain of acute myocardial infarction normally has a more gradual onset than that of acute dissection. In dissection the onset of

Table 36-2. Site of External Rupture in Relation to Site of Intimal Tear

Site	Ascending aortic (%) (n = 227)	Aortic arch (%) (n = 37)	Descending aorta (%) (n = 97)
Pericardium	70	35	12
Left pleural space	6	32	44
Mediastinum	6	8	15
Esophagus	—	8	1

n = number of patients studied.

pain is characteristically sudden, and severity is maximal at the onset. The patient often describes the quality of pain as very sharp, only rarely using the words *tearing* or *ripping*. The pain may be migratory and actually follow the path of the spreading dissection. Patients with ascending aorta dissection are somewhat more likely to present within 24 hours of the onset of symptoms than are patients with dissection of the descending aorta [44]. Presenting symptoms in addition to chest pain include syncope, usually due to cardiac tamponade; congestive heart failure, due to acute aortic insufficiency; stroke or limb ischemia, due to arterial compression; abdominal pain; restlessness; acute myocardial infarction, due to involvement of a coronary artery; fever; anterior spinal artery ischemia with motor and sensory deficits; disseminated intravascular coagulopathy; renal failure, and renovascular hypertension [1,5,6,8,53].

Pertinent history includes history of hypertension, history of previous aortic valve disease, known aortic regurgitation murmurs, previous pulse deficit, and existence of prior chest radiographs.

PHYSICAL EXAMINATION. Hypertension (systolic blood pressure >160 mm Hg) is present in more than half of patients who present with dissection of the descending aorta [19] (Table 36-3). Although as many as 50 percent of patients with dissection of the ascending aorta have a history of hypertension, at the time of presentation only 10 to 30 percent are hypertensive [5,44]. Because of the complications of ascending aortic dissection, 20 to 25 percent of patients present with hypotension (systolic blood pressure <100 mm Hg) [5,19,44]. Hypotension is rare (1%) at the time of presentation of dissection of the descending aorta [5,19].

Absent or markedly diminished arterial pulses are the hallmark of aortic dissection, noted in as many as 50 percent of patients with ascending aortic dissection [5]. Only 10 to 15 percent of patients with descending aortic dissection have demonstrable pulse deficits at the time of presentation. In most cases the pulse deficit is asymptomatic, although stroke, limb ischemia, and neurologic syndromes due to spinal artery involvement may be seen. Pulses must be routinely carefully examined in all patients with suspected myocardial infarction, and the presence of a pulse deficit should alert to the possible presence of aortic dissection rather than myocardial infarction.

Aortic regurgitation is found in the majority of patients with ascending aortic dissection. Rarely, retrograde dissection from the arch or descending aorta may involve the aortic valve, but in general aortic regurgitation indicates dissection originating in the ascending aorta. If acute severe aortic regurgitation results in left ventricular failure, the wide pulse pressure typically associated with aortic regurgitation will not be present. Evidence of left ventricular failure due to acute aortic insufficiency may be found in dissection of the ascending aorta. Occasionally, a preexisting murmur of aortic regurgitation will cause diagnostic confusion in a patient with either ascending or descending dissection.

Cardiac tamponade due to rupture of ascending aortic dissection into the pericardial sac causes syncope and hypotension in a significant proportion of cases. Distended neck veins, elevated central venous pressure, tachycardia, pulsus paradoxus, and hypotension are typical of tamponade. A pericardial friction rub has occasionally been described. In a patient presenting with features suggestive of tamponade, a history of abrupt onset of pain, as well as the presence of pulse deficits or the murmur of aortic regurgitation, should lead to the correct diagnosis.

External rupture of descending aortic dissection may occur into the left pleural space and cause dullness to percussion at the left base [52].

Neurologic deficits may be due to carotid compromise resulting in hemiplegia or to spinal artery occlusion leading to paraplegia. In major limb ischemia, loss of deep tendon reflexes, anesthesia, and paralysis may result [1,52].

LABORATORY FINDINGS. Tables 36-4A and 36-4B list the usual laboratory findings in aortic dissection.

Electrocardiography. There are no electrocardiographic findings specific to aortic dissection. Left ventricular hypertrophy with pressure overload due to hypertension or left ventricular diastolic overload due to prior chronic aortic regurgitation may be present. With cardiac tamponade, electrical alternans may be seen. In the case of dissection involving a coronary artery, typical ECG changes of ischemia or infarction are present. A normal ECG in a patient with ongoing severe chest pain is extremely useful in helping to exclude the major differential diagnosis—acute myocardial infarction.

Chest Radiograph. The most common finding on plain chest radiography, seen in more than 80 percent of patients with aortic dissection, is widening of the superior mediastinum due to the increased diameter of the aorta (Fig. 36-1) [1,9,53,54,55]. Unfortunately, this finding is nonspecific and is frequently seen in hypertension, aortic aneurysm, and aging. It is difficult to assess the size of the mediastinum on a portable anteroposterior chest radiograph; therefore, it is important to obtain posteroan-

Table 36-3. Physical Findings in Aortic Dissection

Finding	Ascending	Descending
Hypertension	+	+ +
Absent or changing pulses	+ +	±
Aortic regurgitation murmur	+ +	±
Left ventricular failure	+	±
Stroke	+ +	−
Shock	+ +	±
Elevated central venous pressure with pulsus paradoxus	+ +	±
Dullness at left lung base	−	+
Pericardial friction rub	±	−
Arterial compromise	+ +	±

+ = occasionally present; + + often present; ± = rarely present; − = never present.

Table 36-4A. Laboratory Findings in Acute Aortic Dissection

A. Electrocardiogram
  1. Nonspecific
     a. LVH
     b. ST–T abnormalities
  2. Absence of MI (usual)
  3. If coronary ostium involved, MI or ischemia may be seen
B. Chest radiograph
  1. Widened superior mediastinum
  2. Haziness or enlargement of aortic knob
  3. Irregular aortic contour
  4. Double density of descending aorta
  5. Separation (>5 mm) of intimal calcium from outer aortic contour
  6. Rightward displacement of trachea
  7. Enlargement of cardiac silhouette due to pericardial effusion
  8. Left pleural effusion

LVH = left ventricular hypertrophy; MI = myocardial infarction.

Table 36-4B. Laboratory Findings in Acute Aortic Dissection

	Echo/Doppler TTE and TEE	Angiography	Contrast CT	MRI
Anatomic findings				
Two lumens	+	+	+	+
Intimal flap	+	+	+	+
Aortic valve involvement	+	+	−	+
Pericardial effusion	+	−	+	+
Physiologic findings				
Site (flow through) intimal tear	+	+ cine	−	+ cine
Aortic insufficiency	+	+	−	+ cine

TTE = transthoracic echocardiography; TEE = transesophageal echocardiography; CT = computed tomography; MRI = magnetic resonance imaging

terior and lateral chest radiographs when aortic dissection is suspected. When the radiographic findings are equivocal, it is vital to obtain prior chest films for comparison.

In a small number of cases of dissection involving only the most proximal ascending aorta, the posteroanterior or anteroposterior chest radiograph may appear normal [56]. In these cases a lateral or lateral oblique film often demonstrates the dilated aorta [57]. Another explanation for the occasional normal chest film is that the false lumen may compress the true lumen, and the combined diameters may be nearly equal to the original diameter of the true lumen [9,56].

Enlargement or haziness of the aortic knob, irregularity of the aortic shadow, and/or double density of the descending aorta are seen in the majority of cases [37]. A less common but nearly diagnostic finding is the separation of intimal calcification from the outer contour of the descending aorta in the frontal plane film by more than 5 mm (calcium sign) [58]. Dilation of the aorta with intimal calcification less than 5 mm from the outer contour is more suggestive of atherosclerotic aneurysmal dilation of the aorta than of acute dissection. As Nusbacher et al. described, however, calcification of the neointima of the false lumen of dissection may occur in chronic, healed dissection and may give an appearance identical to that of atherosclerotic aneurysm [59]. Other chest radiograph findings include rightward displacement of the trachea, enlargement of cardiac silhouette due to hemopericardium, and left pleural effusion.

In summary, the chest radiograph in aortic dissection is usually abnormal if examined in light of the clinical diagnosis. The importance of obtaining posteroanterior and lateral films and comparing them to previous films cannot be overemphasized.

Echocardiography. Shortly after the first reported echocardiographic diagnosis of aortic dissection by Millward et al. [60], Nanda and co-workers published the M-mode criteria for aortic root dissection [61]. Identification of an oscillating intimal flap by Nicholson et al. in 1976 led to the description of the first specific M-mode echocardiographic finding in aortic dissection [62]. In 1981, Victor et al. published a study in which the intimal flap was demonstrated by two-dimensional echocardiography (2-D echo) in 12 of 15 patients with angiographically confirmed aortic dissection [63].

Two-dimensional echo has greatly improved identification of structures and accuracy of dimension measurements [64,65,66]. Although identification of an oscillating flap is specific for aortic dissection, the sensitivity of this finding by transthoracic echo is only 60 to 80 percent [63–67]. Using multiple transducer positions to visualize the aorta, 2-D transthoracic echo has been shown to have a 91 percent positive predictive accuracy [68,69]. False negatives occur primarily in descending aortic dissection. Color-flow Doppler study allows the demonstration of intimal tears and reentry sites as well as semiquantitation of aortic regurgitation [70].

Multiplane transesophageal echocardiography (TEE) represents a major advance in diagnosing aortic dissection by allowing visualization of the ascending aorta, aortic arch, and descending aorta [71]. After a screening transthoracic echo (mandatory in virtually all cases) to assess the proximal ascending aorta, the presence of wall motion abnormalities, pericardial effusion, and aortic insufficiency, a transesophageal echo can be performed rapidly in the emergency room or at the bedside. Local pharyngeal anesthesia and intravenous sedation with midazolam (1–2 mg) allow safe, rapid introduction of the esophageal transducer in nearly all patients. Sedation is important to prevent increases of blood pressure during intubation. Examination time averages 10 to 15 minutes. The speed and accuracy of testing has made TEE the diagnostic test of choice in a growing number of centers [72]. Several recent studies have demonstrated the technique to be fast and accurate [73–76]. Comparison with angiography and computed tomography (CT) in a large cooperative trial in 162 patients showed superior sensitivity and specificity of TEE [77].

Computed Tomography. Since the first reported cases of aortic dissection in 1979 [78,79], a number of studies have demonstrated the CT findings in aortic dissection [80–86]. These include identification of two lumens, detection of intimal flap, compression between lumens due to clotted blood in false lumen, pleural or pericardial fluid, quantification of lumen diameter, and displacement of intimal calcium. Differentiation from atherosclerotic aneurysm is not always possible, especially if the false lumen is thrombosed [84,87]. In Egan and co-workers' series of 24 cases of dissection or atherosclerotic aneurysm, CT scan was diagnostic in 15 (62.5%) [84]. However, in the eight cases ultimately proved to be dissection, only two scans were considered diagnostic.

Contrast enhancement has resulted in improved diagnostic accuracy [79,86]. Excellent results were reported in the series by Gross et al. and Heiberg et al. (11 cases in each report), with accurate diagnosis in 80 to 100 percent [82,83]. As Gross et al. pointed out, the studies reported include few patients with acute dissection of the ascending aorta. The diagnostic accuracy in two recent reports is comparable to that of aortography [88,89].

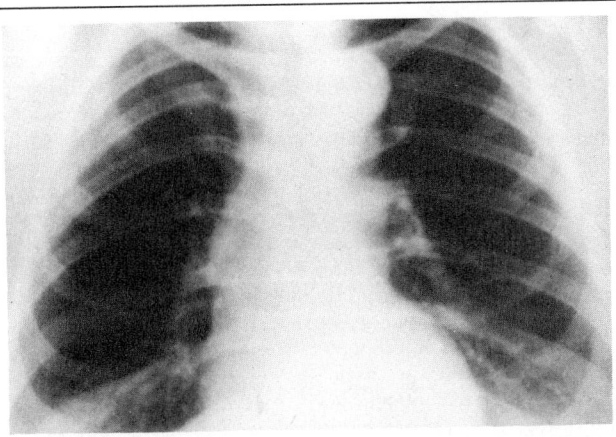

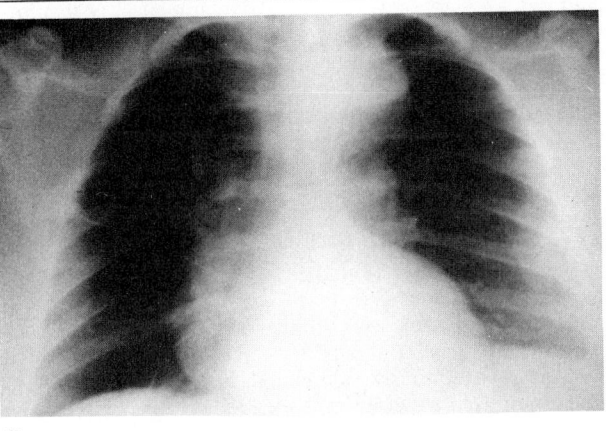

Fig. 36-1. Chest radiographs taken in a 57-year-old woman. When film taken 3 years previously (*A*) is compared with film taken at presentation with acute dissection of the ascending aorta (*B*), widening of the mediastinum is noted.

The chief limitation of CT would seem to be in dissection of the ascending aorta. Computed tomography does not demonstrate aortic valve disruption and insufficiency, which occurs in more than 50 percent of patients with ascending aortic dissection. Other problems include mistaking other structures for false lumens, streak artifacts, and poor resolution due to thick slices, giving a false impression of aortic wall thickness [90,91].

Magnetic Resonance Imaging. Magnetic resonance imaging provides superb anatomic detail of the aorta, intimal tear, and false channel. Sensitivity and specificity are as high as 98 percent [92,93]. Differences in blood flow between true and false channels may be detected through gated images. The ability to image in different planes increases anatomic definition. Another advantage is that no contrast is required for imaging. Cine MRI (cardiac-gated) is necessary to assess aortic insufficiency but significantly lengthens scanning time [93].

The major disadvantage of MRI is that because of inaccessibility to the patient and relatively long scanning times (average 30–40 minutes), unstable patients cannot be examined [94,95,96]. Nienaber et al. recently reported results of MRI, CT, and TEE in 110 patients with suspected aortic dissection. The diagnostic sensitivity and specificity of MRI were 98.3 percent and 97.8 percent, confirming the accuracy of this technique [92].

Angiography. Aortography using the transfemoral approach has historically been the definitive diagnostic procedure in the evaluation of suspected aortic dissection [97,98]. Angiographic diagnosis depends on demonstration of both the true and false lumens within the aorta [9,98,99,100]. Deformity of the true lumen by the false lumen is also seen in nearly all cases and may be the only angiographic finding suggestive of dissection in cases where the false lumen is not opacified [9]. In patients treated medically and in whom the false lumen is not opacified and is presumably thrombosed, survival appears to be enhanced. One study of patients in whom both lumens were seen in long-term follow-up study (9 months to 5 years) showed 90 percent survival in patients without false lumen opacification compared with 43 percent survival in patients in whom both lumens were seen [45].

Properly sequenced films reveal altered flow patterns between true and false lumens or in branch vessels [58]. Visualization of the intimal flap, aortic valvular incompetence, and involvement of aortic branches may likewise be demonstrated. Additional injections and use of biplane technique increase the likelihood of demonstrating the intimal tear [9,55]. Other angiographic features of aortic dissection include apparent thickening of the aortic wall by the nonopacified hematoma and abnormal catheter position. An early angiographic sign of aortic dissection may be ulcerlike projections of contrast from the lumen [101].

Problems may arise in making the diagnosis of dissection by aortography, chiefly when one fails to define the dissection adequately [48]. Occasionally the diagnosis of aortic dissection is missed if the false lumen is thrombosed and therefore not opacified. Contrast injection within the false lumen does not seem to be a cause of problems [97]. In cases of Marfan's syndrome or idiopathic cystic medionecrosis with localized dissection, extreme dilation of the ascending aorta may make angiographic diagnosis more difficult [57].

The technique of biplane cineangiography has been compared favorably to results obtained using cut-film aortography [102]. Nonrandomized studies indicate that cineangiography better defines the intimal tear and reentry sites, aortic valve morphology, and retrograde dissection [102,103]. Because of the better definition of the aortic valve leaflets and an overall superior definition of proximal aortic dissection, we employ cineangiography in patients with suspected dissection of the ascending aorta. Conventional cut-film aortography is reserved for patients with clinical evidence of dissection limited to the descending aorta.

Comparison of Imaging Techniques. The right diagnostic strategy for suspected acute aortic dissection depends on the availability of imaging techniques and experienced personnel. If all techniques are available, a screening transthoracic echocardiogram followed by TEE should be performed in all cases of suspected acute aortic dissection. In most cases of acute ascending dissection, the combined echo/Doppler techniques provide sufficient information to bring the patient to surgery without other diagnostic procedures. In some institutions the surgeons prefer confirmatory angiography and in some cases coronary angiography. Where TEE is not available, a screening transthoracic echo alone, if positive, can quickly provide important diagnostic information in many patients. The transthoracic echo may demonstrate aortic insufficiency, pericardial effusion, and, often, a proximal intimal flap. It is extremely important to recognize the sensitivity limitations of transthoracic echo, however, and perform more definitive tests if the screening transthoracic study is negative.

In many community hospitals CT scan is the primary imaging technique available and remains extremely useful in the diagnosis of aortic dissection, with high sensitivity and specificity. Visualization of the descending aorta by contrast CT is far superior to that obtained by transthoracic echo. The chief limitation of CT is in its inability to identify the intimal tear and to assess aortic insufficiency. Most patients transferred to our tertiary care center have had the diagnosis of dissection made at their community hospital by CT scan and then undergo TEE in our emergency room as the confirmatory procedure prior to surgery.

Despite strikingly superior image quality and extremely high accuracy, MRI remains the imaging procedure of choice only when patient instability is not an issue. Therefore, MRI is not employed for most acute dissections. It is especially useful for complete evaluation and close follow-up study of patients being treated medically.

Differential Diagnosis

The chest pain of dissection is most often mistaken for angina or acute myocardial infarction. In a review by Eagle and colleagues of 55 patients presenting with a clinical picture of aortic dissection but negative aortograms, 9 proved to have myocardial infarction [104]. Unlike the pain of myocardial ischemia, which usually comes on gradually and increases in severity over several minutes, the pain of aortic dissection usually begins suddenly; its severity is maximal at onset. Radiation to the back is also a frequent feature of the pain of dissection. The diagnosis of dissection rather than myocardial infarction is usually suggested when physical examination reveals pulse deficits or the murmur of aortic regurgitation, ECG fails to show evidence of myocardial infarction, and/or chest radiograph shows a wide mediastinum.

Reports of patients inadvertently receiving thrombolytic therapy for unrecognized aortic dissection thought to be acute myocardial infarction highlight the importance of accurate diagnosis. Nine of the 11 reported cases had a fatal outcome [105,106,107]. In the four cases reported by Butler and colleagues the chest radiograph was abnormal and ECG abnormalities were absent or minimal. Because of the potential consequences of thrombolytic therapy in patients with severe chest pain and equivocal ECG abnormalities in whom the diagnosis of myocardial infarction is not clear, the diagnosis of acute aortic dissection should be carefully considered.

Other causes that must be excluded when diagnosing severe chest pain include acute pulmonary embolism and spontaneous pneumothorax. Arterial blood gases, chest radiograph, and perfusion lung scan should help distinguish acute pulmonary embolism and spontaneous pneumothorax from dissection. Other causes of severe chest pain are acute pancreatitis, penetrating duodenal ulcer, pleurodynia, and pericarditis. Rarely, in patients with pulmonary hypertension, dissection of the pulmonary artery may occur and mimic aortic dissection or acute myocardial infarction [108].

Pulse deficits without chest or back pain should suggest another diagnosis. Pulse deficits alone are usually due to chronic atherosclerotic peripheral vascular disease, in which the presence of vascular bruits and a history of claudication suggest the diagnosis. Arterial embolism may cause acute vascular insufficiency and should lead to a search for the presence of predisposing conditions, such as atrial fibrillation, mitral valve disease, or myocardial infarction. Although vascular compromise is common in dissection, it is usually asymptomatic and often detected only by physical examination and confirmed by angiography. Therefore, although pulse deficits are highly sug-

gestive when found, the lack of pulse deficits should not be weighed too heavily as evidence against the diagnosis of dissection, particularly when the clinical picture is suggestive of dissection limited to the descending aorta.

When cerebral ischemia or infarction is caused by dissection, there is still usually chest pain and other evidence of dissection. In 272 consecutive patients treated surgically at Stanford, only 7 (of 128 type A dissections) had a new stroke before surgery [109]. In the rare case where stroke is the presenting symptom (2 of 124 patients in the Massachusetts General Hospital series and 3 of 236 in the Mayo Clinic series), careful examination of the chest radiograph should be helpful [5,34].

Acute cardiac tamponade with severe chest pain due to aortic dissection must be differentiated from other causes of tamponade with chest pain, such as acute viral or idiopathic pericarditis or acute myocardial infarction with external myocardial rupture. The history of fever or gradual onset of pleuritic pain would suggest pericarditis. Electrocardiographic evidence of infarction would point toward acute myocardial infarction. It is also important to look for an aortic diastolic murmur, since ascending aortic dissection causing tamponade will cause aortic insufficiency in most cases.

Syncope, shock, or collapse is the presenting symptom in a significant number of cases and is usually caused by cardiac tamponade due to rupture of the dissection into the pericardial cavity. The differential diagnosis of hypotension with elevated central venous pressure includes cardiac tamponade, acute massive pulmonary embolism, right ventricular infarction, and cardiogenic shock.

A normal aortic contour on chest radiograph is extremely useful in helping to exclude the diagnosis of aortic dissection in cases where the clinical picture is unclear. In any case where the diagnosis is seriously entertained, further diagnostic tests must be performed to confirm or exclude dissection.

Treatment

In few medical conditions is survival as dependent on rapid diagnosis and institution of treatment as in acute aortic dissection. Untreated, acute dissection has an extremely rapid, usually fatal clinical course. In Jamieson and co-workers' series of 43 patients diagnosed at autopsy as having acute dissection of the ascending aorta, the time from presentation to death was less than 24 hours in 72 percent [8]. In contrast, in Roberts and Roberts' report of 40 necropsy patients with entrance tears in the descending thoracic aorta the interval from aortic dissection to death was more than 30 days in 18 (58%) of 31 patients not treated with surgery. Twenty-two of the 31 were diagnosed at necropsy [46]. We know from Hirst et al.'s collected series that the mortality rate for untreated acute aortic dissection is 21 percent at 24 hours and 74 percent at 2 weeks [1]. McCloy et al. reported similar data from the Mayo Clinic: 30 percent at 24 hours and 63 percent at 2 weeks [3]. The term *acute dissection* has been generally applied to cases presenting within 2 weeks of the onset of symptoms.

In 1955, DeBakey and co-workers published results of the first surgical correction of aortic dissection [110]. Subsequent results in 1965 showed a surgical mortality rate of 40 percent for acute ascending dissection (10 cases) [42]. Dissatisfied with poor surgical results, Wheat and associates developed an aggressive medical approach [111]. The rationale for medical treatment, sometimes called "anti-impulse" therapy, has been supported by results of laboratory investigations of the effects of dp/dt (myocardial contractility) and blood pressure on the propagation of dissection [47,48,112]. Wheat et al. originally recommended that all patients receive medical therapy unless contraindicated by the presence of severe congestive heart failure due to aortic insufficiency, significant arterial compromise, or significant hemorrhage. These complications occur, however, in most patients with dissection of the ascending aorta, making them ineligible for purely medical management treatment. Dalen et al. reviewed the treatment of aortic dissection at the Peter Bent Brigham Hospital between 1963 and 1973 and found that 84 percent of patients with dissection of the ascending aorta had contraindications to medical therapy, compared with none of the patients with dissection of the descending aorta [7]. Surgery is now widely accepted as the primary treatment for dissection of the ascending aorta. Treatment for dissection of the descending aorta, on the other hand, in the absence of complications is usually medical [4,7,113–116]. The results of surgery for aortic dissection have improved over time [8,10,30,42,43,117–124].

One of the main goals in surgical treatment of ascending aortic dissection is to repair or replace the ascending aorta, thereby preventing retrograde dissection into the pericardial space and cardiac tamponade, the chief cause of death [125,126]. Preliminary results using surgical glue instead of replacement in 15 patients with type A dissection suggest this technique may become an alternative in selected patients [127]. Aortic valve resuspension or reconstruction is preferred to replacement and is usually possible except in cases of Marfan's syndrome or aortic root dilatation [10,117,118,128,129,130]. The operative mortality rate for acute ascending dissection is now reported to be in the range of 8 to 25 percent [8,10,44,117,118,120,131]. From 1976 to 1981, the Stanford group's operative mortality rate for 24 patients with acute ascending dissection was 8 percent, with actuarial 5-year survivals of 75 percent [132].

While there is general agreement on the choice of surgical therapy for the treatment of acute dissection of the ascending aorta, there is some controversy regarding treatment of dissection confined to the descending aorta [133]. With medical therapy, the short-term survival rate for acute dissection of the descending aorta is reported as high as 80 percent [43,44,121]; however, as many as 30 to 50 percent of patients have progression of dissection despite intensive drug therapy and require either emergency or elective surgery [9,44,113,134]. Examination of late survival of patients treated for acute dissection of the descending aorta reveals a high complication rate in patients treated medically in some series [135]. Results of the medical and surgical management of descending aortic dissection continue to be studied and published in efforts to define optimal therapy [136–142]. As operative mortality for acute descending dissection has fallen, some groups propose early elective surgical intervention after initial stabilization [10,135]. Definite indications for surgical treatment include failure to control pain, progressive dissection, expansion, and rupture or arterial compromise (Table 36-5). Miller and co-workers pointed out the paradox of using the same markers of high operative mortality as indicators for surgery. Patients with failed medical treatment of acute descending dissection have a predicted surgical mortality of 75 percent, compared with 11 to 39 percent [143].

In all patients except those who are hypotensive, initial management of acute aortic dissection is directed at lowering myocardial contractility and systemic arterial pressure, the two factors most important in the progression of dissection. Intensive medical treatment should be instituted as soon as the clinical diagnosis of acute dissection is made and should not be delayed prior to definitive testing (Table 36-6).

Initial management of patients with suspected acute aortic dissection includes establishing venous access and continuous

Table 36-5. Indications for Surgery

1. Ascending aorta involvement
2. Contraindications to myocardial depressants
   a. Aortic insufficiency
   b. Left ventricular failure
3. External rupture
   a. Hemopericardium
   b. Hemothorax
   c. Other
4. Arterial compromise
   a. Limb ischemia
   b. Renal failure
   c. Cerebral ischemia or infarction
5. Progression
   a. Continued pain
   b. Expansion of dissecting hematoma as seen on chest radiograph, computed tomography, or magnetic resonance imaging

Table 36-6. Initial Medical Therapy for Acute Aortic Dissection

Drug	Dosage
One of: Propranolol hydrochloride	0.5 mg IV test dose; 1.0 mg q5 min until HR<60/min; repeat as needed q2–3h
Esmolol	500 mg/kg/min IV for 1 min followed by 50 mg/kg/min for 4 min; titrate upward by repeat of same loading dose with 50 mg/kg/min incremental increases in maintenance dose
Labetalol	0.25 mg/kg IV over 2 min; 40–80 mg q10 min up to 300 mg; continuous infusion 2 mg/min according to BP
In combination with: Sodium nitroprusside	25 mg/min IV; titrate by 25 mg/min increments q3–5 min to achieve systolic BP 100–120 mm Hg (Caution: urine output and mental status must be monitored)
Alternate treatment to above combination: Trimethaphan	1–2 mg/min IV; titrate

HR = heart rate.

blood pressure and urine output monitoring. A Foley catheter should be inserted to monitor urine output. The goal of therapy is to lower the blood pressure. Despite adequate blood pressure lowering, nitroprusside increases myocardial contractility and thereby causes progression of dissection in some cases. To avoid this undesired effect of nitroprusside, adequate beta blockade is essential and should be initiated prior to infusing nitroprusside. Intravenous propranolol, labetalol, or esmolol may be administered to achieve beta blockade (Table 36-6). After a test dose of 0.5 mg propranolol given intravenously, doses in further increments of 1 mg are given every 5 minutes until the heart rate is slowed, usually to 60 to 72 beats per minute. As soon as this is accomplished, intravenous sodium nitroprusside administration is begun at 25 µg per minute and titrated upward to a maximum of 1 mg per minute to reduce systolic blood pressure to 100 to 120 mm Hg. More recently, intravenous labetalol and alpha- and beta-adrenergic blockers have been used in acute treatment of aortic dissection. The very short-acting beta-blocker esmolol has the potential advantage of nearly immediate elimination of effect when the infusion is stopped. In patients with contraindications (e.g., asthma) to beta-blocking drugs, calcium-blocking drugs may be considered, although few data are available. One report of the successful use of nifedipine to control severe hypertension suggests these drugs may be useful [144]. Careful monitoring of urine output and mental status is important to determine how low a systolic pressure can be safely tolerated. The goal is to maintain vital organ perfusion at the lowest possible pressures. In patients with hypotension, a Swan-Ganz catheter may be used to evaluate filling pressures and cardiac output.

An alternative regimen employs trimethaphan, 1 to 2 mg per minute, as an initial intravenous infusion. Unlike nitroprusside, trimethaphan does not increase, but rather tends to decrease, myocardial contractility. Rapid development of tachyphylaxis has led to trimethaphan becoming second-choice therapy in most centers.

Patients who present with hypotension are likely to have hemopericardium with tamponade or rupture into the left pleural space. In these patients, intravenous volume should be expanded with saline, colloid, or lactated Ringer's solution. Beta blockade and nitroprusside should not be used until hemodynamic stability is restored. In patients with aortic regurgitation and congestive heart failure, myocardial depressants should not be given.

The goals of medical therapy are to stop the spread of the intramural hematoma and prevent rupture. Control of pain is one of the best indications that these goals have been attained. Continued pain usually means ongoing dissection. Other indications of ongoing dissection and failure of medical therapy are enlargement of aneurysm on chest radiograph, loss of a pulse, development of a stroke, renal failure, aortic insufficiency, or congestive heart failure. Hypotension may signal rupture, as may the development of a pericardial friction rub. Inability to control blood pressure is considered a relative failure.

Immediate surgery as previously discussed is recommended in all ascending aortic dissections in the absence of contraindications (Table 36-5). Patients with uncomplicated dissection limited to the descending aorta should be managed with intensive parenteral drug therapy in the intensive care unit for 48 to 72 hours, then treated with an oral regimen of beta-blockers and other antihypertensive medication as necessary. Careful monitoring is essential in this group. Even if asymptomatic, patients who develop evidence of expansion, complications, or continued dissection should immediately undergo surgery.

References

1. Hirst AE Jr, Johns VJ Jr, Kime SW Jr: Dissecting aneurysm of the aorta: A review of 505 cases. *Medicine* 37:217, 1958.
2. Levinson DC, Edmeades DT, Griffith GC: Dissecting aneurysm of aorta: Its clinical, electrocardiographic and laboratory features: Report of fifty-eight autopsied cases. *Circulation* 1:360, 1950.
3. McCloy RM, Spittell JA Jr, McGoon DC: The prognosis in aortic dissection (dissecting aortic hematoma or aneurysm). *Circulation* 31:665, 1965.
4. Anagnostopoulos CE, Prabhakar MJS, Kittle CF: Aortic dissections and dissecting aneurysms. *Am J Cardiol* 30:263, 1972.
5. Slater EE, DeSanctis RW: The clinical recognition of dissecting aortic aneurysm. *Am J Med* 60:629, 1975.
6. Lindsay J Jr, Hurst JW: Clinical features and prognosis in dissecting aneurysm of the aorta: A re-appraisal. *Circulation* 35:880, 1967.
7. Dalen JE, Alpert JS, Cohn LH, et al: Dissection of the thoracic aorta: Medical or surgical therapy? *Am J Cardiol* 34:803,1974.
8. Jamieson WRE, Munro AI, Miyagishima RT, et al: Aortic dissection: Early diagnosis and surgical management are the keys to survival. *Can J Surg* 25:145, 1982.
9. Earnest F IV, Muhm JR, Sheedy PF II: Roentgenographic findings in thoracic aortic dissection: *Mayo Clin Proc* 54:43, 1979.
10. Miller DC, Stinson EB, Oyer PE, et al: Operative treatment of aortic dissections: Experience with 125 patients over a sixteen-year period. *J Thorac Cardiovasc Surg* 78:365, 1979.
11. Doroghazi RM, Slater EE, DeSanctis RW, et al: Long-term survival of patients with treated aortic dissection. *J Am Coll Cardiol* 3:1026, 1984.
12. DeBakey ME, McCollum CH, Crawford ES, et al: Dissection and dissecting aneurysms of the aorta: Twenty-year follow-up of five hundred twenty-seven patients treated surgically. *Surgery* 92:1118, 1982.
13. Crawford ES, Svensson LG, Coselli JS, et al: Aortic dissection and dissecting aortic aneurysms. *Ann Surg* 208:254, 1988.
14. Nakashima Y, Kurozumi T, Sueishi K, et al: Dissecting aneurysm. *Hum Pathol* 21:291, 1990.
15. Murdoch JL, Walker BA, Halpern BL, et al: Life expectancy and causes of death in the Marfan syndrome. *N Engl J Med* 286:804, 1972.
16. Wilson SK, Hutchins GM: Aortic dissecting aneurysms: Causative factors in 204 subjects. *Arch Pathol Lab Med* 106:175, 1982.
17. Rottino A: Medial degeneration of the aorta: A study of two hundred and ten routine autopsy specimens by a serial block method. *Arch Pathol* 28:377, 1939.
18. Hirst AE, Johns VJ: Experimental dissection of media of aorta by pressure: Its relation to spontaneous dissecting aneurysm. *Circ Res* 10:897, 1962.
19. Murray CA, Edwards JE: Spontaneous laceration of ascending aorta: *Circulation* 47:848, 1973.
20. Braunstein H: Pathogenesis of dissecting aneurysm. *Circulation* 28:1071, 1963.
21. Larson EW, Edwards WD: Risk factors for aortic dissection: A necropsy study of 161 cases. *Am J Cardiol* 53:849, 1984.
22. Schlatmann TJM, Becker AE: Pathogenesis of dissecting aneurysm of aorta: Comparative histopathologic study of significant medial changes. *Am J Cardiol* 39:21, 1977.
23. Schlatmann TJM, Becker AE: Histologic changes in the normal aging aorta: Implications for dissecting aortic aneurysm. *Am J Cardiol* 39:13, 1977.
24. Carlson RG, Lillehei CW, Edwards JE: Cystic medial necrosis of the ascending aorta in relation to age and hypertension. *Am J Cardiol* 25:411, 1970.
25. Boucek RJ, Nobel NL, Gunja-Smith Z, et al: The Marfan syndrome: A deficiency in chemically stable collagen cross links. *N Engl J Med* 305:988, 1981.
26. Roberts WC: Aortic dissection: Anatomy, consequences, and causes. *Am Heart J* 101:195, 1981.
27. Whittle MA, Haselton PS, Anderson JC, et al: Collagen in dissecting aneurysms of the human thoracic aorta. *Am J Cardiovasc Pathol* 4: 311, 1990.
28. Francomano CA, Streeter EA, Meyers DA, et al: Exclusion of fibrillar procollagens as causes of the Marfan syndrome. *Am J Med Genet* 29:457, 1988.
29. Nakashima Y, Sueishi K: Alteration of elastic architecture in lathyritic rat aorta implies the pathogenesis of aortic dissecting aneurysm. *Am J Pathol* 140:959, 1992.
30. St John Sutton M, Oldershaw PJ, Miller GAH, et al: Dissection of the thoracic aorta: A comparison between medical and surgical treatment. *J Cardiovasc Surg* 22:195, 1981.
31. Leonard JC, Haselton PS: Dissecting aortic aneurysms: Clinicopathological study. I. Clinical and gross pathologic findings. *Q J Med* 48:55, 1979.
32. Comino A, Ciravegna G, Mollo F: Aortic dissection at autopsy: A fifty-four year survey in Torino. *Giornale Italiano Di Cardiologia* 16:510, 1986.
33. Roberts CS, Roberts WC: Dissection of the aorta associated with congenital malformation of the aortic valve. *J Am Coll Cardiol* 17:712, 1991.
34. Spittell, PC, Spittell JA, Joyce JW, et al: Clinical features and differential diagnosis of aortic dissection experience with 236 cases (1980 through 1990) *Mayo Clin Proc* 68:642, 1993.
35. Fukuda T, Tadavarthy SM, Edwards JE: Dissecting aneurysm of aorta complicating aortic valvular stenosis. *Circulation* 53:169, 1976.

36. Edwards WD, Leaf DS, Edwards JE: Dissecting aortic aneurysm associated with congenital bicuspid aortic valve. *Circulation* 57:1022, 1978.

37. Hainer JW, Hamilton GW: Aortic abnormalities in relapsing polychondritis. Report of a case with dissecting aortic aneurysm. *N Engl J Med* 280:1166, 1969.

38. Simons AJ, Arazoza E, Hare CL, et al: Circumferential aortic dissection in a young woman. *Am Heart J* 123:1077, 1992.

39. Erbel R, Bednarczyk I, Pop T, et al: Detection of dissection of the aortic intima and media after angioplasty of coarctation of the aorta. *Circulation* 81:805, 1990.

40. Orszulak TA, Pluth JR, Schaff HV: Results of surgical treatment of ascending aortic dissections occurring late after cardiac operation. *J Thorac Cardiovasc Surg* 83:538, 1982.

41. Still RJ, Hilgenberg AD, Akins CW, et al: Intraoperative aortic dissection. *Ann Thorac Surg* 53:374, 1992.

42. DeBakey ME, Henly WS, Cooley DA, et al: Surgical management of dissecting aneurysms of the aorta. *J Thorac Cardiovasc Surg* 49:130, 1965.

43. Daily PO, Trueblood HW, Stinson EB, et al: Management of acute aortic dissections. *Ann Thorac Surg* 10:237, 1970.

44. Dalen JE, Pape LA, Cohn LH, et al: Dissection of the aorta: Pathogenesis, diagnosis, and treatment. *Prog Cardiovasc Dis* 23:237, 1980.

45. Dinsmore RE, Willerson JT, Buckley MJ: Dissecting aneurysm of the aorta: Aortographic features affecting prognosis. *Radiology* 105:567, 1972.

46. Roberts CS, Roberts WC: Aortic dissection with the entrance tear in the descending thoracic aorta. *Ann Surg* 213:356, 1990.

47. Prokop EK, Palmer RF, Wheat MW Jr: Hydrodynamic forces in dissecting aneurysm: In vitro studies in a Tygon model and in dog aortas. *Circ Res* 27:121, 1970.

48. Carney WI Jr, Rheinlander HF, Cleveland RJ: Control of acute aortic dissection. *Surgery* 78:114, 1975

49. Cipriano PR, Griepp RB: Acute retrograde dissection of the ascending thoracic aorta. *Am J Cardiol* 43:520, 1979.

50. Prendes JL: Neurovascular syndromes of aortic dissection. *Am Fam Physician* 23:175, 1981.

51. Cambria RP, Brewster DC, Gertler J, et al: Vascular complications associated with spontaneous aortic dissection (review). *J Vasc Surg* 7:199, 1988.

52. Gore I, Hirst AE Jr: Dissecting aneurysm of the aorta. *Cardiovasc Clin* 5:239, 1973.

53. Smith DC, Jang GC: Radiological diagnosis of aortic dissection, in Doroghazi RM, Slater EE (eds): *Aortic Dissection*. New York, McGraw-Hill, 1983.

54. Beachley MC, Ranniger K, Roth FJ: Roentgenographic evaluation of dissecting aneurysms of the aorta. *Am J Roentgenol Radium Ther Nucl Med* 121:617, 1974.

55. Itzchak Y, Rosenthal T, Raphael A, et al: Dissecting aneurysm of thoracic aorta: Reappraisal of radiologic diagnosis. *Am J Roentgenol Radium Ther Nucl Med* 125:559, 1975.

56. Dinsmore RE, Rourke JA, DeSanctis RW: Angiographic findings in dissecting aortic aneurysm. *N Engl J Med* 275:1152, 1966.

57. Eisen S, Elliott LP: The roentgenology of cystic medial necrosis of the ascending aorta. *Radiol Clin North Am* 6:437, 1968.

58. Eyler WR, Clark MD: Dissecting aneurysm of the aorta: Roentgen manifestations including a comparison with other types. *Radiology* 85:1047, 1965.

59. Nusbacher N, Bockel R, Byrk D: Chronic calcified aortic dissection. *Chest* 69:235, 1976.

60. Millward DK, Robinson NJ, Craig E: Dissecting aortic aneurysm diagnosed by echocardiography in a patient with rupture of the aneurysm into the right atrium. *Am J Cardiol* 30:427, 1972.

61. Nanda NC, Gramiak R, Shah PM: Diagnosis of aortic root dissection by echocardiography. *Circulation* 48:506, 1973.

62. Nicholson WJ, Cobbs BW Jr: Echocardiographic oscillating flap in aortic root dissecting aneurysm. *Chest* 70:305, 1976.

63. Victor MF, Mintz GS, Kotler MN, et al: Two-dimensional echocardiographic diagnosis of aortic dissection. *Am J Cardiol* 48:1155, 1981.

64. DeMaria AN, Bommer W, Neuman A, et al: Identification and localization of aneurysms of the ascending aorta by cross-sectional echocardiography. *Circulation* 59:755, 1979.

65. Come PC: Improved cross-sectional echocardiographic technique for visualization of the retrocardiac descending aorta in its long axis: Normal findings and abnormalities in saccular and/or dissecting aneurysms. *Am J Cardiol* 51:1029, 1983.

66. Roudaut RP, Billes MA, Gosse P, et al: Accuracy of M-mode and two-dimensional echocardiography in the diagnosis of aortic dissection: An experience with 128 cases. *Clin Cardiol* 11:553, 1988.

67. Smuckler AL, Nomeier AM, Watts LE, et al: Echocardiographic diagnosis of aortic root dissection by M-mode and two-dimensional techniques. *Am Heart J* 103:897, 1982.

68. Khandheria BK, Tajik AJ, Taylor CL, et al: Aortic dissection: Review of value and limitations of two-dimensional echocardiography in a six-year experience. *J Am Soc Echo* 2:17, 1989.

69. Granato JE, Dee P, Gibson RS: Utility of two-dimensional echocardiography in suspected aortic dissection. *Am J Cardiol* 56:123, 1985.

70. Iliceto S, Nanda NC, Rizzon P, et al: Color Doppler evaluation of aortic dissection. *Circulation* 75:748, 1987.

71. Seward JB, Khandheria BK, Oh JK, et al: Transesophageal echocardiography: Technique, anatomic correlations, implementation, and clinical applications. *Mayo Clin Proc* 63:649, 1988.

72. Kotler MN: Is transesophageal echocardiography the new standard for diagnosing aortic aneurysms? (editorial). *J Am Coll Cardiol* 14:1263, 1989.

73. Engberding R, Bender F, Grosse-Heitmeyer W, et al: Identification of dissection or aneurysm of the descending thoracic aorta by conventional and transesophageal two-dimensional echocardiography. *Am J Cardiol* 59:717, 1987.

74. Hashimoto S, Kumada T, Osakada G, et al: Assessment of transesophageal Doppler echography in dissecting aortic aneurysm. *J Am Coll Cardiol* 14:1253, 1989.

75. Adachi H, Kyo S, Takamoto S, et al: Early diagnosis and surgical intervention of acute aortic dissection by transesophageal color flow mapping. *Circulation* 82:IV-19, 1982.

76. Ballal RS, Nanda NC, Gatewood R, et al: Usefulness of transesophageal echocardiography in assessment of aortic dissection. *Circulation* 84:1903, 1991.

77. Erbel R, Engberding R, Daniel W, et al: Echocardiography in diagnosis of aortic dissection. *Lancet* 1:457, 1989.

78. Harris RD, Usselman JA, Vint VC, et al: Computerized tomographic diagnosis of aneurysms of the thoracic aorta. *Comput Tomogr* 3:81, 1979.

79. Guthaner DF, Ricci M, Brody WR, et al: The use of computed tomography in the evaluation of aortic dissection, abstract. *Circulation* 60(suppl II):27, 1979.

80. Sanders JH, Malare S, Nieman HL, et al: Thoracic aortic imaging without angiography. *Arch Surg* 14:1326, 1979.

81. Larde D, Belloir C, Vasile N, et al: Computed tomography in dissection of the thoracic aorta. *Radiology* 136:147, 1980.

82. Gross SC, Barr I, Eyler WR, et al: Computed tomography in dissection of the thoracic aorta. *Radiology* 136:135, 1980.

83. Heiberg E, Wolverson M, Sundaram M, et al: CT findings in thoracic aortic dissection. *Am J Roentgenol* 136:13, 1981.

84. Egan TJ, Neiman HL, Herman RJ, et al: Computed tomography in the diagnosis of aortic aneurysm, dissection or traumatic injury. *Radiology* 136:141, 1980.

85. Suchato C, Pekanan P, Singjaroen T, et al: Indication of dissecting aortic aneurysm on noncontrast computed tomography. *J Comput Assist Tomogr* 4:115, 1980.

86. Moncada R, Churchill R, Reynes C, et al: Diagnosis of dissecting aortic aneurysm by computed tomography. *Lancet* 1:238, 1981.

87. Machida K, Tasaka A: CT patterns of mural thrombus in aortic aneurysms. *J Comput Assist Tomogr* 4:840, 1980.

88. Thorsen MK, San Dretto MA, Lawson TL, et al: Dissecting aortic aneurysms: Accuracy of computed tomographic diagnosis. *Radiology* 148:773, 1983.

89. White RD, Lipton MJ, Higgins CB, et al: Noninvasive evaluation of suspected thoracic aortic disease contrast-enhanced computed tomography. *Am J Cardiol* 57:282, 1986.

90. Godwin JD, Breiman RS, Speckman JM: Problems and pitfalls in the evaluation of thoracic aortic dissection by computed tomography. *J Comput Assist Tomogr* 6:750, 1982.

91. Godwin JD, Herfkens RJ, Skioldebrand CG, et al: Evaluation of

dissections and aneurysms of the thoracic aorta by conventional dynamic CT scanning. *Radiology* 136:125, 1980.

92. Nienaber CA, Vondlitsch Y, Nicolas V, et al: The diagnosis of thoracic aortic dissection by noninvasive imaging procedures. *N Engl J Med* 328:1, 1993.

93. Nienaber CA, Spielmann RP, von Kodolitsch Y, et al: Diagnosis of thoracic aortic dissection. *Circulation* 85:434, 1992.

94. Amparo EG, Higgins CB, Hricak H, et al: Aortic dissection: Magnetic resonance imaging. *Radiology* 155:399, 1985.

95. Geisinger MA, Risius B, O'Donnell JA, et al: Thoracic aortic dissections: Magnetic resonance imaging. *Radiology* 155:407, 1985.

96. Kersting-Sommerhoff BA, Higgins CB, White RD: Aortic dissection: Sensitivity and specificity of MR imaging. *Radiology* 166:651, 1988.

97. Shuford WH, Sybers RG, Weens HS: Problems in the aortographic diagnosis of dissecting aneurysm of the aorta. *N Engl J Med* 280:225, 1969.

98. Soto B, Harman MA, Ceballos R, et al: Angiographic diagnosis of dissecting aneurysm of the aorta. *Am J Roentgenol* 116:146, 1972.

99. Hemley SD, Kanick V, Kittredge RD, et al: Dissecting aneurysms of the thoracic aorta: Their angiographic demonstration. *Am J Roentgenol* 91:1263, 1964.

100. Guthaner DF, Brody WR, Miller DC: Intravenous aortography after aortic dissection repair. *Am J Radiol* 137:1019, 1981.

101. Tisnado J, Cho SR, Beachley MC, et al: Ulcerlike projections: A precursor angiographic sign to thoracic aortic dissection. *Am J Radiol* 135:719, 1980.

102. Gutierrez FR, Gowda S, Ludbrok PA, et al: Cineangiography in the diagnosis and evaluation of aortic dissection. *Radiology* 135:759, 1980.

103. Arciniegas JG, Soto B, Little WC, et al: Cineangiography in the diagnosis of aortic dissection. *Am J Cardiol* 47:890, 1981.

104. Eagle KA, Quertermous T, Kritzer GA, et al: Spectrum of conditions initially suggesting acute aortic dissection but with negative aortograms. *Am J Cardiol* 57:322, 1986.

105. Wilcox RG, Olsson CG, Skene AM, et al: Trial of tissue plasminogen activator for mortality reduction in acute myocardial infarction: Anglo-Scandinavian study of early thrombolysis. *Lancet* 2:525, 1980.

106. Butler J, Davies AH, Westaby S: Streptokinase in acute aortic dissection. *Br Med J* 300:517, 1990.

107. Kahn JK: Inadvertent thrombolytic therapy for cardiovascular diseases masquerading as acute coronary thrombosis. *Clin Cardiol* 16:67, 1993.

108. Steurer J, Jenni R, Medici TC, et al: Dissecting aneurysm of the pulmonary artery with pulmonary hypertension. *Am Rev Respir Dis* 142:1219, 1990.

109. Fann JI, Sarris GE, Miller DC, et al: Surgical management of acute aortic dissection complicated by stroke. *Circulation* 80(suppl I):I-257, 1989.

110. DeBakey ME, Cooley DA, Creech O Jr: Surgical considerations of dissecting aneurysm of the aorta. *Ann Surg* 142:586, 1955.

111. Wheat MW Jr, Palmer RF, Bartley TD: Treatment of dissecting aneurysms of the aorta without surgery. *J Thorac Cardiovasc Surg* 50:364, 1965.

112. Moran JF, Derkac WM, Conkle DM: Pharmacologic control of acute aortic dissection in hypertensive dogs. *Surg Forum* 39:74, 1971.

113. Wolfe WG, Moran JF: The evolution of medical and surgical management of acute aortic dissection (editorial). *Circulation* 56:503, 1977.

114. Kolff J, Bates RJ, Balderman SC: Acute aortic arch dissection: Reevaluation of the indications for medical and surgical therapy. *Am J Cardiol* 39:727, 1977.

115. Sanderson CJ, Rich S, Beere PA: Clotted false lumen: Reappraisal of indications for medical management of acute aortic dissection. *Thorax* 36:194, 1981.

116. McFarland J, Willerson JT, Dinsmore RE: The medical treatment of dissecting aortic aneurysm. *N Engl J Med* 286:116, 1972.

117. Cachera JP, Vouhe PR, Loisance DY, et al: Surgical management of acute dissections involving the ascending aorta: Early and late results in 38 patients. *J Thorac Cardiovasc Surg* 82:576, 1981.

118. Wolfe WG: Acute ascending aortic dissection. *Ann Surg* 192:658, 1980.

119. Reul GJ Jr, Cooley DA, Hallman GL, et al: Dissecting aneurysm of the descending aorta: Improved surgical results in 91 patients. *Arch Surg* 110:632, 1975.

120. Doroghazi RM, Slater EE: Long-term survival for 184 patients with treated aortic dissection (abstract). *Am J Cardiol* 45:489, 1980.

121. Thomas CJ Jr, Alford WC Jr, Burrus GR: The effectiveness of surgical treatment of acute aortic dissection. *Ann Thorac Surg* 26:42, 1978.

122. Austen WG, DeSanctis RW: Surgical treatment of dissecting aneurysm of the thoracic aorta. *N Engl J Med* 272:1314, 1965.

123. Culliford AT, Ayvaliotis B, Shemin R: Aneurysms of the ascending aorta and transverse arch. *J Thorac Cardiovasc Surg* 83:701, 1982.

124. Mills SE, Teja K, Crosby IK: Aortic dissection: Surgical and nonsurgical treatments compared: Analysis of 74 cases at the University of Virginia. *Am J Surg* 137:240, 1979.

125. Cabrol C, Pavie A, Gandjbakhch I, et al: Complete replacement of the ascending aorta with reimplantation of the coronary arteries. *J Thorac Cardiovasc Surg* 81:309, 1981.

126. Bentall M, DeBono A: A technique for complete replacement of ascending aorta. *Thorax* 23:338, 1968.

127. Fabiani J-N, Jebara VA, Deloche A, et al: Use of surgical glue without replacement in the treatment of type A aortic dissection. *Circulation* 80(suppl I):I-264, 1989.

128. Svensson LG, Crawford ES, Coselli JS, et al: Impact of cardiovascular operation on survival in the Marfan patient. *Circulation* 80(suppl I):I-233, 1989.

129. Collins JJ, Cohn LH: Reconstruction of the aortic valve: Correcting valve incompetence due to acute dissecting aneurysm. *Arch Surg* 106:35, 1973.

130. Koster JK Jr, Cohn LH, Mee RBB, et al: Late results of operation for acute aortic dissection producing aortic insufficiency. *Ann Thorac Surg* 26:461, 1978.

131. Meng RL, Najafi H, Javid H: Acute ascending aortic dissection: Surgical management. *Circulation* 64(suppl II):231, 1981.

132. Miller DC: Surgical management of aortic dissections: Indications, perioperative management and long term results, in Doroghazi RM, Slater EE (eds): *Aortic Dissection.* New York, McGraw-Hill, 1983.

133. Jex RK, Schaff HV, Piehler JM, et al: Early and late results following repair of dissections of the descending thoracic aorta. *J Vasc Surg* 3:226, 1986.

134. Crawford ES, Walker HSJ III, Saleh SA: Graft replacement of aneurysm in descending thoracic aorta: Results without bypass or shunting. *Surgery* 89:73, 1981.

135. Appelbaum A, Karp RB, Kirklin JW: Ascending vs descending aortic dissections. *Ann Surg* 183:296, 1976.

136. Glower DD, Fann JI, Speier RH, et al: Comparison of medical and surgical therapy for uncomplicated descending aortic dissection. *Circulation* 82(suppl IV):IV-39, 1990.

137. Svensson LG, Crawford ES, Hess KR, et al: Dissection of the aorta and dissecting aortic aneurysms. *Circulation* 82(suppl IV):IV-24, 1990.

138. Tanaka K, Takano T, Sasaki K, et al: Medical vs surgical treatment of acute aortic dissection in an intensive care unit. *Jp Circ J* 55:815, 1991.

139. Cooley DA: Panel 3: Aortic dissection. *Semin Thorac Cardiovasc Surg* 3:251, 1991.

140. Masuda Y, Yamada Z, Morooka N, et al: *Circulation* 84(supp III):III-7, 1991.

141. Hara K, Yamaguchi T, Wanibuchi Y, et al: The roles of medical treatment of distal type aortic dissection. *Int J Cardiol* 32:231, 1991.

142. Neya K, Omoto R, Kyo S, et al: Peripheral and thoracic aortic disease: Outcome of Stanford type B acute aortic dissection. *Circulation* 86(suppl II):II-1, 1992.

143. Miller DC, Mitchell RS, Oyer PE, et al: Independent determinants of operative mortality for patients with aortic dissections. *Circulation* 70(suppl I):I-153, 1984.

144. White SR, Hall JB: Control of hypertension with nifedipine in the setting of aortic dissection. *Chest* 88: 780, 1985.

37. Acute Aortic Insufficiency

Joseph S. Alpert and Joseph R. Benotti

Aortic insufficiency (AI) manifests in a variety of ways (Fig. 37-1). At one end of the spectrum is the patient with chronic hemodynamically significant AI who may be asymptomatic, with only a heart murmur and/or evidence of progressive cardiac enlargement. He or she may subsequently develop symptoms of congestive heart failure. This patient is usually easily recognized because in the absence of congestive heart failure, he or she displays the often described findings of chronic severe AI, recognized since the time of Corrigan [1,2]. At the opposite end of the spectrum is the patient who presents with acute, severe AI resulting from destruction or disruption of a previously normal aortic valve. Acute AI is usually the result of infective endocarditis, dissection of the ascending aorta, trauma, or spontaneous rupture of a myxomatous valve. Such patients invariably develop congestive heart failure, which is often refractory to medical therapy; they require urgent aortic valve replacement. The patient with acute, severe AI, despite the presence of congestive heart failure, may be very difficult to identify. In such cases, torrential AI pours into a normal left ventricle lacking dilatation, hypertrophy, and the usually associated increase in ventricular compliance. Because forward stroke output is not increased, the secondary physical signs (increased arterial pulse pressure, hyperdynamic precordial activity) are usually lacking [3]. With advances in cardiovascular diagnostic techniques, cardiac surgery, and critical care over the past 15 years, the syndrome of acute, severe AI has been more thoroughly described and is consequently more frequently recognized [4].

Definition and Etiology

Acute, severe AI is defined as hemodynamically significant AI of sudden onset, occurring across a previously competent aortic valve into a left ventricle not previously subjected to volume overload. The causes of acute AI are enumerated in Table 37-1.

INFECTIVE ENDOCARDITIS. Bacterial or fungal organisms infecting and damaging a native or prosthetic aortic valve are the most common cause of acute, severe AI. Acute bacterial endocarditis is commonly the result of *Staphylococcus aureus*. It often produces necrosis and perforation and/or detachment of one or more aortic valve leaflets. Infection of the aortic annulus, often with necrosis and abscess formation, can cause weakening and progressive dilation of that structure so that the aortic valve commissures fail to coapt properly during diastole. An annular abscess may distort the annulus, resulting in one or more aortic commissures failing to coapt or prolapsing into the left ventricular outflow tract during diastole. One or more large valvular vegetations may prevent proper diastolic coaptation of the aortic valve commissures. Although present in staphylococcal endocarditis, such bulky vegetations are characteristic of fungal endocarditis caused by *Aspergillus, Candida albicans, Histoplasma capsulatum,* or other such species.

Acute endocarditis with an organism of sufficient virulence to cause valve destruction or perforation can infect a previously normal valve. Although common in narcotic addicts as a result of intravenous injections, acute endocarditis may also occur secondary to abscess formation complicating subcutaneous drug use (skin popping). More commonly, infection involves an anatomically bicuspid aortic valve. Usually there is no significant aortic stenosis or AI prior to the onset of infective endocarditis. Patients with a congenitally bicuspid aortic valve are at increased risk for aortic valve endocarditis because (1) the bicuspid valve is associated with turbulent flow, (2) the valve lesion is commonly asymptomatic and may have escaped detection, and (3) antibiotic prophylaxis was not prescribed for dental or other surgical procedures [5–9].

Infective endocarditis resulting in acute, severe AI may cause several life-threatening cardiac complications [6,10,11].

Annular abscess, nearly always associated with hemodynamically severe AI, may result in gradual or sudden onset of first- or second-degree atrioventricular (A-V) block, left bundle branch block, or complete heart block secondary to inflammation and necrosis of the A-V node and proximal His-Purkinje region of the conduction system. Infection may erode into the pericardium, resulting in purulent pericarditis, hemopericardium, and cardiac tamponade. Annular abscess extending into the membranous intraventricular septum may cause septal rupture and a left-to-right shunt. Extension of infection into the muscular septum can cause ventricular irritability in conjunction with a variety of infranodal heart block patterns. Infection may extend from the aortic valve and annulus into the contiguous right ventricle or anterolaterally situated right atrium, resulting in the development of an aorto-right ventricular or right atrial fistula. These complications are associated with the development of a machinelike murmur (related to the substantial left-to-right shunt) and severe congestive heart failure. Superior extension of infection can cause a mycotic aneurysm involving the sinus of Valsalva or proximal ascending aorta. The development of any of these complications in the setting of acute endocarditis mandates urgent aortic valve replacement.

In addition to the presence of acute, severe AI with or without one or more of the above-enumerated complications, the diagnosis of infective endocarditis is suggested by one or more large- or small-vessel embolic events as well as by systemic signs of infection (e.g., fever, hypotension). Blood cultures demonstrating the causative organism confirm the diagnosis [6,11,12,13]. (See Chap. 88.)

DISSECTION. Dissection of the ascending aorta with medial hematoma may involve the aortic valve (see Chap. 36). The hematoma can displace the attachments of the aortic valve cusps downward and medially, such that one or more cusps prolapse or evert into the outflow tract of the left ventricle during diastole, thereby leading to incompetence of the valve. Aortic insufficiency occurs in approximately 65 percent of patients with dissection of the ascending aorta [14–17].

It is important to recognize that aortic dissection has caused acute, severe AI, since it mandates urgent aortography followed by operative intervention [18,19,20]. Additional suggestive clinical features of aortic dissection include severe chest pain and evidence of vascular compromise to the head, upper or lower extremities, gut, or kidney.

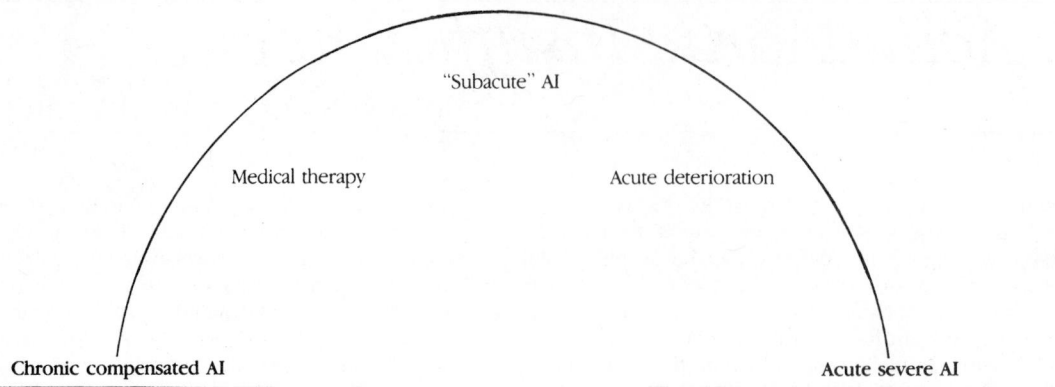

Fig. 37-1. Clinical spectrum of aortic insufficiency (AI). A patient with chronic compensated AI is hemodynamically stable, has an enlarged left ventricle and widened pulse pressure, and is asymptomatic. A patient with acute, severe AI is hemodynamically unstable, has a normal-sized left ventricle and normal pulse pressure, and presents with acute pulmonary edema and cardiogenic shock.

CONNECTIVE TISSUE DISEASES. There are reports of acute, severe AI complicating systemic lupus erythematosus [21,22]. This complication results from sterile perforation of one or more aortic valve cusps secondary to fibrinoid necrosis of the valve parenchyma. Aortitis, with inflammation and furling of the aortic valve leaflet, extraarticular manifestations of ankylosing spondylitis, or Whipple's disease, can also result in progressive severe AI [23]. In idiopathic giant cell aortitis [24] and Takayasu's arteritis, the inflammatory process can result in severe AI [25]. It is likely that some cases of "spontaneous" acute, severe AI are related to noninfectious inflammatory processes involving the aortic valve. Simultaneous acute aortic and mitral insufficiency have been reported as complications of ankylosing spondylitis [26].

TRAUMA. Acute disruption of the aortic valve may result from closed chest or abdominal trauma, such as that caused by automobile accidents, crush injuries, or falls [27]. Sudden compression of the thoracoabdominal aorta during diastole when the aortic valve is closed can elevate intravascular pressure and cause aortic cuspal tearing, perforation, or detachment [28,29]. Trauma can damage a previously normal aortic valve; however, it is likely that myxomatous degenerated valves are more susceptible to physical injury [30]. Although more frequently a consequence of high-energy closed chest or abdominal impact, traumatic AI has also been reported as a consequence of very strenuous physical activity, such as that associated with shoveling snow [31] or parturition [32].

The detection of traumatic AI requires careful and thorough cardiovascular evaluation (1) initially, when the trauma victim presents to the hospital, (2) after resuscitative and initial ther-

Table 37-1. Causes of Acute Aortic Insufficiency

1. Infective endocarditis
2. Dissection of the ascending aorta
3. Connective tissue diseases
4. Trauma
5. "Spontaneous" or idiopathic aortic insufficiency
6. Prosthetic or bioprosthetic valve aortic insufficiency

apeutic interventions are complete, and (3) after several weeks of recovery, so that any delayed manifestations of aortic valve damage are not neglected [28].

"SPONTANEOUS" AORTIC INSUFFICIENCY. Sudden eversion of an aortic cusp may result in spontaneous acute, severe AI. This may occur with a myxomatous valve or, occasionally, with a previously normal aortic valve. A myxomatous valve may spontaneously perforate [30,33] or an intrinsically redundant leaflet may prolapse [34]. Spontaneous acute, severe AI has also been reported as a result of cuspal eversion affecting a bicuspid aortic valve [35]. Because of the asymmetric nature of a bicuspid valve, the greater valve leaflet faces an abnormally large total force in diastole. With an asymmetric and deformed raphe, the larger valve leaflet may not be sufficiently buttressed by the smaller leaflet along the line of coaptation. Under such circumstances a valve cusp may spontaneously evert, resulting in acute, severe AI.

PROSTHETIC VALVE AORTIC INSUFFICIENCY. Sudden, partial dehiscence of the sewing ring of a prosthetic valve from the aortic annulus causes acute AI. This is an occasional complication of emergency aortic valve replacement for bacterial endocarditis with the valve implanted into an infected annulus. It may also occur in the absence of infection [36]. Pannus ingrowth, thrombus formation, or a vegetation may impede proper seating of the ball or poppet during diastole, resulting in severe aortic insufficiency. Poppet wear and failure may also precipitate AI, which is frequently chronic and progressive and only occasionally acute and catastrophic. Acute AI is particularly dangerous in the patient who has undergone aortic valve replacement for aortic stenosis. Here, the ventricle is hypertrophied and noncompliant; it cannot increase stroke volume without a marked elevation in filling pressure, with resultant pulmonary congestion [3]. Homograft valves and porcine bioprostheses fixed in formaldehyde undergo progressive degeneration that frequently culminates in severe AI. Glutaraldehyde-fixed porcine valves can also spontaneously degenerate after a number of years of flawless performance [37]; however, this complication fortunately occurs much less frequently than is the case with formaldehyde-fixed valves. Chronic, progressive or acute, catastrophic AI may result from bland leaflet disruption secondary to degenerative changes in bioprostheses [38,39,40]. Acute, severe AI may also result from sudden tearing of a porcine valve leaflet resulting from trauma or endocarditis.

Pathophysiology

The left ventricular response elicited by the volume-overload state characteristic of AI is conditioned by the severity of the hemodynamic insult and the rapidity with which it develops [41,42]. Helpful in appreciating the hemodynamic impact of acute, severe AI is a thorough grasp of the fundamental hemodynamic derangement and compensatory mechanisms evoked in chronic severe AI [2].

In chronic, severe AI, the volume of blood regurgitating back into the left ventricle during diastole increases slowly over time. To accommodate this regurgitant volume, the left ventricle slowly dilates, its walls undergoing minimal thickening and its compliance increasing. This pattern of increased chamber radius with little or no increase in septal and posterior wall thickness is called eccentric hypertrophy. It allows the ventricle to operate at a larger end-diastolic volume with little or no rise in end-diastolic pressure. As long as systolic function is preserved, the ventricle is capable of ejecting the abnormally large total volume (stroke volume and regurgitant stroke volume), so that organ perfusion is maintained, ejection fraction is preserved [43,44,45], left ventricular diastolic pressure does not rise, and symptoms of cardiac decompensation do not ensue. In effect, the ventricle operates at a much greater end-diastolic volume with a normal end-diastolic pressure (i.e., its compliance has increased). Ejection of the large total stroke volume results in a widened arterial pulse pressure.

Although a basal, blowing, decrescendo diastolic murmur is the specific hallmark of chronic AI, it is the widened arterial pulse pressure of brisk upstroke and rapid fall-off with its associated peripheral manifestations (e.g., head and uvular bobbing, Quincke's pulses) that attest to the hemodynamic severity of the regurgitant lesion. Equally important but not as well appreciated is that these findings also indicate reasonable preservation of ventricular systolic function in chronic AI. At a later stage of the illness, congestive cardiomyopathy gradually develops secondary to volume overload and/or some other intercurrent myocardial insult; systolic function deteriorates and left ventricular diastolic pressure rises. The inevitable reduction in organ perfusion and pulmonary congestion leads to symptoms of cardiac decompensation: fatigue, decreased exercise capacity, and dyspnea. As forward cardiac output declines, arterial resistance rises to preserve blood pressure. Concomitantly, the peripheral manifestations of chronic compensated AI are no longer seen, although the patient is now severely ill with cardiac decompensation. The dramatic clinical, radiographic, and echocardiographic evidence of biventricular enlargement testify to the chronicity of the volume-overload state.

Contrasted with the above situation is the hemodynamic and clinical scenario seen with acute perforation or destruction of the aortic valve in the setting of normal left ventricular function. Lacking eccentric hypertrophy, ventricular compliance is not increased and, indeed, remains normal despite the sudden regurgitant load. This is poorly tolerated because the ventricle is operating on a steep or noncompliant portion of its diastolic pressure-volume relationship [41]. If the acute AI is severe, end-diastolic left ventricular pressure may approach aortic diastolic pressure. The normal ventricle, neither hypertrophied nor dilated, cannot acutely increase its total left ventricular stroke volume sufficiently to maintain forward stroke volume. There is a precipitous rise in left ventricular end-diastolic pressure without an improvement in total cardiac output [46]. The noncompliant left ventricle and even the pericardium limit the increase in left ventricular volume in acute, severe AI [42]. The impact of declining cardiac output on arterial blood pressure is somewhat mitigated by a reflex increase in systemic vascular resistance. This tends to maintain adequate perfusion pressure to the heart and brain.

The acute regurgitant volume refluxing back into the relatively noncompliant left ventricle has several consequences. The rise in left ventricular diastolic pressure rapidly elevates left atrial and pulmonary capillary pressures to levels that produce pulmonary edema. Early in diastole, left ventricular pressure rises rapidly, causing the mitral leaflets to drift toward the closed position. Blood entering the left ventricle from the left atrium and flowing through these relatively coapted mitral leaflets may give rise to a low-pitched, mid- to late-diastolic (Austin Flint) rumble. Tumultuous acute AI may elevate left ventricular diastolic pressure so rapidly that it exceeds left atrial pressure and causes premature closure of the mitral valve [33]. Moreover, the mitral valve may open late in diastole because the ejection period of the acutely volume-loaded ventricle is prolonged. Finally, compensatory tachycardia shortens diastole. These factors taken together appreciably reduce the time during which the mitral valve is open in diastole [47–50]. Premature mitral closure results in absence or marked softening of the first heart sound.

The patient with acute, severe AI and reduced cardiac output has impaired regional arterial flow, oliguria, pallor and coolness of the skin, deranged temperature regulation secondary to reduced cutaneous blood flow, and gastrointestinal and hepatic dysfunction. With extreme reduction in tissue perfusion, there may be cardiogenic shock and lactic acidosis. Table 37-2 compares and contrasts the hemodynamic features of chronic, severe and acute, severe AI.

Table 37-2. Comparison of Major Hemodynamic Features of Acute and Chronic Aortic Regurgitation

Hemodynamic feature	Acute	Chronic*
Left ventricular compliance	Not increased	Increased
Regurgitant volume	Increased	Increased
Left ventricular end-diastolic pressure	Markedly increased	May be normal
Left ventricular ejection velocity (dp/dt)	Not significantly increased	Markedly increased
Aortic systolic pressure	Not increased	Increased
Aortic diastolic pressure	Normal to decreased	Markedly decreased
Systemic arterial pulse pressure	Slightly to moderately increased	Markedly increased
Ejection fraction	Not increased	Normal to increased
Effective stroke volume	Decreased	Normal
Effective cardiac output	Decreased	Normal
Heart rate	Increased	Normal
Peripheral vascular resistance	Increased	Not increased

*Without left ventricular failure.
Source: Adapted from Morganroth J, Perloff JK, Zeldis SM, et al: Acute, severe aortic regurgitation. *Ann Intern Med* 87:223, 1977.

Clinical Presentation

HISTORY. The patient with acute, severe AI presents with symptoms of rapid onset due to the precipitous rise in left atrial pressure (pulmonary congestion) and an abrupt reduction in forward cardiac output. Symptoms attributable to progressive, severe pulmonary congestion include:

1. Dyspnea with exertion
2. Orthopnea and a dry or minimally productive cough aggravated by recumbency
3. Paroxysmal nocturnal dyspnea
4. Dyspnea at rest even while sitting upright

Symptoms reflecting the reduction in cardiac output are more subtle and often overshadowed by those due to pulmonary congestion. There may be fatigue on exertion, apathy, agitation, and/or a deterioration in intellectual function reflecting impaired skeletal muscle and cerebral perfusion.

Also important in establishing an etiologic diagnosis are associated symptoms. Severe chest and/or back pain, abrupt in onset, characterizes aortic dissection. Fever, chills, malaise, and evidence of peripheral arterial emboli implicate infective endocarditis. A history of recent chest and/or abdominal trauma raises the likelihood of traumatic disruption of the aortic valve. The abrupt onset of cardiac decompensation in the absence of ancillary symptoms or known heart disease suggests sudden disruption or perforation of an aortic valve intrinsically weakened by myxomatous degeneration.

PHYSICAL EXAMINATION. Physical findings in the patient with acute, severe AI relate to severity of pulmonary congestion and impairment in forward cardiac output and tissue perfusion. It is imperative to perform a complete and thorough examination, actively seeking findings that convey more specific information with respect to the etiology of AI.

An understanding of the pathophysiology of acute, severe AI as previously outlined is mandatory for thorough recognition and proper interpretation of the physical findings, particularly with respect to their prognostic and therapeutic implications. The most important features (in contradistinction to chronic, severe, compensated AI) are the manifestations of pulmonary congestion and reduced cardiac output as well as the relative paucity of findings reflecting left ventricular volume overload with augmentation of stroke output. Because of the acute nature of the AI, the left ventricle has not undergone eccentric hypertrophy; widened arterial pulse pressure and dramatic peripheral arterial findings characteristic of chronic compensated AI are absent.

In acute, severe AI, forward ventricular stroke output is reduced. The pulse pressure is not appreciably widened, systolic blood pressure is normal or only slightly elevated, and diastolic arterial pressure is usually slightly elevated [41,42]. Tachycardia is the rule. The precordium is relatively quiet; conspicuously lacking is the laterally displaced, heaving, apical impulse reflecting volume overload and eccentric hypertrophy of chronic, compensated AI. The first heart sound is usually soft as the regurgitant volume rapidly fills the ventricle and pushes the mitral leaflets toward the closed position at the time of ventricular activation. With severe, acute AI, left ventricular diastolic pressure exceeds left atrial pressure prior to ventricular activation; mitral valve closure occurs late in diastole, actually preceding ventricular and even atrial systole. Occasionally, the first heart sound is absent.

The second heart sound is also soft and may be absent if one or more aortic valve leaflets have been destroyed to the point that there is little or no diastolic coaptation. An ejection-type murmur of variable intensity is often heard, localized to the base. This reflects turbulent flow across the aortic valve resulting from augmented stroke output across the damaged valve. The diastolic murmur of aortic insufficiency (high-pitched, decrescendo, and lasting throughout most of diastole in patients with chronic AI) may be rather nondescript and of mixed frequencies in acute, severe AI. A flail cusp may evoke a musical (narrow-frequency band) and very intense diastolic murmur [30]. If there is free AI with rapid diastolic equilibration of aortic and left ventricular pressures, the murmur may end well before the end of diastole. An Austin Flint murmur is often present in acute, severe AI [51]. A third heart sound is also frequently present, reflecting rapid, early diastolic ventricular filling. The cacophony of sounds and murmurs may mimic the two- or three-component rub of pericarditis. The clinical findings in acute AI and the important differences between chronic and acute AI with respect to the overall presentation are presented in Table 37-3.

Important ancillary physical findings may provide clues to the cause of the aortic valve dysfunction leading to acute, severe AI. Fever, petechiae, purpura, and/or small or large arterial embolic events implicate infective endocarditis. Excruciating chest or back discomfort and/or an inequality of pulses in the neck, upper, or lower extremities suggest aortic dissection. Aortic insufficiency in a tall thin patient with a long arm span, hyperextensile joints, and/or ectopia lentis points to the diagnosis of annuloaortic ectasia and/or aortic dissection complicating Marfan's syndrome [52]. Figure 37-2 is an algorithm that directs the clinician to the etiology of AI as a function of associated ancillary clinical information.

Laboratory Findings

CHEST RADIOGRAPH. The chest radiograph usually reveals bilateral patchy interstitial infiltrates that progress to confluent alveolar infiltrates emanating from the hilar regions as pulmonary congestion progresses to fulminant pulmonary edema. The lung fields may be reasonably clear if the hemodynamic insult is so acute (<36 hours) that there has been insufficient time for the accumulation of extravascular lung water. There is usually apical redistribution of flow in the pulmonary veins. The cardiac silhouette is not enlarged unless there is preexisting chronic valvular, myocardial, or pericardial dysfunction. The absence of cardiomegaly essentially rules out the presence of chronic AI of hemodynamic consequence. Table 37-3 details the chest radiographic findings in acute AI. If aortic dissection is suspected, it is imperative to obtain a good quality posteroanterior chest film. This study facilitates the detection of true mediastinal widening and/or displacement of calcium in the wall of the aortic knob—findings highly suggestive of dissecting hematoma involving the thoracic aorta [53].

ELECTROCARDIOGRAM. Electrocardiographic findings in acute, severe AI are neither sensitive nor specific. Sinus tachycardia is the rule, but it is indicative only of the severity of cardiac decompensaton. Left ventricular hypertrophy is absent unless there is a preexisting cardiac condition resulting in chronic volume and/or pressure overload. Acute, severe AI may evoke compensatory ventricular dilation and an increase in muscle mass such that electrocardiographic criteria for left ventricular hypertrophy are manifest as early as 2 weeks after the

Table 37-3. Comparison of Clinical Findings in Acute and Chronic Aortic Insufficiency

Clinical finding	Acute	Chronic*
Congestive heart failure	Early and sudden	Late and insidious
Arterial pulse		
Rate per minute	Increased	Normal
Rate of rise	Not increased	Increased
Systolic pressure	Normal to decreased	Increased
Diastolic pressure	Normal to decreased	Decreased
Pulse pressure	Near normal	Increased
Contour of peak	Single	Bisferiens
Pulsus alternans	Common	Uncommon
Left ventricular impulse	Near normal to laterally displaced, not hyperdynamic	Laterally displaced, hyperdynamic
Auscultation		
First heart sound	Soft to absent	Normal
Aortic component of second heart sound	Soft	Normal or decreased
Pulmonic component of second heart sound	Normal or increased	Normal
Fourth heart sound	Consistently absent	Usually absent
Third heart sound	Common	Uncommon
Aortic systolic murmur	Grade 3 or less	Grade 3 or more
Aortic regurgitant murmur	Short, medium-pitched	Long, high-pitched
Austin Flint murmur	Mid-diastolic	Presystolic, mid-diastolic, or both
Peripheral arterial auscultatory signs	Absent	Present
Electrocardiogram	Normal left ventricular voltage with minor repolarization abnormalities	Increased left ventricular voltage with major repolarization abnormalities
Chest radiograph		
Left ventricle	Normal to slightly increased	Markedly increased
Aortic root and arch	Usually normal	Prominent
Pulmonary venous pattern	Redistributed to upper lobes	Normal
Interstitial and alveolar fluid	Usually present	Usually absent, unless terminally decompensated

*Without left ventricular failure.
Source: Adapted from Benotti JR: Acute aortic insufficiency, in Alpert JS, Dalen JE (eds): *Valvular Heart Disease.* 2nd ed. Boston, Little, Brown, 1987.

onset of severe AI [54]. There may be nonspecific S–T segment and T wave abnormalities related to subendocardial ischemia, hypoxemia, acidosis, and/or other metabolic-electrolyte abnormalities. The pattern of left ventricular hypertrophy and prominent upright left precordial T waves (diastolic-volume overload pattern) characteristic of chronic AI is absent in acute, severe AI.

ECHOCARDIOGRAM. M-mode, two-dimensional, and Doppler echocardiography are exceedingly important in evaluating the patient with acute, severe AI [49,50,55]. These studies should be performed at the time of initial presentation and at regular intervals during the course of the illness. The initial echocardiogram and Doppler study provide information concerning the hemodynamic severity of the regurgitation, involvement of other valves, and presence of preexisting heart disease. The echocardiogram may also provide information regarding the cause of AI (e.g., infective endocarditis, aortic dissection). During treatment, serial evaluations assess the patient's therapeutic response and permit prompt detection of cardiac complications. Echocardiographic findings suggestive of acute, severe AI are, for the most part, nonspecific. Systolic motion of the septum and posterior wall is usually normal, unless there is such a profound degree of afterload mismatch that systolic function is depressed. The pattern of well-compensated left ventricular volume overload (increased end-diastolic dimension, augmented septal and posterior wall shortening velocity, and a near normal end-systolic dimension) suggestive of

chronic AI is not present in acute AI unless there is preexisting chronic aortic and/or mitral insufficiency. In acute AI, the end-diastolic and end-systolic dimensions are normal or slightly increased. The left atrial dimension is normal or slightly increased unless there is chronic disease of the mitral valve, aortic valve, or myocardium. The right ventricular end-diastolic and end-systolic dimensions are normal or slightly increased.

The mitral valve echocardiogram usually reveals anterior and posterior leaflets of normal thickness and mobility unless there is preexisting mitral valvular disease. Large redundant mitral leaflets with exaggerated opening and closing motion and/or mitral valve prolapse implicate myxomatous degeneration of the mitral valve. This may be present in cases of acute, severe AI resulting from annuloaortic ectasia, Marfan's syndrome, and/or spontaneous perforation of an inherently "normal" aortic valve. There is usually a reduction in the diastolic rate of mitral valve closure, since the overloaded ventricle is relatively noncompliant. If AI is very severe, the mitral valve may close prior to the onset of the QRS complex [48,49,50]. Premature closure of the mitral valve in conjunction with tachycardia results in profound abbreviation of the diastolic filling period. On the echocardiogram, this is evident as shortening of the interval during which the anterior and posterior mitral valve leaflets are separated during diastole. Premature closure of the mitral valve and appreciable shortening of the interval of diastolic flow across the mitral valve are important diagnostic and prognostic echocardiographic findings. They are associated with severe aortic insufficiency and left ventricular diastolic hypertension.

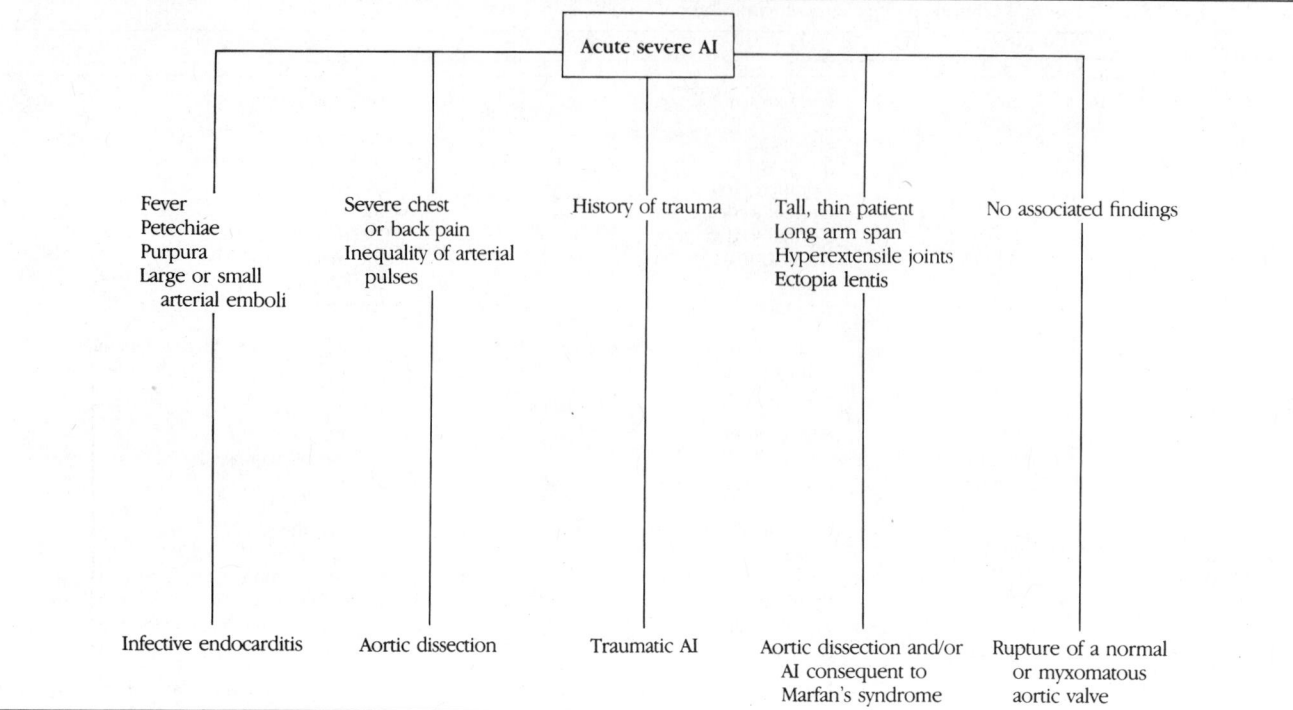

Fig. 37-2. Etiology of acute, severe aortic insufficiency (AI) as determined by ancillary clinical findings.

Under such circumstances, procrastination delays potentially lifesaving aortic valve replacement. Figure 37-3 (left) is a mitral valve echogram depicting premature closure of the mitral valve, diastolic mitral valve fluttering, and shortening of the diastolic filling period in a patient with acute, severe AI. The right-hand panel of Figure 37-3 depicts the left ventricular echogram in the same patient. It demonstrates slight left ventricular dilatation and normal to mildly reduced septal and posterior wall excursion characteristic of acute, severe AI. The aortic valve echogram may demonstrate opening of the aortic valve late in diastole. As ventricular pressure rises and aortic pressure falls late in diastole, the aortic cusps may float into the open position. Late diastolic recoil of the acutely overdistended ventricular myocardium together with atrial systole further elevate ventricular pressure and may facilitate late diastolic opening of the aortic valve [56]. Table 37-4 summarizes and contrasts the echocardiographic manifestations of acute, severe, and chronic AI.

The echocardiogram of the aortic valve and proximal aortic root may also provide specific information regarding etiology of acute AI [57–64]. A shaggy, large, irregular, echo-dense mass in association with the aortic valve leaflets is virtually diagnostic of a vegetation resulting from infective endocarditis. Figures 37-4 and 37-5 illustrate aortic valve bacterial vegetations of varying echodensity and mobility in two patients with acute AI resulting from infective endocarditis. Valvular vegetations are more accurately identified with transesophageal as compared with transthoracic echocardiography [61,62].

Chronic, nonspecific thickening of one or more aortic valve leaflets due to rheumatic disease, acquired degenerative changes involving a bicuspid valve, calcification and fibrosis of a normal valve, or an organized sterile vegetation secondary to previous endocarditis may sometimes mimic vegetations characteristic of infective endocarditis.

A fine, linear structure moving in a to-and-fro fashion into the aortic root during systole and into the outflow tract of the left ventricle during diastole suggests bland perforation or detachment of an aortic valve cusp. This may be related to trauma, myxomatous degeneration, or congenital malformation of the valve. The echogram of the aortic root may demonstrate dilatation with the characteristic spadelike deformity of Marfan's syndrome.

The echocardiographic diagnosis of intimal detachment due to dissection is suggested by the identification of a relatively redundant echo-dense band located centrally or eccentrically in the proximal aortic root, originating at or just above the aortic annulus and partitioning the aorta into two channels of equal or unequal size [65,66]. Figure 37-6, an echogram of the aortic root in a patient with dissection of the ascending aorta, illustrates the intimal flap that has partitioned the aortic root into a true and false lumen. Transesophageal echocardiography is more accurate than transthoracic echo in diagnosing dissection of the aorta [66].

Doppler echocardiography is now the principal noninvasive means of identifying aortic insufficiency [55]. It yields a semiquantitative estimate of the severity of the aortic regurgitant hemodynamic burden. Good correlation with angiographic estimation of aortic regurgitant severity has been demonstrated [55]. Color flow Doppler studies are of particular value in identifying and quantifying aortic regurgitation.

CARDIAC CATHETERIZATION. Often when high-quality Doppler and two-dimensional (2-D) echocardiograms are obtained and interpreted by experienced cardiologists, cardiac catheterization is required to confirm the diagnosis of acute, severe AI. If there is clear-cut Doppler and 2-D echocardiographic evidence of aortic valve leaflet destruction, severe aortic insufficiency, and premature closure of the mitral valve in a patient previously free of cardiac disease and presenting with

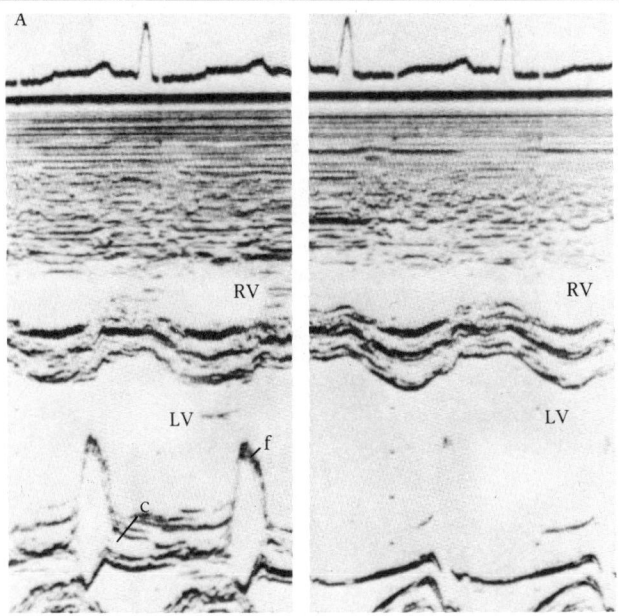

Fig. 37-3. Representative echocardiogram showing features of acute, severe aortic insufficiency, including slight left ventricular dilatation, normal to mildly reduced septal and posterior wall excursion, diastolic fluttering, and premature closure of the mitral valve. RV = right ventricle; LV = left ventricle; f = flutter of anterior mitral valve leaflet; C = closure point of mitral valve. (Adapted from Benotti JR: Acute aortic insufficiency, in Alpert JS, Dalen JE (eds): *Valvular Heart Disease*. Boston, Little, Brown, 1980. With permission.)

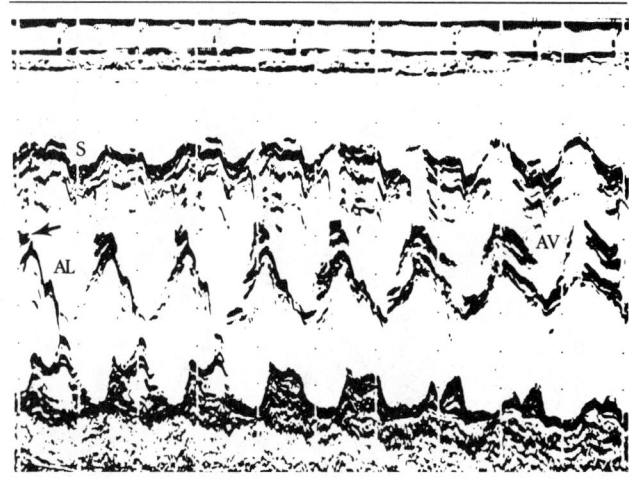

Fig. 37-4. Echocardiogram of the mitral and aortic valves in a patient with acute, severe aortic insufficiency secondary to bacterial endocarditis. It demonstrates an abnormally thickened structure contiguous with the aortic valve prolapsing into the left ventricular outflow tract at the onset of diastole (*arrow*) and displaying high-frequency diastolic vibrations. At surgery, this structure was identified as a staphylococcal vegetation attached to a necrotic and partially dehisced aortic valve leaflet. S = ventricular septum; AL = anterior leaflet of mitral valve; AV = aortic valve. (Adapted from Benotti JR: Acute aortic insufficiency, in Alpert JS, Dalen JE (eds): *Valvular Heart Disease*. Boston, Little, Brown, 1980. With permission.)

shock and/or pulmonary edema refractory to inotropic and afterload reduction therapy, urgent aortic valve replacement may be lifesaving. Here, the inevitable delay and the hemodynamic stress associated with cardiac catheterization and angiography put the patient at added risk and may reduce the likelihood of a successful surgical outcome. However, cardiac catheterization, left ventricular angiography, and coronary arteriography are usually required in patients with clinical and/or echocardiographic evidence of preexisting heart disease. Specific questions may relate to the presence of mitral insufficiency, whether there has been prior myocardial infarction or evidence of coronary artery disease.

Table 37-4. Comparison of Echocardiographic Manifestations of Acute and Chronic Aortic Regurgitation

Echocardiographic variable	Acute	Chronic*
Mitral valve		
Closure	Early	Normal
Opening	Late	Normal
Anterior leaflet E/F slope	Reduced	Normal
Diastolic fluttering	Yes	Yes
Aortic valve presystolic opening	Yes	No
Septal wall motion	Normal	Hyperkinetic
Posterior wall motion	Normal	Hyperkinetic
End-diastolic dimension	Normal	Increased
End-systolic dimension	Normal	Normal
Shortening fraction	Normal	Increased

*Without left ventricular failure.
Source: Adapted from Benotti JR: Acute aortic insufficiency, in Alpert JS, Dalen JE (eds): *Valvular Heart Disease*. 2nd ed. Boston, Little, Brown, 1987.

In patients with aortic insufficiency and suspected aortic dissection, angiographic assessment of the ascending thoracic aorta is required to confirm (1) the presence and extent of dissection and (2) the presence and severity of AI.

Hemodynamic findings associated with acute, severe AI include (1) an arterial pulse pressure that is slightly increased or of normal amplitude, (2) equilibration of left ventricular and aortic pressures late in diastole, and (3) marked elevation in left ventricular diastolic pressure, which may exceed left atrial (pulmonary artery wedge) pressure in late diastole [4]. Other hemodynamic findings not specific for acute AI but indicative of the resultant left ventricular failure include (1) elevation in the pulmonary artery wedge pressure to a level often exceeding 25 to 30 mm Hg; (2) mild to modest elevation in mean pulmonary artery pressure such that the pressure gradient across the lungs does not usually exceed 10 to 12 mm Hg; and (3) mild elevation in mean right atrial pressure (8–10 mm Hg) with pulmonary artery and right ventricular systolic pressure in excess of 35 to 45 mm Hg. The hemodynamic findings in acute, severe AI are summarized in Table 37-2.

Ventriculographic findings in acute, severe AI include the following:

1. Normal or near normal systolic function (ejection fraction ≥ 0.50) with normal left ventricular segmental wall motion
2. Slight increase in left ventricular end-diastolic and end-systolic volumes
3. Thickening of one or more aortic leaflets or a filling defect at the level of the aortic valve suggestive of a vegetation in patients with acute endocarditis
4. Thickening of the anterior mitral valve leaflet and mitral insufficiency of variable severity if infective endocarditis of the aortic valve causes septic involvement of the anterior leaflet of the mitral valve
5. High-frequency vibrations of the anterior mitral leaflet as it

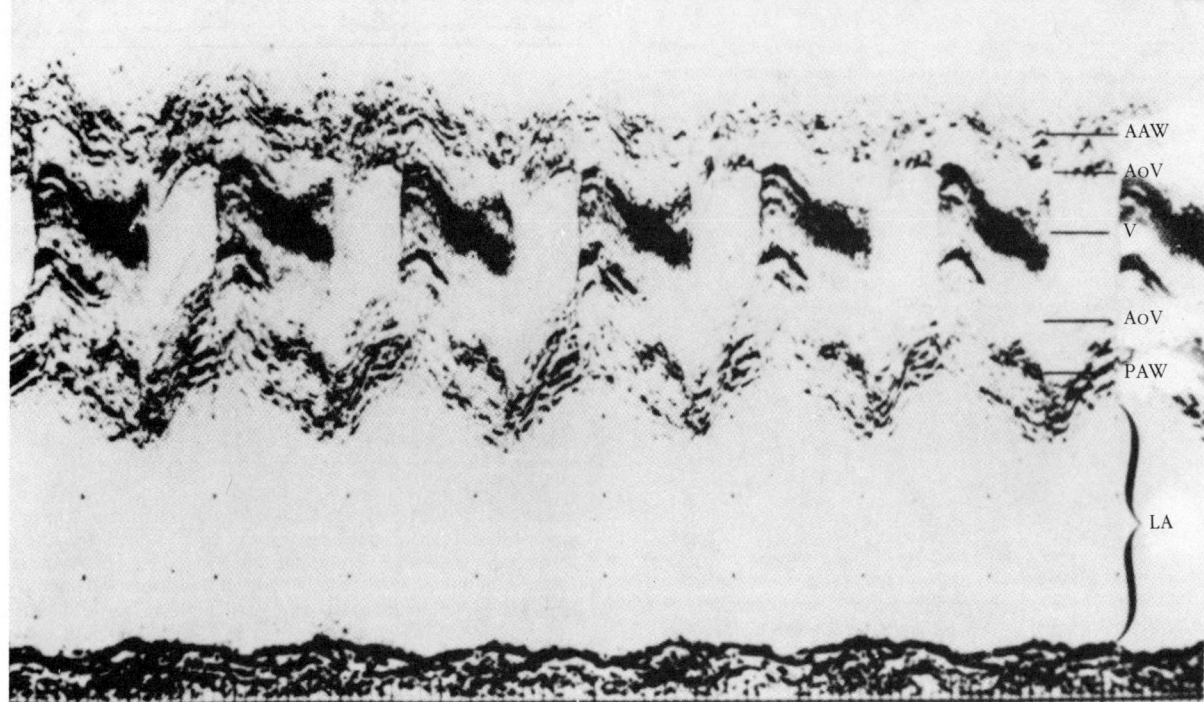

Fig. 37-5. Aortic valve echocardiogram in a patient with acute, severe aortic insufficiency secondary to bacterial endocarditis. It demonstrates a dense bacterial vegetation on a leaflet of the aortic valve, which vibrates with a high frequency in diastole as it is buffeted by the high-velocity regurgitant jet. AAW = anterior wall of aorta; AoV = aortic valve leaflet in systole; V = vegetation; PAW = posterior wall of aorta; LA = left atrium.

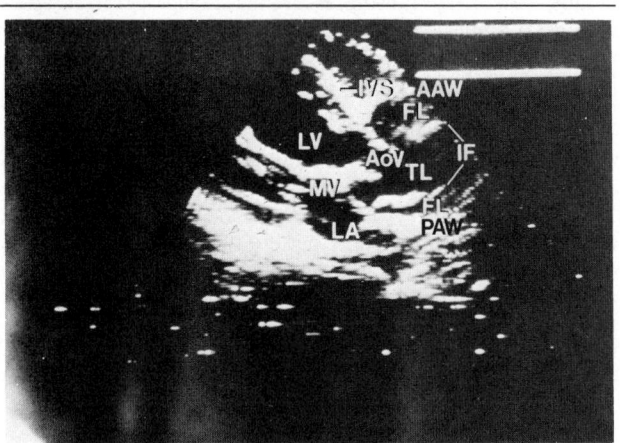

Fig. 37-6. Long axis, M-mode (*left*) and sweeping, two-dimensional (*right*) echocardiograms of the left ventricle and aortic root in a patient with proximal aortic dissection. The circumferential dissection beginning just above the sclerotic aortic valve (AoV) has partitioned the aortic root into true and false lumens. The false lumen (FL), bounded by the aortic media and intimal flap, envelops the true lumen (TL) in a coaxial fashion. The aortic root is markedly dilated and the left atrium (LA) is compressed. AAW = anterior aortic wall; IVS = interventricular septum; IF = intimal flap; LV = left ventricle; MV = mitral valve; PAW = posterior aortic wall.

is pushed toward the closed position in late diastole by the aortic regurgitant stream
6. Abnormal "filling defects" projecting into the left ventricular outflow tract at the level of the aortic annulus, membranous, or muscular ventricular septum, suggesting vegetations and/or abscess formation in patients with infective endocarditis.

The risk of cardiac catheterization and angiography relates to additional hemodynamic stresses imposed by these procedures on a critically ill patient. Concern is often expressed regarding the risk of arterial embolization secondary to catheter-induced traumatic disruption of one or more friable aortic valve vegetations as the catheter crosses the aortic valve during retrograde left ventricular catheterization in patients with infective endocarditis. Although this has not been reported to be a problem for a large number of patients with infective endocarditis, it remains a source of major concern [64].

Treatment

The treatment of patients with acute, severe AI may be categorized as follows:

1. General supportive cardiovascular measures
2. Pharmacologic (medical) management
3. Surgical management

These measures are carried out simultaneously to ensure a satisfactory outcome by stabilizing the patient promptly and optimally. It must be emphasized that medical and surgical therapeutic modalities are mutually complementary, rather than mutually exclusive, in the total management of these critically ill patients.

General supportive cardiovascular measures include supplementary inspired oxygen to maintain the arterial PaO_2 in excess of 65 mm Hg and/or arterial oxygen saturation in excess of 95 percent. If pulmonary congestion progresses to pulmonary edema and acidosis, bicarbonate administration and/or intubation and assisted mechanical ventilation are required. Pulmonary edema is also managed by the intravenous administration of a potent loop diuretic (furosemide, 10–40 mg IV, or ethacrynic acid, 25–50 mg IV) as well as with morphine sulfate (2–4 mg IV) and positioning the patient with the head and thorax elevated at least 45 degrees above the horizontal plane.

Acute pulmonary edema often improves dramatically following 1 to 4 mg of morphine administered intravenously. This can be repeated at 10- to 15-minute intervals to reduce preload and afterload and to allay anxiety. Significant hypotension and alveolar hypoventilation may complicate morphine administration and may require the use of fluids, pressor agents, intubation, and assisted ventilation. Nonetheless, fear of respiratory depression should not prevent the use of morphine in the management of acute pulmonary edema.

Evidence of peripheral organ hypoperfusion in the setting of acute AI mandates pulmonary artery catheterization and intraarterial cannulation so that right and left heart filling pressures, cardiac output, and arterial blood pressure can be monitored continuously. A cardiac index less than 2.0 L/min/m², mean pulmonary artery pressure greater than 20 mm Hg, arterial systolic pressure less than 90 mm Hg, oliguria (urine output <30 ml/hr), and other indirect evidence of impaired tissue perfusion (e.g., decreased mental acuity, cool moist skin, pallor) substantiate the presence of cardiogenic shock. Bedside hemodynamic assessment not only confirms the presence of cardiogenic shock but also provides a rational guide for the selection and administration of appropriate vasopressors, diuretics, and vasodilators [67–75].

Vasodilator therapy may stabilize and improve the patient's tenuous clinical and hemodynamic status. Nitroprusside in a total dose of 3 to 6 μg/kg/min (starting at 0.5 μg/kg/min) with titration can produce a 30 to 50 percent increase in cardiac output, a similar decline in pulmonary artery wedge pressure, and only a modest reduction in arterial pressure. This direct arteriolar and venous smooth muscle relaxant reduces impedance to left ventricular ejection (afterload) as well as left ventricular end-diastolic volume (preload). Nitroprusside reduces the regurgitant volume per beat, improves forward cardiac output, and lowers ventricular filling pressure, thereby promoting resolution of pulmonary edema. The use of nitroprusside in patients with acute, severe AI is associated with a greater than 50 percent reduction in ventricular filling pressure, a 20 percent increase in forward cardiac index, and a 36 percent decline in systemic vascular resistance. This is associated with a statistically significant but clinically insignificant increase in heart rate [72,73].

Should the cardiac index not rise above 2.0 to 2.2 L/min/m² in response to nitroprusside infusion despite a dose sufficient to lower systolic blood to 90 mm Hg and/or reduce mean blood pressure by at least 15 mm Hg, a sympathomimetic agent should be added. This is necessary to increase cardiac output and keep the blood pressure at a level sufficient to maintain adequate coronary and cerebral perfusion. Dobutamine, a relatively pure beta₁ myocardial stimulant, selectively augments myocardial contractility, thereby raising cardiac index with little or no increase in heart rate. Because dobutamine, unlike dopamine, has no intrinsic alpha-adrenergic agonist activity, it neither elevates arterial resistance (increased afterload) nor augments venous tone (increased preload). Dobutamine infusion is instituted at 3 to 5 μg/kg/min and is increased by 2 to 4 μg/kg/min every 15 to 30 minutes to maintain the cardiac index above 2.0 to 2.2 L/min/m² and/or systolic arterial pressure in excess of 90 mm Hg. Side effects at high doses (> 15–20 μg/kg/min) include tachycardia, ventricular premature contractions, nervousness, anxiety, nausea, and vomiting [74,75]. Patients with acute, severe AI who require parenteral inotropic and vasodilator therapy to reverse cardiogenic shock require prompt aortic valve replacement.

Patients with acute AI are critically ill and require frequent monitoring of renal function, serum electrolytes, and arterial blood gases. Hypoxemia, initially related to ventilation-perfusion imbalance resulting from pulmonary congestion, may be paradoxically worsened by vasodilator therapy with nitroprusside despite a substantial decline in the pulmonary capillary wedge pressure. Thiocyanate levels also must be monitored in the patient with low cardiac output, impaired hepatic perfusion, and impaired renal function if nitroprusside is given. Downward dosage adjustments must be made to avoid toxicity from accumulation of this nitroprusside metabolite.

Definitive management of acute AI resulting from infective endocarditis often requires early aortic valve replacement. Aortic valvular insufficiency with congestive heart failure complicating infective endocarditis carries a mortality rate of 50 to 90 percent. Patients with severe heart failure from aortic valve endocarditis have a higher mortality rate than patients with heart failure from mitral valve endocarditis. Although it is desirable to delay aortic valve replacement until antibiotic therapy is completed, this luxury may, at any moment, be precluded by a precipitous deterioration in the patient's condition. The risk of early aortic valve replacement prior to completion of antibiotic therapy relates to the possibility of residual infection: aortic valve replacement may be complicated by infection of the prosthetic valve or by mycotic aneurysm. Nevertheless, valve replacement can be performed emergently or after only a few days of antibiotic therapy with an acceptably low risk of reinfection (usually less than 10%). If the patient presents with cardiogenic shock from acute aortic insufficiency, aortic valve replacement should be undertaken immediately even though there is little or no time for antibiotic administration. All patients should receive 4 to 6 weeks of parenteral antibiotic therapy following aortic valve replacement.

The major risk of valve replacement in these patients relates to the severity of heart failure at the time of surgery. In patients with active endocarditis complicated by severe heart failure, surgery should not be delayed. The increased operative risk consequent to delaying surgery exceeds the potential benefit of completing a full course of antibiotic therapy prior to valve replacement [76,77,78].

Other indications for surgery in acute AI complicating infective endocarditis include infection of a prosthetic valve, infection with an organism refractory to antibiotic therapy, continued sepsis despite appropriate antimicrobial therapy, recurrent large-vessel emboli, fungal endocarditis, and myocardial abscess as manifested by the development of high-grade atrioventricular block and/or inability to sterilize the blood with appropriate antibiotics.

AORTIC DISSECTION. Hypertension and severe pain require analgesia and rapid control of blood pressure with at least one agent that depresses shear force in the ascending aorta (left ventricular dp/dt). Morphine (3–6 mg IV) is administered intravenously every 5 to 10 minutes and titrated carefully to produce analgesia while avoiding respiratory depression and/or excessive hypotension (systolic blood pressure below 85–90 mm Hg). Intravenous propranolol is effective in lowering aortic shear force by reducing heart rate and left ventricular dp/dt. Propranolol is contraindicated in patients with decompensated heart failure and patients with reactive airways disease. Propranolol can be given as a slow intravenous bolus, using heart rate and blood pressure response to titrate therapeutic efficacy. It is desirable to slow the heart rate to 50 to 70 beats per minute and to lower the blood pressure to 90 to 110 mm Hg systolic with an intravenous propranolol dose not exceeding 0.1 mg per kilogram administered over 45 minutes to 1 hour. This can be repeated every 4 to 6 hours. Patients may be refractory to effective beta blockade (because of very high levels of sympathetic tone and circulating catecholamines) unless effective pain control is achieved. Furthermore, satisfactory analgesia cannot be obtained in patients with active aortic dissection unless control of blood pressure terminates propagation of the dissecting medial hematoma. This invariably requires the addition of a potent antihypertensive drug, usually a ganglionic blocking agent (trimethaphan) or a vasodilator (nitroprusside). Trimethaphan has generally been replaced by nitroprusside as the preferred hypotensive agent in the treatment of aortic dissection. Nitroprusside lowers arterial blood pressure by reducing systemic vascular resistance and increasing venous capacitance. It has a very rapid onset of action and a very short half-life. Nitroprusside must be administered intravenously; the starting dose is 0.5 to 1 μg/kg/min. The infusion rate should be increased by 0.5 μg/kg/min every 5 minutes. When administered at a precise rate through a constant infusion pump, prompt blood pressure control with minimal overshoot can be achieved. Because of variable and unpredictable individual sensitivity to nitroprusside, this agent requires continuous monitoring of the arterial pressure through an indwelling arterial cannula. Nitroprusside should always be used in conjunction with propranolol or another beta-adrenergic blocking agent.

Proximal aortic dissection with or without AI usually requires immediate surgical repair unless the patient has a serious, unrelated illness (e.g., metastatic cancer, severe chronic obstructive lung disease, dementia) that precludes a successful surgical outcome (see Chap. 36).

References

1. Willis FA, Keys TE: *Classics of Cardiology*. New York, Dover, 1941, p 422.
2. Alpert JS: Chronic aortic regurgitation, in Alpert JS, Dalen JE (eds): *Valvular Heart Disease*. Boston, Little, Brown, 1980.
3. Benotti JR: Acute aortic insufficiency, in Alpert JS, Dalen JE (eds): *Valvular Heart Disease*. 2nd ed. Boston, Little, Brown, 1987.
4. Morganroth J, Perloff JK, Zeldis SM, et al: Acute, severe aortic regurgitation. *Ann Intern Med* 87:223, 1977.
5. Cohen L, Friedman LR: Damage to aortic valve as a cause of death in bacterial endocarditis. *Ann Intern Med* 55:562, 1961.
6. Weinstein L, Rubin RH: Infective endocarditis. *Prog Cardiovasc Dis* 16:239, 1973.
7. Robinson MJ, Rendy J: Sequellae of bacterial endocarditis. *Am J Med* 32:922, 1962.
8. Roberts WC: The congenitally bicuspid aortic valve. *Am J Cardiol* 26:72, 1970.
9. Perloff JK: Innocent or normal murmurs, in Russek HI (ed): *Cardiovascular Problems*. Baltimore, University Park Press, 1976, p 27.
10. Dinuble MJ: Surgery in active endocarditis. *Ann Intern Med* 96:650, 1982.
11. Braniff BA, Shumway NE, Harrison DC: Valve replacement in active bacterial endocarditis. *N Engl J Med* 276:1464, 1967.
12. Dorney ER: Endocarditis, in Hurst JW, Logue, RB, Schlant RC, et al (eds): *The Heart*. New York, McGraw-Hill, 1978, p 1497.
13. Weinstein L: Infective endocarditis, in Braunwald E (ed): *Heart Disease: A Textbook of Cardiovascular Medicine*. Philadelphia, WB Saunders, 1980, p 1166.
14. Dalen JE, Pape LA, Cohn LH, et al: Dissection of the aorta: Pathogenesis, diagnosis and treatment. *Prog Cardiovasc Dis* 23:237, 1980.
15. Koster JK, Cohn LH, Meer BB, et al: Late results of operation for acute aortic dissection producing aortic insufficiency. *Ann Thorac Surg* 26:461, 1978.
16. Anagnostopoulos CE, Prabhakar MJS, Kittle CF: Aortic dissections and dissecting aneurysms. *Am J Cardiol* 30:263, 1972.
17. Cipriano PR, Griepp RB: Acute retrograde dissection of the ascending thoracic aorta. *Am J Cardiol* 43:520, 1978.
18. Liddicoat JE, Bekassy SM, Rubio PA, et al: Ascending aortic aneurysms: Review of 100 cases. *Circulation* 51,52(suppl I):I-202, 1975.
19. Dalen JE, Alpert JS, Cohen LH, et al: Dissection of the thoracic aorta, medical or surgical therapy? *Am J Cardiol* 34:803, 1974.
20. Kainuma Y, Sakamoto T, Shimakuna T, et al: Successful surgical management of a dissecting aneurysm of the ascending and transverse aorta with heart failure due to sudden, severe aortic valve insufficiency. *J Cardiovasc Surg* 19:387, 1978.
21. Thandroyen FT, Matisonn RE, Weir EK: Severe aortic incompetence caused by systemic lupus erythematosus. *S Afr Med J* 54:166, 1978.
22. Rawsthorne L, Ptacin MJ, Choi H, et al: Lupus valvulitis necessitating double valve replacement. *Arthritis Rheum* 24:561, 1981.
23. Wright CB, Hiratzka LF, Crosslands TE, et al: Aortic insufficiency requiring valve replacement in Whipple's disease. *Ann Thorac Surg* 25:466, 1978.
24. Honig HS, Weintraub AN, Gomes MN, et al: Severe aortic regurgitation secondary to idiopathic aortitis. *Am J Med* 63:623, 1977.
25. Soorae AS, McKeown F, Cleland J: Aortic valve replacement for severe aortic regurgitation caused by idiopathic giant cell aortitis. *Thorax* 35:60, 1980.
26. Stewart SR, Robbins DL, Castles JJ: Acute fulminant aortic and mitral insufficiency in ankylosing spondylitis. *N Engl J Med* 299:1448, 1978.
27. Levene RJ, Roberts WC, Morrow AG: Traumatic aortic regurgitation. *Am J Cardiol* 10:752, 1962.
28. Parmley LF, Manion WC, Mattingly TW: Non-penetrating injury to aorta. *Circulation* 17:1086, 1958.
29. Scully RE (ed): Case records of the Massachusetts General Hospital (case 3-1976). *N Engl J Med* 294:152, 1976.
30. O'Brien KP, Hitchcock GC, Banat-Boges BG, et al: Spontaneous aortic cusp rupture associated with valvular myxomatous transformation. *Circulation* 37:273, 1968.
31. Howard CP: Aortic insufficiency due to rupture by strain of a normal aortic valve. *Can Med J* 18:12, 1920.
32. Sainani GS, Szatkowski J: Rupture of a normal aortic valve after physical strain. *Br Heart J* 31:653, 1969.
33. Esteves CM, Dillon JC, Walker JD, et al: Echocardiographic manifestations of aortic cusp rupture in a myxomatous aortic valve. *Chest* 69:685, 1976.
34. Olenger GN, Korus ME, Bonchek LI: Acute aortic valvular insufficiency due to isolated myxomatous degeneration. *Ann Intern Med* 88:807, 1978.
35. Becker AE, Duren DR: Spontaneous rupture of a bicuspid aortic valve. *Chest* 72:361, 1977.
36. Salem BI, Pechacek LW, Leachman RD: Major dehiscence of a prosthetic aortic valve. *Chest* 75:513, 1979.
37. Cohn LH, Mudge GH, Pratter F, et al: Five to eight year followup of patients undergoing porcine heart valve replacement. *N Engl J Med* 304:258, 1981.
38. Housman LB, Pitt WA, Mazur JH, et al: Mechanical failure (leaflet disruption) of a porcine aortic heterograft. *J Thorac Cardiovasc Surg* 76:212, 1978.
39. Cohn LH: Durability of mechanical and biologic prosthetic valves for aortic valve replacement, in Davila JC (ed): *The Second Henry Ford Hospital International Symposium on Cardiac Surgery*. New York, Appleton-Century-Crofts, 1977, chap 61, p 380.
40. Gore JM, Haffajee CI, Collins JJ, et al: Acute spontaneous failure of a porcine aortic valve. *Arch Intern Med* 142:1553, 1982.
41. Welch GH, Braunwald E, Sarnoff SJ: Hemodynamic effects of quantitatively varied experimental aortic regurgitation. *Circ Res* 5:546, 1957.
42. Wigle ED, Labrosse CJ: Sudden, severe aortic insufficiency. *Circulation* 32:708, 1965.
43. Miller GA, Kirklin JW, Swan HJ: Myocardial function and left ventricular volumes in acquired valvular insufficiency. *Circulation* 31:374, 1965.

44. Engloff E: Aortic incompetence: Clinical, hemodynamic and angiographic evaluation. *Acta Med Scand* 193(suppl 538):3, 1972.

45. Grant C, Greene DG, Bunnell IL: Left ventricular enlargement and hypertrophy. *Am J Med* 39:895, 1965.

46. Parke TO, Case RB: Normal left ventricular function. *Circulation* 60:4, 1979.

47. Wise JR, Cleland WP, Hallidie-Smith KA, et al: Urgent aortic valve replacement for acute aortic regurgitation due to infective endocarditis. *Lancet* 2:115, 1971.

48. Mann T, McLaurin L, Grossman W, et al: Assessing the hemodynamic severity of acute aortic regurgitation due to infective endocarditis. *Lancet* 2:115, 1971.

49. Sareli P, Klein Ho, Schamroth CL, et al: Contribution of echocardiography and immediate surgery to the management of severe aortic regurgitation from active infective endocarditis. *Am J Cardiol* 57:413, 1986.

50. Meyer T, Sareli P, Pocock WA, et al: Echocardiographic and hemodynamic correlates of diastolic closure of mitral valve and diastolic opening of aortic valve in severe aortic regurgitation. *Am J Cardiol* 59:1144, 1987.

51. Fortuin NJ, Craige E: On the mechanism of the Austin Flint murmur. *Circulation* 45:558, 1972.

52. Freiden J, Hurwitt ES, Leader E: Ruptured aortic cusp associated with a heritable disorder of connective tissue. *Am J Med* 33:615, 1962.

53. Baron MG: Dissecting aneurysm of the aorta. *Circulation* 43:933, 1971.

54. Goldschlager N, Pfeifer J, Cohn K, et al: The natural history of aortic regurgitation, a clinical and hemodynamic study. *Am J Med* 54:577, 1973.

55. Feigenbaum H: *Echocardiography*. 4th ed. Philadelphia, Lea & Febiger, 1986.

56. Weaver WF, Wilson CS, Rourke T, et al: Mid-diastolic aortic valve opening in severe acute aortic regurgitation. *Chest* 55:145, 1977.

57. Jackson DH, Murphy GW, Stewart S, et al: Delayed appearance of left-to-right shunt following aortic valvular replacement. *Chest* 75:184, 1979.

58. Wann LS, Dillon JC, Weyman AE, et al: Echocardiography in bacterial endocarditis. *N Engl J Med* 295:135, 1976.

59. Roy P, Tajik AJ, Giuliani ER, et al: Spectrum of echocardiographic findings in bacterial endocarditis. *Circulation* 53:474, 1976.

60. Alann LS, Hallam CC, Dillon JC, et al: Comparison of M-mode and cross-sectional echocardiography in infective endocarditis. *Circulation* 60:728, 1979.

61. Castello R, Fagan L, Lenzen P, et al: Comparison of transthoracic and transesophageal echocardiography for assessment of left-sided valvular regurgitation. *Am J Cardiol* 68:1677, 1991.

62. Mugge A, Daniel WG, Frank G, Lichtlen PR: Echocardiography in infective endocarditis: Reassessment of prognostic implications of vegetation size determined by the transthoracic and the transesophageal approach. *J Am Coll Cardiol* 14:631, 1989.

63. Melver ET, Berger M, Lutzker LG: Noninvasive methods for detection of valve regurgitations in infective endocarditis. *Am J Cardiol* 47:271, 1981.

64. Welton DE, Young JB, Raizner AE, et al: Value and safety of cardiac catheterization during active endocarditis. *Am J Cardiol* 44:1306, 1978.

65. Moothart RW, Spangler RD, Blount SG: Echocardiography in aortic root dissection and dilation. *Am J Cardiol* 36:17, 1975.

66. Chan KL: Impact of transesophageal echocardiography on the treatment of patients with aortic dissection. *Chest* 101:406, 1992.

67. Biddle TL, Yu PN: Effect of furosemide on hemodynamics and lung water in acute pulmonary edema secondary to myocardial infarction. *Am J Cardiol* 43:86, 1979.

68. Hutter AM Jr, DeSanctis RW, Nathan MJ, et al: Aortic valve surgery as an emergency procedure. *Circulation* 41:623, 1970.

69. Alpert JS, Rippe JM: *Manual of Cardiovascular Diagnosis and Therapy*. Boston, Little, Brown, 1980, pp 73–74.

70. Cohn JN, Franciosa JA: Vasodilator therapy of cardiac failure. *N Engl J Med* 297:27, 254, 1977.

71. Miller RR, Awan NA, Joye JA, et al: Combined dopamine and nitroprusside therapy in congestive heart failure. *Circulation* 55:881, 1977.

72. Miller RR, Vismara LA, DeMara AN, et al: Afterload reduction therapy with nitroprusside in severe aortic regurgitation: Improved cardiac performance and reduced regurgitant volume. *Am J Cardiol* 38:564, 1976.

73. Warner RA, Bowser M, Zuehlhe S, et al: Treatment of acute aortic insufficiency with sodium nitroferricyanide. *Chest* 72:375, 1977.

74. Goldberg LI: Dopamine: Clinical use of an endogenous catecholamine. *N Engl J Med* 291:707, 1974.

75. Sonnenblick EM, Frishman WH, LeJemtel TH: Dobutamine: A new synthetic cardioactive sympathetic amine. *N Engl J Med* 300:17, 1979.

76. Wilson WR, Danielson GK, Giuliani ER, et al: Cardiac valve replacement in congestive heart failure due to infective endocarditis. *Mayo Clin Proc* 54:223, 1979.

77. Larbalestier RI, Kinchla NM, Aranki SF, et al: Acute bacterial endocarditis: Optimizing surgical results. *Circulation* 86(Suppl 2):II-68, 1992.

78. Krishnaswami V, Sudhaker PR, Curtiss EI, et al: Surgical treatment of acute aortic regurgitation in infective endocarditis. *Ann Thorac Surg* 22:464, 1976.

38. Acute Mitral Regurgitation

Robert A. Harrington and James M. Rippe

Acute mitral regurgitation (MR) may result from sudden disruption of any portion of the mitral valve apparatus [1,2]: the valve leaflets, chordae tendineae, papillary muscle, or attachments of the papillary muscles to the left ventricular wall. Acute MR may occur in a variety of situations commonly treated in the intensive care unit (ICU). In the prethrombolytic era, life-threatening, acute MR caused by papillary muscle rupture was estimated to occur in 1 percent of acute myocardial infarctions [3]. Recently, Tcheng and co-workers, in an analysis of 1480 patients at Duke University Medical Center undergoing acute cardiac catheterization within 6 hours of myocardial infarction, reported a 17.9 percent incidence of mitral regurgitation and a 3.4 percent incidence of moderately severe (3+) or severe MR (4+); 90 percent of these patients had received thrombolytic therapy prior to the acute catheterization [4]. Moderately severe or severe MR was associated with higher mortality rates: 24 percent at 30 days, 42 percent at 6 months, and 52 percent at 1 year. When the presence of MR was added to a regression model that included age, sex, acute ejection fraction, congestive heart failure class, and severity of coronary artery disease as variables, it approached statistical significance (p = 0.06) as an independent predictor of mortality following acute infarction. Similar findings were reported by the Thrombolysis in Myocardial Infarction (TIMI) study group [5]. In 206 patients enrolled in TIMI I who underwent catheterization within 7 hours of acute infarction, MR was diagnosed by ventriculography in 13 percent. Early MR was associated with cardiovascular mortality at 1 year (relative risk 7.5, 95% CI 2.0–28.6, p = 0.0008).

Ischemia to the papillary muscles sufficient to cause dysfunction and the resultant clinically apparent transient murmur may occur in up to 30 percent of patients with coronary artery disease [6] and may imply a poorer prognosis [7,8], the presence of MR being the sixth most important factor of survival in patients with coronary artery disease [9]. Over the past 25 years the underlying etiologies, natural history, physical examination, and hemodynamic findings of this entity have been elucidated [10–14]. Earlier diagnosis, aggressive use of reperfusion therapy with either thrombolytic agents or percutaneous transluminal coronary angioplasty, and improved surgical techniques, with emphasis on valvular repair, have allowed many individuals to survive a previously fatal condition.

Clinical suspicion, careful auscultation, echocardiography, including modalities such as color flow Doppler and transesophageal studies [13,14,15], and right heart catheterization (frequently at the bedside) are essential to the early diagnosis of acute MR [16]. The differential diagnosis includes aortic stenosis, hypertrophic obstructive cardiomyopathy, acute ventricular septal defect, and an innocent flow murmur. Right and left heart catheterization is generally required to establish the diagnosis firmly and, in the case of ischemic MR, possibly to provide reperfusion therapy [9,17–20]. Thrombolytic therapy is considered an essential part of initial medical management of acute ischemic MR [9,17], though recent evidence suggests it may not provide the definitive therapy suggested by early observations. Vasodilators [21,22] and the intraaortic balloon pump [23,24] remain mainstays of ICU treatment as stabilizing measures prior to surgery. Adjuvant use of reperfusion therapy may eliminate the need for surgery or at least make it a less urgent and safer procedure [9,17,18]. In the Duke series, the MR patients with the lowest in-hospital mortality were those with an already patent infarct related artery at the time of acute catheterization and patients with the highest in-hospital mortality were those who required reperfusion therapy at the time of the acute catheterization (17% vs. 50%) [17]. In a separate report from the TIMI group, Lehmann et al. showed that the resolution of MR noted on acute catheterization occurred independently of infarct vessel patency [25]. One group reported, in a randomized trial of first inferior myocardial infarctions, that treatment with thrombolytic therapy was associated with less MR, as assessed by color flow Doppler, at 24 hours, 7 to 10 days, and 28 to 30 days [25]. The study population, however, was very small (104 patients) and the 90 percent confidence intervals on the odds ratios very close to zero (meaning no significant difference). The Duke study and the TIMI report suffer from problems of observational bias, since neither was a randomized trial designed to compare treatments of acute MR; however, both suggest that neither thrombolytic therapy nor angioplasty successfully treats all patients with acute MR. These patients need to be closely followed with a low threshold for more definitive surgical therapy. Valvular repair is emerging as the procedure of choice when sugery is required [17,26–30].

Etiology

The mitral valve apparatus consists of the valve leaflets, annulus, chordae tendineae, and papillary muscles. Normal function of the mitral valve depends on coordinated interplay of all these structures [1,2]. Disruption of any element in this delicate network can result in acute MR. A partial listing of the causes of acute MR, according to the anatomic site of disruption, is found in Table 38-1.

GENERAL ANATOMIC CONSIDERATIONS. In contrast to the other three cardiac valves, which have three cusps, the mitral valve has two leaflets, designated anterior and posterior. The surface area of the two leaflets is approximately equal, although the anterior leaflet has a greater basal-to-margin length and the posterior leaflet a longer annular attachment. Together the surface area of the leaflets is greater than 2.5 times the area of the annulus. The anterior leaflet is continuous with the wall of the ascending aorta and aortic valve, whereas the posterior leaflet is an extension of the posterior and lateral left atrial walls.

Table 38-1. Causes of Acute Mitral Regurgitation

A. Disorders of the mitral valve leaflets
   1. Infective endocarditis
   2. Trauma
   3. Left atrial myxoma
   4. Methysergide (Sansert) therapy
   5. Ankylosing spondylitis
   6. Severe myxomatous degeneration
   7. Trauma of mitral vulvuloplasty
B. Disorders of the mitral valve annulus
   1. Connective tissue disorders
   2. Severe calcification
C. Disorders of the chordae tendineae
   1. Infective endocarditis
   2. Rheumatic valvulitis
   3. Trauma
   4. Myxomatous degeneration
   5. Marfan's syndrome
   6. Systemic lupus erythematosus
   7. Congenital aortic valve disease
   8. Libman-Sacks endocarditis
   9. Acute rheumatic fever
  10. Pregnancy
  11. "Spontaneous"
D. Disorders of the papillary muscles
   1. Dysfunction
     a. Ischemia
     b. Myocardial infarction
     c. Left ventricular dilatation
     d. Left ventricular aneurysm
     e. Amyloidosis
     f. Sarcoidosis
     g. Other infiltrative cardiomyopathies
     h. Trauma and myocardial contusion
     i. Papillary muscle cryoablation
   2. Rupture
     a. Trauma
     b. Acute myocardial infarct
     c. Myocardial abscess
     d. Syphilis
     e. Periarteritis nodosa
E. Prosthetic valve malfunction
   1. Deterioration of Silastic disc
   2. Lodging of the ball or disc in the open position
   3. Dislodgement of the ball or disc
   4. Ring or strut fracture
   5. Paravalvular leak
   6. Suture or pledget dislodgement
   7. Deterioration of leaflets of tissue valve
   8. Prosthetic valve endocarditis
   9. Porcine valve cuspal tear

The leaflets are tethered to the papillary muscles by a complex array of collagenous strands, the *chordae tendineae*. Chordae from both papillary muscles attach to both leaflets. Approximately 12 chordae attach to each papillary muscle and form a progressive branching network, so that approximately 120 chordae attach to the leaflets (Fig. 38-1).

The two papillary muscles are designated anterolateral and posteromedial to correspond with their anatomic positions. The anterolateral papillary muscle is generally larger and protrudes more into the left ventricular cavity. Both papillary muscles have relatively poor blood supplies, owing to their considerable distances from the origins of the coronary arteries. The posteromedial papillary muscle derives its blood supply from branches of the posterior descending artery, while the anterolateral is supplied by the left anterior descending artery and often by the left circumflex coronary artery as well.

MITRAL VALVE LEAFLETS. Disruption of the mitral valve leaflets, although a common cause of chronic MR (in rheumatic valvular disease), is a rare cause of acute MR. Recent work by Kono et al. in a canine model of acute myocardial ischemia and MR demonstrates that hypokinesia of the myocardium overlying the papillary muscle may lead to abnormal retraction of the leaflets and resultant regurgitation [31]. Acute MR may occur after infective endocarditis, when vegetations may inhibit nor-mal leaflet closure; actual leaflet destruction may occur [32,33,34]. Leaflet disruption has also been reported after trauma [35] and with left atrial myxoma [36], where impact of the swinging mass on the leaflets may prevent proper closure. Percutaneous mitral valvuloplasty frequently results in hemo-dynamically insignificant MR [37]; however, a case of severe acute MR resulting from a large tear in the anterior leaflet fol-lowing valvuloplasty has been reported [38]. Both methysergide therapy [39] and ankylosing spondylitis [40] have been reported to cause fibrous thickening of the leaflets severe enough to result in acute regurgitation. Connective tissue disorders in-volving the leaflets, such as the severe myxomatous degener-ation occasionally seen in floppy valve syndrome [41,42] or Marfan's syndrome, may result in acute MR, although other portions of the mitral valve apparatus, such as the annulus or chordae tendineae, are also typically involved.

ANNULUS. Early reports suggested that MR could result from dilatation of the valve annulus, particularly in conditions caus-ing left ventricular failure and dilatation [43]. It now appears that acute MR is rarely caused by annular dilatation except in the setting of a connective tissue disorder involving the heart's fibrous skeleton (floppy valve syndrome, Marfan's syndrome) [43]. There is a subgroup of patients with ischemic MR on the basis of generalized ventricular and annular dilatation caused by diffuse left ventricular ischemic dysfunction [18,30]. Contin-ued ischemia may lead to acute decompensation of the valvular lesion. Calcification of the annulus, seen frequently in older women, may cause regurgitation because of loss of normal sphincteric contraction, but it does not lead to acute decom-pensation [44].

CHORDAE TENDINEAE. Ruptured chordae tendineae is a common cause of acute MR and may complicate infective en-docarditis [45] (either active or healed) or rheumatic valvulitis [46]. Other causes of ruptured chordae include trauma [47], myxomatous degeneration [42], Marfan's syndrome [48], sys-temic lupus erythematosus [49], congenital aortic valve disease with aortic regurgitation [50], Libman-Sacks endocarditis [49,51], acute rheumatic fever [52], and pregnancy [53,54]. In most cases of ruptured chordae, no underlying etiology can be determined, and it is termed *spontaneous* [55]. Fibrosis of the papillary mus-cles is typically present in this setting, suggesting that ineffectual contraction of these supports leads to thinning and, ultimately, rupture of the chordae [55,56]. Ruptured chordae tendineae always lead to acute MR [57].

PAPILLARY MUSCLES. Acute MR due to papillary muscle dysfunction may be caused by ischemia [9,17,30,58,59] and be transient or permanent [60], by altered geometry of a dilated ventricle that inhibits normal leaflet coaptation [60,61], or by blunt chest trauma with subsequent myocardial contusion caus-ing transient papillary muscle dysfunction [62]. Because the papillary muscles are supplied by the most distal portions of the coronary arterial tree, these muscles are vulnerable to tran-sient ischemia and/or infarction [63]; hence, during episodes of angina, temporary ischemia may result in acute MR. Intense ischemia during myocardial infarction may lead to papillary muscle necrosis [59] and permanent MR or the catastrophic complication of papillary muscle rupture [64]. The patient's abil-ity to survive papillary muscle rupture depends on the amount of tissue infarcted (Fig. 38-2). Rupture of one of the six heads of the muscle is analogous to several ruptured chordae tendi-neae and allows short-term survival. Rupture of the entire trunk

Fig. 38-1. Average number of chordae tendineae normally origi-nating from each left ventricular papillary muscle. Although greater variation exists, each left ventricular papillary muscle contains about six "heads," each of which contains two primary or first-order chor-dae tendineae. Each primary cord subdivides into two secondary chordae, each of which divides into two or three tertiary or third-order chordae. The number of chordae attached to each left ventric-ular papillary muscle thus averages 12, and the number of chordae inserting directly into the mitral leaflets from a single papillary muscle averages 62. (These numbers were found by counting chordae and papillary muscle heads in 12 normal hearts.) LA = left atrium; LV = left ventricle. (From Roberts WC, Perloff JK: Mitral valve disease. *Ann Intern Med* 77:939, 1972. With permission.)

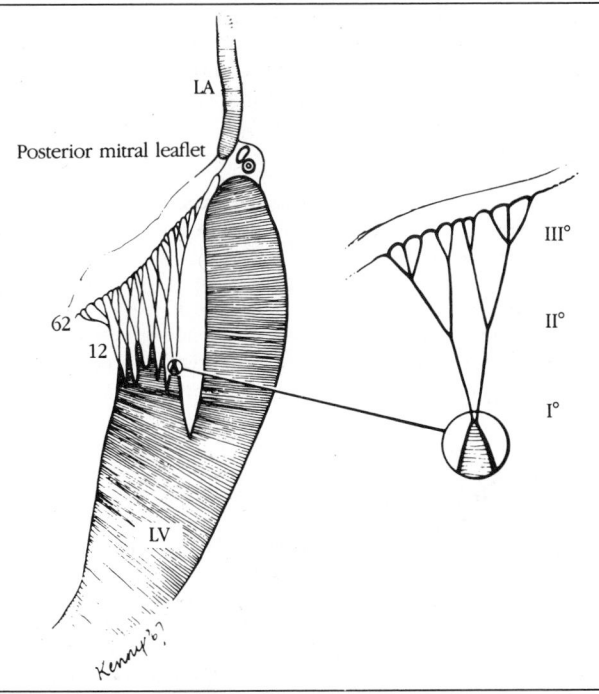

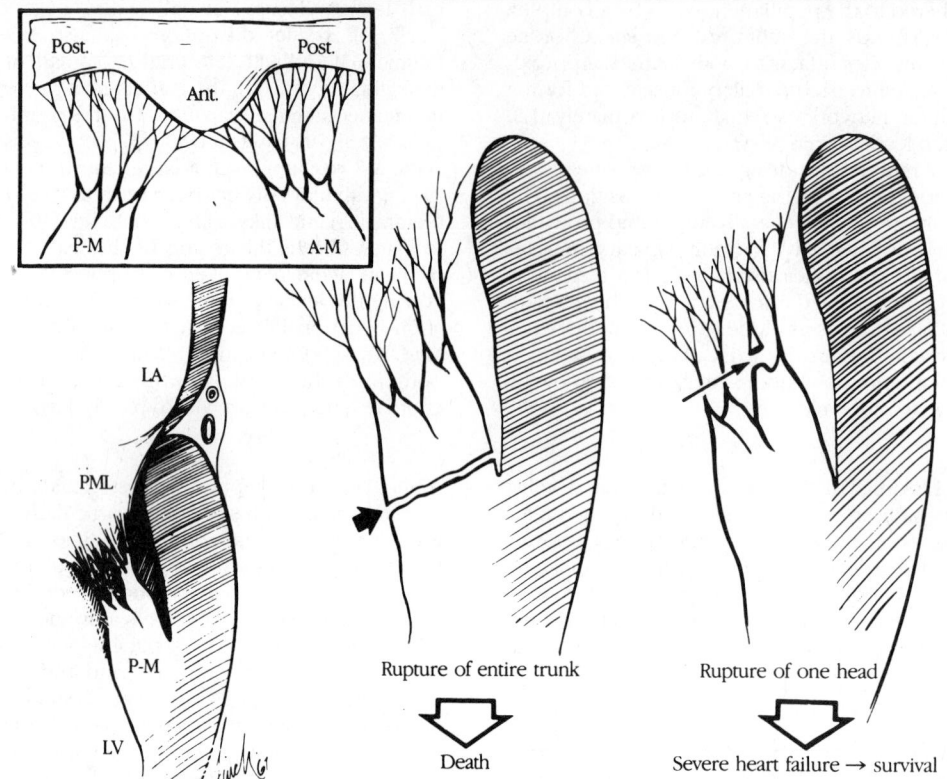

Fig. 38-2. Syndromes arising from rupture of various portions of the papillary muscle. Both the posterior (P-M) and anterior (A-M) papillary muscles give rise to branching chordae tendineae that attach to both anterior and posterior leaflets (*inset*). Rupture of the entire central body (trunk) of the papillary muscle (*center*) leads to overwhelming mitral regurgitation, shock, and death, while rupture of one head (*right*) leads to pulmonary edema and survival if promptly treated. PML = papillary muscle leaflet; LA = left atrium; LV = left ventricle. (From Perloff JK, Roberts WC: The mitral apparatus. *Circulation* 46:277, 1972. With permission.)

of a papillary muscle leads to torrential regurgitation and rapid hemodynamic deterioration. Because its entire blood supply comes from branches of the posterior descending artery, the posteromedial papillary muscle is more vulnerable to ischemia than is the anterolateral. In a recent report by Sharma et al. of 50 consecutive patients presenting with severe ischemic MR, 14 of 15 patients requiring surgery for valve repair or replacement had pathologic documentation of posteromedial papillary muscle dysfunction and involvement [65].

Dilatation of the left ventricle may lead to acute MR by altering the geometric relationship of the papillary muscles to the leaflets [66]. This may occur in left ventricular failure of any etiology, in dilated cardiomyopathies, or in left ventricular aneurysm. Occasionally, infiltrative diseases may cause sufficient papillary muscle dysfunction to result in acute MR. This complication has been described in amyloidosis [67], sarcoidosis [68], and infiltrative cardiomyopathies [69]. Permanent papillary muscle dysfunction with MR requiring valve replacement has been reported following cryoablation for refractory ventricular tachycardia [70].

PROSTHETIC VALVE. Prosthetic mitral valve deterioration can occur in a variety of ways and should be strongly consid-

ered when a patient with a prosthetic mitral valve presents with new-onset pulmonary edema. Deterioration of Silastic discs can produce acute MR [69]. The discs may lodge in the supporting cage in the open position [71], intermittently stick in the open position, occasionally break free, and lodge elsewhere in the arterial circulation [72]. Deterioration of the outer margins of the disc has also been described. Pledgets from the sewing ring may erode, particularly in patients with connective tissue disease. Paravalvular leaks have been reported in up to 10 percent of patients receiving mitral valve prostheses and may be severe enough to cause acute MR [73]. This complication is particularly common with a heavily calcified mitral annulus or ruptured chordae tendineae. Prosthetic valve endocarditis occurs in approximately 2 percent of patients with a mitral valve prosthesis and may lead to acute MR [74]. Porcine valves have reduced the incidence of thromboembolic phenomena but have shown a disturbing tendency to disintegrate, with studies reporting up to a 16 percent incidence of degenerative failure at 7 years, particularly in patients younger than 35 years old [75]. Although the majority of these patients manifest chronic rather than acute MR [76], recent reports note the occurrence of hemodynamic decompensation from acute MR resulting from cuspal tears, either spontaneous or calcific [77,78].

Pathophysiology

Acute MR provides the left ventricle with an additional orifice parallel with the aortic valve. The hemodynamic effect is that of sudden, dramatic afterload reduction, allowing the left ventricle to eject blood into the relatively low-pressure left atrium during both isometric contraction and early ejection. Approximately 50 percent of the regurgitant volume is ejected into the left atrium prior to opening of the aortic valve [79]. Rapid ejection of blood acutely allows the left ventricle to function at lower end-systolic volumes and partially explains experimental findings that acute MR is better tolerated than acute aortic insufficiency [80,81]. In acute MR, the increased myocardial oxygen consumption essential for increased fiber shortening is offset by decreases in ventricular wall tension [82].

Two factors determine the volume of regurgitant flow: the regurgitant orifice size and the pressure gradient between the left ventricle and left atrium [83,84]. In conditions in which the mitral valve annulus is not calcified, left ventricular size may exert profound influence on the orifice size [85]; hence, interventions that decrease left ventricular volume (diuretics or vasodilators) or increase inotropy (digitalis glycosides) will diminish regurgitant volume. Interventions that decrease left ventricular systolic pressure, such as arterial dilators (nitroprusside, hydralazine, or angiotensin converting enzyme inhibitors) or the intraaortic balloon pump, decrease regurgitant volume by reducing the left ventricular to left atrial pressure gradient.

The hemodynamic syndromes caused by MR may be viewed as a spectrum, with acute MR at one end and chronic MR at the other [86]. Patients with severe, chronic MR show the effects of long-term volume overload of both the left ventricle and the left atrium. Marked dilatation of both chambers occurs (Fig. 38-3). While left atrial pressures become elevated, the left atrial pressure tracing rarely shows tall regurgitant (CV) waves in chronic MR. In contrast, patients with acute, severe MR have minimal or no left atrial or left ventricular dilatation, [1,13,86]. Rather, compensatory hypertrophy of a small, vigorously contracting left atrium occurs, and high pressures are reflected back into the pulmonary circulation, causing pulmonary hypertension and right ventricular hypertrophy (Fig. 38-3) [1]. These patients frequently display tall regurgitant waves (giant V waves) indicative of blood ejected into a noncompliant left atrium [1,86], although the appearance of giant V waves is not limited to acute MR [87]. Most patients with acute MR fall somewhere between these pathophysiologic extremes, depending on acuteness and degree of regurgitation, volume status, and associated cardiac disease.

Although MR is the most common cause of large CV waves, they may also occur in any condition that impairs left atrial emptying (mitral stenosis), when a mitral prosthesis is present, in combined aortic and mitral disease, with coronary artery disease, and with ventricular septal defect; furthermore, patients with severe MR may exhibit trivial CV waves [88]. This is particularly common in patients with low left atrial pressure. The presence or absence of large CV waves at bedside right heart catheterization is still a useful finding [16], but it should be interpreted cautiously, particularly in patients with associated mitral stenosis or coronary artery disease and those who have recently undergone diuresis and are volume-depleted [88].

Initially patients with acute MR generally exhibit slight increases in ejection fraction; therefore, a normal ejection fraction in a patient with severe MR suggests impaired myocardial function, whereas moderate decreases in ejection fraction (e.g., <50%) may signify severe dysfunction [89,90]. Patients with acute MR and ejection fractions less than 40 percent generally have such severe left ventricular dysfunction that mitral valve replacement may not result in either significant symptomatic improvement [91] or increased long-term survival [30].

Diagnosis

HISTORY. The natural history of acute MR varies according to the underlying etiology of the lesion and the severity of regur-

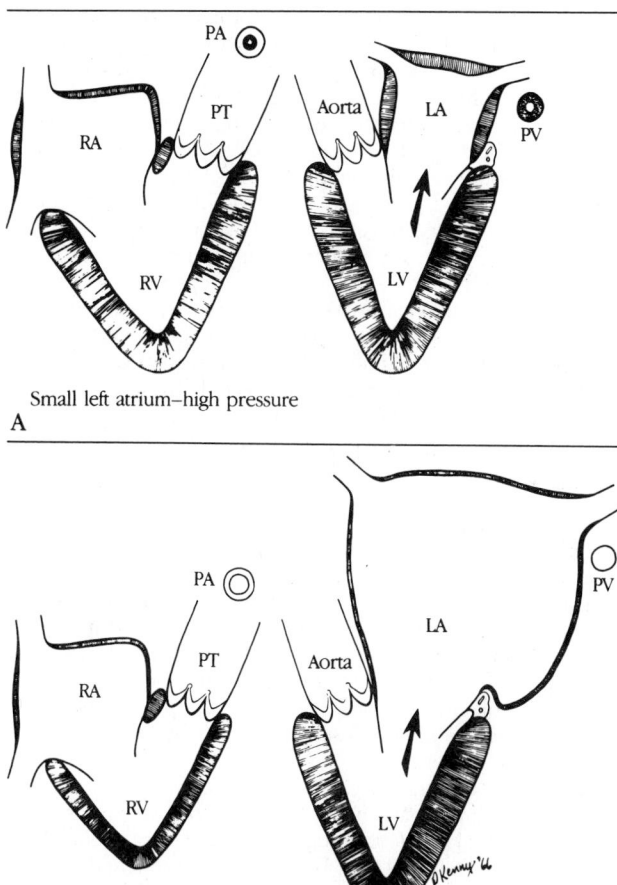

Fig. 38-3. The two extremes of severe acute and chronic mitral regurgitation. A. In acute mitral regurgitation, disruption of a portion of the valvular apparatus occurs suddenly. The left atrial and left ventricular sizes remain small. Hypertrophy begins to occur rapidly, and high pressures are transmitted back into the pulmonary vasculature. B. In chronic mitral regurgitation, left atrial dilatation occurs and the chamber functions at lower pressures. LA = left atrium; LV = left ventricle; PA = pulmonary artery; PV = pulmonary vein; RA = right atrium; RV = right ventricle. (From Perloff JK, Roberts WC: The mitral apparatus. *Circulation* 46:227, 1972, with permission.)

gitation [92]. In contrast to chronic MR patients, who become symptomatic slowly as left ventricular failure develops, patients with acute MR can generally pinpoint a date when symptoms began [77]. A typical clinical picture of acute MR includes relatively good health, sudden onset of symptoms, and a new or markedly changed murmur. The severity of symptoms depends on the underlying cause of acute MR; these symptoms may vary from dyspnea on exertion with ruptured chordae tendineae to overwhelming pulmonary edema and shock with a ruptured papillary muscle [93].

Symptoms related to the underlying causes of acute MR (Table 38-1) should be explored. Patients with ruptured chordae may give a history of previous rheumatic fever and/or long-standing asymptomatic murmur complicated by a sudden exacerbation of symptoms [12]. A history of mitral valve prolapse also should suggest ruptured chordae as a cause of acute decompensation [42]. The patient may give a history of infective endocarditis or trauma. Although the severity of symptoms depends on the number of chordae ruptured, patients typically remember exactly when symptoms began.

In contrast, rupture of a papillary muscle is a catastrophic event, generally occurring during acute myocardial infarction and resulting in pulmonary edema and shock [93]. Without prompt surgical repair, 75 percent of patients die within 24 hours and 95 percent die within 2 weeks [64].

The symptoms of acute MR are those of pulmonary edema and pulmonary hypertension [94]. The acute volume load presented to the relatively noncompliant left atrium results in abrupt elevation of left atrial pressures. Depending on the volume of regurgitation, the patient may experience symptoms ranging from dyspnea on exertion to acute pulmonary edema. Abrupt elevation of pulmonary vascular pressures may cause acute right heart failure, with its attendant signs and symptoms (i.e., hepatomegaly, ascites, peripheral edema, and evidence of low output congestive heart failure).

PHYSICAL EXAMINATION. A summary of the physical examination findings in acute MR is found in Table 38-2. It is a spectrum of findings, ranging from the presence of a new systolic murmur with hemodynamic stability to cardiogenic shock. Evidence of systemic manifestations of entities known to cause acute MR should be carefully sought. Fever and occasionally Roth spots, Janeway lesions, or splinter hemorrhages may be present in infective endocarditis. Skeletal, ophthalmologic, or dermatologic abnormalities suggestive of connective tissue disease may be present.

A cluster of findings on cardiac auscultation helps distinguish acute from chronic MR [9,12]. Patients with chronic MR are typically in atrial fibrillation, suggesting a chronically dilated left atrium. S_1 is often soft and blowing; a high-pitched murmur heard best at the apex and radiating to the axilla is present. The murmur begins with S_1 and extends throughout systole, often obscuring A_2 (reflecting the persistence of a gradient between the left ventricle and left atrium throughout systole). The murmur changes little in response to changes in left ventricular volume typical of atrial fibrillation, and the intensity of the murmur correlates poorly with the severity of regurgitation.

In contrast, in acute MR the underlying rhythm is typically sinus tachycardia. A prominent, often palpable presystolic gallop is frequently present as the hypertrophied left atrium forcefully ejects blood into the left ventricle [95,96]. S_2 may be widely split (reflecting early closure of the aortic valve), and if pulmonary hypertension is present P_2 may be accentuated. The murmur of acute MR often suggests dysfunction of a specific portion of the valvular apparatus [97,98]. When chordae tendineae to the posterior leaflet rupture, the regurgitant jet may be

directed anteriorly and may impact on the atrial septum adjacent to the aortic root [99]. The resultant murmur, best heard at the base of the heart, may be confused with aortic stenosis. When chordae to the anterior leaflet rupture, the regurgitant jet is directed toward the posterior wall of the left atrium, and the murmur may radiate to the patient's back or top of the head. Since left atrial pressures rise abruptly in acute MR, the systolic gradient between the left ventricle and left atrium may be abolished during the latter part of systole, resulting in a crescendo-decrescendo murmur ending well before A_2. It is important to remember that overwhelming MR may present without an audible murmur. No murmur is audible in 50 percent of patients with acute papillary muscle rupture, probably because of left ventricular power failure [51]. In the Duke series, Tcheng et al. noted that a systolic murmur consistent with MR was present only 56 percent of the time in cases of 3+ or 4+ MR and only 7 percent of the time in cases of 1+ or 2+ MR [4]. When right ventricular failure follows acute MR, the murmur of tricuspid insufficiency may be present.

Palpation of the apical impulse may also be helpful. In acute MR, the left ventricular impulse is hyperdynamic [100] and nondisplaced, while in chronic MR evidence of left ventricular dilatation is present [101].

The murmur of acute MR may be difficult to distinguish from that of aortic stenosis, hypertrophic obstructive cardiomyopathy, or ventricular septal defect. Other physical examination findings may be helpful. The pulse pressure is typically increased in acute MR and decreased in aortic stenosis. The carotid arterial upstroke is sharp in acute MR and usually delayed in aortic stenosis. On dynamic auscultation, the murmur of acute MR is increased with isometric exercise (e.g., handgrip) and transient arterial occlusion (simultaneous inflation of bilateral sphygmomanometers 20–40 mm Hg above the patient's systolic blood pressure) [102], whereas those of aortic stenosis and hypertrophic obstructive cardiomyopathy are diminished. The murmur of acute MR may usually be distinguished from that of ventricular septal defect by location, since the latter is typically best heard at the left sternal border and is often accompanied by a palpable thrill.

LABORATORY EXAMINATION. A summary of laboratory findings pertinent to acute MR is found in Table 38-3.

Electrocardiogram. Although there are no electrocardiographic findings specific for acute MR, the ECG may be helpful in distinguishing possible underlying etiologies [103]. Sinus tachycardia is typical in acute MR, while atrial fibrillation suggests a chronic condition. Occasionally, a biphasic P wave with large terminal forces in lead V_1 suggests left atrial volume overload [104]. Acute papillary muscle infarction may be accompanied by electrocardiographic changes typical of acute myocardial infarction (see Chap. 33), whereas the location of particular ischemic changes may identify the involved papillary muscle. Evidence of right ventricular hypertrophy is occasionally present.

Radiology. The chest radiograph in acute MR typically reveals the striking findings of interstitial or alveolar edema with a normal-sized cardiac silhouette [105]. Occasionally left atrial enlargement is present, but more often the left atrium is normal in size [106]. Fluoroscopy is rarely used to observe the systolic expansion of the left atrium, since MR is easily and more sensitively viewed with echocardiography [107].

Echocardiogram. M-mode and two-dimensional (2-D) echocardiography, including pulse Doppler and Doppler color flow

Table 38-2. Physical Examination Findings in Acute Mitral Regurgitation

1. Evidence of systemic manifestations of any disorder listed in Table 38-1
   a. Fever, Roth spots, Janeway lesions
   b. Evidence of blunt chest trauma
2. Cardiovascular findings
   a. Prominent (often palpable) S_4
   b. Sinus tachycardia
   c. Widely split S_2
   d. Systolic murmur (may mimic murmur of aortic stenosis)
3. Other findings
   a. Evidence of pulmonary congestion
   b. Evidence of shock

Table 38-3. Laboratory Findings in Acute Mitral Regurgitation

1. Electrocardiogram
   a. Sinus tachycardia
   b. Large terminal forces in P wave in V_1
   c. Acute ischemic changes
2. Chest radiograph
   a. Pulmonary congestion without cardiomegaly
   b. Left atrial enlargement (rare)
3. Echocardiogram
   a. Systolic expansion of left atrium (two-dimensional echocardiogram)
   b. Flail leaflet
   c. Vegetation
   d. Flattened septal or posterior wall motion (infarction)
   e. Hyperdynamic septal and posterior wall motion (acute volume overload)
   f. Increased E/F slope
   g. Demonstration of regurgitant flow by pulse and/or color flow Doppler
   h. Absence of evidence of AS, HOCM, or VSD
4. Gated cardiac blood pool scan
   a. Left-to-right stroke volume index of greater than 1.5–2.0 : 1.0
   b. Elevated left ventricular ejection fraction
5. Cardiac catheterization
   a. Giant CV waves (see text)
   b. Absence of oxygen content step-up between right atrium and right ventricle
   c. Angiographic evidence of regurgitation
   d. Presence or absence of other cardiac abnormalities

AS = aortic stenosis; HOCM = hypertrophic obstructive cardiomyopathy; VSD = ventricular septal defect.

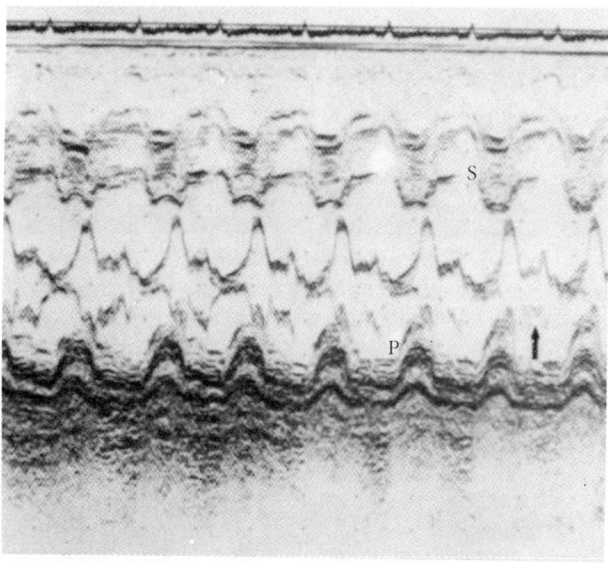

Fig. 38-4. M-mode echocardiograms, showing typical findings in ruptured chordae tendineae. The septum (S) and left ventricular posterior wall (P) show hyperdynamic motion. The coarse oscillations of the posterior mitral valve leaflet are typical for ruptured chordae tendineae. (From Howe JP III, Alpert JS: Acute mitral regurgitation, in Dalen JE, Alpert JS (eds): *Valvular Heart Disease.* Boston, Little, Brown, 1981, p 145. With permission.)

techniques, make several important contributions to the diagnosis of acute MR [108]. First, these studies help differentiate the many possible underlying conditions causing acute MR [109]. Second, they can rule out conditions that may mimic acute MR [103]. In acute MR, because neither left ventricular nor left atrial chamber enlargement may be apparent on 2-D echocardiogram, use of Doppler techniques greatly aids in confirming the diagnosis. Although it has well-described limitations, secondary mainly to technical problems and to the complexity of regurgitant jet dynamics [110], Doppler color flow is quite impressive in its ability to image and quantitate regurgitant flow [15,110,111,112]. Although it has not replaced angiography as the gold standard, Doppler color flow is very useful in making the initial diagnosis and for noninvasively following patients to determine progression or regression of disease and timing of surgical intervention. Color flow may be useful in identifying the specific mitral leaflet responsible for the regurgitation by delineating the direction of the jet [113]. Two-dimensional echocardiography may reveal marked systolic expansion of the left atrium in severe MR with a characteristic convex bowing of the interatrial septum toward the right atrium at end-systole [114,115]. In addition, 2-D echocardiography may allow direct visualization of the papillary muscles and any abnormalities of contraction seen with ischemic dysfunction [116].

In ruptured chordae tendineae, a characteristic flail motion of either the anterior or posterior leaflet as well as hyperdynamic left ventricular wall motion may be present (Fig. 38-4) [117]. In contrast, in papillary muscle rupture, leaflet fluttering may be present, but the motion of the infarcted interventricular septum or posterior wall of the left ventricle is flattened [118]. Early closure of the aortic valve may reflect decreased forward cardiac output and/or severe MR.

In patients with infective endocarditis, echocardiography may visualize vegetations as small as 2 mm in diameter [119]. Larger vegetations causing acute MR may present with dramatic

findings (Fig. 38-5) and may be difficult to distinguish from a flail leaflet [34]. Left atrial myxoma may be revealed by a dense cluster of echoes attached to a leaflet and prolapsing into the left atrium during systole. Papillary muscle dysfunction may be suggested by decreased diastolic E/F velocity of the mitral valve and increased left ventricular cavity size.

Echocardiography provides important information for distinguishing acute MR from aortic stenosis, hypertrophic obstructive cardiomyopathy, and ventricular septal defect [109]. In aortic stenosis, redundant, calcific echoes are present in the aortic valve region, together with decreased systolic opening and concentric left ventricular hypertrophy. In hypertrophic obstructive cardiomyopathy, asymmetric septal hypertrophy as well as systolic anterior motion of the mitral valve may be observed [120]. Pulsed Doppler echocardiography has been demonstrated to distinguish reliably between acute MR and ventricular septal defect by localizing the site of turbulent flow [121,122]. Finally, the use of intraoperative transesophageal Doppler echocardiogram during volume loading may allow identification of the patient with volume-dependent MR requiring surgical repair [18,30].

Gated Cardiac Blood Pool Scan. This radionuclide technique has been demonstrated to be reasonably accurate in assessing the severity of both aortic regurgitation and MR [15,123,124]. The technique compares right and left ventricular stroke volume indices. In normal individuals, the left-to-right ventricular stroke index is near unity, whereas in regurgitant lesions it is typically greater than 1.5 and often greater than 2.0. Comparison of left ventricular to right ventricular stroke volume can suggest the total amount of regurgitation; if cardiac catheterization data are available for validation, gated cardiac blood pool scanning can be used to follow the patient sequentially, because reproducibility is good [15]. The gated blood pool scan can also be used to measure cardiac output [125].

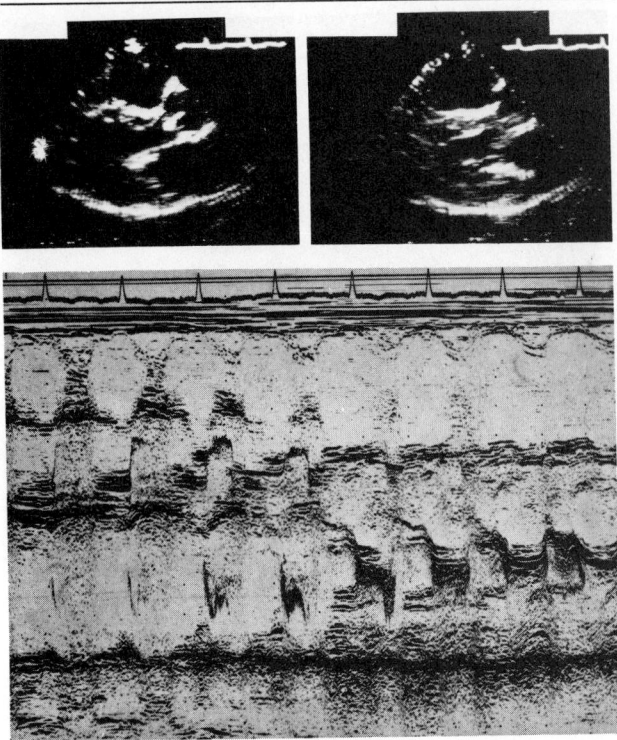

Fig. 38-5. M-mode (*top*) and 2-dimensional (*bottom*) echocardiograms in a patient with acute mitral regurgitation caused by infective endocarditis. A large mass of shaggy echoes from the mitral valve vegetation can be seen to prolapse into the left atrium during systole. (From Rippe JM, Curley F, Paraskos JA, et al: Triple valve endocarditis with unusual echocardiographic findings. *Am Heart J* 107:598, 1984. With permission.)

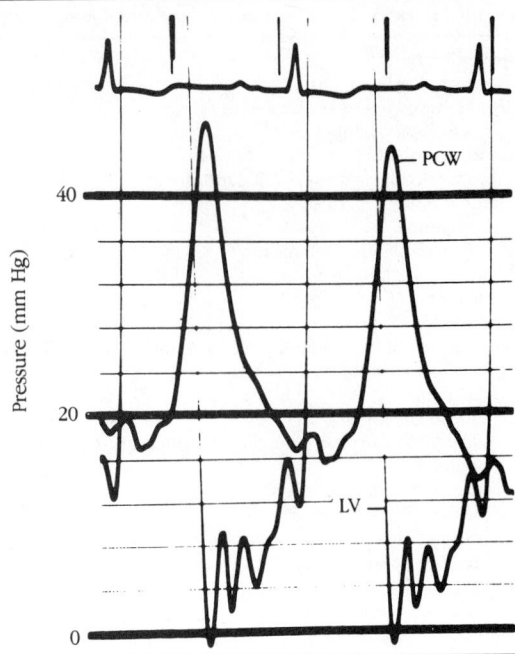

Fig. 38-6. Pressure tracings obtained during cardiac catheterization from a patient with acute mitral regurgitation caused by ruptured chordae tendineae. The top tracing is the patient's ECG. Large CV waves are present in the pulmonary capillary wedge (PCW) pressure tracing. LV = left ventricular diastolic pressure. (From Howe JP III, Alpert JS: Acute mitral regurgitation, in Dalen JE, Alpert JS (eds): *Valvular Heart Disease.* Boston, Little, Brown, 1981, p 147. With permission.)

Cine Magnetic Resonance Imaging. This technique, which relies on identification of a changing signal intensity, its intracardiac location, and its relationship to the cardiac cycle, can reliably demonstrate and quantitate regurgitant valvular lesions [126,127]. Correlation with echocardiography is good, but at present there are major limitations, not the least of which are patient transportation problems and prolonged imaging times, which make its use in acute MR impractical. At this time cine magnetic resonance imaging may be best used to study more chronic valvular lesions.

Cardiac Catheterization

RIGHT HEART CATHETERIZATION. This technique provides important diagnostic information in the patient with suspected acute MR and is useful in optimizing vasodilation therapy [128]. The procedure may be performed at the bedside in an unstable patient, using a balloon-tipped, flow-directed catheter (insertion techniques and interpretation of hemodynamic data are discussed in Chap. 4) [16]. Despite the limitations of the finding of giant CV waves (already discussed), their presence still suggests acute MR (Fig. 38-6) [88]. Bedside right heart catheterization is particularly helpful in distinguishing acute MR from rupture of the interventricular septum. In the latter condition, a step-up in oxygen content of greater than 1 vol% between the right atrium and right ventricle is present with a hemodynamically significant left-to-right shunt [16]. Pulmonary artery pressures are typically elevated in acute MR, although this finding

is nonspecific. Oxygen saturation in pulmonary arterial blood is often diminished, resulting from low cardiac output [16].

LEFT HEART CATHETERIZATION. Although angiography is still far from ideal in its ability to quantify regurgitation absolutely [129], left heart catheterization provides useful information about the severity of regurgitation, the degree of coexisting coronary artery disease, left ventricular function, and the presence or absence of any other valvular lesions. The diagnosis of MR is established during left ventricular cineangiography by the appearance of contrast material in the left atrium after its injection into the left ventricle [130,131]. Both qualitative and quantitative determinations of the severity of regurgitation may be made. Prompt opacification of the entire left atrium (within 1 or 2 systoles) indicates severe MR. By simultaneous measurement of the forward cardiac output by the Fick method and cardiac output estimated angiographically, the regurgitant volume may be estimated. A number of studies document that the regurgitant volume may equal or exceed forward output [132]. The functional status of the left ventricle is important when considering surgical intervention, because patients with diffuse left ventricular dysfunction and poor residual myocardium have an extremely high in-hospital mortality, regardless of the therapy chosen [18,30]. These patients may be more appropriate candidates for cardiac transplantation, rather than a procedure meant to restore valvular competence [30]. The presence of high-grade obstructive lesions of the coronary arteries leads to revascularization at the time of mitral valve replacement, and the finding of a discrete ventricular aneurysm may lead to simultaneous aneurysmectomy [133].

Differential Diagnosis

As already described, patients with acute MR present with signs and symptoms of left ventricular failure and pulmonary hypertension. The clinical presentation depends on the severity of acute regurgitation and ranges from chest pain with dyspnea on exertion to florid pulmonary edema with cardiogenic shock. The onset of symptoms is typically abrupt. Patients with acute MR typically demonstrate sinus tachycardia, a prominent S_4, and a new apical systolic murmur. A normal heart size and pulmonary vascular congestion are present on chest radiograph.

The symptoms of chest pain and dyspnea may suggest angina or pulmonary embolism. Here, the presence of a new systolic murmur and a loud S_4 should point to acute MR [7]. The murmur may be difficult to distinguish from that of aortic stenosis, hypertrophic obstructive cardiomyopathy, acute rupture of the interventricular septum, or decompensated chronic MR [134]. Delayed carotid upstroke and diminished S_2 should point to the diagnosis of aortic stenosis. Left ventricular hypertrophy on ECG should suggest either aortic stenosis or hypertrophic obstructive cardiomyopathy. The ECG may also demonstrate ischemic changes or an acute myocardial infarction, making the diagnosis of ischemic MR more likely. Echocardiography should reliably distinguish both of these conditions from acute MR. Bedside right heart catheterization provides information essential for distinguishing acute MR from an acute ventricular septal defect. The presence of atrial fibrillation and an enlarged heart on chest radiograph favors chronic, rather than acute, MR. Information from the history, physical examination, ECG, echocardiogram, and bedside right heart catheterization should distinguish acute MR from these other entities.

Treatment

INTENSIVE CARE UNIT MANAGEMENT. Medical therapy in the ICU should focus on hemodynamic stabilization and rapid identification of the mechanical defect and underlying etiology. If the acute MR is ischemic in origin with papillary muscle dysfunction, reperfusion therapy, with either thrombolytic agents or percutaneous transluminal coronary angioplasty (PTCA), may be indicated [9,17–20]. Successful reperfusion may provide rapid hemodynamic stabilization and may obviate the need for emergent surgery or at least allow surgery under less urgent circumstances [9]. Successful reperfusion preserves the mitral structures (and thus left ventricular function) and avoids the long-term problems associated with prosthetic valve replacement. While early case reports suggested that early reperfusion was quite successful in its ability to restore valvular competence, more recent studies have not been as promising. Tcheng et al. [4] reported that of the 50 patients with moderately severe or severe MR, 18 had a patent infarct vessel at the time of catheterization. Twenty-two of the remaining patients underwent rescue PTCA, with 18 being successful. Thirty-eight patients left the lab with a patent vessel, and despite this the mortality rate remained exceedingly high. In fact, the highest in-hospital mortality (50%) was in patients who required reperfusion therapy in the catheterization lab. Seven of 10 patients who had PTCA of the infarct vessel and who were alive at 6 months underwent follow-up cardiac catheterization. Four of these patients continued to have 3+ or 4+ MR despite successful initial reperfusion and sustained 6-month arterial patency. The TIMI group also recently reported that the resolution of acute MR appears to ber independent of infarct vessel patency [5].

The mainstays of medical therapy are vasodilating drugs [135] and the intraaortic balloon pump (see Chap. 11) [23,24]. Afterload reducing agents, such as nitroprusside, hydralazine, and angiotensin converting enzyme inhibitors, improve hemodynamics in acute MR by several mechanisms. First, by lowering systemic vascular resistance and impedance to left ventricular ejection, forward cardiac output is increased and regurgitant volume diminished [136,137]. Second, by decreasing left ventricular volume, these agents decrease the size of the regurgitant orifice [136,137]. While oral angiotensin converting enzyme inhibitors, hydralazine, or prazosin therapy is often sufficient for long-term management of patients with chronic MR, nitroprusside is the agent of choice for acute MR [138]. Systemic arterial pressures and pulmonary artery pressures should be continuously monitored with an indwelling arterial catheter (see Chap. 3) and pulmonary artery catheter (see Chap. 4) in patients receiving nitroprusside therapy. The nitroprusside infusion is titrated to maintain pulmonary capillary wedge pressure in the range of 15 to 18 mm Hg and systolic blood pressure in the range of 90 to 100 mm Hg. We typically initiate therapy with an infusion rate between 3 and 6 µg/kg/min and increase the dosage until symptoms are relieved or systolic pressure falls below 100 mm Hg. Evidence of thiocyanate toxicity from nitroprusside infusion includes mental confusion and gastrointestinal distress [138]. Toxicity is unusual during the first 24 hours of therapy. Thiocyanate levels may be monitored when infusions are employed for longer time periods, although thiocyanate toxicity is unusual.

Patients with acute MR should be loaded with digoxin. Other measures used in the treatment of heart failure should be employed. A Foley catheter should be inserted to monitor urine output. Arrhythmias should be treated aggressively to prevent additional cardiac dysfunction, although antiarrhythmic agents that cause myocardial depression, such as disopyramide, should be avoided if possible.

Patients with low systemic arterial pressures (systolic pressure <90 mm Hg, diastolic pressure <60 mm Hg) may benefit from judicious use of inotropic agents such as dopamine or dobutamine [21]. Dopamine can, however, carry the disadvantage of elevating systemic vascular resistance and may result in increased MR and/or myocardial ischemia. Such patients are probably best managed with a combination of vasodilator drugs and intraaortic balloon pump therapy. Patients with low arterial pressures or in whom systemic pressures fall prior to a decrease in pulmonary artery pressures are candidates for prompt insertion of the intraaortic balloon pump (see Chap. 11) [23].

While these measures to improve hemodynamic stability are being undertaken in the ICU, personnel should be mobilized to perform emergency cardiac catheterization. The timing of this procedure reflects the etiology of the acute MR and the patient's clinical status. In ischemic MR, administration of a thrombolytic agent or performance of PTCA may be indicated to reperfuse the dysfunctional papillary muscle, though it should be recognized that surgery may still be needed to provide optimal and definitive therapy. If cardiogenic shock is present (even if hemodynamic improvement occurs after insertion of the intraaortic balloon pump), emergency catheterization should be performed as soon as possible so that coronary anatomy can be delineated and infarct vessel reperfusion attempted. Recent work by Bengston and co-workers demonstrates that survival in cardiogenic shock is significantly associated with infarct vessel patency [140]. In anticipation of possible emergency surgery, the cardiac surgical team should be placed on standby as soon as catheterization is scheduled [139].

SURGICAL THERAPY. Once the diagnosis of acute MR is secure, and if reperfusion therapy of ischemic disease fails, surgical therapy is the treatment of choice. A variety of techniques for repair of specific portions of the valve apparatus may be employed, including leaflet or annulus plication, Carpentier ring annuloplasty, placement of artificial chordae, and direct suture repair of chordae or papillary muscle head; however, repair of the valve is emerging as the surgical therapy of choice [9,18,26–30]. The pathology of the valvular disease can suggest the indicated therapy [18,27,28,29], but repair seems to be contraindicated only when there is severe damage to the anterior leaflet or unreparable calcific fusion of mitral structures [27]. Given that an emergent procedure combining mitral valve replacement with coronary artery bypass surgery has an in-hospital mortality approaching 50 percent [18], the arguments for repair, particularly in the emergency setting, are compelling. With repair there is shortened operating time, preservation of the mitral apparatus and left ventricular function, and a decrease in the complications associated with prosthetic valves [18]. One study reports a 26 percent in-hospital mortality for valve repair in ischemic MR, compared with a 53 percent in-hospital mortality for valve replacement [30]. Durability of repair is excellent, with a reported 90 percent 5-year freedom from early or late valve replacement [29].

The results of surgical intervention depend on the age of the patient; the cause of acute regurgitation; existence of other cardiac lesions (e.g., coronary artery disease, ventricular aneurysm); functional capacity of the left ventricle; presence of pulmonary hypertension; presence of cardiogenic shock; coexistence of hepatic, renal, or pulmonary disease; need for intraaortic balloon pump therapy; and urgency of surgery [9,18,27,140–144].

Surgical intervention to correct acute MR causing acute left ventricular failure is associated with much greater surgical risk than valve replacement in chronic regurgitation. Without surgical intervention, however, chances of survival are very small. If MR results from acute myocardial infarction, reperfusion therapy should be considered as initial therapy. If reperfusion is successful, valvular competence can be assessed serially with echocardiography and surgery considered if the MR persists. Otherwise, an attempt should be made to stabilize the patient and, if possible, to defer surgery for 4 to 6 weeks after infarction. Patients with acute MR caused by prosthetic valve dysfunction or left ventricular failure following infectious endocarditis also carry higher-than-average surgical risk; however, early surgical intervention is warranted for both indications [145,146]. Patients with generalized ventricular dilatation secondary to diffuse ischemia and multiple infarcts with resultant MR have a very low probability of in-hospital survival despite surgery, because the valve procedure may be inadequate given the residual dysfunctional myocardium [17,18,30]. Surgery in this group should be carefully considered and other alternatives, such as comfort measures only, discussed with the patient and family.

Long-term results of surgical intervention to correct acute MR also vary according to the underlying etiology. The 5-year survival rate in patients with acute MR caused by myocardial ischemia is 30 percent, whereas 5-year survival of valve replacement in the absence of an acute coronary event is much better [134].

References

1. Roberts WC, Perloff JK: Mitral valvular disease. *Ann Intern Med* 77:939, 1972.

2. Perloff JK, Roberts WC: The mitral apparatus: Functional anatomy of mitral regurgitation. *Circulation* 46:227, 1972.

3. Morrow AG, Cohen LS, Roberts WC, et al: Severe mitral regurgitation following acute myocardial infarction and ruptured papillary muscle: Hemodynamic findings and results of operative treatment in four patients. *Circulation* 37(suppl II):124, 1968.

4. Tcheng JE, Jackman JD, Nelson CL, et al: Outcome of patients sustaining acute ischemic mitral regurgitation during myocardial infarction. *Ann Intern Med* 117:18, 1992.

5. Lehmann KG, Francis CK, Dodge HT: Mitral regurgitation in early myocardial infarction: Incidence, clinical detection and prognostic implications. TIMI Study Group. *Ann Intern Med* 117:10, 1992.

6. Gahl K, Sutton R, Pearson M, et al: Mitral regurgitation in coronary heart disease. *Br Heart J* 39:13, 1977.

7. Maisel AS, Gilpin EA, Klein L, et al: The murmur of papillary muscle dysfunction in acute myocardial infarction: Clinical features and prognostic implications. *Am Heart J* 112:705, 1986.

8. Barzilai B, Gessler C, Perez JE, et al: Significance of Doppler-detected mitral regurgitation in acute myocardial infarction. *Am J Cardiol* 61:220, 1988.

9. Hickey MStJ, Smith LR, Muhlbaier LH, et al: Current prognosis of ischemic mitral regurgitation: Implications for future management. *Circulation* 78(suppl I):I-51, 1988.

10. Pizzarello RA, Gulotta SJ: Cardiology: Acute severe mitral regurgitation. *Postgrad Med J* 60:215, 1976.

11. Johnson A: The natural history of valvular disease: Implications regarding medical and surgical management of aortic and mitral regurgitation. *Med Times* 106:77, 1978.

12. Roberts WC, Braunwald E, Morrow AG: Acute severe mitral regurgitation secondary to ruptured chordae tendineae. *Circulation* 33:58, 1966.

13. DePace NL, Nestico PF, Morganroth J: Acute severe mitral regurgitation: Pathophysiology, clinical recognition, and management. *Am J Med* 78:293, 1985.

14. Kusiak V, Brest AN: Acute mitral regurgitation: Pathophysiology and management. *Cardiovasc Clin* 16:257, 1986.

15. Iskandrian AS, Hakki A, Kotler MN: Value of echocardiography and nuclear techniques in assessment of valvular heart lesions. *Cardiovasc Clin* 17:181, 1986.

16. Meister SG, Helfant RH: Rapid bedside differentiation of ruptured interventricular septum from acute mitral insufficiency. *N Engl J Med* 287:1024, 1972.

17. Rankin JS, Hickey MStJ, Smith LR, et al: Ischemic mitral regurgitation. *Circulation* 79(suppl I):I-116, 1989.

18. Rankin JS, Hickey MStJ, Smith LR, et al: Current management of mitral valve incompetence associated with coronary artery disease. *J Cardiac Surg* 4:25, 1989.

19. Shawl FA, Forman MB, Punja S, et al: Emergent coronary angioplasty in the treatment of acute ischemic mitral regurgitation: Long-term results in five cases. *J Am Coll Cardiol* 14:986, 1989.

20. Heuser RR, Maddoux GL, Goss JE, et al: Coronary angioplasty for acute mitral regurgitation due to myocardial infarction: A nonsurgical treatment preserving mitral valve integrity. *Ann Intern Med* 107:852, 1987.

21. Massie BM, Chatterjee K: Vasodilator therapy of pump failure complicating acute myocardial infarction. *Med Clin North Am* 63:25, 1979.

22. Greenberg BH, Massie BM, Brundage BH, et al: Beneficial effects of hydralazine in severe mitral regurgitation. *Circulation* 58:273, 1978.

23. Quaal SJ: Extended medical indications for balloon pumping, in Quaal SJ: *Comprehensive Intra-aortic Balloon Pumping*. St. Louis, CV Mosby, 1984.

24. Replogle RL, Campbell CD: Surgery for mitral regurgitation associated with ischemic heart disease: Results and strategies. *Circulation* 79(suppl I):I-122, 1989.

25. Leor J, Feinberg MS, Vered Z, et al: Effect of thrombolytic therapy on the evolution of significant mitral regurgitation in patients with a first inferior myocardial infarction. *J Am Coll Cardiol* 21:1661, 1993.

27. Galloway AC, Colvin SB, Baumann FG, et al: Current concepts of mitral valve reconstruction for mitral insufficiency. *Circulation* 78:1087, 1988.

28. Cohn LM: Surgery for mitral regurgitation. *JAMA* 260:2883, 1988.

29. Galloway AC, Colvin SB, Baumann FG, et al: Long-term results of mitral valve reconstruction with Carpentier techniques in 148 patients with mitral insufficiency. *Circulation* 78(suppl I):I-97, 1988.

30. Rankin JS, Feneley MP, Hickey MStJ, et al: A clinical comparison of mitral valve repair versus valve replacement in ischemic mitral regurgitation. *J Thorac Cardiovasc Surg* 95:165, 1988.

31. Kono T, Sabbah HN, Rosman H, et al: Mechanism of functional mitral regurgitation during acute myocardial ischemia. *J Am Coll Cardiol* 19:1101, 1992.

32. Castleman B, McNeeley BU: Case records of the Massachusetts General Hospital: Weekly clinicopathological exercises (case 29-1971). *N Engl J Med* 285:220, 1971.

33. Greenland P, Murphy GW: Acute valvular insufficiency complicating hypertrophic obstructive cardiomyopathy. *Chest* 75:182, 1979.

34. Rippe JM, Curley F, Paraskos JA, et al: Triple valve endocarditis with unusual echocardiographic findings. *Am Heart J* 107:598, 1984.

35. McLaughlin JS, Cowley RA, Smith G, et al: Mitral valve disease from blunt trauma. *J Thorac Cardiovasc Surg* 48:261, 1974.

36. Penny JL, Gregory JJ, Ayres SM, et al: Calcified left atrial myxoma simulating mitral insufficiency. *Circulation* 36:417, 1967.

37. Abascal VM, Wilkins GT, Choong CY, et al: Mitral regurgitation after percutaneous balloon mitral valvuloplasty in adults: Evaluation by pulsed Doppler echocardiography. *J Am Coll Cardiol* 11:257, 1988.

38. Cequier A, Bonan R, Crepeau J, et al: Massive mitral regurgitation caused by tearing of the anterior leaflet during percutaneous mitral balloon valvuloplasty. *Am J Med* 85:100, 1988.

39. Munroe DS, Allen P, Cox AR: Mitral regurgitation occurring during methysergide (Sansert) therapy. *Can Med Assoc J* 101:536, 1969.

40. Stewart SR, Robbins DL, Castles JJ: Acute fulminant aortic and mitral insufficiency in ankylosing spondylitis. *N Engl J Med* 299:1448, 1967.

41. Turri M, Thiene G, Bortolotti U, et al: Surgical pathology of disease of the mitral valve, with special reference to lesions promoting valvular incompetence. *Int J Cardiol* 22:213, 1989.

42. Rippe JM, Fishbein MC, Carabello B, et al: Primary myxomatous degeneration of cardiac valves: A clinical, pathologic, hemodynamic and echocardiographic profile. *Br Heart J* 44:621, 1980.

43. Bulkley BH, Roberts WC: Dilatation of the mitral annulus: A rare cause of mitral regurgitation. *Am J Med* 59:457, 1975.

44. Korn D, DeSanctis RW, Sell S: Massive calcification of the mitral annulus. *N Engl J Med* 267:900, 1962.

45. Sanders CA, Austen WG, Hawthorne JW, et al: Diagnosis and surgical treatment of mitral regurgitation secondary to ruptured chordae tendineae. *N Engl J Med* 276:943, 1967.

46. Caulfield JB, Page DL, Kaster JA, et al: Dissolution of connective tissue in ruptured chordae tendineae. *Circulation* 40:57, 1969.

47. Bircks W, Korfer R: Traumatic mitral incompetence. *J Cardiovasc Surg* 19:557, 1978.

48. Simpson JW, Nora JJ, McNamara DG: Marfan's syndrome and mitral valve disease: Acute surgical emergencies. *Am Heart J* 77:96, 1969.

49. Murray FT, Fuleihan DS, Cornwall CS, et al: Acute mitral regurgitation from ruptured chordae tendineae in systemic lupus erythematosus. *J Rheumatol* 2:454, 1975.

50. Joseph S, Emanuel R, Sturridge M, et al: Congenital aortic valve disease with rupture of mitral chordae tendineae. *Br Heart J* 38:665, 1976.

51. Luther RR, Meyers SN: Acute mitral insufficiency secondary to ruptured chordae tendineae. *Arch Intern Med* 134:568, 1974.

52. Hwang WS, Lam KL: Rupture of chordae tendineae during acute rheumatic carditis. *Br Heart J* 30:429, 1968.

53. Daves RK, Paneth M: Acute mitral regurgitation in pregnancy due to ruptured chordae. *Br Heart J* 34:541, 1972.

54. Castillo RA, Llado I, Adamsons K: Ruptured chordae tendineae complicating pregnancy: A case report. *J Reprod Med* 32:137, 1987.

55. Cuasay RS, Morse DP, Spagna P, et al: Massive mitral regurgitation from chordal rupture and coronary artery disease. *Ann Thorac Surg* 25:438, 1978.

56. Gallagher PJ, Caves PK, Stinson EB: Pathological changes in spontaneous rupture of chordae tendineae. *Ann Chir Gynaecol* 66:135, 1977.

57. Osmundson PJ, Callahan JD, Edwards JE: Ruptured mitral chordae tendineae. *Circulation* 23:42, 1961.

58. Burch GE, DePasquale NP, Phillips JH: Clinical manifestations of papillary muscle dysfunction. *Arch Intern Med* 112:158, 1963.

59. DePasquale NP, Burch GE: The necropsy incidence of gross scars or acute infarction of the papillary muscles of the left ventricle. *Am J Cardiol* 17:169, 1966.

60. Heikkila J: Acute mitral incompetence in myocardial infarction. *Geriatrics* 24:150, 1969.

61. Felner JM, Arensheng D, Meyer TP, et al: Ventricular septal rupture and mitral regurgitation in a patient with an acute myocardial infarction. *Chest* 75:614, 1979.

62. Dodd DA, Johns JA, Graham TP: Transient severe mitral and tricuspid regurgitation following blunt chest trauma. *Am Heart J* 114:652, 1987.

63. Estes EH Jr, Dalton FM, Eastman ML, et al: The anatomy and blood supply of the papillary muscle of the left ventricle. *Am Heart J* 71:356, 1966.

64. Wei JY, Hutchins GM, Bulkley BH: Papillary muscle rupture in fatal acute myocardial infarction. *Ann Intern Med* 90:149, 1979.

65. Sharma SK, Seckler J, Israel DH, et al: Clinical, angiographic and anatomic findings in acute severe ischemic mitral regurgitation. *Am J Cardiol* 70:277, 1992.

66. Kremkau EL, Gilbertson PR, Bristow ID: Acquired, nonrheumatic mitral regurgitation: Clinical management with emphasis on evaluation of myocardial performance. *Prog Cardiovasc Dis* 15:414, 1973.

67. Cohen LS, Roberts WC: The clinical and pathologic spectrum of mitral regurgitation caused by malfunction of the papillary muscles or fibrosis of the left ventricular free wall. *Circulation* 38(suppl VI):57, 1968.

68. Zoneraich S, Gupta MP, Mehta J, et al: Myocardial sarcoidosis presenting as acute mitral insufficiency. *Chest* 66:452, 1974.

69. Vasko JS, Leighton RF: Acute massive mitral regurgitation resulting from disc-valve malfunction. *Ann Thorac Surg* 6:564, 1968.

70. Piccione W, Goldin MD: Mitral valve dysfunction following papillary muscle cryoablation. *Ann Thorac Surg* 46:347, 1988.

71. Samaan HA: Acute massive mitral regurgitation resulting from disc valve replacement of mitral valve. *J Cardiovasc Surg* 36:477, 1969.

72. Carlson CJ, Collins JJ, Ockene IS, et al: Mitral regurgitation due to intermittent prosthetic valvular dysfunction. *Chest* 71:90, 1977.

73. Duvoisin GE, Wallace RB, Ellis FH, et al: Late results of cardiac-valve replacement. *Circulation* 37,38(suppl II):75, 1968.

74. Bailey IK, Richards JG: Infective endocarditis in a Sydney teaching hospital—1962–1971. *Aust NZ J Med* 5:413, 1975.

75. Magilligan DJ, Lewis JW, Java FM, et al: Spontaneous degeneration of porcine bioprosthetic valves. *Ann Thorac Surg* 30:259, 1980.

76. Brown JW, Quinn JM, Spooner E, et al: Late spontaneous disruption of a porcine xenograft mitral valve. *J Thorac Cardiovasc Surg* 75:606, 1978.

77. Voyce SJ, Gore JM, Murphy KR, et al: Accurate patient diagnosis of acute porcine valve failure. *Arch Intern Med* 147:585, 1987.

78. Pomar JL, Bosch X, Chaitman BR, et al: Late tears in leaflets of porcine bioprostheses in adults. *Ann Thorac Surg* 37:78, 1984.

79. Eckberg DL, Gault JH, Bouchard RL, et al: Mechanics of left ventricular contraction in chronic severe mitral regurgitation. *Circulation* 47:1252, 1973.

80. Braunwald E: Mitral regurgitation: Physiological, clinical and surgical considerations. *N Engl J Med* 281:425, 1969.

81. Urshel CW, Covell JW, Sonnenblick EH, et al: Myocardial mechanics in aorta and mitral valvular regurgitation: The concept of instantaneous impedance as a determinant of the performance of the intact heart. *J Clin Invest* 47:867, 1968.

82. Braunwald E: Control of myocardial oxygen consumption: Physiologic and clinical considerations. *Am J Cardiol* 27:416, 1971.

83. Braunwald E, Welch GH Jr, Sarnoff SJ: Hemodynamic effects of quantitatively varied experimental mitral regurgitation. *Circ Res* 5:539, 1957.

84. Yoran C, Yellin EL, Becher RM, et al: Dynamic aspects of acute mitral regurgitation: Effects of ventricular volume, pressure, and

contractility on the effective regurgitant orifice area. *Circulation* 60:170, 1979.

85. Howe JP III, Alpert JS: Acute mitral regurgitation, in Dalen JE, Alpert JS (eds): *Valvular Heart Disease*. Boston, Little, Brown, 1981.

86. Schwinger M, Cohen M, Fuster V: Usefulness of onset of the pulmonary wedge V wave in predicting mitral regurgitation. *Am J Cardiol* 62:646, 1988.

87. Fuchs RM, Heuser RR, Yin FCP, et al: Limitations of pulmonary wedge V waves in diagnosing mitral regurgitation. *Am J Cardiol* 49:849, 1982.

88. Sasayama S, Takahashi M, Osakada G, et al: Dynamic geometry of the left atrium and left ventricle in acute mitral regurgitation. *Circulation* 60:177, 1979.

89. Rosenblatt A, Clark R, Burgess J, et al: Echocardiographic assessment of the level of cardiac compensation in valvular heart disease. *Circulation* 54:509, 1976.

90. Schuler G, Peterson KL, Johnson A, et al: Temporal response of left ventricular performance to mitral valve surgery. *Circulation* 59:1218, 1979.

91. Simpson PC Jr, Bristow JD: Recognition and management of emergencies in valvular heart disease. *Med Clin North Am* 63:155, 1979.

92. Becker AE, Anderson RH: Mitral insufficiency complicating acute myocardial infarction. *Eur J Cardiol* 2:351, 1975.

93. Raftery EB, Oakley CM, Goodwin JF: Acute subvalvular mitral incompetence. *Lancet* 1:360, 1966.

94. Armstrong TG, Meeran MK, Gotsman MS: The left atrial lift. *Am Heart J* 82:764, 1971.

95. Basta LL, Wolfson P, Eckberg DL, et al: The value of left parasternal impulse recordings in the assessment of mitral regurgitation. *Circulation* 48:1055, 1973.

96. Izumi S, Miyatake K, Beppu S, et al: Mechanism of mitral regurgitation in patients with myocardial infarction: A study using real-time two-dimensional Doppler flow imaging and echocardiography. *Circulation* 76:777, 1987.

97. Nellen M, Maurer B, Goodwin JF: Value of physical examination in acute myocardial infarction. *Br Heart J* 35:777, 1973.

98. Antman EM, Angoff GH, Gloss LJ: Demonstration of the mechanism by which mitral regurgitation mimics aortic stenosis. *Am J Cardiol* 42:1044, 1978.

99. Sutton GC, Craig E: Clinical signs of severe acute mitral regurgitation. *Am J Cardiol* 20:141, 1967.

100. Reichek N, Shelburne JC, Perloff JK: Clinical aspects of rheumatic valvular disease. *Prog Cardiovasc Dis* 15:491, 1973.

101. Lembo NJ, Dell'Italia LJ, Crawford MH, et al: Bedside diagnosis of systolic murmurs. *N Engl J Med* 318:1572, 1988.

102. Heikkila J: Electrocardiography in acute papillary muscle dysfunction and infarction: A clinicopathologic study. *Chest* 57:510, 1970.

103. Cooksey J, Parker BM, Aker U, et al: Mitral regurgitation secondary to ruptured chordae tendineae: Clinical hemodynamic and electrocardiographic findings. *South Med J* 69:864, 1976.

104. Raphael MJ, Steiner RE, Raftery ED: Acute mitral incompetence. *Clin Radiol* 18:126, 1967.

105. Lerona P: Acute mitral regurgitation due to rupture of the chordae tendineae: Status of the left atrium. *Radiology* 113:593, 1974.

106. Auger P, Wigle ED: Sudden, severe mitral insufficiency. *Can Med Assoc J* 96:1493, 1967.

107. Parisi AF, Tour DE, Felix WR, et al: Noninvasive cardiac diagnosis. *N Engl J Med* 296:368, 1977.

108. Silverman B, Kozma G, Silverman M, et al: Echocardiographic manifestations of postinfarction ventricular septal rupture. *Chest* 68:778, 1975.

109. Bolger AF, Eigler NL, Maurer G: Quantifying valvular regurgitation: Limitations and inherent assumptions of Doppler techniques. *Circulation* 78:1316, 1988.

110. Spain MG, Smith MD, Grayburn PA, et al: Quantitative assessment of mitral regurgitation by Doppler color flow imaging: Angiographic and hemodynamic correlations. *J Am Coll Cardiol* 13:585, 1989.

111. Shah PM: Quantitative assessment of mitral regurgitation. *J Am Coll Cardiol* 13:591, 1989.

112. Tei C, Tanaka H, Nakao S, et al: Motion of the interatrial septum in acute mitral regurgitation. *Circulation* 62:1080, 1980.

113. Smyllie JH, Sutherland GR, Geuskens R, et al: Doppler color flow mapping in the diagnosis of ventricular septal rupture and acute mitral regurgitation after myocardial infarction. *J Am Coll Cardiol* 15:1449 1990.

114. Gehl LG, Mintz GS, Kotler MN, et al: Left atrial volume overload in mitral regurgitation: A two dimensional echocardiographic study. *Am J Cardiol* 49:33, 1982.

115. Ogawa S, Dupler DA, Pauletto FJ, et al: Flail mitral valve in rheumatic heart disease. *Chest* 74:88, 1978.

116. Kisanuki A, Otsuji Y, Kuroiwa R, et al: Two-dimensional echocardiographic assessment of papillary muscle contractility in patients with prior myocardial infarction. *J Am Coll Cardiol* 21:932, 1993.

117. Ahmad S, Kleiger RE, Connors J, et al: The echocardiographic diagnosis of rupture of a papillary muscle. *Chest* 73:232, 1978.

118. DeMaria AN, Neumann A, Lee G, et al: Mitral valve disease revisited. *Cardiovasc Clin* 9:59, 1978.

119. Shah PM, Gramiak R, Kramer DH: Ultrasound localization of left ventricular outflow obstruction in hypertrophic obstructive cardiomyopathy. *Circulation* 40:3, 1969.

120. Stevenson JG, Kawabori I, Guneroth WG: Differentiation of ventricular septal defects from mitral regurgitation by pulsed Doppler echocardiography. *Circulation* 56:14, 1977.

121. Abbasi AS, Allen MW, DeCristofaro D, et al: Detection and estimation of the degree of mitral regurgitation by range-gated pulsed Doppler echocardiography. *Circulation* 61:154, 1980.

122. Rigo P, Alderson PO, Robertson RM, et al: Measurement of aortic and mitral regurgitation by gated cardiac blood pool scans. *Circulation* 60:306, 1979.

123. Sorenson SG, O'Rourke RA, Chaudhuri TK: Noninvasive quantitation of valvular regurgitation by gated equilibrium radionuclide angiography. *Circulation* 62:1089, 1980.

124. Konstain MA, Wynne J, Holman BL, et al: Use of equilibrium (gated) radionuclide ventriculography to quantitate left ventricular output in patients with and without left-sided valvular regurgitation. *Circulation* 64:578, 1981.

125. Sechtem V, Pflugfelder PW, Cassidy MM, et al: Mitral or aortic regurgitation: Quantification of regurgitant volumes with cine MR imaging. *Radiology* 167:425, 1988.

126. Utz JA, Herfkens RJ, Heinsimer JA, et al: Valvular regurgitation: Dynamic MR imaging. *Radiology* 168:91, 1988.

127. Gore JM, Alpert JS, Benotti JR, et al: *Handbook of Hemodynamic Monitoring*. Boston, Little, Brown, 1985, p 5.

128. Lopez JF, Hanson S, Orchard RC, et al: Quantification of mitral valve incompetence. *Cath Cardiovasc Diagn* 11:139, 1985.

129. Wexler L, Silverman JF, DeBusk RF, et al: Angiographic features of rheumatic and nonrheumatic mitral regurgitation. *Circulation* 44:1080, 1971.

130. Kisslo KB, Bashore TM: Common disease states, in Bashore TM: *Invasive Cardiology: Principles and Techniques*. Philadelphia, BC Decker, 1990.

131. Kennedy JW, Yarnall SR, Murray JA, et al: Quantitative angiography. IV. Relationships of left atrial and ventricular pressure and volume in mitral valve disease. *Circulation* 41:817, 1970.

132. Miller DC, Stinson ED, Rossiter SJ, et al: Impact of simultaneous myocardial revascularization on operative risk, functional result, and survival following mitral valve replacement. *Surgery* 84:848, 1978.

133. Sanders CA, Armstrong PW, Willerson JT, et al: Etiology and differential diagnosis of acute mitral regurgitation. *Prog Cardiovasc Dis* 14:129, 1971.

134. Harshaw CW, Grossman W, Munro AB, et al: Reduced systemic vascular resistance as therapy for severe mitral regurgitation of valvular origin. *Ann Intern Med* 83:312, 1975.

135. Lehmann KG, Francis CK, Sheehan FH, et al: Effect of thrombolysis on acute mitral regurgitation during evolving myocardial infarction: Experience from the Thrombolysis in Myocardial Infarction (TIMI) Trial. *J Am Coll Cardiol* 22:714, 1993.

136. Yorna C, Yellin EL, Becker RM, et al: Mechanism of reduction of mitral regurgitation with vasodilator therapy. *Am J Cardiol* 43:773, 1979.

137. Greenberg BH, DeMots H, Murphy E, et al: Arterial dilators in mitral regurgitation: Effects on rest and exercise hemodynamics and long-term clinical follow-up. *Circulation* 65:181, 1982.

138. Chatterjee K, Swan HJC: Vasodilator therapy in acute myocardial infarction. *Mod Concepts Cardiovasc Dis* 43:119, 1974.

139. Weldon CS, Krause AH, Parker BM, et al: Clinical recognition and surgical management of acute disruption of the mitral valve. *Ann Surg* 175:1000, 1972.

140. Bengston JR, Kaplan AJ, Peiper KS, et al: Prognosis in cardiogenic shock after acute myocardial infarction in the intervention era. *J Am Coll Cardiol* 20:1482, 1992.

141. Buckley MJ, Mundth ED, Daggett WM, et al: Surgical management of ventricular septal defects and mitral regurgitation complicating acute myocardial infarction. *Ann Thorac Surg* 16:598, 1973.

142. Lamberti J, Cohn LH, Collins JJ Jr: Management of papillary muscle dysfunction after acute myocardial infarction. *J Thorac Cardiovasc Surg* 67:349, 1974.

143. Cohn LH: Surgical treatment of valvular heart disease. *Am J Surg* 135:444, 1978.

144. Salomon NW, Stinson EB, Griepp RB, et al: Patient-related risk factors as predictors of results following isolated mitral valve replacement. *Ann Thorac Surg* 24:519, 1977.

145. Kensley RH, Colsen PR, Bakst A: Emergency valve replacement for primary infective endocarditis. *S Afr Med J* 53:86, 1978.

146. Young JB, Welton DE, Raizner AE, et al: Surgery in active infective endocarditis. *Circulation* 60(suppl I):77, 1979.

39. Syncope

Carlos Cuello, Gregory J. Bonavita, Alan B. Wagshal, and Shoei K. Stephen Huang

Syncope is defined as a sudden transient loss of consciousness associated with loss of postural tone and spontaneous recovery, primarily a manifestation of transient neurologic dysfunction as a consequence of significantly reduced cerebral blood flow. Thirty to 50 percent of the general population suffers from one or more episodes of syncope in their lifetime, with the incidence rising in the elderly. Syncope accounts for 1 to 3 percent of all emergency room visits (300,000 visits per year), 1 to 3 percent of physician office visits, and 6 percent of hospital admissions, frequently to an intensive care unit (ICU) setting to allow for cardiac monitoring or to rule out a serious underlying condition [1,2,3].

The prognostic significance of a syncopal event depends on the presence and degree of underlying structural heart disease. Syncope of new onset unassociated with structural disorders in younger patients usually reflects a disorder of autonomic tone, carries minimal morbidity, and has a high remission rate. However, when structural heart disease is present, a more serious cause, such as ventricular tachycardia, is likely, and the 1-year mortality may be as high as 30 percent [4,5,6].

Syncope of unknown etiology has become a focus of special attention in the past decade. By historical accounts, up to 47 percent of patients presenting with syncope have no cause established. However, the use of newer diagnostic techniques, such as tilt-table testing, event recorders with memory loop, signal-averaged electrocardiography, and electrophysiologic testing, allows an etiology to be established in up to 75 to 80 percent of patients for whom an initial evaluation is negative [4].

Classification of Syncope

Syncope can be classified into *cardiovascular syncope,* which accounts for up to 85 perent of all cases, and *noncardiovascular syncope* (Table 39-1). Cardiovascular syncope may be further divided into *neurally mediated* and *neurally independent* mechanisms. Neurally mediated syncope includes neurocardiogenic syncope and similar phenomena as well as syncope resulting from the effect of a wide variety of diseases and medications on the autonomic nervous system. Neurally independent syncope is not dependent on specific cardiovascular receptors nor the autonomic system. It includes mechanical (e.g., obstructive and ischemic) cardiac disease and arrhythmias. Noncardiovascular syncope is the result of psychiatric or central nervous system disorders or hypovolemia.

NEURALLY MEDIATED CARDIOVASCULAR SYNCOPE
Syncope Associated with Autonomic Augmentation

NEUROCARDIOGENIC SYNCOPE. Approximately 10 years ago, several cases of bradycardia or even prolonged periods of asystole occurring in association with exercise, particularly in the immediate postexercise period, in otherwise healthy persons were reported. Several of these occurrences were documented on treadmill exercise tests [7–10]. These patients were subsequently shown to develop syncope during tilt-table testing, and since then neurocardiogenic syncope has been shown to be an important mechanism of recurrent syncope in young, otherwise healthy individuals [11–14], particularly athletes who develop syncope in the immediate postexercise period [15,16].

Neurocardiogenic syncope is mediated by the Bezold-Jarisch reflex (named for Von Bezold, who first speculated on its existence in 1867 [17], and Jarisch, who revived the concept in 1958 [18]). The afferent signals for neurocardiogenic syncope are inhibitory nonmyelinated neurons (C fibers) localized predominantly in the posterobasal wall of the left ventricle. These neurons detect the overvigorous ventricular contraction resulting from a combination of the relative volume depletion of the upright state and sympathetic stimulation from exercise or emotional stress; they initiate a reflex control mechanism involving activation of vasomotor centers in the brainstem. This leads to an output of vagal and spinal vasodilatory neural activity, resulting in bradycardia and peripheral vasodilatation, which, in susceptible patients, can result in hypotension and syncope (Fig. 39-1).

Tilt-table testing provides a laboratory model of this hyperactive reflex, during which susceptible patients exhibit severe

Table 39-1. Causes of Syncope

I. Cardiovascular
  A. Neurally mediated cardiovascular syncope
    1. Autonomic augmentation
      a. Neurocardiogenic
      b. Situational
        (1) Fright and pain
        (2) Oculovagal
        (3) Glossopharyngeal neuralgia
        (4) Valsalva associated with:
          Defecation
          Weight lifting
          Micturition
          Cough
          Sneeze
          Trumpet playing
          Diving
        (5) Deglutition
        (6) Supine hypotensive syndrome of near term
        (7) pregnancy
        (8) Instrumentation
          Postprandial
      c. Carotid hypersensitivity syndrome
    2. Autonomic insufficiency
      a. Primary
        (1) Bradbury-Eggleston syndrome
        (2) Shy-Drager syndrome
      b. Secondary
        (1) Drugs—pharmacologic agents, cocaine
        (2) Diabetes
        (3) Alcoholic
        (4) Amyloid
        (5) Tabes dorsalis
  B. Neurally independent cardiovascular syncope
    1. Mechanical
      a. Valvular stenosis (aortic, mitral, pulmonary)
      b. Aortic dissection
      c. Hypertrophic cardiomyopathy
      d. Left atrial myxoma
      e. Cardiac tamponade
      f. Global myocardial ischemia
      g. Pulmonary hypertension
      h. Tetralogy of Fallot
      i. Pulmonary embolism
    2. Dysrhythmic
      a. Sick sinus syndrome
      b. Atrioventricular block
      c. Pacemaker syndrome
      d. Ventricular tachycardia/fibrillation
        (1) Secondary to coronary heart disease and other forms of structural heart disease
        (2) Idiopathic right and left ventricular tachycardia and catecholamine-sensitive ventricular tachycardia
        (3) Long Q–T syndrome and *Torsades de pointes*
          Primary
          Romano-Ward syndrome
          Jervell-Lange-Nielsen syndrome
          Secondary (electrolytes, drugs, etc.)
      e. Supraventricular tachycardia
        (1) Wolff-Parkinson-White syndrome
        (2) Other supraventricular tachycardia
II. Noncardiovascular
  A. Primary neurologic disorders
    1. Ischemic
      a. Vertebrobasilar transient ischemic attacks
      b. Subclavian steal syndrome
      c. Takayasu's disease
    2. Normal pressure hydrocephalus
    3. Metabolic
      a. Hypoglycemia
      b. Hypoxia
      c. Hyperventilation
  B. Psychogenic
    1. Panic disorders
    2. Hysteria
    3. Major depression
  C. Hypovolemic
    1. Hemorrhagic
    2. Dehydration
    3. Idiopathic hypovolemia

bradycardia, hypotension, or syncope, and allows definitive diagnosis of what was once only a diagnosis of exclusion (Fig. 39-2). In addition, serial tilt-table tests predict drug efficacy without relying on recurrent syncope as the only marker for drug failure. A variety of protocols are available; most include tilting at 60 to 80 degrees of upright tilt for 20 to 45 minutes both at baseline and with isoproterenol provocation [13,19,20].

Because of the vagal activation, a majority of patients experience brief premonitory symptoms, such as diaphoresis, nausea, or pallor, prior to complete loss of consciousness, which can help suggest the diagnosis. Effective treatments for neurocardiogenic syncope are beta-blockers and disopyramide, presumably based on their potent negative inotropic effects, and theophylline, presumably based on its ability to antagonize the intracardiac effects of adenosine on the muscarinic system [21,22,23].

SITUATIONAL SYNCOPE. In addition to the Bezold-Jarisch reflex, a variety of receptors with their own triggering mechanisms can lead to a parasympathetic outflow and potentially to so-called situational syncope. These include micturition syncope (triggered by sudden bladder decompression and the accompanying Valsalva maneuver performed with voiding) [24] and syncope associated with coughing, defecation, sneezing, weight-lifting, trumpet playing, and so on [25–28], in which syncope is related to the associated Valsalva maneuver. Post-prandial hypotension is not infrequently the cause of hypotension in elderly patients with impaired baroreflex function and poor hemodynamic compensation for splanchnic venous pooling during digestion [29]. Glossopharyngeal and trigeminal neuralgia may present with syncope [30–33].

CAROTID SINUS HYPERSENSITIVITY. Carotid sinus hypersensitivity may be found in 5 to 25 percent of the adult population, particularly in the elderly patient with ischemic heart disease [34,35,36], and may be associated with episodes of clinical syncope in 10 to 20 percent of these patients. The carotid sinus baroreceptors are located in the internal carotid artery along the bifurcation of the common carotid artery: afferent impulses travel to the brainstem via the nerve of Hering through the glossopharyngeal nerve. It is typically divided into cardioinhibitory and vasodepressor forms, depending on whether the parasympathetic outflow results in predominant bradycardia/asystole or hypotension, respectively.

Carotid sinus massage may be performed at bedside with the patient in the supine position while obtaining simultaneous electrocardiographic and (if possible) blood pressure monitoring. The carotid pulse is first lightly palpated adjacent to the angle of the mandible. Pressure is then applied for approximately 5 seconds while monitoring; a sinus pause of greater than 3 seconds is considered abnormal. It is important to rule out carotid bruits before performing carotid sinus massage, and

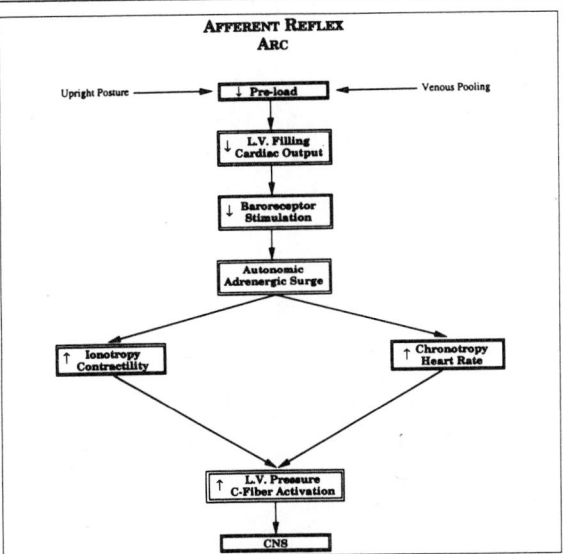
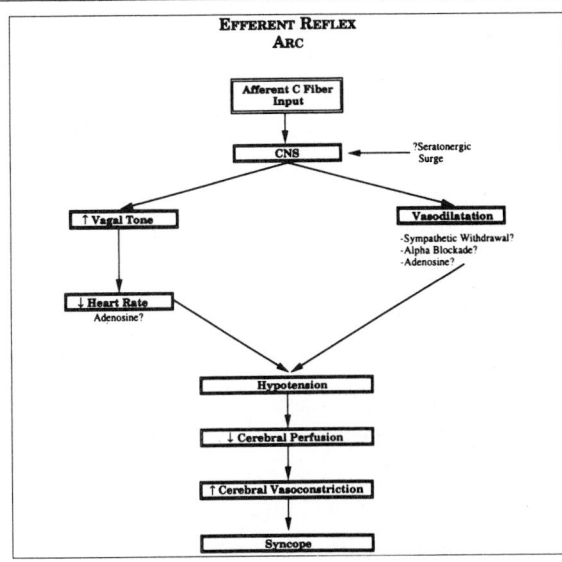

Fig. 39-1. Afferent and efferent reflex arcs involved in neurocardiogenic syncope. (From Kosinski DJ, Wolfe DA, Grubb BP: Neurocardiogenic syncope: A review of pathophysiology, diagnosis, and treatment. *Cardiovasc Rev Rep* 14:22, 1993, with permission.)

bilateral carotid sinus pressure should never be applied. Atropine and a defibrillator should be available in the event of an emergency.

A positive response to carotid sinus massage does not necessarily constitute an explanation of syncope, since the incidence of carotid sinus hypersensitivity is relatively high in the elderly. Careful evaluation for other causes of syncope should be performed before a permanent pacemaker is implanted.

Syncope Associated with Autonomic Insufficiency. Dysautonomic (orthostatic) syncope is observed in patients with an impaired autonomic pressor regulation mechanism. Normally upon standing, peripheral venous pooling causes a decreased cardiac output and blood pressure, resulting in compensatory reflex tachycardia and vasoconstriction mediated by sympathetic stimulation. A persistent drop in systolic blood pressure greater than 20 to 30 mm Hg (sometimes accompanied by a drop in diastolic blood pressure >10 mm Hg) indicates a failure of the reflex mechanism. Dysautonomic syncope is seen in various forms of primary and secondary autonomic insufficiency, including Bradbury-Eggleston syndrome and Shy-Drager syndrome associated with Parkinson's disease; amyloidosis; porphyria; syringomyelia; tabes dorsalis (syphilis); spinal cord lesions; alcoholic and diabetic polyneuropathy; paraneoplastic syndromes; and pernicious anemia [37,38]. Surgical sympathectomy is frequently associated with orthostatic hypotension that may lead to syncope. Many vasoactive drugs, such as antihypertensives, phenothiazines, antidepressants, and tranquilizers, may cause postural hypotension and syncope from either central nervous system effects or altered autonomic control of vascular tone [39,40].

NEURALLY INDEPENDENT CARDIOVASCULAR SYNCOPE

Mechanical Causes. Primary cardiovascular causes of syncope are shown in Table 39-1. Syncope due to obstructive disorders

in the heart typically occurs during exercise during which the limited cardiac output is unable to meet the increased demand and overcome associated peripheral vasodilatation. Syncope is one of the classic presenting signs of aortic stenosis and usually suggests that valve replacement is required [41,42]. Left atrial myxoma also presents commonly with syncope, often associated with change of position, during which the pedunculated tumor plops into and occludes the mitral valve orifice, preventing diastolic filling of the left ventricle [43,44]. Thrombosis of a prosthetic valve not infrequently presents with cardiovascular collapse and syncope and requires emergent treatment.

Hypertrophic cardiomyopathy is a particularly important cause of syncope to consider, since its physical signs may be subtle and it frequently involves younger patients and athletes. Patients with hypertrophic cardiomyopathy and a history of syncope have been shown to be at increased risk of sudden cardiac death [45,46]. In a necropsy study of 29 young athletes who died suddenly, Maron et al. [47] confirmed the diagnosis of hypertrophic cardiomyopathy in 14, only 6 of whom had clinical suspicion of structural heart disease despite the fact that most patients had been evaluated by a physician. In only one patient was the diagnosis of hypertrophic cardiomyopathy made before death. Older patients may develop hypertrophic cardiomyopathy of the elderly, presenting with syncope and features similar to the congenital form [48] (see Chap. 33).

A variety of mechanisms have been shown to cause syncope in hypertrophic cardiomyopathy patients, among them a sudden increase in the outflow tract obstruction (e.g., that which results from the increased inotropy and peripheral vasodilatation associated with exercise). Due to the increased wall thickness there is a susceptibility to myocardial ischemia even in the absence of coronary artery disease, which can also lead to ventricular arrhythmias. Any form of tachycardia, including sinus tachycardia, can lead to a sudden fall in ventricular filling due to diastolic dysfunction and an inability to maintain cardiac output at high heart rates. In addition, these patients have been shown to exhibit a fall in peripheral vascular resistance during or shortly after exercise, resulting in a significant fall in blood pressure, as well as a high incidence of abnormal tilt-table responses. This suggests that they may also be prone to neurocardiogenic syncope, presumably as a consequence of the

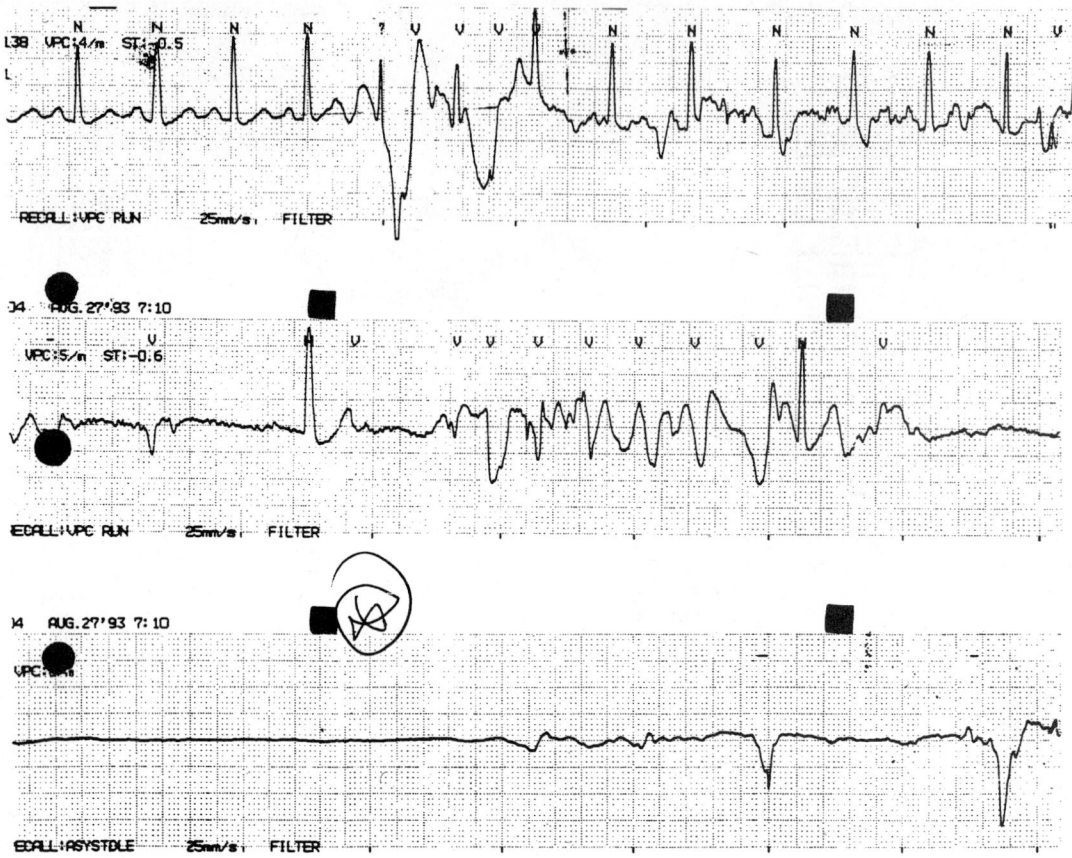

Fig. 39-2. Continuous telemetry strip recorded during a syncopal spell in the emergency room on a previously healthy 27-year-old woman who presented after a syncopal spell at home. While awaiting a chest x-ray, the patient suddenly became dizzy and nauseous, followed by complete loss of consciousness. Subsequent tilt-table testing reproduced the symptoms and prolonged period of asystole. Following treatment with theophylline, the tilt-table test became negative and the patient has remained syncope-free for several months. The longest asystolic period lasted for 7.5 seconds. There is also motion artifact present, particularly on the middle panel.

increased left ventricular wall tension, resulting in activation of the same intramyocardial receptors responsible for neurocardiogenic syncope [49,50]. The same mechanism has been suggested to play a role in some patients with aortic stenosis [51].

Pulmonary hypertension with acute crisis of pulmonary arteriolar spasm and marked decrease in left ventricular preload may lead to recurrent syncope and sudden death, usually associated with exertion since the constricted pulmonary vasculature precludes adequate left ventricular filling [52]. Large pulmonary emboli can also present with syncope; this is a particularly important cause to keep in mind, since syncope may be the only presenting symptom in some patients with this potentially fatal disorder. The presence of syncope in association with pulmonary embolus usually implies that 50 percent or more of the pulmonary circulation is obstructed. In one study, 15 percent of patients with pulmonary embolism experienced syncope early in the course [53]. Associated signs and symptoms of hypoxemia, hypotension, dyspnea, chest pain,

tachycardia, and acute cor pulmonale should be sought on physical examination and electrocardiogram.

Acute myocardial ischemia can also present with syncope from various mechanisms. Global ischemia and severe three-vessel coronary artery disease or left main disease can present with syncope purely from cardiac dysfunction [54,55,56]. In fact, Heberden's original classic description of angina mentioned syncope as one of the signs [57]. However, syncope and hypotension associated with a severe episode of acute coronary ischemia usually suggest either associated ventricular arrhythmias, conduction system disease, or a mechanical complication such as myocardial rupture or ventricular septal defect. Acute coronary occlusion can also activate the Bezold-Jarisch reflex, particularly during inferior ischemia or infarction [58]. In younger patients, coronary artery anomalies, particularly anomalous origin of the left main coronary artery from the anterior sinus of Valsalva, may present with syncope or sudden cardiac death [59]. Coronary vasospasm can also present with syncope related to associated ventricular arrhythmias, even in patients with angiographically normal coronary arteries [60,61,62]. Finally, acute myocardial infarction can present with ventricular tachycardia or fibrillation, usually a result of triggered automaticity reflecting the effects of acute ischemia on the membrane potential [63]. Such arrhythmias that occur within the first 48 hours of myocardial infarction have been shown to be unrelated to the development of later arrhythmic events [64,65]. This is in distinct contrast to the reentrant arrhythmias associated with prior myocardial infarction and left ventricular dysfunction (discussed below), which are due to a reentry circuit and usually recur if not treated definitively.

Cyanotic congenital heart disease, aortic dissection (see Chap. 36), and cardiac tamponade can also manifest with syncope. Aortic dissection can occur either in older patients as a result of cystic medial necrosis of the aorta, usually the result of chronic hypertension, or in younger patients with Marfan's syndrome, a congenital disorder of connective tissue affecting the aortic wall and producing the characteristic physical stigmata (e.g., excessively tall stature, long arms and fingers, pectus excavatum, and an extremely thin body habitus) [66]. Severe tearing chest and/or back pain and unilateral pulse deficits suggest this disease, which can be confirmed by a variety of tests, including transesophageal echocardiography, chest computed tomography scanning, or magnetic resonance imaging.

Dysrhythmic Causes

BRADYARRHYTHMIAS. Many young patients, particularly if athletically trained, can exhibit bradycardia and/or atrioventricular nodal conduction system disturbances as a result of exaggerated vagal tone. Although this physiologic adaptation is usually asymptomatic, occasionally syncope can result [67,68]. In the elderly patient, however, bradyarrhythmias are usually reflective of an underlying degenerative cardiac process affecting the conduction system. Lev's disease is a primary disorder affecting the fibrous skeleton of the heart and conduction system [69]. Lenegre's disease is a primary degenerative disorder of the conduction system [70]. Secondary causes of conduction disease include coronary artery disease; idiopathic dilated cardiomyopathy; calcific aortic stenosis; mitral annular calcification; myocardial abscess from endocarditis; intramural tumors; and infiltrative diseases of the heart, such as sarcoidosis, amyloidosis, Chagas disease, scleroderma, and polymyositis.

Sick sinus syndrome is characterized by impaired sinoatrial impulse formation or propagation, manifesting as sinus pauses or arrest resulting in syncope. When accompanied by supraventricular tachycardia (commonly atrial fibrillation) it is referred to as bradycardia-tachycardia syndrome. Sinus node dysfunction is frequently unmasked by relatively low concentrations of drugs such as digoxin, beta-blockers, and calcium channel blockers [71–75]. Enhanced sensitivity to endogenous adenosine appears closely related to the development of sick sinus syndrome. This has been the rationale for the occasionally successful use of theophylline (an adenosine antagonist) in this disorder [76], although essentially all patients with syncope secondary to sick sinus syndrome require permanent pacemaker implantation.

Survivors of acute myocardial infarction, usually of the anterior wall, complicated by the appearance of Mobitz type II second-degree A-V block or concomitant bifascicular bundle branch block and first-degree A-V block, are usually left with severe residual conduction system disease and are usually considered for prophylactic permanent pacemaker implantation. If the patients do not receive a pacemaker they may be at high risk for third-degree A-V block and syncope. This disruption of the conduction system is associated with a slow, lower-level ventricular pacemaker focus. One study reported that 45 percent of patients with bifascicular block following acute myocardial infarction developed sudden death or syncope within 12 months of hospital discharge [77].

Pacemaker syndrome may cause recurrent syncope in patients with ventricular pacemakers [78]. Loss of A-V synchrony with subsequent impaired ventricular filling and decreased cardiac output appears to be the principal mechanism. However, reflex vasodilatation caused by atrial distention during atrial

contraction against closed A-V valves may also contribute to syncope in these patients [79].

TACHYARRHYTHMIAS. Both ventricular and supraventricular tachyarrhythmias may present with syncope due to marked decrease in stroke volume. Ventricular tachycardia is particularly important to document because there is a definite risk of degeneration to ventricular fibrillation and cardiac arrest in most forms of ventricular tachycardia. In most patients with ventricular tachycardia, arrhythmia is secondary to either coronary artery disease with prior myocardial infarction or the other forms of structural heart disease discussed above (e.g., valvular heart disease, hypertrophic cardiomyopathy). Five other recognized causes of ventricular arrhythmias are native or repaired congenital heart disease (particularly tetralogy of Fallot) [80]; myocarditis; idiopathic dilated cardiomyopathy; severe mitral valve prolapse, usually in association with a severely damaged mitral valve and mitral regurgitation [81–84]; and arrhythmogenic right ventricular dysplasia. Right ventricular dysplasia is a form of cardiomyopathy affecting the right ventricle with fatty infiltration and atrophy of the myocytes. It often presents with ventricular tachycardia, but sudden cardiac death with degeneration to ventricular fibrillation has also been described [85,86]. Common to all these diseases is the development of myocardial fibrosis, creating areas of slow conduction and differing refractory periods, providing the setup for reentrant ventricular tachycardia [87,88]. Patients with structural heart disease, particularly coronary artery disease, associated with ventricular tachycardia usually can have their arrhythmia induced with programmed ventricular stimulation (see below).

The risk of developing ventricular tachycardia following myocardial infarction has been shown to correlate well with the extent of impairment of ventricular function and an abnormal signal-averaged ECG [89,90]. Patients with prior myocardial infarction and reduced left ventricular ejection fraction, even if asymptomatic but with nonsustained ventricular tachycardia on Holter monitoring, who have inducible ventricular tachycardia on electrophysiologic testing have been shown to be at substantial risk of sudden cardiac death within 2 years unless appropriately treated [91]. This certainly emphasizes the importance of making the diagnosis of ventricular tachycardia when it is associated with syncope.

Despite the usual association of ventricular tachycardia with structural heart disease, a few relatively rare forms of ventricular tachycardia can affect young patients with no evidence of organic heart disease. These include idiopathic left and right ventricular tachycardia, which originate from specific sites, mostly in the inferior apical wall of the left ventricle and the right ventricular outflow tract, respectively. Each form is associated with a characteristic tachycardia morphology on the ECG: right bundle branch block with left axis deviation and left bundle branch block with right axis deviation, respectively [92, 93] (Fig. 39-3). Patients often complain of palpitations, and the arrhythmia often is diagnosed before episodes of true syncope occur. A variant of idiopathic ventricular tachycardia triggered by stress or exercise (so-called catecholamine-sensitive ventricular tachycardia) responds to adenosine [94]. All of these forms of tachycardias usually have a fairly benign prognosis and respond well to antiarrhythmic medications, including verapamil or beta-blockers. Alternatively, catheter ablation of the arrhythmogenic focus is often successful [95].

Two other causes of tachyarrhythmias that typically present in young patients without structural cardiac disease, because of their potential serious consequences, should be specifically sought on the ECG of all patients with syncope. First is the idiopathic long Q–T syndrome, which can result in repetitive episodes of true syncope and/or episodes of cardiac arrest due

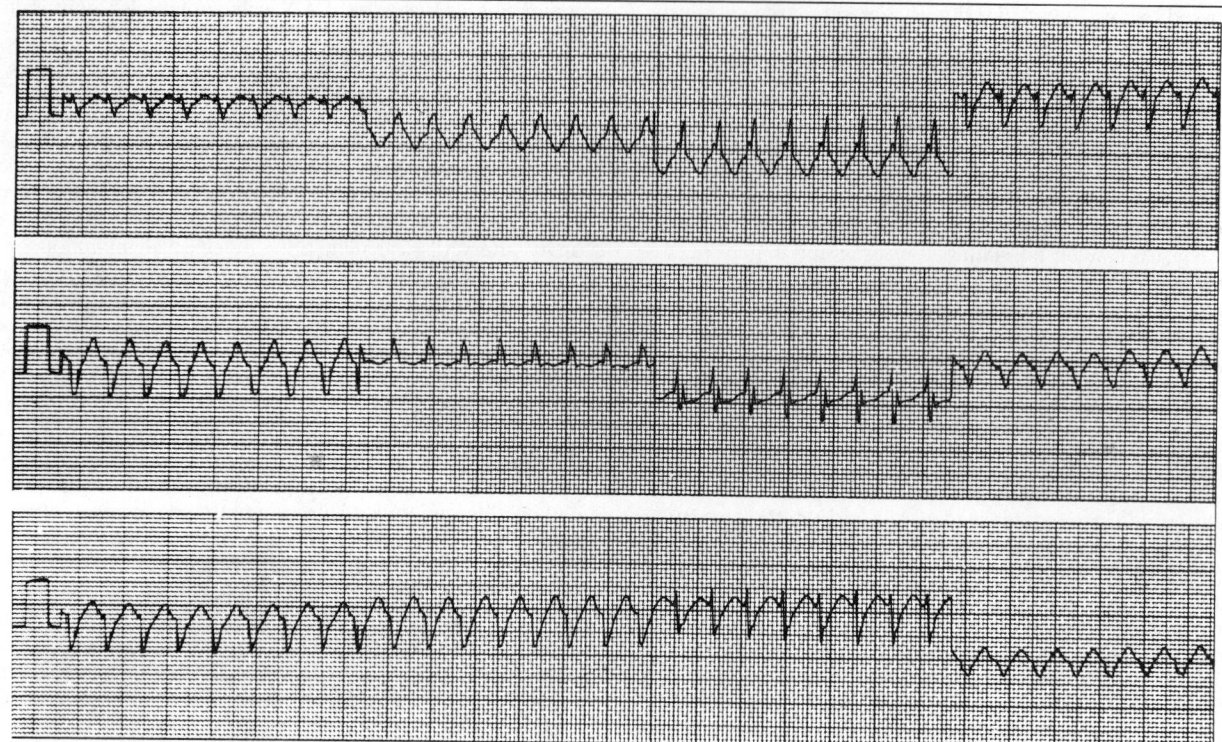

Fig. 39-3. A 12–lead ECG, revealing ventricular tachycardia with a right bundle branch block and left axis deviation morphology recorded during an emergency room visit for syncope. The patient was a 37-year-old man who complained of frequent palpitations and several syncopal spells occurring with exertion. He had no prior cardiac history, and cardiac work-up, including a stress test and echocardiography, was normal. Electrophysiologic testing confirmed the diagnosis of verapamil-sensitive idiopathic left ventricular tachycardia, and the patient underwent successful ablation of the ventricular tachycardia focus in the inferior septal wall of the left ventricle with complete reversal of symptoms. (From Wagshal AB, Huang SKS: Syncope in athletes. *J Musculoskeletal Med* 10:21, 1993. With permission.)

to runs of polymorphic ventricular tachycardia (*Torsades de pointes*) or ventricular fibrillation [96]. Family history is particularly important in recognizing this syndrome, as is the prolonged Q–T interval (a Q–T interval corrected for heart rate ≥460 msec) on routine ECG, although in some patients the Q–T interval abnormality may not be marked. Although this is congenital, patients can be asymptomatic for long periods of time and develop their first symptoms at any age (Fig. 39-4).

In some patients with long Q–T syndrome, but not the majority, associated congenital deafness is present (Jervell-Lange-Nielson syndrome) [97, 98]. The more common variant, without associated hearing loss, is Romano-Ward syndrome [99,100]. These patients classically present with syncope in association with sympathetic stimulation, such as during exercise, extreme anger, or fright. This disorder is believed to be related to a primary abnormality affecting the potassium ion channels in the ventricular myocardium, resulting in delayed and disordered repolarization, leading to early after-depolarizations. There may also be an associated primary imbalance in the sympathetic nervous system [96,101].

A variety of successful therapeutic options includes beta-blockers and left stellate ganglionectomy. Because long Q–T syndromes are often familial, screening of all family members is an important part of management. Since sympathetic stimulation is the key factor in triggering arrhythmias, all patients with long Q–T syndrome, even if treated, must avoid strenuous athletic activity.

A long Q–T interval and associated *Torsades de pointes* can also result from hypomagnesemia and hypokalemia (sometimes resulting from liquid protein diets) [102,103] and a variety of medications, including tricyclic antidepressants, class Ia and class III antiarrhythmics, long-acting antihistamines, and erythromycin. *Torsades de pointes* in these circumstances is usually associated with bradycardia and triggered by an early premature ventricular contraction falling on a particularly long and often bizarre T wave following a prior pause (so-called pause-dependent mechanism) [104,105]. This form of *Torsades* responds to interventions that increase heart rate (atrial or ventricular pacing or isoproterenol infusion) or to intravenous magnesium [106].

The second important cause of tachycardias, particularly in young patients, is Wolff-Parkinson-White (WPW) syndrome, which can also be diagnosed on routine ECG by the appearance of characteristic delta waves (a slur on the upstroke of the QRS) and a short P–R interval. Patients with WPW syndrome exhibit two major arrhythmias. The first is orthodromic A-V reciprocating tachycardia, which uses the A-V node for antegrade conduction and the accessory pathway for retrograde conduction. The electrocardiographic appearance is that of a regular supraventricular tachycardia with a normal narrow QRS complex, sometimes with retrograde P waves visible, at rates up to 200 beats per minute or more (Fig. 39-5). This arrhythmia, although a troublesome cause of palpitations or syncope, is usually not life-threatening.

The second, most feared, arrhythmia in patients with WPW syndrome is atrial fibrillation. In the presence of an accessory

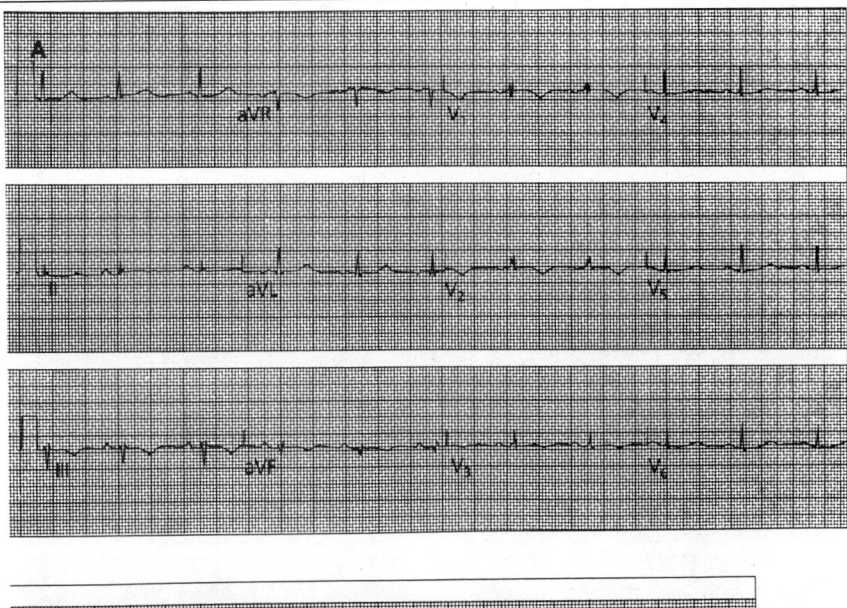

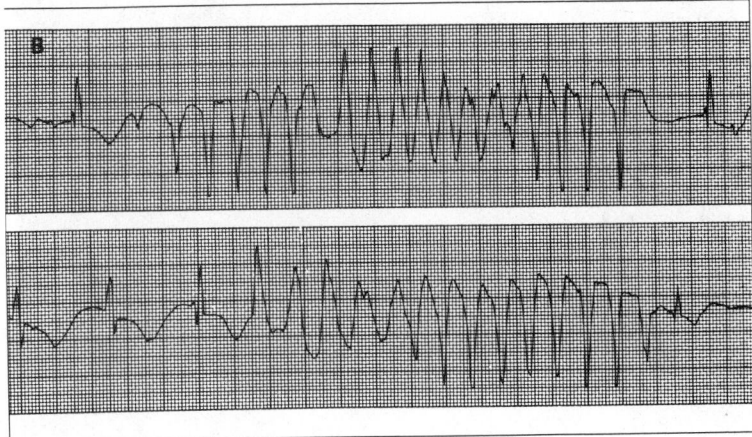

Fig. 39-4. An 80-year-old woman with no known heart disease or use of medications suddenly lost consciousness while at church. A. The ECG recorded in the emergency room revealed a long Q–T interval (520 msec, Q–Tc 530 msec). B. The patient's ECGs from up to 7 years earlier revealed an equally long Q–T interval. During subsequent hospitalization, runs of polymorphic ventricular tachycardia consistent with *Torsades de pointes* and compatible with the diagnosis of idiopathic long Q–T syndrome were documented. (From Wagshal AB, Huang SKS: Syncope in athletes. *J Musculoskeletal Med* 10:21, 1993. With permission.)

pathway with a short antegrade refractory period, atrial fibrillation may produce a very rapid wide QRS complex (preexcited) ventricular response, which may lead to ventricular fibrillation. For the symptomatic patient with WPW syndrome and documented episodes of atrial fibrillation or supraventricular tachycardia, the preferred treatment is catheter ablation. This avoids the problems of lifelong treatment with antiarrhythmic medications and allows full resumption of activities.

While supraventricular arrhythmias (particularly rapid preexcited atrial fibrillation) secondary to WPW syndrome are the most likely to result in severe symptoms, others, such as paroxysmal atrial fibrillation/flutter and A-V nodal reentrant tachycardia, may also result in syncope—particularly if they occur during exercise when maximal cardiac output is needed—or even cardiac arrest [107]. Although atrial fibrillation usually is associated with underlying heart disease, it may also appear without any associated heart disease (lone atrial fibrillation), and A-V nodal reentrant tachycardia in the younger population is seldom associated with underlying heart disease. Syncope results from the sudden change in heart rate as well as loss of coordinated atrial and ventricular contraction, resulting in a sudden dramatic decrease in cardiac output. Vasomotor factors (activation of cardiac mechanoreceptors from the vigorous ventricular contraction accompanying tachycardia) may also be important in producing syncope [108].

NONCARDIOVASCULAR SYNCOPE

Neurologic Disorders. Pure neurologic syncope represents less than 5 percent of syncope cases. External compression due to intracranial tumors or atherosclerosis may cause vertebrobasilar insufficiency with transient ischemic attacks. Associated symptoms of vertebrobasilar insufficiency include temporary bilateral cerebral dysfunction accompanied by brainstem dysfunction (vertigo, diplopia, ataxia, dysarthria, weakness or numbness of bilateral limbs) and syncope. Pure carotid artery

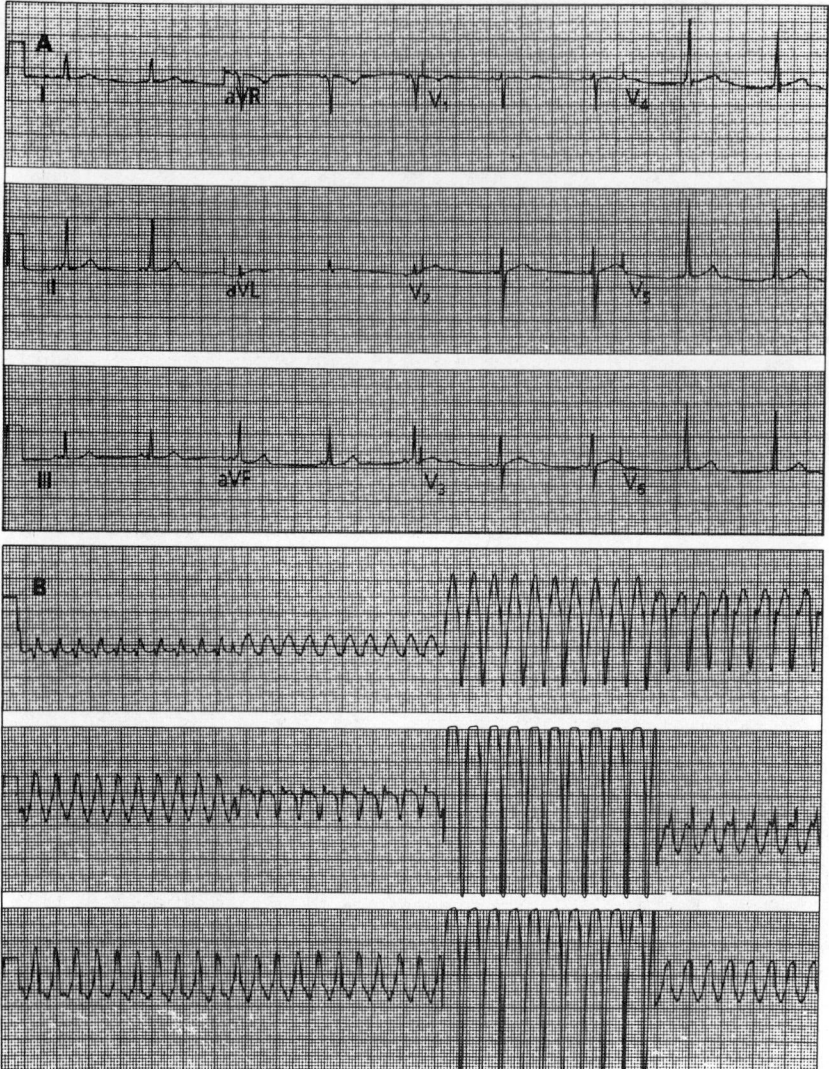

Fig. 39-5. Sudden onset of severe palpitations followed by syncope developed in a previously healthy 17-year-old varsity high school pitcher while he was pitching. A. The 12-lead ECG revealed a short P–R interval and delta waves diagnostic of the Wolff-Parkinson-White syndrome with a right free wall bypass tract. B. During electrophysiologic study a rapid orthodromic atrioventricular reciprocating tachycardia utilizing a second, concealed posteroseptal accessory bypass tract was induced. This pathway was successfully ablated using radiofrequency catheter ablation. The patient resumed full athletic activities and has remained asymptomatic for 2 years. (From Wagshal AB, Huang SKS: Syncope in athletes. *J Musculoskeletal Med* 10:21, 1993. With permission.)

disease is an extremely rare cause of syncope, since simultaneous bilateral occlusions would be required. Patients with normal pressure hydrocephalus present with a triad of ataxia, incontinence, and dementia but may also suffer true syncope [109]. Epilepsy may be indistinguishable from true syncope on presentation, as tonic-clonic movements may in fact be a feature of both, although incontinence and tongue biting are usually diagnostic for epilepsy, as is a prolonged postictal state.

Extrinsic compression of vertebral arteries can occur with cervical spondylosis, osteoarthritis, or a cervical rib, resulting in syncope during lateral rotation or hyperextension of the head. Subclavian steal syndrome is an infrequent cause of syncope seen during arm exercise in the presence of major occlusive disease to the proximal subclavian artery [110]. Occasionally, syncope is associated with severe migraine headaches [111,112].

Alcoholics may suffer syncopal events due to various causes, most of which are organic, such as chronic orthostatic hypotension due to autonomic failure, cardiomyopathy with arrhythmias, or withdrawal seizures [113]. Syncope can also be related to recreational drug use [114]. Severe hypoglycemia and hypoxemia and/or hypercapnea secondary to severe pulmonary disease are other potential causes of syncope.

Psychogenic Syncope. Patients with mental disorders frequently present with symptoms suggestive of syncope. For this reason, psychiatric illness should be entertained in the young, otherwise healthy patient presenting with recurrent syncope. Anxiety disorders may present with syncope due to motor tension, apprehension, and hyperventilation, since the resulting alkalosis can cause cerebral vasoconstriction. Autonomic hyperactivity may accompany anxiety attacks, with vasodepressor reactions, hypotension, and loss of consciousness [115]. Epidemics of fainting described in young individuals have been attributed to transitory anxiety attacks [116,117]. Patients with somatization during panic disorders or with severe depression may present with syncope [118,119,120]. These patients often complain of neurologic, gastrointestinal, cardiopulmonary, psychoneural, and other physical symptoms.

Hypovolemia. Even with a structurally normal heart and circulatory system, severe hypovolemia, particularly if acute, may also result in syncope. Volume changes sufficient to cause syncope usually occur in the setting of acute hemorrhage or acute fluid loss. Blood extravasation may be internal (hematoma, gastrointestinal bleed, bloody pleural effusion) or external (laceration). Fluid losses may accompany a variety of illnesses, including gastrointestinal diseases, ascites, and third-degree burns. Finally, syncope can result from idiopathic hypovolemia [121].

Approach to the Patient with Syncope

Syncope is a symptom, not a disease, and therefore the approach to the patient presenting with syncope is a search for clues from the history, physical examination, ECG, and electrolytes for the underlying disease process.

HISTORY. The history of the syncopal event from the patient usually needs supplementation from witnesses. Syncope needs to be differentiated from conditions such as epilepsy and vertigo, and the specific initiating factors leading to syncope need to be discovered. Although both syncope and seizures can be associated with tonic-clonic movements, in syncope loss of consciousness precedes any tonic-clonic movements, and any such movements are usually very brief in syncope. Such features as incontinence or tongue biting are not associated with syncope. Finally, seizures are usually associated with a prolonged postictal state, unlike most cases of syncope, where recovery is usually quite rapid. As mentioned earlier, neurocardiogenic syncope is often preceded by premonitory symptoms reflecting vagal activation, and situational syncope is associated with certain activities. Associated symptoms together with the syncopal event need to be sought. The use of medications can also furnish important clues. Determining evidence of cardiac disease or cardiac symptoms is particularly important.

PHYSICAL EXAMINATION. Clues to underlying acute or chronic diseases should be sought, with particular attention to clues suggesting a potentially life-threatening disease presenting as syncope, such as aortic dissection, cardiac tamponade, ventricular arrhythmia, or pulmonary embolus. A major effort should be put on discerning evidence for underlying structural heart disease such as aortic stenosis, hypertrophic cardiomyopathy, or any cause of decreased ventricular function. The finding of significant structural heart disease makes underlying ventricular tachycardia more likely. Accordingly, electrophysiologic testing should be considered in patients with significant underlying heart disease and unexplained syncope (see below).

ELECTROCARDIOGRAM. The ECG should be analyzed for clues to such disorders as WPW syndrome, long Q–T syndrome, acute cor pulmonale suggesting pulmonary embolus, acute or prior myocardial ischemia or infarction, arrhythmias, or conduction system disease.

LABORATORY TESTS. Routine laboratory tests can document such causes as acute blood loss. Hypokalemia or hypomagnesemia may suggest a propensity to arrhythmias. Cardiac enzymes can help confirm the diagnosis of acute myocardial infarction.

FURTHER STUDY. Other studies depend on the provisional diagnosis. For suspected bradycardia as the cause of syncope, Holter monitoring and 30-day event monitoring with a memory loop recorder are useful. All causes of bradycardia may appear only intermittently, which can make diagnosis difficult even with 24-hour Holter monitoring. Formal electrophysiologic testing may be normal even in the presence of documented severe intermittent sick sinus syndrome or conduction system disease [122]. Event recorders with memory loops used for a month or more may be more helpful [123,124].

New devices are available that constantly store and update the last 30 to 60 seconds of heart rhythm recordings until the patient feels symptoms, at which point pressing a button stores the rhythm strip for 30 to 60 seconds both before and after the event button is triggered. The stored rhythm strip can then be transmitted via telephone to a receiving station, where it is recorded in hard copy for later retrieval. These devices can also be useful in detecting ventricular arrhythmias. For both bradyarrhythmias and tachyarrhythmias, one strong advantage of these devices over other techniques is that they allow a definitive correlation between the rhythm disorder and the patient's symptoms of syncope or near syncope.

Signal-averaged ECG can suggest the likelihood of ventricular arrhythmia as a cause of syncope. Approximately 250 consecutive QRS complexes are obtained and summed by computer, allowing random electrical noise to be filtered out, so that low-amplitude and high-frequency electrical deflections at the end of the QRS (late potentials) can be detected (Fig. 39-6). Late potentials indicate the presence of areas in the heart with slow conduction; they are present in a significant number of patients with prior myocardial infarction, particularly with significantly reduced left ventricular ejection fraction. Their presence correlates well with clinical episodes of ventricular tachycardia and with the ability to induce ventricular tachycardia during electrophysiologic testing [90,125]. More recently, signal averaging was shown to correlate with the incidence of ventricular tachycardia in patients with idiopathic dilated cardiomyopathy as well [126]. Finally, signal averaging is useful in predicting the likelihood of patients developing serious ventricular arrhythmias following acute myocardial infarction; studies are underway to assess whether such patients should be treated prophylactically [127,128].

Electrophysiologic study remains the gold standard for diagnosing the likelihood of ventricular arrhythmias as the cause of syncope. Electrophysiologic study can also be used to assess sinus node, A-V node, and His-Purkinje system function to help confirm the diagnosis of syncope in patients with suspected bradyarrhythmias, although the sensitivity of this testing in these circumstances is quite low [122]. To diagnose ventricular tachycardia as the cause of syncope, electrophysiologic study routinely includes up to three extrastimuli during ventricular pacing at two different cycle lengths from two different right ventricular sites, in an effort to induce sustained ventricular

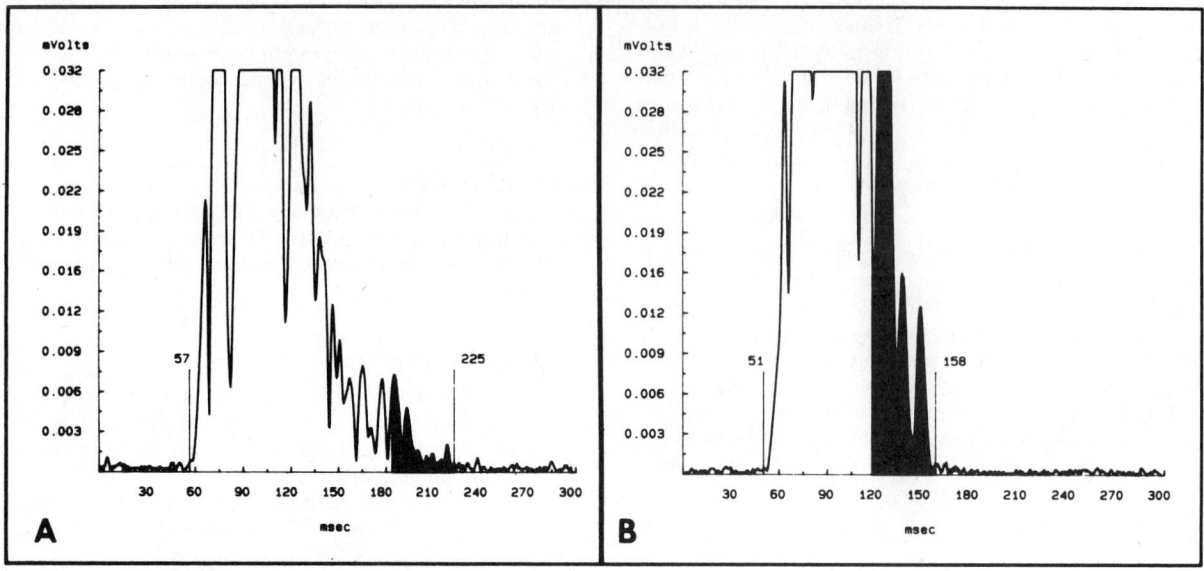

Fig. 39-6. Abnormal (*A*) and normal (*B*) signal-averaged ECGs. The abnormal tracing is of longer duration, with characteristic features of a late potential (prolonged duration of the low-amplitude signal and presence of only the low-amplitude signal during the last 40 msec of the QRS, as shown in black).

tachycardia. The sensitivity and specificity of the ability to induce sustained monomorphic ventricular tachycardia during electrophysiologic study in patients with clinical episodes of ventricular tachycardia are quite high, particularly in patients with underlying ischemic heart disease [129–132]. Electrophysiologic study is also useful in hypertrophic cardiomyopathy [46] but is often falsely negative in patients with dilated cardiomyopathy or ventricular arrhythmias from other forms of structural heart disease. Electrophysiologic testing is seldom able to induce ventricular tachycardia in patients without underlying heart disease, with the exception of the rare forms of idiopathic right and left ventricular tachycardia discussed earlier. Guidelines for the use of intracardiac electrophysiologic studies, including their role in patients with syncope of unknown etiology, were published by the American College of Cardiology and American Heart Association [133].

Treatment

Treatment depends on the diagnosis and is usually directed at the underlying disease process (e.g., pulmonary embolus, dissection of the aorta) rather than the resulting syncope per se. Bradyarrhythmias that result in syncope are usually managed with pacemaker insertion, with the notable exception of neurocardiogenic syncope, which responds well to a variety of medications (see earlier discussion) but poorly to pacemaker therapy [134]. Indications for use of pacemakers were published by the American College of Cardiology and American Heart Association [135]. One option for the management of ventricular arrhythmias is antiarrhythmic drug therapy, guided by either serial Holter monitoring in the presence of a large amount of background ventricular ectopy or serial electrophysiologic

studies to find a drug capable of rendering the patient noninducible [136]. Other alternatives include catheter ablation, surgical resection, or an implantable defibrillator. The latter technique is becoming more popular with the advent of transvenous lead systems, which avoid the significant morbidity of a thoracotomy in the typical patient with severe underlying heart disease [137,138]. Unfortunately, catheter ablation in patients with ventricular tachycardia secondary to coronary artery disease has been successful in only highly selected patients to date [139]. Surgical approaches usually carry a relatively high degree of morbidity and mortality in all but the most ideal candidates [140], although surgical therapy offers the potential benefit of combining endocardial resection with aneurysmectomy, coronary bypass grafting, ventricular remodeling, and/or valve replacement [141].

References

1. Gendelman HE, Linzer M, Gabelman M, et al: Syncope in a general hospital patient population. *NY State J Med* 83:1161, 1980.
2. Silverstein MD, Singer DE, Mulley AG, et al: Patients with syncope admitted to medical intensive care units. *JAMA* 248:1185, 1982.
3. Kapoor W, Karpf M, Levey GS: Issues in evaluating patients with syncope. *Ann Intern Med* 100:755, 1984.
4. Eagle KA, Black HR, Cook EF, et al: Evaluation of prognostic classifications for patients with syncope. *Am J Med* 79:455, 1985.
5. Kapoor WN, Karpf M, Wieand S, et al: A prospective evaluation and follow-up of patients with syncope. *N Engl J Med* 309:198, 1983.
6. Day SC, Cook EF, Funkelstein H, et al: Evaluation and outcome of emergency room patients with transient loss of consciousness. *Am J Med* 73:15, 1982.
7. Fleg JL, Asante AVK: Asystole following treadmill exercise in a man without organic heart disease. *Arch Intern Med* 20:1821, 1983.
8. Hirata T, Yano K, Ohui T, et al: Asystole with syncope following strenuous exercise in a man without organic heart disease. *J Electrocardiol* 20:280, 1987.
9. Huycke EC, Card HG, Sobol SM, et al: Postexertional cardiac asystole in a young man without organic heart disease. *Ann Intern Med* 106:844, 1987.

10. Tamura Y, Onodera O, Kodera K, et al: Atrial standstill after treadmill exercise test and unique response to isoproterenol infusion in recurrent postexercise syncope. *Am J Cardiol* 65:533, 1990.

11. Abi-Samra F, Maloney J, Fouad FM, et al: The usefulness of head-up tilt table testing and hemodynamic investigations in the workup of syncope of unknown origin. *PACE* 10:406, 1987.

12. Almquist A, Goldenberg IF, Milstein S, et al: Provocation of bradycardia and hypotension by isoproterenol and upright posture in patients with unexplained syncope. *N Engl J Med* 320:346, 1989.

13. Benditt DG, Remole S, Bailin S, et al: Tilt table testing for evaluation of neurally-mediated (cardioneurogenic) syncope: Rationale and proposed protocols. *PACE* 14:1528, 1991.

14. Milstein S, Buetikofer J, Lesser J: A manifestation of neurally mediated hypotension-bradycardia. *J Am Coll Cardiol* 14:1626, 1989.

15. Wagshal AB, Huang SKS: Syncope in athletes. *J Musculoskel Med* 10:21, 1993.

16. Grubb BP, Temesy-Armos PN, Samoil D, et al: Tilt table testing in the evaluation and management of athletes with recurrent exercise induced syncope. *Med Sci Sports Exercise* 25:25, 1993.

17. Von Bezold A, Hirt L: Uber die physiologischen Wirungen des essigsauren veratrins. *Untersuchungen Physiologischen Laboratoruim Wurzburg* 1:75, 1867.

18. Mark AL: The Bezold-Jarisch reflex revisited: Clinical implications of inhibitory reflexes originating in the heart. *J Am Coll Cardiol* 1:90, 1983.

19. Sheldon R, Killam S: Methodology of isoproterenol tilt-table testing in patients with syncope. *J Am Coll Cardiol* 19:773, 1992.

20. Fitzpatrick AP, Theodorakis G, Vardas P, et al: Methodology of head-up tilt testing in patients with unexplained syncope. *J Am Coll Cardiol* 17:125, 1991.

21. Favale S, DiBiase M, Rizzo U, et al: Effect of adenosine and adenosine-5'-triphosphate on atrioventricular conduction in patients. *J Am Coll Cardiol* 5:1212, 1985.

22. Milstein S, Buetikofer J, Dunnigan A, et al: Usefulness of disopyramide for prevention of upright tilt-induced hypotension-bradycardia. *Am J Cardiol* 65:1339, 1990.

23. Sra J, Murthy VS, Jazayeri MR: Use of intravenous esmolol to predict efficacy of oral beta-adrenergic blocker therapy in patients with neurocardiogenic syncope. *J Am Coll Cardiol* 19:402, 1992.

24. Kapoor WN: Diagnostic evaluation of syncope. *Am J Med* 90:91, 1991.

25. Aicardi J, Gastaut H, Mises J: Syncopal attacks compulsively self-induced by Valsalva's maneuver associated with typical absence seizures. *Arch Neurol* 45:923, 1988.

26. Kapoor WN, Peterson J, Karpf M: Defecation syncope. *Arch Intern Med* 146:2377, 1986.

27. Kadish AH, Wechsler L, Marchlinski FE: Swallowing syncope: Observations in the absence of conduction system or esophageal disease. *Am J Med* 81:1098, 1986.

28. Baron SB, Huang SK: Cough syncope presenting as Mobitz type II atrioventricular block: An electrophysiologic correlation. *PACE* 10:65, 1987.

29. Lipsitz LA, Nyquist R Jr, Wei JY, et al: Postprandial reduction in blood pressure in the elderly. *N Engl J Med* 309:81, 1983.

30. Thompson JL: Glossopharyngeal neuralgia accompanied by unconsciousness. *J Neurosurg* 11:511, 1954.

31. Richburg PL, Kern CE: Glossopharyngeal neuralgia with syncope and convulsions. *JAMA* 152:703, 1953.

32. Hassam AB, Abindar EG, Goldhammer EI, et al: Complete heart block and trigeminal neuralgia. *Neurology* 37:1089, 1987.

33. Kapoor WN, Jannetta PJ: Trigeminal neuralgia associated with seizure and syncope. *J Neurosurg* 61:594, 1984.

34. Stryjer D, Friedensohn A, Schlesinger Z: Carotid sinus hypersensitivity: Diagnosis of vasodepressor type in the presence of cardioinhibitory type. *PACE* 5:793, 1982.

35. Almquist A, Gornick C, Benson DW Jr, et al: Carotid sinus hypersensitivity: Evaluation of the vasodepressor component. *Circulation* 71:927, 1985.

36. Walter PF, Crawley IS, Dorney ER: Carotid sinus hypersensitivity and syncope. *Am J Cardiol* 42:396, 1978.

37. Lipsitz L: Orthostatic hypotension in the elderly. *N Engl J Med* 321:952, 1989.

38. Atkins D, Sefcik T, Kapoor W: Orthostatic hypotension and syncope. *Clin Res* 38:701A, 1990.

39. White WB: Hypotension with postural syncope secondary to the combination of chlorpromazine and captopril. *Arch Intern Med* 146:1833, 1986.

40. Manolis AS, Estes NA III: Orthostatic hypotension due to quinidine and atenolol (letter). *Am J Med* 82:1083, 1987.

41. Lombard JT, Selzer A: Valvular aortic stenosis. *Ann Intern Med* 106:292, 1987.

42. Richards AM, Nicholls MG, Ikram H, et al: Syncope in aortic valvular disease. *Lancet* 2:1113, 1984.

43. Yufe R, Karpati G, Carpenter S: Cardiac myxoma: A diagnostic challenge for the neurologist. *Neurology* 26:1060, 1976.

44. Ghahramani AR, Arnold JR, Holdner FJ, et al: Left atrial myxoma. *Am J Med* 52:525, 1972.

45. McKenna W, Harris L, Deanfield J: Syncope in hypertrophic cardiomyopathy. *Br Heart J* 47:177, 1982.

46. Fananapazir L, Chang AC, Epstein SE, et al: Prognostic determinants in hypertrophic cardiomyopathy: Prospective evaluation of a therapeutic strategy based on clinical, Holter, hemodynamic, and electrophysiologic findings. *Circulation* 86:218, 1992.

47. Maron BJ, Roberts WC, McAllister HA, et al: Sudden death in young athletes. *Circulation* 62:218, 1980.

48. Topol EJ, Traill TA, Fortuin NJ: Hypertensive hypertrophic cardiomyopathy of the elderly. *N Engl J Med* 312:277, 1985.

49. Frenneaux MP, Counihan PJ, Caforio AL, et al: Abnormal blood pressure response during exercise in hypertrophic cardiomyopathy. *Circulation* 82:1995, 1990.

50. Gilligan DM, Nihoyannopoulos P, Chan WL, et al: Investigation of a hemodynamic basis for syncope in hypertrophic cardiomyopathy: Use of a head-up tilt test. *Circulation* 85:2140, 1992.

51. Mark AL, Kioschos JM, Abboud FM, et al: Abnormal vascular responses to exercise in patients with aortic stenosis. *J Clin Invest* 52:1138, 1973.

52. Dressler W: Effort syncope as an early manifestation of primary pulmonary hypertension. *Am J Sci* 233:131, 1952.

53. Thames D, Alpert JS, Dalen JE: Syncope due to massive pulmonary embolism. *JAMA* 238:2509, 1977.

54. Pathy MS: Clinical presentation of myocardial infarction in the elderly. *Br Heart J* 29:190, 1967.

55. Dixon MS, Thomas P, Sheridan DJ: Syncope at the presentation of unstable angina. *Int J Cardiol* 19:125, 1988.

56. Irving JB, Kifchin AH: Syncopal attacks as symptoms of severe coronary artery disease. *Br Heart J* 1:155, 1975.

57. Heberden W: Some account of a disorder of the breast. *M Tr R Coll Physicians (London)* 2:59, 1772.

58. Uchida Y, Murao S: Excitation of afferent cardiac sympathetic nerve fibers during coronary occlusion. *Am J Physiol* 226:1094, 1974.

59. Roberts WC: Major anomalies of coronary arterial origin seen in adulthood. *Am Heart J* 111:941, 1986.

60. MacAlpin R: Cardiac arrest and sudden unexpected death in variant angina: Complications of coronary spasm that can occur in the absence of severe organic coronary stenosis. *Am Heart J* 125:1011, 1993.

61. Myerburg RJ, Kessler KM, Mallon SM, et al: Life-threatening ventricular arrhythmias in patients with silent myocardial ischemia due to coronary artery spasm. *N Engl J Med* 326:1451, 1992.

62. Beltran P, Lichstein E, Sanders M: Coronary artery spasm appearing as syncope. *Arch Intern Med* 142:192, 1982.

63. Fozzard HA, Makielski JC: The electrophysiology of acute myocardial ischemia. *Ann Rev Med* 36:275, 1985.

64. Lie KI, Wellens HJJ, Downar E, et al: Observations on patients with primary ventricular fibrillation complicating acute myocardial infarction. *Circulation* 52:755, 1975.

65. Lawrie DM, Higgins MR, Goodman MJ, et al: Ventricular fibrillation complicating acute myocardial infarction. *Lancet* 2:523, 1968.

66. Slater EE, DeSanctis RW: The clinical recognition of dissecting aortic aneurysm. *Am J Med* 60:625, 1976.

67. Rubenstein JJ, Schulman CL, Yurchak PM, et al: Clinical spectrum of the sick sinus syndrome. *Circulation* 46:5, 1972.

68. Rasmussen V, Haunso S, Skagen K: Cerebral attacks due to excessive vagal tone in heavily trained persons. *Acta Med Scand* 204:401, 1978.

69. Lev M: The pathology of complete atrioventricular block. *Prog Cardiovasc Dis* 6:317, 1964.

70. Lenegre J: Etiology and pathology of bilateral bundle branch block in relation to complete heart block. *Prog Cardiovasc Dis* 6:409, 1964.

71. Simon AB, Zloto AE: Symptomatic sinus node disease: Natural history after permanent ventricular pacing. *PACE* 2:305, 1979.

72. Rosenqvist M, Vallin H, Edhag O: Clinical and electrophysiological course of sinus node disease: Five-year follow-up study. *Am Heart J* 109:513, 1985.

73. Strauss HC, Bigger JT, Saroff LA, et al: Electrophysiologic evaluation of sinus node function in patients with sinus node dysfunction. *Circulation* 53:763, 1976.

74. Bigger JT, Reiffel JA: Sick sinus syndrome. *Annu Rev Med* 30:91, 1979.

75. Albin G, Hayes DL, Holmes DR Jr: Sinus node dysfunction in pediatric and young adult patients: Treatment by implantation of a permanent pacemaker in 39 cases. *Mayo Clin Proc* 60:667, 1985.

76. Saito D, Matsubara K, Yamanari H, et al: Effects of oral theophylline on sick sinus syndrome. *J Am Coll Cardiol* 21:1199, 1993.

77. Waugh R, Wagner J, Haney T, et al: Immediate and remote prognostic significance of fascicular block during acute myocardial infarction. *Circulation* 47:705, 1973.

78. Ausubel K, Furman S: The pacemaker syndrome. *Ann Intern Med* 103:420, 1985.

79. Erlebacher JA, Danner RL, Steizer PE: Hypotension with ventricular pacing: An atrial vasodepressor reflex in human beings. *J Am Coll Cardiol* 4:550, 1984.

80. Vetter V, Horowitz L: Electrophysiologic residua and sequelae of surgery for congenital heart defects. *Am J Cardiol* 50:588, 1982.

81. Devereux RB, Kramer-Fox R, Kligfield D: Mitral valve prolapse: Causes, clinical manifestations and management. *Ann Intern Med* 111:305, 1989.

82. Boudoulax H, Kolibagh AJ, Baker P, et al: Mitral valve prolapse and the mitral valve prolapse syndrome: A diagnostic classification and pathogenesis of symptoms. *Am Heart J* 118:796, 1989.

83. Swartz MH, Teichholz LE, Donoso E: Mitral valve prolapse: A review of associated arrhythmias. *Am J Med* 62:377, 1977.

84. Taylor D, Horenstein S, Williams G, et al: Syncope, seizure, and stroke in the mitral valve prolapse syndrome. *Trans Am Neurol Assoc* 104:114, 1979.

85. Thiene G, Nava A, Corrado D, et al: Right ventricular cardiomyopathy and sudden death in young people. *N Engl J Med* 318:129, 1988.

86. Blomstrom-Lundqvist C, Sabel KG, Olsson SB: A long term follow up of 15 patients with arrhythmogenic right ventricular dysplasia. *Br Heart J* 58:477, 1987.

87. Wellens HJJ, Duren DR, Lie KI: Observations on mechanisms of ventricular tachycardia in man. *Circulation* 54:237, 1976.

88. Akhtar M: Clinical spectrum of ventricular tachycardia. *Circulation* 82:1561, 1990.

89. Kuchar DL, Thorburn CW, Sammel NL: Prediction of serious arrhythmic events after myocardial infarction: Signal-averaged electrocardiogram, Holter monitoring and radionuclide ventriculography. *J Am Coll Cardiol* 9:531, 1987.

90. Gomes JA, Winter SL, Steward D, et al: A new noninvasive index to predict sustained ventricular tachycardia and sudden death in the five years after myocardial infarction based on signal-averaged electrocardiograms, radionuclide ejection fraction, and Holter monitoring. *J Am Coll Cardiol* 10:349, 1987.

91. Wilber DJ, Olshansky B, Moran JF, et al: Electrophysiological testing and nonsustained ventricular tachycardia: Use and limitations in patients with coronary artery disease and impaired ventricular function. *Circulation* 82:350, 1990.

92. Ohe T, Shimomura K, Aihara N, et al: Idiopathic sustained left ventricular tachycardia: Clinical and electrophysiologic characteristics. *Circulation* 77:560, 1988.

93. Buxton A, Waxman H, Marchlinski F, et al: Right ventricular tachycardia: Clinical and electrophysiologic characteristics. *Circulation* 68:917, 1983.

94. Lerman BB, Belardinelli L, West GA, et al: Adenosine-sensitive ventricular tachycardia: Evidence suggesting cyclic AMP-mediated triggered activity. *Circulation* 74:270, 1986.

95. Klein LS, Shih HT, Hackett FK, et al: Radiofrequency catheter ablation of ventricular tachycardia in patients without structural heart disease. *Circulation* 85:1666, 1992.

96. Schwartz PG, Periti M, Malliani A: The idiopathic long QT syndrome: Progress and questions. *Am Heart J* 109:399, 1985.

97. Jervell A, Lange-Nielsen F: Congenital deaf mutism, functional heart disease with prolongation of the Q–T interval and sudden death. *Am Heart J* 54:59, 1957.

98. Fraser GR, Froggatt P, James TN: Congenital deafness associated with electrocardiographic abnormalities, fainting attacks, and sudden deaths. *Q J Med* 33:361, 1964.

99. Ward OC: New familial cardiac syndrome in children. *J Irish Med Assoc* 54:103, 1964.

100. Romano C, Gemme G, Pongiglione R: Aritmie cardiache rare dell'eta pediatrica. *Clin Pediatr* 45:656, 1963.

101. Jackman WM, Friday KJ, Anderson JL, et al: The long QT syndromes: A critical review, new clinical observations and a unifying hypothesis. *Prog Cardiovasc Dis* 31:115, 1988.

102. Singh B, Goardner T, Kanegae T: Liquid protein diets and torsade de pointes. *JAMA* 240:115, 1978.

103. Isner JM, Sours HE, Paris AL, et al: Sudden, unexpected death in avid dieters using the liquid-protein-modified fast diet. *Circulation* 60:1401, 1979.

104. Smith WM, Gallagher JJ: Les "torsades de pointes": An unusual ventricular arrhythmia. *Ann Intern Med* 93:578, 1980.

105. Kay GN, Plumb VJ, Arciniegas JG: Torsade de pointes: The long-short initiating sequence and other clinical faeatures: Observations in 32 patients. *J Am Coll Cardiol* 2:806, 1983.

106. Tzivoni D, Banai S, Schuger CD, et al: Treatment of torsade de pointes with magnesium sulfate. *Circulation* 77:392, 1988.

107. Wang Y, Scheinman MM, Chien WW, et al: Patients with supraventricular tachycardia presenting with aborted sudden death: Incidence, mechanism, and long-term follow-up. *J Am Coll Cardiol* 18:1711, 1991.

108. Leitch JW, Klein GJ, Yee R, et al: Syncope associated with supraventricular tachycardia: An expression of tachycardia rate or vasomotor response? *Circulation* 85:1064, 1992.

109. Haan J, Jansen EN, Oostrom J, et al: Falling spells in normal pressure hydrocephalus: A favorable prognostic sign? *Eur Neurol* 27:216, 1987.

110. Fields WS, Lemak NA: Joint study of extracranial arterial occlusion. VII. Subclavian steal—A review of 168 cases. *JAMA* 222:1139, 1972.

111. Lees F, Watkins SM: Loss of consciousness in migraine. *Lancet* 2:647, 1963.

112. Bickerstaff ER: Impairment of consciousness in migraine. *Lancet* 2:647, 1961.

113. Johnson RH, Eisenhofer G, Lambie DG: The effects of acute and chronic ingestion of ethanol on the autonomic nervous system. *Drug Alcohol Depend* 18:319, 1986.

114. Lowenstein DH, Massa SM, Rowbotham MC, et al: Acute neurologic and psychiatric complications associated with cocaine abuse. *Am J Med* 83:841, 1987.

115. Engel GL: Psychologic stress, vasodepressor (vasovagal) syncope, and sudden death. *Ann Intern Med* 89:403, 1978.

116. Small GW, Borus JF: Outbreak of illness in a school chorus. *N Engl J Med* 308:632, 1983.

117. Levine RJ: Epidemic faintness and syncope in a school marching band. *JAMA* 238:2373, 1977.

118. Escobar JI, Burnam A, Karno M, et al: Somatization in the community. *Arch Gen Psychiatry* 1987:713, 1987.

119. Katon W: Panic disorder and somatization: Review of 55 cases. *Am J Med* 77:101, 1984.

120. Linzer M, Felder A, Hackel A, et al: Psychiatric syncope: A new look at an old disease. *Psychosomatics* 31:181, 1990.

121. Fouad FM, Tadena-Thome L, Bravo EL, et al: Idiopathic hypovolemia. *Ann Intern Med* 104:298, 1986.

122. Fujimura O, Yee R, Klein GJ, et al: The diagnostic sensitivity of electrophysiologic testing in patients with syncope caused by transient bradycardia. *N Engl J Med* 321:1703, 1989.

123. Linzer M, Pritchett E, Pontinen M, et al: Incremental diagnostic yield of loop electrocardiographic recorders in unexplained syncope. *Am J Cardiol* 66:214, 1990.

124. Brown AP, Dawkins KD, Davies JG: Detection of arrhythmias: Use of a patient-activated ambulatory electrocardiogram device with a solid-state memory loop. *Br Heart J* 58:251, 1987.

125. Winters SL, Stewart D, Gomes JA: Signal averaging of the surface QRS complex predicts inducibility of ventricular tachycardia in

patients with syncope of unknown origin: A prospective study. *J Am Coll Cardiol* 10:775, 1987.

126. Mancini DM, Wong KL, Simson MB: Prognostic value of an abnormal signal-averaged electrocardiogram in patients with nonischemic congestive cardiomyopathy. *Circulation* 87:1083, 1993.

127. Pires LA, Huang SKS: Nonsustained ventricular tachycardia: Identification and management of high-risk patients. *Am Heart J* 126:189, 1993.

128. Nisam S, Thomas A, Mower M, et al: Identifying patients for prophylactic automatic implantable cardioverter defibrillator therapy: Status of prospective studies. *Am Heart J* 122:607, 1991.

129. Gulamhusein S, Naccarelli GV, Ko PT, et al: Value and limitations of clinical electrophysiology study in assessment of patients with unexplained syncope. *Am J Med* 73:700, 1982.

130. DiMarco JP, Garan H, Harthorne JW, et al: Intracardiac electrophysiologic techniques in recurrent syncope of unknown cause. *Ann Intern Med* 95:542, 1981.

131. DiMarco JP: Electrophysiological studies in patients with unexplained syncope. *Circulation* 75 (suppl III):III-140, 1987.

132. McAnulty JH: Syncope of unknown origin: The role of electrophysiologic studies. *Circulation* 75 (suppl III):144, 1987.

133. Zipes DP, Akhtar M, Denes P, et al: ACC/AHA Task Force Report: Guidelines for clinical intracardiac electrophysiologic studies. *J Am Coll Cardiol* 14:1827, 1989.

134. Sra JS, Jazayeri MR, Avitall B, et al: Comparison of cardiac pacing with drug therapy in the treatment of neurocardiogenic (vasovagal) syncope with bradycardia or asystole. *N Engl J Med* 328:1085, 1993.

135. Dreifus LS, Fisch C, Griffin JC, et al: ACC/AHA Task Force Report: Guidelines for implantation of cardiac pacemakers and antiarrhythmia devices. *J Am Coll Cardiol* 18:1, 1991.

136. ESVEM Investigators: Determinants of predicted efficacy of antiarrhythmic drugs in the electrophysiologic study versus electrocardiographic monitoring trial. *Circulation* 87:323, 1993.

137. Lehmann MH, Steinman RT, Schuger CD, et al: The automatic implantable cardiac defibrillator as antiarrhythmic therapeutic modality of choice for survivors of cardiac arrest unrelated to acute myocardial infarction. *Am J Cardiol* 62:803, 1988.

138. Bardy GH, Hofer B, Johnson G, et al: Implantable transvenous cardioverter-defibrillators. *Circulation* 87:1152, 1993.

139. Morady F, Harvey M, Kalbfleisch SJ, et al: Radiofrequency catheter ablation of ventricular tachycardia in patients with coronary artery disease. *Circulation* 87:363, 1993.

140. Horowitz LN, Harken AH, Kastor JA, et al: Ventricular resection guided by epicardial and endocardial mapping for treatment of recurrent ventricular tachycardia. *N Engl J Med* 302:589, 1980.

141. Manolis AS, Rastegar H, Estes NA III: Effects of coronary artery bypass grafting on ventricular arrhythmias. *PACE* 16:984, 1993.

40. Systemic Embolism

James E. Dalen

The exact incidence of systemic embolism is difficult to determine. Emboli to the abdominal viscera may cause nonspecific signs or symptoms not recognized as being the result of embolism. In nearly all studies, the incidence of systemic embolism as detected at postmortem study is far greater than the number detected clinically. For example, in patients with mitral valve disease, the incidence of emboli recognized clinically is 16 to 18 percent [1,2], whereas at postmortem study 50 percent of patients have evidence of systemic embolism [3].

The most common site of systemic embolism is the cerebral circulation, specifically the middle cerebral artery [4]. Sixty to 70 percent of systemic emboli that are recognized clinically are to the brain [2,5]. It has been estimated that approximately 20 percent of all ischemic strokes are due to systemic embolism [6]. In a postmortem study of 333 patients who had been in atrial fibrillation, Hinton et al. found that 32 percent had evidence of systemic embolism. Seventy-three percent of the emboli were to the brain [7]. Estimates of the true incidence of systemic embolism are further compromised by the fact that whereas stroke is readily recognized, it is often difficult to distinguish clinically between embolic and nonembolic stroke.

Of systemic emboli that do not involve the cerebral circulation, the vast majority affect the lower extremities. In a review of 974 noncerebral emboli at the Massachusetts General Hospital, Abbott et al. reported that 63 percent affected the legs, 20 percent the arms, 9 percent the viscera, and 9 percent other sites [8]. The majority of emboli lodge where there is an abrupt arterial narrowing, especially at a bifurcation or at the site of an atherosclerotic plaque.

The most frequent sites of embolism in the lower extremity in Abbott's series were the femoral artery (44%), aortoiliac arteries (29%), and popliteal artery (27%) [8]. Emboli to the upper extremities are most likely to involve the radial (61%), axillary (23%), or subclavian artery (12%), as reported by Haimovici in a collected series of 572 patients [9].

Pathophysiology

Emboli to the systemic circulation nearly always originate as thrombi within the left heart (Table 40-1). In a literature review of 1575 patients with systemic emboli, Heiskell and Conn reported that 89 percent of the emboli originated as thrombi within the heart [10]. In less than 1 percent, the source was an aortic aneurysm. Paradoxical embolism of the systemic circulation by venous thrombi crossing a patent foramen ovale or intracardiac defect was recognized in 0.3 percent of cases. In 6.5 percent, the source of the systemic embolism was not determined.

The three disorders that cause thrombi in the left heart most frequently are atrial fibrillation, coronary artery disease, and valvular heart disease, including prosthetic heart valves. Of these three disorders, atrial fibrillation is of prime importance, being present in more than 50% of patients with systemic embolism. Coronary artery disease and valvular heart disease are most likely to be complicated by systemic embolism when atrial fibrillation is present.

Many investigators have reported that the number of patients with systemic embolism associated with rheumatic heart disease has decreased over the past 30 years, while the number of patients with coronary heart disease has increased. Hight et al. compared the experience with arterial embolism at the Peter Bent Brigham Hospital from 1964 to 1973 to an earlier review from 1948 to 1963 at the same hospital by Edwards [11]. From

Table 40-1. Sources of Systemic Emboli

Nonvalvular heart disease with atrial fibrillation	45%
Acute myocardial infarction	15%
Ventricular aneurysm	10%
Mitral valve disease	10%
Prosthetic heart valves	10%
All other	10%

1948 to 1963, 59 percent of patients with systemic embolism had rheumatic heart disease, versus only 33 percent from 1964 to 1973. The percentage of patients with atherosclerotic heart disease increased from 41 percent in the 1948 to 1963 review to 67 percent in the 1964 to 1973 study. Similar findings were noted by Abbott et al. in a review of systemic embolism at Massachusetts General Hospital (MGH) from 1937 to 1979 [8]. The percentage of patients with rheumatic heart disease decreased from 46 percent in 1937 to 1953, to 36 percent in 1959 to 1963, to only 20 percent in 1964 to 1979. This decrease is due to the progressive decrease in the incidence of rheumatic fever and rheumatic heart disease over the past decades.

Whereas the number of patients with systemic embolism who have rheumatic heart disease has decreased and the number of patients with coronary artery disease has increased, the incidence of atrial fibrillation has remained nearly constant. The incidence of atrial fibrillation in all patients with systemic embolism at MGH was 80 percent in 1937 to 1953, 75 percent in 1954 to 1963, and 74 percent in 1964 to 1979 [8]. These observations indicate that although the primary cause of atrial fibrillation has shifted from rheumatic heart disease to coronary artery disease over the past decades, atrial fibrillation is clearly the dominant cause of systemic embolism.

VALVULAR HEART DISEASE. The incidence of systemic embolism in patients with valvular heart disease is greatest in those who have rheumatic mitral valve disease, particularly mitral stenosis. Sixteen to 18 percent of patients being followed for mitral stenosis have a history of systemic embolism [1,2]. The incidence of emboli at postmortem examination is much higher, in the range of 50 percent [3]. Of the emboli, 60 to 70 percent are cerebral [2,5].

The incidence of emboli in patients with valvular heart disease increases with age and is especially increased in patients with atrial fibrillation. Coulshed et al. reported an incidence of systemic embolism of 11 percent in patients with mitral stenosis with normal sinus rhythm, as compared to 32 percent in patients with mitral stenosis complicated by atrial fibrillation [12]. Systemic emboli in patients with valvular heart disease usually originate as left atrial thrombi. In a postmortem study of 136 patients with valvular heart disease complicated by atrial fibrillation, Aberg found left atrial thrombi in 28 percent [13]. Given the high risk of systemic embolism in patients with mitral valve disease complicated by paroxysmal or chronic atrial fibrillation, long-term anticoagulation with warfarin, at a dose sufficient to prolong the prothrombin time to an international normalized ratio (INR) of 2.5 to 3.5, is indicated [14].

Systemic embolism is the most common late complication of valve replacement with mechanical prosthetic valves. The incidence is greatest in patients with mitral valve replacement, in large part due to the high incidence of chronic atrial fibrillation. The annual rate of embolism in patients with prosthetic mitral valves even with chronic anticoagulation varies from 6.1 to 10 percent per year [15,16]. All patients with mechanical heart valves require chronic anticoagulation with warfarin at a dose sufficient to prolong the INR to 2.0 to 3.0 [17].

The incidence of systemic embolism in patients with bioprosthetic valves is much less, illustrating the importance of atrial fibrillation in the etiology of systemic embolism in patients with valvular heart disease. Whereas the overall annual incidence of systemic embolism in patients with bioprosthetic valves is 5.4 percent per year, the incidence is much higher in patients with chronic atrial fibrillation [18]. In the absence of atrial fibrillation, a history of systemic embolism, or the finding of thrombus in the left atrium at surgery, the risk of systemic embolism in patients with bioprosthetic valves is small. Antithrombotic therapy is therefore not indicated [19].

CORONARY ARTERY DISEASE. Systemic embolism in patients with coronary artery disease (CAD) may originate as thrombus in the left ventricle or left atrium. The factors that lead to thrombus formation in patients with coronary heart disease are myocardial infarction, ventricular aneurysm, cardiomyopathy, and atrial fibrillation.

As shown in Table 40-2, in a collected series of 1080 patients with systemic embolism in the 1960s and 1970s, 24 percent had acute myocardial infarction [8,20–24]. A high incidence of left ventricular mural thrombus in patients dying of acute myocardial infarction has long been recognized. In a series of 100 patients dying of acute myocardial infarction, 37 percent had left ventricular thrombi [25]; in another series of 210 cases, the incidence was 39 percent; and in yet another series, the incidence was 44 percent [26].

Studies utilizing two-dimensional echocardiography (2-D echo) have confirmed the high incidence of left ventricular thrombus in patients with acute myocardial infarction. Asinger et al. detected left ventricular mural thrombi in 12 of 35 patients with anterior myocardial infarction and none of 35 patients with inferior myocardial infarction [27]. Friedman et al. reported similar findings: 2 thrombi in 13 patients with inferior myocardial infarction, and 8 in 21 patients with anterior myocardial infarction [28]. In both series, left ventricular mural thrombi originated in the apex of the left ventricle at the site of dyskinesis or akinesis.

In contrast to the high incidence of left ventricular mural thrombus, systemic embolism is uncommon in patients with acute myocardial infarction. None of the 12 patients with left ventricular thrombus reported by Asinger et al. had evidence of systemic embolism [27]; 2 patients of Friedman et al. embolized [28]. Large series of patients with acute myocardial infarction report an incidence of systemic embolism of 3 to 5 percent detected clinically [29,30,31]. This low incidence does not justify full-dose anticoagulation of all patients with acute myocardial infarction. However, patients with acute transmural anterior myocardial infarction are at a particularly high risk. A recent study [32] demonstrated that full-dose heparin decreased the incidence of left ventricular thrombi from 32 to 11 percent. The

Table 40-2. Incidence of Atrial Fibrillation (AF) and Myocardial Infarction (MI) in Systemic Embolism

Study	Years	No. patients	AF (%)	MI (%)
Abbott et al. [8]	1964–1979	313	74	33
Szczepanski [20]	1963–1973	260	51	17
Green et al. [21]	1963–1973	149	49	17
Silvers et al. [22]	1964–1979	106	75	22
Lorentzen et al. [23]	1969–1978	130	37	24
Satiani et al. [24]	1965–1977	122	43	25
Total		1080	(57)	(24)

American College of Chest Physicians conference on antithrombotic therapy recommended that patients with acute transmural anterior myocardial infarction be treated with full-dose heparin during hospitalization, followed by warfarin for 1 to 3 months after discharge [33].

In patients who recover from acute myocardial infarction, the incidence of systemic embolism is highest in those who develop a ventricular aneurysm. In a review of 5 postmortem series, Simpson et al. reported that 49 percent of patients with postmyocardial infarction left ventricular aneurysm had mural thrombi [34]. In a collected series of 674 patients undergoing left ventricular aneurysmectomy, 53 percent were noted at surgery to have mural thrombi [34].

As in the case of acute myocardial infarction, systemic embolism is much less common than mural thrombi. In the 674 patients undergoing left ventricular aneurysmectomy, only 4 percent had a history of clinically recognized systemic embolization. In patients with left ventricular aneurysm at postmortem study, 32 percent had evidence of systemic embolism [34]. This discrepancy between the clinical and postmortem study incidence of systemic embolism in patients with coronary heart disease underscores the fact that most episodes of systemic embolism are not recognized clinically.

Left ventricular thrombi may occur in patients with dilated cardiomyopathy without left ventricular aneurysm. Roberts and Ferrans reported an incidence of left ventricular thrombus of 47 percent in patients with dilated cardiomyopathy [35]. Using 2-D echo, Gottdiener et al. detected left ventricular thrombus in 36 percent of 123 patients with dilated cardiomyopathy [36]. The incidence was essentially the same in patients with ischemic versus idiopathic cardiomyopathy. Events compatible with systemic embolism occurred in 11 percent of the patients; however, the occurrence of systemic embolism was not different in patients with or without left ventricular thrombus as detected by 2-D echo.

In addition to acute anterior myocardial infarction, postinfarction left ventricular aneurysm, and dilated cardiomyopathy, the other factor that predisposes to systemic embolism in patients with CAD is atrial fibrillation. In the MGH series, as reported by Abbott et al., 67 percent of patients with systemic emboli from 1963 to 1979 had coronary artery disease [8]. Atrial fibrillation occurred in 80 percent of these patients. Hinton et al. studied the incidence of systemic embolism at postmortem study in 333 patients with atrial fibrillation [7]. As expected, the incidence of systemic embolism was high (42%) in patients with mitral valve disease; however, in 171 patients with coronary artery disease with atrial fibrillation, 35 percent had evidence of systemic embolism at postmortem study, as compared to only 7 percent in CAD patients without atrial fibrillation. The increased incidence of systemic embolism when CAD is complicated by atrial fibrillation may reflect an increased incidence of left atrial thrombi in such patients. In a postmortem study of 506 patients with nonvalvular heart disease complicated by atrial fibrillation, Aberg found left atrial thrombi in 13 percent [13]. Of the patients with nonvalvular heart disease complicated by atrial fibrillation, 42 percent had evidence of systemic embolism. The incidence of left atrial clot in 642 controls without atrial fibrillation was 2 percent.

ATRIAL FIBRILLATION. It is clear that atrial fibrillation is the dominant factor leading to systemic embolism in patients with valvular or coronary artery disease. A controversial question is whether atrial fibrillation in and of itself, without associated heart disease, may lead to systemic embolism.

One reason this question is difficult to answer is that most patients with atrial fibrillation have overt heart disease. As

Table 40-3. Heart Disease in Patients with Atrial Fibrillation

Disease	Clinical series (%)[a]	Postmortem series (%)[b]
Coronary artery disease	46	51
Valvular heart disease	20	30
Hypertension	11	10
Other heart disease	15	4
Total	92	95

[a] 230 patients were studied.
[b] 333 patients were studied.
Source: Data on clinical series from Hurst JW, Paulk EA Jr, Proctor HD, et al: Management of patients with atrial fibrillation *Am J Med* 37:728, 1964; data on postmortem series from Hinton RC, Kistler JP, Fallon JT, et al: Influence of etiology of atrial fibrillation on incidence of systemic embolism. *Am J Cardiol* 40:509, 1977.

shown in Table 40-3, in a clinical series of 230 patients with atrial fibrillation, Hurst et al. found that 92 percent had heart disease [37]. Coronary artery disease was found in 46 percent and valvular heart disease in 20 percent. In a postmortem series of 333 patients with atrial fibrillation, Hinton et al. noted nearly identical findings: 95 percent had heart disease [7]. The predominant cardiac disease associated with atrial fibrillation in Hinton's series was coronary heart disease (51%)—87 percent of the patients studied had old or recent myocardial infarction.

Highly suggestive evidence that atrial fibrillation in and of itself may predispose to systemic embolism is derived from a study of the incidence of stroke in the Framingham study [38]. In this study, the incidence of stroke in those with atrial fibrillation without valvular heart disease was 5.6 times greater than in patients with normal sinus rhythm matched for age and blood pressure. This and other studies [7] demonstrating a significant increased risk of stroke in patients with atrial fibrillation without valvular heart disease has led to a recommendation that anticoagulation should be considered in all patients with chronic atrial fibrillation [39].

Further evidence of the importance of atrial fibrillation in the etiology of systemic embolism emerges from studies of systemic embolism in patients with thyrotoxicosis [40,41,42]. As shown in Table 40-4, the incidence of atrial fibrillation in patients with thyrotoxicosis ranges from 10 to 28 percent. The incidence of systemic embolism in thyrotoxic patients with atrial fibrillation averages 14 percent. In Bar-Sela's series, there were no systemic emboli in 112 patients with thyrotoxicosis who were in normal sinus rhythm [40]. In each of these three series, the majority of emboli were strokes.

In the series reported by Staffurth et al., 3 of the 26 emboli occurred when the patient reverted to normal sinus rhythm and 11 occurred in patients who were in chronic atrial fibrillation despite becoming euthyroid [41]. Each of these three groups of investigators recommended that anticoagulation be considered in all patients with thyrotoxicosis complicated by atrial fibrillation. The ability to measure left atrial size noninvasively by echocardiogram has helped elucidate the pathophysiology of

Table 40-4. Thyrotoxicosis, Atrial Fibrillation (AF), and Systemic Embolism

Study	No. patients with thyrotoxicosis	AF (%)	Emboli in patients with AF (%)
Bar-Sela et al. 1981 [40]	142	21	40
Yuen et al. 1979 [42]	210	10	24
Staffurth et al. 1977 [41]	845	28	10
Total	1197	(24)	(14)

atrial fibrillation. Studies by Henry et al. have shown that the incidence of atrial fibrillation increases when left atrial size exceeds 40 mm [43]; furthermore, successful cardioversion is less likely, and recurrence to atrial fibrillation is more likely when left atrial size exceeds 45 mm. The critical factor, however, that leads to left atrial thrombus formation and systemic embolism is the occurrence of atrial fibrillation. Enlargement of the left atrium predisposes to left atrial thrombus because it predisposes to atrial fibrillation.

Most studies of systemic embolism in patients with atrial fibrillation have involved patients with chronic atrial fibrillation; however, in Aberg's postmortem studies, he noted an incidence of systemic embolism of 38 percent in patients who had been in atrial fibrillation for less than 1 week, compared to 56 percent in patients with chronic atrial fibrillation (>1 week) [13]. In a series of patients with rheumatic heart disease with atrial fibrillation, Szekely reported that 13 of 37 episodes of embolism occurred within 1 month of the onset of atrial fibrillation [44].

There is considerable evidence that patients with paroxysmal atrial fibrillation are at increased risk of systemic embolism. In Bar-Sela's study of systemic embolism in patients with thyrotoxicosis, 11 episodes occurred in patients with paroxysmal atrial fibrillation, and 6 in patients with chronic atrial fibrillation [40]. In a study of 100 patients with stroke who had atrial fibrillation, 37 percent had paroxysmal atrial fibrillation [45]. Embolism may occur when patients convert from atrial fibrillation to normal sinus rhythm, as evidenced by the occurrence of systemic embolism after cardioversion. Morris et al. [46] reported three emboli after 90 cardioversions and Hurst et al. reported two episodes of embolism at 3 and 8 days after cardioversion in 186 patients [37]. In a larger series, Bjerkelund and Orning noted an incidence of systemic embolism of 5.3 percent 1 to 6 days after cardioversion of 209 patients who were not anticoagulated [47].

The aspect of atrial fibrillation that most likely leads to thrombus formation in the left atrium is the loss of normal atrial contraction. Restoration of atrial contraction after cardioversion, or spontaneously in patients with paroxysmal atrial fibrillation, may dislodge a left atrial clot, with resultant systemic embolism. The importance of the lack of normal atrial contraction in the etiology of systemic embolism is illustrated by the increased incidence of systemic embolism in patients with the sick sinus syndrome [48].

It has long been recognized that the risk of systemic embolism in patients with atrial fibrillation complicated by mitral valve disease is sufficiently high to warrant long-term anticoagulation with warfarin [14]. Four recent randomized clinical trials [49–52] have compared warfarin to placebo, or no therapy, in patients with atrial fibrillation without mitral valve disease. The annual incidence of stroke or other systemic embolism ranged from 3.0 to 7.4 percent in the placebo and control groups. In patients treated with warfarin, the annual incidence of stroke or other systemic embolism was decreased to 0.4 to 2.3 percent. The decrease in the incidence of stroke and systemic embolism was significantly decreased in each of these four trials. On the basis of these clinical trials, the Third ACCP Consensus Conference on Antithrombotic Therapy recommended that in the absence of contraindications, all patients with atrial fibrillation should receive chronic anticoagulation with warfarin (INR 2.0–3.0) unless they have no associated cardiovascular disease or evidence of thyrotoxicosis *and* are younger than 60 years [53].

OTHER CARDIAC SOURCES. As noted, most systemic emboli originate as left atrial thrombi in patients with atrial fibrillation, mitral valve disease, prosthetic heart valves, or as left ventricular thrombi in patients with coronary artery disease. In addition to these intracardiac sources, emboli may originate on the aortic or mitral valves in patients with infective or marantic endocarditis. The incidence of systemic embolism has decreased with the advent of antibiotic therapy; however, emboli are noted in up to one-third of patients dying of endocarditis. The most frequent site of embolism is the brain [54].

In addition to emboli originating as left atrial thrombi in patients with valvular heart disease, calcific emboli may occur in patients with calcific aortic stenosis [55] and microthrombi may originate from the aortic or mitral valve. Emboli in patients with prosthetic or bioprosthetic valves may originate as thrombi on the valve apparatus or as left atrial thrombi. Myxoma is another potential, but rare, intracardiac source of systemic embolism. The majority of myxomas occur in the left atrium and arise from the atrial septum in the region of the fossa ovalis [56].

EXTRACARDIAC SOURCES. The prime extracardiac source of systemic embolism is the aorta. Thrombi may form within aortic aneurysms or may occur as mural thrombi in atherosclerotic segments of the aorta. Such thrombi may dislodge, with resultant embolism of the distal arterial circulation. Williams et al. reported 20 patients with visceral or lower extremity embolism in whom the source was judged to be aortic thrombus as demonstrated by angiography [57]. They urged a wider use of aortography in patients with unexplained systemic embolism, because they believe these patients may require aortotomy to remove intraaortic thrombus to prevent recurrent embolism. In addition to emboli arising as thrombus in the aorta, smaller emboli composed of atheromatous material (cholesterol emboli) may originate in an atherosclerotic aorta.

Finally, systemic emboli may originate as thrombi in the venous circulation. Paradoxical embolism of the systemic circulation by venous thrombi may occur in patients with an intracardiac defect (atrial or ventricular septal defect, patent ductus arteriosus, or pulmonary arterial-venous fistula). The vast majority of cases of paradoxical embolism, however, occur in patients who have a patent foramen ovale [58], which occurs in 27 percent of all adults [59] and does not cause cardiac symptoms or findings. In patients with a foramen ovale, shunting of blood or emboli from the right atrium to the left atrium does not normally occur because the higher pressure in the left atrium compresses a flap valve across the patent foramen, thereby preventing right-to-left flow; however, if right atrial pressure exceeds that in the left atrium, right-to-left shunting across the patent foramen occurs [60]. In the vast majority of cases of paradoxical embolism, the circumstance that causes right atrial pressure to exceed left atrial pressure and thereby permit passage of a venous thrombus across the patent foramen ovale is acute pulmonary embolism [58]. To cause elevation of right atrial pressure, pulmonary embolism must be sufficiently massive to obstruct more than 60 to 75 percent of the pulmonary circulation with consequent acute cor pulmonale [61]. Other than massive pulmonary embolism, conditions that may lead to paradoxical embolism in patients with venous thrombosis who have a patent foramen ovale include cor pulmonale secondary to chronic lung disease and the performance of a Valsalva maneuver [58]. Paradoxical embolism is usually first suspected at postmortem exam.

Diagnosis

Arterial embolism is recognized by the sudden occurrence of signs and symptoms of ischemia due to the abrupt interruption of arterial flow to the affected organ. It may occur at any time of the day and is unrelated to exertion or other specific activity [45].

CEREBRAL EMBOLISM. Since cerebral embolism is the most frequent type of arterial embolism, its recognition is critical to prevent further arterial embolism. As noted, the middle cerebral artery is the most frequent site of arterial embolism. The abrupt onset of motor sensory hemiplegia or monoplegia typically occurs without prodrome. Recognition of the embolic etiology of stroke is enhanced by the presence of atrial fibrillation or acute myocardial infarction.

Differentiation of embolic stroke from hemorrhagic stroke is vital to determine which patients with stroke require anticoagulation. In patients with embolic stroke, the computed tomography (CT) scan is negative for hemorrhage. Angiography demonstrates an abrupt occlusion of an otherwise normal artery or is normal due to migration or lysis of the embolus [62].

CORONARY ARTERY EMBOLISM. Since the original postmortem description of coronary artery embolism by Virchow in 1856 [63], its recognition, even at postmortem examination, has remained difficult. The signs and symptoms of coronary artery embolism are the same as those due to coronary occlusion in patients with coronary atherosclerosis.

The primary clinical clue that myocardial infarction may be due to coronary embolism rather than a complication of coronary atherosclerosis is its occurrence in young patients who have no prior angina pectoris and no risk factors for premature coronary atherosclerosis. The diagnosis of coronary embolism is further suggested when the patient has one or more conditions predisposing to arterial embolism: atrial fibrillation, valvular heart disease, prosthetic heart valves, or endocarditis. Indeed, it was the postmortem examination of patients with endocarditis that led Virchow to hypothesize that fragments from the heart valves could detach and embolize to the systemic circulation that constituted the first description of arterial embolism in 1847 [64].

The diagnosis of coronary embolism is particularly difficult in the setting where it may be very common, that is, in patients with coronary artery disease complicated by left ventricular or left atrial clot. In this circumstance, even at postmortem examination it would be difficult or impossible to determine whether the clot obstructing an atherosclerotic coronary artery was due to in situ thrombus or to embolism from the left ventricle or left atrium. Coronary embolism must be far more common than clinically recognized. In a postmortem study of 419 patients with myocardial infarction, Charles et al. found a 13 percent incidence of embolic infarcts [65].

Coronary angiography performed acutely will demonstrate occlusion or obstruction of the affected artery; however, if performed more than 4 weeks after the event, the occlusion may resolve completely, with a resultant normal coronary angiogram [66]. The left ventriculogram usually demonstrates segmental akinesis or dyskinesis corresponding to the electrocardiographic site of infarction; thus, coronary embolism must be considered in the differential diagnosis of myocardial infarction with normal coronary arteries. As with embolic stroke, it is important to recognize coronary embolism as the cause of myocardial infarction in order to prevent recurrent episodes of systemic embolism.

OTHER SITES OF ARTERIAL EMBOLISM. In addition to the cerebral and coronary arteries, emboli may affect the renal and mesenteric arteries. Emboli to the visceral arteries are far less likely to be recognized clinically than emboli to the brain, heart, or extremities.

In a review of 974 patients with noncerebral arterial emboli, Abbott et al. reported that 63 percent were to the leg and 20 percent involved the arm [8]. Arterial embolism is most readily recognized when it involves the upper extremity. Patients present with sudden onset of pain in the hand or forearm, often accompanied by paresthesias. On physical examination, the arm is cold, pale, and pulseless. The most frequent sites of occlusion are the brachial (61%), axillary (23%), or subclavian artery (12%) [9]. Occlusion of arteries in the upper extremity rarely causes complete ischemia because of collateral flow, therefore tissue necrosis and its metabolic complications are rare [67].

Once embolic arterial occlusion of the upper extremity is recognized, anticoagulation with intravenous heparin should be instituted. Embolectomy using the Fogarty catheter technique should be performed [68]. Arteriography is rarely needed. The results of embolectomy are excellent. In a review of 322 patients undergoing Fogarty embolectomy of the upper extremity, 79 percent of the arms were salvaged; the amputation rate was 9 percent [9]. The hospital mortality was 12 percent, due to underlying heart disease or recurrent embolism. Embolectomy may be successful even when performed more than 48 hours after the onset of symptoms [67]. The salvage rate is related to the severity of preoperative ischemia rather than to its duration [21]. As with all cases of systemic embolism, long-term anticoagulation with warfarin (INR 2.0–3.0) should be prescribed unless there are contraindications, and the conditions predisposing to systemic embolism should be evaluated.

Of all arterial emboli that do not enter the cerebral circulation, the vast majority lodge in the lower extremities. In the MGH series reported by Abbott et al., the most frequent site of embolism in the lower extremities was the femoral arteries (44%), followed by the aortoiliac (29%) and the popliteal (27%) [8]. Patients with embolism to the lower extremities present with a painful, cold, pulseless lower extremity. Embolic occlusion of arteries in the lower extremities may lead to irreversible ischemia with resultant tissue necrosis. The stages of ischemia secondary to peripheral arterial embolism were categorized by Gregg et al. as follows: stage 1, loss of pulse without muscle weakness or tenderness and without loss of proprioception; stage 2, varying degrees of paresis, loss of proprioception, or muscle tenderness; stage 3, stage 1 and 2 signs and symptoms plus some areas of muscle rigidity; and stage 4, stage 1 to 3 signs and symptoms plus extensive muscle rigidity or obvious necrosis [68].

The principal differential diagnosis of arterial embolism to the lower extremities is arterial thrombosis superimposed on atherosclerotic disease. Arterial thrombosis is a more likely cause of arterial occlusion when the onset is not abrupt and the level of demarcation is vague, especially in patients with a history of claudication or diffuse atherosclerotic disease. Embolism is more likely when symptoms occur abruptly in a previously healthy patient without a history of claudication and with atrial fibrillation, coronary artery disease, or valvular heart disease.

Embolic arterial occlusion in the lower extremities may cause severe muscle ischemia with resultant acidosis, myoglobinuria, hypokalemia, and potential renal shutdown [70]. Anticoagulation with intravenous heparin should be started when the diagnosis of acute embolic occlusion is suspected. When there is uncertainty as to the presence of underlying atherosclerotic disease or the differential diagnosis between arterial thrombus and embolism is uncertain, arteriography may be performed.

Embolectomy is performed by the Fogarty technique, using

the femoral artery approach with local anesthesia [68]. The overall results of embolectomy from the standpoint of limb salvage are good, in the range of 75 to 85 percent (Table 40-5); however, the 30-day mortality is high, in the range of 20 to 25 percent.

The high mortality of patients having embolectomy for embolic occlusion in the lower extremities has not significantly decreased since the introduction of the Fogarty catheter technique in 1963. In the MGH series, the hospital mortality was 23 percent from 1954 to 1963 and 19 percent from 1964 to 1979 [8]. In Green's series, the mortality rate before the use of the Fogarty technique was 20 percent, compared to 24 percent after 1963 [21]. In the Peter Bent Brigham series, mortality before 1963 was 43 percent; after 1963 hospital mortality was 30 percent [11]. The lack of a significant drop in hospital mortality since the introduction of the Fogarty catheter has been attributed to the fact that patients with systemic embolism are currently older and more likely to have advanced atherosclerotic disease than in earlier decades, when they were more likely to be young patients with rheumatic heart disease.

The limb salvage rate with or without embolectomy is clearly related to the severity of ischemia. The importance of the severity of ischemia as opposed to its duration is illustrated by a series of 14 patients who underwent embolectomy more than 48 hours after the onset of symptoms of acute limb ischemia [71]. The limb salvage rate was 88 percent, and only 2 patients died (14%).

The severity of limb ischemia also may affect the mortality rate following embolectomy. Blaisdell et al. believe the high mortality rate after embolectomy in patients with advanced ischemia is due to the release of toxic materials from the revascularized limb, with deleterious effect on the heart, lungs, and kidneys [71]. They believe embolectomy is contraindicated in patients with Gregg's stage 3 or 4 ischemia, that is, when there is paralysis and/or muscle rigidity [69]. In this circumstance, they believe the limb is not viable and that treatment should consist of high-dose heparin or amputation [72]. In a review of their experience, Gregg et al. also concluded that embolectomy is contraindicated when there is advanced muscle injury as evidenced by muscle rigidity or necrosis [68]. Embolectomy in this circumstance does not increase limb salvage and may contribute to death.

INITIAL TREATMENT. Once the diagnosis of systemic embolism is suspected, therapy with intravenous heparin should begin unless there are contraindications to anticoagulation. In patients with suspected embolic stroke, anticoagulation should be delayed until hemorrhage has been excluded by CT scan performed at least 24 hours after stroke onset. Heparin should be given only in nonhypertensive patients with small to moderate-sized embolic strokes [6]. A baseline partial thromboplastin time (PTT) should be obtained and then a bolus of 5000 units of heparin given intravenously. Heparin should then be given by continuous intravenous infusion, beginning at a rate of 1200 units per hour in a patient of average size. The PTT should be repeated in 4 to 6 hours to determine whether it is elevated to 1.5 times the control level; if it is below this level, the infusion rate should be adjusted upward. Periodic checks of the PTT should be performed to be certain the patient is adequately anticoagulated. Warfarin should then be given orally in a daily dose of 5 to 10 mg; the warfarin dose is regulated to keep the prothrombin time prolonged to an INR of 2.0 to 3.0. Heparin should be given for a total of 7 to 10 days, and then warfarin should be continued for a period of time dependent on the clinical circumstances. In addition to anticoagulation, embolectomy using the Fogarty technique should be performed when indicated, as noted above.

SEARCH FOR UNDERLYING CAUSE. When indicated, anticoagulation with heparin and embolectomy represent the initial therapy for systemic embolism. Further therapy depends on the conditions that predispose to systemic embolism. Patients with systemic embolism are subject to recurrent embolism. Green et al. reported a recurrence rate of 31 percent in 128 patients with systemic embolism treated with embolectomy [21]. In a series of 106 patients, Silvers et al. noted a 32 percent recurrence rate [22]. Of the 34 recurrences, 28 occurred while the patient was still in the hospital. In both series, the recurrence rate was lower in patients who were anticoagulated [21,22]. The risk of recurrence and the duration of risk depend on the factors that led to systemic embolism. For this reason, it is critical that the clinician search for the underlying cause of systemic embolism in each case. The appropriate long-term therapeutic plan depends on the results of that search.

In the majority of cases, the underlying conditions that predispose to systemic embolism are evident on evaluation of the history, physical examination, ECG, and chest radiograph. The two most common predispositions, chronic atrial fibrillation and acute myocardial infarction, are self-evident and account for more than 70 to 80 percent of all cases of systemic embolism (see Table 40-2). The other cardiac causes, chronic CAD with aneurysm or ischemic cardiomyopathy, prosthetic heart valves, and valvular heart disease, should also be identified by standard clinical examination.

The remaining identifiable causes of systemic embolism include paroxysmal atrial fibrillation or other atrial arrhythmias in the absence of heart disease, thrombi from an atherosclerotic aorta or aortic aneurysm, endocarditis, myxoma, and paradoxical embolism. Paroxysmal atrial fibrillation or other atrial arrhythmia is suggested by a history of palpitations or the presence of thyrotoxicosis. Holter monitoring in this setting is appropriate. Holter monitoring is unlikely to be productive when there are no clinical clues to the presence of a paroxysmal arrhythmia. Come et al. performed Holter monitoring in 150 patients with suspected systemic embolism [72]. Atrial fibrillation was detected in 15 patients, all of whom had prior ECG documentation of atrial fibrillation. Mural thrombi from an atherosclerotic aorta or aneurysm should be considered in patients with evidence of aortic aneurysm or widespread atherosclerotic disease. Aortography should confirm the diagnosis by demonstrating nonocclusive mural thrombi [57]. Endocarditis should be considered on the basis of clinical findings. Echocardiography may confirm the presence of valvular vegetations [73]. Myxoma, a rare but treatable cause of systemic embolism, is difficult to recognize clinically. The diagnosis is most likely to be established by pathologic examination of an embolectomy specimen or by echocardiography [74].

Venous thrombus as a cause of paradoxical embolism should be suspected when a patient with unexplained systemic em-

Table 40-5. Results of Fogarty Embolectomy in Systemic Embolism of the Extremities

Study	Year	No. patients	Limb salvage (%)	30-day mortality (%)
Green et al. [21]	1975	149	87	24
Hight et al. [11]	1976	124	78	30
Szczepanski [20]	1979	260	79	29
Abbott et al. [8]	1982	303	88	19
Silvers et al. [22]	1980	106	87	22
Lorentzen et al. [23]	1980	130	77	14

bolism has findings consistent with venous thromboembolism [58,75]. The diagnosis is confirmed by demonstrating right-to-left intracardiac shunting by means of indicator dilution curves [60], angiography, or echocardiography [76].

DEFINITIVE THERAPY. The most common cause of systemic embolism, atrial fibrillation, is also the condition most likely to lead to recurrent systemic embolism. In a study of 69 patients with rheumatic heart disease complicated by systemic embolism, Szekely reported that the recurrence rate in 46 patients not treated with chronic anticoagulation was 9.6 percent per year [44], compared with 3.4 percent per year in 23 patients maintained on chronic anticoagulation. Forty percent of the recurrences were within 1 month and 66 percent within 1 year [44].

The most appropriate treatment (Table 40-6) of atrial fibrillation is reversion to normal sinus rhythm [77]. Since conversion to normal sinus rhythm, whether spontaneous or induced by antiarrhythmic drugs or electrical cardioversion, can lead to systemic embolism [37,46,47], patients should be maintained on chronic anticoagulation for 3 to 4 weeks before cardioversion is performed [78]. Quinidine should be given in a dose of 400 mg twice per day beginning 24 hours prior to cardioversion [78]. Quinidine should not be given if the ECG shows prolongation of the Q–T interval, because of the risk of precipitating ventricular tachycardia or ventricular fibrillation [79].

If cardioversion is successful, digoxin and quinidine should be continued indefinitely to decrease the risk of recurrent atrial fibrillation. Anticoagulation with warfarin should be continued. If 1 to 2 months after cardioversion the patient continues to be in normal sinus rhythm, anticoagulation should be discontin-

Table 40-6. Definitive Treatment to Prevent Recurrent Systemic Embolism

Underlying condition	Definitive treatment*
Chronic AF	Cardioversion after 3–6 wk of anticoagulation; if unsuccessful, chronic anticoagulation
Acute MI	Anticoagulation for 6 mo
Chronic CAD with aneurysm or cardiomyopathy	Chronic anticoagulation
Valvular heart disease	Chronic anticoagulation; surgical correction if hemodynamic compromise
Prosthetic heart valves	Optimize anticoagulation, add platelet active agents, possible valve replacement with bioprosthetic valve
Paroxysmal AF or other atrial arrhythmia	Antiarrhythmic agents; if unsuccessful, chronic anticoagulation
Atherosclerotic aorta or aneurysm with mural thrombi	Surgical correction ± chronic anticoagulation
Endocarditis	Antibiotic treatment ± valve replacement ± anticoagulation
Myxoma	Surgical removal
Paradoxial embolism	Chronic anticoagulation ± IVC interruption ± closure of intracardiac defect

* See text for further details.
AF = atrial fibrillation; MI = myocardial infarction; CAD = coronary artery disease; IVC = inferior vena cava.

ued. If cardioversion is unsuccessful, quinidine should be discontinued, but warfarin must be continued because of the persistent risk of systemic embolism in patients with chronic atrial fibrillation.

In patients in whom systemic embolism is associated with paroxysmal atrial fibrillation, attempts should be made with antiarrhythmic drugs to prevent paroxysms of atrial fibrillation. Warfarin should be continued until it is clear by history and/or Holter monitor that the patient is in persistent normal sinus rhythm. If therapy is unsuccessful, the patient should be kept on long-term warfarin therapy.

The second most frequent precipitant of systemic embolism is acute myocardial infarction. In this circumstance, the duration of the risk of recurrence is less than in patients with atrial fibrillation. Carter reported that most recurrent emboli in patients with acute myocardial infarction occur within the first 6 months [80]. In another study [81], all embolic events occurred within 4 months of acute myocardial infarction; therefore, it is appropriate to continue warfarin therapy for 6 months in patients who have systemic embolism as a complication of acute myocardial infarction. If, however, the myocardial infarction is complicated by chronic ischemic cardiomyopathy, ventricular aneurysm, or atrial fibrillation, chronic anticoagulation is appropriate.

Most episodes of systemic embolism in patients with valvular heart disease occur in the presence of atrial fibrillation; however, systemic embolism may occur in patients with mitral valve disease who are in normal sinus rhythm, especially in those older than 35 years [12]. In this circumstance, chronic anticoagulation is indicated. In the absence of hemodynamic compromise, surgical correction of valvular heart disease to prevent recurrent embolism is not indicated if the surgical treatment would consist of valve replacement with a prosthetic valve. Prosthetic heart valves predispose to systemic embolism even with chronic anticoagulation [15,16]. If the procedure were mitral valvuloplasty rather than mitral valve replacement, surgical correction to prevent recurrent embolism may be indicated in an otherwise asymptomatic patient with mitral stenosis; that is, if there were no evidence of mitral regurgitation or mitral valve calcification, and a surgeon experienced in mitral valvuloplasty were at hand. Mitral valvuloplasty in this subset of patients with mitral stenosis has been shown to decrease the incidence of recurrent systemic embolism [82]. When systemic embolism occurs in patients with prosthetic heart valves despite adequate anticoagulation, dipyridamole (225–400 mg/day) or low-dose aspirin should be added to the regimen. If medical therapy to prevent recurrent embolism is unsuccessful, reoperation using a bioprosthetic valve may be indicated.

As noted, embolism occurs in approximately one-third of patients with endocarditis, with the majority of emboli affecting the cerebral circulation [54]. The role of anticoagulation in patients with endocarditis complicated by embolism is controversial. Some believe that anticoagulation is contraindicated because of an increase of hemorrhage, particularly intracranial hemorrhage [83]; however, cerebral thromboemboli in patients with endocarditis should be treated as other embolic strokes. It is important to distinguish between embolism due to thromboemboli and embolism due to vegetations. If vegetations are the source of embolism, anticoagulation is not indicated. Examination of coexistent conditions helps determine whether emboli are thromboemboli or vegetations. The presence of atrial fibrillation increases the probability of thromboembolism. The detection of vegetations by echocardiography increases the likelihood that the emboli originated as vegetations.

Recurrent embolism in patients with infective endocarditis is one of the indications for emergency valve replacement. Emboli to large arteries in the extremities are a strong indication for valve replacement, because they suggest large vegetations due to fungal endocarditis, which is less likely to respond to medical therapy.

When emboli are manifestations of intracardiac myxoma, surgical removal is the definitive therapy of choice. This procedure, performed with cardiopulmonary bypass, is quite effective. Follow-up echocardiography should be performed to detect recurrence of myxoma.

Since paradoxical embolism is in reality a complication of venous thromboembolism, definitive therapy depends on the factors predisposing to venous thromboembolism and the nature of the intracardiac defect. If the patient with paradoxical embolism is chronically predisposed to venous thrombosis, chronic anticoagulation or venous interruption is indicated. In this circumstance, ligation of the inferior vena cava may be indicated, rather than the placement of a filter in the vena cava, which may permit small emboli to reach the systemic circulation. In patients who are not chronically predisposed to venous thrombosis and in whom the defect permitting paradoxical embolism is a patent foramen ovale, a short course of anticoagulation is indicated until the conditions leading to venous thrombosis have resolved.

When the defect permitting paradoxical embolism is a congenital cardiac defect such as an atrial or ventricular septal defect, patent ductus arteriosus, or pulmonary atrioventricular fistula, definitive therapy depends on the status of the pulmonary circulation. In most such cases, the congenital defect has led to pulmonary hypertension, and chronic right-to-left shunting across the defect occurs. When these cardiac defects are complicated by pulmonary vascular disease, the risk of surgical correction is very high and surgical correction is thus contraindicated [84]. The most appropriate definitive therapy for preventing recurrent systemic embolism is chronic anticoagulation. Inferior vena caval interruption is not indicated in the presence of pulmonary vascular disease because of a greatly increased surgical risk.

References

1. Ellis LB, Harken DE: Arterial embolization in relation to mitral valvuloplasty. *Am Heart J* 62:611, 1961.
2. Deverall PB, Olley PM, Smith DR, et al: Incidence of systemic embolism before and after mitral valvotomy. *Thorax* 23:530, 1968.
3. Graham GK, Taylor JA, Ellis LB, et al: Studies in mitral stenosis. *Arch Intern Med* 88:532, 1951.
4. Easton JD, Sherman DG: Management of cerebral embolism of cardiac origin. *Stroke* 5:433, 1980.
5. Selzer A, Cohn KE: Natural history of mitral stenosis: A review. *Circulation* 45:878, 1972.
6. Sherman DG, Dyken ML, Fisher M, et al: Antithrombotic therapy for cerebrovascular disorders. *Chest* 95:140S, 1989.
7. Hinton RC, Kistler JP, Fallon JT, et al: Influence of etiology of atrial fibrillation on incidence of systemic embolism. *Am J Cardiol* 40:509, 1977.
8. Abbott WM, Maloney RD, McCabe CC, et al: Arterial embolism: A 44 year perspective. *Am J Surg* 143:460, 1982.
9. Haimovici H: Cardiogenic embolism of the upper extremity. *J Cardiovasc Surg* 23:209, 1982.
10. Heiskell CA, Conn J Jr: Aortoarterial emboli. *Am J Surg* 132:4, 1976.
11. Hight DW, Tileny NL, Couch NP: Changing clinical trends in patients with peripheral arterial emboli. *Surgery* 79:172, 1976.
12. Coulshed N, Epstein EJ, McKendrick CS, et al: Systemic embolism in mitral valve disease. *Br Heart J* 32:26, 1970.
13. Aberg H: Atrial fibrillation. *Acta Med Scand* 185:373, 1969.
14. Levine HJ, Pauker SG, Salzman EW: Antithrombotic therapy in valvular heart disease. *Chest* 95:98S, 1989.
15. Starr A, Grunkemeier G, Lambert L, et al: Mitral valve replacement. *Circulation* 54:47, 1976.
16. Salomon NW, Stinson EB, Griepp RB, et al: Mitral valve replacement: Long-term evaluation of prosthesis-related mortality and morbidity. *Circulation* 56:94, 1977.
17. Stein PD, Alpert JS, Copeland J, et al: Antithrombotic therapy in patients with mechanical and biological prosthetic heart valves. *Chest* 102(Suppl):445S, 1992.
18. Hetzer R, Hill JD, Kerth WJ, et al: Thromboembolic complications after mitral valve replacement with Hancock xenograft. *J Thorac Cardiovasc Surg* 75:651, 1978.
19. Stein PD, Kantrowitz A: Antithrombotic therapy in mechanical and biological prosthetic heart valves and saphenous vein bypass grafts. *Chest* 95(Suppl):107S, 1989.
20. Szczepanski KP: Results of surgical treatment of arterial embolism. *Scand J Thorac Cardiovasc Surg* 13:71, 1979.
21. Green RM, DeWeese JA, Rob CG: Arterial embolectomy before and after the Fogarty catheter. *Surgery* 77:24, 1975.
22. Silvers LW, Royster TS, Mulcare RJ: Peripheral arterial emboli and factors in their recurrence rate. *Ann Surg* 192:232, 1980.
23. Lorentzen JE, Roder OC, Hansen HJB: Peripheral arterial embolism. *Acta Chir Scand* 502:111, 1980.
24. Satiani B, Evans WE: Immediate prognosis and five year survival after arterial embolectomy following myocardial infarction. *Surg Gynecol Obstet* 150:41, 1980.
25. Jordan RA, Miller RD, Edwards JE, et al: Thromboembolism in acute and in healed myocardial infarction: Intracardiac mural thrombosis. *Circulation* 6:1, 1952.
26. Hellerstein HK, Martin JW: Incidence of thromboembolic lesions accompanying myocardial infarction. *Am Heart J* 33:443, 1947.
27. Asinger RW, Mikell FL, Elsperger J, et al: Incidence of left ventricular thrombosis after acute transmural myocardial infarction. *N Engl J Med* 305:297, 1981.
28. Friedman MJ, Carlson K, Marcus FI, et al: Clinical correlations in patients with acute myocardial infarction and left ventricular thrombus detected by two-dimensional echocardiography. *Am J Med* 72:894, 1982.
29. Assessment of short-term anticoagulant administration after cardiac infarction: Report of the working party on anticoagulant therapy in coronary thrombosis to the Medical Research Council. *Br Med J* 1:335, 1969.
30. Drapkin A, Merskey C: Anticoagulant therapy after acute myocardial infarction. *JAMA* 222:541, 1972.
31. Anticoagulants in acute myocardial infarction: Results of a cooperative clinical trial. *JAMA* 225:724, 1973.
32. Turpie AGG, Robinson JG, Doyle DJ, et al: Comparison of high-dose with low-dose subcutaneous heparin to prevent left ventricular mural thrombosis in patients with acute transmural anterior myocardial infarction. *N Engl J Med* 320:352, 1989.
33. Cairns JA, Hirsh J, Lewis HD, et al: Antithrombotic agents in coronary artery disease. *Chest* 102(Suppl):456S, 1992.
34. Simpson MT, Oberman A, Kouchoukos NT, et al: Prevalence of mural thrombi and systemic embolization with left ventricular aneurysm. *Chest* 77:463, 1980.
35. Roberts WC, Ferrans VJ: Pathologic anatomy of the cardiomyopathies: Idiopathic dilated and hypertrophic types, infiltrative types, and endomyocardial disease with and without eosinophilia. *Hum Pathol* 6:287, 1975.
36. Gottdiener JS, Gay JA, VanVoorhees L, et al: Frequency and embolic potential of left ventricular thrombus in dilated cardiomyopathy: Assessment by 2-dimensional echocardiography. *Am J Cardiol* 52:1281, 1983.
37. Hurst JW, Paulk EA Jr, Proctor HD, et al: Management of patients with atrial fibrillation. *Am J Med* 37:728, 1964.
38. Wolf PA, Dawber TR, Thomas HE Jr, et al: Epidemiologic assessment of chronic atrial fibrillation and risk of stroke: The Framingham study. *Neurology* 28:973, 1978.
39. Milliken JA: Atrial fibrillation and embolism. *Can Med Assoc J* 128:1370, 1983.
40. Bar-Sela S, Ehrenfeld M, Eliakim M: Arterial embolism in thyrotoxicosis with atrial fibrillation. *Arch Intern Med* 141:1191, 1981.
41. Staffurth JS, Gibberd MC, Fui SNT: Arterial embolism in thyrotoxicosis with atrial fibrillation. *Br Med J* 2:688, 1977.
42. Yuen RWM, Gutteridge DH, Thompson PL, et al: Embolism in thyrotoxic atrial fibrillation. *Med J Aust* 1:630, 1979.

43. Henry WL, Morganroth J, Pearlman AS, et al: Relation between echocardiographically determined left atrial size and atrial fibrillation. *Circulation* 53:273, 1976.

44. Szekely P: Systemic embolism and anticoagulant prophylaxis in rheumatic heart disease. *Br Med J* 1:1209, 1964.

45. Fisher CM: Reducing risks of cerebral embolism. *Geriatrics* 59:66, 1979.

46. Morris JJ Jr, Kong Y, North WC, et al: Experience with "cardioversion" of atrial fibrillation and flutter. *Am J Cardiol* 94:100, 1964.

47. Bjerkelund CJ, Orning OM: The efficacy of anticoagulant therapy in preventing embolism related to D.C. electrical conversion of atrial fibrillation. *Am J Cardiol* 23:208, 1969.

48. Fairfax AJ, Lambert CD, Leatham A: Systemic embolism in chronic sinoatrial disorder. *N Engl J Med* 295:190, 1976.

49. Petersen P, Godtfredsen J, Boysen G, et al: Placebo-controlled, randomized trial of warfarin and aspirin for prevention of thromboembolic complications in chronic atrial fibrillation. *Lancet* 1:175, 1989.

50. The Stroke Prevention in Atrial Fibrillation Investigators: The stroke prevention in atrial fibrillation trial: Final results. *Circulation* 85:527, 1991.

51. The Boston Area Anticoagulation Trial for Atrial Fibrillation Investigators: The effect of low-dose warfarin on the risk of stroke in patients with nonrheumatic atrial fibrillation. *N Engl J Med* 323:1505, 1990.

52. Ezekowitz MD, Bridgers SL, James KE, et al: Interim analysis of VA co-operative study, Stroke Prevention in Nonrheumatic Atrial Fibrillation (SPINAF). American Heart Association Abstracts, November 11–14, 1991.

53. Laupacis A, Albers G, Dunn M, Feinberg W: Antithrombotic therapy in atrial fibrillation. *Chest* 102(Suppl):426S, 1992.

54. Pruitt AA, Rubin RH, Karchmer AW, et al: Neurologic complications of bacterial endocarditis. *Medicine* 57:329, 1978.

55. Brockmeier LB, Adolph RJ, Gustin BW, et al: Calcium emboli to the retinal artery in calcific aortic stenosis. *Am Heart J* 101:32, 1981.

56. Bulkley BH, Hutchins GM: Atrial myxomas: A fifty year review. *Am Heart J* 97:639, 1979.

57. Williams GM, Harrington D, Burdick J, et al: Mural thrombus of the aorta. *Ann Surg* 194:737, 1981.

58. Meister SG, Grossman W, Dexter L, et al: Paradoxical embolism. *Am J Med* 53:292, 1972.

59. Hagen PT, Scholz DG, Edwards WD: Incidence and size of patent foramen ovale during the first 10 decades of life: An autopsy study of 965 normal hearts. *Mayo Clin Proc* 59:17, 1984.

60. Banas JS, Meister SG, Gazzaniga AB, et al: A simple technique for detecting small defects of the atrial septum. *Am J Cardiol* 28:467, 1971.

61. Dalen JE, Banas JS Jr, Brooks HL, et al: Resolution rate of acute pulmonary embolism in man. *N Engl J Med* 280:1194, 1969.

62. Virchow R: Ueber capillare Embolie. *Virchows Arch [Pathol Anat]* 9:307, 1856.

63. Virchow R: *Arch Pathol Anat Physiol* I:134, 1847.

64. Prizel KR, Hutchins GM, Bulkley BH: Coronary artery embolism and myocardial infarction: A clinicopathologic study of 55 patients. *Ann Intern Med* 88:155, 1978.

65. Charles RG, Epstein EJ, Holt S, et al: Coronary embolism in valvular heart disease. *Q J Med* 202:147, 1982.

66. Wirsing P, Andriopoulos A, Botticher R: Arterial embolectomies in the upper extremity after acute occlusion. *J Cardiovasc Surg* 24:40, 1983.

67. Fogarty TJ, Carnley JJ, Drause RJ: A method for extraction of arterial emboli and thrombi. *Surg Gynecol Obstet* 116:241, 1963.

68. Gregg RO, Chamberlain BE, Myers JK, et al: Embolectomy or heparin therapy for arterial emboli? *Surgery* 93:377, 1983.

69. Campbell HC, Hubbard SG, Ernst CB: Continuous heparin anticoagulation in patients with arteriosclerosis and arterial emboli. *Surg Gynecol Obstet* 150:54, 1980.

70. Jarrett F, Dacumos GC, Crummy AB, et al: Late appearance of arterial emboli: Diagnosis and management. *Surgery* 86:898, 1979.

71. Blaisdell FW, Steele M, Allen RE: Management of acute lower extremity arterial ischemia due to embolism and thrombosis. *Surgery* 84:822, 1978.

72. Come PC, Riley MF, Bivas NK: Roles of echocardiography and arrhythmia monitoring in the evaluation of patients with suspected systemic embolism. *Ann Neurol* 13:527, 1983.

73. Melvin ET, Berger M, Lutzker BG, et al: Noninvasive methods for detection of valve vegetations in infective endocarditis. *Am J Cardiol* 47:271, 1981.

74. Lappe DL, Bulkley BH, Weiss JL: Two dimensional echocardiographic diagnosis of left atrial myxoma. *Chest* 74:55, 1978.

75. Padula RT, Camishion RC: Paradoxical embolization. *Ann Surg* 167:598, 1968.

76. Kronik G, Mosslacher H: Positive contrast echocardiography in patients with patent foramen ovale and normal right heart hemodynamics. *Am J Cardiol* 49:1806, 1982.

77. DeSilva RA, Graboys TB, Podrid PJ, et al: Cardioversion and defibrillation. *Am Heart J* 100:881, 1980.

78. Mancini BJ, Goldberger AL: Cardioversion of atrial fibrillation: Consideration of embolization, anticoagulation, prophylactic pacemaker, and long-term success. *Am Heart J* 104:617, 1982.

79. Bauman JL, Bauernfeind RA, Hoff JV, et al: Torsades des pointes due to quinidine: Observations in 31 patients. *Am Heart J* 107:425, 1984.

80. Carter AB, Cantab MD: Prognosis of cerebral embolism. *Lancet* 2:514, 1965.

81. Weinreich DJ, Burke JF, Pauletto FJ: Serial echocardiographic evaluation of mural thrombi. *J Am Coll Cardiol* 3:614, 1984.

82. Ellis LB, Singh JB, Morales DD, et al: Fifteen to twenty-year study of one thousand patients undergoing closed mitral valvuloplasty. *Circulation* 48:357, 1973.

83. Kanis JA: The use of anticoagulants in bacterial endocarditis. *Postgrad Med J* 50:312, 1974.

84. Dalen JE, Haynes FW, Dexter L: Life expectancy with atrial septal defect. *JAMA* 200:112, 1967.

41. Supraventricular Tachycardias

Steven P. Beaudette and
Robert S. Mittleman

Supraventricular tachycardias (SVTs) are frequently encountered in the intensive care setting. With the availability of invasive electrophysiologic studies and other techniques, insight into the mechanisms responsible for these arrhythmias continues to improve [1,2,3]. By understanding these mechanisms, one can in most cases systematically identify the arrhythmia and tailor pharmacologic therapy.

Definition

A tachycardia is considered supraventricular in origin if the atrium or atrioventricular (A-V) junction participates in the arrhythmia, either as the origin of the abnormal impulse or as an essential part of a reentry circuit. The QRS is usually narrow. However, if the rate is fast, aberrant ventricular conduction is not uncommon, which produces a wide QRS complex.

Pathophysiology

Three general mechanisms account for the generation of supraventricular arrhythmias [4,5]. First is increased automaticity. The sinus node is normally the dominant pacemaker, because it has faster phase 4 depolarization than the other heart tissues, causing a faster rate of discharge. When another area of myocardium exhibits an enhanced rate of spontaneous depolarization (i.e., faster than the sinus node), it becomes the dominant pacemaker. When this occurs in the atria or A-V junction it produces a SVT. This type of arrhythmia can be suppressed by pacing the heart faster than the spontaneous rate of discharge, but the automatic focus resumes its role after pacing is terminated. Programmed electrical stimulation fails to initiate or terminate an automatic SVT [6].

An example of an arrhythmia presumed to occur as a result of increased automaticity is atrial tachycardia occurring in a patient with severe emphysema and resultant high catecholamine levels. This causes different parts of the atrium to have a more rapid discharge rate and consequently allows that focus to become the dominant pacemaker, resulting in atrial tachycardia.

A second mechanism, which is responsible for many SVTs, is reentry. In contrast to increased automaticity, there is no problem with impulse formation, but rather a problem with abnormal conduction. Although a variety of phenomena may account for reentry tachycardias, they have classically been described as requiring an area of slow conduction and unidirectional block. When a premature impulse occurs or is produced by a pacing catheter, it propagates into the reentry circuit. However, because of differences in refractory state, the impulse blocks in one limb of the circuit and proceeds through the alternate limb. It can then conduct retrograde through the original site of block, which is no longer refractory. If the relationship between conduction velocity and refractory periods is appropriate, a perpetuating reentry loop is established that

leads to atrial and ventricular depolarization. By understanding the specific reentry circuit, one can predict the electrocardiographic characteristics of the atrial and ventricular depolarizations and the interventions needed to change its conduction properties and thus terminate the arrhythmia. Reentry circuits can be reproducibly induced and terminated with premature extrastimuli such as are produced in the electrophysiology lab. Those extrastimuli conduct into the reentry circuit and alter the critical timing necessary to perpetuate the conduction in the region. Spontaneous atrial or ventricular premature beats sometimes act in this fashion as well. Consequently, arrhythmias caused by reentry tend to start and stop abruptly.

A third mechanism that may contribute to the genesis of some atrial arrhythmias is triggered activity. This is pacemaker activity that occurs as a result of a preceding impulse or series of impulses. This is in contrast to automaticity, which occurs spontaneously. The impulse that initiates triggered activity is an afterdepolarization, classified as either early (EAD) or delayed (DAD). There are only a limited number of SVTs for which the mechanism is currently thought to be triggered automaticity. For example, some of the SVTs associated with digoxin toxicity are thought to be produced in this way [7].

Diagnosis

A direct recording of the arrhythmia is the most important initial information for diagnosis. For a patient who is hemodynamically stable, a 12-lead electrocardiogram (ECG) obtained as rapidly as possible is essential information. If a 12-lead ECG cannot be obtained because of the patient's hemodynamic status, the transient nature of the arrhythmia, or some other reason, a telemetry recording can still be of enormous value. Special attention should be given to identifying the P waves. Usually leads II and V_1 are the best leads to identify atrial activity. If P waves are not clearly visible, atrial activity can be recorded using Lewis leads, where the right and left arm leads are placed along the sternal borders and lead I is monitored. Alternately, when P waves cannot be clearly distinguished and a diagnosis is important for management, an esophageal or intraatrial recording electrode can be used. After open heart surgery epicardial recording electrodes are commonly placed; when available, they can be of enormous value in identifying atrial activity. The presence of P waves and their morphology, regularity, rate, and relationship to ventricular depolarization (QRS) should all be noted [8] (Figs 41-1 and 41-2).

Other available diagnostic modalities, although generally not indicated in a critically ill patient, may be of value after the patient recovers. A Holter monitor, which records two or three modified ECG leads continuously for 1 or more days, can be used to record a patient's arrhythmia when the symptoms occur frequently [9]. Transtelephonic event monitors can be used when symptoms are less frequent [10]. They can be worn for prolonged periods of time. When the symptom occurs, the arrhythmia can be directly transmitted by telephone or can be recorded on tape for subsequent analysis.

Type	P-Wave Morphology	P-Wave Location	Presumed Mechanism
Sinus Tachycardia	Normal	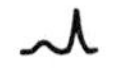 ⁀ᴧ	↑ Automaticity
Sinus Node Re-entry	Normal	⁀ᴧ	Re-entry
Automatic Atrial Tachycardia	Abnormal	⁀ᴧ	↑ Automaticity
Intra-atrial Re-entry	Abnormal	⁀ᴧ	Re-entry
AV Nodal Re-entry	ABN (not seen)	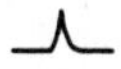 ⁀ᴧ	Re-entry
AV-Reciprocating Tachycardia	Abnormal	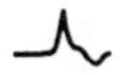 ⁀ᴧ	Re-entry
Multifocal Atrial Tachycardia	Varying	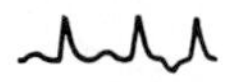 ⁀ᴧᴧᴧ	↑ Automaticity
Atrial Fibrillation	Chaotic	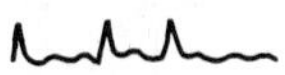 ᴧᴧᴧᴧ	Re-entry
Atrial Flutter	Sawtooth	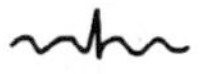 ᴧᴧᴧᴧ	Re-entry

Fig. 41-1. Characteristics of supraventricular tachyarrhythmias.

The cardiac electrophysiology study can provide detailed information about an arrhythmia [11,12]. Specialized multipolar temporary pacing catheters are positioned at multiple sites in the heart by the transvenous route. The catheters are used to record and stimulate selectively to provide information about the sequence of cardiac conduction and depolarization.

Reproducing the arrhythmia in the electrophysiology lab often provides a more accurate diagnosis of the mechanism than that obtained by routine ECG. For example, with a wide-complex tachycardia, P waves are often not visualized on the routine ECG. Reproduction of the tachycardia in the laboratory allows analysis of the relationship between atrial and ventricular activity, which should yield a definitive diagnosis. Reentry circuits can be initiated by programmed stimulation using premature extrastimuli. Once the tachycardia has been initiated, termination can be attempted with pacing or insertion of premature beats. The ability of a medication to suppress a previously inducible tachycardia can also be evaluated.

Vagal maneuvers can provide important insight into the mechanisms of an SVT, often leading to a diagnosis without the need for invasive electrophysiologic testing. Carotid sinus massage or the Valsalva maneuver transiently increase vagal tone, prolonging sinoatrial (SA) and A-V nodal conduction time and refractoriness [13]. Sometimes SVTs with reentry circuits involving the SA or A-V nodes, such as A-V node reentry tachycardia (AVNRT), A-V reciprocating tachycardia (AVRT), or sinus node reentry tachycardia (SNRT), terminate with these maneuvers. With SVTs caused by reentry circuits that do not involve the SA or A-V nodes, such as atrial flutter, atrial tachycardia, or atrial fibrillation, there is often an increase in the ratio of A-V conduction, leading to a decrease in the ventricular rate. The increased vagal tone does not affect the reentry circuit. For example, in atrial flutter the atrial rate is unchanged. When atrial flutter presents with 2:1 A-V block, the increased A-V block produced by the increased vagal tone may allow recognition of the flutter waves, leading to the diagnosis. Similarly, auto-matic tachycardias in which the automatic focus is above the A-V node, such as automatic atrial tachycardia, will manifest an increase in conduction ratio and consequently a slowing of the ventricular rate in response to vagal maneuvers. In sinus tachycardia there is a gradual progressive slowing of the sinus rate, with a return to the former rate once the maneuver is discontinued. To summarize, vagal maneuvers act either to terminate an SVT or to slow the ventricular response and allow atrial activity to be more clearly distinguished, often without the need for more invasive procedures (Table 41-1).

The increased vagal tone can also be mimicked pharmacologically. Adenosine, an endogenous nucleoside, produces SA and A-V nodal block when administered in an intravenous bolus [14]. The advantage of using adenosine is its very short half-life of 10 to 15 seconds. Similar to vagal maneuvers, adenosine can lead to termination of the SVT or an increase of the ratio of A-V conduction, allowing atrial activity to be more easily distinguished. Its use is outlined below.

Treatment

The treatment of an SVT is geared to the underlying mechanism [15,16]. In general, the primary treatment of arrhythmias produced by enhanced automaticity is to remove the stimulus or treat the underlying process. The ectopic automaticity can sometimes be diminished by agents that slow depolarization. In addition, the ventricular rate can be controlled by using agents to increase the degree of A-V block. These arrhythmias will not terminate in response to pacing or cardioversion. Arrhythmias utilizing reentry circuits that involve the SA or A-V nodes may terminate in response to agents that change the refractoriness or slow conduction in these regions. Drugs that slow atrial myocardial or accessory pathway conduction are effective in treating rhythms with a reentry circuit involving these structures (Table 41-2, Figure 41-3).

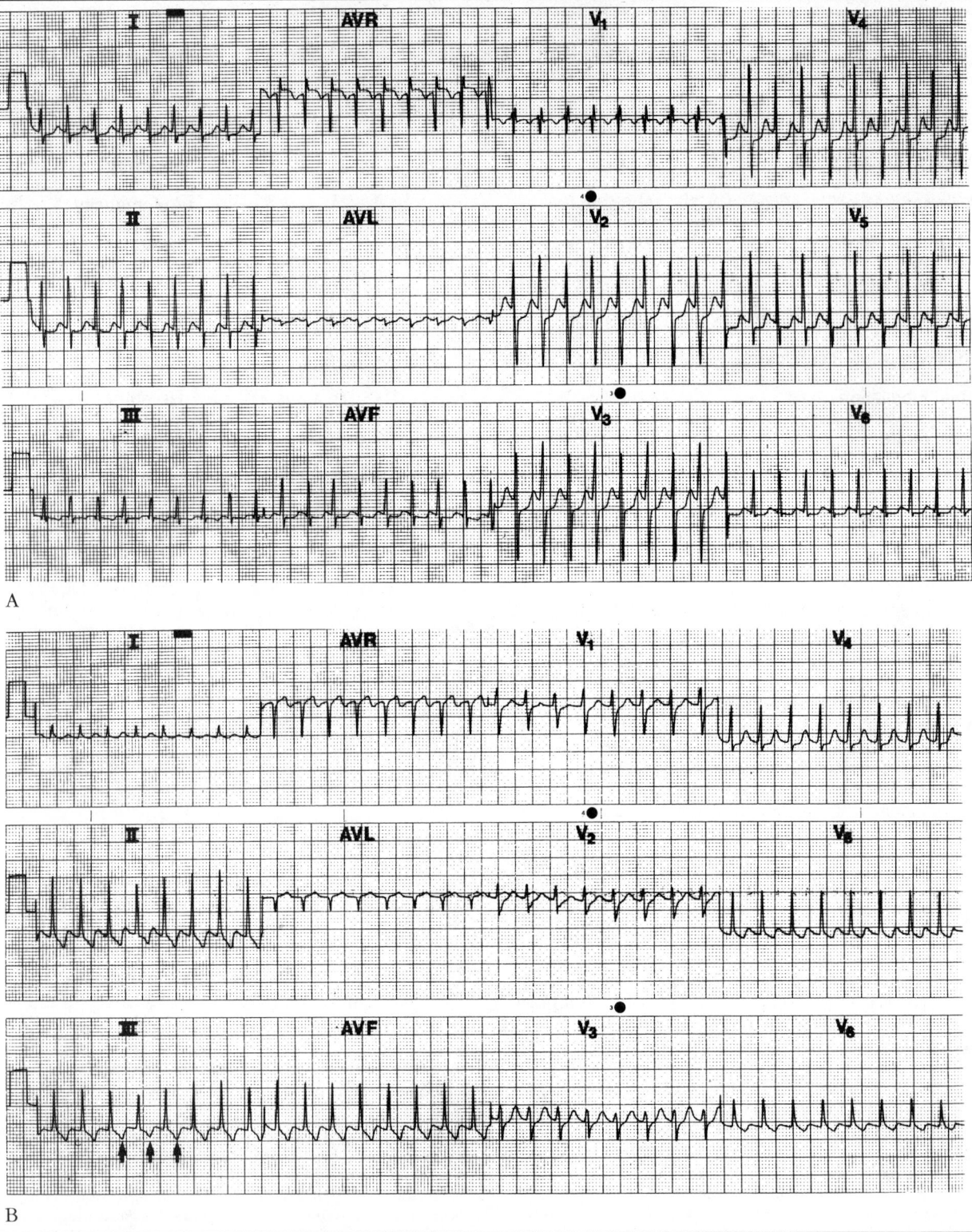

Fig. 41-2. Standard 12-lead ECG from two young patients with paroxysmal palpitations. A. There is a narrow complex rhythm with no visible P waves. By electrophysiologic testing, this patient was found to have an A-V nodal reentry tachycardia. B. Patient with an A-V reciprocating tachycardia. Note the P waves, which occur immediately after the QRS complex and are best seen in the inferior leads (*arrows*).

Table 41-1. Effect of Vagal Maneuvers or Adenosine on Supraventricular Tachycardias

Arrhythmia	Response to maneuver
A-V nodal reentry tachycardia	No effect or abrupt conversion to NSR
A-V reciprocating tachycardia	No effect or abrupt conversion to NSR
Intraatrial reentry tachycardia	No effect or increase in A-V block
Sinus node reentry tachycardia	No effect or abrupt conversion to NSR
Atrial fibrillation	Increased A-V block, with slowing of the ventricular rate
Atrial flutter	Increased A-V block, with slowing of the ventricular rate
Sinus tachycardia	Gradual slowing, then gradual acceleration
Automatic atrial tachycardia	Increased A-V block, with slowing of the ventricular rate
Multifocal atrial tachycardia	Increased A-V block, with slowing of the ventricular rate

A-V = atrioventricular; NSR = normal sinus rhythm.

CARDIOVERSION. When the patient is hemodynamically compromised, DC cardioversion is the treatment of choice, although only reentrant tachycardias will respond to this. In addition, DC cardioversion can be performed in the hemodynamically stable patient to restore sinus rhythm. For the procedure, the patient should have an intravenous catheter in place, along with supplemental oxygen and continuous oximetry monitoring. If possible, an intravenous short-acting benzodiazepine is administered for sedation and amnesia. The cardioverting equipment is set on the synchronous mode, with confirmation of adequate synchronization. The paddles are covered with conductive gel and placed in the anteroposterior or anterolateral position. The shock is delivered after ascertaining that all personnel are clear from the bed. The amount of energy is titrated up from the lowest amount thought likely to revert the rhythm. In atrial fibrillation, the starting dose is usually 100 joules. Often 25 joules is sufficient for atrial flutter, AVNRT, and AVRT. The benefit of cardioverting a patient with atrial fibrillation has to be weighed against the risk of embolization. A full discussion of cardioversion is found in Chapter 6.

ADENOSINE. Adenosine can be effective in both diagnosis and treatment of SVTs. This endogenous nucleoside causes adenosine receptor stimulation with a resultant hyperpolarization of the cells. When given by intravenous bolus, it produces profound conduction slowing in the sinus and A-V nodal tissue. Due to its extraordinarily rapid metabolism, these effects resolve within several seconds. Therefore, SVTs with reentry circuits that involve these structures can be terminated with immediate return to normal conduction. The injection is often associated with symptoms of dyspnea, flushing, and chest discomfort [17,18]. Chest pain is felt to be mediated by adenosine receptors. The symptoms last 15 to 20 seconds. Preexisting second- or third-degree A-V block and sick sinus syndrome are relative contraindications. Adenosine can produce bronchoconstriction and should therefore be used with extreme caution in patients with asthma.

For adult patients the initial dose is 6 mg by rapid intravenous bolus, followed by a rapid saline flush [19]. If this is ineffective, a dose of 12 mg can be used. If central access is available the initial dose can be reduced to 3 mg [20]. Methyl xanthines, such as caffeine and theophylline, are competitive antagonists. Larger dosages may be needed in the presence of these compounds, or the adenosine may not be effective. Dipyridamole is a nucleoside transport blocker, thus smaller dosages of adenosine should be used in patients receiving this medication.

DRUGS FOR RATE CONTROL

Cardiac Glycosides. The cardiac glycosides, long used in the treatment of SVTs, cause conduction slowing and increased refractoriness in the SA and A-V nodes, mainly indirectly by hypersensitizing the carotid baroreceptors [21]. This leads to an increased vagal and decreased sympathetic cardiac neural tone. It also can shorten refractoriness and accelerate conduction in atrial tissue and accessory pathways [22]. It is useful in acute or chronic treatment of SVTs with a reentry circuit involving the SA or A-V node or in slowing the ventricular rate by increasing A-V block, as in atrial flutter.

Digoxin can be given orally or intravenously. Its onset of action after an intravenous dose is 30 minutes, which is slow compared to adenosine or the calcium entry blockers. It must be loaded regardless of the route of administration. Oral absorption can be variable. Digoxin is excreted primarily by the kidneys, therefore the maintenance dose must be adjusted in patients with renal failure or if used in conjunction with medications that raise its serum level.

Digoxin toxicity is not uncommon, given its narrow therapeutic window. Signs of toxicity include fatigue, nausea, visual disturbances, and confusion. It can also lead to multiple arrhythmias. The increased vagal tone can produce sinus bradycardia or A-V block. In addition, there can be increased atrial and ventricular excitability, leading to premature atrial and ventricular beats, ectopic atrial tachycardia, ventricular tachycardia, or fibrillation. Digoxin toxicity should always be considered when an SVT does not respond to increasing doses of digoxin. This is particularly true with atrial tachycardia associated with A-V block.

The therapy for digitalis toxicity depends on the arrhythmia and clinical condition. Often stopping the digitalis and correcting any underlying hypokalemia is sufficient. Temporary pacing may be needed for severe bradycardia or complete heart block. Digoxin specific Fab antibody fragments can be used in life-threatening cases to bind and neutralize the digitalis.

Beta-Blockers. Beta-blockers exert their effect by competitively inhibiting catecholamine binding to beta-adrenergic receptors. The beta-blockers can be separated into those that nonselectively block receptors in the heart (beta$_1$) and bronchi and blood vessels (beta$_2$) and those that selectively inhibit beta$_1$-receptors. At higher dosages the selective beta$_1$-blockers also block beta$_2$-receptors. Propranolol, nadolol, and timolol are all nonselective. Metoprolol, atenolol, and esmolol offer beta$_1$ specificity.

Beta-blockers, by blocking beta-adrenergic receptor sites, slow normal and abnormal automaticity and slow conduction time and refractoriness through the A-V node [23]. They are useful in acute or chronic treatment of SVTs caused by a reentry circuit involving the SA or A-V node and in slowing the ventricular response by increasing A-V block.

Beta-blockers exert negative inotropy and can precipitate congestive heart failure in patients with depressed left ventricular function. They also can produce sinus bradycardia or A-V block. Asthma and claudication can be exacerbated. The symptoms of hypoglycemia in an insulin-dependent diabetic can be masked. In addition, they can impair sexual function or cause mental depression.

Table 41-2. Drugs Commonly Used for Treatment of Supraventricular Tachycardias

Drug	Most commonly used dosage	Half-life	Route of elimination	Major adverse effects	Comments
Adenosine	IV bolus: 6–12 mg (3 mg if given centrally)	10 sec	Erythrocytes	Transient dyspnea, flushing, chest pain, SA and A-V block	Larger dose may be needed in the presence of caffeine and theophylline. Reduce dose with concomitant dipyridamole use.
Digoxin	IV loading: 1–1.25 mg over 24 hr po: 0.125–0.5 mg/day	36–48 hr	Renal	Fatigue, nausea, visual disturbances, arrhythmias	Adjust maintenance dose in renal failure. Accelerates accessory bypass tract conduction.
Propranolol	IV: 1–3 mg po: 10–80 mg q6hr	4–6 hr	Hepatic	CHF, bronchospasm, SA and A-V block, hypotension, masks hypoglycemia, depression	Nonselective beta receptor blocker.
Metoprolol	IV: 5 mg q5min (to 15 mg) po: 50–200 mg/qd; 2-4 times/day	3–7 hr	Hepatic	See propranolol	Beta$_1$-selective.
Esmolol	IV loading: 500 μg/kg over 1 min, then 25 μg/kg/min; increase by 25–50 μg/kg/min q4min to desired effect	9 min	Erythrocytes	See propranolol	Beta$_1$-selective. Very short half-life.
Verapamil	IV bolus: 0.10–0.15 mg/kg po: 40–120 mg q8hr	3–7 hr	Hepatic	Hypotension, bradycardia, A-V block, CHF, constipation	Increases digoxin levels. Accelerates accessory bypass tract conduction.
Diltiazem	IV bolus: 0.25 mg/kg; 0.35 mg/kg if ineffective IV maintenance: 10–20 mg/hr po: 30–120 mg q8hr	4–5 hr	Hepatic	Hypotension, bradycardia, A-V block, CHF	
Quinidine	po: 300–600 mg q6hr	6–7 hr	Hepatic	Gastrointestinal distress, diarrhea, thrombocytopenia, anemia, rash, *Torsades de pointes*	Frequent early toxicity causing drug termination.
Procainamide	IV loading: 15 mg/kg IV maintenance: 2–5 mg/min	3–5 hr	Hepatic, renal	Lupuslike syndrome, nausea, diarrhea, rash, confusion, myalgias, *Torsades de pointes*	60% develop antinuclear antibodies, with 20–30% developing clinical lupuslike syndrome. NAPA (active metabolite) formed in the liver.
Disopyramide	po: 100–200 mg q6hr	6–7 hr	Renal	Anticholinergic effects: urinary retention, constipation, dry mouth; CHF; *Torsades de pointes*	Greater negative inotropy than other class IA agents.
Flecainide	po: 100–200 mg q12hr	20 hr	Hepatic	Dizziness, visual disturbances, bradycardia, sustained ventricular tachycardia	Increases mortality in patients with depressed ejection fraction and prior myocardial infarction.
Propafenone	po: 150–300 mg q8hr	5–8 hr	Hepatic	Bradycardia, bronchospasm, CHF, sustained ventricular tachycardia	Beta-blocker activity 1/40 that of propranolol, on mg per mg basis.
Amiodarone	po loading: 800–1600 mg/day for 1–3 wk, then 600–800 mg/day for 4 wk po maintenance: 200–400 mg/day	50 days	Hepatic	Pulmonary fibrosis, hepatitis, hypo- and hyperthyroidism, neuropathy, corneal deposits, photosensitivity	Possesses class I, II, III, and IV activity. Use limited by frequent side effects. Most side effects dose-related.
Sotolol	po: 80–160 mg q12hr	6–18 hr	Renal	Bronchospasm, CHF, A-V block, bradycardia, hypotension, *Torsades de pointes*	Potent beta-blocker in addition to class III activity.

A-V = atrioventricular; CHF = congestive heart failure; SA = sinoatrial.

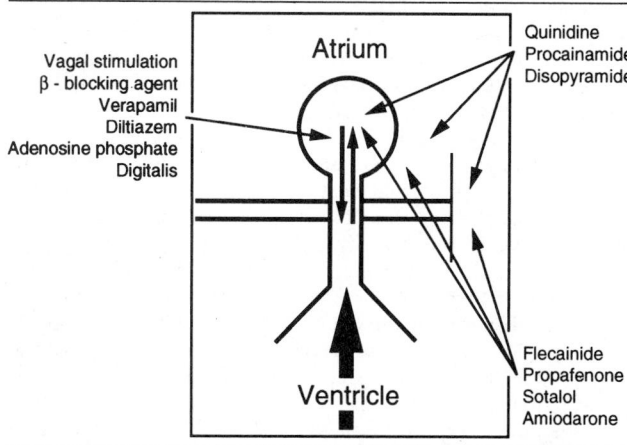

Fig. 41-3. Site of action of antiarrhythmic drugs. The class I and III antiarrhythmic agents affect the atrial and ventricular myocardium and accessory pathway as well as the A-V node, while the class II (beta-blockers) and class IV (calcium channel blockers) agents and digoxin primarily affect the atrioventricular node. (Modified from Falk RH, Podrid PT: *Atrial Fibrillation Mechanisms and Management.* New York, Raven, 1992, Chap. 12. With permission.)

Calcium Channel Blockers. Verapamil and diltiazem block the slow calcium channels, leading to slowed conduction and refractoriness in the sinus and A-V nodes. They can be used to suppress reentry arrhythmias that involve the sinus or A-V node. They are also effective in slowing ventricular rates in atrial arrhythmias, by increasing the ratio of A-V conduction.

Both verapamil and diltiazem can cause hypotension, bradycardia, A-V block, and worsening of congested heart failure through their negative inotropic effects. In addition, though verapamil has no direct effects on accessory bypass tract conduction, by lowering blood pressure and causing an increase in sympathetic tone it indirectly accelerates conduction through the tract.

DRUGS USED FOR PROPHYLAXIS AND CONVERSION TO NORMAL SINUS RHYTHM

Class I Antiarrhythmic Agents. Class IA and IC agents are effective for terminating and preventing recurrences of certain SVTs. Class IA drugs block fast sodium channels and therefore reduce the maximal rate of rise of the action potential upstroke (V_{max}), slowing conduction in atrial and ventricular myocardium. They also prolong refractoriness, which is manifested as QRS and Q–T prolongation on the surface ECG. Agents in this class are quinidine, procainamide, and disopyramide.

Quinidine can be administered orally as quinidine sulfate or, more commonly, as quinidine gluconate, which is somewhat better tolerated. Quinidine has little negative inotropy and if initially well tolerated can be taken long term without additional side effects. However, initial side effects are frequent and can lead to cessation of treatment in 30 to 40 percent of patients. The most common side effect is gastrointestinal distress, including nausea and diarrhea. Approximately 1 percent of patients may have syncope, most often caused by a polymorphic ventricular tachycardia associated with a prolonged Q–T (*Torsades de pointes*) [24]. For this reason, patients should be hospitalized and continuously monitored during initiation of quinidine and the other type IA agents. Other disadvantages of quinidine therapy are that it is administered three times per day and its ability to increase conduction through the A-V node.

Procainamide is acetylated in the liver to n-acetyl procainamide (NAPA), which is excreted by the kidney. The metabolite NAPA also is effective for SVTs, since it possesses type III antiarrhythmic properties. Procainamide can be given orally or intravenously. Although fairly well tolerated initially, side effects frequently lead to cessation of long-term treatment. Sixty to 70 percent of patients on procainamide eventually develop antinuclear antibodies and 20 to 30 percent develop clinical symptoms of a lupuslike syndrome, with arthralgias, fever, pericarditis, and pleuritis. The symptoms resolve once the drug is stopped. *Torsades de pointes* can also occur, necessitating monitoring during initiation of therapy.

Disopyramide has a greater negative inotropic effect than quinidine or procainamide and therefore must be used with caution in patients with depressed left ventricular function. It also has more anticholinergic effect, which can lead to urinary retention, dry mouth, constipation, and exacerbation of glaucoma. As is true for the other agents, it can precipitate *Torsades de pointes.*

Class IC drugs markedly decrease V_{max}, leading to a slowing of conduction in atrial and ventricular myocardial tissue. On ECG this appears as a widening of the QRS complex. Agents currently available in this class are flecainide and propafenone. In general they are well tolerated, but they may carry a risk of proarrhythmia in certain patient populations. In the Cardiac Arrhythmia Suppression Trial, in which the class IC drugs flecainide, encainide, and moricizine were administered to a population with frequent spontaneous ventricular ectopy, a previous myocardial infarction, and a depressed ejection fraction, there was a 2.5-fold higher mortality compared with patients who received placebo [25]. Although this raises concerns about drugs in this class, these data cannot necessarily be extrapolated to propafenone or to patients with an SVT who have other forms of heart disease or no structural heart disease at all. Telemetry monitoring is recommended during initiation of therapy.

Propafenone, in addition to having the type IC antiarrhythmic actions, has weak beta-blocker effect of approximately 1/40 that of propranolol, milligram per milligram. Therefore it is often effective in controlling the ventricular response as well as in terminating an SVT.

Class III Antiarrhythmic Agents. Class III antiarrhythmic agents block potassium channels, prolonging repolarization. These drugs, however, have additional electrophysiologic effects. The class III agents current clinically available to treat SVTs are amiodarone and sotolol.

Amiodarone has class III as well as class I, II, and IV activity. It prolongs action potential duration and refractoriness throughout the heart [26] and leads to a slowing of the sinus rate and P–R, QRS, and Q–T interval prolongation. It therefore is effective in the treatment of a wide variety of arrhythmias. Its use, however, is limited by its high potential for adverse effects: It can cause pulmonary fibrosis, elevation of liver enzymes, hyper- and hypothyroidism, neuropathy, photosensitivity, and corneal microdeposits [27–30]. Although it appears to be very efficacious, its toxicity increases with higher doses and longer duration of treatment. Its use should therefore be reserved at this time for life-threatening arrhythmias or after other conventional treatments have been attempted.

Sotolol has both type III and beta-blocker properties and therefore provides rate control in addition to maintenance of sinus rhythm. Other advantages include twice per day dosing and a relatively low incidence of toxicity. Side effects—negative inotropy and bradycardia—are mainly due to its beta-blocker activity. *Torsades de pointes* also can be precipitated, necessitating telemetry monitoring during initiation [31].

Ablation Therapy. Over the past decade, safe, effective catheter ablation techniques have added a new dimension to the treatment of supraventricular arrhythmia. Initially ablations were performed using high-energy DC current as an energy source. Radiofrequency energy has since become the dominant energy source for multiple reasons, including the possibility of more controlled lesion formation. The procedure involves invasive electrophysiologic evaluation to localize the origin and/or reentry pathways of the arrhythmia. Radiofrequency energy is then delivered directly through the mapping catheter to create a thermally mediated lesion and permanently inactivate the tissue responsible for the arrhythmia. Therefore, it can be used as definitive treatment, with ablation of the accessory bypass tracts in AVRT and ablation of the slow A-V node pathway in AVNRT (Fig. 41-4). In addition, complete A-V block can be readily achieved with radiofrequency catheter ablation. This is particularly advantageous in selected patients with atrial fibrillation or flutter whose ventricular rate cannot be adequately controlled pharmacologically. It necessitates the placement of a permanent pacemaker. Early investigation suggests that radiofrequency ablation will also be effective for ablation of the atrial pathway responsible for atrial flutter [32].

Catheter ablation can be used as definitive treatment for patients with Wolff-Parkinson-White syndrome, orthodromic A-V reciprocating tachycardia associated with a concealed accessory pathway, and slow pathway ablation for A-V nodal reentry. It is currently recommended for patients with significant symptoms who do not respond to or are unable to tolerate medications. Many physicians advocate its use as first-line therapy or for patients who prefer to avoid chronic medical therapy.

Prior to development of catheter ablation techniques, surgical ablation of a portion of the reentry circuit in AVNRT or AVRT, or an ectopic atrial focus, was possible through a variety of surgical approaches involving direct incision or cryoinjury from a cryoprobe [33]. With the advent of closed chest tranvenous catheter ablation, which obviates the morbidity of a thoracotomy, these techniques are largely used when catheter ablation is unsuccessful. Surgical techniques have been developed for atrial flutter [34] and atrial fibrillation [35], and may be an option in some centers for difficult cases of those arrhythmias.

Individual Supraventricular Tachycardias

REENTRANT SUPRAVENTRICULAR TACHYCARDIAS
Atrioventricular Nodal Reentry Tachycardia. Atrioventricular nodal reentry tachycardia is the most common form of paroxysmal SVT. It often presents in young patients without structural heart disease but can present at any age. The reentry circuit, located within the A-V node, consists of two pathways: a slow pathway with a long conduction time and a short refractory time, and a fast pathway with a short conduction time and a long refractory time [36,37]. Normally, in a patient with dual-pathway A-V node physiology, an impulse arrives from the sinus node and travels over both pathways, reaching the His bundle (and the ventricle) faster via the fast pathway. When a critically timed premature impulse arrives, either from a premature atrial beat (PAC) or from a paced beat introduced with programmed stimulation during electrophysiologic study, it arrives at the A-V node when the fast pathway is still refractory. Consequently, conduction proceeds selectively over the slow pathway. There is a "jump" in the A-V nodal conduction time for this beat, manifested on the surface ECG as a prolonged

P–R interval [38]. The delay in conduction allows the fast pathway to recover excitability, and the impulse then travels retrograde up that pathway to activate the atrium. The reentry loop is perpetuated as the impulse travels down the slow pathway and up the fast pathway, activating both the atrium and the ventricle on each circuit.

The initiation sequence often seen on the surface ECG consists of a premature atrial beat followed by a prolonged P–R interval, indicating conduction over the slow pathway. This is followed by initiation of a regular, usually narrow complex tachycardia with a rate generally between 150 and 220 beats per minute. In the vast majority of patients (90%), the retrograde P wave is obscured by the QRS complex. Rarely, the P wave is after the QRS, with an R–P interval less than 50 percent of the R–R interval. The retrograde activation of the atrium produces P waves that are inverted in leads II, III, and aVF.

In the rare atypical form of AVNRT, the direction of impulse propagation is reversed, with anterograde conduction over the fast pathway and retrograde conduction over the slow pathway [39]. This results in a retrograde P wave with a long R–P interval.

Therapy for AVNRT is aimed at altering the refractoriness of the reentry circuit. Acutely vagal maneuvers, which the patient can learn, can frequently terminate the tachycardia. Alternatively, agents that increase A-V conduction time and refractoriness, such as adenosine [40], calcium channel antagonists (verapamil and diltiazem) [41,42], beta-blockers [43], and digitalis can be used. Adenosine has the advantage of a very short half-life and has been shown to have an efficacy comparable to that of verapamil [44]. Atrial, ventricular, or esophageal pacing can also be effective in penetrating the reentrant circuit and altering the critical timing necessary for perpetuation of the arrhythmia [45]. This can be accomplished with overdrive pacing, at a rate faster than the tachycardia, or with programmed delivery of premature beats. If there is hemodynamic compromise, synchronized direct current cardioversion with 25 to 50 joules is usually successful.

In patients who have frequent, severely symptomatic, or hemodynamically compromising attacks, chronic therapy is required. Verapamil [46], diltiazem [47], beta-blockers, or digitalis can be used. Class IA [48] and class IC agents [49] are effective in preventing recurrences. Because of the potential for proarrhythmia, class IC agents should be used with caution in patients with coronary artery disease and depressed ventricular function.

Patients refractory to drug therapy, who have poorly tolerated tachyarrhythymias, or who are intolerant of medications should be considered for ablation therapy. This can be performed surgically [50] or, more commonly, with closed chest radiofrequency catheter. Current radiofrequency slow pathway ablation techniques have a high success rate (>90%) and low incidence of A-V block (<2%) or other serious morbidity [51,52]. Many investigators now advocate the use of radiofrequency ablation as first-line therapy for patients whose symptoms are severe enough to require drug therapy.

Atrioventricular Reciprocating Tachycardia. Atrioventricular reciprocating tachycardia is the second most common form of paroxysmal SVT; like AVNRT, it often occurs in young patients without structural heart disease. An A-V bypass tract (accessory pathway) is required to complete a reentry circuit. If the accessory pathway has anterograde conduction properties, the baseline surface ECG shows evidence of preexcitation (Fig. 41-4). In pathways without anterograde (atrial to ventricular) conduction, there is no preexcitation on the ECG, consequently the ECG in normal sinus rhythm is without any abnormalities. These accessory pathways are therefore designated "concealed."

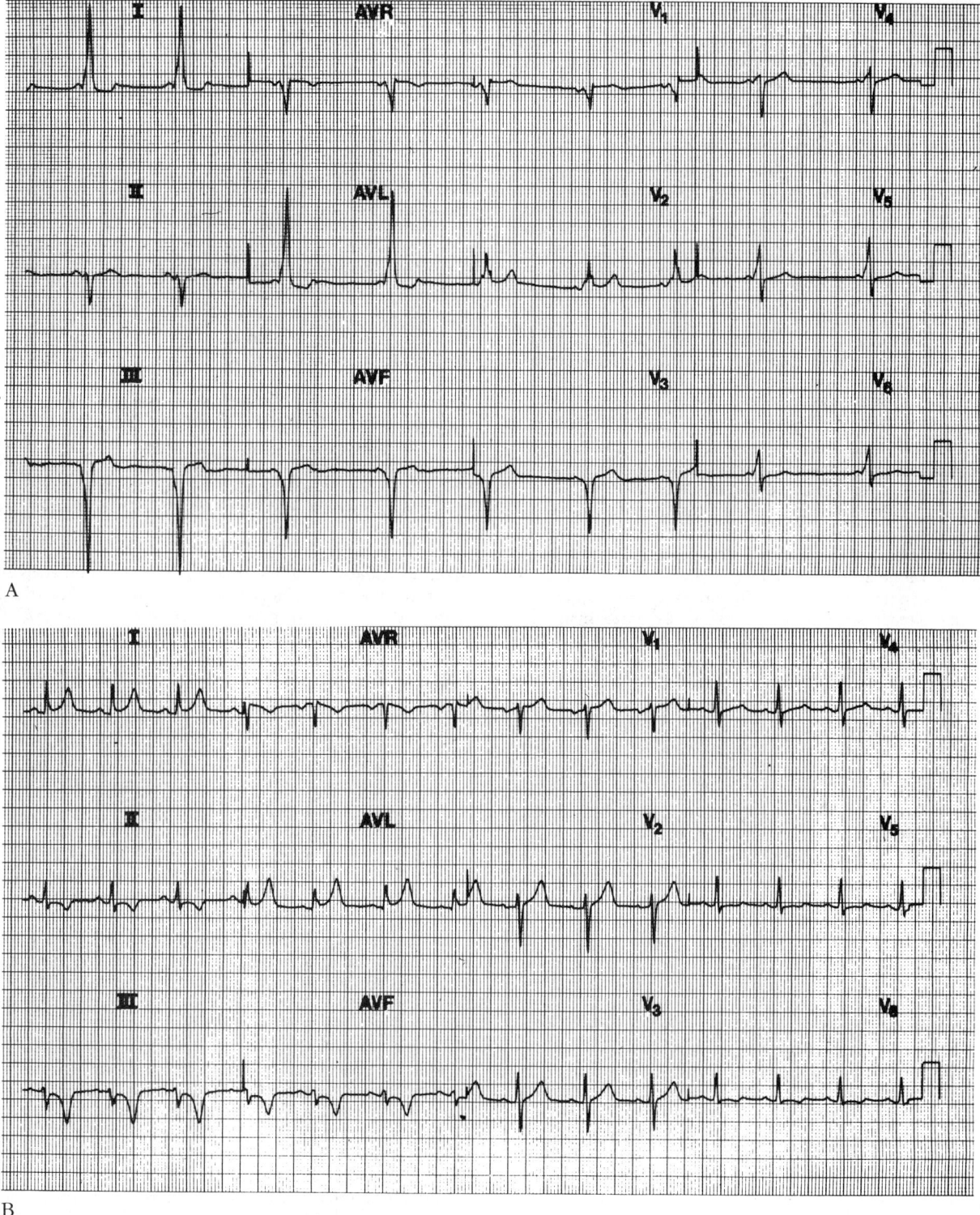

Fig. 41-4. Standard 12-lead ECG from a young woman prior to and immediately after radiofrequency catheter ablation of a right-sided accessory pathway producing the Wolff-Parkinson-White syndrome. A. The P–R interval is short, with a prominent upright delta wave in the lateral leads and a negative delta wave in leads III, aV$_F$, and V$_1$. B. Immediately after ablation, the P–R interval and QRS complexes have reverted to normal. There are persistent ST–T wave abnormalities, which also returned to normal within the next few weeks.

In orthodromic AVRT, the most common type, anterograde conduction occurs over the A-V node and retrograde conduction through the accessory pathway. Since the ventricular activation is over the normal conduction system, the QRS complex is usually narrow. With each retrograde conduction through the accessory pathway there is retrograde activation of the atrium. This results in a P wave after each QRS complex, with an R–P interval usually less than 50 percent of the R–R interval. Because atrial activation is retrograde, the P wave is inverted in leads II, III, and aVF [53]. The rate is generally 150 to 240 beats per minute. In antidromic AVRT, which is much less common, there is anterograde conduction over the accessory pathway and retrograde conduction over the A-V node, with a resultant wide preexcited QRS. This arrhythmia consequently is only seen in patients with the Wolff-Parkinson-White syndrome or Mahaim-type conduction (see below).

Acute therapy for orthodromic AVRT is similar to that for AVNRT. Therapy is aimed at altering the refractoriness of the reentry circuit. If there is hemodynamic compromise, synchronized direct current cardioversion, beginning at 50 joules, should be performed. Adenosine, calcium channel antagonists, and beta-blockers, as previously described, all prolong A-V node conduction time and refractoriness. Adenosine, because of its extremely short half-life, is the drug of choice.

In patients with orthodromic AVRT who do not respond to A-V node blocking agents, intravenous procainamide can be administered. Class IA antiarrhythmic agents prolong the refractoriness of the accessory pathway [54,55].

Chronic therapy is necessary if the episodes are frequent or cause hemodynamic compromise. Type IA antiarrhythmics (procainamide, quinidine, disopyramide) can be used for chronic prophylaxis [56]. They can be used alone or in combination with an A-V node blocking medication, such as quinidine, and a beta-blocker to affect both limbs of the reentry circuit. Type IC antiarrhythmics (flecainide, propafenone) affect both limbs by increasing conduction time and refractoriness in the A-V node and accessory bypass tract [57,58]. They are generally well tolerated. As previously indicated, they should be used with caution in patients with coronary artery disease and depressed ventricular function. Amiodarone also increases the conduction time and refractoriness in the A-V node and accessory bypass tract [59,60], but its use is limited by its prominent side effects [61].

Electrophysiologic testing can characterize the mechanism of the tachycardia and the location and conduction properties of the bypass tract. An electrophysiologic study should be considered in patients not controlled with empiric drug therapy or with life-threatening episodes or if ablation therapy is contemplated. Ablation therapy should be considered in patients who have recurrent episodes despite drug therapy, who have life-threatening episodes, or who wish to avoid lifelong drug therapy. Closed chest catheter ablation can be successfully performed in 93 to 97 percent of patients with an overall complication rate of less than 2 percent [62,63,64]. Surgical ablation of the accessory bypass tract is also highly effective, though it carries the morbidity and other disadvantages of open heart surgery [65].

Intraatrial Reentry Tachycardia. In intraatrial reentry tachycardia the reentry circuit is confined to the atrium [66]. The reentry circuit is frequently initiated with a premature atrial extrastimulus, occurring while a portion of the atrium is still refractory. This leads to the critical delay needed for establishing the reentry circuit. Since atrial activation is not from the sinus node, the P wave has a different morphology than when in sinus rhythm. The impulse is then conducted in the usual fashion, through the A-V node to the ventricles. Thus, the QRS

morphology is unchanged from that in sinus rhythm. Since the sinus and A-V nodes are not involved in the circuit, A-V block can be seen without termination of the tachycardia. Similarly, vagal maneuvers may produce such block, but they do not affect the circuit and therefore do not terminate the tachycardia. Termination can occur with a spontaneous or programmed premature atrial stimulus or with atrial pacing. Intraatrial reentry tachycardias often occur in patients with heart disease. Type IA and IC antiarrhythmics, which prolong the atrial conduction time and refractoriness, can be used. Acutely, the ventricular rate can be slowed by increasing the A-V block with calcium antagonists, beta-blockers, or digoxin.

Sinus Node Reentry Tachycardia. Sinus node reentry tachycardia is an uncommon cause of SVT but when it does occur it is often in patients with underlying heart disease. Because the reentry circuit is within the sinus node, the P waves are identical to those occurring in sinus rhythm; in fact, on ECG SNRT can look identical to sinus tachycardia. However, in contrast to sinus tachycardia, which has a slow onset and termination, with SNRT there is a sudden onset and termination. Vagal maneuvers can abruptly terminate the tachycardia by prolonging conduction and refractoriness in the sinus node. Drugs that do the same, such as calcium antagonists, beta-blockers, or digitalis, can be used for both acute and chronic management.

Atrial Fibrillation. Atrial fibrillation is a common arrhythmia, occurring in approximately 1 percent of people older than 65 years and 5 percent of people older than 75 years [67,68]. As with atrial flutter, it usually occurs in the setting of underlying structural heart or pulmonary disease. Hypertensive heart disease and coronary artery disease are the most common risk factors, accounting for approximately 60 percent of cases [69]. It is also associated with valvular heart disease, cardiomyopathies, pericarditis, pulmonary embolism, ethanol excess, and thyrotoxicosis. It occurs in 16 percent of patients with acute myocardial infarction and is associated with a higher in-hospital and long-term mortality [70].

Atrial fibrillation is thought to be a reentrant arrhythmia with multiple wavelets of depolarization traveling in a random sequence [71,72]. This results in disorganized atrial depolarization with ineffective atrial contraction. Electrocardiographically atrial depolarizations are manifested as irregular fine undulations at a rate of 400 to 600 beats per minute. The ventricular response is irregularly irregular, with a variable rate that depends on the conduction time through the A-V node. In untreated patients with normal A-V node function, the rate is usually 120 to 180 beats per minute.

Since depolarization of the ventricles is through the normal conduction system, the QRS complex is narrow unless there is a baseline bundle branch block. Occasionally, especially at faster ventricular rates, the QRS can be widened because of aberrant conduction. This most often occurs when a short R–R interval is immediately preceded by a long R–R interval, most often with a right bundle branch block morphology. The resulting aberration in this beat is termed Ashman's phenomenon. The QRS may also be wide in patients with Wolff-Parkinson-White syndrome when ventricular depolarization occurs through anterograde conduction through an accessory bypass tract. Rapid conduction over the bypass tract can lead to ventricular rates greater than 300 beats per minute and degenerate into ventricular fibrillation [73].

The symptoms in atrial fibrillation are variable, depending on the ventricular rate and underlying heart disease. Some patients are asymptomatic. Palpitations or irregular pulse are often noted. The increased rate can lead to angina in patients with coronary artery disease. The loss of atrial contraction along with the increased rate can lead to a drop in cardiac output and resultant congestive heart failure. The hemodynamic compromise is often worse in patients with disorders reliant on the atrial component of ventricular filling, such as dilated and hypertrophic cardiomyopathies and aortic stenosis.

The initial presenting symptom may be systemic embolization or stroke. The possibility of intermittent atrial fibrillation should be considered in every patient who presents with these findings. The risk of stroke among patients with nonrheumatic atrial fibrillation is 5 times greater than for comparable patients in sinus rhythm [74]. The risk is even higher in patients with mitral stenosis and atrial fibrillation, with a 4 to 6 percent annual incidence of embolic events [75].

On clinical examination there is an absence of a waves in the jugular venous pulse and an irregularly irregular rhythm. The intensity of the peripheral pulse varies with each beat, depending on the ventricular filling time. Physical examination should be directed at finding a possible cause of the atrial fibrillation, such as murmurs indicative of valvular disease, a pericardial friction rub, or signs of hyperthyroidism. An echocardiogram should be performed on every patient with new onset atrial fibrillation. Information on valvular function, left ventricular systolic and diastolic dysfunction, and left atrial size can help guide management. Transesophageal echocardiography (TEE) offers improved resolution and visualization of the atria and appendages, allowing improved visualization of atrial thrombi. Early studies suggest that the lack of visualized thrombi by TEE may allow safe cardioversion without precardioversion anticoagulation [76]. Thyroid function tests should also be performed in patients with new onset atrial fibrillation to rule out occult hyperthyroidism. A sensitive thyroid stimulating hormone (TSH) assay is usually sufficient.

A number of acute management strategies depend on the clinical status of the patient, duration of atrial fibrillation, and anticoagulation status. If the patient is hemodynamically compromised, immediate synchronized DC cardioversion, beginning at 100 joules, should be performed. Immediate DC cardioversion can also be performed in the hemodynamically stable patient known to have been in atrial fibrillation for less than 2 days and likely to maintain sinus rhythm without medication. An alternative approach in patients in atrial fibrillation for less than 2 days is to achieve rate control and attempt pharmacologic cardioversion with electrical cardioversion if the rhythm remains. The patient who has been in atrial fibrillation longer than 2 days or for an indeterminate time should be acutely treated with agents to slow the ventricular rate. If there are no contraindications Coumadin should be given for 3 weeks prior to electrical or chemical cardioversion, to minimize the risk of embolization. The therapy must be individualized and weighed against the potential toxicity of pharmacologic therapy, including proarrhythmia. Some patients, particularly the elderly or those unlikely to maintain sinus rhythm, may be left in atrial fibrillation.

Acute slowing of conduction through the A-V node, and thus the ventricular rate, can be accomplished with intravenous digoxin, verapamil [77], diltiazem [78], or a beta-blocker [79]. Digoxin has traditionally been the initial drug used for rate control. An initial intravenous load of 1 to 1.25 mg over 24 hours, as previously outlined, is administered, followed by a daily oral maintenance dose. Digoxin takes at least 1 hour to achieve peak effect. Also, since it slows A-V node conduction indirectly by increasing vagal tone, its effect may be minimal in patients with high sympathetic tone [80]. Intravenous diltiazem, verapamil, and beta-blockers have a quicker onset of action and can be used in place of, or in addition to, digoxin to slow the ventricular rate [81,82]. Their administration is outlined in the

therapy section. The additional benefits of the various agents, such as anginal or hypertensive control, or the detriments of negative inotropy or bronchospasm can be used to guide a specific choice.

Patients with suspected conduction over an accessory bypass tract with a wide QRS complex without a known preexisting bundle branch block should receive intravenous procainamide if they are hemodynamically stable or be immediately electrically cardioverted if they are not. Verapamil or digoxin should not be given because of their tendency to increase accessory pathway conduction time [83,84]. This can lead to an acceleration of the ventricular rate, with a potential for hemodynamic compromise [85]. (See the section on arrhythmias associated with Wolff-Parkinson-White-syndrome.)

Once the rate is controlled, an antiarrhythmic agent can be started to attempt cardioversion to normal sinus rhythm, if there is an acceptable risk of thromboembolism (see below). Procainamide is the only agent currently available for intravenous use. For oral use, a type IA [86], IC [87,88], or III [89,90] antiarrhythmic can be used. Therapeutic levels of most of these agents can be achieved in most cases within 24 to 36 hours, with electrical cardioversion performed if conversion does not occur pharmacologically. Although the rationale for the selection of oral antiarrhythmic agents is beyond the scope of this chapter, a thorough understanding of their pharmacology aids immeasurably in drug selection. For example, a type IC antiarrhythmic agent would not be an optimal choice in a patient with coronary artery disease and a depressed ejection fraction given its proarrhythmia in this group of patients. It should be stressed that normally the rate should be controlled prior to initiation of a type IA antiarrhythmic, since their vagolytic properties can lead to an acceleration of the rate. If cardioversion is successful, the antiarrhythmic agent is frequently continued for 3 to 6 months, then stopped if the patient remains in sinus rhythm. However, this has to be individualized and weighed against the risk of future episodes. In patients who have atrial fibrillation due to an acute condition that has resolved, the risk of future episodes may be low enough that the potential risk of antiarrhythmic agents outweighs the benefit. On the other hand, in high-risk patients, such as one with mitral stenosis and a large left atrium, it would be reasonable to continue the agent indefinitely.

If sinus rhythm cannot be maintained, rate control should be the goal of therapy. The antiarrhythmic should be discontinued and the rate controlled with digoxin, verapamil, diltiazem, or a beta-blocker. In cases where rate control is difficult to achieve pharmacologically, radiofrequency A-V node ablation with pacemaker implantation can be performed [91,92].

Patients who have been in atrial fibrillation longer than 2 days should, if there are no contraindications, receive 3 weeks of anticoagulation prior to attempted cardioversion to minimize the risk of embolization [93,94]. Coumadin should be given, maintained at an INR of 2.0 to 3.0. Anticoagulation should be continued until sinus rhythm has been maintained for 4 weeks, since atrial contractile activity can lag behind electrical evidence of sinus rhythm [95]. Early reports indicate that cardioversion can be performed safely on patients who have no demonstrable thrombus on TEE [76]. Further prospective randomized studies are needed before this can be recommended as standard care. Numerous studies support the use of long-term anticoagulation with warfarin in patients with chronic atrial fibrillation, showing a reduction in the incidence of stroke [96,97,98]. The current American College of Chest Physicians recommendation is to initiate long-term warfarin therapy (INR 2–3) in all patients with chronic atrial fibrillation who do not have contraindications to anticoagulation, except patients younger than 60 years without associated cardiovascular disease ("lone a fib") [91]. In patients in the intensive care setting who are having multiple invasive procedures performed, normally intravenous heparin would be substituted for warfarin.

Atrial Flutter. Atrial flutter is thought to be caused by a reentry mechanism [99,100]. It usually occurs in patients with underlying structural heart disease or in the setting of pulmonary embolus, pericarditis, ethanol consumption, or thyrotoxicosis. It tends to be an unstable rhythm, reverting to sinus rhythm or degenerating into atrial fibrillation, though it can also be chronic. The atrial rate during flutter is usually 250 to 350 beats per minute, though it may slow to 200 beats per minute after antiarrhythmic therapy. There is usually 2:1 block in the A-V node, with a resultant ventricular rate of around 150 beats per minute. With enhanced A-V node conduction, anterograde accessory bypass tract conduction, or in children, atrial flutter rarely conducts to the ventricle in a 1:1 fashion, which usually results in hemodynamic compromise. With 2:1 A-V block, it can be difficult to distinguish atrial flutter from other regular narrow QRS complex SVTs. Vagal maneuvers or adenosine can be used to increase the degree of A-V block, unmasking the characteristic "sawtooth" flutter waves, which are normally inverted in the inferior leads. Since the reentry circuit does not involve the sinus or A-V node, vagal maneuvers do not affect the atrial flutter rate.

Therapy is twofold, aimed at controlling the ventricular response and converting to sinus rhythm. If there is hemodynamic compromise, synchronized DC cardioversion should be performed. Low energies (25–50 joules) are often effective. If cardioversion results in atrial fibrillation, a higher energy (100–200 joules) can be used. Rapid atrial pacing for 15 seconds at a rate 10 to 15 percent faster than the flutter also often leads to conversion to sinus rhythm [101]. This is particularly useful in the postcoronary artery bypass surgery setting, where the patient typically has temporary atrial and ventricular epicardial pacing wires.

Acute and chronic management strategies are similar to those for atrial fibrillation, but the use of anticoagulation for atrial flutter is controversial. It is clear that there is a lower risk of thromboembolism with atrial flutter than with atrial fibrillation. Current guidelines do not call for anticoagulation with atrial flutter [93]. However, since some patients with atrial flutter may also have significant periods of atrial fibrillation, in some cases a more prudent approach is warranted. It is important to control the rate prior to initiating a type IA antiarrhythmic, because the combination of slowing the flutter rate and their vagolytic properties can lead to 1:1 A-V conduction [102].

Special mention should be made of atrial flutter with suspected conduction over an accessory bypass tract. In these cases there is a wide QRS, often 1:1 A-V conduction, and possibly a history of Wolff-Parkinson-White syndrome. Vagal maneuvers fail to cause increased A-V block. If there is hemodynamic compromise, synchronized DC cardioversion should be performed. Pharmacologic treatment is geared at prolonging conduction and refractory time over the accessory pathway. Acutely, intravenous procainamide should be used. (See the section on arrhythmias associated with Wolff-Parkinson-White syndrome.)

Given the potential for proarrhythmia with type I antiarrhythmics, they should be withdrawn if recurrences cannot be prevented. Therapy is then directed toward controlling the ventricular rate.

AUTOMATIC SUPRAVENTRICULAR TACHYCARDIAS

Sinus Tachycardia. Sinus tachycardia is the most common etiology of an atrial tachyarrhythmia and thus must be considered in the differential diagnosis of every tachyarrhythmia. It is a result of increased automaticity of the sinus node. The P wave morphology is normal, with a rate greater than 100 beats per minute. The maximum sinus rate for any patient is normally approximately 220 minus their age, though in high catecholamine states it can be even higher. Each P wave is followed by a normal QRS complex. As with other arrhythmias caused by increased automaticity, there is a gradual onset and termination. There is normally a subtle change in the rate associated with the respiratory cycle. Vagal maneuvers cause a gradual slowing with slow acceleration once the maneuver is completed.

Sinus tachycardia is the normal physiologic reaction to a number of stressors. Fever, hypovolemia, hypoxia, anemia, pain, anxiety, exertion, and beta-blocker withdrawal all can cause sinus tachycardia. It is commonly seen in myocardial ischemia, left ventricular dysfunction, pulmonary embolus, and thyrotoxicosis. Medications with sympathomimetic activity, including most pressor and inotropic agents, also can be responsible.

Treatment is aimed at identifying and correcting the underlying cause, such as fluid replacement in a patient who is hypovolemic or analgesics for a patient in pain. In patients with an acute myocardial infarction or ischemia, if no other cause can be identified and there are no clinical contraindications, the heart rate can be slowed with beta-blocker therapy to decrease myocardial oxygen demand.

Automatic Atrial Tachycardia. Also referred to as atrial ectopic tachycardia, this SVT occurs when an atrial focus undergoes spontaneous phase 4 depolarization at a rate faster than the sinus node, becoming the dominant pacemaker. The P wave morphology differs from that during sinus rhythm in that there is a "warm-up" period, at the onset, with rate acceleration until a stable rate is reached. As with other arrhythmias caused by increased automaticity, vagal maneuvers do not terminate automatic atrial tachycardia, but may cause A-V block. Programmed stimulation does not initiate or terminate the arrhythmia.

Automatic atrial tachycardias occur most often in patients with chronic obstructive pulmonary disease, pneumonia, myocardial infarction, cardiomyopathy, or drug toxicity, particularly digoxin toxicity. In patients with digoxin toxicity, the tachycardia often occurs in association with A-V block and often is exacerbated by sympathomimetic agents.

The management of automatic atrial tachycardia involves first identifying episodes caused by drug toxicity. If A-V block is also present in the patient on digoxin, intoxication should be suspected. Often the toxicity is precipitated by hypokalemia. The digoxin should be withheld and, if necessary, the potassium should be repleted. The need for sympathomimetic agents, if they are in use, must be weighed against the likelihood that they are contributing to the tachycardia. In those not caused by drug toxicity, type IA antiarrhythmics are the treatment of choice. Type IC [103] and III [104] antiarrhythmics have also been used. In patients refractory to pharmacologic treatment, there is the possibility of catheter radiofrequency [105,106] or surgical ablation [107], although experience with these therapies in this setting is limited.

Multifocal Atrial Tachycardia. In multifocal atrial tachycardia (MAT) there are, by definition, at least three different P wave morphologies representing different atrial foci. The atrial rate is greater than 100 beats per minute. The P–P and resultant R–R intervals are irregularly irregular. Therefore, MAT can sometimes be confused with atrial fibrillation. Vagal maneuvers do not affect the atrial rate, though they occasionally cause A-V block.

This tachycardia occurs commonly in patients who are acutely ill with chronic obstructive pulmonary disease, congestive heart failure, or other causes of hypoxia or acidosis or with theophylline toxicity. The treatment is directed toward the underlying disease. Intravenous verapamil has been shown to be effective in causing a reduction in atrial and ventricular rates [108]. Beta-blockers are effective but are contraindicated in a large percentage of patients with MAT who also have obstructive pulmonary disease [109].

Automatic Junctional Tachycardia. Automatic junctional tachycardia occurs when a focus in the A-V junctional tissue depolarizes and discharges faster than the sinus node, becoming the dominant pacemaker. The atria usually continue to be depolarized from the sinus node, which may result in A-V dissociation with an atrial rate slower than the ventricular rate. Alternatively, there may be retrograde activation of the atria from the junctional focus. Onset and termination are gradual. Vagal maneuvers can have no effect or can produce gradual slowing of the ventricular rate with a return to the previous rate once the maneuver is terminated.

This tachycardia often occurs in patients with chronic obstructive lung disease or structural heart disease, after cardiac surgery, or with digoxin toxicity. Regularity of the ventricular rhythm in a patient with atrial fibrillation on digoxin may indicate that digoxin toxicity is the underlying cause.

Therapy is directed toward the underlying disease process. If digoxin toxicity is the cause, the drug should be stopped and potassium should be repleted if needed. If there is hemodynamic compromise, atrial pacing at a rate exceeding that of the tachycardia will occasionally restore A-V synchrony and improve cardiac output. This can be of value after open heart surgery, when atrial pacing is readily accomplished.

WOLFF-PARKINSON-WHITE SYNDROME. The arrhythmias associated with preexcitation are discussed individually above. The different approach to acute therapy with them, however, warrants a focused review. Preexcitation occurs when atrial impulses activate all or part of the ventricle earlier than expected by traveling through accessory pathways faster than normal conduction through the A-V node. This early activation of the ventricle, referred to as the Wolff-Parkinson-White syndrome, produces the classic ECG findings (see below). The incidence is approximately 0.3 percent [110]. The accessory tracts are congenital. These tracts are usually atrioventricular, though they can also be atriofascicular or A-V nodoventricular (Mahaim fibers). They are usually associated with a normal heart but can be associated with Ebstein's anomaly. Diagnosis is made with a 12-lead ECG showing the hallmarks of preexcitation: (1) P–R interval less than 120 msec while in sinus rhythm; (2) QRS of greater than 120 msec duration with a delta wave; and (3) secondary ST–T wave changes (Fig. 41-3).

Patients with preexcitation may be asymptomatic but are prone to a number of SVTs. Approximately 80 percent are due to A-V reciprocating tachycardia, 15 percent to atrial fibrillation, and 5 percent to atrial flutter. In atrial fibrillation and flutter, the accessory bypass tract does not participate in the genesis of the arrhythmia but facilitates rapid conduction to the ventricle. The mechanisms of and treatments for the specific arrhythmias are outlined in their respective sections. Some key points common to treatment of all the arrhythmias associated with preexcitation are reviewed here.

In orthodromic and antidromic AVRT, therapy is geared at changing the refractoriness in the reentry circuit. In the management of orthodromic AVRT, special care should be used with verapamil in patients with known preexcitation, since it can accelerate conduction over the accessory pathway [111]. This becomes significant if there is spontaneous conversion of the AVRT to atrial fibrillation or flutter with anterograde conduction over the bypass tract, which occurs occasionally [112]. Digitalis can also accelerate conduction over the accessory pathway, leading to a fast ventricular rate and possible degeneration into ventricular fibrillation if atrial fibrillation or flutter develops [113,114]. Given the availability of other agents, digitalis should generally be avoided in patients with Wolff-Parkinson-White syndrome. In patients with antidromic AVRT, manifested on ECG as a wide preexcited QRS, intravenous procainamide is the initial treatment of choice.

In atrial fibrillation or flutter with preexcitation on the ECG, the concern for rapid conduction alters the approach to acute management. As mentioned above, verapamil and digoxin can lead to accelerated conduction over the bypass tract, with resultant hemodynamic compromise and degeneration into ventricular fibrillation. For this reason the treatment of choice for any patient with suspected preexcitation and atrial fibrillation or flutter is intravenous procainamide if the patient is hemodynamically stable or immediate cardioversion if not.

Differential Diagnosis

Acute management of an SVT is geared at determining the underlying mechanism, which allows a more directed approach to therapy. A number of clues can be rapidly obtained from a direct recording and bedside maneuvers. It is very helpful to record the initiation and termination sequence of the tachycardia. Arrhythmias from a reentry mechanism are often initiated or terminated by a PAC, with abrupt onset and termination. Arrhythmias caused by increased automaticity are often gradual in onset and termination. If the P–R interval of the initial PAC is prolonged (reflecting selective conduction through the slow pathway of the A-V node), the reentry circuit likely involves the A-V node (AVNRT or AVRT). Atrioventricular block present during the tachycardia for all practical purposes rules out a reentry circuit that involves the A-V node.

In sinus tachycardia, sinus node reentry tachycardia, intraatrial reentry tachycardia, automatic atrial tachycardia, and multifocal atrial tachycardia the P wave is in front of the QRS complex, with a P–R interval less than the R–P interval. In sinus tachycardia and SNRT, the P wave morphology and P–R interval are identical to the patient's baseline sinus rhythm. However, since SNRT is generated by a reentry mechanism, it may be initiated and terminated by a PAC, and it starts and stops abruptly. Vagal maneuvers or adenosine can terminate SNRT, but will only transiently slow sinus tachycardia.

In intraatrial reentry tachycardia (IART) and automatic atrial tachycardia (AAT) the P wave morphology usually differs from that in sinus rhythm. The two may be difficult to distinguish. An IART, however, may exhibit the signs of a reentry mechanism, with initiation and termination by a PAC and abrupt onset and termination. Vagal maneuvers and adenosine may lead to a slowing of the ventricular rate by causing A-V block in both. Since the reentry circuit does not involve the SA or A-V nodes in IART, it will not be terminated.

In MAT there will be multiple (at least three) P wave morphologies, with a resultant irregularly irregular rhythm. If the P waves are not appreciated a diagnosis of atrial fibrillation can inadvertently be made. Vagal maneuvers may cause A-V block but will not slow the atrial rate.

Retrograde P waves are often seen with AVRT, as the impulse travels through the concealed bypass tract from the ventricle to depolarize the atrium, and can occasionally be seen with AVNRT. Since atrial activation is retrograde, the P wave is inverted in leads II, III, and aVF. An AVRT and AVNRT can often be differentiated with an esophageal electrode or intraatrial recording. One rule of thumb is that if the R–P interval is less than 70 msec when recorded with an esophageal lead or less than 95 msec on a high right atrial electrogram, AVNRT is the diagnosis [115,116]. Vagal maneuvers or adenosine can alter the refractoriness of the reentry circuit terminating the arrhythmia.

The absence of a clear P wave during a regular SVT suggests an AVNRT. However, at rapid heart rates it can sometimes be difficult clearly to identify the P waves associated with other SVTs (i.e., atrial flutter with 2:1 A-V block). Therefore, vagal maneuvers or adenosine should be used to increase A-V block, enabling identification of the P waves if it is not an AVNRT and possible termination if it is.

In atrial fibrillation there is no organized atrial activity on ECG, with irregular undulations at a rate of 400 to 600 beats per minute. This produces an irregularly irregular rhythm. This must be distinguished from MAT.

In atrial flutter there are flutter waves, with an atrial rate of 250 to 350 beats per minute. The atrial activity can often be better appreciated after vagal maneuvers or after adenosine is administered to increase A-V block. Occasionally the A-V block can be variable, resulting in an irregularly irregular rhythm.

Wide QRS Supraventricular Tachycardia

The QRS width during an SVT is occasionally greater than 120 msec. When confronted with a wide QRS tachycardia, the first distinction is whether it is supraventricular or ventricular in origin. This is crucial, given the very different prognosis and therapy associated with each. Findings suggestive of ventricular tachycardia include A-V dissociation, fusion beats, positive QRS concordance (positive deflections in all precordial leads), QRS duration of greater than 140 msec with a right bundle branch block and 160 msec with a left bundle branch block, left axis deviation greater than minus 90 degrees, and a different QRS morphology during tachycardia compared to a baseline preexisting bundle branch block [117]. In addition, ventricular tachycardia is statistically likely if the patient has structural heart disease or a history of myocardial infarction. A QRS complex identical to that in sinus rhythm is highly suggestive of SVT [118]. If the above criteria are not present, an SVT is likely. The wide QRS may be attributed to a preexisting bundle branch block, aberrant conduction, or antidromic bypass tract conduction. Vagal maneuvers or adenosine can be given if the diagnosis is uncertain and there is no hemodynamic compromise [119,120]. If the rhythm is ventricular in origin there will be no effect. If the rhythm is an SVT with conduction through the A-V node it may terminate or produce A-V block, allowing identification of the P waves. Verapamil should be avoided in the treatment of wide QRS tachycardias, since it can lead to marked hypotension if inadvertently administered to a patient with ventricular tachycardia or an antidromically conducted SVT. In addition, it can reflexly decrease the refractory time of the accessory bypass tract, leading to an acceleration of the ventricular rate and degeneration into ventricular fibrillation. If there is hemodynamic compromise, synchronized DC cardioversion should be performed regardless of its origin. If the patient is hemodynamically stable and the diagnosis remains uncertain, intravenous procainamide can be administered, since it will be effective for both ventricular tachycardia and

SVT. Finally, if necessary an electrophysiologic study can be performed for differentiation.

References

1. Gilmour RF, Zipes DP: Basic electrophysiologic mechanisms for the development of arrhythmias: Clinical applications. *Med Clin North Am* 68:795, 1984.
2. Zipes DP: Genesis of cardiac arrhythmias: Electrophysiological considerations. In Braunwald E (ed): *Heart Disease: A Textbook of Cardiovascular Medicine* 4th ed. Philadelphia, WB Saunders, 1992.
3. Zipes DP: Specific arrhythmias: Diagnosis and treatment. In Braunwald E (ed): *Heart Disease: A Textbook of Cardiovascular Medicine*. 4th ed. Philadelphia, WB Saunders, 1992.
4. Josephson ME, Kastor JA: Supraventricular tachycardia: Mechanisms and management. *Ann Intern Med* 87:346, 1977.
5. Manolis AS, Estes AM: Supraventricular tachycardias: Mechanism and therapy. *Arch Intern Med* 147:1706, 1987.
6. Gillette PC, Garson A: Electrophysiologic and pharmacologic characteristics of automatic ectopic atrial tachycardia. *Circulation* 56:571, 1977.
7. Ferrier GR: Digitalis arrhythmias: Role of oscillatory afterpotentials. *Prog Cardiovasc Dis* 19:459, 1977.
8. Kalbfleisch SJ, Atassi R, Calkins H, et al: Differentiation of paroxysmal narrow QRS complex tachycardias using the 12 lead electrocardiogram. *J Am Coll Cardiol* 21:85, 1993.
9. Mandel WJ, Peter LT, Bleifer SB: Holter monitor recording. In Mandel WJ (ed): *Arrhythmias: Their Mechanisms, Diagnosis, and Management*. 2nd ed. Philadelphia, JB Lipincott, 1987.
10. Linzer M, Prystowsky EN, Brunnetti LL, et al: Recurrent syncope of unknown origin diagnosed by ambulatory continuous loop ECG recording. *Am Heart J* 16:1632, 1988.
11. Ross TF, Mandell WJ: Invasive cardiac electrophysiologic testing. In Mandel WJ (ed): *Arrhythmias: Their Mechanisms, Diagnosis, and Management*. 2nd ed. Philadelphia, JB Lippincott, 1987.
12. Leitch J, Klein GJ, Yee R, Murdock C: Invasive electrophysiologic evaluation of patients with supraventricular tachycardia. *Cardiol Clin* 8:465, 1990.
13. Mehta D, Wafa S, Ward DE, Camm AJ: Relative efficacy of various physical manoeuvres in the termination of junctional tachycardia. *Lancet* 1:1181, 1988.
14. DiMarco JP, Sellers TD, Berne RM, et al: Adenosine: Electrophysiologic effects and therapeutic use for terminating paroxysmal supraventricular tachycardia. *Circulation* 68:1254, 1983.
15. Haines DE, Dimarco JP: Current therapy for supraventricular tachycardia. *Curr Prob Cardiol* 17:414, 1992.
16. Ornato JP: Management of paroxysmal supraventricular tachycardia. *Circulation* 74:IV-108, 1986.
17. Sylven C, Jonzon B, Brandt R, Beerman B: Adenosine provoked angina pectoris-like pain: Time characteristics, influence of autonomic blockade, and naloxone. *Eur Heart J* 8:738, 1987.
18. Sylven C, Jonzon B, Edlund A: Angina pectoris-like pain provoked by IV bolus of adenosine: Relationship to coronary sinus blood flow, heart rate and blood pressure in healthy volunteers. *Eur Heart J* 10:48, 1989.
19. Camm AJ, Garratt CL: Adenosine and supraventricular tachycardia. *N Engl J Med* 325:1621, 1991.
20. McIntosh-Yellin NL, Drew BJ, Scheinman MM: Safety and efficacy of central intravenous bolus administration of adenosine for termination of supraventricular tachycardia. *J Am Coll Cardiol* 22:741, 1993.
21. Chai CY, Wang HH, Hoffman BF, et al: Mechanisms of bradycardia induced by digitalis substances. *Am J Physiol* 212:26, 1967.
22. Mendez C, Mendez R: The action of cardiac glycosides in the excitability and conduction velocity of the mammalian atrium. *J Phamacol Exp Ther* 121:402, 1957.
23. Duff H, Rosen DM, Brorson L, et al: Electrophysiologic actions of high plasma concentrations of propranolol in human subjects. *J Am Coll Cardiol* 2:1134, 1983.

24. Selzer A, Wray HW: Quinidine syncope: Paroxysmal ventricular fibrillation occurring during treatment of chronic atrial arrhythmias. *Circulation* 30:17, 1964.
25. Echt DS, Liebson PR, Mitchell LB, et al: Mortality and morbidity in patients receiving encainide, flecainide, or placebo: The Cardiac Arrhythmia Suppression Trial. *N Engl J Med* 324:781, 1991.
26. Gallagher JD, Bianchi J, Gessman LJ: A comparison of the electrophysiologic effects of acute and chronic amiodarone administration on canine Purkinje fibers. *J Cardiovasc Pharmacol* 13:723, 1989.
27. Greene HL, Graham EL, Werner JA, et al: Toxic and therapeutic effects of amiodarone in the treatment of cardiac arrhythmias. *J Am Coll Cardiol* 2:1114, 1983.
28. Raeder EA, Podrid PJ, Lown B: Side effects and complications of amiodarone therapy. *Am Heart J* 109:975, 1983.
29. Martin WJ, Rosenow EC: Amiodarone pulmonary toxicity: Recognition and pathogenesis (part 1). *Chest* 93:1067, 1988.
30. Martin WJ, Rosenow EC: Amiodarone pulmonary toxicity: Recognition and pathogenesis (part 2). *Chest* 93:1242, 1988.
31. Mason JW, for the Electrophysiologic Study Versus Electrocardiographic Monitoring Investigators: A comparison of seven antiarrhythmic drugs in patients with ventricular tachyarrhythmias. *N Engl J Med* 329:452, 1993.
32. Saoudi N, Atallah G, Kirkorian G, Touboul P: Catheter ablation of the atrial myocardium in human type I atrial flutter. *Circulation* 81:762, 1990.
33. Gallagher JJ, Selle JG, Svenson RH: Surgical treatment of arrhythmias. *Am J Cardiol* 61:27A, 1988.
34. Klein GJ, Guiraudon GM, Sharma AD, et al: Demonstration of macro-reentry and feasibility of operative therapy in the common type of atrial flutter. *Am J Cardiol* 57:587, 1986.
35. Cox JL, Schuessler RB, D'Agostino HJ, et al: The surgical treatment of atrial fibrillation: Development of a definitive surgical procedure. *J Thorac Cardiovasc Surg* 101:569, 1991.
36. Denes P, Wu D, Dhingra RC, et al: Demonstration of dual AV nodal pathways in patients with paroxysmal supraventricular tachycardia. *Circulation* 48:549, 1973.
37. Rosen KM, Mehta A, Miller RA: Demonstration of dual atrioventricular nodal pathways on man. *Am J Cardiol* 33:291, 1974.
38. Akhtar M, Jazayeri R, Sra J, et al: Atrioventricular nodal reentry: Clinical, electrophysiological, and therapeutic considerations. *Circulation* 88:282, 1993.
39. Akhtar M, Damato AN, Ruskin JN, et al: Anterograde and retrograde conduction characteristics in three patterns of paroxysmal atrioventricular junctional reentry tachycardia. *Am Heart J* 95:22, 1978.
40. DiMarco JP, Sellars T, Berne RM, et al: Adenosine: Electrophysiologic effects and therapeutic use for terminating paroxysmal supraventricular tachycardia. *Circulation* 68:1254, 1983.
41. Reddy CP, McAllister RF: Effect of verapamil on retrograde conduction in atrioventricular nodal reentrant tachycardia. *Am J Cardiol* 54:535, 1984.
42. Dougherty AH, Jackman WM, Naccarelli GV, et al: Acute conversion of paroxysmal supraventricular tachycardia with intravenous diltiazem. *Am J Cardiol* 70:587, 1992.
43. Wu D, Denes P, Dhingra R, et al: The effects of propranolol on induction of AV nodal reentrant paroxysmal tachycardia. *Circulation* 50:665, 1974.
44. DiMarco JP, Miles W, Akhtar M, et al: Adenosine for paroxysmal supraventricular tachycardias: Dose ranging and comparison with verapamil. *Ann Intern Med* 113:104, 1990.
45. Gallagher JJ, Smith WM, Kerr CR, et al: Esophageal pacing: A diagnostic and therapeutic tool. *Circulation* 65:336, 1982.
46. Mauritson DR, Winniford MD, Walker WS, et al: Oral verapamil for paroxysmal supraventricular tachycardia. *Ann Intern Med* 96:409, 1982.
47. Clair WK, Wilkinson WE, McCarthy EA, Pritchett EL: Treatment of paroxysmal supraventricular tachycardia with oral diltiazem. *Clin Pharmacol Ther* 51:562, 1992.
48. Wu D, Hung JS, Kuo CT, et al: Effects of quinidine on atrioventricular nodal reentrant paroxysmal tachycardia. *Circulation* 64:823, 1981.
49. Anderson JL: Long-term safety and efficacy of flecainide in the treatment of supraventricular tachyarrhythmias: The United States experience. *Am J Cardiol* 70:11A, 1992.
50. Cox JL, Holman WL, Cain ME: Cryosurgical treatment of atrioventricular node reentrant tachycardia. *Circulation* 76:1329, 1987.
51. Jackman WM, Beckman KJ, McClelland JH, et al: Treatment of supraventricular tachycardia due to atrioventricular nodal reentry by radiofrequency catheter ablation of slow-pathway conduction. *N Engl J Med* 327:313, 1992.
52. Kay GN, Epstein AE, Dailey SM, Plump VJ: Selective radiofrequency ablation of the slow pathway for the treatment of atrioventricular nodal reentrant tachycardia. *Circulation* 85:1675, 1992.
53. Prystowsky EN: Diagnosis and management of the preexcitation syndromes. *Curr Probl Cardiol* 13:227, 1988.
54. Mandel WJ, Laks MM, Obayasi K, et al: The Wolff-Parkinson-White syndrome: Pharmacologic effects of procainamide. *Am Heart J* 90:744, 1975.
55. Kerr CR, Prystowsky EN, Smith WM, et al: Electrophysiologic effects of disopyramide phosphate in patients with Wolff-Parkinson-White syndrome. *Circulation* 65:869, 1982.
56. Sellars T, Cambell RWF, Bashore TM, et al: Effects of procainamide and quinidine sulfate in the Wolff-Parkinson-White syndrome. *Circulation* 55:15, 1977.
57. Neus H, Buss J, Schlepper M, et al: Effects of flecainide on electrophysiological properties of accessory pathways in the Wolff-Parkinson-White syndrome. *Eur Heart J* 4:347, 1983.
58. Breithardt G, Borggrefe M, Wiebringhaus E, et al: Effect of propafenone in the Wolff-Parkinson-White syndrome: Electrophysiologic findings and long term follow-up. *Am J Cardiol* 54:29D, 1984.
59. Rosenbaum MB, Chiale PA, Ryba D, et al: Control of tachyarrhythmias associated with Wolff-Parkinson-White syndrome by amiodarone hydrochloride. *Am J Cardiol* 34:215, 1974.
60. Wellens HJJ, Lie KI, Bar FW, et al: Effect of amiodarone in Wolff-Parkinson-White syndrome. *Am J Cardiol* 38:189, 1976.
61. Mason JW: Drug therapy: Amiodarone. *N Engl J Med* 316:455, 1987.
62. Calkins H, Sousa J, Atassi R, et al: Diagnosis and cure of the Wolff-Parkinson-White syndrome or paroxysmal supraventricular tachycardia during a single electrophysiologic test. *N Engl J Med* 324:1612, 1991.
63. Jackman WM, Wang XZ, Friday KJ, et al: Catheter ablation of accessory atrioventricular pathways (Wolff-Parkinson-White syndrome) by radiofrequency current. *N Engl J Med* 424:1605, 1991.
64. Morady F: Catheter ablation of accessory pathways. *Cardiol Clin* 8:557, 1990.
65. Cox JL, Gallagher JJ, Cain ME: Experience with 118 consecutive patients undergoing surgery for the Wolff-Parkinson-White syndrome. *J Thorac Cardiovasc Surg* 90:490, 1985.
66. Wu D, Amat-Y-Leon F, Denes P, et al: Demonstration of sustained sinus and atrial reentry as a mechanism of paroxysmal supraventricular tachycardia. *Circulation* 51:234, 1975.
67. Rose G, Baxter PJ, Reid DD, et al: Prevalence and prognosis of electrocardiographic findings in middle-aged men. *Br Heart J* 40:636, 1978.
68. Cambell A, Caird FI, Jackson TF: Prevalence of abnormalities of electrocardiogram in old people. *Br Heart J* 36:1005, 1974.
69. Kannel WB, Abbott RD, Savage DD, et al: Epidemiologic features of chronic atrial fibrillation: The Framingham Study. *N Engl J Med* 306:1018, 1982.
70. Goldberg RJ, Seeley D, Becker RC, et al: Impact of atrial fibrillation on the in-hospital and longterm survival of patients with acute myocardial infarction: A community-wide perspective. *Am Heart J* 119:996, 1990.
71. Moe GK, Rheinboldt WC, Abildskov JA: A computer model of atrial fibrillation. *Am Heart J* 67:200, 1964.
72. Allessie MA, Bonke FLM, Schopman FJ: Circus movement in rabbit atrial muscle as a mechanism of tachycardia. III. The "leading circle" concept: A new model of circus movement in cardiac tissue without the involvement of an anatomical obstacle. *Circ Res* 41:9, 1977.
73. Klein GJ, Bashore TM, Sellers T, et al: Ventricular fibrillation in the Wolff-Parkinson-White syndrome. *N Engl J Med* 301:1080, 1979.
74. Wolf PA, Dawber TR, Thomas HE, Kannel WB: Epidemiologic assessment of chronic atrial fibrillation and risk of stroke: The Framingham Study. *Neurology* 28:973, 1978.
75. Stein B, Halperin JL, Fuster M: Should patients with atrial fibrillation be anticoagulated prior to and chronically following cardioversion? *Cardiovasc Clin* 21:231, 1990.

76. Manning WJ, Silverman DI, Gordon SPF, et al: Cardioversion from atrial fibrillation without prolonged anticoagulation with use of transesophageal echocardiography to exclude the presence of atrial thrombi. *N Engl J Med* 328:750, 1993.

77. Waxman HL, Myerburg RJ, Appel R, et al: Verapamil for control of ventricular rate in paroxysmal supraventricular tachycardia and atrial fibrillation or flutter: A double- blind randomized cross-over study. *Am Intern Med* 94:1, 1981.

78. Salerno DM, Dias VC, Kleiger RE, et al: Efficacy and safety of intravenous diltiazem for treatment of atrial fibrillation and atrial flutter: The Diltiazem Atrial Fibrillation/Flutter Study Group. *Am J Cardiol* 63:1046, 1989.

79. Platia EV, Michelson EL, Porterfield JK, Das G: Esmolol versus verapamil in the acute treatment of atrial fibrillation or atrial flutter. *Am J Cardiol* 63:925, 1989.

80. Goldman S, Probst P, Selzer A, et al: Inefficacy of "therapeutic" serum levels of digoxin in controlling the ventricular rate in atrial fibrillation. *Am J Cardiol* 35:651, 1975.

81. Lewis RV, Laing E, Moreland TA, et al: A comparison of digoxin, diltiazem, and their combination in the treatment of atrial fibrillation. *Eur Heart J* 9:279, 1988.

82. David D, Di Segni E, Klein HO, et al: Inefficacy of digitalis in the control of heart rate in patients with chronic atrial fibrillation: Beneficial effects of an added beta blocking agent. *Am J Cardiol* 44:1378, 1979.

83. Gulamhusein S, Ko P, Carruthers SG, et al: Acceleration of the ventricular response during atrial fibrillation in the Wolff-Parkinson-White syndrome after verapamil. *Circulation* 65:348, 1982.

84. Sellers T, Bashore TM, Gallagher JJ: Digitalis in the preexcitation syndrome: Analysis during atrial fibrillation. *Circulation* 56:260, 1977.

85. Garratt C, Antoniou A, Ward D, et al: Misuse of verapamil in preexcited atrial fibrillation. *Lancet* 1:367, 1989.

86. Fernster P, Comess KA, Marsh R, et al: Conversion of atrial fibrillation to sinus rhythm by acute intravenous procainamide infusion. *Am Heart J* 106:501, 1983.

87. Borgeat A, Goy J, Maendlt R, et al: Flecainide versus quinidine for conversion of atrial fibrillation to sinus rhythm. *Am J Cardiol* 58:496, 1986.

88. Bianconi L, Boccadomo R, Pappalardo A, et al: Effectiveness of intravenous propafenone for conversion of atrial fibrillation and flutter of recent onset. *Am J Cardiol* 64:335, 1989.

89. Campbell TJ, Gavaghan TP, Morgan JJ: Intravenous sotalol for the treatment of atrial fibrillation and flutter after cardiopulmonary bypass: Comparison with disopyramide and digoxin in a randomized trial. *Br Heart J* 54:86, 1985.

90. Horowitz LN, Spielman SR, Greenspan AM, et al: Use of amiodarone in the treatment of persistent and paroxysmal atrial fibrillation resistant to quinidine therapy. *J Am Coll Cardiol* 6:1402, 1985.

91. Gallagher JJ, Svenson RH, Kasell JH, et al: Catheter technique for closed-chest ablation of the atrioventricular conduction system. *N Engl J Med* 306:194, 1982.

92. Klein GJ, Sealy WL, Pritchett ELC, et al: Cryosurgical ablation of the atrioventricular node-His bundle: Long term follow up and properties of the junctional pacemaker. *Circulation* 61:8, 1980.

93. Laupacis A, Albers G, Dunn M, Feinberg W: Antithrombotic therapy in atrial fibrillation. *Chest* 102:426S, 1992.

94. Bjerkeland CJ, Orning OM: The effect of anticoagulant therapy in preventing embolism related to DC electrical cardioversion of atrial fibrillation. *Am J Cardiol* 23:208, 1969.

95. Manning WJ, Leeman DE, Gotch PJ, et al: Pulsed Doppler evaluation of atrial mechanical function after electrical cardioversion of atrial fibrillation. *J Am Coll Cardiol* 13:617, 1989.

96. The Boston Area Anticoagulation Trial for Atrial Fibrillation Investigators: The effect of low-dose warfarin on the risk of stroke in patients with nonrheumatic atrial fibrillation. *N Engl J Med* 323:1505, 1990.

97. Ezekowitz M, Bridgers S, James K, et al, for the Veterans Affairs Stroke Prevention in Nonrheumatic Atrial Fibrillation Investigators: Warfarin in the prevention of stroke associated with nonrheumatic atrial fibrillation. *N Engl J Med* 327:1406, 1992.

98. Connolly SJ, Laupacis A, Gent M, et al, for the CAFA study coinvestigators: Canadian Atrial Fibrillation Anticoagulation (CAFA) Study. *J Am Coll Cardiol* 18:349, 1991.

99. Disertori M, Inama G, Vergara G, et al: Evidence of a reentry circuit in the common type of atrial flutter in man. *Circulation* 67:434, 1983.

100. Klein GJ, Guiraudon GM, Sharma AD, et al: Demonstration of macroreentry and feasibility of operative therapy in the common type of atrial flutter. *Am J Cardiol* 57:587, 1986.

101. Haft J, Kosowsky B, Lau S, et al: Termination of atrial flutter by rapid pacing of the atrium. *Am J Cardiol* 20:239, 1967.

102. Robertson CE, Miller HC: Extreme tachycardia complicating the use of disopyramide in atrial flutter. *Br Heart J* 44:602, 1980.

103. Kunze KP, Kuck KH, Schluter M, Bleifeld W: Effect of encainide and flecainide on chronic ectopic atrial tachycardia. *J Am Coll Cardiol* 7:1121, 1986.

104. Colloridi V, Perri C, Ventriglia F, Critelli G: Oral sotalol in pediatric atrial ectopic tachycardia. *Am Heart J* 123:254, 1992.

105. Walsh EP, Saul JP, Hurse JE, et al: Transcatheter ablation of ectopic atrial tachycardia in young patients using radiofrequency current. *Circulation* 86:1138, 1992.

106. Case CL, Gillette PC, Oslizlok PC, et al: Radiofrequency catheter ablation of incessant, medically resistant supraventricular tachycardia in infants and small children. *J Am Coll Cardiol* 20:1405, 1992.

107. Prager NA, Cox JL, Lindsay BD, et al: Long-term effectiveness of surgical treatment of ectopic atrial tachycardia. *J Am Coll Cardiol* 22:85, 1993.

108. Levine JH, Michael JR, Guarnieri T: Treatment of multifocal atrial tachycardia with verapamil. *N Engl J Med* 312:21, 1985.

109. Arsura E, Lefkin AS, Scher DL, et al: A randomized, double-blind, placebo-controlled study of verapamil and metoprolol in treatment of multifocal atrial tachycardia. *Am J Med* 85:519, 1988.

110. Munger TM, Feldman BJ, Hammill SC, et al: The natural history of Wolff-Parkinson-White syndrome: A population study—Olmsted County, Minnesota: 1953–1989 (abstract). *Circulation* 82(suppl III):317, 1990.

111. Gulamhusein S, Ko P, Carruthers SG, et al: Acceleration of the ventricular response during atrial fibrillation in the Wolff-Parkinson-White syndrome. *Circulation* 56:409, 1977.

112. Sung RJ, Castellanos A, Mallon SM, et al: Mechanisms of spontaneous alternation between reciprocating tachycardia and atrial flutter-fibrillation in the Wolff-Parkinson-White syndrome. *Circulation* 56:409, 1977.

113. Sellers T, Cambell RWF, Bashore TM, et al: Effects of procainamide and quinidine sulfate in the Wolff-Parkinson-White syndrome. *Circulation* 56:260, 1977.

114. Klein GJ, Bashore TM, Sellers T, et al: Ventricular fibrillation in the Wolff-Parkinson-White syndrome. *N Engl J Med* 301:1080, 1979.

115. Gallagher JJ, Smith WM, Kassell J, et al: Use of the esophageal lead in diagnosis of mechanisms of reciprocating supraventricular tachycardias. *PACE* 3:440, 1980.

116. Benditt DG, Pritchett ELC, Smith WM, et al: Ventriculoatrial intervals: Diagnostic use in paroxysmal supraventricular tachycardia. *Ann Intern Med* 91:161, 1979.

117. Akhtar M, Shenasa M, Jazayeri M, et al: Wide QRS complex tachycardia: Reappraisal of a common clinical problem. *Ann Intern Med* 109:905, 1988.

118. Dongas J, Lehman MH, Mahmud R, et al: Value of preexisting bundle branch block in the electrographic differentiation of supraventricular from ventricular origin of wide complex tachycardia. *Am J Cardiol* 55:717, 1985.

119. Griffith MJ, Linker NJ, Ward DE, Camm AJ: Adenosine in the diagnosis of broad complex tachycardias. *Lancet* 1:672, 1988.

120. Crankin A, Goldroyd K, Chong E, et al: Value and limitations of adenosine in the diagnosis and treatment of narrow and broad complex tachycardias. *Br Heart J* 62:195, 1989.

III. Coronary Care

Section Editor
Richard C. Becker

42. Acute Heart Failure

Ronald Caputo and Roger Laham

Heart failure is a common disorder in Western society. Despite advances in the diagnosis and treatment of congestive heart failure, the incidence and prevalence of this devastating syndrome continue to increase. In 1970 the National Center for Health Statistics reported that 155,000 patients were discharged from hospitals in the United States with the diagnosis of congestive heart failure [1]. By 1982, this number had increased to 1.5 million, nearly a tenfold rise over one decade. Congestive heart failure afflicts two to four million Americans, or approximately 2 percent of the U.S. population, and 400,000 patients are diagnosed with congestive heart failure annually [2].

Heart failure may be defined as occurring when the heart is unable to either receive adequate venous return from or pump blood into the arterial system at a sufficient rate and/or quantity to meet the metabolic demands of the body. Heart failure must be differentiated from circulatory failure. The latter has been defined as inadequacy of the cardiovascular system in performing the basic functions of providing nutrition to, removing metabolic waste materials from, and providing communication between the various cells of the body. Circulatory disorders thus include aberrations in the normal structure and function of the blood vessels, those systems regulating blood vessels, blood hemoglobin content and function, blood volume, and so on, as well as disorders of the heart.

Acute heart failure must also be defined. The gradual development of chronic heart failure allows time for the body to respond through several compensatory mechanisms. Rapidly developing heart failure outpaces the body's ability to compensate through many of these mechanisms. Thus, given equal impairment of ventricular function, patients with acute heart failure would be expected to present with more impressive symptoms than patients with chronic heart failure (Table 42-1). In such patients there is an inherent need for rapid diagnostic and therapeutic intervention. Physicians caring for these patients must therefore have knowledge of the pathophysiology underlying the various forms of this disease and the rapidly available options for management. Patients with well-compensated heart failure often present with an acute exacerbation, most often due to mild disruptions or imbalances in these compensatory mechanisms. This chapter focuses on new symptoms of uncompensated heart failure, rather than decompensated chronic heart failure.

Pathophysiology

The heart may fail by several mechanisms, which may be classified according to three etiologic categories (Table 42-2). The first category includes structural abnormalities of the heart valves, pericardium, endocardium, great vessels that impede cardiac filling and emptying. The second category encompasses pathologic situations of primary myocyte dysfunction. The third category consists of alterations in the organization or signaling of cardiac contraction (i.e., dysrhythmias).

The pathophysiology of left ventricular (LV) dysfunction is described in terms of pressure or volume overload (afterload or preload). The mechanisms and consequences of these insults differ at both the macroscopic and the cellular level. The manifestations of each differ according to the duration of the insult. Pressure overload results in increased ventricular systolic wall stress, as illustrated by Laplace's law (wall stress = $P \times r/2h$, where P = pressure, r = LV radius, and h = LV wall thickness). An *acute* increase in wall stress is associated with increased myocardial oxygen consumption and a decrease in the rate and extent of sarcomere shortening [3]. This translates into impaired ventricular systolic performance and decreased cardiac output.

Table 42-1. Common Causes of Acute Heart Failure

Pressure overload	Systemic hypertension
	Aortic stenosis
	Hypertrophic cardiomyopathy
	Pulmonary embolism
	Cessation of afterload therapy
	Dysfunctional prosthetic aortic valve
Volume overload	Aortic insufficiency (trauma, dissection, ABE)
	High-output failure (thyrotoxicosis, beriberi, severe anemia)
	Cessation of diuretic therapy
Impaired ventricular filling	Mitral stenosis (RHD, MAC, myxoma)
	Tamponade (neoplasm, viral, uremia)
	Constriction (post-XRT, post-surgery)
	Restriction (amyloid, hemochromatosis)
Myocardial diseases	Myocarditis (viral, etc.)
	Dilated cardiomyopathy (ischemic, ETOH, idiopathic)
	Metabolic diseases (hypocalcemia, hypophosphatemia)
	Toxic insult (cocaine, lead, antineoplastic therapy)
Dysrhythmias	Ischemia
	Bradyarrhythmias (heart block, sick sinus, iatrogenic)
	Tachyarrhythmias (VT, SVT)

ABE = acute bacterial endocarditis; RHD = rheumatic heart disease; XRT = external beam radiation therapy; ETOH = ethanol induced; VT = ventricular tachycardia, SVT = supraventricular tachycardia.

Table 42-2. Etiologic Categories of Cardiac Failure

Impediments to cardiac filling and emptying
    Valvular disease
    Pericardial disease
    Restrictive disease
    Pulmonary embolism
    Extreme hypertension
Primary myocyte dysfunction
    Myocarditis
    Cardiomyopathies
    Toxic injury
    Metabolic disturbances
    Ischemic disease
Abnormal organization or signaling of cardiac contraction
    Tachyarrythmias
    Bradyarrhythmias
    Asystole

In the *chronic* situation the left ventricle undergoes compensatory hypertrophy (h) (through replication of sarcomeres in parallel), and there is a reduction in left ventricular cavity size (r), which leads to a normalization of systolic wall stress [4,5]. However, this compensatory hypertrophy may ultimately result in decreased left ventricular compliance and impaired diastolic filling, which may lead to elevated left-sided pressures and pulmonary edema. *Acute* volume overload results in dilatation of the compliant left ventricular cavity at low or slightly increased intraventricular pressures. Wall stress is increased. Stroke volume is enhanced due to increased sarcomere stretch and a favorable shift along the Starling curve. In *chronic* volume overload there is normalization of left ventricular wall stress through compensatory hypertrophy (replication of sarcomeres in series), which is of a lesser degree than that seen in pressure overload [6,7,8]. Compliance of the left ventricular chamber eventually decreases, leading to greater changes in left ventricular end-diastolic pressure per unit change in left ventricular end-diastolic volume and worsening of diastolic function.

The terms commonly used to describe the pathophysiologic basis and clinical manifestations of heart failure are gross descriptions at best, often incomplete and somewhat inaccurate; however, they allow for efficient interphysician communication. These descriptions help physicians to conceptualize a treatment plan targeted at ameliorating the fundamental hemodynamic abnormalities.

Systolic and *diastolic dysfunction* are frequently used to describe the abnormal function of the left ventricle in patients with heart failure (see Chap. 45). *Systolic dysfunction* refers to heart failure occurring as a result of poor contractility, while *diastolic dysfunction* generally refers to heart failure that occurs despite normal or supernormal contractility, presumably on the basis of impaired ventricular filling. The two dysfunctions usually coexist in both chronic and acute heart failure, although in acute heart failure usually one predominates.

Forward and *backward heart failure* are used to depict patients with symptomatic heart failure. *Forward failure* describes the clinical symptoms resulting from decreased forward cardiac output and tissue perfusion, including fatigue, exercise intolerance and decreased mental status. *Backward failure* describes the syndrome of tissue congestion resulting from, at least in the acute setting, increased venous hydrostatic pressure. The most notable symptom of backward failure is pulmonary edema. In acute heart failure, patients may manifest symptoms of forward failure, backward failure, or both, depending on the nature and extent of the cardiac injury.

Similarly, *right* and *left heart failure* are used to describe signs and symptoms of either right or left ventricular dysfunction. Classically, signs of right ventricular dysfunction include ascites, edema, and hepatic congestion, whereas signs of left ventricular dysfunction include pulmonary congestion and decreased tissue perfusion. Over time, because of ventricular interdependence, these isolated signs and symptoms become less distinct, and eventually signs and symptoms of both left and right ventricular dysfunction coexist. Therefore, it is more common to see signs of isolated left or right ventricular dysfunction in acute, rather than chronic, heart failure.

the insult. When faced with decreased cardiac output several mechanisms are employed to maintain tissue perfusion and oxygen delivery by increasing contractility, increasing blood volume, optimizing available perfusion to critical organs, and facilitating oxygen transfer. The duration of the insult often determines the compensatory response.

The Frank-Starling mechanism is a well-described phenomenon in which an increase in end-diastolic volume results in increased cardiac wall stretch, increased myofibril stretch, and more optimal alignment of myofibrils for cross-bridge cycling [9]. This results in an increased force of contraction; it occurs in both acute and chronic situations. In chronic heart failure myocyte hypertrophy occurs in a pattern characteristic of the hemodynamic insult (see above). This results in decreased wall tension and decreased myocardial oxygen consumption. Plasma levels of norepinephrine and epinephrine are increased systemically in acute and chronic heart failure [10,11,12]. This initially results in decreased perfusion of the peripheral tissues, increased blood flow to the central organs, increased heart rate, and increased contractility; however, these effects are modified over time due to a decrease in beta$_1$-adrenergic receptors [13] and a depletion of intramyocardial norepinephrine [11,14]. Increased extraction of oxygen by the peripheral tissues occurs immediately, resulting in a widened arteriovenous oxygen difference. Hemoglobin rapidly displays a decreased affinity for oxygen, therefore oxygen tissue delivery is enhanced. This is due to an increase in 2,3-DPG (diphosphoglycerate) and a mild lactic acidosis (resulting in part from decreased peripheral tissue perfusion and a shift to anaerobic metabolism). Over time, through the retention of sodium via activation of the renin-angiotensin-aldosterone system, blood volume is increased. This increases cardiac preload and optimizes cardiac function through the Starling mechanism.

On a cellular level heart failure induces changes in energy production and utilization and in the structure and composition of various cellular components. One variable that helps to determine these responses is duration of the insult. Chronic heart failure due to pressure overload is associated with an increase in mitochondrial mass and increased respiratory activity, without a change in the ratio of ATP produced per molecule of oxygen [13,14]. Ultrastructurally, chronic heart failure is associated with a reduction in myocyte myofibrillar ATPase [15,16]. Another ultrastructural change noted in chronic heart failure due to pressure overload is the shift in heavy chain myoglobin isoforms from predominantly A (fast) to B (slow) forms [17,18,19]. This results in reduced oxygen consumption per unit of tension developed at the expense of decreased force of contraction. This mechanism is probably not operable to a significant degree in the case of acute heart failure. Other changes, such as alterations in calcium homeostasis (prolonged calcium transient) [20,21], alteration in the regulatory G proteins (increased Gi:Gs ratio), and downregulation of adrenergic receptors, are also seen in chronic heart failure [22]. The extent of these alterations in acute heart failure is unknown; however, as these changes require altered gene expression and translation, they may not be operative to a significant degree in the acute situation.

Compensatory Mechanisms

As with any insult, when confronted with cardiac failure, the body reacts through programmed compensatory responses. These responses occur at both macroscopic and microscopic levels and vary according to the type, severity, and duration of

Diagnostic Tools

Multiple diagnostic tools are available to help decipher the etiologic problem of acute heart failure. A physician must know the strengths and weaknesses of each test before they are implemented. This is especially true in acute heart failure, as the time available to make a diagnosis is often short, and therefore the optimal test must be quickly performed. This section describes some of the common tests used assessing patients with acute heart failure and the indications for which they are best used. (See also Chapter 48.)

PULMONARY ARTERY CATHETERIZATION. Recently there has been some discussion regarding the utility of the balloon-tipped pulmonary artery catheter [23,24,25]. While debate continues, we believe hemodynamic monitoring is unequivocally useful in the following clinical circumstances:

1. When the diagnosis of cardiogenic versus noncardiogenic pulmonary edema is unclear from data obtained from the history, physical examination, or chest radiograph
2. In instances where knowledge of the patient's intravascular volume status is critical but not discernible by noninvasive means
3. For diagnostic purposes in cases of acute cardiac failure (i.e., tamponade or left-to-right shunt)
4. To assess the therapeutic efficacy of cardiotonics, vasopressors, or vasodilators by means of cardiac output and intracardiac pressures.

Descriptions and techniques for insertion of these catheters are covered in Chapter 4. Data derived from these catheters include intracardiac pressures (right atrium, right ventricle, pulmonary artery, pulmonary capillary wedge) and the oxygen saturation of blood from the various right-sided cardiac structures (superior and inferior venae cavae as well as the right heart structures mentioned above). From these data estimations of the cardiac output (by the Fick or thermodilution method), systemic vascular resistance, and peripheral vascular resistance can be made.

The pulmonary artery catheter is useful in the diagnosis of cardiac tamponade, pericardial constriction, left-to-right shunt, noncardiogenic shock or noncardiogenic pulmonary edema, and cardiogenic shock due to severe left ventricular dysfunction. In addition, the diagnosis of pulmonary embolism, severe mitral or tricuspid regurgitation, and right ventricular infarction may be suggested.

INDWELLING ARTERIAL CATHETER. The indwelling arterial catheter has a low diagnostic yield and should mainly be used for blood pressure monitoring or frequent blood gas sampling. Situations where close observation of blood pressure is indicated include hypertensive crisis, vasodilator therapy, and severe hemodynamic derangement (shock). If an arterial line is in place for the above reasons, the diagnosis of hypertensive crisis is supported by a diastolic blood pressure greater than 130 mm Hg. Cardiac tamponade may be suggested by the presence of a paradoxical pulse. Aortic insufficiency often results in a widened pulse pressure.

ECHOCARDIOGRAPHY. Transthoracic cardiac ultrasound is an extremely useful tool in patients with acute heart failure. It provides an abundance of information at little risk to the patient (see Chap. 7). A transthoracic echocardiogram provides information regarding atrial and ventricular size and function, valvular structure and function, intracardiac blood flow, anatomy of the ascending and transverse aorta, pericardium, and intracardiac masses, and right-sided cardiac pressures [26–34]. The usefulness of this test, however, is directly proportional to the quality of the study. If the study is performed by a less skilled

operator or on patients who are uncooperative or obese, have chronic obstructive pulmonary disease (COPD), or are on a ventilator, it has a lower yield. Echocardiography is justified in almost any case of acute heart failure. It is particularly helpful in assessing for the presence of cardiac tamponade, regional wall motion abnormalities (especially in patients with a history consistent with cardiac ischemia but without diagnostic ECG changes), valvular disease (especially acute mitral regurgitation or aortic regurgitation), intracardiac shunts, ventricular free wall rupture, right ventricular infarction, pulmonary embolism, and pathology of the aortic root, such as dissection [26–34]. Echocardiography is less helpful in the diagnosis of hypertensive crisis or high output failure.

TRANSESOPHAGEAL ECHOCARDIOGRAPHY. Transesophageal echocardiography (TEE) provides similar information to that provided by transthoracic studies, but it is a more technically involved procedure (see Chap. 7). For this reason, a transthoracic study should generally be performed before TEE is considered. This study may be indicated before transthoracic echocardiography in patients with suspected acute dissection of the ascending or transverse aorta. While TEE provides superior visualization of the aortic root, all heart valves, intraatrial structures, and the atrial/basal ventricular septum, the apical portion of the heart and the upper portion of the ascending aorta are not well seen [35–38]. Therefore, if pathology is suspected in these areas of the heart (ventricular septal defect, apical thrombus) TEE may not be helpful. Moreover, before TEE is seriously considered, the patient must be screened for contraindications to the procedure, primarily esophageal pathology.

CARDIAC CATHETERIZATION. By utilizing intracardiac pressure measurements, oxygen saturation data, ventriculography, aortography, and angiography, cardiac catheterization provides information regarding right and left ventricular function, valvular function, pulmonary-systemic-intracardiac hemodynamics, intracardiac shunting, aortic pathology, and coronary anatomy. In addition, the catheterization laboratory is an appropriate setting for treatment of acute heart failure because of the availability of procedures such as coronary angioplasty, intraaortic balloon counterpulsation, and pericardiocentesis (see Chap. 8 and 9). This study is appropriate for the diagnosis of ischemic cardiac failure, pericardial tamponade or constriction, valvular disease, ventricular or atrial septal defect, aortic dissection, or pulmonary embolism (pulmonary arteriogram) [39]. The evaluation of patients with cardiogenic shock should include cardiac catheterization, as it affords an opportunity for therapy in situations of ischemia and visualization of the coronary anatomy in patients who are best treated surgically. There are several *relative* contraindications to elective cardiac catheterization, such as baseline renal dysfunction, peripheral vascular disease, and allergy to radiographic contrast agents. However, in the presence of life-threatening acute heart failure it must be remembered that these are *relative* contraindications only.

COMPUTED TOMOGRAPHY. Computed tomography (CT), including ultrafast CT and gated CT, has been studied regarding its usefulness in cardiac diagnostics. It is effective in assessment of wall thickness (global and regional), myocardial mass, left ventricular volumes and ejection fraction, myocardial perfusion, the anterior and lateral pericardium, and the aorta [40,41]. However, in most of these areas information obtained through other tests is superior. In acute heart failure, the only valid indication for CT is in the assessment of aortic pathology, specifically proximal dissection. The diagnosis of aortic dissection requires demonstration of an intimal flap and is supported by the demonstration of differential enhancement of the true and false lumens and by compression of the true lumen by the thrombosed false channel [42]. It may be difficult to differentiate thrombus in the false channel from mural thrombus in an aneurysm; however, dissection is more likely if the thrombus extends more than 10 cm longitudinally. The sensitivity of this test has been reported at greater than 90 percent when compared to angiography [41]. It appears that CT is less sensitive for this diagnosis in the setting of blunt chest trauma.

MAGNETIC RESONANCE IMAGING. Magnetic resonance imaging (MRI) is rapidly developing as an important tool for the diagnosis of cardiac pathology. Wall thickness, wall motion, regional perfusion, ejection fraction, and even proximal coronary anatomy can be assessed. However, currently this information is more easily and accurately obtained using other modalities. The main strengths of MRI at this time are in the diagnosis of pericardial disease and effusion, cardiac masses, and aortic pathology [43,44,45]. In acute heart failure, the only possible indication for MRI is in the diagnosis of aortic dissection, for which it is probably superior to CT. Again, the visualization of an intraluminal flap is required, and the diagnosis is supported by a flow differential between the true and false lumens on velocity-encoded cine MRI [44]. One factor that may limit the use of MRI in the acute setting is the contraindication to magnetic objects present during the study, which prohibits its use in any patient with a metallic prosthesis, an embedded metallic foreign body, or intravenous infusion pumps.

Therapy

The general principles of therapy for acute heart failure are not different from those of any other disease. Initially, nonspecific treatment strategies aimed at short-term symptomatic benefit are employed. Next, the specific aberration responsible for the acute illness should be identified. A more directed therapeutic plan is then formed. Finally, a long-term treatment strategy is employed and plans for chronic follow-up are made. This chapter focuses on the initial stages of this paradigm.

NONSPECIFIC THERAPY. Several simple therapeutic maneuvers are beneficial in the majority of cases of acute heart failure (Table 42-3). Proper positioning of the patient is essential but often overlooked. If the patient is not hypotensive, it is helpful to position him or her in the semi-upright or sitting position. This decreases venous return from the lower extrem-

Table 42-3. Nonspecific Therapy of Acute Heart Failure

1. Place patient in proper position
2. Ensure adequate oxygenation
3. Obtain sufficient venous access
4. Optimize blood pressure
5. Rapidly determine heart rhythm (antiarrhythmic, cardioversion, pacemaker)
6. Sedate patient
7. Consider fluid restriction/diuresis
8. Rapidly diagnose cardiac pathology

ities, reducing cardiac preload. Also, ventilation perfusion mismatch due to pulmonary edema may be somewhat lessened because of a decrease in intravascular hydrostatic pressure in the upper lung fields. A hypotensive patient may achieve some benefit from the Trendelenburg position, which increases venous return from the lower extremities and enhances volume in the central circulation.

Adequate oxygenation is imperative. The increased oxygen demands of a failing heart must be met. Inadequate oxygen delivery further exacerbates pump failure, and a self-perpetuating downward spiral of poor oxygenation and depressed pump function will ensue. Immediate attempts to break this cycle must be made with the administration of supplemental oxygen. Unless the patient is known to have obstructive airway disease (and carbon dioxide retention), it is advisable to place the patient on high fraction of inspired oxygen initially and taper downward, rather than the reverse. Mechanical ventilation is occasionally necessary to deliver a high fraction of inspired oxygen or to rest fatigued respiratory muscles. Positive end-expiratory pressure (PEEP) has been used in patients placed on a ventilator in an attempt to decrease venous return to the left heart [9,46,47]. This technique is unproved, however, and should be avoided due to the possibilities of barotrauma or hypotension due to inadequate left ventricular filling and depressed cardiac output.

Adequate venous access must be obtained to administer pharmacologic therapy and/or intravenous fluids. Two large-bore (16 or 18-gauge) peripheral lines are the necessary minimum in terms of venous access, and central venous access is often needed to administer vasoactive medicine safely. If central access is obtained, initial placement of a venous sheath is recommended (see Chap. 2). This allows rapid placement of a diagnostic pulmonary artery catheter in the event it is needed.

Careful attention must be paid to correcting abnormalities in blood pressure. There is evidence that a mean arterial pressure of 70 to 80 mm Hg or greater is required for optimal perfusion of the coronary vascular bed, especially in the setting of an acute myocardial infarction [48]. At lower pressures, myocardial dysfunction due to ischemia may occur. To maintain an appropriate blood pressure, proper positioning of the patient, intravenous fluids (normal saline), or vasopressors may be utilized. Severe elevations in blood pressure may also impair cardiac function (see below) by imposing a pressure load on the left ventricle and, as mentioned previously, increasing wall stress (and MVO_2). Rapid correction of hypertension, with intravenous vasodilators if necessary, may greatly improve left ventricular systolic performance.

The cardiac rhythm must be determined rapidly and accurately. Cardiogenic shock due to ventricular fibrillation, ventricular tachycardia, or asystole is obvious. Less obvious is low cardiac output (CO = heart rate [HR] × stroke volume [SV]) secondary to bradycardia (low HR) or a supraventricular tachycardia (low SV), with or without organized atrial function. Prompt and careful attention to the 12-lead ECG (preferably) or a monitored rhythm strip may give a clue as to the etiology of the acute cardiac decompensation and help direct initial therapeutic measures.

In patients with congestive heart failure, the decrease in cardiac output and sometimes mean arterial pressure may be associated with a reduction of the renal fraction of the cardiac output. This results in a decrease of both renal plasma flow and glomerular filtration rate [49–52]. This, in addition to complex activation or inhibition of several neurohumoral systems, including the renin-angiotensin-aldosterone axis, sympathetic nervous system, hypothalamic-pituitary axis, and atrial natriuretic peptide system [53–56], leads to sodium and water retention and the inability to excrete a sodium load. Accordingly, the patient with congestive heart failure should have a diet low in salt. In the United States, the average adult consumes about 10 gm per day of sodium chloride [57]. In patients with acute heart failure, a strict low-salt diet is needed and restriction of fluid intake to less than 2 liters per day may be necessary [57]. At our institution, restriction of sodium to 2 gm per day is routine. Further fluid restriction is added as necessary.

Sedation is often an important adjunctive therapy in patients experiencing high levels of discomfort or anxiety, as in the setting of acute pulmonary edema. In this regard morphine has long been recommended [58,59]. Narcotics dull the subjective symptoms of heart failure and may thereby decrease the circulating levels of catecholamines, which themselves may increase blood pressure and MVO_2. Morphine also acts as a vasodilator, increasing venous capacitance and decreasing cardiac preload [58,59,60]. We recommend administering morphine in 2-mg increments every 10 minutes to achieve the desired effects. The main side effects of morphine are hypotension, depression of central respiratory drive, nausea, and an idiosyncratic allergic reaction [58,59] (see Chap. 155).

A therapy previously used for decreasing cardiac preload but rarely used today is the application of tourniquets to each extremity in rotating fashion for a period of 15 minutes [60]. This may be effective therapy in extreme emergencies or when optimal medical support is delayed or unavailable.

IDENTIFICATION OF A SPECIFIC PROCESS. Once these general measures of therapy have been implemented, a search for the specific cause of the acute heart failure must be immediately undertaken. Information obtained from patient history, physical examination, chest radiography, and electrocardiography often narrows the differential diagnosis to the extent that a single confirmatory test may be utilized. When the diagnosis remains vague after expedient but careful examination of the initial data, it is advisable to perform a test that yields information regarding several aspects of cardiac function, such as cardiac catheterization or echocardiography (see above). Such tests obviously have a higher diagnostic yield than more selective tests. Even if a specific diagnosis is not made, one might be suggested, and therapy along those lines may be initiated while the patient awaits a more definitive diagnostic test. Once a secure diagnosis is made, therapy can be directed at the underlying pathology with the hope of reversing or ameliorating the disease process.

PHARMACOLOGIC THERAPY. The concept of using single or combined pharmacologic agents to improve the hemodynamic status of patients with uncompensated heart failure is fairly straightforward (Table 42-4). One strategy is to improve the pumping function of the heart directly; another strategy is

Table 42-4. Pharmacologic Therapies

Diuretics	Thiazide (metolazone, chlorthiazide)
	Loop (furosemide, bumetanide)
Nitrates	
Inotropic agents and vasopressors	Sympathomimetic amines (dopamine, etc.)
	Phosphodiesterase inhibitors (amrinone)
	Cardiac glycosides (digitalis)
	Miscellaneous inotropic agents
Afterload reducers	ACE inhibitors
	Hydralazine
	Nitroprusside

to optimize or normalize hemodynamic status by altering other components of the circulatory system. An oversimplified but useful description of the altered hemodynamics that occur secondary to acute congestive heart failure will help illustrate the possible utility of the pharmacologic agents now in use. Decreased cardiac output occurs as a result of a diminution in the stroke volume that is not completely compensated for by an increase in heart rate. Systemic arterial pressure becomes low, causing reflex activation of the sympathetic nervous system and fluid retention; this, in turn, results in increased systemic vascular resistance (SVR) and increased central venous pressure (CVP) [57,61]. Left ventricular filling pressures rise due to increased left ventricular end-diastolic volume (LVEDV), impaired left ventricular relaxation, and increased plasma volume. This pressure is transmitted back to the left atrium and pulmonary venous bed, resulting in an increase in pulmonary capillary wedge pressure (PCWP). If the PCWP exceeds the combined plasma oncotic pressure and tissue hydrostatic pressure and the rate of fluid extravasation into the extravascular space exceeds the rate of pulmonary drainage, then pulmonary edema will ensue. In addition, increased right-sided filling pressures may impair the drainage of the coronary veins, resulting in decreased myocardial perfusion and increased myocardial turgor, which further decreases left ventricular and right ventricular compliance. Furthermore, elevation in right ventricular pressure and volume may alter left ventricular function because of the interdependence of both ventricles, which is determined by the common interventricular septum and surrounding pericardium. Treatment strategies for acute congestive heart failure include (1) decreasing cardiac preload, (2) inotropic support, (3) circulatory support, and (4) afterload reduction.

Decreasing Cardiac Preload

DIURETICS. The importance of diuretics in the treatment of congestive heart failure relates to the central role of the kidneys as the target organ of many of the neurohumoral and hemodynamic changes that occur in response to the failing myocardium [49,57,62]. Diuresis results in fluid loss and a decline in ventricular filling pressures in most patients with congestive heart failure.

A variety of diuretic agents are available. Overtreatment must be avoided, since the resultant hypovolemia may further decrease cardiac output. The acute use of these agents is occasionally associated with untoward effects such as hypokalemia, hypomagnesemia, hyponatremia, hypotension, allergic reactions, hearing impairment, and gouty attacks.

Thiazide Diuretics. The thiazide diuretics include a number of chemically and pharmacologically similar agents, the prototype of which is chlorothiazide (Diuril) (see Chap. 210) [61,63]. The usual dose of chlorothiazide is 500 to 1000 mg orally or intravenously once or twice daily. Metolazone (Zaroxolyn) is a quinazololine diuretic with properties generally similar to those of the thiazide diuretics and is effective in combination with loop diuretics in refractory congestive heart failure [64]. The adult dose is 5 to 10 mg orally once daily.

Loop Diuretics. Ethacrynic acid was the first available loop diuretic, followed by furosemide (Lasix) and bumetanide (Bumex) [65,66] (see Chap. 210). The drugs can be administered orally or intravenously. Both bumetanide and furosemide have reduced natriuretic effect when administered orally in patients with congestive heart failure, in part because of delayed intestinal absorption and delivery of the drug to its tubular site of action [65–68]. In acute congestive heart failure, these agents should be administered intravenously. The intravenous dose of ethacrynic acid is 0.5 to 1 mg per kilogram not to exceed 100 mg up to twice daily. The intravenous dose of furosemide is 20 to 200 mg every 2 hours up to 1000 mg daily. The intravenous dose of bumetanide is 0.5 to 2 mg every 2 to 3 hours up to a total daily dose of 20 mg. These agents acutely reduce venous capacitance; the initial benefit of these drugs may result from reduction in cardiac preload. Rapid administration of these agents may precipitate or exacerbate hypotension.

NITRATES. Nitroglycerin produces a striking reduction in right and left ventricular filling pressures [69,70] (see Chap. 210). The pulmonary vasodilating and slight systemic arteriolar dilating effects are sufficient to cause a modest increase in cardiac output in patients with congestive heart failure [70]. Nitrates can be used intravenously, orally, or topically. Arteriolar vasodilation may be more significant with intravenous administration [71]. Pharmacologic tolerance may develop with prolonged use, blunting the beneficial hemodynamic effects [72,73]. This may be due to a combination of depletion of sulfhydryl groups in vascular smooth muscle and to countervailing neurohormonal activation [71]. Intermittent therapy can effectively obviate this problem. A recommended starting dose of intravenous nitroglycerine for the treatment of acute congestive heart failure is 10 μg per minute, titrated to the desired effect.

Increasing Contractility. Inotropic agents play an important role in the pharmacologic management of patients with acute congestive heart failure. We divide them into sympathomimetic amines, phosphodiesterase inhibitors, and cardiac glycosides.

SYMPATHOMIMETIC AMINES. Catecholamines and other sympathomimetic amines exert potent inotropic effects by interacting with myocardial beta-adrenoreceptors.

Dopamine. Dopamine, a naturally occurring catecholamine, is the immediate biosynthetic precursor of norepinephrine. Dopamine increases cardiac contractility by a direct stimulation of myocardial beta$_1$-adrenergic receptors and indirectly through sympathetic nerve terminal release of norepinephrine [74,75,76]. Dopamine stimulates dopamine$_1$-receptors, resulting in coronary, renal, mesenteric, and cerebral arterial vasodilation, through activation of the adenylyl cyclase enzyme [76,77,78]. In addition, it stimulates the dopamine$_2$-receptors, resulting in vasodilation by inhibiting sympathetic nerve terminals [78]. When larger doses are administered, vasoconstriction results from activation of alpha$_1$-adrenergic and serotonin receptors [79].

The effects of dopamine are dose-dependent. With infusion rates below 2 μg/kg/min, the major effect of dopamine is to vasodilate the renal, coronary, and mesenteric circulation. Doses of 2 to 5 μg/kg/min exert a positive inotropic effect with little change in heart rate and variable effect on the vascular beds. With infusion rates higher than 5 μg/kg/min, there is an increase in arterial pressure, peripheral vascular resistance, and heart rate [74,75,76]. We have occasionally noted a predominant vasodilatory effect at doses up to 12–14 μg/kg/min. Dopamine increases coronary blood flow secondary to the increase in myocardial oxygen consumption and in part due to a direct coronary vasodilation at lower doses [80].

Thus, dopamine can be useful in patients with acute congestive heart failure who are hypotensive or have decreased urine output. Care must be taken, however, to avoid an excessive increase in heart rate and peripheral vascular resistance (seen at higher infusion rates). In normotensive patients, dopamine should be started at low rates and gradually increased to achieve the desired response. In the presence of hypotension, higher infusion rates may be appropriately used.

Dobutamine. Dobutamine (Dobutrex) is a synthetic sympathomimetic amine composed of two stereoisomers, levodobutamine and dextrodobutamine, in a 1:1 racemic mixture. Levodobutamine is primarily an alpha$_1$-adrenergic agonist having vasoconstrictive effects, and dextrodobutamine stimulates beta$_1$- and beta$_2$-adrenergic receptors, thus increasing myocar-

dial contractility and promoting vasodilation. Dextrodobutamine also appears to have some alpha-adrenergic receptor blocking activity [81,82,83]. The adrenergic agonist effects of dobutamine are such that beta$_1$ selectivity is greater than beta$_2$ selectivity, which is greater than alpha$_1$ selectivity, with a net effect of increasing contractility while producing vasodilation. In clinically effective doses of up to 40 μg/kg/min, dobutamine directly stimulates myocardial beta$_1$-adrenergic receptors and is almost devoid of clinically relevant beta$_2$ or alpha-adrenergic effects [82]. Dobutamine increases renal blood flow by increasing cardiac output [83]. In patients with heart failure, the hemodynamic profile of dobutamine is characterized by a consistent increase in cardiac output and stroke volume and decrease in peripheral and pulmonary vascular resistance and pulmonary capillary wedge pressure [84]. Dobutamine has been administered to patients with acute myocardial infarction without provoking undesirable side effects and without increasing the extent of myocardial injury [85]. Improvement in cardiac index (mean increase 54%) and stroke work index (mean increase 65%) has also been reported in response to dobutamine infusion in patients with heart failure secondary to ischemic heart disease, with infrequent precipitation of overt myocardial ischemia [86,87].

The usual dosage ranges from 2.5 to 20 μg/kg/min, although occasionally doses as low as 0.5 or as high as 40 μg/kg/min have been used. Vasodilation, through direct alpha adrenergic blockade or reflex mechanisms, can sometimes result in hypotension. It is important to be certain by clinical examination or invasive monitoring that hypovolemia is not present. Sinus tachycardia and other cardiac arrhythmias are important adverse effects.

Norepinephrine. Norepinephrine (Levophed) is the naturally occurring cardiac catecholamine. It stimulates both alpha- and beta$_1$-adrenergic receptors and thus has both vasoconstrictive and positive inotropic properties. Its hemodynamic effects are variable, depending on the dosage and clinical setting. With small doses, cardiac output and arterial blood pressure are increased. With larger doses, vascular resistance is markedly increased and cardiac output may actually fall, despite the positive inotropic effect of the drug. However, norepinephrine increases myocardial oxygen consumption and causes further vasoconstriction in a syndrome where excessive vasoconstriction has already occurred. Accordingly, norepinephrine, if needed, should be administered in the smallest effective dose, with frequent attempts at withdrawal. It is usually started at an intravenous rate of 1 to 2 μg per minute in refractory cardiogenic shock, after other therapeutic modalities have failed [88].

PHOSPHODIESTERASE INHIBITORS. The mechanism of action of this class of agents is through the inhibition of phosphodiesterase III, an enzyme responsible for the breakdown of cyclic AMP [88,89]. This raises intracellular cyclic AMP concentration, which in turn is responsible for both the positive inotropic and vasodilator effects of these agents [90]. Increased cyclic AMP levels activate a protein kinase that enhances the slow calcium inward current [90,91].

Amrinone. Amrinone is a bipyridine derivative that exerts both direct positive inotropic effect and direct systemic vasodilator actions. In patients with heart failure it causes dose-dependent increases in cardiac output and reductions in right- and left-sided filling pressures and systemic vascular resistance [92]. Its effects are additive to those of the digitalis glycosides and are synergistic with sympathomimetic amines. The vasodilator action of amrinone tends to offset the effects of the positive inotropic action, resulting in little change in myocardial oxygen consumption [93]. Amrinone facilitates atrioventricular conduction, resulting in an acceleration of ventricular rate in patients with atrial fibrillation [94].

· Intravenous amrinone is useful in the treatment of acute heart failure as an alternative or adjunctive to dobutamine. After an initial bolus of 0.75 mg per kilogram, it is administered as an infusion at the rate of 5 to 10 μg/kg/min [95]. It is particularly useful in patients with postcardiac surgical myocardial depression [94] and in some patients with acute myocardial infarction and left ventricular failure [95,96]. The vasodilator effect of amrinone may induce hypotension in patients with hypovolemia.

DIGITALIS GLYCOSIDES. Digitalis has been used for more than 200 years. Its role in the treatment of chronic heart failure has been highly controversial, particularly among patients with normal sinus rhythm. Digoxin is the most widely used digitalis glycoside. Recent controlled studies showed that digoxin improves the symptoms and exercise tolerance of patients with normal sinus rhythm and impaired ventricular systolic function [97,98]. The use of digitalis in acute congestive heart failure is limited by its delayed onset of action, except in patients with atrial fibrillation and a rapid ventricular rate, in whom it may help control the ventricular response. Patients with acute heart failure related to ventricular systolic dysfunction who are already on digitalis should be continued on it to prevent worsening of their heart failure [98,99].

Decreasing Cardiac Afterload

SODIUM NITROPRUSSIDE. Sodium nitroprusside is probably the most widely used vasodilator in the treatment of acute congestive heart failure [100] (see Chap. 210). It is particularly useful in patients with severe hypertension associated with left ventricular failure, severe heart failure with mitral and/or aortic regurgitation, acute myocardial infarction, and heart failure after cardiac surgery [101]. The initial infusion rate in adults is usually 10 μg per minute, increased to achieve the desired effect, and the maximum dose is 300 μg per minute. Sodium nitroprusside has a rapid onset of action and a short half-life of 1 to 3 minutes. Its main side effect is excessive hypotension. In addition, sodium nitroprusside may lead to hypoxemia in patients with pulmonary disease secondary to the perfusion of poorly ventilated alveoli. If sodium nitroprusside is used for a prolonged period, particularly in patients with renal insufficiency, thiocyanate toxicity may ensue (thiocyanate, the metabolite of nitroprusside, is excreted by the kidneys). Accordingly, thiocyanate levels should be monitored and maintained below 6 mg per deciliter if sodium nitroprusside is used for more than 2 to 3 days.

ANGIOTENSIN-CONVERTING ENZYME (ACE) INHIBITORS. In patients with heart failure, ACE inhibition causes a decrease in left and right ventricular filling pressure and a modest increase in cardiac output [103] (see Chap. 210). The ACE inhibitors are becoming the agents of choice for the treatment of chronic congestive heart failure, with an improvement in symptoms, hemodynamic parameters, and mortality [102–105]. Their use in acute heart failure has not been adequately studied, although they appear to be beneficial in patients with an acute myocardial infarction and an ejection fraction less than 40 percent. Of the numerous approved ACE inhibitors, the ones most extensively studied in heart failure are captopril and enalapril. Captopril (Capoten) is started at 6.25 mg three times daily and increased as tolerated to 50 mg three times daily. The starting dose of enalapril (Vasotec) is 2.5 mg daily, increased to 10 to 20 mg twice daily. Enalaprilat (Vasotec I.V.), the active metabolite of the orally administered enalapril, has been approved for the treatment of hypertension and is administered in doses of 1.25 mg every 6 hours. The major side effects of ACE inhibitors are hypotension, renal insufficiency, and hyperkalemia.

HYDRALAZINE AND OTHER VASODILATORS. In congestive heart failure, hydralazine increases cardiac output with a minor reduction in ventricular filling and arterial pressure and a minor increase in heart rate [106] (see Chap. 210). The usual dosage is 25 to 100 mg three to four times daily. The combined use of nitrates appears to add to its benefit. It is a second-line agent in the treatment of chronic heart failure and should be used only when ACE inhibitors are not tolerated [107]. Other vasodilators include prazocin, calcium antagonists, and flosequinan.

CIRCULATORY SUPPORT

Vasopressors. In patients whose mean arterial pressure is less than 70 mm Hg, norepinephrine or high-dose dopamine should be used promptly to restore blood pressure and perfusion to the vital organ and the coronary circulation. Their vasoconstrictive effects, particularly in the case of norepinephrine, with its unopposed alpha-mediated vasoconstrictive effects, reduce peripheral tissue perfusion and greatly increase the afterload determinant of myocardial oxygen consumption. These effects are detrimental in what may already be a state of severe organ hypoperfusion [108]; this necessitates limiting the use of these agents and instituting other measures for circulatory support. The hemodynamic effects of dopamine at moderate doses (5–15 μg/kg/min) are dependent on the net interactions of $beta_1$- and alpha-adrenergic stimulation; mean arterial pressure, pulmonary capillary wedge pressure, stroke volume, and heart rate often rise. In doses above 15 to 20 μg/kg/min, dopamine predominantly produces peripheral alpha-adrenergic effects, increasing total peripheral resistance and blood pressure. Cardiac irritability and increased myocardial oxygen consumption are not uncommon at these high doses [77]. Norepinephrine increases blood pressure primarily by its potent alpha-adrenergic effects, which increase systemic arterial and venous pressure and total peripheral resistance.

Intraaortic Balloon Counterpulsation. Intraaortic balloon pumping reduces S–T segment abnormalities in patients with acute myocardial infarction or unstable angina, and it is effective in the treatment of angina unresponsive to medical therapy [109] (see Chap. 9). In patients with cardiogenic shock due to acute myocardial infarction, intraaortic balloon pumping improved left ventricular function and systemic hemodynamics and prevented ventricular dilation at 2 weeks, but had no mortality benefit [110]. Intraaortic balloon pumping may be useful in rescue angioplasty following failed thrombolysis [111]. Other indications include mechanical complications of acute myocardial infarction, such as acute ventricular septal defect and mitral regurgitation [112,113], inability to wean from cardiopulmonary bypass support [114], and prophylactic applications, including patients with left main stenosis awaiting surgery [115].

Vascular complications remain the major risk of intraaortic balloon pumping. Presence of peripheral vascular disease, female gender, diabetes mellitus, and prolonged support are risk factors for vascular complications [116]. Other complications include platelet reduction, hemolysis, aortic damage, embolic events, and balloon rupture.

Left Ventricular Assist Devices. External pulsatile assist devices have been used successfully in both bridge-to-transplant and postcardiotomy cardiogenic shock patients [117,118] (see Chap. 10). Except as a bridge to transplant, the use of these devices in acute heart failure has not been adequately studied.

The femorofemoral ECMO (extracorporeal membrane oxygenator) and the Hemopump have not been studied in acute heart failure. Advances in immunosuppression and transplant management have made cardiac transplantation an established and accepted treatment for end-stage heart failure.

Diagnosis and Management in Specific Scenarios

PRESSURE OVERLOAD

Hypertension. The magnitude of hypertension required to precipitate acute heart failure depends on a patient's baseline cardiac function. In the case of malignant hypertension-hypertensive crisis (defined as a diastolic pressure > 130 mm Hg and evidence of end organ compromise) left ventricular dysfunction and acute heart failure may occur in patients with normal baseline function [119] (see Chap. 52).

Initial management of a patient with hypertension and acute heart failure centers on rapid reduction of blood pressure, using intravenous medications (nitroglycerin, enalapril, or nitroprusside) if necessary. If baseline cardiac function is unknown, then an echocardiogram is helpful in providing information regarding the most appropriate pharmacologic therapy. For example, a patient with left ventricular hypertrophy and normal or supernormal systolic function may achieve maximum benefit from an antihypertensive that improves diastolic function. A patient with a dilated left ventricle and low ejection fraction might improve dramatically with a drug that reduces cardiac afterload. If hypertension precipitates ischemic left ventricular dysfunction, then an agent with antihypertensive and antiischemic properties is ideal. Long-term therapy should, of course, include the resolution of any condition predisposing to secondary hypertension [119,120].

Aortic Stenosis. Aortic stenosis does not develop acutely, except in the case of prosthetic valve dysfunction. Patients with aortic stenosis can, however, present with acute heart failure [121]. This occurs when there is a sudden alteration in the compensatory balance on which these patients depend. The gradient across the valve varies proportionately to the cardiac output and in inverse proportion to heart rate and systolic ejection period:

$$\sqrt{P} = \frac{CO/(SEP \times HR)}{AVA}$$

(P = pressure gradient, CO = cardiac output, SEP = systolic ejection period, HR = heart rate, and AVA = aortic valve area) [122]; anything that alters these parameters will increase the transvalvular gradient. Common examples include myocardial infarction, hypertension, or tachycardia secondary to a noncardiac stress or atrial fibrillation with a rapid ventricular response [123]. In many such cases these patients have been previously diagnosed with aortic stenosis. In other cases, the diagnosis is suspected when physical examination reveals findings typical of aortic stenosis (delayed carotid upstrokes, a harsh systolic crescendo decrescendo murmur at the upper right sternal border, laterally displaced precordial impulse; see Chap. 33).

Acute heart failure associated with aortic stenosis is best managed by treating the precipitating event. By correcting heart rate, rhythm, contractility, and blood pressure toward normal, the pressure/wall stress mismatch is also normalized and left ventricular function is consequently improved. In the case of atrial fibrillation, for example, cardioversion can restore sinus rhythm, control heart rate, and eventually restore atrial systole [124]. All of these changes have a favorable effect on left ventricular function and systemic hemodynamics. Rarely, symptoms persist despite treatment of the acute precipitants. In these cases balloon aortic valvuloplasty or aortic valve replacement must be considered.

Hypertrophic Cardiomyopathy. There are several forms of cardiac hypertrophy (see Chap. 33). Therapy for acute heart failure that occurs in the setting of hypertrophic cardiomyopathy centers an improving diastolic left ventricular function and reducing the ventricular gradient if present. This is best accomplished using medicines that slow heart rate, enhance ventricular relaxation, and decrease the force of contraction. Beta-blockers (such as metoprolol, 25 mg q12h, titrated up to a maximal dose of 400 mg/day) and calcium channel blockers, particularly verapamil (maximal tolerated dose: starting with 40 mg q8h, up to a maximal dose of 480 mg/day) [125], have been shown to be effective. Disopyramide (Disopyramide immediate-release, 100 mg q8h, titrated up to a maximal dose of Disopyramide extended-release, 300 mg q12h) has also been used with some success [126], and ventricular pacing may provide some benefit [127]. A critical mistake is the use of inotropic agents in these patients. These drugs speed the heart rate, impair diastolic relaxation, and exacerbate the intraventricular gradient. Diuretics must be used cautiously as volume depletion also increases the intraventricular gradient. It may be worthwhile to perform an echocardiogram to rule out hypertrophic cardiomyopathy in patients with left ventricular hypertrophy who present with acute heart failure and do not respond to inotropic support.

Pulmonary Embolism. Pulmonary embolism is not an uncommon medical problem and is probably underdiagnosed [128,129] (see Chap. 60). Acute pulmonary embolism results in decreased flow across the pulmonary bed, decreased left ventricular filling, and diminished cardiac output. Severe pressure overload of the right ventricle occurs when more than 50 percent of the cross-sectional area of the pulmonary vascular bed is occluded by embolus. Because of ventricular interdependence, left ventricular diastolic pressure may increase, resulting in a further decrease in left ventricular filling. Oxygenation is compromised due to the development of ventilation/perfusion mismatch [130].

The diagnosis of pulmonary embolism may be suspected from the history, which should include a careful search for factors that predispose to pulmonary embolism. Therapy for pulmonary embolism is discussed in detail in Chapter 60. It must be emphasized that if life-threatening pulmonary embolism is suspected, definitive therapy must be initiated immediately, even without the benefit of pulmonary angiography in extreme cases. Surgical embolectomy remains the most definitive treatment, although thrombolytic agents and catheter embolectomy have been used with some success.

Acute Cessation of Afterload Therapy. Since afterload reduction (with ACE inhibitors or hydralazine) has been shown to be an important and effective therapy for left ventricular pressure overload, many patients suffering from long-standing heart failure are maintained on these medicines chronically. Abrupt cessation of such therapy can often precipitate an acute exacerbation of heart failure. The possibility of nonadherence to a medical regimen must therefore be examined when such patients present with these symptoms.

Dysfunction of Prosthetic Aortic Valve. The syndrome of a thrombosed prosthetic aortic valve is exceptionally rare (<0.5% per 100 patient years) and is almost always associated with mechanical valves and suboptimal systemic anticoagulation [131,132,133]. Patients present with acute heart failure due to acute pressure overload and/or syncope as well as altered prosthetic heart sounds. The diagnosis should be immediately suspected and confirmed by an echocardiogram. Immediate surgical therapy is indicated.

VOLUME OVERLOAD

Aortic Regurgitation. There are several causes of acute aortic insufficiency, the most common being dissection of the aortic root, trauma, infective endocarditis, rheumatic fever, rupture of a sinus of Valsalva aneurysm, or prosthetic valve dysfunction (see Chap. 37). Acute exacerbation of chronic aortic insufficiency can occur in many situations, including syphilis, collagen vascular diseases, rheumatic diseases, Marfan's syndrome, cystic medial necrosis, aortitis (Takayasu's syndrome), and myxomatous degeneration. The diagnosis should be entertained in patients known to have a history of, or consistent with, any of the above diseases and new onset heart failure. The management of acute aortic insufficiency must be expedient, because often these patients quickly decompensate (see Chap. 37).

High-Output Heart Failure. There are certain circumstances in which heart failure can occur in the setting of a "supernormal" cardiac output, termed *high-output failure*. Increased cardiac output is due mainly to either increased circulatory volume (preload) or decreased peripheral resistance (afterload), although heart rate and contractility are also mildly increased. Specific causes of high-output failure include anemia, thyrotoxicosis, beriberi, arteriovenous fistulas, Paget's disease, polyostotic fibrous dysplasia (Albright's syndrome), cirrhosis, and carcinoid. Pathophysiologically, pulmonary or systemic congestion occurs secondary to a sustained rise in left ventricular diastolic pressure. This is due to increased end-systolic volume and a shortened diastolic filling period that is a consequence of tachycardia [134,135].

High-output failure should be suspected in patients with a mild to moderate tachycardia, a flow murmur, an S_3 gallop, bounding pulses, and other physical findings similar to those of aortic insufficiency (e.g., Derozier's syndrome, Quincke's syndrome). Hemodynamic measurements reveal increased cardiac index, normal or reduced arteriovenous oxygen differential, low SVR, and increased right and left heart pressures.

Although the development of high-output failure is not an acute process, the congestive symptoms may appear abruptly. Typically, symptoms appear when cardiac output, although remaining at supernormal levels, begins to decline slightly [135]. The time frame in which this happens depends partially on baseline ventricular function. Initial therapy includes reduction of circulatory volume with diuretics and, in some instances (thyrotoxicosis), controlling heart rate with beta-blockers. Long-term therapy is focused on treating the underlying pathologic process, for example thyroid ablation, correction of anemia, and thiamine supplementation.

Acute Cessation of Diuretic Therapy. Acute exacerbation of heart failure secondary to volume overload frequently occurs in patients who fail to adhere to chronic diuretic therapy or low-salt diet. Patients with known left ventricular dysfunction should thus be questioned in a nonjudgmental manner regarding adherence to their medical regimen and regarding the specific side effects known to occur with their medicines. If a particular medicine is not well tolerated it should be stopped and another substituted, in the hope of improving compliance and preventing future episodes of heart failure.

IMPAIRED LEFT VENTRICULAR FILLING

Mitral Stenosis. Mitral stenosis (MS) is occasionally associated with acute heart failure. The incidence in the United States is declining. Rheumatic heart disease remains the most common cause of valvular MS; other etiologies include congenital malformations (cor triatriatum), carcinoid, collagen vascular diseases (lupus, rheumatoid), methysergide therapy, severe calcification of the mitral annulus, and obstruction due to myxoma or thrombus [9]. Mitral stenosis is usually considered mild when the valve area is approximately 2.0 cm² and severe when the valve area reaches 1.0 cm² or less [39]. Symptoms of MS other than pulmonary congestion are uncommon but include hemoptysis, chest pain, and thromboembolic phenomena (see Chaps. 60 and 61).

Acute heart failure is typically precipitated by tachycardia or increased circulatory volume. When heart rate increases, the portion of the cardiac cycle that shortens most is diastole. This allows less time for blood flow across the stenotic orifice, and consequently left atrial pressure and pulmonary capillary pressure rise. The Gorlin formula:

$$\sqrt{P}\,\frac{CO/(HR \times DFP)}{MVA}$$

(P = pressure gradient, CO = cardiac output, DFP = diastolic filling period, HR = heart rate, and MVA = mitral valve area) suggests that for any increase in cardiac output the pressure gradient across the mitral valve increases by a power of 2 [122]. This explains why an increased cardiac output precipitates symptoms in the setting of MS.

The diagnosis of MS can be strongly suspected in patients who give a history of rheumatic fever and develop pulmonary edema in situations associated with an increased heart rate (exertion, fever, atrial fibrillation) or increased circulatory volume (pregnancy) [136]. Physical examination reveals a normal precordial impulse or right ventricular heave, accentuated S_1, and characteristic diastolic opening snap and low-pitched apical rumbling murmur. The ECG shows left atrial enlargement in the 90 percent of patients with significant MS who remain in sinus rhythm [39]. Atrial fibrillation is common. Patients with long-standing MS and pulmonary hypertension often manifest right ventricular hypertrophy on ECG. Chest radiography reveals a normal left ventricle, enlarged left atrium, and often right ventricular hypertrophy. Echocardiography provides information regarding the thickness of the mitral valve and subvalvular apparatus, leaflet mobility, degree of calcification of the mitral valve and annulus, and presence of regurgitation. These are all components of the balloon mitral valvuloplasty score, which has been shown to correlate with short- and long-term outcome following this procedure [137]. Valve area, left atrial size, and presence of left atrial thrombus can also be determined. Transesophageal echocardiography seems to provide fairly accurate results regarding the latter. Cardiac catheterization, with exercise if indicated, provides invaluable information regarding intracardiac pressures, valve size, and presence and degree of pulmonary hypertension.

Acute and chronic medical therapy centers on controlling heart rate and reducing circulatory volume. Beta-blockers or digoxin combined with diuretics are an effective time-tested combination. Anticoagulation should be strongly considered, as there is a high incidence of thromboembolic complications in these patients irrespective of the presence of atrial fibrillation. Antibiotic prophylaxis for endocarditis must be administered before any procedure associated with a high likelihood of a transient bacteremia. Definitive therapy such as balloon mitral valvuloplasty, mitral valve repair, or mitral valve replacement (in that order) should be considered for patients with significant pulmonary hypertension or severe recurrent symptoms.

Prosthetic (Mitral) Valve Dysfunction. Thrombosis of the mechanical prosthetic valve is more common in the mitral than in the aortic position. The particular type of device affects the rate of thrombosis, with the Bjork Shiley valve having a significantly higher incidence than other tilting disc, or even ball-and-cage, prostheses [138]. A characteristic clinical syndrome associated with thrombosis of the prosthetic mitral valve consists of 1 to 3 days of progressive dyspnea, orthopnea, malaise, and altered prosthetic heart sounds. These symptoms are caused by a hemodynamic situation similar to mitral stenosis, with decreased left ventricular filling and increased left atrial pressures. Therefore, on patient presentation this syndrome should be rapidly suspected and a diagnostic echocardiogram performed. Cardiac catheterization is not usually needed. Immediate reoperation is the therapy of choice.

Pericardial Diseases. Pericardial tamponade is fairly common in the intensive care setting (see Chap. 34). Acute tamponade is usually secondary to infection, pericardial hemorrhage (often due to perforation), trauma, or proximal aortic dissection and can be caused by as little as 150 to 200 ml of fluid [9]. Chronic tamponade is caused by collagen vascular diseases, uremia, infection, neoplasm, and hypothyroidism. It can be associated with fluid accumulations of 1 to 2 liters or more. However, these patients can present acutely, as their ability to compensate for a decreased cardiac output chronically is rapidly outstripped by a progressive increase in pericardial pressure or sudden volume depletion. The diagnosis and treatment of pericardial tamponade are discussed in Chapter 34.

Constrictive Heart Disease. Pericardial constriction impairs diastolic filling and causes heart failure due to rising intracardiac pressures, even though systolic function is normal. Although this is not an acute process, patients can present with new symptoms of dyspnea and orthopnea secondary to progressive disease or an acute volume load. See Chapter 34 for a complete discussion of diagnosis and treatment.

Restrictive Heart Disease. The hallmark of the restrictive cardiomyopathies is abnormal diastolic function. A variety of specific pathologic processes, such as amyloidosis, hemochromatosis, scleroderma, carcinoid, or Hurler's disease, may result in restrictive cardiomyopathy, although the cause often remains unknown [124,139]. The clinical and hemodynamic features of restrictive cardiomyopathy resemble those of chronic constrictive pericarditis, as impaired ventricular filling is characteristic of both diseases [124,140].

These two processes can sometimes be differentiated at cardiac catheterization, because in restrictive disease left ventricular end-diastolic pressure is often greater than right ventricular end-diastolic pressure. Also, the magnitude of elevation of right heart pressures is often greater in restrictive disease (RV systolic > 60 mm Hg) [39]. Exercise intolerance, resulting from the inability to increase cardiac output without compromising ventricular filling, is a frequent symptom. Patients with restrictive cardiomyopathy may occasionally present with acute congestive heart failure. Treatment consists of cautious preload reduction (i.e., diuresis). Afterload reduction may be useful in the presence of systolic left ventricular dysfunction. Digitalis glycosides and calcium channel blockers [141] should be used with great caution in patients with cardiac amyloidosis because of the increased risk of toxicity probably related to selective binding to amyloid fibrils.

MYOCARDIAL DISEASES

Myocarditis. Myocarditis is an inflammatory process that involves the myocardium, may be an acute or a chronic process, and may occcur in the peripartum period. Acute heart failure can occur with acute fulminant myocarditis [142,143]. In North America, viruses are presumed to be the most common agents producing myocarditis, while in South America, Chagas disease (*Trypanosoma cruzi*) is far more common [144]. Among viruses, Coxsackie B virus is the most frequent cause of viral myocarditis [145]. The diagnosis is usually clinical. The ECG may show S–T segment and T wave abnormalities as well as various conduction abnormalities. Echocardiography demonstrates some degree of left ventricular dysfunction, which can be regional [146]. Radionuclide scanning using ^{67}Ga, [11]In antimyosin antibody, or ^{99}Tc pyrophosphate may identify inflammatory and necrotic changes in the myocardium [147]. Endomyocardial biopsy is used to confirm the diagnosis, though a borderline or negative biopsy does not exclude the diagnosis because of the focal nature of the disease [148].

Therapy is usually supportive, with prolonged bed rest, digitalis, diuretics, and afterload reduction with ACE inhibitors. The use of corticosteroids is controversial. Antimicrobial agents may be used with susceptible infections.

Cardiomyopathies

IDIOPATHIC DILATED CARDIOMYOPATHY. Dilated cardiomyopathy is a syndrome characterized by cardiac enlargement and impaired systolic function of one or both ventricles. This condition most probably represents the end result of a variety of disease processes involving the myocardium. The disease is most common in middle age and is more frequent in men than in women. The course of dilated cardiomyopathy is usually one of progressive deterioration [149]. Symptoms commonly develop gradually and are usually the result of left ventricular failure with weakness, easy fatiguability, and dyspnea on exertion [149,150]. Patients with dilated cardiomyopathy can present with acute congestive heart failure.

Treatment usually consists of diuretics, digitalis, and afterload reduction with ACE inhibitors. Only cardiac transplantation and specific vasodilator therapy have been shown to decrease mortality [151]. Oral anticoagulation, if not contraindicated, should be used for severe left ventricular dysfunction. Beta-adrenergic blockade has been studied in dilated cardiomyopathy and is thought to prevent the deleterious cardiac effects of the sympathetic nervous system activation [152]. Results to date have been generally favorable [152,153].

ALCOHOLIC CARDIOMYOPATHY. Chronic excessive alcohol consumption may be associated with a dilated cardiomyopathy, which may lead to congestive heart failure. Possible mechanisms include a direct toxic effect of alcohol or its metabolites, nutritional deficiencies (thiamine), and toxic effect due to additives (cobalt) [154]. Congestive heart failure secondary to alcoholic cardiomyopathy is treated similarly to other forms of congestive heart failure, except for the use of thiamine. However, the key long-term treatment is immediate and total abstinence. Ceasing consumption of alcohol early in the couse of alcoholic cardiomyopathy may halt the progression or even reverse the ventricular dysfunction [155].

Metabolic Disturbances. Severe hypophosphatemia may result in a reversible left ventricular dysfunction that resolves with restoration of serum phosphate to normal levels [156]. Severe chronic hypocalcemia may rarely cause congestive heart failure [157], which resolves when the serum calcium is raised. Severe hypomagnesemia may result in focal myocardial necrosis. Thiamine deficiency can cause a reversible myocardial dysfunction (beri beri). Carnitine [158] and selenium [159] deficiencies may also lead to dilated cardiomyopathy.

Toxic Injury. A wide variety of substances may act on the heart and damage the myocardium. Cocaine increases myocardial oxygen demand by increasing heart rate and blood pressure, causes coronary vasoconstriction, may accelerate atherosclerosis, and can lead to thrombotic occlusion of the coronary arteries, with resultant acute myocardial infarction [160,161]. Treatment consists of beta- and alpha-adrenergic blockers and calcium channel blockers [152] and abstinence from cocaine. Lead poisoning may lead to overt congestive heart failure secondary to left ventricular dysfunction that is reversible with chelation therapy [162]. The venom of the scorpion may lead to severe left ventricular dysfunction and resultant acute congestive heart failure [163]. Treatment includes adrenergic blocking agents and specific antivenom. Arsenicals can lead to a dilated cardiomyopathy that is reversible with chelation therapy [164].

Antineoplastic agents can have a deleterious effect on the heart. Interferon alpha treatment has been reported to cause a dilated cardiomyopathy that resolves with discontinuation of therapy [165]. High doses of cyclophosphamide have been associated with heart failure secondary to a hemorrhagic myocarditis [166]. Anthracycline cardiotoxicity may be early or late. The early cardiotoxicity is not dose-dependent and includes electrocardiographic abnormalities, left ventricular dysfunction, and myopericarditis [167]. The late cardiotoxicity is related to the development of dose-dependent degenerative cardiomyopathy.

Acute Myocardial Infarction. In the United States, nearly 1.5 million patients suffer from acute myocardial infarction (MI) annually, and approximately one-fourth of all deaths are due to acute MI [168]. Three decades ago, hospital mortality of AMI was as high as 30 percent. The introduction of coronary care units in the early 1960s substantially reduced mortality, but it remained in the range of 15 to 20 percent. Subsequently, the use of aspirin, thrombolytics, and beta-adrenergic blockers lowered that mortality even further, with a mortality of 5 percent or less reported in several clinical trials [169]. Clinical heart failure accompanies loss of 25 percent of left ventricle and cardiogenic shock accompanies loss of more than 40 percent of the left ventricular myocardium [170]. Early reperfusion of the infarct-related artery is the major link to improve survival after myocardial infarction [169].

Invasive hemodynamic monitoring is essential to guide therapy of patients with severe heart failure. Therapy includes avoiding hypoxemia, preload and afterload reduction, and inotropes or intraaortic balloon pumping if necessary. Successful coronary reperfusion is essential for improvement of survival of patients with acute MI associated with cardiogenic shock [170–175]. Thrombolysis alone does not seem sufficient to improve survival [170,171,172]. Primary angioplasty or rescue angioplasty after failed thrombolysis may improve survival in patients with acute MI and cardiogenic shock [173,174,175]. Surgery is necessary in patients with failed angioplasty or patients with acute MI and cardiogenic shock secondary to multivessel coronary artery disease, ventricular septal rupture, acute mitral regurgitation, or cardiac rupture [176,177].

Clinically significant right ventricular infarction is treated by intravascular volume loading, inotropes, and atrioventricular sequential pacing when complete heart block is present [178–182]. See Chapters 44 and 45 for detailed discussions of acute MIs.

ARRHYTHMIAS

Bradyarrhythmias. Bradyarrhythmias may result from sinus bradycardia, sinus arrest, or complete atrioventricular block with a slow junctional or ventricular escape rhythm (see Chap. 49). Sinus bradycardia or sinus arrest may be iatrogenic, most commonly secondary to excessive dosages of beta-adrenergic blockers, calcium channel blockers, or a combination. Other

causes of severe sinus bradycardia include excessive vagal tone, sick sinus syndrome, sinoatrial (exit) block, and ischemia of the sinus node in acute myocardial infarction. Complete heart block may also be iatrogenic, commonly secondary to digitalis toxicity, beta-adrenergic blockers, calcium channel blockers, or a combination. Other causes of atrioventricular block include congenital atrioventricular block, degenerative changes of the conduction system, excessive vagal tone, and ischemic injury in the setting of acute MI. Severe bradyarrhythmias may lead to congestive heart failure and hemodynamic compromise.

Treatment is usually started with intravenous atropine at doses of 0.5 mg, to a total dose of 2 mg. If bradycardia persists with hemodynamic compromise, transcutaneous or transvenous pacing should be initiated. Atrial pacing is preferred in sinus bradycardia without atrioventricular block to maintain atrioventricular synchrony. Isuprel may be used but should be avoided, if possible, in patients with ischemic heart disease.

Tachyarrhythmias. Tachyarrhythmias, whether due to ventricular or supraventricular tachycardia, can lead to acute congestive heart failure. Treatment is directed at immediate termination of the arrhythmia and its prevention (see Chaps. 41 and 49).

References

1. Kannel WB: Epidemiologic aspects of heart failure, in Weber KT (ed): *Heart Failure: Current Concepts and Management.* Philadelphia, WB Saunders, 1989.
2. Kannel WB, Savage D, Castelli WP: Cardiac failure in the Framingham study: Twenty year follow up. In Braunwald E, et al (ed): *Congestive Heart Failure: Current Research and Clinical Applications.* New York, Grune & Stratton, 1982, pp 15–30.
3. Gunther S, Grossman W: Determinants of ventricular function in pressure overload hypertrophy in man. *Circulation* 59:679, 1979.
4. Grossman W, Jones D, McLaurin LP: Wall stress and patterns of hypertrophy in the human left ventricle. *J Clin Invest* 56:56, 1975.
5. Sasayama S, Ross J Jr, Franklin D, et al: Adaptations of the left ventricle to chronic pressure overload. *Circ Res* 38:172, 1976.
6. McCullagh WH, Corell JW, Ross J Jr: Left ventricular dilatation and diastolic compliance changes during chronic volume overloading. *Circulation* 45:943, 1972.
7. Meerson F: The myocardium in hyperfunction hypertrophy and heart failure. *Cir Res* 28:49, 1971.
8. Carabello BA, Nakano K, Corin W, et al: Left ventricular function in experimental volume overload hypertrophy. *Am J Physiol* 223:1150, 1989.
9. Braunwald E (ed): *Heart Disease.* 4th ed. Philadelphia, WB Saunders, 1992, p 397.
10. Minami M, Yasuda H, Yamazaki N, et al: Plasma norepinephrine concentration and plasma dopamine beta hydroxylase activity in patients with congestive heart failure. *J Am Coll Cardiol* 5:832, 1985.
11. Viquerat CE, Daly P, Swedberg K, et al: Endogenous catecholamine levels in chronic heart failure: Relation to the severity of hemodynamic abnormalities. *Am J Med* 78:455, 1985.
12. Chidsey CA, Braunwald E, Morrow AG: Catecholamine excretion and cardiac stores of norepinephrine in congestive heart failure. *Am J Med* 39:442, 1965.
13. Bristow MR, Ginsburg R, Minabe W, et al: Decreased catecholamine sensitivity and beta adrenergic receptor density in failing human hearts. *N Engl J Med* 307:205, 1982.
14. Schaffer J, Tews A, Langes K, et al: Relationship between myocardial norepinephrine content and left ventricular function: An endomyocardial biopsy study. *Eur Heart J* 8:748, 1987.
15. Alpert NR, Gordon MS: Myofibrillar adenosine triphosphate activity in congestive heart failure. *Am J Physiol* 202:940, 1962.
16. Gordon MS, Brown AL: Myofibrillar adenosine triphosphate activity of human heart tissue in congestive failure: Effects of ouabain and cancium. *Circ Res* 19:534, 1966.

17. Geenen DL, Malhotra A, Scheuer J: Ventricular function and contractile proteins in the infarcted rat heart exposed to chronic pressure overload. *Am J Physiol* 256:H745, 1989.

18. Izumo S, Lampre AM, Matsouka R, et al: Myosin heavy chain messenger RNA and protein isoform transitions during cardiac hypertrophy. *J Clin Invest* 79:970, 1987.

19. Bouvagnet P, Leter J, Deschesne CA, et al: Local changes in myosin types in diseased human atrial myocardium: A quantitative immunofluorescence study. *Circulation* 72:272, 1985.

20. Gwathmey JK, Copelas L, Mackinnon R, et al: Abnormal intracellular calcium handling in myocardium from patients with end stage heart failure. *Circ Res* 61:70, 1987.

21. Keung EC: Calcium current is increased in isolated adult myocytes from hypertrophied rat myocardium. *Circ Res* 64:753, 1989.

22. Neumann J, Schmitz W, Schalz H, et al: Increase in myocardial G1 proteins in heart failure. *Lancet* 2:936, 1988.

23. Matthay MA, Chatterjee K: Bedside catheterization of the pulmonary artery: Risks compared with benefits. *Ann Intern Med* 109:826, 1988.

24. Sibbald WJ, Sprung CL: The pulmonary artery catheter: The debate continues. *Chest* 94:899, 1988.

25. Dalen JE: Does pulmonary artery catheterization benefit patients with acute myocardial infarction? *Chest* 98:1313, 1990.

26. Godley RW, Wann LS, Rogers EW, et al: Incomplete mitral leaflet closure in patients with papillary muscle dysfunction. *Circulation* 63:565, 1981.

27. Ballester M, Foale R, Presbitero P, et al: Cross sectional echocardiographic features of ruptured chordae tendinae. *Eur Heart J* 4:795, 1983.

28. Grayburn PA, Smith MD, Handshoe R, et al: Detection of aortic insufficiency by standard echocardiography, pulsed Doppler echocardiography and auscultation. *Ann Intern Med* 104:599, 1986.

29. Barchard A, Yock P, Schiller NB, et al: Value of color Doppler estimation of regurgitant volume in patients with chronic aortic insufficiency. *Am Heart J* 117:1099, 1989.

30. Sutherland GS, Smylie JH, Ogilvie BL, et al: Color flow imaging in the diagnosis of multiple ventricular septal defects. *Br Heart J* 62:43, 1989.

31. Pollick C, Sullivan H, Cujec B, Wilansky S: Doppler color flow imaging assessment of shunt size in atrial septal defect. *Circulation* 78:522, 1988.

32. Buda AJ, Zotz RJ, Pace DP, Krause LC: Comparison of two dimensinal echocardiographic wall motion and wall thickening abnormalities in relation to the myocardium at risk. *Am Heart J* 111:587, 1986.

33. Birstow DJ, Oh JK, Barley KR, et al: Cardiac tamponade: Characteristic Doppler observations. *Mayo Clin Proc* 64:312, 1989.

34. Horowitz MS, Schultz CS, Stinson EB, et al: Sensitivity and specificity of echocardiographic diagnosis of aortic dissection. *Am J Cardiol* 56:123, 1985.

35. Seward JB, Khandheria BK, Oh JK, et al: Transesophageal echocardiography: Technique, anatomic correlations, implementation and clinical applications. *Mayo Clin Proc* 63:649, 1988.

36. Bansal RC, Shakudo M, Shah PM: Biplane transesophageal echocardiography: Technique, image orientation, and preliminary experience in 131 patients. *J Am Soc Echocardiogr* 3:348, 1990.

37. Hashimoto S, Kumada T, Osakada G, et al: Assessment of transesophageal Doppler echocardiography in dissecting aortic aneurysm. *J Am Coll Cardiol* 14:1252, 1989.

38. Erbel R, Borner N, Steller D, et al: Detection of aortic dissection by transesophageal echocardiography. *Br Heart J* 58:45, 1987.

39. Grossman W, Baim DS (eds): *Cardiac Catheterization, Angiography and Intervention.* 4th ed. Philadelphia, Lea & Febiger, 1991.

40. Wlofkiel CJ, Ferguson JL, Chamka EV, et al: Measurement of myocardial blood flow by ultrafast computed tomography. *Circulation* 76:1262, 1987.

41. Doherty PW, Lipton MJ, Berninger WH, et al: The detection and quantitation of myocardial infarction in vivo using transmission tomography. *Circulation* 63:597, 1981.

42. White RC, Lipton MJ, Higgins CB, et al: Noninvasive evaluation of suspected thoracic aortic disease by contrast enhanced computed tomography. *Am J Cardiol* 57:282, 1986.

43. Stork DD, Higgins CB, Lanzer P, et al: Magnetic resonance imaging of the pericardium: Normal and pathologic findings. *Radiology* 150:469, 1984.

44. Kersting-Sommerhoff BA, Higgins CB, White RD, et al: Aortic dissection: Sensitivity and specificity of MR imaging. *Radiology* 3:651, 1988.

45. Didier D, Higgins CB: Identification and localization of ventricular septal defects by gated magnetic resonance imaging *J Am Coll Cardiol* 57:1636, 1986.

46. Jardin F, Farcot JC, Boisante L, et al: Influence of positive end expiratory pressure on left ventricular performance. *N Engl J Med* 304:387, 1981.

47. Rizk NW, Murray JF: PEEP and pulmonary edema. *Am J Med* 72:381, 1982.

48. Judgutt BI, Warnica JW: Intravenous nitroglycerin therapy to limit myocardial infarct size. *Circulation* 78:906, 1988.

49. Dzau VJ: Renal and circulatory mechanisms in congestive heart failure. *Kidney Int* 31:1402, 1987.

50. Thompson DD: Salt and water excretion in heart failure. *Prog Cardiovasc Dis* 3:520, 1961.

51. Cody RJ, Ljungman S, Covit AB, et al: Regulation of GFR in chronic congestive heart failure patients. *Kidney Int* 34:361, 1988.

52. Ljungman S, Laragh JH, Cody RJ: Role of the kidney in congestive heart failure: Relationship of cardiac index to kidney function. *Drugs* 39(suppl 4):10, 1990.

53. Riegger GAJ, Lieban G, Kochsiek K: Antidiuretic hormone in congestive heart failure. *Am J Med* 72:49, 1982.

54. Kirchheim H, Ehmke H, Persson P: Physiology of the renal baroreceptor mechanism of renin release and its role in congestive heart failure. *Am J Cardiol* 62:68E, 1988.

55. Hirsch AT, Pinto YM, Schunkert H, Dzau VJ: Potential role of the tissue renin-angiotensin system in the pathophysiology of congestive heart failure. *Am J Cardiol* 66:22D, 1990.

56. Burnett JC: Atrial natriuretic factor: Is it physiologically important? *Circulation* 82:1523, 1990.

57. Ledley GS, Lowell FS, Rackley C: Therapeutic options in congestive heart failure. *J Crit Illness* 4:39, 1989.

58. Zelis R, Monsour EJ, Capone RJ, et al: The cardiovascular effects of morphine: The peripheral capacitance and resistance vessels in human subjects. *J Clin Invest* 54:1247, 1974.

59. Vismora LA, Leaman DM, Zelis R: Effects of morphine on venous tone in patients with acute pulmonary edema. *Circulation* 54:335, 1976.

60. Hurst JW (ed): *The Heart*. New York, McGraw-Hill, 1974, p 487.

61. Channer KS, Richardson M, Crook R, Jones JV: Thiazide with loop diuretics for severe congestive heart failure. *Lancet* 1:922, 1990.

62. Anand I, Ferrari R, Kalra G, et al: Congestive heart failure: Edema of cardiac origin. *Circulation* 80:299, 1989.

63. Masterson BJ, Epstein M: Thiazide diuretics, chlorthalidone and metolazone, in Messerli FH (ed): *Cardiovascular Drug Therapy*. Philadelphia, WB Saunders, 1990, p 337.

64. Kiyingi A, Field MJ, Pawsey CC, et al: Metolazone in treatment of severe refractory congestive heart failure. *Lancet* 1:29, 1990.

65. Epstein M, Masterson BJ: Loop diuretics: Furosemide, in Messerli FH (ed): *Cardiovascular Drug Therapy*. Philadelphia, WB Saunders, 1990, p 318.

66. Whelton A, Whelton PK: Loop diuretics: Butenamide, in Messerli FH (ed): *Cardiovascular Drug Therapy*. Philadelphia, WB Saunders, 1990, p 328.

67. Shammas FV, Dickstein K: Clinical pharmacokinetics in heart failure: An updated review. *Clin Pharmacokinet* 15:94, 1988.

68. Cook JA, Smith DE, Cornish LA, et al: Kinetics, dynamics and bioavailability of butenamide in healthy subjects and patients with congestive heart failure. *Clin Pharmacol Ther* 44:487, 1988.

69. Cohn JN: Nitrates for congestive heart failure. *Am J Cardiol* 56:19A, 1985.

70. Packer M: Mechanisms of nitrate action in patients with severe left ventricular failure. *Am Heart J* 110:259, 1985.

71. Cohn JN, Archibald DG, Ziesche S, et al: Effects of vasodilator therapy on mortality in chronic congestive heart failure: Results of a Veterans Administration cooperative study. *N Engl J Med* 314:1547, 1986.

72. Packer JO: Nitrate tolerance. *Am J Cardiol* 60:44H, 1987.

73. Packer M, Lee-Wai H, Kessler PD, et al: Prevention and reversal

of nitrate tolerance in patients with congestive heart failure. *N Engl J Med* 317:799, 1987.

74. Goldberg LI: Cardiovascular and renal actions of dopamine: Potential clinical applications. *Pharmacol Rev* 24:1, 1972.
75. Port JD, Gilbert EM, Larrabee P, et al: Neurotransmitter depletion compromises the ability of indirect-acting amines to provide inotropic support in the failing human heart. *Circulation* 81:929, 1990.
76. Dasta JF, Kirby MG: Pharmacology and therapeutic use of low-dose dopamine. *Pharmacotherapy* 6:304, 1986.
77. Goldberg LI: Dopamine: Clinical uses of an endogenous catecholamine. *N Engl J Med* 291:707, 1974.
78. Goldberg LI, Rajfer SI: Dopamine receptors: Applications in clinical cardiology. *Circulation* 72:245, 1985.
79. Gilbert JC, Goldberg LI: Characterization by cyproheptadine of the dopamine induced contraction in canine isolated arteries. *J Pharmacol Exp Ther* 193:435, 1975.
80. Toda N, Goldberg LI: Effect of dopamine on isolated canine coronary arteries. *Cardiovasc Res* 9:384, 1975.
81. Tuttle RR, Mills J: Dobutamine: Development of a new catecholamine to selectively increase cardiac contractility. *Circ Res* 36:185, 1975.
82. Ruffolo RR, Spradlin TA, Pollack GD, et al: Alpha and beta adrenergic effects of the stereoisomers of dobutamine. *J Pharmacol Exp Ther* 219:447, 1981.
83. Sonnenblick EH, Frishman WH, Lejemtel TH: Dobutamine: A new synthetic cardioactive sympathetic amine. *N Engl J Med* 300:17, 1979.
84. Leier CV, Webel J, Bush CA: The cardiovascular effects of the continuous infusion of dobutamine in patients with severe cardiac failure. *Circulation* 56:468, 1977.
85. Gillespie JA, Ambros HD, Sobel BE, Roberts R: Effects of dobutamine in patients with acute myocardial infarction. *Am J Cardiol* 39:588, 1977.
86. Leer CV, Heban PT, Huss P, et al: Comparative systemic and regional hemodynamic effects of dopamine and dobutamine in patients with cardiomyopathic heart failure. *Circulation* 58:466, 1978.
87. Bendersky R, Chatterjee K, Parmley WW, et al: Dobutamine in chronic ischemic heart failure: Alterations in left ventricular function and coronary hemodynamics. *Am J Cardiol* 48:554, 1981.
88. Bourdarias JP, Dubourg O, Gueret P, et al: Inotropic agents in the treatment of cardiogenic shock. *Pharmacol Ther* 22:53, 1983.
89. Colucci WS, Wright RF, Braunwald E: New positive inotropic agents in the treatment of congestive heart failure: Mechanisms of action and recent clinical developments. *N Engl J Med* 314:349, 1986.
90. Katz AM: Changing strategies in the management of heart failure. *Am J Cardiol* 63:12A, 1989.
91. Evans DB: Modulation of cAMP: Mechanism for positive inotropic action. *J Cardiovasc Pharmacol* 8(suppl 9):22, 1986.
92. Brauwald E: A symposium on amrinone. *Am J Cardiol* 56:1B, 1985.
93. Benotti JR, Grossman W, Braunwald E, et al: Hemodynamic assessment of amrinone: A new inotropic agent. *N Engl J Med* 299:1373, 1978.
94. Naccarelli GV, Gray EL, Dougherty AH, et al: Amrinone: Acute electrophysiologic and hemodynamic effects in patients with congestive heart failure. *Am J Cardiol* 54:600, 1984.
95. Goenen M, Pedemonte O, Baele P, Col J: Amrinone in the management of low cardiac output after open heart surgery. *Am J Cardiol* 56:33B, 1985.
96. Taylor SH, Verma SP, Hussain M, et al: Intravenous amrinone in left ventricular failure complicated by acute myocardial infarction. *Am J Cardiol* 56:29B, 1985.
97. Lee DC-S, Johnson RA, Bingham, et al: Heart failure in outpatients: A randomized trial of digoxin versus placebo. *N Engl J Med* 306:699, 1982.
98. Guyatt GH, Sullivan MJJ, Fallen EL, et al: A controlled trial of digoxin in congestive heart failure. *Am J Cardiol* 61:371, 1988.
99. Packer M, Gheorghiade M, Young JB, et al: Withdrawal of digoxin from patients with chronic heart failure treated with angiotensin-converting-enzyme inhibitors. *N Engl J Med* 329:1, 1993.
100. Miller RM, Fennell WH, Young JB, et al: Differential systemic arterial and venous actions and consequent cardiac effects of vasodilator drugs. *Prog Cardiovasc Dis* 24:353, 1982.
101. Leier CV: Regional blood flow in congestive heart failure: Regional blood flow responses to vasodilators and inotropes in congestive heart failure. *Am J Cardiol* 62:86E, 1988.
102. Massie BM, Kramer BL, Topic N: Long-term captopril therapy for chronic congestive heart failure. *Am J Cardiol* 53:1316, 1984.
103. Packer M: Vasodilator and inotropic therapy for the treatment of chronic congestive heart failure: Distinguishing hype from hope. *J Am Coll Cardiol* 12:1299, 1988.
104. Newman TJ, Maskin CS, Dennick LG, et al: Effects of captopril on survival in patients with heart failure. *Am J Med* 84:140, 1988.
105. Massie B, Ports T, Chatterjee K, et al: Long-term vasodilator therapy for heart failure: Clinical response and its relationship to hemodynamic measurements. *Circulation* 63:269, 1981.
106. Packer M, Meller J, Medina N, et al: Dose requirements of hydralazine in patients with severe chronic congestive heart failure. *Am J Cardiol* 45:655, 1980.
107. Packer M, Meller J, Medina N, et al: Hemodynamic characterization of tolerance to long-term hydralazine therapy in severe chronic heart failure. *N Engl J Med* 306:57, 1982.
108. Weil MH, Shubin H, Carlson R: Treatment of circulatory shock: Use of sympathomimetic and related vasoactive agents. *JAMA* 231:1280, 1975.
109. Weintraub RM, Voukydis PC, Aroesty JM: Treatment of preinfarction angina with intraaortic balloon counterpulsation and surgery. *Am J Cardiol* 34:809, 1974.
110. Flaherty JT, Becker LC, Weiss JL, et al: Results of a randomized prospective trial of intraaortic balloon counterpulsation and intravenous nitroglycerin in patients with acute myocardial infarction. *J Am Coll Cardiol* 6:434, 1985.
111. McEnany MT, Kay HR, Buckley MJ, et al: Clinical experience with intraaortic balloon pump support in 728 patients. *Circulation* 58:124, 1978.
112. Gold HK, Leinbach RC, Sanders CA, et al: Intraaortic balloon pumping for ventricular septal defect or mitral regurgitation complicating acute myocardial infarction. *Circulation* 47:1191, 1973.
113. Buckley MJ, Craver JM, Gold HK, et al: Intraaortic ballon pump assist for cardiogenic shock after cardiopulmonary bypass. *Circulation* 48:90, 1973.
114. Rajai HR, Hartman CW, Innes BJ, et al: Prophylactc use of intraaortic balloon pump in aortocoronary bypass for patients with left main coronary artery disease. *Ann Surg* 187:118, 1978.
115. Gottlieb SO, Brinker JA, Borkon AM, et al: Identification of patients at high risk for complications of intraaortic balloon counterpulsation: A multivariate risk factor analysis. *Am J Cardiol* 53:1135, 1984.
116. Alderman JD, Gabliani GI, McCabe CH, et al: Incidence and management of limb ischemia with percutaneous wire-guided intraaortic balloon catheters. *J Am Coll Cardiol* 9:524, 1987.
117. Farrar DJ, Hill DJ, Gray LA, et al: Heterotopic prosthetic ventricles as a bridge to cardiac transplantation. *N Engl J Med* 318:333, 1988.
118. Pennington DG, McBride LR, Swartz MT, et al: Use of the Pierce-Danachy ventricular assist device in patients with cardiogenic shock after cardiac operations. *Ann Thorac Surg* 47:130, 1989.
119. Rom CVS, Hyman D: Hypertensive crisis. *J Intensive Care Med* 2:151, 1987.
120. Koch-Weser J: Hypertensive emergencies. *N Engl J Med* 290:211, 1974.
121. Ross J Jr, Braunwald E: Aortic stenosis. *Circulation* 38(suppl 5):61, 1968.
122. Gorlin R, Gorlin SG: Hydrolic formula for calculation of the area of stenotic mitral valve, other cardiac valves and central circulatory shunts. *Am Heart J* 41:1, 1951.
123. Stott DK, Marpole DG, Bristow M, et al: The role of left atrial transport in aortic and mitral stenosis. *Circulation* 41:1031, 1970.
124. Child JS, Perloff JK: The restrictive cardiomyopathies. *Cardiol Clin* 6:289, 1988.
125. Bonow RO, Dilsezean V, Rosing D, et al: Verapamil induced improvement in left ventricular diastolic filling and increased exercise tolerance in patients with hypertrophic cardiomyopathy: Short and long term effects. *Circulation* 72:853, 1985.
126. Sherrid M, Delia E, Dwyer E: Oral disopyramide therapy for obstructive hypertrophic cardiomyopathy. *Am J Cardiol* 62:1085, 1985.
127. McDonald KM, Mauner B: Permanent pacing as treatment for hypertrophic cardiomyopathy. *Am J Cardiol* 68:853, 1991.

128. Dalen JE, Alpert JS: Natural history of pulmonary embolism. *Prog Cardiovasc Dis* 17:259, 1975.

129. Dalen JE, Haffajee CI, Alpert JS, et al: Pulmonary embolism, pulmonary hemorrhage and pulmonary infarction. *N Engl J Med* 296:1431, 1977.

130. Kelley MA, Garson JL, Polevsky HI, et al: Diagnosing pulmonary embolism: New facts and strategies. *Ann Intern Med* 114:300, 1991.

131. Kloster FE: Diagnosis and management of complications of prosthetic heart valves. *Am J Cardiol* 35:872, 1975.

132. Nitter-Hauge S, Abdelnoor M: Ten year experience with the Medtronic Hall valvular prosthesis: A study of 1,104 patients. *Circulation* 80:I43, 1989.

133. Arom KV, Nicoloff DM, Kersten TE, et al: Ten years experience with the St. Jude medical valve prosthesis. *Ann Thorac Surg* 47:831, 1989.

134. Braunwald E: On the difference between the heart's output and its contractile state. *Circulation* 43:171, 1971.

135. Ingram CW, Satler LF, Rackley CE: Progressive heart failure secondary to a high output state. *Chest* 92:1117, 1987.

136. Stott DK, Marpole DG, Bristow JD, et al: The role of left atrial transport in aortic and mitral stenosis. *Circulation* 41:1031, 1970.

137. Cohen DJ, Kuntz RE, Gordon SP, et al: Predictors of long term outcome after percutaneous balloon mitral valvuloplasty. *N Engl J Med* 327:1329, 1992.

138. Karp RB, Cyrus RJ, Blackstone EH, et al: The Bjork Shiley valve: Intermediate term follow-up. *J Thorac Cardiovasc Surg* 81:602, 1981.

139. Benotti JR, Grossman W, Cohn PF: Clinical profile of restrictive cardiomyopathy. *Circulation* 61:1206, 1986.

140. Plehn JF, Friedman BJ: Diastolic dysfunction in amyloid heart disease: Restrictive cardiomyopathy or not? *J Am Coll Cardiol* 13:54, 1989.

141. Gertz MA, Falk RH, Skinner M, et al: Worsening of congestive heart failure in amyloid heart disease treated by calcium channel blocking agents. *Am J Cardiol* 55:1645, 1985.

142. Peters NS, Poole-Wilson PA: Myocarditis: Continuing clinical and pathologic confusion. *Am Heart J* 121:942, 1991.

143. Marboe CC, Feneglio JJ: Pathology and natural history of human myocarditis. *Pathol Immunopathol Res* 7:226, 1988.

144. Weinstein C, Fenoglio JJ: Myocarditis. *Hum Pathol* 18:613, 1987.

145. Reyes MP, Lerner AM: Coxsackie virus myocarditis: With special reference to acute and chronic effect. *Prog Cardiovasc Dis* 27:373, 1985.

146. Pinamonti B, Alberti E, Cigalotto A, et al: Echocardiographic findings in myocarditis. *Am J Cardiol* 62:285, 1988.

147. Khaw BA, Haber E: Imaging necrotic myocardium: Detection with 99m Tc-pyrophosphate and radiolabeled antimyosin. *Cardiol Clin* 7:577, 1989.

148. Chow LH, Radio SJ, Sears TD et al: Insensitivity of right ventricular endomyocardial biopsy in the diagnosis of myocarditis. *J Am Coll Cardiol* 14:915, 1989.

149. Juilliere Y, Danchin N, Briancon S, et al: Dilated cardiomyopathy: Long-term follow-up and predictors of survival. *Int J Cardiol* 21:269, 1988.

150. Roubin GS, Anderson SD, Shen WF, et al: Hemodynamic and metabolic basis of impaired exercise tolerance in patients with severe left ventricular dysfunction. *J Am Coll Cardiol* 15:986, 1990.

151. Massin EK: Current treatment of dilated cardiomyopathy. *Texas Heart Inst J* 18:41, 1991.

152. Waagstein F, Caidahl K, Wallentin I, et al: Long-term beta-blockade in dilated cardiomyopathy: Effects of short- and long-term metoprolol treatment followed by withdrawal and readministration of metoprolol. *Circulation* 80:551, 1989.

153. Gilbert EM, Anderson JL, Deitchman D, et al: Long-term beta-blocker vasodilator therapy improves cardiac function in idiopathic dilated cardiomyopathy: A double-blind, randomized study of bucindolol versus placebo. *Am J Med* 88:223, 1990.

154. Davidson MD: Cardiovascular effects of alcohol. *West J Med* 151:430, 1989.

155. Pavan D, Nicolosi GL, Lestuzzi C, et al: Normalization of variables of left ventricular function in patients with alcoholic cardiomyopathy after cessation of excessive alcohol intake: An echocardiographic study. *Eur Heart J* 8:535, 1987.

156. Venditti FJ, Marotta C, Panezai FR, et al: Hypophosphatemia and cardiac arrhythmias. *Miner Electrolyte Metab* 13:19, 1987.

157. Feldman AM, Fivush B, Zahka KG, et al: Congestive cardiomyopathy in patients on continuous ambulatory peritoneal dialysis. *Am J Kidney Dis* 11:76, 1988.

158. Ino T, Sherwood WG, Benson LN, et al: Cardiac manifestations in disorders of fat and carnitine metabolism in infancy. *J Am Coll Cardiol* 11:1301, 1988.

159. Reeves WC, Marcuard SP, Willis SE, et al: Reversible cardiomyopathy due to selenium deficiency. *J Parenter Enteral Nutr* 13:663, 1989.

160. Lange RA, Cigarroa RG, Yancy CW, et al: Cocaine-induced coronary-artery vasoconstriction. *N Engl J Med* 321:1557, 1989.

161. Isner JM, Chokshi SK: Cocaine and vasospasm. *N Engl J Med* 321:1604, 1989.

162. Kopp SJ, Barron JT, Tow JP: Cardiovascular actions of lead and relationship to hypertension: A review. *Environ Health Perspect* 78:91, 1988.

163. Brand A, Keren A, Kerem E, et al: Myocardial damage after a scorpion sting: Long-term echocardiographic follow-up. *Pediatr Cardiol* 9:59, 1988.

164. Zaloga GP, Deal J, Spurling T, et al: Unusual manifestations of arsenic intoxication. *Am J Med Sci* 289:210, 1985.

165. Cohen MC, Huberman MS, Nesto RW: Recombinant alpha$_2$ interferon-related cardiomyopathy. *Am J Med* 85:549, 1988.

166. Cazin B, Gorin NC, Laporte JP, et al: Cardiac complications after bone marrow transplantation: A report on a series of 63 consecutive transplantations. *Cancer* 57:2061, 1986.

167. Porembka DT, Lowder JN, Orlowski JP, et al: Etiology and management of doxorubicin cardiotoxicity. *Crit Care Med* 17:569, 1989.

168. American Heart Association: 1990 heart facts. Dallas, American Heart Association National Center, 1990, p. 1.

169. Mueller HS: Reperfusion therapy in acute myocardial infarction: Present status and controversy. *Clin Cardiol* 13:239, 1990.

170. Rackley CE, Russel RO Jr, Mantle JA, et al: Modern approach to the patient with acute myocardial infarction. *Curr Probl Cardiol* 1:49, 1977.

171. Gruppo Italiano per lo Studio della Streptochinasi nell'Infarto Miocardico (GISSI): Effectiveness of intravenous thrombolytic treatment in acute myocardial infarction. *Lancet* 1:397, 1986.

172. Topol EJ, Califf RM, George BS, et al: Insights derived from the thrombolysis and angioplasty in myocardial infarction (TAMI) trials. *J Am Coll Cardiol* 12(suppl A):24A, 1988.

173. Kennedy JW, Gensini GG, Timmis GC, et al: Acute myocardial infarction treated with intracoronary streptokinase: A report of the Society for Cardiac Angiography. *Am J Cardiol* 55:871, 1985.

174. Lee L, Bates ER, Pitt B, et al: Percutaneous transluminal coronary angioplasty improves survival in acute myocardial infarction complicated by cardiogenic shock. *Circulation* 78:1345, 1988.

175. Rothbaum DA, Linnemeier TJ, Landin RJ, et al: Emergency percutaneous transluminal angioplasty in acute myocardial infarction: A 3 year experience. *J Am Coll Cardiol* 10:264, 1987.

176. Ellis SG, O'Neil WW, Bates ER, et al: Implications for patient triage from survival and left ventricular functional recovery analyses in 500 patients treated with coronary angioplasty for acute myocardial infarction. *J Am Coll Cardiol* 13:1251, 1989.

177. Stack RS, Califf RM, Hinohara T, et al: Survival and cardiac event rates in the first year after emergency coronary angioplasty for acute myocardial infarction. *J Am Coll Cardiol* 11:1141, 1988.

178. Jones MT, Schofield PM, Dark JF, et al: Surgical repair of acquired ventricular septal defects: Determinant of early and late outcome. *J Thorac Cardiovasc Surg* 93:680, 1987.

179. Miller DC, Stinson EB: Surgical management of acute mechanical defects secondary to myocardial infarction. *Am J Surg* 141:677, 1981.

180. Cohn JN, Giuka NH, Brodeur MI, et al: Right ventricular infarction. *Am J Cardiol* 33:209, 1974.

181. Manfred Z, Wolfgang K, Elisabeth K, et al: Right ventricular infarction as an independent predictor of prognosis after acute myocardial infarction. *N Engl J Med* 328:981, 1993.

182. Lopez-Sendon J, Coma-Canella I, Adanez JV: Volume loading in patients with ischemic right ventricular dysfunction. *Eur Heart J* 2:329, 1981.

43. Thrombotic Disorders of the Arterial and Venous Circulatory Systems

Richard C. Becker

Arterial thrombotic and thromboembolic disorders are responsible for life-threatening cardiovascular events, including acute myocardial infarction (MI), unstable angina, and ischemic stroke. Venous thrombosis and thromboembolism causing deep venous occlusion and pulmonary embolism also may lead to serious disability or death. As a result, the diagnosis, treatment, prevention, and monitoring of arterial and venous thrombotic events are of considerable importance in modern day medicine.

In most hospitals and major medical centers, thrombotic disorders of the arterial and venous circulatory systems account for a considerable proportion of treated patients. At the University of Massachusetts Medical Center, fully three of every four patients admitted to the coronary care unit fall into this diverse category. Considering 1200 to 1400 yearly admissions, this translates to a total of approximately 1000 patients with serious or life-threatening arterial and venous thromboembolic disease.

Vascular Thrombosis: Basic Principles

Under normal physiologic conditions, blood components do not interact with an intact vascular endothelium. The exposure of circulating blood to disrupted or dysfunctional surfaces initiates a series of complex yet orderly mechanisms that give rise to the rapid deposition of platelets, erythrocytes, leukocytes, and insoluble fibrin, producing a mechanical barrier to blood flow.

In most instances, thrombosis ocurring in the arterial system is comprised of platelets and fibrin in a tightly packed network (white thrombus). In contrast, venous thrombi consist of a loosely packed network of erythrocytes, leukocytes, and fibrin (red thrombus).

The process of vascular thrombosis, particularly in the arterial system, is dynamic, with clot formation and dissolution occurring almost simultaneously. The overall extent of thrombosis and ensuing circulatory compromise is therefore determined by a predominant force, in essence pushing the balance in one direction or another. If local stimuli exceed the vessel's own thromboresistant mechanisms, thrombosis will occur. If, on the other hand, the stimulus toward thrombosis is not strong and the intrinsic defenses are intact, clot formation of physiologic importance is unlikely. In some circumstances, systemic factors may contribute to or magnify local prothrombotic factors, pushing the balance toward thrombosis.

Overall, the site, size, and composition of thrombi forming within the arterial and venous circulatory systems are determined by (1) alterations in blood flow; (2) thrombogenicity of endovascular surfaces; (3) concentration and reactivity of plasma cellular components; and (4) effectiveness of physiologic protective mechanisms.

Critical Steps in Thrombosis

PLATELET DEPOSITION. Platelets attaching to nonendothelialized or disrupted surfaces undergo adherence by activation and distribution along the involved area and subsequent recruitment to form a rapidly enlarging platelet mass. Under physiologic conditions this represents the primary step in hemostasis. In pathologic thrombosis, however, platelet adherence initiates a process ultimately leading to circulatory compromise (Fig. 43-1).

The process of platelet deposition involves (1) platelet attachment to collagen or exposed surface adhesive proteins; (2) platelet activation and intracellular signaling; (3) the expression of platelet receptors for adhesive proteins; (4) platelet aggregation; and (5) platelet recruitment mediated by thrombin, thromboxane A_2, and adenosine diphosphate (ADP) [1–5].

ACTIVATION OF COAGULATION FACTORS. Thrombin is rapidly generated in response to vascular injury. It also plays a central role in platelet recruitment and the formation of an insoluble fibrin network. The thrombotic process is localized, amplified, and modulated by a series of biochemical reactions driven by the reversible binding of circulating proteins (coagulation factors) to damaged vascular cells, elements of exposed subendothelial connective tissue (especially collagen), platelets (which also express receptor sites for coagulation factors), and macrophages. These events lead to an assembly of enzyme complexes that increases local concentrations of procoagulant material; in this way, a relatively minor initiating stimulus can be greatly amplified to yield a thrombus (Fig. 43-2).

FIBRIN FORMATION. The final phase in thombus formation involves the generation of a stable fibrin network that provides the structural support for the circulating blood's cellular elements and the scaffolding for vascular remodeling. In this pivotal process, thrombin cleaves two small peptides, fibrinopeptide A and fibrinopeptide B, to form fibrin monomers, which in turn polymerize to form soluble fibrin strands. An orderly assembly, branching, and lateral association of fibrillar strands follows, terminating with factor XIII-mediated covalent cross-linking to form a mature fibrin network (mature thrombus).

Vascular Thromboresistance

The vascular endothelium is structurally simple yet functionally complex. Its integrity is essential for normal vessel responsiveness and thromboresistance.

In most vertebrates, vascular endothelial cells form a single layer of simple squamous lining cells 0.1 to 0.5 μm thick, joined by intercellular junctions. The cells themselves are polygonal,

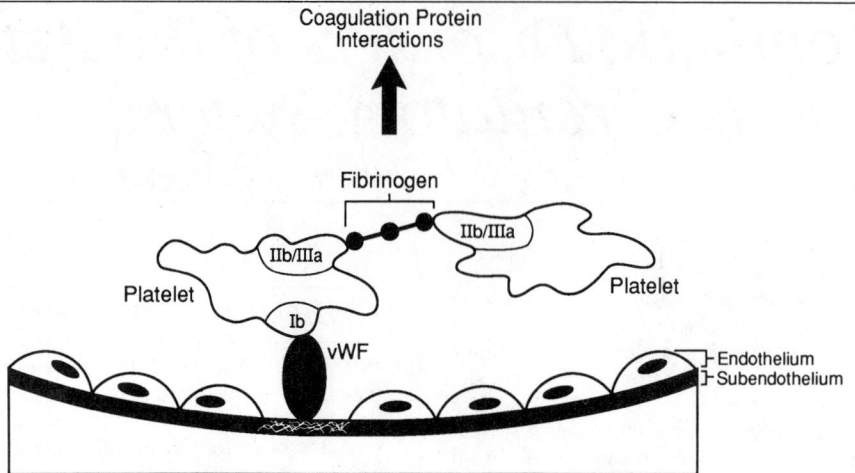

Fig. 43-1. Platelets adhere to areas of damaged or dysfunctional endothelium. With more extensive (deep) vascular injury, the subendothelium is exposed, providing a strong stimulus for platelet adherence and activation. Platelet-vessel wall interactions are mediated by von Willebrand factor (vWF), which also binds to the platelets glycoprotein (GP) Ib receptor. Platelet-platelet interactions are mediated by fibrinogen, which binds to the GPIIb/IIIa receptor. The surface of aggregated platelets subsequently provides a platform for assembling coagulation proteins (platelet-clotting factor interactions).

varying between 10 and 50 μm, and are elongated in the long axis of the vessel (direction of blood flow).

The endothelial cell layer has three surfaces: nonthrombogenic (luminal), adhesive (subluminal), and cohesive (abluminal). The luminal surface, under normal circumstances, is entirely nonthrombogenic and devoid of electron-dense connective tissue. The luminal membrane itself adds significantly to the thromboresistant properties of the vessel, carrying a negative charge that effectively repels similarly charged circulating blood components.

As an active site of protein synthesis, the vascular endothelium could be considered the largest and most productive organ system in the human body. Endothelial cells synthesize, secrete, modify, and regulate connective tissues, vasodilators, vasoconstrictors, anticoagulants, procoagulants, fibrinolytic compounds, and prostanoids (Fig. 43-3).

Normal endothelial cell structure and function must be maintained for vasoactivity and thromboresistance to be preserved [6–19].

Pathology of Thrombotic Events

ARTERIAL CIRCULATORY SYSTEM

Acute Myocardial Infarction. Occurring in upwards of 1.25 million individuals yearly in the United States, MI represents the most commonly observed arterial thrombotic event in clinical practice. In a vast majority of cases, fissuring or rupture of an atherosclerotic plaque within a major epicardial coronary artery is followed by occlusive thrombosis, typically anchored to the damaged vascular surface and exposed plaque components.

Although hard collagenous material (sclerosis) contributes the most voluminous component of a coronary arterial plaque,

the soft, lipid-rich component (atherosis) is the portion that determines a plaque's vulnerability to rupture. Pathologic specimens reveal that ruptured plaques contain less collagen and connective tissue matrix, more extracellular lipid, half as many smooth muscle cells, and twice as many macrophages than nonruptured atherosclerotic plaques. Of interest and clinical importance, plaque rupture does not occur randomly throughout the coronary tree. Instead, there are "vulnerable" sites located in (1) the proximal portion of the left anterior descending coronary artery, (2) the right coronary artery near the origin of its marginal branch, and (3) the left circumflex coronary artery at the origin of the first obtuse marginal branch [20–28] (Fig. 43-4).

In general terms, the severity of vessel wall injury determines the extent of thrombosis. Mild injury (type I) is typically associated with the deposition of platelets in a single (nonocclusive) layer. Moderate injury (type II) yields a loosely adherent platelet mass that can quickly be dispersed by normal blood flow. Severe injury (type III) leads to platelet adherence, activation, and stimulation of the coagulation cascade, producing an occlusive thrombus. Type III injury is present in a majority of patients with MI.

Unstable Angina/Non-Q Wave Myocardial Infarction. Angiographic, angioscopic, and pathologic studies have shown that atherosclerotic plaque rupture accompanied by varying degrees of intraluminal thrombosis is the primary pathologic event in unstable angina/non-Q wave MI [29–34]. Although considered an intermediate step in a continuum of advanced atherosclerosis and acute coronary syndromes, unstable angina or non-Q wave MI may, in fact, represent a unique cardiac event. Mounting evidence suggests that chronic, recurrent plaque rupture of mild to moderate severity may be responsible. Thrombosis occurs with each episode but typically is not sufficiently extensive to compromise coronary arterial blood flow. Over time, however, plaque growth occurs, obstructing the coronary lumen. Thus, the obstructive lesion is a combination of mature plaque and layers of aged thrombus, consisting primarily of platelets in a tightly packed fibrin network.

In some patients, non-Q wave MI has clinical features reminiscent of acute Q-wave MI, progressing suddenly because of plaque rupture and occlusive intracoronary thrombosis. Experience has shown that these patients frequently have multives-

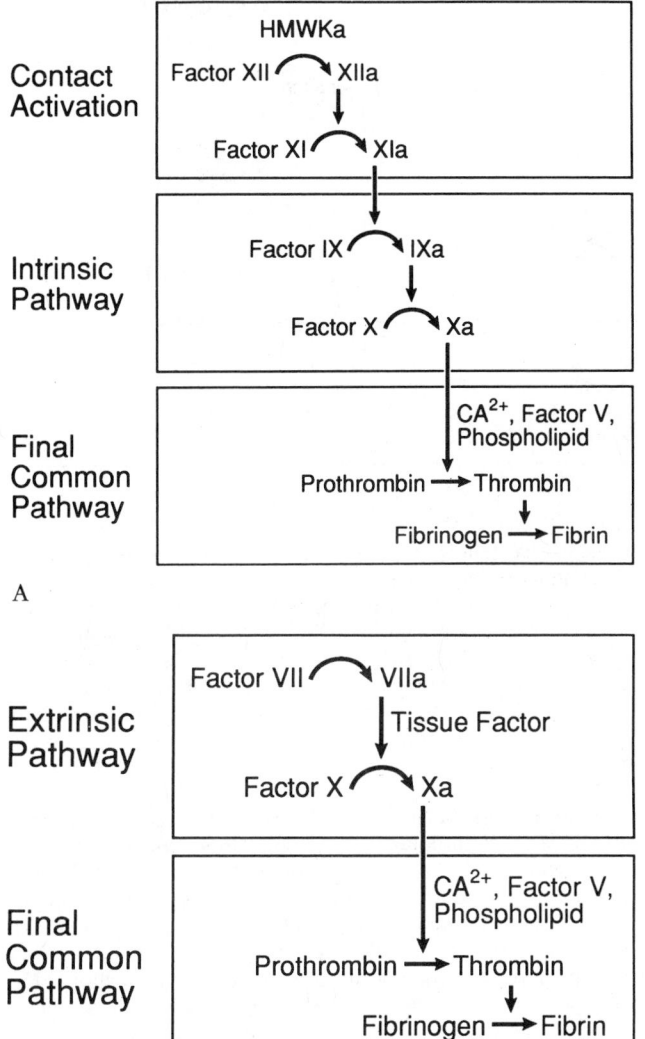

Contact Activation

HMWKa

Factor XII → XIIa

Factor XI → XIa

Intrinsic Pathway

Factor IX → IXa

Factor X → Xa

Final Common Pathway

CA²⁺, Factor V, Phospholipid

Prothrombin → Thrombin

Fibrinogen → Fibrin

A

Extrinsic Pathway

Factor VII → VIIa

Tissue Factor

Factor X → Xa

Final Common Pathway

CA²⁺, Factor V, Phospholipid

Prothrombin → Thrombin

Fibrinogen → Fibrin

B

Fig. 43-2. A. The intrinsic coagulation cascade is initiated by contact activation, predominantly through factor XII in the presence of high-molecular-weight kininogen (HMWKa). B. The extrinsic coagulation cascade is initiated by factor VIIa in the presence of tissue factor.

sel coronary artery disease and, therefore, represent a high-risk group. (See Chapter 44 for more on this subject.)

Plaque Rupture: Triggers. Plaque rupture is not a random event, nor is it part of the natural history of coronary atherosclerosis. Instead, plaque rupture results from a combination of factors, both internal and external to the plaque itself.

As previously described, plaques prone to rupture contain a considerable amount of extracellular lipid and macrophages and are separated from the vessel's lumen by a thin fibrous cap. Epidemiologic studies have consistently shown that acute cardiac events, including unstable angina and MI, occur more frequently between 6 A.M. and 12 P.M. than at other times. Moreover, symptom onset not uncommonly begins soon after

the patient awakes and assumes an upright posture, suggesting that heightened sympathetic activity may contribute. Most authorities feel, however, that sympathetic activity alone is not enough to cause plaque rupture. Instead, an appropriate environment (increased sympathetic activity, heightened platelet aggregability, decreased fibrinolytic activity) and a vulnerable plaque are both prerequisites [35–41].

Thrombosis: Risk Factors. Clearly, the severity of vessel wall damage in a majority of cases is the major determinant of thrombosis. However, beyond local events, systemic factors favoring thrombosis may also contribute and, at least in part, determine the overall response to a given level of injury. Systemic risk factors for thrombosis include smoking, plasma total cholesterol, fibrinogen, plasma viscosity, increasing age, diabetes mellitus, factor VII activity, and genetically determined factors [42–54].

Thrombosis in Cardiac Chambers. Thromboembolic events involving the arterial circulatory system are a major source of morbidity and mortality in current clinical practice. Cardiac cerebral embolism is responsible for more than 100,000 strokes yearly in the United States alone and upward of 1 million strokes worldwide. Nonvalvular atrial fibrillation is thought to be responsible for nearly 50 percent of all embolic strokes of cardiac origin and ventricular mural thrombi almost one-third. Therefore, between them, nearly 80 percent of thromboembolic strokes originating from the heart are accounted for.

Sixty percent of all left ventricular mural thrombi are associated with acute MI. In an overwhelming majority of cases, the affected territory involves the anterior myocardial wall and apex. On occasion, mural thrombosis complicates a large inferoapical infarction with apical involvement or multiple infarctions with poor left ventricular function (ejection fraction <35%). The remainder are found in patients with chronic ventricular dysfunction resulting from coronary artery disease, hypertensive heart disease, or dilated cardiomyopathy.

Overall, left ventricle thrombi developed in 15 to 20 percent of all patients with acute MI, 40 percent of anterior infarctions, and 60 percent of large anterior infarctions involving the ventricular apex. On occasion, right ventricular mural thrombosis complicates an inferior MI with right ventricular extension. As one would anticipate, the risk of embolic stroke is highest in patients with large anteroapical infarctions, occurring in 10 to 20 percent of cases (Table 43-1) [55–73].

The two-dimensional (2-D) echocardiogram is the most widely used imaging technique for diagnosing left ventricular mural thrombosis. The sensitivity and specificity are on the order of 80 percent when compared with autopsy studies [59]. Approximately one-fourth of all ventricular thrombi can be identified within the first 24 hours after infarction; 50 percent can be visualized within 48 to 72 hours, and 75 percent within the first week [60,61]. Although a consensus has not been reached, most studies have shown that thrombus protrusion and mobility are associated with an increased risk of thromboembolism [74].

Other methods for diagnosing ventricular mural thrombosis include contrast ventriculography, computed tomography, magnetic resonance imaging, and ¹¹¹In-labeled platelet scintigraphy. However, none of these techniques has been shown to be superior to echocardiography [75].

Atrial Fibrillation. It is currently estimated that 1 to 1.5 million individuals in the United States have experienced atrial fibrillation. The Framingham Heart Study and other large epidemiologic databases have shown that the prevalence of atrial fib-

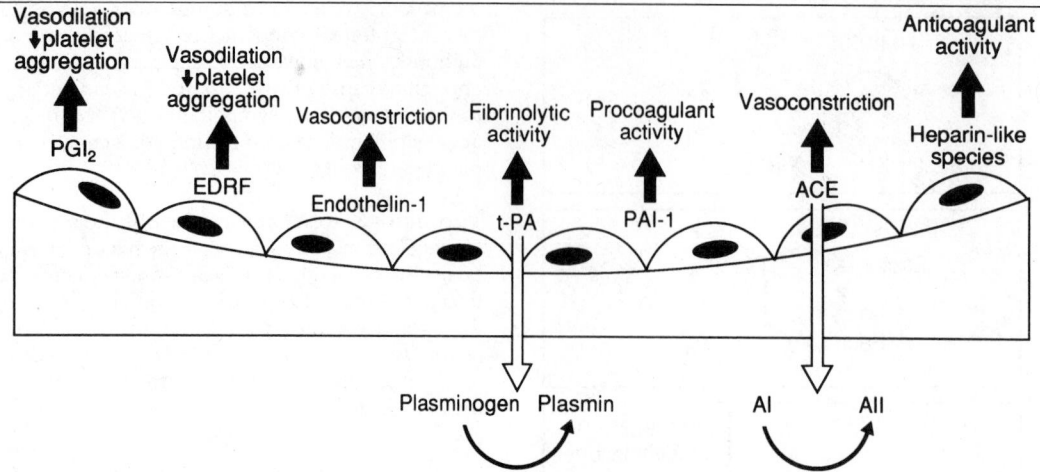

Fig. 43-3. The vascular endothelium is responsible for controlling both hemostasis and thromboresistance. Under normal circumstances, this delicate balance is maintained. Atherosclerosis, however, can shift the balance, increasing the propensity toward thrombosis. PGIG = prostacyclin; EDRF = endothelium-derived relaxing factor; t-PA = tissue plasminogen activator; PAI-1 = plasminogen activator inhibitor-1; ACE = angiotensin-converting enzyme.

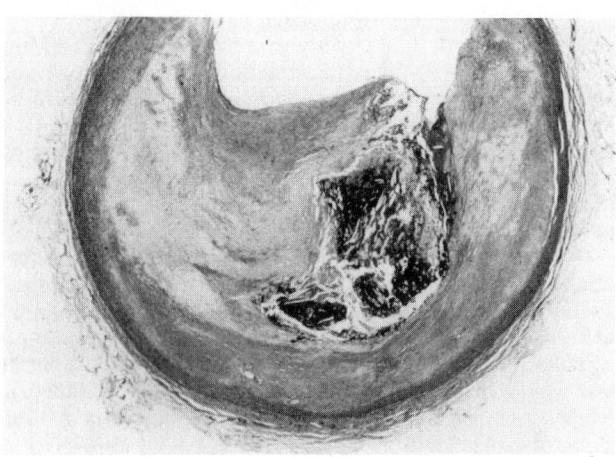

Fig. 43-4. Acute atheromatous plaque rupture in a major epicardial coronary artery. The plaque constituents and vascular subendothelium are exposed to circulating blood components, providing the necessary elements for thrombus formation.

rillation increases with advancing age, affecting 0.4 percent of patients younger than 60 years and 2 to 4 percent of patients older than 60 years. It is commonly associated with other disease processes (Table 43-2).

The risk of stroke and systemic embolism among patients with atrial fibrillation is widely recognized and attributed to a propensity for thrombus formation in a noncontracting left atrium [76]. In the Framingham Heart Study, the risk ratio for stroke was 17.56 among patients with rheumatic atrial fibrillation and 5.6 for those with nonrheumatic atrial fibrillation [77]. Current data suggest that the annual incidence of stroke among individuals with nonvalvular atrial fibrillation is 4 to 5 percent [78]. Although other contributors to stroke, including hyperten-

sion, cardiac failure, and advanced age, often coexist, a majority of central nervous system events are cardioembolic in nature.

The consequences of thromboembolic stroke in the setting of atrial fibrillation are often devastating. In fact, nearly two-thirds result in either death or significant neurologic deficit. Patient groups at highest risk for stroke include women older than 75 years and those with recent thromboembolism, rheumatic atrial fibrillation, hypertension, or left ventricular dysfunction.

Cardioversion. Several clinical series have cited a high incidence of stroke following successful cardioversion among patients with atrial fibrillation. Although the data are difficult to interpret because of the high incidence of rheumatic valvular heart disease in earlier studies, pooled data suggest that cardioversion (pharmacologic or electrical) is associated with a 2 to 4 percent incidence of thromboembolic complications. The risk persists for upward of 3 to 4 weeks, as atrial contractile activity is frequently delayed after the restoration of electrical activity [79–89].

Transesophageal echocardiography (TEE) may be of value in identifying high-risk individuals as well as guiding anticoagulant therapy [90]. This is currently being explored in a multicenter clinical trial.

Prosthetic Heart Valves. Patients with prosthetic heart valves are at moderate to high risk for experiencing thromboembolic events. In general, mechanical valves are more thrombogenic than bioprosthetic valves, and valve replacement in the mitral position is associated with a greater risk of thromboembolism

Table 43-1. Prevalence of Mural Thrombosis and Thromboembolic Events Following Acute Myocardial Infarction and in Other Cardiac Conditions

Cardiac condition	Mural thrombosis %	Embolic events (per 100 patient years)
Myocardial infarction		
Overall	10–20	2–4
Anteroapical	60–70	10–20
Anterior	20–30	5
Inferior	3–5	1
Chronic ventricular aneurysm	40–50	1–2
Dilated cardiomyopathy	30	3–5

Table 43-2. Diseases and Conditions Associated with Atrial Fibrillation

Disease/condition	Prevalence in patients with atrial fibrillation (%)
Rheumatic heart disease	20–30
Coronary artery disease	30–40
Hypertension	40–50
Postoperative state	<5
Hyperthyroidism	2–4
Cardiomyopathy	1–2
Pulmonary embolism	1–2
Pericarditis	<1
Alcohol abuse	<1
"Lone" absence of organic heart disease	3–5

Table 43-3. Clinical Conditions and Prothrombotic States Associated with Venous Thromboembolism

Trauma
Malignancy
Indwelling venous catheters
Immobilization
Surgery
Pregnancy
Oral contraceptives
Systemic lupus erythematosus
Polycythemia rubra vera
Circulating lupus anticoagulant
Paroxysmal nocturnal hemoglobinuria
Hyperviscosity states
Spinal cord injury
Congestive heart failure
Stroke
Protein C deficiency
Protein C resistance
Protein S deficiency
Antithrombin III deficiency
Plasminogen deficiency
Dysfibrinogenemia
Heparin-induced thrombocytopenia with thrombosis
Plasminogen activator inhibitor excess

than in the aortic position. Three factors contribute to thrombosis: (1) perioperative damage of paravalvular tissue; (2) stasis of blood flow; and (3) inherent thrombogenicity of prosthetic materials [91–97]. Patient-related factors contributing to the development of thrombosis include (1) left atrial enlargement, (2) atrial fibrillation, (3) previous thromboembolism, and (4) left ventricular dysfunction.

Among patients with mechanical prosthetic valves, the highest risk of thromboembolism occurs during the first postoperative year. During this period, the level of systemic anticoagulation is more variable, fresh tissue injury exists, and the prosthetic surface is not fully endothelialized. Overall, the St. Jude mechanical valve has the lowest rate of thromboembolism, but valve thrombosis may occur. The Bjork-Shiley prosthetic valve has the highest rate of thromboembolic events.

Thromboembolism after bioprosthetic valve replacement is much less frequent than with mechanical valves; however, events can occur, particularly in the first three postoperative months. The risk is influenced not only by the prosthetic valve itself, but by patient factors as well. Therefore, even among potentially low-risk clinical conditions (e.g., bioprosthetic valve replacement in the aortic position) thromboembolism may be observed, originating from either the left atrial appendage or the left ventricle in the setting of atrial fibrillation and left ventricular dysfunction, respectively [98]. It is vital to assess thromboembolic risk carefully in each patient.

Valve thrombosis occurs most commonly in the first three postoperative months in patients with mechanical prosthetic valves. In a majority of cases, inadequate anticoagulation contributes directly. Clearly, prosthetic valve thrombosis represents a medical emergency that carries a high mortality rate if not diagnosed and treated promptly. The most commonly employed diagnostic modalities include echocardiography with Doppler flow measurements and biplane cinefluoroscopy [99–104].

VENOUS CIRCULATORY SYSTEM

Deep Venous Thrombosis. Venous thromboembolism may be encountered in a variety of clinical conditions and prothrombotic states (Table 43-3). In each, the delicate balance of coagulation and anticoagulation is shifted toward the former, and often intrinsic fibrinolysis is defective as well.

The clinical settings associated with venous thromboembolism have been of interest to physicians for more than a century. In 1856, Rudoth Virchow suggested that changes in blood elements (hypercoagulable state), reduced blood flow velocity (stasis), and vascular injury (endothelial damage) combined to produce an environment suitable for thrombosis.

Six primary sites of venous thrombosis have been recognized: (1) iliac veins, (2) common femoral veins, (3) termination of the deep femoral veins, (4) popliteal veins distal to the adductor ring, (5) posterior tibial veins, and (6) soleal arcade of the calf. Although venous thrombosis can occur at other sites, including the periprostatic plexus, parovarian veins, and uterine veins, they are rarely a source of embolism.

Pulmonary Embolism. When venous thrombi dislodge, they are carried through the venous system to the pulmonary arterial circulation. One or more major vessels may be partially or completely occluded. Occasionally, the thrombus is large enough to occlude the pulmonary arterial bifurcation, a life-threatening condition known as saddle embolism.

A majority of pulmonary emboli lodge in arterial vessels supplying the lower lobes, particularly the posterior basal and apical segments. Embolism to the right lung is more common than to the left.

Nonfatal emboli may undergo complete lyses, extend or migrate distally, or organize to form webs. In addition to abrupt mechanical obstruction, neurohumoral-mediated vasoconstriction and bronchoconstriction can add significantly to the overall clinical manifestations of pulmonary embolism. See Chapter 60 for a complete discussion of pulmonary embolism and deep venous thrombosis.

Anticoagulants

HEPARIN. Heparin is the most widely tested and clinically used anticoagulant. A complete discussion of heparin appears in Chapter 121.

Intravenous nitroglycerin given in high doses (>350 μg/min) can decrease the anticoagulant activity of heparin; a functional abnormality of antithrombin III has been suggested [105]. Heparin's anticoagulant effect may also be modified by circulating plasma proteins, including histidine-rich glycoprotein, platelet factor IV, and vitronectin [106,107].

The most common adverse effect of heparin is hemorrhage, the incidence of which is influenced by total dose, anticoagulant response, method of administration, and patient-related factors, including age and body weight. Other adverse effects associated with heparin use include thrombocytopenia (with or without thrombosis), hyponatremia, allergic reactions, anaphylactic shock, and osteopenia (only with long-term use).

LOW-MOLECULAR-WEIGHT HEPARIN. The development of low-molecular-weight heparin fractions was prompted by the occurrence of adverse reactions (primarily bleeding) with use of unfractionated heparin, introducing a new dimension to the prevention and treatment of thromboembolic diseases. Although it was originally anticipated that low-molecular-weight heparin preparations would cause less bleeding than unfractionated heparin, increasing clinical experience has not clearly borne this out. They do, however, have the advantage of being almost completely absorbed following subcutaneous administration, allowing for once a day dosing in many instances. See Chapter 121 for a discussion of low-molecular-weight heparin.

NEWER ANTICOAGULANTS. While heparin remains the anticoagulant of choice in the coronary care unit, several potential limitations have been recognized: (1) heparin may be partially inactivated by neutralizing proteins released by activated platelets, including platelet factor IV and thrombospondin; (2) heparin is inaccessible to clot-bound thrombin, factor X_a, and thrombin located in the subendothelial matrix; and (3) fibrin II monomers have heparin-neutralizing properties [108–116]. Translated directly to clinical terms, these limiting features compromise heparin's ability to work effectively in the setting of arterial thrombosis, particularly coronary artery thrombosis. Accordingly, several alternative anticoagulants are undergoing extensive investigation.

Hirudin. The anticoagulant properties of leech head extracts were recognized over a century ago, but it was not until the 1950s that the active agent, hirudin, was isolated and characterized. Hirudin, from the leech *Hirudo medicinalis,* is the most potent and specific thrombin inhibitor known.

Recombinant hirudin, a single peptide of 65 amino acid residues, does not require antithrombin III to exert its anticoagulant effects. Biochemical studies suggest that two specific binding sites mediated hirudin's interaction with thrombin. The C terminal residues 54 to 65 adhere to the fibrinogen binding site of thrombin, while residue 47 binds to a specificity pocket near thrombin's catalytic site [117].

Hirudin prevents not only fibrinogen clotting, but other thrombin-catalyzed reactions, including activation of factors V, VIII, and XII. After forming a complex with hirudin, thrombin-mediated platelet aggregation and release are inhibited, although platelet reactions induced by other activators are not influenced [118].

Due to the commercial production of sufficient quantities of r-hirudin, it has been possible to carry out comprehensive experimental studies. Models of venous and arterial thrombosis suggest that hirudin may offer distinct advantages over heparin. Clinical trials, including TIMI-5 (Thrombolysis in Myocardial Infarction Phase 5) also have yielded encouraging results; however, further research is necessary [119]. Two large studies, TIMI-9 and GUSTO-II (Global Use of Strategies to Open Occluded Arteries in Acute Coronary Syndromes) will provide much-needed information for using hirudin either alone in the treatment of unstable angina or adjunctively with tissue plasminogen activator or streptokinase in treating patients with MI.

Hirulog. Hirulog is a 20-amino acid synthetic peptide derived from hirudin. Like hirudin, it selectively binds to thrombin and is a direct, specific, and reversible inhibitor. However, hirulog is unique for several reasons: (1) It is a smaller peptide (20 vs. 65 amino acids) than hirudin. (2) Hirulog binds directly to the thrombin active site via a d-phe-pro-arg-pro sequence in a substratelike fashion, whereas hirudin binds the active site with a divergent, unique orientation. (3) The circulating half-life of hirulog (40 minutes) is shorter than that of hirudin (120 minutes).

Anticoagulation with hirulog can be achieved rapidly following a bolus dose. Preliminary studies have shown that it has a potent, yet well-tolerated, anticoagulant profile [120,121].

Hirugen. Hirugen is a synthetic dodecapeptide containing residues 53 to 64 of the carboxy-terminus of hirudin. Unlike hirudin, hirugen binds only to the thrombin substrate recognition site (anion binding exosite). To date, clinical studies using this specific thrombin inhibitor have not been performed [122].

WARFARIN. Vitamin K is an essential cofactor for the carboxylation of coagulation factors II, VII, IX, and X, enabling them to bind negatively charged phospholipid surfaces in the presence of calcium. Oral anticoagulants such as warfarin inhibit this critical step, preventing the synthesis of functional vitamin K-dependent coagulation factors [123,124,125]. Crystalline sodium warfarin is the predominant coumarin anticoagulant used in North America. For a complete discussion of warfarin, see Chapter 121.

The major adverse effect associated with warfarin administration is hemorrhage. Experience accumulated over many years of clinical use has shown that the risk of hemorrhage increases with increasing prothrombin times. The concomitant administration of antiplatelet agents, particularly when prolonged and in high doses (> 325 mg daily), also increases the risk. Skin necrosis is a rare but serious complication of warfarin therapy. In a majority of cases, it occurs during the initiation phase of treatment, typically in areas of subcutaneous fat.

ANTICOAGULATION MONITORING. The anticoagulant effects of heparin are typically monitored using the activated partial thromboplastin time (aPTT) (see Chap. 121).

A direct relationship between a failure to achieve a therapeutic aPTT (1.5–2.5 times control) and recurrent thromboembolic events has been observed in several clinical studies [126–131]. Unfortunately, different commercial aPTT reagents vary in their responsiveness to heparin [132–135]; with very sensitive reagents the therapeutic range may, in fact, be higher than a ratio of 1.5 to 2.5 times control, while for insensitive reagents the therapeutic range may be lower. Technical variables, including the clot detection system, contact activator, and phospholipid composition of the reagent, may also affect the aPTT response to heparin. There are ongoing efforts to develop standards for the aPTT system; however, an international standard is not available at this time. Hospital laboratories are encouraged to establish a therapeutic range using protamine titration heparin levels of 0.2 to 0.4 unit per milliliter as a reference standard.

BEDSIDE (NEAR PATIENT) COAGULATION MONITORING. Because of the complex pharmacokinetics and pharmacodynamics of heparin, frequent monitoring of the aPTT is required during the course of treatment. In this regard, current laboratory methods have several shortcomings that impact directly on the widescale challenge of achieving and maintaining therapeutic states of systemic anticoagulation in heparinized patients. One of the most concerning is excessive time delay for aPTT availability.

In 1991, the University of Massachusetts Medical Center Coronary Care Unit began using a bedside coagulation monitor to follow all heparinized patients. It is a battery-powered, portable, laser photometer that uses a phospholipid (soybean phosphatide) and an activator of intrinsic coagulation (bovine brain phosphatide) to determine the aPTT in microliter samples of capillary (fingerstick), venous, or arterial whole blood.

Several studies performed at our institution have demonstrated the accurate, reliable and convenient features of bedside coagulation monitoring [136,137]. In essence, a reliable aPTT is obtained within 3 minutes, allowing prompt "real-time" decisions to be made.

HEPARIN DOSE TITRATION. The primary aim of heparin therapy is to prevent recurrent thromboembolic events while minimizing the chance of bleeding. Despite the importance of careful heparin monitoring and dose titration, few guidelines are available. Our experience has shown that "physician-guided" heparin titration frequently results in subtherapeutic anticoagulation [138]. Heparin titration nomograms have been developed to improve on current clinical practices. Initially, not unlike physician-guided titration, they failed to recommend adequate heparin doses [139]. Recent improvements have resulted in a high proportion of therapeutically anticoagulated patients within 24 hours of heparin initiation [140].

Our current practice utilizes a weight-adjusted heparin titration nomogram and bedside coagulation monitoring (Table 43-4).

MONITORING OF NEW ANTICOAGULANTS. Low-molecular-weight heparin does prolong the aPTT, but it does so to a lesser degree than unfractionated heparin. In studies performed to date, monitoring of the anti-X_a activity heparin concentration has been followed [108].

Hirudin and hirulog prolong most in vitro coagulation tests. Because of their potent thrombin-inhibiting potential, the thrombin time assay is markedly prolonged. In contrast, the prothrombin time (PT; INR) is minimally prolonged; therefore the aPTT is used to follow the anticoagulant effects of hirudin and hirulog. Preliminary evidence suggests that the therapeutic range may be lower for these new agents (favorable antithrombotic-antihemostatic profile) and that frequent monitoring may not be required because of their predictable anticoagulant effects [119].

MONITORING OF WARFARIN. The PT is the most commonly used test to monitor the anticoagulant effects of warfarin, although others have been evaluated [141–144] (see Chap. 121). The PT is responsive to depressions of three of the four vitamin K-dependent clotting factors—factors II, VII, and X. Each is reduced by warfarin at a rate proportional to its circulating half-life, ranging from 6 hours with factor VII to 60 hours with factor II.

The PT is influenced directly by the reagent used in the testing procedure. A greater elevation is seen with human brain thromboplastin compared with rabbit brain thromboplastin. Therefore, a similar degree of PT prolongation would require larger warfarin doses when using a rabbit brain thromboplastin reagent [145,146].

One of the major challenges of warfarin treatment is the potential for large fluctuations between and within patients.

Table 43-4. Intravenous Heparin Titration Nomogram: University of Massachusetts Medical School Coronary Care Unit*

aPTT (sec)	Bolus (units)	Discontinue infusion (min)	Rate change (units/hr)	Repeat aPTT (hr)
Initial Bolus: 80U/kg (not to exceed 10,000U)				
<40	5000	0	↑ 200	6
40–54	2000	0	↑ 100	6
55–80	0	0	No change	6
81–120	0	0	↓ 100	4
>120	0	30	↓ 200	4

Body weight	Initial infusion (15–17 units/kg/hr) (not to exceed 2000 units/hr)
≥55 kg	800 units/hr
56–60 kg	900
61–68 kg	1000
69–75 kg	1100
76–82 kg	1200
83–89 kg	1300
90–96 kg	1400
97–102 kg	1500
103–109 kg	1600
110–116 kg	1700
117–123 kg	1800
124–130 kg	1900
131–137 kg	2000
138–144 kg	2000
≥145 kg	2000

* Patients greater than 65 years of age may require lower heparin doses.

The PT varies with the warfarin dose (vitamin K inhibition) and vitamin K availability (intestinal and food sources). Drug interactions are also extremely important (Table 43-5).

Clinical Guidelines: Current Recommendations for Management

DEEP VENOUS THROMBOSIS (DVT) PROPHYLAXIS. It is estimated that pulmonary embolism is responsible for more than 100,000 deaths annually in the United States and contributes directly to an additional 100,000 deaths (see Chap. 60). The silent nature of DVT, coupled with the morbidity of acute pulmonary embolism, has set a precedent for prophylaxis among moderate- to high-risk patients (Table 43-6). Moderate-risk patients have a risk of DVT between 10 and 40 percent, a risk of proximal DVT of 2 to 10 percent, and a risk of fatal pulmonary embolism of 1 to 2 percent. Patients included in this category include those greater than 40 years of age undergoing major surgery. High-risk patients have a 40 to 80 percent risk of DVT, a 10 to 25 percent risk of proximal DVT, and a 2 to 10 percent risk of fatal pulmonary embolism. Patients included in this category include those with major trauma to the hip and/or knee, extensive pelvic or abdominal surgery, and previous DVT or pulmonary embolism [147–172].

Specific prophylactic methods provide a reduction in venous stasis, a change in blood components (reduce coagulability), or a change in the blood vessel wall. Thus, one or more aspects of Virchow's triad are addressed (Tables 43-7 and 43-8) (see Chap. 60).

Table 43-5. Clinical Conditions and Drug Effects Influencing Warfarin Response

Mechanism	PT (INR) effect	Example
Vitamin K malabsorption		Malabsorption syndromes
Vitamin K administration		Nutritional supplements, total parenteral nutrition
Decreased synthesis of vitamin K-dependent factors		Liver disease
Increased catabolism of coagulation factors		Hyperthyroidism
Decreased vitamin K absorption		Antibiotics, cholestyramine, mineral oil
Displaces warfarin from protein binding sites		Nonsteroidal antiinflammatory agents, amiodarone
Decreased catabolism of warfarin		Allopurinol, metronidazole, cimetidine, disulfiram
Increased catabolism of warfarin		Barbiturates, griseofulvin, anticonvulsants
Increased receptor affinity		Quinidine

Table 43-6. Patients at Increased Risk for Deep Venous Thrombosis/Pulmonary Embolism: Candidates for Prophylaxis

General surgery
Orthopaedic surgery (hip, knee)
Hip fracture
Hip replacement
Elective intracranial neurosurgery
Acute spinal cord injury
Multiple trauma
Burns
Stroke
Congestive heart failure
Puerperium
Congenital or acquired antithrombin III, protein C, or protein S deficiency
Previous deep venous thrombosis/pulmonary embolism

DEEP VENOUS THROMBOSIS/PULMONARY EMBOLISM. In venous thrombosis, stasis of blood flow and alterations in circulating blood elements are the predominant pathogenetic factors. Drugs that inhibit coagulation, such as heparin and warfarin, are therefore the agents of choice in treatment. These drugs are, in essence, prophylactic, preventing thrombus progression and embolization. Unlike thrombolytic drugs, heparin and warfarin do not dissolve thrombus. See Chapters 60 and 121 for management and treatment of DVT and pulmonary embolism.

There has been some debate concerning the potential for thrombi within the calf veins to embolize. Clearly, embolization of these clots is a rate event; however, nearly one of every four calf vein thrombi have proximal extension to the deep veins of the thigh and pelvis, and of these, 10 percent will embolize. Unfortunately, proximal extension is difficult to diagnose with accuracy based on physical findings alone. Therefore, we recommend treatment of calf vein thrombosis. Alternatively, serial noninvasive testing for 10 to 14 days can be performed to exclude extension. If observed, treatment should be initiated.

In cases of suspected pulmonary embolism, we recommend that heparin, 5000 units intravenously followed by a continuous

Table 43-7. Prophylactic Methods: Mechanism of Action

Method	Beneficial effects
1. Mechanical: pneumatic compression boots, graded compression stockings	Reduces venous stasis Prostacyclin release t-PA release
2. Warfarin	Inhibits coagulation cascade Primarily extrinsic pathway
3. Unfractionated heparin	Inhibits amplification of coagulation cascade
4. Low-molecular-weight heparin	Inhibits factor Xa/prothrombinase complex
5. Dihydroergotamine	Reduces venous stasis
6. Dextran	blood viscosity platelet function weakens fibrin architecture of thrombus

infusion, be given while confirmation is obtained through appropriate diagnostic testing.

Thrombolytic therapy for massive pulmonary embolism is discussed in Chapter 46.

Patients with proximal DVT with or without pulmonary embolism in whom anticoagulation is either contraindicated or ineffective (i.e., recurrent thrombotic events despite a therapeutic level of anticoagulation) should be considered for inferior vena cava interruption. The most common method employed at our institution is placement of a Greenfield filter [173].

UNSTABLE ANGINA. Heparin and oral anticoagulants have been used in the treatment of unstable angina and non-Q wave MI for over five decades [173–177]. The first major clinical trial of anticoagulation was performed by Théroux and colleagues [177a]. In their study of 479 patients with unstable angina, these investigators observed a marked benefit (reduced incidence of MI and refractory angina) in patients treated with either aspirin (325 mg twice per day) or intravenous heparin (continuous infusion to maintain the aPTT between 1.5 and 2 times the laboratory control). There was a trend favoring heparin over aspirin. A study by the RISC group [178] subsequently showed that a combination of heparin and aspirin may be more beneficial than either agent used alone.

We currently recommend that all patients with unstable angina receive aspirin, 160 to 325 mg, starting as soon as possible. Patients with an aspirin allergy should receive ticlopidine, 250 mg twice per day. In addition to antiplatelet therapy, anticoagulation with heparin is recommended for patients with ischemic chest pain at rest accompanied by electrocardiographic abnormalities. Heparin should be given intravenously as a bolus, followed by a continuous infusion for a total of 3 to 5 days. We recommend achieving and maintaining an aPTT of 1.5 to 2.5 times the laboratory control. An alternative to intravenous heparin is subcutaneous administration given at a dose of 17,500 units every 12 hours. As in other acute clinical settings, we prefer bedside coagulation monitoring and a heparin titration nomogram. When intravenous heparin is to be discontinued, we recommend a "pseudo" wean to prevent a rebound prothrombotic state. Our current practice is to decrease the heparin infusion by 50 percent for 12 hours prior to discontinuation. All patients should receive either aspirin or an alternative antiplatelet agent for at least 24 hours prior to heparin discontinuation. Antiplatelet therapy should be continued thereafter for at least 1 year and possibly indefinitely [179,180,181]. At present, thrombolytic therapy cannot be recommended routinely in the care of patients with unstable angina [182]. The potential benefit of the alternative thrombin antagonist hirudin is currently being explored in GUSTO-II.

Table 43-8. Deep Venous Thrombosis Prophylaxis: Suggested Regimens

Condition	Prophylactic agent/method	Dose	Dosing strategy	Alternatives
Low-risk general surgery	Early ambulation	—	—	Graded compression stockings
Moderate-risk general surgery	Unfractionated heparin	5000 units	q8–12h (SC)	Intermittent pneumatic compression
	LMW heparin	5000 XaI	q day (SC)	
High-risk general surgery	Unfractionated heparin	5000 units	q8h (SC)	Intermittent pneumatic compression
	LMW heparin	5000 XaI	q day (SC)	Dextran
Very-high-risk general surgery	Unfractionated heparin plus intermittent pneumatic compression	5000 units —	q8° (SC) —	LMW heparin plus intermittent pneumatic compression IVC filter (other forms of prophylaxis contraindicated or ineffective)
Total hip replacement	Unfractionated heparin (adjusted dose)	5000–7500 units (Achieve aPTT upper limits of normal)	q8°–12° (SC)	Warfarin (adjust to INR 2.0–3.0) LMW heparin
Hip fracture	Warfarin	Adjust to INR 2.0–3.0 (PO)		LMW heparin Adjusted unfractionated heparin
Knee surgery	Intermittent pneumatic compression	—	—	Unfractionated heparin
Intracranial neurosurgery	Intermittent pneumatic compression	—	—	Low-dose unfractionated heparin
Acute spinal cord injury	Unfractionated heparin (adjusted dose)	5000–7500 units (maintain aPTT upper) (limits of normal)	q8°–12° (SC)	Low-dose unfractionated heparin plus Intermittent compression pneumatic
Myocardial infarction	Unfractionated heparin LMW heparin	5000 units 5000 XaI	q8°–12° (SC) q day (SC)	Intermittent pneumatic compression
Ischemic stroke with lower extremity paralysis	Unfractionated heparin LMW heparin	5000 units 5000 XaI	q8°–12° (SC) q day (SC)	Intermittent pneumatic compression Warfarin (INR 2.0–3.0)
Congestive heart failure	Unfractionated heparin LMW heparin	5000 units 5000 XaI	q8°–12° (SC) q day (SC)	Intermittent pneumatic compression

XaI = Factor Xa inhibiting units; LMW = low-molecular-weight; IVC = inferior vena cava; INR = international normalized ratio.

MYOCARDIAL INFARCTION. The use of antithrombotic therapy among patients sustaining MI is based on the established pathology, placing intracoronary thrombosis at the center of attention. The risk of DVT, pulmonary embolism, and thromboembolic stroke in this setting also provides a strong rationale for antithrombotic strategies. Furthermore, the thrombolytic era has provided new insights, stressing the importance of thrombin antagonists and platelet inhibitors to reduce coronary arterial reocclusion, recurrent ischemia, reinfarction, and death.

A review of approximately 30 reports on the topic of anticoagulant use in MI indicates that mortality may be reduced by approximately 25 percent [183,184,185]. Several studies have also shown that thromboembolic events in high-risk patients (e.g., anterior Q wave infarction) can be reduced significantly by early institution of anticoagulant therapy with heparin [186,187].

ANTITHROMBOTIC THERAPY: CORONARY THROMBOLYSIS. The importance of plaque rupture and intraluminal thrombosis is discussed earlier in this chapter. Although thrombolytic therapy is a mainstay of treatment, several limitations have been recognized: (1) patency is achieved in only 80 to 85 percent of patients; (2) complete perfusion (TIMI grade 3 flow) is achieved in only 50 percent of patients; and (3) reocclusion occurs in nearly 10 percent of patients within the first 3 to 4 days of treatment. Anatomically, the postthrombolytic coronary artery consists of the following components: (1) ruptured/fissured atheromatous plaque; (2) retained mural and intraluminal thrombus; and (3) residual luminal narrowing. Each predisposes to thrombosis and recurrent ischemic events.

While thrombolytic therapy effectively lyses intracoronary thrombus in a majority of patients, dissolution is rarely complete. In fact, incomplete lysis is the rule rather than the exception. As a result, it is common to have residual thrombus at the original site of plaque rupture [188–191]. There is mounting evidence that the thrombolytic process itself may predispose to thrombus formation. Clot lysis, in essence, reexposes the original thrombogenic substrate to circulating blood [192,193]. Furthermore, thrombin is released during lysis, stimulating platelets and coagulation [192–197]. Factor X may also be activated on the thrombus surface, contributing directly to continued thrombus growth. Beyond the ability to activate and/or release thrombin, thrombolytic therapy, through the production of plasmin, also can activate platelets and the intrinsic coagulation cascade [198,199,200]. Reperfusion injury of the vascular endothelium

[201–204] and the presence of circulating procoagulant factors [205–210] may also provoke recurrent cardiac events.

Several recently completed clinical trials have shown that intravenous heparin, dosed sufficiently to elevate the aPTT to at least 1.5 times control, can reduce the incidence of coronary reocclusion among patients given tissue plasminogen activator. Pooled analyses suggest that mortality may also be reduced, and the findings of GUSTO-I (Global Utilization of Streptokinase and t-PA for Occluded Coronary Arteries) strongly support the adjunctive use of intravenous heparin with accelerated tPA and aspirin [211].

The adjunctive use of heparin among patients treated with streptokinase has been more difficult to establish. The available data point in favor of heparin administration, although the benefits appear modest. Anticipating that a therapeutic level of anticoagulation must be achieved and maintained to observe any benefit, intravenous heparin is the preferred route of administration. In GUSTO-I, intravenous heparin given for at least the initial 48 hours was not associated with an excess of transfusions, major hemorrhagic events, or intracerebral hemorrhage [212]. Pooled data from the GISSI-2/International Study, the International Study of Infarct Survival (ISIS-3), and GUSTO support adjunctive heparin to reduce in-hospital reinfarction and early mortality. More substantial benefits can be expected in select high-risk groups, including patients with previous MI or large anterior Q-wave infarctions and insulin-requiring diabetics [212,213].

Little information is available concerning heparin use among patients treated with APSAC (anisoylated plasminogen streptokinase activator complex). As with streptokinase, the benefits are probably modest [214].

In the setting of MI, antiplatelet therapy, primarily with aspirin, has been shown to reduce vascular mortality by one-fourth [215]. A 50 percent reduction in mortality was observed in ISIS-2 when aspirin, given immediately on hospital presentation, was combined with a thrombolytic [215]. Recurrent infarction and stroke can also be reduced with aspirin. Long-term antiplatelet therapy has been advocated strongly based on the pooled results of clinical trials [216–221].

The potential advantages of combining aspirin and low-dose warfarin are currently being explored in the Coumadin Aspirin Reinfarction Study (CARS).

MYOCARDIAL INFARCTION/CORONARY THROMBOLYSIS.
Patients with MI, particularly those considered to be at high risk for venous or arterial thromboembolism because of severe left ventricular dysfunction, congestive heart failure, history of thromboembolism, large anterior Q wave MI, or atrial fibrillation, should receive heparin given initially as a 5,000- to 10,000-unit bolus (60–80 units/kg) followed by a continuous infusion to maintain the aPTT at 1.5 to 2.0 times control. Treatment should be continued for 3 days (or longer for high-risk patients). If subcutaneous heparin is given, a dose of 17,500 units twice per day is recommended. Warfarin, administered for 3 months at a dose sufficient to elevate the international normalized ratio (INR—see Chap. 121) between 2.0 and 3.0 should be considered strongly for high-risk patients.

All patients should receive, at the very least, prophylaxis for DVT and pulmonary embolism with unfractionated heparin (or a suitable alternative) at a dose of 5000 to 7500 units given subcutaneously two to three times per day until daily ambulation is achieved.

All patients should receive 325 mg of non-enteric-coated aspirin (preferably chewed) as soon as possible and 160 to 325 mg daily thereafter. For patients subsequently started on warfarin, the aspirin dose should be reduced to 80 mg daily. Anti-platelet therapy should be discontinued if the potential for bleeding is considered high. Ticlopidine (250 mg twice a day) is recommended as an alternative in the case of either aspirin allergy or intolerance.

Thrombolytic therapy also may be initiated. All patients given thrombolytic therapy should receive adjunctive antiplatelet treatment, as follows.

t-PA. Heparin should be given intravenously (bolus, maintenance infusion) for at least 72 hours or longer (for patients at high risk).

Streptokinase. Heparin should be given intravenously (without a bolus) beginning 6 hours after treatment initiation. A maintenance infusion is recommended for at least 72 hours. As an alternative heparin can be given subcutaneously at a dose of 17,500 units twice per day.

APSAC. Heparin should be given intravenously beginning 6 to 12 hours after treatment initiation. A maintenance infusion is recommended for at least 72 hours. As an alternative, heparin can be given subcutaneously at a dose of 17,500 units twice per day.

ATRIAL FIBRILLATION.
It is strongly recommended that long-term anticoagulation with warfarin (INR 2.0–3.0) be offered to patients with chronic valvular or nonvalvular atrial fibrillation. Patients younger than 65 years without organic heart disease (lone atrial fibrillation) do not require anticoagulation. The role of aspirin therapy has not been determined fully; however, it is possible that patients with atrial fibrillation without systemic hypertension (systolic >160 mm Hg), left ventricular dysfunction (ejection fraction < 40%), clinical congestive heart failure, or previous thromboembolism can be treated with aspirin, 325 mg daily. The safety and efficacy of combined warfarin and aspirin for high-risk patient groups are currently under investigation [222–226].

Anticoagulation is not recommended for atrial fibrillation of brief duration (<48 hours) unless there are other features associated with a high risk of thromboembolism (cardiomyopathy, severe left ventricular dysfunction, significant valvular heart disease, or previous thromboembolism). If the duration of atrial fibrillation is unknown, anticoagulation should be instituted unless contraindications exist.

Hospitalized patients with confirmed or suspected atrial fibrillation greater than 48 hours in duration should be anticoagulated with heparin given intravenously to maintain the aPTT between 1.5 and 2.5 times control. If elective chemical or electrical cardioversion is planned, anticoagulation with heparin or warfarin should be continued for 2 to 3 weeks prior to and 4 weeks after establishing normal sinus rhythm. Anticoagulation with heparin is also recommended for emergency cardioversion, when feasible, if the duration of atrial fibrillation is unknown and additional thromboembolic risk factors are present.

Anticoagulation is not recommended for patients with atrial flutter or other atrial tachyarrhythmias unless they are considered to be at high risk for thromboembolism.

The role of TEE in determining the need for anticoagulation among patients with atrial fibrillation of unknown duration is currently being investigated.

MECHANICAL HEART VALVES.
Patients with mechanical heart valves, including Bjork-Shiley, St. Judes, Starr-Edwards, and Medtronic-Hall valves, in either the aortic or mitral position should receive long-term (lifelong) anticoagulation with warfarin titrated carefully to an INR of 2.5 to 3.5. Hemorrhagic complications increase with an INR greater than 4.5 and throm-

boembolic rates increase with an INR less than 1.8. In high-risk patients, dipyridamole (375–400 mg daily) or aspirin (100 mg daily) can be added without increased bleeding complications [227–230]. Higher doses of aspirin are not recommended because of the low likelihood of deriving additional benefit and the recognized risk of excessive hemorrhagic events [231]. It must be understood that aspirin or alternative antiplatelet therapy alone does not provide adequate protection against thromboembolism.

Patients with mechanical prosthetic valves admitted to the intensive care unit should be anticoagulated with intravenous heparin titrated to an aPTT of 1.5 to 2.5 times control. Heparin is preferred over warfarin in most instances to allow better control of the state of anticoagulation.

BIOPROSTHETIC HEART VALVES. Patients with bioprosthetic heart valves, including Hancock and Carpentier-Edwards valves, are less prone to thromboembolism than patients with mechanical prosthetic valves. Despite this recognized advantage, anticoagulation is recommended for at least the first 3 postoperative months. Heparin given intravenously can be used initially, followed by oral warfarin titrated to an INR of 2.0 to 3.0. Anticoagulation for longer periods may be required in patients at increased risk for thromboembolism (e.g., clonic atrial fibrillation, left ventricular dysfunction, previous thromboembolism) [232–236].

INTERRUPTION OF ANTICOAGULANT THERAPY. Occasionally existing circumstances (e.g., noncardiac surgery) necessitate interruption of anticoagulation. Among patients in an intensive care unit setting receiving intravenous heparin this can be achieved by discontinuing the infusion 2 to 4 hours before the scheduled procedure. The heparin can then be restarted after surgery when hemostasis has been achieved. Often heparin is restarted without a bolus at relatively low infusion rates (400–500 units/h) to maintain the aPTT at the upper limits of normal. The infusion is then increased when clinically feasible. When minimally invasive procedures are performed, heparin can be continued while maintaining an aPTT at the lower limits of therapeutic (1.5 times control).

Patients at high risk for thromboembolism present a clinical challenge. In most instances, heparin is not interrupted. Instead, the infusion is continued at low infusion rates and dipyridamole is added for further protection. Life-threatening hemorrhage may necessitate complete discontinuation for variable periods of time. In this situation, potential risks and benefits must be weighed carefully [237–238].

HEMORRHAGIC COMPLICATIONS OF ANTITHROMBOTIC THERAPY. Bleeding is the most common complication of antithrombotic therapy. In most cases, bleeding is minor and can be controlled with local measures, including manual pressure or pressure dressings. The aPTT should be determined for patients receiving heparin, while the INR should be checked when warfarin is given. Adjustments can be made as needed. The platelet count should also be assessed.

Moderate bleeding can often be observed without discontinuing antithrombotic therapy; however, the risk-benefit ratio must be assessed carefully. Clearly, the threshold for stopping therapy would be high among patients at high risk for thromboembolism. As with minor bleeding, responsible sites should be identified and local measures for control instituted. The aPTT, INR, and platelet count should be determined.

Major or life-threatening bleeding presents a unique clinical dilemma, particularly when it occurs in the setting of a major or life-threatening thrombolic event. The site of bleeding must be identified and appropriate measures undertaken. If a decision to discontinue antithrombotic therapy is made, the heparin infusion should be stopped immediately. Residual heparin effect can be neutralized with protamine sulfate (1 mg per 100 units heparin given during the prior 4 hours). The anticoagulant effect of warfarin can be reversed by replacing vitamin K-dependent coagulation factors. Administration of vitamin K (0.5–1 mg intravenously or 10 mg subcutaneously) can reduce the INR within 12 to 24 hours. Larger doses (5–10 mg intravenously or 20–30 mg subcutaneously) can reduce the INR within 6 to 8 hours. Rapid reversal can be achieved with fresh frozen plasma or prothrombin concentrates.

Major or life-threatening hemorrhage in patients given thrombolytic therapy within the prior 24 to 48 hours is especially challenging because of the broad array of potential hemostatic abnormalities. If heparin is being administered, it should be discontinued immediately. Residual heparin effect can then be neutralized with protamine. If bleeding persists and the plasma fibrinogen concentration is less than 1 g per liter, replacement with fresh frozen plasma (15 ml/kg) is recommended. Cryoprecipitate (10 units) is also an excellent source of fibrinogen (200–250 mg per 10–15 ml) and provides factor VIII (80 units per 10–15 ml), capable of generating thrombin via the intrinsic coagulation cascade, as well. If bleeding persists despite heparin neutralization and supplementation with plasma coagulation factors and the platelet count is less than 100×10^9 per liter, platelet transfusions (10 units) should be given to correct plasmin-mediated platelet dysfunction. Amicar or tranexamic acid, potent inhibitors of plasmin and plasminogen activator, should be considered only when all other measures have failed [239,240].

RECOMMENDATIONS FOR INCREASED INR WITHOUT BLEEDING. Patients receiving warfarin must be monitored closely to maintain an acceptable level of systemic anticoagulation. Occasionally, an excessive level occurs that may or may not be associated with overt bleeding. Regardless, considerable experience suggests that an INR greater than 4.5 is associated with an increased risk of hemorrhage; therefore efforts to lower the INR should be undertaken. The following guidelines were derived by the American College of Chest Physicians Committee on Antithrombotic Therapy [241].

1. INR >3.5 but <6.0 without evidence of bleeding or a need for rapid reversal (e.g., surgical procedure). Hold warfarin for 1 to 3 days. Follow INR daily and restart warfarin when the therapeutic range is achieved.
2. INR >6.0 but <10.0 without evidence of bleeding; however, nonemergent surgical procedure pending. Give vitamin K 0.5 to 1.0 mg intravenously, recheck INR in 6 to 8 hours. Repeat dose if needed. Alternatively, give vitamin K 10 mg subcutaneously, recheck INR in 24 hours. Repeat dose as needed.
3. INR >10.0 but <20.0 without evidence of bleeding. Give vitamin K 3 to 5 mg intravenously. Repeat INR 6 hours later. Repeat dose as needed to lower INR below 6.0.
4. INR >20.0 without evidence of bleeding. Give vitamin K 10 mg intravenously. Repeat INR in 6 hours. Repeat dose as needed to lower INR below 6.0.

References

1. Harker LA: Pathogenesis of thrombosis, in Williams WJ (ed): *Hematology*. 4th ed. New York, McGraw-Hill, 1990, pp 1559–1569.

2. Turrito VT, Baumgartner JR: Platelet-surface interactions, in Colman RW, Hirsh J, Marder VJ, Salzman EW (eds): *Haemostasis and Thrombosis: Basic Principles and Clinical Practice*. 2nd ed. Philadelphia, JB Lippincott, 1987, pp 555–571.

3. Kieffer N, Phillips DR: Platelet membrane glycoproteins: Functions in cellular interactions. *Ann Rev Cell Biol* 6:329, 1990.

4. Ruoslahti E: Integrins. *J Clin Invest* 87:1, 1991.

5. Moncada S, Palmer RMJ, Higgs EA: Prostacyclin and endothelium-derived relaxing factor: Biological interactions and significance, in Cerstarete M, Vermylen J, Lijnen R, Arnout J (eds): *Thrombosis and Haemostasis*. Leuven, Leuven University Press, 1987, pp 505–523.

6. Ludmer PL, Selwyn AP, Shook TL, et al: Paradoxical vasoconstriction induced by acetylcholine and atherosclerotic coronary arteries. *N Engl J Med* 315:1046, 1986.

7. Nabel EG, Selwyn AP, Ganz P: Paradoxical narrowing of atherosclerotic coronary arteries induced by increases in heart rate. *Circulation* 81:850, 1990.

8. Vita JA, Treasure CB, Ganz P, et al: Control of shear stress in the epicardial coronary arteries of humans: Impairment by atherosclerosis. *J Am Coll Cardiol* 14:1193, 1989.

9. Coupe MO, Mak JCW, Yacoub M, et al: Autoradiographic mapping of calcitonin gene-related polypeptide receptors in human and guinea pig hearts. *Circulation* 81:741, 1990.

10. Yatani A, Yokoyama M, Akita H, Fakuzak H: Endothelium dependent vasodilating effect of substance P during flow-reducing coronary stenosis in the dog. *J Am Coll Cardiol* 15:1374, 1990.

11. Schwartz JS, Carlyle PF, Cohn JN: Effect of dilation of the distal coronary bed on flow and resistance in severely stenotic coronary arteries in the dog. *Am J Cardiol* 43:219, 1979.

12. Jelke FW, Quillen JE, Brooks LA, Harrison DG: Endothelial modulation of the coronary vasculature in the vessels perfused via mature collaterals. *Circulation* 81:1938, 1990.

13. Peters KG, Marcus ML, Harrison DG: Vasopressin and the mature coronary collateral circulation. *Circulation* 79:1324, 1989.

14. Yamamoto H, Bossaller C, Cartwright J Jr, et al: Videomicroscopic demonstration of defective cholinergic arteriolar vasodilation in atherosclerotic rabbit. *J Clin Invest* 81:1752, 1988.

15. Harrison DG, Armstrong ML, Freiman PC, Heistad DD: Restoration of endothelium dependent relaxation by dietary treatment of atherosclerosis. *J Clin Invest* 80:1808, 1987.

16. Saellke FW, Armstrong ML, Harrison DG: Endothelium-dependent vascular relaxation is abnormal in the coronary microcirculation of atherosclerotic primates. *Circulation* 81:1586, 1990.

17. Kwaan HC: Possible effects of risk factors on fibrinolysis, in Chandler AB (ed): *Thrombotic Processes in Atherosclerosis*. New York, Plenum, 1978, pp 235–300.

18. Walker ID, Davidson JF, Hutton I, et al: Disordered fibrinolytic potential in coronary heart disease. *Thromb Res* 10:509, 1977.

19. Chakrabarti R, Hocking ED: Fibrinolytic activity and coronary heart disease. *Lancet* 1:987, 1968.

20. Kragel AH, Reddy SG, Wittes JT, Roberts WC: Morphometric analysis of the composition of atherosclerotic plaques in the four major epicardial coronary arteries in acute myocardial infarction and in sudden coronary death. *Circulation* 80:1747, 1989.

21. Kragel AH, Reddy SG, Wittes JT, Roberts WC: Morphometric analysis of the composition of coronary arterial plaques in isolated unstable angina pectoris with pain at rest. *Am J Cardiol* 66:562, 1990.

22. Dollar AL, Kragel AH, Fernicola DJ, et al: Composition of atherosclerotic plaques in coronary arteries in women <40 years of age with fatal coronary artery disease and implications for plaque reversibility. *Am J Cardiol* 67:1223, 1991.

23. Gertz SD, Malekzadeh S, Dollar AL, et al: Composition of atherosclerotic plaques in the four major epicardial coronary arteries in patients ≥90 years of age. *Am J Cardiol* 67:1228, 1991.

24. Lendon C, Davies MJ, Richardson PH, Born GVR: Pathogenesis of fissuring in human atherosclerotic plaques, in Chamerlain DA, Julain DG, Sleight P (eds): *The Management of Acute Myocardial Ischemia*. London, Chapman & Hall, 1990, pp 9–11.

25. Davies MJ, Woolf N, Katz DR: Structure and cellular composition of aortic atherosclerotic plaques undergoing ulceration (abstract). *Br Heart J* 66:92, 1991.

26. Falk E: Plaque rupture with severe pre-existing stenosis precipi-tating coronary thrombosis: Characteristics of coronary atherosclerotic plaques underlying fatal occlusive thrombi. *Br Heart J* 50:127, 1983.

27. Ridolfi RL, Huchins GM: The relationship between coronary artery lesions and myocardial infarcts: Ulceration of atherosclerotic plaques precipitating coronary thrombosis. *Am Heart J* 93:468, 1977.

28. Hore T, Sekiguchi M, Hirosawa K: Coronary thrombosis in pathogenesis of acute myocardial infarction: Histopathological study of coronary arteries in 108 necropsied cases using serial section. *Br Heart J* 40:153, 1978.

29. Falk E: Why do plaques rupture? *Circulation* 86(suppl III):III-30, 1991.

30. Davies MJ, Thomas AC: Plaques fissuring: The cause of acute myocardial infarction, sudden ischemic death, and crescendo angina. *Br Heart J* 53:363, 1985.

31. Badimon L, Chesebro JH, Badimon JJ: Thrombus formation on ruptured atherosclerotic plaques and rethrombosis on evolving thrombi. *Circulation* 86(suppl III):III-74, 1992.

32. Ambrose JA, Winters SL, Stern A, et al: Angiographic morphology and the pathogenesis of unstable angina pectoris. *J Am Coll Cardiol* 5:609, 1985.

33. Moise A, Theroux P, Taeymans Y, et al: Unstable angina and progression of coronary atherosclerosis. *N Engl J Med* 309:685, 1983.

34. Mizuno K, Satomura K, Miymoto A, et al: Angioscopic evaluation of coronary artery thrombi in acute coronary syndromes. *N Engl J Med* 326:287, 1992.

35. Master AM, Dack S, Jaffe HL: Activities associated with the onset of acute coronary artery occlusion. *Am Heart J* 18:434, 1939.

36. Master AM: The role of effort and occupation (including physicians) in coronary occlusion. *JAMA* 174:84, 1960.

37. Muller JE, Stone PH, Turi ZG, et al: Circadian variation in the frequency of onset of acute myocardial infarction. *N Engl J Med* 313:1315, 1985.

38. Tofler GH, Stone PH, Maclure M, et al: Analysis of possible triggers of acute myocardial infarction (the MILIS Study Group). *Am J Cardiol* 66:22, 1990.

39. Stone PH: Triggers of transient myocardial ischemia: Circadian variation and relation to plaque rupture and coronary thrombosis in stable coronary artery disease. *Am J Cardiol* 66:32G, 1990.

40. Kubota K, Sakurai T, Tamura J, et al: Is the circadian change in hematocrit and blood viscosity a factor triggering cerebral and myocardial infarction? (letter) *Stroke* 18:812, 1987.

41. Gertz SD, Uretzky G, Wajnberg RS, et al: Endothelial cell damage and thrombus formation after partial arterial constriction: Relevance to the role of coronary artery spasm in the pathogenesis of myocardial infarction. *Circulation* 63:476, 1981.

42. Wihelmsen L, Svardsudd K, Korsan-Bengsten K, et al: Fibrinogen as a risk factor for stroke and myocardial infarction. *N Engl J Med* 311:501, 1984.

43. Kannel WB, Castelli WP, Meeks SL: Fibrinogen and cardiovascular disease. Abstract of paper for 34th Annual Scientific Session of the American College of Cardiology, March 1985, Anaheim, California.

44. Kannel WB, Wolf PA, Castelli WP, et al: Fibrinogen and risk of cardiovascular disease. *JAMA* 258:1183, 1987.

45. Yarnell JWG, Baker IA, Sweetnam PM, et al: Fibrinogen, viscosity and white blood cell count are major risk factors for ischemic heart disease: The Cearphilly and Speedwell Collaborative Heart Disease Studies. *Circulation* 83:836, 1991.

46. Miller GJ, Martin JC, Webster J, et al: Association between dietary fat intake and plasma factor VII coagulant activity: A predictor of cardiovascular mortality. *Atherosclerosis* 60:269, 1986.

47. Simpson HCR, Mann JI, Meade TW: Hypertriglyceridemia and hypercoagulability. *Lancet* 1:786, 1983.

48. Humpries SE, Cook M, Dubowitz M, et al: Role of genetic variation at the fibrinogen locus in determination of plasma fibrinogen concentrations. *Lancet* 1:1452, 1987.

49. Thomas AE, Green FR, Kelleher CH, et al: Variation in the promoter region of the β fibrinogen gene is associated with plasma fibrinogen levels in smokers and non-smokers. *Thromb Haemost* 65:487, 1991.

50. Green FR, Kelleher CK, Wilkes HC, et al: A common genetic

polymorphism associated with lower coagulation factor VII levels in healthy individuals. *Arterioscler Thromb* 11:540, 1991.

51. Thompson WD, Smith EB, et al: Atherosclerosis and the coagulation system. *J Pathol* 159:97, 1989.

52. Lowe GDO: Blood rheology in arterial disease. *Clin Sci* 71:137, 1986.

53. Meade TW, Vickers MV, Thompson SG, et al: Epidemiological characteristics of platelet aggregability. *Br Med J* 290:428, 1985.

54. Gurewich V, Lipinski B, Hyde E, et al: The effect of the fibrinogen concentration and the leukocyte count on intravascular fibrin deposition from soluble fibrin monomer complexes. *Thromb Haemost* 36:605, 1976.

55. Benjamin EJ, Levy D, Plehn JF, et al: Left atrial size: an independent risk factor for stroke: The Framingham Heart Study (abstract). *Circulation* 80(suppl IV):615, 1989.

56. Daniel WG, Angermann C, Engberding G, et al: Transeophageal echocardiography in patients with cerebral ischemic events and arterial embolism: A European multicenter study (abstract). *Circulation* 80(suppl IV):II-473, 1989.

57. Nellessen U, Daniel WG, Matheis G, et al: Impending paradoxical embolism from atrial thrombus: Correct diagnosis by transesophageal echocardiography and prevention by surgery. *J Am Coll Cardiol* 5:1002, 1985.

58. Aschenberg W, Schluter M, Kremer P, et al: Transesophageal two-dimensional echocardiography for the detection of left atrial appendage thrombus. *J Am Coll Cardiol* 7:163, 1986.

59. Visser CA, Kan G, Meltzer RS, et al: Long term follow up of left ventricular thrombus after acute myocardial infarction: A two-dimensional echocardiography study in 96 patients. *Chest* 86:532, 1984.

60. Stratton JR, Resnick AD: Increased embolic risk in patients with left ventricular thrombi. *Circulation* 75:1004, 1987.

61. Funke Kupper AJ, Verheugt FWA, Peels CH: Left ventricular thrombus incidence and behavior studied by serial two-dimensional echocardiography in acute anterior myocardial infarction: Left ventricular wall motion, systemic embolism and oral anticoagulation. *J Am Coll Cardiol* 13:1514, 1989.

62. Penny WJ, Chesebro JG, Heras M, et al: Antithrombotic therapy for patients with cardiac disease. *Curr Probl Cardiol* 13:464, 1988.

63. Sechtem U, Theissen P, Heindel W, et al: Diagnosis of left ventricular thrombi by magnetic resonance imaging and comparison with angiocardiography, computerized tomography and echocardiography. *Am J Cardiol* 64:1195, 1989.

64. Mikell F, Asinger R, Elperger J, et al: Long term prospective evaluation of left ventricular thrombus in acute myocardial infarction (abstract). *Circulation* 64(suppl 4):93, 1989.

65. Visser CA, Kan G, Lie KI, et al: Long term follow up of left ventricular thrombus following acute myocardial infarction: A prospective serial echocardiography study of 96 patients. *Eur Heart J* 4:333, 1983.

66. Visser CA, Kan G, Meltzer RS, et al: Long term follow up of left ventricular thrombus after acute myocardial infarction: A two-dimensional echocardiographic study in 96 patients. *Chest* 86:532, 1984.

67. Tramarin R, Pozzoli M, Vecchio C: Tromboli ventricolare sinistra nell'infarto miocardio recente: studio ecocardiografico. *G Ital Cardiol* 12:397, 1982.

68. McEntee CW, VanReet RE, Winters WL, et al: Incidence and natural history of mural thrombi in acute myocardial infarction by two-dimensional echocardiography (abstract). *Circulation* 68(suppl 3):331, 1983.

69. Friedman MJ, Carlson K, Marcus FI, et al: Clinical correlations in patients with acute myocardial infarction and left ventricular thrombus detected by two dimensional echocardiography. *Am J Med* 72:894, 1982.

70. Keating EC, Gross SA, Schlamowitz RA, et al: Mural thrombi in myocardial infarctions: Prospective evaluation by two-dimensional echocardiography. *Am J Med* 74:989, 1983.

71. Haugland JM, Asinger RW, Mikell FL, et al: Embolic potential of left ventricular thrombus detected by two-dimensional echocardiography. *Circulation* 70:588, 1984.

72. Visser CA, Kan G, Meltzer RS, et al: Embolic potential of left ventricular thrombi after myocardial infarction: A two-dimen-

sional echocardiographic study of 119 patients. *J Am Coll Cardiol* 5:1276, 1985.

73. Cabin HS, Roberts WC: Left ventricular aneurysm, intraaneurysmal thrombus and systemic embolus in coronary heart disease. *Chest* 77:586, 1980.

74. Stratton JR, Nemanich JW, Johannessen K-A, et al: Fate of left ventricular thrombi in patients with remote myocardial infarction or idiopathic cardiomyopathy. *Circulation* 78:1388, 1988.

75. Stratton JR, Ritchie JL: In platelet imaging of left ventricular thrombi. *Circulation* 81:1182, 1990.

76. Kumagai, K, Fukunami M, Ohmori M, et al: Increased intracardiovascular clotting in patients with chronic atrial fibrillation. *J Am Coll Cardiol* 16:377, 1990.

77. Kannel WB, Abbott RD, Savage DD, et al: Epidemiologic features of chronic atrial fibrillation: The Framingham Study. *N Engl J Med* 306:1018, 1982.

78. Wolf PA, Abbott RD, Kannel WB: Atrial fibrillation: A major contributor to stroke in the elderly. *Arch Intern Med* 147:1561, 1987.

79. Sokolow M, Ball RE: Factors influencing conversion of chronic atrial fibrillation with special reference to serum quinidine concentration. *Circulation* 14:568, 1956.

80. Goldman MJ: The management of chronic atrial fibrillation indications for and method of conversion to sinus rhythm. *Prog Cardiovasc Dis* 2:465, 1960.

81. Lown B, Perlroth MG, Kaidbey S, et al: "Cardioversion" of atrial fibrillation: A report on the treatment of 65 episodes in 50 patients. *N Engl J Med* 269:325, 1963.

82. Killip T: Synchronized DC precordial shock for arrhythmias: Safe new techniques to establish normal rhythm may be utilized on an elective or an emergency basis. *JAMA* 186:1, 1963.

83. Freeman I, Wexler J: Anticoagulation for treatment of atrial fibrillation. *JAMA* 184:1007, 1963.

84. Rokseth R, Storstein O: Quinidine therapy of chronic auricular fibrillation: The occurrence and mechanism of syncope. *Arch Intern Med* 111:184, 1963.

85. Morris JJ, Kong Y, North WC, et al: Experience with "cardioversion" of atrial fibrillation and flutter. *Am J Cardiol* 14:94, 1964.

86. Oram S, Davies JPH: Further experience of electrical conversion of atrial fibrillation to sinus rhythm: Analysis of 100 patients. *Lancet* 1:1294, 1964.

87. Hurst JW, Paulk EA, Proctor HD, et al: Management of patients with atrial fibrillation. *Am J Med* 37:728, 1964.

88. Selzer A, Kelly JJ, Johnson RB, et al: Immediate and long term results of electrical conversion of arrhythmias. *Prog Cardiovasc Dis* 9:90, 1966.

89. Hall JI, Wood DR: Factors affecting cardioversion of atrial arrhythmias with special reference to quinidine. *Br Heart J* 30:84, 1968.

90. Manning WJ, Silverman DI, Gordon SP, et al: Cardioversion from atrial fibrillation without prolonged anticoagulation with use of transesophageal echocardiography to exclude the presence of atrial thrombi. *N Engl J Med* 328:750, 1993.

91. Dewanjee MK, Trastek VF, Tago M, et al: Radiotropic techniques for noninvasive detection of platelet deposition in bovine tissue mitral-valve prostheses and in vitro quantification of visceral microembolism in dogs. *Invest Radiol* 6:535, 1984.

92. Pipkin RD, Buch WAS, Fogarty TS: Evaluation of aortic valve replacement with a porcine xenograft without long term anticoagulants. *J Thorac Cardiovasc Surg* 71:179, 1976.

93. Stinson EB, Griepp RB, Oyer PE, et al: Long term experience with porcine aortic valve xenografts. *J Thorac Cardiovasc Surg* 73:54, 1977.

94. Ionescu MI, Pakrashi BC, Mary DAS, et al: Long term evaluation of tissue valves. *J Thorac Cardiovasc Surg* 68:361, 1974.

95. Cevese PG: Long term results of 212 xenograft valve replacement. *J Cardiovasc Surg* 16:639, 1975.

96. Davila JC, Magilligan DJ, Lewis JW: Is the Hancock porcine valve the best cardiac valve substitute today? *Ann Thorac Surg* 26:303, 1978.

97. Heras M, Chesebro JH, Grill DE, et al: Chronic risk of thromboembolism after bioprosthetic valve replacement (abstract). *Eur Heart J* 10(suppl C):260, 1989.

98. Turpie AGG, Gunstensen J, Hirsh J, et al: Randomized comparison of two intensities of oral anticoagulant therapy after tissue heart valve replacement. *Lancet* 1:1242, 1988.

99. Lorient Roudant M-F, Ledain L, Roudant R, et al: Thrombolytic treatment of acute thrombotic obstruction with disk valve prostheses: Experience with 26 cases. *Semin Thromb Hem* 13:201, 1987.

100. Deviri E, Sareli P, Wisenbaugh T, et al: Obstruction of mechanical heart valve prostheses: Clinical aspects and surgical management. *J Am Coll Cardiol* 17:646, 1991.

101. Massad M, Gahl M, Slim M, et al: Thrombosed Bjork-Shiley standard disc mitral valve prosthesis. *J Cardiovasc Surg* 30:976, 1989.

102. Balram A, Kaul U, Rao R, et al: Thrombotic obstruction of Bjork-Shiley valves: Diagnostic and surgical considerations. *Int J Cardiol* 6:61, 1984.

103. Quintanilla MA, Haque AK: Thrombotic obstruction of prosthetic aortic valve presenting as acute myocardial infarction. *Am Heart J* 117:1378, 1989.

104. Tapanainen J, Ikaheimo M, Jouppila P, et al: Thrombosis in a mechanical aortic valve prosthesis during subcutaneous heparin therapy in pregnancy: A case report. *Eur J Obstet Gynecol Reprod Biol* 36:175, 1990.

105. Rosenberg RD, Lam L: Correlation between structure and function of heparin. *Proc Natl Acad Sci USA* 76:1218, 1979.

106. Rosenberg RD: The heparin-antithrombin system: A natural anticoagulant mechanism, in Colman RW, Hirsh J, Marder VJ, Salzman EW (eds): *Hemostasis and Thrombosis*. Philadelphia, JB Lippincott, 1987, pp 1373–1392.

107. Lindahl U, Backstrom G, Hook M, Thunberg L: Structure of antithrombin-binding site of heparin. *Proc Natl Acad Sci USA* 76:3198, 1979.

108. Harker LA, Malpass TW, Branson HE, et al: Mechanisms of abnormal bleeding in patients undergoing cardiopulmonary bypass: Acquired transient platelet dysfunction associated with selective α-granule release. *Blood* 56:824, 1980.

109. Massel DR, Hudoba M, Weitz JI: Clot bound thrombin is protected from heparin inhibition: A potential mechanism for rethrombosis after lytic therapy. *Circulation* 80(suppl):II-420, 1989.

110. Salzma EW, Rosenberg RD, Smith MH, et al: Effect of heparin and heparin fractions of platelet aggregation. *J Clin Invest* 65:64, 1980.

111. Anderson WH, Mohammad SF, Chuang HYK, et al: Heparin potentiates synthesis of thromboxane A2 in human platelets. *Adv Prostaglandin Thromboxane Leukot Res* 6:287, 1980.

112. Bock PE, Luscombe M, Marshall SE, et al: The multiple complexes formed by the interaction of platelet factor 4 with heparin. *Biochem J* 191:769, 1980.

113. Weitz JI, Hudoba M, Massel D, et al: Clot bound thrombin is protected from inhibition by heparin antithrombin III but is susceptible to inactivation by antithrombin III independent inhibitors. *J Clin Invest* 86:385, 1990.

114. Bar-Shavit R, Eldor A, Vlodavsky I: Binding of thrombin to subendothelial extracellular matrix: Protection and expression of functional properties. *J Clin Invest* 84:1096, 1989.

115. Teitel JM, Rosenberg RD: Protection of factor X$_a$ from neutralization by the heparin antithrombin complex. *J Clin Invest* 71:1383, 1983.

116. Hogg PH, Jackson CM: Fibrin monomer protects thrombin from inactivation by heparin antithrombin III: Implications for heparin efficacy. *Proc Natl Acad Sci USA* 86:3619, 1989.

117. Kaiser B: Anticoagulant and antithrombotic actions of recombinant hirudin. *Semin Thromb Hemost* 17:130, 1991.

118. Homeister JW, Michelson JK, Hoff PT, et al: Recombinant hirudin reduces the incidence of thrombotic occlusion in a canine model of coronary vascular injury. *Cor Art Dis* 2:237, 1991.

119. Cannon CP, McCabe CH, Henry TD, et al: A pilot trial of recombinant Desulfatohirudin compared with heparin in conjunction with tissue-type plasminogen activator and aspirin for acute myocardial infarction. Results of the TIMI 5 trial. *Am Coll Cardiol* 23:993, 1994.

120. Cannon CP, Maraganore JM, Lascalzo J, et al: Anticoagulant effects of hirulog, a novel thrombin inhibitor, in patients with coronary artery disease. *Am J Cardiol* 71:778, 1993.

121. Topol EJ, Bonan R, Jewitt D, et al: Use of a direct antithrombin, hirulog, in place of heparin during coronary angioplasty. *Circulation* 87:1622, 1993.

122. Maraganore JM, Bourdon P, Jablonski J, et al: Design and characterization of hirulogs: A novel class of bivalent peptide inhibitors of thrombin. *Biochemistry* 29:7095, 1990.

123. Stenflo J, Fernlund P, Egan W, et al: Vitamin K dependent modifications of glumatic acid residues in prothrombin. *Proc Natl Acad Sci USA* 71:2730, 1974.

124. Nelsesteun GL, Zytkovicz TH, Howard JB: The mode of action of vitamin K: Identification of gamma caboxyglytamic acid as a component of prothrombin. *J Biol Chem* 249:6347, 1974.

125. Lian JB, Hauschka PV, Gallop PM: Properties and biosynthesis of a vitamin K dependent calcium binding protein in bone. *Fed Proc* 37:2615, 1978.

126. Hsia J, Hamilton WP, Kleiman N, et al: A comparison between heparin and low-dose aspirin as adjunctive therapy with tissue plasminogen activator for acute myocardial infarction. *N Engl J Med* 323:1433, 1990.

127. de Bono DP, Simoons ML, Tijssen J, et al: Effect of early intravenous heparin on coronary patency, infarct size, and bleeding complications after alteplase thrombolysis: Results of a randomized double blind European Cooperative Study Group trial. *Br Heart J* 67:122, 1992.

128. Hull RD, Raskob GE, Hirsh J, et al: Continuous intravenous heparin compared with intermittent subcutaneous heparin in the initial treatment of proximal-vein thrombosis. *N Engl J Med* 315:1109, 1986.

129. Arnout J, Simoons M, de Bono D, et al: Correlation between level of heparinization and patency of the infarct-related coronary artery after treatment of acute myocardial infarction with alteplase (rt-PA). *J Am Coll Cardiol* 20:513, 1992.

130. Hsia J, Kleiman N, Aguirre F, et al: Heparin-induced prolongation of partial thromboplastin time after thrombolysis: Relation to coronary artery patency. *J Am Coll Cardiol* 20:31, 1992.

131. Basu D, Gallus A, Hirsh J, Cade J: A prospective study of the value of monitoring heparin treatment with the activated partial thromboplastin time. *N Engl J Med* 287:324, 1972.

132. Bain B, Forster T, Sleigh B: Heparin and the activated partial thromboplastin time: A difference between the in vitro and in vivo effects and implications for the therapeutic range. *Am J Clin Pathol* 74:668, 1980.

133. Barrowcliffe TW, Gray E: Studies of phospholipid reagents used in coagulation II: Factors influencing their sensitivity to heparin. *Thromb Haemost* 46:634, 1981.

134. Shapiro G, Huntzinger SW, Wilson JE: Variation among commercial activated partial thromboplastin time reagents in response to heparin. *Am J Clin Pathol* 67:477, 1977.

135. Banez EI, Triplett DA, Koepke J: Laboratory monitoring of heparin therapy: The effect of different salts of heparin on the activated partial thromboplastin time. *Am J Clin Pathol* 74:569, 1980.

136. Ansell J, Tiarks C, Hirsh J, et al: Measurement of the activated partial thromboplastin time from a capillary (fingerstick) sample of whole blood. *Am J Clin Pathol* 95:222, 1991.

137. Becker R, Cyr J, Corrao J, et al: Bedside aPTT monitoring: A convenient, rapid, and accurate assessment of systemic anticoagulation in heparinized patients. *J Am Coll Cardiol* 21:219A, 1993.

138. Becker RC, Corrao JM, Ball SP, Gore JM: A comparison of heparin strategies following thrombolytic therapy. *Am Heart J* 126:750, 1993.

139. Cruickshank MK, Levine MN, Hirsh J, et al: A standard heparin nomogram for the management of heparin therapy. *Arch Intern Med* 151:333, 1991.

140. Hull RD, Raskob GE, Rosenbloom D, et al: Optimal therapeutic level of heparin therapy in patients with venous thrombosis. *Arch Intern Med* 152:1589, 1992.

141. Owren PA: Thrombotest: A new method for controlling anticoagulant therapy. *Lancet* 2:754, 1959.

142. Paulssen MMP, Kolhorn A, Rothuizen J, et al: An automated aminolytic assay for thrombin generation: An alternative for the prothrombin time test. *Clin Chim Acta* 92:465, 1979.

143. Furie B, Duiguid CF, Jacobs M, et al: Randomized prospective trial comparing the native prothrombin antigen with the prothrombin time for monitoring oral anticoagulant therapy. *Blood* 75:344, 1990.

144. Lammle B, Vainnamlaux H, Market GA, et al: Monitoring of oral anticoagulation by an aminolytic factor X assay. *Thromb Haemost* 44:150, 1980.

145. Hirsh J: Is the dose of warfarin prescribed by American physicians unnecessarily high? *Arch Intern Med* 147:769, 1987.

146. Hull R, Hirsh J, Jay R, et al: Different intensities of anticoagulation in the long term treatment of proximal venous thrombosis. *N Engl J Med* 307:1676, 1982.

147. Coe NP, Collins REC, Klein LA, et al: Prevention of deep vein thrombosis in urological patients: A controlled, randomized trial of low dose heparin and external pneumatic compression boots. *Surgery* 83:230, 1978.

148. Covey TH, Sherman L, Baue AE: Low dose heparin in postoperative patients: A prospective, coded study. *Arch Surg* 110:1021, 1975.

149. Gallus AS, Hirsh J, Tuttle RJ, et al: Small subcutaneous doses of heparin in prevention of venous thrombosis. *N Engl J Med* 288:5455, 1983.

150. Vandendris M, Kutnowski M, Futeral B, et al: Prevention of postoperative deep vein thrombosis by low dose heparin in open prostatectomy. *Urol Res* 8:219, 1980.

151. Kiil J, Axelsen F, Anderson D: Prophylaxis against postoperative pulmonary embolism and deep vein thrombosis by low dose heparin. *Lancet* 1:1115, 1978.

152. Sagar S, Massey J, Sanderson JM: Low dose heparin prophylaxis against fatal pulmonary embolism. *Br Med J* 4:257, 1975.

153. Koppenhagen K, Wiechman A, Zuhlke HV, et al: Effectiveness and risk of thromboembolism prophylaxis in surgery: A comparison study of heparin-dihydroergot and low dose heparin. *Therapiewoche* 29:5920, 1979.

154. Moser G, Krahenbuhl B, Barroussel R, et al: Mechanical versus pharmacologic prevention of deep venous thrombosis. *Surg Gynecol Obstet* 152:448, 1981.

155. Veth G, Meuwissen OJ, can Houwelingen HC, et al: Prevention of postoperative deep vein thrombosis by a combination of subcutaneous heparin with subcutaneous dihydroergotamine or oral sulfinpyrazone. *Thromb Haemost* 54:570, 1985.

156. Wille-Jorgensen P, Kjaergaard J, Thorup J, et al: Heparin with or without dihydroergotamine in prevention of thromboembolic complications of major abdominal surgery: A randomized trial. *Arch Surg* 118:926, 1983.

157. Speziale F, Ceradi S, Taurino M, et al: Low molecular weight heparin prevention of post operative deep vein thrombosis in vascular surgery. *Pharmatherapeutica* 5:261, 1988.

158. Caen JP: A randomized double blind study between a low molecular weight heparin Kabi 2165 and standard heparin in the prevention of deep vein thrombosis in general surgery: A French multicenter trial. *Thromb Haemost* 59:216, 1988.

159. Wille-Jorgensen P, Thorup J, Fischer A, et al: Heparin with and without graded compression stockings in the prevention of thromboembolic complications of major abdominal surgery: A randomized trial. *Br J Surg* 72:579, 1985.

160. Torngren S: Low dose heparin and compression stockings in the prevention of postoperative deep venous thrombosis. *Br J Surg* 67:482, 1980.

161. Poller L, McKernan A, Thomson JM, et al: Fixed minidose warfarin: A new approach to prophylaxis against venous thrombosis after major surgery. *Br Med J* 295:1309, 1987.

162. Leyvraz PF, Bachmann F, Hoek J, et al: Prevention of deep venous thrombosis after hip replacement: Randomized comparison between unfractionated heparin and low molecular weight heparin. *Br Med J* 303:531, 1991.

163. Cerrato D, Ariano C, Fiacchino F: Deep vein thrombosis and low dose heparin prophylaxis in neurosurgical patients. *J Neurosurg* 49:378, 1978.

164. Green D, Lee MY, Ito VY, et al: Fixed vs adjusted dose heparin in the prophylaxis of thromboembolism in spinal cord injury. *JAMA* 260:1255, 1988.

165. Shackford SR, Davies JW, Hollingsword-Fridlund P, et al: Venous thromboembolism in patients with major trauma. *Am J Surg* 159:365, 1990.

166. Wray R, Maurer B, Shillingford J: Prophylactic anticoagulant therapy in the prevention of calf-vein thrombosis after myocardial infarction. *Br Med J* 2:436, 1972.

167. McCarthy ST, Turner JJ, Robertson D, et al: Low dose heparin as a prophylaxis against deep vein thrombosis after acute stroke. *Lancet* 2:800, 1977.

168. Cade JF: High risk of the critically ill for venous thromboembolism. *Crit Care Med* 10:448, 1982.

169. Bonnar J, Walsh J: Prevention of thrombosis after pelvic surgery by British dextran 70. *Lancet* 1:1614, 1972.

170. Clarke-Pearson DL, Synan IS, Hinshaw WM et al: Prevention of postoperative venous thromboembolism by external pneumatic calf compression in patients with gynecologic malignancy. *Obstet Gynecol* 63:92, 1984.

171. Harris WH, Salzman EW, Athanasoulis CA, et al: Aspirin prophylaxis of venous thromboembolism after total hip replacement. *N Engl J Med* 297:1246, 1977.

172. Harris WH, Salzman EW, Athanasoulis C, et al: Comparison of warfarin, low molecular weight dextran, aspirin and subcutaneous heparin in prevention of venous thromboembolism following total hip replacement. *J Bone Joint Surg* 56:1552, 1974.

173. Greenfield LJ, Michna BA: Twelve year clinical experience with the Greenfield vena cava filter. *Surgery* 104:706, 1988.

174. Gifford RH, Feinstein AR: A critique of methodology in studies of anticoagulant therapy for acute myocardial infarction. *N Engl J Med* 280:351, 1969.

175. Chapman I: The cause-effect relationship between recent coronary artery occlusion and acute myocardial infarction. *Am J Heart* 87:267, 1974.

176. Drapkin A, Merskey C: Anticoagulant therapy after acute myocardial infarction: Relation of therapeutic benefit to patient's age, sex and severity of infarction. *JAMA* 222:541, 1972.

177. Telford AM, Wilson C: Trial of heparin versus atenolol in prevention of myocardial infarction in intermediate coronary syndrome. *Lancet* 1:1225, 1981.

177a. Théroux P, Ouimet H, McCans J, et al: Aspirin, heparin, or both to treat acute unstable angina. *N Engl J Med* 319:1105, 1988.

178. The RISC Group: Risk of myocardial infarction and death during treatment with low dose aspirin and intravenous heparin in men with unstable coronary artery disease. *Lancet* 336:827, 1990.

179. Gold HK, Torres FW, Garabedian HD, et al: Evidence for a rebound coagulation phenomenon after cessation of a 4-hour infusion of a specific thrombin inhibitor in patients with unstable angina pectoris. *J Am Coll Cardiol* 21:1039, 1993.

180. Lewis HD, Davis JW, Archibald DG, et al: Protective effects of aspirin against acute myocardial infarction and death in men with unstable angina: Results of a Veterans' Administration Cooperative Study. *N Engl J Med* 309:396, 1983.

181. Cairns JA, Gent M, Singer J, et al: Aspirin, sulfinpyrazone, or both, in unstable angina: Results of a Canadian multicenter trial. *N Engl J Med* 313:1369, 1985.

182. The TIMI IIIA Investigators: Early effects of tissue type plasminogen activator added to conventional therapy on the culprit coronary lesion in patients presenting with ischemic cardiac pain at rest. *Circulation* 87:38, 1993.

183. Report of the 60+ reinfarction study research group: A double-blind trial to assess long term anticoagulant therapy in elderly patients after myocardial infarction. *Lancet* 2:989, 1980.

184. Smith P, Aresen H, Holme I: The effect of warfarin on mortality and reinfarction artery myocardial infarction. *N Engl J Med* 323:147, 1990.

185. McMahon S, Collins R, Knight C, et al: Reduction in major morbidity and mortality by heparin in acute myocardial infarction (abstract). *Circulation* 78(suppl 2):98, 1988.

186. Turpie AGG, Robinson JG, Doyle DJ, et al: Comparison of high dose with low dose subcutaneous heparin to prevent left ventricular mural thrombosis in patients with acute transmural anterior myocardial infarction. *N Engl J Med* 320:352, 1989.

187. The SCATI (Studio Sulla Calciparina Nell'Angina e Nella Thrombosi Ventriculare Nell'Infarto) Group: Randomized controlled trial of subcutaneous calcium heparin in acute myocardial infarction. *Lancet* 2:182, 1989.

188. Ouyang P, Shapiro EP, Gottlieb SO: Thrombolysis in postinfarction angina. *Am J Cardiol* 68:124B, 1991.

189. Shapito EP, Brinker JA, Gottlieb SO, et al: Intracoronary thrombolysis 3 to 13 days after acute myocardial infarction for post infarction angina pectoris. *Am J Cardiol* 55:1453, 1985.

190. Brown BG, Gallery CA, Badger RS, et al: Incomplete lysis of thrombus in the moderate underlying atherosclerotic lesion during intracoronary infusion of streptokinase for acute myocardial

infarction: quantitative angiographic observations. *Circulation* 73:653, 1986.

191. Lierde JV, DeGeest H, Verstraete M, van de Werf F: Angiographic assessment of the infarct-related residual coronary stenosis after spontaneous or therapeutic thrombolysis. *J Am Coll Cardiol* 16:1545, 1990.

192. Davies MJ: Successful and unsuccessful coronary thrombolysis. *Br Heart J* 61:381, 1986.

193. Richardson SG, Callen D, Morton P, et al: Pathological changes after intravenous streptokinase treatment in eight patients with acute myocardial infarction. *Br Heart J* 61:390, 1989.

194. Badimon L, Badimon JJ, Turitto VT, et al: Platelet thrombus formation collagen type I. *Circulation* 78:1431, 1988.

195. Eisenberg PR, Miletich JP: Induction of marked thrombin activity by pharmacologic concentrations of plasminogen activators in nonanticoagulated whole blood. *Thromb Res* 55:635, 1989.

196. Francis CW, Markham RF, Barlow GH, et al: Thrombin activity of fibrin thrombi and soluble plasmic derivatives. *J Lab Clin Med* 102:200, 1983.

197. Weitz JI, Cruickshang MK, Thong B, et al: Human tissue-type plasminogen activator releases fibrinopeptides A and B from fibrinogen. *J Clin Invest* 82:1700, 1988.

198. Griffen JT, Cochran LHG: Recent advances in the understanding of contact activation reactions. *Semin Thromb Hemost* 5:254, 1979.

199. Munkvad S, Jespersen J, Gram J, Kluft C: Depression of factor XII-dependent fibrinolytic activity characterized patients with early myocardial reinfarction after recombinant tissue-type plasminogen activator therapy. *J Am Coll Cardiol* 18:454, 1991.

200. Munkvad S, Jespersen J, Gram J, Kluft C: Long-lasting depression of the factor XII-dependent fibrinolytic system in patients with myocardial infarction undergoing thrombolytic therapy with recombinant tissue-plasminogen activator: A randomized placebo-controlled study. *J Am Coll Cardiol* 17:957, 1991.

201. Tsao PS, Aoki N, Leger DJ, et al: Time course of endothelial dysfunction and myocardial injury during myocardial ischemia and reperfusion in the cat. *Circulation* 82:1402, 1990.

202. Pelc LR, Garancis JC, Gross GJ, Warltier DC: Alteration of endothelium-dependent distribution of myocardial blood flow after coronary occlusion and reperfusion. *Circulation* 81:1928, 1990.

203. Forman MB, Puett DW, Virmani R: Endothelial and myocardial injury during ischemic and reperfusion: Pathogenesis and therapeutic implication. *J Am Coll Cardiol* 13:450, 1989.

204. Pearson PJ, Schaff HV, Vanhoutte PM: Long-term impairment of endothelial-dependent relaxations to aggregating platelets after reperfusion injury in canine coronary arteries. *Circulation* 81:1921, 1990.

205. Badimon JJ, Badimon L, Turitto VT, Fuster V: Platelet deposition at high shear rates is enhanced by high plasma cholesterol levels: In vivo study in the rabbit model. *Arteriosclerosis* 11:395, 1991.

206. Carvalho ACA, Colman RW, Lees RS: Platelet function in hyperlipoproteinemia. *N Engl J Med* 290:434, 1974.

207. Stuart MJ, Gerrard JM, White JG: Effect of cholesterol on production of thromboxane B2 by platelets in vitro. *N Engl J Med* 302:6, 1980.

208. Muller JE, Stone PH, Turi ZG, et al: The MILIS Study Group: Circadian variation in the frequency of onset of acute myocardial infarction. *N Engl J Med* 313:1315, 1985.

209. Trip MD, Cats VM, Can Capell FJL, Vreeken J: Platelet hyperreactivity and prognosis in survivors of myocardial infarction. *N Engl J Med* 322:1549, 1990.

210. Lowe GDO, Wood DA, Douglas JT, et al: Relationships of plasma viscosity, coagulation and fibrinolysis to coronary risk factors and angina. *Thromb Haemost* 65:339, 1991.

211. The GUSTO investigators. An international randomized trial comparing four thrombolytic strategies for acute myocardial infarction. *N Engl J Med* 329:673, 1993.

212. ISIS-3 (Third International Study of Infarct Survival) Collaborative Group: A randomized comparison of streptokinase vs tissue plasminogen activator vs anistreplase and of aspirin plus heparin vs aspirin alone among 41,299 cases of suspected acute myocardial infarction. *Lancet* 339:1, 1992.

213. The International Study Group: In-hospital mortality and clinical course of 20,891 patients with suspected acute myocardial in-

farction randomized between alteplase and streptokinase with or without heparin. *Lancet* 33:71, 1990.

214. O'Conner CM, Meese R, Carney R, et al, for the Duke University Clinical Cardiology Study (DUCCS) Group: A randomized trial of intravenous heparin in conjunction with anistreplase (APSAC) in acute myocardial infarction. *J Am Coll Cardiol* 23:11, 1994.

215. ISIS-2 (Second International Study of Infarct Survival) Collaborative Group: Randomized trial of intravenous streptokinase, oral aspirin, both or neither among 17,187 cases of suspected acute myocardial infarction: ISIS-2. *Lancet* 2:349, 1988.

216. Elwood PC, Cochrane AL, Burr ML, et al: A randomized controlled trial of acetylsalicylic acid in the secondary prevention of mortality from myocardial infarction. *Br Med J* 1:436, 1974.

217. The Coronary Drug Project Research Group: Aspirin in coronary heart disease. *J Chron Dis* 29:625, 1976.

218. Breddin K, Loew D, Lechner K, et al: Secondary prevention of myocardial infarction: Comparison of acetylsalicylic acid, phenprocoumon and placebo. *Hemostasis* 9:325, 1980.

219. Aspirin Myocardial Infarction Study Research Group: A randomized controlled trial of aspirin in persons recovered from myocardial infarction. *J Am Coll Cardiol* 243:661, 1980.

220. The Presantin-Aspirin Reinfarction Study Research Group: Persantine and aspirin in coronary heart disease. *Circulation* 62:449, 1980.

221. Klimt CR, Knatterud GL, Stamler J, Meier P: Persantine-Aspirin Reinfarction Study. II. Secondary coronary prevention with persantine and aspirin. *J Am Coll Cardiol* 7:251, 1986.

222. The Copenhagen AFASAK Study: Placebo controlled randomized trial of warfarin and aspirin for prevention of thromboembolic complications in chronic atrial fibrillation. *Lancet* 1:175, 1989.

223. Stroke Prevention in Atrial Fibrillation Investigators: Stroke prevention in atrial fibrillation study. *Circulation* 84:527, 1991.

224. The Boston Area Anticoagulation Trial for Atrial Fibrillation Investigators: The effect of low dose warfarin on the risk of stroke in patients with nonrheumatic atrial fibrillation. *N Engl J Med* 323:1505, 1990.

225. Connolly SJ, Laupacis A, Gent M, et al: Canadian Atrial Fibrillation Anticoagulation (CAFA) study. *J Am Coll Cardiol* 18:349, 1991.

226. Ezekowitz MD, Bridgers SL, James KE, et al: Warfarin in the prevention of stroke associated with nonrheumatic atrial fibrillation. *N Engl J Med* 327:1406, 1992.

227. Sullivan JM, Harken DE, Gorlin R: Effect of dipyridamole on the incidence of arterial emboli after cardiac valve replacement. *Circulation* 39-40(suppl 1):I-49, 1969.

228. Kasahara T: Clinical effect of dipyridamole ingestion after prosthetic heart valve replacement—Especially on the blood coagulation system. *Nippon Kyobu Geka Gakkai Zasshi* 25:1007, 1977.

229. Raha SM, Sreeharan N, Joseph A, et al: Perspective trial of dipyridamole and warfarin in heart valve patients (abstract). *Act Ther (Brussels)* 6:54, 1980.

230. Turpie AGG, Gent M, Laupacis A, et al: Reduction in mortality by adding aspirin (100 mg) to oral anticoagulants in patients with heart valve replacement (abstract). *J Am Coll Cardiol* 19(suppl A):103A, 1992.

231. Chesebro JH, Fuster V, Elveback LR, et al: Trial of combined warfarin plus dipyridamole or aspirin therapy in prosthetic valve replacement: Danger of aspirin compared with dipyridamole. *Am J Cardiol* 51:1537, 1983.

232. Cohn LH, Allred EN, DiSesa VJ, et al: Early and late risk of aortic valve replacement: A 12-year concomitant comparison of the porcine bioprosthetic and tilting disc prosthetic aortic valves. *J Thorac Cardiovasc Surg* 88:695, 1984.

233. Bolooki H, Kaiser GA, Mallon SM, et al: Comparison of long term results of Carpentier-Edwards and Hancock bioprosthetic valves. *Ann Thorac Surg* 42:494, 1986.

234. Bloomfield P, Kitchin AH, Wheatly DJ, et al: A prospective evaluation of the Bjork-Shiley, Hancock and Carpentier-Edwards heart valve prostheses. *Circulation* 73:1213, 1986.

235. Williams JB, Karp RB, Kirklin JW, et al: Considerations in selection and management of patients undergoing valve replacement with glutaraldehyde-fixed porcine bioprostheses. *Ann Thorac Surg* 30:247, 1980.

236. Gonzalez-Lavin L, Tandon AP, Chi S, et al: The risk of thrombo-

embolism and hemorrhage following mitral valve replacement. *J Thorac Cardiovasc Surg* 87:340, 1984.
237. Tinker JH, Tarhan S: Discontinuing anticoagulant therapy in surgical patients with cardiac valve prostheses. *J Am Coll Cardiol* 239:738, 1978.
238. Bodnar AG, Hutter AM: Anticoagulation in valvular heart disease preoperatively and postoperatively. *Cardiovasc Clin* 14:247, 1984.
239. Sane DC, Califf RM, Topol EJ, et al: Bleeding during thrombolytic

therapy for acute myocardial infarction: Mechanisms and management. *Ann Intern Med* 111:1010, 1989.
240. Johnstone MT, Andrews T, Ware A, et al: Bleeding time prolongation with streptokinase and its reduction with 1-desamino-8-D-Arginine vasopressin. *Circulation* 82:2142, 1990.
241. Hirsh J, Dalen JE, Deykin D, et al: Oral anticoagulants: Mechanism of action, clinical effectiveness, and optional therapeutic range. *Chest* 10:3125, 1992.

44. Unstable Angina

Pierre Théroux and Felix Pérez-Villa

Unstable angina, once considered a harbinger to myocardial infarction, stands now as a well-defined clinical entity with specific causes, pathophysiologic mechanisms, symptoms, laboratory findings, and treatment. The original concept, derived from retrospective observations of frequent symptoms preceding an acute myocardial infarction [1,2,3], was confirmed by prospective studies [4,5,6]. The terminology of unstable angina was adopted in 1971 [7]. Subsequent investigation looked at the natural history of the syndrome [8,9,10], its mechanisms [11,12], and the results of various therapeutic measures [13,14]. In the mid-1980s, thrombus formation on a complicated atherosclerotic plaque was recognized as the cause of unstable angina [15,16] and the efficacy of antithrombotic therapy was confirmed [17,18]. The field of therapeutic interventions is now rapidly expanding.

Pathogenic Mechanisms

MYOCARDIAL ISCHEMIA. Myocardial ischemia is caused by an imbalance between myocardial oxygen demand and supply. In stable angina, the ischemia is induced by an excess in demand relative to the capability of supply. In acute ischemic syndromes, ischemia occurs without the increase in myocardial oxygen demand and is caused by a primary decrease in coronary artery blood flow and, typically, an occluding thrombus. The ischemia can be more or less severe to cause transmural or subendocardial ischemia and more or less sustained to result or not in myocardial necrosis.

The formation of endovascular thrombus has been documented by a variety of methods. Pathologic studies in patients dying suddenly have identified their presence in 72 percent of cases, with 89 percent overlying a plaque rupture or fissure [19]. Thrombi are often of varying age, indicating the cyclic nature of the disease [20]. Coronary angiographic studies have documented the presence of occluding thrombi in 90 percent of patients catheterized within 6 hours after the onset of a Q wave myocardial infarction [21] and partially occluding thrombi in 75 percent of patients catheterized early during the evolution of unstable angina and of non-Q wave myocardial infarction [22]. Coronary angioscopy is more sensitive and can detect thrombi more frequently [23]. Clots are reddish in myocardial infarction and greyish white in unstable angina [24].

PLAQUE RUPTURE. The rupture of a plaque triggering thrombus formation is influenced by its composition, making it more friable, and its tridimensional structure, increasing shear stress. The plaque that ruptures is histologically younger, rich in cholesterol and cholesterol esters, and has a thin, fibrous cap infiltrated by monocytes/macrophages [25]. It possesses angiographic features favoring blood flow separation [26–28] with abrupt edges and often a division branch in its vicinity. It is of moderate severity, typically with 40 to 60 percent lumen diameter reduction. More severe stenoses occlude more often but the occlusion is less commonly associated with a clinical syndrome [29].

PLAQUE ACTIVATION. Platelets interact with adhesive proteins of the vessel's subendothelium, leading to platelet adhesion, secretion, recruitment, and activation. In this process, the glycoprotein receptors IIb/IIIa are activated. These receptors represent the final and obligatory pathway to platelet aggregation [30]. They possess a three-amino acid sequence, arginine-glycine-aspartic acid (RGD sequence), which is the minimal chain required to bind fibrinogen. These receptors can also bind von Willebrand factor at high shear rate [31].

THROMBIN FORMATION. Activated platelets act as a template for intravascular coagulation. Tissue factor present in a variety of tissues combines with factor VII of the extrinsic system and factor IX of the intrinsic system to activate factor X and form the prothrombinase complex to generate thrombin [32]. Thrombin has several key roles in thrombus formation: it converts fibrinogen to fibrin, activates platelet, and self-amplifies its reaction by feedback stimulation of factors V, VIII, and XI. A unique thrombin receptor was recently described [33]. Thrombin cleaves this receptor at arginine-41 in a LDPR/S sequence, unmasking a new amino acid terminus that in turn acts as a tethered ligand to activate the receptor. The molecule of thrombin remains free to activate other receptors. Thrombin generated in the prothrombinase complex and thrombin-bound to fibrin is relatively protected from inactivation by circulating antithrombins. Their subsequent release in the circulation extends the thrombogenic stimulation beyond the initial insult [34].

VASCULAR REACTIVITY. Vascular reactivity is impaired in diseased endothelium, and paradoxic vasoconstriction can occur in response to physiologic stimuli that would normally be vasodilators [35]. The normal endothelium modulates coronary artery tone by releasing the endothelium-derived relaxing factor (EDRF) among many other vasoactive agents; this function is impaired with hypercholesterolemia and early atherosclerosis

[36]. Endothelium-derived reducing factor has been identified as nitric oxide or a similar substance [37]. It increases cyclic guanylate cyclase (cyclic GMP) to cause vascular relaxation and inhibit platelet adhesion and aggregation. Activated platelets release thromboxane A_2, a potent vasoconstrictor. Thrombin also stimulates platelets to release large amounts of thromboxane A_2. In the intact but not in the diseased endothelium, this effect of thrombin is overcome by stimulation of nitric oxide and prostacyclin production [38]. Prostacyclin and thromboxane A_2 are formed via the enzyme cyclooxygenase and act by modulating the intracellular cyclic AMP content [39].

Diagnosis

SYMPTOM RECOGNITION. The diagnosis of unstable angina is based mainly on symptom recognition. The symptoms may be severe or mild; they may be typical but also atypical and manifested as angina equivalents. A high index of suspicion results in more frequent but less accurate diagnosis and a low index to the opposite. When the diagnosis is not clear, close observation for a few days is recommended, with use of appropriate diagnostic measures.

The essential diagnostic feature of unstable angina is recognition that the symptoms are becoming more severe and departing from the usual pattern of angina for a given patient. Unstable angina is routinely classified as (1) new onset or crescendo angina, with chest pain occurring at rest or at a progressively lower threshold of exercise, and (2) prolonged chest pain, poorly relieved with nitroglycerin [10]. The usefulness of more recently suggested classifications is under evaluation [40].

DIFFERENTIAL DIAGNOSIS. Pain of cardiac origin must first be suspected and differentiated from noncardiac pain (see Chap. 51), recognizing that chest pain from different causes may often coexist in the same patient. Noncardiac pain may be of various causes but most often is musculoskeletal. It can also be of pulmonary or gastrointestinal nature; the differential diagnosis with esophageal spasm is at times difficult. When cardiac pain is the likely diagnosis, secondary causes of unstable angina must be ruled out. These include conditions leading to excessive myocardial oxygen needs: inappropriate heart rate acceleration by various etiologies, including anemia, fever, hypoxia, tachyarrhythmias, thyrotoxicosis; high afterload due to aortic valve stenosis, hypertrophic cardiomyopathy, and hypertension with left ventricular hypertrophy; high preload with cardiac chamber dilatation and congestive heart failure; and high cardiac output conditions observed in arteriovenous fistula, beriberi heart disease, Paget's disease; and an inappropriately high inotropic state due to sympathicomimetic drugs, cocaine intoxication, and various other causes. When none of these contributing factors is present, unstable angina is primarily caused by an intracoronary disease process.

SPECIFIC FORMS OF UNSTABLE ANGINA
Unstable Angina following Coronary Angioplasty. Restenosis within 6 months following balloon angioplasty occurs in 30 to 50 percent of patients successfully dilated [41] and is frequently manifest as pain at rest. This syndrome rarely results in myocardial infarction, however, as it is caused by muscle cell proliferation at the angioplasty site. When unstable angina occurs more than 6 months after the procedure, it is most likely related to a new active lesion [42].

Unstable Angina following Bypass Surgery. Unstable angina occurring in the first few years following coronary artery bypass surgery may be related to a single active lesion; later it is frequently associated with more extensive graft disease. The short-term prognosis is similar to that in other patients with unstable angina, but the long-term prognosis is less favorable, with twice as many cardiac events. One explanation for this finding is more extensive coronary artery lesions less amenable to corrective revascularization procedures [43].

Non-Q Wave Myocardial Infarction. Non-Q wave myocardial infarction is manifested by prolonged chest pain, 30 minutes or more in duration, with usually more persisting ST–T changes. The diagnosis is confirmed by elevation of the cardiac enzymes in serial plasma samples obtained in the first 12 hours. Non-Q wave myocardial infarction is generally considered similar to unstable angina, since the pathophysiology, treatment, and prognosis are very much alike in the two conditions [44]. The non-Q wave infarctions can sometimes be large and involve a sizable amount of myocardium with associated regional wall motion abnormalities.

Prinzmetal's Variant Angina. Prinzmetal's variant angina is a specific, well-defined entity representing the extreme manifestation of coronary artery vasomotion [45]. The primary spasm is usually focal at the site of a coronary artery stenosis, which can be mild or severe. In some instances, the coronary arteries are angiographically normal [46]. Most patients with variant angina are smokers, but their risk factor profiles are otherwise similar to those of other coronary patients. Those with angiographically normal coronary arteries tend to be younger and women and do not have more risk factors than noncoronary patients [47]. Migraine headache or Raynaud's phenomenon is observed in 25 percent of affected patients [48]. The pain typically occurs at rest, often at night and more frequently in the early morning hours. The spasm is usually severe enough to create transmural myocardial ischemia resulting in S–T segment elevation; severe arrhythmias and syncope may also occur. The spasm and associated symptoms are usually relieved promptly by nitroglycerin but may recur in a repetitive fashion in some patients.

Laboratory Studies

The presence of ST–T changes on the presenting electrocardiogram aids in the diagnosis of unstable angina. Their absence, however, does not rule out the disease. The ECG obtained during an episode of chest pain is more informative. The ST–T changes can further help evaluate the severity and location of the ischemic process [44]. Thus, deep T wave inversions involving the anterior and lateral leads are characteristic of significant narrowing in the proximal left anterior descending coronary artery.

Other, more specialized diagnostic procedures can be used, but these are currently performed only in some clinical centers developing special expertise. Myocardial scintigraphy obtained during an episode of chest pain can detect transient myocardial ischemia with high sensitivity; thallium 201 has been used for this purpose, but ^{99m}Tc Sestamibi may offer distinct advantages since it can be injected during an episode of chest pain and the image obtained several hours later, when the patient is stable [49]. Radionuclide and echocardiographic imaging can also document the presence of transient wall motion abnormalities during an episode of myocardial ischemia. Cardiac enzymes and, more specifically, creatine kinase and creatine kinase MB activity should be determined in all patients with unstable angina and more particularly when the acute chest pain is prolonged. Elevated levels indicate that myocardial necrosis and non-Q wave myocardial infarction have occurred. More recently, plasma levels of troponin T were documented as more sensitive and elevated in 40 percent of patients [49a]; these high levels were associated with an impaired prognosis, possibly by indicating cell necrosis and more severe coronary artery disease. Troponin T and troponin I have a similar specificity and sensitivity; myoglobin plasma levels are sensitive but not specific.

An interesting new diagnostic approach consists in markers of an inflammatory state. The inflammatory process associated with plaque rupture and thrombus formation may result in activated leukocytes and acute phase reactants in the blood [49b]. Elevated plasma levels of C-reactive protein and of amyloid A protein have been documented in 65 percent of patients with severe unstable angina and were associated with an impaired prognosis.

Markers of an active thrombogenic state exist and can be detected in plasma or urine. Thus, elevated urinary levels of 2,3-dinor thromboxane A_2 and of 2,3-dinor $PGF_{1\alpha}$ have been described, with peak elevations coinciding with episodes of ischemia [50]. Plasma and urinary fibrinopeptide A levels, cleaved from fibrinogen on its conversion to fibrin by thrombin, can be elevated [51], as can fibrin(ogen) degradation products [52]. The clinical usefulness of these tests is hampered by their low sensitivity and specificity when applied to individual patients. Assays of other surrogate markers of blood coagulation, such as prothrombin fragment F_{1+2} and the activation peptide of factor X, have been developed; their utility is now under investigation.

Holter monitor recordings allow detection of silent ischemia in approximately 20 percent of patients with unstable angina [44]. Recognition of silent ischemia adds information on the presence of more severe coronary artery disease and has prognostic implications [53]. Its overall prognostic value is enhanced when episodes of S–T segment shifts last for 1 hour or more in a 24-hour recording [54]. The information obtained, however, usually adds little to simple clinical observation [55]. Holter monitoring has been used to evaluate treatment response and disease control [56].

PROVOCATIVE TESTING. Provocative testing using either an exercise treadmill or a pharmacologic agent, such as dipyridamole or dobutamine, allows the detection of ischemia in the presence of a significant coronary narrowing. However, the results of these tests can be influenced by the presence of a dynamic stenosis such as that caused by an endovascular thrombus or vasospasm. Indeed, an occlusive clot can lyse within a few days, leaving a residual nonsignificant coronary narrowing. Conversely, the arterial segment at risk may not be significantly narrowed when the test is performed but still be prone to rapid progression, causing clinical complications and myocardial infarction. Thus, provocative testing is performed acutely only when the diagnosis is in doubt. Diagnostic procedures performed during the acute phase of unstable angina are associated with some risk, and cautious interpretation of the results is required. These tests, however, should be routinely performed before hospital discharge, to evaluate the patient's exercise capacity and to detect the presence of residual zones of ischemia that may indicate more severe and more extensive coronary artery disease.

Prinzmetal's variant angina represents a special diagnostic challenge. It is usually recognized by transient S–T segment elevation appearing during episodes of chest pain. Ergonovine testing is highly sensitive for the diagnosis when performed during an active phase of the disease [57]. To minimize risk, it is done only in patients with angiographically documented non-severe coronary artery disease. Occasionally, in higher-risk patients, it is performed to document that the disease is well-controlled by treatment. Intracoronary acetylcholine can also serve as a provocative agent, with a very high sensitivity [58]. It induces mild vasoconstriction in patients with abnormal endothelial function, but severe coronary artery spasm of 20 to 30 seconds' duration may occur in patients with Prinzmetal's angina.

CORONARY ANGIOGRAPHY. The most useful diagnostic procedure in unstable angina is coronary angiography. This procedure is performed with minimal risk, especially when the disease process has been controlled for a few days. Coronary angiography provides information on the extent, severity, and location of coronary atherosclerosis and is most useful in guiding long-term orientation of treatment. As many as 20 percent of patients with unstable angina have no coronary artery disease, whereas 10 percent have left main disease and 30 percent three-vessel disease [59]. In many patients, numerous but nonsignificant coronary narrowings can be demonstrated. These patients with a greater extent of disease are at risk of progression and recurrent coronary events [60]. Coronary angiography should be performed in patients with recurrent or refractory angina in the hospital and in patients with a low tolerance to exercise before hospital discharge to evaluate the feasibility of balloon angioplasty and bypass surgery.

Prognosis

The major early complication of unstable angina is myocardial infarction. The second major complication is recurrence of chest pain despite optimal therapy; this situation requires aggressive intervention, sometimes supported by intraaortic balloon counterpulsation. These events clearly represent treatment failure related to the unstable state. Accordingly, they are valid endpoints in natural history studies and in clinical trials testing the efficacy of various interventions. Residual ischemia manifested during exercise is also a frequent sequela of unstable angina but is less specific, since it can also be related to fixed severe coronary artery lesions. Unstable angina is indeed one of the causes of rapid progression of coronary artery disease [61].

Beyond the acute phase, the prognosis for patients with unstable angina is mainly influenced by left ventricular function and the extent of coronary artery disease. In addition, the patient who has experienced an episode of unstable angina is at higher risk of recurrence, for the same reasons that triggered the initial event. The variable prognosis reported in clinical series is not unexpected, considering that unstable angina occurs in patients at various stages in the evolution of coronary artery disease. A review of natural history studies, including the control groups of recent intervention trials, provides consistent figures, allowing a fair appraisal of prognosis [62,63]. The cumulative risk of fatal and nonfatal myocardial infarction is approximately 10 percent in the hospital, 15 percent at 3 months, and 20 percent at 1 year. The risk of early death is 4 percent and of death at 1 year is 10 percent. In addition, 20 to 25 percent of patients will manifest early recurrent refractory angina and 50 percent other forms of residual ischemia.

Factors associated with a worse prognosis are older age [64], white race [65], female gender [65], more severe clinical presentation [66], presence of electrocardiographic changes at admission and during chest pain [63,67], poorer left ventricular function [64], and more severe coronary artery disease [68]. The single greatest independent predictor of prognosis is the recurrence of chest pain in the hospital [10,63,64,67,69]. This situation is analogous to early postinfarction ischemia and marks an ongoing, uncontrolled disease process [70]. Data consistently show that persisting ischemia following the onset of acute coronary syndromes marks an active uncontrolled disease process and a worse prognosis.

Medical Therapy

The therapeutic options in unstable angina have expanded following the recognition of its thrombogenic cause and of the efficacy of antiplatelet and anticoagulant drugs, as documented in Table 44-1. The use of thrombolytic therapy, however, has been deceptive. Antianginal therapy with nitroglycerin beta-blockers and calcium antagonists are also useful.

When formulating a treatment plan, it should be realized that unstable angina is a dynamic condition with an acute, a subacute, and a chronic phase.

PLATELET INHIBITORS. One trial of patients with unstable angina has documented the effectiveness of aspirin during the acute phase [71]. Others have shown benefit during the subacute phase [18,72] and the chronic phase [73]. The relative risks for occurrence of fatal or nonfatal myocardial infarction were reduced by 71 percent at 1 week, 55 and 64 percent at 3 months, and 52 percent at 2 years. Doses of aspirin used in these trials have varied from 75 mg to 1.3 g daily with as much benefit observed with lower as with higher doses, but with fewer side effects. Aspirin had no effect on the incidence of early severe recurrent ischemia [71], but did reduce the long-term need for coronary angiography and bypass surgery [74]. A bolus dose of 160 to 325 mg is recommended, followed by maintenance doses of 80 to 160 mg per day.

Ticlopidine is an acceptable alternative in patients who do not tolerate aspirin. In one study comparing ticlopidine, 250 mg given twice per day, and placebo, the risk of fatal or nonfatal myocardial infarction at 6 months was reduced by 53 percent

[75]. Sulfinpyrazone is not recommended in the treatment of unstable angina [73].

ANTICOAGULANTS. Heparin use has been evaluated in fewer clinical trials than aspirin use but has been associated with greater benefit [17,76] (see Chap. 121). Risk reductions for the occurrence of myocardial infarction exceeded 80 percent. Heparin also significantly decreased early recurrent ischemia [71] and episodes of S–T segment depression detected by Holter monitoring [56]. In these trials, intravenous therapeutic doses were used early after hospital admission for 1 to 5 days with an intravenous bolus of 5000 units, followed by an infusion of 1000 units per hour titrated to an activated partial thromboplastin time 2 to 2.5 times control. The optimal duration of treatment remains empirical; it should probably be individualized, from 48 hours in patients with no recurrent angina to the time of an intervention in patients with persisting symptoms. The most critical issue could be the initiation of aspirin therapy before the discontinuation of heparin to prevent early disease reactivation, which occurs in up to 14 percent of patients receiving no concomitant aspirin [77]. This reaction usually occurs early, 3 to 18 hours after the discontinuation of heparin.

Large-scale clinical trials have not evaluated the clinical usefulness of long-term oral anticoagulants after an episode of unstable angina; these drugs are generally not used for this purpose except in a few high-risk patients. The early literature on unstable angina, however, reported impressive success with anticoagulants. Wood prematurely stopped randomization in a clinical trial because of the marked benefits observed with anticoagulants after the first 40 patients [76]. Vakil described a reduction in mortality at 3 months from 23.7 percent in control patients to 9.5 percent in treated patients [5]. More recently, Williams et al. reported a risk reduction of 65 percent in cardiac events at 6 months with anticoagulants in a randomized, placebo-controlled study [78]. The target INR for an optimal risk-benefit ratio has not been determined in this condition but should probably be 2 to 2.5 without aspirin; target INR of 1.3 to 2 with concomitant aspirin is now under investigation.

NITROGLYCERIN. Nitroglycerin and the other nitrovasodilators produce their biologic effects by releasing nitric oxide (NO), the metabolic equivalent of EDRF [37] (see Chap. 210).

Table 44-1. Clinical Trials in Unstable Angina with Antiplatelet, Antithrombin and Thrombolytic Therapy

Agent + daily dose	Duration of follow-up	Fatal and nonfatal myocardial infarction			
		Control (%)	Therapy (%)	Risk reduction	p value
Antiplatelets					
Lewis et al. [18] ASA, 324 mg	3 mo	10.1	5	51	0.0005
Cairns et al. [73] ASA, 1300 mg	24 mo	17	8.6	51	0.008
Théroux et al. [71] ASA, 650 mg	6 days	12	3.3	72	0.01
RISC [72] ASA, 75 mg	30 days	13.4	4.3	68	0.0001
Balsano [75] Ticlopidine, 500 mg	6 mo	13.6	7.6	53	0.009
Anticoagulants					
Telford and Wilson [17] Heparin, 30,000–40,000 units	7 days	15	3	80	<0.05
Williams et al. [78] Heparin 40,000 units + warfarin	6 mo	12	34	65	<0.05
Théroux et al. [71] Heparin, aPTT titrated to 2 ×	6 days	7.5	1.2	85	<0.05
RISC [72] Heparin, 14,000–20,000 units	5 days	4.9	3.4	30	NS
Thrombolytics					
Bär et al. [103] APSAC	30 days	28	40	+73	NS
Schreiber [108] Urokinase	90 days	3.8	8.3	+132	NS
TIMI-3 [102] t-PA + heparin	40 days	5	7.5	+52	0.04

NS = not significant.

Thus, nitroglycerin possesses pharmacologic effects similar to those of EDRF with the potential of correcting some vicious pathophysiologic defects involved in unstable angina. However, studies published to date have been of limited sample size, involving fewer than 100 patients, and were neither controlled nor randomized [78–86]. One study did not show a benefit of intravenous compared to oral or transdermal nitroglycerin [85]. Despite the paucity of clinical data, intravenous nitroglycerin is widely used in unstable angina, with a general consensus that the drug is highly effective in preventing recurrent chest pain, probably by its antiplatelet [87] and local vasodilatory effects. The significance of nitrate tolerance in unstable angina has not been well studied. Nitroglycerin is generally started at an infusion rate of 50 µg per minute and increased in increments of 5 µg per minute as needed or until side effects or hypotension develop. Interruption of an infusion of nitroglycerin can be associated with recurrence of chest pain [88].

BETA-BLOCKERS. Beta-blockers, by reducing heart rate, blood pressure, and myocardial contractility, are useful antianginal agents (see Chap. 210). They also possess myocardial protective effects. In a subset of patients presenting with chest pain suggestive of myocardial infarction, beta-blockers reduced by 13 percent the risk of developing a myocardial infarction [89]. Studies in a more general population of patients with unstable angina have not documented a reduction in death or myocardial infarction but have shown their effectiveness in controlling recurrent chest pain [44]. The initial dose may be administered intravenously, followed by oral administration. The dose is titrated to the individual response to maintain a basal heart rate of approximately 60 beats per minute. Beta-blockers are associated with unopposed alpha-adrenergic vasoconstriction and may occasionally exacerbate coronary artery spasm in patients with Prinzmetal's variant angina [90].

CALCIUM ANTAGONISTS. Calcium antagonists are the treatment of choice, along with nitrates, for the management of Prinzmetal's variant angina [91] (see Chap. 210). They are potent peripheral and coronary vasodilators. Diltiazem also induces a variable degree of heart rate reduction, and verapamil has a negative inotropic effect. Calcium antagonists do not prevent myocardial infarction in unstable angina but can be useful in controlling recurrent angina. The dihydropiridines, such as nifedipine, nicardipine, and isradipine, can exacerbate ischemia and lead to myocardial infarction and death [92,93,94]. These drugs should be used cautiously in unstable angina and preferably in combination with a beta-blocker [94].

Indications for Revascularization

REFRACTORY ANGINA. Many patients remain unstable despite optimal medical therapy, representing a clinically disturbing and high-risk situation [44]. Attempts should be made to correct this situation by coronary angioplasty or bypass surgery. These procedures are associated with a higher risk when performed in the acute setting but may be extremely rewarding when successful. Early balloon angioplasty carries a 10 percent risk of myocardial infarction, urgent surgery, repeat angioplasty, or death [95,96,97]. Primary success is achieved in 75 to 90 percent of patients. With early bypass surgery, operative mortality is 4 percent, perioperative myocardial infarction 10 percent, and low cardiac output 16 percent [97]. The survival rate after 10 years is 80 percent and the annual rate of myocardial infarction is 3 to 4 percent [97].

Bypass surgery is indicated when left main disease or "left main equivalent" disease is present; it is preferred over coronary angioplasty in patients with three-vessel disease. Angioplasty limited to the culprit coronary artery lesion can be useful as an initial procedure to stabilize the patient [98]. Some studies suggest that a 3- to 6-day period of heparin treatment prior to the procedure (in the presence of a thrombus) can reduce the incidence of abrupt vessel closure from 10 to 2 percent [99]. Use of intracoronary fibrinolytic agents has also been suggested [100].

SEVERITY OF CORONARY ARTERY DISEASE. The two most important randomized trials comparing surgical versus medical therapy for unstable angina are the National Cooperative Study, published in 1978 [14], and the Veterans Administration Cooperative study, published in 1987 [101]. The TIMI-3B study has compared an early invasive strategy to an early conservative strategy [102]. The medical groups of these trials, except for the TIMI-3B, have been at a disadvantage, since antithrombotic therapy was not used. The surgical groups were also at a disadvantage because the myocardial protection techniques have improved since then, internal mammary implants have become first treatment choice, and coronary angioplasty is widely used.

None of the three studies showed that routine surgery can reduce the rate of fatal and nonfatal myocardial infarction. All three, however, document an important cross-over from medical to surgical therapy. In the National Cooperative Study of 288 patients, mortality at 1 year was 8 percent in surgical patients and 7 percent in medical patients. In the Veterans Administration Study, which included 468 men, the rate of nonfatal myocardial infarction in surgical patients was 11.7 percent at 2 years and in medical patients was 12.2 percent. Cross-over rates to surgery were 19 percent at 1 year in the former study and 34 percent at 2 years in the latter.

Important subsets of patients in the Veterans Administration Study benefitted in the long term from surgery. The 5-year survival in patients with three-vessel disease was 89 percent, compared to 75 percent with medical treatment (p <0.02). Mortality in patients with an ejection fraction between 30 and 49 percent was reduced from 27 to 14 percent with surgical intervention. Patients with an ejection fraction of 50 percent or more did better with medical therapy (patients with an ejection fraction lower than 30 percent were not included in this trial).

The TIMI-3B study is the largest trial performed in unstable angina, including 1473 well-characterized patients to compare treatment strategies modeled on actual practice. The inclusion criteria included ischemic chest discomfort at rest within the previous 24 hours diagnosed as unstable angina or non-Q wave myocardial infarction. The trial had a factorial design with randomization to t-PA or placebo and to an early invasive versus an early conservative strategy. Aspirin and heparin were administered to all patients. The early invasive strategy required coronary arteriography 18 to 48 hours after randomization, with rapid coronary angioplasty when feasible. Coronary artery bypass surgery was to be performed as soon as possible but before 6 weeks in the presence of left main coronary stenosis, three-vessel disease, and an ejection fraction less than 40 percent or recurrent angina in a patient not considered a suitable candidate for coronary angioplasty. Failure of therapy in the early conservative group was an indication for coronary angiography and revascularization, if suitable. Failure was defined as recurrent chest pain with S–T segment changes, a 20-minute or longer period of ischemic S-T segment shifts on a 24-hour Holter monitor, or a positive stress thallium exercise test before completion of stage 2 of the Bruce protocol. In this study cardiac catheterization was performed in 98 percent of patients randomized to the early invasive group and in 65 percent randomized to the early conservative strategy, angioplasty in 38 and 26 percent and surgery in 25 and 24 percent of patients, respectively. Endpoint events included death, nonfatal myocardial infarction, and a positive treadmill test at 6 weeks. They were observed as follows: death in 2.4 percent of early invasive patients and 2.5 percent of early conservative patients; myocardial infarction in 5.1 percent and 5.7 percent; a positive treadmill in 8.5 percent and 10.2 percent; and any of the three in 16.1 and 18.4 percent, respectively (p = .24).

The TIMI-3B trial is a clinically realistic description of actual management of unstable angina; many therapeutic options are available, and they are used in various combinations for optimal patient care. The acute treatment includes antithrombotic ther-

apy with aspirin and heparin to protect against death and myocardial infarction. Treatment failure manifested by spontaneous or inducible ischemia is frequent and may suggest the presence of more severe coronary artery disease.

Thrombolytic Therapy

Early angiographic studies have shown a reduction in the severity of stenosis of the culprit coronary artery lesion with the use of thrombolysis [22,103,104,105] (see Chap. 46). However, clinical benefits have been inconsistent [106,107] and the three largest trials reported an increased risk of fatal and nonfatal myocardial infarction with thrombolysis, suggesting that its use could be harmful in unstable angina (Table 44-1) [102,103,108,109]. These studies have tested t-PA, anistreplase (APSAC), and urokinase. Subset analysis of patients with non-Q wave myocardial infarction in TIMI-3B [102] and also in the large GISSI-1 and ISIS-2 trials [110] have not documented a trend to a benefit. The reasons for a lack of benefit of thrombolysis in unstable angina are numerous. Thrombolytic agents dissolve clots but have procoagulant effects by exposing fibrin-bound thrombin with feedback activation of coagulation, by activating platelets, and also by increasing plasminogen activator inhibitor activity. The goal of treatment in Q wave myocardial infarction

Fig. 44-1. Schematic representation of the potential advantages of new versus standard antiplatelet therapy (*top*) and of new direct thrombin inhibitors versus heparin (*bottom*). Inhibition of the glycoprotein IIb/IIIa receptors does not prevent platelet adhesion, activation, and the release reaction. However, it inhibits platelet aggregation to all aggregation pathways. Hirudin has no known circulating inhibitors and does not require a cofactor for its effects. It is active on fibrin-bound thrombin as well as on fluid-phase thrombin. TxA_2 = thromboxane A_2.

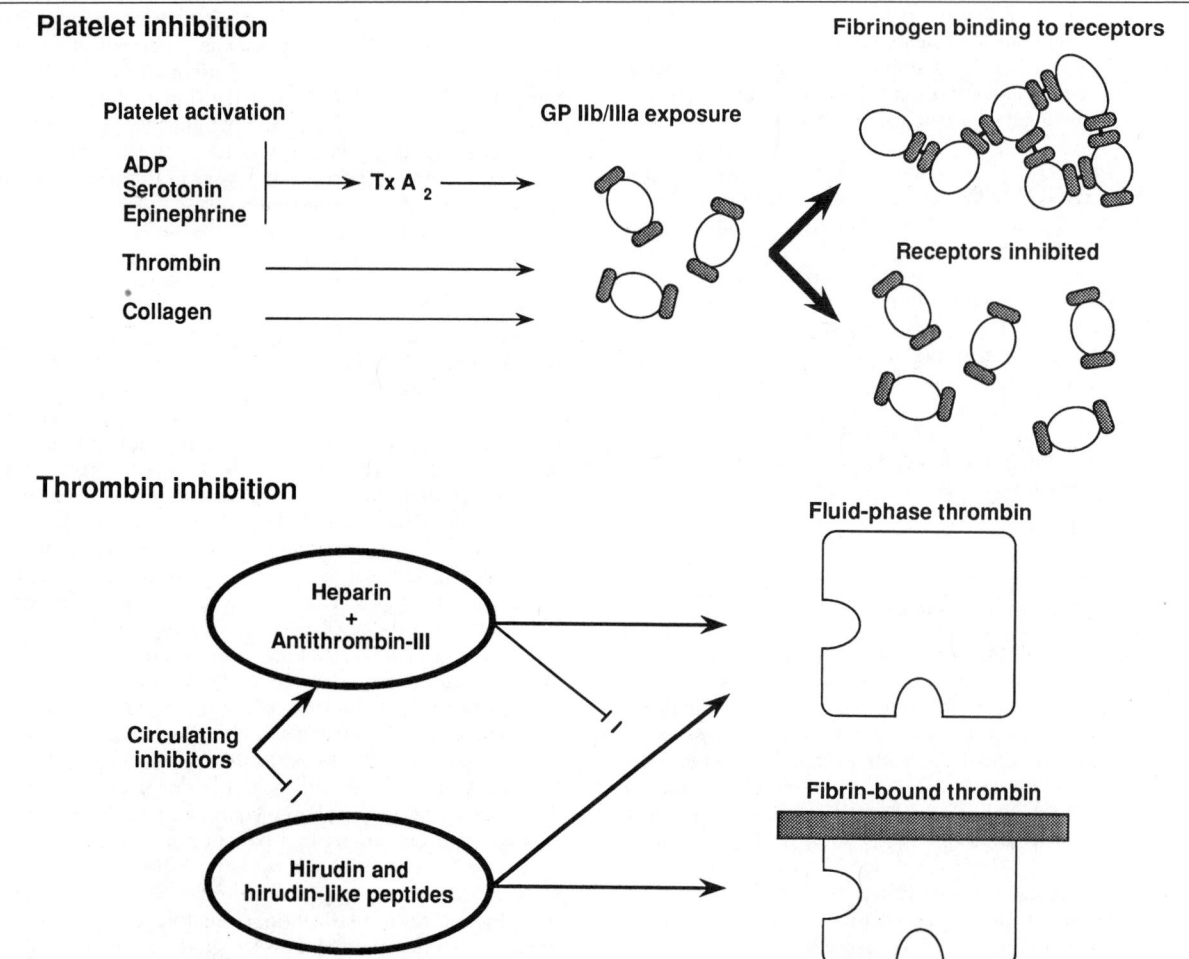

is to open the artery; in unstable angina and non-Q wave myocardial infarction it is to prevent blood clot progression and thrombotic occlusion. Aspirin and heparin are useful in this regard and a newer antithrombotic therapy may further improve benefits by overcoming some of their limitations.

New Antithrombotic Agents

Aspirin, ticlopidine, and other agents exert their benefits by blocking one of the many pathways of platelet aggregation. These pathways, however, all converge to activation of the glycoprotein receptor IIb/III, which is the final and obligatory step in platelet aggregation. Monoclonal antibodies against glycoprotein IIb/IIIa and peptide and nonpeptide inhibitors of the fibrinogen recognition sites are now available (Fig. 44-1). Similarly, the active sites of thrombin can be directly and specifically inhibited by agents that do not encounter circulating inhibitors. These agents are active on clot-bound thrombin as well as on fluid phase thrombin (Fig. 44-1). Hirudin is the salivary gland product of the medicinal leech (*Hirudo medicinalis*) and is now undergoing clinical investigation. Other small peptides blocking the active sites of thrombin are also under clinical investigation.

Unstable angina, myocardial infarction, and coronary balloon angioplasty are the three clinical situations most frequently associated with acute thrombosis. Accordingly, trials of the new antithrombotic drugs are performed in these conditions. c7E3, the monoclonal antibody to platelet membrane receptor GP IIb/IIIa, reduced by 40 percent the acute complication rate of high-risk angioplasty in the EPIC trial that has enrolled 2099 patients [111]. MK-383 (tyrafiban) and RO-44-9883 (lamifiban), two nonpeptidic inhibitors of the receptor, favorably influenced the event rate in unsable angina [112,113]. r-hirudin, argatroban, hirulog and efegetran are direct thrombin inhibitors actually investigated. Other blood active products acting at various sites of platelet and thrombin activation are at earlier phases of clinical investigation.

References

1. Sampson JJ, Eliaser M Jr: The diagnosis of impending acute coronary artery occlusion. *Am Heart J* 13:675, 1937.
2. Feil H: Preliminary pain in coronary thrombosis. *Am J Med Sci* 193:42, 1937.
3. Master AM, Dack S, Jaffe HL: Premonitory symptoms of acute coronary occlusion: A study of 260 cases. *Ann Intern Med* 14:1115, 1941.
4. Levy H: The natural history of changing pattern of angina pectoris. *Ann Intern Med* 44:1123, 1956.
5. Vakill RJ: Intermediate coronary syndrome. *Circulation* 24:557, 1961.
6. Beamish RE, Storrie VM: Impending myocardial infarction: Recognition and management. *Circulation* 21:1107, 1960.
7. Fowler NO: "Preinfarctional" angina: A need for an objective definition and for a controlled clinical trial of its management. *Circulation* 44:755, 1971.
8. Krauss KR, Hutter AM, De Sanctis RW: Acute coronary insufficiency course and follow-up. *Circulation* 45(suppl I):66, 1972.
9. Fulton M, Lutz W, Donald KM, et al: Natural history of unstable angina. *Lancet* 1:800, 1972.
10. Gazes PC, Mobly FM, Faris HM, et al: Pre-infarctional (unstable angina): A prospective study—10 year follow-up. Prognostic significance of electrocardiographic changes. *Circulation* 48:331, 1973.
11. Maseri A, L'Abbate A, Baroldi G, et al: Coronary vasospasm as a possible cause of myocardial infarction: Conclusion derived from the study of "pre-infarction angina." *N Engl J Med* 299:1271, 1978.
12. Alison HW, Russell RO, Mantle JA, et al: Coronary anatomy and arteriography in patients with unstable angina pectoris. *Am J Cardiol* 41:204, 1978.
13. Selden R, Neill WA, Rizmann LW, et al: Medical versus surgical therapy for acute coronary insufficiency: A randomized study. *N Engl J Med* 293:1329, 1975.
14. Russel RO, Moraski RE, Kouchoukos N, et al: Unstable angina pectoris: National Cooperative Study Group to compare surgical and medical therapy. II. In-hospital experience and initial follow-up results in patients with one, two and three vessel disease. *Am J Cardiol* 42:839, 1978.
15. Davies MJ, Thomas AC: Plaque fissuring: The cause of acute myocardial infarction, sudden ischemic death, and crescendo angina. *Br Heart J* 53:363, 1985.
16. Fuster V, Badimon L, Badimon JJ, et al: Mechanisms of disease: The pathogenesis of coronary artery disease and the acute coronary syndromes. *N Engl J Med* 326:310, 1992.
17. Telford AM, Wilson C: Trial of heparin vesus atenolol in prevention of myocardial infarction in intermediate coronary syndrome. *Lancet* 1:1225, 1981.
18. Lewis HD, Davis JW, Archibald DG, et al: Protective effects of aspirin against myocardial infarction and death in men with unstable angina. *N Engl J Med* 309:396, 1983.
19. Falk E: Plaque rupture with severe pre-existing stenosis precipitating coronary thrombosis: Characteristics of coronary atherosclerotic plaques underlying fatal occlusive thrombi. *Br Heart J* 50:127, 1983.
20. Falk E: Unstable angina with fatal outcome: Dynamic coronary thrombosis leading to infarction and/or sudden death—Autopsy evidence of recurrent mural thrombosis with peripheral embolization culminating in total vascular occlusion. *Circulation* 50:127, 1985.
21. De Wood M, Spores J, Notske R, et al: Prevalence of total coronary occlusion during the early hours of transmural myocardial infarction. *N Engl J Med* 303:897, 1980.
22. The TIMI Investigators: Early effects of tissue-type plasminogen activator added to conventional therapy on the culprit lesion in patients presenting with ischemic chest pain at rest: Results of the Thrombolysis in Myocardial Ischemia (TIMI IIIA) trial. *Circulation* 87:38, 1993.
23. Sherman CT, Litvack F, Grundfest W, et al: Coronary angioscopy in patients with unstable angina pectoris. *N Engl J Med* 315:913, 1986.
24. Mizuno K, Satomura K, Miyamoto A, et al: Angioscopic evaluation of coronary-artery thrombi in acute coronary syndromes. *N Engl J Med* 326:287, 1992.
25. Davies MJ, Woolf N, Rowles PM, et al: Morphology of the endothelium over atherosclerotic plaques in human coronary arteries. *Br Heart J* 60:459, 1988.
26. Taeymans Y, Théroux P, Lespérance J, et al: Quantitative angiographic morphology of the coronary artery lesions at risk of thrombotic occlusion. *Circulation* 85:78, 1992.
27. Jost S, Deckers JW, Nikutta P, et al: Progression of coronary artery disease is dependent on anatomic location and diameter. *J Am Coll Cardiol* 21:1339, 1993.
28. Ellis S, Alderman EL, Cain K, et al: Morphology of left anterior descending coronary territory lesions as a predictor of anterior myocardial infarction: A CASS registry study. *J Am Coll Cardiol* 13:1481, 1989.
29. Waters D, Lespérance J, Hudon G: Progression of coronary atherosclerosis: A prospective, quantitative angiographic study (abstract). *Circulation* 82(suppl III):III-251, 1990.
30. Harviger J: Formation and regulation of platelet and fibrin hemostatic plug. *Hum Pathol* 18:111, 1987.
31. Ruoslahti E, Pierschbacher MD: New perspectives in cell adhesion: RGD and integrins. *Science* 238:491, 1987.
32. Rapaport SI, Rao VM: Initiation and regulation of tissue-factor dependent blood coagulation. *Arterioscl Thromb* 12:1111, 1992.
33. Coughlin SR, Vu TKH, Wheaton VI: Characterization of a functional thrombin receptor: Issues and opportunities. *J Clin Invest* 89:351, 1992.

34. Weitz JI, Huboch M, Massel D, et al: Clot-bound thrombin is protected from inhibition by heparin-antithrombin III but is susceptible to inactivation by antithrombin III-independent inhibitors. *J Clin Invest* 86:385, 1990.

35. Ludmer PL, Selwyn AP, Shook TL, et al: Paradoxical vasoconstriction induced by acetylcholine in atherosclerotic human coronary arteries. *N Engl J Med* 315:1046, 1986.

36. Lerman A, Edwards BS, Hallett JW, et al: Circulating and tissue endothelin immunoreactivity in advanced atherosclerosis. *N Engl J Med* 325:997, 1991.

37. Palmer RMJ, Ferrige AG, Moncada S: Nitric acid release accounts for the biological activity of endothelium-derived relaxing factor. *Nature* 327:524, 1987.

38. Lüscher TF, Diederich D, Siebenmann R, et al: Difference between endothelium-dependent relaxations in arterial and in venous coronary bypass grafts. *N Engl J Med* 319:462, 1988.

39. Moncada S, Vane JR: Pharmacology and endogenous roles of prostaglandin endoperoxides, thromboxane A_2 and prostacyclin. *Pharmacol Rev* 30:293, 1979.

40. Braunwald E: Unstable angina: A classification. *Circulation* 80:410, 1989.

41. Nobuyoshi M, Kimura T, Nosaka H, et al: Restenosis after successful percutaneous transluminal coronary angioplasty: Serial angiographic follow-up of 229 patients. *J Am Coll Cardiol* 12:616, 1988.

42. Joelson JM, Most AS, Williams DO: Angiographic findings when chest pain recurs after successful percutaneous transluminal coronary angioplasty. *Am J Cardiol* 60:792, 1987.

43. Waters DD, Walling A, Roy D, et al: Previous coronary artery bypass grafting as an adverse prognostic factor in unstable angina pectoris. *Am J Cardiol* 58:465, 1986.

44. Théroux P, Lidón RM: Unstable angina: Pathogenesis, diagnosis and treatment. *Curr Probl Cardiol* 13:159, 1993.

45. Prinzmetal M, Kennamer R, Merliss R, et al: Angina pectoris. I. A variant form of angina pectoris. *Am J Med* 27:375, 1959.

46. MacAlpin RN, Kattus AA, Alvaro AB: Angina pectoris at rest with preservation of exercise capacity: Prinzmetal's variant angina. *Circulation* 47:946, 1973.

47. Scholl JM, Benacerraf A, Ducimetiere P, et al: Comparison of risk factors in vasospastic angina without significant fixed coronary narrowing to significant fixed coronary narrowing and no vasospastic angina. *Am J Cardiol* 57:199, 1986.

48. Miller D, Waters DD, Warnica W, et al: Is variant angina the coronary manifestation of a generalized vasospastic disorder? *N Engl J Med* 304:763, 1981.

49. Bilodeau L, Théroux P, Grégoire J, et al: Technetium-99m Sestamibi tomography in patients with spontaneous chest pain: Correlations with clinical, electrocardiographic and angiographic findings. *J Am Coll Cardiol* 18:1684, 1991.

49a. Hamm CW, Ravkilde J, Gerhardt W, et al: The prognostic value of troponin T in unstable angina. *N Engl J Med* 327:146, 1992.

49b. Liuzzo G, Biasucci LM, Gallimore JR, et al: The prognostic value of C-reactive protein and serum amyloid A protein in severe unstable angina. *N Engl J Med* 331:417, 1994.

50. Fitzgerald DJ, Roy L, Catella F, et al: Platelet activation in unstable coronary disease. *N Engl J Med* 315:983, 1986.

51. Théroux P, Latour JG, De Lara J, et al: Fibrinopeptide A and platelet factor levels in unstable angina pectoris. *Circulation* 75:156, 1987.

52. Alexopoulos D, Ambrose JA, Stump D, et al: Thrombosis-related markers in unstable angina pectoris. *J Am Coll Cardiol* 17:866, 1991.

53. Gottlieb SO, Weisfeldt ML, Ouyang P, et al: Silent ischemia as a marker for early unfavorable outcome in patients with unstable angina. *N Engl J Med* 314:1214, 1986.

54. Langer A, Freeman MR, Armstrong PW: ST segment shift in unstable angina: Pathophysiology and association with coronary anatomy and hospital outcome. *J Am Coll Cardiol* 13:1495, 1989.

55. Romeo F, Rosano GMC, Martuscelli E, et al: Unstable angina: Role of silent ischemia and total ischemic time (silent plus painful ischemia)—A 6 year follow-up. *J Am Coll Cardiol* 19:1173, 1992.

56. Neri Serneri GG, Gensini GR, Poggesi L, et al: Effect of heparin, aspirin or alteplase in reduction of myocardial ischemia in refractory unstable angina. *Lancet* 335:615, 1990.

57. Heupler FA Jr, Proudfit WL, Razavi M, et al: Ergonovine maleate provocative test for coronary arterial spasm. *Am J Cardiol* 41:631, 1978.

58. Okumura K, Yasue H, Matsuyama K, et al: Sensitivity and specificity of intracoronary injection of acetylcholine for the induction of coronary artery spasm. *J Am Coll Cardiol* 12:883, 1988.

59. Rafflenbeul W, Russell RO, Lichtlen PR: Angiographic anatomy of coronary arteries in unstable angina pectoris, in Rafflenbeul W, Lichtlen PR, Balcon R (eds): *Unstable Angina Pectoris.* New York, Thieme, 1981, p 51.

60. Moise A, Théroux P, Taeymans Y, et al: Clinical and angiographic factors associated with progression of coronary artery disease. *J Am Coll Cardiol* 3:659, 1984.

61. Moise A, Théroux P, Taeymans Y, et al: Unstable angina and progression of coronary atherosclerosis. *N Engl J Med* 309:695, 1983.

62. Betriu A, Heras M, Cohen M, et al: Unstable angina: Outcome according to clinical presentation. *J Am Coll Cardiol* 19:1659, 1992.

63. Théroux P: Unstable angina: Prognosis and risk factors, in Kapoor AS, Singh BN (eds): *Prognosis and Risk Assessment in Cardiovascular Disease,* New York, Churchill Livingstone, 1993, pp 139–152.

64. Théroux P, Ouimet H, Latour JG, et al: Prediction and prevention of myocardial infarction during the acute phase of unstable angina (abstract). *J Am Coll Cardiol* 13:192A, 1989.

65. Stone P, Kleiman N, Kronenberg M, et al: Effect of gender, race and age on the natural history of unstable angina and non-Q wave MI: The T3 Registry (abstract). *J Am Coll Cardiol* 21:453A, 1993.

66. Fahri JI, Cohen M, Fuster V: The broad spectrum of unstable angina pectoris and its implications for future clinical trials. *Am J Cardiol* 58:547, 1986.

67. Cohen M, Hawkins L, Greenberg S, et al: Usefulness of ST-segment changes in >2 leads on the emergency room electrocardiograms in either unstable angina or non-Q-wave myocardial infarction in predicting outcome. *Am J Cardiol* 67:1368, 1991.

68. Roberts KB, Califf RM, Harrel F, et al: The prognosis to patients with new onset angina who have undergone cardiac catheterization. *Circulation* 68:970, 1983.

69. Mulcahy R, Daly L, Graham I, et al: Unstable angina: Natural history and determinants of prognosis. *Am J Cardiol* 48:525, 1981.

70. Bosch X, Théroux P, Waters D, et al: Early post-infarction ischemia: Clinical, angiographic and prognostic significance. *Circulation* 75:988, 1987.

71. Théroux P, Ouimet H, McCans J, et al: Aspirin, heparin, or both to treat acute unstable angina. *N Engl J Med* 319:1105, 1988.

72. The RISC Group: Risk of myocardial infarction and death during treatment with low dose aspirin and intravenous heparin in men with unstable coronary disease. *Lancet* 336:827, 1990.

73. Cairns JA, Gent M, Singer J, et al: Aspirin, sulfinpyrazone, or both in unstable angina. *N Engl J Med* 313:1369, 1985.

74. Wallentin LC and the Research Group on Instability in Coronary Artery Disease in Southeast Sweden: Aspirin (75 mg/day) after an episode of unstable coronary artery disease: Long-term effect on the risk for myocardial infarction, occurrence of severe angina and the need for revascularization. *J Am Coll Cardiol* 18:1587, 1991.

75. Balsano F, Rizzon P, Violi F, et al: Antiplatelet treatment with ticlopidine in unstable angina: A controlled multicenter clinical trial. *Circulation* 82:17, 1990.

76. Wood P: Acute and subacute coronary insufficiency. *Br Med J* 1:1779, 1961.

77. Théroux P, Waters D, Lam J, et al: Reactivation of unstable angina following discontinuation of heparin. *N Engl J Med* 327:141, 1992.

78. Williams DO, Kirby MG, McPherson K, et al: Anticoagulant treatment in unstable angina. *Br J Clin Pract* 40:114, 1986.

79. Dauwe F, Affaki G, Waters DD, et al: Intravenous nitroglycerin in refractory unstable angina (abstract). *Am J Cardiol* 43:416, 1979.

80. Mikolich JR, Nicoloff MB, Robinson PH, et al: Relief of refractory angina with continuous intravenous infusion of nitroglycerin. *Chest* 77:375, 1980.

81. Page A, Gateau P, Ohayon J, et al: Intravenous nitroglycerin in unstable angina, in Lichtlen PR, Engel HJ, Schrey A, Swan JHC (eds): *Nitrates III. Cardiovascular Effects.* Berlin, Springer Verlag, 1981, p 371.

82. Curfman GD, Heinsimer JA, Lozner EC, et al: Intravenous nitro-

glycerin in the treatment of spontaneous angina pectoris: A prospective randomized trial. *Circulation* 67:276, 1983.

83. Roubin GS, Harris PJ, Eckhardt I, et al: Intravenous nitroglycerin in refractory unstable angina pectoris. *Aust NZ J Med* 12:598, 1982.

84. Squire A, Cantor R, Packer M: Limitations of continuous intravenous nitroglycerin prophylaxis in patients with refractory angina at rest (abstract). *Circulation* 66(suppl II):120, 1982.

85. Kaplan K, Davison R, Parker M, et al: Intravenous nitroglycerin for the treatment of angina at rest unresponsive to standard nitrate therapy. *Am J Cardiol* 51:694, 1983.

86. DePace NL, Herling IM, Kotler MN, et al: Intravenous nitroglycerin in refractory unstable angina: Potential pathophysiologic mechanisms of action. *Arch Intern Med* 142:1806, 1982.

87. Diodati J. Théroux P, Latour JG, et al: Effects of nitroglycerin at therapeutic doses on platelet aggregation in unstable angina pectoris and acute myocardial infarction. *Am J Cardiol* 66:683, 1990.

88. Figueras J, Lidón R, Cortadellas J: Rebound myocardial ischemia following abrupt interruption of intravenous nitroglycerin infusion in patients with unstable angina at rest. *Eur Heart J* 12:405, 1991.

89. Yusuf S, Ramsdale D, Peto R, et al: Early intravenous atenolol treatment in suspected acute myocardial infarction. *Lancet* 2:273, 1980.

90. Tilmant PY, Lablanche JM, Thieuleux FA, et al: Detrimental effect of propranolol in patients with coronary arterial spasm countered by combination with diltiazem. *Am J Cardiol* 52:230, 1983.

91. Waters DD, Théroux P, Szlachcic J, et al: Provocative testing with ergonovine to assess the efficacy of treatment with nifedipine, diltiazem and verapamil in variant angina. *Am J Cardiol* 48:123, 1981.

92. Gottlieb SO, Weisfeldt ML, Ouyang P, et al: Effect of the addition of propranolol to therapy with nifedipine for unstable angina pectoris: A randomized, double-blind, placebo-controlled trial. *Circulation* 73:331, 1986.

93. Holland Inter-University Nifedipine-Metoprolol Trial (HINT) Research Group: Early treatment of unstable angina in the coronary care unit: A randomized, double-blind, placebo-controlled comparison of recurrent ischemia in patients treated with nifedipine, metoprolol or both. *Br Heart J* 56:400, 1986.

94. Waters D: Proischemic complications of dihydropyridine calcium channel blockers. *Circulation* 84:2598, 1991.

95. de Feyter PJ, Suryapranata H, Serruys PW, et al: Coronary angioplasty for unstable angina: Immediate and late results in 200 consecutive patients with identification of risk factors for unfavorable early and late outcome. *J Am Coll Cardiol* 12:324, 1988.

96. Myler RK, Shaw RE, Stertzer SH, et al: Unstable angina and coronary angioplasty. *Circulation* 82(suppl II):II-88, 1990.

97. Kaiser GC, Schaff HV, Killip T: Myocardial revascularization for unstable angina pectoris. *Circulation* 79(suppl I):1-60, 1989.

98. de Feyter PJ, Serruys PW, van den Brand M, et al: Emergency coronary angioplasty in refractory unstable angina. *N Engl J Med* 313:342, 1985.

99. Lukas MA, Deutsch E, Hirshfeld JW Jr, et al: Influence of heparin therapy on percutaneous transluminal coronary angioplasty outcome in patients with coronary arterial thrombus. *Am J Cardiol* 65:179, 1990.

100. Suryapranata H, de Feyter PJ, Serruys PW: Coronary angioplasty in patients with unstable angina: Is there a role for thrombolysis? *J Am Coll Cardiol* 12:69A, 1988.

101. Luchi RJ, Scott SM, Deupree RH, et al: Comparison of medical and surgical treatment for unstable angina pectoris. *N Engl J Med* 316:977, 1987.

102. The TIMI IIIB Investigators: Effects of tissue plasminogen activator and a comparison of early and conservative strategies in unstable angina and non-Q-wave myocardial infarction. Results of the TIMI IIIB trial. *Circulation* 89:1545, 1994.

103. Bär FW, Verheugt FW, Col J, et al: Thrombolysis in patients with unstable angina improves the angiographic but not the clinical outcome: Results of UASEM, a multicenter, randomized, placebo-controlled, clinical trial with anistreplase. *Circulation* 86:131, 1992.

104. Gold HK, Johns JA, Leinbach RC, et al: A randomized, placebo-controlled trial of recombinant human tissue-type plasminogen activator in patients with unstable angina pectoris. *Circulation* 75:1192, 1987.

105. Nicklas JM, Topop EJ, Kander N, et al: Randomized double-blind placebo-controlled trial of tissue plasminogen activator in unstable angina. *J Am Coll Cardiol* 13:434, 1989.

106. Ambrose JA, Hjemdahl-Monsen C, Borrico S, et al: Quantitative and qualitative effects of intracoronary streptokinase in unstable angina and non-Q wave infarction. *J Am Coll Cardiol* 9:1156, 1987.

107. Freeman MR, Langer A, Wilson RF, et al: Thrombolysis in unstable angina: Randomized double-blind trial of t-PA and placebo. *Circulation* 85:150, 1992.

108. Schreiber TL, Rizik D, White C, et al: Randomized trial of thrombolysis versus heparin in unstable angina. *Circulation* 86:1407, 1992.

109. Waters D, Lam JYT: Is thrombolytic therapy striking out in unstable angina? *Circulation* 86:1642, 1992.

110. ISIS-2 (Second International Study of Infarct Survival) Collaborative Group: Randomized trial of intravenous streptokinase, oral aspirin, both or neither among 17,187 cases of suspected acute myocardial infarction. *Lancet* 2:349, 1988.

111. The EPIC Investigators: Use of a monoclonal antibody directed against the platelet glycoprotein IIb/IIIa receptor in high-risk coronary angioplasty. *N Engl J Med* 330:956, 1994.

112. Theroux P, White H, David D, et al: A heparin-controlled study of MK-383 in unstable angina (abstract). *Circulation* 90(suppl I):I-231, 1994.

113. Théroux P, Kouz S, Knudston ML, et al: A randomized double-blind controlled trial with the non-peptidic GP IIb/IIIa antagonist RO 44-9883 in unstable angina (abstract). *Circulation* 90(suppl I):I-232, 1994.

45. *Complicated Myocardial Infarction*

Christopher P. Cannon,
Leonard I. Ganz, and Peter H. Stone

Patient care following acute myocardial infarction (MI) initially focuses on limiting the acute event but then turns to preventing, identifying, and treating complications. The majority of complications and the highest mortality occur in the first months following the acute event [1] (Fig. 45-1), thus prompt identification and treatment of any established or potential complications are necessary.

It has been well established that the proximate cause of acute MI in the vast majority of patients is an acute coronary occlusion due to thrombosis [2]. The sequelae of coronary occlusion are depicted in Figure 45-2. After a period of prolonged ischemia, myocardial necrosis occurs, leading to myocardial dysfunction and, in some cases, death [3]. A number of major processes play a significant role in determining the prognosis following

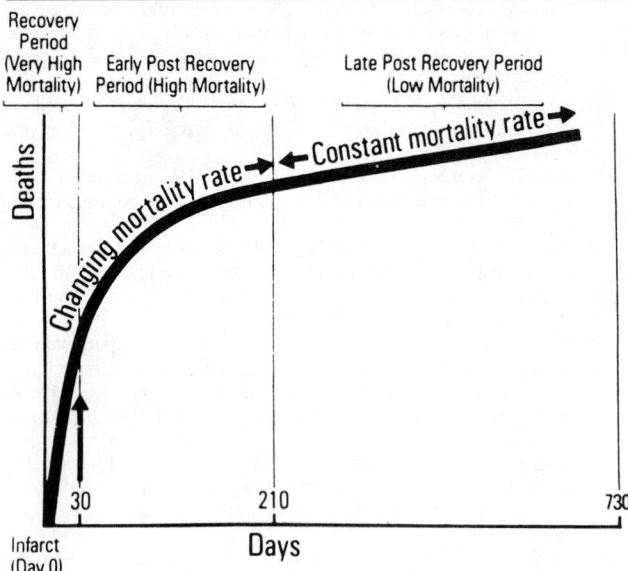

Fig. 45-1. Cumulative mortality after an acute myocardial infarction. (From Sherry S: The Anturane Reinfarction Trial. *Circulation* 62(suppl V):V-73, 1980. Reproduced with permission. Copyright 1980 American Heart Association.)

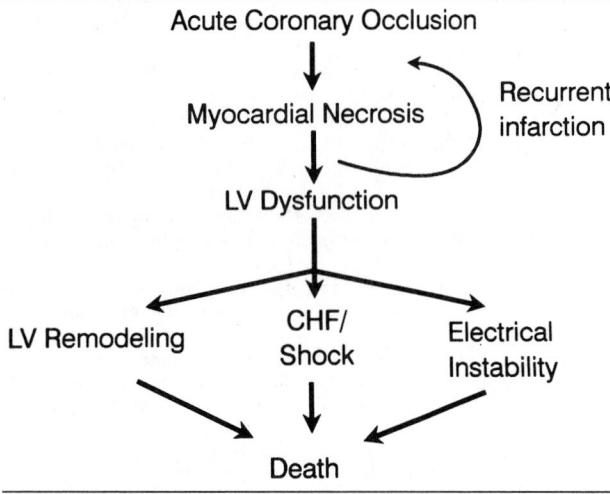

Fig. 45-2. Sequelae following acute myocardial infarction. LV = left ventricular; CHF = congestive heart failure.

acute MI: (1) persistent ischemic jeopardy with the potential for recurrent infarction and further loss of myocardial function; (2) left ventricular (LV) dysfunction occurring either in the acute setting or as part of a more insidious process of left ventricular remodeling [4,5]; and (3) electrical disturbances that can lead to significant arrhythmias and/or conduction disorders [6,7].

The categorizes of complications that may follow acute MI are shown in Table 45-1. Great efforts have been made over the past two decades to interrupt the cascade of events that follow acute MI and to reduce subsequent complications. This chapter reviews the many sequelae of acute MI and discusses diagnostic and therapeutic modalities for patients with these complications and those who manifest difficult management issues.

Table 45-1. Complications following Acute Myocardial Infarction

1. Recurrent infarction or ischemia
   a. Q-wave or non-Q wave
   b. Right ventricular infarction
2. Left ventricular dysfunction
   a. Diastolic dysfunction
   b. Systolic dysfunction
   c. Left ventricular dilatation and remodelling
   d. Left ventricular aneurysm
3. Disruption of cardiac structures
   a. Rupture of left ventricular free wall
   b. Rupture of intraventricular septum
   c. Rupture of papillary muscle
4. Miscellaneous
   a. Thromboembolism
   b. Pericarditis
5. Electrical disturbances and conduction disorders
   a. Ventricular arrhythmias
   b. Supraventricular arrhythmias
   c. Conduction disorders and bradyarrhythmias

Recurrent Ischemia/Infarction

Recurrent ischemic events following acute MI are a major cause of subsequent mortality [8,9]; therefore, prompt identification and therapy are needed. Recurrent ischemia may be due to a variety of causes. There may be an "unstable" coronary plaque or thrombus initially recanalized by pharmacologic or endogenous thrombolysis but which remains in jeopardy of spontaneous reocclusion (Fig. 45-3). Recurrent ischemia in this setting often manifests itself as rest angina and postinfarction unstable angina and requires urgent coronary angiography and revascularization. Alternatively, there may be a stable but persistently stenotic lesion in the infarct-related artery or another coronary artery, which may lead to ischemia only during an exercise test or with physical activities performed as part of in-hospital rehabilitation. This form of recurrent ischemia is often more stable than rest angina; although coronary angiography and revascularization are indicated [10], they may be performed less urgently.

INCIDENCE AND CLINICAL CONSEQUENCES. Recurrent infarction may occur in patients whose initial MI was treated with thrombolytic agents and in those whose MI evolved without such therapy. Reinfarction occurs in 4 to 10 percent of patients following thrombolytic therapy [11–14], which is slightly higher than in patients not treated with thrombolytic therapy (approximately 3%) [15,16,17]. There appears to be no difference between the thrombolytic agents in the rate of reinfarction [12,17]. Among patients treated with thrombolytic therapy, the incidence of reinfarction appears to be greater in those treated within 2 hours of onset of pain. However, this adverse effect is offset by a more substantial salvage of myocardium, leading to a net effect of a lower mortality in this group [18].

The consequences of reinfarction with regard to short- and long-term mortality are great. In the MILIS study patients who experienced an infarct extension had an in-hospital mortality more than fourfold higher than those patients without an extension (30% vs. 7%, p<0.01) [19]. In the TIMI-2 and TIMI-4 trials, patients who experienced reinfarction had a 2.6 times higher mortality at 1- to 3-year follow-up compared to those who did not [8,9]. In a series of 1253 patients not treated with thrombolytic therapy, mortality was greater in patients experi-

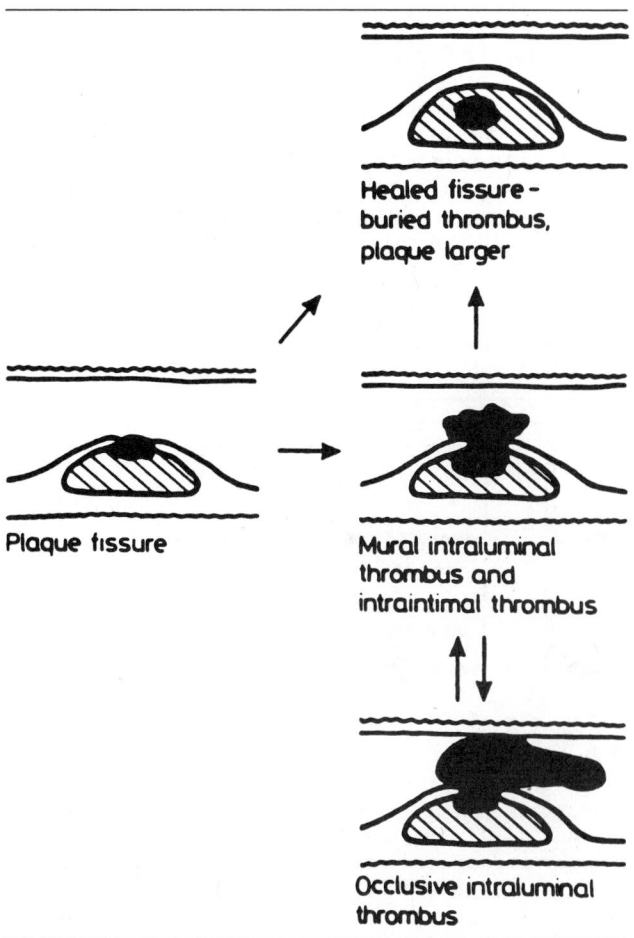

Fig. 45-3. "Unstable" coronary plaque with superimposed thrombus, which may stabilize and undergo reendothelialization or undergo further thrombosis and totally occlude the artery. (From Davies MJ, et al: Plaque fissuring: The cause of acute myocardial infarction, sudden ischemic death, and crescendo angina. *Br Heart J* 53:363, 1985. With permission.)

encing reinfarction, especially in patients who initially had a non-Q wave MI [14].

The angiographic equivalent of reinfarction is reocclusion of the infarct-related artery. This has been documented in angiographic trials of thrombolytic therapy, where all patients undergo early angiography and have follow-up angiography. In the largest series, 12.4 percent of patients treated with thrombolytic therapy experienced reocclusion prior to hospital discharge; the majority of them were symptomatic, with recurrent ischemic pain with S–T segment changes [20]. The consequences of reocclusion were significant: there was a 2.7-fold increase in mortality in those experiencing reocclusion compared to those who did not (11.0% vs. 4.5%, p = 0.01) [20]. In addition, patients experiencing reocclusion had an increased incidence of pulmonary edema, congestive heart failure, and second- or third-degree heart block.

Recurrent ischemia (without infarction) is a pathophysiologically related although less severe event, mainly because it is transient and does not permanently impair myocardial function. The incidence of recurrent ischemia at rest (without infarction) following MI ranges from 20 to 30 percent [11], with approximately the same incidence with or without thrombolytic therapy [21]. After primary PTCA or thrombolytic therapy fol-

lowed by an invasive strategy, as in TIMI-2, recurrent ischemia at rest appears to be reduced, likely because of the reduction in lesion stenosis achieved with percutaneous transluminal coronary angioplasty (PTCA) [11,22]. The consequences of recurrent ischemia are not as clearly defined. One study suggested that patients experiencing recurrent ischemia had a worse in-hospital prognosis, but this group included patients with recurrent infarction [23]. In an analysis from the TIMI-4 and TIMI-5 trials, the 1-year mortality of patients experiencing recurrent ischemia without infarction was similar to that of patients without recurrent ischemia [8].

PREVENTION. The management of recurrent ischemic events falls into two categories: prevention and treatment of the acute event. The two components shown to be important for prevention are effective antithrombotic therapy (see Chap. 121) and beta-blockade (see Chap. 210).

Antithrombotic Therapy. The first component of antithrombotic therapy is aspirin, which has been shown to be of benefit across the spectrum of ischemic heart disease [24]. Evidence for the benefit of aspirin in acute MI comes from three sources: the ISIS-2 trial, which showed a mortality benefit of nearly 25 percent [15]; the PARIS-2 study, which showed a reduction in death or MI following MI [25]; and a meta-analysis that showed a reduction by one-half in the rate of reocclusion [26]. In addition, four trials of patients with unstable angina, a clinical syndrome pathophysiologically related to acute MI, showed reduced reinfarction with aspirin treatment [27–30]. The dose of aspirin ranged from 1300 [29] to 75 mg per day [30], indicating that any dose of aspirin appears to confer benefit. The ISIS-2 trial used 160 mg daily; with the mortality benefit observed, this is generally considered the standard minimum dose in acute MI [15].

The second component of antithrombotic therapy for prevention of recurrent infarction after MI is heparin. Following thrombolytic therapy with tissue plasminogen activator, intravenous heparin has been clearly shown to improve infarct-related artery patency at 18 hours [31] and at 48 to 120 hours [32,33]. No difference in initial patency was observed at 90 minutes with or without heparin [34], suggesting that the effect of intravenous heparin was mainly in preventing reocclusion. The effect of heparin was greatest when anticoagulation was effective, with a therapeutic aPTT (≥60 seconds) [35,36]. Following streptokinase or anistreplase (APSAC) the role of heparin is less clear. Because reocclusion appears to be less frequent in patients treated with these two agents, which have a longer half-life, heparin may not be needed. Patients treated with streptokinase with intravenous or subcutaneous heparin in the GUSTO trial had similar infarct-related artery patency at 90 minutes and 24 hours, but those receiving intravenous heparin had significantly higher patency at 5 to 7 days (84% vs. 72%, p = 0.04) [37]. Nonetheless, the overall mortality and the rate of clinical reinfarction were the same between these two groups [12]; therefore intravenous heparin may be considered optional in streptokinase-treated patients. Subcutaneous heparin has been shown to be of no benefit in preventing reinfarction or death compared to placebo [38,39].

Warfarin received great attention in the 1970s, but aspirin appears to have overshadowed the possible benefits of warfarin, possibly because of the relative ease of use of aspirin compared to warfarin. However, there is a strong rationale that long-term anticoagulation would prevent new thrombotic coronary events. Merlini and colleagues demonstrated that, as expected, in the acute phase of unstable angina or MI, thrombin activity, prothrombin activity, and other activated clotting factors are elevated [40]. The levels decrease in the recovery phase but do

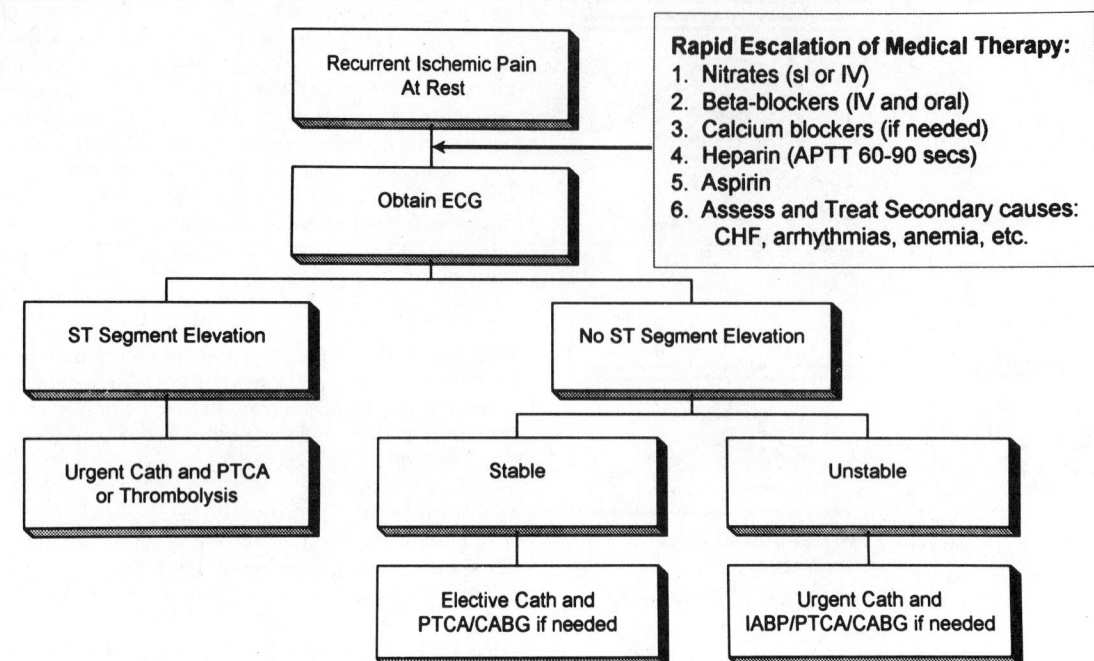

Fig. 45-4. Treatment of recurrent ischemic events.

not return to normal, thus maintaining a "prethrombotic" state [40,41]. Warfarin, which decreases the levels of clotting factors, would therefore eliminate the tendency for thrombosis. The WARIS trial supports this hypothesis: MI patients randomized to warfarin had a 34 percent reduction in reinfarction and a 24 percent reduction in mortality [42]. The combination of warfarin and low-dose aspirin is currently being compared to aspirin alone [43].

Beta-Adrenergic Blockade. Beta blockade in the setting of acute MI and after MI has been studied extensively and found almost uniformly to be beneficial. Several studies have shown that in patients with acute MI not treated with thrombolytic therapy, beta-blockers administered within 12 hours of the onset of pain result in smaller infarct size, less frequent ventricular fibrillation, and lower mortality than in patients not treated with a beta-blocker [44–49]. In TIMI-2B, early intravenous blockade with metoprolol was shown to reduce reinfarction in thrombolytic-treated patients if administered within 2 hours and to reduce recurrent ischemia in all patients [11]. In current practice, early intravenous, followed by oral, beta blockade should be used in all patients without contraindications (bradycardia, atrioventricular block, hypotension, pulmonary edema, history of bronchospasm).

TREATMENT. After preventative antithrombotic and anti-ischemic medical therapy, the treatment of an acute ischemic event depends on whether acute reocclusion is occurring. Figure 45-4 outlines an approach to the acute evaluation and treatment of a recurrent ischemic event. General measures aimed at controlling heart rate and blood pressure, preventing coronary vasoconstriction and coronary thrombosis, as well as ameliorating ischemic pain include: (1) sublingual and/or intravenous nitroglycerin, a potent agent that improves coronary blood flow, reduces myocardial oxygen demand by venous dilatation and reducing preload, and has been shown to reduce the incidence of early reocclusion [50]; (2) intravenous beta blockade,

if no contraindications are present; (3) calcium channel blockers, if tolerated, to prevent episodic coronary vasoconstriction; (4) intravenous heparin or verification that anticoagulation is adequate (aPTT ≥ 60 seconds); (5) aspirin; and (6) morphine or other analgesics to relieve ischemic pain. The goals of this therapy are to reduce the systolic blood pressure to approximately 110 to 120 mm Hg and the heart rate to 50 to 60 beats per minute. In clinically unstable patients with evidence of congestive heart failure, volume status must be assessed carefully and treated appropriately. Electrocardiography should be performed to identify the presence of S–T segment elevation, a reliable marker for acute coronary occlusion [2]. Although the presence of S–T segment deviation indicates the need for rapid treatment, S–T segment elevation in particular indicates that urgent coronary reperfusion therapy is needed.

Reperfusion can be achieved with urgent revascularization with PTCA or coronary artery bypass grafting (CABG) or administration of a thrombolytic agent (a second dose in some cases) (see Chap. 46). In a large series of patients in the TAMI trials, Ellis et al. demonstrated the importance of rapid treatment of evolving reocclusion/reinfarction [23]. In-hospital mortality was 0 percent in patients treated within 90 minutes of the onset of symptoms (usually with PTCA), compared to 21 percent for patients with successful reperfusion achieved *after* 90 minutes and 24 percent for patients with failed reperfusion [23]. These data emphasize the need for rapid reperfusion when reinfarction/reocclusion with S–T segment elevation occurs.

Similar results have been found when thrombolytic therapy is used to treat acute reocclusion. Barbash et al. demonstrated clinical success in 85 percent of patients treated with repeat thrombolysis for reinfarction; nearly one-half of patients needed no further intervention [51]. The agent used in most series is t-PA, because of its rapid action and because allergic reactions are avoided in patients previously treated with streptokinase [52]. Barbash et al. recently extended their observations, noting that patients treated with repeat thrombolysis within 20 minutes of the onset of recurrent chest pain had significantly better left ventricular function than patients treated later. This reemphasizes the benefit of early reperfusion [53].

This strategy is gaining acceptance: in the recently completed GUSTO trial, approximately 40 percent of patients with re-infarction were treated with repeat thrombolysis [13].

If S–T segment elevation is not present, medical therapy should be rapidly escalated until the ischemic pain resolves. Thrombolytic therapy in patients with unstable angina and non-Q wave MI (i.e., those whose ischemia is generally not associated with S–T segment elevation) was recently found *not* to be of benefit; in fact, it may be detrimental [54]. Thrombolytic therapy is therefore recommended only for patients with recurrent S–T segment elevation.

If ischemia cannot be controlled with medical therapy, use of an intraaortic balloon pump (IABP) may be necessary, usually in concert with urgent coronary angiography and revascularization.

INDICATIONS FOR CORONARY ANGIOGRAPHY FOLLOWING ACUTE MYOCARDIAL INFARCTION. The decision to perform coronary angiography and/or coronary revascularization following acute MI is generally based on a standard approach to risk stratification (Fig. 45-5) [10,55,56]. Patients who develop rest ischemia or ischemia occurring with the gradual progression of physical activities during early in-hospital rehabilitation should undergo coronary angiography. Those who develop ischemia only as part of a prehospital discharge exercise test are also candidates for coronary angiography to define their risk more clearly [10,56]. Coronary revascularization (PTCA or CABG) is recommended for patients with recurrent ischemia

Fig. 45-5. Prognostic stratification after acute myocardial infarction (MI). Patients who develop ischemia after MI, whether spontaneous or induced by exercise (box in center of figure), are candidates for coronary angiography. (From DeBusk RF, et al: Identification and treatment of low-risk patients after acute myocardial infarction and coronary-artery bypass graft surgery. *N Engl J Med* 314:161, 1986. Reprinted by permission.)

in the early post-MI period if the coronary anatomy is suitable [10]. This strategy of catheterization and revascularization for recurrent spontaneous or provokable post-MI ischemia has been the standard of practice in the United States, although it should be noted that rates of revascularization outside the United States are much lower [57,58].

Type of Infarction

Once the infarct has occurred, there are different outcomes that can be anticipated based on the electrocardiographic characteristics of the acute and evolving event. These different patterns often present difficult management issues.

Q WAVE VERSUS NON-Q WAVE MYOCARDIAL INFARCTION. The ECG is the most widely used tool in the evaluation of patients with acute MI, and the presence or absence of Q waves provides valuable information regarding the extent of infarction as well as the patient's prognosis. Although the clinicopathologic correlation is poor between the development of Q waves and the transmural or nontransmural extent of myocardial necrosis, the natural history of patients following an MI may be quite different based on whether or not Q waves develop. Patients with Q wave infarctions have been found to have higher peak creatine kinase (CK) and lower ejection fraction than those without Q waves and at autopsy were found to have larger infarctions [1].

In a pooled analysis of 45 studies of patients with acute MI in the prethrombolytic therapy era, patients with Q wave MI had an in-hospital mortality nearly twice that of patients with non-Q wave MI [59]. On the other hand, patients with non-Q wave MI had higher postdischarge reinfarction rates and higher

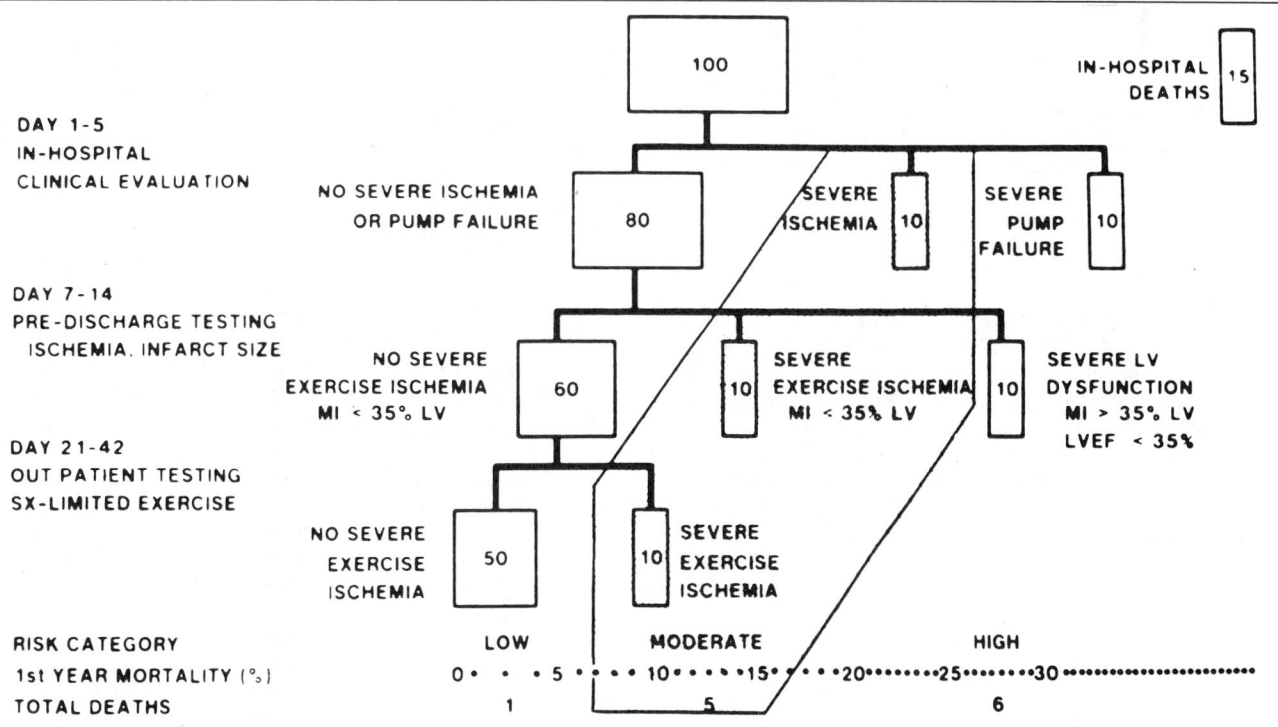

mortality [59]. This finding was recently noted in the large International TPA/SK Mortality Trial [60]. When in-hospital and late mortality of MI patients are considered together, however, overall prognosis appears to be related more to the size and location of infarction (i.e., anterior vs. inferior) rather than to the presence or absence of Q waves [61]. In patients with their first infarction, those with non-Q wave MI were found to have a significantly higher rate of reinfarction through 10 years than those with Q-wave MI (44.8% vs. 27.4%, p = 0.02) [62]. Mortality was similar, however, indicating that the smaller infarct size and better left ventricular function associated with a first MI offsets the higher rate of reinfarction. Thus, non-Q wave MI has generally been considered an incomplete event and specific medical and revascularization strategies have been sought for these patients (see Chap. 44).

Medical therapy for patients with Q wave MI and non-Q wave MI is generally similar, since the pathophysiology underlying both entities may be quite similar. All patients should receive aspirin, which has been found to be beneficial in all aspects of coronary artery disease [24]. Beta-blockers have been shown in several studies to reduce reinfarction and mortality after MI and are generally recommended following MI regardless of type [45–49]. Diltiazem may have a beneficial effect on non-Q wave MI in particular. Diltiazem was found in two studies to reduce the rate of early reinfarction after non-Q wave MI [63,64]; however, neither mortality nor long-term reinfarction rate was improved [65]. Therefore, diltiazem can be recommended in the early treatment following non-Q wave MI, but longer-term therapy should be with a beta-blocker. Because beta blockade has been shown to be of benefit following acute MI in secondary prevention [44–49], in unstable angina [66], and even in those with only risk factors for coronary artery disease (e.g., hypertension, [67]) beta-blockers should be used routinely after MI.

Some investigators suggest that coronary angiography and coronary revascularization should be performed routinely in patients with non-Q wave MI, since these patients remain at increased risk for reinfarction and late mortality. The TIMI-3B study demonstrated no difference in the rate of death or nonfatal MI in patients with non-Q wave MI treated medically, compared with similarly treated patients who were also randomized to early routine coronary angiography and revascularization [54]. However, the latter patients experienced lower rates of rehospitalization, shorter duration of rehospitalization, and required fewer antiischemic medications than those receiving medical therapy alone [54]. It may therefore be reasonable to recommend early coronary angiography and revascularization if the patient with a non-Q wave MI has no contraindications to such invasive therapy and has access to a facility with high-quality PTCA and CABG.

MYOCARDIAL INFARCTION PRESENTING WITH VERSUS WITHOUT S–T SEGMENT ELEVATION. Although differences in management strategy based on the presence of Q waves are important, Q waves characteristically do not develop until many hours or days after onset of MI. From an *acute* treatment perspective, a more relevant dichotomy is whether the MI initially presents with S–T segment elevation. While there is often a concordance between the direction of S–T segment deviation on admission and the development of Q waves as the MI evolves, the direction of S–T segment deviation may prompt critical management decisions long before Q waves can be detected.

Complete coronary occlusion occurs in at least 87 percent of patients with symptoms of acute MI who present early with S–T segment elevation [2], compared with only 26 percent of those without S–T segment elevation [68]. Similar findings were observed in the TIMI-3A trial [69]. Consistent with these fundamental differences in coronary pathology associated with the direction of S–T segment deviation, differences in the efficacy of reperfusion therapy have been noted. Patients with S–T segment elevation uniformly benefit from early reperfusion therapy with thrombolysis or direct angioplasty (see Chap. 46), while those without S–T segment elevation, who usually have a patent artery on presentation, do not benefit from thrombolysis [54]. Early management of the MI patient with S–T segment *elevation*, therefore, includes aggressive efforts to restore coronary patency with thrombolytic therapy or direct PTCA, while early management of the MI patient with S–T segment *depression* focuses on reducing myocardial oxygen demand and administering antithrombotic therapy.

Right Ventricular Infarction

Right ventricular infarction occurs in 35 to 50 percent of patients with inferior MI (themselves accounting for over half of MIs) [70,71] and therefore requires special diagnostic evaluation and therapy (Fig. 45-6). A small percentage (roughly 5%) of patients have isolated right ventricular infarction without inferior MI. Clinical recognition of right ventricular infarction is frequently lower [72], because special (although simple) diagnostic tests are needed to diagnose it.

IDENTIFICATION. The simplest test to investigate the presence of a right ventricular infarction utilizes right precordial ECG leads placed in the usual positions except beginning in the *left* second intercostal space and moving over to the *right* chest. The acute presence of S–T segment elevation in lead V_{4R} has a sensitivity and specificity of 85 to 90 percent for the diagnosis of right ventricular infarction, compared with the "gold standard"—a technetium pyrophosphate scan [70,71]. The presence of a Q wave in lead V_{4R} does *not* indicate an old or evolving right ventricular infarction, but is rather a normal finding (electrical forces of the left ventricle move away from the right precordium and generate a Q wave in V_{4R}). Other modalities used to diagnose right ventricular infarction are thallium or sestamibi perfusion imaging, coronary arteriography, echocardiography or hemodynamic measurements with a pulmonary artery catheter. An elevated right atrial pressure equal or nearly equal to pulmonary capillary wedge pressure indicates right ventricular dysfunction and hence probable acute infarction [71]. The ready availability of echocardiography has made it very useful in the evaluation of acute MI. A right ventricular wall motion abnormality or decreased right ventricular ejection fraction on echocardiography is a concrete sign of right ventricular infarction.

The differential diagnosis for right ventricular infarction includes hypotension due to left ventricular infarction, pericardial tamponade, constrictive pericarditis, and pulmonary embolus [72] (see below and Chaps. 34 and 60).

CLINICAL MANIFESTATIONS. Right ventricular infarction may be suggested by characteristic ECG, echocardiographic, or scintigraphic findings, but these abnormalities are most meaningful if they occur in the setting of clinical manifestations of right ventricular infarction, typically including a characteristic hemodynamic profile and sinoatrial (SA) or atrioventricular (A-V) nodal conduction disturbances. Initial descriptions of right ventricular infarction focused on hemodynamic complications, namely decreased performance of the right ventricle with consequent increased filling pressures and isolated right-

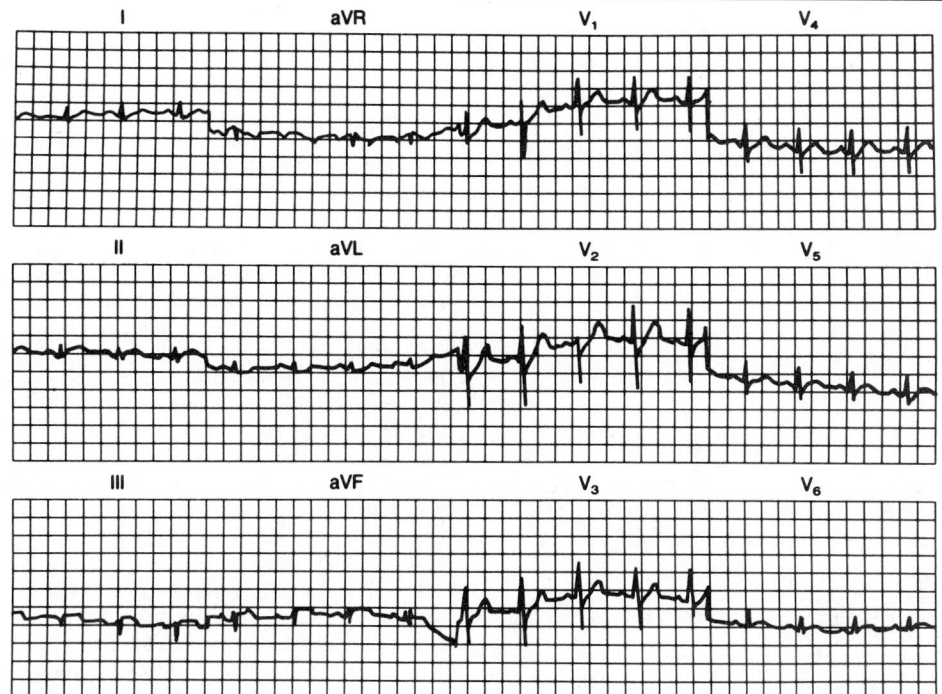

Fig. 45-6. Electrocardiogram from a patient with a right ventricular infarct. Note the true posterior left ventricular involvement.

sided congestion [71]. Jugular venous distention and clear lungs distinguish right ventricular infarction from combined right- and left-sided congestion due to left ventricular dysfunction. Systemic hypotension is a frequent complication of right ventricular infarction, in which poor right ventricular output leads to decreased filling of the left ventricle. In this setting, the right atrial pressure is characteristically equal to or greater than the pulmonary capillary wedge pressure, and the wedge pressure is often low (<12 mm Hg). Encroachment of the left ventricle by a volume-overloaded right ventricle may decrease left ventricular stroke volume and cardiac output [71].

Atrioventricular and/or sinoatrial nodal block occurs in 10 to 15 percent of patients with inferior MI but is particularly prevalent in those with right ventricular infarction; nearly 25 percent of inferior MI patients with right ventricular infarction exhibit complete atrioventricular block, compared with 4 percent of those without right ventricular infarction [70]. The need for temporary pacing closely parallels the incidence of complete atrioventricular block, as does the occurrence of complications including ventricular fibrillation, sustained ventricular tachycardia, and cardiogenic shock [70]. A more thorough discussion of bradycardia and atrioventricular block in inferior MI and right ventricular infarction is presented below.

The prognostic importance of right ventricular infarction is underscored by the recent report of 200 patients with an inferior MI treated between 1985 and 1990 (in whom 35% were eligible for and received thrombolytic therapy). In-hospital mortality was significantly and dramatically higher in those whose inferior MI included right ventricular infarction (31%) than in those whose inferior MI was not complicated by right ventricular infarction (5%) [70].

MANAGEMENT. Initial treatment of right ventricular infarction involves early reperfusion therapy directed at limiting infarct size (see Chap. 121). If hemodynamic compromise is present, measures should be used to increase forward output of the right ventricle. Volume expansion is the mainstay of therapy, aiming for a right atrial or central venous pressure as high as necessary to fill the left ventricle adequately. Acute boluses of 250 to 500 ml of normal saline should be used; many liters of fluid may be required to elevate right ventricular filling pressures sufficiently to increase forward flow. If right ventricle volume expansion is sufficient to increase right ventricular output so that the left ventricle is adequately filled, systemic hemodynamics may stabilize and invasive monitoring with a pulmonary artery catheter may not be necessary. If acute volume loading does not correct the hemodynamic disturbance, however, usually a pulmonary catheter is indicated to determine the filling pressures of the left and right ventricles and to guide optimal management. If the infarct is large, there may be dysfunction of both the right and left ventricles; volume expansion may improve the right ventricular function to the degree that the left ventricular dysfunction then becomes evident, manifested by rales and pulmonary edema. A pulmonary artery catheter is essential for optimal management of these patients with combined ventricular failure.

If volume expansion alone does not restore systemic blood pressure to greater than 90 mm Hg, dobutamine or dopamine should be used to increase right ventricular output. In contrast to left-sided heart failure, in right-sided heart failure venous vasodilators, such as nitrates, should be avoided, because they decrease right ventricular filling pressures and, hence, output. If hemodynamically significant sinus bradycardia or atrioventricular block develops, temporary ventricular pacing may be necessary (see below).

Left Ventricular Dysfunction

It has long been recognized that the severity of MI relates directly to the amount of myocardium that is damaged [73]. The

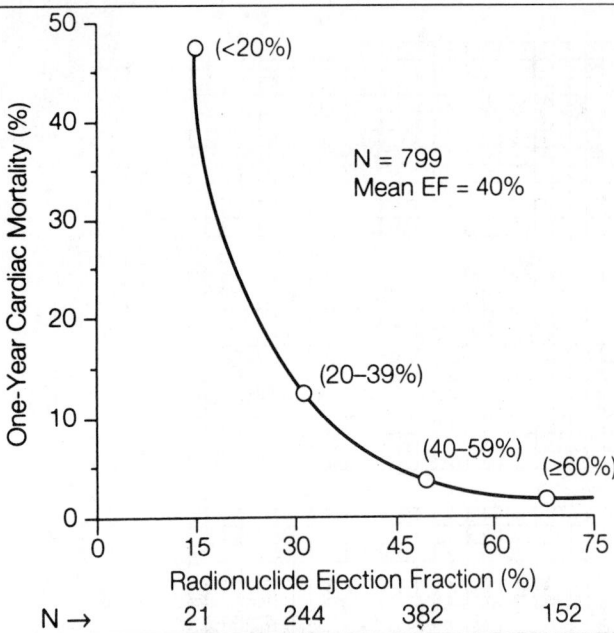

Fig. 45-7. Relationship between left ventricular ejection fraction (EF) determined before discharge and 1-year mortality. (From Multicenter Postinfarction Research Group: Risk stratification and survival after myocardial infarction. *N Engl J Med* 309:331, 1983. Reprinted by permission.)

most important determinant of prognosis after MI is the degree of left ventricular dysfunction [6] (Fig. 45-7), even when reperfusion with thrombolysis is achieved [74]. Many factors influence residual ventricular function: (1) left ventricular function prior to the acute MI; (2) infarct size; and (3) location of the MI. Patients with a prior MI have a worse prognosis than those without prior MI [11]. Infarct size is measured by the amount of CPK released, the presence or absence of Q waves on the ECG [59], or by imaging techniques that estimate the percentage of left ventricle which has been damaged [75]. Anterior location of the MI has been noted to have a worse prognosis than other locations [11,61].

CONGESTIVE HEART FAILURE. The clinical consequence of left ventricular dysfunction is congestive heart failure. There may be systolic dysfunction, manifested by reduced systemic perfusion and evidence of pulmonary congestion, or diastolic dysfunction, manifested by increases in left ventricular filling pressures and pulmonary congestion, but no evidence of reduced systemic perfusion.

Diastolic Dysfunction. Diastolic dysfunction occurs almost uniformly in patients with acute MI, although it becomes clinically significant in only one-fourth to one-third of such patients. It is the most common cause of early mild congestive heart failure in the setting of acute MI and can be responsible for acute or "flash" pulmonary edema (Fig. 45-8). The pathophysiology of diastolic dysfunction begins with increased wall stiffness from ischemia and infarction. This decreased compliance results in higher filling pressures in the left ventricle and consequently in the left atrium and pulmonary vasculature. Clinical signs of elevated pulmonary venous congestion are shortness of breath, dyspnea on exertion, orthopnea, rales on physical examination, and pulmonary vascular redistribution on chest

radiograph. Diastolic dysfunction is usually associated with an S_4, indicating decreased compliance of the left ventricle, but not an S_3, which is associated with syndromes of systolic dysfunction. Systolic function may be entirely normal in these patients.

TREATMENT. The treatment goals in patients with diastolic dysfunction include treatment of the pulmonary congestion, which involves diuresis, and treatment of the ischemia. Furosemide is most commonly used as a diuretic, beginning with very small doses (5–10 mg intravenously in patients not previously receiving furosemide or higher doses in patients previously receiving diuretics). Since pulmonary congestion is due to a transiently stiff left ventricle from ischemia, and not to increased intravascular volume, it is important to avoid overdiuresis. Transient hypotension may result from overdiuresis since left ventricular volume and filling pressures may become excessively low once the ischemia is resolved and the left ventricular compliance has returned to baseline (see Fig. 45-8).

Acute afterload and preload reducing agents also help reduce pulmonary congestion. Intravenous nitroglycerin and nitroprusside have been used widely because they can be rapidly titrated in response to blood pressure. Nitroglycerin is most active in producing venous dilatation (preload reduction) and thus is most suitable to reducing pulmonary congestion; nitroprusside is a balanced vasodilator, producing arterial vasodilatation (afterload reduction) as well as preload reduction. It is most suitable to reducing ischemia and pulmonary congestion in the setting of marked arterial hypertension.

Beta-blockers may be invaluable in patients whose pulmonary congestion is due to isolated diastolic dysfunction. These agents reduce ischemia and thereby improve left ventricular compliance and reduce left ventricular filling pressures. Pulmonary congestion often then rapidly resolves. If the diagnosis of isolated diastolic dysfunction is not secure and there is concern that a beta-blocker may exacerbate systolic dysfunction, then cautious administration of an ultra-short-acting beta-blocker, such as esmolol, may be particularly useful.

Because left ventricular systolic function is often quite preserved in patients with isolated diastolic dysfunction, prognosis after MI is relatively good compared to patients with systolic dysfunction. However, patients with systolic or diastolic congestive heart failure have a worse long-term outcome than patients without such manifestations [76]. Patients whose acute MI is complicated by congestive heart failure have an increased mortality (28%) compared to those whose acute MI is not complicated by heart failure (5.5%) [77]. Furthermore, patients whose congestive heart failure is due to systolic dysfunction have a significantly worse outcome than those whose congestive heart failure is due to diastolic dysfunction [76].

Systolic Dysfunction. Congestive heart failure due to systolic dysfunction is the most serious complication following acute MI. In a recent large series of patients, approximately one-fourth of patients had evidence of left ventricular dysfunction, defined as an ejection fraction of 40 percent or less [76]. While approximately two-thirds of these patients had clinical evidence of congestive heart failure, only one-third (9% of the total population) had documented left ventricular failure on chest radiograph in addition to reduced ejection fraction [76]. In another series, approximately 25 percent of patients showed clinical evidence of left ventricular failure during initial hospitalization [78]. The cause of systolic dysfunction is usually impaired left ventricular contractility due to a large MI. More than two-thirds of patients who develop congestive heart failure from systolic dysfunction have anterior MI (Fig. 45-9), and approximately one-third of patients with congestive heart failure have large inferior infarctions.

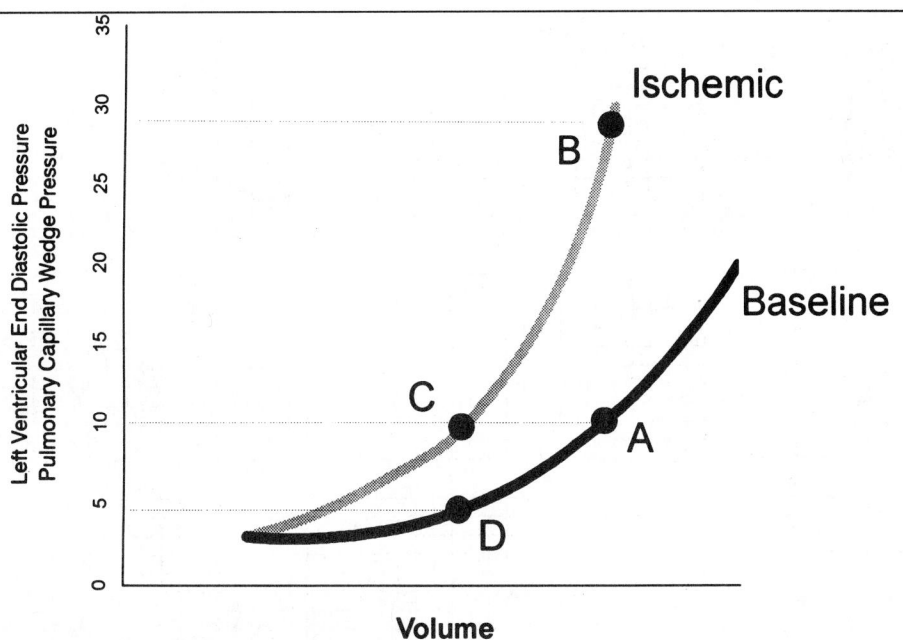

Fig. 45-8. Relationship between left ventricular end-diastolic pressure (LVEDP) and volume at baseline and during acute ischemia. A representative example of "flash" pulmonary edema. At baseline (point A) the LVEDP (or PCWP) is 10 mm Hg. If ischemia acutely develops, the pressure-volume curve is shifted upwards and to the left. At the same left ventricular (LV) volume, the LVEDP then becomes elevated to 30 mm Hg (point B) and pulmonary edema develops. Optimal antiischemia treatment, often with minimal diuresis, restores the ischemia-induced change in LV compliance back to baseline and returns the patient from point B to point A. If the diuresis is excessive (point C), the LVEDP may become too low when the ischemia resolves (point D) and the patient may become tachycardic and hypotensive.

Systolic dysfunction, even severe pump failure, may be due to myocardial "stunning" [79], not necessarily to frank infarction. Myocardial stunning is a reversible process of myocardial dysfunction due to an episode of ischemia (often in border zones surrounding a central zone of infarction). Though necrosis in this ischemic zone does not occur, the dysfunction may persist for a number of days before more normal function is restored. The dysfunctional, stunned myocardium can respond to inotropic stimulation, such as infusion of dopamine or dobutamine [80]. Stunned myocardium may be suspected when the degree of myocardial failure (i.e., congestive heart failure) seems disproportionate to the size of the documented MI (i.e., peak creatine kinase levels). The results of aggressive and continued inotropic support of dysfunctional myocardium for a few days will indicate whether the early congestive heart failure was due to stunned myocardium, in which case the congestive heart failure and wall motion will improve, or to actual infarction, in which case no improvement will be evident.

Transient mitral regurgitation may also complicate and exacerbate left ventricular dilatation and dysfunction. This form of reversible mitral regurgitation occurs when the subvalvular apparatus and the two leaflets are pulled apart by the dilated walls of the ventricle, making it impossible for the two valve leaflets to coapt properly. The incompetent mitral valve usually resolves quickly with diuresis: as the dilated left ventricular chamber decreases in size, the subvalvular apparatus comes into more normal position and the mitral valve leaflets can coapt normally again.

Cardiogenic Shock. The most malignant end of the spectrum of congestive heart failure is cardiogenic shock, in which congestive heart failure is manifested by frank systemic hypotension and pulmonary congestion. Patients with cardiogenic shock have the highest risk of acute MI patients, and evaluation and treatment must be aggressive.

The hemodynamic characteristics of cardiogenic shock include an elevated pulmonary capillary wedge pressure and a reduced cardiac index [81]. Clinically, there is evidence of peripheral organ hypoperfusion, with oliguria, cool extremities, and mottled skin. Mortality in this patient population is very high—50 to 80 percent in the original series in the early 1970s [81,82] and still high in more modern series, 53% [83].

TREATMENT. The initial treatment goal for patients with severe congestive heart failure is to assure adequate oxygenation with supplemental oxygen (and endotracheal intubation, if necessary) and to maintain systolic blood pressure at 90 mm Hg or greater, to provide adequate perfusion of vital organs.

Preload and afterload reduction and inotropic support are necessary for patients with marked systolic function and cardiogenic shock. As shown in Figure 45-10, the Frank-Starling curve in patients with severe congestive heart failure becomes flattened and depressed. As left ventricular end-diastolic pressure rises (representing a means of increasing cardiac output via the Starling mechanism), pulmonary congestion develops. If cardiac output becomes excessively reduced, oliguria, mental clouding, and other symptoms of low-output state ensue. Inotropic agents such as digitalis will increase cardiac output associated with a slight decrease in ventricular end-diastolic pressure (preload). Diuretics and/or nitrates will diminish pulmonary congestion, but there will be no major improvement in cardiac output. A balanced vasodilator such as nitroprusside will reduce both preload and afterload, thereby increasing cardiac output, reducing left ventricular end-diastolic pressure, and alleviating pulmonary congestion. Most effective is administration of both inotropic and vasodilator therapies, with nitroprusside to reduce afterload and dopamine or dobutamine to act as an inotropic cardiac stimulant.

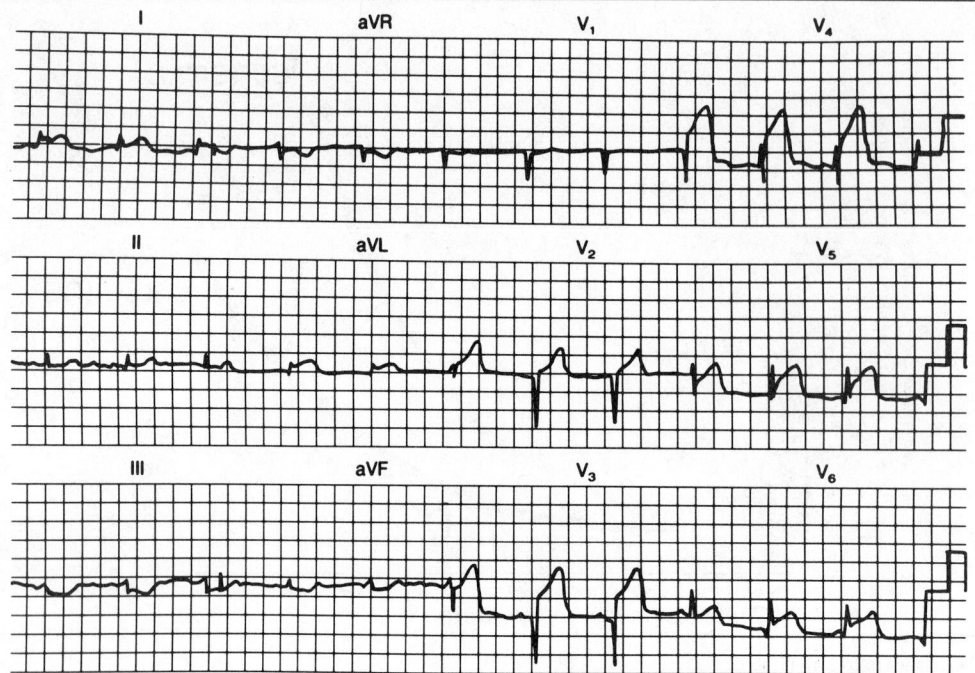

Fig. 45-9. Electrocardiogram from a patient with a large antero-lateral myocardial infarction and impending cardiogenic shock.

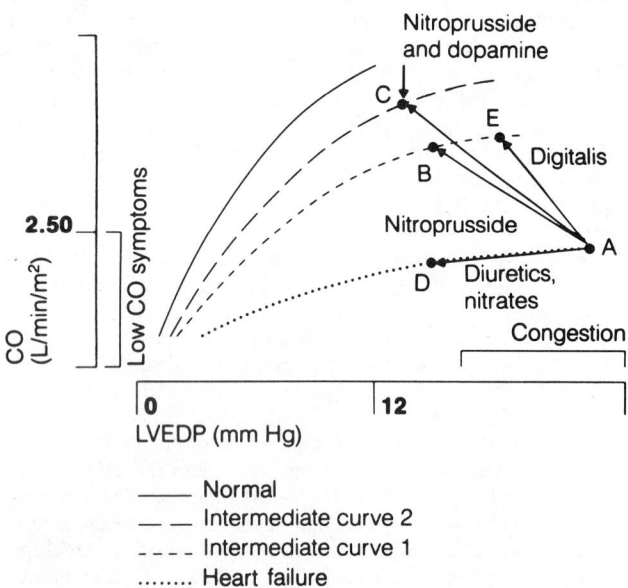

Fig. 45-10. Cardiac performance with preload reduction, afterload reduction, and inotropic support. LVEDP = left ventricular end-diastolic pressure.

Dopamine is an extremely useful inotropic agent, its effects depending on the dose delivered. Lower doses (<5 μg/kg/min) improve renal and mesenteric perfusion, and medium-range doses (5–10 μg/kg/min) exert the additional effect of improving contractility. Higher doses have both effects and also produce peripheral vasoconstriction. Dobutamine, in contrast, has no direct effect on the peripheral vasculature. A beta-adrenergic agonist, dobutamine improves myocardial contractility and, to a degree, lowers peripheral vascular resistance secondarily by decreasing the stimulus for vasoconstriction. It is considered less arrhythmogenic than dopamine and therefore may be somewhat better tolerated if inotropic stimulation is the goal of therapy. If a peripheral vasoconstrictor is also needed, however, dopamine may be a better choice.

In addition to agents such as dopamine and dobutamine that stimulate the production of intracellular cyclic AMP via beta-adrenergic stimulation, phosphodiesterase inhibitors, such as milrinone and amrinone, can be used to increase intracellular cyclic AMP by reducing its metabolism, and thereby improve contractility and vasodilatation. Since the beta-adrenergic agonists and phosphodiesterase inhibitors act via different pathways, their beneficial effects are additive (see also Chap. 210).

Table 45-2 lists the vasodilating agents used in preload and afterload reduction therapy. Nitroglycerin is predominantly a venous vasodilator and is most effective for lowering pulmonary artery wedge pressure. Hydralazine, an arterial vasodilator, is most helpful for reducing afterload and improving cardiac output. Drugs such as nitroprusside and angiotensin-converting enzyme (ACE) inhibitors, as well as combination regimens such as hydralazine plus isosorbide dinitrate, are balanced vasodilators and act by both decreasing wedge pressure and improving cardiac output.

High-risk patients with cardiogenic shock may require insertion of an intraaortic balloon counterpulsation pump as an adjunct in the treatment of severe systolic dysfunction (see Chap. 9). Early studies of intraaortic balloon pumps failed to show improvement in mortality [82], but more recent series suggest that intraaortic balloon counterpulsation is of benefit [83].

Table 45-2. Major Actions of Vasodilating Agents Used in Preload and Afterload Reduction

	Major sites of Action	Chief hemodynamic effects		
		↓ PAW	↑ CO	↓ BP
Intravenous				
Sodium nitroprusside	A + V	+ +	+ +	+
Nitroglycerin	V	+ + +	+	+
Oral				
Isosorbide dinitrate (ISO)	V	+ + +	+	+
Hydralazine or nifedepine	A	±	+ +	+
ISO + hydralazine	A + V	+ +	+ +	+
Captopril	A + V	+ +	+ +	+

A = arterioles; V = veins; PAW = pulmonary artery wedge pressure; CO = cardiac output; HR = heart rate; BP = systemic blood pressure.

More important in the treatment of patients with cardiogenic shock is angioplasty, to achieve reperfusion of the infarct-related artery. In a large series from Duke [83], the strongest predictor of in-hospital mortality was infarct-related artery patency. The mortality rate was 75 percent for those with a closed artery compared to 33 percent for those with an open artery (p < 0.01). Several other series have demonstrated a relatively good prognosis in patients treated with acute angioplasty [84,85,86]. Thus, an aggressive approach with emergent angioplasty (or coronary artery bypass surgery) is indicated in these patients if feasible (see Chap. 46).

The use of thrombolytic therapy in patients with cardiogenic shock has been debated [87]. Despite some limitations, overall mortality appears to be better in patients receiving thrombolysis. Although revascularization appears to be the best management strategy, when not available, thrombolysis is a reasonable alternative.

Echocardiography in Managing Congestive Heart Failure

Echocardiography can provide important information for the management of acute MI complicated by congestive heart failure, including the location and size of the infarct, global and regional systolic and diastolic function, presence of concomitant valvular disease or mural thrombus, and disruption of cardiac structures (see below). In the patient with hypotension, the diagnosis of systolic dysfunction versus hypovolemia can be corroborated accurately and quickly. Early assessment of left ventricular function by noninvasive means is invaluable early in an acute infarct to guide management and identify complications. Because most patients with MI experience some improvement in myocardial function as the "stunned," but not infarcted, myocardium recovers, repeat echocardiogram is generally indicated prior to discharge for more accurate assessment of long-term risk and tailoring of medical therapy (e.g., the need for anticoagulation or ACE inhibitors) [10].

Left Ventricular Dilatation and Remodeling After Myocardial Infarction

Following acute MI there are often changes in left ventricular size and shape that may occur either acutely or insidiously and

progressively and which have an important influence on subsequent prognosis. Infarct "expansion" is an acute process consisting of dilatation and thinning of the infarcted segment occurring in the first few days following acute MI [88]. The expansion consists of an abrupt slippage of myocardial fibers, leading to a change in the architecture of the ventricular chamber that may be associated with chest pain, new S–T segment changes, and hemodynamic disturbances [88]. This event may be difficult to distinguish from an infarct extension (or reinfarction), except that there is not reelevation of cardiac enzymes associated with infarct expansion [19]. Infarct expansion occurs in the setting of transmural MI, especially in an anterior location, and is correlated with the size of the MI [88]. This process adversely affects prognosis and is associated with increased mortality and incidence of heart failure and ventricular aneurysm. Therapy is directed at optimizing hemodynamic disturbances that may have occurred as a consequence of altered ventricular shape and size (see above).

Left ventricular dilatation and remodeling after MI is a more insidious and progressive process that begins shortly after acute MI and continues over the following weeks and months [89,90] (Fig. 45-11). A vicious cycle develops that may culminate in congestive heart failure and, ultimately, death. Following a discrete insult of loss of myocardial tissue from the MI, the left ventricle dilates according to the Starling mechanism in an effort to increase forward cardiac output. The ventricle becomes enlarged and more spheric than ellipsoid, and wall stress consequently increases. The increased wall stresses lead to more ventricular enlargement in an effort to improve pump function. This progressive enlargement continues to lead to progressive dysfunction, and ultimately manifestations of congestive heart failure may develop [91]. This process occurs primarily in large, anterior infarcts [73,89].

This vicious cycle can be interrupted by therapies that reduce wall stress on the left ventricle by reducing both afterload and preload. Ventricular dilatation after MI has been attenuated by early treatment with intravenous nitroglycerin [92] or ACE inhibitors [57,58,93,94,95]. While intravenous nitroglycerin was shown to improve survival in small trials in the prethrombolytic era [94], GISSI-3 trial failed to show any benefit on mortality of intravenous followed by oral nitroglycerin [58]. On the other hand, ACE inhibitors have been shown to improve survival. In the SAVE study, MI patients with an ejection fraction of 40 percent or less but without overt congestive heart failure experienced a 19 percent improvement in survival when captopril was started 3 to 16 days after MI [93] (Fig. 45-12). Captopril prevented the development and consequences of congestive heart failure and also appeared to reduce reinfarction. Of note, these benefits of captopril occurred *in addition to* the benefits of aspirin, beta blockade, and thrombolysis. The AIRE study confirmed these findings in acute MI patients who manifested signs of congestive heart failure [94]. Preliminary results from the ISIS-4, GISSI-3, and Chinese studies demonstrated a small but significant improvement in survival from ACE inhibitors in an unselected population of acute MI patients [57,58,95]. These trials estimated that five lives per 1000 patients treated would be saved [57,58,95]. However, in patients with anterior MI, approximately 10 lives per 1000 patients treated were saved with early ACE inhibition, and only 1 life per 1000 patients with inferior MI [57,58,95]. All of these studies noted, however, that patients with a systolic blood pressure of 100 mm Hg or less did not benefit from ACE inhibitors.

At present, ACE inhibition is clearly indicated in MI patients with evidence of congestive heart failure or with an ejection fraction of 40 percent or less. Therapy can be started several days after MI. In the acute MI setting, ACE inhibitors are indicated on the first day of MI for hypertensive patients, those with

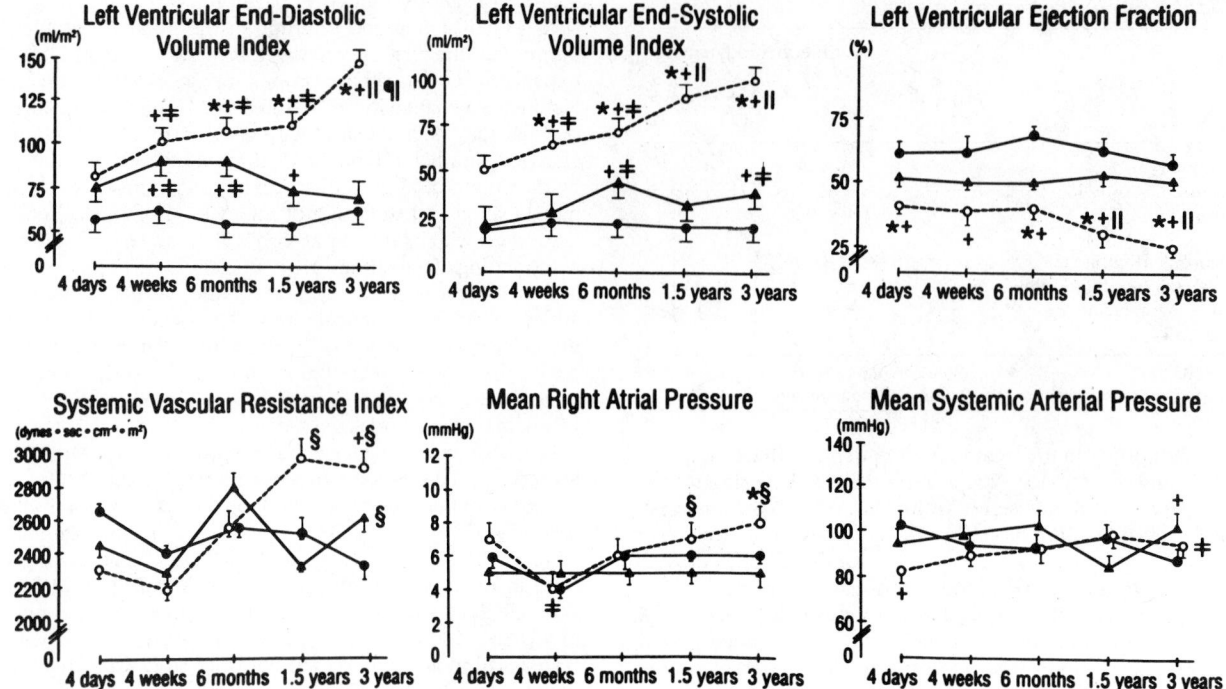

Fig. 45-11. The course of left ventricular end-diastolic and end-systolic volume indices, ejection fraction, systemic vascular resistance index, and mean right atrial and systemic arterial pressures in patients with progressive (O), limited (▲), and no (●) left ventricular dilatation from 4 days to 3 years after myocardial infarction. Values are given as mean ± SEM; p<0.05, * vs. limited dilatation; † vs. no dilatation; ‡ vs. 4 days, § vs. 4 weeks, ¶ vs. 4 days, 4 weeks, and 6 months; ‖ vs. 1.5 years. (From Gaudron P, et al: Progressive left ventricular dysfunction and remodelling after myocardial infarction: Potential mechanism and early prediators. *Circulation* 87:755, 1993. With permission. Copyright 1993 American Heart Association.)

congestive heart failure and on left ventricle dysfunction, and patients with anterior MI (provided that systolic pressure is >100 mm Hg). They may be indicated in all acute MI patients, but final recommendations await review of the full, published results of the large trials and results from current, ongoing trials (see Chap. 210).

LEFT VENTRICULAR ANEURYSM. At the extreme end of the spectrum of left ventricular dilation is the development of a true aneurysm, a bulging saccular structure emanating from the left ventricular cavity and composed of myocardial tissue. While mild degrees of infarct zone expansion can be seen in 8 to 10 percent of patients [96], significant aneurysms are more rare. An aneurysm is characterized by persistent S–T segment elevation in the infarct zone and may be asymptomatic or associated with angina, arrhythmias, or congestive heart failure. Diagnosis is made by echocardiography or left ventriculography. Surgical resection of an aneurysm is rarely performed in the absence of a revascularization procedure and is usually reserved for large aneurysms and those associated with refractory symptoms. Medical treatment consists of routine care for patients with poor left ventricular function (i.e., ACE inhibition, digitalis, etc.) and anticoagulation if there is a severe wall mo-

tion abnormality or ejection fraction less than 30 percent (see Chap. 42).

Disruption of Cardiac Structures

Rupture of the myocardial wall is one of the most serious complications following acute MI. Rupture can occur in the free wall, the intraventricular septum, or a papillary muscle (Fig. 45-13) (Table 45-3). Free wall rupture occurs in approximately 10 percent of patients who die of acute MI; those at highest risk are women, acutely hypertensive patients, and those with large infarctions [97]. Dilation and expansion of necrotic myocardium appears to be the substrate for rupture [98], which is frequently a serpiginous dissection through the myocardium [97]. Rupture usually occurs 3 to 5 days after MI but may occur earlier in patients treated with thrombolytic therapy.

The clinical presentation of patients with free wall rupture can range from sudden electromechanical dissociation and death to congestive heart failure. Frequently patients develop hypotension with evidence of poor peripheral perfusion, jugular venous distension, a pulsus paradoxus, and distant heart sounds. Diagnosis is made by emergent echocardiography or pericardiocentesis, which may temporarily relieve the hemopericardium and improve hemodynamics. In some cases, leaking of blood into the pericardium is only gradual or episodic, leading to the development of a small hemopericardium or a pseudoaneurysm, in which the pericardium and organized clot act as the retaining structure for blood. The prognosis is grave in cases of free wall rupture, although emergent surgical repair can be successful [99].

Ventricular septal rupture is less common than free wall rupture, and the clinical presentation is frequently less acute, al-

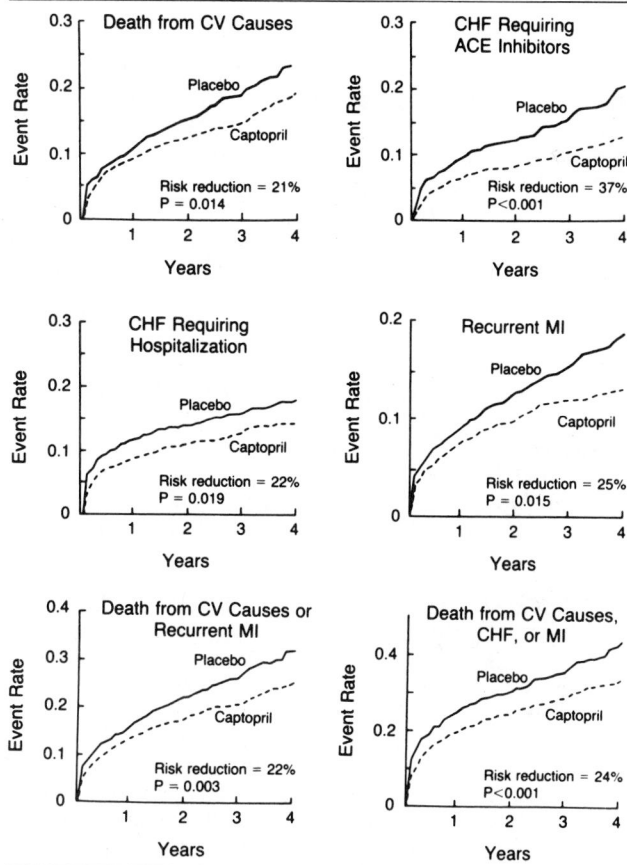

Fig. 45-12. Life tables for cumulative fatal and nonfatal cardiovascular events in the SAVE trial. (From Pfeffer MA, et al: Effect of captopril on mortality and morbidity in patients with left ventricular dysfunction after myocardial infarction: Results of the survival and ventricular enlargement trial. *N Engl J Med* 327:669, 1992. Reproduced by permission.)

lowing for more careful consideration of surgical therapy. Rupture can occur in two regions of the septum: in the midapex in anterior infarctions and in the inferobasal region in inferior infarctions. The clinical presentation of septal rupture is frequently characterized by new-onset congestive heart failure associated with the development of a new, harsh systolic murmur (Table 45-3). Diagnosis can be made by careful Doppler echocardiographic study or detection of an oxygen saturation step-up between the right atrium and right ventricle or pulmonary artery during right heart catheterization. The prognosis is related to the size and site of the rupture.

Ventricular septal rupture occurring in the setting of an inferior MI is associated with a mortality of approximately 75 percent and rupture following an anterior MI approximately 35 percent [100]. Acute treatment involves inotropic support with dopamine or dobutamine in combination with afterload reduction with intravenous nitroglycerin, nitroprusside, and an intraaortic balloon pump. Surgical repair should be performed as quickly as possible to avoid the multisystem complications that result from prolonged medical and intraaortic balloon pump management. There have been isolated reports of transcatheter placement of umbrella-shaped devices to reduce the shunt across the septal defect in critically ill, inoperable patients [101].

The papillary muscle is the cardiac structure that ruptures

least frequently (Table 45-3). This event is often associated with very high early mortality, because of the large volume load imposed on a compromised left ventricle that is incapable of adequate compensation [102]. Papillary muscle rupture occurs more frequently in inferior MIs involving the posteromedial papillary muscle, and the infarct may be nontransmural. Patients with partial rupture present with congestive heart failure and a harsh mitral regurgitation murmur [102]. Treatment is similar to that for ventricular septal rupture and involves inotropic support, afterload reduction, and early surgical repair (usually valve replacement) [99].

Severe papillary muscle ischemic dysfunction may occur without frank anatomic rupture. If the dysfunctional papillary muscle is only "stunned," then mitral valve function may become competent after a number of days. In permanent dysfunction due to infarction, however, valve replacement may become necessary.

The differential diagnosis between ventricular septal rupture and ruptured papillary muscle can generally be readily made by physical examination and echocardiography (Table 45-3). Diagnosis can also be made using a pulmonary artery catheter: ventricular septal rupture is identified by a marked step-up in oxygen saturation from the right atrium to the right ventricle and pulmonary artery, and ruptured papillary muscle is associated with marked V waves in the pulmonary capillary wedge tracing (Fig. 45-14).

Thromboembolism

Thromboembolism is a recognized complication of acute MI, occurring in 5 to 10 percent of patients. Both arterial and venous emboli can occur, with left ventricular mural thrombi accounting for most arterial emboli and right ventricular or deep venous thrombi leading to pulmonary emboli.

The development of mural thrombi in patients with acute MI is common, occurring in up to 20 percent of patients, especially those with large anterior infarctions [103]. Thrombi tend to form in areas of stagnant blood flow and are usually adherent to infarcted areas of myocardium. Diagnosis is usually made by echocardiography, whether routine or following thromboembolism. The incidence of arterial embolism from a documented mural thrombus is in the range of 5 percent [104], and it usually occurs within 4 months after MI. Anticoagulants appear to decrease mural thrombi and thromboembolic events [103,104,105]; their use is recommended for 3 to 6 months if a mural thrombus is found on echocardiogram (see Chaps. 60 and 121).

Pericarditis

Pericardial irritation occurs in approximately one-fourth of patients with acute MI and usually begins 2 to 4 days following MI [1]. It may present as an asymptomatic pericardial effusion, early symptomatic pericarditis with or without effusion, or late pericarditis [106]. Pericardial irritation is more common in larger infarcts, notably Q wave infarcts [107]. In patients with an asymptomatic effusion no treatment is necessary; the effusion usually resorbs within 1 to 3 months [1]. Early pericarditis occurs 2 days to 6 weeks after MI. Patients present with chest pain, usually pleuritic in nature but sometimes difficult to discriminate from ischemic pain. Classically, pain improves when the patient sits up and is worse when lying down [108]. Effusions

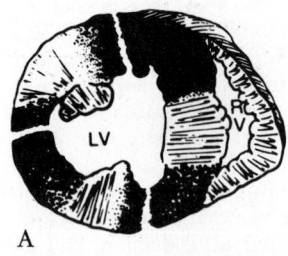 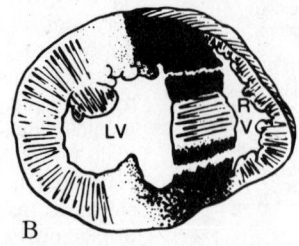 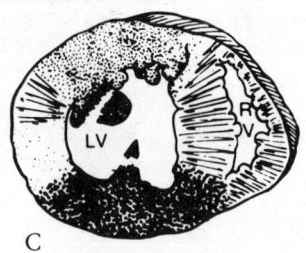

Fig. 45-13. Sites of rupture of cardiac structures after myocardial infarction. *A,* Rupture of left ventricular free wall; *B,* rupture of interventricular septum; *C,* rupture of papillary muscle. LV = left ventricle; RV = right ventricle. (From Vlodaver Z, Edwards JE: Rupture of ventricular septum or papillary muscle complicating myocardial infarction. *Circulation* 55:815, 1977. With permission. Copyright 1977 American Heart Association.)

can be seen, but their absence does not exclude pericarditis. Aspirin is given to relieve pain and decrease inflammation, up to 650 mg every 4 hours and decreasing as symptoms permit. Other nonsteroidal antiinflammatory medications relieve pain but may lead to infarct thinning [109] and thus should be avoided. In severe cases the use of anticoagulants is relatively contraindicated, since they may lead to the development of a hemorrhagic effusion. Cardiac tamponade is rare but can occur in patients with hemorrhagic effusions [110] (see Chap. 34).

Dressler's syndrome, or postmyocardial infarction syndrome [111], occurs 2 weeks to 3 months after MI. It is thought to be mediated by an immune mechanism. Treatment is the same as for early pericarditis, although in severe cases steroids are sometimes needed.

Electrical Disturbances

Cardiac arrhythmias are an important complication during acute MI. In the prehospital phase, ventricular tachycardia and fibrillation probably account for the majority of sudden deaths.

Tachyarrhythmias and bradyarrhythmias are seen in the phase of in-hospital MI. Arrhythmias in the setting of acute MI may be due to reentry, abnormal automaticity, or conduction block; these mechanisms are modulated by ischemia, left ventricular failure, and variations in autonomic tone. Table 45-4 outlines the treatment objectives as well as therapeutic options for the various arrhythmias [112] (see also Chaps. 41 and 49).

VENTRICULAR ARRHYTHMIAS DURING ACUTE MYOCARDIAL INFARCTION. The metabolic milieu accompanying acute infarction predisposes to arrhythmogenesis; the rapid movement of intracellular potassium out of cells and subsequent membrane depolarization may be the predominant factor [113]. In addition, increased sympathetic tone can trigger both ventricular and supraventricular tachyarrhythmias; high parasympathetic tone appears to protect from ventricular tachyarrhythmias but can cause bradycardia and atrioventricular block.

Early ventricular arrhythmias probably result from reentry arising in the region of infarction. Beginning 6 hours into the infarct and continuing for approximately 48 hours, Purkinje fibers in the infarct zone may develop abnormal automaticity [113]. This period of electrical instability provides the rationale for continuous electrocardiographic monitoring during the first 48 hours of acute MI. Ventricular arrhythmias occurring more than 48 hours into the infarct may reflect the development of a scar, the anatomic substrate for recurrent ventricular arrhythmias after hospital discharge.

Table 45-3. Clinical Profile of Mechanical Complications of Acute MI

Variable	Ventricular septal defect	Free wall rupture	Papillary muscle rupture
Age (mean, years)	63	69	65
Days post-MI	3–5	3–5	3–5
Anterior MI	66%	50%	25%
New murmur	90%	25%	50%
Palpable thrill	Yes	No	Rare
Previous MI	25%	25%	30%
Echocardiographic findings			
2-D	Visualize defect may have pericardial—effusion		Flail or prolapsing leaflet
Doppler	Detect shunt	—	Regurgitant jet in LA
PA catheterization	Oxygen step-up in RV	Equalization of diastolic	Prominent V wave in PCW pressure tracing
Incidence	2–4%	≤ 10%	1%
Mortality			
Medical	90%	90%	90%
Surgical	50%	Case reports	40–90%

MI = myocardial infarction; VSD = ventricular septal defect; 2-D = two dimensional; LA = left atrium; PA = pulmonary artery; RV = right ventricle; PCW = pulmonary capillary wedge.
Source: Pasternak RC, Braunwald E, Sobel BE: Acute myocardial infarction, in Braunwald E (ed): *Heart Disease.* 4th ed. Philadelphia, WB Saunders, 1992, p 1257; and Labovitz AJ, et al: Mechanical complications of acute myocardial infarction. *Cardiovasc Rev Rep* 5:948, 1984. With permission.

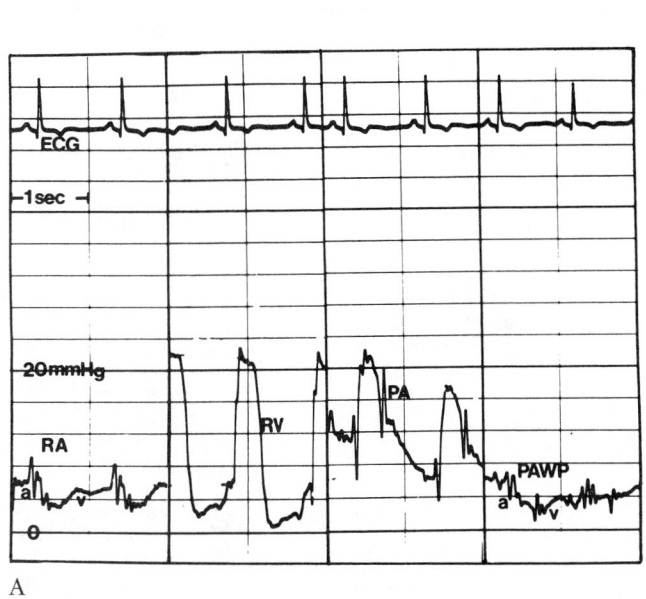

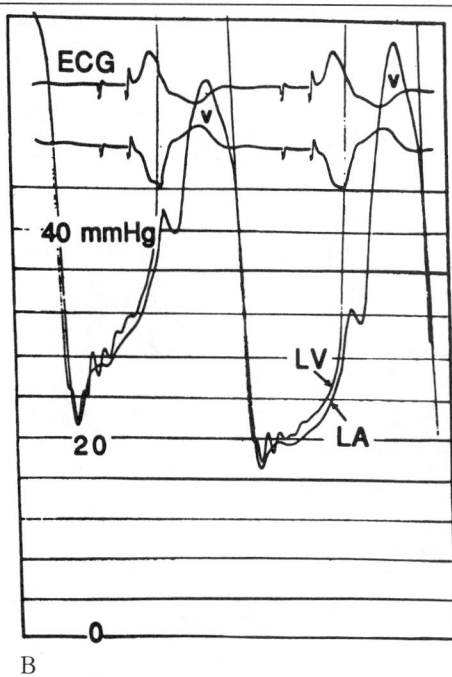

Fig. 45-14. A. Right heart catheterization tracings from a normal patient. B. Left atrial pressure tracing from a patient with mitral regurgitation. Note the elevated pressure, with a marked V wave, indicating the presence of severe mitral regurgitation. (Courtesy of Dr. John A. Bittl.)

Ventricular Fibrillation

INCIDENCE AND PROGNOSIS. Ventricular fibrillation (VF), the cause of most prehospital deaths in acute MI, remains a serious in-hospital complication. It occurs most frequently in the first few hours of an acute MI; the incidence drops sharply thereafter [114]. Secondary VF, in contrast to primary VF, occurs in the setting of significant congestive heart failure or cardiogenic shock. The likelihood of VF increases with the extent of infarction; it is rare in non-Q wave MI. In GISSI-1, the incidences of primary and secondary VF were 2.8 percent [115] and 2.7 percent [116], respectively; patients receiving streptokinase had less secondary but as much primary VF as did control patients. Moreover, the incidence of primary ventricular fibrillation appears to have decreased over the last 20 years [117].

Although primary VF has historically been considered a transient event without prognostic significance, recent studies have documented a significantly higher in-hospital mortality (up to 18%) in acute MI patients who are resuscitated from VF [115,118]. It remains uncertain, however, whether VF directly causes or is simply a marker of poor outcome. Secondary VF occurring in the setting of congestive heart failure or cardiogenic shock is associated with an extremely poor prognosis [116,119]. Of note, patients who sustain primary or secondary VF and survive to hospital discharge have the same long-term prognosis as patients who do not experience VF [120,121].

PROPHYLAXIS. For years, lidocaine has been used prophylactically in acute MI patients to prevent primary VF [122]. While intravenous lidocaine reduces the incidence of VF by about one-third, an *increased* mortality in lidocaine-treated patients has been observed in meta-analyses [123,124]. This excess mor-

tality may be related to an increased incidence of bradyarrhythmias and heart failure. "Warning arrhythmias" (frequent ventricular premature beats [VPBs], R on T VPBs, multifocal VPBs, ventricular couplets, or short runs of VT) do not reliably predict the later occurrence of VF [125]. Thus, selective prophylaxis of patients who manifest such ventricular ectopy has not been an effective strategy [126]. Prophylactic lidocaine, therefore, should not be used routinely in acute MI [127].

Many randomized studies have documented that early intravenous beta-blockers reduce mortality in acute MI [128]. Part of this benefit is due to prevention of VF. Several beta-blockers have been tested, including propranolol [129], metoprolol [130], and atenolol [49]. The beneficial effects of intravenous beta blockers are greatest when given early [48] and appear also to occur in patients treated with concomitant thrombolysis [11]. Because of the improvements in ventricular arrhythmias, recurrent ischemia, reinfarction, and mortality, early administration of intravenous followed by oral beta-blockers in acute MI patients is strongly recommended in the absence of contraindications (significant bradycardia, hypotension, advanced atrioventricular block, history of bronchospasm, severe left ventricular systolic dysfunction, or pulmonary edema).

Hypokalemia during acute MI has been associated with increased frequency of VF [131], ventricular tachycardia [132], and cardiac arrest [120]. Aggressive potassium repletion to greater than 4.0 mEq per liter is therefore recommended in patients with acute MI. High doses of magnesium sulfate have not been documented to reduce mortality or incidence of VF [57], but repletion to greater than 2.0 mEq per liter is reasonable in hypomagnesemic patients.

Although animal studies raised concern, a high incidence of VF has not been noted in patients treated with thrombolytic agents. In fact, the GISSI-1 [16] and ISIS-2 [15] megatrials, as well as a recent meta-analysis [133], showed a slightly lower incidence of VF in patients receiving thrombolytic therapy. So-called "reperfusion arrhythmias" (i.e., low-grade ventricular ec-

Table 45-4. Arrhythmias during Acute Myocardial Infarction

Category	Arrhythmia	Objective of therapy	Therapeutic options
Ventricular tachyarrhythmias	Ventricular fibrillation	Urgent reversion to sinus rhythm	Defibrillation; lidocaine; bretylium
	Ventricular tachycardia	Restoration of hemodynamic stability	Cardioversion/defibrillation; lidocaine; procainamide; bretylium
	Accelerated idioventricular rhythm	Observation unless hemodynamic compromise	Atropine; atrial pacing
	Ventricular premature beats	None	Observation
Supraventricular tachyarrhythmias	Sinus tachycardia	Reduce heart rate to diminish myocardial work/oxygen demand	Identify and treat underlying cause; beta-blockers
	Atrial fibrillation/flutter	Reduce ventricular rate; restore sinus rhythm	Cardioversion if unstable; beta-blockers, calcium blockers; digoxin; rapid atrial pacing (for flutter); consider antiarrhythmic therapy
	Paroxysmal supraventricular tachycardia	Reduce ventricular rate; restore sinus rhythm	Vagal maneuvers; adenosine; beta-blockers, calcium blockers; cardioversion if unstable
	Nonparoxysmal junctional tachycardia	Search for precipitating cause (e.g., digitalis toxicity); observation unless hemodynamic compromise	Consider overdrive atrial pacing; consider suppressive antiarrhythmic therapy
Bradyarrhythmias and conduction disturbances	Sinus bradycardia	Increase heart rate only if hemodynamic compromise	Atropine; temporary pacing
	Junctional escape rhythm	Increase heart rate only if hemodynamic compromise	Atropine; temporary pacing
	Atrioventricular block or intraventricular conduction block	Increase heart rate; prophylax against progression to high grade A-V block	Atropine; aminophylline; ventricular pacing

Source: Ganz LI, Antman EM: Cardiac arrhythmias during acute myocardial infarction, in Antman EM, Rutherford JD (eds): *Coronary Care Medicine: A Practical Approach.* 2nd ed. Boston, Martinus Nijhoff, in press. Reprinted by permission of Kluwer Academic Publishers.

topy and accelerated idioventricular rhythms) are more common after thrombolytic therapy, perhaps relating to improved infarct-related artery perfusion.

In summary, early intravenous beta blockade and potassium repletion reduces the risk of VF in patients with acute MI. Lidocaine prophylaxis is not recommended but is indicated following an episode of VF or significant ventricular tachycardia (see below). Patients should have continuous electrocardiographic monitoring for at least 48 hours in uncomplicated acute MI and longer if complications occur. Finally, a plan for prompt defibrillation, if necessary, is vital to the management of acute MI patients.

TREATMENT. Treatment of VF requires a prompt resuscitation effort, beginning with immediate electrical defibrillation with an unsynchronized discharge of 200 joules; up to 360 joules should be used if initial efforts are unsuccessful [134] (see Chap. 6). Successfully resuscitated patients with primary VF should receive a bolus and then a continuous infusion of lidocaine. If no further arrhythmias or complications occur, lidocaine can usually be tapered after 24 hours. Further evaluation should be considered for patients with VF occurring late after MI (see Chap. 48). Lidocaine toxicity, common in elderly patients and those with hepatic or left ventricular dysfunction, is manifested by lethargy, confusion, slurred speech, and seizures. Thus, serum lidocaine levels and clinical status should be carefully mon-

itored. Careful attention should also be paid to metabolic and hemodynamic derangements that may have precipitated the VF. Patients with recurrent VF despite lidocaine therapy should be treated with bretylium tosylate [135].

Ventricular Tachycardia

INCIDENCE AND PROGNOSIS. Because of the potential for hemodynamic collapse and degeneration to VF, ventricular tachycardia (VT) is a potentially life-threatening complication of acute MI. Ventricular tachycardia has been defined as three or more consecutive ventricular beats at a rate greater than 100. With this broad definition, the incidence of VT ranges from 10 to 30 percent [1,136]. Thrombolytic therapy seems to increase the incidence of VT defined as such [133], but much of this VT is likely low-grade ectopy of no clinical significance. Ventricular ectopy in the first 24 hours is frequently benign [1], but late ventricular ectopy is associated with (though not necessarily causative of) increased late mortality [7,137]. *Sustained* VT, lasting more than 30 seconds or causing hemodynamic collapse, is much less common. In the SPRINT trial, less than 1.0 percent of patients had sustained primary VT, but those who did had a substantially higher in-hospital cardiac mortality than patients with nonsustained or no VT [138].

TREATMENT. Acute management of sustained VT depends on the patient's hemodynamic status. For unstable patients, immediate countershock is necessary. If no pulse is present, VT should be treated like VF, with an unsynchronized discharge of 200 joules as quickly as possible. If a pulse is present but the episode is accompanied by hypotension, ischemia, or significant heart failure, urgent synchronized cardioversion should be performed. Because VT often responds to low energies, a chest thump (which delivers approximately 1 joule) may be administered as the paddles are being prepared. Monomorphic VT may revert with 25 joules, but higher energies may be used as needed. If synchronization is impossible or delayed, an unsynchronized defibrillatory discharge should be used. After successful resuscitation from VT, patients should receive lidocaine as for VF. Procainamide may be used if VT recurs on lidocaine.

Hemodynamically tolerated VT should be initially treated with intravenous lidocaine or procainamide. If pharmacologic therapy fails, low-energy synchronized cardioversion should be performed. Refractory or recurrent cases of VT may respond to intravenous bretylium tosylate. As with VF, a diligent search should be made for hemodynamic and metabolic precipitants to the VT.

Short salvos of nonsustained VT do not require specific therapy. Longer episodes, however, can cause transient hemodynamic compromise and symptoms. In addition, the rapid heart rate increases myocardial oxygen demand. It is thus reasonable to use lidocaine to try to suppress relatively long runs of nonsustained VT.

Polymorphic VT is an occasional complication of acute MI. Unlike *Torsades de pointes,* these episodes tend not to be associated with a long Q–T interval but rather are generally preceded by electrocardiographic signs and symptoms of myocardial ischemia [139]. Sustained episodes should be treated with electrical countershock. Antiarrhythmic agents are unreliable in suppressing this arrhythmia. As ischemia seems to be the trigger, myocardial revascularization seems to provide the most definitive therapy [139].

Late VT (>48 hours postinfarction) frequently reflects the presence of a scar from which recurrent ventricular arrhythmias may originate. An invasive electrophysiologic evaluation may be helpful in such patients [140] (see Chap. 48).

Accelerated Idioventricular Rhythm and Ventricular Premature Beats.
Accelerated idioventricular rhythm (AIVR), or slow VT, is a ventricular rhythm occurring at 60 to 100 beats per minute. Often, AIVR occurs as an escape rhythm in the setting of sinus bradycardia; however, earlier in the infarct abnormal automaticity in the Purkinje fibers can give rise to AIVR. Usually nonsustained and well tolerated, AIVR is of uncertain prognostic significance; clear links to VF and sustained VT have not been demonstrated [112]. While AIVR frequently accompanies reperfusion after thrombolytic therapy, careful studies suggest it is not a reliable marker [141].

Ventricular premature beats occur frequently during acute MI and appear to be of no prognostic significance. Suppression of VPBs with class I antiarrhythmic agents following MI has been associated with an adverse outcome (see below). Specific treatment of VPBs is therefore not indicated.

Ventricular Arrhythmias Occurring Late after Myocardial Infarction.
Malignant ventricular arrhythmias that occur late in the course of acute MI suggest a high rate of recurrence, but optimal management strategies for these patients remain elusive. Efforts continue to identify patients at high risk for arrhythmia recurrence after MI. While inducible VT during electrophysiologic study predicts a high rate of arrhythmic events [142], such a specialized, invasive study is not a feasible screening test. Several noninvasive tests, including Holter monitoring, heart rate variability, baroreflex sensitivity, and signal-averaged

ECG, in combination with left ventricular ejection fraction may eventually yield a useful noninvasive prediction of risk [112,143].

Although VPBs are associated with an increased mortality after MI, the CAST I and II trials documented that VPB suppression with class I agents worsens survival after MI [144,145]. Other conventional antiarrhythmic agents have also failed to improve outcome after MI [146]. Several randomized trials, however, suggest that amiodarone reduces long-term mortality in MI survivors with asymptomatic ventricular ectopy [146–149]. Several ongoing trials will further evaluate the use of amiodarone in this setting.

At present, indefinite administration of oral beta-blockers, shown to reduce the risk of sudden death in MI survivors [150], is recommended in all patients with no contraindications.

SUPRAVENTRICULAR ARRHYTHMIAS DURING ACUTE MYOCARDIAL INFARCTION.
Supraventricular arrhythmias complicating acute MI are frequently associated with increased sympathetic tone (see Chaps. 41 and 49). Ongoing ischemia, hypoxia, pain, fever, pericarditis, and anxiety all may play a role, and management of these arrhythmias requires careful attention to these issues.

Sinus Tachycardia.
Many factors can cause sinus tachycardia during acute MI. Refractory sinus tachycardia increases myocardial oxygen demand and can therefore lead to infarct extension. If no specific causes can be found and treated, cautious administration of beta-blockers may be helpful in the absence of hypotension or heart failure. Persistent sinus tachycardia without obvious cause generally accompanies large infarcts and is therefore a poor prognostic sign [151].

Atrial Fibrillation and Flutter.
Atrial fibrillation (AF) and flutter (AFL) occur in up to 16 percent of cases of acute MI [152]. Patients who develop AF during acute MI have a higher in-hospital mortality, but this seems entirely attributable to a higher incidence of congestive heart failure [11,153]. Chronic AF, however, does not seem to affect survival during acute MI [154]. In addition to heart failure, atrial infarction, pericarditis, and pulmonary embolus can cause episodes of AF during acute MI. As with VF, early beta blockade reduces the incidence of AF during acute MI [130].

The rapid ventricular rate associated with AF and AFL increases the oxygen demand of the myocardium and reduces the time available for diastolic perfusion of the coronary arteries. In addition, the loss of the atrial contribution to ventricular filling, especially in the setting of an ischemic, noncompliant left ventricle, may compromise cardiac output. For these reasons, AF during acute MI requires prompt treatment; the specific therapy depends on whether hemodynamic compromise accompanies the AF.

Hypotension, heart failure, or angina pectoris mandates urgent synchronized cardioversion; initial energies should be 100 joules for AF and 25 joules for AFL. Higher energies may be used if initial attempts are unsuccessful. Patients with AF who are hemodynamically stable should be treated medically, with initial efforts aimed at controlling the ventricular rate. Beta-blockers are an ideal first-line therapy because of the potential contributions of ischemia and high sympathetic tone in triggering AF. Esmolol, an ultra-short-acting beta-blocker, may be useful when it is unclear whether a beta-blocker will be tolerated. Diltiazem and verapamil, available in both intravenous and oral formulations, are also quite effective. Digoxin may be used but has a delayed onset of action, whereas beta-blockers and calcium channel blockers act promptly at the atrioventricular node.

Antiarrhythmic therapy to convert AF or prevent recurrences during acute MI has not been carefully examined. Class IA-induced proarrhythmia, including *Torsades de pointes* (see Chaps. 35 and 41), may be more common in the setting of acute ischemia [155]. In addition, CAST I and II have raised concern about the safety of type I agents in MI patients. Thus, the potential risks and benefits of antiarrhythmic therapy must be considered in each individual patient. Anticoagulation should also be considered if AF lasts longer than 24 to 48 hours or recurs.

Atrial flutter, a macroreentrant circuit, can frequently be terminated by rapid atrial pacing. A standard temporary bipolar pacing electrode is positioned in the right atrium under either electrocardiographic or fluoroscopic guidance, and an external pulse generator capable of rapid stimulation is used.

Paroxysmal Supraventricular Tachycardia. Regular, narrow-complex paroxysmal supraventricular tachycardia (PSVT) occurs infrequently during acute MI (see Chap. 41). The most common PSVTs are atrioventricular nodal reentrant tachycardia and atrioventricular reentrant tachycardia using an accessory pathway. Vagal maneuvers are frequently effective at terminating episodes [156]. If drug therapy is necessary, adenosine is probably the drug of choice in the non-MI setting [157], but few data exist describing the use of adenosine during the course of acute MI. Intravenous verapamil is very effective but may cause systemic hypotension. Diltiazem and beta-blockers have also been used. In unstable patients, synchronized cardioversion should be considered.

Junctional Rhythms. Like AIVR, a junctional escape rhythm (rate < 60) may emerge at times of sinus node slowing. Relatively common during inferior MI and probably not indicative of poor outcome, a junctional bradycardia should be treated with atropine or temporary pacing only if hemodynamic compromise is present. Accelerated junctional rhythm (rate > 70) called nonparoxysmal junctional tachycardia (NPJT; rate >100) reflect enhanced automaticity of the atrioventricular junction. This arrhythmia is also seen in the setting of digitalis toxicity. In the prethrombolytic era, NPJT accompanied roughly 10 percent of acute MIs [158] and was associated with a poor outcome during anterior but not inferior MI [159]. Similar data are unavailable for patients treated with thrombolytic therapy.

BRADYARRHYTHMIAS AND CONDUCTION DISTURBANCES. The pathophysiology, prognosis, and management of bradyarrhythmias and conduction disturbances during acute MI depend on the blood supply to the specialized conduction system (Table 45-4). In most patients, the sinoatrial and atrioventricular nodes are perfused by branches of the right coronary artery and are therefore affected more commonly in inferior MI, while the bundle branches receive blood from septal branches of the left anterior descending artery and tend to be damaged more in anteroseptal MI. The His bundle receives blood from both the right coronary and left anterior descending arteries [160]. Much of the data regarding bradyarrhythmias and conduction block derive from the era in which aspirin, thrombolytic agents, and beta-blockers were not routinely used. The impact of these therapies on the incidence, prognosis, and management of these dysrhythmias remains unclear.

Sinus Bradycardia. Sinus bradycardia occurs in up to 40 percent of acute MIs and is especially common within the first hours of infarction and in inferior MI [161]. Sinus bradycardia occurs more commonly in patients treated with beta-blockers [150] and streptokinase [162], though a more frequent need for treatment with atropine or temporary pacing has not been noted. The mechanism of bradycardia with or without associated hypotension early during acute MI is likely a manifestation of the Bezold-Jarisch (vasovagal) reflex, which accompanies both ischemia and reperfusion of the inferior wall more than the anterior wall [163]. In addition, sinus node ischemia may occasionally cause sinus bradycardia.

The proper management strategy for sinus bradycardia is a function of the patient's hemodynamic status. Asymptomatic sinus bradycardia without hypotension should be observed. In fact, use of beta blockade to achieve a resting heart rate of 50 to 60 beats per minute may be ideal during acute MI. For more severe asymptomatic sinus bradycardia, beta-blockers should be reduced or withheld.

If sinus bradycardia causes hypotension, angina, or heart failure, small doses of atropine (0.3–0.5 mg) should be given intravenously. Early in the course of infarction, when much of the bradycardia observed is due to heightened vagal tone, atropine is very effective. If sinus bradycardia persists or recurs despite a maximal total dose of atropine (2.0 mg), a temporary transvenous pacemaker should be placed (Table 45-5). Rare cases of atropine-induced VF have been reported [164].

Late sinus bradycardia, occurring more than 6 hours into infarction, is frequently due to sinus node ischemia rather than the Bezold-Jarisch reflex and is therefore less responsive to atropine. In atropine refractory patients, a temporary pacemaker is preferable to the use of isoproterenol, which causes a substantial increase in myocardial oxygen demand.

Atrioventricular Block. Like sinus bradycardia, atrioventricular block occurs more commonly in inferior MI than anterior MI. Significant atrioventricular block has not been documented to occur more frequently in patients treated with beta-blockers or thrombolytic agents.

FIRST-DEGREE AND MOBITZ I (WENKEBACH) SECOND-DEGREE ATRIOVENTRICULAR BLOCK. First-degree and Mobitz I second-degree atrioventricular block occur frequently, especially during inferior MI [165]. The P–R interval should be monitored carefully and beta-blocker therapy reduced or even discontinued if further P–R prolongation occurs. Low-grade atrioventricular block during anterior MI is usually well tolerated and not associated with a poor outcome; occasionally, patients with hypotension respond to atropine.

MOBITZ II SECOND-DEGREE AND THIRD-DEGREE ATRIOVENTRICULAR BLOCK. High-grade atrioventricular block during acute MI can be more ominous. Mobitz II second-degree atrioventricular

Table 45-5. Atrioventricular Block during Acute Myocardial Infarction

	Approximate incidence	Anterior MI	Inferior MI
Sinus bradycardia	40%	Observe[a]	Observe[a]
First-degree A-V block	7–13%	Observe	Observe
Second-degree A-V block—Mobitz I	5–10%		Observe[b]
Second-degree A-V block—Mobitz II	1%	Temporary pacemaker	
Third-degree A-V block	11–13% (IMI) 5% (ASMI)	Temporary pacemaker	Observe[b]

[a] If symptomatic, treat with atropine and temporary pacing if necessary.
[b] If symptomatic, treat with atropine and temporary pacing if necessary. Late A-V block in inferior MI may respond to intravenous aminophylline.
A-V = atrioventricular; MI = myocardial infarction.
Source: Ganz LI, Antman EM: Cardiac arrhythmias during acute myocardial infarction, in Antman EM, Rutherford JD (eds): *Coronary Care Medicine: A Practical Approach.* 2nd ed. Boston, Martinus Nijhoff, in press. Reprinted by permission of Kluwer Academic Publishers.

block is rare, occurring almost exclusively in patients with anterior MI. Complete heart block accompanies 11 to 13 percent of inferior MI and frequently lasts only several hours [119,166]. Inferior MI patients with complete heart block have a higher in-hospital mortality, but the long-term prognosis is unaffected in those who survive to discharge. In anterior MI, complete heart block occurs less frequently but is associated with an extremely high in-hospital mortality [119]. The long-term prognosis of hospital survivors is unaffected, however. For anterior MI and probably inferior MI as well, complete heart block appears to be a marker for extensive infarction, rather than an independent poor prognostic indicator, but this has not been documented definitively. Beta-blockers should be withheld in patients with high-grade atrioventricular block until a temporary pacemaker has been placed (Table 45-5).

The location of infarction dictates the pathophysiology of complete heart block. In inferior MI, block occurs within the atrioventricular node; many patients progress from first-degree to Mobitz I second-degree atrioventricular block prior to the development of complete heart block. The QRS complex is typically narrow, suggesting an escape focus proximal in the specialized conducting system. The escape rhythm is usually fast enough to maintain hemodynamic stability. Early in infarction, such complete heart block is frequently due to the Bezold-Jarisch reflex and responds to atropine. Later in the course of inferior MI, however, atrioventricular nodal ischemia can cause complete heart block; these patients do not usually respond to atropine. Because adenosine may be the cellular mediator, preliminary reports suggest that intravenous aminophylline, an adenosine antagonist, improves such complete heart block [167] (see Table 45-4).

Conversely, in anterior MI, complete heart block usually reflects ischemia or infarction *below* the atrioventricular node in the distal conducting system. The escape complex is generally wide, slow, and poorly responsive to atropine. Complete heart block typically develops in anterior MI patients who have already manifested an intraventricular conduction block (most commonly right bundle branch block) rather than lower-grade atrioventricular block as in inferior MI. Thus, in anterior MI, complete heart block is indicative of extensive infarction, and a temporary pacemaker is needed (see Table 45-5).

Intraventricular Conduction Block. Because of the blood supply to the distal conducting system, intraventricular conduction disturbances frequently accompany anterior MI, reflect large infarctions, and carry a high in-hospital mortality [168,169]. Isolated fascicular block occurs infrequently and rarely progresses to complete heart block. Bundle branch block progresses more frequently, and patients with bifascicular and trifascicular block are at very high risk for development of complete heart block [170,171]. Beta-blockers should be withheld in high-risk patients, pending placement of a temporary pacemaker (Table 45-6).

INDICATIONS FOR PACEMAKER PLACEMENT DURING MYOCARDIAL INFARCTION. Whether a temporary pacemaker is necessary during acute MI is a function of the particular conduction disturbance and its hemodynamic sequelae, as well as the site of infarction (Tables 45-5 and 45-6). For relatively low-risk patients, having a transcutaneous pacing system available may be adequate, though not all patients can be reliably paced in this manner. For pacemaker-dependent patients, however, a transvenous system should be placed. The risks of the procedure, which include right ventricular perforation, infection, vascular complications, and bleeding, should be considered, especially if thrombolytic therapy has already been administered.

Table 45-6. Intraventricular Block during Acute Myocardial Infarction

	Incidence	Progression to CAB	Management
LAHB	3–5%	Low	Observe
LPHB	1–2%	Low	Observe
LBBB	4.5%	13–16%	Observe*
RBBB	2.3%	14–23%	Observe*
1° AVB and LBBB or RBBB		Approx. 20%	Consider temporary pacemaker*
RBBB/LAHB	4.0%	27–34%	Temporary pacemaker
RBBB/LPHB	0.8%	29–31%	Temporary pacemaker
Trifascicular block		38%	Temporary pacemaker
Alternating BBB		44%	Temporary pacemaker

* Optimal management in these patients remains unclear
LAHB = left anterior hemiblock; LPHB = left posterior hemiblock; LBBB = left bundle branch block; RBBB = right bundle branch block; AVB = atrioventricular block.
Source: Ganz LI, Antman EM: Cardiac arrhythmias during acute myocardial infarction, in Antman EM, Rutherford JD (eds): *Coronary Care Medicine: A Practical Approach.* 2nd ed. Boston, Martinus Nijhoff, in press. Reprinted by permission of Kluwer Academic Publishers.

Patients who develop permanent complete (third-dgree) heart block as a result of acute MI should generally receive a permanent pacemaker prior to discharge. Patients with permanent bundle branch block and transient Mobitz II second-degree or third-degree atrioventricular block may benefit from permanent pacemaker implantation, but the lack of randomized data necessitates an individualized approach to each patient.

References

1. Pasternak RC, Braunwald E, Sobel BE. Acute myocardial infarction, in Braunwald E (ed): *Heart Disease.* 4th ed. Philadelphia, WB Saunders, 1992, pp. 1200–1291.
2. DeWood MA, Spores J, Notske R, et al: Prevalence of total coronary occlusion during the early hours of transmural myocardial infarction. *N Engl J Med* 303:897, 1980.
3. Braunwald E: Myocardial reperfusion, limitation of infarct size, reduction of left ventricular dysfunction, and improved survival: Should the paradigm be expanded? *Circulation* 79:441, 1989.
4. Pfeffer MA, Braunwald E: Ventricular remodeling after myocardial infarction: Experimental observations and clinical implications. *Circulation* 81:1161, 1990.
5. Pfeffer MA, Pfeffer JM, Steinberg C, Finn P: Survival after an experimental myocardial infarction: Beneficial effects of long-term therapy with captopril. *Circulation* 72:406, 1985.
6. Multicenter Postinfarction Research Group: Risk stratification and survival after myocardial infarction. *N Engl J Med* 309:331, 1983.
7. Bigger JT Jr, Weld FM, Rolnitzky LM: Prevalence, characteristics and significance of ventricular tachycardia (three or more complexes) detected with ambulatory electrocardiographic recording in the late hospital phase of acute myocardial infarction. *Am J Cardiol* 48:815, 1981.
8. Cannon CP, McCabe CH, Schweiger MJ, et al: Prospective validation of a composite end point for evaluation of new thrombolytic regimens for acute MI: Results from the TIMI 4 trial (abstract). *Circulation* 88:I-60, 1993.
9. Mueller HS, Forman SA, Manegus MA, et al: Prognostic significance of nonfatal reinfarction in TIMI II (abstract). *Circulation* 88:I-490, 1993.
10. Gunnar RM, Bourdillon PDV, Dixon DW, et al: Guidelines for the

early management of patients with acute myocardial infarction: A report of the American College of Cardiology/American Heart Association Task Force on the assessment of diagnostic and therapeutic cardiovascular procedures (Subcommittee to develop guidelines for the early management of patients with acute myocardial infarction). *Circulation* 82:664, 1990.

11. TIMI Study Group: Comparison of invasive and conservative strategies after treatment with intravenous tissue plasminogen activator in acute myocardial infarction. Results of the Thrombolysis in Myocardial Infarction (TIMI) Phase II Trial. *N Engl J Med* 320:618, 1989.

12. The GUSTO Investigators: An international randomized trial comparing four thrombolytic strategies for acute myocardial infarction. *N Engl J Med* 329:673, 1993.

13. Ohman EM, Armstrong PW, Guerci AD, Vahanian A, for the GUSTO Trial Investigators: Reinfarction after thrombolytic therapy: Experience from the GUSTO trial (abstract). *Circulation* 88:I-490, 1993.

14. Maisel AS, Ahnve S, Gilpin E, et al: Prognosis after extension of myocardial infarct: The role of Q wave or non-Q wave infarction. *Circulation* 71:211, 1985.

15. ISIS-2 (Second International Study of Infarct Survival) Collaborative Group: Randomized trial of intravenous streptokinase, oral aspirin, both, or neither among 17,187 cases of suspected acute myocardial infarction: ISIS-2. *Lancet* 2:349, 1988.

16. Gruppo Italiano per lo Studio della Streptochinasi nell'Infarto Miocardico (GISSI): Effectiveness of intravenous thrombolytic treatment in acute myocardial infarction. *Lancet* 1:397, 1986.

17. Rivers JT, White HD, Cross DB, et al: Reinfarction after thrombolytic therapy for acute myocardial infarction followed by conservative management: Incidence and effect of smoking. *J Am Coll Cardiol* 16:340, 1990.

18. Timm TC, Ross R, McKendall GR, et al and the TIMI Investigators: Left ventricular function and early cardiac events as a function of time to treatment with t-PA: A report from TIMI II (abstract). *Circulation* 84:II-230, 1991.

19. Muller JE, Rude RE, Braunwald E, et al: Myocardial infarct extension: Occurrence, outcome, and risk factors in the Multicenter Investigation of Limitation of Infarct Size. *Ann Intern Med* 108:1, 1988.

20. Ohman EM, Califf RM, Topol EJ, et al: Consequences of reocclusion after successful reperfusion therapy in acute myocardial infarction. *Circulation* 82:781, 1990.

21. Simoons ML, Serruys PW, van den Brand M, et al: Improved survival after early thrombolysis in acute myocardial infarction: A randomized trial by the Interuniversity of Cardiology Institute in the Netherlands. *Lancet* 2:578, 1985.

22. Grines CL, Browne KF, Marco J, et al: A comparison of immediate angioplasty with thrombolytic therapy for acute myocardial infarction. *N Engl J Med* 328:673, 1993.

23. Ellis SG, Debowey D, Bates ER, Topol EJ: Treatment of recurrent ischemia after thrombolysis and successful reperfusion for acute myocardial infarction: Effect on in-hospital mortality and left ventricular function. *J Am Coll Cardiol* 17:752, 1991.

24. Willard JE, Lange RA, Hillis LD: The use of aspirin in ischemic heart disease. *N Engl J Med* 327:175, 1992.

25. Klimt CR, Knatterud GL, Stamler J, Meier P, for the PARIS II Investigator Group: Persantine-Aspirin Reinfarction Study. II. Secondary coronary prevention with persantine and aspirin. *J Am Coll Cardiol* 7:251, 1986.

26. Roux S, Christeller S, Ludin E: Effects of aspirin on coronary reocclusion and recurrent ischemia after thrombolysis: A meta-analysis. *J Am Coll Cardiol* 19:671, 1992.

27. Theroux P, Ouimet H, McCans J, et al: Aspirin, heparin or both to treat unstable angina. *N Engl J Med* 319:1105, 1988.

28. Lewis HD, Davis JW, Archibald DG, et al: Protective effects of aspirin against acute myocardial infarction and death in men with unstable angina. *N Engl J Med* 309:396, 1983.

29. Cairns JA, Gent M, Singer J, et al: Aspirin, sulfinpyrazone, or both in unstable angina. *N Engl J Med* 313:1369, 1985.

30. The RISC Group: Risk of myocardial infarction and death during treatment with low dose aspirin and intravenous heparin in men with unstable coronary artery disease. *Lancet* 336:827, 1990.

31. Hsia J, Hamilton WP, Kleiman N, et al: A comparison between heparin and low-dose aspirin as adjunctive therapy with tissue plasminogen activator for acute myocardial infarction. *N Engl J Med* 323:1433, 1990.

32. de Bono DP, Simoons MI, Tijssen J, et al: Effect of early intravenous heparin on coronary patency, infarct size, and bleeding complications after alteplase thrombolysis: Results of a randomized double blind European Cooperative Study Group trial. *Br Heart J* 67:122, 1992.

33. Bleich SD, Nichols T, Schumacher RR, et al: Effect of heparin on coronary patency after thrombolysis with tissue plasminogen activator in acute myocardial infarction. *Am J Cardiol* 66:1412, 1990.

34. Topol EJ, Califf RM, George BS, et al: A randomized trial of immediate versus delayed elective angioplasty after intravenous tissue plasminogen activator in acute myocardial infarction. *N Engl J Med* 317:581, 1987.

35. Hsia J, Kleiman N, Aguirre F, et al: Heparin-induced prolongation of partial thromboplastin time after thrombolysis: Relationship to coronary artery patency. *J Am Coll Cardiol* 20:31, 1992.

36. Arnout J, Simoons M, de Bono D, et al: Correlation between level of heparinization and patency of the infarct-related coronary artery after treatment of acute myocardial infarction with alteplase (rt-PA). *J Am Coll Cardiol* 20:513, 1992.

37. The GUSTO Angiographic Investigators: The comparative effects of tissue plasminogen activator, streptokinase, or both on coronary artery patency, ventricular function and survival after acute myocardial infarction. *N Engl J Med* 329:1615, 1993.

38. Gruppo Italiano per lo Studio della Sopravvivenza nell'Infarto Miocardico: GISSI-2: A factorial randomized trial of alteplase versus streptokinase and heparin versus no heparin among 12,490 patients with acute myocardial infarction. *Lancet* 336:65, 1990.

39. ISIS-3 (Third International Study of Infarct Survival) Collaborative Group: ISIS-3: A randomized comparison of streptokinase vs tissue plasminogen activator vs anistreplase and of aspirin plus heparin vs aspirin alone among 41,299 cases of suspected acute myocardial infarction. *Lancet* 339:753, 1992.

40. Merlini PA, Bauer KA, Oltrona L, et al: Persistent activation of coagulation mechanism in unstable angina and myocardial infarction. *Circulation* 90:61, 1994.

41. Handin RI, Loscalzo J: Hemostasis, thrombosis, fibrinolysis, and cardiovascular disease, in Braunwald E (ed): *Heart Disease*. 4th ed. Philadelphia, WB Saunders, 1992, pp. 1767–1789.

42. Smith P, Arnesen H, Holme I: The effect of warfarin on mortality and reinfarction after myocardial infarction. *N Engl J Med* 323:147, 1990.

43. Fuster V, Badimon L, Badimon JJ, Chesebro JH: The pathophysiology of coronary artery disease and the acute coronary syndromes. *N Engl J Med* 326:242, 1992.

44. The Norwegian Multicenter Study Group: Timolol-induced reduction in mortality and reinfarction in patients surviving acute myocardial infarction. *N Engl J Med* 304:801, 1981.

45. Hjalmarson A, Elmfeldt D, Herlitz J, et al: Effect on mortality of metoprolol in acute myocardial infarction: A double-blind randomized trial. *Lancet* 2:823, 1981.

46. Beta-Blocker Heart Attack Trial Research Group: A randomized trial of propranolol in patients with acute myocardial infarction. 1. Mortality results. *JAMA* 247:1707, 1982.

47. Hjalmarson A, Herlitz J, Holmberg S, et al: The Gotenborg metoprolol trial: Effects on mortality and morbidity in acute myocardial infarction. *Circulation* 67 (suppl I):I-26, 1983.

48. The MIAMI Trial Research Group: Metoprolol in acute myocardial infarction (MIAMI): A randomized placebo-controlled international trial. *Eur Heart J* 6:199, 1985.

49. ISIS-1 (First International Study of Infarct Survival) Collaborative Group: Randomized trial of intravenous atenolol among 16,027 cases of suspected acute myocardial infarction. *Lancet* 2:57, 1986.

50. Hackett D, Davies G, Chierchia S, Maseri A: Intermittent coronary occlusion in acute myocardial infarction: Value of combined thrombolytic and vasodilator therapy. *N Engl J Med* 317:1055, 1987.

51. Barbash GI, Hod H, Roth A, et al: Repeat infusions of recombinant tissue-type plasminogen activator in patients with acute myocardial infarction and early recurrent myocardial ischemia. *J Am Coll Cardiol* 16:779, 1990.

52. Becker RC: Recurrent myocardial ischemia following thrombolytic therapy: Guidelines for practicing clinicians. *Am Heart J* 124:183, 1992.

53. Barbash GI, for the Israeli Investigators: Rescue thrombolysis in reinfarction (abstract). *Circulation* 88(Pt.2):I-491, 1993.
54. The TIMI IIIB Investigators: Effects of tissue plasminogen activator and a comparison of early invasive and conservative strategies in unstable angina and non-Q-wave myocardial infarction: Results of the TIMI IIIB Trial. *Circulation* 89:1545, 1994.
55. DeBusk RF, Blomqvist CG, Kouchoukos NT, et al: Identification and treatment of low-risk patients after acute myocardial infarction and coronary bypass surgery. *N Engl J Med* 314:161, 1986.
56. Ross J Jr, Gilpin EA, Madsen EB, et al: A decision scheme for coronary angiography after acute myocardial infarction. *Circulation* 79:292, 1989.
57. ISIS Collaborative Group: ISIS-4: Randomized study of oral captopril in over 50,000 patients with suspected acute myocardial infarction (abstract). *Circulation* 88(Pt.2):I-394, 1993.
58. Gruppo Italiano per lo Studio della Sopravvivenza nell'Infarto Miocardico. GISSI-3: Effect of lisinopril and transdermal glyceryl trinitrate singly and together on 6-week mortality and ventricular function after acute myocardial infarction. *Lancet* 343:1115, 1994.
59. Gibson RS: Non-Q wave myocardial infarction: Prognosis, changing incidence, and management, in Gersh BJ, Rahimtoola SH (eds): *Acute Myocardial Infarction.* New York, Elsevier, 1991, pp 284–307.
60. Tajer CD, Diaz R, Paolasso EA, Van de Werf F, on behalf of the investigators of the TPA/SK Mortality Trial: Non Q wave myocardial infarction after thrombolytic therapy treatment predicts a high rate of reinfarction and death during follow up (abstract). *Circulation* 88(Pt.2):I-490, 1993.
61. Stone PH, Raabe DS, Jaffe AS, et al: Prognostic significance of location and type of myocardial infarction: Independent adverse outcome associated with anterior location. *J Am Coll Cardiol* 11:453, 1988.
62. Berger CJ, Murabito JM, Evans JC, et al: Prognosis after first myocardial infarction: Comparison of Q wave and non-Q wave myocardial infarction in the Framingham Heart Study. *JAMA* 268:1545, 1992.
63. Gibson RS, Boden WE, Théroux P, et al: Diltiazem and reinfarction in patients with non-Q wave myocardial infarction: Results of a double-blind, randomized, multicenter trial. *N Engl J Med* 315:423, 1986.
64. The Multicenter Diltiazem Postinfarction Trial Research Group: The effect of diltiazem on mortality and reinfarction after myocardial infarction. *N Engl J Med* 319:385, 1988.
65. Wong S-C, Greenberg H, Hager WD, Dwyer EM: Effects of diltiazem on recurrent myocardial infarction in patients with non-Q wave myocardial infarction. *J Am Coll Cardiol* 19:1421, 1992.
66. Muller J, Morrison J, Stone P, et al: Nifedipine therapy for patients with threatened and acute myocardial infarction: A randomized, double blind comparison. *Circulation* 69:740, 1984.
67. Wikstrand J, Warnold I, Olsson G, et al: Primary prevention with metoprolol in patients with hypertension: Mortality results from the MAPHY study. *JAMA* 259:1976, 1988.
68. DeWood MA, Stifter WF, Simpson CS, et al: Coronary arteriographic findings soon after non-Q wave myocardial infarction. *N Engl J Med* 315:417, 1986.
69. The TIMI IIIA Investigators: Early effects of tissue-type plasminogen activator added to conventional therapy on the culprit lesion in patients presenting with ischemic cardiac pain at rest: Results of the Thrombolysis in Myocardial Ischemia (TIMI IIIA) trial. *Circulation* 87:38, 1993.
70. Zehender M, Kasper W, Kauder E, et al: Right ventricular infarction as an independent predictor of prognosis after acute inferior myocardial infarction. *N Engl J Med* 328:981, 1993.
71. Cohn JN, Guiha NH, Broder MI, Limas CJ: Right ventricular infarction: Clinical and hemodynamic features. *Am J Cardiol* 33:209, 1974.
72. Lorell B, Leinbach RC, Pohost GM, et al.: Right ventricular infarction: Clinical diagnosis and differentiation from cardiac tamponade and pericardial constriction. *Am J Cardiol* 43:465, 1979.
73. Braunwald E: The path to myocardial salvage by thrombolytic therapy. *Circulation* 76(suppl II):II-2, 1987.
74. Zaret BL, Wackers FJ, Terrin M, et al: Does left ventricular ejection fraction following thrombolytic therapy have the same prognostic impact described in the prethrombolytic era? Results of the TIMI II trial (abstract). *J Am Coll Cardiol* 17:214A, 1991.
75. Cerqueira MD, Maynard C, Ritchie JL, et al: Long-term survival in 618 patients from the Western Washington Streptokinase in Myocardial Infarction Trials. *J Am Coll Cardiol* 20:1452, 1992.
76. Nicod P, Gilpin E, Dittrich H, et al: Influence on prognosis and morbidity of left ventricular ejection fraction with and without signs of left ventricular failure after acute myocardial infarction. *Am J Cardiol* 61:1165, 1988.
77. Dwyer EM, Greenberg HM, Steinberg G, and the Multicenter Postinfarction Research Group: Clinical characteristics and natural history of survivors of pulmonary congestion during acute myocardial infarction. *Am J Cardiol* 63:1423, 1989.
78. Maynard C, Weaver D, Litwin PE, et al: Hospital mortality in acute myocardial infarction in the era of reperfusion therapy (the Myocardial Infarction Triage and Intervention Project). *Am J Cardiol* 72:877, 1993.
79. Braunwald E, Kloner RA: The stunned myocardium: Prolonged postischemic ventricular dysfunction. *Circulation* 66:1146, 1982.
80. Scott BD, Kerber RE: Clinical and experimental aspects of myocardial stunning. *Prog Cardiovasc Dis* 35:61, 1992.
81. Forrester JS, Diamond G, Chatterjee K, Swan HJC: Medical therapy of acute myocardial infarction by application of hemodynamic subsets (first of two parts). *N Engl J Med* 295:1356, 1976.
82. Scheidt S, Wilner G, Mueller H, et al: Intra-aortic balloon counterpulsation in cardiogenic shock: Report of a co-operative clinical trial. *N Engl J Med* 288:979, 1973.
83. Bengston JR, Kaplan AJ, Pieper KS, et al: Prognosis in cardiogenic shock after acute myocardial infarction in the interventional era. *J Am Coll Cardiol* 20:1482, 1992.
84. Lee L, Bates ER, Pitt B, et al: Percutaneous transluminal coronary angioplasty improves survival in acute myocardial infarction complicated by cardiogenic shock. *Circulation* 78:1345, 1988.
85. Ellis SG, O'Neill WW, Bates ER, et al: Implications for patient triage from survival and left ventricular functional recovery analysis in 500 patients treated with coronary angioplasty for acute myocardial infarction. *J Am Coll Cardiol* 13:1251, 1989.
86. Lee L, Erbel R, Brown TM, et al: Multicenter Registry of Angioplasty Therapy of Cardiogenic Shock: Initial and long-term survival. *J Am Coll Cardiol* 17:599, 1991.
87. Bates ER, Topol EJ: Limitations of thrombolytic therapy for acute myocardial infarction complicated by congestive heart failure and cardiogenic shock. *J Am Coll Cardiol* 18:1077, 1991.
88. Hutchins GM, Bulkley BH: Infarct expansion versus extension: Two different complications of acute myocardial infarction. *Am J Cardiol* 41:1127, 1978.
89. Gaudron P, Eilles C, Kugler I, Ertl G: Progressive left ventricular dysfunction and remodeling after myocardial infarction. *Circulation* 87:755, 1993.
90. Jeremy RW, Allman KC, Bautovitch G, Harris PJ: Patterns of left ventricular dilation during the six months after myocardial infarction. *J Am Coll Cardiol* 13:304, 1989.
91. Pfeffer MA, Pfeffer JM: Ventricular enlargement and reduced survival after myocardial infarction. *Circulation* 75(suppl IV):IV-93, 1987.
92. Jugdutt BI, Warnica JW: Intravenous nitroglycerin therapy to limit myocardial infarct size, expansion, and complications: Effect of timing, dosage, and infarct location. *Circulation* 78:906, 1988.
93. Pfeffer MA, Braunwald E, Moye LA, et al: Effect of captopril on mortality and morbidity in patients with left ventricular dysfunction after myocardial infarction. *N Engl J Med* 327:669, 1992.
94. The Acute Infarction Ramipril Efficacy (AIRE) Study Investigators: Effect of ramipril on mortality and morbidity of survivors of acute myocardial infarction with clinical evidence of heart failure. *Lancet* 342:821, 1993.
95. Liu L, for the Chinese ACE-AMI Trial Collaborative Group: Chinese Infarction-ACE Inhibitor Trial. George Washington University Symposium on Thrombolysis and Interventional Therapy in Acute Myocardial Infarction. Atlanta, November 1993.
96. Abrams DL, Edelist A, Luria MH, Miller AJ: Ventricular aneurysm: A reappraisal based on a study of 65 consecutive autopsied cases. *Circulation* 27:164, 1963.
97. Bates RJ, Beutler S, Resnekov L, Anaguostopoulos CE: Cardiac rupture: Challenges in diagnosis and management. *Am J Cardiol* 40:429, 1977.
98. Schuster EJ, Bulkley BH: Expansion of transmural myocardial in-

farction: A pathophysiologic feature in cardiac rupture. *Circulation* 60:1532, 1979.

99. Bolooki H: Surgical treatment of complications of acute myocardial infarction. *JAMA* 263:1237, 1990.

100. Radford MJ, Johnson RA, Daggett WMJ, et al: Ventricular septal rupture: A review of clinical and physiologic features and an analysis of survival. *Circulation* 64:545, 1981.

101. Lock JE, Block PC, McKay RG, et al: Transcatheter closure of ventricular septal defects. *Circulation* 78:361, 1988.

102. Nishimura RA, Schaff HV, Shub C, et al: Papillary muscle rupture complicating acute myocardial infarction. *Am J Cardiol* 51:373, 1983.

103. Weinreich DJ, Burke JF, Pauletto FJ: Left ventricular mural thrombi complicating acute myocardial infarction: Long-term follow-up with serial echocardiography. *Ann Intern Med* 100:789, 1984.

104. Gueret P, Dubourg O, Ferrier A, et al: Effects of full-dose heparin anticoagulation on the development of left ventricular thrombosis in acute myocardial infarction. *J Am Coll Cardiol* 8:419, 1986.

105. Turpie AGG, Robinson JG, Doyle DJ, et al: Comparison of high-dose with low-dose subcutaneous heparin to prevent left ventricular mural thrombosis in patients with acute transmural anterior myocardial infarction. *N Engl J Med* 320:352, 1989.

106. Pierard LA, Albert A, Henrad L, et al: Incidence and significance of pericardial effusion in acute myocardial infarction as determined by two-dimensional echocardiography. *J Am Coll Cardiol* 8:517, 1986.

107. Sugiura T, Iwasaka T, Takayama Y, et al: Factors associated with pericardial effusion in acute Q wave myocardial infarction. *Circulation* 81:477, 1990.

108. Tofler GH, Muller JE, Stone PH, et al: Pericarditis in acute myocardial infarction: Characterization and clinical significance. *Am Heart J* 117:86, 1989.

109. Brown EJ, Kloner RA, Schoen FJ, et al: Scar thinning due to ibuprofen administration following experimental myocardial infarction. *Am J Cardiol* 51:877, 1983.

110. Guberman BA, Fowler NO, Engel PJ, et al: Cardiac tamponade in medical patients. *Circulation* 64:633, 1981.

111. Dressler W: A post-myocardial-infarction syndrome: Preliminary report of a complication resembling idiopathic recurrent, benign pericarditis. *JAMA* 160:1379, 1956.

112. Ganz LI, Antman EM: Cardiac arrhythmias during acute myocardial infarction, in Antman EM, Rutherford JD (eds): *Coronary Care Medicine: A Practical Approach*. 2nd ed. Boston, Martinus Nijhoff (in press).

113. Weiss JN, Nademanee K, Stevenson WG, Singh B: Ventricular arrhythmias in ischemic heart disease. *Ann Intern Med* 114:784, 1991.

114. Lawrie DM, Higgins MR, Godman MJ, et al: Ventricular fibrillation complicating acute myocardial infarction. *Lancet* 2:523, 1968.

115. Volpi A, Cavalli A, Santoro E, Tognoni G, and GISSI Investigators: In-hospital prognosis of patients with acute myocardial infarction complicated by primary ventricular fibrillation. *N Engl J Med* 317:257, 1987.

116. Volpi A, Cavalli A, Santoro E, Tognoni G, and GISSI Investigators: Incidence and prognosis of secondary ventricular fibrillation in acute myocardial infarction. *Circulation* 82:1279, 1990.

117. Antman EM, Berlin JA: Declining incidence of ventricular fibrillation in myocardial infarction: Implications for prophylactic use of lidocaine. *Circulation* 86:764, 1992.

118. Behar S, Goldbourt U, Reicher-Reiss H, Kaplinsky E, and the Principal Investigators of the SPRINT Study: Prognosis of acute myocardial infarction complicated by primary ventricular fibrillation. *Am J Cardiol* 66:1208, 1990.

119. Behar S, Zissman, E, Zion M, et al: Complete atrioventricular block complicating inferior wall myocardial infarction: Short and long-term prognosis. *Am Heart J* 125:1622, 1993.

120. Tofler GH, Stone PH, Muller JE, et al: Prognosis after cardiac arrest due to ventricular tachycardia or ventricular fibrillation associated acute myocardial infarction. *Am J Cardiol* 60:755, 1987.

121. Volpi A, Cavali A, Franzosi MG, et al: One year prognosis of primary ventricular fibrillation complicating acute myocardial infarction. *Am J Cardiol* 63:1174, 1989.

122. Lie KI, Wellens HJ, van Capelle FJ, Durrer D: Lidocaine in the prevention of primary ventricular fibrillation. *N Engl J Med* 291:1324, 1974.

123. MacMahon S, Collins R, Peto R, et al: Effects of prophylactic lidocaine in suspected acute myocardial infarction: An overview of results of the randomized, controlled trials. *JAMA* 260:1910, 1988.

124. Hine LK, Laird N, Hewitt P, Chalmers TC: Meta-analytic evidence against prophylactic use of lidocaine in acute myocardial infarction. *Arch Intern Med* 149:2694, 1989.

125. El-Sharif N, Myerberg RJ, Scherlag BJ, et al: Electrocardiographic antecedents of primary ventricular fibrillation: Value of the R-on-T phenomenon in myocardial infarction. *Br Heart J* 38:415, 1976.

126. Wyse DG, Kellen J, Rademaker AW: Prophylactic versus selective lidocaine for early ventricular arrhythmias of myocardial infarction. *J Am Coll Cardiol* 12:507, 1988.

127. Singh BN: Routine prophylactic lidocaine administration in acute myocardial infarction: An idea whose time has come and gone? *Circulation* 86:1033, 1992.

128. Yusuf S, Sleight P, Rossi P, et al: Reduction in infarct size, arrhythmias and the chest pain by early intravenous beta blockade in suspected myocardial infarction. *Circulation* 67(suppl I):I-32, 1983.

129. Norris RM, Brown MA, Clark ED, et al: Prevention of ventricular fibrillation during acute myocardial infarction by intravenous propranolol. *Lancet* 2:833, 1984.

130. Ryden L, Ariniego R, Arnman K, et al: A double-blind trial of metoprolol in acute myocardial infarction: Effects on ventricular tachyarrhythmias. *N Engl J Med* 308:614, 1983.

131. Nordrehaug JE, von der Lippe G: Hypokalemia and ventricular fibrillation in acute myocardial infarction. *Br Heart J* 50:525, 1983.

132. Nordrehaug JE, Johannessen K-A, von der Lippe G.: Serum potassium as a risk factor of ventricular arrhythmias early in acute myocardial infarction. *Circulation* 86:774, 1985.

133. Solomon SD, Ridker PM, Antman EM: Ventricular arrhythmias in trials of thrombolytic therapy for acute myocardial infarction: A meta-analysis. *Circulation* 88:2575, 1993.

134. Emergency Cardiac Care Committee and Subcommittees AHA: Guidelines for cardiopulmonary resuscitation and emergency cardiac care. III. Adult advanced cardiac life support. *JAMA* 268:2172, 1992.

135. Bacaner MB: Treatment of ventricular fibrillation and other acute arrhythmias with bretylium tosylate. *Am J Cardiol* 21:530, 1968.

136. Bigger JT, Fleiss JL, Kleiger R, et al and the Multicenter Postinfarction Research Group: The relationships between ventricular arrhythmias, left ventricular dysfunction, and mortality in the 2 years after myocardial infarction. *Circulation* 69:250, 1984.

137. Willems AR, Tijsseen JG, van Capelle FJL, et al: Determinants of prognosis in symptomatic ventricular tachycardia or ventricular fibrillation late after myocardial infarction. *J Am Coll Cardiol* 16:521, 1990.

138. Eldar M, Sievner Z, Godbourt U, et al: Primary ventricular tachycardia in acute myocardial infarction: Clinical characteristics and mortality. *Ann Intern Med* 117:31, 1992.

139. Wolfe CL, Nibley C, Bhandari A, et al: Polymorphous ventricular tachycardia associated with acute myocardial infarction. *Circulation* 84:1543, 1991.

140. Josephson ME: *Clinical Cardiac Electrophysiology: Techniques and Interpretations*. Philadelphia, Lea & Febiger, 1993.

141. Califf RM, O'Neill W, Stack RS, et al: Failure of simple clinical characteristics to predict perfusion status after intravenous thrombolysis. *Ann Intern Med* 108:658, 1988.

142. Bourke JP, Richards DAB, Ross DL, et al: Routine programmed electrical stimulation in survivors of acute myocardial infarction for prediction of spontaneous ventricular tachyarrhythmias during follow-up: Results, optimal stimulation protocol, and cost-effective screening. *J Am Coll Cardiol* 18:780, 1991.

143. Farrell TG, Bashir Y, Cripps T, et al: Risk stratification for arrhythmic events in postinfarction patients based on heart rate variability, ambulatory electrocardiographic variables and the signal-averaged electrocardiogram. *J Am Coll Cardiol* 18:687, 1991.

144. Echt DS, Liebson PR, Mitchell LB, et al: Mortality and morbidity in patients receiving encainide, flecainide, or placebo: The Cardiac Arrhythmia Suppression Trial. *N Engl J Med* 324:782, 1991.

145. The Cardiac Arrhythmia Suppression Trial II Investigators: Effect of the antiarrhythmic agent moricizine on survival after myocardial infarction. *N Engl J Med* 327:227, 1992.

146. Teo KT, Yusuf S, Furberg CD: Effects of prophylactic antiarrhythmic drug therapy in acute myocardial infarction: An over-

view of results from randomized controlled trials. *JAMA* 270:1589, 1993.

147. Burkart F, Pfisterer M, Kiowski W, et al: Effect of antiarrhythmic therapy on mortality in survivors of myocardial infarction with asymptomatic complex ventricular arrhythmias: Basel Antiarrhythmic Study of Infarct Survival (BASIS). *J Am Coll Cardiol* 16:1711, 1990.

148. Cairns JA, Connolly SJ, Gent M, Roberts R: Post-myocardial infarction mortality in patients with ventricular premature depolarizations: Canadian Amiodarone Myocardial Infarction Arrhythmia Trial Pilot Study. *Circulation* 84:550, 1991.

149. Ceremuzynski L, Kleczar E, Krzeminska-Pakula M, et al: Effect of amiodarone on mortality after myocardial infarction: A double-blind, placebo-controlled, pilot study. *J Am Coll Cardiol* 20:1056, 1992.

150. Yusuf S, Peto R, Lewis J, et al: Beta-blockade during and after myocardial infarction: An overview of the randomized trials. *Prog Cardiovasc Dis* 27:335, 1985.

151. Crimm A, Severance HW, Coffey K, et al: Prognostic significance of isolated sinus tachycardia during the first three days of acute myocardial infarction. *Am J Med* 76:983, 1984.

152. Goldberg RJ, Seeley D, Becker RC, et al: Impact of atrial fibrillation on the in-hospital and long-term survival of patients with acute myocardial infarction: A community-wide perspective. *Am Heart J* 119:996, 1990.

153. Behar S, Zahavi Z, Goldbourt U, Reicher-Reiss H, and the SPRINT Study Group: Long-term prognosis of patients with paroxysmal atrial fibrillation complicating acute myocardial infarction. *Eur Heart J* 13:45, 1992.

154. Behar S, Tanne D, Zion M, et al: Incidence and prognostic significance of chronic atrial fibrillation among 5,839 consecutive patients with acute myocardial infarction. *Am J Cardiol* 70:816, 1992.

155. Falk RH: Proarrhythmia in patients treated for atrial fibrillation or flutter. *Ann Intern Med* 117:141, 1992.

156. Mehta D, Ward DE, Wafa S, Camm AJ: Relative efficacy of various physical manoeuvres in the termination of junctional tachycardia. *Lancet* 1:1181, 1988.

157. Ganz LI, Friedman PL: Supraventricular tachycardia. *N Engl J Med* 332:162, 1995.

158. Konecke LL, Knoebel SB: Non-paroxysmal junctional tachycardia complicating acute myocardial infarction. *Circulation* 45:367, 1972.

159. Fishenfeld J, Dessen KB, Benchimol A: Non-paroxysmal junctional tachycardia complicating acute myocardial infarction. *Am J Cardiol* 86:754, 1973.

160. Scheinman MM, Gonzales RP: Fascicular block in acute myocardial infarction. *JAMA* 244:2646, 1980.

161. Lown B, Klein MD, Hershberg PI: Coronary and precoronary care. *Am J Med* 46:705, 1969.

162. The ISAM Study Group: A prospective trial of Intravenous Streptokinase in Acute Myocardial infarction (ISAM): Mortality, morbidity, and infarct size at 21 days. *N Engl J Med* 314:1465, 1986.

163. Koren G, Weiss AT, Ben-David J, et al: Bradycardia and hypotension following reperfusion with streptokinase (Bezold-Jarish reflex): A sign of coronary thrombolysis and myocardial salvage. *Am Heart J* 112:468, 1986.

164. Cooper MJ, Abinader EG: Atropine-induced ventricular fibrillation: Case report and review of the literature. *Am Heart J* 97:225, 1979.

165. Johansson BW: Atrioventricular and bundle branch block in acute myocardial infarction: Natural history and prognosis, in Meltzer LE, Dunning AJ (eds): *Textbook of Coronary Care*. Mount Kisco, Futura, 1972, pp 283–324.

166. Clemmensen P, Bates ER, Califf RM, et al: Complete atrioventricular block complicating inferior wall acute myocardial infarction treated with reperfusion therapy. *Am J Cardiol* 67:225, 1991.

167. Strasberg B, Bassevich R, Mager A, et al: Effects of aminophylline on atrioventricular conduction in patients with late atrioventricular block during inferior wall acute myocardial infarction. *Am J Cardiol* 67:527, 1991.

168. Klein RC, Vera Z, Mason DT: Intraventricular conduction defects in acute myocardial infarction: Incidence, prognosis and therapy. *Am Heart J* 108:1007, 1984.

169. Hollander G, Nadiminti V, Lichstein E, et al: Bundle branch block in acute myocardial infarction. *Am Heart J* 105:738, 1983.

170. Hindman MC, Wagner GS, JaRo M, et al: The clinical significance of bundle branch block complicating acute myocardial infarction. 1. Clinical characteristics, hospital mortality, and one-year follow-up. *Circulation* 58:679, 1978.

171. Hindman MC, Wagner GS, JaRo M, et al: The clinical significance of bundle branch block complicating acute myocardial infarction. 2. Indications for temporary and permanent pacemaker insertion. *Circulation* 58:689, 1978.

46. Thrombolytic Therapy: A Coronary Care Unit Perspective

George R. McKendall

The role of thrombus in the pathogenesis of acute myocardial infarction (MI) has been firmly established. Despite historical controversies, it is now accepted that intracoronary thrombus formation on a ruptured or fissured atherosclerotic plaque is the precipitating pathophysiologic event in acute MI. The abrupt, complete occlusion of a coronary artery results in regional myocardial ischemia and subsequent tissue necrosis. With the recognition of a central role of thrombus, treatment in the coronary care unit (CCU) has focused on the use of thrombolytic therapy for patients with acute MI. Timely administration of thrombolytic therapy to appropriate acute MI patients significantly influences outcome and has dramatically changed the focus of the CCU. This chapter addresses issues related to the use of thrombolytic therapy for acute MI from a CCU perspective.

Mortality Reduction

When administered to selected patients with acute MI, thrombolytic therapy reduces infarct mortality. This benefit has been associated with both intracoronary (IC) and intravenous (IV) administration of first- and second-generation thrombolytic agents. One of the earliest trials to demonstrate mortality reduction following thrombolytic therapy was the Western Washington Intracoronary Streptokinase Study [1]. Patients with acute MI randomly assigned to receive IC streptokinase following angiographic identification of an occluded infarct artery had a 30-day mortality rate of 3.7 percent, compared to 11.2 percent for those treated with a placebo infusion.

Similarly, IV streptokinase was demonstrated to have an important reduction in mortality in the Gruppo Italiano per Lo Studio Della Streptochinasi Nell' Infarcto Miocardico (GISSI) study, one of the earliest large trials of thrombolytic therapy for acute MI [2]. In this trial 11,806 patients with acute MI were treated with 1.5 million units of IV streptokinase or with usual care without thrombolytic therapy. Mortality at 21 days was significantly reduced in the streptokinase group (10.7%) compared to the control group (13.0%). Furthermore, this trial demonstrated that mortality reduction was greatest when treatment was given early in the course of MI, with almost a 50 percent reduction for those treated in the first hour. No significant benefit was conferred if treatment was given after 6 hours.

A large trial of patients with suspected acute MI by the International Study of Infarct Survival (ISIS-2) investigators demonstrated a powerful reduction in total vascular mortality with the use of either 1.5 million units of streptokinase or 162 mg of oral aspirin. Moreover, the salutary effects of streptokinase and aspirin are additive, as the mortality reduction was greatest when the two agents were given together. In this study of 17,187 patients, mortality was 9.2 percent for those treated with streptokinase, 9.4 percent for those treated with aspirin, 8.0 percent for those treated with both, and 13.2 percent for those treated with neither [3].

Mortality reduction has also been demonstrated with other thrombolytic agents. In the APSAC Intervention Mortality Study (AIMS) 1258 patients received either 30 units of anisoylated plasminogen streptokinase activator complex (APSAC) or placebo. Mortality at 30 days and 12 months was 6 percent and 11 percent for the APSAC group, compared to 12 percent and 18 percent placebo [4].

Lastly, recombinant tissue plasminogen activator (t-PA) has been shown to reduce mortality in acute MI. In the Anglo-Scandinavian Study of Early Thrombolysis (ASSET), 5011 patients were treated with either 100 mg of IV t-PA or placebo. One month mortality was 7.2 percent in the t-PA group compared to 9.8 percent in the control group [5].

It is well accepted, then, that thrombolytic therapy for acute MI significantly reduces early and late mortality. Moreover, the improvement in mortality is influenced by the timing of treatment. That is, the greatest reduction in mortality occurs when treatment is given early in the course of acute MI.

Preservation of Left Ventricular Function

In addition to its positive influence on mortality, thrombolytic therapy limits infarct size and is associated with improved left ventricular function. The latter occurs both globally and regionally at the infarct zone. Enhancement of left ventricular function has been demonstrated to occur following treatment with streptokinase, APSAC, and t-PA. Improvement can be identified when ejection fraction is measured either early or late in the postinfarct course. Although improvement of left ventricular function appears to be greatest in patients with anterior wall MI, recovery has also been demonstrated for infarcts of the inferior wall.

The Tissue Plasminogen Activator: Toronto (TPAT) Study measured left ventricular ejection fraction 9 days after acute MI in 115 patients randomly assigned to t-PA or placebo [6]. In the treatment group, global ejection fraction improved by 4.0 ± 2.4 percent units while regional infarct zone ejection fraction improved by 4.3 ± 2.6 percent units. Also using t-PA, the National Heart Foundation of Australia Coronary Thrombolysis

Group measured 1-week ejection fraction of 57.7 percent in 73 patients randomly assigned to receive t-PA, compared to an ejection fraction of 51.7 percent in 71 patients randomly assigned to placebo [7].

Ejection fraction enhancement with APSAC was demonstrated by the APSAC dans l'Infarctus du Myocarde [APSIM] Study Investigators [8]. This study randomly assigned 231 patients to receive 30 units IV of APSAC or conventional therapy with IV heparin (as a control) and subsequently undergo catheterization at 4 days. The ejection fraction was 53 percent in the APSAC group compared to 47 percent in the control group. Improvement in ejection fraction occurred for the entire group as well as for subgroups of patients with anterior and inferior infarctions.

Using IV streptokinase, the Intravenous Streptokinase in Acute Myocardial Infarction (ISAM) investigators measured ejection fraction later (3–4 weeks) in the course of acute MI in 848 patients who were randomly assigned to receive 1.5 million units of streptokinase or placebo [9]. Ejection fraction was 56.8 percent in the streptokinase group compared to 53.9 percent in the placebo group. The impact of thrombolysis could be identified regardless of infarct location.

As with mortality reduction, the greatest improvement in left ventricular function is measured when treatment occurs early in the course of acute MI. O'Rourke et al. measured 21-day ejection fraction of 61 percent in a study of patients with first MI who could be treated within 2.5 hours of symptom onset [10]. The ejection fraction of the placebo group in the same study was 54 percent. Similar dependence of improvement on time to treatment was demonstrated in a review of all patients enrolled in the Thrombolysis in Myocardial Infarction (TIMI) Study [11]. In this review of 3924 patients, Timm et al. reported that 38 percent of patients treated within 1 hour of symptom onset had an ejection fraction greater than 55 percent measured 6 weeks following treatment. By contrast, only 28 percent of patients treated later than 1 hour from symptom onset had an ejection fraction greater than 55 percent. Moreover, the proportion of patients with an ejection fraction less than 35 percent was lowest in those who were treated within the first hour.

Importance of Coronary Reperfusion

The presumed mechanism for reduction of mortality and infarct size is achievement of reperfusion of the infarct-related coronary artery. Pioneering work from DeWood et. al. in 1980 (later confirmed by many other angiographic trials) identified the presence of a total coronary occlusion in 87 percent of acute MI patients evaluated within 4 hours of symptom onset [12]. In patients studied 6 to 12 hours after symptom onset the frequency of occlusion was 68 percent. For those presenting between 12 and 24 hours, total occlusions were detected in 65 percent. This work established primary coronary occlusion as the underlying pathophysiology of acute MI; furthermore, it demonstrated that spontaneous reperfusion occurred in a small proportion of patients in a manner that appeared to be time-dependent. Acute MI treatment, therefore, has been directed at relieving coronary occlusion, by either pharmacologic or mechanical means.

Reperfusion of an infarct-related artery requires recanalization and patency. Recanalization is the establishment of anterograde blood flow in an artery demonstrated to be occluded angiographically prior to treatment. Patency is demonstrated by identification of anterograde flow following treatment without knowledge of the perfusion status before initiating therapy. Patency rates are higher than recanalization rates because of the added contribution of spontaneous reperfusion.

Angiographic trials have traditionally measured patency rates 90 minutes following initiation of therapy. Despite likely fluctuations in flow during the course of therapy, the 90-minute patency rate has become the standard for comparing various thrombolytic regimens. The Thrombolysis in Myocardial Infarction (TIMI) investigators defined coronary artery blood flow according to a semiquantitative scale [13]: grade 0 indicates no anterograde flow beyond the culprit lesion; grade 1 is penetration of contrast beyond the culprit lesion without perfusion of the distal vessel; grade 2 is partial perfusion, whereby the contrast enters or clears from the distal vessel at a sluggish rate; and grade 3 is complete and normal filling and clearance of the vessel distal to the culprit stenosis. Until recently, grade 2 or 3 flow has been considered to indicate achievement of patency, and outcome was believed to be similar for the two grades. New reports indicate that normal anterograde flow (grade 3) is superior to flow grade 2 and that infarct size and mortality are reduced if grade 3 flow is established [14,15].

Reperfusion following acute MI with or without thrombolytic therapy is associated with improved left ventricular function and mortality as well as with other markers of outcome, including left ventricular volume. In a retrospective analysis of 179 patients with recent acute MI and single-vessel disease at the time of catheterization, Cigarroa et al. demonstrated a significant impact of anterograde perfusion on mortality and morbidity during long-term follow-up regardless of whether treatment with thrombolytic therapy had occurred [16]. Patients with anterograde reperfusion had a lower incidence of subsequent unstable angina, congestive heart failure, and death compared to a comparable group of patients who did not demonstrate infarct artery reperfusion.

Similarly, in reports of patients treated with thrombolytic therapy, improved survival is associated with establishment of infarct artery patency. The Western Washington Study reported a 1-year mortality of 2.5 percent in patients with reperfusion compared to 23.1 percent and 14.6 percent in patients with partial or no reperfusion [17]. In TIMI-1, patients with infarct-related artery patency at 90 minutes had 6- and 12-month mortalities of 5.6 percent and 8.1 percent compared to 12.5 percent and 14.8 percent for those patients without patency [18]. This difference was independent of the agent used to achieve patency.

Reperfusion is also associated with improved left ventricular volume and function. Jeremy et al., in a study of 40 patients not treated with thrombolytic therapy, found that the degree of perfusion of the infarct artery was a significant predictor of left ventricular dilatation as measured by change in left ventricular volume during the first month following infarction [19]. In this report perfusion status of the infarct artery was more important than infarct size in determining degree of left ventricular dilatation.

In patients treated with thrombolytic therapy, infarct-related artery perfusion status correlates with left ventricular function. The TIMI investigators measured left ventricular function by contrast ventriculography before and after treatment with either t-PA or streptokinase. Increases in ejection fraction were limited to patients who had achieved reperfusion by 90 minutes after treatment or who initially demonstrated subtotal occlusions [20]. Similarly, the ISAM investigators determined infarct artery patency and measured left ventricular ejection fraction in 368 patients 1 month after treatment with either IV streptokinase or placebo [21]. Regardless of treatment, patients with patency of the infarct-related artery had an ejection fraction of 56 percent,

compared to 50 percent in patients who did not demonstrate patency.

The importance of reperfusion of the coronary artery is illustrated by evaluating the impact of infarct-related artery reocclusion in patients who demonstrate initial success to reperfusion therapy. Ohman et al. reviewed the consequences of reocclusion in a large series of consecutive patients enrolled in the Thrombolysis and Myocardial Infarction (TAMI) trials who underwent 90-minute and predischarge coronary angiography of the infarct artery [22]. Reocclusion of the infarct artery was identified in 12.4 percent of patients, 58 percent of whom were asymptomatic. Patients with reocclusion had less left ventricular recovery and higher in-hospital morbidity. The mortality rate was 11.0 percent in patients with reocclusion, compared to only 4.5 percent in those without reocclusion.

Despite the importance of establishing and maintaining infarct artery reperfusion, it is extremely difficult to evaluate efficacy of treatment without coronary angiography. An approach that includes routine coronary angiography, however, is not practical for clinical management. Consequently, great attention has been focused on the use of noninvasive clinical markers to predict the perfusion status of the infarct artery. Relief of symptoms, resolution of electrocardiographic changes, presence of arrhythmias, and early peaking of creatinine kinase have all been evaluated as noninvasive methods to detect reperfusion. The accuracy of these parameters is mixed, with no highly sensitive and specific marker identified to date.

Califf et al. correlated noninvasive events with 90-minute patency in 386 patients treated with t-PA who subsequently underwent coronary angiography [23]. Complete resolution of S–T segment elevation was identified in only 6 percent of patients but was associated with a 96 percent angiographic patency rate. Partial resolution of S–T segment elevation occurred in 38 percent of patients and was associated with patency in 84 percent. Complete relief of chest pain was reported in 29 percent of patients and was associated with patency in 84 percent. Arrhythmias alone did not correlate with infarct artery patency. Of note, 56 percent of patients with no S–T segment or symptom resolution nevertheless demonstrated infarct artery patency.

Hohnloser et al. evaluated 82 patients treated with thrombolytic therapy and identified sensitivity and specificity for early peaking of creatinine kinase, reduction of S–T segment elevation by at least 50 percent, and presence of arrhythmias [24]. Although the presence of all three parameters was associated with 100 percent sensitivity, 90 percent specificity, and 97 percent positive predictive value for identifying reperfusion, no single noninvasive marker alone was both highly sensitive and highly specific. Furthermore, enzyme peaking cannot be identified in the early hours of MI, when determination of perfusion status may significantly alter immediate management.

Risks and Complications

The major complication associated with the use of thrombolytic therapy is bleeding. Rates of hemorrhage reported in major thrombolytic trials have varied, mainly because of differences in definition, data collection, and protocol use of invasive procedures and anticoagulants. Major bleeding events occurred in 4.2 percent of 1395 patients in the TIMI-2 trial who did not have routine invasive procedures. Minor bleeding occurred in 8.7 percent in the same group. By contrast, 7.0 percent of 1424 patients routinely undergoing cardiac catheterization exhibited major bleeding, while 11.5 percent developed minor bleeding [25]. While the majority of bleeding events are related to vascular puncture sites and can be controlled with local pressure and reduction of associated anticoagulants, bleeding can occur at other sites. These most commonly include the gastrointestinal tract, genitourinary system, sites of recent surgery or trauma, and the central nervous system.

The most serious and devastating complication of thrombolytic therapy is intracranial bleeding. Almost half of all intracranial bleeds are fatal, and severe morbidity is common in patients who survive. Although the incidence of combined cerebrovascular events following thrombolytic therapy is similar to that associated with placebo treatment, there is an increased incidence of intracranial bleeding with thrombolytic therapy. Fortunately, the overall incidence with careful patient selection is low. Alpert et al. pooled rates of intracranial bleeding from available randomized trials and identified rates of 0.22 percent with streptokinase, 0.56 percent with t-PA, 0.51 percent with APSAC, and 0.02 percent with placebo [26].

Because of relatively small event rates in published studies and the absence of randomized trials assessing risk for intracranial bleeding, it is difficult to identify accurately absolute risk factors predisposing to intracranial bleeding. For patients treated with t-PA, the risk of intracranial bleeding increases if the administered dose exceeds 100 mg. Regardless of the agent, there appears to be an increased rate of intracranial bleeding in patients who are elderly or hypertensive, or with a history of previous cerebrovascular events [27,28].

The management of bleeding complications related to the use of thrombolytic therapy depends on severity. Major bleeding involving the central nervous system or bleeding associated with large blood loss necessitates discontinuation of the thrombolytic agent and any associated anticoagulant. If heparin has been used, protamine may be necessary to reverse its effects. The clinical situation may warrant blood replacement or administration of plasma products. Rarely, antifibrinolytic agents may be required. Minor bleeding episodes can usually be managed with reduction of concomitant anticoagulant therapy, compression of vascular access sites, or other local supportive therapy [29].

Thrombolytic Agents

Several thrombolytic agents are beneficial for the treatment of acute MI (see Chap. 121). These include streptokinase, urokinase, t-PA, APSAC, combinations of t-PA with streptokinase or urokinase, and several other agents. Perhaps the greatest controversy in the field of thrombolysis lies in the agent of choice for MI. The two most widely used agents, streptokinase and t-PA, differ in degree of fibrin specificity as well as cost.

Angiographic trials comparing streptokinase and t-PA have established that t-PA is associated with a higher reperfusion rate. The TIMI investigators required pretreatment angiograms before administering either IV streptokinase or IV t-PA to 290 patients with acute MI [13]. The recanalization rate was 62 percent in those treated with t-PA, compared to 31 percent in those treated with streptokinase. Similarly, the European Cooperative Study Group measured infarct artery patency in 123 patients treated with either t-PA or streptokinase. Patency rates at 90 minutes after treatment were 70 percent in the t-PA group, compared to 55 percent in the streptokinase group [30].

Despite wide acceptance that t-PA is superior to streptokinase in achieving infarct artery patency, great debate exists about whether this ability to open more arteries confers benefit in regard to measurable clinical outcome, such as mortality reduction and preservation of left ventricular function. The open artery hypothesis suggests that outcome is better with those

agents with higher reperfusion rates. Until recently, however, data supporting this hypothesis have been lacking.

Because left ventricular ejection fraction may be a crude measure of thrombolytic efficacy and mortality differences with various agents may be small, large clinical trials have been necessary for adequate comparison of thrombolytic agents with different patency rates. The first large comparative trial, GISSI-2 randomly assigned 12,490 patients to receive t-PA or streptokinase [31]. Patients were also assigned to receive subcutaneous heparin beginning 12 hours after therapy or to receive no heparin. This trial identified no difference in a combined endpoint of death and severe left ventricular damage between the two thrombolytic agents. These findings were later corroborated by the International Study Group, which combined patients from GISSI-2 and evaluated a total of 20,891 patients treated with t-PA or streptokinase with and without subcutaneous heparin [32]. Hospital mortality was 8.9 percent in the t-PA group and 8.5 percent in the streptokinase group, a difference that is not statistically significant. Of note, there was a greater incidence of overall stroke in the tissue plasminogen activator group (1.3% vs. 1.0%) and more bleeding in the streptokinase group (0.6% vs. 0.9%).

Another large trial comparing thrombolytic agents was undertaken by ISIS-3 [33], which randomly assigned 41,299 patients with suspected acute MI to receive streptokinase, t-PA, or APSAC. Patients were also randomly assigned to subcutaneous heparin starting 4 hours after enrollment or to no heparin. All patients were treated with aspirin commencing with enrollment. This trial showed no difference in mortality associated with the three agents. There was a greater incidence of allergic reactions and hypotension in those receiving APSAC and streptokinase compared to t-PA. As in other comparative trials, t-PA was associated with a slight increase in stroke compared to either streptokinase or APSAC.

The results of these large clinical trials questioned the validity of the open artery hypothesis, which would have predicted better outcome among those patients treated with t-PA. These findings, however, have been strongly challenged on the basis of the methodology employed by the investigators. The ISIS-3 trial used a preparation of t-PA (duteplase) that is not commercially available and may differ from the standard single-chain preparation (alteplase), which has been investigated more thoroughly in both angiographic and clinical trials. Moreover, GISSI-2 and ISIS-3 investigators used a standard infusion of t-PA, rather than one of several accelerated regimens associated with higher patency rates [34,35].

The greatest challenge regarding the findings of these trials, however, has been associated with the use of adjuvant subcutaneous heparin. Heparin administered subcutaneously has not been used routinely as an adjuvant to treatment with thrombolytic therapy. Most large trials using t-PA have employed early IV heparin as adjuvant therapy. Hsia et al. reported a significantly higher early patency rate with IV heparin as an adjuvant to t-PA compared to the use of 80 mg of oral aspirin alone (82% vs. 52%) [36]. Similarly, Bleich et al. demonstrated a 3-day patency rate of 71 percent in acute MI patients receiving both t-PA and IV heparin, compared to 43 percent in patients receiving t-PA alone [37]. An additional trial evaluating the routine use of t-PA and aspirin with or without adjuvant heparin demonstrated a 48- to 120-hour patency rate of 83.4 percent in those treated with both heparin and aspirin, compared to 74.7 percent in those treated with aspirin alone [38]. Based on these studies, it is clear that optimal use of thrombolytic therapy with IV t-PA includes adjuvant use of IV heparin and aspirin. Other, more potent direct thrombin inhibitors may prove to be useful as adjuvant agents.

The role of IV heparin as an adjuvant to streptokinase has

been less intensely investigated. Small reports have suggested enhancement of infarct artery patency as well as reduction of infarct size when IV heparin has been used as an adjuvant to IV streptokinase [39,40]. As noted previously, the use of subcutaneous heparin with streptokinase has been studied extensively by the GISSI-2 and ISIS-3 investigators, who employed twice daily regimens of 12,500 units starting 12 and 4 hours after streptokinase, respectively [31,33]. In both trials, subcutaneous heparin did not influence mortality, although greater bleeding was noted with its use.

The Global Utilization of Streptokinase and t-PA for Occluded Coronary Arteries Trial (GUSTO) was a multicenter international study designed to address the issues raised by the GISSI-2 and ISIS-3 trials. In this study, 41,021 patients were randomly assigned to receive one of four treatment strategies: (1) accelerated IV t-PA with IV heparin; (2) IV t-PA and streptokinase with IV heparin; (3) IV streptokinase with subcutaneous heparin; or (4) IV streptokinase with IV heparin. Results of this trial were reported recently [41]. Thirty-day mortality rates for patients in the t-PA group, t-PA plus streptokinase group, streptokinase plus subcutaneous heparin group, and streptokinase plus IV heparin group were 6.3 percent, 7.0 percent, 7.2 percent, and 7.4 percent, respectively. The incidence of total stroke was 1.55 percent, 1.64 percent, 1.22 percent, and 1.40 percent, respectively. Hemorrhagic strokes occurred in 0.72 percent, 0.94 percent, 0.49 percent, and 0.54 percent, respectively. Net clinical benefit, defined as the incidence of death or nonfatal disabling stroke, was 6.9 percent, 7.6 percent, 7.7 percent, and 7.9 percent, respectively. Combining data from the streptokinase groups, then, revealed that t-PA was superior in terms of mortality reduction and net clinical benefit of death or nonfatal stroke.

Based on these results, it appears that the initial premise of the open artery hypothesis is valid. Thrombolytic regimens achieving the greatest infarct artery patency are associated with mortality reduction. t-PA, when used with intravenous heparin, is associated with lower mortality than IV streptokinase. The slightly greater incidence of hemorrhagic stroke with t-PA partially offsets the mortality benefit. The large difference in cost between streptokinase and t-PA is an important issue that must be factored into the decision regarding the agent of choice. This subject, however, is beyond the scope of this chapter.

Although various dosing regimens of thrombolytic agents have been employed in clinical trials, experience from GUSTO with an accelerated regimen of t-PA is helpful in dosing this agent. A total dose not exceeding 100 mg was used. This was administered as a 15-mg bolus followed by 0.75 mg per kilogram over 30 minutes (not to exceed 50 mg) and 0.50 mg per kilogram over 60 minutes (not to exceed 35 mg). The IV streptokinase was dosed as a 1.5 million unit infusion over 60 minutes. Standard dosing for APSAC is a 30 unit injection over 2 to 3 minutes.

More important than the choice of thrombolytic agent for acute MI is the impact of early identification and treatment of appropriate patients. The benefits of thrombolytic therapy are inversely related to the time of treatment. As discussed previously, the greatest benefit in terms of mortality reduction and left ventricular salvage is measured when treatment occurs early in the course of MI. In spite of the importance of early treatment, several studies have indicated long delays prior to administration of thrombolytic therapy [42,43,44]. These delays occur at several stages, including the time required for patients to recognize the symptoms of acute MI and seek assistance, the time required to transport the patient to the hospital, and the time to initiate treatment following hospital arrival. Total elapsed time from symptom onset to treatment can exceed several hours, with a large component of this delay occurring after

hospital arrival. To optimize the benefits of thrombolytic therapy, efforts to reduce these delays must be directed at patient education to seek assistance sooner and at prompt identification and treatment following hospital arrival.

Role of Mechanical Intervention

Another important issue related to the use of thrombolytic therapy is the role of adjuvant mechanical revascularization following thrombolysis. In instances where the infarct artery remains occluded despite thrombolytic therapy, salvage or "rescue" percutaneous transluminal coronary angioplasty (PTCA) may achieve coronary reperfusion. Despite the presumed benefit of this approach, it has not been uniformly adopted. Several reports have associated rescue PTCA with a less than favorable clinical outcome, particularly when improvement in coronary obstruction was not achieved with the procedure [45].

A less controversial and more intensely studied issue relates to routine use of cardiac catheterization and PTCA following treatment with thrombolytic therapy in uncomplicated MI. The data are quite conclusive and do not demonstrate a need for routine cardiac catheterization and subsequent PTCA in patients treated with thrombolytic therapy who do not have recurrent symptoms of angina or provocable ischemia on exercise stress testing [46]. Based on these results, a "watchful waiting" approach to patients who respond clinically to therapy is most prudent.

Recently, treatment of acute MI by primary or direct PTCA as a means of achieving reperfusion has been proposed as an alternative to thrombolytic therapy. Observational trials as well as those comparing primary PTCA to thrombolytic therapy have demonstrated that this approach is reasonable for patients who have ready access to a catheterization laboratory with skilled PTCA operators [47]. It remains to be seen whether specific subgroups of patients with acute MI will benefit more or less from one of these two approaches. At this time, then, thrombolytic therapy remains the treatment of choice for patients who are eligible and have no contraindications. Direct or primary PTCA can be considered a reasonable alternative for patients with immediate access to this treatment. The optimal treatment of patients with acute MI who are not eligible to receive thrombolytic therapy remains uncertain.

Patient Selection

Although various trials have established the benefits of thrombolytic therapy, selection and treatment criteria have often varied, making extrapolation to clinical practice difficult. For these reasons patient selection can remain a clinical dilemma (Table 46-1). In current practice indications and contraindications for treatment are often relative, requiring case-by-case assessment.

Indications for treatment are based primarily on the presenting electrocardiogram (ECG) and the duration of symptoms. There is general agreement that treatment is indicated for patients with acute MI who present with S–T segment elevation on ECG. Although treatment is probably indicated for patients presenting with S–T depression in the right precordial leads suggestive of a true posterior infarct, no data exist to support the general use of thrombolytic therapy in patients with S–T segment depression or nondiagnostic ECG changes. Patients presenting with left bundle branch block on ECG have uncertain indications for treatment. Although patients with bundle

Table 46-1. Patient Selection Criteria for Thrombolytic Therapy

Indications
  Clinical syndrome consistent with acute myocardial infarction
  S–T segment elevation
  Presentation within 12 hours
  New left bundle branch block

Contraindications
  Active bleeding
  Recent head trauma or cerebrovascular accident
  Uncontrolled hypertension
  Pregnancy
  Recent surgery
  Underlying bleeding diathesis

Relative contraindications
  Inactive peptic ulcer disease
  Remote nonhemorrhagic cerebrovascular accident

branch block in the ISIS-2 trial had lower mortality rates with either aspirin, streptokinase, or both compared to placebo [32], most trials rigorously evaluating thrombolytic therapy have excluded left bundle branch block, therefore definitive data regarding treatment in this circumstance are not available. Decisions regarding administration of thrombolytic agents to patients with left bundle branch block must be made on an individual basis.

Based on multiple trials, there is strong agreement that otherwise eligible patients presenting within the first 6 hours of symptom onset should be treated with thrombolytic therapy. Data supporting treatment beyond 6 hours, however, are mixed. Results from the first GISSI trial showed no significant difference in mortality when streptokinase was administered beyond 6 hours [2]. The Late Assessment of Thrombolytic Efficacy (LATE) trial was designed to evaluate the benefit of thrombolytic therapy given beyond the first 6 hours of infarction. Patients were randomly assigned to receive either t-PA or placebo. The results indicate lower mortality for the group treated with t-PA up to 12 hours from symptom onset [48]. Based on this study, the treatment window for thrombolytic therapy should be extended to 12 hours.

Just as there are relatively few absolute indications for treatment with thrombolytic therapy, there are few absolute contraindications to its use. These include instances where active bleeding or potential hemorrhagic complications make administration prohibitive. Therefore, patients with aortic dissection, ongoing internal bleeding, recent intracranial surgery, intracranial neoplasm, head trauma, or history of hemorrhagic stroke should not be treated with thrombolytic therapy. Sustained uncontrolled hypertension is also an absolute contraindication to thrombolytic therapy, although the value of blood pressure beyond which thrombolysis is contraindicated is uncertain. Because of varying blood pressure criteria employed by major trials, no standards exist regarding limits of acceptable blood pressure prior to treatment. The American College of Cardiology/American Heart Association (ACC/AHA) Task Force on the Management of Acute Myocardial Infarction has recommended that a recorded blood pressure greater than 200/120 mm Hg is an absolute contraindication to thrombolytic therapy [49]. Few data exist, however, to support the choice of these specific readings. Small observational reports have associated an increased rate of intracranial bleeding in patients with a history of hypertension or poorly controlled blood pressure [27,28].

Other contraindications to thrombolytic therapy are pregnancy, recent surgery or trauma that could be a potential source of uncontrolled bleeding, prolonged cardiopulmonary resuscitation, and previous allergic reaction to or recent (6–9 months)

exposure to streptokinase or APSAC (where antibody titers may inhibit thrombolysis by these specific agents). Patients with a reaction to or recent treatment with APSAC or streptokinase can be treated with t-PA or urokinase.

Relative contraindications include inactive peptic ulcer disease, previous remote nonhemorrhagic cerebrovascular accident, and an underlying bleeding diathesis without active hemorrhage at the time of evaluation.

The use of thrombolytic therapy in the elderly remains a great dilemma in clinical practice. Although elderly patients with acute MI have a high infarct-related mortality, this group of patients has generally been excluded from thrombolytic trials. Elderly patients, particularly those with other relative contraindications, appear to be at greater risk for intracranial bleeding from thrombolytic therapy [50]. Until further data are available from large clinical trials, age must be considered a relative contraindication for treatment, and patients should be judged on a case-by-case basis.

The ACC/AHA Task Force has made recommendations for treatment of patients who present with no apparent contraindications [49]. Standard indications for treatment include acute MI patients younger than 70 years presenting within 6 hours with S–T segment elevation. The Task Force also favors treating patients between 70 and 75 years who present in a similar fashion. Patients presenting more than 6 hours from symptom onset but who demonstrate ongoing "stuttering" symptoms may also benefit from treatment, as may patients with suspected reinfarction following thrombolysis. Circumstances considered to be of uncertain benefit but probably helpful include symptom duration of 6 to 24 hours, age greater than 75 years with large impending infarction when treatment can be initiated early, and acute MI associated with borderline S–T segment elevation.

The Task Force agreed that there was no indication to treat chest pain of unclear etiology or uncertain onset or that occurring after 24 hours in duration.

References

1. Kennedy J, Ritchie J, Davis K, Fritz J: Western Washington Randomized Trial of Intracoronary Streptokinase in Acute Myocardial Infarction. *N Engl J Med* 309:1477, 1983.
2. Gruppo Italiano per Lo Studio Della Streptochinasi Nell 'Infarto Miocardico (GISSI): Effectiveness of intravenous thrombolytic treatment in acute myocardial infarction. *Lancet* 1:397, 1986.
3. ISIS-2 : Randomised trial of intravenous streptokinase, oral aspirin, both, or neither among 17,187 cases of suspected acute myocardial infarction: ISIS-2. *Lancet* 2:349, 1988.
4. AIMS Trial Study Group: Long-term effects of intravenous anistreplase in acute myocardial infarction: Final report of the AIMS study. *Lancet* 335:427, 1990.
5. Anglo-Scandinavian Study of Early Thrombolysis Study Group: Trial of tissue plasminogen activator for mortality reduction in acute myocardial infarction. *Lancet* 2:525, 1988.
6. Armstrong P, Baigrie R, Daly P, et al: Tissue plasminogen activator: Toronto (TPAT) Placebo-Controlled Randomized Trial in acute myocardial infarction. *J Am Coll Cardiol* 13:1469, 1989.
7. National Heart Foundation of Australia Coronary Thrombolysis Group: Coronary thrombolysis and myocardial salvage by tissue plasminogen activator given up to 4 hours after onset of myocardial infarction. *Lancet* 1:203, 1988.
8. Bassand J, Machecourt J, Cassagnes J: Multicenter trial of intravenous anisoylated plasminogen streptokinase activator complex (APSAC) in acute myocardial infarction: Effects on infarct size and left ventricular function. *J Am Coll Cardiol* 13:988, 1989.
9. The I.S.A.M. Study Group: A prospective trial of intravenous streptokinase in acute myocardial infarction. *N Engl J Med* 314:1465, 1986.

10. O'Rourke M, Baron D, Keogh A, et al: Limitation of myocardial infarction by early infusion of recombinant tissue-type plasminogen activator. *Circulation* 77:1311, 1988.

11. Timm TC, Ross R, McKendall GR, et al: Left ventricular function and early cardiac events as a function of time to treatment with t-PA: A report from TIMI II. *Circulation* 84 (suppl II):230, 1991.

12. DeWood M, Spores J, Notske R, et al: Prevalence of total coronary occlusion during the early hours of transmural myocardial infarction. *N Engl J Med* 303:897, 1980.

13. Chesebro JH, Knatterud G, Roberts R, et al: Thrombolysis in Myocardial Infarction (TIMI) Trial, phase I: A comparison between intravenous tissue plasminogen activator and intravenous streptokinase. *Circulation* 76:142, 1987.

14. Anderson JL, Karagounis LA, Becker LC, et al: TIMI Perfusion grade 3 but not grade 2 results in improved outcome after thrombolysis for myocardial infarction. *Circulation* 87:1829, 1993.

15. Vogt A, Rainer von Essen, Tebbe U, et al: Impact of early perfusion status of the infarct-related artery on short-term mortality after thrombolysis for acute myocardial infarction: Retrospective analysis of four German multicenter studies. *J Am Coll Cardiol* 21:1391, 1993.

16. Cigarroa R, Lange R, Hillis D: Prognosis after acute myocardial infarction in patients with and without residual anterograde coronary blood flow. *Am J Cardiol* 64:155, 1989.

17. Kennedy J, Ritchie J, Davis K: The Western Washington Randomized Trial of Intracoronary Streptokinase in Acute Myocardial Infarction: A 12-month follow-up report. *N Engl J Med* 312:1073, 1985.

18. Dalen J, Gore J, Braunwald E, et al: Six- and twelve-month follow-up of the phase I Thrombolysis in Myocardial Infarction (TIMI) Trial. *Am J Cardiol* 62:179, 1988.

19. Jeremy R, Hackworthy R, Bautovich G, et al: Infarct artery perfusion and changes in left ventricular volume in the month after acute myocardial infarction. *J Am Coll Cardiol* 9:989, 1987.

20. Sheehan F, Braunwald E, Canner P, et al: The effect of intravenous thrombolytic therapy on left ventricular function: A report on tissue-type plasminogen activator and streptokinase from the Thrombolysis in Myocardial Infarction (TIMI Phase I) trial. *Circulation* 75:817, 1987.

21. Schröder R, Neuhaus K, Linderer T, et al: Impact of late coronary artery reperfusion on left ventricular function one month after acute myocardial infarction (results from the ISAM study). *Am J Cardiol* 64:878, 1989.

22. Ohman E, Califf R, Topol E, et al: Consequences of reocclusion after successful reperfusion therapy in acute myocardial infarction. *Circulation* 82:781, 1990.

23. Califf R, O'Neil W, Stack R, et al: Failure of simple clinical measurement to predict perfusion status after intravenous thrombolysis. *Ann Intern Med* 108:658, 1988.

24. Hohnloser S, Zabel M, Kasper M, et al: Assessment of coronary artery patency after thrombolytic therapy: Accurate prediction utilizing the combined analysis of three noninvasive markers. *J Am Coll Cardiol* 18:44, 1991.

25. Bovill E, Terrin M, Stump D, et al: Hemorrhagic events during therapy with recombinant tissue-type plasminogen activator, heparin, and aspirin for acute myocardial infarction: Results of the Thrombolysis in Myocardial Infarction (TIMI), phase II trial. *Ann Intern Med* 115:256, 1991.

26. Alpert JS, Becker RC, Gore JM: Hemorrhagic events and intracranial bleeding in patients receiving thrombolytic therapy for acute myocardial infarction. *Am J Cardiol* 15, 1993.

27. Anderson JL, Karagounis L, Allen A, et al: Older age and elevated blood pressure are risk factors for intracerebral hemorrhage after thrombolysis. *Am J Cardiol* 68:166, 1991.

28. Gore JM, Sloan M, Price TR, et al: Intracerebral hemorrhage, cerebral infarction, and subdural hematoma after acute myocardial infarction and thrombolytic therapy in the Thrombolysis in Myocardial Infarction Study. *Circulation* 83:448, 1991.

29. Sane D, Califf R, Topol E, et al: Bleeding during thrombolytic therapy for acute myocardial iInfarction: Mechanisms and management. *Ann Intern Med* 111:1010, 1987.

30. Vestraete M, Bory M, Collen D, et al: Randomised trial of intravenous recombinant tissue-type plasminogen activator versus intravenous streptokinase in acute myocardial infarction. *Lancet* 1:842, 1985.

31. Gruppo Italiano per Lo Studio Della Sopravvivenza Nell 'Infarto Miocardico. GISSI-2: A factorial randomised trial of alteplase versus streptokinase and heparin versus no heparin among 12,490 patients with acute myocardial infarction. *Lancet* 336:65, 1990.

32. The International Study Group: In-hospital mortality and clinical course of 20,891 patients with suspected acute myocardial infarction randomised between alteplase and streptokinase with or without heparin. *Lancet* 336:71, 1990.

33. Third International Study of Infarct Survival Collaborative Group. ISIS-3: A randomised comparison of streptokinase vs tissue plasminogen activator vs anistreplase and of aspirin plus heparin vs aspirin alone among 41,299 cases of suspected acute myocardial infarction. *Lancet* 339:753, 1992.

34. McKendall GR, Attubato MJ, Drew TM, et al: Safety and efficacy of a new regimen of intravenous recombinant tissue-type plasminogen activator potentially suitable for either prehospital or in-hospital administration. *J Am Coll Cardiol* 18:1774, 1991.

35. Neuhaus KL, Feuerer W, Jeep-Tebbe S, et al: Improved thrombolysis with a modified dose regimen of recombinant tissue-type plasminogen activator. *J Am Coll Cardiol* 14:1566, 1989.

36. Hsia J, Hamilton W, Kleiman N, et al: A comparison between heparin and low-dose aspirin as adjunctive therapy with tissue plasminogen activator for acute myocardial infarction. *N Engl J Med* 323:1433, 1990.

37. Bleich SD, Nicholas TC, Schumacher RR, et al: Effect of heparin on coronary arterial patency after thrombolysis with tissue plasminogen activator in acute myocardial infarction. *Am J Cardiol* 66:1412, 1990.

38. de Bono DP, Simoons ML, Tijssen J, et al: Effect of early intravenous heparin on coronary patency, infarct size, and bleeding complications after alteplase thrombolysis: Results of a randomised double blind European cooperative study group trial. *Br Heart J* 67:122, 1992.

39. Melandri G, Branzi A, Semprini F, et al: Enhanced thrombolytic efficacy and reduction of infarct size by simultaneous infusion of streptokinase and heparin. *Br Heart J* 64:118, 1990.

40. Mahan EF, Chandler JW, Rogers WJ, et al: Heparin and infarct coronary artery patency after streptokinase in acute myocardial infarction. *Am J Cardiol* 65:967, 1990.

41. The GUSTO Investigators: An international randomized trial comparing four thrombolytic strategies for acute myocardial infarction. *N Engl J Med* 329:673, 1993.

42. Sharkey SW, Brunette DD, Ruise E, et al: An analysis of time delays preceding thrombolysis for acute myocardial infarction. *JAMA* 262:3171, 1988.

43. McKendall GR, McDonald MJ, Woolard R, et al: Characterization of the time course from infarction onset to thrombolytic therapy: Identification of delays and remedies. *Ann Emerg Med* 19:479, 1990.

44. Kereiakes DJ, Weaver WD, Anderson JL, et al: Time delays in the diagnosis and treatment of acute myocardial infarction: A tale of eight cities. *Am Heart J* 120:773, 1990.

45. Califf RM, Topol EJ, George BS, et al: Characteristics and outcome of patients in whom reperfusion with intravenous tissue-type plasminogen activator fails: Results of the Thrombolysis and Angioplasty in Myocardial Infarction (TAMI) I Trial. *Circulation* 77:1090, 1988.

46. The TIMI Study Group: Comparison of invasive and conservative strategies after treatment with intravenous tissue plasminogen activator in acute myocardial infarction. *N Engl J Med* 320:618, 1989.

47. Grines CL, Browne KF, Marco J, et al: A comparison of immediate angioplasty with thrombolytic therapy for acute myocardial infarction. *N Engl J Med* 328:673, 1993.

48. LATE Study Group: Late Assessment of Thrombolytic Efficacy (LATE) study with alteplase 6–24 hours after onset of acute myocardial infarction. *Lancet* 342:759, 1993.

49. Gunnar RM, Bourdillon PDV, Dixon DW, et al: ACC/AHA guidelines for the early management of patients with acute myocardial infarction. *Circulation* 82:664, 1990.

50. Lew AS, Hod H, Cercek B, et al: Mortality and morbidity rates of patients older and younger than 75 years with acute myocardial infarction treated with intravenous streptokinase. *Am J Cardiol* 59:1, 1987.

47. Secondary Prevention After Acute Myocardial Infarction: A Coronary Care Unit Perspective

Michael Vredenburg and Steven Borzak

Management of the patient with acute myocardial infarction (MI) has undergone radical transformation over the past three decades. Once guided by "the tincture of time" coupled with rest and relaxation, therapy is now based on mortality data from large-scale clinical trials in thousands of patients, whose outcomes may be joined by meta-analysis [1]. This chapter reviews the current understanding of secondary prevention measures and prioritizes their use for individual patients.

Secondary Prevention as a Treatment Strategy

The modern paradigm of acute MI management typically involves several stages. First, acute management focuses on the early and sustained restoration of coronary patency, combined with efforts to limit infarct size and treat early ventricular arrhythmias. This stage begins with the patient's decision to seek medical attention, continues in the ambulance and emergency department, and may extend to the coronary care unit (CCU) or catheterization laboratory. The next stage, which may begin in the emergency department or CCU, involves early risk stratification, monitoring and treatment of complications, and consideration of adjunctive therapy designed to reduce the risk of death and morbidity during hospitalization and in early recovery.

The final stage involves efforts to restore the patient to the highest possible functional capacity and to modify cardiac risk through prevention strategies. Such efforts initiated after an MI are referred to as secondary prevention. In distinction, primary prevention is directed toward the population at large or high-risk subgroups without overt manifestations of coronary heart disease. For the practitioner caring for the post-MI patient, secondary prevention efforts have a higher yield than primary prevention, since the risk of events is substantially higher [1], though fewer total deaths are prevented and the aggregate value to society may be less. The CCU is the appropriate setting in which to begin making therapeutic choices of secondary prevention.

A diverse array of drugs and other interventions is currently available for the patient experiencing an acute MI [1]. The selection of treatment depends on an understanding of the physiologic principles governing adverse outcome after MI (Table 47-1). However, choices must be firmly grounded by the results of large-scale mortality trials, since there is often a lack of correlation of the known or presumed mechanism of a drug and its effect on survival. Interventions for the patient after MI are also appropriately guided by the risk factor profile (Table 47-2). Patients at higher risk clearly have the most to gain from a secondary prevention strategy [2–9].

This chapter focuses primarily on measures that depend on early initiation and only briefly reviews measures more appropriately considered somewhat later during hospitalization or after hospital discharge.

Antiplatelet Agents

Platelet aggregation, adhesion, and the subsequent formation of intracoronary thrombus in response to atherosclerotic plaque rupture are pivotal events in the pathophysiology of MI [10,11] (see Chap. 43). Aspirin irreversibly inhibits the cyclooxygenase reaction necessary for the production of thromboxane A_2, a potent stimulator of vasoconstriction and platelet aggregation

Table 47-1. Mechanistic Strategies Linking Acute Treatment and Secondary Prevention in Acute Myocardial Infarction

Physiologic variable	Presumed mechanism	Potentially applicable intervention
Interruption of triggering mechanism of infarction	Plaque rupture, platelet aggregation, coronary thrombosis	Antiplatelet agents, antihypertensives, beta-blockers, smoking cessation, anticoagulants
Achievement of coronary patency	Mechanical revascularization, spontaneous or thrombolysis-induced recanalization	Thrombolytic agents, antiplatelet agents, anticoagulants, acute revascularization
Reinfarction	Increase in myocardial oxygen demand or reduction in supply, reocclusion of infarct artery or new site of occlusion	Beta-blockers, calcium channel blockers, nitrates, antihypertensives, revascularization, antiplatelet agents, anticoagulants, ACE inhibitors
Sudden death	Ventricular arrhythmia	Beta-blockers, antiarrhythmic agents
Progression of coronary artery disease	Atherosclerosis	Cholesterol-lowering strategies, antihypertensives, smoking cessation, calcium channel blockers, ACE inhibitors, exercise training
Development of congestive heart failure	Ventricular expansion or remodeling	ACE inhibitors, nitrates, antihypertensives, revascularization
Comorbid events	Cardiogenic embolus	Anticoagulants, antiplatelet agents

Table 47-2. Features of Myocardial Infarction Associated with Increased 1-Year Mortality

	Approximate odds ratio
Left ventricular dysfunction	
Ejection fraction < 40%	4.2
Congestion on chest radiograph	0.0
Increased ventricular volume	6.0
Previous infarction	1.8
Residual myocardial ischemia	
Angina before discharge	1.3
Angina on exercise test	2.5
Persistent S–T segment depression on ECG	2.5
Electrical instability, autonomic dysfunction	
More than 10 VPB/hr	2.7
Abnormal signal-averaged ECG	8.0
Diminished heart rate variability	3.8
Occluded infarct artery	2.5

Adapted from Krone RJ: The role of risk stratification in the early management of a myocardial infarction. *Ann Intern Med* 116:223, 1992; Bodenheimer MM: Risk stratification in coronary disease: A contrary viewpoint. *Ann Intern Med* 116:927, 1992; Cigarroa RG, Lange RA, Hills LD: Prognosis after acute myocardial infarction in patients with and without residual anterograde blood flow. *Am J Cardiol* 64:155, 1989; Gheorghiade M, Shivkumar K, Schultz L, et al: Prognostic significance of electrocardiographic persistent ST depression in patients with their first myocardial infarction in the placebo arm of the Beta-Blocker Heart Attack Trial. *Am Heart J* 126:271, 1993; White HD, Norris RM, Brown MA, et al: Left ventricular end-systolic volume as the major determinant of survival after recovery from myocardial infarction. *Circulation* 76:44, 1987.

[10]. Ticlopidine exerts its effect primarily by inhibition of the adenosine diphosphate (ADP) pathway of platelet aggregation [12]. A new strategy, not yet available to clinicians, employs a murine-derived monoclonal antibody Fab fragment, 7E3, directed at the platelet glycoprotein IIb/IIIa receptor [13]. This approach leads to nearly complete platelet inhibition, since binding to IIb/IIIa receptors is the final step in platelet aggregation by any mechanism [14].

The most convincing evidence for the routine use of aspirin during and after MI comes from the results of the Second International Study of Infarct Survival (ISIS-2), in which 17,187 patients with suspected MI were randomized to placebo, aspirin 160 mg per day for 30 days, streptokinase 1.5 million units, or aspirin plus streptokinase. This trial demonstrated a 23 percent reduction in 5-week vascular mortality with aspirin, 25 percent with streptokinase, and 42 percent with the combination of aspirin and streptokinase. The beneficial effect on survival persisted in follow-up analysis (mean 15 months) [15]. These findings are supported by pooled results from smaller trials [16].

Most trials prior to ISIS-2 used 300 to 1500 mg per day of aspirin. Analysis of earlier trials found 900 to 1200 mg per day of aspirin no more effective than 300 to 325 mg per day [16]. Recent trials have shown 75 mg of aspirin per day to be effective in reducing cardiovascular events in patients with angina [17] and those with cerebrovascular ischemic events [18]. In the Dutch TIA trial, 30 mg of aspirin per day was as effective as 283 mg per day in reducing subsequent vascular events in patients with transient ischemic attack or minor ischemic stroke [19]. However, with lower doses (<160 mg) the benefit of aspirin may not be fully achieved for several days [20,21]. It is therefore currently recommended that patients with MI receive 160 to 325 mg of aspirin on hospital admission and 160 to 325 mg daily thereafter.

Ticlopidine was shown to decrease the incidence of MI in an open study of patients with unstable angina [22] and to decrease the incidence of death or recurrent stroke in patients with stroke

or TIA [23]. Post-MI trials have not been conducted; however, ticlopidine, 250 mg given twice per day, might be considered for patients with aspirin allergy or intolerance.

Warfarin therapy is covered in depth in Chapters 43 and 121. In the largest trial of warfarin after MI, there was a 24 percent reduction in mortality and a 34 percent reduction in reinfarction [24], but aspirin was prohibited. Because of the risk of cardioembolic stroke, warfarin should be strongly considered when MI is complicated by atrial fibrillation, extensive anterior wall MI, or left ventricular thrombus or aneurysm [25]. The combination of aspirin and warfarin is largely unstudied, though aspirin (160 mg/day) is being given with or without low-dose warfarin (1 or 3 mg) in the ongoing Coumadin-Aspirin Reinfarction Study.

Early Beta-Adrenergic Blockade

The role of long-term oral administration of beta-adrenergic blocking agents (beta-blockers) for secondary prevention after MI is well established from individual trials and pooled results revealing a 20 to 25 percent reduction in long-term mortality [26].

Early intravenous (IV) beta-blockade in the absence of thrombolytic therapy has been studied in more than 28,000 patients. Pooled data show that its use can reduce short-term mortality by approximately 15 percent [26,27]; therefore, IV beta-blockers should be strongly considered in all patients without contraindications (bradyarrhythmias, conduction disturbances, severe congestive heart failure, bronchospastic airway disease).

Early thrombolytic treatment in combination with IV beta-blockade is appealing, since those agents offer benefit by complementary mechanisms and the peak effects occur at slightly different times during the early clinical course of MI. In the ISIS-1 trial, early intravenous atenolol reduced mortality primarily during the initial 24 to 48 hours of presentation [27]. Review of the GISSI [28] and ISIS-2 [15] trials of IV streptokinase showed an "early hazard" of 20 to 33 percent excess deaths during the first 24 hours, though overall 1-week and 1-month vascular mortality were significantly reduced [29,30]. Furthermore, beta-blockers have been shown to reduce in vitro platelet aggregation [31].

Despite the theoretical appeal of combining thrombolytic agents and IV beta-blockers, few clinical trials have addressed this strategy. The Thrombolysis in Myocardial Infarction (TIMI-2) trial treated 3534 patients with MI presenting within 4 hours from symptom onset with aspirin, intravenous heparin, and t-PA. They were then randomized to angiography (and prophylactic percutaneous transluminal coronary angioplasty (PTCA), where appropriate) within 18 to 48 hours—the invasive strategy—or no angiography in the absence of symptomatic recurrent ischemia occurring either spontaneously or on predischarge exercise testing—the conservative strategy. In 13 of the 20 clinical centers, patients were further eligible for randomization to receive IV metoprolol followed by oral treatment (the immediate group) or to oral metoprolol begun on day 6 (the deferred group).

The primary endpoint of the trial was left ventricular ejection fraction on a predischarge radionuclide angiogram. Secondary endpoints included other parameters of left ventricular function and clinical events. The global ejection fraction at hospital discharge was 51.0 percent in immediately treated patients and 50.1 percent in the deferred metoprolol group, a difference that was not significant. Mortality was nearly identical in the immediate and deferred groups at 6 days, 6 weeks, and 1 year.

Recurrent ischemia and nonfatal MI were reduced in patients receiving immediate intravenous beta-blockade.

The incidence of intracranial hemorrhage was less in the immediate group compared with the deferred group (2 patients and 10 patients, respectively). Of clinical importance, the two events occurring in the immediate beta-blocker groups were among 89 patients who received 150 mg of t-PA. In the deferred group, 5 events occurred in the 97 patients who received 150 mg and 5 occurred in the 617 patients who received 100 mg [32].

In a separate study of 292 patients receiving alteplase and heparin for MI who were subsequently randomized to IV and oral atenolol, IV and oral alinidine, a specific bradycardic agent, or placebo, Van de Werf and colleagues found no difference in the primary endpoint, global and regional ejection fraction [33]. Further, differences were not observed in infarct size or in-hospital events, including death, reinfarction, stroke, and revascularization, although both active treatments were associated with a greater incidence of bradycardia, and an increase in pulmonary edema occurred in patients receiving atenolol.

It has been hypothesized that the increased mortality seen on days 0 to 1 with thrombolytic therapy is due to an excess of left ventricular rupture and intracranial hemorrhage [29]. A meta-analysis of thrombolytic therapy trials has suggested that early treatment, in fact, protects against rupture, and treatment initiated after 7 to 11 hours, while increasing the incidence of rupture, still improves all-cause survival [34]. Intravenous beta-blockers offer the greatest benefit during the first several days after MI and may protect against rupture [35]. Grines et al. [36] showed that among patients receiving thrombolytic therapy (and PTCA, if necessary to achieve early coronary patency), IV metoprolol both improved infarct zone hypokinesis and reduced compensatory hyperkinesis of the noninfarct zone without changing left ventricular ejection fraction or intracavity pressures. In contrast, however, the TIMI-2 study failed to show a difference in rupture between the beta-blocker treatment groups [32].

The combination of thrombolytic therapy and IV beta-blockade is a safe and well-tolerated regimen among patients presenting early with signs and symptoms of MI [32,37]. Insufficient data are available, however, to determine whether the combination lowers mortality beyond that for either agent given alone. Despite this limitation, early beta-blockade should be considered in all eligible patients.

Smoking

Approximately 30 percent of all adults in the United States smoke cigarettes. Many studies have examined the incidence of coronary heart disease (CHD) events and mortality among smokers who have suffered an MI and subsequently discontinued smoking. These studies have demonstrated a dramatic and consistent reduction in CHD mortality—nearly 50 percent among smokers who have been able to quit [38–43]. The design of most studies has been observational and the findings may have been confounded by concurrent behavioral changes in the study population. Still, smoking cessation offers one of the most significant opportunities for secondary prevention of CHD and therefore must be given a high priority.

Admission to the CCU offers a unique opportunity to assist patients with smoking cessation. There is evidence that an organized approach to assist those who wish to quit smoking can achieve cessation rates of 40 to 70 percent [44], far in excess of similar programs for healthy outpatients [45]. Many patients cite the advice of their physicians as the most important factor in their decision to quit smoking [46]. Kottke et al. reviewed trials of smoking cessation methods and concluded that individualized intervention programs utilizing more than one modality and involving both physicians and nonphysicians were most successful [47]. The role of nursing intervention cannot be overemphasized [48].

Patients admitted to the CCU commonly experience anxiety. Smokers may experience several troubling effects from the abrupt cessation of smoking. Nicotine withdrawal includes craving for nicotine, irritability, anxiety, difficulty with concentration, restlessness, increased heart rate, and increased appetite [49]. These signs and symptoms can increase myocardial oxygen demand. We have noted an increased occurrence of sinus tachycardia and arrhythmias among active smokers admitted to the CCU [50].

Treatment of nicotine withdrawal is based on the patient's symptom profile, utilizing supportive care and sedation with benzodiazepines. Nicotine replacement therapy may be dangerous in patients with active myocardial ischemia [51], although some have suggested that it may be used safely [52].

It has been suggested that smokers have a better prognosis after MI than nonsmokers [53]. Closer inspection, however, reveals that as a group, smokers who experience MI are 5 to 7 years younger and have fewer CHD risk factors than nonsmokers. After adjusting for these differences, some studies have demonstrated a worse prognosis for patients who smoke [40,54,55].

When considering magnitude of risk reduction, potential benefit, and side effects for various interventions after MI, smoking cessation may be the most beneficial. Health care providers' recommendations to quit smoking, initiated in the CCU to all patients who smoke and reinforced during cardiac rehabilitation, offer a cost-effective, convenient, safe, and vitally important intervention for the secondary prevention of CHD.

Magnesium

Magnesium has several effects on the myocardium that might be protective following MI. Magnesium antagonizes the effect of calcium at the cellular level and causes both systemic and coronary vasodilation [56,57]. Platelet aggregation and adhesion may be reduced [58]. Magnesium also suppresses some types of ventricular arrhythmias [59] and in experimental animals limits ischemic injury to the myocardium following reperfusion [60].

Several small trials of magnesium administration after MI demonstrated a striking decrease in mortality—nearly 55 percent—by meta-analysis [59,61]. The Second Leicester Intravenous Magnesium Intervention Trial (LIMIT-2) included 2316 and randomized patients to receive magnesium administration or placebo. A 24 percent reduction in 28-day mortality and 25 percent reduction in left ventricular failure were associated with magnesium administration, although the confidence interval for mortality reduction was wide [62].

The Fourth International Study of Infarct Survival (ISIS-4) randomized 58,000 patients to IV magnesium or control [63]. Patients received 8 mM of magnesium sulfate IV over 15 minutes and then 72 mM IV over 24 hours. In contrast to the earlier studies, magnesium administration led to no improvement in 35-day mortality, which was 7.3 percent in magnesium-treated patients versus 6.9 percent in control patients, a difference that was not significant [64]. While IV magnesium was associated with a slight excess of flushing and hypotension, there was no difference in the rates of confirmed infarction, reinfarction, postinfarction angina, ventricular fibrillation, or heart block. Unlike LIMIT-2, which suggested heart failure prevention, congestive heart failure during hospitalization was slightly more prevalent in magnesium-treated patients (17.9% in magnesium vs. 16.6% in control groups). No interaction was seen with captopril or nitrates, the other study medications, nor with aspirin or thrombolytic agents, both of which were used widely.

When the ISIS-4 and LIMIT-2 results were combined, mortality was not significantly affected [64]. The most likely explanation for the discrepancy between the promising meta-analysis and negative "megatrial" is that studies of smaller groups of patients, even when pooled, may still be susceptible to the play of chance. However, some workers have maintained that, given differences in study design between LIMIT-2 and ISIS-4, magnesium may have a role in certain high-risk subgroups [64a,64b].

Angiotensin-Converting Enzyme (ACE) Inhibitors

LEFT VENTRICULAR FUNCTION AND REMODELING AFTER MI. One of the most powerful predictors of death after MI is the extent of left ventricular systolic dysfunction [6] (Table 47-2). The ejection fraction is commonly used to measure left ventricular performance, with 1-year mortality rising precipitously as the left ventricular ejection fraction falls below 40 percent. A more powerful predictor of death, however, is the extent of left ventricular dilation. White and colleagues [65] showed that among patients with MI stratified for left ventricular ejection fraction, a further prognostic discrimination is possible by separating patients with larger ventricles from those with smaller ventricles (Fig. 47-1). Ventricular enlargement occurs after MI by ventricular remodeling [66–71]. Clinical studies have defined both the adaptive and maladaptive processes that reshape the ventricle following an MI. Factors that have been causally linked to ventricular remodeling and dilation include degree of wall stress, presence of trophic growth factors, activation of the sympathetic nervous system, and persistent occlusion of the infarct-related coronary artery [8,71,72]. The extent and timing of ventricular dilation are difficult to predict, but some series have documented progressive changes within the first 10 days after MI [73,74], progressing over the ensuing 6 to 12 months in some patients [69,70,72]. Since ventricular dilation is associated with increased patient morbidity and mortality, considerable interest exists in preventing maladaptive remodeling as a means to improve clinical outcome [67,75].

ANGIOTENSIN-CONVERTING ENZYME INHIBITION AND VENTRICULAR REMODELING. Pfeffer and colleagues laid the groundwork for clinical studies of ACE inhibition after MI [76]. Using a rat model of coronary ligation, they demonstrated that ventricular expansion could be attenuated and mortality reduced in captopril-treated rats. In a pilot study [75], captopril given to patients with asymptomatic left ventricular dysfunction following an anterior infarction led to reduced end-diastolic and end-systolic volumes. This was followed by the Survival and Ventricular Enlargement (SAVE) study, which compared captopril treatment begun 3 to 16 days after MI with placebo in 2200 patients followed for an average of 42 months [77]. Inclusion criteria included an ejection fraction less than 40 percent without signs of ischemia or overt congestive heart failure. Captopril treatment resulted in a 19 percent reduction

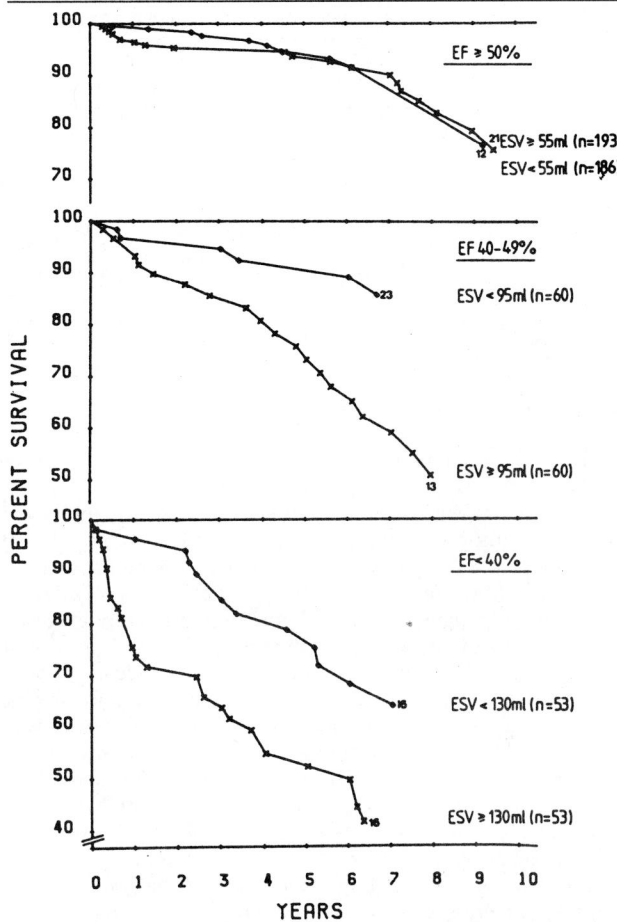

Fig. 47-1. Effect of ventricular size on survival after myocardial infarction. Survival curves are shown for three groups of patients with ejection fractions (EF) > 50% (*top*), 40–49% (*middle*), and < 40% (*bottom*). Patients are further stratified according to end-systolic volume (ESV) of the left ventricle. (From White HD, Norris RM, Brown MA, et al: Left ventricular end-systolic volume as the major determinant of survival after recovery from myocardial infarction. *Circulation* 76:44, 1987. With permission. Copyright 1987 American Heart Association.)

in total mortality, significant reductions in congestive heart failure requiring the addition of open-label ACE inhibitor treatment or hospitalization, and a 25 percent reduction in reinfarction. The latter finding is consistent with observations made in the Studies of Left Ventricular Dysfunction (SOLVD) trials [78] and support the evidence in animal models [79,80] that ACE inhibition may have an antiatherosclerotic effect. The experimental observations of Ridker and colleagues [81] suggest that chronic ACE inhibition may lower endogenous levels of plasminogen activator inhibitor (PAI-1), which has been identified as a potential trigger for coronary arterial thrombosis.

The SAVE study results are similar to those of the Acute Infarction Ramipril Efficacy (AIRE) study, in which ramipril or placebo was given 3 to 10 days after an acute MI to 2006 patients with clinical evidence of heart failure. After an average of 15 months of follow-up study, mortality was reduced 27 percent, as was the combined incidence of death, reinfarction, stroke, or development of severe or resistant heart failure [82].

These two long-term secondary prevention studies beginning at least 3 days after MI are complemented by a set of emerging

Table 47-3. Studies of Angiotensin-Converting Enzyme Inhibitors after Myocardial Infarction

Trial	Publication date	Agent	No. of patients	Initiation of treatment	Duration of treatment	Average follow-up	Mortality reduction	Reinfarction reduction
SAVE	1992	Captopril	2,231	3–16 days	>2 yr	42 mo	19%	25%
AIRE	1993	Ramipril	2,006	3–10 days	15 mo	15 mo	27%	0
CONSENSUS II	1992	Enalapril	6,090	<24 hr	6 mo	6 mo	+10%	0
ISIS-4	*	Captopril	54,824	<24 hr	30 days	35 days	6.3%	0
GISSI-3	1994	Lisinopril	18,895	<24 hr	NA	42 days	12%	0
Chinese study	*	Captopril	11,345	NA	NA	28 days	3.4%	NA

* Preliminary findings, as of November 1993.
NA = Information not available

trials of earlier intervention begun within 24 hours of MI onset and a shorter course of treatment (Table 47-3).

The effects of intravenous followed by oral enalapril were studied in an unselected, and therefore lower-risk, population than that in SAVE or AIRE. The Cooperative Northern Scandinavian Enalapril Survival Study (CONSENSUS-II) enrolled nonhypotensive patients within 24 hours from MI symptom onset [83]. The initial 1 mg dose given intravenously over 2 hours was lengthened to 3 hours and blood pressure exclusions were made stricter when a trend toward a higher mortality among patients with early hypotension was observed. Treatment was to continue for 6 months, but the study was terminated on the recommendation of the Safety and Data Monitoring Committee [84] after a trend toward death persisted in patients with early hypotension despite changes in the protocol, and because benefit was increasingly unlikely to be demonstrated.

The value of early ACE inhibition after MI has been further addressed by the results of two large randomized trials including more than 76,000 patients. In ISIS-4, 58,000 patients were randomized to receive placebo or captopril, at a starting dose of 6.25 mg orally and then increased to 50 mg twice per day as tolerated [63]. The 35-day vascular mortality was significantly less in the captopril group (6.9%) than the placebo group (7.3%), with a reduction of 5 percent [85]. Hypotension was reported more frequently in the captopril group—approximately 10 percent of patients required adjustment or termination of captopril secondary to hypotension—but there was no difference in the rate of reinfarction or the need for revascularization between the two groups [85].

In the Gruppo Italiano per lo Studio della Sopravvivenza nell'Infarto Miocardico study (GISSI-3), 19,000 patients were randomized to receive either lisinopril, 5 mg per day and increased to 10 mg per day at 48 hours (half the dose if systolic blood pressure was less than 120 mm Hg), or placebo. The main outcomes were mortality at 6 weeks and the combined 6-month endpoint of death or severe left ventricular dysfunction. The 6-week mortality was significantly reduced in the lisinopril group (6.3%) compared to the control group (7.1%) [86]. The ISIS-4 investigators presented the pooled preliminary results from the megatrials of early ACE inhibition, including ISIS-4, GISSI-3, and a Chinese study of early captopril. Together, in more than 85,000 patients, early ACE inhibition was shown to lower absolute 28- to 35-day mortality by 5 lives per 1000 patients treated, a modest clinical benefit that was highly statistically significant. Early ACE inhibition was safe and independent of aspirin, thrombolysis, and beta-blockers. The early and late starting trials suggest that ACE inhibition started early is a safe but only modestly effective intervention in the unrestricted MI population. The ACE inhibitors are preferred in patients with extensive MI, heart failure, or left ventricular dysfunction and

have the most impact when continued long-term [77,82] (see Chap. 210).

Nitrates

Nitrates have been used for more than a century in the treatment of angina. Hemodynamic benefits include a reduction in preload and ventricular filling pressures and coronary vasodilatation [87]. Recent evidence supports an antiplatelet effect [88,89,90].

Several small clinical trials performed prior to the widespread use of thrombolytic therapy examined the benefits of nitrate preparations [91–97]. In the majority of studies, intravenous nitroglycerin was given for 48 hours and titrated to reduce mean arterial blood pressure by 10 percent, or up to 30 percent in hypertensive patients. The available evidence suggests that intravenous nitroglycerin reduces ischemic pain and lessens morphine requirements [93].

Early nitrate administration may favorably influence left ventricular architecture and remodeling. In a relatively large trial, Judgutt and Warnica [97] assessed left ventricular size and architecture by echocardiography in 310 MI patients on presentation, prior to randomization to either intravenous nitroglycerin or control. Repeat echocardiography was performed at 10 days. Patients in the control group were shown to have an increase in left ventricular end-diastolic volume, while those allocated to intravenous nitroglycerin had no increase in left ventricular size. The nitroglycerin group also had less infarct expansion and a greater improvement in left ventricular ejection fraction than the control patients. These improved indices of left ventricular function were also accompanied by a lower incidence of congestive heart failure, cardiogenic shock, and death.

Nitroglycerin administration after MI has been studied in two large randomized trials to date. In ISIS-4, a once daily controlled-release mononitrate or placebo was given to 58,000 patients [63]. Intravenous nitroglycerin was permitted in the initial phase of management. The 35-day mortality was 7.0 percent in the nitroglycerin group and 7.2 percent in the placebo group, a difference that was not significant. Similarly, the GISSI-3 trial randomized 19,000 patients to IV and then transdermal nitroglycerin or placebo. The 42-day mortality was 6.5 percent in the nitroglycerin group and 6.9 percent in control patients [86]. Combining the results of ISIS-4 and GISSI-3, there was no survival benefit for the use of nitroglycerin [98].

The negligible effect of prophylactic nitrate administration studied in large trials was a disappointment compared to the promising results of smaller trials and meta-analysis [99–102].

Nitrates can be considered for symptom relief of angina or heart failure (see Chap. 210). Since oral and topical nitrates are safe early in the course of MI [86,98], the expense of an intravenous preparation can be obviated by oral administration in those patients who receive treatment.

Calcium Channel Blockers

Cellular calcium overload has been identified as a final common pathway of cellular injury in MI [103]. This observation, coupled with several promising animal studies, led to the widespread application of calcium channel blockers to reduce infarction size, lower mortality, and reduce reinfarction in MI patients.

The available agents are grouped according to chemical structure. Although all agents bind to the L-type calcium channel in the sarcolemmal membrane, the agents differ with respect to pharmacokinetics, affinity for the open state of the channel, lipophilicity, and tissue specificity (see Chap. 210). Clinical manifestations of these different properties include variations in the extent of negative inotropism, sinus rate slowing, atrioventricular conduction block, coronary vasodilatation, and peripheral vasodilatation with accompanying reflex sympathetic activation [104].

NIFEDIPINE AND DIHYDROPYRIDINES. A number of trials have examined the effect of nifedipine in patients with acute or threatened MI [105–113]. A consistent finding was the overall lack of benefit; in fact, several studies revealed evidence of harm [109,112]. Adverse effects included a trend toward higher reinfarction rates as well as higher mortality (Fig. 47-2). These effects were termed "proischemic" by Waters and have been

Fig. 47-2. Comparative effects of several agents on death and reinfarction after myocardial infarction. Odds ratios of death (*top*) and reinfarction (*bottom*) following treatment with several agents for secondary prevention. Strength of evidence is estimated qualitatively from the size of the populations studied, consistency across studies, and quality of trials. (Data derived from Yusuf et al. [26,78,125], Pfeffer et al. [77], Held et al. [126].)

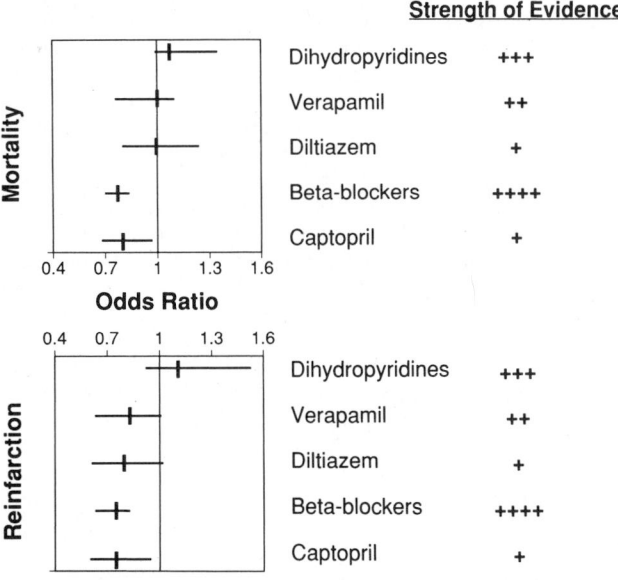

seen in nifedipine trials of unstable angina as well as in nicardipine studies designed to examine the potential antiatherosclerotic effect of the drug on coronary disease progression [114].

One leading hypothesis to explain the adverse effects of dihydropyridines is that their potent peripheral vasodilatory properties simultaneously reduce coronary perfusion pressure and trigger reflex catecholamine release [114]. In support of this hypothesis are findings from the Holland Interuniversity Nifedipine Trial [105], in which nifedipine and metoprolol alone and in combination were given to patients with unstable angina. Nifedipine alone was associated with a trend toward higher event rates, while the combination tended to lower events to the same degree as metoprolol alone. In patients already receiving a beta-blocker, the addition of nifedipine reduced the incidence of recurrent ischemia or infarction. Some investigators have argued that a sustained-release formulation of nifedipine, which leads to a more gradual onset of drug effect, might obviate harm [115], but these preparations have not been investigated in patients with unstable coronary syndromes.

VERAPAMIL AND DILTIAZEM. These agents tend to depress atrioventricular nodal conduction and sinus node activity to a greater degree than dihydropyridines [104] and are considered rate-slowing. At recommended doses, most investigators have also found a more potent negative inotropic effect.

Two major and several minor studies have examined the effect of verapamil on secondary prevention following MI. In the first Danish Verapamil Trial (DAVIT-I) [116], 3498 patients with suspected MI and without severe heart failure, conduction block, or prior beta-blocker or calcium blocker use were randomized to intravenous followed by oral verapamil or matched placebo for 6 months. For patients in whom MI was excluded, treatment was stopped. Therefore, 1436 patients were included in the final analyses. Mortality was 12.8 percent in the verapamil group and 13.9 percent in the placebo group. Seven percent of verapamil-treated patients and 8.3 percent of placebo-treated patients experienced reinfarction. These differences were not statistically significant.

In a subsequent trial (DAVIT-II) [117], 1775 patients with confirmed MI were randomized between 7 and 15 days after presentation to verapamil or placebo, using inclusion and exclusion criteria similar to those in DAVIT-I. Treatment was continued for a mean of 16 months. Eighteen-month mortality was not significantly reduced by verapamil (11.1% vs. 13.8%, respectively), nor was reinfarction significantly lowered (11.0% vs. 13.2%, respectively). The pooled results from these and several smaller studies are shown in Figure 47-2.

The Multicenter Diltiazem Postinfarction Trial (MDPIT) [118] randomized 2466 patients within 3 to 15 days after MI to diltiazem or placebo. The average length of follow-up study was 25 months. Unlike the Danish verapamil trials, beta-blockers were permitted and administered to just over half of patients. Mortality was 13.5 percent in both groups. Nonfatal reinfarction was 8.0 percent in diltiazem-treated patients and 9.4 percent in placebo-treated patients, a difference that failed to reach statistical significance. The Diltiazem Reinfarction Study [119] was the only acute treatment and secondary prevention trial to limit enrollment to patients with non-Q wave MI, a subset of MI patients expected to have a similar long-term mortality but a higher reinfarction rate than patients with Q wave infarctions. In this study, 576 patients received diltiazem (90 mg three times daily) or placebo within 72 hours of admission and continued treatment for up to 14 days or to hospital discharge. Nearly two-thirds of patients received beta-blockers. Reinfarction at 2 weeks, defined by a reelevation in surveillance creatine kinase measurements (the primary endpoint), was 9.3 percent in the placebo group and 5.2 percent in diltiazem-treated patients, a statistically significant reduction by a one-tailed test of significance. Mortality was 3.8 percent in the diltiazem group and 3.1 percent in the placebo group, a difference that was not significant (Fig. 47-2).

CALCIUM BLOCKERS AND SUBSET ANALYSES. A consistent finding, particularly in studies including rate-slowing calcium channel antagonists, has been the increased incidence of clinical congestive heart failure [116,117,118]. Thus, the benefit of calcium blockers after MI appears to be limited to a lower-risk subset of patients in whom signs or symptoms of congestive heart failure are not present. This observation is in contrast to beta-adrenergic blockers, where the effect on late mortality, and particularly sudden death, is greater in the setting of heart failure [120].

Some investigators have argued for the use of rate-slowing calcium channel antagonists after non-Q wave MI [121]. Patients with non-Q wave MI included in the Diltiazem Reinfarction Study, as well as those included in MDPIT and DAVIT-II, were recently analyzed [122]. A pooled analysis supports a reduction in reinfarction without a significant impact on mortality. Fewer data are available on patients with non-Q wave MI participating in beta-blocker trials [121,123]. All subset analyses, however, must be interpreted cautiously, since post hoc conclusions are more susceptible to the play of chance than are prospectively defined (prespecified) hypotheses [124].

Nifedipine and other dihydropyridines are associated with an increased risk of infarction and death, particularly when they are used without prior beta-blockade [105] or during periods of active ischemia [114]. Rate-slowing agents may approach the efficacy of beta-blockers in reducing reinfarction, but they do not offer the benefit of beta-blockers in lowering patient mortality [124,125,126]. Overall, rate-slowing calcium channel antagonists should not be used in the presence of overt heart failure or subclinical left ventricular dysfunction.

Antiarrhythmic Drugs and Devices

Ventricular arrhythmias are frequently seen in patients with decreased left ventricular function after MI and contribute independently to the increased risk of overall mortality and sudden cardiac death [6,127]. This observation has led to trials of antiarrhythmic agents to suppress both benign and symptomatic ventricular arrhythmias in an attempt to decrease sudden death after MI. The results, compiled by Teo et al. [128] and other investigators [129], reveal several interesting findings.

Class I antiarrhythmics are associated with an increased mortality. The Cardiac Arrhythmia Suppression Trial (CAST) demonstrated an increased mortality with class IC antiarrhythmics compared to placebo. This trial had a substantial impact on clinical practice, since it directly challenged the assumption that suppression of premature ventricular contractions decreases the likelihood of sudden death [130,131].

Beta-blockers, class II antiarrhythmic agents, are discussed in a previous section. One of the primary benefits of beta-blocker therapy after MI is its ability to reduce ventricular arrhythmias and sudden cardiac death [26], particularly among high-risk patients [120].

Recent trials with amiodarone, an agent with primarily class III antiarrhythmic properties, offer promising results [129]. Ceremuzynski et al. [132] studied the effect of amiodarone administration in patients who were ineligible for beta-blockers. The

1-year cardiac mortality was reduced from 10.7 percent in the placebo group to 6.9 percent in the amiodarone group. A Swiss study included survivors of MI with ventricular arrhythmias and randomized them to receive individualized therapy, amiodarone (200 mg/day), or placebo. The 1-year mortality was 10 percent in the individualized therapy group, 5 percent in the amiodarone group, and 13 percent in the placebo group [133]. The benefit appeared to persist despite discontinuation of the study drugs at 1 year [134]. The Canadian Amiodarone Myocardial Infarction Trial (CAMIAT) pilot study demonstrated an acceptable side effect profile with amiodarone therapy and a trend toward reduced arrhythmic deaths and all causes of mortality [135]. The CAMIAT study is continuing, as is a European trial. An investigation of another class III agent, D-sotalol, has been halted because of increased mortality in the treatment group [135a].

Several studies are underway to examine the effect of prophylactic implantable cardioverter-defibrillators on mortality among patients with coronary disease who may have sustained an MI. These include the Multicenter Automatic Defibrillator Intervention Trial (MADIT) in patients with decreased ejection fraction, the Multicenter Unsustained Tachycardia Trial (MUSTT) in patients with decreased ejection fraction and non-sustained ventricular tachycardia unresponsive to drug treatment, and the Coronary Artery Bypass Grafting Patch (CABG Patch) trial in patients with decreased ejection fraction undergoing bypass surgery.

Beta-adrenergic blockers are considered the first line treatment of high-risk patients after MI. Because of potential proarrhythmic effects and toxicity, conventional antiarrhythmic agents should be reserved at present for patients who demonstrate sustained or symptomatic ventricular arrhythmias prior to hospital discharge.

Antihypertensive Treatment

Hypertension is associated with increased risk of coronary heart disease, cerebrovascular disease, left ventricular hypertrophy, congestive heart failure, and renal failure [137,138]. There are no trials of antihypertensive therapy for secondary prevention of MI, and most primary prevention trials selectively excluded patients with known coronary disease.

Data from primary prevention trials demonstrate the value of antihypertensive therapy for prevention of cerebrovascular disease, with a consistent reduction in stroke of about 40 percent [137]. Most studies have shown small (10%) reductions in coronary heart disease incidence [138,139]. Recent studies that have included elderly patients, a population at higher risk for MI, support the value of antihypertensive therapy in the reduction of cardiac-related and total mortality [136,140,141]. Despite several adverse metabolic side effects of diuretics (increased cholesterol, decreased potassium) and beta-blockers (increased triglycerides, glucose intolerance), these agents have been endorsed as first-line therapy because of considerable data supporting a mortality reduction [142].

Some investigators have reported increased mortality with low diastolic pressure (the J-shaped curve), particularly in patients with preexisting heart disease when diastolic pressure is lowered below 85 mm Hg [143,144,145]. There is considerable debate over the existence and clinical significance of this observation.

The selection of an antihypertensive regimen in patients after MI should be individualized. beta-blockers and ACE inhibitors, as discussed previously, reduce mortality and should therefore be considered in all patients without contraindications.

Cholesterol-Lowering Strategies

Elevated total cholesterol, elevated low-density lipoprotein (LDL) cholesterol, and decreased high-density lipoprotein (HDL) cholesterol are associated with an increased risk of coronary heart disease [146,147,148]. After MI, elevated cholesterol levels are strongly associated with recurrent cardiac events [149] and cardiovascular mortality [150,151,152]. Several studies have demonstrated that lowering cholesterol by behavioral intervention, drug therapy, or a combination can retard and even reverse progression of atherosclerotic plaques seen on angiography in both native arteries [153,154] and bypass grafts [155].

Ornish and colleagues provided a program of life-style change incorporating a low-fat vegetarian diet, smoking cessation, stress management training, and moderate exercise. Twenty-eight patients enrolled in a life-style change program had a regression in average percent stenosis at 1 year compared with baseline, while 20 control patients had a progression [153]. In motivated, compliant patients, a multiple intervention approach may offer an alternative to coronary revascularization [153].

Rossouw et al. reviewed several secondary prevention trials of cholesterol lowering [151]. The combined results demonstrated a 22 percent reduction in total reinfarction and a 9 percent reduction in mortality. Although pooled data have shown a limited impact on total mortality due to an increase in accidental and violent deaths offsetting reduction in coronary heart disease death [151], Smith and others have shown that treatment causes a net benefit when expected mortality is at least 30 deaths per 1000 person-years (i.e., a high-risk population) [152]. Many, but not all, MI patients fall into this category. Recent National Cholesterol Education Program II guidelines recommend a lower optimum LDL cholesterol level in patients with documented coronary disease than in individuals without coronary disease [156].

The first study to evaluate the effect on mortality of a newer class of cholesterol-lowering agents, the HMG Co-A reductase inhibitors, has just been completed. In the Scandinavian Simvastatin Survival Study (4S) patients with coronary disease, documented by previous myocardial infarction or angina pectoris, were randomized to either simvastatin or placebo in addition to a low-fat diet. In a mean follow-up of 5.4 years, total mortality was reduced 30 percent, cardiovascular deaths were reduced 42 percent, and there was a 34 percent reduction in cardiovascular events [152a].

Total cholesterol, LDL cholesterol, and HDL cholesterol have been shown to decrease in the days following an MI. Several studies have demonstrated that cholesterol levels in the first 24 hours do not differ significantly from preinfarction levels [157] or from levels at 3 to 4 months after infarction [158,159]. Thus, levels obtained in the first 24 hours after acute MI may be utilized to assess a patient's cholesterol level, which may prevent delay in instituting appropriate therapy.

Cardiac Rehabilitation

As recently as the 1960s, some patients with MI were kept in the hospital with limited activity for 3 to 6 weeks. This practice was based on early pathologic descriptions of infarct evolution from initial ischemic damage to scar formation [160,161]. As early as the 1940s, however, physicians began recognizing the adverse physiologic and psychologic effects of prolonged bed rest; as a result, a trend toward early mobilization began [162–165].

Current therapy of patients with MI includes commode privileges on the first or second CCU day, progressing gradually to ambulation upon CCU discharge and performance of tasks simulating those required at home prior to hospital discharge [166]. Cardiac rehabilitation programs have evolved from primary emphasis on exercise training to programs that emphasize reduction in coronary disease risk factors, including smoking cessation, exercise, nutritional counseling, and psychosocial support [161,167].

Most trials of cardiac rehabilitation have been either too small or of insufficient duration to allow statistical evaluation of benefit, but pooled data support a 20 percent reduction in mortality associated with cardiac rehabilitation. An increase in nonfatal reinfarction, not statistically significant, was also noted, stressing the importance of close monitoring [166,168,169].

Patients at high risk for complications of exercise training include those with unstable angina or ischemia demonstrated by electrocardiographic changes at low-level stress testing and, in one study, patients who exceeded their prescribed exercise heart rate [167,170,171]. Jugdutt et al. observed that in six patients with extensive anterior myocardial infarctions, exercise training was accompanied by infarct expansion and deterioration in ventricular function, compared to a nonrandomized control group not undergoing training [172]. However, another group examining 49 patients randomized to exercise training or control found similar changes in left ventricular function determined echocardiographically [173].

The available evidence supports early mobilization and ambulation after MI, with further benefit to those enrolled in a program of cardiac rehabilitation. Patients at high risk for complications of exercise training require individual assessment of potential risks and benefits.

Estrogen

Estrogen is believed to prevent coronary disease by mediating a favorable change in serum lipids (increased HDL, reduced LDL). It may also reduce vasomotor tone and decrease platelet aggregation [174,175]. Epidemiologic studies have suggested a 40 to 50 percent reduction in risk of CHD in general populations with estrogen therapy [176,177]. Three observational studies examined the effect of postmenopausal estrogen replacement therapy on angiographically defined coronary artery stenosis. All three found that estrogen therapy was associated with less severe coronary artery disease [178,179,180].

In addition to its effect on coronary disease, postmenopausal estrogen replacement therapy reduces the risk of osteoporosis and hip fracture and decreases the symptoms associated with menopause. However, it may also increase the risk of endometrial cancer and possibly breast cancer [181]. Using the existing primary prevention data, Goldman and Tosteson concluded that although the relative risk reduction in coronary disease was about 40 percent, compared with a sixfold increase in the relative risk of endometrial cancer, the calculated change in mortality was nil: the effect on absolute risk was similar in magnitude and in opposite directions, since coronary disease has a higher fatality rate [182]. A similar balance was seen with estrogen's prevention of lethal hip fracture and promotion of death from breast cancer. An important limitation to this analysis is the absence of randomized data [182]. Furthermore, after an MI, the effect of estrogen therapy may have a greater impact on subsequent cardiovascular death than in a primary prevention setting.

The addition of progestin to estrogen may reduce the chance of endometrial cancer but could obviate cardiovascular benefit as well [182]. Among women who have had a hysterectomy, the balance would favor a greater benefit.

Estrogen replacement has great potential for reducing coronary disease death, but widespread recommendations must await the results of prospective, randomized trials.

Conclusions

A tremendous number of effective agents are available to lower risk after MI, and the selection changes continuously as meta-analyses and mega-trials are completed. The recent failure of large trials to confirm promising meta-analyses of magnesium and nitrates demonstrates the incomplete nature of mechanistic and physiologic trials in predicting the ultimate effect of interventions on survival. While the allure of statistical power is compelling, not all agents are right for all patients. The most rational approach considers the patient's expected risk, concomitant therapy, and other individualized concerns to derive the best treatment or combination of treatments. It must be remembered that more is not necessarily better, and that the interaction of multiple effective agents is the least well-studied aspect of post-MI management [183].

References

1. Antman EM, Lau J, Kupelnick B, et al: A comparison of results of meta-analyses of randomized control trials and recommendations of clinical experts. *JAMA* 268:240, 1992.
2. Moss AJ, Benhorin J: Prognosis and management after a first myocardial infarction. *N Engl J Med* 322:743, 1990.
3. O'Rourke RA: Risk stratification after myocardial infarction. *Circulation* 84(suppl I):I-177, 1991.
4. Krone RJ: The role of risk stratification in the early management of a myocardial infarction. *Ann Intern Med* 116:223, 1992.
5. Bodenheimer MM: Risk stratification in coronary disease: A contrary viewpoint. *Ann Intern Med* 116:927, 1992.
6. Bigger JT, Fleiss JL, Kleiger R, et al and the Multicenter Post-Infarction Research Group: The relationships among ventricular arrhythmias, left ventricular dysfunction, and mortality in the 2 years after myocardial infarction. *Circulation* 69:250, 1984.
7. Kleiger RE, Miller JP, Bigger JT, Moss AJ, and the Multicenter Post-Infarction Research Group: Decreased heart rate variability and its association with increased mortality after acute myocardial infarction. *Am J Cardiol* 59:256, 1987.
8. Cigarroa RG, Lange RA, Hills LD: Prognosis after acute myocardial infarction in patients with and without residual anterograde coronary blood flow. *Am J Cardiol* 64:155, 1989.
9. Gheorghiade M, Shivkumar K, Schultz L, et al: Prognostic significance of electrocardiographic persistent ST depression in patients with their first myocardial infarction in the placebo arm of the Beta-Blocker Heart Attack Trial. *Am Heart J* 126:271, 1993.
10. Moncada S, Vane JR: Arachidonic acid metabolites and interactions between platelets and blood vessel walls. *N Engl J Med* 300:1142, 1979.
11. Forrester JS, Litvack F, Grundfest W, Hickey A: A perspective of coronary disease seen through the arteries of living man. *Circulation* 75:505, 1987.
12. McTavish D, Faulds D, Goa KL: Ticlopidine: An updated review of its pharmacology and therapeutic use in platelet-dependent disorders. *Drugs* 40:238, 1990.
13. Kleiman NS, Ohman EM, Califf RM, et al: Profound inhibition of platelet aggregation with monoclonal antibody 7E3 Fab after thrombolytic therapy: Results of the Thrombolysis and Angioplasty in Myocardial Infarction (TAMI) 8 pilot study. *J Am Coll Cardiol* 22:381, 1993.
14. Weiss HJ, Hawiger J, Ruggeri ZM, et al: Fibrinogen-independent platelet adhesion and thrombus formation on subendothelium mediated by glycoprotein IIb-IIIa complex at high shear rate. *J Clin Invest* 83:288, 1989.
15. ISIS-2 Collaborative Group: Randomized trial of intravenous streptokinase, oral aspirin, both, or neither among 17,187 cases of suspected acute myocardial infarction: ISIS-2. *Lancet* 2:349, 1988.
16. Antiplatelet Trialists' Collaboration: Secondary prevention of vascular disease by prolonged antiplatelet treatment. *Br Med J* 296:320, 1988.
17. Juul-Moller S, Edvardsson N, Jahnmatz B, et al: Double-blind trial of aspirin in primary prevention of myocardial infarction in patients with stable chronic angina pectoris. *Lancet* 340:1421, 1992.
18. SALT Collaborative Group: Swedish Aspirin Low-Dose Trial (SALT) of 75 mg aspirin as secondary prophylaxis after cerebrovascular ischemic events. *Lancet* 338:1345, 1991.
19. Dutch TIA Trial Study Group: A comparison of two doses of aspirin (30 mg vs. 283 mg a day) in patients after a transient ischemic attack of minor ischemic stroke. *N Engl J Med* 325:1261, 1991.
20. Patrignani P, Filabozzi P, Patrono C: Selective cumulative inhibition of platelet thromboxane production by low-dose aspirin in healthy subjects. *J Clin Invest* 69:1366, 1982.
21. Reilly I, FitzGerald GA: Inhibition of thromboxane formation in vivo and ex vivo: Implications for therapy with platelet inhibitory drugs. *Blood* 69:180, 1987.
22. Balsano F, Rizzon P, Violi F, et al: Antiplatelet treatment with ticlopidine in unstable angina. *Circulation* 82:17, 1990.
23. Hass WK, Easton JD, Adams HP, et al: A randomized trial comparing ticlopidine hydrochloride with aspirin for the prevention of stroke in high risk patients. *N Engl J Med* 321:501, 1989.
24. Smith P, Arnesen H, Holme I, et al: The effect of warfarin on mortality and reinfarction after myocardial infarction. *N Engl J Med* 323:147, 1990.
25. Cairns JA, Hirsh J, Lewis HD, et al: Antithrombotic agents in coronary artery disease. *Chest* 102:456S, 1992.
26. Yusuf S, Peto R, Lewis J, et al: Beta blockade during and after myocardial infarction: An overview of the randomized trials. *Prog Cardiovasc Dis* 27:335, 1985.
27. ISIS-1 (First International Study of Infarct Survival) Collaborative Group: Randomised trial of intravenous atenolol among 16 027 cases of suspected acute myocardial infarction: ISIS-1. *Lancet* 2:57, 1986.
28. Mauri F, DeBiase AM, Franzosi MG, et al: G.I.S.S.I.: Analisi delle cause di morte intraospedaliera. *G Ital Cardiol* 17:37, 1987.
29. Popma JJ, Topol EJ: Adjuncts to thrombolysis for myocardial reperfusion. *Ann Intern Med* 115:34, 1991.
30. Baigent C, for the Fibrinolytic Therapy Trialists' Collaboration: Late benefit and early hazard associated with fibrinolytic therapy for acute myocardial infarction: Results from six large randomized controlled trials (abstract). *Circulation* 86(suppl I):I-643, 1992.
31. Hjemdahl P, Larsson PT, Wallen NH: Effects of stress and β-blockade on platelet function. *Circulation* 84(suppl VI):44, 1991.
32. Roberts R, Rogers WL, Mueller HS, et al: Immediate versus deferred β-blockade following thrombolytic therapy in patients with acute myocardial infarction. *Circulation* 83:422, 1991.
33. Van de Werf F, Janssens L, Brzostek T, et al: Short-term effects of early intravenous treatment with a beta-adrenergic blocking agent or a specific bradycardiac agent in patients with acute myocardial infarction receiving thrombolytic therapy. *J Am Coll Cardiol* 22:407, 1993.
34. Honan MB, Harrell FE, Reimer KA, et al: Cardiac rupture, mortality and the timing of thrombolytic therapy: A meta-analysis. *J Am Coll Cardiol* 16:359, 1990.
35. ISIS-1 (First International Study of Infarct Survival) Collaborative Group: Mechanisms for the early mortality reduction produced by beta-blockade started early in acute myocardial infarction: ISIS-1. *Lancet* 2:921, 1988.
36. Grines C, Booth DC, Nissen SE, et al: Acute effects of parenteral beta-blockade on regional ventricular function of infarct and non-infarct zones after reperfusion therapy in humans. *J Am Coll Cardiol* 17:1382, 1991.
37. Vlay SC, Lawson WE: The safety of combined thrombolysis and β-adrenergic blockade in patients with acute myocardial infarction: A randomized study. *Chest* 93:716, 1988.
38. Sparrow D, Dawber TR: The influence of cigarette smoking on prognosis after a first myocardial infarction. *J Chron Dis* 31:425, 1978.

39. Gordon T, Kannel WB, McGee D: Death and coronary attacks in men after giving up cigarette smoking. *Lancet* 2:1345, 1974.

40. Ronnevik PK, Gundersen T, Abrahamsen AM: Effect of smoking habits and timolol treatment on mortality and reinfarction in patients surviving acute myocardial infarction. *Br Heart J* 54:134, 1985.

41. Wilhelmsson C, Vedin JA, Elmfeldt D, et al: Smoking and myocardial infarction. *Lancet* 1:415, 1975.

42. Aberg A, Bergstrand R, Johansson S, et al: Cessation of smoking after myocardial infarction: Effects on mortality after 10 years. *Br Heart J* 49:416, 1983.

43. Salonen J: Stopping smoking and long-term mortality after acute myocardial infarction. *Br Heart J* 43:463, 1980.

44. Tullio MD, Granata D, Taioli E, et al: Early predictors of smoking cessation after myocardial infarction. *Clin Cardiol* 14:809, 1991.

45. Fiore MC, Jorenby DE, Baller TB, Kenford SL: Tobacco dependence and the nicotine patch: Clinical guidelines for effective use. *JAMA* 268:2687, 1992.

46. Russel MA, Wilson C, Taylor C, Baker CD: Effect of general practitioners' advice against smoking. *Br Med J* 2:231, 1979.

47. Kottke TE, Battista RN, DeFriese GH, Brekke ML: Attributes of successful smoking cessation interventions in medical practice. *JAMA* 259:2883, 1988.

48. Taylor CB, Houston-Miller N, Killen JD, DeBusk RF: Smoking cessation after acute myocardial infarction: Effects of a nurse-managed intervention. *Ann Intern Med* 113:118, 1990.

49. American Psychiatric Association: *Diagnostic and Statistical Manual of Mental Disorders.* 3rd ed. Washington, D.C.: American Psychiatric Association, 1987, pp 150–151.

50. Borzak S, Havstad S, Ketterer M, Joseph C: Effect of smoking or smoking withdrawal or complications of myocardial infarction (abstract). *Chest* 104(suppl):1S, 1993.

51. Fiore MC, Jorenby DE, Baker TB, Kenford SL: Tobacco dependence and the nicotine patch. *JAMA* 268:2687, 1992.

52. Benowitz NL: Smoking-induced coronary vasoconstriction: Implications for therapeutic use of nicotine (editorial). *J Am Coll Cardiol* 22:648, 1993.

53. Mueller HS, Cohen LS, Braunwald E, et al: Predictors of early morbidity and mortality after thrombolytic therapy of acute myocardial infarction. *Circulation* 85:1254, 1992.

54. Jafri SM, Tilley BC, Peters R, et al: Effects of cigarette smoking and propranolol in survivors of acute myocardial infarction. *Am J Cardiol* 65:271, 1990.

55. Kelly TL, Gilpin E, Ahnve S, et al: Smoking status at the time of acute myocardial infarction and subsequent prognosis. *Am Heart J* 110:535, 1985.

56. Altura BM, Altura BT: Magnesium, electrolyte transport and coronary tone. *Drugs* 28 (suppl 1):120, 1984.

57. Turlapaty PDMV, Altura BM: Magnesium deficiency produces spasms of coronary arteries: Relationship to etiology of sudden death ischemic heart disease. *Science* 208:198, 1980.

58. Adams JH, Mitchell JRA: The effect of agents which modify platelet behavior and of magnesium ions on thrombus formation in vivo. *Thromb Haemost* 42:603, 1979.

59. Horner SM: Efficacy of intravenous magnesium in acute myocardial infarction in reducing arrhythmias and mortality: Meta-analysis of magnesium in acute myocardial infarction. *Circulation* 86:774, 1992.

60. Borchgrevink PC, Bergan AS, Bakoy OE, Jynge P: Magnesium and reperfusion of ischemic rate heart as assessed by ^{31}P-NMR. *Am J Physiol* 256:H195, 1989.

61. Teo KK, Yusuf S, Collins R, et al: Effects of intravenous magnesium in suspected acute myocardial infarction: Overview of randomised trials. *Br Med J* 303:1499, 1991.

62. Woods KL, Fletcher S, Roffe C, Haider Y: Intravenous magnesium sulphate in suspected acute myocardial infarction: Results of the Second Leicester Intravenous Magnesium Intervention Trial (LIMIT-2). *Lancet* 339:1553, 1992.

63. ISIS-4 Collaborative Group: Fourth International Study of Infarct Survival: Protocol for a large, simple study of the effects of oral mononitrate, oral captopril, and intravenous magnesium. *Am J Cardiol* 68:87D, 1991.

64. ISIS-4 Collaborate Group: Randomized study of intravenous magnesium in over 50,000 patients with suspected acute myocardial infarction (abstract). *Circulation* 88(suppl I):I-242, 1993.

64a. Shechter M, Hod H, Chouragin P, et al: Magnesium therapy in acute myocardial infarction when patients are not candidates for thrombolytic therapy. *Am J Cardiol* 75:321, 1995.

64b. Autman EM: Randomized trials of magnesium in acute myocardial infarction: Big numbers do not tell the whole story (editorial). *Am J Cardiol* 75:391, 1995.

65. White HD, Norris RM, Brown MA, et al: Left ventricular end-systolic volume as the major determinant of survival after recovery from myocardial infarction. *Circulation* 76:44, 1987.

66. Hutchins GM, Bulkley BH: Infarct expansion versus extension: Two different complications of acute myocardial infarction. *Am J Cardiol* 41:1127, 1978.

67. McKay RG, Pfeffer MA, Pasternak RC, et al: Left ventricular remodeling after myocardial infarction: A corollary to infarct expansion. *Circulation* 74:693, 1986.

68. Picard MH, Wilkins GT, Ray PA, Weyman AE: Natural history of left ventricular size and function after acute myocardial infarction. *Circulation* 82:484, 1990.

69. Gaudron P, Eilles C, Kugler I, Ertl G: Progressive left ventricular dysfunction and remodeling after myocardial infarction. *Circulation* 87:755, 1993.

70. Jeremy RW, Allman KC, Bautovitch G, Harris PJ: Patterns of left ventricular dilation during the six months after myocardial infarction. *J Am Coll Cardiol* 13:304, 1989.

71. Pfeffer MA, Pfeffer JM, Lamas GA: Development and prevention of congestive heart failure following myocardial infarction. *Circulation* 87:IV-120, 1993.

72. Warren SE, Royal HD, Markis JE, et al: Time course of left ventricular dilation after myocardial infarction: Influence of infarct-related artery and success of coronary thrombolysis. *J Am Coll Cardiol* 11:12, 1988.

73. Sharpe N, Murphy J, Smith H, Hannan S: Treatment of patients with symptomatic left ventricular dysfunction after myocardial infarction. *Lancet* 1:255, 1988.

74. Sharpe N, Smith H, Murphy J, et al: Early prevention of left ventricular dysfunction after myocardial infarction with angiotensin-converting-enzyme inhibition. *Lancet* 337:872, 1991.

75. Pfeffer MA, Lamas GA, Vaughan DE, et al: Effect of captopril on progressive ventricular dilatation after anterior myocardial infarction. *N Engl J Med* 319:80, 1988.

76. Pfeffer JM, Pfeffer MA, Braunwald E: Influence of chronic captopril therapy on the infarcted left ventricle of the rat. *Circ Res* 57:84, 1985.

77. Pfeffer MA, Braunwald E, Moye LA, et al on Behalf of the SAVE Investigators: Effects of captopril on mortality and morbidity in patients with left ventricular dysfunction after myocardial infarction. *N Engl J Med* 327:669, 1992.

78. Yusuf S, Pepine CJ, Garces C, et al: Effect of enalapril on myocardial infarction and unstable angina in patients with low ejection fractions. *Lancet* 340:1173, 1992.

79. Chobanian AV, Haudenschild CC, Nickerson C, Drago R: Antiatherogenic effect of captopril in the Watanabe heritable hyperlipidemic rabbit. *Hypertension* 15:327, 1990.

80. Aberg G, Ferrer P: Effects of captopril on atherosclerosis in cynomolgus monkeys. *J Cardiovasc Pharmacol* 15:565, 1990.

81. Ridker PM, Gaboury CL, Conlin PR, et al: Stimulation of plasminogen activator inhibitor in vivo by infusion of angiotensin II. *Circulation* 87:1969, 1993.

82. The Acute Infarction Ramipril Efficacy (AIRE) Study Investigators: Effect of ramipril on mortality and morbidity of survivors of acute myocardial infarction with clinical evidence of heart failure. *Lancet* 342:821, 1993.

83. Swedberg K, Held P, Kjekshus J, et al on Behalf of the CONSENSUS II Study Group: Effects of the early administration of enalapril on mortality in patients with acute myocardial infarction. *N Engl J Med* 327:678, 1992.

84. Furberg CD, Campbell RWF, Pitt B: CONSENSUS II study (letter). *N Engl J Med* 328:967, 1993.

85. ISIS-4 Collaborative Group: ISIS-4: Randomized study of oral captopril in over 50,000 patients with suspected acute myocardial infarction (abstract). *Circulation* 83(supp I):I-394, 1993.

86. Tagnoni G, for the GISSI-3 Investigators: Lisinopril and nitrates after acute myocardial infarction: Introduction and results–GISSI-3. Presented at the 66th Scientific Sessions of the American Heart Association, Atlanta, November 1993.

87. McGregor M: The nitrates and myocardial ischemia. *Circulation* 66:689, 1982.

88. Stamler JS, Loscalzo J: The antiplatelet effects of organic nitrates and related nitroso compounds in vitro and in vivo and their relevance to cardiovascular disorders. *J Am Coll Cardiol* 18:1529, 1991.

89. Stamler J, Cunningham M, Loscalzo J: Reduced thiols and the effect of intravenous nitroglycerin on platelet aggregation. *Am J Cardiol* 62:377, 1988.

90. Diodati J, Theroux P, Latour J-G, et al: Effects of nitroglycerin at therapeutic doses on platelet aggregation in unstable angina pectoris and acute myocardial infarction. *Am J Cardiol* 66:683, 1990.

91. Lis Y, Bennett D, Lambert G, Robson D: A preliminary double-blind study of intravenous nitroglycerin in acute myocardial infarction. *Intensive Care Med* 10:179, 1984.

92. Flaherty JT, Becker LC, Bulkley BH, et al: A randomized prospective trial of intravenous nitroglycerin in patients with acute myocardial infarction. *Circulation* 68:576, 1983.

93. Bussmann W-D, Passek D, Seidel W, Kaltenbach M: Reduction of CK and CK-MB indexes of infarct size by intravenous nitroglycerin. *Circulation* 63:615, 1981.

94. Chiche P, Baligadoo SJ, Derrida JP: A randomised trial of prolonged nitroglycerin infusion in acute myocardial infarction (abstract). *Circulation* 60(suppl II):11, 1979.

95. Jaffee AS, Geltman EM, Tiefenbrunn AJ, et al: Reduction of infarct size in patients with inferior infarction with intravenous glyceryl trinitrate: A randomised study. *Br Heart J* 49:452, 1983.

96. Borer JS, Redwood DR, Levitt B, et al: Reduction in myocardial ischemia with nitroglycerin or nitroglycerin plus phenylephrine administered during acute myocardial infarction. *N Engl J Med* 293:1008, 1975.

97. Jugdutt BI, Warnica JW: Intravenous nitroglycerin therapy to limit myocardial infarct size, expansion, and complications. *Circulation* 78:906, 1988.

98. ISIS-4 Collaborative Group: ISIS-4: Randomised study of oral isosorbide mononitrate in over 50,000 patients with suspected acute myocardial infarction (abstract). *Circulation* 83(suppl I):I-394, 1993.

99. Yusuf S, MacMahon S, Collins R, Peto R: Effect of intravenous nitrates on mortality in acute myocardial infarction: An overview of the randomised trials. *Lancet* 1:1088, 1988.

100. Hochman JS, Choo H: Limitation of myocardial infarct expansion by reperfusion independent of myocardial salvage. *Circulation* 75:299, 1987.

101. Hildebrandt P, Torp-Pedersen C, Joen T, et al: Reduced infarct size in nonreperfused myocardial infarction by combined infusion of isosorbide dinitrate and streptokinase. *Am Heart J* 124:1139, 1992.

102. Rapaport E: Influence of long-acting nitrate therapy on the risk of reinfarction, sudden death, and total mortality in survivors of acute myocardial infarction. *Am Heart J* 110:276, 1985.

103. Murphy JG, Marsh JD, Smith TW: The role of calcium in ischemic myocardial injury. *Circulation* 75 (suppl V):V-15, 1987.

104. Snyder SH, Reynolds IJ: Calcium antagonist drugs: Receptor interactions that clarify therapeutic effects. *N Engl J Med* 313:995, 1985.

105. Report of the Holland Interuniversity Nifedipine/Metoprolol Trial (HINT) Research Group: Early treatment of unstable angina in the coronary care unit. A randomised, double blind, placebo controlled comparison of recurrent ischaemia in patients treated with nifedipine or metoprolol or both. *Br Heart J* 56:400, 1986.

106. Walker JE, MacKenzie G, Adgey AAJ: Effect of nifedipine on enzymatically estimated infarct size in the early phase of acute myocardial infarction. *Br Heart J* 59:403, 1988.

107. Gottlieb SO, Becker LC, Weiss JL, et al: Nifedipine in acute myocardial infarction: An assessment of left ventricular function, infarct size, and infarct expansion—A double blind, randomised, placebo controlled trial. *Br Heart J* 59:411, 1988.

108. Wilcox I, Hampton JR, Banks DC, et al: Trial of early nifedipine in acute myocardial infarction: The Trent study. *Br Med J* 293:1204, 1986.

109. Muller JE, Morrison J, Stone PH, et al: Nifedipine therapy for patients with threatened and acute myocardial infarction: A randomized, double-blind, placebo-controlled comparison. *Circulation* 69:740, 1984.

110. Sirnes PA, Overskeid K, Pedersen TR, et al: Evolution of infarct size during the early use of nifedipine in patients with acute myocardial infarction: The Norwegian Nifedipine Multicenter Trial. *Circulation* 70:638, 1984.

111. Walsh BK, Kelly P, Collins WC, et al: Effect of early treatment with nifedipine in suspected acute myocardial infarction. *Eur Heart J* 7:859, 1986.

112. The Israeli Sprint Study Group: Secondary Prevention Reinfarction Israeli Nifedipine Trial (SPRINT): A randomized intervention trial of nifedipine in patients with acute myocardial infarction. *Eur Heart J* 9:354, 1988.

113. Goldbourt U, Behar S, Reicher-Reiss H, et al for the SPRINT Study Group: Early administration of nifedipine in suspected acute myocardial infarction. *Arch Intern Med* 153:345, 1993.

114. Waters D: Proischemic complications of dihydropyridine calcium channel blockers. *Circulation* 84:2598, 1991.

115. Parmley WW, Nesto RN, Singh BN, et al: Alteration of circadian patterns of myocardial ischemia with nifedipine GITS in patients with chronic stable angina: N-CAP Study. *J Am Coll Cardiol* 19:1380, 1992.

116. The Danish Study Group on Verapamil in Myocardial Infarction: Verapamil in acute myocardial infarction. *Eur Heart J* 5:516, 1984.

117. The Danish Study Group on Verapamil in Myocardial Infarction: Effect of verapamil on mortality and major events after acute myocardial infarction (The Danish Verapamil Infarction Trial II—DAVIT II). *Am J Cardiol* 66:779, 1990.

118. The Multicenter Diltiazem Postinfarction Trial Research Group: The effect of diltiazem on mortality and reinfarction after myocardial infarction. *N Engl J Med* 319:385, 1988.

119. Gibson RS, Boden WE, Theroux P, et al and the Diltiazem Reinfarction Study Group: Diltiazem and reinfarction in patients with non-Q-wave myocardial infection. *N Engl J Med* 315:423, 1986.

120. Chadda K, Goldstein S, Byington R, Curb JD: Effect of propranolol after acute myocardial infarction in patients with congestive heart failure. *Circulation* 73:503, 1986.

121. Gheorghiade M, Schultz L, Tilley B, Kao W, et al: Effects of propranolol in non-Q-wave acute myocardial infarction in the Beta Blocker Heart Attack trial. *Am J Cardiol* 66:129, 1990.

122. Boden WE: Meta-analysis in clinical trials reporting: Has a tool become a weapon? *Am J Cardiol* 69:681, 1992.

123. The MIAMI Trial Research Group: Mortality. *Am J Cardiol* 56:15G, 1985.

124. Yusuf S, Wittes J, Probstfield J: Evaluating effects of treatment in subgroups of patients within a clinical trial: The case of non-Q-wave myocardial infarction and beta blockers. *Am J Cardiol* 66:220, 1990.

125. Yusuf S, Held P, Furberg C: Update of effects of calcium antagonists in myocardial infarction or angina in light of the Second Danish Verapamil Infection Trial (DAVIT-II) and other recent studies. *Am J Cardiol* 67:1295, 1991.

126. Held PH, Yusuf S, Furburg CD: Calcium channel blockers in acute myocardial infarction and unstable angina: An overview. *Br Med J* 299:1187, 1989.

127. Kostis JB, Byington R, Friedman LM, et al: Prognostic significance of ventricular ectopic activity in survivors of acute myocardial infarction. *J Am Coll Cardiol* 10:231, 1987.

128. Teo K, Yusuf S, Furgerg C: Effect of antiarrhythmic drug therapy on mortality following myocardial infarction (abstract). *Circulation* 82:197, 1990.

129. Nademanee K, Singh BN, Stevenson WG, Weiss JN: Amiodarone and post-MI patients. *Circulation* 88:764, 1993.

130. Echt SD, Liebson PR, Mitchell B, et al: Mortality and morbidity in patients receiving encainide, flecainide, or placebo: The Cardiac Arrhythmia Suppression Trial. *N Engl J Med* 324:781, 1991.

131. The Cardiac Arrhythmia Suppression Trial II Investigators: Effect of the antiarrhythmic agent moricizine on survival after myocardial infarction. *N Engl J Med* 327:227, 1992.

132. Ceremuzynski Y, Kleczar E, Krzeminska-Pakula M, et al: Effect of amiodarone on mortality after myocardial infarction. *J Am Coll Cardiol* 20:1056, 1992.

133. Burkart F, Pfisterer M, Kiowski W, et al: Effect of antiarrhythmic therapy on mortality in survivors of myocardial infarction with asymptomatic complex ventricular arrhythmias: Basel Antiarrhythmic Study of Infarct Survival (BASIS). *J Am Coll Cardiol* 16:1711, 1990.

134. Pfisterer ME, Kiowski W, Brunner H, et al: Long-term benefit of

1-year amiodarone treatment for persistent complex vehicular arrhythmias after myocardial infarction. *Circulation* 87:309, 1993.

135. Cairns JA, Connolly SJ, Gent M, Roberts R: Post-myocardial infarction mortality in patients with ventricular premature depolarizations: Canadian Amiodarone Myocardial Infarction Arrhythmia Trial Pilot Study. *Circulation* 84:550, 1991.

135a. Waldo AL, Camm AJ, de Ruyter M, et al: Preliminary mortality results from the Survival with Oral D-Sotalol (SWORD) trial (abstract). *J Am Coll Cardiol* 25:15A, 1995.

136. SHEP Cooperative Research Group: Prevention of stroke by anti-hypertensive drug treatment in older persons with isolated systolic hypertension. *JAMA* 265:3255, 1991.

137. MacMahon S, Peto R, Cutler J, et al: Blood pressure, stroke, and coronary heart disease. 1: Prolonged differences in blood pressure: Prospective observational studies corrected for the regression dilution bias. *Lancet* 335:765, 1990.

138. Collins R, Peto R, MacMahon S, et al: Blood pressure, stroke, and coronary heart disease. 2. Short-term reductions in blood pressure: Overview of randomized drug trials in their epidemiological context. *Lancet* 335:827, 1990.

139. Hebert PR, Fiebach NH, Eberlein KA, et al: The community-based randomized trials of pharmacologic treatment of mild-to-moderate hypertension. *Am J Epidemiol* 127:581; 1988.

140. MRC Working Party: Medical Research Council Trial of Treatment of Hypertension in Older Adults: Principal results. *Br Med J* 304:405, 1992.

141. Dahlof B, Lindholm LH, Hansson L, et al: Morbidity and mortality in the Swedish Trial in Old Patients With Hypertension (STOP-Hypertension). *Lancet* 338:1281, 1991.

142. *The Fifth Report of the Joint National Committee on Detection, Evaluation and Treatment of High Blood Pressure.* NIH publication 93-108, 1993.

143. Farnett L, Mulrow CD, Linn WD, et al: The J-curve phenomenon and the treatment of hypertension. *JAMA* 265:489, 1991.

144. Cruickshank JM: Coronary flow reserve and the J curve relation between diastolic blood pressure and myocardial infarction. *Br Med J* 297:1227, 1988.

145. D'Agostino RB, Belanger AJ, Kannel WB, Cruickshank JM: Relation of low diastolic blood pressure to coronary heart disease death in presence of myocardial infarction: The Framingham Study. *Br Med J* 303:385, 1991.

146. Anderson KM, Castelli WP, Levy D: Cholesterol and mortality: 30 years of follow-up from the Framingham Study. *JAMA* 257:2176, 1987.

147. Stamler J, Wentworth D, Neaton JD: Is relationship between serum cholesterol and risk of premature death from coronary heart disease continuous and graded? *JAMA* 256:2823, 1986.

148. Castelli WP, Garrison RJ, Wilson WF, et al: Incidence of coronary heart disease and lipoprotein cholesterol levels. *JAMA* 256:2835, 1986.

149. Coronary Drug Project Research Group: Clofibrate and niacin in coronary heart disease. *JAMA* 231:360, 1975.

150. Pekkanen J, Linn S, Heiss G, et al: Ten-year mortality from cardiovascular disease in relation to cholesterol level among men with and without preexisting cardiovascular disease. *N Engl J Med* 322:1700, 1990.

151. Rossouw JE, Lewis B, Rifkind BM: The value of lowering cholesterol after myocardial infarction. *N Engl J Med* 323:1112, 1990.

152. Smith GD, Song F, Sheldon TA: Cholesterol lowering and mortality. *Br Med J* 306:1367, 1993.

152a. Scandinavian Simvastatin Survival Study Group: Randomised trial of cholesterol lowering in 4444 patients with coronary heart disease: the Scandinavian Simvastatin Survival Study (4S). *Lancet* 344:1383, 1994.

153. Ornish D, Brown SE, Scherwitz LW, et al: Can lifestyle changes reverse coronary heart disease? *Lancet* 336:129, 1990.

154. Brown G, Albers JJ, Fisher LL, et al: Regression of coronary artery disease as a result of intensive lipid lowering therapy in men with high levels of apolipoprotein B. *N Engl J Med* 323:1989, 1990.

155. Blankenhorn DH, Nessim SA, Johnson RL, et al: Beneficial effects of combined colestipol-niacin therapy on coronary atherosclerosis and coronary venous bypass grafts. *JAMA* 257:3233, 1987.

156. Summary of the second report of the National Cholesterol Education Program (NCEP) expert panel on detection, evaluation, and treatment of high blood cholesterol in adults (Adult Treatment Panel II). *JAMA* 269:3015, 1993.

157. Ronnemaa T, Irjala VK, Peltola O: Marked decrease in serum HDL cholesterol level during acute myocardial infarction. *Acta Med Scand* 207:161, 1980.

158. Ryder REJ, Hayes TM, Mulligan IP, et al: How soon after myocardial infarction should plasma lipid values be assessed? *Br Med J* 289:1651, 1984.

159. Gore JM, Goldberg RJ, Matsumoto AS, et al: Validity of serum total cholesterol level obtained within 24 hours of acute myocardial infarction. *Am J Cardiol* 54:722, 1984.

160. Mallory G, White P, Salcedo-Salgar J: The speed of healing of myocardial infarction: A study of the pathological anatomy in seventy-two cases. *Am Heart J* 18:647, 1939.

161. Pashkow FJ: Issues in contemporary cardiac rehabilitation: A historical perspective. *J Am Coll Cardiol* 21:822, 1993.

162. Levine SA: Some harmful effects of recumbency in the treatment of heart disease. *JAMA* 126:80, 1944.

163. Taylor H, Henschel A, Borzek J: Effects of bed rest on cardiovascular function and work performance. *J Appl Physiol* 2:223, 1949.

164. Levine S, Lown B: The "chair" treatment of acute coronary thrombosis. *Trans Assoc Am Physicians* 64:316, 1953.

165. Levine S, Lown B: The armchair treatment of acute coronary thrombosis. *JAMA* 148:1365, 1952.

166. Oldridge NB, Guyatt GH, Fischer ME, Rimm AA: Cardiac rehabilitation after myocardial infarction. *JAMA* 260:945, 1988.

167. Greenland P, Chu JS: Efficacy of cardiac rehabilitation services. *Ann Intern Med* 109:650, 1988.

168. O'Connor GT, Buring JE, Yusuf S, et al: An overview of randomized trials of rehabilitation with exercise after myocardial infarction. *Circulation* 80:234, 1989.

169. Collins R, Yusuf S, Peto R: Exercise after myocardial infarction reduces mortality: Evidence from randomized trials (abstract). *J Am Coll Cardiol* 3:622, 1984.

170. Hossack KF, Hartwig R: Cardiac arrest associated with supervised cardiac rehabilitation. *J Cardiac Rehab* 2:402, 1982.

171. Williams RS, Miller H, Koisch FP Jr, et al: Guidelines for unsupervised exercise in patients with ischemic heart disease. *J Cardiac Rehab* 3:213, 1981.

172. Jugdutt BI, Michorowski BL, Kappagoda CT: Exercise training after Q wave myocardial infarction: Importance of regional left ventricular function and topography. *J Am Coll Cardiol* 12:362, 1988.

173. Giannuzzi P, Tavazzi L, Temporelli PL, et al: Long-term physical training and left ventricular remodeling after anterior myocardial infarction: Results of the Exercise in Anterior Myocardial Infarction (EAMI) trial. *J Am Coll Cardiol* 22:1821, 1993.

174. Hong MK, Romm PA, Reagan K, et al: Effects of estrogen replacement therapy on serum lipid values and angiographically defined coronary artery disease in postmenopausal women. *J Am Coll Cardiol* 69:176, 1992.

175. Williams JK, Adams MR, Klopfenstein HS: Estrogen modulates responses of atherosclerotic coronary arteries. *Circulation* 81:1680, 1990.

176. Stampfer MJ, Colditz GA: Estrogen replacement therapy and coronary heart disease: A quantitative assessment of the epidemiologic evidence. *Prev Med* 20:47, 1991.

177. Barrett-Connor E, Bush TL: Estrogen and coronary heart disease in women. *JAMA* 265:1861, 1991.

178. Sullivan JM, Vander Zwaag R, Lemp GF, et al: Postmenopausal estrogen use and coronary atherosclerosis. *Ann Intern Med* 108:358, 1988.

179. McFarland KF, Boniface ME, Hornung CA, et al: Risk factors and noncontraceptive estrogen use in women with and without coronary disease. *Am Heart J* 117:1209, 1989.

180. Gruchow HW, Anderson AJ, Barboriak JJ, Sobocinski KA: Postmenopausal use of estrogen and occlusion of coronary arteries. *Am Heart J* 115:954, 1988.

181. Grady D, Rubin SM, Pelilli DB, et al: Hormone therapy to prevent disease and prolong life in post-menopausal women. *Ann Intern Med* 117:1016, 1992.

182. Goldman L, Tosteson ANA: Uncertainty about postmenopausal estrogen: Time for action, not debate (editorial). *N Engl J Med* 325:800, 1991.

183. Borzak S, Rosman HS: Cumulative meta-analyses and the problem of multiple drug effects (letter). *JAMA* 269:214, 1993.

48. Diagnostic Testing in the Coronary Care Unit

Jeffrey R. Smith and Robert C. Hendel

A myriad of diagnostic procedures are available in the coronary care unit (CCU). In addition to procedures that may be performed at the patient's bedside or in a nearby procedure room, the intensivist must be familiar with procedures that critically ill patients might require. This chapter outlines the diagnostic procedures most often required for patients in the CCU.

Electrocardiography

Developed in the early 1900s, the electrocardiogram (ECG) remains one of the most informative and least expensive diagnostic procedures available in the CCU. The ECG displays the sum total of cardiac electrical vectors at a particular point in time as recorded from the body surface. From this electrical activity, information on chamber size, ischemia, injury, dysrhythmias, conduction, and electrolyte disturbances can be obtained.

MORPHOLOGY OF THE ELECTROCARDIOGRAM

Normal Electrocardiogram. Atrial depolarization originates in the sinus node and activates the atria from right to left, resulting in a positive P wave in the inferior and lateral electrocardiographic leads. The normal P wave is less than 0.2 mV (2 mm) in amplitude and less than 0.12 seconds in duration. The P–R interval includes the time for intraatrial, atrioventricular nodal, and His-Purkinje conduction; it is typically 0.12 to 0.20 seconds (Fig. 48-1).

Ventricular activation proceeds symmetrically outward from the septum and from endocardium to epicardium. Septal activation produces initial Q waves in leads I, II, III, aV$_L$, V$_5$, and V$_6$ and R waves in V$_1$ to V$_4$. Right and left ventricular depolarization next result in R waves in leads I, II, III, aV$_L$, aV$_F$, and V$_3$ to V$_6$. Terminal forces produced by the activation of the left ventricular septum result in a terminal S wave in leads I, V$_5$, and V$_6$.

The S–T segment is normally isoelectric. The T wave represents ventricular repolarization, which usually produces upright T waves in all leads except aV$_R$ and V$_1$. The juvenile T wave, inverted in the right precordial leads, is a normal variant that may persist into adulthood [1].

Measured from the beginning of the QRS to the end of the T wave, the Q–T interval reflects the duration of ventricular depolarization and repolarization. The duration of the Q–T interval varies with the cardiac cycle length. Bazett [2] proposed the corrected Q–T interval: Q–T$_c$ = Q–T/(square root of RR). The upper limit of Q–T$_c$ is 0.39 second for men and 0.41 second for women [3], but many accept a Q–T$_c$ as long as 0.44 seconds as normal [4]. The causes of Q–T prolongation include idiopathic long Q–T interval syndrome, myocardial ischemia, cardiomyopathy, central nervous system disease, autonomic nervous system dysfunction, hypocalcemia, hypokalemia, antiarrhythmic drugs, and psychotropic drugs [4].

Atrial Abnormalities. P wave abnormalities may represent atrial enlargement or hypertrophy or altered intraatrial pressure, volume, or conduction. Right atrial abnormality is manifest by a low P wave amplitude in lead I and a tall peaked P wave in leads II, III, and aV$_F$ (P pulmonale). In adults the most common cause of right atrial abnormality is chronic obstructive pulmonary disease (COPD). However, the correlation of an abnormal P wave with echocardiographic findings of right atrial enlargement is low [5].

Left atrial abnormality is manifest by prolongation and notching of the P wave with shortening of the P–R segment (P mitrale). The duration of the P wave is 0.12 seconds or longer in lead II, with an interpeak duration more than 0.04 seconds. The negative deflection of the P wave in lead V$_1$ is 0.04 seconds in duration and 0.1 mV in depth. The most frequent cause of P mitrale is left ventricular disease with increased left ventricular end-diastolic pressure.

P–R segment depression may be seen in pericarditis, atrial infarction, and atrial injury due to penetrating wounds or may be secondary to atrial depolarization abnormalities.

Ventricular Hypertrophy. Electrocardiographic (ECG) manifestations of left ventricular hypertrophy (LVH) include increased voltage, delayed terminal forces, S–T and T wave abnormalities, and left atrial abnormalities. The QRS voltage

Fig. 48-1. Schematic representation of the surface electrocardiogram. P = atrial depolarization; QRS = ventricular depolarization; T = ventricular repolarization. See text for further description of intervals and normal values. (From Chung EK (ed): *Principles of Cardiac Arrhythmias.* 2nd ed. Baltimore, Williams & Wilkins, 1977. With permission.)

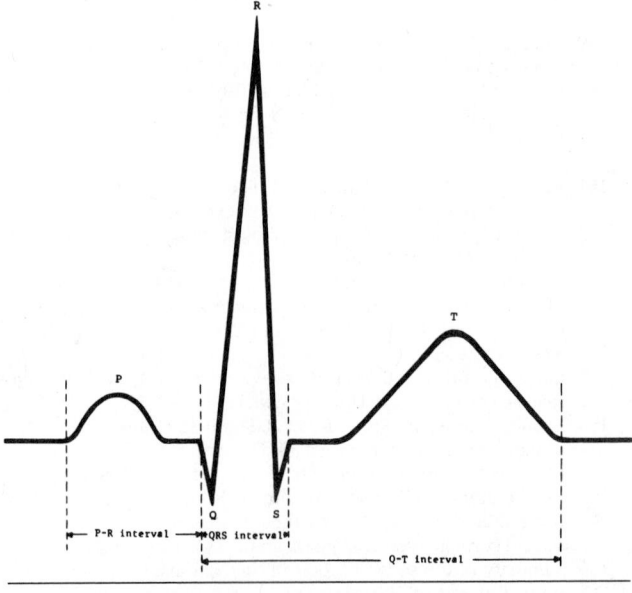

Table 48-1. Voltage Criteria for the Diagnosis of Left Ventricular Hypertrophy

One or more of the following:
    R wave in lead I + S wave in lead III > 25 mm
    R wave in aV_L > 11 mm
    R wave in aV_F > 20 mm
    S wave in aV_R > 14 mm
    R wave in V_5 or V_6 > 26 mm
    R wave in V_5 or V_6 + S wave in V_1 > 35 mm
    largest R wave + largest S wave in precordial leads > 45 mm

Table 48-2. Scale for the Diagnosis of Left Ventricular Hypertrophy

Amplitude	3 points
Largest R or S wave in limb leads ≥ 20 mm	
S wave in V_1 or V_2 ≥ 30 mm	
R wave in V_5 or V_6 ≥ 30 mm	
Strain pattern	
With digitalis	1 point
Without digitalis	3 points
Left atrial abnormality	3 points
Left axis deviation more than −30°	2 points
QRS ≥ 90 msec	1 point
Intrinsicoid deflection in V_5 and V_6 ≥ 50 msec	1 point

Left ventricular hypertrophy is diagnosed if the points total 5 or greater and is considered probable if the point total is 4.
Source: Adapted from Romhilt DW, Estes EH: Point-score system for the ECG diagnosis of left ventricular hypertrophy. *Am Heart J* 75:752, 1968.

criteria for LVH [6–9] are listed in Table 48-1. A more precise method for the ECG diagnosis of LVH than QRS voltage criteria was developed by Romhilt and Estes [10] using a point-score system (Table 48-2). Left ventricular hypertrophy is diagnosed if the points total 5 or greater and is considered probable if the points total 4. Right ventricular hypertrophy (RVH) produces right axis deviation, an R:S ratio in lead V_1 of 1 or greater and an R wave of 0.5 mV or greater [11].

Pulmonary Embolus. The most common ECG features of acute pulmonary embolus are sinus tachycardia and nonspecific repolarization abnormalities. The S_1–Q_3–T_3 (Fig. 48-2) pattern described by McGinn and White [12], right bundle branch block, right axis deviation, and P pulmonale are seen in only one-fourth of patients [13]. Other ECG findings include an S_1, S_2, S_3 pattern, RVH, right axis deviation, and atrial dysrhythmias.

Chronic Obstructive Pulmonary Disease. Chronic obstructive pulmonary disease often results in a peaked P wave in lead II, right axis deviation, and clockwise rotation of the QRS axis. Absence of R waves in the precordial leads may simulate anterior myocardial infarction.

Myocardial Ischemia. Subepicardial ischemia is often manifest by T wave inversion, but subendocardial ischemia may maintain a positive T wave. S–T segment depression is usually seen with myocardial ischemia, although S–T segment elevation may be seen with coronary arterial spasm. Most important is evidence of changes in the ECG when compared to prior tracings.

Myocardial Infarction. The ECG changes of myocardial infarction (Fig. 48-3) are caused by ischemia, injury, and cellular death identified by T wave changes, S–T segment displacement, and the appearance of Q waves [14]. An early tracing in acute myocardial infarction may show increased magnitude of T waves (hyperacute), either upright or inverted [15]. This is followed within minutes by upright displacement of the S–T segment in the leads facing the area of injury. Q waves usually occur within hours to days but may be present initially. The time of appearance of the ECG changes varies from patient to patient, and often a single ECG is not diagnostic.

The ECG is of critical importance for the early confirmation of acute myocardial infarction. Typical chest pain and characteristic ECG changes of 1 mm or greater S–T segment elevation in two contiguous leads establishes the diagnosis of acute myocardial infarction. This enables the institution of immediate therapy directed toward reperfusion, with either thrombolytic therapy or primary angioplasty.

Right ventricular infarction may significantly complicate the course of an acute myocardial infarction and is an independent risk factor for a poor prognosis. Right ventricular involvement with an acute inferior wall myocardial infarction may be accurately diagnosed by the presence of S–T segment elevation in the fourth right precordial lead (V_{4R}) [16]. Therefore, a right-sided ECG should be routinely performed in patients with acute inferior wall myocardial infarction. It should be performed early, as this finding may be transient [17].

A myocardial infarction may also be associated with atypical ECG patterns, including normal ECG, subtle T wave and S–T

Fig. 48-2. 12-lead electrocardiogram from a patient with acute pulmonary embolism. Note the $S_1Q_3T_3$ pattern. (From Chou T-C (ed): *Electrocardiography in Clinical Practice.* 3rd ed. Philadelphia, WB Saunders, 1991. With permission.)

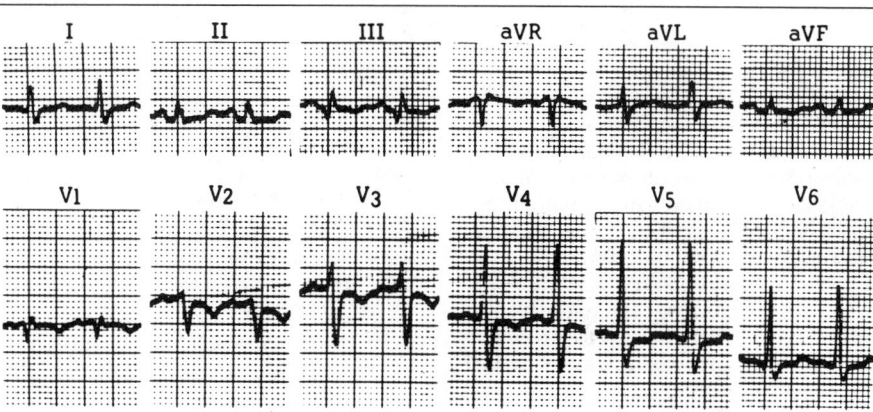

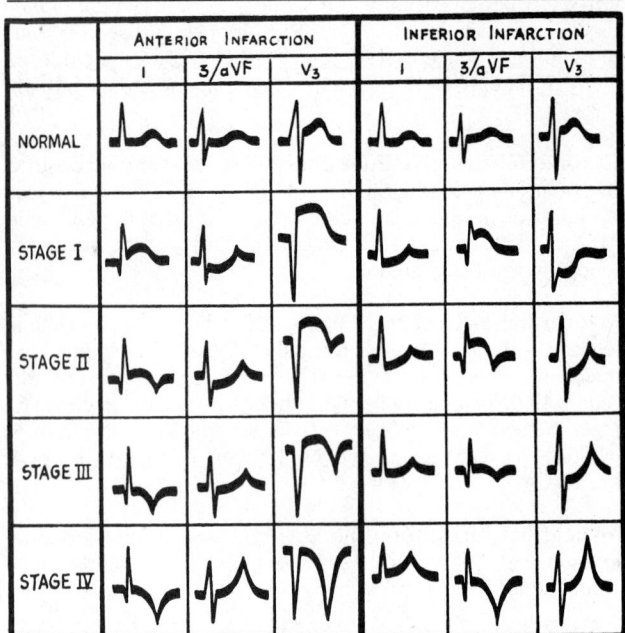

	ANTERIOR INFARCTION			INFERIOR INFARCTION		
	I	3/aVF	V₃	I	3/aVF	V₃
NORMAL						
STAGE I						
STAGE II						
STAGE III						
STAGE IV						

Fig. 48-3. Succession of 12-lead electrocardiograms, demonstrating evolution of an acute anterior wall myocardial infarction (*left*) and inferior wall myocardial infarction (*right*). Note the progression from isoelectric S–T segments to S–T elevation in stage I, T wave inversion in stage II, resolution of S–T elevation in stage III, and deep T wave inversion in stage IV. (From Marriott HJL: *Practical Electrocardiography.* 8th ed. Baltimore, Williams & Wilkins, 1988. With permission.)

segment changes, isolated T wave abnormalities, or transient normalization of previously abnormal portions of the ECG. Conversely, conditions that can mimic or mask an acute myocardial infarction by causing S–T elevation include pericarditis, early repolarization, bundle branch blocks, hyperkalemia, ventricular aneurysm, ventricular hypertrophy, and variant angina. Q waves in the absence of myocardial necrosis (noninfarction Q waves) have been recorded during transient ischemia (transmural), stunning, myocarditis, amyloidosis, neuromuscular disorders, sarcoidosis, cardiomyopathy, left venticular hypertrophy, and intraventricular conduction disturbances. Noninfarction Q waves are common in hypertrophic cardiomyopathy [18]. It is important to obtain serial ECGs to document evolving changes and to compare observed changes with prior tracings.

DYSRHYTHMIAS

Bradyarrhythmias and Heart Block. Sinus bradycardia is a regular rhythm of normal morphology with a rate less than 60 beats per minute and may be well tolerated even at rates below 50 beats per minute. This is common during sleep and in well-conditioned athletes [4]. Thus, a low heart rate must be correlated with the patient's symptoms and blood pressure. When the sinus rate is not adequate to maintain cardiac output, as evidenced by hypotension, ischemia, oliguria, or depressed mental status, emergency treatment is often necessary.

Atrioventricular heart block is diagnosed on ECG. A P–R interval greater than 0.20 seconds defines first-degree A-V block. In second-degree A-V block, some P wave are not followed by a QRS complex. Although the nonconducted P wave may be intermittent or frequent, at regular or irregular intervals, a distinguishing feature is that conducted P waves relate to the QRS

complex with recurring P–R intervals. Mobitz type I second-degree A-V block is characterized by progressive P–R prolongation leading up to a nonconducted P wave. In Mobitz type II second-degree A-V block, the P–R interval remains constant prior to the blocked P wave. Complete A-V block is recognized when P waves are not conducted to the ventricles.

An accurate diagnosis of A-V block is important to determine whether or not a patient should receive a pacemaker. Second-degree type I A-V block nearly always occurs at the level of the A-V node and seldom progresses to complete heart block. High-grade A-V block (second-degree type II or third-degree A-V block) often involves the His-Purkinje system, especially when the resultant QRS complex is wide, and not infrequently requires pacemaker therapy.

Tachyarrhythmias

NARROW COMPLEX TACHYCARDIAS. Narrow complex tachycardias are nearly always of supraventricular origin. If the P wave is buried in the QRS (short R–P), the tachycardia is most likely A-V nodal reentrant tachycardia (AVNRT). When the P wave lands within the S–T segment, A-V reentrant tachycardia (AVRT) using an accessory pathway as well as atypical AVNRT must be considered. If the P wave lands beyond the T wave (very long R–P) the most common causes are atrial tachycardia, sinus tachycardia, and sinus node reentrant tachycardia.

Atrial fibrillation and atrial flutter are distinguished from other supraventricular tachyarrhythmias by the absence of discernible P waves and by the irregular ventricular response in the former and sawtooth atrial activity in the latter. Vagal maneuvers, carotid sinus massage, or intravenous adenosine (6–12 mg bolus) may block A-V conduction, unmasking atrial activity in those tachycardias in which the diagnosis is unclear, and may also terminate tachycardias dependent on the A-V node (A-V nodal reentrant and most A-V reentrant tachycardias utilizing an accessory pathway).

WIDE COMPLEX TACHYCARDIAS. The origin of a wide complex tachycardia is often difficult to determine. Brugada et al. [19] recently proposed criteria for distinguishing supraventricular tachycardia with aberrant conduction from ventricular tachycardia and found them to be more sensitive (98%) and specific (96%) than the older Wellens criteria [20] (Table 48-3).

The intensivist caring for patients in the CCU should be familiar with diagnostic tests used to identify patients at risk of a clinically significant ventricular arrhythmia or sudden cardiac death. The single best predictor of spontaneous ventricular

Table 48-3. Criteria for the Differential Diagnosis of Wide-Complex Tachycardias

Absence of an R–S complex in all precordial leads
R–S interval > 100 msec in one precordial lead
A-V dissociation
Morphology criteria for VT present in precordial leads V₁–V₂ and V₆
  LBBB
    R > 30 msec
    R–S interval > 60 msec in V₁ or V₂
    Q in V₆
  RBBB
    Monophasic R, Rr, qS, or RS in V₁
    rS or monophasic S in V₆

If any of the above criteria are satisfied, the rhythm is classified as ventricular tachycardia. If no criteria are satisfied, the rhythm is classified as supraventricular with aberrant conduction.

A-V = atrioventricular; VT = ventricular tachycardia; LBBB = left bundle branch block; RBBB = right bundle branch block

Source: Adapted from Brugada P, Brugada J, Mont L, et al: A new approach to the differential diagnosis of a regular tachycardia with a wide QRS complex. *Circulation* 83:1649, 1991.

tachycardia and sudden death following a myocardial infarction is the ability to induce monomorphic ventricular tachycardia at the time of invasive electrophysiologic testing [21]. Since an invasive electrophysiologic study is not practical in all patients with myocardial infarction, noninvasive markers are of clinical importance.

The left ventricular ejection fraction is a powerful predictor of survival following myocardial infarction. The incidence of clinically significant ventricular tachycardia following a myocardial infarction is 4.8 times greater for patients with ejection fractions of less than 0.40 when compared to patients with ejection fractions greater than 0.40 [21]. The significance of asymptomatic nonsustained ventricular tachycardia detected by 24-hour Holter monitoring and myocardial late potentials as determined by a signal-averaged ECG in predicting arrhythmic events is still being defined [21,22]. Patients with one or more noninvasive predictors of ventricular arrhythmias should be considered for an invasive electrophysiologic study. Survivors of sudden cardiac death have such a high likelihood of recurrence that they are often treated with an implantable defibrillator regardless of the results of diagnostic testing.

Cardiac Enzyme Analysis

The measurement in serum of cardiac enzymes released from damaged myocytes has proven invaluable in the diagnosis of myocardial infarction and may also be useful in the detection of reperfusion. Unfortunately, the most widely used enzyme assays do not provide definitive information early enough to guide intervention. Lactate dehydrogenase isoenzyme inversion (fraction 1 > fraction 2) has a 90% efficiency in diagnosing myocardial infarction but has an effective "window" that occurs 18 to 36 hours after the onset of symptoms (Table 48-4). Creatine kinase-MB (CK-MB) has an efficiency of 95 percent, but its window occurs at 10 to 24 hours. Accurate but earlier markers of infarction are needed to direct attempts toward reperfusion and to assess noninvasively the success of attempted reperfusion.

In patients who present with only moderate suspicion for acute myocardial infarction, the rapid bedside fingerstick assay for creatine kinase increases diagnostic yield for acute myocardial infarction and may lead to appropriate thrombolytic therapy for patients in whom it might otherwise be denied [23]. However, CK-MB is not specific for myocardial damage and may be elevated after acute or chronic skeletal muscle injury, chronic renal failure, or hypothyroidism [24].

Creatine kinase isoforms have been identified with different electrophoretic properties. Creatinine kinase-MM (CK-MM) isoforms may be detected early after myocardial damage and

allow more rapid determination of acute myocardial infarction. When a ratio of $MM_3:MM_1$ of greater than 0.5 is used to diagnose patients who present early and the CK-MB is used to diagnose patients presenting late, 94 percent sensitivity is obtained on the first blood sample drawn at presentation [25]. Rapid assays for CK-MB subform 2 (tissue) and subform 1 (plasma-modified) are also available. An $MB_2:MB_1$ ratio greater than 2:1 obtained 4 to 6 hours after the onset of symptoms is 92 percent sensitive for detecting acute myocardial infarction [26]. For the detection of reperfusion following therapy, a rate of rise of MM_3 of 0.18 percent per minute or greater suggests successful reperfusion [27]. MB isoforms have also been used to detect reperfusion, using a ratio of MB_2 to $MB_1 \geq 3.8$ as the threshold [28].

Myoglobin, a low-molecular-weight heme protein, is a sensitive but not specific marker of myocardial infarction and is present in the first blood sample of 65 percent of patients. When used for the early detection of coronary reperfusion, a rate of change greater than 2.6 ng/mL-min over 60 minutes or a 4.6-fold increase over 2 hours following reperfusion therapy is 85 percent sensitive and 100 percent specific for predicting successful reperfusion [29].

Myosin light chains are elevated in plasma from 6 hours to 7 days following myocardial infarction. Their prolonged elevated levels make myosin light chains sensitive markers for myocardial injury, allowing detection of infarction for up to 2 weeks [30]. Myosin heavy chains, on the other hand, have limited cardiac specificity, because of the existence of multiple cross-reacting variants in the atria, ventricles, and skeletal muscle [31].

Troponins are proteins that regulate the calcium-mediated interaction of actin and myosin. Cardiac troponin I is not present outside of the heart in adults. Thus, cardiac troponin I is highly specific for myocardial injury and may also be used to distinguish CK-MB elevations caused by skeletal muscle injury from those caused by myocardial injury [32]. Cardiac troponin I is not elevated in acute or chronic muscle disease or renal failure in the absence of myocardial damage. Like troponin I, cardiac troponin T is confined to the myocardium. Troponin T is a more sensitive indicator than CK-MB of myocardial cell injury in patients with unstable angina and is also a useful prognostic indicator. In a recent study, 10 of 11 in-hospital myocardial infarctions occurred in patients whose serum was positive for troponin T, while the hospital course was uneventful in 50 of 51 patients who had no measurable troponin T during the first 2 days after admission for unstable angina [33].

For the routine diagnosis of myocardial infarction, measurement of CK-MB remains the test of choice. A retrospective diagnosis can be made by lactate dehydrogenase detection but will probably be replaced by more specific long-lived markers, such as troponins, in the future. When skeletal muscle injury is present, cardiac troponin I may be more specific in making the diagnosis of concomitant myocardial damage. Very early diagnosis may be improved by CK-MB isoforms or combined CK-MB isoforms and myoglobin. Isoforms of CK-MM and CK-MB and myoglobin hold promise for noninvasively diagnosing coronary recanalization following thrombolysis. The science of determining serum markers of myocardial damage is rapidly growing; however, the choice of the best marker for each clinical situation remains to be determined.

Table 48-4. Biochemical Markers of Myocardial Damage

Enzyme	Rise (hours)	Peak (hours)	Nadir (days)
CK	3–8	10–24	2–3
CK-MB	3–8	10–24	3–4
LD	8–12	72–144	8–14
Myoglobin	2–3	6–9	1–2
MLC	3–8	24–100	10–15
Troponin	4–6	10–24	10–15
Isoforms	1–6	4–8	1–4

CK = total creatine kinase; CK-MB = MB isoenzyme of CK; LD = lactate dehydrogenase; MLC = myosin light chains; Isoforms = CK-MB and CK-MM isoforms.

Chest Radiography

INTERPRETATION OF THE PORTABLE CHEST FILM
Pulmonary Vasculature. In normal pulmonary flow the pulmonary arteries and veins branch outward from each hilum

with gradual peripheral tapering. As pulmonary flow increases to twice normal, the enlarged arteries and veins become apparent on chest radiographs. High-output states, such as anemia, pregnancy, thyrotoxicosis, volume overload, intracardiac shunts, and fever, result in symmetric increases in vascularity. Pulmonary venous hypertension, caused by left ventricular dysfunction, mitral stenosis, or other obstructions to blood flow between the pulmonary capillaries and left ventricle, results in increased flow to the apices, followed by interstitial edema with Kerley's lines, and finally alveolar edema [34]. Pulmonary arterial hypertension causes the radiographic appearance of dilated central arteries, with abrupt tapering or distal "pruning." Causes of pulmonary arterial hypertension are chronic pulmonary emboli, primary arterial hypertension, pulmonary fibrosis, COPD, chronic hypoxia, and Eisenmenger's syndrome.

Causes of diffuse undercirculation of the pulmonary vessels are right ventricular tumor, Addison's disease, hemorrhage, and COPD. Asymmetric decreases in pulmonary vascularity may be seen with pulmonary embolism (Westermark's sign), segmental COPD, partial pneumonectomy, and branch pulmonary artery stenoses or compression.

Cardiac Silhouette. The cardiac silhouette is a function of cardiac pathology, body habitus, age, respiratory phase, cardiac cycle, and patient position. Cardiac enlargement is usually evaluated subjectively, since objective measures are subject to much variation [35]. Nonetheless, the normal cardiothoracic ratio—the ratio of transverse cardiac diameter to the maximum internal diameter of the thorax—is defined as less than 0.5. Left ventricular enlargement may be secondary to hypertrophy, dilatation, or both. Classically, LVH causes downward and lateral displacement without cardiac enlargement. Left ventricular dilatation causes an increase in cardiothoracic ratio together with an inferior displacement of the cardiac apex. Left ventricular aneurysm resulting from prior myocardial infarction may cause a localized bulge or angulation in the left ventricular contour [36].

Left atrial enlargement is easily identified on the chest radiograph as a prominence of the left superior heart border, double density behind the right atrial margin, and splaying of the carina due to upward displacement of the left main bronchus. Isolated left atrial enlargement is most commonly due to mitral stenosis.

Right atrial enlargement is evidenced by increased fullness and convexity of the right cardiac contour and a filling in of the retrosternal clear space. Marked right atrial enlargement may simulate left atrial enlargement. Right ventricular enlargement displaces the whole heart rotationally to the left. This displacement causes increased convexity of the left upper heart border and elevation of the cardiac apex. Right ventricular enlargement may also obliterate the retrosternal clear space.

SPECIFIC DISEASES DETECTED BY CHEST RADIOGRAPHY

Coronary Artery Disease. Although the radiograph may be normal in a patient with severe coronary artery disease, when extensive myocardial scarring occurs there is usually left ventricular dilatation, often accompanied by left atrial enlargement, pulmonary venous hypertension, and, if chronic, pulmonary arterial hypertension and enlarged right-sided chambers. This radiographic appearance may be indistinguishable from that of a dilated cardiomyopathy. Acute left ventricular failure associated with ischemia or acute myocardial infarction is often manifest as pulmonary congestion in the presence of a normal size heart. Similarly, congestive heart failure due to diastolic dysfunction may appear radiographically as a normal-sized heart in the presence of increased pulmonary vascularity [37].

Valvular Heart Disease. Calcific aortic stenosis is suggested by radiopaque calcifications at the level of the aortic cusps and poststenotic dilatation of the ascending aorta (seen as a localized bulge in the right superior contour) [38,39]. In aortic insufficiency, chest radiograph demonstrates left ventricular elongation and downward apical displacement with enlargement of the ascending aorta or aortic unfolding.

The radiographic appearance of mitral stenosis consists of calcified mitral valve leaflets, left atrial or left atrial appendage enlargement, and pulmonary congestion. Mitral regurgitation results in left ventricular and left atrial enlargement. The left atrial enlargement is often greater than that seen in mitral stenosis, but the pulmonary vascular changes in mitral regurgitation are usually less severe. Interstitial and alveolar edema are uncommon except when onset of mitral regurgitation is acute, as occurs in papillary muscle ischemia or ruptured chordae tendineae.

Pulmonary stenosis causes poststenotic dilatation of the pulmonary trunk and left pulmonary artery. Heart size and contour are typically normal, but right atrial enlargement may follow if there is stretching and regurgitation of the tricuspid valve.

Pericardial Disease. The normal pericardium is seldom evident on plain chest radiographs. A pericardial stripe greater than 2 mm along the inferior heart border seen on the lateral projection suggests pericardial effusion. A small effusion may increase the size of the heart compared to prior films, while a large effusion may produce the classic "water flask" heart. Pericardial calcification supports the diagnosis of constrictive pericarditis, which may be further evaluated by magnetic resonance imaging (MRI) or computed tomogaphy (CT).

Aortic Disease. The most common finding in aortic aneurysm is widening of the superior mediastinum. Other findings include displacement of the trachea or esophagus and displacement of intimal calcification from the outer aortic contour by more than 4 to 10 mm. [40]. Transesophageal echocardiography, CT, and MRI are frequently useful for further assessment of aortic dissection.

Cardiac Catheterization and Angiography

Although not performed at the bedside, invasive radiographic procedures are often necessary in cardiac patients. The intensivist should be familiar with the applications of such techniques as well as the potential for procedural complications, including cardiac perforation, vascular intimal dissection, myocardial infarction, thromboembolic events, induction of dysrhythmias, and hemodynamic changes. Renal toxicity [41] and allergic reactions related to the iodinated contrast material are also observed but may be reduced in frequency or severity with appropriate patient preparation. The nephrotoxicity of contrast agents may be reduced by hydrating the patient prior to the study [42]. Allergic reactions may be reduced by pretreatment with 50 mg of oral prednisone given 13, 7, and 1 hour prior to the procedure and 50 mg of oral diphenhydramine given 1 hour prior to the procedure [43]. Patients should be kept in a fasting state for 8 hours prior to all invasive procedures.

AORTOGRAPHY. The indications for aortography are suspected acute aortic dissection or acute aortic regurgitation. In the latter, aortography may be performed as part of a complete angiographic assessment of the heart, including coronary arteriography and left ventriculography. In suspected aortic dissection, the predictive value and delineation of aortic anatomy afforded by aortography must be weighed against the availability, ease, and safety of noninvasive modalities of visualizing the aorta. Aortography, despite its associated risks and long time to perform the procedure, may be necessary in some patients considered for surgery, especially in patients with evidence of involvement of major arterial trunks of the aorta.

PULMONARY ANGIOGRAPHY. In suspected pulmonary embolism, the pulmonary angiogram remains the gold standard for diagnosis. Perfusion lung scanning is the initial screen to exclude the diagnosis of pulmonary embolus, but often it is not definitive. Pulmonary angiography is reserved for patients with moderate probability or indeterminate lung scans [44] or when clinical suspicion for pulmonary embolus is high despite normal lung scan results. Pulmonary angiography also may be used when thrombolytic therapy or caval interruption is considered [45]. Selective and subselective injections, with use of balloon occlusion, help minimize the amount of contrast needed and the risk of the procedure [46].

LEFT VENTRICULOGRAPHY. Cardiac catheterization and left ventriculography, with or without arteriography, is used to confirm acute mitral regurgitation or ventricular septal defect prior to emergent surgical repair. It is also used to determine left ventricular function by hemodynamics and contrast angiography, the latter for assessment of global and regional systolic function.

CORONARY ARTERIOGRAPHY. Selective cannulation of the coronary arteries and contrast administration is the standard for determining the presence and extent of critical coronary stenoses (Fig. 48-4). Emergent or urgent coronary arteriography is indicated in patients with unstable angina or postinfarction angina so that emergency therapy with angioplasty or coronary bypass grafting may be considered prior to the development of irreversible myocardial damage. Likewise, in patients who present with acute myocardial infarction who are hemodynamically unstable or in whom thrombolytic therapy is contraindicated, cardiac catheterization with a view toward angioplasty or immediate surgical revascularization may decrease infarct size and reduce mortality [47]. In some centers, primary coronary arteriography with an intention to perform angioplasty has become the preferred treatment for acute myocardial infarction [48].

Echocardiography

Echocardiography uses ultrasound waves to examine the heart and record information in the form of reflected sound waves [49,50]. Echocardiography is a safe, convenient, and efficient method of evaluating cardiac structure and motion and in conjunction with Doppler techniques may be used to assess blood flow through cardiac structures (see Chap. 7).

CARDIAC FUNCTION. One of the most important uses of echocardiography in the CCU is assessment of left ventricular function. The detection of systolic dysfunction and assessment of its severity impact on therapeutic decisions in the CCU and afterward. Left ventricular systolic function may be assessed using the M-mode technique of recording the diastolic and

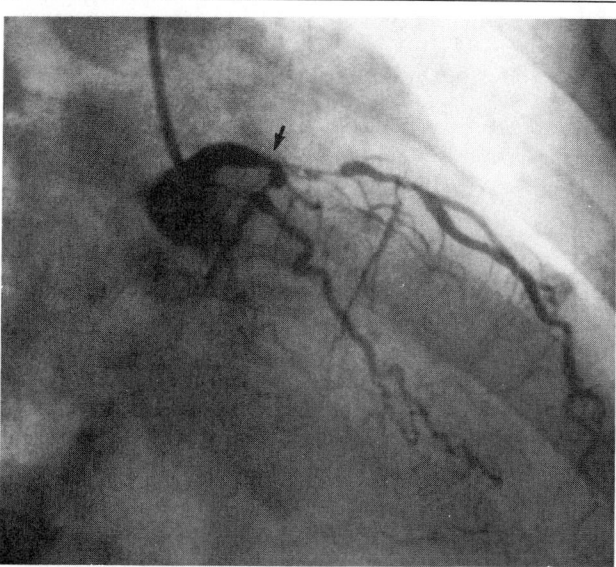

Fig. 48-4. Right anterior oblique projection of the left coronary artery demonstrated by selective coronary arteriography. The patient had an 80% luminal narrowing of the left main coronary artery (*arrow*), a subtotal occlusion of the proximal left anterior descending artery, and an occluded circumflex artery. (Courtesy of C. J. Davidson.)

systolic internal dimensions of the left ventricle (LVIDd and LVIDs, respectively) [51]. The fractional shortening of the left ventricle ([LVIDd − LVIDs] / LVIDd) provides useful information about LV systolic function and is normally 0.18 to 0.42 [52]. However, these echocardiographic measurements reflect the motion of only a small portion of the left ventricle and must be viewed with caution in patients with segmental wall motion abnormalities, left bundle branch block, dilated right ventricle, or unusual cardiac window [53].

Two-dimensional echocardiography has been used to provide qualitative and quantitative assessment of left ventricular volumes and function. Segments of myocardium that contract less vigorously than normal are termed hypokinetic and those that fail to contract are akinetic (Fig. 48-5). When regional segments expand or bulge during systole, they are described as dyskinetic. Several geometric formulas have been suggested for calculating left ventricular volumes [54,55,56] and estimating cardiac output. Other signs of reduced cardiac output include a poorly moving aorta, reduced opening of the mitral valve, and slow closure of the aortic valve. Left ventricular wall thickening as demonstrated by M-mode and two-dimensional echocardiography also indicates myocardial function. Normally, the left ventricular wall thickens during systole, but during ischemia or infarction it thickens less or may actually become thinner [57].

Diastolic dysfunction can also be suggested by echocardiography. The rapidity with which the left ventricular size increases in early diastole is an estimate of left ventricular relaxation. Doppler echocardiography demonstrates reduced early diastolic mitral inflow and increased velocity following atrial contraction in the presence of left ventricular diastolic dysfunction [58]. Distinguishing systolic from diastolic dysfunction is crucial for the appropriate treatment of the patient in heart failure, as the medications for one may be contraindicated in the other. Systolic dysfunction is treated with afterload reducing agents,

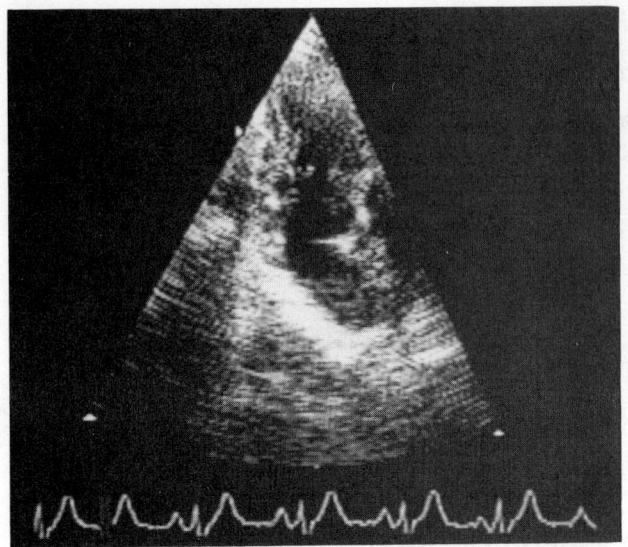

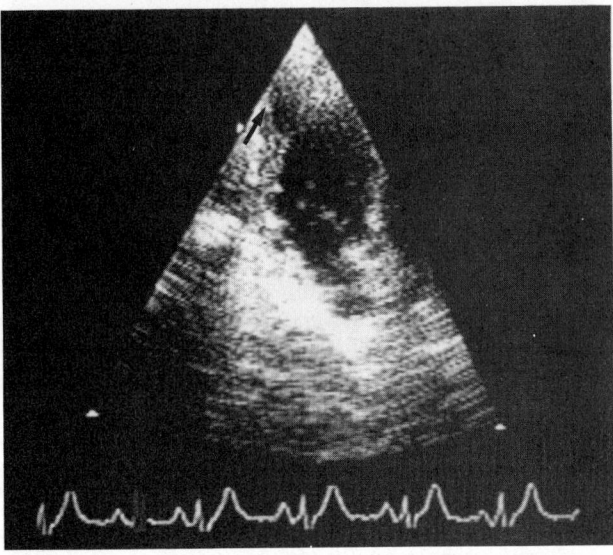

Fig. 48-5. Two-dimensional echocardiographic image of a patient with segmental left ventricular apical akinesis secondary to a prior anterior wall myocardial infarction. A. Diastolic frame. B. Systolic frame, demonstrating thinning and failure of contraction (*arrow*) of the left ventricular apex. (Courtesy of J. V. Talano and P. M. Mowbray.)

diuretics, and possibly digoxin, while the mainstays of treatment of diastolic dysfunction are calcium channel antagonists and beta-blockers.

HYPERTROPHIC CARDIOMYOPATHY. Hypertrophic cardiomyopathy (HCM) is readily evaluated using echocardiographic techniques. Systolic anterior motion of the mitral valve (SAM) is associated with left ventricular outflow tract obstruction. However, SAM may also be seen in patients who are hypovolemic or in a hyperdynamic state [59]. Midsystolic closure of the aortic valve usually indicates a significant amount

of outflow tract obstruction. Asymmetric or concentric left ventricular hypertrophy is demonstrated by echocardiography in patients with HCM. In the asymmetric form of this disease the ratio of the thickness of the septum to the free wall exceeds 1.3:1.0 [60]. In the concentric form of HCM the echocardiogram often demonstrates left ventricular cavity obliteration during systole. Doppler echocardiography in HCM demonstrates an abnormal pattern of midsystolic cessation of left ventricular outflow or increased subvalvular velocity, and hence subvalvular pressure gradient [61]. Reduced left ventricular compliance in HCM results in the typical Doppler findings of diastolic dysfunction [62].

CORONARY ARTERY DISEASE

Myocardial Ischemia. Normally functioning myocardium thickens and contracts during ventricular systole. Echocardiographic findings of ischemic myocardium consist of abnormalities of left ventricular wall thickness, thickening, and motion [63,64]. Echocardiography may be used to confirm the diagnosis of ischemia and determine which areas of myocardium are at risk. A more recent application of echocardiography is the assessment of inducible ischemia. In conjunction with exercise [65] or pharmacologic [66] stress, echocardiography has been shown to be a reliable diagnostic tool for the detection of coronary artery disease, with diagnostic accuracy similar to that of other noninvasive techniques [67]. A comparison of dobutamine stress echocardiography with perfusion scintigraphy in the detection of coronary artery disease found comparable accuracy overall and better specificity by echocardiography in patients with left ventricular hypertrophy [68].

Myocardial Infarction. There exists a strong correlation between the extent of echocardiographically determined wall motion abnormalities and the size of a myocardial infarction [69]. Usually, the extent of regional dyskinesis seen with echocardiography is larger than the infarct size, due to a "tethering" effect on adjacent nonischemic tissue. Echocardiography may not be sensitive enough to detect small or nontransmural infarcts [70]. Although regional hypokinesia may be a manifestation of a condition other than infarction, two-dimensional echocardiographic evidence of impaired wall motion in a patient with characteristic chest pain should raise the index of suspicion for myocardial infarction [71]. Furthermore, myocardial stunning, the delayed recovery of myocardial function that may persist for more than 10 days after an ischemic episode, results in an overestimation of infarct size after reperfusion [72]. Therefore, accurate assessment of left ventricular function after a myocardial infarction requires a delay of 1 to 2 weeks after the acute event.

Echocardiography may also be used to diagnose many of the complications associated with acute myocardial infarction. Ventricular septal rupture or papillary muscle rupture (with or without a flail mitral valve leaflet) may be detected at the bedside [73]. The latter results in mitral regurgitation, which may also be seen with an ischemic papillary muscle. Doppler study may show the abnormal flow pattern of mitral regurgitation or ventricular septal defect. Left ventricular aneurysms, pseudoaneurysms, and thrombi may also be identified using two-dimensional echocardiography and may suggest changes in treatment. For example, mural thrombus and anterior wall akinesis are indications for anticoagulation. Likewise, patients with significant left ventricular dysfunction after acute myocardial infarction should probably be started on an angiotensin-converting-enzyme inhibitor [74].

Valvular Heart Disease. The bedside echocardiogram is valuable in confirming suspected valvular disease in the CCU patient with severe congestive heart failure or other symptomatology. Acute aortic insufficiency or acute mitral regurgitation complicating a myocardial infarction can be quickly recognized using color flow Doppler echocardiography as a turbulent retrograde jet through the valve. In addition, Doppler echocardiography may be used to assess the presence and degree of valvular stenosis. Transesophageal echocardiography (TEE) may provide a more detailed image of the valve apparatus and function.

Endocarditis may be suggested by echocardiography, especially with the enhanced diagnostic capability of TEE [75]. In addition, complications of endocarditis, including abscesses, aneurysms, or perforations involving the anterior mitral valve leaflet or mitral-aortic intervalvular fibrosa, may be identified.

Aortic Dissection. Transesophageal echocardiography is likely the noninvasive diagnostic method of choice in suspected aortic dissection because of its accuracy, safety, speed, and convenience [76] (Fig. 48-6). Although TEE has a sensitivity of 97 to 100 percent for detecting an intimal flap and 77 to 87 percent for identifying the site of entry of an aortic dissection, it is associated with a lack of specificity [76,77]. In this respect, MRI may be superior, but logistical constraints limit its application in many patients.

Source of Embolus. Two-dimensional echocardiography can be used to identify the source of embolus. Perhaps the most common source of embolus in a cardiac patient is an intracavitary thrombus. Patients with atrial fibrillation, left ventricular aneurysm, or dilated cardiomyopathy are prone to develop mural thrombi and subsequent embolism. Transthoracic and transesophageal echocardiograms are therefore helpful not only in identifying a thrombus, but also in identifying those characteristics that predispose to cardiac thrombus formation. Transesophageal echocardiography is superior to transthoracic echocardiography in detecting left atrial thrombi prior to cardioversion for atrial fibrillation and may be used to determine

which patients may safely undergo cardioversion without prolonged anticoagulation [78].

Paradoxical embolism from the venous system across a right-to-left shunt may be suggested by identification of a patent foramen ovale or atrial septal defect by Doppler and color flow Doppler examination. Further demonstration of a right-to-left shunt is afforded by bubble contrast echocardiography in which agitated D_5W or albumin is injected rapidly into a peripheral intravenous line. In normal patients the microcavitary bubbles are extracted by the lung, but in patients with right-to-left intracardiac shunts contrast bubbles may be visualized in the left-sided cardiac chambers.

Pericardial Disease. Two-dimensional echocardiography is the method of choice for detecting pericardial effusions. In the hemodynamically compromised patient with clinical evidence of cardiac tamponade, the echocardiogram may be performed quickly and at the bedside with a high sensitivity for pericardial effusion. Echocardiographic findings of a hemodynamically significant pericardial effusion (cardiac tamponade) include a large effusion, right atrial or right ventricular diastolic collapse, and increased respiratory variation in transvalvular flow velocities [79]. Real-time echocardiography may be used to guide needle aspiration of the pericardial effusion at the bedside.

Nuclear Cardiology

Imaging with radioisotopes is used to assess a wide variety of cardiac physiologic properties, including myocardial perfusion and ventricular function. In addition to establishing the diagnosis and determining prognosis of coronary artery disease, nuclear cardiology techniques provide reproducible measurements of left ventricular volume and ejection fraction and a quantitative assessment of the severity and extent of perfusion abnormalities. Furthermore, thallium scintigraphy may provide a highly accurate assessment of myocardial viability, and a variety of techniques may demonstrate cardiac injury. Nuclear studies demonstrate physiologic, rather than anatomic, properties of the heart.

MYOCARDIAL PERFUSION IMAGING. Although the coronary arteriogram is accurate in defining vessel morphology, radionuclide studies to assess myocardial perfusion are superior in determining the physiologic significance of a coronary stenosis. Furthermore, scintigraphy may function as a noninvasive predictor for the presence of and prognosis from such stenoses.

Thallium 201 is a cationic potassium analog whose myocardial uptake is dependent on cell membrane integrity and is proportional to blood flow. Imaging is performed shortly after intravenous injection at maximum exercise and reveals the pattern of blood flow during maximal stress. Imaging repeated several hours later provides a determination of the resting blood flow. Perfusion defects seen both during rest and during stress represent areas of myocardial scar, while areas that are hypoperfused during stess but have improved perfusion during rest represent regions of myocardial ischemia. The enhanced detection of viable myocardium is possible with late imaging (24 hours) [80] or thallium reinjection [81] (Fig. 48-7). In patients unable to exercise, other forms of stress or vasodilation may be used in lieu of walking on a treadmill. These include dipyridamole, adenosine, dobutamine, and other newer agents [82,83,84]. Patients preparing for pharmacologic stress imaging should fast and avoid caffeine prior to an adenosine or dipyri-

Fig. 48-6. Transesophageal echocardiographic image of an aortic dissection. The dissected intimal flap (*) can be seen separating the true and false lumens. (Courtesy of S. P. Wiet.)

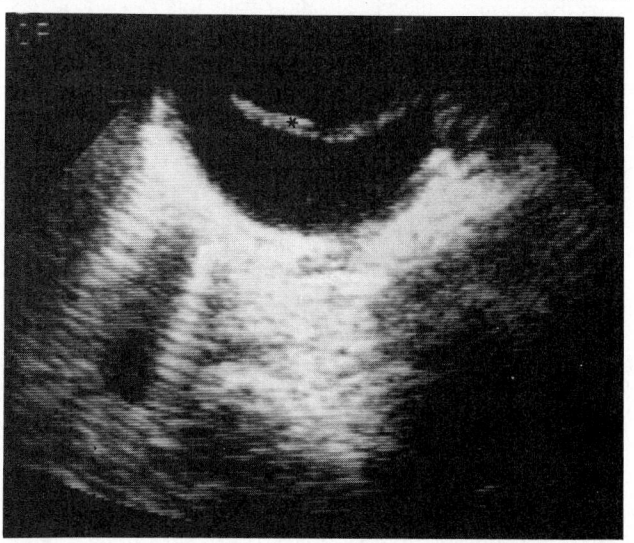

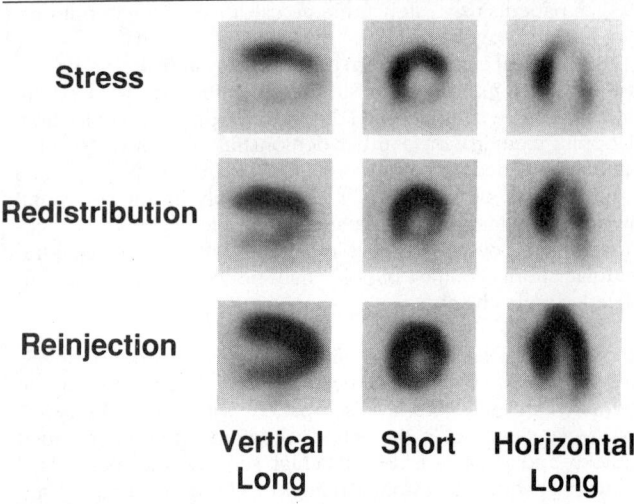

Fig. 48-7. Thallium-201 images of the heart at peak stress, after 4 hours of redistribution, and following reinjection of thallium. This patient had ischemic, but viable, myocardium, as demonstrated by the decreased perfusion in the inferolateral and apical left ventricle during stress (*top*), which shows modest improvement with redistribution (*middle*) and marked improvement following reinjection (*bottom*). (Courtesy of R. C. Hendel.)

damole infusion test. If dobutamine is used, beta blockade should be discontinued prior to the procedure.

Exercise or other forms of stress are important for accurate detection of coronary stenosis by perfusion scanning but are contraindicated in the critically ill patient. Fortunately, the redistribution properties of thallium make it useful for detecting coronary blood flow even in the absence of exercise studies. Perfusion imaging at rest may be used to detect myocardial infarction. A large defect on early imaging during an acute myocardial infarction portends a poorer prognosis [85,86].

Ischemic but viable myocardium may also be suggested by imaging thallium injected at rest and 4 hours later (redistribution) in patients too ill to stress. Viability assessment with thallium is highly concordant with positron emission tomography (PET) [87]. Viability demonstrated by PET imaging in regions of known wall motion abnormalities or decreased perfusion is highly predictive of reversible myocardial ischemia or "hibernating" myocardium [88]. These areas of "blood flow metabolism mismatch" are likely to improve with revascularization and lead to improved left ventricular function and possibly prolonged survival. The presence of numerous asynergic but viable myocardial segments demonstrated by rest-redistribution thallium imaging before coronary bypass surgery is correlated with improvement of left ventricular function after surgery [89]. Thus, determination of viable myocardium using thallium techniques may help select patients with left ventricular dysfunction for revascularization.

In addition to its diagnositic utility, thallium stress imaging is helpful in determining prognosis from coronary artery disease in unselected patients [90], patients with recent myocardial infarction [91,92], and patients undergoing preoperative evaluation for vascular surgery [93,94]. Thallium scintigraphy after infusion of dipyridamole has been shown to have independent and significant prognostic utility in unselected patients referrred for diagnostic work-up, with an abnormal scan, especially the presence of multiple transient thallium defects, elevating the relative risk of myocardial infarction or cardiac-related death

[90]. Gibson et al. [91] demonstrated that patients who have survived an uncomplicated myocardial infarction may be separated into high- and low-risk groups based on results of submaximal exercise thallium scintigraphy. High-risk patients were identified by the presence of two or more vascular regions of thallium defect, redistribution of thallium, or increased lung uptake. Dipyridamole thallium scintigraphy following myocardial infarction has also proven a safe and sensitive predictor of subsequent cardiac events [92]. Perioperative and late cardiac risk assessment for noncardiac surgery may be obtained with thallium scintigraphy following the administration of dipyridamole [93,94].

Despite the many applications and widespread use of thallium, the physical characteristics of this agent are far from ideal. The higher photon energy and favorable dosimetry of ^{99m}Tc agents allow for improved image quality. Currently, ^{99m}Tc sestamibi (Cardiolite) and ^{99m}Tc teboroxime (Cardiotec) are available, and other agents are under development. Sestamibi, the most frequently used technetium agent, demonstrates stable myocardial distribution [95] and images may be obtained long after injection, during which time therapeutic maneuvers may be instituted.

Resting sestamibi imaging has a sensitivity for detecting myocardial infarction of 94 percent and a normalcy rate of 100 percent in normal volunteers [96]. Excellent concordance between the scintigraphic infarct size and that determined at necropsy with histochemical staining has been shown [97]. Since little redistribution occurs with sestamibi, it is a promising agent for perfusion imaging during acute ischemic syndromes. The patient may be injected during the acute episode and imaged later, when stable. This provides information on the presence of ischemia [98] and the amount of myocardium salvaged during an acute myocardial infarction treated with thrombolytic agents [99].

INFARCT AVID IMAGING. Although most acute myocardial infarctions can be diagnosed by the combination of clinical history, ECG, and cardiac enzymes, there are situations when the diagnosis may still be in doubt. The ECG may be nondiagnostic in a non-Q wave infarct or in the presence of left bundle branch block. Cardiac enzymes may not be interpretable due to recent cardioversion, open heart surgery, or hypothyroidism or may not be available at the approptiate time intervals. Scintigraphic visualization with infarct avid agents may be used to identify, localize, and size myocardial infarcts.

Irreversibly damaged myocardial cells accumulate deposits of calcium. Technetium pyrophosphate (^{99m}Tc-PPi) complexes with the calcium deposits in the infarcted myocardium and can be used to detect a recent myocardial infarction [100]. These scans may become abnormal anytime from less than 1 day to more than 5 days after the myocardial infarction, depending on how rapidly and successfully reperfusion was obtained [101], and have a sensitivity of up to 90 percent [102].

A radiolabeled monoclonal antibody to human cardiac myosin, ^{111}In antimyosin, has recently been developed. The sarcolemma disruption that occurs with myocardial necrosis allows for the binding of the intravenous antibody to the myosin filaments. After intravenous injection of radiolabeled fragments of antibodies (Fab) specific for cardiac myosin, localized areas of uptake have been demonstrated (Fig. 48-8). When the tracer is injected within 24 hours of onset of symptoms, detection of Q wave acute myocardial infarctions is more than 90 percent [103]. Antimyosin may also be used to detect necrosis secondary to cardiac contusion or myocarditis [104,105].

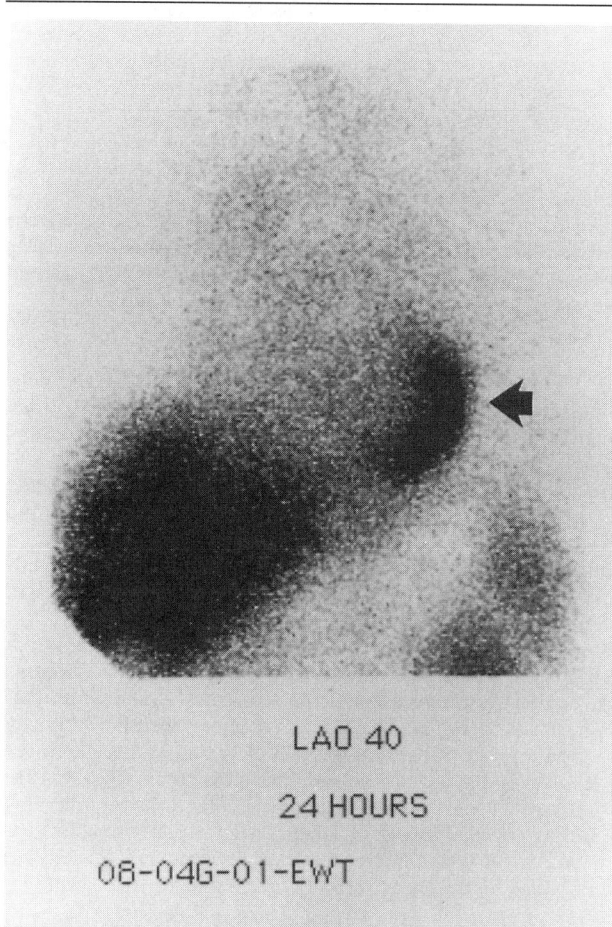

LAO 40

24 HOURS

08-04G-01-EWT

Fig. 48-8. Indium-123 antimyosin antibody-tagged image in a patient with a 5-day-old myocardial infarction. In this 40 degree left anterior oblique view, note the increased tracer uptake (*arrow*) in the infarcted posterolateral wall, compatible with left circumflex pathology. (Courtesy of R. C. Hendel.)

CARDIAC PERFORMANCE. Right and left ventricular ejection fractions and regional wall motion may be safely and reproducibly determined noninvasively using radionuclide techniques. In addition, ventricular volumes, indices of diastolic dysfunction, indices of valvular regurgitation, and intracardiac shunts may be determined. First-pass radionuclide studies measure the initial transit of radiotracer through the heart, while equilibrium studies (gated blood pool scan [MUGA], radionuclide ventriculogram [RVG], radionuclide angiogram [RNA]) rely on counts of tracer within the intravascular space during multiple cardiac cycles.

Left ventricular function is the most important noninvasive predictor of reinfarction and sudden death following myocardial infarction [106]. From time-activity curves generated from left ventricular activity following intravenous injection of radiolabeled tracer, the count rates during end diastole and end systole are determined. The ejection fraction (EF) is determined by dividing the difference in count rates at end diastole (ED) and end systole (ES) by the count rate at end diastole (EF = [ED − ES]/ED). Excellent correlation between radionuclide and contrast ventriculographically determined ejection fractions has been achieved. Since no geometric assumptions are used to determine ejection fraction by radionuclide angi-

ography, it may be the most accurate and reproducible technique.

Methods have been developed to assess regional left ventricular ejection fraction [107]. Radionuclide angiocardiography has sensitivity comparable to that of contrast ventriculography in detecting ventricular aneurysms and regional wall motion.

Computed Tomography

Computed tomography has been successfully employed to detect intracardiac masses, pericardial disease, and aortic dissections [108]. The size, location, and movement of atrial myxomas, the most common intracardiac tumor, are demonstrated by CT. Less common primary cardiac tumors, such as rhabdomyomas, fibromas, and lipomas, are also identifiable by CT.

Pericardial effusions may be identified by CT if the effusion does not have a high protein content, in which case it may be mistaken for thickened pericardium. Computed tomography may differentiate the normal-thickness pericardium and poorly contracting ventricle of cardiomyopathy from the thickened pericardium and impaired diastolic left ventricular filling of constrictive pericarditis.

Computed tomography also permits noninvasive assessment of suspected aortic dissection. It offers a reasonable imaging alternative to angiography with decreased radiation and avoids the risks of aortic cannulation. In hospitals lacking emergent TEE, CT scanning is an alternative for the rapid screening of patients with suspected acute aortic dissection [76].

Magnetic Resonance Imaging

Nuclei with an odd number of neutrons or protons have angular momentum or spin. The energy emitted as protons within a magnetic field returns to an equilibrium state after being perturbed by a radiofrequency pulse is used to produce magnetic resonance images. High-resolution MRI can define abnormal cardiac anatomy (Fig. 48-9). Unfortunately, MRI is not performed at the bedside and may require transport of the patient and support equipment to an off-site imaging facility.

Magnetic resonance imaging may be the most accurate procedure for the detection of aortic dissection, with the highest sensitivity and specificity compared to aortography, CT, and TEE [76,77]. It is also very accurate in determining the site of intimal tear, presence of thrombus, and presence of associated pericardial effusion. The major drawbacks to the routine use of MRI are cost, relative inavailability, and the need for patient and equipment transport to the MRI facility.

Magnetic resonance imaging allows excellent visualization of pericardial effusions and pericardial thickness. Although echocardiography is a more convenient and less expensive method of visualizing pericardial effusions, it does not identify pericardial thickening as accurately as MRI.

Preliminary reports have demonstrated the ability of magnetic resonance coronary angiography to detect left main and proximal coronary stenoses accurately [78]. Although much work remains to be done before this technique becomes clinically useful, MRI does hold the promise of being a comprehensive noninvasive test capable of providing information on coronary anatomy, coronary perfusion, left ventricular function, and cardiac anatomy.

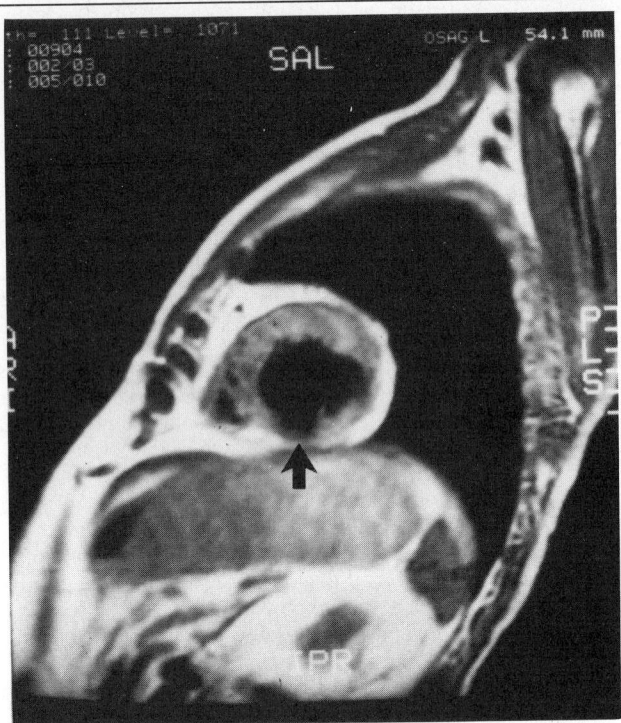

Fig. 48-9. Magnetic resonance image of an inferior wall myocardial infarction. In this left sagittal section, note the thinning of the inferior wall (*arrow*) of the left ventricle. (Courtesy of R. C. Hendel.)

Right Heart Catheterization

Hemodynamic monitoring via pulmonary artery catheterization allows measurement of pressures in the right-sided cardiac chambers and pulmonary artery, estimates of the left atrial pressure from the pulmonary capillary wedge pressure (PCWP), and calculation of cardiac output and pulmonary and systemic vascular resistance.

PULMONARY EDEMA. Pulmonary edema may be classified as cardiogenic or noncardiogenic, with the former type resulting from increased hydrostatic pressure in the pulmonary venous system secondary to left heart failure or obstruction of blood flow. The PCWP must be greater than 18 mm Hg for pulmonary edema to be considered cardiac in origin [109]. Serial calculations of the PCWP and cardiac output during treatment serve to determine optimal loading conditions.

DETERMINATION OF CARDIAC OUTPUT. The most common method of cardiac output determination in the CCU is thermodilution, which relies on the rate at which an unknown volume of blood is cooled by a known volume of saline injectate at a known temperature to determine the volume of that blood. Cardiac output determination by thermodilution has a reproducibility of plus or minus 5 percent. The thermodilution method has the greatest error in the presence of low cardiac output, severe mitral or aortic regurgitation, or intracardiac shunts [110].

In the setting of low cardiac output, the PCWP is irreplaceable

for determining left ventricular loading conditions. The increased PCWP seen in left ventricular failure may be optimized by use of the pulmonary artery catheter. Results of interventions to optimize left ventricular loading conditions may be determined by monitoring the PCWP, systemic vascular resistance, and cardiac output. The pulmonary artery catheter is also diagnostic in hypovolemic shock when the filling pressures (right atrial and wedge) are low.

In the setting of low cardiac output, a right atrial pressure greater than or equal to the PCWP suggests right ventricular dysfunction. A steep *y* descent and right ventricular diastolic dip and plateau (square root sign) may also be present.

COMPLICATIONS OF MYOCARDIAL INFARCTION. Ventricular septal rupture is a complication of acute myocardial infarction that may be suspected by the presence of a new systolic murmur in the setting of acute worsening of heart failure. Blood samples for oxygen saturation should be obtained from the superior vena cava and the pulmonary artery during pulmonary artery catheter insertion. A difference in oxygen saturation between the superior vena cava and pulmonary artery of greater than 7 percent indicates a possible left-to-right shunt [111].

Another complication of acute myocardial infarction, papillary muscle ischemia or ruptured chordae tendineae, presents as acute onset pulmonary edema and a new systolic murmur. In addition to elevated PCWP, acute mitral insufficiency may cause a tall, late V wave in the PCWP tracing as the left atrium fills with regurgitant blood from the left ventricle (Fig. 48-10).

Physiologic assessment of left ventricular function following acute myocardial infarction gives prognostic information. Patients found to have decreased cardiac output or elevated left ventricular filling pressure following an acute myocardial in-

Fig. 48-10. Pulmonary capillary wedge pressure tracing in a patient with mitral insufficiency. Note the tall late V wave of mitral insufficiency when the catheter is wedged. The timing of the mitral V wave relative to the QRS is later than the simultaneously displayed left ventricular systolic pressure waveform. (From Grossman W (ed): *Cardiac Catheterization, Angiography and Intervention.* 4th ed. Baltimore, Williams & Wilkins, 1991. With permission.)

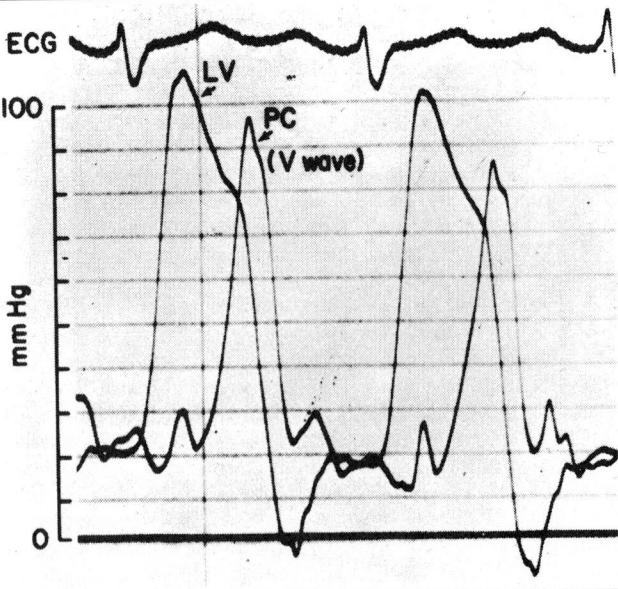

farction have a worse prognosis [112]. A cardiac index below 2.2 L/min/m² or PCWP greater than 18 mm Hg has been shown to be associated with an increased mortality [113].

PERICARDIAL DISEASE. Cardiac tamponade should be suspected when the PCWP and right atrial pressures are elevated and equal (less than 5 mm Hg difference). There is also a loss of the descending limb of the V wave in the right atrial pressure tracing.

Elevation and equalization of pressures may also be present in constrictive heart disease. In the presence of constrictive pericarditis the right heart catheter may reveal prominent descent of the right atrial A and V waves and an early diastolic dip (square root sign) in the right ventricular waveform.

Conclusions

Each of the wide variety of diagnostic modalities available to the intensivist in the CCU offers unique information. Factors to consider in deciding which diagnostic test to perform should include, foremost, the utility of a given test to make the correct diagnosis and guide therapy. When faced with the choice of more than one diagnostic option for a given clinical situation, the relative risk of an invasive procedure must be weighed against the possible lack of specificity or sensitivity of noninvasive alternatives. The ability to perform a test rapidly at the patient's bedside has obvious advantages for a critically ill patient. Finally, in the current era of cost containment, one must critically assess the benefit to be gained by performing a more expensive study compared to its less expensive counterpart. A familiarity with each type helps the physician choose those tests most likely to provide the diagnosis and impact on the management of the critically ill patient.

References

1. Friedman NH: *Diagnostic Electrocardiography and Vectorcardiography.* New York, McGraw-Hill, 1977.
2. Bazett HC: An analysis of the time-relations of electrocardiograms. *Heart* 7:353, 1920.
3. Lepeschkin E: Physiological basis of the U wave, in Schlant RC, Hurst JW (eds): *Advances in Electrocardiography.* New York, Grune & Stratton, 1972.
4. Chou T: *Electrocardiography in Clinical Practice.* 3rd ed. Philadelphia, WB Saunders. 1991.
5. Reeves WC, Hallahan W, Schwiter EJ, et al: Two-dimensional echocardiographic assessment of electrocardiographic criteria for right atrial enlargement. *Circulation* 64:387, 1981.
6. Hamer J, Shinebourne E, James F: Significance of electrocardiographic changes in hypertension. *Br Med J* 1:79, 1969.
7. Noth PH, Myers GB, Klein HA: The precordial electrocardiogram in left ventricular hypertrophy: A study of autopsied cases. *J Lab Clin Med* 32:1517, 1947.
8. Schack JA, Rosenman RH, Katz LN: The AV limb leads in the diagnosis of left ventricular strain. *Am Heart J* 40:696, 1950.
9. Sokolow M, Lyon TP: The ventricular complex in ventricular hypertrophy as obtained by unipolar precordial and limb leads. *Am Heart J* 37:161, 1949.
10. Romhilt DW, Estes EH: Point-score system for the ECG diagnosis of left ventricular hypertrophy. *Am Heart J* 75:752, 1968.
11. Scott RC: The electrocardiographic diagnosis of right ventricular hypertrophy: Correlation with anatomic findings. *Am Heart J* 60:659, 1960.
12. McGinn S, White PD: Acute cor pulmonale resulting from pulmonary embolism: Its clinical recognition. *JAMA* 104:1473, 1960.
13. National Cooperative Study: The Urokinase-Pulmonary Embolism Trial. *Circulation* 47(suppl II):1, 1973.
14. Pardee HEB: An electrocardiographic sign of coronary artery obstruction. *Arch Intern Med* 26:244, 1920.
15. Madias JE: The earliest electrocardiographic signs of acute transmural myocardial infarction. *J Electrocardiol* 10:193, 1977.
16. Zehender M, Kasper W, Kauder E, et al: Right ventricular infarction as an independent predictor of prognosis after acute inferior myocardial infarction. *N Engl J Med* 328:981, 1993.
17. Chou T-C, Van Der Bel-Kahn J, Allen J, et al: Electrocardiographic diagnosis of right ventricular infarction. *Am J Med* 70:1175, 1981.
18. Frank S, Braunwald E: Idiopathic hypertrophic subaortic stenosis: Clinical analysis of 126 patients with emphasis on the natural history. *Circulation* 37:759, 1968.
19. Brugada P, Brugada J, Mont L, et al: A new approach to the differential diagnosis of a regular tachycardia with a wide QRS complex. *Circulation* 83:1649, 1991.
20. Wellens HJJ, Bar FWHM, Lie KI: The value of the electrocardiogram in the differential diagnosis of a tachycardia with a widened QRS complex. *Am J Med* 64:27, 1978.
21. Richards DAB, Byth K, Ross DL, et al: What is the best predictor of spontaneous ventricular tachycardia and sudden death after myocardial infarction? *Circulation* 83:756, 1991.
22. Shen W, Hammill SC: Survivors of acute myocardial infarction: Who is at risk for sudden cardiac death? *Mayo Clin Proc* 66:950, 1991.
23. Downie AC, Frost PG, Fielden P, et al: Bedside measurement of creatine kinase to guide thrombolysis in the coronary care unit. *Lancet* 341:452, 1993.
24. Jaffe AS, Ritter C, Meltzer V, et al: Unmasking artifactual increases in creatine kinase isoenzymes in patients with renal failure. *J Lab Clin Med* 104:193, 1984.
25. Abendschein D, Seacord LM, Hohara R, et al: Prompt detection of myocardial injury by assay of creatine kinase isoforms in initial plasma samples. *Clin Cardiol* 11:661, 1988.
26. Puleo PR, Guadagno PA, Roberts R, et al: Early diagnosis of acute myocardial infarction based on assay for subforms of creatine kinase-MB. *Circulation* 82:759, 1990.
27. Abendschein DR, Ellis AK, Eisenberg PR, et al: Prompt detection of coronary recanalization by analysis of rates of change of concentrations of macromolecular markers in plasma. *Cor Artery Dis* 88:101, 1993.
28. Puleo PR, Peryman B: Noninvasive detection of reperfusion in acute myocardial infarction based on plasma activity of creatine kinase MB subforms. *J Am Coll Cardiol* 17:1047, 1991.
29. Ellis AK, Little T, Nasud ARZ, et al: Early noninvasive detection of successful reperfusion in patients with acute myocardial infarction. *Circulation* 78:1352, 1988.
30. Katus HA, Yasuda T, Gold H, et al: Diagnosis of acute myocardial infarction by detection of circulating cardiac myosin light chains. *Am J Cardiol* 54:964, 1984.
31. Bouvagnet P, Leger JOC, Pons F, et al: Fiber types and myosin types in human atrial and ventricular myocardium. *Circ Res* 55:794, 1984.
32. Adams JE, Bodor GS, Davila-Roman VG, et al: Improved detection of perioperative myocardial infarction with cardiac troponin I (abstract). *J Am Coll Cardiol* 21:88A, 1993.
33. Hamm CW, Ravkilde J, Gerhardt W, et al: The prognostic value of serum troponin T in unstable angina. *N Engl J Med* 327:146, 1992.
34. Simon M: The pulmonary vessels: Their hemodynamic evaluation using routine radiographs. *Radiol Clin North Am* 11:363, 1963.
35. Glover L, Baxley WA, Dodge HT: A quantitative evaluation of heart size measurements from chest roentgenograms. *Circulation* 47:1289, 1973.
36. Baron MG: Postinfarction aneurysm of the left ventricle. *Circulation* 43:762, 1971.
37. Bonow RO, Udelson JE: Left ventricular diastolic dysfunction as a cause of congestive heart failure: Mechanisms and management. *Ann Intern Med* 117:502, 1992.
38. Amplatz K: The roentgenographic diagnosis of mitral and aortic valvular disease. *Am Heart J* 64:556, 1962.
39. Klatte EC, Tampas JP, Campbell JA, et al: The roentgenographic

manifestations of aortic stenosis and aortic valvular insufficiency. *Am J Radiol* 88:57, 1962.

40. Eyler WR, Clark MD: Dissecting aneurysm of the aorta: Roentgen manifestations including a comparison with other types. *Radiology* 85:1047, 1965.

41. D'Elia JA, Gleason RE, Alday M, et al: Nephrotoxicity from angiographic contrast material: A prospective study. *Am J Med* 72:719, 1982.

42. Giammona ST, Lurie PR, Segar WE: Hypertonicity following selective angiocardiography. *Circulation* 28:1096, 1963.

43. Greenberger PA, Patterson R, Tapio CM: Prophylaxis against repeated radiocontrast media reactions in 857 cases. *Arch Intern Med* 145:2197, 1985.

44. The PIOPED Investigators: Value of ventilation/perfusion scan in acute pulmonary embolism: Results of the Prospective Investigation of Pulmonary Embolism Diagnosis (PIOPED). *JAMA* 263:2753, 1990.

45. Cheely R, McCartney WH, Perry JR, et al: The role of noninvasive tests versus pulmonary angiography in the diagnosis of pulmonary embolism. *Am J Med* 70:17, 1981.

46. Ferris EJ, Hobler JL, Lim WH, et al: Angiography of pulmonary emboli: Digital studies and balloon-occlusion cineangiography. *Am J Roentgenol* 142:369, 1984.

47. Guidelines for the early management of patients with acute myocardial infarction: A report of the American College of Cardiology/American Heart Association task force on assessment of diagnostic and therapeutic cardiovascular procedures (subcommittee to develop guidelines for the early management of patients with acute myocardial infarction). *J Am Coll Cardiol* 16:249, 1990.

48. Grines CL, Browne KF, Marco J, et al: A comparison of immediate angioplasty with thrombolytic therapy for acute myocardial infarction. *N Engl J Med* 328:673, 1993.

49. Feigenbaum H: *Echocardiography*. 4th ed. Philadelphia, Lea & Febiger, 1986.

50. Seward JB, Khandheria BK, Oh JK, et al: Transesophageal echocardiography: Technique, anatomic correlations, implementation, and clinical applications. *Mayo Clin Proc* 63:649, 1988.

51. Feigenbaum H, Popp RL, Wolfe SB, et al: Ultrasound measurements of the left ventricle: A correlative study with angiography. *Arch Intern Med* 129:461, 1972.

52. Erbel R, Schweizer P, Herrn G, et al.: Apical two-dimensional echocardiography: Normal values for single and bi-plane determination of left ventricular volume and ejection fraction. *Dtsch Med Wochenschr* 107:1872, 1982.

53. Feigenbaum H: Echocardiographic examination of the left ventricle. *Circulation* 51:1, 1975.

54. Gordon EP, Schnittger I, Fitzgerald PJ, et al: Reproducibility of left ventricular volumes by two-dimensional echocardiography. *J Am Coll Cardiol* 2:506, 1983.

55. Wyatt HL, Meerbaum S, Heng MK, et al: Cross-sectional echocardiography. III. Analysis of mathematic models for quantifying volume of symmetric and asymmetric left ventricles. *Am Heart J* 100:821, 1980.

56. Quinones MA, Waggoner AD, Reduto LA, et al: A new, simplified and accurate method for determining ejection fraction with two-dimensional echocardiography. *Circulation* 64:744, 1981.

57. Corya BC, Rasmussen S, Feigenbaum, et al: Systolic thickening and thinning of the septum and posterior wall in patients with coronary artery disease, congestive cardiomyopathy, and atrial septal defect. *Circulation* 55:109, 1977.

58. Spirito P, Maron BJ, Bonow RO: Noninvasive assessment of left ventricular diastolic function: Comparative analysis of Doppler echocardiographic and radionuclide angiographic techniques. *J Am Coll Cardiol* 7:518, 1986.

59. Maron BJ, Gottdiener JS, Perry LW: Specificity of systolic anterior motion of anterior mitral leaflet for hypertrophic cardiomyopathy. *Br Heart J* 45:206, 1981.

60. Henry WL, Clark CE, Roberts WC, et al: Difference in distributions of myocardial abnormalities in patients with obstructive and non-obstructive asymmetric septal hypertrophy (ASH): Echocardiographic and gross anatomic findings. *Circulation* 50:447, 1974.

61. Maron BJ, Gottdiener JS, Arce J, et al: Dynamic subaortic obstruction in hypertrophic cardiomyopathy: Pulsed Doppler echocardiography. *J Am Coll Cardiol* 6:1, 1985.

62. Spirito P, Maron BJ, Chiarella F, et al: Diastolic abnormalities in patients with hypertrophic cardiomyopathy: Relation to magnitude of left ventricular hypertrophy. *Circulation* 72:310, 1985.

63. Jacobs JJ, Feigenbaum H, Corya BC, et al: Detection of left ventricular asynergy by echocardiography. *Circulation* 48:263, 1973.

64. Buda AJ, Zotz RJ, Pace DP, et al: Comparison of two-dimensional echocardiographic wall motion and wall thickening abnormalities in relation to the myocardium at risk. *Am Heart J* 111:587, 1986.

65. Ryan T, Vasey CT, Presti CF, et al: Exercise echocardiography: Detection of coronary artery disease in patients with normal left ventricular wall motion at rest. *J Am Coll Cardiol* 11:993, 1988.

66. Sawada SG, Segar DS, Ryan T, et al: Echocardiographic detection of coronary artery disease during dobutamine infusion. *Circulation* 83:1605, 1991.

67. Quinones MA, Verani MS, Haichin RM, et al: Exercise echocardiography versus ²⁰¹Tl single-photon emission computed tomography in evaluation of coronary artery disease: Analysis of 292 patients. *Circulation* 85:1026, 1992.

68. Marwick T, D'Hondt A, Baudhuin T, et al: Optimal use of dobutamine stress for the detection and evaluation of coronary artery disease: Combination with echocardiography or scintigraphy, or both? *J Am Coll Cardiol* 22:159, 1993.

69. Weiss JL, Buckley BH, Hutchins GM, et al: Two-dimensional echocardiographic recognition of myocardial injury in man: Comparison with post-mortem studies. *Circulation* 63:401, 1981.

70. Pandian NG, Skorton DJ, Collins SM, et al: Myocardial infarct size threshold for two-dimensional echocardiographic detection: Sensitivity of systolic wall thickening and endocardial motion abnormalities in small vs. large infarctions. *Am J Cardiol* 55:551, 1985.

71. Reeder GS, Seward JB, Tajik AJ: The role of two-dimensional echocardiography in coronary artery disease: A critical appraisal. *Mayo Clin Proc* 57:247, 1982.

72. Taylor AL, Kieso R, Melton J, et al: Echocardiographically detected dyskinesis, myocardial infarct size, and coronary risk region relationships in reperfused canine myocardium. *Circulation* 71:1292, 1985.

73. Mintz GS, Victor MF, Kotler MN, et al: Two-dimensional echocardiographic identification of surgically correctable complications of acute myocardial infarction. *Circulation* 64:91, 1981.

74. Pfeffer MA, Braunwald E, Moye LA, at al: Effect of captopril on mortality and morbidity in patients with left ventricular dysfunction after myocardial infarction. *N Engl J Med* 327:669, 1992.

75. Karalis DG, Bansal RC, Hauck AJ, et al: Transesophageal echocardiographic recognition of subaortic complications in aortic valve endocarditis: Clinical and surgical implications. *Circulation* 86:353, 1992.

76. Cigarroa JE, Isselbacher EM, DeSanctis RW, et al: Diagnostic imaging in the evaluation of suspected aortic dissection: Old standards and new directions. *N Engl J Med* 328:35, 1993.

77. Nienaber CA, vonKodolitschY, Nicolas V, et al: The diagnosis of thoracic aortic dissection by noninvasive imaging procedures. *N Engl J Med* 328:1, 1993.

78. Manning WJ, Silverman DI, Gordon SPF, et al: Cardioversion from atrial fibrillation without prolonged anticoagulation with use of transesophageal echocardiography to exclude the presence of atrial thrombi. *N Engl J Med* 328:750, 1993.

79. Appleton CP, Hatle LK, Popp RL: Cardiac tamponade and pericardial effusion: Respiratory variation in transvalvular flow velocities studied by Doppler echocardiography. *J Am Coll Cardiol* 11:1020, 1988.

80. Kiat H, Berman DS, Maddahi J, et al: Late reversibility of tomographic myocardial thallium-201 defects: An accurate marker of myocardial viability. *J Am Coll Cardiol* 12:1456, 1988.

81. Dilsizian V, Rocco TP, Freedman NMT, et al: Enhanced detection of ischemic but viable myocardium by the reinjection of thallium after stress-redistribution imaging. *N Engl J Med* 323:141, 1990.

82. Leppo JA: Dipyridamole-thallium imaging: The lazy man's stress test. *J Nucl Med* 30:281, 1989.

83. Pennell DJ, Underwood SR, Swanton RH, et al: Dobutamine thallium myocardial perfusion tomography. *J Am Coll Cardiol* 18:1471, 1991.

84. Nishimura S, Mahmarian JJ, Boyce TM, et al: Equivalence between adenosine and exercise thallium-201 myocardial tomography: A multicenter, prospective, crossover trial. *J Am Coll Cardiol* 20:265, 1992.

85. Wackers FJ, Becker AE, Samson G, et al: Location and size of acute transmural myocardial infarction estimated from thallium-201 scintiscans: A clinicopathological study. *Circulation* 56:72, 1977.

86. Silverman KJ, Becker LC, Bulkley BH, et al: Value of early thallium-201 scintigraphy for predicting mortality in patients with acute myocardial infarction. *Circulation* 61:996, 1980.

87. Bonow RO, Dilsizian V, Cuocolo A, et al: Identification of viable myocardium in patients with chronic coronary artery disease and left ventricular dysfunction: Comparison of thallium scintigraphy with reinjection and PET imaging with ^{18}F-fluorodeoxyglucose. *Circulation* 83:26, 1991.

88. Tillisch J, Brunken R, Marshall R, et al: Reversibility of cardiac wall motion abnormalities predicted by positron tomography. *N Engl J Med* 314:884, 1986.

89. Ragosta M, Beller GA, Watson DD, et al: Quantitative planar rest-redistribution ^{201}Th imaging in detection of myocardial viability and prediction of improvement in left ventricular function after coronary bypass surgery in patients with severely depressed left ventricular function.

90. Hendel RC, Layden JJ, Leppo JA: Prognostic value of dipyridamole thallium scintigraphy for evaluation of ischemic heart disease. *J Am Coll Cardiol* 15:109, 1990.

91. Gibson RS, Watson DD, Craddock GB, et al: Prediction of cardiac events after uncomplicated myocardial infarction: A prospective study comparing predischarge exercise thallium-201 scintigraphy and coronary angiography. *Circulation* 68:321, 1983.

92. Leppo JA, O'Brian J, Rothendler JA, et al: Dipyridamole-thallium-201 scintigraphy in the prediction of future cardiac events after acute myocardial infarction. *N Engl J Med* 310:1014, 1984.

93. Leppo J, Plaja J, Gionet M, et al: Noninvasive evaluation of cardiac risk before elective vascular surgery. *J Am Coll Cardiol* 9:269, 1987.

94. Hendel RC, Whitfield SS, Villegas BJ, et al: Prediction of late cardiac events by dipyridamole thallium imaging in patients undergoing elective vascular surgery. *Am J Cardiol* 70:1243, 1992.

95. Okada R, Glover D, Gaffney T, et al: Myocardial kinetics of Tc-99m-hexakis-2-methoxy-2-methylpropylisonitrile. *Circulation* 77:491, 1988.

96. Boucher CA: Detection and location of myocardial infarction using technetium-99m sestamibi imaging at rest. *Am J Cardiol* 66:32E, 1988.

97. Verani MS, Jeroudi MO, Jahmarian JJ, et al: Quantification of myocardial infarction during coronary occlusion and myocardial salvage after reperfusion using cardiac imaging with technetium-99m hexakis 2-methoxyisobutyl isonitrile. *J Am Coll Cardiol* 12:1573, 1988.

98. Gibbons RJ, Verani MS, Behrenbeck T, et al: Feasibility of tomographic Tc-99m-2-methoxy isobutyl isonitrile tomoscintigraphic imaging for the assessment of myocardial area at risk and the effect of treatment in acute myocardial infarction. *Circulation* 80:1277, 1989.

99. Gregoire J, Theroux P: Detection and assessment of unstable angina using myocardial perfusion imaging: Comparison between technetium-99m-sestamibi SPECT and 12-lead electrocardiogram. *Am J Cardiol* 66:42E, 1990.

100. Willerson JT, Parkey RW, Bonte FJ, et al: Technetium stannous pyrophosphate myocardial scintigrams in patients with chest pain of varying etiology. *Circulation* 51:1046, 1975.

101. Falkoff M, Parkey RW, Bonte FJ, et al: Technetium-99m stannous pyrophosphate myocardial scintigraphy: Serial imaging to detect myocardial infarcts in patients. *Clin Cardiol* 1:163, 1978.

102. Rutherford JD, Roberts R, Muller JE, et al: Multicenter investigation of the limitation of infarct size (MILIS): Comparison on enzymatic, scintigraphic and electrocardiographic methods of detecting acute myocardial infarction. *Circulation* 64(suppl IV):IV-84, 1981.

103. Johnson LL, Seldin DW, Becker LC, et al: Antimyosin imaging in acute transmural myocardial infarction: Results of a multicenter clinical trial. *J Am Coll Cardiol* 13:27, 1989.

104. Hendel RC, Cohn S, Aurigemma G, et al: Focal myocardial injury following blunt chest trauma: A comparison of indium-111 antimyosin scintigraphy with other noninvasive methods. *Am Heart J* 123:1208, 1992.

105. Dec GW, Palacios I, Yasuda T, et al: Antimyosin antibody imaging: Its role in the diagnosis of myocarditis. *J Am Coll Cardiol* 16:92, 1990.

106. Norris RM, Barnaby PF, Brandt PW, et al: Prognosis after recovery from first acute myocardial infarction: Determinants of reinfarction and sudden death. *Am J Cardiol* 53:23, 1984.

107. Steckley RA, Kronenberg MW, Born ML, et al: Radionuclide ventriculography: Evaluation of automated and visual methods for regional wall motion analysis. *Radiology* 142:179, 1982.

108. Stanford W, Rooholamini SA, Galvin JR: Assessment of intracardiac masses and extracardiac abnormalities by ultrafast computed tomography, in Marcus ML (ed): *Cardiac Imaging*. Philadelphia, WB Saunders, 1990.

109. Sibbald WJ, Cunningham DR, Chin DN: Noncardiac or cardiac pulmonary edema: A practical approach to clinical differentiation in critically ill patients. *Chest* 84:460, 1983.

110. Van Grondelle A, Ditchey RV, Groves BM, et al: Thermodilution method overestimates low cardiac output in humans. *Am J Physiol* 245:H690, 1983.

111. Antman EM, Marsh JD, Green LH, et al: Blood oxygen measurement in the assessment of intracardiac left to right shunts: A critical appraisal of methodology. *Am J Cardiol* 46:265, 1980.

112. Rackley CE, Satler LF, Pearle DL, et al: Use of hemodynamic measurements for management of acute myocardial infarction, in Rackley CE (ed): *Advances in Critical Care Cardiology*. Philadelphia, FA Davis, 1986.

113. Forrester JS, Diamond G, Chatterjee K, et al: Medical therapy of acute myocardial infarction by application of hemodynamic subsets. *N Engl J Med* 295:1356, 1976.

49. Clinical Management of Cardiac Arrhythmias in the Coronary Care Unit

Christopher A. Clyne
and Carey Kimmelstiel

Cardiovascular-related disease accounts for more American deaths and health care dollars than all other causes of death combined, and within this group arrhythmic-related sudden cardiac death in patients with coronary artery disease accounts for nearly 50 percent of deaths [1]. Identification of the coronary care unit (CCU) patient at risk for significant arrhythmias and management of these arrhythmias are fundamental to the health care provider's role in an intensive care unit setting.

Historical Perspective

The British physician John MacWilliam is credited as the first to identify ventricular fibrillation as a cause of sudden death [2,3]. It was not until half a century later that Harris and Rojas described the association between coronary artery disease, ischemia, and ventricular tachyarrhythmias. This seminal report helped change the approach to patients with cardiovascular-related disease, a process that is still evolving. Recognition of the important relationship between myocardial ischemia and ventricular tachyarrhythmias in the pathophysiology of sudden cardiac death sparked intensive investigation in areas of basic cellular mechanisms of ventricular arrhythmias; clinical epidemiology, which has helped define the natural history of this disorder and enabled recognition of high-risk subgroups; and treatment/outcome studies, which have shaped our approach to managing patients with cardiovascular disease to prevent arrhythmic-related deaths.

Mechanisms of Arrhythmias

TACHYARRHYTHMIAS. An understanding of the basic mechanisms responsible for tachyarrhythmias in the human heart (Table 49-1) is imperative to the management of the CCU patient with cardiac arrhythmias. The easiest mechanism to understand may be *automaticity*. This is because the normal rhythm of the heart, initiated and controlled in the healthy state by the sinoatrial (SA) node, is an example of normal automaticity (Fig. 49-1). Under normal conditions, pacemaker cells

Table 49-1. Mechanisms of Tachyarrhythmias

Disorders of impulse propagation
  Re-entry
Disorders of impulse generation
  Automaticity
    Normal—enhanced, depressed
    Abnormal
  Triggered activity
    Early afterdepolarizations
    Delayed afterdepolarization

Adapted from Hoffman BF, Cranefield PF: The physiological basis of cardiac arrhythmias. *Am J Med* 37:670–675, 1964.

depolarize slowly due to slow inward movement of positive ions [4]. Under conditions of ischemia, myocardial injury, and due to various neurogenic and pharmacologic influences, the pattern of automaticity may change. Cells that retain their normal resting membrane potentials may fire at an increased or decreased rate. This altered *normal automaticity* is due to influences on the rate of inward positive ion movement, as well as changes in the threshold potentials for each cell. The same influences may result in *abnormal automaticity*, which occurs at more depolarized (less negative) resting membrane potentials than normal automaticity. Normal resting membrane potential is between −80 and −90 mV, while abnormal automaticity may be seen when cell resting membrane potentials change to between −60 and −70 mV. These cells show altered action potential contours, that is, the rapid initial upstroke (phase 0) decreases in slope (rate of rise), as well as in amplitude. This is most likely due to a change in cellular mechanism, which includes a decrease in fast inward sodium channel conductance and an increased influence by the slow calcium inward channels [5].

In the CCU, accelerated normal automatic tachyarrhythmias may be due to high catecholamine states produced by discomfort, low cardiac output, or infusion of drugs with sympathomimetic activity. The resulting tachyarrhythmia is usually sinus tachycardia and does not require treatment. The precipitating condition responsible for the tachycardia should be treated. Abnormal automatic tachyarrhythmias may be quite difficult to suppress and management can be quite complex, including removal of the underlying etiology (e.g., ischemia) or stabilization until the precipitating insult (coronary reperfusion, myocardial infarction) has subsided. Specific management strategies are discussed later in this chapter.

Triggered activity is a second accepted mechanism for arrhythmogenesis in cardiac tissues. Triggered activity differs from automaticity in that action potentials generated by a triggered mechanism are dependent on the previous action potential. Automatically generated action potentials are not dependent on previous action potentials. Triggered activity arises from afterdepolarizations that occur during (early afterdepolarizations) or following (delayed afterdepolarizations) action potential repolarization [6].

Both early and delayed afterdepolarizations appear to be calcium channel-dependent. Models for early afterdepolarizations (EADs) have been produced using cesium in a number of preparations and are considered a leading explanation for the clinical tachyarrhythmia seen in *Torsades de pointes* [7]. Delayed afterdepolarizations (DADs) have been studied in digitalis-intoxicated canine Purkinje fibers and catecholamine superfused preparations from canine coronary sinus cells [8,9].

Both EAD- and DAD-related triggered activity appear to be due to calcium overloading of the cell [7,8,9]. Triggered activity, although not believed to be a predominant mechanism for tachyarrhythmias in patients with coronary artery disease, does help explain some clinically important arrhythmias. Digitalis-induced junctional and ventricular tachycardia may be ex-

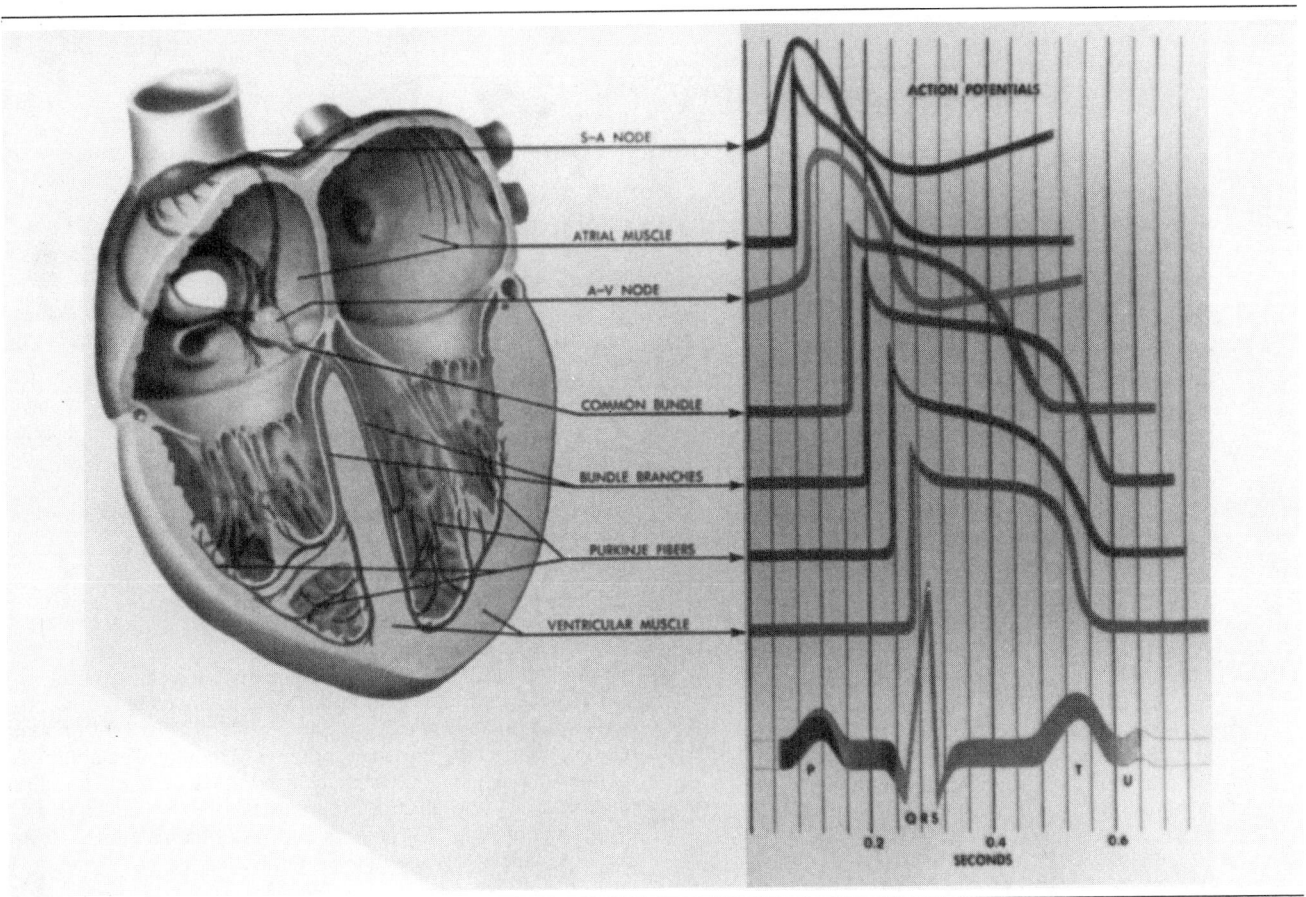

Fig. 49-1. The electrocardiogram.

plained by DAD-related triggered activity. Some forms of ventricular tachycardia occurring in patients without evidence of organic heart disease have also been attributed to triggered activity [10].

Reentry is the third mechanistic model for tachyarrhythmias and represents the mechanism for most ventricular and supraventricular tachyarrhythmias in the CCU setting. The majority of available data that point to reentry as the principal mechanism for supraventricular and ventricular tachyarrhythmias are from patients with chronic coronary artery disease and prior myocardial infarction [11,12]. The original model of reentry described by Mines in 1913 and 1914 is the foundation for our understanding of this mechanism of tachyarrhythmias [13,14]. Mines's early descriptions are of a reentrant circuit around an anatomically defined central obstacle (Figs. 49-2 and 49-3A). The conditions for reentry are: (1) that conduction down the nonblocked limb of the circuit is slow enough to allow the myocardium in the blocked limb of the circuit to recover its excitability and that the impulse can reenter the circuit retrogradely traveling up the previously blocked limb, resulting in reexcitation at the point of origin of the impulse (slow conduction) (Fig. 49-2A); (2) that a premature impulse can block in one direction and propagate down another direction (unidirectional block) (Fig. 49-2B); and (3) that the cycle length (time in milliseconds of one full movement around this circuit) is long enough to allow recovery of previously refractory tissue. This last condition is referred to as an *excitable gap* between the tail of the circulating wavefront (x) and the arrival of the head of the reentering impulse (x + 1) (Fig. 49-2B). If the circuit is so large that a portion of the tissue within the circuit may be fully

repolarized, the gap is referred to as *fully excitable* (white section, Fig. 49-3A). If the tissue has not completely recovered but is still excitable with somewhat altered conduction properties (stippled section, Fig. 49-3A) this is referred to as a *partially excitable gap*. An entrance and exit for the electrical impulse is present within the circuit.

The ability to initiate arrhythmias in the electrophysiology laboratory using programmed electrical stimulation helps define the tachyarrhythmia as *reentrant*. The ability to terminate the same arrhythmia by placing appropriately timed extrastimuli into the circuit during the tachyarrhythmia also defines the arrhythmia as reentrant. Further, this observation that properly timed extrastimuli may create bidirectional block and terminate reentrant arrhythmias has led to pacing as an important treatment strategy for reentrant arrhythmias.

A second model of reentry was described some 75 years after by Allessie et al. [15]. These investigators described reentry around a *functional barrier* composed of excitable tissue that was refractory due to continued impulse bombardment from the periphery. Reentrant impulses circulate around the path on the tail of their own refractoriness; therefore an excitable gap is absent (Fig. 49-3B). These small circuits of reentering impulses may be mobile and move throughout excitable myocardial tissue, producing nonuniform, rapid, inhomogeneous depolarization and repolarization of myocardial tissue. The clinical description of this mechanistic behavior is *fibrillation* [16]. This model of reentry, called the leading circle model, has been used to describe the mechanisms of atrial and ventricular fibrillation in vivo where the ability to enter the circuit and terminate the tachycardia with properly timed premature stimuli is not possible.

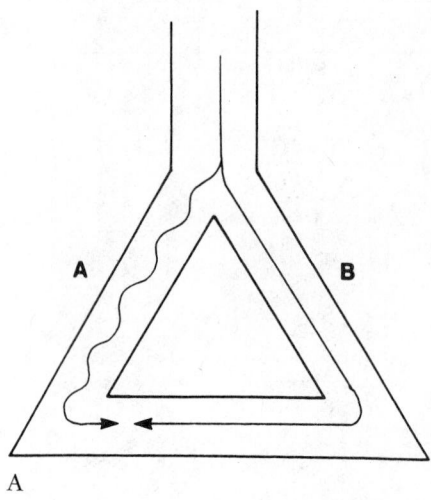

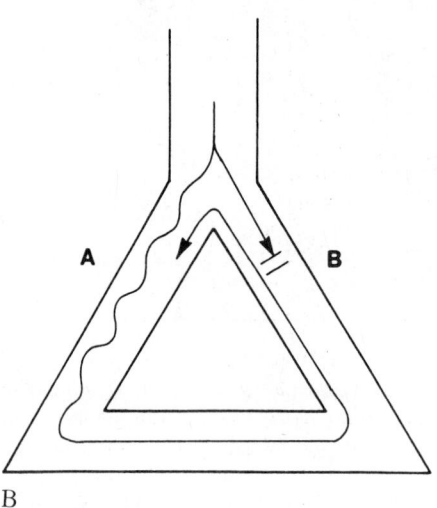

Fig. 49-2. Mechanisms of reentry. A. Prerequisites for reentry. B. Initiation of reentry. (From Fogoros RN: *Practical Cardiac Diagnosis: Electrophysiologic Testing.* Cambridge, MA, Blackwell, 1991. With permission.)

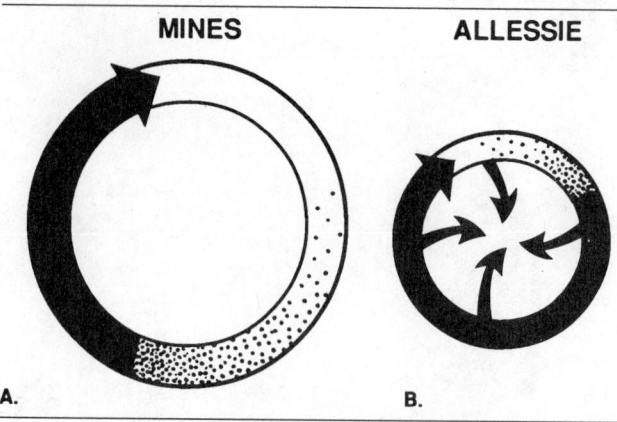

Fig. 49-3. Types of reentry. (From Zipes D: Genesis of cardiac arrhythmias: Electrophysiological considerations, in Braunwald E (ed): *Heart Disease: A Textbook of Cardiovascular Medicine.* 4th ed. Philadelphia, WB Saunders, 1992. With permission.)

Examples of important reentrant arrhythmias in the CCU include uniform and polymorphic ventricular tachycardia, supraventricular tachycardias due to atrioventricular (A-V) nodal reentry, and bypass tract-dependent A-V reentry. The ability to induce and terminate these tachyarrhythmias in the controlled environment of an electrophysiology laboratory has led to the development of pharmacologic and nonpharmacologic treatment modalities, discussed later in this chapter.

BRADYARRHYTHMIAS. While bradyarrhythmias are infrequent causes of sudden cardiac death, they are frequently seen in the CCU setting related to ischemia, autonomic nervous system influences, drugs, and primary disorders of the conduction system (Table 49-2).

In the CCU setting the most common cause of significant bradyarrhythmias is ischemically and pharmacologically related. Acute ischemia involving the right coronary artery, which supplies the sinus node artery (in 55%) and A-V nodal arteries (in 90%), may cause both sinus bradycardia and periods of varying A-V block. Myocardial infarction may cause bundle branch blocks, A-V nodal block, and periods of symptomatic sinus slowing or arrest. The majority of these ischemic or infarct-related bradyarrhythmias resolve over the first several days or weeks after infarction. Many of the medications used to treat patients with acute and chronic coronary artery disease in the intensive care unit can cause significant bradycardias. These include calcium blockers, digitalis preparations, beta-blockers, and antiarrhythmic drugs. Patients who experience periods of exaggerated vagal tone due to discomfort, pericarditis, bowel obstruction, or cerebral vascular accident may experience bradycardia due to hypervagotonia.

Treatment of Cardiac Arrhythmias Unrelated to Acute Myocardial Infarction/Ischemia

Sudden cardiac death, defined as unexpected death that occurs within 1 hour of the onset of signs of instability, is believed to

Application of these models and principles of reentry to the patient with acute and chronic coronary artery disease is not difficult. The presence of myocardial scar from an infarction or anatomic abnormality (atrial septal defect) may easily explain how reentrant circuits fulfilling requirements for reentry occur in the human heart. The leading circle model of reentry dependent on a central functional area of inexcitable myocardium may be explained by the principle of *anisotropy,* the differential ability of a tissue to conduct an impulse, depending on the direction from which the impulse approaches. Normal cardiac muscle is depolarized more rapidly when the impulse travels parallel to the long fiber orientation (longitudinal) rather than perpendicular (transverse) (Fig. 49-4). In chronically infarcted tissue, nonuniform anisotropy may result due to the presence of scar tissue between surviving myofibrils. Mapping of reentrant activation wavefronts in animal models during ventricular tachycardia reveals a pattern of conduction block consistent with nonuniform anisotropy [17].

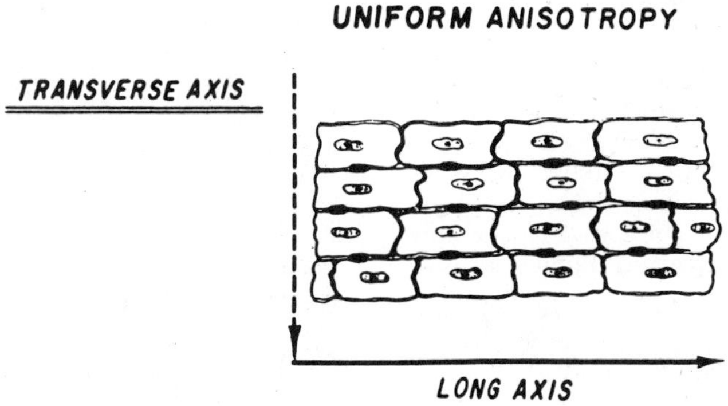

UNIFORM ANISOTROPY

Fig. 49-4. Uniform anisotropy.

occur in patients with ventricular dysfunction secondary to previous myocardial infarction in the majority of cases [18] (see Chap. 35). Many events begin as ventricular tachycardia, then degenerate into ventricular fibrillation, and most are not associated with an acute ischemic syndrome (myocardial ischemia or infarction) [18,19]. Chronic coronary artery disease may be associated with both supraventricular and ventricular arrhythmias. Ventricular arrhythmias may be due to electrical instability secondary to increased myocardial oxygen demand from areas with fixed and inadequate blood supply. Autonomic tone may also serve as an etiology for ventricular arrhythmias by increased sympathetic activity. This change may be responsible for decreasing the fibrillation threshold, leading to ventricular fibrillation in animal models as well as in humans [20].

Symptomatic or asymptomatic acute ischemia may also result in changes in refractoriness between ischemic and nonischemic zones of ventricular myocardium. Acute ischemia shortens the effective refractory period of Purkinje fibers and ischemic myocardial cells. Normal cells adjacent to the ischemic zone remain unchanged. Further, ischemia results in an abrupt reduction (toward zero potential) in transmembrane resting potential as well as in the amplitude and duration of the action potential. Ischemic cells depolarize to a resting membrane potential of less than -60 mV and exhibit reduced excitability and upstroke velocity, thus providing two key elements for reentrant tachyarrhythmias: slow conduction and unidirectional block [21]. In the ischemic border zone, islets of injured cells, interspersed with normal cells, produce fragmented and slowed electrical impulses during diastole. These slowly conducting electrical impulses can then reenter and reactivate excitable tissue, initiating a reentrant beat. If this reentrant circuit remains fixed and perpetuates around an anatomic barrier (scar), the product is ventricular tachycardia (VT). These fragmented, irregular, low-amplitude electrical impulses may create multiple electrical circuits due to changing conduction and refractory properties of interspersed normal and ischemic myocardial cells. The result of these mobile multiple microwavelets of reentry is ventricular fibrillation (VF).

An important determinant of impulse propagation within myocardial tissue is the axial and transverse resistances that are determined by the degree of *intercellular coupling*. The higher the degree of coupling between cells (parallel), the lower the resistance to current flow and the faster the conduction velocity. Uncoupling of cells and slowing of conduction occurs with ischemia, acidosis, and calcium overload [21].

The occurrence of ventricular arrhythmias in the late or posthospital phase correlates with an increased risk of sustained ventricular arrhythmias, sudden cardiac death, and total mortality during the first year after discharge [22,23]. Early studies on the natural history of patients following acute myocardial infarction revealed that in addition to ventricular arrhythmias, low ejection fraction served as an independent predictor of increased risk of death [23]. More recent data show that signal-averaged electrocardiogram (SAECG) and invasive electrical programmed stimulation (EPS) may enhance left ventricular ejection fraction and noninvasive ambulatory recording of ventricular premature complexes in predicting outcome [24,25].

In the study by Dennis et al., 403 survivors of myocardial infarction underwent invasive electrical programmed stimulation for the induction of ventricular arrhythmias [25]. These patients were followed for a mean of 12 months, with the primary endpoint being an arrhythmic event. Ventricular arrhythmias were induced in 34 percent of the study population. Twelve percent of patients with an inducible sustained (>30 seconds) ventricular arrhythmia had a spontaneous arrhythmic event during the follow-up period, compared to 4 percent in the group without an inducible ventricular arrhythmia (p<0.05).

Risk stratification of patients with coronary artery disease and previous myocardial infarction should include an assessment of

Table 49-2. Causes of Bradyarrhythmias

A. Ischemia
B. Autonomic nervous system (parasympathetic)
C. Drugs—calcium blockers, beta-blockers, antiarrhythmic drugs, digitalis
D. Disorders of conduction
  1. Degenerative
    a. Lev's disease
    b. Lenegre's disease
  2. Infectious
    a. Lyme disease
    b. Viral (HIV)
    c. Chagas disease
  3. Muscular disorders
    a. Myotonic dystrophy
    b. Emory-Dreiffus syndrome
    c. Kearns-Sayer syndrome
  4. Inflammatory
    a. Sarcoid
    b. Rheumatoid arthritis
    c. SLE
  5. Congenital

left ventricular function by echocardiography, radionuclide angiography, or cardiac catheterization; noninvasive ambulatory monitoring to quantify ventricular ectopic activity and presence of nonsustained ventricular tachycardia; and signal-averaged ECG to detect the presence of late potentials, which indicate areas of slow conduction in the myocardium. Patients in the high-risk subset (ejection fraction < 40%; > 10 PVCs per hour, and/or salvos of greater than 3 ventricular beats; and/or an abnormal signal-averaged ECG) should be considered for more intense investigation, including exercise testing and invasive electrical programmed stimulation.

Cardiac Arrhythmias Associated with Acute Ischemic Syndrome

In the first 48 hours after myocardial infarction, the incidence of ventricular arrhythmias ranges from 34 to 100 percent [26, 27,28]. Ventricular arrhythmias tend to be associated with larger infarcts, congestive heart failure, and previous or resultant conduction disturbances. Some forms of ventricular arrhythmias are considered benign and need no treatment, while others may be malignant and require prompt treatment. In the early postinfarction phase of the CCU patient, ventricular arrhythmias may be divided into four categories: (1) warning arrhythmias, (2) accelerated idioventricular rhythm, (3) paroxysmal ventricular tachycardia (unsustained and sustained), and (4) ventricular fibrillation.

WARNING ARRHYTHMIAS. Warning arrhythmias may occur at any time during the early or late postinfarction phase. Early experimental studies showed that a single ventricular stimulus delivered in late systole or during late diastole could result in ventricular fibrillation [29]. Subsequent experience in CCUs revealed an association between premature ventricular depolarizations and development of significant life-threatening ventricular arrhythmias [30,31,32]. Warning arrhythmias include ventricular ectopic beats at a frequency of at least 3 per hour and salvos of 3 or more beats of ventricular tachycardia [23]. Although warning arrhythmias do predict high risk for symptomatic sustained ventricular arrhythmias and sudden cardiac death, it is unclear whether these asymptomatic arrhythmias should be treated.

ACCELERATED IDIOVENTRICULAR RHYTHMS. Accelerated idioventricular rhythm (AIVR) is defined as ventricular rhythm with rates of 50 to 100 beats per minutes. This rhythm is not uncommon within the first 24 hours after acute myocardial infarction [33]. It is equally common in patients with anterior and inferior myocardial infarctions and is not affected by size of the infarct or presence of left ventricular dysfunction. It is not associated with a higher incidence of sustained lethal ventricular arrhythmias, in-hospital mortality, or sudden cardiac death. Accelerated idioventricular rhythm is most commonly seen in association with restoration of antegrade flow after coronary occlusion, which may occur spontaneously or as the result of thrombolytic therapy [34,35]. This arrhythmia occurs in more than 80 percent of patients who have had successful recanalization of an occluded artery. It has been used as a marker for successful thrombolysis when it occurs soon after administration of the thrombolytic agent.

VENTRICULAR TACHYCARDIA. Ventricular tachycardia is defined as 3 or more consecutive ventricular depolarizations at a rate of greater than 100 beats per minute. Sustained ventricular tachycardia lasts longer than 30 seconds, while unsustained ventricular tachycardia lasts from 3 beats to less than 30 seconds and terminates spontaneously. Ventricular tachycardia can be further distinguished as uniform (i.e., of constant morphology and rate) or polymorphic (i.e., nonuniform morphology and rate). Polymorphic ventricular tachycardia and ventricular fibrillation are generally distinguished on the basis of rate: ventricular tachycardia is less than 250 beats per minute, while ventricular fibrillation occurs at rates greater than 250 beats per minute.

Ventricular tachycardia has been reported to occur on average in 10 percent (range 6–40%) of patients with acute myocardial infarction [27,28,36]. Most episodes of ventricular tachycardia are asymptomatic nonsustained events that occur within the first 48 hours following acute myocardial infarction. Sustained ventricular tachycardia is relatively infrequent in the first 48 hours following myocardial infarction and is associated with extensive infarction and congestive heart failure. Unsustained and sustained ventricular tachycardia within the 48 hours after myocardial infarction is associated with a higher in-hospital mortality but has not been found to affect adversely long-term prognosis [28,32,37].

The distinction between uniform and polymorphic ventricular tachycardia is important. It is thought that the mechanisms, and therefore management of, these two types of ventricular arrhythmias are different. Polymorphic ventricular tachycardia unrelated to a long Q–T interval is believed to be related to ongoing severe myocardial ischemia and may be treated effectively with antiischemic management strategies, including nitrates and beta-blockers, treatment of congestive heart failure, and intraaortic balloon pump or emergent coronary artery bypass surgery [38,39]. Sustained uniform ventricular tachycardia is infrequently seen in the first 48 hours following acute myocardial infarction. When found, it is thought to be due to reperfusion arrhythmias or related to underlying scar from previous myocardial infarction. A previous scar may serve as an anatomic barrier around which the reentry tachycardia propagates. Unstable myocardium in the area of the scar distant to this barrier may produce premature ventricular depolarizations, which can initiate the reentrant tachycardia.

VENTRICULAR FIBRILLATION. Ventricular fibrillation, described as a sustained polymorphic ventricular tachycardia with rates greater than 250 beats per minute, is almost always associated with hemodynamic compromise. Primary ventricular fibrillation occurs within the first 48 hours after acute myocardial infarction or severe coronary ischemia and is not preceded by heart failure, hypotension, or cardiogenic shock. Secondary ventricular fibrillation develops as a terminal complication of these unstable clinical situations. The distinction is important clinically, since the long-term prognosis for patients with primary ventricular fibrillation who are resuscitated successfully is quite favorable, while those who suffer a secondary ventricular fibrillatory event have an extremely high mortality.

Primary ventricular fibrillation occurs most frequently in the first hour after myocardial infarction and declines rapidly over the next 4 to 12 hours [37]. Primary ventricular fibrillation has been reported to occur within the first 48 hours in 1 to 10 percent of patients suffering from an acute myocardial infarction or severe unstable angina. It is preceded by warning ventricular arrhythmias in half of patients and is the first manifestation of underlying electrical instability in the other half [40].

The long-term prognosis of patients who are resuscitated from a primary ventricular fibrillatory event is not adversely affected. There is controversy about the in-hospital mortality. Early studies suggested an unaffected in-hospital mortality, while later studies indicate a higher in-hospital mortality for patients resuscitated from primary ventricular fibrillation [37,41,42].

Nonventricular Arrhythmias Associated with Acute Ischemic Syndrome

SUPRAVENTRICULAR TACHYCARDIAS. The tachycardia most frequently associated with unstable coronary syndromes is sinus tachycardia (see Chap. 41). This is usually a response to the physiologic stresses of pain, anxiety, products of tissue injury, and medications. It may also be due to the presence of underlying heart failure, persistent ischemia and hypotension, or shock. Because of the broad range of associated conditions that elicit this physiologic tachycardia, it is probably the supraventricular tachycardia most associated with poor outcome. Presence of persistent sinus tachycardia should alert the clinician to possible high-risk situations, including persistent ischemia, impending heart failure, and hypotension, which can severely and adversely affect in-hospital and postdischarge mortality. Treatment of the primary disorder is recommended, as is treatment of the sinus tachycardia with beta-blocking agents to decrease myocardial oxygen consumption. Acute beta blockade should be undertaken only in patients without signs of congestive heart failure and bronchospastic pulmonary diseases.

Atrial fibrillation and flutter are frequently seen in CCU patients (see Chap. 41). These forms of supraventricular tachycardias may be due to elevated catecholamine levels, increased left atrial pressure and dilatation of the left atrium, or atrial infarction associated with coronary artery occlusion. The occurrence of atrial fibrillation in the acute myocardial infarction setting does not appear to affect in-hospital prognosis adversely, though it may make patient management much more difficult. Rapid rates result in increased myocardial oxygen consumption, and persistence of ischemia may contribute to extension of the myocardial infarction. Loss of atrial contribution to ventricular filling also may result in a low cardiac output state and precipitate congestive heart failure and hypotension. This may be especially evident in patients with right ventricular infarction, where right ventricular end-diastolic pressures are elevated and the compliant properties of the ventricle are severely reduced, thereby limiting diastolic filling. Loss of the atrial contribution to right ventricular filling may result in clinically significant reduction in blood flow to the left heart and consequent hypotension and shock.

Management of atrial fibrillation resulting in persistent ischemia, heart failure, or hypotension includes control of the ventricular response by various A-V nodal blocking agents (beta- or calcium blockers, digoxin), antiarrhythmic agents (procainamide) for conversion to normal rhythm in stable patients, or rapid synchronized DC cardioversion in the unstable patient [16]. Other forms of supraventricular arrhythmias that may occur in the CCU include automatic or reentrant atrial tachycardias, A-V nodal reentry, and A-V reentry tachycardias. These are not necessarily associated with acute myocardial infarction or ischemia but when present may complicate the course of patients in the throes of an acute ischemic event. These tachyarrhythmias may increase myocardial oxygen consumption and should be swiftly treated (see Chap. 41).

BRADYARRHYTHMIAS AND ATRIOVENTRICULAR BLOCK ASSOCIATED WITH ACUTE MYOCARDIAL INFARCTION. The bradyarrhythmia most commonly associated with myocardial infarction is sinus bradycardia, which occurs in 15 to 40 percent of patients within the first 48 hours of myocardial infarction [43,44]. Reflex vagotonia is the most common etiology of sinus bradycardia during myocardial infarction. The lower aspects of the intraatrial septum and the inferior posterior wall of the left ventricle have a dense supply of vagal afferent receptors [45]. Sinus bradycardia is, therefore, more commonly associated with inferior rather than anterior infarctions. It is thought that ischemia and injury during inferior wall infarction cause stimulation of these receptors, with subsequent increased vagal tone, resulting in inhibition of sinus and A-V nodal automaticity and conduction [45]. Other mechanisms responsible for sinus bradycardia include infarction involving the sinus node artery, which originates from the right coronary artery in 55 percent of normal patients and from the left circumflex artery in the remaining 45 percent, and release of products of tissue injury, which may have negative chronotropic effects.

Sinus arrest and sinus exit block are infrequently observed during acute infarction. Sinus arrest is differentiated from sinus exit block by the presence of an atrial pause that is a noninteger multiple of the sinus cycle length. The sinus pause in sinus exit block is a whole number multiple of the sinus cycle length. Both of these manifestations of sinus node dysfunction may be secondary to either ischemia of the SA node or increased vagal tone. These phenomena are most commonly found in the first 4 to 6 hours of the acute myocardial infarction phase [43,44]. Treatment is directed to patients with symptoms related to these arrhythmias, including congestive heart failure, central nervous system alteration, and/or hypotension due to low cardiac output. In patients with significant symptoms, intravenous atropine is usually effective in the early stages by reversing the overriding vagal tone and correcting the bradyarrhythmia. Atropine should be given in small doses of 0.4 to 0.6 mg intravenously. Caution should be exercised in administering this agent, as sinus tachycardia may result, causing an increase in myocardial oxygen consumption, resulting in ischemia and infarct extension. For patients with continuing and/or unstable angina, temporary pacing of the ventricle (in patients with associated A-V block) and/or atrium may be necessary.

Atrioventricular block occurs in 3 to 15 percent of patients with acute myocardial infarction [44,46]. A-V is characterized as first-degree, second-degree, and third-degree. First-degree A-V block exists when the P–R interval is greater than 200 msec, with maintenance of 1:1 A-V conduction. The site of conduction delay is within the A-V node in the great majority of patients. Therapy is usually not necessary, as these patients are generally asymptomatic. In patients with very prolonged P–R intervals and an underlying tachycardia, the P wave (atrial contraction) may occur during ventricular systole (P wave found in T wave). This may result in an increase in left atrial and pulmonary capillary wedge pressures, resulting in pulmonary congestion and hypotension. This unusual situation may require treatment with temporary A-V sequential pacing and a shorter A-V delay in unstable patients. Watchful waiting is usually sufficient in the asymptomatic patient, although some forms of first-degree A-V block may progress to higher forms of A-V block. Judicious use of pharmacologic agents that may impair A-V nodal conduction, such as calcium blockers, digoxin, and beta-blockers, is advised.

Second- and third-degree A-V block is considered to occur when the sinus rate is constant and atrial depolarization fails to conduct to the ventricle. Second-degree block may be type I (Mobitz I or Wenckebach block), which is associated with progressive lengthening in P–R interval and shortening of successive R–R intervals until the dropped QRS complex occurs. The P–R interval after the dropped beat is shorter than the P–R interval just prior to the dropped beat. Type II (Mobitz II) second-degree block occurs when there is no P–R prolongation prior to the dropped beat. The QRS complex in Mobitz I second-degree heart block is generally narrow (in patients without preexisting bundle branch block) and the site of block is usually within the A-V node. Mobitz II second-degree heart block is often associated with a wide-complex QRS, as the site of block is most often within the His-Purkinje system. The distinction QRS morphology between the two types of second-degree A-V block is helpful in differentiating the site of block and, therefore, risk for progression to complete heart block in patients with 2:1 A-V block, where it is not possible to distinguish between types I and II second-degree heart block.

While any patient with acute first- or second-degree A-V block may progress to third-degree A-V block (complete heart block), those with Mobitz II second-degree heart block are at greatest risk. The risk of developing high-degree A-V block is also dependent on the location of the myocardial infarction and the time period during which block occurs. Patients with inferior wall myocardial infarction usually develop Mobitz I second-degree A-V block [47]. In one study of patients who developed high-degree A-V block in the setting of acute myocardial infarction, complete heart block was preceded by the development of first- or second-degree A-V block in nearly three-fourths of patients [47]. Complete heart block resolved in almost all patients with inferior myocardial infarction. Those patients who developed high-degree A-V block within the first 6 hours usually responded to atropine, suggesting exaggerated vagotonia as the major etiologic factor. In patients who develop later A-V block, the mechanisms may be quite different and include atrial infarction, edema or infarction of the A-V node, and metabolic alterations, which are unlikely to respond to atropine [47].

The presence of higher degrees of A-V block, including second- and third-degree (complete) heart block, appears to be associated with a greater short-term mortality, even when the block is transient. This may be secondary to an increased incidence of hypotension and shock and an association with more frequent anterior myocardial infarctions [48,49].

Mobitz II second-degree block and complete heart block occur in approximately 5 percent of patients with anterior myocardial infarctions [33]. These blocks are almost always below the level of the A-V node and are caused by infarction or ischemia of the lower conduction system. They are generally associated with large amounts of injured myocardium. Complete heart block is associated with mortality in the setting of acute anterior myocardial infarction as high as 70 to 85 percent [33,49]. Cause of death in these patients is usually associated with cardiogenic shock.

INTRAVENTRICULAR CONDUCTION BLOCKS. Intraventricular conduction blocks are found in 8 to 15 percent of patients with acute myocardial infarction [33,50]. The conduction defects are caused by ischemia or infarction of the bundle branches and are directly related to the anatomy of the conduction system and its blood supply. Table 49-3 describes the association of coronary artery and bundle branch anatomy. Bundle branch blocks are significantly more common in anterior than inferior myocardial infarctions. The clinical significance of intraventricular conduction defects during infarction

Table 49-3. Coronary Artery Supply to the Conduction System

Sinus (SA) node: SA nodal artery from:
  a. RCA in 55%
  b. LCX in 45%
Atrioventricular (A-V) node: A-V nodal artery from:
  a. RCA in 90%
  b. LCX in 10%
His bundle:
  Common bundle:
    a. Septal perforating arteries of the left anterior descending artery
    b. A-V nodal artery
  Right bundle branch:
    a. Proximal third from the A-V nodal artery (RCA/LCX)
    b. Distal third from the septal perforating branches of the LAD
  Left bundle branch:
    a. Anterior fascicle from the septal perforators of the LAD
    b. Posterior fascicle from the posterior descending artery of the RCA and branches of the LAD

A-V = atrioventricular; LAD = left anterior descending artery; LCX = left circumflex artery; RCA = right coronary artery; SA = sinoatrial.

is the progression to higher degrees of heart block and higher mortalities. Table 49-4 lists the relative incidence of various types of bundle branch blocks during acute myocardial infarction and the relative progression to complete heart block and associated in-hospital mortalities.

Many patients with bundle branch blocks and acute myocardial infarction are known to have previous conduction defects. The risk of progression to complete heart block appears to be higher if the conduction defect is new or of indeterminant age compared to those in whom the defect is known to have preceded the myocardial infarction [51]. Alternating bundle branch block is due to trifascicular block and has a very high rate of progression to complete heart block (45%) [51]. While patients with bifascicular block and first-degree A-V block have a higher incidence of progression to complete block, as compared to patients with normal P–R intervals (35% vs. 11%), this is not considered to be true trifascicular block [52].

Indications for prophylactic temporary cardiac pacing are listed in Table 49-5. While temporary cardiac pacing may be effective in treating the bradycardia associated with high-degree A-V block and trifascicular block, mortality does not appear to be affected, as the high mortality rates are associated with cardiogenic shock and pump failure secondary to large areas of infarction [33,51,52]. The introduction of the external noninvasive temporary cardiac pacemaker by Zoll et al. has made it possible to defer the placement of a transvenous temporary pacemaker in patients at intermediate risk of developing high-degree heart block [53]. The external cardiac pacer should be demonstrated to be effective and well tolerated in the individual patient if it is to be used instead of transvenous pacing. Patients at high risk for developing complete heart block should have a 4 or 5 Fr. pacing catheter placed in the right ventricular apex under sterile conditions to protect from symptomatic complete heart block.

Management of Tachyarrhythmias in the Coronary Care Unit

Although supraventricular and ventricular tachyarrhythmias share the same mechanisms, management may vary considerably. Supraventricular arrhythmias are usually not associated

Table 49-4. Bundle Branch Blocks during Acute Myocardial Infarction

Bundle branch block	Incidence (%)	Progression to CHB (%)	Hospital mortality (%)
None	0	4	12
LPFB	1	1	40
LAFB	4	2	20
LBBB	4	13	23
RBBB	2	13	23
RBBB + LAFB	5	27	28
RBBB + LPFB	1	29	45
ABBB	1	45	45

MI = myocardial infarction; CHB = complete heart block; LPFB = left posterior fascicle block; LAFB = left anterior fascicle block; LBBB = left bundle branch block; RBBB = right bundle branch block, ABBB = alternating bundle block.
Adapted from Bhandau AK, Sager PT: Management of peri-infarctional ventricular and conduction disturbances, in Nacarrelli GV (ed): *Cardiac Arrhythmias: A Practical Approach*. New York, Futura, 1991, p 313. With permission.

with hemodynamic compromise and rarely require emergent intervention. Ventricular arrhythmias, on the other hand, are frequently associated with hemodynamic compromise and death and may require emergent intervention. As with all medical therapies, that rationale for treatment is based on a risk-benefit analysis. Many antiarrhythmic agents may be proarrhythmic and should be preserved for treatment of life-threatening and/or symptomatic arrhythmias in CCU patients.

Pharmacologic management of, and/or prophylaxis against, unstable arrhythmias is a critical part of CCU management. In the last two decades, several nonpharmacologic approaches to the management of supraventricular and ventricular arrhythmias in the CCU setting have been added to our armamentarium. These include the use of intraaortic balloon counterpulsation, emergent coronary artery bypass grafting, or coronary angioplasty to relieve ischemic burden in patients with recalcitrant polymorphic ventricular tachycardia or fibrillation associated with acute ischemia; electrocardiographic, intracardiac, and intraesophageal recording techniques to differentiate supraventricular from ventricular tachycardias in patients with wide-complex tachycardias; various pacing techniques to terminate symptomatic arrhythmias and prevent lethal arrhythmias; and catheter and surgical mapping and ablation techniques for control of incessant and recalcitrant supraventricular and ventricular tachyarrhythmias. These developments, when combined with beat-to-beat monitoring with storage capability, rapid DC cardioversion and defibrillation, and other forms of acute intervention, have improved management of the CCU patient with cardiac arrhythmias.

Appropriate management of the patient with a tachyarrhythmia requires accurate identification of the arrhythmia and its underlying mechanism. The diagnosis of supraventricular tachycardia is almost always certain when the QRS complex of the tachycardia is identical to that of the sinus rhythm. Proper identification of the mechanism underlying a wide QRS tachycardia may be very difficult but is critical to safe and effective treatment of the arrhythmia and future patient management.

Table 49-5. Indications for Temporary Cardiac Pacing

	Indicated
SA + A-V blocks	
Sinus node dysfunction without Sx ± medications	No
Sinus node dysfunction with hemodynamic Sx despite medical Rx	Yes
First-degree A-V block	No
Mobitz I without Sx	No
Mobitz I with Sx without adequate response to pharmacologic agents	yes
Mobitz II	Yes
Complete heart block, AWMI	Yes
Complete heart block, IWMI with narrow escape rhythm without Sx	No
Complete heart block, IWMI with hemodynamic Sx or new wide complex escape rhythm	Yes
Bundle branch blocks	
New unifascicular block or isolated RBBB	No
New LBBB	Possible
New first-degree A-V block and RBBB or LBBB	Possible
New bilateral BBB	Yes
Alternating BBB	Yes
Old bilateral BBB, RBBB, LBBB	No

A-V = atrioventricular; AWMI = anterior wall myocardial infarction; BBB = bundle branch block; IWMI = inferior wall myocardial infarction; LBBB = left bundle branch block; RBBB = right bundle branch block; Rx = treatment; Sx = symptoms.
From Bhandair AK, Sager PT: Management of peri-infarctional ventricular and conduction disturbances, in Nacarrelli GV (ed): *Cardiac Arrhythmias: A Practical Approach*. New York, Futura, 1991, p 316. With permission.

DIAGNOSTIC APPROACH FOR SUPRAVENTRICULAR ARRHYTHMIAS IN THE CORONARY CARE UNIT.

The cornerstone to diagnosing and treating tachyarrhythmias in the CCU is the surface ECG recording. Single- and multiple-lead monitoring and storage systems should be available in all intensive care unit settings. A chest lead (V_1 or modified chest lead) and/or limb lead II generally allows for the best identification of atrial activity during supraventricular tachycardia. The relationship between atrial and ventricular activity (i.e., ratio of conduction—1:1, 2:1, 1:2, or disassociation) is critical to proper diagnosis. P wave morphology is also very helpful in identifying the mechanism of the supraventricular tachycardia. Sinus node reentry and atrial tachycardias in the area of the sinus node (high right atrium) have P waves with a morphology similar or identical to that in sinus rhythm. Tachycardias originating from the lower atrium or A-V node and circus movement tachycardias involving antegrade conduction through the A-V node may be identified when the P wave morphology is inverted in the inferior leads. For A-V reentrant tachycardias utilizing a left-sided accessory pathway for conduction from the ventricle to the atrium, the P wave in limb leads aVL and lead I is negative and in aVR is positive. The timing of atrial and ventricular complexes must then be determined. Supraventricular tachycardias are classified as short P–R–long R–P, or long P–R–short R–P tachycardias (see Chap. 41). Short P–R–long R–P tachycardias include sinus tachycardias, atrial tachycardias, and circus movement tachycardias with slowly conducting retrograde pathways (atypical A-V nodal reentry, A-V reentry tachycardias with slowly conducting retrograde bypass tracts). Long P–R–short R–P tachycardias include typical A-V nodal reentry and ortho-dromic A-V reentrant tachycardias, and some atrial tachycardias with delayed A-V nodal conduction.

The rate and regularity of the ventricular response can also be very helpful in determining the mechanism of the arrhyth-mia. Atrial fibrillation is usually an irregularly irregular rhythm (except when complete A-V nodal block is present). P waves are not identifiable. Multifocal atrial tachycardia can also be irregularly irregular, but multiple P wave morphologies can be identified. Other supraventricular tachycardias are regular. De-termination of the rate of the tachycardias can be helpful in determining their mechanisms: sinus tachycardia occurs usually at rates of 100 to 140 beats per minute, while atrial flutter with 2:1 block is commonly seen, with a ventricular response rate of 140 to 160 beats per minute. Typical A-V nodal reentry tachy-cardia is commonly seen with rates of 140 to 200 beats per minute, while A-V reentrant tachycardia is generally found with rates of 140 to 240 beats per minute.

Frequently occurring and prolonged episodes of supraven-tricular tachycardias should be recorded on a 12-lead ECG for proper identification of the above features. A 30- to 60-second strip should also be recorded to characterize the degree of oscillation in rate, changes in morphology of the P and QRS, varying P–R–R–P intervals, and the effect of premature atrial and ventricular depolarizations on the arrhythmia. Changing surface lead position can aid in identification of difficult-to-visualize P waves. Placing the skin terminal for aVr at the sternal notch and aVl at the xyphoid (Lewis lead configuration) some-times allows identification of an otherwise hidden P wave. Use of the intracardiac electrogram recording in patients with atrial and ventricular pacing wires enables accurate identification of the pattern of atrial and ventricular association. This is most easily done in patients recovering from cardiothoracic surgery who may have epicardial pacing wires in place. The use of esophageal lead recording of atrial activity simultaneously re-corded with a surface ECG lead also permits accurate identifi-cation of atrioventricular timing and association. Interventions that may alter the rate or terminate the tachycardia are quite useful in determining mechanism. Carotid sinus massage and/or use of the Valsalva maneuver while recording a rhythm strip may permit diagnosis by increasing block at the A-V node, resulting in termination of the arrhythmia (A-V nodal and A-V reentrant tachyarrhythmias) or altering the relationship be-tween atrium and ventricle, permitting the identification of P waves not otherwise seen: 1:1 and 2:1 atrial flutter or atrial tachycardia with increased A-V nodal block so that atrial activity can clearly be seen between QRS complexes.

If the patient is unstable and requires immediate intervention or if manipulation of the autonomic nervous system with carotid sinus pressure or Valsalva maneuver is not effective, various pharmacologic interventions may be safely attempted. Adeno-sine is a purine nucleoside with a half-life of approximately 10 seconds. It can be given into a large peripheral vein or central vein as a 6.0- to 12.0-mg bolus followed by a 10-cc normal saline push while recording a rhythm strip. Block in the A-V node occurs in approximately 90 percent of patients, permitting identification of an underlying atrial mechanism disassociated from the ventricle in atrial fibrillation, atrial flutter, and atrial tachycardias. Termination of arrhythmias relying on A-V nodal conduction (A-V nodal and A-V reentrant tachycardias) occurs in more than 90 percent of patients. Verapamil in doses of 1 to 10 mg given as an intravenous bolus while monitoring blood pressure is also effective in creating block in the A-V node for identification and termination of supraventricular tachycardias. Use of intravenous verapamil is reserved for patients with narrow-complex tachycardias.

DIFFERENTIAL DIAGNOSIS OF WIDE QRS TACHYCAR-DIAS. Differentiation between supraventricular and ventricular tachyarrhythmias is essential if appropriate therapy is to be instituted. Misdiagnosis can lead to inappropriate therapy that may be ineffective or detrimental to the patient. The electro-cardiographic diagnosis of wide QRS tachycardias can be dif-ficult, but several electrocardiographic criteria are useful in differentiating supraventricular from ventricular tachyarrhyth-mias.

Supraventricular tachycardias may appear wide on the sur-face ECG due to an underlying conduction defect or a func-tional bundle branch block (left or right bundle branch block). The latter situation may occur during rapid rates, where the effective refractory period of part or all of one bundle branch is encroached on, producing a wide QRS. Antiarrhythmic drugs may also result in wide QRS supraventricular tachycardia. Some antiarrhythmic agents produce a wider QRS complex with faster rates (use-dependency). This can occur with type IA and type IC agents, including quinidine, procainamide, and encainide/flecainide. Electrolyte imbalances (hypokalemia, hypomagne-semia) also may result in wide-complex supraventricular tachy-arrhythmias. Tachycardias traveling from the atrium to the ven-tricle over an accessory pathway may also manifest as a wide-complex QRS.

In patients with a bundle branch block during sinus rhythm, comparing the 12-lead ECG during the tachycardia with sinus rhythm ECG should reliably distinguish between ventricular and supraventricular tachycardia. The latter should have a QRS morphology identical to that of sinus rhythm QRS complexes in all 12 leads. If there are significant differences in any one lead, the tachycardia is probably ventricular in origin [54].

QRS morphology can be quite helpful in differentiating su-praventricular tachycardia with aberrancy from ventricular tachycardia. When the QRS duration is greater than 140 msec, ventricular tachycardia is the more likely diagnosis. QRS axis is also an important differentiating feature: an extreme left axis ($-90°$ to $-180°$) usually indicates ventricular tachycardia. A left bundle branch block with right axis deviation is also highly suggestive of ventricular origin, while the presence of a typical right bundle branch block with an rsR pattern and a deep S wave is most consistent with supraventricular origin. [55,56]. An approach to the differential diagnosis of wide-complex tachycardias using a combination of morphologic and conduc-tion characteristics in a stepwise fashion with a specificity of greater than 95 percent was recently proposed [57] (Fig. 49-5). Both lead V_1-V_2 *and* lead V_6 criteria for the different bundle branch block-like tachycardias must be met to fulfill the mor-phologic requirements for diagnosis. Further, these criteria should not be used for patients with known or suspected an-tegradely (atrium to ventricle) conducting bypass tracts. Using this approach, it was possible correctly to differentiate ventric-ular tachycardia from supraventricular tachycardia with aber-rancy in greater than 80 percent of cases, using the initial three steps (nonmorphologic) alone.

Although the surface ECG is an important tool for differen-tiating ventricular tachycardia from supraventricular tachycardia with aberrancy in the CCU, intracardiac electrograms obtained through temporary pacing electrodes or esophageal electrodes or during electrophysiologic study still represent the gold stan-dard for diagnosing supraventricular versus ventricular tachy-cardia. If the clinical situation permits intracardiac electrogram evaluation of the tachycardia, this approach should be under-taken at an early stage.

DRUG THERAPY. Administration of parenteral and oral an-tiarrhythmic agents is the cornerstone of tachyarrhythmia man-

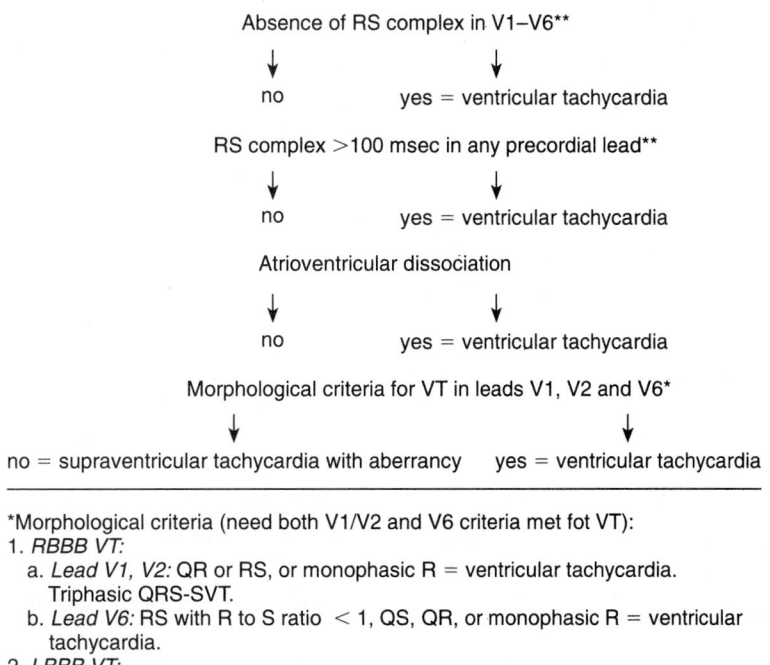

Absence of RS complex in V1–V6**

no   yes = ventricular tachycardia

RS complex >100 msec in any precordial lead**

no   yes = ventricular tachycardia

Atrioventricular dissociation

no   yes = ventricular tachycardia

Morphological criteria for VT in leads V1, V2 and V6*

no = supraventricular tachycardia with aberrancy   yes = ventricular tachycardia

*Morphological criteria (need both V1/V2 and V6 criteria met fot VT):
1. *RBBB VT:*
   a. *Lead V1, V2:* QR or RS, or monophasic R = ventricular tachycardia.
      Triphasic QRS-SVT.
   b. *Lead V6:* RS with R to S ratio < 1, QS, QR, or monophasic R = ventricular
      tachycardia.
2. *LBBB VT:*
   a. *Lead V1 or V2:* R wave >30 msec in duration; or >60 msec from beginning of
      R to nadir of S; knotched S = ventricular tachycardia.
   b. *Lead V6:* QR or QS = ventricular tachycardia.
**Beginning of R wave to nadir of S wave

Fig. 49-5. Wide-complex tachycardias, supraventricular versus ventricular tachycardia, the stepwise approach. (From Brugada P, Brugada J, Mont L, et al: A new approach to the differential diagnosis of a regular tachycardia with a wide QRS complex. *Circulation* 83:1649, 1991. With permission.

agement. A complete discussion of the pharmacokinetics and pharmacodynamics of antiarrhythmic drugs appears in Chapter 207; antiarrhythmic poisoning is discussed in Chapter 131. A general discussion of pharmacologic principles appears in Chapter 205.

The classification developed by Vaughn-Williams and modified by Harrison has contributed greatly to our understanding of arrhythmia mechanisms and drug interactions [58,59]. The classification of antiarrhythmic agents is changing rapidly with the development of many new agents (moricizine) and techniques that allow for the investigation of newly recognized ion channels. (See Table 207-1 for the Vaughn-Williams classification.) Many antiarrhythmic agents have drug effects that cross classes. For example, amiodarone has potassium channel blocking effects and prolongs the repolarization phase of the action potential (class III), sodium channel blocking activity (class I), and sympatholytic effects (class II). Nevertheless, an understanding of the overall effects of an antiarrhythmic agent on the ECG can be helpful in guiding drug therapy. Table 49-6 shows the effects of antiarrhythmic agents on the ECG, and Table 49-7 shows the basic electrophysiologic effects of antiarrhythmic agents. See Chapter 207 for a pharmacokinetic summary and important drug interactions for most of the antiarrhythmic agents currently available. Tables 49-8 to 49-11 list negative inotropic effects, proarrhythmic potential, and comparative toxicity of antiarrhythmic drugs.

Narrow-Complex Tachycardias. Identification of a tachycardia that is narrow and/or of identical morphology to the pa-

tient's QRS during normal sinus rhythm indicates a supraventricular tachycardia that relies on the A-V node for conduction to the ventricles. Atrioventricular nodal blocking agents, including beta-blockers, calcium antagonists, and digoxin, have been the mainstay for rate controlling such tachycardias in the stable patient. For patients who are unstable during a rapid tachycardia, DC synchronized cardioversion (50–200 joules) is the treatment of choice.

Antiarrhythmic drugs may be useful for cardioversion to and maintenance of normal sinus rhythm in some reentrant supraventricular tachycardias, including sinus node reentry, intraatrial reentry, A-V nodal and A-V reentry. Atrial fibrillation and atrial flutter, automatic atrial and junctional tachycardias, and some reentrant arrhythmias may be recalcitrant to the effects of A-V nodal blocking drugs. Class IA, IC, or III antiarrhythmic agents may be useful in converting to normal rhythm and preventing recurrences in these cases. For patients with rapidly conducting atrial fibrillation and flutter, a combination of an

Table 49-6. Electrocardiographic Effects of Antiarrhythmic Agents

	P–R	QRS	Q–T	J–T
IA				
IB	0	0	0	0
IC				0
II		0	0	0
III*				
IV		0	0	0

* Amiodarone, sotalol.
From Albarran-Sotelo R, et al: *Textbook of Advanced Cardiac Life Support*. 2nd ed. Dallas, American Heart Association, 1987, p 420. With permission.

Table 49-7. Basic Electrophysiologic Effects of Antiarrhythmic Agents

	APD	dV/dT and conduction velocity	Use dependence	ERP	ERP/ADP	Sinus node automaticity	Phase 4 automaticity	VFT	MSA
IA			intermediate			0			+
IB			fast			0			+
IC			slow			0			+
II		0	NA	0					+
III		0	intermediate					NA	0
IV	0	0	NA	0	0	0*		0	0

APD = action potential duration; dv/dt = rate of rise phase 0 of action potential; EPR = effective refractory period; VFT = ventricular fibrillation threshold; MSA = membrane stabilizing activity.
* Decreases spontaneous depolarization in calcium channel, slow-response tissue.
= increased;   = moderately increased;   = decreased;   = moderately decreased;   = greatly decreased; 0 = no effect; + = present.
From Nacarrelli GV (ed) *Cardiac Arrhythmias: A Practical Approach.* New York, Futura, 1991, p 420. With permission.

Table 49-8. Comparative Efficacy in Ventricular Arrhythmias

	PVC/VT-NS (Holter)	Sustained VT/VF (PES)
Quinidine	65%	20–25%
Procainamide	60%	20–25%
Disopyramide	60%	20–25%
Tocainide	50%	10–15%
Mexiletine	50%	10–20%
Moricizine	65%	20%
Flecainide	75%	20–25%
Encainide	75%	20–25%
Propafenone	70%	20–25%
Recainam	65%	20%
Propranolol	45%	5%
Acebutolol	45%	5%
Amiodarone	75%	20%(60%)*
Sotalol	55%	30%

* Higher spontaneous efficacy rates despite PES inefficacy.
VT-NS = nonsustained ventricular tachycardia; PES = programmed electrical stimulation; PVC = premature ventricular contraction; VF = ventricular fibrillation; VT = ventricular tachycardia.
From Nacarrelli GV (ed): *Cardiac Arrhythmias: A Practical Approach.* New York, Futura, 1991, p 423. With permission.

A-V nodal blocking agent and class I antiarrhythmic agent may be necessary to limit recurrences of the arrhythmia and to control ventricular response during periods of breakthrough supraventricular tachycardia. In these cases, the ventricular response should be slowed with an A-V nodal blocking agent prior to the initiation of a class IA agent. This is because the ventricular response during atrial fibrillation or atrial flutter (or rapid atrial tachycardia) may increase due to some vagolytic activity of the class IA antiarrhythmic agent on the A-V node and slowing of the atrial rate, thereby decreasing the amount of block at the A-V node. Atrioventricular nodal blocking drugs help maintain a higher degree of A-V block while the antiarrhythmic agent is initiated.

Wide-Complex Tachycardias. Differentiation of supraventricular from ventricular tachycardias in the patient with a wide-complex tachycardia is critical to proper management. As discussed above, ECG criteria should be applied when possible in the stable patient to differentiate these arrhythmias. In the unstable patient, synchronized DC cardioversion (100–360 joules) is the treatment of choice. In patients with well-tolerated wide-complex supraventricular tachycardias where a 12-lead ECG is not helpful in differentiating supraventricular from ven-

Table 49-9. Comparative Oral Efficacy and Electrophysiologic Properties in Supraventricular Arrhythmias

	PACS	AFIB	AVNant	AVNRT	AP	WPW-PSVT
Quinidine	+ +	+ +	±	+	+	+
Procainamide	+ +	+ +	±	+	+	+
Disopyramide	+ +	+ +	±	+	+ +	+ +
Tocainide	0	0	0	0	±	0
Mexiletine	0	0	0	0	±	0
Moricizine	+	NE	0	NE	+	NE
Flecainide	+ +	+ +	+	+ +	+ + +	+ + +
Encainide	+ +	+ +	+ +	+ +	+ + +	+ + +
Propafenone	+ +	+ +	+ +	+ +	+ +	+ +
Recainam	+	+ +	+	+ +	+ +	+ +
Beta-blockers	+	+	+ +	+	0	+
Amiodarone	+ +	+ + +	+ +	+ +	+	+ +
Sotalol	+	+ +	+ +	+ +	+	+
Digoxin	0	+ *	+ +	+	±	+
Verapamil	0	+ *	+ +	+	±	+
Diltiazem	0	+ *	+ +	+	±	+

* Rate control only
AFIB = atrial fibrillation; AVNant = antegrade slowing of A-V nodal conduction; AVNRT = A-V node reentrant tachycardia; AP = effects of accessory pathway conduction; NE = not established.
+ + + = very effective; + + = moderately effective; + = effective; ± = minimal or inconsistent efficacy; 0 = not effective.
From Nacarrelli GV (ed): *Cardiac Arrhythmias: A Practical Approach.* New York, Futura, 1991, p 424. With permission.

Table 49-10. Negative Inotropic Potential of Antiarrhythmic Drugs

Most negative inotropy	Disopyramide
	Verapamil
	Propranolol
	Acebutolol
	Flecainide
	Propafenone
	Sotalol
	Diltiazem
	Encainide
	Recainam
	Lidocaine
	Quinidine
	Procainamide
	Tocainide
Least negative inotropy	Mexiletine
	Moricizine
	Amiodarone
	Bretylium

From Nacarrelli GV (ed): *Cardiac Arrhythmias: A Practical Approach.* New York, Futura, 1991, p 425. With permission.

Table 49-11. Proarrhythmic Potential

	Proarrhythmia nonsustained VT patients	Proarrhythmia sustained VT patients	TDP
Quinidine	+	+ +	+ + +
Procainamide	+	+ +	+ +
Disopyramide	+	+ +	+ +
Tocainide	±	+	0
Mexiletine	±	+	0
Moricizine	+	+	0
Flecainide	+	+ + +	±
Encainide	+	+ + +	±
Propafenone	+	+ +	±
Recainam	+	+ +	±
Beta-blockers	±	+	0
Amiodarone	±	+	+
Sotalol	+	+	+ + +

TDP = *Torsades de pointes;* VT = ventricular tachycardia; + + + = very high potential; + + = moderate potential; + = minimal potential; ± = inconsistent potential; 0 = no potential.
From Nacarrelli GV: *Cardiac Arrythmias: A Practical Approach.* New York, Futura, 1991, p 426. With permission.

tricular tachycardias, intravenous adenosine given as a bolus of 6.0 to 12.0 milligrams, followed by a 10-cc normal saline bolus, may be useful in differentiating supraventricular from ventricular tachyarrhythmias. Tachycardias that do not depend on the A-V node usually do not break with intravenous adenosine. When a bypass tract is suspected but cannot be differentiated from ventricular tachycardia, the treatment of choice is intravenous procainamide (load 15 mg/kg at 20 mg/min with maintenance infusion of 0.11 mg/kg/min). Intravenous verapamil and other A-V nodal blocking agents should not be used in these patients, as conduction down the bypass tract may increase, resulting in a faster ventricular response and more unstable rhythm.

Lidocaine is the initial treatment of choice for patients with symptomatic or sustained ventricular tachycardia [60]. This drug should be given as a bolus of 1 to 1.5 mg per kilogram rapid infusion with a maintenance drip of 1 to 4 mg per minute. A second bolus of 50 percent of the initial bolus should be repeated after 20 minutes. If lidocaine is judged ineffective or the patient is intolerant to this drug, procainamide should be loaded at 10 to 20 mg per kilogram at 20 mg per minute with a maintenance infusion of 1 to 4 mg per minute. The drug dose should ultimately be determined by measuring both procainamide and N-acetyl procainamide (NAPA) levels once steady state is reached. Intravenous bretylium with a loading dose of 5 to 30 mg per kilogram and a maintenance infusion of 1 to 4 mg per minute may also be used in cases of drug refractory ventricular tachycardia. Acute intravenous therapy with beta-blockers may be helpful in managing ventricular tachycardia, especially in patients with ongoing ischemia. The short-acting beta-blocker esmolol may be particularly useful in this patient population because of its rapid elimination properties (elimination half-life 10–20 seconds). Combination drug therapy or mechanical intervention to relieve ongoing ischemia in unstable patients who are recalcitrant to pharmacologic therapy may be quite useful in treating refractory ventricular tachycardia. The use of an intraaortic balloon pump to relieve wall stress, promote vasodilation, and relieve ischemia may be necessary in patients with ischemically induced incessant ventricular tachycardia. These patients may benefit from early coronary revascularization.

All antiarrhythmic agents have the potential to produce arrhythmias, both bradyarrhythmic and tachyarrhythmic. Polymorphic ventricular tachycardia in the setting of drug-induced long Q–T interval (*Torsades de pointes*) may be most effectively treated by discontinuing drugs that can predispose to this situation. These drugs include type IA antiarrhythmics, erythromycin, phenothiazine derivatives, pentamidine, and sotalol. Electrolyte imbalances, including hypokalemia and hypomagnesemia, are frequently seen in patients on chronic diuretics and may also be responsible for the initiation of pause-dependent long Q–T polymorphic ventricular tachycardia. Treatment should involve prompt replacement of potassium and magnesium. Repletion of potassium to levels greater than 4.0 mEq per liter, and magnesium levels greater than 2.0 mg per deciliter is advised. It should be remembered, however, that the total body and intracellular content of both of these ions is poorly reflected by measured serum potassium and magnesium levels. The use of intravenous catecholamines or rapid pacing to prevent pauses that can initiate *Torsades de pointes* may be necessary to stabilize patients until the predisposing condition (drugs or electrolyte imbalance) has been reversed. Target heart rate should be 90 to 120 beats per minute and should eliminate pauses [61].

References

1. American Hospital Association, Health Care Financing Administration, American Health Information Management Association, et al.: Statistics. *JAMA* 267:335, 1992.
2. MacWilliam JA: Cardiac failure in sudden death. *Br Med J* 1:6, 1989.
3. Harris AS, Rojas AJ: Initiation of ventricular fibrillation due to coronary occlusion. *Exp Med Surg* 1:105, 1945.
4. Franchesco D: A new interpretation of the pacemaker current in cat-Purkinje fibers. *J Physiol (Lond)* 314:359, 1981.
5. Gilmour RF, Zipes DP: Abnormal automaticity and related phenomena, in Fozzard H, Haber E, Jennings R (eds): *The Heart and Cardiovascular System.* New York, Raven, 1986.
6. Johnson NG, Rosen MR: The distinction between triggered activity and other cardiac arrhythmias, in Brugada P, Wellens H (eds): *Cardiac Arrhythmias: Where to Go from Here?* Mt. Kisco, Futura, 1987.
7. El-Sherif N, Zeiler RH, Craelius W, et al: QTU prolongation and

polymorphic ventricular tachyarrhythmias due to bradycardia-dependent early afterdepolarizations. *Circ Res* 63:286, 1988.

8. Rosen MR, Danilo P: Digitalis-induced delayed afterdepolarizations, in Zipes D, Bailey J, Elhawar V (eds): *The Slow Inward Current in Cardiac Arrhythmias*. The Hague, Martinus Nijhoff, 1980.

9. Wit AL, Cranefield PF: Triggered and automatic activity in the canine coronary sinus. *Circ Res* 41:435, 1977.

10. Lerman BB, Belardinelli L, West GA, et al: Adenosine sensitive ventricular tachycardia: Evidence suggesting cyclic AMP-mediated triggered activity. *Circulation* 74:270, 1986.

11. Wellens HJ, Düren DR, Lie KI: Observations on mechanisms of ventricular tachycardia in man. *Circulation* 54:237, 1976.

12. Harris L, Downar E, Michleborough L, et al: Activation sequence of ventricular tachycardia: Endocardial and epicardial mapping studies in the human ventricle. *J Am Coll Cardiol* 10:1040, 1987.

13. Mines GR: Dynamic equilibrium in the heart. *J Physiol (Lond)* 46:349, 1913.

14. Mines GR: On circulating excitations in heart muscles and their possible relation to tachycardia and fibrillation. *Trans R Soc Can* 4:43, 1914.

15. Allessie MA, Bonke FIM, Schopman FIG: Circus movement in rabbit atrial muscle as a mechanism of tachycardia: The "leading circle" concept—A new model of circus movement in cardiac tissue without the involvement of an anatomic obstacle. *Circ Res* 41:9, 1977.

16. Olshansky B, Waldo AL: Atrial fibrillation: Update on mechanism, diagnosis and management. *Mod Concepts Cardiovasc Dis* 56:23, 1987.

17. Wit AL, Dillon SM, Coromilas J, et al: Anisotropic reentry in the epicardial border zone of myocardial infarcts: Mathematical approaches to cardiac arrhythmias. *Ann NY Acad Sci* 591:86, 1990.

18. Rapaport E: Sudden cardiac death. *Am J Cardiol* 62:31, 1988.

19. Kemph FC, Josephson ME: Cardiac arrest recorded on ambulatory electrocardiograms. *Am J Cardiol* 53:1577, 1984.

20. Verrier RI: Behavioral stress, myocardial ischemia and arrhythmias, in Zipes D, Jalife J (eds): *Cardiac Electrophysiology and Arrhythmias: From Cell to Bedside*. Philadelphia, WB Saunders, 1990.

21. DeMello WC: Intracellular communication in cardiac muscle: Physiological and pathological implications, in Zipes D, Jalife J (eds): *Cardiac Electrophysiology and Arrhythmias*. New York, Grune & Stratton, 1985.

22. Moss A, Davis HT, DeCamilla J, et al: Ventricular ectopic beats and their relation to sudden and nonsudden cardiac death after myocardial infarction. *Circulation* 60:998, 1979.

23. Bigger JAT, Fleiss JL, Kleiger K, et al: The Multi-Center Post-Infarction Research Group: The relationship between ventricular arrhythmias, left ventricular dysfunction and mortality in the two years after myocardial infarction. *Circulation* 69:250, 1984.

24. Gomes GA, Winters SL, Stewart D, et al: A new non-invasive index to predict sustained ventricular tachycardia and sudden death in the first year after myocardial infarction, based on signal averaged electrocardiogram, radionuclide ejection fraction and Holter monitoring. *J Am Coll Cardiol* 10:349, 1987.

25. Dennis AR, Richards DA, Cody DV, et al: Prognostic significance of ventricular tachycardia and fibrillation induced at programmed stimulation and delayed potentials detected on the signal averaged electrocardiograms of survivors of acute myocardial infarction. *Circulation* 74:731, 1986.

26. Julian DG, Valentine PA, Miller GG: Disturbances of rate, rhythm, and conduction in acute myocardial infarction: A prospective study of 100 consecutive unselected patients with the aid of electrocardiographic monitoring. *Am J Med* 37:915, 1964.

27. Meltzer LE, Kitchell JR: The incidence of arrhythmias associated with myocardial infarction. *Prog Cardiovasc Dis* 9:50, 1966.

28. Bigger JT, Dresdale RJ, Heissenvutte I, et al: Ventricular arrhythmias in ischemic heart disease: Mechanism, prevalence, significance in management. *Prog Cardiovasc Dis* 19:255, 1977.

29. Wiggers CJ, Wégria R: Ventricular fibrillation due to single, localized induction and condensor shocks applied during the vulnerable phase of ventricular systole. *Am J Physiol* 128:500, 1940.

30. Jewitt D: The genesis of cardiac arrhythmias in acute myocardial infarction. *Prog Cardiol* 1:61, 1972.

31. Naito M, Michelson EL, Kaplinsky E, et al: Role of early cycle ventricular extrasystoles in initiation of ventricular tachycardia and fibrillation: Evaluation of the R-on-T phenomenon in myocardial infarction. *Am J Cardiol* 49:317, 1982.

32. Lown B, Kosowsky BD, Klein MD: Pathogenesis, prevention and treatment of arrhythmias in myocardial infarction. *Circulation* 40(supp 4):261, 1969.

33. Norris RM, Mercer CJ: Significance of idioventricular rhythms in acute myocardial infarction. *Prog Cardiovasc Dis* 16:455, 1974.

34. Cerek B, Lew AS, Laramee E, et al: Time course and characteristics of ventricular arrhythmias after reperfusion in acute myocardial infarction. *Am J Cardiol* 60:214, 1987.

35. Gorgels APM, Vos MA, Letsch IS, et al: Usefulness of the accelerated idioventricular rhythm as a marker for myocardial necrosis and reperfusion during thrombolytic therapy in acute myocardial infarction. *Am J Cardiol* 61:231, 1988.

36. Lawrie DM, Greenwood TW, Goddard M, et al: A coronary care unit in the routine management of acute myocardial infarction. *Lancet* 2:109, 1967.

37. Lawrie DM: Longterm survival after ventricular fibrillation complicating acute myocardial infarction. *Lancet* 2:1085, 1969.

38. Hansen EC, Levine FH, Kay HR, et al: Control of post-infarction ventricular irritability with an intra-aortic balloon pump. *Circulation* 62(supp 1):130, 1980.

39. Grenadier E, Alpan G, Maor N, et al: Polymorphous ventricular tachycardia in acute myocardial infarction. *Am J Cardiol* 53:1280, 1984.

40. Lie KL, Wellens HJJ, Downar E, et al: Observations on patients with primary ventricular fibrillation complicating acute myocardial infarction. *Circulation* 52:755, 1975.

41. Conley MJ, McNeer JF, Lie KL, et al: Cardiac arrest complicating acute myocardial infarction: Predictability in prognosis. *Am J Cardiol* 39:7, 1977.

42. Goldberg RJ, Gore JM, Haffajee CCI, et al: Outcome of the cardiac arrest during acute myocardial infarction. *Am J Cardiol* 59:251, 1987.

43. Adgey AAJ, Geddes JS, Mulholland HC, et al: Incidence, significance, and management of early bradyarrhythmia complicating acute myocardial infarction. *Lancet* 2:1097, 1968.

44. James TN: The coronary circulation and conduction system in acute myocardial infarction. *Prog Cardiovasc Dis* 10:410, 1968.

45. Mark AL: Bezold-Jarisch reflex revisited: Clinical implications of inhibitory reflexes originating in the heart. *J Am Coll Cardiol* 1:90, 1983.

46. Feigl D, Ashkenazy J, Kishon Y: Early and late atrioventricular block in acute myocardial infarction. *J Am Coll Cardiol* 4:35, 1984.

47. Tans AC, Lie KL, Düren D: Clinical setting and prognostic significance of high degree atrioventricular block in acute inferior myocardial infarction: A study of 144 patients. *Am Heart J* 99:4, 1980.

48. Strasberg B, Pinchas A, Arditti A, et al: Left and right ventricular function in inferior acute myocardial infarction and significance of advanced atrioventricular block. *Am J Cardiol* 54:985, 1984.

49. Nicod P, Gilpin E, Diettrich H, et al: Long-term outcome in patients with inferior myocardial infarction in complete atrioventricular block. *J Am Coll Cardiol* 12:589, 1988.

50. Klein RC, Vera Z, Mason DT: Intraventricular conduction defects in acute myocardial infarction: Incidence, prognosis, and therapy. *Am Heart J* 108:1007, 1984.

51. Hindman MC, Wagner GS, Jaro M, et al: The clinical significance of bundle branch block complicating acute myocardial infarction. 2. Indications for temporary and permanent pacemaker insertion. *Circulation* 58:689, 1978.

52. Waugh RA, Wagner GS, Haney TL, et al: Immediate and remote prognostic significance of fascicular block during acute myocardial infarction. *Circulation* 47:765, 1973.

53. Zoll PM, Zoll RH, Falk RH, et al: External non-invasive temporary cardiac pacing: Clinical trials. *Circulation* 71:937, 1985.

54. Dongas J, Lehmann MH, Mahmud R, et al: Value of preexisting bundle branch block in the electrocardiographic differentiation of supraventricular from ventricular origin of wide QRS tachycardia. *Am J Cardiol* 55:717, 1985.

55. Wellens HJJ, Bar FW, Lie KL: The value of the electrocardiogram in the differential diagnosis of a tachycardia with a widened QRS complex. *Am J Med* 64:27, 1978.

56. Akhtar M, Shenasa M, Jazayeri M, et al: Wide QRS complex tachycardia: Reappraisal of a common clinical problem. *Ann Intern Med* 109:905, 1988.

57. Brugada P, Brugada J, Mont L, et al: A new approach to the differential diagnosis of a regular tachycardia with a wide QRS complex. *Circulation* 83:1649, 1991.

58. Vaughn-Williams EM: A classification of antiarrhythmic actions reassessed after a decade of new drugs. *J Clin Pharmacol* 24:129, 1984.

59. Harrison DC: Antiarrhythmic drug classification: New science in practice applications. *Am J Cardiol* 56:185, 1985.

60. Albarran-Sotelo R, Atkins JM, Bloom RS, et al: *Textbook of Advanced Cardiac Life Support.* 2nd ed. Dallas, American Heart Association, 1987.

61. Jackman WM, Friday KJ, Anderson JL, et al: The long-QT syndromes: A critical review—New clinical observation and a unifying hypothesis. *Prog Cardiovasc Dis* 31:115, 1988.

50. *Mechanisms of Acute Myocardial Ischemia and Infarction*

Carey D. Kimmelstiel,
Christopher Clyne, and
Richard C. Becker

The heart is an aerobic organ that relies almost exclusively on the oxidation of substrates for the generation of energy; therefore it tolerates only a small oxygen debt. Since the heart does not contain oxygen stores, its high rate of energy expenditure, required to meet the needs of actively functioning tissues and organs throughout the body, causes a striking decline in oxygen (O_2) tension within seconds of coronary arterial occlusion, followed by a loss of myocardial contractility.

At rest, the heart's O_2 consumption is 6 to 8 ml/min/100 gm tissue, increasing with physical activity and increased metabolic demands. Coronary arterial blood flow averages 60 to 80 ml/min/100 gm tissue and O_2 extraction is 12 to 15 ml/100 ml blood.

The quantity of oxygen required to maintain physiologic processes is determined by heart rate, myocardial contractility/inotropic state, and afterload (wall stress).

Normal Coronary Anatomy

Blood and essential substrate are carried to the myocardium through the major epicardial coronary arteries, their branches, intramural and subendocardial extensions, and the collateral circulation.

RIGHT CORONARY ARTERY. The right coronary artery (RCA), typically 2.5 to 3.0 mm in diameter, originates within the right coronary sinus of Valsalva (Fig. 50-1). It extends between the right atrium and right ventricle in the atrioventricular groove. When the RCA reaches the acute margin of the heart it turns posteriorly, following the atrioventricular (A-V) groove to the crux cordis. An acute marginal branch is typically given off immediately before the RCA takes its posterior course. In approximately 80 percent of individuals, the RCA reaches the crux cordis and gives rise to posterior descending, A-V node, and left ventricular branches. In 10 to 20 percent of individuals the RCA does not reach the crux cordis.

The first branch of the RCA is the conus branch. In nearly 50 percent of individuals this branch originates from a separate ostium in the right coronary sinus of the Valsalva. The second branch is the sinus node branch. This branch arises from the left circumflex coronary artery in 40 percent of individuals. Rarely, two sinus node branches exist, one from the RCA and one from the left circumflex coronary artery.

In its course along the anterolateral aspect of the atrioventricular groove, the RCA gives off one or more ventricular branches that serve the free wall of the right ventricle. The acute marginal branch arises from the RCA at the lower aspect of the right atrium and is typically the largest of the right ventricular branches serving the inferior and diaphragmatic surfaces of the right ventricle and, occasionally, the posteroapical intraventricular septum as well.

The right atrial branch of the RCA originates at the same level as the acute marginal branch but travels superiorly. This branch is an important collateral source of blood supply to the proximal and midsections of the RCA, including the sinus node artery.

Following its course between the acute margin and the crux

Fig. 50-1. Anatomy of the right coronary artery.

RIGHT CORONARY ARTERY

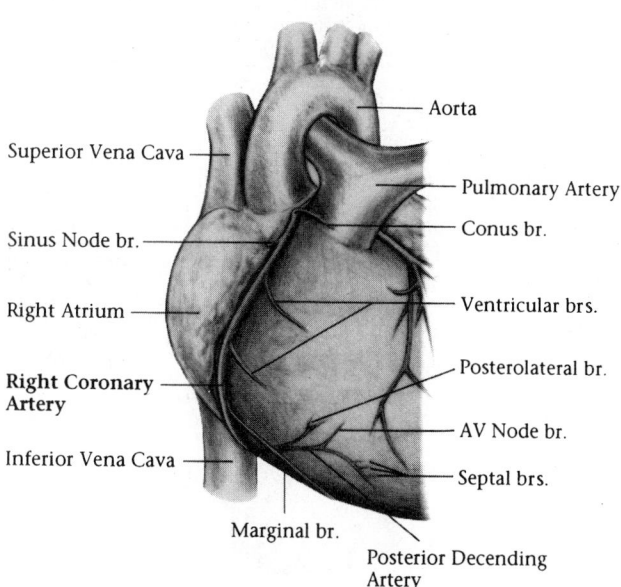

cordis, the RCA gives rise to several small to moderate-sized posterior left ventricular branches. It also gives rise to the A-V node artery, which courses vertically. The posterior descending branch of the RCA, with its septal branches, is the sole source of blood supply to the posterosuperior aspect of the intraventricular septum. In nearly 70 percent of individuals, the posterior descending artery does not reach the heart's apex. As a result, this portion of the posterior interventricular septum is typically supplied by the recurrent branch of the left anterior descending coronary artery.

The most distal branch of the RCA is the left atrial branch. When present, it courses along the left posterior atrioventricular groove toward the left atrium.

LEFT CORONARY ARTERY. The left coronary artery originates in the left coronary sinus of the Valsalva. The ostium is typically located at the level of the aortic ring, up to 1.0 cm higher than the ostium of the RCA (Fig. 50-2). The left main coronary artery, which may be up to 4.5 mm in diameter, divides into two major branches—the left anterior descending (LAD) coronary artery and the left circumflex coronary artery. Rarely, these vessels may arise from separate ostia located within the left coronary sinus.

The LAD begins as a continuation of the left main coronary artery. It passes to the left of the pulmonic valve and courses along the anterior interventricular sulcus. The LAD is an important vessel that perfuses the interventricular septum, anterior wall, lateral wall, and apex of the left ventricle. In some individuals, the LAD is of relatively small caliber, reaching the midportion of the anterior wall. In others, however, the LAD reaches the apex or extends around the apex to the diaphragmatic aspect of the left ventricle.

In order of origin, the major branches of the LAD are the first diagonal, first septal, minor septal, second diagonal, right ventricular, and apical. The first diagonal branch of the LAD is typically a large vessel that perfuses the high lateral (free) wall of the left ventricle. On rare occasions, the first diagonal branch may have a separate ostium in the left main coronary artery. The septal branches of the LAD, varying in number from one to five, perfuse approximately 60 percent of the superior portion and nearly 100 percent of the inferior portion of the anterior interventricular septum. The septum is an important area of collaterals between the LAD and RCA.

One or more branches to the right ventricle originate in the midportion of the LAD. The most superior branch courses toward the conus branch of the RCA at the level of the pulmonic valve.

The terminal branches of the LAD are the apical branches, serving both the anterior and diaphragmatic aspects of the left ventricular apex. Typically, at least two branches are present—the recurrent posterior branch and the recurrent lateral-apical branch.

The left circumflex coronary artery commonly takes off at a sharp angle from the left main coronary artery and courses posteriorly in the A-V groove toward the crux cordis. In 80 percent of individuals, the left circumflex artery does not reach the posterior interventricular sulcus. When it does, however, the left circumflex artery gives rise to a posterior descending branch that is the sole source of blood supply to the posterior interventricular septum and the A-V node. In 40 percent of individuals, the left circumflex artery provides a branch to the sinus node.

The longest and most consistent branches of the left circumflex artery are those to the acute margin of the heart—the obtuse marginal branches. These vessels course posteriorly along the left ventricular wall toward the apex. Varying in number from one to four, the obtuse marginal branches perfuse the lateral wall of the ventricle above the diaphragmatic surface.

The coronary circulation has been divided anatomically into dominant and nondominant, depending on which blood vessel reaches and crosses the crux cordis of the heart. In this instance the posterior descending artery and often the A-V nodal artery originate from the dominant vessel. Accordingly, the RCA is considered the dominant vessel in approximately 80 percent of individuals. However, the left coronary artery system provides blood flow to the largest area of myocardium and is therefore the *predominant artery* in most individuals.

CORONARY ARTERY ANOMALIES. For oxygen to be delivered to metabolically active myocardial cells, coronary arterial blood flow must be adequate. Clearly, normal coronary arterial blood flow requires normal coronary artery anatomy. In some cases, anatomic variations (anomalies) preclude normal delivery of essential substrate, compromising myocardial function (Table 50-1).

CORONARY OSTIAL ABNORMALITIES. The coronary ostium can be abnormal with respect to its intrinsic anatomy (proper aortic sinus origin), size (ostial hyperplasia, fibrous endoproliferation, atresia), or orientation (tangential orientation, intussusception) [1–6].

ECTOPIC CORONARY ARTERY ORIGINATION. One or more of the ectopic coronary arteries originate from the pulmonic trunk [7–12]. There may be anomalous origin from an atypical site—a noncoronary cusp, the aortic wall above the coronary sinus, or the descending aorta.

The RCA, left main coronary artery, left anterior descending coronary artery, or left circumflex coronary artery may have anomalous origins. The course taken can be posterior to the aorta, between the aorta and pulmonary trunk, within the ventricular septum, or anterior to the pulmonary infundibulum [13–19]. Other arteries may have ectopic origins, arising from an extracardiac vessel (subclavian artery, internal thoracic artery,

Fig. 50-2. Anatomy of the left coronary artery, including the left main, left anterior descending, and left circumflex coronary arteries.

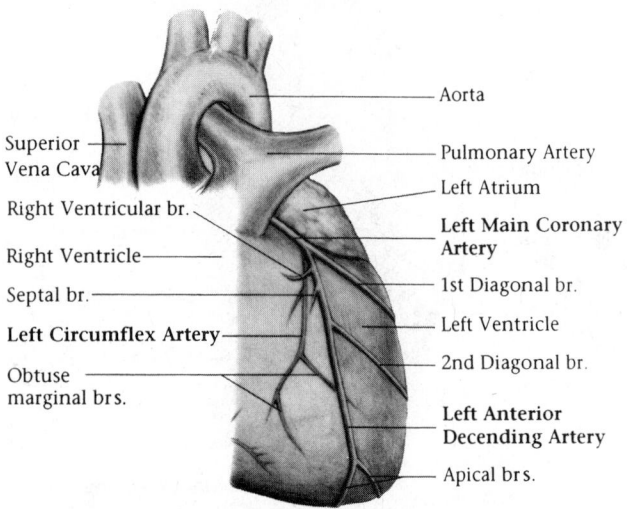

Aorta

Superior Vena Cava

Pulmonary Artery

Left Atrium

Right Ventricular br.

Left Main Coronary Artery

Right Ventricle

1st Diagonal br.

Septal br.

Left Ventricle

Left Circumflex Artery

2nd Diagonal br.

Obtuse marginal brs.

Left Anterior Decending Artery

Apical brs.

Table 50-1. Classification of Anomalous Coronary Arteries

Ostial abnormality
  Origin
  Size
  Orientation
Ectopic coronary artery origination
  Pulmonic trunk
  Opposite coronary sinus
  Opposite coronary artery
  Aortic wall
  Extracardial vessels
  Cardiac chamber
Abnormal connections
  Arteriovenous fistula
  Coronary-cameral fistula
  Coronary to extracardiac artery or vein
Intramuscular coursing (muscular bridge)
  Subepicardial
  Subendocardial
  Intracavitary
Coronary artery size
  Hypoplastic
  Ectasic

brachiocephalic artery, carotid artery) [20–25] or from a heart chamber (left ventricle, right ventricle) [26].

ABNORMAL CONNECTIONS. Abnormal connections between a coronary artery and an adjacent vascular structure tend to enlarge with time because of the persistence of a pressure gradient. Examples are a coronary-cameral fistula (right ventricle, left ventricle, right atrium, left atrium) [27,28,29], coronary arteriovenous fistula [30,31], and coronary to extracardiac artery or vein (coronary-pulmonary, coronary-bronchial, coronary-caval) fistula [32,33].

INTRAMURAL COURSING (MUSCULAR BRIDGE). The main coronary arteries and their branches course on the epicardial surface of the heart. Occasionally, the vessels take a subepicardial course. On rare occasions, the coronary arteries become intracavitary or subendocardial. An exception is the LAD coronary artery, which in its midportion takes a subepicardial course in nearly 50 percent of individuals (and is therefore considered a normal anatomic variant) [34–38].

CORONARY ARTERY SIZE. The diameter of a coronary artery can be too small (hypoplastic) or too large (ectasic). Either may be a congenital or acquired abnormality. Coronary artery ectasia with aneurysm formation is seen with coronary arteritis and atherosclerosis, as well as following trauma.

Collateral Circulation

Vascular connections between two or more coronary arteries that are larger than capillaries are considered collaterals. The presence of a collateral circulation in the human heart is firmly established. A majority, ranging in size from 50 to 1500 mm, are located subendocardially; however, epicardial collaterals can be found at the ventricular apex [34].

There is evidence that the coronary collateral circulation typically develops from a preexisting subendocardial network. In contrast, bridging collaterals (intersegmental anastomoses) represent enlargement of the vasa vasorum located on the vessel's adventitial surface.

Pathologic descriptions suggest that the human heart can develop collateral vessels when and where they are needed. There is active growth of collaterals, which appears to be governed by mechanical forces, chemical influences, and genetic factors [35]. The mechanical forces influencing collateral growth include the intravascular pressure and pressure gradient, the velocity of blood flow, and tangential wall stress. The major chemical influence is tissue hypoxia. Although the mechanisms have not been defined fully, hypoxia may cause growth factors to diffuse from compromised myocytes toward the arteriolar beds. As cellular growth requires oxygen (and other substrate) it has been difficult to explain how collateral vessels form in a hypoxemic environment. Recent evidence suggests that the hexose monophosphate shunt (which requires less oxygen and ATP for enzymatic reactions) may be involved. Another consideration involves DNA salvage from surrounding damaged or necrotic tissue [35].

Differences in the growth, development, and physiologic capabilities of the collateral circulation in human hearts compared with other species suggest a genetic influence. The preexisting collateral circulation in humans may also be genetically determined, explaining, at least in part, differences between individuals as well as the observation that collaterals not infrequently overlap both normal and ischemic myocardial zones.

Oxygen Carrying Capacity of Blood

The complex structural and functional properties of hemoglobin allow erythrocytes to bind, transport, and release oxygen with great efficiency. The interior of a normal erythrocyte contains nearly 300 million molecules of hemoglobin. Each molecule is a tetramer composed of polypeptide chains, to which four heme moieties are bound. Hemoglobins found in normal adults include hemoglobin A (97% total), hemoglobin A_2 (2%), and hemoglobin F (1%).

The heme groups are in four hydrophobic pockets. An iron atom is located at the center of each, bound in a square array by nitrogen atoms within pyrrole rings. The nonaqueous environment around the iron atom allows it to remain in the ferrous state even in the presence of oxygen molecules and imparts to the iron-oxygen bond a strength intermediate between a covalent and noncovalent bond. This property allows reversible oxygen binding.

The unique physiologic role of hemoglobin in tissue metabolism is fostered by the sigmoidal shape of its oxygen-binding curve. In reality, hemoglobin has a relatively low oxygen affinity. With decreasing pH and increasing 2,3-diphosphoglyceric acid (DPG) concentrations or temperature, a further decrease in hemoglobin's affinity for oxygen occurs, causing more oxygen to be released at the tissue level for a given PO_2 (Fig. 50-3).

Hemoglobin's ability to function as an oxygen transporter depends on its ability to bind oxygen and release it at the tissue level. An increased affinity for oxygen reduces tissue PO_2 and may compromise cellular function and viability. A decreased affinity may significantly affect oxygen transport. Genetic and acquired abnormalities of hemoglobin do occur. Although a majority of individuals are asymptomatic, anemia (in patients with decreased oxygen affinity) and erythrocytosis (in patients with increased oxygen affinity) may be seen.

The reversible binding and unbinding of oxygen by hemoglobin requires that heme iron remain in its ferrous (Fe^{2+}) form.

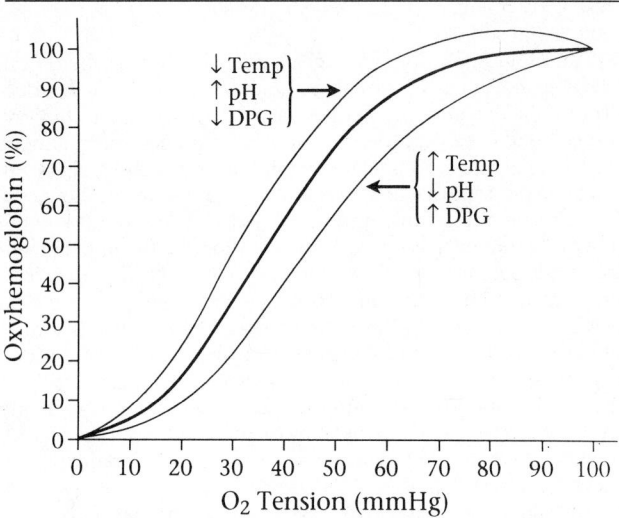

Fig. 50-3. The oxygen binding curve for human hemoglobulin under physiologic conditions. The affinity of hemoglobin for oxygen varies with changes in pH, temperature, and 2,3-diphosphoglyceric acid (DPG) concentrations.

In methemoglobinemia, the iron atom is in its oxidized form (Fe^{3+}), rendering the molecule incapable of binding oxygen (Table 50-2).

Coronary Blood Flow

With increasing myocardial demands, oxygen consumption increases three to fourfold. Since myocardial oxygen extraction cannot increase substantially, coronary blood flow must increase to meet the demands placed on the heart (Table 50-3).

During diastole, when the aortic valve is in the closed position, aortic diastolic blood pressure is transmitted through the dilated sinuses of Valsalva to the coronary ostia. The coronary sinuses act as reservoirs, facilitating uniform blood flow through diastole. Coronary blood flow, to a lesser degree, can also take place during systole, particularly when diastolic pressure is attenuated (e.g., aortic insufficiency). Typically, coronary arterial blood flow proceeds from the epicardial vessels to the intramural vessels and terminates in the subendocardial plexus.

PERFUSION PRESSURE. Coronary arterial blood flow is determined, to a large extent, by the pressure gradient (driving pressure) between the aorta (in diastole) and coronary sinus. This relationship is influenced by atherosclerotic narrowings and elevations in left ventricular end-diastolic and right atrial pressure. Coronary blood flow is maintained when the mean arterial pressure exceeds 65 mm Hg. Below this level, myocardial perfusion is significantly reduced.

EXTRINSIC COMPRESSION. Left ventricular pressure is considerably higher in systole than in diastole. Therefore, myocardial compressive forces act on intramural vessels to a greater extent during the systolic phase of the cardiac cycle. Accordingly, coronary blood flow is facilitated during diastole. The impact of systolic compression on coronary arterial blood flow is of particular importance in states of increased left ventricular

Table 50-2. Methemoglobinemia

Hereditary
Drug-related
   Nitrates
   Dapsone
   Chloroquine, primaquine
   Lidocaine
   Naphthalene
   Trinitrotoluene
   Nitrobenzene
   Sulfanilamide

Table 50-3. Factors Influencing Coronary Arterial Blood Flow

Duration of diastole
Perfusion pressure
Extrinsic coronary arterial compression
Neurohormonal-mediated vasodilation/vasoconstriction
Autoregulation

mass (hypertrophic states) and when the diastolic interval is shortened (tachycardia) [36,37,38].

NEUROHUMORAL INFLUENCES. Coronary arterial resistance and blood flow are regulated by autonomic mechanisms (beta-receptors). The coronary bed contains adrenergic receptors that initiate vasodilation and those that cause vasoconstriction (alpha-receptors) [39]. Parasympathetic-mediated vasodilation and baroreceptor activity also influence coronary arterial resistance.

AUTOREGULATION. Coronary arterial blood flow is linked to myocardial oxygen consumption over a wide range of arterial blood pressure and cardiac output. The matching of blood flow and myocardial oxygen demand is, by definition, autoregulation [40,41,42].

Coronary blood flow can be maintained in the face of decreased perfusion pressure by a reduction in coronary arterial resistance. When mean coronary arterial perfusion pressure is reduced below 65 mm Hg, however, vasodilatory reserve is exhausted and coronary blood flow is linearly related to pressure.

Autoregulatory control is linked directly to local metabolic factors that alter resistance to the arteriolar bed [43]. Several mediators have been implicated, including oxygen, carbon dioxide, and adenosine [44]. Adenosine appears to act on the surface of vascular smooth muscle cells, blocking the entry of calcium and, as a result, promoting coronary vasodilation. Other mediators likely involved in autoregulation include histamine, prostacyclin, and leukotrienes.

Abnormalities in coronary artery flow reserve may be caused by abnormal tonus or vasoconstriction of intramural prearterioles, resulting in a drop in perfusion pressure during maximal or near-maximal vasodilation of the endocardial arteriolar bed [45,46,47].

Disorders of Myocardial Oxygen Supply

CORONARY ATHEROSCLEROSIS. In the vast majority of patients with documented myocardial ischemia or infarction, coronary atherosclerosis is the underlying pathologic lesion [48,49]. Clinical manifestations of coronary atherosclerosis occur due to chronic as well as acute reductions in myocardial blood flow from epicardial coronary arteries. Atherosclerotic narrowing of the epicardial coronary vessel tends to be a focal disease with a propensity for the more proximal arterial segments.

Blood flow limitation due to an obstructive atherosclerotic lesion is mitigated by a compensatory reduction in resistance in the arteriolar vessels inherent to coronary autoregulation. This mechanism, in concert with dilatation of the uninvolved smooth muscle of eccentric atherosclerotic stenoses, acts to maintain coronary perfusion to myocardium in the resting state, even with an 80 percent reduction in luminal cross-sectional area [50,51].

Bernoulli's principle emphasizes the greater importance of lesion severity compared with length in determining the drop in perfusion pressure across a stenosis, the pressure reduction varying directly with stenosis length but inversely with the fourth power of vessel radius [52,53]. Resistance to blood flow induced by an atherosclerotic lesion rises hyperbolically at greater stenosis severities such that small increases in critical stenoses, as may occur when thrombus or platelet clumps adhere to a fractured plaque, are poorly tolerated. In addition, functional stenosis severity can be aggravated by reduction in the distending pressure seen by the stenotic region; such a mechanism is seen, for example, by distal coronary vasodilatation in response to exercise [52,54]. In general, with normal myocardial function in the region of a diseased artery, in the absence of collateral blood supply, lumen reduction in excess of 90 percent eventuates in rest ischemia [54].

Dilatation of the arteriolar resistance vessels in the presence of a high-grade coronary stenosis can prevent ischemia, but once maximum vasodilation has occurred any increase in myocardial oxygen demand will eventuate in ischema, with the duration of insult and participation of potential mitigating factors (e.g., medical therapy, collateral blood supply) determining whether or not ischemia goes on to infarction. As this autoregulation reaches its maximum, the subendocardial layer of myocardium is the first to experience ischemic changes. Indeed, a transmural gradient of blood flow favoring epicardial layers of myocardium is a hallmark of the ischemic process [55,56].

Patients with a history of angina are often admitted to the hospital with an acceleration of their symptomatology with clinical syndromes of unstable angina or frank myocardial infarction. A large body of evidence suggests the conversion from stable to unstable angina is heralded by plaque rupture or fissuring, which exposes the atherosclerotic matrix and subendothelium to circulating blood products [57]. Evidence for plaque rupture comes from angiographic studies in unstable angina patients showing a higher prevalence of eccentric, irregular, narrow-necked stenoses with overhanging edges (type II lesion) when compared to patients with stable angina, who are more likely to exhibit concentric, symmetric stenoses or eccentric broad-necked (type I) stenoses [58,59] (Fig. 50-4). Coronary angiography performed in previously studied unstable angina patients has shown that culprit lesions often arise at the site of a previously minimally diseased arterial segment. Restudy frequently documents a type II stenosis, probably representing a recently fissured plaque [60,61].

The precise cause of plaque fissuring is unknown, but most frequently soft plaques and those with a high concentration of cholesterol and its esters tend to rupture [62]. The site of rupture often is the junction of the lesion's fibrous cap with uninvolved endothelium. Possible inciting events leading to plaque rupture are shear forces caused by the stenosis itself, coronary spasm,

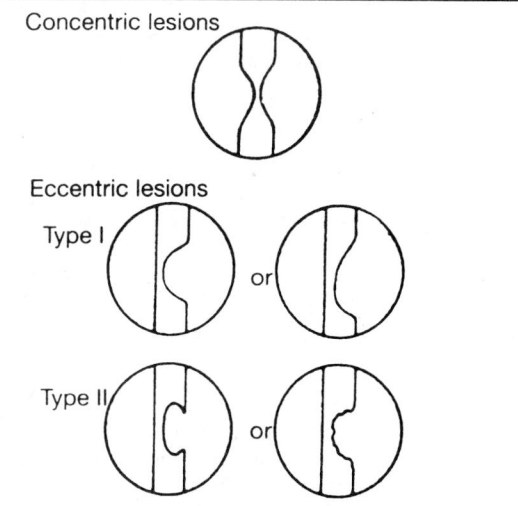

Fig. 50-4. Stenosis morphology in unstable and stable coronary syndromes. (Adapted from Ambrose JA, Winters SL, Stern A, et al: Angiographic morphology in the pathogenesis of unstable angina pectoris. *J Am Coll Cardiol* 5:609, 1985. With permission from the American College of Cardiology.)

and twisting of the coronary artery during the cardiac cycle [63,64]. In addition, macrophages metabolizing lipids within a plaque could facilitate its rupture through release of enzymatic products [62]. Recent data implicate augmented white blood cell activation in the coronary tree of unstable angina patients; this could conceivably enhance coronary thrombosis and vasoconstriction [65].

DeWood and co-workers' initial report documenting intracoronary thrombus in acute myocardial infarction [66] raised interest in thrombosis as an etiologic factor in unstable angina. Several authors have subsequently documented the presence of intracoronary thrombus in unstable angina, with an average frequency of approximately 40 percent [67–72]. The angiographic appearance of thrombus in unstable angina has been confirmed by direct visualization via angioscopy [73]. Thrombolytic therapy in unstable angina patients has resulted in a reduction in stenosis severity [74]. The importance of thrombosis in myocardial infarction and unstable angina is underscored by the presence of an elevated concentration of fibrin and its degradation products, which is not found in patients with stable angina [75].

Platelets attracted to a ruptured atherosclerotic plaque and its adherent thrombus perpetuate ischemic episodes through a variety of mechanisms. Their clinical importance is underscored by the finding of platelet clumps downstream from stenotic coronary segments in unstable angina patients succumbing to sudden death [76]. Platelets episodically occlude or markedly reduce coronary flow through stenotic segments by aggregation, which is enhanced by elevated levels of catecholamines, lipoproteins, and plasminogen-activator inhibitor [77,78]. Thromboxane A_2 promotes further platelet aggregation, in part by inhibiting platelet formation of anti-aggregatory cyclic AMP. Metabolites of thromboxane A_2 are found in elevated concentration in plasma and urine near the time of episodes of unstable angina but not in relation to exercise-induced ischemia in patients with stable angina [79,80]. Spontaneous resolution of anginal episodes may be due in part to endothelial elaboration of prostacyclin and other mediators that limit platelet aggregation and promote vasorelaxation. However, endogenous fibrinolytic activity may be handicapped in unstable coronary syndromes, as elevated plasminogen activator inhibitor has been documented [81].

CORONARY VASOSPASM. The majority of ischemic episodes occur due to an increase in myocardial oxygen demand, but reduction in coronary flow can be associated with ischemic episodes, and in a small percentage of cases vasospasm is the sole etiology [82]. Interest in vasospasm in the pathogenesis of acute coronary syndromes stemmed in part from the documentation of silent ischemia in patients with known atherosclerotic disease when there was no escalation in myocardial oxygen demand.

Coronary vasospasm most often occurs at the site of arterial segments containing atherosclerotic plaque [83,84,85]. In addition, atherosclerosis has been documented to cause endothelial dysfunction. Normal coronary arteries dilate in response to mental and physical exercise and the cold pressor test, whereas diseased vessels constrict [84,86–91]. The mechanism for these abnormal responses is in large measure due to deranged endothelial function. Nondiseased endothelium mediates vasodilation in response to a variety of agents, including acetylcholine, histamine, bradykinin, and thrombin, while mitigating vasoconstriction in response to other substances, such as white blood cells, serotonin, and catecholamines [47,92,93,94]. It is thought that endothelial mediated vasodilatation is accomplished via endothelium-derived relaxing factor-stimulated increases in cyclic GMP concentration leading to smooth muscle relaxation.

Diseased coronary vasculature loses the ability to manifest endothelial-dependent vasodilatation [95,96,97]. One group of investigators documented paradoxical vasoconstriction in diseased coronaries in response to the endothelium-dependent vasodilator acetylcholine [98]. Further evidence indicates that such paradoxical responses to what are normally vasodilatory stimuli occur early in the natural history of the atherosclerotic process, probably prior to angiographic recognition of the disease [98–101]. Not surprisingly, diseased endothelium exhibits unopposed vasoconstriction in response to catecholamines and serotonin, a response not seen in healthy vasculature [102,103].

The precise cause of altered vasomotion in atherosclerotic vessels is not clear, but a quantitative defect in the elaboration of endothelium-derived relaxing factor has been postulated [47]. Diffuse hypersensitivity in response to vasoconstricting stimuli such as ergonovine throughout the coronary circulation has been demonstrated in Prinzmetal's or variant angina [104]. Some investigators have postulated that the underlying abnormality in these patients is hypercontractility of arterial smooth muscle as a result of atherosclerosis [105]. Cations also may play a role in the pathogenesis of coronary spasm, as administration of magnesium has been demonstrated to either prevent or terminate exercise and cold pressor-induced spasm in patients with variant angina [106,107].

Finally, there is an intriguing interaction between thrombosis and coronary spasm. Spasm may induce stasis, thereby leading to enhanced thrombin activity and fibrin production [108]. These effects appear to be the result, rather than the etiology, of symptomatic episodes in patients with Prinzmetal's angina. In addition, diseased endothelium may exhibit impaired production of endogenous plasminogen activators such as t-PA. When the thrombolytic potential of diseased endothelium is combined with abnormal vasomotion as described above, the stage is set for a vicious circle that results in severe ischemia or frank myocardial necrosis. Finally, it should be noted that vasomotor tone may be augmented by exogenous factors such as

cigarettes and cocaine, which inhibits presynaptic uptake of norepinephrine and dopamine [109,110].

While the vast majority of patients exhibiting myocardial ischemia and infarction have atherosclerotic disease as an etiology, several causes of nonatherosclerotic coronary disease (Table 50-4) may lead to symptoms of angina or precipitation of myocardial necrosis. A comprehensive review is beyond the scope of this chapter, but several are reviewed briefly below.

CONGENITAL ABNORMALITIES. Isolated congenital anomalies of the coronary arteries are uncovered in somewhat less than 1 percent of adults undergoing coronary angiography. A wide array of these anomalies exist [111]. Most common is origination of the left circumflex artery from the right sinus of Valsalva or as a branch of the right coronary artery [112]. In general, only a few anomalies cause spontaneous symptoms of ischemia or infarction. Origin of the left coronary artery from the pulmonary artery (Bland-White-Garland syndrome) is extremely uncommon in adults. It is associated with ongoing ischemia and necrosis [111], and most afflicted patients die during early childhood of heart failure [113].

Aberrant origin of the left or right coronary artery from the "wrong" sinus of Valsalva is rare but is associated with sudden death, presumably due to ischemia-induced ventricular fibrillation [113]. Sudden death in this setting often occurs after strenuous physical exercise [114,115] and in patients in whom the aberrantly arising vessel courses between the aorta and pulmonary artery [113–116]. The orifice of the vessels is frequently underdeveloped and slitlike, and early in its course it is at an acute angle, which compromises proximal lumen size [113,116]. Expansion of the great vessels during exercise is thought to lead to occlusion of the vessel in its already narrowed proximal extent [116]. Anomalous vessels are at significantly greater risk for development of atherosclerosis, but the long-term importance of this finding is not clear [112].

Coronary arteriovenous (AV) fistulas can result in myocardial ischemia [117] through a "steal" phenomenon, in which left-to-right shunting of blood deprives the myocardium distal to the fistula of adequate blood flow [118]. However, the large majority of patients with this rare abnormality are asymptomatic. Most AV fistulas are congenital, but acquired forms can occur after trauma [119] or bypass surgery [120].

TRAUMA. Penetrating and blunt trauma can cause myocardial infarction. Penetrating trauma such as stab and gunshot wounds can cause coronary laceration, although the primary clinical presentation in this setting is that of pericardial tamponade. Blunt trauma can cause myocardial infarction even in the absence of preexisting atherosclerotic disease [119]. Whether the myocardial infarction is related to intimal tear, coronary rupture, myocardial contusion, or some combination of these mechanisms is uncertain.

EMBOLISM. Embolism to the coronary arteries can lead to myocardial infarction by acute occlusion of the involved vessel, usually the LAD [121]. Potential sources of coronary embolism include left ventricular mural thrombus, endocarditis (either native or prosthetic valve), neoplasia, air and calcium during cardiac surgery or cardiac catheterization, paradoxical embolization across a patent foramen ovale, and atrial septal defect. Fortunately, coronary embolism is rare given the relatively sequestered position of the coronary ostia in the sinuses of Valsalva and that coronary orientation is at approximately right angles to aortic flow.

DISSECTION. Coronary dissection causes ischemia and infarction when intima separates from media and the resultant flap obstructs blood flow through the vessel lumen. Such obstructive dissections occur most commonly as a complication of coronary angioplasty and rarely as a result of diagnostic angiography. Aortic dissection also may extend proximally to involve the coronary circulation. Spontaneous coronary dissections occur very infrequently. The vast majority of cases occur in young women, one-third in the peripartum period. The clinical presentation of spontaneous coronary dissection usually is acute myocardial infarction, most frequently related to the LAD territory [122].

NONATHEROSCLEROTIC CORONARY DISEASE. Vasculitic involvement of coronary arteries can lead to ischemia and infarction (Table 50-4). In Takayasu's arteritis, pathologic examination reveals panarteritis with intimal proliferation and fibrosis. Coronary arteritis, when present, usually involves the ostium of the epicardial vessels [123]. Coronary involvement is more common in polyarteritis nodosa, seen in approximately two-thirds of patients. Necrotizing inflammation can lead to aneurysm formation and myocardial infarction is common [124]. Giant cell arteritis is most frequently seen in elderly patients, in whom a noncontinuous granulomatous inflammation leads to thrombosis, with resultant ischemia or infarction [125]. Kawaski's disease usually afflicts children. Inflammatory change is first seen in the vasa vasorum; eventually panarteritis with marked intimal thickening and thrombosis ensues, with vessel occlusion to varying degrees [126]. When healing occurs, calcification and scarring of involved arteries and recanalization of occluded vessels are seen.

Thoracic radiation, used to treat a variety of neoplastic disorders, seems to be associated with an excess incidence of coronary artery disease, with a propensity for isolated involvement of the left main coronary artery [127]. Radiation-induced arteritis leading to vascular fibrosis potentiated by hypercholesterolemia has been suggested as the mechanism of ischemia induction in this setting [127].

ANEMIA. Chronic anemia induces a high-output state, due in large measure to a reduction in blood viscosity [128]. Ischemia induction is facilitated in this condition primarily in patients with existing coronary artery disease.

PROCOAGULANT STATES. Ischemia and infarction occasionally occur as a result of one of the so-called hypercoagulable states. Inappropriate thrombosis occurs in these disorders, usually due to a breakdown in thromboregulation at the level of the vascular endothelium. These states have recently been elegantly reviewed [129]. Primary hypercoagulable states include entities such as antithrombin III deficiency, protein C and S deficiency, and homocystinuria. Antithrombin III deficiency is usually associated with venous thrombosis, but arterial thrombosis can occur [129]. Protein C and S mitigate thrombus formation at the capillary level [129]. Hereditary and acquired deficiency of these proteins is usually associated with venous thrombosis, but myocardial infarction has been reported [130,131]. Homocystinuria is associated with premature atherosclerosis in virtually the entire arterial circulation, including the coronary vasculature [132,133]. Elevated levels of homocysteine have been postulated to facilitate thrombogenesis and atherogenesis via a downregulation of endothelial thrombomodulin function, inhibition of tissue plasminogen activator bind-

Table 50-4. Nonatherosclerotic Coronary Artery Disease: Etiologies

Congenital coronary artery anomalies
Coronary AV fistulas
Trauma
Coronary embolism
Coronary dissection
Coronary vasculitis
Radiation arteritis
Anemia
Hypercoagulable states
Hypotension
Aortic stenosis and insufficiency
Left ventricular hypertrophy
Hypertrophic cardiomyopathy
High-output states
Dilated cardiomyopathy

ing to endothelial cells, and facilitated deposition of lipoprotein$_a$ to the vascular endothelium [134,135,136].

Secondary hypercoagulable states include hyperlipidemias, antiphospholipid syndrome, the myeloproliferative disorders, and many others [129]. Hypertriglyceridemia has been postulated to promote a "prothrombotic state" due to the triglyceride-induced enhanced conversion of prothrombin to thrombin and augmentation in activity of both factor X and plasminogen activator inhibitor [137]. A prothrombotic state was recently postulated to account for differences in presentation in patients with unheralded acute myocardial infarction and those with chronic stable angina [138]. The antiphospholipid syndrome includes patients with autoimmune syndromes who produce antibodies against anionic phospholipids [139]. Myocardial infarction has been documented in this patient population [139]. One group has documented that the cause of myocardial necrosis in this syndrome is myocardial microvasculopathy [140]. The myeloproliferative syndromes, such as polycythemia vera and essential thrombocytosis, are associated with a propensity to thrombosis, including that in the coronary circulation. Thrombosis in these disorders is thought to occur due to elevated blood viscosity, thrombocytosis, and platelet aggregability.

HYPOTENSION. Ischemia, especially of the subendocardium, can manifest during periods of hypotension. In this setting, coronary perfusion is reduced. In patients with atherosclerotic disease, the diastolic coronary pressure distal to the obstruction is already compromised, hence hypotension is more apt to induce ischemia. Coexistent elevation in left ventricular diastolic pressure can obviously perpetuate the ischemic process. The clinical syndrome responsible for hypotension may further predispose the patient to ischemia, depending on associated factors, such as the tachycardia associated with systemic sepsis.

Disorders of Myocardial Oxygen Demand

AORTIC STENOSIS. Angina pectoris is a common clinical manifestation of acquired aortic stenosis. Even in the absence of coronary disease, myocardial oxygen demand may exceed supply due to myocardial hypertrophy, prolongation of the systolic ejection period, and elevated left ventricular systolic pressure, a triad that in concert greatly augments myocardial oxygen consumption [141]. In addition, the high left ventricular systolic pressure can compress intramyocardial coronary vessels, disrupting flow, especially to the subendocardium [142]. Coronary perfusion in aortic stenosis is also diminished by a reduction in the transmyocardial perfusion pressure due to the characteristic elevated left ventricular end-diastolic pressure [142,143].

AORTIC INSUFFICIENCY. Although a less common clinical problem, ischemia can be expressed as a symptom of aortic insufficiency in which increased myocardial oxygen demand and diminished supply coexist. Myocardial oxygen demand is increased due to left ventricular dilatation. Diminished systemic diastolic pressure, a hallmark of chronic aortic insufficiency, reduces coronary perfusion, thereby compromising myocardial oxygen supply.

HYPERTENSIVE HEART DISEASE. Hypertension is well known to be a risk factor for the development of left ventricular hypertrophy as well as coronary artery disease. Left ventricular hypertrophy in the absence of coronary stenoses may precipitate ischemia as a consequence of greater myocardial mass combined with diminished perfusion pressure secondary to elevated ventricular end-diastolic pressure. In addition, abnormal coronary flow reserve has been reported in hypertensive patients without atherosclerotic disease [144].

HYPERTROPHIC CARDIOMYOPATHY. In hypertrophic obstructive cardiomyopathy, mechanisms similar to those mentioned above may result in ischemia. In addition, myocardial oxygen demand may be especially high in patients with outflow gradients. Systolic compression of a coronary artery (so-called myocardial bridging) has been suggested as a cause of ischemia in this syndrome. In this instance, an epicardial vessel travels subepicardially for a variable distance before returning to the epicardial surface [145]. Systolic compression of the intramural vessel has been suggested as a cause of ischemia [146,147,148], despite the fact that the majority of coronary flow occurs in diastole. Some case reports have reported improvement in anginal symptoms after surgical bridge resection [149]. Intramural vessels in this disorder have been reported commonly to have a narrowed lumen and thickened media; the areas perfused by these abnormal vessels tend to be fibrotic, implicating ischemia due to abnormal vascular architecture [150].

HIGH-OUTPUT STATES. In high-output states such as hyperthyroidism, ischemic symptoms most often occur in patients with underlying coronary artery disease as a consequence of elevated myocardial oxygen demand via augmented contractility and heart rate. It has been suggested that the hyperthyroid state predisposes afflicted patients to coronary spasm [151].

Patients with left ventricular dysfunction often have ischemia as an etiology of cardiomyopathy; consequently ischemic symptoms are frequently noted. In addition, as left ventricular dilatation ensues, wall stress rises along with myocardial oxygen demand. Therefore, anginal symptoms can be seen in patients with decompensated congestive heart failure.

References

1. Harada K, Fujiseki Y, Usami H, et al: Myocardial infarction and left coronary ostial stenosis in infancy simulating anomalous origin of the left coronary artery: A case report. *Jpn Heart J* 21:435, 1980.

2. Josa M, Danielson GK, Weidman WH, Edwards WD: Congenital ostial membrane of the left coronary artery. *J Thorac Cardiovasc Surg* 81:338, 1981.

3. MacMahon HE, Dickinson PC: Occlusive fibroelastosis of coronary arteries in the newborn. *Circulation* 35:3, 1967.

4. Blackman MS, Schneider B, Sondheimer HM: Absent proximal left main coronary artery in association with pulmonary atresia. *Br Heart J* 46:449, 1981.

5. Kurosawa H, Wagenaar SS, Becker AE: Sudden death in a youth: A case of quadricuspid aortic valve with isolation of origin of left coronary artery. *Br Heart J* 46:211, 1981.

6. Gittenberger de Groot AC, Sauer U, Quaegebeur J: Aortic intramural coronary artery in three hearts with transposition of the great arteries. *J Thorac Cardiovasc Surg* 91:566, 1986.

7. Roberts WC: Anomalous origin of both coronary arteries from the pulmonary artery. *Am J Cardiol* 10:595, 1962.

8. Abbot ME: Anomalous origin from the pulmonary arteries, in Osler W (ed): *Osler's Modern Medicine. Its Theories and Practice.* Philadelphia, Lea & Febiger, 1908, p. 420.

9. Bland EF, White PD, Garland J: Congenital anomalies of the coronary arteries: Report of an unusual case associated with cardiac hypertrophy. *Am Heart J* 8:787, 1933.

10. Edwards JE: Anomalous coronary arteries with special reference to arteriovenous-like communications. *Circulation* 17:1001, 1958.

11. Edwards JE: The direction of blood flow in coronary arteries arising from the pulmonary trunk. *Circulation* 29:163, 1964.

12. Moodie DS, Fyfe D, Gill CC, et al: Anomalous origin of the left coronary artery from the pulmonary artery (Bland-White-Garland syndrome) in adult patients: Long-term follow-up after surgery. *Am Heart J* 106:381, 1983.

13. Meyers DG, McManus BM, McCall D, et al: Single coronary artery with the right coronary artery arising from the first septal perforator. *Cathet Cardiovasc Diagn* 10:479, 1984.

14. Banch A: Morfoglia della arterae coronariae cordis. *Arch Ital Anat Embriol* 3:89, 1903.

15. Ogden JA, Goodyear AVN: Patterns of distribution of the single coronary artery. *Yale J Biol Med* 43:11, 1970.

16. Smith JC: Review of single coronary artery with report of 2 cases. *Circulation* 1:1168, 1950.

17. Lipton MJ, Barry WH, Obrez I, et al: Isolated single coronary artery: Diagnosis, angiographic classification and clinical significance. *Radiology* 130:39, 1979.

18. Vuthoori S, Waisser E, Angelini P: Triple origin of left coronary arteries from right coronary artery: Unusual case of single coronary artery. *Clin Cardiol* 3:67, 1980.

19. Murphy ME: Single coronary artery. *Am Heart J* 74:557, 1967.

20. Davis JS, Lie JT: Anomalous origin of a single coronary artery from the innominate artery. *Angiology* 28:775, 1977.

21. Robicsek F, Sanger PW, Daugherty HK, Gallucci V: Origin of the anterior interventricular (descending) coronary artery and vein from the left mammary vessels: A previously unknown anomaly of the coronary system. *J Thorac Cardiovasc Surg* 53:602, 1967.

22. Cheatham JP, Ruyle NA, McManus BM, Bammel GE: Origin of the right coronary artery from the descending thoracic aorta: Angiographic diagnosis and unique coronary artery anatomy at autopsy. *Cathet Cardiovasc Diagn* 13:321, 1987.

23. Ott DA, Cooley DA, Pinsky WW, Mullins CE: Anomalous origin of circumflex coronary artery from right pulmonary artery: Report of a rare anomaly. *J Thorac Cardiovasc Surg* 76:190, 1978.

24. Bharati S, Chandra N, Stephenson LW, et al: Origin of the left coronary artery. *J Am Coll Cardiol* 3:1565, 1984.

25. Kragel AH, Roberts WC: Anomalous origin of either the right or left main coronary artery from the aorta with subsequent coursing between the aorta and pulmonary trunk: Analyses of 32 necropsy cases. *Am J Cardiol* 62:771, 1988.

26. Waldman JD, Lamberti JJ, Mathewson JW, George L: Surgical closure of the tricuspid valve for pulmonary atresia, intact ventricular septum, and right ventricle to coronary artery communications. *Pediatr Cardiol* 5:221, 1984.

27. Kiso I, Itih T, Morishita M, et al: Blood flow and pressure measurements of right coronary to left ventricle fistula. *Thorax* 33:253, 1978.

28. Adams P, Morris L, Ross I: Congenital left coronary artery-right ventricle fistula. *Aust Paeditr* 19:47, 1983.

29. Croom RD III, Wilcox BR, Abney RL III: Right coronary artery: Coronary sinus arteriovenous fistula. *Ann Thorac Surg* 4:182, 1967.

30. Ogden JA, Stansel HC Jr: Coronary arterial fistulas terminating in the coronary venous system. *J Thorac Cardiovasc Surg* 63:172, 1972.

31. Kimbiris D, Kasparian H, Knibbe P, Brest AN: Coronary artery-coronary sinus fistula. *Am J Cardiol* 56:997, 1985.

32. Dark JH, Pollack JC: Coronary artery-pulmonary artery fistula in tetralogy of Fallot with pulmonary atresia. *Eur Heart J* 6:714, 1985.

33. Baim DS, Kline H, Silverman JF: Bilateral coronary artery-pulmonary artery fistulas: Report of five cases and review of the literature. *Circulation* 65:810, 1982.

34. Cohen MV (ed): *Coronary Collaterals: Clinical and Experimental Observations*. Mount Kisco, Futura, 1985.

35. Schnaper W: *The Collateral Circulation of the Heart*. London, North Holland, 1971.

36. Sabiston DC Jr, Gregg DE: Effect of cardiac contraction on coronary flow. *Circulation* 15:14, 1975.

37. Downey JM, Downey HF, Kirk ES: Effects of myocardial strains on coronary blood flow. *Circ Res* 34:286, 1974.

38. Snyder R, Downey JM, Kirk ES: The active and passive components of extravascular coronary resistance. *Cardiovasc Res* 9:161, 1975.

39. Feigl EO: Sympathetic control of coronary circulation. *Circ Res* 20:262, 1967.

40. Berne RM: Cardiodynamics and the coronary circulation in hyperthermia. *Ann NY Acad Sci* 80:365, 1959.

41. Mosher P, Ross J Jr, McFate PA, et al: Control of coronary blood flow by an autoregulatory mechanism. *Circ Res* 14:250, 1964.

42. Rouleau J, Boerboom LE, Surjadhana A, et al: The role of autoregulation and tissue diastolic pressures in the transmural distribution of left ventricular blood flow in anesthetized dogs. *Circ Res* 45:804, 1979.

43. Berne RM, Rubio R: Coronary circulation, in Berne RM, Sperelakis N, Geiger SR (eds): *Handbook of Physiology: The Cardiovascular System*. Baltimore, Williams & Wilkins, 1979, pp 873–952.

44. Hoffman JIE: Determinants and prediction of transmural myocardial perfusion. *Circulation* 58:381, 1978.

45. Epstein SE, Cannon RO: Site of increased resistance to coronary flow in patients with angina pectoris and normal epicardial arteries. *J Am Coll Cardiol* 8:459, 1986.

46. Cannon RO, Watson RM, Rosing DR, et al: Efficacy of calcium channel blocker therapy for angina pectoris resulting from small vessel coronary artery disease and abnormal vasodilator reserve. *Am J Cardiol* 56:242, 1985.

47. Sax FL, Cannon RO, Hanson C, et al: Forearm flow in patients with microvascular angina: Evidence of a generalized disorder of vascular tone? *N Engl J Med* 317:1366, 1987.

48. Selwyn AP, Yeung AC, Ryan TJ Jr, et al: Pathophysiology of ischemia in patients with coronary artery disease. *Prog Cardiovasc Dis* 35:27, 1992.

49. Alpert JS: The pathophysiology of acute myocardial infarction. *Cardiology* 76:85, 1989.

50. Mosher P, Ross PJ Jr, McFate PA, et al: Control of coronary blood flow by an autoregulatory mechanism. *Circ Res* 14:250, 1964.

51. Gould KL, Lipscomb K: Effects of coronary stenoses on coronary flow reserve and resistance. *Am J Cardiol* 34:78, 1974.

52. Gould KL: Assessing coronary stenosis severity: A recurrent clinical need. *J Am Coll Cardiol* 8:91, 1986.

53. Epstein SE, Talbot TL: Dynamic coronary tone in precipitation, exacerbation and relief of angina pectoris. *Am J Cardiol* 48:797, 1981.

54. Braunwald E, Sobel BE: Coronary blood flow and myocardial ischemia, in Braunwald E (ed): *Heart Disease*. 4th ed. Philadelphia: WB Saunders, 1992, p. 1161.

55. Factor SM, Kirk ES: Pathophysiology of myocardial ischemia, in Hurst JW, Logue RB, Rackley CE, et al (eds): *The Heart*. 6th ed. New York, McGraw-Hill, 1986, p 856.

56. Forman R, Kirk ES, Downey JM, et al: Nitroglycerin and heterogeneity of myocardial blood flow: Reduced subendocardial blood flow and ventricular contractile force. *J Clin Invest* 52:905, 1973.

57. Davies MJ, Thomas AC, Shah PK, et al: Plaque fissuring: The cause of acute myocardial infarction, sudden ischemic death, and crescendo angina. *Br Heart J* 53:363, 1985.

58. Ambrose JA, Winters SL, Stern A, et al: Angiographic morphology in the pathogenesis of unstable angina pectoris. *J Am Coll Cardiol* 5:609, 1985.

59. Ahmed WH, Bittl JA, Braunwald E: Relation between clinical presentation and angiographic findings in unstable angina pectoris, and comparison with that and stable angina. *Am J Cardiol* 72:544, 1993.

60. Fuster V, Stein B, Ambrose JA, et al: Atherosclerotic plaque rupture and thrombosis: Evolving concepts. *Circulation* 82(suppl II):47, 1990.

61. Ambrose JA, Winters SL, Arora RR, et al: Angiographic evolution of coronary artery morphology in unstable angina. *J Am Coll Cardiol* 7:472, 1986.

62. Chesebro JH, Zoldhelyi P, Fuster Z: Plaque disruption and thrombosis in unstable angina pectoris. *Am J Cardiol* 68:9C, 1991.

63. Davies MJ: A macro and micro view of coronary vascular insult in ischemic heart disease. *Circulation* 82(suppl II):38, 1990.

64. Richardson PD, Davies MJ, Born GBR: Influence of plaque configuration and stress distribution on fissuring of coronary atherosclerotic plaques. *Lancet* 2:941, 1989.

65. Mazzone A, De Servi S, Ricevuti G, et al: Increased expression of neutrophil and monocyte adhesion molecules in unstable coronary artery disease. *Circulation* 88:358, 1993.

66. DeWood MA, Spores J, Notske R, et al: Prevalence of total coronary occlusion during the early hours of transmural myocardial infarction. *N Engl J Med* 303:897, 1980.

67. Bresnahan DR, Davis JL, Holmes DR, et al: Angiographic occurrence and clinical correlates of intraluminal coronary artery thrombus: Role of unstable angina. *J Am Coll Cardiol* 6:285, 1985.

68. Vetrovec GW, Cowley MJ, Overton H, et al: Intracoronary thrombus in syndromes of unstable myocardial ischemia. *Am Heart J* 102:1202, 1981.

69. Freeman MR, Williams AE, Chisholm RJ, et al: Intracoronary thrombus and complex morphology in unstable angina: Relation to timing of angiography and in-hospital cardiac events. *Circulation* 8:17, 1989.

70. Holmes DR, Hartzler GO, Smith HC, et al: Coronary artery thrombosis in patients with unstable angina. *Br Heart J* 45:411, 1981.

71. Zack PM, Ichinger T, Aker UT, et al: The occurrence of angiographically detected intracoronary thrombus in patients with unstable angina pectoris. *Am Heart J* 108:1408, 1984.

72. Capone G, Wolf NM, Meyer B, et al: Frequency of intracoronary filling defects by angiography in angina pectoris at rest. *Am J Cardiol* 56:403, 1985.

73. Sherman CT, Litvack F, Grundfest W, et al: Coronary angioscopy in patients with unstable angina pectoris. *N Engl J Med* 315:913, 1986.

74. Bar FW, Verheugt FW, Col J, et al: Thrombolysis in patients with unstable angina improves the angiographic but not the clinical outcome: Results of UNASEM, a multicenter, randomized, placebo-controlled, clinical trial with anistreplase. *Circulation* 86:131, 1992.

75. Kruskal JB, Commerford PJ, Franks JJ, et al: Fibrin and fibrinogen related antigens in patients with stable and unstable coronary artery disease. *N Engl J Med* 317:1361, 1987.

76. Davies MJ, Thomas AC, Knapman PA, et al: Intramyocardial platelet aggregation in patients with unstable angina suffering sudden ischemic cardiac death. *Circulation* 73:418, 1986.

77. Folts JD, Crowell EB, Rowe GG: Platelet aggregation in partially obstructed vessels and its elimination with aspirin. *Circulation* 54:365, 1976.

78. Gerstenblith G: Treatment of unstable angina pectoris. *Am J Cardiol* 70:32G, 1992.

79. Grande P, Grauholt AM, Madsen JK: Unstable angina pectoris: Platelet behavior and prognosis in progressive angina and immediate coronary syndrome. *Circulation* 81(suppl I):16, 1990.

80. Fitzgerald DJ, Roy MBL, Catella F, et al: Platelet activation in unstable coronary disease. *N Engl J Med* 315:983, 1986.

81. Zalewski A, Nardone D, Bravette B, et al: Evidence for reduced fibrinolytic activity in unstable angina at rest: Clinical, biochemical and angiographic correlates. *Circulation* 83:1685, 1991.

82. Deedwania PC: Increased demand vs. reduced supply and the circadian variations in ambulatory myocardial ischemia—therapeutic implications. *Circulation* 81:850, 1990.

83. Nabel EG, Selwyn AP, Ganz P: Paradoxical narrowing of athero-

sclerotic coronary arteries induced by increases in heart rate. *Circulation* 81:850, 1990.

84. Gordon JB, Ganz P, Nabel EG, et al: Atherosclerosis influences the vasomotor response of epicardial coronary arteries to exercise. *J Clin Invest* 83:1946, 1989.

85. Yeung AC, Vekstein VI, Krantz DS, et al: The effect of atherosclerosis on the vasomotor response of coronary arteries to mental stress. *N Engl J Med* 325:1551, 1991.

86. Gaglione A, Hess OM, Corin WJ, et al: Is there coronary vasoconstriction after intracoronary beta-adrenergic blockade in patients with coronary artery disease? *J Am Coll Cardiol* 10:299, 1987.

87. Nabel EG, Ganz P, Gordon JB, et al: Dilation of normal and constriction of atherosclerotic coronary arteries caused by the cold pressor test. *Circulation* 77:43, 1988.

88. Ganz P, Abben RP, Barry WH: Dynamic variations in resistance to coronary arterial narrowings in angina pectoris at rest. *Am J Cardiol* 59:66, 1987.

89. Gage JE, Hess OM, Murakamni T: Vasoconstriction of stenotic coronary arteries during dynamic exercise in patients with classic angina pectoris: Reversibility by nitroglycerin. *Circulation* 73:865, 1986.

90. Mudge GH Jr, Grossman W, Mills RM Jr, et al: Reflex increase in coronary vascular resistance in patients with ischemic heart disease. *N Engl J Med* 295:1333, 1976.

91. Malacoff RF, Mudge GH Jr, Holman BL, et al: Effect of the cold pressor test on regional myocardial blood flow in patients with coronary artery disease. *Am Heart J* 106:78, 1983.

92. Griffith TM, Edwards EH, Lewis MJ, et al: The nature of endothelium-derived vascular relaxant factor. *Nature* 3088:645, 1984.

93. Palmer RMJ, Ferrige AG, Moncada S: Nitric oxide release accounts for the biological activity of endothelium-derived relaxing factor. *Nature* 327:524, 1987.

94. Hutchinson PJA, Palmer RMJ, Moncada S: Comparative pharmacology of EDRF and nitric oxide on vascular strips. *Eur J Pharmacol* 141:145, 1987.

95. Ginsburg R, Bristow MR, Davies K, et al: Quantitative pharmacologic responses of normal and atherosclerotic isolated human epicardial coronary arteries. *Circulation* 69:430, 1984.

96. Chester AH, O'Neil GS, Moncada S, et al: Low basal and stimulated release of nitric oxide in atherosclerotic epicardial coronary arteries. *Lancet* 330:897, 1990.

97. Bossaller C, Habib GB, Yamamoto H, et al: Impaired muscarinic endothelium-dependent relaxation and cyclic guanosine 5' monophosphate formation in atherosclerotic human coronary artery and rabbit aorta. *J Clin Invest* 79:170, 1987.

98. Ludmer PL, Selwyn AP, Shook TI, et al: Paradoxical vasoconstriction induced by acetyl choline in atherosclerotic coronary arteries. *N Engl J Med* 315:1046, 1986.

99. McLenahan JM, William JK, Fish RD, et al: Loss of flow mediated endothelium-dependent dilation occurs early in the development of atherosclerosis. *Circulation* 84:1273, 1991.

100. Okumara K, Morikami Y, Ogawa H: Responses of angiographically normal coronary arteries to intracoronary injection of acetylcholine by age and segment: Possible role of early coronary atherosclerosis. *Circulation* 81:482, 1990.

101. Vita JA, Treasure CB, Nabel EG, et al: The coronary vasomotor response to acetylcholine relates to risk factors for coronary artery disease. *Circulation* 81:491, 1990.

102. Vita JA, Treasure CB, Fish RD, et al: Endothelial dysfunction leads to increased coronary constriction to catecholamines in patients with early atherosclerosis. *J Am Coll Cardiol* 15:158, 1990.

103. Golino P, Piscione F, Willerson JT, et al: Divergent effects of serotonin on coronary artery dimensions and blood flow in patients with coronary atherosclerosis and control patients. *N Engl J Med* 324:641, 1991.

104. Hoshio A, Kotare H, Mashiba H: Significance of coronary artery tone in patients with vasospastic angina. *J Am Coll Cardiol* 14:604, 1989.

105. Ganz P, Alexander RW: New insights into the cellular mechanisms of vasospasm. *Am J Cardiol* 56:11E, 1985.

106. Cohen L, Kitzes R: Prompt termination and/or prevention of cold pressor-stimulus-induced vasoconstriction of different vascular beds by magnesium sulfate in patients with Prinzmetal's angina. *Magnesium* 5:144, 1986.

107. Kugiyama K, Yasu EH, Okumura K, et al: Suppression of exercise induced angina by magnesium sulfate in patients with variant angina. *J Am Coll Cardiol* 12:1177, 1988.

108. Irie T, Imaizumi T, Matuguchi T, et al: Increased fibrinopeptide A during angina attacks in patients with variant angina. *J Am Coll Cardiol* 14:589, 1989.

109. Lange RA, Cigarroa RG, Yancey CW, et al: Cocaine-induced coronary artery vasoconstriction. *N Engl J Med* 321:1557, 1989.

110. Winniford MD, Jansen DE, Reynolds GA, et al: Cigarette smoking-induced coronary vasoconstriction in atherosclerotic coronary artery disease and prevention by calcium antagonists and nitroglycerin. *Am J Cardiol* 59:203, 1987.

111. Cieslinski G, Rapprich B, Kober G: Coronary anomalies: Incidence and importance. *Clin Cardiol* 16:711, 1993.

112. Click RL, Holmes DR Jr, Vlietstra RE, et al: Anomalous coronary arteries: Location, degree of atherosclerosis and effect on survival—A report from the coronary artery surgery study. *J Am Coll Cardiol* 13:531, 1989.

113. Liberthson RR: Case records of the Massachusetts General Hospital: Case 22-1989. *N Engl J Med* 320:1475, 1989.

114. Liberthson RR, Dinsmore RE, Bharati S, et al: Aberrant coronary artery origin from the aorta: Diagnosis and clinical significance. *Circulation* 50:774, 1974.

115. Liberthson RR, Dinsmore RE, Fallon JT: Aberrant coronary artery from the aorta: Report of 18 patients, review of literature and delineation of natural history and management. *Circulation* 59:748, 1979.

116. Cheitlin MD, DeCastro, CM, McAllister HA: Sudden death as a complication of anomalous left coronary origin from the anterior sinus of the valsalva: A not so minor congenital anomaly. *Circulation* 50:780, 1974.

117. Levin DC, Fellows KE, Abrams HL: Hemodynamically significant primary anomalies of the coronary arteries: Angiographic aspects. *Circulation* 58:25, 1978.

118. Houghton JL, Saxena R, Frank MJ: Angina and ischemic electrocardiographic changes secondary to coronary arteriovenous fistula with abnormal basal and reserve coronary blood flow. *Am Heart J* 125:886, 1993.

119. Cohn PF, Braunwald E: Traumatic heart disease, in Braunwald E (ed): *Heart Disease.* Philadelphia: WB Saunders, 1992, p 1517.

120. Kimmelstiel CD, Udelson J, Salem D, et al: Recurrent angina due to a left internal mammary artery to pulmonary artery fistula. *Am Heart J* 125:234, 1993.

121. Miller RD, Burchell HB, Edwards JE: Myocardial infarction with and without acute coronary occlusion: A pathologic study. *Arch Intern Med* 88:597, 1951.

122. Alvarez J, Deal CW: Spontaneous dissection of the left main coronary artery: Case report and review of the literature. *Aust NZ J Med* 21:891, 1991.

123. Amano J, Suzuki A: Coronary artery involvement in Takayasu's arteritis: Collective review and guideline for surgical treatment. *J Thorac Cardiovasc Surg* 102:554, 1991.

124. Holsinger DR, Osmundson PJ, Edwards JE: The heart in periarteritis nodosa. *Circulation* 25:610, 1962.

125. Huston KA, Hunder GG: Giant cell (cranial arteritis): A clinical review. *Am Heart J* 100:99, 1980.

126. Hiraishi S, Yashiro K, Oguchi K, et al: Clinical course of cardiovascular involvement in mucocutaneous lymph node syndrome. *Am J Cardiol* 47:323, 1981.

127. Om A, Ellahham S, Vetrovec GW: Radiation-induced coronary artery disease. *Am Heart J* 124:1599, 1992.

128. Fowler NO, Holmes JC: Blood viscosity and cardiac output in acute experimental anemia. *J Appl Physiol* 39:453, 1975.

129. Nachman RL, Silverstein R: Hypercoagulable states. *Ann Intern Med* 119:819, 1993.

130. Hacker SM, Williamson BD, Lisco S, et al: Protein C deficiency and acute myocardial infarction in the third decade. *Am J Cardiol* 68:137, 1991.

131. Coller BS, Owen J, Jesty J, et al: Deficiency of plasma protein S, protein C, or antithrombin III in arterial thrombosis. *Arteriosclerosis* 7:456, 1987.

132. Mudd SH, Skovby F, Levy HL, et al: The natural history of homocystinuria due to cystathionine beta-synthase deficiency. *Am J Hum Genet* 37:1, 1985.

133. Genest JJ Jr, McNamara JR, Upson B, et al: Prevalence of familial hyperhomocysteinemia in men with premature coronary disease. *Arterioscler Thromb* 11:1129, 1991.

134. Hayashi T, Honda G, Suzuki K: An atherogenic stimulus homocysteine inhibits cofactor activity of thrombomodulin and enhances expression in human umbilical vein endothelial cells. *Blood* 79:2930, 1992.

135. Hajjar KA: Homocysteine-induced modulation of tissue plasminogen activator binding to its endothelial cell receptor. *J Clin Invest* 91:2873, 1993.

136. Harpel PC, Chang VT, Borth W: Homocysteine enhances the binding of lipoprotein (a) to plasmin-modified fibrin providing a potential link between thrombosis and atherogenesis. *Blood* 76:10A, 1990.

137. Becker RC: Seminars in thrombosis, thrombolysis and vascular biology. II. Coagulation and thrombosis. *Cardiology* 78:257, 1991.

138. Bogaty P, Brecker SJ, White SE, et al: Comparison of coronary angiographic findings in acute and chronic first presentation of ischemic heart disease. *Circulation* 87:1938, 1993.

139. Rosove MH, Brewer PMC: Antiphospholipid thrombosis: Clinical course after the first thrombotic event in 70 patients. *Ann Intern Med* 117:303, 1992.

140. Kattwinkel N, Villanueva AG, Labib SB, et al: Myocardial infarction caused by cardiac microvasculopathy in a patient with the primary antiphospholipid syndrome. *Ann Intern Med* 116:974, 1992.

141. Smucker ML, Tedesco CL, Manning SB: Demonstration of an imbalance between coronary perfusion and excessive load as a mechanism of ischemia during stress in patients with aortic stenosis. *Circulation* 78:573, 1988.

142. Vinten-Johansen J, Weiss HR: Oxygen consumption in subepicardial and subendocardial regions of the canine left ventricle: The effect of experimental acute valvular aortic stenosis. *Circ Res* 46:139, 1980.

143. Braunwald E: Valvular heart disease, in Braunwald E (ed): *Heart Disease*. Philadelphia, WB Saunders, 1992, p 1007.

144. Houghton JL, Frank MJ, Carr AA, et al: Relations among impaired coronary flow reserve, left ventricular hypertrophy and thallium perfusion defects in hypertensive patients without obstructive coronary artery disease. *J Am Coll Cardiol* 15:43, 1990.

145. Virmani R, Farb A, Burke AP: Ischemia from myocardial coronary bridging: Fact or fancy? *Hum Pathol* 24:687, 1993.

146. Morales AR, Romanelli R, Tate LG, et al: Intramural left anterior descending coronary artery: Significance of the depth of the muscular tunnel. *Hum Pathol* 24:693, 1993.

147. Noble J, Bourassa MG, Petitclerc R, et al: Myocardial bridging and milking effect of the left anterior descending coronary artery: Normal variant or obstruction? *Am J Cardiol* 37:993, 1976.

148. Furniss SS, Williams DO, McGregor GA: Systolic coronary occlusion due to myocardial bridging: A rare cause of ischemia. *Int J Cardiol* 26:116, 1990.

149. Faragui AMA, Maloy WC, Felner JM, et al: Symptomatic myocardial bridging of coronary artery. *Am J Cardiol* 41:1305, 1978.

150. Maron BJ, Wolfson JK, Epstein SE, et al: Intramural ("small vessel") coronary artery disease in hypertrophic cardiomyopathy. *J Am Coll Cardiol* 8:545, 1986.

151. Featherstone HJ, Stewart DK: Angina in thyrotoxicosis: Thyroid-related coronary artery spasm. *Arch Intern Med* 143:554, 1983.

51. Nonischemic Chest Pain

Donald G. Love, Richard C. Becker, and John A. Paraskos

Chest pain is a common complaint among patients undergoing evaluation in most major medical centers. It may be observed in cardiac, vascular, gastrointestinal, pulmonary, musculoskeletal, psychologic, neurologic, and dermatologic disease entities (Table 51-1). Chest pain accounts for an estimated 2 to 4 percent of all emergency room visits in the United States [1,2,3]. Similarly, more than 1.5 million Americans are admitted to intensive care units (ICUs) for suspected ischemic heart disease yearly [4,5].

Due to earlier recognition and treatment of life-threatening complications such as ventricular arrhythmias, congestive heart failure, acute mitral regurgitation and shock, patients with myocardial infarction (MI) and unstable angina have an improved prognosis if cared for in an ICU setting [2,6–10]. However, only 15 to 30 percent of those admitted to ICUs for possible MI are determined to have infarction [7,11–24]. Still, approximately 3 to 8 percent of acute MI patients may be sent home inappropriately from emergency rooms [2,15]. Those discharged are younger, have atypical symptoms, and are less likely to have had prior MI or angina [2].

It may be in the patient's best interest to err on the side of overdiagnosis of **acute** chest pain. Failure to recognize acute coronary syndromes and other life-threatening causes of chest pain (e.g., pulmonary embolism, aortic dissection, perforating peptic ulcer, and pneumothorax) could result in premature death. In addition, recent advances in techniques of myocardial salvage (thrombolysis and angioplasty) have improved survival for patients with acute MI [25–31]. Expeditious diagnosis of acute coronary syndromes is essential for optimal patient outcome [31]. In contrast, chronic chest pain syndromes are seldom life-threatening, and an erroneous diagnosis can cause undue emotional stress and financial burden.

Numerous studies have evaluated multivariate analytic techniques to improve physicians' ability to limit "unnecessary" hospital and ICU admissions [5,24,32–35] and to decrease the length of ICU stay once patients are admitted [36–40]. Computerized protocols converge in the emphasis placed on a carefully obtained history, cardiac enzymes, and electrocardiogram (ECG) [4,5,24,32,33,36]. These protocols, however, may not improve clinician judgment [35,41].

Accurate diagnosis of chest pain can be lifesaving, cost-saving, and anxiety-relieving. Although many diagnostic tests are available to the clinician evaluating patients with chest pain, the history and physical examination are the most important diagnostic tools. In an angiographic study of 4952 patients with chest pain, "typical angina" was associated with angiographically significant coronary disease in 89 percent of cases while those with "atypical angina" had an incidence of only 16 percent [42].

Table 51-1. Differential Diagnosis of Chest Pain

A. Cardiac
  1. Ischemic
    Atherosclerosis
    Coronary spasm
    Systemic hypertension
    Pulmonary hypertension
    Aortic stenosis
    Aortic insufficiency
    Hypertrophic cardiomyopathy
    Severe anemia
    Severe hypoxia
    Polycythemia
    Nonatherosclerotic epicardial disease
  2. Nonischemic
    Aortic dissection
    Aortic aneurysm
    Pericarditis
    Mitral valve prolapse
    Myocarditis
    Cardiomyopathy
B. Noncardiac
  1. Pulmonary
    Pulmonary embolism
    Pneumothorax
    Pneumonia
    Pleuritis
    Bronchospasm
    Pulmonary hypertension
    Tracheitis and tracheobronchitis
    Intrathoracic tumor
  2. Gastrointestinal
    Motility disorders
      Nutcracker esophagus
      Diffuse esophageal spasm
      Lower esophageal sphincter hypertension
      Nonspecific motility disorder
      Achalasia
    Gastroesophageal reflux
    Esophageal rupture (Boerhaave's syndrome)
    Esophageal tear (Mallory-Weiss syndrome)
    Esophagitis

      Candida
      Herpes
      Irradiation induced
    Esophageal foreign body
    Peptic ulcer disease
    Pancreatitis
    Biliary disease—cholecystitis or biliary colic
    Splenic infarction
    Gaseous bowel distention
  3. Neuromusculoskeletal
    Thoracic outlet syndrome
      Anterior scalene hypertrophy
      Cervical rib
    Cervical disc disease
    Costochondritis/Tietze's syndrome
    Chest wall trauma—rib fracture
    Malignancy
    Herpes zoster
    Precordial catch syndrome
    Sternal wire nerve entrapment
    Xiphodynia
    Slipping rib syndrome
    Ostalgia due to neoplasm, inflammation, or infarction
    Sternal marrow pain (acute leukemia)
    Intercostal neuritis
    Reflex autonomic dysfunction
  4. Psychiatric
    Depression
    Anxiety
    Panic attacks
    Malingering
  5. Other
    Cocaine
    Lymphoma
    Diabetes
    Uremia
    Renal stones
    Superficial thrombophlebitis (Mondor's syndrome)
    Mediastinitis
    Mediastinal emphysema
    Mediastinal neoplasms

Unfortunately, there is considerable overlap in signs and symptoms of myocardial ischemia and other cardiac and noncardiac causes of chest pain. For instance, atypical chest pain described as sharp, pleuritic, burning, and "indigestion" may represent infarction or ischemia in up to 20 percent of emergency room patients [17,43]. Atypical symptoms are particularly common in elderly patients. Often, patients must be approached with a high index of suspicion for myocardial ischemia until the diagnosis is either confirmed or negated by further observation, diagnostic studies, or response to therapy (Table 51-2).

During the evaluation, the clinician must answer basic questions such as whether the pain is typical for ischemic heart pain, atypical but possibly due to ischemic heart pain, or clearly not ischemic in origin and whether the pain is likely to be of a serious nature. Typical angina does not always indicate a serious prognosis. Alternatively, atypical chest pain may be associated with other life-threatening entities (e.g., aortic dissection, critical aortic stenosis, pulmonary embolism, and accelerated hypertension).

History

When evaluating patients with chest pain the history should focus on risk factors for atherosclerosis (age, gender, family history, smoking, cholesterol, hypertension, diabetes, peripheral vascular disease, prior coronary artery disease or MI, type A personality), precipitating factors, alleviating factors, quality, location, intensity, duration, frequency, radiation, pattern, setting, and associated symptoms. It is important not to lead the patient during the interview.

Physical Examination

The physical examination may be completely normal during an episode of life-threatening ischemia or infarction, but careful examination may provide important clues to the correct diagnosis. The examination must include vital signs (temperature, blood pressure in both upper extremities, heart rate, respiratory rate), general appearance (for evidence of diaphoresis, anxiety, cyanosis), gestures (Levine sign), skin examination (for evidence of xanthoma/xanthelasma), chest palpation, lung examination (for evidence of wheezing, consolidation, tympany), heart sounds and murmurs, abdominal examination (for evidence of epigastric tendernous), vascular examination, and special maneuvers (Adson's).

Electrocardiogram

When present, specific electrocardiographic changes are extremely useful in the diagnosis of chest pain. Emergency room patients with chest pain and both S–T elevation and Q waves on the ECG have about an 85 percent chance of having an acute MI [44]. Unfortunately, the sensitivity of ECG for serious disorders is too low to allow reassurance in the abscence of abnormalities [21,22]. Only 13 percent of patients with acute MI have S–T elevation and Q waves on their presenting ECG [35]. In a study of acute MI patients discharged from the emergency ward, 62 percent had a normal ECG on careful review [2]. Serial ECGs, however, are abnormal in 83 to 93 percent of cases of acute MI [21,22,45,46,47].

Chest Radiograph

Chest radiographs are routinely obtained in patients admitted to the ICU with a complaint of chest pain. They are abnormal in 14 to 44 percent [3]. Helpful findings include infiltrates, pneumothorax, vascular redistribution, widened mediastinum, cardiomegaly, atelectasis, rib fracture, free air under the diaphragm, hiatal hernia, pleural effusions, cervical ribs, abnormal calcifications, and mass lesions.

Other Diagnostic Tests

Two-dimensional (2-D) echocardiography may show wall motion abnormalities before chest pain or electrocardiographic findings. Echocardiography at the time of presentation with chest pain is sensitive (92%) but less specific (53%) for MI [48].

Ischemic Chest Pain

Chest pain is part of the symptom complex of most patients with acute ischemic heart disease. The pain of angina pectoris has a diverse presentation (see Chap. 50). Some episodes of ischemia or infarction may be painless but produce "angina equivalents," including profound weakness, diaphoresis, nausea, malaise, dyspnea, and localized discomfort in areas more commonly affected by radiating pain. The incidence of atypical presentation increases with older age [49], diabetes, history of stroke, spinal cord disease, coronary artery bypass surgery, and cardiac transplant. Up to 25 percent of MI may be clinically silent [50].

Ischemic chest pain is not synonymous with chest pain due to atherosclerosis. In addition to atherosclerotic epicardial coronary artery disease, a variety of cardiac abnormalities can manifest similar symptoms (Table 51-3).

A classic description of ischemic chest pain is provided.

LOCATION/RADIATION. Ischemic pain is typically located in the lower substernal area. It may radiate to one or both arms, the shoulders, anterior neck, lower jaw, and, less often, the teeth, wrists, and back. The extreme limits of radiation are from the occiput to the epigastrium.

QUALITY. Ischemic cardiac pain is typically a deep visceral sensation [51,52] and is therefore frequently described as choking, constricting, heaviness, squeezing, suffocating, strangling, pressure, burning, viselike, bandlike, discomfort, not pain, like someone standing on the patient's chest. The intensity ranges from mild to crushing. Rarely is ischemic chest pain well-localized, sharp, stabbing, knifelike, or tearing in quality. Associated symptoms include diaphoresis, hiccoughing, dyspnea, and nausea.

The patient's description of discomfort may be influenced by socioeconomic, educational, cultural, and historical variables as well as emotional state.

DURATION. In most instances ischemic chest pain lasts 2 to 20 minutes. Persistent pain lasting greater than 30 minutes should raise the suspicion of acute MI or a nonischemic etiology.

PRECIPITANTS/ALLEVIANTS. Ischemic chest pain is often precipitated by exertion and can be provoked by emotional stress, a large meal, the supine position (angina decubitus), sexual intercourse, cold weather, and use of the upper extremities. The intensity of effort necessary to incite angina often varies from day to day and throughout a given day; often the threshold is lower in the morning, after large meals, in the cold, and with emotional upset. It may be relieved by rest within 2 to 10 minutes, nitrates within 2 to 5 minutes, standing, carotid sinus massage [53], oxygen, or beta blockade.

Chest pain associated with MI frequently is more severe and radiates more widely. Although it may be, it is not typically triggered by exertion or emotional stress, is not relieved by rest, and is often associated with diaphoresis, nausea, fatigue, vomiting, dyspnea, and a sense of impending doom.

PHYSICAL EXAMINATION. The heart rate and blood pressure may be increased, normal, or decreased [54]. A transient mitral regurgitation murmur may be audible in patients with ischemia. In addition, signs of left ventricular dysfunction, such as pallor, cool clammy skin, an S_3 gallop, rales, and a dyskinetic PMI, may be found. Funduscopic examination may reveal signs of hypertension or diabetes. Peipheral pulses may reveal bruits or diminished pedal pulses consistent with coexisting peripheral vascular disease.

Nonischemic Chest Pain

An estimated 10 to 30 percent of patients with angina in whom coronary angiography is performed have normal-appearing coronaries [54–58]. This results in the diagnosis of greater than 100,000 new cases of "noncardiac" chest pain in the United States each year. These patients have a survival rate equal to that of age- and sex-matched controls [59–66]. Unfortunately, functional limitation often persists [60,62,63,66–70]. They continue to experience chest pain, still believe they have heart disease, use prescription cardiac medications, visit physicians, and become hospitalized for chest pain [62,70,71,72].

Table 51-2. Differential Diagnosis for Chest Discomfort

Diagnosis	Duration	Quality	Provocation	Relief	Location	Comments
Effort angina	2–15 min	Visceral Pressure Dull Crushing Intensity builds Tightness	Effort Emotion	Rest (2–10 min) NTG (1–5 min)	Substernal Radiates	First episode vivid
Infarction	>20 min	Visceral	Spontaneous Exertional	Rest Oxygen Nitrates Calcium blocker Beta-blocker	Substernal Radiates	Risk factors are age, male gender, hypertension, diabetes, smoking, cholesterol, postmenopause
Mitral valve prolapse	Minutes to hours	Superficial Variable Often atypical	No pattern Can be exertional Emotion	Time Beta-blocker Anxiolytic	Left anterior	Often with associated anxiety, palpitations, depression, hyperventilation. Female Transient ischemic attack, family history
Gastroesophageal reflux	10 min to hours	Visceral	Bending Recumbency Cigarettes Alcohol Methylxanthines	Food Antacids Elevated head of bed	Substernal Epigastric May radiate to back	Associated heartburn, regurgitation, dysphagia, nocturnal cough, hiatal hernia
Esophageal spasm	Seconds to 60 min	Visceral	Spontaneous Cold liquid ingestion Exercise	NTG Calcium blockade	Substernal	Often associated with dysphagia, reflux, odynophagia May be associated with foreign body, irradiation, systemic sclerosis
Peptic ulcer	30 min to hours	Visceral Dull Burning Boring	Lack of food Acid foods Salicylates Nonsteroidals	Food Antacid Carafate H2 blocker	Epigastric Substernal	Associated with smoking, alcohol, stress, renal failure, COPD
Biliary	Hours	Visceral Waxes and wanes Colicky	Spontaneous Food ingestion	Time Analgesia Anticholinergics Nasogastric suction	Epigastric Right upper quadrant	Associated with obesity, female gender, North American Indian race, cirrhosis, cholesterol, cystic fibrosis, estrogens, ileal resection, clofibrate
Pericarditis	Variable	Pleuritic	Swallowing Deep breath Supine position	Sitting forward	Left chest Radiates to shoulder	Etiology is viral, tuberculosis, recent MI, uremia, sarcoid, mononucleosis, systemic lupus erythematosus, rheumatoid arthritis, drugs, irradiation Physical exam reveals rub, fever
Esophageal rupture	Persistent	Pleuritic	Vomiting Foreign body Trauma Instrumentation	Analgesics	Left side Substernal	Dyspnea, shock, fever
Pancreatitis	Persistent	Visceral Boring	Supine position Alcohol Vomiting	Sitting forward Analgesics NPO Nasogastric suction	Epigastric Periumbilical Radiates to back	Associated with alcohol abuse, biliary disease, viral illness, hyperlipidemia, spider bite, connective tissue disease
Pulmonary embolism		Pleuritic Anginal			Substernal	Associated with immobilization, cancer, prior pulmonary embolism, prior deep venous thrombosis, oral contraceptives, postpartum
Aortic dissection	Persistent	Severe Tearing Ripping Migratory Steady Maximal at onset			Substernal Radiates to back	Associated with Marfan's, Ehlers-Danlos hypertension, pregnancy, Turner's, coarctation

Table 51-2. (continued)

Diagnosis	Duration	Quality	Provocation	Relief	Location	Comments
Cervical disc disease	Variable	Superficial	Head and neck movement	Time Analgesics Traction	Arm Neck Anterior chest Radiates to arm	No improvement with rest Associated paresthesia
Hyperventila-tion	2 min to days Accentuating brief stabs	Dull ache	Emotion Tachypnea	Stimulus removal Variable response to many interventions	Substernal Cardiac apex	Associated with facial paresthe-sias, headache, lightheaded-ness, nervousness, weakness, sighing, fatigue Reproduced by voluntary hyperventilation
Musculoskel-etal disorder	Variable Seconds to days	Superficial Sharp Stabbing Well-localized	Movement Palpation Deep breath Sneeze Cough Lifting	Time Analgesia	Multiple	Recent unaccustomed or exces-sive exertion
Aortic stenosis	2–15 min	Anginal	Exertion	Rest Nitrates	Substernal	Associated with dyspnea, syn-cope, murmur
IHSS	2–15 min					Associated with dyspnea, syn-cope, fatigue, sudden death, family history

Cardiac Causes of Nonischemic Chest Pain

ABNORMAL CARDIAC SENSITIVITY. Cannon et al. reported on a group of patients with a low threshold for cardiac pain perception [73]. These investigators found right ventricle catheter manipulation, right atrium pacing, and intracoronary contrast injection to be perceived as chest pain significantly more frequently in patients with chest pain syndromes and normal coronaries than in those with angiographically significant coronary disease (29 of 36, or 81%, vs. 2 of 33, or 6%, respectively; p<0.001). Similar results have been found by other investigators [74]. These studies suggest that cardiac hypersensitivity may be either causal or contributory in some chest pain syndromes. Alternatively, cardiac hypersensitivity may be a marker of generalized visceral hypersensitivity.

MITRAL VALVE PROLAPSE. A chest pain syndrome has been described in patients with mitral valve prolapse [75–79]. It is sometimes indistinguishable from angina pectoris but usually has atypical features [80,81,82]. It may be substernal but is more typically located in the left anterior precordium. It may be precipitated by exertion but not always in a reproducible manner. Rest pain is not uncommon. The duration is variable, lasting from seconds to hours. The location, response to nitrates, and pattern of radiation may vary from one episode to the next. Palpitations are frequently reported. Light-headedness, syncope, chronic fatigue, anxiety, depression, and hyperventilation may be reported [80,83,84].

The pathophysiology of chest pain among patients with mitral valve prolapse is unknown but may be due to tension on the chordae tendineae and papillary muscle apparatus. Conversely, the discomfort may be esophageal in origin [85,86].

Auscultation of a typical midsystolic click and late systolic murmur is helpful, but these findings may be evanescent. Repeat examination, including auscultation in the standing, squatting, and supine positions, may be required. There may be associated musculoskeletal abnormalities, such as pectus excavatum, Marfan's syndrome, and a straight back.

The ECG may display S–T depression, T wave flattening, or T wave inversion. These changes may vary with heart rate and treatment with beta-adrenergic blockers [82,87].

ACUTE PERICARDITIS. The chest pain associated with pericarditis is most commonly pleuritic, sharp, stabbing, left-sided, and referred to the trapezius ridge and neck if the diaphragmatic surface is involved [88]. It can, at times, be relieved by sitting forward and aggravated by turning in bed, swallowing, coughing, and twisting. The pain often lasts for hours and is changed little by exertion. However, it can sometimes closely mimic angina, particularly when it occurs in the post-MI setting.

Patients with pericarditis are often younger and have fewer risk factors for atherosclerosis than those with myocardial ischemia. Pericarditis has many underlying causes, including MI (Dressler's syndrome), aortic dissection, viral syndrome, uremia, tuberculosis, and collagen vascular disease.

The auscultation of a three-component pericardial friction rub is pathognomonic. It should be sought with the patient in multiple positions and at various times.

The ECG may be confusing, but careful examination may reveal typical evolution of diffuse, concave upward S–T elevation, P–R segment depression, and T wave inversion [89]. Echocardiography may be helpful if a pericardial effusion is seen. Other laboratory evaluations should include CPK, ANA, PPD, BUN, creatinine, and erythrocyte sedimentation rate. Elevation of the CPK-MB and ECG abnormalities may occasionally lead to an erroneous diagnosis of MI.

Pulmonary Causes of Chest Pain

PULMONARY HYPERTENSION. The discomfort experienced among patients with pulmonary hypertension may be identical to that described above for typical angina [90,91]. The pain may be caused by right ventricular ischemia or dilation of the pulmonary arteries. Underlying causes include massive pulmonary embolism, primary pulmonary hypertension, severe chronic obstructive lung disease, mitral stenosis, and severe

Table 51-3. Nonatherosclerotic Epicardial Coronary Artery Diseases

Arteritis
  Syphilis
  Tuberculosis
  Takayasu's
  Giant cell
  Kawasaki's
  Polyarteritis nodosa
Collagen vascular
  Rheumatoid arthritis
  Systemic lupus erythematosus
  Systemic sclerosis
Coronary mural thickening
  Mucopolysaccharidosis (Hunter's)
  Homocysteinuria
  Fabry's disease
  Amyloidosis
  Juvenile intimal sclerosis
  Pseudoxanthoma elasticum
External compression
  Tumor
  Amyloidosis
  Sinus of Valsalva aneurysm
Coronary aneurysms
  Congenital
  Atherosclerotic
  Traumatic
Coronary embolism
  Cardiomyopathy
  Mitral stenosis
  Mural thrombosis (left ventricular)
  Iatrogenic
  Infectious endocarditis
  Marantic endocarditis
  Thromboembolism
  Fibromyxoma of aortic valve
  Atrial myxoma
Coronary spasm
  Prinzmetal's
  Cocaine
  Industrial nitroglycerin withdrawal
Coronary ostial occlusion
  Takayasu's
  Syphilis
  Aortic Starr-Edwards prosthetic valve
  Congenital supravalvular aortic stenosis
Coronary artery anomalies
  Coronary AV fistula
  Anomalous left coronary from the pulmonary trunk
Trauma
  Coronary artery laceration
  Coronary artery thrombosis
  Myocardial contusion
  Coronary artery dissection
  Electrical, thermal, or radiation trauma
Arterial dissection
  Aortic dissection
  Spontaneous coronary dissection

long-standing left ventricular failure. There is usually little diagnostic confusion, since accompanying history, physical findings, ECG, chest x-ray, and other tests are diagnostic. Similarly, severe pulmonic stenosis can cause anginal chest pain, presumably due to right ventricular subendocardial ischemia.

PLEURA. Inflammation or distention of the pleura causes chest pain that is worsened by deep inspiration and coughing. Movement and palpation have little effect. Physical examination may reveal fever, pleural rub, pleural effusion, and pulmonary consolidation. Pleural inflammation can have many causes (see Chap. 65).

PNEUMONIA. When infectious pneumonia extends from the lung parenchyma to the pleural surface, pleuritic pain may occur. Usually, the accompanying fever, cough, dyspnea, sputum production, elevated white blood cell count, and radiographic findings eliminate diagnostic confusion. Bronchospasm and cough-induced chest trauma may also cause chest pain.

PLEURODYNIA. A self-limited disease associated with Coxsackie B infection, pleurodynia causes pleuritic chest pain. Usually, there is a viral prodrome. This may occur in either an epidemic or cluster setting.

PNEUMOTHORAX. Spontaneous pneumothorax with attendant lung collapse stretches the pleura, causing pleuritic chest pain and dyspnea. There may be underlying emphysema, a history of prior pneumothorax, or connective tissue abnormality, such as Marfan's syndrome or Ehlers-Danlos syndrome. Hyperresonance and decreased breath sounds are found on physical examination. If there is a tension pneumothorax, there may be tracheal deviation, hypotension, and shock. The chest radiograph is usually diagnostic.

PULMONARY EMBOLISM. Chest pain is a common presenting complaint among patients with pulmonary embolism [92]. Pulmonary emboli may cause pleuritic, localized pain or deep, vague, visceral, substernal discomfort. Pleuritic pain is associated with smaller emboli, which cause pulmonary infarction and atelectasis [93]. Substernal pain is more common with massive pulmonary emboli producing right ventricular strain, hypotension, and shock. Frequently, there is marked dyspnea, tachypnea, and tachycardia [93]. There may be hemoptysis, a pleural rub, a pleural effusion, low-grade fever, and cyanosis [92]. Predispositions to deep venous thrombosis and pulmonary embolism include recent surgery, immobilization, pregnancy, prior deep venous thrombosis or pulmonary embolism, oral contraceptive use, congenital procoagulant states, and congestive heart failure (see Chap. 60).

Vascular Causes of Chest Pain

AORTIC DISSECTION. Aortic dissection may be misdiagnosed as myocardial ischemia or infarction. In addition, MI is a possible complication of aortic dissection from proximal extension involving the coronary ostia. Dissection of the aorta is suggested by severe persistent pain radiating to the back or interscapular or lumbar regions. It is often described as sudden, maximal at onset, tearing, ripping, boring, and migratory. There may be associated stroke, transient ischemic attacks, paralysis, ischemic limbs, gastrointestinal ischemia, and/or acute renal failure.

Especially in younger patients, aortic dissection is associated with Marfan's syndrome, Ehlers-Danlos syndrome, and other connective tissue abnormalities causing aortic medial degeneration [94]. In older patients hypertension is nearly always present. Aortic dissection is also associated with blunt chest trauma, pregnancy, coarctation of the aorta, and Turner's syndrome [88].

Emphasis during the physical examination should be on the equality of distal pulses and blood pressure, the presence of aortic insufficiency, markers of underlying abnormalities, and a full neurologic examination. Signs of tamponade, such as elevated jugular venous pressure, pulsus paradoxus, and muffled heart sounds, should be sought.

A chest radiograph may show a widened mediastinum, pleural effusion, and enlarged cardiac silhouette.

The ECG may show acute ischemic changes, especially if proximal extension of the dissection compromises coronary blood flow. The diagnostic algorithm for aortic dissection was revised recently by the advent of transesophageal echocardiography (TEE) [95], computed tomography (CT) [96], and magnetic resonance imaging (MRI) [97,98]. In a stable patient, MRI probably offers the advantage of superior specificity. However, TEE is also very sensitive and specific as well as widely available, portable, and safe. It is therefore often the diagnostic test of choice, especially in hemodynamically unstable patients [99].

A complete blood cell count may reveal a decreased hematocrit. The CPK may be elevated in up to 64 percent of patients with aortic dissection but is typically >95 percent MM isoenzyme [100] (see Chap. 36).

AORTIC ANEURYSM. Expansion of an aortic aneurysm may cause chest pain by eroding or impinging on nearby structures. Erosion of vertebral bodies may cause boring, aching, throbbing, or localized pain. Common causes of aortic aneurysms include atherosclerosis, syphilis, annuloaortic ectasia, and aortic valve disease. Perforation of an aortic aneurysm may also simulate ischemic chest pain.

A dilated aortic contour or a pleural effusion on a standard chest radiograph may prompt further confirmatory tests, including TEE, CT scan, MRI, ultrasound, or angiography.

Musculoskeletal Causes of Chest Pain

CHEST WALL PAIN. Musculoskeletal thoracic pain is generally of short duration (< 1 minute) but can last for days. It may be precipitated by abrupt movement, turning of the head or thorax, or direct palpation. Unlike ischemic pain, which occurs with exercise, musculoskeletal pain often occurs after exercise and subsides over a longer period (hours to days). However, musculoskeletal pain on rare occasion can be exertional and relieved by nitroglycerin [101,102].

Costochondritis is a common cause of chest discomfort in patients with a fear of heart disease. The discomfort is usually sharp and well localized to the costochondral or costosternal junctions, at times is pleuritic, and may be associated with coughing or movement. There may be a history of recent strenuous or unaccustomed physical activity. Relief can be obtained with local heat, nonsteroidal antiinflammatory agents, injection of Xylocaine or steroids, and, most important, reassurance.

Tietze's syndrome, a rare cause of chest pain, is associated with swelling and erythema of the costochondral and costosternal junctions [80,103–106].

Rib fracture causes a well-localized tenderness usually preceded by a history of trauma, malignancy, or severe osteoporosis. Radiography is diagnostic.

Cervical and upper thoracic osteoarthritis and herniated discs may cause chest pain similar to angina pectoris [103,107]. Distinguishing characteristics of radicular pain include worsening with bending and body movement, accompanying neurologic signs and symptoms (e.g., numbness, weakness, stiffness, vertigo, tingling, paresthesias), radiation to the radial aspect of the arm or fingers, pain with coughing and sneezing, and pain with prolonged bed rest [102,107,108]. The discomfort may be traced to a specific initiating event and be elicited by rotating the head, bending the neck, hyperextending the upper spine, and applying pressure to the top of the head. There may be tenderness to deep palpation of the spine [108]. Relief is obtained with cervical traction, nonsteroidals, and analgesics. Radiography, MRI, and myelography are useful adjunctive tests.

Thoracic outlet syndrome, including anterior scalene muscle and cervical rib syndromes [109], may be confused with ischemic chest pain. Compression of the brachial plexus may cause motor and sensory deficits in the arm in an ulnar distribution. Obliteration of the radial pulse with the chin elevated and rotated toward the affected side (Adson's maneuver) is an important clinical finding. Chest radiography reveals an underlying cervical rib.

Chest pain may also occur with ankylosing spondylitis, rheumatoid arthritis, psoriatic arthritis, infectious arthritis, xiphoidalgia, precordial catch syndrome, metastatic cancer, chest trauma, osteochondroma, osteosarcoma, multiple myeloma, slipping rib syndrome, and fibromyalgia.

Precordial catch (Texidor's twinge) is believed to result from muscle spasm and causes acute sharp anterior chest pain in young adults that is worse with breathing and relieved by taking a very deep breath or stretching [103,110].

After open heart surgery patients may complain of chest discomfort. In addition to concerns about adequate revascularization and technical difficulties, possibilities to consider include nerve entrapment [111], postpericardiotomy syndrome, mediastinitis, costochondritis, and superficial wound infections.

HERPES ZOSTER. Herpes zoster (shingles) can affect the anterior chest and mimic angina pectoris. However, the pain is dermatomal and does not cross the midline. Associated neurologic complaints include hyperesthesia, hypoesthesia, and dysesthesia. In addition, the pain is not relieved by nitrates or rest. The ultimate appearance of the pathognomonic vesicular rash is diagnostic, but discomfort may precede the rash by several days. In the elderly, a chronic syndrome of postherpetic neuralgia may occur.

Psychiatric Causes of Chest Pain

Since the Civil War, chest pain has been recognized as a feature of anxiety (Dacosta syndrome, soldier's heart, neurocirculatory asthenia) [112,113]. The discomfort is more commonly located in the inframammary region, near the cardiac apex. It is variably described as dull and aching or sharp and stabbing. It can last seconds to hours. It is not typically exertional but is related more often to emotional strain. Associated symptoms of numbness, tingling, dizziness, perioral numbness, lightheadedness, inability to get a full breath, generalized weakness, headache, palpitations, depression, and fatigue are helpful clinical signs. Reproduction of the chest discomfort with voluntary hyperventilation may be diagnostic. The discomfort is seldom resolved without analgesics. Patients often have few risk factors for coronary atherosclerosis.

Panic attacks, hyperventilation, and depression often include chest discomfort as one of many symptoms. Panic disorders affect 1 to 2 percent of the total population [114]. Up to 60 percent of panic disorder patients complain of chest pain [115].

In studies of noncardiac chest pain, 10 to 43 percent of patients fit the criteria for panic attacks [116–119]. Panic attacks are frequently associated with substance abuse, agoraphobia, depression, and anxiety. Lactate infusion and carbon dioxide inhalation challenge tests are sensitive but not specific for evaluating patients with panic disorders [120]. Panic disorders can be succesfully treated with polycyclic antidepressant medications or benzodiazepines.

Patients with noncardiac chest pain have been found to exhibit somatization, anxiety, and hypochondriacal traits [61,121–124]. Psychiatric disorders may be associated with esophageal causes of chest pain [119,122,125].

Gastrointestinal Causes of Chest Pain

ESOPHAGUS. Esophageal chest pain is described as a visceral discomfort and may be misdiagnosed as angina pectoris. Among patients with chest pain and angiographically normal-appearing coronary arteries, 20 to 60 percent have esophageal abnormalities [125–134].

Common descriptors of esophageal pain include heartburn, acid, warmth, fullness, pressure, and gnawing. The symptoms may be provoked by ingestion of food, especially at the extremes of temperature, of large quantity, or immediatly before recumbency. Esophageal pain is often substernal but may extend to the right or left chest and radiate to the back. It is frequently associated with other gastrointestinal complaints, such as odynophagia, dysphagia, regurgitation, bloating, and dyspepsia [125,126,132,134,135,136]. Esophageal pain can last for hours, may interrupt sleep, and can be relieved with antacids [134]. It can be precipitated by swallowing, exercise, or emotion [137,138] and relieved by rest and nitroglycerin [80,128,139,140]. The presenting history alone may not differentiate esophageal pain from cardiac pain.

GASTROESOPHAGEAL REFLUX. Recent studies with ambulatory monitoring suggest that the most common esophageal cause of chest pain is gastroesophageal reflux. Up to 10 percent of patients with gastroesophageal reflux have chest pain as their only symptom [141]. Overall, gastroesophageal reflux is found in 30 to 50 percent of patients with noncardiac chest pain [142,143].

ESOPHAGEAL MOTILITY DISORDERS. Motility disorders have long been recognized as a cause of chest pain. They include "nutcracker" esophagus (high-amplitude, peristaltic contractions of long duration), diffuse esophageal spasm (frequent simultaneous contractions in the distal esophagus) [144], nonspecific abnormalities, lower esophageal sphincter hypertension [145], and achalasia [126,146].

The specific mechanisms of esophageal pain are poorly understood but are thought to be mediated by chemo- and mechanicoreceptors. Some believe that altered motility causes esophageal ishemia [126,147]. However, ischemic necrosis has not been reported [146].

The diagnostic examinations available for evaluating patients with esophageal disorders include barium swallow, esophagogastroduodenoscopy, resting manometry, ambulatory pH monitoring [148], and ambulatory manometry. Provocative maneuvers include the Bernstein acid infusion test [149], challenges with edrophonium, ergonovine, bethanechol, pentagastrin, balloon distention, and ingestion of hot or cold liquids.

Erosive esophagitis, hiatal hernia, and gastroesophageal reflux can be diagnosed with barium swallow and endoscopy [150,151]. However, only 25 percent of patients with "acid-related" chest pain can be diagnosed with these techniques.

The Bernstein acid infusion test is performed through a nasogastric tube positioned midway in the esophagus and alternately infusing 0.1N HCl and normal saline at 6 to 8 ml per minute. For a positive test, acid, not saline, must reproduce the patient's pain. The prevalence of a positive test varies from 6.7 to 100 percent, depending on patient selection [130,132,151–154]. Using ambulatory pH monitoring as a standard, acid infusion testing is specific (90%) but not sensitive for acid-related chest pain.

Ambulatory pH monitoring involves a 2-mm probe placed nasally and positioned 5 cm above the lower esophageal sphincter. The probe is attached to a recorder on the patient's waist. A diary of symptoms is recorded. A symptom index is then tabulated, which is the percentage of perceived chest pain episodes correlated with acid reflux. Some investigators also account for the number of reflux episodes in calculating a symptom index [155]. Ambulatory pH monitoring may be more sensitive and specific than the acid infusion test [150]. The incidence of chest pain associated with acid reflux during ambulatory monitoring is 14 to 50 percent among patients with noncardiac chest pain [126,136,153,156,157].

Baseline manometry may, at times, uncover an esophageal cause of chest pain. Unfortunately, patients usually do not have their typical chest pain during baseline manometry. An observed motility disorder could be merely coincident with a true abnormality. The detection of a motility disorder at the time of clinical chest pain or a provocative test reproducing the identical pain is generally required as proof of an esophageal etiology [148,155,156,158,159]. The availability of ambulatory 24-hour manometry may improve diagnostic certainty. Currently there is no gold standard for the diagnosis of esophageal chest pain.

Due to higher sensitivity and specificity and safety, the preferred provocative test for motility disorders is edrophonium (Tensilon) (80 µg/kg or 10 mg) [160–163]. Ergonovine is as sensitive but may be less specific than edrophonium due to the possible provocation of coronary spasm [161]. Bethanechol, too, has troubling side effects [164]. Recently, balloon distention (<8 cc) of the esophagus has been used to diagnose esophageal chest pain [165]. Relief of chest pain with antacid/analgesic mixtures must not be relied on for securing a diagnosis.

In a retrospective review of 910 patients referred for evaluation of noncardiac chest pain, Katz et al. [132] reported a 28 percent (225 of 910) incidence of abnormal baseline manometry. Of the motility disorders observed, "nutcracker" esophagus was detected in 40 percent (123 of 255), nonspecific motility disorders in 36 percent, diffuse esophageal spasm in 10 percent, and achalasia in only 2 percent. Provocation with acid infusion reproduced chest pain in 6.7 percent (61 of 910), while provocation with edrophonium reproduced chest pain in 23 percent (210 of 910). Overall, a definite esophageal cause of chest pain was diagnosed in 27 percent (243 of 910) of patients and a probable cause in another 21 percent (192 of 910). In another study, the combination of edrophonium and acid infusion testing reproduced chest pain in 35 percent of patients with chest pain and normal coronary arteries [161].

The causative association of esophageal abnormalities and chest discomfort is often poor. Patients with severe reflux or motility disorders may not have pain [166]. Conversely, pain may be clearly associated with reflux or a motility disorder during one episode but not during another [155,167]. Unfortunately, alleviation of motility disorders may not alleviate chest discomfort [168].

There are some important interactions of angina pectoris and pain of esophageal origin. Since the prevalence of both syndromes increases with age, the two may coexist. Esophageal disease has been found in up to 50 percent of patients with coronary disease [146,169] Reflux may lower the ischemic threshold [140] or even precipitate angina [170]. Therapy for angina (nitrates, calcium channel blockers, and beta-blockers) may decrease the lower esophageal sphincter pressure and hence worsen reflux. Furthermore, exercise can trigger gastroesophageal reflux, leading to chest pain [157]. Patients who clearly understand their chest discomfort to be esophageal in origin are less limited by their continued pain and less likely to visit a doctor for chest pain [67].

Other esophageal causes of chest pain include esophageal rupture (Boerhaave's syndrome), esophageal tear (Mallory-Weiss syndrome), infectious esophagitis (e.g., herpes, *Candida*), and irradiation-induced esophagitis.

Biliary tract disease, including sphincter of Oddi spasm, cholelithiasis, and cholecystitis, can mimic ischemic chest pain. The discomfort with these diseases may present substernally and respond to nitroglycerin. Furthermore, ECG changes have been reported with biliary tract disorders.

Pancreatitis may mimic myocardial ischemia or infarction. A history of alcohol abuse or biliary tract disease may be elicited. The discomfort associated with pancreatitis is often transmitted to the back.

Peptic ulcer disease may be confused with myocardial ischemic syndromes. The relationship between symptoms and either food intake or relief with antacids is an important clinical feature.

Other Causes of Chest Pain

MYOCARDITIS. The clinical spectrum of viral myocarditis ranges from asymptomatic ECG abnormalities to fulminant heart failure, cardiogenic shock, and death. Dec et al. reported on a subset of young patients with chest pain and ECG findings suggestive of MI [171,172]. Thirty-four patients with clinical signs and symptoms of acute MI but normal coronary angiograms underwent endomyocardial biopsy. Eleven were found to have evidence of myocarditis. A preceding viral illness was discernible in 6 of 11 (54%) patients [172].

COCAINE. Cocaine use has been associated with MI [173–180]. Cocaine increases myocardial oxygen demand and decreases coronary artery blood flow. In a study of 101 cocaine abusers presenting to the Hennipen County Medical Center [174], chest pain was frequently suggestive of ischemia (pressure with radiation to the arms), dyspnea was common, and the onset of pain occurred during or up to 1 hour after use. Electrocardiographic abnormalities were common (only 21% interpreted as normal). The muscle creatine kinase level was often elevated with normal MB fraction. Chest pain occurred with inhalation, smoking, or intravenous routes of administration [173,174]. Chest pain was reported in some patients who used less than 1 gm of cocaine. Measurement of urinary cocaine metabolites may provide useful information.

Diagnostic Algorithm for Evaluation of Chest Pain

This overview of noncardiac chest pain should make it clear that multiple organ systems can be the source of chest pain and frequently there is overlap in the clinical presentation of serious acute and more benign disorders. The possibility of life-threatening illness must be the initial concern when evaluating a patient with chest pain. Based on the initial clinical impression and aided by the ECG, screening blood tests, and chest radiograph one can make a reasonable estimate of the probability of serious disorders, including MI, arrhythmias, aortic dissection, pulmonary embolism, perforating peptic ulcer, and pneumothorax. The immediate use of thrombolysis, emergent cardiac catheterization and angioplasty, TEE, aortography, pulmonary angiography, chest tube insertion, and emergency surgery is guided by the clinician's initial assessment.

Most patients admitted to the ICU with chest pain, however, do not have an immediately life-threatening illness. Once MI and other life-threatening entities have been excluded, further evaluation hinges on the clinical estimate of diagnostic probability. Modern cardiology includes an impressive armamentarium of invasive and noninvasive diagnostic tests to identify and quantitate cardiac diseases. One must proceed logically through the evaluation of each patient, integrating each test result with the available clinical data. A careful and complete history and physical examination may either eliminate or minimize unnecessary or expensive procedures.

An in-depth review of the possible diagnostic evaluations and decision analyses is beyond the scope of this chapter. Decisions regarding the use of exercise and pharmacologic stress testing, radionuclide imaging, echocardiography, esophageal manometry, provocative esophageal testing, ambulatory pH monitoring, ambulatory manometry, and cardiac catheterization must be individualized for each patient. Which tests and in which order they are performed depends on the pretest likelihood of a given disease or outcome.

References

1. Hedges JR, Rouan GW, Toltzis R, et al: Use of cardiac enzymes identifies patients with acute myocardial infarction otherwise unrecognized in the emergency department. *Ann Emerg Med* 16:248, 1987.
2. Lee TH, Rouan GW, Weisberg MC, et al: Clinical characteristics and natural history of patients with acute myocardial infarcton sent home from the emergency room. *Am J Cardiol* 60:219, 1987.
3. Templeton WA, McCallion LA, McKinney HK, et al: Chest pain in the accident and emergency department: Is chest radiography worthwhile? *Arch Emerg Med* 8:91, 1991.
4. Paraskos JA: Approach to the patient with chest pain, in Rippe JM, Irwin RS, Alpert JS, Fink MP (eds): *Intensive Care Medicine*. Boston, Little, Brown, 1991, pp. 359–364.
5. Pozen MW, D'Agostino RB, Mitchell JB, et al: The usefulness of a predictive instrument to reduce inappropriate admissions to the coronary care unit. *Ann Intern Med* 92:238, 1980.
6. Adgey AAJ, Geddes JS, Webb SW, et al: Acute phase of myocardial infarction. *Lancet* 1:501, 1971.
7. Schroeder JS, Lamb IH, Harrison DC: Patients admitted to the coronary care unit for chest pain: High-risk subgroup for subsequent cardiovascular death. *Am J Cardiol* 39:829, 1974.
8. Lopes MG, Spivack AP, Harrison DC: Prognosis in coronary care unit noninfarction cases. *JAMA* 228:1558, 1974.
9. Krauss KR, Hutter AM, DeSanctis RW: Acute coronary insufficiency: Course and follow-up. *Arch Intern Med* 129:808, 1972.

10. Gazes PC, Mobley EM Jr, Faris HM, et al: Preinfarctional (unstable) angina: A prospective study—ten years follow-up. *Circulation* 48:331, 1973.

11. Bloom B, Peterson O: End results, cost, and productivity of coronary care units. *N Engl J Med* 288:77, 1973.

12. Bennett JR, Atkinson M: The differentiation between esophageal and cardiac pain. *Lancet* 2:1123, 1966.

13. Alacalay M, Bontous D: Les syndrome douloureux de les paroi thoracique apres infarctus du myocarde et apre cherugie cardiovasculaire. *Coeur Med Int* 13:99, 1974.

14. Fuchs R, Scheidt S: Improved criteria for admission to cardiac care units. *JAMA* 246:2037, 1981.

15. Schor S, Behar S, Modan B, et al: Disposition of presumed coronary patients from an emergency room: A followup study. *JAMA* 236:941, 1976.

16. Sanders CA: The coronary care unit: Necessity or luxury? *N Engl J Med* 288:101, 1973.

17. Lee TH, Cook F, Weisburg MC, et al: Acute chest pain in the emergency room: Identification and examination of low-risk patients. *Arch Intern Med* 145:65, 1985.

18. Lown B, Fakhro AM, Hood WB Jr, et al: The coronary care unit: new perspectives and directions. *JAMA* 199:188, 1967.

19. Hofvendahl S: Influence of treatment in a coronary care unit on prognosis in acute myocardial infarction: A controlled sudy. *Acta Med Scand* 519(suppl):9, 1971.

20. Christiansen I, Iversen K, Skouby AP: Benefits obtained by introduction of a coronary care unit: A comparative study. *Acta Med Scand* 189:285, 1971.

21. Behar S, Schor S, Kariv I, et al: Evaluation of the electrocardiogram in emergency room as a decision making tool. *Chest* 71:486, 1977.

22. McGuinness JB, Begg TB, Semple T: First electrocardiogram in recent myocardial infarction. *Br Med J* 2:449, 1976.

23. Eisenberg JM, Horowitz LN, Busch R, et al: Diagnosis of acute myocardial infarction in the emergency room: Prospective assessment of clinical decision making and the usefulness of immediate cardiac enzyme determination. *J Community Health* 4:190, 1979.

24. Goldman L, Weinberg M, Weisberg MC, et al: A computer derived protocol to aid in the diagnosis of emergency room patients with acute chest pain. *N Engl J Med* 307:588, 1982.

25. Gruppo Italiano Per Lo Studio Della Streptochinase Nell 'Infarto Miocadico (GISSI): Long term effects of intravenous thrombolysis in acute myocardial infarction: Final report of the GISSI study. *Lancet* 2:871, 1987.

26. Simoons ML, Serruys PW, van den Brand M, et al: Early thrombolysis in acute myocardial infarction: Limitation of infarct size and improved survival. *J Am Coll Cardiol* 7:717, 1986.

27. Kennedy JW, Martin GV, Davis KB, et al: The western Washington intravenous streptokinase in acute myocardial infarction randomized trial. *Circulation* 77:345, 1988.

28. ISIS2 (Second International Study of Infarct Survival) Collaborative Group: Randomized trial of intravenous streptokinase, oral aspirin, both or neither among 17 187 cases of suspected acute myocardial infarction: ISIS-2. *Lancet* 2:349, 1988.

29. Anderson JL, Rothbard RL, Hackworthy RA, et al: Multicenter reperfusion trial of intravenous anisoylated plasminogen activator complex (APSAC) in acute myocardial infarction: Controlled comparison with intracoronary streptokinase. *J Am Coll Cardiol* 11:1153, 1988.

30. The I.S.A.M. Study Group: A prospective trial of intravenous streptokinase in acute myocardial infarction (I.S.A.M.): Mortality, morbidity, and infarct size at 21 days. *N Engl J Med* 314:1465, 1986.

31. The GUSTO Investigators: An international randomized trial comparing four thrombolytic strategies for acute myocardial infarction. *N Engl J Med* 329:673, 1993.

32. Pipberger HV, Klingeman JD, Cosma J: Computer evaluation of statistical properties of clinical information in the differential diagnosis of chest pain. *Methods Inf Med* 7:79, 1968.

33. Lubsen J, Pool J, van der Does E: A practical device for the application of a diagnostic or prognostic function. *Methods Inf Med* 17:127, 1978.

34. Patrick EA, Margolin G, Sanghiv V: Pattern recognition applied to early diagnosis of heart attacks. Proceedings of the International Medical Information Processing Conference, Toronto, 1977.

35. Goldman L, Cook EF, Brand DA, et al: A computer protocol to predict myocardial infarction in emergency department patients with chest pain. *N Engl J Med* 318:797, 1988.

36. Mulley AG, Thibault GE, Hughes RA, et al: The course of patients with suspected myocardial infarction: The identification of low risk patients for early transfer from intensive care. *N Engl J Med* 302:943, 1980.

37. Weingarten S, Ermann B, Bolus R, et al: Early "step down" transfer of low-risk patients with chest pain: A controlled interventional trial. *Ann Intern Med* 113:283, 1990.

38. Lee TH, Rouan GW, Weisberg MC, et al: Sensitivity of routine clinical criteria for diagnosing myocardial infarction within 24 hours of hospitalization. *Ann Intern Med* 106:181, 1987.

39. Lee TH, Juarez G, Cook EF, et al: Ruling out acute myocardial infarction: A prospective multicenter validation of a 12–hour strategy for patients at low risk. *N Engl J Med* 324:1239, 1991.

40. Weingarten S, Agocs L, Tankel N, et al: Reducing length of stay for patients hospitalized with chest pain using medical practice guidelines and opinion leaders. *Am J Cardiol* 71:259, 1993.

41. Tierney WM, Fitzgerald J, McHenry R: Physicians' estimates of the probablility of myocardial infarction in emergency room patients with chest pain. *Med Decis Making* 6:12, 1986.

42. Diamond GA, Forrester JS: Analysis of probability as an aid in the clinical diagnosis of coronary artery disiease. *N Engl J Med* 300:1350, 1979.

43. Hedges J, Kobernick MS: Detection of myocardial ischemia/infarction in the emergency department patient with chest discomfort. *Emerg Med Clin North Am* 6:317, 1988.

44. McCarthy BD, Wong JB, Selker HP: Detecting acute cardiac ischemia in the emergency department: A review of the literature. *J Gen Intern Med* 5:365, 1990.

45. Zarling EJ, Sexton H, Milnor P: Failure to diagnose acute myocardial infarction: The clinicopathologic experience at a large community hospital. *JAMA* 250:1177, 1983.

46. Madias JE, Gorlin R: The myth of acute "mild" myocardial infarction. *Ann Intern Med* 86:347, 1977.

47. Gunraj DR, Rajapakse DA: Daily ECG confirmation in acute myocardial infarction. *Practitioner* 213:361, 1974.

48. Peels CH, Visser CA, Funke Kupper AJ, et al: Usefulness of two-dimensional echocardiography for immediate detection of myocardial ischemia in the emergency room. *Am J Cardiol* 65:687, 1990.

49. Solomon CG, Lee TH, Cook EF, et al: Comparison of clinical presentation of acute myocardial infarction in patients older than 65 years of age to younger patients: The multicenter chest pain study experience. *Am J Cardiol* 63:772, 1989.

50. Kannel WB, Abbott RD: Incidence and prognosis of unrecognized myocardial infarction: An update from the Framingham Study. *N Engl J Med* 311:1144, 1984.

51. White JC, Sweet WH: Pain in disease of the thoracic viscera, in White JC, Sweet WH (eds): *Pain and the Neurosurgeon.* Springfield, IL, Charles C Thomas, 1969, pp 525–559.

52. Christie LG, Conti CR: Systematic approach to evaluation of angina-like chest pain: Pathophysiology and clinical testing with emphasis on objective documentation of myocardial ischemia. *Am Heart J* 102:897, 1981.

53. Lown B, Levine SA: The carotid sinus: Clinical value of its stimulation. *Circulation* 23:766, 1961.

54. Kapoor AS, Dang NS: Reliance on physical signs in acute myocardial infarction and its complications. *Heart Lung* 7:1020, 1978.

55. Proudfit WL, Shirey EK, Sones FM: Selective cine coronary arteriography: Correlation with clinical findings in 1000 patients. *Circulation* 33:901, 1966.

56. CASS Principal Investigators: Coronary Artery Surgery Study (CASS): A randomized trial of coronary artery bypass surgery. *Circulation* 68:939, 1983.

57. Mahrer PR, Eshoo N: Outpatient cardiac catheterization and coronary angiography. *Cathet Cardiovasc Diagn* 7:355, 1981.

58. Phibbs B, Fleming T, Ewy GA, et al: Frequency of normal coronary arteriograms in three academic medical centers and one community hospital. *Am J Cardiol* 62:472, 1988.

59. Kemp HG, Vokonas PS, Cohn PF, et al: The anginal syndrome associated with normal coronary arteriograms: Report of six years experience. *Am J Med* 54:735, 1973.

60. Bemiller CR, Pepine CJ, Rogers AK: Long term observations in

patients with angina and normal coronary arteriograms. *Circulation* 47:36, 1973.

61. Wielgosz AT, Fletcher RH, McCants CB, et al: Unimproved chest pain in patients with minimal or no coronary disease: A behavioral phenomenon. *Am Heart J* 108:67, 1984.

62. Papanicolaou MN, Califf RM, Hlatky MA, et al: Prognostic implications of angiographically normal and insignificantly narrowed coronary arteries. *Am J Cardiol* 58:1181, 1986.

63. Proudfit Wl, Bruschke AVG, Sones FM: Clinical course of patients with normal or slightly or moderately abnormal coronary arteriograms: 10-year follow-up of 521 patients. *Circulation* 62:712, 1980.

64. Humphries JO, Kuller L, Ross RS, et al: Natural history of ischemic heart disease in relation to arteriographic findings: A 12-year study of 224 patients. *Circulation* 49:489, 1974.

65. Marchandise B, Bourassa MG, Chartman BR, et al: Angiographic evaluation of the natural history of normal coronary arteries and mild coronary atherosclerosis. *Am J Cardiol* 41:216, 1978.

66. Day LJ, Sowton E: Clinical features and follow-up of patients with angina and normal coronary arteries. *Lancet* 2:334, 1976.

67. Faxon DP, McCabe CH, Kreigel DE, Ryan TJ: Therapeutic and economic value of a normal coronary angiogram. *Am J Med* 73:500, 1982.

68. Lavey EB, Winkle RA: Continuing disability of patients with chest pain and normal coronary arteriograms. *J Chron Dis* 41:216, 1978.

69. Isner JM, Salem DN, Banas JS, et al: Long term clinical course of patients with normal coronary arteriography: Follow-up of 121 patients with normal or near normal arteriograms. *Am Heart J* 102:645, 1981.

70. Pasternak HC, Thibault GE, Savaoia, et al: Chest pain with angiographically insignificant coronary arterial obstruction. *Am J Med* 68:813, 1980.

71. Ward BW, Wu WC, Richter JF, et al: Long-term follow-up of symptomatic status of patients with noncardiac chest pain: Is diagnosis of esophageal etiology helpful? *Am J Gastroenterol* 82:215, 1987.

72. Ockene IS, Shay MJ, Alpert JS, et al: Unexplained chest pain in patients with normal coronary arteriograms: A follow-up study of functional status. *N Engl J Med* 303:1249, 1980.

73. Cannon RO, Quyyumi AA, Schenke WH, et al: Abnormal cardiac sensitivity in patients with chest pain and normal coronary arteries. *J Am Coll Cardiol* 16:1359, 1990.

74. Shapiro LM, Crake T, Poole-Wilson PA: Is altered cardiac sensation responsible for chest pain in patients with normal coronary arteries? Clinical observation during cardiac catheterization. *Br Med J* 296:170, 1988.

75. Cheng TO: Mitral valve prolapse. *Dis Mon* 33:481, 1987.

76. de Leon AC Jr: Mitral valve prolapse: Etiology and management. *Postgrad Med* 67:66, 1980.

77. Beton DC, Brear SG, Edwards JD, et al: Mitral valve prolapse: An assessment of clinical features, associated conditions and prognosis. *Q J Med* 52:150, 1983.

78. Devereaux RB, Kranz-Fox R, Kligfield P: Mitral valve prolapse: Causes, clinical manifestations, and management. *Ann Intern Med* 111:305, 1989.

79. Wynne J: Mitral valve prolapse. *N Engl J Med* 314:577, 1986.

80. Levine HJ: Difficult problems in the diagnosis of chest pain. *Am Heart J* 100:108, 1980.

81. Rutledge JC, Amsterdam EA: Differential diagnosis and clinical approach to the patient with acute chest pain. *Cardiol Clin* 2:257, 1984.

82. Jeresaty RM: *Mitral Valve Prolapse.* New York, Raven, 1979, pp 38–44.

83. Cheitlin MD, Byrd RC: The click-murmur syndrome. *JAMA* 245:1357, 1981.

84. Markiewicz W, Stoner J, London E, et al: Mitral valve prolapse in one hundred presumably healthy young females. *Circulation* 53:464, 1976.

85. Koch KL, Davidson WR, Day FP, et al: Esophageal dysfunction and chest pain in patients with mitral valve prolapse: A prospective study utilizing provocative testing during esophageal manometry. *Am J Med* 86:32, 1989.

86. Abbasi AS, DeCristofaro D, Anabtawi J, et al: Mitral valve prolapse: Comparative value of M-mode, two-dimensional and Doppler echocardiography. *J Am Coll Cardiol* 2:1219, 1983.

87. Abinader EG: Adrenergic beta blockade and ECG changes in the systolic click murmur syndrome. *Am Heart J* 91:297, 1976.

88. Kleiger RE: Chest pain in patients seen in emergency clinics. *JAMA* 236:595, 1976.

89. Spodick D: Pericarditis, pericardial effusion, cardiac tamponade, and constriction. *Crit Care Clin* 5:455, 1989.

90. Moser KM: Diagnosis and management of pulmonary embolism. *Hosp Pract* 15:57, 1980.

91. Parris WC, Lin S, Frist W: Use of stellate ganglion blocks for chronic chest pain associated with primary pulmonary hypertension. *Anesth Analg* 67:993, 1988.

92. Bell WR, Simon TL, DeMets DL: The clinical features of submassive and massive pulmonary emboli. *Am J Med* 62:355, 1977.

93. Moser KM: State of the art: Pulmonary embolism. *Am Rev Respir Dis* 115:829, 1977.

94. Larson EW, Edwards WD: Risk factors for aortic dissection: A necropsy study of 161 cases. *Am J Cardiol* 53:849, 1984.

95. Ballal RS, Nanda NC, Gatewood R, et al: Usefulness of transesophageal echocardiography in assessment of aortic dissection. *Circulation* 84:1903, 1991.

96. Godwin JD, Herfkens RL, Skoldebrand CG, et al: Evaluation of dissections and aneurysms of the thoracic aorta by conventional and dynamic CT scanning. *Radiology* 136:125, 1980.

97. Herfkins RJ, Higgins CB, Hricak H, et al: Nuclear magnetic resonance imaging of the cardiovascular system: Normal and pathologic findings. *Radiology* 147:749, 1983.

98. Goldman AP, Kotler MN, Scanlon MH, et al: Magnetic resonance imaging and two-dimensional echocardiography: Alternative approach to aortography in diagnosis of aortic dissecting aneurysm. *Am J Med* 80:1225, 1986.

99. Nienaber CA, von Kodolitsch Y, Nicolas V, et al: The diagnosis of thoracic aortic dissection by noninvasive imaging procedures. *N Engl J Med* 328:1, 1993.

100. Davidson E, Weinberger I, Rotenberg Z, et al: Elevated serum creatine kinase levels: An early diagnostic sign of acute dissection of the aorta. *Arch Intern Med* 148:2184, 1988.

101. Epstein SE, Garber LH, Borer JS: Chest wall syndrome: A common cause of unexplained chest pain. *JAMA* 241:2793, 1979.

102. Myers G, Freeman R, Scharf D, et al: Cervicoprecordial angina: Diagnosis and management (abstract). *Am J Cardiol* 39:287, 1977.

103. Calabro JJ, Jeghers H, Miller KA: Classification of anterior chest wall syndrome. *JAMA* 243:1420, 1980.

104. Kayser HL: Tietze's syndrome: A review of the literature. *Am J Med* 21:982, 1956.

105. Wehrmacher WH: The painful anterior chest wall syndromes. *Med Clin North Am* 38:111, 1958.

106. Fam AG, Smythe HA: Musculoskeletal chest wall pain. *Can Med Assoc J* 133:379, 1985.

107. Mitchell LC, Schafermeyer RW: Herniated cervical disk presenting as ischemic chest pain. *Am J Emerg Med* 9:457, 1991.

108. Davis D: *Radicular Syndrome: With Emphasis on Chest Pain Simulating Coronary Disease.* Chicago, Year Book, 1980.

109. Urschel HD, Paulson DL, McNamara JJ: Thoracic outlet syndrome. *Ann Thorac Surg* 6:1, 1968.

110. Sparrow MJ, Bird EL: 'Precordial catch': A benign syndrome of chest pain in young persons. *Aust N Z Med J* 88:325, 1978.

111. Eastridge CE, Mahfood SS, Walker WA, et al: Delayed chest wall pain due to sternal wire sutures. *Ann Thorac Surg* 51:56, 1991.

112. Jarcho S: Functional heart disease in the Civil War (DaCosta, 1871). *Am J Cardiol* 29:809, 1959.

113. Wood P: DaCosta's syndrome (or effort syndrome). *Br Med J* 1:767, 1941.

114. Weissman MM, Merikangas KR: The epidemiology of anxiety and panic disorders: An update. *J Clin Psychiatry* 47(suppl):11, 1986.

115. Ballenger J: Pharmacotherapy of panic disorder. *J Clin Psych* 47:27, 1986.

116. Beitman BD, Mukerji V, Lamberti, et al: Panic disorder in patients with chest pain and angiographically normal coronary arteries. *Am J Cardiol* 63:1399, 1989.

117. Bass C, Wade C, Hand D, et al: Patients with angina with normal and near normal coronary arteries: Clinical and psychosocial state 12 months after angiography. *Br Med J* 287:1505, 1983.

118. Katon W, Hall ML, Russo J, et al: Chest pain: Relationship of psy-

chiatric illness to coronary arteriography results. *Am J Med* 84:1, 1988.

119. Carney RM, Freedland KE, Ludbrook PA, et al: Major depression, panic disorder, and mitral valve prolapse in patients who complain of chest pain. *Am J Med* 89:757, 1990.

120. Beitman BD: Panic disorder in patients with angiographically normal coronary arteries. *Am J Med* 92(suppl 5A):33S, 1992.

121. McLaurin LP, Raft D, Tate SC: Chest pain with normal coronaries: A psychosomatic illness? *Circulation* 56(suppl III):III-174, 1977.

122. Clouse RE: Psychiatric disorders in patients with esophageal disease. *Med Clin North Am* 75:1081, 1991.

123. Clouse RE, Lustman PJ: Psychiatric illness and contraction abnormalities of the esophagus. *N Eng J Med* 309:1337, 1983.

124. Lantinga LJ, Sprafkin RP, McCroskery JH, et al: One year psychological follow-up of patients with chest pain and angiographically normal coronary arteries. *Am J Cardiol* 62:209, 1988.

125. Anderson KO, Dalton CB, Bradley LA, Richter JE: Stress: A modulator of esophageal pressures in healthy volunteers and noncardiac chest pain patients. *Dig Dis Sci* 34:83, 1989.

126. DeMeester TR, O'Sullivan GC, Bermudez G, et al: Esophageal function in patients with angina type chest pain and normal coronary angiograms. *Ann Surg* 196:488, 1982.

127. Kline M, Chesne R, Studevant RL, McCallum RW: Esophageal disease in patients with angina like chest pain. *Am J Gastroenterol* 75:116, 1981.

128. Davies HA, Jones DB, Rhodes J: Esophageal angina as the cause of chest pain. *JAMA* 248:2274, 1982.

129. Benjamin SB, Gerhardt DC, Castell DO: High amplitude, peristaltic esophageal contractions associated with chest pain and/or dysphagia. *Gastroenterology* 77:478, 1979.

130. Schofield PM, Whorwell PJ, Jones PE, et al: Differentiation of "esophageal" and "cardiac" chest pain. *Am J Cardiol* 62:315, 1988.

131. Brand DL, Martin D, Pope CE: Esophageal manometry in patients with angina-like chest pain. *Dig Dis Sci* 22:300, 1977.

132. Katz PO, Dalton CB, Richter JE, et al: Esophageal testing in patients with non-cardiac chest pain or dysphagia: Results of three years' experience in 1161 patients. *Ann Intern Med* 106:593, 1987.

133. Eypasch EP, Stein HJ, DeMeester TR, et al: A new technique to define and clarify esophageal motor disorders. *Am J Surg* 159:144, 1990.

134. Beitman BD, Basha I, Flaker G, et al: Atypical or nonanginal chest pain: Panic disorder or coronary artery disease? *Arch Intern Med* 147:1548, 1987.

135. Patterson DR: Diffuse esophageal spasm in patients with undiagnosed chest pain. *J Clin Gastroenterol* 4:415, 1982.

136. Hewson EG, Sinclair JW, Dalton CB, et al: Twenty-four hour esophageal pH monitoring: The most useful test for evaluating noncardiac chest pain. *Am J Med* 90:576, 1991.

137. Schmidt CD, Jones, Hunt JC, et al: The value of the esophageal motility test in evaluation of thoracic pain problems. *Dis Chest* 42:303, 1962.

138. Clark CS, Kraus BB, Sinclair J, et al: Gastroesophageal reflux induced by exercise in healthy volunteers. *JAMA* 261:3599, 1989.

139. Henderson RD, Wigle ED, Sample K, et al: Atypical chest pain of cardiac and esophageal origin. *Chest* 73:24, 1978.

140. Davies HA, Rush EM, Lewis MJ, et al: Oesophageal stimulation lowers exertional angina threshold. *Lancet* 1:1011, 1985.

141. Lawrence L, National Center for Health Statistics: Detailed diagnoses and procedures for patients discharged from short-stay hospitals, United States, 1984. Hyattsville, MD, U.S. Dept. of Health and Human Services, Public Health Services, National Center for Health Statistics, 1986. (Vital and Health Statistics series 13, no. 86)

142. Richter JE, Bradley LA: Chest pain with normal coronary arteries: Another perspective. *Dig Dis Sci* 35:1441, 1990.

143. VanTrappen G, Janssens J: What is irritable esophagus? Another point of view. *Gastroenterology* 94:1092, 1988.

144. Richter JE, Castell DO: Diffuse esophageal spasm: A reappraisal. *Ann Intern Med* 100:242, 1984.

145. Code CF, Schlegel JF, Kelley ML, et al: Hypertensive gastroesophageal sphincter. *Mayo Clin Proc* 35:391, 1986.

146. Richter JE, Bradley LA, Castell DO: Esophageal chest pain: Current controversies in pathogenesis, diagnosis, and therapy. *Ann Intern Med* 110:66, 1989.

147. Mellow M: Symptomatic diffuse esophageal spasm: Manometric

148. Janssens J, Vantrappen G, Ghillebert G: 24-hour recording of esophageal pressure and pH in patients with noncardiac chest pain. *Gastroenterology* 90:1978, 1986.

149. Bernstein LM, Baker LA: A clinical test for esophagitis. *Gastroenterology* 34:760, 1958.

150. Richter JE, Castell DO: Gastroesophageal reflux: Pathogenesis, diagnosis and therapy. *Ann Intern Med* 97:93, 1982.

151. Ott DJ, Wu WC, Gelfand DW: Reflux esophagitis revisited: Prospective analysis of radiographic accuracy. *Gastrointest Radiol* 6:1, 1981.

152. Behar J, Binacini P, Sheahan DG: Evaluation of esophageal tests in the diagnosis of reflux esophagitis. *Gastroenterology* 71:9, 1976.

153. DeCaestecker JS, Brown J, Blackwell JN, et al: The oesophagus as a cause of recurrent chest pain: Which patients should be investigated and which tests should be used? *Lancet* 11:1143, 1985.

154. Areskog M: Angina-like chest pain: A study with special reference to oesophageal dysfunction and ischemic heart disease (dissertation). Linköping Sweden, Linköping University medical dissertation no. 90, 1980.

155. Ghillebert G, Janssens J, Vantrappen G, et al: Ambulatory 24-hour intraesophageal pH and pressure recordings v. provocation tests in the diagnosis of chest pain of esophageal origin. *Gut* 31:738, 1990.

156. Breumelhof R, Nadrop JHSM, Akkermans LMA, et al: Analysis of 24-hour esophageal pressure and pH data in unselected patients with noncardiac chest pain. *Gastroenterology* 99:1257, 1990.

157. Schofield PM, Bennett DH, Whorwell PJ, et al: Exertional gastroesophageal reflux: A mechanism for symptoms in patients with angina pectoris and normal coronary angiograms. *Br Med J* 294:1459, 1987.

158. Hewson EG, Dalton CB, Richter JE: Comparison of esophageal manometry, provocative testing and ambulatory monitoring in patients with unexplained chest pain. *Dig Dis Sci* 35:302, 1990.

159. Soffer EE, Scalabrini P, Wingate DL: Spontaneous non-cardiac chest pain: Value of ambulatory esophageal pH and motility monitoring. *Dig Dis Sci* 34:1651, 1989.

160. London RL, Ouyang A, Snape WJ, et al: Provocation of esophageal pain by ergonovine or edrophonium. *Gastroenterology* 81:10, 1981.

161. Richter JE, Hacksaw BTR, Wu WC, Castell DO: Edrophonium: A useful provocative test for esophageal chest pain. *Ann Intern Med* 103:14, 1985.

162. Benjamin SB, Richter JE, Cordova CM, et al: Prospective manometric evaluation with pharmacologic provocation of patients with suspected esophageal motility dysfunction. *Gastroenterology* 84:893, 1983.

163. Lee CA, Reynolds JC, Ouyang A, et al: Esophageal chest pain: Value of high-dose provocative testing with edrophonium chloride in patients with normal esophageal manometries. *Dig Dis Sci* 32:682, 1987.

164. Nostrant TT, Saves J, Haber T: Bethanechol increases the diagnostic yield in patients with esophageal chest pain. *Gastroenterology* 91:1141, 1986.

165. Richter JE, Barish CF, Castell DO: Abnormal sensory perception in patients with esophageal chest pain. *Gastroenterology* 91:845, 1986.

166. Johnson LF, DeMeester TR: 24-hour pH monitoring of the distal esophagus. *Am J Gastroenterol* 62:325, 1974.

167. Baldi F, Ferrarini F, Longanesi A, et al: Acid gastroesophageal reflux and symptom occcurrence: Analysis of some factors influencing their association. *Dig Dis Sci* 34:1890, 1989.

168. Ellis FH, Crozier RE, Shea JA: Long esophagomyotomy for diffuse esophageal spasm and related disorders, in Siewert JR, Holscher AH (eds): *Diseases of the Esophagus: Pathophysiology, Diagnosis, Conservative and Surgical Treatment.* New York, Springer-Verlag, 1988, pp 913–917.

169. Svensson O, Stenport G, Tibbling L, et al: Oesophageal function and coronary angiograms in patients with disabling chest pain. *Acta Med Scand* 204:173, 1978.

170. Mellow MH, Simpson AG, Watt L, et al: Esophageal acid perfusion in coronary artery disease: Induction of myocardial ischemia. *Gastroenterology* 85:306, 1983.

171. Dec G, Waldman H, Southern J, et al: Is it myocardial infarction or infection? *Cardiol Board Rev* 10:26, 1993.
172. Dec G, Waldman H, Southern J, et al: Viral myocarditis mimicking acute myocardial infarction. *J Am Coll Cardiol* 20:85, 1992.
173. Zimmerman JL, Dellinger RP, Majid PA: Cocaine-associated chest pain. *Ann Emerg Med* 20:611, 1991.
174. Gitter MJ, Goldsmith SR, Dunbar DN, Sharkey SW: Cocaine and chest pain: Clinical features and outcome of patients hospitalized to rule out myocardial infarction. *Ann Intern Med* 115:277, 1991.
175. Isner JM, Estes M, Thompson PD, et al: Acute cadiac events temporally related to cocaine abuse. *N Engl J Med* 315:1438, 1986.
176. Coleman DL, Ross TF, Naughton JL: Myocardial ischemia and infarction related to recreational cocaine use. *West J Med* 135:444, 1982.
177. Wilkins CE, Mathur VS, Ty RC, et al: Myocardial infarction associated with cocaine abuse. *Tex Heart Inst J* 12:385, 1985.
178. Mathias DW: Cocaine-associated myocardial ischemia. *Am J Med* 81:675, 1986.
179. Zimmerman FH, Gustafson GM, Kemp HG: Recurrent myocardial infarction associated with cocaine abuse in a young man with normal coronary arteries: Evidence for coronary artery spasm culminating in thrombosis. *J Am Coll Cardiol* 9:964, 1987.
180. Smith HWB, Liverman HA, Brody SL, et al: Acute myocardial infarction temporally related to cocaine use. *Ann Intern Med* 107:13, 1987.

52. *Evaluation and Management of Hypertension in the Intensive Care Unit*

Robert J. Heyka

Management of hypertension in an intensive care unit (ICU) usually involves one of four situations: hypertensive urgencies and emergencies (hypertensive crises); the need for treatment of chronic hypertension in patients unable to continue their usual oral regimens; new onset of short-lived hypertension; and hypertension unique to the perioperative setting. In these clinical situations, hypertension may complicate and worsen the status of patients with several coexistent medical conditions. This chapter reviews these aspects of hypertensive evaluation and treatment in the ICU and gives guidelines for the use of parenteral and oral agents.

Hypertensive Urgencies and Emergencies

DEFINITIONS. The most dreaded clinical situations in relation to blood pressure control are hypertensive crises. These are classified, depending on patient status, as emergencies, requiring immediate decrease in blood pressure, usually with parenteral agents; or urgencies, requiring a decrease in blood pressure over 24 to 48 hours, possibly with parenteral or oral agents. Usually there is severe elevation of blood pressure with diastolic blood pressure above 120 to 130 mm Hg in either case [1]. The level of systolic, diastolic, or mean arterial pressure (MAP) itself does not distinguish these two entities. Rather, they are differentiated by the presence or absence of acute and progressive target organ damage [2]. Hypertensive emergency refers to a level of blood pressure elevation associated with ongoing target organ demage. Hypertensive urgency means the potential for target organ damage is great and likely to occur if blood pressure is not controlled. Accelerated and malignant hypertension are often used interchangeably but should be defined more narrowly. Both terms refer to the occurrence of diffuse target organ damage and vascular damage with fibrinoid necrosis and myointimal proliferation [3]. They may occur against the background of a sudden worsening of chronic essential hypertension, with secondary forms of hypertension [4] or may develop de novo. The hemodynamic changes are a markedly increased systemic vascular resistance with hypovolemia secondary to pressure-induced diuresis [5]. Vascular resistance is increased in response to elevated levels of vasoactive constricting substances [3]. The clinical manifestations are seen in diffuse organ dysfunction and best diagnosed by funduscopic examination, which provides a "window" to similar damage in other vascular beds. Accelerated hypertension is manifest as grade III Keith-Wagener-Barker retinopathy—constriction and sclerosis (grades I and II) as well as hemorrhages and exudates. The presence of exudate is more worrisome than hemorrhage alone [6]. Accelerated hypertension may be an urgency or emergency, depending on involvement of other target organs. Malignant hypertension, on the other hand, is diagnosed by the presence of Keith-Wagener-Barker grade IV retinopathy involving the above findings as well as papilledema; most often it is a true hypertensive emergency. Malignant hypertension is frequently associated with hypertensive encephalopathy and sometimes with microangiopathic hemolytic anemia, but it can occur independent of either manifestation. Use of the term *malignant* reflects the dismal survival among these patients before effective therapy was available—about 60 percent survival at 2 years after diagnosis and less than 7 percent survival at 10 years [6]. Death was usually due to cardiovascular disease, such as myocardial infarction and stroke, or end-stage kidney disease. Presumably, accelerated and malignant hypertension are a continuum, with the former progressing into the latter if appropriate therapy is not begun. Both should therefore be treated vigorously [7].

IMPORTANCE OF TARGET ORGAN DAMAGE. Table 52-1 lists common examples of target organ damage seen in conjunction with hypertensive crises in the ICU. The heart, brain, and kidneys (in fact, most organ beds) can adjust the amount of blood flow and pressure they receive by the process of autoregulation. That is, small arteries and arterioles constrict or dilate in response to local myogenic effectors that in turn re-

Table 52-1. Examples of Hypertensive Crises

Generalized	Cardiovascular	Neurologic	Renal
Accelerated and malignant hypertension	Acute left ventricular failure	Hypertensive encephalopathy	Acute renal failure
Microangiopathic hemolytic anemia/disseminated intravascular coagulation	Unstable angina pectoris	Subarachnoid hemorrhage	Acute glomerulonephritis
Eclampsia	Myocardial infarction	Intracerebral hemorrhage	Scleroderma crisis
Vasculitis	Aortic dissection	Cerebrovascular accident	
Catecholamine excess (drugs, rebound syndrome, pheochromocytoma)	Suture integrity after surgery		

spond to transmural (perfusion) pressure gradients [8]. A decrease in perfusion pressure leads to vasodilation and increased flows, whereas an increase in perfusion pressure leads to vasoconstriction. This serves to maintain blood flows with decreased systemic pressure and to limit pressure-induced damage when systemic pressures rise [9]. Target organ damage occurs when systemic pressures exceed the usual autoregulatory range and "breakthrough," or loss of autoregulation, occurs [8,9]. Subsequently, endothelial damage, platelet and fibrin deposition, and end organ ischemia with fibrinoid necrosis occur [1]. Tolerance to elevated pressures varies in individual patients. Patients with chronic hypertension have an improved tolerance to hypertension due to an upward shift in the autoregulation curve but a diminished tolerance to hypotension due to functional and structural changes in their vessel walls [10].

Although patients with chronic hypertension are more tolerant of elevated pressures, they are still at greatest risk of developing a hypertensive crisis. Patients without antecedent hypertension who have, for example, acute vasculitis, unstable angina, or eclampsia can still develop a hypertensive crisis. The crisis tends to occur at lower pressure levels in these patients than in those with chronic hypertension.

Individual organs vary in sensitivity to a rise or fall in blood pressure, with the cerebral circulation the most sensitive to breakthrough and ischemia, especially if atherosclerotic disease is present [1]. Renal perfusion can also be affected if underlying atherosclerotic disease is present. Renal blood flow and urine output can be exquisitely sensitive to maintenance of a critical perfusion pressure, and a decline in blood pressure below this level can lead to renal ischemia and oliguria [12]. The heart can tolerate more pronounced drops in blood pressure, even with underlying atherosclerotic disease, since myocardial oxygen demands decrease so dramatically when pressures decrease [2].

APPROACH TO THE PATIENT. In the ICU, therapy must often begin before a comprehensive patient evaluation is completed. A systematic approach offers the opportunity to be both expeditious and inclusive (Table 52-2).

A brief history and physical should be initiated to assess the degree of target organ damage and rule out obvious secondary causes of hypertension [13,14]. Important historical data include any symptoms attributable to changes in target organ perfusion and function. The history should include inquiries about prior hypertension; other significant medical disease; medication use and compliance; recent neurologic symptoms, such as headache, nausea, and vomiting, visual changes, seizures, focal deficits, confusion, and other evidence of mental status changes; cardiac symptoms, such as chest pain, edema, or orthopnea; and changes in urine output or other urinary symptoms. This history must sometimes be obtained from family members as

Table 52-2. Initial Evaluation of Hypertensive Crisis in the ICU

1. Continuous blood pressure monitoring
   1. Direct (intraarterial) preferred
   2. Indirect (cuff)
2. Brief initial evaluation—history and physical exam with attention to:
   a. Neurologic, cardiac, pulmonary, renal symptoms
   b. Organ perfusion and function
   c. Blood and urine studies: electrolytes, BUN, creatinine, CBC with differential, urinalysis with sediment; if indicated, serum catecholamines, cardiac enzymes
   d. ECG
   e. Chest radiograph
3. Initiation of therapy
4. Further evaluation of etiology once stabilized

Adapted from Gifford RW: Management of hypertensive crises. *JAMA* 266:829, 1991; Vidt DG, Gifford RW: A compendium for the treatment of hypertensive emergencies. *Cleve Clin Q* 51:421, 1984; Garcia JY, Vidt DG: Current management of hypertensive emergencies. *Drugs* 34:263, 1987.

well as the patient. Physical examination should include verification of blood pressure readings in both arms, supine and standing if possible, and elimination of pseudohypertension with Osler's maneuver [15]. Intraarterial monitoring may be necessary. Signs of neurologic ischemia, such as altered mental status or focal neurologic deficits, should be sought. A quick, direct ophthalmologic examination for hemorrhages, exudates, and papilledema; auscultation of the lungs and heart for the presence of rales, S_3, murmur, or rub; evaluation of the abdomen and peripheral pulses for bruits, masses, or deficits; and assessment of recent urine output can all be quickly accomplished. As this continues, ancillary and laboratory evaluation should include electrolytes for hypokalemia and acidosis; BUN and creatinine for assessment of renal function; CBC and differential for anemia, sepsis, disseminated intravascular coagulation, or microangiopathic hemolytic anemia; and assessment of cardiac function with electrocardiogram (ECG), cardiac enzymes (if indicated), and chest radiograph.

The last phase of management involves initiation of therapy. This usually requires placement of an intravenous or possibly an intraarterial access. The intensity of intervention is determined by the clinical situation. The patient may need only continuous ECG monitoring or may require placement of a Swan-Ganz catheter to monitor central pressures. Regular monitoring of urine output, with placement of a Foley catheter if necessary, is also important to follow the effects of treatment.

As the patient's condition stabilizes, further evaluation of unexplored reasons for the hypertensive crisis can be considered and pursued [13]. It is important when initiating therapy to choose agents that will not complicate or interfere with further evaluation of secondary causes for the hypertensive crisis. For example, converting enzyme inhibitors (CEI) would be avoided when renal artery stenosis is suspected and an angiogram with renal vein renin levels is planned. If pheochromocytoma is suspected, antihypertensive agents that might interfere with serum catecholamine measurement would be avoided.

TREATMENT. Depending on the target organ involved, interventions such as intubation, control of seizures, hemodynamic monitoring, and maintenance of urine output can be as important as prompt control of blood pressure. The goal of initial therapy is to terminate ongoing target organ damage, *not* to return blood pressure to normal levels. The lower limit of cerebral autoregulation determines the floor for initial therapy. In both hypertensive and normotensive patients, this floor is approximately 25 percent below the initial MAP [2,8] or a diastolic blood pressure in the range of 110 to 100 mm Hg. Therefore, a reasonable target for blood pressure reduction is to decrease MAP by 20 to 25 percent, taking into consideration the patient's medical history, initiating events, and sites of ongoing target organ damage. Exceptions are hypertensive crises associated with acute left ventricular failure, myocardial ischemia, or aortic dissection, when treatment should be more aggressive and blood pressure decreased to lower target levels within 15 to 30 minutes [2]. In most patients with true hypertensive emergencies, the pathophysiologic abnormality is an increase in systemic vascular resistance (SVR), not an increased cardiac output (CO) (MAP = CO × SVR). It is the increased SVR that overrides local autoregulation and leads to organ ischemia necrosis [3]. Cardiac emergencies such as aortic dissection or myocardial ischemia represent exceptions to the general rule, in that both SVR and CO must be decreased. In these situations, agents that cause reflex tachycardia or increased cardiac work, such as hydralazine, minoxidil, or diazoxide, should be avoided.

Once the patient has been evaluated and the decision to treat has been made, there are a large number of options among available agents. With the availability of newer, more potent oral agents, the decision to use oral or parenteral therapy depends on whether the patient is suffering from a true hypertensive emergency, how rapidly the onset of hypotensive response is needed, how rapidly the pressure must be lowered, and, perhaps most important, whether the patient is at risk for new complications from overaggressive treatment of the elevated pressure (Table 52-3). Patients with preexisting atherosclerotic disease comprise the bulk of this latter group. Evidence of a prior myocardial infarction or cerebrovascular accident or presence of renovascular hypertension put the patient at high risk if therapy "overshoots the mark." Volume depletion from diuretics or pressure diuresis and prior antihypertensive therapy place patients at risk for rapid drops in blood pressure. Except for the cardiac situations mentioned above, a strong argument exists for the more gradual reduction of blood pressure in most cases of hypertensive crisis [16].

The answers to the questions in Table 52-3 will guide the choices of parenteral versus oral therapy. Table 52-4 lists recommendations and precautions for therapeutic agents, and Table 52-5 lists proper dosing for each agent [17,18]. Since most patients are volume-depleted secondary to pressure diuresis, diuretics are reserved for patients with acute left ventricular failure and volume overload; patients with oliguric acute renal failure, in an effort to convert oliguric to nonoliguric ATN (once central volumes are filled and prerenal azotemia excluded); and in conjunction with agents known to cause secondary fluid retention, such as minoxidil, hydralazine, and methyldopa. The

Table 52-3. Parenteral versus Oral Therapy of Hypertension in the ICU

Is this a hypertensive emergency?
Is rapid onset of effect needed?
Is rapid lowering of blood pressure needed?
Is a shorter duration of action important?
Is the patient at risk for overshoot hypotension?
  Atherosclerotic heart disease
  Renovascular hypertension
  Cerebrovascular disease
  Dehydration
  Other recent antihypertensive therapy

patient should be closely monitored to avoid new onset of target organ damage and induction of organ ischemia secondary to an overshoot in target blood pressure reduction. In patients with hypertensive urgency or emergency, stabilizing the hemodynamic status allows diagnostic studies (if necessary) to proceed. Over the course of several days to weeks, the blood pressure can be fine-tuned to levels usually no lower than 160/90 mm Hg The patient can be changed to an oral regimen as the situation stabilizes. Since the ICU represents an artificial environment with regard to such factors as salt and water intake, pain, activity level, and proper timing of medication doses, attempts to "normalize" blood pressure, especially if this requires large doses of medications, should be avoided. Efforts to keep blood pressure levels around 160/90 mm Hg at discharge are adequate in the vast majority of patients, with further fine-tuning once the patient resumes his or her usual diet and activity at home. Close follow-up study is necessary, as blood pressures may rise or fall outside the ICU setting and hospital.

HYPERTENSIVE CRISES IN THE CARDIAC ICU

Acute Left Ventricular Failure in the Failing Heart. A decrease in blood pressure and SVR has a significant effect on improving left ventricular (LV) function by decreasing cardiac work, LV wall tension, and thus oxygen demand [2]. Nitroprusside (NTP) is the agent of choice, due to its balanced effects on venous and arterial circulation with a decrease in both preload and afterload [19]. Usually NTP is administered in conjunction with other acute therapy for pulmonary edema, such as intravenous loop diuretics, oxygen, and possibly morphine. Nitroglycerine (NTG) is an alternative (or additive) choice, but it has a greater effect on the venous (preload) side than the arterial side [2]. An intravenous CEI, such as enalaprilat, can also be used to decrease afterload and serve as a bridge in the transition from acute intravenous therapy to chronic oral therapy.

Myocardial Ischemia or Infarction. In this situation, treatment of elevated blood pressure is only part of overall therapy, with the main objective of preserving or restoring cardiac perfusion. Therapy is usually combined with other medications, anticoagulation, thrombolytic therapy, angioplasty, or surgery. Left ventricular function improves dramatically with decreased systemic pressures. Therapy should maintain local coronary arterial flow and not induce a steal syndrome with relaxation of arterial vessels [20]. The effects of NTP are mostly on arteriolar resistance vessels. Since NTP can actually divert flow away from poststenotic areas [21], NTG is the therapy of choice in this situation. It can be started via sublingual or transcutaneous administration while the intravenous solution is being prepared. Compared to NTP, NTG appears better to preserve regional blood flow to poststenotic areas by increasing collateral

Table 52-4. Treatment of Hypertensive Emergency

Etiology		Recommended drugs	Drugs to avoid
Neurologic	Hypertensive encephalopathy	Nitroprusside, labetalol, diazoxide	M-Dopa, clonidine, beta-bockers
	Intracerebral hemorrhage or subarachnoid hemorrhage	Nitroprusside, labetalol	M-Dopa, clonidine, beta-blockers
	Cerebral infarction	Nitroprusside, labetalol	M-Dopa, clonidine, beta-blockers
	Head injury	Nitroprusside	M-Dopa, clonidine, beta-blockers
Cardiovascular	Myocardial ischemia, infarction	Nitroglycerin, nitroprusside, labetalol, calcium antagonists, beta-blockers	Minoxidil, hydralazine, diazoxide
	Aortic dissection	Nitroprusside, beta-blockers, labetalol, trimethaphan	Minoxidil, hydralazine, diazoxide, nitroglycerin
	Acute left ventricular failure	Nitroprusside, nitroglycerin, loop diuretics, converting enzyme inhibitors	Minoxidil, hydralazine, diazoxide, labetalol, beta-blockers
Renal failure	Acute renal failure	Nitroprusside, labetalol, calcium antagonists	
Other	Microangiopathic hemolytic anemia	Nitroprusside, labetalol, calcium antagonists	
	Malignant hypertension	As with encephalopathy— oral agents may be considered	
	Eclampsia	Hydralazine, diazoxide, labetalol, calcium antagonists	Diuretics, beta-blockers

Adapted from Calhoun DA, Oparil S: Treatment of hypertensive crisis. *N Engl J Med* 323:1177, 1990; Gifford RW: Management of hypertensive crises. *JAMA* 266:829, 1991; Garcia JY, Vidt DG: Current management of hypertensive emergencies. *Drugs* 34:263, 1987.

circulation [21]. Beta-blockers or labetalol given intravenously also act to maintain coronary perfusion in the face of decreased systemic pressures and are acceptable adjunctive agents [13]. As with any hypertensive crisis, the goal of therapy is cessation of target organ damage and improvement of organ function, not a predetermined level of blood pressure (see Chap. 50).

Aortic Dissection. Once the diagnosis of proximal or distal aortic dissection is made, it is imperative to begin therapy immediately to prevent extension of the dissection. Therapy involves both a decrease in SVR and a decrease in cardiac sheer stress (dp/dt) [22]. Blood pressure should be lowered rapidly to the lowest level that allows continued good organ perfusion (i.e., no change in mental status or new neurologic symptoms and continued urine output). Therapy of choice has been either trimethaphan or NTP with a beta-blocker. More recently, labetalol has also been used. Any acute therapy that decreases SVR without also decreasing dp/dt or that tends to induce reflex tachycardia can extend the dissection and should be avoided. Appropriate surgical consultation should be initiated while therapy is introduced (see Chap. 36).

Continued Therapy of Chronic Hypertension

Patients in the ICU often have a prior history of hypertension requiring medication for control. Blood pressure levels may rise if the patient is unable to continue his or her usual antihypertensive regimen. Evaluation of these patients is similar to that for patients with hypertensive crises, again with emphasis on any evidence of target organ damage or risk. Blood pressure elevation in patients who have discontinued chronic therapy can sometimes be severe; this entity has been characterized as a rebound or discontinuation syndrome [23]. In this situation, blood pressure levels not only rise, but actually overshoot those seen in the prehospitalization setting. Rebound hypertension probably represents a rapid return of catecholamine secretion suppressed by therapy [24]. These syndromes therefore represent a situation of catecholamine excess, as seen in illicit drug intoxication or pheochromocytoma. Although any antihypertensive agent can be associated with rebound hypertension, adrenergic inhibitors, such as beta-blockers, and central agonists, such as clonidine or methyldopa, are most commonly described [23]. The likelihood of rebound hypertension occurring is proportional to the dose of medication used. For example, with a daily dose of clonidine below 1.2 mg, rebound syndrome is very unlikely [24]. Patients with more severe hypertension and patients with increased plasma renin activity (PRA) are at greater risk for rebound. If the patient is taking both beta-blockers and central agonists, the former should be weaned and stopped first to avoid unopposed vasoconstriction if the vasodilatory peripheral beta-receptors remain blocked. All rebound syndromes respond rapidly to reinstitution of the initial therapy. If the initial medication cannot be reinstituted, another sympathetic inhibitor may be given intravenously to lower blood pressure.

To treat chronic hypertension and avoid rebound hyperten-

Table 52-5. Proper Dosing for Agents to Treat Hypertensive Crisis

	Administration	Onset	Duration
Direct vasodilators			
Nitroprusside	IV infusion: 0.25–10.0 mg/kg/min	Immediate	3–5 min
Nitroglycerin	IV infusion: 5–100 mg/min	1–2 min	3–5 min
Diazoxide	IV bolus 50–100 mg q10–15 (total 600 mg)	1–5 min	6–12 hr
	IV infusion 10–30 mg/min		
Beta-blockers			
Labetalol	IV bolus: 20–80 mg q10 min	5–10	—
Calcium antagonists			
Nicardipine HD	IV infusion 2–5 mg/hr; increase by 1–2.5 mg/hr q15 min (maximum 15 mg/hr)	1–5 min	3–6 hr
Nifedipine	PO 10–20 mg (reg)	Same for SL	3–5 hr
	BUBQ	and PO	
	Intranasal 10–20 mg*	as long	
		as "bite	
		and swal-	
		low" PO,	
		15–20	
		min	
Verapamil	IV bolus: 5–10 mg over 1–5 min	1–5 min	30–60 min
	IV infusion: 3–25 mg/hr (maximum 90 mg/hr)		
Diltiazem	IV bolus: 5–20 mg (repeat q15–30 min if no λ) up to 20 mg	15–30 min	3 hr
	IV infusion: 5–10 mg/hr ↑ by 5 mg/hr, up to 15 mg q30 min	—	3 hr
Nimodipine	60 mg q4 hr × 2 days; repeat	Hours	
Converting enzyme inhibitors			
Captopril	PO 6.25–25 mg, repeat q30 min if necessary	15–30 min	4–6 hr
Enalaprilat	IV 1.25–5.0 mg (over 5 min) q6 hr	15 min	6 hr
Central agonists			
Clonidine	PO 0.2 mg initially; 0.2 mg/hr (total 0.7 mg)	30–120 min	8–12 hr
Methyldopa	IV infusion: 250–500 mg	30–60 min	3–6 hr
Miscellaneous			
Phentolamine	IV bolus: 5–10 mg q5–15 min		
	1–5 min		
	10 min		
Trimethaphan	IV infusion: 0.5–5 mg/min	1–5 min	10 min
Fenoldopam	0.1 mg/kg/min; increase by 0.05–0.2 mg/kg/min at 20-min intervals	20–30 min	1–3 hr

* Not available in the U.S.
SL = sublingual

sion, the same agent or class of agents as that used chronically should be continued, in approximately the same doses. If the patient cannot take medication by mouth, tablets, capsules, or liquids may be given via nasogastric tube or sublingually. In general, medications from the same class are available in intravenous preparations and can be used if necessary. For example, labetalol can be used in lieu of other beta-blockers, intravenous verapamil or nicardipine for calcium antagonists, enalaprilat for CEI, intravenous methyldopa or clonidine patch for central agonists, and intravenous loop diuretics as needed.

It is usually better to choose short-acting medication rather than timed-release preparations (e.g., nifedipine capsules over nifedipine extended release form), since onset of effect is more predictable with the former and if the patient's status changes the antihypertensive effects are short-lived. A patient who has been noncompliant with several medications may experience a dramatic drop in blood pressure when all medications are taken as prescribed. If this is suspected, it is better to start with lower doses and adjust as necessary. As the patient improves, prehospitalization therapy is slowy reintroduced to keep blood pressure levels around 160/90 mm Hg.

New Onset of Hypertension

New, unexpected, temporary increases in blood pressure may be seen in the ICU. In a patient without a prior history of chronic hypertension, secondary causes should be sought. For example, pain, anxiety, new onset of angina, hypercarbia or hypoxia, hypothermia, rigors, excessive arousal after sedation, or fluid mobilization with overload can all lead to short-term elevations in blood pressure (Table 52-6).

The patient should be evaluated to exclude incipient or established target organ damage. Often, a repeated history and physical examination will uncover a history of chronic hypertension, discontinued medication, or rebound hypertension. Evidence of undiagnosed chronic hypertension can be sought if it is suspected. Retinal changes, especially those of arteriolar constriction and sclerosis [6], or evaluation for concentric left ventricular hypertrophy (LVH) on ECG or two-dimensional (2-D) echocardiogram may establish the (new) diagnosis of chronic hypertension with chronic target organ damage [24]. In the absence of the effects of chronic hypertension, therapy

Table 52-6. New Onset of Hypertension in the ICU

Situational
  Pain
  Anxiety
  New-onset angina
  Hypocarbia
  Hypoxemia
  Hypothermia with shivering
  Rigors
  Volume overload
Rebound or discontinuation syndrome
Prior, undiagnosed, untreated hypertension
  Fundus examination
  2-D echocardiogram for concentric left ventricular hypertrophy

Table 52-7. Hypertension with Cardiovascular Surgery

Preoperative period
  Anxiety
  Pain
  Angina
  Discontinuation of antihypertensive or cardiac therapy
  Rebound hypertension
Intraoperative period
  Induction of anesthesia
    Drug effects—vasodilation, inotropic changes
    Manipulation of viscera or trachea, urethra, and rectum
    Sternotomy, chest retraction
  With initiation of cardiopulmonary bypass
Postoperative period
  Early (0–2 hr)
    Hypoxemia, hypercarbia, hypothermia with shivering, post-anesthetic excitement or pain
    After myocardial revascularization, valve replacement, repair of aortic coarctation
  Intermediate (12–36 hr)
    As above
    Fluid overload, mobilization
    Reaction to endotracheal, nasogastric, chest, or bladder tube

Adapted from Estafanous FG: Hypertension in the surgical patient: Management of blood pressure and anesthesia. *Cleve Clin J Med* 56:385, 1989; Estafanous FG, Tarazi RC: Systemic arterial hypertension associated with cardiac surgery. *Am J Cardiol* 46:685, 1985.

should be directed at the secondary causes mentioned above. If antihypertensive agents are necessary, therapy should be with low doses of short-acting agents to avoid sharp drops in blood pressure in this usually limited situation.

Perioperative Hypertension

The patient who arrives in the ICU from surgery or whose course in the ICU is marked by the need for surgery presents unique problems for the control of blood pressure. Elevated blood pressure can induce new target organ damage, increase the risk of vascular suture breakdown and bleeding, and worsen the overall prognosis. In this setting, blood pressure above 160/100 mm Hg in a previously normotensive patient or an increase of more than 30 mm Hg (systolic or diastolic) above preoperative levels in a known hypertensive patient is worrisome. This definition excludes elevations that are easily controlled with sedation or other simple changes in therapy [25]. Hypertension does not represent a major risk factor for surgery in patients with chronic hypertension who are otherwise stable [26]. About 25 percent of these patients will have worsening perioperative blood pressure and 20 to 30 percent will need intraoperative treatment to raise or lower blood pressure, independent of the degree of preoperative blood pressure control [27]. Any routine oral or intravenous blood pressure therapy should be continued up to the morning of surgery, as regularly scheduled. This approach has been shown to decrease blood pressure lability in the operating room, with a concomitant decreased risk of myocardial or cerebral ischemia [25]. A useful classification of hypertension associated with cardiovascular surgery considers the clinical situation, rather than the specific pathologic mechanism [28] (Table 52-7).

Prior to surgery, acute rises in blood pressure may be seen with anxiety or pain. Acute angina pectoris may be precipitated by or necessitate surgery and lead to a cycle of hypertension with chest pain. Inattention to regular antihypertensive medication with an acute rebound can also occur. The ICU team should achieve good blood pressure control prior to surgery. In general, that means blood pressures should be no higher than 160/90 mm Hg. Attention should also be given to atherosclerotic risk factors, volume status, adequacy of renal function, and presence of hyperkalemia. The induction of anesthesia represents a serious threat to circulatory stability. Almost all anesthetic agents, premedications, and muscle relaxants can have hemodynamic effects and alter blood pressure, sometimes significantly. Three intraoperative periods represent the greatest risk for severe hypertension: intubation, median ster-

notomy with retraction of the chest wall, and initiation of cardiopulmonary bypass [25]. Although it is the anesthesiologist's responsibility to monitor and adjust therapy at these times, blood pressure during the operative course will be less labile if the ICU team has controlled blood pressure well prior to the surgery. Once the patient returns to the ICU, the immediate postoperative period (up to 2 hours) represents a time of significant patient instability, and blood pressures can vary widely. Cardiac surgery is associated with worsening blood pressure in up to 50 percent of patients [29]. There is an increase in pressor reflexes from the heart and increased central nervous system activity [25]. Pain, hypothermia with shivering, hypercarbia and hypoxia, or reflex excitement after anesthesia can lead to changes in blood pressure that require minute-to-minute adjustment. The goal is to avoid both overshoot hypotension and inadequate control. As in the preoperative period, blood pressure should be maintained at about 160/90 mm Hg. Since hypertension in this setting is usually neither severe nor long-lasting and is usually quite sensitive to small doses of antihypertensive medications, intravenous infusions or bolus therapy allow the most controlled approach to blood pressure regulation [13]. Nitroprusside is effective in most situations. In the patient with fixed coronary lesions, NTG can be used to improve poststenotic collateral flow, especially if blood pressure elevation is not severe. Rate-controlled infusion pumps can help deliver these agents. A pressure-responsive, rate-regulating infusion device has been developed for use with short-acting drugs [30]. Labetalol as minibolus or infusion therapy can provide a longer duration of action, extending beyond the immediate period of drug administration, if necessary. Over the next 36 hours, hypertension may develop for any of the previously mentioned reasons. If the patient is unable to take medication by mouth for several days after surgery, blood pressure control can be maintained with parenteral medication of the same class as that used before surgery. Many postoperative patients develop intravascular volume expansion during the first 36 to 72 hours secondary to extravascular fluid mobilization, intraoperative fluid administration, antidiuretic effects of anesthetic agents, or decreased capacity for excretion of water secondary to transient renal insufficiency. Increases in blood pressure may respond well to intravenous loop diuretics and fluid restriction. If the patient becomes refractory to medication regimens that were previously effective, volume expansion with "pseudoresistance" to medications should be considered. The treatment, again, is initiation of diuretic therapy.

Pharmacologic Agents

Therapeutic options for treatment of hypertension in the ICU setting are expanding rapidly. In particular, new calcium antagonists, especially the dihydropyridines, should soon become available as intravenous preparations [31] and compare favorably with such standards as NTP [32,33]. The choice between parenteral and oral therapy rests on the answers to several questions, as mentioned above (Table 52-3). In a true hypertensive emergency, parenteral therapy, which offers the advantage of a more rapid onset and offset of effect, is recommended. Nifedipine and other oral agents have been associated with prolonged hypotension and new target organ damage after oral administration [34]. Most agents ingested orally have a 3- to 6-hour duration of effect. If blood pressure is excessively low over this time, the ICU team is forced to support the patient with volume expansion and vasopressor agents until the effect of the medication wanes (Table 52-8). Additional information on the pharmacology of available agents is found in references 1, 2, 13, 14, 17, 18, and 24.

DIRECT VASODILATORS

Sodium Nitroprusside. Sodium nitroprusside is the most predictable and effective agent for the treatment of severe hypertension. It acts to dilate both arterioles and venules, reduces both afterload and preload, and myocardial oxygen demands. Its effects are mediated by intracellular cyclic GMP in an endothelial-independent mechanism that it shares with other nitrovasodilators [35] (see Chap. 210). The advantage of NTP is its rapid onset and offset, which allow minute-to-minute titration. Drug resistance is rarely observed but is more likely to occur in the presence of hypovolemia. The disadvantages of NTP also are related to its rapid onset and offset: Continuous monitoring of infusion rates is required and is best obtained with a variable rate infusion pump [30]. Nitroprusside is degraded by light and must be wrapped in aluminum foil, which is replaced when solutions are replaced.

Nitroglycerin. Nitroglycerin dilates predominantly the venous system, except with very large doses, when it also acts as an arterial dilator. As with NTP, nitroglycerin works via cyclic GMP [35] (see Chap. 210). Left ventricular filling pressure and MAP are reduced without any significant change in stroke volume or cardiac output. Nitroglycerin increases flow via collateral coronary blood vessels and can improve coronary perfusion to poststenotic lesions. Nitroglycerin is an agent of choice in the management of postcoronary bypass hypertension. It is also effective in coronary ischemia with unstable angina. It is not as potent an antihypertensive agent as NTP [17] but can be effective when blood pressures are not severely elevated. The major disadvantage of NTG is the rapid onset and offset of action, which necessitate careful monitoring. It can adsorb to plastic containers and tubing, and therefore must be administered via glass containers and nonadsorbent infusion tubing. Nitroglycerin should be avoided in patients who have increased intracranial pressure or aortic or subaortic stenosis.

Table 52-8. Complications of Treatment of Hypertension in the ICU

Complication	Causes
Overshoot hypotension	Too-rapid infusion Additive drug effects New cardiac disease (MI, tamponade) Volume depletion or redistribution Unsuspected secondary cause of hypertension (renal artery stenosis with CEI) Prolonged duration of effect
Worsening neurologic status	Cerebral ischemia secondary to too rapid a fall in blood pressure Thiocyanate toxicity (with NTP) Worsened hypertensive encephalopathy secondary to inadequate treatment Medication side effect Worsened intracranial hypertension New metabolic abnormality
Worsening of hypertension	Volume overload or redistribution Pseudotolerance Unsuspected secondary cause of hypertension (e.g., catecholamine excess) Poor medical regimen Poor compliance with regimen
Metabolic acidosis	Cyanide toxicity Tissue hypoperfusion—secondary to inappropriately low blood pressure
Worsening renal function	Tissue hypoperfusion Volume depletion ATN Transient—secondary to treatment (do not stop therapy)

ATN = acute tubular necrosis; CEI = converting enzyme inhibitor; NTP = nitroprusside.

Diazoxide. Diazoxide is a potent arterial vasodilator that has no effect on the venous system (see Chap. 210). Its effects, therefore, are to reduce cardiac afterload but not preload, and it tends to induce reflex tachycardia. It is a congener of thiazide diuretics but has no direct diuretic or natriuretic effects. Renal and coronary blood flow are unchanged, but cerebral blood flow may be decreased. Reflex tachycardia can increase cardiac output and myocardial oxygen demands. Precipitous decreases in blood pressure have been observed, especially following larger doses. The drop in blood pressure seems to be related to pretreatment blood pressure levels. Hypotensive effects may be worsened in the presence of renal insufficiency. The advantages of diazoxide are that administration in small doses or by slow infusion enables a controlled reduction in blood pressure with a decreased risk of overshoot hypotension. It can be administered via pulse or minibolus, and effects are observed within 1 or 2 minutes. Hypotensive effects may last up to 12 hours after infusion. Diazoxide is not associated with mental status changes. Disadvantages relate to the risk of a precipitous drop in blood pressure with larger doses. Reflex tachycardia can induce angina in patients with underlying coronary artery disease. It is therefore contraindicated in patients with coronary artery disease, recent myocardial infarction, aortic dissection, coarctation of the aorta, intracerebral hemorrhage, or pulmonary edema. Diazoxide causes sodium and water retention and usually necessitates the use of loop diuretics, particularly with longer administration periods. Hyperglycemia can be observed with continued administration due to inhibition of insulin release. Diazoxide is also contraindicated in the treatment of hypertension during pregnancy. Other side effects include weakness, flushing, nausea, and vomiting.

Hydralazine. As of early 1993, hydralazine is no longer available for parenteral administration.

BETA-BLOCKERS. Although several beta-blockers, such as propranolol and the ultra-short-acting cardioselective beta-blocker esmolol, can be given parenterally, labetalol is the beta-blocker used most commonly in the ICU (see Chap. 210).

Labetalol is a racemic mixture of a nonselective beta-blocker and a selective $alpha_1$-antagonist. It produces prompt reduction in peripheral vascular resistance and blood pressure. The beta-blocker component prevents reflex tachycardia or significant changes in cardiac output. Myocardial oxygen consumption is reduced and coronary hemodynamics are improved in patients with coronary artery disease. Cerebral blood flow is not significantly affected. There is no change in glomerular filtration rate or renal blood flow. It may be administered either as a mini-bolus or as an infusion. Labetalol undergoes first-pass hepatic metabolism. There is no dosage adjustment necessary with renal failure, but some adjustment may be needed in patients with severe hepatic disease. The onset of action is within 5 to 10 minutes.

The advantages of labetalol (compared to NTP or NTG) include safer titration with minibolus technique and less intense supervision required by nursing personnel. Labetalol is effective in many situations, including postoperative hypertension and most hypertensive emergencies. It has been used to treat pheochromocytoma crisis because of it $alpha_1$-blocking properties and in aortic dissection because of its beta-blocking properties [36]. The disadvantages of labetalol relate to several factors. Its alpha-blocking effects can cause orthostatic hypotension. Other side effects include nausea, vomiting, flushing, tingling of the scalp and groin, dizziness, and headache.

The ratio of beta-blocking effects to alpha-blocking effects is approximately 7:1. For this reason, any contraindication to the use of a beta-blocker also applies to the use of labetalol. Its use can be problematic in patients with asthma (since it induces a decrease in FEV_1), obstructive pulmonary disease, congestive heart failure, or heart block greater than first-degree.

CALCIUM ANTAGONISTS. Calcium antagonists, particularly the dihydropyridines, have become more widely used in the ICU setting (see Chap. 210). Several dihydropyridine agents, such as isradipine, are available in intravenous form in Europe and may become available for use in the United States in the near future [31]. Calcium antagonists have been used for hypertensive urgencies and emergencies and are given via the parenteral and enteral routes [37]. The calcium antagonists also have a general advantage of producing a drop in blood pressure that is proportional to pretreatment levels. For this reason, they tend to induce less overshoot hypotension as a class than may be seen with other agents.

Nifedipine. Nifedipine is widely used to treat hypertension in the emergency room or hospital setting. It is administered orally, although an intranasal preparation is being tested in Europe. Nifedipine's potency and rapid onset of action are the reasons for the rapid growth in its popularity. It decreases peripheral vascular resistance and increases collateral coronary blood flow. These effects result in a decreased myocardial oxygen consumption, despite a tendency to reflex tachycardia and

increased cardiac output and stroke volume. As with most calcium antagonists, the response is proportional to the pretreatment blood pressure level. That is, the greater the blood pressure prior to treatment, the greater the decline following administration.

The advantages of nifedipine include ease of administration, rapid onset, effectiveness, and relatively low incidence of serious side effects. It can be administered sublingually or as a bite-and-swallow oral preparation. The onset of action is within 15 to 30 minutes, and in at least one study was faster with the bite-and-swallow technique [38]. Adverse effects are as those seen with any vasodilator, mainly flushing, tachycardia, and headache. There is an uncontrolled reduction in blood pressure following oral administration. Serious complications, such as myocardial infarction, myocardial ischemia, acute worsening of renal failure, and cerebral ischemia, have been reported due to the sudden reduction in blood pressure below the level of autoregulatory bounds [34]. This is more likely to occur in patients who are volume-depleted, have received prior therapy, or have underlying renal vascular disease.

Verapamil. Verapamil is a nondihydropyridine calcium antagonist that induces arterial vasodilation. It has a greater effect on atrioventricular conduction than the dihydropyridine subgroup. It also has a more pronounced negative inotropic effect if left ventricular ejection fraction is already impaired. Multiple studies, especially in Europe [37], have shown its effectiveness in treating hypertensive urgencies and emergencies.

The advantages of verapamil include a decrease in blood pressure proportional to baseline blood pressure. It has a rapid onset of action with a relatively low incidence of serious side effects. It can be given as repeated small boluses or a continuous intravenous infusion. The disadvantages include induction of various degrees of heart block, especially in the patients receiving concomitant beta-blocker therapy, and worsening of congestive heart failure due to its negative inotropic effects.

Nicardipine. Nicardipine is a dihydropyridine calcium antagonist that is a rapid-acting systemic and coronary artery vasodilator. It has minimal effects on cardiac conductivity or inotropy. Its advantages include rapid onset, potency, and ability to titrate versus blood pressure levels [39]. Nicardipine has been used particularly in the setting of postoperative hypertension and has been found in comparison studies to have effects comparable to those of NTP [32]. Disadvantages of nicardipine include tachycardia, hypotension, nausea, and vomiting. There is minimal cardiac depression, and, as with any continuous infusion, administration requires continuous monitoring.

Diltiazem. Diltiazem is available as an intravenous preparation. It is a nondihydropyridine calcium antagonist with effects intermediate between those of verapamil and of the dihydropyridine group. It is a recent addition to the therapy of hypertension in the ICU, although several recent studies have shown it to be as effective as other calcium antagonists or NTP [40]. Its mechanism of action, metabolism, advantages, and disadvantages are as with the other calcium antagonists. It tends to cause less atrioventricular conduction delay than verapamil but more than the dihydropyridines. It should be used with caution in patients taking beta-blockers.

Nimodipine. Nimodipine is a dihydropyridine calcium antagonist that crosses the blood-brain barrier and has recently been used in the ICU [2]. It is currently recommended only for patients with subarachnoid hemorrhage on a 21-day oral dosing schedule. It is also being investigated for acute cerebral infarction. Its metabolism, advantages, and disadvantages are the same as for the other dihydropyridines.

CONVERTING ENZYME INHIBITORS

Captopril. Captopril is the first converting enzyme inhibitor (CEI) available in the United States (see Chap. 210). Captopril is rapidly absorbed, with peak blood levels reached 30 minutes after administration [41]. Unlike some CEIs, captopril is not ingested as a prodrug and is therefore active as soon as it is absorbed.

The advantages of captopril include a rapid onset of effect after oral administration. There is no change in cardiac output, heart rate, or central pressures. There is no reflex tachycardia, as CEIs have a balanced effect on preload and afterload. There is recent evidence that CEIs are particularly effective in patients with congestive heart failure or recent myocardial infarction. A disadvantage of all CEIs is the risk of acute hypotension in patients who are volume-depleted. Patients with bilateral high-grade renal artery stenosis or high-grade stenosis in a solitary functioning kidney are also at risk for severe hypotension. Other acute side effects include bronchospasm, nausea, and vomiting. Converting enzyme inhibitors interfere with potassium excretion, and some potassium retention is expected. This can be more problematic in patients taking potassium supplements or using nonsteroidal anti-inflammatory drugs (NSAIDs). The NSAIDs also attenuate the hypotensive effect of CEIs, possibly by interference with prostaglandin synthesis. Angioedema, a maculopapular rash, and dysgeusia have been reported rarely.

Enalaprilat. Enalaprilat is the only CEI that can be administered parenterally (see Chap. 210). It is the active form of the oral agent enalapril, which is ingested as a prodrug and must be activated in the liver if given in the oral form. Enalaprilat is probably most useful in the ICU when oral therapy is impractical in patients who have been previously treated with a CEI. It is also effective in patients with underlying left ventricular dysfunction or recent myocardial infarction. Disadvantages are as with captopril. A limited dose titration response restricts the use of enalaprilat in a severe hypertensive crisis.

CENTRAL AGONISTS

Clonidine. Clonidine is a central agonist that activates central alpha$_2$-adrenergic receptors and suppresses sympathetic nervous function (see Chap. 210). It acts to decrease peripheral vascular resistance. There is a decrease in venous return and bradycardia that can contribute to reduction in cardiac output at rest. It is available in the United States as an oral preparation. Clonidine is also available as a transdermal patch with an effectiveness of approximately 1 week. The patch should not be used to initiate therapy since it takes several days to achieve a steady state. However, patients previously on clonidine who are unable to take oral medications may be converted to a patch to avoid the possibility of rebound syndrome. Clonidine has been administered in an oral titration regimen to achieve blood pressure control in a period of 2 to 3 hours [42].

The advantages of clonidine include ease of administration and oral titration schedule, which allow gradual reduction in blood pressure with decreased risk for overshoot hypotension. It is also useful in postoperative hypertension, and patients may be converted to a transdermal patch before surgery. Major disadvantages are sedation and dry mouth as well as increased risk of orthostatic hypotension. Since it can cause some sedation, it should be used with caution in patients who require

careful monitoring of central nervous system function. Rebound hypertension may be observed if oral medication, particularly at higher doses, is abruptly discontinued.

Alphamethyldopa. Alphamethyldopa is also a central agonist acting at alpha$_2$-receptors (see Chap. 210). It depresses central sympathetic nervous system outflow and decreases peripheral vascular resistance with little effect on cardiac output. There is no effect on glomerular filtration rate or renal blood flow.

The advantages of methyldopa include slow onset of action with intravenous administration. This makes it better suited for managing hypertensive urgencies than emergencies. It can also be used in postoperative hypertension. The disadvantages are similar to those with clonidine. It can induce drowsiness and should therefore be avoided when mental status must be periodically evaluated. Its effects are less predictable, even with intravenous infusion, than those of other parenteral agents. Long-term oral use has been associated with drug-induced fever, hepatitis, and hemolytic anemia, although these are rarely seen in the ICU setting with short-term use.

ALPHA-ADRENERGIC INHIBITORS. Several alpha-adrenergic inhibitors are available for oral administration. These can be used in situations of catecholamine excess or as therapy for chronic hypertension. The only available intravenous agent with alpha-adrenergic blocking properties is phentolamine, a nonselective alpha-receptor blocking agent. Its use is reserved for treatment of hypertensive emergencies or urgencies associated with excess catecholamine states. These excess states include pheochromocytoma-induced hypertension, rebound hypertension due to withdrawal of clonidine or guanabenz, and catecholamine excess state related to drug ingestion. The hypotensive effect of a single intravenous bolus lasts less than 15 minutes and is associated with significant reflex tachycardia. The drug is metabolized in the liver, with only 10 percent excreted in the urine.

The advantages of phentolamine include its specific effects in patients with pheochromocytoma. It is used as part of the anesthetic regimen in perioperative control of these patients. It has been used as a diagnostic test for suspected pheochromocytoma, but, this use is limited by a high incidence of both false positive and false negative results. Disadvantages include abdominal cramping and pain, vomiting, diarrhea, tachycardia, and dizziness. Rarely, death has occurred with acute cardiac arrhythmias or acute myocardial infarction.

GANGLIONIC BLOCKERS. Trimethaphan camsylate is a ganglion blocking agent that blocks both adrenergic and cholinergic ganglia. It also has a direct vascular dilation effect, which increases its hypotensive effects. Since there is venous dilation, there is no reflex tachycardia or change in cardiac output. It must be administered via an infusion pump, as continued infusion is essential for it to produce antihypertensive effects. There have been reports of late refractoriness. It is metabolized by the kidney. There is some biotransformation, possibly by pseudocholinesterase, with a duration of action of 10 to 15 minutes. Trimethaphan is effective in all forms of hypertension and will reduce blood pressure. Its effects are dependent on the rate of infusion and the concentration used.

The drug is optimally effective when the patient's head is elevated. It requires carefully controlled infusion rates, as it has very rapid onset and offset of effects. Disadvantages include orthostatic hypotension. There is also a risk of paresis of the bowel and bladder, blurry vision, dry mouth, and bladder retention. The response to trimethaphan may be markedly increased if the patient is hypovolemic or if there is concomitant use of diuretics.

FENOLDOPAM. Fenoldopam is a specific dopamine I receptor agonist that is free of alpha- and beta-adrenergic receptor effects [33]. It reduces blood pressure by a marked reduction in peripheral resistance and the renal, splanchnic, and skeletal muscle beds. It increases renal blood flow, fractional excretion of sodium, and water clearance. It is metabolized in the liver to multiple metabolites with uncertain clinical activity. Renal clearance is approximately 15 percent of an intravenous dose.

The advantages of fenoldopam include titration of the infusion. The increased salt and water excretion can be important in patients who would otherwise require diuretics. Fenoldopam may be particularly effective in patients with impaired renal function. The disadvantages are related to vasodilation and include flushing, headache, hypotension, nausea, and occasional ECG changes. These changes may be explained by acute alterations in cardiac chamber volumes.

DIURETICS. Diuretics are usually not considered primary agents in managing hypertensive crises, as most patients are hypovolemic. However, patients with postoperative hypertension, cardiac target organ damage with left ventricular dysfunction, or poor attention by the ICU team to imput and output may have volume overload. In addition, many parenteral antihypertensive agents tend to induce fluid retention, which can lead to pseudoresistance to the drug. In these instances, loop diuretics, such as furosemide or bumetanide, can help control inravascular volume, maintain urine output, and prevent resistance to antihypertensive therapy. They can be given intravenously as a bolus or as a slow infusion. They exhibit a threshold effect whereby the response, which is increased urine output, is not seen unless the dosage reaching the renal tubules exceeds a threshold level. For this reason, the best therapy is with upward dosage titration in 30-minute increments until urine output is seen or until maximum doses are achieved (see Chap. 210).

References

1. Calhoun DA, Oparil S: Treatment of hypertensive crisis. *N Engl J Med* 323:1177, 1990.
2. Gifford RW: Management of hypertensive crises. *JAMA* 266:829, 1991.
3. Vidt DG: Practical management of patients with severe hypertension and hypertensive emergencies. *Am Heart J* 3:205, 1986.
4. Davis BA, Crook JE, Vestal RE, Oates JA: Prevalence of renovascular hypertension in patients with grade III or IV hypertensive retinopathy. *N Engl J Med* 301:1273, 1979.
5. Dzau VJ, Siwek LG, Rosen S, et al: Sequential renal hemodynamics in experimental benign and malignant hypertension. *Hypertension* 3(suppl I):I-63, 1981.
6. Breslin DJ, Gifford RW, Fairbairn JF, Kearns TP: Prognostic importance of ophthalmoscopic findings in essential hypertension. *JAMA* 195:91, 1966.
7. Ahmed MEK, Walker JM, Beevers DG, Beevers M: Lack of difference between malignant and accelerated hypertension. *Br Med J* 292:235, 1986.
8. Phillipa SJ, Whisnant JP: Hypertension and the brain. *Arch Intern Med* 152:938, 1992.
9. Strandgaard S, Olesen J, Skinhøj E, Lassen NA: Autoregulation of brain circulation in severe arterial hypetension. *Br Med J* 1:507, 1973.
10. Strandgaard S, Paulson OB: Cerebral autoregulation (progress review). *Stroke* 15:413, 1984.
11. Ruff RL, Talman WT, Petito F: Transient ischemic attacks associated with hypotension in hypertensive patients with carotid artery stenosis. *Stroke* 12:353,1981.
12. Textor SC, Novick AC, Tarazi RC, et al: Critical perfusion pressure for renal function in patients with bilateral atherosclerotic renal vascular disease. *Ann Intern Med* 102:308, 1985.
13. Vidt DG, Gifford RW: A compendium for the treatment of hypertensive emergencies. *Cleve Clin Q* 51:421, 1984.
14. Garcia JY, Vidt DG: Current management of hypertensive emergencies. *Drugs* 34:263, 1987.
15. Messerli FH: Osler's maneuver, pseudohypertension, and true hypertension in the elderly. *Am J Med* 80:906, 1986.
16. Hurtig HI: The case for gradual reduction of blood pressure, in Narins RG (ed): *Controversies in Nephrology and Hypertension.* New York, Churchill Livingstone, 1984, pp 213–239.
17. Rubenstein EB, Escalante C: Hypertensive crisis. *Crit Care Clin* 5:477, 1989.
18. McRae RP, Liebson PR: Hypertensive crisis. *Med Clin North Am* 70:749, 1986.
19. Cohn JN, Burke LP: Diagnosis and treatment—Drugs five years later: Nitroprusside. *Ann Intern Med* 91:752, 1979.
20. Mann T, Cohn PF, Holman BL, et al: Effect of nitroprusside on regional myocardial blood flow in coronary artery disease: Results in 25 patients and comparison with nitroglycerin. *Circulation* 57:732, 1978.
21. Flaherty JT: Comparison of intravenous nitroglycerin and sodium nitroprusside in acute myocardial infarction. *Am J Med* 74(suppl 6B):53, 1983.
22. Asfoura JY, Vidt DG: Acute aortic dissection. *Chest* 99:724, 1991.
23. Houston C: Abrupt cessation of treatment in hypertension: Consideration of clinical natures, mechanisms, prevention and management of the discontinuation syndrome. *Am Heart J* 102:415, 1981.
24. Kaplan NM, Lieberman E: *Clinical Hypertension.* 4th ed., Baltimore, Williams and Wilkins, 1986.
25. Estafanous FG: Hypertension in the surgical patient: Management of blood pressure and anesthesia. *Cleve Clin J Med* 56:385, 1989.
26. Goldman L: Cardiac risks and complications of noncardiac surgery. *Ann Intern Med* 98:504, 1983.
27. Goldman L, Caldera DL: Risks of general anesthesia and elective operation in the hypertensive patient. *Anesthesiology* 50:285, 1979.
28. Estafanous FG, Tarazi RC: Systemic arterial hypertension associated with cardiac surgery. *Am J Cardiol* 46:685, 1989.
29. Roberts AJ, Niarchos AP, Subramanian VA, et al: Systemic hypertension associated with coronary artery bypass surgery. *J Thorac Cardiovasc Surg* 74:846, 1977.
30. deAsla RA, Benis AM, Jurado RA, Litwak RS: Management of postcardiotomy hypertension by microcomputer-controlled administration of sodium nitroprusside. *J Thorac Cardiovasc Surg* 89:115, 1985.
31. Ziegler M: Advances in the acute therapy of hypertension. *Crit Care Med* 20:1630, 1992.
32. Halpern NA, Goldberg M, Neely C, et al: Postoperative hypertension: A multicenter, prospective, randomized comparison between intravenous nicardipine and sodium nitroprusside. *Crit Care Med* 20:1637, 1992.
33. Shusterman NH, Elliot WJ, White WB: Fenoldopam, but not nitroprusside, improves renal function in severely hypertensive patients with impaired renal function. *Am J Med* 95:161, 1993.
34. Schwartz M, Naschitz JE, Yeshurun D, Sharf B: Oral nifedipine in the treatment of hypertensive urgency: Cerebrovascular accident following a single dose. *Arch Intern Med* 150:686, 1990.
35. Lewicki J: Cellular actions of atrial natriuretic peptide, in Brenner BM, Stein JH (eds): *Atrial Natriuretic Peptides.* New York, Churchill Livingstone, 1989, pp 79–103.
36. Cressman JD, Vidt DG, Gifford RW, et al: Intravenous labetalol in the management of severe hypertension and hypertensive emergencies. *Am Heart J* 107:980, 1984.
37. Frishman WH, Weinberg P, Peled HB, et al: Calcium entry blockers

for the treatment of severe hypertension and hypertensive crisis. *Am J Med* 75:35, 1984.

38. McAllister RG: Kinetics and dynamics of nifedipine after oral and sublingual doses. *Am J Med* 81(suppl 6A):2, 1986.

39. Wallin JD: Intravenous nicardipine hydrochloride: Treatment of patients with severe hypertension. *Am Heart J* 119:434, 1990.

40. Mullen JC, Miller DR, Weisel RD, et al: Postoperative hypertension: A comparison of diltiazem, nifedipine, and nitroprusside. *J Thorac Cardiovasc Surg* 96:122, 1988.

41. Williams G: Converting enzyme inhibitors in the treatment of hypertension. *N Engl J Med* 319:1517, 1988.

42. Anderson RJ, Hart GR, Crumpler CP, et al: Oral clonidine loading in hypertensive urgencies. *JAMA* 246:848, 1981.

IV. Pulmonary Problems in the Intensive Care Unit

Section Editor
Richard S. Irwin

53. A Physiologic Approach to Managing Respiratory Failure

Richard S. Irwin and Melvin R. Pratter

Overview

Respiratory failure occurs when gas exchange becomes substantially impaired, resulting in significant alterations in arterial blood gases. Respiratory failure is delineated by abnormalities in arterial blood gas (ABG) values (i.e., arterial carbon dioxide tension [$PaCO_2$] >49 mm Hg and/or arterial oxygen tension [PaO_2] <50–60 mm Hg) [1,2]. The arterial blood values for PaO_2, $PaCO_2$, pH_a, and bicarbonate (HCO_3^-) are used to assess the adequacy of gas exchange and acid-base homeostasis. Correct interpretation of these values requires a working knowledge of

1. The Henderson or Henderson-Hasselbach equation [3]
2. The simplified form of the alveolar air equation [4]
3. The alveolar-arterial oxygen tension (PO_2) gradient concept [5]
4. The calculation of $\Delta H^+/\Delta PCO_2$ ratios and their application in making therapeutic decisions [5,6]
5. The differential diagnoses for various acid-base disorders [3].

Normal Gas Exchange

ARTERIAL OXYGEN TENSION. Proper interpretation of the PaO_2 requires an understanding of "normal" values. The normal PaO_2 depends on the position of the patient at the time the sample is obtained and the patient's age. Two formulas that can be used to predict normal PaO_2 are [7]:

In the upright position, $PaO_2 = 104.2 - 0.27 \times age\ (yr)$
In the supine position, $PaO_2 = 103.5 - 0.42 \times age\ (yr)$

ALVEOLAR-ARTERIAL OXYGEN TENSION DIFFERENCE.
To interpret a decrease in PaO_2, one must know the difference between the alveolar and arterial PO_2 values, or $P(A\text{-}a)O_2$ gradient. A patient with a decreased PaO_2 can then be additionally categorized as having a normal or abnormally elevated A-a gradient.

To calculate the $P(A\text{-}a)O_2$ gradient, one must first determine the alveolar PO_2 (PAO_2). The PAO_2 can be calculated from the simplified form of the alveolar air equation [4]:

$$PAO_2 = PIO_2 - \frac{PaCO_2}{R}$$

PIO_2, partial pressure of inspired oxygen, is obtained by multiplying the atmospheric pressure of dry inspired air by the fraction of inspired oxygen being breathed (FIO_2). At sea level and breathing room air (21% oxygen) this value can be assumed to be 150 mm Hg. R represents the respiratory exchange ratio. This can be assumed to be 0.8, even in patients with significant

lung disease [4]. Therefore, substituting into the alveolar air equation and assuming a normal $PaCO_2$ of 40 mm Hg:

$$PAO_2 = 150 - \frac{40}{0.8} = 100$$

The $P(A\text{-}a)O_2$ gradient is affected by age and position. In the upright position [7]:

$$P(A\text{-}a)O_2\ gradient = 2.5 + 0.21 \times age\ (yr)$$

In the supine position the (A-a) gradient is slightly higher [7]. Therefore, assuming the normal PaO_2 in a young, healthy 20-year-old person is 90 to 95 mm Hg, the normal (A-a) gradient will be 5 to 10 mm Hg. It will be closer to 5 mm Hg in the upright position and closer to 10 mm Hg in the supine position. The $P(A\text{-}a)O_2$ gradient is a sensitive indicator of respiratory disease that interferes with gas exchange. It can almost always differentiate extrapulmonary from pulmonary causes of hypercapnia and hypoxemia (Table 53-1) [5] but to do so it must be measured on room air ($FIO_2 = 0.21$) [5]. At any age, a $P(A\text{-}a)O_2$ gradient exceeding 20 mm Hg should be considered abnormal and indicative of pulmonary dysfunction [8].

Although arterial hypercapnia in the presence of a normal gradient breathing air has been considered the sine qua non of pure extrapulmonary respiratory failure, a recent study suggests that the gradient can narrow to normal with increasing hypercapnia in patients with chronic obstructive pulmonary disease (COPD) [9]. This finding was explained by substantial changes in the position of the alveolar and arterial points on the oxyhemoglobin dissociation curve related to ventilation-perfusion inequalities. Therefore, while arterial hypercapnia with a normal $P(A\text{-}a)O_2$ gradient is consistent with pure extrapulmonary respiratory failure, it cannot by itself rule out severe COPD.

ARTERIAL CARBON DIOXIDE TENSION. Normal $PaCO_2$ is 37 to 43 mm Hg. This value is determined by the level of alveolar ventilation for a given level of CO_2 produced by the

Table 53-1. Causes of Hypercapnia and Their Pathophysiologic Mechanisms

Cause	Mechanism

Pulmonary disorders of
  Lower airways
  Lung parenchyma
  Pulmonary vasculature
	Severe $\dot{V}/\dot{Q}$ mismatch

Extrapulmonary disorders of
  Central nervous system
  Peripheral nervous system
  Respiratory muscles
  Chest wall
  Pleura
  Upper airways
	Hypoventilation

body. The following equation demonstrates how $PaCO_2$ is determined [10]:

$$PaCO_2 = (K) \frac{CO_2 \text{ production}}{\text{Alveolar ventilation}}$$

where K = proportionality constant. The constant K has the value of 0.863 mm Hg when CO_2 production is expressed in milliliters per minute under standard conditions and alveolar ventilation is expressed in liters per minute under body conditions [11].

Unlike PaO_2, the $PaCO_2$ is unaffected by age or position [7].

Abnormal Gas Exchange

HYPOXEMIA. There are five pathophysiologic mechanisms that can cause hypoxemia [1]: (1) low PIO_2; (2) hypoventilation; (3) low ventilation-perfusion mismatch; (4) right-to-left shunting; and (5) diffusion impairment. In a clinical setting, hypoventilation, low ventilation-perfusion mismatch, and right-to-left shunting are essentially the only important pathophysiologic causes of hypoxemia. In the two latter settings, decreased cardiac output resulting in a decreased mixed venous O_2 content can have a considerable effect on the ultimate composition of arterial blood. A low PIO_2 is generally seen only at high altitude. Diffusion impairment alone is never the major cause of hypoxemia [1]. In patients with hypoxemia, calculating the $P(A-a)O_2$ gradient is vital to determining whether the cause of hypoxemia is hypoventilation only (normal $P(A-a)O_2$ gradient) or low ventilation-perfusion mismatch or right-to-left shunting (both characterized by an elevated $P(A-a)O_2$ gradient). The mechanism(s) responsible for hypoxemia is identified because different mechanisms have different diagnostic and therapeutic implications.

Hypoventilation. *Hypoventilation* is a decrease in alveolar ventilation for a given level of CO_2 production due to a decrease in minute ventilation from extrapulmonary dysfunction. This decrease in minute ventilation leads to a proportional decrease in alveolar ventilation, resulting in an increase in $PaCO_2$. From the alveolar air equation—$PAO_2 = PIO_2 - (PaCO_2/R)$—it is clear that for any constant PIO_2 and R values, an increase in $PaCO_2$ will cause PaO_2 to decrease. Since there is no abnormality of distal gas exchange (i.e., no intrapulmonary dysfunction), the $P(A-a)O_2$ gradient remains normal. While the PAO_2 and PaO_2 decrease, the (A-a) gradient remains normal.

EXAMPLE. A 30-year-old unconscious heroin addict breathing room air is brought into the emergency department with the following arterial blood gas values: pH_a 7.27, $PaCO_2$ 56 mm Hg, PaO_2 70 mm Hg, HCO_3^- 25 mEq per liter. The PAO_2 equals 150 minus (56/0.8), or 80. Consequently, the $P(A-a)O_2$ gradient equals 80 minus 70, or 10. This is a classic example of drug-induced hypoventilation causing hypoxemia due to respiratory center depression without lung disease.

Ventilation-Perfusion Mismatch. Low ventilation (V)-perfusion (Q) mismatch leads to hypoxemia. In areas where there is inadequate ventilation for a given level of perfusion (low $\dot{V}/\dot{Q}$ mismatch), the blood leaving the pulmonary capillary will have a decrease in both PO_2 and oxygen content (decreased % oxyhemoglobin saturation) [10]. In areas of the lung where there is excessive ventilation for the amount of perfusion (high $\dot{V}/\dot{Q}$ mismatch), the blood leaving the pulmonary capillary will

have a higher than normal PO_2 but only a minimal improvement, if any, in oxygen content. This is due to the sigmoid shape of the oxyhemoglobin dissociation curve [10]. At the flat, top portion of the curve, where hemoglobin is already totally saturated, an additional increase in PO_2 has little effect on oxygen content or percent oxyhemoglobin saturation. Consequently, areas of low $\dot{V}/\dot{Q}$ mismatch decrease oxygen transfer into the blood far more than areas of high $\dot{V}/\dot{Q}$ mismatch increase it. The overall net result is that PaO_2 is decreased and the $P(A-a)O_2$ gradient is increased [10].

Right-to-Left Shunting. Right-to-left shunting refers to mixed venous blood going directly into the arterial circulation, without having first been exposed to alveolar gas. When the shunted blood mixes with the rest of the arterial blood, it lowers the average oxygen content and therefore the average PaO_2 [7]. The $P(A-a)O_2$ gradient is always significantly increased. There are three basic types of right-to-left shunts [12]: (1) cardiac or great vessel, (2) pulmonary vascular, and (3) pulmonary parenchymal. Cardiac shunts occur from an atrial septal (or patent foramen ovale) or ventricular septal defect with elevated right-sided pressures. A pulmonary vascular shunt generally occurs through an arteriovenous malformation or fistula. A pulmonary parenchymal shunt occurs whenever blood goes through the normal anatomic lung pathways but the surrounding alveoli are either collapsed or filled with something other than air (e.g., in consolidated pneumonia or edema from adult respiratory distress syndrome [ARDS]).

Effect of Decreased Cardiac Output. In patients with hypoxemia due to marked $\dot{V}/\dot{Q}$ abnormalities and/or a large right-to-left shunt, decreases in cardiac output can worsen hypoxemia by further reducing mixed venous O_2 content [13].

Differential Diagnosis of Hypoxemia. To determine whether hypoventilation, $\dot{V}/\dot{Q}$ mismatch, or right-to-left shunting of blood is the cause of hypoxemia, one must look at the $PaCO_2$, $P(A-a)O_2$ gradient, and, occasionally, the response to 100% oxygen. During hypoventilation, the $PaCO_2$ is elevated, the $P(A-a)O_2$ gradient is normal, and the decrease in PaO_2 is accounted for solely by the low PAO_2. If the patient in this setting is given 100% oxygen to breathe (rarely necessary), there will be a dramatic increase in PaO_2 (i.e., PaO_2 >500 mm Hg) [1]. During $\dot{V}/\dot{Q}$ mismatch and right-to-left shunting, the decreased PaO_2 is typically accompanied by an elevated $P(A-a)O_2$ gradient. During $\dot{V}/\dot{Q}$ mismatch the $PaCO_2$ may or may not be elevated, whereas it is almost never elevated in a right-to-left shunt [1]. The PaO_2 in the patient with $\dot{V}/\dot{Q}$ mismatch will show a dramatic rise in response to 100% oxygen (i.e., PaO_2 >500 mm Hg) [1]. The patient with right-to-left shunting, on the other hand, will show a much smaller response, or, in severe cases, no response at all to 100% oxygen [1]. One hundred percent oxygen can be delivered to the nonintubated patient only with the use of a mouthpiece, noseclips, and a known 100% oxygen source, and the patient must breathe this concentration through a one-way breathing valve.

Differentiating low $\dot{V}/\dot{Q}$ mismatch from right-to-left shunting as the cause of hypoxemia is crucial in terms of both cause and therapy. For instance, a large right-to-left shunt secondary to a pulmonary arteriovenous malformation or a massive pulmonary embolus with a right-to-left shunt through a patent foramen ovale will not respond to oxygen therapy, whereas the low PaO_2 seen in patients with COPD is generally easily corrected with supplemental oxygen. To differentiate the right-to-left shunt of cardiac, great vessel, or pulmonary vascular origin from a pulmonary parenchymal cause, contrast echocardiography [14,15] or a quantitative nuclear medicine perfusion lung scan should be obtained. Transesophageal contrast echocardiography is more sensitive and accurate than transthoracic [14]. When a perfusion lung scan is used, the brain and kidneys should be scanned as well, because early appearance of the radionuclide in the brain and kidneys documents an abnormal vascular pathway, allowing quantitation of the shunt [12].

Right-to-left shunts at the cardiac level through a patent foramen ovale in the critically ill are due to the presence of elevated right atrial pressures from loculated pericardial effusion [16], adult respiratory distress syndrome [17], massive pulmonary embolism [17], mechanical ventilatory support with positive end-expiratory pressure [18], right pneumonectomy [19], and right ventricular infarction [15]. Although orthodeoxia (i.e., arterial desaturation accentuated by the upright position and improved by lying down) is an uncommon clinical event, its presence most commonly suggests a right-to-left vascular or cardiac shunt [20]. The mechanism is unclear.

HYPERCAPNIA. There are three pathophysiologic mechanisms that can lead to an elevated $PaCO_2$ (hypercapnia) [21]: (1) breathing a gas containing CO_2, (2) hypoventilation caused by extrapulmonary disorders (Table 53-1), and (3) severe $\dot{V}/\dot{Q}$ mismatch. Clinically, one can dismiss the first and consider only the last two. As previously discussed, hypoventilation-induced arterial hypercapnia occurs when the level of alveolar ventilation is inadequate for the level of CO_2 production because of an extrapulmonary limitation on minute ventilation. It is typically identified by the combination of an elevated $PaCO_2$ and a normal $P(A-a)O_2$ gradient. The major pathophysiologic mechanism responsible for the development of arterial hypercapnia in patients with pulmonary disease (i.e., intrinsic lung disease) is severe (low) $\dot{V}/\dot{Q}$ mismatch. A substantially greater amount of low $\dot{V}/\dot{Q}$ mismatch must be present to cause arterial hypercapnia than to cause hypoxemia. In addition, secondary respiratory muscle overload (resulting from the increased work of breathing and mechanical disadvantage of the inspiratory muscles associated with severe lung derangement) is commonly a significant contributing factor. The reason $\dot{V}/\dot{Q}$ mismatch must be more severe to cause hypercapnia than hypoxemia relates to the different shapes of the CO_2 and oxygen dissociation curves. The CO_2 dissociation curve is more nearly linear than the oxyhemoglobin dissociation curve. Consequently, areas of high $\dot{V}/\dot{Q}$ mismatch can increase CO_2 elimination much more effectively than they can increase pulmonary capillary blood oxygen content. The compensatory process fails when $\dot{V}/\dot{Q}$ mismatch becomes very severe (too few areas of high $\dot{V}/\dot{Q}$ remain to be effective) and/or when respiratory muscle overload limits the necessary increase (in minute) ventilation to these high $\dot{V}/\dot{Q}$ areas. In this setting, the PaO_2 is significantly reduced; and, while the $P(A-a)O_2$ gradient may occasionally normalize with increasing $PaCO_2$ [9], it typically is substantially elevated at a time when the $PaCO_2$ becomes elevated.

Hypercapnia may occur or worsen in patients unable to increase their ventilation appropriately in response to increases in CO_2 production [11]. For instance, in end-stage COPD patients, hypercapnic respiratory failure may worsen due to fever (CO_2 production increases 13% for each 1°C temperature elevation above normal) or nutritional support with excessive total calories or high carbohydrate loads [22]. Since nonprotein calories in the form of fat cause lower production of CO_2 from tissues than isocaloric quantities of carbohydrate, modifying nutritional supplementation in selected patients may influence the degree of hypercapnia.

Respiratory Acid-Base Disorders

Acid-base balance is assessed clinically from the arterial hydrogen ion (H^+) concentration and may be expressed in nanoequivalents per liter or as its negative logarithm, pH_a. The ratio of the relative availability of acid versus base determines the hydrogen ion concentration. The Henderson version of the Henderson-Hasselbalch equation [3], $H^+ = 24 \times (PaCO_2/HCO_3^-)$, reflects the net availability of acid versus base and the resultant hydrogen ion concentration in the body, where $PaCO_2$ represents the acid level and HCO_3^- is an index of the availability of base. Clinically, all acid-base disorders can be evaluated in terms of this basic equation [3].

To manage an acid-base disturbance properly, it should be decided whether it is (1) a respiratory or metabolic disturbance, (2) a simple or complicated disturbance, or (3) an acute or chronic process. A respiratory disturbance is defined by a primary change in $PaCO_2$, whereas a metabolic disorder involves a primary change in the HCO_3^- (see Chap. 80). The simple disorder is characterized by a primary change in only one parameter, whereas a complicated or mixed disorder is characterized by a primary change in both. An acute process is measured in minutes to hours, but a chronic process is measured in days to weeks or longer.

RESPIRATORY ACIDOSIS. The $PaCO_2$ is elevated in primary respiratory acidosis because of respiratory system dysfunction. Under normal circumstances a typical compensatory change occurs in the HCO_3^- level to help minimize the effect of the elevated PCO_2 on hydrogen ion concentration [3].

Duration of Disturbance. When a primary respiratory acidosis occurs, one must determine how long the $PaCO_2$ has been elevated to manage the patient correctly. The relation between the change in hydrogen ion concentration (ΔH^+) and the change in $PaCO_2$ (ΔPCO_2) is considered and the ratio $\Delta H^+/\Delta PCO_2$ computed [3,6]. In the absence of previous pH_a and $PaCO_2$ determinations, pH_a is assumed to have started at 7.40 ($H^+ = 40$ nEq/L), and $PaCO_2$ at 40 mm Hg. (See Table 53-2 to convert H^+ to pH, or vice versa.) The changes in H^+ and $PaCO_2$

Table 53-2. Relation Between pH and [H^+] Shown over a Small Range of Values*

pH	[H^+](nM/L)
7.36	44
7.37	43
7.38	42
7.39	41
7.40	40
—	—
7.41	39
7.42	38
7.43	37
7.44	36

*Note that pH 7.40 corresponds to hydrogen ion concentration of 40 nM/L and that each deviation in pH of 0.01 unit corresponds to opposite deviation in [H^+] of 1 nM/L. For pH values between 7.28 and 7.45, [H^+] calculated empirically in this fashion agrees with the actual value obtained by means of logarithms to the nearest nM/L (nearest 0.01 pH unit). Below pH 7.28 and above pH 7.45, estimated [H^+] is always lower than the actual value, the discrepancy reaching 11% at pH 7.10 and 5% at pH 7.50.

Source: Kassirer JP, Bleich HL: Rapid estimation of plasma carbon dioxide tension from pH and total carbon dioxide content. Reprinted by permission of *The New England Journal of Medicine* 272:1067, 1965.

are calculated by subtracting 40 from the most recently measured values.

Any acute change in HCO_3^- reflects nonrenal body buffering. An acute respiratory acidosis indicates that the elevated $PaCO_2$ has been present for minutes to hours. During a chronic, simple, respiratory acid-base disturbance, the kidneys gradually readjust the HCO_3^- level in the appropriate direction to bring H^+ back toward normal. Chronic respiratory acidosis indicates that the elevated $PaCO_2$ has been present for several days or longer [3]. When there is an acute increase in $PaCO_2$ in the face of chronic hypercapnia, an intermediate degree of compensation should be expected [23]. In the presence of chronic hypercapnia, nonrenal compensation (in the form of increased body buffers) moderates the change in H^+ that occurs for any additional acute change in $PaCO_2$.

The $\Delta H^+/\Delta PCO_2$ ratios for acute, chronic, and acute-on-chronic respiratory acidosis are 0.8, 0.3, and greater than 0.3 but less than 0.8, respectively [6].

Differential Diagnosis and Therapeutic Implications. The differential diagnosis of respiratory acidosis is the same as that of hypercapnic respiratory failure (Table 53-3). The therapeutic approach is also the same.

RESPIRATORY ALKALOSIS. Primary respiratory alkalosis is defined by a decrease in $PaCO_2$ with an accompanying compensatory decrease in HCO_3^-.

Duration of Disturbance. The duration of respiratory alkalosis is analyzed just as for duration of respiratory acidosis [6]. The $\Delta H^+/\Delta PCO_2$ ratios are determined in a similar manner. The ratios for acute and chronic respiratory alkalosis are 0.8 and 0.17 [6].

Differential Diagnosis and Therapeutic Implications. The differential diagnosis of respiratory alkalosis is presented in Table 53-4. Note that a primary respiratory alkalosis may have a normal or elevated $P(A-a)O_2$ gradient. The differential diagnosis of respiratory alkalosis with an elevated $P(A-a)O_2$ gradient is the same as that of nonhypercapnic, hypoxemic respiratory failure.

The general approach to a respiratory alkalosis is to direct therapy at the underlying disorder. However, when respiratory alkalosis continues to worsen in critically ill patients on mechanical ventilatory support, it may become necessary to treat the respiratory alkalosis directly. In such a setting, sedation with or without paralysis of skeletal muscles can be useful.

Physiologic Approach to Respiratory Failure

Respiratory failure occurs when gas exchange becomes significantly impaired. As it is impossible to predict PaO_2 and $PaCO_2$ accurately using clinical criteria [24,25], the diagnosis of respiratory failure depends on ABG analysis. Various clinical signs and symptoms, including those reflecting the effects of hypoxemia and/or hypercapnia on the central nervous system and cardiovascular system (see Chap. 15), may lead to suspicion of the diagnosis, and the ABG is obtained for confirmation.

HYPERCAPNIC VERSUS NONHYPERCAPNIC RESPIRATORY FAILURE. Because respiratory failure is diagnosed

Table 53-3. Differential Diagnosis of Respiratory Acidosis*

Site of abnormality	Disease
Pulmonary disorders of	
Lower airways	Chronic obstructive pulmonary disease, asthma, cystic fibrosis
Lung parenchyma	Industrial lung disease
Pulmonary vasculature	Pulmonary embolism (rare)
Extrapulmonary disorders of	
Central nervous system	Respiratory center depression due to overdose, primary alveolar hypoventilation, myxedema
Peripheral nervous system	Spinal cord disease, amyotrophic lateral sclerosis, Guillain-Barré syndrome
Respiratory muscles	Myasthenia gravis, polymyositis, hypophosphatemia
Chest wall	Ankylosing spondylitis, flail chest, thoracoplasty
Pleura	Restrictive pleuritis
Upper airways	Tracheal obstruction, epiglottitis, adenoidal and tonsillar hypertrophy, peripheral sleep apnea

*This table is not an exhaustive listing; it includes the more common causes for each involved compartment of the respiratory system.

Table 53-4. Causes of Respiratory Alkalosis*

Normal $P(A-a)O_2$ gradient	Elevated $P(A-a)O_2$ gradient
CNS disorders	Sepsis and capillary leak syndrome (ARDS)
Hormones, drugs	Hepatic failure
Salicylates	Chronic interstitial lung diseases
Catecholamines	Pulmonary edema
Progesterone	Cardiogenic
Analeptic overdose	Noncardiogenic (ARDS)
Thyroid hormone excess	Pulmonary emboli
Pregnancy	Pneumonia
High altitude	Asthma
Severe anemia (~ 3 gm/dl hemoglobin)	
Psychogenic hyperventilation	
Endotoxemia	
Mechanical hyperventilation with normal lungs	
During menses after ovulation	

*The differential diagnosis of respiratory alkalosis with an elevated $P(A-a)O_2$ gradient is the same as that of nonhypercapnic, hypoxemic respiratory failure.

based on ABG and because the presence or absence of arterial hypercapnia has both diagnostic and therapeutic implications, it should be determined whether hypercapnic or nonhypercapnic respiratory failure is present.

In hypercapnic respiratory failure the $PaCO_2$ is elevated and PaO_2 is decreased. The $P(A-a)O_2$ gradient may or may not be increased. When hypercapnic respiratory failure results from hypoventilation from dysfunction in the extrapulmonary compartment [5,26,27], the $P(A-a)O_2$ gradient is normal. When it results from severe $\dot{V}/\dot{Q}$ mismatch from abnormalities of the pulmonary compartment [21], the $P(A-a)O_2$ gradient is typically (but not always) very increased (e.g., > 40 mm Hg). When it results from a combination of the two [27], the $P(A-a)O_2$ gradient is typically only modestly increased (e.g., >15–20 mm Hg).

Table 53-5. Salient Features of Hypercapnic and Nonhypercapnic Respiratory Failure

Type of failure	Compartment involved	P($_{A-a}$)O$_2$ gradient	Specific disease
Hypercapnic	Pure extrapulmonary	Normal	Guillain-Barré, CNS depression due to drug overdose
	Pure pulmonary	Very increased (>40 mm Hg)	End-stage pulmonary fibrosis, severe COPD, severe cystic fibrosis
	Combined pulmonary and extrapulmonary	Increased (>15–20 mm Hg)	Kyphoscoliosis
Nonhypercapnic	Pure pulmonary	Increased to very increased	Moderate COPD, asthma, ARDS, cardiogenic pulmonary edema, pulmonary embolism

In nonhypercapnic (hypoxemic) respiratory failure the PaCO$_2$ is normal or decreased, PaO$_2$ is decreased, and P($_{A-a}$)O$_2$ gradient is increased. The condition results from disorders of the pulmonary compartment from either low $\dot{V}/\dot{Q}$ mismatch or a right-to-left shunt [1]. It does not occur from extrapulmonary respiratory disease [1]. Table 53-5 summarizes the salient features of hypercapnic and nonhypercapnic failure.

The cause of respiratory failure can also be approached in terms of which site of the system is malfunctioning [5,26] and the specific disease responsible [5].

RESPIRATORY FAILURE SITE ANALYSIS. The various parts of the respiratory system can be categorized into two major compartments: *extrapulmonary* and *pulmonary* (Table 53-3) [26]. Significant dysfunction in any part in either compartment can lead to impaired gas exchange (i.e., respiratory failure).

The extrapulmonary compartment includes the central nervous system, peripheral nervous system, respiratory muscles, chest wall, pleura, and upper airway. Dysfunction in this compartment causes decreased gas exchange between the atmosphere and the distal airways and alveoli of the lung [26].

The pulmonary compartment includes the lower airway, pulmonary vasculature, and lung parenchyma. Dysfunction in this compartment causes a decrease in gas exchange between the distal airway-alveoli and the pulmonary capillary blood [26].

It is not uncommon for a given disease process to affect components in both compartments and/or for an abnormality in one compartment to cause secondary abnormalities in the other [28].

SPECIFIC DISEASES. The major diseases associated with respiratory failure are listed in Tables 53-3 and 53-4.

Treatment

Respiratory failure can be managed by supportive or specific treatment, which are approached clinically in parallel. The purpose of supportive therapy is to stabilize the clinical situation by improving gas exchange, thereby correcting blood gas and acid-base abnormalities. The purpose of specific therapy is to reverse the basic pathophysiologic process, permanently if possible.

SUPPORTIVE THERAPY. In hypercapnic respiratory failure the major problem is the elevated PaCO$_2$ and resultant respiratory acidosis. The following formula indicates that the PaCO$_2$ may be decreased either by increasing CO$_2$ elimination (i.e.,

increasing alveolar ventilation) or by decreasing the metabolic production of CO$_2$ (decreasing the demand for alveolar ventilation) [26,28]:

$$PaCO_2 = (K) \frac{CO_2 \text{ production}}{\text{Alveolar ventilation}}$$

The increase in ventilation can be achieved by improving work production by the respiratory muscles (i.e., increased force generation and/or decreased respiratory system impedance) [26,28] or, if this is ineffective, by placing the patient on a mechanical ventilator. The key initial decision in hypercapnic respiratory failure is whether or not the patient requires intubation and ventilation [5]. In general, intubation should be strongly considered in the face of a $\Delta H^+/\Delta PCO_2$ ratio that indicates an acute respiratory acidosis that has not rapidly responded to medical therapy [5]. The patient with a ratio that signifies a chronic respiratory acidosis would very rarely be intubated [5]. In the acute-on-chronic situation, the trend of the acidosis is most crucial in deciding whether intubation is necessary [5]. Although these ratios are strictly correct only for simple respiratory acid-base disturbances, we believe they should be applied therapeutically even in a complicated disturbance. If the ratio is consistent with an acute respiratory acidosis, the patient who fails to improve with treatment must be intubated.

In nonhypercapnic (hypoxemic) respiratory failure the major problem is a low PaO$_2$. If the mechanism is low $\dot{V}/\dot{Q}$ mismatch, supportive therapy primarily involves the use of supplemental oxygen [29]. If the problem is a right-to-left cardiac or pulmonary vascular shunt, supplemental oxygen is of only limited benefit; the emphasis is on specific therapy (i.e., surgical repair of an atrial septal defect or obliteration of a pulmonary arteriovenous fistula by interventional radiology, if feasible). If the process involves a diffuse pulmonary intraparenchymal shunt, as in ARDS, positive end-expiratory pressure (PEEP) with or without mechanical ventilation in addition to supplemental oxygen is the major supportive therapeutic modality.

SPECIFIC THERAPY. Since specific therapy varies greatly by disease, no broad generalizations can be made. Examples of specific therapy include the use of naloxone in respiratory center depression from narcotic overdose, the respiratory center-stimulant progesterone in primary alveolar hypoventilation, a diaphragmatic pacemaker for diaphragmatic paralysis secondary to permanent cervical cord injury, nasal continuous positive airway pressure (CPAP) or tracheostomy for peripheral obstructive sleep apnea, bronchodilators and corticosteroids for asthma, and bronchodilators and antibiotics for conditions such as cystic fibrosis. Details of therapy for the most common of these diseases are presented in subsequent chapters.

Summary

A working knowledge of the Henderson or Henderson-Hasselbalch equation, the alveolar air equation, the concept of the $P(A-a)O_2$ gradient, and calculation of $\Delta H^+/\Delta PCO_2$ ratios and their application in therapeutic decision-making allows for systematic management of respiratory failure.

For patients with hypercapnic respiratory failure, it should be quickly determined whether acute respiratory acidosis is present. If it is and treatment does not improve the situation promptly, the patient should be intubated. If chronic respiratory acidosis is present, intubation is not usually required. If acidosis is acute-on-chronic, intubation is not always necessary; the $PaCO_2$ and pH_a should be closely monitored and the endotracheal tube kept ready at the bedside. A useful general guideline is that one should not intubate for the absolute value of any $PaCO_2$ but rather the relationship between $PaCO_2$ and pH_a.

In a patient with hypercapnic respiratory failure, once the decision has been made whether to intubate immediately it should be determined whether the cause is extrapulmonary (e.g., CNS, peripheral nervous system, respiratory muscles, chest wall, or upper airway) or pulmonary. This is done by calculating the $P(A-a)O_2$ gradient on room air (Table 53-5). The next step is to consider the likely specific diseases (Table 53-3).

For patients with respiratory alkalosis and an increased $P(A-a)O_2$ gradient (i.e., nonhypercapnic, hypoxemic respiratory failure), likely specific diseases should be considered (Table 53-4).

References

1. West JB: *Pulmonary Pathophysiology: The Essentials*. 2nd ed. Baltimore, Williams & Wilkins, 1982.
2. Pontoppidan H, Geffin B, Lowenstein E: Acute respiratory failure in the adult (first of three parts). *N Engl J Med* 287:690, 1972.
3. Narins RG, Emmett M: Simple and mixed acid-base disorders: A practical approach. *Medicine* 59:161, 1980.
4. Begin R, Renzetti AO Jr: Alveolar-arterial oxygen pressure gradient. I. Comparison between an assumed and actual respiratory quotient in stable chronic pulmonary disease. II. Relationship to aging and closing volume in normal subjects. *Respir Care* 22:491, 1977.
5. Demers RR, Irwin RS: Management of hypercapnic respiratory failure: A systematic approach. *Respir Care* 24:328, 1979.
6. Bear RA, Gribik M: Assessing acid-base imbalances through laboratory parameters. *Hosp Pract* November 1974, p 157.
7. Bates DV: *Respiratory Function in Disease,* third edition. Toronto, WB Saunders, 1989.
8. Mellemgaard K: The alveolar-arterial oxygen difference: Its size and components in normal man. *Acta Physiol Scand* 67:10, 1966.
9. Gray BA, Blalock JM: Interpretation of the alveolar-arterial oxygen difference in patients with hypercapnia. *Am Rev Respir Dis* 143:4, 1991.
10. Murray JF: *The Normal Lung: The Basis for Diagnosis and Treatment of Pulmonary Disease*. Philadelphia, WB Saunders, 1976.
11. Weinberger SE, Schwartzstein RM, Weiss SW: Hypercapnia. *N Engl J Med* 321:1223, 1989.
12. Robin ED, Laman PD, Goris ML, et al: A shunt is (not) a shunt is (not) a shunt. *Am Rev Respir Dis* 115:553, 1977.
13. Murray JF: Pathophysiology of acute respiratory failure. *Respir Care* 28:531, 1983.
14. Chen W-J, Kuan P, Lien W-P, Lin F-Y: Detection of patent foramen ovale by contrast transesophageal echocardiography. *Chest* 101:1515, 1992.
15. Cox D, Taylor J, Nanda NC: Refractory hypoxemia in right ventricular infarction from right-to-left shunting via a patent foramen ovale: Efficacy of contrast transesophageal echocardiography. *Am J Med* 91:653, 1991.
16. Adolph EA, Lacy WO, Hermoni YK, et al: Reversible orthodeoxia and platypnea due to right-to-left intracardiac shunting related to pericardial effusion. *Ann Intern Med* 116:138, 1992.
17. Dewan NA, Gayasaddin M, Angelillo VA, et al: Persistent hypoxemia due to patent foramen ovale in a patient with adult respiratory distress syndrome. *Chest* 89:611, 1986.
18. Ravenscraft SA, Marinelli WA, Johnson T, Henke CA: Profound hypoxemia precipitated by positive end-expiratory pressure: Induction of an intracardiac shunt. *Crit Care Med* 20:434, 1992.
19. Holtzman J, Lippmann M, Nakhjavan F, Kimbel P: Postpneumonectomy interatrial right-to-left shunt. *Thorax* 35:307, 1980.
20. Tenholder MF, Russell MD, Knight E, Rajagopal KR: Orthodeoxia: A new finding in interstitial fibrosis. *Am Rev Respir Dis* 136:170, 1987.
21. West JB: Causes of carbon dioxide retention in lung disease. *N Engl J Med* 284:1232, 1971.
22. Talpers SS, Romberger DJ, Bunce SB, Pingleton SK: Nutritionally associated increased carbon dioxide production: Excess total calories vs high proportion of carbohydrate calories. *Chest* 102:551, 1992.
23. Ingram RH, Miller RB, Tate LA: Acid-base response to acute carbon dioxide changes in chronic obstructive pulmonary disease. *Am Rev Respir Dis* 108:225, 1973.
24. Mithoefer JC, Bossman OG, Thibeault DW, et al: The clinical estimation of alveolar ventilation. *Am Rev Respir Dis* 98:868, 1968.
25. Comroe JH Jr, Botelho S: The unreliability of cyanosis in the recognition of arterial anoxemia. *Am J Med Sci* 214:1, 1947.
26. Pratter MR, Corwin RW, Irwin RS: An integrated analysis of lung and respiratory muscle dysfunction in the pathogenesis of hypercapnic respiratory failure. *Respir Care* 27:55, 1982.
27. Bergofsky B: Respiratory failure in disorders of the thoracic cage. *Am Rev Respir Dis* 119:643, 1979.
28. Roussos C, Macklem PT: The respiratory muscles. *N Engl J Med* 307:786, 1982.
29. West JB: Ventilation-perfusion relationships. *Am Rev Respir Dis* 116:919, 1977.

54. Pulmonary Edema: Etiologies and Pathogenesis

Daniel P. Schuster

Certainly one of the most common problems the intensivist faces is respiratory failure from pulmonary edema. Clinically, its presentation can be explosive, even life-threatening. Yet pulmonary edema is never a primary problem; it always represents a disturbance in the forces designed to maintain the principal function of the lung: efficient and effective gas exchange. Therefore, although treating pulmonary edema may be a critically important first step, searching for a cause can be the most important determinant of outcome. Structuring this search by considering the pathophysiology of pulmonary edema is a useful and comprehensive approach.

Definition

Pulmonary edema is the abnormal accumulation of extravascular water in both lungs. Normal gas exchange is critically dependent on maintaining an ultrathin barrier at the air-blood interface. In normal alveoli, this barrier consists of little more than the basement membrane of the alveolar epithelium (covered by a thin layer of surfactant) apposed to the basement membrane of the capillary endothelium (Fig. 54-1). When alveolar edema develops, this barrier is widened and gas exchange suffers accordingly.

The normal extravascular water content of the lung is less than 500 ml [1]. At first, any additional extravascular water accumulates within the interstitium (Fig. 54-2). Since interstitial widening does not seriously compromise the thin portion of the alveolocapillary interface, interstitial edema alone generally has little effect on gas exchange. However, the interstitial compartment cannot expand indefinitely. When the extravascular lung water content approximately doubles, alveolar edema usually develops and gas exchange is compromised [2,3].

Pulmonary edema is usually first suspected when any patient with acute onset of tachypnea and respiratory distress also has crackles (rales) by auscultation of the chest. When severe, gurgles (rhonchi) and even sounds of parenchymal consolidation may be heard. In patients with airway hyperresponsiveness, wheezing can develop, even with relatively trivial amounts of interstitial edema.

Disturbances in gas exchange depend on the amount of pulmonary edema, the presence or absence of bronchospasm, the effectiveness of hypoxic vasoconstriction, and the presence or absence of underlying lung disease. With severe pulmonary edema, cyanosis is common. In the absence of underlying lung disease, most patients are hypocapneic, despite the disturbance in ventilation-perfusion matching.

If the cause of pulmonary edema is due to heart failure, signs of myocardial or valvular dysfunction or of right ventricular failure may also be present, along with a third and fourth heart sound. If pulmonary edema is noncardiogenic in origin, then signs of commonly associated disorders (e.g., sepsis, shock) may be present.

Clinical recognition of pulmonary edema, however, ultimately depends on evaluating a standard or portable chest radiograph. The abnormalities on chest radiograph consist of some combination of linear and less well-defined densities that may eventually coalesce to form a so-called alveolar pattern (Fig. 54-3). The pattern and temporal development of these densities are characteristically associated with certain etiologies. These different patterns are considered in detail in Chapter 70. Although other methods exist for measuring or detecting pulmonary edema, they have little clinical application [4]. Under very carefully controlled conditions, the extensiveness of abnormalities on the chest radiograph can correlate reasonably well with quantitative estimates of extravascular water content by some of these other methods [5]. However, since lung density is affected not only by the extravascular water content of the lung but also by blood content, amount of underlying parenchyma, and state of inflation, it is not surprising that other studies have not been able to confirm this relationship between measurements of extravascular water content and abnormalities on chest radiograph [6,7]. Technical differences in obtaining the chest radiograph among different patients undoubtedly contribute to this poor clinical correlation.

Pathogenesis

Starling is generally credited as the first person to describe the forces controlling the movement of water across a biologic semipermeable membrane [8]. The interrelationship among these forces is embodied in the Starling equation. When applied to the lung and modified to account for the total surface area over which filtration might occur, as well as mechanisms by which fluid may be returned to the vascular space, the equation might be written as follows:

$$EVLW = ((SA \times L_p)[(P_{mv} - P_{pmv}) - \sigma(\pi_{mv} - \pi_{pmv})]) - \text{lymph flow} \quad (1)$$

where EVLW = extravascular lung water content; SA = surface area; L_p = the hydraulic conductivity for water; P_{mv} and P_{pmv} = the hydrostatic pressure within the microvascular and perimicrovascular spaces, respectively; σ = the reflection coefficient for protein; π_{mv} and π_{pmv} = the oncotic pressure within the microvascular and perimicrovascular spaces; and lymph flow summarizes those mechanisms responsible for returning fluid to the vascular compartment. The term *microvascular* is used because filtration can occur in small arterioles and venules in the lung, in addition to capillaries.

Note that $SA \times L_p = K_{fc}$, the filtration coefficient for the conductance of water. Although it is difficult to measure SA and L_p separately, expressing the equation this way emphasizes the importance of SA on overall fluid balance in the lung. The reflection coefficient σ is a mathematical expression for vascular permeability to protein. When a semipermeable membrane is completely impermeable to those proteins responsible for producing oncotic pressure, σ has a value of 1.0. Conversely, if the membrane provides no resistance to protein diffusion, σ has a value of zero. Thus, σ in effect expresses how changes in vas-

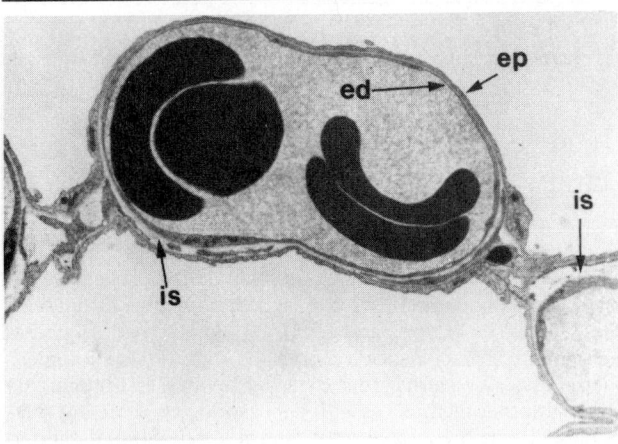

Fig. 54-1. Electron micrograph of a normal dog alveolar capillary. Note the "thin" portion of the alveolar-capillary interface, where endothelium (ed) and epithelium (ep) basement membrane are directly apposed to one another. Also note the "thick" portion of the interface, consisting of normal interstitium (is). (×3000) (From Velazquez et al: PET evaluation of pulmonary vascular permeability: A structure-function correlation. *J Appl Physiol* 70:2206–2216, 1991. With permission.)

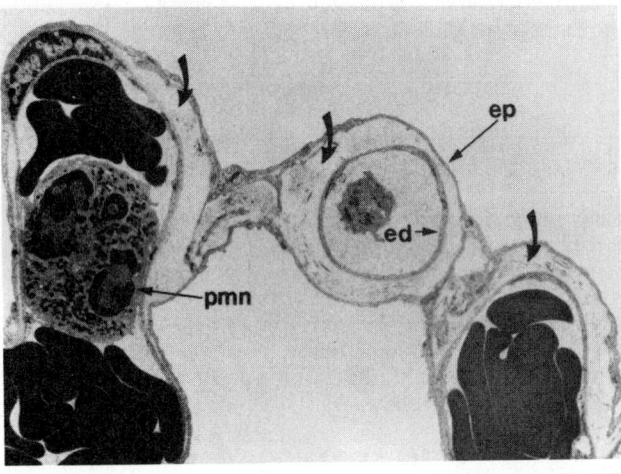

Fig. 54-2. Electron micrograph of interstitial edema (*arrows*) in dog lung. Note interstitial widening compared with Figure 54-1. pmn = polymorphonuclear leukocyte; ep = epithelium; ed = endothelium. (×3000) (From Velazquez et al: PET evaluation of pulmonary vascular permeability: A structure-function correlation. *J Appl Physiol* 70:2206–2216, 1991. With permission.)

cular permeability modify the impact of an oncotic pressure gradient on EVLW accumulation. In the lung, σ for the endothelium is estimated to be about 0.9. For the alveolar epithelium, σ is closer to 1.0 [9]. Thus, the alveolar epithelia are somewhat less "leaky" than the endothelia, resulting in the tendency for interstitial edema to develop before alveolar edema.

The Starling equation is a useful paradigm for evaluating which forces or, more commonly, which *combination* of forces are responsible for the development of pulmonary edema. Note that increases in SA, L_p (i.e., K_{fc}), P_{mv}, and π_{pmv} all result in increased EVLW, assuming other factors remain unchanged. Decreases in P_{pmv}, σ, π_{mv} and lymph flow have a similar effect. Neither P_{mv} nor P_{pmv} is uniform throughout the lung [10].

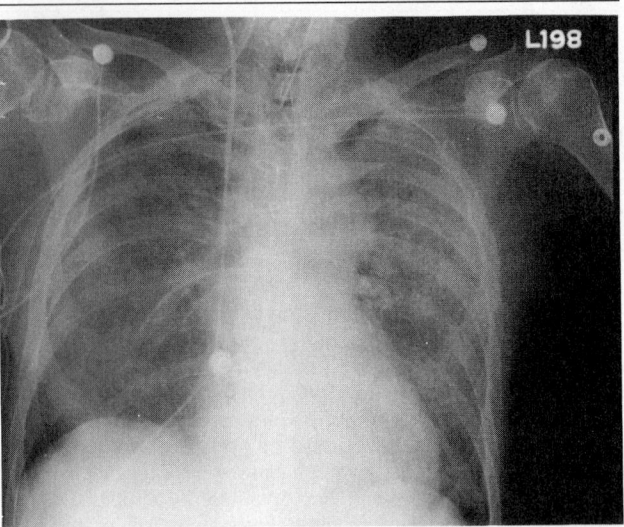

Fig. 54-3. Portable chest radiograph of a patient with noncardiogenic pulmonary edema, showing both interstitial (linear) and alveolar (coalescent) infiltrates.

Both vary as a result of gravity and mechanical properties of the lung. However, P_{mv} apparently increases to a greater extent than P_{pmv} in regions below the level of the left atrium, which helps explain why pulmonary edema tends to develop first in the most gravity-dependent portions of the lung.

In experiments, increases in P_{mv} do not cause proportionate increases in EVLW [11,12]. Indeed, P_{mv} can increase over a reasonably broad physiologic range without causing pulmonary edema. This observation has been explained by the countervailing effect of so-called "safety factors" [13]. Actually, these safety factors simply represent compensatory changes in the other variables of Equation 1 as P_{mv} changes. For instance, as P_{mv} increases, the flux of relatively protein-free fluid into the interstitial compartment increases. As a result, pressure within the interstitial compartment (P_{pmv}) also increases, interstitial oncotic pressure decreases (because of dilution), and lymph flow increases. These changes all tend to oppose further fluid flux or EVLW accumulation. When permeability increases (i.e., when L_p increases and σ decreases), the benefit of diluting interstitial oncotic proteins is reduced. As a result, any increase in hydrostatic pressure will go unopposed. Therefore, reducing hydrostatic pressure is as—if not more—important in limiting EVLW accumulation when permeability is increased as it is when hydrostatic pressures are increased.

When the interstitial compartment cannot expand further and other safety factors also cannot keep up with the increased flux of fluid from the vascular space, alveolar flooding develops (Fig. 54-4). The term *flooding* is used because experimental evidence indicates that filling of the alveolar compartment seems to be an all-or-none phenomenon [14]. The exact site at which flooding occurs is still unknown, although the most likely point is at terminal airways "upstream" from the alveoli [15].

One consequence of flooding is that the protein content of alveolar and interstitial edema is the same. This feature is useful in distinguishing increased hydrostatic pressure forms of pulmonary edema from those due to increased vascular permeability in the first few hours after presentation [16]. In the former, interstitial protein content has been diluted, therefore the protein content of any alveolar fluid recovered is also less than that of plasma (usually less than half). When edema develops pri-

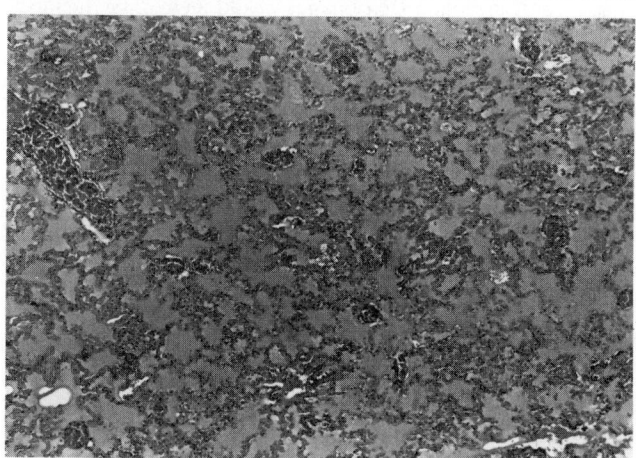

Fig. 54-4. Light micrograph of alveolar flooding with proteinaceous edema in dog lung. (×100) (From Velazquez et al: PET evaluation of pulmonary vascular permeability: A structure-function correlation. *J Appl Physiol* 70:2206–2216, 1991. With permission.)

Table 54-1. Changes in the Variables of the Starling Equation Associated with Pulmonary Edema

Variable	Change	Clinical examples
L_p	↑	ARDS
σ	↓	ARDS
P_{mv}	↑	CHF, volume overload, pulmonary venous hypertension (any cause)
P_{pmv}	↓	UAO, reexpansion pulmonary edema*
π_{mv}	↓	Severe hypoalbuminemia
π_{pmv}	↑	None known

L_p = hydraulic conductivity for water; σ = reflection coefficient for protein; P_{mv} and P_{pmv} = microvascular and perimicrovascular hydrostatic pressures, respectively; π_{mv} and π_{pmv} = microvascular and perimicrovascular oncotic pressures, respectively; ARDS = acute respiratory distress syndrome; CHF = congestive heart failure; UAO = upper airway obstruction [20]. UAO may also cause pulmonary edema by increasing vascular permeability by unknown mechanisms [21].

*Reexpansion pulmonary edema may actually be a form of ischemia-reperfusion injury, resulting in increased vascular permeability.

marily because of increased vascular permeability, the protein content of alveolar fluid is closer to that of plasma. After several hours, and certainly after several days, the protein concentration of the alveolar fluid is affected by the effectiveness of mechanisms responsible for edema resolution [17].

Etiology

Clinical examples of disturbances in the variables of Equation 1 are listed in Table 54-1. There are no known instances of primary increases in π_{pmv} as a cause of pulmonary edema. Also, there are no known instances of changes in vascular permeability that affect L_p but not σ.

The vast majority of cases of pulmonary edema are caused by increased hydrostatic pressures or increased vascular permeability. Undoubtedly, the most common cause of increased pulmonary microvascular hydrostatic pressure is left ventricular failure (congestive heart failure; considered in detail in Chap. 42). By itself, intravascular volume expansion (overload) is probably an unusual cause of pulmonary edema. However, in combination with renal failure, myocardial dysfunction, or increased vascular permeability, intravascular volume expansion commonly leads to pulmonary edema.

The incidence of pulmonary venous hypertension as a cause of or contributor to pulmonary edema is unknown, although many mediators (e.g., thromboxane, histamine) are capable of specifically increasing pulmonary venous resistance. Unfortunately, there is no simple bedside technique for measuring the effect of increased pulmonary venous resistance per se on pulmonary microvascular pressure. Wedge pressure is a measure of the pressure at the junction of the stagnant column of blood caused by pulmonary artery balloon occlusion and flowing blood (see Chap. 4). Typically, this point is in the large pulmonary veins near the left atrium. When left atrial pressure is normal but pulmonary venous resistance is increased, the pulmonary microvascular pressure is increased but wedge pressure is normal. Thus, many clinically relevant cases of increased hydrostatic pressure pulmonary edema due specifically to increased pulmonary venous hypertension may go unrecognized

or be misdiagnosed as increased permeability pulmonary edema. For instance, pulmonary edema associated with tocolytic therapy seems to behave like pulmonary edema associated with other causes of increased hydrostatic pressure [18]. However, wedge pressures, though measured infrequently in this condition, often are normal [18]. Although this observation would generally imply increased permeability, pulmonary venous hypertension (perhaps from thromboxane release) would also explain this finding.

The possibility of increased pulmonary venous pressures should be considered whenever there is a significant gradient between pulmonary artery mean and wedge pressures. However, the gradient could be due to either increased pulmonary arterial or increased pulmonary venous resistance. Although Holloway et al. proposed a method for measuring pulmonary capillary pressures (not wedge pressures) at the bedside [19], clinical application in the intubated, tachypneic, mechanically ventilated patient is difficult.

According to Equation 1, decreases in π_{mv} should cause pulmonary edema. The clinically relevant example would be hypoalbuminemia. However, although hypoalbuminemia permits edema to develop at lower P_{mv} [11], it is rarely by itself a cause of pulmonary edema. In part this is because as π_{mv} decreases, so does π_{pmv}. Furthermore, hypoalbuminemia rarely develops very acutely. Therefore, other compensatory mechanisms (e.g., increased lymphatic function) have time to become effective. Nevertheless, hypoalbuminemia often complicates other clinical circumstances in which intravascular hydrostatic pressures are increased by volume overload or myocardial dysfunction or in which permeability is increased (e.g., by sepsis).

Also according to Equation 1, decreases in P_{pmv} should cause pulmonary edema. In normal lungs, P_{pmv} approximates pleural pressure and typically is slightly negative relative to atmospheric pressure [20]. Two clinical examples where P_{pmv} probably decreases suddenly and significantly are reexpansion pulmonary edema (i.e., associated with rapid expansion of a collapsed lung) and pulmonary edema associated with upper airway obstruction (e.g., near hanging). However, other evidence indicates that reexpansion pulmonary edema is characterized by an increased protein concentration in alveolar edema fluid [21], suggesting a change in permeability, plausibly related to a kind of ischemia-reperfusion injury. The pathogenesis of pulmonary edema in association with upper airway obstruction is probably more complex than simply the result of an increased hydrostatic gradient secondary to a decrease in P_{pmv} [22].

The most common cause of increased permeability pulmonary edema is the acute respiratory distress syndrome (ARDS). Indeed, some would probably consider *any* case of increased permeability edema an example of ARDS. The pathogenesis and pathophysiology of ARDS are discussed in Chapter 55.

Of course, more than one cause of pulmonary edema may be present. In many cases, pulmonary edema during ARDS is probably due to both increased permeability and increased intravascular hydrostatic pressures, the latter from a combination of volume overload due to therapy for shock and/or increased pulmonary venous resistance from the release of mediators such as thromboxane and histamine.

Resolution

Despite the importance of pulmonary edema, much less is known about how it resolves than how it is generated. Several important new insights into its resolution have been reported. For one, it is clear that the resolution of pulmonary edema is not simply a reversal of how it developed. Pulmonary edema can and probably does resolve via several pathways: lymphatics, pulmonary circulation, bronchial circulation, airways, and pleural space. The quantitative importance of each probably depends on the rapidity with which edema develops, the nature of the edema fluid, the amount of edema that develops, whether vascular permeability is normal, and therapeutic factors (e.g., mechanical ventilation with PEEP) that might interfere with resolution by certain routes (e.g., the lymphatics).

Normally, a small amount of fluid moves across the alveolocapillary membrane and is carried back to the central circulation via lymphatics [23]. In experimental animals, however, interstitial *edema* apparently is not cleared by lymphatics, and instillation of fluid into the alveolar space seems to resolve primarily into the pulmonary circulation [24,25,26]. The relevance of this observation is uncertain because clinically pulmonary edema is always first accompanied by interstitial edema and/or increased vascular permeability. Changes in pulmonary blood flow do not affect the *rate* of edema clearance, implying that the pulmonary circulation serves simply as a reservoir for fluid clearance.

The clearance of proteinaceous alveolar edema (as in ARDS) is especially interesting. Matthay and co-workers have shown that as the edema leaves the alveolar compartment, the protein concentration increases; further clearance is slower but not absent [27,28]. The fact that clearance continues despite the unfavorable oncotic pressure gradient suggests that it is to some degree dependent on an active transport process [29,30]. Indeed, the alveolar epithelia do actively transport sodium ion into the interstitium (with water following passively). Furthermore, Matthay et al. have reported that patients with ARDS who can increase the protein concentration in alveolar lavage fluid (implying intact epithelial transport) have a better prognosis than those patients who cannot do so [27]. It remains to be determined whether these observations can be confirmed and are generalizable, but they do hold promise that therapeutic interventions to improve edema resolution are plausible.

Even less clear is how the protein in the alveolar space is cleared. Although potential mechanisms include diffusion, mucociliary clearance, and transcellular transport, it seems likely that much of the protein will be incorporated as hyaline membranes into the rest of the inflammatory exudate that accompanies the increased permeability edema of ARDS. Accordingly,

clearance by alveolar macrophages would seem to be the most likely, albeit still unproven, route.

References

1. Sivak ED, Wiedemann HP: Clinical measurement of extravascular lung water. *Crit Care Clin* 2:511, 1986.
2. Bongard FS, Matthay M, Mackersie RC, Lewis FR: Morphologic and physiologic correlates of increased extravascular lung water. *Surgery* 96:395, 1984.
3. Gabel JC, Drake RE, Arens JF: Oxygenation as an indicator of lung fluid accumulation. *Anesthesiology* 51:S156, 1979.
4. Lily CM, Ishizaka A, Raffin TA: The measurement of lung water. *J Crit Care* 5:252, 1990.
5. Milne ENC, Pistolesi M, Miniati M, Giuntini C: The radiographic distinction of cardiogenic and noncardiogenic edema. *Am J Roentgenol* 144:879, 1985.
6. Eisenberg PR, Hansbrough JR, Anderson D, Schuster DP: A prospective study of lung water measurements during patient management in an intensive care unit. *Am Rev Respir Dis* 136:662, 1987.
7. Smith RC, Mann H, Greenspan RH, et al: Radiographic differentiation between different etiologies of pulmonary edema. *Invest Radiol* 22:859, 1987.
8. Starling EH: On the absorption of fluids from the connective tissue spaces. *J Physiol (Lond)* 19:312, 1896.
9. Matthay MA: Pathophysiology of pulmonary edema. *Clin Chest Med* 6:301, 1985.
10. Camp MA, Gray BA: Pulmonary edema: Lung water balance in relation to physiologic monitoring and clinical outcome in the critically ill, in Carlson RW, Geheb MA (ed): *Principles and Practice of Medical Intensive Care*. Philadelphia, WB Saunders, 1993.
11. Guyton AC, Lindsey AW: Effect of elevated left atrial pressure and decreased plasma protein concentration on the development of pulmonary edema. *Circ Res* 7:649, 1959.
12. Brigham KL, Woolverton WC, Blake LH, et al: Increased sheep lung vascular permeability caused by *Pseudomonas* bacteria. *J Clin Invest* 54:792, 1974.
13. Guyton AC, Taylor AE, Ganger JR: Dynamics of edema and the safety factor against edema, in Guyton AC, Taylor AE, Ganger JR (eds): *Circulatory Physiology. II. Dynamics and Control of the Body Fluids*. Philadelphia, WB Saunders, 1975.
14. Staub NC, Nagano H, Pearce ML: Pulmonary edema in dogs, especially the sequence of fluid accumulation in the lungs. *J Appl Physiol* 22:227, 1967.
15. Staub NC: The pathogenesis of pulmonary edema. *Prog Cardiovasc Dis* 23:53, 1980.
16. Fein A, Grossman RF, Jones JG, et al: The value of edema fluid protein measurements in patients with pulmonary edema. *Am J Med* 67:32, 1979.
17. Matthay MA: Resolution of pulmonary edema: Mechanisms of liquid, protein, and cellular clearance from the lung. *Clin Chest Med* 6:521, 1985.
18. Pisani RJ, Rosenow EC: Pulmonary edema associated with tocolytic therapy. *Ann Intern Med* 110:714, 1989.
19. Holloway H, Perry M, Downey J, et al: Estimation of effective pulmonary capillary pressure in intact lungs. *J Appl Physiol* 54:846, 1983.
20. Meyer BJ, Meyer A, Guyton AC: Interstitial fluid pressure. V. Negative pressure in the lung. *Circ Res* 22:263, 1968.
21. Jackson RM, Veal CF: Re-expansion, re-oxygenation, and rethinking. *Am J Med Sci* 298:44, 1989.
22. Kollef MH, Pluss J: Noncardiogenic pulmonary edema following upper airway obstruction. *Medicine* 70:91, 1991.
23. Staub NC: "State-of-the-art" review: Pathogenesis of pulmonary edema. *Am Rev Respir Dis* 109:358, 1974.
24. Sakuma T, Pittet JF, Jayr C, Matthay MA: Alveolar liquid and protein clearance in the absence of blood flow or ventilation in sheep. *J Appl Physiol* 74:176, 1993.
25. Kambara K, Longworth E, Serikov VB, Staub NC: Effect of interstitial edema on lung lymph flow in goats in the absence of filtration. *J Appl Physiol* 72:1142, 1992.

26. Pearse DB, Wagner EM, Sylvester JT: Edema clearance in isolated sheep lungs. *J Appl Physiol* 74:126, 1993.
27. Matthay MA, Weiner-Kronish JP: Intact epithelial barrier function is critical for the resolution of alveolar edema in humans. *Am Rev Respir Dis* 142:1250, 1990.
28. Matthay MA, Berthiaume Y, Staub NC: Long-term clearance of liquid and protein from the lungs of unanesthetized sheep. *J Appl Physiol* 59:928, 1985.
29. Berthiaume Y, Broaddus VA, Gropper MA, Tanita T, et al: Alveolar liquid and protein clearance from normal dog lungs. *J Appl Physiol* 65:585, 1988.
30. Goodman BE, Brown JEJ, Crandall ED: Regulation of transport across pulmonary alveolar epithelial cell monolayers. *J Appl Physiol* 57:703, 1984.

55. *Acute Respiratory Distress Syndrome*

Daniel P. Schuster and Marin H. Kollef

Intensivists maintain a passionate interest in the acute respiratory distress syndrome (ARDS) even though it comprises only a small fraction of the total intensive care unit (ICU) patient population. Undoubtedly, this interest is sustained by the need to be familiar with many aspects of caring for the critically ill patient. A "complete" approach to managing the ARDS patient involves a broad-based knowledge of various etiologies; of lung, heart, brain, liver, and other organ pathophysiology; of disordered interactions between organ systems; and of the support of vital organs with complicated machinery and potent medications for prolonged periods while monitoring for complications of nosocomial infection, malnutrition, drug toxicity, and so on. It is a formidable task, but there are few rewards in critical care medicine as great as bringing a patient with ARDS through such a devastating illness, because full recovery of lung and other organ system function—while not as common as one would like—is still quite possible.

Definition

Although ARDS was first described more than a quarter century ago [1], in retrospect it was not a new entity even then [2]. Many names have been used to describe this clinical entity, but ARDS is now used almost exclusively to characterize acute respiratory failure in association with new bilateral radiographic infiltrates. Acute lung injury, noncardiogenic pulmonary edema, and diffuse alveolar damage are also commonly used in connection with, if not synonymously with, ARDS. Acute lung injury refers to some acute change in the lung's function, typically either for gas exchange and/or as a barrier to abnormal water or solute accumulation in the air spaces. As the term is typically used, this *functional* injury is the result of *structural* changes in the alveolocapillary unit, identified histologically as diffuse alveolar damage. Diffuse alveolar damage is defined as endothelial, and especially type I alveolar epithelial, cell necrosis associated with hyaline membranes and proteinaceous alveolar edema. Thus, abnormalities in lung function (e.g., bronchospasm) or purely inflammatory conditions (e.g., pneumonia) that leave the alveolar-capillary unit intact are not usually considered forms of acute lung injury.

Inevitably, a breakdown in endothelial barrier function leads to the development of noncardiogenic pulmonary edema via increased vascular "permeability" (see Chap. 54). As the air spaces fill with edema, the gas exchange and mechanical properties of the lung deteriorate. When severe, the clinical manifestations are those of ARDS.

Thus, ARDS can be defined as the clinical manifestations of severe acute lung injury, characterized pathologically as diffuse alveolar damage and pathophysiologically by the development of noncardiogenic pulmonary edema due to increased microvascular permeability. It is quite possible, if not likely, that lesser degrees of injury result in less disturbed physiology—even to the point that patients may not require ventilatory or ICU support [3]. The extent to which this more moderate form of acute lung injury may exist, or may be clinically relevant, is not known.

Etiology

Given that the lungs are exposed to an enormous number of air pollutants, are at risk for airway contamination by aspiration, and filter nearly the entire cardiac output every minute, it is not surprising that a long list of agents, mediators, and conditions have been reported as causes of both diffuse alveolar damage and ARDS [4,5,6] (Table 55-1). However, many isolated case reports of "ARDS" may simply be examples of noncardiogenic pulmonary edema without diffuse alveolar damage (DAD). In many of these cases DAD has not been reported, and often recovery is relatively rapid and benign.

Although Murray et al. [7] and others have made a useful distinction between "direct" and "indirect" causes of ARDS, perhaps it is better to say that ARDS is *associated* with the underlying condition, as opposed to being *caused* by it, when ARDS is the result of indirect mechanisms. Since many patients do not develop ARDS even after exposure to an agent thought to cause direct lung injury, all of these conditions are sometimes referred to even more indefinitely as risk factors, rather than as causes per se.

Direct causes of lung injury lead to ARDS more frequently than indirect ones. In one study, 36 percent of patients with apparent pulmonary aspiration developed ARDS, as opposed to only 5 percent of patients who required multiple blood transfusions [5]. On the other hand, indirect mechanisms cause ARDS much more frequently overall than do direct ones. Fully 47 to 63 percent of all ARDS cases are associated with sepsis syndrome [4,5,6] (now generally referred to as systemic inflammatory response syndrome, or SIRS) (see Chap. 173).

The risk of developing ARDS increases as the number of potential causes (risk factors) increase [4,5,6]. Indeed, since sepsis is so often suspected as an underlying contributor, many physicians begin treatment for possible infectious etiologies immediately after considering the diagnosis of ARDS. When

Table 55-1. Causes of Acute Respiratory Distress Syndrome

Shock: Any type, especially septic shock

Infection: Any pneumonia or sepsis from any cause, especially viral pneumonia, *P. carinii* pneumonia, or gram-negative pneumonia/ sepsis

Trauma: Burns, fat emboli, lung contusion, head trauma

Toxic gas inhalation: Prolonged hyperoxia, smoke, NO_2, NH_3, Cl_2, cadmium, phosgene

Aspiration: Gastric contents, near drowning

Drug ingestion*: Barbiturates, chlordiazepoxide, colchicine, dextran-40, ethchlorvynol, fluorescein, heroin, methadone, salicylates, thiazides

Miscellaneous: Pancreatitis, post-cardiopulmonary bypass, multiple blood transfusions, leukoagglutinin reaction, eclampsia, air emboli, amniotic fluid emboli, bowel infarction, carcinomatosis, high altitude, neurogenic causes other than head trauma, radiologic contrast media, protamine, diffuse alveolar hemorrhage

*Diffuse alveolar damage has not been documented for all of these conditions when associated with ARDS; therefore, some may simply be examples of noncardiogenic pulmonary edema.

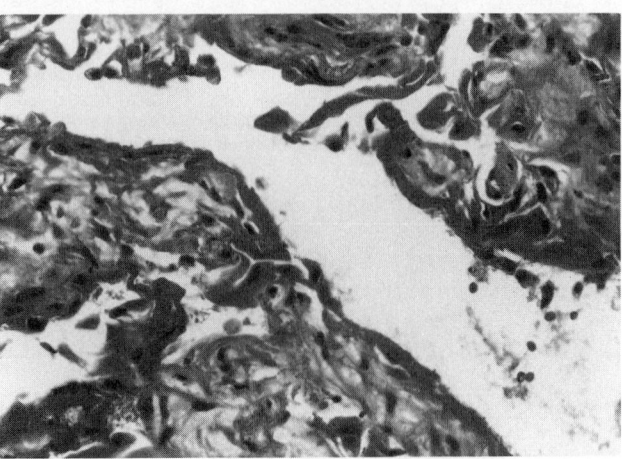

Fig. 55-1. Example of diffuse alveolar damage with prominent hyaline membranes within a bronchiole.

sepsis precedes ARDS, the abdomen is often the source of infection (see Chap. 159). In contrast, when sepsis develops in a patient with established ARDS, the source is usually nosocomial pulmonary infection [8,9,10].

Virtually all the major classes of infectious agents have been associated with the development of sepsis (and ARDS), although gram-negative organisms are still responsible for the majority of cases that develop in hospitalized patients. When ARDS develops outside the hospital because of infection, viral infection is the most likely cause. However, *Pneumocystis carinii* infection can also cause ARDS [11]. It should be suspected in patients with AIDS and those at risk for human immunodeficiency virus (HIV) infection (see Chaps. 74 and 93).

In the absence of obvious massive trauma or burns, if ARDS develops in an otherwise healthy subject outside the hospital, the most likely causes are viral infection, illicit drug ingestion, toxic gas inhalation, or gastric aspiration after some other event that caused a change in the level of consciousness (e.g., seizure or cardiac arrest). In contrast, when ARDS develops in a hospitalized patient, the most likely cause is either sepsis syndrome or gastric aspiration.

Pathology

The initial pathologic lesions are interstitial swelling, proteinaceous intraalveolar edema, alveolar hemorrhage, and fibrin deposition [12,13]. Complete alveolar flooding characteristically occurs in some regions next to alveoli that are otherwise apparently normal. On electron microscopy degenerative cellular changes, including basement membrane disruption and denudation, are found among both endothelial and alveolar epithelial cells, although damage to epithelial cells is usually much more prominent. After 1 to 2 days, hyaline membranes are commonly observed within alveoli (Fig. 55-1). These bands of eosinophilic material represent cellular debris from alveolar lining cells that have sloughed and mixed with fibrin. At this point, cellular infiltrate may be minimal or may be dominated by neutrophils. Fibrin thrombi can be seen in some of the alveolar capillaries and small pulmonary arteries.

Type I alveolar epithelial cells, which cover 95 percent of the alveolar surface, are terminally differentiated cells that cannot regenerate. It is type II cells (those responsible for surfactant production) that several days after the onset of ARDS proliferate and eventually differentiate into new type I cells to reline the alveolar walls.

After approximately 1 week, usually most of the alveolar edema has resolved and hyaline membranes are much less prominent. In the absence of complicating pneumonia, the neutrophilic infiltrate is replaced by mononuclear cells and interstitial fibroblast proliferation and new collagen deposition becomes increasingly prominent. Although lung fibrosis may develop subsequently, the extent of involvement is enormously variable. Some patients seem to resolve lung injury with little if any fibrosis, while others go on to develop severe parenchymal remodeling and so-called honeycombing. When parenchymal fibrosis does develop, intimal fibrosis and medial hypertrophy of pulmonary arterioles, along with complete obliteration of portions of the vascular bed, are also common. Why some patients recover so uneventfully and others develop disastrous degrees of scarring is unknown. Many potentially confounding variables may play a role, including the severity and extent of initial injury, the possibility of ongoing injury, the coexistence of sepsis, the development of nosocomial infection, and the consequences of treatment (e.g., oxygen toxicity and barotrauma).

Lung fibrosis in ARDS is often referred to as interstitial because structures between air spaces appear to be markedly widened by fibrotic material. Newer immunohistochemical techniques have revealed, however, that this fibrosis is often the result of either alveolar collapse or *intra*alveolar fibrosis, in which the proteinaceous edema and cellular debris of the exudative stage have been incorporated into the alveolar wall. Deposition of new collagen within the interstitial space per se appears to be relatively uncommon [14,15].

Pathogenesis

There is a temporal component to DAD that can be divided into an exudative phase (days 1–3), a proliferative phase (days 3–7 or so), and a fibrotic phase (after 1 week).

EXUDATIVE PHASE. Even when injury is initiated by so-called direct means, the exact mechanism of damage to the pulmonary endothelium and epithelium is still unknown. Explaining increased vascular permeability is especially interesting, since histologic evidence of damage to the endothelium, unlike the alveolar epithelium, is relatively difficult to find, even in early ARDS [12,13].

The most likely proximate agents of damage to the lungs are various reactive oxygen species and proteases [16,17]. Many of these reactive oxygen species interact and combine to form new reactive molecules, or they initiate chain reactions in which the total number of reactive molecules becomes greatly amplified. Numerous studies have shown that reactive oxygen species and proteases can cause cell damage in both in vitro and in vivo systems [16,17,18].

Normally, cells are protected from damage by reactive oxygen species by potent intravascular scavengers, such as superoxide dismutase, catalase and glutathione [18]. Extracellular defenses, however, are not as efficient or as effective. Likewise, antiproteases normally protect lung tissue from proteolytic digestion, but during ARDS these defenses are either overwhelmed or inactivated.

If oxidants and proteolytic enzymes are the most likely agents of cellular damage, then the most likely source of production is the neutrophil [19–23]. The mechanism(s) by which neutrophils attach to endothelial cells (via adhesion molecules) has been the focus of enormous interest recently, because if adhesion can be prevented, injury might be reduced or eliminated [24]. Neutrophils (and other cells) can also release a number of arachidonic acid metabolites [25]. Although these eicosanoids can markedly affect the development and course of lung injury (as chemoattractants, by their vasoactive effects, or by modulating the inflammatory response), they probably are not themselves responsible for increased permeability or cell damage per se.

It is interesting that ARDS can develop in patients with severe neutropenia [26,27]. It is possible, if not likely, that other cells residing in the lungs (e.g., tissue macrophages) are also responsible for the increased production of toxic molecules. Alternatively, some molecules (e.g., endotoxin, tumor necrosis factor, the interleukins, or platelet activating factor) may be able to initiate membrane damage directly, by as yet uncertain mechanisms.

The increased expression of these toxic molecules by their cellular sources is probably initiated by complement, endotoxin (lipopolysaccharide), and various cytokines (especially tumor necrosis factor-alpha and interleukin-1) [28]. Endotoxin can also stimulate the production of cytokines from blood as well as alveolar and lung tissue macrophages, which may serve as a source for producing reactive oxygen species and eicosanoids in neutropenic patients. How complement or cytokine production might be stimulated in the absence of infection or endotoxemia is not known.

Many of these processes are not specific for ARDS but are present during any septic state or, more locally, during pneumonia. Yet pneumonia, even gram-negative pneumonia, generally does not cause alveolar damage per se. Apparently, pneumonia remains a *regulated* response to infection, whereas ARDS represents, to some extent, a breakdown in this regulation. Which elements of the normal regulatory process are uncontrolled in ARDS is still unknown.

FIBROPROLIFERATIVE PHASE. After neutrophils are activated, they not only release potentially toxic products along endothelial surfaces but also migrate into the lung interstitium, where they can damage resident cells and release mediators (e.g., leukotriene B$_4$) that act as chemoattractants for other inflammatory cells. These cells, along with alveolar macrophages, are in part responsible for the orderly removal of cellular debris and for the orderly repair of damaged alveolar epithelium. In some patients, however, the repair process is disordered, resulting in an exuberant fibrosis that makes gas exchange ineffective and inefficient.

Why one patient completely resolves lung injury and another develops extensive fibrosis is unknown. Using normal wound healing as a paradigm, it seems likely that an intact basement membrane is essential for normal repair [14]. An intact basement membrane acts as a scaffold on which replicating type II pneumocytes can migrate and differentiate into new type I cells to reestablish a normal alveolar lining. Thus, one factor determining the development of fibrosis may be the severity of the initial injury; that is, with severe basement membrane disruption, normal cells cannot breach the large gaps that develop, and the spaces are filled by scar tissue instead [14].

Another factor may be the presence of ongoing or repetitive injuries, such as persistent endotoxemia, toxic effects of oxygen therapy, or barotrauma from high airway pressures. These additional insults may also disrupt or overwhelm the normal repair process.

The molecular and cell-cell signals that control this whole process are poorly understood [29]. It seems likely that platelet-derived growth factor, fibronectin, TGF-α, EGF, IGF, PGE, IL-6, TGF-β, proteases, and antiproteases and their regulation are important factors in the ARDS repair process. Indeed, some have speculated that wound healing, idiopathic pulmonary fibrosis, and ARDS are simply variations on the same theme, differing principally in acuteness, severity, and extensiveness of the process rather than on fundamental differences in regulation of the processes as a whole [14,15]. In ARDS, the impact of nosocomial lung infection on the normal regulation of this fibroproliferative response also is probably important.

In addition to repair of the alveolar epithelium, changes in the microvasculature can have a significant impact on the effectiveness of overall repair from lung injury [30]. Endothelial injury causes platelets to be sequestered, the coagulation cascade to be initiated, and microthrombi to develop. Experimentally, different types of microemboli can cause acute lung injury, while more proximal occlusions of the pulmonary artery seem to have less of an immediate effect [31,32]. The natural history of microthrombi in ARDS is unknown. With resolution and reperfusion of still injured areas, a type of reperfusion injury might develop [33]. On the other hand, severe fibrosis is associated with concomitant progressive occlusion and obliteration of the pulmonary vascular bed. Pulmonary arterial filling defects have been found in ARDS, but how they resolve and/or affect the resolution of the injured lung parenchyma is unknown [30]. Finally, the balance (or imbalance) between procoagulant and fibrinolytic systems in the alveolar space may be important factors affecting fibroproliferative repair [34].

Pathophysiology

ACCUMULATION AND RESOLUTION OF PULMONARY EDEMA. This process is considered in detail in Chapter 54.

GAS EXCHANGE. At the time of onset, the hallmarks of ARDS are severe tachypnea and hypoxemia. The hypoxemia in ARDS is primarily the result of extensive right-to-left intrapulmonary shunting of blood flow, which may approach 25 to 50 percent of cardiac output [35]. Since blood flowing through a shunt is not exposed to alveolar gas, supplemental oxygen per se is of little or no value in improving the hypoxemia of ARDS, thus accounting for the "refractory" nature of the hypoxemia. The shunt in ARDS is due to persistent perfusion of atelectatic and fluid-filled alveoli. Perfusion to poorly ventilated lung regions is usually reduced by hypoxic pulmonary vasoconstriction, which limits the amount of shunt for any given amount of poorly ventilated lung. In ARDS, however, hypoxic vasoconstriction may be ineffective or absent in some patients, thereby actually increasing (in relative terms) the magnitude of shunt [36]. Endotoxemia and the increased production of eicosanoids such as prostacyclin may be responsible (at least in part) for this compensatory failure. Another factor may be differences among patients in the mixed venous oxygen concentration of blood perfusing the injured lung regions, caused by differences in cardiac output or tissue oxygen consumption (see Chaps. 58 and 181).

As alveolar edema resolves during the first week, the amount of shunt and the need for supplemental oxygen and airway pressure therapy decrease and stabilize. At this point, further improvements in oxygenation depend on whether the fibroproliferative response can restore normal lung architecture for gas exchange.

Increased physiologic dead space ventilation and intrapulmonary shunt are both responsible for the tachypnea and high minute ventilation required to achieve effective carbon dioxide excretion in ARDS. One cause of increased dead space ventilation is hyperventilation of still normal or relatively normal alveolar units, a process exaggerated by differences in the distribution of ventilation with mechanical ventilatory support (see Chap. 66) and by overinflation of lung units when mean airway pressure is increased by PEEP or other maneuvers. The dead space-to-tidal volume ratio is normally 0.3, but in ARDS this ratio can increase to 0.6 to 0.9. In other words, in severe ARDS, as much as 90 percent of each tidal volume is "wasted"—it does not participate in gas exchange. As a consequence, a minute ventilation of 30 liters per minute or more may be necessary to achieve eucapnia (not necessarily a desirable goal; see section on management). The normal minute ventilation is only 6 to 8 liters per minute.

In patients who resolve ARDS relatively rapidly (over 10–14 days), minute ventilation and dead space ventilation decrease in tandem with improvements in oxygenation. In patients with more severe ARDS (i.e., those who go on to develop significant lung fibrosis), minute ventilatory requirements stay high even as oxygenation improves. Presumably, as fibrosis develops progressive amounts of the vascular bed are obliterated, contributing to the increase in dead space ventilation even as alveolar edema and shunt fraction resolve.

LUNG MECHANICS. Because high airway pressures are almost always required when usual tidal volumes are used for ventilation in ARDS, lung compliance is often said to be reduced. (Actually this is a misnomer, since this method of evaluating static pressure-volume relationships is a measure of *respiratory system* chest wall-lung compliance.) For instance, the normal respiratory system compliance is greater than 100 ml per cm H_2O, for a tidal volume of about 8 ml per kilogram. Thus, when delivered by mechanical ventilation with no end-expiratory pressure, the static inflation pressure for this tidal volume should be less than 6 cm H_2O. With ARDS, it is not unusual to see static inflation pressures of more than 28 cm H_2O (i.e., compliance < 20 ml/cm H_2O).

To reflect the actual intrinsic elastic properties of lung tissue, compliance must be calculated for a given volume of aeratable lung. In ARDS, the volume of aeratable lung is reduced as alveoli fill with edema [37,38]. Thus, surfactant function may be abnormal in ARDS, and some of the reduction in aeratable lung may be due to atelectasis [39]. The increase in inflation pressure is really a measure of the amount of edema and atelectasis that is present and not a measure of the lung injury per se. When and if fibrosis develops, the elastic properties of the lung parenchyma can change and result in true reductions in lung compliance.

Peak airway pressures are also increased during mechanical ventilation of ARDS patients, sometimes out of proportion to the increase in static inflation pressures. This finding suggests an increase in airways resistance. Given the potential presence of airway secretions, edema, and mediators that might provoke bronchospasm, increases in airway resistance are plausible [38,40]. Of course, any intrinsic increase in airways resistance would be amplified by the additional resistance provided by narrow endotracheal tubes and the rest of the mechanical apparatus needed for ventilatory support. However, airways resistance, like compliance, should be normalized for the amount of aeratable lung volume available. Since such data are not available, the extent to which airway resistance is increased in ARDS is unknown.

WORK OF BREATHING. The work of breathing in ARDS is increased by all of the changes in pulmonary mechanical properties just discussed [38]. This effect is multiplied by the effect of tachypnea. In ARDS, work of breathing may be responsible for 25 to 50 percent of the body's total oxygen consumption. To supply the energy necessary to sustain this level of work, resources such as relative blood flow may have to be diverted from other vital organ systems. Thus, one of the chief benefits of mechanical ventilatory support in ARDS is to reduce the patient's work of breathing so that blood flow can be redirected to other vital organs.

HEMODYNAMICS. There is no hemodynamic pattern that is characteristic of ARDS, which should not be surprising given the variety of conditions associated with the development of acute lung injury. Indeed, the hemodynamic pattern in any particular patient is more likely to reflect the underlying condition itself (Table 55-1).

A low wedge pressure in the presence of pulmonary edema, of course, strongly suggests that noncardiogenic forces are responsible for the development of edema. However, as previously discussed, it is not unusual for the wedge pressure to be elevated because of concomitant volume overload or complications that may confuse the clinical picture (e.g., myocardial dysfunction). Since it is unusual for pulmonary edema to develop from elevated hydrostatic forces alone until the pulmonary microvascular pressure is greater than 18 mm Hg, this level of pressure is often used as a benchmark for diagnosing ARDS [7]. As a result, many ARDS studies are biased toward the inclusion of patients with low wedge pressures [3]. The actual incidence of higher microvascular pressures when ARDS is diagnosed without relying on pressure measurements is unknown.

One hemodynamic feature that has generated much attention is the development of pulmonary vascular hypertension in ARDS [41]. In general, pulmonary blood pressure is only mildly to moderately elevated, but some patients develop right ventricular failure, and the prognosis of patients with significant elevations in pulmonary vascular resistance is worse than of those with lesser degrees of pulmonary hypertension. This observation has led to attempts at therapeutic reductions in pulmonary vascular resistance (see section on management).

The cause of pulmonary hypertension in ARDS is multifactorial (e.g., the effects of pulmonary vasoconstriction due to alveolar hypoxia or other vasoactive mediators such as thromboxane, intravascular obstruction from platelet thrombi or perivascular edema, and vascular obliteration from developing lung fibrosis). In the first few days, vasoactive mechanisms and platelet thrombi are probably of greatest importance. Reducing pulmonary perfusion to injured lung regions may actually have beneficial effects, by improving ventilation-perfusion matching and by reducing the accumulation of alveolar edema. At a later stage, sustained or worsening pulmonary hypertension probably reflects the degree to which fibrosis is responsible for the obliteration of the vascular bed. Thus, the poor prognosis associated with late pulmonary hypertension in ARDS probably simply reflects the severity of the fibrotic process.

Finally, the normal relationship between oxygen consumption and oxygen delivery may be disturbed in ARDS because peripheral tissue oxygen extraction may be abnormal [32]. Specifically, oxygen consumption may be linearly dependent on oxygen delivery over the entire clinical range of oxygen deivery (see Chap. 181). This so-called pathologic dependency of oxygen consumption on oxygen delivery is in contrast to the normal circumstance, in which oxygen consumption is constant over the physiologic range of oxygen delivery. Whether this disturbance is due to ARDS per se or to the effects of SIRS with which ARDS is so often associated is not clear. Also, pathologic dependency itself may be an artifact of measurement (see Chap. 181). As a result, the therapeutic implications of these observations remain very controversial (see Chap. 181).

Presentation

Like many other clinical syndromes, ARDS is easy to recognize when it presents without preexisting or coexisting conditions that can mimic or obscure otherwise typical symptoms and signs. When the cause of ARDS occurs outside the hospital or before hospital admission and the tissue injury that develops is limited to the lung, the clinical presentation is often very reproducible. Inhalation of a toxic gas or ingestion of certain drugs in toxic doses, severe viral pneumonia, aspiration of gastric contents during resuscitation from a cardiac arrest—these are examples of well-defined events that can lead to ARDS in otherwise healthy individuals. When such events are followed by the rapid development of respiratory distress and bilateral alveolar infiltrates on a chest radiograph, little else but ARDS can explain these findings.

It is interesting that the onset of respiratory distress is almost always delayed by at least a few hours (and sometimes by as many as 1–3 days) from the inciting event. No explanation for this delay or its variation among individuals has been supported with evidence, although it is widely suspected that time is needed for upregulation of inflammatory mediators in some cases. Even so, 80 percent of patients who develop ARDS do so within 24 hours of the inciting event [5].

Another interesting and still inadequately explained aspect of presentation is that respiratory symptoms often precede the full development of infiltrates on the chest radiograph. Dyspnea and tachypnea are often severe, even while the chest radiograph shows relatively little infiltrate. However, alveolar infiltrates invariably develop within the next several hours. Thus, the chest radiograph seems to lag behind the clinical picture. The disparity between the chest radiograph and the magnitude of dyspnea might be due to superimposed abnormalities in

airways resistance (although severe bronchospasm is rare), interstitial edema per se (by stimulating so-called interstitial J receptors), or the poor correlation of the chest radiograph with the actual content of extravascular lung water [42]. None of these possibilities, however, is supported by data in ARDS patients.

Respiratory symptoms other than dyspnea are uncommon. Obviously, significant fever, cough, and purulent sputum suggest a primary pneumonia instead of ARDS. Audible wheezing and pleuritic pain are also unexpected. And, of course, symptoms of heart failure suggest a different etiology altogether for pulmonary edema.

The most dramatic and consistent findings of physical examination include tachypnea, tachycardia, increased work of breathing (intercostal muscle retraction and use of other accessory muscles of respiration during inspiratory effort), and, occasionally, cyanosis. With such signs, the patient may be extremely agitated, even in the absence of a primary neurologic condition. Hypotension and signs of shock are present only if they are due to an associated condition, such as sepsis or massive trauma. Likewise, fever may not be prominent unless the associated condition is related to infection. On pulmonary examination, "dry" crackles (rales) and scattered gurgles (rhonchi) may be heard throughout the lung fields. Not uncommonly, however, the chest examination may be remarkably normal, despite severe alveolar infiltrates on the chest radiograph. End-expiratory wheezes can often be heard, but frank airway obstruction with prolonged expiratory times is not expected. Pleural friction rubs are also rare. At the time of presentation, the rest of the physical examination is usually normal unless other organ systems are involved due to preexisting or coexisting disease.

DIAGNOSIS. The diagnosis of ARDS ideally would be made by documenting both diffuse alveolar damage and increased vascular permeability in any patient with severe respiratory distress (dyspnea), diffuse radiographic infiltrates, and hypoxemia. However, obtaining lung tissue in these critically ill patients is often impractical. And while pulmonary vascular permeability can be evaluated noninvasively, the information is not useful therapeutically because at present there is no specific treatment for abnormal vascular permeability. The diagnosis of ARDS is therefore made by inference (Table 55-2).

Lung injuries can be direct (e.g., inhalation of a toxic gas or aspiration of gastric acid) or indirect (i.e., the initiating mediator is unknown or uncertain and a host response seems to be required for injury to develop). When the mode of injury is indirect, ARDS develops in association with other readily identifiable clinical problems, such as sepsis, pancreatitis, or severe trauma.

Although the distribution of injury in ARDS is diffuse [43], the radiographic distribution of pulmonary edema may not be. As imaged by computed tomography [37], gravity-dependent lung may be the only region in which edema accumulates in some patients, despite "diffuse" (i.e., bilateral) infiltrates as judged on anteroposterior chest radiograph. Presumably, edema develops in gravity-dependent lung first where hydrostatic pressures are greatest.

Although severe hypoxemia is generally included as a diagnostic criterion for ARDS, the appropriate threshold for defining the abnormality in PaO_2 has never been studied. Murray et al [7] suggested that a PaO_2/FIO_2 ratio less than 300 mm Hg (normal > 500 mm Hg) is a reasonable minimum criterion. Sometimes abnormal respiratory system "compliance" is also included as a criterion (e.g., compliance < 80 ml/cm H_2O; normal > 100 ml/cm H_2O) in recognition of the high airway pressures

Table 55-2. Diagnostic Criteria for Acute Respiratory Distress Syndrome

1. Identifiable cause or associated condition
2. Dyspnea (usually severe)
3. Hypoxemia (usually refractory to supplemental oxygen)
4. Bilateral radiographic infiltrates (interstitial and alveolar)
5. Reduced respiratory system compliance (optional)
6. No evidence for cardiac factors as the principal cause of pulmonary edema

Table 55-3. Lung Injury Score

Score:	0	1	2	3	4
Chest radiograph*	0	1	2	3	4
PaO$_2$/FiO$_2$	≥300	225–299	175–224	100–174	<100
PEEP (cm H$_2$O)	≥5	6–8	9–11	12–14	≥15
CRS (ml/cm H$_2$O)	≥80	60–79	40–59	20–39	≥19
Final value = aggregate sum divided by number of components used					

*Number of quadrants with alveolar consolidation
PaO$_2$/FiO$_2$ = arterial oxygen to inspired oxygen concentration ratio [(plateau pressure − PEEP)/tidal volume]; PEEP = positive end-expiratory pressure; CRS = respiratory system compliance.

often required during mechanical ventilatory support. However, since it is unlikely that respiratory system compliance would be normal when oxygenation is severely impaired in the presence of diffuse roentgenographic infiltrates, compliance measurements are not always included as inclusion criteria for ARDS studies. Indeed, none of the abnormalities in the most popular method of quantifying injury in ARDS (Table 55-3) (degree of hypoxemia, extent of pulmonary infiltration on chest radiograph, and respiratory system compliance measurement) are mutually exclusive [7]. For instance, as edema develops (represented radiographically by alveolar infiltrates), oxygenation will worsen. Since recruitable air space for ventilation is reduced as alveolar edema develops, higher-than-normal airway pressures will develop during mechanical ventilatory support (reduced compliance).

It may sometimes be necessary to exclude a cardiogenic or hydrostatic pressure component for the etiology of pulmonary edema by obtaining data with a pulmonary artery flotation catheter. Demonstrating increased protein in edema fluid suctioned from the airways [44] or an increased rate of pulmonary uptake of radiolabeled proteins by gamma scintigraphy or other means (suggesting increased vascular permeability) [45] would also support a diagnosis of ARDS. However, these results would not be specific for ARDS, since other inflammatory conditions also increase vascular permeability [45]. In the appropriate setting, a lung biopsy demonstrating diffuse alveolar damage would also support a diagnosis of ARDS. Usually, however, a lung biopsy is performed to exclude other treatable conditions (e.g., infection, vasculitis) rather than to make the diagnosis of ARDS per se.

Chest Radiography and Other Laboratory Tests

Although the chest radiograph may be normal for some hours after the inciting event, full progression to a bilateral alveolar filling pattern ordinarily takes place within 4 to 24 hours after the first abnormal radiographic signs. Thus, whether the full radiographic sequence of events is appreciated or not depends on the frequency with which the radiographs are obtained. The initial abnormal radiograph may show only a bilateral perihilar haze with linear opacities extending from the hilum. This pattern is consistent with interstitial edema. However, many technical factors—especially shallow, rapid breathing—may mask this appearance on portable radiographs of suboptimal quality. As alveolar flooding develops in some areas, the linear opacities coalesce radiographically into areas consistent with alveolar filling. The appearance of radiographic shadows in the lung parenchyma can be identical to those seen in congestive heart failure, although at least one group has concluded that the densities tend to be more peripheral and less gravitationally oriented (from apex to base in the semirecumbent or supine position) than in typical heart failure [46]. More important, in the absence of preexisting or coexisting heart disease or intravascular fluid overload, other radiographic signs of congestive failure (cardiomegaly, perfusion redistribution, peribronchial cuffing, peripheral septal lines, and pleural effusions) will be absent. As alveolar filling progresses in ARDS, more and more of the lung parenchyma is involved radiographically, occasionally progressing to near total "whiteout" of both lung fields (Fig. 55-2). When regions of lung become consolidated, air bronchograms can be seen on the radiograph (Fig. 55-2). Although always bilateral, the actual extent of lung involvement in many cases is much less dramatic.

Whether noncardiogenic and cardiogenic forms of pulmonary edema can be distinguished radiographically has been controversial. Milne et al. suggested that the distribution of vascular markings, the distribution of alveolar edema in the lung parenchyma, the width of the vascular pedicle, and the absence or presence of such signs as cardiomegaly, peribronchial cuffing, pleural effusions, and septal lines usually allows these entities to be differentiated [46]. However, others have not been able to reproduce these results [42,47].

The radiographic appearance in ARDS can also be strongly influenced by the effects of therapy. Aggressive intravascular fluid administration for shock or hypotension may worsen the accumulation of alveolar edema, whereas diuretics may limit or reduce edema accumulation. Mechanical ventilation, especially with positive end-expiratory pressure (PEEP) or any mode that

Fig. 55-2. Portable chest radiograph in a patient with severe ARDS. Note the presence of air bronchograms, especially in the left lung. A chest tube is present in the right chest.

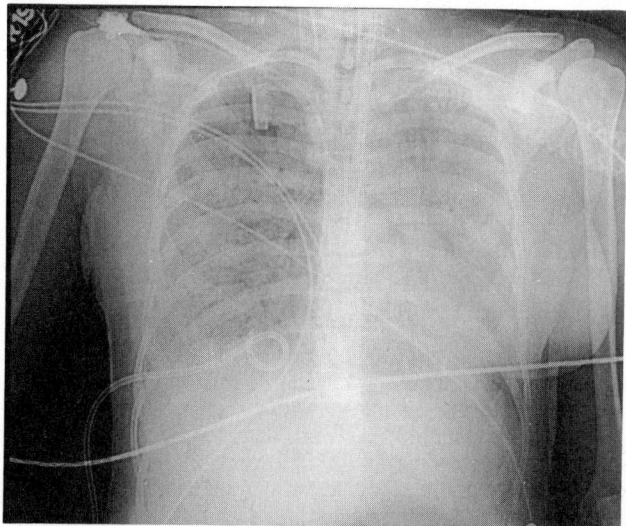

significantly increases mean airway pressure (e.g., inverse ratio ventilation), may reduce regional lung density by increasing lung inflation, giving the appearance of radiographic improvement despite continued severe abnormalities in gas exchange. In addition, when high airway pressures are required for effective ventilation, a wide spectrum of other radiographic signs of barotrauma may quickly become evident (especially subcutaneous and mediastinal emphysema and pneumothorax).

Measurements of gas exchange, although absolutely vital to management, are rarely of much diagnostic use. Not uncommonly, initial arterial blood studies show a respiratory alkalosis and varying degrees of hypoxemia. Finger pulse oximetry shows arterial desaturation in proportion to the extent of arterial hypoxemia. The hypoxemia is often resistant to supplemental oxygen administration, as discussed previously. This classic sign of ARDS indicates that intrapulmonary shunting is the principal cause of the hypoxemia. As alveolar edema accumulates, hypoxemia continues to worsen and mechanical ventilatory support becomes necessary. Other routine laboratory tests are not expected to be abnormal unless they reflect abnormalities due to associated conditions.

Ideally, acute lung injury would be detected by some specific test of lung function. As mentioned in the previous section, techniques are available to evaluate the integrity of the pulmonary microvascular membrane by measuring the protein content of fluid suctioned from the airways or when obtained during bronchoalveolar lavage [23,48] or by measuring the flux of radiolabeled proteins from blood to lung tissue [49]. When abnormal, these tests support the inference that pulmonary edema is noncardiogenic in etiology. However, because these tests can be cumbersome, time-consuming, and expensive, and because therapy is rarely affected by the information they provide, they are rarely obtained outside research settings.

Extravascular lung water can be quantified at the bedside by the thermal indocyanine green dye indicator-dilution technique or other methods [50]. These tests are also cumbersome, time-consuming, and expensive and are rarely performed except for research purposes. On average, the extravascular water content of the lung is about 3 times the normal upper limit of 500 ml, but may be as high as 6 to 8 times the normal value [51].

Bronchoalveolar lavage is performed occasionally in patients with ARDS to rule out opportunistic infection. Even in the absence of infection, however, the most prominent finding is increased polymorphonuclear leukocytes, comprising as much as 80 percent of the total cell population (normal < 5%) [23]. Occasionally, eosinophilia is also prominent, with important implications for therapy (see section on management).

Tests of endothelial "metabolic" function instead of barrier function (e.g., pulmonary uptake of small peptides) or blood assays of potential markers of endothelial damage (e.g., angiotensin-converting enzyme or factor VIII-related antigen) have also been studied as diagnostic markers of ARDS [52]. Again, there is no evidence that these tests are sensitive, specific, easy to perform, or inexpensive to obtain or that their results affect management.

In contrast, hemodynamic monitoring via pulmonary artery catheterization is one of the most commonly performed procedures in ARDS, often accomplished within hours of presentation. Although the issues relevant to hemodynamic monitoring are dealt with at length in Chapters 2 to 4, several points concerning its use in ARDS are important. First, and most important, there is no hemodynamic profile that is diagnostic of ARDS. Pulmonary edema, high cardiac output, and low ventricular filling pressures are certainly characteristic of ARDS, but partially treated intravascular volume overload and so-called flash pulmonary edema (in which filling pressures are elevated only during a period of coronary ischemia and then resolve

before pulmonary artery catheterization is performed) are examples of situations that can cause confusion with the expected hemodynamics of ARDS. Equally important, filling pressures can be elevated either artifactually (e.g., by increased intrathoracic pressures or therapeutically (as with volume administration for hypotension), and cardiac function can be depressed (e.g., by acidosis, hypoxia, or depressant factors associated with sepsis). In our opinion, while hemodynamic monitoring can be quite valuable for *therapeutic* decision-making (and even this point is controversial), it is rarely of value *diagnostically*.

Overlap Syndromes

Any process that is associated with alveolar filling can mimic the clinical manifestations of ARDS. For instance, any of the alveolar hemorrhage syndromes (see Chap. 61), any acute inflammatory process (especially pneumonia), and any other condition that causes pulmonary edema can be confused with ARDS. Conversely, alveolar hemorrhage (apart from the distinct alveolar hemorrhage syndromes) is often a component of diffuse alveolar damage, volume overload is not uncommon as a complication during the early stages of therapy, and the incidence of nosocomial pneumonia increases steadily if ARDS does not resolve quickly.

Often the diagnosis of ARDS can be made definitively only once these other processes have been excluded or when pulmonary infiltrates fail to clear despite treatment for these other conditions. Even so, this indirect approach to diagnosis must mean that some cases of ARDS are inappropriately excluded because other alveolar filling processes are present, or that some cases of ARDS are diagnosed rather late in their natural history. Although the clinical implications of this imprecision may not be substantial as long as there is no specific therapy for ARDS, the situation could change as soon as more specific treatments are developed. In the meantime, studies of ARDS may be biased by misrepresentative patient sampling [3].

Management

Since there are no specific measures to correct either the permeability abnormality or the injurious inflammatory reaction in ARDS, clinical management primarily involves supportive measures aimed at maintaining cellular and physiologic functions (e.g., gas exchange, organ perfusion, aerobic metabolism) while the acute lung injury resolves. These measures should include mechanical ventilation, oxygen administration, antibiotics for infection, nutritional support and hemodynamic monitoring when necessary to guide fluid management, and cardiovascular support. Few specific therapeutic approaches have been evaluated in a rigorous scientific fashion; therefore many therapeutic strategies in ARDS are controversial. To make explicit the basis for our own recommendations, we have graded them (Table 55-4) whenever possible according to the quality of the currently available scientific information (using only investigations specifically involving ARDS patients or patients with sepsis).

NONPHARMACOLOGIC THERAPIES
Mechanical Ventilation. The overall goals of mechanical ventilation in ARDS are (1) to maintain acceptable gas exchange and (2) to minimize the occurrence of adverse effects associated

Table 55-4. Recommendations for the Treatment of Acute Respiratory Distress Syndrome

Intervention	Recommended	Grade*	References	Level*
Tidal volume: ≤ 8 ml/kg	Yes	B	58,59	2
Least PEEP with $SaO_2 \geq 0.9$ and $FiO_2 \leq 0.6$	Yes	Ungraded	—	—
Permissive hypercapnia (pressure-targeted ventilation) for plateau pressure > 30–35 cm H_2O	Yes	B	67	2
Inverse ratio ventilation for persistent hypoxemia or plateau pressure > 30–35 cm H_2O	Yes	B	69–72	2
High-frequency ventilation	No	A	76–78	1,2
ECMO	No	A	79	1
$ECCO_2R$	No	A	81	1
Patient repositioning (excluding prone position)	Yes	B	82–84	2
Early fluid restriction/diuresis	Yes	A	51,85–88	1,2
Oxygen transport optimization	P	—	—	—
Early corticosteroids	No	A	97–99	1,4
Late corticosteroids	P	—	—	—
N-acetylcysteine	No	A	103	1
Nitric oxide	P	—	—	—
Ibuprofen	No	C	108,109	3
PGE_1	No	A	112	1
Pentoxifylline	P	—	—	3
Antiendotoxin and anticytokine therapy	No	C	117–122	
Surfactant	No	A	94	1

*Quality of evidence and recommendation of grade was determined by the level of clinical investigation: grade A = randomized, prospective, controlled investigations of ARDS (level 1); grade B = nonrandomized concurrent cohort investigations, historical cohort investigations, and case series of ARDS (level 2); grade C = randomized, prospective, controlled investigations of sepsis with potential application to ARDS (level 3); grade D = case reports of ARDS (level 4); ungraded = no available clinical investigations (level 5).

PEEP = positive end-expiratory pressure; SaO_2 = arterial oxygen saturation; FiO_2 = inspired concentration of oxygen; ECMO = extracorporeal membrane oxygenation; $ECCO_2R$ = extracorporeal CO_2 removal; P = pending current or anticipated clinical trials; PGE_1 = prostaglandin E_1; SDD = selective digestive decontamination.

with its application. A growing consensus currently supports the use of patient-specific physiologically targeted goals to guide ventilator settings, instead of "routine" ordering strategies [53,54,55] (see Chap. 66). In the absence of data, such an approach is logical.

We recommend that patients with ARDS initially be managed with a volume-cycled mechanical ventilator in the assist-control (AC) mode. Theoretically, the intermittent mandatory ventilation (IMV) mode could be used as an alternative to the AC mode because mean airway pressures are usually lower, with potentially favorable effects on hemodynamics and the incidence of barotrauma. However, in our experience, the differences in airway pressures in the early stages of ARDS are small. Furthermore, patient work of breathing is usually greater in the IMV mode compared to the AC mode, since the patient provides a greater fraction of the ventilatory effort.

We recommend other initial ventilator settings as follows: FiO_2 = 1.0; tidal volume (TV) = ≤ 8 ml per kilogram; PEEP = 0 cm H_2O; inspiratory flow rate = 60 liters per minute. The rationale for these recommendations is given in the following sections and in Chapter 66. Our priorities in formulating these suggestions were (1) to preserve arterial oxygen saturation (i.e., $SaO_2 \geq 0.9$) and (2) to prevent complications from elevated alveolar pressures (reflected by end-inflation hold pressure or plateau pressure >30–35 cm H_2O) or high inspired oxygen concentrations (i.e., $FiO_2 > 0.6$). (See Chap. 66 for further discussion of predicting barotrauma with peak airway and plateau pressures.)

TIDAL VOLUME. Large tidal volumes and peak airway pressures have been implicated as causes of gross lung injury (so-called volotrauma or barotrauma in the form of pneumomediastinum or pneumothorax) [56] and of injury to the alveolar-endothelial barrier [57]. Traditionally, tidal volumes between 12 and 15 ml per kilogram have been recommended for patients receiving mechanical ventilation. This range may be inappropriate for many patients with ARDS due to their smaller aeratable lung volume [37,38]. Indeed, several recent studies [58,59] have found improved hemodynamic performance and fewer pulmonary complications using tidal volumes as low as 6 ml per kilogram in patients with ARDS.

Therefore, we recommend that tidal volumes of ≤ 8 ml per kilogram be used to keep plateau pressures below 30 to 35 cm H_2O. Because lung impedances (i.e., airway resistance and tissue compliance) change frequently in ARDS, it may be necessary to change the tidal volume regularly to maintain this preselected goal. As an alternative to using plateau pressures, effective static lung compliance (C_{ES}) has been advocated as a way to optimize tidal volume selections in ARDS [60].

POSITIVE END-EXPIRATORY PRESSURE. The use of prophylactic PEEP (i.e., 5 cm H_2O) in patients at risk for developing ARDS is ineffective in preventing this syndrome [61]. However, routine use of low levels of PEEP may still be valuable as a means of reducing the development of atelectasis and in any case is probably a harmless maneuver.

For more than two decades PEEP has been used to improve arterial oxygenation in patients with ARDS. However, despite complex changes in ventilatory and hemodynamic variables that can occur when extrinsically applied end-expiratory pressure (extrinsic PEEP) is used to improve oxygenation in ARDS, there are no prospective studies of its use in ARDS. Therefore, we recommend that PEEP be applied in increments of 3 to 5 cm H_2O (to a maximum of 15 cm H_2O) to achieve acceptable arterial oxygenation (i.e., $SaO_2 \geq 0.9$) with nontoxic levels of FiO_2 (i.e., $FiO_2 \leq 0.6$) and acceptable plateau pressure (i.e., < 30–35 cm H_2O) (Figs. 55-3 and 55-4). This recommendation is based on the association of barotrauma with higher plateau pressures and evidence suggesting that elevated plateau pressure [53] and high inspired oxygen concentrations [62] may interfere with normal repair of lung injury. Alternative approaches to determining the optimal level of PEEP are problematic, since some potentially detrimental effects of PEEP (e.g., reduction in cardiac output) may also be beneficial (i.e., PEEP-associated improvements in oxygenation via PEEP-induced decreases in blood flow through pulmonary shunt units [63]. The debate over the appropriate PEEP level has recently been further complicated by data suggesting that PEEP-induced changes in oxygen transport may adversely influence patient outcome in ARDS [64].

VENTILATORY RATE (INCLUDING AUTO PEEP AND PERMISSIVE HYPERCAPNIA). Patient ventilatory rates have traditionally been set to avoid hypercapnia and respiratory acidosis. With normal lungs, this goal can usually be achieved with respiratory rates of 8 to 14 breaths per minute. Due to the increased physiologic dead space and smaller aeratable lung volumes of patients with ARDS, ventilatory rates greater than 20 to 25 breaths per minute are often required to normalize $PaCO_2$ and pH. These rates are usually well tolerated, unless excessive intrathoracic gas trapping occurs, leading to the development of auto-PEEP (i.e., intrinsic PEEP).

Auto PEEP occurs primarily in the setting of obstructive airways disease (i.e., asthma and COPD); however, it has also been described in patients with ARDS [65]. Potentially adverse effects of auto PEEP include barotrauma and hemodynamic instability, increased work of breathing, and decreased efficiency of diaphragmatic contractility [38]. The level of auto-PEEP can be decreased by allowing adequate time for the exhalation of trapped intrathoracic gases (e.g., by decreasing delivered minute volume or increasing inspiratory flow rate). Occasionally, the hemodynamic sequelae of auto-PEEP are so severe that shock or electromechanical dissociation can occur [66]. In these circumstances a *brief* trial of hypoventilation (i.e., respiratory rate $\geq$ 6 breaths/min) or even apnea may be indicated to reverse these sequelae.

Another strategy to adjust minute ventilation in ARDS is so-called controlled hypoventilation with permissive hypercapnia, also termed pressure-targeted ventilation. With this strategy, hypoventilation and hypercapnia are allowed so that detrimental increases in alveolar pressure can be avoided. Pressure-targeted ventilation has been successfully used in patients with ARDS [67]. As the respiratory rate and tidal volume are adjusted to prevent increases in plateau pressure, the $PaCO_2$ rises. (See Chap. 56 for further discussion of permissive hypercapnia and whether bicarbonate infusions are necessary.) Extracorporeal carbon dioxide removal has also been used to remove carbon dioxide during pressure-targeted ventilation [68]. We recommend that pressure-targeted ventilation with permissive hypercapnia be considered in patients developing plateau pressures greater than 30 to 35 cm H_2O despite other appropriate interventions.

INVERSE RATIO VENTILATION. Inverse ratio ventilation (IRV) is a mode of mechanical ventilation in which the inspiratory time is prolonged, increasing mean airway pressures. Therefore, IRV is another ventilatory strategy to improve oxygenation while maintaining acceptable peak airway pressures in ARDS [69]. An advantage of IRV over the conventional use of extrinsic-PEEP is that unacceptable increases in peak airway pressures and peak alveolar pressures can be avoided. The fact that pulmonary infiltrates can be distributed inhomogeneously in the lungs of ARDS patients [37] has also been offered as a rationale for using IRV. Sustained inspiratory pressures might have their greatest incremental effect on these unrecruited lung regions, especially if sustained traction is required to achieve their recruitment [70]. Several hours may be required to achieve the maximal benefits of IRV on gas exchange, supporting a role for sustained inspiratory traction with IRV [71].

Growing clinical experience with the use of IRV suggests it is a useful strategy for salvaging gas exchange in ARDS patients whose oxygenation cannot be maintained with more conventional approaches [69–72]. Therefore, we recommend that IRV be used when acceptable arterial oxygenation cannot be achieved with PEEP less than 15 cm H_2O or when the use of PEEP is associated with excessive plateau pressures. A computerized protocol for adjusting IRV parameters in a systematic fashion has been published [73]. To date, no studies have been performed comparing IRV to pressure-targeted ventilation with permissive hypercapnia.

OTHER MODES. Clinical experience with airway pressure release ventilation is too limited to allow any recommendations on its use in ARDS [74]. Likewise, studies of high-frequency ventilation in patients with ARDS [75–78] show no significant advantage over conventional forms of mechanical ventilation. We do *not* recommend the routine use of high-frequency ventilation in ARDS.

Extracorporeal Respiratory Support. Two forms of extracorporeal respiratory support have been evaluated in ARDS patients: extracorporeal membrane oxygenation (ECMO) and extracorporeal carbon dioxide removal ($ECCO_2R$). A prospective trial of ECMO has shown it is not superior to conventional mechanical ventilation in terms of patient survival [79]. However, in specific patient situations ECMO could still be a useful support mode, such as while awaiting lung transplantation in selected patients [80]. We recommend, however, that ECMO *not* be used for routine treatment of ARDS.

Still frequently used in Europe [68], $ECCO_2R$ was evaluated in a recently completed NIH-sponsored investigation involving a computerized management design [81]. To date, no survival advantage has been reported for the $ECCO_2R$-treated group. We therefore recommend that $ECCO_2R$ *not* be used in the routine management of ARDS.

Patient Positioning. Because of the nonuniform distribution of lung infiltrates in ARDS [37], positional changes can improve oxygenation by improving the distribution of perfusion [82,83,84]. Indeed, despite obvious impracticality, the prone position significantly improves oxygenation in some patients with ARDS [84]. Accurate predictors of patient response to repositioning are currently unavailable. We recommend that repositioning (i.e., lateral decubitus positioning) be attempted in patients with hypoxemia that is unresponsive to other medical interventions, especially if radiographic infiltrates are not uniformly distributed between the two lungs. Use of the prone position should be limited to institutions familiar with its use and potential complications.

Fluid Management. Though pulmonary edema in ARDS is due to increased vascular permeability [45], intravascular hydrostatic forces may still be a contributing factor in ARDS (see Chap. 54). Several clinical studies [85,86,87] indicate that pulmonary function and outcome are better in patients who lose weight or in whom wedge pressure falls as a result of diuresis

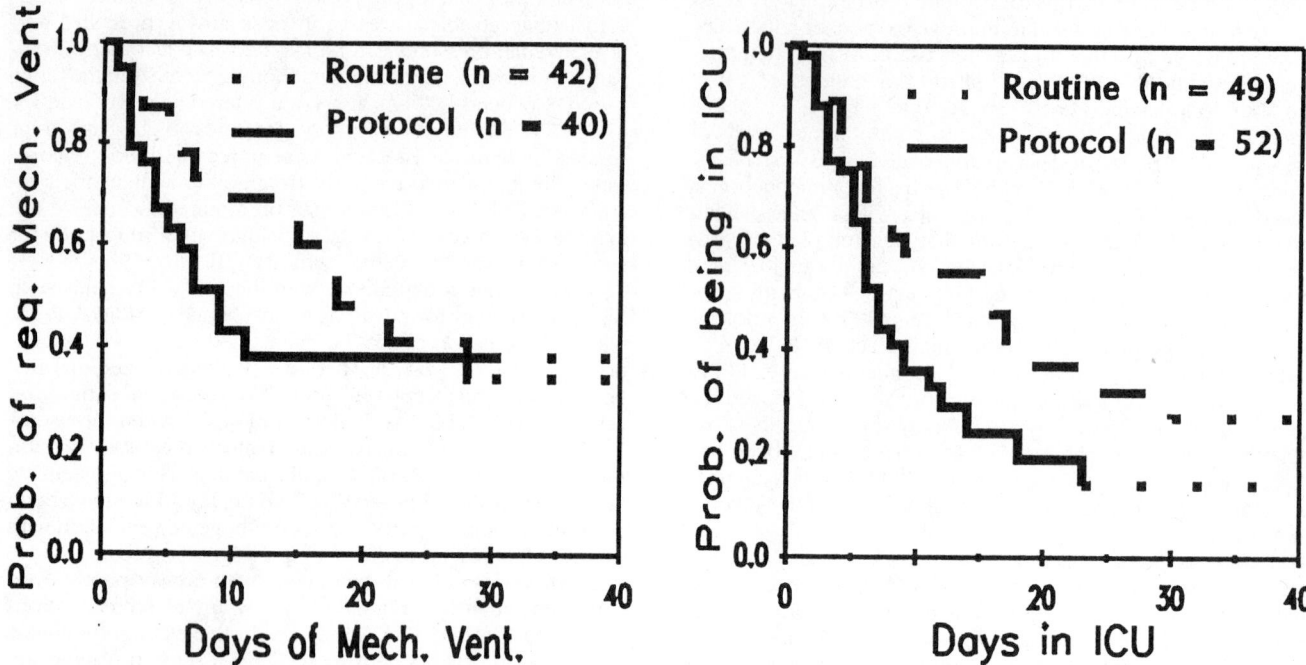

Fig. 55-3. Kaplan-Meier plots of days on mechanical ventilation (left) or days in the ICU (right) for 89 patients with pulmonary edema. Data are the Kaplan-Meier estimates of the probability of still requiring mechanical ventilation or still being alive in the ICU as a function of time. Patients who died on mechanical ventilation were treated as censored observations. Patients managed according to a protocol that emphasized fluid restriction/diuresis had a significantly shorter median requirement for mechanical ventilation and shorter ICU stay. Modified from reference 17, with permission.

or fluid restriction. A recent prospective trial [51,88] arrived at a similar conclusion (Fig 55-3), although it included both patients with congestive heart failure as well as ARDS. Importantly, the strategy of early diuresis/fluid restriction was not associated with a higher incidence of complications, such as renal failure or hemodynamic compromise. Therefore, we recommend that patients with ARDS be fluid-restricted and even diuresed, especially during the first few days after onset, while carefully monitoring (and correcting) any compromise in end-organ function. Subsequently (after 3–4 days), the benefits of fluid restriction/diuresis are unclear.

Oxygen Transport Optimization. Although the basic mechanisms underlying the pathophysiology of cellular injury in ARDS are unresolved, clinical evidence suggests that tissue perfusion may be an important factor. Russell and colleagues [89] reported that nonsurvivors of ARDS have significantly lower values for oxygen delivery (DO_2) and oxygen consumption (VO_2) than survivors. Although highly controversial, many studies indicate that oxygen consumption is dependent on oxygen delivery in ARDS [90], and two prospective interventional studies aimed at optimizing oxygen transport found a favorable impact on patient outcome. However, they were performed in postoperative [91] or septic [92] patients. The number of patients with ARDS was either few or unclear. Furthermore, some measures often used to improve cardiac performance (e.g., nitroprusside) often seem to be ineffective in ARDS [93]. Therefore, specific recommendations for ARDS cannot be made with confidence. At present, it is not our practice to attempt to achieve "supranormal" values for oxygen delivery. When evidence for

end-organ hypoperfusion is present (i.e., oliguria, metabolic acidosis, hypotension) we prefer to reverse organ hypoperfusion with the administration of inotropes if possible (e.g., dobutamine) and to administer fluids secondarily (unless there is significant clinical evidence for hypovolemia).

PHARMACOLOGIC THERAPIES

Exogenous Surfactant. Although surfactant is present in normal amounts in ARDS, it may be dysfunctional [39]. Exogenous surfactant replacement in ARDS might improve air space stability and have antibacterial and immunologic properties, resulting in reduced airway pressures, improved ventilation, and reduced incidence of nosocomial pneumonia. The only available prospective trial of exogenous surfactant administration in patients with ARDS was not encouraging [94], but different prospective clinical trials of more than one preparation (synthetic or prepared from mammalian lungs) are currently in progress. Specific recommendations await the results of these investigations.

Corticosteroids. Although preliminary trials in patients with sepsis and ARDS indicated some benefit from steroid administration [95,96], subsequent prospective multicenter placebo-controlled studies demonstrated that patients with ARDS do not benefit from high-dose corticosteroids administered early in the disease process [97,98,99].

Despite the lack of proved efficacy in early ARDS, other indications are being considered for this class of drugs. Anecdotal reports [100,101,102] suggest that corticosteroids may be useful if administered during the fibroproliferative phase (7–10 days after onset). Also, a few patients with ARDS have high numbers of eosinophils in their blood and lungs (as assayed by bronchoalveolar lavage) [52]. These patients may have a form of eosinophilic pneumonia, and some have developed the syndrome after inhalation of crack cocaine. In any case, some of these patients seem to respond to the use of early corticosteroids.

We recommend that corticosteroids *not* be used in patients at risk for ARDS or during the first few days of ARDS (unless blood or BAL eosinophilia is documented). The use of corticosteroids in later phases of ARDS has not been adequately investigated. If a prolonged course of corticosteroids is to be administered for established ARDS, we recommend (ungraded) that systemic infection *first* be excluded or adequately treated. We have used 250 to 500 mg twice per day for 3 days with a rapid taper to 60 mg methylprednisolone daily over the next week. When a clinical response seems to occur (improved oxygenation, clearing of chest radiographic infiltrates), this dose was continued until extubation was possible.

N-Acetylcysteine. When used in ARDS, N-acetylcysteine apparently has no benefit on gas exchange, amelioration of ARDS, or patient survival [103]. Based on these results, we recommend that N-acetylcysteine *not* be administered for ARDS.

Nitric Oxide. Inhaled nitric oxide can act as a selective pulmonary vasodilator in both animals and humans when inspired in concentrations of 5 to 80 ppm [104]. Animal studies have demonstrated that nitric oxide in concentrations of 10 to 40 ppm can be inhaled safely for up to 6 months without apparent significant systemic toxicity [105]. The rapid binding of nitric oxide to hemoglobin, for which it has a high affinity, prevents occurrence of any significant systemic vasodilation.

Rossaint and co-workers [106] administered nitric oxide in a concentration of 18 ppm to 10 patients with severe ARDS. Statistically significant reductions in pulmonary artery pressures and intrapulmonary shunt occurred, while the PaO_2/FiO_2 ratio increased and mean arterial pressure and cardiac output remained unchanged. Continuous administration of nitric oxide consistently (although modestly) lowered pulmonary artery pressures and increased the PaO_2/FiO_2 ratio (modestly) for 3 to 53 days in individual patients. Nitric oxide, unlike intravenous prostacyclin, produced no systemic hypotension. At present, the experience with inhaled nitric oxide is too meager to recommend its routine use in ARDS.

Eicosanoids and Their Inhibitors. Although nonsteroidal antiinflammatory drugs (e.g., ibuprofen, indomethacin) have been shown to improve outcome in experimentally induced sepsis [107], two clinical trials of ibuprofen in patients with sepsis [108,109] have failed to show any significant benefit on patient outcome. Clinical trials in healthy humans show that ibuprofen inhibits endotoxin-induced rises in circulating tumor necrosis factor (TNF) and attenuates patient symptoms following the administration of *Escherichia coli* endotoxin [110]. Although patients with ARDS were not specifically studied, we recommend that ibuprofen not yet be used routinely in ARDS.

Holcroft and colleagues [111] found that prostaglandin E_1 (PGE_1) improved the PO_2/FiO_2 ratio and patient survival in a study of 41 surgical patients with ARDS. However, in a larger multicenter study of PGE_1 involving 100 patients with ARDS (surgical and medical patients), no survival advantage from the use of PGE_1 was found [112]. Therefore, we recommend that PGE_1 *not* be used in the treatment of ARDS.

Other Vasodilators and Vasoconstrictors. Vasoactive drugs such as nitroprusside are frequently used to improve cardiac performance. In ARDS, however, this may worsen gas exchange by inhibiting vasoconstriction to edematous lung units [36]. Indeed, enhanced vasoconstriction can actually improve gas exchange in ARDS [113,114]. The long-term benefits of such a therapeutic strategy, however, although promising, have not been demonstrated [115].

Pentoxifylline. Montravers and colleagues evaluated the administration of a large initial dose of pentoxifylline followed by a constant infusion of the drug in six patients with severe ARDS [116]. They demonstrated no significant detrimental effects from the administration of pentoxifylline on respiratory and hemodynamic parameters. Recommendations for the clinical use of pentoxifylline in ARDS await the results of further clinical investigations.

Antiendotoxin and Anticytokine Therapy. Since ARDS is often associated with sepsis, it is reasonable to assume that therapy directed against putative mediators of sepsis (endotoxin, tumor necrosis factor, and interleukin-1) might reduce the incidence of ARDS. At least one clinical trial suggested this might well be the case [117]. However, none of the agents tested to date in prospective trials have shown any benefit in terms of overall mortality [117–120]. None have been approved for use in sepsis or ARDS. Furthermore, decreased circulating levels of some cytokines during sepsis could actually result in poorer patient outcome [121,122]. Thus, the safety of these therapies must be thoroughly addressed before recommendations about their use can be made.

MANAGEMENT DURING THE RECOVERY PHASE. Most patients who die with ARDS do so within the first 2 weeks of the illness [9]. However, for those who survive, recovery often takes 2 weeks or longer. Thus, for most survivors of ARDS, many issues of general supportive care must be addressed.

In general, after 7 to 10 days much of the alveolar edema has resolved and infiltrates on the chest radiograph represent inflammatory infiltrate and/or new collagen deposition as a precursor to developing fibrosis [12,13]. Thus, it is not unusual for oxygenation to have improved significantly during this first week, while minute ventilatory demands remain high. Typically, all but the most severely affected patients will have improved to the point where oxygenation can be supported by 40 to 60 percent FiO_2 and 5 to 8 cm H_2O PEEP. In arriving at this point, and even afterward, it can be quite tempting to reduce airway pressure support quickly. Since terminal airways are still quite unstable, this tendency should be avoided so that precipitous deterioration in oxygenation can be averted. We recommend that in general PEEP (or other modes of increasing mean airway pressure, such as inverse ratio ventilation) be reduced gradually, so that mean airway pressure is decreased only 2 to 3 cm H_2O every 12 hours [53]. Only rarely will such a conservative approach unnecessarily prolong the patient's dependency on mechanical ventilation.

Since most patients with ARDS require at least 10 to 14 days of mechanical ventilatory support, decisions about the timing of a tracheostomy are common. However, issues concerning eventual extubation or need for tracheostomy are not unique to the ARDS patient (see Chap. 16). In general, we believe that if a patient will require more than 2 weeks of ventilatory support, a tracheostomy is warranted. This decision can usually be made after 7 to 10 days into the illness.

Many patients with ARDS develop a syndrome of multiorgan dysfunction (see Chap. 99). Recovery depends on adequate support of vital organ systems. Complications of management are common among ARDS patients (Table 55-5) [123]. Chief among these are barotrauma (see Chap. 66), nosocomial pneumonia (see Chap. 76), and so-called stress-related gastrointestinal bleeding (see Chap. 99).

Prognosis

The outcome for an individual patient with ARDS is difficult to predict. General scoring systems, such as APACHE III (Acute

Table 55-5. Complications Associated with Acute Respiratory Distress Syndrome

Pulmonary
   Barotrauma (volutrauma)
   Pulmonary emboli
   Pulmonary fibrosis
   Ventilator-associated pneumonia
Gastrointestinal
   Hemorrhage
   Dysmotility
   Pneumoperitoneum
   Bacterial translocation (interstitial barrier dysfunction)
Cardiac
   Arrhythmias
   Myocardial dysfunction
Renal
   Acute renal failure
   Positive fluid balance
Mechanical (due to medical devices)
   Vascular injury
   Pneumothorax
   Tracheal injury/stenosis
Nutritional
   Malnutrition (protein-calorie)
   Electrolyte deficiency
   Elevated CO_2 production (excess carbohydrates)
Systemic
   Bacteremia/sepsis
   Multiple organ system failure

Physiology and Chronic Health Evaluation), provide an estimate of the probability of mortality after the first 24 hours of intensive care [124]. A specific scoring system for ARDS [7] has been developed, but its predictive accuracy has not been validated. The number of acquired organ system failures is often the most important prognostic indicator for patients requiring intensive care, including patients with ARDS. In addition, liver failure in association with ARDS carries a particularly poor prognosis [125].

For most of the two decades since ARDS was first reported, mortality has remained relatively constant, at 60 to 70 percent [4,5,6]. Recent reports, however, suggest that mortality may be falling to about 40 percent [126,127]. The explanation for this apparent improvement is not clear, but it could be due to differences in patient populations, use of less corticosteroids in early ARDS, use of more corticosteroids in late ARDS, greater attention to fluid management, improving hemodynamic or nutritional support, improved antibiotics for nosocomial infection, changes in ventilator support strategies, or the benefits of protocol-driven management in recent clinical trials [51,73].

More specific predictors of outcome for patients with ARDS have been sought from measurements of various serum and lung lavage factors. The concentration of von Willebrand factor antigen in serum [128] and of neutrophil activating factor-1/interleukin-8 in air space lavage fluid [129] seem to correlate with outcome of ARDS. The integrity of the epithelial barrier in relation to resolution of alveolar edema also appears to be a determinant of outcome in patients with ARDS [130]. Similarly, the change in the PaO_2/FIO_2 ratio following initial treatment of ARDS can discriminate between survivors and nonsurvivors [131]. At present, none of these markers has been validated as an accurate method of predicting outcome in the individual ARDS patient.

The long-term functional outlook for survivors of ARDS has also been evaluated. Elliot found that if an elevated FIO_2 is necessary for more than 24 hours, a reduced D_LCO is likely a

year after recovery from ARDS [132]. Similarly, Peters and colleagues [133] showed that long-term abnormalities in pulmonary function could be directly related to the persistence of impaired lung function more than 3 days after the onset of ARDS. Ghio and co-workers [134] found that physiologic indices of the severity of ARDS (e.g., maximal pulmonary artery pressure, lowest static thoracic compliance, and maximal level of PEEP) were the best predictors of impaired lung function 1 year or more after ARDS survival.

References

1. Ashbaugh DG, Petty TL, Bigelow DB, et al: Acute respiratory distress in adults. *Lancet* 2:319, 1967.
2. Petty TL: Adult respiratory distress syndrome: Definition and historical perspective. *Clin Chest Med* 3:3, 1982.
3. Rinaldo JE: The prognosis of the adult respiratory distress syndrome: Inappropriate pessimism? *Chest* 90:470, 1990.
4. Pepe PE, Potkin RT, Reus DH, et al: Clinical predictors of the adult respiratory distress syndrome. *Am J Surg* 144:124, 1982.
5. Fowler AA, Hamman RF, Good JT, et al: Adult respiratory distress syndrome: Risk with common predispositions. *Ann Intern Med* 98:593, 1983.
6. Sloane PJ, Gee MH, Gottlieb JE, et al: A multicenter registry of patients with acute respiratory distress syndrome. *Am Rev Respir Dis* 146:419, 1992.
7. Murray JF, Matthay MA, Luce JM, Flick MR: An expanded definition of the adult respiratory distress syndrome. *Am Rev Respir Dis* 138:720, 1988.
8. Bell RC, Coalson J, Smith JD, et al: Multi organ failure and infection in adult respiratory distress syndrome. *Ann Intern Med* 99:293, 1983.
9. Montogomery AB, Stager MA, Carrico CJ, Hudson LD: Cause of mortality in patients with the adult respiratory distress syndrome. *Am Rev Respir Dis* 132:485, 1985.
10. Seidenfeld JJ, Pohl DF, Bell RC, et al: Incidence, site, and outcome of infections in patients with the adult respiratory distress syndrome. *Am Rev Respir Dis* 134:12, 1986.
11. Maxfield RA, Sorkin IB, Fazzini EP, et al: Respiratory failure in patients with acquired immunodeficiency syndrome and *Pneumocystis carinii* pneumonia. *Crit Care Med* 14:443, 1986.
12. Meyrick B: Pathology of the adult respiratory distress syndrome. *Crit Care Clin* 2:405, 1986.
13. Tomashefski JF Jr: Pulmonary pathology of the adult respiratory distress syndrome. *Clin Chest Med* 11:593, 1990.
14. Crouch E: Pathobiology of pulmonary fibrosis. *Am J Physiol* 259:L159, 1990.
15. McDonald JA: Idiopathic pulmonary fibrosis: A paradigm for lung injury and repair. *Chest* 99:87S, 1991.
16. Henson PM, Johnston RB: Tissue injury in inflammation: Oxidants, proteinases, and cationic proteins. *J Clin Invest* 79:669, 1987.
17. Deby-Dupont G, Lamy M, Faymonville ME, et al: Proteases and antiproteases in the adult respiratory distress syndrome, in Zapol WM, Lemaire F (eds): *Adult Respiratory Distress Syndrome*. New York, Marcel-Dekker, 1991, pp 305–352.
18. Frank L: Oxidant injury to pulmonary endothelium, in Said SI (ed): *The Pulmonary Circulation and Acute Lung Injury*. Mt. Kisco, NY, Futura, 1985.
19. Tate RM, Repine JE: Neutrophils and the adult respiratory distress syndrome. *Am Rev Respir Dis* 128:552, 1985.
20. Zimmerman GA, Renzetti AD, Hill HR: Functional and metabolic activity of granulocytes from patients with adult respiratory distress syndrome: Evidence for activated neutrophils in the pulmonary circulation. *Am Rev Respir Dis* 127:290, 1983.
21. Heflin AC, Brigham KL: Prevention by granulocyte depletion of increased vascular permeability of sheep lung following endotoxemia. *J Clin Invest* 68:1253, 1981.
22. Parker JC, Martin DJ, Rutili G, et al: Prevention of free radical mediated vascular permeability increase in lung using superoxide dismutase. *Chest* 83:52S, 1983.

23. Idell S, Cohen AB: Bronchoalveolar lavage in patients with the adult respiratory distress syndrome. *Clin Chest Med* 6:459, 1985.

24. Bevilacqua MP: Endothelial-leukocyte adhesion molecules. *Ann Rev Immunol* 11:767, 1993.

25. Malik AB, Perlman MB, Cooper JA, et al: Pulmonary microvascular effects of arachidonic acid metabolites and their role in lung vascular injury. *Fed Proc* 44:36, 1985.

26. Laufe MD, Simon RH, Flint A, Keller JB: Adult respiratory distress syndrome in neutropenic patients. *Am J Med* 80:1022, 1986.

27. Maunder RJ, Hackman RC, Riff E, et al: Occurrence of the adult respiratory distress syndrome in neutropenic patients. *Am Rev Respir Dis* 133:313, 1986.

28. Rinaldo JE, Christman JW: Mechanisms and mediators of the adult respiratory distress syndrome. *Clin Chest Med* 11:621, 1990.

29. Marinelli WA, Henke CA, Harmon KR, et al: Mechanisms of alveolar fibrosis after acute lung injury. *Clin Chest Med* 11:657, 1990.

30. Jones R, Reid LM, Zapol WM, et al: Pulmonary vascular pathology: Human and experimental studies, in Falke KJ (ed): *Lung Biology in Health and Disease.* New York, Marcel Dekker, 1985.

31. Ferro TJ, Malik AB: Mechanisms of lung vascular injury and edema after pulmonary microembolism. *J Crit Care* 4:118, 1989.

32. Wickershan NE, Johnson JJ, Meyrick BO, et al: Lung ischemia-reperfusion injury in awake sheep: Protection with verapamil. *J Appl Physiol* 71:1554, 1991.

33. Bishop MJ, Cheney FW: Lung reperfusion in dogs causes bilateral lung injury. *J Appl Physiol* 63:942, 1987.

34. Idell S, James KK, Levin EG, et al: Local abnormalities in coagulation and fibrinolytic pathways predispose to alveolar fibrin deposition in the adult respiratory distress syndrome. *J Clin Invest* 84:695, 1989.

35. Dantzker DR, Brook CJ, Dehart P, et al: Ventilation-perfusion distribution in the adult respiratory distress syndrome. *Am Rev Respir Dis* 120:1039, 1979.

36. Dantzker DR: Pulmonary gas exchange, in Dantzker DR (ed): *Cardiovascular Critical Care.* 2nd ed. Philadelphia, WB Saunders, 1992.

37. Gattinoni L, Pesenti A: Computed tomography scanning in acute respiratory failure, in Zapol WM, Lemaire F (eds): *Adult Respiratory Distress Syndrome.* New York, Marcel-Dekker, 1991, pp 199–222.

38. Marini JJ: Lung mechanics in the adult respiratory distress syndrome: Recent conceptual advances and implications for management. *Clin Chest Med* 11:673, 1990.

39. Lewis JF, Jobe AH: Surfactant and the adult respiratory distress syndrome. *Am Rev Respir Dis* 147:218, 1993.

40. Wright PE, Bernard GR: The role of airflow resistance in patients with the adult respiratory distress syndrome. *Am Rev Respir Dis* 139:1169, 1989.

41. Zapol WM, Rie NA, Frikker M, et al: Pulmonary circulation during acute respiratory distress syndrome, in Falke KJ (ed): *Lung Biology in Health and Disease,* New York, Marcel Dekker, 1985.

42. Eisenberg PR, Hansbrough JR, Anderson D, Schuster DP: A prospective study of lung water measurements during patient management in an intensive care unit. *Am Rev Respir Dis* 136:662, 1987.

43. Sandiford P, Province MA, Schuster DP: Distribution of regional density and vascular permeability in the adult respiratory distress syndrome. *Am J Respir Crit Care Med* 151:737, 1995.

44. Fein A, Grossman R, Jones JG, et al: The value of edema fluid protein measurements in patients with pulmonary edema. *Am J Med* 67:32, 1979.

45. Kaplan JD, Calandrino FS, Schuster DP: A positron emission tomographic comparison of pulmonary vascular permeability during the adult respiratory distress syndrome and pneumonia. *Am Rev Respir Dis* 143:150, 1991.

46. Milne ENC, Pistolesi M, Miniati M, Giuntini C: The radiographic distinction of cardiogenic and noncardiogenic edema. *Am J Roentgenol* 144:879, 1985.

47. Smith RC, Mann H, Greenspan RH, et al: Radiographic differentiation between different etiologies of pulmonary edema. *Invest Radiol* 22:859, 1987.

48. Sprung CL, Rackow EC, Fein IA, et al: The spectrum of pulmonary edema: Differentiation of cardiogenic, intermediate, and noncardiogenic forms of pulmonary edema. *Am Rev Respir Dis* 124:718, 1981.

49. Drake RE, Liane GA: Pulmonary microvascular permeability to fluid and macromolecules. *J Appl Physiol* 64:487, 1988.

50. Lily CM, Ishizaka A, Raffin TA: The measurement of lung water. *J Crit Care* 5:252, 1990.

51. Mitchell JP, Schuller D, Calandrino FS, Schuster DP: Improved outcome based on fluid management in critically ill patients requiring pulmonary artery catheterization. *Am Rev Respir Dis* 145:990, 1992.

52. Wiedemann HP, Matthay MA, Gillis CN: Pulmonary endothelial cell injury and altered lung metabolic function: Early detection of the adult respiratory distress syndrome and possible functional significance. *Clin Chest Med* 11:723, 1990.

53. Schuster DP: A physiologic approach to initiating, maintaining, and withdrawing mechanical ventilatory support during acute respiratory failure. *Am J Med* 88:268, 1990.

54. MacIntyre NR: Building consensus on the use of mechanical ventilation. *Chest* 104:334, 1993.

55. Marini JJ, Kelsen SG: Re-targeting ventilatory objectives in adult respiratory distress syndrome. *Am Rev Respir Dis* 146:2, 1992.

56. Gammon RB, Shin MS, Buchalter SE: Pulmonary barotrauma in mechanical ventilation: Patterns and risk factors. *Chest* 102:568, 1992.

57. Dreyfuss D, Soler P, Basset G, Saumon G: High inflation pressure pulmonary edema: Respective effects of high airway pressure, high tidal volume, and positive end-expiratory pressure. *Am Rev Respir Dis* 137:1159, 1988.

58. Leatherman JW, Lari RL, Iber C, Ney AL: Tidal volume reduction in ARDS: Effect on cardiac output and arterial oxygenation. *Chest* 99:1227, 1991.

59. Kiiski R, Takala J, Kari A, Milic-Emili J: Effect of tidal volume on gas exchange and oxygen transport in the adult respiratory distress syndrome. *Am Rev Respir Dis* 146:1131, 1992.

60. Stoller JK, Kacmarek RM: Ventilatory strategies in the management of the adult respiratory distress syndome. *Clin Chest Med* 11:755, 1990.

61. Pepe PE, Hudson LD, Carrico CJ: Early application of positive end-expiratory pressure in patients at risk for the adult respiratory distress syndrome. *N Engl J Med* 311:281, 1984.

62. Elliott CG, Rasmusson BY, Crapo RO, et al: Prediction of pulmonary function abnormalities after adult respiratory distress syndrome. *Am Rev Respir Dis* 135:634, 1987.

63. Lynch JP, Myhre JG, Dantzker DR: Influence of cardiac output on intrapulmonary shunt. *J Appl Physiol* 46:315, 1987.

64. Ranieri VM, Giuliani R, Eissa NT, et al: Oxygen delivery-consumption relationship in septic adult respiratory distress syndrome patients: The effects of positive end-expiratory pressure. *J Crit Care* 75:150, 1992.

65. Eberhard L, Guttman J, Wolff G, et al: Intrinsic PEEP monitored in the ventilated ARDS patient with a mathematical method. *J Appl Physiol* 73:479, 1992.

66. Kollef MH: Lung hyperinflation caused by inappropriate ventilation resulting in electromechanical dissociation: A case report. *Heart Lung* 21:74, 1992.

67. Hickling DG, Henderson SJ, Jackson R: Low mortality associated with low volume, pressure limited ventilation with permissive hypercapnia in severe adult respiratory distress syndrome. *Intensive Care Med* 16:372, 1990.

68. Presenti A, Gattinoni L, Bombino M: Long term extracorporeal respiratory support: 20 years of progress. *Intensive Crit Care Dig* 12:15, 1993.

69. Gurevitch MJ, Van Dyke J, Young ES, Jackson K: Improved oxygenation and lower peak airway pressure in severe adult respiratory distress syndrome: Treatment with inverse ratio ventilation. *Chest* 89:211, 1986.

70. Marcy TW, Marini JJ: Inverse ratio ventilation in ARDS: Rationale and implementation. *Chest* 100:494, 1991.

71. Tharratt RS, Allen RP, Albertson TE: Pressure controlled inverse ratio ventilation in severe adult respiratory failure. *Chest* 94:755, 1988.

72. Lain D, DiBenedetto R, Morris S, et al: Pressure control inverse ratio ventilation as a method to reduce peak inspiratory pressure

and provide adequate ventilation and oxygenation. *Chest* 95:1081, 1989.

73. East TD, Bohm SH, Wallace J, et al: A successful computerized protocol for clinical management of pressure control inverse ratio ventilation in ARDS patients. *Chest* 101:697, 1992.

74. Downs JB, Stock MC: Airway pressure release ventilation: A new concept in ventilatory support. *Crit Care Med* 15:459, 1987.

75. Villar J, Winston B, Slutsky AS: Non-conventional techniques of ventilatory support. *Crit Care Clin* 6:579, 1990.

76. Schuster DP, Klain M, Snyder JV: Comparison of high frequency jet ventilation to conventional mechanical ventilation during severe acute respiratory failure in humans. *Crit Care Med* 10:625, 1982.

77. Holzapfel L, Robert D, Perrin F, et al: Comparison of high frequency jet ventilation to conventional ventilation in adults with respiratory distress syndrome. *Intensive Care Med* 13:100, 1987.

78. Carlon GC, Howland WS, Ray C, et al: High-frequency jet ventilation: A prospective randomized evaluation. *Chest* 84:551, 1983.

79. Zapol WM, Snider MT, Hill JD, et al: Extracorporeal membrane oxygenation in severe acute respiratory failure. *JAMA* 242:2193, 1979.

80. Brichon PY, Barnoud D, Pison C, et al: Double lung transplantation for adult respiratory distress syndrome after recombinant interleukin 2. *Chest* 104:609, 1993.

81. Morris AH, Menlove RL, Rollins RJ, et al: A controlled clinical trial of a new 3-step therapy that includes extracorporeal CO_2 removal for ARDS. *Trans Am Soc Artif Intern Organs* 11:48, 1933.

82. Piehl M, Brown R: Use of extreme position changes in acute respiratory failure. *Crit Care Med* 4:13, 1976.

83. Douglas W, Rehder K, Beynen F, et al: Improved oxygenation in patients with acute respiratory failure: The prone position. *Am Rev Respir Dis* 115:559, 1977.

84. Langer M, Mascheroni D, Macolin R, Gattinoni L: The prone position in ARDS patients: A clinical study. *Chest* 94:103, 1988.

85. Bone RC: Treatment of adult respiratory distress syndrome with diuretics, dialysis, and positive end-expiratory pressure. *Crit Care Med* 6:136, 1978.

86. Simmons RS, Berdine GG, Seidenfeld JJ, et al: Fluid balance and the adult respiratory distress syndrome. *Am Rev Respir Dis* 135:924, 1987.

87. Humphrey H, Hall J, Sznajder I, et al: Improved survival in ARDS patients associated with a reduction in pulmonary capillary wedge pressure. *Chest* 97:1176, 1990.

88. Schuller D, Mitchell JP, Calandrino FS, Schuster DP: Fluid balance during pulmonary edema: Is fluid gain a marker or a cause of poor outcome? *Chest* 100:1068, 1991.

89. Russell JA, Ronco JJ, Lockhat D, et al: Oxygen delivery and consumption and ventricular preload are greater in survivors than in nonsurvivors of the adult respiratory distress syndrome. *Am Rev Respir Dis* 141:659, 1990.

90. Schumacker PT, Samsel RW: Oxygen supply and consumption in the adult respiratory distress syndrome. *Clin Chest Med* 11:715, 1990.

91. Shoemaker WC, Appel PL, Kram HB: Role of oxygen debt in the development of organ failure, sepsis, and death in high-risk surgical patients. *Chest* 102:208, 1992.

92. Tuchschmidt J, Fried J, Astiz M, Rackow E: Elevation of cardiac output and oxygen delivery improves outcome in septic shock. *Chest* 102:216, 1992.

93. Sibbald WJ, Driedger AA, McCallum D, et al: Nitroprusside infusion does not improve biventricular performance in patients with acute hypoxemic respiratory failure. *J Crit Care* 1:197, 1986.

94. Weg JG, Balk RA, Tharratt S, et al: Safety and potential efficacy of an aerosolized surfactant in human sepsis-induced adult respiratory distress syndrome. *JAMA* 272:1433, 1994.

95. Sibbald WJ, Anderson R, Reid B, et al: Alveocapillary permeability in human septic ARDS. *Chest* 79:133, 1981.

96. Sprung C, Caralis P, Marcial E, et al: The effects of high dose corticosteroids in patients with septic shock: A prospective controlled study. *N Engl J Med* 311:1137, 1984.

97. Bernard GR, Luce JM, Sprung CL, et al: High dose corticosteroids in patients with the adult respiratory distress syndrome. *N Engl J Med* 317:1565, 1987.

98. Luce JM, Montgomery AB, Marks JD, et al: Ineffectiveness of high-dose methylprednisolone in preventing parenchymal lung injury and improving mortality in patients with septic shock. *Am Rev Respir Dis* 138:62, 1988.

99. Bone RC, Fisher CJ, Clemmer TP, et al: Early methylprednisolone treatment for septic syndrome and the adult respiratory distress syndrome. *Chest* 92:1032, 1987.

100. Ashbaugh DG, Maier RV: Idiopathic pulmonary fibrosis in adult respiratory distress syndrome: Diagnosis and treatment. *Arch Surg* 120:530, 1985.

101. Hooper RG, Kearl RA: Established ARDS treated with a sustained course of adrenocortical steroids. *Chest* 97:138, 1990.

102. Meduri GU, Belenchia JM, Estes RJ, et al: Fibroproliferative phase of ARDS: Clinical findings and effects of corticosteroids. *Chest* 100:943, 1991.

103. Jepsen S, Herlevsen P, Knudsen P, et al: Antioxidant treatment with N-acetylcysteine during adult respiratory distress syndrome: A prospective, randomized, placebo-controlled study. *Crit Care Med* 20:918, 1992.

104. Frostell CG, Blomqvist H, Hedenstierna G, et al: Inhaled nitric oxide selectively reverses human hypoxic pulmonary vasoconstriction without causing systemic vasodilation. *Anesthesiology* 78:427, 1993.

105. Oda H, Nogami H, Kusumoto S, et al: Long-term exposure to nitric oxide in mice. *Jpn J Soc Air Pollut* 11:150, 1976.

106. Rossaint R, Falkle KJ, Lopez F, et al: Inhaled nitric oxide for the adult respiratory distress syndrome. *N Engl J Med* 328:399, 1993.

107. Fletcher JR, Ramwell PW: Indomethacin treatment following baboon endotoxin shock improves survival. *Adv Shock Res* 4:103, 1980.

108. Bernard GR, Reines HD, Halushka PV, et al: Prostacyclin and thromboxane A2 formation is increased human sepsis syndrome: Effects of cyclooxygenase inhibition. *Am Rev Respir Dis* 144:1095, 1991.

109. Haupt MT, Jastremski MS, Clemmer TP, et al: Effect of ibuprofen in patients with severe sepsis: A randomized double-blind, multicenter study. *Crit Care Med* 19:1339, 1991.

110. Michie HR, Manogue KR, Spriggs DR, et al: Detection of circulating tumor necrosis factor after endotoxin administration. *N Engl J Med* 318:1481, 1988.

111. Holcroft JW, Vassar MJ, Weber CJ: Prostaglandin E_1 and survival in patients with the respiratory distress syndrome. *Ann Surg* 203:371, 1986.

112. Bone RC, Slotman G, Maunder R, et al: Randomized double-blind, multicenter study of prostaglandin E_1 in patients with the adult respiratory distress syndrome. *Chest* 96:114, 1989.

113. Reyes An Roca J, Rodriguez-Roisin R, Torres A, et al: Effect of almitrine on ventilator-perfusion distribution in adult respiratory distress syndrome. *Am Rev Respir Dis* 137:1062, 1988.

114. Melot C, Naeije R, Mols P, et al: Pulmonary vascular tome improves pulmonary gas exchange in the adult respiratory distress syndrome. *Am Rev Respir Dis* 136:1232, 1987.

115. Schuster DP: ARDS: Clinical lessons from the oleic acid model of acute lung injury. *Am J Respir Crit Care Med* 149:245, 1994.

116. Montravers P, Fagon JY, Gilbert C, et al: Pilot study of cardiopulmonary risk from pentoxifylline in adult respiratory distress syndrome. *Chest* 103:1017, 1993.

117. Ziegler EJ, Fisher CJ, Sprung CL, et al: Treatment of gram negative bacteremia and septic shock with HA-1A human monoclonal antibody against endotoxin. *N Engl J Med* 324:429, 1991.

118. Greenman RL, Schein RM, Martin MA, et al: A controlled clinical trial of E5 murine monoclonal IgM antibody to endotoxin in the treatment of gram negative sepsis. *JAMA* 266:1097, 1991.

119. Wenzel R, Bone R, Fein A, et al: Results of a second double-blind randomized, controlled trial of antiendotoxin antibody E5 in gram-negative sepsis (abstract 1170), in *Program and Abstracts of the 31st Interscience Conference on Antimicrobial Agents and Chemotherapy.* Washington DC, American Society for Microbiology, 1991, p 294.

120. Fisher CJ, Opal SM, Dhainaut JF, et al: Influence of an anti-tumor necrosis factor monoclonal antibody on cytokine levels in patients with sepsis. *Crit Care Med* 21:318, 1993.

121. Luger A, Graf H, Schwarz HP, et al: Decreased serum interleukin 1 activity and monocyte interleukin 1 production in patients with fatal sepsis. *Crit Care Med* 14:458, 1986.

122. Munoz C, Misset B, Fitting C, et al: Dissociation between plasma and monocyte associated cytokines during sepsis. *Eur J Immunol* 21:2177, 1991.

123. Pingleton SK: Complications of acute respiratory failure. *Am Rev Respir Dis* 137:1463, 1988.

124. Knaus WA, Wagner DP, Draper EA, et al: The Apache III prognostic system: Risk prediction of hospital mortality for critically ill hospitalized adults. *Chest* 100:1619, 1991.

125. Matuschak GM, Rinaldo JE, Pinsky MR, et al: Effect of end-stage liver failure on the incidence and resolution of the adult respiratory distress syndrome. *J Crit Care* 2:162, 1987.

126. Suchyta MR, Clemmer TP, Elliott CG, et al: The adult respiratory distress syndrome: A report of survival and modifying factors. *Chest* 101:1074, 1992.

127. Suchyta MR, Clemmer TP, Orme JF, et al: Increased survival of ARDS patients with severe hypoxemia (ECMO criteria). *Chest* 99:951, 1991.

128. Rubin DB, Weiner-Kronish JP, Murray JF, et al: Elevated von Willebrand factor antigen is an early plasma predictor of impending acute lung injury in nonpulmonary sepsis syndrome. *J Clin Invest* 86:474, 1990.

129. Miller EJ, Cohen AB, Nagao S, et al: Elevated levels of NAP-1/interleukin-8 are present in the airspaces of patients with the adult respiratory distress syndrome and are associated with increased mortality. *Am Rev Respir Dis* 146:427, 1992.

130. Matthay MA, Wiener-Kronish JP: Intact epithelial barrier function is critical for the resolution of alveolar edema in humans. *Am Rev Respir Dis* 142:1250, 1990.

131. Bone RC, Maunder R, Slotman G, et al: An early test of survival in patients with the adult respiratory distress syndrome: The PaO₂/FiO₂ ratio and its differential response to conventional therapy. *Chest* 96:849, 1989.

132. Elliott CG: Pulmonary sequelae in survivors of the adult respiratory distress syndrome. *Clin Chest Med* 11:789, 1990.

133. Peters JI, Bell RC, Prihoda TJ, et al: Clinical determinants of abnormalities in pulmonary functions in survivors of the adult respiratory distress syndrome. *Am Rev Respir Dis* 139:1163, 1989.

134. Ghio AJ, Elliott CG, Crapo RO, et al: Impairment after adult respiratory distress syndrome: An evaluation based on American Thoracic Society recommendations. *Am Rev Respir Dis* 139:1158, 1989.

56. Status Asthmaticus

J. Mark Madison and Richard S. Irwin

Asthma is an inflammatory disease of the airways that results in reversible airway obstruction [1,2]. Inflammation in the airways causes airway obstruction by making airway smooth muscle more sensitive to contractile stimuli [3], by thickening the airway wall with edema and inflammatory cell infiltration, by stimulating glands to secrete mucus into the airway lumen, and by damaging the airway epithelium [4]. Typically, intermittent worsening or exacerbation of asthma is triggered by exposure to environmental factors. These exacerbations represent acute or subacute episodes of increased airflow obstruction that may be mild to life-threatening in severity. Moderate to severe exacerbations that fail to respond rapidly to sympathomimetic treatment constitute status asthmaticus [5,6]. Assessment, management, and prevention of status asthmaticus are the critical challenges of caring for adult patients with asthma.

Epidemiology

Asthma ranks among the most common chronic diseases, affecting 4 percent of the U.S. population [7]. Many patients with asthma have mild disease and are never hospitalized, but a minority of patients have moderate to severe disease that is potentially life-threatening. In 1987, the rate of hospitalization for asthma approached 20 per 10,000 population in the United States, and 4360 people died from the disease [7].

There has been worldwide concern that the prevalence, severity, and mortality of asthma increased during the 1980s. In the United States, this trend has been most prominent among children and young adults, especially for females and minorities. From 1980 to 1987, overall hospitalization and mortality rates for asthma increased 6 percent and 31 percent, respectively. The factors underlying these trends in morbidity and mortality are controversial and may be partially accounted for by changing definitions of asthma, increased physician awareness, and improved reporting methods. However, poor patient access to medical care [8], failure of physicians and patients to recognize worsening airway obstruction promptly [9,10], over-utilization of beta-adrenergic agonists alone or in combination with methylxanthines [11,12], and delays in the institution of corticosteroids [9] all have been considered potential contributors.

Pathophysiology

Pathology. Bronchial biopsies of patients with even mild asthma are pathologically abnormal [13,14], with collagen deposition beneath the epithelial basement membranes, mucosal infiltration by eosinophils, mast cell degranulation, and epithelial damage. These findings occur in mild asthma, supporting the concept that airway inflammation is of primary importance in the pathogenesis of asthma.

Much of our understanding about the pathology of asthma stems from autopsies of patients who died from status asthmaticus [4]. Macroscopically, the lungs are hyperinflated and thick tenacious mucus fills the lumens of the airways. Microscopically, there is an eosinophilic bronchitis, with pronounced areas of mucosal edema and desquamation of the epithelium. The basement membrane beneath the epithelium is thickened. Typically, there is hypertrophy and hyperplasia of smooth muscle and the muscle appears contracted.

PATHOGENESIS. The causes of airway inflammation in asthma are not understood entirely [15]. Inhaled allergens [16], pollutants [17], smoke, and viral infections [18] all may play a role in establishing or augmenting inflammation in the asthmatic airway. In many patients, exposure to inhaled allergen is responsible for establishing the inflammatory process by binding to IgE on mast cells and macrophages to incite the release of potent inflammatory mediators such as histamine, platelet activating factor, leukotrienes, and thromboxanes. These mediators attract other inflammatory cells to the airway, especially eosinophils, and also have potent effects on other cell types in the airways. Mediators alter smooth muscle cell function, cause microvascular leakage, participate in neural regulation of the airways, and stimulate glands to secrete. The eosinophils that invade the airway wall release potent epithelial cell toxins that cause the epithelial damage typical in asthma.

These complex inflammatory events produce the multiple causes of airway obstruction of asthma. One consequence of inflammation is the development of the bronchial hyperresponsiveness that is the hallmark of asthma and the basis for methacholine challenge testing for asthma [3]. Mediators released during the inflammatory process render airway smooth muscle abnormally sensitive to contractile stimuli such as inhaled allergens, smoke, pollutants, cold air, fog, exercise, emotional stress, dusts, powders, and irritant fumes. These environmental stimuli contract airway smooth muscle, narrow airway caliber, and increase obstruction to airflow. In general, airway smooth muscle contraction is rapidly reversed by beta-adrenergic agonists. However, alleviating the underlying state of bronchial hyperresponsiveness itself is more slowly reversed by antiinflammatory therapy in the form of corticosteroids.

The other major causes of airway obstruction in asthma are less rapidly reversible than smooth muscle contraction; they are due to the effects of inflammation on cells other than smooth muscle cells. These slowly reversible causes of obstruction assume paramount importance during status asthmaticus. Inflammation damages the epithelium, causing cells to slough into the airway lumen, and stimulates gland cells to secrete mucus that obstructs the airway lumen [19]. Finally, edema and inflammatory cell infiltration of the airway wall diminish the caliber of the airway lumen by thickening the mucosa and submucosa. These other causes of airway obstruction do not respond well to beta-adrenergic agonists but do respond slowly to corticosteroid treatment.

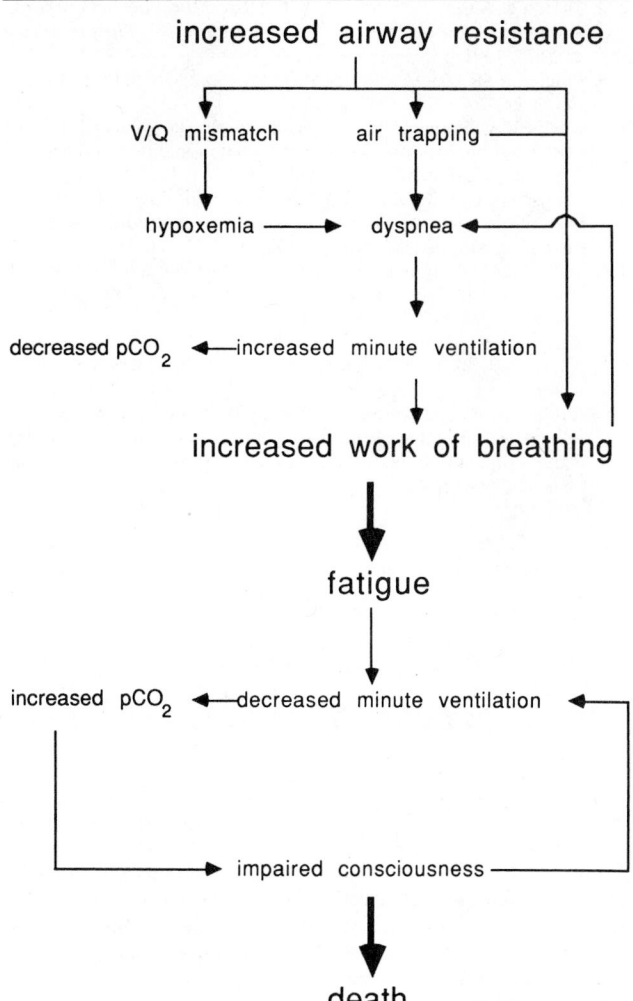

Fig. 56-1. The physiologic consequences of airway obstruction.

PHYSIOLOGY. The major physiologic consequences of airway obstruction are hypoxemia and increased work of breathing (Fig. 56-1). Understanding these physiologic disturbances is important for the assessment and management of status asthmaticus.

Narrowing the caliber of airway lumens causes hypoxemia by two mechanisms. First, increases in the resistance to flow in the conducting airways result in uneven distribution of ventilation to the alveoli. Hypoxic vasoconstriction of vessels supplying underventilated alveoli partially compensates for this uneven ventilation, but overall ventilation/perfusion ($\dot{V}/\dot{Q}$) ratios remain abnormal and are the principal cause of hypoxemia in asthma [20]. Consequently, even patients with severe exacerbations of asthma usually respond well to supplemental oxygen. A second, less common, cause of hypoxemia in asthma is shunt due to atelectasis of lung distal to airways completely occluded by mucus. This mechanism of hypoxemia may be significant in some patients.

The second physiologic consequence of severe airway obstruction is increased work of breathing. During status asthmaticus, respiratory muscles must expend increased energy, generating large changes in pleural pressure to overcome high airway resistance [21]. The resulting discordance between respiratory effort and the change in thoracic volume also plays a role in the patient's sensation of dyspnea and central drive to increase minute ventilation. The ensuing rapid respirations further increase the work of breathing and worsen air trapping behind narrowed airways that prematurely close during expiration. The air trapping itself leads to increased respiratory muscle energy costs because it restricts vital capacity to high thoracic volumes where alveolar dead space is increased, the respiratory muscles are at suboptimal mechanical advantage, and the lung is much less compliant. Thus, the respiratory muscles must expend more energy to achieve the same alveolar ventilation. All of these factors contribute to the enormous increase in the work of breathing.

Respiratory muscles may be able to exert the force needed to maintain alveolar ventilation initially but will fatigue if airway resistance increases rapidly or if there is inadequate delivery of energy supplies to the skeletal muscles. High respiratory frequencies and the prolonged contraction of accessory inspiratory muscles at high lung volumes interfere with blood flow to the muscles [22]. Similarly, high intraabdominal pressures during expiration may limit blood delivery to the diaphragm [23]. As severe hypoxemia develops, the blood that reaches the respiratory muscles carries inadequate oxygen content. Eventually, the respiratory muscles are unable to generate the force required to sustain alveolar ventilation.

Differential Diagnosis

Not all acute dyspnea with wheezing is due to asthma (Table 56-1). Congestive heart failure commonly causes wheezing, because edema in the bronchovascular interstitial space compresses the airways. Cardiac abnormalities on physical examination and radiographic changes in the cardiac silhouette and lung fields distinguish congestive heart failure from asthma. Acute pulmonary thromboembolism also can masquerade as an exacerbation of asthma, because the mediators released by platelets in thromboemboli cause bronchoconstriction and wheezing. However, hemoptysis, pleuritic pain, and pleural effusions rarely are seen in acute exacerbations of asthma. Foreign bodies in the airways may result in wheezing, although typically the wheezing is localized rather than diffuse. Inspiratory wheezing (stridor) due to extrathoracic airway obstruction sometimes is confused with the wheezing of acute asthma. Causes of stridor are multiple, but among those most commonly confused with acute asthma is laryngeal dysfunction [24].

Less common diseases mimicking asthma have distinctive chest radiographic findings. Chronic eosinophilic pneumonia can present with dyspnea and wheezing, but the chest radiograph shows an interstitial and alveolar filling pattern, predominantly at the lung periphery. Allergic bronchopulmonary aspergillosis may complicate chronic asthma and features upper lobe retraction and fibrosis with or without central cystic bronchiectasis. Allergic granulomatosis (Churg-Strauss disease) may mimic asthma, but there is characteristically a diffuse, mixed interstitial and alveolar pattern on chest radiograph.

Assessment

Physician failure to appreciate the severity of airway obstruction in acute asthma probably contributes to mortality [9]. Patients who die from asthma often have been evaluated by medical personnel who underestimated the severity of airway obstruction. Patient-reported symptoms and the amount of wheezing heard by auscultation of the chest are inadequate assessments of airway obstruction. The cornerstone of evaluation of patients with asthma exacerbations is the objective measurement of airflow. Since some patients may be unable to perform the necessary maneuvers, the physician also must be adept at recognizing certain historical features and physical findings that strongly suggest high risk for severe airway obstruction.

HISTORY. Historical details important for identifying patients at high risk for life-threatening airway obstruction include identification of current medications and coexisting illness, especially cardiopulmonary disease. A history of known coronary artery disease is important since the patient may be more sensitive to the stimulatory effects of beta-adrenergic agonists and to the cardiac complications of hypoxemia. The physician should discern the time of onset of the current exacerbation and what triggered the attack. In general, the longer an exacerbation has been active, the more severe the attack and the slower the resolution.

Patient complaints of severe breathlessness or chest tightness

Table 56-1. Differential Diagnosis of Wheezing

Upper respiratory tract
  Amyloid
  Angioedema
  Foreign body
  Goiter
  Infection
  Neuromuscular disease
  Relapsing polychondritis
  Tracheal stenosis
  Tumor
  Vocal cord paralysis
Lower respiratory tract
  Adenopathy
  Amyloid
  Asthma
  Aspiration
  Bronchiolitis
  Chronic obstructive pulmonary disease
  Cystic fibrosis
  Foreign body
  Pulmonary infiltrates with eosinophilia
  Sarcoidosis
Vascular
  Acute respiratory distress syndrome
  Congestive heart failure
  Pulmonary embolism
  Vasculitis
Extrathoracic
  Carcinoid
  Factitious

or difficulty walking more than 100 feet suggest severe airway obstruction. Prior endotracheal intubation for asthma, frequent or recent (within the month) emergency department visits or hospitalizations for asthma, current or recent use of systemic corticosteroids, and a history of syncope or seizures during prior asthma exacerbations should alert the physician to a patient's tendency to develop severe airway obstruction [25]. In general, patients are somewhat better judges of the severity of airway obstruction during an attack of asthma than are physicians eliciting their history [26]. However, patient assessment of airway obstruction should never be the exclusive means of assessing the severity of airway obstruction.

PHYSICAL EXAMINATION. Physical examination is important for excluding other causes of dyspnea (see Differential Diagnosis) and assessing the degree of airway obstruction [27]. Tachycardia (>120 beats/min), tachypnea (>30 breaths/min), diaphoresis [28], bolt upright posture in bed, pulsus paradox greater than 10 mm Hg, and accessory muscle use all should be regarded as signs of severe airway obstruction [29]. However, since the absence of these signs does not rule out severe obstruction, physical examination cannot be relied on exclusively to estimate the severity of airway obstruction. The amount of wheezing heard on auscultation of the chest is a notoriously poor method of assessing airway obstruction because expiratory wheezing is a function not only of the amount of airway obstruction but also of the volume of air exhaled. Therefore, even a patient with severe obstruction may have minimal wheezing on auscultation of the chest [30]. Cyanosis is a late, insensitive finding of severe hypoxemia. Respiratory muscle alternans, abdominal paradox, and depressed mental status due to hypoxemia and hypercapnia are ominous indicators of muscle fatigue and often herald the necessity for endotracheal intubation and mechanical ventilation [31].

Table 56-2. Objective Assessment of Airway Obstruction

	PEFR or FEV$_1$	Interpretation
Initial assessment	70%-nl predicted	Mild obstruction
	40–70% predicted	Moderate obstruction
	<40% predicted	Severe obstruction
Assessment after intensive bronchodilator therapy	>70% predicted	Good response
	40–70% predicted	Incomplete response
	<40% predicted	Poor response

PEFR = peak expiratory flow rate; FEV$_1$ = forced expired volume of air in 1 second; nl = normal.

PULMONARY FUNCTION TESTS. To evaluate patients for the presence of severe airway obstruction reliably, an objective measure of maximal expiratory airflow should be performed whenever possible. Peak expiratory airflow rate (PEFR) and the forced expired volume of air in 1 second (FEV$_1$) are equally good bedside measures to quantify the degree of airway obstruction [32]. These tests are invaluable for the initial assessment and for following responses to therapy [33]. In general, a PEFR or FEV$_1$ less than 40 percent of baseline (either the predicted value or the patient's best known value) is regarded as severe airway obstruction (Table 56-2).

The PEFR and FEV$_1$ do have limitations in assessing airway function. Both are most sensitive to obstruction of central airways, which have rapid increases in resistance during an asthma exacerbation. Obstructions in small peripheral airways develop and resolve more slowly, and these changes are less well reflected by PEFR and FEV$_1$ [34]. These factors may explain the occasional clinical dissociation between improvement in flow rates and persistence of abnormal gas exchange.

ARTERIAL BLOOD GASES. Arterial blood gas (ABG) analysis is important for assessing and managing acute asthma exacerbations (see Chap. 15) and should be performed whenever the history, physical findings, or spirometric measures of airflow suggest high risk for severe airway obstruction. Also, any patient failing to respond to the first 30 to 60 minutes of intensive bronchodilator therapy should have an ABG performed. Although ABGs are not predictive of overall patient outcome [32], there is some correlation between hypoxemia and the degree of airway obstruction measured by FEV$_1$ [35]. Also, ABGs aid in management of severely obstructed patients, because the degree of hypoxemia and hypercapnia is important in deciding when to institute mechanical ventilation.

During acute exacerbations of asthma, hypoxemia primarily is due to $\dot{V}/\dot{Q}$ mismatch (see Physiology). Areas of atelectasis due to mucus plugging presumably account for instances of increased shunt fraction in asthma. A PaO$_2$ less than 60 mm Hg or a pulse oximeter value less than 90 percent on room air should be regarded as additional evidence of severe airway obstruction [25].

Understanding the changes in PaCO$_2$ expected during asthma exacerbation is important for recognition of a rapidly deteriorating course. With modest airway obstruction, the central nervous system detects a discordance between respiratory effort and changes in thoracic volume. This results in the sensation of mild dyspnea and stimulates an increase in minute ventilation that meets or exceeds the level required to maintain normal alveolar ventilation. Thus, patients with modest obstruction have a normal or slightly below normal PaCO$_2$. As airway obstruction worsens, dyspnea becomes more severe and the central nervous system drive to increase minute ventilation becomes intense. Typically, the increase in minute ventilation exceeds the level required to maintain constant alveolar ventilation; consequently, patients with moderate to severe obstruction have lower than normal PaCO$_2$ and respiratory alkalosis. As the airway obstruction becomes more severe or prolonged enough to cause fatigue of the respiratory muscles, high minute ventilation can no longer be maintained and alveolar ventilation decreases. As a result, the PaCO$_2$ rises toward normal and then continues to climb, resulting in hypercapnia and respiratory acidosis. A normal or high PaCO$_2$ ($\geq$ 40 mm Hg) during a severe exacerbation of asthma signifies fatigue, impending respiratory failure, and the need for prompt attention. In general, patients presenting with hypercapnia have a longer duration of chronic asthma and are frequently steroid-dependent. Of course, any coexisting conditions (malnutrition, advanced age) or medications (sedatives) that weaken respiratory muscle function or depress respiratory drive should be expected to accelerate the onset of hypercapneic ventilatory failure during acute exacerbations of asthma [36].

OTHER LABORATORY STUDIES. For status asthmaticus, routine chest radiographs reveal few abnormalities other than hyperinflation [37]. However, chest radiography is useful for identifying other causes of dyspnea and wheezing (see Differential Diagnosis) and detecting complications of severe airway obstruction. Chest radiographs should be examined carefully for evidence of enlarged cardiac silhouette, upper lung zone redistribution of blood flow, pleural effusions, and alveolar or interstitial infiltrates, since any of these findings suggests a diagnosis other than or in addition to acute asthma. For example, radiographic evidence suggestive of pneumonia, congestive heart failure, or pulmonary embolism would lead to changes in diagnostic and therapeutic plans. In addition, chest radiography allows the early detection of common complications of airway obstruction, including pneumothorax, pneumomediastinum, and atelectasis.

In the elderly, in patients with severe hypoxemia, and in patients with suspected cardiac ischemia or dysrhythmia, an electrocardiogram should be performed. Sinus tachycardia is common during acute exacerbations of asthma [27]. Other, less common and transient, findings include right axis deviation, right ventricular dominance, P pulmonale, S–T and T wave abnormalities, right bundle branch block, and ventricular ectopic beats [27,38]. The acute development of P pulmonale suggests severe airway obstruction and has been attributed to transmission of markedly negative pleural pressures to the right atrium [39].

Therapeutic Agents

Optimal management of status asthmaticus begins with a careful assessment of the degree of airway obstruction. This initial

Table 56-3. Treatment of Status Asthmaticus

Pharmacologic agents
  Antiinflammatory agents
  Bronchodilators

  Systemic corticosteroids
  Inhaled beta-adrenergic agonists
  Oral or intravenous methylxanthines
  Cholinergic antagonists (not routine)
  Systemic beta-adrenergic agonists (not routine)
  MgSO₄ (not routine)
  General anesthetics (not routine)

Supportive measures
  Frequent reassessment
  Supplemental oxygen
  Fluid management
  Mechanical ventilation if needed (controlled hypoventilation)
  Helium-oxygen mixtures (not routine)
  Lavage by bronchoscopy (not routine)
Education
  Avoidance of asthma triggers
  Medication use
  Access to medical follow-up
  Home monitoring of airway obstruction

assessment and repeated objective measures of airway obstruction guide treatment that combines supportive measures, bronchodilator therapy, and antiinflammatory therapy (Table 56-3).

Because the dominant causes of airway obstruction in status asthmaticus are the result of airway inflammation, the cornerstone of treatment is antiinflammatory therapy with systemic corticosteroids. Since corticosteroids take at least 4 to 6 hours to have a beneficial effect and the inflammatory causes of airway obstruction may take days to resolve, the medical challenge is to support patients until the inflammatory processes have responded to corticosteroids.

Bronchodilator therapy with beta-adrenergic agonists to relieve the bronchospasm due to airway smooth muscle contraction is an important therapeutic maneuver in initial treatment. Although bronchodilators relieve only one component of the airway obstruction in status asthmaticus, even small improvements in airflow lead to important clinical benefits. Of the available bronchodilators, beta-adrenergic agonists are the most effective and rapidly acting and therefore most useful during that critical time before the onset of corticosteroid action. Other measures that support the patient until the inflammatory processes in the airways have resolved include supplemental oxygen, judicious fluid administration, and, when indicated, mechanical ventilation.

BETA-ADRENERGIC AGONISTS. On a molecular level, beta-adrenergic agonists bind to beta₂-adrenergic receptors on airway smooth muscle cells and stimulate adenylyl cyclase to synthesize 3′,5′-cyclic adenosine monophosphate (cyclic AMP). Cyclic AMP activates the cytosolic enzyme protein kinase A, which phosphorylates proteins to foster a decrease in cytosolic calcium and relaxation of the muscle cell [40].

The primary cellular targets of beta-adrenergic agonists are airway smooth muscle cells. However, other cells in the airways also express beta-adrenergic receptors. For example, acute administration of beta-adrenergic agonists may limit mediator release by stimulating beta-adrenergic receptors on mast cells [41]. Beta-adrenergic agonists also enhance mucociliary clearance by stimulating epithelial cells [42] and may inhibit cholinergic neurotransmission [43]. In the acute setting, however, these effects on nonmuscle cells probably are of minor importance.

Two different classes of beta-adrenergic agonists have emerged. Short-acting beta-adrenergic agonists have bronchodilatory effects that last approximately 3 to 5 hours. They include epinephrine, isoproterenol, terbutaline, metaproterenol, albuterol, and fenoterol. It is these short-acting agents that are the mainstay of bronchodilator therapy for acute asthma. These agents differ in their selectivity for beta₂-adrenergic receptors, the rank order of selectivity being epinephrine < isoproterenol < metaproterenol < fenoterol, terbutaline, and albuterol [44]. However, all of these agents have approximately equal efficacy in the treatment of asthma. A newer class of drugs, the long-acting beta-adrenergic agonists, have bronchodilatory effects that last at least 12 hours. Two examples are salmeterol and formotero [45]. Notably, salmeterol has a slow onset of bronchodilatory action [46] and is not recommended for the treatment of acute exacerbations of asthma. More information is needed regarding the potential role of formoterol in the treatment of acute asthma.

The major side effects of beta-adrenergic agonists during the treatment of status asthmaticus are tremor, cardiac stimulation, and hypokalemia [47]. These side effects are potentially serious, especially in the elderly, who frequently have underlying cardiac disease. Cardiac toxicity can be minimized by using agonists with improved beta₂-adrenergic receptor selectivity and by avoiding the systemic administration of beta-adrenergic agonists.

Beta-adrenergic agonists can be administered to patients by inhalational, subcutaneous, or intravenous routes. Numerous studies have shown that the bronchodilator effects of inhaled beta-adrenergic agonists are rapid in onset and equal to that achieved by systemic delivery [48,49,50]. Because the inhalational route allows administration of small doses directly to the airways with minimal systemic toxicity, this route is almost always preferable to systemic delivery.

Several options exist for the delivery of inhaled beta-adrenergic agonists (see Chapter 69). A small-volume nebulizer is widely used. Recent studies have shown that metered-dose inhalers (MDIs) equipped with spacing devices are as effective as small-volume nebulizers in the treatment of acute asthma, although some patients may have difficulty with MDI use [51,52,53]. Four puffs of albuterol by MDI have been given at 1-minute intervals and repeated every 30 minutes up to six doses [54]. Frequent inhalations may allow for progressively deeper penetration of drug into peripheral airways [55]. Powdered aerosols also have recently become available, but the data are insufficient to define their role in the treatment of status asthmaticus. Intermittent positive-pressure breathing (IPPB) devices to deliver aerosols were once popular but are rarely used today because many patients with severe asthma cannot tolerate the device and because the devices are no more effective than small-volume nebulizers [56]. Furthermore, the risk of barotrauma is significantly increased with IPPB, and pneumothorax resulting in death has been reported [57].

Subcutaneous administration is an alternative to inhalational delivery. Theoretically, systemic administration could deliver drugs to obstructed airways poorly accessible to inhaled aerosols. However, this theoretical advantage has not been supported by most studies [48,49,50].

Subcutaneous epinephrine (adults 0.3 ml and children 0.01 ml/kg of a 1:1000 solution every 20 min for 3 doses) has been a traditional therapy for acute asthma in emergency departments [58,59]. A major concern with the use of subcutaneous epinephrine in adults has been cardiac toxicity [60,61]. More selective beta$_2$-adrenergic agonists, such as terbutaline, are available for subcutaneous use, but cardiac toxicity in the elderly is still a significant concern. A theoretical advantage of the nonselective drug epinephrine is that it has considerable alpha-adrenergic activity that constricts pulmonary vasculature normally dilated by selective beta-adrenergic agonists. Thus, the decrease in PaO$_2$ sometimes seen with selective beta-adrenergic agonist administration does not occur with epinephrine [62].

Formerly, intravenous isoproterenol (0.05–1.5 μg/kg/min) was commonly used to treat status asthmaticus [63,64]. However, intravenous delivery of beta-adrenergic agonists is no longer recommended for the routine treatment of status asthmaticus. No convincing evidence has shown intravenous administration to be superior to inhaled delivery of beta-adrenergic agonists. The lack of enhanced efficacy and the potential cardiac toxicity of intravenous beta-adrenergic agonists have led most to reserve intravenous delivery for those rare patients who continue to deteriorate on mechanical ventilation despite maximal routine therapy with inhaled beta-adrenergic agonists. Some reports have described patients who had significantly greater bronchodilation to intravenous rather than inhaled beta-adrenergic agonists [63]. The intravenous route should be used only in closely monitored adults, because myocardial ischemia can occur [65].

CHOLINERGIC ANTAGONISTS. The muscarinic cholinergic antagonists ipratropium and atropine are effective bronchodilators but more slowly acting and less effective than the beta-adrenergic agonists [66,67,68]. In general, these agents should not be the primary therapy for acute asthma. Exceptions may be bronchospasm induced by acetylcholinesterase inhibitors or beta-adrenergic antagonists and rare patients with severe cardiac disease unable to tolerate any systemic effects of beta-adrenergic agonists [69].

Some data suggest that cholinergic antagonists may be a useful adjunct to beta-adrenergic agonists in the initial treatment of status asthmaticus [70,71]. Patients treated with ipratropium plus fenoterol had a larger mean increase in FEV$_1$ during the first 45 to 90 minutes of treatment compared to patients treated with either agent alone [71]. However, the benefit of adding ipratropium to beta-adrenergic agonists was relatively small in these studies. Additional studies are needed to define what role, if any, cholinergic antagonists have in the routine treatment of acute asthma.

METHYLXANTHINES. Methylxanthines are potentially toxic medications long used in the treatment of status asthmaticus. A reanalysis of trials examining the use of aminophylline in the therapy of status asthmaticus compared patients treated with aminophylline versus those treated with beta-adrenergic agonists [72]. Seven trials reported no differences in spirometric values between aminophylline and beta-adrenergic agonist treatment [73–79], three found aminophylline treatment superior [80,81,82], and three favored beta-adrenergic agonists [83,84,85]. When these results are pooled, there is no difference between aminophylline and beta-adrenergic agonist therapy. Because of these findings and because of the toxicity of methylxanthines, beta-adrenergic agonists have supplanted methylxanthines as the primary bronchodilators used to treat status asthmaticus.

The risks and benefits of routinely combining methylxanthines with beta-adrenergic agonists in the treatment of status asthmaticus have not been adequately reassessed since superior beta-adrenergic agonists and early corticosteroid use have become standard therapy. In the emergency department setting

it appears that routinely adding methylxanthines to beta-adrenergic agonists does not enhance bronchodilation but does increase the incidence of serious drug toxicity [79]. However, in hospitalized patients it is recommended that methylxanthines be routinely used in the treatment of status asthmaticus [25]. One rationale for this recommendation is the possibility that methylxanthines prolong the bronchodilator effects of beta-adrenergic agonists, thereby minimizing nocturnal symptoms of asthma in the recovering patient. Other theoretic beneficial effects include its positive inotropic and diuretic effects [86], induction of catecholamine release from adrenal glands [87], vagolytic effects [88], pulmonary and systemic vasodilation [89], central respiratory drive stimulation [90], and enhanced diaphragmatic contractility [91,92].

For patients not already taking methylxanthines, a loading dose of aminophylline (6 mg/kg lean body weight) is administered over 20 to 30 minutes, followed by an intravenous infusion rate of 0.6 mg/kg/hr. This infusion rate should be decreased if there are conditions that decrease methylxanthine clearance, especially congestive heart failure, cirrhosis, and use of cimetidine, ranitidine, allopurinol, oral contraceptives, erythromycin, ciprofloxacin, or norfloxacin [93,94,95]. Six hours after initiation of the infusion the serum theophylline level should be checked and the infusion rate adjusted accordingly, with 10 to 15 μg per milliter being therapeutic. Serum concentrations greater than 20 μg per milliliter are toxic.

Patients already taking theophylline as an outpatient may be continued on an oral sustained-release preparation. For hospitalized patients already taking theophylline who are unable to tolerate oral intake for any reason, a continuous infusion of aminophylline may be started but no loading dose should be administered.

Methylxanthine toxicity should be suspected when nausea, vomiting, diarrhea, tachycardia, cardiac dysrhythmias, or seizures are present. Because seizures can occur suddenly in the absence of other symptoms, serum levels should be monitored closely [86,96] (see Chap. 148).

CORTICOSTEROIDS. Numerous studies have documented the safety and effectiveness of short courses of corticosteroids in the treatment of status asthmaticus [97,98,99]. Their beneficial effects are attributed to their many potent antiinflammatory effects. Corticosteroids decrease synthesis of leukotrienes, prostaglandins, and thromboxanes [100]; inhibit cytokine release by macrophages and T cells [101]; decrease expression of endothelial cell adhesion molecules to inhibit migration of inflammatory cells into the airway [102]; increase neutral endopeptidase expression to enhance degradation of neuropeptides that regulate inflammation [103]; and decrease secretions from gland cells [104]. These effects on multiple cell types are mediated by glucocorticoid receptors in the cell cytosol that bind the corticosteroid and then translocate to the nucleus to bind at specific DNA sequences known as glucocorticoid response elements (GREs) [105]. The GREs are located near or adjacent to promoter sites for specific genes, and occupancy of the GRE either inhibits or stimulates gene synthesis. For example, corticosteroids inhibit the transcription of the genes encoding interleukins-1, 2, 4, and 8, gamma interferon, and tumor necrosis factor. Alternatively, transcription of the gene encoding lipocortin is stimulated by corticosteroids [100]. Lipocortin is a potent inhibitor of phospholipase A$_2$ activity, the enzyme that regulates arachidonic acid availability for leukotriene and prostaglandin synthesis. In addition to these many antiinflammatory effects, corticosteroids also may inhibit airway smooth muscle tachyphylaxis to beta-adrenergic agonists [98].

Systemic corticosteroids are the principal therapy for status asthmaticus [106]. Prednisone and methylprednisolone are the preferred agents. Compared with betamethasone and dexamethasone, prednisone and methylprednisolone do not contain metabisulfites and have shorter half-lives. Although hydrocortisone has the shortest half-life, it has more mineralocorticoid effect and may cause idiosyncratic bronchospasm in some aspirin-sensitive individuals [107].

The optimal route of corticosteroid administration in the treatment of status asthmaticus is not well established by double-blind, placebo-controlled clinical studies. Currently, aerosolized corticosteroids do not have an established role in the treatment of status asthmaticus and may exacerbate bronchospasm. For initial treatment of status asthmaticus, several studies suggest that oral administration of corticosteroids is as effective as intravenous therapy [108,109]. However, because absorption of orally administered drugs may be variable in critically ill patients, it is currently recommended that intravenous therapy be used for initial treatment [25]. Additional clinical trials are needed better to define the role of intravenous, oral, and inhaled corticosteroids in the treatment of status asthmaticus.

Intravenous administration of corticosteroids, either as a continuous infusion or as an intermittent bolus, is effective [97]. The optimum dose of intravenous corticosteroids is not well established. One study compared 15, 40 and 125 mg of methylprednisolone every 6 hours and suggested that patients improved most rapidly with the 125-mg dose [99]. However, most studies have failed to show a dose-response relationship for doses this high [110]. The current recommendation is that patients receive 60 to 80 mg of methylprednisolone every 6 to 8 hours [25].

Once a patient with status asthmaticus shows objective evidence of daily improvement, corticosteroids can be administered orally. Usually prednisone is started at 60 mg per day, gradually tapered by 2.5 to 5 mg per day [110,111]. As the oral prednisone dose is being tapered successfully, the recovering patient should be started on a corticosteroid aerosol.

OXYGEN. Supplemental oxygen therapy should be the initial intervention in the emergency department. Because $\dot{V}/\dot{Q}$ mismatch is the dominant cause of hypoxemia in asthma, the partial pressure of arterial oxygen readily increases in response to low levels (2–4 L/min O_2 by nasal prongs) of supplemental oxygen therapy. In addition to mitigating the cardiac and neurologic complications of severe hypoxemia, supplemental oxygen minimizes potential episodes of hypoxemia due to the acute administration of beta-adrenergic agonists, decreases elevated pulmonary vascular pressures due to hypoxic vasoconstriction, decreases bronchospasm due to hypoxia, and improves oxygen delivery to respiratory muscles.

FLUIDS. There is no convincing evidence that fluid administration hastens mobilization of inspissated secretions in the airways; thus fluid therapy should be used conservatively unless there is convincing evidence of significant dehydration. Excessive fluid administration may increase pulmonary capillary hydrostatic pressures and decrease plasma oncotic pressures. Combined with the markedly negative pleural pressures transmitted to the bronchovascular interstitium, these changes in vascular pressure gradients promote pulmonary edema formation, which might further complicate management [112].

OTHER. Some therapeutic agents used in the treatment of outpatients with asthma have no established role in the treatment of status asthmaticus. These include aerosolized cortico-steroids and sodium cromolyn as well as oral beta-adrenergic agonists, which cause significant systemic toxicities.

Intravenous magnesium sulfate has acute bronchodilator properties [113,114]. However, because the bronchodilatory effect is transient, is less than that of beta-adrenergic agonists [113,115], and does not augment the response to beta-adrenergic agonists [116], administration is not currently recommended for routine use (see Additional and Unconventional Management Measures).

Although mucus is an important cause of airway obstruction, mucolytics are not recommended. No convincing evidence suggests that acetylcysteine or potassium iodide has a role in treating status asthmaticus, and these agents may worsen cough and bronchospasm [117].

In general, status asthmaticus is not triggered by bacterial infections of the airways. Therefore, antibiotics are not routinely given [118]. Microscopic evaluation of purulent sputum in status asthmaticus reveals abundant eosinophils, not the neutrophils of an acute bacterial process. Institution of antibiotics is warranted only when there is strong suspicion of an active infectious process, particularly pneumonia and bacterial sinusitis.

Unless a patient is mechanically ventilated, sedatives and narcotics have absolutely no role in the treatment of status asthmaticus [6,119]. These agents depress the respiratory central drive to breathe that is critical for maintaining adequate minute ventilation. Theoretically, narcotics also may cause mast cell degranulation and worsen bronchospasm [120].

TREATMENT DURING PREGNANCY. Pregnancy does not alter treatment of uncomplicated status asthmaticus. Because severe asthma attacks have been associated with increased perinatal mortality, probably due to maternal hypoxia and respiratory alkalosis [121,122], pregnancy should not result in the withholding of agents usually used to treat status asthmaticus [123,124] (see Chap. 59).

Management

EMERGENCY DEPARTMENT. The National Asthma Education Program, conducted under the auspices of the National Institutes of Health, recently published guidelines for the assessment and management of patients with status asthmaticus [25]. Initial management of a patient with an acute exacerbation of asthma is based on the physician's assessment of the degree of airway obstruction and the patient's response to initial bronchodilator therapy using beta-adrenergic agonists. If in the initial assessment the patient is in extreme distress and has evidence of fatigue, impaired consciousness, or hypercapnia such that respiratory arrest is judged imminent, endotracheal intubation and mechanical ventilation should be the first priorities and then systemic corticosteroids and beta-adrenergic agonists (either aerosolized or parenteral) started immediately. On the other hand, if respiratory arrest is not impending within minutes, then 2 to 4 liters per minute of supplemental oxygen should be initiated and beta-adrenergic agonists delivered by aerosol for three doses over 60 to 90 minutes (e.g., albuterol 2.5 mg every 20–30 minutes by small-volume nebulizer or albuterol 0.4 mg—four puffs—every 20–30 minutes by MDI with spacer) [53,54]. After these treatments are initiated, a more detailed history and physical and laboratory examination can be completed. Close monitoring and repeated airflow measurements are critical for detecting further deterioration during this initial period of treatment.

If in response to initial bronchodilator therapy there is resolution of symptoms and wheezing and the PEFR or FEV_1 increases to 70 percent of baseline or greater (either the patient's predicted value or best known previous value), the patient has had a "good response," indicating that the airway obstruction was due primarily to airway smooth muscle contraction (i.e., the patient did not have status asthmaticus). Most of these patients will not require hospitalization. Exceptions might be patients with a history strongly suggestive of high risk for mortality from asthma. If the patient is discharged from the emergency department, strong consideration should be given to initiating a short course of oral prednisone and attention directed to close medical follow-up and patient education.

If after initial bronchodilator therapy the patient has persistent wheezing and shortness of breath and PEFR or FEV_1 is less than 70 percent of predicted, the patient still has active inflammation and edema of the airways and requires further treatment. Hourly inhaled beta-adrenergic agonists should be administered and systemic corticosteroids begun. During the next 4 hours of treatment, the patient's symptoms, physical findings, and expiratory flow should be monitored at least hourly, and then a decision is made either to hospitalize or to discharge the patient. Some evidence suggests that decisions regarding hospitalization may be made after only 1 hour of intensive bronchodilator therapy [33,54].

Patients who have resolved their wheezing and shortness of breath and have expiratory flow rates 70 percent of predicted or greater (good response) may be discharged with close medical follow-up, patient education, and a course of corticosteroids. Patients with flow rates 40 to 70 percent of predicted after 4 hours of therapy (incomplete response) present a difficult triage decision. Some patients do well if discharged with detailed instructions, close medical follow-up, and oral corticosteroids. However, other patients do poorly if discharged. Currently, it is recommended that a patient with an incomplete response should be hospitalized when there is any clinical feature to suggest he or she is at high risk for asthma mortality (Table 56-4) [25]. Severe symptoms, severe airflow obstruction, past history of severe asthma, prior history of intubation for asthma, prolonged duration of symptoms before presentation, steroid use at the time of exacerbation, poor access to medical follow-up, poor home conditions, or presence of psychiatric conditions that impair adherence to medical advice all suggest the potential for a poor outcome on discharge. Finally, patients with a PEFR less than 40 percent of predicted after 4 hours of bronchodilator therapy (poor response) should be hospitalized.

ROUTINE INPATIENT MANAGEMENT. Most patients with status asthmaticus who are admitted to the hospital can be monitored and managed safely on a hospital ward that is well-staffed by experienced nursing personnel and respiratory therapists. However, patients with severe airway obstruction who are at high risk for mortality from asthma, especially those with an elevated $PaCO_2$ despite initial intensive bronchodilator therapy, need the close monitoring often available only in an intensive care unit (IUC) setting. Successful management of all patients with status asthmaticus depends on repeated history, physical examination, and measures of expiratory airflow to guide adjustments in therapy.

Pharmacotherapy for hospitalized patients includes a continuation of the inhaled beta-adrenergic agonists and systemic corticosteroids begun in the emergency department and initiation of methylxanthine therapy [25]. For patients with severe airway obstruction and only transient relief from treatment, inhaled beta-adrenergic agonists may be administered fre-

Table 56-4. Factors Favoring Hospitalization

Poor response to 4 hr of bronchodilator therapy

or

Incomplete response to 4 hr of bronchodilator therapy and one or more of the following:
    Recent emergency department visit for asthma
    Recent hospitalization for asthma
    Multiple hospitalizations for asthma in last year
    Multiple emergency department visits for asthma in last year
    Past history of endotracheal intubation for asthma
    Duration of current exacerbation >1 wk
    Current use of oral corticosteroids
    Home situation inadequate for follow-up
    Psychiatric conditions that may interfere with medical compliance

quently—as often as every 10 to 30 minutes in severe cases [125,126]. For patients with less severe obstruction or those with intolerable side effects, frequency may be reduced accordingly. Most patients require beta-adrenergic agonists a minimum of every 4 hours. Evidence indicates that delivery of beta-adrenergic agonists by small-volume nebulizer and delivery by MDI with spacer give equivalent results [51,52,53].

Most hospitalized patients begin to show improvement in expiratory airflow after 6 to 12 hours of systemic corticosteroid therapy, but improvement sufficient for hospital discharge frequently takes 2 to 7 days [127]. Expiratory airflow should be measured at least twice daily to assess the patient's progress [25]. In general, the more severe the obstruction at presentation and the longer an exacerbation of asthma has been developing before treatment, the longer it takes to resolve. Patient exercise tolerance and PEFR usually improve incrementally during hospitalization, but it is not uncommon for patients recovering from status asthmaticus to have a hospital course punctuated by periods of worsening dyspnea, especially at night. These episodes of nocturnal worsening require patient assessment but generally respond well to inhaled beta-adrenergic agonists. When the expiratory flow rate does not improve over the initial days of hospitalization, additional or alternative diagnoses, especially congestive heart failure and pulmonary thromboembolism, should be considered.

As the hospitalized patient recovers, the intensity of therapy is decreased gradually. As airway obstruction resolves, the frequency of beta-adrenergic agonist administration is decreased to four times daily by MDI; oral theophylline is substituted for intravenous aminophylline; and oral prednisone (60 mg daily) is substituted for intravenous corticosteroids. When the patient has minimal or no wheezing, is no longer awakened by dyspnea at night, can tolerate activity without oxygen desaturation of hemoglobin, and has expiratory flow rates greater than 70 percent of baseline, he or she is ready for hospital discharge.

Discharge planning is important for preventing future episodes of status asthmaticus (Table 56-5). Patients need to be educated about asthma and the importance of seeking medical advice early in the course of exacerbations. Particularly important are detailed instructions on MDI use and routine measurement of PEFR at home. On discharge, the patient is given instructions for tapering oral prednisone in 2.5- to 5.0-mg decrements over 1 to 2 weeks and is instructed to begin regular use of an aerosol corticosteroid preparation or cromolyn [110]. Subsequent outpatient follow-up should include reassessment of bronchodilator needs. Patients who have recovered from status asthmaticus should be instructed to use inhaled beta-adrenergic agonists on an as-needed basis only [25]. Many patients with asthma do not require long-term treatment with methylxanthines.

MANAGEMENT OF RESPIRATORY FAILURE

Assessment. When alveolar ventilation is severely compromised by respiratory muscle fatigue, mechanical ventilation is potentially lifesaving. Even severely obstructed patients can be supported with mechanical ventilation for the vital hours needed for corticosteroid action. However, mechanical ventilation for status asthmaticus is complicated by morbidity and mortality [6,128,129], with mortality ranging from 0 to 38 percent [129,130].

The decision to initiate mechanical ventilation for status asthmaticus should be based on a number of considerations individualized for each patient. For patients in severe distress in whom respiratory arrest has already occurred or is imminent [6,117,131–134], the need for intubation and mechanical ventilation is obvious. The possibility of pneumothorax should be promptly addressed in these patients. Patients not *in extremis* should be monitored closely during initial bronchodilator therapy and the physician should be prepared to perform intubation in case of substantial deterioration. The decision to intubate for status asthmaticus is a clinical judgment based on whether the patient is responding to therapy, whether hypercapnia is worsening, whether there are signs of muscle fatigue as evidenced by paradoxical abdominal wall motion during inspiration, and whether the patient's mental status is deteriorating, factors that should be repeatedly assessed. In severely obstructed patients with decreasing objective measures of airflow, worsening mental status, or signs of respiratory muscle fatigue despite bronchodilator therapy, intubation and mechanical ventilation should be strongly considered. Any patient who responds poorly to initial bronchodilator therapy and has an initial $PaCO_2$ of 40 mm Hg or more in association with moderately severe hypoxemia should have close serial ABG monitoring. In patients with $PaCO_2$ greater than 55 to 70 mm Hg, increasing $PaCO_2$ (>5 mm Hg/hr) in association with a PaO_2 of less than 60 mm Hg, or presence of metabolic acidosis, intubation and mechanical ventilation should be strongly considered [27,29,128,135].

Endotracheal Intubation. Airway control should be established by the most experienced personnel available, because even minor manipulation of the larynx and trachea can precipitate vagal reflexes that elicit laryngospasm and bronchospasm. Atropine may be given before intubation to attenuate these vagally mediated reflexes. Lidocaine can be used to achieve topical anesthesia of the hypopharynx and larynx, but even lidocaine has been associated with bronchospasm [136]. Administration of a short, rapid-acting intravenous benzodiazepine [137] often can facilitate patient relaxation and preoxygenation, allowing time for a controlled intubation that minimally irritates the larynx and trachea. Opiates are not used for intubation or sedation in asthmatics because narcotics can provoke nausea and vomiting and theoretically can provoke histamine release that worsens bronchospasm [120].

Oral, rather than nasal, intubation is preferred in patients with status asthmaticus because nasal polyps and sinusitis are common in asthma and because the oral route allows a larger endotracheal tube (internal diameter ≥8 mm). A large endotracheal tube preserves the option of therapeutic bronchoscopy.

Mechanical Ventilation. See Chapter 66 on initiating mechanical ventilation. The guiding principle for mechanical ventilation in status asthmaticus is to provide adequate oxygenation while minimizing the risk of barotrauma (Table 56-6). Because the risk of barotrauma is related to dynamic hyperinflation of the lungs and high airway pressures, a ventilatory strategy that minimizes lung volumes and airway pressures should be utilized [25].

Table 56-5. Discharge Planning

Medications
  Inhaled beta-adrenergic agonists
  Oral theophylline
  Inhaled corticosteroids
  Oral corticosteroids tapered over 1–2 wk
Education
  Avoidance of asthma triggers
  Home monitoring of peak expiratory flow rates
  Metered dose inhaler techniques
  Action plan if relapse starts
  Appointment for medical follow-up

Table 56-6. Goals of Mechanical Ventilation*

Maintain oxygen saturation of hemoglobin >90%
Minimize dynamic hyperinflation
  Decrease minute ventilation
  Increase expiratory time
  Accept hypercarbia
Monitor closely for complications of mechanical ventilation

* See Chapter 66 for specific recommendations on how to accomplish these goals.

With conventional mechanical ventilation strategies, delivering a high minute ventilation to normalize the $PaCO_2$ usually requires high tidal volumes and rapid frequencies of ventilation that increase air trapping and result in high airway pressures [6,117,129,131,133,134,138,139]. Some have advocated the rapid correction of respiratory acidosis to reduce the need for sedation [140], but many believe high airway pressures are to be avoided as a major cause of serious morbidity and mortality during mechanical ventilation of asthmatics [129].

The increasingly popular strategy for mechanical ventilation in status asthmaticus is controlled hypoventilation [129,141] (see Chap. 66). Proponents of this strategy argue that as long as the minute ventilation and fraction of inspired oxygen maintain tissue oxygenation, a normal $PaCO_2$ should not be a goal of therapy. Physician acceptance of hypercapnia in this setting has been termed *permissive hypercapnia* [141a].

While the use of sodium bicarbonate to treat acidosis is controversial, advocates for its use in severe acute respiratory acidosis have regarded a pH of 7.20 to be the minimum safe level [141]. This impression and the practice of infusing sodium bicarbonate to maintain a pH of >7.2 is based on two uncontrolled studies in which stuporous and comatose patients with acute respiratory acidosis markedly and quickly improved when infusion of sodium bicarbonate increased the pH to greater than 7.2 [142,142a]. However, no controlled studies of respiratory acidosis support the use of sodium bicarbonate to maintain a specific pH value.

The physiologic responses to metabolic and respiratory acidosis include cardiac output, pulmonary arterial pressure, and heart rate increase, whereas systemic vascular resistance decreases and mean systemic arterial pressure remains unchanged [142b,142c,142d]. In diseased lungs, PaO_2 improves [142b]. The hemodynamic changes are mediated directly by endogenous secretion of catecholamines, primarily norepinephrine, stimulated by decreases in pH. The effects of sodium bicarbonate infusions on these hemodynamic responses and gas exchange have been studied. As the acidosis lessens, cardiac output and PaO_2 worsen [142b,142c]. Moreover, sodium bicarbonate infusions have been shown neither to improve survival nor enhance bronchodilatation. While studies from the 1950s and 1960s suggested that endogenous epinephrine release was depressed in acidosis, recent studies have conclusively shown that it is either unchanged or augmented [142c]. Because carbon dioxide is generated when infused sodium bicarbonate buffers hydrogen ions, infusion of sodium bicarbonate will predictably raise carbon dioxide tensions in blood [142e]. Because carbon dioxide readily diffuses across cell membranes, sodium bicarbonate therapy may therefore cause paradoxical intracellular acidosis [142f], and this may adversely affect survival.

In managing patients during mechanical controlled hypoventilation with permissive hypercapnia, the minimum safe pH is not known. In three recent uncontrolled studies, pH values were not maintained at >7.2, and outcomes did not appear to be adversely affected. Sodium bicarbonate was not given in one study unless pH was <7.15 [142g]; in the other two studies, it was not given to any patient even when pH was 7.02 and <7.00 [142h,142i].

Neuromuscular blocking agents, such as pancuronium and vecuronium, are commonly used to help maintain low airway pressures during delivery of mechanical ventilation (see Chap. 208). Paralyzing skeletal muscles prevents patients from developing high airway pressures due to bucking or fighting the ventilator. Recent reports, however, suggest that patients who undergo even brief neuromuscular blockade in conjunction with corticosteroid administration have a significant risk of developing a prolonged and sometimes severe myopathic illness manifest as significant skeletal muscle weakness [143]. Since all patients with status asthmaticus are treated with corticosteroids, paralyzing agents should be avoided whenever possible [144]. For patients who cannot be managed without neuromuscular blockade, continuous infusions of neuromuscular blocking agents probably should be avoided and muscle function allowed to recover partially between repetitive boluses.

Mechanical ventilation usually can be discontinued after 1 to 3 days, once weaning guidelines are met [6,140,145,146,147] (see Chap. 67). Some patients may require 2 to 4 weeks of mechanical ventilation, especially when pneumonia complicates status asthmaticus.

Complications of Mechanical Ventilation. Serious complications have been reported due to mechanical ventilation in status asthmaticus (see Chap. 66) [6,129,131,133]. Most of these are preventable or treatable if detected early. Problems with airway control, including traumatic and esophageal intubation, should always be anticipated [128]. Intubation of the right mainstem bronchus is a serious problem of airway control because delivery of tidal volumes to one lung increases the risk of barotrauma. Once an airway is established and mechanical ventilation initiated, transient hypotension may occur because the high intrathoracic pressures that occur during mechanical ventilation in status asthmaticus impede venous return of blood to the right ventricle of the heart [128]. This is treated by administering intravenous fluids and adjusting tidal volumes, respiratory frequency, and inspiratory flow rates to decrease hyperinflation and intrinsic positive end-expiratory pressure [148].

Barotrauma is the main cause of morbidity and mortality among patients receiving mechanical ventilation for status asthmaticus [132,147]. High airway pressures are associated with overdistended alveoli that rupture. Air may dissect along the bronchovascular interstitium and sometimes is evident on chest radiograph as parenchymal air cysts, linear air streaks emanating from the hila, and perivascular air halos [149]. As the air dissects centrally, mediastinal and subcutaneous emphysema develop. Alternatively, air from ruptured alveoli may dissect through the pleural surfaces into the pleural space to create a pneumothorax [150]. For patients on mechanical ventilation, pneumothorax progresses to tension pneumothorax rapidly and always should be treated immediately with tube thoracos-

tomy. It must be assumed that any pneumothorax during mechanical ventilation is under tension [151].

Mucus plugging commonly occurs in status asthmaticus. Large mucus plugs occluding the endotracheal tube should be considered when there is insurmountable difficulty in ventilating a patient with status asthmaticus. Large mucus plugs also may cause lobar or lung atelectasis that impairs gas exchange and increases airway pressures. Therapeutic bronchoscopy may be necessary to relieve large mucus plugs if conservative measures, steroids, and bronchodilators are not effective. Retained secretions and atelectasis also contribute to the significant risk of nosocomial pneumonia during mechanical ventilation for status asthmaticus [152].

Other complications are indirectly related to mechanical ventilation. Thromboembolism and gastric stress ulcers may occur with greater frequency in patients with status asthmaticus [6,153]. Dysrhythmias may occur during status asthmaticus because of therapy with sympathomimetic drugs. Hypophosphatemia may develop when phosphates shift from blood to intracellular compartments secondary to alkalosis.

Additional and Unconventional Management Measures. Even after bronchodilators, corticosteroids, sodium bicarbonate, and mechanical ventilation, airway obstruction sometimes may be sufficiently severe to prevent maintenance of an acceptable arterial pH or adequate tissue oxygenation. In these rare cases, additional, sometimes unconventional, measures may be used to support the patient until corticosteroids have had time to suppress the underlying inflammatory process. Many of these measures are not established and are based on anecdotal experience (Table 56-7).

A small improvement in airway resistance may be achieved by delivering a mixture of helium and oxygen (heliox) to the ventilated patient (see Chap. 69) [154]. The decreased density of the gas mixture reduces resistance to turbulent gas flow in the large airways. Sometimes this small improvement buys critical time.

Because inhaled beta-adrenergic agonists and methylxanthines are excellent smooth muscle relaxants, bronchospasm usually is not the major factor limiting airflow in patients already being treated for status asthmaticus. However, for patients who fail to respond to maximal conventional therapy, a variety of strategies have been advocated to maximize bronchodilation. For a deteriorating patient many clinicians add empiric therapy with inhaled cholinergic antagonists. Also, some reports suggest that intravenous isoproterenol (0.05–1.5 μg/kg/min) or salbutamol (0.1 μg/kg/min) may significantly improve airway obstruction [63,64,155]. Another bronchodilator sometimes advocated for treatment of severe status asthmaticus is intravenous magnesium sulfate (1.2 gm $MgSO_4$ in 50 ml saline over 20 min) [114]. However, the bronchodilator effect of magnesium ion is only transient, and repeat administration of magnesium sulfate has potentially serious toxicities [156,157]. Finally, general anesthetics are excellent bronchodilators and an important option for patients refractory to maximal routine therapy. Halothane [158,159], thiopental [160], and ketamine [161] all have been

Table 56-7. Special and/or Unconventional Therapeutic Measures

Intravenous beta-adrenergic agonists
Intravenous $MgSO_4$
Helium-oxygen mixtures
General anesthetics
Bronchoscopy with therapeutic lavage
Hypothermia
Extracorporeal life support

used successfully to treat patients with status asthmaticus. If general anesthetics are used, an anesthesiologist should be consulted.

Since a major cause of airway obstruction during status asthmaticus is mucus plugging, therapeutic bronchoscopy with lavage has been used as an additional supportive measure [162,163]. Therapeutic bronchoscopy is not done routinely in asthma because worsening bronchospasm that is refractory to conventional therapy is a recognized complication in asthmatics. A fiberoptic bronchoscope with a large suction channel should be used, and the mechanically ventilated patient should be heavily sedated for the procedure. Acetylcysteine, a mucolytic agent, is associated with bronchospasm in asthmatics, but it has been used cautiously and successfully during therapeutic bronchoscopy by delivering a dilute solution (<1%) through the bronchoscope to dissolve mucus plugs [162].

Recent reports describe unconventional measures that might be considered for the management of exceedingly difficult cases. One report described the use of hypothermia to manage status asthmaticus. The decreased metabolic rate associated with hypothermia resulted in decreased carbon dioxide production, which permitted adequate ventilation at lower airway pressures [164]. Another report described a case of status asthmaticus with markedly elevated airway pressures and a severe respiratory acidosis refractory to sodium bicarbonate administration. To support the patient until airway inflammation responded to corticosteroids, extracorporeal life support was employed successfully [165]. In the future, these unconventional modalities may prove important in managing those rare cases of status asthmaticus that are refractory to conventional measures.

References

1. Farr RS: Definition and heterogeneity in asthma. *Semin Respir Med* 8:195, 1987.
2. American Thoracic Society: Chronic bronchitis, asthma, and pulmonary emphysema. *Am Rev Respir Dis* 136:224, 1987.
3. Boushey HA, Holtzman MJ, Sheller JR, et al: Bronchial hyperreactivity. *Am Rev Respir Dis* 121:389, 1980.
4. Dunnill MS: The pathology of asthma, with special reference to changes in the bronchial mucosa. *J Clin Pathol* 13:27, 1960.
5. Busey JF, Fenger EPK, Hepper NG, et al: Management of status asthmaticus. *Am Rev Respir Dis* 97:735, 1968.
6. Scoggin CH, Sahn SA, Petty TL: Status asthmaticus: A nine-year experience. *JAMA* 238:1158, 1977.
7. Centers for Disease Control: Asthma: United States, 1980–1987. *MMWR* 39:493, 1990.
8. Weiss KB, Gergen PJ, Crain EF: Inner-city asthma. *Chest* 101:362S, 1992.
9. Glazebrook KN, Sutherland DC: Management of acute asthma attacks in Auckland A & E departments. *Aust NZ Med J* 98:590, 1985.
10. FitzGerald JM, Hargreave FE: The assessment and management of acute life-threatening asthma. *Chest* 95:888, 1989.
11. Spitzer WO, Suissa S, Ernst P, et al: The use of β-agonists and the risk of death and near death from asthma. *N Engl J Med* 326:501, 1992.
12. Sears MR, Taylor DR, Print CG, et al: Regular inhaled beta-agonist treatment in bronchial asthma. *Lancet* 336:1391, 1990.
13. Beasley R, Roche WR, Roberts JA, et al: Cellular events in the bronchi in mild asthma and after bronchial provocation. *Am Rev Respir Dis* 139:806, 1989.
14. Bousquet J, Chanez P, Lacoste JY, et al: Eosinophilic inflammation in asthma. *N Engl J Med* 323:1033, 1990.
15. Barnes PJ: New concepts in the pathogenesis of bronchial hyperresponsiveness and asthma. *J Allergy Clin Immunol* 83:1013, 1989.
16. Cockcroft DW, Murdock KY: Comparative effects of inhaled salbutamol, sodium cromoglycate, and beclomethasone dipropionate on allergen-induced early asthmatic response, late asthmatic responses and increased bronchial responsiveness to histamine. *J Allergy Clin Immunol* 79:734, 1987.
17. Golden JA, Nadel JA, Boushey HA: Bronchial hyperirritability in healthy subjects after exposure to ozone. *Am Rev Respir Dis* 118:287, 1978.
18. Empey DW, Laitinen LA, Jacobs L, et al: Mechanisms of bronchial hyperreactivity in normal subjects after upper respiratory tract infection. *Am Rev Respir Dis* 113:131, 1976.
19. Shelhamer JH, Marom Z, Kaliner M: Immunologic and neuropharmacologic stimulation of mucous glycoprotein release from human airways in vitro. *J Clin Invest* 66:1400, 1980.
20. Rubinfield AR, Wagner PD, West JB: Gas exchange during acute experimental canine asthma. *Am Rev Respir Dis* 118:525, 1978.
21. Freedman AR, Lavietes MH: Energy requirements of the respiratory musculature in asthma. *Am J Med* 80:215, 1986.
22. Martin JG, Powell E, Shore S, et al: The role of the respiratory muscles in the hyperinflation of bronchial asthma. *Am Rev Respir Dis* 121:441, 1980.
23. Bellemare F, Grassino A: Evaluation of human diaphragm fatigue. *J Appl Physiol* 53:1196, 1982.
24. Christopher KL, Wood RP, Eckert RC, et al: Vocal-cord dysfunction presenting as asthma. *N Engl J Med* 308:1566, 1983.
25. U.S. Dept of Health and Human Services, Public Health Service, National Institutes of Health: Expert Panel Report: *Guidelines for the Diagnosis and Management of Asthma.* Publication No. 91–3042, August 1991.
26. Shim CS, Williams MH: Evaluation of the severity of asthma: patients versus physicians. *Am J Med* 68:11, 1980.
27. Rebuck AS, Read J: Assessment and management of severe asthma. *Am J Med* 51:788, 1971.
28. Brenner BE, Abraham E, Simon RR: Position and diaphoresis in acute asthma. *Am J Med* 74:1005, 1983.
29. Sahn SA, Mountain RD: Clinical features and outcome in patients with acute asthma presenting with hypercapnia. *Am Rev Respir Dis* 138:535, 1988.
30. Shim CS, Williams MH: Relationship of wheezing to the severity of obstruction in asthma. *Arch Intern Med* 143:890, 1983.
31. Cohen CA, Zagelbaum G, Gross D, et al: Clinical manifestations of inspiratory muscle fatigue. *Am J Med* 73:308, 1982.
32. Nowak RM, Pensler MJ, Sarkar DD, et al: Comparison of peak expiratory flow and FEV_1 admission criteria for acute bronchial asthma. *Ann Emerg Med* 11:64, 1982.
33. Fanta CH, Rossing TH, McFadden ER: Emergency room treatment of asthma. *Am J Med* 72:416, 1982.
34. McFadden ER, Lyons HA: Airway resistance and uneven ventilation in bronchial asthma. *J Appl Physiol* 25:365, 1968.
35. McFadden ER, Lyons HA: Arterial blood gas tensions in asthma. *N Engl J Med* 278:1027, 1968.
36. Palmer KNV, Diament ML: Spirometry and blood gas tensions in bronchial asthma and chronic bronchitis. *Lancet* 2:383, 1967.
37. Findley LJ, Sahn SA: The value of chest roentgenograms in acute asthma in adults. *Chest* 80:535, 1981.
38. Siegler D: Reversible electrocardiographic changes in severe acute asthma. *Thorax* 32:328, 1977.
39. Gelb AF, Lyons HA, Fairshter RD, et al: P pulmonale in status asthmaticus. *J Allergy Clin Immunol* 64:18, 1979.
40. Rasmussen H, Kelley G, Douglas JS: Interactions between Ca^{+2} and cAMP messenger systems in regulation of airway smooth muscle. *Am J Physiol* 258:L279, 1990.
41. Butchers PR, Skidmore IF, Vardey CJ, et al: Characterization of the receptor mediating the anti-anaphylactic effects of beta-adrenoceptor agonists in human lung tissue in vitro. *Br J Pharmacol* 71: 663, 1980.
42. Knowles M, Murray G, Shallal J, et al: Bioelectric properties and ion flow across excised human bronchi. *J Appl Physiol* 56:868, 1984.
43. Vermiere PA, Vanhoutte PM: Inhibitory effects of catecholamines in isolated canine bronchial smooth muscle. *J Appl Physiol* 46:787, 1979.
44. Tashkin DP, Jenne JW: Alpha and beta adrenergic agents, in

Weiss EB, Segal MS, Stein M (eds): *Bronchial Asthma*. Boston, Little, Brown, 1985.

45. Lofdahl CG, Chung KF: Long-acting β2-adrenoceptor agonists: A new perspective in the treatment of asthma. *Eur Respir J* 4:218, 1991.

46. Brogden RN, Faulds D: Salmeterol xinafeate. *Drugs* 42:895, 1991.

47. Nograsdy SG, Hartley JPR, Seaton A: Metabolic effects of intravenous salbutamol in the course of acute severe asthma. *Thorax* 32:559, 1977.

48. Lawford P, Jones BJM, Milledge JS: Comparison of intravenous and nebulized salbutamol in initial treatment of severe asthma. *Br Med J* 1:84, 1978.

49. Hetzel MR, Clark IJH: Comparison of intravenous and aerosol salbutamol. *Br Med J* 1:919, 1976.

50. Williams SJ, Winner SJ, Clark TJH: Comparison of inhaled and intravenous terbutaline in acute severe asthma. *Thorax* 36:629, 1981.

51. Shim CS, Williams MH Jr: Effect of bronchodilator administered by canister versus jet nebulizer. *J Allergy Clin Immunol* 73:387, 1984.

52. Morley TF, Marozsan E, Zappasodi SJ, et al: Comparison of beta-adrenergic agents delivered by nebulizer vs metered dose inhaler with InspirEase in hospitalized asthmatic patients. *Chest* 94:1205, 1988.

53. Colacone A, Afilalo M, Wolkove N, et al: A comparison of albuterol administered by metered dose inhaler (and holding chamber) or wet nebulizer in acute asthma. *Chest* 104:835, 1993.

54. Idris AH, McDermott MF, Raucci JC, et al: Emergency department treatment of severe asthma. *Chest* 103:665, 1993.

55. Brittan J, Tattersfield NA: Comparison of cumulative and noncumulative techniques to measure dose-response curves for β-agonist in patients with asthma. *Thorax* 39:597, 1984.

56. Cherniack RM, Goldberg I: The effect of nebulized bronchodilator delivered with and without IPPB on ventilatory function in chronic obstructive emphysema. *Am Rev Respir Dis* 91:13, 1965.

57. Karetsky MS: Asthma mortality associated with pneumothorax and intermittent positive-pressure breathing. *Lancet* 1:828, 1975.

58. Fanta CH, Rossing TH, McFadden ER: Treatment of acute asthma: Is combination therapy with sympathomimetics and methylxanthines indicated? *Am J Med* 80:5, 1986.

59. Spiteri MA, Millar AB, Pavia D, et al: Subcutaneous adrenaline versus terbutaline in the treatment of acute severe asthma. *Thorax* 43:19, 1988.

60. Bendkowski B: Effects of adrenaline injections on ECG in elderly asthmatics. *J Coll Gen Pract* 8:66, 1964.

61. Laaban JP, Iung B, Chauvet JP, et al: Cardiac arrhythmias during the combined use of intravenous aminophylline and terbutaline in status asthmaticus. *Chest* 94:496, 1988.

62. Coupe MD, Guly U, Brown E, et al: Nebulized adrenaline in acute severe asthma: Comparison with salbutamol. *Eur J Respir Dis* 71:227, 1987.

63. Parry WH, Martorano F, Colton EK: Management of life-threatening asthma with intravenous isoproterenol infusion. *Am J Dis Child* 130:39, 1976.

64. Herman JJ, Noah ZL, Moody RR: Use of intravenous isoproterenol for status asthmaticus in children. *Crit Care Med* 11:716, 1983.

65. Kurland G, Williams J, Lewiston NJ: Fatal myocardial toxicity during continuous infusion intravenous isoproterenol therapy of asthma. *J Allergy Clin Immunol* 63:407, 1979.

66. Karpel JP, Appel D, Breidbart D, et al: A comparison of atropine sulfate and metaproterenol sulfate in the emergency treatment of asthma. *Am Rev Respir Dis* 133:727, 1986.

67. Gross NJ, Skorodin MS: Anticholinergic, antimuscarinic bronchodilators: State of the art. *Am Rev Respir Dis* 129:856, 1984.

68. Storms WW, Bodman SF, Nathan RA, et al: Use of ipratropium bromide in asthma. *Am J Med* 81:61, 1986.

69. Bethel RA, Irvin CG: Anticholinergic drugs and asthma. *Semin Respir Dis* 8:366, 1987.

70. Higgins RM, Stradling JR, Lane DJ: Should ipratropium bromide be added to beta-agonists in treatment of acute severe asthma? *Chest* 94:718, 1988.

71. Rebuck AS, Chapman KR, Abboud R, et al: Nebulized anticholinergic and sympathomimetic treatment of asthma and chronic obstructive airways disease in the emergency room. *Am J Med* 82:59, 1987.

72. Littenberg B: Aminophylline treatment in severe, acute asthma. *JAMA* 259:1678, 1988.

73. Josephson GW, MacKenzie EJ, Lietman PS, et al: Emergency treatment of asthma: A comparison of 2 treatment regimens. *JAMA* 242:639, 1979.

74. Rose CC, Murphy JG, Schwartz JS: Performance of an index predicting the response of patients with acute bronchial asthma to intensive emergency department treatment. *N Engl J Med* 310:573, 1984.

75. Beswick K, Davies J, Daveys AJ: A comparison of intravenous aminophylline and salbutamol in the treatment of severe bronchospasm. *Practitioner* 214:561, 1975.

76. Femi-Pearse D, George WO, Ilecukukwu SI, et al: Comparison of intravenous aminophylline and salbutamol in severe asthma. *Br Med J* 1:491, 1977.

77. Williams SJ, Parrish RW, Seaton A: Comparison of intravenous aminophylline and salbutamol in severe asthma. *Br Med J* 4:685, 1975.

78. Tribe AE, Wong RM, Rolunson JS: A controlled trial of intravenous salbutamol and aminophylline in acute asthma. *Med J Aust* 2:749, 1976.

79. Siegal D, Sheppard D, Gelb A, et al: Aminophylline increases the toxicity but not the efficacy of an inhaled beta-adrenergic agonist in the treatment of acute exacerbations of asthma. *Am Rev Respir Dis* 132:283, 1985.

80. Rossing T, Fanta CH, McFadden ER, et al: A controlled trial of the use of single versus combined-drug therapy in the treatment of acute episodes of asthma. *Am Rev Respir Dis* 123:190, 1981.

81. Evans MV, Monie RDH, Gimmins J, et al: Aminophylline, salbutamol and combined intravenous infusions in acute severe asthma. *Br J Dis Chest* 74:385, 1980.

82. Pierson WE, Bierman CW, Stamm SJ, et al: Double-blind trial of aminophylline in status asthmaticus. *Pediatrics* 48:642, 1971.

83. Appel D, Shim C: Comparative effect of epinephrine and aminophylline in the treatment of asthma. *Lung* 159:243, 1981.

84. Sharma TN, Gupta RB, Gupta PR, et al: Comparison of intravenous aminophylline, salbutamol and terbutaline in acute asthma. *Indian J Chest Dis Allied Sci* 26:155, 1984.

85. Rossing T, Fanta CH, Goldstein DH, et al: Emergency therapy of asthma: Comparison of the acute effects of parenteral and inhaled sympathomimetics and infused aminophylline. *Am Rev Respir Dis* 122:365, 1980.

86. Zwillich CW, Sutton FD, Neff TA, et al: Theophylline-induced seizures. *Ann Intern Med* 82:784, 1975.

87. Matthay RA, Berger HJ, Loke J, et al: Effects of aminophylline upon right and left ventricular performance in chronic obstructive pulmonary disease. *Am J Med* 65:903, 1978.

88. MacKay AD, Baldwin CJ, Tattersfield AE: Action of intravenously administered aminophylline on normal airways. *Am Rev Respir Dis* 127:609, 1983.

89. Vozeh S, Kewitz G, Perruchoud A, et al: Theophylline serum concentration and therapeutic effect in severe acute bronchial obstruction: The optimal use of intravenously administered aminophylline. *Am Rev Respir Dis* 125:181, 1982.

90. Eldridge FL, Millhorn DE, Waldrop TG, et al: Mechanism of respiratory effects of methylxanthines. *Respir Physiol* 53:239, 1983.

91. Lakshminarayan S, Sahn SA, Weil JV, et al: The effect of aminophylline on ventilatory responses in normal man. *Am Rev Respir Dis* 117:33, 1978.

92. Aubier M, DeTroyer A, Sampson M, et al: Aminophylline improves diaphragmatic contractility. *N Engl J Med* 305:249, 1981.

93. Powell JR, Vozek S, Hopewell P, et al: Theophylline disposition in acutely ill hospitalized patients. *Am Rev Respir Dis* 118:229, 1978.

94. Roy AK, Cuda MP, Levine RA: Induction of theophylline toxicity and inhibition of clearance rates by ranitidine. *Am J Med* 85:525, 1988.

95. Tietze KJ, Hussar DA: Avoiding drug interactions in respiratory medicine. *J Respir Dis* 13:1669, 1992.

96. Sessler CN: Theophylline toxicity: Clinical features of 116 consecutive cases. *Am J Med* 88:567, 1990.

97. Fanta CH, Rossing TH, McFadden ER: Glucocorticosteroids in acute asthma: A critical control trial. *Am J Med* 74:845, 1983.

98. Kaliner M: Mechanism of glucocorticosteroid action in bronchial asthma. *J Allergy Clin Immunol* 76:321, 1985.

99. Haskell RJ, Wang BM, Hansen JE: A double-blind, randomized trial of methylprednisolone in status asthmaticus. *Arch Intern Med* 143:1324, 1983.

100. Flower RJ: Lipocortin and the mechanism of action of the glucocorticoids. *Br J Pharmacol* 94:987, 1988.

101. Robinson D, Hamid Q, Ying S, et al: Prednisolone treatment in asthma is associated with modulation of bronchoalveolar lavage cell interleukin4, interleukin5, and interferon-gamma cytokine gene expression. *Am Rev Respir Dis* 148:401, 1993.

102. Schleimer RP, Rutledge BK: Inhibition of attachment of PMNs to vascular endothelial cells by dexamethasone. *Fed Proc* 44:1185, 1985.

103. Borson DB, Gruenert DC: Glucocorticoids induce neutral endopeptidase in transformed human tracheal epithelial cells. *Am J Physiol* 260:L83, 1991.

104. Lundgren JD, Hirata F, Marom Z, et al: Dexamethasone inhibits respiratory glycoconjugate secretion from feline airways in vitro by the induction of lipocortin (lipomodulin) synthesis. *Am Rev Respir Dis* 137:353, 1988.

105. Miesfeld RL: Molecular genetics of corticosteroid action. *Am Rev Respir Dis* 141:S11, 1990.

106. Siegel SC: Overview of corticosteroid treatment. *J Allergy Clin Immunol* 76:312, 1985.

107. Partridge MR, Gibson GJ: Adverse bronchial reactions to intravenous hydrocortisone in two aspirin-sensitive asthmatic patients. *Br Med J* 1:1521, 1978.

108. Ratto D, Alfaro C, Sipsey J, et al: Are intravenous cortico-steroids required in status asthmaticus? *JAMA* 260:527, 1988.

109. Harrison BDW, Hart GJ, Ali NJ, et al: Need for intravenous hydrocortisone in addition to oral prednisolone in patients admitted to hospital with severe asthma without ventilatory failure. *Lancet* 1: 181, 1986.

110. McFadden ER: Dosages of corticosteroids in asthma. *Am Rev Respir Dis* 147:1306, 1993.

111. King TE, Chang S: Corticosteroid therapy in the management of asthma. *Semin Respir Med* 8:387, 1987.

112. Stalcup SA, Mellins RB: Mechanical forces producing pulmonary edema in acute asthma. *N Engl J Med* 297:592, 1977.

113. Okayama H, Takashi A, Okayama M, et al: Bronchodilating effect of intravenous magnesium sulfate in bronchial asthma. *JAMA* 257:1076, 1987.

114. Skobeloff EM, Spivey WH, McNamara RM, et al: Intravenous magnesium sulfate for the treatment of acute asthma in the emergency department. *JAMA* 262:1210, 1989.

115. Rolla G, Bucca C, Caria E, et al: Acute effect of intravenous magnesium sulfate on airway obstruction of asthmatic patients. *Ann Allergy* 61:388, 1988.

116. Tiffany BR, Berk WA, Todd IK, et al: Magnesium bolus or infusion fails to improve expiratory flow in acute asthma exacerbations. *Chest* 104:831, 1993.

117. Bernstein IL, Ausdenmoore RW: Iatrogenic bronchospasm occurring during clinical trials of a new mucolytic agent, acetylcysteine. *Dis Chest* 46:469, 1964.

118. Graham VAL, Milton AF, Knowles GK, et al: Routine antibiotics in hospital management of acute asthma. *Lancet* 2:418, 1982.

119. Williams MH Jr: Life-threatening asthma. *Arch Intern Med* 140:1604, 1980.

120. Jaffe JH, Martin WR: Opioid analgesics and antagonists, in Gilman AG, Goodman LS, Gilman A (eds): *The Pharmacologic Basis of Therapeutics*. 4th ed. New York, Macmillan, 1980, p 494.

121. Gordon M, Wiswander KR, Berendes H, et al: Fetal morbidity following potentially anoxic obstetric conditions. VII: Bronchial asthma. *Am J Obstet Gynecol* 106:421, 1970.

122. Motoyama EK, Acheson F, Rivard G, et al: Adverse effects of maternal hyperventilation on the fetus. *Lancet* 1:286, 1966.

123. Schatz M, Zeiger RS, Harden KM, et al: The safety of inhaled beta-agonist bronchodilators during pregnancy. *J Allergy Clin Immunol* 82:686, 1988.

124. Turner ES, Greenberger PA, Patterson R: Management of the pregnant asthmatic. *Ann Intern Med* 93:905, 1980.

125. Black PN, Woodhouse A, Burmeister S, et al: How frequently should nebulised salbutamol be administered in acute asthma. *Am Rev Respir Dis* 147:A57, 1993.

126. Newhouse MT, McCallum AL, Abboud RT, et al: A multi-centre clinical trial to compare the safety profiles of fenoterol MDI and albuterol MDI in acute severe adult asthmatics treated in the emergency room. *Am Rev Respir Dis* 147:A57, 1993.

127. Benfield GFA, Smith AP: Predicting rapid and slow response to treatment in acute severe asthma. *Br J Dis Chest* 77:249, 1983.

128. Dales RE, Munt PW: Use of mechanical ventilation in adults with severe asthma. *Can Med Assoc J* 130:391, 1984.

129. Darioli R, Perret C: Mechanical controlled hypoventilation in status asthmaticus. *Am Rev Respir Dis* 129:385, 1984.

130. James OF, Mills RM, Allen KM: Severe bronchial asthma: Factors influencing intensive care management and outcome. *Anaesth Intensive Care* 5:11, 1977.

131. Westerman DE, Benatar SR, Potgieter PD, et al: Identification of the high-risk asthmatic patient: Experience with 39 patients undergoing ventilation for status asthmaticus. *Am J Med* 66:565, 1979.

132. MacDonald JB, Seaton A, Williams DA: Asthma deaths in Cardiff, 1963–74: 90 deaths outside hospital. *Br Med J* 1:1493, 1976.

133. Webb AK, Bilton RH, Hanson G: Severe bronchial asthma requiring ventilation: A review of 20 cases and advice on management. *Postgrad Med J* 55:161, 1979.

134. Picado JM, Montserrat JM, Roca J, et al: Mechanical ventilation in severe exacerbation of asthma. *Eur J Respir Dis* 64:102, 1983.

135. Bondi E, Williams MH Jr: Severe asthma: Course and treatment in hospital. *NY State J Med* 77:350, 1977.

136. Weiss EB, Patwardham AV: The response of lidocaine in bronchial asthma. *Chest* 72:429, 1977.

137. Simons FE, Pierson WE, Bierman CW: Respiratory failure in childhood status asthmaticus. *Am J Dis Child* 131:1097, 1977.

138. Sheehy AF, Dibenedeto R, Lefrak S, et al: Treatment of status asthmaticus. *Arch Intern Med* 130:37, 1972.

139. Santiago SM, Klaustermeyer WB: Mortality in status asthmaticus: A nine-year experience in a respiratory intensive care unit. *J Asthma Res* 17:75, 1980.

140. Higgins B, Greening AP, Crompton GK: Assisted ventilation in severe asthma. *Thorax* 41:464, 1986.

141. Menitove SM, Goldring RM: Combined ventilator and bicarbonate strategy in the management of status asthmaticus. *Am J Med* 74:898, 1983.

141a. Feihl F, Perret C: Permissive hypercapnia. *Am J Respir Crit Care Med* 150:1722, 1994.

142. Westlake EK, Simpson T, Kaye M: Carbon dioxide narcosis in emphysema. *Q J Med* 24:155, 1955.

142a. Addis GJ: Bicarbonate buffering in acute exacerbation of chronic respiratory failure. *Thorax* 20:337, 1965.

142b. Brimioulle S, Vachiery J-L, Lejeune P, et al: Acid-base status affects gas exchange in canine oleic acid pulmonary edema. *Am J Physiol* 260:H1080, 1991.

142c. Brofman JD, Leff AR, Munoz NM, et al: Sympathetic secretory response to hypercapnic acidosis in swine. *J Appl Physiol* 69:710, 1990.

142d. Ebata T, Watanabe Y, Amaha K, et al: Haemodynamic changes during the apnoea test for diagnosis of brain death. *Can J Anaesth* 38:436, 1991.

142e. Cooper DJ, Walley KR, Wiggs BR, et al: Bicarbonate does not improve hemodynamics in critically ill patients who have lactic acidosis. *Ann Intern Med* 112:492, 1990.

142f. Shapiro JI, Whalen M, Kucera R, et al: Brain pH responses to sodium bicarbonate and carbicarb during systemic acidosis. *Am J Physiol* 69:710, 1990.

142g. Williams TJ, Tuxen DV, Scheinkestel CD, et al: Risk factors for morbidity in mechanically ventilated patients with acute severe asthma. *Am Rev Respir Dis* 146:607, 1992.

142h. Bellomo R, McLaughlin P, Tai E, et al: Asthma requiring mechanical ventilation: A low morbidity approach. *Chest* 105:891, 1994.

142i. Hickling KG, Henderson SJ, Jackson R: Low mortality associated with low volume pressure limited ventilation with permissive hypercapnia in severe adult respiratory distress syndrome. *Intensive Care Med* 16:372, 1990.

143. Hansen-Flaschen J, Cowen J, Raps EC: Neuromuscular blockade in the intensive care unit. *Am Rev Respir Dis* 147:234, 1993.

144. Shapiro JM, Condos R, Cole RP: Myopathy in status asthmaticus: Relation to neuromuscular blockade and corticosteroid administration. *J Intensive Care Med* 8:144, 1993.

145. Braman SS, Kaemmerlen JT: Intensive care of status asthmaticus: A 10-year experience. *JAMA* 264:366, 1990.

146. Mansel JK, Stogner SW, Petrini MF, et al: Mechanical ventilation in patients with acute severe asthma. *Am J Med* 89:42, 1986.

147. Williams TJ, Tuxen DV, Scheinkestel CD, et al: Risk factors for morbidity in mechanically ventilated patients with acute severe asthma. *Am Rev Respir Dis* 146:607, 1992.

148. Pepe PE, Marini JJ: Occult positive end-expiratory pressure in mechanically ventilated patients with airflow obstruction: The "auto-PEEP" effect. *Am Rev Respir Dis* 126:166, 1982.

149. Johnson TH, Altman AR: Pulmonary interstitial gas: First sign of barotrauma due to PEEP therapy. *Crit Care Med* 7:532, 1979.

150. Haake R, Schlichtig R, Ulstad DR, et al: Barotrauma. *Chest* 91:608, 1987.

151. Albelda SM, Giefter WB, Kelley MA, et al: Ventilator-induced subpleural air cysts: Clinical, radiographic, and pathologic significance. *Am Rev Respir Dis* 127:360, 1983.

152. Zwillich CW: Complications of assisted ventilation: A prospective study of 354 consecutive episodes. *Am J Med* 57:161, 1974.

153. Pingleton SK, Bone RC, Pingleton WW, et al: The efficacy of low-dose heparin in prevention of pulmonary emboli in a respiratory intensive care unit. *Chest* 79:647, 1981.

154. Gluck EH, Onorato DJ, Castriotta R: Helium-oxygen mixtures in intubated patients with status asthmaticus and respiratory acidosis. *Chest* 98:693, 1990.

155. Williams S, Seaton A: Intravenous or inhaled salbutamol in acute asthma. *Thorax* 32:555, 1977.

156. Burrow GN, Ferris TF (eds): *Medical Complications During Pregnancy.* Philadelphia, WB Saunders, 1975, p 82.

157. Rizzo MA, Fisher M, Lock JP: Hypermagnesemic pseudocoma. *Arch Intern Med* 153:1130, 1993.

158. O'Rourke PP, Crone RK: Halothane in status asthmaticus. *Crit Care Med* 10:341, 1982.

159. Schwartz SH: Treatment of status asthmaticus with halothane. *JAMA* 251:2688, 1984.

160. Grunberg G, Cohen JD, Keslin J, et al: Facilitation of mechanical ventilation in status asthmaticus with continuous intravenous thiopental. *Chest* 99:1216, 1991.

161. Sarma VJ: Use of ketamine in acute severe asthma *Acta Anaesthesiol Scand* 36:106, 1992.

162. Millman M, Goldman AH, Goldstein IM: Status asthmaticus: Use of acetylcysteine during bronchoscopy and lavage to remove mucus plugs. *Ann Allergy* 50:85, 1983.

163. Smith DL, Deshazo RD: Bronchoalveolar lavage in asthma. *Am Rev Respir Dis* 148:523, 1993.

164. Browning D, Goodrum DT: Treatment of acute severe asthma assisted by hypothermia. *Anaesthesia* 47:223, 1992.

165. Shapiro, MB, Kleaveland AC, Bartlett RH: Extracorporeal life support for status asthmaticus. *Chest* 103:1651, 1993.

57. Chronic Obstructive Pulmonary Disease

Stephen E. Lapinsky and
Ronald F. Grossman

Chronic obstructive pulmonary disease (COPD) is a disease not easily defined. The definition proposed by Snider [1] is the one we prefer: "Chronic obstructive pulmonary disease (COPD) may be defined as a process characterized by the presence of chronic bronchitis or emphysema that may lead to the development of airways obstruction; airways obstruction need not be present at all stages of the process and may be partially reversible." While a variety of conditions characterized by chronic airflow obstruction have been termed COPD, the presence of largely irreversible chronic airflow obstruction predominantly in current or former cigarette smokers is the meaning commonly used in the subsequent discussion.

Emphysema is the underlying disease process mainly responsible for severe airflow obstruction [1]. The distinction between chronic obstructive bronchitis, bronchiolitis, and emphysema is difficult to make with precision and is usually clinically unimportant. Thus no attempt is made to distinguish these patients in this chapter.

Respiratory failure secondary to COPD leads to 75,000 deaths annually in the United States and is the fifth most common cause of death [2]. While the death rate for coronary heart disease has decreased 45 percent during the last two decades, COPD deaths have increased 71 percent, the greatest percentage increase among the major causes of death in the United States [2]. Chronic obstructive pulmonary disease is also the second most common cause of permanent disability in people older than age 40 (exceeded only by coronary artery disease) [2], and more than $14 billion in direct and indirect health care costs can be attributed to this illness [2].

Etiology

The major risk factor associated with the development of COPD is cigarette smoking [3,4,5]. The total number of pack-years of smoking correlates best with development of COPD [6,7], although the total length of time spent smoking probably contributes as well [7]. The amount of current cigarette smoking [6], use of filtered cigarettes [7], tar content of the cigarette smoke [8], and positive or negative history for inhalation [7] do not correlate. Smokers as a group are unreliable in determining the extent to which they inhale cigarette smoke [9], which may explain this lack of correlation. A relatively small minority of even heavy cigarette smokers develop significant COPD [5,6,10], which means that some cofactor(s) (e.g., host susceptibility) in addition to cigarette smoking must be important. While exposure and susceptibility to the effects of cigarette smoking are the major factors involved in the development of COPD, other factors have been identified. Homozygous alpha$_1$-antitrypsin deficiency is a risk factor for the development of

COPD [11,12] even in the absence of cigarette smoking; however, the presence of this condition accounts for only a fraction of cases of COPD [11]. Moreover, nonsmoking patients with alpha$_1$-antitrypsin deficiency may not necessarily develop COPD. There are conflicting views on the relative importance of heterozygous alpha$_1$-antitrypsin deficiency in the pathogenesis of COPD [13–17]. Other factors that may increase the risk of COPD, particularly in cigarette smokers, include a history of significant childhood respiratory illnesses [18,19], air pollution [20], the presence of increased airway reactivity [21,22], and heavy alcohol consumption [23]. Occupational exposure to grain dust [24,25], mineral dusts (silica, coal, iron) [26], and textile material such as cotton or hemp [27] may be a risk factor for the development of COPD, even in the absence of cigarette smoking.

Pathophysiology

PATHOGENESIS. Three zones of the lung are involved in the pathologic changes of COPD: the central airways (bronchi), the peripheral airways (bronchioles), and the lung parenchyma. Respiratory bronchiolitis is the initial lesion seen in smokers [28]. The inflammatory process may progress, in susceptible people, to glandular enlargement and mucous plugging in bronchi, goblet cell metaplasia, smooth muscle hypertrophy, inflammation in the walls of membranous bronchioles, worsening respiratory bronchiolitis, and parenchymal involvement with emphysema [1,29]. Studies utilizing autopsy or surgical specimens and chest computed tomography (CT) scanning have reached conflicting conclusions regarding the importance of small airways disease and emphysema in causing irreversible airflow obstruction. While pathologic studies have suggested that changes in bronchi or bronchioles correlate weakly with chronic airflow obstruction and that irreversible airflow obstruction requires the presence of emphysema [1], chest CT scanning demonstrates a poor correlation between emphysema and airflow limitation [30]. Since less than 10 percent of heavy cigarette smokers develop significant COPD [3], other factor(s) in addition to the presence of cigarette smoke must be involved. Factors influencing the inflammatory response in the lung appear to be most important [3]. Normally, a relative balance exists between destructive proteolytic enzymes, which are released in the lung as a result of inflammation, and various inhibitory, antiproteolytic substances, which act to dampen the response and limit the damage (the protease-antiprotease hypothesis) [31–35]. In some cigarette smokers there may be a genetic tendency favoring a greater inflammatory and destructive response to certain elements of cigarette smoke. Population studies show a definite familial tendency toward COPD [13,36], and pulmonary function comparison studies of identical twins suggest a genetic susceptibility [37].

PHYSIOLOGIC DERANGEMENTS. Expiratory airflow obstruction results from structural airway narrowing as well as functional narrowing due to loss of radial distending forces on the airways. Inflammatory edema, excessive mucus, and glandular hypertrophy are responsible for intrinsic obstruction of airways. Destruction of alveolar walls causes loss of elastic recoil and airflow obstruction, which increases in a dynamic fashion with expiratory effort.

The pathophysiologic consequences of severe, chronic airflow obstruction in the lung include (1) reduced flow rates that limit minute ventilation [38]; (2) maldistributed ventilation, resulting in both wasted ventilation (high ventilation-perfusion [$\dot{V}/\dot{Q}$] mismatch) and impaired gas exchange (low $\dot{V}/\dot{Q}$ mismatch) [39,40]; (3) increased airway resistance, which causes increased work of breathing [41]; and (4) air trapping and hyperinflation, which alter the geometry of the respiratory muscles and place them at a mechanical disadvantage. The maximum force they are capable of generating is decreased, which may predispose them to fatigue [41,42].

In addition to the above factors, some patients with COPD may have a blunted respiratory center drive, which further predisposes them to CO_2 retention [43].

Diagnosis

The diagnosis of COPD is based on clinical grounds but confirmed by pulmonary function tests (PFTs). Arterial blood gases (ABGs) determine the diagnosis of respiratory failure. These tests are objective and quantifiable and reflect the pathogenic mechanisms. In contrast, findings on clinical examination are often subjective, difficult or impossible to quantitate, and nonspecific. Clinical findings are used primarily to suggest the diagnosis, which must be then confirmed on the basis of laboratory findings.

HISTORY. It is essential to inquire about a history of cigarette smoking, and a negative history makes the diagnosis of COPD unlikely. A chronic productive cough and dyspnea on exertion are the two symptoms most commonly associated with COPD. However, a history of a chronic productive cough is of limited value in the diagnosis of COPD because conditions such as asthma, bronchiectasis, postnasal drip from sinusitis, and gastroesophageal reflux with aspiration [44] may be present. There is little correlation between a chronic productive cough (reflecting large-airway mucus hypersecretion) and the development of significant airflow limitation (predominantly a manifestation of disease of small airways less than 2 mm in diameter) [45]. Chronic exertional dyspnea, the cardinal symptom of COPD, is associated with a large variety of other respiratory and nonrespiratory causes. Nevertheless, a history of dyspnea on exertion in a heavy cigarette smoker should always raise the possibility of COPD, which can then be confirmed by objective investigations.

PHYSICAL EXAMINATION. The physical examination can distinguish those patients who should undergo objective laboratory testing, but it is less accurate than pulmonary function testing in detecting and quantifying the severity of COPD [45,46,47]. The most useful physical finding is a definite decrease in breath sound intensity [49,50]. Other suggestive clinical signs include hyperinflation, prolonged forced expiratory time, and wheezing.

The physical examination aids in the assessment of a patient with respiratory distress. A combative, confused, or obtunded patient should alert the physician to the possibility of hypercapnia or hypoxia. Respiratory muscle fatigue is a poor prognostic sign indicating that mechanical ventilatory support may be required and is heralded by new onset of paradoxical respiratory motion or respiratory alternans [41,51,52]. During normal inspiration, the rib cage moves upward and outward and the anterior abdominal wall moves outward [41,52]. With diaphragmatic fatigue, the anterior abdominal wall may move inward during inspiration and outward during expiration. Respiratory alternans describes alternate abdominal (diaphragmatic) breathing and rib cage (intercostal) breathing. When overt, this condition can be detected clinically by observing dramatic shifts in relative movement of the abdomen and rib cage every few breaths.

RADIOLOGY. Posteroanterior and lateral chest radiographs are useful for evaluation of the patient with COPD. Radiographic findings may include (1) hyperinflation with flattened diaphragmatic domes and increased retrosternal and retrocardiac air space, (2) one of two distinctly different bronchovascular patterns—vascular attenuation or prominence of lung markings, (3) enlarged hilar pulmonary arteries and right ventricular enlargement, and (4) regional hyperlucency and bullae [53]. Although one or more of these findings is common in patients with severe COPD, radiographic studies have low sensitivity for the diagnosis of mild COPD [53].

In the patient presenting with an acute exacerbation, a chest radiograph may exclude reversible conditions such as pneumonia, pleural effusion, pneumothorax, atelectasis, and pulmonary edema. However, the diagnostic yield of routine radiographs is low [54]. In the intensive care unit (ICU), technical factors limit the quality of the chest films, making interpretation of a portable anteroposterior film even more difficult. These studies nevertheless provide valuable information, particularly in ventilated patients [55].

PULMONARY FUNCTION TESTS. It is the demonstration of expiratory airflow obstruction [5,45] in the laboratory that determines the diagnosis of COPD. A decrease in the ratio of forced expiratory volume in 1 second (FEV_1) to forced vital capacity (FVC) is the hallmark of obstructive airways disease and is useful in the diagnosis of mild disease. However, it is the FEV_1 that is correlated with clinical outcome and mortality [5,45]. Hypercapnic respiratory failure from COPD is extremely unlikely unless FEV_1 is less than 1.3 liters [56] and is usually not observed unless FEV_1 is less than 1 liter; it becomes increasingly more likely as the FEV_1 progressively falls below 1 liter [57]. An absent or poor forced expiratory flow response to bronchodilators may be indicative of fixed airway obstruction and could differentiate COPD from asthma, in which reversibility is a prominent feature.

Chronic obstructive pulmonary disease is also associated with an increase in total lung capacity and residual volume [58] and a reduction in carbon monoxide diffusing capacity (DLCO) [59]. These investigations are helpful in the initial assessment of the patient with suspected COPD, but spirometry alone usually suffices for subsequent follow-up study.

Impaired exercise performance is commonly found in patients with COPD. The patient with significant airflow obstruction or ABG abnormalities does not require routine exercise testing. However, such an evaluation may be useful to assess a patient with dyspnea out of proportion to the degree of airflow obstruction or when considering oxygen therapy to improve exercise performance [60].

Pulmonary function tests are essential in diagnosing and quantitating the severity of COPD; on the other hand, ABGs provide the data necessary to diagnose and quantitate the severity of respiratory failure. The patient with severe COPD typically presents with an elevated $PaCO_2$, a substantially decreased PaO_2, and a $P(A-a)O_2$ gradient that is substantially increased [39,56,57,61]. Abnormalities in the ABG do not always correlate closely with abnormalities in PFTs [61].

The ABG is also useful in predicting the evolution of CO_2 retention. The relation between the change in $PaCO_2$ and the

change in hydrogen ion concentration allows one to determine whether hypercapnia is due to an acute, acute-on-chronic, or chronic process [62]. See Chapter 53 for further discussion on computing these ratios and their therapeutic implications, which are considerable.

Differential Diagnosis

Chronic obstructive pulmonary disease usually must be distinguished from other conditions that cause expiratory airflow limitation and hypercapnia. Asthma, cystic fibrosis, bronchiectasis, and bronchiolitis obliterans can cause expiratory airflow obstruction. A previous PFT demonstrating reversibility of the airflow obstruction suggests asthma. Younger age, presence of blood or sputum eosinophilia, absence of cigarette smoking, and presence of expiratory and inspiratory monophonic wheezing are all suggestive of asthma. In doubtful cases a trial of bronchodilators and corticosteroids for a predetermined time interval (e.g., 3 weeks) with objective measurement of lung function may be useful. The patient with chronic asthma will have a substantial improvement (i.e., reversibility) in function with systemic corticosteroids, whereas the patient with COPD will not. Cystic fibrosis is diagnosed on the basis of a positive sweat chloride test in a patient with obstructive lung disease, positive family history for cystic fibrosis, or pancreatic insufficiency [63]. Bronchiectasis may be suggested by a history of copious sputum production, recurrent chest infections or hemoptysis, or from the chest radiograph [53]. Lung markings that are increased in size and crowded together, bronchial wall thickening, and the presence of cystic spaces, often containing air-fluid levels, are highly suggestive of this diagnosis [53], which may be confirmed by CT.

Since the differential diagnosis of hypercapnic respiratory failure is extensively covered in Chapters 53 and 58, it is only briefly summarized here. The initial step in sorting out the possibilities is to compute the $P(A-a)O_2$ gradient on room air. With extrapulmonary causes of respiratory failure, the $P(A-a)O_2$ gradient is normal. Pulmonary diseases, which cause an increased $P(A-a)O_2$, can be distinguished clinically and radiographically.

Exacerbations of Chronic Obstructive Pulmonary Disease

While many factors may be associated with acute decompensation (Table 57-1), the most commonly identified cause is an acute viral upper or lower respiratory tract infection [64,65]. It has not been proved conclusively that secondary bacterial infection plays a consistent role in most exacerbations of COPD.

With an acute exacerbation the patient complains of increased dyspnea and increased cough and sputum production, often accompanied by a change in the color and consistency of the expectorated sputum [64]. Expiratory airflow obstruction is worsened, the work of breathing increases, and mucus production and/or mucociliary clearance are altered. The PFTs show worsened expiratory airflow obstruction [66], while ABGs usually show an additional decrease in the PaO_2 and, in patients with severe COPD, development or worsening of arterial hypercapnia [51]. Systemic effects such as fever and neutrophilia may or may not be found, and most often the chest radiograph shows no new abnormality.

Some of the other factors listed in Table 57-1 may be easily

Table 57-1. Differential Diagnosis of Acute Decompensation in Chronic Obstructive Pulmonary Disease

Air pollution
Aspiration
Cardiac arrhythmia
Chest wall injury (e.g., rib fracture)
Cigarette smoking
Metabolic derangements (e.g., hypophosphatemia)
Pleural effusion
Pneumonia
Pneumothorax
Pulmonary edema
Pulmonary embolism
Sedation
Surgery
Systemic illness
Tracheobronchial infection
Upper respiratory tract infection

recognizable, such as a large pneumothorax or pneumonia, but others may be subtle, such as an electrolyte abnormality or unrecognized use of drugs that can cause respiratory center depression. Furthermore, events such as pulmonary emboli may go totally unrecognized because clinical findings such as dyspnea or tachypnea may be attributed to the underlying COPD itself. In this setting, the only hint of pulmonary emboli may be an unexplained drop in PaO_2 accompanied by the unexpected finding of an acute respiratory alkalosis [67]. Despite the increase in wasted ventilation, hypercapnia in thromboembolic disease is unusual even in COPD. When it has occurred, it was associated with massive embolization [68] or inability to increase minute ventilation, as might occur with controlled mechanical ventilation.

Treatment

Treatment of the patient with COPD involves chronic management of the stable patient, treatment of acute exacerbations, and treatment of respiratory failure.

CHRONIC MANAGEMENT. Once COPD is diagnosed, smoking cessation is the obvious first step in management. The annual decline in FEV_1 has been demonstrated to be less in ex-smokers than in current smokers [4]. However, the success of smoking cessation programs is limited, with a 70 percent to 80 percent relapse rate in the first year [69]. Annual influenza vaccination is a useful, cost-effective preventative measure [70] and is generally recommended [71]. Data regarding the benefit of pneumococcal vaccination are limited to bacteremic pneumococcal infection, and their value in patients with respiratory tract infection alone have not been demonstrated. However, some authorities have recommended vaccination of patients with COPD [72].

Inhaled bronchodilators have a definite role in the chronic management of patients with COPD, improving airflow obstruction, although to a less marked degree than in asthmatics, and improving exercise capacity and quality of life [73]. Both beta-agonists and the anticholinergic agent ipratropium bromide are useful, with similar efficacy [74]. Ipratropium could be

considered first-line therapy, as it is associated with fewer side effects [75]. In addition to some bronchodilator effect, theophylline may have beneficial effects on diaphragmatic strength, resistance to fatigue, and CNS respiratory drive [76-81]. This agent produces a clinical benefit in some patients with COPD [82,83], but the potential for toxicity must be recognized.

Although the role of oral corticosteroids in the chronic management of patients with COPD remains controversial, a small subgroup of patients do benefit [84,85]. A steroid trial, with pulmonary function testing before and after a 2-week course of 20 to 40 mg prednisone daily, will identify most of these patients. Inhaled steroids may be of value for patients with documented reversibility, although not all such patients show a response [86]. Their role in chronic management remains unclear [87].

Long-term oxygen therapy used for at least 15 hours per day is associated with prolonged survival and improved quality of life, increasing life span by 6 to 7 years [87–90]. Oxygen therapy is recommended for patients with PaO_2 less than 55 mm Hg and those with a PaO_2 of 55 to 59 mm Hg who have polycythemia or right heart failure [69]. Significant increases in $PaCO_2$ usually do not occur as a result of this therapy [91].

A number of other modes of therapy may be beneficial in certain patients with COPD. Iodinated glycerol may decrease cough and increase ease in bringing up sputum [92], but its use remains controversial and has not been widely adopted. Pulmonary rehabilitation programs have been demonstrated to improve exercise tolerance and reduce dyspnea [93,94], which may be useful in patients who remain significantly symptomatic on maximum medical therapy. Although endurance training of ventilatory muscles alone has been associated with increased exercise tolerance in these patients [95,96], the usefulness of this therapy remains controversial [97,98]. Phlebotomy to reduce the hematocrit from greater than 55 percent to approximately 50 percent is associated with a significant decrease in mean pulmonary artery pressure [99] and a significant increase in exercise tolerance [100]. Since respiratory muscle fatigue plays a prominent part in the development of respiratory failure, nocturnal negative-pressure ventilatory assistance has been used to rest respiratory muscles [101]. Whether this intervention is, in fact, beneficial is unclear, as a recent large controlled trial failed to demonstrate improvement in exercise tolerance, ABGs, or quality of life [102].

ACUTE EXACERBATION. Treatment of acute exacerbation may be divided into two primary methods: supportive and specific.

Supportive Therapy

OXYGEN THERAPY. Supplemental oxygen therapy should be administered to all hypoxemic or hypercapnic patients presenting with an acute exacerbation. The $PaCO_2$ commonly rises somewhat when a patient with COPD receives supplemental oxygen [103], but CO_2 narcosis due to oxygen therapy is uncommon [104]. Patients should not be kept hypoxemic, for fear that oxygen therapy will aggravate CO_2 retention, but ABGs should be closely monitored. Supplemental oxygen therapy is discussed under Respiratory Failure and in Chapter 69.

BRONCHODILATORS. Although COPD is characterized by irreversible airflow obstruction, there is often a reversible component, particularly in the setting of an acute exacerbation [66]. A significant percentage of patients with acute exacerbations of COPD respond to these agents with some improvement in airflow obstruction [105,106,107]. Inhaled beta-agonists and ipratropium appear to be equally effective bronchodilators in patients with acute exacerbations [108]. These agents may be administered by nebulizer or, with equal efficacy, by metered-dose inhaler using a spacer device [109]. A metered-dose inhaler with an aerosol holding chamber also may be used effectively for patients on mechanical ventilation [110]. For specific details on the use of these agents, see Chapters 56 and 69.

Theophylline may have some additional benefit in patients with COPD by increasing CNS respiratory drive, respiratory muscle contractility, and resistance to respiratory muscle fatigue [75–79] (see Chap. 211). The role of theophylline in acute exacerbations is, however, even less well accepted than in chronic management. A double-blind placebo-controlled trial demonstrated no additional benefit of aminophylline over standard therapy, but increased adverse effects were noted [111].

ANTIBIOTICS. There is no evidence that antibiotics given routinely, as is frequently done, are beneficial in all exacerbations of COPD. Therefore, the importance of bacterial infection in COPD is still open to question [65,112,113]. Although the results of a number of studies are inconclusive (Table 57-2), a recent double-blind, placebo-controlled study on the effects of broad-spectrum antibiotics on exacerbations of COPD demonstrated significant benefit [114]. Antibiotic treatment produced significantly earlier resolution of symptoms and prevented clinical deterioration [114]. The difference in success rates between antibiotic and placebo was small. Clinical benefits from antibiotic therapy are most likely to occur in patients with more serious exacerbations, particularly those with fever and grossly purulent sputum [114]. The organisms usually responsible for bacterial infection in acute exacerbations include *Haemophilus influenzae, Streptococcus pneumoniae,* and *Moraxella catarrhalis.* As many as 30 percent of strains of *H. influenzae* and 70 to 80 percent of strains of *M. catarrhalis* are beta-lactamase producing and will be resistant to beta-lactam antibiotics such as amoxicillin [72,115]. Appropriate antibiotics are ampicillin-clavulanate, second- or third-generation cephalosporins, trimethoprim-sulfamethoxazole, tetracyclines, quinolones, and clarithromycin [72,116].

CORTICOSTEROIDS. Short-term use of corticosteroids is generally advocated in acute exacerbations, although not all patients benefit [105,117]. A paucity of literature exists in this regard (Table 57-3). One prospective double-blind, randomized study showed that COPD patients given 0.5 mg per kilogram of methylprednisolone intravenously every 6 hours exhibited more improvement in lung function within the first 72 hours than did a control placebo group [118]. The short-term risk of relapse may be reduced if initial treatment of an acute exacerbation includes a course of corticosteroids [119]. Additional studies to confirm these beneficial effects would be desirable.

OTHER INTERVENTIONS. In stable patients with COPD, chest percussion and postural drainage produce no significant improvement in airflow or gas exchange [120]. Moreover, there is no evidence to suggest that these modalities are effective in the COPD patient in exacerbation in the absence of bronchiectasis and/or bronchorrhea (expectoration of sputum >30 ml/24 hr).

Patients with severe COPD are frequently nutritionally depleted, contributing to their overall poor status and decreased respiratory muscle strength [121–124]. Nutritional support should be instituted early in the course of hospitalization [125]. A high carbohydrate load via parenteral alimentation may, however, result in increased CO_2 production [126]. In a patient with a limited ability to increase ventilation, significant worsening of arterial hypercapnia can result, even requiring the institution of mechanical ventilatory support. Since nonprotein calories in the form of fat cause a lower production of CO_2 compared to isocaloric amounts of carbohydrate, a higher fat and reduced carbohydrate supplement may lessen the degree of hypercapnia in selected patients [127] (see Chap. 202).

Patients with acute respiratory failure may have elevated levels of antidiuretic hormone, decreased renal blood flow, and right-sided heart failure [128]. These factors tend to increase fluid retention and may lead to increased extravascular lung water (pulmonary edema). Diuretics are helpful in correcting this problem [128,129] but a complicating metabolic alkalosis may follow. In patients with COPD, digitalis preparations are of little benefit in the routine treatment of cor pulmonale unless concomitant left ventricular dysfunction is found [130,131]. Furthermore, since patients with acute decompensation of COPD tend to be at increased risk of digitalis toxicity [130], digitalis should be avoided in this setting.

Respiratory stimulants such as doxapram and nikethamide have not been shown to be beneficial, using clinically relevant endpoints [105,132], and are associated with substantial toxicity [105]. Almitrine may increase ventilation and improve ventilation-perfusion relationships in patients with COPD [133], but there is a high incidence of significant side effects [134].

Specific Therapy. Exacerbations of COPD are usually due to upper and/or lower airway infections (e.g., viral). However, should a specific condition listed in Table 57-1 be discovered and specific treatment exists (e.g., anticoagulation for pulmonary embolism), it should be instituted. (See chapters that deal with the specific condition listed in Table 57-1.)

RESPIRATORY FAILURE. Administration of supplemental low-flow oxygen is probably the single most useful treatment in COPD-induced hypercapnic respiratory failure. The decision to intubate and mechanically ventilate is often complicated by concerns that the patient may be difficult to wean from the ventilator. It is difficult to predict the outcome of ventilated patients with COPD [135], but most patients with an acute reversible process are successfully separated from the ventilator [135,136]. Patients with progressive end-stage lung disease should be identified and carefully assessed to determine whether a reversible component exists.

Supplementary Oxygen. Patients with exacerbations of COPD may present with profound hypoxemia with a PaO_2 in the 30s or even 20s [50,103]. A PaO_2 below 34 mm Hg in otherwise normal animals is associated with the development of lactic acidosis [137]. Any concomitant decrease in cardiac output will lead to the development of lactic acidosis at even higher levels of PaO_2 [137]. A low alveolar PO_2 (PAO_2) leads to the development of pulmonary arterial vasoconstriction and pulmonary hypertension [138]. Renal function, particularly the excretion of a free water load, may be significantly impaired when PaO_2 falls below 40 mm Hg [139]. The mechanism appears to be CNS release of antidiuretic hormone in response to severe hypoxemia [140]. Other consequences include CNS dysfunction [141] and cardiac arrhythmias and/or ischemia [142].

The use of supplemental oxygen leads to (1) a decrease in anaerobic metabolism and lactic acid production, (2) an improvement in brain function, (3) a decrease in cardiac arrhythmias and ischemia, (4) a decrease in pulmonary hypertension, (5) an improvement in right heart function with improvement in right heart failure, (6) a decrease in the release of antidiuretic hormone and an increase in the kidneys' ability to clear free water, (7) a decrease in the formation of extravascular lung water (i.e., pulmonary edema), (8) an improvement in survival, and (9) a decrease in red blood cell mass and hematocrit [88,143].

Table 57-2. Summary of Placebo-Controlled Trials of Antibiotic Use in Exacerbations of COPD

Reference	Patients	Antibiotic	Regimen	Outcome
Anthonisen et al, 1987 [114]	173	TMP-SMZ* or amoxicillin or doxycycline	Ambulatory 10 d course	Earlier resolution of symptoms; prevented deterioration
Nicotra et al 1982 [112]	40	Tetracycline	Hospitalized 7 d course	No benefit over placebo
Pines et al, 1972 [164]	259	Tetracycline or chloramphenicol	Ambulatory 12 d course	Earlier recovery; no difference at 1 month
Pines et al, 1968 [165]	30	Penicillin + streptomycin	Hospitalized parenteral therapy	Prevented deterioration
Elmes et al, 1965 [166]	56	Ampicillin	Hospitalized 7 d course	No benefit over placebo

* TMP-SMZ = trimethoprim-sulfamethoxazole; d = day.

Table 57-3. Summary of Clinical Trials of Corticosteroid Use in Exacerbations of COPD

Reference	Number of patients	Study design	Therapeutic regimen	Outcome
Murata et al, 1990 [119]	30*	Retrospective	IV in ED[+] followed by oral	Decreased relapse rate at 48 hrs
Emerman et al, 1989 [167]	96	Randomized controlled	Single dose IV in ED[+]	No difference in FEV_1[#] at 5 hrs, or relapse at 48 hrs
Albert et al, 1980 [118]	44	Randomized controlled	IV q6h— hospitalized	Improved FEV_1[#] at 18 hrs up to 72 hrs

* 30 patients with 90 acute exacerbations treated with or without steroids; [+]ED = emergency department; [#]FEV_1 = forced expiratory volume in 1 second; IV = intravenous; q6h = every 6 hours.

A simple relation between PaO_2 and oxygen delivery often does not exist in these patients. In patients with an acute exacerbation of COPD with severe arterial hypoxemia, the administration of supplemental oxygen results in a direct increase in oxygen delivery with no change in cardiac output [144]. On the other hand, in patients with acute exacerbations of COPD and moderate degrees of arterial hypoxemia, the result of supplemental oxygen is no change in oxygen delivery but a decrease in previously elevated cardiac output [144].

Administration of supplemental oxygen is often associated with an additional rise in the $PaCO_2$ [103]. This is probably due to a change in dead space or shift of the hemoglobin-oxygen binding curve, rather than decreased respiratory drive [145]. This rise is expected and should not be specifically treated unless it is excessive, resulting in a trend toward acute respiratory acidosis on serial ABGs, with CNS or cardiovascular side effects. Should this occur, the supplemental oxygen should not be discontinued abruptly, but rather decreased slowly until the $PaCO_2$ returns to a more acceptable level [104] and the situation stabilizes. Since abrupt discontinuation of supplemental oxygen may not be associated with a prompt increase in ventilation, the $PaCO_2$ may not fall. Withdrawal of supplemental oxygen will therefore additionally depress the already low PaO_2, causing arterial hypoxemia [104]. Carbon dioxide narcosis may occur with excessive oxygen therapy but is much less likely with low flow-controlled oxygen therapy [105].

Some variability in ABG determinations is to be expected in patients in the ICU, even if they are clinically stable [146]. In a group of stable ICU patients on a fixed FIO_2 of 0.50, serial ABGs drawn every 10 minutes for a 50-minute period showed an average intrapatient variation of 5 ± 3 percent in PaO_2 and 3 ± 1.5 percent in $PaCO_2$. Therefore, small changes in consecutive ABG values should not be overinterpreted; rather, it is the overall trend of serial ABGs that should be acted on.

Intubation and Ventilation. Whether or not to intubate the patient and institute mechanical ventilatory support is often a difficult decision in hypercapnic respiratory failure associated with COPD. This decision reflects a continuous reassessment of the patient's status, including the trend of ABG values and determining whether the patient is strong and alert enough to clear his or her secretions and protect the airway. Assessing and reassessing the relation between the arterial hydrogen ion and $PaCO_2$ values can often be singularly helpful in indicating whether the patient has acute, acute-on-chronic, or chronic respiratory acidosis, which helps determine whether immediate intubation is required (e.g., acute acidosis), should be prepared for expectantly (e.g., acute-on-chronic), or can be delayed for the present (e.g., chronic).

The presence of acute respiratory acidosis with a low arterial pH (e.g., <7.2) and inadequate PaO_2 (e.g., <55 mm Hg) or CNS and cardiovascular dysfunction dictates the need for assisted ventilation. Difficulty arises when the data are not as definitive.

While it is prudent to avoid intubating the patient with COPD whenever possible, the development of stupor or coma may necessitate emergency intubation, a potentially disastrous complication. The index of suspicion of which patients are likely to require mechanical ventilation should be high. Predictors of which patients ultimately require mechanical ventilation during hospitalization include the presence of asynchronous or paradoxical breathing with an initial $PaCO_2$ greater than 60 mm Hg [51], and marked deterioration in ABGs from previous outpatient baseline [103]. A significant drop in pH following the administration of low-flow oxygen is also predictive of the ultimate need for mechanical ventilation [103].

The objectives of ventilation are to support gas exchange and rest the muscles of respiration, enabling the patient to resume spontaneous breathing once the excessive mechanical loads of breathing have been corrected. Respiratory muscle function should nevertheless be maintained, but the level of workload required to achieve this goal is not known. Triggering the ventilator during assisted ventilation does require significant respiratory work [147], and this may be sufficient. Adequate nutrition also is essential to maintain respiratory muscle function [148], and early introduction of feeding is recommended [125].

A particular problem in ventilating patients with airflow obstruction is the development of intrinsic or auto PEEP, the difference between the alveolar pressure and proximal airway pressure measured by the ventilator at the end of exhalation [149]. Auto PEEP is the result of air trapping due to low expiratory flow through obstructed airways. It is aggravated by rapid respiratory rates, slow inspiratory flow rates, and ventilation through narrow endotracheal tubes. The consequences of auto PEEP include elevation of peak inspiratory and plateau pressures, hypotension, and increased workload for spontaneous or triggered breaths [150]. To develop a negative airway pressure to initiate respiration, the patient must first create negative intrapleural pressure to reverse the positive auto PEEP and then further the negative intrapleural pressure before inspiratory flow can begin [151]. This effect can be overcome by applying external PEEP equivalent to or slightly less than auto PEEP. The only effect of this externally applied PEEP is to reduce inspiratory work; therefore it is of no value in paralyzed patients [149]. Applied PEEP of up to 85 percent of intrinsic PEEP does not aggravate hyperinflation or compromise hemodynamics [152].

Ventilatory rate and tidal volume on mechanical ventilation should be regulated to return pH toward normal. Hyperventilation of a patient with chronic CO_2 retention may cause a marked respiratory alkalosis, resulting in seizures [153] and difficulty in weaning. In the patient with marked airflow obstruction, excessive peak and plateau airway pressures and elevated auto PEEP may result from attempts to normalize pH and correct $PaCO_2$. In this situation, reduction of the ventilator rate and controlled hypoventilation will decrease the risk of barotrauma [154]. Adequate oxygenation must be maintained, but the $PaCO_2$ may be allowed to rise. Acidosis due to this permissive hypercapnia may require treatment with bicarbonate [155], but blood gases should correct when the airflow obstruction improves. (See Chap. 56 for further discussion of the bicarbonate issue.)

Further details on the mechanical ventilation of the patient with COPD are found in Chapter 66.

Noninvasive Ventilation. Although intubation and mechanical ventilation are lifesaving measures, they carry significant risks [156]. Noninvasive modalities have been successfully used to support gas exchange and prevent intubation in patients with acute exacerbation of COPD. Pressure support ventilation administered by tight-fitting face mask [157] or nasal mask [158] may obviate the need for conventional mechanical ventilation. Mask ventilation is generally well tolerated by most patients but should not be used in patients who are excessively agitated or unable to clear secretions or protect their airway. As the mask may be easily reapplied, this mode of support may be used to provide intermittent or nocturnal ventilation after the acute period [159]. Continuous positive airway pressure without ventilation may be effective in improving gas exchange in acutely hypercapnic patients with COPD [160].

Prognosis

The prognosis for COPD patients with respiratory failure varies depending on the need for mechanical ventilation. Hospital survival can be as high as 94 percent [161] and 2-year survival can be 72 percent [161] in patients not requiring mechanical ventilation. As the decision to ventilate a patient with respiratory failure is largely subjective, data concerning the survival of patients requiring mechanical ventilation vary. The outcome of patients surviving an episode of respiratory failure requiring mechanical ventilation is dependent on the state of the underlying COPD [162], with a mortality of 51 to 82 percent in the first year [135,136,162]. These results are considerably better than figures reported from the early 1970s, which may indicate improved patient selection [162] or improved care. Long-term survival has been reported to be 16 percent at 5 years and 9 percent at 8.5 years [163].

References

1. Snider GL: Chronic obstructive pulmonary disease: A definition and implications of structural determinants of airflow obstruction for epidemiology. *Am Rev Respir Dis* 140(3 Suppl):S3, 1989.
2. Higgins MW: Chronic airways disease in the United States: Trends and determinants. *Chest* 96(suppl):328S, 1989.
3. Macklem PT, Permutt S: Lung biology in health and disease, in Macklem PT, Permutt S (eds): *The Lung in Transition Between Health and Disease.* New York, Marcel Dekker, 1979.
4. Fletcher C, Peto R: The natural history of chronic airflow obstruction. *Br Med J* 1:1645, 1977.
5. Higgins MW, Keller JB, Becker M, et al: An index of risk for obstructive airways disease. *Am Rev Respir Dis* 125:144, 1982.
6. Burrows B, Knudson RJ, Cline MG, et al: Quantitative relationships between cigarette smoking and ventilatory function. *Am Rev Respir Dis* 115:195, 1977.
7. Beck GJ, Doyle CA, Schacter EN: Smoking and lung function. *Am Rev Respir Dis* 123:149, 1981.
8. Sparrow D, Stefos T, Bosse R, et al: The relationship of tar content to decline in pulmonary function in cigarette smokers. *Am Rev Respir Dis* 127:56, 1983.
9. Tobin MJ, Jenouri G, Sackner MA: Subjective and objective measurement of cigarette smoke inhalation. *Chest* 82:696, 1982.
10. Bates DV: The fate of the chronic bronchitic: A report of the ten year followup in the Canadian Department of Veterans Affairs coordinated study of chronic bronchitis. *Am Rev Respir Dis* 108:1043, 1973.
11. Kueppers F, Black LF: Alpha₁-antitrypsin and its deficiency. *Am Rev Respir Dis* 110:176, 1974.
12. Morse JO: Alpha₁-antitrypsin deficiency (second of two parts). *N Engl J Med* 299:1099, 1978.
13. Madison R, Mittman C, Afifi AA, et al: Risk factors for obstructive lung disease. *Am Rev Respir Dis* 124:149, 1981.
14. Lam S, Abboud RT, Chan-Yeung M, et al: Neutrophil elastase and pulmonary function in subjects with intermediate alpha₁-antitrypsin deficiency (MZ phenotype). *Am Rev Respir Dis* 119:941, 1979.
15. Morse JO, Lebowitz MD, Knudson RJ, et al: Relation of protease inhibitor phenotypes to obstructive lung diseases in a community. *N Engl J Med* 296:1190, 1977.
16. Morse JO, Lebowitz MD, Knudson RJ, et al: A community study of the relation of alpha₁-antitrypsin levels to obstructive lung diseases. *N Engl J Med* 292:278, 1975.
17. Buist AS, Sexton GJ, Azzam AH, et al: Pulmonary function in heterozygotes for alpha₁-antitrypsin deficiency: A case-control study. *Am Rev Respir Dis* 120:759, 1979.
18. Burrows B, Knudson RJ, Lebowitz MD: The relationship of childhood respiratory illness to adult obstructive airway disease. *Am Rev Respir Dis* 115:751, 1977.

19. Samet JM, Tager IA, Speizer FE: State of the art: The relationship between respiratory illness in childhood and chronic air-flow obstruction in adulthood. *Am Rev Respir Dis* 127:508, 1983.

20. Detels R, Sayre JW, Coulson AH, et al: The UCLA population studies of chronic obstructive respiratory disease. IV. Respiratory effect of long-term exposure to photochemical oxidants, nitrogen dioxide, and sulfates on current and newer smokers. *Am Rev Respir Dis* 124:673, 1981.

21. Gertner A, Bromberger-Barnea B, Traystman R, et al: Airway reactivity in the periphery of the lung in mongrel dogs: Male and female differences. *Am Rev Respir Dis* 126:1020, 1982.

22. Gerrard JW, Cockcroft DW, Mink JT, et al: Increased nonspecific bronchial reactivity in cigarette smokers with normal lung function. *Am Rev Respir Dis* 122:577, 1980.

23. Lebowitz MD: Respiratory symptoms and disease related to alcohol consumption. *Am Rev Respir Dis* 123:16, 1981.

24. Chan-Yeung M, Wong R, MacLean L: Respiratory abnormalities among grain workers. *Chest* 75:461, 1979.

25. Dosman JA, Cotton DJ, Graham BL, et al: Chronic bronchitis and decreased forced expiratory flow rates in lifetime nonsmoking grain workers. *Am Rev Respir Dis* 121:11, 1980

26. Becklake MR: Occupational exposures: Evidence for a causal association with chronic obstructive pulmonary disease. *Am Rev Respir Dis* 140(3 Suppl):S85, 1989.

27. Beck GJ, Schachter EN, Maunder LA, et al: A prospective study of chronic lung disease in cotton textile workers. *Ann Intern Med* 97:645, 1982.

28. Niewoehner DE, Kleinerman J, Rice DB: Pathologic changes in the peripheral airways of young cigarette smokers. *N Engl J Med* 291:755, 1974.

29. Hogg JC, Macklem PT, Thurlbeck WM: Site and nature of airway obstruction in chronic obstructive lung disease. *N Engl J Med* 278:1355, 1968.

30. Gelb AF, Schein M, Kuei J, et al: Limited contribution of emphysema in advanced chronic obstructive pulmonary disease. *Am Rev Respir Dis* 147:1157, 1993.

31. Janoff A, Carp H: Possible mechanisms of emphysema in smokers: Cigarette smoke condensate suppresses protease inhibition in vitro. *Am Rev Respir Dis* 116:65, 1977.

32. Lam S, Chan-Yeung M, Abboud R, et al: Interrelationships between serum chemotactic factor inactivator, alpha$_1$-antitrypsin deficiency, and chronic obstructive lung disease. *Am Rev Respir Dis* 121:507, 1980.

33. Kramps JA, Bakker W, Dijkman JH: A matched-pair study of the leukocyte elastase-like activity in normal persons and in emphysematous patients with and without alpha$_1$-antitrypsin deficiency. *Am Rev Respir Dis* 121:253, 1980.

34. Martin WJ II, Taylor JC: Abnormal interaction of alpha$_1$-antitrypsin and leukocyte elastolytic activity in patients with chronic obstructive pulmonary disease. *Am Rev Respir Dis* 120:411, 1979.

35. Galdston M, Melnick ER, Goldring RM, et al: Interactions of neutrophil elastase, serum trypsin inhibitory activity, and smoking history as risk factors for chronic obstructive pulmonary disease in patients with MM, MZ, and ZZ phenotypes for alpha$_1$-antitrypsin. *Am Rev Respir Dis* 116:837, 1977.

36. Tager IB, Rosner B, Tishler PV, et al: Household aggregation of pulmonary function and chronic bronchitis. *Am Rev Respir Dis* 114:485, 1976.

37. Webster PM, Lorimer EG, Man SFP, et al: Pulmonary function in identical twins: Comparison of nonsmokers and smokers. *Am Rev Respir Dis* 119:223, 1979.

38. West JB: *Pulmonary Pathophysiology: The Essentials.* 2nd ed. Baltimore, Williams & Wilkins, 1982.

39. West JB: Causes of carbon dioxide retention in lung disease. *N Engl J Med* 284:1232, 1971.

40. Davidson FF, Glazier JB, Murray JF: The components of the alveolar-arterial oxygen tension difference in normal subjects and in patients with pneumonia and obstructive lung disease. *Am J Med* 52:754, 1972.

41. Roussos C, Macklem PT: The respiratory muscles. *N Engl J Med* 307:786, 1982.

42. Luce JM, Culver BH: Respiratory muscle function in health and disease. *Chest* 81:82, 1982.

43. Gelb AF, Klein E, Schiffman P, et al: Ventilatory response and drive in acute and chronic obstructive pulmonary disease. *Am Rev Respir Dis* 116:9, 1977.

44. Irwin RS, Corrao WM, Pratter MR: Chronic persistent cough in the adult: The spectrum and frequency of causes and successful outcome of specific therapy. *Am Rev Respir Dis* 123:413, 1981.

45. Peto R, Speizer FE, Cochrane AL, et al: The relevance in adults of airflow obstruction, but not of mucus hypersecretion, to mortality from chronic lung disease: Results from 20 years of prospective observation. *Am Rev Respir Dis* 128:491, 1983.

46. Schneider IC, Anderson AE Jr: Correlation of clinical signs with ventilatory function in obstructive lung disease. *Ann Intern Med* 62:477, 1965.

47. Pardee NE, Winterbauer RH, Morgan EH, et al: Combinations of four physical signs as indicators of ventilatory abnormality in obstructive pulmonary syndromes. *Chest* 77:354, 1980.

48. Stubbing DG, Mathur PN, Roberts RS, et al: Some physical signs in patients with chronic airflow obstruction. *Am Rev Respir Dis* 125:549, 1982.

49. Badgett RG, Tanaka DJ, Hunt DK et al: Can moderate chronic obstructive pulmonary disease be diagnosed by historical and physical findings alone? *Am J Med* 94:188, 1993.

50. Pardee NE, Martin CJ, Morgan EH: A test of the practical value of estimating breath sound intensity: Breath sounds related to measured ventilatory function. *Chest* 70:341, 1976.

51. Gilbert R, Ashutosh K, Auchincloss JH Jr, et al: Prospective study of controlled oxygen therapy: Poor prognosis of patients with asynchronous breathing. *Chest* 71:456, 1977.

52. Cohen CA, Zagelbaum G, Gross D, et al: Clinical manifestations of inspiratory muscle fatigue. *Am J Med* 73:308, 1982.

53. Fraser RG, Pare JAP: *Diagnosis of Diseases of the Chest.* 2nd ed. Philadelphia, WB Saunders, 1979, vol 3.

54. Sherman S, Skoney JA, Ravikrishnan KP: Routine chest radiographs in exacerbations of chronic obstructive pulmonary disease: Diagnostic value. *Arch Intern Med* 149:2493, 1989.

55. Swensen SJ, Peters SG, LeRoy AJ, et al: Radiology in the intensive-care unit. *Mayo Clin Proc* 66:396, 1991.

56. Gilbert R, Keighley J, Auchincloss JH Jr: Mechanisms of chronic carbon dioxide retention in patients with obstructive pulmonary disease. *Am J Med* 38:217, 1965.

57. Burrows B, Strauss RH, Niden AH: Chronic obstructive lung disease. 3. Interrelationships of pulmonary function data. *Am Rev Respir Dis* 91:861, 1965.

58. West WW, Nagai A, Hodgkin JE, Thurlbeck WM: The National Institutes of Health Intermittent Positive Pressure Breathing trial: Pathology studies. *Am Rev Respir Dis* 135:123, 1987.

59. Morrison NJ, Abboud RT, Ramadan F, et al: Comparison of single breath carbon monoxide diffusing capacity and pressure-volume curves in detecting emphysema. *Am Rev Respir Dis* 139:1179, 1989.

60. Loke J, Mahler DA, Man SFP, et al: Exercise impairment in chronic obstructive pulmonary disease. *Clin Chest Med* 5:121, 1984.

61. Parot S, Miara B, Milic-Emili J, et al: Hypoxemia, hypercapnia, and breathing pattern in patients with chronic obstructive pulmonary disease. *Am Rev Respir Dis* 126:882, 1982.

62. Bear RA, Gribik M: Assessing acid-base imbalances through laboratory parameters. *Hosp Pract* 9:157, 1974.

63. Stern RC, Boat TF, Doershuk CF, et al: Cystic fibrosis diagnosed after age 13: Twenty-five teenage and adult patients including three asymptomatic men. *Ann Intern Med* 87:188, 1977.

64. Gump DW, Phillips CA, Forsyth BR, et al: Role of infection in chronic bronchitis. *Am Rev Respir Dis* 113:465, 1976.

65. Smith CB, Golden CA, Kanner RE, et al: Association of viral and *Mycoplasma pneumoniae* infections with acute respiratory illness in patients with chronic obstructive pulmonary diseases. *Am Rev Respir Dis* 121:225, 1980.

66. Irwin RS, Corrao WM, Erickson AD, et al: A true exacerbation of chronic obstructive bronchitis can be objectively defined. *Am Rev Respir Dis* 123(suppl):57, 1981.

67. Lippman M, Fein A: Pulmonary embolism in the patient with chronic obstructive pulmonary disease. *Chest* 79:39, 1981.

68. Bouchama A, Curley W, Al-Dossary S, Elguindi A: Refractory hypercapnia complicating massive pulmonary embolism. *Am Rev Respir Dis* 138:466, 1988.

69. American Thoracic Society: Standards for the diagnosis and care

of patients with chronic obstructive pulmonary disease (COPD) and asthma. *Am Rev Respir Dis* 136:225, 1987.

70. Riddiough MA, Sisk JE, Bell JC: Influenza vaccination: Cost-effectiveness and public policy. *JAMA* 249:3189, 1983.

71. Center for Disease Control: Prevention and control of influenza. *MMWR* 33:253, 1984.

72. Murphy TF, Sethi S: Bacterial infections in chronic obstructive pulmonary disease. *Am Rev Respir Dis* 146:1067, 1992.

73. Guyatt GH, Townsend M, Pugsley SO, et al: Bronchodilators in chronic airflow limitation: Effects on airway function, exercise capacity and quality of life. *Am Rev Respir Dis* 135:1069, 1987.

74. Easton PA, Jadue C, Dhingra S, Anthonisen NR: A comparison of bronchodilatory effects of a beta-2 adrenergic agent (albuterol) and an anticholinergic agent (ipratroprium bromide) given by aerosol alone or in sequence. *N Engl J Med* 315:735, 1986.

75. Gross NJ: Anticholinergic agents in COPD. *Chest* 91(suppl 5):52S, 1987.

76. Eaton ML, Green BA, Church TR, et al: Efficacy of theophylline in "irreversible" airflow obstruction. *Ann Intern Med* 92:758, 1980.

77. Sanders JS, Berman TM, Bartlett MM, et al: Increased hypoxic ventilatory drive due to administration of aminophylline in normal men. *Chest* 78:279, 1980.

78. Lakshminarayan S, Sahn SA, Weil JV: Effect of aminophylline on ventilatory responses in normal man. *Am Rev Respir Dis* 117:33, 1978.

79. Aubier M, DeTroyer A, Sampson M, et al: Aminophylline improves diaphragmatic contractility. *N Engl J Med* 305:249, 1981.

80. Sigrist S, Thomas D, Howell S, et al: The effect of aminophylline on inspiratory muscle contractility. *Am Rev Respir Dis* 126:46, 1982.

81. Murciano D, Aubier M, Lecocguic Y, Pariente R: Effects of theophylline on diaphragmatic strength and fatigue in patients with chronic obstructive pulmonary disease. *N Engl J Med* 311:349, 1984

82. Murciano D, Auclair M-H, Pariente R, Aubier M: A randomized, controlled trial of theophylline in patients with severe chronic obstructive pulmonary disease. *N Engl J Med* 320:1521, 1989.

83. Thomas P, Pugsley JA, Stewart JH: Theophylline and salbutamol improve pulmonary function in patients with irreversible chronic obstructive pulmonary disease. *Chest* 101:160, 1992.

84. Mendella LA, Manfreda J, Warren CPW, Anthonisen NR: Steroid response in stable chronic obstructive pulmonary disease. *Ann Intern Med* 96:17, 1982.

85. Callahan CM, Dittus RS, Katz BP: Oral corticosteroid treatment for patients with stable chronic obstructive pulmonary disease: A metaanalysis. *Ann Intern Med* 114:216, 1991.

86. Shim CS, Williams MH: Aerosol beclomethasone in patients with steroid-responsive chronic obstructive pulmonary disease. *Am J Med* 78:655, 1985.

87. Chung KF: Long-term inhaled corticosteroid therapy in chronic airways obstruction. *Eur Respir J* 5:913, 1992.

88. Anthonisen NR: Long-term oxygen therapy. *Ann Intern Med* 99:519, 1983.

89. Nocturnal Oxygen Therapy Trial Group: Continuous or nocturnal oxygen therapy in hypoxemic chronic obstructive lung disease: A clinical trial. *Ann Intern Med* 93:391, 1980

90. Stuart-Harris C, Bishop JM, Clark TJH, et al: Long-term domiciliary oxygen therapy in chronic hypoxemic cor pulmonale complicating chronic bronchitis and emphysema: Report of the Medical Research Council Working Party. *Lancet* 1:681,1981.

91. Goldstein RS, Ramcharan V, Bowes G, et al: Effect of supplemental nocturnal oxygen on gas exchange in patients with severe obstructive lung disease. *N Engl J Med* 310:425, 1984.

92. Petty TL: The national mucolytic study: Results of a randomized, double-blind, placebo-controlled study of iodinated glycerol in chronic obstructive bronchitis. *Chest* 97:75, 1990.

93. Lertzman MM, Cherniak RM: Rehabilitation of patients with chronic obstructive pulmonary disease. *Am Rev Respir Dis* 114:1145, 1976.

94. Mertens OJ, Shephard KJ, Kavanagh T: Long term exercise therapy for chronic obstructive lung disease. *Respiration* 35:96, 1978.

95. Belman MJ, Mittman C: Ventilatory muscle training improves exercise capacity in chronic obstructive lung disease patients. *Am Rev Respir Dis* 121:273, 1980.

96. Pardy RL, Rivington RN, Despas PJ, Macklem PT: Inspiratory muscle training compared with physiotherapy in patients with chronic airflow limitation. *Am Rev Respir Dis* 123:421, 1981.

97. Guyatt G, Keller J, Singer J, et al: Controlled trial of respiratory muscle training in chronic airflow obstruction. *Thorax* 47:598, 1992.

98. Smith K, Cook D, Guyatt GH, et al: Respiratory muscle training in chronic airflow imitation: A meta-analysis. *Am Rev Respir Dis* 145:533, 1992.

99. Weisse AB, Moschos CB, Frank MJ, et al: Hemodynamic effects of staged hematocrit reduction in patients with stable cor pulmonale and severely elevated hematocrit levels. *Am J Med* 58:92, 1975.

100. Chetty KG, Brown SE, Light RW: Improved exercise tolerance of the polycythemic lung patient following phlebotomy. *Am J Med* 74:415, 1983.

101. Cropp A, Dimarco AF: Effects of intermittent negative pressure ventilation on respiratory muscle function in patients with severe chronic obstructive lung disease. *Am Rev Respir Dis* 135:1056, 1987.

102. Shapiro SH, Ernst P, Gray-Donald K, et al: Effect of negative pressure ventilation in severe chronic obstructive pulmonary disease. *Lancet* 340:1425, 1992.

103. Bone RC, Pierce AK, Johnson RL Jr: Controlled oxygen administration in acute respiratory failure in chronic obstructive pulmonary disease: A reappraisal. *Am J Med* 65:896, 1978.

104. Bone RC: Treatment of respiratory failure due to advanced chronic obstructive lung disease. *Arch Intern Med* 140:1018, 1980.

105. Schmidt GA, Hall JB: Acute on chronic respiratory failure: Assessment and management of patients with COPD in the emergency setting. *JAMA* 261:3444, 1989.

106. Patterson JW, Woolcock AJ, Shenfield GM: State of the art: Bronchodilator drugs. *Am Rev Respir Dis* 120:1149, 1979.

107. Gross NJ: Ipratropium bromide. *N Engl J Med* 319:486, 1988.

108. Karpel JP, Pesin J, Greenberg D, Gentry E: A comparison of the effects of ipratropium bromide and metaproterenol sulfate in acute exacerbations of COPD. *Chest* 98:835, 1990.

109. Berry RB, Shinto RA, Wong FH, et al: Nebulizer vs spacer for bronchodilator delivery in patients hospitalized for acute exacerbations of COPD. *Chest* 96:1241, 1989.

110. Fuller HD, Dolovich MB, Posmituck G, et al: Pressurized aerosol versus jet aerosol delivery to mechanically ventilated patients: Comparison of dose to the lungs. *Am Rev Respir Dis* 141:440, 1990.

111. Rice KL, Leatherman JW, Duane PG, et al: Aminophylline for acute exacerbations of chronic obstructive pulmonary disease: A controlled trial. *Ann Intern Med* 107:305, 1987.

112. Nicotra MB, Rivera M, Awe RJ: Antibiotic therapy of acute exacerbations of chronic bronchitis: A controlled study using tetracycline. *Ann Intern Med* 97:18, 1982.

113. Tager I, Speizer FE: Role of infection in chronic bronchitis. *N Engl J Med* 292:563, 1975.

114. Anthonisen NR, Monfreda J, Warren CPW, et al: Antibiotic therapy in exacerbations of chronic obstructive pulmonary disease. *Ann Intern Med* 106:196, 1987.

115. Jorgensen JH, Doern GV, Maher LA, et al: Antimicrobial resistance among respiratory isolates of *Haemophilus influenzae, Moraxella catarrhalis,* and *Streptococcus pneumoniae* in the United States. *Antimicrob Agents Chemother* 34:2075, 1990.

116. Chodosh S: Treatment of acute exacerbations of chronic bronchitis: State of the art. *Am J Med* 91(Suppl GA):87S, 1991.

117. Sahn SA: Critical review: Corticosteroids in chronic bronchitis and pulmonary emphysema. *Chest* 73:389, 1978.

118. Albert RK, Martin TR, Lewis SW: Controlled clinical trial of methylprednisolone in patients with chronic bronchitis and acute respiratory insufficiency. *Ann Intern Med* 92:753, 1980.

119. Murata GH, Gorby MS, Chick TW, Halperin AK: Intravenous and oral corticosteroids for the prevention of relapse after treatment of decompensated COPD: Effect on patients with a history of multiple relapses. *Chest* 98:845, 1990.

120. May DB, Munt PW: Physiologic effects of chest percussion and postural drainage in patients with stable chronic bronchitis. *Chest* 75:29, 1979.

121. Hunter AMB, Carey MA, Larsh HW: The nutritional status of patients with chronic obstructive pulmonary disease. *Am Rev Respir Dis* 124:376, 1981.

122. Openbrier DR, Irwin MM, Rogers RM, et al: Nutritional status and lung function in patients with emphysema and chronic bronchitis. *Chest* 83:17, 1983.

123. Arora NS, Rochester DF: Respiratory muscle strength and maximal voluntary ventilation in undernourished patients. *Am Rev Respir Dis* 126:5, 1982.

124. Driver AG, McAlevy MT, Smith JL: Nutritional assessment of patients with chronic obstructive pulmonary disease and acute respiratory failure. *Chest* 82:568, 1982.

125. Driver AG, LeBrun M: Iatrogenic malnutrition in patients receiving ventilatory support. *JAMA* 244:2195, 1980.

126. Covelli HD, Black JW, Olsen MS, et al: Respiratory failure precipitated by high carbohydrate loads. *Ann Intern Med* 95:579, 1981.

127. Weinberger SE, Schwartzstein RM, Weiss JW: Hypercapnia. *N Engl J Med* 321:1223, 1989.

128. Heinemann HO: Right-sided heart failure and the use of diuretics. *Am J Med* 64:367, 1978.

129. Gertz I, Hedenstierna G, Western PO: Improvement in pulmonary function with diuretic therapy in the hypervolemic and polycythemic patient with chronic obstructive pulmonary disease. *Chest* 75:146, 1979.

130. Green LH, Smith TW: The use of digitalis in patients with pulmonary disease. *Ann Intern Med* 87:459, 1977.

131. Mathur PN, Powles ACP, Pugsley SO, et al: Effect of digoxin on right ventricular function in severe chronic airflow obstruction: A controlled clinical trial. *Ann Intern Med* 95:283, 1981.

132. Derenne J-P, Fleury B, Pariente R: Acute respiratory failure of chronic obstructive pulmonary disease. *Am Rev Respir Dis* 138:1006, 1988.

133. Powles ACP, Tuxen DV, Mahood CB, et al: The effect of intravenously administered almitrine, a peripheral chemoreceptor agonist, on patients with chronic air-flow obstruction. *Am Rev Respir Dis* 127:284, 1983.

134. Bardsley PA, Howard P, DeBacker W, et al: Two years treatment with almitrine bismesylate in patients with hypoxic chronic obstructive airways disease. *Eur Respir J* 4:308, 1991.

135. Kaelin RM, Assimacopoulos A, Chevrolet J-C: Failure to predict six-month survival with COPD requiring mechanical ventilation by analysis of simple indices: A prospective study. *Chest* 92:971, 1987.

136. Menzies R, Gibbons W, Goldberg P: Determinants of weaning and survival among patients with COPD who require mechanical ventilation for acute respiratory failure. *Chest* 95:398, 1989.

137. Simmons DH, Alpas AP, Tashkin DP, et al: Hyperlactacidemia due to arterial hypoxemia or reduced cardiac output, or both. *J Appl Physiol* 45:195, 1978.

138. Harvey RM, Enson Y, Ferrer MI: A reconsideration of the origins of pulmonary hypertension. *Chest* 59:82, 1971.

139. Kilburn KH, Dowell AR: Renal function in respiratory failure: Effects of hypoxia, hyperoxia, and hypercapnia. *Arch Intern Med* 127:754, 1971.

140. Anderson RJ, Pluss RG, Berns AS, et al: Mechanism of effect of hypoxemia on renal water excretion. *J Clin Invest* 62:769, 1978.

141. Gibson GE, Pulsinelli W, Blass JP, et al: Brain dysfunction in mild to moderate hypoxia. *Am J Med* 70:1247, 1981.

142. Tirlapur VG: Nocturnal hypoxemia and associated electrocardiographic changes in patients with chronic obstructive airways disease. *N Engl J Med* 306:125, 1982.

143. Findley LJ, Whelan DM, Moser KM: Long-term oxygen therapy in COPD. *Chest* 83:671, 1983.

144. Degaute JP, Domenighetti G, Naeije R, et al: Oxygen delivery in acute exacerbation of chronic obstructive lung disease: Effects of controlled oxygen therapy. *Am Rev Respir Dis* 124:26, 1981.

145. Aubier M, Murciano D, Fournier M, et al: Effects of the administration of O_2 on ventilation and blood gases in patients with chronic obstructive pulmonary disease during acute respiratory failure. *Am Rev Respir Dis* 122:747, 1980.

146. Thorson SH, Marini JJ, Pierson DJ, et al: Variability of arterial blood gas values in stable patients in the ICU. *Chest* 84:14, 1983.

147. Marini JJ, Copps JS, Culver BH: The inspiratory work of breathing during assisted mechanical ventilation. *Chest* 87:612, 1985.

148. Pingleton SK: Nutritional support in the mechanically ventilated patient. *Clin Chest Med* 9:101, 1988.

149. Marini JJ: Should PEEP be used in airflow obstruction? *Am Rev Respir Dis* 140:1, 1989.

150. Hinson JR, Marini JJ: Principles of mechanical ventilator use in respiratory failure. *Annu Rev Med* 43:341, 1992.

151. Smith TC, Marini JJ: Impact of PEEP on lung mechanics and work of breathing in severe airflow obstruction. *J Appl Physiol* 65:1488, 1988.

152. Ranieri VM, Giuliani R, Cinnella G, et al: Physiological effects of positive end-expiratory pressure in patients with chronic obstructive pulmonary disease during acute ventilatory failure and controlled mechanical ventilation. *Am Rev Respir Dis* 147:5, 1993.

153. Kilburn KH: Shock, seizures and coma with alkalosis during mechanical ventilation. *Ann Intern Med* 65:977, 1966.

154. Darioli R, Perret C: Mechanical controlled hypoventilation in status asthmaticus. *Am Rev Respir Dis* 129:385, 1984.

155. Menitove SM, Goldring RM: Combined ventilator and bicarbonate strategy in the management of status asthmaticus. *Am J Med* 74:898, 1983.

156. Pingleton SK: Complications of acute respiratory failure. *Am Rev Respir Dis* 137:1463, 1988.

157. Brochard L, Isabey D, Piquet J, et al: Reversal of acute exacerbations of chronic obstructive lung disease by inspiratory assistance with a face mask. *N Engl J Med* 323:1523, 1990.

158. Pennock BE, Kaplan PD, Carlin BW, et al: Pressure support ventilation with a simplified ventilatory support system administered with a nasal mask in patients with respiratory failure. *Chest* 100:1371, 1991.

159. Benhamou D, Girault C, Faure C, et al: Nasal mask ventilation in acute respiratory failure: Experience in elderly patients. *Chest* 102:912, 1992.

160. Miro AM, Shivaram U, Hertig I: Continuous positive airway pressure in COPD patients in acute hypercapnic respiratory failure. *Chest* 103:266, 1993.

161. Martin TR, Lewis SW, Albert RK: The prognosis of patients with chronic obstructive pulmonary disease after hospitalization for acute respiratory failure. *Chest* 82:310, 1982.

162. Hudson LD: Survival data in patients with acute and chronic lung disease requiring mechanical ventilation. *Am Rev Respir Dis* 140(3 Suppl):S19, 1989.

163. Asmundsson T, Kilburn KA: Survival after acute respiratory failure: 145 patients observed 5 to 8½ years. *Ann Intern Med* 80:54, 1974.

164. Pines A, Raafat H, Greenfield JSB, et al: Antibiotic regimens in moderately ill patients with purulent exacerbations of chronic bronchitis. *Br J Dis Chest* 66:107, 1972.

165. Pines A, Raafat H, Plucinski K, et al: Antibiotic regimens in severe and acute purulent exacerbations of chronic bronchitis. *Br Med J* 2:735, 1968.

166. Elmes PC, King TKC, Langlands JHM, et al: Value of ampicillin in the hospital treatment of exacerbations of chronic bronchitis. *Br Med J* 2:904, 1965.

167. Emerman CL, Connors AF, Lukens TW, et al: A randomized controlled trial of methylprednisolone in the emergency treatment of acute exacerbations of COPD. *Chest* 95:563, 1989.

58. Extrapulmonary Causes of Respiratory Failure

Helen M. Hollingsworth and
Richard S. Irwin

The conditions that cause respiratory failure exclusively or primarily by their effect on structures other than the lungs are discussed in this chapter. Because severe impairment of the extrapulmonary compartment produces respiratory failure through the mechanism of hypoventilation (see Chap. 53), the resultant respiratory failure is always hypercapnic in nature. Extrapulmonary causes can account for up to an estimated 17 percent of all cases of hypercapnic respiratory failure [1].

Etiology and Pathophysiology

The following components make up the extrapulmonary compartment: (1) central nervous system (CNS), (2) peripheral nervous system, (3) respiratory muscles, (4) chest wall, (5) pleura, and (6) upper airway [2,3,4]. Because many conditions can cause extrapulmonary respiratory failure, it is helpful to categorize them according to the specific component affected by the disease process (Fig. 58-1). In the discussion that follows, descriptions of the individual diseases and conditions are limited to the features that are most important to the topic of respiratory failure. They are summarized in Tables 58-1 to 58-4. A more general discussion of each entity is beyond the scope of this chapter.

The pathophysiology of extrapulmonary respiratory failure is described in Chapter 53. Functionally, extrapulmonary disorders can lead to hypercapnic respiratory failure due to (1) a decrease in normal force generation (e.g., central nervous system dysfunction, peripheral nervous system abnormalities, or respiratory muscle dysfunction) or (2) an increase in impedance to bulk flow ventilation (e.g., chest wall and pleural disorders or upper airway obstruction) [5].

Diagnosis

GENERAL CONSIDERATIONS.
Arterial hypercapnia in the presence of a normal $P(A-a)O_2$ gradient on room air is the sine qua non of pure extrapulmonary respiratory failure [6]. The normal gradient reflects the fact that in pure extrapulmonary failure distal gas exchange is entirely normal, and the decrease in PaO_2 directly reflects the decrease in PAO_2. A $P(A-a)O_2$ gradient less than 20 mm Hg in the presence of an elevated $PaCO_2$ is, with few exceptions, diagnostic of extrapulmonary respiratory failure [7–13]. The alveolar-arterial gradient can narrow to normal in patients with chronic obstructive pulmonary disease (COPD) who have increasing hypercapnia [14]. The normal $P(A-a)O_2$ gradient in this setting is likely related to substantial changes in the position of the alveolar and arterial points on the oxyhemoglobin dissociation curve related to ventilation-perfusion inequalities [14]. Therefore, while arterial hypercapnia with a normal $P(A-a)O_2$ gradient is consistent with pure extrapulmonary respiratory failure, it cannot by itself rule out severe COPD.

Pulmonary parenchymal disease can also exist concomitantly with extrapulmonary respiratory failure. For example, polymyositis can cause respiratory muscle fatigue in addition to interstitial pulmonary fibrosis. This may be suggested by the combination of hypercapnia and only mild to moderate widening of the $P(A-a)O_2$ gradient. A gradient between 20 and 30 mm Hg in the presence of arterial hypercapnia should raise the suspicion that a significant element of extrapulmonary dysfunction may be present. It is also important to realize that even when the $P(A-a)O_2$ gradient exceeds 30 mm Hg, some degree of extrapulmonary dysfunction may be present concomitantly with significant pulmonary impairment. For example, this is commonly the case in hypercapnic respiratory failure, which results from an acute exacerbation of COPD. In this situation, respiratory muscle fatigue often develops and significantly contributes to the development of carbon dioxide retention [15]. A much rarer example is the presence of a large abdominal ventral hernia in a patient with COPD. The resultant paradoxical breathing pattern may significantly contribute to abnormal gas exchange and increased dyspnea [16].

DECREASE IN NORMAL FORCE GENERATION.
Because the inspiratory respiratory muscles generate the force that results in ventilation, any condition that directly or indirectly impairs respiratory muscle function can result in decreased force generation [5]. Dysfunction of the respiratory center, peripheral nervous system pathways, or the respiratory muscles themselves will decrease the force available to produce ventilation. If this impairment of force generation is severe enough, the level of minute ventilation is insufficient for the level of (metabolic) production of carbon dioxide, and hypercapnic respiratory failure results.

As described later, an acute decrease in CNS output sufficient to result in hypercapnic respiratory failure (e.g., acute narcotic overdose) is usually accompanied by obvious evidence of generalized CNS depression. In contrast, a chronic (e.g., primary alveolar hypoventilation) or episodic (e.g., central sleep apnea) cause of decreased impulse formation may present a much more difficult diagnostic dilemma. Tests to evaluate respiratory center drive, such as voluntary hyperventilation, carbon dioxide stimulation test, or monitored sleep study (e.g., polysomnography), may be necessary to define the problem.

The diagnosis of impaired peripheral nervous system function or primary weakness of the respiratory muscles is often facilitated by the presence of certain suggestive clinical findings, which vary depending on the specific entity present (see following discussion). Respiratory muscle fatigue/weakness may be suspected clinically and documented using a number of tests specifically designed to evaluate respiratory muscle function.

Symptoms are usually nonspecific; patients may complain of dyspnea on exertion, when supine (bilateral diaphragmatic paralysis) or when upright (C_5, C_6 quadriplegia). Complaint of

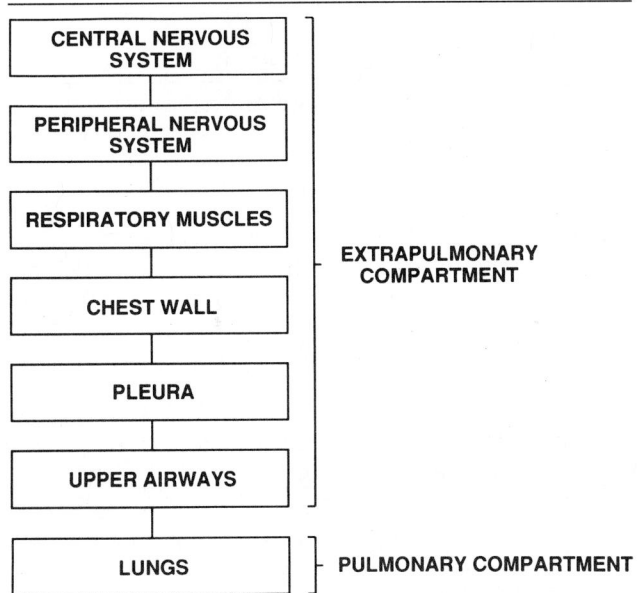

Fig. 58-1. Schematic representation of the anatomy of the respiratory system.

weakness in other muscle groups, difficulty swallowing, and change in voice volume or tone may be other important clues. Physical findings of stressed, fatigued, or weakened respiratory muscles may be manifested by changes in the rate, depth, and pattern of breathing. Respiratory rate may be increased and tidal volume decreased. Paradoxical inward motion of the anterior abdominal wall may occur during inspiration. This indicates a failure of the diaphragm to contract sufficiently to descend and move the abdominal contents downward, which normally results in an outward motion of the abdominal wall during inspiration. Cyclic changes in breathing patterns with either predominantly chest wall or predominantly abdominal wall motion, called respiratory alternans, represent the cyclic contractions of intercostal and accessory muscles on the one hand and the diaphragm on the other. We infer that these different muscle groups are alternating in their contribution to the work of breathing and allowing each other to "rest."

Three laboratory tests can be useful diagnostically. First, measurement of maximal inspiratory and expiratory pressures at the mouth are easy to perform, noninvasive, and highly predictive of the development of hypercapnic respiratory failure when the problem is decreased respiratory muscle force generation [17,18]. Arterial hypercapnia as a result of respiratory muscle weakness is generally not seen until the maximal inspiratory pressure is reduced to 30 percent of normal or less [17,18]. Although normal predicted values vary (primarily on the basis of age and sex [19,20]), a maximal inspiratory pressure less negative than -30 cm H_2O is likely to be associated with arterial hypercapnia [18,21]. Maximal expiratory pressures at the mouth are also reduced when there is respiratory muscle weakness, and in a number of neuromuscular disorders the decrease may be even greater than that of the corresponding inspiratory pressure [18]. A maximal expiratory pressure of less than 40 cm H_2O is generally associated with a poor cough and difficulty clearing secretions [21].

Second, measurements of vital capacity are valuable in predicting the development of arterial hypercapnia and can be performed at the bedside [17,21]. Although a vital capacity of less than 1 liter or less than 15 ml per kilogram body weight in a patient with neuromuscular weakness is commonly associated with arterial hypercapnia [1,21,22], this is a less sensitive predictor of arterial hypercapnia than the maximal inspiratory pressure, particularly in patients with chest wall disorders such as kyphoscoliosis [18]. Although significant arterial hypercapnia with an inspiratory pressure more negative than -30 cm H_2O is rare, it may be present with a vital capacity as high as 55 percent or as low as 20 percent of predicted [17,18].

Third, measurements of transdiaphragmatic pressures (P_{di}) and diaphragmatic electromyograms (EMGs), although not commonly used clinically, may be helpful. An inspiratory effort associated with a P_{di} consistently greater than 40 percent of maximum predictably results in diaphragmatic fatigue [23]. It therefore follows that patients with diaphragmatic weakness and a reduced maximum P_{di} are at risk of developing diaphragmatic fatigue and respiratory failure even in the face of normal inspiratory resistance [23]. Similarly, a decrease of more than 20 percent from baseline in the high- to low-frequency ratio for the diaphragmatic EMG indicates diaphragmatic fatigue and portends subsequent development of hypercapnic failure [24,25].

CENTRAL NERVOUS SYSTEM DYSFUNCTION. The respiratory center, located in the brainstem, is composed of two main parts [26,27]: The medullary center is responsible for initiation and maintenance of spontaneous respiration; and the pneumotaxic center in the pons helps coordinate cyclic respiration. A decrease in central drive can occur from a direct central loss of sensitivity to changes in PCO_2 and pH and/or a peripheral chemoreceptor loss of sensitivity to hypoxia as a result of several different CNS insults: CNS depressants, metabolic abnormalities, structural lesions, primary alveolar hypoventilation, and central sleep apnea (Table 58-1).

PERIPHERAL NERVOUS SYSTEM DYSFUNCTION. Disruption in impulse transmission from the respiratory center to the respiratory muscles can eventuate in respiratory failure. Disrupted impulse transmission may be caused by spinal cord disease [28], anterior horn cell disease [29,30], peripheral neuropathy [22], or neuromuscular junction blockade [21] (Table 58-2). The innervation of the inspiratory respiratory muscles may be involved as part of a generalized process (e.g., Guillain-Barré syndrome [22], myasthenia gravis [21]) or as an isolated abnormality (e.g., phrenic nerve palsy secondary to hypothermic cardioplegia during cardiac surgery [31,32]).

Peripheral nervous system dysfunction severe enough to produce hypercapnic respiratory failure is always associated with pulmonary function test findings of a reduced vital capacity (usually <50 percent of predicted value [17,21]) and markedly decreased maximal inspiratory and expiratory pressures at the mouth (usually ≤30% of predicted [17,21,30]). Clinically, this type of respiratory failure is characterized by an ineffective cough and a high incidence of aspiration, atelectasis, and pneumonia [7].

Interruption of CNS impulses resulting from spinal cord abnormalities affects the respiratory system in a variable way that depends on the level of the injury [28,33]. A lesion at the C_3 level or above abolishes both diaphragmatic and intercostal activity, leaving only some residual accessory muscle function [33]. The result is severe hypercapnic respiratory failure. Acute spinal cord lesions at the C_5 and C_6 levels produce an immediate fall in the vital capacity to 30 percent of the predicted value [28]. Within approximately 3 months of injury, however, the vital capacity will have increased to 50 to 60 percent of normal [28]. High thoracic lesions affect the intercostal as well as the

Table 58-1. Respiratory Failure Caused by Central Nervous System Dysfunction

Causes	Salient clinical features	Diagnostic tests	Treatment
CNS depressant drugs [39,173,174]	Pupillary changes Needle marks	Toxicology screen ECG in tricyclic overdose	See Chapters 128–158
Hypothyroidism [175]	Myxedema	Thyroid function tests	Cautious thyroid replacement
Starvation [176]	Cachexia Diarrhea	↓ Albumin ↓ Cholesterol	Nutrition
Metabolic alkalosis [177]	Lethargy Confusion	Arterial blood gases Serum electrolytes	See Chapter 80
Structural brainstem damage [174,178,179]	Localizing neurologic findings		
Neoplasm	Headache	CT, MRI, CSF cytology	Radiation, chemotherapy
Infection	Headache, fever	CT, MRI	Antimicrobial therapy
Infarct		CT, MRI, cardiac echo	
Primary alveolar hypoventilation (Ondine's curse) [123,180–187]	Daytime hypersomnolence Headache Rarely dyspneic Polycythemia Cor pulmonale	Blunted or absent ventilatory response to ↑ CO_2, ↓ O_2 in inspired gas Normal PFTs	Nighttime ventilatory support Electrophrenic pacing Medroxyprogesterone acetate Supplemental oxygen
Central sleep apnea [161,179,187,188]	Same as primary alveolar hypoventilation	Polysomnography: apnea without respiratory effort Normal CO_2, O_2 response curves while awake	Nighttime ventilatory support Electrophrenic pacing Nasal CPAP Supplemental oxygen

CNS = central nervous system; ECG = electrocardiogram; CT = computed tomography; MRI = magnetic resonance imaging; CSF = cerebrospinal fluid; PFT = pulmonary functional test; CPAP = continuous positive airway pressure.

abdominal muscles, resulting in a limitation of both inspiratory capacity and active expiration. Midthoracic spinal cord lesions have relatively little impact on respiratory muscle function because they principally affect the abdominal muscles, resulting in only a limitation of active expiration and cough [7,33].

Although the pathophysiologic mechanism of most spinal cord diseases is interruption of impulse transmission (which results in respiratory muscle weakness), two notable exceptions exist: tetanus and strychnine poisoning. In both conditions there is a decrease in inhibitory influences at the spinal cord and anterior horn cell level [34,35,36], causing a simultaneous increase in motor activity to groups of muscles that are normally antagonistic to one another. This results in intense muscle spasms, including involvement of the upper airway muscles, diaphragm, and intercostal muscles. Consequently, repetitive spasms and episodes of apnea occur, resulting in severe arterial hypoxemia, hypercapnia, and metabolic acidosis [34,35,36]. Tetanus and strychnine poisoning are therefore characterized by hypercapnic respiratory failure from dysfunction of the inspiratory muscles, upper airway obstruction, and CNS respiratory center depression (secondary to hypoxia).

Interruption of efferent impulse transmission may result from diseases that specifically involve the anterior horn cells of the spinal cord. Amyotrophic lateral sclerosis (ALS) is now the most common example, surpassing poliomyelitis, of an anterior horn cell disease causing respiratory failure [7,29,30]. In most cases of ALS, the patient suffers from segmental muscular atrophy, weakness of the distal extremities, hyperreflexia, fasciculations, and/or bulbar paralysis [29]. Although respiratory failure usually develops late in the course of the disease, it may be the presenting manifestation [29]. Repetitive episodes of aspiration secondary to bulbar dysfunction are often a contributing factor [7].

It has been speculated that antecedent poliomyelitis may be involved in some cases of ALS [37]. A "postpolio" syndrome, characterized by new, slowly progressive muscle weakness, may develop years after recovery from acute poliomyelitis [38]. The syndrome can vary from simple nonprogressive deterio-

ration in function to atypical forms of spinal muscular atrophy or a condition that appears to be an atypical presentation of ALS. This new syndrome does not appear to be life-threatening and is most likely due to a dysfunction of the postpolio surviving motor neurons [38].

Polyneuropathies with prominent motor neuron involvement frequently involve the respiratory nerves and can lead to respiratory failure [39]. The typical clinical picture is that of a symmetric, predominantly distal muscle weakness with absent tendon reflexes [39]. Guillain-Barré syndrome is probably the most common example (see Chap. 189). Severe respiratory muscle involvement is common. In one series of patients with Guillain-Barré syndrome, 28 percent required mechanical ventilatory assistance. The average duration of mechanical ventilation was 9 weeks (range 3 weeks to 7 months) [22]. Although the mortality rate is generally low [22], in one series 21 percent of hospitalized patients died [40]. Concomitant autonomic dysfunction associated with increased mortality has been described [40], including new onset hypertension (57%), sinus tachycardia (50%), postural hypotension (43%), and facial flushing (25%).

Critical illness polyneuropathy commonly occurs in the setting of sepsis and multiorgan failure (e.g., up to 30% by clinical examination and up to 70% by electrophysiologic testing) [40a,40b,40c]. When it causes profound generalized muscle weakness, it is a major reason why patients remain on prolonged mechanical ventilatory support. Like Guillain-Barré syndrome, patients with critical illness polyneuropathy have areflexia; however, they more commonly have prominent sensory nerve findings and a normal cerebrospinal fluid examination. Electrophysiologic testing distinguishes critical illness polyneuropathy from the Guillain-Barré syndrome. The findings in critical illness polyneuropathy show evidence of axon degeneration rather than demyelination. While the etiology of critical illness polyneuropathy is not known, it is predominantly a disease of older patients who stay in the ICU for more than 28 days and who have had elevated serum glucose and lowered albumin levels at the time of diagnosis. Approximately 53 percent of patients with sepsis, multiorgan system failure, and critical illness polyneuropathy survive; their prognosis for significant improvement from the neuropathy is very good.

Paralytic shellfish poisoning (red tide) is a dramatic but uncommon cause of respiratory failure from a peripheral neuropathy [41–44]. The responsible agent is a heat-stable neurotoxin that interferes with action potential propagation along peripheral nerves. During the warm summer months, the dinoflagellates that produce the toxin proliferate and are ingested by shellfish. Certain shellfish (mainly clams, mussels, oysters, and scallops) concentrate the neurotoxin and, when ingested, cause illness. The clinical picture is virtually pathognomonic. Within 30 minutes of ingesting contaminated shellfish, tingling and numbness of the face, lips, and tongue develop. Paresthesias and muscle weakness follow, with rapid progression to limb and respiratory muscle paralysis [43,44]. Multiple-case presentations from one source of exposure are common.

Peripheral phrenic nerve palsies can contribute to or cause hypercapnic respiratory failure, particularly if they are bilateral [45]. Bilateral phrenic nerve palsies have been described as an uncommon complication resulting from hypothermia used for cardioplegia during cardiac surgery (particularly where ice slush is used) [31], trauma [31,45], a variety of neurologic diseases (e.g., poliomyelitis and Guillain-Barré syndrome) [31,45,46], intrathoracic malignancies [47], and even as a part of a paraneoplastic endocrinopathy [48]. Severe orthopnea, marked abdominal paradoxical breathing in the supine position, and minimal or absent transdiaphragmatic pressure gradient are hallmarks of bilateral diaphragmatic paralysis [31,32,49]. Bilateral diaphragmatic paralysis also may be idiopathic [50] or may rarely be due to Charcot-Marie-Tooth disease [51]. This hereditary motor and sensory neuropathy, characterized by chronic degeneration of peripheral nerves and roots beginning in the feet and legs and later involving the hands, was recently reported to involve the phrenic nerves as well [51]. Bilateral diaphragmatic paralysis should also be considered in the postoperative cardiac surgery patient who cannot be weaned from mechanical ventilation [31,32]. Fluoroscopy and transcutaneous phrenic nerve stimulation with surface diaphragmatic EMG recordings can help confirm the diagnosis [45].

Other peripheral neuropathies that can involve the efferent pathways to the respiratory muscles include diphtheria, herpes zoster infection and tick paralysis (as a result of the production of a neurotoxin), acute intermittent porphyria, beriberi, and a variety of metabolic disorders [39]. Respiratory failure associated with diphtheria is of delayed onset, usually 4 to 6 weeks after the onset of illness [39]. Tick paralysis is seen mainly in children in whom the presence of the tick goes unnoticed for 5 to 6 days [39]. In acute intermittent porphyria, respiratory involvement may be a slowly progressive process or may cause an abrupt deterioration in respiratory function [39]. Bilateral diaphragmatic (phrenic nerve) dysfunction is usually the major problem.

Myasthenia gravis [21], botulism [52–55], organophosphate poisoning [39], and a variety of drugs can produce neuromuscular blockade that results in respiratory failure [56] (Table 58-2). Although acute respiratory failure may occasionally be a presenting manifestation [39,57], patients with myasthenia gravis typically show signs of obvious muscle weakness and rapid fatigability of muscles, particularly the cranial muscles, prior to the development of respiratory failure. More commonly, respiratory failure develops following surgical procedures, on the institution of corticosteroid therapy, or, in some cases, as a result of undertreatment or overtreatment with anticholinesterase medications [21].

Although the diagnosis is suspected on clinical grounds and a positive response to edrophonium chloride (Tensilon) is supportive, generally the diagnosis is confirmed by a typical EMG (decremental responses on repetitive nerve stimulation) and elevated serum level of antibodies to acetylcholine receptors [58]. Because patients with myasthenia gravis may rapidly deteriorate, it is helpful to follow serial maximum inspiratory pressures at the mouth and vital capacity measurements to detect high risk for respiratory failure [21,39]. A decrease in maximum inspiratory pressure to a value less negative than -30 cm H_2O or vital capacity to 1 liter or less is a warning sign of impending respiratory failure [21].

Eaton-Lambert syndrome, a form of neuromuscular blockade similar to myasthenia gravis, occurs in association with certain carcinomas, particularly small cell carcinoma of the lung [59]. The neuromuscular blockade in most cases precedes other evidence of the carcinoma [59], and the EMG shows an incremental pattern unlike that in true myasthenia.

Organophosphates, commonly used in insecticides, inhibit the enzyme cholinesterase, resulting in accumulation of acetylcholine at neurosynaptic junctions. The symptoms of organophosphate poisoning are those of cholinergic toxicity, including blurred vision, weakness, vomiting, diarrhea, cramps, sweating, increased secretions, incoordination, twitching, ataxia, mental status changes, and, if severe enough, respiratory failure and death [60]. Respiratory muscle paralysis along with respiratory center depression, excessive secretions, and possibly bronchoconstriction appear to combine to cause respiratory failure [60] (see Chaps. 137 and 153).

In botulism, neuromuscular blockade develops as a result of a neurotoxin produced by the bacteria *Clostridium botulinum*. Most cases are caused by neurotoxin-contaminated food [52,53,61], but occasionally botulism develops as a result of a wound infection with *C. botulinum* [54] (see Chap. 96). A variety of findings in botulism helps predict whether respiratory failure requiring mechanical ventilatory assistance will develop. A vital capacity of 30 percent or less of predicted value is generally associated with evidence of hypercapnic failure [53]. Other clinical clues are the presence of nausea, vomiting, diarrhea, dyspnea, ptosis, or extremity weakness on initial examination.

Prolonged neuromuscular blockade is occasionally seen following the administration of succinylcholine in individuals with pseudocholinesterase deficiency [39]. In contrast to the usual duration of paralysis of approximately 3 minutes, the effect in these individuals usually lasts 4 to 6 hours, during which time they require mechanical ventilatory support [39].

Prolonged administration (>2 days) of neuromuscular blocking agents such as pancuronium and vecuronium in intensive care units has been associated with two distinct patterns of neuromuscular dysfunction [62]: (1) persistent neuromuscular junction blockade in patients with renal insufficiency who accumulate the parent drug and its active metabolites; and (2) an acute noninflammatory myopathy that becomes apparent as neuromuscular transmission improves. The myopathy appears to be a consequence of an interaction between neuromuscular blocking agents and corticosteroids and seems to be related to the total dose of neuromuscular blocking agent [63]. This has been particularly dramatic in previously healthy asthmatic patients who became quadriparetic for days to weeks after concomitant treatment with high-dose corticosteroids and a neuromuscular blocking agent [62].

Neuromuscular blockade also may occur as a result of administration of a variety of drugs [56]. Certain cardiovascular drugs (e.g., lidocaine, quinidine, procainamide, and propranolol), anticonvulsants (e.g., phenytoin and trimethadione), D-penicillamine, and a number of antibiotics (most notably the

Table 58-2. Respiratory Failure Caused by Peripheral Nervous System Dysfunction

Causes	Salient clinical features	Diagnostic tests	Specific treatment
Spinal cord disease [7,28,33,147–149] Traumatic Neoplasm Hemorrhage Syrinx Infarct Transverse myelitis	Above C_5, diaphragm, intercostal, and abdominal activity abolished Below C_5, diaphragm preserved, intercostal and abdominal activity abolished Below T_5, abdominal activity diminished, impaired force expiration	Spinal x-ray film, CT, MRI	Support, VC tends to improve over 3 mo in traumatic lesions C_5 and below Phrenic nerve pacing for high cervical cord lesions with intact phrenic nerves
Tetanus [34,35]	Intense muscle spasms Trismus Apnea Metabolic acidosis History of penetrating wound	Clinical setting Gram stain, anaerobic culture of wound History of inadequate immunization	Human antitetanus antiglobulin Wound debridement Penicillin, high dose Tetanus toxoid vaccination to prevent recurrence
Strychnine [36]	Intense muscle spasms Apnea Metabolic acidosis	Toxicology screen Clinical picture	Gastric lavage Activated charcoal Barbiturates or diazepam for seizures
Anterior horn cell disease Amyotrophic lateral sclerosis [7,29,30,37] Poliomyelitis [38]	Segmental muscle atrophy Hyperreflexia Fasciculations Distal extremity weakness	EMG	Supportive Prevention with vaccine
Polyneuropathy [22,36,39] Guillain-Barré syndrome [22,39,40,150–153]	Viral illness, symmetric ascending distal muscle weakness Areflexia Autonomic dysfunction	Elevated CSF protein without pleocytosis Demylination by electrophysiology tests	Early plasmapheresis Prophylactic low-dose heparin Intravenous gammaglobulin
Shellfish poisoning (red tide) [41–44]	Paresthesias of face, progressive muscle weakness starting 30 min after ingestion of shellfish	History of fish ingestion	Supportive No specific antidote
Bilateral phrenic nerve palsy [31,32,45,47–50]	Severe orthopnea Abdominal paradoxical respiration	Fluoroscopy of diaphragm Surface EMG of diaphragm Transdiaphragmatic pressure	Diaphragmatic pacing
Charcot-Marie-Tooth disease [51]	Peripheral muscle weakness and wasting, hereditary PES cavus, hammertoes	EMG	Supportive
Diphtheria [39]	Numbness of lips Paralysis of pharyngeal and laryngeal muscles	Throat culture	Prevention with vaccine
Tick paralysis [39]	Tick exposure	Find tick	Remove tick
Acute intermittent porphyria [39]	Acute polyneuropathy like Guillain-Barré syndrome Mental disturbance Abdominal pain	Urine for porphobilinogen, delta-aminolevulinic acid	Avoid exacerbating drugs such as phenytoin, barbiturates, ethosuximide
Pseudocholinesterase deficiency [39]	Prolonged paralysis following succinylcholine Family history	Serum pseudocholinesterase	Avoid succinylcholine
Myasthenia gravis [21,39,56–58,189] (autoimmune and drug-induced)	Muscle weakness Rapid fatigability Antecedent surgery, corticosteroid, or aminoglycoside	EMG Tensilon test Antibodies to acetylcholine receptors	Anticholinesterase Calcium gluconate Thymectomy Steroids Immunosuppressants Plasmapheresis — See Chapter 190
Persistent drug-induced neuromuscular blockade [62,63]	Renal insufficiency Corticosteroids	Creatinine kinase	Limit use of pancuronium and vecuronium
Eaton-Lambert syndrome [59,190]	Muscle wasting, hyporeflexia Associated cancer (e.g., small cell of lung)	Incremental pattern on EMG Chest film	Treatment of associated cancer 3,4-diaminopyridine Anticholinesterase
Botulism [52–55,61]	Wound infection: fever Ingestion of contaminated food: nausea and vomiting Dysphagia, diplopia, ptosis, dysarthria	Gram stain and culture of stool, wound, or suspected food Demonstrate toxin in stool, serum, or food by mouse neutralization test	Trivalent antitoxin Wound debridement, penicillin Nasogastric lavage

Table 58-2. (continued)

Causes	Salient clinical features	Diagnostic tests	Specific treatment
Organophosphates [60]	Use of insecticides Cholinergic toxicity (vomiting, diarrhea, weakness, cramps, sweating, ataxia, mental status changes)	History of exposure	Anticholinergics Pralidoxime
Neuralgic amyotrophy [46]	Shoulder and neck pain, upper extremity weakness, breathlessness, orthopnea	Fluoroscopy of diaphragm, chest film, EMG	Analgesics, possibly corticosteroids
Critical illness polyneuropathy	Sepsis multiorgan failure, generalized weakness, areflexia	Normal CSF, axonal degeneration by electrophysiology tests	Supportive

CT = computed tomography; MRI = magnetic resonance imaging; VC = vital capacity; EMG = electromyography; CSF = cerebrospinal fluid.

aminoglycosides) can prolong postoperative respiratory depression, unmask underlying myasthenia gravis, and cause a drug-induced form of myasthenia gravis [56]. The definitive diagnosis of drug-induced neuromuscular blockade is usually made in retrospect, if the abnormality reverses following elimination of the offending agent. The administration of calcium gluconate has in some cases been reported to result in prompt improvement in neuromuscular transmission [56].

Neuralgic amyotrophy, a disorder of the peripheral nervous system affecting the brachial plexus, has recently been associated with diaphragmatic dysfunction and dyspnea [46]. Neuralgic amyotrophy usually presents with acute severe shoulder pain that may extend to the neck, back, and arm. Motor weakness of the ipsilateral shoulder and arm usually develops within a month of the onset of pain. A sensory defect may be present in one-fourth of patients. Electromyographic studies suggest axonal degeneration affecting the brachial plexus. In one study [46], 12 of 16 patients had bilateral diaphragm paralysis and 4 of 16 had unilateral diaphragm paralysis. Mild nocturnal desaturation, hypopneas, and obstructive sleep apneas were found in some patients, but alveolar hypoventilation was not found. However, as in other patients with bilateral diaphragm paralysis, superimposed pulmonary parenchymal disease could potentially cause respiratory failure.

RESPIRATORY MUSCLE DYSFUNCTION. A number of systemic myopathies feature prominent respiratory muscle involvement, including muscular dystrophies, myotonic disorders, inflammatory myopathies, periodic paralyses, metabolic storage diseases, endocrine myopathies, infectious myopathies, toxic myopathies, rhabdomyolysis, and electrolyte disturbances [18,39,64–69] (Table 58-3). The clinical presentation generally is widespread skeletal muscle weakness. Respiratory muscle involvement and respiratory failure usually develop only as the disease progresses. On occasion, however, respiratory failure may be the presenting manifestation of a generalized myopathy [65]. As is the case in primary neurologic disorders, myopathy-induced hypercapnic respiratory failure is almost invariably accompanied by a severely impaired cough mechanism and an inability to clear respiratory tract secretions effectively [7]. Typical pulmonary function findings of primary respiratory muscle weakness are a decrease in maximum inspiratory and expiratory pressures that can be generated at the mouth and, as the disease progresses, a decrease in lung volumes [70].

The muscular dystrophies are inherited disorders that present with evidence of proximal muscle weakness and atrophy [39,71]. The myotonic dystrophies are also hereditary or congenital in origin. Their most prominent clinical features are myotonia (i.e., sustained contraction of muscles in response to

direct stimulation) and the findings of ptosis, prominent distal and facial muscle weakness, and atrophy [39,71]. The periodic paralyses are genetic disorders characterized by attacks of muscle weakness in response to a variety of precipitating factors, such as exercise, emotional upset, exposure to cold, and, in some cases, exposure to alcohol [39]. Patients may exhibit hypokalemia or normokalemia.

Glycogen storage diseases result from defects in muscle glycogenolysis or glycogen storage. The most common example is McArdle's disease. Clinically, these patients exhibit exercise-induced muscle cramping and slowly progressive muscle weakness and atrophy [39,65,71]. On occasion, respiratory failure may be the presenting manifestation [65]. The diagnosis is confirmed by pathologic examination of a muscle biopsy sample and chemical assay for muscle acid maltase levels [65].

Polymyositis is a collagen vascular disease the primary abnormality of which is skeletal muscle inflammation. Proximal muscle weakness is prominent and develops over a period of weeks to months. Patients may have difficulty swallowing secondary to pharyngeal muscle involvement. The diagnosis is confirmed by typical EMG and muscle biopsy findings and an elevation in serum muscle enzyme levels [72,73]. Respiratory muscle failure is an uncommon complication of polymyositis but is more common than previously thought [18,74].

Patients with polymyositis may also develop interstitial pulmonary fibrosis, which can present with dyspnea and should be considered in the differential diagnosis of dyspnea in these patients [74]. In this situation, crackles are usually present on physical examination, the $P_{(A-a)}O_2$ gradient is increased, and the carbon monoxide diffusing capacity of the lung is decreased.

Eosinophilia-myalgia syndrome, strongly associated with oral ingestion of l-tryptophan, presents with severe muscle pain, muscle weakness, mouth ulcers, and peripheral eosinophilia (>2000 cells/mm^3) [75,76]. Although some patients improve with discontinuation of tryptophan, others progress to develop sclerodermiform skin changes, profound muscle weakness, and an ascending polyneuropathy. Respiratory findings include dyspnea, cough, aspiration, and respiratory failure [75,76]. Similarities with toxic oil syndrome have been noted, but the specific etiologic agent has not been identified in either syndrome [77].

Procainamide has been reported to cause a necrotizing myopathy with diaphragm involvement that results in respiratory failure [78]. Although anti-double-stranded DNA and anti-histone antibodies were positive, antinuclear antibodies were absent and the muscle biopsy did not reveal an inflammatory infiltrate. Neuromuscular junction transmission was normal, suggesting that this was not a drug-induced myasthenic syn-

Table 58-3. Respiratory Failure Caused by Respiratory Muscle Dysfunction

Causes	Salient features	Diagnostic tests	Specific treatment
Muscular dystrophies [39,71]	Proximal muscle weakness and atrophy Hereditary	Muscle biopsy	Supportive
Myotonic dystrophies [39,71]	Myotonia, ptosis Distal and facial muscle weakness and atrophy Hereditary	Muscle biopsy EMG	Supportive
Periodic paralyses [39,154]	Hypokalemic or hyperkalemic Genetic Muscle weakness associated with exercise, emotional upset, cold, alcohol	Serum potassium Family history	Avoid precipitating factors Carbonic anhydrase inhibitor
Glycogen storage diseases [39,65,71] (McArdle's disease)	Exercise-related muscle cramping Slowly progressive muscle weakness and atrophy	Muscle biopsy and assay for acid maltase level	Supportive
Polymyositis [18,72–74]	Proximal muscle weakness Difficulty swallowing	EMG Muscle biopsy Elevated CPK, aldolase	Corticosteroids Immunosuppressants
Hyperthyroidism [191]	Thyrotoxicosis, heat intolerance, tachycardia, hyperreflexia	TSH, TFTs	Propylthiouracil, methimazole See Chapter 112
Hypothyroidism [39]	Myxedema, cold intolerance, hyporeflexia, bradycardia	TSH, TFTs	Replace thyroid hormone See Chapter 112
Hyperadrenocorticolism [39,155]	Cushingoid appearance	Serum cortisol Dexamethasone suppression test Adrenal CT	Depends on cause
Rhabdomyolysis 2° colchicine or chloroquine toxicity [39]	Muscle pain, swelling, myoglobinuria	$\uparrow$ CPK	Supportive
Infectious myositis Trichinosis [39,159] Viral [39]	Muscle tenderness, weakness, fever	Serology Muscle biopsy	Rest, corticosteroids Thiabendazole
Hypophosphatemia [66–68,156,192]	Weakness Difficulty weaning	$\downarrow$ Phosphate	Replete
Hypermagnesemia or hypomagnesemia [68,157,158]	Weakness Difficulty weaning	$\uparrow$ or $\downarrow$ MG	See Chapter 114
Hypokalemia [68]	Weakness	$\downarrow$ K$^+$	Replete
Hypercalcemia [68,158]	Lethargy, confusion	$\uparrow$ Ca^{2+}	See Chapter 114
Eosinophilia-myalgia [75–79]	L-tryptophan ingestion Muscle tenderness and weakness Fasciitis	Eosinophilia Muscle biopsy	Discontinue L-tryptophan Supportive
Procainamide-induced myopathy [78]	Weakness Respiratory failure	Muscle biopsy, $\uparrow$ CPK	Discontinue procainamide

EMG = Electromyography; CPK = creatinine phosphokinase; TSH = thyroid-stimulating hormone; TFT = thyroid function test.

drome. Slow improvement in muscle strength followed discontinuation of procainamide.

INCREASED IMPEDANCE TO BULK FLOW. In a number of pulmonary disorders, the development of hypercapnic respiratory failure is, to a considerable extent, the result of a marked increase in intrinsic impedance to ventilation (e.g., increased airflow resistance in COPD or asthma or increased elastic recoil in interstitial fibrosis), which even normal respiratory muscle force generation cannot overcome [5]. It may be less widely appreciated that increases in extrapulmonary impedance to ventilation also can result in hypercapnic respiratory failure. These disorders can be divided into those that involve a decrease in chest wall or pleural compliance (e.g., kyphoscoliosis or pleural fibrosis) and those that involve an increase in airflow resistance resulting from upper airway obstruction (e.g., tracheal stenosis or laryngeal edema) (Table 58-4).

Chest Wall and Pleural Disorders. Kyphoscoliosis is a common cause of extrapulmonary respiratory failure [7]. Scoliosis (i.e., lateral curvature of the spine) is more commonly associated with the development of respiratory failure than is kyphosis (i.e., dorsal curvature of the spine). When the two conditions coexist, usually the severity of the scoliosis determines the probability of respiratory failure [7]. Although most cases of scoliosis are idiopathic, a significant number result from poliomyelitis, congenital abnormalities, and, to a lesser extent, chronic infectious diseases of the spine such as tuberculosis [7]. Individuals with severe deformity at a relatively young age are at the greatest risk for eventual development of respiratory failure [7]. In idiopathic kyphoscoliosis, chronic hypercapnic respiratory failure generally occurs when the angle of curvature is 120 degrees or greater [7]. In contrast, in paralytic kyphoscoliosis (e.g., as a result of poliomyelitis), the angle of curvature does not reliably predict either vital capacity or hypercapnic respiratory failure [79]. This appears to reflect the fact

Table 58-4. Respiratory Failure Caused by Chest Wall, Pleural, and Upper Airway Diseases

Causes	Salient features	Diagnostic tests	Specific treatment
Chest wall and pleural disorders			
Kyphoscoliosis [7,79–83,160]	Spinal curvature ≥120° Progressive dyspnea on exertion over several years	Spinal x-ray films Restriction on PFTs	Nighttime ventilatory support
Obesity-hypoventilation [84–88,193]	Massive chest wall obesity ± sleep apnea	Polysomnography ↓ CO_2 response curve ↓ chest wall compliance	Weight loss Medroxyprogesterone acetate Nasal CPAP for sleep apnea
Flail chest [194]	Multiple rib fractures, paradoxical respiration	Chest film Observation of chest wall	Mechanical positive pressure ventilation
Fibrothorax [174,195–199]	± pleuritic chest pain Asbestos exposure, pleural infection, pleural hemorrhage, uremia, collagen vascular disease	Restriction on PFTs Decreased maximum static elastic recoil pressure	Decortication
Thoracoplasty [7]	Chest wall deformity 2° resection of ribs	Restriction on PFTs Chest film	Supportive
Ankylosing spondylitis [7]	Limited chest expansion Apical pulmonary fibrosis Limited lumbar mobility Chronic low back pain	PFTs (↑ FRC, ↓ TLC) HLA-B27 Spine and sacroiliac x-ray films	Antiinflammatory agents Flexibility exercises
Upper airway obstruction			
Acute epiglottitis [89,90,111,200,201]	Fever, sore throat, stridor, dysphagia	Soft tissue films of neck	See Chapter 75
Acute laryngeal edema Anaphylactic [91,111,202–208]	Stridor in setting of *Hymenoptera* sting, contrast media, or drug administration	Other evidence of angioedema/anaphylaxis	Epinephrine-parenteral Cricothyroidotomy
Traumatic [209]	Stridor following endotracheal extubation	History	Racemic inhaled epinephrine Heliox
Foreign body aspiration [92–96,210]	Unable to speak Stridor or apnea	X-ray film helpful when foreign body below cords	Heimlich maneuver Bronchoscopy Cricothyroidotomy
Retropharyngeal hemorrhage [97]	Associated with anticoagulation or head and neck surgery Sore throat	Soft tissue film of neck CT scan or tomography	Reverse anticoagulation
Bilateral vocal cord paralysis [98–101,110,113–115]	Stridor Aspiration	Flow volume loop Laryngoscopy	See text
Tracheal stenosis [106,107,110,209,211] Tracheomalacia [106,107]	Progressive dyspnea after endotracheal intubation	Flow volume loop Tomography Laryngotracheoscopy	Tracheostomy Stent, resection of stenosis
Laryngeal and tracheal tumors [102–104,111,112]	Dyspnea Hoarseness Stridor	Flow volume loop Tomography Laryngotracheoscopy	Laser or surgical resection, radiation
Idiopathic obstructive sleep apnea [116–122,124–127,129, 131–140,161–172]	Snoring Daytime hypersomnolence Pulmonary hypertension Cor pulmonale	Polysomnography	Nasal CPAP Protriptyline Uvulopalatopharyngoplasty Tracheostomy Nocturnal oxygen Weight loss
Adenotonsillar hypertrophy [130]	Daytime hypersomnolence Obstructive sleep apnea	Direct visualization Lateral x-ray film	Resection
Obstructive goiter [108]	Stridor Enlarged thyroid	Tomography CT	Suppression with exogenous thyroid hormone Resection

PFT = pulmonary function test; CPAP = continuous positive airway pressure; FRC = functional residual capacity; TLC = total lung capacity; CT = computed tomography that in paralytic kyphoscoliosis there is a greater element of muscle weakness [79]. Even in idiopathic kyphoscoliosis, however, the presence of markedly decreased chest wall compliance is further complicated by inspiratory muscle weakness, which significantly contributes to the development of hypercapnic respiratory failure [80]. In addition, a modest element of pulmonary gas exchange abnormality is usually present [7].

Patients with kyphoscoliosis usually complain of progressive dyspnea on exertion and exercise limitation for a period of years before actual arterial hypercapnia develops [7]. Once chronic hypercapnia is present, these patients often require chronic, intermittent mechanical ventilatory support, which can be accomplished by nocturnal mechanical ventilation [81,82].

It is also important to recognize that patients with moderately advanced kyphoscoliosis can develop acute hypercapnic respiratory failure as a result of acute reversible complications, such as pulmonary congestion, retained secretions, or pulmonary infection [83]. In many of these patients, mechanical ventilation may not be required even during acute decompensation [83].

Massive chest wall obesity may be associated with significant hypoventilation and the development of hypercapnic respiratory failure [84]. This is termed the obesity-hypoventilation or pickwickian syndrome. The pathogenesis of respiratory failure appears to be multifactoral and includes significant reduction in chest wall compliance, decreased respiratory muscle efficiency, reduced carbon dioxide responsiveness, and impaired pulmonary gas exchange as a result of pulmonary congestion [84–87]. The pulmonary congestion is believed to be related to the abnormal blood gas values associated with hypoventilation [84,87] as well as concomitant obstructive sleep apnea, frequently seen in these patients [88].

Upper Airway Obstruction. A variety of causes of upper airway obstruction involving the extrathoracic upper airway or intrathoracic trachea can result in the development of respiratory failure (Table 58-4). These include acute epiglottitis [89,90], acute laryngeal edema [91], foreign body aspiration [92–96], retropharyngeal hemorrhage [97], bilateral vocal cord paralysis [98,99,100], tumors of the upper airway [101–105], tracheal stenosis or malacia [106,107], and intrathoracic goiter [108].

Significant upper airway obstruction should be considered in the patient who complains of dyspnea in association with inspiratory stridor (extrathoracic obstruction) or expiratory wheezing (intrathoracic obstruction), particularly if other symptoms suggest an upper airway process (e.g., dysphagia in epiglottitis). Unless the patient is acutely ill, the diagnosis can usually be confirmed in the pulmonary function laboratory from the results of flow-volume loop analysis [109]. This technique not only demonstrates the presence of an upper airway obstruction but usually also helps determine whether it is extrathoracic or intrathoracic and variable or fixed [109]. Studies such as soft tissue neck radiographs, laryngoscopy, and bronchoscopy can identify the exact nature of the structural abnormality.

Upper airway obstruction from bilateral vocal cord paresis or paralysis may result from a variety of causes. Most common is trauma, particularly related to thyroid surgery [101] and, occasionally, following endotracheal intubation [110]. Other causes include tumors [102–105,111,112]; cricoarytenoid arthritis [100]; herpes simplex viral infection [113]; and neurologic conditions, including Guillain-Barré syndrome [100], extrapyramidal disorders such as Parkinson's disease [114], and myasthenia gravis [99]. Bilateral vocal cord paralysis should be considered when one of these conditions is present and the patient complains of aspiration, dyspnea, or stridor [101]. Hoarseness is usually absent during normal speech in bilateral adductor paralysis. The results of flow-volume loop analysis can help confirm the presence of the typical extrathoracic variable obstruction associated with bilateral vocal cord paralysis [115].

Peripheral, obstructive sleep apnea is increasingly recognized as a relatively common cause of intermittent functional upper airway obstruction [116–122]. It is most commonly seen in men and may go unrecognized for years. Although obesity is a common finding in these patients, obstructive sleep apnea can occur in its absence [123,124]. It is postulated that episodic loss of pharyngeal muscle tone caused by decreased respiratory center motor output, which occurs particularly during rapid eye movement (REM) sleep, results in the intermittent airway obstruction [116,125]. It is also believed that this disturbance in respiratory center control accounts for the mixed apneas (i.e., combination obstructive and central apneas) frequently seen in these patients [125].

The major clues to the diagnosis are history of snoring, frequent nocturnal awakenings or arousals, and apneic episodes (usually reported by the patient's partner) [126]. Daytime hypersomnolence is frequently [124,127] but not always present [128]. Other common findings include systemic hypertension [128], pulmonary hypertension, cor pulmonale, polycythemia, cardiac arrhythmias, and morning headaches [120,121,122,124–127,129]. These findings are believed to result primarily from severe hypoxemia, which occurs during apneic episodes [120,124,126,127,129].

The diagnosis of obstructive sleep apnea can be definitively established by a sleep study (polysomnography) that demonstrates frequent, severe apneic episodes associated with vigorous respiratory efforts that do not result in airflow [119,120,121,126]. It is also important to evaluate whether other conditions that can cause or exacerbate obstructive sleep apnea are present. These include intermittent upper airway obstruction caused by adenotonsillar hypertrophy [130], deviated nasal septum [131], retrognathia or micrognathia [132,133], and macroglossia from acromegaly [134]. Endocrine and metabolic abnormalities such as hypothyroidism [31,135,136]; CNS depressants such as ethanol, barbiturates, and benzodiazepines [137,138]; and exogenous androgen administration [139,140] can precipitate or exacerbate this syndrome.

Differential Diagnosis

The major differential diagnosis of extrapulmonary respiratory failure is hypercapnic respiratory failure from intrinsic lung diseases (e.g., COPD or asthma) (Fig. 58-1). These latter conditions can be readily distinguished because they are almost always associated with a markedly elevated $P(A-a)O_2$ gradient when calculated on room air, which reflects the severe derangement of distal gas exchange that is present. Hypercapnic respiratory failure may also result from a combination of pulmonary and extrapulmonary abnormalities. This diagnosis is also suggested by the $P(A-a)O_2$ gradient. A $P(A-a)O_2$ gradient of 25 to 30 mm Hg suggests significant pulmonary and extrapulmonary disease. If the extrapulmonary abnormality is predominant, the gradient, although abnormal, is generally less than 25 mm Hg [7]. When primary pulmonary disease is severe enough to cause hypercapnia, the gradient is generally above 30 mm Hg.

Treatment

The treatment of extrapulmonary respiratory failure can be divided into specific and supportive therapy. Supportive therapy involves the use of mechanical ventilatory assistance (see Chap.

66), supplemental oxygen, and techniques of airway hygiene (see Chap. 69). In addition, regardless of the primary cause of respiratory muscle weakness, malnutrition exacerbates muscle weakness, and proper nutritional replacement can be beneficial in increasing respiratory muscle strength and function [141,142] (see Chap. 67). In selected circumstances, inspiratory resistive training of the respiratory muscles and the use of theophylline as a positive respiratory muscle inotrope have been reported to improve respiratory muscle function and associated hypercapnic respiratory failure [143–146]. Only specific forms of therapy are discussed here and in Tables 58-1 to 58-4.

CENTRAL NERVOUS SYSTEM DEPRESSION. A description of specific treatment modalities for CNS depression is given in Table 58-1.

PERIPHERAL NERVOUS SYSTEM DYSFUNCTION. Treatment for peripheral nervous system disorders is outlined in Table 58-2. In general, there is little in the way of specific therapy for established spinal cord or anterior horn cell disease. The use of phrenic nerve pacemakers for high cervical cord transection or bilateral phrenic nerve palsies is feasible to help treat the resultant respiratory failure when nerve conduction studies have determined that the phrenic nerves are intact and functioning [45,147,148,149]. If obstructive sleep apnea is brought on by pacing, tracheostomy or nasal continuous positive airway pressure (CPAP) may be necessary.

The availability and value of specific therapy for peripheral neuropathy vary depending on the cause. In the case of acute Guillain-Barré syndrome, plasmapheresis has been found to be helpful when administered according to the following guidelines [150,151,152]:

1. Begin pheresis promptly for patients who reach or appear to be approaching the inability to walk without help, substantial decrease in ventilatory capacity, or bulbar insufficiency.
2. Pheresis is not likely to help in patients who are no longer progressing 21 days or more after the disease has begun.
3. Pheresis can be of benefit when used again for relapses.
4. Pheresis is indicated for human immunodeficiency virus (HIV)-seropositive patients with Guillain-Barré syndrome [151].

Intravenous infusion of pooled gamma globulin has been found to compare favorably to plasmapheresis [152a,152b] and may be preferred based on greater ease of administration [152b]. Corticosteroids [151,152,152b] and immunosuppressive agents [151] have not been found to be beneficial.

Patients with severe respiratory muscle weakness due to Guillain-Barré syndrome require supportive mechanical ventilatory assistance, usually for weeks to months [22] and occasionally for longer than a year [153]. If cranial nerve involvement is prominent, intubation for airway protection should be strongly considered even in the absence of overt respiratory failure. Management is complicated by autonomic nervous system dysfunction, commonly present and now the leading cause of death in this syndrome [40]. Abnormalities of increased or decreased sympathetic and parasympathetic nervous system activity, such as hypertension, hypotension, bradyarrhythmias, tachyarrhythmias, flushing, diaphoresis, and ileus, frequently occur [40]. Because these events are often transient and changeable, minor fluctuations in heart rate or blood pressure should not be treated. When intervention is deemed necessary, short-acting and easily titratable drugs should be used [40]. Because

patients are at increased risk of deep venous thrombosis and pulmonary embolism, low-dose heparin should be administered prophylactically [22]. See Chapter 189 for more details on treating Guillain-Barré syndrome.

Treatment of patients with respiratory failure caused by myasthenia gravis is directed primarily at the myasthenia (see Chap. 190).

Drug-induced neuromuscular blockade often improves simply by discontinuing the offending agent [56]. There is some evidence that intravenous calcium gluconate may help shorten the recovery time by reversing the presynaptic component of the neuromuscular blockade [56]. If this fails and the patient improves following a Tensilon test, neostigmine bromide may be effective by reversing the postsynaptic component [56]. When myasthenia gravis is exacerbated or made manifest by a drug, therapy directed specifically at the myasthenic symptoms may be required [56].

Treatment of botulism is primarily directed at minimizing further binding of toxin to nerve endings while supporting the patient until the toxin that is bound dissipates [55] (see Chap. 96). Recovery of ventilatory and upper airway muscle strength in type A botulism occurs slowly; patients recover most of their strength in the first 12 weeks, but full recovery may take a year [61].

RESPIRATORY MUSCLE DYSFUNCTION. The treatment of myopathy depends on the etiology (Table 58-3). Specific therapy is currently unavailable for muscular dystrophy or myotonia.

Some patients with each of the different subtypes of periodic paralyses have responded well to acetazolamide, a carbonic anhydrase inhibitor that is kaliuretic [154]. Acetazolamide is often dramatically effective in preventing acute attacks of hypokalemic periodic paralysis, perhaps by causing a metabolic acidosis that in turn protects against sudden decreases in potassium that provoke attacks. Certain patients benefit from low-carbohydrate or low-sodium diets in addition to acetazolamide. Inhalation of the beta-adrenergic agonist albuteral alleviates acute attacks of weakness in some patients [154].

Polymyositis often responds to corticosteroids or other immunosuppressants [72,73]. Muscle weakness from hypothyroidism, hypophosphatemia, hypomagnesemia, or hypokalemia responds to replacement therapy [39,155–158]. The specific treatment of trichinosis is less than satisfactory [159]. Thiabendazole may eliminate intestinal worms, but only if initiated within 1 day of ingestion of larvae. Thiabendazole has no effect on the larvae that have reached the muscle and also does not appear to alter the course of established infections. The mainstays of treatment are bed rest, corticosteroids, and antiinflammatory analgesic agents.

CHEST WALL AND PLEURAL DISORDERS. Scoliosis is best treated orthopedically (e.g., by Milwaukee brace or Harrington rod) prior to the development of a severe deformity and respiratory failure [7] (Table 58-4). If acute respiratory failure develops, reversible factors such as pulmonary congestion, infection, retained secretions, and other intercurrent illnesses should be carefully sought and treated [83]. A recent study suggests that episodes of acute respiratory failure in patients with kyphoscoliosis can sometimes be managed without mechanical ventilatory assistance [83]. The study emphasized the importance of diuretics for pulmonary congestion and supplemental oxygen for hypoxemia. In severe kyphoscoliosis associated with significant chronic hypercapnic respiratory failure, nocturnal mechanical ventilation using a conventional positive pressure ventilator necessitating a permanent tracheostomy, positive pressure ventilation by nasal mask, or a variety of negative pressure ventilators often results in marked improvement in daytime function and gas exchange off the ventilator [81,82,160].

UPPER AIRWAY OBSTRUCTION. The first step in treating acute upper airway obstruction is to establish an adequate airway. Specific definitive therapy can then be used. In acute bacterial epiglottitis associated with significant respiratory distress, immediate steps are mandatory to prevent development of total obstruction. Although tracheostomy has been the standard traditional approach, recent evidence suggests that in skilled hands endotracheal intubation is an acceptable and perhaps preferable alternative [89]. Chapter 75 provides a complete discussion of this and other treatment issues.

In peripheral, obstructive sleep apnea complicated by life-threatening arrhythmias, severe arterial hypoxemia, or severe functional impairment [117,119,120,121], a permanent tracheostomy is generally curative [117,119,120,121,161]. However, because tracheostomy is not always well tolerated on a long-term basis, a variety of other treatment modalities have been attempted, with varying success rates [162]. These modalities have included weight loss [163], nasal CPAP [164,165], continuous nasal airflow using nasal prongs [166], upper airway surgery other than tracheostomy (primarily uvulopalatopharyngoplasty) [167], and, in selected cases, deviated nasal septum repair [131]. Nasal CPAP is usually effective if the patient can tolerate it (up to 85% can; see Chap. 69). Avoidance of alcohol and other sedative drugs may improve the severity of obstructive sleep apnea [132]. The drug protriptyline has been reported to decrease the degree of obstructive apnea, particularly during REM sleep [132], and may be a reasonable alternative to tracheostomy in selected cases [168,169]. Nocturnal oxygen may also be beneficial by decreasing the severity of arterial desaturation that occurs during apneas [170,171]. In cases of obstructive sleep apnea in which an identifiable cause is present (e.g., hypothyroidism), correction of the problem may be curative [135,136].

In patients suffering from a combination of severe obstructive sleep apnea and central hypoventilation, combined treatment with tracheostomy and phrenic nerve diaphragmatic pacing may be necessary [172].

References

1. Williams MH Jr, Shim CS: Ventilatory failure. *Am J Med* 48:477, 1970.
2. Bates DV, Macklem PT, Christie RV: *Respiratory Function in Disease.* Philadelphia, WB Saunders, 1971, p 442.
3. Pontoppidan H, Geffin B, Lowenstein E: Acute respiratory failure in the adult. *N Engl J Med* 287:690, 1972.
4. Asmundsson T, Kilburn KH: Survival after acute respiratory failure. *Ann Intern Med* 80:54, 1974.
5. Pratter MR, Irwin RS: Extrapulmonary causes of respiratory failure. *J Intensive Care Med* 1:197, 1986.
6. Demers RR, Irwin RS: Management of hypercapnic respiratory failure: A systematic approach. *Respir Care* 24:328, 1979.
7. Bergofsky EH: Respiratory failure in disorders of the thoracic cage. *Am Rev Respir Dis* 119:643, 1979.
8. Aubier M, Murciano D, Fournier M, et al: Central respiratory drive in acute respiratory failure of patients with chronic obstructive pulmonary disease. *Am Rev Respir Dis* 122:191, 1980.
9. Bone RC, Pierce AK, Johnson RL Jr: Controlled oxygen administration in acute respiratory failure in chronic obstructive pulmonary disease. *Am J Med* 65:896, 1978.
10. Degaute JP, Domenighetti G, Naeije R, et al: Oxygen delivery in acute exacerbation of chronic obstructive pulmonary disease. *Am Rev Respir Dis* 124:26, 1981.
11. Weitzenblum E, Sautegeau A, Ehrhart M, et al: Long-term oxygen therapy can reverse the progression of pulmonary hypertension in patients with chronic obstructive pulmonary disease. *Am Rev Respir Dis* 131:493, 1985.
12. Marthan R, Castaing Y, Manier G, Guenard H: Gas exchange alterations in patients with chronic obstructive lung disease. *Chest* 87:470, 1985.
13. Lejeune P, Mols P, Naeije R, et al: Acute hemodynamic effects of controlled oxygen therapy in decompensated chronic obstructive pulmonary disease. *Crit Care Med* 12:1032, 1984.
14. Gray BA, Blalock JM: Interpretation of the alveolar-arterial oxygen difference in patients with hypercapnia. *Am Rev Respir Dis* 143:4, 1991.
15. Braun NMT, Rochester DF: Respiratory muscle strength in obstructive lung disease. *Am Rev Respir Dis* 115:91, 1977.
16. Celli BR, Rassulo J, Berman JS, Make B: Respiratory consequences of abdominal hernia in a patient with severe chronic obstructive pulmonary disease. *Am Rev Respir Dis* 131:178, 1985.
17. O'Donohue WJ Jr, Baker JP, Bell GM, et al: Respiratory failure in neuromuscular disease: Management in a respiratory intensive care unit. *JAMA* 235:733, 1976.
18. Braun NMT, Arora NS, Rochester DF: Respiratory muscle and pulmonary function in polymyositis and other proximal myopathies. *Thorax* 38:616, 1983.
19. Smyth RJ, Chapman KR, Rebuck AS: Maximal inspiratory and expiratory pressures in adolescents: Normal values. *Chest* 86:568, 1984.
20. Black LF, Hyatt RE: Maximal respiratory pressures: Normal values and relationship to age and sex. *Am Rev Respir Dis* 99:696, 1969.
21. Gracey DR, Divertie MB, Howard FM Jr: Mechanical ventilation for respiratory failure in myasthenia gravis. *Mayo Clin Proc* 58:597, 1983.
22. Moore P, James O: Guillain-Barré syndrome: Incidence, management and outcome of major complications. *Crit Care Med* 9:549, 1981.
23. Roussos CS, Macklem PT: Diaphragmatic fatigue in man. *J Appl Physiol* 43:189, 1977.
24. Gross D, Grassino A, Ross WRD, Macklem PT: Electromyogram pattern of diaphragmatic fatigue. *J Appl Physiol* 46:1, 1979.
25. Cohen CA, Zabelbaum G, Gross D, et al: Clinical manifestations of inspiratory muscle fatigue. *Am J Med* 73:308, 1982.
26. Mitchell RA, Berger AJ: Neural regulation of respiration. *Am Rev Respir Dis* 111:206, 1975.
27. Berger AJ, Mitchell RA, Severinghaus JW: Regulation of respiration. *N Engl J Med* 297:138, 1977.
28. Ledsom JR, Sharp JM: Pulmonary function in acute cervical cord injury. *Am Rev Respir Dis* 124:41, 1981.
29. Fromm GB, Wisdom PJ, Block AJ: Amyotrophic lateral sclerosis presenting with respiratory failure. *Chest* 71:612, 1977.
30. Hill R, Martin J, Hakim A: Acute respiratory failure in motor neuron disease. *Arch Neurol* 40:30, 1983.
31. Chandler KW, Rozas CJ, Kory RC, Goldman AL: Bilateral diaphragmatic paralysis complicating local cardiac hypothermia during open heart surgery. *Am J Med* 77:243, 1984.
32. Kohorst WR, Schonfeld SA, Altman M: Bilateral diaphragmatic paralysis following topical cardiac hypothermia. *Chest* 85:65, 1984.
33. Luce J: Medical management of spinal cord injury. *Crit Care Med* 13:126, 1985.
34. Weinstein L: Tetanus. *N Engl J Med* 289:1293, 1973.
35. Weinstein L: Tetanus. *Infect Dis Pract* 4:1, 1980.
36. Boyd RE, Brennan PT, Deng JF, et al: Strychnine poisoning. *Am J Med* 74:507, 1983.
37. Mulder DW, Rosenbaum RA, Layton DD Jr: Late progression of poliomyelitis or forme fruste amyotrophic lateral sclerosis? *Mayo Clin Proc* 47:756, 1972.
38. Dalakas MC, Elder G, Hallett M, et al: A long-term follow-up study of patients with post-poliomyelitis neuromuscular symptoms. *N Engl J Med* 314:959, 1986.
39. Ringel SP, Carroll JE: Respiratory complications of neuromuscular

disease, in Weiner WJ (ed): *Respiratory Dysfunction in Neurologic Disease*. Mt. Kisco, NY, Futura, 1980, p 113.

40. Lichtenfeld P: Autonomic dysfunction in Guillain-Barré syndrome. *Am J Med* 50:772, 1971.

40a. Zochodne DW, Bolton CF, Wells GA, et al: Critical illness polyneuropathy: A complication of sepsis and multiple organ failure. *Brain* 110:819, 1987.

40b. Witt NJ, Zochodne DW, Bolton CR, et al: Peripheral nerve function in sepsis and multiple organ failure. *Chest* 99:176, 1991.

40c. Gorson KC, Ropper AH: Acute respiratory failure neuropathy: A variant of critical illness polyneuropathy. *Crit Care Med* 21:267, 1993.

41. Massachusetts Department of Public Health: The red tide: A public health emergency. *N Engl J Med* 288:1126, 1973.

42. Ahles MD: Red tide: A recurrent health hazard. *Am J Public Health* 64:807, 1974.

43. Merson MH, Hughes JM, Gangaros EJ: Miscellaneous food poisoning, in *Practice in Medicine*. vol. III. U.S. Department of Health, Education, and Welfare, Public Health Service, 1976, p 17.

44. Paralytic sellfish poisoning: Massachusetts and Alaska, 1990. *MMWR* 40:157, 1991.

45. Moorthy SS, Markand ON, Mahomed Y, Brown JW: Electrophysiologic evaluation of phrenic nerves in severe respiratory insufficiency requiring mechanical ventilation. *Chest* 88:211, 1985.

46. Mulvey DA, Aquilina RJ, Elliot MW, et al: Diaphragmatic dysfunction in neuralgic amyotrophy: An electrophysiologic evaluation of 16 patients presenting with dyspnea. *Am Rev Respir Dis* 147:66, 1993.

47. Piehler JM, Pairolero PC, Gracey DR, Bernatz PE: Unexplained diaphragmatic paralysis: A harbinger of malignant disease? *J Thorac Cardiovasc Surg* 84:861, 1982.

48. Thomas NE, Passamonte PM, Sunderrajan EV, et al: Bilateral diaphragmatic paralysis as a possible paraneoplastic syndrome from renal cell carcinoma. *Am Rev Respir Dis* 129:507, 1984.

49. Kreitzer SM, Feldman NT, Saunders NA, Ingram RH Jr: Bilateral diaphragmatic paralysis with hypercapnic respiratory failure. *Am J Med* 65:89, 1978.

50. Spitzer SA, Korczyn AD, Kalaci J: Transient bilateral diaphragmatic paralysis. *Chest* 64:355, 1973.

51. Chan CK, Mohsenin V, Loke J, et al: Diaphragmatic dysfunction in siblings with hereditary motor and sensory neuropathy (Charcot-Marie-Tooth disease). *Chest* 91:567, 1987.

52. Hughes JM, Blumenthal JR, Merson MH, et al: Clinical features of types A and B food-borne botulism. *Ann Intern Med* 95:442, 1981.

53. Schmidt-Nowara WW, Samet JM, Rosario PA: Early and late pulmonary complications of botulism. *Arch Intern Med* 143:451, 1983.

54. Lewis SW, Pierson DJ, Cary JM, Hudson LD: Prolonged respiratory paralysis in wound botulism. *Chest* 75:59, 1979.

55. Morris JA Jr, Hathaway CL: Botulism, in Hoeprick PD (ed): *Botulism in Infectious Diseases*. 3rd ed. Philadelphia, Harper & Row, 1983, p 1115.

56. Argov Z, Mastaglia FL: Disorders of neuromuscular transmission caused by drugs. *N Engl J Med* 301:409, 1979.

57. Dushay KM, Zibrak JD, Jensen WA: Myasthenia gravis presenting as isolated respiratory failure. *Chest* 97:232, 1990.

58. Drachman DB: Myasthenia gravis. *N Engl J Med* 298:186, 1978.

59. Hyde L, Hyde CI: Clinical manifestations of lung cancer. *Chest* 65:299, 1974.

60. Arena JM: *Poisoning*. Springfield, IL, Charles C. Thomas, 1979, p 126.

61. Wilcox PC, Morrison NJ, Pardy RL: Recovery of the ventilatory and upper airway muscles and exercise performance after type A botulism. *Chest* 98:620, 1990.

62. Hansen-Flaschen J, Cowen J, Raps EC: Neuromuscular blockade in the intensive care unit: More than we bargained for. *Am Rev Respir Dis* 147:234, 1993.

63. Douglass JA, Tuxen DV, Horne M, et al: Myopathy in severe asthma. *Am Rev Respir Dis* 146:517, 1992.

64. Chausow AM, Kane T, Levinson D, Szidon JP: Reversible hypercapnic respiratory insufficiency in scleroderma caused by respiratory muscle weakness. *Am Rev Respir Dis* 130:142, 1984.

65. Rosenow RC III, Engel AG: Acid maltase deficiency in adults presenting as respiratory failure. *Am J Med* 64:485, 1978.

66. Newman JH, Neff TA, Ziporin P: Acute respiratory failure associated with hypophosphatemia. *N Engl J Med* 296:1101, 1977.

67. Stoff JS: Phosphate homeostasis and hypophosphatemia. *Am J Med* 72:489, 1982.

68. Knochel JP: Neuromuscular manifestations of electrolyte disorders. *Am J Med* 72:521, 1982.

69. Begin R, Bureau MA, Lupien L, et al: Pathogenesis of respiratory insufficiency in myotonic dystrophy. *Am Rev Respir Dis* 125:312, 1982.

70. Black LF, Hyatt RE: Maximal static respiratory pressures in generalized neuromuscular disease. *Am Rev Respir Dis* 103:641, 1971.

71. Adams RD, Victor M: *Principles of Neurology*. New York, McGraw-Hill, 1981, p 961.

72. Bohan A, Peter JB: Polymyositis and dermatomyositis. *N Engl J Med* 292:344, 1975.

73. Strongwater SL: Overview and clinical manifestations of inflammatory myositis: Polymyositis and dermatomyositis. *Mt Sinai J Med* 55:435, 1988.

74. Dickey BF, Myers AR: Pulmonary disease in polymyositis/dermatomyositis. *Semin Arthritis Rheum* 14:60, 1984.

75. Hertzman PA, Blevins WL, Mayer J, et al: Association of the eosinophilia-myalgia syndrome with the ingestion of tryptophan. *N Engl J Med* 322:869, 1990.

76. Silver RM, Heyes MP, Maize JC, et al: Scleroderma, fasciitis, and eosinophilia associated with the ingestion of tryptophan. *N Engl J Med* 322:874, 1990.

77. Medsger TA Jr: Tryptophan-induced eosinophilia-myalgia syndrome. *N Engl J Med* 322:926, 1990.

78. Ventayya RV, Poole RM, Pentz WH: Respiratory failure from procainamide-induced myopathy. *Ann Intern Med* 119:345, 1993.

79. Kafer ER: Respiratory failure in paralytic scoliosis. *Am Rev Respir Dis* 110:450, 1974.

80. Lisboa C, Moreno R, Fava M, et al: Inspiratory muscle function in patients with severe kyphoscoliosis. *Am Rev Respir Dis* 132:48, 1985.

81. Hoeppner VH, Cockcroft DW, Dosman JA, Cotton DJ: Nighttime ventilation improves respiratory failure in secondary kyphoscoliosis. *Am Rev Respir Dis* 129:240, 1984.

82. Fulkerson WJ, Wilkins JK, Esbenshade AM, et al: Life threatening hyperventilation in kyphoscoliosis: Successful treatment with a molded body brace-ventilator. *Am Rev Respir Dis* 129:185, 1984.

83. Libby DM, Briscoe WA, Boyce B, Smith JP: Acute respiratory failure in scoliosis or kyphosis. *Am J Med* 73:532, 1982.

84. Rochester DF, Enson Y: Current concepts in the pathogenesis of the obesity-hypoventilation syndrome. *Am J Med* 57:402, 1974.

85. Sampson MG, Grassino A: Neuromechanical properties in obese patients during carbon dioxide rebreathing. *Am J Med* 75:81, 1983.

86. Luce JM: Respiratory complications of obesity. *Chest* 78:626, 1980.

87. Kaltman AJ, Goldring RM: Role of circulatory congestion in the cardiorespiratory failure of obesity. *Am J Med* 60:645, 1976.

88. Kryger M, Quesney LF, Holder D, et al: The sleep deprivation syndrome of the obese patient. *Am J Med* 56:531, 1974.

89. Black MJ, Harbour J, Remsen KA, Baxter JD: Acute epiglottitis in adults. *J Otolaryngol* 10:23, 1981.

90. Lederman MM, Lowder J, Lerner PI: Bacteremic pneumococcal epiglottitis in adults with malignancy. *Am Rev Respir Dis* 125:117, 1982.

91. Hunt KJ, Valentine MD, Sobotka AK, et al: A controlled trial of immunotherapy in insect hypersensitivity. *N Engl J Med* 299:157, 1978.

92. Mittleman RE, Wetli CV: The fatal cafe coronary. *JAMA* 247:1285, 1982.

93. Irwin RS, Ashba JK, Braman SS, et al: Food asphyxiation in hospitalized patients. *JAMA* 237:2744, 1977.

94. Gelperin A: Sudden death in an elderly population from aspiration of food. *J Am Geriatr Soc* 22:135, 1974.

95. Haugen RK: The cafe coronary. *JAMA* 186:142, 1963.

96. Heimlich HJ: A life-saving maneuver to prevent food choking. *JAMA* 234:398, 1975.

97. Rosenbaum L, Thurman P, Krantz SB: Upper airway obstruction

as a complication of oral anticoagulation therapy. *Arch Intern Med* 139:1151, 1979.

98. Rodrigues JF, York EL, Nair CPV: Upper airway obstruction in Guillain-Barré syndrome. *Chest* 86:147, 1984.

99. Schmidt-Nowara WW, Marder EJ, Feil PA: Respiratory failure in myasthenia gravis due to vocal cord paresis. *Arch Neurol* 41:567, 1984.

100. Libby DM, Schley WS, Smith JP: Cricoarytenoid arthritis in ankylosing spondylitis. *Chest* 80:641, 1981.

101. Proctor DF: The upper airways. II. The larynx and trachea. *Am Rev Respir Dis* 115:315, 1977.

102. Fleetham JA, Lynn RB, Munt PW: Tracheal leiomyosarcoma: A unique cause of stridor. *Am Rev Respir Dis* 116:1109, 1977.

103. Olmedo G, Rosenberg M, Fonseca R: Primary tumors of the trachea. *Chest* 81:701, 1982.

104. Braman SS, Whitcomb ME: Endobronchial metastasis. *Arch Intern Med* 135:543, 175.

105. Weber AL, Grillo HC: Tracheal tumors: A radiological clinical and pathological evaluation of 84 cases. *Radiol Clin North Am* 16:227, 1976.

106. Gamsu G, Borson DB, Webb WR, Cunningham JH: Structure and function in tracheal stenosis. *Am Rev Respir Dis* 121:519, 1980.

107. Feist JH, Johnson TH, Wilson RJ: Acquired tracheomalacia: Etiology and differential diagnosis. *Chest* 68:340, 1975.

108. Torres A, Arroyo J, Kastanos N, et al: Acute respiratory failure and tracheal obstruction in patients with intrathoracic goiter. *Crit Care Med* 11:265, 1983.

109. Acres JC, Kryger MH: Clinical significance of pulmonary function tests: Upper airway obstruction. *Chest* 80:207, 1981.

110. Kastanos N, Miro RE, Perez AM, et al: Laryngotracheal injury due to endotracheal intubation: Incidence, evolution, and predisposing factors—A prospective long-term study. *Crit Care Med* 11:362, 1983.

111. Schecter WP, Wilson RS: Management of upper airway obstruction in the intensive care unit. *Crit Care Med* 9:577, 1981.

112. Kvale PA, Eichenhorn MS, Radke JR, Miks V: YAG laser photoresection of lesions obstructing the central airways. *Chest* 87:283, 1985.

113. Magnussen CR, Patanella HP: Herpes simplex virus and recurrent laryngeal nerve paralysis. *Arch Intern Med* 139:1423, 1979.

114. Vincken WG, Gauthier SG, Dollfuss RE, et al: Involvement of upper-airway muscles in extrapyramidal disorders: A cause of airflow limitation. *N Engl J Med* 311:438, 1984.

115. Cormier Y, Kashima H, Summer W, Menkes H: Upper airway obstruction with bilateral vocal cord paralysis. *Chest* 75:423, 1979.

116. Sharp JT, Druz WS, Foster JR, et al: Use of the respiratory magnetometer in diagnosis and classification of sleep apnea. *Chest* 77:350, 1980.

117. Walsh RE, Michaelson ED, Harkleroad LE, et al: Upper airway obstruction in obese patients with sleep disturbance and somnolence. *Ann Intern Med* 76:185, 1972.

118. Cherniack NS: Respiratory dysrhythmias during sleep. *N Engl J Med* 305:325, 1981.

119. Orr WC, Martin RJ, Imes NK, et al: Hypersomnolent and nonhypersomnolent patients with upper airway obstruction during sleep. *Chest* 75:418, 1979.

120. Miller WP: Cardiac arrhythmias and conduction disturbances in the sleep apnea syndrome. *Am J Med* 73:317, 1982.

121. Tilkian AG, Guilleminault C, Schroeder JS, et al: Hemodynamics in sleep-induced apnea: Studies during wakefulness and sleep. *Ann Intern Med* 85:714, 1976.

122. Bradley TD, Rutherford R, Grossman RF, et al: Role of daytime hypoxemia in the pathogenesis of right heart failure in the obstructive sleep apnea syndrome. *Am Rev Respir Dis* 131:835, 1985.

123. Strohl KP, Hensley MJ, Saunders NA, et al: Progesterone administration and progressive sleep apneas. *JAMA* 245:1230, 1981.

124. Tilkian AG, Guilleminault C, Schroeder JS, et al: Sleep-induced apnea syndrome: Prevalence of cardiac arrhythmias and their reversal after tracheostomy. *Am J Med* 63:348, 1977.

125. Onal E, Lopata M, O'Connor T: Pathogenesis of apneas in hypersomnia: Sleep apnea syndrome. *Am Rev Respir Dis* 125:167, 1982.

126. Phillipson EA: Breathing disorders during sleep. *Basics of RD-ATS News* 7:18, 1979.

127. Motta J, Guilleminault C, Schroeder JS, Dement WC: Tracheostomy and hemodynamic changes in sleep-induced apnea. *Ann Intern Med* 89:454, 1978.

128. Fletcher EC, DeBehnke RD, Lovoi MS, Gorin AB: Undiagnosed sleep apnea in patients with essential hypertension. *Ann Intern Med* 103:190, 1985.

129. Shepard JW Jr, Garrison MW, Grither DA, Dolan GF: Relationship of ventricular ectopy to oxyhemoglobin desaturation in patients with obstructive sleep apnea. *Chest* 88:335, 1985.

130. Orr WC, Martin RJ: Obstructive sleep apnea associated with tonsillar hypertrophy in adults. *Arch Intern Med* 141:990, 1981.

131. Heimer D, Scharf SM, Lieberman A, Lavie P: Sleep apnea syndrome treated by repair of deviated nasal septum. *Chest* 84:184, 1983.

132. Bradley D, Phillipson EA: The treatment of obstructive sleep apnea. *Am Rev Respir Dis* 128:583, 1983.

133. Davies SF, Iber C: Obstructive sleep apnea associated with adult-acquired micrognathia from rheumatoid arthritis. *Am Rev Respir Dis* 127:245, 1983.

134. Mezon BJ, West P, Maclean JP, Kryger MH: Sleep apnea in acromegaly. *Am J Med* 69:615, 1980.

135. Rajagopal KR, Abbrecht PH, Derderian SS, et al: Obstructive sleep apnea in hypothyroidism. *Ann Intern Med* 101:491, 1984.

136. Orr WC, Males JL, Imes NK: Myxedema and obstructive sleep apnea. *Am J Med* 70:1061, 1981.

137. Bonora M, St. John WM, Bledsoe TA: Differential elevation by protriptyline and depression by diazepam of upper airway respiratory motor activity. *Am Rev Respir Dis* 131:41, 1985.

138. Remmers JE: Obstructive sleep apnea: A common disorder exacerbated by alcohol. *Am Rev Respir Dis* 130:153, 1984.

139. Sandblom RE, Matsumoto AM, Schoene RB, et al: Obstructive sleep apnea syndrome induced by testosterone administration. *N Engl J Med* 308:508, 1983.

140. Johnson MW, Anch AM, Remmers JE: Induction of the obstructive sleep apnea syndrome in a woman by exogenous androgen administration. *Am Rev Respir Dis* 129:1023, 1984.

141. Rochester DF, Esau SA: Malnutrition and the respiratory system. *Chest* 85:411, 1984.

142. Kelly SM, Rosa A, Field S, et al: Inspiratory muscle strength and body composition in patients receiving total parenteral nutrition therapy. *Am Rev Respir Dis* 130:33, 1984.

143. Aldrich TK, Karpel JP: Inspiratory muscle resistive training in respiratory failure. *Am Rev Respir Dis* 131:461, 1985.

144. Gross D, Ladd HW, Riley EJ, et al: The effect of training on strength and endurance of the diaphragm in quadriplegia. *Am J Med* 68:27, 1980.

145. Howell S, Fitzgerald RS, Roussos CH: Effects of aminophylline, isoproterenol, and neostigmine on hypercapnic depression of diaphragmatic contractility. *Am Rev Respir Dis* 132:241, 1985.

146. Vires N, Aubier M, Murciano D, et al: Effects of aminophylline on diaphragmatic fatigue during acute respiratory failure. *Am Rev Respir Dis* 129:396, 1984.

147. Glenn WWL, Hogan JF, Loke JSO, et al: Ventilatory support by pacing of the conditioned diaphragm in quadriplegia. *N Engl J Med* 310:1150, 1984.

148. McMichan JC, Piepgras DG, Gracey DR, et al: Electrophrenic respiration. *Mayo Clin Proc* 54:662, 1979.

149. Young RF: Diaphragm pacing as an adjunct in respiratory insufficiency. *Neurosurgery* 2:43, 1978.

150. French cooperative group on plasma exchange in Guillain-Barré syndrome: Role of replacement fluids. *Ann Neurol* 22:753, 1987.

151. McKhann GM, Griffin JW: Plasmapheresis and the Guillain-Barré syndrome. *Ann Neurol* 22:762, 1987.

152. Mendell JR, Kissel JT, Kennedy MS, et al: Plasma exchange and prednisone in Guillain-Barré syndrome: A controlled randomized trial. *Neurology* 35:1551, 1985.

152a. van der Meche FGA, Schmitz PIM, Dutch Guillain-Barré Study Group. A randomized trial comparing intravenous immune globulin and plasma exchange in Guillain-Barré syndrome. *N Engl J Med* 326:1123, 1992.

152b. Ropper AH: The Guillain-Barre Syndrome. *N Engl J Med* 326:1130, 1992.

153. Sunderrajan EV, Davenport J: The Guillain-Barré syndrome: Pulmonary-neurologic correlations. *Medicine* 64:333, 1985.

154. Griggs RC, Ptacek LJ: The periodic paralyses. *Hosp Pract* 15, 1992, p 123.
155. Gold EM: The Cushing syndromes: Changing views of diagnosis and treatment. *Ann Intern Med* 90:829, 1979.
156. Varsano S, Shapiro M, Taragan R, Bruderman I: Hypophosphatemia as a reversible cause of refractory ventilatory failure. *Crit Care Med* 11:908, 1983.
157. Dhingra S, Solven F, Wilson A, McCarthy DS: Hypomagnesemia and respiratory muscle power. *Am Rev Respir Dis* 129:497, 1984.
158. Agus ZS, Wasserstein A, Goldfarb S: Disorders of calcium and magnesium homeostasis. *Am J Med* 72:473, 1982.
159. Grove DI, Warren KS, Mahmoud AAF: Algorithms in the diagnosis and management of exotic diseases. VII. Trichinosis. *J Infect Dis* 132:485, 1975.
160. Garay SM, Turino GM, Goldring RM: Sustained reversal of chronic hypercapnia in patients with alveolar hypoventilation syndromes: Long-term maintenance with noninvasive nocturnal mechanical ventilation. *Am J Med* 70:269, 1981.
161. Guilleminault C, Tilkian A, Dement WC: The sleep apnea syndromes. *Am Rev Med* 27:465, 1976.
162. Conway WA, Victor LD, Magilligan DJ Jr, et al: Adverse effects of tracheostomy for sleep apnea. *JAMA* 246:347, 1981.
163. Browman CP, Sampson MG, Yolles SF, et al: Obstructive sleep apnea and body weight. *Chest* 85:435, 1984.
164. Remmers JE, Sterling JA, Thorarinsson B, Kuna ST: Nasal airway positive pressure in patients with occlusive sleep apnea. *Am Rev Respir Dis* 130:1152, 1984.
165. Sanders MH: Nasal CPAP effect on patterns of sleep apnea. *Chest* 86:839, 1984.
166. Wilhoit SC, Brown ED, Suratt PM: Treatment of obstructive sleep apnea with continuous nasal airflow delivered through nasal prongs. *Chest* 85:170, 1984.
167. Conway W, Fugita S, Zorick F, et al: Uvulopalato-pharyngoplasty. *Chest* 88:385, 1985.
168. Brownell LG, West P, Sweatman P, et al: Protriptyline in obstructive sleep apnea. *N Engl J Med* 307:1037, 1982.
169. Smith PL, Haponik EF, Allen RP, Bleecker ER: The effects of protriptyline in sleep-disordered breathing. *Am Rev Respir Dis* 127:8, 1983.
170. Smith PL, Haponik EF, Bleecker ER: The effects of oxygen in patients with sleep apnea. *Am Rev Respir Dis* 130:958, 1984.
171. Martin RJ, Sanders MH, Gray BA, Pennock BE: Acute and long-term ventilatory effects of hyperoxia in the adult sleep apnea syndrome. *Am Rev Respir Dis* 125:175, 1982.
172. Glenn WWL, Gee JBL, Cole DR, et al: Combined central alveolar hypoventilation and upper airway obstruction. *Am J Med* 64:50, 1978.
173. Weil JV, McCullough RE, Kline JS, Sodal IE: Diminished ventilatory response to hypoxia and hypercapnia after morphine in normal man. *N Engl J Med* 292:1103, 1975.
174. Santiago TV, Pugliese AC, Edelman NH: Control of breathing during methadone addiction. *Am J Med* 62:347, 1977.
175. Skatrud J, Iber C, Ewart R, et al: Disordered breathing during sleep in hypothyroidism. *Am Rev Respir Dis* 124:325, 1981.
176. Doekel RC Jr, Zwillich CW, Scoggin CH, et al: Clinical semistarvation depression of hypoxic ventilatory response. *N Engl J Med* 295:358, 1976.
177. Tuller MA, Mehdi F: Compensatory hypoventilation and hypercapnia in primary metabolic alkalosis. *Am J Med* 50:281, 1971.
178. Farmer WC, Glenn WWL, Gee JBL: Alveolar hypoventilation syndrome: Studies of ventilatory control in patients selected for diaphragm pacing. *Am J Med* 64:39, 1978.
179. Phillipson EA: Control of breathing during sleep. *Am Rev Respir Dis* 118:909, 1978.
180. Comroe JH Jr: Frankenstein, Pickwick and Ondine. *Am Rev Respir Dis* 111:689, 1975.
181. Hunt CE, Matalon SV, Thompson TR, et al: Central hypoventilation syndrome: Experience with bilateral phrenic nerve pacing in 3 neonates. *Am Rev Respir Dis* 118:23, 1978.
182. Wolkove N, Altose MD, Kelsen SG, Cherniack NS: Respiratory control abnormalities in alveolar hypoventilation. *Am Rev Respir Dis* 122:163, 1980.
183. Sugar O: In search of Ondine's curse. *JAMA* 240:236, 1978.
184. Butler J: Clinical problems of disordered respiratory control. *Am Rev Respir Dis* 110:695, 1974.
185. Skatrud JB, Dempsey JA, Kaiser DG: Ventilatory response to medroxyprogesterone acetate in normal subjects: Time course and mechanism. *J Appl Physiol* 44:939, 1978.
186. Hyland RH, Jones NL, Powles ACP, et al: Primary alveolar hypoventilation treated with nocturnal electrophrenic respiration. *Am Rev Respir Dis* 117:165, 1978.
187. Bubis MJ, Anthonisen NR: Primary alveolar hypoventilation treated by nocturnal administration of O_2. *Am Rev Respir Dis* 118:947, 1978.
188. Tilkian AG, Guilleminault C, Schroeder JS, et al: Sleep-induced apnea syndrome: Prevalence of cardiac arrhythmias and their reversal after tracheostomy. *Am J Med* 63:348, 1977.
189. Gracey DR, Howard FM Jr, Divertie MB: Plasmapheresis in the treatment of ventilator-dependent myasthenia gravis patients. *Chest* 85:739, 1984.
190. McEvoy KM, Windebank AJ, Daube JR, et al: 3,4-diaminopyridine in the treatment of Lambert-Eaton myasthenic syndrome. *N Engl J Med* 321:1567, 1989.
191. Siafakas NM, Milona I, Salesiotou V, et al: Respiratory muscle strength in hyperthyroidism before and after treatment. *Am Rev Respir Dis* 146:1025, 1992.
192. Aubier M, Murciano D, Lecocguic Y, et al: Effect of hypophosphatemia on diaphragmatic contractility in patients with acute respiratory failure. *N Engl J Med* 313:420, 1985.
193. Sutton FD Jr, Zwillich CW, Creagh CE, et al: Progesterone for outpatient treatment of pickwickian syndrome. *Ann Intern Med* 83:476, 1975.
194. Trinkle JK, Richardson JD, Franz JL, et al: Management of flail chest without mechanical ventilation. *Ann Thorac Surg* 19:355, 1975.
195. Colp C, Reichel J, Park SS: Severe pleural restriction: The maximum static pulmonary recoil pressure as an aid in diagnosis. *Chest* 67:658, 1975.
196. Miller LR, Greenberg SD, McLarty JW: Lupus lung. *Chest* 88:265, 1985.
197. Hunninghake GW, Fauci AS: Pulmonary involvement in the collagen vascular diseases. *Am Rev Respir Dis* 119:471, 1979.
198. Miller A, Teirstein AS, Selikoff IJ: Ventilatory failure due to asbestos pleurisy. *Am J Med* 75:911, 1983.
199. Gilbert L, Ribot S, Frankel H, et al: Fibrinous uremic pleuritis: A surgical entity. *Chest* 67:53, 1975.
200. Phelan DM, Love JB: Adult epiglottitis: Is there a role for the fiberoptic bronchoscope? *Chest* 86:783, 1984.
201. Stauffer JL, Olson DE, Petty TL: Complications and consequences of endotracheal intubation and tracheotomy: A prospective study of 150 critically ill adult patients. *Am J Med* 70:65, 1981.
202. Austen KF: Systemic anaphylaxis in man. *JAMA* 192:108, 1965.
203. Sonin L, Grammer LC, Greenberger PA, Patterson R: Idiopathic anaphylaxis: A clinical summary. *Ann Intern Med* 99:634, 1983.
204. Greenberger PA, Patterson R, Simon R, et al: Pretreatment of high risk patients requiring radiographic contrast media studies. *J Allergy Clin Immunol* 67:185, 1981.
205. Sheffer AL, Austen KF: Exercise-induced anaphylaxis. *J Allergy Clin Immunol* 66:106, 1980.
206. Rothbach C, Green RL, Levin MI, Fireman P: Prophylaxis of attacks of hereditary angioedema. *Am J Med* 66:681, 1979.
207. Gelfand JA, Boss GR, Conley CL, et al: Acquired C1 esterase inhibitor deficiency and angioedema: A review. *Medicine* 58:321, 1979.
208. Matthews KP: Management of urticaria and angioedema. *J Allergy Clin Immunol* 66:347, 1980.
209. Harley HRS: Laryngotracheal obstruction complicating tracheostomy or endotracheal intubation with assistesd respiration. *Thorax* 26:493, 1971.
210. Abdulmajid OA, Ebeid AM, Motaweh MM, Kleibo IS: Aspirated foreign bodies in the tracheobronchial tree: Report of 250 cases. *Thorax* 31:635, 1976.
211. Bergstrom B, Ollman B, Lindholm CE: Endotracheal excision of fibrous tracheal stenosis and subsequent prolonged stenting: An alternative method in selected cases. *Chest* 71:6, 1977.

59. Acute Respiratory Failure in Pregnancy

Helen M. Hollingsworth

Maternal mortality decreased from 15.3 to 7.8 for every 100,000 live births from 1975 to 1985 [1,2]. However, acute respiratory failure remains an important cause of maternal and fetal morbidity and mortality. Thromboembolism, amniotic fluid embolism, and venous air embolism together account for approximately 20 percent of maternal deaths, [2] and other causes of respiratory failure probably account for another 10 to 15 percent [2]. Several researchers have discussed the effects of pregnancy on chronic respiratory insufficiency as well as the effects of chronic respiratory insufficiency on pregnancy [3–7]. This chapter focuses on the causes of acute respiratory failure that are increased in frequency during pregnancy, are unique to pregnancy, or present special management requirements during pregnancy. The spectrum of problems associated with eclampsia [8,9] is discussed in Chapter 170. Management of the acute respiratory distress syndrome caused by sepsis, trauma, or other etiologies unrelated to pregnancy is discussed in Chapter 55. Table 59-1 gives a list of causes of acute respiratory failure in pregnancy.

Because the management of acute maternal respiratory failure requires management of gas exchange derangements in both the woman and the fetus, the normal gestational changes in maternal gas transfer, respiratory mechanics, and maternal circulation, as well as the determinants of fetal oxygen delivery, are reviewed first. Having set general guidelines for protection of fetal development, the various causes of acute respiratory failure are then considered, and, finally, supportive and specific therapies are discussed, concentrating on how pregnancy would influence management decisions. Aspects of diagnostic procedures such as hemodynamic monitoring, fetal monitoring, and radiologic testing that are unique to respiratory failure in pregnancy are reviewed.

pregnancy is 30 to 34 mm Hg, suggesting chronic mild hyperventilation. The degree of hyperventilation has been found to be in excess of the amount needed to compensate for increased oxygen consumption; in fact, hyperventilation develops early in gestation, before any significant increase in oxygen consumption occurs [3,6]. This has been attributed to elevation in levels of progesterone, which has a known respiratory stimulating effect. The exact mechanism by which it produces this effect is not known [4–7]. In addition, pregnancy is associated with increased sensitivity to CO_2 as measured by CO_2 ventilatory response curves [5,6], reflecting the new, lower setpoint in $PaCO_2$.

Changes in lung volumes associated with gestation are relatively small: total lung capacity decreases 4 to 6 percent, functional residual capacity decreases approximately 15 to 25 percent, and residual volume remains constant [5,10]. Despite the decrease in functional residual capacity, early airway closure has not been demonstrated and specific airway conductance remains constant [11]. Diffusing capacity is elevated in the first trimester but then declines, despite continued increases in cardiac output and plasma volume [6,11].

Studies of lung mechanics during pregnancy have shown that as gestation progresses the resting level of the diaphragm rises, but diaphragmatic excursion with tidal breathing actually increases [5,12]. In fact, increased tidal volume accounts for much of the increased minute ventilation and mild respiratory alkalosis that is characteristic of early to midpregnancy [5]. Increased respiratory rate becomes more important late in pregnancy [5] (Fig. 59-1).

Numerous circulatory changes occur during gestation to supply oxygen-rich blood to the placenta and to accommodate the stress of labor and delivery. Cardiac output begins to rise in the

Normal Alterations in Cardiopulmonary Physiology during Pregnancy

Maternal respiratory alterations during pregnancy include changes in control of respiration, lung volumes, and mechanics of ventilation. Normal carbon dioxide tension ($PaCO_2$) during

Table 59-1. Causes of Acute Respiratory Failure in Pregnancy

Thromboembolism
Amniotic fluid embolism
Venous air embolism
Aspiration of gastric contents
Respiratory infections
Asthma
Beta-adrenergic tocolytic therapy
Pneumomediastinum and pneumothorax
Eclampsia (see Chap. 170)
Acute respiratory distress syndrome (see Chap. 55)

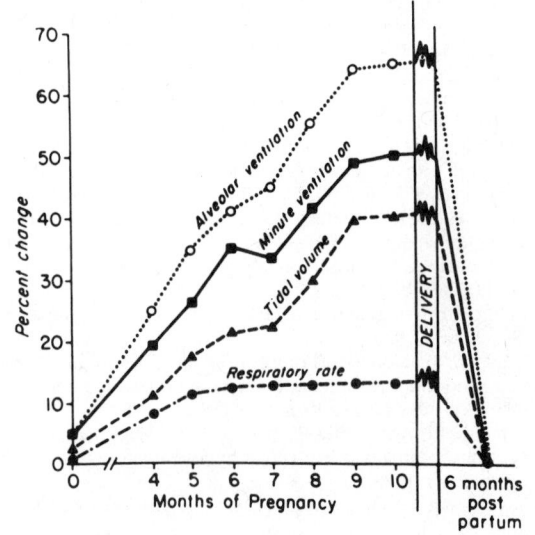

Fig. 59-1. Changes in respiratory function during pregnancy. (From Leontic EA: Respiratory disease in pregnancy. *Med Clin North Am* 61:111, 1977. With permission.)

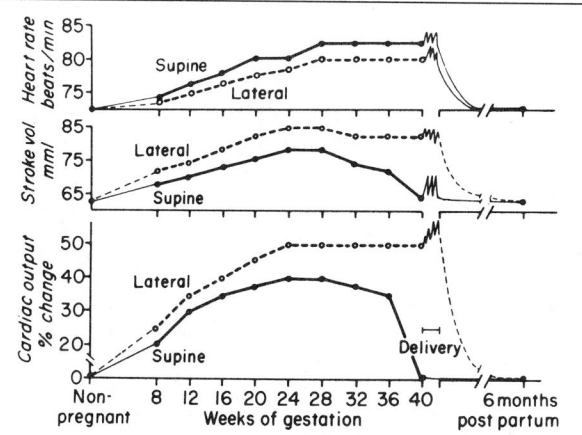

Fig. 59-2. Changes in maternal heart rate, stroke volume, and output during pregnancy with the gravida in the supine and lateral positions. (From Cheek TG, Gutsche BB: Maternal physiologic alterations during pregnancy, in Shnider SM, Levinson G (eds): *Anesthesia for Obstetrics*. Baltimore, Williams & Wilkins, 1987, p 3. With permission.)

first trimester and peaks around the 20th week of gestation at 30 to 45 percent above resting, nonpregnant levels (Fig. 59-2) [7]. Thus, measured cardiac output during gestation that is in the normal range for a nonpregnant patient would signify significant hemodynamic compromise for the pregnant patient and potentially decreased oxygen delivery for the fetus. As pregnancy progresses, cardiac output becomes quite dependent on body position, because the gravid uterus interferes with venous return from the lower extremities. As shown in Figure 59-2, this effect is most marked in the supine position and least in the left lateral decubitus position. Estimates of expected cardiac output during gestation should be revised upward for intercurrent stresses such as fever, infection, and pain.

Heart rate increases progressively throughout gestation, reaching a 20 percent or a 15 beat per minute increase over nonpregnant levels [13]. Stroke volume increases more rapidly at first and then stabilizes. Left ventricular compliance must increase in pregnancy, because the increased stroke volume appears to be related more to left ventricular enlargement than to increased emptying [7]. Thus, the cardiac silhouette on chest radiogram may appear enlarged as a result of mild normal left ventricular enlargement and lateral and upward displacement by the gravid uterus.

During labor, cardiac output increases up to 45 percent over nonpregnant values, and during uterine contraction cardiac output transiently increases another 10 to 15 percent because of increased venous return [14]. Another factor that may be important in patients who are sensitive to left ventricular afterload is inhibition of circulation to the uterus during labor contractions. Because uterine blood flow at term accounts for a significant proportion of the cardiac output, marked increases in afterload during contractions and immediately postpartum may occur. During labor, contractions are associated with increased blood return from the uterus. These "autotransfusions" may reach 500 ml when the uterus contracts after parturition. This effect, however, may be offset by blood loss. Cardiac output may increase as much as 80 percent over prelabor levels in the first few minutes postpartum, then decrease to 40 to 50 percent over prelabor values by 1 hour postpartum, and finally return to nearly prepregnant levels by 1 to 2 weeks postpartum.

Systemic vascular resistance is reduced in pregnancy, possibly as a result of increased synthesis of the vasodilator prostacyclin. Thus, mean blood pressure remains relatively constant despite increases in cardiac output [7]. Pressures in the right ventricle, pulmonary artery, and pulmonary capillaries are no different from nonpregnant values [15].

Blood volume starts increasing in the first trimester, increases 40 percent above prepregnant levels by the beginning of the third trimester, and then remains stable until term. The extent of blood volume increase is dependent on the number of fetuses present. One to two extra liters of extracellular water is normal in pregnancy, as is peripheral edema in 50 to 80 percent of pregnancies.

Colloid osmotic pressure measurements during gestation reveal a mean decrease of 5 mm Hg, which reaches a plateau at 26 weeks [16]. This parallels a decrease in serum albumin concentrations from approximately 4 to 3.4 gm per deciliter. A further decline in colloid osmotic pressure of roughly 4 mm Hg occurs immediately postpartum, probably as a result of a combination of factors, such as recumbency, crystalloid administration, and blood loss [16]. These changes may be even more marked in patients with pregnancy-induced hypertension. Unfortunately, neither the absolute value of colloid osmotic pressure nor the colloid osmotic pressure-pulmonary capillary wedge pressure gradient is an accurate predictor of pulmonary edema because of the multiplicity of contributing variables. However, these trends in colloid osmotic pressure should be considered when interpreting pulmonary capillary wedge pressures, especially in patients who have received large amounts of crystalloid.

Determinants of Fetal Oxygen Delivery

One of the major questions that arises in the care of pregnant patients with respiratory failure, especially when maternal oxygenation is a major problem, is what level of maternal oxygenation should be maintained to prevent adverse consequences in the fetus. Studies of women at high altitudes have suggested a correlation between decreased inspired oxygen concentration and low-birth-weight infants [17]. Women with higher hemoglobin levels and relative hyperventilation delivered normal-sized infants, suggesting that oxygen content is more important than oxygen tension (PaO_2) [18]. Case reports of women with hypoxemia caused by bronchiectasis [19] and pulmonary alveolar proteinosis [20] suggest a correlation between hypoxemia and intrauterine growth retardation and intrauterine death. It is not clear whether these generalizations about hypoxemia throughout gestation can be extended to insults that last only a few hours or days. Because assessment of fetal oxygenation is possible only at the time of delivery, little objective data exist to answer this question, but an understanding of maternal-fetal gas exchange helps somewhat in predicting the margin of safety.

Oxygen delivery to fetal tissues can be affected at many levels: maternal oxygen delivery to the placenta, placental transfer, and fetal oxygen transport from the placenta to fetal tissues [21,22]. The major determinants of oxygen delivery to the placenta are the oxygen content of uterine artery blood, which is determined by maternal PaO_2; hemoglobin concentration and saturation; and uterine artery blood flow, which is dependent on maternal cardiac output [23]. Thus, a decreased PaO_2 can be offset somewhat by increased blood hemoglobin concentration or by increased cardiac output. One would expect that the converse also holds true: the combination of maternal hypoxemia and decreased cardiac output likely has a profoundly deleterious effect on fetal oxygenation.

Variations in maternal pH also influence oxygen delivery [6,23]. Alkalosis causes vasoconstriction of the uterine artery, resulting in decreased fetal oxygen delivery. This effect is magnified by a leftward shift in the maternal oxyhemoglobin saturation curve, which increases oxygen affinity and consequently decreases oxygen transfer to the umbilical vein. Although mild maternal acidosis does not enhance uterine blood flow because the uterine vasculature is already maximally dilated, it shifts the maternal oxyhemoglobin saturation curve to the right, which leads to decreased oxygen affinity and increased fetal oxygen delivery [6]. Maternal hypotension and increased sympathetic stimulation (exogenous or endogenous) both cause uterine arterial vasoconstriction [23].

The importance of maternal cardiac output is supported by the observation that women with left ventricular outflow obstruction have an increased incidence of fetal death and surviving infants have an increased incidence of congenital heart disease [6]. Data from a sheep model, however, suggest that a decrease in uterine blood flow up to 50 percent for brief periods does not appreciably decrease fetal and placental oxygen uptake [24]. Chronically decreased maternal cardiac output may have other effects, perhaps on placental development, that explain the results in women with left ventricular outflow obstruction. The sheep data are reassuring, however, in terms of brief fluctuations in uterine blood flow.

The interaction of maternal and fetal circulations in the placenta most likely follows a concurrent exchange mechanism [22,23,25]. This is less efficient than a countercurrent exchange mechanism and partly explains why fetal umbilical vein PO_2 is in the range of 32 mm Hg, far lower than uterine vein PO_2, and why increased maternal inspired oxygen increases uterine artery oxygen tension but does not cause major increases in umbilical vein PO_2. Other placental factors that determine fetal oxygenation are amount of intraplacental shunt, degree of matching of maternal and fetal blood flows, and presence of any placental abnormalities, such as placental infarcts. There seem to be no placental autoregulatory mechanisms that adjust to decreased maternal PaO_2 [7].

Despite low umbilical vein PO_2, fetal oxygen content is actually quite close to maternal oxygen content, because of the shape of the oxyhemoglobin saturation curve for fetal hemoglobin (Fig. 59-3) [7,26]. This is one of the major protective mechanisms for fetal oxygenation. In addition, the fetal oxyhemoglobin saturation curve is relatively unaffected by changes in pH; although acidosis may decrease maternal oxygen affinity, fetal oxygen affinity is unchanged.

Mathematical models predicting the optimal apportionment of fetal cardiac output between umbilical (to collect oxygen) and systemic (to deliver oxygen) circulations have yielded values surprisingly close to those measured under normal physiologic conditions [27]. This appears to be another compensation mechanism for the apparent inefficiency (concurrent exchange mechanism) of the placenta [27]. One disadvantage in terms of oxygen delivery to fetal tissues is that oxygenated umbilical vein blood is mixed in the fetal inferior vena cava with deoxygenated systemic venous blood before delivery to the systemic circulation. Thus, fetal arterial blood has an even lower PO_2 than umbilical vein blood. This is compensated in part by a high fetal cardiac output relative to oxygen consumption, thus enhancing oxygen delivery to fetal tissues [27]. In addition, the fetal circulation appears to have the ability to autoregulate in

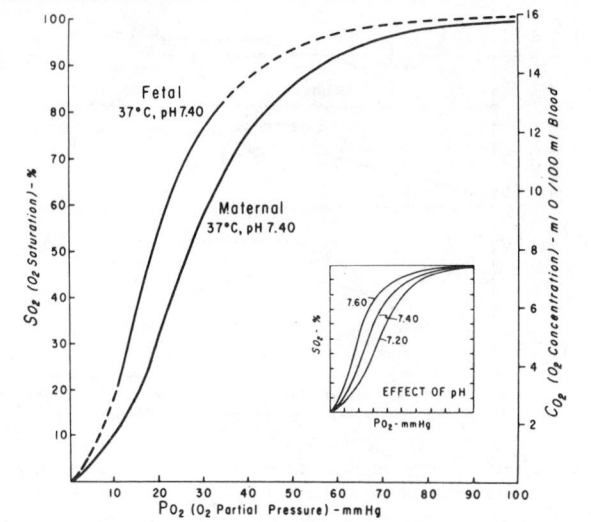

Fig. 59-3. Oxygen dissociation (equilibrium) curves of human fetal and maternal blood. The effect of pH on the position of the curve (Bohr effect) is shown on the insert. The oxygen capacity of 16 ml/100 ml blood on the right-hand ordinate refers to maternal blood. (From Novy MJ, Edwards MJ: Respiratory problems in pregnancy. *Am J Obstet Gynecol* 99:1024, 1967. With permission.)

the face of hypoxemia to protect the brain, adrenal glands, and heart [28]. How long this adaptation can be depended on safely before organ damage occurs in underperfused areas is not known.

How well do the compensatory mechanisms that provide adequate oxygen supply to the fetus under normal conditions manage during maternal hypoxia? Calculation of oxygen stores in the term infant with 60 percent hemoglobin saturation yields a total oxygen content of 40 ml. Given an oxygen consumption of 6 ml/kg/min, or about 18 ml per minute at term, this reserve will last barely 2 minutes when maternal oxygen supply is completely interrupted [29]. One study that specifically measured the influence of variations in maternal inspired oxygen concentration on fetal oxygenation was conducted during labor [30]; fetal umbilical artery and vein PO_2 were measured immediately after delivery (Table 59-2). Fetal umbilical vein PO_2 decreased to 25.6 mm Hg when the mother's inspired oxygen concentration (FiO_2) decreased to 15 percent, corresponding to a maternal PaO_2 of 64.7 mm Hg [30]. At an FiO_2 of 10 percent, the fetal umbilical vein PO_2 actually increased slightly to 27.1 mm Hg. The range of variation was significant, making it difficult to predict the exact fetal umbilical vein PO_2 for a given maternal PaO_2. Maternal ventilation with 100 percent oxygen led to a maternal PaO_2 of 583 mm Hg, but fetal umbilical vein PO_2 increased only from 32 to 40 mm Hg. The shape of the fetal oxyhemoglobin dissociation curve places umbilical vein PO_2 values below 30 mm Hg on the steep part of the curve, so small changes in maternal PO_2 may cause significant changes in fetal oxygen content. Therefore, it seems reasonable to aim for a maternal PaO_2 greater than 65 mm Hg (the usual goal of mechanical ventilation and supplemental oxygenation in patients with respiratory failure). Concern regarding fetal oxygen supply would be further reduced, if a normal maternal PaO_2 of 90 mm Hg, or greater, could be achieved without too great a risk of barotrauma or oxygen toxicity. This assumes that maternal cardiac output, hemoglobin concentration, and pH are not adversely affected.

Table 59-2. Influence of Maternal Oxygen Partial Pressure on Fetal Partial Pressures of Oxygen and Carbon Dioxide

Vessel	Oxygen content of inspired air[a]			
	10%	15%	21%	100%
Maternal brachial artery				
PO_2 (mm Hg)	47.3 ± 3.0	64.7 ± 7.8	90.7 ± 14.7	583.0 ± 16.8
PCO_2 (mm Hg)	37.0 ± 6.2	38.9 ± 6.2	36.4 ± 7.4	37.2 ± 2.2
Fetal umbilical vein				
PO_2 (mm Hg)	27.1 ± 5.3	25.6 ± 8.5	31.9 ± 8.1	39.8 ± 7.1
PCO_2 (mm Hg)	51.7 ± 5.7	46.7 ± 8.2	49.5 ± 7.4	48.0 ± 3.2

[a] Values are mean ± standard deviation.
PO_2 = oxygen tension; PCO_2 = carbon dioxide tension.
Source: Wulf KH, Kunzel W, Lehman V: Clinical aspects of placental gas exchange, in Longo LD, Bartels H (eds): *Respiratory Gas Exchange and Blood Flow in the Placenta.* Bethesda, MD, Public Health Service, 1972, p. 505.

Causes of Acute Respiratory Failure

This section describes the more common causes of acute respiratory failure in pregnancy in terms of frequency, clinical presentation, pathophysiology, and diagnosis.

THROMBOEMBOLIC DISEASE. Pulmonary embolism follows ectopic pregnancy as the second leading cause of maternal mortality, with a death rate of 0.1 to 0.7 for every 100,000 deliveries [31]. Thromboembolic complications have been estimated to occur in 2 to 5 of every 1000 deliveries [31,32]. The increased frequency of thromboembolic disease associated with pregnancy has been attributed to an increase in clotting factors VII, VIII, and X as well as to an increased fibrinogen level and decreased fibrinolytic activity [32]. Depression in antithrombin III activity may also have a role, if one can extrapolate from data on estrogen therapy [33]. Venous stasis caused by uterine pressure on the inferior vena cava may also be a contributing factor. Factors that further increase the risk of thromboembolic disease during pregnancy and the puerperium include (1) cesarean section, which has a 10 times greater risk of fatal pulmonary embolism compared with vaginal delivery; (2) increased maternal age; (3) multiparity; (4) obesity, especially in association with bed rest; (5) suppression of lactation with estrogens; and (6) surgical procedures during pregnancy and early puerperium [31].

The appropriate diagnostic steps and treatment of venous thrombosis and pulmonary embolism in nonpregnant patients are reviewed in Chapter 60. Other authors [31,32] have discussed the management of submassive thromboembolic disease in pregnancy and the puerperium. This chapter therefore focuses on the diagnosis and management of massive pulmonary embolism associated with severe respiratory and hemodynamic compromise. Respiratory failure may ensue in pulmonary embolism when extensive occlusion of the pulmonary vasculature or concomitant pulmonary edema occurs. Pulmonary edema has been associated with pulmonary embolism in areas of intact blood flow [34,36] and has been attributed to increased hydrostatic forces in nonoccluded vessels, vigorous crystalloid resuscitation, and increased microvascular permeability caused by platelet-derived mediators [36].

Although none of the symptoms, physical signs, laboratory, radiographic, or electrocardiographic findings frequently attributed to pulmonary embolic disease are specific, these investigations can help rule out other diseases in the differential diagnosis. Likewise, hemodynamic data obtained at pulmonary artery catheterization are more helpful in excluding other processes and in guiding hemodynamic management than in making a definitive diagnosis of pulmonary embolism.

The typical hemodynamic findings in nonpregnant patients with massive pulmonary embolism are delineated in Chapter 60. Although there are no data for pregnant patients with massive pulmonary embolism, one would anticipate similar findings, as pregnancy does not significantly alter right heart and pulmonary artery pressures. Thus, pulmonary capillary wedge pressure should be normal or low, mean pulmonary artery pressure moderately elevated (≥35 mm Hg), and right atrial pressure moderately elevated (>8 mm Hg).

In the evaluation of patients with suspected pulmonary embolism without hemodynamic compromise, relatively noninvasive tests, such as impedance plethysmography, venography, and perfusion lung scanning, should be performed first. Pulmonary angiography should be reserved for patients in whom pulmonary embolism cannot be excluded by these studies. However, in massive pulmonary embolism, pulmonary angiography (rather than perfusion lung scanning) frequently is the diagnostic procedure of choice to document the presence of pulmonary embolism and the extent of obstruction. The most efficient system may be to combine pulmonary artery catheterization and hemodynamic monitoring with angiography in an angiography suite, rather than transporting a patient first to the intensive care unit, then to nuclear medicine facilities, and finally to the angiography laboratory (see Chap. 60).

Lung scanning and pulmonary angiography obviously expose the fetus to radiation, but the dose from angiography can be minimized by abdominal shielding and by using brachial access (see Diagnostic Testing). If a main pulmonary artery embolus is not found, selective balloon occlusion angiography can be used to diminish the total volume of contrast needed and to improve sensitivity and specificity (see Chap. 60).

AMNIOTIC FLUID EMBOLISM. Amniotic fluid embolism is a rare but usually catastrophic complication of pregnancy and delivery that accounts for 11 to 13 percent of maternal deaths [37]. Its frequency has been estimated at 1 in every 8000 to 80,000 deliveries; in a review of 272 patients the mortality rate was 86 percent [37,38]. Although the majority of reported cases predated modern critical care techniques, 25 percent of the deaths occurred within 1 hour of the onset of symptoms, suggesting that even optimal management will continue to be associated with a high mortality rate.

It is unknown why amniotic fluid enters the maternal circulation in some patients, although certain potential predisposing clinical factors have been identified. These factors include older maternal age (mean 32 years), multiparity (88% of cases), amniotomy, cesarean section, insertion of intrauterine fetal or pressure monitoring devices, and term pregnancy in the presence of an intrauterine device [38]. Other factors previously suggested to be associated with amniotic fluid embolism, such as short or tumultuous labor, large fetal size, and intrauterine fetal death, were not found in increased frequency in the largest review [38]. Although most of these proposed etiologic factors are related to labor and delivery, 10 percent of reported cases occur before labor, including one case at 20 weeks gestation without uterine manipulation [38].

Presumably, amniotic fluid enters the maternal circulation through one of three ports: endocervical veins; uterine tears (small tears may occur in the lower uterine segment as a part of normal labor); and uterine injury secondary to iatrogenic manipulation, such as cesarean section, insertion of monitoring devices, or membrane rupture [38].

The two life-threatening consequences of amniotic fluid embolism are cardiorespiratory collapse and disseminated intravascular coagulation (DIC), which may occur simultaneously or in sequence. The pathophysiology of cardiorespiratory collapse remains controversial. Initially it was thought to be due to pulmonary hypertension caused by obstruction of the pulmonary vasculature. Another theory is that the vasoconstrictor prostaglandin F_2 (PGF$_2$), known to be increased in concentration in amniotic fluid at the time of labor, might be responsible for the development of pulmonary hypertension [39]. Animal models of amniotic fluid embolization show conflicting results: some investigators have produced pulmonary hypertension with injection of cell- and debris-free filtrates of amniotic fluid, but others have not [38].

Although Morgan [38] described only a 24 percent incidence of pulmonary edema, Peterson and Taylor [40] noted in an autopsy review that most lungs exhibited pulmonary edema (10% severe, 60% moderate). Because most cases are rapidly fatal, radiographs have been infrequently obtained, which perhaps explains the low incidence of edema reported by Morgan [38]. The cause of pulmonary edema has variably been ascribed to vigorous fluid resuscitation; increased permeability pulmonary edema; and cardiac decompensation caused by hypoxia and tachycardia. Based on reported hemodynamic measurements and an elevated respiratory secretion protein content, it seems likely that pulmonary parenchymal shunting as a result of increased permeability pulmonary edema has an important role in both the initial gas exchange abnormality and its duration [41,42].

It has been suggested that the cardiovascular collapse associated with amniotic fluid embolism might be due to an anaphylactic reaction. However, the absence or rarity of pruritus, urticaria, laryngospasm, or wheezing in case reports is evidence against a mast cell-mediated mechanism [38].

The other major consequence of amniotic fluid embolism is coagulation failure. In 10 to 15 percent of patients, excessive bleeding, particularly uterine bleeding, may be the first sign of amniotic fluid embolism. Up to 50 percent of patients who survive the first 30 to 60 minutes have clinical evidence of coagulopathy, and most of the remaining patients will have laboratory evidence of DIC [38]. Whether a specific activator of factor X that has been demonstrated in amniotic fluid, the activation of fibrinolysis by intravascular amniotic fluid, or other factors are the initiators of DIC is not known [38,43].

The abrupt onset of severe dyspnea, tachypnea, and cyanosis during labor or the early puerperium is the classic presentation of amniotic fluid embolism, characterizing more than half of cases. Shock, which is out of proportion to blood loss, is the first manifestation in another 10 to 15 percent. Bleeding is the forerunning sign in 10 to 15 percent of patients, and the longer

the survival, the greater the likelihood the patient will manifest respiratory failure, cardiovascular collapse, and DIC. Whatever the presenting symptom complex, 90 percent of cases occur prior to or during labor [38]. Other complications, such as acute renal failure and signs of central nervous system injury, are probably secondary to hypotension and hypoxemia. Prodromal symptoms, such as vomiting and shivering, are nonspecific and frequently associated with otherwise uneventful deliveries.

Definitive diagnosis of amniotic fluid embolism rests on demonstration of fetal elements in the maternal circulation. At autopsy, special stains are used to demonstrate epithelial squames from fetal skin, lanugo hairs, fat from the vernix caseosa, mucin from fetal gut, and bile-containing meconium [44,45]. It has been reported that a definitive diagnosis can be made antemortem by demonstrating fetal squames in sputum samples [38] and fetal squames, mucin, and hair in buffy coat preparations of blood aspirated from central venous [37] and right heart catheters [41,42]. However, a recent study found it virtually impossible to eliminate exogenous squamous cell contamination: pulmonary artery samples from 42 nonpregnant cardiac patients had 1 to 50 squames per slide [46]. Therefore, the antemortem diagnosis of amniotic fluid embolism still rests predominantly on the clinical setting and the exclusion of other causes of acute respiratory failure.

VENOUS AIR EMBOLISM. Venous air embolism has been described during normal labor, delivery of patients with placenta previa, criminal abortions using air, orogenital sex, and insufflation of the vagina during gynecologic procedures and may account for as many as 1 percent of maternal deaths [47–50]. Presumably, the subplacental venous sinuses are the site of air entry when antepartum or peripartum air embolism occurs [47]. More commonly, venous air embolism occurs during head and neck surgery, during neurosurgical procedures, and in association with central venous catheter placement [49,51].

Sudden, profound hypotension is the most common presenting sign of venous air embolism. Cough, dyspnea, dizziness, tachypnea, tachycardia, and diaphoresis also may be noted. Hypotension is usually followed quickly by respiratory arrest. The classic sign associated with air embolus is the mill wheel murmur, which is audible over the precordium [46,48]; a drumlike or bubbling sound may also be heard. There are occasional reports of air shown radiographically in the right side of the heart or the main pulmonary artery [46,52]. Electrocardiographic evidence of ischemia, right heart strain, and arrhythmias has been described [46,52], and metabolic acidosis, presumably caused by lactic acid production, may be present [49].

The volume of air that is likely to be lethal seems to vary with the rate of infusion and patient position. Any amount greater than 100 ml may cause death, but some patients have survived after infusion of up to 1600 ml [46,48]. It was initially thought that the bolus of air formed a block in the apical tract of the right ventricle, thus preventing pulmonary blood flow [46]. Animal studies have suggested two further mechanisms that probably have a role. First, turbulent blood flow from the whipping action of the heart appears to make an air-blood interface that produces platelet damage and fibrin formation, which then leads to fibrin microemboli [53]. These microemboli may then cause obstruction of the pulmonary arterioles and capillaries. Second, polymorphonuclear leukocytes may be recruited and activated by denatured, aggregated proteins at the air-blood interface, as evidenced by polymorphonuclear leukocyte infiltration found in animal models of air embolism [53]. In a sheep model, a dramatic increase in lung lymph flow was demonstrated during air emboli. This increase in lymph fluid flow can be diminished by depleting the sheep of circulating leukocytes before injection of the air emboli or by treatment with the enzyme superoxide dismutase, a scavenger of toxic oxygen radicals [53].

Increased permeability pulmonary edema has been described in a few patients who survived initial cardiorespiratory collapse [52,53]. Pulmonary edema in these patients seemed to be fairly short-lived, because extubation was accomplished after 30 to 72 hours. Of note, one of the patients underwent open lung biopsy, which revealed mild, scattered perivascular interstitial infiltration of polymorphonuclear leukoyctes. This is similar to the histology previously described in sheep and dog models of venous air embolism, suggesting a similar mechanism.

ASPIRATION OF GASTRIC CONTENTS. Aspiration of acidic gastric contents into the tracheobronchial tree was first described in 1946 by Mendelson [54] in women in labor and delivery. Since then, it has been estimated that 2 percent of maternal deaths in the United States result from aspiration of liquid vomitus [55]. Acid aspiration is usually followed several hours later by development of chemical pneumonitis and increased permeability pulmonary edema. However, massive aspiration of stomach contents leading to immediate asphyxia and bacterial pneumonia from aspiration of oropharyngeal bacteria may also occur [56].

At term, several factors contribute to an increased risk of aspiration of stomach contents: (1) increased intragastric pressure caused by external compression by the gravid uterus; (2) progesterone-induced relaxation of the lower esophageal sphincter; (3) delayed gastric emptying during labor; (4) analgesia-induced decreased mental status and decreased vocal cord closure; and (5) rarely, increased production of low pH gastric juice when intravenous ethanol is used as a tocolytic agent [55,57]. One study found that 55 percent of intrapartum patients had more than 45 ml of gastric juice in the stomach; a pH of 2.5 or less was found in 45 percent of patients [55].

The volume of acid aspiration determines, in part, the rapidity of symptom onset. Aspiration of smaller volumes may go unnoticed clinically until 6 to 8 hours later, when tachypnea, tachycardia, hypoxemia, hypotension, bronchospasm, and production of frothy pink sputum are noted in association with diffuse infiltrates on chest radiograph. Progression of chest radiographic findings may continue for up to 36 hours. The clinical course may follow one of three patterns: (1) rapid improvement over 4 to 5 days; (2) initial improvement followed by deterioration caused by supervening bacterial pneumonia, with a fatal outcome in up to 60 percent; and (3) early death as a result of intractable hypoxia [58]. The bacterial pathogens in this setting are usually oropharyngeal anaerobes, although the longer the patient is in the hospital before clinical development of pneumonia, the greater the likelihood of facultative, gram-negative bacillary and *Staphylococcus aureus* infections [59].

Mendelson [54] first proposed that the low pH of gastric contents precipitates chemical pneumonitis. Although a pH of 2.5 has been thought to be the dividing point in humans between aspiration that produces pneumonitis (pH < 2.5) and benign aspiration (pH > 2.5) [60,61], a pH greater than 2.5 is not always benign. Aspiration of gastric contents containing small food particles with a pH as high as 5.9 has been reported to cause hypoxemia and hypercapnia [60]. The hypercapnia was likely due to airway obstruction by food particles and a peribronchial, mononuclear inflammatory response. Clear gastric juice with a pH of 5.9 caused transient alterations in gas exchange, but no pathologic changes were evident after 48 hours [60].

RESPIRATORY INFECTIONS. Community-acquired pneumonia complicates approximately 1 in every 2300 deliveries [62]. In the preantibiotic era, bacterial pneumonia was associated with a 20 to 30 percent maternal mortality rate and a 75 percent fetal mortality rate. However, recent reports note 0 to 8 percent maternal mortality and less than 10 percent fetal mortality [62]. The major factors in improving fetal and maternal outcome seem to have been earlier presentation and prompt institution of antibiotic therapy. Although these infections rarely develop into respiratory failure, it is advisable to assess maternal oxygenation in all cases of maternal pneumonia. The spectrum of organisms to consider is similar to that in the nonpregnant population; the most common organisms are *Streptococcus pneumoniae, Haemophilus influenzae,* and *Mycoplasma pneumoniae. Legionella* pneumonia accounts for up to 22 percent of community-acquired pneumonia [63] and has been reported to cause respiratory failure in pregnancy [64].

Certain other respiratory infections (e.g., influenza, varicella, coccidioidomycosis, tuberculosis, and listeriosis) have been associated with increased maternal and fetal morbidity and mortality. The traditional association of these infections with patients who have defective cell-mediated immune responses has raised the question of whether immune function is altered in pregnancy [65]. This has been supported by in vitro studies of the maternal immune response. During the second and third trimesters, maternal lymphocytes show diminished proliferative responses to soluble antigens and allogeneic lymphocytes [66,67]. Decreased cell-mediated cytotoxicity and decreased numbers of T-helper lymphocytes have also been found [68,69]. The reported increases in maternal morbidity and mortality from these infections have occurred in the second and third trimesters in concordance with the time course of diminished maternal in vitro immune response [67]. Fortunately, the impairment in maternal immune response is mild and the increase in maternal morbidity small.

In both the 1918–1919 and 1957–1958 influenza pandemics, an excess incidence of influenza pneumonia was noted among pregnant women. A 50 percent incidence of influenza pneumonia and an overall mortality of 27 percent for influenza in pregnancy were found in the 1918–1919 season [65]. In the 1957–1958 pandemic, several studies noted that 50 percent of deaths from influenza in women of childbearing age were in pregnant patients [65]. Autopsy reports noted that the cause of death in pregnant women was respiratory insufficiency caused by fulminant influenza pneumonia, rather than secondary bacterial infection, the more common cause of death in nonpregnant influenza victims. Other than during these pandemic years, pregnancy has not been demonstrated to be a risk factor for severe influenza infection [70,71].

Primary varicella-zoster infections progress to pneumonia more commonly in adults than in children, though only 20 percent of varicella cases occur in adults [72,73]. Progression to pneumonia has also been noted more frequently in pregnant women in their second and third trimesters; 10 percent of reported cases of varicella pneumonia have occurred in pregnant women. In the past, maternal varicella-zoster pneumonia was associated with a maternal mortality rate of 45 percent, in comparison with an overall adult mortality rate of 15 to 20 percent [72]. However, these statistics predate modern critical care technology and do not reflect the current experience. Paryani and Arvin [74] reported 4 cases of pneumonia among 43 women with varicella during pregnancy. One woman died and one required ventilatory support; premature delivery occurred in 4 of the remaining 42 pregnancies.

Respiratory symptoms usually develop 2 days after the onset of fever, rash, and malaise. Typical symptoms are cough (89%), dyspnea (70%), hemoptysis (38%), and chest pain (21%) [75].

Generalized varicella-zoster infections may also be associated with hepatitis, myocarditis, nephritis, thrombocytopenia, and adrenal hemorrhage [75]. Although fetal infection with the virus is uncommon, high frequencies of prematurity, spontaneous abortion, and stillbirth have been reported, suggesting that maternal hypoxia and fever may have had an important role [72,76]. In the absence of dissemination, herpes zoster does not appear to be associated with significant maternal morbidity or evidence of fetal infection [74].

Of the fungal infections reported during pregnancy, coccidioidomycosis has been most commonly associated with an increased risk of dissemination during pregnancy [3,77]. Case reports of cryptococcosis, blastomycosis, and sporotrichosis in pregnancy are rare enough to suggest that there is no increased susceptibility to these infections [77]. By contrast, coccidioidal infections during pregnancy have a 20 percent rate of dissemination, compared with 0.2 percent in nonpregnant patients. Higher rates have been noted when infection is contracted in the second or third trimester [3]. Catanzaro [77] suggested that increased serum 17 β-estradiol levels during pregnancy are a growth stimulant to *Coccidioides immitis*, which may be as or more important than the mild suppression of host immune responsiveness in pregnancy. Maternal *C. immitis* infections are rare (<1 in every 1000 pregnancies), but third trimester infections are associated with a high mortality rate [77].

Disseminated coccidioidal infection should be suspected in patients with primary or chronic progressive coccidioidal pneumonia in whom rapidly progressive respiratory failure and a clinical picture resembling miliary tuberculosis develop. Unfortunately, diagnosis is sometimes difficult because sputum is positive in less than 40 percent of cases and complement fixation titers may be low [77]. Evaluation of these patients should include a careful search for extrapulmonary disease (e.g., lumbar puncture, urinalysis, culture of skin lesions) [77].

Respiratory failure due to *Mycobacterium tuberculosis* is rare in the general population and even rarer in pregnancy, although before the advent of effective chemotherapy, maternal and infant mortality in cases of advanced disease approached 40 percent [78]. Reports on the rates of reactivation of tuberculosis during pregnancy and the first postpartum year have shown variable results [3], suggesting that any increased risk is slight. Similarly, the literature contains conflicting reports concerning the risk of active tuberculosis developing during pregnancy in patients with a positive purified protein derivative (PPD) skin test and a normal chest radiograph [78]. The most recent study suggests that the new active case rate is identical in women of childbearing age, whether pregnant or not [78]. It is also now accepted that PPD skin testing is probably valid throughout the course of pregnancy, because the rate of false negative reactions is more dependent on other factors, such as nutritional status and other intercurrent diseases [65].

Eighty percent of all women with acquired immunodeficiency syndrome (AIDS) are of childbearing age [79]. As the number of women infected with the human immunodeficiency virus (HIV) grows, the spectrum of respiratory disease in pregnancy will include an increasing proportion of opportunistic infections and other respiratory complications related to AIDS. Already, it appears that pregnancy may accelerate the course of AIDS and that maternal survival after pregnancy is short [79]. Infection with HIV even without comorbid conditions, such as substance abuse and poor nutrition, may adversely affect fetal maturation and preterm delivery [80]. Fetal HIV infection can lead to a distinct fetal AIDS syndrome, with growth failure, microcephaly, a prominent boxlike forehead, prominent eyes, and a flattened nasal bridge [80].

Death during pregnancy in women with AIDS is usually associated with *Pneumocystis carinii* pneumonia (PCP)

[79,81,82]. Diagnostic evaluation follows the same protocol as in a nonpregnant patient with suspected PCP. Induced sputum should be examined for the presence of pneumocystis; if this is negative fiberoptic bronchoscopy with bronchoalveolar lavage should be performed. As prophylactic therapy for PCP during pregnancy has not been recommended, the yield of bronchoalveolar lavage should be high.

Listeria monocytogenes, a cause of meningitis and sepsis in immunocompromised hosts, also has a predilection for pregnant women, most commonly resulting in abortion or neonatal sepsis. The usual sporadic incidence is 2 to 3 for every 1 million of the population each year, but local outbreaks may occur as a result of ingestion of contaminated cheese, cabbage, or milk [83]. In a recent outbreak that caused 29 fetal and neonatal deaths, maternal morbidity was limited to fever and gastrointestinal symptoms [83]. However, in a few reported cases of maternal sepsis caused by *Listeria* acute respiratory distress syndrome developed [84]. In these cases, the fetal outcome was excellent despite *Listeria* sepsis. Diagnosis may be problematic because of difficulties in isolating the organism from respiratory tract secretions. When *Listeria* sepsis is suspected cultures should be obtained from the blood, sputum, rectum, cervix, and amniotic fluid [84].

ASTHMA. Asthma occurs in 0.4 to 1.3 percent of pregnant women [11], making it the most common cause of respiratory difficulties during pregnancy. Several excellent reviews of the general management of asthma during pregnancy have been published [11,85]. The scope of this section is limited to the rarer asthmatic exacerbations that lead to respiratory failure.

Early reports of the outcome of pregnancies complicated by asthma noted an increased frequency of infant prematurity, increased perinatal mortality, and increased maternal mortality [86,87]. More recent studies have reported outcomes to be as favorable for pregnant patients as for the general population, suggesting that close monitoring and consistent control of asthma are crucial to maternal and fetal well-being [85,88,89]. This was emphasized by a study that found a statistically increased incidence of low birth weight and small size for gestational age in infants born to women who experienced status asthmaticus when compared to infants born to women who may have required prednisone or beclomethasone dipropionate but did not require emergency department therapy or experience status asthmaticus [90]. However, even with the most careful outpatient management, patients occasionally present with severe exacerbations.

The initial clinical assessment of a pregnant woman with asthma should include personal history (detailing etiologic factors and prior therapy), physical examination, and either peak expiratory flow rate or spirometric pulmonary function testing (see Chap. 56). Although asthma may be the most common cause of airway obstruction during pregnancy, wheezing, shortness of breath, coughing, and sensation of chest tightness are suggestive, but not diagnostic, of asthma, and several other entities may mimic asthma (see Chap. 56) [91]. Assuming the diagnosis of asthma is secure, certain findings taken together can be used to predict which patients are likely to require hospitalization [92]. These include diaphoresis, use of accessory muscles, assumption of upright posture, altered level of consciousness, pulse rate greater than 120 beats per minute, respiratory rate greater than 30 per minute, pulsus paradoxus greater than 18 mm Hg, and peak expiratory flow rate less than 120 liters per minute. When the forced expiratory volume in 1 second (FEV_1) is less than or equal to 15 percent predicted or is less than 0.5 liter, both a pulsus paradoxus of 10 mm Hg or greater and use of accessory muscles of respiration are almost always found [93,94]. Conversely, the absence of both an elevated pulsus paradoxus and use of accessory muscles generally correlates with an FEV$_1$ greater than 40 percent predicted or greater than 1.25 liter [93,94]. Peak flows have been used in the evaluation of nonpregnant patients with asthma to predict the need for arterial blood gas determination. Flows greater than 200 liters per minute (50% predicted) are virtually never associated with significant hypoxemia or hypercapnia (see Chap. 56). However, just as alveolar-arterial oxygen tension gradients are known to be widened in pregnancy [11], it seems prudent to document adequacy of oxygenation in pregnant women with asthma who do not show a significant improvement (>20%) in peak expiratory flow rate after an initial inhaled bronchodilator treatment.

During acute asthma attacks, arterial blood gas measurements typically reveal mild hypocapnia (PaCO$_2$ = 35 mm Hg) and moderate hypoxemia. In pregnancy, as noted previously, the baseline PaCO$_2$ is usually already depressed [3,30] and probably decreases further with an acute asthma attack. The importance of this is twofold: (1) a PaCO$_2$ of 35 mm Hg during an acute attack may actually represent "pseudonormalization" caused by fatigue, inability to meet the increased work of breathing, and impending respiratory failure; and (2) persistent hypocapnia with associated respiratory alkalosis (pH > 7.48) may result in uterine artery vasoconstriction and decreased fetal perfusion [6].

BETA-ADRENERGIC TOCOLYTIC THERAPY. Beta-adrenergic agents have become accepted therapy for inhibition of preterm labor. The use of relatively beta$_2$-selective agents, such as ritodrine, terbutaline, and isoxsuprine hydrochloride, has diminished the frequency of unacceptable maternal tachycardia, but maternal pulmonary edema has remained a serious side effect. The published results of hemodynamic monitoring are conflicting, leaving the pathophysiologic mechanism of pulmonary edema in these cases obscure [95,96].

The typical symptoms and signs of beta-adrenergic tocolytic-induced pulmonary edema are chest discomfort, dyspnea, tachypnea (24–40 breaths/min), rales, and pulmonary edema on chest radiograph. Evidence of pulmonary edema develops relatively acutely, occasionally after only 24 hours and usually after 48 hours of beta-adrenergic tocolytic therapy. A nonproductive cough is occasionally present. Wheezes in addition to rales were noted in one case [95]. The size of the heart has been difficult to assess on radiographs because of the normal increase in diameter with pregnancy. Of 11 recently reported cases, 5 had concurrent evidence of infection, such as fever, elevated white blood cell counts, and/or amnionitis [95,96,97]. One of the 11 had mild preeclampsia. These characteristics are similar to those reported in earlier cases. The relatively rapid improvement that occurs with discontinuation of beta-adrenergic tocolytic therapy (usually in less than 24 hours), the absence of hypotension and clotting abnormalities, as well as the lack of need for mechanical ventilation support the possibility that these cases represent a separate syndrome related to beta-adrenergic tocolytic therapy. However, in individual cases the lack of specificity of symptoms and clinical findings makes it crucial to consider alternative diagnoses, such as thromboembolic disease, amniotic fluid embolism, aspiration, and increased permeability pulmonary edema caused by septicemia.

Several possible mechanisms to explain beta-adrenergic tocolytic-induced edema have been proposed based on certain known effects of parenteral beta-adrenergic agents. These include fluid overload, myocardial toxicity, reduced colloid osmotic pressure, and increased pulmonary capillary permeability [95,97]. Fluid overload is suggested by the known increased

release of antidiuretic hormone, which occurs 30 minutes after initiation of intravenous therapy and is associated with decreased renal excretion of sodium [98]. This observation is supported by the clinical evidence of a decrease in hematocrit consistent with an increase in plasma volume shortly after the drug is administered [97]. This effect may be accentuated by infusion of large volumes of crystalloids in an attempt to counteract hypotension caused by decreased peripheral vascular resistance. Concomitant use of glucocorticoids to enhance fetal lung maturation may further contribute to salt and water retention, because of their mineralocorticoid effects. However, pulmonary artery catheterization data have documented an elevated pulmonary capillary wedge pressure in only one patient [96], normal pressures in another [95], and normal pressures after administration of furosemide and morphine sulfate in three others [97]. Several patients improved without diuretic therapy [95], whereas in others improvement was associated with diuresis [96,98].

The possibility of direct myocardial toxicity was raised by the finding of myocardial changes in patients with pheochromocytoma and the known chronotropic and inotropic effects of these beta-adrenergic agents [98]. However, this possibility has not been supported by any pathologic correlation in patients receiving beta-adrenergic tocolytic therapy. In addition, echocardiograms in two patients showed no evidence of left ventricular dysfunction [96], and cardiac output values have not shown decreased left ventricular function [97]. In one patient, however, cardiac output was 6.0 liters per minute, which is relatively low for 1 hour postpartum [97].

Reduction in colloid osmotic pressure alone seems unlikely, because the few measurements that have been taken have not revealed any greater decrease than would be expected with bed rest alone. Increased permeability pulmonary edema was suggested by the findings of a normal pulmonary capillary wedge pressure in some [96,97], but why beta-adrenergic agents would cause increased capillary permeability is not known. The rapid improvement associated with discontinuation of therapy seen in some patients contradicts the hypothesis that increased permeability is the predominant mechanism. A small increase in capillary permeability could result in a large transudation of fluid when accompanied by increased hydrostatic pressures caused by relative volume overload and a slightly reduced colloid osmotic pressure. Nevertheless, the pathogenetic mechanism remains unknown.

PNEUMOMEDIASTINUM AND PNEUMOTHORAX. Pneumomediastinum is another rare complication of pregnancy. Estimates of incidence range from 1 in 2000 to 1 in 100,000 patients [99]. It occurs most commonly in the second stage of labor and is associated with chest or shoulder pain that radiates to the neck and arms, mild dyspnea, and subcutaneous emphysema. Prolonged, dysfunctional labor seems to be a predisposing factor, although frequently no predisposing factor is identified. Of the reported cases in pregnancy, only one patient required decompression of the mediastinum for treatment of venous obstruction.

Spontaneous pneumothorax with tension may occur with or without associated pneumomediastinum. It occurs rarely during pregnancy but should be considered in the differential diagnosis of respiratory failure during pregnancy.

Diagnostic Testing

RADIOLOGY. Evaluation of patients with respiratory failure usually requires at least one, if not sequential, chest radiographs. Potential adverse fetal effects include congenital malformation, intrauterine growth retardation, and increased risk of leukemia and other malignancies [100,101,102]. One report [15] suggested a 1 to 3 percent increase in the risk of congenital anomalies associated with a pelvic radiation exposure of 5 to 10 rad during the first trimester. Other studies have concluded that no appreciable increased risk of gross congenital abnormalities or intrauterine growth retardation exists with exposure to less than 5 to 10 rads [15,99]. The risk of childhood leukemia before age 10 in children whose mothers underwent pelvimetry is increased from 1 in every 3000 children in the general population to 1 in every 2000 [100,102]. The overall risk of any adverse effect from exposure to 1 rad is estimated to be 0.1 percent when the greatest reported oncogenic risk is included. To put radiation risk to the fetus in perspective, the natural risk of intrauterine growth retardation is 2 to 3 percent, which increases to 4 to 6 percent when maternal smoking is a factor and to 30 to 50 percent when chronic alcohol consumption is a factor [99]. The risk of developmental anomalies in otherwise normal pregnancies is approximately 2 to 4 percent [103]. Based on this assessment of relative risks, fetal exposure to less than 5 rad is considered insufficient reason to recommend termination of a desired pregnancy [15,100,101,104].

A posteroanterior chest radiograph exposes the lungs to 10 to 30 mrad and the female gonads to 5 mrad. Careful shielding of the abdomen reduces this. Thus, portable chest radiographs performed daily for 2 weeks to assess location of endotracheal tubes and central venous catheters as well as response of the underlying illness to treatment would expose the fetus to about 70 mrad. Chest fluoroscopy has been estimated to expose the fetus to 70 mrad, although this obviously varies with the operator, shielding, and reason for fluoroscopy [15]. Pulmonary angiography using the brachial route with abdominal shielding should result in a fetal absorbed dose of less than 0.05 rad [101].

Estimates of fetal radiation exposure during perfusion lung scanning with ^{99m}Tc macroaggregated albumin are 0.018 rad with 3 mCi and 0.006 rad with 1 mCi [105]. Although the biologic effects of this type of radiation on the fetus are not known, the risk seems acceptable when compared with the increased risk of prematurity and stillbirth attributed to long-term heparin anticoagulation [106].

HEMODYNAMIC MONITORING. Cardiopulmonary monitoring in critically ill patients has advanced rapidly since the introduction of flow-directed pulmonary artery catheters in 1970 [107–112]. Although the vast majority of pregnancies and deliveries proceed well without invasive monitoring, Berkowitz and Rafferty [109] estimated that at an active referral obstetric hospital the management of approximately 70 patients each year would be markedly improved by monitoring central pressures using pulmonary artery catheterization. This estimate seems high, but it suggests a growing utilization of central hemodynamic monitoring.

Several articles have described in detail how to insert pulmonary artery catheters, how to obtain dependable values for pressures and cardiac output, and how to diminish the risk of complications [110,111,112]. There are no reports of specific complications of pulmonary artery catheterization pertaining to obstetric patients. Presumably, they are at equal risk for reported complications such as hematoma or pneumothorax at the time of insertion, balloon rupture, catheter knotting, pulmonary infarct, pulmonary artery rupture, thrombosis, embolism, arrhythmias, right bundle branch block, valvular damage, and infection (see Chap. 4).

The changes that occur in maternal hemodynamics during pregnancy, labor, and delivery have already been described.

Although cardiac output is quite different during gestation and parturition (Fig. 59-2), normal values for central pressures should not be significantly different for pregnant and nonpregnant patients [15]. However, pulmonary edema may occur at a lower pulmonary capillary wedge pressure, especially in the immediate postpartum period, because of a lower colloid osmotic pressure [16].

Reasonable indications for pulmonary artery catheterization in obstetric patients are the diagnosis or management of septic shock, class 3 and 4 cardiac patients in labor, severe preeclampsia or eclampsia during labor, pulmonary edema that does not quickly respond to diuretic therapy, and pulmonary hypertension in patients in labor and to optimize positive end-expiratory pressure (PEEP) in the adult respiratory distress syndrome.

Because of the complications that may accompany pulmonary artery catheterization, the expense of the procedure, and the lack of formal demonstration of improved morbidity or mortality related to the technique, it has been suggested that more caution be exercised when choosing to proceed with pulmonary artery catheterization [113,114,115]. However, it is also clear that clinical assessment is frequently inadequate to differentiate between cardiogenic and noncardiogenic pulmonary edema in nonobstetric patients [116,117]. The task does not appear any easier in obstetric patients, because both increased permeability pulmonary edema and pulmonary edema caused by volume overload are common causes of respiratory failure in pregnancy. In addition, careful hemodynamic management is needed to maintain adequate uterine blood flow in compromised patients. Obviously, maintaining a good risk-to-benefit ratio depends on obtaining accurate information, interpreting this information in the context of the stage of pregnancy or labor, and determining the specific situations when the information will contribute significantly to patient management.

FETAL MONITORING. When respiratory failure occurs early in gestation, before fetal viability is assured, and when early delivery is not an option, the best course is to focus on optimizing care for the woman, and not on minute-to-minute variations in fetal heart rate. However, it is reasonable to measure and record a daily fetal heart rate to document that the fetus is alive. When able, the woman can report whether fetal movement is present. If respiratory failure persists for several weeks, fetal growth measurement by ultrasound may be indicated. When gestation has progressed enough for delivery by cesarean section, amniocentesis may be helpful to determine fetal maturity [118]. Continuous external fetal heart rate monitoring may be helpful during surgical procedures to alert the anesthesiologist to problems with maternal ventilation or cardiac output [119,120]. More detailed information about fetal monitoring has been published elsewhere [118,121].

Treatment

SUPPORTIVE THERAPY. Mechanical ventilation, nutritional support, and maintaining an adequate blood pressure are important considerations in respiratory insufficiency during pregnancy.

Mechanical Ventilation. The guidelines for intubation and mechanical ventilation are essentially the same for pregnant patients as for nonpregnant patients: (1) inability to maintain a minimal PaO$_2$ of 60 to 65 mm Hg with supplemental oxygen,

(2) uncompensated respiratory acidosis, and (3) inability to clear secretions and need to protect the airway because of altered mental status (see Chaps. 1 and 66).

Intubation of pregnant patients differs only slightly from that of nonpregnant patients [122]. One difference is that hyperemia associated with pregnancy can narrow the upper airway sufficiently that patients are at increased risk for upper airway trauma during intubation [14], and relatively small (interior diameter >6–7 mm) endotracheal tubes may be required. Nasotracheal intubation should probably be avoided because of upper airway narrowing.

The decreased functional residual capacity in pregnancy [14] may lower the oxygen reserve such that at the time of intubation a short period of apnea may be associated with a precipitous decrease in PaO_2 [14]. Therefore, before any attempt at endotracheal intubation, 100 percent oxygen should be administered, either by mask when the patient is able to ventilate spontaneously or by hand resuscitation bag when the patient requires assisted ventilation. However, overenthusiastic hyperventilation to increase the PaO_2 before intubation should be avoided, because the associated respiratory alkalosis may actually decrease uterine blood flow. During assisted ventilation and intubation, cricoid pressure with the head and neck extended can help decrease gastric inflation and prevent regurgitation into the hypopharynx [122].

Initiating mechanical ventilation follows the same general principles for pregnant patients as for nonpregnant patients [123] (see Chap. 66). In general, the minute ventilation should be adjusted to aim for a $PaCO_2$ of 30 to 32 mm Hg, the normal level in pregnancy. Respiratory rate and tidal volume may be increased when oxygenation is a problem, but marked respiratory alkalosis should be avoided because of the resultant decrease in uterine blood flow. When only small increases in the fraction of inspired oxygen are necessary (<40%), it is reasonable to aim for the usual gestational PaO_2 of greater than 95 mm Hg.

In patients with asthma, respiratory rate and tidal volume should be no greater than necessary to maintain oxygenation. Lower respiratory rates and tidal volumes help reduce airway pressures, thereby reducing barotrauma [123]. Inspiratory flow rates can be increased to allow adequate time for expiration. Increasing the inspiratory flow rate decreases the inspiratory-to-expiratory ratio and mitigates air trapping. (See Chaps. 56 and 66 for further discussion of mechanical ventilatory support of the asthmatic.)

In patients with acute respiratory distress syndrome (ARDS) who require a fraction of inspired oxygen greater than 50 percent to maintain a PaO_2 of 65 mm Hg or greater or an oxygen saturation greater than 90 percent, consideration should be given to adding PEEP. As in nonpregnant patients, the goals are to reduce FIO_2 to less than 50 percent, if possible, and to maintain adequate oxygen delivery without compromising cardiac output or risking further lung damage caused by excess intraalveolar pressure [124] (see Chap. 55).

When fluid is required to support cardiac output, blood products are preferred, especially if the hematocrit is less than 30 percent [124]. Blood cell transfusion should help improve oxygen-carrying capacity and limit further leakage of fluid through leaky capillaries associated with crystalloid administration [124]. However, increasing the hematocrit over 38 percent may actually decrease oxygen delivery because of increased blood viscosity [124]. Albumin infusion may increase extravascular lung water because it equilibrates with the extravascular space within hours, causing an increase in tissue oncotic pressure that potentiates further extravasation of fluid. Hetastarch and dextran are more likely to remain intravascular, but both have adverse effects on clotting and should not be used peripartum.

Dextran can also cause anaphylaxis in sensitive patients (see Chap. 217).

Lowering oxygen consumption by lowering elevated temperature and suppressing spontaneous respiration is also helpful. Temperature regulation may be particularly important during gestation, because an increased rate of congenital malformations has been associated with maternal fever, especially during the first few months of pregnancy [104,125]. Sedation and muscle paralysis, when indicated, are best accomplished with morphine sulfate and pancuronium bromide [126], which appear to be without adverse fetal effects except when used at the time of delivery or when used excessively, as in narcotic addiction [127]. Whether benzodiazepine use results in an increased risk of cleft lip remains controversial, so this class of drugs is best avoided until more definite data are available [128].

Although sitting is usually the most advantageous position for weaning nonpregnant patients from mechanical ventilation, in patients near term it may result in inferior vena cava compression, and the lateral decubitus position is preferable. Weaning parameters for pregnant patients are not well established, but it seems reasonable to follow the same guidelines as for nonpregnant patients (see Chap. 67) [129].

Nutrition. The importance of adequate nutrition during gestation is well recognized in that maternal weight gain correlates with fetal weight gain and a successful outcome. In addition, maternal malnutrition has been shown to correlate in certain cases with intrauterine growth retardation and development of preeclampsia [130]. It is also well recognized that hospitalized patients suffering from prolonged starvation have greater problems with wound healing and that diminished protein stores are associated with increased susceptibility to infection [131].

Problems remain in assessing the degree of nutritional depletion and the resting and stressed energy requirements in an individual patient, as well as in determining the best proportions of fat, glucose, branched-chain amino acids, and essential amino acids [131–136]. These questions are even less understood in obstetric patients, but until further studies are done it seems reasonable in most cases to follow the suggestions for nonobstetric patients.

Animal studies have shown that during starvation the mother is favored over the fetus and that this preferential trend continues with refeeding [130]. In humans, it appears true as well that maternal body stores are protected at the expense of fetal growth during semistarvation [130]. The duration of starvation or semistarvation that can be tolerated without ill effects on the fetus is unknown. In animal models, protein restriction begun immediately after conception results in diminished expansion of plasma volume, which may result in decreased placental blood flow and abnormal fetal development [130]. Significant growth restriction occurring before 26 weeks' gestation is more likely to lead to permanent stunting of brain growth and clear neurologic impairment than later growth restriction [130].

Thus, in critically ill obstetric patients, nutritional support is important for both maternal and fetal outcome (see Chaps. 200, 201, and 202). As with nonobstetric patients, enteral nutrition is preferred over parenteral nutrition to avoid the risk of complications associated with central venous catheters, to reduce expense, and to minimize gastric mucosal atrophy [134,136]. The various methods of tube placement and choices of enteric diet formulation have been reviewed for nonobstetric patients [136]. One caveat is that pregnancy is associated with decreased lower esophageal sphincter tone and decreased gastric motility; therefore nasoduodenal tubes are preferred over nasogastric tubes to decrease the likelihood of reflux and aspiration.

Several case reports have described successful implementation of total parenteral nutrition (TPN) in patients whose pregnancies were complicated by inflammatory bowel disease [137], prolonged hyperemesis gravidarum [130], and postoperative ileus [130]. Given the stress of respiratory failure and its underlying causes, it seems reasonable to extend this experience with TPN to patients with respiratory failure who will be unable to eat for more than a couple of days and whose gastrointestinal system cannot be used. The methods of catheter placement have been described by other authors [134,135].

Because TPN has been used only in a small number of pregnancies, much is still unknown about optimal concentrations of carbohydrates, amino acids, and fat. Animal studies suggest that when fat emulsions provide greater than 50 percent of caloric intake, fatty infiltration of the placenta and premature uterine contractions may occur [130]. When the amount of fat was decreased to 20 percent of total caloric intake, neither of these occurred [130,137]. Pulmonary fat infiltration has been noted in neonates receiving TPN but not in infants of mothers receiving TPN [130]. Use of fat emulsions to provide 20 percent of total calories seems reasonable based on these observations, on maternal requirements for essential fatty acids, and on fetal need for linoleic acid [130]. Fat is also considered the favored energy source in sepsis [134,135]. An excess of carbohydrates may hamper weaning because of increased carbon dioxide production, resulting in increased respiratory work to eliminate the carbon dioxide [138]. Thus, within limits the carbohydrate-to-fat ratio should be kept low in patients with weaning difficulties.

Although some case reports have described using caloric intakes that surpassed the Recommended Daily Allowance, the question has been raised whether this will lead to fetal side effects similar to those seen in infants of diabetic mothers [130]. Further study is needed to explore this question and to determine whether cyclic hyperalimentation would be preferable. Vitamins should probably be replaced according to the Recommended Daily Allowances for pregnancy [130].

Blood glucose levels should be measured frequently at first, then once or twice weekly, along with serum electrolyte concentrations and renal and hepatic function. Measurement of trace element concentrations is needed for prolonged TPN. Periodic nutritional assessment should include evaluation of nitrogen balance, lymphocyte counts, transferrin, maternal weight, and fetal growth by ultrasound. If delivery occurs while the woman is receiving TPN, the neonate should be observed closely for hypoglycemia.

Reversal of Hypotension. Supine recumbency may cause a significant decrease in venous return in women in their second or third trimesters. To counteract this, the right hip should be elevated 10 to 15 cm (15 degrees) to move the uterus off the inferior vena cava, or the lateral decubitus position should be used. As a corollary to this, if patients in the second or third trimester become hypotensive, placing them in the Trendelenburg position is unlikely to help and may actually decrease venous return because of vena cava compression.

When hypotension does not respond to reduction of uterine pressure on the vena cava or fluid resuscitation, vasopressor therapy is indicated. The ideal vasopressor would restore maternal blood pressure without compromising uterine blood flow. Ephedrine, which has both alpha- and beta-stimulating effects, tends to preserve uterine blood flow while reversing systemic hypotension [139]. Although metaraminol restores uterine blood flow when used to treat hypotension during spinal anesthesia [139], it decreases uterine blood flow in normotensive pregnant ewes. Therefore, it may not be an ideal vasopressor for hypotension during human pregnancy. Isoproterenol and other predominantly beta-adrenergic drugs de-

crease mean maternal blood pressure and uterine blood flow [139]. Predominantly alpha-adrenergic agents, such as norepinephrine, improve maternal blood pressure but decrease uterine blood flow because of uterine artery vasoconstriction. If maternal hypotension remains refractory, drugs with more alpha-adrenergic activity, such as epinephrine, norepinephrine, and dopamine, which do not preserve uterine blood flow, should be tried [139]. Dobutamine may also be added for life-threatening maternal hypotension when pulmonary artery pressure and cardiac output values indicate it is appropriate. Improvement in blood pressure may also follow reversal of lactic acidosis by bicarbonate administration. This therapy should be guided by arterial blood gas values.

SPECIFIC THERAPY

Thromboembolism. When massive pulmonary embolism is strongly suspected (greater than 50% occlusion of pulmonary vascular bed or systemic hypotension), the major immediate goals of therapy are to (1) provide adequate oxygenation as dictated by arterial blood gas analysis, (2) treat hypotension and organ hypoperfusion by elevating right ventricular preload with colloid or crystalloid administration and vasopressor therapy if necessary, and (3) interrupt clot propagation by immediate anticoagulation with intravenous heparin. Heparinization should be instituted immediately in all patients without clear contraindications, such as active bleeding, rather than delay therapy pending conclusive diagnostic studies. In patients without a detectable blood pressure or pulse, closed chest compression may break up large proximal pulmonary emboli, thus improving pulmonary perfusion and reducing right ventricular afterload, which may restore adequate circulation (see Chap. 60). In patients with massive and submassive pulmonary embolic disease and no contraindication to anticoagulation, heparin is the initial drug of choice. Because heparin does not cross the placenta, it is not teratogenic. Fetal and maternal outcomes in heparin-treated patients are similar to outcomes in the normal population when the contribution of comorbid conditions is accounted for [140,141].

When hemodynamic and angiographic information is available for patients with massive pulmonary embolism, it must be decided whether thrombolytic therapy or embolectomy is indicated and whether inferior vena cava interruption is indicated to provide immediate and reliable prophylaxis against recurrent thromboembolism. Because large studies have failed to document that thrombolytic therapy results in any significant improvement in mortality or morbidity compared with heparinization, it is not indicated for submassive pulmonary embolism [142,143]. However, in patients with massive pulmonary embolism and significant hemodynamic compromise despite vasopressor therapy, it is appropriate to consider thrombolytic therapy as an alternative to pulmonary endarterectomy [142,143]. Specific circumstances for which thrombolytic therapy might be preferable include (1) lack of immediate availability of surgery and cardiopulmonary bypass, (2) emboli that are inaccessible to the surgeon without dissection of the lung parenchyma, (3) absence of large vessel puncture sites, and (4) surgery that would increase the risk of bleeding (see Chap. 60). One problem with instituting thrombolytic therapy is that if it is unsuccessful in achieving clot lysis sufficient to improve the hemodynamic function, subsequent endarterectomy may be impossible because of the lytic state. Obviously, endarterectomy, associated with a 30 percent mortality rate in nonpregnant patients, is not an easy choice (see Chap. 60).

Pregnancy and the immediate postpartum state are relative contraindications to thrombolytic therapy because of the risk of hemorrhage during labor, delivery, and the first several days postpartum [144,145]. However, streptokinase was used successfully in 24 pregnant patients with deep venous thrombosis and pulmonary embolism [146]. These patients received streptokinase for varying lengths of time (36 hours to 5 days) with no significant hemorrhage and with delivery of normal infants. Patients in each of the trimesters were included, but none of the patients were receiving streptokinase at the time of parturition. Animal studies suggest that minimal amounts of streptokinase, if any, cross the placenta to enter the fetal circulation [146]. Peripartum use of streptokinase for massive pulmonary embolism with hemodynamic collapse resulted in persistent uterine hemorrhage following vaginal delivery [147]. Hemorrhage was finally controlled with discontinuation of streptokinase, infusion of oxytocin and ergometrine, uterine massage, and a dose of aminocaproic acid. It was suggested that thrombolytic therapy contributed to uterine atony, thus slowing labor and causing excessive uterine bleeding. There is no published experience on the use of tissue plasminogen activator in pregnancy.

If thrombolytic therapy with streptokinase or urokinase is used during pregnancy, it seems reasonable to limit the duration of therapy to the time needed for restoration of acceptable hemodynamic function, to discontinue therapy at least 4 to 6 hours antepartum, and to use continuous uterine massage and methylergonovine maleate postpartum if thrombolytic therapy was only recently discontinued. Because aminocaproic acid crosses the placenta readily and is teratogenic, aprotinin (Trasylol), which does not cross the placenta, should be used when rapid reversal of the lytic state is needed before delivery [147]. Cryoprecipitate can also be used and is preferred over fresh frozen plasma [145].

Monitoring the lytic state is complicated because clot lysis and risk of bleeding do not correlate well with laboratory measurement of the lytic state [143]. The activated partial thromboplastin time, prothrombin time, thrombin time, or fibrinogen levels can be used to document presence of a lytic state [145]. The first two values help document the lytic state but are not helpful in guiding dosage. Doses of thrombolytic agents should be adjusted to maintain the thrombin time at a value less than 5 times the normal value [145]. Difficulty in attaining a lytic state with streptokinase may be due to the presence of antistreptococcal antibodies. In this situation, urokinase should be substituted. Administration of heparin should follow thrombolysis in all patients. After discontinuing streptokinase or urokinase, heparin therapy should be delayed until the activated thromboplastin time is less than 2 times the normal value [145].

Inferior vena cava interruption should be strongly considered in any patient with cardiopulmonary compromise caused by pulmonary embolus who does not receive thrombolytic therapy and in those who have a contraindication to heparin or recurrent emboli despite heparin anticoagulation. The best method now available is transvenous placement of a vena cava filter, which has a long-term patency rate greater than 95 percent (see Chap. 60).

Once the patient has been stabilized and has received 7 to 10 days of heparin by continuous intravenous infusion, heparin should be administered subcutaneously in doses adjusted to prolong the aPTT to 1.5 to 2.5 times control when measured 6 hours after a dose of heparin [148]. Anticoagulant therapy should be continued throughout pregnancy and for an additional 4 to 6 weeks postpartum [148]. If the pulmonary embolism occurs late in pregnancy or in the postpartum period, anticoagulant therapy should be continued for at least 3 months [148], perhaps longer if impedance plethysmography or venous duplex studies remain abnormal.

Amniotic Fluid Embolism. Treatment of amniotic fluid embolism is currently limited to supportive measures aimed at providing adequate ventilation and oxygenation, blood pressure support, and management of bleeding.

Most patients require intubation and mechanical ventilation. Positive end-expiratory pressure has seemed helpful for oxygenation in some patients [41,42]. Currently, no particular drug regimen has been used with any clear success to reverse pulmonary hypertension. If pulmonary capillary wedge pressures are elevated, it seems reasonable to use a diuretic to reduce hydrostatic pressures across the injured capillary endothelium. Measurement of changes in cardiac output can be used to guide this.

In addition to fluid resuscitation to reverse hypotension, vasopressor therapy is frequently required. Ephedrine should be tried first (see Supportive Therapy). If this fails, isoproterenol [39] and dopamine [41] should be used, both of which have been used with success.

Treatment of coagulopathy is likewise nonspecific. Some authors favor early use of heparin because it was associated with survival in a few cases [149]. More recent case reports have noted survival without heparin infusion [37,42,44]. For active bleeding, transfusion with fresh frozen plasma, cryoprecipitate, and platelets is indicated. Also important are reduction of uterine bleeding by manual massage, oxytocin infusion, and, when necessary, methylergonovine maleate therapy. When uterine bleeding is refractory to these interventions, exploration for uterine tears or retained placenta should be considered.

Venous Air Embolism. When venous air embolism is suspected, certain specific therapies should be instituted promptly. Placing the patient in the left lateral decubitus position has been helpful in some cases by causing the bubble of air to migrate away from the right ventricular outflow tract [49]. Closed chest cardiac compression has also been reported to be helpful [49]. Aspiration of air from the right atrium, right ventricle, or pulmonary outflow tract can be attempted with a central venous or pulmonary artery catheter [49]. Air emboli that have migrated into the pulmonary vasculature can be decreased in size by ventilating the patient with 100 percent oxygen to facilitate removal of nitrogen, which may comprise as much as 80 percent of the embolus. When air embolism occurs during general anesthesia, nitrous oxide should be discontinued, because it has a high solubility and tends to increase the size of air bubbles in the pulmonary vasculature [49].

Use of anticoagulation with heparin has been suggested in the treatment of fibrin microemboli [49]. High doses of corticosteroids administered at the time of air embolism or immediately thereafter have been shown to decrease pulmonary edema formation in sheep [53]. In theory, corticosteroids might prevent some of the inflammatory reaction caused by oxygen radicals. Whether this will be clinically useful is not known. Hyperbaric oxygen therapy, if readily available, has also been proposed [48].

Aspiration of Gastric Contents. Prophylactic antibiotics have not been found to be beneficial [150] in aspiration pneumonitis; rather, antibiotics should be prescribed only when infection complicates the initial chemical pneumonitis. If the patient's clinical course suggests development of bacterial pneumonia, the choice of antibiotic should be guided by appropriate bacteriologic evaluation of respiratory secretions, pleural fluid (if present), and blood cultures. For patients who have been in the hospital for 48 hours or less, either penicillin or cefuroxime is a reasonable empiric choice. Most recent studies have not supported an ameliorative role for corticosteroids [151,152] despite early anecdotal suggestions of success [153]. Lung lavage with normal saline or alkaline solutions is not helpful and may worsen the patient's condition [155].

Respiratory Infections. Antibacterial agents to treat pneumonia during pregnancy should be selected according to the same principles used for nonpregnant patients [63]; however, consideration should be given to choosing drugs with the least risk to the fetus and woman (see Chap. 85). The following comments about antibiotic safety are derived from a recent review [155].

For community-acquired pneumonias in pregnancy, penicillins and erythromycin (excluding the estolate that is associated with an increased risk of cholestatic jaundice in pregnancy) are probably safe. Tetracycline is contraindicated because it is teratogenic and causes hepatic toxicity when administered intravenously in pregnancy. The aminoglycosides have the potential of causing eighth nerve toxicity in the fetus and should be used only when strong clinical indications exist. Serum drug levels should then be monitored closely. Sulfonamides are considered contraindicated at term because of the risk of neonatal kernicterus. Clindamycin has no reported adverse fetal effects, but experience is limited and it should be used with caution. Vancomycin hydrochloride may cause fetal renal and auditory toxicity and should be used with caution, following careful monitoring of serum drug levels.

For specific treatment of respiratory failure as a result of influenza pneumonia, most effective is prevention by vaccination of women during the second trimester if their second or third trimester is likely to coincide with the influenza season. The influenza vaccine is made from inactivated virus and thus is considered safe after the first trimester (excluding recipients who are allergic to eggs) [70,71,156]. Amantadine hydrochloride interferes with replication and shedding of influenza A virions, thus limiting spread of the virus within the respiratory tract [71]. It has also been shown to hasten resolution of symptoms and small airway dysfunction [156]. Amantadine use in pregnancy has not been studied in humans; it was teratogenic in rats at 12 but not 9 times the recommended human dose [157]. Rabbits were unaffected when 25 times the human dose was administered. Thus, the use of amantadine during pregnancy should probably be limited to patients with evidence of influenza pneumonia or unvaccinated patients with other significant respiratory impairment and influenza A infection. The usual dose is 200 mg per day; mild central nervous system toxicity can be limited by using a split-dosage schedule [71]. Supportive therapy should follow the same guidelines as outlined for other causes of respiratory failure in pregnancy.

The antiviral agents vidarabine and acyclovir have been demonstrated to be effective in treating primary and reactivation cases of varicella-zoster in immunocompromised children and adults [157,158]. A patient suffering from varicella pneumonia who developed rapidly progressive respiratory failure at 21 weeks' gestation was treated in our hospital with intravenous acyclovir and mechanical ventilation with PEEP, with good maternal and fetal outcome. New vesicle formation stopped 72 hours after initiation of acyclovir, and extubation was successfully accomplished on day 16. A normal infant was delivered at term. In an animal study of acyclovir, no teratogenicity, embryotoxicity, or increased incidence of fetal malformations was noted [159]. Similar results have been reported with acyclovir used in other pregnant patients with varicella [160,161]. Impairment of renal function as a result of accumulation of acyclovir in the renal collecting system has been noted in inadequately hydrated patients [162]. Therefore, good urine output should be maintained and the dose of acyclovir adjusted for any fall in creatinine clearance. The importance of early initiation of acyclovir and vidarabine to ensure a favorable outcome has been stressed [158,162]. Thus, it seems reasonable to initiate acyclovir at the first evidence of respiratory system involvement in pregnant patients with cutaneous varicella infection. Infants born to women who developed varicella infection within 4 days of delivery should receive zoster immune globulin within 72 hours of birth [160].

Amphotericin B remains the drug of choice for severe disseminated coccidioidal infections, although ketoconazole has shown promise in the treatment of chronic progressive coccidioidal pneumonia. Amphotericin B has been used with success in pregnancy [77]. It has been shown to cross the placenta and to be present in umbilical cord serum at concentrations one-third that of maternal serum concentrations. However, it does not appear to have an adverse effect on fetal development; normal, full-term infants have been born to women who received amphotericin B during the first trimester as well as later in gestation. Because anemia often occurs during the course of amphotericin B therapy, blood cell counts and renal function should be monitored closely. Ketoconazole has not yet been studied in pregnancy but is known to be teratogenic when given to rats in high doses. Its use should therefore be reserved for cases in which amphotericin B cannot be used because of hypersensitivity or nephrotoxicity. Although placental involvement is common in disseminated disease, fetal infection is reportedly rare, so successful treatment of the mother should be associated with good fetal outcome [77].

Active tuberculosis has been treated with modern chemotherapeutic agents with excellent maternal and fetal outcome. Because the most extensive experience has been with isoniazid and ethambutol, these agents should be used preferentially in pregnancy unless there is risk of isoniazid resistance [4]. Rifampin does cross the placenta, so it should be used with caution until more data are available [78]. Streptomycin has been associated with fetal hearing loss and vestibular dysfunction and should be avoided [78]. Little is known about the specific effects of the other antituberculosis agents in pregnancy, except that ethionamide has been identified as a teratogen [54] (see Chap. 95).

Treatment of PCP during pregnancy includes trimethoprim-sulfamethoxazole (TMP-SMX), as well as corticosteroids if the oxygen saturation is less than 90 percent [163]. Two neonates born to women receiving TMP-SMX for PCP [81] and a third neonate born approximately 1 month after the mother completed a course of TMP-SMX [82] did not appear to have any adverse consequences from that medication.

For *Listeria*-associated pneumonia in pregnancy, prompt treatment with penicillin has been associated with a favorable outcome [86]. Penicillin G and ampicillin are the recommended antibiotics for *Listeria* infections, although sensitivity of the organism to erythromycin and cephalothin has also been reported [164].

Asthma. The first priority of therapy for pregnant women with asthma is to prevent or reverse the hypoxemia that to some degree accompanies virtually every exacerbation of asthma. Because hypoxemia may worsen initially when bronchodilator therapy is instituted, oxygen should be used in all asthmatic patients who present to the hospital with exacerbation [165].

The three groups of drugs that are most effective in reversing acute asthmatic attacks are beta-adrenergic agents, methylxanthines, and corticosteroids. Despite the lack of adequate, well-controlled studies delineating the ideal pharmacotherapy of severe exacerbations of asthma during pregnancy, the consensus is that these agents should be used in pregnant asthmatics as in nonpregnant asthmatics [85a] (see Chap. 56). One protocol for emergency room management suggests epinephrine 0.3 ml of a 1:1000 solution subcutaneously, repeated twice with concomitant administration of theophylline and corticosteroids [89,90]. Epinephrine is suggested because of the long experience with it in pregnancy and its efficacy [89,90]. However, one of these studies [90] found a greater incidence of infants with low birth weight and small size for gestational age in women whose asthma had required such emergency treatment. The other study [89] had a smaller sample size (28 vs. 56 pregnancies) and did not find this association. If this association is true, it remains unclear whether it was the nature of the treatment or a consequence of the exacerbation itself. Epinephrine has also been reported to decrease uterine blood flow in animals [85,139] and to result in an increase in human fetal malformations when given in the first trimester [5,85]; however it is unknown whether the fetal malformations were due to epinephrine or comorbid conditions.

An alternative approach is to use the more selective beta-agonists, which have the theoretic advantage of not decreasing uterine flow unless there is a decrease in maternal systemic vascular resistance. In addition, the effects of inhaled agents are predominantly local, which should decrease the amount of fetal exposure. Terbutaline is the only beta$_2$-agonist with a pregnancy category B rating (Alupent and epinephrine are category C); it was not teratogenic in rodents at 42 times the recommended human dose [166]. Category B is defined as no evidence of risk in humans: either animal studies show a risk but human studies do not, or, if no adequate human studies have been done, animal studies are negative. Category C includes drugs for which a risk in humans cannot be ruled out: human studies are lacking and animal studies are either positive or lacking. Parenteral terbutaline has also been used as a tocolytic agent without evidence of specific adverse fetal effect. However, it carries the risk of hypokalemia and pulmonary edema if used at high doses for more than 24 to 48 hours (see Tocolytic Therapy). Metaproterenol sulfate has been found to be teratogenic in rats and mice, but not rabbits, at doses many times greater than recommended for humans. However, inhaled metaproterenol sulfate does not significantly increase the incidence of congenital malformation, preterm birth, low birth weight, or small size for gestational age [167]. Studies in nonpregnant asthmatics have shown inhaled beta$_2$-adrenergic agents to be as effective as epinephrine in terms of rapidity and degree of reversal of airflow obstruction [168], with the advantage of decreased cardiovascular side effects. On the other hand, some patients who become refractory to inhaled nebulized metaproterenol sulfate respond to a 0.3 ml subcutaneous injection of 1:1000 solution epinephrine [169]. At this point, reasonable therapy of acute asthma in pregnancy could include inhaled nebulized metaproterenol sulfate, subcutaneous terbutaline, or subcutaneous epinephrine.

In addition, intravenous theophylline can be given. This recommendation is based on long-published experience in humans [11,85,89,90,170], despite theophylline's listing as a category C drug. Since theophylline toxicity can develop in the fetus when theophylline is administered at the time of delivery [170], serum levels should be kept below 15 μg/ml to avoid this. Theophylline dosing is similar to the usual nonpregnant adult dosing: no loading dose if a patient is already on maintenance therapy, otherwise an intravenous loading dose of 5.6 mg per kilogram lean pregnant body weight up to a maximum of 400 mg over 20 to 30 minutes [5]. Maintenance infusion is usually 0.5 mg/kg/hr. Concurrent cimetidine, viral infection, liver disease, heart disease, or erythromycin dictates a downward adjustment to 0.3 mg/kg/hr, and smoking or adolescence dictates an upward adjustment to 0.7 mg/kg/hr. Clearly, serum levels should be closely followed. During the second and third trimesters, the volume of distribution and half-life both increase, but clearance remains unchanged [171], suggesting that the dosage on a milligram per kilogram basis should remain constant but the total dose would increase as weight increases. Presumably, the proportion of weight gain due to increased blood

volume and uterine-fetal weight compared with fat would have to be considered.

Prednisone and prednisolone cross the placenta poorly, and few if any untoward fetal effects can be attributed to maternal steroid treatment [11,85,90]. The increased prevalence of spontaneous abortions, placental insufficiency, and cleft palate found in rodents given corticosteroids during gestation has not been substantiated in humans [11,85,90].

Institution of corticosteroids should be rapid to help reverse airflow obstruction and thereby decrease the amount of high-dose beta-adrenergic therapy needed. One study suggests that the onset of action may be more rapid [172] than previously appreciated [173]. A high-dose regimen of intravenous methylprednisolone (125 mg every 6 hours) is recommended because it is associated with more rapid improvement in pulmonary function than lower-dose regimens [174].

For patients who are extremely difficult to manage even with therapeutic levels of bronchodilators, high-dose corticosteroids, and mechanical ventilation, a few less-studied therapeutic interventions can be considered. These include controlled hypoventilation [175], intravenous isoproterenol [176], magnesium sulfate [177], and inhaled halothane [178]. None have been studied in pregnancy, so their use should be limited to situations where the woman's life is in danger and all other forms of therapy have failed. For a full discussion see Chapter 56.

Intravenous infusion of isoproterenol has been used successfully in children with severe status asthmaticus [176]; its use in adults has been more limited because of the concern of increased risk of cardiac arrhythmias. Experience with isoproterenol in pregnancy is limited: there are no known teratogenic effects of isoproterenol in humans, but it does decrease uterine blood flow. All other parenteral sympathomimetics should be stopped while intravenous isoproterenol is used [176]. Theophylline levels may fall during isoproterenol infusion and rise with discontinuation of isoproterenol. A pulmonary artery catheter should be in place for management because of the association in pregnancy of pulmonary edema and beta-adrenergic tocolytic therapy, particularly after 24 to 48 hours of intravenous therapy (see Beta-Adrenergic Tocolytic Therapy). Patients should also be monitored for hypoglycemia and fetal tachycardia.

Intravenous magnesium sulfate has been shown to have a bronchodilating effect in asthma, although not as potent an effect as albuteral [177]. It may be a helpful adjunct in the treatment of refractory asthma. A reasonable dose is 0.615 mM per minute (3 gm over 20 minutes) [177]. Magnesium sulfate has been used extensively in pregnancy for treatment of pre-eclampsia and as a tocolytic agent and should have a similar safety profile when used to treat asthma in pregnancy.

Some of the inhalational anesthetics have a bronchodilator effect and have occasionally been used in life-threatening refractory asthma. Halothane, for instance, has been reported to diminish refractory bronchospasm [178]. Its use has been recommended in patients requiring general anesthesia for cesarean section because it does not appear to affect neonatal neurobehavior [180]. It does have a myocardial depressant effect that may limit its use in pregnant women with cardiac disease. Arrhythmias have also been reported in patients with abnormal arterial blood gas values and/or ongoing sympathomimetic therapy.

Once a pregnant woman reaches this point of life-threatening refractory asthma, emergent delivery of the fetus by cesarean section should be considered. Obviously, this is a difficult decision that is in part dependent on the age and viability of the fetus. Topilsky and colleagues [180] reported a case of dramatic abatement in bronchospasm 12 hours after removal of a stillborn fetus from a 22-year-old primigravida whose condition had been deteriorating despite treatment with mechanical ventilation and high-dose steroids. Whether this dramatic response to delivery of a stillborn would also apply to live infants is not known. Depending on the gestational age of the fetus, emergent delivery might be a reasonable consideration.

Pneumomediastinum and Pneumothorax. Pneumomediastinum does not usually require drainage in adults, because the air usually dissects out of the mediastinum into the subcutaneous tissues of the neck. Thus, treatment should be directed at any underlying cause, such as asthma, if present.

A spontaneous pneumothorax occupying less than 20 percent of the hemithorax in an asymptomatic patient not on mechanical ventilation can be monitored closely without immediate insertion of a chest tube. In symptomatic patients, patients on mechanical ventilation, or patients with an enlarging pneumothorax, chest tube placement is mandatory (see Chap. 11). Patients whose pneumothorax develops as a complication of barotrauma during mechanical ventilation require not only chest tube insertion but also adjustments in the ventilator settings to reduce peak airway pressures and further barotrauma [124].

Prevention

THROMBOEMBOLIC DISEASE. Preventing deep venous thrombosis is probably the most important intervention to reduce maternal mortality caused by pulmonary embolism. Patients who require bed rest or surgery during pregnancy should be treated prophylactically with low-dose heparin, 5000 units subcutaneously every 12 hours [31,32] or external pneumatic calf compression [33]. Warfarin crosses the placenta and is teratogenic: it is contraindicated in pregnancy [31]. Heparin does not cross the placenta and appears safe for the fetus [181]. Long-term heparin therapy (>20 weeks) is associated with maternal bone demineralization [182]. External pneumatic calf compression may therefore be preferred but should probably be accompanied by weekly impedance plethysmography or venous duplex studies. Another alternative is pulsatile subcutaneous heparin administration through a portable infusion pump, which resulted in no thromboembolic events or evidence of osteoporosis in a small group of pregnant patients [183].

Patients who are receiving ongoing warfarin therapy for prior thromboembolic disease should be changed to subcutaneous heparin therapy before conception or at least before the sixth week of pregnancy.

Patients with a history of deep venous thrombosis or pulmonary embolism during a prior pregnancy should have some form of surveillance or prophylaxis during subsequent pregnancies [31,148]. Unfortunately, insufficient data exist to help predict the timing of thrombotic events in future pregnancies [148]. Until more definitive data are available, patients should be considered to be at risk for the entire course of subsequent pregnancies [148]. One recommended regimen is to administer 5000 units of heparin subcutaneously every 12 hours during the first and second trimesters, followed in the third trimester by adjusted-dose heparin administered subcutaneously every 12 hours and the dose adjusted to maintain the aPTT at 1.5 to 2.5 times control when measured 4 to 6 hours after injection [141,148,184]. Once the correct dose is identified, aPTTs can be measured weekly or as the patient's condition warrants. Although nonpregnant patients do not require weekly aPTT monitoring, heparin requirements change as pregnancy progresses, so weekly measurements are recommended in pregnancy [31].

The platelet count should also be measured periodically, because some patients develop heparin-induced thrombocytopenia.

In patients receiving subcutaneous heparin prophylaxis during pregnancy, heparin should be withheld at the onset of labor or discontinued with induction of labor 24 hours later [148]. Once adequate hemostasis has been accomplished postpartum, subcutaneous heparin therapy can be resumed and continued until 6 weeks postpartum. Alternatively, warfarin can be added to subcutaneous heparin and the heparin stopped when therapeutic prolongation of the prothrombin time is achieved.

ASPIRATION OF GASTRIC CONTENTS. It seems reasonable to try to reduce the risk of acid aspiration sequelae by prophylactic antacid administration or H_2 blockade in pregnant women who require general anesthesia or analgesic therapy other than local or epidural anesthetics, despite the lack of complete protection achieved with gastric pH values greater than 2.5. Some authors recommend that all women in labor receive nothing by mouth except medications. This should probably be individualized, in view of the low risk of aspiration during spontaneous vaginal delivery in unsedated patients and the small proportion of patients who require emergent general anesthesia. Other preventive measures that have been proposed are the use of regional anesthesia when possible, cuffed endotracheal tubes, and application of cricoid pressure during intubation [55].

BETA-ADRENERGIC TOCOLYTIC THERAPY. A multicenter, randomized study comparing ritodrine to placebo for tocolysis found that ritodrine had no significant beneficial effect on perinatal mortality, frequency of prolongation of pregnancy to term, or birth weight [185]. Alternatively, tocolysis has been achieved with intravenous infusion of magnesium sulfate, yielding a mean serum level of 6.6 mg per deciliter [184]. Side effects appear to be dose-related and include lethargy, diplopia, impaired deep tendon reflexes, depressed respirations, hypocalcemia, and cardiac arrhythmias [186]. If fetal outcome studies confirm that magnesium has a beneficial effect on perinatal mortality, prolongation of pregnancy to term, and birth weight, the ability to monitor serum levels and the reported low incidence of side effects may make magnesium sulfate preferable to beta-adrenergic agents.

When beta-adrenergic agents are used, awareness of certain epidemiologic associations may help prevent pulmonary edema. The epidemiologic factors that may help identify patients at increased risk [97] include longer duration of intravenous beta-adrenergic tocolytic therapy (>24–48 hours), large volume of crystalloid infusion, multiple gestation, concomitant sepsis, and possibly preeclampsia. It seems wise, therefore, to limit at least the intravenous phase of therapy to less than 24 to 48 hours and to adjust the dose to keep the maternal heart rate under 120 beats per minute. The beta-adrenergic agent should be discontinued immediately at the earliest sign of respiratory distress, such as chest pain, tachypnea, and dyspnea. Careful fluid balance records should be maintained, and fluid restriction and possibly diuresis should be considered when intake exceeds output by greater than 500 ml. If supplemental oxygenation, discontinuation of the drug, and gentle diuresis do not result in improvement after one hour, insertion of a pulmonary artery catheter to guide fluid management should be considered.

Patients with underlying cardiac disease, particularly structural defects causing outflow obstruction, should be excluded from beta-adrenergic tocolytic therapy. Patients with multiple gestation should either be excluded or undergo prophylactic pulmonary artery catheterization. Patients with severe preeclampsia would likely benefit more from early delivery than from combining the increased risks of tocolytic therapy with those of continuing pregnancy-induced hypertension.

References

1. United States Public Health Service: Progress toward achieving the 1990 objectives for pregnancy and infant health. *MMWR* 37:405, 1988.

2. Kaunitz AM, Hughes JM, Grimes DA, et al: Causes of maternal mortality in the United States. *Obstet Gynecol* 65:605, 1985.

3. Weinberger SE, Weiss ST, Cohen WR, et al: Pregnancy and the lung. *Am Rev Respir Dis* 121:559, 1980.

4. Gaensler EA, Patton WE, Verstracten JM, et al: Pulmonary function in pregnancy. III. Serial observations in patients with pulmonary insufficiency. *Am Rev Respir Dis* 67:779, 1953.

5. Niederman MS, Matthay RA: Asthma and other severe respiratory diseases during pregnancy, in Berkowitz RL (ed): *Critical Care of the Obstetric Patient*. New York, Churchill Livingstone, 1983, p 355.

6. Novy MJ, Edwards MJ: Respiratory problems in pregnancy. *Am J Obstet Gynecol* 99:1024, 1967.

7. Sullivan JM, Ramanathan: Management of medical problems in pregnancy: Severe cardiac disease. *N Engl J Med* 313:304, 1985.

8. Ferris TF: How should hypertension during pregnancy be managed? An internist's approach. *Med Clin North Am* 66:491, 1984.

9. Sibai BM: Pitfalls in diagnosis and management of preeclampsia. *Am J Obstet Gynecol* 159:1, 1988.

10. Cugell DW, Frank NR, Gaensler EA, et al: Pulmonary function in pregnancy. I. Serial observations in normal women. *Am Rev Respir Dis* 67:568, 1953.

11. Greenberger PA, Patterson R: Management of asthma during pregnancy. *N Engl J Med* 312:897, 1985.

12. Gilroy RJ, Mangura BT, Lavietes MH: Rib cage and abdominal volume displacements during breathing in pregnancy. *Am Rev Respir Dis* 137:668, 1988.

13. Lotgering FK, Gilbert RD, Longo LD: Maternal and fetal responses to exercise during pregnancy. *Physiol Rev* 65:1, 1985.

14. Cheek TG, Gutsche BB: Maternal physiologic alterations during pregnancy, in Shnider SM, Levinson G (eds): *Anesthesia for Obstetrics*. Baltimore, Williams & Wilkins, 1987, p 3.

15. Barron WM: The pregnant surgical patient: Medical evaluation and management. *Ann Intern Med* 101:683, 1984.

16. Berkowitz RL: The Swan-Ganz catheter and colloid osmotic pressure determinations, in Berkowitz RL (ed): *Critical Care of the Obstetric Patient*. New York, Churchill Livingstone, 1983, p 1.

17. Moore LG, Rounds SS, Jahnigen D, et al: Infant birth weight is related to maternal arterial oxygenation at high altitude. *Arch Environ Health* 32:36, 1977.

18. Moore LG, Jahnigen D, Rounds SS, et al: Maternal hyperventilation helps preserve arterial oxygenation during high-altitude pregnancy. *J Appl Physiol* 52:690, 1982.

19. Templeton A: Intrauterine growth retardation associated with hypoxia due to bronchiectasis. *Br J Obstet Gynecol* 84:389, 1977.

20. Matuschak GM, Owens GR, Rogers RM, et al: Progressive intrapartum respiratory insufficiency due to pulmonary alveolar proteinosis. *Chest* 68:104, 1983.

21. Metcalfe J: Oxygen supply and fetal growth. *J Reprod Med* 30:301, 1985.

22. Meschia G: Supply of oxygen to the fetus. *J Reprod Med* 23:160, 1979.

23. Parer JT: Uteroplacental circulation and respiratory gas exchange, in Shnider SM, Levinson G (eds): *Anesthesia for Obstetrics*. Baltimore, Williams & Wilkins, 1987, p 14.

24. Greiss FC: A clinical concept of uterine blood flow during pregnancy. *Obstet Gynecol* 30:595, 1967.

25. Meschia G: Transfer of oxygen across the placenta, in Gluck L (ed): *Intrauterine Asphyxia and the Developing Fetal Brain*. Chicago, Year Book, 1977, p 107.

26. Metcalfe J, Dhindsa DS, Novy MJ: General aspects of oxygen transport in maternal and fetal blood, in Longo LD, Bartels H (eds): *Respiratory Gas Exchange and Blood Flow in the Placenta*. Bethesda, MD, Public Health Service, 1972, p 63.

27. Longo LD, Hill EP, Power GG: Oxygen transfer, in Longo LD, Bartels H (eds): *Respiratory Gas Exchange and Blood Flow in the Placenta*. Bethesda, MD, Public Health Service, 1972, p 380.

28. Peeters LLH, Sheldon RE, Jones MD, et al: Blood flow to fetal organs as a function of arterial oxygen content. *Am J Obstet Gynecol* 135:637, 1979.

29. Meschia G: Safety margin of fetal oxygenation. *J Reprod Med* 30:308, 1985.

30. Wulf KH, Kunzel W, Lehman V: Clinical aspects of placental gas exchange, in Longo LD, Bartels H (eds): *Respiratory Gas Exchange and Blood Flow in the Placenta*. Bethesda, MD, Public Health Service, 1972, p 505.

31. Bonnar J: Venous thromboembolism and pregnancy. *Clin Obstet Gynecol* 8:455, 1981.

32. Bolan JC: Thromboembolic complications of pregnancy. *Clin Obstet Gynecol* 26:913, 1983.

33. Benotti JR, Pratter MR, Dalen JE: Pulmonary embolism. *Cur Pulmonol* 6:91, 1984.

34. Hyers TM, Fowler AA, Wicks AB: Focal pulmonary edema after massive pulmonary embolism. *Am Rev Respir Dis* 123:232, 1981.

35. Meth RF, Tashkin DP, Hansen KS, et al: Pulmonary edema and wheezing after pulmonary embolism. *Am Rev Respir Dis* 111:693, 1975.

36. Staub NC: Pulmonary edema due to increased microvascular permeability to fluid and protein. *Circ Res* 43:143, 1978.

37. Turner R, Gusack M: Massive amniotic fluid embolism. *Ann Emerg Med* 13:359, 1984.

38. Morgan M: Amniotic fluid embolism. *Anaesthesia* 34:20, 1979.

39. Sterner S, Campbell B, Davies S: Amniotic fluid embolism. *Ann Emerg Med* 13:343, 1984.

40. Peterson EP, Taylor HB: Amniotic fluid embolism. *Obstet Gynecol* 35:787, 1970.

41. Duff P, Engelsgjerd B, Zingery LW, et al: Hemodynamic observations in a patient with intrapartum amniotic fluid embolism. *Am J Obstet Gynecol* 146:112, 1983.

42. Masson RG, Ruggieri J, Siddiqui MM: Aminiotic fluid embolism: Definitive diagnosis in a survivor. *Am Rev Respir Dis* 120:187, 1979.

43. Lumley J, Owen R, Morgan M: Amniotic fluid embolism. *Anaesthesia* 34:33, 1979.

44. Shapiro SH, Wessely Z: Rhodamine B fluorescence as a stain for amniotic fluid squames in maternal pulmonary embolism and fetal lungs. *Ann Clin Lab Sci* 18:451, 1988.

45. Garland IWC, Thompson WD: Diagnosis of amniotic fluid embolism using an antiserum to human keratin. *J Clin Pathol* 36:625, 1983.

46. Giampaolo C, Schneider V, Kowalski BN, et al: The cytologic diagnosis of amniotic fluid embolism: A critical reappraisal. *Diagn Cytopathol* 3:126, 1987.

47. Gottlieb JD, Ericsson JA, Sweet RB: Venous air embolism. *Anaesth Analg* 44:773, 1965.

48. Bray P, Myers RAM, Cowley RA: Orogenital sex as a cause of nonfatal air embolism in pregnancy. *Obstet Gynecol* 61:653, 1983.

49. O'Quinn RJ, Lakshminarayan S: Venous air embolism. *Arch Intern Med* 142:2173, 1982.

50. Fyke FE, Kazmier FJ, Harms RW: Venous air embolism: Life-threatening complication of orogenital sex during pregnancy. *Am J Med* 78:333, 1985.

51. Campkin TB, Perks JS: Venous air embolism. *Lancet* 1:235, 1973.

52. Ence TJ, Gong H Jr: Adult respiratory distress syndrome after venous air embolism. *Am Rev Respir Dis* 119:1033, 1979.

53. Clark MC, Flick MR: Permeability pulmonary edema caused by venous air embolism. *Am Rev Respir Dis* 129:633, 1984.

54. Mendelson CL: The aspiration of stomach contents into the lungs during obstetric anesthesia. *Am J Obstet Gynecol* 52:191, 1946.

55. Baggish MS, Hooper S: Aspiration as a cause of maternal death. *Obstet Gynecol* 43:327, 1974.

56. Bartlett JG, Gorbach SL: The triple threat of aspiration pneumonia. *Chest* 68:560, 1975.

57. Huxley EJ, Viroslav J, Gray WR, et al: Pharyngeal aspiration in normal adults with depressed consciousness. *Am J Med* 64:564, 1978.

58. Bynum LJ, Pierce AK: Pulmonary aspiration of stomach contents. *Am Rev Respir Dis* 114:1129, 1976.

59. Lorber B, Swenson RM: Bacteriology of aspiration pneumonia. *Ann Intern Med* 81:329, 1974.

60. Schwartz DJ, Wynne JW, Gibbs CP, et al: The pulmonary consequences of aspiration of gastric contents at pH values greater than 2.5. *Am Rev Respir Dis* 121:119, 1980.

61. Bond VK, Stoelting RK, Gupta CO: Pulmonary aspiration syndrome after inhalation of gastric juice containing antacid. *Anesthesiology* 51:452, 1979.

62. Benedetti TJ, Valle R, Ledger WJ: Antepartum pneumonia in pregnancy. *Am J Obstet Gynecol* 144:413, 1982.

63. Donowitz GR, Mandell GL: Acute pneumonia, in Mandell GL, Douglas RG, Bennett JE, (eds): *Principles and Practices of Infectious Diseases.* New York, Wiley, 1985, p 394.

64. Soper DE, Melone PJ, Conover WB: Legionnaire disease complicating pregnancy. *Obstet Gynecol* 67:10S, 1986.

65. Lederman MM: Cell-mediated immunity and pregnancy. *Chest* 86:6S, 1984.

66. Birkeland SA, Kristofferson K: Lymphocyte transformation with mitogens and antigens during pregnancy: A longitudinal study. *Scand J Immunol* 11:321, 1980.

67. Gehrz RC, Christianson WR, Linner KM, et al: A longitudinal analysis of lymphocyte proliferative responses to mitogens and antigens during pregnancy. *Am J Obstet Gynecol* 104:665, 1981.

68. Sridama V, Pacini F, Yang S, et al: Decreased levels of helper T cells: A possible cause of immunodeficiency in pregnancy. *N Engl J Med* 307:352, 1982.

69. Thong YH, Steele RW, Vincent MM, et al: Impaired *in vitro* cell-mediated immunity to rubella virus during pregnancy. *N Engl J Med* 289:604, 1973.

70. Advisory Committee on Immunization Practices: Prevention and control of influenza. *MMWR* 34:261, 1985.

71. Centers for Disease Control: Recommendations for prevention and control of influenza. *Ann Intern Med* 105:399, 1986.

72. Harris RE, Rhoades ER: Varicella pneumonia complicating pregnancy. *Obstet Gynecol* 25:734, 1965.

73. Weber DM, Pellecchia JA: Varicella pneumonia. *JAMA* 192:228, 1965.

74. Paryani SG, Arvin AM: Intrauterine infection with varicella-zoster virus after maternal varicella. *N Engl J Med* 314:1542, 1986.

75. Triebwasser JH, Harris RE, Bryant RE, et al: Varicella pneumonia in adults. *Medicine* 46:409, 1967.

76. Stagno S, Whitley RJ: Herpes virus infections of pregnancy. *N Engl J Med* 313:1327, 1985.

77. Catanzaro A: Pulmonary mycosis in pregnant women. *Chest* 86:14S, 1984.

78. Snider D: Pregnancy and tuberculosis. *Chest* 86:10S, 1984.

79. Koonin LM, Ellerbrock TV, Atrash JK, et al: Pregnancy-associated deaths due to AIDS in the United States. *JAMA* 261:1306, 1989.

80. Dinsmoor MJ: HIV infection and pregnancy. *Med Clin North Am* 73:701, 1989.

81. Minckoff H, deRegt RH, Landesman S, et al: *Pneumocystis carinii* pneumonia associated with acquired immunodeficiency syndrome in pregnancy: A report of three maternal deaths. *Obstet Gynecol* 67:284, 1986.

82. Hicks ML, Nolan GH, Maxwell SL, et al: Acquired immunodeficiency syndrome and *Pneumocystis carinii* infection in a pregnant woman. *Obstet Gynecol* 76:480, 1990.

83. Centers for Disease Control: Listeriosis outbreak associated with Mexican style cheese: California. *MMWR* 34:357, 1985.

84. Boucher M, Yonekura ML, Wallace RJ, et al: Adult respiratory distress syndrome: A rare manifestation of *Listeria monocytogenes* infection in pregnancy. *Am J Obstet Gynecol* 149:686, 1984.

85. Turner ES, Greenberger PA, Patterson R: Management of the pregnant asthmatic patient. *Ann Intern Med* 6:905, 1980.

85a. Working Group on Asthma in Pregnancy: Management of asthma during pregnancy. NIH Publication No. 93-3279, 1993, pp. 1–59.

86. Bahna SL, Berkedal T: The course of pregnancy and outcome of pregnancy in women with bronchial asthma. *Acta Allerg* 27:397, 1972.

87. Gordon M, Niswander KR, Berendes H, et al: Fetal morbidity following potentially anoxic obstetric conditions. VII. Bronchial asthma. *Am J Obstet Gynecol* 106:421, 1970.

88. Schatz M, Patterson R, Zeitz S, et al: Corticosteroid therapy for the pregnant asthmatic patient. *JAMA* 233:804, 1975.

89. Apter AJ, Greenberger PA, Patterson R: Outcome of pregnancy in adolescents with severe asthma. *J Allergy Clin Immunol* 149:2571, 1989.

90. Fitzsimmons R, Greenberger PA, Patterson R: Outcome of pregnancy in women requiring corticosteroids for severe asthma. *J Allergy Clin Immunol* 78:349, 1986.

91. Hollingsworth HM: Wheezing and stridor. *Clin Chest Med* 8:231, 1987.

92. Fischl MA, Pitchenik A, Gardner LB: An index predicting relapse and hospitalization in patients with acute bronchial asthma. *N Engl J Med* 305:783, 1981.

93. Rebuck AS, Read J: Assessment and management of severe asthma. *Am J Med* 51:788, 1971.

94. McFadden ER Jr, Kiser R, DeGroot WJ: Acute bronchial asthma: Relations between clinical and physiologic manifestations. *N Engl J Med* 288:221, 1973.

95. Benedetti TJ, Hargrove JC, Rosene KA: Maternal pulmonary edema during premature labor inhibition. *Obstet Gynecol* 59:33S, 1982.

96. Nimrod CA, Beresford P, Frais M, et al: Hemodynamic observations on pulmonary edema associated with a β-mimetic agent. *J Reprod Med* 29:341, 1984.

97. Mabie WC, Pernoll ML, Witty JB, et al: Pulmonary edema induced by betamimetic drugs. *South Med J* 76:1354, 1983.

98. Jacobs MM, Arias F: Cardiopulmonary complications associated with beta-adrenergic tocolytic therapy, in Berkowitz RL (ed): *Critical Care of the Obstetric Patient.* New York, Churchill Livingstone, 1983, p 505.

99. Karson EM, Saltzman D, David MR: Pneumomediastinum in pregnancy: Two case reports and a review of the literature, pathophysiology and management. *Obstet Gynecol* 64:39S, 1984.

100. Mossman KL, Hill LT: Radiation risks in pregnancy. *Obstet Gynecol* 60:237, 1982.

101. Brent RL: The effects of embryonic and fetal exposure to x-ray, microwaves and ultrasound. *Clin Obstet Gynecol* 26:484, 1983.

102. Swartz HM, Reichling BA: Hazards of radiation exposure for pregnant women. *JAMA* 239:1907, 1978.

103. Stewart A, Kneale GW: Radiation dose effects in relation to obstetric x-rays and childhood cancers. *Lancet* 1:1185, 1970.

104. Kalter H, Warkany J: Congenital malformations. *N Engl J Med* 308:424, 1983.

105. Ginsberg JS, Hirsh J, Rainbow AJ, et al: Risks to the fetus of radiologic procedures used in the diagnosis of maternal venous thromboembolic disease. *Thromb Haemost* 61:189, 1989.

106. Hall JG, Pauli RM, Wilson KM: Maternal and fetal sequelae of anticoagulation in pregnancy. *Am J Med* 68:122, 1980.

107. Keefer JR, Strauss RG, Ciretta JM, et al: Noncardiogenic pulmonary edema and invasive cardiovascular monitoring. *Obstet Gynecol* 58:46, 1981.

108. Cotton DB, Benedetti TJ: Use of the Swan-Ganz catheter in obstetrics and gynecology. *Obstet Gynecol* 56:641, 1980.

109. Berkowitz RL, Rafferty TD: Pulmonary artery flow-directed catheter use in the obstetric patient. *Obstet Gynecol* 55:507, 1980.

110. Weidemann HP, Matthay MA, Matthay RA: Cardiovascular-pulmonary monitoring in the intensive care unit. *Chest* 85:537, 1984.

111. Weidemann HP, Matthay MA, Matthay RA: Cardiovascular-pulmonary monitoring in the intensive care unit. *Chest* 85:656, 1984.

112. Matthay MA: Invasive hemodynamic monitoring in critically ill patients. *Clin Chest Med* 4:233, 1983.

113. Robin ED: The cult of the Swan-Ganz catheter. *Ann Intern Med* 103:445, 1985.

114. Dalen JE: Bedside hemodynamic monitoring. *N Engl J Med* 301:1176, 1979.

115. Robin ED: Death by pulmonary artery flow-directed catheter. *Chest* 92:727, 1987.

116. Fein AM: Is pulmonary artery catheterization necessary for the diagnosis of pulmonary edema? *Am Rev Respir Dis* 129:1006, 1984.

117. Eisenbert PR, Jatte AS, Schuster DP: Clinical evaluation compared to pulmonary artery catheterization in hemodynamic assessment of critically ill patients. *Crit Care Med* 12:533, 1984.

118. Parer JT: Diagnosis and management of fetal asphyxia, in Shnider SM, Levinson G (eds): *Anesthesia for Obstetrics*. Baltimore, Williams & Wilkins, 1987, pp 474–488.

119. Biehl DR: Foetal monitoring during surgery unrelated to pregnancy. *Can Anaesth Soc J* 32:455, 1985.

120. Liu PL, Warren TM, Ostheimer GW, et al: Foetal monitoring in parturients undergoing surgery unrelated to pregnancy. *Can Anaesth Soc J* 32:525, 1985.

121. Laros RK Jr: Evaluation of the fetus, in Shnider SM, Levinson G (eds): *Anesthesia for Obstetrics*. Baltimore, Williams & Wilkins, 1987, p 461.

122. Sellick BA: Cricoid pressure to control regurgitation of stomach contents during induction of anesthesia. *Lancet* 2:404, 1961.

123. Grum CM, Morganroth ML: Initiating mechanical ventilation. *J Intensive Care Med* 3:6, 1988.

124. Broddus VC, Berthiaume Y, Biondi JW, et al: Hemodynamic management of the adult respiratory distress syndrome. *J Intensive Care Med* 2:190, 1987.

125. Milunsky A, Ulcickas M, Rothman KJ, et al: Maternal heat exposure and neural tube defects. *JAMA* 268:882, 1992.

126. Roizen MF, Feeley TW: Pancuronium bromide. *Ann Intern Med* 88:64, 1978.

127. Kalter H, Warkany J: Congenital malformations. *N Engl J Med* 308:491, 1983.

128. Niebyl JR: Therapeutic drugs in pregnancy. *Postgrad Med J* 75:165, 1984.

129. Morganroth ML, Grum CM: Weaning from mechanical ventilation. *J Intensive Care Med* 3:109, 1988.

130. Martin R, Blackburn GL: Hyperalimentation during pregnancy, in Berkowitz RL (ed): *Critical Care of the Obstetric Patient*. New York, Churchill Livingstone, 1983, p 133

131. Silk DBA: Nutrition. *Curr Opin Gastroenterol* 1:279, 1985.

132. Bartlett RH, Deschert RE, Mault JR, et al: Metabolic studies in chest trauma. *J Thorac Cardiovasc Surg* 87:503, 1984.

133. Detsky AS, Baker JP, Mendelson RA, et al: Evaluating the accuracy of nutritional assessment techniques applied to hospitalized patients: Methodology and comparisons. *J Parenter Enteral Nutr* 8:153, 1984.

134. D'Attellis NP, Bursztein S, Askanazi J, et al: Tailoring nutritional support: What, when, and why. *J Crit Illness* 3:49, 1988.

135. Wright PD: Nutritional requirements in parenteral nutrition. *Curr Opin Gastroenterol* 1:302, 1985.

136. Silk DBA: Enteral nutrition. *Curr Opin Gastroenterol* 1:295, 1985.

137. Tresadern JC, Falconer GF, Turnberg LA, et al: Successful completed pregnancy in a patient maintained on home parenteral nutrition. *Br Med J* 286:602, 1983.

138. Covelli HD, Black JW, Olsen MS, et al: Respiratory failure precipitated by high carbohydrate loads. *Ann Intern Med* 95:579, 1981.

139. Cosmi EV, Shnider SM: Obstetric anesthesia and uterine blood flow, in Shnider SM, Levinson G (eds): *Anesthesia for Obstetrics*. Baltimore, Williams & Wilkins, 1987, p 22.

140. Ginsberg JS, Hirsh J, Turner DC, et al: Risks to fetus of anticoagulant therapy during pregnancy. *Thromb Haemost* 61:197, 1989.

141. Ginsberg JS, Kowalchuk G, Hirsh J, et al: Heparin therapy during pregnancy. *Arch Intern Med* 149:2233, 1989.

142. Marder VJ: The use of thrombolytic agents: Choice of patient, drug administration, laboratory monitoring. *Ann Intern Med* 90:802, 1979.

143. Kinasewitz GT, George RB: Management of thromboembolism: Anticoagulants, thrombolytics, or surgical intervention. *Chest* 86:106, 1984.

144. Bell WR, Meek AG: Guidelines for the use of thrombolytic agents. *N Engl J Med* 301:1266, 1979.

145. Shafer KE, Santoro SA, Sobel BE, et al: Monitoring activity of fibrinolytic agents. *Am J Med* 76:879, 1984.

146. Ludwig H: Results of streptokinase therapy in deep venous thrombosis during pregnancy. *Postgrad Med J* 49(suppl):66, 1973.

147. Hall RJC, Young C, Sutton GC, et al: Treatment of acute massive pulmonary embolism by streptokinase during labor and delivery. *Br Med J* 4:647, 1972.

148. Demers C, Ginsberg JS: Deep venous thrombosis and pulmonary embolism in pregnancy. *Clin Chest Med* 13:645, 1992.

149. Chung AF, Merkatz IR: Survival following amniotic fluid embolism with early heparinization. *Obstet Gynecol* 46:809, 1973.

150. Murray HW: Antimicrobial therapy in pulmonary aspiration. *Am J Med* 66:188, 1979.

151. Bernard GR, Luce JM, Spring CL, et al: High-dose corticosteroids in patients with the adult respiratory distress syndrome. *N Engl J Med* 317:1565, 1987.

152. Wolfe JE, Bone RC, Ruth WE: Effects of corticosteroids in the treatment of patients with gastric aspiration. *Am J Med* 63:719, 1977.

153. Downs JB, Chapman RL Jr, Modell JH, et al: An evaluation of steroid therapy in aspiration pneumonitis. *Anesthesiology* 40:129, 1974.

154. Taylor G, Pryse-Davies J: Evaluation of endotracheal steroid therapy in acid pulmonary aspiration syndrome (Mendelson's syndrome). *Anesthesiology* 29:17, 1968.

155. Chow AW, Jewesson RJ: Pharmacokinetics and safety of antimicrobial agents in pregnancy. *Rev Infect Dis* 7:278, 1985.

156. Little JW, Hall WJ, Douglas RG, et al: Amantadine effect on peripheral airways abnormalities in influenza. *Ann Intern Med* 85:177, 1976.

157. DuPont Pharmaceuticals: Symmetrel (amantadine hydrochloride), in Huff BB (ed): *Physicians' Desk Reference*. Oradell, NJ, Medical Economics, 1990, p 929.

158. Whitley R, Hilty M, Haynes R: Vidarabine therapy of varicella in immunosuppressed patients. *J Pediatr* 101:125, 1982.

159. Moore HL, Szczech GM, Rodwell DE, et al: Preclinical toxicology studies with acyclovir. *Fundam Appl Toxicol* 3:560, 1983.

160. Lansberger EJ, Hager WD, Grossman JH: Successful management of varicella pneumonia complicating pregnancy. *J Reprod Med* 31:311, 1986.

161. Eder SE, Apuzzio JJ, Weiss G: Varicella pneumonia during pregnancy. *Am J Perinatol* 5:16, 1988.

162. Balfour HH: Intravenous acyclovir therapy for varicella in immunocompromised children. *J Pediatr* 104:134, 1984.

163. Montaner JSG, Lawson LM, Levitt N, et al: Corticosteroids prevent early deterioration in patients with moderately severe *Pneumocystis carinii* pneumonia and the acquired immunodeficiency syndrome (AIDS). *Ann Intern Med* 113:14, 1990.

164. Armstrong D: *Listeria monocytogenes,* in Mandell GL, Douglas RG, Bennett JE (eds): *Principles and Practice of Infectious Diseases*. New York, Wiley, 1985, p 1177.

165. Gazioglu K, Condemi JJ, Hyde RW, et al: Effect of isoproterenol on gas exchange during air and oxygen breathing in patients with asthma. *Am J Med* 50:185, 1971.

166. Geigy Pharmaceuticals. Brethaire (terbutaline sulfate), in Huff BB (ed): *Physicians' Desk Reference*. Oradell, NJ, Medical Economics, 1990, p 974.

167. Schatz M, Zeiger RS, Harden KM, et al: The safety of inhaled β-agonist bronchodilators during pregnancy. *J Allergy Clin Immunol* 82:686, 1988.

168. Rossing TH, Fanta CH, Goldstein DH, et al: Emergency therapy of asthma: Comparison of the acute effects of parenteral and inhaled sympathomimetics and infused aminophylline. *Am Rev Respir Dis* 122:365, 1980.

169. Appel D, Karpel JP, Sherman M: Epinephrine improves expiratory flow rates in patients with asthma who do not respond to inhaled metaproterenol sulfate. *J Allergy Clin Immunol* 84:90, 1989.

170. Spector SL: Reciprocal relationship between pregnancy and pulmonary disease. *Chest* 86:1S, 1984.

171. Sutton PL, Koup JR, Ros JQ, et al: The pharmacokinetics of theophylline in pregnancy. *J Allergy Clin Immunol* 61(suppl):174, 1978.

172. Littenberg B, Gluck EH: A controlled trial of methylprednisolone in the emergency treatment of acute asthma. *N Engl J Med* 314:150, 1986.

173. Fanta CH, Rossing TH, McFadden ER Jr: Glucocorticoids in acute asthma: A critical controlled trial. *Am J Med* 74:845, 1983.

174. Haskell RJ, Wong BM, Hansen JE: A double-blind, randomized clinical trial of methylprednisolone in status asthmaticus. *Arch Intern Med* 143:1324, 1983.

175. Menitove SM, Goldring RM: Combined ventilator and bicarbonate strategy in the management of status asthmaticus. *Am J Med* 74:898, 1983.

176. Parry WH, Martorano F, Cotton EK: Management of life-threatening asthma with intravenous isoproterenol infusions. *Am J Dis Child* 130:39, 1976.
177. Noppen M, Vanmaele L, Impens N, et al: Bronchodilating effect of intravenous magnesium sulfate in acute severe bronchial asthma. *Chest* 97: 373, 1990.
178. O'Rourke PP, Crone RK: Halothane in status asthmaticus. *Crit Care Med* 10:341, 1982.
179. Brooks GZ: Anaesthesia for the critical care obstetric patient, in Berkowitz RL (ed): *Critical Care of the Obstetric Patient*. New York, Churchill Livingstone, 1983, p 73.
180. Topilsky M, Levo Y, Spitzer SA, et al: Status asthmaticus in pregnancy: A case report. *Ann Allergy* 32:151, 1974.
181. Ginsberg JS, Hirsh J, Turner DC, et al: Risks to the fetus of anticoagulant therapy during pregnancy. *Thromb Haemost* 61:197, 1989.

182. Loa TT, DeSwiet M, Letsky E, et al: Prophylaxis of thromboembolism in pregnancy: An alternative. *Br J Obstet Gynaecol* 92:202, 1985.
183. Hahn CLA: Pulsatile heparin administration in pregnancy: A new approach. *Am J Obstet Gynecol* 155:283, 1982.
184. Hull R, Delmore T, Carter C, et al: Adjusted subcutaneous heparin versus warfarin sodium in the long-term treatment of venous thrombosis. *N Engl J Med* 306:189, 1982.
185. Canadian Preterm Labor Investigations Group: Treatment of preterm labor with the beta-adrenergic agonist ritodrine. *N Engl J Med* 327:308, 1992.
186. Hollander DI, Nagey DA, Pupkin MJ: Magnesium sulfate and ritodrine hydrochloride: A randomized comparison. *Am J Obstet Gynecol* 156:631, 1987.

60. Pulmonary Embolism and Deep Vein Thrombosis

John G. Weg

Pulmonary Thromboembolism

INCIDENCE AND NATURAL HISTORY. The incidence of pulmonary thromboembolism (PE) in the United States is estimated to be in excess of 600,000 per year [1]. Untreated, PE has a mortality of about 30 percent. In striking contrast the 1 year mortality due to treated PE is 2.5 percent, a greater than a 10-fold reduction in mortality [2–5]. Determining the true incidence of pulmonary emboli is problematic because of the immense difficulty of clinical diagnosis, the inherent bias in populations studied, and the intensity with which PE is sought at postmortem examination. In one study careful dissection identified PE in 52 percent of right lungs, while general autopsy found only 12 percent in the left lungs [6]. Pulmonary thromboembolism has accounted for 6 to 26 percent of hospital deaths. The mortality rate appears to be decreasing somewhat in North America [7]. However, in one study PE was the most frequently missed diagnosis in patients in whom therapy was likely to prevent death, 9 of 34 (26%) in 300 autopsies and missed overall in 15 of 24 (63%) [8]. Even in the mid 1970s, only 16 of 54 (30%) of patients with major emboli at autopsy had the diagnosis of PE before they died. Accuracy of diagnosis was greater in postoperative patients and in patients with autopsy proved venous thrombosis. Strikingly, the diagnosis was not made in any of 21 patients with pneumonia [9].

PATHOGENESIS. The development of venous thrombosis is primarily related to stasis of blood flow, vascular wall damage, activation of the clotting system, and a hypercoagulable state. In a vein, stasis permits red blood cells, platelets, white cells, and fibrin to adhere, usually in a valve pocket; this aggregation enlarges in the direction of blood flow, producing a "red" thrombus. With further growth the thrombus continues to enlarge and obstruct blood flow. Trauma or surgery may produce a hypercoagulable state and the activation of factor X; there is release of thromboplastins, an increase in factor VIII and fibrinogen, and a decrease of antithrombin III.

It is believed that more than 90 percent of PEs originate in the lower extremities [10]. There is evidence that the initial site is most often in the calf veins, but thrombi can form in the more proximal (thigh) veins or even the internal iliac veins of patients undergoing gynecologic surgery, parturition, or prostate surgery. Thrombus formation is often bilateral and frequently asymptomatic. Thrombi may also occur in the upper extremities and form around central venous or pulmonary artery balloon catheters. The frequency and morbidity of such thrombi have not been systematically prospectively studied. Septic PEs may develop from infected peripheral thrombi, a common occurrence in intravenous drug abusers (IVDAs), with endometritis, and from right-sided endocarditis, also common in IVDAs.

PATHOPHYSIOLOGY. The cardinal pulmonary effect is altered gas exchange, a ventilation/perfusion ($\dot{V}/\dot{Q}$) mismatch. There is also an increased $\dot{V}/\dot{Q}$ in the local area of the clot, due to obstruction of blood flow. The major abnormalities are intrapulmonary shunt areas with no ventilation versus blood flow ($0\ \dot{V}/\dot{Q}$) and areas of decreased ventilation to blood flow ($\downarrow\dot{V}/\dot{Q}$), resulting in a reduced arterial oxygen tension (hypoxemia) in approximately 85 percent of patients and a widened alveolar to arterial oxygen tension gradient $P(A-a)O_2$ in 90 percent. Thus the PaO_2 and $P(A-a)O_2$ can be normal in patients with acute PE. An additional, almost consistent, finding is hypocarbia, a reduced arterial carbon dioxide tension. The arterial to alveolar PCO_2 $P(A-a)CO_2$ should be increased because of the increased physiologic dead space in the local area of the clot. However, this is extremely difficult to measure in acutely ill patients and is probably quite transient because the decreased to absent alveolar carbon dioxide tension ($PACO_2$) in the area of the clot decreases blood flow to this area [11–15]. Although it occurs very infrequently, there can be an increased $PaCO_2$ in patients with chronic obstructive pulmonary diseases who have baseline hypercarbia, and there are reported cases of de novo hypercarbia with overwhelming PE [16,17].

Concomitant physiologic changes include: (1) increased minute ventilation ($\dot{V}E$); (2) decreased vital capacity (VC) due to pain and splinting, atelectasis, increased lung water, and decreased compliance; (3) increased airways resistance (R_{aw}) or decreased FEV_1 due to decreased $PaCO_2$, serotonin, histamine, kinins, and other vasoactive polypeptides (the increased resistance responds to heparin and, in part, to bronchodilators); and (4) decreased diffusing capacity due to obstruction of the pulmonary capillary bed, decreased pulmonary capillary blood volume and uneven $\dot{V}/\dot{Q}$ relationships [11,12,13].

The hemodynamic response to obstruction or reduction of the pulmonary vascular bed is remarkably variable. Pulmonary vascular resistance (R_{pulm}) equals the mean pulmonary artery pressure P_{pa} minus the pulmonary capillary wedge pressure (PCW) divided by the cardiac output ($\dot{Q}$) or $R_{pulm} = P_{pa} - PCW/\dot{Q}$. This low-resistance circuit can accommodate a four to sixfold increase in $\dot{Q}$ due to strenuous activity with little or no change in P_{pa} because of distention and recruitment of the pulmonary vascular bed. Even with a pneumonectomy, P_{pa} does not increase with a twofold increase in $\dot{Q}$ if the remaining lung is normal. However, pulmonary vascular resistance is also increased by hypoxia, acidosis, hypercarbia, vasoactive substances, and interstitial edema. In patients with PE without underlying cardiopulmonary disease, P_{pa} is usually increased if the obstruction is 25 percent or more, but some patients display increases with less than 20 percent obstruction and others have normal pressures with greater than 50 percent obstruction. Mean P_{pa} in patients without underlying cardiopulmonary disease generally remains at or below 40 to 45 mm Hg with acute PE, although there are exceptions. Usually with pressures above this level, right ventricular failure occurs, manifest by a rise in mean right atrial pressure, right ventricular dilation, decreased ejection fraction, and decreased cardiac index to less than 2.5 liters per minute. In patients with preexisting cardiopulmonary disease, especially mitral stenosis, or left ventricular failure P_{pa} may be much higher, 40 to 60 mm Hg or greater [13,18,19,20]. In a prospective evaluation of patients with suspected PE, P_{pa}, R_{pulm}, $\dot{Q}$, and systemic vascular resistance (SVR) could not distinguish between individuals with or without PE and did not correlate with the extent of pulmonary vascular obstruction [21,22]. This lack of correlation is likely due to the varying degree of underlying cardiopulmonary disease(s), the effects of hypoxia, and the possible release of vasoactive substances.

CLINICAL MANIFESTATIONS.

To date no clinical findings for the diagnosis of PE alone or in combination are sufficiently sensitive to identify PE when present or sufficiently specific to exclude PE when absent. Nonetheless, most patients with acute PE can be identified on the basis of a brief history and simple physical examination. Dyspnea or tachypnea (respiratory rate ≥ 20) have been found in 347 of 383 (91%) of patients with PE, dyspnea or tachypnea or pleuritic pain in 371 of 383 (97%), and dyspnea or tachypnea or pleuritic pain or signs and symptoms of deep venous thrombosis (however inaccurate in making that diagnosis) in 373 of 383 (97%) [23,24,25]. The obvious difficulty is that these signs and symptoms are very common, almost a constant in patients in the intensive care unit [26]. They are also frequent manifestations of other serious diseases that can mimic PE [26,27].

Over the last 25 years three large prospective studies have produced data on the clinical findings in patients with acute PE. These are the Streptokinase-Urokinase Trials (SK-SD), phases I and II, and the Prospective Investigation of Pulmonary Embolism Diagnosis (PIOPED) study [23,24,25,28–31]. PIOPED is the only study to collect information prospectively on clinical findings in patients with suspected PE prior to $\dot{V}/\dot{Q}$ scans or pulmonary angiograms and to evaluate the sensitivity and specificity of $\dot{V}/\dot{Q}$ scans versus pulmonary angiography. These three studies, conducted almost two decades apart, provide remarkably similar clinical data. The PIOPED study reflects the lack of specificity of clinical data. These studies are used as the primary source of the following section. It should be noted at the outset that the time-honored (perhaps hoary) classic clinical manifestations of acute PE occur quite infrequently and often are nonspecific. Since the diagnosis of PE is so difficult, and untreated, the mortality rate is high (30%), it is of the utmost importance that individual and group risk factors for thromboembolic disease (TED) be identified, allowing prompt and effective prophylaxis against TED.

A practical approach to the diagnosis of PE is to consider the constellation of predisposing factors, symptoms and signs, "routine" laboratory studies, chest radiographs, electrocardiograms, and arterial blood gases [2]. They provide sufficient information to judge whether the patient should have further studies, such as $\dot{V}/\dot{Q}$ scans, duplex ultrasound or impedance plethysmography (IPG) of the lower extremities, and/or pulmonary angiography.

Predisposing Factors. The most common predisposing factors in PIOPED were immobilization (PE 56% vs. no PE 33%; p<0.001) and surgery within 3 months (PE 54% vs. 31%; p<0.001) [23], factors that are clearly interactive. The same predisposing factors were identified in the SK-SD study (Table 60-1) [28–31]. In the SK-SD study, thrombophlebitis (40%), the combination of nonspecific congestive heart failure and chronic vague pulmonary disease (38%), and obesity (30%) were fairly frequent findings. In contrast, in PIOPED malignancy (PE 23% vs. no PE 15%; n.s.) joined this list [23,24]. Other factors thought to predispose to PE were quite infrequent in both studies. Recent surgery, bed rest, and age greater than 40 years stand out as predisposing factors for PE and identify a high-risk group requiring prophylaxis against TED.

Patients with the antiphospholipid-antibody (anticardiolipin antibody or lupus anticoagulant syndrome) are also at high risk of recurrent venous and arterial thrombosis along with fetal loss [31a–31c]. Approximately 50 percent of such patients have systemic lupus erythematosus or a lupus-like disease. Activated protein C resistance due to a specific point mutation in the gene coding for coagulation factor V in which adenine is subtituted for guanine at nucleotide 1691 has recently been associated with an increase in venous thrombosis. Reports from northern Europe document its occurrence in families. It has been found in 2 percent of the normal population and 20 to 60 percent of patients with venous thrombosis. In the Physicians Health Study the prevalence for heterozygosity in men with venous thromboembolism or pulmonary embolism was 11.6 percent (p=0.02) but not for arterial occlusive disease. The relative risk for primary venous thromboembolism was 3.5; 95 percent confidence interval, 1.5 to 8.4; p = 0.004; and in men over 60 the relative risk was 7.0; 95 percent confidence interval, 2.6 to 19.1; (p<0.001). This risk factor appears to be the most common inherited predisposing factor for venous thrombosis. Other less common risk factors include acquired deficiency of antithrombin III, protein C, and protein S; abnormalities in plasminogen and tissue plasminogen activator; perhaps factor VII deficiency; and thrombocytopenia, particularly in systemic lupus erythematosus and acute leukemia.

Table 60-1. Predisposing Factors or Coexisting Conditions in Pulmonary Embolism

Urokinase/Streptokinase Trial (UK-SK) Phase I (N = 327) Predisposing Factors	PE (%)	Prospective Investigation of Pulmonary Embolism Diagnosis (PIOPED) Predisposing Factors—No history of Cardiopulmonary Disease	PE (%) (N = 117)	No PE (%) (N = 248)
Immobilization	55	Immobilization	56	33*
Current venous disease	49	Surgery (3 months)	54	31*
Congestive heart failure and		Malignancy	23	15
Chronic pulmonary disease	38	Thrombophlebitis (ever)	14	8
		Trauma-Lower Extremities	10	10
		Estrogen	9	10
		Stroke	7	4
		Postpartum ≤ 3 mo	4	3
Urokinase/Streptokinase Trial (UK/SK) Phase II (N = 167) Coexisting conditions				
Thrombophlebitis	40			
Bed Rest	32			
Recent Surgery	31			
Recent Immobilization	15			
Obesity	30			
Venous Varicosity/Insufficiency	15			
Congestive Heart Failure	17			
Arrhythmia	16			
No predisposing factor	6			

In UK-SK, the following were identified in less than 10%: other heart disease, primary pulmonary disease; diabetus mellitus, malignancy, pelvic disease, angina, rheumatic heart disease, peripheral arterial disease, and recent termination of pregnancy.
* p<0.001

In a recent report of a kindred with antithrombin III deficiency the prevalence of symptomatic venous thrombosis was approximately 50 percent; however more than 80 percent of subjects did not have objective testing. Thrombotic events were often associated with a risk factor. It was concluded that lifelong anticoagulant prophylaxis does not appear to be warranted in asymptomatic carriers. More than 50 percent of patients with protein S deficiency, an autosomal dominant trait, have TED episodes, with frequent recurrences. Protein S deficiency is common in long-term HIV-infected individuals and may predispose to thromboembolic complications.

Signs and Symptoms. The primacy of dyspnea, pleuritic chest pain, and tachypnea in identifying patients in whom PE should be considered is evident in Table 60-2. Crackles were found in 51 percent of PIOPED patients with PE versus 40 percent without PE (p<0.001); this was the only statistically significant difference found in a majority. An increased pulmonary second heart sound (23% vs. 13%) and a fourth heart sound (24% vs. 14%) were also statistically more common (p<0.001)[32–42].

Chest Radiographs and Electrocardiograms. The chest radiograph is abnormal in more than 80 percent of patients with PE (Table 60-3). Areas of consolidation or atelectasis are found in 68 percent of patients with PE versus 48 percent of those without PE (p<0.001). Pleural effusion is present in 48 percent with PE versus 31 percent of those without PE (p<0.01). The combination of a prominent central pulmonary artery with decreased pulmonary vascularity, although uncommon, occurred more frequently in patients with PE; however, these findings are difficult to define on a standard posteroanterior chest radiograph and unreliable on portable anteroposterior studies [23,24,25,29,31].

The electrocardiogram is abnormal in 70 percent or more of patients with PE, but the common findings are tachycardia and ST–T wave changes, which are not helpful. Left axis deviation is more common in patients with PE and is perhaps a reflection of underlying cardiac disease. The classic $S_1 S_2 S_3$ and $S_1 Q_3 T_3$ patterns are quite uncommon [23,24,25,29,31].

Radiographic and electrocardiographic abnormalities are very common in patients with PE but lack specificity. Absence of either or both lowers the likelihood of PE.

Other Laboratory Studies. The usual hematologic and chemical laboratory studies are not helpful in evaluation for PE. Elevation of the MB isoenzyme fraction of creatine kinase (CK-MB) is useful in identifying an acute myocardial infarction as the cause of the presenting symptoms. However, recent data provide evidence that right ventricular infarction without electrocardiographic evidence of acute myocardial ischemia (S–T elevations) may occur, as evidenced by elevated CK-MB and echocardiographic changes [43]. Thus an acute PE cannot be excluded if the CK-MB levels are elevated.

Arterial Blood Gases. In 10 to 15 percent of patients with angiographically documented PE breathing air, the PaO_2 may be 85 mm Hg or greater and $P(A-a)O_2$ 20 mm Hg or less [23,33]. In the PIOPED study, there were no differences in PaO_2, with values of 70 ± 16 mm Hg in patients with PE versus 72 ± 18 mm Hg in those without PE and/or $P(A-a)O_2$ with values of 37 ± 17 mm Hg and 35 ± 18 mm Hg in the two groups, respectively. In this study arterial blood gases while breathing air were obtained in only 75 percent of patients with PE and 81 percent of patients without PE. The absence of any differences between patients with or without PE is a reflection of the similarity in gas exchange abnormalities in conditions that commonly mimic PE. The 10 to 15 percent of patients with PE who have a normal PaO_2 or $P(A-a)O_2$ may be a function of embolic size or rapid reversal of $\dot{V}/\dot{Q}$ abnormalities. In summary, arterial blood gas analysis, too, is not specific and not sufficiently sensitive. An abnormal PaO_2 or $P(A-a)O_2$ is compatible with a PE, but normal

Table 60-2. Signs and Symptoms in Pulmonary Embolism

UK/SK trials (N=327)	PE (%)	PIOPED (no prior cardiopulmonary disease)	PE (N=117) (%)	No PE (N=248) (%)
Respiration (>16/min)	92	Respirations (>20/min)	70	68
Dyspnea	84		73	72
Chest pain	88		66	59
Pleuritic	74			
Apprehension	59			
Crackles	58		51	40*
Cough	53		37	36
Hemoptysis	30		13	8
S2P	53		23	13*
Pulse > 100	44		30	24
Sweats	27		11	8
Syncope	13	Leg pain	26	24
Temperature (≥37.8°)	43		7	12
Diaphoresis	36			
Gallop	34	S3	3	4
		S4	24	14*
Phlebitis	32			
Edema	24			
Murmur	23			
Cyanosis	19			
		Holman's sign	4	2
		Palpitations	10	18
		Wheezing	9	11
		Anginalike pain	4	6
		Right ventricular lift	4	2
		Pleural friction rub	3	2

* $p < 0.001$

values do not exclude the diagnosis, they only lower its likelihood [25,29,31,44].

VENTILATION/PERFUSION ($\dot{V}/\dot{Q}$) SCANS VERSUS PULMONARY ANGIOGRAPHY. In 1990 the PIOPED trial reported on the value of $\dot{V}/\dot{Q}$ scans in acute PE in 931 patients who underwent scintigraphy. Pulmonary angiography was performed in 755 of these patients (81%) and revealed PE in 251 (33%). The study design identified all patients in whom a $\dot{V}/\dot{Q}$ scan or angiogram was ordered for the diagnosis of acute PE. A standardized history, physical examination, chest radiograph, and electrocardiogram were obtained prior to the $\dot{V}/\dot{Q}$ scan. The $\dot{V}/\dot{Q}$ scans and chest radiograph were read by two nuclear medicine specialists at institutions other than the one where the scan was performed and without knowledge of the history, physical examination, other laboratory studies, or angiogram. The angiograms with $\dot{V}/\dot{Q}$ scans were read in a similar fashion. If there was disagreement between the two nuclear medicine or the two angiographic readers, an adjudication process was established for resolution [28].

A fairly complex set of criteria for interpretation of the $\dot{V}/\dot{Q}$ scans was established by the PIOPED nuclear medicine investigators. High probability was defined as two or more large (> 75% of a segment) perfusion defects without corresponding ventilation or radiographic abnormalities or substantially larger than either matching ventilation or chest radiographic abnormality; two or more moderate segmental (≥ 25% and ≤ 75% of a segment) perfusion defects without matching ventilation or chest radiographic abnormalities and one large mismatched segmental defect; or four or more moderate segmental perfusion defects without ventilation or chest radiographic abnor-

malities. Normal was defined as without perfusion defects and with perfusion outlines exactly the shape of the lungs as seen on the chest radiograph. They also established a new category of very low probability, defined as three or less small segmental perfusion defects with a normal chest radiograph—usually considered normal. Low probability was defined as nonsegmental perfusion defects, or a single moderate mismatched segmental perfusion defect with normal chest radiograph, or any perfusion defect with a substantially larger chest radiographic abnormality, or large or moderate segmental perfusion defects involving no more than four segments in one lung and no more than three segments in one lung region with matching ventilation defects either equal to or larger in size and chest radiograph either normal or with abnormalities substantially smaller than perfusion defects, or more than three small segmental perfusion defects less than 25 percent of a segment with a normal chest radiograph. Indeterminate (intermediate probability) was used for abnormalities between high and low. In practice, the investigators had considerable difficulty in separating normal, very low probability, and low probability, and therefore developed the category near normal/normal, which included variations on readings within the categories of low probability, very low probability, and normal. A perfectly normal scan was found in only 21 of the 931 scans, making this a clinically useless category. The generally interpreted, very low probability and near normal/normal categories are probably generally read as normal. The PIOPED nuclear medicine working group reported in great detail on the data collection and tabulation of $\dot{V}/\dot{Q}$ scintigraphy and have suggested alternative criteria for interpretation. In my opinion, the modest changes suggested are based on small numbers and add little to the original interpretation [28,45,46].

Table 60-3. Chest Radiographic and Electrocardiographic Change in Pulmonary Embolism

	Urokinase PE (N=128) (%)	PIOPED PE (N=117) (%)	No PE (N=247) (%)
Chest Radiographs			
Lung parenchyma	47	68	48[a]
Consolidation	41	48	31[b]
Atelectasis	20		
Pleural effusion	28	48	31[b]
Diaphragmatic elevations	41	35	21[b]
Decreased pulmonary vascularity+	21	21	12[c]
Prominent central pulmonary artery++	23	15	11
Both + and ++		19	11
Pulmonary edema		4	13[c]
Cardiomegaly	19	12	

	PE (N=132) (%)	PE (N=117) (%)	No PE (N=248) (%)
Electrocardiograms			
Abnormal	87	70	—
ST–T wave changes	64	49	42
Left axis deviation	12	6	1*
Complete right bundle branch block	11	6	7
Premature ventricular beats	9		
$S_1 S_2 S_3$	9		
$S_1 Q_3 T_3$	11		
Low voltage	16		

The following were found in PIOPED in less than 4% of patients with or without PE: incomplete right bundle branch block, acute myocardial infarction pattern, low-voltage QRS, P pulmonale, right axis deviation, and right ventricular hypertrophy.

The following were found in the UK study in 5% or less: premature atrial beats, atrial fibrillation, P pulmonale, right axis deviation, incomplete right bundle branch block, and right ventricular hypertrophy.

[a] $p<0.001$
[b] $p<0.01$
[c] $p<0.05$

Only 124 of 931 (13%) patients had high-probability $\dot{V}/\dot{Q}$ scans; these had a positive predictive value of 88 percent. Indeterminate (intermediate) $\dot{V}/\dot{Q}$ scans were found in 39 percent and had a positive predictive value of 33 percent, the same as the incidence of PE in the entire study population. Low-probability $\dot{V}/\dot{Q}$ scans were found in 34 percent and had a positive predictive value of 16 percent. Near normal/normal scans were found in only 14 percent and had a positive predictive value of 9 percent. When patients with low-probability and normal/near normal scans who did not receive anticoagulation therapy and had no evidence of pulmonary thromboembolic events in a year of follow-up study were added, the incidence of PE in the low-probability group could be no less than 12 percent and in the normal/near normal no less than 4 percent [5,28]. Thus, $\dot{V}/\dot{Q}$ scan probability readings that permit clinical decision-making are only high probability (13%) and near normal/normal scan, (14%), representing a total of 27 percent of the population.

The clinicians involved in the study assigned patients to categories of estimated likelihood of PE of 80 to 100 percent, 20 to 79 percent, and 0 to 19 percent. High clinical likelihood (80–100%) was assigned to only 10 percent of patients and low likelihood to only 26 percent. In patients with a high clinical likelihood and a high-probability scan, PE was present in 28 of 29 (96%). For those with low clinical likelihood (0–19%) and low-probability $\dot{V}/\dot{Q}$ scan (90 patients), the incidence was 4 percent. Efforts to create decision rules using multivariate analysis based on history, physical examination, chest radiograph,

electrocardiogram, and $\dot{V}/\dot{Q}$ scans to develop scores in a retrospective series of angiographically proved PE followed by application to a different set of patients with angiographically proven PE did not perform as well as this information and the intuitive clinical probability of the PIOPED investigators. Very few patients were given a high negative predictive value and even fewer were given a high positive predictive value [28,47].

The 1-year follow-up evaluation of all patients improved the negative predictive value of the low-probability scan from 84 to approximately 88 percent and of the near normal/normal scan from 91 to 96 percent. It also substantiated the gold standard of angiography: only four (0.6%) patients who had an angiogram interpreted as negative had subsequent evidence of a pulmonary embolism [5].

Hull and colleagues reported on 305 consecutive patients with abnormal lung perfusion scans [48,49]. Of 59 patients with one or more segmental or greater mismatched defects (perfusion absent, ventilation present; high probability), 51 (86%) had angiographically proved PE. In 28 patients with one or more segmental or greater matched defects, 10 (36%) had PE. Of 40 patients with one or more subsegmental defects and a mismatch, 16 (40%) had PE; in 24 patients with matched defects, 6 (25%) had PE. The frequency of PE in these latter two categories was roughly comparable to that in the low-probability group in PIOPED. In Hull and colleagues' study, 57 percent of patients did not have adequate ventilation scans and only 66 percent (202 of 305) had angiograms. Eighty-one of those who did not have angiograms were excluded because they were judged clinically to be critically ill or angiography was thought to be contraindicated. In an additional 29 patients angiography was inadequate. Therefore, satisfactory angiography was performed in only 173 of 305 patients (57%). Overall, 51 percent of patients who had angiograms had PEs. In a subsequent report, 515 of 1420 (36%) consecutive patients had normal perfusion scans [50]. It is evident that the population studied by Hull and associates differs considerably from that in the PIOPED study in that the number of patients with normal scans was much larger and the percentage of patients with PE in the low probability groups (25–40%) was higher. Impedance plethysmography (IPG) was performed on 83 patients who had a positive angiogram, and the results were negative in 47 (57%).

Subgroup Analyses. A *past history of PE* was noted in 60 patients, 20 of whom were found to have pulmonary emboli on angiography; in this group, the positive predictive value of a high-probability scan dropped from 88 to 74 percent [28]. Ninety-eight patients were randomly selected from the PIOPED group, 67 of whom had angiographic proof of presence or absence of PE. When perfusion scans alone were read with the chest radiograph, versus $\dot{V}/\dot{Q}$ scans with chest radiograph, there were no differences in this small series in positive predictive value, high probability $\dot{V}/\dot{Q}$ (94%), and $\dot{Q}$ 93%. The frequency of PE in the low-probability group did not differ significantly (5 of 25 with $\dot{V}/\dot{Q}$, 0 of 25 with $\dot{Q}$ alone). The $\dot{V}/\dot{Q}$ combination resulted in more low-probability interpretations (38% vs. 23%, $p < 0.05$) [51]. In contrast to older reports, there was no significant difference in the diagnostic features of acute pulmonary embolism among 72 of the PIOPED patients *70 years of age or older* when compared with 140 patients 40 to 69 years of age and 44 patients younger than 40 years [52]. When all patients in the PIOPED study *without preexisting cardiac or pulmonary disease* were compared to those *with any cardiac or pulmonary disease*, there were no statistically significant differences. However, the positive predictive value of a high-probability scan in patients without previous cardiac or pulmonary disease was 93 percent (50 of 54) versus 83 percent (55 of 66) in patients with cardiopulmonary disease. The incidence of PE in patients without cardiopulmonary disease was 32 percent (117 of 365) versus 27 percent (140 of 526) in patients with cardiopulmonary disease [53]. In the overall PIOPED population, the prevalence of PE was 28 percent (252 of 887) versus 19 percent (21 of 108) in patients with chronic obstructive pulmonary disease (COPD) ($p < 0.02$). The frequency of a reading of indeterminate matched the prevalence of PE in the total PIOPED population, those with or without cardiopulmonary disease, and those with COPD [17,28,53].

The scan was interpretated as high-probability in only five patients with *COPD*, all of whom had pulmonary emboli. The interpretation was near normal/normal in only five patients (5%) (none of whom had PE) versus 10 percent of persons with cardiac or pulmonary disease and 22 percent of those without any cardiac or pulmonary disease. Of the 10 patients with a low clinical probability and a low-probability scan (9%), none had PE. There were no normal lung scans in individuals with moderate or more severe airways obstruction, defined as an FEV_1 less than 65 percent of predicted. Thus, in patients with even moderate airways obstruction a near normal/normal lung scan interpretation was not found. As in the general population, the presence of predisposing factors was not different in those with or without PE. Immobilization and surgery led the list of predisposing factors. There were no differences in presenting symptoms: dyspnea (90% of patients with PE vs. 92% of those without), cough (62% vs. 55%), pleuritic chest pain (43% vs. 37%) and leg swelling (43% vs. 26%). Chest radiograph abnor-

malities also did not differentiate. There was no difference in the $P(A-a)O_2$ gradient among patients with PE (64 ± 59 mm Hg) versus those without PE (89 ± 116 mm Hg). In patients with prior $P(A-a)O_2$ measurements, it increased from 47 ± 18 to 96 ± 71 mm Hg in patients with PE and from 51 ± 31 mm Hg to 106 ± 117 mm Hg in those without PE ($p < 0.01$). The $PaCO_2$ was 34 ± 6 mm Hg in patients breathing air with PE versus 38 ± 11 mm Hg in those without PE. Changes in $PaCO_2$ from prior values also were not helpful. In patients with at least moderate airways obstruction ($FEV_1 < 65\%$ of predicted), the lung scan was clinically useful in only the 5 percent of patients with a high-probability interpretation. The signs and symptoms of PE and an exacerbation of COPD mimic each other so closely that they cannot be clinically distinguished; in all likelihood this accounts for the appreciably lower incidence of PE in the PIOPED patients with COPD. Documentation of PE in this group is less than that reported in prior postmortem studies (28–51%). One patient with PE had an increase of $PaCO_2$ from 51 mm Hg to 68 mm Hg [17]. Several other cases of increased $PaCO_2$ developing despite an increase in minute ventilation have been reported [16].

Normal chest radiographs in the PIOPED study were found in 20 of 260 (8%) patients with PE and 113 of 642 (18%) without PE. In 17 patients with a PaO_2 of 70 mm Hg or less, dyspnea, and a normal chest radiograph, PE was found in 9 of 17 (53%) versus 18 of 93 (19%) such patients with a PaO_2 greater than 70 mm Hg ($p<0.01$). Pulmonary thromboembolism was found in only six of nine (67%) patients with a high-probability scan. Thus, the scan did not perform better in patients with a normal chest radiograph [23].

In a retrospective study of 617 consecutive *patients admitted to a respiratory intensive care unit because of respiratory insufficiency* or failure ($PaO_2 < 50$ mm Hg or $PaCO_2 > 40$ mm Hg), PE was found in 18 of 66 (27%) patients at autopsy. Though the diagnosis of PE was strongly suspected in 10 of the 18, therapeutic action was taken in only 8. During the same period, lung scans were performed on 88 consecutive patients (14%). Despite this attention to possible PE, the diagnosis was not entertained in 44 percent of patients with PE at postmortem and therapeutic intervention was not initiated in 66 percent. There was no correlation between lung scans and pulmonary angiograms in the 12 patients who had both. In the 11 patients in whom autopsy correlation with lung scans was possible, only 1 had a high-probability scan that correlated with the presence of PE. Thus, it is clear that in patients in respiratory failure and in a respiratory intensive care unit or other similar unit, the clinical, radiographic, arterial blood gas, and $\dot{V}/\dot{Q}$ scan findings are unsatisfactory in making a diagnosis. The usual clinical criteria for the diagnosis of PE are almost a constant in each patient in such a situation. Therefore, when the diagnosis of PE is considered, an angiogram is almost invariably required; indeed, it is reasonable to proceed with angiography immediately in such patients [26]. The efficacy of prophylaxis against venous thromboembolic disease has been shown in a prospective randomized trial and a trial with historical controls [54,55].

The value of a *normal lung scan* in excluding clinically important pulmonary emboli has been reported in a retrospective study of 68 patients from a Veterans Administration hospital who were followed over 2 to 97 months (mean 30.2 months). In only one of these patients was a small basilar pulmonary infarct noted at postmortem. There was no clinical evidence of PE in this group, based on record review [56]. In a much larger prospective study of 515 consecutive patients with normal lung perfusion scans, concurrent IPG in 493 of patients in whom the test could be performed revealed proximal vein thrombosis in 5 (1%). Three additional patients had objectively documented venous thromboembolism in a 3-month follow-up [50].

PULMONARY ANGIOGRAPHY. In the overall PIOPED study, 1111 patients had angiography. Five of these (0.5%) died within 24 hours [57], but it is believed that three of the deaths were not related to either catheterization or angiography, and all five patients had severe cardiopulmonary disease. These patients all were clinically unstable. One patient died following a ventilation scan. Major nonfatal complications occurred in nine patients (respiratory distress requiring cardiopulmonary resuscitation or intubation in 4, renal failure requiring dialysis in 3, hematoma requiring transfusion of two or more units of blood in 2). Less significant complications occurred in 60 patients (5%). In this series, the angiographic catheters used had a pigtail-shaped tip, which eliminated entirely the complication of myocardial perforation and resulted in a decrease in major cardiac arrhythmias. More fatal or major nonfatal complications occurred in patients in the medical intensive care unit. There was no correlation with pulmonary artery pressures, amount of contrast material, or presence or absence of PE. Renal dysfunction after angiography was more likely to occur in older patients (74 ± 13 years vs. 57 ± 17 years; $p < 0.001$). Angiograms were nondiagnostic in 35 of 1111 (3%) and studies were incomplete in 12 of 1111 (1%), usually because of complications. On the basis of the angiograms and other data, a correct diagnosis of the presence or absence of PE was made in 96 percent of the 1111 patients. The mortality rate was similar to that reported by pooling nine series (91 of 3074; 0.3%) [57]. A negative angiogram excludes the diagnosis of PE [58]. Although prompt angiography is desirable, circumstances might lead to unavoidable delays. Very rarely do emboli lyse within 1 or 2 days; in fact, slow resolution, over weeks, is the norm, as detected by both angiography and $\dot{V}/\dot{Q}$ scans [29,60].

A PRUDENT ALGORITHM FOR THE DIAGNOSIS OF PULMONARY EMBOLISM. The criteria selected for the PIOPED interpretation of $\dot{V}/\dot{Q}$ scans were exceptionally complex to enhance interpretation and subsequent analysis. In daily clinical use the following criteria are satisfactory. A *high-probability* scan is one with two or more segmental or near segmental (> 75%) perfusion defects without corresponding ventilation scan or radiographic abnormalities or with the perfusion defect being substantially larger than the ventilation or chest radiograph abnormality. A *low-probability* scan is one with a single moderate mismatched segmental perfusion defect with a normal chest radiograph; any perfusion defect with a substantially larger chest radiographic abnormality; or matching segmental perfusion and ventilation defects. The indeterminate (intermediate) category is used for abnormalities between high and low. A normal scan is one with no perfusion defects or with small (< 25%) perfusion defects ("rat bites") [59].

The diagnosis of pulmonary embolism rests on the clinical evaluation (Fig. 60-1). Most patients who have acute PE have one or more risk factors or are a member of one of the risk groups previously described. The characteristics and symptoms of PE have been detailed. Dyspnea or tachypnea is present in 91 percent of people with PE; dyspnea, tachypnea, or pleuritic pain in 97 percent; and dyspnea, tachypnea, pleuritic pain, or clinical evidence of DVT in 97 percent. Data from many studies indicate that 85 to 90 percent of patients with PE have a decreased PaO_2 and/or increased $P(A-a)O_2$. The $PaCO_2$ is also decreased in a great majority of patients. Nonspecific abnormalities of the chest radiograph and electrocardiogram are present in 70 to 80 percent of patients with PE. The decision to order a $\dot{V}/\dot{Q}$ scan must be based on these factors. Clearly, it would be inappropriate to order a $\dot{V}/\dot{Q}$ scan on every person evaluated because of dyspnea or tachypnea, such as the 22-year-old asthmatic with clearcut polyphonic wheezing [2].

Thus, the decision to order a $\dot{V}/\dot{Q}$ lung scan is based on the clinical evaluation, especially the presence of predisposing factors. There is no such thing as a positive or negative lung scan; rather, probabilities are assigned.

Only a high-probability $\dot{V}/\dot{Q}$ scan warrants treatment for PE without further diagnostic studies if the clinical impression is high or uncertain. The positive predictive value with a high clinical suspicion is 96 percent and with an uncertain (20–79%) clinical probability is 88 percent. The only $\dot{V}/\dot{Q}$ scan finding that warrants a decision not to treat and not to obtain further diagnostic studies is a normal scan interpretation. A normal scan with very high clinical suspicion might rarely lead to IPG or duplex ultrasound. In my opinion, both low-probability and indeterminate (intermediate) lung scan findings require further objective evaluation. A reasonable approach is to perform IPG or duplex ultrasound. If positive, the patient should be treated; if negative, the patient should have an angiogram. The PIOPED data show that the positive predictive value in individuals with a low-probability lung scan and a low clinical probability (present in about 10% of the patients) was 4 percent (4 of 90). However, unless the clinical probability is extremely low, the combination should also lead to IPG or ultrasound. If the results are positive, the patient should be treated; if negative, an angiogram should be performed.

This algorithm mates data from studies of IPG, duplex ultrasonography, and PIOPED. Impedance plethysmography or ultrasound studies have been negative in up to 57 percent of patients with angiographically proven PE. Therefore, the percentage of patients with symptoms of PE and negative noninvasive studies is sufficiently high that they should have angiography. Treating the patient for PE with a positive IPG or ultrasound should reduce the need for angiography about 50 percent. See further discussion under Deep Venous Thrombosis (DVT) for recent data indicating that ultrasound outperforms IPG but is insensitive to asymptomatic DVT in high-risk patients [61,62]. Clearly, in an intensive care unit setting, serial IPGs or ultrasound studies would rarely, if ever, be appropriate. Other diagnostic algorithms are available [63,64,65].

Treatment

Heparin. Acute PE is treated immediately with intravenous heparin (Fig. 60-2) [66,67,68]. Heparin interrupts the progression of the thrombotic process (see Chap. 121). The initial loading dose should be 5000 to 10,000 units given on the basis of strong clinical suspicion, unless there is a high risk or contraindication to the use of anticoagulants. If PE is believed to be massive, some would give 15,000 to 25,000 units as a loading dose. Prior to giving this dose, baseline activated partial thromboplastin time (aPTT) or thrombin clotting time (TCT), prothrombin time (PT) to determine the international normalized ratio (INR), complete blood count (CBC), and platelets should be drawn. If the baseline INR is more than 1.5 or the aPTT more than 1.5 × the midrange of the control value, they should be repeated and evaluation for a potential coagulopathy should be considered. The CBC and platelets should be repeated daily while heparin is continued. Following the loading dose, intravenous heparin at 1300 units per hour should be started [69]. In an elderly or frail individual some would reduce this dose, but for most patients it is a minimum. The goal is to obtain an aPTT that is 1.5 to 2.5 times the mean of the normal range. An aPTT of 1.5 to 2.5 times the midrange of the control was selected in the algorithm in Figure 60-2 as ideal, providing adequate anticoagulation to prevent recurrence of thromboembo-

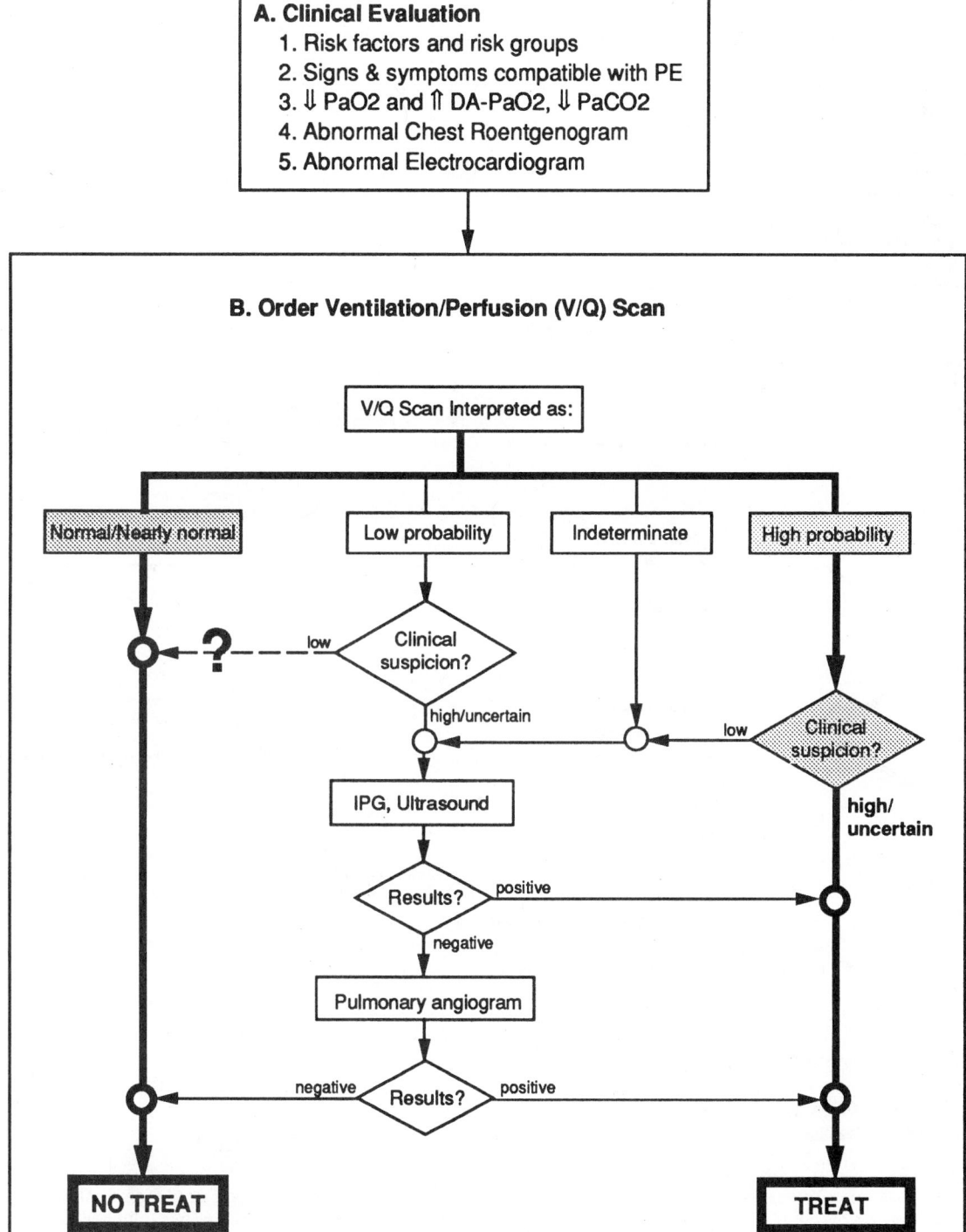

Fig. 60-1. An Algorithm for the diagnosis of pulmonary embolism.

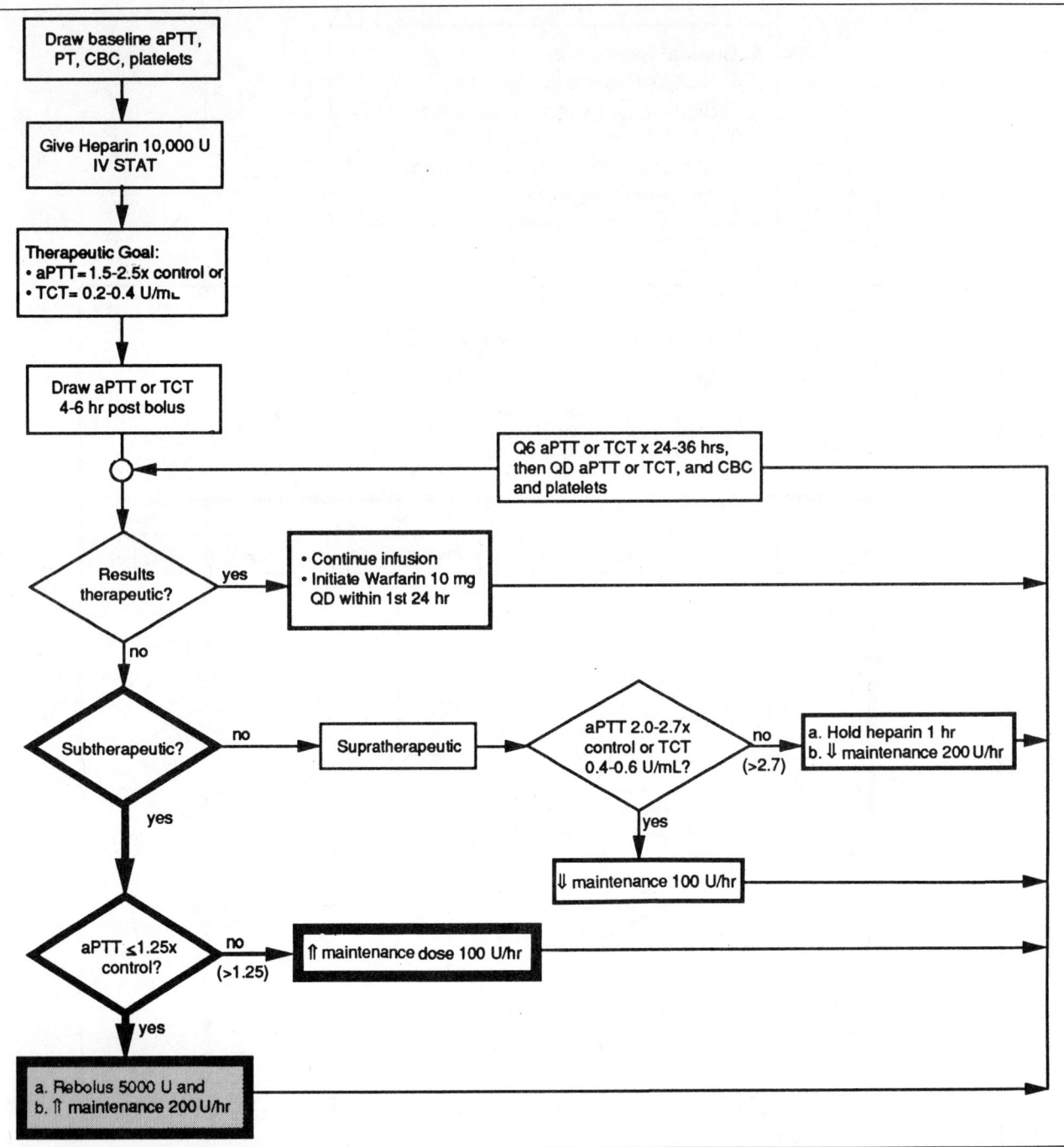

Fig. 60-2. An algorithm for initiating anticoagulation for pulmonary embolism or deep venous thrombosis. Initial inadequate anticoagulation should be avoided.

lism with the least likelihood of bleeding. Alternatively, a TCT that is 0.2 to 0.4 heparin units per milliliter can be used. It is most important that the aPTT not fall below 1.5 times the mean of the control. However, an aPTT somewhat on the high side poses appreciably less risk than one that falls below 1.5 times the mean range of the control. In subanalyses of two prospective studies of the treatment of deep venous thrombosis, the relative risk of recurrence of a thromboembolic event ranged from 10.7 to 15 times that of those in the therapeutic range [57,58]. The aPTT or TCT should be repeated at 4 to 6 hours and then every 6 hours for the first 24 to 36 hours or until it is clear a therapeutic range has been established.

If the aPTT or TCT is subtherapeutic (≤ 1.25 times the mean of the control), the patient should receive a rebolus of 5000 units of heparin and the maintenance dose should be increased 200 units per hour. If the subtherapeutic level is more than 1.25 but less than 1.5 times the mean of the control, the maintenance dose should be increased 100 units per hour.

If the aPTT or TCT is supratherapeutic (2.0–2.7 or more than 0.4–0.66, respectively), the maintenance dose of heparin should be reduced 100 units per hour. If the aPTT is more than 2.7 times the mean of the control or the TCT is more than 0.66, the heparin infusion should be held for 1 hour and the maintenance dose reduced to 200 units per hour. Since the average half-life of heparin is approximately 60 minutes when given in therapeutic doses intravenously, generally it should not be discontinued for more than 1 hour unless the aPTT or TCT remains very high. The goal is to avoid a subtherapeutic level less than 1.5 times the mean of the control. Heparin may be given intravenously intermittently. Studies show that heparin may be given subcutaneously, but the onset of action is delayed for approximately 1 hour and a peak level generally occurs at approximately 3 hours. If the subcutaneous route is to be used, the patient should receive initial doses in the range of 35,000 units per 24 hours in two doses. In addition, an intravenous bolus of 5000 units should be given initially. The aPTT or TCT should be monitored midway between the every 12-hour doses.

There are variations in the responsiveness of the various commercial aPTT reagents to heparin, and the aPTT is also altered by the type of clot detection system, contact activator, and phospholipid composition of the reagent. There may be differences between batches of the same brand of aPTT. An approximation of the therapeutic range of 0.2 to 0.4 units of heparin by protamine titration should be made by testing the aPTT reagent in a plasma system, or aPTT ratios can be prepared with measured heparin levels by protamine titration [70].

There is a diurnal variation of aPTT and TCT, with a peak around 3:20 A.M. and a trough around 3:20 P.M. The mean peak-to-trough difference is 9.5 seconds (range 5.9–13.2 seconds). This should be taken into account when evaluating the aPTT or TCT, and once a therapeutic level is obtained the test should be performed close to the same time each day [69].

Heparin should not be given when there is a history of heparin thrombocytopenia, active bleeding, or recent brain, eye, spinal cord, or other surgery with a high risk of bleeding. A positive test for occult blood from the gastrointestinal tract is not a contraindication to anticoagulation.

COMPLICATIONS. The most common complication of heparin therapy is bleeding [66,67,70] (see Chap. 121). Clinically important bleeding has been reported in 5 to 20 percent of patients, as either identifiable hemorrhage or a decrease in hematocrit [71,72]. A recent review of bleeding related to heparin reported a frequency of fatal, major, and major or minor bleeding as 0.05, 0.8, and 2.0 percent, respectively, approximately 2 times the expected bleeding without heparin [73]. In the PIOPED study, a decrease in hemoglobin of 2 gm or more or bleeding into the central nervous system or a joint was found in 16 of 238 (7%) patients treated with anticoagulants [5]. There is a general association between bleeding and higher levels of anticoagulation. In the Urokinase Pulmonary Embolism Trial, blood clotting times greater than 60 minutes resulted in bleeding in 9 of 44 (20%) of patients [29] versus only 1 of 28 (4%) with blood clotting times less than 60 minutes. A retrospective identification of predictors of major bleeding in hospitalized patients who were anticoagulated identified intensity of anticoagulation as an important predictor. If the aPTT was prolonged to 2 to 2.9 times the control value, complications increased threefold. If the aPTT was 3 times or longer that of control, the bleeding complication was increased to eightfold. Other comorbid factors were identified: acute myocardial infarction, systolic blood pressure less than 90 mm Hg, need for

intraaortic balloon pump, bilirubin level greater than 1 mg per deciliter, macrocytosis, increase in creatinine of greater than 50 percent to greater than 1.5 mg per deciliter, cancer, or hematocrit of less than 30 without recent bleeding [74]. In general, the risk of bleeding has been shown to be decreased by the use of continuous infusion of heparin versus intermittent injection.

Heparin-induced thrombocytopenia is relatively uncommon (see Chap. 120). Many patients have a modest decrease in platelets with no overt ill effects, but some develop what appears to be an IgG heparin immune complex involving the Fab and Fc portions of the IgG molecule. In these patients, the platelet count usually falls precipitously to less than 100,000, often in the range of 40,000 to 60,000 per cubic milliliter. In such patients, there is a major risk of thrombotic events on both the arterial and venous sides, including thrombotic cerebral vascular accidents and myocardial infarction. With a decrease in platelet count to less than 100,000 or a precipitous drop in that direction, heparin must be discontinued. If the patient is adequately anticoagulated with warfarin or nearly so, no other intervention is necessary. However, if anticoagulation is inadequate, insertion of a vena cava filter should be considered the standard of therapy. Alternative therapies under consideration are a heparinoid (Org 10172 or danaparoid or orgaran) manufactured by Organon, which does not cross-react in vitro with plasma samples of patients with heparin-induced thrombocytopenia. Alternatively, ancrod may be substituted to obtain anticoagulation. (This agent can be made available for compassionate use by Knoll pharmaceutical.) Ancrod's long-term use is limited by antibody development [70,75–82].

Long-term use of high-dose heparin may result in osteoporosis. The vast majority of cases have been reported in individuals receiving at least 20,000 units per day for more than 6 months [70,83]. Skin necrosis, which may or may not be associated with thrombocytopenia, and urticaria have also been reported. Rare cases of hypoaldosteronism leading to hyperkalemia, other metabolic derangements, and death have been reported [70].

The effects of heparin may be reversed with protamine sulfate, which should be given by very slow intravenous injection over 10 minutes to avoid hypotension. One milligram of protamine sulfate neutralizes approximately 100 units of heparin. An individual dose should not exceed 50 mg.

Warfarin. The following is a reasonable set of guidelines for treating with warfarin [66,84,85] (see Chap. 121). Initiate therapy with 5 mg per day, starting within the first 24 hours. The INR should be checked daily after the first 2 days, until it stabilizes in the range of 2 to 3. The mean half-life of warfarin is approximately 35 hours (range 15–44 hours). It is therefore helpful to give warfarin in the afternoon, so that the morning INR 36 hours later will reflect the dose. If dosage adjustments are necessary, they should be modest (e.g., ≤ 5 mg). After a stable INR in the range of 2 to 3 for 48 hours has been achieved, the interval of checking can gradually be lengthened. An INR of 2 to 3 is appropriate for venous thromboembolism, including recurrent evidence of embolism. Higher ranges in TED have not been shown to improve efficacy but increase the risk of bleeding.

Warfarin acts by interfering with the cyclic interconversion of vitamin K to vitamin K epoxide. This leads to the depletion of the vitamin K-dependent coagulant proteins—factors II (prothrombin), VII, IX, and X. It also limits the carboxylation of the anticoagulants protein C and protein S. The biologic half-life of the clotting factors is quite variable: factor VII, 4 to 6 hours; factors IX and X, 20 to 65 hours; and factor II (prothrombin), longer than 100 hours. Thus, the INR may promptly reach the therapeutic range because of the decrease in factor VII, but factors II, IX, and X may still be present in sufficient amounts to generate thrombin. Therefore, this accounts for the general guidelines of a 4- to 5-day overlap of heparin with warfarin and a 48- to 72-hour period in which the INR is within the therapeutic range [66,67,69,70,84–87].

INTERNATIONAL NORMALIZED RATIO. The effect of anticoagulation therapy has been reported as the prothrombin time in seconds or the prothrombin time ratio—the patient's prothrombin time divided by the mean control. Over the last two decades an International Standardized Thromboplastin reagent has been developed and adapted by the World Health Organization. Its use in the United States was recommended by the Committee on Antithrombotic Therapy of the American College of Chest Physicians and the National Heart, Lung and Blood Institute in 1986, 1989, and 1992 [66,84,85]. The international reference preparation (IRP) for thromboplastin permits comparison of the thromboplastin used in an individual laboratory with the international standard. The international sensitivity index (ISI) is calculated as a measure of the responsiveness of a given thromboplastin to that of the IRP, which has an ISI of 1.0. One can then calculate the INR:

$$INR = \left(\frac{PT(patient)}{PT(control)}\right)^{ISI}$$

The necessity for this form of reporting has become increasing evident. A recent survey of 53 laboratories and 140 additional laboratories involved in a stroke prevention and atrial fibrillation trial found the ISI to range from 1.8 to 2.8, with a few as low as 1.4. The manufacturers indicated they were marketing thromboplastins with ISI values from 1.2 to 2.8 [88]. Under these circumstances, the prothrombin time as a measure of coagulation is unacceptable. Use of the INR eliminates variations related to the activity of various thromboplastins and permits accurate comparison of values from one laboratory or thromboplastin to another. The more sensitive the thromboplastin, (the closest the ISI is to 1) the higher will be the patient's prothrombin time. If a sample of one patient's blood is taken and prothrombin times are measured with various thromboplastins, this patient's PT with a thromboplastin having an ISI of one would be 38 seconds, with an ISI of 2.0 would be 21 seconds, and with an ISI of 3.2 would be 16 seconds. If it is reported as the INR in each of these patients, the INR would be the same (2.6). A thromboplastin with an ISI of 1.2 or less is recommended.

The generally accepted duration of warfarin therapy is 3 months. If a second episode of thromboembolic disease occurs after anticoagulants have been discontinued, most recommend therapy for at least 6 months and some would continue warfarin indefinitely. If a high-risk factor for thromboembolic disease persists, one should consider continuing anticoagulation therapy indefinitely or inserting a vena cava filter (see below).

An alternative to oral anticoagulation with warfarin is the use of subcutaneous heparin twice a day with a dose adjusted to achieve an aPTT of 1.5 times the mean control value midway between doses. This is somewhat more expensive than warfarin therapy and carries the morbidity of multiple subcutaneous injections [66,70,89,90]. Some would discontinue warfarin in less than 3 months if the risk factor can be eliminated, such as with a period of immobilization or use of estrogens, although there are not sufficient well-controlled prospective studies [66].

The effects of excess warrfarin can be reversed slowly by stopping treatment, more quickly by administering vitamin K, and still more rapidly using fresh frozen plasma or factor concentrates. For an INR greater than 3 but less than 6 in a patient who is not bleeding, withholding the next several doses of warfarin suffices. With an INR in the range of 6 to 10 and a patient who is not bleeding, vitamin K_1 at a low dose (0.5–1 mg) intravenously usually reduces the INR within 8 hours and results in a INR of 2 to 3 over 24 hours. If the INR is still higher (10–20) and the patient is not bleeding, the dose should be increased to 2 mg intravenously. If the INR is greater than 20 or there is serious bleeding, vitamin K in a dose of 2 mg can be given; the INR should be checked every 6 hours. Vitamin K can be given every 12 hours. Some authors prefer subcutaneous injections of 3 to 5 mg to avoid the occurrence of an anaphylactoid reaction, which has been reported only very rarely. If there is serious or life-threatening bleeding, fresh frozen plasma or plasma concentrates can be given along with vitamin K_1. If large doses of vitamin K have been given, anticoagulation with heparin may be necessary to protect the patient adequately from recurrent thromboembolic events [84].

Many factors may affect the anticoagulant activity of warfarin. Its effect may be potentiated by low vitamin K intake (a likely setting in the ICU), a host of drugs—phenylbutazone, metronidazole, trimethoprim-sulfamethoxazole, amiodarone, erythromycin, clofibrate, cimetidine, omeprazole, ketoconazole, fluconazole, isoniazid, proxican, tamoxifen, quinidine, and phenytoin, liver disease, and hypermetabolic states, such as pyrexia and thyrotoxicosis. The effect of warfarin can be reduced by absorption by cholestyramine, barbiturates, rifampin, griseofulvin, carbamazepine, and penicillin and by alterations in other aspects of coagulation [66,84,85].

Rare instances of hereditary resistance to warfarin have been reported. Such patients may require doses 5 to 20 times greater than usual [91,92].

ADVERSE EFFECTS. Bleeding is the most common complication of warfarin therapy. This risk is markedly influenced by the intensity of anticoagulant therapy. An INR in the range of 2 to 3 reduces the clinically important bleeding to the range of 4.3 to 6 percent, compared with 14 to 42 percent when the INR is in the range of 3 or greater. These data are derived from four randomized prospective studies [89,90]. Bleeding is also increased with the use of high doses of aspirin and by the risk factors previously cited for heparin [23,66,74,84,85]. A literature review reported that during warfarin therapy, the average annual frequency of fatal, major, and major or minor bleeding was 0.6 percent, 3.0 percent, and 9.6 percent, respectively, approximately 5 times the expected bleeding without warfarin [73]. The most common sites of bleeding are the gastrointestinal and urinary tracts; in about one-third of these cases an unknown lesion is identified. The risk of bleeding is also increased with serious comorbid diseases involving the central nervous system, kidney, heart, and liver. Old age may also contribute. Warfarin skin necrosis may occur and has been associated with malignancy and protein C and protein S deficiency; it usually appears on day 3 to 8 [93].

PREGNANCY. Heparin is the drug of choice for the treatment and prophylaxis of TED in pregnancy (see Chap. 59). It is clear that heparin is safer for the fetus. In a retrospective cohort study of 100 pregnancies in 77 women treated with heparin, 98 for the prevention or treatment of venous thromboembolism, the rates of prematurity, abortions, stillbirths, neonatal deaths, and congenital abnormalities were similar to those in a normal population [94,95]. Warfarin may result in an embryopathy characterized by nasal hypoplasia, stippling of bone, optic atrophy, and mental retardation. Cleft lip, cleft palate, and cataracts and microphthalmia have also been reported [96,97]. Other central nervous system abnormalities associated with warfarin include dorsal midline dysplasia, ventral midline dysplasia, and hemorrhage. The incidence of warfarin embryopathy in 72 pregnant women with prosthetic heart valves was 29 percent (10 of 35) when treated between weeks 7 and 12 of gestation: this did not occur in the infants of mothers whose warfarin was discontinued between weeks 6 and 12 [94].

Thrombolytic Therapy. Thrombolytic agents activate plasminogen to plasmin, which degrades fibrin in a thrombus or hemostatic plug to soluble peptides. The older agents, streptokinase and urokinase, are not specific for thrombi; they may lyse any fresh platelet-fibrin hemostatic plug. Tissue plasminogen activator (t-PA) is more specific against thrombi or hemostatic plugs versus circulating plasminogen. However, there is no difference in the incidence of bleeding with any of these agents. With urokinase, there has been a 72 to 81 percent reduction in plasminogen and a reduction of approximately 50 percent in fibrinogen. With streptokinase, the reduction in plasminogen in the Urokinase Streptokinase Pulmonary Embolism Trial was 94 percent, with a 58 percent reduction in fibrinogen. In various studies with t-PA, there has been a reduction in plasminogen in the range of 34 to 45 percent [29,30,98–101].

Uncontrolled trials of streptokinase were first reported in 1959, of urokinase in 1967, and of t-PA in 1985. At least 18 controlled clinical trials of urokinase, streptokinase, and t-PA in more than 750 patients have yet to show any improvement in mortality, hemodynamics beyond 24 hours, or perfusion lung scans beyond 1 and 3 days. A clinically unimportant increase in carbon monoxide diffusing capacity was shown at 2 weeks and 1 year in patients treated with thrombolytic therapy compared to those with conventional therapy [66].

We recommend the use of thrombolytic therapy for patients with acute massive pulmonary embolism who are hemodynamically unstable (in shock) despite fluid resuscitation and use of vasopressors (see Chap. 46). However, many patients in whom thrombolytic therapy might be of value are excluded because of absolute contraindications, such as active internal bleeding; uncontrolled hypertension (diastolic blood pressure > 110); a bleeding disorder; increased risk of intracranial hemorrhage, such as malignancy, abscess, arteriovenous malformation, aneurysm or recent head trauma, or neurosurgery within 2 months; or relative contraindications, such as severe recent trauma within 2 months, any surgical or invasive procedure, including parturition, deep biopsies within 10 days, hemorrhagic retinopathy, ophthalmologic surgery within 6 weeks, and extended cardiopulmonary resuscitation. In a collaborative effort by the PIOPED investigators over 7 months, in their six hospitals with more than 5000 beds, and all patients in whom PE was suspected strongly enough to request a $\dot{V}/\dot{Q}$ scan or pulmonary angiogram, only 13 patients were entered in a double-blind dose comparison of t-PA. The criteria for entry were occlusion of a lobar artery or at least two segmental arteries, and patients in shock were excluded. The study was discontinued because of the very low enrollment. This was most likely due to the very few patients who did not have a contraindication to thrombolytic therapy [101].

The selection of patients who are hemodynamically unstable (in shock) is based on the mortality rate in this group (32 percent) compared to others with PE including those with more than 50 percent obstruction but with normal blood pressure (6%) [102]. In addition to the increased risk of bleeding and potential mortality with the use of thrombolytic agents, the expense should be considered—recent charges for urokinase approximate $4000, for t-PA approximately $2000, and for streptokinase approximately $280. In addition, all patients still require heparin and subsequent warfarin for treatment of PE.

When thrombolytic therapy is to be used, heparin is discontinued until the aPTT is 1.5 times control or less. Streptokinase is given, with a 250,000 IU loading dose and then 100,000 IU per hour for 24 hours. Urokinase is given in a loading dose of 4400 IU per kilogram followed by a maintenance dose of 4400 IU per hour. Tissue plasminogen activator is given as 100 mg (56 million IU) over 2 hours. Heparin is restarted when the aPTT has returned to 1.5 times control or less. An aPTT 2 to 4 hours into treatment can be obtained to document fibrinolysis; prolongation by 10 seconds or more is an indicator of fibrinolysis. No laboratory monitoring of t-PA is recommended [66].

Inferior Vena Cava Interruption. The major indications for inferior vena cava interruption are a contraindication or complication of anticoagulation in a patient with or at high risk of venous thromboembolic disease of the lower extremity; documented recurrent thromboembolism despite adequate anticoagulation; a large free-floating caval thrombus; chronic recurrent embolism with pulmonary hypertension; and pulmonary embolectomy [53,66,103–106]. Filter insertion has been recently documented to be effective in primary prophylaxis of thromboembolism in patients at high risk of bleeding, such as extensive trauma, visceral cancer, spinal cord injury, hip fracture, and hip and knee surgery [107–114]. The largest experience to date has been with the Greenfield filter, which can be inserted through the femoral vein or an internal jugular vein. The filter patency rate is in the range of 98 percent. If the filter is inserted in the absence of a contraindication or complication of anticoagulant therapy or in a patient at high risk of such a complication, many authorities recommend resuming anticoagulation. In a review of 24 case series encompassing more than 2500 patients, recurrence of PE was extremely rare and mortality due to PE occurred in only 8 (0.0003%) [103]. Other filters in use include the Simon-Nitinol, the Bird's Nest, and the Amplatz [115].

Complications of filter placement include thrombus at the site of insertion, migration of the filter, improper filter deployment, formation of a clot proximal to the filter with proximal propagation, inferior vena cava obstruction, and venous insufficiency. Rare complications include myocardial infarction, pericardial tamponade, and cardiac arrhythmias [103–115]. The filter may be inserted above the renal vessels in individuals with renal vein or ovarian vein thrombi or IVC thrombi extending to or above the renal veins [116].

Pulmonary Embolectomy. There is considerable dispute concerning the role of emergency pulmonary embolectomy. If it is to be considered, the patient should meet the following criteria: (1) massive PE (angiographically documented, if possible); (2) hemodynamic instability (i.e., shock) despite heparin therapy and resuscitative efforts; and (3) failure of thrombolytic therapy or a contraindication to its use. In addition, an experienced open heart surgery team should be available for the procedure. Even with immediately available cardiopulmonary bypass, reported mortality has ranged from 10 to 75 percent. If the patient has had a cardiopulmonary arrest mortality has ranged from 50 to 94 percent. Cardiac arrest, shock, and cardiopulmonary disease are predictors of mortality. Complications of pulmonary embolectomy include the acute respiratory distress syndrome, acute renal failure, mediastinitis, and severe neurologic sequelae [117–122].

Transvenous Catheter Extraction of Emboli. Use of a balloon-tipped catheter under fluoroscopy has been recently reported to be successful in extraction of the embolus in 23 of 26 patients (88%), with a mortality of 27 percent; 2 of the patients subsequently had open embolectomy. The institutional mortality rate for open embolectomy was 33 percent. In another report of catheter embolectomy in 18 patients the mortality rate was 28 percent. Better results were obtained with a shorter period from the first episode of PE and a shorter duration of hemodynamic impairment. This procedure deserves continued evaluation. A vena cava filter is inserted following catheter extraction of the PE [122–123].

COURSE AND PROGNOSIS OF PULMONARY EMBOLISM. Untreated PE have a hospital mortality of approximately 30 percent. In a recent report on 399 patients, 375 of whom received treatment for PE, 10 patients (2.5%) died of PE, 9 of whom had clinically suspected recurrent emboli [5]. The recurrence rate of PE in this series was 8.3 percent (33 patients). The overall mortality was 23.8 percent (95 of 399). Conditions that predicted death were cancer (relative risk 3.8; 95% confidence interval 2.3–6.4), left-sided congestive heart failure (relative risk 2.7; 95% confidence interval 1.5–4.6), and chronic lung disease (relative risk 2.2; 95% confidence interval 1.2–4.0). The most frequent causes of death in patients with PE were cancer (34.7%), infection (22.1%), and cardiac disease (16.8%). Twenty-two percent of the deaths occurred within 1 week of entry and 23 percent within 2 weeks. The hospital mortality rate for patients with PE was 9.5 percent. Eight of the 10 deaths due to PE occurred within one week of entry into the study and 9 within two weeks. This in all likelihood is related to the continued difficulty in obtaining adequate anticoagulation with heparin promptly. These data are similar to those reported in 1976; 12 of 144 (8%) patients died of PE and PE was the primary cause of death in only 4 of these patients (2.7%); each of these patients had a massive PE with acute right ventricular failure [102]. Three were hypotensive and two died within 1 hour of diagnosis. In the other eight, PE was a final event in patients with serious underlying diseases. In the urokinase trial and the urokinase streptokinase trials, 8 percent of 327 patients died of PE and the 6-month mortality rate was 13 percent [29,30]. Other studies have reported a mortality rate between 3 and 9 percent without pre-existing cardiac disease. A poorer long-term outcome is related to underlying disease [124,125,126]. The mortality rate due to PE can be reduced 10-fold with treatment, from approximately 30 percent to 2.5 to 3 percent.

Other Emboli

SEPTIC EMBOLI. Pulmonary septic emboli generally present as multiple peripheral nodules, often with a feeding vessel sign, evidence of cavitation, or a wedge-shaped pleural lesion. Air bronchograms within nodules and extension into the pleural space are also seen. These may be identified with greater sensitivity with the use of computed tomography (CT) scan [127,128].

AMNIOTIC FLUID EMBOLISM. Amniotic fluid embolism is characterized by the abrupt onset of profound shock, central nervous system irritability, hyperreflexia; convulsions, altered mental status, restlessness, cyanosis, dyspnea, and vomiting (see Chap. 59). This is a rare complication of pregnancy with a high mortality rate. It occurs more frequently in older multiparous patients with a large fetus, and hard labor. The amniotic fluid, containing fetal urine, membrane secretions, particulate matter from the fetus, such as squames and lanugo hairs, fat, mucin, bile, and meconium enters the maternal circulation via small tears in the endocervix, lower uterine segment, or at the placental site. It causes pulmonary vascular obstruction. Disseminated intravascular coagulation is common. The chest radiograph shows bilateral diffuse infiltrates compatible with the acute respiratory distress syndrome. Although identification of squames and aspirates from a pulmonary artery catheter has been considered diagnostic, this is generally not accepted. Amniotic fluid material has also been recovered from the lungs antemortem in pregnant patients without amniotic fluid embolism. In one case report the administration of cryoprecipitate resulted in survival of the patient [129–132].

FAT EMBOLI. Fat emboli occur following long bone fractures and large joint replacement. It is estimated that they may occur in a subclinical fashion in 90 percent of such patients. The classic fat embolism syndrome consists of the following: progressive respiratory insufficiency; petechial rash; and altered mental status; it is estimated to occur in 0.5 to 2 percent of patients with long bone fractures. Its onset is usually 24 to 72 hours after injury. The patient develops hypoxemia, a widened $P(A-a)O_2$ and diffuse bilateral infiltrates on chest radiograph. The petechiae may appear about the head, neck, or axillae, in the conjunctiva, and in mucous membranes. There are no specific laboratory tests for fat embolism. Fat may be found in serum, urine, and sputum following long bone fractures with or without the fat embolism syndrome. The syndrome is generally mild and responds to supportive measures. Although corticosteroids have been used, there are no controlled studies to support their use. Prophylactic corticosteroids have been shown to reduce the incidence of the syndrome but are generally not recommended [133–138].

TUMOR EMBOLI. Tumor emboli may present with the characteristic signs and symptoms of PE, although this is uncommon. More often tumor emboli are microscopic or seen in association with lymphangitic spread of carcinoma. Tumor emboli are common with breast, liver, kidney, stomach, and choriocarcinoma. Tumor emboli presenting as PE have been reported with hepatoma, renal cell carcinoma, and right atrial myxoma [139–142].

AIR EMBOLISM. See Chapter 68.

Deep Venous Thrombosis

INCIDENCE AND NATURAL HISTORY. Using data from the Tecumseh Community Health Study extrapolated to the 1970 U.S. census figures, it is estimated that there are 250,000 cases of clinically recognized deep venous thrombosis (DVT) in the United States annually [143]. Extrapolating from necropsy studies with complete leg vein dissection, the estimated incidence of DVT in the United States approaches 1 million [103]. In autopsy studies, six sites of primary venous thrombosis have been identified: the iliac, common femoral, deep femoral, popliteal, posterior tibial, and soleal veins [144]. In older postmortem series, thrombi were found in the calf in approximately 50 percent, in the calf and femoral vein in 40 percent, and in the femoral vein only in 10 percent or less of cases.

PREDISPOSING CAUSES. Since PE is in essence a complication of DVT, the predisposing causes are the same. Rarely does DVT occur in the absence of such predisposing causes. The most common of these are immobilization or surgery followed by malignancy. Other predisposing factors include a previous history of venous thromboembolism, heart disease, congestive heart failure, atrial arrhythmias, trauma, especially multiple trauma and trauma to pelvis, hips, or lower extremity, the puerperium, paralysis, age more than 40, oral contraceptive use, estrogen therapy, and obesity (> 20% above life insurance tables). Utilizing IPG in 1464 consecutive patients suspected of having DVT, 4 percent had DVT. The incidence of DVT was 11 percent when no major risk factors were present, 24 percent with one risk factor, 36 percent with two major risk factors, 50 percent with three major risk factors, and 100 percent when four or more risk factors were present [145].

SYMPTOMS AND SIGNS. There are two quite distinct presentations of DVT. It is estimated that 50 to 85 percent, of patients with DVT present *without symptoms*. In the PIOPED study, only 15 percent of patients had clinical evidence of DVT [65]. In various studies of postoperative patients, especially following hip and knee surgery, DVT was identified using objective testing in 40 to 70 percent of these high-risk patients without symptoms [66,146]. Clearly, this presentation of DVT is not subject to clinical diagnosis. It is also evident that it is important to screen high-risk patients. Therefore, patients with a substantial risk of DVT require prophylactic therapy to prevent it and, in particular, PE, which may lead to death when untreated.

In juxtaposition to the high frequency of asymptomatic DVT is the large percentage of patients with signs and symptoms compatible with DVT who have another diagnosis; this has ranged to 80 or 95 percent. Leg or thigh swelling, proximal extension of symptoms, and tenderness are the most commonly recorded signs of DVT [107]. In a retrospective study of 355 symptomatic patients who had venography, DVT was found in 96 (27%). Five independent clinical correlates of proximal DVT were found: (1) swelling above the knees; (2) swelling below the knees; (3) recent immobility; (4) cancer; and (5) fever. When none, one, two, or more of these findings were present, proximal DVT was identified in 5 percent, 15 percent, and 42 percent, respectively. In this study, 21 percent of the venograms were read as equivocal (which included calf-only thrombi). In patients with proven DVT, cancer was present in 45 percent, fever in 59 percent, recent immobility in 39 percent, swelling above the knee in 42 percent, and swelling below the knee in 32 percent. In those with a normal venogram, cancer was present in 28 percent, fever in 18 percent, recent immobility in 33 percent, swelling above the knee in 32 percent, and swelling below the knee in 48 percent [147]. Thus, in the diagnosis of DVT, as with PE, there are no highly sensitive or specific signs and symptoms. Diagnosis depends on objective studies. In another study of 53 patients, 58 percent of whom had DVT, 85 percent had pain in the leg, 96 percent had ankle edema, and 70 percent had a palpable difference in temperature, versus 81 percent, 66 percent, and 52 percent, respectively, in patients with normal venograms [148].

OBJECTIVE DIAGNOSTIC TESTING. Venography is the reference standard for the diagnosis of DVT. However, it is difficult to perform and interpretation requires extensive experience. It may cause appreciable foot and calf pain, superficial phlebitis, DVT, hypersensitivity reactions to the radiopaque medium, and local skin necrosis due to extravasation of dye. A positive venogram is generally defined as a constant intraluminal filling defect on multiple films in different projections. Artifacts are fairly common due to nonfilling of venous segments and blood flow from venous tributaries not filled with dye. In addition, even in centers with considerable experience in evaluating

DVT, some 7 to 20 percent of patients have a technically inadequate venogram or the venogram cannot be performed. Despite these difficulties, the venogram is considered the most sensitive and specific test available [149].

In many large series reported in the mid-1970s and 1980s IPG had a cumulative sensitivity of 95 percent and specificity of 96 percent [109–113]. Changes in blood volume of the calf produced by inflation and deflation of a pneumatic thigh cuff are recorded as changes in electrical resistance (impedance). The preferred technique is to use a cuff occlusion period of 2 minutes with repeated testing. False positive results may arise if (1) there is compression (tensing) of leg muscles; (2) the vein is compressed by an extravascular mass; (3) venous outflow is obstructed by raised central pressure; or (4) there is reduced arterial flow. Impedance plethysmography is not sensitive to calf vein thrombi. Several studies have demonstrated an initial negative IPG in 6 to 26 percent of symptomatic patients who then developed an abnormal test (DVT) with serial testing [150–151]. However in a recent study IPG was abnormal in only 37 of 56 (66%) patients and DVT was found in only 37 of 57 (65%) patients with an abnormal IPG; this is from the same center that previously reported a sensitivity of 92 to 98 percent and specificity of 95 to 98 percent. [152]. In addition, the IPG may be abnormal bilaterally. This was found in 19 percent of 425 patients in one study and accounted for 55 percent of all abnormal IPG's. Acute proximal DVT was found in 26 percent of these patients with further diagnostic testing [153].

Duplex ultrasound is another noninvasive test that has been used for more than a decade. It utilizes high-resolution, high-frequency transducers, usually in the range of 5 to 10 mHz. Real-time imaging permits direct visualization of major vascular channels and Doppler provides an audible/graphic depiction of blood flow. The best duplex ultrasound criterion for thrombosis is failure to collapse the vascular lumen completely with gentle probe pressure. Another sign is intraluminal echogenic material due to the clot. Less specific is loss of variation in Doppler signals with respiration. In devices with color-flow displays, blood flowing toward the transducer is depicted in red, blood flowing away is depicted in blue, and color intensity is proportional to blood flow [149]. In an extensive review the cumulative sensitivity of duplex ultrasound for proximal thrombi was 95 percent (confidence interval 92–98%) and specificity was 99 percent (confidence interval 98–100%) [154,155,156]. It may also identify other causes of leg swelling, including muscle tear, calf hematoma, popliteal cyst, and unusual causes of extrinsic compression. False negative tests may result from missing small clots or misinterpreting total occlusion of the femoral vein due to dilated collateral veins. False positive tests may result from inability to compress the femoral vein because of pregnancy (lack of positioning) or a pelvic tumor. The study may be difficult to interpret in extremely obese people or very well-muscled individuals. Duplex ultrasound is less sensitive in identifying isolated calf vein thrombosis, with reported sensitivity of 36 percent in one study.

Color Doppler ultrasound is insensitive to proximal DVT in asymptomatic high-risk patients. In a comparison of color Doppler ultrasound and venograms in 319 high-risk patients participating in a low-molecular-weight heparin trial for prevention of DVT, DVT was identified by contrast venography in 80 patients (prevalence 25%, 95% confidence interval 20–30%) and involved the proximal veins in 21 patients (prevalence 7%, confidence interval 4–10%); for proximal DVT color Doppler ultrasound showed poor sensitivity (38%, confidence interval 18–62%), moderately good specificity (92%, confidence interval 89–95%) and a poor positive predictive value for this population (26%) [62].

In a randomized prospective trial in 985 consecutive outpatients with clinically suspected DVT, serial IPG was performed in 494 patients and serial compression ultrasonography in 491 patients. The positive predictive value of an abnormal ultrasonogram was 94 percent (95% confidence interval 87–98%) versus the predictive value of IPG of 83 percent (95% confidence interval 75–90%) (p<0.02). In patients with repeatedly normal results the incidence of venous thromboembolism over 6 months was 1.5 percent (95% confidence interval 0.5–3.3%) for serial compression ultrasonography versus 2.5 percent (95% confidence interval 1.2–4.6%) for serial impedance plethysmography [61].

Although both IPG and compression ultrasonography have been reported to have excellent sensitivity, specificity, and positive predictive values in large series of patients, recent reports, some from the centers that provided the original material, cast some doubt on the excellent results in earlier studies. It is thus prudent periodically to evaluate the performance of IPG or ultrasound locally to assure acceptable performance. When ordering a Doppler ultrasound test it is important to indicate that it is for venous disease. Doppler technique is also used for arterial disease, which involves measuring arterial pressure by inflating the blood pressure cuff. This could result in dislodgment of a thrombus.

Although ^{125}I-fibrinogen scanning had been used as a screening technique to detect postoperative thrombi, it has generally fallen out of favor. It has a high false positive rate compared with venography and a 24-hour delay in interpretation of results. Recent concern over the spread of hepatitis B or HIV infection with the use of fibrinogen has contributed to the discontinuation of this study.

SYNDROMES

Phlegmasia Cerulea Dolens. Phlegmasia cerulea dolens is characterized by the acute onset of severe edema, cyanosis, and pain of a lower extremity. It is due to ischemic venous thrombosis brought about by obstruction of the iliofemoral and/or femoral or popliteotibial veins. This uncommon presentation of DVT is usually seen in the postoperative period and is often associated with neoplasia. The lower extremity becomes blue (cerulea), often following a period when the leg appears white (phlegmasia alba dolens). The nonpitting edema is hard, woody, or rubbery to touch. Marked extravasation of fluid into the limb commonly results in hypovolemic shock. About 15 percent of patients develop PE. Without treatment gangrene usually develops over 4 to 8 days after the onset of ischemia. Included in the differential diagnosis are reflex arteriospasm and peripheral arterial emboli. Initial management includes elevation of the extremity, fluid replacement, and intravenous heparin. Some advocate early thrombolytic therapy. Insertion of an inferior vena cava filter has also been recommended. If the condition does not resolve over 24 to 72 hours, surgical thrombectomy should be considered [157,158,159].

Calf Vein Thrombosis. Substantial evidence exists that calf vein thrombi may migrate to the proximal venous system or be the source of PE even without proximal vein thrombosis. In a study using clinical findings and ^{125}I-fibrinogen testing for up to 6 days after surgery with venographic confirmation of DVT, 23 percent of patients with distal (calf) thrombi had proximal extension and 10 percent had clinical evidence of PE [160]. In another study, 10 percent of patients with calf vein thrombosis had evidence of PE [161]. There was no clinical evidence of DVT in about one-half of the patients in each of these studies. In a smaller study without objective testing beyond 7 days, clinical evaluation at 3 months did not identify extension in 21

patients who were initially asymptomatic [162]. In a prospective, postmortem study, the venous system from the planta pedis to the right heart and into the lungs was examined both grossly and microscopically in 261 patients [163]. Eighty percent of the population was 60 years of age or older. Deep vein thrombi were defined to include microthrombi, fresh valve pocket thrombi, and small fibrous remnants of DVT and PE. On gross examination, DVT was present in 62 percent of patients. With microscopic examination, this increased to 72 percent. Pulmonary embolism was present in 69 percent of patients. It was concluded that emboli that arose from below the knee (no evidence of proximal vein thrombosis) accounted for 25 percent of patients with serious PE—contributing to or causing death—and 45 percent of patients whose PE was less serious. Fresh PE were found in 20 percent of healthy people who had a sudden death [93]. In a prospective randomized study of 51 patients with symptomatic calf DVT, all received intravenous heparin for 5 days. Subsequently, 23 were treated with warfarin for 3 months, during which period there was no recurrence. At 1 year, there was a recurrence in only 1 of the 23. Twenty-eight were randomized to no warfarin treatment. At 3 months, there was a recurrence in 8 of 28 (29%); 5 had proximal extension and 1 had PE. At the end of 1 year, recurrence in the untreated group was 19 of 28 (68%) (p< 0.02) [164]. In a retrospective study, 13 percent of fatal pulmonary emboli originated only from the calf veins [165]. Two studies document an approximately 6 to 20 percent propagation of clot from the leg in symptomatic patients over 2 weeks after the initial evaluation [150,151]. On the basis of the above, we believe all patients with identified calf thrombosis must be anticoagulated for 3 months. In venues other than the intensive care unit, serial noninvasive tests for 10 to 14 days could be considered as an alternative [151,167].

Upper Extremity DVT. Upper extremity DVT, involving the cephalic, basilic, brachial, axillary, or subclavian vein, has generally been divided into primary DVT (also called idiopathic, spontaneous, stress, traumatic, effort, strain, or Paget-Schroetter syndrome) or secondary DVT. Primary DVT is usually seen in young, physically active men and involves the right upper extremity more than the left. It is sometimes attributed to cervical rib, thoracic outlet syndrome, musculoskeletal abnormalities, or aberrant arteries. Secondary upper extremity DVT, is most commonly associated today with central venous catheter-induced thrombosis. It has also been associated with malignancy, particularly breast carcinoma, intravenous drug abuse, thrombocytosis, heart failure, trauma, immunocompromise, and local infection. In a review of studies in which subclavian venous catheterization was prospectively examined with the use of objective means of diagnosis, 28 percent developed upper extremity venous thrombosis; this was often subclinical. However, the incidence of PE in this review was 12.4 percent; it often occurred during anticoagulation treatment [168–172].

The clinical presentation is that of pain, tenderness, swelling, and/or a palpable cord. These findings, however, have not distinguished between patients with or without axillary/subclavian venous thrombosis (ASVT). Swelling was the most common finding. Just as with lower extremity DVT, objective diagnostic studies must be used. The upper extremity venogram remains the criterion standard. However, duplex scanning has an acceptable accuracy [170,171,172]. In a retrospective review of 693 consecutive upper extremity duplex scans, a diagnosis of acute venous thrombosis was made in 123; 85 involved the axillary or subclavian vein and 5 (8%) had PE, 2 of whom died. It should be noted that two of these patients did not have a central venous catheter in place [170].

Of concern in attributing PE to DVT of the upper extremity are the extensive data identifying DVT in the lower extremities in 90 percent or more of patients with PE. Most patients in whom PE has been related to upper extremity DVT have not had thorough objective testing of the lower extremities and inferior vena cava. Despite this, the evidence indicates that upper extremity DVT may lead to PE and, rarely, death due to PE.

Of considerable concern with upper extremity DVT is a residual postthrombotic syndrome characterized by chronic pain, tenderness, swelling, numbness, heaviness, weakness or limited motion, color changes, and even ulceration; these symptoms and signs may be exacerbated by exercise. Subclavian vein thrombosis can originate in peripheral sites with extension to the subclavian vein. One-third of patients have one or more signs or symptoms of postphlebitic syndrome [170].

Anticoagulation with heparin followed by warfarin for 3 months is generally recommended. Some authors recommend thrombolytic therapy to eliminate the clot, but there are no prospective studies to document its value. Supportive care includes elevation of the arm and removal of any offending intravenous devices. In primary or idiopathic ASVT, surgical intervention to remove the clot or correct anatomic abnormalities has been recommended.

Identification of infected thrombi and septic thrombophlebitis requires the identification of organisms in the involved area or from the catheter through this area unless there is extensive local inflammation with purulence. If infection is documented, appropriate antibiotic therapy should be instituted. Various authors have indicated that the risk of infection from central venous catheters is related to the duration of catheterization, type of catheter, single versus multiple lumen, transparent versus occlusive dressings, and catheter material. Recent prospective, randomized studies have shown no difference in the rate of infection between single- or triple-lumen catheters, with the latter requiring peripheral venous access in 1 of 61 (0.016%), versus 37 percent for the former [173]. Tunneling the catheter also has been recommended, but a recent study shows no difference in infection rate or durability with the use of nontunneled Silastic catheters [174]. In another prospective controlled trial of scheduled replacement of central venous and pulmonary artery catheters, there was no difference in infection rates between replacement every 3 days versus replacement for clinical indications. However, insertion every 3 days over a guidewire was more likely to result in a bloodstream infection and insertion every 3 days at a new site was more likely to result in mechanical complications [175].

Postphlebitic Syndrome. Postphlebitic syndrome (i.e., venous insufficiency and venous ulcers following DVT) is a result of varicose veins (superficial veins), incompetent venous perforators, and deep venous obstruction. Varicose veins primarily involve the tortuous dilated branches of the greater and lesser saphenous veins or these veins themselves. They are associated with valvular incompetency and dilatation. The perforating veins between the superficial and deep veins become similarly dilated and have incompetent valves. Patients develop discomfort, described as aching or heaviness in the leg, and edema of the lower extremity is evident. Over time edema becomes more firm and is described as woody or brawny induration. It is usually associated with brown pigmentation, dermatitis, and, ultimately, venous ulcers, usually in the lower third of the leg above and behind the malleoli. Treatment is directed at reducing edema with the use of elevation, pressure gradient stockings, and, in selected cases, ligation and stripping of the greater or lesser saphenous veins [176].

TREATMENT. The treatment of DVT is in general the same as that for PE. In addition, it is recommended that the leg be elevated in an attempt to reduce edema. Rethrombosis following heparin therapy with or without lytic therapy is in the range of 8 to 14 percent. Many recommend the use of thrombolytic therapy for 3 days with a large thigh clot with major swelling to reduce the risk of postphlebitic syndrome. However, there is no consensus on the use of thrombolytic therapy [177–180]. Low-molecular-weight heparin is also used but has not been approved for treatment (only prophylaxis) in the United States [180–183].

Prevention

Critically ill patients in an intensive care unit manifest on a continuing basis a plethora of the signs, symptoms, and laboratory and radiographic findings of PE. This makes identification of the patient with acute PE nearly impossible. There is strong evidence that such patients are at increased risk of venous thromboembolic disease, including PE [26,184]. Two studies, one using a historic control and the other randomized prospectively, show a reduction in DVT/PE with the prophylactic use of low-dose heparin (5000 units subcutaneously twice a day) [55,56].

The mean incidence of DVT in multiple trauma patients by autopsy or venography has been reported as 48 percent (95% confidence interval 43–53%) [146]. The mean incidence of DVT diagnosed by venography in patients with acute spinal cord injury is reported as 38 percent (95% confidence interval 31–46%) [146]. In patients with multiple trauma or acute spinal cord injury, anticoagulant therapy may be impossible. While there are no large randomized prospective studies of DVT prophylaxis, there is some evidence to support the use of low-molecular-weight heparin in patients with acute spinal cord injury and the use of intermittent pneumatic compression in those with acute spinal cord trauma. Again without the benefit of controlled studies, inferior vena cava filters are being used with increasing frequency in high-risk patients for DVT with multiple trauma [108,114,185,186].

Other patients at increased risk of DVT are those with hip fractures or requiring hip replacement, with an incidence of DVT in the range of 40 to 70 percent and an incidence of fatal PE in the range of 1 to 5 percent. Total knee arthroplasty falls in the same category, with an estimated incidence of fatal PE of 5 percent. Urologic, general, gynecologic, and neurologic surgery have a risk of DVT in the range of 15 to 20 percent, with an incidence of fatal PE in the range of 1 to 5 percent. Medical patients (excluding ICU patients) have a slightly lower incidence of venous thrombosis of 15 percent, with a 1 percent incidence of fatal PE [66,146].

Current recommendations for prophylaxis of patients following total hip arthroplasty are the use of warfarin, INR of 2 to 3 or low-molecular-weight heparin; graduated compression stockings should be used as well (see Chap. 43). A further decrease in DVT can be obtained with the use of epidural anesthesia. It seems reasonable to add intermittent pneumatic compression to either warfarin or low-molecular-weight heparin. Recommendations are the same for patients with hip fracture, although there may be increased concern for excessive bleeding with the use of either warfarin or low-molecular-weight heparin. Similar recommendations are in order for knee surgery. In a recent study using transesophageal echocardiography in 29 patients undergoing total knee arthroplasty, showers of substantial echogenic material for 3 to 15 minutes were visible in the right atrium and ventricle within 10 to 15 seconds after tourniquet deflation [187]. Satisfactory prophylaxis of other patients in the intensive care unit can be achieved with low-dose heparin (5000 units twice or three times per day) or low-molecular-weight heparin; the cost of low molecular heparin currently mitigates its general use [188]. In patients following general and usual gynecologic surgery this same prophylaxis is effective. Intermittent pneumatic compression is recommended for patients who have had neurologic or urologic surgery [66,146].

References

1. Consensus Conference: Prevention of venous thrombosis and pulmonary embolism. *JAMA* 256:744, 1986.
2. Weg JG: Pulmonary embolism: Diagnosis and treatment. *Appl Cardiopulm Pathophysiol* 2:23, 1988.
3. Dalen JE, Alpert JS: Natural history of pulmonary embolism. *Prog Cardiovasc Dis* 17:259, 1975.
4. Coon WW: Venous thromboembolism, prevalence, risk factors and prevention. *Clin Chest Med* 3:391, 1984.
5. Carson JL, Kelley MA, Terrin ML, et al: The clinical course of pulmonary embolism: One year follow-up of PIOPED patients. *N Engl J Med* 326:1240, 1992.
6. Morrell MT, Dunhill MS: The post-mortem incidence of pulmonary embolism in a hospital population. *Br J Surg* 55:347, 1968.
7. Dismuke SE, Wagner EH: Pulmonary embolism as a cause of death. *JAMA* 255:2039, 1986.
8. Goldman L, Sayson R, Robbins S, et al: The value of the autopsy in three medical eras. *N Engl J Med* 308:1000, 1983.
9. Goldhaber SZ, Hennekens CH, Evans DA, et al: Factors associated with correct antemortem diagnosis of major pulmonary embolism. *Am J Med* 73:822, 1982.
10. Nicolaides AN, O'Connell JD: Origin and distribution of thrombi in patients presenting with clinical deep venous thrombosis, in Nicolaides AN (ed): *Thromboembolism Etiology, Advances in Preventional and Management* Baltimore, University Park Press, 1975, pp 177–180.
11. Riedel M, Stanek V, Widimsky J: Spirometry and gas exchange in chronic pulmonary thromboembolism. *Physiopath Resp* 17:209, 1981.
12. Wilson JE III, Pierce AK, Johnson RL, et al: Hypoxemia in pulmonary embolism, a clinical study. *J Clin Invest* 50:481, 1971.
13. Sasahara AA, Cannilla JE, Morse RL, et al: Clinical and physiologic studies in pulmonary thromboembolism. *Am J Cardiol* 20:10, 1967.
14. D'Alonzo GE, Bower JS, DeHart P, et al: The mechanisms of abnormal gas exchange in acute massive pulmonary embolism. *Am Rev Respir Dis* 128:170, 1983.
15. D'Alonzo GE, Dantzker G: Gas exchange alterations following pulmonary thrombo-embolism. *Clin Chest Med* 5:411, 1984.
16. Boochama D, Curley W, Al-Dossary S, et al: *Am Rev Resp Dis* 138:466, 1988.
17. Lesser BA, Leeper KV Jr, Stein PD, et al: The diagnosis of acute pulmonary embolism in patients with chronic obstructive pulmonary disease. *Chest* 102:17, 1992.
18. McIntyre KM, Sasahara AA: The hemodynamic response to pulmonary embolism in patients without prior cardiopulmonary disease. *Am J Cardiol* 28:288, 1971.
19. McIntyre KM, Sasahara AA: Determinants of right ventricular function and hemodynamics after pulmonary embolism. *Chest* 65:534, 1974.
20. McIntyre KM, Sasahara AA: The ratio of pulmonary arterial pressure to pulmonary vascular obstruction, index of pre-embolic cardiopulmonary status. *Chest* 7:692, 1971.
21. Weg JG, Cho K, Stevens A: Pulmonary hemodynamics are not helpful in identifying pulmonary emboli (abstract). *Am Rev Resp Dis* 133:A221, 1986.

22. Marsh JD, Glynn M, Torman HA: Pulmonary angiography: Application and new spectrum of patients. *Am J Med* 75:763, 1983.
23. Stein P, Alavi A, Gottschalk A, et al: Usefulness of non-invasive diagnostic tools for diagnosis of acute pulmonary embolism in patients with a normal chest radiograph. *Am J Cardiol* 67:1117, 1991.
24. Stein PD, Terrin ML, Hales CA, et al: Clinical, laboratory, roentgenographic and electrocardiographic findings in patients with acute pulmonary embolism and no pre-existing cardiac or pulmonary disease. *Chest* 100:598, 1991.
25. Stein PD, Saltzman HA, Weg JG: Clinical characteristics of patients with acute pulmonary embolism. *Am J Cardiol* 68:1723, 1991.
26. Neuhaus A, Bentz RR, Weg JG: Diagnosis of pulmonary embolism in respiratory failure. *Chest* 73:460, 1978.
27. Modan B, Sharan E, Jelin N: Factors contributing to the incorrect diagnosis of pulmonary embolic disease. *Chest* 62:388, 1972.
28. The PIOPED Investigators: Value of the ventilation/perfusion scan in acute pulmonary embolism: Result of the prospective investigators of pulmonary embolism diagnosis (PIOPED). *JAMA* 263:2753, 1990.
29. The Urokinase Pulmonary Embolism Trial: A national cooperative study. *Circulation* 47(suppl):1, 1973.
30. Urokinase-Streptokinase Pulmonary Embolism Trial: A national cooperative study. *JAMA* 229:1606, 1974.
31. Bell WR, Simon TL, DeMets DL: The clinical features of submassive and massive pulmonary emboli. *Am J Med* 62:355, 1977.
31a. Lockshin MD: Antiphospholipid antibody syndrome. *Rheum Dis Clin North Am* 20:45, 1994.
31b. Khamashta MA, Cuadrado MJ, Mujic F, et al: The management of thrombosis in the antiphospholipid-antibody syndrome. *N Engl J Med* 332:993, 1995.
31c. Lockshin MD: Answers to the antiphospholipid-antibody syndrome? Editorial. *N Engl J Med* 332:1025, 1995.
31d. Ridker PM, Hennekens CH, Lindpaintner K, et al: Mutation in the gene coding for coagulation factor V and the risk of myocardial infarction, stroke, and venous thrombosis in apparently healthy men. *N Engl J Med* 332:912, 1995.
31e. Koeleman BPC, Reitsma PH, Allaart CF, et al: Activated protein C resistance as an additional risk factor for thrombosis in protein C-deficient families. *Blood* 84:1031, 1994.
31f. Koster, T, Rosendaal FR, de Ronde H, et al: Venous thrombosis due to poor anticoagulant response to activated protein C: Leiden thrombophilia study. *Lancet* 342:1503, 1993.
31g. Svensson PJ, Dahlback B: Resistance to activated protein C as a basis for venous thrombosis. *N Engl J Med* 330:517, 1994.
31h. Dahlback B, Hildebrand B: Inherited resistance to activated protein C is corrected by anticoagulant cofactor activity found to be a property of factor V. *Proc Natl Acad Sci USA* 91:1396, 1994.
31i. Bertina RM, Koeleman BP, Koster T, et al: Mutation in blood coagulation factor V associated with resistance to activated protein C. *Nature* 359:64, 1994.
32. Kaufmann RH, Veltkamp JJ, Van Tilburg NH, et al: Acquired antithrombin III deficiency and thrombosis in the nephrotic syndrome. Am J Med 65:607, 1968.
33. Demers C, Ginsberg JS, Hirsh J, et al: Thrombosis in antithrombin II deficient persons: Report of a large kindred and literature review. *Ann Intern Med* 116:754, 1992.
34. Mitchell CA, Rowell JA, Hau L, et al: A fatal thrombotic disorder associated with an acquired inhibitor of protein C. *N Engl J Med* 317:1638, 1987.
35. Matsuda M, Sugo T, Sakata Y, et al: A thrombotic state due to an abnormal protein C. *N Engl J Med* 319:1265, 1988.
36. Engesser L, Broekmans AW, Breit E, et al: Hereditary protein S deficiency: Clinical manifestations. *Ann Intern Med* 106:677, 1987.
37. Stahl CP, Wideman CS, Spira TJ, et al: Protein S deficiency in men with long-term human immunodeficiency virus infection. *Blood* 81:1801, 1993.
38. Comp PC, Esmon CT: Recurrent venous thromboembolism in patients with a partial deficiency of protein S. *N Engl J Med* 311:1525, 1984.
39. Peck B, Hoffman GS, Franck WA: Thrombophlebitis in systemic lupus erythematosus. *JAMA* 240:1728, 1978.

40. Shifter T, Machtey I, Creter D: Thromboembolism in congenital factor VII deficiency. *Acta Haematol* 71:60, 1984.
41. Gershwin ME, Grude JK: Deep venous thrombosis in pulmonary embolism in congenital factor VII deficiency. *N Engl J Med* 288:141, 1973.
42. Heijboer H, Brandjes DPM, Buller HR, et al: Deficiencies of co-agulation-inhibiting and fibrinolytic proteins in outpatients with deep-vein thrombosis. *N Engl J Med* 323:1512, 1990.
43. Adams JE III, Siegel BA, Goldstein JA, et al: Elevations of CK-MB following pulmonary embolism: A manifestation of occult right ventricular infarction. *Chest* 101:1203, 1992.
44. Menzioan JO, Williams LF: Is pulmonary angiography essential in the diagnosis of acute pulmonary embolism? *Am J Surg* 137:543, 1979.
45. Gottschalk A, Juni JE, Sostman HD, et al: Ventilation-perfusion scintigraphy in the PIOPED study. I. data collection and tabulation. *J Nucl Med* 34:1109, 1993.
46. Gottschalk A, Sostman HD, Coleman RE, et al: Ventilation-perfusion scintigraphy in PIOPED study. II. evaluation of the scinti-graphic criteria and interpretations. *J Nucl Med* 34:1119, 1993.
47. Hoellerich VL, Wigton RS: Diagnosing pulmonary embolism using clinical findings. *Arch Intern Med* 146:1699, 1986.
48. Hull RD, Hirsh J, Carter CJ, et al: Pulmonary angiography, venti-lation lung scanning, and venography for clinically suspected pul-monary embolism with abnormal perfusion lung scan. *Ann Intern Med* 98:891, 1983.
49. Hull RD, Hirsh J, Carter CJ, et al: Diagnostic value of ventilation perfusion lung scanning in patients with suspected pulmonary embolism. *Chest* 88:818, 1985.
50. Hull RD, Raskob GF, Coates G, et al: Clinical validity of a normal perfusion lung scan in patients with suspected pulmonary embo-lism. *Chest* 97:23, 1990.
51. Stein PD, Terrin ML, Gottschalk A: Value of ventilation/perfusion scans versus perfusion scans alone in acute pulmonary embolism. *Am J Cardiol* 69:1239, 1992.
52. Stein PD, Gottschalk A, Saltzman HA, et al: Diagnosis of acute pulmonary embolism in the elderly. *J Am Coll Cardiol* 18:1452, 1991.
53. Stein PD, Coleman RE, Gottschalk A, et al: Diagnostic utility of ventilation/perfusion lung scans in acute pulmonary embolism is not diminished by pre-existing cardiac or pulmonary disease. *Chest* 100:604, 1991.
54. Cade JF: High risk of the critically ill for venous thromboembolism. *Crit Care Med* 10:448, 1982.
55. Pingleton SK, Bone RC, Pingleton WW, et al: Prevention of pul-monary emboli in a respiratory intensive care unit: Efficacy of low-dose heparin. *Chest* 79:647, 1979.
56. Kipper MS, Moser KM, Kartman KE, Ashbarn WL: Long-term fol-low-up of patients with suspected pulmonary embolism and nor-mal lung scan. *Chest* 82:411, 1982.
57. Stein PD, Athanasoulis C, Alavi A, et al: Complications and validity of pulmonary angiography in acute pulmonary embolism. *Circu-lation* 85:462, 1992.
58. Novelline RH, Baltarowich OH, Athanasoulis CA, et al: The clinical course of patient with suspected pulmonary embolism and a neg-ative pulmonary angiogram. *Radiology* 126:561, 1978.
59. Biello DR, Mattar AG, McKnight RC, et al: Ventilation perfusion studies in suspected pulmonary embolism. *Am J Radiol* 133:1033, 1979.
60. Dalen JE, Banas JS Jr, Brooks HL, et al: Resolution rate of acute pulmonary embolism in man. *N Engl J Med* 280:1194, 1969.
61. Heijboer H, Buller HR, Lensing AWA: A comparison of real-time compression ultrasonography with impedance plethysmography for the diagnosis of deep-vein thrombosis in symptomatic outpa-tients. *N Engl J Med* 329:1365, 1993.
62. Davidson BL, Elliott CG, Lensing AWA, et al: Low accuracy of color Doppler ultrasound in the detection of proximal leg vein thrombosis in asymptomatic high-risk patients. *Ann Intern Med* 117:735, 1992.
63. Hull RD, Raskob GE, Coates G, et al: A new noninvasive manage-ment strategy for patients with suspected pulmonary embolism. *Arch Intern Med* 149:2549, 1989.
64. Kelley MA, Carson JL, Palevsky HI, et al: Diagnosing pulmonary embolism: New facts and strategies. *Ann Intern Med* 114:300, 1991.
65. Stein PD, Hull RD, Saltzman HA, et al: Strategy for diagnosis of patients with suspected acute pulmonary embolism. *Chest* 103:1553, 1993.
66. Hyers TM, Hull RD, Weg JG: Antithrombotic therapy for venous thrombolitic disease. *Chest* 102:408S, 1992. (The ACCP Consensus Conference on Antithrombotic Therapy, *Chest* 303S–550S, 1992 is an excellent resource.)
67. Hirsch J: Heparin. *N Engl J Med* 324:1565, 1991.
68. Barrit DW, Jordan SC: Anticoagulant drugs in the treatment of pulmonary embolism: A controlled clinical trial. *Lancet* 1:1309, 1960.
69. Hull Rd, Raskob GE, Rosenbloom D, et al: Optimal therapeutic level of heparin therapy in patients with venous thrombosis. *Arch Intern Med* 152:1589, 1992.
70. Hirsh J, Dalen JE, Deykin D, et al: Heparin: Mechanism of action, pharmacokinetics, dosing considerations, monitoring, efficacy, and safety. *Chest* 102:337S, 1992.
71. Hull RD, Raskob GE, Hirsh J, et al: Continuous intravenous heparin compared with intermittent subcutaneous heparin in the initial treatment of proximal-vein thrombosis. *N Engl J Med* 315:1109, 1986.
72. Basu D, Gallus A, Hirsch J, et al: A prospective study of value of monitoring heparin treatment with the activated partial thrombo-plastin time. *N Engl J Med* 287:324, 1972.
73. Landefeld CS, Beyth RJ: Anticoagulant-related bleeding: Clinical epidemiology, prediction, and prevention. *Am J Med* 95:315, 1993.
74. Landefeld CS, McGuire E III, Rosenblatt MW: A bleeding risk index for estimating the probability of major bleeding in hospitalized patients starting anticoagulant therapy. *Am J Med* 89:569, 1990.
75. Warkentin TE, Kelton JG: Heparin-induced thrombocytopenia. *Prog Hemost Thromb* 10:1, 1991.
76. Arthur CK, Isbister JP, Aspery EM: The heparin induced throm-bosis-thrombocytopenia syndrome (H.I.T.T.S.): A review. *Pathol-ogy* 17:82, 1985.
77. Sandler RM, Seifer DB, Morgan K, et al: Heparin induced throm-bocytopenia and thrombosis: Detection and specificity of a plate-let-aggregating IgG. *Am J Clin Pathol* 83:760, 1985.
78. Sheridan D, Carter C, Kelton JG: A diagnostic test for heparin-induced thrombocytopenia. *Blood* 67:27, 1986.
79. Leroy J, Leclerc MH, Delahousse B, et al: Treatment of heparin-associated thrombocytopenia and thrombosis with low molecular weight heparin (cy 216). *Semin Thromb Hemost* 11:326, 1985.
80. Ansell J, Deykin K: Heparin-induced thrombocytopenia and re-current thromboembolism. *Am J Hematol* 8:325, 1980.
81. Bell WR, Tomasulo PA, Alving BM, et al: Thrombocytopenia oc-curring during the administration of heparin: A prospective study in 52 patients. *Ann Intern Med* 85:155, 1976.
82. Cines DB, Tomaski A, Tannenbaum S: Immune endothelial-cell injury in heparin-associated thrombocytopenia. *N Engl J Med* 316:581, 1987.
83. Squires JW, Pinch LW: Heparin-induced spinal fractures. *JAMA* 241:2417, 1979.
84. Hirsh J, Dalen JE, Deykin D, et al: Oral anticoagulants: Mechanism of action, clinical effectiveness, and optimal therapeutic range. *Chest* 102:312S, 1992.
85. Hirsch J: Oral anticoagulant drugs. *N Engl J Med* 324:1865, 1991.
86. Hull RD, Raskob GE, Rosenbloom D, et al: Heparin for 5 days as compared with 10 days in the initial treatment of proximal venous thrombosis. *N Engl J Med* 322:1260, 1990.
87. Gallus A, Jackman J, Tillett J, et al: Safety and efficacy of warfarin started early after submassive venous thrombosis or pulmonary embolism. *Lancet* 2:1293, 1986.
88. Bussey HI, Force RW, Bianco TM, et al: Reliance on prothrombin time ratios causes significant errors in anticoagulation therapy. *Arch Intern Med* 152:278, 1992.
89. Hull RD, Delmore TJ, Carter C, et al: Adjusted subcutaneous hep-arin versus warfarin sodium in the long-term treatment of venous thrombosis. *N Engl J Med* 306:189, 1982.
90. Hull RD, Raskob GE, Hirsh J, et al: A cost-effectiveness analysis of alternative approaches for long-term treatment of proximal venous thrombosis. *JAMA* 252:235, 1984.

91. O'Reilly RA, Pool JG, Aggeler PM: Hereditary resistance to coumarin anticoagulant drugs in man and rat. *Ann NY Acad Sci* 151:913, 1968.

92. Alving BM, Strickler MP, Knight RD, et al: Hereditary warfarin resistance. *Arch Intern Med* 145:499, 1985.

93. Faraci PA, Deterling RA, Stein AM, et al: Warfarin induced necrosis of the skin. *Surg Gynecol Obstet* 146:695, 1978.

94. Ginsberg JS, Kowalchuk G, Hursh J, et al: Heparin therapy during pregnancy: Risks to the fetus and mother. *Arch Intern Med* 149:2233, 1989.

95. Ginsberg JS, Hirsh J: Anticoagulants during pregnancy. *Ann Rev Med* 40:79, 1989.

96. Wong V, Cheng CH, Chan KC: Fetal and neonatal outcome of exposure to anticoagulants during pregnancy. *Am J Med Genet* 145:17, 1993.

97. Zakzouk MS: The congenital warfarin syndrome. *J Laryngol Otol* 100:215, 1986.

98. Cella G, Palla A, Sasahara A: Controversies of different regimens of thrombolytic therapy in acute pulmonary embolism. *Semin Thromb Hemost* 13:163, 1987.

99. Goldhaber SZ, Vaughan DE, Markis JE, et al: Acute pulmonary embolism treated with tissue plasminogen activator. *Lancet* 2:886, 1986.

100. Goldhaber SZ, Kessler CM, Heit J, et al: Randomized controlled trial of recombinant tissue plasminogen activator versus urokinase in the treatment of acute pulmonary embolism. *Lancet* 2:293, 1988.

101. PIOPED Investigators: Tissue plasminogen activator for the treatment of acute pulmonary embolism. *Chest* 97:528, 1990.

102. Alpert JS, Smith R, Carlson CJ, et al: Mortality in patients treated for pulmonary embolism. *JAMA* 236:1477, 1976.

103. Becker DM, Philbrick JT, Selby JB: Inferior vena cava filters: Indications, safety, effectiveness. *Arch Intern Med* 152:1985, 1992.

104. Norris CS, Greenfield LJ, Herrmann JB: Free-floating iliofemoral thrombosis. *Arch Surg* 120:806, 1985.

105. Greenfield LJ, Michna BA: Twelve year clinical experience with the Greenfield vena cava filter. *Surgery* 104:706, 1988.

106. Greenfield LJ, Cho KJ, Proctor M, et al: Results of a multicenter study of the modified hook-titanium Greenfield filter. *J Vasc Surg* 14:253, 1991.

107. Radomski JS, Jarrell BE, Carabasi RA, et al: Risk of pulmonary embolus with inferior vena cava thrombosis. *Am Surg* 53:97, 1987.

108. Fink JA, Jones BT: The Greenfield filter as the primary means of therapy in venous thromboembolic disease. *Surg Gynecol Obstet* 172:253, 1991.

109. Rohrer MJ, Scheidler MG, Wheeler B, et al: Extended indications for placement of an inferior vena cava filter. *J Vasc Surg* 10:44, 1989.

110. Golueke PJ, Garrett WV, Thompson JE, et al: Interruption of the vena cava by means of the Greenfield filter: Expanding the indications. *Surgery* 103:11, 1988.

111. Cohen JR, Tenenbaum N, Citron M: Greenfield filter as primary therapy for deep venous thrombosis and/or pulmonary embolism in patients with cancer. *Surgery* 109:12, 1991.

112. Calligaro KD, Bergen WS, Haut MJ, et al: Thromboembolic complications in patients with advanced cancer; anticoagulation versus Greenfield filter placement. *Ann Vasc Surg* 5:186, 1991.

113. Emerson RH, Cross R, Head WC: Prophylactics and early therapeutic use of the Greenfield filter in hip and knee joint arthroplasty. *J Arthroplasty* 6:129, 1991.

114. Vaughn BK, Knezevich S, Lombardi AV, et al: Use of the Greenfield filter to prevent fatal pulmonary embolism associated with total hip and knee arthroplasty. *J Bone Joint Surg* 71A:1542, 1989.

115. Dorfman GS: Percutaneous inferior vena caval filters. *Radiology* 174:987, 1990.

116. Orsini RA, Jarrell BE: Suprarenal placement of vena caval filters: Indications, techniques, and results. *J Vasc Surg* 1:124, 1984.

117. Meyer G, Tamisier D, Sors H, et al: Pulmonary embolectomy: A 20 year experience at one center. *Ann Thorac Surg* 51:232, 1991.

118. Mattox KL, Feldtman RW, Beall AC, et al: Pulmonary embolectomy for acute massive pulmonary embolism. *Ann Surg* 195:726, 1982.

119. Meyer G, Tamisier D, Sors H, et al: Pulmonary embolectomy: A 20 year experience at one center. *Ann Thorac Surg* 51:232, 1991.

120. Gray HH, Morgan JM, Paneth M, et al: Pulmonary embolectomy for acute massive pulmonary embolism: An analysis of 71 cases. *Br Heart J* 60:196, 1988.

121. Clarke DB, Abrams LD: Pulmonary embolectomy: A 25 year experience. *J Thorac Cardiovasc Surg* 92:442, 1986.

122. Stewart JR, Greenfield LJ: Transvenous vena caval filtrations and pulmonary embolectomy. *Surg Clin North Am* 62:411, 1982.

123. Timsit J-F, Reynaud P, Meyer G, et al: Pulmonary embolectomy by catheter device in massive pulmonary embolism. *Chest* 100:655, 1991.

124. Paraskos JA, Adelstein SJ, Smith RE, et al: Late prognosis of acute pulmonary embolism. *N Engl J Med* 289:55, 1973.

125. Hall RJC, Sutton GC, Kerr IH: Long-term prognosis of treated acute massive pulmonary embolism. *Br Heart J* 39:1128, 1977.

126. Riedel M, Stanek V, Widimsky J, et al: Longterm follow-up of patients with pulmonary thromboembolism: Late prognosis and evolution of hemodynamic and respiratory data. *Chest* 81:151, 1982.

127. Huang RM, Naidich DP, Lubat E, et al: Septic pulmonary emboli: CT-radiographic correlation. *Am J Roentgenol* 153:41, 1989.

128. Kuhlman JE, Fishman EK, Teigen C: Pulmonary septic emboli: Diagnosis with CT. *Radiology* 174:211, 1990.

129. Ratnoff OD, Vosburgh GJ: Observations on the clotting defect in amniotic fluid embolism *N Engl J Med* 247:270, 1952.

130. Rodgers GP, Heymach GJ, Peterson EP, et al: Amniotic fluid embolism: An analysis of 40 cases. *Obstet Gynecol* 35:787, 1970.

131. Lee KR, Catalono PM, Ortiz-Giroux S: Cytologic diagnosis of amniotic fluid embolism: Report of a case with a unique cytologic feature and emphasis on the difficulty of eliminating squamous contamination. *Acta Cytol* 30:177, 1986.

132. Clark SL: Amniotic fluid embolism. *Clin Perinatol* 13:801, 1986.

133. Gunter CA, Braun TE: Fat embolism syndrome: Changing prognosis. *Chest* 79:143, 1981.

134. Chan KM, Tham KT, Chiu HS, et al: Post traumatic fat embolism: Its clinical and subclinical presentations. *J Trauma* 24:45, 1984.

135. McCarthy B, Mammen E, LeBlanc LP, et al: Subclinical fat embolism: A prospective study of 50 patients with extremity fractures. *J Trauma* 13:9, 1973.

136. Schonfeld SA, Ploy Song Sang Y, Di Lisio R, et al: Fat embolism prophylaxis with corticosteroids. *Ann Intern Med* 99:438, 1983.

137. Fabian TC, Hoots AV, Stanford DS, et al: Fat embolism syndrome: Prospective evaluation in 92 fracture patients. *Crit Care Med* 18:42, 1990.

138. Burgher LW, Dines DE, Linscheid RL, et al: Fat embolism in the adult respiratory distress syndrome. *Mayo Clin Proc* 49:107, 1974.

139. Graham JP, Rotman H, Weg JG: Tumor emboli presenting as pulmonary hypertension: A diagnostic dilemma. *Chest* 69:229, 1976.

140. Winterbauer RH, Elfenbein IB, Ball WC Jr: Incidence in clinical significance of tumor embolization to the lungs. *Am J Med* 45:271, 1968.

141. Goldhaber SZ, Dricker E, Buring JE, et al: Clinical suspicion of autopsy proven thrombotic and tumor pulmonary embolism in cancer patients. *Am Heart J* 114:1432, 1987.

142. Soares FA, Landell GAM, DeOliveira JAM: Pulmonary tumor embolism to alveolar septal capillaries: A prospective study of 12 cases. *Arch Pathol Lab Med* 115:127, 1991.

143. Coon WW: Thromboembolism, prevalence risk factors, and prevention. *Clin Chest Med* 5:391, 1984.

144. Coon WW, Willis PW III, Keller JB: Venous thromboembolism and other venous disease in the Tecumseh Community Health Study. *Circulation* 48:839, 1973.

145. Wheeler HB, Anderson FA Jr, Cardullo PA, et al: Suspected deep vein thrombosis: Management by impedance plethysmography. *Arch Surg* 117:1206, 1982.

146. Clagett GP, Anderson FA, Levine MN, et al: Prevention of venous thromboembolism. *Chest* 102:391S, 1992.

147. Landefeld CS, McGuire E, Cohen AM: Clinical findings associated with acute deep vein thrombosis: A basis for quantifying clinical judgment. *Am J Med* 92:582, 1990.

148. Nicolaides AN, Meadway J, Irving D: The value of clinical signs in the diagnosis of deep venous thrombosis, in Nicolaides AN (ed): *Thromboembolism Etiology, Advances in Preventional and Management.* Baltimore, University Park Press, 1975, pp 243–248.

149. Hull RD, Raskob GE, Leclerc JR, et al: The diagnosis of clinically suspected venous thrombosis. *Clin Chest Med* 5:439, 1984.

150. Hull RD, Hirsch J, Carter CJ, et al: Diagnostic efficacy of impedance plethysmography for clinically suspected deep vein thrombosis: A randomized trial. *Ann Intern Med* 102:21, 1985.

151. Huisman MV, Buller HR, ten Cate JW, et al: Serial impedance plethysmography for clinically suspected deep venous thrombosis in outpatients: The Amsterdam General Practitioner Study. *N Engl J Med* 314:823, 1986.

152. Anderson DR, Lensing AWA, Wells PS, et al: Limitations of impedance plethysmography in the diagnosis of clinically suspected deep-vein thrombosis. *Ann Intern Med* 118:25, 1993.

153. Curley FJ, Pratter MR, Irwin RS, et al: The clinical implications of bilaterally abnormal impedance plethysmography. *Arch Intern Med* 147:125, 1987.

154. White RH, McGahan JP, Daschbach MM, et al: Diagnosis of deep-vein thrombosis using duplex ultrasound. *Ann Intern Med* 111:297, 1989.

155. Heijboer H, Cogo A, Buller HR, et al: Detection of deep vein thrombosis with impedance plethysmography and real-time compression ultrasonography in hospitalized patients. *Arch Intern Med* 152:1901, 1992.

156. Lensing AWA, Prandoni P, Brandjes DPM, et al: Detection of deep-vein thrombosis by real-time b-mode ultrasonography. *N Engl J Med* 320:342, 1989.

157. Haimovici H: Ischemic venous thrombosis: Phlegmasia cerulea dolens and venous gangrene, in *Vascular Surgery: Principles and Techniques.* 3rd ed. New York, McGraw-Hill, 1976.

158. Brockman SK, Vasko JS: Plegmasia cerulea dolens. *Surg Gynecol Obstet* 121:1347, 1965.

159. Wilson B, Hawkins ML, Mansberger AR Jr: Post-traumatic phlegmasia cerulea dolens: An indication for the Greenfield filter. *South Med J* 82:780, 1989.

160. Kakkar VV, Howe CT, Flanc C: Natural history of postoperative deep vein thrombosis. *Lancet* 2:230, 1969.

161. Kakkar VV, Howe CT, Nicolaides AN, et al: Deep vein thrombosis of the legs: Is there a high risk group? *Am J Surg* 120:527, 1970.

162. Moser KM, LeMoine JR: Is embolic risk conditioned by location of deep venous thrombosis? *Ann Intern Med* 94:435, 1981.

163. Havig O: Deep vein thrombosis and pulmonary embolism. *Acta Chir Scand (Suppl)* 478:1, 1977.

164. Lagerstedt CI, Olsson CG, Fagher BO, et al: Need for long-term anticoagulant treatment in symptomatic calf-vein thrombosis. *Lancet* 2:515, 1985.

165. Giachino A: Relationship between deep vein thrombosis in the calf and fatal pulmonary embolism. *Can J Surg* 31:129, 1988.

166. Philbrick JT, Becker DM: Calf deep venous thrombosis: A wolf in sheep's clothing? *Arch Intern Med* 148:2131, 1988.

167. Horratas MC, Wright DJ, Fenton AH, et al: Changing concepts of deep venous thrombosis of the upper extremity: Report of a series and review of the literature. *Surgery* 104:561, 1988.

168. Corona ML, Peters SG, Narr BJ, et al: Infections related to central venous catheters. *Mayo Clin Proc* 65:979, 1990.

169. Kerr TM, Lutter KS, Moeller DM, et al: Upper extremity venous thrombosis diagnosed by duplex scanning. *Am J Surg* 160:202, 1990.

170. Brismar B, Nystrom B: Thrombophlebitis in septicemia: Complication related to intravascular devices and their prophylaxis: A review. *Acta Chir Scand* 530:73, 1986.

171. Cronan JJ: State of the art venous thromboembolic disease: The role of US. *Radiology* 186:619, 1993.

172. Bern MM, Lokich JJ, Wallach SR, et al: Very low doses of warfarin can prevent thrombosis in central venous catheters. *Ann Intern Med* 112:423, 1990.

173. Farkas JC, Liu N, Bleriot JP, et al: Single versus triple lumen central catheter related sepsis: A prospective randomized study in a critically ill population. *Am J Med* 93:277, 1992.

174. Raad I, Davis S, Becker N, et al: Low infection rate and long durability of nontunneled Silastic catheters: A safe and cost effective alternative for long term venous access. *Arch Intern Med* 153:1791, 1993.

175. Cobb DK, High KP, Sawyer RG, et al: A controlled trial of schedule replacement of central venous and pulmonary artery catheters. *N Engl J Med* 327:1062, 1992.

176. Immelman EJ, Jeffery PC: The postphlebitic syndrome: Pathophysiology prevention and management. *Clin Chest Med* 5:537, 1984.

177. Elliot MS, Immelman EJ, Jeffery P, et al: A comparative randomized trial of heparin versus streptokinase in the treatment of acute proximal venous thrombosis: Interim report of a prospective trial. *Br J Surg* 66:838, 1979.

178. Common HH, Seaman AJ, Rosch J, et al: Deep vein thrombosis treated with streptokinase or heparin. *Angiology* 27:645, 1976.

179. Rogers LQ, Lutcher CL: Streptokinase therapy for deep vein thrombosis: A comprehensive review of the English literature. *Am J Med* 88:389, 1990.

180. A Collaborative European Multicentre Study: A randomized trial of subcutaneous low molecular weight heparin (CY216) compared with intravenous unfractionated heparin in the treatment of deep vein thrombosis. *Thromb Haemost* 65:251, 1991.

181. Albada J, Nieuwenhuis HK, Sixma JJ: Treatment of acute venous thromboembolism with low molecular weight heparin (Fragmin): Results of double-blind randomized study. *Circulation* 80:935, 1989.

182. Prandoni P, Lensing AWA, Buller HR, et al: Comparison of subcutaneous low molecular weight heparin with intravenous standard heparin in proximal vein thrombosis. *Lancet* 339:441, 1992.

183. Hull RD, Raskob GE, Pineo GF, et al: Subcutaneous low-molecular weight heparin compared with continuous intravenous heparin in the initial treatment of proximal-vein thrombosis. *N Engl J Med* 326:975, 1992.

184. Sevitt S, Gallagher N: Venous thrombosis and pulmonary embolism: A clinico-pathological study in injured and burned patients. *Br J Surg* 48:475, 1961.

185. Shackford SR, Davis JW, Hollingsworth-Fridlund P, et al: Venous thromboembolism in patients with major trauma. *Am J Surg* 159:365, 1990.

186. Collins R, Scrimgeour A, Yusuf S, et al: Reduction in fatal pulmonary embolism and venous thrombosis by perioperative administration of subcutaneous heparin: Overview of results of randomized trials in general, orthopedic, and urologic surgery. *N Engl J Med* 318:1162, 1988.

187. Parmet JL, Berman AT, Horrow JC, et al: Thrombolism coincident with tourniquet inflation during total knee arthroplasty. *Lancet* 341:1057, 1993.

188. Hull R, Raskob G, Pineo G, et al: A comparison of subcutaneous low-molecular-weight heparin with warfarin sodium for prophylaxis against deep-vein thrombosis after hip or knee implantation. *N Engl J Med* 329:1370, 1993.

61. Managing Hemoptysis

Richard S. Irwin and Frederick J. Curley

Overview

Hemoptysis is defined in *Stedman's Medical Dictionary* as "the spitting of blood derived from the lungs or bronchial tubes." This common symptom may be the primary reason for seeking consultation in approximately 8 to 15 percent of an average chest clinic population [1,2]. It elicits great apprehension in the patient and is likely to prompt early medical attention. The basis for this fear is the presumption that the hemoptysis is caused by a serious disease such as cancer and that it signals impending massive bleeding [3]. The patient may describe an associated burning pain, vague discomfort, or bubbling sensation in the chest and shortness of breath. Hemoptysis may be scant, producing the appearance of streaks of bright red blood in the sputum, or profuse, with expectoration of a large volume of blood. *Massive hemoptysis* is defined as the expectoration of 600 ml of blood within 24 to 48 hours [4,5] and occurs in 3 to 10 percent of all patients with hemoptysis [4,6]. *Gross* or *frank hemoptysis* produces a quantity smaller than massive hemoptysis and greater than blood streaking. Dark red clots may also be expectorated when blood has been present in the lungs for days.

Pseudohemoptysis, on the other hand, is the expectoration of blood from a source other than the lower respiratory tract. It may cause diagnostic confusion when patients cannot clearly describe the source of their bleeding. Pseudohemoptysis may occur when blood from the oral cavity [7,8], nares [2,8], pharynx [8], or tongue [8,9] drains to the back of the throat and initiates the cough reflex; when blood is aspirated into the lower respiratory tract in patients who have hematemesis [9]; and when the oropharynx is colonized with a red, pigment-producing, aerobic, gram-negative rod, *Serratia marcescens* [10]. This colonization may occur in hospitalized patients who have received broad-spectrum antimicrobial agents and mechanical ventilatory support. Other rare causes of pseudohemoptysis are self-inflicted injuries [11] or other bizarre tactics in the malingering patient seeking hospitalization [12,13] and rifampin overdose

[14] (red man syndrome). The causes and distinguishing features of pseudohemoptysis are listed in Table 61-1.

This chapter deals with managing hemoptysis in the intensive care unit (ICU) within the context of a general discussion of hemoptysis. The management of tracheoartery fistula, traumatic rupture of the pulmonary artery due to balloon flotation catheters, and diffuse intrapulmonary hemorrhage are highlighted.

Etiology

Hemoptysis can be caused by a wide variety of disorders (Table 61-2) [15–108]. Although the incidences of the causes of hemoptysis have been described in several populations of patients, no study has ever reported the most frequent causes of hemoptysis in critically ill patients.

The etiology of hemoptysis is considered here in three general categories: nonmassive, massive, and idiopathic. Patients in the ICU frequently have nonmassive hemoptysis, and the spectrum of the causes of hemoptysis in these patients probably differs little from that reported in major series. Because of the nature of ICUs, one would suspect that iatrogenic causes of hemoptysis (e.g., due to anticoagulation or tracheal ulceration secondary to suctioning) might be more frequent. Hemoptysis due to trauma and infection might also be frequent, depending on the population of the individual ICU. Unlike the general ICU patient, patients with massive hemoptysis are frequently in the ICU because of their hemoptysis and thereby constitute a different subgroup of patients.

NONMASSIVE HEMOPTYSIS. Although bronchitis, bronchiectasis, lung carcinoma, and tuberculosis have always been among the most common causes of hemoptysis [9,105,109,110], their incidence varies depending on the study group population. For example, at King's County Hospital in Brooklyn, the

Table 61-1. Differential Features of Pseudohemoptysis

Cause	History	Physical examination	Laboratory tests
Upper respiratory tract	Little or no cough: epistaxis, bleeding from gums when brushing teeth	Gingivitis, telangiectasias, ulcerations, lacerations, or varices of the tongue, nose, or naso-, oro-, or hypopharynx	None
Upper gastrointestinal tract	Coffee-ground appearance of blood due to mixture with HCl; usually lacks the bubbly, frothy appearance of bloody sputum; nausea, vomiting, or history of GI disease	Epigastric tenderness; signs of chronic liver disease	Acid pH of blood; blood in nasogastric aspirate; barium swallow, esophagoscopy, and gastroscopy
Serratia marcescens	Previous hospitalization, broad-spectrum antibiotics, mechanical ventilation	Normal	No red blood cells in red sputum; culture of organism
Malingering	Psychiatric illness; unconfirmed history of massive hemoptysis at midnight	Normal unless self-induced lesions seen; patients unable to cough up blood on command (patients with true hemoptysis will)	True hemoptysis usually must be ruled out (see Table 61-4)

Table 61-2. Causes of Hemoptysis

1. Tracheobronchial disorders
   a. Acute tracheobronchitis [15]*
   b. Amyloidosis [16]
   c. Aspiration of gastric contents [17]
   d. Bronchial adenoma [15,18]
   e. Bronchial endometriosis [19]
   f. Bronchial telangiectasia [20]
   g. Bronchiectasis [21–23]*
   h. Bronchogenic carcinoma [15,22,24]
   i. Broncholithiasis [15,25]
   j. Chronic bronchitis [22]*
   k. Cystic fibrosis [26]*
   l. Endobronchial hamartoma [27]
   m. Endobronchial metastases [28]
   n. Endobronchial tuberculosis [29]
   o. Foreign body aspiration [30,32]
   p. Mucoid impaction of the bronchus [33]
   q. Thyroid cancer [34]
   r. Tracheobronchial trauma [35]
   s. Tracheoesophageal fistula [36–38]
   t. Tracheoartery fistula [39]
2. Cardiovascular disorders
   a. Aortic aneurysm [41]
   b. Bronchial artery rupture [42]
   c. Congenital heart disease [43,44]
   d. Congestive heart failure [29,45]*
   e. Coronary artery bypass graft [46]
   f. Fat embolization [47]
   g. Hughes-Stovin syndrome [48]
   h. Mitral stenosis [49,50]*
   i. Neonatal intrapulmonary hemorrhage [51]
   j. Postmyocardial infarction syndrome [52]
   k. Pulmonary arteriovenous fistula [53]
   l. Pulmonary artery aneurysm [54]
   m. Pulmonary embolus [55,56]
   n. Pulmonary venous varix [57]
   o. Schistosomiasis [58]
   p. Subclavian artery aneurysm [59]
   q. Superior vena cava syndrome [60]
   r. Tumor embolization [61]
3. Hematologic disorders
   a. Anticoagulant therapy [64]
   b. Disseminated intravascular coagulation [65]
   c. Leukemia [66]
   d. Thrombocytopenia [67]

4. Localized parenchymal diseases
   a. Acute and chronic nontuberculous pneumonia [15,22]*
   b. Actinomycosis [69]
   c. Amebiasis [70]
   d. Ascariasis [71]
   e. Aspergilloma [72]
   f. Bronchopulmonary sequestration [73]
   g. Coccidioidomycosis [74]
   h. Congenital and acquired cyst [75]
   i. Cryptococcosis [76]
   j. Exogenous lipoid pneumonia [77]
   k. Histoplasmosis [78]
   l. Hydatid mole [79]
   m. Lung abscess [80]
   n. Lung contusion [81]
   o. Metastatic cancer [82]
   p. Mucormycosis [83]
   q. Nocardiosis [84]
   r. Paragonimiasis [85]*
   s. Pulmonary endometriosis [86]
   t. Pulmonary tuberculosis [29]*
   u. Sporotrichosis [87]
5. Diffuse parenchymal diseases
   a. Disseminated angiosarcoma [88]
   b. Farmer's lung [89]
   c. Goodpasture's syndrome [90]
   d. Idiopathic pulmonary hemosiderosis [91]
   e. IgA nephropathy [92]
   f. Inhaled isocyanates [93]
   g. Charcoal lighter fluid injection [94]
   h. Legionnaires' disease [95]
   i. Mixed connective tissue disease [96]
   j. Mixed cryoglobulinemia [97]
   k. Polyarteritis nodosa [98]
   l. Scleroderma [99,100]
   m. Systemic lupus erythematosus [101]
   n. Trimellitic anhydride toxicity [102]
   o. Viral pneumonitis [103]
   p. Wegener's granulomatosis [104]
6. Other
   a. Idiopathic [105]*
   b. Iatrogenic (e.g., bronchoscopy [106], cardiac catheterization [107], needle biopsy of lung [108]

*Common causes

causes of hemoptysis reported in 1976 were tuberculosis in 61 percent of patients, bronchiectasis in 21 percent, bronchogenic carcinoma in 12 percent, lung abscess in 4 percent, and unknown in 2 percent [9]. At the Veterans Administration Hospital in Boston, the causes of hemoptysis reported in 1973 were bronchitis in 32 percent of patients, bronchogenic carcinoma in 25 percent, granulation tissue at tracheostomy stoma in 6 percent, tuberculosis in 2 percent, metastatic cancer in 3 percent, and unknown in 32 percent [109]. At the National Naval Medical Center in Bethesda, Maryland, the causes of hemoptysis reported in 1973 were chronic bronchitis or bronchiectasis in 56 percent of patients, carcinoma in 21 percent, tuberculosis in 6 percent, pneumonia in 6 percent, aspiration in 5 percent, pulmonary embolus in 3 percent, and trauma in 3 percent [110].

More recent studies have shown that the causes may have shifted slightly, bronchiectasis and tuberculosis being less common and bronchitis being more common. In 148 urban, adult, mostly indigent patients studied in Kansas City between 1977 and 1985, the causes of hemoptysis were bronchitis in 37 percent, bronchogenic carcinoma in 19 percent, tuberculosis in 7

percent, pneumonia in 5 percent, and bronchiectasis in 1 percent [111]. In 59 patients with hemoptysis of more than 200 ml per day studied at Duke University between 1972 and 1981, the causes included bronchitis or bronchiectasis in 28 percent, cancer in 36 percent, cystic fibrosis in 7 percent, anticoagulation in 7 percent, and tuberculosis in 5 percent [6]. Because of increasing frequency of human immunodeficiency virus (HIV) infection and of tuberculosis in HIV-infected patients, however, the incidence of hemoptysis due to tuberculosis may increase again during the next decade [112].

While bleeding from tracheoartery fistula complicating tracheostomy, rupture of pulmonary artery from a balloon flotation catheter, and diffuse intrapulmonary hemorrhage may be submassive, they are discussed under massive hemoptysis.

MASSIVE HEMOPTYSIS. The more frequent causes of massive hemoptysis likely to present in the ICU are listed in Table 61-3. Virtually all causes of hemoptysis may result in massive hemoptysis, but it is most frequently caused by infection and

Table 61-3. Common Causes of Massive Hemoptysis

Infectious
    Bronchitis
    Bronchiectasis
    Tuberculosis
    Cystic fibrosis
    Aspergilloma
    Sporotrichosis
    Lung abscess
Malignant
    Bronchogenic cancer
    Metastatic cancer
    Leukemia
Cardiovascular
    Arteriobronchial fistula
    Congestive heart failure
    Pulmonary arteriovenous fistula
Diffuse parenchymal disease
Diffuse intrapulmonary hemorrhage
Trauma
Iatrogenic
    Pulmonary artery rupture
    Malposition of chest tube
    Tracheoartery fistula

Table 61-4. Routine Evaluation of Hemoptysis

History
Physical examination
CBC
Urinalysis
Coagulation studies
ECG
Chest radiographs
± FBB*

*Although flexible fiberoptic bronchoscopy (FBB) should not be performed in some conditions (e.g., pulmonary embolism, aortopulmonary fistula), it should be routinely considered (see text).

Table 61-5. Special Evaluation of Hemoptysis

1. Tracheobronchial disorders
    a. Expectorated sputa for tubercle bacilli, parasites, fungi, and routine cytologic testing
    b. Bronchoscopy
    c. Bronchography
2. Cardiovascular disorders
    a. Echocardiogram
    b. Arterial blood gases on 21% and 100% oxygen
    c. Ventilation and perfusion lung scans
    d. Pulmonary angiogram
    e. Aortogram, CT scan with contrast
    f. Cardiac catheterization
3. Hematologic disorders
    a. Coagulation studies
    b. Bone marrow
4. Localized parenchymal diseases
    a. Expectorated sputa for parasites, tubercle bacilli, fungi, and routine cytologic testing
    b. Tomogram, CT scan
    c. *Aspergillus* precipitins in serum
    d. Lung biopsy with special stains
5. Diffuse parenchymal diseases*
    a. Expectorated sputa for cytologic testing
    b. BUN, creatinine, ANA, rheumatoid factor, complement, cryoglobulins, LE prep
    c. Serum for circulating antiglomerular basement membrane antibody and antineutrophilic cytoplasmic antibody
    d. Serum for precipitins for hypersensitivity pneumonitis screen
    e. Acute and convalescent serum antibody studies for Legionnaires' disease and respiratory viruses
    f. Lung and/or kidney biopsy with special stains, including immunofluorescence

*Diffuse implies involvement of all lobes.
ANA = antinuclear antibody; LE = lupus erythematosus.

cancer. Several series report that more than 60 percent of cases are due to tuberculosis, bronchiectasis, and lung abscess [4,113,114]. Infection is also the cause of bleeding from aspergilloma [72] and cystic fibrosis [26]. In one series of 22 patients, 27 percent of cases were due to bronchitis, 18 percent to tuberculosis, 9 percent to aspergilloma, 4 percent to bronchiectasis, and 4 percent to sporotrichosis [111]. In a series from Duke University, 17 of 42 (40%) patients with massive hemoptysis had cancer and only 8 (19%) had bronchitis, bronchiectasis, or tuberculosis as a cause [6]. Idiopathic hemoptysis is less frequent in patients with massive hemoptysis and usually constitutes less than 5 percent of cases [111].

Rupture of a pulmonary artery complicates balloon flotation catheterizations in less than 0.2 percent of cases [62,63]. It is fortunate that it is rare, since it carries a mortality approximating 40 percent [63]. *Tracheoartery fistula* is also an unusual but devastating condition, complicating approximately 0.7 percent of tracheostomies [39]. These two complications of procedures commonly performed in ICU populations and *diffuse intrapulmonary hemorrhage,* usually due to an immunologically mediated disease, are most likely to be considered in the differential diagnosis of massive rather than submassive hemoptysis in the ICU.

IDIOPATHIC HEMOPTYSIS. Using the systemic diagnostic approach outlined below and in Tables 61-4 and 61-5, the cause of hemoptysis can be found in most instances. In 2 to 32 percent of patients [9,109] (average 12%), the cause cannot be determined. This condition, called *idiopathic* or *essential hemoptysis,* is seen most commonly in men between the ages of 30 and 50 years. Prolonged follow-up study almost always fails to reveal the source of bleeding, even though 10 percent continue to have occasional episodes of hemoptysis [3,105].

Pathogenesis

To appreciate fully the pathogenesis of hemoptysis, it is necessary to review briefly the normal anatomy of the nutrient blood supply to the lungs [115,116]. The bronchial arteries are the chief source of blood of the airways (from mainstem bronchi to terminal bronchioles); the supporting framework of the lung that includes the pleura, intrapulmonary lymphoid tissue; and large branches of the pulmonary vessels and nerves in the hilar regions. The pulmonary arteries supply the pulmonary parenchymal tissue, including the respiratory bronchioles. Communications between these two blood supplies (Fig. 61-1), bronchopulmonary arterial and venous anastomoses, occur in the proximity of the junction of the terminal and respiratory bronchioles. These anastomoses allow the two blood supplies to complement each other. For instance, if flow through one system is increased or decreased, a reciprocal change occurs in the amount of blood supplied by the other system [117]. Arte-

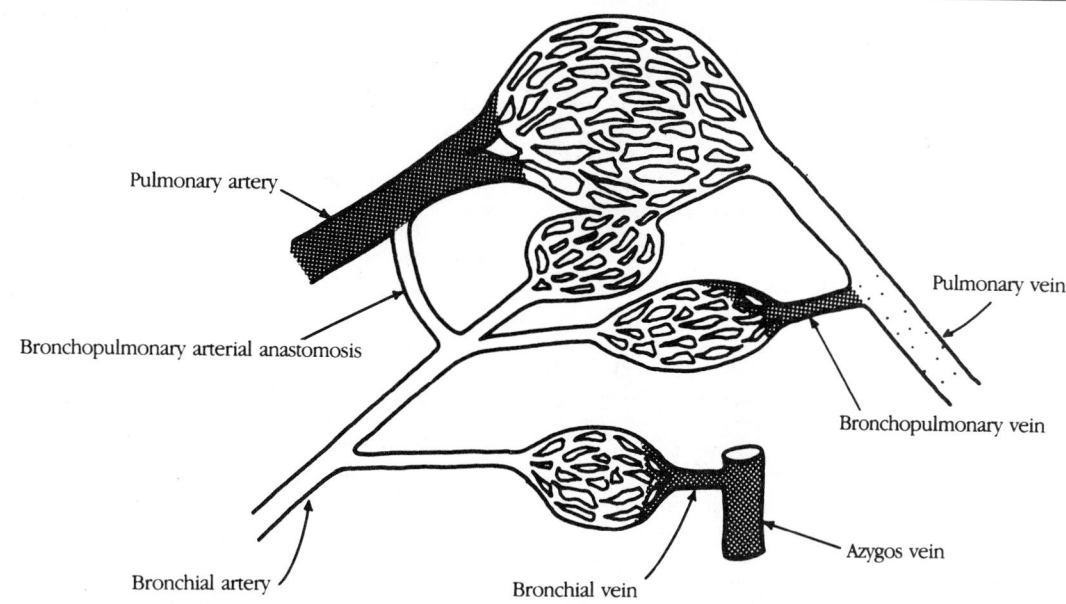

Fig. 61-1. Relation between bronchial and pulmonary circulations. (From Murray JF: Postnatal growth and development of the lung, in Murray JF: *The Normal Lung: The Basis for Diagnosis and Treatment of Pulmonary Disease.* Philadelphia, WB Saunders, 1976, p 42. With permission.)

riographic studies in patients with active hemoptysis have shown that the systemic circulation is primarily responsible for the bleeding in about 92 percent of cases [118].

The pathogenesis of hemoptysis depends on the type and location of the disease [29]. In general, if the lesion is endobronchial the bleeding is from the bronchial circulation, and if the lesion is parenchymal the bleeding is from the pulmonary circulation. Moreover, in chronic diseases, repetitive episodes are most likely due to increased vascularity in the involved area [119].

In bronchogenic carcinoma, hemoptysis results from necrosis of the tumor, with its increased blood supply from bronchial arteries or from local invasion of a large blood vessel [29]. In bronchial adenomas, bleeding is usually from rupture of the prominent surface vessels [29]. In bronchiectasis, hemoptysis is usually due to irritation by infection of the granulation tissue that has replaced the normal bronchial wall [28]. In acute bronchitis, bleeding results from irritation of the unusually friable and vascular mucosa [29].

The mechanism of hemoptysis in mitral stenosis is controversial, but the most likely explanation is rupture of the dilated varices of the bronchial veins in the submucosa of large bronchi [120] due to pulmonary venous hypertension. Pulmonary venous hypertension may also be responsible for the bleeding in congestive heart failure, since it is associated with widening of the capillary anastomoses between bronchial and pulmonary arteries [119].

Hemoptysis in pulmonary embolism may be due to infarction [56], with necrosis of parenchymal tissue or hemorrhagic consolidation due to an excessive influx of bronchial arterial blood at systemic pressures through the bronchopulmonary anastomoses into the pulmonary circulation distal to the obstructing clot [56].

In tuberculosis, bleeding can occur for a variety of reasons [28]. In the acute parenchymal exudative lesion, scant hemoptysis may result from necrosis of a small branch of a pulmonary

artery or vein. In the chronic, parenchymal fibroulcerative lesion, massive hemoptysis may result from rupture of a pulmonary artery aneurysm [121] bulging into the lumen of a cavity. The aneurysm occurs from tuberculous involvement of the adventitia and media of the vessel [122]. When a healed and calcified tuberculous lymph node erodes the wall of a bronchus because of pressure necrosis, the patient may cough up blood as well as the calcified node (broncholith). In endobronchial tuberculosis, hemoptysis may result from acute tuberculous ulceration of the bronchial mucosa. In healed and fibrotic parenchymal areas of tuberculosis, bleeding may arise from irritation of granulation tissue in the walls of bronchiectatic airways in the same areas.

In traumatic *rupture of the pulmonary artery* by a balloon flotation catheter, risk factors include pulmonary hypertension, distal location of the catheter tip, excessive catheter manipulation in an attempt to obtain a pulmonary artery occluded pressure measurement, a large catheter loop in the right ventricle, and advanced age [63].

In *tracheoartery fistula* complicating tracheostomy, bleeding is due to trauma from the tracheostomy cannula and/or balloon [39]. Bleeding is usually due to rupture of the innominate artery. The fistula can form at three tracheal locations: the stoma, the intratracheal cannula tip, and the balloon. Trauma at the stoma is caused by pressure necrosis, usually because the tracheostomy was created too low (below the fourth tracheal ring); at the cannula tip because of excessive angulation of the cannula; and at the balloon site due to pressure necrosis due to use of excessive inflation pressures.

Diffuse intrapulmonary hemorrhage due to immunologic diseases is due to an inflammatory lesion, usually of capillaries. Lung biopsies of patients with hemorrhage due to systemic lupus erythematosus (SLE) or Wegener's granulomatosis have shown a pulmonary capillaritis [123,124].

Diagnosis

GENERAL CONSIDERATIONS. The success rate in determining the cause of hemoptysis is excellent but variable. If one accepts the diagnosis of idiopathic (essential) hemoptysis as a distinct entity, the cause of hemoptysis can be determined in close to 100 percent of cases [9,109]. If one does not accept this diagnosis in patients with hemoptysis from an unknown cause, the cause can be determined in 68 to 98 percent of cases [9,109,111] (average about 88%).

The diagnostic work-up of hemoptysis involves routine (Table 61-4) as well as special evaluations (Table 61-5). Routine evaluations are initially performed in every patient, whereas special studies are ordered only when the clinical setting suggests they are indicated. In general, each category of disease (Table 61-2) has its special studies (Table 61-5).

ROUTINE EVALUATION. As in any diagnostic problem, a detailed history and physical examination must be performed. These should be performed in a systematic fashion not only to rule in the common causes of hemoptysis but also to rule in the category of the cause (Table 61-2).

Although the amount of bleeding is generally not indicative of the seriousness of the underlying disease process, a history of the frequency, timing, and duration of hemoptysis may be helpful. For example, repeated episodes of hemoptysis occurring over months to years suggest bronchial adenoma and bronchiectasis [29], whereas small amounts of hemoptysis occurring every day for weeks are more likely to be caused by bronchogenic carcinoma [125]. Bleeding due to bronchogenic carcinoma usually is of short duration, since it is generally a late finding in these patients [29]. In addition to having an abnormal chest radiograph, these patients are usually older than 40 years and are almost invariably cigarette smokers [125].

Hemoptysis that coincides with the menses suggests the rare diagnostic possibility of pulmonary endometriosis [19,86], whereas bleeding associated with sexual intercourse [126] or other forms of exertion [127] suggests passive congestion of the lungs. Although hemoptysis may be a symptom at any age, it is distinctly uncommon in the young. When hemoptysis is present before the third decade of life, it suggests an acute tracheobronchitis, a congenital cardiac or lung defect, an unusual tumor, cystic fibrosis, a blood dyscrasia, or infectious pneumonia. No matter what the age, if a patient with pneumonia who is undergoing appropriate therapy has hemoptysis that persists for more than the usual 24 hours, an endobronchial lesion or coagulopathy should be suspected [127].

A travel history can often be helpful in bringing certain endemic diseases to mind. This is true of coccidioidomycosis and histoplasmosis in the United States, of paragonimiasis and ascariasis in the Far East, and of schistosomiasis in South America, Africa, and the Far East. Chronic sputum production before hemoptysis suggests a diagnosis of chronic bronchitis, bronchiectasis, and cystic fibrosis. The presence of orthopnea and paroxysmal nocturnal dyspnea makes likely the diagnoses of passive congestion of the lungs from mitral stenosis and left ventricular failure. A history of anticoagulant therapy suggests an intrapulmonary bleed from too large a dose or recurrent pulmonary embolism from too small a dose. The possibility of pulmonary embolism should always be considered when a patient who presents with hemoptysis has been at increased risk for deep venous thrombosis [55].

The possibility of traumatic rupture of a pulmonary artery due to balloon flotation catheterization should always be considered when these catheters are utilized [62,63].

Although tracheoartery fistula must be considered in the differential diagnosis of hemoptysis in every patient with a tracheostomy, it is fortunately an infrequent cause in this setting. When it occurs, the onset is almost always at least 48 hours following the procedure [39]. While the peak incidence is be-

tween the first and second week and 72 percent of fistulas will bleed during the first 21 days following tracheostomy, hemorrhage from this complication can also occur as late as 18 months following the procedure [39]. There is a sentinel bleed in 34 to 50 percent of cases [39]. Prior to 48 hours, bleeding from the stoma is usually due to capillary bleeding from inadequate hemostasis. Whenever hemoptysis occurs in a patient with an endotracheal tube or tracheostomy in place, trauma from suctioning, especially when coagulation is abnormal, should be considered a likely cause.

Although patients with diffuse intrapulmonary hemorrhage typically have hemoptysis, they may occasionally not expectorate at all but just complain of dyspnea [128] or the abrupt onset of fever, dyspnea, cough, and malaise. Therefore, lack of hemoptysis does not rule out a substantial intrapulmonary hemorrhage [128].

The diagnosis of trimellitic anhydride (TMA)-induced pulmonary hemorrhage should be suspected in workers exposed to high-dose TMA fumes. Exposure occurs when heated metal surfaces are sprayed with corrosion-resistant epoxy resin coatings. The syndrome requires a latent period of exposure and appears to be antibody-mediated [129–133]. Respiratory failure with pulmonary infiltrates and hemoptysis have also been reported, in a patient with a documented exposure and antibodies to isocyanates [134].

In a patient with the triad of known upper airway disease, lower airway disease, and renal disease, systemic Wegener's granulomatosis should be suspected. Although the diagnosis of SLE is readily considered in a patient known to have this disease, pulmonary hemorrhage can be the presenting manifestation [101]. Goodpasture's syndrome (antibasement membrane antibody-mediated disease) typically occurs in young men [135], and it has been reported to be associated with influenza infection [136], inhalation of hydrocarbons [137], and penicillamine ingestion [138]. Therefore, it should be considered in these historical contexts.

Physical examination may be helpful in several ways. Inspection of the skin and mucous membranes may show telangiectasias (Fig. 61-2), suggesting hereditary hemorrhagic telangiectasia, or ecchymoses and petechiae, suggesting a hematologic abnormality. Pulsations transmitted to a tracheostomy cannula should heighten suspicion of a tracheoartery fis-

Fig. 61-2. Localized arteriovenous capillary connections on lower lip and tip of tongue. These lesions are characteristic of hereditary telangiectasia. They also occur on the face, in the nailbeds, on the skin of the body, and in nearly all organs.

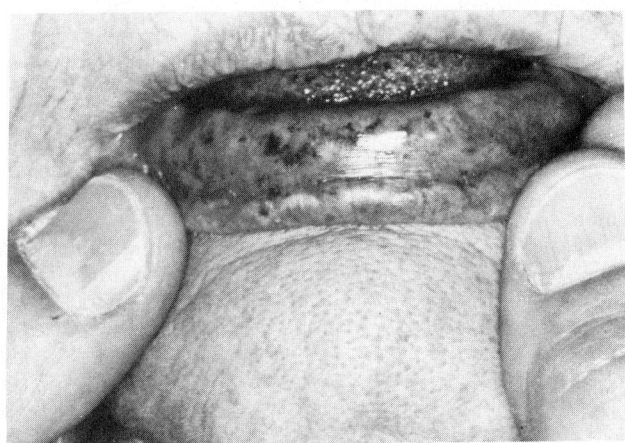

tula or risk of one. Inspection of the thorax may show evidence of recent or old chest trauma, and unilateral wheeze or rales may herald localized disease such as bronchial adenoma or carcinoma. Although pulmonary embolism is not definitively diagnosed on physical examination, tachypnea, phlebitis, and pleural friction rub suggest this disorder. If crackles are heard diffusely on chest examination, passive congestion as well as other diseases causing diffuse intrapulmonary hemorrhage should be considered (Table 61-2). Careful cardiovascular examination may rule in mitral stenosis, pulmonary artery stenosis, or pulmonary hypertension.

The routine laboratory studies listed in Table 61-4 are useful for the following reasons. The CBC results may suggest presence of an infection, hematologic disorder, or chronic blood loss. Idiopathic hemosiderosis or other causes of diffuse intrapulmonary hemorrhage (Table 61-2) may present only with diffuse pulmonary infiltrates and iron deficiency anemia from chronic bleeding into the lungs. Urinalysis may reveal hematuria and suggest the presence of a systemic disease associated with diffuse parenchymal disease (e.g., pulmonary renal hemorrhage syndrome due to SLE, Goodpasture's syndrome, systemic Wegener's granulomatosis, and other systemic vasculitides) (Table 61-2). While there is simultaneous evidence of clinical involvement of the lungs and kidneys in 33 percent of cases of Goodpasture's syndrome, there can be clinical lung involvement without renal disease in 33 percent and clinical renal involvement without lung disease in 33 percent [139,140,141].

Coagulation studies may uncover a hematologic disorder that is primarily responsible for the hemoptysis or that contributes to excessive bleeding from another disease. The ECG may help suggest the presence of a cardiovascular disorder. Although as many as 30 percent of patients with hemoptysis have normal chest radiographs [15], routine posteroanterior and lateral films may be diagnostically valuable.

When pulmonary tumor or infection is not readily apparent, other radiographic signs that may suggest the cause and source of bleeding include radiopaque foreign bodies, which may give rise to hemoptysis even years after entry into the lungs; the disappearance of a calcified mediastinal lymph node after it has eroded the bronchial wall and is expectorated as a broncholith; aortic (Fig. 61-3) or pulmonary (Fig. 61-4) aneurysms, which by dissection may erode into the bronchial tree; single or multiple pulmonary cavities, which suggest pulmonary tuberculosis, fungal disease, parasitic disease, acute or chronic lung abscess, primary or metastatic neoplasm, septic pulmonary emboli, or Wegener's granulomatosis; an intracavitary mass lesion that is indicative of a fungus ball (Fig. 61-5) (aspergilloma) or blood clot; and localized honeycombing, which is consistent with bronchiectasis. The presence of a new infiltrate localized to the area subtending a balloon flotation catheter suggests a rupture of the pulmonary artery [62,63]. The appearance of a new air-fluid level in a preexisting cavity (Fig. 61-6) [80] or cyst suggests the location of the source of bleeding, as does a nonsegmental alveolar pattern that clears within a few days. A solitary pulmonary nodule with vessels going toward it suggests an arteriovenus fistula (Fig. 61-7). In patients with hemoptysis due to pulmonary embolism, a parenchymal density abutting a pleural surface with evidence of pleural reaction and/or effusion is usually present [55]. The cardiac silhouette, vascular or parenchymal patterns (Fig. 61-8), and presence of Kerley B lines may be useful in documenting cardiovascular disease.

When the chest radiograph shows diffuse pulmonary infiltrates, hemorrhage from bleeding disorders (e.g., thrombocytopenia in the compromised host), lung contusion from blunt chest trauma, free-base cocaine use, and passive congestion of the lungs should be considered, in addition to the diseases

listed in Table 61-2. In the earliest stages of diffuse intrapulmonary hemorrhage, chest radiographs may appear normal but usually it initially appears in a diffuse alveolar pattern. This progresses to a mixed alveolar-interstitial pattern and then, when bleeding ceases entirely, an interstitial pattern, as hemosiderin deposition accumulates.

Even if the history, physical examination, and chest radiograph are normal or there is an "obvious" cause of hemoptysis on chest radiograph, bronchoscopy is invaluable for not only accurate diagnosis but also precise localization of the pulmonary hemorrhage. It is not uncommon for bronchoscopy to establish sites of bleeding different from those suggested by chest radiograph [100,110]. Bronchoscopy may not be needed in patients with stable chronic bronchitis with one episode of blood streaking, particularly if associated with an exacerbation of acute tracheobronchitis; in whom the site of bleeding was recently documented by bronchoscopic examination; with acute lower respiratory tract infections; and patients with obvious cardiovascular causes of hemoptysis, such as congestive heart failure and pulmonary embolism. In localizing the bleeding site, the best results are obtained when bronchoscopy is performed during or within 24 hours of active bleeding. The bleeding site can be localized in 93 percent of patients [110,142] with a flexible fiberoptic bronchoscope and in 86 percent with the rigid instrument [1]. When rigid bronchoscopy is done after bleeding has ceased, however, accurate localization is reduced to 50 to 52 percent of patients [12,142]. Although the fiberoptic bronchoscope is usually the instrument of choice in diagnosing lower respiratory tract problems, rigid bronchoscopy is preferred in cases of massive uncontrolled hemorrhage because patency of the airway is maintained more effectively during the procedure (see Chap. 12). With the exception of tracheoartery fistula, the tracheobronchial disorders that can be diagnosed by a bronchoscopic examination are listed in Table 61-2.

Bedside bronchoscopy should not be performed to rule in the diagnosis of tracheoartery fistula [39]. In tracheostomized patients with hemoptysis, bronchoscopy should be performed to rule out other causes, such as bleeding from suction ulcers, tracheitis, or lower respiratory tract disorders. If no other cause for hemoptysis can be found and bleeding has stopped or anterior and downward pressure on the cannula on the stomal site or overinflation of the tracheostomy balloon slows down or stops the bleeding, a surgical consultation should be sought immediately and the patient brought to the operating room for examination in a more controlled environment. In this setting, balloon deflation and removal of the tracheostomy tube is not advised unless airway protection with an endotracheal tube can be performed nearly simultaneously, followed by a definitive vascular repair should the diagnosis be correct. *As long as tracheoartery fistula remains a diagnostic possibility, the tracheostomy balloon should not be deflated and the tracheostomy tube should not be removed without protecting the airway below the tracheostomy tube.*

When there is no active bleeding, bronchoscopy with bronchoalveolar lavage can be helpful in suggesting diffuse intrapulmonary hemorrhage. Return of bright red or blood-tinged lavage fluid from multiple lobes from both lungs suggests an active, diffuse intrapulmonary hemorrhage; hemosiderin-laden macrophages on cytologic analysis from these same specimens suggest bleeding that has been ongoing.

Although the diagnosis of bronchiectasis can be made without question only with the aid of the bronchogram [143] or high-resolution chest computed tomography (CT) scan, a presumptive diagnosis can be made without bronchography. Bronchiectasis is visible on routine chest radiographs in well over 90 percent of cases [143], and bronchoscopy can localize the bleeding to the corresponding abnormal areas.

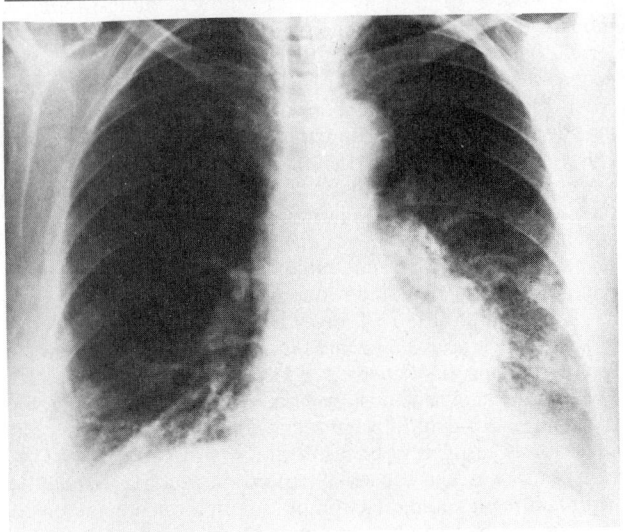

A

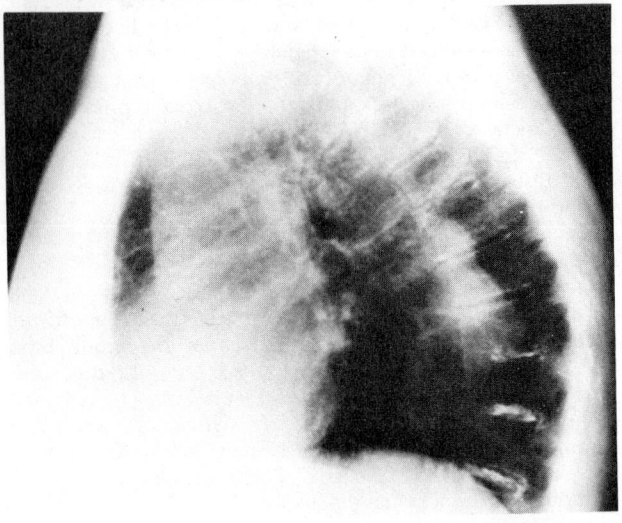

B

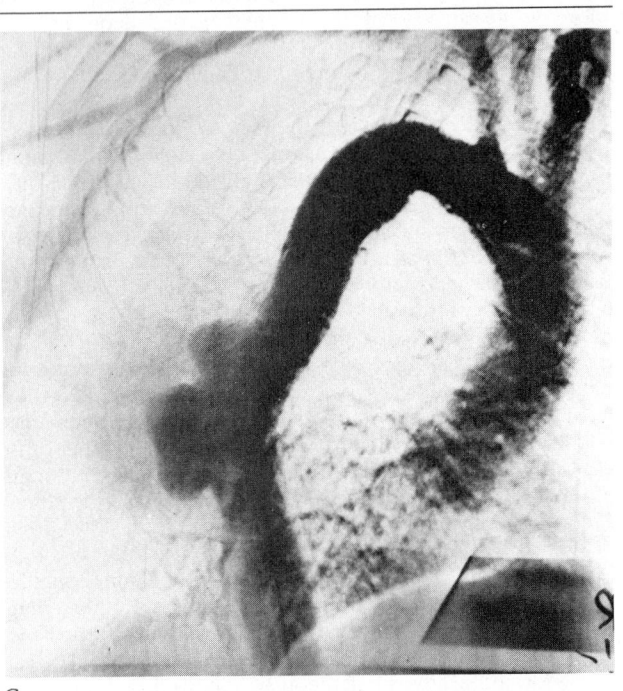

C

Fig. 61-3. Hemoptysis due to dissecting aneurysm of the aorta with aortopulmonary fistula. The possibility of a cardiovascular cause of hemoptysis is suggested by the ill-defined lobulated density on the posteroanterior view (A) and the lobulated density contiguous with the descending aorta on the lateral view (B). The aortogram (C) demonstrates the aneurysm as well as extravasation of dye into the left lower lobe.

Angiography can determine the site of bleeding in 90 to 93 percent of cases [142]. When performed routinely, diagnostic angiography establishes a diagnosis not identified by bronchoscopy in only 4 percent of patients [142]. Technetium-labelled colloid and red blood cell studies have been shown to be accurate and may be positive in 6 to 10 minutes [143]. While angiography may not be initially helpful in confirming rupture of the pulmonary artery due to balloon flotation catheterization if the rent has sealed, it can be extremely helpful in detecting a pseudoaneurysm that has formed in the healing process [63]. Identification of an unstable lesion is important because it should be obliterated to prevent future rupture and death [63]. Angiography has not been useful in diagnosing tracheoartery fistula [39].

SPECIAL EVALUATION. Depending on the results of the initial evaluation and the possible categories of cause of hemoptysis (Table 61-2), additional diagnostic evaluations should be systematically performed (Table 61-5).

The diagnosis of Goodpasture's syndrome is made by demonstrating linear deposition of IgG along the basement membrane of the lung [144] or kidney [145] and the presence of high titers of circulating antibasement membrane antibody in the blood [146]. The choice of lung or kidney biopsy depends on the clinical setting. However, anti-IgG immunofluorescent staining of the kidney may be positive even in the absence of clinical evidence of renal disease [141]. Although Goodpasture's syndrome is typically associated with IgG, there is also a report of a pulmonary-renal hemorrhagic syndrome associated with IgA [147]. The importance of this observation is that the immunoserologic testing must be designed to include both immunoglobulins [147].

Definitive diagnosis of the pulmonary vasculitides depends on histologic examination, including special stains and cultures that rule out tuberculosis and fungal diseases. Pulmonary capillaritis with hemorrhage has been described in Wegener's granulomatosis, systemic necrotizing vasculitis, and SLE [123,124]. The diagnosis can sometimes be made on transbronchial biopsy, thus avoiding the need for open lung biopsy [123], but care must be taken to exclude infectious etiologies by using special stains. In SLE, intraalveolar hemorrhage carries a 50 to 70 percent mortality rate and requires prompt institution of pulse methylprednisolone [124] (see Chap. 219). Antineutrophil cytoplasmic autoantibodies are helpful in diagnosing Wegener's granulomatosis and following disease activity [148]. The complete evaluation of Wegener's granulomatosis, SLE, and mixed cryoglobulinemia is reviewed in Chapters 219 and 220. The diagnostic features of polyarteritis nodosa, the hypersensitivity vasculitides, giant cell and Takayasu's arteritis, and Beh-

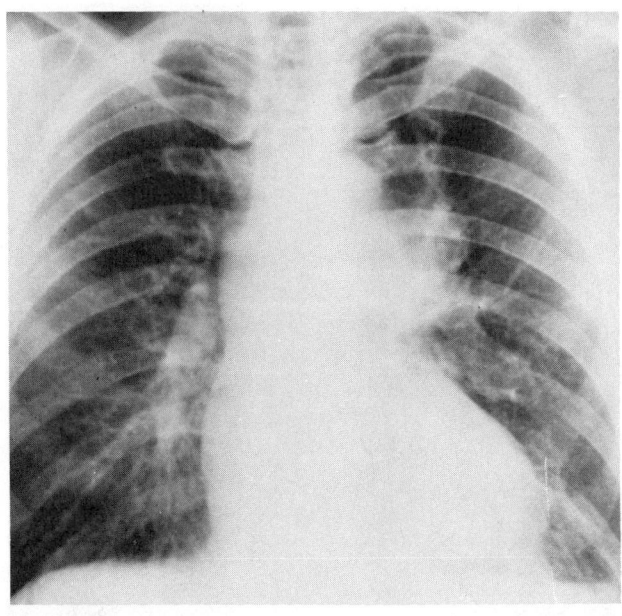

A

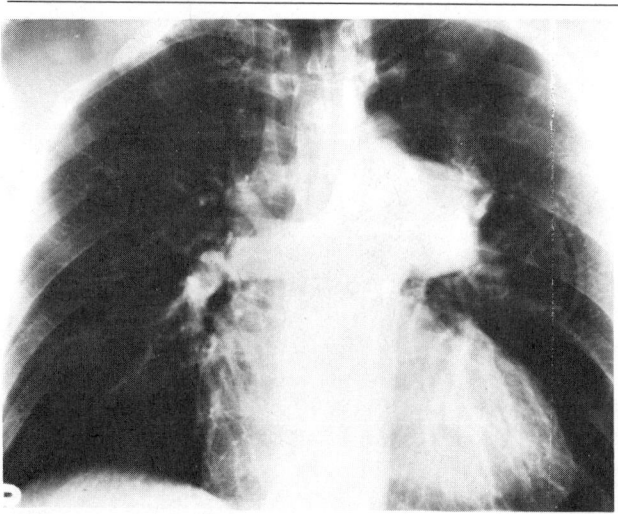

B

Fig. 61-4. Main pulmonary artery aneurysm. The poorly defined left hilar density seen on the posteroanterior view of the chest (A) was demonstrated by pulmonary angiography to be of a vascular nature (B).

çet's disease are presented in detail in Chapter 220. In all of the these, pulmonary involvement is rare. Several cases of Henoch-Schonlein syndrome, one of the hypersensitivity vasculitides, have been reported with severe alveolar hemorrhage, including one in which immunofluorescent stains of the lung revealed granular deposits of IgA consistent with an immune complex mediation [149]. Alveolar hemorrhage has also been reported with Behçet's syndrome [150]. Giant cell arteritis involvement of the lung is centered on the upper respiratory tract, with clinical symptoms of sore throat and hoarseness [151].

While high levels of IgG, IgA, and IgM antibody to trimellitic-coupled protein and trimellitic-conjugated erythrocytes have been found in patients with TMA-induced pulmonary disease

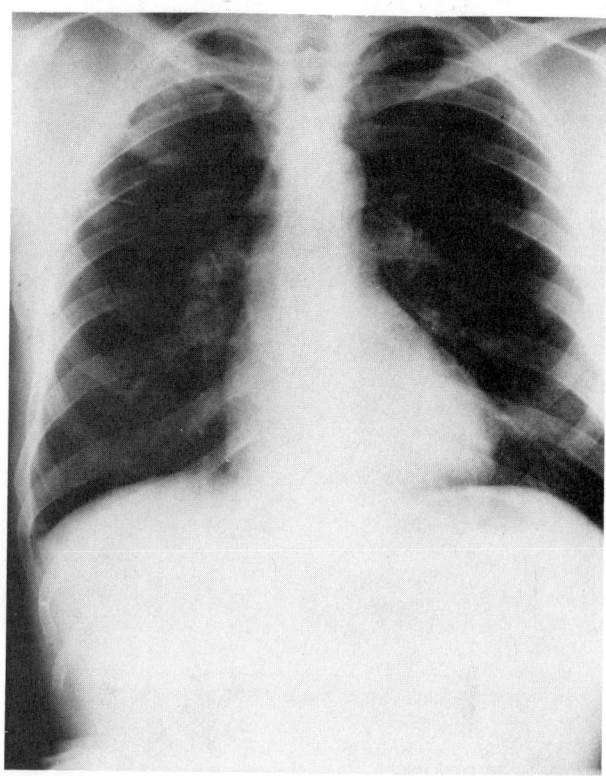

A

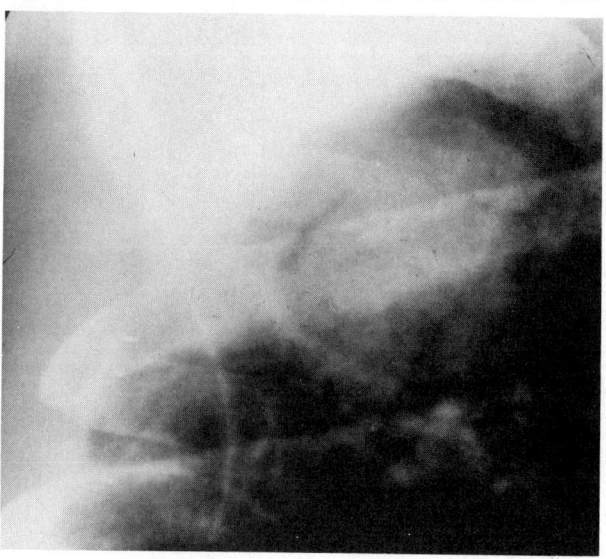

B

Fig. 61-5. Aspergilloma colonizing a preexisting, old, healed, and treated tuberculous cavity. A. The intracavitary nature of the lesion is suggested by the rim of air seen over the superior aspect of the lesion on the routine posteroanterior view. B. This suspicion was confirmed when the rim of air appeared on the lateral margin of the lesion when the patient was rolled onto his left side.

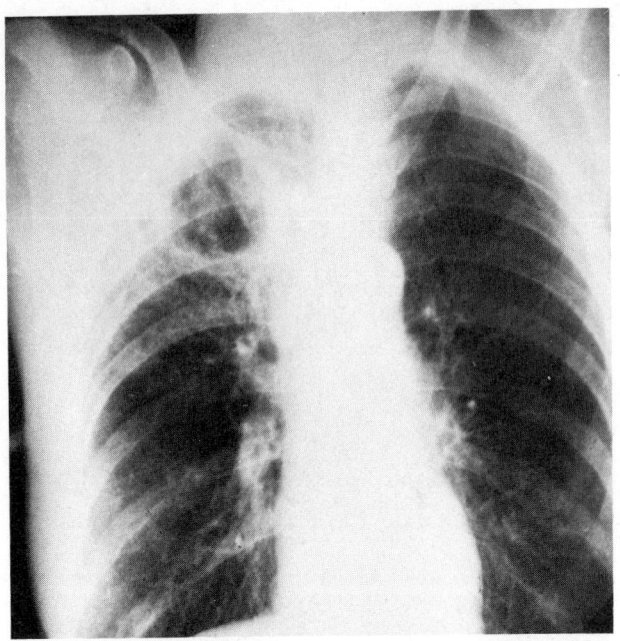

A

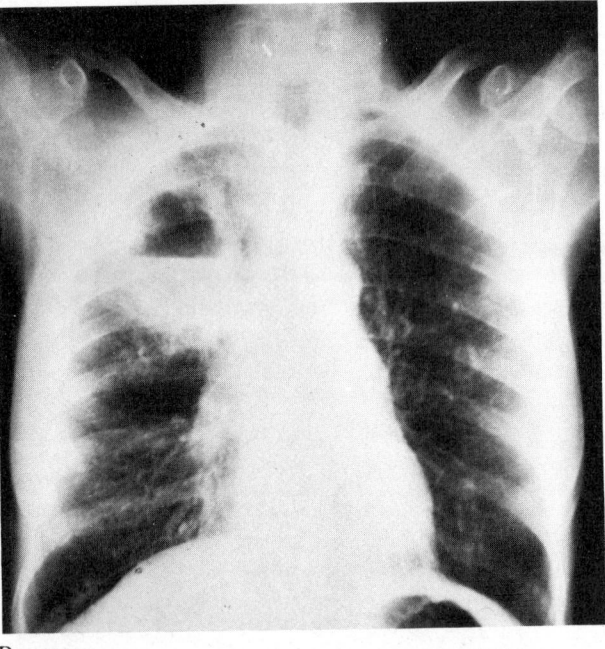

B

Fig. 61-6. Hemoptysis originating from a lung abscess. The emptying (A), refilling (B) pattern is indicative of life-threatening hemoptysis in a primary lung abscess.

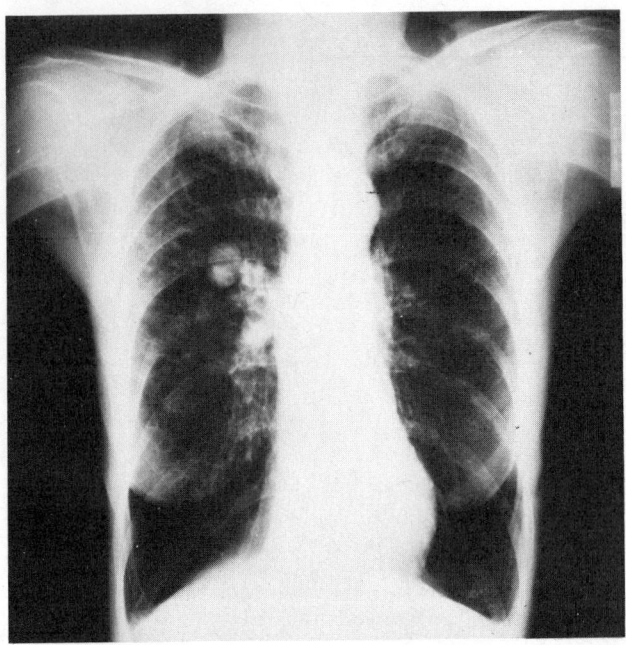

A

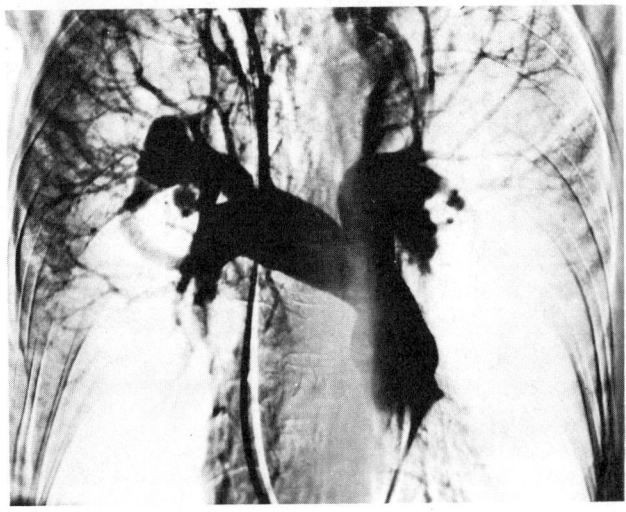

B

Fig. 61-7. Arteriovenous fistula presenting as a solitary pulmonary nodule. The vascular nature of the lesion seen on the posteroanterior view of the chest (A) was confirmed by pulmonary angiography (B). This patient with hereditary telangiectasia had the characteristic mucous membrane lesions shown in Figure 61-2.

[129,131,132,133], the diagnosis can be made clinically by obtaining a history of the exposure and ruling out other diseases (Table 61-2).

It is important to be aware that diseases may be considered and therefore evaluated in more than one category. For instance, a patient with hemoptysis due to overzealous anticoagulation may be evaluated in three categories; it is (1) a hematologic disorder that may cause (2) localized and (3) diffuse parenchymal disease [152]. A patient with chronic bleeding from the tracheobronchial disorder of diffuse bronchial telan-

giectasis [153] could present with diffuse as well as localized parenchymal disease (aspiration hemosiderosis [154]). A patient with long-standing passive congestion of the lungs—a cardiovascular disorder—might present with diffuse pulmonary hemosiderosis [155], whereas a patient with acute pulmonary edema usually presents with diffuse pulmonary infiltrates.

Differential Diagnosis

In evaluating patients with hemoptysis, it is necessary to rule out the causes of pseudohemoptysis. Features that can help to

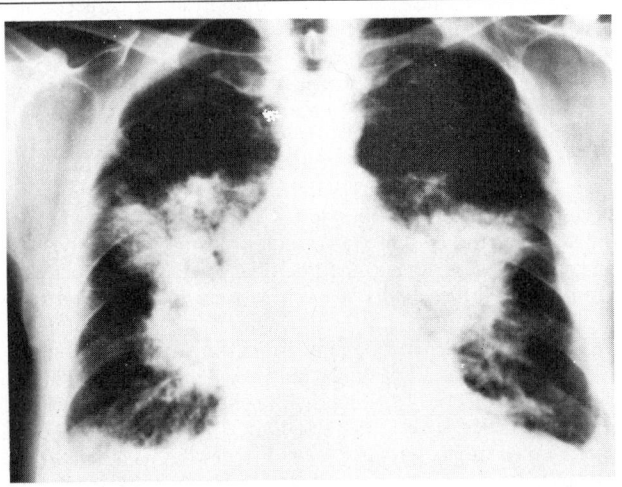

Fig. 61-8. "Butterfly" alveolar filling pattern. This pattern, in association with bilateral pleural effusions and an enlarged cardiac silhouette, is almost diagnostic of a cardiovascular cause of concomitant hemoptysis.

differentiate the causes of pseudohemoptysis from one another and pseudohemoptysis from true hemoptysis are found in Table 61-1. (See Chapter 168 for an in-depth discussion of epistaxis.) In addition to history and routine physical examination, it is important to perform a meticulous examination of the nose and entire pharynx, preferably with a nasopharyngoscope. Unless the cause of pseudohemoptysis is definitively determined, the spitting up of blood must be assumed to be true hemoptysis. An upper airway lesion must not be assumed to be the cause of the bleeding unless it is seen bleeding actively at the time of examination.

Treatment

The treatment of hemoptysis can be divided into supportive and definitive categories. In prescribing definitive therapy, it is important to consider the cause, amount of bleeding, and patient's underlying lung function.

SUPPORTIVE CARE. Supportive care usually includes bed rest and mild sedation. Drugs with antitussive effects (all narcotics) should not be used. An effective cough may be necessary to clear blood from the airways and avoid asphyxiation. Drugs with antiplatelet effects also should not be used. Depending on the results of arterial blood gas analysis, supplemental oxygen should be given (see Chap. 69). If bleeding continues and gas exchange becomes further compromised, endotracheal intubation and mechanical ventilation may become necessary. To facilitate fiberoptic bronchoscopy with a sufficiently large suction port, an endotracheal tube with an internal diameter of 8.5 mm or greater should be used, if possible. Other respiratory adjunctive therapy, such as chest physiotherapy and postural drainage [156], should be avoided. Fluid and blood resuscitation should be given when indicated.

The amount of hemoptysis should be continuously quantitated until it stops. The amount helps determine the patient's subsequent care [4,9].

DEFINITIVE CARE

Nonmassive Hemoptysis. In patients with scant or frank (submassive) hemoptysis, treatment is directed at the specific cause. For instance, suppurative bronchiectasis is treated with antibiotics plus a mucociliary escalator drug (e.g., theophylline [157], beta-adrenergic agonists [158]). Chronic bronchitis associated with cigarette smoking is treated with a mucociliary escalator and cessation of cigarette smoking. Although the role of antibiotics has not been proved, it is not unreasonable to give them [159] (see Chap. 57). Cystic fibrosis is treated with antibiotics (mucoid *Pseudomonas aeruginosa* and *Staphylococcus aureus* should be covered [160]) plus a mucociliary escalator. Bronchial adenoma and bronchogenic carcinoma should be resected whenever possible. Congestive heart failure is treated with combinations of drugs for preload and afterload reductions and digitalis when appropriate, mitral stenosis with diuretics, and pulmonary embolism with heparin. The effects of overzealous anticoagulation are treated with cessation of blood thinning and perhaps fresh frozen plasma and vitamin K. Tuberculosis is treated with antituberculous drugs (see Chap. 95). Appropriate antibiotic therapy is prescribed for acute infectious pneumonias (see Chap. 76).

Massive Hemoptysis. In patients with massive hemoptysis, treatment is directed not only at the specific cause but also at abrupt cessation of bleeding. Death from massive hemoptysis is predominantly due to asphyxiation [4], and the likelihood of death appears directly related to the rate of bleeding [4,6,9].

Urgent management in all cases of massive hemoptysis must emphasize protecting the uninvolved lung from aspiration of blood and tamponading the bleeding site. When tracheoartery fistula may be present, the following steps should be considered. If bleeding is immediate and profuse, there may be time only to overinflate the balloon, tamponading the potential bleeding site at the balloon, and apply downward and forward pressure on the top of the tracheostomy tube, tamponading the potential bleeding site at the stoma. If the arterial rupture is at the cannula tip, these efforts will not be helpful. If bleeding stops or slows either by these efforts or spontaneously, an endotracheal tube should be placed distal to the tip of the tracheostomy tube and a surgical consultation requested. Ideally, a surgeon should be present when the tracheostomy tube is removed; should crisp bleeding start again, the surgeon can attempt to finger tamponade/compress the bleeding artery (e.g., usually the innominate) by bluntly dissecting down the anterior tracheal wall and behind the sternum to the vessel. The vessel, once reached, can be compressed against the back of the sternum [39]. When the situation has been stabilized, clots can be gently suctioned from the distal trachea and the patient taken to the operating room for definitive repair. A review of the definitive surgical options can be found elsewhere [39].

When bleeding originates from below the primary carina, the bleeding lung should be kept dependent to minimize aspiration of expectorated blood. Numerous techniques have been advocated to help minimize aspiration and have proved helpful. A bronchoscopically positioned endobronchial balloon may provide effective tamponade [162,163]. Hemoptysis due to bleeding from all but the right upper lobe has been managed with balloon occlusion [164]. Placement of a Carlen's tube, which intubates each mainstem bronchus separately, is helpful, but the tubes can be difficult to place, and once in position their small diameter may prevent subsequent diagnostic fiberoptic bronchoscopy [165]. In cases of persistent massive hemoptysis, diagnostic considerations may need to be delayed because placement of a Carlen's tube may be necessary to ensure patient survival.

Urgent treatment to stop massive hemoptysis may involve laser bronchoscopy, iced saline lavage, angiographic embolization, supportive treatment only, or surgical resection. Use of laser to stop hemoptysis has been successful in more than 90 percent of patients with cancer [166], but recurrence of bleeding within a few weeks is typical. No large studies of patients with massive hemoptysis have been reported. Because laser is useful only in patients with proximal airway lesions and is difficult to use during massive hemoptysis, laser therapy will probably not evolve into a common therapeutic tool for these patients.

Bronchoscopically directed iced saline lavage of the bronchi leading to the site of hemorrhage has been reported to be successful in stopping hemorrhage in an uncontrolled series [167].

Angiography can identify the bleeding site in more than 90 percent of cases [118,142] and when combined with an embolization procedure has been successful in stopping bleeding in massive hemoptysis in more than 90 percent of cases [118]. Several angiographic sessions may be required, and both systemic and pulmonary vessels may need to be studied. Fourteen percent of patients bleed again within 1 to 4 days, and multiple procedures are frequently necessary [118,168]. Once active bleeding ceases, 20 percent of patients bleed again during the next 6 months [169] and 22 percent by 3 to 5 years [118]. Angiographic embolization may be achieved with the use of Gelfoam or polyurethane particles and is aided by temporary balloon occlusion of the involved vessel [118,170,171]. Sclerosing agents have led to subsequent massive lung necrosis and should be avoided [118]. Although early studies included several cases complicated by embolization of spinal arteries with subsequent paresis or paralysis, this complication appears rare when the procedure is performed by experienced angiographers [118]. Other complications, such as pleurisy or hematoma formation, are infrequent and usually minor [118].

In patients with hemoptysis due to trauma, urgent thoracotomy has been advocated, with the recommendation that it be performed with the patient in the supine position to minimize aspiration and that the bronchovascular trunk of the involved lung be clamped while the patient is stabilized to minimize the chance of air embolism while on positive-pressure ventilation [172].

Survival from iatrogenic rupture of the pulmonary artery has been reported. Several urgent maneuvers may prove helpful, and balloon tamponade and selective intubation should always be attempted. Balloon tamponade of the ruptured vessel with the Swan-Ganz balloon has been helpful [173]. With the balloon deflated, the catheter should be withdrawn 5 cm, the balloon inflated with 2 ml of air, and the balloon allowed to float back into the hemorrhaging vessel to occlude it. Ideally, patients should immediately be intubated in the mainstem bronchus opposite the involved lung to minimize aspiration. In most patients, death from pulmonary artery rupture occurs before the bleeding lung can be identified. Because the catheter usually floats to the right pulmonary artery, when it is not known which pulmonary artery has been ruptured selective intubation of the left mainstem bronchus or placement of a Carlen's tube should be attempted. Selective intubation of the left mainstem bronchus might be facilitated by using a bronchoscope or suction catheter designed specifically to enter the left lung. All patients who stop bleeding require angiographic evaluation to help localize the arterial tear and check for the formation of a pseudoaneurysm [63]. At the time of angiography, embolization of the affected vessel should be performed if a pseudoaneurysm or a tear is found. Hemoptysis from a pseudoaneurysm usually occurs in the first day after formation but may occur weeks later [62,63].

Aside from repairing lesions such as a tracheoartery fistula,

the role of emergency surgery for hemoptysis remains controversial. Several studies have advocated emergency surgery for all patients with massive hemoptysis when feasible, citing statistics that patients who have had surgery have a 19 percent mortality compared with 54 percent in the nonoperative group [4]. A more recent study challenges this, finding that in 84 patients with hemoptysis of more than 200 ml per day, (1) there was no mortality in patients with less than 1 liter of hemoptysis per day, even when not operated on; (2) mortality varied more with whether the patient was operable than with whether the patient underwent surgery (mortality in operable patients with hemoptysis of more than 1 liter per day was 30 percent vs. 65% in inoperable patients); and (3) mortality was greatly affected by diagnosis, in that no patient died from hemoptysis due to bronchitis, tuberculosis, bronchiectasis, or anticoagulation whereas 80 percent of patients with cancer and hemoptysis of more than 1 liter per day died [6]. Others have advocated conservative nonsurgical treatment when hemoptysis is due to infectious causes [176]. In patients with cystic fibrosis, even with normal lung function, resection should be avoided because repeated episodes in other areas are likely to occur. A patient with an FEV_1 of less than 2 liters or a maximum voluntary ventilation of less than 50 percent of predicted should not undergo surgery unless split lung function studies reveal that he or she is not likely to be left a respiratory cripple.

With respect to surgery, it is clear that no treatment preference can be recommended for all patients on the basis of reported studies. The trials of therapy span different decades of practice, have widely differing causes of hemoptysis in their populations, and employ several different definitions for massive hemoptysis. A review of the literature suggests the following strategy: (1) patients who are not candidates for surgery because of their pulmonary function, general medical condition, or diffuse nature of their lesions should be treated with selective embolization; (2) resectional surgery should be performed in operable patients when surgery is the definitive treatment for the underlying disease; and (3) all potentially operable patients who continue to bleed at rates of more than 1 liter per day despite supportive, conservative care should undergo either surgical resection or embolization. The correct therapy in a given patient depends on the cause of the bleeding, lung function, availability of resources, and local expertise.

In patients with diffuse intrapulmonary hemorrhage, selective arterial embolization and surgery are not options. For immunologically mediated diseases, corticosteroids, cytotoxic agents, and other interventions are available.

With respect to corticosteroid and cytotoxic drug therapies, the following generally apply [151]: (1) corticosteroids are used alone if the syndrome is self-limited; (2) cytotoxic therapy should be added when the disease is known to respond to cytotoxic therapy (e.g., Wegener's granulomatosis, Goodpasture's syndrome); (3) cytotoxic agents can be used as steroid-sparing agents in patients whose disease has responded to corticosteroids but who are having side effects caused by corticosteroids; (4) cytotoxic agents may be considered in immunologic lung disease that has not responded as expected to corticosteroids and no intercurrent disease process can be identified.

When corticosteroid therapy is given alone for critically ill patients with immunologic lung diseases, the dose is 1 mg/kg/day of intravenous methylprednisolone or the equivalent dose of another corticosteroid. Larger doses, on the order of 7 to 15 mg/kg/day for 1 to 3 days, have been recommended to control progressive pulmonary hemorrhage and hypoxemia of Goodpasture's syndrome, SLE, and some of the vasculitides (see specific chapters) [135]. In general, corticosteroids should be administered initially in round-the-clock divided doses until substantial improvement has occurred [175]. They can then be given once per day and tapered as the patient's condition dictates.

When combined corticosteroid and cytotoxic drug therapy is given, it is usually prescribed for immunologic lung diseases due to the vasculitides [151,176] (e.g., Wegener's granulomatosis [176], rheumatoid vasculitis [177]) and Goodpasture's syndrome [178]. In the critically ill patient with vasculitis *without* fulminant disease, methylprednisolone (1 mg/kg/day in divided doses) and cyclophosphamide (1–2 mg/kg/day) are given [151]. If the clinical response is favorable, these doses are maintained unless readjustments are needed to keep the total leukocyte count greater than 3000 per cubic millimeter with total neutrophil count of 1000 to 1500 per cubic millimeter [151]. If there is no evidence of a favorable response, the daily dose of cyclophosphamide should be increased by 25 mg and kept at this level for 2 weeks [151]. This rate of increment should be continued until evidence of a clinical response is seen or until drug toxicity, such as leukopenia, occurs [151]. In critically ill patients with vasculitis *with* fulminant disease [151], the initial dose of cyclophosphamide is 4 mg/kg/day, given either orally or intravenously for 3 days, followed by rapid dose reduction during a subsequent 3-day period, until a dose of 1 to 2 mg/kg/day is reached. This dose is maintained until evidence of a favorable therapeutic response or leukopenia occurs; toxicity of course necessitates dose reduction. After 5 to 7 days of daily corticosteroid therapy (1 mg/kg/day) [151], the dose can usually be tapered rapidly to a single daily dose and then to alternate-day therapy to minimize cushingoid and infectious complications [175]. After a few weeks to months, corticosteroids may be totally withdrawn, depending on the individual clinical response [151]. Recommendations for the long-term management of patients with Wegener's granulomatosis can be found elsewhere [176].

In general, patients with Goodpasture's syndrome are treated in the same manner, with the following exceptions: (1) if patients present with severe pulmonary hemorrhage, methylprednisolone is initially administered at a higher dose of 7 to 15 mg/kg/day for 1 to 3 days; (2) plasmapheresis may be useful for the immediate and long-term reduction of antiglomerular basement membrane antibody levels [135,179]; and (3) short-term and long-term cyclophosphamide and plasmapheresis therapy are guided by the results of serially obtained serum antiglomerular basement membrane antibody [135,179]. If pharmacologic doses of corticosteroids control severe pulmonary hemorrhage and the plasmapheresis and cyclophosphamide therapy makes circulating antiglomerular basement membrane antibody disappear, bilateral nephrectomy is unnecessary [135,179].

References

1. Pursel SE, Lindskog GE: Hemoptysis. *Am Rev Respir Dis* 84:329, 1961.
2. Chaves AD: Hemoptysis in chest clinic patients. *Am Rev Tuberc* 63:194, 1951.
3. Selecky PA: Evaluation of hemoptysis through the bronchoscope. *Chest* 73(suppl):741, 1978.
4. Crocco JA, Rooney JJ, Fankushen DS, et al: Massive hemoptysis. *Arch Intern Med* 121:496, 1968.
5. Gourin A, Garzon AA: Operative treatment of massive hemoptysis. *Ann Thorac Surg* 18:52, 1974.
6. Corey R, Hla KM: Major and massive hemoptysis: Reassessment of conservative management. *Am J Med Sci* 294:301, 1987.
7. Thomson SC: Hemorrhage from the throat (hemoptysis not of pulmonary origin). *Ann Otol Rhinol Laryngol* 37:209, 1928.
8. Stiernberg C: Hemoptysis of undetermined etiology. *Tex State J Med* 60:630, 1964.
9. Lyons HA: Differential diagnosis of hemoptysis and its treatment. *Basics RD* 5:26, 1976.
10. Gale D: Overgrowth of *Serratia marcescens* in respiratory tract, simulating hemoptysis. *JAMA* 164:1328, 1957.
11. Barrett NR, Hoyle C: A case of haemoptysis. *Br J Tuberc* 36:172, 1942.
12. Gupta SK: Midnight haemoptysis. *Br Med J* 1:1505, 1960.
13. Chapman JS: Peregrinating problem patients: Munchausen's syndrome. *JAMA* 165:927, 1957.
14. Newton RW, Forrest ARW: Rifampicin overdosage: "The red man syndrome." *Scott Med J* 20:55, 1975.
15. Jackson CL, Diamond S: Hemorrhage from the trachea, bronchi and lungs of nontuberculous origin. *Am Rev Tuberc* 46:126, 1942.
16. Domm BM, Vassalio CL, Adams CL: Amyloid deposition localized to the lower respiratory tract. *Am J Med* 38:151, 1965.
17. Kennedy JH: "Silent" gastroesophageal reflux: An important but little known cause of pulmonary complications. *Dis Chest* 42:42, 1962.
18. Foster-Carter AF: Bronchial adenoma. *Q J Med* 10:139, 1941.
19. Rodman MH, Jones CW: Catamenial hemoptysis due to bronchial endometriosis. *N Engl J Med* 266:805, 1962.
20. Libman E, Ottenberg R: Hereditary hemoptysis. *JAMA* 81:2030, 1923.
21. Lindskog GE, Hubbell DS: An analysis of 215 cases of bronchiectasis. *Surg Gynecol Obstet* 100:643, 1955.
22. Seppala AJ: Clinical significance of hemoptysis: A study of 505 cases examined bronchoscopically. *Acta Otolaryngol* 47:172, 1957.
23. Ogilvie AG: The natural history of bronchiectasis: A clinical, roentgenologic and pathologic study. *Arch Intern Med* 68:395, 1941.
24. Emerson GL, Emerson MS, Sherwood CE: The natural history of carcinoma of the lung. *J Thorac Cardiovasc Surg* 37:291, 1959.
25. Schmidt HW, Clagett OT, McDonald JR: Broncholithiasis. *J Thorac Surg* 19:226, 1950.
26. Stern RC, Wood RE, Boat TF, et al: Treatment and prognosis of massive hemoptysis in cystic fibrosis. *Am Rev Respir Dis* 117:825, 1978.
27. Blair TC, McElvein RB: Hamartoma of the lung: A clinical study of 25 cases. *Dis Chest* 44:296, 1963.
28. Gerle R, Felson B: Metastatic endobronchial hypernephroma. *Dis Chest* 44:225, 1963.
29. Souders CR, Smith AT: The clinical significance of hemoptysis. *N Engl J Med* 247:791, 1952.
30. McManis AG, Windsor HM: The intrabronchial foreign body. *Med J Aust* 2:57, 1954.
31. Gardner AMN: Aspiration of food and vomit. *Q J Med* 27:227, 1958.
32. Pattison CW, Leaming AJ, Townsend ER: Hidden foreign body as a cause of recurrent hemoptysis in a teenage girl. *Ann Thorac Surg* 45:330, 1988.
33. Greer AE: Mucoid impaction of the bronchi. *Ann Intern Med* 46:506, 1957.
34. Weiland JE, delos Santos ET, Mazzaferri EL, et al: Hemoptysis as the presenting manifestation of thyroid carcinoma. *Arch Intern Med* 149:1693, 1989.
35. Guest JL Jr, Anderson JN: Major airway injury in closed chest trauma. *Chest* 72:63, 1977.
36. Halasz HA, Lindskog GE, Liebow AA: Esophago-bronchial fistula and bronchopulmonary sequestration. *Am Surg* 155:215, 1962.
37. Mellins RB: Acquired fistula between the esophagus and the respiratory tract: Report of a case, review of the literature and discussion of the pathogenesis. *N Engl J Med* 246:896, 1952.
38. Wychulis AR, Ellis FH Jr, Anderson HA: Acquired non-malignant esophagotracheobronchial fistula: Report of 36 cases. *JAMA* 196:117, 1966.
39. Schaefer OP, Irwin RS: Tracheo-artery fistula. *J Intensive Care Med* 10:64, 1995.
40. Gouley BA, Anderson E: Chronic dissecting aneurysm of the aorta, simulating syphilitic cardiovascular disease: Notes on the associated aortic murmurs. *Ann Intern Med* 14:978, 1940.
41. Coblentz CL, Sallee DS, Chiles C: Aortobronchopulmonary fistula complicating aortic aneurysm: Diagnosis in four cases. *Am J Radiol* 150:535, 1988.
42. Sheffield BA, Moore-Gillon J, Murday AR, et al: Short reports:

Massive haemoptysis caused by spontaneous rupture of a bronchial artery. *Thorax* 43:71, 1988.

43. Brown JW, Heath D, Whitaker W: Eisenmenger's complex. *Br Heart J* 17:273, 1955.

44. Whitaker W, Heath D, Brown JW: Patent ductus arteriosus with pulmonary hypertension. *Br Heart J* 17:121, 1955.

45. Hurst JW: Symptoms due to diseases of the heart and blood vessels, in Hurst JW, Logue RB, Schlant RC, et al (eds): *The Heart*. 4th ed. New York, McGraw-Hill, 1978, p 158.

46. Nielsen JF, Stentoft J, Aunsholt NA: Haemoptysis caused by aneurysm of saphenous bypass graft to a coronary artery. *Scand J Thorac Cardiovasc Surg* 22:189, 1988.

47. Carreau EP, Higgins GA: Fat embolism. *Arch Intern Med* 88:692, 1951.

48. Hughes JP, Stovin PGI: Segmental pulmonary artery aneurysms with peripheral venous thrombosis. *Br J Dis Chest* 53:19, 1959.

49. Greenwood WF, Aldridge HE, McKelvey AD: Effect of mitral commissurotomy on duration of life, functional capacity, hemoptysis and systemic embolism. *Am J Cardiol* 11:348, 1963.

50. Wolff L, Levine HB: Hemoptysis in rheumatic heart disease. *Am Heart J* 21:163, 1941.

51. Castile RG, Kleinberg F: The pathogenesis and management of massive pulmonary hemorrhage in the neonate: Case report of a normal survivor. *Mayo Clin Proc* 51:155, 1976.

52. Weiser NJ, Kantor M, Russell HK: Postmyocardial infarction syndrome. *Circulation* 20:371, 1959.

53. Hodgson CH, Burchell HB, Good CA, et al: Hereditary hemorrhagic telangiectasia and pulmonary arteriovenous fistula: Survey of a large family. *N Engl J Med* 261:625, 1959.

54. Deterling RA Jr, Clagett OT: Aneurysm of the pulmonary artery: Review of the literature and report of a case. *Am Heart J* 34:471, 1947.

55. Moser KM: Pulmonary embolism. *Am Rev Respir Dis* 115:829, 1977.

56. Dalen JE, Haffajee CI, Alpert JS, et al: Pulmonary embolism, pulmonary hemorrhage, and pulmonary infarction. *N Engl J Med* 296:1431, 1977.

57. Neiman BH: Varix of the pulmonary vein. *Am J Roentgenol Radium Ther* 32:608, 1934.

58. Rodriguez HF, Rivera E: Pulmonary schistosomiasis. *N Engl J Med* 258:1196, 1958.

59. Boundy K, Bignold LP: Syphilitic aneurysm of the right subclavian artery presenting with hemoptysis. *Aust NZ J Med* 17:533, 1987.

60. Henshaw DB: Obstructions of the superior vena cava: A review of the literature with two case reports. *Am Heart J* 37:958, 1949.

61. Winterbauer RH, Elfenbein IB, Ball WC Jr: Incidence and clinical significance of tumor embolization to the lungs. *Am J Med* 45:271, 1968.

62. Dieden JD, Friloux LA III, Renner JW: Pulmonary artery false aneurysms secondary to Swan-Ganz pulmonary artery catheters. *AJR* 149:901, 1987.

63. Bartter T, Irwin RS, Phillips DA, et al: Pulmonary artery pseudoaneurysm: A potential complication of pulmonary artery catheterization. *Arch Intern Med* 148:471, 1988.

64. Chakraborty AK, Dreisin RB: Pulmonary hematoma secondary anticoagulant therapy. *Ann Intern Med* 96:67, 1982.

65. Robboy SJ, Minna JD, Colman RW, et al: Pulmonary hemorrhage syndrome as a manifestation of disseminated intravascular coagulation: Analysis of ten cases. *Chest* 63:718, 1973.

66. Smith LJ, Katzenstein AA: Pathogenesis of massive pulmonary hemorrhage in acute leukemia. *Arch Intern Med* 142:2149, 1982.

67. Buchanan GR, Moore GC: Pulmonary hemosiderosis and immune thrombocytopenia: Initial manifestations of collagen-vascular disease. *JAMA* 246:861, 1981.

68. Connolly JP: Hemoptysis as a presentation of mild hemophilia A in an adult. *Chest* 103:1281, 1993.

69. Smith LR, Heaton CL: Actinomycosis presenting as Wegener's granulomatosis. *JAMA* 240:247, 1978.

70. Abdel-Hakim M, Higazi AM: Bronchopulmonary amoebiasis. *Dis Chest* 34:607, 1958.

71. Gelpi AP, Mustafa A: *Ascaris* pneumonia. *Ann Intern Med* 44:377, 1968.

72. Glimp RA, Bayer AS: Pulmonary aspergilloma: Diagnostic and therapeutic considerations. *Arch Intern Med* 143:303, 1983.

73. Gallagher PG, Lynch JP, Christian HJ: Intralobar bronchopulmonary sequestration of the lung. *N Engl J Med* 257:643, 1957.

74. Drutz DJ, Catanzaro A: Coccidiodomycosis: Part II. *Am Rev Respir Dis* 117:727, 1978.

75. Cooke FN, Blades B: Cystic disease of the lungs. *J Thorac Surg* 23:546, 1952.

76. Kerkering TM, Duma RJ, Shadomy S: The evolution of pulmonary cryptococcosis: Clinical implications from a study of 41 patients with and without compromising host factors. *Ann Intern Med* 94:611, 1981.

77. Volk BW, Nathanson L, Losner S, et al: Incidence of lipoid pneumonia in a survey of 389 chronically ill patients. *Am J Med* 10:316, 1951.

78. Goodwin RA, Des Prez RM: Histoplasmosis. *Am Rev Respir Dis* 117:929, 1978.

79. Savage MB: Trophoblastic lesions of the lungs following benign hydatid mole. *Am J Obstet Gynecol* 62:346, 1951.

80. Thoms NW, Wilson RF, Puro HE, et al: Life-threatening hemoptysis in primary lung abscess. *Ann Thorac Surg* 14:347, 1972.

81. Fraser RG, Pare JAP, Pare PD, et al: Diseases of the thorax caused by external physical agents, in *Diagnosis of Diseases of the Chest*. Third edition. Edited by RG Fraser, JAP Pare, PD Pare, et al. Toronto, WB Saunders, 1991, vol 4, pp 2480–2597.

82. Crow NE, Brogdon BG: Cystic lung lesions from metastatic sarcoma. *Ann J Roentgenol Rad Ther Nucl Med* 81:303, 1959.

83. Record NB Jr, Ginder DR: Pulmonary phycomycosis without obvious predisposing factors. *JAMA* 235:1256, 1976.

84. Curry WA: Human nocardiosis: A clinical review with selected case reports. *Arch Intern Med* 140:818, 1980.

85. Roque FT, Ludwick RW, Bell JC: Pulmonary paragonimiasis: A review with case reports from Korea and the Philippines. *Ann Intern Med* 38:1206, 1953.

86. Lattes R, Shepard F, Tovell H, et al: A clinical and pathologic study of endometriosis of the lung. *Surg Gynecol Obstet* 103:552, 1956.

87. Ridgeway NA, Whitcomb FC, Erickson EE, et al: Primary pulmonary sporotrichosis: Report of two cases. *Am J Med* 32:153, 1962.

88. Rajdev N, Green R, Crosby WH: Angiosarcoma with pulmonary siderosis and persistent reticulocytosis: Steroid responsiveness suggests an immune basis. *Arch Intern Med* 138:1549, 1978.

89. Emanuel DA, Wenzel FJ, Bowerman CI: Farmer's lung: Clinical, pathologic and immunologic study of twenty-four patients. *Am J Med* 37:392, 1964.

90. Briggs WA, Johnson JP, Teichman S, et al: Antiglomerular basement membrane antibody-mediated glomerulonephritis and Goodpasture's syndrome. *Medicine* 58:348, 1979.

91. Irwin RS, Cottrell TS, Hsu KC, et al: Idiopathic pulmonary hemosiderosis: An electron microscopic and immunofluorescent study. *Chest* 65:41, 1974.

92. Border WA, Baehler RW, Bhathena D, et al: IgA antibasement membrane nephritis with pulmonary hemorrhage. *Ann Intern Med* 91:21, 1979.

93. Patterson R, Nugent KM, Harris KE, Eberle ME: Immunologic hemorrhagic pneumonia caused by isocyanates. *Am Rev Respir Dis* 141:226, 1990.

94. Vaziri ND, Jeminson-Smith P, Wilson AF: Hemorrhagic pneumonitis after intravenous injection of charcoal lighter fluid. *Ann Intern Med* 90:794, 1979.

95. Relman AS: CPC conference. *N Engl J Med* 298:1014, 1978.

96. O'Donohue WJ Jr: Idiopathic pulmonary hemosiderosis with manifestations of multiple connective tissue and immune disorders. *Am Rev Respir Dis* 109:473, 1974.

97. Gorevic PD, Kassab HJ, Levo Y, et al: Mixed cryoglobulinemia: Clinical aspects and long-term followup of 40 patients. *Am J Med* 69:287, 1980.

98. Schmidt HW: Lung purpura and pulmonary hemosiderosis. *Med Clin North Am* 48:1011, 1964.

99. Kallenbach J, Prinsloo I, Zwi S: Progressive systemic sclerosis complicated by diffuse pulmonary hemorrhage. *Thorax* 32:767, 1977.

100. Kim JH, Follett JV, Rice JR, et al: Endobronchial telangiectasias and hemoptysis in scleroderma. *Am J Med* 84:173, 1988.

101. Gould DB, Soriano RZ: Acute alveolar hemorrhage in lupus erythematosus. *Ann Intern Med* 83:836, 1975.

102. Herbert FA, Orford R: Pulmonary hemorrhage and edema due to

inhalation of resins containing trimellitic anhydride. *Chest* 76:546, 1979.

103. Wilson CB, Smith RC: Goodpasture's syndrome associated with influenza A$_2$ virus infection. *Ann Intern Med* 76:91, 1972.

104. Hensley MJ, Feldman NT, Lazarus JM, et al: Diffuse pulmonary hemorrhage and rapidly progressive renal failure: An uncommon presentation of Wegener's granulomatosis. *Am J Med* 66:894, 1979.

105. Barrett RJ, Tuttle WM: A study of essential hemoptysis. *J Thorac Cardiovasc Surg* 40:468, 1960.

106. Lukomsky GI, Ovchinnikov AA, Bilal A: Complications of bronchoscopy: Comparison of rigid bronchoscopy under general anesthesia and flexible fiberoptic bronchoscopy under topical anesthesia. *Chest* 79:316, 1981.

107. Pape LA, Haffajee CI, Markis JE, et al: Fatal pulmonary hemorrhage after use of the flow-directed balloon-tipped catheter. *Ann Intern Med* 90:344, 1979.

108. vanSonnenberg E, Casola G, Ho M, et al: Difficult thoracic lesions: CT-guided biopsy experience in 150 cases. *Radiology* 167:457, 1988.

109. Rath GS, Schaff JT, Snider GL: Flexible fiberoptic bronchoscopy: Techniques and review of 100 bronchoscopies. *Chest* 63:689, 1973.

110. Smiddy JF, Elliott RC: The evaluation of hemoptysis with fiberoptic bronchoscopy. *Chest* 64:158, 1973.

111. Johnston H, Reiza G: Changing spectrum of hemoptysis: Underlying causes in 148 patients undergoing diagnostic flexible fiberoptic bronchoscopy. *Arch Intern Med* 149:1666, 1989.

112. Wasser J, Talavera W, Villamena P, et al: Massive haemoptysis in the acquired immunodeficiency syndrome. *Br J Dis Chest* 82:421, 1988.

113. American Thoracic Society statement on the management of hemoptysis. *Am Rev Respir Dis* 93:471, 1966.

114. Johnston RN, Lockhart W, Ritchie RT, et al: Hemoptysis. *Br Med J* 1:592, 1960.

115. Remy J, Arnaud A, Fardou H, et al: Treatment of hemoptysis by embolization of bronchial arteries. *Radiology* 122:33, 1977.

116. Murray JF: Postnatal growth and development of the lung, in Murray JF (ed): *The Normal Lung: The Basis for Diagnosis and Treatment of Pulmonary Disease.* Philadelphia, WB Saunders, 1976, p 21.

117. Auld PA, Rudolph AM, Golinko RJ: Factors affecting bronchial collateral flow in the dog. *Am J Physiol* 198:1166, 1960.

118. Rabkin JE, Astafjev VI, Gothman LN, et al: Transcatheter embolization in the management of pulmonary hemorrhage. *Radiology* 163:361, 1987.

119. Wood DA, Miller M: Role of dual pulmonary circulation in various pathologic conditions of lungs. *J Thorac Surg* 7:649, 1938.

120. Ferguson FC, Kobilak RE, Deitrick JE: Varices of bronchial veins as source of hemoptysis in mitral stenosis. *Am Heart J* 28:445, 1944.

121. Rasmussen V: On hemoptysis, especially when fatal, in its anatomical and clinical aspects. *Edinb Med J* 14:385, 1968.

122. Auerbach O: Pathology and pathogenesis of pulmonary arterial aneurysm in tuberculous cavities. *Am Rev Tuberc* 39:99, 1939.

123. Imoto EM, Lombard CM, Sachs DPL: Pulmonary capillaritis and hemorrhage: A clue to the diagnosis of systemic necrotizing vasculitis. *Chest* 96:927, 1989.

124. Myers JL, Katzenstein AA: Microangiitis in lupus-induced pulmonary hemorrhage. *Am J Clin Pathol* 85:552, 1986.

125. Soll B, Selecky PA, Chang R, et al: The use of the fiberoptic bronchoscope in the evaluation of hemoptysis. *Am Rev Respir Dis* 115:165, 1977.

126. Fagin ID: Hemoptysis with intercourse. *JAMA* 240:22, 1978.

127. Pratt LW: Hemoptysis. *Ann Otol Rhinol Laryngol* 63:296, 1954.

128. Thomas HM III, Irwin RS: Classification of diffuse intrapulmonary hemorrhage. *Chest* 68:483, 1975.

129. Zeiss CR: Reactive chemicals as inhalant allergens. *Immunol Allerg Clin N Am* 9:235, 1989.

130. Ahmad D, Patterson R, Morgan WKC, et al: Pulmonary hemorrhage and haemolytic anemia due to trimellitic anhydride. *Lancet* 2:238, 1979.

131. Patterson R, Addington W, Banner AS, et al: Antihapten antibodies in workers exposed to trimellitic anhydride fumes: A potential immunopathogenetic mechanism for the trimellitic anhydride pul-

monary disease-anemia syndrome. *Am Rev Respir Dis* 120:1259, 1979.

132. Leach CL, Hatoum NS, Ratajczak HV, et al: Evidence of immunologic control of lung injury induced by trimellitic anhydride. *Am Rev Respir Dis* 137:186, 1988.

133. Zeiss CR, Leach CL, Smith LJ, et al: A serial immunologic and histopathologic study of lung injury induced by trimellitic anhydride. *Am Rev Respir Dis* 137:191, 1988.

134. Patterson R, Nugent KM, Harris KE, et al: Immunologic hemorrhagic pneumonia caused by isocyanates. *Am Rev Respir Dis* 141:226, 1990.

135. Briggs WA, Johnson JP, Teichman S, et al: Antiglomerular basement membrane antibody-mediated glomerulonephritis and Goodpasture's syndrome. *Medicine* 58:348, 1979.

136. Wilson CB, Smith RC: Goodpasture's syndrome associated with an influenza A2 virus infection. *Ann Intern Med* 76:91, 1972.

137. Kleinknecht D, Morel-Maroger L, Callard P, et al: Antiglomerular basement membrane nephritis after solvent exposure. *Arch Intern Med* 140:230, 1980.

138. Sternlieb I, Bennett B, Scheinberg H: D-penicillamine induced Goodpasture's syndrome in Wilson's disease. *Ann Intern Med* 82:673, 1975.

139. Wilson CB, Dixon FJ: Anti-glomerular basement membrane antibody-induced glomerulonephritis. *Kidney Int* 3:74, 1973.

140. Mathew TH, Hobbs JB, Kalowski S, et al: Goodpasture's syndrome: Normal renal diagnostic findings. *Ann Intern Med* 82:215, 1975.

141. Zimmerman SW, Varanasi UR, Hoff B: Goodpasture's with normal renal function. *Am J Med* 66:163, 1979.

142. Saumench J, Escarrabill J, Padro L, et al: Value of fiberoptic bronchoscopy and angiography for diagnosis of the bleeding site in hemoptysis. *Ann Thorac Surg* 48:272, 1989.

143. Fraser RG, Pare JAP, Pare PD, et al: Diseases of the airways, in Fraser RG, Pare JAP, Pare PD, et al (eds): *Diagnosis of Diseases of the Chest.* 3rd ed. Toronto, WB Saunders, 1990, vol 3, pp 2186–2206.

144. Koffler D, Sandson J, Carr R, et al: Immunologic studies concerning the pulmonary lesions in Goodpasture's syndrome. *Am J Pathol* 54:293, 1969.

145. Wilson CB, Dixon FJ: Diagnosis of immunopathologic renal disease. *Kidney Int* 5:389, 1974.

146. McPhaul JJ, Dixon FJ: The presence of anti-glomerular basement membrane antibodies in peripheral blood. *J Immunol* 103:1168, 1969.

147. Border WA, Baehler RW, Bhathena D, et al: IgA anti-basement membrane nephritis with pulmonary hemorrhage. *Ann Intern Med* 191:21, 1979.

148. Nolle B, Specks U, Ludemann J, et al: Anticytoplasmic autoantibodies: Their immunodiagnostic value in Wegener's granulomatosis. *Ann Intern Med* 111:28, 1989.

149. Kathuria S, Chejfec G: Fatal pulmonary Henoch-Schonlein syndrome. *Chest* 82:654, 1982.

150. Raz I, Okon E, Chajek-Shaul T: Pulmonary manifestations in Behcet's syndrome. *Chest* 95:585, 1989.

151. Fauci AS, Haynes BF, Katz P: The spectrum of vasculitis: Clinical, pathologic, immunologic, and therapeutic considerations. *Ann Intern Med* 89:660, 1978.

152. Finley TN, Aronow A, Cosentino AM, et al: Occult pulmonary hemorrhage in anticoagulated patients. *Am Rev Respir Dis* 112:23, 1975.

153. Masson RG, Altose MD, Mayock RL: Isolated bronchial telangiectasia. *Chest* 65:450, 1974.

154. Green RA: Nodular aspirational pulmonary hemosiderosis. *Am J Radiol* 92:561, 1964.

155. Lendrum AC: Pulmonary hemosiderosis of cardiac origin. *J Pathol Bacteriol* 62:555, 1950.

156. Tyler ML: Complications of positioning and chest physiotherapy. *Respir Care* 27:458, 1982.

157. Sutton PP, Pavia D, Bateman JRM, et al: The effect of oral aminophylline on lung mucociliary clearance in man. *Chest* 80(suppl):889, 1981.

158. Sackner MA: Effect of respiratory drugs and mucociliary clearance. *Chest* 73(suppl):958, 1978.

159. Nicotra MB, Rivera M, Awe RJ: Antibiotic therapy of acute exac-

erbations of chronic bronchitis: A controlled study using tetracycline. *Ann Intern Med* 97:18, 1982.

160. Wood RE, Boat TF, Doershuk CF: Cystic fibrosis. *Am Rev Respir Dis* 113:833, 1976.

161. Winzelberg GG: Patients with hemoptysis examined with Tc-99 sulfur colloid and Tc-99m-labeled red blood cells: A preliminary appraisal. *Radiology* 153:523, 1984.

162. Skwersky RB, Chang JB, Wisoff BG, et al: Endobronchial balloon tamponade of hemoptysis in patients with cystic fibrosis. *Ann Thorac Surg* 27:262, 1979.

163. Saw EC, Gottlieb LS: Flexible fiberoptic bronchoscopy and endobronchial tamponade in the management of massive hemoptysis. *Chest* 70:589, 1976.

164. Garzon AA, Cerruti MM, Golding ME: Exsanguinating hemoptysis. *J Thorac Cardiovasc Surg* 84:829, 1982.

165. Winter SM, Ingbar DH: Massive hemoptysis: Pathogenesis and management. *J Intensive Care Med* 3:171, 1988.

166. Clarke CP, Jackson KA, Moreland M, et al: Bronchoscopic use of the neodymium-yttrium-aluminum-garnet laser for lesions of the trachea and bronchus. *Med J Aust* 150:260, 1989.

167. Conlan AA: Massive hemoptysis: Review of 123 cases. *J Thorac Cardiovasc Surg* 85:120, 1983.

168. Hickey NM, Peterson RA, Leech JA, et al: Percutaneous embolotherapy in life-threatening hemoptysis. *Cardiovasc Intervent Radiol* 11:270, 1988.

169. Stoll JF, Bettmann MA: Bronchial artery embolization to control hemoptysis: A review. *Cardiovasc Intervent Radiol* 11:263, 1988.

170. Uflacker R: Bronchial artery embolization in the management of hemoptysis: Technical aspects and long-term results. *Radiology* 157:637, 1985.

171. Jardin M, Remy J: Control of hemoptysis: Systemic angiography and anastomoses of the internal mammary artery. *Radiology* 168:377, 1988.

172. Wilson RF, Soullier GW, Wiencek RG: Hemoptysis in trauma. *J Trauma* 27:1123, 1987.

173. Remy T, Siproudhis L, Laurent JF, et al: Massive hemoptysis from iatrogenic balloon catheter rupture of pulmonary artery: Successful early management by balloon tamponade. *Crit Care Med* 15:272, 1987.

174. Bobrowitz ID, Ramakrishna S, Shim Y-S: Comparison of medical vs. surgical treatment of major hemoptysis. *Arch Intern Med* 143:1343, 1983.

175. Fauci AS, Dale DC, Balow JE: Glucocorticosteroid therapy: Mechanisms of action and clinical considerations. *Ann Intern Med* 84:304, 1976.

176. Fauci AS, Haynes BF, Katz P, et al: Wegener's granulomatosis: Prospective clinical and therapeutic experience with 85 patients for 21 years. *Ann Intern Med* 98:76, 1983.

177. Abel T, Andrews BS, Cunningham PH, et al: Rheumatoid vasculitis: Effect of cyclophosphamide on the clinical course and levels of circulating immune complexes. *Ann Intern Med* 93:407, 1980.

178. Johnson JP, Whitman W, Briggs WA, et al: Plasmapheresis and immunosuppressive agents in antibasement membrane antibody induced Goodpasture's syndrome. *Am J Med* 64:354, 1978.

179. Johnson JP, Moore J, Austin AA, et al: Therapy of anti-glomerular basement membrane antibody disease: Analysis of prognostic significance of clinical, pathologic and treatment factors. *Medicine* 64:219, 1985.

62. Aspiration

Richard S. Irwin

Overview

Aspiration is defined in *Webster's New Collegiate Dictionary* as "taking a foreign material into the lungs with the respiratory current." The foreign material can be particulate matter, irritating fluids (e.g., HCl, mineral oil, animal fat), or oropharyngeal secretions containing infectious agents. Although infectious pneumonias can be caused by inhaling air containing organisms (i.e., infectious aerosols), aspiration of oropharyngeal contents is the primary way bacterial pathogens are introduced into the lower respiratory tract. This chapter discusses the wide spectrum of syndromes caused by aspiration of foreign matter [1].

Tracheostomy with a standard uncuffed metal tube or a large-volume, low-pressure cuff may be associated with aspiration in up to 87 percent [2,3] or 15 percent [4] of patients, respectively, but the incidence or prevalence of all clinically significant aspirations is not known. However, a review of Table 62-1 suggests that aspiration syndromes can be very common causes of pulmonary disease in the critically ill. An in-depth discussion of near drowning can be found in Chapter 63.

Pathogenesis

Syndromes caused by aspiration are determined by (1) what is aspirated, (2) the amount aspirated, and (3) the state of the patient's defenses against inhaled fluid and food and infectious assaults. An understanding of these normal defenses and how and when they become impaired is the basis for an understanding of the pathogenesis of all the aspiration syndromes.

NORMAL UPPER GASTROINTESTINAL DEFENSES AGAINST ASPIRATION OF FLUID AND FOOD. The following upper gastrointestinal mechanisms normally work in a coordinated, synchronized fashion [4,5,6]. The teeth break up large food particles into smaller ones, and the tongue propels both fluid and masticated food into the hypopharynx. As the hypopharyngeal muscles prepare to thrust food into the esophagus, the epiglottis covers the laryngeal inlet while the vocal cords close and the upper esophageal sphincter (cricopharyn-

Table 62-1. Aspiration Syndromes

Mendelson's syndrome
Foreign body aspiration
Bacterial pneumonia and lung abscess
Exogenous lipoid pneumonia
    Recurrent pneumonias
    Chronic interstitial fibrosis
    Bronchiectasis
    Mycobacterium fortuitum or *chelonei* pneumonia
Tracheobronchitis
    Chronic persistent cough
    Bronchorrhea
    "Asthma"
Near drowning

geus muscle) relaxes. Pharyngeal swallowing initiates primary peristaltic waves in the esophagus, which carry fluid and food through a relaxed lower esophageal sphincter into the stomach. The lower esophageal sphincter then contracts and prevents, though not entirely, gastroesophageal reflux. Even in normal persons, some of the above defenses may become impaired with increasing age [5,7,8] or during sleep [9]. The vocal cords close much more slowly after the age of 50 years [8] and may not close at all during sleep or with sedation [9], no matter what the patient's age. The older, sleeping, and/or sedated patient is therefore particularly vulnerable to development of an aspiration syndrome, since the cough response to airway irritation is decreased during sleep compared to the waking state [10]. During REM sleep, the normal cough reflex may be totally absent [10], which explains the fact that normal people may silently aspirate oropharyngeal contents [9].

NORMAL RESPIRATORY DEFENSES AGAINST ASPIRATION OF INFECTIOUS AGENTS, FLUID, AND FOOD.

These defenses can be categorized as nonimmunologic and immunologic mechanisms. For infectious agents to enter the lower respiratory tract (below the vocal cords), they must first escape aerodynamic filtration in the nose, mouth, and larynx. Here particles that are larger than 10 μ in diameter never reach the lower respiratory tract, because they are filtered out of the airstream [11]. Particles between 2 and 10 μ in diameter can reach the airways, and those between 0.5 and 2 μ in diameter can reach the alveoli [11]. Normally, mucociliary clearance removes the larger particles [12] and the alveolar macrophage (primarily) and neutrophil clear the smaller ones [13–19]. Cough is not a primary defense mechanism; it provides a clearance function only when mucociliary clearance is inefficient or overwhelmed (e.g., by aspiration of large amounts of fluid and food) [20]. As clearance is taking place, the infectious particles are detoxified by lysozyme [21] and other proteases in mucus and by the alveolar macrophage and neutrophil enzymes [13]. Immunologic mechanisms augment the nonimmunologic mechanisms. For instance, complement and immunoglobulins opsonize bacteria for the alveolar phagocytes [22,23].

IMPAIRMENT OF UPPER GASTROINTESTINAL DEFENSES.

The risk of aspiration of fluid and food is increased when the normal mechanisms fail to work in a coordinated, synchronized manner. This can occur when the bolus cannot readily be cleared from the pharynx due to neuromuscular disorders (e.g., electrolyte disorders [24], debilitation [25], mal-

nutrition [26,27], myasthenia gravis [4], parkinsonism [4], polymyositis [4], demyelinating diseases [4], congenital and degenerative disorders [4], disorders of the brainstem [4], alcoholism [28], cricopharyngeal achalasia [5], and Zenker's diverticulum [29]). The risk of aspiration becomes prohibitive in these settings, when patients do not adequately masticate their food [30] (e.g., poor or absent dentition, sedation), and in settings in which vocal cord closure becomes excessively delayed (e.g., old age [8], debilitation [25], sedation [1,9], tracheostomy [31], and after extubation [32]). Aspiration of stomach contents is also predictable in elderly, sedated, or sleeping patients with gastroesophageal reflux [33], especially when their upper and lower esophageal sphincters have been rendered incompetent by a nasogastric tube [1,31]. Moreover, the risk of aspiration with a nasogastric tube in place is enhanced by the supine position [34].

IMPAIRMENT OF RESPIRATORY TRACT DEFENSES.

Aspirated material will cause pulmonary disease if it cannot be effectively cleared and detoxified or it is irritating (e.g., HCl).

Mucociliary clearance may become overwhelmed with aspirated fluid and food or with large amounts of inhaled infectious material when aerodynamic filtration by the upper airways is bypassed (e.g., endotracheal intubation). It may also become ineffective in the following settings: inhalational or systemic general anesthesia, endotracheal intubation with a cuffed balloon, endotracheal suctioning, hypercapnia and hyperoxia, smoking, asthma, chronic bronchitis, cystic fibrosis and bronchiectasis, and respiratory infections with viruses and *Mycoplasma pneumoniae* [12]. Even in the absence of mucociliary clearance, however, the airways can be cleared of excessive secretions and foreign bodies if the patient has an effective cough [35]. For instance, an effective cough and rapid closure of the vocal cords might limit the consequences of gastroesophageal reflux of gastric contents to a chemical laryngitis. An effective cough with slow closure of the vocal cords might limit the consequences of gastroesophageal reflux of gastric contents with aspiration to a chemical tracheobronchitis [36]. A consequence of an ineffective cough in the latter setting might be the acute respiratory distress syndrome ARDS [31]. Since an effective cough is determined by both good expiratory flow rates and respiratory muscle strength [36], cough may be ineffective in patients with severe asthma, chronic obstructive pulmonary disease (COPD), or respiratory neuromuscular disorders (e.g., myasthenia gravis and malnutrition); patients with painful incisions; and those receiving excessive sedation and analgesia with antitussive effects.

Aspirated material is cleared from the airways by mucociliary clearance and cough, whereas alveolar phagocytes clear the alveoli [11,13]. Since the most important bactericidal mechanism of the lung resides in the alveolar phagocytes [11,13], aspirated bacteria cause infectious pneumonia only when the alveolar phagocytes become impaired [11,13,37] (e.g., alcoholism, pH <7.2, acute alveolar hypoxia with PO_2 <25 mm Hg, alveolar hyperoxia, corticosteroid therapy, respiratory viral infections, hypothermia, starvation, and exposures to nitrogen dioxide, sulfur dioxide, ozone, and cigarette smoke on a long-term basis).

Although the role of immunologic defenses against infectious particles is sketchy, it is believed they are important in augmenting and occasionally directing the alveolar phagocytes [11,13]. For instance, patients with hereditary and acquired immunologic abnormalities (e.g., IgG and complement deficiencies) are susceptible to frequent and often severe bacterial pneumonias.

Diagnosis

GENERAL CONSIDERATIONS. The possibility that an aspiration syndrome is causing any pulmonary problem should be considered in every patient, but especially in the elderly, debilitated, or sedated patient with unexplained deterioration in pulmonary status and any patient presenting with one of the syndromes listed in Table 62-1. Aspiration syndromes are underdiagnosed. Failure to make the diagnosis probably stems from the glut of articles in the 1970s stressing the importance of anaerobic aspiration infections, a widespread tendency to consider all pulmonary complications of aspiration to be infectious, overreliance on inaccurate sputum sampling techniques such as expectorated sputum, and the misconception that aspiration must be witnessed before it can be assumed to have occurred.

DIAGNOSTIC PROTOCOL. Table 62-2 outlines all the studies that may be necessary to diagnose aspiration syndromes accurately (see Differential Diagnosis). In addition to taking a history and performing a physical examination to uncover impairment of the normal defenses against aspiration of fluid, food, and infectious agents, the physician should watch the patient swallow a glass of water [4,5]. A pharyngeal problem may be uncovered by watching the patient cough and sputter and tilt his or her neck and head in an unnatural posture. For instance, cricopharyngeus achalasia may be suggested by an inability to swallow despite multiple efforts. While observing patients can be useful when there is obvious difficulty during swallowing, the positive and negative predictive values for the potential for aspirating of this diagnostic observation are not known. A recent study [38] has begun to address this issue and suggests that observing patients swallow may not have high sensitivity in tracheotomized patients for exposing the potential to aspirate. Eighty-three tracheotomized, ventilator-dependent patients had videofluoroscopic barium esophagography prior to beginning oral feeding. Fifty percent aspirated at least once, and the aspiration event was "silent" (i.e., no cough or respiratory distress) in 79 percent of these.

If history and physical examination uncover a swallowing defense defect, routine expectorated sputum smears and cultures may be totally inadequate (see Chap. 13). Transtracheal aspiration and quantitative bacterial cultures obtained with telescoping plugged catheters at bronchoscopy not only identify

Table 62-2. Diagnostic Protocol for Aspiration Syndromes

History
Physical examination
    Baseline examination
    Observation of patient drinking water
Chest radiographs
Lower respiratory studies
    Expectorated samples
    Transtracheal aspiration
    Protected specimen brush with quantitative cultures
    Bronchoalveolar lavage
    Lung biopsy
Upper gastrointestinal studies
    Contrast films
    Endoscopy
    Motility
    Scintiscan
    24-hour esophageal pH monitoring

the lower respiratory tract infectious agent more accurately but also may rule out a bacterial problem. For instance, negative transtracheal aspiration Gram smear and aerobic and anaerobic cultures plus bronchoalveolar lavage showing food particles may help diagnose an exogenous lipoid pneumonia. Lung biopsy may be necessary to confirm this. Fat stains performed on unfixed expectorated sputum and bronchoalveolar lavage specimens may reveal numerous lipid-laden alveolar macrophages consistent with an exogenous lipoid pneumonia, but these lipid-laden cells may also represent nothing more than a nonspecific response of the lung to acute injury of any nature [39]. Although radionuclide scintiscanning using ^{99m}Tc-sulfur colloid and barium swallow appear to be insensitive techniques for documenting pulmonary disorders as a consequence of gastroesophageal reflux, when findings are abnormal they are specific for demonstrating aspiration of stomach contents [40]. A discussion of why these studies are likely to be insensitive can be found elsewhere [41].

Differential Diagnosis

MENDELSON'S SYNDROME. This syndrome [1,31,42,43] is due to the parenchymal inflammatory reaction caused by a large volume of aspirated liquid gastric contents. After aspiration, patients develop ARDS (see Chap. 55). They have tachypnea, fever, crackles, severe hypoxemia, and localized or diffuse chest radiograph abnormalities that progress within the next 24 to 36 hours. Contrary to the general view that gastric aspirates with pH greater than 2.5 are benign, the same syndrome can occur at a pH of 5.9 [44]. The important clues to the diagnosis are the situations that interfere with swallowing defenses. Patients invariably have a marked disturbance of consciousness (e.g., sedative drug overdose, general anesthesia) interfering with vocal cord protection and/or a nasogastric tube in place, making the upper and lower esophageal sphincters incompetent (Fig. 62-1). Subsequent clinical courses are death in 30 to 62 percent of cases, progressive improvement, and an initial improvement followed by worsening due to secondary bacterial infection.

FOREIGN BODY ASPIRATION. Aspiration of solid particles causes varying degrees of respiratory obstruction [45]. Most cases occur in children. When foreign bodies are inhaled into the tracheobronchial tree, 38 percent of patients give a clear diagnostic history, 22 percent give a history of an acute choking and coughing episode, and 40 percent complain of cough and dyspnea and are heard to wheeze. Although the chest radiograph may demonstrate the foreign object, atelectasis, or obstructive emphysema, it is normal in 80 percent of the cases.

Food asphyxiation is due to obstruction by food of the upper respiratory tract, usually at the level of the hypopharynx (Fig. 62-2). It occurs whenever and wherever people eat, including in hospitalized patients [46]. In restaurants it is called the "cafe coronary" because it is often mistaken for a heart attack [47]. Food asphyxiation should be suspected in middle-aged or elderly patients with poor dentition or dentures who are sedated by alcohol or other drugs and who attempt to swallow solid food. The key to the diagnosis is that the patient cannot speak. The inability to chew adequately, impairment of good judgment by sedation, and impairment of swallowing defenses by sedation and advancing age all contribute to the occurrence of this syndrome.

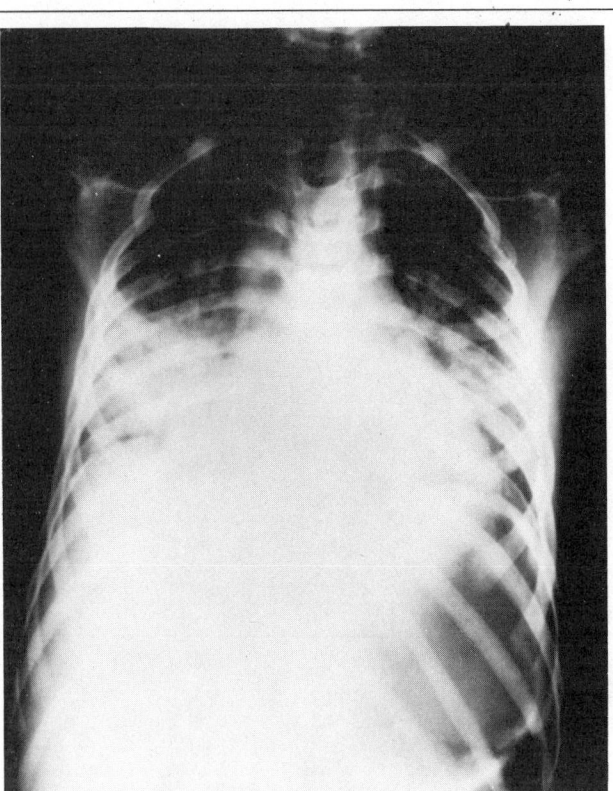

Fig. 62-1. Acute respiratory distress syndrome due to massive aspiration of gastric contents. This 15-year-old patient with marked disturbance of consciousness due to aspirin overdose aspirated during gastric lavage with a nasogastric tube. Prophylactic endotracheal intubation could have prevented this complication.

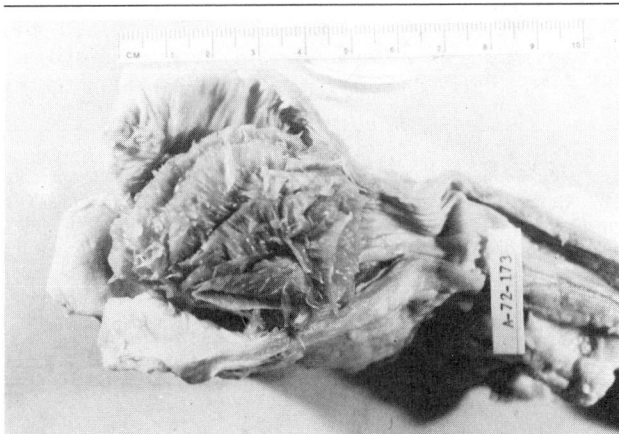

Fig. 62-2. Foreign body (food) aspiration obstructing the upper airway. An incredibly large piece of unchewed meat, 5 cm long, is lodged in the hypopharynx (the vocal cords appear as the ridge to the right of the meat). The patient died from asphyxiation.

BACTERIAL PNEUMONIA AND LUNG ABSCESS. Normal respiratory defenses prevent lower respiratory tract infection. Though not widely appreciated, most bacterial pneumonias are a consequence of aspiration of oropharyngeal infectious material. Pneumococcal pneumonia probably occurs because the aspirated *Pneumococcus* cannot be cleared and detoxified by mucociliary clearance and the alveolar phagocytes have been rendered ineffective (e.g., by a preceding viral infection) [11,13,48]. Anaerobic pneumonia or lung abscess probably occurs in alcoholics with pyorrhea (Fig. 62-3) because an overwhelming amount of anaerobes is aspirated [1,49,50]. Since cough is suppressed, the aspirate is not readily cleared and airways are temporarily obstructed. Distal to this, anaerobes may not be killed by alveolar macrophages that are probably rendered ineffective due to alcohol and acute local hypoxia [11,13,37]. While aspirational bacterial pneumonias that are community-acquired are most commonly due to the *Pneumococcus* [51] and anaerobes [52], nosocomial aspiration bacterial pneumonias are most commonly (50–74% of cases) due to facultative, enteric gram-negative bacilli [53,54,55]. The intubated patient is particularly susceptible to pneumonia because the tube bypasses the aerodynamic filtration protection of the upper respiratory tract and stops mucociliary clearance [12]. The intubated patient who requires a narcotic is at greater risk because cough is also suppressed.

EXOGENOUS LIPOID PNEUMONIA. This condition can be caused by aspiration of mineral oil, animal oil (e.g., cod liver oil, milk products), vegetable oil [56], or formula feedings [57]. Conditions more likely to be complicated by exogenous lipoid pneumonia include pharyngeal swallowing disorders, Zenker's diverticulum, cricopharyngeal achalasia, scleroderma involving the esophagus, epiphrenic diverticulum, esophageal carcinoma and achalasia, and gastroesophageal reflux disease [4,5,58]. Although patients with exogenous lipoid pneumonia usually do not appear toxic [59], their clinical presentation occasionally cannot be distinguished from that of acute bacterial pneumonia. (The varying clinical presentation depends in part on the type of oil aspirated [56].) The important clues to the diagnosis must

Fig. 62-3. Poor oral hygiene. The periodontal disease demonstrated here is typical of the patient with anaerobic aspiration bacterial infection.

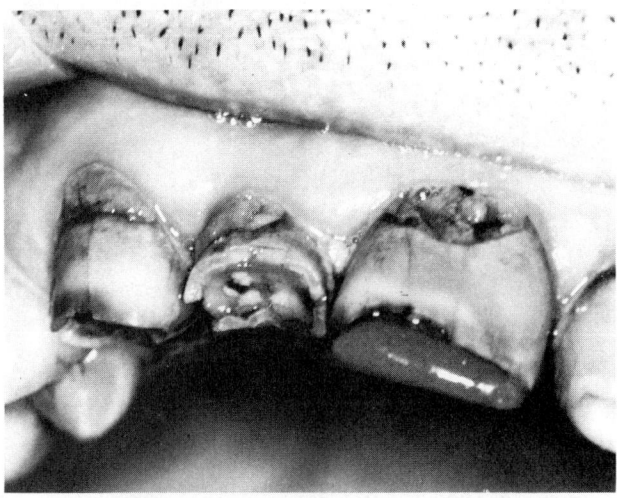

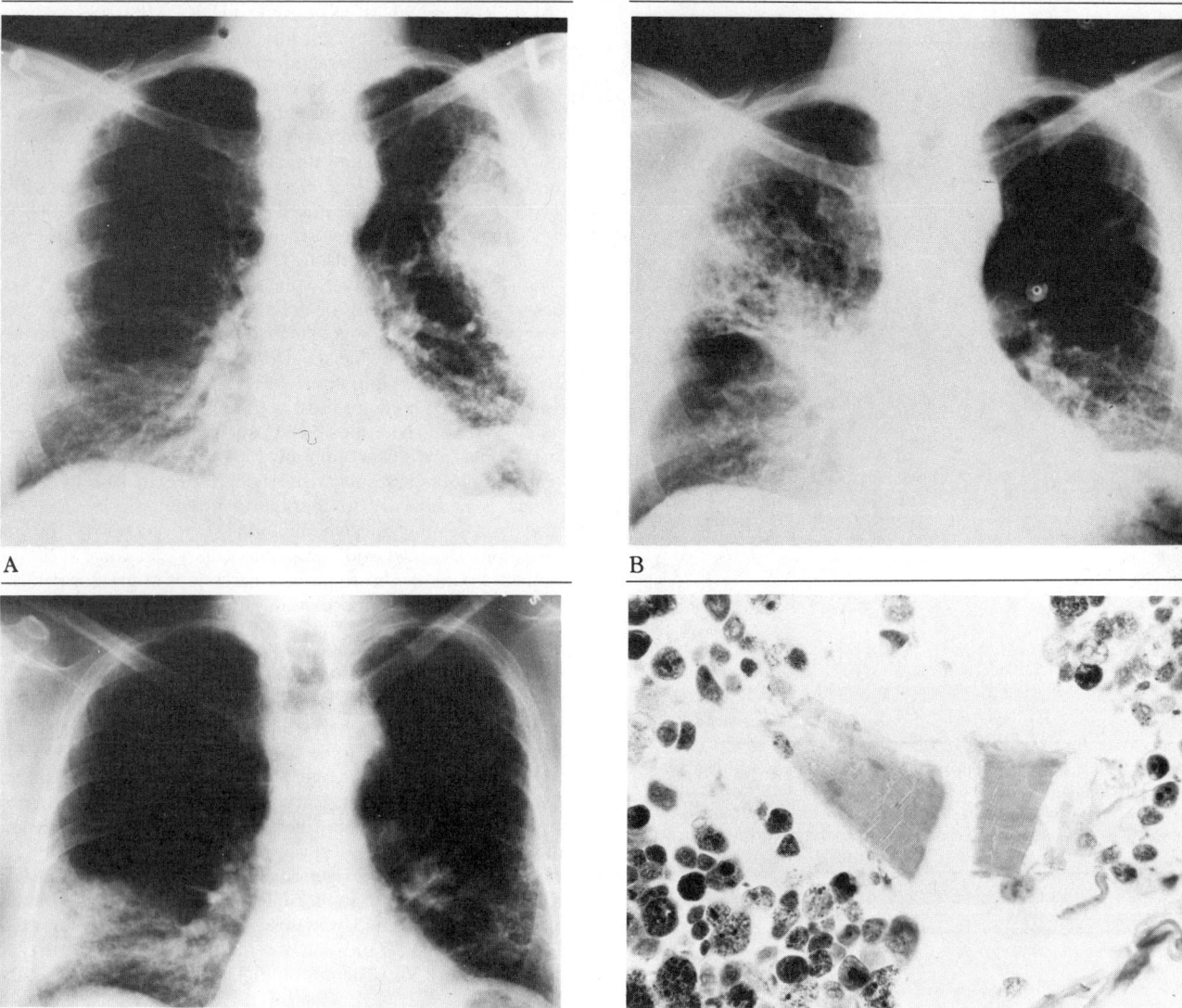

Fig. 62-4. Recurrent exogenous lipoid pneumonias. This patient with chronic myelogenous leukemia and esophageal swallowing dysfunction due primarily to alcoholism and gastroesophageal reflux disease repeatedly aspirated gastroesophageal contents, causing clinical pictures indistinguishable from recurrent bacterial infections (A–C). The diagnosis was made when bronchoalveolar lavage revealed meat fibers (D) and numerous lipid-laden and hemosiderin-laden macrophages and when recurrent pneumonias ceased (E) with cessation of alcohol ingestion and treatment for gastroesophageal reflux disease.

come from the history and physical examination (see Diagnostic Protocol) and upper gastrointestinal studies. Transtracheal aspiration in nonintubated patients and quantitative cultures obtained with telescoping plugged catheters at bronchoscopy may be needed to rule out a bacterial infection, and lung biopsy may be needed to rule out cancer and rule in the diagnosis. Lower respiratory tract secretions obtained by transtracheal aspiration may be sterile in this condition, since alveolar macrophages appear to be quite capable of clearing and detoxifying bacteria when exogenous lipid and bacteria are aspirated together [60]. If not diagnosed promptly, recurrent aspirations of lipid and/or small amounts of liquid gastric contents can present

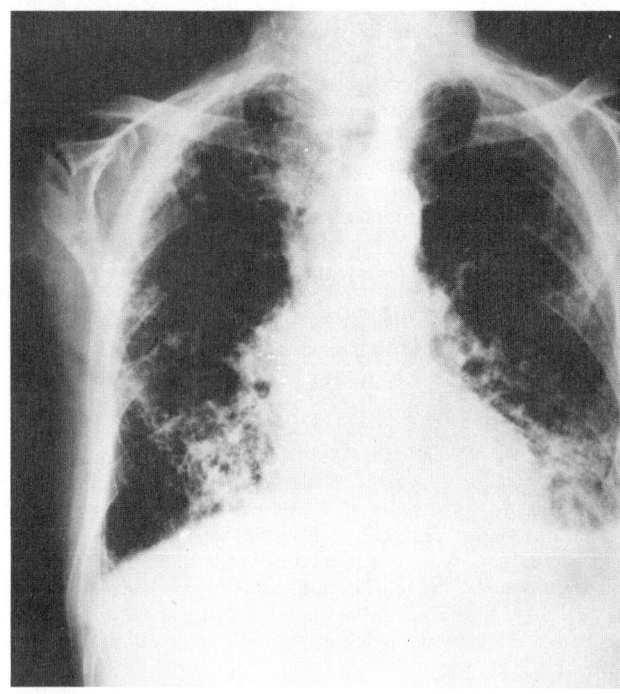

A

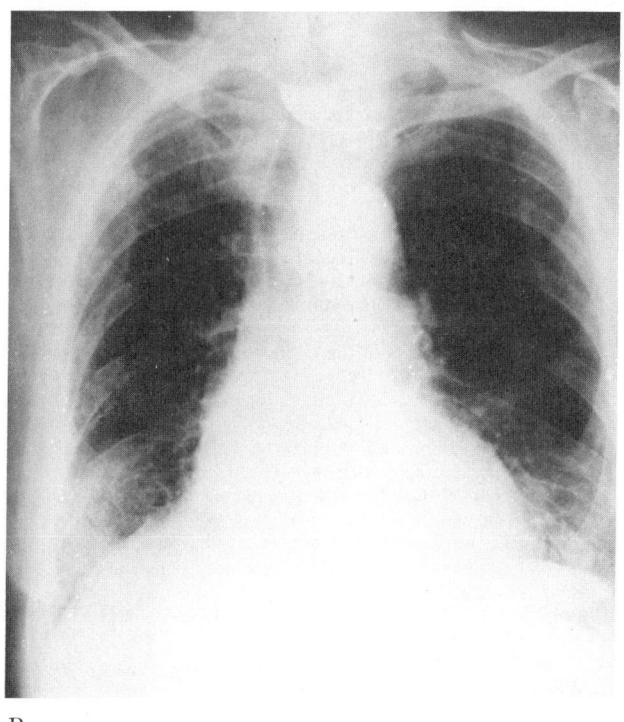

B

Fig. 62-5. Chronic interstitial fibrosis (A) due to chronic aspiration from Zenker's diverticulum (B).

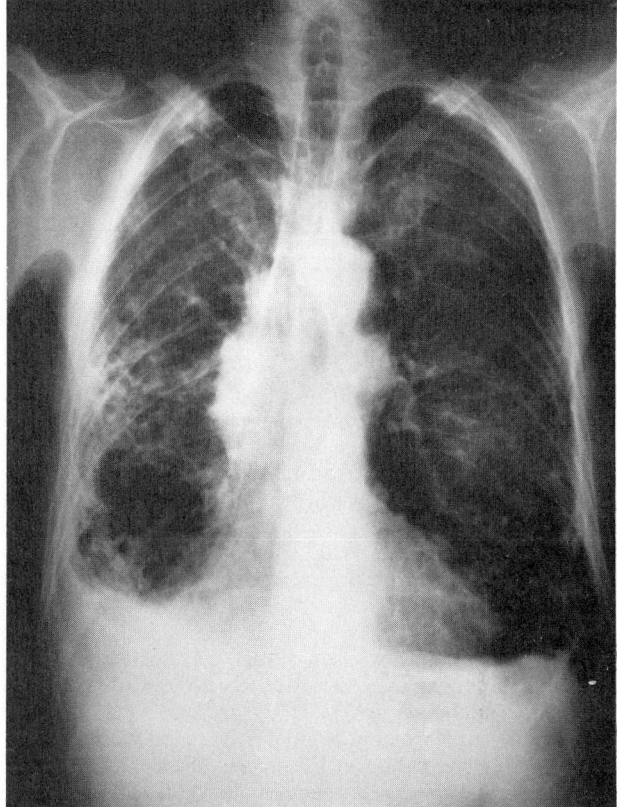

Fig. 62-6. Cystic bronchiectasis due to chronic aspiration from gastroesophageal reflux disease.

as recurrent hemoptysis [61] or recurrent pneumonias (Fig. 62-4) [56] or can lead to chronic interstitial fibrosis (Fig. 62-5) [56,62] and/or bronchiectasis (Fig. 62-6) [56,63,64]. Rarely, exogenous lipoid pneumonias are complicated by organisms of the *Mycobacterium fortuitum* complex [65,66,67].

TRACHEOBRONCHITIS. Aspiration of small amounts of liquid gastric contents [36], oral feedings, or formula feeding solutions administered through small nasogastric tubes [57] may cause airway consequences. Tracheobronchitis must be considered, not only in outpatients with gastroesophageal reflux disease and chronic persistent cough [68], but also in hospitalized patients (e.g., debilitated, postoperative, intubated, or recently extubated patients or those with neuromuscular diseases) who have cough and wheeze ("asthma") and/or bronchorrhea. Bronchorrhea is defined as expectoration of more than 30 ml of phlegm in 24 hours. Swallowing defenses have been shown to be impaired in all of these hospitalized patients [1,4,9,24–27,31,32]. If bronchorrhea is due to aspiration of oral feedings, the diagnosis can be suggested by merely watching the patient having difficulty swallowing water [4]. Aspiration can occur up to 38 percent of the time with small-bore nasogastric tube feedings, even with cuffed endotracheal tubes in place [57]. Unfortunately, tracheal secretion glucose determinations have not been shown to be useful in predicting aspiration of enteral feedings. They were shown to be similar in intubated patients whether they were enterally or non-enterally fed [68a]. While aspiration can be mitigated in this setting by placing the patient in the semirecumbent rather than supine position (i.e., 45 degree angle) [34], the placement of the end of the feeding tube has not been shown consistently to affect aspiration rates. A recent study revealed equal aspiration rates from postpylorus and intragastric-placed small-bore nasoenteric feeding tubes [69].

Treatment

Treatment for the aspiration syndromes should be prophylactic as well as specific.

MENDELSON'S SYNDROME. This syndrome should be anticipated in all patients with a marked disturbance of consciousness, especially if a nasogastric tube has been placed. Consequently such patients, whenever possible, should be prophylactically intubated for airway protection until they are awake. Elevation of the head of the bed also decreases gastroesophageal reflux [70] and aspiration [34]. Once liquid gastric content aspiration has occurred and ARDS has supervened, adequate oxygenation is essential. Mechanical ventilation with positive end-expiratory pressure (PEEP) may be necessary. Despite their frequent use, parenteral corticosteroids have not been shown to be helpful [71,72,73]. Antibiotics are indicated only when the chemical pneumonitis is complicated by infection [74]. On the other hand, intratracheal instillations of corticosteroids or alkaline and saline solutions consistently worsen the condition [75,76].

FOREIGN BODY ASPIRATION. Aspiration of foreign bodies other than food can be prevented by not putting them in one's mouth. Particles that reach the lower respiratory tract and do not totally obstruct the trachea can be removed by bronchoscopy [43]. Those that totally obstruct the trachea must be removed immediately by subdiaphragmatic abdominal thrusts and finger sweeps in the unconscious individual and/or chest thrusts in the markedly obese person and women in advanced stages of pregnancy [77].

Food asphyxiation should be anticipated in the elderly sedated hospitalized patient with poor dentition [46]. Large pieces of meat should not be ordered, sedation should be minimized, and mealtimes should be supervised. If food asphyxiation occurs, the obstructed airway is managed with the techniques mentioned above [77].

BACTERIAL PNEUMONIA AND LUNG ABSCESS. The causative organism(s) should be identified and appropriate antibiotic therapy given (see Chaps. 76 and 85).

To help prevent future anaerobic infections, periodontal disease must be definitively treated by a dentist. Moreover, attempts must be made to persuade the alcoholic to stop drinking.

EXOGENOUS LIPOID PNEUMONIA. Although corticosteroids may be helpful [78] in cases of acute lipid aspiration, acute exogenous lipoid pneumonias usually resolve on their own. The key to therapy is to prevent recurrences. Cricopharyngeus and esophageal achalasia and Zenker's diverticulum should be surgically repaired. Gastroesophageal reflux with aspiration can

be treated with a variety of measures, including 8-inch head-of-the-bed elevation, antacids/histamine-2 blockers or omeprazole, a high-protein, low-fat antireflux diet, nothing to eat or drink for 2 hours before bedtime and no snacking between meals, and metoclopramide or cisapride and/or bethanechol in the nonasthmatic; or, if these measures fail, surgery [70]. Patients receiving formula feedings by nasogastric tube should be positioned at a 45-degree angle [34]. The constipated patient must stop nocturnal mineral oil ingestion. To prevent aspiration in patients with swallowing problems due to neuromuscular diseases, it may be necessary to stop all oral feedings and feed through a gastrostomy or jejunostomy. If life-threatening aspiration of saliva occurs, it may become necessary to perform a tracheostomy and close off the laryngeal inlet with a pursestring suture [79].

TRACHEOBRONCHITIS. Aspirations of small amounts of oral feedings, liquid gastric contents, or formula feeding solutions are treated as described in Exogenous Lipoid Pneumonia. In general, postoperative, debilitated, and recently extubated patients will stop aspirating and their bronchorrhea will disappear when oral feeding and drinking are stopped. An oral diet should not be resumed until the patient has had a contrast study demonstrating the ability to swallow without aspirating [38].

References

1. Bartlett JG: The triple threat of aspiration pneumonia. *Chest* 68:560, 1975.
2. Bone DK, Davis JL, Zuidema GD, et al: Aspiration pneumonia: Prevention of aspiration in patients with tracheostomies. *Ann Thorac Surg* 18:30, 1974.
3. Cameron JL, Reynolds J, Zuidema GD: Aspiration in patients with tracheostomies. *Surg Gynecol Obstet* 136:68, 1973.
4. Donner MW, Silbiger ML: Cinefluorographic analysis of pharyngeal swallowing in neuromuscular disorders. *Am J Med Sci* 251:134, 1966.
5. Palmer ED: Disorders of the cricopharyngeus muscle: A review. *Gastroenterology* 7:510, 1976.
6. Cohen S: Motor disorders of the esophagus. *N Engl J Med* 301:184, 1979.
7. Soergel KH, Zboralske F, Amberg JR: Presbyesophagus: Esophageal motility in nonagenarians. *J Clin Invest* 43:1472, 1964.
8. Pontoppidan H, Beecher HK: Progressive loss of protective reflexes in the airway with the advance of age. *JAMA* 174:2209, 1960.
9. Huxley EJ, Viroslav J, Gray WR, et al: Pharyngeal aspiration in normal adults and patients with depressed consciousness. *Am J Med* 64:564, 1978.
10. Phillipson EA: Breathing disorders during sleep. *Basics of Respiratory Disease* 7:18, 1979.
11. Green GM: Pulmonary clearance of infectious agents. *Ann Rev Med* 19:315, 1968.
12. Wanner A: Clinical aspects of mucociliary transport. *Am Rev Respir Dis* 116:73, 1977.
13. Green GM, Jakab GJ, Low RB, et al: Defense mechanisms of the respiratory membrane. *Am Rev Respir Dis* 115:479, 1977.
14. Green GM, Kass EH: The role of the alveolar macrophage in the clearance of bacteria from the lung. *J Exp Med* 119:167, 1964.
15. Jackson AE, Southern PM, Pierce AK, et al: Pulmonary clearance of gram-negative bacilli. *J Lab Clin Med* 69:833, 1967.
16. Pierce AK, Reynolds RC, Harris G: Leukocytic response to inhaled bacteria. *Am Rev Respir Dis* 116:679, 1977.
17. Toews GB, Gross GN, Pierce AK: The relationship of inoculum size of lung bacterial clearance and phagocytic cell response in mice. *Am Rev Respir Dis* 120:559, 1979.

18. Rehm SR, Gross GN, Pierce AK: Early bacterial clearance from murine lung: Species-dependent phagocyte response. *J Clin Invest* 66:194, 1980.

19. Onofrio JM, Shulkin AN, Heidbrink PJ: Pulmonary clearance and phagocytic cell response to normal pharyngeal flora. *Am Rev Respir Dis* 123:222, 1981.

20. Loudon RG: Cough in health and disease, in *Current Research in Chronic Obstructive Lung Disease: Proceedings of Tenth Emphysema Conference.* Washington DC, US Department of Health, Education and Welfare, 1967, p 41.

21. Konstan MW, Chen PW, Sherman JM, et al: Human lung lysozyme: Sources and properties. *Am Rev Respir Dis* 123:120, 1981.

22. Hof DG, Repine JE, Peterson PK, et al: Phagocytosis by human alveolar macrophages and neutrophils: Qualitative differences in the opsonic requirements for uptake of *Staphylococcus aureus* and *Streptococcus pneumoniae* in vitro. *Am Rev Respir Dis* 121:65, 1980.

23. Heidbrink PJ, Toews GB, Gross GN, et al: Mechanisms of complement-mediated clearance of bacteria from the murine lung. *Am Rev Respir Dis* 125:517, 1982.

24. Knochel JP: Neuromuscular manifestations of electrolyte disorders. *Am J Med* 72:521, 1982.

25. Arms RA, Dines DE, Tinstman TC: Aspiration pneumonia. *Chest* 65:136, 1974.

26. Weinsier RL, Hunker EM, Krumdieck CL, et al: Hospital malnutrition: A prospective evaluation of general medical patients during the course of hospitalization. *Am J Clin Nutr* 32:418, 1979.

27. Willard MD, Gilsdorf RB, Price RA: Protein-calorie malnutrition in a community hospital. *JAMA* 243:1720, 1980.

28. Weber LD, Nashel DJ, Mellow MH: Pharyngeal dysphagia in alcoholic myopathy. *Ann Intern Med* 95:189, 1981.

29. Hawes LE, Walker JH: Severe pulmonary disease subsequent to Zenker's diverticulum. *N Engl J Med* 253:209, 1955.

30. Mittleman RE, Wetli CV: The fatal cafe coronary: Foreign-body airway obstruction. *JAMA* 247:1285, 1982.

31. Wynne JW, Modell JH: Respiratory aspiration of stomach contents. *Ann Intern Med* 87:466, 1977.

32. Burgess GE, Cooper JR Jr, Marino RJ, et al: Laryngeal competence after tracheal extubation. *Anesthesiology* 51:73, 1979.

33. Chernow B, Johnson LF, Janowitz WR: Pulmonary aspiration as a consequence of gastroesophageal reflux: A diagnostic approach. *Dig Dis Sci* 24:839, 1979.

34. Terres A, Serra-Batlles J, Ros E, et al: Pulmonary aspiration of gastric contents in patients receiving mechanical ventilation: The effect of body position. *Ann Intern Med* 116:540, 1992.

35. Irwin RS, Rosen MJ: Cough: A comprehensive review. *Arch Intern Med* 137:1186, 1977.

36. Wynne JW, Ramphal R, Hood CI: Tracheal mucosal damage after aspiration: A scanning electron microscope study. *Am Rev Respir Dis* 124:728, 1981.

37. Cohen AB, Cline MJ: The human alveolar macrophage: Isolation, cultivation in vitro, and studies of morphologic and functional characteristics. *J Clin Invest* 50:1390, 1971.

38. Elpern EH, Scott MG, Petro L, et al: Pulmonary aspiration in mechanically ventilated adults with tracheostomies. *Am Rev Respir Dis* 147:A409, 1993.

39. Corwin RW, Irwin RS: The lipid-laden alveolar macrophage as a marker of aspiration in parenchymal lung disease. *Am Rev Respir Dis* 132:576, 1985.

40. Barish CF, Wu WC, Castell DO: Respiratory complications of gastroesophageal reflux. *Arch Intern Med* 145:1882, 1985.

41. Irwin RS, Doherty PW, Bartter T, et al: Evaluation of technetium pertechnetate as a radionuclide marker of pulmonary aspiration of gastric contents in rabbits. *Chest* 93:1270, 1988.

42. Mendelson CL: The aspiration of stomach contents into the lungs during obstetric anesthesia. *Am J Obstet Gynecol* 52:191, 1946.

43. Bynum LJ, Pierce AK: Pulmonary aspiration of gastric contents. *Am Rev Respir Dis* 114:1129, 1976.

44. Schwartz DJ, Wynne JW, Gibbs CP, et al: The pulmonary consequences of aspiration of gastric contents at pH values greater than 2.5. *Am Rev Respir Dis* 121:119, 1980.

45. Abdulmajid OA, Ebeid AM, Motaweh MM, et al: Aspirated foreign bodies in the tracheobronchial tree: Report of 250 cases. *Thorax* 31:635, 1976.

46. Irwin RS, Ashba JK, Braman SS, et al: Food asphyxiation in hospitalized patients. *JAMA* 237:2744, 1977.

47. Eller WC, Haugen RK: Food asphyxiation: Restaurant rescue. *N Engl J Med* 289:81, 1973.

48. Hof DG, Repine JE, Peterson PK, et al: Phagocytosis by human alveolar macrophages and neutrophils: Qualitative differences in the opsonic requirements for uptake of *Staphylococcus aureus* and *Streptococcus pneumoniae* in vitro. *Am Rev Respir Dis* 121:65, 1980.

49. Kannangara DW, Thadepalli H, Bach VT, et al: Animal model for anaerobic lung abscess. *Infect Immun* 31:592, 1981.

50. Gorbach SL, Bartlett JG: Anaerobic infections (second of three parts). *N Engl J Med* 290:1237, 1974.

51. Fick RB Jr, Reynolds HY: Changing spectrum of pneumonia: News media creation or clinical reality? *Am J Med* 74:1, 1983.

52. Lorber B, Swenson RM: Bacteriology of aspiration pneumonia: A prospective study of community—and hospital—acquired cases. *Ann Intern Med* 81:329, 1974.

53. LaForce FM: Hospital-acquired gram-negative rod pneumonias: An overview. *Am J Med* 70:664, 1981.

54. Stamm WE, Martin SM, Bennett JV: Epidemiology of nosocomial infections due to gram-negative bacilli: Aspects relevant to development and use of vaccines. *J Infect Dis* 136(suppl):5151, 1977.

55. Pierce AK, Sanford JP: Aerobic gram-negative bacillary pneumonias. *Am Rev Respir Dis* 110:647, 1974.

56. Spencer H: *Pathology of the Lung.* 3rd ed. Elmsford, NY: Pergamon, 1977, vol 1, p 468.

57. Winterbauer RH, Durning RB Jr, Barron E, et al: Aspirated nasogastric feeding solution detected by glucose strips. *Ann Intern Med* 95:67, 1981.

58. Hughes RL, Frelich RA, Bytell DE, et al: Aspiration and occult esophageal disorders. *Chest* 80:489, 1981.

59. Schwindt WD, Barbee RA, Jones RJ: Lipoid pneumonia. *Arch Surg* 95:652, 1967.

60. Corwin RW, DeVine K, Irwin RS: The effects of oil ingestion on rabbit alveolar macrophage function. *Am Rev Respir Dis* 127(suppl):202, 1983.

61. Belsey R: The pulmonary complications of esophageal disease. *Br J Dis Chest* 54:342, 1960.

62. Pearson JEG, Wilson RSE: Diffuse pulmonary fibrosis and hiatus hernia. *Thorax* 26:300, 1971.

63. Schacter EN, Basta W: Bronchiectasis following heroin overdose: A report of two cases. *Chest* 63:363, 1973.

64. Banner AS, Muthuswamy P, Shah RS, et al: Bronchiectasis following heroin-induced pulmonary edema: Rapid clearing of pulmonary infiltrates. *Chest* 69:552, 1976.

65. Burke DS, Ullian RB: Megaesophagus and pneumonia associated with *Mycobacterium chelonei*: A case report and a literature review. *Am Rev Respir Dis* 116:1101, 1977.

66. Hutchins GM, Boitnott JK: Atypical mycobacterial infection complicating mineral oil pneumonia. *JAMA* 240:539, 1978.

67. Irwin RS, Pratter MR, Corwin RW, et al: Pulmonary infection with *Mycobacterium chelonei*: Successful treatment with one drug based on disk diffusion susceptibility data. *J Infect Dis* 145:772, 1982.

68. Irwin RS, Corrao WM, Pratter MR: Chronic persistent cough in the adult: The spectrum and frequency of causes and successful outcome of specific therapy. *Am Rev Respir Dis* 123:413, 1981.

68a. Kinsey GC, Murray MJ, Swensen SJ, et al: Glucose content of tracheal aspirates: Implications for the detection of tube feeding aspiration. *Crit Care Med* 22:1557, 1994.

69. Strong RM, Condon SC, Solinger MR, et al: Equal aspiration rates from postpylorus and intragastric-placed small-bore nasoenteric feeding tubes: A randomized, prospective study. *J Parenter Enter Nutr* 16:59, 1992.

70. Richter JE, Castell DO: Gastroesophageal reflux: Pathogenesis, diagnosis, and therapy. *Ann Intern Med* 97:93, 1982.

71. Wolfe JE, Bone RC, Ruth WE: Effects of corticosteroids in the treatment of patients with gastric aspiration. *Am J Med* 63:719, 1977.

72. Chapman RL Jr, Modell JH, Ruiz BC, et al: Effect of continuous positive-pressure ventilation and steroids on aspiration of hydrochloric acid (pH 1.8) in dogs. *Anesth Analg* 53:556, 1974.

73. Downs JB, Chapman RL Jr, Modell JH, et al: An evaluation of

steroid therapy in aspiration pneumonitis. *Anesthesiology* 40:129, 1974.

74. Murray HW: Antimicrobial therapy in pulmonary aspiration. *Am J Med* 66:188, 1979.

75. Taylor G, Pryse-Davies J: Evaluation of endotracheal steroid therapy in acid pulmonary aspiration syndrome (Mendelson's syndrome). *Anesthesiology* 29:17, 1968.

76. Bannister WK, Sattilaro AJ, Otis RD: Therapeutic aspects of aspiration pneumonitis in experimental animals. *Anesthesiology* 22:440, 1961.

77. National Research Council: Standards and guidelines for cardiopulmonary resuscitation (CPR) and emergency cardiac care (ECC). *JAMA* 255:2905, 1986.

78. Ayvazian LF, Steward DS, Merkel CG, et al: Diffuse lipoid pneumonitis successfully treated with prednisone. *Am J Med* 43:930, 1967.

79. Montgomery WW: Surgical laryngeal closure to eliminate chronic aspiration. *N Engl J Med* 292:1390, 1975.

63. Near-Drowning

Nicholas A. Smyrnios and
Richard S. Irwin

Overview

Drowning is one of the most common causes of accidental death in the world, but confusion often arises when the terms *drowning* and *near-drowning* are used together. The definitions proposed by Modell in 1981 [1] are the simplest and most accurate available and should be used in any discussion on the subject. He defines *drown* as "to die from suffocation by submersion in water." *Near-drown* means "to survive, at least temporarily, after suffocation by submersion in water." These are the definitions used in this chapter.

Drowning is the fourth most common cause of accidental injury death in the United States [2]. An average of 5363 persons drowned in the United States each year between 1983 and 1989. Fortunately, the incidence of drowning declined from 2.7 per 100,000 to 1.9 per 100,000 during that period. Drowning is most common in young children (<5 years) and young adults (15–29 years). It is also more common in Native Americans, blacks, and males and in the southern states [3,4,5].

Statistics on near-drowning are less exact because many near-drowning victims do not seek medical attention. In South Carolina alone between 1968 and 1972, an estimated 15,400 near-drowning episodes occurred, in comparison to 182 deaths from drowning [6]. Extrapolation of these figures to the national drowning statistics quoted earlier implies a near-drowning incidence of more than 450,000 per year. Of these, some 45,000 would be expected to seek medical attention [6]. The magnitude of this problem is seriously underappreciated.

Etiology and Pathogenesis

The following factors are associated with an increased risk of drowning and near-drowning.

SEIZURES. A history of seizure disorder was found in 17 of the 293 cases of drowning in Sacramento County, California, between 1974 and 1985 [5]. This contrasts with the prevalence of seizures of 6 per 1000 in the general population. Detectable anticonvulsant levels were found in only eight of these persons. This implies either lack of compliance with medication regi-

mens or inadequate dosing or monitoring. Both Pearn [7] and Livingston and colleagues [8] reported that all drownings among epileptic children occurred in the bathtub. This implies the need for closer supervision in the homes of epileptics with active seizures.

BOATING ACCIDENTS. Twenty-nine percent of all drowning victims in Maryland in 1972 were boaters [9]. Similarly, 18 percent of the cases in the Sacramento group were victims of boating mishaps [5]. Most of these individuals were passengers on outboard motorboats or smaller vessels that sank or capsized. Both alcohol intake and failure to use personal flotation devices contributed to these deaths [5,9,10].

AQUATIC SPORTS. Water-related activities produce about 140,000 injuries annually. Diving, surfing, and waterskiing account for 77 percent of the 700 spinal cord injuries produced annually by aquatic sports. Diving and sliding head first produce the most serious injuries as a result of striking the bottom or side of a shallow body of water [10]. Although the exact number of near-drownings produced by these accidents is uncertain, aquatic sport injuries place the victim at substantial risk. Four of seven swimming pool drowning victims in the Maryland series had various abrasions and contusions consistent with diving accidents [9]. Although only 3 percent of drownings of children in New Mexico were observed to follow diving, an unspecified number of additional episodes associated with swimming, boating, and water activities probably were actually due to diving accidents [11].

VOLUNTARY HYPERVENTILATION. Young men who swim underwater often hyperventilate before submersion. This decreases their $PaCO_2$ and extends the time during which they can function underwater before reaching the point at which they must surface [12,13]. These persons may reach a critical level of hypoxia and lose consciousness before this "breaking point," because the contribution of hypoxic drive to the urge to breathe is much weaker than the hypercapnic drive [12,13]. Therefore, voluntary hyperventilation places an underwater swimmer at risk for near-drowning. There are reports of swimmers continuing their swimming movements and surfacing even after losing consciousness [12].

INADEQUATE ADULT SUPERVISION. The backyard pool and family bathtub are common sites of pediatric near-drowning [10,14–17]. Lack of appropriate precautions and supervision play a major role in many of these cases. Studies have shown lower rates of immersion accidents in areas where residential pools are required by law to be surrounded by a fence [18,19]. Appropriate sign posting in hazardous areas, effective educational programs on the dangers of water recreation, and the presence of lifeguards also lessen risk and improve survival [10,20,21].

Inattentive guardians and child abuse also contribute to bathtub-related drownings. In one study, all bathtub-related submersions in children younger than 5 years old occurred while the child was bathing unattended or with another young child [22]. The practice of leaving infants to bathe in the custody of a toddler is inappropriate and should be discouraged [14,15,23].

Another newly recognized site where young children may be injured is in 5-gallon industrial buckets used for home cleaning. Children climb into the bucket partially but are unable to extricate themselves because of their undeveloped coordination and high center of gravity. In one study these cases represented 24 percent of drownings of infants and toddlers [24].

DRUGS. Of 247 drug screens of adult Sacramento County victims, 22 were positive for one or more central nervous system (CNS) active drugs. Ten samples contained drugs other than anticonvulsants [5]. Among these were diazepam, amphetamine, morphine, codeine, hydroxyzine, doxepin, and desipramine. Centrally acting drugs can not only cloud the sensorium, causing disorientation and inducing sleep, but also impair coordination and reduce the ability to swim.

ALCOHOL. Ethanol use is the major risk factor in immersion accidents. Thirty-seven to 47 percent of drownings are associated with alcohol consumption [9,11,25]. Alcohol use is highly associated with drowning in men 30 to 64 years of age and in adolescents. However, significant blood alcohol levels are frequently found in drowned males of all ages [16,25]. Alcoholic beverages reduce the ability to deal with emergency situations by depressing conditioned reflexes and decreasing awareness of stimuli. Furthermore, alcohol consumption by a potential rescuer can destroy that person's ability to function effectively, often resulting in a double tragedy [25]. The availability of alcoholic beverages in water recreation areas and increased risk taking among drinkers both contribute to alcohol-related drownings. In addition, alcohol is frequently a factor in drownings that result from automobile accidents [5].

Pathophysiology

GENERAL CONSIDERATIONS. Two mechanisms produce the major pathologic changes responsible for morbidity in near-drowning: anoxia and hypothermia.

Anoxia. Controlled human experiments are obviously impossible, but most drownings and near-drownings are thought to follow a common pattern. The drowning sequence begins with a period of panic followed by a vigorous attempt at breath holding [26,27,28]. There is frequently a struggle to surface, and gasping may occur. During this period, large amounts of water may be swallowed that are eventually regurgitated and often are aspirated with gastric contents.

Eventually, the breaking point is reached and breath holding is no longer possible because of hypercarbia and hypoxia. Involuntary breaths are taken, with aspiration of varying amounts of water. So-called dry near-drowning occurs in 10 to 15 percent of cases, with aspiration of little or no fluid [29]. In these cases, a small amount of fluid aspirated into the trachea is thought to produce intense laryngospasm. The laryngospasm protects the lungs from further aspiration of fluid at the expense of preventing ventilation. In most cases, however, fluid reaches the lung and causes a variety of pathologic changes. The common factor in both wet and dry near-drowning is a severe degree of hypoxemia. Eventually, the victim becomes unconscious and cardiac arrest occurs.

Hypothermia. Humans tolerate hypothermia poorly. Survival is generally decreased in cold water immersions, despite the occasional spectacular reports of prolonged survival in ice water [30,31,32]. Several major disasters involving drowning, such as the deaths after the sinking of the *Titanic,* occurred not because of inability to float in most cases but because of hypothermia caused by exposure to extremely cold water.

Changes in human metabolism in response to hypothermia occur in two phases: the shivering phase and the nonshivering phase. A more detailed discussion on hypothermia is found in Chapter 72. Shivering involves contractions of both small and large muscle groups, resulting in increased heat production, oxygen consumption, and metabolic rate. These changes occur at a central temperature of 30 to 35°C. The nonshivering phase occurs below 30°C, when muscle contractions nearly cease and oxygen consumption and metabolic rate decrease.

Shivering is frequently accompanied by voluntary muscular movements. In a dry environment, both shivering and voluntary movements are effective in increasing heat production with minimal increase in heat loss, thereby preventing a severe drop in core temperature [33]. They are not nearly as effective in cold water. Both shivering and voluntary muscular movement increase blood flow to the extremities, thereby increasing conductive heat loss [26]. Exercise also stirs the surrounding water and can increase heat loss from convection [34]. Body type may also play a major role. Obese men tolerate immersion in cold water longer than thin men due to increased insulation from body fat [35]. Water reduces the insulative function of clothing by replacing the air between the fibers, thereby increasing heat conductance.

Immersion in very cold water can acutely lead to death three ways. First, a vagally mediated asystolic cardiac arrest may occur (immersion syndrome) [36]. Second, hypothermia produces an increased tendency toward malignant arrhythmias separate from this immediate response. Cardiac arrest from ventricular fibrillation is common at core temperatures below 25°C and asystole occurs at less than 18°C [37]. These arrhythmias may be refractory to resuscitative efforts until the body temperature has been increased. Third, a decrease in core temperature can cause loss of consciousness and aspiration from the victim's inability to keep the head above water. This can result in the sequence of events described above.

PULMONARY EFFECTS. Many of the most important pathophysiologic effects of near-drowning occur in the respiratory system. Controlled studies have been performed on animal models. Much information can be extrapolated from these experiments to the injury in humans.

The effects of aspiration of various water solutions on lung injury have been studied in animals [38,39]. Sterile water was found to be the most disruptive of pulmonary function. Normal and hypertonic saline solutions also cause significant increases in (P_A-a)O_2 gradient and shunt fraction, with a decrease in PaO_2:FiO_2. Decreases in arterial oxygen saturation and dynamic compliance as well as increases in minute ventilation, mean pulmonary artery pressure, and shunt fraction are seen in sheep after bilateral aspiration of either fresh or sea water [39]. Hypoxemia appears to be due to increased venous admixture.

Freshwater and saline solutions cause their effects via several mechanisms. Atelectasis due to increased surface tension, bronchoconstriction, and noncardiogenic pulmonary edema all play a role in the development of hypoxemia at different times after freshwater aspiration [39,40]. Fresh water acts partly by inactivating surfactant in the alveoli. Surfactant activity is decreased in both chlorinated and nonchlorinated freshwater aspirations [41]. In addition, the presence of water in the alveolus may damage type II pneumocytes, thereby preventing the production of surfactant for up to 24 hours [42]. The combination of these effects may damage the alveolar capillaries and interstitium and lead to the acute respiratory distress syndrome (ARDS).

The mechanism of development of hypoxemia in saltwater near-drowning is different. Electrolyte-containing solutions do not appear to inactivate surfactant. Hypertonic sea water, however, may draw additional fluid from the plasma into the alveoli, thereby causing pulmonary edema despite a decreased intravascular volume [38]. The fluid-filled alveoli are then unavailable for efficient gas transfer, and a ventilation-perfusion mismatch occurs and causes hypoxemia. This fluid may also damage the type II pneumocytes by hypoxic and osmotic effects [40]. Particulate matter in the aspirate may combine with these effects to damage the alveolar membrane and lead to ARDS.

Several other mechanisms of lung injury may occur with near-drowning. Bacterial pneumonia, barotrauma, mechanical damage from cardiopulmonary resuscitation (CPR), chemical pneumonitis, centrally mediated apnea, and oxygen toxicity can cause respiratory deterioration in the postresuscitation period [40]. These must be considered along with noncardiogenic pulmonary edema in cases of respiratory distress occurring 1 to 48 hours after the near-drowning event.

NEUROLOGIC EFFECTS. The pathologic effects that most affect prognosis in near-drowning are related to the CNS. Cerebral injury is produced as a result of anoxia due to gas exchange impairment and subsequent cardiopulmonary arrest.

Anoxic damage begins 4 to 10 minutes after cessation of cerebral blood flow in most situations [43]. The time course of anoxia in near-drowning is uncertain, for several reasons. First, the duration of submersion is often unclear because of the emotional condition of the witnesses [44]. Second, although the diving reflex sometimes may act to slow the heart rate and shunt blood preferentially to the heart and brain and thereby protect the most oxygen-sensitive structures, the importance of this reflex in humans has been cast in doubt [45,46]. Third, hypothermia may also have a direct protective effect on cerebral tissue. This may be particularly effective in children, whose relatively large surface area and small layer of insulating fat predispose them to rapid cooling. Several case studies report neurologic recovery after submersion in cold water even up to 66 minutes [30,32,47,48]. Rapid onset of hypothermia may protect the brain by slowing biochemical reactions that require oxygen. The protective effect is limited by the frequent induction of fatal dysrhythmias when core temperature drops below 28°C.

Despite these factors, many near-drowning victims suffer neurologic impairment. Victims of near-drowning display pathologic features similar to those of patients with anoxic encephalopathy from other causes. Macroscopic changes can include diffuse cerebral edema as well as focal areas of necrosis. Early histologic changes consist of mitochondrial swelling and ischemic changes with altered staining characteristics [49]. These changes occur primarily in the cerebral cortex, hippocampus, and cerebellum.

In a series of 30 consecutive cases of near-drowning, Conn et al. [44] reported 9 cases of permanent brain damage and 1 death. Although Modell and coauthors [29] found a much lower rate of residual neurologic damage in survivors, all of their patients who presented with fixed, dilated pupils and coma eventually died. In another study, all children who required cardiotonic drugs to restore a perfusing rhythm suffered poor neurologic outcomes [50]. Only patients who present with hypothermia seem occasionally to survive intact [51]. Severe anoxic encephalopathy with persistent coma, seizures, delayed language development, spastic quadriplegia, aphasia, and cortical blindness have been reported as sequelae of immersion accidents [28,30,52–55]. Prognosis is probably related to the time needed to reestablish a perfusing rhythm [50].

MUSCULOSKELETAL EFFECTS. Children who develop anoxic encephalopathy due to near-drowning frequently develop musculoskeletal problems [56]. These problems result from spasticity, which appears to be more aggressive in these children than in those with other forms of spastic disorder. The most common of these are lower extremity contractures, hip subluxation or dislocation, and scoliosis [56].

SERUM ELECTROLYTES. The effects of aspirating large quantities of hypotonic or hypertonic fluid have traditionally been emphasized as a cause of serum electrolyte changes and a potential cause of death. Although differing effects of aspirating large volumes of fresh water and sea water in animals can be demonstrated experimentally, the actual clinical effect of electrolyte changes is minimal [29,57,58,59]. Humans rarely aspirate enough fluid to cause most of the serious changes seen in experimental situations [59]. In addition, the body may rapidly correct the electrolyte changes that do occur, making medical therapy of them unnecessary.

HEMATOLOGIC EFFECTS. Near normal hemoglobin values and hematocrits have been demonstrated in patients who nearly drowned in either sea water or fresh water [28,29,60]. This refutes the previously held assumption that freshwater near-drowning causes clinically significant hemolysis whereas saltwater aspiration causes hemoconcentration [55,61].

Three cases of disseminated intravascular coagulation (DIC) complicating freshwater near-drowning have been described [62]. All three patients eventually died. Although the precipitating mechanisms are unclear, routine coagulation studies should probably be part of the initial and ongoing evaluation of the near-drowning victims.

Because polymorphonuclear leukocyte counts are significantly lower in patients treated with therapeutic hypothermia [63], cold water immersion may be associated with increased susceptibility to infection.

RENAL EFFECTS. Near-drowning can adversely affect the kidneys. Acute tubular necrosis, hemoglobinuria, and albuminuria all have been reported as consequences of submersion accidents [55,61,64,65]. Diuresis may occur as a result of changes in renal tubular function due to hypothermia [66]. Near-drowning victims also frequently present with metabolic acidosis as a result of lactate accumulation. In general, the pathologic effects seen in the kidney are the secondary result of anoxia and hypothermia.

CARDIAC EFFECTS. Hypoxia and hypothermia can induce dysrhythmias in near-drowning victims. Atrial fibrillation and sinus dysrhythmias are most common but rarely require therapy [67]. P–R, QRS, and Q–T interval prolongations as well as J point elevation (Osborn wave) can be seen as in other causes of hypothermia [68,69]. More severe cases may result in death due to ventricular fibrillation or asystole. Autopsy studies of drowned patients demonstrate focal myocardial necrosis that may be similar to findings in pheochromocytoma and other situations of high adrenergic output [70,71]. These areas of necrosis may provide an ectopic focus or induce a malignant reentry syndrome.

Near-drowning can also have an effect on hemodynamics. Orlowski and co-workers found transient increases in central venous and pulmonary capillary wedge pressures following experimental near-drowning [72]. In addition there was a persistent decrease in cardiac output, which lasted more than 4 hours. These findings were independent of the tonicity of the solutions used and no different from those of anoxic controls. It is therefore postulated that the hemodynamic effects of near-drowning are the result of induced anoxia.

Diagnosis and Clinical Presentation

The diagnosis of near-drowning is usually obvious from the clinical presentation.

HISTORY. Although it is often impossible to take a detailed history, minimum background information to be obtained includes the patient's age, underlying cardiac, respiratory, or neurologic diseases, and medications used. It is also important to determine the activities precipitating the immersion, such as boating, diving, and ingestion of drugs or alcohol; the duration of submersion; and the temperature and type of water in which it occurred.

PHYSICAL EXAMINATION. Initial physical examination is often hurried, with more detailed assessment delayed until resuscitative efforts have been established. Tachypnea has been described as the most frequent physical finding, and tachycardia is also common [28,60]. Patients may also be apneic and pulseless. Hypothermia is common and depends on the temperature of the water and duration of submersion. When there is hypothermia, resuscitation efforts must not be discontinued until the patient is adequately rewarmed. It is important that an appropriate thermometer, such as a flexible probe or telethermometer, be used; standard thermometers record only to 34.4°C and can underestimate the degree of hypothermia, which could cause caregivers to abandon their efforts prematurely. Other physical findings include fever and signs of pulmonary edema [28,65]. Any physical findings seen in cases of cerebral anoxia or severe hypothermia also may be seen in near-drowning. In addition to revealing the consequences of hypoxia/anoxia and hypothermia, the major importance of the physical examination

is to uncover coexisting injuries that may have caused or resulted from the immersion.

A simple classification scale has been developed to guide the initial neurologic assessment of patients who have nearly drowned [73]. Modell and Conn adapted commonly used triage classifications of near-drowning victims for formal prognostic use. Category A describes patients who are fully alert within 1 hour of presentation to the emergency department. These patients uniformly do well neurologically. Category B includes patients who are obtunded and stuporous but arousable at the time of evaluation. Eighty-nine to 100 percent of these patients survive, and severe permanent neurologic deficit was not seen in any of these patients in two studies [74,75]. Category C involves patients who are comatose with abnormal respirations and abnormal response to pain. These patients have a much higher mortality, and survivors, particularly children, have a higher rate of neurologic dysfunction. A great deal of research has been done on methods of improving neurologic recovery in category C patients by reducing intracranial pressure and cerebral metabolism [44,76,77]. This is discussed later in this chapter.

LABORATORY STUDIES. Hemoglobin, hematocrit, and serum electrolytes are usually normal on arrival in the emergency department whether the near-drowning occurred in fresh water or salt water [78]. Arterial blood gas analysis frequently shows metabolic acidosis and hypoxemia. The blood alcohol level, PT, PTT, serum creatinine, urinalysis, and drug screen should also be obtained to help determine the cause of the accident and assess for complications of near-drowning. Cervical spine films should be performed whenever there is evidence of trauma [79]. An electrocardiogram (ECG) should be obtained and continuous monitoring performed whenever there is a significant chance of dysrhythmia.

Up to 20 percent of initial chest radiographs in near-drowning victims are normal [29,60,80,81,82]. The remainder show evidence of varying degrees of pulmonary edema. Two patterns are commonly seen in these films. Whereas many display confluent alveolar densities, primarily in the perihilar regions, others exhibit a diffuse, almost homogeneous nodular pattern bilaterally.

One to 48 hours after the event the patient may develop ARDS [40,81]. Most patients display clearing on chest radiographs within 5 to 6 days, but some radiographs performed at this point reflect the delayed complications of near-drowning (e.g., localized consolidations, pneumothorax, interstitial fibrosis) [83].

Therapy

All near-drowning patients should be admitted to the hospital for 24 to 48 hours to be observed for the development of respiratory distress [29,40,84]. Patients who show no evidence of hypoxemia or neurologic compromise can then be discharged with careful follow-up. Treatment of the others should be approached in the following four phases.

INITIAL RESUSCITATION. Resuscitation of apneic or pulseless near-drowning victims should be initiated immediately. Mouth-to-mouth resuscitation must be begun in the water and not delayed until the victim is brought to shore [79,85,86]. The rescuer should carefully support the victim's neck to prevent exacerbation of undiagnosed vertebral injuries. Full CPR with chest compressions should begin immediately on arrival on shore and proceed according to standard guidelines [87]. Although the Heimlich maneuver has been advocated as a method of removing water from the airways of nearly drowned patients to facilitate external respiration, it should be used only when a foreign body is obstructing the airway [79,85,88,89,90]. Subdiaphragmatic pressure can cause chest trauma and aspiration of gastric contents.

Resuscitation must be continued in victims of cold water submersion at least until the patient has been rewarmed. Core temperature should be obtained immediately on arrival at the emergency department and monitored carefully during the first several hours. All near-drowning victims with cardiopulmonary arrest and hypothermia should be rewarmed as aggressively as possible. In the field, passive external rewarming or inhalation of heated oxygen is commonly used [91,92]. In the hospital, cardiopulmonary bypass should be used in cases of severe hypothermia from near-drowning, especially with circulatory collapse [30,92–96]. This method has the advantage of rapidly and directly rewarming the core. It can also correct the metabolic acidosis that commonly occurs. The disadvantage is that it requires highly specialized equipment that may be unavailable. When this technique is not possible, rewarming with warmed peritoneal lavage, hemodialysis, or heated oxygen can be attempted. (See Chapter 72 for an in-depth discussion of rewarming techniques.)

A more difficult question is when and how long to resuscitate victims of warm water submersion. Although the need for cardiotonic medications to restore pulse is uniformly associated with a poor outcome in children, the decision to terminate resuscitation must be based on a variety of factors particular to the individual case until more information is available [50].

THERAPY OF THE UNDERLYING CAUSE. Serum alcohol levels and a drug screen can detect potential intoxicants and prompt administration of necessary antidotes or other measures. Anticonvulsant levels can help tailor therapy in known epileptic patients. If there is any question of possible head or neck trauma, the neck should be immobilized in a brace until cervical spine films are available. Hypoglycemia and severe electrolyte abnormalities can be detected on routine serum testing and corrected rapidly in the emergency department.

TREATMENT OF RESPIRATORY AND OTHER ORGAN FAILURE. The pathophysiologic changes caused by near-drowning have been described. The main treatment issue involves the management of noncardiogenic pulmonary edema and related complications.

The initial management of all pulmonary edema states involves monitoring PaO_2 and providing appropriate supplemental oxygen. Mechanical ventilation with positive end-expiratory pressure (PEEP) should be instituted if refractory hypoxic or hypercapnic respiratory failure develops [29,40, 50,78,97,98]. (See Chapter 66 on mechanical ventilation for details.) Because controlled studies have not demonstrated benefit from their use in ARDS, intravenous steroids should be used only if there are other specific indications [99,100]. Diuretics may be beneficial to keep the lungs "dry," but their use must be determined by the patient's volume status. (See Chapter 55 for an in-depth discussion of the treatment of ARDS.) Although the incidence of lobar pneumonia after near-drowning is substantial, no evidence suggests a reduction with routine use of prophylactic antibiotics. Therefore, we limit the use of antibiotics to cases in which the clinical suspicion of infection is particularly high.

Treatment of other end-organ damage must be approached systematically. Serum electrolytes tend to be normal and rarely require therapy. The treatment of renal failure in near-drowning focuses on optimizing fluid status and renal blood flow. This can be difficult to achieve on a clinical basis, often requiring placement of a pulmonary artery catheter. Severe cases may require temporary dialysis. Lactic acidosis should be corrected by restoration of adequate ventilation and circulation.

Clinically significant hematologic effects are limited to leukopenia and DIC. Leukopenia exists in this context only as a complication of hypothermia used for cerebral protection and should therefore not occur if this treatment is not used (see below). The treatment of DIC is addressed in Chapter 118.

The cardiac dysrhythmogenic effects of hypothermia are corrected by rewarming. Sinus and atrial dysrhythmias as well as most interval prolongations rarely require additional therapy [67]. For a discussion of the treatment of hypothermia-related malignant ventricular dysrhythmias, see Chapter 72.

Musculoskeletal complications of near-drowning are treated in standard fashion. Contractures are treated with casts or splints; subluxed or dislocated hips can be approached with various operative procedures; and scoliosis is treated with bracing or spinal instrumentation [56]. The relative success of these interventions in this population is unclear.

NEUROLOGIC SALVAGE. Patients in Modell and Conn's categories A and B regain neurologic function almost uniformly if they do not die of an unrelated complication. Previous work on the resuscitation of category C (comatose) patients focused on the reduction of intracranial pressure and cerebral metabolism. Conn et al. [44,75,101] once advocated an aggressive treatment protocol for comatose near-drowning patients, but various components have not been found to be effective. Their protocol involved sedation with barbiturates, intracranial pressure monitoring, external cooling, muscle paralysis, hyperventilation, and forced diuresis. Barbiturates failed to show a benefit in multiple studies [63,76,102]. Intracranial pressure monitoring has similarly failed to show any improvement in neurologic outcome among comatose near-drowning victims [103]. Therapeutic hypothermia has no clear role in the treatment of near-drowning and may decrease neutrophil number and function, predisposing the patient to infection [63]. Muscle paralysis occasionally improves ventilation and oxygenation but must be addressed on a case-by-case basis. Hyperventilation is an effective and readily reversible means of decreasing intracranial pressure temporarily by decreasing cerebral blood flow, but its clinical value is unproved [77]. Forced diuresis can decrease cardiac output and therefore decrease cerebral blood flow, but its value also has not been shown.

On the basis of this information, maintaining adequate oxygenation and cerebral blood flow are the central foci of appropriate therapy for comatose victims of near-drowning [77]. Therefore, measures such as effective mechanical ventilation, vasopressors, and hemodynamic monitoring with careful fluid management assume primary importance. Decisions on fluid management must be made based on the individual patient's volume status. Hypothermic patients must be warmed to near-normal core temperature. Seizures should be treated with phenytoin or phenobarbital as required. Further advances in restorative therapy for damaged neurons must be made before specific effective therapy for cerebral salvage can be developed [77]. Until then, the responsibility of the intensive care physician is to provide effective resuscitative and supportive care for victims of near-drowning.

Summary

The course of the postimmersion syndrome, or near-drowning, is variable. The 10 to 15 percent of victims who do not aspirate because of submersion laryngospasm or loss of spontaneous ventilation and who survive because of prompt CPR have dramatic and complete recoveries. On the other hand, patients who aspirate fresh water or sea water may exhibit ARDS after resuscitation. Only about 11 percent of those who nearly drown and are brought to the hospital for treatment die [29]. Because ARDS may not become clinically apparent for hours, all near-drowning victims should be hospitalized and observed for 24 to 48 hours. Although freshwater and seawater near-drownings cause different clinical pictures in animals, they cannot be distinguished in humans, with the possible exception of DIC, which has been reported only in freshwater submersion. In general, patients who aspirate water present with hypoxemia and metabolic acidosis. They usually do not aspirate enough fluid to produce changes in blood volume, electrolytes, hemoglobin, and hematocrit sufficient to be life-threatening. Although prolonged neurologic deficits may exist after resuscitation, patients submerged in cold water for up to 66 minutes may recover fully.

Treatment varies with the severity of the illness. Initial hospital treatment for patients with no or minimal hypoxemia involves observation. Therapy for patients with severe hypoxemia includes institution of all the supportive modalities used in ARDS. Abnormalities of multiple organ systems—most commonly metabolic acidosis—should be addressed immediately. In hypothermic patients, rewarming methods should be instituted immediately also. These include removing wet clothing, covering with warm blankets, infusing warm fluids (37–38°C) intravenously, and performing gastrointestinal irrigation with warm fluids. If the patient's temperature is less than 32°C, core rewarming may be most easily accomplished by cardiopulmonary bypass or peritoneal dialysis with a potassium-free dialysate warmed to 54°C. Neither prophylactic antibiotic therapy nor corticosteroid administration has shown to be helpful.

References

1. Modell JH: Drown versus near-drown: A discussion of definitions. *Crit Care Med* 9:351, 1981.
2. National Safety Council: *Accident Facts,* 1992 edition. Itasca, IL, 1992.
3. Baker SP, O'Neil B, Ginsburg MJ, Li G: *The Injury Fact Book.* New York, Oxford, 1992.
4. Gulaid JA, Sattin RW: Drownings in the United States, 1978–1984. *MMWR* 37:27, 1988.
5. Wintemute GJ, Kraus JF, Teret SP, et al: The epidemiology of drowning in adulthood: Implications for prevention. *Am J Prev Med* 4:343, 1988.
6. Schuman SH, Rowe JR, Glazer HM, et al: The iceberg phenomenon of near-drowning. *Crit Care Med* 4:127, 1976.
7. Pearn JH: Epilepsy and drowning in childhood. *Br Med J* 1:1510, 1977.
8. Livingston S, Paul LL, Pruce I: Epilepsy and drowning in childhood. *Br Med J* 2:515, 1977.
9. Dietz PE, Baker S: Drowning. *Am J Public Health* 64:303, 1974.
10. Aquatic deaths and injuries: United States. *MMWR* 31:417, 1982.
11. Davis S, Ledman J, Kilgore J: Drownings of children and youth in a desert state. *West J Med* 143:196, 1985.
12. Craig AB: Underwater swimming and loss of consciousness. *JAMA* 176:255, 1961.
13. Craig AB: Causes of loss of consciousness during underwater swimming. *J Appl Physiol* 16:583, 1961.
14. Pearn JH, Brown J, Wong R, et al: Bathtub drownings: Report of seven cases. *Pediatrics* 64:68, 1979.
15. Budnick LD, Ross DA: Bathtub-related drownings in the United States, 1979–81. *Am J Public Health* 75:630, 1985.
16. Wintemute GJ, Kraus JF, Teret SP, et al: Drowning in childhood and adolescence: A population-based study. *Am J Public Health* 77:830, 1987.
17. O'Carroll PW, Alkon E, Weiss B: Drowning mortality in Los Angeles County, 1976–1984. *JAMA* 260:380, 1988.
18. Pearn JH, Thompson J: Drowning and near-drowning in the Australian Capital Territory: A five-year total population study of immersion accidents. *Med J Aust* 1:130, 1988.
19. Pearn J, Wong RYK, Brown J: Drowning and near-drowning involving children: A 5-year total population study from the city and county of Honolulu. *Am J Public Health* 69:450, 1979.
20. Manolios N, Mackie I: Drowning and near-drowning on Australian beaches patrolled by life-savers: A 10-year study, 1973–1983. *Med J Aust* 148:165, 1988.
21. Pearn J: Drowning, the sea and life-savers: A clinical audit. *Med J Aust* 148:164, 1988.
22. Quan L, Gore EJ, Wentz K, et al: Ten-year study of pediatric drownings and near-drownings in Kings County, Washington: Lessons in injury prevention. *Pediatrics* 83:1035, 1989.
23. Livingston S, Pauli LL, Pruce I, et al: Drowning in epilepsy. *Ann Neurol* 7:495, 1980.
24. Jumbelic MI, Chambliss M: Accidental toddler drowning in 5-gallon buckets. *JAMA* 263:1952, 1990.
25. Plueckhahn VD: Alcohol and accidental drowning: A 25-year study. *Med J Aust* 141:22, 1984.
26. Martin TG: Near-drowning and cold water immersion. *Ann Emerg Med* 13:263, 1984.
27. Pearn J: Pathophysiology of drowning. *Med J Aust* 142:586, 1985.
28. Fandel I, Bancalari E: Near-drowning in children: Clinical aspects. *Pediatrics* 58:573, 1976.
29. Modell JH, Graves SA, Ketover A: Clinical course of 91 consecutive near-drowning victims. *Chest* 70:231, 1976.
30. Bolte RG, Black PG, Bowers RS, et al: The use of extracorporeal rewarming in a child submerged for 66 minutes. *JAMA* 260:377, 1988.
31. Hervey GR: The physiology of cold/wet survival. *J R Nav Med Serv* 58:161, 1972.
32. Sekar TS, Macdonnell KF, Namsirikul P, et al: Survival after prolonged submersion in cold water without neurologic sequelae. *Arch Intern Med* 140:775, 1980.
33. Reuler JB: Hypothermia: Pathophysiology, clinical settings, and management. *Ann Intern Med* 89:519, 1978.
34. Keatinge WR: The effect of work and clothing on the maintenance of the body temperature in water. *Q J Exp Physiol* 46:69, 1961.
35. Pugh LGC: The physiology of channel swimmers. *Lancet* 2:761, 1955.
36. Goode RC, Duffin J, Miller R, et al: Sudden cold water immersion. *Respir Physiol* 23:301, 1975.
37. Hegnauer AH, Angelakos ET: Excitable properties of the hypothermic heart. *Ann N Y Acad Sci* 80:336, 1959.
38. Orlowski JP, Abulliel MM, Phillips JM: Effects of tonicities of saline solutions on pulmonary injury in drowning. *Crit Care Med* 15:126, 1987.
39. Halmagyi DFJ, Colebatch HJH: Ventilation and circulation after fluid aspiration. *J Appl Physiol* 116:35, 1961.
40. Pearn JH: Secondary drowning in children. *Br Med J* 281:1103, 1980.
41. Giammona ST, Modell JH: Drowning by total immersion: Effects on pulmonary surfactant of distilled water, isotonic saline, and sea water. *Am J Dis Child* 114:612, 1967.
42. Modell JH, Calderwood HW, Ruiz BC, et al: Effects of ventilatory patterns on arterial oxygenation after near-drowning in sea water. *Anesthesiology* 40:376, 1974.
43. Peterson B: Morbidity of childhood near-drowning. *Pediatrics* 59:364, 1977.
44. Conn AW, Edmonds JF, Barker GA: Cerebral resuscitation in near-drowning. *Pediatr Clin North Am* 26:691, 1979.
45. Gooden BA: Drowning and the diving reflex in man. *Med J Aust* 2:583, 1972.
46. Ramey CA, Ramey DN, Hayward JS: Dive response of children in

relation to cold water near-drowning. *J Appl Physiol* 63:665, 1987.

47. Young RSK, Zalneraitis EL, Dooling EC: Neurologic outcome in cold water drowning. *JAMA* 244:1233, 1980.

48. Fritz KW, Kasperczyk W, Galaske R: Successful resuscitation in accidental hypothermia after drowning. *Anaesthetist* 37:331, 1988.

49. Griggs RC, Satran R: Metabolic encephalopathy, in Rosenberg RN (ed): *The Clinical Neurosciences.* New York, Churchill Livingstone, 1983.

50. Nichter MA, Everett PB: Childhood near-drowning: Is cardiopulmonary resuscitation always indicated? *Crit Care Med* 17:993, 1989.

51. Biggart MJ, Bohn DJ: Effect of hypothermia and cardiac arrest on outcome of near-drowning accidents in children. *J Pediatr* 117:179, 1990.

52. Reilly K, Ozanne A, Murdoch BE, et al: Linguistic status subsequent to childhood immersion injury. *Med J Aust* 148:225, 1988.

53. Sibert JR, Webb E, Cooper S: Drowning and near-drowning in children. *Practitioner* 232:439, 1988.

54. King RB, Webster IW: A case of recovery from drowning and prolonged anoxia. *Med J Aust* 1:919, 1964.

55. Kvittingen TD, Naess A: Recovery from drowning in fresh water. *Br Med J* 1:1315, 1963.

56. Abrams RA, Mubarak S: Musculoskeletal consequences of near-drowning in children. *J Pediatr Orthop* 11:168, 1991.

57. Modell JH, Weibly TC, Ruiz BC, et al: Serum electrolyte concentrations after freshwater aspiration: A comparison of species. *Anesthesiology* 30:421, 1969.

58. Modell JH, Moya F, Newby EJ, et al: The effects of fluid volume in seawater drowning. *Ann Intern Med* 67:68, 1967.

59. Modell JH, Davis JH: Electrolyte changes in human drowning victims. *Anesthesiology* 30:414, 1969.

60. Hasan S, Avery WG, Fabian C, et al: Near-drowning in humans: A report of 36 patients. *Chest* 59:191, 1971.

61. Munroe WD: Hemoglobinuria from near-drowning. *J Pediatr* 64:57, 1964.

62. Ports TA, Deuel TF: Intravascular coagulation in fresh-water submersion: Report of three cases. *Ann Intern Med* 87:60, 1977.

63. Bohn DJ, Biggar WD, Smith CR, et al: Influence of hypothermia, barbiturate therapy, and intracranial pressure monitoring on morbidity and mortality after near-drowning. *Crit Care Med* 14:529, 1986.

64. Grausz H, Amend WJC, Earley LE: Acute renal failure complicating submersion in seawater. *JAMA* 217:207, 1971.

65. Fuller RH: The clinical pathology of near-drowning. *Proc R Soc Med* 56:33, 1963.

66. Segar WE, Riley PA, Barila TG: Urinary composition during hypothermia. *Am J Physiol* 185:528, 1956.

67. Gunton RW, Scott JW, Lougheed WM, et al: Changes in cardiac rhythm in the form of the electrocardiogram resulting from induced hypothermia in man. *Am Heart J* 52:419, 1956.

68. Trevino A, Razi B, Beller BM: The characteristic electrocardiogram of accidental hypothermia. *Arch Intern Med* 127:470, 1971.

69. Vandam LD, Burnap TK: Hypothermia. *N Engl J Med* 261:546, 1959.

70. Karch SB: Pathology of the heart in drowning. *Arch Pathol Lab Med* 109:176, 1985.

71. Lunt DWR, Rose AG: Pathology of the heart in drowning. *Arch Pathol Lab Med* 111:939, 1987.

72. Orlowski JP, Abulleil MM, Phillips JM: The hemodynamic and cardiovascular effects of near-drowning in hypotonic, isotonic, hypertonic solutions. *Ann Emerg Med* 18:1044,1989.

73. Modell JH, Conn AW: Current neurological considerations in near-drowning. *Can Anaesth Soc J* 3:197, 1980.

74. Modell JH, Graves SA, Kuck EJ: Near-drowning: Correlation of level of consciousness and survival. *Can Anaesth Soc J* 27:211, 1980.

75. Conn AW, Montes JE, Barker GA, et al: Cerebral salvage in near-drowning following neurological classification by triage. *Can Anaesth Soc J* 27:201, 1980.

76. Nussbaum E, Maggi JC: Pentobarbital therapy does not improve neurologic outcome in nearly drowned, flaccid-comatose children. *Pediatrics* 81:630, 1988.

77. Modell JH: Treatment of near-drowning: Is there a role for H.Y.P.E.R. therapy? *Crit Care Med* 14:593, 1986.

78. Sirik Z, Lev A, Ruach M, et al: Freshwater near-drowning: Our experience in life-supportive treatment. *Israel J Med Sci* 20:523, 1984.

79. Kizer KW: Resuscitation of submersion casualties. *Emerg Med Clin North Am* 1:643, 1983.

80. Wunderlich P, Rupprecht E, Trefftz F, et al: Chest radiographs of near-drowned children. *Pediatr Radiol* 15:297, 1985.

81. Hunter TB, Whitehouse WM: Fresh-water near-drowning: Radiologic aspects. *Radiology* 112:51, 1974.

82. Rosenbaum HT, Thompson WL, Fuller RH: Radiographic pulmonary changes in near-drowning. *Radiology* 83:306, 1964.

83. Glauser FL, Smith WR: Pulmonary interstitial fibrosis following near-drowning and exposure to short-term high oxygen concentrations. *Chest* 68:373, 1975.

84. Simcock AD: Treatment of near-drowning: A review of 130 cases. *Anaesthesia* 41:643, 1986.

85. Ornato JP: The resuscitation of near-drowning victims. *JAMA* 256:75, 1986.

86. Orlowski JP: Drowning, near-drowning, and ice-water submersions. *Pediatr Clin North Am* 34:75, 1987.

87. American Heart Association: *Textbook of Advanced Cardiac Life Support.* Dallas, American Heart Association, 1987.

88. Heimlich HJ: Subdiaphragmatic pressure to expel water from the lungs of drowning persons. *Ann Emerg Med* 10:476, 1981.

89. Ruben A, Ruben H: Artificial respiration: Flow of water from the lung and the stomach. *Lancet* 1:780, 1962.

90. Ornato JP: The Heimlich maneuver and the resuscitation of near-drowning victims (letter). *JAMA* 256:2960, 1986.

91. Hayward JS, Steinman AM: Accidental hypothermia: An experimental study of inhalation rewarming. *Aviat Space Environ Med* 46:1236, 1975.

92. Wickstrom P, Ruiz E, Lilja GP, et al: Accidental hypothermia: Core rewarming with partial bypass. *Am J Surg* 131:622, 1976.

93. Kugelberg J, Schuller H, Berg B, et al: Treatment of accidental hypothermia. *Scand J Cardiovasc Surg* 1:142, 1967.

94. Towne WD, Geiss P, Yanes HO, et al: Intractable ventricular fibrillation associated with profound accidental hypothermia: Successful treatment with cardiopulmonary bypass. *N Engl J Med* 287:1135, 1972.

95. Truscott DG, Firor WB, Clein LJ: Accidental profound hypothermia: Successful resuscitation by core rewarming and assisted circulation. *Arch Surg* 106:216, 1973.

96. Husby P, Anderson KS, Owen-Falkenberg A, et al: Accidental hypothermia with cardiac arrest: Complete recovery after prolonged resuscitation and rewarming by extracorporeal circulation. *Intensive Care Med* 16:69,1990.

97. van Heringen JR, Blokzijl EJ, van Dyl W, et al: Treatment of the respiratory distress syndrome following nondirect pulmonary trauma with positive end expiratory pressure with special emphasis on near-drowning. *Chest* 66(suppl):30S, 1979.

98. Rutledge RR, Flor RJ: The use of mechanical ventilation with positive end-expiratory pressure in the treatment of near-drowning. *Anesthesiology* 38:194, 1973.

99. Calderwood HW, Modell JH, Ruiz BC: The ineffectiveness of steroid therapy for treatment of freshwater near-drowning. *Anesthesiology* 43:642, 1975.

100. Bernard GR, Luce JM, Sprung CL, et al: High dose corticosteroids in patients with the adult respiratory distress syndrome. *N Engl J Med* 317:1565, 1987.

101. Conn AW, Edmonds JF, Barker GA: Near-drowning in cold fresh water: Current treatment regimens. *Can Anaesth Soc J* 25:259, 1978.

102. Rockoff MA, Marshall LF, Shapiro HM: High-dose barbiturate therapy in humans: A clinical review of 60 patients. *Ann Neurol* 6:194, 1979.

103. Dean JM, McComb JG: Intracranial pressure monitoring in severe pediatric near-drowning. *Neurosurgery* 9:627, 1981.

64. Pulmonary Hypertension

Lewis J. Rubin

The pulmonary circulation has four major functions: (1) it provides a means for effective gas exchange between air and blood (external respiration); (2) it serves as a filter for particulates in the systemic venous system; (3) it plays a role in the synthesis and degradation of a variety of biologically active substances; and (4) as the bridge between the two sides of the heart, it serves as a reservoir of blood for the left ventricle. This chapter is concerned with pulmonary hypertension, an abnormality of the reservoir function of the pulmonary circulation. Pulmonary hypertension is considered to be present when mean pulmonary artery pressure exceeds 25 mm Hg at rest or 35 mm Hg during exercise. *Cor pulmonale,* a term that is often equated with right heart failure, is most accurately used to describe the presence of pulmonary hypertension in the setting of parenchymal lung disease. Cor pulmonale can be an acute process, as in the acute respiratory distress syndrome (ARDS), or during exacerbations of long-standing lung disease, or chronic, as a complicating factor in chronic obstructive or restrictive lung diseases.

Etiology

The causes of pulmonary hypertension can be grouped into three major pathophysiologic categories (Table 64-1). Pulmonary artery hypertension may be passive, due to postcapillary pressure elevations; active, due to the constriction or obstruction of capillary and precapillary vessels, resulting in increased resistance to flow; and reactive, in which pulmonary hypertension is initially passive but the upstream pulmonary vasculature responds to chronic passive congestion by developing an active-superimposed-on-passive component.

Pathogenesis

ANATOMIC CONSIDERATIONS. The pulmonary circulation begins at the main pulmonary artery and ends where the four main pulmonary veins enter the left atrium. It has a pump (the right ventricle), a system of conduit arteries and arterioles, mechanisms by which it can transfer substances between air and blood (blood-air barrier), and a collecting system of veins and venules. This system is unique among regional circulations: It is the only one that accepts the equivalent of the entire cardiac output, and does so at a pressure which is a fraction of that in the systemic circulation (Fig. 64-1).

The pulmonary circulation possesses several unique structural characteristics: (1) The pulmonary arteries have more elastic tissue and less muscle than systemic arteries of equivalent size [1]; (2) the precapillary arterioles (vessels in the systemic circulation that probably determine systemic blood pressure) and small veins are almost devoid of smooth muscle [1]; (3) veins and venules have no valves [1]; and (4) the rich peripheral nervous system supplying the circulation [2] appears to play a relatively small role in controlling resistance, flow, and pressure [3,4]. For all these reasons, the normal pulmonary circulation can accommodate large volumes of blood with a remarkably low vascular resistance.

Biophysical Considerations. The central function of any circulation is to supply sufficient blood to meet the demands of the peripheral tissues. The pulmonary circulation must do this and also return blood to the left ventricle. By applying Ohm's law and the Poiseuille-Hagan formula to the pulmonary circulation, it is possible not only to understand its blood flow and pressure characteristics but also to appreciate its remarkable distensibility.

Ohm's law (Equation 1) can be applied to the study of fluids (Equation 2), since current is equivalent to flow and electromotive force is equivalent to pressure.

$$\text{Current} = \frac{\text{Electromotive force}}{\text{Resistance}} \tag{1}$$

$$\text{Flow} = \frac{\text{Pressure (P)}}{\text{Resistance (R)}} \tag{2}$$

Ohm's law theoretically can be applied to the study of the pulmonary circulation (Equation 3), since flow equals the cardiac output of the right ventricle and pressure is a pressure differential (ΔP) that drives blood from the main pulmonary artery to the left atrium.

$$F = \frac{\Delta P}{R} \tag{3}$$

Table 64-1. Causes of Pulmonary Hypertension

1. Passive pulmonary hypertension [1,12]
   a. Left ventricular failure
   b. Mitral valve disease
   c. Congenital cardiac malformations (e.g., cor triatriatum)
   d. Congenital pulmonary vein stenosis
   e. Acquired obstruction of major pulmonary veins
   f. Left atrial myxoma or thrombus
2. Active pulmonary hypertension [5,15,20]
   a. Pulmonary embolism
   b. Schistosomiasis
   c. Primary pulmonary hypertension
   d. Congenital heart disease (Eisenmenger's reaction)
   e. Disorders of ventilation
   f. Collagen-vascular diseases
   g. Sickle hemoglobinopathies
   h. Portal hypertension
   i. Ingestion of drugs and herbal remedies
   j. Diffuse pulmonary vascular amyloidosis
   k. Pulmonary vasculitis
3. Reactive pulmonary hypertension [20]
   a. Mitral valve disease
   b. Other causes of pulmonary venous hypertension, including pulmonary veno-occlusive disease
   c. Pulmonary capillary hemangiomatosis
   d. Toxic oil syndrome due to rapeseed oil ingestion
   e. Eosinophilia-myalgia syndrome due to contaminated L-tryptophan ingestion

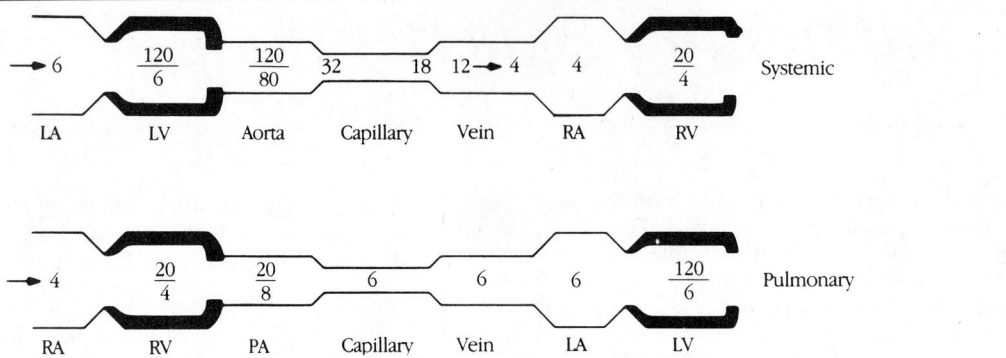

Fig. 64-1. Comparison of pressures (mm Hg) in systemic and pulmonary circulations. LA = left atrium; LV = left ventricle; RA = right atrium; RV = right ventricle; PA = pulmonary artery. (From Robin ED, Gaudio R: Cor pulmonale. *Disease a Month* May:6 1970. With permission.)

Although this modification of Ohm's law allows us to understand that flow to the tissues and left ventricle is determined by a driving pressure and resistance, it does not allow an appreciation of the complexity of the resistance factor. By applying the Poiseuille-Hagan formula to the pulmonary circulation and combining it with the hydraulic extrapolation of Ohm's law, it is possible to conceive of multiple factors that might affect the resistance to blood flow. The Poiseuille-Hagan formula (Equation 4) states that continuous, laminar flow through a rigid tube is influenced directly by a driving pressure ($P_A - P_B$), a geometric factor ($\pi/8$), and the radius of the tube (R^4), and inversely by a viscosity factor ($1/n$) of the fluid and the length of the tube (L).

$$F = (P_A - P_B) \times \pi/8 \times 1/n \times R^4/L \qquad (4)$$

Since $F = (P_A - P_B)/R$, Equation 4 can be substituted for F and resistance can be solved for (Equation 5):

$$R = \frac{8nL}{\pi R^4} \qquad (5)$$

It follows that resistance in the pulmonary circulation theoretically might be affected by the viscosity of the blood and the cross-sectional diameter of the vascular bed. (The length of the pulmonary circulation should not change.) Therefore, flow through the pulmonary circulation might be determined by pressure, viscosity, and cross-sectional diameter of the vascular bed.

The preceding biophysical considerations are useful in understanding what controls the overall behavior of the pulmonary circulation. However, these formulas cannot be applied directly for an accurate or reliable prediction of function in health or disease, since blood is not a perfect fluid, the pulmonary circulation is not a rigid tube, and flow is not necessarily laminar or continuous. This point can be emphasized in normal adults by increasing cardiac output and measuring pulmonary arterial pressure (Fig. 64-2); until cardiac output increases more than two and one-half fold, the pulmonary arterial pressure remains unchanged and resistance decreases [5]. Pressure remains unchanged due to both dilatation of the pulmonary vascular bed and the additional recruitment of previously closed vessels. Only when the pulmonary vascular bed has already been restricted, as in a patient with a pneumonectomy, does pulmonary artery pressure acutely rise concomitant with an increase in blood flow (Fig. 64-2) [5]. On the other hand, chronic increases in pulmonary blood flow may lead to pulmonary hypertension (see "Active" Pulmonary Hypertension) [6].

DETERMINANTS OF NORMAL PULMONARY VASCULAR PRESSURES. By performing cardiac catheterization, knowing the anatomy of the pulmonary circulation, and appreciating and applying the preceding biophysical considerations, it is possible to measure and understand the determinants of pulmonary vascular pressures. The following discussion considers only the overall behavior of the pulmonary circulation to allow clear exposition. It is not meant to imply that the entire pulmonary vasculature participates homogeneously.

Pulmonary artery end-diastolic pressure (PA_{ed}), measured in the main pulmonary artery, has been shown to be equal to the left atrial and left ventricular end-diastolic pressures, as long as the diastolic pressure in the left ventricle equals or exceeds 5 mm Hg [7]. When the left ventricular end-diastolic pressure is

Fig. 64-2. The relation between cardiac output (pulmonary blood flow) and mean pulmonary artery pressure. (From Robin ED, Gaudio R: Cor pulmonale. *Disease a Month* May:7 1970. With permission.)

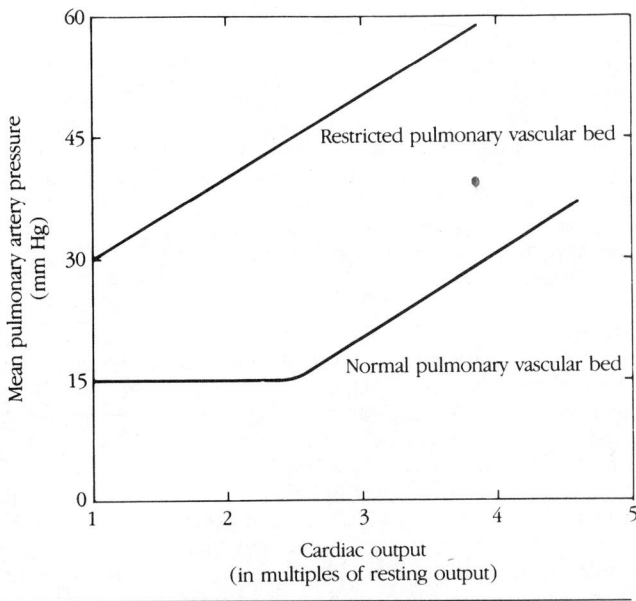

less than 5 mm Hg, pulmonary arterial pressure exceeds left ventricular end-diastolic pressure by a few millimeters of mercury [7]. Studies have suggested that this gradient represents the critical closing pressure of the pulmonary vasculature, since it can be abolished by increasing left atrial pressure [8]. Presumably, the increase in pulmonary blood volume associated with the increase in left atrial pressure increases the cross-sectional area of the pulmonary vascular bed by dilating existing vessels or opening previously closed ones. It is not surprising that PA_{ed} is equal to left ventricular end-diastolic pressure, because pulmonary blood flow is not appreciable at the end of diastole [9,10,11] and no structures during end diastole interrupt the stream of blood between the pulmonary artery and left ventricle. (The mitral valve is open; there are no valves in the pulmonary veins or venules; there is no smooth muscle in the precapillary arterioles; and there is little, if any, neural control over the circulation.) Consequently, PA_{ed} is determined by the volume of blood that distends the pulmonary vascular bed, and this volume is determined by the function of the right and left ventricles.

The pressure recorded from a catheter tip wedged in a distal pulmonary artery (pulmonary capillary wedge pressure; PCW) is also equal to left atrial and left ventricular end-diastolic pressures, because it does not allow any additional blood to flow into the wedged vessel that is still part of the continuous stream. Since PCW accurately reflects pulmonary venous pressure, it is possible to evaluate precapillary and capillary as well as post-capillary pressure events by passing a catheter through systemic veins into the right heart.

Pulmonary artery systolic and mean pressures are determined by the stroke volume of the right ventricle and the volume of blood already distending the elastic arteries at the end of diastole. This has been demonstrated by predicting mathematically what the systolic and mean pressures should be for given stroke volumes and diastolic pressures and then measuring by cardiac catheterization almost identical values [12].

The resistance to blood flow across the normal pulmonary circulation is very low. This can be appreciated in two ways. Calculated traditionally, pulmonary vascular resistance is approximately one-tenth of the resistance across the systemic vascular bed. Since mean pulmonary arterial pressure is approximately 15 mm Hg and mean left atrial pressure or PCW pressure is approximately 5 mm Hg, the pressure gradient across the normal pulmonary circulation is only about 10 mm Hg. Thus, a normal cardiac output of approximately 6 liters per minute flows from the right ventricle to the left atrium with a pressure drop of only 10 mm Hg, as opposed to a pressure drop in the systemic circulation, between the left ventricle and the right atrium, of approximately 100 mm Hg. In numbers, the pulmonary vascular resistance equals $(15 - 5)/6$, or about 1.7 mm Hg/L/min (approximately 100 dyne/sec/cm^{-5}). However, since pulmonary arterial mean pressure measurements reflect stroke volume—a ventricular function—pulmonary vascular resistance calculated in the traditional manner may not be the most sensitive indicator of intrinsic pulmonary vascular disease. The PA_{ed} to the mean atrial or PCW (PA_{ed}-PCW) gradient is another way of looking at pulmonary vascular resistance to flow [13]. Normally, as long as left atrial pressure equals or exceeds 5 mm Hg, there should be no gradient [13,14]. If there is active pulmonary vascular disease, as in chronic obstructive pulmonary disease (COPD), there is a gradient, with PA_{ed} greater than PCW [13]. If pulmonary hypertension is caused by passive congestion from left ventricular failure, PA_{ed} and PCW are both elevated but there is not a gradient [13].

Using the concept of a (PA_{ed}-PCW) gradient, it is possible to distinguish a postpulmonary capillary from a capillary or pre-pulmonary capillary origin of pulmonary hypertension and,

therefore, a "passive" from an "active" or "reactive" mechanism. The exception is pulmonary veno-occlusive disease (PVOD), in which pulmonary hypertension is due in large part to obliteration of the pulmonary venules and small veins but the pulmonary wedge pressure is usually normal. This is because the catheter tip in the wedged position will measure downstream reflected pressure in the larger veins, which drain blood from vascular beds that are not affected, while those beds that are affected "drop out" of the communication between the upstream and downstream vascular beds.

"PASSIVE" PULMONARY HYPERTENSION. Pulmonary hypertension may be due to elevation of PCW, which reflects postpulmonary capillary pressure (Table 64-1). The PA_{ed} rises passively due to the increased pulmonary blood volume (passive congestion) that can occur in left ventricular failure, mitral stenosis, cor triatriatum, and obstruction of the major pulmonary veins from mediastinitis. Since PA_{ed} and PCW are both elevated, the PA_{ed}-PCW gradient remains normal. Data from patients with mitral stenosis and left ventricular disease [3] support this.

"ACTIVE" PULMONARY HYPERTENSION. Pulmonary hypertension may be due to vasoconstriction and/or anatomic restriction in the total cross-sectional area of the pulmonary vascular bed. The restriction can be at precapillary or capillary sites. In active pulmonary hypertension, the PA_{ed}-PCW gradient is 5 mm Hg or greater and the PCW is within normal limits.

Diseases that commonly cause active pulmonary hypertension (Table 64-1) are pulmonary embolism [15,16,17]; schistosomiasis [18]; primary (idiopathic) pulmonary hypertension [19,20]; congenital heart lesions characterized initially by a left-to-right shunt, such as ventricular septal defect (VSD) [6,21], patent ductus arteriosus (PDA) [6,22], and secundum atrial septal defect (ASD) [6]; connective tissue diseases; and disorders of ventilation.

In pulmonary embolism, pulmonary hypertension occurs from mechanical obstruction of precapillary vessels due to thromboemboli and factors such as hypoxemia and the release of vasoactive substances [15]. In schistosomiasis, pulmonary hypertension may be caused by obstruction of embolized ova or allergic arteritis [1]. In primary pulmonary hypertension, pulmonary vascular resistance probably increases initially from an unknown vasospastic or vasoconstrictive tendency and subsequently from primary vascular injury ranging histologically from concentric intimal thickening and fibrosis and smooth muscle hypertrophy to plexiform lesions and arteritis with necrosis [20,23,24].

In patients with ventricular septal defect, patent ductus arteriosus, and secundum atrial septal defect, pulmonary vascular resistance increases due to intimal thickening and fibrosis and smooth muscle hypertrophy that presumably occurs in response to chronic increases in pulmonary blood flow from the left-to-right shunt [1]. Eventually, flow through these shunts becomes bidirectional or predominantly right-to-left, with resultant hypoxemia and polycythemia. The development of severe pulmonary hypertension with shunt reversal in patients with congenital cardiac defects is called Eisenmenger syndrome.

Pulmonary hypertension from ventilatory respiratory diseases can be caused by vasoconstriction of the pulmonary vascular bed, anatomic restriction of the pulmonary vascular bed, or a combination (Table 64-2).

The most potent and clinically important vasoconstrictive stimulus in chronic respiratory disease is alveolar hypoxia [25].

Table 64-2. Active Pulmonary Hypertension Due to Disorders of Ventilation

A. Vasoconstriction of the precapillary and capillary vascular bed
  1. Structurally normal pulmonary parenchyma and vascular bed [25,29]
    a. High-altitude pulmonary hypertension (residence >3000 m)
    b. Primary central hypoventilation
    c. Peripheral obstructive sleep apnea
    d. Obesity-hypoventilation syndrome
    e. Paralytic poliomyelitis
    f. Myasthenia gravis
  2. Pulmonary parenchymal disease [56]
    a. Chronic obstructive pulmonary disease
    b. Cystic fibrosis
B. Anatomic restriction of the pulmonary capillary vascular bed [31,54,55]
  1. Diffuse parenchymal lung disease*
    a. Sarcoidosis
    b. Progressive systemic sclerosis
    c. Idiopathic interstitial fibrosis
    d. Acute respiratory distress syndrome
  2. Extensive lung resection
  3. Extensive fibrothorax
C. Vasoconstriction plus anatomic restriction of the vascular bed [32,57]
  1. Kyphoscoliosis
  2. Chronic fibrotic tuberculosis

*Any disease that leads to diffuse interstitial fibrosis may be complicated by pulmonary hypertension.

Although the mechanism of hypoxic vasoconstriction is not well understood, it appears to be an intrinsic function of pulmonary vascular smooth muscle cells [26]. Alveolar hypoxia occurs in a number of different pulmonary diseases as a consequence of high altitude, alveolar hypoventilation alone (e.g., central hypoventilation, paralytic poliomyelitis), or ventilation-perfusion inequalities (e.g., COPD, cystic fibrosis). In addition, increases in plasma hydrogen ion concentration (acidemia) or carbon dioxide tension (hypercarbia) not only cause pulmonary vasoconstriction [27] but also augment the effect of alveolar hypoxia. High-altitude pulmonary hypertension is due to the hypoxic vasoconstrictive effects of chronic alveolar hypoxia and occurs in humans born and raised at high altitude. As long as these persons reside at altitudes above 3000 m, pulmonary hypertension remains sustained. It can be reversed on return to sea level, however, since alveolar hypoxia is no longer present [28,29].

Ventilatory diseases such as idiopathic interstitial fibrosis, sarcoidosis, progressive systemic sclerosis, and, rarely, extensive fibrothorax can cause pulmonary hypertension by anatomically restricting the pulmonary vascular bed [1]. These diseases replace, destroy, or compress vessels. Compression of the vasculature by hyperinflated lungs also may contribute to the development of pulmonary hypertension in patients with emphysema. Although pulmonary hypertension is virtually a universal feature of severe acute respiratory distress syndrome (ARDS) [30], the pathogenesis is unknown. The pathologic picture, however, is characterized by partial or complete disruption and even disappearance of much of the pulmonary vascular bed [31].

A combination of anatomic restriction and hypoxic vasoconstriction is involved in the pathogenesis of pulmonary hypertension in kyphoscoliosis [32] and long-standing fibrotic tuberculosis complicated by fibrothorax, thoracoplasty, or acute respiratory infection.

"REACTIVE" PULMONARY HYPERTENSION. Pulmonary hypertension may be due to a combination of passive and active mechanisms (Table 64-1). Although initially it is due to passive congestion, pulmonary artery pressures subsequently rise out of proportion to postcapillary pressures as passive congestion becomes chronic. In reactive pulmonary hypertension, the PA_{ed}-PCW gradient is 5 mm Hg or greater and PCW is greater than normal. Reactive pulmonary hypertension is most likely to occur in patients with mitral valvular disease, particularly mitral stenosis [21]. It is quite uncommon in patients with ventricular failure secondary to aortic valve disease, coronary heart disease, or systemic hypertension [21]. Reactive pulmonary hypertension also may be present in pulmonary veno-occlusive disease [33,34].

CONSEQUENCES OF PULMONARY HYPERTENSION. Pulmonary hypertension leads to hypertrophy and, ultimately, dilation of the right ventricle. As the right ventricle becomes unable to sustain normal contractile function faced with a markedly increased downstream vascular resistance, right heart failure—the most ominous prognostic finding of chronic pulmonary hypertension—ensues. Chronic pulmonary hypertension may also lead to life-threatening hemorrhage as the result of ruptured arteriosclerotic or aneurysmal pulmonary arteries [35].

THE RIGHT VENTRICLE IN HEALTH: GENERAL CONSIDERATIONS. Cardiac output of the right ventricle (RV) equals that of the left ventricle (LV) [36], despite the fact that pressures are normally much lower in the former. These facts reveal that the RV is more distensible than the LV. The following anatomic and physiologic observations of the normal adult ventricles support this: (1) The outer wall of the RV is much thinner (4–5 mm) than that of the LV (8–15 mm) [37], and (2) the pressure-volume characteristics of both ventricles demonstrate that the RV is more compliant (Fig. 64-3) [38]. That is, for the same ventricular volume, chamber pressure is greater in the LV.

The explanation for the equality of RV and LV outputs is not related to distensibility but rather to Starling's law of the heart [36]. The RV and LV function according to the same ventricular function curve theory (Fig. 64-4): cardiac output depends on the volume of blood present before contraction (preload). Since the two pumps are in series and pump according to the same principle, they pass the same volume of blood between each other. According to Figure 64-4, it is possible, on a beat-to-beat

Fig. 64-3. Pressure-volume characteristics of right and left ventricles. LV = left ventricle; RV = right ventricle.

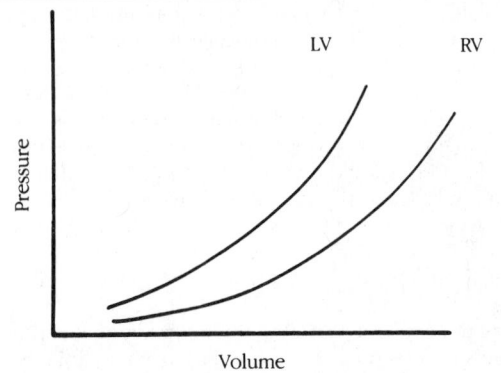

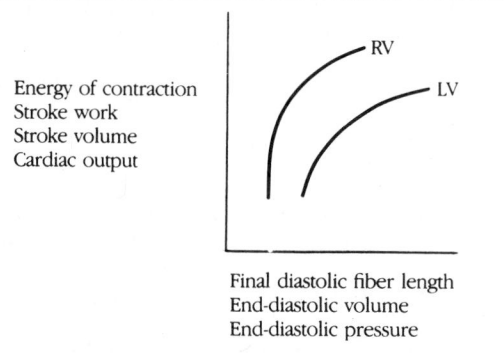

**Energy of contraction
Stroke work
Stroke volume
Cardiac output**

**Final diastolic fiber length
End-diastolic volume
End-diastolic pressure**

Fig. 64-4. RV and LV function curves. Although they have similar shapes, the LV curve is shifted to the right because it is less compliant (i.e., for the same volume, LV end-diastolic pressure is greater). RV = right ventricle; LV = left ventricle.

basis, to move up and down the corresponding ventricular function curves by varying the volume of blood returned to each pump. For instance, if the recumbent position is assumed, venous return to the RV increases. This increases RV preload and is responsible for increasing RV output. Left ventricular preload and output then increase by the same amount.

Although the RV and LV function curves have essentially the same shape, the LV curve is shifted to the right because it is less compliant (i.e., for the same volume, LV end-diastolic pressure is greater).

A brief review of the anatomy and physiology of the fetal cardiovascular system [39] makes possible (1) an understanding of why LV muscle mass is greater than that of RV and (2) an appreciation that ventricular output, in addition to preload, may be influenced by the resistance the ventricle has to eject against (i.e., circulation peripheral to the pump). Before birth, the ductus arteriosus is patent. Since approximately 90 percent of RV output is pumped through the patent ductus into the same conduit (aorta) the LV is pumping into, both ventricles empty into the same circulation, which exposes both ventricles to the same systemic vascular resistance. Not surprisingly, RV and LV chamber pressures and muscle masses are similar. At birth, when the ductus closes and the lungs become aerated, the RV pumps blood into the pulmonary circulation with a low vascular resistance to flow. Consequently, the RV no longer needs to be as strong as the LV; RV chamber pressures and muscle mass decrease.

CARDIAC COMPENSATORY MECHANISMS. To maintain cardiac output in the face of functional abnormalities, the RV can compensate acutely, subacutely, and chronically [40]. Acutely, increased sympathetic nervous system activity increases heart rate and myocardial contractility (inotropic effect). Subacutely, RV dilatation occurs, due to the inability of the chamber to empty completely in afterload heart failure. According to the law of Laplace, RV dilatation makes afterload worse (resistance increases). Since preload also increases, however, RV output increases by Starling's law. In other words, at the expense of elevating RV end-diastolic pressure and potentially causing passive congestion of the systemic venous system (RV congestive heart failure), the RV can eject more blood.

Chronically, if RV end-diastolic pressure gradually rises, RV hypertrophy occurs before congestive heart failure. According to the law of Laplace, RV hypertrophy decreases afterload because of the increased muscle thickness. On the basis of the

above considerations, compensated RV failure is manifested clinically by tachycardia and cardiomegaly (hypertrophy and/or dilatation).

RELATION BETWEEN RIGHT AND LEFT VENTRICULAR FAILURE. Since the ventricles share common muscle bundles, it is not surprising that RV failure can cause LV abnormalities. In clinically stable patients with COPD, however, LV abnormalities are generally only subtle [41,42,43]. In these patients RV failure does not appear to cause LV failure; if LV failure occurs in the presence of cor pulmonale, it appears to be due to intrinsic LV disease. On the other hand, in critically ill, unstable patients, there is some evidence that the extreme RV volume overloading can be partially responsible for LV failure [44].

DETERMINANTS OF NORMAL RIGHT VENTRICULAR FUNCTION. Normal RV and LV cardiac outputs are determined by the same two factors: (1) stroke volume, a function of preload, myocardial contractility, and afterload; and (2) heart rate. Preload (Fig. 64-3) is the amount of blood present before contraction takes place. *Contractility* defines the performance of the ventricular muscle. Although contractility can be described in terms of how quickly the muscle contracts, the effects on cardiac output perhaps can be best appreciated by studying a family of RV function curves (Fig. 64-5). For the same preload, increased contractility shifts the curve upward and decreased contractility shifts the curve downward. Afterload can be described by the law of Laplace:

$$T = \frac{P \times R}{2 \text{ (Wall thickness)}} \qquad (6)$$

It is the tension (T) that must be developed in the ventricular muscle before the muscle fibers shorten and eject blood. Afterload is directly proportional to the intraventricular pressure (P) (equivalent to the pressure within the circulation that the ventricle has to push against) times the radius (R) of the chamber, and it is indirectly proportional to twice the muscle wall thickness. The effect of afterload on cardiac output is negative. When afterload increases, cardiac output tends to decrease. For in-

Fig. 64-5. Effect of myocardial contractility on stroke work (stroke volume). For the same preload (A), increased contractility increases cardiac output by shifting the curve upward (B), and decreased contractility decreases cardiac output by shifting the curve downward (C).

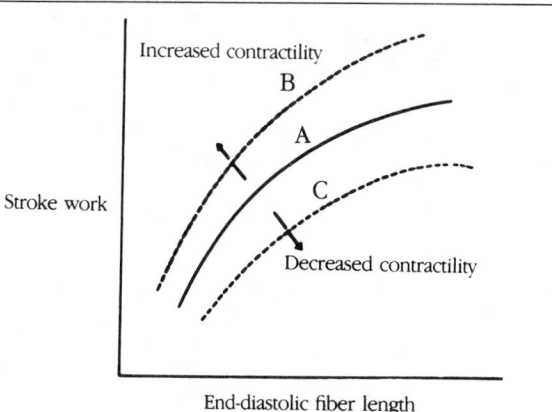

Increased contractility

B

A

C

Stroke work

Decreased contractility

End-diastolic fiber length

stance, before the RV will eject blood into the pulmonary circulation when pulmonary hypertension is present, a greater tension must be generated in the myocardium. Because of the extra time it may take to reach this greater tension, systole may be over before the ventricle empties entirely.

Since cardiac output is equal to stroke volume times heart rate, at any given stroke volume cardiac output is linearly related to heart rate. Should stroke volume be reduced for any reason, a compensatory increase in heart rate can usually maintain an appropriate cardiac output.

THE RIGHT VENTRICLE IN DISEASE. Potentially, RV failure is mediated functionally by disturbances of contractility, heart rate, preload, and afterload. Although primary or predominant contractility disturbances of the RV and LV may occur concomitantly in cardiomyopathies and acute myocardial infarctions of the inferior wall of the LV, it is not common for RV failure to occur from a selective contractility abnormality of the RV alone. Such an abnormality can occur during an infarction localized to the RV. Right ventricular failure due to an isolated disturbance of heart rate is extremely unlikely theoretically as well as clinically.

By reconsidering Starling's law, it is theoretically possible to volume underload the RV to such an extent that cardiac output is markedly reduced. Although underloading causes concomitant LV and RV failure during cardiac tamponade, RV failure alone from this mechanism may be seen rarely in tricuspid stenosis.

Diagnosis

SIGNS AND SYMPTOMS. Symptoms that can be attributed solely to pulmonary hypertension occur in patients with the very rare condition of primary pulmonary hypertension [19,20]. These patients typically complain of exertional dyspnea (without orthopnea or paroxysmal nocturnal dyspnea), fatigue, exertional substernal chest pain, and exertional or postexertional syncope. While patients with other forms of pulmonary hypertension may have similar symptoms, they may well be overshadowed by other manifestations of the underlying disease (Tables 64-1 and 64-2), such as pleuritic pain and hemoptysis in pulmonary embolism; cough and sputum expectoration and nonspecific central nervous system complaints in COPD; acute and catastrophic respiratory distress in ARDS; and daytime hypersomnolence and nighttime snoring in patients with obstructive sleep apnea. On the other hand, patients with passive pulmonary hypertension usually complain of orthopnea and paroxysmal nocturnal dyspnea as well as dyspnea on exertion.

Physical findings that can be attributed solely to pulmonary hypertension are usually indicative of RV pressure overload [19,20,45] and are usually not appreciated before pulmonary artery systolic pressures approach 55 mm Hg [46]. These findings may include a large A wave in the jugular venous pulse, left parasternal (RV) heave, pulmonic ejection click and flow murmur, prominent pulmonic component of the second heart sound, RV fourth heart sound, and signs of RV failure (hepatomegaly, peripheral edema, and ascites). Patients with severe pulmonary hypertension may also have a prominent V wave in the jugular venous pulse, an RV third heart sound, and murmurs of tricuspid and/or pulmonic regurgitation. When pulmonary hypertension is not primary, many of these signs are overshadowed by other manifestations of the underlying cardiac or pul-

monary disease, causing pulmonary hypertension (Tables 64-1 and 64-2) such as the auscultatory findings of wheezing in COPD and cystic fibrosis; crackles in idiopathic interstitial fibrosis and passive congestion of the lungs; and massive obesity in obesity-hypoventilation syndrome and chest wall distortion in severe kyphoscoliosis.

CHEST ROENTGENOGRAPHY. The routine chest roentgenogram, consisting of posteroanterior (PA) and lateral projections, is a useful test to screen for abnormalities of the pulmonary circulation. The normal pulmonary circulation is seen in Figure 64-6A.

Certain characteristic roentgenographic changes may be produced in the pulmonary vascular patterns of the lungs and in the size of the heart. These changes are qualitatively similar in all forms of pulmonary hypertension (cogenital and acquired) that are due to increased vascular resistance [47], although they are most marked in patients with left-to-right shunts due to congenital defects. They include marked enlargement of the main pulmonary artery segment, dilatation of the central hilar pulmonary artery branches down to the origin of the segmental vessels, and constriction of the segmental arteries (Fig. 64-6B) [47]. These changes correlate with the decreased cross-sectional area of the pulmonary vascular bed. The pulmonary veins will not be enlarged. The following measurements on routine inspiratory upright PA films suggest the presence of active pulmonary hypertension: (1) protrusion of the main pulmonary artery segment is present when the width of the main pulmonary artery from the midline is greater than 35 percent of half of the internal diameter of the hemithorax and (2) dilatation of the central pulmonary arteries is present when the width of the descending branch of the right pulmonary artery is greater than 16 mm [48]. Although slight elevations of pulmonary arterial pressures may not produce any abnormal clinical or roentgenographic signs, some or all of the changes described are usually present in active hypertensive states when the pressures reach the range of 55/25 mm Hg.

The characteristic roentgenographic signs of passive pulmonary hypertension are the signs of pulmonary venous hypertension (Fig. 64-7A). On routine inspiratory upright PA films, prominence of upper lobe vessels (veins) over lower lobe vessels due to redistribution of pulmonary blood flow suggests the presence of pulmonary venous hypertension [49]. The presence of interstitial edema (Figs. 64-7B, C, and D) and alveolar edema (Fig. 64-7E) are indicative of edema accumulation; they are not specific for pulmonary venous hypertension. When pulmonary vascular congestion is acute, roentgenographic signs of passive pulmonary hypertension begin to appear at PCW pressures of 18 mm Hg [50]. The size and shape of the left ventricle and left atrium depend on the cause(s) of the passive pulmonary hypertension.

ELECTROCARDIOGRAPHY. While the ECG is reliable in predicting the presence of severe pulmonary hypertension due to primary pulmonary hypertension, congenital heart disease, and interstitial fibrosis (right axis deviation, right ventricular hypertrophy), it is less reliable in pulmonary embolism and COPD. Because of the downward displacement of the heart in the thorax due to lung hyperinflation and the less severe pulmonary hypertension in COPD, ECG evidence of overt RV hypertrophy is uncommon. Serial changes are most often seen [51]. There may be a rightward shift of the mean QRS axis; T wave abnormalities in right precordial leads; S–T depressions in leads II, III, and aVF; transient right bundle branch block; and prominent P waves, particularly in the inferior and right precordial leads

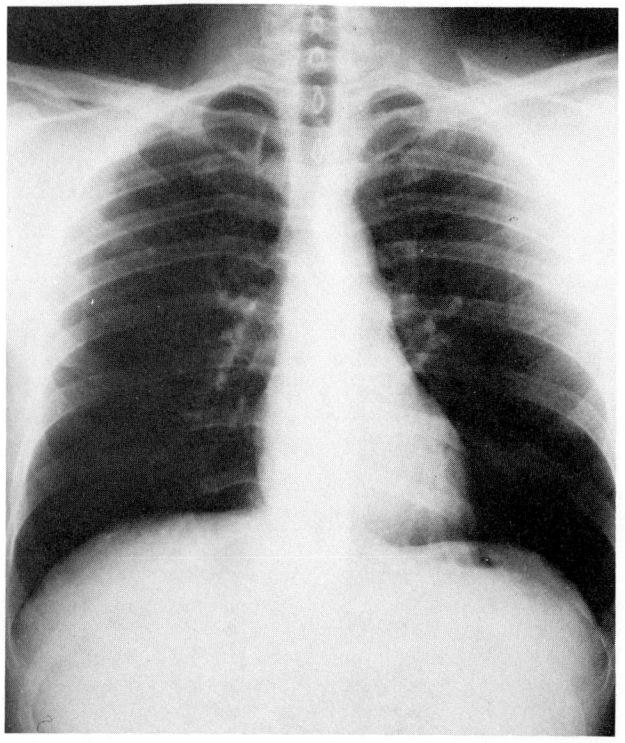

A

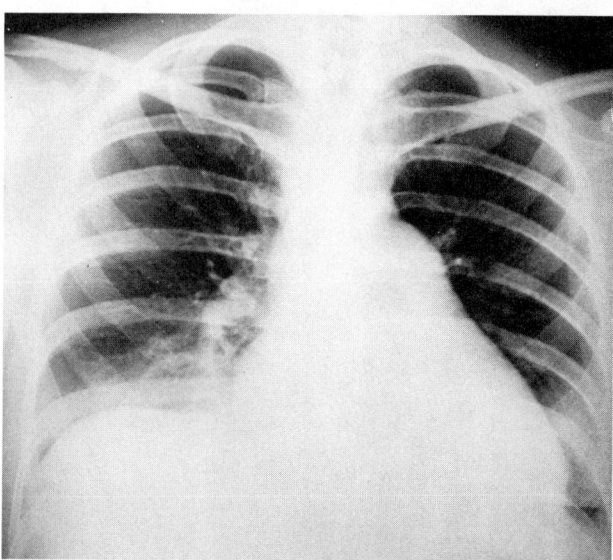

B

Fig. 64-6. A. Normal chest radiograph. Along the left side of the mediastinum, there are three normal convexities: the aorta at the level of the carina, the main pulmonary artery just above the left mainstem bronchus, and the left ventricle just above the left hemidiaphragm. B. Chest radiograph of a patient with primary pulmonary hypertension. The main pulmonary artery is enlarged and the right main pulmonary artery is quite prominent and rapidly tapers.

(p pulmonale). All of these changes may subside with improvement in gas exchange and hyperinflation.

ECHOCARDIOGRAPHY. This diagnostic modality can be used to evaluate right heart morphology and function, exclude LV and congenital heart disease, assess for the presence of mitral valve disease and left atrial myxoma, and estimate the severity of pulmonary hypertension by the Doppler examination of the tricuspid regurgitant jet [52]. Predictions of pulmonary systolic pressures correlate well with catheterization values in the studies reported to date [52]. Transesophageal echocardiography promises to be useful for comprehensive imaging of the right heart structures, particularly in patients with lung disease, in whom transthoracic echocardiography is often technically difficult.

RADIONUCLIDE ANGIOGRAPHY. This technique allows noninvasive assessment of biventricular function. Normal LV and reduced RV ejection fraction are present in active pulmonary hypertensive states. However, not all passive pulmonary hypertensive states demonstrate a reduced LV ejection fraction (e.g., mitral stenosis, severe mitral regurgitation). Radionuclide angiography is most useful in evaluating the course of the disease once it is known and the response to therapy [53].

PULMONARY FUNCTION TESTS. Lung volumes, flow rates, diffusing capacity, and arterial blood gases can be excellent predictors of pulmonary hypertension. In diffuse interstitial lung diseases such as sarcoidosis and idiopathic interstitial fibrosis, the vital capacity may be a useful predictor [54]. When it is between 50 and 80 percent of predicted, pulmonary hypertension may develop with exercise; when it is 50 percent of predicted in these diseases, pulmonary hypertension may well be present at rest. In pulmonary hypertension due to progressive systemic sclerosis, a diffusing capacity less than 43 percent of predicted was a better predictor than a vital capacity less than 50 percent of predicted in one study; diffusing capacity had a sensitivity of 67 percent in predicting definite pulmonary hypertension [55]. The pulmonary hypertension that occurs in COPD and cystic fibrosis is due in large part to the effects of hypoxia; it predictably occurs in these patients when PaO_2 is less than 50 mm Hg and $PaCO_2$ is greater than 45 mm Hg. Furthermore, these degrees of hypercapnia and hypoxemia become predictable in COPD patients when the absolute value of FEV_1 is less than 1 liter [56]. It is also possible to predict when pulmonary hypertension is present at rest in patients with idiopathic kyphoscoliosis [57]. Pulmonary hypertension at rest should not be anticipated unless the vital capacity is less than 60 percent of predicted.

CARDIAC CATHETERIZATION. This is the single most important study in evaluating pulmonary hypertension. In the critically ill patient, right heart catheterization with a Swan-Ganz catheter can not only help document the presence of pulmonary hypertension but also help categorize it as active, passive, or reactive according to the PA_{ed}-PCW gradient or calculation of vascular resistance, as described previously. This is the first crucial step in determining the cause of pulmonary hypertension (Table 64-1). It is important to be aware of the potential limitations of the flotation device for right heart catheterization in critically ill patients [58]. For instance, it may not always be possible to obtain a wedge pressure by balloon occlusion in a

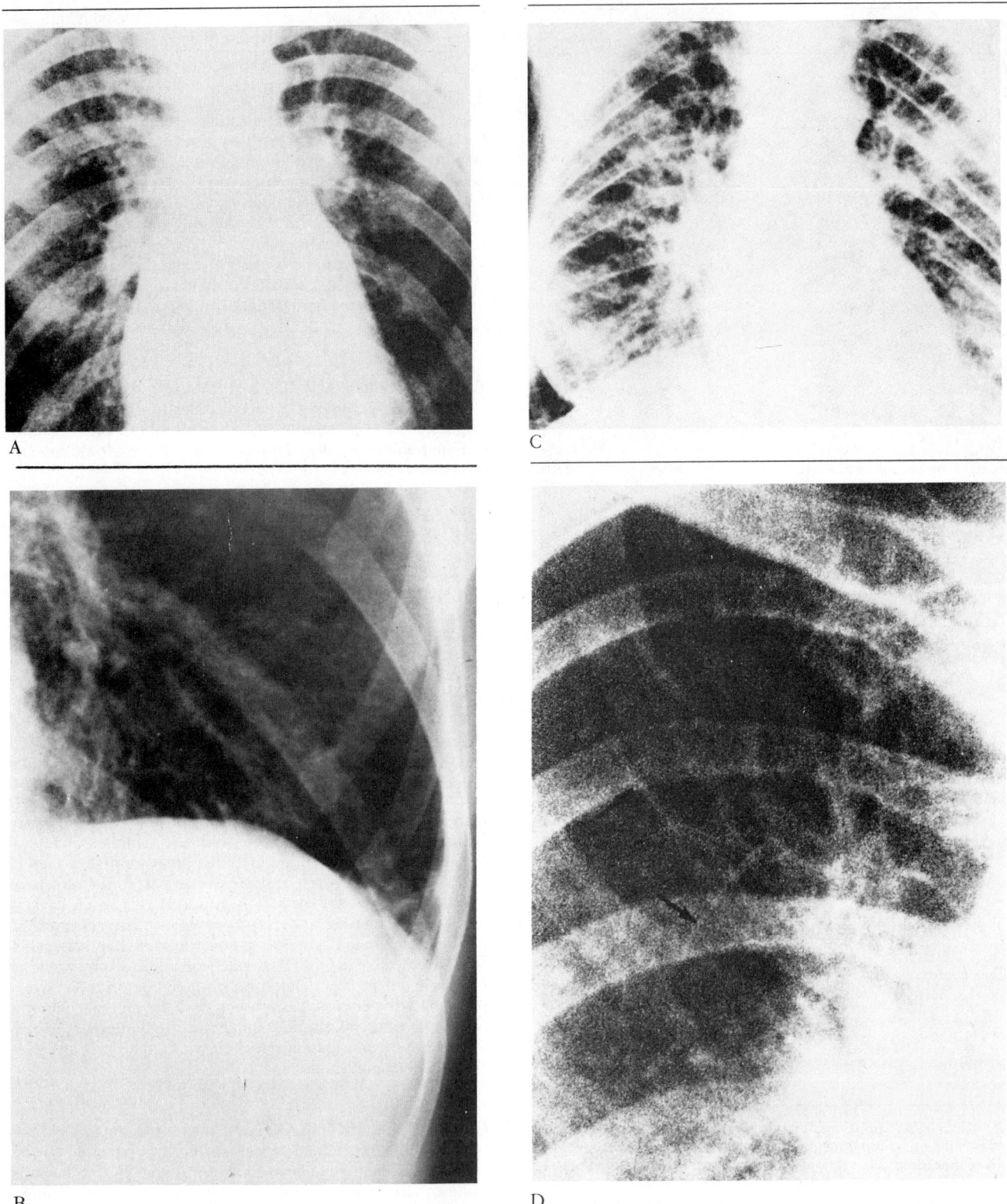

Fig. 64-7. Pulmonary venous hypertension. A. The diameter of the blood vessels in the upper lung zones is greater than that of the vessels in the lower lung zones. B. Kerley B lines are seen in the cardiophrenic angle; they are no more than 1 mm in diameter and usually no more than 1–2 cm long. C. Kerley C lines appear as a diffuse spiderweb pattern. D. Kerley A lines (*arrow*) are long, sometimes sharply angulated lines that appear to arise from hilar shadows. E. Alveolar edema appears as a characteristic bat wing alveolar filling pattern.

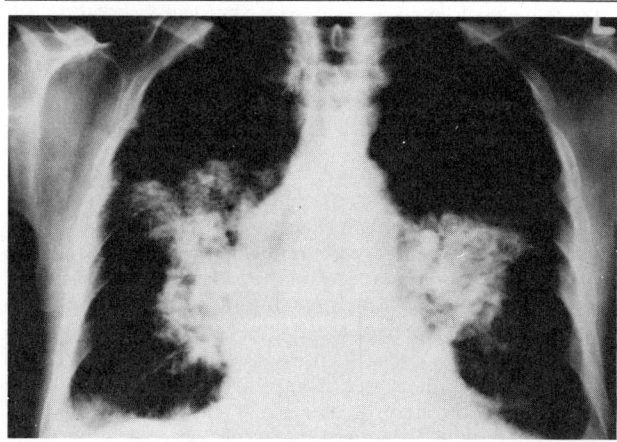

E

patient with pulmonary hypertension, and if it can be obtained, it may not accurately reflect LV end-diastolic volume [58].

Differential Diagnosis

After determining the presence of pulmonary hypertension and the operant pathophysiologic type (passive, active, or reactive), it is crucial from a therapeutic standpoint to establish the specific cause. Special diagnostic studies are used to accomplish this.

PASSIVE PULMONARY HYPERTENSION. If the history, physical examination, echocardiography, and right heart catheterization do not elucidate the cause of passive pulmonary hypertension (Table 64-1), left heart catheterization in the cardiac catheterization laboratory may be necessary. For instance, angiography and measurements of shunts may be necessary to elucidate the specific anatomic abnormalities in congenital heart disease, and left atrial pressure measurements may be needed to diagnose the presence of acquired obstruction of the main pulmonary veins (i.e., PA_{ed} and PCW pressures will be increased, PA_{ed}-PCW gradient will be normal, and left atrial pressure will be normal).

ACTIVE PULMONARY HYPERTENSION. Special studies may be needed to determine the specific cause of active pulmonary hypertension (Tables 64-1 and 64-2). Ventilation-perfusion lung scans and, on occasion, pulmonary angiography are necessary to make the diagnosis of chronic thromboembolic disease (see Chap. 60). A history of wading or swimming in fresh water contaminated with the snail host in an endemic area is important in considering the diagnosis of schistosomiasis. Ova may be demonstrable [59] in urine (*Schistosoma haematobium*), in stool (*Schistosoma mansoni* or *Schistosoma japonicum*), on rectal biopsy (all three types), or rarely, in sputum. Lung biopsy may be required for definitive diagnosis [6]. The diagnosis of congenital shunts can often be made by echocardiography, particularly with color Doppler or contrast studies, and confirmed by complete cardiac catheterization [60]. Although the clinical findings and symptoms of ventricular septal defect and patent ductus arteriosus usually lead to their detection in childhood, a secundum atrial septal defect is more likely to go undetected until adult life. Although history, physical examination, chest radiographs (e.g., diffuse pulmonary infiltrates, scoliosis, bilateral fibrothoraces), and pulmonary function studies usually predict the ventilatory cause of pulmonary hypertension, other investigations, such as sleep studies and thoracoscopic lung biopsy, may be necessary. Since the cause of primary pulmonary hypertension is unknown, the diagnosis is one of exclusion, made when all other causes of active pulmonary hypertension have been ruled out. There can be a close clinical similarity between primary pulmonary hypertension and chronic thromboembolic pulmonary hypertension, and perfusion lung scans can help distinguish between them [61,62]. A normal or low-probability study virtually excludes the diagnosis of chronic thromboembolic disease. If chronic thromboembolic disease is suggested by perfusion lung scan, pulmonary angiography should be performed, both to confirm the diagnosis and to determine the sites and extent of clot. Lung biopsy is not required for the diagnosis of primary pulmonary hypertension. Readers interested in primary pulmonary hypertension are referred to two recent articles [19,20].

REACTIVE PULMONARY HYPERTENSION. Elevated PA_{ed} and PCW and increased PA_{ed}-PCW gradient suggest a reactive pulmonary hypertensive condition (Table 64-1) or a cause of active precapillary pulmonary hypertension such as pulmonary embolism superimposed on a passive pulmonary hypertensive disorder such as LV failure from coronary artery disease.

Although it is usually not difficult to diagnose the presence and cause of reactive pulmonary hypertension when it is due to mitral and aortic valve disease or coronary and systemic hypertensive heart disease, this may not be the case with veno-occlusive disease. Because of the patchiness of the venular lesions, PCW are not always helpful; they may be normal, high, or low [20]. When PCW are not elevated, it may be extremely difficult to distinguish pulmonary veno-occlusive disease from primary pulmonary hypertension. A clinical clue to differentiating the two diseases in this setting is chest radiograph findings (e.g., Kerley B lines) consistent with pulmonary venous hypertension in veno-occlusive disease.

Treatment

The treatment of pulmonary hypertension varies with the cause and state of the disease. A basic principle of the management is to identify and treat the underlying condition, if a specific treatment exists.

PASSIVE PULMONARY HYPERTENSION. Passive pulmonary hypertension is clearly reversible if the underlying cause of pulmonary venous hypertension is corrected. Treatment of systemic hypertension, surgical removal of left atrial myxoma, and surgical correction of aortic and mitral valve disease, cor triatriatum, and congenital pulmonary vein stenosis lower pulmonary venous pressure, thereby reversing passive pulmonary hypertension.

Passive pulmonary hypertension may be controllable in other settings (e.g., coronary artery disease) only with combinations of an inotropic agent, a diuretic, preload and/or afterload reducing drugs, pacemakers, or even surgery. For comprehensive discussions of the treatment of the above disorders, see Chapters 33, 37, 38, and 42.

ACTIVE PULMONARY HYPERTENSION. Pulmonary embolism is the most common cause of acute, active pulmonary hypertension. In general, the pulmonary hypertension due to pulmonary embolism is reversible with anticoagulation or thrombolytic agents [63]. As the degree of embolic obstruction and hypoxemia decreases, pulmonary artery pressures return to normal [16]. Patients with chronic pulmonary hypertension may have had repeated attacks of silent pulmonary embolism or multiple symptomatic episodes of pulmonary embolism that were not adequately treated [64,65]. Patients with unresolved proximal vessel obstruction should be referred to a center experienced in performing pulmonary thromboendarterectomy [65].

The most effective treatment for pulmonary hypertension due to schistosomiasis is preventive: avoiding wading and swimming in fresh water contaminated with the snail host. Once pulmonary hypertension occurs, medical treatment will not reverse the process. However, additional damage caused by additional egg emboli can be prevented with praziquantel, an effective, relatively nontoxic oral drug [59].

Rarely, primary pulmonary hypertension may spontaneously regress [66] and may respond to vasoactive agents [67]. However, there is no uniformly effective medical therapy for the majority of these patients. Mortality is largely determined by the severity of pulmonary artery pressure elevation and the state of function of the RV [68].

While vasoactive drug therapy is not consistently effective in primary pulmonary hypertension, it is the only hope at present for reversing elevated pulmonary vascular resistance. Recent reports on the use of oxygen [69], prostacyclin [70,71], prostaglandin E_1 [70], and chronic oral medications such as the calcium channel blocking agents nifedipine and diltiazem [72,73,74] have shown that these agents as well as others can improve hemodynamics in certain patients. However, since all of these agents can produce serious adverse reactions, they should not be given empirically. Careful monitoring and initial evaluation with a Swan-Ganz catheter in place are necessary to determine which patients will benefit from initial and continued therapy. When assessing the response to vasodilators, the overall effects of a drug on pulmonary and systemic hemodynamics, gas exchange, and oxygen transport must be considered [67]. The goal of a decrease in pulmonary artery pressure accompanied by an increase in cardiac output with little or no change in systemic pressure or gas exchange occurs in approximately 25 to 30 percent of patients [73]. A decrease in pulmonary vascular resistance greater than 20 percent is considered by some to represent a favorable response as long as gas exchange and systemic blood pressure are not adversely effected [72]. Since (1) prostacyclin and prostaglandin E_1 are powerful pulmonary vasodilators with very short half-lives (minutes) when given intravenously [70,71], (2) substantial data show that they can be given safely to patients with primary pulmonary hypertension [70,71], and (3) the acute response to these agents has predictive value for subsequent oral vasodilator therapy [75,76], these agents may become an integral part of the routine management of patients with primary pulmonary hypertension as test drugs. In addition, continuous intravenous infusion of prostacyclin has been used in some patients for periods ranging from months to years [71]. If vasoactive agent therapy is ineffective, symptomatic treatment consisting of salt restriction, oxygen, digitalis, and diuretics is usually prescribed. Oral anticoagulant therapy with coumarin derivatives is also commonly undertaken and may prolong survival [74,77]. Lung or combined heart-lung transplantation should be considered in patients who are unresponsive to vasodilators and who have low cardiac output [78,79].

The treatment of choice for the pulmonary hypertensive re-action that develops in patients with ventricular septal defect, patent ductus, and secundum atrial septal defect [80] is surgical correction. The best results are obtained before severe (systemic level) pulmonary hypertension occurs. Once Eisenmenger's syndrome has developed, these patients should be evaluated for transplantation.

Pulmonary hypertension due to ventilatory disorders may be treated in a variety of ways. For primary central hypoventilation, a respiratory center stimulant such as progesterone may suffice. For the morbidly obese, weight reduction is the primary mode of therapy. For peripheral obstructive sleep apnea, nasal continuous positive airway pressure (CPAP) or a permanent tracheostomy may be curative. Continuous supplemental oxygen therapy prolongs survival in patients with severe COPD [81] and should be administered using flow rates that achieve an arterial oxygen saturation greater than 90 percent. Decortication may be curative in pulmonary hypertension caused by fibrothorax, and corticosteroids or other immunomodulator drugs may be beneficial in idiopathic interstitial fibrosis and sarcoidosis. Treatment of ARDS includes supportive as well as specific measures (see Chap. 55). Finally, since the vasoconstrictive disorder is the only element that can be reversed, alveolar hypoxia must always be considered and treated aggressively with supplemental oxygen. Although prostaglandin E_1 and nifedipine [82,83] can acutely inhibit hypoxic pulmonary vasoconstriction, it is not known what role the long-term administration of these agents will play in the treatment of pulmonary hypertension. The endothelium-derived vasodilator nitric oxide was recently used to treat patients with pulmonary hypertension complicating ARDS [84]. This agent, which is administered by inhalation, has selective pulmonary vasodilator effects because it rapidly binds to circulating hemoglobin and is inactivated. However, the safety of long-term administration has not been evaluated, and delivery and monitoring are cumbersome.

REACTIVE PULMONARY HYPERTENSION. While pulmonary veno-occlusive disease appears to have at best a negligible response to various therapeutic measures, including anticoagulants and corticosteroids [20], it is important to stress that patients with mitral stenosis must not be considered inoperable merely because they have reactive pulmonary hypertension. Both components of pulmonary hypertension should resolve after mitral valve replacement. Passive pulmonary hypertension resolves immediately after surgery, although the PA_{ed}-PCW gradient remains increased. Follow-up catheterizations months to years after mitral valve replacement demonstrate a progressive decrease in the gradient, with a return of pulmonary artery pressure to near normal levels.

References

1. Harris P, Heath D: The structure of the normal pulmonary blood vessels after infancy, in Harris P, Heath D (eds): *The Human Pulmonary Circulation.* 2nd ed. London, Churchill Livingstone, 1977, pp 22–42.
2. Richardson JB: Nerve supply to the lungs. *Am Rev Respir Dis* 119:785, 1979.
3. Harvey RM, Enson Y, Ferrer MI: A reconsideration of the origins of pulmonary hypertension. *Chest* 59:82, 1971.
4. Kadowitz PJ, Joiner PD, Hyman AL: Effect of sympathetic nerve stimulation on pulmonary vascular resistance in the intact spontaneously breathing dog. *Proc Soc Exp Biol Med* 147:68, 1974.
5. Robin ED, Gaudio R: Cor pulmonale. *DM* May 1970.
6. Wagenvoort CA, Moo WI: *Biopsy Pathology of the Pulmonary Vasculature.* London, Chapman and Hall, 1989, pp 114–125.

7. Kaltman AJ, Herbert WH, Conroy RJ, et al: The gradient in pressure across the pulmonary vascular bed during diastole. *Circulation* 34:377, 1966.

8. Borst HG, McGregor M, Whittenberger JL, et al: Influence of pulmonary arterial and left atrial pressures on pulmonary vascular resistance. *Circ Res* 4:393, 1956.

9. Morkin E, Collins JA, Goldman HS, et al: Pattern of blood flow in the pulmonary veins of the dog. *J Appl Physiol* 20:1118, 1965.

10. Karatzas NB, Lee G: Propagation of blood flow pulse in the normal human pulmonary arterial system. *Circ Res* 25:11, 1969.

11. Gabe IT, Gault JH, Ross J Jr, et al: Measurement of instantaneous blood flow velocity and pressure in conscious man with a catheter tip velocity probe. *Circulation* 40:603, 1969.

12. Harvey RM, Enson Y, Ferrer MI: A reconsideration of the origins of pulmonary hypertension. *Chest* 59:82, 1971.

13. Enson Y, Schmidt DH, Ferrer MI, et al: The effect of acutely induced hypervolemia on resistance to pulmonary blood flow and pulmonary arterial compliance in patients with chronic obstructive lung disease. *Am J Med* 57:395, 1974.

14. Kaltman AJ, Herbert WH, Conroy RJ, et al: The gradient in pressure across the pulmonary vascular bed during diastole. *Circulation* 34:377, 1966.

15. McIntyre KM, Sasahara AA: Hemodynamic and ventricular responses to pulmonary embolism. *Prog Cardiovasc Dis* 17:175, 1974.

16. Dalen JE, Banas JS Jr, Brooks HL, et al: Resolution rate of acute pulmonary embolism in man. *N Engl J Med* 280:1194, 1969.

17. Alpert JS, Godtfredsen J, Ockene IS, et al: Pulmonary hypertension secondary to minor pulmonary embolism. *Chest* 73:795, 1978.

18. Cavalcanti IL, Thompson G, De Souza N, et al: Pulmonary hypertension in schistosomiasis. *Br Heart J* 24:363, 1962.

19. Rich S, Dantzker DR, Ayres SM, et al: Primary pulmonary hypertension: A national prospective study. *Ann Intern Med* 107:216, 1987.

20. Rubin LJ: ACCP Consensus statement on primary pulmonary hypertension. *Chest* 104:236, 1993.

21. Dalen JE, Dexter L, Ockene IS, et al: Precapillary pulmonary hypertension: Its relationship to pulmonary venous hypertension. *Trans Am Clin Climatol Assoc* 86:207, 1974.

22. Gordon AJ, Donoso E, Kuhn CLA, et al: Patent ductus arteriosus with reversal of flow. *N Engl J Med* 251:923, 1954.

23. Reeves JT: Hope in primary pulmonary hypertension. *N Engl J Med* 302:112, 1980.

24. Wagenvoort CA, Wagenvoort N: Primary pulmonary hypertension: A pathologic study of the lung vessels. *Circulation* 42:1163, 1970.

25. Fishman AP: Chronic cor pulmonale. *Am Rev Respir Dis* 114:775, 1976.

26. Yuan XJ, Tod ML, Rubin LJ, Blaustein MP: Contrasting effects of hypoxia on tension in rat pulmonary and mesenteric arteries. *Am J Physiol* 28:H281, 1990.

27. Enson Y, Giuntini C, Lewis ML, et al: The influence of hydrogen ion concentration and hypoxia on the pulmonary circulation. *J Clin Invest* 43:1146, 1964.

28. Lenfant C, Sullivan K: Adaptation to high altitude. *N Engl J Med* 284:1298, 1971.

29. Penaloza D, Sime F: Chronic cor pulmonale due to loss of altitude acclimatization (chronic mountain sickness). *Am J Med* 50:728, 1971.

30. Zapol WM, Snider MT: Pulmonary hypertension in severe acute respiratory failure. *N Engl J Med* 296:476, 1977.

31. Snow RL, Davies P, Pontoppidan H, et al: Pulmonary vascular remodeling in adult respiratory distress syndrome. *Am Rev Respir Dis* 126:887, 1982.

32. Bergofsky EH: Respiratory failure in disorders of the thoracic cage. *Am Rev Respir Dis* 119:643, 1979.

33. Wagenvoort CA: Pulmonary veno-occlusive disease: Entity or syndrome. *Chest* 69:82, 1976.

34. Clinical Pathologic Conference: Rapidly progressive dyspnea in a teenage boy. *JAMA* 223:1243, 1973.

35. Bartter T, Irwin RS, Nash G: Aneurysms of the pulmonary arteries. *Chest* 94:1065, 1988.

36. Sarnoff SJ, Berglund E: Ventricular function. I. Starling's law of the heart studied by means of simultaneous right and left ventricular function curves in the dog. *Circulation* 9:706, 1954.

37. Silverman ME, Schlant RC: Anatomy of the normal heart and blood vessels, in Hurst JW, Logue RB, Schlant RC, et al (eds): *The Heart.* 4th ed. New York, McGraw-Hill, 1978, p 22.

38. Weber KT, Janicki JS, Shroff SG, et al: The right ventricle: Physiologic and pathophysiologic considerations. *Crit Care Med* 11:323, 1983.

39. Schlant RC: Altered cardiovascular function of congenital heart disease, in Hurst JW, Logue RB, Schlant RC, et al (eds): *The Heart.* 4th ed. New York, McGraw-Hill, 1978, p 813.

40. Mason DT: The failing heart. *Disease a Month* xxiii:2, 1977.

41. Bahler RC: Assessment of left ventricular function in chronic obstructive pulmonary disease. *Chest* 68:132, 1975.

42. Steele P, Ellis JH Jr, Van Dyke D, et al: Left ventricular ejection fraction in severe chronic obstructive airways disease. *Am J Med* 59:21, 1975.

43. Slutsky RA, Ackerman W, Karliner JS, et al: Right and left ventricular dysfunction in patients with chronic obstructive lung disease: Assessment by first-pass radionuclide angiography. *Am J Med* 68:197, 1980.

44. Caldwell EJ: The left ventricle in chronic lung disease, in Rubin LJ (ed): *Pulmonary Heart Disease.* Boston, Martinus Nijhoff, 1984, pp 247–272.

45. Kanemoto N, Furuya H, Etoh T, et al: Chest roentgenograms in primary pulmonary hypertension. *Chest* 76:45, 1979.

46. Weens HS, Gay BG Jr: The chest roentgenogram, in Hurst JW, Logue RB, Schlant RC, et al (eds): *The Heart.* 4th ed. New York, McGraw-Hill, 1978, p 324.

47. Felson B: The hila and pulmonary vessels, in Felson B: *Chest Roentgenology.* Philadelphia, WB Saunders, 1973, p 216.

48. Simon G: The anterior view chest radiograph-criteria for normality derived from a basic analysis of shadows. *Clin Radiol* 26:429, 1975.

49. Meszaros WT: Lung changes in left heart failure. *Circulation* 47:859, 1973.

50. McHugh TJ, Forrester JS, Adler L, et al: Pulmonary vascular congestion in acute myocardial infarction: Hemodynamic and radiologic correlations. *Ann Intern Med* 76:29, 1972.

51. Kilcoyne MM, Davis AL, Ferrer MI: A dynamic electrocardiographic concept useful in the diagnosis of cor pulmonale: Result of a survey of 200 patients with chronic obstructive pulmonary disease. *Circulation* 42:903, 1970.

52. Yock PG, Popp RL: Noninvasive estimation of right ventricular systolic pressure by Doppler ultrasound in patients with tricuspid regurgitation. *Circulation* 70:657, 1984.

53. Matthay RA, Berger JH: Noninvasive assessment of right and left ventricular function in acute and chronic respiratory failure. *Crit Care Med* 11:329, 1983.

54. Enson Y, Thomas HM III, Bosken CH, et al: Pulmonary hypertension in interstitial lung disease: Relation of vascular resistance to abnormal lung structure. *Trans Assoc Am Physicians* 88:248, 1975.

55. Ungerer RG, Tashkin DP, Furst D, et al: Prevalence and clinical correlates of pulmonary arterial hypertension in progressive systemic sclerosis. *Am J Med* 75:65, 1983.

56. Burrows B, Strauss RH, Niden AH: Chronic obstructive lung disease. 3. Interrelationships of pulmonary function data. *Am Rev Respir Dis* 91:861, 1965.

57. Bergofsky EH, Turino GM, Fishman AP: Cardiorespiratory failure in kyphoscoliosis. *Medicine* 38:263, 1959.

58. Raper R, Sibbald WJ: Misled by the wedge? *Chest* 89:427, 1986.

59. Barrett-Connor E: Parasitic pulmonary disease. *Am Rev Respir Dis* 126:558, 1982.

60. Brinsfield DE, Plauth WH Jr: Clinical recognition and medical management of congenital heart disease, in Hurst JW, Logue RB, Schlant RC, et al (eds): *The Heart.* 4th ed. New York, McGraw-Hill, 1978, p 831.

61. Fishman AJ, Moser KM, Fedullo PF: Perfusion lung scans vs pulmonary angiography in evaluation of suspected primary pulmonary hypertension. *Chest* 84:679, 1983.

62. D'Alonzo GE, Bower JS, Dantzker DR: Differentiation of patients with primary and thromboembolic pulmonary hypertension. *Chest* 85:457, 1984.

63. Dalen JE, Alpert JS: Natural history of pulmonary embolism. *Prog Cardiovasc Dis* 16:259, 1975.

64. de Soyza NDB, Murphy ML: Persistent post-embolic pulmonary hypertension. *Chest* 62:665, 1972.

65. Moser KM, Spragg RG, Utley J, et al: Chronic thrombotic obstruction

of major pulmonary arteries: Results of thromboendarterectomy in 15 patients. *Ann Intern Med* 99:299, 1983.

66. Bourdillon PDV, Oakley CM: Regression of primary pulmonary hypertension. *Br Heart J* 38:264, 1976.

67. Rubin LJ: Approach to the diagnosis and treatment of pulmonary hypertension. *Chest* 96:659, 1989.

68. D'Alonzo GG, Barst RJ, Ayres SM, et al: Survival in patients with primary pulmonary hypertension: Results from a national prospective registry. *Ann Intern Med* 115:343, 1991.

69. Nagasaka Y, Akutsu H, Lee YS, et al: Longterm favorable effect of oxygen administration on a patient with primary pulmonary hypertension. *Chest* 74:299, 1978.

70. Long WA, Rubin LJ: Prostacyclin and PGE$_1$ treatment of pulmonary hypertension. *Am Rev Respir Dis* 136:773, 1987.

71. Rubin LJ, Mendoza J, Hood M, et al: Treatment of primary pulmonary hypertension with continuous intravenous prostacyclin (epoprostenol). *Ann Intern Med* 112:485, 1990.

72. Weir EK, Rubin LJ, Ayres SM, et al: The acute administration of vasodilators in primary pulmonary hypertension: Experience from the NIH registry on PPH. *Am Rev Respir Dis* 140:1623, 1989.

73. Rich S, Brundage BH: High dose calcium channel blocking therapy for primary pulmonary hypertension: Evidence for long-term reduction in pulmonary arterial pressure and regression of right ventricular hypertrophy. *Circulation* 76:135, 1987.

74. Rich S, Kaufmann E, Levy PS: The effect of high doses of calcium channel blockers on survival in primary pulmonary hypertension. *N Engl J Med* 327:76, 1992.

75. Barst RJ: Pharmacologically induced pulmonary vasodilation in chil-

dren and young adults with primary pulmonary hypertension. *Chest* 98:497, 1986.

76. Groves BM, Rubin LJ, Reeves JT, et al: Comparable hemodynamic effects of prostacyclin and hydralazine in primary pulmonary hypertension. *Am Heart J* 110:1200, 1985.

77. Fuster V, Steele PM, Edwards WD, et al: Primary pulmonary hypertension: Natural history and the importance of thrombosis. *Circulation* 70:580, 1984.

78. Reitz BA, Wallwork JL, Hunt SA, et al: Heart-lung transplantation: Successful therapy for patients with pulmonary vascular disease. *N Engl J Med* 306:557, 1982.

79. Pasque MK, Trulock EP, Kaiser LD, Cooper JD: Single lung transplantation for pulmonary hypertension: Three month hemodynamic follow-up. *Circulation* 84:2275, 1991.

80. Dalen JE, Haynes FW, Dexter L: Life expectancy with atrial septal defect. *JAMA* 200:112, 1967.

81. Nocturnal Oxygen Therapy Trial Group: Continuous or nocturnal oxygen therapy in hypoxemic chronic obstructive lung disease: A clinical trial. *Ann Intern Med* 93:391, 1980.

82. Naeije R, Melot C, Mols P, et al: Reduction in pulmonary hypertension by prostaglandin E$_1$ in decompensated chronic obstructive pulmonary disease. *Am Rev Respir Dis* 125:1, 1982.

83. Simonneau G, Escourrou P, Duroux P, et al: Inhibition of hypoxic pulmonary vasoconstriction by nifedipine. *N Engl J Med* 304:1582, 1981.

84. Rossaint R, Folke KJ, Lopez F, et al: Inhaled nitric oxide for the adult respiratory distress syndrome. *N Eng J Med* 328:399, 1993.

65. *Pleural Disease in the Critically Ill Patient*

Steven A. Sahn

Pleural disease itself is an unusual cause for admission to the intensive care unit (ICU). Exceptions are a large hemothorax for monitoring the rate of bleeding and hemodynamic status, a secondary spontaneous pneumothorax, and large unilateral or bilateral pleural effusions that have caused acute respiratory failure.

Pleural disease may be overlooked in the critically ill patient because it is usually overshadowed by the major presenting illness that is the reason for admission to the ICU. Furthermore, it is often a subtle finding, especially on clinical examination, and even on the chest radiograph. A pleural effusion may not be seen on the supine chest radiograph because a diffuse alveolar filling process can mask the posterior layering of fluid or because bilateral effusions without parenchymal infiltrates are misinterpreted as an underexposed film or objects outside the chest. Pneumothorax may not be detected in the supine patient because the pleural air tends to be situated anteriorly and does not produce the diagnostic visceral pleural line seen on an upright radiograph. When the patient on mechanical ventilation is at increased risk for barotrauma because peak airway pressure is high, the index of suspicion for pneumothorax should be heightened; if there is evidence of pulmonary interstitial gas (infra vide) or subcutaneous emphysema, appropriate radiologic studies should be obtained.

Radiologic Signs of Pleural Disease in the Intensive Care Unit

As the distribution of fluid and air in the normal pleural space tends to follow gravitational influences, and since the lung has a tendency to maintain its normal shape as it becomes smaller, fluid initially accumulates between the bottom of the lung and the diaphragm and air between the top of the lung and the apex of the thorax in the upright patient. When chest radiographs are obtained in other than the erect position, free pleural fluid and air change position. In most critically ill patients, radiographs are taken in the supine or semi-erect positions, thereby changing the radiographic appearance of free pleural fluid and air.

Pleural Fluid

STANDARD CHEST RADIOGRAPH. In normal humans, the anteroposterior diameter of the hemithorax is greatest at the lung base, therefore in the supine position, the radiolucency of the lung base is equal to or greater than that in the lung apex [1]. Furthermore, in the supine patient, breast and pectoral tissue tend to fall laterally away from the lung base. Thus, a pleural effusion should be suspected if there is increased homogeneous density over the lower lung fields compared to the upper lung fields. As the pleural effusion increases in size, the increased radiodensity involves the upper hemithorax as well. However, failure of chest wall tissue to move laterally, cardiomegaly, prominent epicardial fat pad, and lung collapse or consolidation may obscure a pleural effusion on a supine radiograph. The unilateral homogeneous density can be mimicked by patient rotation or an off-center x-ray beam [2]. An absent pectoral muscle, prior mastectomy, unilateral hyperlucent lung, scoliosis, previous lobectomy, hypoplastic pulmonary artery, or pleural or chest wall mass may lead to unilateral homogeneous increased density and mimic an effusion.

Approximately 175 to 525 ml of pleural fluid results in blunting of the costophrenic angle on an erect chest radiograph [3]. In most instances, this quantity of pleural fluid can be detected on a supine radiograph as an increased density over the lower lung zone. Failure to visualize the hemidiaphragm, absence of the costophrenic angle meniscus, and apical capping are less likely to be seen with effusions of less than 500 ml but are more likely to be recognized as the volume of fluid increases [1]. The major radiographic finding of a pleural effusion in a supine position is increased homogeneous density over the lower lung field that does not obliterate normal bronchovascular markings, does not show air bronchograms, and does not show hilar or mediastinal displacement until the effusion is massive. If a pleural effusion is suspected in the supine patient, an erect or lateral decubitus radiograph should be performed for confirmation or exclusion.

OTHER RADIOGRAPHIC IMAGING. Underlying diffuse parenchymal lung disease, as is commonly found in the critically ill patient, makes the diagnosis of pleural effusion problematic and may require ultrasonography or computed tomography (CT) scanning.

Sonography. Chest sonography provides good characterization for pleural diseases and is a useful diagnostic modality for critically ill patients when they cannot be transported for CT. Sonographic examination takes less time and is less expensive than CT, can be done at the bedside, and can be repeated serially. Disadvantages include hindrance of the ultrasonic wave by air, either in the lung or pleural space, a restricted field of view, inferior evaluation of the lung parenchyma compared to CT, and operator dependence [4]. Chest sonography was helpful in diagnosis in 27 of 41 (66%) and in treatment in 37 of 41 (90%) critically ill patients. It had an important influence on treatment planning in 17 of 41 (41%) patients [5]. In the same study, sonography excluded an effusion in five patients with suspected pleural fluid, confirmed the presence of effusion in eight patients, found unsuspected effusion in three patients, and provided additional information in seven patients with effusion. Sonographic bedside thoracentesis was successful in 24 of 25 critically ill patients in the same study [5].

Computed Tomography. Computed tomography is recognized as providing increased resolution compared with more conventional radiographic techniques. Although moving a critically ill patient for a CT scan has potential risks, the diagnostic advantage can be justified in the stable patient when the clinical course is not congruent with the proposed diagnosis suggested by the portable chest radiograph. In selected patients with multisystem trauma, chest CT often provides additional diagnostic

information and positively affects patient management and outcome [6,7].

Pneumothorax

In the supine patient, pneumothorax gas migrates along the anterior surface of the lung, making detection on the anteroposterior radiograph problematic. The base, lateral chest wall, and juxtacardiac area should be carefully visualized for evidence of pneumothorax [8]. Accumulation of air along the mediastinal parietal pleura may simulate pneumomediastinum [9]. An erect or decubitus (suspected hemithorax up) radiograph should be obtained to assess for the presence of a pneumothorax.

The most common radiographic signs of tension pneumothorax are contralateral mediastinal shift, ipsilateral diaphragmatic depression, and ipsilateral chest wall expansion. Underlying lung disease may prevent total lung collapse even if tension is present, and in patients on mechanical ventilation little or no midline mediastinal shift may result from the tension [10,11]. In the latter, a depressed ipsilateral diaphragm is a more reliable sign of tension than mediastinal shift.

In patients with the acute respiratory distress syndrome (ARDS), barotrauma can result in a localized tension pneumothorax with a subtle contralateral mediastinal shift, flattening of the cardiac contour, and depression of the ipsilateral hemidiaphragm [12]. Pleural adhesions and relative compressibility and mobility of surrounding structures, in addition to the supine position, probably account for these loculated tension pneumothoraces.

In a study of 88 critically ill patients with 112 pneumothoraces, the anteromedial and subpulmonic recesses were involved in 64 percent of patients in the supine and semi-erect position [13]. Furthermore, in 30 percent of the pneumothoraces in this study not initially detected by the clinician or radiologist, half of the patients progressed to tension pneumothorax. Therefore, a high index of suspicion is necessary in these critically ill patients to avoid catastrophic situations.

Familiarity with atypical locations of pneumothoraces in critically ill patients, usually due to the supine or semi-erect position, the consequence of underlying cardiopulmonary disease, and knowledge of other risk factors contributing to misdiagnosis (e.g., mechanical ventilation, altered mental status, prolonged ICU stay, and development of pneumothorax after peak physician staffing hours) may contribute to an improved ability to diagnose this potentially lethal problem [14].

DIGITAL RADIOGRAPHY. Digital radiography offers some potential advantages over standard portable chest radiography in the critically ill patient. Some of the problems with portable radiographs are caused by the patient and some by technical limitations. These include uncontrolled respiratory and gross body motion; limited kilovoltage and milliamperage, leading to long exposure and excessive image contrast; unavailability of phototiming, causing a reduction in image quality; and difficulty in interpreting sequential images because of technical variations [15]. In an evaluation of 3500 portable digital chest radiographs in an ICU, it was found that no major problems were encountered in visualization of tubes or catheters or detection of pneumothoraces. Assessment of volume status or presence of bilateral effusions was initially problematic but improved with further experience [15]. Other studies found that radiologists detected pneumothoraces equally well on conventional radiographs and digital images printed on film but less well on electronic viewing consoles [16,17]. When comparing conventional to digital images, the parameters of the systems being compared must be clearly defined, as the system itself may impact on the quality of the image produced [17].

Evaluations of the Patient with a Pleural Effusion in the Intensive Care Unit

DIAGNOSTIC THORACENTESIS

Indications. Patients with a pleural effusion provide the opportunity to diagnose, at least presumptively, the underlying process responsible for pleural fluid accumulation. Pleural effusions are most commonly caused by primary lung disease but may also result from a systemic illness that has its focus in the gastrointestinal tract, liver, kidney, heart, or reticuloendothelial system [18].

While disease of any organ system can cause a pleural effusion in critically ill patients, the diagnoses listed in Table 65-1 represent the majority of the etiologies seen in ICUs. The types of pleural effusions seen in medical and surgical ICUs are similar, but some etiologies related to surgical (coronary artery bypass grafting [CABG], chylothorax, abdominal surgery) and nonsurgical trauma (hemothorax) represent a substantial percentage of surgical ICU effusions.

When a pleural effusion is suspected on physical examination and confirmed radiologically, a diagnostic thoracentesis should be performed in an attempt to establish the etiology. Exceptions might be patients with a secure clinical diagnosis and only a small amount of pleural fluid, as in atelectasis, or patients with uncomplicated congestive heart failure [18]. Ob-

Table 65-1. Causes of Pleural Effusions

In the Medical ICU
   Atelectasis
   Congestive heart failure
   Pneumonia
   Hypoalbuminemia
   Pancreatitis
   ARDS
   Pulmonary embolism
   Hepatic hydrothorax
   Esophageal sclerotherapy
   Postmyocardial infarction
   Iatrogenic
In the Surgical ICU
   Atelectasis
   Congestive heart failure
   Pneumonia
   Pancreatitis
   Hypoalbuminemia
   Coronary artery bypass surgery
   ARDS
   Pulmonary embolism
   Esophageal rupture
   Hemothorax
   Chylothorax
   Abdominal surgery
   Iatrogenic

ARDS = acute respiratory distress syndrome.

servation may be warranted in these situations but thoracentesis should be performed if there are adverse changes.

When there is less than 1 cm from the pleural fluid line to the inside of the chest wall on the lateral decubitus view, the risk of thoracentesis probably outweighs the usefulness of pleural fluid analysis. If the underlying disease or pleural effusion becomes clinically important, the effusion will increase in size and allow for safer thoracentesis. When sampling of fluid is indicated clinically and the volume of the effusion is small, thoracentesis should be performed under ultrasound guidance, which can be done at the bedside [19]. The indications for diagnostic thoracentesis do not change simply because the patient is in the ICU or on mechanical ventilation. In fact, establishing the diagnosis quickly in these critically ill patients may be more important and lifesaving than in non-critically ill patients. It has been well documented that even in patients on mechanical ventilation, diagnostic thoracentesis is safe if there is strict adherence to the general principles of the procedure (see Chap. 14) [20]. Pneumothorax, the most clinically important complication of thoracentesis [21,22], is no more likely to occur in the patient on mechanical ventilation than in the patient who is not; however, if a pneumothorax does develop, the patient on mechanical ventilation will likely develop a tension pneumothorax.

Contraindications. There are no absolute contraindications to diagnostic thoracentesis. If clinical judgment dictates that the information gained from the pleural fluid analysis may help in diagnosis and therapy, thoracentesis should be performed [23] (see Chap. 14). Diagnostic thoracentesis with a small-bore needle can be performed safely in virtually any patient if meticulous technique is employed. The major relative contraindications to thoracentesis are a bleeding diathesis or anticoagulation. A patient with a small amount of pleural fluid and a low benefit-risk ratio also represents a relative contraindication. Thoracentesis should not be attempted through an area of active skin infection.

Complications. Complications of diagnostic thoracentesis include pain at the needle insertion site, bleeding (local, intrapleural, or intraabdominal), pneumothorax, empyema, and spleen or liver puncture (see Chap. 14). Pneumothorax has been reported in prospective studies to occur in 4 to 30 percent of patients [21,24,25,26]. However, the pneumothorax rate is inversely correlated with the experience of the operator [24]. Pneumothorax caused by diagnostic thoracentesis is usually small and often can be treated expectantly. Liver or spleen puncture tends to occur when the patient is not sitting absolutely upright, because movement toward recumbency causes cephalad migration of the abdominal viscera. Even if the liver or spleen is punctured with a small-bore needle, generally the outcome is favorable if the patient is not receiving anticoagulants and does not have a bleeding diathesis.

THERAPEUTIC THORACENTESIS
Indications and Contraindications. The primary indication for therapeutic thoracentesis is relief of dyspnea. Contraindications to therapeutic thoracentesis are similar to those for diagnostic thoracentesis. However, there appears to be an increased risk of pneumothorax [21], therefore making a therapeutic thoracentesis in patients on mechanical ventilation potentially hazardous.

The technique for therapeutic thoracentesis is essentially the same as for diagnostic thoracentesis, except that either a blunt-tip needle or plastic catheter, rather than a sharp tip needle, should be used (see Chap. 14). This reduces the risk of pneumothorax, which may occur as fluid is removed and the lung expands toward the chest wall.

The amount of fluid that can be removed safely from the pleural space at one session is controversial. Ideally, monitoring pleural pressure should dictate the amount of fluid that can be removed. As long as intrapleural pressure does not fall to less than -20 cm H_2O, fluid removal can continue [27]. However, intrapleural pressure monitoring is not done routinely. In the patient with contralateral mediastinal shift on chest radiograph who tolerates thoracentesis without chest tightness, cough, or lightheadedness, probably several liters of pleural fluid can be removed safely. However, neither the patient nor the operator may be aware of a precipitous drop in pleural pressure. In patients without a contralateral mediastinal shift or with ipsilateral shift, the likelihood of a precipitous drop in intrapleural pressure is increased, and either pleural pressure should be monitored during thoracentesis or less than 1 liter should be removed.

Physiologic Effects and Complications. Improvement in lung volumes up to 24 hours following therapeutic thoracentesis does not correlate with the amount of fluid removed, despite relief of dyspnea in those patients [28,29,30]. However, in some patients maximum spirometric improvement may not occur for several days. Patients with initial negative pleural pressures and those with more precipitous falls in pleural pressure with thoracentesis tend to have the least improvement in pulmonary function after therapeutic thoracentesis, because many have a trapped lung or major endobronchial obstruction [27]. The mechanism of dyspnea from a large pleural effusion probably is related to decreased chest wall compliance, contralateral mediastinal shift, and loss of ipsilateral lung volume, in addition to neurogenic factors of the lung parenchyma [29].

Complications of therapeutic thoracentesis are the same as those seen with diagnostic thoracentesis (see Chap. 14). Three complications that are unique to therapeutic thoracentesis are hypoxemia, unilateral pulmonary edema, and hypovolemia [23]. After therapeutic thoracentesis, hypoxemia may occur despite relief of dyspnea [31,32]. It may result from worsening $\dot{V}/\dot{Q}$ relationships in the ipsilateral lung or clinically occult unilateral pulmonary edema.

Some investigators have concluded that the change in PaO_2 following therapeutic thoracentesis is unpredictable [32], some have observed a characteristic increase in PaO_2 within minutes to hours [28], and others suggest a systematic decrease in PaO_2 that returns to prethoracentesis values by 24 hours [31]. In the largest study, encompassing 33 patients with various causes of unilateral pleural effusions, a significant increase in PaO_2 was found 20 minutes, 2 hours, and 24 hours following therapeutic thoracentesis [33]. This was in conjunction with a decrease in the $P(A-a)O_2$ and was accompanied by a small but significant decrease in shunt, while V_D/V_T did not change. Data suggest an improved ventilation-perfusion relationship following therapeutic thoracentesis, with an increase in ventilation of parts of the lung that were previously poorly ventilated but well perfused. The relief of dyspnea in these patients cannot completely be explained by improved arterial oxygen tension. The increases have been modest, and in some cases there has been a fall in PaO_2. Improvement in lung volumes is a constant finding following therapeutic thoracentesis but may take days or even weeks to maximize; immediate changes are usually modest and highly variable. No significant change in expiratory flow rates has been observed. Therefore, the relief of dyspnea cannot be adequately explained by changes in either lung volume or in the mechanics of breathing but may be the result of decreased stimulation of lung or chest wall receptors or both [29].

Pleural Effusions in the Intensive Care Unit

The types of pleural effusions in critically ill patients are listed in Table 65-2.

ATELECTASIS. Atelectasis is a common cause of small pleural effusions in comatose, immobile, pain-ridden patients in ICUs and following upper abdominal surgery [34,35]. Other causes include major bronchial obstruction from lung cancer, a mucous plug, or a foreign body. Atelectasis causes pleural fluid because of decreased pleural pressure. With alveolar collapse, the lung and chest wall separate further, creating local areas of increased negative pressure. This decrease in pleural pressure favors the movement of fluid into the pleural space, presumably from the parietal pleural surface. The fluid accumulates until the pleural space-parietal pleural capillary pressure gradient returns to normal [18].

Pleural fluid from atelectasis is a serous transudate with a low number of mononuclear cells, normal glucose concentration, and pH in the range of 7.45 to 7.55. When atelectasis resolves, pleural fluid dissipates over several days.

CONGESTIVE HEART FAILURE. Congestive heart failure is the most common cause of all transudative pleural effusions and a common cause of pleural effusions in ICUs. Pleural effusions due to congestive heart failure are significantly associated with increases in pulmonary venous pressure [36]. Most patients with subacute or chronic elevation in pulmonary venous pressure (PCWP >24 mm Hg) have evidence of pleural effusion at least on ultrasonography or lateral decubitus radiograph. Isolated increases in systemic venous pressure, even right atrial pressures of 25 mm Hg in the chronic state, tend not to produce pleural effusions. Thus, patients with chronic obstructive pulmonary disease (COPD) and cor pulmonale rarely have pleural effusions, and the presence of pleural fluid implies another etiology.

Most patients with pleural effusions secondary to congestive heart failure (CHF) have the classic signs and symptoms. The chest radiograph shows cardiomegaly and bilateral small to moderate pleural effusions of similar size (right slightly greater than left). There is usually radiographic evidence of pulmonary congestion, with the severity of pulmonary edema correlating with the presence of pleural effusions [36]. Patients in the ICU usually have intake greater than output for several days, weight gain, worsening $P(A-a)O_2$ gradient, and, in those on mechanical ventilators, a decrease in static compliance.

The effusion is a classic transudate, with mesothelial cells and lymphocytes accounting for the majority of the less than 1000 cells per microliter [18]. Acute diuresis changes the transudate to an exudate in 8 percent [37] and 38 percent [38] of patients. In the afebrile patient with clinical CHF and bilateral pleural effusions of relatively equal size and an enlarged cardiac silhouette on chest radiograph, the diagnosis is reasonably secure and observation is appropriate. Thoracentesis should be performed if the patient is febrile, has pleural effusions of disparate size, has a unilateral pleural effusion, does not have

Table 65-2. Differential Diagnosis of Pleural Effusions in Critically Ill Patients

	Clinical presentation	Chest radiograph	Pleural fluid analysis	Diagnosis	Comments
Transudates					
Congestive heart failure	Usual signs and symptoms plus I > O, weight gain, worsening P(A-a)O$_2$, ↓ C$_{ST}$	Bilateral effusions, R > L, cardiomegaly, extravascular lung water	Serous, nucleated cells <1000/μl, lymphocytes, mesothelial, pH 7.45–7.55	Presumptive	Associated with ↑ PCWP, acute diuresis may result in an exudate
Atelectasis	Asymptomatic or dyspnea, worsening P(A-a)O$_2$	Small unilateral or bilateral effusions, volume loss	Serous, nucleated cells <1000/μl, lymphocytes, mesothelial cells, pH 7.45–7.55	Presumptive	Common after upper abdominal surgery, also with PE, mucous plug
Hepatic hydrothorax	Stigmata of liver disease, clinical ascites, asymptomatic or dyspnea, worsening P(A-a)O$_2$, poor response to low-flow O$_2$	Unilateral R or bilateral effusions, small to massive, normal heart size, no other CXR abnormalities	Serous-serosanguinous nucleated cells <1000/μl, lymphocytes, mesothelial cells, pH 7.40–7.55	Presumptive, PF protein and LDH similar to ascitic fluid	6% of patients with clinical ascites, fluid movement from abdomen to chest via diaphragm defect
Hypoalbuminemia	Asymptomatic or dyspnea, anasarca	Small to moderate bilateral effusions, normal heart size, no other CXR abnormalities	Serous, nucleated cells <1000/μl, lymphocytes, mesothelial cells, pH 7.45–7.55	Presumptive	Serous albumin <1.5 g/dl, never have isolated pleural effusion
Iatrogenic: extravascular migration of central venous catheter	Chest pain, dyspnea	Abnormal position of catheter, widening of mediastinum, small to large unilateral effusion	Serous-hemorrhagic, may contain PMNs, chemistries similar to infusate, PF/S glucose >1.0	Presumptive	Highest incidence with L external jugular vein placement, aspiration or retrograde flow of blood confirms intravascular placement
Exudates					
Parapneumonic effusions: uncomplicated	Fever, chest pain ↑ WBC, purulent sputum	New alveolar infiltrate, moderate to large ipsilateral free-flowing effusion	Turbid, PMNs, glucose >60 mg/dl, LDH <700 IU/L, pH ≥7.30	Presumptive	Effusion resolves without sequelae on antibiotics only
Parapneumonic effusion: complicated	Fever, chest pain, ↑ WBC, purulent sputum	New alveolar infiltrate, moderate to large ipsilateral effusion with or without loculation	Pus, positive bacteriology, pH <7.10, glucose <40 mg/dl, LDH >1000 IU/L	Based on PFA, positive bacteriology, aspiration of pus, loculation	Putrid odor, anaerobic empyema, requires pleural space drainage for resolution
Pancreatitis	Acute abdominal pain, nausea, vomiting, fever	Small, unilateral, L effusion (60%), atelectasis	Turbid, nucleated cells 10,000–50,000/μl PMNs, pH 7.30–7.35, PF/S amylase >1.0	PF/S amylase >1.0 or > upper limits of normal for serum	Effusion resolves as pancreatitis resolves without need for pleural space drainage
Pulmonary embolism	Acute dyspnea, tachypnea, chest pain, ↑ P(A-a)O$_2$	Unilateral, small to moderate effusion, peripheral infiltrate, atelectasis	Serous-bloody nucleated cells 100–50,000/μl, PMNs or lymphocytes	Presumptive	20% transudates, effusion present on admission, reaches maximum volume by 72 hr
Postcardiac injury syndrome	Chest pain, pericardial rub, fever, dyspnea 3 days to 3 wk after cardiac injury, ↑ WBC, ↑ ESR	L or bilateral small to moderate effusion, L lower lobe infiltrates	Serosanguinous-bloody, nucleated cells 500–39,000/μl, PMNs or lymphocytes, pH >7.30	Presumptive	Effusion resolves in 1–3 wk, may require steroids
Esophageal sclerotherapy	Chest pain following sclerotherapy with large sclerosant volume, effusion appears by 48–72 hr	Small, unilateral or bilateral effusion	Serosanguinous, nucleated cells 100–38,000/μl, PMNs or mononuclear, pH >7.30	Presumptive	Requires no specific therapy, resolves over days to weeks

Table 65-2. (continued)

	Clinical presentation	Chest radiograph	Pleural fluid analysis	Diagnosis	Comments
Exudates (continued)					
ARDS	Depends on cause	Bilateral alveolar infiltrates tend to mask small bilateral effusions	Serous-serosanguinous, PMNs	Presumptive	Requires no specific therapy, effusions resolve as ARDS resolves
Spontaneous esophageal rupture	Severe retching or vomiting followed by thoracoabdominal pain, fever, subcutaneous air	Subcutaneous/mediastinal air, L pneumothorax, followed by L effusion	Early: serous, pH >7.30; later: turbid-purulent effusion, PMNs, pH approaches 6.00, ↑amylase	Pleural fluid pH <7.00, with ↑salivary amylase and positive bacteriology	With early diagnosis prognosis good with primary closure and drainage
Hemothorax	Following blunt and penetrating chest trauma, invasive procedures, malignancy, anticoagulation	Small to massive unilateral effusion, other abnormalities depending on cause of hemothorax	Gross blood, PF/blood Hct >50%	PF/blood Hct >50%	Often not appreciated on initial radiograph in setting of trauma; should be drained with chest tube
Coronary artery bypass graft	Asymptomatic, dyspnea	Small to moderate L effusion without parenchymal infiltrates, L lower lobe atelectasis, elevation of L hemidiaphragm	Hemorrhagic PF/blood Hct <5%, nucleated cells <10,000/μl, pH >7.40	Presumptive	May require weeks for resolution, rarely results in trapped lung
Abdominal surgery	Asymptomatic 48–72 hr following upper abdominal surgery	Small bilateral effusions, atelectasis	Serous nucleated cells <10,000/μl (75%), pH usually >7.40	Presumptive	Larger L effusions following splenectomy, most commonly found with atelectasis and diaphragmatic irritation, resolves spontaneously
Chylothorax (traumatic)	Asymptomatic or dyspnea following intrathoracic surgery, especially coarctation and esophagectomy	Small to massive L, R, or bilateral effusion	Milky fluid, nucleated cells <7000/μl almost all lymphocytes, pH 7.40–7.80, ↑triglycerides	Triglycerides >110 mg/dl, chylomicrons on lipoprotein electrophoresis	Defect in thoracic duct frequently closes spontaneously with tube drainage and minimizing chyle formation

ARDS = acute respiratory distress syndrome; CXR = chest radiograph; ESR = erythrocyte sedimentation rate; I = input; L = left; LDH = lactate dehydrogenase; O = output; PCWP = pulmonary capillary wedge pressure; PF = pleural fluid; PFA = pleural fluid acidosis; PF/S = pleural fluid/serum; PMN = polymorphonuclear leukocyte; R = right; WBC = white blood cell.

cardiomegaly, has pleuritic chest pain, or has a PaO_2 inappropriate for the degree of pulmonary edema.

Treatment consists of decreasing venous hypertension and improving cardiac output with diuretics, digitalis, and afterload reduction. In successfully managed heart failure the effusions resolve over days to weeks.

HEPATIC HYDROTHORAX. Pleural effusions occur in approximately 6 percent of patients with cirrhosis of the liver and clinical ascites [39,40]. The effusions result from movement of ascitic fluid through diaphragmatic defects or diaphragmatic lymphatics [39]. An effusion may occur acutely following rupture of a diaphragmatic bleb, which is formed because of defects in the muscle and collagen bundle structure at their base.

The patient usually has the classic stigmata of cirrhosis and clinically apparent ascites. With a large to massive pleural effusion the patient may present with acute dyspnea, but with a smaller effusion its presence may be detected only on routine chest radiograph. Rarely, a massive pleural effusion may be found without clinical ascites (demonstrated only by ultrasonography), implying the presence of a large diaphragmatic defect. The usual chest radiograph shows a normal cardiac silhouette and a right-sided pleural effusion in 70 percent of patients, which can vary from small to massive; effusions are less likely isolated to the left pleural space (15%) or are bilateral (15%) [39,40]. The pleural fluid is a serous transudate with a low nucleated cell count and a predominance of mononuclear cells, pH greater than 7.40, a glucose level similar to that of serum, and an amylase less than serum amylase [18]. The fluid can be hemorrhagic due to an underlying coagulopathy. The diagnosis is substantiated by demonstrating that pleural fluid and ascitic fluid have similar protein and LDH concentrations [39]. If the diagnosis is still problematic, injection of a radiolabeled tracer into the ascitic fluid with detection on chest imaging within 1 to 2 hours supports a pleuroperitoneal communication through a diaphragmatic defect [41]; delayed demonstration of the tracer suggests that the pathogenesis of the effusion is via the diaphragmatic lymphatics.

Treatment of hepatic hydrothorax is directed at the ascites, with sodium restriction and diuresis. The effusion frequently persists unchanged until all of the ascites is mobilized. If the patient is acutely dyspneic or in respiratory failure, therapeutic thoracentesis should be done. Care should be exercised with paracentesis or thoracentesis, as hypovolemia can occur with rapid evacuation of fluid.

HYPOALBUMINEMIA. Many patients in a medical ICU who have a chronic illness or prolonged stay have or develop hypoalbuminemia. When the albumin levels are less than 1.5 gm per deciliter, pleural effusions are likely. Since the pleural space has an effective lymphatic drainage system, pleural fluid tends to be the last collection of extravascular lung water that occurs in patients with low oncotic pressure. It is unusual to find a pleural effusion solely due to hypoalbuminemia in the absence of anasarca, which is invariably present at an albumin level less than 1.0 gm per deciliter [42]. Patients with hypoalbuminemic pleural effusions tend not to have pulmonary symptoms unless the effusions are large and there is underlying lung disease. Chest radiograph shows small to moderate bilateral effusions and a normal heart size. The pleural fluid is a serous transudate with less than 1000 nucleated cells per microliter, predominantly lymphocytes and mesothelial cells. The pleural fluid glucose level is similar to that of blood and the pH is in the range of 7.45 to 7.55. Diagnosis is presumptive if other causes of transudative effusions can be excluded. The effusions resolve when hypoalbuminemia is corrected.

IATROGENIC. Extravascular migration of a central venous catheter can cause pneumothorax, hemothorax, and chylothorax but also can be a cause of a transudative pleural effusion [43,44,45]. Its incidence is estimated at less than 1 percent but may be considerably higher. Malposition of the catheter on placement should be suspected if there is absence of blood return or questionable central venous pressure measurements. The immediate postprocedure chest radiograph should be assessed for proper catheter placement; a catheter placed from the right side should not cross the midline. If the catheter is not in the appropriate vessel, phlebitis, perforation of a vein or the heart, or instillation of fluid into the mediastinum or pleural space may occur. In the alert patient, acute infusion of intravenous fluid into the mediastinum usually results in new onset chest discomfort and dyspnea. Depending on the volume and the rate with which it is introduced into the mediastinum, tachypnea, worsening respiratory status, and cardiac tamponade may ensue. The classic chest radiograph shows the catheter tip in an abnormal position [46], a widened mediastinum, and evidence of unilateral or bilateral pleural effusions. The effusion can have characteristics similar to those of the infusate (milky if lipid is being given) and may be hemorrhagic and neutrophil-predominant due to trauma and inflammation. The pleural fluid-to-serum glucose ratio is greater than 1.0 [44]. The pleural fluid glucose concentration can fall rapidly following glucose infusion into the pleural space, probably explaining the relatively low glucose concentrations in pleural fluid compared to the infusate [47]. Extravascular migration of a central venous catheter appears to be more common with placement in the external jugular vein, particularly on the left side. Left-sided catheters appear to put the patient at increased risk of perforation because of the horizontal orientation of the left compared to the right brachiocephalic vein.

Free flow of fluid and proper fluctuation in central venous pressure during the respiratory cycle may not be reliable indicators of intravascular placement. This is probably because intrathoracic pressure changes are transmitted to the mediastinum

and, thus, the venous pressure catheter. Aspiration of blood or retrograde flow of blood when the catheter is lowered below the patient's heart level should confirm intravascular catheter placement. If blood cannot be aspirated and the effusate is aspirated instead, extravascular migration is assured. The central venous catheter should be removed immediately. If there is a small effusion, observation is warranted. If the effusion is large, causing respiratory distress, or a hemothorax is discovered, thoracentesis or tube thoracostomy should be performed.

PARAPNEUMONIC EFFUSIONS. Community-acquired or nosocomial pneumonia is common in critically ill patients. The classic presentation is fever, chest pain, leukocytosis, purulent sputum, and a new alveolar infiltrate on chest radiograph. In the elderly, debilitated patient, however, many of these findings may not be present. The chest radiograph usually shows a small to large ipsilateral pleural effusion. When the effusion is free-flowing, as demonstrated by lateral decubitus view, and thoracentesis shows a turbid, polymorphonuclear (PMN) predominate exudate with a glucose level greater than 60 mg per deciliter, LDH less than 700 IU per liter, and a pH of 7.30 or greater, the patient has an uncomplicated effusion, which should be treated with antibiotics alone at the usual dose recommended for the causative organism [48]. The effusion usually resolves over 7 to 14 days without sequelae. If the chest radiograph demonstrates loculation and pus is aspirated, the diagnosis of empyema is established and immediate drainage is needed. In the nonpurulent fluid, if Gram stain or culture is positive or pH is less than 7.10, the glucose is less than 40 mg per deciliter, and LDH is greater than 1000 IU per liter, the fluid tends to behave like an empyema and requires drainage [48]. This can be accomplished by standard chest tube or radiographic-guided catheter with or without the use of fibrinolytic agents. Failure to respond to drainage or the presence of multiple loculations requires more aggressive drainage, usually empyemectomy and decortication [49]. Some thoracic surgeons now routinely perform thoracoscopy in the latter situation and if not successful proceed immediately to empyemectomy and decortication through a standard thoracotomy [50].

PANCREATITIS. Pleuropulmonary abnormalities are commonly associated with pancreatitis, largely due to the close proximity of the pancreas to the diaphragm. About half of patients with pancreatitis have an abnormal chest radiograph, with pleural effusions in 3 to 17 percent [51]. Mechanisms that may be involved in the pathogenesis of pancreatic pleural effusion include direct contact of pancreatic enzymes with the diaphragm (sympathetic effusion), transfer of ascitic fluid via diaphragmatic lymphatics or defects, communication of a fistulous tract between a pseudocyst and the pleural space, and retroperitoneal movement of fluid into the mediastinum with mediastinitis or rupture into the pleural space [51,52]. Ascitic amylase moves into the pleural space via diaphragmatic lymphatics or through a diaphragmatic defect. The pleural fluid-to-serum amylase ratio is greater than unity in pancreatitis because of impaired lymphatic drainage from the pleural space compared with more rapid amylase clearance by the kidney.

The effusion associated with acute pancreatitis is usually small and left-sided (60%), but may be isolated to the right (30%) or bilateral (10%) [51]. The patient usually presents with abdominal symptoms of acute pancreatitis. The diagnosis is confirmed by an elevated pleural fluid amylase concentration that is greater than that in serum. A normal pleural fluid amylase may be found initially in acute pancreatitis but increases on serial measurements. The fluid is a PMN predominant exudate with glucose values approximating those of serum. Leukocyte counts may reach 50,000 cells per microliter. The pleural fluid pH is usually 7.30 to 7.35 [18].

No specific treatment is necessary for the pleural effusion of acute pancreatitis; the effusion resolves as the pancreatic inflammation subsides. Drainage of the pleural space does not appear to affect residual pleural damage. If the pleural effusion does not resolve in 2 to 3 weeks, pancreatic abscess or pseudocyst should be excluded.

PULMONARY EMBOLISM. The presence of a unilateral pleural effusion may suggest pulmonary embolism or obscure the diagnosis by directing attention to a primary lung or cardiac process. Pleural effusions occur in up to 50 percent of patients with pulmonary embolism [53]. These effusions result from several different mechanisms, including increased pleural capillary permeability, imbalance in microvascular and pleural space hydrostatic pressures, and pleuropulmonary hemorrhage [53,54]. Ischemia from pulmonary vascular obstruction, in addition to release of inflammatory mediators from platelet-rich thrombi, can cause capillary leak into the lung and subsequently pleural space, explaining the usual finding of an exudative effusion. Transudates, described in approximately 20 percent of patients with pulmonary embolism, result from atelectasis [54].

With pulmonary infarction, necrosis and hemorrhage into the lung and pleural space may result. More than 80 percent of patients with infarction have bloody pleural effusions, but more than 35 percent of patients with pulmonary embolism without radiographic infarction also have hemorrhagic fluid [53]. The presence of a pleural effusion does not alter the signs or symptoms in patients with pulmonary embolism. Chest pain, usually pleuritic, occurs in most patients with pleural effusions complicating pulmonary embolism and is invariably ipsilateral [53]. The chest radiograph typically shows a small, unilateral pleural effusion with a volume less than one-third of the hemithorax [53]. An associated pulmonary infiltrate is seen in approximately half of patients with pulmonary embolism and effusion.

Pleural fluid analysis is highly variable and nondiagnostic [54]. However, a bloody pleural effusion suggests pulmonary embolism in the absence of blunt chest trauma, recent cardiac injury, or malignancy [55]. The pleural fluid is bloody in two-thirds of patients, but the number of red blood cells exceeds 100,000 per microliter in less than 20 percent [54]. The nucleated cell count ranges from less than 100 (presumably atelectatic transudates) to greater than 50,000 per microliter (pulmonary infarction) [54]. There is a predominance of PMN when a thoracentesis is performed near the time of the acute injury and of lymphocytes with later thoracentesis. The effusion due to pulmonary embolism is usually apparent on the initial chest radiograph and reaches a maximum volume during the first 72 hours [53]. Patients with pleural effusions that progress with therapy should be evaluated for recurrent embolism, hemothorax secondary to anticoagulation, an infected infarction, or an alternate diagnosis. When consolidation is absent on chest radiograph, effusions resolve in less than 1 week; with consolidation there is a longer resolution time [53].

The association of pleural effusion with pulmonary embolism does not alter therapy. Furthermore, the presence of a bloody effusion is not a contraindication to full-dose anticoagulation, since hemothorax is a rare complication of heparin therapy [56]. An enlarging pleural effusion on therapy necessitates thoracentesis to exclude hemothorax, empyema, or another etiology. Active pleural space hemorrhage necessitates discontinuation of anticoagulation, tube thoracostomy, and consideration of vena caval interruption.

POSTCARDIAC INJURY SYNDROME. Postcardiac injury syndrome (PCIS) is characterized by the onset of fever, pleuropericarditis, and parenchymal infiltrates 3 weeks (2–86 days) following injury to the myocardium or pericardium [57,58,59]. Postcardiac injury syndrome has been described following myocardial infarction, cardiac surgery, blunt chest trauma, percutaneous left ventricular puncture, and pacemaker implantation. The incidence following myocardial infarction has been estimated at up to 4 percent [57] but with more extensive myocardial and pericardial involvement it may be higher. It occurs with greater frequency (up to 30%) following cardiac surgery [60]. The pathogenesis of PCIS remains obscure but is probably on an autoimmune basis in patients with myocardial or pericardial injury and possibly concomitant viral illness.

The diagnosis remains one of exclusion, for no specific criteria exist. It is important to diagnose or exclude PCIS presumptively. Failure to institute prompt therapy could lead to iatrogenic complications from inappropriate therapy, such as cardiac tamponade from anticoagulation for presumed pulmonary embolism and adverse effects related to antimicrobial therapy for presumed pneumonia.

Pleuropulmonary manifestations are the hallmark of PCIS. The most common presenting symptoms are pleuritic chest pain, found in virtually all patients, and fever, pericardial rub, dyspnea, and rales, which occur in half [59]. Rarely, hemoptysis occurs, an important differential point when pulmonary embolism with infarction is in the differential diagnosis. Fifty percent of patients have leukocytosis and almost all have an elevated erythrocyte sedimentation rate [59].

The chest radiograph is abnormal in almost all patients, with the most common abnormality being left-sided and bilateral pleural effusions; a unilateral right effusion is unusual [59]. Pulmonary infiltrates are present in 75 percent of patients and are most commonly seen in the left lower lobe [59].

The pleural fluid is a serosanguinous or bloody exudate with a glucose level greater than 60 mg per deciliter and pleural fluid pH greater than 7.30. Nucleated cell counts range from 500 to 39,000 per microliter, with a predominance of PMNs early in the course [59]. Pericardial fluid on echocardiogram is an important finding suggesting PCIS. The pleural fluid characteristics should help differentiate PCIS from a parapneumonic effusion or CHF but do not exclude pulmonary embolism.

Postcardiac injury syndrome is usually self-limited and may not require therapy if symptoms are trivial. It usually responds to aspirin or nonsteroidal antiinflammatory agents, but some patients require corticosteroid therapy for resolution. In those who respond, the pleural effusion resolves within 1 to 3 weeks.

ESOPHAGEAL SCLEROTHERAPY. Pleural effusions are found in approximately 50 percent of patients 48 to 72 hours following esophageal sclerotherapy [61,62]. Effusions may be unilateral or bilateral, with no predilection for side. Effusion appears more likely with larger total volumes of sclerosant injected and larger volume injected per site [61,62]. The type of sclerosant does not appear to be a factor. The effusions tend to be small-volume, serous exudates with variable nucleated (90–38,000/μl) and red cell counts (126–160,000/μl) and glucose concentration similar to that of blood [61]. These effusions probably result from an intensive inflammatory reaction following extravasation of the sclerosant into the esophageal mucosa, resulting in mediastinal and pleural inflammation. The effusion not associated with fever, chest pain, or evidence of perforation is of little consequence, requires no specific therapy, and resolves over several days to weeks [61,62]. However, late perforation may evolve in patients with apparent innocuous effusions. In patients with symptomatic effusions for 24 to 48 hours, diagnostic thoracentesis should be done and an esophagram considered.

ACUTE RESPIRATORY DISTRESS SYNDROME. The presence of pleural effusions in ARDS has not been well appreciated. In a retrospective study of 25 patients with ARDS, a 36 percent incidence of pleural effusions was found, a percentage similar to that found with hydrostatic pulmonary edema [63]. All patients had extensive alveolar pulmonary edema and endotracheal tube fluid that was compatible with increased permeability edema. Several experimental models of increased permeability pulmonary edema, including alpha-naphthyl-thiourea [64], oleic acid [65], and ethchlorvynol [66], have been shown to produce pleural effusions. In both the oleic acid and ethchlorvynol model, the development of pleural effusions lagged behind interstitial and alveolar edema by several hours. In the oleic acid model, 35 percent of the excess lung water collected in the pleural spaces. It appears that the pleura acts as a reservoir for excess lung water in both increased permeability and hydrostatic pulmonary edema. These effusions tend to be underdiagnosed clinically, because the patient has bilateral alveolar infiltrates and the radiograph is taken with the patient in a supine position. Experimentally, the effusion is serous to serosanguinous, with a predominance of PMNs [66]. These effusions require no specific therapy and resolve as ARDS resolves.

SPONTANEOUS ESOPHAGEAL RUPTURE. Esophageal rupture, a potentially life-threatening event, requires immediate diagnosis and therapy. The history in spontaneous esophageal rupture is usually severe retching or vomiting or a conscious effort to resist vomiting. In some patients the perforation may be silent. Early recognition of spontaneous rupture depends on interpretation of the chest radiograph. Several factors influence chest radiograph findings: the time between perforation and chest radiograph examination, site of perforation, and mediastinal-pleural integrity [67]. A chest radiograph taken within minutes of the acute injury is usually unremarkable. Mediastinal emphysema probably takes at least 1 to 2 hours to be demonstrated radiographically and is present in less than half of patients; mediastinal widening may take several hours [68]. Pneumothorax, present in 75 percent of patients with spontaneous rupture, indicates violation of the mediastinal pleura; 70 percent of pneumothoraces are on the left, 20 percent are on the right, and 10 percent are bilateral [68]. Mediastinal air is seen early if pleural integrity is maintained, while pleural effusion secondary to mediastinitis tends to occur later. Pleural fluid, with or without associated pneumothorax, occurs in 75 percent of patients. A presumptive diagnosis should be confirmed radiographically immediately. Esophagrams are positive in about 90 percent of patients [69]. In the upright patient, rapid passage of the contrast material may not demonstrate a small rent; therefore, the study should be done with the patient in the appropriate lateral decubitus position [70].

Pleural fluid findings depend on the degree of perforation and the timing of thoracentesis from injury. Early thoracentesis without mediastinal perforation shows a serous, sterile exudate with a predominance of PMNs and a normal pleural fluid amylase and pH [71]. Once the mediastinal pleura tears, amylase of salivary origin appears in the fluid in high concentrations [72]. As the pleural space is seeded with anaerobic organisms from the mouth, the pH falls rapidly and progressively to approach 6.00 [71,73]. Other pleural fluid findings suggestive of esophageal rupture include the presence of squamous epithelial cells and food particles. The diagnosis of spontaneous esophageal rupture dictates immediate operative intervention. If diagnosed and treated appropriately within the first 24 hours with primary closure, survival is greater than 90 percent [69]. Delay from the time of initial symptoms to diagnosis results in a reduced survival with any form of therapy.

HEMOTHORAX. Hemothorax (blood in the pleural space) should be differentiated from a hemorrhagic pleural effusion, as the latter can be the result of only a few drops of blood in pleural fluid. A practical definition of a hemothorax with regard to therapy is a pleural fluid-to-blood hematocrit ratio greater than 50 percent [74]. A majority of hemothoraces result from penetrating or blunt chest trauma [75]. Hemothorax can also result from invasive procedures, such as placement of central venous catheters, thoracentesis, and pleural biopsy, and pulmonary embolism, malignancy, or ruptured aortic aneurysm. Bleeding can occur from vessels of the chest wall, lung, diaphragm, or mediastinum. Blood that enters the pleural space clots, rapidly undergoes fibrinolysis, and becomes defibrinogenated; thus it rarely causes significant pleural fibrosis.

Hemothorax should be suspected in any patient with blunt or penetrating chest trauma. If a pleural effusion is found on the admitting chest radiograph, thoracentesis should be performed immediately and the hematocrit measured on the fluid. The hemothorax may not be apparent on the initial chest radiograph, which may be due to supine position of the patient [76]. Because bleeding may be slow and not appear for several hours [76], it is imperative that serial radiographs be performed in these patients. The incidence of concomitant pneumothorax is high (approximately 60 percent) [75,76]. Patients with traumatic hemothorax should be treated with immediate tube thoracostomy [75–78]. Large-diameter chest tube drainage will evacuate the pleural space, may tamponade the bleeding (especially if the origin is from a pleural laceration), will allow monitoring of the bleeding, and will decrease the likelihood of subsequent fibrothorax [78,79]. If bleeding continues without signs of slowing, thoracotomy should be performed, depending on the individual circumstances [78]. Pleural effusions occasionally occur following removal of the chest tube from traumatic hemothoraces [80]. A diagnostic thoracentesis is indicated to exclude empyema. If empyema is excluded, the pleural effusion usually resolves without specific treatment and without residual pleural fibrosis.

Hemothorax is a rare complication of anticoagulation and has been reported in patients receiving heparin and warfarin [81]. Coagulation studies are usually within the acceptable therapeutic range. The hemothorax tends to occur on the side of the pulmonary embolism. Anticoagulation should be discontinued immediately, a chest tube inserted to evacuate the blood, and a vena cava filter considered.

CORONARY ARTERY BYPASS SURGERY. A small left pleural effusion is virtually always present following coronary artery bypass surgery. This is associated with left lower lobe atelectasis and elevation of the left hemidiaphragm on chest radiograph. Left diaphragm dysfunction is secondary to intraoperative phrenic nerve injury from cold cardioplegia, stretch injury, or surgical trauma [82,83,84]. The larger and grossly bloody effusions tend to be associated with internal mammary artery grafting, which causes marked exudation from the bed where the internal mammary artery was harvested [85]. Furthermore, the larger and more persistent pleural effusions appear to be associated with left pleurotomy. Pleurotomy may increase pleural fluid accumulation by increasing production of fluid and decreasing lymphatic drainage from the pleural space.

The pleural fluid is a hemorrhagic exudate with a low nucleated cell count, a glucose level similar to that of blood, and a pH greater than 7.40. Rarely, a loculated hemothorax may develop with trapped lung, resulting in clinically significant restriction [86]. Some cardiovascular surgeons suggest avoiding pleurotomy, minimizing chest wall distortion during internal mammary artery harvesting, and taking special care not to injure the phrenic nerve, in an attempt to decrease the volume and persistence of left pleural effusions. If there is a large effusion that qualifies as a hemothorax (supra vide), the fluid should be drained by tube thoracostomy. It is unclear whether a large hemorrhagic effusion (pleural fluid/blood hematocrit <50%) needs to be drained with a needle. It is probably prudent to drain moderately large, bloody effusions to avoid later necessity for decortication.

ABDOMINAL SURGERY. Approximately half of patients who undergo abdominal surgery have been documented to develop small unilateral or bilateral pleural effusions within 48 to 72 hours of surgery [34,35]. The incidence is higher following upper abdominal surgery, in patients with postoperative atelectasis, and in patients who have free ascitic fluid at the time of surgery [34]. Larger left-sided pleural effusions are common following splenectomy [34]. The effusion is usually an exudate with less than 10,000 nucleated cells per microliter. The glucose level is similar to that of blood and pH is usually greater than 7.40 [34]. The effusion is usually related to diaphragmatic irritation or atelectasis. Small effusions generally do not require diagnostic thoracentesis, are of no clinical significance, and resolve spontaneously. Pleural effusion from subphrenic abscess or pulmonary embolism is unlikely to occur within 2 to 3 days of surgery. The only indication for diagnostic thoracentesis in this setting would be to exclude infection if the effusion is relatively large or loculated.

CHYLOTHORAX. Trauma from surgery accounts for approximately 25 percent of cases of chylothorax, second only to lymphoma [87]. Most series estimate an incidence of chylothorax less than 1 percent following thoracic surgery [88], but a 3 percent incidence has been reported following esophagectomy [89]. Virtually all intrathoracic procedures, including lobectomy and pneumonectomy and coronary artery bypass grafting, have been reported to cause chylothorax. Other iatrogenic chylothoraces can be caused by complications of prolonged central vein catheterization [90]. Nonsurgical trauma, such as penetrating and nonpenetrating neck, thoracic, and upper abdominal injuries, also has been associated with chylothorax.

When the thoracic duct is torn by stretching during surgery, chyle leaks into the mediastinum and subsequently ruptures through the mediastinal pleura [91]. In the nonsurgical setting, penetrating injuries and fractures may directly tear the thoracic duct. Chylothorax from a central venous catheter usually involves venous thrombosis [90].

The patient may be asymptomatic if the effusion is small and unilateral or present with dyspnea with a large unilateral or bilateral effusions. The pleural fluid is usually milky, but 12 percent can be serous or serosanguinous [92], with less than 7000 nucleated cells, virtually all lymphocytes [18]. The pH is alkaline (7.40–7.80) and triglyceride levels are greater than plasma levels. The diagnosis can be established by a triglyceride concentration in the pleural fluid of greater than 110 mg per deciliter [92]. If the triglyceride level is less than 50 mg per deciliter, chylothorax can be virtually excluded. Triglyceride levels of 50 to 110 mg per deciliter indicate the need for lipo-

Table 65-3. Classification of Pneumothorax

Spontaneous
  Primary: no clinical lung disease
  Secondary: clinical presence of lung disease
Traumatic
Iatrogenic
  Barotrauma
  Invasive procedures: central line, thoracentesis
  Misplacement of an enteral feeding tube

Table 65-4. Causes of Pneumothorax in the Intensive Care Unit

Secondary spontaneous
  COPD
  Status asthmaticus
  Interstitial lung disease
    Pulmonary histiocytosis X
    Stage IV sarcoidosis
  Pneumocystis carinii pneumonia
  Cystic fibrosis
  Necrotizing pneumonia
Iatrogenic
  Barotrauma
    ARDS
    COPD
    Necrotizing pneumonia
  Invasive procedures
    Central venous catheters
    Thoracentesis
    Placement of narrow-bore enteral feeding tubes

ARDS = acute respiratory distress syndrome; COPD = chronic obstructive pulmonary disease.

protein electrophoresis [92]. Demonstration of chylomicrons on electrophoresis confirms the diagnosis of chylothorax. The thoracic duct defect following trauma usually closes spontaneously within 10 to 14 days with chest tube drainage as well as bed rest and total parenteral nutrition to minimize chyle formation. A pleuroperitoneal shunt also relieves dyspnea, recirculates chyle, and prevents malnutrition and immunocompromise [93].

Pneumothorax

DEFINITIONS AND CLASSIFICATION. *Pneumothorax* literally means "presence of air within the thorax," but it actually refers to the presence of free air within the confines of the chest. Most use *pneumothorax* to mean free air within the pleural space, but free air may be found in the adventitial planes of the lung or the mediastinum (pneumomediastinum).

The classification of pneumothorax is shown in Table 65-3. Spontaneous pneumothorax occurs without an obvious cause as a consequence of the natural course of a disease process. Primary spontaneous pneumothorax occurs without clinical findings of lung disease. Secondary spontaneous pneumothorax occurs as a consequence of clinically manifest lung disease (Table 65-4). Traumatic pneumothorax results from penetrating or blunt chest injury. Iatrogenic pneumothorax occurs as an inadvertent consequence of diagnostic or therapeutic procedures (Table 65-4).

PATHOPHYSIOLOGY. Pressure in the pleural space is subatmospheric throughout the normal respiratory cycle, averaging approximately −9 mm Hg during inspiration and −5 mm Hg during expiration. Due to lung elasticity, pressure in the airways is positive during expiration (+3 mm Hg) and negative (−2 mm Hg) during inspiration [94]. Thus, in normal breathing airway pressure is greater than pleural pressure throughout the respiratory cycle. Airway pressure may be increased markedly with coughing or strenuous exercise; however, pleural pressure rises concomitantly so that the transpulmonary pressure gradient is usually not substantially changed. When there are rapid fluctuations in intrathoracic pressure, however, a large transpulmonary pressure gradient occurs transiently. Bronchial and bronchiolar obstruction, resulting in air trapping, can significantly increase the transpulmonary pressure gradient. The alveolar walls and visceral pleura maintain the pressure gradient between the airways and pleural space. When the pressure gradient is transiently increased, alveolar rupture may occur; air will enter the interstitial tissues of the lung and may enter the pleural space, resulting in a pneumothorax. If the visceral pleura remains intact, the interstitial air moves toward the hilum, resulting in pneumomediastinum [95,96]. Since mean pressure within the mediastinum is always less than in the periphery of the lung, air would move proximally along the bronchovascular sheaths to the hilum and mediastinal soft tissues. The development of pneumomediastinum following alveolar rupture requires continual cyclic respiratory efforts, which result in slow movement of air from the ruptured alveolus along a pressure gradient to the mediastinum [96]. Mediastinal air may decompress into the cervical and subcutaneous tissues or the retroperitoneum. With abrupt rise in mediastinal pressure or insufficient decompression to subcutaneous tissue, the mediastinal pleura may rupture, causing pneumothorax. Inadequate decompression of the mediastinum, rather than direct rupture of subpleural blebs into the pleural space, may be the major cause of pneumothorax [95].

When pneumothorax occurs, the elasticity of the lung causes it to collapse. Lung collapse continues until the pleural defect seals or pleural and alveolar pressures equalize. When a ball-valve effect occurs at the site of communication between the pleural space and the alveolus, permitting only egress of air from the lung, there is a progressive accumulation of air within the pleural space, which can result in markedly increased positive pleural pressure, producing a tension pneumothorax. Tension pneumothorax compresses mediastinal structures, resulting in impaired venous return to the heart, decrease in cardiac output, and, at times, fatal cardiovascular collapse [97,98]. Rarely, tension along the bronchovascular sheaths and in the mediastinum can cause collapse of the pulmonary arteries and veins, resulting in cardiovascular collapse [95].

Patients with primary spontaneous pneumothorax have a decrease in vital capacity and an increase in the $P(A-a)O_2$ gradient and usually present with hypoxemia due predominantly to the development of an intrapulmonary shunt and areas of low $\dot{V}/\dot{Q}$ in the atelectatic lung [99,100]. Hypercapnia does not occur, because there is adequate function in the uninvolved lung to maintain necessary alveolar ventilation. Patients with secondary spontaneous pneumothorax, in contrast, commonly develop hypercapnia because the gas exchange abnormality caused by the pneumothorax is superimposed on lungs with preexisting abnormal pulmonary gas exchange [101,102].

PNEUMOTHORAX IN THE INTENSIVE CARE UNIT. Patients with secondary spontaneous pneumothorax may be admitted to an ICU because they develop severe hypoxemic and, at times, hypercapnic respiratory failure. Patients with primary spontaneous pneumothorax rarely require ICU admission, as the contralateral lung can maintain necessary alveolar ventila-

tion and the hypoxemia can be managed with supplemental oxygen. The most common causes of pneumothoraces in ICU patients are invasive procedures and barotrauma.

Iatrogenic Pneumothorax

CENTRAL VENOUS CATHETERS. Central venous catheters are used routinely in critically ill patients for volume resuscitation, parenteral nutrition, and drug administration. Approximately 3 million central venous catheters are placed annually in the United States, and this procedure continues to be associated with clinically relevant morbidity and some mortality [103]. The morbidity and mortality associated with central venous catheter use are most commonly physician-related [43]. Pleural complications of both acquisition of venous access and the indwelling phase of central venous catheters include pneumothorax, hydrothorax, hemothorax, and chylothorax. In a recent study of mechanical complications of central venous catheters, 1.1 percent of 534 patients had pneumothorax [104]. This translates into approximately 36,000 pneumothoraces per year from central venous catheter insertions in critically ill patients in the United States. In the same study, none of the 405 patients developed pneumothorax when the central venous catheter was replaced over a guidewire. Both the subclavian and internal jugular routes have been associated with pneumothorax, hemothorax, chylothorax, and catheter placement into the pleural space. Cannulation of the subclavian vein is associated with a higher risk of pneumothorax (1–5%) [105] than cannulation of the internal jugular vein (0–0.2%) [106]; with the external jugular venous approach pneumothorax is avoided. There is a greater risk of pneumothorax with the infraclavicular compared to the supraclavicular approach to the subclavian vein. All complications of insertion, regardless of approach, can be reduced by appropriate physician training and experience. Operator inexperience appears to increase the number of complications with the internal jugular approach. It probably does not have as much impact as on the incidence of pneumothorax with the subclavian vein approach, which accounts for 25 to 50 percent of all complications [106].

Most pneumothoraces occur at the time of the procedure from direct lung puncture, but delayed pneumothoraces have been noted; therefore it is prudent to view a chest radiograph 12 to 24 hours after the procedure. Up to half of patients with needle puncture pneumothorax may be managed expectantly without the need for tube drainage. Bilateral pneumothoraces have been reported to occur from unilateral attempts [107], and death can occur when there is a delay in the diagnosis of pneumothorax [108]. As stated previously, a pneumothorax may be more difficult to detect while the patient is supine. Additional views should be taken, especially if the venous cannulation does not proceed as anticipated. With any newly placed central venous catheter, a postprocedure chest radiograph should be obtained, regardless of the site cannulated, to assure that the catheter tip is properly positioned. If a small pneumothorax is diagnosed by chest radiograph and the patient is asymptomatic and not on mechanical ventilation, the patient can be followed expectantly with repeat chest radiographs to assure that the leak has ceased. If the patient is on mechanical ventilation or the pneumothorax is large or has caused significant symptoms or gas exchange abnormalities, then tube thoracostomy should be performed as soon as possible.

BAROTRAUMA. Pulmonary barotrauma is an important clinical problem because of the widespread use of mechanical ventilation. Barotrauma occurs in about 10 percent of patients on mechanical ventilation and includes parenchymal interstitial gas, pneumomediastinum, subcutaneous emphysema, pneumoperitoneum, and pneumothorax [11,109,110,111]. The form most clinically important is pneumothorax, occurring in 1 to

15 percent of patients on mechanical ventilation. The number of ventilation days, underlying disease (ARDS, COPD, necrotizing pneumonia), and use of positive end-expiratory pressure (PEEP) impact on the incidence of pneumothorax [109, 110–115]. When a pneumothorax develops in the setting of mechanical ventilation, 30 to 97 percent of patients develop tension [11,110,112,116,117].

The initial radiographic sign of barotrauma is often pulmonary interstitial gas [116]. However, in the early stages interstitial gas may be difficult to detect radiographically. This harbinger of pneumothorax may be detected as distinct subpleural air cysts, linear air streaks emanating from the hilum, and perivascular air halos. Subpleural air cysts, most commonly seen in ARDS, tend to appear abruptly on the chest radiograph as single or multiple thin-walled, round lucencies and are most often visualized at the lung bases, medially or diaphragmatically [118]. The cysts, which may expand rapidly, are usually 3 to 5 cm in diameter. Differentiating between peripheral subpleural air cysts and a localized basilar pneumothorax may be problematic. Pleural air cysts appear to be more common in younger patients, possibly because connective tissue planes of the lung are looser in younger than in older patients [119]. The risk of tension pneumothorax is substantial in patients who have developed subpleural lung cysts with continued mechanical ventilation. When mechanical ventilation is discontinued, the cyst may resolve spontaneously or become secondarily infected.

When evidence of barotrauma without pneumothorax is observed in any patient requiring continued mechanical ventilation, immediate attempts should be made to lower the plateau airway pressure. In ARDS, tidal volumes [120,121] and inspiratory flow rates should be lowered, an attempt should be made to reduce or remove PEEP, and neuromuscular blockers and sedation should be given [122]. In status asthmaticus, in addition to the aforementioned maneuvers, controlled hypoventilation should be accomplished [123,124]. There is no evidence supporting the use of prophylactic chest tubes. However, the patient should be monitored closely for tension pneumothorax and provisions made for emergency bedside tube thoracostomy.

Tension Pneumothorax. Pneumothorax in the mechanically ventilated patient usually presents as an acute cardiopulmonary emergency, beginning with respiratory distress and, if unrecognized and untreated, progressing to a cardiovascular collapse. In one report of 74 patients, the diagnosis of pneumothorax was made clinically in 45 (61%) patients based on hypotension, hyperresonance, diminished breath sounds, and tachycardia [115]. The mortality rate was 7 percent in these patients diagnosed clinically. In the remaining 29 patients, diagnosis was delayed between 30 minutes and 8 hours, and 31 percent of these patients died of pneumothorax. Other series of barotrauma in the setting of mechanical ventilation have reported mortality rates from 58 to 77 percent [11,111,113,114].

Tension pneumothorax is lethal if diagnosis and treatment are delayed. The diagnosis should be made clinically at the bedside in the patient on mechanical ventilation who develops a sudden deterioration characterized by apprehension, tachypnea, cyanosis, decreased ipsilateral breath sounds, subcutaneous emphysema, tachycardia, and hypotension. The diagnosis may be problematic in the unconscious patient, the elderly, and the patient with bilateral tension, which may be more protective of the mediastinal structures and lessen the impact on cardiac output.

In the unconscious or critically ill patient, hypoxemia may be one of the earlier signs of tension pneumothorax. In the patient on mechanical ventilation, increasing peak and mean airway pressure, decreasing compliance, and auto PEEP should raise the possibility of tension pneumothorax. Difficulty in bagging the patient and delivering adequate tidal volumes may be noted.

When the clinical signs and symptoms are noted in mechanically ventilated patients, treatment should not be delayed to obtain radiographic confirmation. If a chest tube is not immediately available, placement of a large-bore needle into the anterior second intercostal space will be lifesaving and confirm the diagnosis, as a rush of air will be noted on entering the pleural space. An appropriately large chest tube can then be placed and connected to an adequate drainage system that can accommodate the large air leak which may develop in mechanically ventilated patients [125].

On relief of the tension, there is a rapid improvement in oxygenation, increase in blood pressure, decrease in heart rate, and fall in peak airway pressure. In experimental tension pneumothorax, it has been observed that the inability to raise cardiac output in response to hypoxemia leads to a reduction in systemic oxygen transport and a decrease in mixed venous PO_2, partially explaining the cardiovascular collapse seen in these patients [98].

Bronchopleural Fistula

DEFINITION AND CAUSES. Communication between the bronchial tree and the pleural space is a dreaded complication of mechanical ventilation [126,127]. There are three presentations of bronchopleural fistula (BPF): (1) failure to reinflate the lung despite chest tube drainage or continued air leak after evacuation of the pneumothorax in the setting of chest trauma; (2) complication of a diagnostic or therapeutic procedure, such as thoracic surgery; and (3) complication of mechanical ventilation, usually for ARDS [128]. In ARDS, often a pneumothorax occurs under tension and is later associated with empyema, multiple sites of leakage, and a poor prognosis. A large air leak through a BPF can result in failure of lung reexpansion, loss of a significant amount of each delivered tidal volume, loss of the ability to apply PEEP, inappropriate cycling of the ventilator [129], and inability to maintain alveolar ventilation (Table 65-5).

If there is a continued air leak for greater than 24 hours following the development of pneumothorax, then a BPF exists. The main factors that perpetuate BPF are high airway pressures that increase the leak during inspiration, increased mean intrathoracic pressures throughout the respiratory cycle (PEEP, inflation hold, high inspiratory/expiratory ratio) that increase the leak throughout the breath, and high negative suction [128]. In severe ARDS, all of these factors are present, because they usually are necessary to support gas exchange and lung inflation.

MANAGEMENT. Given the frequency of barotrauma in BPF in mechanically ventilated patients, intensivists will be called to advise on the management of these difficult patients. Definitive therapy of BPF frequently involves invasive surgical approaches that include thoracoplasty, mobilization of the pec-

Table 65-5. Consequences of a Large Bronchopleural Fistula

Failure of lung reexpansion
Loss of delivered tidal volume
Inability to apply PEEP
Inappropriate cycling of ventilator
Inability to maintain alveolar ventilation

toralis or intercostal muscles, bronchial stump stapling, and decortication [130–135]. While some of these techniques are still used today, there is a trend toward more conservative management of both acute and chronic BPF, using innovations of standard techniques and new modalities that include chest tube management, drainage systems, ventilatory support, and definitive nonoperative therapy (Table 65-6). Nonoperative therapy provides an alternative to the surgical approaches in patients who are poor operative candidates. Each patient with a BPF is unique and requires individual management based on the specific clinical setting. Attention to the basics of medical care of patients with BPF should not be neglected in the face of the potentially dramatic events related to the BPF. Nutritional status must be maintained, appropriate antibiotics used for the infected pleural space, and the space adequately drained [136].

Chest Tubes. The initial therapy for pneumothorax in a patient on mechanical ventilation is placement of a chest tube in an attempt to reexpand the lung (see Chap. 11). The chest tube is initially necessary, can be detrimental later, and may play a role more important than that of a passive conduit. Air leaks in the setting of BPF range from less than 1 to 16 liters per minute [137]; therefore, a chest tube that permits prompt and efficient drainage of this level of airflow is required. Gas moves through a tube in a laminar fashion and is governed by Poiseuille's law ($v = [\pi r^4 \, P/8lV] \, t$). In the clinical setting, the gas moving through a chest tube is moist; it is therefore subject to turbulent flow and governed by the Fanning equation ($v = [\pi^2 r^5 \, P/fl]$) [137–140]. Therefore, both the length (l) and, more important, the radius (r) are important when choosing a chest tube and connecting tubing to evacuate a BPF adequately (as flow varies exponentially to the fifth power of the radius of the tube). The smallest internal diameter that will allow a maximum flow of 15.1 liters per minute at -10 cm H_2O suction is 6 mm [137,139] (a 32 Fr. chest tube has an internal diameter of 9 mm). A chest tube with a diameter adequate to convey the potentially large airflow of the BPF must be considered. A chest tube with too small a diameter can lead to lung collapse and tension pneumothorax in the setting of a mobile mediastinum.

Not only can the chest tube be used to drain pleural air, it can also be used to limit the air leak in certain situations. One modality is the application of intrapleural pressure equivalent to the level of PEEP during the expiratory phase of ventilation [141,142,143]. With positive intrapleural pressure applied through the chest tube, the air leak persists during the inspiratory phase of ventilation but decreases during expiration, allow-

Table 65-6. Management of Bronchopleural Fistula in Patients Requiring Mechanical Ventilation

Conservative
    Adequate-size chest tube
    Use of drainage system with adequate capabilities
    Mechanical ventilation
        Conventional (controlled, assist control, intermittent mandatory ventilation)
        High-frequency
        Independent lung
    Fiberoptic bronchoscopy
        Direct application of sealant
Invasive
    Mobilization of intercostal or pectoralis muscles
    Thoracoplasty
    Bronchial stump stapling
    Pleural abrasion and decortication

ing maintenance of PEEP in patients in whom it is necessary for adequate oxygenation. Synchronized closure of the chest tube during the inspiratory phase has also been used to control the air leak [144]. A combination of these techniques has been suggested for patients with significant BPF air leaks during both the inspiratory and expiratory phases of mechanical ventilation [126,145]. These techniques pose potential hazards, including increased pneumothorax and tension pneumothorax [126,128,144], necessitating extremely close patient monitoring when such manipulations are used.

Instillation of chemical agents through the chest tube may potentially help close the BPF if the anatomic defect is small and single, but it is unlikely to be successful if the fistula is large or if there are multiple fistulas. Various agents have been successful in preventing recurrent pneumothoraces in patients not on mechanical ventilation [146–150], but BPF in the setting of mechanical ventilation is a different situation. One study compared the recurrence of pneumothorax in 39 patients with BPF randomized to intrapleural tetracycline or placebo groups [151]. There was no evidence that intrapleural tetracycline facilitated closure of the BPF. No adverse effects were encountered from the instillation of tetracycline in patients with persistent air leaks.

The chest tube may be associated with adverse effects in patients with BPF. The gas escaping through the chest tube represents part of the minute ventilation delivered to the patient and makes maintenance of an effective tidal volume problematic [152,153]. Maintenance of a specific level of ventilation is not only affected by the amount of gas escaping through the fistula. The escaping gas does not passively flow from the airways into the BPF but is involved in physiologic gas exchange [152,153]. Approximately 25 percent of the minute ventilation has been found to escape via the BPF in patients with ARDS, with more than 20 percent of CO_2 excretion occurring by this route in half of patients [153]. The role of the BPF in active CO_2 exchange is complex: proposed mechanisms include drainage of gas from alveoli in the area of the BPF and removal of gas from remote alveolar areas by pressure gradients created by the BPF [53].

Carbon dioxide excretion and a reduction in minute ventilation occur to a lesser extent in BPF trauma victims [152]. In these patients, variable CO_2 excretion and loss of minute ventilation were dynamic and dependent on the level of chest tube suction. The difference between trauma and ARDS patients may have been due to the variability of lung compliance and the use of different ventilators [153]. Also, BPF may affect oxygen utilization, which generally decreases the utilization of inspired oxygen before it escapes through the fistula [152]. This relationship is variable but requires consideration in patients with oxygenation problems.

Negative pressure applied to the chest tube may be transmitted beyond the pleural space and into the airways, creating inappropriate cycling of the ventilator [129,154]. The increased flow through a BPF can occur with increased negative pleural pressure and may interfere with closure and healing of the fistulous site [126,128]. Therefore, the least amount of chest tube suction that will keep the lung inflated should be maintained in patients with BPF. The chest tube is a potential source of infection, both at the insertion site and within the pleural space [138].

Drainage Systems. As with the chest tube, the resistance of flow of gases is a consideration in the choice of the drainage system for the patient with a BPF [137,138]. The size of the air leak and the flow that the drainage system can accommodate are necessary considerations. In an experimental model of BPF that simulated the type of air leak seen clinically (mean maximal flow 5 L/min), four pleural drainage units (PDU) (Emerson Post-Operative Pump, Pleur-Evac, Sentinel Seal, and Thora-Klex) were tested at water seal, -20 cm H_2O, and -40 cm H_2O suction [137]. Compared to the water seal, -20 cm H_2O suction significantly increased the ability of all four PDUs to evacuate air via the chest tube, but an increase in suction to -40 cm H_2O did not significantly alter flow. When the air leak reached 4 to 5 liters per minute, use of the Thora-Klex or Sentinel Seal become clinically impractical. The Pleur-Evac can handle flow rates up to 34 liters per minute, but its use with rates greater than 28 liters per minute is impractical due to intense bubbling in the suction control chamber [137]. Air leaks of this magnitude are infrequent clinically in BPF and are likely to be seen only with major airway disruption or diffuse parenchymal leak secondary to ARDS with severe barotrauma [128,154]. In the latter situations, the low-pressure, high-volume Emerson suction pump remains the only PDU capable of handling the air leak [137]. The choice of PDU should be influenced by its physiologic capabilities and the type of BPF air leak that is encountered.

Mechanical Ventilation

CONVENTIONAL VENTILATION. The dilemma with a BPF in a mechanically ventilated patient is between achieving adequate ventilation and oxygenation while allowing repair of the BPF to occur. Because air flow escaping through a BPF theoretically delays healing of the fistulous site, reducing flow through the fistula has been a major goal in promoting repair. The BPF provides an area of low resistance to flow and acts as a conduit for the escape of a variable percentage of delivered tidal volume during conventional positive-pressure mechanical ventilation. Thus, the goal of management is to maintain adequate ventilation and oxygenation while reducing the fistula flow [126,128]. This can be done by using the lowest possible tidal volume, fewest mechanical breaths per minute, lowest level of PEEP, and shortest inspiratory time (see Chap. 66). Avoidance of expiratory retard also reduces airway pressures. Using the greatest number of spontaneous breaths per minute, thereby reducing use of positive pressure, may also be advantageous. Intermittent mandatory ventilation may have an advantage over assist control ventilation in BPF.

In a retrospective study of 39 patients with BPF who were maintained on conventional ventilation, only 2 patients developed a pH less than 7.30 despite air leaks of up to 900 ml per breath [154]. Overall, mortality was higher when the BPF developed late in the illness and was higher with larger leaks (>500 ml/breath).

High-Frequency Ventilation.

Despite anecdotal reports, experimental data, and clinical studies involving high-frequency ventilation (HFV) in the setting of BPF, controversy exists. However, there appear to be subgroups of patients with BPF in whom HFV may be beneficial. Both animal [155–158] and human [159,160] studies suggest that HFV is superior to conventional ventilation in controlling PO_2 and PCO_2 when there is a proximal (tracheal or bronchial) unilateral or bilateral fistula in the presence of normal lung parenchyma.

The use of HFV in BPF in patients with parenchymal lung disease such as ARDS is more controversial. While some studies have shown that HFV improves or stabilizes gas exchange in patients with extensive parenchymal lung disease [159,160,161], others have not shown a beneficial effect on gas exchange or a reduction in fistula outflow [162,163]. A trial of HFV appears reasonable in the patient with a proximal BPF and normal lung parenchyma; however, it is unclear whether HFV should be considered the primary mode of ventilation in this setting. Despite discrepancies in clinical results, a trial of HFV in a critically ill patient with a BPF and diffuse parenchymal disease who fails conventional ventilation appears justified. Caution must be exercised, however, with close monitoring of gas exchange parameters and fistula flow whenever HFV is used.

OTHER MODES OF VENTILATION. Other maneuvers during both conventional ventilation and HFV can be potentially helpful in patients with BPF. Selective intubation and conventional ventilation of the unaffected lung in patients with unilateral BPF may be useful but will predispose to the collapse of the nonintubated lung [164,165]. The use of differential lung ventilation with conventional ventilation may be of benefit in some patients [164]. Positioning of the patient such that the BPF is dependent has been shown to decrease fistula flow [166].

Case reports and animal studies suggest other potential applications of HFV in BPF, including the use of independent lung ventilation with HFV applied to the BPF lung and conventional ventilation to the normal lung [167]. Another mode of HFV, ultra-high-frequency jet ventilation, is being explored and has been used with some success in reducing BPF in both humans [168] and animal models [169]. Independent lung ventilation with ultra-high-frequency lung ventilation applied to the BPF lung and conventional ventilation to the normal lung led to rapid BPF closure in two of three patients [168].

Fiberoptic Bronchoscopy.

The fiberoptic bronchoscope can be valuable in the diagnosis of BPF [170,171,172]. Bronchoscopic therapy of BPF has several potential advantages, including low cost, shortened hospital stay, and relative noninvasiveness, particularly in poor operative candidates [170,172] (see Chap. 12). Proximal fistulas, such as those associated with lobectomy or pneumonectomy or stump breakdown, can be directly visualized through the bronchoscope. Distal fistulas cannot be visualized directly and require bronchoscopic passage of an occluding balloon to localize the bronchial segment leading to the fistula [173–176]. A balloon is systematically passed through the working channel of the bronchoscope and into each bronchial segment in question and then inflated; a reduction in air leak indicates localization of a bronchial segment communicating with the BPF. Once the fistula has been localized, various materials can be passed through a catheter in the working channel of the bronchoscope and into the area of the fistula [170–182]. Direct application of a sealant through the working channel catheter onto the fistula site is the method generally used for directly visualized proximal fistulas. For distal fistulas, a multiple-lumen Swan-Ganz catheter has been used to localize the BPF and pass the occluding material of choice [173]. Several agents have been used through the bronchoscope in an attempt to occlude BPF. These include fibrin agents [172,173,181], cyanoacrylate-based agents [170,178,179,182], absorbable gelatin sponge (Gelfoam) [180], blood-tetracycline [174], and lead shot [176]. The reports on all of these agents are limited to only a few patients. The cyanoacrylate-based and fibrin agents have received the most attention but still have had less than 20 total cases reported. These patients have had at least a 50 percent reduction of fistula flow and most had closure of the fistula subsequent to sealant application, although multiple applications were necessary in some patients. These agents appear to work in two phases, with the agent initially sealing the leak by acting as a plug and subsequently inducing an inflammatory process with fibrosis and mucosal proliferation permanently sealing the area [170,178]. They are not useful with large proximal tracheal or bronchial ruptures or multiple distal parenchymal defects [173].

References

1. Woodring JH: Recognition of pleural effusion on supine radiographs: How much fluid is required? *AJR* 142:59, 1984.

2. Christensen EE, Curry TS III, Dowdey JE: *An Introduction to the Physics of Diagnostic Radiology.* 2nd ed. Philadelphia, Lea & Febiger, 1978, pp 101–102.

3. Collins JD, Burwell D, Furmanski S, et al: Minimum detectable pleural effusions: A roentgen pathology model. *Radiology* 105:51, 1975.

4. Wiener ND, Garay SM, Leitman BS, et al: Imaging of the intensive care unit patient. *Clin Chest Med* 12:169, 1991.

5. Yu C-J, Yang P-C, Chang D-B, et al: Diagnostic and therapeutic use of chest sonography: Value in critically ill patients. *AJR* 159:695, 1992.

6. Mirvis SE, Tobin KD, Kostrubiak I, et al: Thoracic CT in detecting occult disease in critically ill patients. *AJR* 148:685, 1987.

7. Peruzzi W, Garner W, Bools J, et al: Portable chest roentgenography and computed tomography in critically ill patients. *Chest* 93:722, 1988.

8. Greene R, McLoud TC, Stark P: Pneumothorax. *Semin Roentgenol* 12:313, 1977.

9. Moskowitz PS, Griscom NT: The medial pneumothorax. *Radiology* 120:143, 1976.

10. Joffe N: The adult respiratory distress syndrome. *AJR* 122:719, 1974.

11. Rohlfing BM, Webb WR, Schlobohm RM: Ventilator-related extra-alveolar air in adults. *Radiology* 121:25, 1976.

12. Gobien RP, Reines HD, Schabel SI: Localized tension pneumothorax: Unrecognized form of barotrauma in adult respiratory distress syndrome. *Radiology* 142:15, 1982.

13. Tocino IM, Miller MH, Fairfax WR: Distribution of pneumothorax in the supine and semirecumbent critically ill adult. *AJR* 144:901, 1985.

14. Kollef MH: Risk factors for the misdiagnosis of pneumothorax in the intensive care unit. *Crit Care Med* 19:906, 1991.

15. Marglin SI, Rowberg AH, Godwin JD: Preliminary experience with portable digital imaging for intensive care radiology. *J Thorac Imaging* 5:49, 1990.

16. Elam EA, Rehm K, Hillman BJ, et al: Efficacy of digital radiography for the detection of pneumothorax: Comparison with conventional chest radiography. *AJR* 158:509, 1992.

17. Humphrey LM, Fitzpatrick K, Paine SS, et al: Physician experience with viewing digital radiographs in an intensive care unit environment. *J Digit Imaging* 6:30, 1993.

18. Sahn SA: The pleura. *Am Rev Respir Dis* 138:184, 1988.

19. Lipscomb DJ, Flower CDR, Hadfield JW: Ultrasound of the pleura: An assessment of its clinical value. *Clin Radiol* 32:289, 1981.

20. Godwin JE, Sahn SA: Thoracentesis: A safe procedure in mechanically ventilated patients. *Ann Intern Med* 113:800, 1990.

21. Collins TR, Sahn SA: Thoracentesis: Clinical value, complications, technical problems, and patient experience. *Chest* 91:817, 1987.

22. Health and Public Policy Committee: American College of Physicians position paper: Diagnostic thoracentesis and pleural biopsy in pleural effusions. *Ann Intern Med* 103:799, 1985.

23. Sahn SA: Thoracentesis and pleural biopsy, in Shelhamer J, Pizzo PA, Parillo JE, Masur H (eds): *Respiratory Disease in the Immunosuppressed Host.* Philadelphia, JB Lippincott, 1991, pp 118–129.

24. Bartter T, Mayo PD, Pratter MR, et al: Lower risk and higher yield for thoracentesis when performed by experienced operators. *Chest* 103:1873, 1993.

25. Seneff MG, Corwin W, Gold LH, et al: Complications associated with thoracentesis. *Chest* 89:97, 1986.

26. Grogan DR, Irwin RS, Channick R, et al: Complications associated with thoracentesis. *Arch Intern Med* 150:873, 1990.

27. Light RW, Jenkinson SG, Minh V, et al: Observations on pleural pressures as fluid is withdrawn during thoracentesis. *Am Rev Respir Dis* 121:799, 1980.

28. Brown NE, Zamel N, Aberman A: Changes in pulmonary mechanics in gas exchange following thoracocentesis. *Chest* 74:540, 1978.

29. Estenne M, Yernault J-C, Detroyer A: Mechanism of relief of dyspnea after thoracentesis in patients with large effusions. *Am J Med* 74:813, 1983.

30. Light RW, Stansbury DW, Brown SE: Changes in pulmonary function following therapeutic thoracentesis. *Chest* 80:375, 1981.

31. Brandstetter RD, Cohen RP: Hypoxemia after thoracentesis: A predictable and treatable condition. *JAMA* 242:1060, 1979.

32. Karetzky M, Kothari GA, Fourre JA, et al: The effect of thoracentesis on arterial oxygen tension. *Respiration* 36:96, 1978.

33. Perpina M, Benlloch E, Marco V, et al: The effect of thoracentesis on pulmonary gas exchange. *Thorax* 38:747, 1983.

34. Light RW, George RB: Incidence and significance of pleural effusion after abdominal surgery. *Chest* 69:621, 1976.

35. Nielsen PH, Jepsan SB, Olsen AD: Postoperative pleural effusion following upper abdominal surgery. *Chest* 96:1133, 1989.

36. Wiener-Kronish JP, Matthay MA, Callen PW, et al: Relationship of pleural effusions to pulmonary hemodynamics in patients with congestive heart failure. *Am Rev Respir Dis* 132:1253, 1987.

37. Shinto RA, Light RW: Effects of diuresis on the characteristics of pleural fluid in patients with congestive heart failure. *Am J Med* 88:230, 1990.

38. Chakko SC, Caldwell SH, Sforza PP: Treatment of congestive heart failure: Its effect on pleural fluid chemistry. *Chest* 95:798, 1989.

39. Lieberman FL, Hidemura R, Peters RL, et al: Pathogenesis and treatment of hydrothorax complicating cirrhosis with ascites. *Ann Intern Med* 64:341, 1966.

40. Johnson RF, Loo RB: Hepatic hydrothorax: Studies to determine the source of the fluid and report of 13 cases. *Ann Intern Med* 61:385, 1964.

41. Frazer IH, Lichtenstein M, Andrews JT: Pleuroperitoneal effusion without ascites. *Med J Aust* 2:520, 1983.

42. Adams DA: The pathophysiology of nephrotic syndrome. *Arch Intern Med* 106:117, 1960.

43. Scott WL: Complications associated with central venous catheters: A survey. *Chest* 94:1221, 1988.

44. Duntley P, Siever J, Korwes ML, et al: Vascular erosion by central venous catheters: Clinical features and outcome. *Chest* 101:1633, 1992.

45. Ellis LM, Vogel SB III, Copeland EM: Central venous catheter vascular erosions. *Ann Surg* 209:475, 1989.

46. Wechsler RJ, Byrne KJ, Steiner RM: The misplaced thoracic venous catheter: Detailed anatomical consideration. *Crit Rev Diagn Imaging* 21:289, 1982.

47. Ball GV, Whitfield CL: Studies on rheumatoid disease pleural fluid. *Arthritis Rheum* 9:846, 1966.

48. Sahn SA: Clinical commentary: Management of complicated parapneumonic effusions. *Am Rev Respir Dis* 148:813, 1993.

49. Ashbaugh DG: Empyema thoracis: Factors influencing morbidity and mortality. *Chest* 99:1162, 1991.

50. Ridley PD, Brainbridge MV: Thoracoscopic debridement and pleural irrigation in the management of empyema thoracis. *Ann Thorac Surg* 51:461, 1991.

51. Kaye MD: Pleuropulmonary complications of pancreatitis. *Thorax* 23:297, 1968.

52. Anderson WJ, Skinner DB, Zuidema GD, et al: Chronic pancreatic pleural effusions. *Surg Gynecol Obstet* 137:827, 1973.

53. Bynum LJ, Wilson JE III: Radiographic features of pleural effusions in pulmonary embolism. *Am Rev Respir Dis* 117:829, 1978.

54. Bynum LJ, Wilson JE III: Characteristics of pleural effusions associated with pulmonary embolism. *Arch Intern Med* 136:159, 1976.

55. Sahn SA: Pleural fluid analysis: Narrowing the differential diagnosis. *Semin Respir Med* 9:22, 1987.

56. Simon HB, Daggett WN, DeSanctis RW: Hemothorax as a complication of anticoagulant therapy in the presence of pulmonary infarction. *JAMA* 208:1830, 1969.

57. Dressler W: The post-myocardial infarction syndrome: A report of 44 cases. *Arch Intern Med* 103:28, 1959.

58. Engle MA, Ito T: The post-pericardiotomy syndrome. *Am J Cardiol* 7:73, 1961.

59. Stelzner TJ, King TE Jr, Antony VB, et al: The pleuro-pulmonary manifestations of the postcardiac injury syndrome. *Chest* 84:383, 1983.

60. Kaminsky ME, Rodan BA, Osborne DR, et al: Post-pericardiotomy syndrome. *AJR* 138:503, 1982.

61. Bacon BR, Bailey-Newton RS, Connors AF Jr: Pleural effusions after endoscopic variceal sclerotherapy. *Gastroenterology* 88:1910, 1985.

62. Saks BJ, Kilby AE, Dietrich PA: Pleural and mediastinal changes following endoscopic injection sclerotherapy of esophageal varices. *Radiology* 149:639, 1983.
63. Aberle DR, Wiener-Kronish JP, Webb WR, et al: Hydrostatic versus increased permeability pulmonary edema: Diagnosis based on radiographic criteria in critically ill patients. *Radiology* 168:73, 1988.
64. Cunningham AL, Hurley JV: Alpha-naphthyl-thiourea-induced pulmonary oedema in the rat: A topographical and electron-microscope study. *J Pathol* 106:25, 1971.
65. Wiener-Kronish JP, Broaddus VC, Albertine KH, et al: Relationship of pleural effusions to increased permeability pulmonary edema in anesthetized sheep. *J Clin Invest* 82:1422, 1988.
66. Miller KS, Harley RA, Sahn SA: Pleural effusions associated with ethchlorvynol lung injury result from visceral pleural leak. *Am Rev Respir Dis* 140:764, 1989.
67. Parkin GJS: The radiology of perforated esophagus. *Clin Radiol* 24:324, 1973.
68. O'Connell ND: Spontaneous rupture of the esophagus. *Am J Roentgenol* 99:186, 1967.
69. Bladergroen MR, Lowe JE, Postlethwait RW: Diagnosis and recommended management of esophageal perforation and rupture. *Ann Thorac Surg* 42:235, 1986.
70. DeMeester TR: Perforation of the esophagus. *Ann Thorac Surg* 42:231, 1986.
71. Maulitz RM, Good JT Jr, Kaplan RL, et al: The pleuropulmonary consequences of esophageal rupture: An experimental model. *Am Rev Respir Dis* 120:363, 1979.
72. Sherr HP, Light RW, Merson MH, et al: Origin of pleural fluid amylase in esophageal rupture. *Ann Intern Med* 76:985, 1972.
73. Abbott OA, Mansour KA, Logan WD Jr, et al: Atraumatic so-called "spontaneous" rupture of the esophagus. *J Thorac Cardiovasc Surg* 59:67, 1970.
74. Light R: *Pleural Diseases.* 2nd ed. Philadelphia, Lea & Febiger, 1990, pp 263–267.
75. Graham JM, Mattox KL, Beall AC Jr: Penetrating trauma of the lung. *J Trauma* 19:665, 1979.
76. Drummond DS, Craig RH: Traumatic hemothorax: Complications and management. *Am Surgeon* 33:403, 1967.
77. Beall AC Jr, Crawford HW, DeBakey ME: Considerations in the management of acute traumatic hemothorax. *J Thorac Cardiovasc Surg* 52:351, 1966.
78. Weil PH, Margolis IB: Systematic approach to traumatic hemothorax. *Am J Surg* 142:692, 1981.
79. Griffith GL, Todd EP, McMillin RD, et al: Acute traumatic hemothorax. *Ann Thorac Surg* 26:204, 1978.
80. Wilson JM, Boren CH, Peterson SR, et al: Traumatic hemothorax: Is decortication necessary? *J Thorac Cardiovasc Surg* 77:489, 1979.
81. Rostand RA, Feldman RL, Block ER: Massive hemothorax complicating heparin anticoagulation for pulmonary embolism. *South Med J* 70:1128, 1977.
82. Iverson L, Mittal A, Dugan D, et al: Injuries to the phrenic nerve resulting in diaphragmatic paralysis with special reference to stretch trauma. *Am J Surg* 132:263, 1976.
83. Marco J, Hahn J, Barner H: Topical cardiac hypothermia and phrenic nerve injury. *Ann Thorac Surg* 23:235, 1977.
84. Wheeler W, Rubis L, Jones C, et al: Etiology and prevention of topical cardiac hypothermia-induced phrenic nerve injury and left lower lobe atelectasis during cardiac surgery. *Chest* 88:680, 1985.
85. Landymore RW, Howell F: Pulmonary complications following myocardial revascularization with the internal mammary artery graft. *Eur J Cardiothorac Surg* 4:156, 1990.
86. Kollef MH: Trapped-lung syndrome after cardiac surgery: A potentially preventable complication of pleural injury. *Heart Lung* 19:671, 1990.
87. Valentine VG, Raffin TA: The management of chylothorax. *Chest* 102:586, 1992.
88. Ferguson MK, Little AG, Skinner DB: Current concepts in the management of postoperative chylothorax. *Ann Thorac Surg* 45:542, 1985.
89. Orringer MB, Bluett M, Deeb GM: Aggressive treatment of chylothorax complicating transhiatal esophagectomy without thoracotomy. *Surgery* 104:720, 1988.
90. Teba L, Dedhia HV, Bowen R, et al: Chylothorax review. *Crit Care Med* 13:49, 1985.
91. Weidner WA, Steiner RM: Roentgenographic demonstration of intrapulmonary and pleural lymphatics during lymphangiography. *Radiology* 100:533, 1971.
92. Staats BA, Ellefson RD, Budhan LL, et al: The lipoprotein profile of chylous and nonchylous pleural effusions. *Mayo Clin Proc* 55:700, 1980.
93. Little AG, Kadowaki MH, Ferguson MK, et al: Pleuroperitoneal shunting: Alternative therapy for pleural effusions. *Ann Surg* 208:443, 1988.
94. Killen DA, Gobbel WG Jr: *Spontaneous Pneumothorax.* Boston, Little, Brown, 1968, pp 1–7.
95. Macklin MT, Macklin CC: Malignant interstitial emphysema of the lungs and mediastinum as an important occult complication in many respiratory diseases and other conditions: An interpretation of the clinical literature in the light of laboratory experiments. *Medicine* 23:281, 1944.
96. Macklin CC: Transport of air along sheaths of pulmonic blood vessels from alveoli to mediastinum: Clinical implications. *Arch Intern Med* 64:913, 1939.
97. Gustman P, Yerger L, Wanner A: Immediate cardiovascular effects of tension pneumothorax. *Am Rev Respir Dis* 127:171, 1983.
98. Hurewitz AN, Sidhu U, Bergofsky B, et al: Cardiovascular and respiratory consequence of tension pneumothorax. *Bull Eur Physiopathol Respir* 22:545, 1986.
99. Norris RM, Jones JG, Bishop JM: Respiratory gas exchange in patients with spontaneous pneumothorax. *Thorax* 23:427, 1968.
100. Moran JF, Jones RH, Wolfe WG: Regional pulmonary function during experimental unilateral pneumothorax in the awake state. *J Thorac Cardiovasc Surg* 74:394, 1977.
101. Dines DE, Clagett OT, Payne WS: Spontaneous pneumothorax and emphysema. *Mayo Clin Proc* 45:41, 1970.
102. George RB, Herbert SJ, Shames JM, et al: Pneumothorax complicating pulmonary emphysema. *JAMA* 234:389, 1975.
103. Food and Drug Administration Task Force: Precautions necessary with central venous catheters. *FDA Drug Bull* July 1989, p 15.
104. Hagley MT, Martin B, Gast P, et al: Infectious and mechanical complications of central venous catheters placed by percutaneous venipuncture and over guide wires. *Crit Care Med* 20:1426, 1992.
105. Eerola R, Kaukinen L, Kaukinen S: Analysis of 13,800 subclavian catheterizations. *Acta Anaesthesiol Scand* 29:193, 1985.
106. Tyden H: Cannulation of the internal jugular vein: 500 cases. *Acta Anaesthesiol Scand* 26:485, 1982.
107. Weiner P, Sznajder I, Plavnick L, et al: Unusual complications of subclavian vein catheterization. *Crit Care Med* 12:538, 1984.
108. Adar R, Mozes M: Fatal complication of central venous catheter. *Br Med J* 3:746, 1971.
109. Kumar A, Pontoppidan H, Falke KJ, et al: Pulmonary barotrauma during mechanical ventilation. *Crit Care Med* 1:1, 1973.
110. Zimmerman JE, Dunbar BS, Klingenmaier CH: Management of subcutaneous emphysema, pneumomediastinum, and pneumothorax during respirator therapy. *Crit Care Med* 3:69, 1975.
111. Cullen DJ, Caldera DL: The incidence of ventilator-induced pulmonary barotrauma in critically ill patients. *Anesthesiology* 50:185, 1979.
112. Zwillich CW, Pierson DJ, Creagh CE, et al: Complications of assisted ventilation: A prospective study of 354 consecutive episodes. *Am J Med* 57:161, 1974.
113. Fleming WH, Bowen MD, Hatcher CR: Early complications of long term respiratory support. *J Thorac Cardiovasc Surg* 64:729, 1972.
114. de Latorre FJ, Tomasa A, Klamburg J, et al: Incidence of pneumothorax and pneumomediastinum in patients with aspiration pneumonia requiring ventilatory support. *Chest* 72:141, 1977.
115. Steier M, Ching N, Roberts EB, et al: Pneumothorax complicating continuous ventilatory support. *J Thorac Cardiovasc Surg* 67:17, 1979.
116. Johnson TH, Altman AR: Pulmonary interstitial gas: First sign of barotrauma due to PEEP therapy. *Crit Care Med* 7:532, 1979.
117. Petersen GW, Baier H: Incidence of pulmonary barotrauma in the medical ICU. *Crit Care Med* 11:67, 1983.
118. Albelda SM, Gefter WB, Kelley MA, et al: Ventilator-induced subpleural air cysts: Clinical, radiographic, and pathologic significance. *Am Rev Respir Dis* 127:360, 1983.
119. Westcott JL, Cole SR: Interstitial pulmonary emphysema in children and adults: Roentgenographic features. *Radiology* 111:367, 1974.

120. Snyder J, Carrol G, Schuster DP, et al: Mechanical ventilation: Physiology and application. *Curr Probl Surg* 21:1, 1984.

121. Suter PM, Fairley HP, Isenberg MD: Effect of tidal volume and positive end-expiratory pressure on compliance during mechanical ventilation. *Chest* 73:158, 1978.

122. Willetts SM: Paralysis of ventilated patients: Yes or no? *Intensive Care Med* 11:2, 1985.

123. Darioli E, Perret C: Mechanical controlled hypoventilation in status asthmaticus. *Am Rev Respir Dis* 129:385, 1984.

124. Menitove SM, Goldring RM: Combined ventilator and bicarbonate strategy in the management of status asthmaticus. *Am J Med* 94:898, 1983.

125. Baumann MH, Sahn SA: Tension pneumothorax: Diagnostic and therapeutic pitfalls. *Crit Care Med* 21:177, 1993.

126. Powner DJ, Grenvik A: Ventilatory management of life-threatening bronchopleural fistulae: A summary. *Crit Care Med* 9:54, 1981.

127. Ratliff JL, Hill JD, Fallat RJ, et al: Complications associated with membrane lung support by venoarterial perfusion. *Ann Thorac Surg* 19:537, 1975.

128. Pierson DJ: Persistent bronchopleural air leak during mechanical ventilation: A review. *Respir Care* 27:408, 1982.

129. Tilles RB, Don HF: Complications of high pleural suction in bronchopleural fistulas. *Anesthesiology* 43:486, 1975.

130. Steiger Z, Wilson RF: Management of bronchopleural fistulas. *Surgery* 158:267, 1984.

131. Shenstone NS: The use of intercostal muscle in the closure of bronchopleural fistulae. *Ann Surg* 4:560, 1936.

132. Beltrami V: Surgical transsternal treatment of bronchopleural fistula postpneumonectomy. *Chest* 95:379, 1989.

133. Barker WL, Faber LP, Ostermiller WE, et al: Management of persistent bronchopleural fistulas. *J Thorac Cardiovasc Surg* 62:393, 1971.

134. Demos NJ, Timmes JJ: Myoplasty for closure of tracheal bronchofistula. *Ann Thorac Surg* 15:88, 1973.

135. Hankins JR, Miller JE, McLaughlin JS: The use of chest wall muscle flaps to close bronchopleural fistulas: Experience with 21 patients. *Ann Thorac Surg* 6:491, 1978.

136. Baumann MH, Sahn SA: Medical management and therapy of bronchopleural fistulas in the mechanically ventilated patient. *Chest* 97:721, 1990.

137. Rusch VW, Capps JS, Tyler ML, et al: The performance of four pleural drainage systems in an animal model of bronchopleural fistula. *Chest* 4:859, 1988.

138. Miller KS, Sahn SA: Chest tubes: Indications, technique, management and complications. *Chest* 91:258, 1987.

139. Batchelder TL, Morris KA: Critical factors in determining adequate pleural drainage in both the operated and nonoperated chest. *Am Surgeon* 28:296, 1962.

140. Swensen EW, Birath G, Ahbeck A: Resistance to airflow in bronchospirometric catheters. *J Thorac Surg* 33:275, 1957.

141. Downes JB, Chapman RL: Treatment of bronchopleural fistula during continuous positive pressure ventilation. *Chest* 69:363, 1976.

142. Phillips YY, Lonigan RM, Joyner LR: A simple technique for managing a bronchopleural fistula while maintaining positive pressure ventilation. *Crit Care Med* 7:351, 1979.

143. Weksler N, Ovadia L: The challenge of bilateral bronchopleural fistula. *Chest* 95:938, 1989.

144. Gallagher TJ, Smith RA, Kirby RR, et al: Intermittent inspiratory chest tube occlusion to limit bronchopleural cutaneous airleaks. *Crit Care Med* 4:328, 1976.

145. Bevelaqua FA, Kay S: A modified technique for the management of bronchopleural fistula in ventilator-dependent patients: A report of 2 cases. *Respir Care* 31:904, 1986.

146. Larrieu AJ, Tyers FO, Williams EH, et al: Intrapleural instillation of quinacrine for treatment of recurrent spontaneous pneumothorax. *Ann Thorac Surg* 28:146, 1979.

147. Goldszer RC, Bennett J, VanCampen J, et al: Intrapleural tetracycline for spontaneous pneumothorax. *JAMA* 241:724, 1979.

148. Nandi P: Recurrent spontaneous pneumothorax: An effective method of talc poudrage. *Chest* 77:493, 1980.

149. Macoviak JA, Stephenson LW, Ochs R, et al: Tetracycline pleurodesis during active pulmonary-pleural airleak for prevention of recurrent pneumothorax. *Chest* 81:78, 1982.

150. Verschoof AC, Vende T, Greve LH, et al: Thoracoscopic pleurodesis in the management of spontaneous pneumothorax. *Respiration* 53:197, 1988.

151. Light RW, O'Hara VS, Moritz TE, et al: Intrapleural tetracycline for the prevention of recurrent of spontaneous pneumothorax. *JAMA* 264:2224, 1990.

152. Powner DJ, Cline CD, Rodman GH: Effect of chest-tube suction on gas flow through a bronchopleural fistula. *Crit Care Med* 13:99, 1985.

153. Bishop MJ, Benson MS, Pierson DJ: Carbon dioxide excretion via bronchopleural fistulas in adult respiratory distress syndrome. *Chest* 91:400, 1987.

154. Pierson DJ, Horton CA, Bates PW: Persistent bronchopleural airleak during mechanical ventilation: A review of 39 cases. *Chest* 90:321, 1986.

155. Kuwik RJ, Glass D, Coombs DW: Evaluation of high-frequency positive pressure ventilation for experimental bronchopleural fistula. *Crit Care Med* 9:164, 1981.

156. Hoff BH, Wilson E, Smith RB, et al: Intermittent positive pressure ventilation and high-frequency ventilation in dogs with experimental bronchopleural fistulae. *Crit Care Med* 11:598, 1983.

157. Carlon GC, Griffin J, Ray C, et al: High-frequency jet ventilation in experimental airway disruption. *Crit Care Med* 11:353, 1983.

158. Mayers I, Long R, Breen PH, et al: Artificial ventilation of a canine model of bronchopleural fistula. *Anesthesiology* 64:739, 1986.

159. Turnbull AD, Carlon GC, Howland WS, et al: High-frequency jet ventilation in major airway or pulmonary disruption. *Ann Thorac Surg* 32:468, 1981.

160. Carlon GC, Ray C, Pierri MK, et al: High-frequency jet ventilation: Theoretical considerations and clinical observations. *Chest* 81:350, 1982.

161. Carlon GC, Kahn RC, Howland WS, et al: Clinical experience with high-frequency jet ventilation. *Crit Care Med* 9:1, 1981.

162. Albeda SM, Hansen-Flaschen JH, Taylor E, et al: Evaluation of high-frequency jet ventilation in patients with bronchopleural fistulas by quantitation of the airleak. *Anesthesiology* 63:551, 1985.

163. Bishop MJ, Benson MS, Sato P, et al: Comparison of high-frequency jet ventilation with conventional mechanical ventilation for bronchopleural fistula. *Anesth Analg* 66:833, 1987.

164. Rafferty TD, Palma J, Motoyama EK, et al. Management of a bronchopleural fistula with differential lung ventilation and positive end-expiratory pressure. *Respir Care* 25:654, 1980.

165. Brown CR: Postpneumonectomy empyema and bronchopleural fistula: Use of prolonged endobronchial intubation: A case report. *Anesth Analg* 52:439, 1973.

166. Lau K: Postural management of bronchopleural fistula. *Chest* 94:1122, 1988.

167. Feeley TW, Keating D, Nishimura T: Independent lung ventilation using high-frequency ventilation in the management of a bronchopleural fistula. *Anesthesiology* 69:420, 1988.

168. Crimi G, Candiani A, Conti G, et al: Clinical applications of independent lung ventilation with unilateral high-frequency jet ventilation (ILV-UHFJV). *Intensive Care Med* 12:90, 1986.

169. Orlando R, Gluck EH, Cohen M, et al: Ultra-high-frequency jet ventilation in a bronchopleural fistula model. *Arch Surg* 123:591, 1988.

170. Torre M, Chiesa G, Ravine M, et al: Endoscopic gluing of bronchopleural fistula. *Ann Thorac Surg* 43:295, 1987.

171. Hoier-Madsen K, Schulze S, Pedersen VM, et al: Management of bronchopleural fistula following pneumonectomy. *Scand J Thorac Cardiovasc Surg* 18:263, 1984.

172. Glover W, Chavis TV, Daniel TM, et al: Fibrin glue application through the flexible fiberoptic bronchoscope: Closure of bronchopleural fistula. *J Thorac Cardiovasc Surg* 93:470, 1987.

173. Regel G, Sturm JA, Neumann C, et al: Occlusion of bronchopleural fistula after lung injury: A new treatment by bronchoscopy. *J Trauma* 29:223, 1989.

174. Lan R, Lee C, Tsai Y, et al: Fiberoptic bronchial blockade in a small bronchopleural fistula. *Chest* 92:944, 1987.

175. Pace R, Rankin RN, Finley RJ: Detachable balloon occlusion of bronchopleural fistulae in dogs. *Investig Radiol* 18:504, 1983.

176. Ratliff JL, Hill JD, Tucker H, et al: Endobronchial control of bronchopleural fistulae. *Chest* 71:98, 1971.

177. Ellis JH, Sequeira FW, Weber TR, et al: Balloon catheter occlusion of bronchopleural fistulae. *AJR* 138:157, 1982.
178. Roksvaag H, Skalleberg L, Nordberg C, et al: Endoscopic closure of bronchial fistula. *Thorax* 38:696, 1983.
179. Menard JW, Prejean CA, Tucker YW: Endoscopic closure of bronchopleural fistulas using a tissue adhesive. *Am J Surg* 155:415, 1980.

180. Jones DP, David I: Gelfoam occlusion of peripheral bronchopleural fistulas. *Ann Thorac Surg* 42:334, 1986.
181. Jessen C, Sharma P: Use of fibrin glue in thoracic surgery. *Ann Thorac Surg* 39:521, 1985.
182. Hartmann W, Rausch V: A new therapeutic application of fiberoptic bronchoscope. *Chest* 71:237, 1977.

66. *Mechanical Ventilation: Initiation*

Rolf D. Hubmayr and Richard S. Irwin

Mechanical ventilation refers to any method of breathing in which a mechanical apparatus is used to augment or satisfy entirely the bulk flow requirements of a patient's breathing. Mechanical ventilation is indicated when the patient's spontaneous ventilation is not adequate to sustain life or when it is necessary to take control of the patient's ventilation to prevent impending collapse of other organ functions; it can be given by negative or positive pressure [1]. Literature on the history of mechanical ventilation can be found elsewhere [1,2]. This chapter discusses the institution and maintenance of mechanical ventilation. Due to the paucity of well-controlled clinical trials defining specific roles for each mode of mechanical ventilation, this chapter deals with mechanical ventilation from a physiologic perspective.

Principles of Operation

NEGATIVE-PRESSURE VENTILATION. Until the mid-1950s, mechanical ventilators used for continuous ventilation were predominantly of the negative-pressure variety. The "iron lung," or tank ventilator, was the most familiar of these. Bulk flow was mobilized into the patient's lungs by cyclically creating a subatmospheric pressure around the chest; actually, only the patient's head was not enclosed in the negative-pressure chamber. Subsequent ventilators applied negative external pressures to the rib cage only to induce inspiratory flow ($\dot{V}_I$) [3]. The original chest-enclosing ventilators of this type, called cuirass ventilators, incorporated a rigid shell that was applied to the chest. Later versions employed a much more flexible housing for the chest that was better tolerated by patients. The logistic problems encountered in providing routine nursing care for unstable patients resulted in an abandonment of negative-pressure ventilators in the acute care setting some 30 years ago. Interest in intermittent nocturnal mechanical ventilation as home therapy for chronic respiratory failure led to a minor resurgence in their use in the 1980s [3–6]. However, because negative-pressure ventilators tend to be bulky, are poorly tolerated, may cause obstructive sleep apnea, and have not proved effective in the rehabilitation of patients with end-stage obstructive lung diseases, they are being replaced by positive-pressure ventilators for home use as well [7,8].

A more in-depth discussion of negative-pressure ventilation, as well as the use of pneumobelts and rocking beds for long-term ventilatory assistance in stable patients, can be found elsewhere [5].

POSITIVE-PRESSURE VENTILATION. Positive-pressure ventilation is operative when a superatmospheric pressure is cyclically created at the upper airway [1]. The resultant pressure gradient between the upper airway and the lungs "pushes" gases through the airways. Although positive-pressure ventilation can be given noninvasively with a face mask, nasal mask, or mouth seal and can be effective in stable patients with neuromuscular diseases, kyphoscoliosis, or central hypoventilation [9], in the acute care setting it is usually delivered through an endotracheal or tracheostomy tube. This practice may change as advances in ventilator technology offer alternative noninvasive means to augment ventilation in patients with impending respiratory pump failure [10–14].

Conventional positive-pressure ventilation has come to be identified with respiratory rates up to 60 breaths per minute; any mode of ventilation administered at higher respiratory rates, specifically in the range of 60 to 100 breaths per minute [15], is considered high-frequency positive-pressure ventilation (HFPPV). High-frequency jet ventilation (HFJV) is a form of HFPPV whereby gases are delivered into the trachea by means of a narrow cannula inserted into an endotracheal tube or percutaneously through the cricothyroid membrane [16]; rates between 100 and 350 breaths per minute are commonly used. High-frequency oscillation (HFO) implies ventilation at frequencies on the order of 20 breaths per second (20 Hz) or 1200 breaths per minute [15,16]. Although HFJV and HFO are forms of HFPPV, they differ in the type of apparatus used and physiologic effects. The purported advantage of all forms of HFPPV is that adequate gas exchange can be maintained with lower mean airway pressure than is possible with conventional positive-pressure ventilation. Theoretically, lower mean airway pressures interfere less with cardiac output, reduce the risk of barotrauma, and reduce the leakage of air through a bronchopleural fistula in patients who may have already sustained a pneumothorax [16]. Unfortunately, these theoretical advantages were not borne out in carefully designed clinical trials, and survival benefits from HFPPV could not be substantiated [17].

Particularly during HFO, mean tracheal pressure may be substantially below mean alveolar pressure and thus provide a misleading estimate of lung volume and the risk of barotrauma [18,19]. In the early 1980s, the mechanisms of gas transport during HFO were hotly debated, but, not unlike conventional ventilation, they have been shown ultimately to involve convection and diffusion [20].

The rest of this chapter deals principally with conventional positive-pressure ventilation. The experimental, nonconventional methods of ventilation (e.g., apneic oxygenation, low-frequency positive-pressure ventilation with extracorporeal removal of CO_2, and constant-flow ventilation [21]) are not discussed. Before discussing different categories and modes of positive-pressure ventilation, it is useful to review the basic mechanical determinants of patient-ventilator interactions.

MECHANICAL DETERMINANTS OF PATIENT-VENTILATOR INTERACTIONS. Despite gross oversimplifications, linear models of the respiratory system have proved useful for the understanding of patient-ventilator interactions [22,23]. In Figure 66-1, a piston pump (the mechanical ventilator) is attached to a rigid tube (the resistive element representing endotracheal tube and airways). An elastic element, a balloon, represents the lung parenchyma and chest wall. The pressure applied at time (t) to the tube inlet ($P_{i(t)}$, near the attachment to the ventilator) is equal to the sum of two pressures, an elastic pressure ($P_{el(t)}$) and a resistive pressure ($P_{res(t)}$).

$$P_{i(t)} = P_{el(t)} + P_{res(t)} \tag{1}$$

The tube outlet pressure at the junction with the balloon is equal to the pressure inside the balloon (P_{el}). P_{res} is the difference in pressure between the tube inlet and the tube outlet. Assuming linear system behavior, the inlet pressure-time profile can be computed for any piston stroke volume (V_{stroke}) and flow ($\dot{V}$) setting, provided the resistive properties of the tube (R) and the elastic properties of the balloon (E) are known:

$$P_{i(t)} = EV_{(t)} + R\dot{V}_{(t)} \tag{2}$$

Elastance, E, is a measure of balloon stiffness and is equal to the ratio of P_{el} and V_{stroke} (assuming 0 volume and pressure at the beginning of balloon inflation). Therefore, $P_{el(t)}$ of Equation 1 can be substituted with $E\dot{V}_{(t)}$ in Equation 2. Because Ohm's law states that the tube resistance, R, is equal to the ratio of pressure and flow, $P_{res(t)}$ of Equation 1 can be substituted with the product $R\dot{V}_{(t)}$ in Equation 2.

Fig. 66-1. Components of inlet pressure. Right. Model of the respiratory system consisting of a resistive element (straight tube) and an elastic element (balloon) connected to a ventilator (piston). During inflation of the model with constant flow (bottom), there is a stepwise increase in inlet pressure (P_i) that equals the loss of pressure across the resistive element (P_{res}) (top). Thereafter, P_i increases linearly and reflects the mechanical properties of the elastic element (P_{el}). P_i is the sum of P_{res} and P_{el}. At end inspiration, when flow has ceased (Insp. Pause), P_i decreases by an amount equal to P_{res}; P_i equals P_{el} during Insp. Pause. T_I = inspiratory time; T_E = expiratory time. (From Hubmayr RD, Abel MD, Rehder K: Physiologic approach to mechanical ventilation. *Crit Care Med* 18:103, 1990. With permission.)

COMPONENTS OF INLET PRESSURE

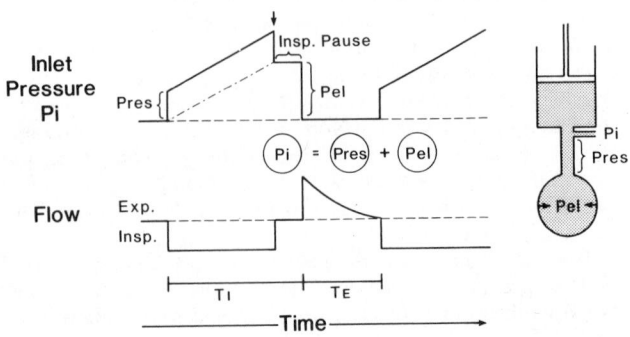

While Equation 2 helps illustrate the determinants of airway (or inlet) pressure during volume or flow/time, preset ventilation is just as valid a predictor of instantaneous flow and volume during pressure preset ventilation (when pressure is an independent variable). Accordingly, instantaneous volume and flow vary in proportion with airway pressure but are inversely related to elastance and resistance. Equations 1 and 2 also explain how a patient's elastance and inspiratory system resistance can be estimated from peak and end-inflation hold pressure measurements. Peak pressure (P_{peak}) reflects both elastic and resistive pressures. After airway occlusion at end inspiration, flow (and with it P_{res}) decline to 0 such that airway plateau pressure (P_{plat}) becomes equal to the elastic recoil pressure of the relaxed respiratory system (P_{el}). In turn, P_{res} can be computed by subtracting P_{peak} from P_{plat}. According to Equation 2, elastance and resistance are simply the ratios of P_{plat} to tidal volume (TV) and P_{res} to flow, respectively. For these calculations to yield meaningful estimates of the mechanical properties of the respiratory system, two important conditions must be satisfied: (1) the respiratory muscles must be relaxed at end inspiration and (2) machine breaths must have been initiated from relaxation volume (V_{rel}) at which P_{el} is 0.

If expiration is passive and is driven by the P_{el} of the respiratory system, then the instantaneous expiratory flow ($\dot{V}_{E(t)}$) is given by

$$\dot{V}_{E(t)} = P_{el}(t)/R \tag{3}$$

Because $P_{el(t)}$ is a function of elastance (E) and of the instantaneous lung volume ($V_{(t)}$), Equation 3 can be rewritten as

$$\dot{V}_{E(t)} = E \times V_{(t)/R} = V_{(t)/R} \times C \tag{4}$$

whereby C (the compliance of the respiratory system) is simply the inverse of E. The product of R and C characterizes the time constant of single-compartment linear systems. The time constant defines the time at which approximately two-thirds of the volume above V_{rel} has emptied passively. From this it should be clear that patients with increased respiratory system resistances and compliances (e.g., patients with emphysema) are prone to dynamic hyperinflation.

Conventional Positive-Pressure Ventilation

Modes. The mode of mechanical ventilation refers to the shape of the inspiratory pressure or flow profile and determines whether a patient can augment TV or rate through his or her own efforts. Descriptors of ventilation mode are conveniently separated into determinants of amplitude, rate, and relative machine breath timing.

Amplitude of Machine Output

VOLUME PRESET VENTILATION. In this mode, the machine delivers a volume set on the control panel and, within limits, delivers that volume irrespective of the pressure generated within the system (Fig. 66-2, A–D). During "conventional" forms of volume preset ventilation, the inspiratory flow profile has a square wave shape (i.e., flow remains constant throughout the inspiratory cycle). Newer ventilators provide options such as increasing or decreasing ramp functions as well as sine waves, but it is not known whether the choice among these is important. Most physicians consider volume preset ventilation to be the mode of choice in the treatment of adults with acute respiratory

Volume preset   Pressure preset

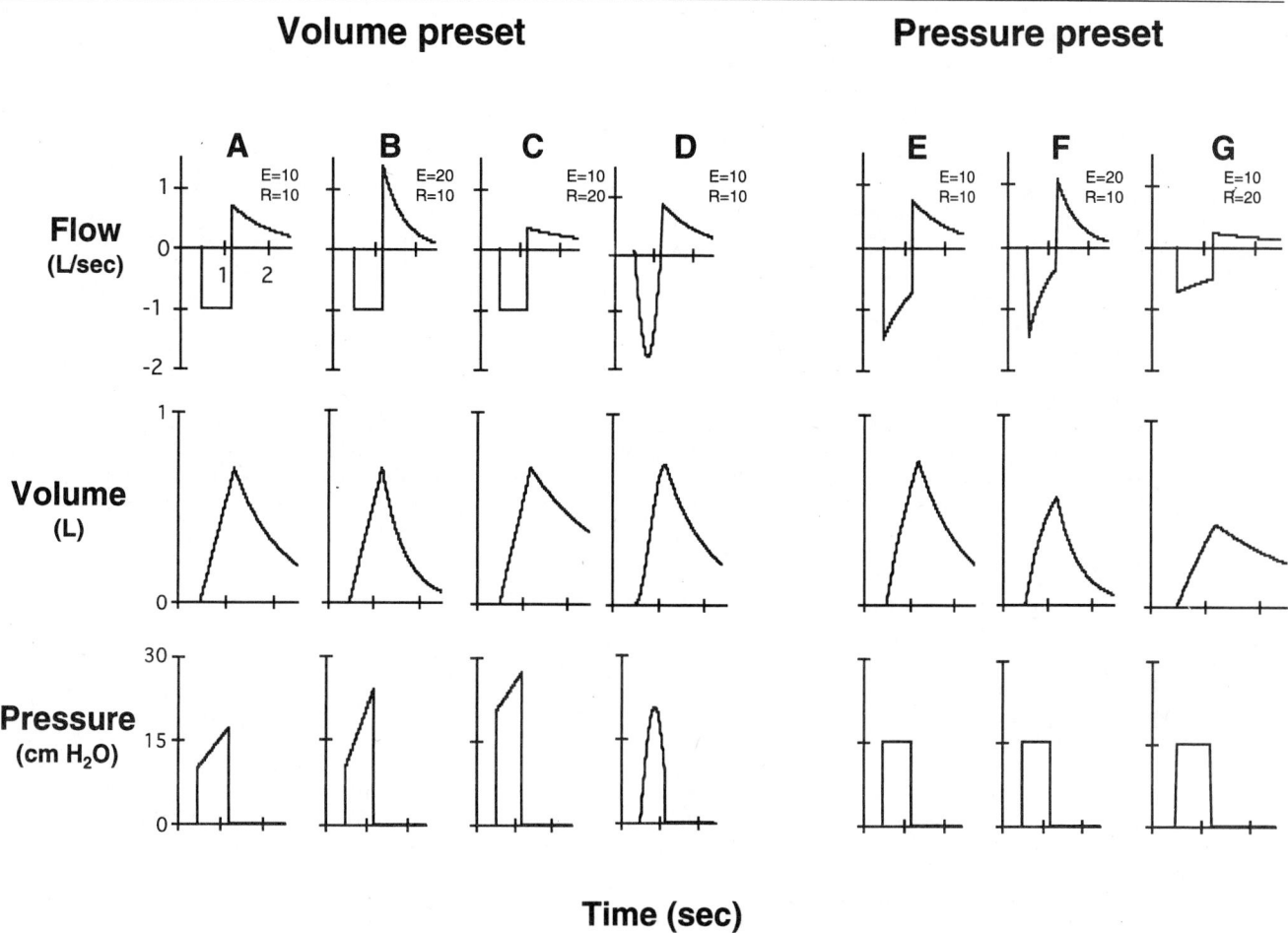

Fig. 66-2. Schematic representation of the interdependence between pressure, volume, and flow during volume preset ventilation (A–D) and pressure preset ventilation (E–G). In the volume preset mode, increases in respiratory elastance (B) and resistance (C) as well as the choice of the inspiratory flow profile (D) affect airway pressure. In the pressure preset mode, the same changes in elastance (F) and resistance (G) compared to control (E) affect volume and flow profiles.

failure, because a predefined minute volume delivery is guaranteed (for exceptions, see pop-off pressures). The disadvantages are that (1) changes in the mechanical properties of the lungs and chest wall may cause the development of high inflation pressures (perhaps increasing the risk of barotrauma) and (2) the patient is unable to adjust the breathing pattern according to changes in ventilatory demand.

PRESSURE PRESET VENTILATION. During pressure preset ventilation, the ventilator applies a predefined target pressure to the endotracheal tube during inspiration (Fig. 66-2, E–G). The resulting TV and inspiratory flow profile vary with the impedance of the respiratory system and the strength of the patient's inspiratory efforts. Therefore, when either lungs or chest wall become stiff, when the airway resistance increases, or when the patient's own inspiratory efforts decline, TV decreases. An increase in respiratory system impedance can lead to a dangerous fall in minute ventilation ($\dot{V}E$), hypoxemia, and CO_2 retention, but, in contrast to volume preset modes, pressure preset ventilation does not predispose the patient to an increased risk of barotrauma. The latter is one reason pressure preset venti-

lation is gaining popularity in the treatment of patients with acute lung injury.

Means to Activate (Trigger) a Machine Breath

CONTROLLED MECHANICAL VENTILATION. Controlled mechanical ventilation (CMV) is a mode during which rate, inspiratory-to-expiratory timing (I:E), and inspiratory flow profile are determined entirely by machine settings and cannot be altered by patient effort. There is never a reason to use this mode unless the patient is apneic from sedation, neuromuscular blockade, or disease. Disabling the machine trigger mechanisms in a patient with phasic inspiratory muscle activity can result in "fighting the ventilator," discomfort, and fatigue.

ASSIST/CONTROL VENTILATION. The ventilator in assist/control (A/C) mode is sensitized to respond to the patient's inspiratory effort, if present; if such efforts are absent, the machine cycles automatically and delivers a controlled breath. Therefore, a patient might conceivably assist at a rate of 12 breaths per minute although the control rate is set at 10 breaths per minute.

Most ventilators operating in A/C mode recognize patient efforts and switch from expiration to inspiration when the airway pressure falls below a predetermined level (usually 1–2 cm H_2O below end-expiratory pressure). During expiration, a valve occludes the inspiratory port of the ventilator. An inspiratory effort against an occluded port lowers the airway opening pressure (P_{ao}), causes the demand valve to open, and initiates a machine breath. Short-lived inspiratory efforts that occur during early expiration are often insufficient to lower P_{ao} below the trigger value. Careful inspection of neck and chest wall motion or intermittent flaring of the alae nasi should alert the physician to this phenomenon, which indicates a dissociation between machine rate and the patient's own intrinsic respiratory rate. Wasted inspiratory efforts are commonly seen in weak, sleeping, or heavily sedated patients and in patients unable to overcome intrinsic (or auto) positive end-expiratory pressure (PEEP) (see below).

Flow-by-trigger mode, which is available on new-generation ventilators, is an alternative to conventional pressure-based machine trigger algorithms (Fig. 66-3) [24].

During flow-by, a continuous flow of gas is presented to the patient and is vented in toto through the expiratory tubing unless the patient makes an inspiratory effort. This so-called "base flow" can be set by the operator between limits of 5 to 20 liters per minute. When the patient makes an inspiratory effort(s), he or she diverts flow into the lungs, resulting in a discrepancy between base flow and the flow of gas through the expiratory circuit. The minimal difference between inspiratory and expiratory flows, which results in a machine breath, is determined by the flow sensitivity setting and can vary from 1 and 3 liters per minute. Compared to pressure triggering, flow-by reduces patient work necessary to initiate a machine breath, because there are no demand valves to be opened. The demand valve-operated trigger mechanisms of older ventilators can be quite "sticky" (i.e., a much larger reduction in P_{ao} is required to open the valve than is indicated on the "trigger" level or sensitivity dial of the ventilator). Therefore, one should *not* force difficult-to-wean patients to breathe unassisted through the ventilator circuits of "old" machines.

The A/C feature has lured many physicians into the erroneous assumption that the machine backup rate setting is unimportant (see discussion on rate settings and troubleshooting). Although only a modest inspiratory effort is required to trigger the ventilator, many patients perform muscular work throughout the entire assisted breath in direct proportion to their ventilatory drive [25]. If the patient's work of breathing is deemed excessive and potentially fatiguing, the physician should lower the trigger sensitivity setting, consider raising $\dot{V}_I$, evaluate oxygenation and alveolar ventilation, assess the adequacy of machine backup rate and PEEP settings, and address sedation and pain control. Only then should neuromuscular blockade be considered as an intervention of last resort.

INTERMITTENT MANDATORY VENTILATION. Intermittent mandatory ventilation (IMV) is a combination of spontaneous ventilation and volume preset assisted ventilation [26]. For example, at an IMV rate of 6 breaths per minute, the ventilator would deliver a positive-pressure breath every 10 seconds. Between these mechanically "controlled" breaths, the patient breathes spontaneously and the ventilator serves as a source of warmed, humidified, potentially oxygen-enriched gas. Virtually all modern ventilators use synchronized IMV algorithms, which prevent the theoretical possibility of the patient getting a "double" breath with IMV (i.e., a mandatory breath plus a spontaneous breath). At intervals determined by the IMV frequency setting, the machine becomes "sensitized" to the patient's inspiratory effort and responds by delivering a mechanical "assisted" breath. Between these assisted cycles, the patient breathes spontaneously at a rate and depth of his or her own choosing. For example, at an IMV rate of 6 breaths per minute, the ventilator allows the patient to breathe spontaneously and is initially refractory to the patient's pattern of breathing. After 10 seconds elapse, the machine is rendered sensitive and waits for the patient's next inspiratory effort. When that effort occurs, the ventilator delivers a positive-pressure "assisted" breath and the patient breathes spontaneously until 10 seconds after the end of the previous refractory period. If the patient does not make an inspiratory effort during the sensitive period, the ventilator delivers a controlled breath after sufficient time elapses. This time varies inversely with the IMV backup rate; it is equal to 60 seconds divided by the IMV rate. In the example given above, the period would be 10 seconds (60 ÷ 6).

Intermittent mandatory ventilation is often used when the patient can perform at least some of the work of breathing and when weaning from mechanical ventilation is contemplated. Compared to T piece weaning, IMV has the advantage that the alarm functions of the ventilator are operational and available at all frequencies (including 0 breaths/min). However, obliging the patient to breathe through the ventilator-humidifier circuit for extended periods may add appreciably to the work of breathing [27,28]. This is true for all but the most advanced new-generation ventilators with ultrafast response times. Although most ventilators offer an IMV option, this mode has not proved superior to other weaning techniques (see Chap. 67).

Another proposed advantage of IMV is the decreased risk of

Fig. 66-3. Schematic representation of flow-triggering principles. (From Dupuis YG. *Ventilators: Theory and Clinical Applications.* 2nd ed. St. Louis, Mosby-Year Book, 1992. With permission.)

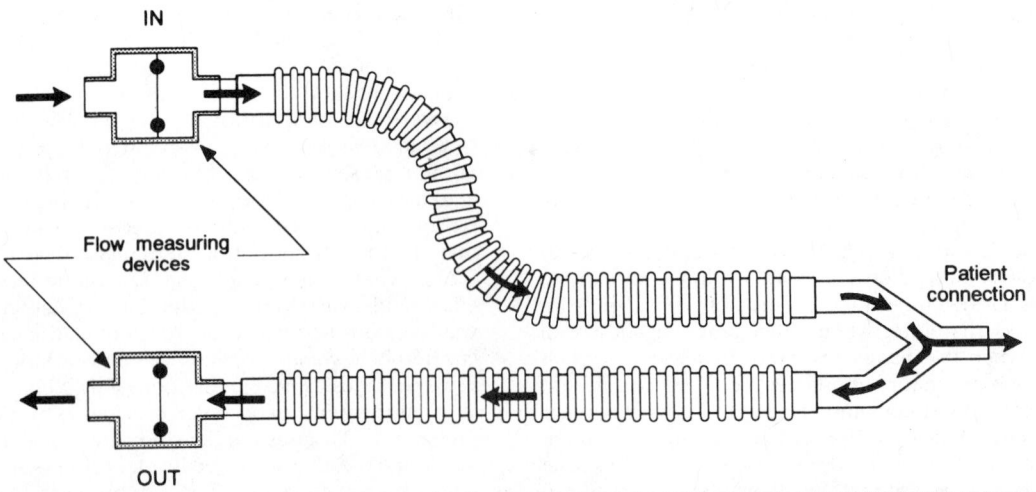

respiratory alkalosis compared with other modes. In several studies, however, $PaCO_2$ was influenced only minimally by switching from volume preset ventilation in A/C to IMV [29,30]. Recent advances in our understanding of the effects of ventilator rate and volume (or pressure) settings on $PaCO_2$ and respiratory motor output are pertinent to this controversy. Particularly during wakefulness, assisted ventilation with high volumes or pressures is apt to diminish or even abolish the influence of inspiratory drive on the regulation of alveolar ventilation [31]. Because respiratory rate is insensitive to $PaCO_2$ in the hypocapnic range, mechanically ventilated, tachypneic, and hypocarbic patients do not lower their respiratory (machine trigger) rate to compensate for alkalemia [32]. Thus, switching from A/C to IMV does not correct respiratory alkalemia unless relatively low machine backup rates and TV settings are used. Also, respiratory alkalemia may be an appropriate ventilatory response to the underlying disease process, in which case correction of hypocarbia with IMV constitutes the undesirable effect of inducing ventilatory pump failure through mechanical loading.

PRESSURE SUPPORT VENTILATION. Pressure support ventilation (PSV) is a form of pressure preset ventilation [33]. It is intermittent positive-pressure breathing with a sensing device that delivers the breath at the time the patient makes an inspiratory effort. As the lungs inflate, $\dot{V}i$ begins to decline because airway pressure and the pressure generated by inspiratory muscles are opposed by rising elastic recoil forces. When $\dot{V}i$ reaches a threshold value (which differs among vendors), the machine switches to expiration [34].

Pressure support ventilation has become a popular weaning mode for adults. Its popularity is based on the premise that weaning from mechanical ventilation should be a gradual process and that the work of unassisted breathing through an endotracheal tube is unreasonably high and could lead to respiratory muscle failure in susceptible patients [35]. However, pulmonary resistance (and, by inference, upper airway resistance) remains very much increased after extubation, weakening the argument that pressure support should be used to "overcome" the resistance of endotracheal tubes [36,37].

PRESSURE CONTROL VENTILATION. Pressure control ventilation (PCV) is a form of pressure preset ventilation. It differs from PSV in two important respects: the operator sets a machine backup rate and determines inspiratory time (Ti). The A/C feature assures ventilation of the lungs in patients who are prone to apneas. Cessation of inspiratory effort can be a problem in sleeping adults who are ventilated in the pressure support mode [38]. On the other hand, PCV does not offer the patient the same control over TV and breathing patterns as PSV. For this reason, PCV with long Ti is usually reserved for use in hypoxic paralyzed patients in whom the need to match ventilator rate and timing with intrinsic respiratory rhythms is not an issue [39].

CHOICE OF VENTILATION MODE. The therapeutic endpoints of mechanical ventilation vary considerably among different respiratory failure syndromes. For example, the ventilatory management of patients with acute lung injury has little in common with that of patients suffering from exacerbation of chronic obstructive pulmonary disease (COPD). However, the need for pathophysiology-based treatment objectives should not be confused with a need to find an optimal ventilation mode for each class of respiratory disorders. With few exceptions, volume preset ventilation in the A/C mode can accomplish therapeutic goals. Therefore, the following discussion of ventilator settings focuses on volume preset modes.

The section on disease-oriented mechanical ventilation strategies that appears later in this chapter summarizes our general approach to managing specific clinical conditions in specific terms.

VOLUME PRESET VENTILATOR SETTINGS

Fraction of Inspired Oxygen. The hazards of indiscriminate administration of oxygen to patients with CO_2 retention and the topic of pulmonary oxygen toxicity are discussed in Chapter 69. Notwithstanding these very real concerns, oxygen must never be withheld from a mechanically ventilated patient. If there is any suspicion that the patient may require oxygen, it should be given. To avoid an initial arterial oxygen tension (PaO_2) less than 60 mm Hg, most adults started on mechanical ventilation should receive an initial concentration of 100 percent [40]. In patients who have received bleomycin, the fraction of inspired oxygen (FIO_2) should be kept as low as possible to avoid potentiating bleomycin pulmonary toxicity [41]. Patients on amiodarone may also be subject to oxygen radical-mediated lung injury, but the data are much less convincing than in the case of bleomycin [42]. Subsequent adjustments in FIO_2 are usually guided by arterial blood gas analyses. It is currently believed that an FIO_2 below 0.6 is not injurious to the lungs even when used for days or weeks. Because the contribution of oxygen to lung injury cannot be separated from that of other agents (e.g., sepsis-related inflammatory mediator release, gastric acid, infectious agents, lung parenchymal stress), oxygen dosing recommendations remain open to debate. It is probably not worth the effort to predict the effects on PaO_2 of reducing FIO_2, assuming a constant P/F ratio, shunt, venous admixture, or alveolar to arterial oxygen tension gradient [40]. This is because the chance of injuring the lungs through inadvertent hyperoxia in the short term is small, the assumptions on which predictions are based are flawed, and pulse oximetry offers a means to screen individuals for inadvertent hypoxemia [43].

Tidal Volume. Most older textbooks and review articles on mechanical ventilation suggest TV settings between 10 and 15 cc per kilogram ideal body weight. This recommendation is appropriate for individuals with normal or minimally impaired lung function, which would include most patients who need assistance during surgery and anesthesia. However, it is not appropriate for patients with acute lung injury, in whom a substantial fraction of lung units are unavailable for ventilation and gas exchange [44]. As a result, the remaining aerated and recruitable lung is smaller than predicted from a patient's weight. There is overwhelming evidence that inflation above total lung capacity (TLC) can damage normal lung units, particularly when this occurs in conjunction with large regional volume excursions [45–49].

Therefore, every attempt should be made to ventilate the lungs of patients with acute lung injury with TV of 8 cc per kilogram ideal body weight or less, and to adjust frequency according to anticipated ventilatory demands. Attention to small TV minimizes the risk of overdistension injury and tissue rupture and guards against local surfactant depletion from large regional volume oscillations [50,51]. In general, TV settings resulting in static inflation pressures (P_{plat}) greater than 35 cm H_2O must be avoided. This is because normal lungs are maximally distended at a respiratory system recoil of approximately 35 cm H_2O [52].

As a group, patients with obstructive lung diseases tend to have greater inspiratory capacities than patients with acute lung injury. They are therefore less prone to overdistension injury when TV settings of approximately 10 cc per kilogram are used. On the other hand, TV is an important determinant of dynamic hyperinflation and, at least initially, TV settings of 8 cc per kilogram or less are recommended when obstruction is severe, as in status asthmaticus [53].

"Sighing." Periodic hyperinflation (the "sigh" or "yawn" maneuver) is a spontaneous reflex in conscious humans. Periodic stretching of the lung is thought to stimulate alveolar type II pneumocyte production of surfactant and therefore prevent atelectasis [54]. Some commercial ventilators incorporate a programmable sigh setting. While it is unknown whether sighs are needed to prevent atelectasis with all modes of ventilation, a recent study suggests that they are not beneficial during PSV [55].

Inflation Pressure

SETTING IN VOLUME PRESET MODES. Although pressure is a dependent variable during volume preset ventilation, generally the cycling pressure should not be allowed to increase without limit. Rather, a pressure limit or pop-off pressure should be imposed to guard against inadvertent overinflation and possible lung rupture. This is set directly on the ventilator's control panel, and when and if it is reached a visual and possibly audible alarm alerts the attendant to the fact that the machine has popped off. That particular cycled breath will have been partially aborted and the patient will have received only part of the volume set on the control panel. A random, infrequent pop-off cycle is most often caused by the patient's coughing or splinting and need not be cause for concern. However, repeated popping off may be an indication that the patient is in acute respiratory distress and should prompt those in attendance to disconnect the patient from the ventilator to determine the cause of the problem. While the patient is manually ventilated, a suction catheter should be passed through the endotracheal tube to determine whether it is plugged, and whether the ventilator should be checked to ensure it is functioning properly. Other factors to consider are whether the patient's airway resistance has markedly increased (e.g., bronchospasm, excessive secretions, mucous plugging), or significant pneumothorax or migration of the endotracheal tube down the right mainstem bronchus has occurred.

By calculating the patient's dynamic effective compliance and static compliance (C_{ST}) on the ventilator, it may be possible to determine why the patient's airway pressures have increased. Dynamic effective compliance is actually a measure of impedance because it includes compliance as well as resistance components. Both compliances are calculated by dividing the TV delivered to the patient (i.e., TV delivered = TV − ventilator compressible volume) by a pressure change [56]. The pressure change for dynamic effective compliance is peak minus end-expiratory pressure; for static compliance, it is plateau pressure minus end-expiratory pressure. Static pressure is determined just before exhalation by occluding the ventilator exhalation tubing. Dynamic effective compliance is reduced by decreases in chest wall or lung compliance or by increases in airway resistance. Static compliance is reduced by a decrease in chest wall or lung compliance but is not affected by airway resistance, if and when the measurement is made while no airflow is occurring. Therefore, a decrease in dynamic effective compliance without a change in static compliance indicates a resistance problem (e.g., bronchospasm, retained secretions, or an obstructed ventilator circuit). Decreases in both static and dynamic effective compliance indicate a problem with lung or chest wall compliance (e.g., tension pneumothorax, right mainstem intubation, pulmonary edema, burn of chest wall, pneumonia, or atelectasis). This analysis is valid only if auto-PEEP is zero or it is accounted for in the calculations.

Pop-off pressures should usually be set at a level slightly above P_{peak} observed during normal cycling and should not be higher than 50 cm H_2O. This is a reasonable safeguard against exceeding inflation hold pressures of 35 cm H_2O when endotracheal tube size is 8 mm or greater in internal diameter. With small endotracheal tube size, resistance to flow increases and P_{peak} does not reflect peak alveolar pressure or P_{plat}. This should trigger an automatic alert if and when the cycling pressure reaches or exceeds 50 cm H_2O. At this point, the patient should be suctioned if retained secretions have caused the increase in pressure, or the cause of the increase in peak airway pressure should be determined.

Although no specific airway pressure is guaranteed to exclude the risk of barotrauma, higher airway pressures appear to impose an increased risk of alveolar overdistention that can lead to permeability pulmonary edema, subcutaneous emphysema, pneumomediastinum, and pneumothorax. There is now a growing consensus that the main determinant of alveolar overdistention is the end-inspiratory volume [57]. Therefore, mechanical ventilation induced pulmonary edema and pneumothorax are more accurately described as being consequences of "volutrauma" rather than barotrauma [57a]. Compared with peak airway pressure, plateau pressure potentially may provide a more reliable estimate of average peak alveolar pressure [57b]. Plateau pressures have been consistently shown to be the best correlate of alveolar transmural pressure and alveolar (overdistention) damage in animals, when pleural pressure is not increased. Based on numerous animal studies and the knowledge that normal human lungs are maximally distended at a respiratory system recoil pressure of approximately 35 cm H_2O, maintaining a plateau pressure less than 35 cm H_2O during mechanical ventilation is recommended as a ventilatory strategy to minimize volutrauma, particularly in ARDS [57].

Maintaining peak airway pressure less than 50 cm H_2O has been advocated by some as another strategy to minimize barotrauma [57c]. However, it has been shown to provide misleading results when greater than 50 cm H_2O in the settings of a small or obstructed endotracheal tube or high machine inspiratory flow settings [57d]. For example, when endotracheal tube size is small (e.g., less than 8 mm in diameter) or its lumen is excessively narrowed due to kinking, resistance to flow increases and peak airway pressure cannot reflect peak alveolar pressure as well as plateau pressure.

While plateau pressure theoretically should more consistently, accurately, and reliably reflect alveolar pressure than peak airway pressure, neither pressure will provide meaningful information about the forces acting to distend the alveoli or volutrauma unless pleural pressure is also considered. This is because the pressure that actually distends the alveoli is the transmural pressure (i.e., alveolar-pleural pressure). For instance, if pleural pressure increases because of excessive expiratory muscle activity or a tensely distended abdomen, peak and plateau pressures will increase even though alveolar transmural pressure remains unchanged.

Because of the increasing risk of barotrauma with rising airway pressures, it is important not only to determine why peak airway pressures are increasing but also to try to reduce them. For instance, if agitation is responsible, the patient should be sedated and, if necessary, paralyzed. Although lower $\dot{V}_I$ rates might help achieve the goal of decreasing peak airway pressure, it is not clear that this prevents susceptible lung units from overdistension injury. Reductions in flow without concomitant reductions in TV may simply reduce the resistive pressure that is dissipated across the endotracheal tube, without lowering peak transpulmonary pressure or lung stress.

SETTING IN PRESSURE PRESET MODES. In these modes the P_{peak} setting is an important determinant of peak lung volume as well as TV [58]. Inflating the respiratory system to static (inflation hold) pressures of 35 cm H_2O or greater must be avoided. Most often, this means inflation pressure settings of 40 cm H_2O or less should be used. In contrast to volume preset modes with constant flow settings, $\dot{V}I$ and resistive pressures during pressure preset ventilation decline as lung volume increases. For this reason, P_{peak} begins to approximate static inflation pressure at end inspiration and should be kept as close as possible to 35 cm H_2O.

Respiratory Rate and Machine Cycle Timing. The choice of rate setting should be made after considering the patient's actual rate demand in conjunction with the TI or I:E setting. Most ventilators are not "smart" enough to vary TI in proportion to the spontaneous respiratory rate (fS) (as opposed to the set machine rate, fM). At an fM setting of 10 breaths per minute (A/C = 10), the total cycle time (TTOT; inspiration plus expiration) equals 6 seconds. If I:E is 1:2, TI is 2 seconds and expiratory time (TE) is 4 seconds. Imagine that the patient actually triggers at 20 breaths per minute (i.e., TTOT declines to 3 seconds). Inspiratory time remains fixed at 2 seconds because it is determined by the preset machine rate and I:E. The TE must decrease from 4 seconds to 1 second and the actual I:E increases from 1:2 to 2:1. At a rate of 30 breaths per minute (TTOT = 2 sec), TE becomes 0 and "fighting the ventilator" results. For these reasons, the machine backup rate should always be set close to the patient's actual rate. If the actual rate is so high that effective ventilation cannot be achieved, the patient may need sedation and/or paralysis.

All ventilators provide the option of maintaining lung volume at end inspiration for a predefined time. This time, also called end inflation hold time or inspiratory pause time, is usually expressed as a percentage of TTOT. For the purpose of defining I:E, the pause time is considered part of the expiratory machine cycle. Long pause times favor the recruitment of previously collapsed or flooded alveoli and offer a means of shortening expiration independent of rate and mean $\dot{V}I$. Although alveolar recruitment is a desired therapeutic endpoint in the treatment of patients with edematous lungs, keeping the lungs expanded at high volumes (and pressures) for an extended period may damage relatively normal units.

Inspiratory Flow. Many ventilators require that $\dot{V}I$, as opposed to I:E or TTOT, be specified. Since $\dot{V}I$ is equal to the ratio of TV and TI, flow cannot be changed without affecting at least one of the other timing variables. Under most clinical circumstances, $\dot{V}I$ is 1 liter per second or less during volume preset ventilation. Increasing flow always raises peak P_{ao}, but this need not be of concern if most of the added pressure is dissipated across the endotracheal tube. Although $\dot{V}I$ is one factor that determines the regional distribution of inspired gas, the effect of flow on pulmonary gas exchange in disease is too unpredictable to warrant general guidelines. Much more important is the realization that the combined effects of flow, volume, and time settings influence the functional residual capacity (FRC) and degree of dynamic hyperinflation (see below) [59].

The $\dot{V}I$ is rarely specified as part of the physician's orders. Rather, the respiratory therapist usually sets the $\dot{V}I$ rate by empirically observing the patient's pressure-flow pattern during positive-pressure inflation and weighing the advantages of high versus low flow rates. A low flow rate prolongs TI, which leads to higher mean airway pressures. Increasing mean airway pressure of patients with acute lung injury promotes alveolar recruitment, but it may also have adverse cardiovascular effects because it may increase right ventricular afterload and impair venous return. Conversely, in patients with obstruction, a reduction in $\dot{V}I$ may lead to excessive hyperinflation [60]. Also, the patient may find flow delivery insufficient and begin to "lead" the ventilator, sustaining the inspiratory effort through-

out much (or all) of the inspiratory cycle [25]. This can cause fatigue and respiratory distress. A high flow rate (100 L/min) shortens TI and improves gas exchange in patients with COPD [61]; however, a high initial flow rate also abruptly mobilizes a bolus of gas into the patient's airway. This may be uncomfortable and may cause the patient to "buck" or splint, a pattern sometimes described as "fighting the ventilator" or "being out of phase." Therefore, an intermediate flow rate should be selected initially.

Mean Expiratory Flow (The "Hidden Variable"). Mean expiratory flow is defined by the ratio of TV and TE. Expiratory time is equal to TTOT minus TI, and TTOT is equal to 60 per minute (60/f). Because the machine backup rate and actual frequency may differ in the A/C mode, assumed and actual TTOT may also differ. Recall from the discussion on rate and timing that TI is defined by both the set machine backup rate (fM) and the set I:E and that TI remains constant irrespective of the actual rate. In contrast, TE is affected by the actual breathing rate (fA) (i.e., TE = 60/fA − TI). Therefore, the choice of volume and timing settings, together with the patient's rate response, determines mean expiratory flow [62].

It is now appreciated that end-expiratory alveolar pressure can remain positive during intermittent positive-pressure ventilation (IPPV) even when PEEP is not intentionally applied [63]; this is called auto-PEEP (or intrinsic PEEP, PEEPi) and is not readily apparent on the ventilator manometer. Mean expiratory flow, TV/TE, is the principal ventilator setting-related determinant of dynamic hyperinflation. A patient with airways obstruction and a maximal forced expiratory flow of 0.2 liter per second in the mid-vital capacity range (FEF 25–75) obviously can not accommodate a TV/TE of 0.3 liter per second without an increase in end-expired lung volume. Dynamic hyperinflation will result.

Although PEEPi may be present in the majority of ventilated patients in intensive care units [64], it is likely to be worse in patients with COPD [63]. Intrinsic PEEP places the patient at risk for the same pulmonary and cardiovascular consequences as intentional external PEEP (PEEPe). When disregarded, PEEPi effects can lead to serious errors in management. For instance, failure to recognize that PEEPi can elevate pulmonary capillary wedge (PCW) pressure or decrease cardiac output and blood pressure may lead to inappropriate fluid restriction or vasopressor therapy. At the bedside, PEEPi should be clinically suspected if exhalation has not ended before the next inhalation (Fig. 66-4). Intrinsic PEEP can be measured using the expiratory port occlusion technique [63] or from the measurement of change of P_{ao} at the onset of $\dot{V}I$ [64]. It can also be estimated by respiratory inductive plethysmography [65]. In Siemens series ventilators, PEEPi can be estimated by pressing the end-expiratory hold button and waiting until P_{ao} reaches a steady value. In patients with spontaneous respiratory efforts at end expiration P_{ao} will not reach a plateau, and in these patients PEEPi cannot be estimated with this technique. It has been proposed that PEEPi be estimated from esophageal pressure measurements in spontaneously breathing patients. Because such estimates rely on subtle inflections in the esophageal pressure tracing and because the determinants of PEEPi in spontaneously breathing subjects are more complex than those during mechanical ventilation and include the contributions of expiratory muscles to intrathoracic pressure, such measurements should be interpreted with caution. Furthermore, the technique is invasive and subject to artifacts in recumbent individuals [66].

Intrinsic PEEP can be minimized by reducing mean expiratory flow requirement or increasing the patient's capacity to generate the required flow near V_{rel}. Examples of the former strategy are reductions in TV, increasing $\dot{V}I$ and thereby increas-

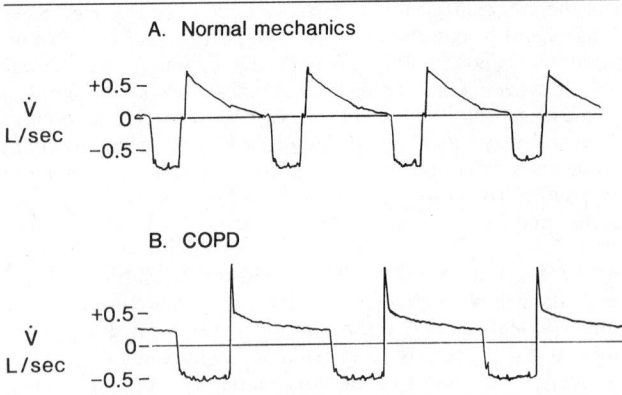

Fig. 66-4. Comparison of flow profiles during mechanical ventilation in a subject with normal mechanics (A) and a subject with chronic obstructive pulmonary disease (B). The presence of expiratory flow prior to machine inflation of the relaxed respiratory system indicates dynamic hyperinflation and intrinsic positive end-expiratory pressure. (From Hubmayr RD, Rehder K: Respiratory muscle failure in critically ill patients. *Semin Respir Med* 13:14–21, 1992. With permission.)

ing T_E, and reducing the actual ventilator rate through manipulations of the set backup rate, sedation and pain control, or imposing neuromuscular blockade. Strategies for increasing the patient's flow generating capacity include bronchodilators [67] and occasionally diuretics when peribronchial edema contributes to obstruction. If subjects with PEEPi make inspiratory efforts while being ventilated in the A/C mode, it is crucial to use extrinsic PEEP to reduce inspiratory work requirements. As a general rule, PEEP settings approaching 75 percent of PEEPi are recommended [68,69].

Minute Ventilation. With the exception of older Siemens series ventilators, minute ventilation ($\dot{V}_E$) is not a primary parameter that must be set directly by the operator. It is rather the consequence of the TV and rate settings. The A/C mode is not a foolproof safeguard for assuring a rate setting independent delivery of an appropriate $\dot{V}_E$. Therefore, a knee-jerk order, such as A/C of 12 and TV of 800, may cause severe alkalemia in a comatose patient with normal lungs yet lead to profound respiratory acidemia in an individual with the acute respiratory distress syndrome (ARDS). As a general rule, the $\dot{V}_E$ setting for patients with hypoxic respiratory failure from ARDS should be 15 to 20 liters per minute until blood gas analyses, airway pressure responses, and cardiovascular status guide further ventilator adjustments. The high ventilatory requirement of such patients reflects hypermetabolic states with increased CO_2 production as well as an increase in physiologic dead space from high ventilation/perfusion ($\dot{V}/\dot{Q}$) mismatch. In contrast to patients with ARDS, patients with COPD tend to have a lower ventilatory requirement, usually 8 to 12 liters per minute unless their disease is exacerbated by left heart failure, sepsis, or pneumonia. Normal individuals maintain normocarbia with a resting ventilation of approximately 5 liters per minute.

Although normocarbia is a desired therapeutic endpoint, it is not essential. Increases in respiratory system impedance combined with increased ventilatory requirements and poor pulmonary gas exchange may necessitate a choice between hypercarbia and risking barotrauma [70,71]. Evidence is mounting that hypercarbia and acidemia are well tolerated provided patients are heavily sedated and paralyzed [72]. It is unclear whether pH levels below 7.20 require administration of bicarbonate or other buffer solutions. (See Chap. 56 for further dis-

cussion of this issue.) It is also unclear whether extracorporeal CO_2 removal or tracheal oxygen insufflation is of benefit in such instances [73].

Positive End-Expiratory Pressure. Positive end-expiratory pressure is the artificial maintenance of positive (superatmospheric) pressure after passive exhalation is complete. This technique is called continuous positive-pressure ventilation (CPPV) when PEEP is added to positive-pressure ventilation; continuous positive airway pressure (CPAP) when the inspiratory and expiratory limbs of the circuit are pressurized to the desired end-expiratory pressure in patients who are breathing without mechanical assistance; and expiratory positive airway pressure (EPAP) when only the expiratory limb is pressurized [74,75,76]. Although mean airway pressure is lower for EPAP compared with CPAP, the work of breathing is greater. This section discusses PEEP primarily applied to patients who are intubated and ventilated with a positive-pressure ventilator. Positive end-expiratory pressure is compatible with positive-pressure mechanical ventilation in any of its modes.

In patients with hypoxic respiratory failure, PEEP is used to raise lung volume to recruit collapsed and flooded alveoli and to improve oxygenation [77,78,79]. In contrast, the goal of PEEP therapy in patients with obstruction is to minimize inspiratory work [68,80,81].

POSITIVE END-EXPIRATORY PRESSURE IN HYPOXIC RESPIRATORY FAILURE. Positive end-expiratory pressure is most useful in the treatment of patients with pulmonary edema resulting from increased alveolocapillary membrane permeability (ARDS) or increased hydrostatic pressure (cardiogenic pulmonary edema) [82]. It increases PaO_2 by diminishing intrapulmonary shunting of blood and improving the matching of ventilation and perfusion. Although it may work by redistributing intraalveolar edema, it does not drive fluid out of the lungs [82].

Most physicians use some measure of blood oxygen content or shunt as endpoints of PEEP therapy. The best PEEP is considered to be the least amount of extrinsic PEEP necessary to achieve adequate blood gas tensions (ordinarily this means arterial O_2 saturation $\geq 90\%$ or $PO_2 \geq 60$ mm Hg with FIO_2 values ≤ 0.6) [79,83]. An alternative approach, which is appealing in a mechanistic sense, is to analyze the shape and the hysteresis area of lung pressure/volume (P/V) loops [84]. The hysteresis of the lung P/V loop is a measure of the energy lost between inflation and deflation [85]. The hysteresis of normal lungs has been attributed to surfactant/surface tension phenomena [52]. In diseases with peribronchial and alveolar edema, the recruitment (opening) and derecruitment (collapse) of alveolar units during lung inflation and deflation are thought to provide an additional source of hysteresis. Positive end-expiratory pressure therapy is instituted to prevent derecruitment of alveoli during lung deflation and thereby reduce pulmonary shunt and $\dot{V}/\dot{Q}$ mismatch [45].

At present, available ICU technology makes it more feasible to base adjustments in PEEPe therapy on measurements of gas exchange than on measurements of lung mechanics. Those who advocate P/V loop-guided therapy focus on the inflection point of the inspiratory P/V relationship as a measure of the critical opening pressure (P_{crit}) of recruitable lung units. Based on this reasoning, they propose to apply an amount of PEEPe equal to P_{crit}. Unfortunately, the evidence in support of this practice is circumstantial and there are no studies in which the efficacy of gas exchange-driven PEEP adjustments and P/V loop-based PEEP management have been compared. There are also technical concerns with the standard techniques used to generate the P/V curve. Measurements made with a large oxygen-filled supersyringe take one minute or more to obtain and may be subject to artifacts from gas uptake. Random airway occlusions during mechanical ventilation have been proposed to circumvent this problem, and automated occlusion algorithms will probably be offered as a diagnostic option in future-generation ventilators.

Reductions in cardiac output and hypotension (see below) occasionally prevent increasing PEEPe sufficiently to reach the therapeutic goal set by gas exchange and lung mechanics criteria. When this happens, it is imperative to stabilize heart and circulation with intravenous fluids and/or inotropic agents before raising PEEPe further [83]. It is inappropriate, however, to consider the therapeutic goal unattainable without attempts at increasing cardiac output.

There are two ways to raise lung volume in the hope of recruiting flooded or partially collapsed alveoli: the judicious use of PEEPe and dynamically raising lung volume. Since it is not uncommon for patients with acute lung injury to be tachypneic, a component of dynamic hyperinflation is often present in mechanically ventilated ARDS patients [86]. Despite the short time constant for lung emptying, the use of PEEP valves that represent resistive as well as threshold loads [74] and ventilator settings that require large mean expiratory flows (TV/TE; see above) contribute to dynamic hyperinflation. Sedation and neuromuscular blockade are useful adjuncts to PEEP therapy insofar as they help raise lung volume by abolishing expiratory muscle activity.

It is unclear whether PEEPe therapy or inducing dynamic hyperinflation with inverse ratio ventilation (IRV) is more effective in recruiting and preventing the collapse of edematous lung regions. Simplistic mathematical models with parallel time constant inhomogeneities suggest that dynamic hyperinflation with IRV is less effective than conventional PEEPe therapy in recruiting low-compliance lung units [87]. Since it may not be appropriate to characterize the mechanical behavior of collapsed and flooded lung units with simple elastic and resistive constants, and because there are no experimental data on the specific values of such constants in disease, it is impossible to assess the relative efficacies of static and dynamic hyperinflation strategies at this point. Whatever the mechanisms, in the short term (minutes) there seems to be little difference in gas exchange when conventional therapy with PEEPe is compared with IRV [88].

EFFECTS OF POSITIVE END-EXPIRATORY PRESSURE ON CIRCULATION. The major cardiovascular complication associated with PEEP is reduction in cardiac output. Although the effect of PEEP on cardiac output is complex, the decrease is caused predominantly by decreasing venous return (right ventricular filling) and direct heart-lung interaction [89,90]. It appears that PEEP affects heart compliance rather than rate or contractility. By increasing lung volume and intrathoracic pressure, PEEP can increase pulmonary vascular resistance and decrease ventricular volume. Decreases in left ventricular diastolic compliance have been attributed either to the direct effect of lung expansion compressing the lateral left ventricular wall or to changes in the position or shape of the interventricular septum related to changes in right ventricular volume. Clinically, a decrease in cardiac output is particularly common with preexisting hypotension or hypovolemia. Although healthy volunteers demonstrate a predictable fall in cardiac output when PEEP is instituted [91], severely ill patients often demonstrate stable hemodynamics or even increased cardiac output [77]. If cardiac output before PEEP is high, a slight reduction may have no adverse consequences; however, a reduction in cardiac output with hypotension should prompt the use of fluid replacement therapy, vasopressor drugs, or discontinuation of PEEP. Also, PEEP may lead to water retention in the lungs [92] by decreasing left atrial volume, thereby stimulating antidiuretic hormone secretion; may alter portal circulatory hemodynamics [93]; and may

decrease perfusion to splanchnic organs that may lead to ischemia of the bowel [94]. All of the cardiovascular complications can be avoided or minimized by adhering to proper indications for use of PEEP and by careful monitoring during its use.

Changes in PEEP can introduce uncertainties in the measurement and interpretation of pulmonary artery pressures. Because left ventricular compliance can be affected by PEEP and because PEEP-induced changes in intrathoracic pressure are transmitted directly to the heart [63,89,90], it is important to appreciate that a change in PCW pressure may not reflect a change in transmural cardiac filling pressure or left ventricular end-diastolic volume. Moreover, if the pulmonary artery catheter is located in a nondependent area of the lung, PCW pressure may not reflect intravascular pressure [95].

Since patients on CPPV have alveolar pressures that are much higher than atmospheric pressure (alveolar pressure will be equal to PEEP at the end of exhalation when there is no airflow), alveolar pressure may be greater than capillary hydrostatic pressure in different regions of the lung. For instance, in a patient with a pulmonary venous pressure of 15 mm Hg on 10 mm Hg PEEP, alveolar pressure will equal 10 mm Hg at the end of exhalation. If the pulmonary artery catheter rests in the upper part of the lung, rather than being in a dependent position, it is conceivable that the catheter is measuring alveolar rather than pulmonary capillary hydrostatic pressure. Although pulmonary venous pressure may be 15 mm Hg in the most dependent lung zones, pulmonary venous pressures at the top of the lung may not be greater than 9 mm Hg because of the effect of gravity (i.e., less blood will flow to the top of the lung). In this situation alveolar pressure, because it is greater than pulmonary venous pressure, will compress the pulmonary capillary; therefore, the PCW pressure in this zone will reflect alveolar pressure.

Although theoretically these problems in measurement and interpretation of pulmonary vascular pressures during PEEP may be avoided by removing PEEP while pulmonary vascular pressures are measured, marked worsening in PaO₂ with resultant persistent hypoxemia can occur and may induce an unsteady state with new hemodynamic changes. Furthermore, hemodynamic measurements off PEEP are of dubious value since they may change as PEEP is reinstituted.

In summary, although it appears that some of the limitations of pulmonary vascular pressure measurements in critically ill patients must be accepted, others can be avoided. For instance, ensuring that the pulmonary artery catheter is in proper position below the level of the left atrium can maximize the time PCW pressure will reflect pulmonary venous rather than alveolar pressure. Pulmonary capillary wedge pressures in patients on PEEP reflect pulmonary venous pressures whenever they are greater than PEEP.

POSITIVE END-EXPIRATORY PRESSURE AND THE OBSTRUCTED PATIENT. Continuous positive airway pressure reduces the inspiratory work of breathing in dynamically hyperinflated patients by two mechanisms: (1) it helps oppose the expiratory action of P$_{el}$ at end expiration (i.e., PEEPi) and (2) it promotes active expiration below the predicted V$_{rel}$ of the respiratory system [80]. As a result, CPAP can inflate the relaxed respiratory system to V$_{rel}$ because of expiratory muscle derecruitment during inspiration even if the inspiratory muscles were to remain inactive. It is crucial to oppose PEEPi with extrinsic PEEP in ventilator-dependent patients with COPD when they make inspiratory triggering efforts. If this is not done, the patient is forced to generate inspiratory pressures slightly above PEEPi before the machine can respond. Such efforts are potentially exhausting and could prevent successful weaning from mechanical ventilation.

"PHYSIOLOGIC" AND PROPHYLACTIC POSITIVE END-EXPIRATORY PRESSURE. While the term "physiologic" PEEP has been applied to the application of 5 to 10 cm H_2O of PEEP in intubated patients with normal lungs [96], it is a misnomer. The term was coined because gas exchange and FRC in these patients were comparable with that in normal nonintubated individuals. Though placement of an endotracheal tube is frequently associated with a decrease in FRC [97], there are no data to suggest that "physiologic PEEP" improves gas exchange in all intubated patients with restrictive lung disease or that it necessarily has any effect on their morbidity or mortality.

There also are no conclusive data to show that prophylactic PEEP reduces the incidence of ARDS in predisposed patients [98]. Moreover, although PEEP is commonly used in the postoperative management of patients who have experienced thoracic, cardiovascular, or abdominal surgery to prevent postoperative atelectasis, there are no data to support this proposed indication. In fact, it has been shown that the routine use of PEEP after open heart surgery has no beneficial prophylactic effect in preventing atelectasis [99]. There also are no data to support the use of PEEP to reduce or control mediastinal bleeding after cardiac surgery [100].

PRESSURE PRESET VENTILATION SETTINGS

Pressure Controlled Ventilation. Because of concerns for barotrauma, PCV is gaining popularity as a support mode for patients with severe hypoxic respiratory failure. Because of the need to recruit flooded or collapsed lung units while avoiding overdistension of alveoli, PCV is often employed in conjunction with I:E ratios of 1 or greater (IRV) and permissive hypercarbia [39,71,101]. In this context, use of PCV requires heavy sedation and neuromuscular blockade. Because such patients have a high ventilatory requirement and need extrinsic PEEP for additional alveolar recruitment, initially the ventilator might be set to deliver a (peak) pressure of 35 cm H_2O at a rate of 20 breaths per minute with an I:E of 1:1 and a PEEPe of 10 cm H_2O. Subsequent adjustments should be guided by measurements of minute volume and blood gas tensions. If PaO_2 is inadequate at these settings, there are two options: increase I:E from 1:1 to 2:1 (apply IRV) or raise PEEPe. The first approach is designed to raise mean lung volume with little or no increase in end-expiratory volume (i.e., FRC). However, we favor the latter approach, because the FRC-independent gas exchange benefits of IRV are marginal [88] and intuitively it makes more sense to prevent airway closure and alveolar derecruitment by raising minimal as well as mean lung volume. Finally, there are theoretical reasons (based on linear mechanics theory) that raising FRC statically with PEEPe might be preferred over dynamic hyperinflation as a recruitment strategy for fast time constant units [87]. The price for raising PEEPe is a reduction in TV and $\dot{V}E$ and thus an increase in $PaCO_2$. Attempts to prevent CO_2 retention by increasing respiratory rate may not be successful because reductions in Ti and further gas trapping (with increased auto PEEP) will cause TV to fall. Raising (peak) inflation pressure much above 35 cm H_2O would defeat the purpose of using PCV to prevent barotrauma. Increases in inflation pressure should be considered only in the presence of a large peak-to-P_{plat} difference. A detailed review of the theory behind patient/ventilator interactions during PCV can be found elsewhere [58].

Pressure Support Ventilation. The use of PSV as a weaning tool is discussed in Chapter 67. Aside from weaning attempts, PSV is occasionally useful in caring for patients with high respiratory rates and drive. Since the goal in these patients is to facilitate patient-ventilator synchrony, as opposed to improving pulmonary gas exchange, the pressure setting should be adjusted at the bedside to minimize signs and symptoms of heightened respiratory effort.

Nonconventional Modes and Alternative Options of Mechanical Ventilation

INVERSE RATIO VENTILATION. Inverse ratio ventilation (IRV) is a technique that uses increased I:E of up to 4:1 [60]. It can be applied by slowing the rate of flow delivery during conventional volume preset ventilation or by maintaining pressure at a controlled volume for a finite interval of time (pressure-control ventilation). This method is designed to improve oxygenation. Inverse ratio ventilation is uncomfortable and usually requires heavy sedation and paralysis and, therefore, controlled ventilation. Improved oxygenation may be attributed to increased mean airway pressure and volume. Because TE is markedly shortened, auto PEEP or PEEPi is a common occurrence. Although dynamic hyperinflation may explain the improved oxygenation, it may also increase the risk of barotrauma and decrease cardiac output [102,103].

AIRWAY PRESSURE RELEASE VENTILATION. Airway pressure release ventilation (APRV) is a form of pressure preset ventilation; essentially it is PCV with IRV. A constant pressure is applied to the airway for approximately 80 percent of the respiratory cycle and then it is released, allowing the lungs to deflate passively [60]. The target population for APRV is identical to that for PCV with IRV (i.e., patients with severe lung injury and hypoxemia). Patients are allowed to take spontaneous breaths with APRV, making heavy sedation and paralysis unnecessary. However, it is uncertain that this is an advantage, because active expiration, which is common in such patients, counteracts efforts to raise end-expiratory lung volume [97].

INDEPENDENT LUNG VENTILATION. Independent lung ventilation has been useful in selected patients with severe unilateral lung disease [104]. Each lung is ventilated separately according to its requirements for TV, PEEP, and so forth. A bifid endotracheal tube separates the lungs with different inflation and gas exchange functions. Differential lung ventilation can be given through this tube by a single ventilator with two distribution circuits or two ventilators that provide asynchronous or synchronous inflation of both lungs. The decision to institute unilateral lung ventilation should not be taken lightly, because as a rule the divided airway needs to be repositioned daily to correct leaks or cuff-related obstruction of mainstem or upper lobe bronchi.

MANDATORY MINUTE VOLUME VENTILATION. Mandatory minute volume ventilation (MMV) is designed to provide a certain $\dot{V}E$ [60]. It provides a safety net for weaning patients in the PSV mode. The physician determines the minimum amount of $\dot{V}E$ to be maintained; when it falls below this target, some ventilators augment pressure support per breath and others switch automatically to volume-controlled assisted ventilation. Although MMV is an appealing feature of newer ventilators, it is not always clear what the minimum $\dot{V}E$ should be. An inappropriately low MMV setting may obscure the presence of respiratory pump failure by blood gas criteria and could theoretically contribute to chronic respiratory muscle fatigue.

VOLUME ASSURED PRESSURE SUPPORT. Volume assured pressure support (VAPS) is fashioned after MMV insofar as the safety net is applied to TV rather than minute volume [105]. The paucity of experimental data and the somewhat limited rationale for VAPS cast doubt on its clinical utility at this point in time.

PROPORTIONAL ASSIST VENTILATION. Proportional assist ventilation (PAV) is a novel mode of mechanical ventilation currently in its early clinical trial stage in Canada. In contrast to any other form of mechanical ventilation, PAV augments machine output in proportion to patient demand. The interested reader is referred elsewhere [14,106].

Disease-Oriented Mechanical Ventilation Strategies

At the risk of redundancy, in the following section we present a disease-oriented approach to ventilator management that emphasizes differences in pathophysiology and therapeutic goals.

MECHANICAL VENTILATION IN INDIVIDUALS WITH (NEAR) NORMAL RESPIRATORY MECHANICS AND PULMONARY GAS EXCHANGE. Most patients who require ventilation during anesthesia, neuromuscular blockade, and surgery, most patients with respiratory failure from CNS depressant drugs, and many patients with diseases of peripheral nerves and muscles have (near) normal respiratory mechanics and pulmonary gas exchange. The goal in these patients is to maintain or restore adequate alveolar ventilation and oxygenation, and therefore the single most important initial ventilator setting is minute volume ($\dot{V}_E$). Minute volume is the product of fM and TV and is an important determinant of the body's CO_2 stores and consequently of $PaCO_2$:

$$PaCO_2 = \frac{\dot{V}CO_2 \times k}{\dot{V}_E (1 - V_D/TV)} \tag{5}$$

$\dot{V}CO_2$ is the volume of CO_2 produced (in liters per minute); V_D/TV is the dead space-to-TV ratio, a variable with which the efficiency of the lung as a CO_2 eliminator can be approximated; k is a constant that equals 0.863 and which scales $\dot{V}CO_2$ and $\dot{V}_E$ to the same temperature and humidity.

In resting patients with normal lungs and metabolic rates, a $\dot{V}_E$ setting between 80 and 100 cc per kilogram usually results in normocapnia. Usual TV settings range between 10 and 12 cc per kilogram, with the occasional neuromuscular disease patient preferring 15 cc per kilogram for comfort. If a subsequent blood gas analysis shows hypercarbia despite seemingly adequate $\dot{V}_E$ delivery, a hypermetabolic state (increased $\dot{V}CO_2$) or $\dot{V}/\dot{Q}$ mismatch (abnormal V_D/TV) should be suspected. It may not be wise to normalize the $PaCO_2$ of patients with chronic CO_2 retention suddenly because of the adverse hemodynamic effects of posthypercapnic alkalosis [107]. Therefore, $\dot{V}_E$ settings of approximately 60 cc per kilogram should be used when the initial $PaCO_2$ and pH targets are approximately 55 mm Hg and 7.35, respectively. It remains unresolved whether patients with chronic CO_2 retention should ever be mechanically ventilated

to normocapnia. Those who argue against this practice assume that a resetting of chemoresponsiveness toward normal elevates ventilatory requirement and prevents weaning. Proponents cite the adverse effects of hypercapnia on respiratory muscle contractility [108].

MECHANICAL VENTILATION IN INDIVIDUALS WITH AIRWAYS OBSTRUCTION. Because of expiratory airflow limitation, patients with obstructive physiology are at risk of having mechanical ventilation cause or worsen dynamic hyperinflation (i.e., PEEPi). This in turn increases the risk of barotrauma (e.g., pneumothorax), hypotension, and death. Therefore, the goal of therapy is to maintain adequate oxygenation while minimizing the thoracic volume about which the lungs are ventilated. The latter can be accomplished by (1) reducing airway inflammation and alleviating bronchoconstriction, (2) decreasing TV, (3) increasing T_E, and (4) accepting hypercapnia.

Status Asthmaticus. The idea of permissive hypercarbia [70] and the contributions of Tuxen's group [53,59,109] have changed both indications and management principles of mechanical ventilation in status asthmaticus. In contrast to patients with chronic airflow obstruction from emphysema or bronchitis, patients with status asthmaticus suffer from airway closure and mucous plugging and have much more severe $\dot{V}/\dot{Q}$ mismatch and a higher ventilatory requirement, and are therefore particularly prone to hyperinflation, barotrauma, cardiovascular collapse, and death (see Chap. 56). Intubation and mechanical ventilation should be viewed as measures of last resort and thus are ideally reserved for patients who require sedation, neuromuscular blockade, and ventilation with permissive hypercarbia.

Since the primary goal is to prevent overdistension of unobstructed lung units, relatively low initial TV settings (e.g., <8 cc/kg) should be used in conjunction with high peak flows (e.g., 60–90 L/min) and a rate of 12 to 16 breaths per minute. Higher rates should be used only if cardiovascular instability is attributed to severe respiratory acidemia rather than dynamic hyperinflation. In practice, it is rarely possible to make this distinction. Because peak airway pressure may not adequately reflect lung parenchymal strain in such patients [53], Tuxen et al. proposed guiding ventilator adjustments on the basis of measurements of "trapped gas volume" [109].

The $\dot{V}_{EI}$ is the volume of air above FRC that is in the patient's lungs after delivery of TV. While P_{peak} and P_{plat} are read directly off the ventilator manometer, $\dot{V}_{EI}$ is measured in a spirometer. For $\dot{V}_{EI}$ measurement, patients must be sedated, paralyzed, and well oxygenated and disconnected from the ventilator immediately after TV is delivered. Expired air must be collected in a spirometer until no more air escapes. In severely obstructed patients, this collection may take, on average, 40 to 60 seconds. Making ventilator changes aimed at keeping $\dot{V}_{EI}$ below 20 ml per kilogram has been shown to protect against barotrauma and hypotension in status asthmaticus [53].

To manage the most severely obstructed patients with status asthmaticus, we recommend making ventilatory changes as needed to stay below the $\dot{V}_{EI}$ threshold of 20 ml/kg. If $\dot{V}_{EI}$ is greater than 20 ml per kilogram after the patient has stabilized on the initial ventilator settings, the TV or rate should be decreased. If $\dot{V}_{EI}$ is greater than 20 ml per kilogram but gas exchange is marginal, ventilating the patient with a helium-oxygen mixture should be considered, as it may reduce lung inflation pressure and improve oxygenation [110]. It must be stressed that there is no single upper $PaCO_2$ or lower pH threshold which has been associated with cardiovascular instability or poor outcome. Therefore, concern for barotrauma usually takes precedence over maintenance of alveolar ventilation. (See Chap. 56 for the role of bicarbonate infusion.)

CHRONIC OBSTRUCTIVE PULMONARY DISEASE. In general, the management principles for COPD are similar to those for asthmatics, except that patients with exacerbations from COPD rarely require neuromuscular blockade or permissive hypercarbia. Patients with COPD are prone to dynamic hyperinflation from expiratory flow limitation rather than airway closure and mucous plugging. The challenge is to minimize hyperinflation and inspiratory work despite limited control over respiratory rate (see Chap. 57). In a patient who is not paralyzed, machine trigger rate, as opposed to machine backup rate and I:E settings, determines TE (see earlier discussion). To the extent to which COPD patients remain tachypneic during MV, changing VI and TI settings may not be effective in reducing gas trapping. Increasing VI under the assumption that it would prolong TE may actually have the opposite effect, since higher flows often increase respiratory rate [111]. Therefore, we initially choose a TV between 8 and 10 cc per kilogram, an intermediate flow of 40 to 60 liters per minute, and a rate close to the patient's spontaneous effort rate. We add 5 cm H$_2$O of CPAP to reduce machine trigger work (see earlier discussion).

Because these patients are not paralyzed, it is not feasible to monitor trapped gas volume, as has been proposed for asthmatics. Rather, one should assure that end-inflation hold pressure remains below 35 cm H$_2$O. If the initial ventilator settings fail to reduce dyspnea and patient effort, we raise CPAP until peak airway pressure starts to rise [68]. At that point, the difference between CPAP and auto PEEP is presumably at a minimum. If adjustments in CPAP fail to reduce patient effort, as judged by symptoms or accessory muscle use, usually sedation must be increased and, rarely, neuromuscular blockade considered.

ACUTE RESPIRATORY DISTRESS SYNDROME. Much of our treatment philosophy and its underpinnings for patients with ARDS are presented in the sections on TV and rate settings, pressure control ventilation, IRV, and the use of PEEP. To summarize, we attempt to increase FRC and mean lung volume through the application of extrinsic PEEP, avoid end-inflation hold pressure in excess of 35 cm H$_2$O, and reduce TV as we raise PEEP to stay within "safe volume" boundaries. In practice, this means TV settings between 5 and 8 cc per kilogram when we use volume preset modes or P$_{peak}$ settings ≤40 cm H$_2$O when we use pressure preset modes. The rate is usually 20 to 30 breaths per minute unless the patient has been paralyzed to tolerate hypercapnia or IRV. There is no upper limit to PEEP as long as the peak lung volume and recoil pressure guidelines are adhered to, but in practice it is rarely possible to deliver sufficient alveolar ventilation at cycling pressures between 20 (PEEP setting) and 35 cm H$_2$O (P$_{plat}$). Patients who cannot be oxygenated at such settings invariably need to be sedated and paralyzed and may be candidates for nonconventional alternative and investigational interventions. These include extracorporeal membrane oxygenators, extracorporeal CO$_2$ removal devices, and high-frequency ventilators. To date, none of these interventions have proved efficacious in clinical trials [112,113,114] (see Chap. 55).

HEAD TRAUMA. The key to the ventilatory management of patients with head trauma is to avoid excessive intrathoracic pressures and at the same time provide sufficient ventilation to lower PaCO$_2$. High intrathoracic pressures are transmitted to the subarachnoid space and may thereby reduce the perfusion pressure of a CNS that is already compromised by intracranial hypertension from bleeding or edema. In practice, this means correcting hypoxemia preferentially with oxygen supplementation rather than PEEP (see Chap. 175).

MYOCARDIAL ISCHEMIA AND CONGESTIVE HEART FAILURE. In addition to the heart-lung interactions already discussed in the context of PEEP therapy, mechanical ventilation reduces systemic as well as myocardial oxygen demands. This may be critical in patients with ischemia and cardiogenic shock and is associated with a redistribution of blood from working respiratory muscles toward vital organs [115].

In principle, the ventilatory management of patients with ischemia and congestive heart failure is similar to that of patients with noncardiogenic forms of pulmonary edema. Positive end-expiratory pressure should be used to recruit flooded lung units and redistribute edema fluid from the alveolar to interstitial spaces. When congestive heart failure complicates active ischemia, premature weaning attempts that focus only on maintenance of blood gas tension and ignore work of breathing and associated increases in myocardial oxygen demand are ill advised (see Chaps. 42 and 50).

MECHANICAL VENTILATION IN INDIVIDUALS WITH A BRONCHOPLEURAL FISTULA. For discussion of the ventilatory strategy of this entity, see Chapter 65.

Complications Associated with Intermittent Positive-Pressure Ventilation

The hazards associated with mechanical ventilation can be divided into five major categories [116,117]: (1) complications attributable to intubation and extubation, (2) complications associated with endotracheal or tracheostomy tubes, (3) complications attributable to operation of the ventilator, (4) medical complications occurring during assisted mechanical ventilation, and (5) psychologic effects.

Complications attributable to intubation and extubation and those associated with endotracheal-tracheostomy tubes [116] include upper airway trauma, inadvertent placement or migration of the endotracheal tube into the right mainstem bronchus, vocal cord edema or granuloma, cuff-related damage to the trachea [118], accidental intubation of the esophagus, induction of vomiting with resultant aspiration, premature extubation, self-extubation, tube malfunction, nasal necrosis, and sinusitis associated with nasotracheal intubation. For a more complete discussion of these complications, see Chapter 1.

Complications attributable to operation of the ventilator [117] include machine failure, alarm failure, alarm inadvertently turned off, inadequate nebulization or humidification, overheating of inspired air [119], ventilator asynchrony or noncapture [120], and bacterial contamination of various components of the mechanical ventilator [121]. All of these can be minimized or eliminated if patients on ventilators are not left unattended and infection control methods are adhered to strictly.

Medical complications occurring during assisted ventilation [117] include inadvertent alveolar hypoventilation and hyperventilation, bronchopulmonary dysplasia [122], hypotension caused by decreased cardiac output from a reduction in venous return [123], vascular insufficiency in patients with arteriosclerotic vascular disease caused by decreased cardiac output, water retention from increased circulating levels of antidiuretic hormone presumably stimulated when positive-pressure ventilation decreases left atrial volume [92], and lung barotrauma [124,125,126].

The classic manifestations of barotrauma are pulmonary interstitial emphysema with pneumomediastinum, subcutaneous emphysema, pneumoretroperitoneum, pneumoperitoneum, and pneumothorax with or without tension. However, in the last decade it has become abundantly clear that there are many more subtle manifestations of ventilator-induced lung injury originally attributed to intrinsic disease. These range from capillary leak and noncardiogenic edema to alveolar hemorrhage and subpleural cyst formations and are thought to be causally related to overdistension and surfactant depletion from excessive regional tidal excursions. Realizing that large TV can be injurious even when lung inflation beyond TLC is avoided invalidates many older studies in which the incidence of barotrauma was related to PEEP. In fact, PEEP protects the lungs from injury as long as TV is reduced while PEEP is increased. The older literature quotes an overall incidence of pneumothorax with IPPV of 3.5 percent [117] with values as high as 30 percent in the status asthmaticus subgroup [127]. It is hoped that an improved understanding of patient-ventilator interactions and lung biology will substantially reduce the incidence of barotrauma. Since 60 to 90 percent of pneumothoraces in patients on positive-pressure ventilation are under tension [128] and mortality increases from 7 to 31 percent when there is a delay from 30 minutes to 8 hours in diagnosing and treating pneumothoraces that occur on ventilators [129], there must be a high index of suspicion for this complication and it must be managed swiftly. For management of this problem, see Chap. 65 and studies by Pierson [130] and Powner and Grenvik [131]. Powner and Grenvik [131] review ventilatory strategies for closing persistent bronchopleural fistulas. These include high-frequency methods to minimize leaks during exhalation and during inspiration. These techniques are investigational because they have not been rigorously studied, but they should be considered when a large bronchopleural fistula causes profound hypoxemia. (See Chap. 65 for further discussion.) Pneumoperitoneum from mechanical ventilation mimicking a perforated viscus can lead to needless laparotomy [124]. Mechanical ventilation can also be complicated by massive gastric distention, gastric ulceration, atelectasis, and pneumonia [117]. A number of studies suggest that nosocomial gram-negative bacillary pneumonia in patients on ventilators results from retrograde gram-negative bacillary colonization of the pharynx and trachea from the stomach and that stomach colonization is associated with the lack of acidity in the stomach. Sucralfate, when given as stress ulcer prophylaxis, is just as effective as antacids or histamine type 2 blockers but is less likely to be associated with pneumonia [132]. See Chapter 76 for further discussion.

References

1. Barach AL, Bickerman HA, Petty TL: Perspectives in pressure breathing. *Respir Care* 20:627, 1975.
2. Snider GL: Historical perspective on mechanical ventilation: From simple life support system to ethical dilemma. *Am Rev Respir Dis* 140:S2, 1989.
3. Holtackers TR, Loosbrock LM, Gracey DR: The use of the chest cuirass in respiratory failure of neurologic origin. *Respir Care* 27:271, 1982.
4. Goldstein RS, Molotiu N, Skrastins R, et al: Reversal of sleep-induced hypoventilation and chronic respiratory failure by nocturnal negative pressure ventilation in patients with restrictive ventilatory impairment. *Am Rev Respir Dis* 135:1049, 1987.
5. Hill NS: Clinical applications of body ventilators. *Chest* 90:897, 1986.
6. Rochester DF, Braun NMT, Laine S: Diaphragmatic energy expenditure in chronic respiratory failure. *Am J Med* 63:223, 1977.
7. Levy RD, Cosio MG, Gibbons L, et al: Induction of sleep apnoea with negative pressure ventilation in patients with chronic obstructive lung disease. *Thorax* 47:612, 1992.
8. Shapiro SH, Ernst P, Gray-Donald K, et al: Effect of negative pressure ventilation in severe chronic obstructive pulmonary disease. *Lancet* 340:1425, 1992.
9. Meduri GU, Conoscenti CC, Menashe P, et al: Noninvasive face mask ventilation in patients with acute respiratory failure. *Chest* 95:865, 1989.
10. Bott J, Carroll MP, Conway JH, et al: Randomised controlled trial of nasal ventilation in acute ventilatory failure due to chronic obstructive airways disease. *Lancet* 341:1555, 1993.
11. Brochard L, Isabey D, Piquet J, et al: Reversal of acute exacerbations of chronic obstructive lung disease by inspiratory assistance with a face mask. *N Engl J Med* 323:1523, 1990.
12. Marino W: Intermittent volume cycled mechanical ventilation via nasal mask in patients with respiratory failure due to COPD. *Chest* 99:681, 1991.
13. Meduri GU, Abou-Shala N, Fox RC, et al: Noninvasive face mask mechanical ventilation in patients with acute hypercapnic respiratory failure. *Chest* 100:445, 1991.
14. Younes M, Puddy A, Roberts D, et al: Proportional assist ventilation: Results of an initial clinical trial. *Am Rev Respir Dis* 145:121, 1992.
15. Froese AB, Bryan AC: High frequency ventilation. *Am Rev Respir Dis* 135:1363, 1987.
16. Keszler M, Klein R, McClellan L, et al: Effects of conventional and high frequency jet ventilation on lung parenchyma. *Crit Care Med* 10:514, 1982.
17. The HIFI Study Group: High-frequency oscillatory ventilation compared with conventional mechanical ventilation in the treatment of respiratory failure in preterm infants. *N Engl J Med* 320:88, 1989.
18. Saari AF, Rossing TH, Solway J, et al: Lung inflation during high frequency ventilation. *Am Rev Respir Dis* 129:333, 1984.
19. Simon BA, Weisman GG, Mitzner W: Mean airway pressure and alveolar pressure during high frequency ventilation. *J Appl Physiol* 57:1069, 1984.
20. Saari AF, Rossing TH, Drazen JM: Physiological bases for new approaches to mechanical ventilation. *Ann Rev Med* 35:165, 1984.
21. Slutsky AS: Nonconventional methods of ventilation. *Am Rev Respir Dis* 138:175, 1988.
22. Bates JH, Rossi A, Milic-Emili J: Analysis of the behavior of the respiratory system with constant inspiratory flow. *J Appl Physiol* 58:1840, 1985.
23. Hubmayr RD, Gay PC, Tayyab M: Respiratory system mechanics in ventilated patients: Techniques and indications. *Mayo Clin Proc* 62:358, 1987.
24. Sassoon CSH: Mechanical ventilation design and function: The trigger variable. *Respir Care* 37:1056, 1992.
25. Marini JJ, Rodriguez RM, Lamb V: The inspiratory work-load of patient-initiated mechanical ventilation. *Am Rev Respir Dis* 134:902, 1986.
26. Weisman IM, Rinaldo JE, Rogers RM, et al: Intermittent mandatory ventilation. *Am Rev Respir Dis* 127:641, 1983.
27. Gibney RTN, Wilson RS, Pontoppidan H: Comparison of work of breathing on high gas flow and demand valve continuous positive airway pressure systems. *Chest* 82:692, 1982.
28. Marini JJ, Smith TC, Lamb VJ: External work output and force generation during synchronized intermittent mechanical ventilation. *Am Rev Respir Dis* 138:1169, 1988.
29. Culpepper JA, Rinaldo JE, Rogers RM: Effect of mechanical ventilator mode on tendency towards respiratory alkalosis. *Am Rev Respir Dis* 132:1075, 1985.
30. Hudson LD, Hurlow RS, Craig KC, et al: Does intermittent mandatory ventilation correct respiratory alkalosis in patients receiving assisted mechanical ventilation? *Am Rev Respir Dis* 132:1071, 1985.
31. Dunn WF, Nelson SB, Hubmayr RD: The control of breathing

during weaning from mechanical ventilation. *Chest* 100:754, 1991.

32. Lofaso F, Isabey D, Lorino H, et al: Respiratory response to positive and negative inspiratory pressure in humans. *Respir Physiol* 89:75, 1993.

33. MacIntyre NR: Respiratory function during pressure support ventilation. *Chest* 89:677, 1986.

34. MacIntyre NR, Ho L-I: Effects of initial flow rate and breath termination criteria on pressure support ventilation. *Chest* 99:134, 1991.

35. Fiastro JF, Habib MP, Quan SF: Pressure support compensation for inspiratory work due to endotracheal tubes and demand continuous positive airway pressure. *Chest* 93:499, 1988.

36. Brochard L, Rua F, Lorino H, et al: Inspiratory pressure support compensates for the additional work of breathing caused by the endotracheal tube. *Anesthesiology* 75:739, 1991.

37. Nathan SD, Ishaaya AM, Koerner SK, et al: Predicting minimal pressure support during weaning from mechanical ventilation. *Chest* 103:1215, 1993.

38. Morrell MJ, Shea SA, Adams L, et al: Effects of inspiratory support upon breathing in humans during wakefulness and sleep. *Respir Physiol* 93:577, 1993.

39. Marcy TW, Marini JJ: Inverse ratio ventilation in ARDS: Rationale and implementation. *Chest* 100:494, 1991.

40. Baigelman W, Bellin SJ, Pearce L, et al: Relation of inspired oxygen fraction to hypoxemia in mechanically ventilated adults. *Crit Care Med* 12:486, 1984.

41. Waid-Jones MI, Coursin DB: Perioperative considerations for patients treated with bleomycin. *Chest* 99:993, 1991.

42. Rosenow EC III, Myers JL, Swensen SJ, et al: Drug-induced pulmonary disease: An update. *Chest* 102:239, 1992.

43. Clark JS: Noninvasive assessment of blood gases: State of the art. *Am Rev Respir Dis* 145:220, 1992.

44. Gattinoni L, Pesenti A: ARDS: The nonhomogeneous lung—Facts and hypothesis. *Intensive Crit Care Dig* 61:1, 1987.

45. Corbridge TC, Wood LDH, Crawford GP, et al: Adverse effects of large tidal volume and low PEEP in canine acid aspiration. *Am Rev Respir Dis* 142:311, 1990.

46. Dreyfuss D, Basset G, Soler P, et al: Intermittent positive-pressure hyperventilation with high inflation pressures produces pulmonary microvascular injury in rats. *Am Rev Respir Dis* 132:880, 1985.

47. Kolobow T, Moretti MP, Fumagalli R, et al: Severe impairment in lung function induced by high peak airway pressure during mechanical ventilation. *Am Rev Respir Dis* 135:312, 1987.

48. Sykes MK: Does mechanical ventilation damage the lung? *Acta Anaesthesiol Scand* 35(suppl):35, 1991.

49. Webb HH, Tierney DF: Experimental pulmonary edema due to intermittent positive pressure ventilation with high inflation pressure. *Am Rev Respir Dis* 110:556, 1974.

50. McClenahan JB, Urtnowski A: Effect of ventilation on surfactant and its turnover rate. *J Appl Physiol* 23:215, 1967.

51. Wyszogrodski I, Kyei-Aboagye K, Taeusch HW Jr, et al: Surfactant inactivation by hyperventilation: Conservation by positive end-expiratory pressure. *J Appl Physiol* 38:461, 1975.

52. Hoppin FG Jr, Stothert JC Jr, Greaves IA, et al: Lung recoil: Elastic and rheological properties, in *Handbook of Physiology. 3. The Respiratory System.* vol. 3. *Mechanics of Breathing, Part 1.* Baltimore, Waverly, 1986, pp 195–215.

53. Williams TJ, Tuxen DV, Scheinkestel CD, et al: Risk factors for morbidity in mechanically ventilated patients with acute severe asthma. *Am Rev Respir Dis* 146:607, 1992.

54. Egbert LD, Laver MB, Bendixen HH: Intermittent deep breaths and compliance during anesthesia in man. *Anesthesiology* 24:57, 1963.

55. Davis K Jr, Branson RD, Campbell RS, et al: The addition of sighs during pressure support ventilation: Is there a benefit? *Chest* 104:867, 1993.

56. Demers RR, Pratter MR, Irwin RS: Use of the concept of ventilator compliance in the determination of static total compliance. *Respir Care* 26:644, 1981.

57. ACCP Consensus Conference: Mechanical ventilation. *Chest* 104:1833, 1993.

57a. Dreyfuss D, Saumon G: Role of tidal volume, FRC, and end-inspiratory volume in the development of pulmonary edema following mechanical ventilation. *Am Rev Respir Dis* 148:1194, 1993.

57b. Manning HL: Peak airway pressure: Why the fuss? *Chest* 105:242, 1994.

57c. Petersen GW, Baier H: Incidence of barotrauma in a medical ICU. *Crit Care Med* 11:67, 1983.

57d. Tuxen DV, Williams TJ, Scheinkestel CD, et al: Use of a measurement of pulmonary hyperinflation to control the level of mechanical ventilation in patients with acute severe asthma. *Am Rev Respir Dis* 146:1136, 1992.

58. Marini JJ, Crooke PS III, Truwit JD: Determinants and limits of pressure-preset ventilation: A mathematical model of pressure control. *J Appl Physiol* 67:1081, 1989.

59. Tuxen DV, Lane S: The effects of ventilatory pattern on hyperinflation, airway pressures, and circulation in mechanical ventilation of patients with severe air-flow obstruction. *Am Rev Respir Dis* 136:872, 1987.

60. Marini JJ: Newer concepts in mechanical ventilation, in Moser KM (ed): *Pulmonary Perspectives.* vol. 5. Park Ridge, IL, American College of Chest Physicians, 1988, p 3.

61. Connors AF, McCaffree DR, Gray BA: Effect of inspiratory flow rate on gas exchange during mechanical ventilation. *Am Rev Respir Dis* 124:537, 1981.

62. Hubmayr RD, Abel MD, Rehder K: Physiologic approach to mechanical ventilation. *Crit Care Med* 18:103, 1990.

63. Pepe PE, Marini JJ: Occult positive end-expiratory pressure in mechanically ventilated patients with airflow obstruction. *Am Rev Respir Dis* 126:166, 1982.

64. Rossi A, Gottfried SB, Zocchi L, et al: Measurement of static compliance of the total respiratory system in patients with acute respiratory failure during mechanical ventilation. *Am Rev Respir Dis* 131:672, 1985.

65. Hoffman RA, Ershowsky P, Krieger BP: Determination of auto-PEEP during spontaneous and controlled ventilation by monitoring changes in end-expiratory thoracic gas volume. *Chest* 96:613, 1989.

66. Mead J, Gaensler EA: Esophageal and pleural pressures in man upright and supine. *J Appl Physiol* 14:81, 1959.

67. Gay PC, Rodarte JR, Tayyab M, et al: The evaluation of bronchodilator responsiveness in mechanically ventilated patients. *Am Rev Respir Dis* 136:880, 1987.

68. Gay PC, Rodarte JR, Hubmayr RD: The effects of positive expiratory pressure on isovolume flow and dynamic hyperinflation in patients receiving mechanical ventilation. *Am Rev Respir Dis* 139:621, 1989.

69. Ranieri VM, Giuliani R, Cinella G, et al: Physiologic effects of positive end-expiratory pressure in patients with chronic obstructive pulmonary disease during acute ventilatory failure and CMV. *Am Rev Respir Dis* 147:5, 1993.

70. Darioli R, Perret C: Mechanical controlled hypoventilation in status asthmaticus. *Am Rev Respir Dis* 129:385, 1984.

71. Hickling KG, Henderson SJ, Jackson R: Low mortality associated with low volume pressure limited ventilation with permissive hypercapnia in severe adult respiratory distress syndrome. *Intensive Care Med* 16:372, 1990.

72. Capellier G, Toth JL, Walker P, et al: Hemodynamic effects of permissive hypercapnia. *Am Rev Respir Dis* 145:A527, 1992.

73. Ravenscraft SA, Burke WC, Nahum A, et al: Tracheal gas insufflation augments CO_2 clearance during mechanical ventilation. *Am Rev Respir Dis* 148:345, 1993.

74. Kacmarek RM, Dimas S, Reynolds J, et al: Technical aspects of positive end-expiratory pressure (PEEP). I. Physics of PEEP devices. *Respir Care* 27:1478, 1982.

75. Kacmarek RM, Dimas S, Reynolds J, et al: Technical aspects of positive end-expiratory pressure (PEEP). II. PEEP with positive-pressure ventilation. *Respir Care* 27:1490, 1982.

76. Kacmarek RM, Dimas S, Reynolds J, et al: Technical aspects of positive end-expiratory pressure (PEEP). III. PEEP with spontaneous ventilation. *Respir Care* 27:1505, 1982.

77. Falke KJ, Pontoppidan H, Kumar A, et al: Ventilation with positive end-expiratory pressure in acute lung disease. *J Clin Invest* 51:2315, 1972.

78. Malo J, Ali J, Wood LDH: How does positive end-expiratory pressure reduce intrapulmonary shunt in canine pulmonary edema? *J Appl Physiol* 57:1002, 1984.

79. Ranieri VM, Eissa NT, Corbeil C, et al: Effects of positive end-

expiratory pressure on alveolar recruitment and gas exchange in patients with the adult respiratory distress syndrome. *Am Rev Respir Dis* 144:544, 1991.

80. Martin JG, Shore S, Engel LA: Effect of continuous positive airway pressure on respiratory mechanics and pattern of breathing in induced asthma. *Am Rev Respir Dis* 126:812, 1982.

81. Petrof BJ, Legare M, Goldberg P, et al: Continuous positive airway pressure reduced work of breathing and dyspnea during weaning from mechanical ventilation in severe chronic obstructive pulmonary disease. *Am Rev Respir Dis* 141:281, 1990.

82. Rizk NW, Murray JF: PEEP and pulmonary edema. *Am J Med* 72:381, 1982.

83. Wood LDH, Prewitt RM: Cardiovascular management in acute hypoxemic respiratory failure. *Am J Cardiol* 47:963, 1981.

84. Matamis D, Lemaire F, Harf A, et al: Total respiratory pressure-volume curves in the adult respiratory distress syndrome. *Chest* 86:58, 1985.

85. Fredberg J, Stamenovic D: On the imperfect elasticity of lung tissue. *J Appl Physiol* 67:2408, 1989.

86. Broseghini C, Brandolese R, Poggi R, et al: Respiratory resistance and intrinsic positive end-expiratory pressure (PEEPi) in patients with the adult respiratory distress syndrome (ARDS). *Eur Respir J* 1:726, 1988.

87. Otis AB, Mckerrow CB, Bartlett RA, et al: Mechanical factors in distribution of pulmonary ventilation. *J Appl Physiol* 8:427, 1956.

88. Cole AGH, Weller SF, Sykes MK: Inverse ratio ventilation compared with PEEP in adult respiratory failure. *Intensive Care Med* 10:227, 1984.

89. Dorinsky PM, Whitcomb ME: The effect of PEEP on cardiac output. *Chest* 84:211, 1983.

90. Van Hook CJ, Carilli AD, Haponik EF: Hemodynamic effects of positive end-expiratory pressure: Historical perspective. *Am J Med* 81:307, 1986.

91. Lutch JS, Murray JF: Continuous positive-pressure ventilation: Effects on systemic oxygen transport an tissue oxygenation. *Ann Intern Med* 76:193, 1972.

92. Sladen A, Laver MB, Pontoppidan H: Pulmonary complications and water retention in prolonged mechanical ventilation. *N Engl J Med* 279:448, 1968.

93. Johnson EE, Hedley-Whyte J: Continuous positive-pressure ventilation and portal flow in dogs with pulmonary edema. *J Appl Physiol* 33:385, 1972.

94. Dorinsky PM, Hamlin RL, Gadek JE: Alterations in regional blood flow during positive end-expiratory pressure ventilation. *Crit Care Med* 15:106, 1987.

95. Tooker J, Huseby J, Butler J: The effect of Swan-Ganz catheter height on the wedge pressure-left atrial pressure relationship in edema during positive-pressure ventilation. *Am Rev Respir Dis* 117:721, 1978.

96. Shapiro BA, Cane RD, Harrison RA: Positive end-expiratory pressure therapy in adults with special reference to acute lung injury: A review of the literature and suggested clinical correlations. *Crit Care Med* 12:127, 1984.

97. Quan SF, Falltrick RT, Schlobohm RM: Extubation from ambient or expiratory positive airway pressure in adults. *Anesthesiology* 55:53, 1981.

98. Weisman IM, Rinaldo JE, Rogers RM: Positive end-expiratory pressure in adult respiratory failure. *N Engl J Med* 307:1381, 1982.

99. Good JT, Wolz JF, Anderson JT, et al: The routine use of positive end-expiratory pressure after open heart surgery. *Chest* 76:397, 1979.

100. Zurick AM, Urzua J, Ghatas M, et al: Failure of positive end-expiratory pressure to decrease postoperative bleeding after cardiac surgery. *Ann Thorac Surg* 34:608, 1982.

101. Reynolds EM, Ryan DP, Doody DP: Permissive hypercapnia and pressure-controlled ventilation as treatment of severe adult respiratory distress syndrome in a pediatric burn patient [corrected and republished article originally printed in *Crit Care Med* 21:468, 1993]. *Crit Care Med* 21:944, 1993.

102. Poelaert JI, Visser CA, Everaert JA, et al: Acute hemodynamic changes of pressure-controlled inverse ratio ventilation in the adult respiratory distress syndrome: A transesophageal echocardiographic and Doppler study. *Chest* 104:214, 1993.

103. Tharratt RS, Allen RP, Albertson TE: Pressure controlled inverse ratio ventilation in severe adult respiratory failure. *Chest* 94:755, 1988.

104. Parish JM, Gracey DR, Southern PA, et al: Differential mechanical ventilation in respiratory failure due to severe unilateral lung disease. *Mayo Clin Proc* 59:822, 1984.

105. Amato MB, Barbas CS, Bonassa J, et al: Volume-assured pressure support ventilation (VAPSV): A new approach for reducing muscle workload during acute respiratory failure. *Chest* 102:1225, 1992.

106. Younes M: Proportional assist ventilation, a new approach to ventilatory support: Theory. *Am Rev Respir Dis* 145:114, 1992.

107. Narins RG, Emmett M: Simple and mixed acid-base disorders: A practical approach. *Medicine* 59:161, 1980.

108. Juan G, Calverley P, Talamo C, et al: Effect of carbon dioxide on diaphragmatic function in human beings. *N Engl J Med* 310:874, 1984.

109. Tuxen DV, Williams TJ, Scheinkestel CD, et al: Use of a measurement of pulmonary hyperinflation to control the level of mechanical ventilation in patients with acute severe asthma. *Am Rev Respir Dis* 146:1136, 1992.

110. Gluck EJ, Onorato DJ, Castriotta R: Helium-oxygen mixtures in intubated patients with status asthmaticus and respiratory acidosis. *Chest* 98:693, 1990.

111. Puddy A, Younes M: Effect of inspiratory flow rate on respiratory output in normal subjects. *Am Rev Respir Dis* 146:787, 1992.

112. Bosken C, Lenfant C: Extracorporeal membrane oxygenation revisited again (editorial). *Ann Thorac Surg* 53:551, 1992.

113. Gluck E, Heard S, Patel C, et al: Use of ultrahigh frequency ventilation in patients with ARDS: A preliminary report. *Chest* 103:1413, 1993.

114. Morris P, Bernard GR: Adult respiratory distress syndrome: Strategies to provide support and enhance oxygen delivery. *Postgrad Med* 90:163, 1991.

115. Aubier M, Trippenbach T, Roussos C: Respiratory muscle fatigue during cardiogenic shock. *J Appl Physiol* 51:499, 1981.

116. Stauffer JL, Silvestri RC: Complications of endotracheal intubation, tracheostomy and artificial airway. *Respir Care* 27:417, 1982.

117. Zwillich CW, Pierson DJ, Creagh CE, et al: Complications of assisted ventilation: A prospective study of 354 consecutive episodes. *Am J Med* 57:161, 1974.

118. Demers RR, Saklad M: Intratracheal inflatable cuffs: A review. *Respir Care* 22:29, 1977.

119. Klein EF Jr, Graves SA: "Hot pot" tracheitis. *Chest* 65:225, 1974.

120. Gurevitch MJ, Gelmont D: Importance of trigger sensitivity to ventilator response delay in advanced chronic obstructive pulmonary disease with respiratory failure. *Crit Care Med* 17:354, 1989.

121. Irwin RS, Demers RR, Pratter MR, et al: An outbreak of *Acinetobacter* infection associated with the use of a ventilator spirometer. *Respir Care* 25:232, 1980.

122. Chung A, Golden J, Fligiel S, et al: Bronchopulmonary dysplasia in the adult. *Am Rev Respir Dis* 127:117, 1983.

123. Cournand A, Motley HL, Werko L, et al: Physiological studies of the effect of intermittent positive pressure breathing on cardiac output in man. *Am J Physiol* 1:148, 1948.

124. Glauser FL, Bartlett RH: Pneumoperitoneum in association with pneumothorax. *Chest* 66:536, 1974.

125. Siemoneit KD: Retroperitoneal air dissection and mechanical ventilation. *Chest* 71:431, 1977.

126. Stein AL, Lane E: A new treatment modality for pneumoperitoneum associated with mechanical ventilation. *Chest* 81:519, 1982.

127. Menitove SM, Goldring RM: Combined ventilator and bicarbonate strategy in the management of status asthmaticus. *Am J Med* 74:898, 1983.

128. Albelda SM, Gefter WB, Kelley MA, et al: Ventilator-induced subpleural air cysts: Clinical, radiographic, and pathologic significance. *Am Rev Respir Dis* 127:360, 1983.

129. Haake R, Schlichtig R, Ulstad DR: Barotrauma: Pathophysiology, risk factors, and prevention. *Chest* 91:608, 1987.

130. Pierson DJ: Persistent bronchopleural air leak during mechanical ventilation: A review. *Respir Care* 27:408, 1982.

131. Powner DJ, Grenvik A: Ventilatory management of life-threatening bronchopleural fistulae: A summary. *Crit Care Med* 9:54, 1981.

132. Driks MR, Craven DE, Celli BR, et al: Nosocomial pneumonia in intubated patients given sucralfate as compared with antacids or histamine type 2 blockers. *N Engl J Med* 317:1376, 1987.

67. Mechanical Ventilation: Weaning

Richard S. Irwin and Rolf D. Hubmayr

Introduction

From a clinical standpoint, weaning is a process by which a patient is removed from a treatment modality on which he or she has become dependent. This chapter focuses on weaning patients from mechanical ventilatory support (MV). The process involves the *gradual* discontinuation of MV and the *gradual* resumption of spontaneous breathing on the part of the patient.

For most patients who require MV, weaning is simple and readily accomplished. In others, weaning is complicated, frustrating, prolonged, and not necessarily ever accomplished.

In the past 5 to 10 years, a great deal of effort has been devoted to developing scientifically based strategies to more consistently achieve successful weaning. This chapter reviews the advances made in four general areas: (1) understanding the problem, (2) using criteria for reliably predicting successful weaning, (3) identifying the most useful methods, and (4) managing weaning failure.

Understanding the Weaning Problem

WHO ARE THE PATIENTS? Patients with or likely to suffer from respiratory failure are the individuals who require MV support. Although there is overlap, respiratory failure can be generally categorized into lung failure and pump failure (Fig. 67-1) [1]. Lung failure is pure gas-exchange failure and is manifested by hypoxemia, usually with hypocapnia. It is commonly due to the acute respiratory distress syndrome (ARDS) or cardiogenic pulmonary edema. Pump failure is pure ventilatory failure and is manifested by hypercapnia and hypoxemia. It is commonly due to CNS depression (e.g., overdose, anesthesia) or respiratory muscle fatigue or weakness. Muscle fatigue is "a condition in which there is loss in the capacity for developing force and/or velocity of a muscle, resulting from muscle activity under load and which is reversible by rest" [2,3,4]. Muscle weakness is "a condition in which the capacity of a rested muscle to generate force is impaired" [2,3,4]. While fatigue and weakness can be experimentally distinguished, this is not usually possible in the clinical setting. Therefore, the term *muscle fatigue* may actually encompass fatigue and/or weakness. Contributors to respiratory muscle fatigue may be (1) CNS depression, (2) mechanical defects, such as flail chest and kyphoscoliosis, that increase the work of breathing, (3) lung disease that increases the work of breathing, and (4) mediators of ongoing active diseases (e.g., sepsis) that adversely affect the respiratory muscles.

WHAT IS THEIR OUTCOME? Survival to discharge in all patients who undergo at least 48 hours of MV is about 50 percent or less [5,6]. For those who recover from the insult that necessitated MV, most (80–90% [7,8]) can be easily weaned and extubated. In this group, 77 percent can be weaned within 72 hours of the initiation of MV [8]. This group is composed predominantly of postoperative patients, patients with overdoses, and patients whose conditions cause pure lung (gas-exchange) failure that reverses rapidly. The minority of patients, probably 10 to 20 percent overall, are difficult to wean. This group is largely composed of patients receiving MV for longer than 1 month [9].

Because most patients who survive the initial reason for MV eventually are weaned and many are alive and at home one year later, it is appropriate to be optimistic about the chances of being weaned. Up to 82 percent of patients on MV for 30 to 100 days may eventually be weaned within 43 days or longer [9]. Moreover, patients weaned from prolonged MV may have a hospital survival of 70 percent [9] and a 1- or 2-year survival between 30 percent [9] and 72 percent [10].

WHAT IS WRONG WITH PATIENTS ON PROLONGED VENTILATOR SUPPORT? The theoretical causes of respiratory failure are presented in Figure 67-1; there are potentially four separate and reversible reasons for prolonged MV (Table 67-1). Inadequate respiratory drive may be due to nutritional deficiencies [11], sedatives, CNS abnormality, or sleep deprivation [12]. Inability of the lungs to carry out gas exchange effectively without the assistance of the ventilator may continue if the underlying cause of respiratory failure has not sufficiently improved. There may be profound inspiratory respiratory muscle fatigue, and psychologic dependency may be an additional factor. While no studies have been performed systematically to determine the relative importance of these factors, and while combinations of these factors may be responsible for prolonged MV, the literature suggests that pump failure due to inspiratory respiratory muscle fatigue is primarily responsible for failure to wean in these patients [7,13–16]. Inadequate respiratory drive alone is unlikely to be responsible for the inability to wean [7,17].

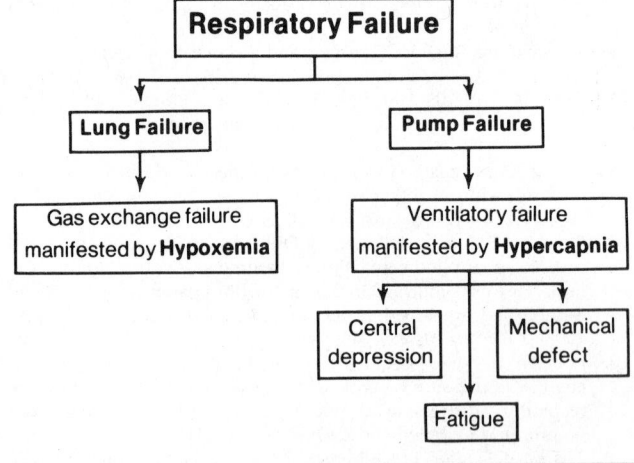

Fig. 67-1. A conceptual framework by which to categorize respiratory failure. (From Roussos C, Macklem PT: The respiratory muscles. Reprinted by permission of *The New England Journal of Medicine* 307:786, 1982.)

Table 67-1. Potentially Reversible Reasons for Prolonged
Mechanical Ventilation

Inadequate respiratory drive
Inability of the lungs to carry out gas exchange effectively
Psychologic dependency
Inspiratory respiratory muscle fatigue
Combinations of the above

Table 67-2. Possible Causes of Inspiratory Respiratory Muscle
Fatigue

Nutritional and metabolic deficiencies [18]
　　Hypokalemia [19]
　　Hypomagnesemia [20]
　　Hypocalcemia [19]
　　Hypophosphatemia [22,23]
　　Hypothyroidism [24,25]
Corticosteroids [26]
Chronic renal failure [28]
Decreased protein synthesis and increased degradation [29,30]
Decreased glycogen stores [31]
Hypoxemia and hypercapnia [32,33]
Anemia [34]
Persistently increased work of breathing (e.g., disease, ventilator)
Failure of the cardiovascular system (e.g., disease, ventilator)
Neuromuscular blocking agents
Critical illness polyneuropathy [35,36]
Combinations of the above

Table 67-3. Comparison of Intermittent Mandatory Ventilation
(IMV) Ventilator Systems with T Piece System*

Ventilator	Inspiratory resistance (cm H_2O/L/sec)	Expiratory resistance (cm H_2O/L/sec)
IMV systems		
Bourns Bear 1	3.6	3.2
Emerson Post Op	4.1	1.2
Bennett MA-1	8.5	5.1
(with demand valve)		
Monaghan 225	2.8	7.5
Siemens Servo	8.3	9.1
T piece system	0.0	0.0

* At a tidal volume of 300 ml and a frequency of 24/min, all IMV ventilator systems
produced inspiratory and expiratory resistances to airflow, whereas the T piece
system produced none. All IMV systems have the potential of increasing the work
of breathing during weaning.
Adapted from Christopher KL, Good JT Jr, Bowman, JL, et al: Should COPD
patients be weaned by T-piece or intermittent mandatory ventilation (IMV)? A
comparison of pressure and resistance in different systems. *Chest* 80:381, 1981.

The cause of inspiratory respiratory muscle fatigue is likely
to be multifactorial (Table 67-2). Muscle strength and endurance
may be compromised because of the factors listed in Table 67-
2 or combinations of those factors.

Animal studies have demonstrated a significant impairment
in diaphragmatic force generation during sepsis, but the mechanism
by which this occurred has yet to be elucidated. While
recent studies have failed to provide evidence that this is a
direct effect of tumor necrosis factor or endotoxin [37], other
data suggest that several free radical species (superoxide ions,
hydrogen peroxide, and hydroxyl ions) may play a role in mediating
injury to diaphragm and intercostal muscles [38].

Although it is assumed that one of the benefits of MV is that
it rests the respiratory muscles, this may not necessarily occur.
Synchronized intermittent mandatory ventilation (SIMV) and
assist ventilation modes both may cause problems in this regard.
Some SIMV systems expose patients to increases in airway
resistance that result from breathing through the ventilator tubing
during spontaneous efforts which occur between volume-cycled
breaths [39,40,41] (Table 67-3). A similar effect can also occur
during machine-assisted breathing with SIMV [42]. Both continuous
flow and demand valve systems have the potential for
increasing the work of breathing. For instance, the continuous
flow may not satisfy the patient's inspiratory flow demands.
Demand valve SIMV systems may increase the work of
breathing because they may require more than a modest effort
by the patient to breathe spontaneously. In assist mode, if tidal
volume and inspiratory flow rate do not meet the patient's
inspiratory demands or requirements the patient's inspiratory
muscles are liable to work throughout the entire inspiratory
cycle, rather than being fully "assisted" [43,44]. If auto-positive
end-expiratory pressure (auto PEEP) is present (see Chap. 66),
the patient may not be able to trigger the ventilator or may be
able to capture it only intermittently while performing a prohibitively
large amount of work during assist ventilation, since

he or she must drop airway pressure below the amount of auto
PEEP before triggering the ventilator [45].

Failure of the cardiovascular system [46] may prolong MV for
a variety of reasons. Gas exchange may continue impaired because
of persistent passive congestion of the lungs, and this
may contribute to an increased work of breathing during spontaneous
breaths. Poor cardiac performance may contribute to
an inadequate supply of oxygen to the respiratory muscles [47].
Although MV may adversely affect cardiac output by increasing
intrathoracic pressure, thereby decreasing venous return and
cardiac output, it is also possible that some cardiovascular patients
cannot be weaned from MV because the ventilator exerts
a beneficial influence on cardiac function (i.e., unloading the
left ventricle in left ventricular failure) [48–51]. Withdrawing MV
from these patients may lead to a deterioration in cardiac function.

Nutritional deficiencies may prolong weaning from MV by
leading to myocardial as well as respiratory muscle dysfunction
[52].

Criteria for Predicting Successful Weaning

**WHEN IS IT APPROPRIATE TO BEGIN THE WEANING
PROCESS?** Because there are no objective, rigorously generated
data to determine when it is prudent or imprudent to
initiate weaning, physicians must rely on their clinical judgment.
In practice, weaning is usually considered when the original
indication for MV has been stabilized or is improving. A
recent study [53] suggests that physicians underestimate the
weaning potential of their patients, at least in the short term.
The investigators asked intensivists to predict whether their
patients would be able to complete a 1-hour T piece trial and
then proceeded to test the accuracy of these predictions using
a weaning protocol of graduated pressure support withdrawal.
Failure criteria had been established prospectively and were
based primarily on the intensity of respiratory sensations (dyspnea
scores $\geq$ 18 using a modified Borg scale), tachypnea (respiratory
rate $\geq$ 35/min) and also included cardiovascular response
parameters indicative of a hyperdynamic state.
Clinically, the intensivists predicted successful completion of
the discontinuation trial with a sensitivity of 79 percent, speci-

ficity of 35 percent, positive predictive value of 50 percent, and negative predictive value of 66 percent.

Although weaning as early as possible is important to avoid muscular weakness and complications related to prolonged endotracheal intubation, tracheostomy, and MV support, there are theoretical concerns (not yet substantiated) that premature attempts may be counterproductive because of adverse physiologic and psychologic effects. Because of potential negative reinforcement that may result from failure of a weaning trial, which may render subsequent attempts more difficult, careful selection of the initial period of spontaneous breathing may be important.

Numerous studies have been performed to develop reliable criteria to predict successful weaning. However, all of these have been utilized not to predict when to initiate the weaning process but rather to predict when MV can be totally withdrawn and the patient extubated.

PREDICTIVE INDICES FOR TOTAL DISCONTINUATION OF MECHANICAL VENTILATION. Numerous studies have evaluated a wide variety of physiologic indices to predict a patient's ability to sustain spontaneous ventilation without MV [7,17,54–65]. They have yielded much conflicting data, due in large part to differences in methodology and experimental design, such as patient population studied, choice of physiologic index threshold value, physiologic measurement techniques, and definition of success and failure. Two recent prospective studies [66,67] that provide a comprehensive account of the sensitivity and specificity of commonly used weaning parameters are discussed in detail here.

In a prospective study involving medical intensive care patients, Yang and Tobin [66] assessed the accuracy of a variety of commonly used physiologic indices of predicting weaning success and failure. Success was defined as ability to sustain spontaneous breathing for 24 hours or longer after extubation; failure was defined as the need for reinstitution of MV at the end of a discontinuation trial or for reintubation within 24 hours. Objective criteria for reinstitution of MV included one or more of the following: $PaCO_2$ of 50 mm Hg or greater, increase in $PaCO_2$ of 8 mm Hg, pH_a of 7.33 or less, decrease in pH_a of 0.07 or greater, PaO_2 of 60 mm Hg or less with an FIO_2 of 0.5 or greater. Clinical criteria for weaning failure included diaphoresis, increasing respiratory effort, tachycardia, arrhythmias, or hypotension. Physiologic measurement techniques were clearly stated. Optimal threshold values for predicting success were prospectively assessed, not chosen by post hoc analysis of data. Table 67-4 shows both threshold values and the accuracy of indices used to predict weaning outcome [66]. Of all the indices, the index of rapid shallow breathing (number of breaths per minute divided by tidal volume in liters [f/TV]) had the highest positive and negative predictive values. Although the authors emphasized the value of f/TV, it should be noted that a TV of 325 ml or less was almost as good a predictor of weaning failure as an f/TV of 105 or greater. By comparing values in patients who required MV for 8 days or longer with those who required it for less time, the authors were able to assess the influence of the duration of MV on the accuracy of their indices. In general, the accuracy was lower by 0.15 or greater in patients on MV for 8 days or longer, especially in terms of positive predictive values.

Yang and Tobin made their measurements with a handheld spirometer after disconnecting patients from the ventilator and allowing them to breathe room air. This may be important since many physicians use ventilator-based instrumentation to measure TV during unassisted breathing on morning rounds before they establish a weaning plan. This is usually done without

Table 67-4. Threshold Values and Accuracy of Indices Used to Predict Weaning Outcome

Index	Value[a]	Positive predictive value[b]	Negative predictive value[b]
Minute ventilation (L/min)	≤ 15	0.55	0.38
Respiratory frequency (breaths/min)	≤ 38	0.65	0.77
Tidal volume (ml)	≥ 325	0.73	0.94
Tidal volume (ml)/weight (kg)	≥ 4	0.67	0.85
Maximum inspiratory pressure (cm/H_2O)[c]	≤ −15	0.59	1.00
Dynamic compliance (ml/cm H_2O)	≥ 22	0.65	0.58
Static compliance (ml/cm H_2O)	≥ 33	0.60	0.53
PaO_2/PAO_2 ratio	≥ 0.35	0.59	0.53
Frequency/tidal volume ratio (breaths/min/L)	≤ 105	0.78	0.95
CROP index (ml/breath/min)[d]	≥ 13	0.71	0.70

[a] Threshold values were those that discriminated best in the training data set between patients who were successfully weaned and those in whom a weaning trial failed; ≥ and ≤ indicate whether the values above the threshold value or those below it are those that predicted a successful weaning outcome.
[b] Values shown were derived from the complete prospective validation data set, comprising 36 successfully weaned patients and 28 patients in whom weaning failed.
[c] To convert value to kilopascals, multiply by 0.09807.
[d] A weaning outcome index that integrates thoracic compliance, respiratory rate, arterial oxygenation, and PI_{max}.
Adapted from Yang KL, Tobin MJ: A prospective study of indexes predicting the outcome of trials of weaning from mechanical ventilation. *N Engl J Med* 324:1445, 1991.

disconnecting the patient or changing the inspired oxygen concentration and may or may not include the use of continuous positive end-expiratory pressure (CPAP) and low levels of pressure support ventilation (PSV). Furthermore, TV measurements derived from ventilator-based instrumentation are certainly not as accurate as those reported in a research paper. For example, in a small survey, 25 percent of ventilator-derived TV estimates (means of 6 breaths) had a greater than 10 percent error (R.W. Stroetz, personal communication).

Figure 67-2 reveals how ventilator settings can influence the sensitivity and specificity of a weaning parameter such as f/TV. It shows that the f/TV ratio is likely to have significantly lower positive and negative predictive values when used in conjunction with PSV weaning. Two sets of receiver operator characteristic (ROC) curves for f/TV are compared: the data of Yang and Tobin [66] on the left; the data of Stroetz and Hubmayr [53] on the right. The latter authors evaluated the discriminative value of f/TV during PSV weaning. These curves offer a means to analyze the discriminative power of tests independent of the choice of threshold values. False positive and true positive rates are plotted against each other over the range of all possible threshold values. The area to the right of this relationship determines the values of the test. When the relationship follows the line of identity, the test is no better than flipping a coin. When the relationship encompasses an area of 1.0, the test provides perfect discriminative power. Note that the area under the ROC curve derived from the data of Stroetz and Hubmayr is smaller than that reported by Yang and Tobin. The reason is the dependence of TV and f/TV on the pressure support setting. When failure occurs while subjects are being ventilated with low levels of pressure support, their TV is usually greater than it would be during unassisted breathing.

In a prospective study of medical ICU patients, Jabour et al. [67] took a different approach, evaluating a new weaning index

Frequency / Tidal Volume Ratio

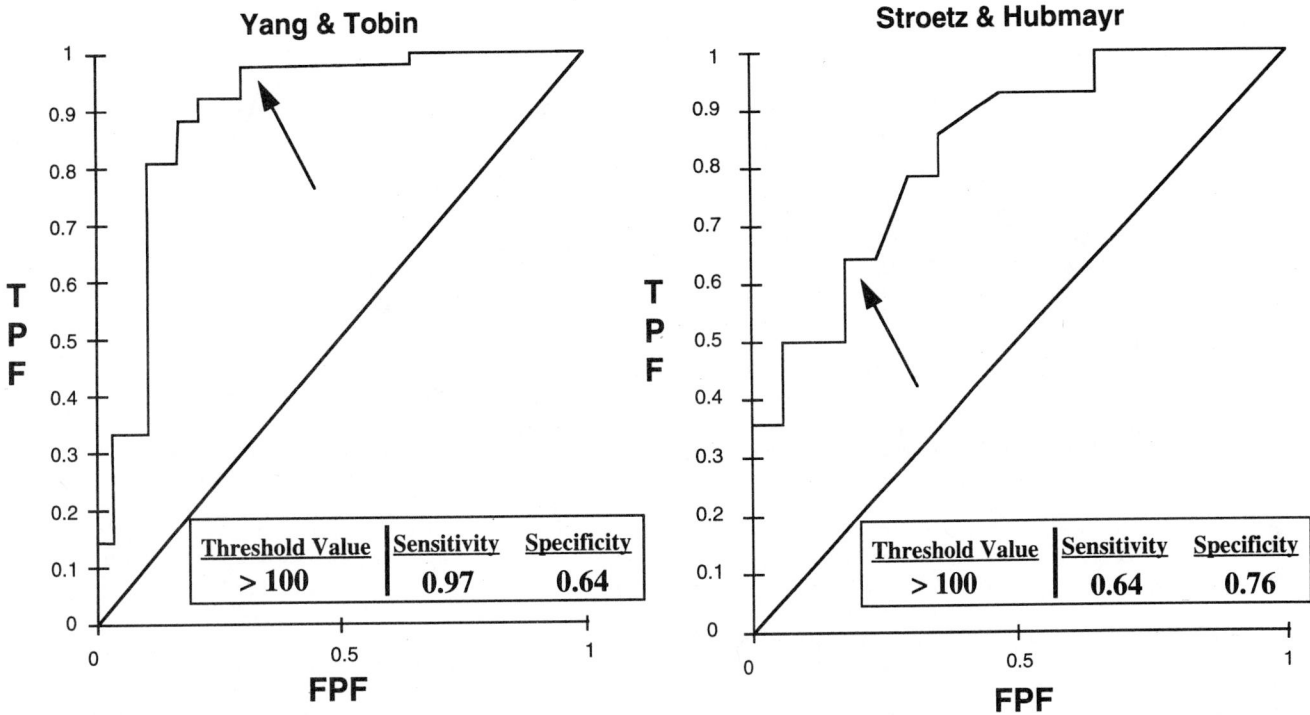

Fig. 67-2. Comparison of two sets of receiver operator characteristics curves (ROC) for f/TV. The curve on the left is derived from data in spontaneously breathing subjects while disconnected from the ventilator and breathing room air. (Adapted from Yang KL, Tobin MJ: A prospective study of indexes predicting the outcome of trials of weaning from mechanical ventilation. *N Engl J Med* 324:1445–1450, 1991). The curve on the right is based on patient data collected during pressure support ventilation.

based on ventilatory endurance and the efficiency of gas exchange. According to their post hoc analysis of weaning responses, this index had positive and negative predictive values of 0.95 and 0.96, respectively. While this index is more complex and therefore not nearly as appealing clinically as the f/TV ratio, the data affirm the pathophysiologic mechanisms of ventilatory pump failure as they have emerged from research from the past 20 years. In the late 1970s, physiologists introduced the idea that ventilatory pump failure was the result of an imbalance between the strength of the respiratory muscles and the load placed on them [1,62]. Later, it was demonstrated that the diaphragm of human volunteers can be fatigued through inspiratory resistive loading and that its fatigue threshold is dependent on diaphragm strength and load, as well as the relative duration of muscle contraction [68,69]. Jabour et al. applied these concepts to the weaning assessment of ventilator-dependent patients and defined a pressure time index (PTI) based on an estimate of the average inspiratory muscle pressure per breath (P_{breath}), maximum voluntarily generated negative inspiratory pressure (NIP), and inspiratory duty cycle, which is the inspiratory time (T_I) normalized by the total breath duration (T_{TOT}).

$$PTI = (P_{breath} / NIP) \times (T_I / T_{TOT}) \qquad (1)$$

P_{breath} was calculated making the following assumptions: (1) the impedance of the respiratory system is independent of the mode of breathing, which means the load on the inspiratory muscles during a spontaneous breath is the same as the load on a mechanical ventilator during a machine breath; (2) differences in inspiratory flow between the modes of breathing can be ignored; (3) there is no inadvertent PEEP; and (4) expiratory muscles do not contribute to the work of breathing. Therefore:

$$P_{breath} = (P_{peak} - PEEP) \times (TV_S / TV_M) \qquad (2)$$

where P_{peak} is the peak airway pressure during mechanical ventilation, PEEP is the extrinsic positive end-expiratory airway pressure, and TV_S and TV_M are the tidal volumes during spontaneous breathing and mechanical ventilation, respectively. Jabour et al. realized that PTI did not fully characterize the load on the inspiratory muscles and that the efficiency of the lungs as CO_2 eliminators also had to be taken into account. Their weaning index (WI), therefore, also contains an estimate of the minute volume ($V_{E_{40}}$, in ml/kg/min) that would have been required to achieve a $PaCO_2$ of 40 mm Hg:

$$WI = PTI \times V_{E_{40}} / TV_S \qquad (3)$$

$V_{E_{40}}$ was linearly interpolated from the actual V_E (in ml/kg body weight) and $PaCO_2$ during mechanical ventilation:

$$V_{E_{40}} = (fM\ TV_M) \times (PaCO_2 M / 40) \qquad (4)$$

TV_M and fM are tidal volume and respiratory rate while on mechanical ventilation in the assist or control mode.

Although most of the assumptions of Jabour et al. are not strictly valid, the discriminative power of WI turned out to be very good. What is interesting about this approach is that patients are not constrained to defend a $PaCO_2$ of 40 mm Hg during spontaneous breathing; thus, this weaning index represents a hypothetical rather than an actual load. Indeed, PTI alone did not distinguish very well between weaning success and weaning failure, an observation previously made by others [70]. In this regard, one could argue that reductions in actual VE, and consequently CO_2 retention, represent attempts of ventilatory control mechanisms to prevent inspiratory muscle overload. This discrepancy between actual and predicted $PaCO_2$ values in patients who fail weaning seems to support such a contention [70].

Although clinical observation of the respiratory muscles during spontaneous breaths was initially thought to be reliable in predicting subsequent weaning failure [57], respiratory inductive plethysmographic studies [63] have shown this to be not necessarily the case. Any time there is a substantial increase in load on the respiratory muscles, a change in the rate, depth, and pattern of breathing may be observed. Because these signs may also be a manifestation of fatigue, it is useful to note them. If these signs never appear, successful weaning is likely. If they do appear, patients must be observed closely for further deterioration, since weaning inevitably fails if these signs are due to fatigue.

In patients whose inspiratory muscles are fatigued or sense the increased load of being taken off the ventilator, the following sequence of events can be observed, not necessarily in this sequence. Both respiratory rate and minute ventilation initially increase [57]. This may be followed by a paradoxical inward motion of the anterior abdominal wall during inspiration (Fig. 67-3) [4,57]. This indicates that the diaphragm fails to contract sufficiently to descend and move the abdominal contents downward, which normally results in an outward motion of the abdominal wall during inspiration. Cyclic changes in breathing patterns with either a chest wall motion or a predominantly abdominal wall motion are another sign potentially indicative of muscle fatigue. This so-called respiratory alternans [57] represents the cyclic contractions of intercostal and accessory muscles on the one hand and of the diaphragm on the other. Presumably, these different muscle groups can alternate in their contribution to the work of breathing and allow each other to "rest."

PERSPECTIVE. Based on ease and simplicity of measurement and prospective, validated data, it appears that the index of rapid shallow breathing (f/TV of ≤ 105) measured under the conditions described by Yang and Tobin [66] can be recommended as an accurate, albeit imperfect, predictor of failure and success in weaning patients totally from MV. However, neither f/TV nor any other predictive index has been evaluated as an aid in deciding when it is appropriate to initiate weaning. It remains to be prospectively determined in rigorously designed studies whether the specificity of f/TV in predicting weaning success can be improved by assessing weaning outcome with a newly derived parameter, f/TV × $P_{0.1}$ [71]. $P_{0.1}$ is the airway occlusion pressure measured 0.1 second from the onset of inspiration. While it is actually an estimate of the pressure generated by inspiratory muscles, it is generally considered to be an estimate of neuromuscular drive to breathe.

When the patient's clinical condition has been stabilized, it is reasonable to consider starting the weaning process even if predictive index thresholds for success have not been met. Since they are not 100 percent accurate and clinical prediction often underestimates when the patient is ready for a short-term

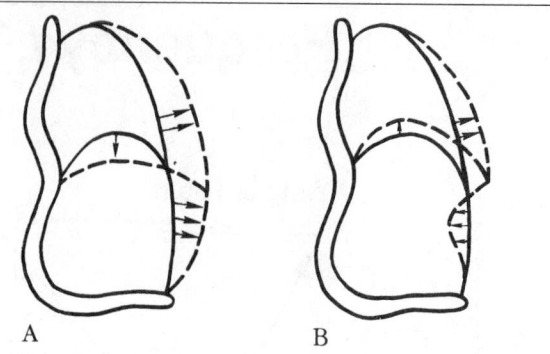

Fig. 67-3. Breathing patterns. Directions of movement of the diaphragm (*single arrow*), rib cage (*double arrows*), and abdominal wall (*triple arrows*) during spontaneous inspiration. A. Normal breathing. B. Asynchronous breathing.

trial [53], valuable time may be lost in liberating patients from the ventilator. Furthermore, we are unaware of any data which show that unsuccessful weaning trials have long-term adverse consequences provided one monitors patients closely and avoids certain pitfalls. For example, it is unwise to impose a weaning stress on patients with active ischemic heart disease, since systemic oxygen demand and cardiac output can increase substantially during transition from controlled mechanical ventilation to spontaneous breathing [58,72]. Patients must be prepared psychologically that failing a weaning trial has no bearing on their ultimate prognosis. Finally, it seems prudent to guarantee sufficient respiratory muscle rest following an episode of weaning-induced ventilatory pump failure. Although there is considerable controversy about the role of respiratory muscle fatigue in the pathogenesis of ventilatory failure syndromes, we usually do not have our patients undergo more than one (failed) weaning trial in any 24-hour time span.

Principles and Methods of Weaning

PRINCIPLES OF WEANING. Weaning should be thought of as a form of structured, progressive respiratory skeletal muscle exercise. It is a time when the load associated with breathing is returned from the MV to the patient's respiratory muscles. Because breathing is a form of continuous muscular exercise, weaning should incorporate the appropriate principles of muscle training. In other words, to elicit adaptive responses, training stimuli must be of the appropriate type, intensity, and timing [73]. These principles may be incorporated into a weaning strategy as follows:

1. Stress the respiratory muscles to early fatigue by making them assume some or all of the load of breathing, then rest them.
2. Progressively increase training stress by increasing more of the load or increasing the duration of the weaning period.
3. Maintain a structured, progressive program, because the effect of conditioning is transient.

There are no consistently reliable predictors of early fatigue. Future studies may reveal typical changes, but until then the physician must rely on clinical findings (e.g., appearance of new dysrhythmia, worsening tachypnea, tachycardia, hypertension/hypotension, diaphoresis, asynchronous breathing patterns) (Fig. 67-3), judgment (e.g., patient complaints of worsening shortness of breath and poor appearance), desaturation, and acute or acute-on-chronic respiratory acidosis. On the other hand, it is important not to terminate a weaning trial before making the patient's muscles work hard enough, because this can markedly prolong the total duration of MV support. It makes no sense to place a patient back on the ventilator after a short interval simply to adhere to a rigid protocol applied to all patients when that particular patient could have stayed off the ventilator for 12 hours or more. The patient who looks good when weaning is started should be observed closely and kept off the ventilator until evidence suggests fatigue or clinical deterioration. In other words, rigid limits should not be arbitrarily established.

In stable patients who are progressing in a weaning program, it is counterproductive to stop weaning for any nonemergency reason (e.g., transporting them for nonemergency computed tomography scans).

CONVENTIONAL METHODS OF WEANING. Three methods of weaning patients from MV are in general use: (1) T piece with or without the addition of CPAP, (2) synchronized intermittent mandatory ventilation, and (3) pressure support ventilation. While most physicians generally use one of these methods alone, some have used them in combination. At this time, studies have not consistently shown one of these methods to be superior to the others. While Bouchard et al showed that pressure support ventilation was associated with a shorter duration of weaning than the other two methods [73a], Esteban et al demonstrated that a once-daily trial of T piece, spontaneous breathing resulted in the shortest duration of successful weaning [73b]. The differing results of these two prospective, randomized clinical trials may be explained by the different populations of patients studied, differences in familiarity of physicians participating in these studies with the methods used, and/or the pace of the weaning protocols.

T Piece Weaning. This consists of the sudden, complete withdrawal of machine support. Patients are closely observed as they breathe humidified gas mixtures delivered by the T-shaped plastic tube that is connected to tubing and the endotracheal or tracheostomy tube (Fig. 67-4). In contrast to techniques that involve the gradual withdrawal of machine support, such as SIMV and PSV, during T piece weaning the patient's cardiorespiratory response patterns can be assessed without the confounding influence of machine settings (Fig. 67-2). While there is no generally agreed upon standard of applying this method of weaning, we begin T piece trials from assisted, not controlled, mechanical ventilation and continue until there are clinical signs consistent with fatigue (see protocol below), rather than arbitrarily stopping at a predetermined time. We usually do not attempt another trial within the same 24-hour period after an unsuccessful attempt.

Irrespective of the underlying disease process, we believe it is physiologically sound to undertake T piece weaning in conjunction with CPAP. Five centimeters of CPAP mitigates the fall in end-expired lung volume that results from having eliminated glottic regulation of upper airway resistance and flow with an endotracheal tube [74]. Furthermore, in patients with airflow obstruction, CPAP can substantially lower the work of breathing by counterbalancing end-expiratory system recoil pressures (i.e., intrinsic positive end-expiratory pressure [PEEPi]) and by shifting loads from inspiratory to expiratory muscles [75,76,77]. These two mechanisms are shown schematically in Figure 67-

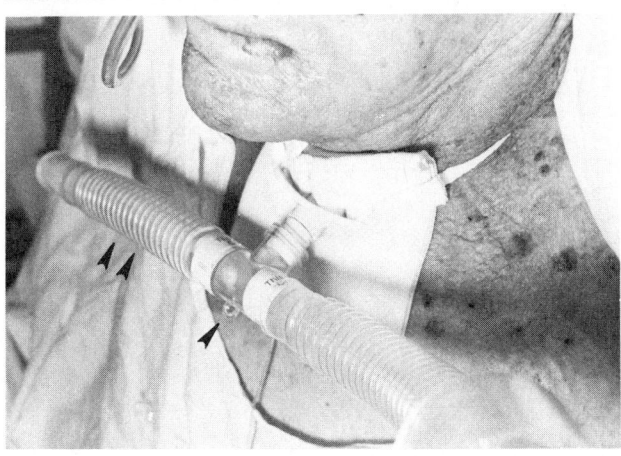

Fig 67-4. Apparatus used for traditional T tube weaning. Humidified gas mixture is delivered to the patient by means of a T-shaped plastic tube connected to a length of disposable tubing and the tracheostomy tube (*single arrow*). The distal tubing ("afterburner") serves as a reservoir for the humidified gas mixture being delivered to the patient (*double arrows*). It prevents retrograde entrainment of room air.

5. Figure 67-5A shows the pressure-volume relationships of the relaxed respiratory system and depicts the elastic work (W_{el}) required to raise lung volume from end expiration to end inspiration (shaded area) in the presence of dynamic hyperinflation. W_{el} has two components: (1) work required to halt expiratory flow by counterbalancing respiratory system recoil at end expiration (W related to PEEPi) and (2) work expended during inflation of the lungs and thorax. In theory, the inspiratory work related to PEEPi (darker shaded area) can be provided externally with CPAP equal to PEEPi. However, as CPAP approaches PEEPi, additional hyperinflation may occur [78]. To guard against this, the physician can monitor the effect of increasing levels of external PEEP on peak or end inflation hold pressure on the ventilator prior to beginning weaning. When too much external PEEP has been applied and hyperinflation worsens, these pressures rise.

An alternative mechanism by which CPAP can reduce inspiratory elastic work in airflow obstruction is shown in Figure 67-5B. Continuous positive airway pressure may result in exhalation below the new static equilibrium volume (SEV) through the recruitment of expiratory muscles. Subsequent relaxation of the expiratory muscles inflates the lungs passively back to the new equilibrium volume. Inspiratory muscles are unloaded because the expiratory muscles do part of the inspiratory work. This is depicted by the lighter shaded area in Figure 67-5B. This mechanism is of limited value in patients with severe obstruction, however, because low maximal flows prevent significant reductions in lung volume below SEV.

In patients who continue to require mechanical ventilation only for oxygenation, CPAP may help maintain the benefits of improved oxygenation provided by PEEP without exposing the patient to the hazards of MV. It may also augment cardiac function during weaning [48,49,50].

T-PIECE WEANING PROTOCOL. General guidelines for weaning by this method are as follows:

1. When it has been decided that the patient is improving and stable, attempt to communicate with the patient, telling him or her weaning is about to begin, why you believe he or she

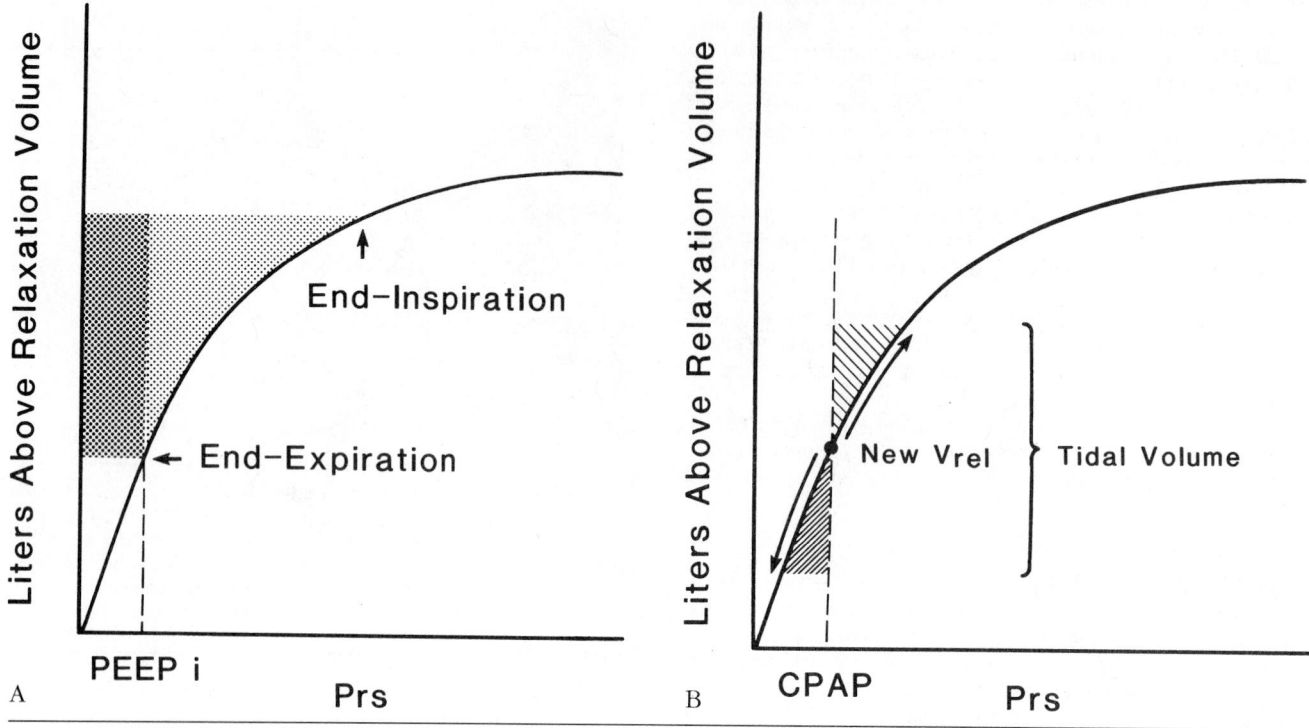

Fig. 67-5. A. Effect of dynamic hyperinflation on elastic inspiratory work. The solid curve shows the relationship between the volume above the relaxation volume (V_{rel}) and the recoil of the respiratory system (P_{rs}). Dynamic hyperinflation exists. The inspiration is now initiated from a volume above V_{rel}. The increase in lung volume necessitates an increase in elastic inspiratory work, which may be considered to have two components: work to halt expiratory flow (dark shaded area) and work required to inflate the respiratory system (light shaded area). B. Effect of continuous positive airway pressure (CPAP) on respiratory work. The solid curve is the pressure-volume curve of the respiratory system. With CPAP, a new relaxation volume (V_{rel}) is achieved. To conserve inspiratory elastic work, the patient recruits expiratory muscles and exhales below the new V_{rel}. The elastic work performed by the expiratory muscles is represented by the dark shaded area. Relaxation of the expiratory muscles inflates the lungs back to the new V_{rel} without inspiratory effort. The inspiratory muscles then increase lung volume further, performing elastic inspiratory work (light shaded area). Hence, CPAP reduced the work of the inspiratory muscles by allowing the expiratory muscles to do part of the inspiratory work. (From Hubmayr RD, Abel MD, Rehder K: Physiologic approach to mechanical ventilation. *Crit Care Med* 18:103–113, 1990. With permission.)

is ready, and what to expect. It is important to allow the patient to express fears whenever possible and to try to alleviate them [79].

2. Obtain baseline values and begin monitoring clinical parameters, such as pulse rate, respiratory rate, blood pressure, and subjective distress (e.g., have patients rate their dyspnea from zero to 10); gas-exchange (e.g., by pulse oximetry); and cardiac rhythm (e.g., by ECG monitoring). Record these values on a weaning flow sheet, which should be maintained and kept at the patient's bedside. We are unaware of any studies that support the need for frequent arterial blood gas analyses during weaning trials. We obtain them routinely only if extubation is considered imminent.

3. Ensure a calm atmosphere by having the nurse, respiratory therapist, or physician remain at the bedside to offer encouragement and support.

4. Avoid sedation to ensure maximal patient cooperation and effort.

5. Whenever possible, sit the patient upright in bed or in a chair.

6. Fit the patient's intratracheal tube with a T tube connected to a heated nebulizer with an inspired oxygen concentration 10 percent greater than that prevailing during the previous course of MV. Ensure that the T tube flow exceeds the patient's peak inspiratory flow and that the inhaled gas is constantly humidified. Add CPAP (see above for determining the amount to be added).

Continue the trial unless clinical findings, judgment, oxygenation, and cardiac monitoring suggest respiratory muscle fatigue or clinical deterioration (e.g., heart rate 30/min above baseline; development of ventricular ectopy and/or supraventricular tachyarrhythmia; mean blood pressure > 15 mm Hg or < 30 mm Hg of baseline; respiratory rate > 35/min for at least 5 minutes; O_2 saturation < 90%; and dyspnea rated by patient as $\geq$ 5/10).

If the trial is terminated, place the patient back on the preweaning MV settings. Rest the patient and try again later. The length of the rest periods and the frequency and duration of subsequent weaning trials are determined by trial and error, keeping in mind the goal of having the patient progressively take over the entire work of breathing. In general, we do not subject patients to more than one failed weaning trial in a 24-hour period. If a patient has no underlying lung disease and has been on an MV for only a short time (e.g., <1 week), appears to be tolerating spontaneous ventilation without dyspnea, and maintains adequate blood gases or level of oxygenation, extubation may be performed.

7. Patients who have received prolonged ventilatory support, for whatever reason, and those with COPD, should continue the weaning trial. We usually observe these patients breathing spontaneously for a long period (e.g., 24 hours) before extubation.

Synchronized Intermittent Mandatory Ventilation Weaning.

Intermittent mandatory ventilation weaning was the first alternative approach to T piece weaning. It consists of gradually reducing the amount of ventilatory assistance and gradually increasing the amount of unassisted work on the part of the patient. Ventilator (mandatory) breaths are regularly interspersed between the patient's spontaneous respirations. This technique necessitates that the interface between the patient and MV be maintained.

In the late 1970s and early 1980s, there was considerable debate among intensivists whether gradual SIMV weaning was superior to intermittent T piece trials [80,81]. Proponents of SIMV argued that intermittent "T piece sprints" might be fatiguing, which implied that sudden, as opposed to gradual, withdrawal of machine support might cause maladaptive responses in breathing strategy. The controversy remains largely unresolved, except that a few important observations regarding SIMV have been made. First, the inexperienced physician may be tempted to seek assurances through frequent arterial blood gas analyses during SIMV weaning, thereby prolonging and adding unnecessary cost to the weaning process. Second, SIMV with low backup machine rates may obscure the presence of impending ventilatory pump failure by blood gas criteria. This is because even a few volume preset breaths per minute may augment alveolar ventilation and CO_2 elimination enough to prevent frank acidemia. This should be suspected in patients with small spontaneous tidal volumes (≤ 3 ml/kg body weight), in those with spontaneous rates of 30 breaths per minute or greater, and when dyspnea and thoracoabdominal paradox (Fig. 67-3) indicate heightened respiratory effort. Third, compared to T piece weaning, breathing through the demand valve of SIMV circuits can increase the work of breathing. This can be mitigated by machines that offer a continuous flow option (Table 67-3).

There is no generally agreed upon standard of applying this method of weaning. We progressively decrease the SIMV rate based on clinical assessment.

SIMV WEANING PROTOCOL. Guidelines for weaning by the SIMV method are as follows.

1. Repeat steps 1 through 5 of the T piece weaning protocol.
2. Switch the MV mode from assist to SIMV or, if the patient is already on SIMV as a ventilatory mode, decrease the rate.
3. For patients who have received prolonged ventilator support for whatever reason and for those with COPD, consider a protocol such as the following. Begin SIMV weaning at a frequency of 8 breaths per minute. Continue the same tidal volume of the mandatory breaths but increase the fraction of inspired oxygen by 10 percent. Decrease the SIMV rate by 2 breaths per minute every hour unless clinical findings, judgment, oxygenation, or cardiac monitoring suggest respiratory muscle fatigue or clinical deterioration (e.g., see step 6 of the T piece weaning protocol). If the patient appears to fail to assume the increased work of breathing at a lower rate, increase the SIMV rate to the previously tolerated level and then higher, if necessary, until the patient is stable again. When the patient is stable for at least 1 hour on an SIMV rate of zero breaths per minute, fit him or her with a T tube and then observe for an extended period (e.g., 24 hours) before extubation.
4. In patients who have no underlying lung disease and who have been on MV for only a short time (e.g., <1 week), decrease the SIMV rate at 30-minute intervals. If a rate of zero is well tolerated without dyspnea and gas exchange is well maintained, perform extubation.

Pressure Support Ventilation Weaning.

This method can also be used to decrease mechanical ventilatory support gradually. The level of pressure support is gradually decreased, making the patient responsible for a gradually increasing amount of ventilation. While it is commonly assumed that (1) pressure support can be decreased to a low level (e.g., 5 cm) which will compensate for endotracheal tube and circuit resistance and (2) patients can be safely extubated at that level, there is no simple way of predicting the level of PSV that will compensate for this resistance (see below).

Pressure support ventilation has become a popular weaning mode for adults. In PSV mode, a target pressure is applied to the endotracheal tube, which augments the inflation pressure exerted by the inspiratory muscles (P_{mus}) on the respiratory system [82]. As the lungs inflate, inspiratory flow begins to decline because airway pressure and P_{mus} are opposed by rising elastic recoil forces. When inspiratory flow reaches a threshold value (which differs among vendors), the machine switches to expiration [83]. Compared to SIMV weaning, during which spontaneous breaths are occasionally augmented by a volume preset machine breath, PSV is thought to offer greater patient autonomy over inspiratory flow, TV, and Ti [84]. As with SIMV, the popularity of PSV is based on the premise that weaning from mechanical ventilation should be a gradual process. In addition, proponents of PSV over T piece trials argue that the work of unassisted breathing though an endotracheal tube is unreasonably high and could lead to inspiratory muscle failure in susceptible patients [85]. For example, it has become popular to assume that PSV is an effective means to overcome the resistance of endotracheal tubes. Conceptually, this is incorrect, because airway pressure during PSV does not vary with flow. Furthermore, a reduction in pulmonary resistance is not demonstrated after extubation [86], and the work of breathing may actually increase [87]. This suggests that, at least immediately after extubation, most patients manifest upper airway resistance that is, in effect, equal to or greater than that of an 8-mm internal diameter endotracheal tube.

While PSV has not been consistently shown to be superior to other weaning modalities [73b], results of a multicenter trial from Europe suggest that it may have advantages over SIMV [73a,88].

Enthusiasm for using PSV in all patients should be tempered by knowledge of its potential adverse patient-ventilator interactions. For example, elderly patients and even normal individuals [89] are susceptible to pressure support setting-induced central apneas. The responsible mechanism appears to be a lung volume-related inhibition of inspiratory motor output. On occasion, lung volume-mediated inhibition of inspiration is strong enough to turn off respiratory muscle activity altogether. Problems may arise when the physician feels compelled to rest susceptible subjects with PSV at night. Unless sufficiently high intermittent mandatory ventilation backup rates are used in combination with PSV, the mechanical inhibition of inspiratory drive may result in apneas, which trigger ventilator alarms and cause arousals and sleep fragmentation that can prolong weaning.

Dyssynchrony between patient and machine breaths is not uncommon in the ICU, particularly during PSV. This is true for patients with high intrinsic respiratory rates, reduced inspiratory pressure output from low drive or respiratory muscle weakness, or airways obstruction and when ventilator support results in greater than normal tidal volumes. However, the diagnostic and prognostic significance of this dyssynchrony is uncertain. When it impairs ventilatory assistance or causes patient discomfort, sedation and adjustments in CPAP, rate, flow, or trigger mode are required. On the other hand, when "wasted" inspiratory efforts are not perceived as uncomfortable, it is not clear that adjustments in ventilator settings are warranted. Increases in machine rate to match the rate of patient efforts may cause worsening dynamic hyperinflation in patients with airflow obstruction and compromise circulation.

PSV WEANING PROTOCOL. General guidelines for weaning by the PSV method are as follows.

1. Repeat steps 1 through 5 of the T piece weaning protocol.
2. Switch the MV mode from volume cycled breathing with assist or SIMV modes to PSV, or, if the patient is already on PSV as a ventilatory mode, decrease the amount of pressure support.
3. For patients who have received prolonged ventilator support for whatever reason and for those with COPD, consider a protocol such as the following. Begin PSV weaning at a pressure of 25 cm H_2O, if switching from another ventilatory mode, or less than the amount previously used during pressure support mechanical ventilation, and increase the fraction of inspired oxygen by 10 percent. Decrease airway inflation pressure by 5 cm every hour unless clinical findings, judgment, oxygenation, and cardiac monitoring suggest respiratory muscle fatigue or clinical deterioration (see step 6 of the T piece weaning protocol). If the patient appears to fail to assume the increased work of breathing at a lower pressure, increase the pressure to the previously tolerated level and then higher, if necessary, until the patient is stable again. When the patient is stable for at least 1 hour on a pressure of zero, fit him or her with a T tube and then observe for an extended period (e.g., 24 hours) before extubation.
4. In patients who have no underlying lung disease and who have been on MV for only a short time (e.g., <1 week), pressure can be decreased at 30-minute intervals. If a pressure of zero is well tolerated without dyspnea and gas exchange is well maintained, extubation can be performed. While some would extubate from a pressure support greater than zero (e.g., 5 cm), thinking the need for the extra pressure support will be eliminated once the endotracheal tube is removed, we are not convinced that this is prudent (see above).

UNCONVENTIONAL METHODS OF WEANING. A variety of unconventional techniques have been tried for weaning patients from MV. These include inspiratory resistive training [90,91,92], mandatory minute volume ventilation [93], and biofeedback [94]. Although these techniques appear to have been helpful in selected patients, their roles remain to be defined by controlled prospective studies.

Uncontrolled reports suggest that inspiratory muscle resistive training [90,91,92] may be useful in preparing patients who are on prolonged ventilatory support for weaning. This method is thought to serve as a means of respiratory muscle endurance training; it is implemented by having patients breathe spontaneously through an adjustable inspiratory resistor.

Mandatory minute volume ventilation is a relatively new concept in weaning from MV [93]. The system ensures a patient a constant, predetermined minute volume. If there is any shortfall in the patient's spontaneous minute volume, the ventilator automatically compensates. This method, unlike SIMV, does not cause the ventilator to provide a predetermined number of fixed breaths. As long as the patient breathes at an adequate rate, the machine stands ready but does not deliver a breath. Although there are few data to support its use, this method may be useful in weaning patients with irregular breathing patterns who may not appear to be doing well from breath to breath but who have adequate spontaneous ventilation over a minute.

Biofeedback, the detection and transmission back to the patient of some biologic function that he or she cannot detect, may be helpful in weaning certain patients [94,95]. For instance, by displaying respiratory volumes on bedside oscilloscopes and having patients make voluntary efforts to push volume tracings beyond limits taped on the screen, Corson et al. [94] allowed two patients with spinal cord lesions, one with a sensory level at C_6 who lacked proprioceptive afferents from the chest wall, to gain control over their breathing. These authors assumed that "the repeated practice of reaching the criteria of feedback increased the strength of the diaphragm and inspiratory muscles and may have had the net effect of enabling the medullary center to reinstate automatic breathing" [94].

Managing Weaning Failure

The respiratory muscles play a pivotal role in the onset and perpetuation of respiratory failure. When patients have met the traditional indications for weaning but fail, it is predominantly due to inspiratory respiratory muscle fatigue. In general, muscle fatigue occurs because there is (1) a decrease in the maximum force the muscles are capable of generating or (2) an increase in the force required of the muscles to sustain ventilatory demand. Because respiratory muscle fatigue is almost always multifactorial in etiology (Table 67-2), ways to increase muscle strength and decrease muscle demand should be systematically considered.

The following measures should be considered to *increase* respiratory muscle strength:

1. Reverse malnutrition [18] and deficiencies in phosphorus [22,23], calcium [19], potassium [19], and magnesium [20]. In the absence of hypomagnesemia, routine administration of magnesium does not appear to be useful [21].
2. In addition to correcting hypoxemia, consider correcting, rather than maintaining, chronic hypercapnia during MV, since hypercapnia may adversely affect muscle strength and endurance [32,33].
3. Reverse hypothyroidism [24,25].
4. Correct anemia [34].
5. Improve cardiovascular function [46,47,51], because poor cardiac performance may contribute to an inadequate supply of oxygen to the respiratory muscles.
6. Although short-acting sedatives may be indicated in selected patients (see strategy 11, below), attempt to discontinue sedative drugs whenever possible, since they may be responsible for central fatigue (Fig. 67-1).
7. Consider using theophylline in the therapeutic doses given for bronchodilatation; it may act as a direct respiratory center and diaphragm stimulator. Although theophylline can increase the strength of contraction and suppress fatigue of the diaphragm [96,97,98], its specific role in weaning has yet to be determined in randomized, prospective studies. If theophylline is shown in future studies to have a salutary affect on weaning, it may become important to consider the drug-drug interaction between theophylline and calcium channel antagonists. Calcium channel antagonists were shown in an animal model to inhibit the beneficial effects of theophylline on diaphragm function [99].
8. Consider the use of progesterone as a respiratory center stimulant [100,101]. The effect of 20 mg of medroxyprogesterone acetate (Provera) three times per day should begin within 2 days and be maximal within 7 days. Theoretically, the effects can be variable; in some patients with severe

respiratory muscle weakness, the additional respiratory center stimulation may have the same effect as "whipping a tired horse" and precipitate worsening muscle fatigue.

9. Consider dopamine infusion (10 μg/kg body weight/min) to increase diaphragmatic blood flow [102].

10. In all cases of recurrent failure to wean, consider and evaluate for the possibilities of polyneuropathy [36,103–106], myopathy [107], and drug-induced neuromuscular dysfunction (e.g, neuromuscular blocking agents and antibiotics, especially aminoglycosides) [108,109].

11. Because sleep deprivation may suppress ventilatory drive [12] and contribute to central fatigue, short-acting sedatives may be considered in sleep-deprived individuals.

12. By taking advantage of gravity and having the patient sit up, the diaphragm may function better.

The following measures should be considered to *decrease* respiratory muscle demand.

1. Maximize treatment of systemic disease (e.g., infection) to decrease metabolic requirements and mitigate production of chemical mediators with adverse effects on muscle [29,30,37,38,110,111].

2. Give bronchodilators for conditions associated with increased airway resistance; discontinue beta-blockers in asthmatic patients.

3. A course of methylprednisolone therapy is helpful in hypercapnic patients who have COPD [112] and who are experiencing an exacerbation as well as in asthmatic patients. A daily dose of 0.5 mg per kilogram every 6 hours, tapered over 1 week in patients with COPD, may reverse inflammatory lesions in airways, thereby decreasing the work of breathing.

4. Use diuretics to keep patients with lung edema on the dry side; this will make the lungs less "stiff."

5. In patients with compromised cardiac function, diagnose and improve underlying cardiac disorders. The increased work of breathing during weaning may "steal" oxygen from the heart as well as other organs and precipitate ischemia and heart failure in susceptible patients [46,48,49,50].

6. In average-size adults, intratracheal tubes less than 8 mm in internal diameter significantly increase airway resistance [113,114]. The increased work of breathing associated with narrow tubes is magnified as minute ventilation increases [115,116]. If a patient fails to wean with a tube with an internal diameter less than 7.5 mm, consider replacing the tube with one of a larger size. However, it is unlikely that tube size (unless prohibitively small, e.g., 6 mm internal diameter) will determine whether the patient can be weaned.

7. Consider CPAP in patients with marginal cardiac function. It may provide support for a failing heart by decreasing left ventricular preload [48–51].

8. Switch from SIMV to T piece weaning if the patient cannot tolerate the increase in airway resistance that may result from breathing through the ventilator tubing during spontaneous efforts (Table 67-3) [39,40,41]. One method of assessing whether SIMV is fatiguing the patient is that of Christopher et al. [41]. Placing an aneroid manometer in line between the patient's intratracheal tube and ventilatory tubing enables measurement of maximal inspiratory pressure. They believe fatigue eventually occurs with SIMV and that SIMV should be discontinued "if the maximal negative pressure recorded at the beginning of inspiration is in excess of 4 cm H_2O or is greater than 30 percent of the standard occluded" MIP. Synchronized intermittent mandatory ventilation weaning should also be terminated if the tidal volumes of the patient's spontaneous breaths are wasted. They should be at least greater than the anatomic dead space (i.e., anatomic dead space approximates ideal weight in pounds).

9. In patients with marginal respiratory reserve and in hypercapnic patients, evaluate for overfeeding as the cause of increased carbon dioxide production. Overfeeding may precipitate respiratory acidosis in patients unable to improve their alveolar ventilation adequately when compensating for increased CO_2 production. While the cause of nutritionally related hypercapnia was initially thought to be excess carbohydrates or glucose calories, it has now been shown that excessive total calories are more likely to influence CO_2 production than percentage of carbohydrate calories [117].

Perspective

Recently, a great deal of effort has been devoted to developing scientifically based strategies to achieve successful weaning more consistently. Many advances have occurred. We now have a better understanding of the problem and of why patients fail to wean readily.

When patients fail to wean and require prolonged MV, it is predominantly the result of inspiratory respiratory muscle fatigue. No matter which physiologic measurements one uses to predict success or failure, or which method one uses to wean, a structured training program should be instituted and factors adversely affecting the respiratory muscles should be corrected. Because respiratory muscle fatigue is almost always multifactorial in etiology, attempts should be made systematically to increase muscle strength and decrease muscle demand, with particular attention to maximizing nutrition, diuresis, and cardiovascular function and minimizing sedation.

When managing patients with weaning failure, it is not likely that they fail for technologic reasons and/or the weaning method but rather because of their diseases and how well their diseases are managed. In a recent study [118], a ventilator management team was able to decrease the number of ventilator and ICU days.

References

1. Roussos C, Macklem PT: The respiratory muscles. *N Engl J Med* 307:786, 1982.
2. NHLBI Workshop Summary: Respiratory muscle fatigue: Report of the Respiratory Muscle Fatigue Workshop Group. *Am Rev Respir Dis* 142:474, 1990.
3. Mador MJ: Respiratory muscle fatigue and breathing pattern. *Chest* 100:1430, 1991.
4. Bryant S, Edwards RHT, Faulkner JA, et al: Respiratory muscle failure: Fatigue or weakness? The role of theophylline. *Chest* 89:116, 1986.
5. Elpern EH, Larson R, Douglass P, et al: Long-term outcomes for elderly survivors of prolonged ventilator assistance. *Chest* 96:1120, 1989.
6. Swinburne AJ, Fedullo AJ, Shayne DS: Mechanical ventilation: Analysis of increasing use and patient survival. *J Intensive Care Med* 3:315, 1988.
7. Tobin MJ, Perez W, Guenther SM, et al: The pattern of breathing during successful and unsuccessful trials of weaning from mechanical ventilation. *Am Rev Respir Dis* 134:1111, 1986.
8. Morganroth ML, Grum CM: Weaning from mechanical ventilation. *J Intensive Care Med* 3:109, 1988.
9. Morganroth ML, Morganroth JL, Nett LM, et al: Criteria for weaning from prolonged mechanical ventilation. *Arch Intern Med* 144:1012, 1984.

10. Davis H, Lefrak S, Miller D, et al: Prolonged mechanical assisted ventilation: Analysis of outcomes and charges. *JAMA* 243:43, 1980.

11. Doekel RC, Zwillich CW, Scoggin CH, et al: Clinical semistarvation: Depression of hypoxic ventilatory response. *N Engl J Med* 295:358, 1976.

12. Schiffman PL, Trontell MC, Mazar MF, et al: Sleep deprivation decreases ventilatory response to CO_2 but not load compensation. *Chest* 84:695, 1983.

13. Macklem PT: Respiratory muscles: The vital pump. *Chest* 78:753, 1980.

14. Belman MJ, Sieck GC: The ventilatory muscles: Fatigue, endurance and training. *Chest* 82:761, 1982.

15. Pratter MR, Corwin RW, Irwin RS: An integrated analysis of lung and respiratory muscle dysfunction in the pathogenesis of hypercapnic respiratory failure. *Respir Care* 27:55, 1982.

16. Tobin MJ: Predicting weaning outcome. *Chest* 94:227, 1988.

17. Sassoon CSH, Te TT, Mahutee CK, et al: Airway occlusion pressure: An important indicator for successful weaning in patients with chronic obstructive pulmonary disease. *Am Rev Respir Dis* 135:107, 1987.

18. Wilson DO, Rogers RM: The role of nutrition in weaning from mechanical ventilation. *J Intensive Care Med* 4:124, 1989.

19. Knochel JP: Neuromuscular manifestations of electrolyte disorders. *Am J Med* 72:521, 1982.

20. Molloy DW, Dhingra S, Solven F, et al: Hypomagnesemia and respiratory muscle power. *Am Rev Respir Dis* 129:497, 1984.

21. Johnson D, Gallagher C, Cavanaugh M, et al: The lack of effect of routine magnesium administration on respiratory function in mechanically ventilated patients. *Chest* 104:536, 1993.

22. Aubier M, Murciano D, Lecocguic Y, et al: Effect of hypophosphatemia on diaphragmatic contractility in patients with acute respiratory failure. *N Engl J Med* 313:420, 1985.

23. Gravelyn TR, Brophy N, Siegert C, et al: Hypophosphatemia-associated respiratory muscle weakness in a general inpatient population. *Am J Med* 84:870, 1988.

24. Laroche CM, Cairns T, Moxham J, et al: Hypothyroidism presenting with respiratory muscle weakness. *Am Rev Respir Dis* 138:472, 1988.

25. Martinez FJ, Bermudez-Gomez M, Celli BR: Hypothyroidism: A reversible cause of diaphragmatic dysfunction. *Chest* 96:1059, 1989.

26. Viires N, Pavlovic D, Pariente R, et al: Effects of steroids on diaphragmatic function in rats. *Am Rev Respir Dis* 142:34, 1990.

27. Shapiro JM, Condos R, Cole RP: Myopathy in status asthmaticus: relation to neuromuscular blockade and corticosteroid administration. *J Intensive Care Med* 8:144, 1993.

28. Tarasuik A, Heimer D, Bark H: Effect of chronic renal failure on skeletal and diaphragmatic muscle contraction. *Am Rev Respir Dis* 146:1383, 1992.

29. Clowes GHA Jr, George BC, Villee CA Jr, et al: Muscle proteolysis induced by a circulating peptide in patients with sepsis or trauma. *N Engl J Med* 308:545, 1983.

30. Baracos V, Rodemann HP, Dinarello C, et al: Stimulation of muscle protein degradation and prostaglandin E_2 release by leukocytic pyrogen (interleukin-1). *N Engl J Med* 308:553, 1983.

31. Gertz I, Hedenstierna G, Hellers G, et al: Muscle metabolism in patients with chronic obstructive lung disease and acute respiratory failure. *Clin Sci Molec Med* 52:395, 1977.

32. Juan G, Calverley P, Talamo C, et al: Effect of carbon dioxide on diaphragmatic function in human beings. *N Engl J Med* 310:874, 1984.

33. Esau SA: Hypoxic, hypercapnic acidosis decreases tension and increases fatigue in hamster diaphragm muscle in vitro. *Am Rev Respir Dis* 139:1410, 1989.

34. Murray JF, Gold P, Johnson BJ Jr: The circulatory effects of hematocrit variations in normovolemic and hypervolemic dogs. *J Clin Invest* 42:1150, 1963.

35. Bolton CE, Gilbert JJ, Brown JD, et al: Polyneuropathy in critically ill patients. *J Neurol Neurosurg Psychiatry* 47:1223, 1984.

36. Zochodne DW, Bolton CF, Wells GA, et al: Critical illness polyneuropathy: A complication of sepsis and multiple organ failure. *Brain* 110:819, 1987.

37. Diaz PT, Julian MW, Wewers MD, et al: Tumor necrosis factor and endotoxin do not directly affect in vitro diaphragm function. *Am Rev Respir Dis* 148:281, 1993.

38. Supinski G, Nethery D, Dimarco A: Effect of free radical scavengers on endotoxin-induced respiratory muscle dysfunction. *Am Rev Respir Dis* 148:1318, 1993.

39. Hillman K, Friedlos J, Davey A: A comparison of intermittent mandatory ventilation systems. *Crit Care Med* 14:499, 1986.

40. Gibney RTN, Wilson RS, Pontoppidan H: Comparison of work of breathing on high gas flow and demand valve continuous positive airway pressure systems. *Chest* 82:692, 1982.

41. Christopher KL, Neff TA, Bowman JL, et al: Demand and continuous flow intermittent mandatory ventilation systems. *Chest* 87:625, 1985.

42. Marini JJ, Smith TC, Lamb VJ: External work output and force generation during synchronized intermittent mechanical ventilation: Effect of machine assistance on breathing effort. *Am Rev Respir Dis* 138:1169, 1988.

43. Marini JJ, Rodriguez RM, Lamb V: The inspiratory workload of patient-initiated mechanical ventilation. *Am Rev Respir Dis* 134:902, 1986.

44. Marini JJ, Capps JS, Culver BH: The inspiratory work of breathing during assisted mechanical ventilation. *Chest* 87:612, 1985.

45. Gurevitch MJ, Gelmont D: Importance of trigger sensitivity to ventilator response delay in advanced chronic obstructive pulmonary disease with respiratory failure. *Crit Care Med* 17:354, 1989.

46. Lemaire F, Teboul J-L, Cinotti L, et al: Acute left ventricular dysfunction during unsuccessful weaning from mechanical ventilation. *Anesthesiology* 69:171, 1988.

47. Aubier M, Viires N, Syllie G, et al: Respiratory muscle contribution to lactic acidosis in low cardiac output. *Am Rev Respir Dis* 126:648, 1982.

48. Vaisanen IT, Rasanen J: Continuous positive airway pressure and supplemental oxygen in the treatment of cardiogenic pulmonary edema. *Chest* 92:481, 1987.

49. Rasanen J, Vaisanen IT, Heikkila J, et al: Acute myocardial infarction complicated by left ventricular dysfunction and respiratory failure: The effects of continuous positive airway pressure. *Chest* 87:158, 1985.

50. Rasanen J, Nikki P, Heikkila J: Acute myocardial infarction complicated by respiratory failure: The effects of mechanical ventilation. *Chest* 85:21, 1984.

51. Bradley TD, Holloway RM, McLaughlin PR, et al: Cardiac output response to continuous positive airway pressure in congestive heart failure. *Am Rev Respir Dis* 145:377, 1992.

52. Ulicny KS, Hiratzka LR: Nutrition and the cardiac surgical patient. *Chest* 101:836, 1992.

53. Stroetz RW, Hubmayr RD: Mechanical load compensation during ventilator weaning. *Chest* 102:59S, 1992.

54. Sahn SA, Lakshminarayan S: Bedside criteria for discontinuation of mechanical ventilation. *Chest* 63:1002, 1973.

55. Sahn SA, Lakshminarayan S, Petty TL: Weaning from mechanical ventilation. *JAMA* 235:2208, 1976.

56. Rochester DF: The diaphragm: Contractile properties and fatigue. *J Clin Invest* 75:1397, 1985.

57. Cohen CA, Zabelbaum G, Gross D, et al: Clinical manifestations of inspiratory muscle fatigue. *Am J Med* 73:308, 1982.

58. Hubmayr RD, Loosbrock LM, Gillespie DJ, et al: Oxygen uptake during weaning from mechanical ventilation. *Chest* 94:1148, 1988.

59. Kemper M, Weissman C, Askanazi J, et al: Metabolic and respiratory changes during weaning from mechanical ventilation. *Chest* 92:979, 1987.

60. Fiastro JF, Habib MP, Shon BY, et al: Comparison of standard weaning parameters and the mechanical work of breathing in mechanically ventilated patients. *Chest* 94:233, 1988.

61. Murciano D, Boczkowski J, Lecocguic Y, et al: Tracheal occlusion pressure: A simple index to monitor respiratory muscle fatigue during acute respiratory failure in patients with chronic obstructive pulmonary disease. *Ann Intern Med* 108:800, 1988.

62. Roussos CS, Macklem PT: Diaphragmatic fatigue in man. *J Appl Physiol* 43:189, 1977.

63. Tobin MJ, Guenther SM, Perez W, et al: Konno-Mead analysis of ribcage-abdominal motion during successful and unsuccessful trials of weaning from mechanical ventilation. *Am Rev Respir Dis* 135:1320, 1987.

64. Krieger BP, Ershowsky P: Non-invasive detection of respiratory failure in the intensive care unit. *Chest* 94:254, 1988.

65. Mohsenifar Z, Hay A, Hay J, et al: Gastric intramural pH as a predictor of success or failure in weaning patients from mechanical ventilation. *Ann Intern Med* 119:794, 1993.

66. Yang KL, Tobin MJ: A prospective study of indexes predicting the outcome of trials of weaning from mechanical ventilation. *N Engl J Med* 324:1445, 1991.

67. Jabour ER, Rabil DM, Truwit JD, et al: Evaluation of a new weaning index based on ventilatory endurance and the efficiency of gas exchange. *Am Rev Respir Dis* 144:531, 1991.

68. Aubier M, Murciano D, Lecocguic Y, et al: Bilateral phrenic stimulation: A simple technique to assess diaphragmatic fatigue in humans. *J Appl Physiol* 58:58, 1985.

69. Bellemare F, Grassino A: Effect of pressure and timing of contraction on human diaphragmatic fatigue. *J Appl Physiol* 53:1190, 1982.

70. Dunn WF, Nelson SB, Hubmayr RD: The control of breathing during weaning from mechanical ventilation. *Chest* 100:754, 1991.

71. Sassoon CSH, Mahutte CK: Airway occlusion pressure and breathing pattern as predictors of weaning outcome. *Am Rev Respir Dis* 148:860, 1993.

72. Field S, Sanci S, Grassino A: Respiratory muscle oxygen consumption estimated by the diaphragm pressure-time index. *J Appl Physiol* 57:44, 1984.

73. Pardy RL, Leith DE: Ventilatory training. *Respir Care* 29:278, 1984.

73a. Brouchard L, Rauss A, Benito S, et al: Comparison of three methods of gradual withdrawal from ventilatory support during weaning from mechanical ventilation. *Am J Respir Crit Care Med* 150:896, 1994.

73b. Esteban A, Frutos F, Tobin MJ, et al: A comparison of four methods of weaning patients from mechanical ventilation. *N Engl J Med* 332:345, 1995.

74. Quan SF, Falltrick RT, Schlobohm RM: Extubation from ambient or expiratory positive airway pressure in adults. *Anesthesiology* 55:53, 1981.

75. Martin JG, Shore S, Engel LA: Effect of continuous positive airway pressure on respiratory mechanics and pattern of breathing in induced asthma. *Am Rev Respir Dis* 126:812, 1982.

76. Milic-Emili J, Gottfried SB, Rossi A: Dynamic hyperinflation: Intrinsic PEEP and its ramifications in patients with respiratory failure. In Vincent JL (ed): *Update in Intensive Care and Emergency Medicine: Update*. New York, Springer-Verlag, 1987, pp 192–198.

77. Petrof BJ, Legare M, Goldberg P, et al: Continuous positive airway pressure reduced work of breathing and dyspnea during weaning from mechanical ventilation in severe chronic obstructive pulmonary disease. *Am Rev Respir Dis* 141:281, 1990.

78. Gay PC, Rodarte JR, Hubmayr RD: The effects of positive expiratory pressure on isovolume flow and dynamic hyperinflation in patients receiving mechanical ventilation. *Am Rev Respir Dis* 139:621, 1989.

79. Bergbom-Engberg I, Haljamae J: Assessment of patients' experience of discomforts during respiratory therapy. *Crit Care Med* 17:1068, 1989.

80. Weisman IM, Rogers RM, Sanders MH: Intermittent mandatory ventilation. *Am Rev Respir Dis* 127:641, 1983.

81. Tomlinson JR, Miller KS, Lorch DG, et al: A prospective comparison of IMV and T-piece weaning from mechanical ventilation. *Chest* 96:348, 1989.

82. MacIntyre NR: Respiratory function during pressure support ventilation. *Chest* 89:677, 1986.

83. MacIntyre NR, Ho L-I: Effects of initial flow rate and breath termination criteria on pressure support ventilation. *Chest* 99:134, 1991.

84. Brochard L, Pluskwa F, Lemaire F: Improved efficacy of spontaneous breathing with inspiratory pressure support. *Am Rev Respir Dis* 136:411, 1987.

85. Fiastro JF, Habib MP, Quan SF: Pressure support compensation for inspiratory work due to endotracheal tubes and demand continuous positive airway pressure. *Chest* 93:499, 1988.

86. Brochard L, Rua F, Lorino H, et al: Inspiratory pressure support compensates for the additional work of breathing caused by the endotracheal tube. *Anesthesiology* 75:739, 1991.

87. Nathan SN, Ishaaya AM, Koerner, SK, et al: Prediction of pressure

88. Brochard L, Rauss A, Benito S, et al: Comparison of three techniques of weaning from mechanical ventilation: Results of a European multicenter trial. *Am Rev Respir Dis* 143:A602, 1991.

89. Morrell MJ, Shea SA, Adams L, et al: Effects of inspiratory support upon breathing in humans during wakefulness and sleep. *Respir Physiol* 93:57, 1993.

90. Aldrich TK, Karpel JP: Inspiratory muscle resistive training in respiratory failure. *Am Rev Respir Dis* 131:461, 1985.

91. Aldrich TK, Uhrlass RM: Weaning from mechanical ventilation: Successful use of modified inspiratory resistive training in muscular dystrophy. *Crit Care Med* 15:247, 1987.

92. Aldrich TK, Karpel JP, Uhrlass RM, et al: Weaning from mechanical ventilation: Adjunctive use of inspiratory muscle resistive training. *Crit Care Med* 17:143, 1989.

93. Hewlett AM, Platt AS, Terry VG: Mandatory minute volume: A new concept in weaning from mechanical ventilation. *Anesthesia* 32:163, 1977.

94. Corson JA, Grant JL, Moulton DP, et al: Use of biofeedback in weaning paralyzed patients from respirators. *Chest* 76:543, 1979.

95. Holliday JE, Hyers TM: The reduction of weaning time from mechanical ventilation using tidal volume and relaxation biofeedback. *Am Rev Respir Dis* 141:1214, 1990.

96. Murciano D, Aubier M, Lecocguic Y, et al: Effects of theophylline on diaphragmatic strength and fatigue in patients with chronic obstructive pulmonary disease. *N Engl J Med* 311:349, 1984.

97. Bryant S, Edwards RHT, Faulkner JA, et al: Respiratory muscle failure: Fatigue or weakness? The role of theophylline. *Chest* 89:116, 1986.

98. Murciano D, Auclair M-H, Pariente R, et al: A randomized, controlled trial of theophylline in patients with severe chronic obstructive pulmonary disease. *N Engl J Med* 320:1521, 1989.

99. Kolbeck RC, Speir WA: Diltiazem, verapamil, and nifedipine inhibit theophylline-enhanced diaphragmatic contractility. *Am Rev Respir Dis* 139:139, 1989.

100. Skatrud JB, Dempsey JA, Kaiser DG: Ventilatory response to medroxyprogesterone acetate in normal subjects: Time course and mechanism. *J Appl Physiol* 44:939, 1978.

101. Goldman AL, Morrison D, Foster LJ: Oral progesterone therapy: Oxygen in a pill. *Arch Intern Med* 141:574, 1981.

102. Aubier M, Murciano D, Menu Y, et al: Dopamine effects on diaphragmatic strength during acute respiratory failure in chronic obstructive pulmonary disease. *Ann Intern Med* 110:17, 1989.

103. Roelofs RI: Critical illness polyneuropathy. *Chest* 99:5, 1991.

104. Coronel B, Mercatello A, Couturier J-C, et al: Polyneuropathy: Potential cause of difficult weaning. *Crit Care Med* 18:486, 1990.

105. Witt NJ, Zochodne DW, Bolton CF, et al: Peripheral nerve function in sepsis and multiple organ failure. *Chest* 99:176, 1991.

106. Gorson KC, Ropper AH: Acute respiratory failure neuropathy: A variant of critical illness polyneuropathy. *Crit Care Med* 21:267, 1993.

107. Shapiro JM, Condos R, Cole RP: Myopathy in status asthmaticus: Relation to neuromuscular blockade and corticosteroid administration. *J Intensive Care Med* 8:144, 1993.

108. Argov Z, Mastaglia FL: Disorders of neuromuscular transmission caused by drugs. *N Engl J Med* 301:409, 1979.

109. Hansen-Flaschen J, Cowen J, Raps EC: Neuromuscular blockade in the intensive care unit: more than we bargained for. *Am Rev Respir Dis* 147:234, 1993.

110. Boczkowski J, Dureuil B, Branger C, et al: Effects of sepsis on diaphragmatic function in rats. *Am Rev Respir Dis* 138:260, 1988.

111. Rochester DF, Esau SA: Critical illness, infection, and the respiratory muscles. *Am Rev Respir Dis* 138:258, 1988.

112. Albert RK, Martin TR, Lewis SW: Controlled clinical trial of methylprednisolone in patients with chronic bronchitis and acute respiratory insufficiency. *Ann Intern Med* 92:753, 1980.

113. Sullivan M, Paliotta J, Saklad M: Endotracheal tube as a factor in measurement of respiratory mechanics. *J Appl Physiol* 41:590, 1976.

114. Demers RR, Sullivan MJ, Paliotta J: Airflow resistances of endotracheal tubes. *JAMA* 237:1362, 1977.

115. Plost GN, Campbell SC, Vagedes RT, et al: The nonelastic work of

breathing by normal humans using different size endotracheal tubes. *J Intensive Care Med* 5:23, 1990.
116. Demers RR, Irwin RS: Importance of the nonelastic resistance of endotracheal tubes. *J Intensive Care Med* 5:3, 1990.
117. Talpers SS, Romberger DJ, Bunce SB, et al: Nutritionally associated

increased carbon dioxide production: Excess total calories vs high proportion of carbohydrate calories. *Chest* 102:551, 1992.
118. Cohen IL, Bari N, Strosberg MA, et al: Reduction of duration and cost of mechanical ventilation in an intensive care unit by use of a ventilatory management team. *Crit Care Med* 19:1278, 1991.

68. Air Embolism and Decompression Sickness

Alfred A. Bove

Introduction

Illness or injury due to the effects of free gas in organs, tissues, or the circulation may occur from exposure to altered barometric pressure; accidental introduction of gas, usually air, into the circulation during medical procedures; and a variety of other accidents related to inappropriate access to the circulation. Persons may be exposed to reduced barometric pressure relative to sea level at high altitude and during space flight and to increased barometric pressure during underwater diving. Oxygen inhalation therapy under pressure (hyperbaric oxygen) is used in the treatment of some medical disorders and has added another dimension to the need for education in the treatment of pressure-related illness.

Physical Considerations

The weight of atmospheric air and water at any point on or above the earth's surface or beneath the surface of the water may be expressed in various units of pressure. The major difference between pressure changes at altitude and at depth is the nonlinear relationship of pressure to altitude compared to the linear relationship of pressure to depth underwater. On ascent, we pass through an air atmosphere that extends from sea level to an altitude of about 430 miles, where pressure is absent. At sea level the atmosphere weighs 14.7 pounds per square inch (psi) or 760 mm Hg (760 torr). Pressure at any altitude results from the weight of air above. However, due to the compressibility of gas, the pressure change per foot of altitude change decreases as altitude increases. For example, with ascent from sea level to 3048 m (10,000 feet), pressure is reduced from 760 to 523 mm Hg, whereas the same 3048 m altitude change from 9146 m (30,000 feet) to 12,192 m (40,000 feet) reduces pressure from 226 to 141 mm Hg. At depth, pressure change is linear. A column of sea water 1 foot tall weighs 0.445 psi; thus one atmosphere pressure equivalent for sea water is: $14.7 \times 0.445 = 33$ feet (about 10 m). The barometric pressure (P_B) at depth can be referred to in terms of gauge pressure (pressure in excess of sea level pressure) or, more commonly, absolute pressure (the total of sea level atmospheric pressure plus the water pressure). The most commonly used pressure units are millimeters of mercury (mm Hg), feet of sea water (fsw), meters of sea water (msw), and atmospheres absolute (atm). Examples are shown in Table 68-1.

Oxygen makes up about 21 percent and nitrogen about 79 percent of air. Traces of carbon dioxide, water vapor, and other inert gases are so small that they are included with the nitrogen percentage for calculation. Dalton's law states that in a mixture of gases, the total pressure is the sum of partial pressures of gases in the mixture. For example, in air at sea level, partial pressure of oxygen (PO_2) equals 0.21×760 mm Hg, or 160 mm Hg, and partial pressure of nitrogen (PN_2) equals 0.79×760 mm Hg, or 600 mm Hg. When ambient pressure increases, gas percentages remain constant but partial pressures of gases change. For example, at 33 feet underwater in the sea, where barometric pressure is 1520 mm Hg or 2 atm, $PO_2 = 0.21 \times 1520$ mm Hg, or 319 mm Hg, and $PN_2 = 1201$ mm Hg. At normal body temperature the vapor pressure of water is 47 mm Hg; thus by the time inspired dry air reaches the trachea, it has equilibrated at a PH_2O of 47 mm Hg, which then remains constant in the alveolar air. Admixture of carbon dioxide diffused across the alveolocapillary membrane into the alveolus results in a $PaCO_2$ of about 40 mm Hg in a normal human. When breathing air at sea level, PaO_2 is about 110 mm Hg, while at 33 feet under the sea it is about 270 mm Hg. The increased PO_2 can reach toxic levels at deeper depths, and reduced oxygen gas mixtures (usually helium-oxygen mixtures) are used at depths below 200 feet. Normally, 97 percent of oxygen is carried by hemoglobin and 3 percent is dissolved in plasma and cells. Under conditions of increased PO_2, additional dissolved oxygen is carried by the blood even though hemoglobin is fully saturated.

Direct Pressure Effects

As pressure increases, the volume of gas in exposed spaces diminishes according to Boyle's law [1]. Volume in the lungs, middle ear, paranasal sinuses, gut, and so forth is reduced as pressure increases (Fig. 68-1). Displacement of tissues into the diminishing volume of these spaces causes the phenomenon called "squeeze," which damages tissues, and may cause dysfunction of the organ involved. Ear squeeze (middle ear barotrauma) occurs when the eustachian tube is blocked and the middle ear space cannot equilibrate with the increasing ambient pressure [2]. The tympanic membrane is displaced inward and ultimately ruptures. The middle ear may fill with blood from engorged mucous membranes. Infection and reduced hearing loss are complications. Middle ear barotrauma has been classified by severity [3]. The mildest form causes only erythema of

Table 68-1. Pressure Equivalents to Altitude and Depth

	Feet	atm	mm Hg	psi
Altitude above sea level	12000	0.636	483	9.3
	8000	0.742	564	10.9
	4000	0.863	656	12.7
Sea level	0	1	760	14.7
Depth in sea water	33	2	1520	29.4
	66	3	2280	44.1
	99	4	3040	58.8
	132	5	3800	73.5

atm = atmospheres absolute, psi = pounds/square inch.

the tympanic membrane, whereas the severe form involves rupture of the tympanic membrane and hemorrhage into the middle ear [3]. Middle ear barotrauma is prevented by assuring that the eustachian tube is patent and the middle ear can be equilibrated at surface pressure before descending. A gentle Valsalva maneuver is commonly used to accomplish this goal [4]. Similar events can occur in a paranasal sinus with a blocked orifice (sinus squeeze), in a small residual air pocket left between a tooth filling and the base of the tooth (tooth squeeze), in the air space within a diving mask (mask squeeze) or between the skin and a fold in a dry diving suit (suit squeeze). All will produce tissue injury due to displacement of tissues into the diminishing air space. Tooth fillings may also be loosened if air has diffused into a space beneath a filling while under pressure and expands on ascent. Although lung squeeze is theoretically possible by breath-hold diving to a depth that reduces the lung volume below the residual volume [5], in practice this has not been observed. A rare form of barotrauma of ascent occurs when gas is trapped in the gastrointestinal (GI) tract while at depth and expands on ascent. Air enters the GI tract from swallowing and from faulty breathing equipment that produces increased pressure of the breathing gas at the mouth. Expanding air in the gut produces intense pain during ascent and may cause rupture of the stomach. Treatment is usually conservative, but if an air leak continues after surfacing surgical intervention may become necessary. Inner ear barotrauma can occur when large pressure differences occur between the endolymph and the middle ear. Usually, the round window ruptures outward, endolymph is lost, and the diver experiences vertigo, hearing loss, and tinnitus [6]. The mechanism is usually excess efforts at ear equalization during descent. A vigorous Valsalva maneuver increases spinal fluid pressure and endolymph pressure, while middle ear pressure remains low due to eustachian tube obstruction. When the pressure difference becomes great the round window ruptures. This injury requires early treatment, which may include surgical repair of the round window. Squeeze is a common, usually minor, consequence of diving. Middle ear barotrauma is the most common diving-related disorder encountered in divers.

Pulmonary Barotrauma and Air Embolism

Injury to the lungs is a potentially lethal complication of poor diving practices. Early studies by Polak and Adams [7], Schilling [8], and Behnke [9] defined the overpressure syndromes related to diving. Gases used for diving are pressurized to the ambient pressure, so that the pressure gradient from breathing supply to the airways is not altered as the diver descends. A diver

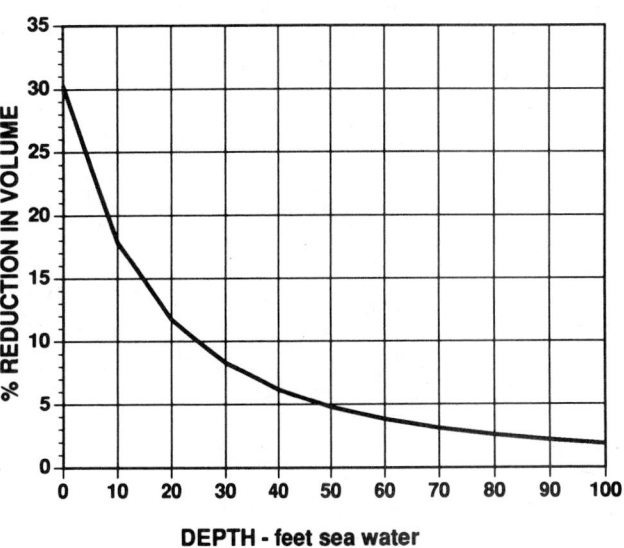

Fig. 68-1. Graphic demonstration of Boyle's law. Volume changes are shown as percentage of initial volume vs. depth at 10-foot increments. The greatest percent change is near the surface.

breathing compressed air at 33 feet (2 atm) will experience expansion of the lung volume on ascent due to Boyle's law. If the diver breathes normally and properly vents the increasing gas volume, no lung expansion will occur; however, if the diver ascends while breath-holding, the lung gas will attempt to expand to twice the volume at 33 feet. When the lung volume expands to the chest capacity, further ascent will cause intrapulmonary pressure to increase to levels which damage lung tissue. Overpressure of 95 to 110 cm H_2O (70–80 mm Hg) initiates damage to the lung [7,10,11]. Pressures of 300 to 400 mm Hg are possible in the lung subjected to gas expansion against a closed glottis. Lung damage occurs immediately on surfacing, and air is injected into the pulmonary veins. Embolization of the heart, brain, and other organs follows [11]. The most commonly involved organ is the brain, where strokelike symptoms are found within minutes of surfacing with a closed glottis. Neurologic abnormalities can range from minor, almost imperceptible changes in behavior to seizures and unconsciousness (Table 68-2). Immediate recompression is lifesaving, but with subtle symptoms, failure to recognize and properly treat this disorder can result in permanent injury to the brain. In some studies 7 to 14 percent of victims of air embolism did not survive [12]. Although most cases of pulmonary barotrauma and air embolism occur because of failure to exhale on ascent, cases have been recorded where no evidence can be found of improper exhalation during ascent from a dive. Thus, breath-holding during ascent is not always necessary to develop a pulmonary overpressure injury.

Poorly ventilated lung segments can result from asthma, chronic bronchitis, lung cysts, and other obstructive airway diseases. Any local airway obstruction can produce air trapping during ascent and increase risk of air embolism. Air embolism has been described from use of scuba equipment in swimming pools. An intrapulmonary pressure of about 80 mm Hg forces air into the pulmonary capillaries. Since 1 foot of water depth is equivalent to about 25 mm Hg pressure, a breath-holding ascent from less than 4 feet of water with full inhalation from a scuba regulator can cause lung damage and air embolism. The greatest danger from gas expansion occurs near the sur-

Table 68-2. Symptoms of Cerebral Air Embolism

Unconsciousness
Dizziness
Chest pain
Convulsions
Paralysis
Nausea
Visual disturbances
Headache
Confusion
Personality changes

Adapted from Kidd DJ, Elliott DH: Decompression disorders in divers, in Bennett PB, Elliott DH (eds): *The Physiology and Medicine of Diving and Compressed Air Work.* 2nd ed. London, Bailliere Tindall, 1982, pp 471–495.

Table 68-3. Diving Injuries Resulting from Pulmonary Barotrauma

Arterial gas embolism
Pneumothorax
Mediastinal emphysema
Subcutaneous emphysema
Ruptured diaphragm

face, where the rate of volume change for a given range of ascent in the water is greatest (Fig. 68-1). Thus, an excursion from 4 feet to the surface produces greater lung volume expansion than an excursion from 100 to 96 feet.

In addition to air embolism, other disorders involving injury to the structures in the chest may occur from lung overpressure. Table 68-3 lists the types of injury that can result from pulmonary barotrauma. Pulmonary overpressure may cause pneumothorax, mediastinal emphysema or subcutaneous emphysema. In severe overpressure accidents, air can distend the diaphragm to the point where air enters the peritoneum.

Blast injury is a unique form of pulmonary barotrauma that produces extensive damage and air embolism [13,14]. An excellent review of the physics of underwater blast is provided by Schilling et al. [15]. When a blast occurs in air or water, there is an initial high-pressure wave that may reach thousands of pounds per square inch, followed within milliseconds by a negative-pressure wave. Underwater blasts are particularly dangerous because of the lack of compressibility of water and the resultant transmission of pressure changes directly to the body. Lung and air containing abdominal viscera are universally injured. Lung injury includes severe barotrauma with pulmonary hemorrhage and pulmonary edema [14]; air embolism results. Rupture of abdominal viscera causes a bacterial peritonitis and often requires surgical intervention. Middle ear and paranasal sinuses are also injured. Air embolism may be extensive, with involvement of cerebral and cardiac vessels. Divers subjected to underwater blast injury should be treated with recompression therapy for both air embolism and decompression sickness, in addition to treatment of direct tissue injuries.

OTHER CAUSES OF AIR EMBOLISM. Air may enter the circulation from crush injury of the chest, vascular injury, or injection during medical procedures, and air may be left in the circulation after surgical procedures in the vascular system. In a review of 34 iatrogenic cases [16], Takahashi et al. found arteriography, open heart surgery, dialysis, surgery on the neck, and craniotomy to be sources of iatrogenic cerebral air embo-

lism. Air can enter the vascular system through vaginal insufflation during oral sex [17]. Hill and Jones [17] described a case of venous air embolism following oral sex in a pregnant woman. Air enters the vascular system via placental sinuses and produces severe venous air embolism. Arterial and venous air embolism produce two distinct clinical patterns. Arterial embolism invariably causes occlusion of cerebral vessels [11], while venous air embolism initially occludes the pulmonary vasculature [18]. Baskin and Wozniak [19] described nine patients who sustained combined venous and arterial air embolism from hemodialysis. All patients complained of chest pain and dyspnea as their first symptoms, and a variety of neurologic symptoms developed. Two patients who sustained a cardiac arrest were successfully resuscitated. All nine patients responded to recompression to 6 atm, using U.S. Navy Treatment Table 6A (Fig. 68-2). In patients with patent foramen ovale, venous air may cross the interatrial septum and embolize the arterial system [20,21,22]. Venous air embolism to the lung becomes symptomatic when significant amounts of air occlude the pulmonary arteries. The lungs ordinarily can tolerate moderate amounts of air before symptoms develop [19]. When air embolizes the brain, a wide spectrum of neurologic abnormalities is possible. Coma, hemiplegia, visual disturbances, disorientation, apnea, and hypotension have been noted [16]. Mader and Hulet [12] found a 30 percent mortality for untreated iatrogenic air embolism, while hyperbaric oxygen therapy reduced mortality to 6 percent. They described a case where treatment was instituted 29 hours after the initial insult, with a good result [12]. We described a successfully treated case of cerebral air embolism following cardiac surgery, with a delay of over 10 hours before institution of hyperbaric oxygen therapy [23].

Although diagnosis of cerebral air embolism depends on the clinical history and physical examination, recent studies using computed tomography (CT) and magnetic resonance imaging have shown air in the cerebral vasculature [24,25]. Kizer [26] found that CT was helpful in the assessment of patients after recompression therapy of air embolism. Cucchiara et al. [27] described echocardiographic evidence of air embolism in neurosurgical patients. In their series of 15 patients who sustained an air embolism during suboccipital craniotomy in the sitting position, 9 showed air using precordial Doppler ultrasound detection, while transesophageal echo (TEE) showed air in all 15. Their results indicated that TEE is a more sensitive indicator of air embolism during surgical monitoring. Also, TEE improved localization of the air in the heart, compared to transthoracic echo.

TREATMENT OF AIR EMBOLISM. Air embolism requires recompression in a hyperbaric chamber, and this should be provided with minimal delay. One hundred percent oxygen (hyperbaric oxygen) is also provided during treatment in the chamber. Protocols for treatment used in the United States were developed by the U.S. Navy based on extensive research and many years of experience in treating diving casualties. U.S. Navy Treatment Tables 6 or 6A, which combine hyperbaric oxygen and pressure therapy at either 2.8 or 6 atm, are commonly used. These tables, from the *U.S. Navy Diving Manual* [28], are a standard reference for treatment of diving injuries. Table 6A involves a rapid excursion in a pressure chamber to 165 feet (6 atm) of equivalent depth on air (Fig. 68-2). After a period of up to 30 minutes at 165 feet, the diver is brought to 60 feet (2.8 atm) equivalent depth and placed on 100 percent oxygen. U.S. Navy Treatment Table 6 (Fig. 68-3) eliminates the initial deep exposure and starts with 100 percent oxygen therapy at 60 feet. If a victim is treated rapidly, there is a striking and dramatic reversal of neurologic symptoms when the patient

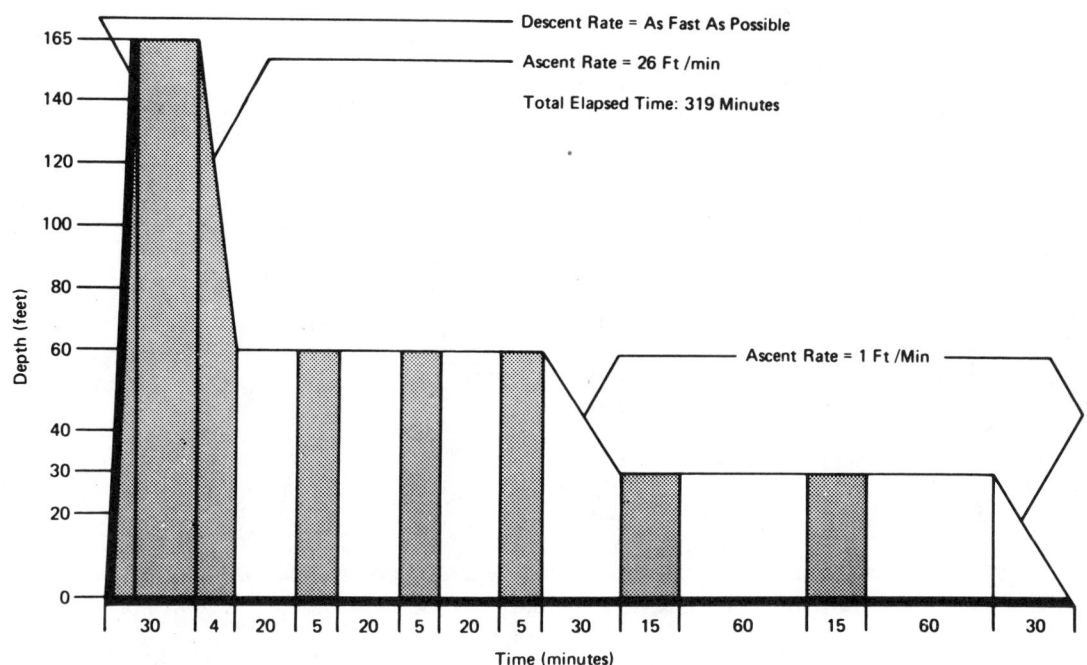

Fig. 68-2. U.S. Navy Treatment Table 6A. The schematic describes the depth and time course of treatment when initial compression to 165 fsw is indicated.

is compressed to 60 or 165 feet, and complete recovery of normal function minutes after recompression is quite possible [9]. When improvement is observed at 60 feet, therapy is usually continued with that described in Figure 68-3; when symptoms are not relieved at 60 feet, treatment can be continued with increased pressure at 165 feet. Failure to treat a cerebral air embolism can result in tragic consequences, including death or permanent neurologic injury. Recent clinical [23] and experimental [29] data indicate that arterial gas embolism can be treated successfully at 60 feet using 100 percent oxygen. This is more practical for many treatment facilities. Catron et al. [30] have also reported experience with successful reversal of cerebral dysfunction using combined pressure and hyperbaric oxygen for therapy of air embolism. The value of pressure and oxygen in this disease has been questioned by Layton [31]. However, the weight of clinical evidence and more than 60 years' experience support the treatment of arterial air embolism with combined pressure and oxygen. An interesting study by Dutka et al. [32] in an animal model of cerebral gas embolism indicates that lidocaine may improve cerebral blood flow after an embolic insult. Combined hyperbaric oxygen therapy and intravenous lidocaine provided a greater improvement of cortical evoked response and cerebral blood flow than did saline in the control group. In addition, the treated animals showed less late deterioration of function. Although access to a hyperbaric chamber immediately following an air embolism is uncommon, there is ample evidence that treatment instituted even after some delay (4–6 hours) can result in significant reversal of the symptoms and reduction of permanent neurologic injury. Bitterman and Melamed [33] treated five patients referred after 15 to 60 hours for cerebral air embolism due to surgical accidents. Significant recovery was observed in three of the five; one died and one did not respond to combined pressure and oxygen therapy. They used U.S. Navy treatment Table 6A (Fig. 68-2) with subsequent daily treatments at 60 feet for 90 minutes.

Emergency care of the patient with cerebral air embolism

should include support of respiration and circulation as needed; 100 percent oxygen should be administered with a tight-fitting mask while the victim is transported to the hyperbaric chamber. Breathing pure oxygen improves oxygen supply to compromised brain tissue and replaces inert gas in the arterial bubbles, thus reducing bubble size as oxygen is consumed from the bubble. An unconscious victim may require endotracheal intubation and ventilatory support. A victim in ventricular fibrillation is likely to have air in the coronary arteries. These patients will not respond to defibrillation while the coronaries are obstructed, and emergency recompression should be undertaken while CPR is provided.

Menasche et al. [34] proposed from animal experiments that fluorocarbons injected into the arterial system may provide a means of rapid treatment of arterial gas embolism. Prevention in upright neurosurgery can be achieved by mild neck compression to increase venous pressure [35,36,37]. Further information on the pathophysiology and therapy of cerebral air embolism can be found in the review by Dutka [38].

Occasionally, even a patient with a severe neurologic disorder from air embolism improves over the first few hours after injury to the point that neurologic abnormalities may be minimal to absent. This "lucid period" is well recognized in air embolism and is usually followed by a return of symptoms, often more severe. Without treatment, permanent neurologic injury results. Occasionally on observing this lucid period medical personnel decide the victim does not need recompression and they resort to conventional medical care. However, patients with a history of neurologic symptoms from suspected cerebral air embolism should undergo recompression treatment, regardless of current clinical status.

Decompression Sickness

INERT GAS KINETICS. Decompression sickness is the disorder that results from damage to various organs and tissues as a result of bubble production and growth [39,40]. Expansion of

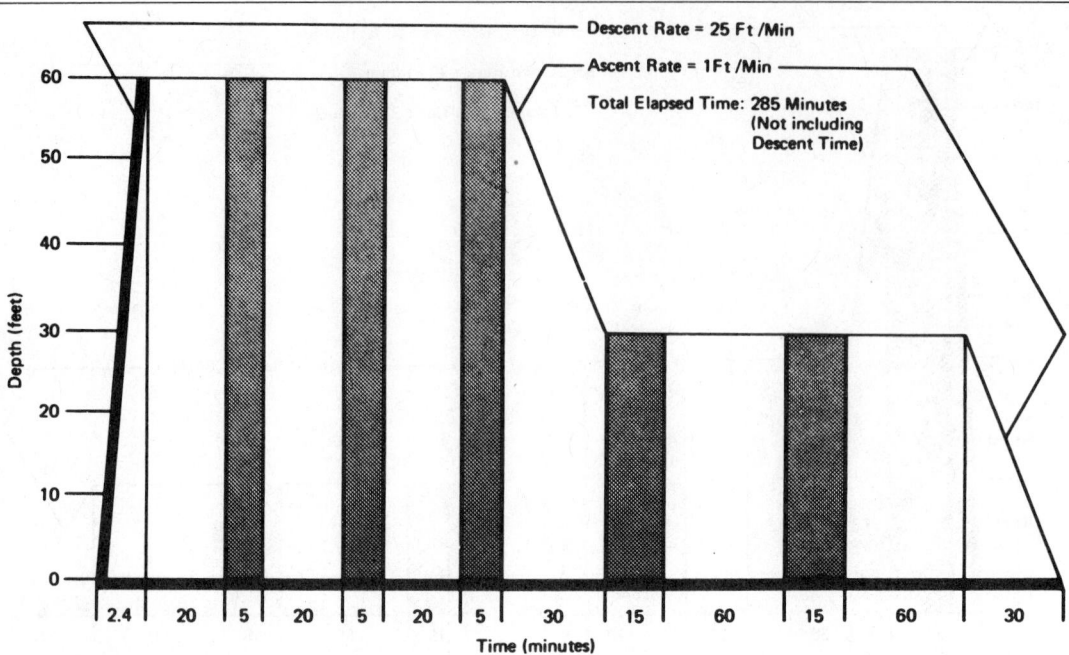

Fig. 68-3. U.S. Navy Treatment Table 6.

gases in blood and tissues on ascent results in damage and dysfunction of the tissues and gas embolism to the lungs [41]. Pressure determines the amount of gas dissolved in the tissues and body fluids. A person subjected to increased ambient pressure will take up gases into the tissues based on an exponential kinetic model [42,43]. Dissolved gas content of tissues depends on the partial pressure of the gas and the solubility of the gas in the specific tissue (Table 68-4). Inert gas (nitrogen, helium), however, is a limiting factor in diving because of its ability to supersaturate quickly as the diver ascends with excess dissolved gas in the tissues. Supersaturation allows dissolved gases to change phase to the gaseous form, and bubbles form in blood and tissues [40]. Of the gases involved in diving, oxygen does not cause a problem in decompression sickness, due to its low partial pressure at the cellular level [44] and CO_2 does not cause concern for decompression sickness because of its high solubility and low partial pressure. Gases dissolve in tissues, fats, and water according to Henry's law:

$$V = K \times P$$

where V is the volume of dissolved inert gas, K is the solubility coefficient, and P is the partial pressure of the gas. Solubility coefficients for water and lipid are provided in Table 68-4. Of interest is the volume of inert gas (nitrogen when breathing air) that is dissolved in various tissues. Although Henry's law determines the amount of gas in the tissue, there is a finite time required for equilibrium to be achieved (Fig. 68-4). Gases entering tissues are thought to follow a first-order differential relationship, where the rate of gas entry into tissue is proportional to the pressure difference between blood and tissue. Factors that affect the rate of entry include blood flow to the tissue and the rate of diffusion of gases into the tissue [45]. In the body, blood flow is the major factor controlling rate of gas exchange. The concentration of gas in tissues follows the kinetic equation:

$$\frac{dC}{dt} = k \times \Delta C$$

where C is the concentration of gas in the tissue at time t, ΔC is the difference in concentration of gas between a tissue and the lungs, and k is a constant that depends on tissue perfusion and gas solubility. This equation describes an asymptotic curve (Fig. 68-4A) in which the tissue gas concentration approaches the maximum concentration for the given pressure after about 5 half-times (time to reach one-half of maximum tissue pressure) have elapsed. There is a family of curves for different values of k. These curves represent different tissue compartments, which have different gas exchange characteristics [42,45]. Similar kinetics control the washout of inert gas from tissues when ambient pressure is reduced (Fig. 68-4B), but washout and uptake are not necessarily symmetric.

Decompression tables are designed to prevent excess supersaturation of tissues and bubble formation [46,47]. Decompression stages are selected to avoid excess supersaturation in specific tissues (Fig. 68-5). Decompression schedules have been designed for different inert gases, continuous or staged decompression, saturation exposure, caisson or tunnel exposure, and types of diving, such as commercial or recreational.

Operations involving exposure to increased partial pressure of inert gas must always consider decompression time as well

Table 68-4. Characteristics of Inert Gases

Gas	Molecular weight	Lipid solubility[a]	Water solubility[a]	Narcotic potential[b]
Helium	4	0.015	0.009	0.23
Neon	20	0.019	0.009	0.28
Hydrogen	2	0.036	0.018	0.55
Nitrogen	28	0.067	0.013	1.00
Argon	40	0.140	0.026	2.32

[a]Expressed as gas volume/solute volume at 1 bar.
[b]Values relative to nitrogen.
Solubility of the various gases in lipid is related to their narcotic potential; helium is the least and argon the most narcotic gas in the list.
Adapted from Bennett PB: Inert gas narcosis, in Bennett PB, Elliott DH (eds): *The Physiology and Medicine of Diving and Compressed Air Work.* Baltimore, Williams & Wilkins, 1975, p. 205.

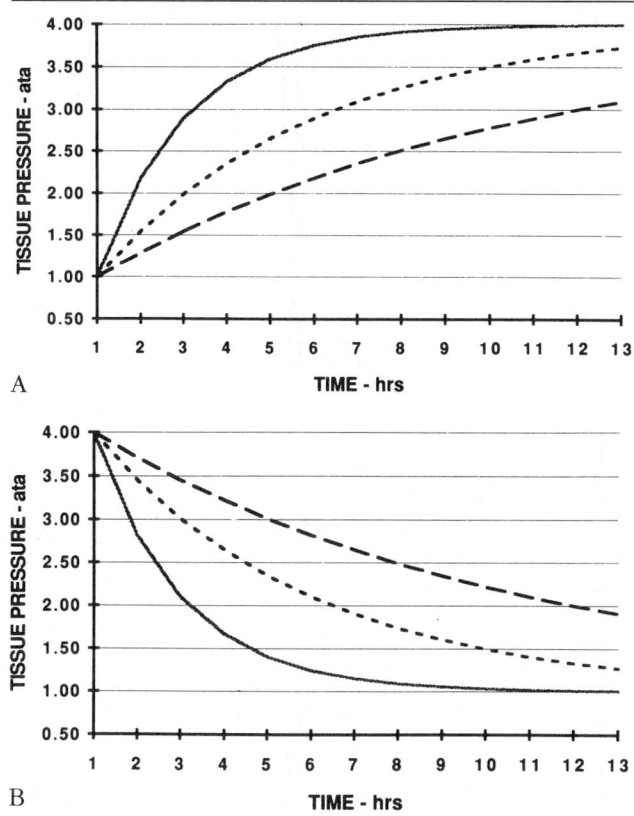

A

B

Fig. 68-4. A. Theoretical inert gas uptake curves for several tissue compartments when the tissues undergo an ambient pressure change from 1 to 4 atms. The upper curve represents a tissue compartment that reaches saturation at 11 hours. The other curves represent slower-filling compartments. B. Washout curves for tissue compartments with the same kinetic properties as shown in A. The curves depict the tissue inert gas content after excursion from 4 to 1 atm ambient pressure. Both figures assume a single excursion with no stops.

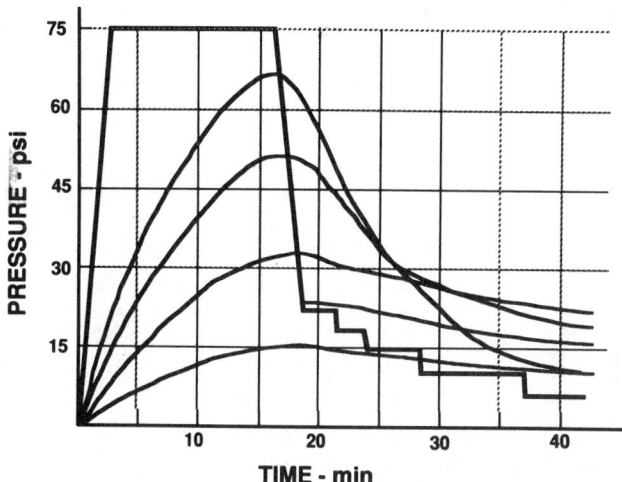

Fig. 68-5. Combined uptake and washout curves of five tissue compartments resulting from a practical pressure exposure and decompression. The heavy line outlines the actual dive profile. Most tissue compartments do not reach saturation at the end of the dive. Stages of decompression are designed to prevent excess supersaturation of any tissue compartment during the decompression. Adapted from Boycott et al [47].

as exposure time. For certain exposures, decompression time far exceeds the exposure time and renders the exposure impractical. For long or deep exposures, the technique of saturation diving is used. In this type of exposure, workers are maintained under pressure for days to weeks until the work is completed. During this time, tissue partial pressures become equilibrated with the ambient pressure, and inert gas reaches its saturation concentration. Once tissues are saturated no further gas uptake occurs, and a single decompression is performed on completion of the work [46]. Pressurized habitats have been constructed specifically to house workers who must live under increased pressure for prolonged periods [48]. Decompression procedures are well defined for air, mixtures of nitrogen and oxygen; helium and oxygen, nitrogen, helium and oxygen (trimix); hydrogen and oxygen; and the noble gases argon and neon, which to date have been used only in experimental exposures.

PATHOPHYSIOLOGIC AND CLINICAL CONSIDERATIONS. In the nineteenth century, Paul Bert described the pathophysiology of decompression sickness [39]. Hill and others [49,50] in the late nineteenth century concluded from autopsies on divers and caisson workers that decompression sick-

ness was caused by inert gas bubbles in the blood and tissues. From their work, clinical symptoms of paresis and unconsciousness were related to bubbles in CNS tissues, and dyspnea was associated with bubbles in the pulmonary circulation. These concepts remain current [51]. The causes of muscle and joint pain associated with decompression sickness are less clear. Pain may be due to bubbles in ligaments, fascia, periosteum, or nerve sheaths. Bubbles also have biochemical effects [51] that are independent of their mechanical effects.

An interesting effect has been recently described in patients with patent foramen ovale [20]. This congenital persistence of a probe-patent foramen may increase the risk of serious decompression sickness by allowing venous bubbles to pass into the arterial circulation. Patency of the foramen ovale occurs in 25 to 30 percent of the normal population [52] and has been related to an increased incidence of stroke [53]. Patients with severe neurologic syndromes from diving that are out of proportion to their diving exposure and who do not appear to have pulmonary barotrauma may have a patent foramen ovale. Testing of all divers for this defect is impractical, but in those who develop severe neurologic injury, echocardiography should be done to evaluate the status of the interatrial septum. Neurologic injury remains the most serious form of diving injury [54].

There is a spectrum of injury in this illness (Table 68-5) that can mimic a variety of other diseases [55–58]. Disorders related to decompression sickness were classified by Golding et al. [59] based on observations of caisson workers. Their classification identified a minor, less serious form of decompression sickness that involved the joints and skin and was manifested by local pain and sometimes associated edema; there were no systemic components in CNS, blood, or other tissue, but a serious form showed evidence of CNS, pulmonary, or other organ injury. Table 68-5 reflects the classification used for diving-related disorders since the original publication of Golding et al. [59]. The disease develops on ascent from depth when a diver does not follow established procedures for returning to the surface. Aviators and astronauts exposed to prolonged periods of reduced pressure also develop decompression sickness.

Table 68-5. Classification of Decompression Sickness

Type I: Pain only decompression sickness
           Limb or joint pain
           Itch
           Skin rash

Type II: Serious decompression sickness
           Central nervous system disorder
           Pulmonary (chokes)
           Systemic (hypovolemic shock)
           Inner ear/vestibular

Adapted from Davis JC: Treatment of decompression sickness and arterial gas embolism, in Bove AA, Davis JC (eds): *Diving Medicine*. Philadelphia, WB Saunders, 1990, pp. 249–260.

Table 68-6. Frequency of Decompression Sickness Symptoms in 100 Cases

Symptom	Percentage of all symptoms
Skin itch	4
Headache	11
Fatigue/malaise	13
Bone/joint pain	54
Spinal/back pain	11
Spinal/neurologic	22
Respiratory	21

Adapted from Yamaki T, Ando S, Ohta K, et al: CT demonstration of massive cerebral air embolism from pulmonary barotrauma due to cardiopulmonary resuscitation. *J Comput Assist Tomogr* 13:313, 1989.

The formation of free gas in the body has several consequences [55–58]. Free gas entering the vascular system from the peripheral tissues transits the veins and causes pulmonary vascular obstruction [18,57]. When the free gas volume is large and significant, pulmonary obstruction occurs. A classical syndrome (chokes) is described [56,58], manifest by chest pain, dyspnea, and cough. Decompression sickness is often associated with free gas in the blood and tissue injury from expanding gas. Bubbles and tissue injury result in activation of acute inflammation [60,61,62]. The inflammatory response alters vascular permeability, causing fluid to leak into the interstitial tissues of the systemic and pulmonary vascular beds [63,64]. In severe cases, pulmonary edema can occur and hypovolemia with significant plasma loss and hemoconcentration results [62,65]. With severe decompression sickness, endothelial damage to blood vessels occurs [65] and significant focal regions of tissue ischemia are evident. A frequent target organ in humans is the spinal cord [66,67]. A common manifestation of decompression sickness in divers is spinal cord injury, usually at levels below the diaphragm [67]. Symptoms include paresthesias, muscle weakness, paralysis of the lower extremities, bowel or bladder incontinence, urinary retention, and sexual impotence. In cases of sudden ascent from the deep depths associated with long or deep diving exposures, a severe decompression sickness syndrome can occur with both cerebral and spinal neurologic symptoms, unconsciousness, hypovolemic shock, pulmonary edema, and a high mortality rate [68].

The less serious form of decompression sickness (type I) is manifest by pains in the extremities and joints [58,69]. The pain is often poorly described, usually spares the hip joints, and may cause diffuse pain in a limb. Symptoms of local pain are often confused with pain from injuries, and the diagnosis of decompression sickness may be missed. A trial of treatment at 60 fsw with 100 percent oxygen may be used to differentiate decompression sickness from mechanical injury, since most type I pain disappears after 5 to 10 minutes of treatment. A high incidence of aseptic bone necrosis is found in some populations of divers who have experienced decompression sickness of the joints in the distant past or deep, prolonged dives in commercial or military operations [70] and in caisson workers [71]. A rare but important symptom of decompression sickness is sudden acute neurologic hearing loss or vestibular dysfunction. Decompression sickness of this type usually occurs from deep, long exposures; if untreated, it will result in permanent deafness or chronic vertigo [72]. Table 68-6 lists the frequency of symptoms in decompression sickness.

We recently described a severe form of decompression injury that results from combined decompression sickness and air embolism. This combination can occur as a diver who has completed a dive develops pulmonary barotrauma during as-

cent. The combination of excess gas in tissues and free gas in the arterial system forms a particularly severe form of gas bubble injury [73].

TREATMENT OF DECOMPRESSION SICKNESS. Treatment of decompression sickness requires knowledge of the use of hyperbaric chambers and hyperbaric oxygen for therapy [28,69] and is usually provided by specialists in diving and hyperbaric medicine. Divers with joint pains or neurologic abnormalities following a diving exposure require consultation with a diving medicine expert and may need recompression treatment in a hyperbaric chamber. Symptoms of decompression sickness may appear up to 24 hours following exposure (Table 68-7). Mistreatments have resulted in permanent brain and spinal cord injury or death because of misdiagnosis. Since only a few centers in the United States can provide expert consultation in this area, it is wise to learn of the treatment facilities available in specific regions of the United States and other countries. Persons suspected of having a diving-related accident involving neurologic abnormalities should not be retained in a hospital without hyperbaric treatment facilities, since prolonging the delay between onset of symptoms and recompression treatment increases the risk of permanent neurologic injury [74].

Bubbles from inadequate decompression form in blood and tissues and activate the inflammatory process [18,62,65]. Adjunctive therapy with drugs has been developed to provide therapy for the secondary (i.e., nonobstructive) effects of bubbles [61]. Individuals with neurologic decompression sickness or arterial gas embolism may benefit from fluid therapy to prevent hemoconcentration, use of intravenous steroids to inhibit cerebral or spinal cord edema, and antiplatelet agents to prevent platelet aggregation by bubble surfaces in the blood [61]. In severe decompression sickness, disseminated intravascular coagulation may develop [64] and anticoagulation may be considered [61,64]. Individuals with permanent neurologic injury from decompression sickness or air embolism require physical therapy to regain musculoskeletal function. Unlike traumatic cord injury or stroke, prompt treatment of neurologic injury from decompression sickness or air embolism often results in excellent recovery of function.

It is sometimes difficult to distinguish between severe decompression sickness and cerebral air embolism. These two conditions may coexist when a diver who has been underwater for a prolonged period ascends rapidly and develops pulmonary barotrauma [73]. Because treatment of both illnesses involves recompression in a hyperbaric chamber, hyperbaric oxygen, and adjunctive drug therapy, it is less important to make a

Table 68-7. Time to Onset of Decompression Sickness
Following Diving

Cumulative percentage	Time of onset
50	30 minutes
85	1 hr
95	3 hr
99	6 hr
100	12–24 hr

Adapted from Yamaki T, Ando S, Ohta K, et al: CT demonstration of massive cerebral air embolism from pulmonary barotrauma due to cardiopulmonary resuscitation. *J Comput Assist Tomogr* 13:313, 1989.

precise diagnosis and more important to institute therapy quickly. Decompression sickness usually develops sometime after diving. Symptoms may develop within minutes of ascent or may appear 12 to 24 hours later. On the other hand, pulmonary barotrauma with arterial gas embolism occurs immediately on ascent and may produce initial unconsciousness. Subtle symptoms of pulmonary barotrauma may go undetected in the initial few hours after ascent; thus, timing of symptom onset should not be the only criterion for differentiating this disorder from decompression sickness.

Recompression therapy involves one of several available protocols for application of pressure and oxygen. Commonly used protocols are U.S. Navy Treatment Table 6 (Fig. 68-3) for decompression sickness and U.S. Navy Treatment Table 6A (Fig. 68-2) for arterial gas embolism [28]. Use of Treatment Table 6 for arterial gas embolism has recently been advocated based on animal studies [29]. Recent clinical experience supports this modification. Patients who do not respond to treatment at 60 fsw should be compressed to deeper depths, using standard treatment protocols such as U.S. Navy Treatment Table 6A. Treatment for all cases of decompression sickness usually follows the Treatment Table 6 protocol: hyperbaric oxygen at 2.8 atm and pressure of 60 feet. All forms of decompression sickness are responsive to this therapy, although U.S. Navy practice provides a shorter treatment schedule for divers with pain in a limb as their only manifestation [24]. In civilian hyperbaric practice, the shorter table is not often used.

Supportive therapy prior to initiation of hyperbaric oxygen includes intravenous infusion of saline to maintain hydration and plasma volume and use of antiplatelet agents (aspirin). Steroid injections have been suggested to prevent cerebral edema, but their efficacy in this application has not been proved. On-site medical supplies for a diving operation should include these medications so that treatment can be instituted while the victim is transported to a treatment facility.

The most important aspect of decompression sickness and air embolism is prevention. The diving environment requires a thorough knowledge of diving physiology and physics and a commitment to safety. Therapy has evolved over more than a century, and treatment protocols are successful in 80 to 90 percent of diving injuries.

References

1. Boyle R: New pneumatic experiments about respiration. *Philos Trans R Soc Lond Biol* 5:2011, 1670.
2. Vail HH: Traumatic conditions of the ear in workers in an atmosphere of compressed air. *Arch Otolaryngol* 10:113, 1929.
3. Farmer JC: Ear and sinus problems in diving, in Bove AA, Davis JC
(eds): *Diving Medicine*. Philadelphia, WB Saunders, 1990, pp 205–208.
4. Taylor GD: The otolaryngologic aspects of skin and scuba diving. *Laryngoscope* 69:809, 1959.
5. Schaefer KE, Allison RD, Dougherty JH, et al: Pulmonary and circulatory adjustments determining the limits of depths in breathhold diving. *Science* 162:1020, 1968.
6. Freeman P, Edmonds C: Inner ear barotrauma. *Arch Otolaryngol* 95:556, 1972.
7. Polak B, Adams H: Traumatic air embolism in submarine escape training. *U.S. Naval Med Bull* 30:165, 1932.
8. Schilling CW: Expiratory force as related to submarine escape training. *U.S. Naval Med Bull* 31:1, 1933.
9. Behnke AR: Analysis of accidents occurring in training with the submarine "lung." *U.S. Naval Med Bull* 30:177, 1932.
10. Schaefer KE, Nulty WP, Carey C, et al: Mechanisms in development of interstitial emphysema and air embolism on decompression from depth. *J Appl Physiol* 13:15, 1958.
11. Malhotra MC, Wright CAM: Arterial air embolism during decompression and its prevention. *Proc R Soc Med* 154B:418, 1960.
12. Mader JT, Hulet WH: Delayed hyperbaric treatment of cerebral air embolism. *Arch Neurol* 36:504, 1979.
13. Ecklund AM: The pathology of immersion blast injuries. *U.S. Naval Med Bull* 41:19, 1943.
14. Clemedson CJ: Blast injury. *Physiol Rev* 36:336, 1956.
15. Schilling CW, Werts MF, Schandelmeier NR: *The Underwater Handbook*. New York; Plenum, 1976, pp 637–646.
16. Takahashi H, Kobayashi S, Hayase H, et al: Iatrogenic air embolism: A review of 34 cases, in Bove AA, Greenbaum LJ, Bachrach AJ (eds): *Proceedings of the 9th International Symposium on Undersea and Hyperbaric Physiology: Undersea and Hyperbaric Medical Society*, Bethesda, 1987, pp 931–948.
17. Hill BF, Jones JS: Venous air embolism following orogenital sex during pregnancy. *Am J Emerg Med.* 11:155, 1993.
18. Bove AA, Hallenbeck JM, Elliott DH: Circulatory responses to venous air embolism and decompression sickness in dogs. *Undersea Biomed Res* 1:207, 1974.
19. Baskin SE, Wozniak RF: Hyperbaric oxygenation in the treatment of hemodialysis-associated air embolism. *N Engl J Med* 293:184, 1975.
20. Moon RE, Camporesi EM, Kisslo JA: Patent foramen ovale and decompression sickness in divers. *Lancet* 1:513, 1989.
21. Cross SJ, Evans SA, Thompson LF, et al: Safety of subaqua diving with a patent foramen ovale. *Br Med J* 304:481, 1992.
22. Wilmshurst PT, Byrne JC, Webb-Peploe MM: Relation between intraatrial shunts and decompression sickness in divers. *Lancet* 2:1302, 1990.
23. Bove AA, Clark JM, Simon AJ, Lambertsen CJ: Successful therapy of cerebral air embolism with hyperbaric oxygen at 2.8 ATA. *Undersea Biomed Res* 9:76, 1982.
24. Yamaki T, Ando S, Ohta K, et al: CT demonstration of massive cerebral air embolism from pulmonary barotrauma due to cardiopulmonary resuscitation. *J Comput Assist Tomogr* 13:313, 1989.
25. Haydon JR, Williamson JA, Ansford AJ, et al: A Scuba-diving fatality. *Med J Aust* 143:458, 1985.
26. Kizer KW: The role of computed tomography in the management of dysbaric diving accidents. *Radiology* 140:705, 1981.
27. Cucchiara RF, Nugent M, Seward JB, Messick JM: Air embolism in upright neurosurgical patients: Detection and localization by two-dimensional transesophageal echocardiography. *Anesthesiology* 60:353, 1984.
28. *U.S. Navy Diving Manual*. NAVSEA 00994–LP001–9010. U.S. Govt. Printing Office, Washington, DC, 1985, p 815.
29. Leitch DR, Greenbaum LJ, Hallenbeck JM: Cerebral air embolism: Is there a benefit in beginning HBO treatment at 6 bar? *Undersea Biomed Res* 11:237, 1984.
30. Catron PW, Dutka AJ, Biondi DM, et al: Cerebral air embolism treated by pressure and hyperbaric oxygen. *Neurology* 41:314, 1991.
31. Layton AJ: Hyperbaric oxygen treatment for cerebral air embolism: Where are the data? *Mayo Clin Proc* 66:641, 1991.
32. Dutka AJ, Mink R, McDermott J, et al: Effect of lidocaine on somatosensory evoked response and cerebral blood flow after canine cerebral air embolism. *Stroke* 23:1515, 1992.

33. Bitterman H, Melamed Y: Delayed hyperbaric treatment of cerebral air embolism. *Isr J Med Sci* 29:22, 1993.
34. Menasche P, Pinard E, Desroches AM, et al: Fluorocarbons: A potential treatment of cerebral air embolism in open-heart surgery. *Ann Thorac Surg* 40:494, 1985.
35. Pfitzner J, McLean AG: Controlled neck compression in neurosurgery: Studies on venous air embolism in upright sheep. *Anaesthesia* 40:624, 1985.
36. Toung TJ, Miyabe M, McShane AJ, et al: Effect of PEEP and jugular venous compression on canine cerebral blood flow and oxygen consumption in the head elevated position. *Anesthesiology* 68:53, 1988.
37. Toung T, Ngeow YK, Long DL, et al: Comparison of the effects of positive end-expiratory pressure and jugular venous compression on canine cerebral venous pressure. *Anesthesiology* 61:169, 1984.
38. Dutka AJ: A review of the pathophysiology and potential application of experimental therapies for cerebral ischemia to the treatment of cerebral arterial gas embolism. *Undersea Biomed Res* 12:403, 1985.
39. Bert P: Barometric pressure: Researches in experimental physiology. Translated by Hitchcock MA, Hitchcock FA. Columbus Book, 1943, reprinted Bethesda, Undersea Medical Society, 1978.
40. Harvey EN, Barnes DK, McElroy WD, et al: Bubble formation in animals. I. Physical factors. *J Cell Comp Physiol* 24:1, 1944.
41. Erdman S: Aeropathy of compressed air illness among tunnel workers. *JAMA* 49:1665, 1907.
42. Kety S: The theory and applications of the exchange of inert gas at the lungs and tissues. *Pharmacol Rev* 3:1, 1951.
43. Perl W, Rackow H, Salanitre E, et al: Intertissue diffusion effect for inert fat-soluble gases. *J Appl Physiol* 20:621, 1965.
44. Duling BR, Berne RM: Longitudinal gradients in periarteriolar oxygen tension. *Circ Res* 27:669, 1970.
45. Piiper J, Meyer M: Diffusion-perfusion relationships in skeletal muscle: Models and experimental evidence from inert gas washout. *Adv Exp Med Biol* 169:457, 1984.
46. Larson RT, Mazzone WF: Excursion diving from saturation exposures at depth, in Lambertsen CJ (ed): *Underwater Physiology III.* Baltimore, Williams & Wilkins, 1966, pp. 241–254.
47. Boycott AE, Damant GCC, Haldane J: The prevention of compressed air illness. *J Hyg* (Cambridge) 8:342, 1908.
48. Miller JW, Koblick IG: *Living and Working in the Sea.* New York, VanNostrand Reinhold, 1984, p. 227.
49. Hill L: *Caisson Sickness and the Physiology of Work in Compressed Air.* London, Arnold, 1912, pp 74–98.
50. Levy E: *Compressed-Air Illness and Its Engineering Importance with a Report of Cases at the East River Tunnels.* Dept. of the Interior, Bureau of Mines, Technical paper 285. Government Printing Office, Washington, DC, 1922.
51. Francis TJR, Dutka AJ, Hallenbeck JM: Pathophysiology of decompression sickness, in Bove AA, Davis JC (eds): *Diving Medicine.* Philadelphia, WB Saunders, 1990, pp 170–187.
52. Lynch JJ, Schuchard GH, Gross CM, Wann LS: Prevalence of right-to-left shunting in a healthy population: Detection by valsalva maneuver contrast echocardiography. *Circulation* 59:379, 1984.
53. Lechat PH, Mas JK, Lascault G, et al: Prevalence of patent foramen ovale in patients with stroke. *N Engl J Med* 318:1148, 1988.
54. Greer HD, Massey EW: Neurologic injury from undersea diving. *Neurol Clin* 10:1031, 1992.
55. Rudge FW, Shafer MR: The effect of delay on treatment outcome in altitude-induced decompression sickness. *Aviat Space Environ Med* 62:687, 1991.
56. Elliott DH, Hallenbeck JM, Bove AA: Acute decompression sickness. *Lancet* 2:1193, 1974.
57. Neuman TS, Spragg RG, Howard R, Moser KM: Cardiopulmonary consequences of decompression stress. *Am Rev Respir Dis* 128:552, 1983.
58. Erde A, Edmonds C: Decompression sickness: A clinical series. *J Ocup Med* 17:324, 1975.
59. Golding FC, Griffiths P, Hempleman HV, et al: Decompression sickness during the construction of the Dartforth tunnel. *Br J Ind Med* 17:167, 1960.
60. Hallenbeck JM, Bove AA, Moquin R, Elliott DE: Accelerated coagulation of whole blood and cell free plasma by bubbling in vitro. *Aerospace Med* 44:712, 1973.
61. Bove AA: Basis for drug therapy in decompression sickness. *Undersea Biomed Res* 9:91, 1982.
62. Cockett TK, Nakamura RM, Kado RT: Physiologic factors in decompression sickness. *Arch Environ Health* 11:760, 1965.
63. Bove AA, Hallenbeck JM: Changes in blood and plasma volumes in dogs during decompression sickness. *Aerospace Med* 45:49, 1974.
64. Philp RB, Inwood MJ, Warren BA: Interaction between gas bubbles and components of the blood: Implications in decompression sickness. *Aerospace Med* 43:946, 1972.
65. Levin LL, Stewart GJ, Lynch PR, Bove AA: Blood and blood vessel wall changes induced by decompression sickness in dogs. *J Appl Physiol* 50:944, 1981.
66. Hallenbeck JM, Bove AA, Elliott DH: Mechanisms underlying spinal cord damage in decompression sickness. *Neurology* 25:308, 1975.
67. Nix WA, Hopf HC: Central nervous system damage after decompression accidents. *Duetsch Med Wochenschr* 105:302, 1980.
68. Norman JN, Childs CM, Jones C, et al: Management of a complex diving accident. *Undersea Biomed Res* 6:209, 1979.
69. Workman RD: Treatment of bends with oxygen at high pressure. *Aerospace Med* 39:1076, 1968.
70. Elliott DH: The role of decompression inadequacy in aseptic bone necrosis of naval divers. *Proc R Soc Med* 64:1278, 1971.
71. McCallum RI, Walder DN: Bone lesions in compressed air workers. *J Bone Joint Surg* 48B:207, 1966.
72. Farmer JC, Thomas WG, Youngblood DG, Bennett PB: Inner ear decompression sickness. *Laryngoscope* 86:1315, 1976.
73. Neuman TS, Bove AA: Combined arterial gas embolism and decompression sickness following no-stop dives. *Undersea Biomed Res* 17:429, 1990.
74. Davis JC: Treatment of decompression sickness and arterial gas embolism, in Bove AA, Davis JC (eds): *Diving Medicine.* Philadelphia, WB Saunders, 1990, pp 249–260.

69. Respiratory Adjunct Therapy

Richard S. Irwin, Cynthia T. French, and
Ronald W. Mike

Introduction

Respiratory adjunct therapy discussed in this chapter includes the delivery of aerosolized drugs, lung expansion techniques, augmentation of mucociliary clearance, augmentation of cough effectiveness, administration of oxygen, administration of helium-oxygen (heliox), and nasal continuous positive airway pressure (CPAP)/ bilevel positive airway pressure (BiPAP).

Aerosol Therapy

An aerosol is a stable suspension of particulates of solid and/ or liquid form in air. Although they can be used in provocative tests in the diagnosis of asthma, administration of contrast substances for radiologic studies, and administration of tagged substances in studies of pulmonary deposition and clearance of particles [1], it is their therapeutic uses that are discussed in this section.

MODE OF DELIVERY. Aerosolized drugs can be delivered by handheld metered-dose inhalers (Fig. 69-1A and B), intermittent positive-pressure breathing (IPPB) devices (Fig. 69-1C), simple aerosol units (nebulizer devices that produce an aerosol by constant gas flow without pressure regulation) (Fig. 69-1D), or inhalation of fine powder. When used by properly trained patients and taken in equivalent doses, bronchodilator aerosols administered by metered-dose inhalers (MDIs) are as effective as those delivered by other aerosol generators. This has been demonstrated in ambulatory chronic obstructive pulmonary disease (COPD) patients and asthmatics [2,3], non-ICU hospitalized patients with airflow obstruction [4,5,6], and acutely ill asthmatics in the emergency department [7,8,9]. For those patients who are unable to use their MDI properly due to poor hand-breath coordination or handicaps, reliable aerosol delivery can usually be achieved with the use of an aerosol holding chamber that attaches to the MDI [3,10] (Fig. 69-1B). Therefore, in spontaneously breathing patients, bronchodilators should be prescribed by MDI whenever possible, since this mode of delivery is less expensive than small-volume nebulizer delivery. While powdered albuterol inhaled from a Rotahaler appears to be as effective as that delivered by MDI and small-volume nebulizer in stable patients when given in equivalent doses, it may not be effective in patients with very low inspiratory flow rates.

In intubated and mechanically ventilated patients, aerosols can also be delivered by small-volume sidestream nebulizers connected to the inspiratory tubing (Fig. 69-1E) as well as MDI with an aerosol holding chamber (Fig. 69-1F). Since studies have either shown these two methods to be equivalent in delivering bronchodilator to the lungs or the MDI holding chamber method to be superior [11,12], we prefer the MDI system.

TYPES OF AEROSOLS

Bland. Water and hypotonic, normotonic, and hypertonic saline are all considered bland aerosols. Theoretical reasons for their use are to (1) humidify inspired gas, (2) hydrate dry mucosal surfaces in patients with inflamed upper airways (vocal cords and above), (3) improve expectoration of lower airway secretions, and (4) induce sputum expectoration for diagnostic purposes [13].

Aerosols of water are effective in humidifying inspired gas. In contradistinction to nonintubated patients, in whom humidification is largely superfluous (gas is adequately humidified by the upper respiratory tract) [14–17], for intubated patients humidification of inspired gases is imperative. This relates to the fact that the endotracheal or tracheostomy tubes bypass the structures of the upper airway, whose function is to warm and humidify inspired gases. Although studies have documented that inspired gases with a relative humidity of 60 percent at room temperature (22-26°C) are sufficiently humidified to prevent mucosal damage during anesthesia [18], gases that are fully saturated at 32°C are required to prevent postoperative complications due to mucosal drying [19].

Although adequate humidification is important and beneficial in intubated patients, routine use of bland aerosols has not been shown to be beneficial in the treatment of upper or lower airway diseases. (This includes mist tent therapy in patients with cystic fibrosis [13].) Moreover, bland aerosols may provoke bronchospasm in nonintubated and intubated asthmatic patients and in intubated nonasthmatic patients [13].

Mucolytic. Theoretically, mucolytic agents facilitate expectoration of excessive lower airway secretions and improve lung function [13]. Although N-acetylcysteine (Mucomyst), the prototypic mucolytic agent, liquifies inspissated mucous plugs when administered by direct intratracheal instillation [20], it is of questionable clinical use when administered as an aerosol to nonintubated patients, since very little of it is actually delivered to the lower respiratory tract. Because mucolytic instillations or aerosols can induce bronchospasm in patients with airway disease [21,22,23] (especially asthma), they should be administered to these patients in combination with a bronchodilator [13]. Recombinant human DNase (rh DNase) (Pulmozyme, Genentech, South San Francisco, CA), when given as an aerosol, in a dose of 2.5 mg once or twice a day to patients with cystic fibrosis, decreased moderately and significantly dyspnea, symptoms of cystic fibrosis, and costs related to exacerbations of respiratory symptoms [23a]. Overall well-being and FEV_1 also modestly improved during this 24-week study.

Antimicrobial. Although endotracheal instillation and aerosolization of antimicrobial solutions has been successfully used in tracheotomized patients and patients with cystic fibrosis with tracheobronchial infections and colonization [24,25], there is little evidence to support the use of aerosolized antibiotics for acute bacterial pneumonia. On the other hand, ribavirin (Virazole) aerosol is recommended for patients with respiratory syncytial virus infection and severe lower respiratory tract disease or infants with chronic underlying conditions such as cardiac disease, pulmonary disease, or a history of prematurity [26]. Because the long-term effects of this drug to health care workers is unknown, conservative safety practices must be followed [27].

Although preliminary studies in patients with acquired im-

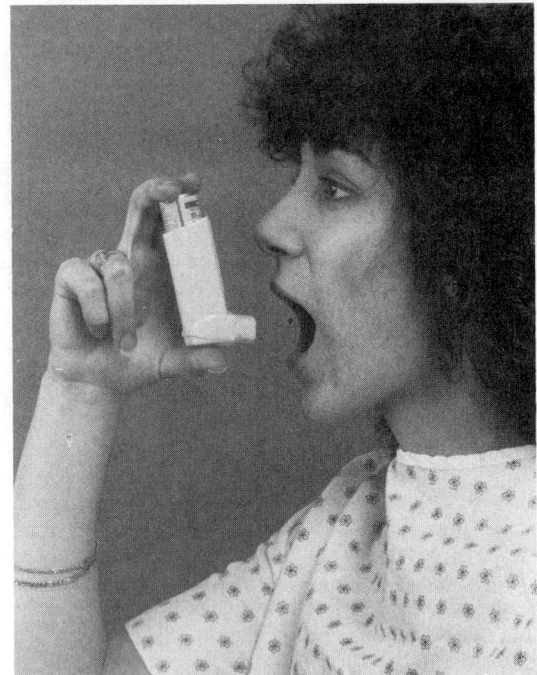

A

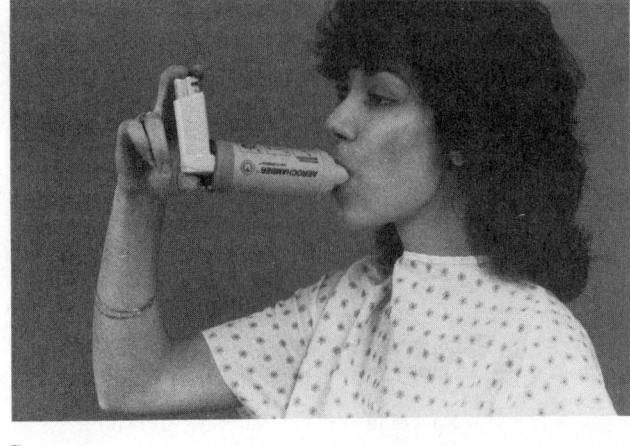

B

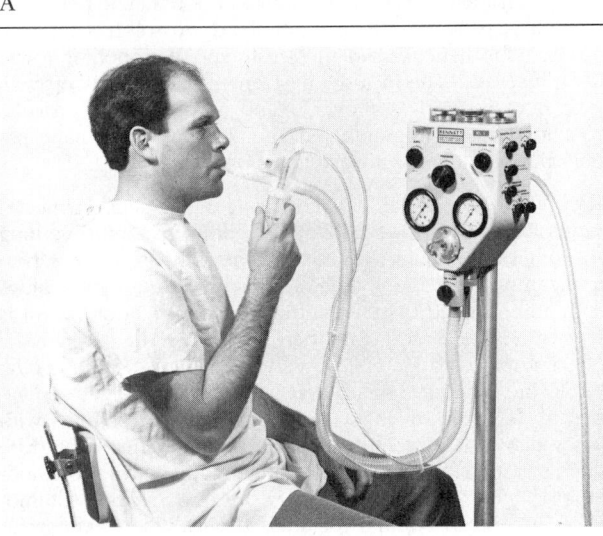

C

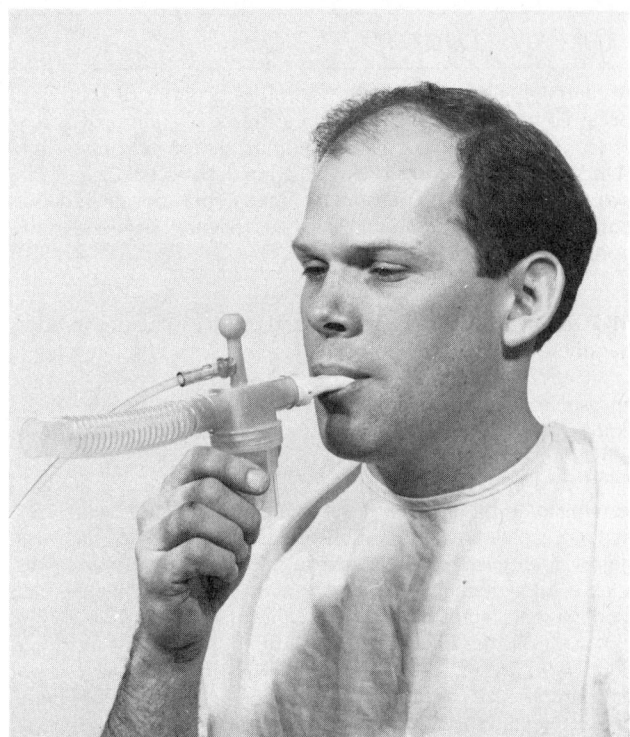

D

Fig. 69-1. Modes of delivering aerosolized drugs. A. Hand-held metered dose dispenser. Proper use requires patient coordination, training, and retraining. B. Hand-held metered dose dispenser attached to reservoir, inhalation aid. The reservoir device assists individuals who have problems with aim and/or coordination. A slow, steady, complete inhalation and 10-second breath hold are required for proper use of metered dose inhaler. The reservoir may also reduce cough and dysphonia secondary to upper airway irritation when the metered dose inhaler is used alone. C. Intermittent positive-pressure breathing (IPPB) device (PR-2, Bennett Respiration Products, Santa Monica, CA). Requires patient coordination and training and the

presence of a respiratory therapist or nurse familiar with the proper use of the machine. D. Simple aerosol unit. Requires patient cooperation and the presence of a respiratory therapist or nurse familiar with its proper use. E. Sidestream nebulizer *(arrow)* is incorporated into disposable tubing that makes up the inspiratory circuit of the ventilator. Nebulizer contents are delivered as a mist to the patient with inspiratory flow. F. Metered dose inhaler cannister with stem (top arrow) inserted into aerosol holding chamber (bottom arrow) (Monaghan Medical Corp., Plattsburgh, NY) that has been incorporated in-line into the inspiratory circuit of the ventilator.

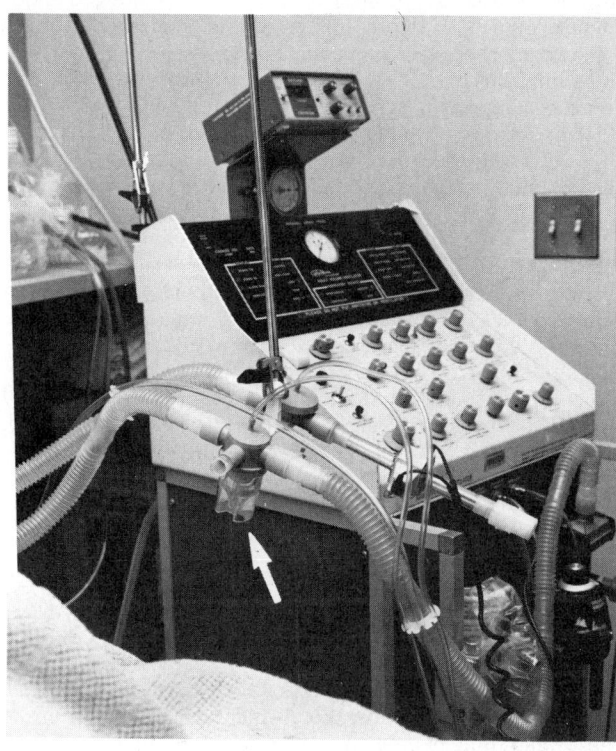

E

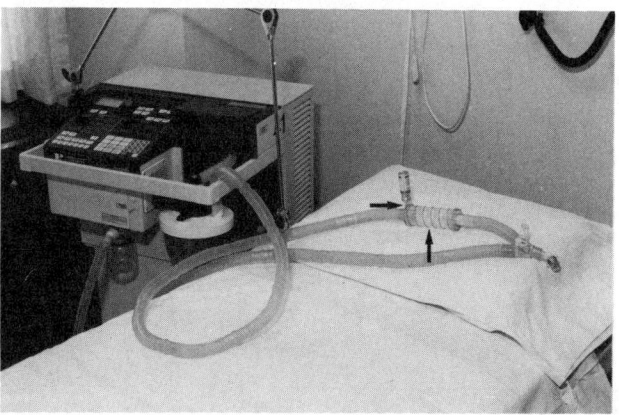

F

munodeficiency syndrome (AIDS) suggest that aerosolized pentamidine can be effective and well tolerated in mild *Pneumocystis carinii* pneumonia (PCP), it is not recommended for routine clinical practice [28]. Trimethoprim-sulfamethoxazole is the preferred therapy for all patients who can tolerate it; parenteral pentamidine has been considered the second therapeutic choice [28]. While aerosolized pentamidine has been used with success for primary and secondary PCP prophylaxis [28], trimethoprim-sulfamethoxazole was recently recommended as the drug of choice for prophylaxis in both situations. Aerosolized pentamidine will still be used but less often. Aerosolized pentamidine (NebuPent; 300 mg reconstituted with sterile water every 4 weeks), delivered by a Respirgard II nebulizer (Marquest) has been approved for PCP prophylaxis [28]. Because toxicity studies on the second-hand effects of aerosolized pentamidine exposure on health care personnel are limited, conservative safety practices must be followed.

Corticosteroid. At present, there is no indication for the use of corticosteroid aerosols in the critically ill patient.

Racemic Epinephrine. Racemic epinephrine (Racepinephrine) is effective in decreasing laryngeal edema by causing vasoconstriction [29]. The usual adult dose is 0.5 ml of a 2.25% solution diluted in 3 ml of normal saline every 4 to 6 hours. Because rebound edema frequently occurs, patients must be observed closely; because tachycardia is common during treatment, it may precipitate angina in patients with coronary artery disease [30]. The role of racemic epinephrine aerosol in epiglottitis is not known. Since racemic epinephrine aerosol is frequently associated with potentially serious side effects, administration by inhalation of mixtures of helium and oxygen should be considered first to decrease airway resistance and therefore the work of breathing associated with laryngeal edema or other upper airway diseases. (See Helium-Oxygen Administration.)

Selective Beta$_2$ Sympathomimetics. Because of their significantly longer bronchodilator effects and far fewer cardiovascular side effects (compared to isoproterenol) [31], beta$_2$ sympathomimetics such as metaproterenol and albuterol are the agents of choice for bronchodilatation and mucociliary escalation. When given by jet nebulizer, the usual adult dose of metaproterenol (Alupent) is 0.3 ml of a 5% solution (15 mg) diluted in 2.5 ml of saline and of albuterol (Proventil) is 0.5 ml of a 0.5% solution (2.5 mg) diluted in 2.5 ml of saline (or 3 ml of 0.083% unit dose nebulizer solution). The frequency of dosing varies depending on the disease and the situation. It can vary from every 4 to 6 hours in patients with COPD and stable asthma to every 20 to 30 minutes for six doses in patients with status asthmaticus [9,32]. Albuterol solution has also been continuously nebulized to patients with acute asthma for 2 hours [33].

Although the usual dosage of bronchodilator by MDI is two puffs (90 micrograms/puff) every 4 to 6 hours in stable hospitalized and ambulatory adult patients, the dosage must be increased up to sixfold in acute, severe asthma to achieve results equivalent to those achieved with small-volume nebulizers [3,7]. In a recently published emergency department treatment study of severe asthma, four puffs of albuteral by MDI every 30 minutes for a total of six dosing intervals (24 puffs) was found to be safe and equivalent to 2.5 mg of albuteral diluted in 2 ml of saline given every 30 minutes for 6 doses [9]. Others have treated acute episodes of asthma in the emergency department in a dose-to-result fashion as follows: initially four puffs of MDI of bronchodilator of choice, followed by one additional puff every minute until the patient subjectively or objectively improves or side effects (e.g., tremor, tachycardia, arrhythmia) occur [7].

If large and frequent doses of beta-agonists are given, ECG and serum potassium monitoring are indicated. Nebulized albuterol can cause a prompt and significant decrease in plasma potassium concentration that is evident at 30 minutes and sustained for at least 2 hours [34]. After 10-mg and 20-mg doses, the maximal decreases can be 0.62 ± 0.09 and 0.98 ± 0.14 mmol per liter, respectively [34]. For further discussion of aerosolized beta-agonists, see Chapters 56 and 57.

Anticholinergics. These agents have a role in acute asthma when combined with sympathomimetic drugs [35]; in exacerbations of COPD when given alone [35]; in intubated patients to prevent bradycardia induced by suctioning [36]; and in selected patients with severe bronchorrhea [37]. The usual adult dose of atropine sulfate is 0.05 mg per kilogram ideal body weight by jet nebulizer every 6 hours and of ipratropium bromide is 500 meg in 2.5 ml normal saline (1 unit 0.02% unit dose vial) or 2 puffs by MDI (18 micrograms/puff) every 6 hours. Ipratropium by MDI can be given to ventilated patients with the same spacer device used for beta-agonist delivery. For further discussion of their use, see Chapters 56 and 57.

Lung Expansion Techniques

A lung expansion technique is any technique that increases lung volume or assists the patient in increasing lung volume above that reached at his or her usual unassisted or uncoached inspiration. Lung expansion techniques are meant to duplicate a normal sigh maneuver [38]. Theoretically, sighs or periodic hyperinflations to near total lung capacity reverse microatelectasis [38].

Lung expansion techniques are indicated to prevent atelectasis and pneumonia in patients who cannot or will not take periodic hyperinflations [38], such as postoperative upper abdominal and thoracic surgical patients and patients with respiratory disorders due to neuromuscular and chest wall diseases. Adequately performed, maximum inspirations 10 times each hour while awake significantly decrease the incidence of pulmonary complications following laparotomy [39]. Whatever technique is used postoperatively (e.g., coached, sustained maximal inspiration with cough; incentive spirometry; volume-oriented IPPB; intermittent CPAP; or positive expiratory pressure (PEP) mask therapy [40]), it should be taught and practiced preoperatively. When properly used, coached, sustained maximal inspiration with cough and incentive spirometry—the least expensive and safest techniques—are as effective as any other method [41]. Of the several commercially available incentive spirometers, the one chosen should combine accuracy, low price, and maximum patient accessibility [42]. Because there are no definitive studies comparing the relative efficacy of volume- and flow-oriented incentive spirometers, the choice of equipment must be based on empiric assessment of patient acceptance, ease of use, and cost. When chest percussion with postural drainage is added to the above expansion techniques in patients without prior lung disease, it has failed to affect the incidence of postoperative pulmonary complications [43].

Augmentation of Mucociliary Clearance

Ineffective mucociliary clearance leads to retention of tracheobronchial secretions. Mucociliary clearance may be ineffective due to depression of the clearance mechanisms and/or oversecretion in the face of normal mucous transport. Mucus is undercleared and overproduced in smokers with or without chronic bronchitis and in asthmatic patients [44,45]. It is undercleared in emphysema, bronchiectasis, and cystic fibrosis; during and 4 to 6 weeks after viral upper respiratory tract infections; during and for an unknown period after general anesthesia due to the inhalation of dry gas and cuffed endotra-

cheal tubes used during surgery; and during prolonged endotracheal intubation due to the presence of the cuffed tube, administration of elevated concentrations of inspired oxygen, and damage to the tracheobronchial tree from suctioning [45]. The most important consideration in improving mucociliary clearance is to remove the above inciting causes of underclearance and overproduction of secretions. Mucociliary clearance can be enhanced pharmacologically and mechanically.

PHARMACOLOGIC AUGMENTATION. Beta agonists [44–48], and aminophylline [49] all speed up mucous transport in patients with various chronic obstructive lung diseases. These drugs should be given in the same dose as given for bronchodilatation. Mucolytics and expectorants (e.g., potassium iodide, glyceryl guaiacolate, ammonium chloride, creosote, cocillana) have not been shown to increase mucociliary clearance [13,50]. While iodinated glycerol (iodopropylidene glycerol) is an effective antitussive drug in patients with chronic bronchitis and asthma [57], it is unclear whether this effect was achieved by augmenting mucociliary clearance.

MECHANICAL AUGMENTATION

Chest Physiotherapy. Usually chest physiotherapy includes a combination of some or all of therapeutic positioning, percussion to the chest wall over the affected area, vibration of the chest wall during expiration, and coughing. Coughing appears to be the most important component of chest physiotherapy (see Augmentation of Couth Effectiveness). It is beneficial in patients with cystic fibrosis and bronchiectasis and in the unusual COPD patient who expectorates more than 30 ml of sputum each day [52] and also is indicated in lobar atelectasis [53]. It is not indicated in asthmatic patients [52] or those with uncomplicated pneumonias [54]. Complications of chest physiotherapy are infrequent yet potentially severe [55]. They include massive pulmonary hemorrhage (perhaps caused by clots dislodged during percussion), decreased PaO_2 from positioning the "bad" lung down in spontaneously breathing patients, rib fractures, increased intracranial pressure, decreased cardiac output, and decreased FEV_1.

Two new alternatives to chest physiotherapy have shown promise in augmenting large volume secretion removal in patients with cystic fibrosis, chronic bronchitis, and bronchiectasis. They are PEP mask therapy and autogenic drainage (AD). In PEP therapy, a mask is applied tightly over the mouth and nose and a variable flow resistor adjusted to achieve a PEP during exhalation between 10 and 20 cm H_2O. This combined with "huff" coughing allows mobilization of peripherally located secretions upward into larger airways. A review of this form of therapy can be found elsewhere [40]. Autogenic drainage is a secretion-clearing technique that combines variable tidal breathing at three distinct lung volume levels, controlled expiratory airflow, and huff coughing [56]. Future studies should better delineate the relative roles of conventional chest physiotherapy, PEP mask therapy, and AD in the removal of excessive secretions. A meta-analysis of randomized trials from 1966 to 1993 in patients with cystic fibrosis revealed that only standard chest physiotherapy resulted in significantly greater sputum expectoration than no treatment [56a].

Suctioning. Mechanical aspiration or suctioning is routine in most hospitals. Unfortunately, many are unaware of the numerous potential complications associated with suctioning, such as tissue trauma, laryngospasm, bronchospasm, hypoxemia, cardiac arrhythmias, respiratory arrest, cardiac arrest, atelectasis, pneumonia, misdirection of catheter, and death [57,58]. Complications are generally avoidable or reversible if proper technique and indications are adhered to strictly.

NASOTRACHEAL. Nasotracheal suctioning is rarely indicated because chest physiotherapy can be used in conscious patients and semicomatose or comatose patients with retained secretions can be intubated. Nasotracheal suctioning has been associated with fatal cardiac arrest [59] and life-threatening arrhythmias [60], presumably due to hypoxemia [61], and with bacteremia [62]. Since quantitative cultures obtained with plugged telescoping catheters at bronchoscopy can be obtained more safely and are definitely more reliable than nasotracheal suction (see Chap. 12) in obtaining uncontaminated lower respiratory tract secretions for culture, nasotracheal suction is not recommended for this purpose.

In those occasional situations in which nasotracheal suctioning may be indicated (conscious patients who cannot or will not cooperate for chest physiotherapy), it should be carried out, preferably in the presence of a physician, as follows:

1. Connect the patient to a source of pure oxygen for a few minutes before and after nasotracheal suctioning. Preoxygenation prevents or minimizes hypoxemia and its risks during the procedure [61]. Postoxygenation minimizes hypoxemia after the procedure and hastens the desaturation recovery period [63].

2. Dip the tip of the suction catheter into a water-soluble anesthetic such as viscous lidocaine (Xylocaine) or lidocaine jelly. Insert the tip of the suction catheter into the nostril and direct it along an inferior and medial path so that it tends to follow the floor of the nasal cavity. Advance the catheter through the nasal cavity with a smooth motion, avoiding poking or prodding the sensitive mucosa. Introduce the catheter along an inferior and medial course and use the catheter's natural droop to facilitate entry.

3. Slight difficulty is sometimes encountered when the catheter tip impinges on the posterior wall of the pharynx. When this occurs, extend the patient's neck and then rotate the catheter between the fingers while gently advancing it to promote inferior deflection toward the vocal cords.

4. Advance the catheter its full length or until it becomes impacted within the bronchus. Place the proximal end of the catheter close to your ear and listen for referred sounds of tidal breathing to confirm that the catheter has entered the trachea instead of the esophagus.

5. Withdraw the catheter a few centimeters, connect it to the suction line, and apply intermittent suction by intermittently occluding the sideport of the catheter.

6. Limit the suctioning attempt to 15 seconds. Perform passive hyperinflation with a manual resuscitator after suctioning to reverse any atelectasis that might have resulted from the procedure. Deliver five such deep breaths, sustaining each breath for about 1 second before allowing the lungs to deflate passively.

7. Rinse the suction line with water and discard the catheter.

NASOPHARYNGEAL. Nasopharyngeal suction is indicated to clear the upper airway. Because the catheter does not reach the vocal cords or enter the trachea, nasopharyngeal suctioning is associated with far less frequent and less serious complications than nasotracheal suctioning [57]. The catheter should not touch or go past the vocal cords. This requires the operator to insert the catheter to a depth that corresponds to the distance between the middle of the patient's chin and the angle of the jaw, just below the earlobe.

ENDOTRACHEAL. Endotracheal suction should be employed only when there is definite evidence of excessive retained se-

cretions. Routine suctioning according to a predetermined schedule causes excessive mucosal damage [64], excessive impairment of mucociliary clearance [65], excessive exposure to the potential risks of hypoxemia associated with the procedure [66,67], atelectasis [68], and bronchoconstriction [69]. The following guidelines should be observed to minimize these complications.

INTERRUPTED VENTILATOR SUCTIONING

1. Preoxygenate the patient with six extra ventilator breaths administered 3 to 5 seconds apart and at the tidal volume set on the ventilator and 100% oxygen [63] before suctioning begins.

2. Strictly observe aseptic technique by donning sterile gloves over freshly washed hands and using a sterile suction catheter.

3. After detaching the ventilator, introduce the catheter smoothly, using firm, gentle pressure without active suction.

4. Withdraw the catheter a few centimeters after it is observed to impact.

5. Apply active suction by intermittently occluding the thumb port.

6. Limit each pass of the catheter to 15 seconds or less.

7. To ensure almost uniform entry of the left bronchial tree, use a curve-tipped catheter properly [70]. Left bronchial tree entry is less reliable if using a straight catheter, but entry is more successful if the patient's head is turned to the right [71].

8. Postoxygenate the patient with the same six extra ventilator breaths with 100% oxygen [63].

9. Reinstate baseline inspired oxygen concentration.

10. Patients on positive end-expiratory pressure (PEEP) ideally should not be taken off the ventilator and therefore off PEEP during suctioning. For this reason and reasons discussed below, consider routine use of a closed suctioning system in patients on ventilators.

CONTINUOUS VENTILATOR SUCTIONING (CLOSED SYSTEM)

1. Attach an adapter (see Chap. 12) that allows insertion of a suction catheter into the endotracheal tube during mechanical ventilation or use a commercially available closed catheter system.

2. Using the technique outlined for interrupted ventilator suctioning, suction through the adaptor while the patient remains connected to the ventilator without any extra breaths or changes in ventilator settings [63]. While suctioning-related arterial oxygen desaturation is minimized when using closed system suctioning with an intermittent mandatory ventilation (IMV) mode with continuous free flow of gas [63], its efficacy with other ventilatory modes is unknown [72]. To ensure adequate oxygenation during suctioning, monitor oxygen saturation. Single-use disposable catheters without protective sheath and multiple-use disposable catheters with protective sheath can be used in closed tracheal suction systems [63,73]. The latter has its own adaptor and can be left in line and discarded after 24 hours [73]. While the multiple-use catheter with protective sheath (TrachCare) also theoretically prevents cross-contamination between patients, prevents contamination of the lower respiratory tract by environment organisms, may protect health care workers from contamination with infected secretions, and lowers cost, these potential advantages await substantiation in prospective, randomized studies [74].

ENDOTRACHEAL EXTUBATION. Just before endotracheal extubation, perform the following suction procedure.

1. Perform naso- and oropharyngeal suction to aspirate secretions that have pooled above the inflated cuff.

2. Replace the catheter with a fresh sterile one.
3. Perform endotracheal suction as described above.
4. In preparation for deflating the cuff, place the endotracheal suction catheter tip just distal to the endotracheal tube to aspirate any secretions that gravitate downward when the cuff is deflated.
5. Deflate the cuff.
6. Intermittently suction while removing the tube and catheter as a unit.

Augmentation of Cough Effectiveness

GENERAL CONSIDERATIONS. While mucociliary transport is the major method of clearing the airway in healthy subjects, cough is an important reserve mechanism, especially in lung disease [75]. Mucociliary clearance is impaired in many lung diseases, and cough is necessary to remove the increased secretions and debris. The role of cough can be assessed by comparing mucociliary clearance of inhaled radiolabelled tracers in patients with cough and in those who cough either spontaneously or voluntarily. For example, Puchelle et al. [76] showed that healthy subjects have twice the rate of mucociliary clearance of that in patients with chronic bronchitis, but that when cough is permitted or encouraged the patients increase their clearance by 20 percent whereas healthy subjects increase clearance by only 2.5 percent. Similar results have been obtained by others. Thus, all studies suggest that cough is effective in causing clearance only if secretions are excessive.

PATHOPHYSIOLOGY OF INEFFECTIVE COUGH. As a defense mechanism, cough has two main functions: to prevent foreign material from entering the lower respiratory tract and to clear foreign material and excessive secretions from the lower respiratory tract. When cough inadequately serves its protective roles, atelectasis, gas-exchange abnormalities, pneumonia, and bronchiectasis may ensue.

The effectiveness of cough in clearing an airway theoretically depends on the presence of secretions of sufficient thickness to be affected by two-phase gas-liquid flow and the linear velocity of air moving through its lumen [77]. The ineffectiveness of voluntary coughing in normal subjects to clear tagged aerosol particles in the lower airways is probably due to the inability of the moving airstream to interact appropriately with the normally thin mucus layer upon which the particles were deposited [78]. Once there is sufficiently thick material in the airways the effectiveness of cough depends on achieving a high flow rate of air and a small cross-sectional area of the airway during the expiratory phase of cough to achieve a high linear velocity. Since

$$Velocity = \frac{Flow}{Cross\text{-}sectional\ area}$$

any condition associated with decreased expiratory flow rates or reduced ability to compress airways dynamically will place affected patients at risk of having an ineffective cough.

All conditions that may lead to an ineffective cough interfere with either the inspiratory or expiratory phases of cough; most conditions affect both. Cough effectiveness is likely to be most impaired in patients with respiratory muscle weakness, since the abilities to take a deep breath in (flow rates are highest at

high lung volumes) and to compress their airways dynamically during expiration are both impaired, placing them at double liability. Disorders or interventions that predominantly affect the compressive phase of cough are probably not clinically important. For instance, although glottic closure is an integral part of the compressive phase, it is not essential for the production of an effective cough pressure [79]. The muscles of expiration appear to be the most important determinant in producing elevated intrathoracic pressures, and they are capable of doing so even with an endotracheal tube in place [80]. Therefore, tracheostomy is not necessary in the intubated patient to increase cough effectiveness.

ASSESSMENT OF COUGH EFFECTIVENESS. Ideally, clinicians would like to predict clinically or physiologically when a given patient is at risk of developing atelectasis, pneumonia, or gas-exchange abnormalities because of an ineffective cough. Unfortunately, there are no such studies. The existing data that relate to assessment of cough effectiveness were generated in patients with muscular dystrophy [81] and myasthenia gravis [82]. These studies suggested that maximum expiratory mouth pressure (MEP) measurements may be useful for assessing cough strength, but they did not correlate these measurements with any clinical outcomes. Using the absence of peak flow transients during cough flow-volume curves as an indication that expiratory muscle strength during coughing was not adequate to compress the airways dynamically, investigators [81] found that MEP was the most sensitive predictor of flow transient production during coughing. All patients who could produce cough transients had MEP values greater than 60 cm H_2O; those who could not produce transients had MEP values of 45 or less. This latter value is consistent with the clinical observations of Gracey et al. [82] in patients with myasthenia gravis that MEP values less than 40 cm H_2O were frequently associated with difficulty in raising secretions without suctioning.

PROTUSSIVE THERAPY. When cough performs a useful function and is inadequate, protussive therapy may be indicated. The goal of protussive therapy is to increase cough effectiveness with or without increasing cough frequency. It can be of a pharmaceutical or mechanical nature.

Only a small number of pharmacologic agents have been adequately evaluated as protussive agents [51]. Of these, aerosolized hypertonic saline in patients with chronic bronchitis and amiloride aerosol in patients with cystic fibrosis have been shown to improve cough clearance [51]. While aerosolized ipratropium bromide diminished the effectiveness of cough for clearing radiolabeled particles from the airways in COPD [51a], aerosolized terbutaline following chest physiotherapy significantly increased cough clearance in patients with bronchiectasis [51b]. The divergent results with these two different types of bronchodilators suggest that terbutaline achieved its favorable effect by increasing hydration of mucus or enhancing ciliary beating, and these overcame any negative effects that bronchodilation had on cough clearance. If bronchodilators result in too much smooth muscle relaxation of large airways, flow rates can actually decrease even in healthy individuals when more complaint large airways narrow too much because they cannot withstand dynamic compression during forced expirations [51c]. Although hypertonic saline, amiloride, and terbutaline by aerosol following chest physiotherapy have been shown to increase cough clearance, their clinical utility remains to be determined in future studies that assess short- and long-term effects of these agents on the patient's condition.

Although several agents, such as inhaled citric acid, have

been used in studies to increase cough frequency to evaluate antitussives [51], these agents have not been studied with respect to their clinical utility.

A variety of mechanical measures have been advocated as possible therapies to improve cough effectiveness [51]. These include positive insufflation followed by manual compression of the lower thorax and abdomen in quadriparetic patients; an abdominal push maneuver that assists expiratory efforts in patients with spinal cord injuries; abdominal binding and muscle training of the clavicular portion of the pectoralis major in tetraplegic patients; and chest physiotherapy in patients with chronic bronchitis. The usefulness of the first three measures in improving clinical outcomes has yet to be studied. In patients with chronic bronchitis, the combination of short bouts of PEP breathing, forced expirations, and chest physiotherapy resulted in reduced coughing, less mucus production, and fewer acute exacerbations compared with patients who received chest physiotherapy alone. There is no clear benefit of combining chest physiotherapy with coughing over vigorous coughing alone [51].

Oxygen Therapy

Administration of supplemental oxygen is indicated for acute myocardial infarction, bronchial asthma, sickle cell crisis, carbon monoxide poisoning, gas gangrene, and cluster headaches, as well as respiratory failure.

HYPERCAPNIC RESPIRATORY FAILURE. In this setting (PaO_2 <55 mm Hg; $PaCO_2$ >46 mm Hg) the goal of oxygen therapy is to increase PaO_2 to 55 to 60 mm Hg [82]. This level of arterial oxygenation is sufficient to achieve an oxyhemoglobin saturation of 88 to 90 percent and to avoid or potentially reverse vasoconstrictive pulmonary hypertension and cor pulmonale [84,85]. However, the presence of hypercapnia should alert one to the possibility that too much oxygen may lead to CO_2 narcosis [86]. The mechanism by which oxygen administration results in CO_2 elevation in patients with COPD is multifactorial. It (1) cannot be explained solely by the effect of oxygen on ventilatory drives, (2) includes an oxygen-induced increase in dead space resulting from relaxation of hypoxic vasoconstriction, and (3) also requires the presence of other abnormalities (e.g., respiratory muscles, hypoxic drive, and/or lung elastic recoil) preventing compensatory hyperventilation [86a,86b,86c]. While CO_2 narcosis uncommonly occurs, the possibility should not be dismissed. Consequently, care should be taken to avoid the administration of excessively rich oxygen mixtures. Barring abrupt decompensation (sudden hypotension or arrhythmias, acute deterioration in mental status, imminent respiratory, or cardiac arrest), for which intubation and mechanical ventilatory support must be employed, controlled low-flow therapy must be used [86,87]. This consists of the provision of gas with a relatively low concentration of oxygen. To minimize the risk of inducing CO_2 narcosis, oxygen must be administered incrementally beginning with low concentrations [88]. (See Chap. 57 for further discussion of oxygen therapy in COPD.)

Devices. Two commonly used devices (Fig. 69-2) can be used for low-flow delivery. The first is the Venturi mask (Table 69-1). This device is driven by pure oxygen and entrains varying amounts of room air. It consequently floods the patient's face with gas of a precisely calibrated concentration of from 24 to 50 percent oxygen [87,89].

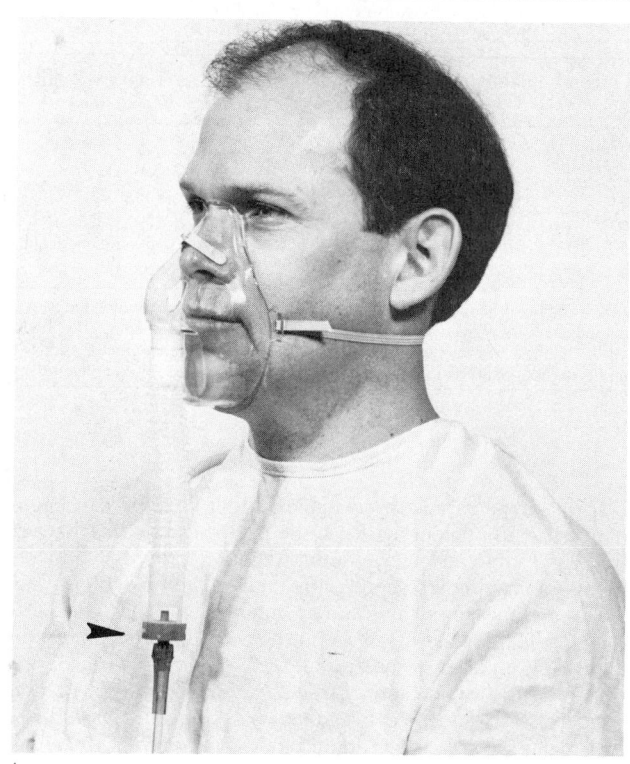

A

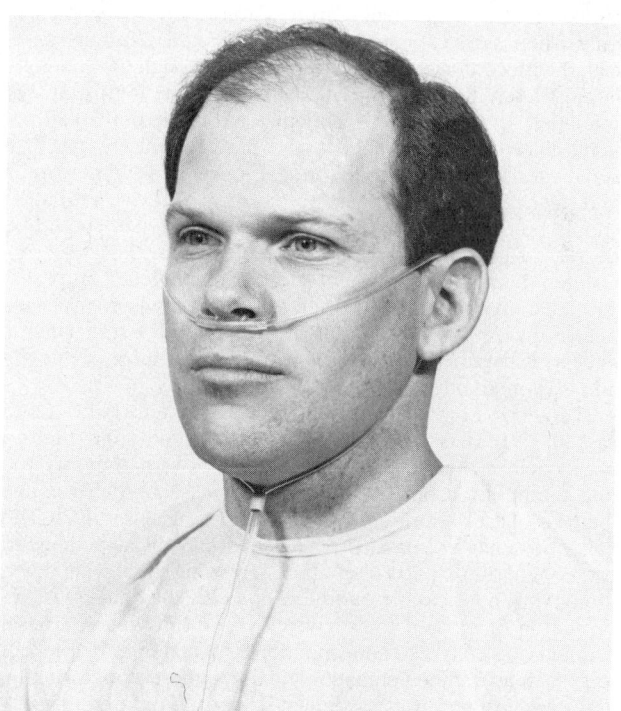

B

Fig. 69-2. A. The Venturi mask. This model (Inspiron Accurox, Rancho Cucamonga, CA) accurately supplies oxygen concentrations of 24% to 50% by means of interchangeable entrainment nozzles (*arrow*) as long as the mask is properly fitted and the patient's inspiratory flow demands are met. B. Nasal cannula (nasal prong). Although this device is less accurate and reliable than Venturi masks, it is more comfortable and allows the patient to eat. It adequately delivers oxygen even in patients who are "mouth breathers."

Table 69-1. Air Entrainment Ratios and Total Gas Outflows of Commercially Available Venturi Masks

O_2 concentration of delivered gas (%)	Liters of air entrained per liter O_2	Total gas outflow (Liter/min)
24	25.3	105 (DF = 4)*
28	10.3	68 (DF = 6)
31	6.9	63 (DF = 8)
35	4.6	56 (DF = 10)
40	3.2	50 (DF = 12)
50	1.7	33 (DF = 12)

* DF = higher driving flow of oxygen, in liters per minute, recommended by the manufacturer for a given concentration. In general, one should employ the highest driving flow to provide the highest total gas outflow. Although 40% and 50% masks do not qualify as low-flow devices, they are included for completeness.

In the hypercapnic, hypoxemic patient, therapy can begin with 24 or 28 percent masks. If the PaO_2 remains less than 55 mm Hg 30 minutes later, administration of progressive increments of inspired oxygen is undertaken. Arterial blood gas levels are measured at frequent intervals, usually every 30 minutes [90], for the first 1 to 2 hours or until it is certain the PaO_2 is 55 mm Hg or greater and CO_2 narcosis is not developing. In the hypercapnic patient, titration of supplemental oxygen is best assessed by arterial blood gas analysis rather than oximetry since the arterial blood gas provides $PaCO_2$ as well as oxygenation data. An initial modest increase in $PaCO_2$ (5–10 mm Hg) is expected in most hypercapnic patients given supplemental oxygen [86]. Carbon dioxide narcosis is present only when hypercapnia and acidemia progress and are associated with confusion, stupor, and coma. Though CO_2 narcosis is most likely to occur in patients with severe hypoxemia or moderate hypoxemia plus acidemia [86], all hypercapnic patients given oxygen must be closely followed clinically and with serial arterial blood gas monitoring. If progressive hypercapnia and mental status changes occur, endotracheal intubation should be considered and/or supplemental oxygen should be decreased in a stepwise fashion (e.g., 31% to 28% to 24%). Oxygen therapy is never completely discontinued. Abrupt discontinuation causes PaO_2 to fall to a level lower than it was before any oxygen was given [87,88], due mostly to the narcotic effects of hypercapnia—the patient breathes more shallowly and less frequently.

The second type of low-flow delivery system is the nasal cannula [91] (nasal prongs) (Fig. 69-2B). Although Venturi masks deliver the most precise doses of oxygen, they may be uncomfortable. Consequently, patients frequently remove them, especially during visiting hours or mealtime [92]. The major advantage of nasal prongs is that they allow patients to eat, cough, drink, and talk without removing the device. Even though it is not possible to predict precisely the delivered concentration of oxygen for a given oxygen flow rate by nasal cannula (the delivered concentration depends on multiple factors, such as minute ventilation, tidal volume, respiratory rate, and peak inspiratory flow demand), oxygen must still be administered by progressive increments starting from a low flow rate [88]. Flow rates of 0.5 to 1 liter per minute by nasal prongs approximate an inspired oxygen concentration of 24 percent and a rate of 2 liters per minute approximates 28%. When switching back and forth between nasal prongs and Venturi mask, arterial blood gas determinations performed after 30 minutes reveal how successful the estimate was, by directly comparing the gases previously obtained on the alternate device [90].

NONHYPERCAPNIC RESPIRATORY FAILURE. The goal of oxygen therapy in this setting (PaO_2 <55 mm Hg) is to increase PaO_2 to 60 mm Hg or greater [83]. This criterion is greater than the minimum acceptable PaO_2 of 55 mm Hg previously cited for hypercapnic patients because acute hypoxemia is less well tolerated than chronic hypoxemia and CO_2 narcosis is not a concern. Therefore, controlled low-flow therapy is not of paramount importance.

Devices. To achieve the desired PaO_2, therapy can be delivered initially by nasal prongs or a Venturi mask. The appropriate flow rate or concentration of inspired oxygen is adjusted based on serial pulse oximetry or arterial blood gas results. When hypoxemia is caused by a lung disease other than COPD pulse oximetry or arterial blood gases should be monitored every 7 rather than every 30 minutes [93]. When oxygen is delivered by nasal prongs at flow rates up to 4 to 5 liters per minute, the gas must be routed through a humidifier or it will be uncomfortable because of its drying effect. If higher flow rates are necessary, higher-concentration Venturi masks (up to 50%) should be given. If a well-fitted 50 percent Venturi mask fails to achieve an oxygen saturation of at least 90 percent or a PaO_2 of 60 mm Hg or greater, the patient usually has severe cardiogenic pulmonary edema, the acute respiratory distress syndrome, overwhelming pneumonia, or a cardiac or pulmonary vascular shunt. In these settings, we recommend a nonrebreathing mask (Fig. 69-3), for two reasons. First, when properly worn, it has the potential to deliver the most predictable oxygen concentration (approximately 90%) of all the high-concentration delivery mask devices (e.g., aerosol masks, partial rebreathing masks, or face tents). Second, it can reveal the presence of a right-to-left shunt. If the PaO_2 is 60 mm Hg or less in the face of an inspired oxygen concentration of approximately 90 percent, a right-to-left shunt of approximately 40 percent of the cardiac output is present (see Chap. 53). If the chest radiograph in this setting demonstrates diffuse pulmonary infiltrates and the patient does not improve rapidly with diuretics, adequate oxygenation is not possible without intubation and mechanical ventilation with positive end-expiratory pressure (PEEP). Although PEEP can be given using a tight-fitting mask (Fig. 69-4) in the absence of intubation [94] (CPAP), it is recommended only for patients who are awake and alert, demonstrate an ability to protect their lower airway, possess adequate respiratory muscle strength, are not retaining CO_2, and have a stable cardiovascular status. Major complications associated with mask CPAP are trauma at the sites of tight mask application and a high likelihood of gastric content aspiration from gastric distention associated with vomiting.

LONG-TERM CONTINUOUS OXYGEN THERAPY. Continuous (24-hour) oxygen therapy significantly prolongs and improves the quality of life in hypoxemic patients with COPD [95,96]. If used for 15 hours per day or more, it decreases mortality 1.5 to 1.9 times for up to 3 years. The following patients should be given continuous oxygen during hospitalization and as outpatients: (1) patients with a PaO_2 of 55 mm Hg or less and (2) those with a PaO_2 of 59 mm Hg or less plus edema, hematocrit of 55 percent or greater, or P pulmonale on ECG. Since many of these patients continue to improve as outpatients, the need for continuous oxygen therapy should be reassessed at 1 month [97].

When prescribing continuous oxygen therapy by nasal prongs initially the lowest flow rate that maintains a resting PaO_2 of 60 to 80 mm Hg should be given. This dose should be increased by 1 liter per minute during exercise and sleep [95]. Three major systems are currently available for delivery of long-

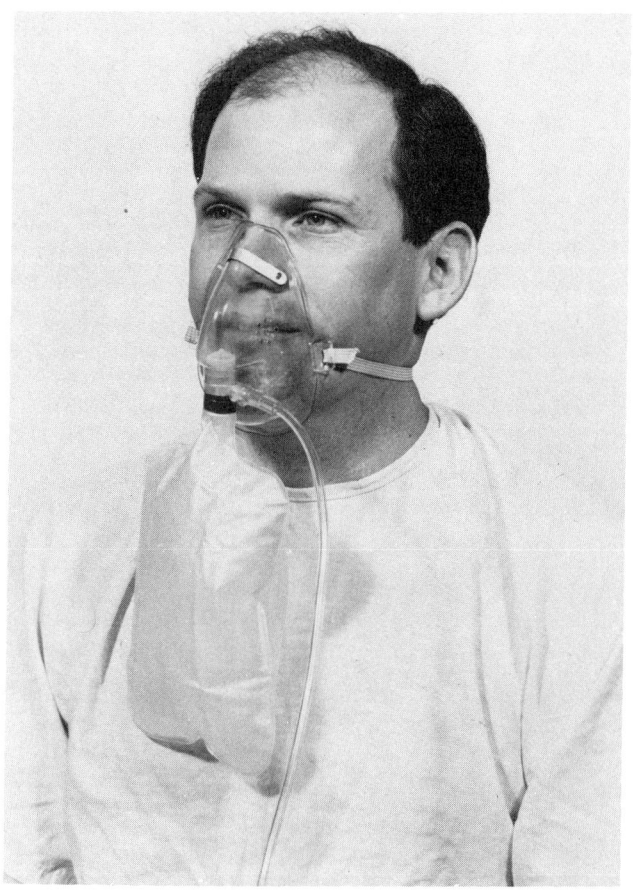

Fig. 69-3. Nonrebreathing mask. This device (Air Life Nonrebreathing Mask, Upland, CA) will deliver approximately 90% oxygen as long as the mask is properly fitted and the patient's inspiratory flow demands are met. The patient's inspiratory flow demand will be met provided the reservoir bag is not allowed to collapse completely.

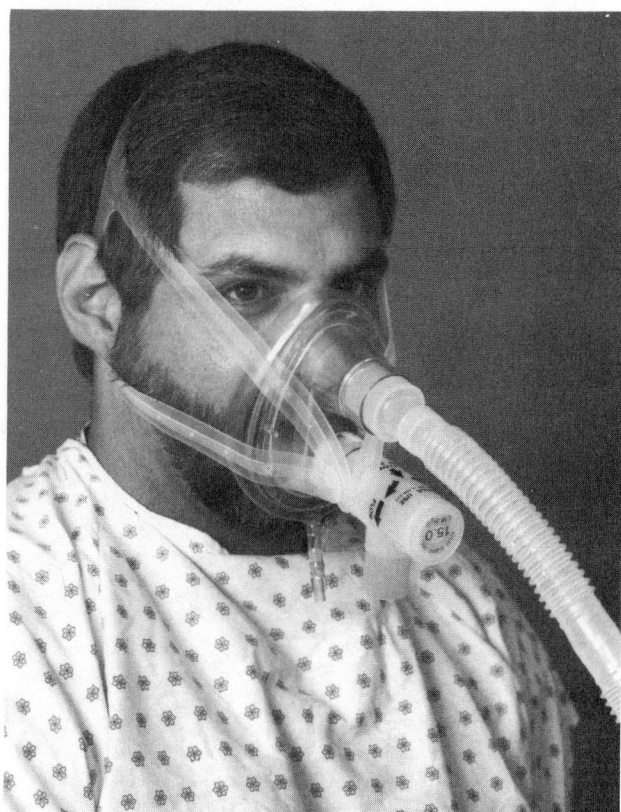

Fig. 69-4. Continuous positive-airway pressure mask. This mask (Vital Signs, Inc., East Rutherford, NJ) is supplied with interchangeable spring-loaded valves that allow for the application of various levels of positive end-expiratory pressure. It must fit tightly to be effective.

term oxygen therapy: compressed oxygen in tanks, liquid oxygen, and oxygen concentrators. The choice for any individual patient must be based on relative cost, the need for portability, and available safety features. To minimize the cost of home oxygen therapy, oxygen concentrators [98] can be prescribed. These machines take in room air and concentrate oxygen, eliminating the need for oxygen tanks or liquid oxygen in patients who are not ambulatory.

New methods of delivery of continuous oxygen are currently undergoing clinical trials [99–102]. The impetus for these developments has been the need for conservation of oxygen to decrease cost and cosmetic improvement to increase patient compliance. Four such methods are transtracheal catheters [103,104,105], reservoir cannulas (Fig. 69-5), demand-pulse oxygen delivery, and oxygen cannulas concealed in eyeglass frames. The first three oxygen-conserving devices are commercially available. When caring for patients with transtracheal catheters in place (Fig. 69-6), it is important to secure them with tape or sutures to prevent accidentally dislodging. There is no need to remove them before or during endotracheal intubation. However, while the patient is intubated, a SCOOP 2 catheter should be changed to a Scoop 1 catheter (if not already in place) and the Scoop 1 catheter capped.

Patients receiving transtracheal oxygen are at risk of developing inspissated secretions, mucus airway casts, and mucus balls, especially when the transtracheally delivered gas is not adequately humidified. Consequently, whenever a patient receiving transtracheal oxygen develops worsening hypoxemia or respiratory distress, mucus obstruction of the airway should be considered. In this setting, nasal cannula oxygen should be instituted and the transtracheal catheter removed. This manuever can often shear off a mucus ball attached to the end of the catheter, allow the patient to expectorate the accumulated mucus, and thereby improve the hypoxemia and eliminate the respiratory distress. The catheter can then be cleaned and reinserted with provision for adequate humidification of the transtracheally delivered gas. Preliminary studies are underway to assess the use of transtracheal air and oxygen mixtures as therapy for obstructive sleep apnea [106] and as a nocturnal mechanical ventilation assist device [107].

ACUTE MYOCARDIAL INFARCTION WITHOUT RESPIRATORY FAILURE. Studies in animals [108] and humans [109] have shown that supplemental oxygen can significantly reduce infarct size, therefore it seems reasonable to treat patients with acute myocardial infarction with modest amounts of oxygen. While the most efficacious dose and duration of therapy are unknown, we recommend oxygen therapy with a 40 percent Venturi mask until the fourth or fifth day after infarction. This recommendation is based on the above studies.

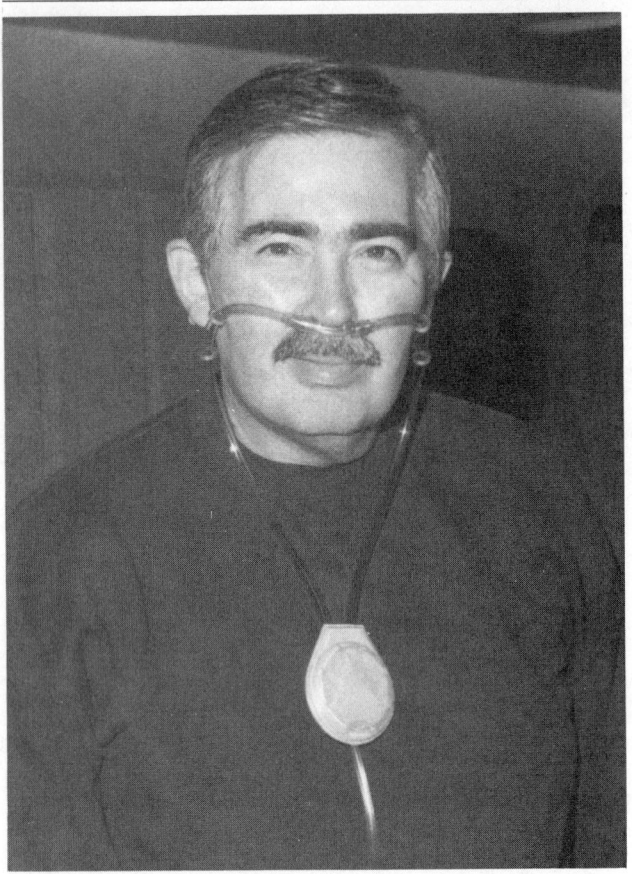

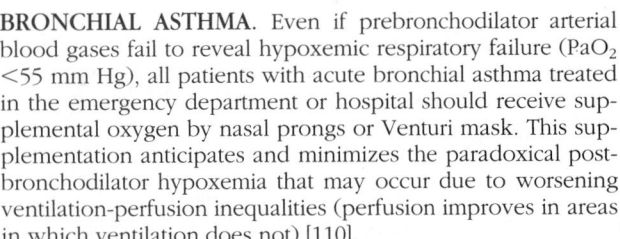

Fig. 69-5. Reservoir cannula. This oxygen-conserving nasal cannula (Oxymizer Pendant, CHAD therapeutics Inc., Chatsworth, CA) stores oxygen during exhalation for delivery during inhalation.

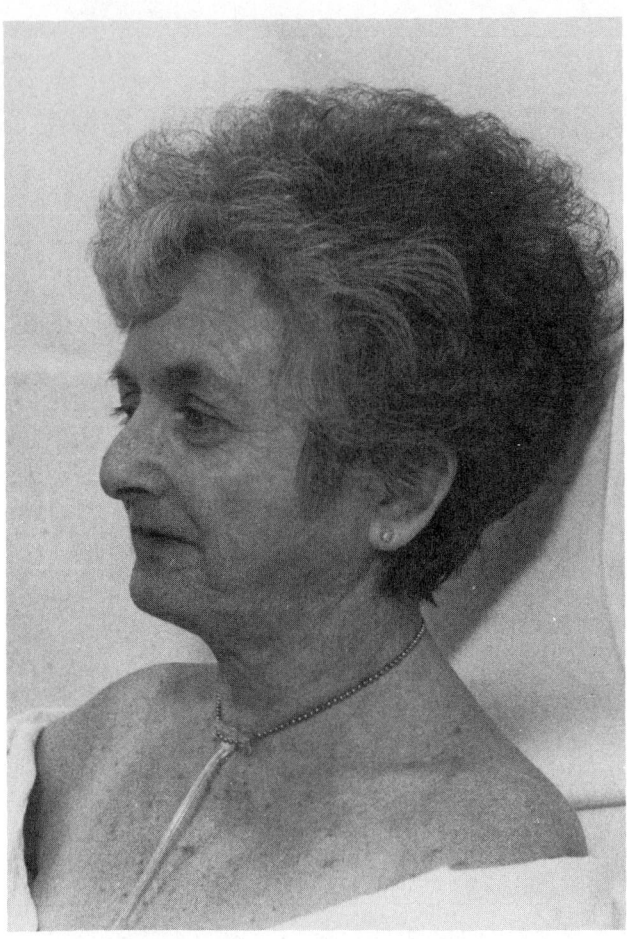

Fig. 69-6. Transtracheal oxygen catheter.

BRONCHIAL ASTHMA. Even if prebronchodilator arterial blood gases fail to reveal hypoxemic respiratory failure (PaO_2 <55 mm Hg), all patients with acute bronchial asthma treated in the emergency department or hospital should receive supplemental oxygen by nasal prongs or Venturi mask. This supplementation anticipates and minimizes the paradoxical postbronchodilator hypoxemia that may occur due to worsening ventilation-perfusion inequalities (perfusion improves in areas in which ventilation does not) [110].

SICKLE CELL CRISIS. The role of oxygen therapy in sickle cell crisis is unknown [111]. Since deoxygenation makes cells sickle, however, it seems reasonable to give supplemental oxygen in this setting. Due to the risk of oxygen toxicity, concentrations in excess of 50 percent should not be given for more than 48 hours.

CARBON MONOXIDE POISONING. Since a PCO of less than 1 mm Hg can saturate 50 percent of hemoglobin and not interfere with lung function, measurements of oxygen tension are not useful in predicting the presence of CO poisoning or in directing oxygen therapy [112]. Carboxyhemoglobin levels must be measured to detect CO poisoning [112]. Administration of

high concentrations of inspiratory oxygen is important in treating carbon monoxide poisoning, for two reasons [112,113]: (1) a substantial amount of oxygen may be placed in solution in the blood to supplement the oxygen already present and (2) a high PaO_2 accelerates the dissociation of carbon monoxide from hemoglobin. In the absence of hyperbaric oxygen, a nonrebreathing mask driven by pure humidified oxygen is the treatment of choice. This should be given immediately and without interruption until it is verified that carboxyhemoglobinemia has fallen to less than 5 percent [112]. Although hyperbaric oxygenation represents a potentially, albeit controversial, more effective alternative [114,115], it is not readily available to most patients. If it is available, patients with carboxyhemoglobin levels greater than 40 percent or with cardiac or neurologic symptoms should be considered for immediate transportation to the hyperbaric oxygen facility for treatment [112]. (See Chap. 71 for further discussion of CO poisoning.)

GAS GANGRENE. If hyperbaric oxygenation is available, it is not unreasonable to use it in the treatment of patients seriously infected with *Clostridium perfringens*. However, although increased oxygen tension in tissues can dramatically inhibit growth of the organism and production of toxin, there does not appear to be a clear-cut improvement in mortality associated with its use [114,115,116].

CLUSTER HEADACHE. High concentrations of oxygen, best delivered by a nonrebreathing mask, appear to be effective treatment for the symptomatic cluster headache [117]. Although oxygen inhalation has not been compared to ergotamine and its mechanism of action is unknown, 75 percent of patients experience headache relief within 15 minutes of oxygen administration.

COMPLICATIONS. In adults, decreased mucociliary clearance, tracheobronchitis, and pulmonary oxygen toxicity are the major complications of oxygen therapy. Mucociliary clearance is decreased by 40 percent when 75 percent oxygen is breathed for 9 hours and by 50 percent when 50 percent oxygen is breathed for 30 hours [45]. Symptomatic tracheobronchitis is caused consistently by the inhalation of high concentrations of oxygen (90% or higher) for 12 hours or more; it is manifested by substernal pain, cough, and dyspnea [118]. To avoid clinically significant pulmonary oxygen toxicity, prolonged administration of concentrations greater than 50 percent should be restricted, whenever possible, to 48 hours [119,120]. The pathology of oxygen toxicity is that of the acute respiratory distress syndrome (ARDS); it can lead to death from refractory and progressive hypoxemia due to interstitial fibrosis. It is best avoided by restricting delivery of oxygen to the lowest concentration and shortest duration absolutely necessary to achieve a satisfactory PaO_2. Therefore, prophylaxis consists of employing any and all measures that allow a decrease in the concentration of inspired oxygen to a subtoxic level. Positive end-expiratory pressure has been shown to be useful in achieving this goal.

Although the complications of retrolental fibroplasia [121] and bronchopulmonary dysplasia [122] from oxygen toxicity have been limited in the past to pediatric patients, reports of adults with bronchopulmonary dysplasia, the eventual result of ARDS, have appeared [123]. Central nervous system dysfunction manifested by myoclonus, nausea, paresthesias, unconsciousness, and seizures is limited to hyperbaric oxygenation at pressures in excess of 2 atm [120].

HYPERBARIC OXYGEN THERAPY. To date, this therapy has been proved efficacious for air embolism and decompression sickness [114,115]. Its efficacy in CO poisoning, has been less well demonstrated. It has decreased morbidity in general and the development of neurologic sequelae in retrospective studies [124,125]. (See Chap. 68 for further discussion of this treatment modality.)

Administration of Helium-Oxygen (Heliox)

Because helium is less dense than nitrogen, it has the potential to improve airflow where airflow is likely to be turbulent (i.e., density-dependent). This is the case in large airways, especially when there is an upper airway obstructing lesion. Heliox has successfully decreased airway resistance in patients with postextubation upper airway obstruction [126], in children with severe croup who were refractory to inhaled racemic epinephrine [126], and in upper airway obstruction due to tracheal tumors or extrinsic compression [127]. Heliox has also enabled fiberoptic bronchoscopy through endotracheal tubes with internal diameters less than 8 mm [128]. The effect of increasing concentrations of helium in decreasing airway resistance is linear, but the majority of the reduction takes place when the

concentration of helium reaches 40 percent [129,130]. Therefore, heliox mixtures should contain a minimum of 40 percent helium, with the balance of the mixture being oxygen. For instance, for patients in respiratory distress with little hypoxemia due to laryngeal edema, a heliox mixture of 80 percent helium and 20 percent oxygen would suffice. For patients in respiratory distress with profound hypoxemia due to pulmonary edema associated with laryngeal edema, a heliox mixture of 40 percent helium and 60 percent oxygen would be most advantageous.

Nasal Continuous Positive Airway Pressure

Since 1981, nasal CPAP has been repeatedly demonstrated to be effective in the treatment of obstructive sleep apnea/hypopnea syndrome and in preventing snoring [131]. A small, uncontrolled case series suggested that nasal CPAP may also be efficacious in some patients with chronic left ventricular failure and Cheyne-Stokes respirations (CSR) [132]. In these patients, nasal CPAP was associated with improvement in CSR, resting left ventricular ejection fraction, and daytime hypersomnolence. The favorable effect on chronic left ventricular failure with CSR was not confirmed in another study [133], however, so the role of nasal CPAP in chronic heart failure is yet to be defined.

Patients with obstructive sleep apnea/hypopnea syndrome who require therapy have, on average, at least 15 apneas and/or hypopneas per hour over an 8-hour overnight sleep study. The site of upper airway occlusion is usually the pharyngeal region. For those patients with obvious anatomic diseases narrowing the oropharynx (e.g., adenotonsillar enlargement, retrognathia and micrognathia, and macroglossia due to myxedema), surgical correction or thyroid replacement therapy can be curative. For the greater majority of patients without gross anatomic disorders or hypothyroidism, other techniques are employed [131,134].

Other treatment modalities [131] include tracheostomy, tongue-retaining prostheses, nocturnal oxygen therapy, deviated nasal septum repair, uvulopalatopharyngoplasty, expan-

Fig. 69-7. Nasal CPAP mask and set-up (Respironics, Inc., Monroeville, PA). A comfortable and properly fitted mask are important for patient tolerance and efficacy.

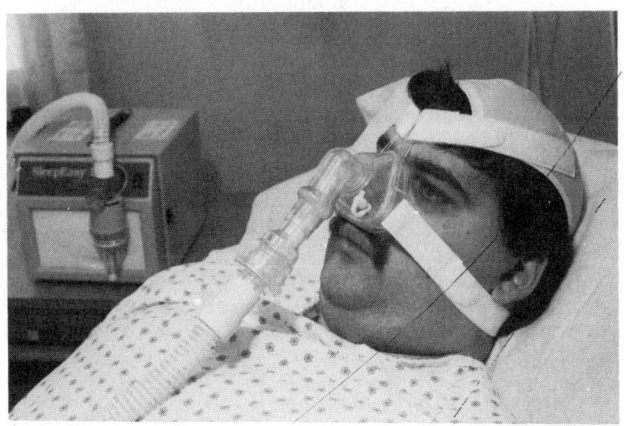

sion hyoidplasty, weight loss in obese patients, and a variety of drugs. Because nasal CPAP is very effective, safe, and reasonably well tolerated, it has become the technique of choice in the treatment of idiopathic obstructive sleep apnea (i.e., no correctable anatomic abnormality identified).

Nasal CPAP acts as a pneumatic splint to prevent upper airway collapse (Fig. 69-7). Patients usually respond rapidly to 3 to 15 cm H_2O. When this fails, it is usually due to a poorly applied mask or patient intolerance [131]. Compliance rates up to 85 percent have been reported [134]. Rare serious complications [134] include bilateral bacterial conjunctivitis, massive epistaxis due to drying of nasal mucosa in a patient with coagulopathy, and worsening obstruction in a patient with a large, lax epiglottis. Nasal CPAP was recently shown to reverse central sleep apneas in some patients [135].

For patients with sleep apnea/hypopnea syndrome who cannot tolerate nasal CPAP because of the sensation of excessive pressure, a nasal ventilator that provides bilevel positive airway pressure (BiPAP) may work and be tolerable. This type of ventilator permits independent adjustments of inspiratory positive airway pressure (IPAP) and expiratory positive airway pressure (EPAP) and has eliminated sleep disordered breathing at lower levels of expiratory airway pressure compared with conventional nasal CPAP therapy in some patients [136].

References

1. Lourenco RV, Cotromanes E: Clinical aerosols. I. Characterization of aerosols and their diagnostic uses. *Arch Intern Med* 142:2163, 1982.
2. Jenkins SC, Heaton RW, Fulton TS: Comparison of domiciliary nebulized salbutamol and salbutamol from a metered-dose inhaler in stable chronic airflow limitation. *Chest* 91:804, 1987.
3. Newhouse MT, Dolovich MB: Control of asthma by aerosols. *N Engl J Med* 315:870, 1986.
4. Summer W, Elston R, Tharpe L, et al: Aerosol bronchodilator delivery methods. *Arch Intern Med* 149:618, 1989.
5. Morley TF, Marozsan E, Zappasodi SJ, et al: Comparison of beta-adrenergic agents delivered by nebulizer vs metered dose inhaler with inspirease in hospitalized asthmatic patients. *Chest* 94:1205, 1988.
6. Morgan MDL, Singh BV, Frame MH, et al: Terbutaline aerosol given through pear spacer in acute severe asthma. *Br Med J* 285:849, 1982.
7. Newhouse M, Dolovich M: Aerosol therapy: Nebulizer vs metered dose inhaler. *Chest* 91:799, 1987.
8. Turner JR, Corkery KJ, Eckman D, et al: Equivalence of continuous flow nebulizer and metered-dose inhaler with reservoir bag for treatment of acute airflow obstruction. *Chest* 93:476, 1988.
9. Idris AH, McDermott MF, Raucci JC, et al: Emergency department treatment of severe asthma: Metered-dose inhaler plus holding chamber is equivalent in effectiveness to nebulizer. *Chest* 103:665, 1993.
10. Konig P: Spacer devices with metered-dose inhalers: Breakthrough or gimmick? *Chest* 88:276, 1985.
11. Fuller HD, Dolovich MB, Posmituck G, et al: Pressurized aerosol vs jet aerosol delivery to mechanically ventilated patients: Comparison of dose to the lungs. *Am Rev Respir Dis* 141:440, 1990.
12. Hess D: How should bronchodilators be administered to patients on ventilators? *Respir Care* 36:377, 1991.
13. Wanner A, Rao A: Clinical indications for and effects of bland, mucolytic, and antimicrobial aerosols. *Am Rev Respir Dis* 122(suppl):79, 1980.
14. Dulfano MJ, Adler K, Wooten O: Physical properties of sputum. IV. Effects of 100 percent humidity and water mist. *Am Rev Respir Dis* 107:130, 1973.
15. Wolfsdorf J, Swift DL, Avery ME: Mist therapy reconsidered: An evaluation of the respiratory deposition of labelled water aerosols produced by jet and ultrasonic nebulizers. *Pediatrics* 43:799, 1969.
16. Bau SK, Aspin N, Wood DE, et al: The measurement of fluid deposition in humans following mist tent therapy. *Pediatrics* 48:605, 1971.
17. Alderson PO, Secker-Walker RH, Strominger DB, et al: Pulmonary deposition of aerosols in children with cystic fibrosis. *J Pediatr* 84:479, 1974.
18. Chalon J, Loew DAY, Malebranche J: Effects of dry anesthetic gases on tracheobronchial ciliated epithelium. *Anesthesiology* 37:338, 1972.
19. Chalon J, Chandrakant P, Ali M, et al: Humidity and the anesthetized patient. *Anesthesiology* 50:195, 1979.
20. Irwin RS, Thomas HM III: Mucoid impaction of the bronchus: Diagnosis and treatment. *Am Rev Respir Dis* 108:955, 1973.
21. Bernstein IL, Ausdenmoore RW: Iatrogenic bronchospasm occurring during clinical trials of a new mucolytic agent, acetylcysteine. *Dis Chest* 46:469, 1964.
22. Rao S, Wilson DB, Brooks RC, et al: Acute effects of nebulization of N-acetylcysteine on pulmonary mechanics and gas exchange. *Am Rev Respir Dis* 102:17, 1970.
23. Hirsch SR, Kory RC: An evaluation of the effect of nebulized N-acetylcysteine on sputum consistency. *J Allergy* 39:265, 1967.
23a. Fuchs HJ, Borowitz DS, Christiansen DH, et al: Effect of aerosolized recombinant human DNase on exacerbations of respiratory symptoms and on pulmonary function in patients with cystic fibrosis. *N Engl J Med* 331:637, 1994.
24. Hodson ME: Antibiotic treatment: Aerosol therapy. *Chest* 94 (suppl):157S, 1988.
25. Ramsey BW, Dorkin HL, Eisenberg JD, et al: Efficacy of aerosolized tobramycin in patients with cystic fibrosis. *N Engl J Med* 328:1740, 1993.
26. Hall CB, Powell KR, MacDonald NE, et al: Respiratory syncytial viral infection in children with compromised immune function. *N Engl J Med* 315:77, 1986.
27. Lee SB: Ribavirin-exposure to health-care workers. *Am Ind Hyg Assoc J* 49:A13, 1988.
28. Masur H: Prevention and treatment of pneumocystis pneumonia. *N Engl J Med* 327: 1853, 1992.
29. Corkey CWB, Barker GA, Edmonds JF, et al: Radiographic tracheal diameter measurements in acute infectious croup: An objective scoring system. *Crit Care Med* 9:587, 1981.
30. Tabachnik E, Levison H: Clinical application of aerosols in pediatrics. *Am Rev Respir Dis* 122(suppl):97, 1980.
31. Leifer KN, Wittig HJ: The beta-2 sympathomimetic aerosols in the treatment of asthma. *Ann Allergy* 35:69, 1975.
32. Schuh S, Parkin P, Rajan A, et al: High-versus low-dose, frequently administered, nebulized albuterol in children with severe, acute asthma. *Pediatrics* 83: 513, 1989.
33. Colacone A, Wolkove N, Stern E, et al: Continuous nebulization of albuterol (salbutamol) in acute asthma. *Chest* 97: 693, 1990.
34. Allon M, Dunlay R, Copkney C. Nebulized albuterol for acute hyperkalemia in patients on hemodialysis. *Ann Intern Med* 110:426, 1989.
35. Rebuck AS, Chapman KR, Abboud R, et al: Nebulized anticholinergic and sympathomimetic treatment of asthma and chronic obstructive airways disease in the emergency room. *Am J Med* 82:59, 1987.
36. Winston SJ, Gravelyn TR, Sitrin RG: Prevention of bradycardic responses to endotracheal suctioning by prior administration of nebulized atropine. *Crit Care Med* 15:1009, 1987.
37. Wick MM, Ingram RH: Bronchorrhea responsive to aerosolized atropine. *JAMA* 235:1356, 1976.
38. Ingram RH Jr: Mechanical aids to lung expansion. *Am Rev Respir Dis* 122(suppl):23, 1980.
39. Bartlett RH: Postoperative pulmonary prophylaxis: Breathe deeply and read carefully. *Chest* 81:1, 1982.
40. Mahlmeister MJ, Fink JB, Hoffman GL, et al: Positive-expiratory pressure mask therapy: Theoretical and practical considerations and a review of the literature. *Respir Care* 36:1218, 1991.
41. Indihar FJ, Forsberg DP, Adams AB: A prospective comparison of three procedures used in attempts to prevent postoperative pulmonary complications. *Respir Care* 27:564, 1982.
42. Demers RR, Irwin RS, Braman SS, et al: Variable accuracy of five commercially available incentive spirometers. *Am Rev Respir Dis* 117(suppl):108, 1978.

43. Torrington KG, Sorenson DE, Sherwood LM: Postoperative chest percussion with postural drainage in obese patients following gastric stapling. *Chest* 86:891, 1984.

44. Sackner MA: Effect of respiratory drugs and mucociliary clearance. *Chest* 73(suppl):95S, 1978.

45. Wanner A: Clinical aspects of mucociliary transport. *Am Rev Respir Dis* 116:73, 1977.

46. Sackner MA, Epstein S, Wanner A: Effect of beta-adrenergic agonists aerosolized by freon propellant on tracheal mucous velocity and cardiac output. *Chest* 69:593, 1976.

47. Wood RE, Wanner A, Hirsch J, et al: Tracheal mucociliary transport in patients with cystic fibrosis and its stimulation by terbutaline. *Am Rev Respir Dis* 111:733, 1975.

48. Cruz RS, Landa J, Hirsch J, et al: Tracheal mucous velocity in normal man and patients with obstructive lung disease: Effects of terbutaline. *Am Rev Respir Dis* 109:458, 1974.

49. Sutton PP, Pavia D, Bateman JRM, et al: The effect of oral aminophylline on lung mucociliary clearance in man. *Chest* 80(suppl):899, 1981.

50. Irwin RS, Curley FJ, Pratter MR: The effects of drugs on cough. *Eur J Respir Dis* 71 (Suppl)153:173, 1987.

51. Irwin RS, Curley FJ, Bennett FM: Appropriate use of antitussives and protussives: A practical review. *Drugs* 46:80, 1993.

51a. Bennett WD, Chapman WF, Mascarella JM. The acute effect of ipratropium bromide bronchodilator therapy on cough clearance in COPD. *Chest* 103:488, 1993.

51b. Sutton PP, Gemmell JG, Innes N, et al: Use of nebulized saline and nebulized terbutaline as an adjunct to chest physiotherapy. *Thorax* 43:57, 1988.

51c. Bouhuys A, Van de Woestijne KP. Mechanical consequences of airway smooth muscle relaxation. *J Appl Physiol* 30:670, 1971.

52. Murray JF: The ketchup bottle method. *N Engl J Med* 300:1155, 1979.

53. Marini JJ, Pierson DJ, Hudson LD: Acute lobar atelectasis: A prospective comparison of fiberoptic bronchoscopy and respiratory therapy. *Am Rev Respir Dis* 119:971, 1979.

54. Graham WGB, Bradley DA, Kleczek R, et al: Efficacy of chest physiotherapy and intermittent positive-pressure breathing in the resolution of pneumonia. *N Engl J Med* 299:624, 1978.

55. Tyler ML: Complications of positioning and chest physiotherapy. *Respir Care* 27:458, 1982.

56. Davidson AGF, McIlwaine PM, Wong LTK, et al: Comparison of positive expiratory pressure and autogenic drainage with conventional percussion and drainage techniques. *Pediatr Pulmonol* Suppl 2:132, 1988.

56a. Thomas J, Cook DJ, Brooks D: Chest physical therapy management of patients with cystic fibrosis: A meta-analysis. *Am J Respir Crit Care Med* 151:846, 1995.

57. Demers RR, Saklad M: Mechanical aspiration: A reappraisal of its hazards. *Respir Care* 20:661, 1975.

58. Demers RR: Complications of endotracheal suctioning procedures. *Respir Care* 27:453, 1982.

59. Fineberg C, Cohn HE, Gibbon JH Jr: Cardiac arrest during nasotracheal aspiration. *JAMA* 174:410, 1960.

60. Jacquette G: To reduce hazards of tracheal suctioning. *Am J Nurs* 71:2362, 1971.

61. Petersen GM, Pierson DJ, Hunter PM: Arterial oxygen saturation during nasotracheal suctioning. *Chest* 76:283, 1979.

62. LeFrock JL, Klainer AS, Wen-Hsien W, et al: Transient bacteremia associated with nasotracheal suctioning. *JAMA* 236:1610, 1976.

63. Brown SE, Stansbury DW, Merrill EJ et al: Prevention of suctioning-related arterial oxygen desaturation. *Chest* 83:621, 1983.

64. Sackner MA, Landa JF, Greeneltch N, et al: Pathogenesis and prevention of tracheobronchial damage with suction procedures. *Chest* 64:284, 1973.

65. Landa JF, Kwoka MA, Chapman GA, et al: Effects of suctioning on mucociliary transport. *Chest* 77:202, 1980.

66. Ehrhart IC, Hofman WF, Loveland SR: Effects of endotracheal suction versus apnea during interruption of intermittent or continuous positive pressure ventilation. *Crit Care Med* 9:464, 1981.

67. Shim C, Fine N, Fernandez R, et al: Cardiac arrhythmias resulting from tracheal suctioning. *Ann Intern Med* 71:1149, 1969.

68. Rosen M, Hillard EK: Effects of negative pressure during tracheal suction. *Anesth Analg* 41:50, 1962.

69. Widdicombe JG: Respiratory reflexes from the trachea and bronchi of the cat. *J Physiol* 200:25, 1969.

70. Freedman AP, Goodman L: Suctioning the left bronchial tree in the intubated adult. *Crit Care Med* 10:43, 1982.

71. Haberman PB, Green JP, Archibald C, et al: Determinants of successful selective tracheobronchial suctioning. *N Engl J Med* 289:1060, 1973.

72. Taggart SA, Dovinsky NL, Sheahan JS: Airway pressures during closed system suctioning. *Heart Lung* 17:536, 1988.

73. Ritz R, Scott LR, Coyle MB, et al: Contamination of a multiple-use suction catheter in a closed-circuit system compared to contamination of a disposable single-use suction catheter. *Respir Care* 31:1086, 1986.

74. Mayhall CG: The trach care(TM) Closed Tracheal Suction System: A new medical device to permit tracheal suctioning without interruption of ventilatory assistance. *Infection Control and Hosptal Epidemiol* 9:125, 1988.

75. Hasani A, Pavia D: Cough as a clearance mechanism, in Braga PC, Allegra L (eds): *Cough*. New York, Raven 1989, pp 39–52.

76. Puchelle E, Zahm JM, Girard F, et al: Mucociliary transport in vivo and in vitro: Relations to sputum properties in chronic bronchitis. *Eur J Respir Dis* 61:254, 1980.

77. Leith DE: Cough, in Brain JD, Proctor DF, Reid LM (eds): *Respiratory Defense Mechanisms. II. Lung Biology in Health and Disease*. New York, Marcel Dekker, 1977, pp 545–592.

78. Camner P: Studies on the removal of inhaled particles from the lungs by voluntary coughing. *Chest* 80(Suppl):824, 1981.

79. McCool FD, Leith DE: Pathophysiology of cough. *Clin Chest Med* 8:189,1987.

80. Gal TJ: Effects of endotracheal intubation on normal cough performance. *Anesthesiology* 52:324, 1980.

81. Szienberg A, Tabachnik E, Rashed N, et al: Cough capacity in patients with muscular dystrophy. *Chest* 94:1232, 1988.

82. Gracey DR, Divertie MB, Howard FM Jr: Mechanical ventilation for respiratory failure in myasthenia gravis: Two-year experience with 22 patients. *Mayo Clin Proc* 58:597, 1983.

83. Snider GL, Rinaldo JE: Oxygen therapy in medical patients hospitalized outside of the intensive care unit. *Am Rev Respir Dis* 122(suppl):29, 1980.

84. Harvey RM, Enson Y, Ferrer MI: A reconsideration of the origins of pulmonary hypertension. *Chest* 59:82, 1971.

85. Ferrer MI: Cor pulmonale (pulmonary heart disease): Present-day status. *Am Heart J* 89:657, 1975.

86. Bone RC, Pierce AK, Johnson RL Jr: Controlled oxygen administration in acute respiratory failure in chronic obstructive pulmonary disease: A reappraisal. *Am J Med* 65:896, 1978.

86a. Aubier M, Murciano D, Fournier M, et al: Central respiratory drive in acute respiratory failure of patients with chronic obstructive pulmonary disease. *Am Rev Respir Dis* 122:191, 1980.

86b. Aubier M, Murciano D, Milic-Emili J, et al: Effects of administration of O_2 on ventilation and blood gases in patients with chronic obstructive pulmonary disease during acute respiratory failure. *Am Rev Respir Dis* 122:747, 1980.

86c. Dunn WF, Nelson SB, Hubmayr RD: Oxygen-induced hypercarbia in obstructive pulmonary disease. *Am Rev Respir Dis* 144:526, 1991.

87. Campbell EJM: The J Burns Amberson Lecture: The management of acute respiratory failure in chronic bronchitis and emphysema. *Am Rev Respir Dis* 96:626, 1967.

88. Bone RC: Treatment of respiratory failure due to advanced chronic obstructive lung disease. *Arch Intern Med* 140:1018, 1980.

89. Cohen JL, Demers RR, Saklad M: Air-entrainment oxygen masks: A performance evaluation. *Respir Care* 22:277, 1977.

90. Woolf CR: Arterial blood gas levels after oxygen therapy. *Chest* 69:808, 1976.

91. Petty TL, Nett LM, Lakshminarayan S: A single nasal prong for continuous oxygen therapy. *Chest* 64:146, 1973.

92. Schiff MM, Massaro D: Effect of oxygen administration by a Venturi apparatus on arterial blood gas values in patients with respiratory failure. *N Engl J Med* 277:950, 1967.

93. Howe JP III, Alpert JS, Rickman FD, et al: Return of arterial PO_2 values to baseline after supplemental oxygen in patients with cardiac disease. *Chest* 67:256, 1975.

94. Kacmarek RM, Dimas S, Reynolds J, et al: Technical aspects of

positive end-expiratory pressure (PEEP). III. PEEP with spontaneous ventilation. *Respir Care* 27:1505, 1982.

95. Nocturnal Oxygen Therapy Trial Group: Continuous or nocturnal oxygen therapy in hypoxemic chronic obstructive lung disease: A clinical trial. *Ann Intern Med* 93:391, 1980.

96. Grant I, Heaton RK, McSweeney AJ, et al: Neuropsychologic findings in hypoxemic chronic obstructive pulmonary disease. *Arch Intern Med* 142:1470, 1982.

97. Timms RM, Kvale PA, Anthonisen NR, et al: Selection of patients with chronic obstructive pulmonary disease for long-term oxygen therapy. *JAMA* 245:2514, 1981.

98. Libby DM, Briscoe WA, King TKC, et al: Oxygen concentration from room air: A new source for oxygen therapy in the home. *JAMA* 241:1599, 1979.

99. Petty TL: Home oxygen therapy. *Mayo Clin Proc* 62:841, 1987.

100. Tiep BL, Lewis MI: Oxygen conservation and oxygen-conserving devices in chronic lung diseases: A review. *Chest* 92:263, 1987.

101. McDonald GJ: Long-term oxygen therapy delivery systems. *Respir Care* 28:898, 1983.

102. Carter R, Tashkin D, Djahed B, et al: Demand oxygen delivery for patients with restrictive lung disease. *Chest* 96:1307, 1989.

103. Christopher KL, Spofford BT, Petrun MD, et al: A program for transtracheal oxygen delivery. *Ann Intern Med* 107:802, 1987.

104. Heimlich HJ, Carr GC: The micro-trach: A seven-year experience with transtracheal oxygen therapy. *Chest* 95:1008, 1989.

105. Johnson LP, Cary JM: The implanted intratracheal oxygen catheter. *Surg Gynecol Obstet* 165:74, 1987.

106. Farney RJ, Walker JM, Elmer JC, et al: Trantracheal oxygen therapy for the treatment of obstructive sleep apnea. *Op Tech Otolaryngol Head Neck Surg* 2:132, 1991.

107. Benditt J, Pollock M, Roa J, et al: Transtracheal delivery of gas decreases the oxygen cost of breathing. *Am Rev Respir Dis* 147:1207, 1993.

108. Maroko PR, Radvany P, Braunwald E, et al: Reduction of infarct size by oxygen inhalation following acute coronary occlusion. *Circulation* 52:360, 1975.

109. Madias JE, Madias NE, Hood WB Jr: Precordial ST-segment mapping. 2. Effects of oxygen inhalation on ischemic injury in patients with acute myocardial infarction. *Circulation* 53(suppl):411, 1976.

110. Gazioglu K, Condemi JJ, Hyde RW, et al: Effect of isoproterenol on gas exchange during air and oxygen breathing in patients with asthma. *Am J Med* 50:185, 1971.

111. Embury SH, Garcia JF, Mohandas N, et al: Effects of oxygen inhalation on endogenous erythropoietin kinetics, erythropoiesis, and properties of blood cells in sickle-cell anemia. *N Engl J Med* 311:291, 1984.

112. Ilano AL, Raffin TA: Management of carbon monoxide poisoning. *Chest* 97:165, 1990.

113. Committee on Medical and Biologic Effects of Environmental Pollutants: *Carbon Monoxide.* Washington, DC, National Academy of Sciences, 1977, p 68.

114. Thom SR: Hyperbaric oxygen therapy. *J Intensive Care Med* 4:58, 1989.

115. Gabb G, Robin ED: Hyperbaric oxygen: A therapy in search of diseases. *Chest* 92:1074, 1987.

116. Weinstein L, Barza MA: Gas gangrene. *N Engl J Med* 289:1129, 1973.

117. Kudrow L: *Cluster headache: Mechanisms and Management.* New York, Oxford, 1980, p 142.

118. Sackner MA, Landa J, Hirsch J, et al: Pulmonary effects of oxygen breathing: A 6-hour study in normal man. *Ann Intern Med* 82:40, 1975.

119. Senior RM, Wessler S, Avioli LV: Pulmonary oxygen toxicity. *JAMA* 217:1373, 1971.

120. Deneke SM, Fanburg BL: Normobaric oxygen toxicity of the lung. *N Engl J Med* 303:76, 1980.

121. Hittner HM, Godio LB, Rudolph AJ, et al: Retrolental fibroplasia: Efficacy of vitamin E in a double-blind clinical study of preterm infants. *N Engl J Med* 305:1365, 1981.

122. Northway WH Jr: Observations on bronchopulmonary dysplasia. *J Pediatr* 95:815, 1979.

123. Chung A, Golden J, Fligiel S, Hogg JC: Bronchopulmonary dysplasia in the adult. *Am Rev Respir Dis* 127:117, 1983.

124. Norkool DM, Kirkpatrick JN: Treatment of acute carbon monoxide poisoning with hyperbaric oxygen: A review of 115 cases. *Ann Emerg Med* 14:168, 1985.

125. Smith G, Sharp GR: Treatment of carbon monoxide poisoning with oxygen under pressure. *Lancet* 2:905, 1960.

126. Duncan PG: Efficacy of helium-oxygen mixtures in the management of severe viral and post-intubation croup. *Can Anesth Soc J* 26:206, 1979.

127. Lu T-S, Ohmura A, Wong KC, et al: Helium-oxygen in treatment of upper airway obstruction. *Anesthesiology* 45:678, 1976.

128. Pingleton SK, Bone RC, Ruth WC: Helium-oxygen mixtures during bronchoscopy. *Crit Care Med* 18:50, 1980.

129. Houck JR, Keamy MF III, McDonough JM, et al: Effect of helium concentration on experimental upper airway obstruction. *Ann Otol Rhinol Laryngol* 99:556, 1990.

130. Vater M, Hanning PG, Aitkenhead AR: Quantitative effects of respired helium and oxygen mixtures on gas flow using conventional oxygen masks. *Anaesthesia* 38:879, 1983.

131. Strohl KP, Cherniack NS, Gothe B: Physiologic basis of therapy for sleep apnea. *Am Rev Respir Dis* 134:791, 1986.

132. Takasaki Y, Orr D, Popkin J, et al: Effect of nasal continuous positive airway pressure on sleep apnea in congestive heart failure. *Am Rev Respir Dis* 140:1578, 1989.

133. Davies RJO, Harrington KJ, Ormerod OJM, et al: Nasal continuous positive airway pressure in chronic heart failure with sleep-disordered breathing. *Am Rev Respir Dis* 147:630, 1993.

134. Strumpf DA, Harrop P, Dobbin J, et al: Massive epistaxis from nasal CPAP therapy. *Chest* 95:1141, 1989.

135. Issa FG, Sullivan CE: Reversal of central sleep apnea using nasal CPAP. *Chest* 90:165, 1986.

136. Sanders MH, Kern N: Obstructive sleep apnea treated by independently adjusted inspiratory and expiratory positive airway pressures via nasal mask: Physiologic and clinical implications. *Chest* 98:317, 1990.

70. The Chest Radiographic Examination

Cynthia B. Umali

Overview

Radiographic examination of the critically ill patient in the intensive care unit (ICU) or coronary care unit (CCU) is often necessary to evaluate clinical status. In this setting, the basic role of radiology is to follow the patient's progress or changes in status after admission or after surgery; the primary diagnosis will already have been established. Radiographic examinations are thus requested both to evaluate the course of the primary disease and to diagnose complications that may ensue. Henscke et al. [1] studied the diagnostic efficacy of bedside chest radiographs and found that in 65 percent of the 1132 consecutive radiographs analyzed, there were new findings or changes affecting patient management. Bekemeyer et al. [2], after analyzing 1354 radiographs from a respiratory ICU, found a 34.5 percent incidence of new or increased abnormalities or tube or catheter malpositions. They concluded that routine morning radiographic examinations frequently demonstrated unexpected or changing abnormalities, many of which prompted changes in diagnostic management.

Critically ill patients in the ICU or CCU often cannot take advantage of numerous radiologic modalities readily available to mobile patients. Because these patients cannot be transported while their circulatory functions are labile and they are connected to ECG monitors, ventilators, catheters, and surgical appliances, usually one is left with the portable bedside radiographic examination. Most often it is a chest examination that is needed; the chest film is especially important because physical examination to determine the presence of a complication such as atelectasis, pneumothorax, pneumonia, or pulmonary edema is difficult in the presence of a ventilator.

Until recently, portable radiographic examinations were restricted by inherent machine limitations in kilovoltage (kV), milliamperage (mA), and x-ray tube currents and by variations in battery charge. The need for adequate penetration to see line and catheter positions necessitated increasing normal exposure time (thereby increasing motion unsharpness) and using a higher kilovoltage (thereby increasing scatter radiation, which increases film fogging). A high kilovoltage also reduces subject contrast. These alterations and limitations cause deterioration of the image, often rendering the film of suboptimal quality for evaluation of subtle changes in the lung parenchyma.

During the last few years, most of the above problems have been practically eliminated with the use of state-of-the-art mobile x-ray units and the new rare earth screen-film combination. New Insight Thoracic Imaging System (Eastman Kodak) is a new film-screen combination that allows improved imaging of both lungs and mediastinum. For portable examinations, a gridded cassette (5:1) uses a thin front screen and a thick back screen. The Insight film is a double-coated film that can be inserted into the cassette only one way, placing the high-contrast emulsion facing front and the low-contrast emulsion facing rear. This system addresses the problem of large differences in x-ray transmission through the mediastinum and the lungs. It consistently shows the details of the mediastinum (the lines of pleural reflection and vertebrae) and tubes and catheters, at the same time providing excellent images (not overexposed) of the lung parenchyma, including the lungs over the diaphragm.

A high-frequency generator mounted on an overhead trolley that can be moved from bed to bed has also been designed specifically for use in the ICU [3]. Well-penetrated films can be obtained with short exposure time, eliminating motion unsharpness. The addition of an automatic exposure device [4], which terminates or prolongs the exposure until the preset film density level is reached, further enhances quality and allows for more consistent lung density between serial examinations [1]. Despite the extreme changes in lung densities due to rapid fluid shifts, the optimal density of serial films can be maintained with automatic exposure. Thus, radiographs of uniformly satisfactory quality, useful in the monitoring of subtle changes in the patient's pulmonary or cardiac status, can now be obtained.

Interpretation of portable examinations is fraught with pitfalls. Magnification of the cardiac silhouette cannot be eliminated because of the short tube-film distance and the often supine position of the patient. Signs used to evaluate postcapillary (pulmonary venous) hypertension are not valid on the supine film and may necessitate use of a horizontal beam (cross-table lateral view) to visualize the discrepancy between the dependent and nondependent vessels, which is far more difficult.

Films are often taken after a poor inspiratory effort due to the patient's inability to cooperate. Unless the type of respirator, phase of cycle, and pressure setting are indicated on the film, the appearance of parenchymal abnormalities is difficult to evaluate. Increased inflation of the lung may cause the opacities to appear less dense, but the apparent improvement secondary to increased aeration does not correspond to a true anatomic improvement. The reverse situation can occur as well. Preferably, therefore, information regarding patient position and ventilator data should be made available to the radiologist before interpretation. Milne [5] fastens adhesive labels to all films, noting mode or type of ventilation (spontaneous respiration, intermittent mandatory ventilation, or assist control ventilation); peak pressure on inspiration; continuous positive airway pressure or positive end-expiratory pressure; patient position; and direction of beam, distance, and technique (maS; kV).

A portable C-arm fluoroscope is often used at the bedside to monitor catheter placement (especially Swan-Ganz). The fluoroscope also may be used to evaluate alignment of fracture fragments during closed reduction and to visualize diaphragmatic motion. Portable ultrasound equipment is particularly useful for detecting fluid collections, including effusions (both pericardial and pleural) and subdiaphragmatic abscesses. Portable gamma cameras are useful for evaluating possible pulmonary embolism in these patients.

Evaluation of Tubes and Catheters

ENDOTRACHEAL TUBES. The location of endotracheal tubes should be checked as soon as possible after insertion (see Chap. 1). To evaluate properly the position of the tube, one must evaluate the head and neck position simultaneously. Goodman et al. showed that when the neck is extended, the inferior border of the mandible lies at or above the fourth cervical vertebral body (C_4) [6]. When the neck is in the neutral position, the inferior border of the mandible lies at the level of C_5-C_6, and when in flexion over the dorsal spine. The level of the tip of the tube should then be evaluated in relation to the neck position. It has been shown that significant change in tube position relative to the trachea occurs with flexion and extension [7]. From extension to flexion and vice versa the tube can travel as much as 4 cm. From the neutral position it can travel 2 cm either way, descending with flexion and ascending with extension. Lateral rotation of the head from the neutral position also causes a 1- to 2-cm ascent of the tube. Thus, to ensure that the tip of the tube is above the carina, it is suggested that the following guidelines be followed.

1. When the inferior border of the mandible is at or above C_4, the tip should be 7 ± 2 cm from the carina.
2. When the inferior border of the mandible is at the C_5-C_6 level, the tip of the tube should be 5 ± 2 cm from the carina.
3. When the inferior border of the mandible is at T_1 or below, the tip of the tube should be 3 ± 2 cm from the carina.

When the tube is too high, it may slip into the pharynx. If it is just below the vocal cords, its inflated cuff can cause glottic or subglottic edema, ulceration, and, ultimately, scarring. If it is too low, it can enter a bronchus and cause atelectasis of the lung supplied by the obstructed bronchus (Fig. 70-1).

Ideally, the tube should be one-half to two-thirds the width of the trachea and the inflated cuff should fill the trachea without causing the lateral walls to bulge. When the ratio of the cuff diameter to the tracheal lumen exceeds 1.5 percent, tracheal damage is likely to result [8]. Ravin et al. observed that repeated overdistention of the cuff on chest film, despite careful cuff inflation to the minimal leak level, should lead to suspicion of tracheomalacia (Fig. 70-2) [9].

Immediately after intubation, and especially after difficult intubation, a film should be obtained to define the position of the tube. The radiologist should also look for signs of perforation of the pharynx, such as marked subcutaneous emphysema, pneumomediastinum, and pneumothorax. There have been reports of dislodging of teeth, dental caps, and portions of dentures into the tracheobronchial tree following intubation. If this is suspected, a foreign body in the tracheobronchial tree should be carefully sought.

Fig. 70-1. Endotracheal tube in right main bronchus. Portable examination, anteroposterior view, shows bilateral pulmonary edema and a dense left lower lobe (*long arrow*). The endotracheal tube is in the bronchus intermedius (*short arrow*), obstructing the left main bronchus and causing left lower lobe atelectasis.

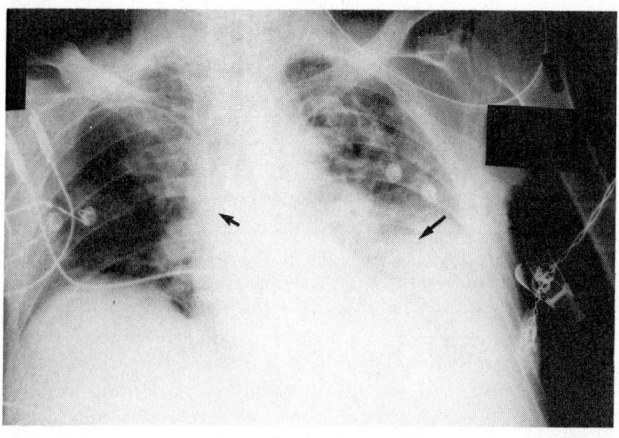

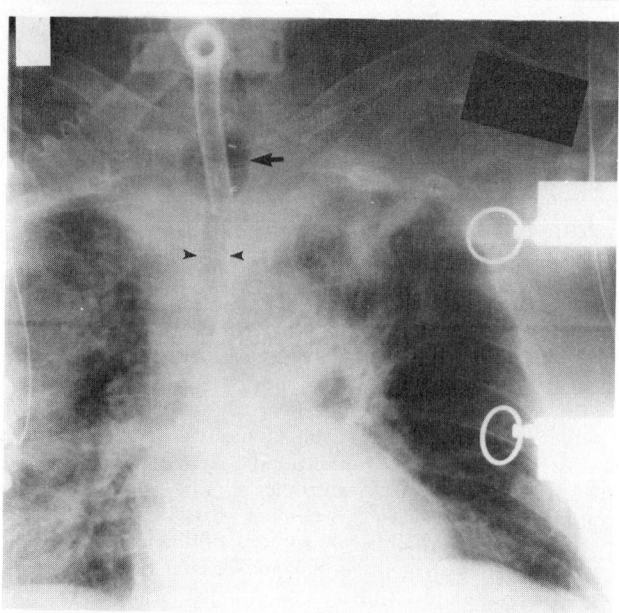

Fig. 70-2. Overdistended tracheostomy tube cuff. Portable examination, anteroposterior view, in a patient with diffuse parenchymal infiltrates from acute respiratory distress syndrome with a tracheostomy tube. Lucent circular area (*arrow*) surrounding the tracheostomy tube is a distended cuff. It markedly exceeds normal tracheal diameter (*arrowheads*). This patient has tracheomalacia and has had the cuff reinflated to this size persistently after deflation and reinflation to the minimal leak level.

TRACHEOSTOMY TUBES. The tip of the tracheostomy tube should be located one-half to two-thirds of the way between the stoma and the carina. Unlike the endotracheal tube, the tracheostomy tube will not change position with flexion and extension of the neck. The tracheostomy tube should be evaluated to determine its inner diameter (which should be two-thirds that of the tracheal lumen), its long axis (which should parallel the tracheal lumen), the location of its distal end (Fig. 70-3) (which should not abut the tracheal wall laterally, anteriorly, or posteriorly), and for development of increasing pneumothorax, pneumomediastinum, or subcutaneous emphysema, which may require immediate attention.

CENTRAL VENOUS CATHETERS. Central venous catheters should be evaluated to ensure that the true central venous pressure (CVP) is measured. The catheter should be located beyond the venous valves, the most proximal of which is just distal to the junction of the internal jugular vein and the subclavian veins. This is found at approximately the level of the first anterior rib (Fig. 70-4) (see Chap. 2) [10].

Brandt et al. found that "the distance to the junction of the superior vena cava and the right atrium is usually the total of the distance from the cutdown site to the suprasternal notch plus one-third the distance from the suprasternal notch to the xyphoid process" [11]. Complications of CVP lines include vascular perforation or dissection (Figs. 70-5A and 70-5B), cardiac perforation leading to cardiac tamponade (Fig. 70-5C), embolization, and infection.

SWAN-GANZ CATHETERS. Swan-Ganz catheters are used to perform right heart catheterizations [12]. Ideally, the tip of the

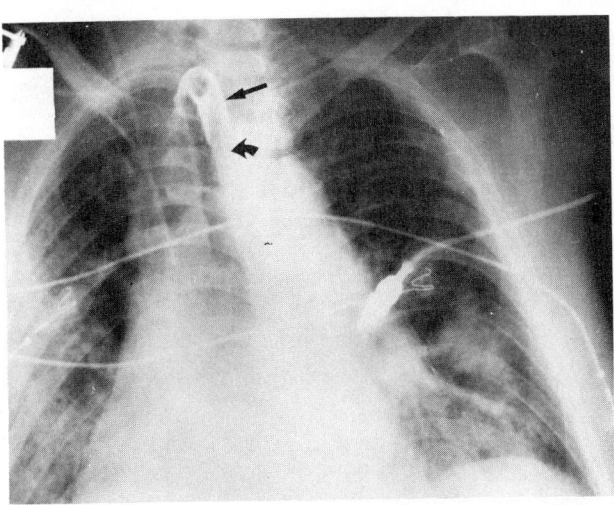

Fig. 70-3. Tracheostomy tube lateral to shadow of trachea. Portable anteroposterior view of a patient with pulmonary edema, with the left lateral edge of the tracheostomy tube (*straight arrow*) lying to the left of the tracheal wall (*curved arrow*). The patient had a history of nasogastric tube feedings being recovered from the tracheostomy tube, which eroded the trachea into the esophagus.

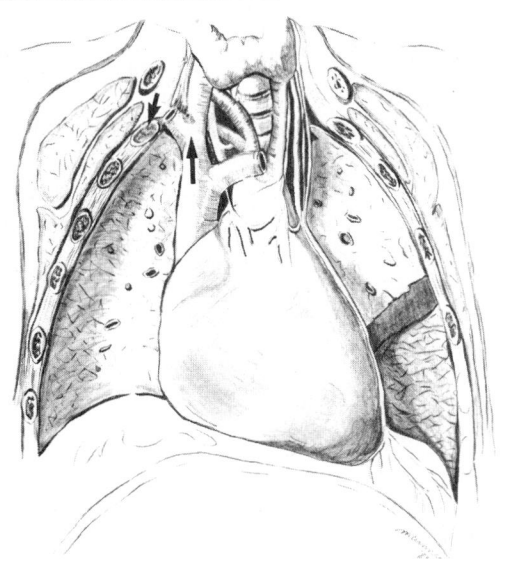

Fig. 70-4. Junction of internal jugular vein and right subclavian vein. Veins shown in relation to the first rib. The junction of the internal jugular and right subclavian veins (*long arrow*) occurs at about the level of the first rib (*short arrow*). The CVP line should be at or beyond this point to measure true venous pressure. (Drawing by Mary Cunnion.)

Swan-Ganz catheter should be located in the right or left branch of the pulmonary artery. Occasionally, the tip may be malpositioned (Fig. 70-6); a film should be routinely taken to check its position. If it is more distal to the above location, the catheter may produce pulmonary infarction (Fig. 70-7) by blocking the artery directly or from a clot in or around the tip. Other, rare complications include perforation of the pulmonary artery, balloon rupture, and pulmonary artery-bronchial tree fistulas.

Similar balloon-tipped flotation catheters equipped with two pairs of electrodes (Chatterjee modification) are used in ICUs for simultaneous monitoring of cardiac rhythm and hemodynamics as well as for temporary emergency atrial, ventricular, or atrioventricular sequential pacing. The catheter tip should be seen in the pulmonary artery, and the distal electrodes should be located in the right ventricle [13].

Swan-Ganz catheters have been used successfully to obtain bedside pulmonary angiograms when pulmonary embolism is suspected [14,15,16]. Bedside pulmonary angiography should be considered when it is inadvisable to move the patient to the angiographic laboratory for definitive studies and an arteriographic study is needed.

INTRAAORTIC COUNTERPULSATION BALLOONS. The intraaortic counterpulsation balloon (IACB) was designed to improve cardiac function in a setting of cardiogenic shock [17], and this remains the major indication for its use (see Chap. 9). The various models all work on the same basic principle: the balloon is inflated during diastole (to increase blood pressure in the proximal aorta and thereby increase coronary artery perfusion) and deflated during systole (to allow the blood to move distally). Ideally, the tip of the IACB should be positioned at the level of the aortic arch just distal to the origin of the left subclavian artery to augment coronary perfusion maximally without occluding the subclavian and cerebral vessels (Fig. 70-8). Complications from IACBs are major vessel obstruction, embolization from a clot formed in or around the catheter, and aortic dissection with balloon rupture.

As with endotracheal tubes, the position of the IACB changes with a change in patient position, moving cephalad 1 to 4.5 cm when the patient moves from a recumbent to a sitting position [18]. The position should therefore be checked periodically.

CHEST TUBES. Chest tubes (thoracostomy or pleural drainage tubes) are used to drain either fluid or air from the pleural space (see Chap. 11). In the ICU patient, who is most often in the supine position, the ideal tube position is dictated by what it is intended to drain. If placed for a pneumothorax, the tube should be seen in the anterosuperior position as the air collects beneath the sternum; if placed to drain a pleural effusion, the tube should be seen in the posteroinferior position. To ascertain that the tube is in the pleural space, one must see both opaque and "nonopaque" sides of the tube. When the nonopaque side is not seen it is because the subcutaneous tissue, which is similar to the tube in density, has silhouetted this nonopaque border and the tube is outside the pleural space [19]. The side hole of the tube (where there is a break in the opaque marker) also should be seen within the pleural space.

Occasionally chest tubes have been placed in an interlobar fissure. A lateral view is necessary to recognize intrafissural positioning. Maurer et al., in a review of 14 cases, noted a 29 percent unsatisfactory drainage rate from tubes in the interlobar fissure, especially in patients who were ill and lying supine and who needed drainage of pleural fluid, which tends to settle in the dependent posterior portion of the chest [20].

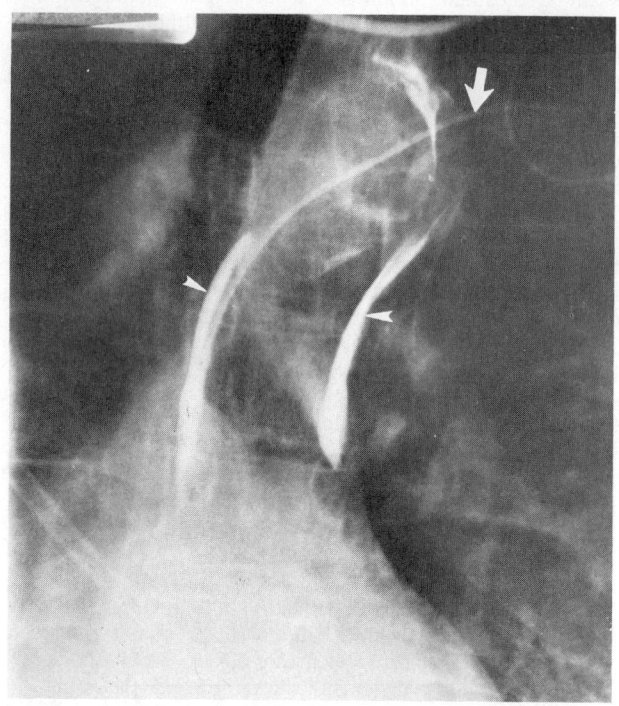

A

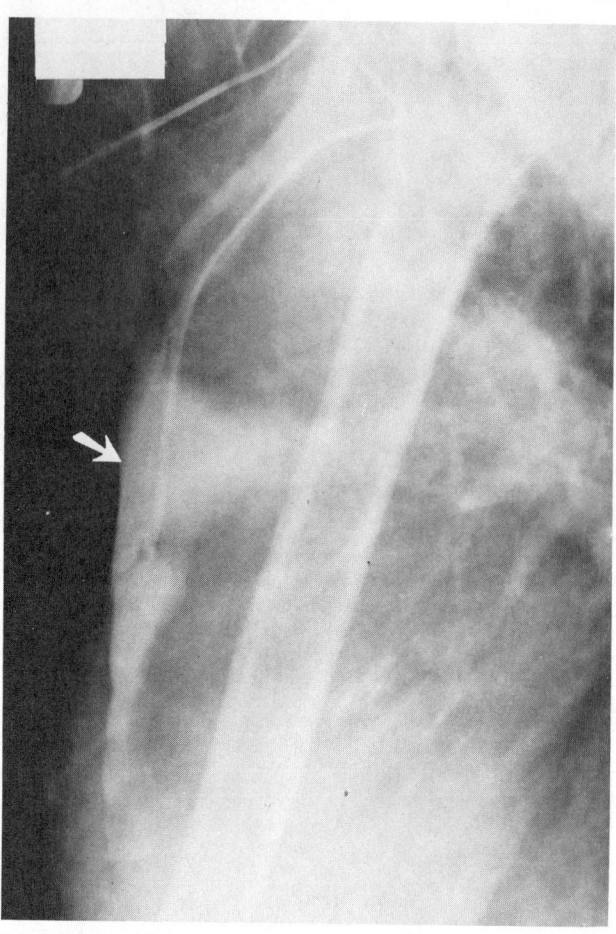

B

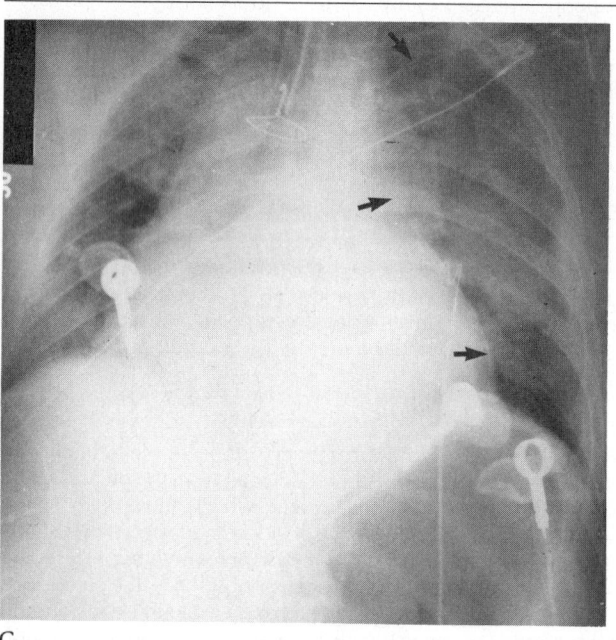

C

Fig. 70-5. Central line complications. A. Anteroposterior spot film of the region of the aorta shows the contrast injected through the CVP line (*arrow*) outlining subintimal dissection of the aorta (*arrowheads*). The CVP line was introduced into the subclavian subintimally. B. Lateral spot film in same patient again shows the contrast pooling in the aortic wall (*arrow*) with absence of rapid flow and washout following injection. C. Portable AP view of a different patient with pulmonary edema in whom a CVP line extends from the left subclavian vein. The line entered the pericardium (*arrows*) and caused tamponade from the bleeding resulting from the vascular perforation.

NASOGASTRIC TUBES. Both the tip of the nasogastric tube and the side hole should be visible below the diaphragm within or past the gastric lumen (Fig. 70-9).

TRANSVENOUS PACEMAKERS. The pacemaker is passed under fluoroscopic guidance to the apex of the right ventricle (see Chap. 5). Films should be checked for breaks or fractures in the wire (Fig. 70-10). A lateral view should be obtained to ascertain that the pacemaker tip is directed anteriorly 3 to 4 mm beneath the epicardial fat stripe [21]. A posteriorly directed tip in the lateral view, coupled with a cephalad direction in the

anteroposterior (AP) view, suggests that the pacer is in the coronary sinus [22]. Projection of the pacemaker tip anterior to the epicardial fat stripe suggests myocardial perforation [21]. Air entrapment in the pulse generator pocket can produce a system malfunction with unipolar pulse generators; this should be kept in mind when examining patients with subcutaneous emphysema [23].

Evaluation of The Lung Parenchyma, Pleura, Mediastinum, and Diaphragm

DENSITIES OF THE LUNG PARENCHYMA. Pulmonary parenchymal densities in the critically ill patient may be caused

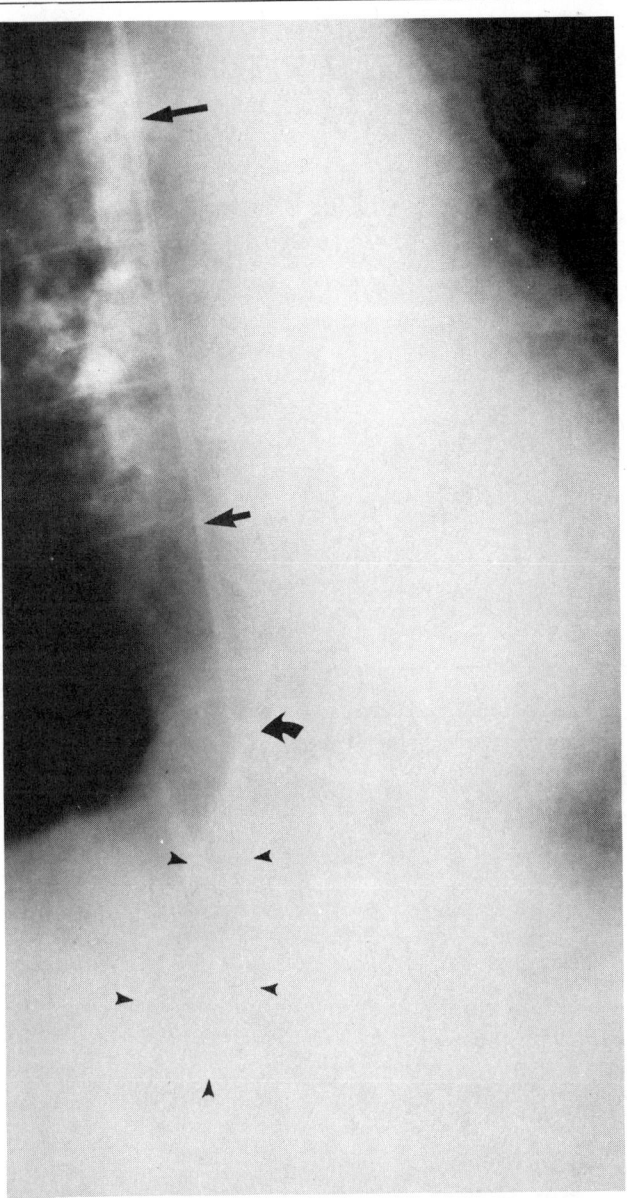

Fig. 70-6. Swan-Ganz catheter looped in inferior vena cava (IVC) and reentering right atrium. Anteroposterior close-up view shows the Swan-Ganz catheter through the superior vena cava (*long arrow*) and right atrium (*short arrow*), looping in the IVC (*arrowheads*) and reentering the right atrium (*curved arrow*).

by either infections or noninfectious conditions, such as atelectasis, cardiogenic pulmonary edema, acute respiratory distress syndrome (ARDS), pulmonary infarction, or contusion. Radiologic evaluation to determine whether parenchymal densities are secondary to pulmonary edema, other causes, or a combination of edema and other causes is often necessary to complement or initiate a clinical search for pneumonia so that proper therapy may be started.

In 1973, Leeming observed gravitational displacement of edema fluid to the dependent lung [24]. He suggested that pulmonary edema could be differentiated from other causes by a positional shift in the infiltrate. Zimmerman et al., in 1982, evaluated the gravitational shift test and concluded that it is a simple, noninvasive method for detecting mobilizable lung water, useful even in the presence of pulmonary damage or an inflammatory process [25].

After baseline films are obtained, the gravitational shift test is performed, using bedside frontal films. The patient is maintained in a lateral decubitus position for 2 to 3 hours before the films are taken. The hemithorax with fewer parenchymal densities is placed in the dependent position. In 85 percent of their patients with pulmonary edema, Zimmerman et al. found that the densities in the up lung shifted toward the dependent lung, while in 78 percent of patients with inflammatory disease no shift was seen [25].

Evaluation of densities in the retrocardiac area may require an overpenetrated film (Fig. 70-11), a 15- to 30-degree left anterior oblique film, or a right lateral decubitus view. The latter position provides better aeration of the left lung and allows greater visualization of the retrocardiac area. In the presence of pleural effusion, a decubitus view may be necessary to displace the pleural fluid and allow better visualization of the parenchyma.

Congestive Failure and Pulmonary Edema Due to Pulmonary Venous Hypertension. Elevation of pulmonary venous pressure, irrespective of cause, produces a sequence of radiologic findings. When pulmonary venous pressures rise above normal, pulmonary vascular gravitational redistribution occurs, producing distention of the upper lobe vessels with a concomitant decrease in caliber of those in the lower lobe, in the upright patient. In patients in the supine position, the equivalents of the upper lobe vessels are the anterior or ventral pulmonary vessels and of the lower lobe vessels are the posterior or dorsal vessels. The change in caliber of the vessels in the supine position is discernible in a good cross-table lateral film of the chest. These changes are also visible with computed tomography (CT); on a CT scan, the dorsal vessels become progressively narrower as venous pressure increases.

The mildest grade of redistribution is difficult to recognize, since only equalization in the caliber of the upper and lower lobe vessels or the ventral and dorsal vessels is visible. Increasing pulmonary venous pressure produces progressive increases in the caliber of the upper lobe ventral vessels compared with lower or dorsal vessels until the difference becomes easily discernible [26].

At pulmonary capillary wedge pressures of 20 to 25 mm Hg, lymphatic drainage is exceeded and the alveolar interstitium, bronchovascular interstitium, interlobular septa, and subpleural tissues become distended with edema fluid. The visible radiologic changes at these pressures are:

1. Thickening of the interlobular septa (Kerley A and B lines) (Fig. 70-12)
2. Peribronchial cuffing, in which hairline, well-defined bronchial walls seen on end increase in thickness and lose their sharp definition (Fig. 70-13A and 70-13B)
3. Blurring or haziness of the perivascular outlines (Fig. 70-13A and 70-13B)
4. Thickening of the interlobular fissures (Fig. 70-13A and 70-13B)
5. Widening of the pleural layer over the convexity of the lungs secondary to the presence of fluid in the subpleural space
6. Pulmonary vascular redistribution (Fig. 70-13C)

Interstitial edema can clear rather rapidly following therapy (Fig. 70-13D). At pulmonary capillary wedge pressures of 25 to 40 mm Hg, edema fluid pours into the alveolar spaces and air space or alveolar edema is seen. The air space consolidation may extend to the subpleural zone, or the more characteristic

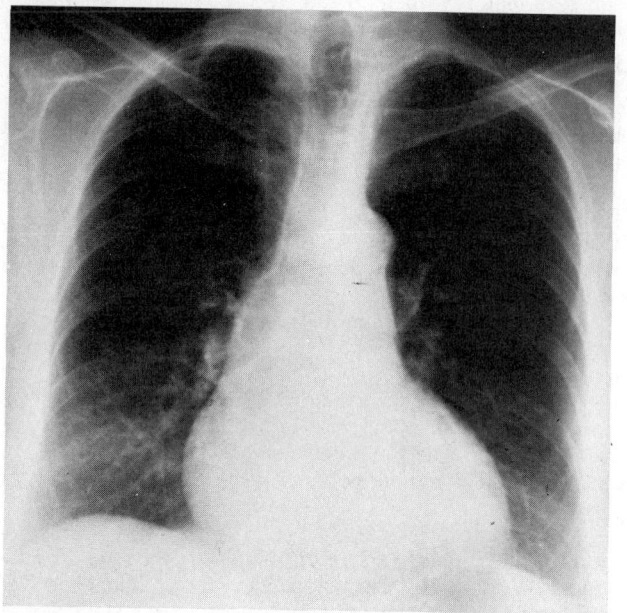

A

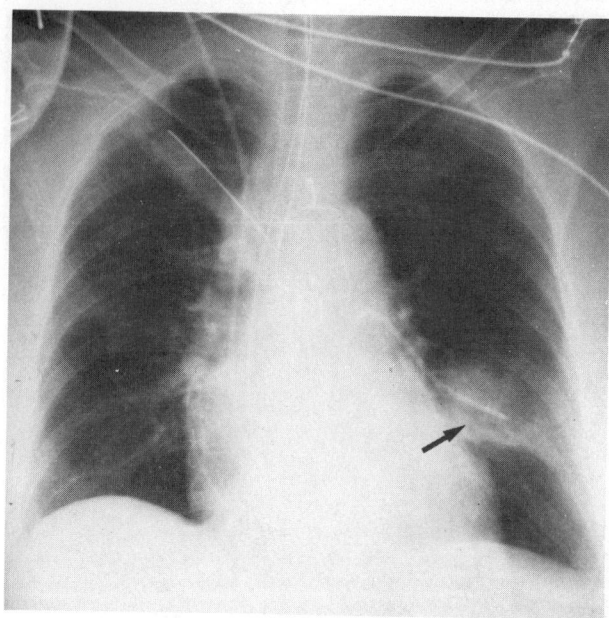

B

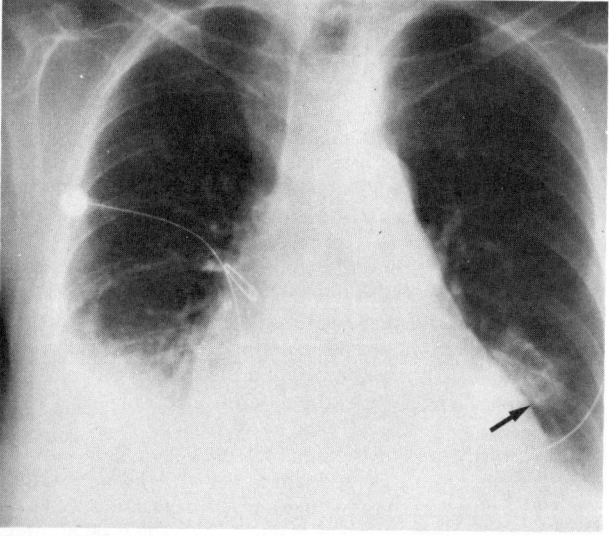

C

Fig. 70-7. Infarction caused by Swan-Ganz catheter. A. Preoperative postercanterior (PA) view of the chest shows bilaterally clear lung parenchyma. B. Postoperative PA view of the chest shows overly distal position of the Swan-Ganz catheter. An area of density (*arrow*) surrounds the tip of the catheter, representing a pulmonary infarct in the area supplied by the occluded artery. C. Posteroanterior film after 5 days shows a persistent left lower lobe density (*arrow*)—the resolving infarct. Right pleural effusion is also present.

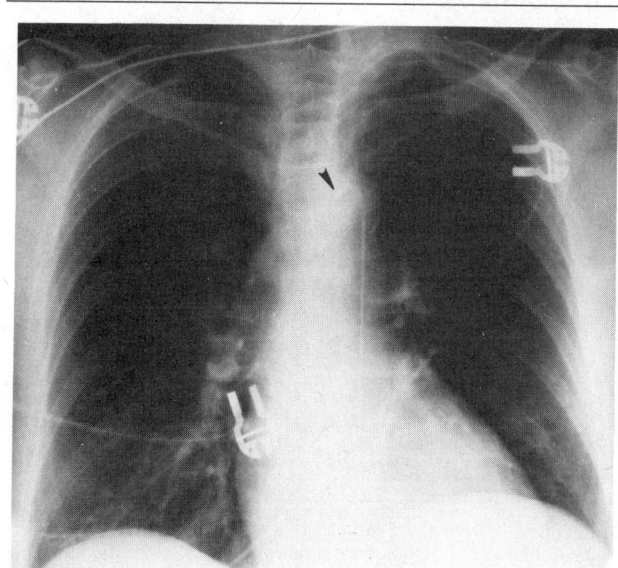

Fig. 70-8. Inaaortic counterpulsation balloon (IACB) occluding left carotid and subclavian arteries. Posteroanterior view shows the tip of the IACB (*arrowhead*) positioned too proximally in the aortic arch, at about the level of the take-off of the left carotid and left subclavian arteries. When inflated during systole, the balloon will occlude these vessels. The tip of the IACB should be distal to the origin of the left subclavian artery.

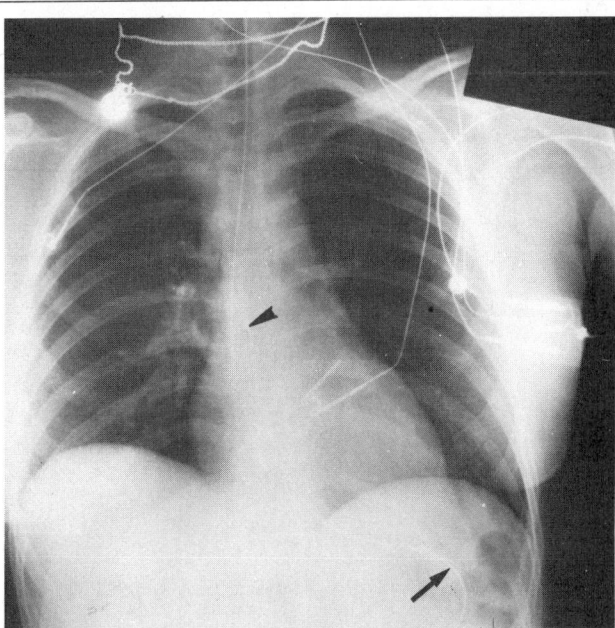

Fig. 70-9. Nasogastric tube tip in midesophagus (*arrowhead*) after looping in stomach (*arrow*).

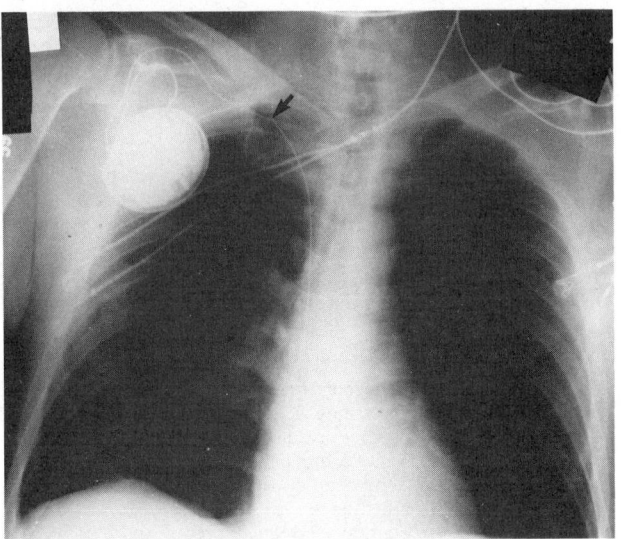

Fig. 70-10. Posteroanterior view of the chest in a patient with a malfunctioning pacemaker. A break in the pacer wire (*arrow*) caused the malfunction.

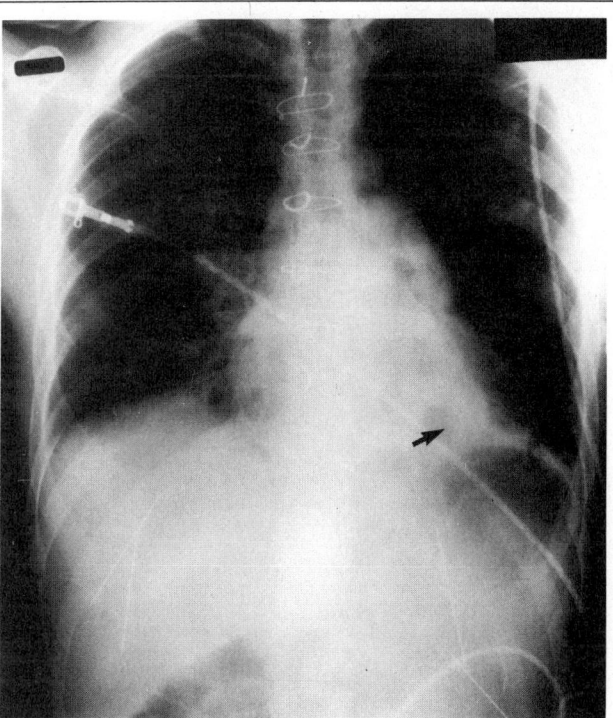

Fig. 70-11. Left lower lobe atelectasis. Overpenetrated Posteroanterior film demonstrates presence of a retrocardiac density (*arrow*) secondary to atelectasis in a patient who had coronary artery bypass surgery.

genital heart disease (e.g., shunts for tetralogy of Fallot)—is another cause of unilateral edema (Fig. 70-15).

Atypical patterns of congestive failure and pulmonary edema were been described by Hublitz and Shapiro in patients with chronic pulmonary disease [27]. Of the four basic patterns they described, two differ in appearance from pulmonary edema in patients with normal lung compliance and vascularity. An asymmetric regional pattern, in which edema occurs only in zones with adequate vascularity, occurs in these patients. The extent of involvement varies greatly from one segment of the lung to another relative to the state of the vascular bed. Another pattern seen is the miliary nodular pattern. Hublitz and Shapiro postulated that the thick-walled spaces in which thickened fibrous septa replace normal alveolar walls impair collateral ventilation and prevent dispersion of edema fluid throughout the lungs [27]. Fluid is then trapped in relatively larger spaces that have replaced normal alveoli. Shadows produced do not coalesce, and the images are seen on radiographs as miliary nodular patterns. The other two patterns, interstitial and reticular, are also seen without chronic lung disease.

Pulmonary edema can be due to cardiac or noncardiac causes. Different radiologic indices distinguish between hydrostatic (cardiac) edema, overhydration pulmonary edema, and edema secondary to increased capillary permeability (see Acute Respiratory Distress Syndrome) [28]. In overhydration edema (e.g., edema secondary to renal failure) the cardiac output is large and, consequently, pulmonary blood flow is large. All of the vessels are recruited, and no redistribution of flow occurs. Because blood volume is also increased, the vascular pedicle, azygos vein, and hilar vessels are large. In pure capillary permeability edema there is no increase in blood volume, so the vascular pedicle and azygos vein remain normal in size; there

"butterfly" or "bat-wing" edema pattern may be seen (Fig. 70-14).

Unilateral pulmonary edema is probably positional, related primarily to a gravitational shift of mobilizable fluids to the dependent lung [24]. It is postulated that asymmetric edema is often right-sided because of cardiac enlargement that impedes blood flow in the left pulmonary arterial system, thereby reducing capillary volume. Unilateral diminution in pulmonary blood flow—as seen in Swyer-James syndrome, main pulmonary artery thromboembolism, and surgical corrections of con-

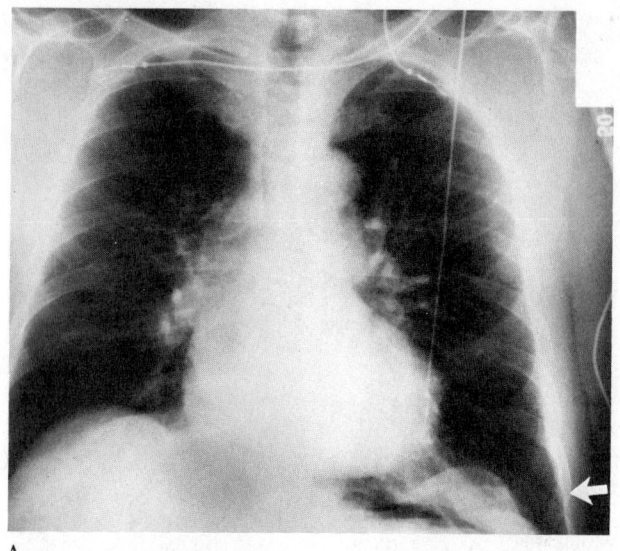

A

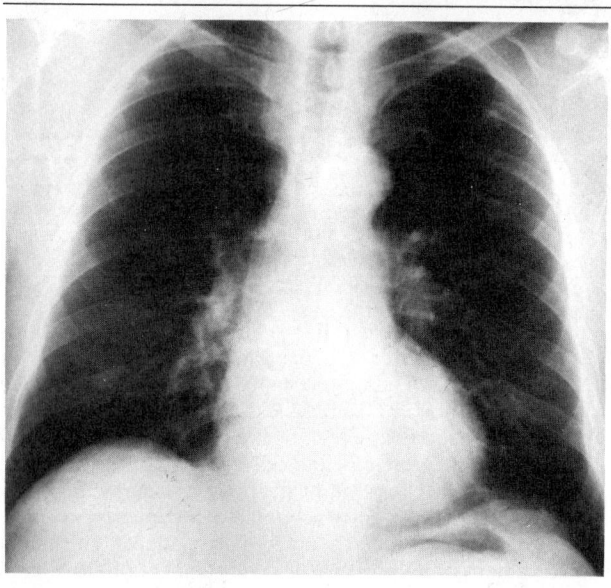

C

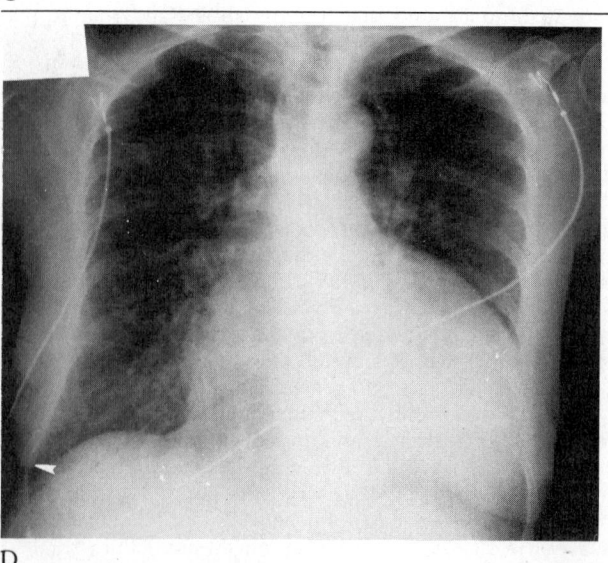

D

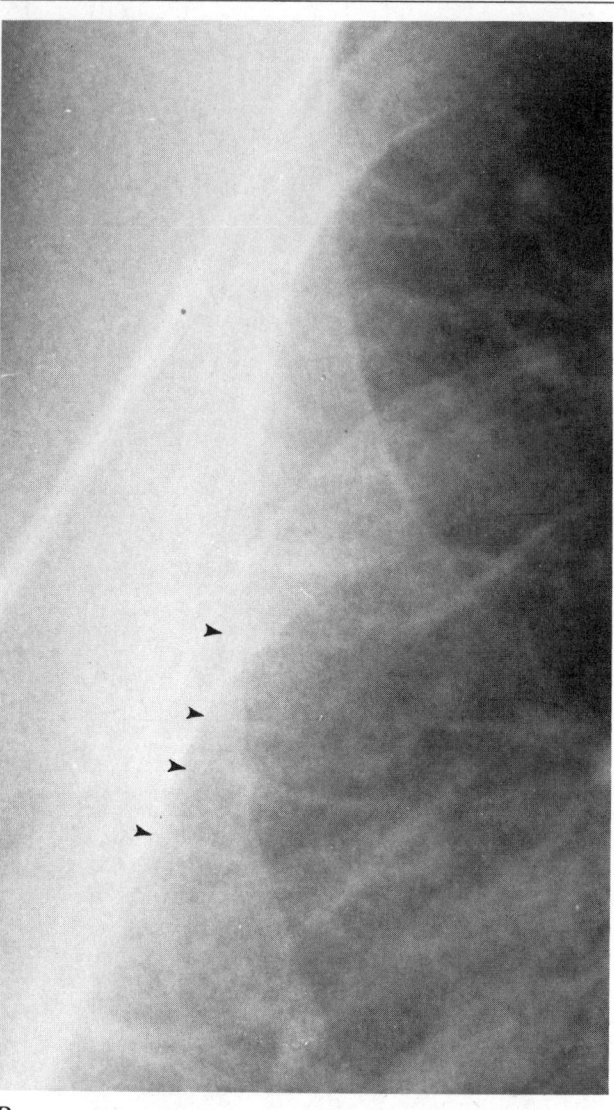

B

Fig. 70-12. Congestive failure. A. Posteroanterior (PA) view of a patient in congestive heart failure. The heart size is at the upper limit of normal. Vascular redistribution and Kerley B lines (*arrow*) are present. B. Enlargment of a PA film of a different patient shows Kerley B lines (*arrowheads*) perpendicular to the lateral chest wall. C. Posteroanterior view of the first patient after therapy shows that pulmonary vascular redistribution is no longer present and Kerley B lines have disappeared. D. Posteroanterior view of a different patient in congestive failure shows cardiomegaly with left ventricular enlargement, numerous Kerley B lines on the right, and a pleural density (*arrowhead*) probably representing subpleural edema (density parallel to the right lower ribs).

are no signs of pulmonary venous hypertension, and heart size is also normal.

When different types of edema coexist, edema may occur at lower left atrial pressures and wedge pressure readings may be low or only slightly elevated [29].

Acute Respiratory Distress Syndrome. Numerous factors can be responsible for ARDS, but the common denominator is always an acute injury to the alveolocapillary unit. The pathologic alterations with corresponding radiologic changes occur

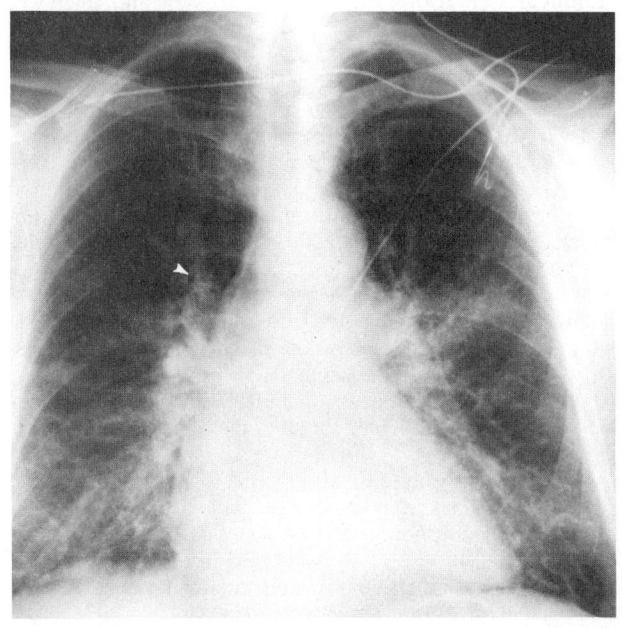

A

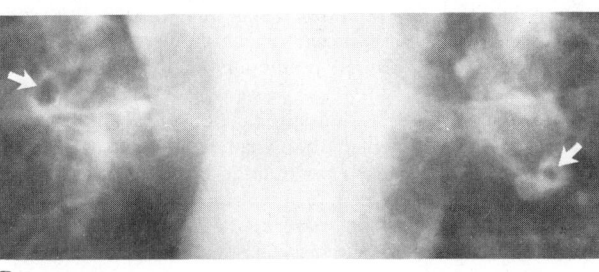

B

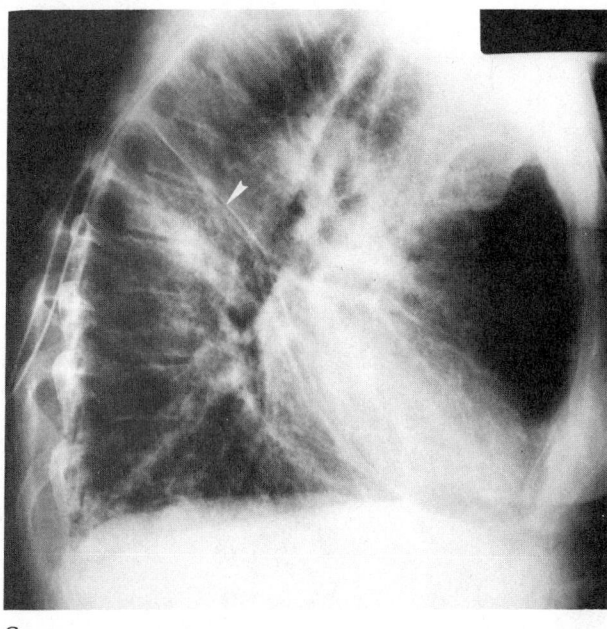

C

Fig. 70-13. Interstitial edema. A. Posteroanterior (PA) film of a patient with congestive heart failure shows cardiomegaly, increased interstitial markings, and right-sided peribronchial cuffing (*arrowhead*) secondary to interstitial edema. B. Enlargement of a PA film of a different patient shows bilateral peribronchial cuffing (*arrows*). C. Lateral view of the first patient shows a small amount of fluid in the fissures (*arrowhead*). D. Follow-up film of the same patient after 6.5 weeks. There is resolution of the congestive heart failure and interstitial edema. The size of the vessels in the upper lobes is greater than that of the vessels in the bases, suggesting that redistribution is still present.

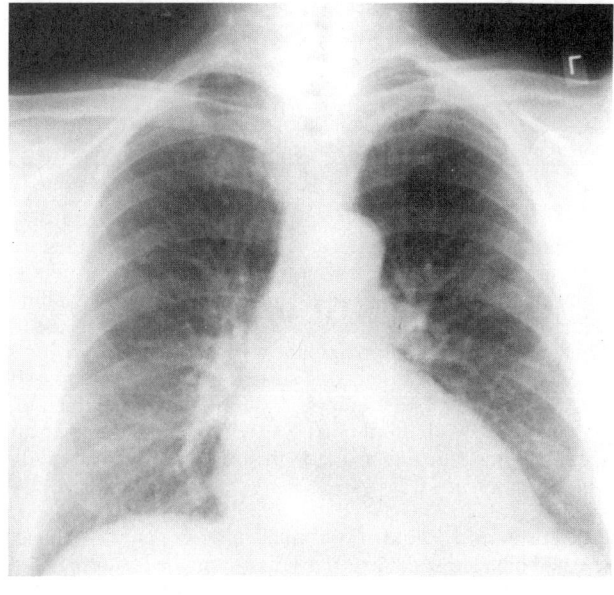

D

12 to 24 hours after the first appearance of respiratory symptoms. Insidious accumulation of edema fluid in the extravascular space occurs. This appears to be confined to the true unrestricted interstitial space, in which the basal laminae of the epithelium and endothelium are separated, not in the restricted interstitial space with fused basal laminae [30].

The corresponding radiologic picture is a perihilar, perivascular haziness with peribronchial cuffing. Only occasionally are Kerley A and B lines seen; in one series, they were noted in only 5 of 75 cases [31]. During the acute stage, the alveoli also become nonhomogeneously filled with a proteinaceous and often hemorrhagic cell-containing fluid. Hyaline membranes form in the alveoli and sometimes in the alveolar ducts. The radiologic picture is one of patchy, ill-defined, confluent miliary nodular or alveolar densities that are not rapidly reversible (Fig. 70-16).

The course of ARDS is highly variable. In some patients reabsorption of the exudates is complete within a few days, thereby producing radiologic clearing of the densities. In some there is a delayed clearing of the exudates, with a corresponding delay in clearing of the radiologic picture. In a third group, progressive fibrosing alveolitis follows. The progression of fibrosis and the degree of tissue derangement do not correlate with the duration of the disease. Radiologically this phase presents a diffuse, fibrotic pattern.

After the first week, the radiologist's main concern is the recognition of superimposed complications, such as pulmonary infections, oxygen toxicity, barotrauma, and pulmonary embolism with infarction. When clinical signs and symptoms of infection are present and the radiographic picture deteriorates,

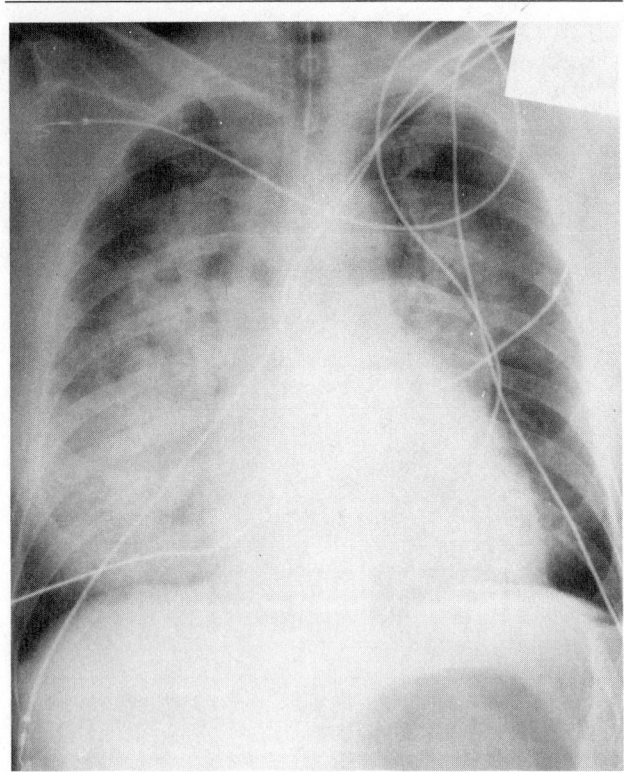

Fig. 70-14. Alveolar pulmonary edema. "Butterfly" pattern of pulmonary edema can be seen in the perihilar areas.

pneumonia should be suspected. Development of cavities and a change in the character of the densities should lead to suspicion of superimposed abscess, infarction, or cardiac failure. Unger et al. showed that only direct hemodynamic measurements of the pulmonary capillary wedge pressure provide a dependable means of detecting superimposed failure in cases of ARDS [32]. Pulmonary embolism, with or without infarction, can be verified with a pulmonary arteriogram using the Swan-Ganz catheter, already in place in most cases, to inject the contrast material.

Atelectasis and Pneumonia. Atelectasis is easily diagnosed when a characteristic linear density or large densities are seen with accompanying signs suggestive of volume loss (shift of fissures and/or mediastinal and diaphragmatic elevation). Densities that fall between these categories, however, such as patchy infiltrates, are often indistinguishable from pneumonic infiltrates on a single study. The presence of air bronchograms makes a mucous plug unlikely; more likely are a pneumonic infiltrate, an atypical pattern of pulmonary edema, or an infarct. In this case treatment for a mucous plug, such as suctioning and bronchoscopy, would be fruitless; rapid improvement following any such procedure suggests the presence of atelectasis due to a mucous plug.

In the presence of densities not readily diagnosed as atelectasis, pneumonia should be strongly considered. Aspirates for culture should be obtained from the lung periphery, with care to bypass the upper airway, as the central airways will become readily colonized after placement of a tracheostomy or endotracheal tube [33]. Open lung biopsy may sometimes be necessary for diagnosis (Fig. 70-17).

Chemical Aspiration Pneumonia. The extent and severity of pulmonary injury following aspiration of gastric contents depend on the volume and character of the aspirated material (see Chap. 62) [34–38]. Pathologically, the lungs show areas of atelectasis within minutes; up to 1 hour after aspiration, however, only mild microscopic abnormalities are present (interstitial edema with capillary congestion). These progress to complete desquamation of the bronchial epithelium and polymorphonuclear leukocyte infiltration of the area (bronchiolitis). Alveolar spaces fill with edema fluid, red blood cells, and polymorphonuclear leukocytes (alveolar infiltrates), progressing to consolidation in 24 to 48 hours. Formation of hyaline membranes occurs by 48 hours, and organization or resolution within 72 hours. Complete resolution, focal parenchymal scars, and/or bronchiolitis obliterans may follow.

From the preceding discussion it is clear that after aspiration, the chest film may show any or all of the following.

1. No finding, if only a small amount is aspirated or if the radiograph is taken too soon after aspiration, before migration of polymorphonuclear leukocytes and edema fluid into the alveoli
2. Increased linear densities secondary to interstitial edema and capillary congestion
3. Nodular alveolar infiltrates, consolidations, and patchy densities (Fig. 70-18) [39] that progress and become confluent secondary to filling of alveolar spaces by edema fluid, red blood cells, and polymorphonuclear leukocytes
4. The pattern of noncardiac pulmonary edema (ARDS)

In ICU patients who aspirate the incidence of complications is increased. In 75 percent of young patients without underlying medical disease, aspiration pneumonia follows an uncomplicated course, and the chest radiograph clears after 7 to 10 days. However, ICU patients are particularly prone to developing infectious complications such as pneumonia, abscess formation, ARDS, and bronchiolitis following aspiration of gastric contents.

Pulmonary Contusion, Hematoma, and Traumatic Lung Cyst. Pulmonary contusion is a frequent cause of posttraumatic pulmonary opacification (Fig. 70-19). It is often seen without evidence of rib or sternal fractures. It may develop in the area of a direct blow or, occasionally, on the opposite side of the trauma (a contrecoup injury). Radiologically it is seen as an area of increased density or a large area of consolidation with poorly defined margins not conforming to the shape of the lobes or lung segments. The lack of sharp demarcation of the margins is due to seepage of blood or edema fluid into the alveoli and probably into the interstitial tissues. The area of increased density or consolidation is usually seen within the first 6 hours. Improvement of the lesion is rapid, occurring within 24 to 48 hours. Complete clearing is usually seen in 3 to 10 days. Secondary infection leads to liquefaction of dead tissues and bronchial communication, producing an air-filled cavity with or without an associated fluid level.

When laceration or tearing of a lung occurs—commonly due to a penetrating injury or surgical resection—a pulmonary hematoma (a collection of blood within a space in the lung) forms. The cavity formed by retraction of the torn elastic tissues may be completely dense or partially air-filled if bronchial communication occurs. The lesion may progressively increase in size in the next few days due to edema or seepage of blood. This is in contrast to a contusion, which regresses in size. The lesion may take weeks or months to clear. Occasionally a clot may form and simulate an intra-

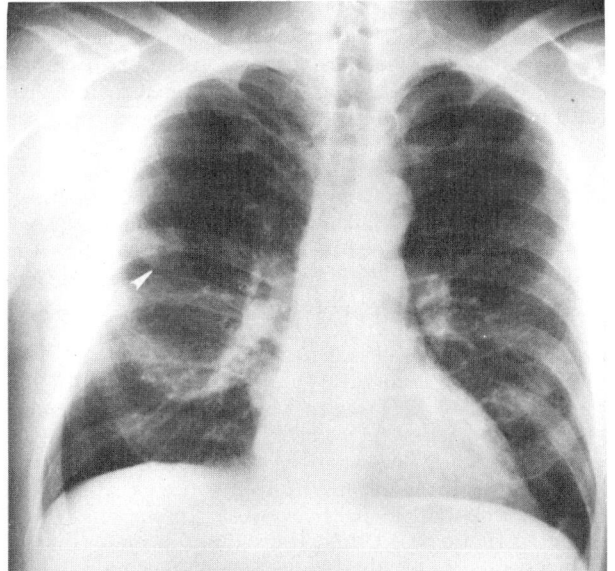

A

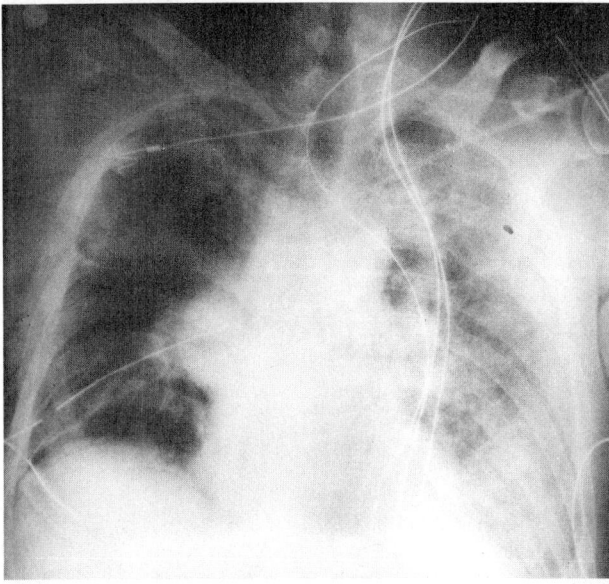

C

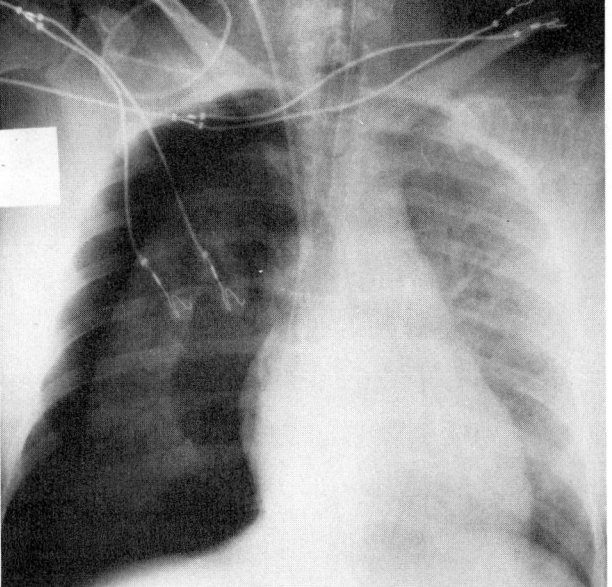

B

Fig. 70-15. Asymmetric pulmonary edema. A. Preoperative posteroanterior film shows a right upper lobe pulmonary nodule (*arrowhead*). B. Anteroposterior film shows changes secondary to the right upper lobe lobectomy. The patient developed a right pulmonary embolus after the film was taken. C. Asymmetric pulmonary edema is seen developing in the left side only, presumably due to the lack of perfusion in the right side.

Fig. 70-16. Acute respiratory distress syndrome with pneumothorax. Portable anteroposterior film shows bilateral alveolar densities. Air bronchograms are seen bilaterally. Note pattern of collapse of the relatively stiff lung when pneumothorax occurred.

cavitary fungus ball. Resolution may be incomplete, resulting in a pulmonary nodule.

Traumatic lung cysts also may occur following trauma. They may appear immediately after blunt trauma or may form after several hours or days. Single, multiple, or multilocular thin-walled, oval to spheric cystic spaces may be seen in the lung periphery or subpleurally. Bleeding into the cyst from ruptured capillaries may occur. The lung cysts persist for long periods, often more than 4 months, but progressively decrease in size during this period.

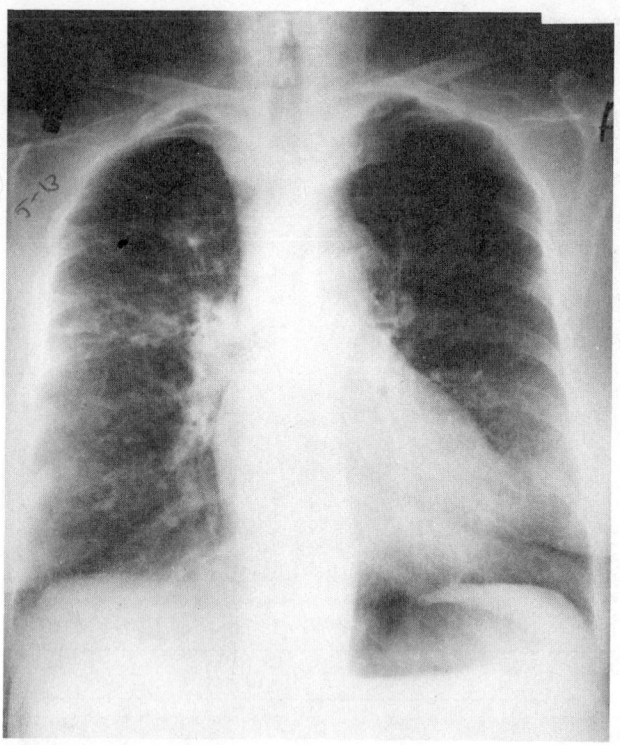

A

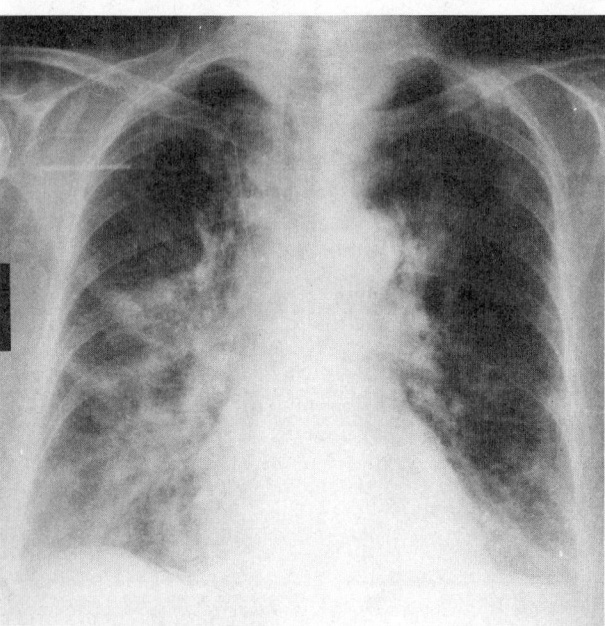

B

Fig. 70-17. Pneumocystis carinii pneumonia. A. Posteroanterior view "baseline" film shows diffuse interstitial infiltrates secondary to Wegener's granulomatosis. (Patient medicated with cyclophospham-ide [Cytoxan] and prednisone.) B. Follow-up film after the patient de-veloped increasing dyspnea and interstitial infiltrates. Appearance of lung parenchyma is indistinguishable from pulmonary edema. Open lung biopsy revealed *Pneumocystis carinii* pneumonia.

Pulmonary Thromboembolism and Infarction. Episodes of pulmonary thromboembolism usually show some changes on plain chest radiographs, such as linear atelectasis, elevation of a hemidiaphragm, or pleural effusion. Most embolic occlusions occur in the lower lobes, the right more often than the left, probably as a result of hemodynamic flow patterns (see Chap. 60).

The radiographic changes can be divided into two categories: those with increased radiographic density (with hemorrhagic consolidation and/or infarction) and those without. Changes without associated hemorrhagic consolidation or infarction are seen only when the thromboembolism is massive. These changes consist of the following.

1. An area of increased radiolucency (local oligemia) of the lung within the distribution of the occluded artery (Wester-mark sign) [40]. This is seen within the first 36 hours after the thromboembolic episode. Oligemia involving an entire lung is recognizable when compared with the pleonemia of the other lung. Generalized oligemia occurs when wide-spread occlusion of smaller arteries or thrombosis of large pulmonary arteries occurs. The diffuse oligemia is almost always associated with pulmonary artery hypertension, cor pulmonale, cardiac decompensation, and dilatation of the superior vena cava and azygos veins.
2. Enlargement of a major hilar vessel secondary to distention of the vessel by the bulk of the thrombus. The size of the left hilum is more difficult to evaluate due to overlying car-diac and main pulmonary artery shadows. To assess enlarge-ment, the size of the right hilum can be determined by meas-uring the diameter of the descending pulmonary artery as it relates to the bronchus intermedius. The maximal diameter is 16 mm in adult males and 15 mm in adult females [41]. Comparison with a previous film showing a significant in-crease in vessel size is a reliable means of detecting enlarge-ment of the hilar vessels. Sudden change in the caliber of the vessel (abrupt tapering or sudden termination) also sug-gests thromboembolism.
3. Signs of volume loss, such as displacement of the hemidia-phragm or fissures, or both. Volume loss is probably caused by a deficit in pulmonary surfactant, resulting from loss of perfusion. It is more frequent in cases accompanied by pul-monary infarction.
4. Cor pulmonale, recognized when right ventricular cardiac enlargement, main pulmonary artery enlargement, increased size of the major hilar vessels with sudden tapering of the vessels, and dilatation of the azygos vein and superior vena cava are seen. These changes occur with widespread mul-tiple peripheral embolism or massive central embolization.

Thromboembolism with increased density or infarction shows the same changes as thromboembolism without in-creased density, except for the sign of peripheral oligemia. The area of oligemia is replaced by parenchymal consolidation from tissue necrosis or hemorrhage and edema. The density is almost always pleurally based. Hampton's hump, a homogeneous, wedge-shaped density with its base contiguous to the pleural surface and apex toward the hilum, is rarely seen but highly suggestive of pulmonary infarction.

The consolidations vary in size, but most are 3 to 5 cm in diameter (Fig. 70-20). Air bronchograms are rarely present; cav-itation is unusual and, if present, suggests septic embolization. If the consolidation is secondary to hemorrhage and edema, it clears in 4 to 7 days without residua; if the infarction leads to necrosis, resolution averages 20 days and may take as long as 5 weeks. This sequence of events is more common in patients with underlying cardiac disease. Linear densities (line shadows)

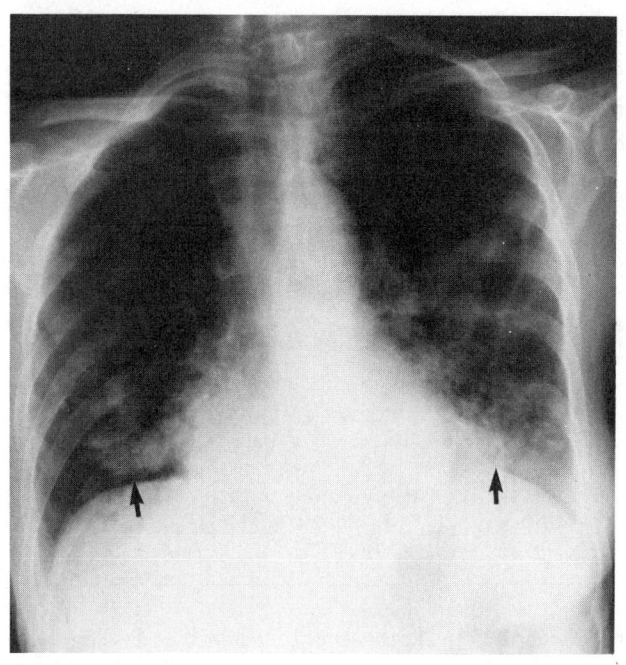

A

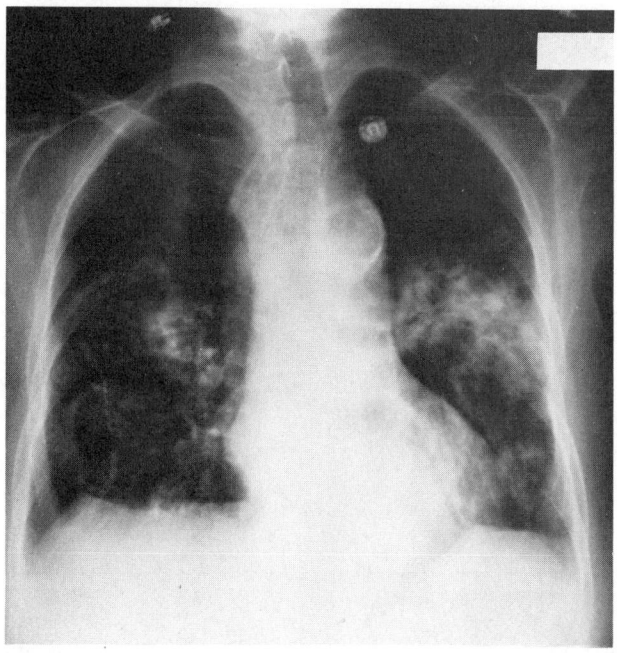

B

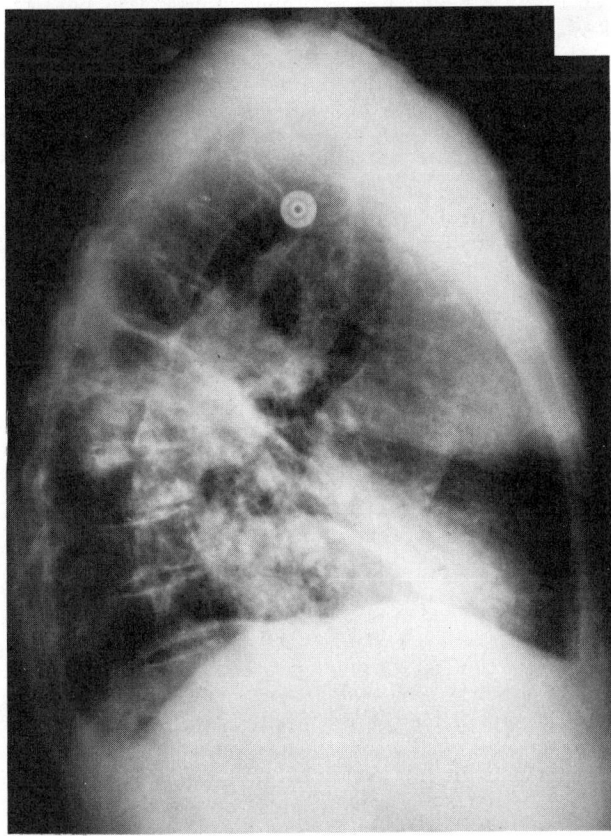

C

Fig. 70-18. Aspiration pneumonia. A. Posteroanterior view of the chest shows bilateral basal densities (*arrows*) in a patient with aspiration pneumonia. B, C. Posteroanterior and lateral views in another patient show patchy densities scattered in both lungs from aspiration pneumonia.

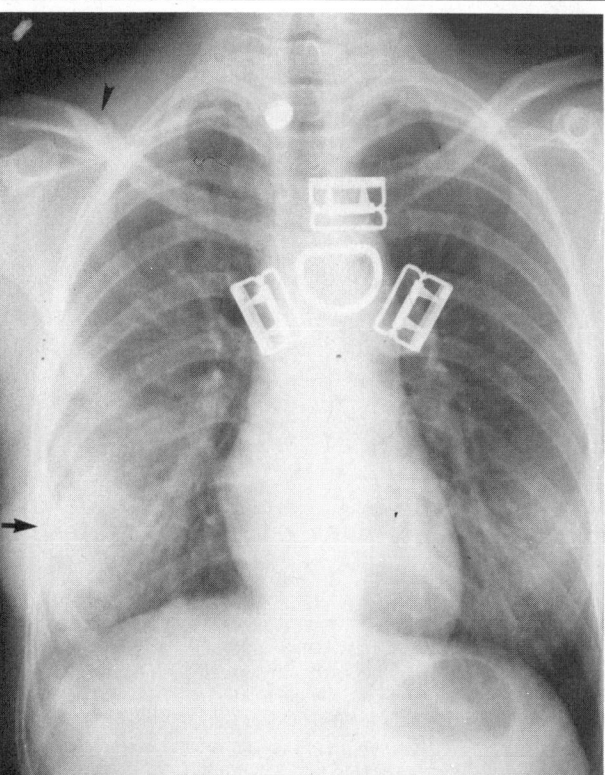

Fig. 70-19. Pulmonary contusion. Opacification ((*arrow*) of the right lower lobe following trauma secondary to lung contusion. Note fracture of the right clavicle (*arrowhead*).

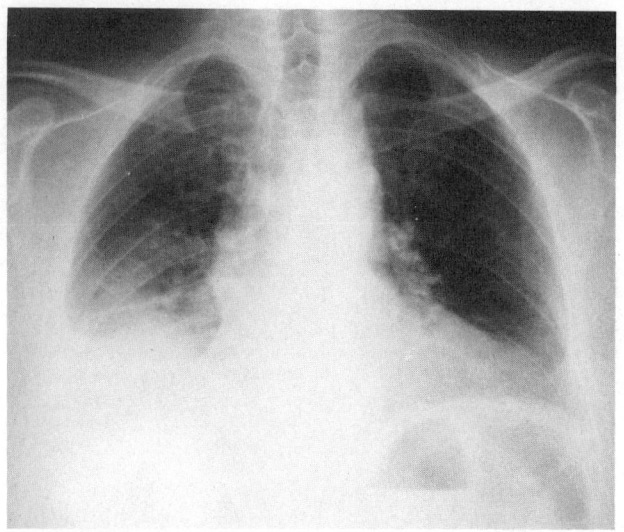

A

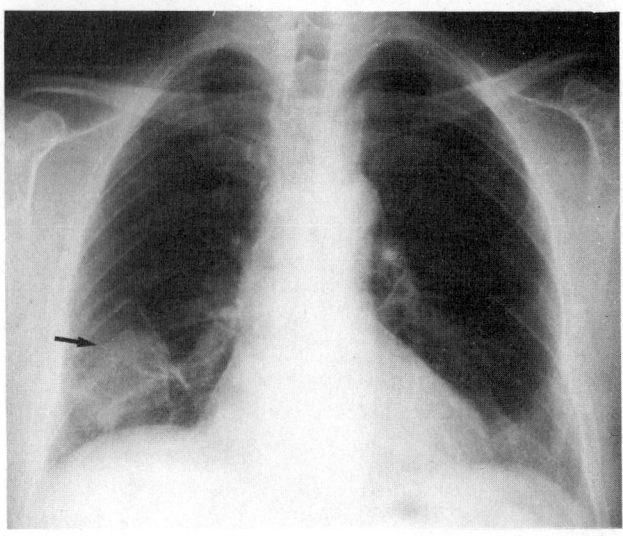

B

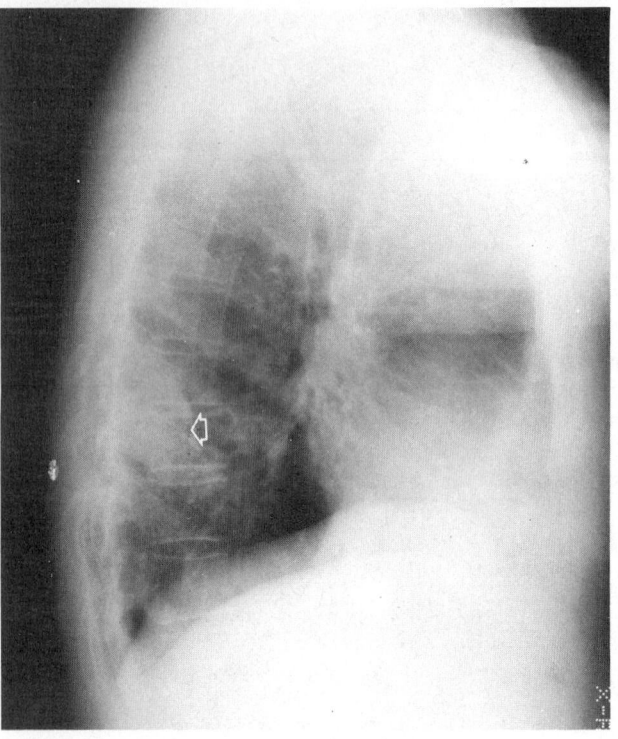

C

Fig. 70-20. Pulmonary embolism and infarction. A. Right pleural effusion, opacification of the lower lobe, and hilar enlargement following a right pulmonary embolic phenomenon. B. Follow-up film 10 days after the initial episode shows a decrease in the right pleural effusion and a rounded density (pulmonary infarct) (*arrow*) in the right lower lobe. C. Corresponding lateral view of the posteroanterior film after 10 days shows that the density is pleurally based (*arrow*).

representing platelike atelectasis, parenchymal scarring, or thrombosed vessels or line shadows of pleural origin (fibrous pleural thickening or interlobular fissure thickening) are also seen radiographically in cases of thromboembolism, but all of these findings are nonspecific. Pleural effusion is at least as common as parenchymal consolidation; the amount of fluid is frequently small, and the fluid is often unilateral.

The frequent presence of underlying chest disorders such as ARDS, pulmonary edema, associated pneumonia, or chronic obstructive lung changes often makes the radiologic diagnosis of pulmonary embolism virtually impossible on plain chest radiographs in the ICU patient. Radioisotopic scanning provides distinctive patterns for pulmonary embolism, congestive heart failure, and emphysema. Ventilation-perfusion ($\dot{V}/\dot{Q}$) scans should be performed whenever pulmonary embolism is suspected. The clearest distinguishing feature of embolism is its focal segmental or local wedge-shaped configuration. An irregular, "moth-eaten" pattern, nonsegmental in nature, is seen in pulmonary congestion and chronic obstructive pulmonary disease. A nonmatched area on a $\dot{V}/\dot{Q}$ scan (a combination of normal ventilation and abnormal perfusion) in the correct temporal setting is highly suggestive of embolism. Ventilation/perfusion scans provide guidelines as to the probability of emboli and serve as an excellent road map for pulmonary arteriography. They also serve as a baseline for future evaluation (see Chap. 60).

The definitive and most specific procedure for the diagnosis of thromboembolism is pulmonary angiography. The primary angiographic finding for pulmonary embolism is an intravascular filling defect. Secondary findings include an abrupt cutoff, tortuosity, and pruning of peripheral vessels localized to select segmental areas, with accompanying slow filling and emptying. These findings are nonspecific but may lead to superselective or magnification arteriograms in suspicious areas.

For the critically ill patient in whom the presence of processes such as ARDS, aspiration pneumonia, or atelectasis complicates the picture, pulmonary angiography is often necessary for diagnosis of pulmonary embolism. Preferably, the examination should be done in an angiography suite with equipment capable of producing high-quality images. For patients who cannot be transferred for selective angiography, however, bedside pulmonary angiograms can be obtained using an already placed Swan-Ganz catheter. When placed, Swan-Ganz catheters are directed toward the areas with highest flow to the right or left lower lobe arteries. Frequently these are the same areas involved in pulmonary thromboembolism, because the same pathophysiologic principles apply. The technique for limited segmental wedge arteriography was first described by Loop et al. [16]. The safety, accuracy, and relative ease of performance of bedside arteriography have been demonstrated in several studies [14,15,16]. It must be emphasized, however, that this procedure should be used only when pulmonary embolism is strongly suspected in a patient who cannot be moved.

Fat Embolism. Fat embolism usually follows trauma with associated fracture, but conditions such as severe burns, diabetes mellitus, fatty liver, pancreatitis, steroid therapy, sickle cell anemia, surgery for prosthetic hip placement, and acute osteomyelitis can also result in fat embolism (see Chap. 177).

Most of the fat is believed to originate as neutral fats released from the marrow, entering the circulation via torn veins in the injured area and, to a lesser extent, through the lymphatic system. Fats are then transported to the lungs in the form of neutral triglycerides. Mechanical occlusion of small vessels occurs, but no significant physiologic abnormality results unless large amounts of fat embolize a great number of vessels. In the lungs, hydrolysis of fat occurs through the action of lipase, converting the triglycerides to unsaturated, chemically toxic fatty acids. Congestion, edema, intraalveolar hemorrhage, and loss of surfactant occur. The fat globules also appear to induce platelet and erythrocyte aggregation and stimulation of intravascular coagulation.

Another probable source of fat is the body fat deposits. Free fatty acids are mobilized and released into the blood following stress. Chylomicrons coalesce into larger fat globules; these fat droplets are then carried into the lungs, where they are hydrolyzed by lipase into the chemically active fatty acids.

Continuous fat embolization, conversion of triglycerides to fatty acids, and intravascular coagulation occur as an ongoing process. Usually within 1 to 3 days the changes are sufficient to produce the full-blown picture of the syndrome. Emboli pass from the pulmonary circulation into the systemic circulation and lodge in different organs, notably the brain, kidney, and skin.

The chest radiograph is normal in 87.5 percent of patients in whom the diagnosis of fat embolism is made based on lipiduria [42]. In those with positive chest findings, widespread or patchy areas of air space consolidation are noted, due to alveolar hemorrhage and edema distributed predominantly in the peripheral and basal areas. The densities clear in 7 to 10 days but may take 4 weeks to resolve completely. Acute cor pulmonale with cardiac failure also may be seen.

ABNORMALITIES OF THE PLEURA, MEDIASTINUM, AND DIAPHRAGM

Pleural Effusion. The appearance of fluid in the pleural space is the same whether the fluid is serous, chylous, purulent, or sanguineous. The degree of opacity of the shadow depends on the amount of fluid and presence or absence of underlying pulmonary disease. Radiologically, pleural fluid is seen as a density that is free from lung markings, displaces the lung, and most often (if free) is located in the dependent portion of the thorax. It is easily identifiable when tangent to the x-ray beam; seen en face, the fluid appears as a homogeneous area of increased density in the thorax. If the amount is not too large or there is no associated parenchymal consolidation, vascular markings may be seen through the area of increased density when the effusion is seen en face.

Free pleural fluid is not confined to any portion of the tho-

racic cavity, and the distribution changes with patient position. Distribution is influenced by gravity, capillary action, and resistance of the underlying lung to expansion. In the upright position, the fluid collects first in the posterior costophrenic sulcus and subsequently in the lateral costophrenic sulcus. The typical meniscal configuration of pleural fluid (Fig. 70-21) is attributed to several factors, including capillary attraction drawing the fluid superiorly between the visceral and parietal pleural surfaces, the relation of the fluid collection to the x-ray beam, the greater retractility of the lung periphery, and the tendency of the lung to preserve its shape while recoiling from the chest.

Subpulmonary collection of pleural fluid is the typical pattern of free fluid collection in the upright position, if no pleural adhesions are present [43]. Radiologically the fluid presents as an opaque density, parallel to the diaphragm and simulating an elevated hemidiaphragm (Fig. 70-22). Subpulmonic effusion is recognized in the posteroanterior (PA) film when the apex of the pseudodiaphragmatic shadow peaks more laterally than usual. The pulmonary vessels in the lung posterior to the subpulmonic collection cannot be seen through the pseudodiaphragmatic contour because of the greater density of the fluid collection. On the left side, there is increased distance between the gastric bubble and the base of the lung. Often the costophrenic sulcus is blunted.

The appearance of interlobar fluid depends on the shape and orientation of the fissure, location of fluid within the fissure, and direction of the x-ray beam. Often an elliptic or rounded, sharply marginated density is identified on PA or lateral films (Fig. 70-23). A "middle lobe step," or step-off appearance, may be seen when the fissures are incomplete laterally [44]. In the supine position, fluid layers may be seen posteriorly, producing a hazy density over the hemithorax. These layers also may produce an apical cap (Fig. 70-24A) or widening of the paravertebral pleural line.

Raasch et al. postulated two explanations for the apical capping [45]. One was that the relatively small capacity of the apex compared with the base allows the fluid to extend between the lung and the superolateral chest wall, a localization tangential to a frontal x-ray beam. The second explanation was that the superior and lateral aspects of the apex are the most dependent parts of the thorax tangential to a frontal x-ray beam. Failure to visualize an apical cap does not rule out pleural effusion in the supine position, however. Trackler and Brinker observed that free pleural effusions in the supine position widen the paravertebral line [46], more often demonstrated on the left side than on the right when an overexposed film with grid is used.

Lateral decubitus views may be obtained to confirm the presence of pleural effusion, rule out a parenchymal process coexisting with an effusion, or quantify grossly the amount of fluid in the pleural cavity. In the lateral decubitus view, fluid forms a shadow parallel to the thoracic wall (Figs. 70-24B and 70-24C). When a decubitus view cannot be obtained for a completely immobile patient, an ultrasonographic evaluation can be performed. Sonographically guided thoracentesis enhances the likelihood of a successful tap in these cases and when the fluid is loculated.

Pleural effusion occurs quite frequently in the first week after thoracic or abdominal surgery (Fig. 70-25). Following pneumonectomy, increasing amounts of fluid are noted to accumulate in the thorax. This accumulation may be rapid or may occur over a period of 1.5 to 2 months following surgery, eventually becoming organized.

Empyema and Peripheral Lung Abscess. An intrathoracic fluid-containing cavitary lesion adjacent to the chest wall may represent either a lung abscess (Fig. 70-26) or an empyema. By conventional radiography, visualization of the three-dimen-

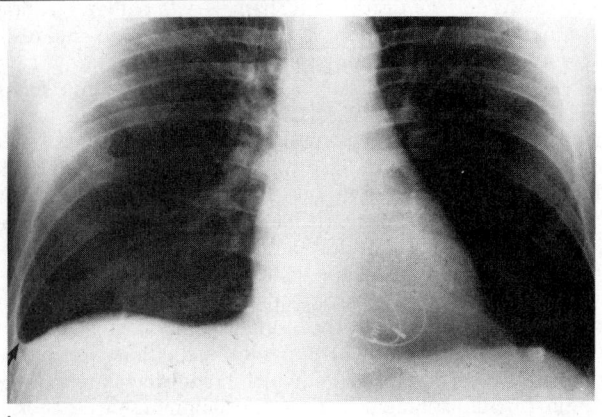

A

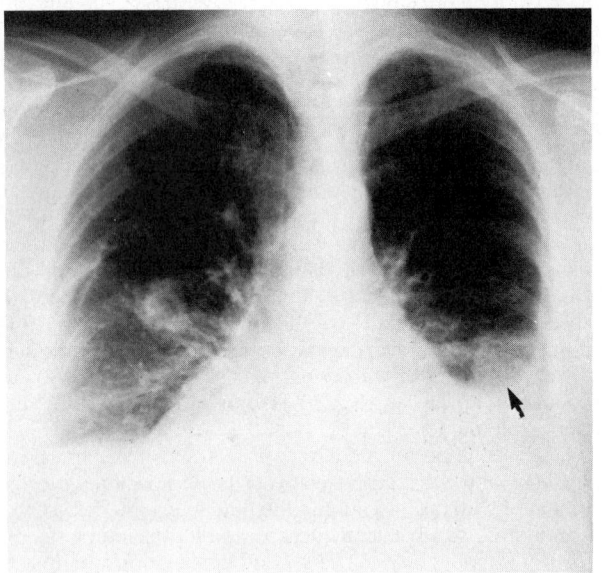

B

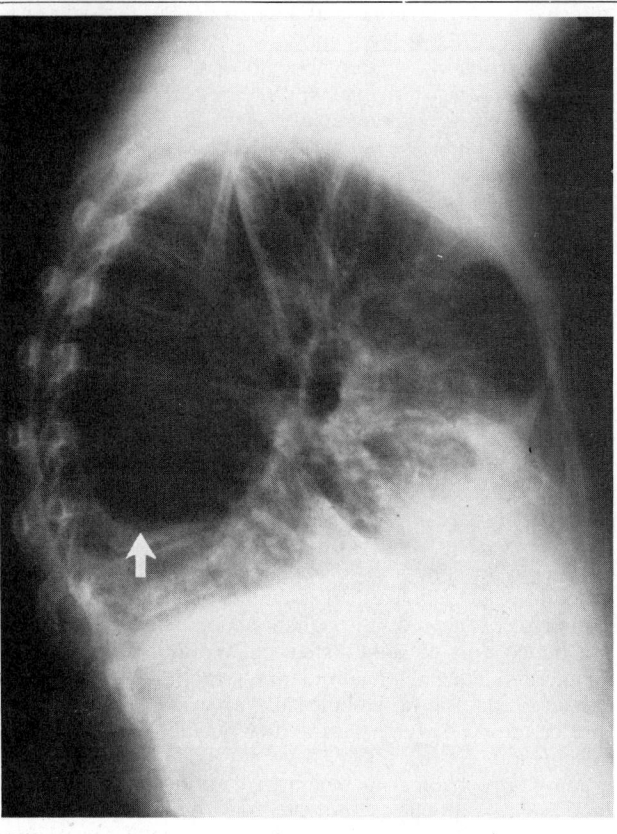

C

Fig. 70-21. Pleural effusion meniscus. A. Anteroposterior film shows minimal blunting of the right costophrenic angle with meniscus (*arrow*). B. Anteroposterior view of a different patient shows meniscus level (*arrow*) in larger pleural effusion. C. Lateral view of meniscus level (*arrow*) in patient shown in B.

sional shape of the pleural lesion as oblong, flattened, and conforming to the shape of the thorax helps differentiate between the two lesions. A discrepancy in the width of the air-fluid levels between two 90-degree projections (i.e., when a wider level is apparent on AP than on lateral view, or vice versa) also suggests a pleural location. Abscesses are more spheric than empyemas and show no significant discrepancy in width on the two projections.

Often, however, one cannot distinguish between abscesses and empyemas by conventional radiography. In these cases, CT should be considered for adequate localization, because there is a radical difference between the appropriate methods of treatment. Empyemas must be drained with a thoracostomy tube, whereas abscesses can be treated medically. Pugatch et al. [47] and, more recently, Baber et al. [48] showed the usefulness of CT in differentiating between empyemas and abscesses. The former group showed that with CT, abscesses appear thick-walled and irregular in shape, with an undulating or ragged

inner wall. They often have multiple loculations, and their shape is unaltered by a change in patient position from supine or prone to decubitus. In contrast, empyemas appear more regular in shape and have smooth inner walls of uniform width. Their margins are sharply defined, with no loculi, and the shape of the cavity often changes with a change in patient position from supine or prone to decubitus.

Postpneumonectomy Space and Bronchopleural Fistula.
After a pulmonary resection, air is seen in the pleural space from small air leaks in the cut surface of the lung. Small amounts of fluid also may be present. There is usually a gradual and continuous reabsorption of air, followed by a reabsorption of fluid, and both may be completely gone within the first 24 to 48 hours. Prolonged persistence of air and fluid may require drainage. Residual spaces may remain indefinitely without untoward effects and do not necessarily suggest bronchopleural fistula. Malamed et al. stated that in 86 percent of cases these residual spaces are obliterated within a year [49].

Air and fluid are always apparent in the basilar zone of the hemithorax after a pneumonectomy (Fig. 70-27) and may be loculated in some cases. There is a variable rate of fluid accumulation, but the space left by a pneumonectomy is usually completely obliterated within 3 weeks to 7 months. If the fluid level decreases rather than increases, one must differentiate between a benign decrease in fluid and a bronchopleural fistula with loss of the fluid through the tracheobronchial tree.

A bronchopleural fistula will displace the mediastinum to the opposite side, due to an increase in the amount of air on the operated side. Benign descent in fluid level without a fistula shows no associated mediastinal shift. Total clearing of fluid from the space and coughing up of fluid and blood suggest a

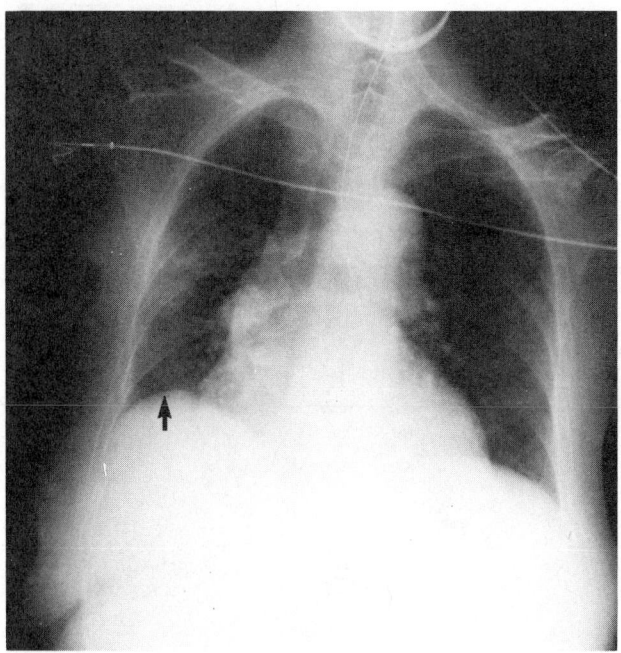

A

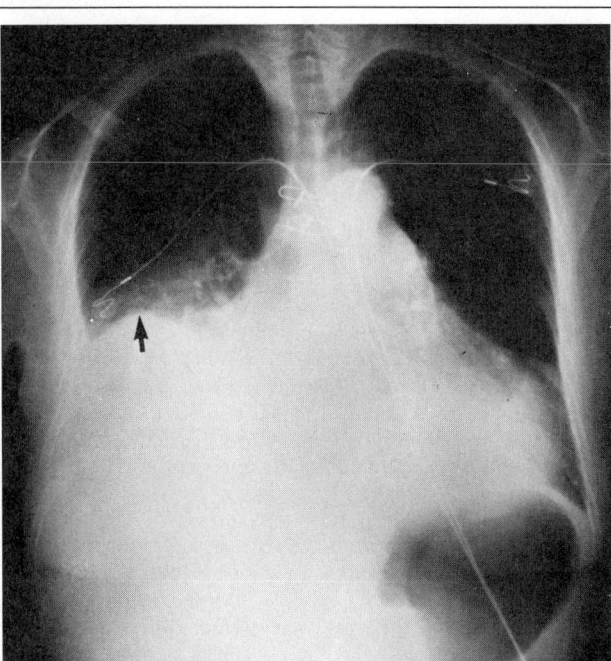

B

Fig. 70-22. Subpulmonic effusion. Anteroposterior views of two different patients with the subpulmonic effusion simulating elevated hemidiaphragms with a more lateral than usual peak (*arrows*).

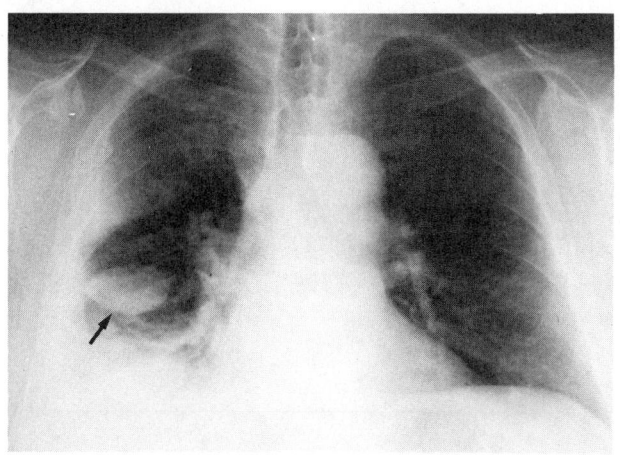

Fig. 70-23. Interlobar effusion. "Pseudotumor" appearance of fluid (*arrow*) within the minor fissure.

bronchopleural fistula (Fig. 70-27). Sudden reappearance of air in an obliterated space suggests either a bronchopleural fistula or a gas-forming infectious process.

A bronchopleural fistula can occur any time during the postoperative period but more often occurs within 8 to 12 days following surgery. If seen within the first 4 postoperative days, it is probably secondary to a mechanical failure of closure of the stump and requires reexploration and reclosure. A bronchopleural fistula also may occur after a suppurative pneumonia or massive pulmonary infarction, or even spontaneously.

Extremely rapid filling of a space with fluid suggests infection, hemorrhage, or malignant effusion. If secondary to infection, the rapid increase in height of the fluid level is usually associated with fever and leukocytosis. Empyema may occur alone or may be associated with a bronchopleural fistula. On the other hand, a bronchopleural fistula can occur without associated empyema, and the fluid in the pleural space in these cases is sterile.

Several methods have been used to diagnose bronchopleural fistulas, including the instillation of methylene blue into the pleural space [50], sinography, and bronchography (Figs. 70-26C, 70-26D, and 70-26E) [51]. Greyson and Rosenthall were the first to report the use of radioactive aerosol inhalation to disclose the presence of a bronchopleural fistula by observing the accumulation of the radiopharmaceutic human serum albumin labeled with ^{99m} in the pleural cavity [52]. Other materials suggested for use were ^{99m}Tc sulfur colloid and ^{131}I albumin. A limitation of these methods is the inability to detect small, slow leaks.

Zelefsky et al. demonstrated small leaks using ^{133}Xe in a gaseous state in a ventilation study [53]. In the presence of a fistula, the ^{133}Xe activity accumulated in the pleural space and remained trapped within the pleural space on the wash-out study. The simplicity and reliability of this procedure make it a useful diagnostic tool.

Pericardial Effusion, Hemopericardium, and Tamponade.
Fluid or blood in the pericardial cavity is suspected when an enlargement of the cardiac silhouette with a water bottle configuration is noted; this typical configuration is not often seen. Fluoroscopy demonstrating diminished pulsations is frequently helpful but not diagnostic. In 1955 Kremens [54] and Torrance [55] using laminography, described the relation of the epicardial fat line to pericardial effusion. In 1968 Lane and Carsky added

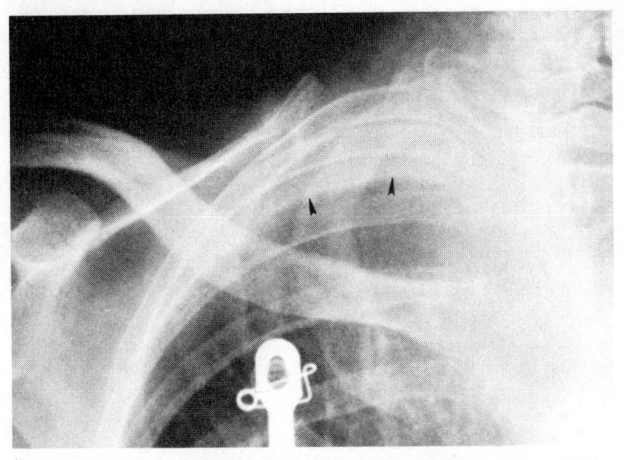

A

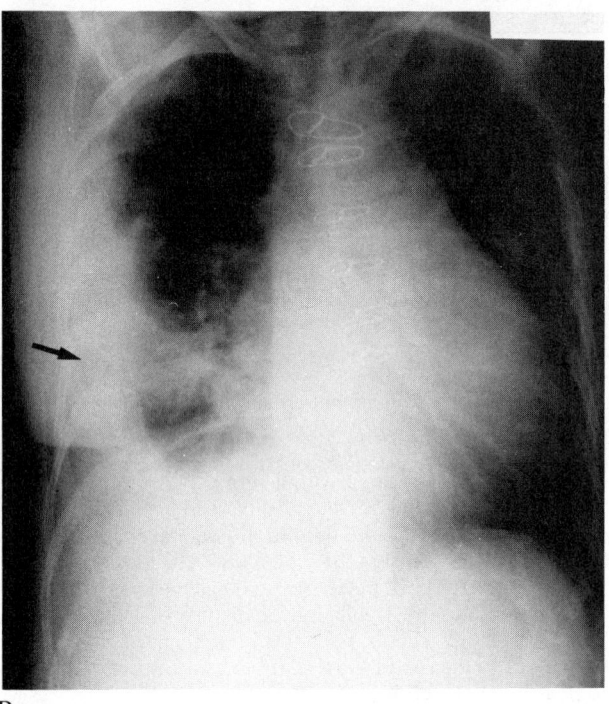

B

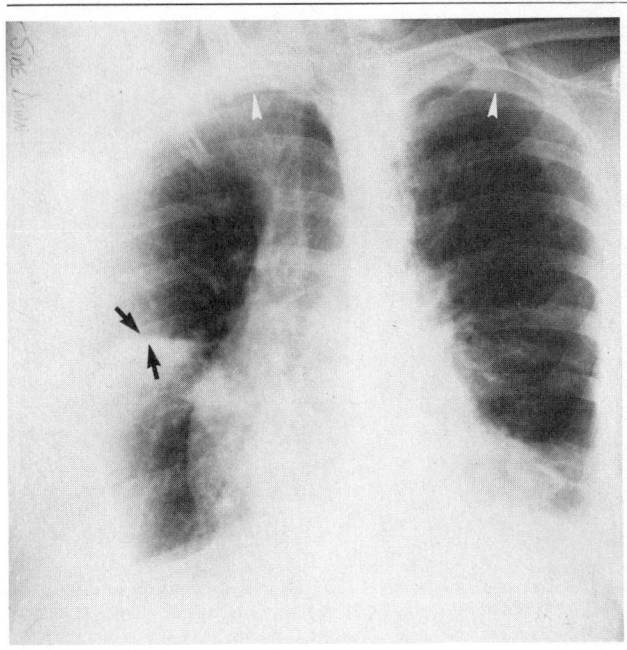

C

Fig. 70-24. Pleural fluid in recumbency. A. Arrowheads show fluid tracking over the lung apex (apical cap) in the recumbent position. B. Right lateral decubitus view (right side down) shows layering of the pleural fluid (*arrow*). C. Right lateral decubitus view shows layering of pleural fluid and tracking into the minor fissure (*arrows*). Note bilateral apical caps (*arrowheads*).

the epicardial fat pad sign as seen in the lateral radiograph as a diagnostic aid [56]. Several authors subsequently described the epicardial fat pad sign in the frontal projection [57,58]. This sign is seen as a strip of soft tissue greater than 2 mm interposed between the anterior mediastinal fat and the epicardial fat (Fig. 70-28).

Chen et al. described widening of the tracheal bifurcation angle in the presence of pericardial effusion [59]. In their series the tracheal bifurcation angle increased to a range of 61.5 to 80.7 degrees in the presence of an effusion, compared with the normal values of 45.3 to 69 degrees set by Alavi et al. [60]. They

also showed a correlation between the increase in tracheal bifurcation angle and the increase in transverse cardiac diameter in patients with pericardial effusion.

Subsequent study of the tracheal bifurcation angle (interbronchial angle and subcarinal angle) by Haskin and Goodman [61], however, showed a wider range of normal (35–87.5 degrees for the interbronchial angle and 35–95.5 degrees for the subcarinal angle), with a mean of 60 degrees and a standard deviation of 10 degrees. This suggests that 95 percent of normal patients would have an angle between 40 and 80 degrees, and only when deviations are severe (>2 standard deviations, especially in an asthenic individual) should it be concluded that the angle is abnormal. If the change in tracheal bifurcation angle is noted as a persistent trend over a series of films, however, it becomes quite significant and is a useful sign for diagnosing pericardial effusion. Ultrasound remains the definitive tool for the diagnosis of pericardial effusion and can be performed at the bedside.

Laceration of the Thoracic Aorta and Brachiocephalic Arteries. The initial diagnosis of injury to the thoracic aorta (Fig. 70-29A) and the brachiocephalic arteries may be suspected on the basis of clinical signs. The presence of fractures of the first and second ribs suggest the possibility of associated vascular injuries. Confirmation by diagnostic imaging is recommended, regardless of a normal radiologic appearance on plain chest films, if the mechanism of injury could potentially affect the thoracic aorta and brachiocephalic vessels.

Laceration of the aorta and brachiocephalic vessels most frequently follows rapid deceleration in vehicular accidents or falls. The differences in the degree of fixation of the different segments of the aorta may cause sufficient stresses between segments in forceful deceleration to cause closed rupture. Flexion stress and a sudden increase in intraluminal pressure also may be the cause of injury.

In 69 to 89 percent of cases, injury to the aorta occurs at the isthmus, the area between the origin of the left subclavian artery and the attachment of the ductus arteriosus. In the remaining cases, injury is equally divided among the ascending aorta,

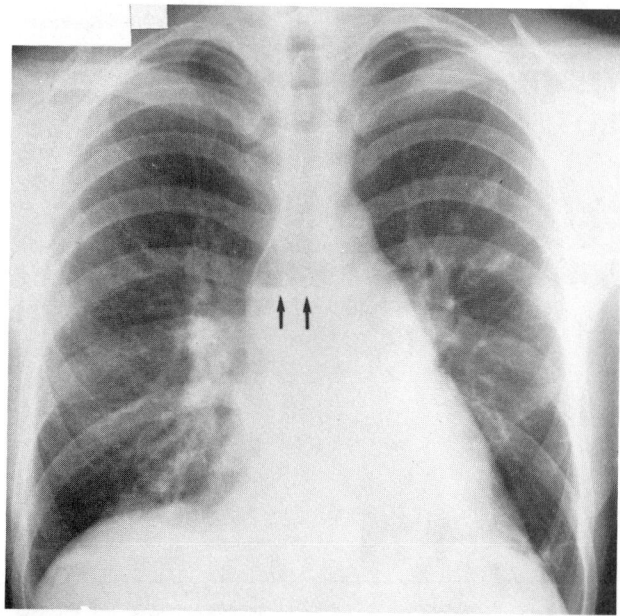

A

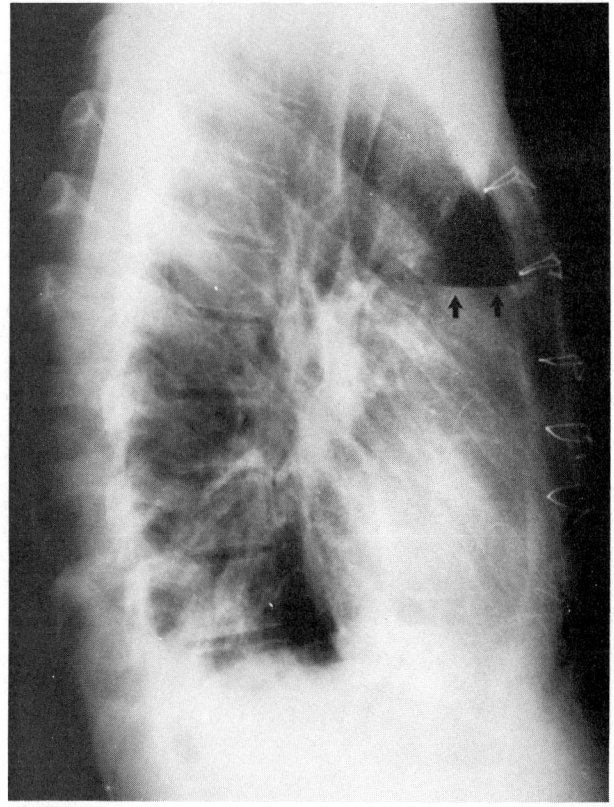

B

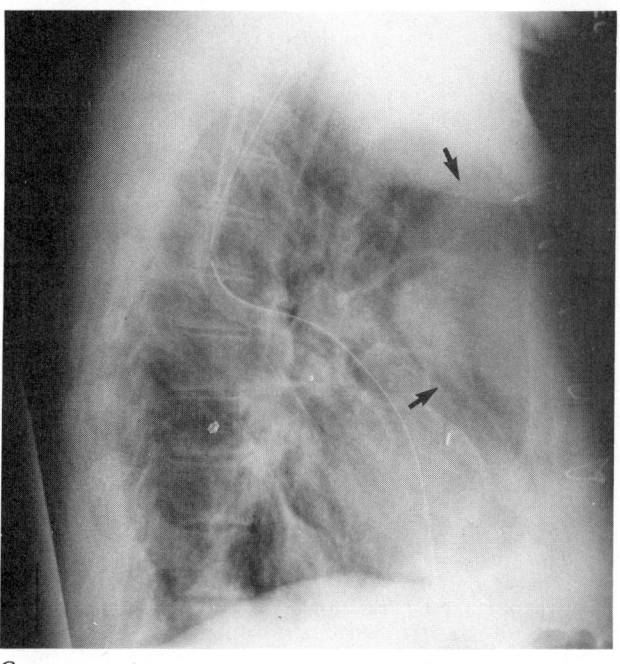

C

Fig. 70-25. Fluid collections after surgery. A. Posteroanterior film of a patient several weeks after coronary artery bypass graft surgery shows an air-fluid level (*arrows*) superimposed on the shadow of the base of the heart. B. Lateral film of the same patient shows the air-fluid level (*arrows*) in the anterior mediastinum. C. Lateral film of a different patient outlines a semicircular soft tissue density (*arrows*) in the anterior mediastinum, representing a loculated fluid collection following surgery.

aortic arch, and descending aorta [62]. Tear is almost always transverse and may involve only one or all of the layers. When all layers are involved, exsanguination occurs; if the tear is only through the intima or the intima and media, the adventitia and the mediastinal pleura can contain the blood at least temporarily. Parmley et al. emphasized that if the diagnosis is missed, up to 90 percent of those who survive the initial impact will die within 4 months [63]. Therefore, the diagnosis must be very aggressively pursued.

In an adequately obtained plain film of the chest, any or all of the following findings suggest a mediastinal hematoma, often secondary to aortic or brachiocephalic injury:

1. Widened superior mediastinum
2. Loss of sharpness of the aortic arch outline
3. Deviation of the nasogastric tube to the right
4. Tracheal deviation to the right on an AP film and anteriorly on a lateral view
5. Downward displacement of the left mainstem bronchus
6. Presence of an apical cap
7. Enlargement or abnormality of the aortic contour
8. Left-sided pleural fluid (hemothorax)
9. Obscured outline of the descending aorta
10. Displacement of the paraspinous line
11. Displacement of the superior vena cava
12. Displacement of intimal calcifications
13. Enlargement of the pericardial outline
14. Obliteration of the aorticopulmonary window

Of all these signs, most of which are nonspecific, mediastinal widening appears to be the most useful [64,65]. A perfectly normal aortic outline without mediastinal widening makes the

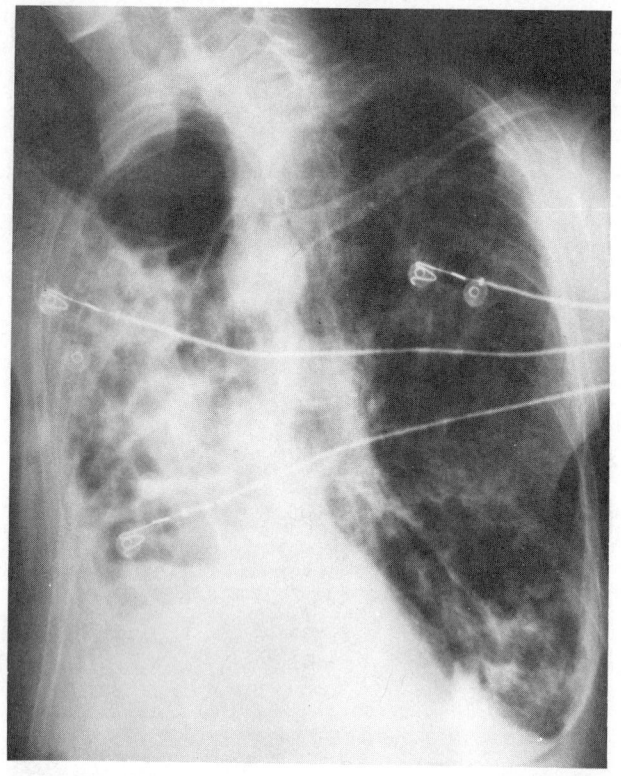

A

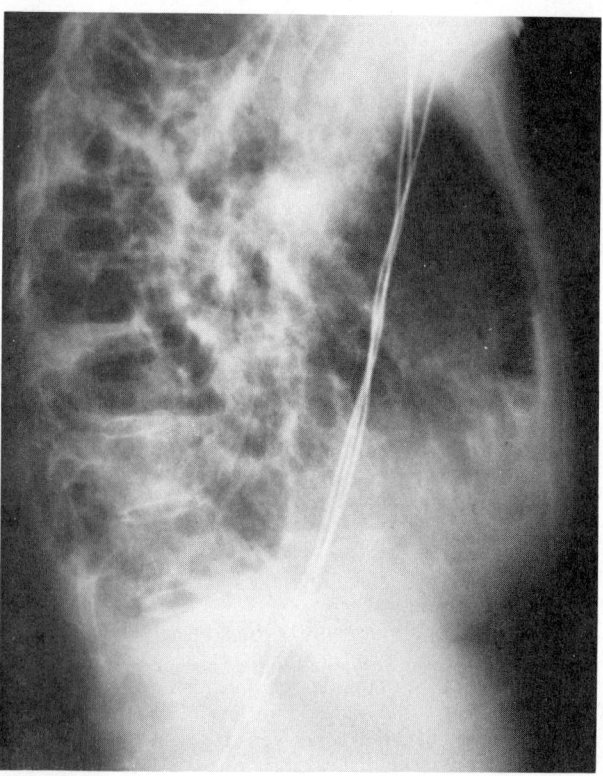

B

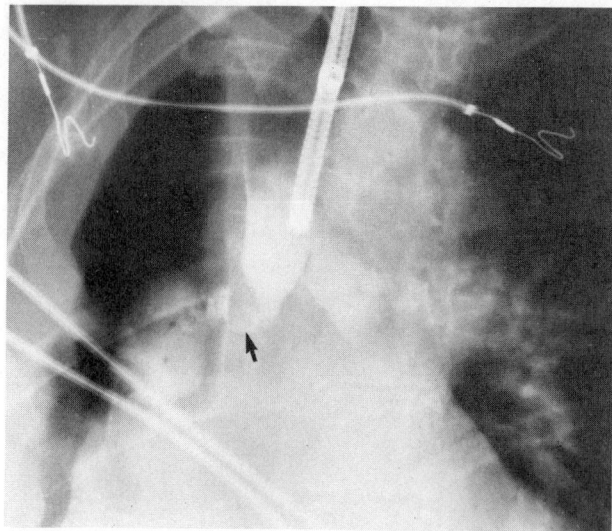

C

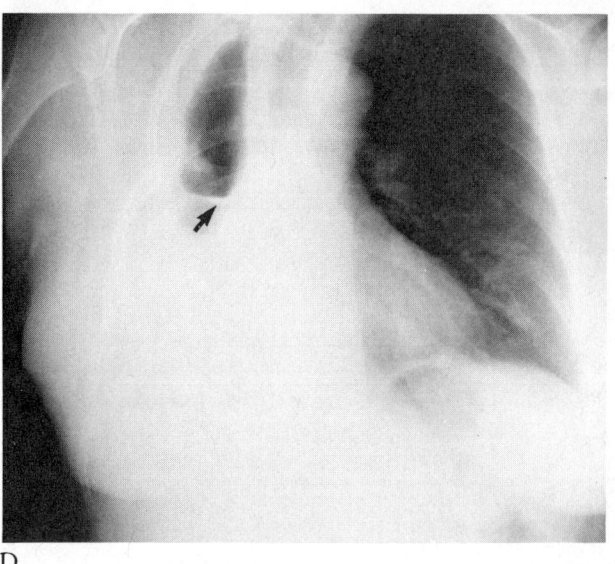

D $\longrightarrow$

Fig. 70-26. Lung abscesses. Posteroanterior (A) and lateral (B) films show multiple cavities with air-fluid levels secondary to staphylococcal pneumonia. C. Following a right-sided pneumonectomy, development of a bronchopleural fistula was suspected. Bronchography reveals contrast material outlining the fistula (*arrow*). Posteroanterior (D) and lateral (E) films after bronchography show the contrast material (*arrows*) forming the upper border of the fluid collection in the pleural space.

diagnosis of aortic or brachiocephalic vessel injury very unlikely.

Aortic and brachiocephalic injuries should be confirmed [66,67]. Magnetic resonance imaging, transesophageal color flow Doppler echocardiography, contrast-enhanced x-ray CT [68], and aortography all have high sensitivities. See Chapter 36 for a complete discussion of the circumstances under which each method is preferred. If static filming is done during aortography, two angiographic series must be obtained, with the right posterior oblique projection as the acceptable standard and the frontal or AP projection as the second view (Figs. 70-29B and 70-29C).

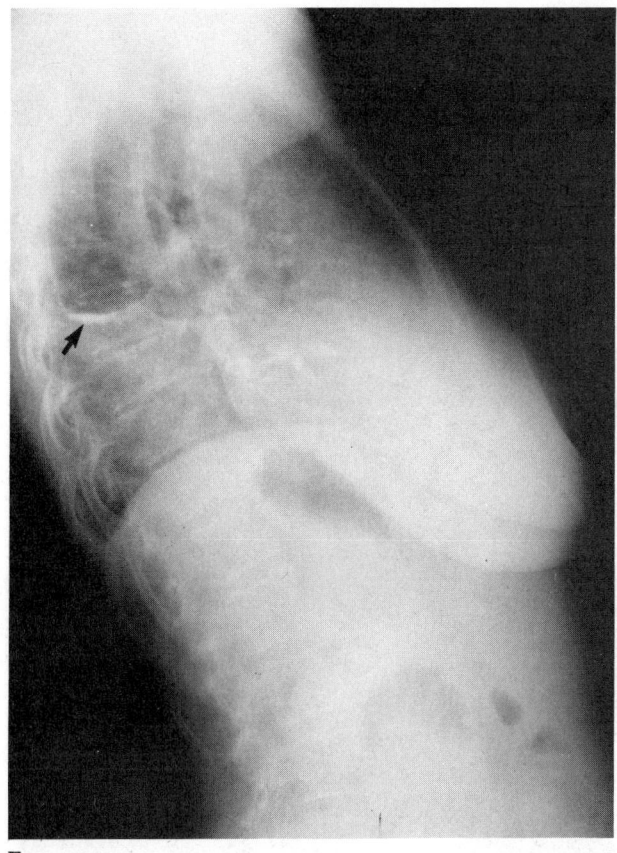

E

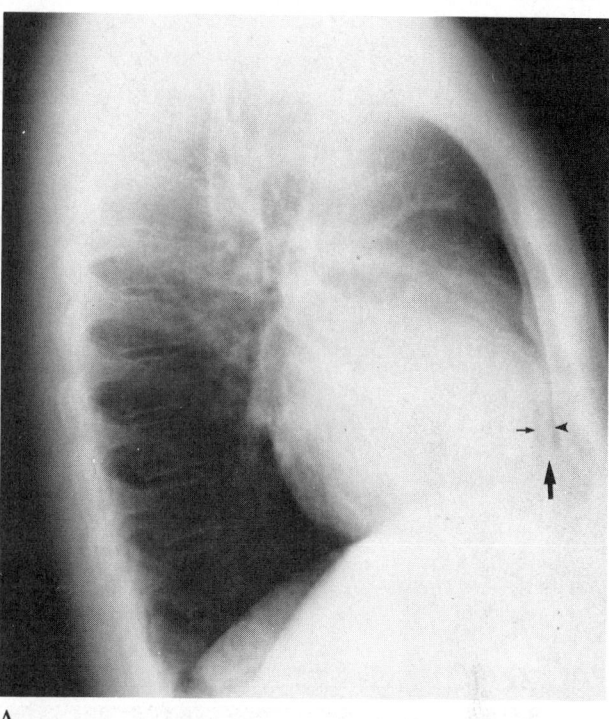

A

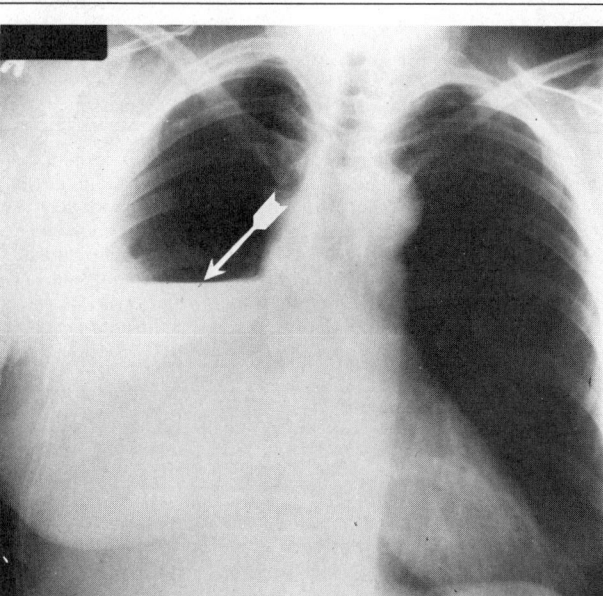

Fig. 70-27. Pleural space with air-fluid level (*arrow*) following pneumonectomy.

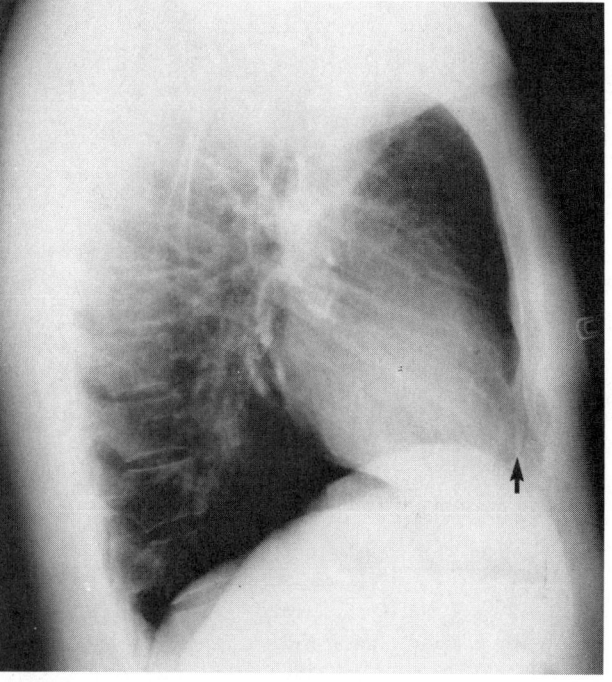

B

Fig. 70-28. Pericardial effusion. A. Lateral view of the chest shows the pericardial effusion as a strip of density (*long arrow*) sandwiched between two strips of lucency. The posterior strip of lucency represents epicardial fat (*short arrow*) and the anterior strip represents mediastinal fat (*arrowhead*). An increase of the density to greater than 2 mm suggests pericardial fluid (effusion or hemopericardium). B. Follow-up lateral view of the same patient after resolution of the pericardial effusion. The cardiac size is smaller, and the width of the strip of density (*arrow*) has returned to normal.

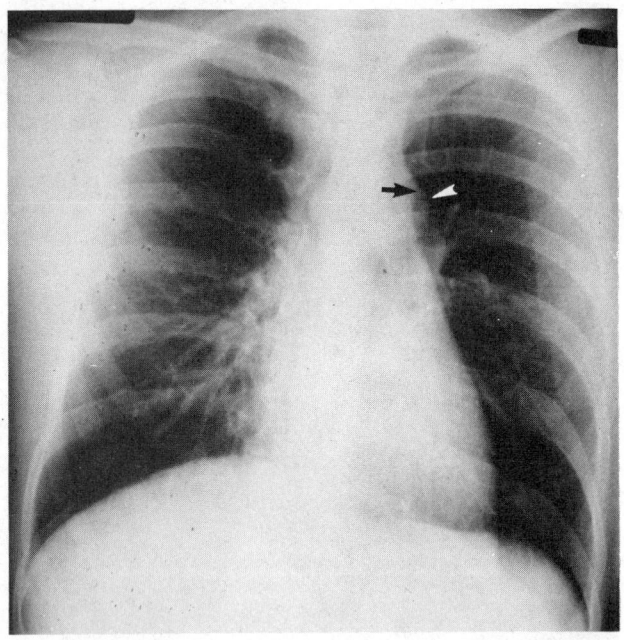

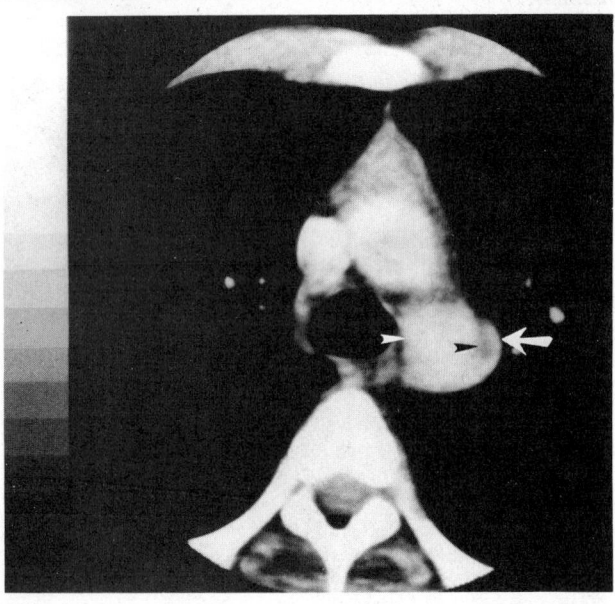

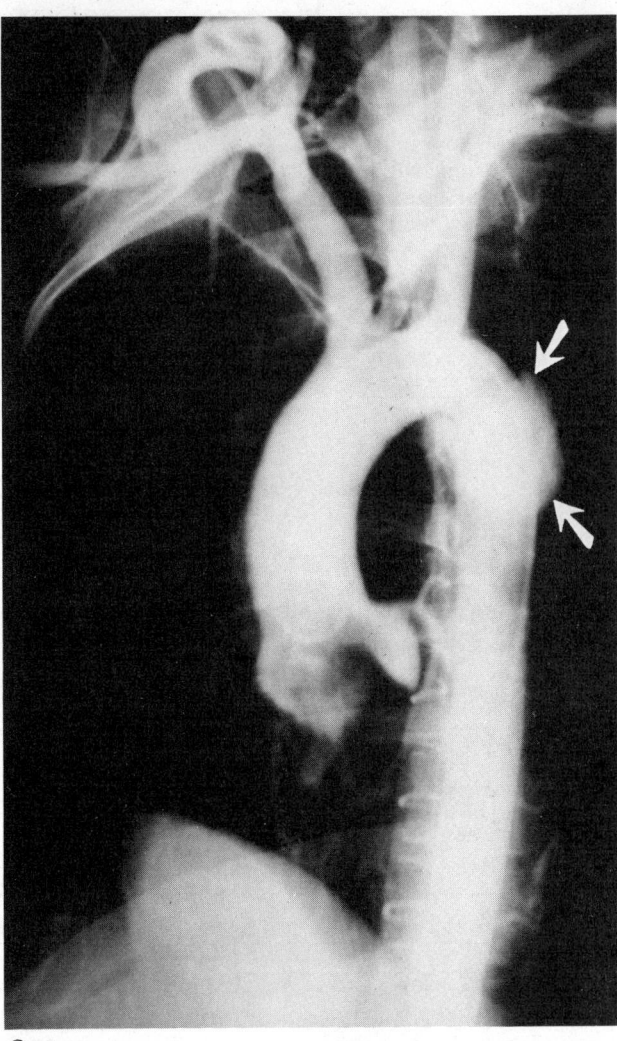

Fig. 70-29. Laceration of aorta. A. Posteroanterior view of the chest shows an abnormal density (*arrowhead*) lateral and to the left of the aortic knob (*arrow*) in a patient who was in a motor vehicle accident. B. "Dynamic" computed angiotomographic section taken at the level of the abnormal density. Contrast medium outlines the lumen of the descending aorta (*white arrowhead*), the aortic intima (*lucent line, black arrowhead*), and the contrast material (*arrow*) lateral to it at the site of the rupture. C. Oblique view of the aortogram shows the aorta and the pseudoaneurysm (*arrows*) at the site of rupture.

Traumatic Diaphragmatic Hernia. Severe diaphragmatic injury following blunt or penetrating trauma to the thoracoabdominal area may allow escape of abdominal contents into the thorax. The presence of a gas-containing viscus within the thoracic cavity is the hallmark of traumatic diaphragmatic rupture with an associated hernia. Most hernias occur on the left side, because the liver acts as a buffer on the right. Very often the condition may be overlooked during the initial phase (the first 14 days). During the "latent period," which varies considerably, patients may have vague chronic symptoms or no symptoms at all. Symptomatic patients may be subjected to numerous diagnostic procedures in an attempt to unravel their vague abdominal complaints, which probably are due to intermittent incarceration of the herniated viscus. The obstructive

phase may occur at any time, the obstruction being secondary to incarceration or strangulation.

Radiologic findings on plain chest films vary from what appears to be merely an arched or elevated diaphragm (with or without platelike atelectasis in the adjacent lung) to visualization of a hollow viscus above the diaphragm with a marked shift in the heart and mediastinum. Ball et al. suggested that the chest film is the most reliable means of determining the correct diagnosis [69]. Additional diagnostic aids include contrast studies with barium to demonstrate the presence of a viscus above the diaphragm, diagnostic pneumoperitoneum to outline the defect with free passage of air from the peritoneum into the pleural or pericardial cavity, and introduction of contrast into the pleural space to demonstrate free passage from the pleura into the peritoneal cavity. Lung and liver-spleen scans also have been used, as has ultrasound.

More recently, Toombs et al. [70] and Heiberg et al. [71] demonstrated the usefulness of CT in recognizing traumatic rupture of the diaphragm. Computed tomography identifies parts of the diaphragm as a separate structure, and a discontinuity in its contour can be recognized. The posterolateral portions of the diaphragm are well demonstrated and tears are easy to see in these areas. Dynamic CT scanning is particularly helpful. We have found direct coronal sections (whenever the patient can be appropriately positioned in the CT gantry) to be extremely helpful in diagnosing diaphragmatic tears with herniation.

Extraalveolar Air and Signs of Barotrauma

PNEUMOTHORAX. The diagnosis of pneumothorax is made when air is seen superior, inferior, lateral, or anterior to the lung and the visceral pleural line is identified. The air creates a zone of radiolucency devoid of lung markings between the lung and the thoracic wall. The lung partially (Fig. 70-30A) or wholly (Fig. 70-30B) collapses and drops to the most dependent position, slung by its fixed attachment at the pulmonary ligament. The density of the partially collapsed lung may not increase when compared with the opposite side because blood flow through it diminishes correspondingly, the degree of diminution of flow progressing with increasing collapse. Thus, the ratio of air to blood is maintained and the lung density remains unaltered [72].

As air accumulates in the pleura, the mediastinum tends to shift to the opposite side. This is best seen in a film taken during the expiratory phase of respiration. For the mediastinum to shift, the intrapleural pressure must become merely less negative, not necessarily positive, on the side of the pneumothorax. If the mediastinum is not fixed, the diminished negative pressure on the side of the pneumothorax creates sufficient imbalance between the pleural pressures of the two sides to cause mediastinal displacement during the expiratory phase of respiration.

If the mediastinum is not fixed, tension pneumothorax will cause a shift of the mediastinum to the opposite side during both inspiratory and expiratory phases of respiration. In addition, flattening, with progression to reversal of the normal curve of the hemidiaphragm, occurs in tension pneumothorax. Rhea et al. [73] described a simple, reproducible means of measuring the percentage of pneumothorax present in upright PA and lateral films. The percentage of pneumothorax is calculated using an average interpleural distance, using the total lung volume of the partially collapsed lung and the total hemithoracic volume as parameters. Pneumothorax size can be predicted using a nomogram based on average interpleural distance (Fig. 70-31).

The distribution of air in the pleural cavity is affected by pleural adhesions and by disease of the underlying lung. Adhesions prevent lung retraction, therefore extensive adhesions may lead to a loculated pneumothorax. A diseased lung, especially one with scarring or atelectasis secondary to bronchial obstruction, tends to retract to a greater degree than the adjacent lung. Obstructive emphysema, consolidation, and interstitial emphysema make the lung rigid and interfere with retraction, keeping the lung or the involved segment expanded. The distribution of air is also influenced by patient position, because air rises to the nondependent portion of the thorax.

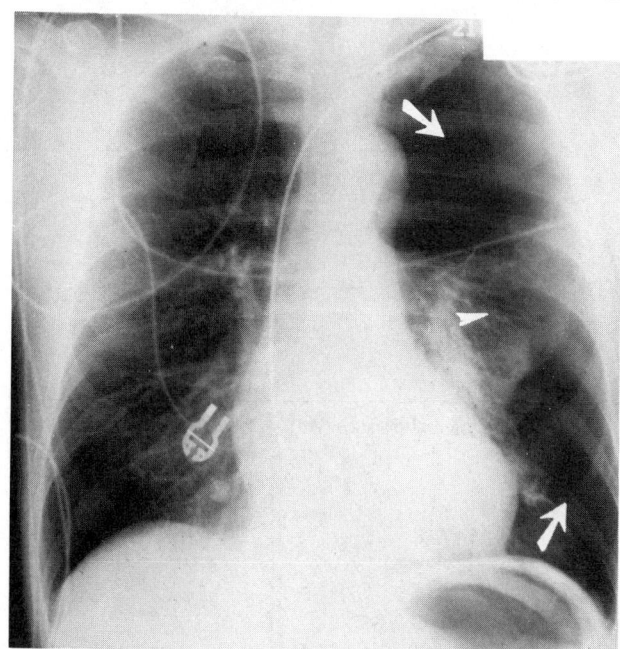

A

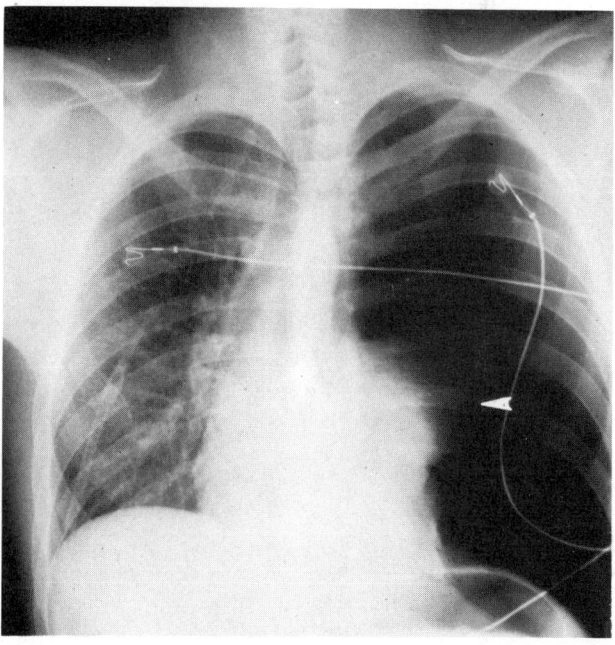

B

Fig. 70-30. Pneumothorax. A. Posteroanterior film of a patient with left pneumothorax. Air in the pleural space (*arrows*) is differentiated from the aerated lung by the absence of bronchovascular markings. Note lack of increased density of the lateral aspect of the partially collapsed lung (*arrowhead*). B. Total collapse of the lung against the mediastinum (*arrowhead*) seen in another patient. Note increase in size of the left hemithorax and slight shift of the mediastinum to the contralateral side.

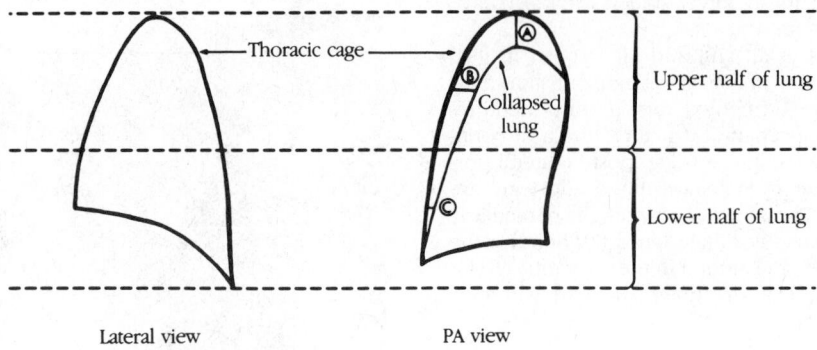

Lateral view   PA view

A

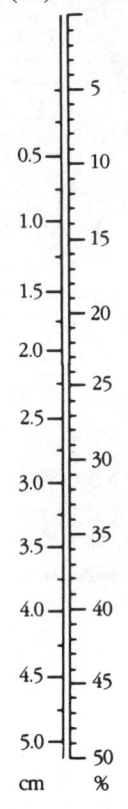

Average interpleural distance (cm) = Pneumothorax size (%)

B

Fig. 70-31. Determining size of pneumothorax in an upright patient. A. Average interpleural distance is obtained on the Posteroanterior view by adding the maximum apical interpleural distance (A), the interpleural distance at the midpoint of the upper half of the lung (B), and the interpleural distance at the midpoint of the lower half of the lung (C) and dividing the sum by 3. B. Nomogram for prediction of pneumothorax size based on average interpleural distance. (From Rhea JT, DeLuca SA, Greene RE: Determining the size of pneumothorax in the upright patient. *Radiology* 144:733, 1982, With permission.)

Early recognition of a pneumothorax is mandatory in ICU patients, especially those on respirators or who are prone to barotrauma or rapid progression to tension pneumothorax. The presence of lower lobe disease, with the lobes resisting reaeration, causes air to collect in the subpulmonic region, simulating a pneumoperitoneum [74]. Thus, in ICU patients the subpulmonic area must be carefully examined, even if the film is obtained in the upright position, because lower lobe disease, consolidation due to ARDS, and pneumonia are frequently present. In the supine patient, air collects in the anterior portion of the thorax, between the medial portion of the lung and the anterior mediastinum, or in the subpulmonic area (Fig. 70-32).

Subpulmonic pneumothorax is seen as a lucent area outlining the anterior costophrenic sulcus projected over the right or left upper quadrant [75] or only as a deep lateral costophrenic sulcus on the involved side [76]. Even with progression to a tension pneumothorax, in a patient with ARDS it is possible for the only finding to be a flattening of the cardiac border or a lateral depression of the hemidiaphragm [77]. These findings should be recognized as signs of tension, because severe cardiovascular and pulmonary compromise can develop rapidly in these patients.

PULMONARY INTERSTITIAL EMPHYSEMA. Pulmonary interstitial emphysema (PIE) results from a rupture of the alveolar wall when the pressure within the alveoli exceeds that within the adjacent vascular bed and perivascular connective tissue. As a result, air dissects along the interstitium of the lungs. Histologically PIE is seen as spaces produced by the dissection of air into the perivascular connective tissues, the interlobular septa, and the subpleural connective tissue, most extensively around the pulmonary veins [78].

Radiologically these spaces are seen as irregular radiolucent mottling in the medial one-half to two-thirds of the lungs or as discrete areas of radiolucency (Fig. 70-33). They are 2 cm or more in diameter (blebs or pneumatoceles) and are best seen at the lung bases. Pulmonary interstitial emphysema also may appear as radiolucent streaks radiating toward the hila or as a lucent halo around vessels on end. Subpleural blebs may be present, most frequently around the hilar areas.

Interstitial emphysema changes rapidly, decreasing in size and disappearing completely in a matter of days. Differentiation of interstitial emphysema from necrotizing bronchopneumonia is sometimes difficult or impossible. Extensive PIE makes the lung appear better aerated than it actually is. Pulmonary interstitial emphysema may progress to pneumothorax, infradiaphragmatic dissection, and/or mediastinal, cervical, or subcutaneous emphysema [79].

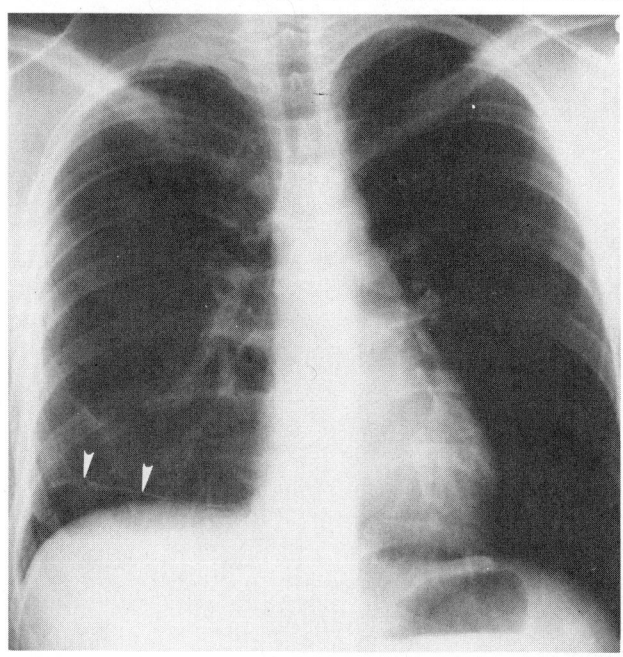

A

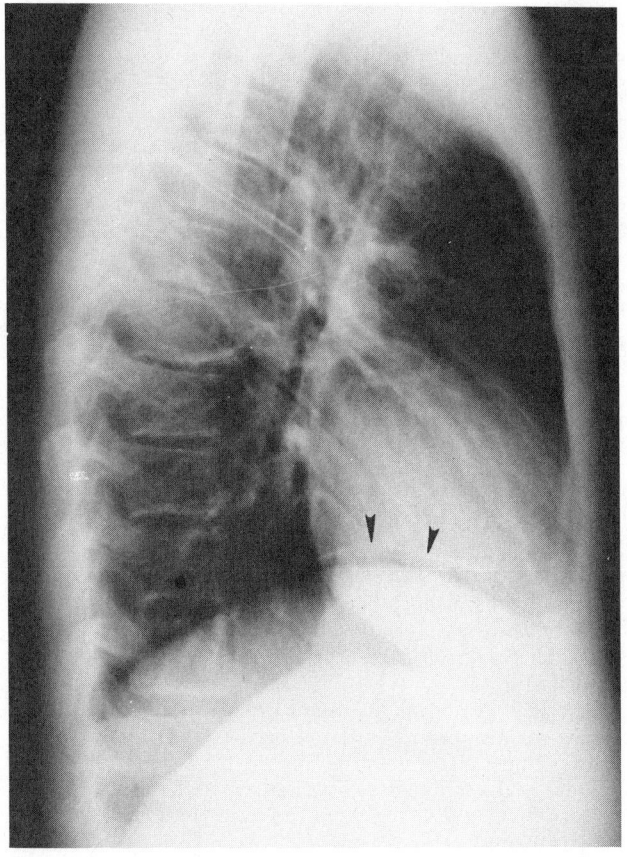

B

Fig. 70-32. Subpulmonic pneumothorax. A. Posteroanterior view of the chest shows a linear density (*arrowheads*) representing the visceral pleura displaced superiorly by the collection of pleural air (subpulmonic pneumothorax) beneath it. B. Lateral view shows the same linear density (*arrowheads*) and subpulmonic pneumothorax.

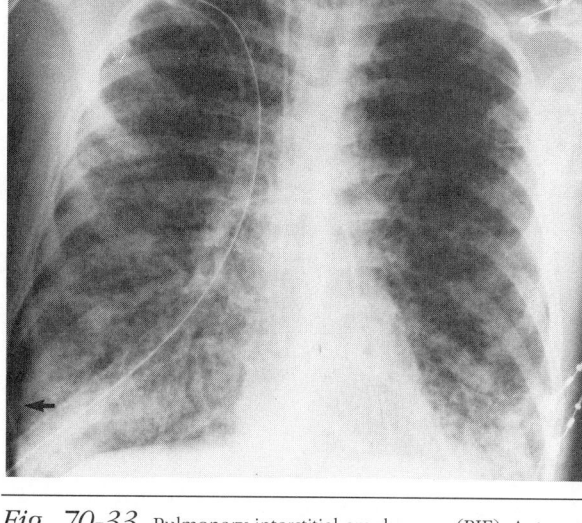

Fig. 70-33. Pulmonary interstitial emphysema (PIE). Anteroposterior film of a patient with acute respiratory distress syndrome and PIE shows the irregular lucent mottling, especially in the medial aspect of both lungs. Pneumothorax (*arrow*) is also seen in the right lower hemithorax.

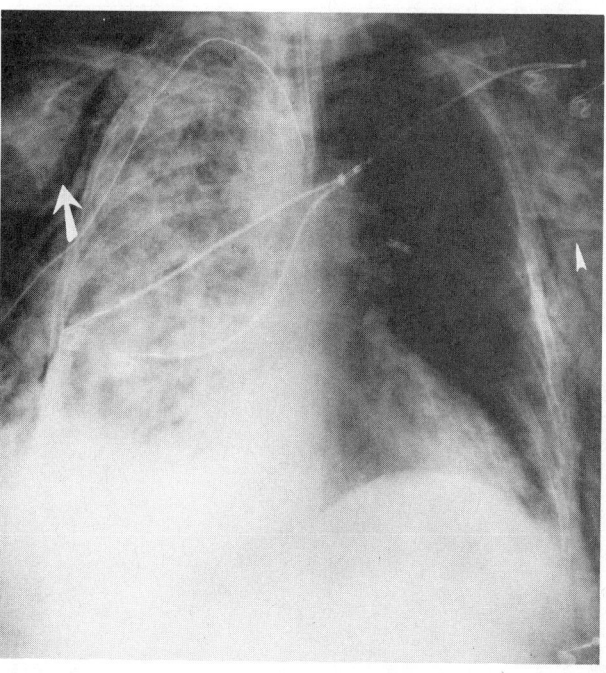

Fig. 70-34. Subcutaneous emphysema. Anteroposterior film of a patient with right lung opacification from a pneumonia with an endotracheal tube and right chest tube in place. The radiating lucencies in the left hemithorax (*arrowhead*) outline the pectoralis muscles. Other air collections (*arrow*) are in the subcutaneous tissues.

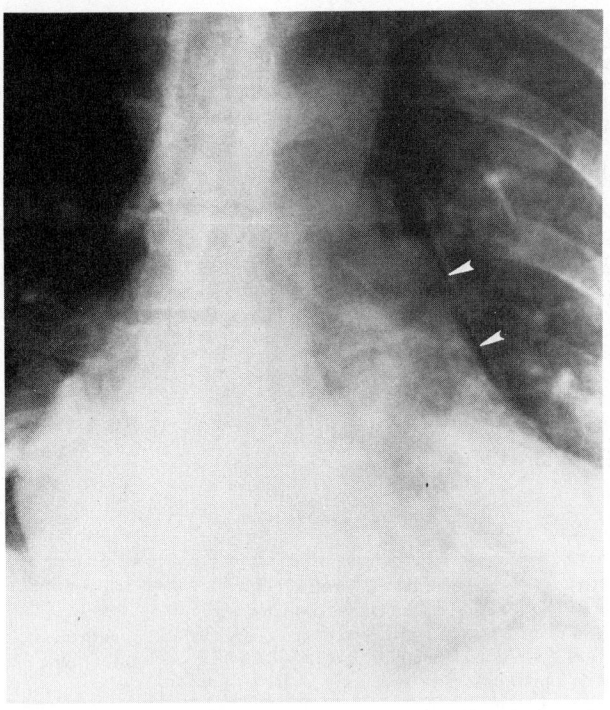

A

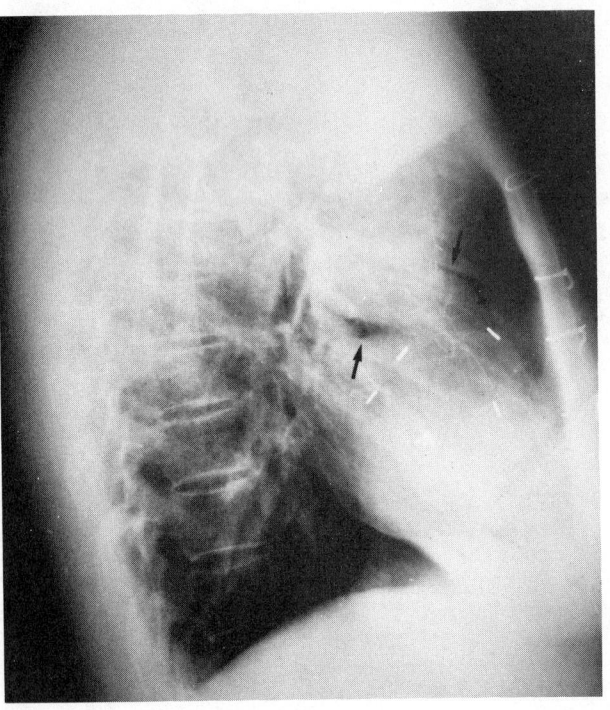

B

Fig. 70-35. Pneumomediastinum. A. Posteroanterior view of the chest shows air in the mediastinum (*arrowheads*). B. Lateral view of chest in a different patient shows lucent areas (*arrows*) representing pneumomediastinum outlining the main pulmonary artery. The patient had previous coronary artery bypass surgery.

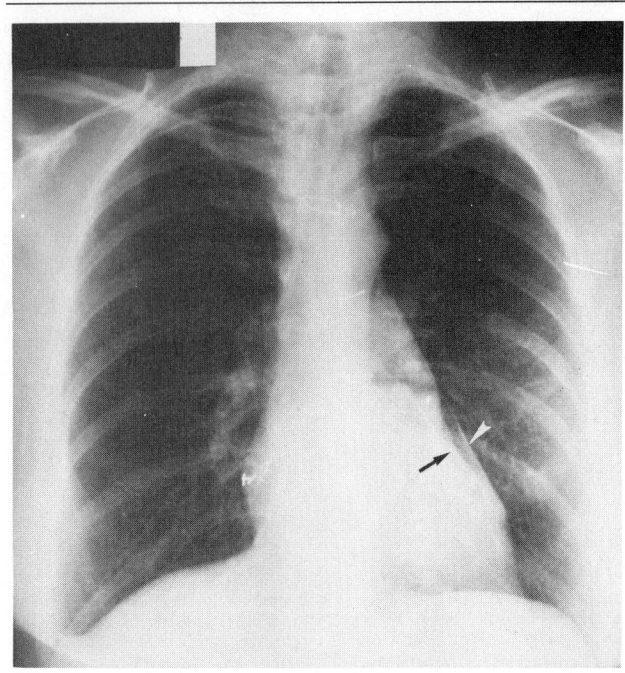

Fig. 70-36. Pneumopericardium. Posteroanterior view of the chest shows a lucent area (pneumopericardium) lateral to the cardiac shadow (*black arrow*) and medial to a strip of density—the pericardium (*arrowhead*). There is also slight blunting of the right costophrenic sulcus from a small pleural effusion. The patient had previous coronary artery bypass surgery.

SUBCUTANEOUS EMPHYSEMA. Air in the subcutaneous tissues is seen as linear streaks of lucency outlining tissue planes or as bubbles of lucency within the soft tissues (Fig. 70-34). Localized subcutaneous emphysema usually follows thoracostomy tube insertions, tracheostomies, and transtracheal aspirations and usually is of no significance. It may also be the earliest sign of pulmonary barotrauma. Extensive air in the subcutaneous tissues may occur in patients on ventilators, those with malfunctioning chest tubes, or those with bronchopleural fistulas.

PNEUMOMEDIASTINUM. Pneumomediastinum is manifested radiologically as vertical streaks of lucency just lateral to the borders of the heart, with the parietal and visceral pleura reflected by the lucent stripe (Fig. 70-35A). Although this condition can be seen in the PA view, the lateral view (Fig. 70-35B), specifically the cross-table lateral view, is more diagnostically useful.

Air can enter the mediastinum from a ruptured bronchus, trachea, or esophagus; from the neck (especially during the course of tracheostomy or line placement, when the negative pressure of the thorax draws air in through the incision); from the retroperitoneum; and from the lungs in association with interstitial emphysema.

Small amounts of pneumomediastinum should be distinguished from the normal lucency of a "kinetic halo" around the heart. This artifactual halo is produced by normal cardiac motion; it is only moderately lucent and does out outline the pleural reflection. When air extends into the soft tissues of the neck or into the retroperitoneum, it is most likely secondary to a pneumomediastinum.

PNEUMOPERICARDIUM. Radiologic diagnosis of a pneumopericardium is made when a lucent stripe is seen around the heart extending to, but not beyond, the proximal pulmonary artery and outlining a thickened pericardium (Fig. 70-36). It may be difficult to differentiate from a pneumothorax or pneumomediastinum; a cross-table lateral film may be necessary. Pneumopericardium is almost always the result of surgery but also may follow trauma or infection.

Extrapulmonary Structures

Evaluation of the chest radiograph is never complete unless the extrapulmonary, extrapleural, and extracardiac structures (extrathoracic soft tissues and bony thorax) are carefully assessed for possible pathology. It is not the purpose of this chapter to deal with these pathologic processes in depth; suffice it to say that one should look for masses, calcifications, and abnormal air collections such as abscesses in the cervical and thoracic soft tissues and subphrenic areas. The bony structures also may provide clues to disease of a systemic nature (e.g., H-shaped vertebrae and bone infarcts in sickle cell anemia) or to metastases in the form of lytic or blastic bone lesions. Fractures following trauma, and occasionally rib fractures following resuscitation procedures after cardiac arrest, may be seen on the chest radiograph.

Fig. 70-37. Arrows point to miliary nodules hardly visible on plain films but well seen by high-resolution computed tomography in a patient with miliary TB. Arrowhead points to an area of tuberculous consolidation.

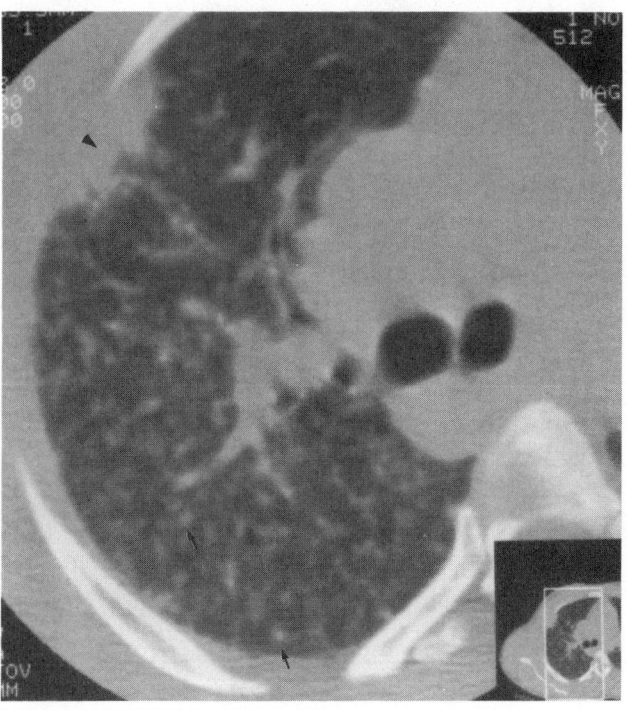

Additional Imaging

As previously stated, most patients cannot be moved from the ICU and CCU areas. For the patient who can be moved and whose clinical conditions demand additional radiologic workup for diagnostic elucidation or therapeutic intervention, other modalities are available. Computed tomography, digital subtraction angiography (DSA), interventional radiography (e.g., catheter placement for pharmacotherapy and drainage of obstructed areas), ultrasonographically guided drainage of abscesses and pleural or pericardial effusions, positron emission tomography (PET), and nuclear magnetic resonance (NMR) all are either available now or will be soon in the armamentarium of radiology departments.

Compute tomography, magnetic resonance imaging (MRI), and ultrasound now form the armamentarium of imaging modalities in addition to plain films available to clinicians for thoracic imaging. The clinical problem to be solved dictates the modality to be used.

The modality of choice for imaging of the lung parenchyma is CT. High-resolution CT (1.5-mm sections at small fields of view and using edge enhancement techniques) allows a very detailed look at the lung parenchyma, allowing imaging early abnormalities of the lungs before they are visible on plain films (Fig. 70-37 and 70-38), assessment of the degree of emphysematous destruction of lung (Fig. 70-39), better characterization of parenchymal and interstitial abnormalities (Figs. 70-40A, 70-41, and 70-42), and even the ability to see through the diffuse opacification of the hemithoraces seen on plain films (Fig. 70-43). The pleura is better assessed by CT than by plain film (Figs. 70-44, 70-45, 70-46 and 70-47). Differentiation between pleural and parenchymal abnormalities is easier using CT (Fig. 70-48).

Fig. 70-38. White arrowheads point to faint areas of alveolar opacification in a patient with *Pneumocystis carinii* pneumonia who had a totally negative chest film.

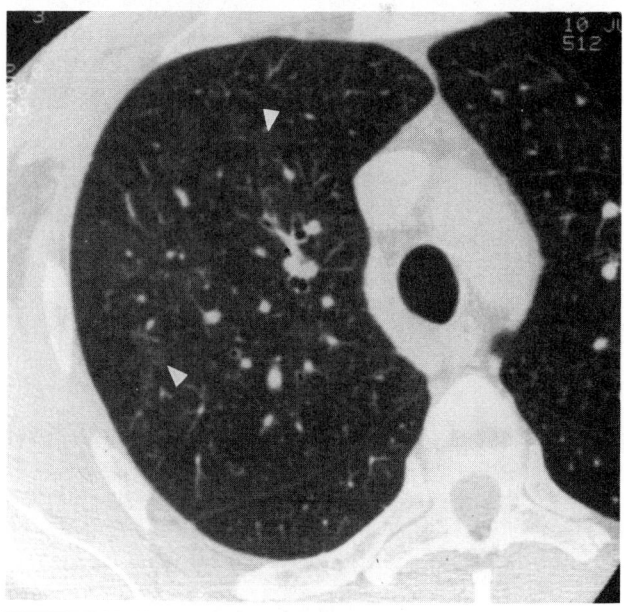

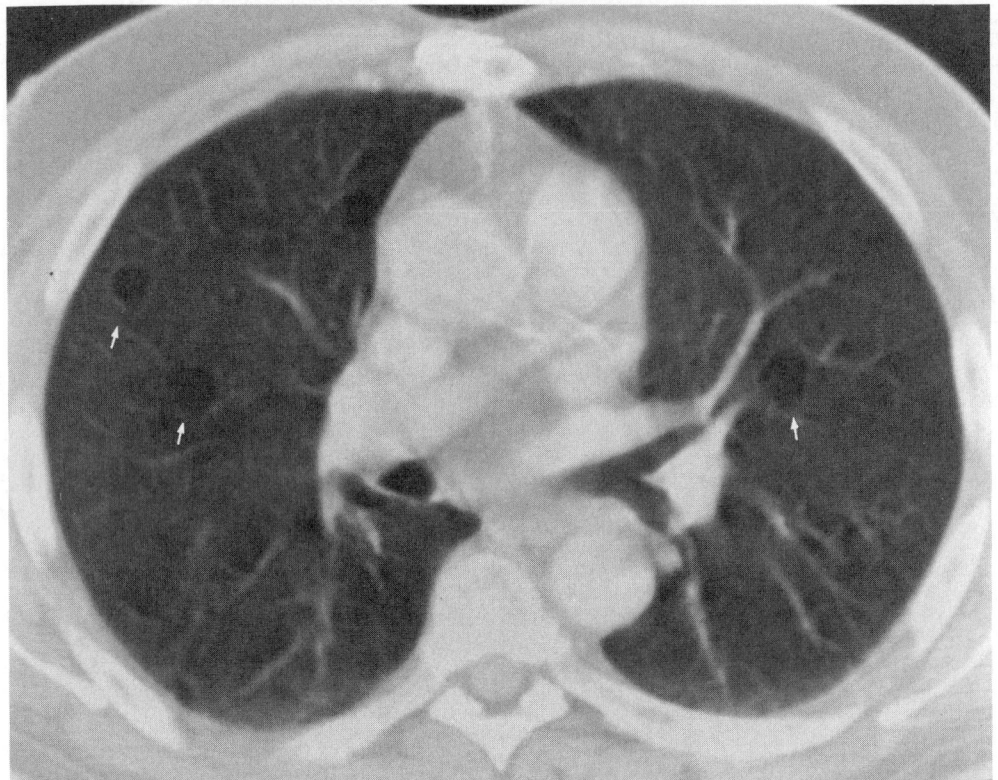

Fig. 70-39. White arrows point to emphysematous areas of lung in a patient with normal chest radiograph.

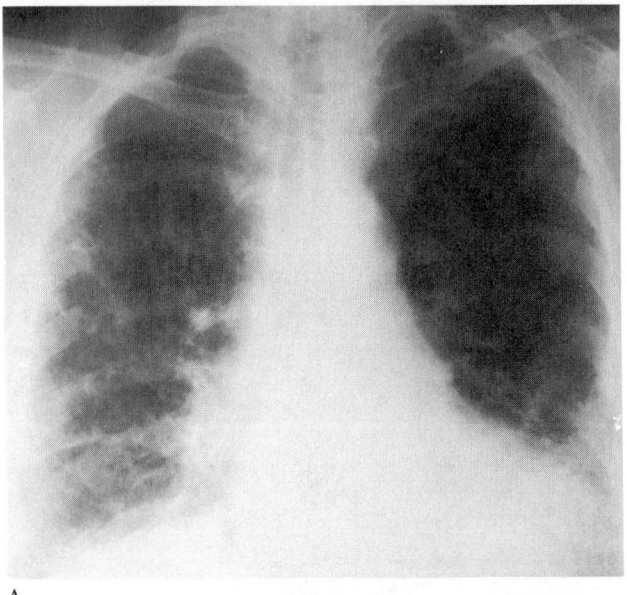

A

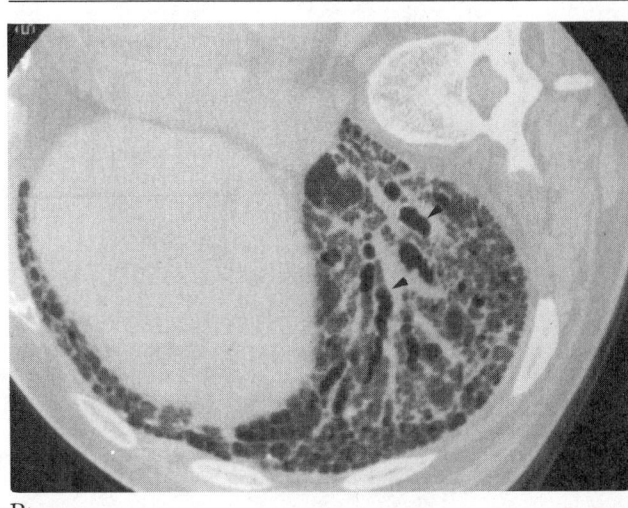

B

Fig. 70-40. A. Patient with interstitial opacities in both lower lobes. B. High-resolution computed tomography shows extremely well the reticular interstitial opacities and the bronchiectasis (*arrowheads*) from the patient's idiopathic pulmonary fibrosis.

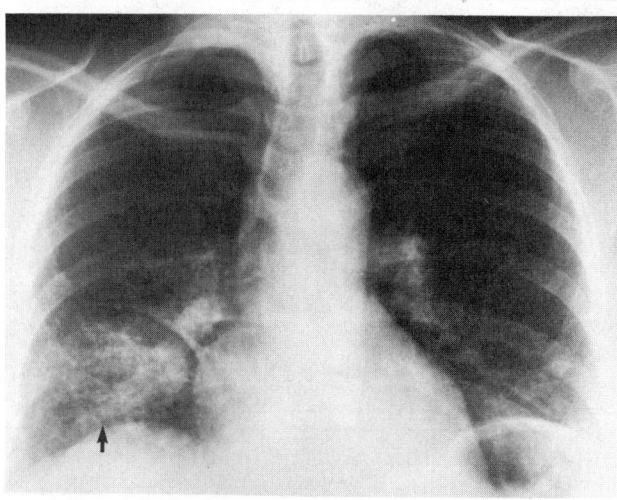

A

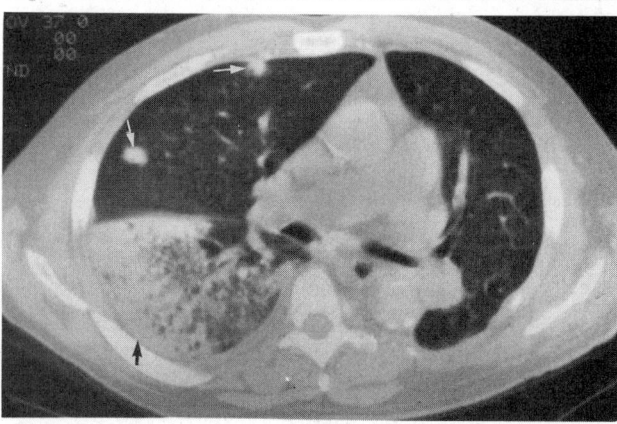

B

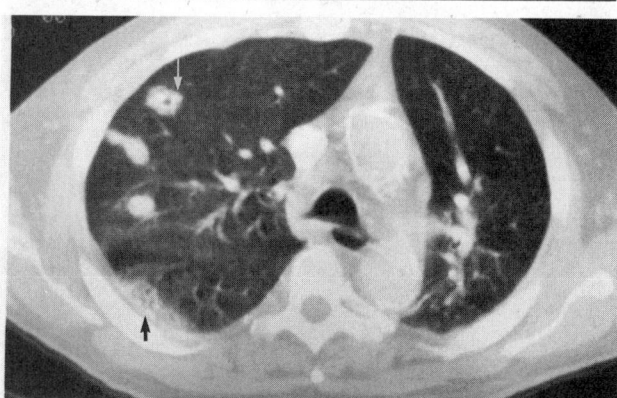

C

Fig. 70-41. A. Posteroanterior film shows confluent opacity (arrow) in the right lower lobe and two nodular opacities in the left lower lobe. B, C. Computed tomography shows the multiple nodular opacities obscured by the area of pneumonia, one of which (C, *arrow*) shows a cavity. The patient is a drug addict with pneumonia and septic emboli.

Computed tomography is the best modality to use when looking for calcification in a lesion, whether it be in lung, mediastinum, or pleura. Small amounts of air are also best seen using CT (Fig. 70-49). Involvement of the arteries and veins most often not identifiable on plain films can be seen using CT (Figs. 70-50 and 70-51). Abnormalities hidden by overlying structures in both PA and lateral views can be seen in CT cross-sectional images (Fig. 70-52).

Mediastinal abnormalities can be imaged using CT, MRI, or ultrasonography. To determine size of mediastinal nodes, CT's resolution would make it superior to MRI—CT can delineate the borders of small nodes lying close to each other or matted together, whereas MRI may make them appear as larger, pathologic-sized nodes. Posterior mediastinal lesions are probably best imaged using MRI to show their relation to an involvement of the spinal canal and spinal cord.

On the other hand, MRI is far superior to CT in imaging vascular structures. It is not within the scope of this chapter to discuss the principles and physics behind MRI. Suffice it to say that using spin-echo technique, flowing blood appears as a signal void (black) and appears as high signal intensity (white) on gradient recall images. The latter provides an angiographic image similar to that achieved using angiography.

The cardiac chambers can be imaged equally well with MRI and ultrasonography but not as well with CT (Fig. 70-53). In the evaluation of the cardiac muscles, however, MRI is superior to CT or ultrasonography.

Aneurysms and dissecting aneurysms of the aorta can be imaged using all four modalities—contrast-enhanced CT, angiography echocardiography for the root of the ascending aorta, transesophageal echo for the descending aorta, and MRI. The advantage of ultrasonography is that it can be done at the bedside if necessary. However, MRI is superior to either CT and ultrasonography because of the ability to do multiplane imaging and delineate the entire extent of the abnormality (Fig. 70-54) noninvasively.

Fig. 70-42. Enlargement of section of high-resolution computed tomography in a patient with lymphangitic metastasis from breast carcinoma. Arrows point to the distended interlobular septae forming the polygonal outline of a secondary lobule. Central density within the secondary lobule represents an arteriole.

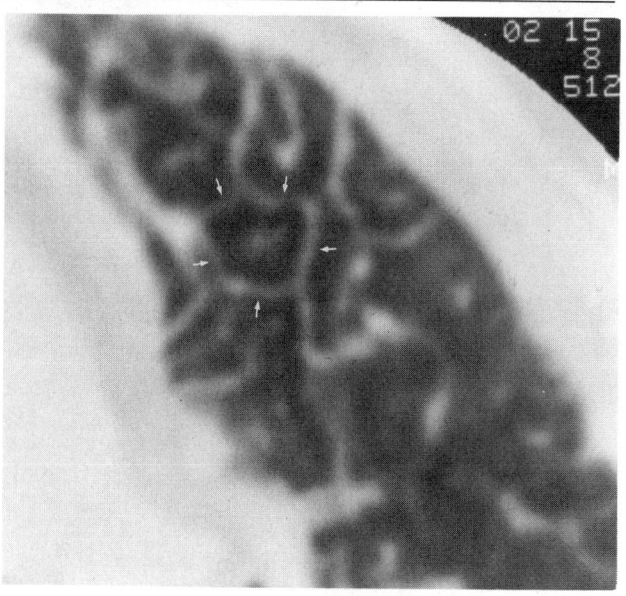

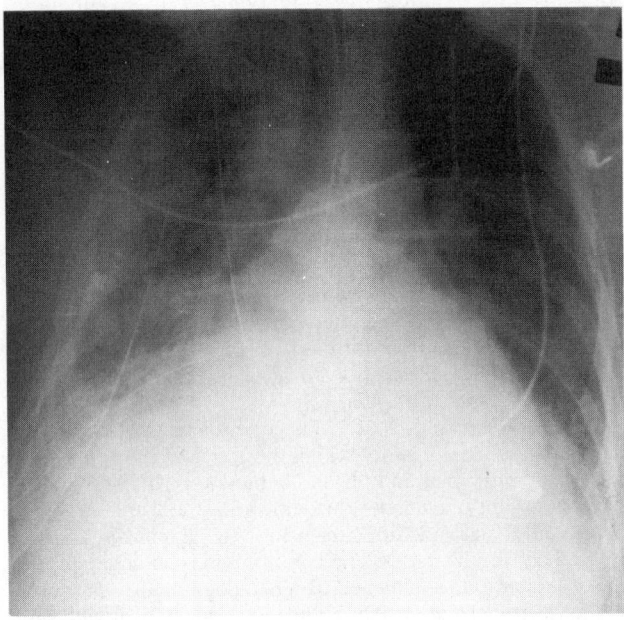

A

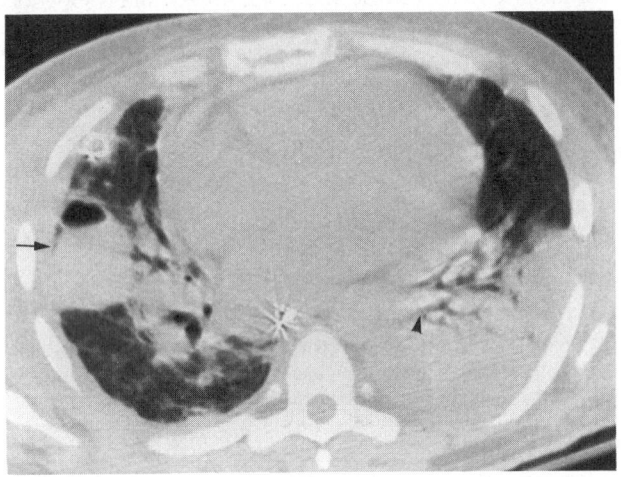

B

Fig. 70-43. A. Posteroanterior (PA) film shows bilateral parenchymal opacification with greater involvement of the right side. B. Computed tomography shows the right lung abscess with air fluid level (*arrow*) and the pneumonia with air bronchograms (*arrowhead*) in the left, defining better the pathology producing the areas of opacification in the PA film.

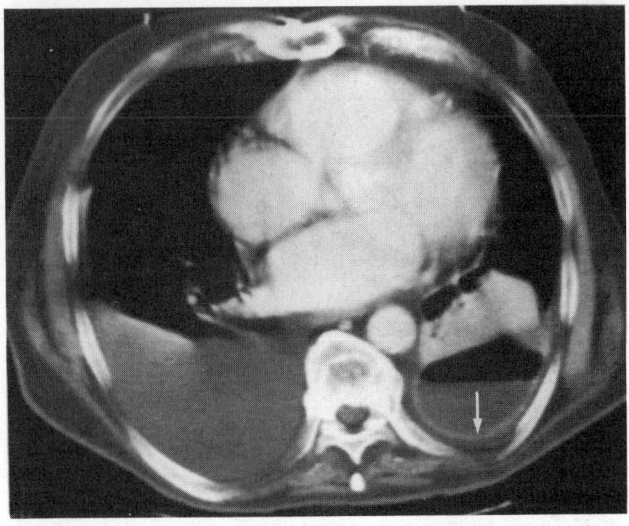

Fig. 70-44. Contrast-enhanced computed tomography distinguishes between a pleural effusion on the right and an empyema on the left by visualization of an enhancing pleura (curvilinear white line, *arrow*).

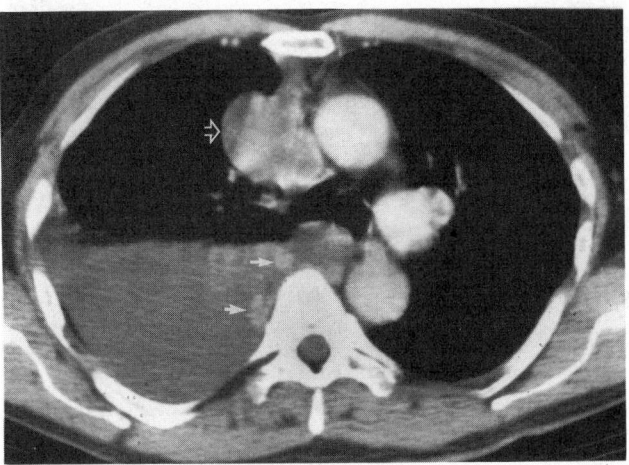

Fig. 70-45. Patient with bronchogenic carcinoma (*open arrow*) with pleural effusion. White arrows point to metastatic pleural deposits that are not visible on plain films.

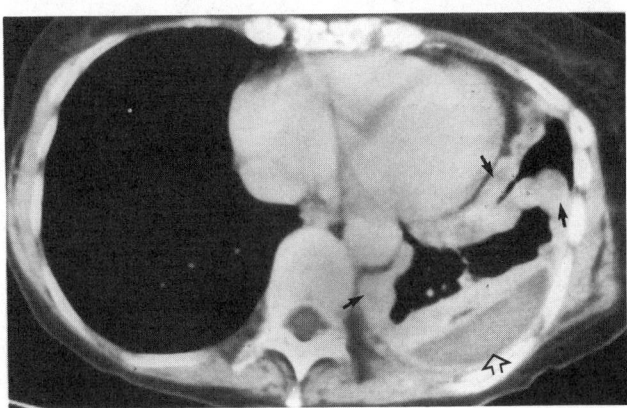

Fig. 70-46. Patient with a densely opacified left hemithorax. Computed tomography shows the lobulated pleural thickening (*arrows*) and pleural effusion (*open arrow*) secondary to mesothelioma.

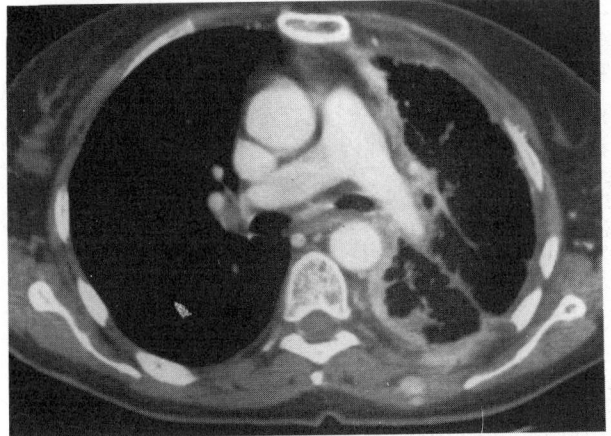

Fig. 70-47. Irregular pleural opacity in the left pleural space from metastatic adenocarcinoma.

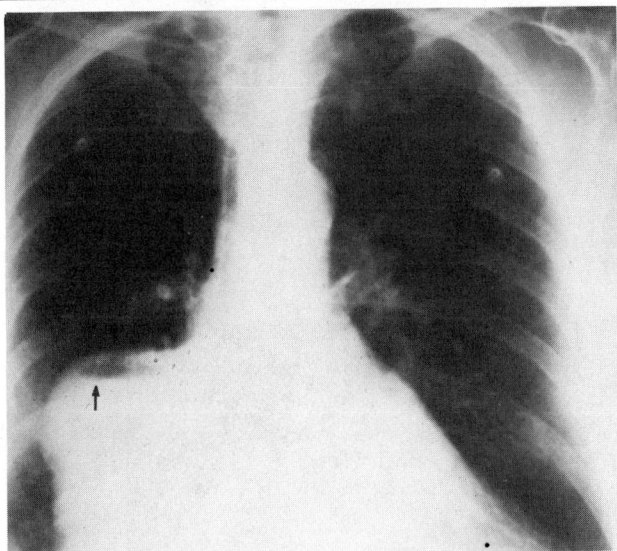

A

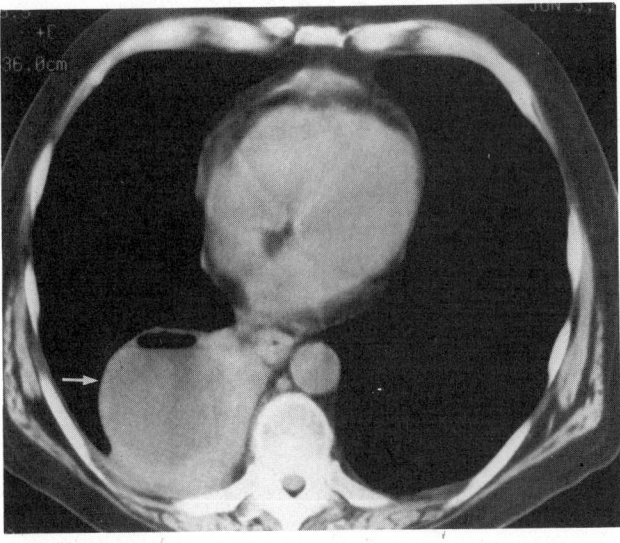

B

Fig. 70-48. Mass opacity with air-fluid level on the posteroanterior view (A), clearly imaged by computed tomography (B) and shown to be a lung abscess.

Esophageal mucosal lesions are best assessed by barium swallow. Submucosal, mural, and serosal lesions and lesions extrinsic to the esophagus can be assessed using CT, ultrasonography, or MRI. Both ultrasonography and MRI are probably superior to CT in delineating the layers of esophagus involved. Transesophageal ultrasonography is the least costly and most efficient modality to use, since the gastroenterologists would probably use a scope anyway in the presence of any esophageal problem. Transesophageal endosonography is superior to CT for staging a tumor, and evaluating depth of tumor infiltration, especially in the early stages (Fig. 70-55). Severe stenosis is the main limiting factor to the use of transesophageal endosonography.

The availability of the various imaging modalities provides clinicians with useful tools in addition to their clinical acumen and laboratory results for diagnostic problem-solving in the ICU patient.

Fig. 70-49. A. Patient with bilateral effusions. Computed tomography (CT) shows air within the effusion (*arrow*) and pleura enhancement (*open arrow*), allowing the diagnosis of an empyema. B. Patient who had coronary bypass surgery several weeks prior to this CT shows mediastinitis with air in the retrosternal area. Empyema is also noted in the posterior left hemithorax.

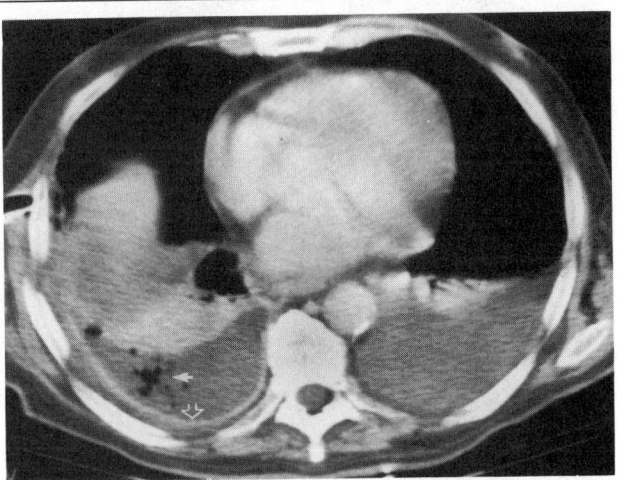

A

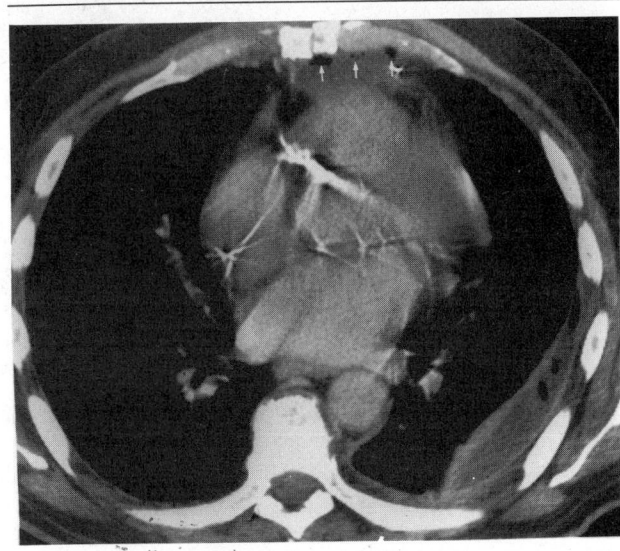

B

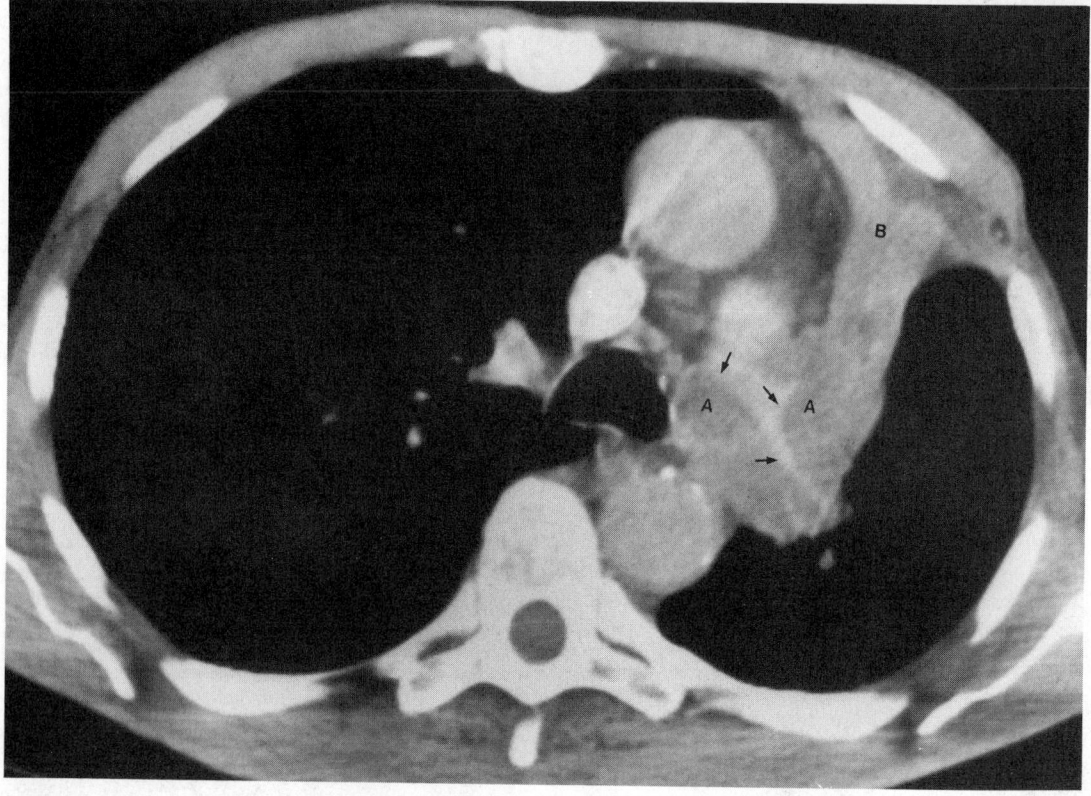

A

B

Fig. 70-50. Contiguous computed tomography sections show
the contrast-enhanced pulmonary artery (*arrows*) encased by and obstructed by the bronchogenic carcinoma (A), which has also produced postobstructive atelectasis (B). The mass and atelectasis, but
not the pulmonary artery's involvement, could be seen on plain films.

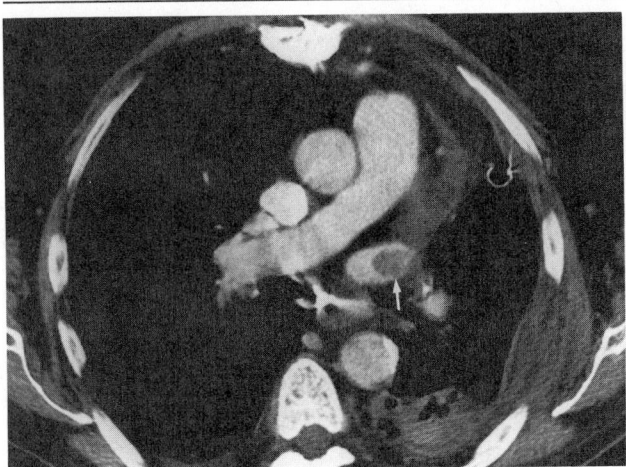

Fig. 70-51. In a patient who had a lobectomy, computed tomography shows a filling defect (*arrow*) representing a thrombus within the contrast-enhanced pulmonary vein.

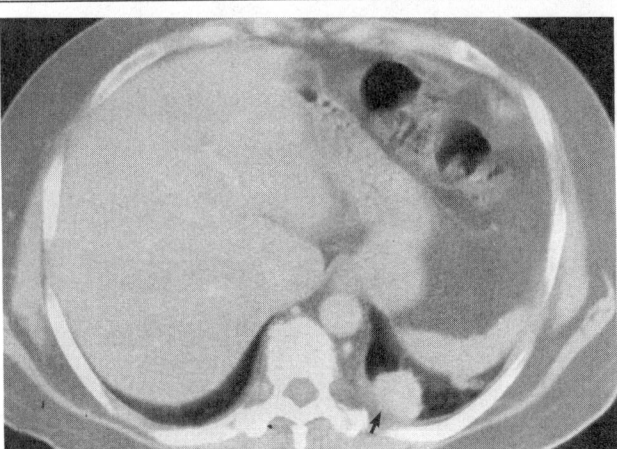

Fig. 70-52. An adenocarcinoma seen only by computed tomography (*arrow*). It was not seen on routine films because it overlies the shadows of the vertebral body on lateral view and is obscured by the spleen and stomach and aorta on the posteroanterior chest film.

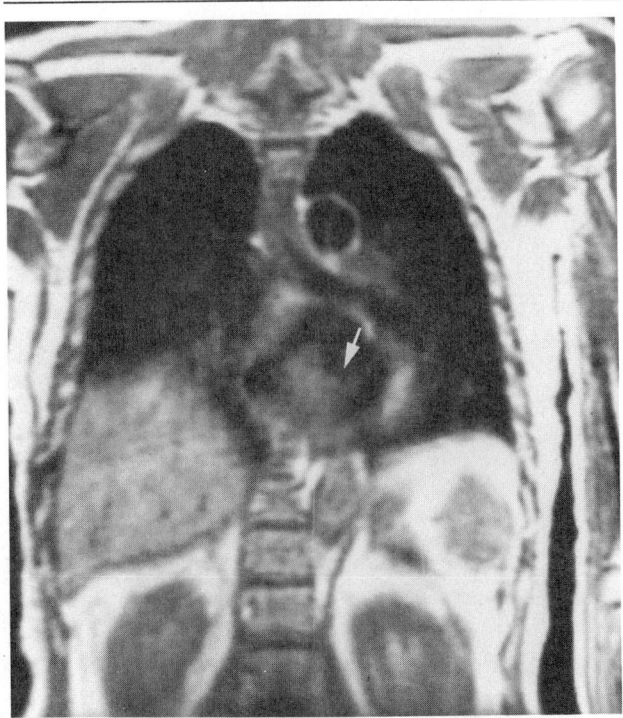

A

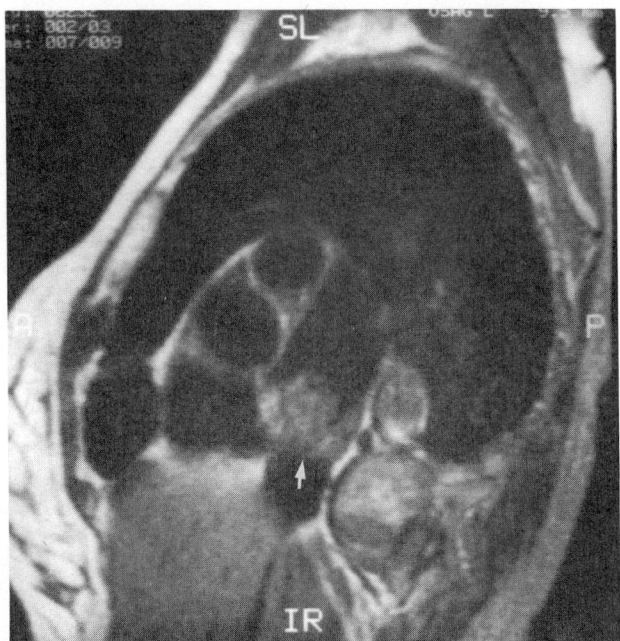

B

Fig. 70-53. A, B. Coronal and sagittal plains on magnetic resonance imagining. Arrow points to an atrial myxoma. Echocardiography demonstrated this lesion also.

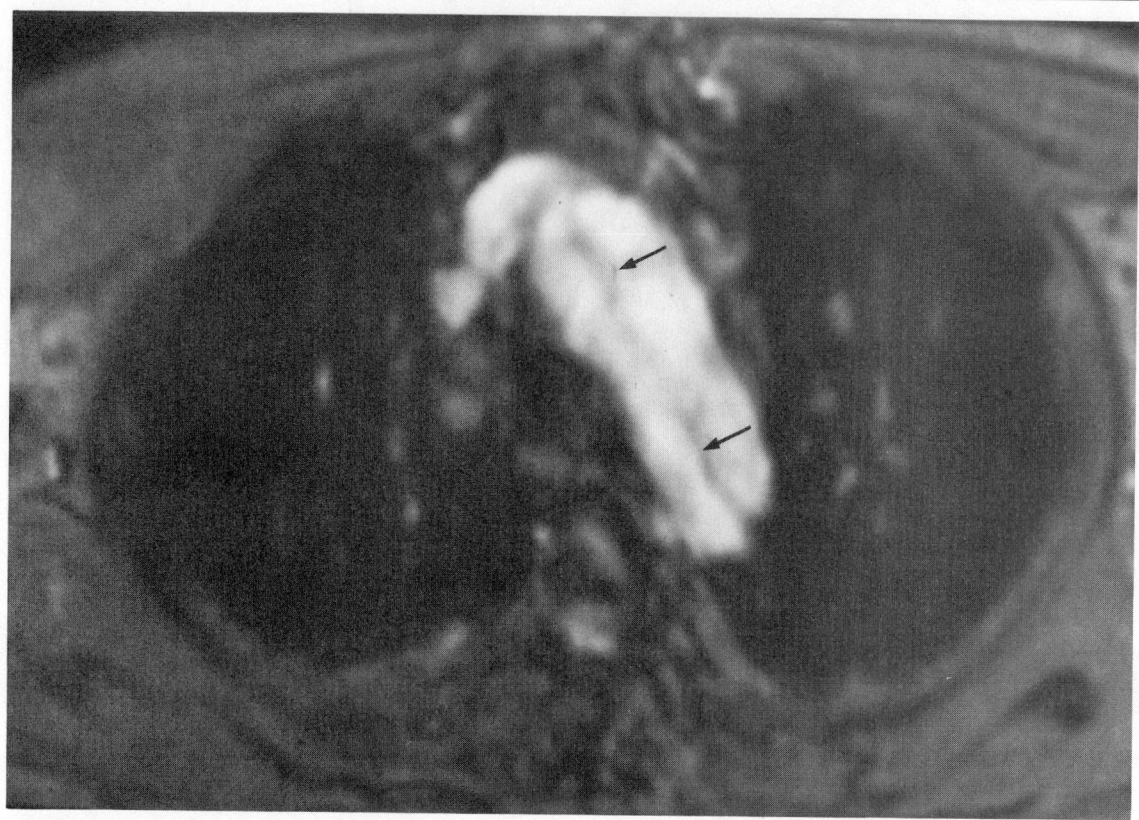

A

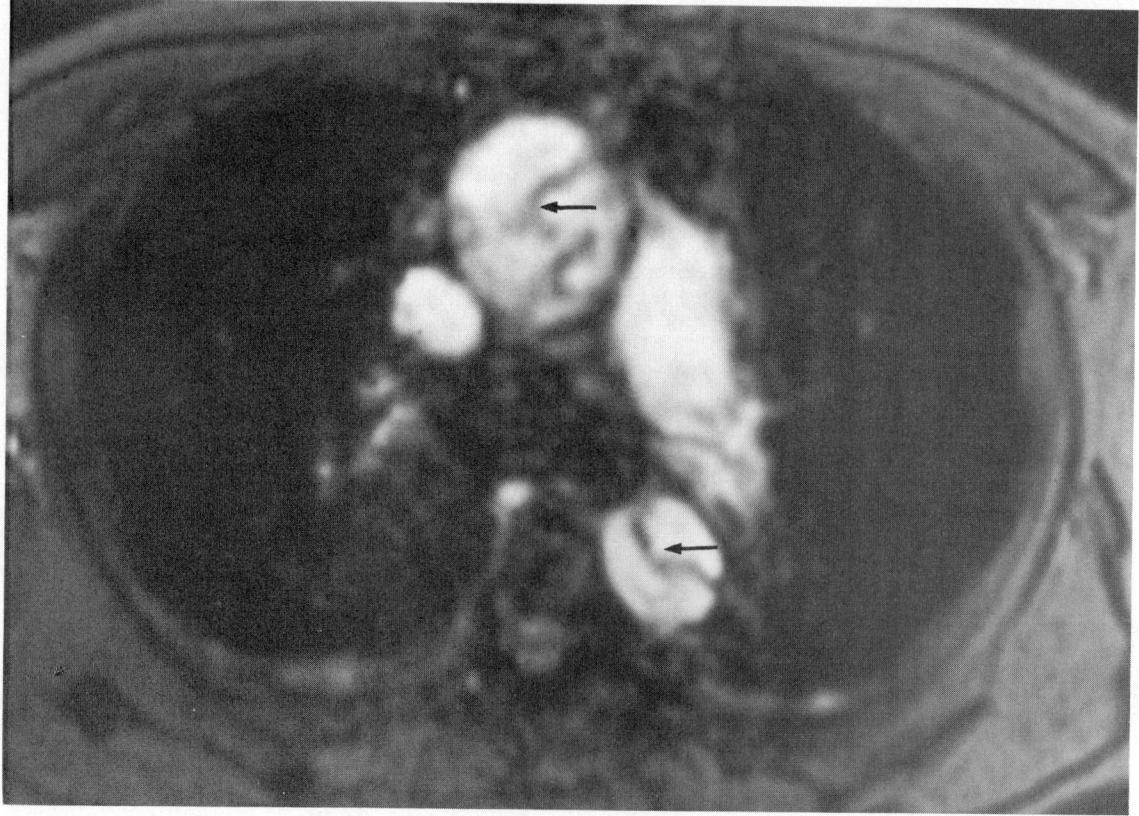

B

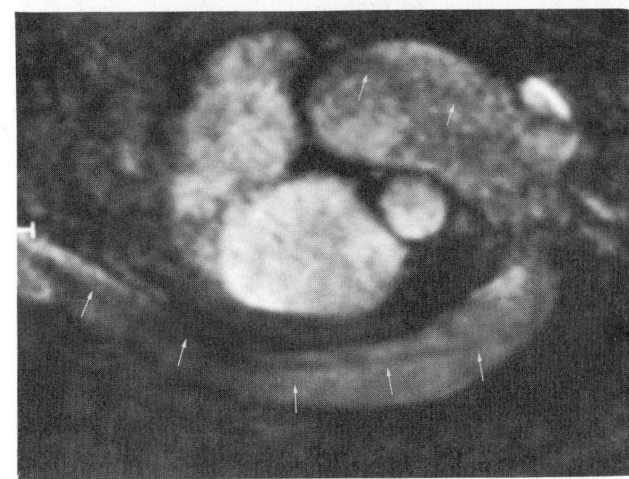

C

Fig. 70-54. A, B, C. Arrows point to the flap in a dissecting aneurysm. Magnetic resonance images well the dissection and its extent in multiple planes.

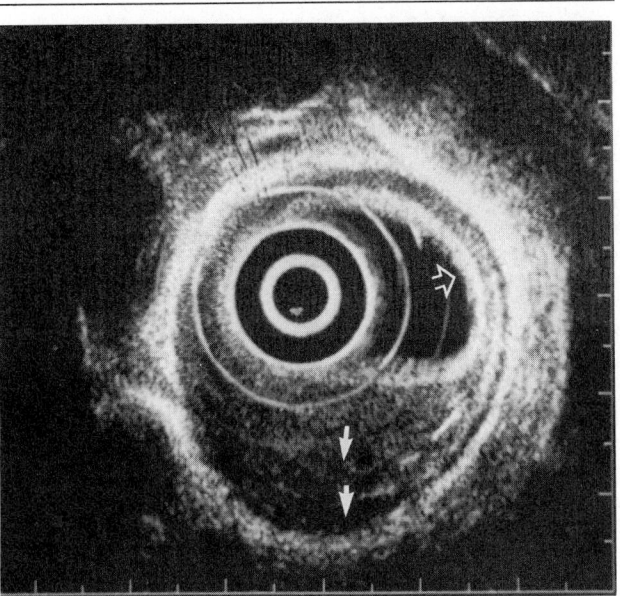

A

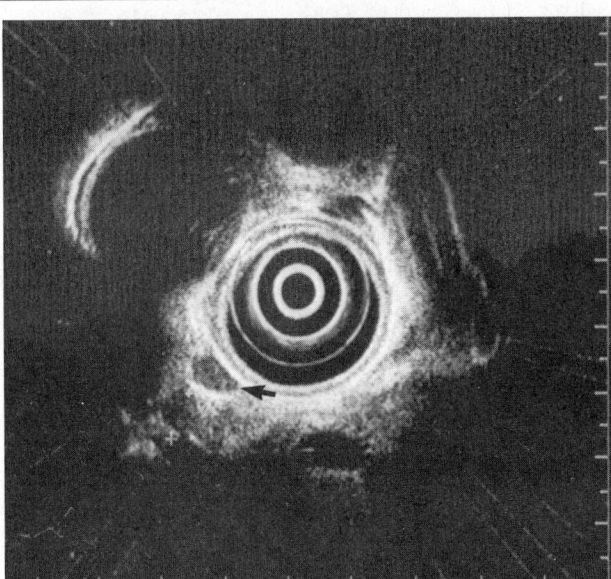

B

Fig. 70-55. Esophageal endosonography in a patient with esophageal carcinoma. Open arrow shows normal thickness of the esophageal wall. White arrows in (A, C) show the extension of the lesion into the adventitia. Black arrow (B) shows metastatic lymphadenopathy.

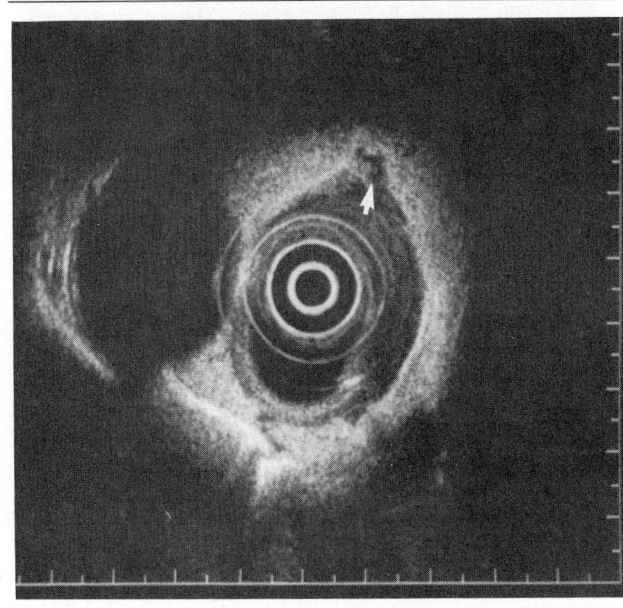

C

References

1. Henscke CI, Pasternak GS, Schroeder S, et al: Bedside chest radiography: Diagnostic efficacy. *Radiology* 149:23, 1983.
2. Bekemeyer WB, Crapo RO, Calhoon S, et al: Efficacy of chest radiography in a respiratory intensive care unit. *Chest* 88:691, 1985.
3. Mirvis SE, Fritz SL, Siegel JH, et al: Radiographic system for use in emergency and intensive care units. *Am J Radiol* 150:691, 1988.
4. Fisher MR, Mintzer RA, Rogers LF, et al: Evaluation of a new mobile automatic exposure control device. *Am J Radiol* 139:1055, 1982.
5. Milne ENC: A physiological approach to reading critical care unit films. *J Thorac Imaging* 1:60, 1986.
6. Goodman LR, Conrardy PA, Laing F, et al: Radiographic evaluation of endotracheal tube position. *Am J Radiol* 127:433, 1976.
7. Conrardy PA, Goodman LR, Laing F, et al: Alteration of endotracheal tube position: Extension and flexion of the neck. *Crit Care Med* 4:7, 1976.
8. Khan F, Reddy NC, Khan A: Cuff/trachea ratio as an indication of tracheal damage (abstract). *Chest* 70:431, 1976.
9. Ravin CE, Handel DB, Kariman K: Persistant endotracheal tube cuff overdistension: A sign of tracheomalacia. *Am J Radiol* 137:408, 1981.
10. Ravin CE, Putnam CE, McLoud TC: Hazards of the intensive care unit. *Am J Radiol* 126:423, 1976.
11. Brandt RL, Foley WJ, Fink GH, et al: Mechanism of perforation of the heart with production of hydropericardium by a venous catheter and its prevention. *Am J Surg* 119:311, 1970.
12. Swan HJC, Ganz W, Forrester J, et al: Catheterization of the heart in man with use of a flow-directed balloon-tipped catheter. *N Engl J Med* 283:447, 1970.
13. Chatterjee K, Swan HJC, Ganz W, et al: Use of a balloon-tipped flotation electrode catheter for cardiac monitoring. *Am J Cardiol* 36:56, 1975.
14. Calinog TA, Magovern GJ, Fisher DL, et al: Newer approaches in the bedside diagnosis of massive pulmonary embolism. *J Thorac Cardiovasc Surg* 63:300, 1972.
15. Dougherty JE, LaSala AF, Fieldman A: Bedside pulmonary angiography utilizing an existing Swan-Ganz catheter. *Chest* 77:43, 1980.
16. Loop JW, Archer G, Northrop CH: Bedside pulmonary arteriography. *Radiology* 114:469, 1975.
17. Moulopoulos SD, Topaz SR, Kolff WJ: Diastolic balloon pumping (with carbon dioxide) in the aorta: A mechanical assistance to the failing circulation. *Am Heart J* 63:669, 1962.
18. Hyson EA, Ravin CE, Kelley MJ, et al: The intraaortic counterpulsation balloon: Radiographic considerations. *Am J Radiol* 128:915, 1977.
19. Webb WR, Godwin JD: The obscured outer edge: A sign of improperly placed pleural drainage tubes. *Am J Radiol* 134:1062, 1980.
20. Maurer JR, Friedman PJ, Wing VW: Thoracostomy tube in an interlobar fissure: Radiologic recognition of a potential problem. *Am J Radiol* 139:1155, 1982.
21. Ormond RS, Rubenfire M, Anbe DT, et al: Radiographic demonstration of myocardial penetration by permanent endocardial pacemakers. *Radiology* 98:35, 1971.
22. Hall WM, Rosenbaum HD: The radiology of cardiac pacemakers. *Radiol Clin North Am* 9:343, 1971.
23. Hearne SF, Maloney JD: Pacemaker system failure secondary to air entrapment within the pulse generator pocket: A complication of subclavian venipuncture for lead placement. *Chest* 82:651, 1982.
24. Leeming BWA: Radiological aspects of the pulmonary complications resulting from intermittent positive pressure ventilation (IPPV). *Australas Radiol* 12:361, 1968.
25. Zimmerman JE, Goodman LR, St Andre AC, et al: Radiographic detection of mobilizable lung water: The gravitational shift test. *Am J Radiol* 138:59, 1982.
26. Heitzman ER Jr, Fraser RG, Proto AV, et al: Radiologic physiologic correlations in pulmonary circulation, in *Chest Disease Syllabus*. 3rd series. Chicago, American College of Radiology, 1981, p 375.
27. Hublitz UF, Shapiro JH: Atypical pulmonary patterns of congestive failure in chronic lung disease: Influence of preexisting disease on appearance and distribution of pulmonary edema. *Radiology* 93:995, 1969.
28. Milne ENC: Some new concepts of pulmonary blood flow and volume. *Radiol Clin North Am* 16:515, 1978.
29. Milne ENC: Chest radiology in the surgical patient. *Surg Clin North Am* 60:1503, 1980.
30. Bachofen M, Weibel ER: Structural alterations of lung parenchyma in the adult respiratory distress syndrome. *Clin Chest Med* 3:35, 1982.
31. Joffe N: The adult respiratory distress syndrome. *Am J Radiol* 122:719, 1974.
32. Unger KM, Shibel EM, Moser KM: Detection of left ventricular failure in patients with adult respiratory distress syndrome. *Chest* 67:8, 1975.
33. Matthew EB, Holstrom FMG, Kaspar RL: A simple method for diagnosing pneumonia in intubated or tracheostomized patients. *Crit Care Med* 5:76, 1977.
34. Mendelsohn CL: The aspiration of stomach contents into the lungs during obstetric anesthesia. *Am J Obstet Gynecol* 52:191, 1946.
35. Exarhos ND, Logan WD Jr, Abbott OA, et al: The importance of pH and volume in tracheobronchial aspiration. *Dis Chest* 47:167, 1965.
36. Roberts RB, Shirley MA: The obstetrician's role in reducing the risk of aspiration pneumonitis: With particular reference to the use of oral antacids. *Am J Obstet Gynecol* 124:611, 1976.
37. Schwartz DJ, Wynne JW, Gibbs CP, et al: The pulmonary consequences of aspiration of gastric contents at pH values greater than 2.5. *Am Rev Respir Dis* 121:119, 1980.
38. Greenfield LJ, Singleton RP, McCaffree DR, et al: Pulmonary effects of experimental graded aspiration of hydrochloric acid. *Ann Surg* 170:74, 1969.
39. Landay MJ, Christensen EE, Bynum LJ: Pulmonary manifestations of acute aspiration of gastric contents. *Am J Radiol* 131:587, 1978.
40. Westermark N: *Roentgen Studies of the Lungs and Heart.* Minneapolis, University of Minnesota, 1948.
41. Chang CH: The normal roentgenographic measurement of the right descending pulmonary artery in 1,085 cases. *Am J Radiol* 87:929, 1962.
42. Glas WW, Grekin TD, Musselman MM: Fat embolism. *Am J Surg* 85:363, 1953.
43. Hessen I: Roentgen examination of pleural fluid: A study of the localization of free effusions, the potentialities of diagnosing minimal quantities of fluid and its existence under physiological conditions. *Acta Radiol* 86(suppl):1, 1951.
44. Fleischner FG: Atypical arrangement of free pleural effusion. *Radiol Clin North Am* 1:347, 1963.
45. Raasch BN, Carsky EW, Lane EJ, et al: Pleural effusion: Explanation of some typical appearances. *Am J Radiol* 139:899, 1982.
46. Trackler RT, Brinker RA: Widening of the left paravertebral pleural line on supine chest roentgenograms in free pleural effusions. *Am J Radiol* 96:1027, 1966.
47. Pugatch RD, Faling LJ, Robbins AH, et al: Differentiation of pleural and pulmonary lesions using computed tomography. *J Comput Assist Tomogr* 2:601, 1978.
48. Baber CE, Hedlund LW, Oddson TA, et al: Differentiating empyemas and peripheral pulmonary abscesses: The value of computed tomography. *Radiology* 135:755, 1980.
49. Malamed M, Hipona FA, Reynes CJ, et al: *The Adult Postoperative Chest.* Springfield, Thomas, 1977.
50. Franz BJ, Murphy JD: Masked broncho-pleural fistula. *J Thorac Surg* 29:512, 1955.
51. Hsu JT, Bennett GM, Wolff E: Radiologic assessment of bronchopleural fistula with empyema. *Radiology* 103:41, 1972.
52. Greyson ND, Rosenthall L: Detection of postoperative bronchopleural fistulas by radionuclide fog inhalation. *Can Med Assoc J* 103:1366, 1970.
53. Zelefsky MN, Freeman LM, Stern H: A simple approach to the diagnosis of bronchopleural fistula. *Radiology* 124:843, 1977.
54. Kremens V: Demonstration of the pericardial shadow on the routine chest roentgenogram: A new roentgen finding—Preliminary report. *Radiology* 64:72, 1955.
55. Torrance DJ: Demonstration of subpericardial fat as an aid in the diagnosis of pericardial effusion or thickening. *Am J Radiol* 74:850, 1955.
56. Lane EJ Jr, Carsky EW: Epicardial fat: Lateral plain film analysis in normals and in pericardial effusion. *Radiology* 91:1, 1968.
57. Carsky EW, Mauceri RA, Azimi F: The epicardial fat pad sign: Anal-

ysis of frontal and lateral chest radiographs in patients with peri-cardial effusion. *Radiology* 137:303, 1980.

58. Spooner EW, Kuhns LR, Stern AM: Diagnosis of pericardial effusion in children: A new radiographic sign. *Am J Radiol* 128:23, 1977.

59. Chen JTT, Putnam CE, Hedlund LW, et al: Widening of the subcarinal angle by pericardial effusion. *Am J Radiol* 139:883, 1982.

60. Alavi SM, Keats TE, O'Brien WM: The angle of tracheal bifurcation: Its normal mensuration. *Am J Radiol* 108:546, 1970.

61. Haskin PH, Goodman LR: Normal tracheal bifurcation angle: A reassessment. *Am J Radiol* 139:879, 1982.

62. Davidson KG: Closed injuries to the aorta and great vessels, in Williams WJ, Smith RE (eds): *Trauma of the Chest*. Bristol, England, John Wright, 1977.

63. Parmley LF, Mattingly TW, Manion WC, et al: Nonpenetrating traumatic injury of the aorta. *Circulation* 17:1086, 1958.

64. Barcia TC, Livoni JP: Indications for angiography in blunt thoracic trauma. *Radiology* 147:15, 1983.

65. Seltzer SE, D'Orsi C, Kirschner R, et al: Traumatic aortic rupture: Plain radiographic findings. *Am J Radiol* 137:1011, 1981.

66. Cigarroa JE, Isselbacher EM, DeSanctis RW, et al: Diagnostic imaging in the evaluation of suspected aortic dissection: Old standards and new directions. *N Engl J Med* 328: 35, 1993.

67. Nienaber CA, von Kodolitsch Y, Nicolas V, et al: The diagnosis of thoracic aortic dissection by noninvasive imaging procedures. *N Engl J Med* 328: 1, 1993.

68. Fabian TM, Raptopoulos V, D'Orsi CJ, et al: Computed body angiotomography: Dynamic scanning with table incrementation. *Radiology* 149:287, 1983.

69. Ball T, McCrory R, Smith JO, et al: Traumatic diaphragmatic hernia: Errors in diagnosis. *Am J Radiol* 138:633, 1982.

70. Toombs BD, Sandler CM, Lester RG: Computed tomography of chest trauma. *Radiology* 140:733, 1981.

71. Heiberg E, Wolverson MK, Hurd RN, et al: CT recognition of traumatic rupture of the diaphragm. *Am J Radiol* 135:369, 1980.

72. Rabin CB, Baron MG: *Radiology of the Chest*. Golden's Diagnostic Radiology Series, Section 3. Baltimore, Williams & Wilkins, 1980.

73. Rhea JT, DeLuca SA, Greene RE: Determining the size of pneumothorax in the upright patient. *Radiology* 144:733, 1982.

74. Kurlander GJ, Helmen CH: Subpulmonary pneumothorax. *Am J Radiol* 96:1019, 1966.

75. Rhea JT, vanSonnenberg E, McLoud TC: Basilar pneumothorax in the supine adult. *Radiology* 133:593, 1979.

76. Gordon R: The deep sulcus sign. *Radiology* 136:25, 1980.

77. Gobien RP, Reines HD, Schabel SI: Localized tension pneumothorax: Unrecognized form of barotrauma in adult respiratory distress syndrome. *Radiology* 142:15, 1982.

78. Westcott JL, Cole SR: Interstitial pulmonary emphysema in children and adults: Roentgenographic features. *Radiology* 111:367, 1974.

79. Johnson TH, Altman AR: Pulmonary interstitial gas: First sign of barotrauma due to PEEP therapy. *Crit Care Med* 7:532, 1979.

71. Acute Inhalation Injury

Peter J. Jederlinic and Richard S. Irwin

Overview

Our lungs play a unique role interfacing with the environment and are at increased risk of injury from natural and manmade alterations in its constituent gases. Exposure to these gases can result in a variety of acute respiratory syndromes (Table 71-1).

Although many environmental respiratory problems result from workplace exposure, individuals living in communities located near industrial centers or along transit routes also can be affected. The 1984 Bhopal disaster claimed 2500 lives, and 200,000 individuals were injured after the town was exposed to a cloud of methyldiisocyanate released accidentally from a nearby chemical plant. Natural disasters may have the same result, such as the asphyxiation of an entire Nigerian village located on the shores of Lake Nyos by a cloud of volcanic gas released from the lake bed.

A simple agent will cause several different syndromes, depending on the intensity and duration of exposure; short heavy exposure causes dramatic and acute symptoms such as pulmonary edema, whereas low-intensity, long-term exposure leads to insidious onset of dyspnea after a prolonged latency period. Problems also arise when the exposure is remote or discontinued but symptoms persist. This problem is encountered, for example, with occupational asthma from toluene diisocyanate exposure. Symptoms of severe asthma can persist indefinitely following one or several accidental exposures, which acts as a sensitizing agent.

In the first part of this chapter acute inhalation injury from gases, fumes, and dusts is discussed in the framework of the resulting systemic, airways, and parenchymal responses. The second part of the chapter deals with the problem of smoke inhalation.

DEFINITIONS AND PREVALENCES. Agents that cause inhalational injury can occur as (1) gases (i.e., in molecular form with no specific volume when unconstrained under ambient conditions), (2) the vapor of a liquid under altered conditions of temperature and pressure, (3) particulates that are further broken down into liquids in the form of mist generated by perturbation, or (4) solids in the form of fumes volatilized during combustion. Under conditions of increasing temperature, combustion and pyrolysis occur in the presence and absence of oxygen, respectively. Both result in production of smoke that consists of a mixture of gases, vapors, fumes, liquid droplets, and carbonaceous particles (soot). Large particles and droplets ($<5.0\ \mu$) deposit in the nose and air passages, whereas smaller particles reach and impact in the terminal bronchioles and alveoli. The smallest particles may not deposit at all but can still exert their toxic effect. Particulates may serve as a carrier for introduction of toxic gases into the lower respiratory tract.

Inhaled agents can cause disease by asphyxia, direct toxicity, or systemic reactions that may be immunologic or nonimmunologically mediated. Combinations of these effects also occur, and different reactions to the same agent can result from varying intensity and duration of exposure. Because carbon monoxide is the most common cause of poisoning, it is highlighted in the

Table 71-1. Differential Features of Environmentally Caused Respiratory Disease

Location	Clinical diagnosis	Major symptoms	Environmental causes	Key to recognition	Differential diagnosis
Upper airway	Rhinitis	Rhinorrhea Postnasal drip Throat clearing Cough	Toxic gases	Exposure history Work-related	Allergic Vasomotor Coryza
	Sinusitis	Sinus drainage Headache Postnasal drip Throat clearing Cough	Toxic gases	Exposure history	Bacterial
	Pharyngitis	Throat pain Throat clearing Cough	Toxic gases	Exposure history	Strep throat Viral pharyngitis
	Laryngitis	Hoarseness Stridor	Toxic gases	Exposure history Recent spill	Viral
	Laryngospasm	Stridor Dyspnea	Chlorine Hydrogen chloride Sulfur dioxide	Exposure history Recent spill	Allergic Angioneurotic edema
Lower airway, small airway	Acute bronchitis (tracheobronchitis)	Productive cough Wheeze	Chlorine Phosgene Ozone Ammonia Sulfur dioxide	Exposure history	Bacterial Asthma Influenza
	Chronic bronchitis	Productive cough Wheeze Dyspnea	Hydrogen sulfide Chlorine Ozone Sulfur dioxide Vanadium-pentox-ide	Chronic exposure history	COPD Chronic asthma
	Asthma	Cough Wheeze Dyspnea	Toluene diisocyan-ate Ammonia	Exposure history Recent onset	Atopic
	Bronchiolitis	Dyspnea Productive cough Wheeze	Oxides of nitrogen Sulfur dioxide Phosgene Organic dusts	Exposure history Recent spills	Viral Collagen vascular disease Postpneumonia
Parenchyma	Pneumonia, acute	Dyspnea Cough Expectoration Cyanosis	Toxic gas Ammonia Chlorine	Massive exposure	Mycoplasma Tuberculosis ARDS (multiple causes)
	Chronic	Dyspnea Dry cough Weight loss	Asbestos Beryllium Hypersensitivity re-action	Long latency Recurrent episodes	Idiopathic pulmonary fibrosis Sarcoidosis Tuberculosis
	Pulmonary edema	Dyspnea Cough Cyanosis Diaphoresis	Toxic gases Hydrogen chloride Hydrogen sulfide Ammonia Chlorine Oxides of nitrogen Sulfur dioxide Ozone Phosgene	Massive exposure	Cardiogenic ARDS (mulitple causes)
Systemic	Viral syndrome	Fever Weakness Myalgia Cough	Polymer fume fever Metal fume fever Organic dust fever	New employee	Influenza
	Cardiopulmonary ar-rest	Unresponsive	Asphyxiants Toxic gases	Massive exposure Closed space	Cardiac etiology

COPD = chronic obstructive pulmonary disease; ARDS = acute respiratory distress syndrome.

following discussion. Smoke inhalation offers such a unique combination of management problems that it merits a separate section.

Asphyxiants. Simple asphyxiants include carbon dioxide (CO_2), nitrogen (N_2), and methane (CH_4), which are normally present in the atmosphere and can be fatal in increased concentration [1]. Toxic asphyxiants are present in the atmosphere in minute amounts or are released by manufacturing processes or combustion; they asphyxiate at low concentration. This category includes carbon monoxide (CO), hydrogen cyanide (HCN), acrylonitrile (vinyl cyanide), hydrogen sulfide (H_2S), and carbon disulfide (CS_2) (Table 71-2) [1].

Approximately 5600 deaths are attributed to CO poisoning in the United States each year [2,3]. Of these, less than one-half are suicides and the rest are accidental [3]. This colorless, odorless, tasteless, nonirritating gas is the most common cause of poisoning, responsible for 80 percent of smoke inhalation-related fatalities, most occurring within the first 24 hours of exposure [4]. Twenty-five percent of fatalities occur in persons with underlying cardiopulmonary disease [5]. Subacute exposure accounts for loss of 1 or more workdays per year in another 10,000 individuals [6].

Toxic Gases. A variety of agents act as toxic irritants to the upper and lower respiratory tract, causing mucosal edema, impairment of mucociliary function, and diffuse alveolar damage with pulmonary edema resulting from exposure to high concentration (Table 71-3) [7,8].

Ammonia (NH_3), a colorless, highly water-soluble gas, forms ammonium hydroxide in solution. This reaction makes it highly irritating to the upper respiratory passages and mucous membranes, but alveolar damage also occurs when exposure is massive [7,9]. Nearly 3 million workers are at risk from exposure, and most inhalational injuries occur as the result of industrial accidents [7]. Increased concentrations of NH_3 in the environment are so irritating to the eyes and mucous membranes that the individual will attempt escape before significant pulmonary injury occurs.

Chlorine (Cl_2) is a heavy, very reactive greenish yellow gas under ambient conditions with an unmistakable pungent odor [7]. Approximately 15,000 workers are at risk; a summary of exposures for 1986 compiled from 57 institutions by the Poison Control Center showed 3174 exposures to chlorine gas with an additional 673 exposures occurring in the home as the result of mixing household products [10].

Phosgene ($COCl_2$) is a heavy, insoluble, colorless gas that imparts the smell of freshly mown hay and hydrolyzes to form hydrochloric acid (HCl). Approximately 10,000 workers are at risk from exposure [7]. Phosgene is responsible for the majority of gas fatalities from World War I.

One million workers are estimated to be at risk from exposure to oxides of nitrogen [7]. Nitrous oxide (N_2O) is an anesthetic agent. Nitric oxide (NO) is oxidized to nitrogen dioxide (NO_2), which exists as an irritating, insoluble, heavy orange-brown gas and its dimer dinitrogen tetroxide [7]. One of the best characterized syndromes of toxic gas exposure is silo-fillers' disease, which results from exposure to NO_2 gas that accumulates just above the silage in recently filled top-loading silos. A recent estimate of 5 cases per 100,000 silo-associated farm workers per year may be an underestimate of this problem [11].

Sulfur dioxide (SO_2) is a colorless, heavy, irritating gas highly soluble in water with an identifiable pungent odor. One-half million workers are exposed from industrial processes [7]. Ozone (O_3), another environmental pollutant, is an allotropic form of oxygen that is colorless, unstable, and reactive [7]. With

indoor levels in the home and office reaching 70 percent of outdoor levels, it is difficult to assess the population at risk.

Other agents require mention because they are so ubiquitous and can cause severe respiratory symptoms. Formaldehyde, a colorless, nonflammable, dense gas, was recognized as a hazard after extensive use of ureaformaldehyde foam insulation in homes [12,13]. Exposure to cadmium as elemental metal, salt, dust, or more toxic vapor poses a risk to 2 million workers [7]. Mercury is dangerous in vapor, dust, and salt forms; nearly 1.1 million workers are at risk [7]. The salts of vanadium and osmium are implicated in the development of bronchitis in exposed workers. Vanadium pentoxide, a catalyst for various industrial processes and residue of crude oil from various sources, may affect approximately 174,000 workers [7]. Osmium tetroxide, another acidic compound, is used by pathologists to process tissue [7]. Paraquat is thought to cause problems by absorption through the skin, although most accidents with this herbicide occur while it is being sprayed on fields; inhalation results in pulmonary fibrosis [14]. Severe reactions are also seen with the metal hydrides, which include arsine (AsH_3), phosphine (PH_3), silane (SiH_3), and diborane (B_2H_6) and are formed by reaction with nascent hydrogen [15].

Asthma Syndromes. The airways can be affected by extreme physical conditions (e.g., heat or cold), by toxic agents based in part on their water solubility and concentration, and via immunologic and nonimmunologic mechanisms. Development of asthma symptoms can be the initial indication of a problem, or it can develop as a sequela of earlier exposure and injury. This discussion emphasizes occupational asthma (OA) and reactive airways dysfunction syndrome (RADS), which are distinctive asthma syndromes. Severe bronchiolitis causing acute airflow obstruction can occur after a variety of exposures (e.g., NH_3 and oxides of nitrogen). Although it may be indistinguishable from asthma syndromes and many of the same treatment considerations apply, bronchiolitis is discussed not here but in the sections on toxic gases. Chronic airflow obstruction as a sequela of environmental exposure is also excluded from further discussion here. Acute respiratory failure in conditions of chronic airflow obstruction is covered in Chapter 57.

It is estimated that 2 to 15 percent of asthma is related to workplace exposures [16]. The rapid turnover of new workers in these occupations leads to an artificially low estimate of the true prevalence (the "healthy worker effect") [16]. Failure to recognize an association between symptoms and workplace can result in progressive disease and disability in the patient and exposure to other workers. Unlike other conditions that result from an acute exposure, OA may persist long after exposure is discontinued [17,18].

Occupational asthma is defined as variable airway narrowing causally related to exposures encountered in the workplace to airborne dusts, fumes, vapors, and gases [19]. Diagnosis requires that the following criteria be met: (1) symptoms consistent with asthma (e.g., cough, wheeze, dyspnea, and chest tightness); (2) identification of the offending agent; (3) proof that the suspected agent can cause asthma; (4) spirometric evidence of airflow obstruction; and (5) immunologic evidence, which may consist of demonstration of specific IgE and skin testing. Preexisting asthma should be considered separate from OA, since the former can be aggravated by a wide variety of industrial irritants.

The number of workers exposed to these agents is variable. Estimates include 8 million farmers, animal handlers, and lumberjacks; 250,000 bakers and beauticians; and 30,000 isocyanates-exposed workers in spray paint, plastics, and rubber industries [20].

Reactive airways dysfunction syndrome may be considered

(*Text continues on p. 830.*)

Table 71-2. Asphyxiant Gases

Agent	Some sources	Uses	Form	TWA	IDLH	Effects	Pathophysiology	Treatment	Sequelae
Simple									
Carbon dioxide	Atmospheric 0.03–0.06%, combustion of organic material in oxygen, foundry work, mining	Carbonization, neutralizing, fire extinguishers, dry ice, refrigeration	Colorless, odorless, inert	5000 ppm	50,000 ppm (5%)	Unconsciousness, asphyxia	Displaces oxygen	Oxygen, supportive care	—
Nitrogen	Atmospheric 78.09%, from ammonia, decomposition of nitrogenous compounds, mining	Fertilizer, ammonia production, inert medium	Colorless, odorless, inert	—	—	Unconsciousness, asphyxia	Displaces oxygen	Oxygen, supportive care	—
Methane	Decomposition or organics, mining, petroleum industry	—	—	—	—	Unconsciousness, asphyxia	Displaces oxygen	Oxygen, supportive care	—
Toxic									
Carbon monoxide	Oxidation of hydrocarbons, combustion of organics in low-oxygen, gas engine exhaust (1–10% of emissions), motor vehicles (55–60% of total), foundry work, refineries, distillation coal and wood, paint strippers	Reducing agent for metallurgy, industrial heating, gases	Colorless, odorless	50 ppm	1500 ppm	(see Table 71-6) 10,000 to 40,000 ppm death in minutes	Carboxyhemoglobin, carboxymyoglobin	High F$_I$O$_2$, hyperbaric oxygen	Persistent memory deficit (43%)

Substance	Uses	Sources	Physical properties	TWA	IDLH	Signs/symptoms	Mechanism	Treatment	Chronic effects
Hydrogen cyanide	Synthetic fibers, plastics, exterminating rodents, electroplating, steel industry	Almonds, combustion of organics, electroplating	Colorless, water-soluble, bitter almond smell	10 ppm	50 ppm	Weakness, headache, cherry red color, confusion, asphyxia	Inhibits cytochrome oxidase and other enzymes, poisons cell respiration	Nitrate therapy, amyl nitrite (IV), thiosulfate (IV), cobalt EDTA (IM), hydroxycyanocobalamin	Chronic exposure dermatitis, motor weakness, headache
Vinyl cyanide (Acrylonitrile)	Synthetic fibers, plastics, resins, and rubber	Oxidation of ammonia and propylene	Colorless, water-soluble, faint odor	4 ppm	4 ppm	Slower than cyanide, weakness, dyspnea, cyanosis, burning throat, nausea, impaired judgment, convulsions, death	Inhibits cytochrome oxidase and other enzymes, poisons cell respiration	—	—
Hydrogen sulfide	Analytic reagent production of sulfides, sulfuric acid, and organic sulfur	Decomposition of organics, sewers, reacting iron sulfide with acid, petroleum products, synthetic materials	Colorless, water-soluble, rotten egg odor	20 ppm	300 ppm	Green face and chest, unconsciousness, asphyxia, membrane irritation, diffuse rales, ronchi, pulmonary edema, 10–500 ppm slight poisoning, 500–700 ppm moderate	Inhibits cytochrome oxidase	Oxygen, supportive care	Chronic bronchitis

TWA = time-weighted average;
IDLH = immediately dangerous to life and health.

Table 71-3. Toxic Irritant Gases

Agent	Sources	Uses	Form	Dose	Persons at risk	Pathophysiology	Effect	Acute	Chronic	Treatment
Ammonia	Combustion sources, wool, silk, nylon, melamine, polyurethane	Fertilizer production, chemical industry, pharmaceuticals, refrigerant, explosives, transport accidents, cleaning agents	Colorless, water-soluble, sharp odor	50 ppm TWA, 500 ppm IDLH, 40–100 ppm acute irritation upper respiratory tract, 700–1700 ppm inflammation	3 million	Forms ammonium hydroxide on contact with membranes	Liquification necrosis of membranes with sloughing predominantly upper tract initially	Airway obstruction, pulmonary edema, bronchopneumonia	Tracheitis, bronchitis, bronchiectasis, small airway disease, ? bronchiolitis, RADS	Oxygen, observation, support, airway maintenance, long-term follow-up
Chlorine	Polyvinylchloride, chlorinated acrylics	Bleaching agent in paper and textiles, disinfectant, polymers, solvents, pesticides, container leakages	Green-yellow heavy, slight water solubility, pungent odor	1 ppm TWA, 25 ppm IDLH 6–15 ppm throat irritation, 30–90 ppm coughing fits, 100–300 ppm may cause lethal damage, 1000–3000 ppm fatal after several breaths	15,000	Forms hydrogen chloride and free radical (0)	Affects entire respiratory tract, can be delay in effects after exposure	Airflow obstruction, pulmonary edema, ulcerative tracheobronchitis	Persistent air flow obstruction, RADS	Oxygen, observation, support, long-term follow-up
Hydrogen chloride	Polyvinylchloride pyrrolysis	Fertilizer, dye, textile and rubber manufacture, polyvinyl chloride, refining metal ore	Colorless, pungent odor	5 ppm TWA, 100 ppm IDLH, 4–10 ppm burning throat	—	—	Upper airways and mucous membranes	Laryngospasm, atelectasis, pulmonary edema	Unknown	Oxygen, airway maintenance, observation, supportive care

Agent	Source	Uses	Physical properties	Exposure limits	Concentration	Mechanism	Site	Acute	Chronic	Treatment
Oxides of nitrogen, nitrous oxide, nitrogen dioxide	Combustion of fabric and nitrocelluose films	Fresh silage, arc welding, combustion nitrogen polymers, chemical industry dyes and lacquers, mining, explosives, gas stoves	Red-brown gas, heavy, insoluble, irritating odor	5 ppm TWA, 50 ppm IDLH, 50 ppm acute respiratory problems	1 million	Forms nitric acid, direct inflammation, peroxidation of lipid, impairs surfactant	Lower tract	Acute pulmonary edema	Bronchiolitis obliterans, chronic bronchitis, ? emphysema, persisting obstruction	Oxygen, observation, support, long-term follow-up
Phosgene	Polyvinylchloride combustion	Isocyanate production, pesticide, dye, and pharmaceutical products, polyvinyl chloride, carbon tetrachloride extinguishers	Colorless gas, heavy, prickling smell, mown hay, poor water solubility	0.1 ppm TWA, 2 ppm IDLH	10,000	Hydrolyzes to HCl and CO_2, sympathetic effects	Lower tract, delayed recognition, fluid shifts, necrosis and sloughing of mucosal surfaces, decrease lung volumes, decrease D_LCO, hypoxemia	Atelectasis, acute pulmonary edema, acute bronchiolitis, ulcerative bronchitis	Air trapping	Oxygen, observation, support, long-term follow-up
Ozone	Photochemical smog, arc welding, high altitude, oxidizing agent		Bluish gas, pungent odor, poor water solubility	0.1 ppm TWA, 10 ppm IDLH, 0.02–0.05 ppm threshold, 2 ppm acute symptoms	Diverse group	Powerful oxidizing agent, cholinergic effects	Lower tract, tolerance with chronic exposure	Acute pulmonary edema, asthma	? COPD	
Sulfur dioxide	Sulfur-containing compounds, wood, oil	Combustion fossil fuels, smelting ores, paper manufacture, food preparation	Colorless gas, heavy, pungent odor, water-soluble	5 ppm TWA, 100 IDLH, 0.5 ppm detectable, 6–10 ppm irritation	500,000	Forms sulfate (SO_3^-) and bisulfite (HSO_3^-)	Bronchoconstriction, extensive sloughing of mucosa, alveolar edema and hemorrhage	Laryngospasm, airway narrowing, pulmonary edema, bronchopneumonia, worsens asthma	? COPD, emphysema bronchiectasis, bronchiolitis obliterans	

TWA = time-weighted average, IDLH = immediately dangerous to life and health, D_LCO = carbon monoxide diffusing capacity of the lung, RADS = reactive airways dysfunction syndrome, COPD = chronic obstructive pulmonary disease.

a form of inflammatory bronchoconstriction, usually resulting from a single massive or multiple accidental high-level exposures to an irritating vapor, fume, or smoke, with symptoms persisting years after exposure. The number at risk is probably as large as that for OA [21].

Hypersensitivity Pneumonitis. In contrast to OA, hypersensitivity pneumonitis (HP) results from an immunologic reaction to inhaled antigens that affects the alveoli and interstitium of the lung but not the airways. Approximately 2.8 million workers are at risk, but the true incidence is difficult to establish because it is usually diagnosed as some other condition [22]. Prevalence rate estimates for some of the more common causes of HP are 0.9 to 9.6 percent for farmer's lung, 6 to 15 percent for pigeon breeder's disease [23], and 1 to 15 percent in populations exposed to contaminated air-cooling systems [23].

Etiology

ASPHYXIANTS. Carbon dioxide accumulates in sealed or poorly ventilated areas (e.g., storage lockers, tanks, mines, and underwater caissons). Nitrogen is found in increased amounts in mines; if present with increased amounts of carbon dioxide it causes significant reductions in ambient partial pressure of oxygen. Methane is a highly explosive asphyxiant gas released during breakdown of organic matter. It occurs naturally in the crust of the earth and is also present in mines. Modern mining methods and improved ventilation have reduced the risk from these simple asphyxiants.

Cyanide is encountered as inorganic salts (sodium and potassium) in metallurgy, electroplating, and photoprocessing; in the combustion of natural (wood, silk) and synthetic polymers (nylon, polyurethane), including polyacrylonitrile with production of hydrogen cyanide and vinyl cyanide (acrylonitrile); and as the agent in suicides [10,24].

Morbidity related to H_2S inhalation is minimal due to the characteristic "rotten egg" odor that is appreciated at low concentration, although paralysis of the olfactory nerve may occur at high concentrations [7]. Significant exposure and fatalities have occurred in workers processing sewage (manure, wastewater, fish), in industrial processing (petrochemical plants and leather and rubber processing), and drilling where this gas is generated [25]. Carbon disulfide is used as a solvent and pesticide.

Carbon monoxide is generated during the combustion of any carbon-containing fuel. The most important source is the internal combustion engine, and high levels of CO develop rapidly in enclosed spaces (car in enclosed garage, 10 minutes) [26,27]. Other sources include smoke from all types of fires, including wood, coal, and kerosene burned in the home; improperly maintained heating systems [28]; combustion of propane gas for heat and by motor vehicles [29]; exposure to fumes of methylene chloride, which is used as a paint stripper [30]; and metabolism of hemoglobin to bilirubin [26]. Cigarette smoke contains about 4 percent CO, and smoking can have a significant impact on the interpretation of levels (see Diagnosis) [2]. Smoke emitted by a burning cigarette tip contains 2.5 times the CO of inhaled smoke [2]. Methylene chloride, present in many paint thinners, is converted in vivo by hepatic metabolism to CO, even after exposure ceases [30].

TOXIC GASES. Workers are exposed to toxic gases during industrial production and use. Other exposures occur in the home from cleaning solvents, pesticides, and other sources. Major uses of NH_3 include fertilizer production, chemicals, plastics, dye manufacture, and refrigeration.

The industrial uses of Cl_2 are in the production of alkali, bleaches, and disinfectants and in paper and textile processing. Most exposures result from industrial spills. The density of Cl_2 causes it to accumulate in dependent areas, and these sites should be avoided during its accidental release [7]. Hydrogen chloride (HCl), much less toxic than chlorine gas, is used in the manufacture of fertilizer, dyes, textiles, and rubber. It is also released by thermal decomposition of polyvinyl chloride film [31]. Current uses of $COCl_2$ include isocyanate, pesticide, dye, and pharmaceutical production. Firefighters, welders, and paint strippers are exposed to heated chlorinated hydrocarbons such as polyvinyl chloride, and $COCl_2$ is also released in these settings [7]. $COCl_2$ is less irritating to the eyes and mucous membranes than Cl_2 or HCl and may be inhaled for prolonged periods without discomfort, thereby greatly increasing the risk of serious injury to the lower respiratory tract.

Oxides of nitrogen are used in dye and fertilizer manufacture and are generated during nitric acid use, arc welding and braziering, engraving, metal work, combustion of nitrogenous compounds including explosives, and in fresh silage [15,32]. Gas stoves, tobacco smoke, and diesel fumes are other commonly encountered sources of intense exposure to NO, NO_2, and N_2O_4 [33]. Silo-fillers' disease, the classic example of a toxic, irritant gas reaction, is related to the atmosphere at the top of a recently filled silo being O_2-depleted and CO_2-enriched. Nitrates in the silage (corn, oats, hay) are anaerobically converted into NO, which then forms NO_2 and N_2O_4, the gases responsible for the acute lung injury in this disease. Rapid accumulation to toxic levels of 200 to 2000 parts per million of NO_2 begins within hours and high levels persist for days [34]. Danger is heightened by the ability of high concentrations of NO_2 to cause rapid unconsciousness. Conversely, as with $COCl_2$, there may be little warning of low levels, resulting in prolonged exposure and delayed lung injury [34].

A common atmospheric pollutant from combustion of coal and gasoline, SO_2 is used in bleaching, refrigeration, paper manufacture, and other processes [7]. Sources of O_3 exposure include arc welding, bleaching, high-flying aircraft, and waste treatment. Industrial uses of formaldehyde include paper products, floor coverings, adhesives, and cosmetics. The volatility of cadmium increases the risk to workers in or near heated environments. Workers in a variety of metal and electronics industries, welders, braziers, solderers, and painters are among those potentially exposed. Mercury is encountered in metal, electronics, battery, drug, and dye manufacture and other occupations.

The metal hydrides are gases used in the production of semiconductors and related manufacturing processes [15]. Arsine, phosphine, silane, and diborane are the most important agents in this class. Arsine, the principal source of industrial arsenic poisoning, is encountered in lead, tin, and zinc processing [15].

ASTHMA SYNDROMES. The classification of OA is based on pathophysiologic considerations (Table 71-4) [35]. Reflex bronchoconstriction is seen with exposure to cold air, exercise, noxious gases, and some inert particulates. Preexisting asthma is also aggravated by these factors. Inflammatory bronchoconstriction results from most of the toxic, irritant asphyxiants discussed earlier and from solvents and fumes of a variety of volatile organic compounds found in household and industrial settings. Pharmacologic agents include cotton and related fiber dusts, organophosphate insecticides, plastic pyrolysis products, and isocyanates.

Table 71-4. Types of Occupational Asthma

Category	Examples (% prevalence)	Occupation	Mechanism	Onset	Duration	Comments
Reflex	Cold air Exercise Lactose powder	Refrigeration Athletics Pharmaceuticals	Direct effect on irritant receptors in bronchial submucosa	Immediate	Ceases after exposure discontinued	Aggravates preexisting asthma
Irritant	Ammonia Chlorine Solvents	Chemical industry	Chemical inflammation Mucosal edema Irritant receptor effect	Late	Prolonged (months)	Reactive airways Dysfunction Syndrome
Pharmacologic	Organophosphates	Farming	Acts as anticholinesterase	Immediate	Ceases after exposure	At high enough concentrations all exposed develop bronchoconstriction
Allergic High-molecular-weight	Cotton dust Biologic enzymes (66%) *Bacillus subtilis*	Linen industry Detergent manufacture	Endotoxin-mediated	Most severe at start of week		Not from domestic use
	Animal products (30%)	Laboratory workers	Type I allergic reaction Positive skin tests Specific IgE	Immediate and late reactions	Ceases after exposure Remain sensitive	Rhinitis common
	Cereal flour (20%)	Bakers				Cross-reactivity among flours
Low-molecular-weight	Diisocyanates (10%)	Plastics	Type I allergic reaction Positive skin tests Specific IgE	Weeks to months after exposure starts	Persists after exposure ceases	Cough syndrome
	Anhydrides (36%)	Epoxy resins				Immediate rhinitis and asthma Late asthma and fever Pulmonary infiltrates
	Wood dusts (4%) Plicatic acid	Carpentry Sawmill		Late onset		More common in smokers Eosinophilia common

The largest, most important, and best understood cause of OA is those agents that act via an allergic mechanism. High-molecular-weight causes include proteins, polysaccharides, glycoproteins, and peptides derived from danders, excreta, feathers, marine animals, insects, grain, and plants during harvesting and processing and during a variety of industrial uses. A number of chemicals, including isocyanates, anhydrides, other organic compounds, pharmaceuticals, and metals and their salts and fumes, comprise the low-molecular-weight agents that cause allergic-type OA.

With certain agents, up to 5 to 10 percent of a given workforce may be affected with OA. Higher prevalences have occasionally resulted from abnormally high exposure intensity, poor ventilation, or unrecognized exposure. Examples include laboratory animal handlers, with a 30 percent prevalence of OA. The prevalence of OA in workers exposed to Western red cedar or isocyanates is 4 to 5 percent, more compatible with the prevalence of atopy in the general population. Those with atopy are more likely to develop sensitization to environmental agents [16].

A number of factors predispose to the development of OA. Environmental determinants include poor ventilation, noncompliance with safety procedures, exposures to spills, and viral respiratory infections. Host factors include smoking history, a history of atopy, and presence of nonspecific bronchial hyperreactivity [16]. Evidence suggests that smokers are more easily sensitized to some agents [36], but the majority of workers with red cedar asthma are lifelong nonsmokers [37]. Although it is commonly assumed that bronchial hyperreactivity preexists in workers who develop OA, the return of bronchial hyperreactivity to normal in some patients following discontinuation of exposure suggests this may not be the case [38].

HYPERSENSITIVITY PNEUMONITIS. Causative agents are encountered in a variety of occupations and also result from indoor (home and office) exposure to antigens dispersed by contaminated humidification and climate control systems [22]. Thermophilic actinomyces are a common cause of HP, responsible for farmer's lung seen in farmers and dairy workers exposed to moldy hay and feedstuffs. Bagassosis, mushroom worker's lung, and HP due to contaminated climate control systems are also caused by this class of antigens. Fungal antigens cause HP in cheese worker's lung, malt worker's lung, maple bark stripper's lung, paprika slicer's lung, sequoisis, and suberosis. Animal antigens include amoeba, insects, and animal excrement and extracts. Chemical causes of HP include isocyanates, phthalic anhydride, and trimellitic anhydride, although these more often cause OA. Some types of HP have unknown antigens but are associated with coffee dust, cereal grain, tap water, tobacco, sawdust, tea, and climate control systems.

Pathophysiology

ASPHYXIANTS. Simple asphyxiants work by displacing oxygen from inspired air (Table 71-5). Cyanide binds to the cytochrome aa3 complex, blocking the final step of oxidative phosphorylation and mitochondrial oxygen utilization. The tricarboxylic acid cycle is blocked, and pyruvate is anaerobically converted to lactate, resulting in severe lactic acidosis. Hydrogen sulfide alters the oxygen-carrying capacity of the blood by binding with hemoglobin to form sulfhemoglobin. It also poisons the respiratory enzymes of the cell by reversibly binding

Table 71-5. Mechanisms of Asphyxiation by Inhalational Gas and Fume Injury

Displacement of oxygen from inspired air
Nitrogen
Carbon dioxide
Methane
Altered oxygen-carrying capacity
Carbon monoxide—carboxyhemoglobin
Oxides of nitrogen—methemoglobin
Hydrogen sulfide—sulfhemoglobin
Poisoning of cell respiratory enzymes
Cyanide
Acrylonitrile
Hydrogen sulfide

to cytochrome oxidase, an action also characteristic of cyanide and acrylonitrile.

The affinity of CO for hemoglobin is 250 times that of oxygen. Carbon monoxide is readily and reversibly bound to hemoglobin after it enters the bloodstream via the alveolar capillary interface. The high affinity for hemoglobin makes even low concentrations of CO toxic, and carboxyhemoglobin (COHb) levels of 50 percent can be seen after a few minutes at 0.1 percent concentration [39]. Furthermore, even at low concentrations of CO increased minute ventilation in response to reduced tissue oxygen delivery further increases uptake. The formation of COHb results in reduction of the total oxygen-carrying capacity of the blood, a shift of the oxyhemoglobin saturation curve to the left, and an increased affinity of hemoglobin for oxygen at the remaining binding sites, due to allosteric modification. Thus, the cumulative effect on peripheral oxygen delivery is greater than that expected from the decreased oxygen-carrying capacity alone [40]. There is also evidence that CO reversibly binds to other heme proteins, including cytochrome oxidase and myoglobin, poisoning respiration at the cellular level much like cyanide and further reducing the amount of oxygen available for metabolism in peripheral and cardiac muscle [41,42,43].

TOXIC GASES. Accidental massive exposure to NH_3, Cl_2, HCl, oxides of nitrogen, $COCl_2$, SO_2, and some of the other irritant gases discussed causes similar pathologic change. Ammonia, SO_2, and HCl have high water solubility and tend to be highly irritating to conjunctivae, mucous membranes, and upper air passages [44]. Laryngospasm, bronchospasm, and mucous membrane necrosis ensue. Less water-soluble agents, such as N_2O, O_3, and $COCl_2$, can penetrate deeper into the respiratory tree and cause damage at the alveolar level, resulting in pulmonary edema and bronchospasm. The absence of immediate symptoms with these less water-soluble agents can prolong exposure. Chlorine has intermediate solubility and has an effect throughout the respiratory tract, but exposure to a heavy concentration of any of these toxic agents causes diffuse involvement [45]. In addition to concentration and solubility, pH and chemical reactivity influence the amount of damage inflicted. Hydrochloric acid, SO_2, and $COCl_2$ are acidic, whereas O_3, Cl_2, and oxides of nitrogen are highly alkaline. Toxicity is enhanced if particulates (soot) are present, which help carry irritants further down the airways. Following acute exposure, there may be residual damage to the respiratory system in the form of reactive airways disease, asthma, bronchitis, bronchiolitis obliterans with and without organizing pneumonia, or bronchiectasis [46]. Most of our understanding concerning these agents is the result of industrial accidents and controlled exposure of normals.

The strong smell associated with NH_3 is present within moments at 50 parts per million (ppm), and few persons can tolerate greater than 100 ppm without experiencing nasal stuffiness and irritating cough [47]. Reaction with H_2O on the mucous membranes, airways, and conjunctivae results in ammonium hydroxide formation and liquefaction necrosis with intense pain of affected areas, choking, cyanosis, aphonia, and suffocation. Death from asphyxiation can occur within one minute with high concentrations (1500 ppm). Findings within hours of acute exposure observed in fatal cases include edema, ulceration, necrosis, and sloughing of mucous membranes and airway mucosa with airway obstruction due to laryngeal edema and plugging of airways by sloughed epithelium [9]. Clinical bronchopneumonia and acute pulmonary edema are seen within 24 hours. Severe airway obstruction is seen within 24 hours, and this may take more than 1 year to improve [8,9]. Long-term sequelae include bronchitis, bronchiectasis, bronchiolitis obliterans, and asthma [9,48].

Chlorine is detectable at levels of 1 ppm. On contact with mucous membranes, HCl, hypochlorous acid (HOCl), and free oxygen radicals are formed; much of the damage results from this last product [45]. Shortly after initial exposure the ability to detect continued exposure is blunted, subjecting the victim to additional risk. Following onset of exposure there is choking and coughing, which stop after removal from exposure. The paucity of symptoms initially belies the true severity of the problem, and the patient may be inappropriately sent home from the emergency room [44,47]. Slight wheezing and erythematous mucous membranes may be the only physical findings. If exposure is severe enough, death can result from laryngospasm or massive pulmonary edema. Hours to days after exposure, upper air passage edema, pulmonary edema, and exudative inflammatory bronchitis cause plugging of medium and small bronchi, leading to atelectasis. Development of stridor reflects upper airway obstruction due to nasal, pharyngeal, and laryngeal edema. Hypoxemia and hypercapnia occur secondary to these changes. Pulmonary edema and bronchopneumonia accompany peripheral airway obstruction. These changes subsequently revert to near normal, but chronic airway problems, including bronchiolitis obliterans with organizing pneumonia and asthma, persist.

Phosgene is only mildly irritating to the eyes and upper airways, increasing the risk of continued exposure. Dyspnea and dry cough develop, followed by pulmonary edema. The increase in airway resistance following inhalation of low levels of ozone is abolished by atropine, suggesting an effect on the neural determinants of bronchomotor tone [49]. Ozone also affects the lower respiratory tract, causing symptoms of chest pain, cough, and dyspnea. Pulmonary edema is seen at 2 ppm, and levels above 5 ppm may be fatal [7].

Exposure to NO_2 at 50 ppm increases the risk of acute respiratory problems such as silo-fillers' disease. Poor water solubility results in a paucity of upper tract and mucous membrane irritation, and exposure may be initially inapparent because of this. The clinical response occurs in three phases [44]. Cough, dyspnea, and hypoxemia develop, followed by noncardiogenic pulmonary edema several hours later. As pulmonary edema clears, slight dyspnea may be present for 3 to 5 weeks. Finally, an illness characterized by cough, dyspnea, and fever with nodular or patchy infiltrates progresses to chronic obstruction, and lung biopsy shows bronchiolitis obliterans of the proximal type without organizing pneumonia [34,46]. Most severe lung injury and mortality occurs in victims suffering high-dose exposure associated with initial loss of consciousness, choking, acute onset of audible wheezing, or chest pain [34]. Most deaths occur during the acute phase [33]. Molecular effects of NO_2 include lipid peroxidation and impairment of surfactant activity [50].

Diborane and PH_3 are extremely irritating and cause pulmonary edema at low doses as well as central nervous system (CNS) depression [20]. Arsine is associated with a distinctive systemic reaction. It combines with hemoglobin, resulting in a clinical picture of fulminant intravascular hemolysis of rapid onset [51].

ASTHMA SYNDROMES. The pathophysiology of asthma is reviewed in Chapter 56. With this as background, how acute inhalation injury further exacerbates or causes asthma is discussed here.

Irritants in low concentration can abruptly precipitate or aggravate airway obstruction in persons with a history of asthma. This is thought to occur via direct stimulation of irritant receptors in the bronchial mucosa of vagal origin, and the reaction can be blocked by atropine. Offending agents include Cl_2, fluorine, $COCl_2$, NH_3, and N_2O in gaseous form, and vapors of strong acids and organic solvents [35].

Accidental exposure to high concentrations of irritant gases, vapors, and combustion products results in airways obstruction from mucosal edema, mucous plugging, epithelial sloughing, and inflammation as a direct effect of mediator release. In contrast to reflex bronchoconstriction, inflammatory bronchoconstriction occurs late, usually several hours after inhalation, reaches a maximum in 1 week, and persists for up to several months [35].

Following recurrent exposures to high concentrations of some agents, including irritants and organic solvents (i.e., spills), airways hyperreactivity persists. This has been attributed to regeneration of bronchial epithelium, resulting in altered innervation of mucosa and smooth muscle. Such a mechanism has been postulated to explain the bronchial hyperreactivity observed with RADS [21].

The dose-response relationship is an important characteristic of pharmacologic bronchoconstriction [35]. These agents release histamine, inhibit beta-adrenergic receptors, act as anticholinesterases, or cause complement activation by the classic or alternate pathways, with release of chemical mediators of inflammation. At a high enough concentration, all exposed persons will demonstrate bronchoconstriction. Although nonspecific bronchial hyperreactivity can be shown during exposure, this finding no longer persists when exposure ceases. An example of pharmacologic bronchoconstriction is that from organophosphate insecticides, which precipitate airflow obstruction by their anticholinesterase action [52].

The majority of agents that cause OA do so by an allergic mechanism [16]. These agents most often affect persons with a history of atopy. High-molecular-weight compounds from animal and plant sources are natural sensitizing agents and cause formation of specific IgE and IgG antibodies over weeks to months. These antibodies can be demonstrated by skin tests and radioimmunoassay and are responsible for the immediate response seen during specific bronchoprovocation testing. Cross-reactivity of antigens exists within classes of agents.

The list of low-molecular-weight agents causing OA is burgeoning and includes inorganic and organic agents [16]. Specific IgE may not be demonstrated to the agent alone, but when it is conjugated to serum protein it acts as a hapten and induces antibodies. Workers exposed to isocyanates develop sensitization weeks or months after exposure is initiated; thereafter an attack of bronchospasm can be induced by very low levels of the agent. Exposure to single or recurrent spills also plays a significant role in sensitization. Most patients with isocyanate asthma have eosinophilia. Cross-reactivity to other diisocyanates occurs. Isocyanate-induced asthma can persist long after exposure has ceased.

HYPERSENSITIVITY PNEUMONITIS. The unifying features of agents causing HP are their ability, based on particle size, to penetrate the distal airways and alveoli, leading to development of alveolitis [22]. Although serum precipitins (IgG) occur in the majority of symptomatic persons, they are also seen in large numbers of exposed asymptomatic persons and thus lack specificity [53]. Current models of pathogenesis invoke nonspecific stimulation by antigen of the alternative pathway of complement, resulting in increased vascular permeability, release of lysosomal enzymes and monokines, neutrophil chemotaxis, and activation of alveolar macrophages with release of enzymes and oxygen products, interleukin-1, and monokines. T and B lymphocyte recruitment results in further magnification of this cellular response and production of immune complexes.

Biopsy study during the acute phase demonstrates infiltration of alveolar walls with neutrophils and some eosinophils, numerous intraalveolar macrophages, foreign body giant cells, and neutrophils [22]. Later, the cellular infiltrate becomes more lymphocytic and includes plasma cells. Granulomas consisting of palisading epithelioid cells develop around areas of liquefaction necrosis. This initial reaction may vary in intensity depending on the dose of antigen [54]. Subsequent changes are influenced by the degree of sensitization, antigen dose, and frequency and number of exposures.

Diagnosis

The patient's occupation can offer important clues to the diagnosis of acute inhalation injury. In farmers, the differential diagnosis of acute dyspnea and cough includes silo-fillers' disease, hypersensitivity pneumonia, grain and barn dust asthma, and organic toxic dust syndrome [55]. Welders can be exposed to an array of toxic inhalants, including cyanide, oxides of nitrogen, phosgene and methylene chloride, and sulfur dioxide, produced by thermal decomposition of components of the local environment.

SIMPLE ASPHYXIANTS. Symptoms of hypoxemia accompany exposure to the simple asphyxiants and vary in severity depending on exposure intensity. These are primarily cardiovascular and CNS symptoms and include breathlessness, tachycardia, headache and diaphoresis, bounding pulse, loss of consciousness, and cardiac arrest.

Symptoms of cyanide exposure include headache, dizziness, tachypnea and tachycardia, nausea, chest and abdominal pain, confusion, and seizures. Victims give off a distinctive bitter almond odor, but its detection is unreliable and the correct diagnosis is better reached by the circumstances involved (e.g., suspected suicide in a dentist or laboratory worker in conjunction with the finding of severe metabolic acidosis). Crackles are present on auscultation in the case of severe exposure to H_2S, the result of pulmonary edema. Otherwise, abnormal physical findings may represent aspiration of gastric contents.

A careful history is important in CO intoxication because the clinical features are protean, dependent on concentration, duration of exposure, and underlying health of the victim [41,56]. A history of cardiopulmonary disease, anemia, extremes of age, and performance of heavy exertion further increase risk [27,57]. Because of the increased affinity of fetal hemoglobin for CO, infants and fetuses are at greater risk for CO poisoning [58]. Increasing severity of symptoms correlates with COHb level [56]. Subacute intoxication frequently results in flulike symptoms. Headache, fatigue, cloudy thinking, dizziness, paresthesias, palpitations, chest pains, nausea, diarrhea, and abdominal pain are initially attributed to other causes and when common to multiple individuals suggest an environmental source [6]. Confusing the recognition of CO intoxication is a more likely occurrence during colder weather and influenza season [29].

Acute CO intoxication causes rapid loss of consciousness without adequate warning. Neurologic and cardiovascular impairment predominate, reflecting the high requirement of these organ systems for oxygen [2,39]. Symptoms, signs, and prognosis of acute poisoning correlate poorly with COHb levels obtained on arrival at the hospital (Table 71-6) [41,59,60]. Carbonaceous sputum and facial and body burns suggest CO intoxication. Breathlessness is uncommon initially, and cyanosis, previously thought to be uncommon, is seen more frequently than cherry red skin color [2,39]. The presence of retinal hemorrhages may suggest the diagnosis [39]. Tachypnea and tachycardia then predominate, as the respiratory and cardiovascular systems try to compensate for decreased peripheral oxygen delivery. Evidence of coronary ischemia, including hypotension, arrhythmias, and electrocardiographic changes, may be present. Severe poisoning is associated with seizures, coma, and cardiac arrest.

A careful baseline neurologic examination is helpful in excluding other causes of altered mental status and serves as a prognostic tool. Extrapyramidal signs and persistent cognitive and behavioral abnormalities have been reported after recovery from CO poisoning [41,61].

Arterial blood gas analysis helps alert the clinician to the possibility of CO or HCN exposure. In both cases metabolic acidosis is present, while arterial oxygen tension is normal or near normal and saturation and content are reduced. Rapid formation of the cytochrome oxidase-cyanide complex results in paralysis of the electron transport system, halting cellular oxygen utilization. Venous PO_2 does not fall, resulting in the arteriolization of venous blood gases [62]. A toxicology screen helps rule out other causes for these presenting symptoms. Carboxyhemoglobin levels are readily available and are essential to the diagnosis of CO intoxication in suspected cases (Table

Table 71-6. Signs and Symptoms Seen with Various Carboxyhemoglobin Concentrations

Carboxyhemoglobin concentration (%)	Signs and symptoms
0.3–0.7	None
2.5–5.0	Decreased blood flow to vital organs; angina with less exertion
10–20	Headache, slight dyspnea, lethal to fetus and severe cardiac patients
20–30	Nausea, increased headache, throbbing temples, flushing, decreased manual dexterity
30–40	Severe headache, vertigo, nausea, vomiting, weakness, irritability, impaired judgment, syncope
40–50	Above but more severe; syncope and collapse likely
50–60	Coma, convulsions, Cheyne-Stokes respiration
60–70	Depressed respiration and cardiac function, death possible
70–80	Weak pulse, slow respiration, CNS depression, death

CNS = central nervous system.

71-6). Urban nonsmokers have baseline COHb levels of 5 to 6 percent, compared with 1 to 2 percent in rural nonsmokers. A one-pack-per-day cigarette smoker can have a COHb level of 6 percent [63], and secondary cigar and pipe smokers (ex-cigarette smokers) up to 38 percent [64] and 6 percent [65], respectively. Interpretation should include consideration of time elapsed since exposure. A COHb of less than 10 percent is not usually associated with symptoms; of less than 20 percent (mild exposure) is associated with headaches, tinnitus, dizziness, nausea, and slight behavioral abnormalities (Table 71-6); and of 20 to 40 percent (moderately severe exposure) can present with coma and convulsions. A level greater than 40 to 60 percent suggests severe exposure and increased risk of cardiac arrest. Continuous electrocardiographic monitoring is indicated.

TOXIC GASES. The need for a careful scene history from rescue personnel, co-workers, witnesses, and plant management cannot be overemphasized. This will help establish which agents are involved, relative concentrations, the site of exposure (closed space or outdoor), and duration. A description of symptoms and odors from those less affected is also useful, and exposures occurring as the result of industrial accidents frequently involve groups of victims.

Evidence of burn injury, skin lesions, and examination of eyes and mucous membranes helps predict intensity of exposure and the likelihood of laryngeal obstruction. Auscultation of the chest reveals crackles, rhonchi, and wheezing, depending on the time elapsed since injury. Arterial blood gas analysis should be obtained early and repeated as necessary to adjust oxygen therapy. A COHb level will assess simultaneous CO poisoning. Toxicology screening may help determine why an accident occurred. A chest radiograph is indicated; the typical bat-wing distribution of cardiogenic pulmonary edema is less likely than diffuse or patchy infiltrates of noncardiogenic pulmonary edema. Other findings include atelectasis, hyperinflation, and aspiration pneumonia.

Arsine exposure is suggested in appropriate industrial settings [51]. Arsine has a garlic odor, and exposures as low as 10 ppm have resulted in delirium, coma, and death. The hemolytic picture develops rapidly, and the hematocrit may drop by 50 percent in minutes. Pulmonary edema has also been reported [15]. Circulating free hemoglobin may result in the development of acute renal failure due to direct toxic effects on the renal tubular cells and sludging. The patient's urine is dark. Free serum hemoglobin should be measured. Ischemia-related problems may also develop as hematocrit continues to drop. Urine arsenic levels may be helpful in later management if available but usually do not have an impact on initial care [51].

Silo-Fillers' Disease. Premature entry into, or improper preparation before entering, the silo are prominent historical features. Alternatively, collapse, sudden death, or a fall from a silo suggest the diagnosis. With milder exposures, symptoms may be delayed in onset. Clinical findings include fever and development of rales and wheezes. The victim may appear to be in pulmonary edema. Moderate to severe hypoxemia is present. Leukocytosis also is common. The chest radiograph can be normal or reveal diffuse fluffy nodular infiltrates.

ASTHMA SYNDROMES. Because most exposed persons develop symptoms within months of onset of exposure, duration of employment is important and exposure to spills or changes in the manufacturing process should be noted. The pattern of symptom development is helpful in diagnosis [35]. Symptoms improve dramatically over weekends and vacations, with maximal symptoms occurring the first day of the week. Other patterns include a progressive increase in symptoms through the week or a similar deterioration each work day. Once the environmental exposure is recognized, it is necessary to establish whether there is a specific or nonspecific irritant effect. A search for other known triggers for asthma also should be undertaken. Other predisposing factors, such as smoking history and medications used, should be sought, since beta-blocker or aspirin use can precipitate bronchospasm in some individuals. Absence of wheezing on examination does not exclude OA. Arterial blood gases and measurement of peak expiratory flow is indicated only as needed in the management of severe asthma or status asthmaticus. The total eosinophil count is elevated in some types of OA.

The principles for evaluation of pulmonary function in acute asthma (see Chap. 56) can be applied to OA. A positive inhalation challenge test with methacholine is consistent with asthma but does not confirm an environmental etiology; moreover, a number of conditions besides asthma can lead to a positive test [66]. A negative challenge may result early on or if the patient has left the workplace months earlier [66]. When a return to the workplace is associated with conversion to a positive methacholine challenge, the result carries considerably more weight and documents that sensitization has occurred. The methacholine challenge test result helps determine how sensitive the patient will be to specific bronchoprovocation testing with the suspected offending agent [16]. The course of the methacholine challenge test result over time can be of use in following the response of OA to removal from the exposure. Several other nonprovocative methods can be used to follow the development of airflow obstruction in relation to the workplace. The patient can carry a portable peak flow meter and make several determinations of peak flow during the day at work, in the evening and early morning, and over weekends and holidays. Alternatively, if malingering is suspected, spirometry can be measured by a qualified technician using a portable apparatus several times each day.

Specific bronchoprovocation challenge testing may be indicated to study a previously unrecognized agent, to determine the causative agent in a complex environment, and occasionally for medicolegal purposes [16,33]. Because there are various patterns of reaction (e.g., immediate, late, dual, and recurrent nocturnal), prolonged monitoring of spirometry is required after challenge is administered, and a control is necessary to determine whether the response is merely nonspecific. The early or immediate response begins within minutes, peaks by 10 to 20 minutes, and resolves by 1 hour. The late response occurs 1 or more hours after exposure, peaks at several hours, and may last 24 to 48 hours. A dual response occurs with both early and late components, and often a single agent, such as plicatic acid, can demonstrate any one of the three in different patients. A prolonged late response, lasting weeks with a nightly decline in flow rates, has occurred following challenge with toluene diisocyanate [67].

Allergy skin prick testing is useful for determining sensitization to suspected antigens and can help determine the dose of allergen for specific bronchoprovocation challenge testing. Although high-molecular-weight agents can be used directly, low-molecular-weight agents may require a carrier protein. Furthermore, many low-molecular-weight chemicals have a direct irritant effect and give confusing results. Specific IgE antibodies can be measured by radioallergosorbent test (RAST) and RAST inhibition or by enzyme-linked immunoabsorbent testing (ELISA) and have been demonstrated to both high-molecular-weight and low-molecular-weight protein conjugates. It should be emphasized that these tests show only sensitization, which can also occur in patients without asthma.

HYPERSENSITIVITY PNEUMONITIS. Clinical presentation of HP varies depending on intensity, duration, and recurrence of exposure [22]. Brief intermittent exposure results in fever, chills, malaise, cough, and dyspnea within 4 to 10 hours after exposure, with severity of symptoms dependent on intensity of exposure. Fever may reach 40°C. On examination, patients appear acutely ill, and chest auscultation demonstrates end-inspiratory crackles. Occasionally, an immediate, late, or dual bronchoconstriction response can be seen in atopic persons. Pulmonary function testing demonstrates restriction with decreased lung compliance. Hypoxemia results from alteration in ventilation-perfusion relationships. With more continuous low-grade exposure, subacute or chronic forms of HP develop. In long-term continuous or intermittent exposure, clinical features of pulmonary fibrosis predominate. Progressive abnormalities of restriction in association with obstruction and abnormal gas exchange lead to unrelenting respiratory failure and cor pulmonale even after exposure is discontinued.

A neutrophilic leukocytosis of up to 25,000 per cubic millimeter with left shift is common; however, eosinophilia is rare [22]. Erythrocyte sedimentation rate is elevated. Arterial blood gas analysis demonstrates mild to moderate hypoxemia and hypocapnia. Serum immunoglobulins are elevated, and IgG precipitins can be demonstrated against the involved antigen; IgE is not elevated. Rheumatoid factor is often nonspecifically elevated. Skin testing with antigen is useful in some cases. Bronchoalveolar lavage in patients with HP showed a lymphocytic alveolitis, with T cells predominating.

The chest radiograph in acute or subacute forms of HP can be normal, show a diffuse nodular or reticulonodular pattern sparing the costophrenic angles and apices, or reveal diffuse patchy infiltrates without associated adenopathy. When the patient is severely affected, the chest radiograph can suggest non-cardiogenic pulmonary edema. In chronic HP, findings are pulmonary fibrosis with reduced lung volumes, coarse linear or reticular interstitial infiltrates, and honeycombing.

In addition to following spirometry after challenge, it is useful to measure diffusing capacity and white blood cell count over time, since these characteristically change in HP, whereas alteration in flow rates may not be demonstrated.

Differential Diagnosis

ASPHYXIANTS. The alternative diagnostic considerations for victims of asphyxiation are entertained only after rapid institution of emergency treatment, including cardiopulmonary resuscitation. Catastrophic conditions of cardiac and respiratory arrest, drug overdose, intracranial hemorrhage, and acute alteration in mental status and coma all should be considered, although the majority can occur with or be sequelae of the exposures being discussed.

TOXIC GASES. The presentation of these disorders as a group is very distinctive and usually occurs in the setting of an industrial or transport-related accident. Patients present in acute respiratory distress with evidence of intense conjunctival and mucous membrane edema, erythema and ulceration, and laryngeal edema causing upper respiratory tract obstruction. The stridor may be associated with the clinical and radiographic picture of

pulmonary edema, with bronchopneumonia occurring later. Anaphylaxis and angioneurotic edema with bronchospasm can have similar presentations, but severe mucous membrane inflammation and ulceration are not prominent features of these disorders.

Because AsH_3 poisoning causes such a dramatic presentation with hemolysis, the differential diagnosis is much broader, including serious infections such as *Clostridia bacteremia* as well as disorders such as thrombotic thrombocytopenic purpura [51]. The other metal hydrides cause abrupt pulmonary edema and altered mental status and require knowledge of workplace exposure (e.g., semiconductor plant) [15].

Silo-Fillers' Disease. The farm environment contains a number of potential exposures capable of provoking acute respiratory distress [55]. Even when dealing with silo exposure-provoked respiratory symptoms, it may be impossible to distinguish between NO_2-induced silo-fillers' disease and organic dust-related disease such as hypersensitivity pneumonia (Farmer's lung) from *Thermophilic actinomyces* species and dust-related asthma. Possible exposures to pesticides and other toxins further complicate the clinical picture.

ASTHMA SYNDROMES. Symptoms and signs of asthma syndromes are consistent with a viral upper respiratory infection, asthma, rhinitis, or bronchitis. Clinically, HP may be suggested in the patient who has onset of dyspnea in a characteristic exposure setting, but in HP the pulmonary response is predominantly restrictive and the immunologic findings those of IgG precipitins and a cell-mediated immune response.

HYPERSENSITIVITY PNEUMONITIS. The presentation of acute HP, with its constitutional and pulmonary symptoms, suggests infectious pneumonia. The lack of a response to antibiotics and recurrent nature are helpful in distinguishing these two disorders. In some instances HP presents with wheezing and may be confused with asthma, and some antigens cause either of these disorders (isocyanates and trimellitic anhydride). Chest radiographic and restrictive pulmonary function changes usually clarify the diagnosis. Allergic bronchopulmonary aspergillosis is a form of hypersensitivity disease in which *Aspergillus* colonizes the airways and precipitins to the fungus are present in the blood. The presentation, with difficult-to-control asthma, peripheral eosinophilia, and specific radiographic findings, distinguishes it from HP. When chronic changes have developed as the result of recurrent exposure to antigen, HP must be distinguished from other chronic interstitial lung diseases. These include sarcoidosis and idiopathic pulmonary fibrosis. Differentiation requires demonstration of exposure to an agent known to cause HP, precipitating antibodies, positive inhalation challenge to the agent, or lung biopsy demonstrating pathognomonic changes. Peripheral, hilar, and mediastinal lymphadenopathy do not occur in HP.

Treatment

ASPHYXIANTS. The principles of management for any asphyxiation include increasing inspired oxygen concentration to 100 percent, providing for cardiopulmonary resuscitation and respiratory and circulatory systems support, and treating complicating conditions, such as burns and alcohol and drug intoxication. A bag-valve-mask device should be used for initial ventilation in patients with cyanide poisoning, since there may be risk of secondary cyanide poisoning when mouth-to-mouth or mouth-to-nose resuscitation is used [68]. Severe metabolic acidosis may require therapy with sodium bicarbonate. Implementation of these simple measures can become complicated when the number of victims is large.

For many years, therapy for cyanide poisoning has been based on the use of other agents that compete with cytochrome oxidase for cyanide. Intravenous or inhaled nitrites (amyl nitrite) form complexes with hemoglobin, resulting in production of methemoglobin which is subsequently converted to thiosulfate by thiosulfate transulfurase. Amyl nitrite pearls, included in the cyanide antidote kit, are broken onto gauze and held over the bag-valve-mask intake valve or endotracheal tube for 30 seconds of each minute. Sodium nitrite can be administered intravenously at a dose of 10 ml of 3 percent solution over 2 to 4 minutes. Nitrite therapy can be complicated by hypotension, which usually responds to fluids and vasopressors [68]. Methemoglobin and cyanide combine to form cyanomethemoglobin, which then reacts with thiosulfate and is converted to nontoxic thiocyanate by transulfurase. Sodium thiosulfate can also be administered directly as 50 ml of a 25 percent solution intravenously. Although methemoglobin alters the oxygen-carrying capacity of the blood and contributes to tissue hypoxemia, the risk of untreated cyanide poisoning is far greater.

Newer therapies focus on the ability of cobalt to combine with cyanide. Hydroxycobalamin (vitamin B_{12}) is given intravenously using an empiric dose of 4 gm, but since the drug comes in 1 mg per millimeter concentration a large volume is required to administer it [69]. Dicobalt edentate, a chelated cobalt, is newer, more effective, and less toxic. It is given intravenously as a 600 mg slowly pushed dose and a repeat dose of 300 mg if there is no improvement [68]. Care at the scene is important for survival. Inhaled amyl nitrate and dicobalt edentate can be given immediately while oxygen is administered and cardiopulmonary resuscitation instituted. Gastric decontamination with activated charcoal and/or 5 percent sodium thiosulfate solution lavage (leave 200 ml in stomach) may be useful for oral ingestion [68].

Treatment for H_2S poisoning includes oxygen, supportive measures, and nitrites but not thiosulfate. Although nitrite therapy causes sulfmethemoglobin formation and increases excretion of oxidized sulfur, it delays excretion of sulfide, which is also toxic.

In carbon monoxide poisoning, the victim should be removed from further exposure and at the same time therapy with 100 percent oxygen should be administered by tight-fitting mask or endotracheal tube if the patient is obtunded. Oxygen is the major therapy for CO poisoning, because it can be rapidly instituted and because it decreases the half-life of COHb to 40 to 60 minutes or less (from 240 minutes breathing room air) by competing with CO for binding sites on hemoglobin [70]. The rate of elimination is related to FIO_2 (and PaO_2) and alveolar ventilation. Metabolic acidosis should not be treated unless severe (<7.2), since the acidosis facilitates oxygen delivery by shifting the oxygen dissociation curve to the right. Prolonged oxygen therapy is required in cases of fetal CO poisoning and in cases caused by methylene chloride exposure. In the latter, levels may rise after exposure has ceased [30]. Serial measurements of COHb and ABG are required.

Hyperbaric oxygen (HBO) therapy has been demonstrated in retrospective reviews of CO poisoning to reduce morbidity in general and the development of neurologic sequelae in particular [59,71]. Oxygen at 2.5 atm reduces the half-life of COHb to 22 minutes and furthermore increases dissolved oxygen in the blood to a level that will supply the body's needs without hemoglobin [70,72]. The limited availability of HBO therapy

limits its applicability, and many patients are treated adequately with significant improvement in COHb level to nonlethal levels within 1 hour using 100 percent oxygen alone [73].

It has been suggested that comatose patients with high COHb levels should be treated at the initial hospital until COHb falls to 5 percent; if coma or neurologic symptoms persist, they should be transferred to an HBO facility while continuing to receive 100 percent oxygen [2]. Other guidelines have been proposed [56]. Mild poisoning (COHb <20%) should be treated with 100 percent oxygen by nonrebreather mask until levels fall to 5 percent. Moderate poisoning (COHb 20–40%) without cardiac or neurologic dysfunction requires monitoring of acid-base status and 100 percent oxygen therapy until COHb is less than 5 percent and symptoms have resolved. Finally, patients with severe poisoning (COHb >40%) or with cardiac or neurologic symptoms should undergo HBO therapy if available; otherwise, 100 percent oxygen should be used. If improvement is not evident within 4 hours, patients should be transferred to an HBO facility for therapy. Admission is required for those with a COHb greater than 25 percent and those with a lower level when signs of cardiac ischemia or neurologic impairment are present [56].

Clinically significant asphyxiation and poisoning with CO and HCN require admission to the intensive care unit for continuation of treatment. Following the acute event, long-term neurologic follow-up and neuropsychologic testing are indicated in survivors of acute CO intoxication.

TOXIC GASES. Exposures are minimized by worker education and by establishing and following certain safety guidelines. For instance, use of protective clothing and self-contained pressure demand or open-circuit respirators in any situation that would require a worker to enter a storage tank with an atmosphere immediately dangerous to life and health to inspect or clean should be mandated. Disaster preparedness programs and drills can reduce the risk to workers in the event of an accident. Positive-pressure respirators and oxygen should be accessible at numerous sites in the workplace, and workers should be fully educated about their use in an emergency. Basic life support training should be part of these safety programs, since it is most effective to institute these measures at the scene. Emergency planning for communities located near industrial installations and transfer facilities, using computer modeling based on the gas or chemical released and varying environmental conditions, can be helpful [74].

The mainstay of management for any gas exposure is removal of the victim from the site of exposure by rescue workers using respirators and protective clothing and immediate administration of oxygen. Airway patency should be assured, because laryngeal edema may lead to complete airway obstruction over several hours. Evidence of upper airway obstruction secondary to edema or the need to control the airway in the unconscious patient are indications for endotracheal intubation, emergency cricothyroidotomy, or tracheostomy. A large endotracheal tube (>8.0 mm internal diameter) is helpful for pulmonary toilet and for anticipated bronchoscopy to remove mucous plugs. Even when there is a delay in the development of respiratory distress, these measures may be required later.

Exposure to Cl_2 and $COCl_2$ is followed by an initial period of well-being or minor distress. This is followed several hours later by acute respiratory failure with clinical and radiographic evidence of pulmonary edema. These patients therefore require prolonged monitoring in the emergency room with a low threshold for admission. Treatment is otherwise largely supportive. Pulmonary edema is treated with oxygen and mechanical ventilation, and positive end-expiratory pressure (PEEP) therapy may be required. Bronchospasm is treated with inhaled and intravenous bronchodilators. Intravenous fluids are necessary because of fluid losses secondary to mucosal edema and sloughing and associated burn injury. Empiric antibiotics are not indicated and have the disadvantage of selecting out resistant pathogens, but their use when convincing evidence for pneumonia exists is not controversial. There has been no systematic study of the use of corticosteroids in Cl_2- or $COCl_2$-related inhalation injury; their use remains controversial and anecdotal and may be associated with a significant increase in early mortality [75,76]. Early use should be limited to the treatment of bronchospasm refractory to conventional bronchodilators and to upper airway obstruction causing postextubation stridor. Conversely, late complications, such as refractory bronchospasm due to asthma or RADS or bronchiolitis obliterans, are an indication for their use. Complete pulmonary function testing should be obtained when the patient is able, since such testing will form the basis for determining the degree of recovery.

With acute, obvious massive exposure, victims will require admission to a respiratory intensive care unit, where they can be treated and closely monitored for increasing respiratory distress and mechanical ventilation can be instituted as needed. After discharge, long-term follow-up care with a pulmonary medicine specialist will be necessary for monitoring of pulmonary function and treatment of sequelae (e.g., bronchiolitis obliterans, asthma).

Treatment of AsH_3 poisoning requires general supportive measures, including exchange transfusion in some cases. Chelation therapy may also be indicated [51].

Silo-Fillers' Disease. Supportive measures for maintaining ventilation and circulation should be instituted and are similar to those outlined for other toxic gas inhalations. The lack of a systematic study has not precluded most authors from recommending high-dose intravenous or oral corticosteroid therapy (oral prednisone 60 mg per day) [11,34]. This therapy is continued for up to 4 weeks after admission to minimize the risk of progressive respiratory impairment and development of late bronchiolitis obliterans [34], which occurs 1 to 6 weeks after exposure.

Most farmers are aware of the dangers of silo gas and avoid unnecessary exposure. The following guidelines are employed [55]:

1. Avoid entering silo for 2 weeks after it is filled
2. Ventilate thoroughly before entering
3. Avoid ascending the silo chute for the first 2 days
4. Avoid descending into low places in the silage
5. Check for gas before entering the silo
6. Learn to recognize gas
7. Never enter alone or without a lifeline or safety equipment during the danger period
8. See a physician if any symptoms develop.

ASTHMA SYNDROMES. Treatment of acute asthma of any cause entails use of beta-sympathomimetics, theophylline, and corticosteroids (see Chap. 56). Once asthma is attributed to a specific environment, every effort should be made to remove the affected person, a complicated process that may involve the physician, worker, union, management, and federal and state agencies. Economic exigencies may make it impossible for the worker to leave a job, increasing the risk of chronic asthma. Improved workplace ventilation, methods of production, and use of a dust mask or respirator may be of some help, but often these measures are inadequate since the worker with OA is sensitized and reacts to a very low level of antigen. Use of disodium cromoglycate and inhaled steroids offers some control of symptoms, but there is no evidence that they protect against the development of chronic asthma and fixed obstruction. Long-term follow-up is also required, because patients with OA demonstrate persistence of asthma and nonspecific bronchial hyperreactivity long after exposure is discontinued.

HYPERSENSITIVITY PNEUMONITIS. Acute management of HP should include supplemental oxygen when hypoxemia is evident. Limited courses of corticosteroids may help speed resolution in acute and subacute forms, but in the chronic stage significant amounts of fibrosis may prevent a recognizable response. Symptomatic recurrences are a more important determinant of progressive disease than continued work in the same occupation [77]. However, only leaving the exposure permanently can help prevent development of disabling pulmonary fibrosis. Less often, methods that improve air quality and remove the antigen from the environment are successful.

Affected patients may require brief hospitalization unless symptoms and hypoxemia are mild. Unless the exposure situation is clearly recognized as a potential cause of HP, corticosteroids should be held pending confirmation of the diagnosis by a pulmonologist or allergist working in conjunction with occupation medicine and environmental engineers.

Smoke Inhalation

OVERVIEW. The victim of smoke inhalation poses a number of unique diagnostic and management problems for intensive care physicians. These are a result of the complex toxic nature of the fire environment and the frequent association with significant surface burns, trauma, and delayed sequelae of infection and multiorgan system failure.

More than one-half of the 130,000 patients hospitalized each year for burns require intensive care, and more than 10,000 die despite the efforts of specialized burn units [73,78]. With improved management of burn wounds, trauma, shock, wound sepsis, and acute renal failure, inhalation injury remains the major impediment to further improvements in burn mortality [79].

Approximately 80 percent of fire-associated deaths are attributed to inhalation injury [80], and smoke inhalation is the most common cause of death in fire victims without surface burns [81]. Inhalation injury exerts a greater influence than burn size or age in determining burn mortality, and there is a synergistic lethal effect when surface burns are present, with a mortality exceeding 50 percent [81].

Although respiratory failure can develop as a complication of large burns or multiorgan system failure, inhalation injury still accounts for two-thirds of those victims requiring mechanical ventilation [82]. The need for prolonged intensive care and hospital stay significantly increases cost.

In 1985, there were 2.4 million fires in the United States, of which 72.4 percent were residential, resulting in 4885 deaths [83]. More than 60 percent of these deaths were victims younger than 9 or greater than 60 years of age, suggesting that impaired mobility from physical obstacles, decreased vision and mobility, inexperience, handicaps, and poor judgment all add to fire-related fatalities, in addition to problems caused by inhalation injury [80].

Smoke consists of a mixture of gases, vapors, fumes, liquid droplets, and carbonaceous particles generated by combustion (oxygen present) or pyrolysis (oxygen absent) during increased temperature. Black smoke results from particles of carbon or soot generated during combustion or pyrolysis of carbon-containing materials. These can adsorb aldehydes and organic acids to their surface [84]. White smoke is released during thermal decomposition of plastic polymers [31]. Toxic gases may be invisible and are more likely to be released during pyrolysis than combustion (Table 71-7) [85].

The causes of injury and death from fires are multiple, including heat resulting in direct consumption or oxygen deficiency, the generation and release of toxic products of incomplete combustion (TPCs), trauma, and fear and panic [86]. It should be clear that smoke and TPCs are responsible for the majority of deaths.

ETIOLOGY. Although cigarettes are the major cause of house fire deaths, carelessness with matches, wood stoves, and heaters as well as appliance and heating system malfunctions also contribute significantly [87]. The TPCs liberated in a given setting are determined by type of fuel, temperature, rate of heating, whether combustion or pyrolysis is occurring, and distance from the source [79,88]. Skyscrapers and basements are generally poorly ventilated. Hypoxemia contributes to ischemic injury and further worsens exposure to TPCs because of hyperventilation due to increased respiratory drive [79].

Combustible materials in the home include wood, paper, plastics, polyurethane, paints, and other polymers present in carpeting and upholstery, and an ever-increasing list of new synthetics that result in a wider variety of TPC. More than 50 chemicals, many unidentified, have been found in tissue analysis performed on fire victims [79]. During 200 residential fires, firefighters were exposed to high concentrations of CO and acrolein; HCL, HCN, NO_2, and CO_2 were also present, albeit at low levels [89]. Nonetheless, synergistic toxicity of a variety of TPCs at low concentration is a problem. During combustion or pyrolysis involving plastic polymers, intense heat is generated in addition to toxic gases and fumes [90]. Particulates and HCl are higher during the initial phase of a fire, whereas CO_2 and CO are elevated during the knockdown, or suppression phase [91].

PATHOPHYSIOLOGY. Respiratory injuries in fire victims with smoke inhalation can be the result of heat, asphyxia, and exposure to TPCs (Table 71-8). Most deaths are the result of asphyxia [92]. Consumption of oxygen by fire can result in a significant decrement in FIO_2 to as low as 0.05 during a flashover [88]. Carbon monoxide and HCN are the two major as-

Table 71-7. Common Toxic Exposures During Fires

Substance	Toxic by-products of incomplete combustion
Polyvinyl chloride	Hydrogen chloride, phosgene, chlorine
Wood, cotton, paper	Acrolein, acetaldehyde, formaldehyde, acetic acid, formic acid
Petroleum products	Acrolein, acetic acid, formic acid
Nitrocellulose film	Oxides of nitrogen, acetic acid, formic acid
Polyurethane	Isocyanate, hydrogen cyanide
Melamine resins	Ammonia, hydrogen cyanide
Polytef (Teflon)	Octafluoroisobutylene

Source: Adapted from Fein A, Leff A, Hopewell PC: Pathophysiology and management of the complications resulting from fire and the inhaled products of combustion: Review of the literature. *Crit Care Med* 8:94, 1980.

Table 71-8. Causes of Respiratory Distress in Fire Victims

Asphyxia
 Respiratory
 Cellular
Upper airway obstruction
Tracheobronchitis
Pulmonary edema
 Cardiogenic
 Noncardiogenic
Acute bronchiolitis
Nosocomial pneumonia

phyxiants (see Chap. 157). These two asphyxiants frequently occur together. Clark et al. [93] found that 27 percent of individuals with serious smoke inhalation and elevated COHb had elevated blood cyanide levels, occasionally to near lethal levels. Carbon monoxide is responsible for 80 percent of smoke inhalation-related fatalities, and nearly one-fourth of these occur in victims with underlying cardiac or pulmonary disease [2]. The combination of heat, CO, and oxygen deficiency in fires probably acts synergistically to increase lethality. Exposure to 200°C, 0.5 to 1.0 percent CO, or 6 percent oxygen results in death within 5 minutes, whereas exposure to 125°C, 0.3 percent CO, or 17 percent oxygen leads to physiologic impairment in 15 minutes [94]. Many of the considerations discussed in Toxic Gases apply here; however, the additional toxins require special discussion.

Proliferating use of synthetic polymers has made the fire environment much more deadly. Firefighters are unable to predict the intensity of exposure based on subjective criteria [95]. Demutation of 1 kg of polyvinyl chloride releases 0.4 kg of HCl gas, along with significant CO generation [78]. Effects of these agents have been discussed. Acrolein is an aldehyde released in fires involving polyethylene, polypropylene, and vinyl materials but is also released during combustion of wood and other organic fuels. At low concentrations (5.5 ppm) acrolein is intensely irritating to the upper respiratory tract; at high concentrations (10 ppm) pulmonary edema and death may ensue [78]. Isocyanates are included among the other toxic products generated (see sections on airways disease). A respiratory rate in the normal range confers some immunity against inhalation injury, because deposition of particles in the respiratory tract is minimal [91]. High and low respiratory rates increase the rate of particle deposition by prolonging contact time with gas containing TPCs. Soot and liquid droplets present in the smoke environment adsorb TPCs and may greatly increase exposure to irritants. Size, water solubility, degree of contamination of particulates, duration of exposure, and minute ventilation all determine site and extent of injury [91]. Particles less than 0.06 μ may completely bypass the upper airway and deposit in the lung parenchyma. Those 2 μ and greater in diameter deposit throughout the respiratory tract, whereas larger particles (>5 μ) deposit predominately in the upper airway. Therefore, large particles (soot in the nasopharynx) are not necessarily associated with damage to the lower respiratory tract [96]. A sufficiently high concentration of soot, however, may cause direct asphyxiation by obstruction of the upper airway.

Although hot particulates, hot gases, and steam can result in injury to the lower respiratory tract [78], direct heat injury is usually limited to the upper respiratory tract, since intense heat can result in reflex apnea [97]. Upper airway obstruction occurs in up to 30 percent of burn patients, and the incidence may be higher when flow volume loops are analyzed [98]. This is the result of heat-soluble and water-soluble TPCs, which cause edema early on (4 hours) [99]. Edema formation is related to release of oxygen-free radicals and thromboxanes [82]. Later, constricting eschars of the neck produce compression; this effect is more common in children [100]. Respiratory tract damage is more severe in burned than nonburned patients with similar smoke inhalation. Tracheobronchitis is due to chemical injury in the majority of cases, with heat injury occurring only after steam exposure [78]. In the tracheobronchial tree and the parenchyma of the lung, injury is mediated by polymorphonuclear leukocytes that migrate to the affected areas and release oxygen-free radicals and chemotactic factors. Frank pulmonary edema is a rare sequela of smoke inhalation, occurring in up to 8.8 percent, but has a high mortality (83%) [101]. Other associations with mortality include large burn surface, renal failure, extremes of age, and overhydration [102].

Pulmonary complications of inhalation injury thus can be subdivided based on time of occurrence as early (CO poisoning, upper airway obstruction, tracheobronchial obstruction), delayed for 2 to 5 days (upper airway obstruction, pulmonary edema, and pneumonia), and late (pulmonary edema, pneumonia, and pulmonary embolism).

With improvements in the management of surface burn wound infections, pneumonia has become the principal fatal complication of inhalation injury. Early pneumonias are more often aerogenous and result from aspiration, immobility, and as a complication of therapy [78]. Penicillin-resistant *Staphylococcus* is a common pathogen, followed later by gram-negative rods [103]. Hematogenous pneumonias tend to occur later as the result of seeding from wound infections, suppurative thrombophlebitis, and other infections [78]. Gram-negative rods are the most common pathogens, but fungal and viral pneumonias also occur.

DIAGNOSIS. Whether or not surface burns are present, it is essential to consider smoke inhalation in any victim retrieved from an accident scene, particularly when there is alteration of mental status. Signs suggesting recent drug or alcohol use may be absent, and therefore a toxicology screen and COHb level should be obtained. The most important differential diagnosis is associated trauma, which requires early recognition to avoid precipitous worsening. All of these patients should be approached as a trauma code.

Classic predictors of smoke inhalation injury include (1) consistent exposure (closed environment, entrapment, loss of consciousness, knowledge of fuels present, as in jetliner or industrial accident); (2) respiratory signs and symptoms (dyspnea, hoarseness, wheezing, stridor, cyanosis); (3) cervical, facial, and oropharyngeal burns, especially between the nose and mouth; and (4) expectoration of carbonaceous sputum [104,105]. Initial evaluation should focus on recognition and treatment of CO poisoning and airway obstruction, the major early problems. However, there may be a delay in symptoms for hours to days [106].

Although facial burns are often identified in inhalation injury, 23 percent of victims without facial burn have respiratory damage [104]. Carbonaceous sputum is present in more than one-third of patients with inhalation injury and persists for up to 2 weeks [104,105]. Hemoptysis and expectoration of bronchial casts may be seen with more severe injury [107]. Cyanosis is an inconsistent finding masked by soot, burns, hemorrhage, or, rarely, the cherry red color of carboxyhemoglobinemia [104]. Lung findings are inconsistent and crackles, wheezes, and rhonchi may not be apparent until 24 hours later. Sputum cytology has not been of demonstrated benefit [108].

Arterial blood gas analysis is essential in management of smoke inhalation victims. Hypoxemia and an increased alveo-lar-arterial oxygen gradient may be present even in the absence of demonstrable radiographic abnormalities, especially with increasing burn surface. When it fails to respond as predicted to supplemental oxygen, right-to-left shunt is probably present, indicating the acute respiratory distress syndrome (ARDS) [109,110]. Delayed development of hypoxemia 48 hours later has also been documented [111]. Measurement of arterial blood oxygen tensions can be misleading in the setting of CO poisoning because arterial oxygen tension can be normal when COHb is elevated. Arteriolization of venous blood has been observed with cyanide poisoning [62]. Cooximetry for COHb level is essential in management of the smoke inhalation victim, because the diagnosis of CO intoxication is impossible without this measurement. High COHb levels suggest the need for immediate measurement and institution of empiric therapy for cyanide poisoning [93] (see Treatment of Asphyxiants). An unexplained metabolic acidosis in the presence of normal or mildly elevated COHb levels and normal PaO_2 also suggests cyanide exposure [112]. A plasma lactate concentration greater than 10 mM per liter is an indicator of cyanide poisoning in victims of smoke inhalation [113]. A chest radiograph should be obtained routinely during initial evaluation of smoke inhalation, but a normal film has little predictive value for subsequent inhalation injury and therefore serial studies are needed [114]. Ventilation-perfusion radionuclide scans of the lung may show segmental retention and delayed clearance of xenon in up to 30 percent of victims with inhalation injury [115,116]. Two-thirds of these will later demonstrate radiographic abnormalities [117]. Increased minute ventilation in the postinhalation injury period may prohibit valid test results.

Early laryngoscopic survey of the upper airway is indicated to confirm the diagnosis of inhalation injury, and the results may also aid management [104]. Bronchoscopic examination of the subglottic airway is not essential in all patients, particularly when laryngoscopic examination is normal, but is easily accomplished with little morbidity in those intubated for upper airway obstruction or other respiratory compromise [104,118]. Findings of inhalational injury in the upper airway include pharyngeal and laryngeal soot, severe edema with obliteration of normal landmarks, erythema, and mucosal blistering [119]. Changes in the lower airway include mucosal edema, erythema, blistering, hemorrhage, ulceration, and necrosis with severe narrowing of the trachea and bronchi and subsequent development of crusts, casts, and mucous plugs of the airway [119]. Although the presence of bronchoscopic abnormalities has been associated with a higher mortality [120], others have noted a lack of correlation with presence of parenchymal injury and prognosis [121].

Physiologic testing with spirometry and flow volume loops, despite limitations, offers an accurate assessment of the risk of pulmonary problems following inhalation injury and can help exclude patients unlikely to develop problems [98,114,117]. The vital capacity may fall by 12 hours after inhalation injury, with the greatest deterioration occurring in patients with associated significant surface burn [117]. The flow volume loop demonstrates a sawtoothing pattern to the inspiratory curve and the expiratory-inspiratory ratio is increased (FEF 50%/FIF 50% > 1) in the presence of significant upper airway edema and injury. Restrictive abnormalities may become apparent when significant intrapulmonary trauma or chest wall burn (eschar) occurs or complications of atelectasis, pneumonia, and cardiogenic and noncardiogenic pulmonary edema develop. Airways obstruction after smoke inhalation may be more common and persist longer than is generally recognized (122).

TREATMENT. Management of smoke inhalation requires application of the principles of respiratory and cardiac support outlined in Chapters 1, 66, 171, and 179 as well as trauma resuscitation and burn wound care. There are a paucity of controlled prospective data in this population. Control of the airway is the initial priority. Endotracheal intubation is indicated for stridor, for facial burns and smoke inhalation with CNS depression, for mucous membrane burns, for full-thickness burns of the nose and lips, for full-thickness burns of the neck, and when signs and symptoms suggest impending obstruction (e.g., drooling, hoarseness) [104]. The procedure should be performed by the most experienced person (see Chap. 1). Nasotracheal intubation may be preferred over orotracheal intubation in the presence of mouth burns, since the latter may predispose to contracture of the mouth. An endotracheal tube 8 mm or greater in internal diameter is preferable, since frequent therapeutic bronchoscopies may be necessary in the presence of inspissated secretions, plugs, and casts that obstruct the airway repetitively. Prolonged intubation of 3 weeks is preferable to tracheostomy, which has been associated with major complications and increased mortality [123,124,125]. Use of supplemental oxygen should follow general guidelines. Humidification of the upper respiratory tract decreases hoarseness, dryness, and discomfort [126]. Chest physiotherapy is of limited value, especially when surface burns are present. Inhaled and parenteral bronchodilators may be useful for management of bronchospasm following smoke inhalation, although proof of this benefit is currently lacking. The inflammatory nature of acute inhalation injury suggests a role for drugs that modify the inflammatory response. Corticosteroids have been associated with increased mortality due to infection, and their use has not been recommended in patients with acute inhalation injury [79,104]. The obvious hazards associated with corticosteroid use in patients with large surface burns may obscure their value in those with small surface burns and smoke inhalation. Some authors have advocated that corticosteroids be reserved for severe bronchospasm resistant to conventional bronchodilator therapy, for severe upper airway obstruction, and for failed extubation due to stridor [127]. Corticosteroids have been of demonstrated benefit in the treatment of bronchiolitis obliterans due to irritant gas injury (oxides of nitrogen), and their use to prevent the same lesion in patients with acute inhalation injury has been suggested [127].

The role of HBO in the management of smoke inhalation has not been studied, and its role in CO intoxication has already been discussed. Anecdotal reports have claimed that use of HBO may limit mucosal edema even in the absence of an elevated COHb [128]. Mechanical ventilation and use of continuous positive airway pressure and PEEP should follow the guidelines outlined in Chapter 66.

The delayed chronic sequelae of smoke inhalation include asthma, bronchiolitis obliterans, chronic obstructive pulmonary disease, and pulmonary fibrosis. However, the role of antiinflammatory drugs when early lung function testing detects increased airway reactivity has not been assessed prospectively [117].

References

1. Seaton A, Morgan WKC: Toxic gases and fumes, in Morgan WKC, Seaton A (eds): *Occupational Lung Diseases*. 2nd ed. Philadelphia, WB Saunders, 1984, p 609.
2. Dolan MC: Carbon monoxide poisoning. *Can Med Assoc J* 133:392, 1985.
3. Cobb N, Etzel RA: Unintentional carbon monoxide-related deaths in the United States, 1979 through 1988. *JAMA* 266:659, 1991.
4. Levine MS, Radford EP: Fire victims: Medical outcomes and demographic characteristics. *Am J Public Health* 67:1077, 1977.
5. Zawacki BE, Azen SP, Imbus SH, et al: Multifactorial probit analysis of mortality in burned patients. *Ann Surg* 189:1, 1979.
6. Kirkpatrick JN: Occult carbon monoxide poisoning. *West J Med* 146:52, 1987.
7. Frank R: Acute and chronic respiratory effects of exposure to inhaled toxic agents, in Marchant JA (ed): *Occupational Respiratory Disease*. Washington, DC, US Department of Health and Human Services, 1986, p 571.
8. Montague TJ, MacNeil AR: Mass ammonia inhalation. *Chest* 77:496, 1980.
9. Walton M: Industrial ammonia gasing. *Br J Ind Med* 30:78, 1973.
10. Litovitz TL, Martin TG, Schmitz B: 1986 Annual report of the American Association of Poison Control Centers National Data Collection System. *Am J Emerg Med* 5:405, 1987.
11. Zwemer FL, Pratt DS, May JJ: Silo-Filler's disease in New York state. *Am Rev Respir Dis* 146:650, 1992.
12. Hanrahan LP, Dally KA, Anderson HA, et al: Formaldehyde vapor in mobile homes: A cross-sectional survey of concentrations and irritant effects. *Am J Public Health* 74:1026, 1984.
13. Frigas E, Filley WV, Reed CE: Asthma induced by dust from urea-formaldehyde foam insulating material. *Chest* 79:706, 1981.
14. Bullivant CM: Accidental poisoning by paraquat: Report of two cases in man. *Br Med J* 1:1272, 1966.
15. Wald PH, Becker CE: Toxic gases used in the microelectronics industry, in LaDou J (ed): *State of the Art Reviews: Occupational Medicine*. Philadelphia, Hanley & Belfus, 1986, p 105.
16. Cham-Yeung M, Lam S: Occupational asthma. *Am Rev Respir Dis* 133:686, 1986.
17. Adams WG: Long term effects on the health of men engaged in the manufacture of toluene diisocyanate. *Br J Ind Med* 32:72, 1975.
18. Chan-Yeung M, Lam S, Koerner S: Clinical features and natural history of occupational asthma due to western red cedar (*Thuja plicata*). *Am J Med* 72:411, 1982.
19. Newman Taylor AJ: Occupational asthma. *Thorax* 35:241, 1980.
20. Salvaggio JE, Taylor G, Weill H: Occupational asthma and rhinitis, in Marchant JA (ed): *Occupational Respiratory Disease*. Washington, DC, US Department of Health and Human Services, 1986, p 461.
21. Brooks SM, Weiss MA, Bernstein IL: Reactive airways dysfunction syndrome (RADS). *Chest* 88:376, 1985.
22. Fink J: Hypersensitivity pneumonitis, in Marchant JA (ed): *Occupational Respiratory Disease*. Washington, DC, US Department of Health and Human Services, 1986, p 481.
23. Banaszak EF, Thiede WH, Fink JN: Hypersensitivity pneumonitis due to contamination of an air conditioner. *N Engl J Med* 283:271, 1965.
24. Symington IS, Anderson RA, Thomson I, et al: Cyanide exposure in fires. *Lancet* 2:91, 1978.
25. Burnett WW, King EG, Grace M, et al: Hydrogen sulfide poisoning: Review of 5 years experience. *Can Med Assoc J* 117:1277, 1977.
26. Stewart RD: The effect of carbon monoxide on humans. *Ann Rev Pharmacol* 15:409, 1975.
27. Baker SP, Fisher RS, Masenore WC, et al: Fatal unintentional carbon monoxide poisoning in motor vehicles. *Am J Public Health* 62:1463, 1972.
28. Kelly JS, Sopholeus GJ: Retinal hemorrhages in subacute carbon monoxide poisoning: Exposure in homes with blocked furnace flues. *JAMA* 239:1515, 1978.
29. Fort L, Griggs P: Carbon monoxide poisoning in North Carolina. *NC Med J* 48:317, 1987.
30. Stewart RD, Baretta ED, Platte LR, et al: Carboxyhemoglobin levels in American blood donors. *JAMA* 229:1187, 1974.
31. Dyer RF, Esch VH: Polyvinyl chloride toxicity in fires: Hydrogen chloride toxicity in fire fighters. *JAMA* 235:393, 1976.
32. Gailitis J, Burns LE, Nally JB: Silo-filler's disease. *N Engl J Med* 258:543, 1958.
33. Dawson SV, Schenker MB: Health effects of inhalation of ambient concentrations of nitrogen dioxide. *Am Rev Respir Dis* 120:281, 1979.
34. Douglas WM, Hyzser NG, Colley TV: Silo-filler's disease. *May Clin Proc* 64:291, 1989.
35. Bernstein IL: Occupational asthma. *Clin Chest Med* 2:255, 1981.

36. Jones JG, Minty BD, Royston D, et al: Carboxyhemoglobin and pulmonary epithelial permeability in man. *Thorax* 38:129, 1983.
37. Chan-Yeung M: Immunologic and nonimmunologic mechanisms in asthma due to western red cedar (*Thuja plicata*). *J Allergy Clin Immunol* 70:32, 1982.
38. Lam S, Wong R, Chem-Yeung M: Nonspecific bronchial reactivity in occupational asthma. *J Allergy Clin Immunol* 63:28, 1979.
39. Olson KR: Carbon monoxide poisoning: Mechanisms, presentation, and controversies in management. *J Emerg Med* 1:233, 1984.
40. Douglas CG, Haldane JS, Haldane JBS: The laws of combination of haemoglobin with carbon monoxide and oxygen. *J Physiol* 44:275, 1912.
41. Meredith T, Vale A: Carbon monoxide poisoning. *Br Med J* 296:77, 1988.
42. Caughey WS: Carbon monoxide bonding in hemeproteins. *Ann NY Acad Sci* 174:148, 1970.
43. Somogyi E, Sotonyi P, Balogh I, et al: New findings concerning the pathogenesis of acute carbon monoxide (CO) poisoning. *Am J Forens Med Pathol* 2:31, 1981.
44. Schwartz DA: Acute inhalation injury, in LaDou J (ed): *State of the Art Reviews: Occupational Medicine*. Philadelphia, Hanley & Belfus, 1986, p 105.
45. Adelson L, Kaufman J: Fatal chlorine poisoning: Report of two cases with clinicopathologic correlation. *Am J Clin Pathol* 56:430, 1971.
46. Epler GR, Colby TV: The spectrum of bronchiolitis obliterans. *Chest* 83:161, 1983.
47. Conner EH, Dubois AB, Comroe JH: Acute chemical injury of the airway and lungs. *Anesthesiology* 23:538, 1962.
48. Leduc D, Gris P, Lheureux P, et al: Acute and long-term respiratory damage following inhalation of ammonia. *Thorax* 47:755, 1992.
49. Dimeo MJ, Glenn MG, Holtzman MJ, et al: Threshold concentrations of ozone causing an increase in bronchial reactivity in humans and adaptation with repeated exposures. *Am Rev Respir Dis* 124:245, 1981.
50. Thomas HV, Mueller PK, Lyman RL: Lipoperoxidation of lung lipids in rats exposed to nitrogen dioxide. *Science* 159:532, 1967.
51. Fowler BA, Weissberg JB: Arsine poisoning. *N Engl J Med* 291:1171, 1974.
52. Weiner A: Bronchial asthma due to organic phosphate insecticide. *Ann Allergy* 19:397, 1961.
53. Fink JN: Hypersensitivity pneumonitis. *J Allergy Clin Immunol* 52:309, 1973.
54. DoPico GA: Occupational lung disease in the rural environment, in Gee JB (ed): *Occupational Lung Disease*. New York, Churchill Livingstone, 1984, p 141.
55. doPico GA: Hazardous exposure and lung disease among farm workers. *Clin Chest Med* 13:311, 1992.
56. Ilano AL, Raffin TA: Management of carbon monoxide poisoning. *Chest* 97:165, 1990.
57. Stewart RD, Stewart RS, Stamm W, et al: Rapid estimation of carboxyhemoglobin level in fire fighters. *JAMA* 235:390, 1976.
58. Cramer CR: Fetal death due to accidental maternal carbon monoxide poisoning. *J Toxicol Clin Toxicol* 19:297, 1982.
59. Norkool DM, Kirkpatrick JN: Treatment of acute carbon monoxide poisoning with hyperbaric oxygen: A review of 115 cases. *Ann Emerg Med* 14:168, 1985.
60. Sokol JA, Kralkowska E: The relationship between exposure duration, carboxyhemoglobin, blood glucose, pyruvate and lactate and the severity of intoxication in 39 cases of acute carbon monoxide poisoning in man. *Arch Toxicol* 57:196, 1985.
61. Smith JS, Brandon S: Morbidity from acute carbon monoxide poisoning at three-year follow-up. *Br Med J* 1:318, 1973.
62. Johnson RP, Mellors JW: Arteriolization of venous blood gases: A clue to the diagnosis of cyanide poisoning. *J Emerg Med* 6:401, 1988.
63. Landow SA: Endogenous production of carbon monoxide: The human body as a cause of air pollution. *Ann Intern Med* 70:1275, 1969.
64. Hebbel RP, Eaton JW, Modler S, et al: Extreme but asymptomatic carboxy hemoglobinemia and chronic lung disease. *JAMA* 239:2584, 1978.
65. Goldman AL: Carboxyhemoglobin levels in primary and secondary cigar and pipe smokers. *Chest* 72:33, 1977.
66. Irwin RS, Pratter MR: The clinical value of pharmacologic bronchoprovocation challenge. *Med Clin North Am* 74:767, 1990.
67. Siracusa A, Curradi F, Abritti G: Recurrent nocturnal asthma due to tolylene diisocyanate: A case report. *Clin Allergy* 8:195, 1978.
68. Goldfrank LR, Bresnitz EA: Toxic inhalants including cyanide, in Goldfrank LR, Flomenbaum NE, Lewin NA, et al (eds): *Toxicologic Emergencies*. Norwalk, Appleton & Lange, 1990, p 737.
69. Keller KH: Hydroxycobalamin, in Olsen KR (ed): *Poisoning and Drug Overdose*. Norwalk, Appleton & Lange, 1990, p 317.
70. Pace N, Strajman E, Walker EL: Acceleration of carbon monoxide elimination in man by high pressure oxygen. *Science* 111:652, 1950.
71. Smith G, Sharp GR: Treatment of carbon monoxide poisoning with oxygen under pressure. *Lancet* 2:905, 1960.
72. Norman JN, Ledingham I McA: Carbon monoxide poisoning: Investigations and treatment. *Prog Brain Res* 24:101, 1967.
73. Markley K: Burn care: Infection and smoke inhalation. *Ann Intern Med* 90:269, 1979.
74. Baxter PJ, Davies PC, Murray V: Medical planning for toxic releases into the community: The example of chlorine gas. *Br J Ind Med* 46:277, 1989.
75. Moylan JA: Supportive therapy in burn care—smoke inhalation: Diagnostic technique and steroids. *J Trauma* 19:917, 1979.
76. Moulick ND, Banavalli S, Abhyanker AD et al: Acute accidental exposure to chlorine fumes: A study of 82 cases. *Indian J Chest Dis Allied Sci* 34:85,1992.
77. Braun SR, doPico GA, Tsiatis A, et al: Farmer's lung disease: Long term clinical and physiologic outcome. *Am Rev Respir Dis* 119:185, 1979.
78. Haponik EF, Summer WR: Respiratory complications in burned patients: Pathogenesis and spectrum of injury. *J Crit Care* 2:49, 1987.
79. Haponik EF: Smoke inhalation. *Am Rev Respir Dis* 138:1060, 1988.
80. Coleman DL: Smoke inhalation: Medical staff conference. *West J Med* 135:300, 1981.
81. Thompson PB, Herndon DN, Traper DL, et al: Effect on mortality of inhalation injury. *J Trauma* 26:163, 1986.
82. Marshall WG, Dimick AR: The natural history of major burns with multiple subsystem failure. *J Trauma* 23:102, 1983.
83. Karter MJ: Fire loss in the United States during 1985. *Fire* 80:26, 1986.
84. Zikria BA, Ferrer JM, Floch HF: The chemical factors contributing to pulmonary damage in "smoke poisoning." *Surgery* 71:704, 1972.
85. Levin BC, Paabo M, Fultz ML, Bailey CS: Generation of hydrogen cyanide from flexible polyurethane foam decomposed under different combustion conditions. *Fire Mater* 9:125, 1985.
86. Kimmerle MG: Aspects and methodology for the evaluation of toxicologic parameters during fire exposure. *JFF/Combust Toxicol* 1:4, 1974.
87. Mierley MC, Baker SP: Fatal house fires in an urban population. *JAMA* 249:1466, 1983.
88. Dressler DP: Laboratory background on smoke inhalation. *J Trauma* 19:913, 1979.
89. Treitman RO, Burgess WA, Gold A: Air contaminants encountered by fire fighters. *Am Ind Hyg Assoc J* 41:796, 1980.
90. Sorenson WR: Polyvinyl chloride in fires. *JAMA* 236:1449, 1976.
91. Shirini KZ, Moylan JA, Pritt BA, in Loke J (ed): *Pathophysiology and Treatment of Inhalation Injury*. New York, Marcel Dekker, 1988, p 239.
92. Cahalane M, Demling RH: Early respiratory abnormalities from smoke inhalation. *JAMA* 251:771, 1984.
93. Clark CJ, Campbell D, Reid WH: Blood carboxyhaemoglobin and cyanide levels in fire survivors. *Lancet* 1:1332, 1981.
94. Terrill JB, Montgomery RR, Reinhardt CF: Toxic gases from fires. *Science* 200:1343, 1978.
95. Levine MS: Respirator use and protection from exposure to carbon monoxide. *Am Ind Hyg Assoc J* 40:832, 1979.
96. Brain JD, Valberg PA: Models of lung retention based on ICRP task group report. *Arch Environ Health* 28:1, 1974.
97. Schwerd W, Shuly E: Carboxyhaemoglobin and methaemoglobin findings in burned bodies. *Forensic Sci Int* 12:233, 1978.
98. Haponik EF, Munster AM, Wise RA, et al: Upper airway function

in burn patients: Correlation of flow volume curves and naso-pharyngoscopy. *Am Rev Respir Dis* 129:251, 1984.

99. Skold G, Brunk U. Respiratory tract inflammation after exposure to fire smoke. *Acta Pathol Microbiol Immunol Scand* 52:19, 1961.

100. Stone HH: Pulmonary burns in children. *J Pediatr Surg* 13:48, 1979.

101. Pruitt BA, DiVincenti FC, Mason AD, et al: The occurrence and significance of pneumonia and other pulmonary complications in burned patients: Comparison of conventional and topical treatments. *J Trauma* 10:519, 1970.

102. Stone HH, Reame DW, Corbitt JD, et al: Respiratory burns: A correlation of clinical and laboratory results. *Ann Surg* 165:157, 1967.

103. Herndon DN, Thompson PB, Traber DL: Pulmonary injury in burned patients. *Crit Care Clin* 1:79, 1985.

104. Haponik EF, Summer WR: Respiratory complications in burned patients: Diagnosis and management of inhalation injury. *J Crit Care* 2:121, 1987.

105. DiVincenti FC, Pruitt BA, Reckler JM: Inhalation injuries. *J Trauma* 11:109, 1971.

106. Fein A, Leff A, Hopewell PC: Pathophysiology and management of the complications resulting from fire and the inhaled products of combustion: Review of the literature. *Crit Care Med* 8:94, 1980.

107. Phillips AW, Tanner JW, Cope O: Burn therapy. IV. Respiratory tract damage (an account of the clinical, x-ray and postmortem findings) and the meaning of restlessness. *Ann Surg* 158:799, 1963.

108. Cooney W, Dzuira B, Harper R, Nash G: The cytology of sputum from thermally injured patients. *Acta Cytol* 16:433, 1972.

109. Richards DW: The circulation in traumatic shock in man: The Harvey Lecture. *Bull New York Acad Med* 20:363, 1944.

110. Epstein BS, Hardy DL, Harrison HN, et al: Hypoxemia in the burned patient: A clinical-pathologic study. *Ann Surg* 158:924, 1963.

111. Hudson L: Delayed hypoxemia in smoke inhalation. *Clin Res* 19:191, 1971.

112. Crapo RO: Smoke inhalation injuries. *JAMA* 246:1694, 1981.

113. Baud FJ, Barriot P, Toffis V, et al: Elevated blood cyanide concentrations in victims of smoke inhalation. *N Engl J Med* 325:1761, 1991.

114. Petroff PA, Hander EW, Clayton WH, Pruitt BA: Pulmonary function studies after smoke inhalation. *Am J Surg* 132:346, 1976.

115. Milstein D, Nusynowitz ML, Lull RJ: Radionuclide diagnosis in chest disease resulting from trauma. *Semin Nucl Med* 4:339, 1974.

116. Moylan JA, Wilmore DW, Mouton DE, et al: Early diagnosis of inhalation injury using xenon lung scan. *Ann Surg* 176:477, 1972.

117. Whitener DR, Whitener LM, Robertson J, et al: Pulmonary function measurements in patients with thermal injury and smoke inhalation. *Am Rev Respir Dis* 122:731, 1980.

118. Robinson L, Miller RH: Smoke inhalation injuries. *Am J Otolaryngol* 7:375, 1986.

119. Hunt JL, Agee RN, Pruitt BA: Fiberoptic bronchoscopy in acute inhalation injury. *J Trauma* 15:641, 1975.

120. Moylan JA, Adib K, Burnbaum M: Fiberoptic bronchoscopy following thermal injury. *Surg Gynecol Obstet* 140:541, 1975.

121. Head JM: Inhalation injury in burns. *Am J Surg* 139:508, 1980.

122. Kinsella J, Carter R, Reid WH, et al: Increased airways reactivity after smoke inhalation. *Lancet* 337:595, 1991.

123. Epstein BS, Rudman HL, Hardy DL, et al: Comparison of orotracheal intubation with tracheostomy for anesthesia in patients with face and neck burns. *Anesth Analg* 45:352, 1966.

124. Moncrief JA: Tracheotomy in burns. *Arch Surg* 79:45, 1959.

125. Via-Reque E, Rattenborg CC. Prolonged oro- or nasotracheal intubation. *Crit Care Med* 9:637, 1981.

126. Finland M, Davidson CS, Levenson SM: Clinical and therapeutic aspects of the conflagration injuries to the respiratory tract sustained by victims of the Cocoanut Grove disaster. *Medicine* 25:215, 1946.

127. Haponik EF: Smoke inhalation injury: Some priorities for respiratory care professionals. *Respir Care.* 37:609, 1992.

128. Wiseman DH, Grossman AR: Hyperbaric oxygen in the treatment of burns. *Crit Care Clin* 1:129, 1985.

72. *Disorders of Temperature Control: Hypothermia*

Frederick J. Curley and Richard S. Irwin

This chapter reviews the normal physiology of temperature regulation and the major hypothermic syndromes. It focuses on the pathogenesis, pathophysiologic factors, diagnosis, and management of unintentional hypothermia. Iatrogenic and intentional hypothermia in the perioperative setting are briefly discussed. Three hyperthermic syndromes—heat stroke, malignant hyperthermia, and neuroleptic malignant syndrome—are reviewed in chapter 73.

Normal Physiology of Temperature Regulation

The equilibrium between heat production and heat loss determines body temperature. In healthy resting individuals, this equilibrium is tightly regulated, producing an average oral temperature of $36.6 \pm 0.38°C$ [1]. Table 72-1 is a conversion chart of temperatures in Celsius to Fahrenheit. Small shifts of this temperature setpoint occur, with a normal diurnal variation producing a peak temperature usually near 6:00 P.M. Minute-to-minute changes in body temperature, however, are quickly sensed, and appropriate changes are made in body heat production and loss to restore a "normal" balance.

HEAT PRODUCTION. In a neutral environment (28°C for humans), humans generate all net body heat from the energy released in the dissociation of high-energy bonds during the metabolism of dietary fats, proteins, and carbohydrates. At rest, the trunk and viscera supply 56 percent of the body heat, but during exercise up to 90 percent may be generated by the muscles. Whereas shivering or an increase in muscle tone may produce a fourfold rise in net heat production [2], vigorous exercise may cause a sixfold increase. Thermogenesis without shivering due to the metabolism of brown fat is unimportant in acute temperature control in adults [3] but may be important in our adaptation to cold environments [4]. Although heat production may also be increased by raising the basal metabolic rate,

Table 72-1. Fahrenheit to Celsius Temperature Conversions

°C	°F
45	113.0
44	111.2
43	109.4
42	107.6
41	105.8
40	104.0
39	102.2
38	100.4
37	98.6
36	96.8
35	95.0
34	93.2
33	91.4
32	89.6
31	87.8
30	86.0
29	84.2
28	82.4
27	80.6
26	78.8
25	77.0
24	75.2
23	73.4
22	71.6
21	69.8
20	68.0

changes in basal metabolic rate usually occur slowly and therefore play only a minor role in the minute-to-minute regulation of temperature.

HEAT LOSS. Heat exchange with the environment follows a thermal gradient. That is, when environmental temperature is lower than body temperature, the body loses heat to the environment; when environmental temperature is higher, the body may gain heat.

Under usual environmental conditions, heat exchange with the environment takes the form of heat loss. Heat may be exchanged by radiation, conduction, convection, or evaporation [5]. *Radiation exchange*—the transfer of thermal energy between objects with no direct contact—accounts for 50 to 70 percent of heat lost by humans at rest in a neutral environment. *Conduction* involves the direct exchange of heat with objects in direct contact with the body. To protect us from excessive heat loss by this mechanism, muscles, fat, and skin act as natural insulators, decreasing conducted heat loss from the warmer tissues in the deep core. Large quantities of heat may be rapidly exchanged when the body is submerged in water; this is due to the much greater thermal conductivity of water as compared with air. *Convection* involves the exchange of heat with the warmer or cooler molecules of air that pass by the skin. Heat exchange by this mechanism increases rapidly with greater temperature differences between the skin and the air and with rapid air flow. The wind chill that one notices on a cold, windy day is due to convection. *Evaporative heat loss* in humans occurs primarily through perspiration. Evaporation of sweat from the skin requires that energy be supplied by the skin, resulting in a net loss of heat from the body of 0.6 kcal per gram of sweat absorbed. Unlike the other methods of heat exchange, evaporation can exchange heat loss even when the skin is surrounded by a warmer environment. Evaporation is therefore the major means by which the body prevents hyperthermia in a warm environment.

TEMPERATURE CONTROL SYSTEMS. A complex system is needed to monitor and regulate the heat exchanges that occur constantly with changes in thermogenesis, radiation, conduction, convection, and evaporation.

The anatomy and regulation of the system that controls body temperature have been reviewed in depth by several investigators [2,5,6,7], and are only briefly described here. Neurons directly responsive to temperature ascend from the skin, the deep viscera, and the spinal cord through the lateral spinothalamic tract to the preoptic anterior hypothalamus. The hypothalamus directly senses local temperature and integrates this information with afferent data to make appropriate adjustments in autonomic tone and perhaps endocrine function to maintain body temperature within normal limits. Baroreceptor data, serum osmolarity, and local calcium and sodium concentrations may also affect hypothalamic regulation. When the hypothalamus perceives a temperature increase, it modulates autonomic tone to produce (1) an increase in evaporative heat loss through increased sweat output by the body's 2.5 million sweat glands; (2) cutaneous vasodilatation that allows direct flow of heat to the skin to increase convective and conductive heat losses; and (3) decreased muscle tone and activity to prevent any unnecessary heat production. When the hypothalamus perceives a temperature decrease, it modulates autonomic tone to cause (1) sweat production to cease or decrease; (2) the cutaneous vasculature to constrict; and (3) muscle tone to increase involuntarily and shivering to begin.

The monoamines are believed to be modulators of the anterior hypothalamic thermostat [8]. Feldberg and Myers [9] first reported on the importance of amines in temperature regulation in the hypothalamus in 1963. Numerous experiments in animals have since demonstrated that marked temperature changes can be produced by the injection of minute quantities of amines such as levophed or dopamine in discrete areas of the third ventricle adjacent to the hypothalamus [10,11]. In rats, for example, injections of 5-hydroxytryptophan, dopamine, l-dopa, and apomorphine produce hypothermia, whereas injections of norepinephrine, epinephrine, and isoproterenol produce hyperthermia [12]. The threshold, degree, and direction of the response vary with species. In humans, decreases in dopaminergic tone may, in the appropriate setting, produce hyperthermia [13–16]. Agents that might cause hypothermia and the roles of 5-hydroxytryptophan, histamine, and epinephrine have yet to be clearly elucidated.

Voluntary responses play an important role in thermoregulation. Humans may respond to thermal stress by (1) adding or removing clothes (affecting evaporative, conductive, and radiant heat exchange); (2) moving to a warmer climate (going indoors on a cold day to obtain a more favorable thermal gradient); (3) changing the level of activity (working more slowly on a hot day to reduce heat production); and (4) changing posture (curling up to reduce radiant losses in a cold environment). Whenever possible, we voluntarily alter our environment, necessitating little autonomic adjustment in temperature regulation. The fur-clad Eskimo and the loin-clothed tropical native in the shade have nearly identical temperatures in the air near their skin. Impairment of voluntary control places an unnecessary stress on autonomic control mechanisms and thereby predisposes to an imbalance in heat exchange and a change in body temperature.

Neuroendocrine changes affect temperature regulation by potentiating responses to autonomic stimuli [17]. Because neuroendocrine changes produce effects slowly, they have little to do with the regulation of acute temperature changes. They may be important, however, in determining the body's acclimatization to chronic changes in metabolism or environment.

The ability to regulate temperature effectively declines with age [18,19], probably as a result of deterioration in sensory afferents. Whereas younger individuals usually notice temperature changes as low as 0.8°C, older individuals may not notice changes of up to 2.3°C. Moreover, because sweat threshold increases and sweat volume decreases with age, an older individual may be more susceptible to hyperthermia than a younger person [20]. Old age may also be a liability for hypothermia because of (1) a lower basal metabolic rate, (2) a higher heat conductance due to a decline in body mass, (3) a decrease in the heat generated by shivering due to a smaller muscle mass, and (4) an inability to vasoconstrict cautaneous vessels in response to cold. Although some elderly patients lose their ability to shiver, loss of the ability to maintain heat by vasoconstriction appears both more common and more important. In addition, if an elderly person has restricted mobility or a deterioration in cortical function, voluntary responses to temperature changes may be impaired. Because of all these impairments, the elderly have a much greater risk of hypothermia or hyperthermia than do the young.

Unintentional Hypothermia

Hypothermia, defined as a core temperature below 35°C, is not uncommon; it occurs at all ambient temperatures and in patients of all ages but more commonly in the elderly. Preliminary data indicate that hypothermia occurs within 24 hours of admission in more than 3 percent of ICU admissions [21]. During the winter in Great Britain, 0.7 percent of all hospital admissions [22], 3 percent of elderly patients admitted [23], and at least 10 percent of otherwise healthy elderly individuals examined at home [24] had core temperatures in the hypothermic range. The occurrence of hypothermia in the United States appears to be much lower; in a survey of mostly poor, chronically ill elderly patients studied in their homes in Maine during the winter, not a single patient was hypothermic [25]. Most agencies responsible for recording vital statistics agree that hypothermia is a diagnosis frequently missed and underreported [26]. Until the recent publication of several hypothermia reviews, many physicians were unaware of the extent or severity of the problem. Review of death certificates in the United States reveals an average mortality rate for hypothermia of 0.22 per 100,000 individuals; white women have the lowest rates, and nonwhite men have the highest [27]. When all data are reviewed, the overall mortality from hypothermia in the United States has been conservatively estimated at 17 deaths per 1 million population per year [28]. The mortality rate for treated hypothermia ranges from 12 percent [29] to 73 percent [30].

CAUSES AND PATHOGENESIS. Although hypothermia can occur in all climates, at nearly all ambient temperatures, and at every age, the most frequent causes appear to be exposure, use of depressant drugs, and hypoglycemia. A brief review of the causes of hypothermia (Table 72-2) and their pathogenesis will help to develop a rational approach to treatment.

Age. The elderly, because of a "normal" impairment of regulatory function, constitute a large portion of the patients who become hypothermic. The reasons the elderly are more susceptible to hypothermia are discussed above.

Exposure to Cold. Although the incidence of hypothermia doubles with every 5°C drop in ambient temperature [31], fatal hypothermia occurs even in healthy young adults who simply have been overexposed to the elements. Wet, wind, and ex-

Table 72-2. Causes of Unintentional Hypothermia

Normal aging
Exposure to cold
Drugs (e.g., alcohol)
Endocrine dysfunction (e.g., hypoglycemia)
CNS disorders
Spinal cord transection
Skin disorders
Debility
Trauma

haustion contribute to increased loss of body heat. Wet clothing loses 90 percent of its insulating value [32], rendering soaked individuals effectively nude. Exposure to rain or snow was believed to contribute greatly to the development of hypothermia in 15 of 23 incidents in hikers discussed in one review [32]. Convective heat loss because of wind may increase to more than five times baseline values, and it increases with wind velocity [33]. The exact mechanism by which exhaustion contributes to hypothermia is unclear, but it probably relates to the effects of a decreased energy supply on heat production or, less likely, on hypothalamic regulatory mechanisms.

Poor selection of clothing and failure to seek appropriate shelter promptly are common factors that result in fatal hypothermia in hikers and campers [33]. Hypothermia may also occur in unprepared individuals who attempt cross-country skiing in unfavorable weather or who run for long periods in cool, rainy weather. Victims of hypothermia that results from exposure frequently display inappropriate behavior that compounds the hypothermia; they may remove their clothing and quickly experience loss of coordination and then stupor or collapse. Death may occur within an hour of the onset of symptoms [33].

Immersion in water at a temperature colder than 24°C leads to extremely rapid heat loss. Core temperature drops at a rate proportional to the temperature of the water [34]. Although survival times of 1 to 2 hours have been reported for individuals immersed in water at 0 to 10°C, death may occur within minutes.

Drugs. Alcohol, phenothiazines, barbiturates, and paralytic agents frequently produce hypothermia by depressing sensory afferents, the hypothalamus, and effector responses.

Depending on the patient population studied, alcohol contributes to hypothermia in 14 to 91 percent of cases [35,36]. Because alcohol has been shown to impair the perception of cold, cloud the sensorium, and act as a direct vasodilator, individuals under the influence of alcohol are less likely to perceive danger and to respond appropriately to cold; moreover, they are unable to conserve heat properly by vasoconstriction [37,38]. Animals given high doses of alcohol are rendered poikilothermic [39]. Alcoholics are also thought to be more susceptible to exposure because of debility (a state of relative starvation), increased conductive losses from decreased subcutaneous fat, and high levels of blood alcohol that potentially impair the metabolic response to hypothermia by decreasing blood sugar and increasing acidosis.

Most sedative-hypnotic drugs, such as barbiturates and phenothiazines, cause hypothermia by inhibiting shivering and impairing capability for voluntary control of temperature. Phenothiazines increase the threshold necessary to produce shivering and lead to hypothalamic depression [21,40]; barbiturates decrease effective shivering [41]. Paralytic agents used to suppress ventilation or during anesthesia also prevent shivering, effectively eliminate all voluntary control mechanisms, and may result in hypothermia [42,43].

Hypothermia has resulted from the administration of common antibiotics, such as penicillin [44] and erythromycin [45]. The mechanism by which this occurs is not understood. Bromocriptine may cause hypothermia by altering central dopaminergic tone [46].

Endocrine Dysfunction. Diabetic ketoacidosis, hyperosmolar coma, and hypoglycemia are frequently reported causes of hypothermia [35,47]. In one survey, 20 percent of patients with blood glucose levels less than 60 mg per deciliter had temperatures of less than 35°C. Hypoglycemia produces hypothermia by lowering cerebral intracellular glucose concentrations and impairing hypothalamic function [48]. The fact that some hypoglycemic patients fail to shiver effectively [21] reflects this dysfunction. In acute hypoglycemia such as that caused by insulin administration, subjects experience hypothermia from peripheral vasodilatation and sweating. At glucose concentrations below 2.5 mM per liter, these subjects fail to perceive cold environments and fail to shiver [49]. This impairment appears transient, because normal regulatory mechanisms and euthermia may be restored when normal serum glucose levels are restored.

The prevalence of hypothyroidism in patients with unintentional hypothermia ranges from 0 to 10 percent [47]. Although mild, untreated hypothyroidism produces a physiologic state similar to heat acclimatization in that the basal metabolic rate is slowed and the response to thyroid-stimulating hormone (TSH) is blunted [50], the thermoregulatory system remains intact and appears to cope well with all but overwhelming thermal challenges. Moreover, several patients with mild hypothyroidism have been safely rewarmed to euthermia without administration of exogenous thyroid hormone. In these cases, hypothyroidism went unrecognized until after the successful treatment of hypothermia [47].

In contrast, myxedema coma, a rare presentation of hypothyroidism, is associated with subnormal temperatures in 82 percent of cases [51]. It has a high mortality if not treated with exogenous TSH. Myxedema coma occurs most frequently in middle-aged to older women, and more than 90 percent of cases occur in winter [51]. Severe hypothermia with temperatures below 30°C occurs in 15 percent of patients [51]. Coma arises because of a cerebral TSH deficiency. Hypothermia then results from a combination of loss of voluntary control mechanisms from stupor or coma, decreased calorigenesis from thyroid deficiency, and decreased shivering, presumably from impaired hypothalamic regulation [51,52].

Panhypopituitarism and adrenal insufficiency [35] are also rare causes of hypothermia. Like hypothyroidism, these factors place the body in a state of relative warmth adaptation and blunt the response to cold stress. Unless profound insufficiency exists, these conditions rarely produce significant hypothermia in the absence of some other insult to the thermoregulatory system.

Central Nervous System Disorders. Diseases such as stroke, primary and metastatic brain tumors, luetic gliosis, and sarcoidosis may produce hypothermia by direct anatomic impingement on the hypothalamus [36,53]. Metabolic derangements from carbon monoxide poisoning or thiamine deficiency can also produce hypothermia, presumably by affecting the hypothalamus. Wernicke-Korsakoff syndrome occurs in alcoholic individuals with thiamine deficiency and may rarely produce coma or hypothermia [54–59]. Most of these patients have temperatures above 30°C. Because involvement of the posterior pituitary is frequently seen after death, these pathologic changes support the hypothesis that patients with Wernicke-

Korsakoff syndrome have permanent changes in their thermoregulatory mechanisms.

Hypothermia occurs with severe thiamine deficiency or when control mechanisms are subjected to additional stresses, such as hypoglycemia, cold, or alcohol. Patients with anorexia nervosa have been shown to have multiple hypothalamic abnormalities. Both shivering and vasoconstriction frequently fail to occur in anorexic patients, leading to a rapid drop in core temperature when they are exposed to cold [60]. Agenesis or lipoma of the corpus callosum has been reported to cause spontaneous periodic hypothermia by an unclear mechanism [41,61,62]. These patients are presumed to have multiple minor congenital neurologic deficits and frequently have lifelong histories of episodic coma or stupor preceded by intense sweating. In this rare cause of hypothermia, regulatory mechanisms appear to remain intact but the euthermic setpoint seems to be lowered. Several patients with multiple sclerosis have experienced transient hypothermia with flares of their neuropathy, suggesting the presence of hypothalamic plaques [63,64].

Spinal Cord Transection. Loss of skin and core temperature afferents, reduced body muscle mass, inability to shiver effectively, and, if mobility is compromised, inability to alter the environment make patients with spinal cord injury susceptible to thermal stress. These impairments frequently result in hypothermia in quadriplegic persons exposed to low ambient temperatures [65,66,67]. The prevalence of hypothermia in these patients is probably grossly underestimated.

Skin Disorders. Skin disorders characterized by vasodilatation or increased transepithelial water loss may lead to hypothermia. The vasodilatation in a patient with erythroderma fails to decrease on exposure to cold, leading to inappropriate conductive and convective heat losses. Because increased blood flow from the warm core preserves skin warmth, shivering may not occur [68]. Psoriasis, ichthyosis, and erythroderma have also been shown to be associated with increased evaporative losses of up to 3 liters per day; this computes to a potential loss of more than 1700 kcal of heat per day [69]. Although hypothermia is usually mild in these patients, temperatures as low as 28°C have been reported [30]. When an additional cause of hypothermia is present, these patients may be in danger of severe drops in temperature. Patients with extensive third-degree burns have been reported to have an even larger evaporative heat loss, losing up to 6 liters of fluid, or more than 3400 kcal a day. Burn patients may shiver to maintain a normal temperature in the face of this extreme heat loss. Heat loss and caloric requirements can be decreased dramatically by covering their skin with impermeable membranes to decrease evaporative losses [70,71,72].

Debility. Case reports suggest that hypothermia may occur in patients with debilitating illnesses such as Hodgkin's disease [73,74], systemic lupus erythematosus [75,76], and severe cardiac, renal, hepatic, or septic failure. The reasons for the predisposition to hypothermia in these cases remains unclear; most likely many mechanisms act in concert to produce a drop in temperature. A decrease in cardiac index from 2.8 to 1.4 liters per minute has been shown to result in a drop in temperature from 37 to 35°C [77]. Temperature promptly rose when cardiac index increased. Hypothermia in hepatic failure might result from intermittent hypoglycemia. Most debilitated patients are also compromised by some degree of immobility or decreased voluntary control. Because many of these patients cannot sustain the high level of catabolism necessary for heat production, they may be similar to patients who experience hypothermia as a result of exhaustion.

Trauma. Trauma patients frequently have hypothermia [78,79,80], most likely because of multiple insults to the thermoregulatory system. Loss of voluntary control in adverse environments, such as cool weather or air-conditioned operating rooms, the presence of alcohol in up to 62 percent of cases in some series [78], and the rapid transfusion of unwarmed blood [80] all predispose to the development of hypothermia in these patients. It is unclear whether the physiologic changes inherent to multiple trauma predispose to hypothermia in the absence of other promoting factors. In patients with moderately elevated injury severity scores, initial temperature may reflect hypothermia in 23 percent of cases [78]; during the first day of hospitalization, 42 percent experience hypothermia, 13 percent having temperatures less than 32°C [79]. The presence of shock [79] and massive transfusion [78,80] significantly contributed to the development of hypothermia in these patients.

PATHOPHYSIOLOGY

General Considerations. Profound metabolic alterations occur in every organ system in response to a core temperature below 35°C. Beyond the immediate cardiovascular changes induced by vasoconstriction, metabolic changes that appear to be temperature-dependent occur in two phases: shivering and nonshivering. The shivering phase, usually occurring in the range of 35 to 30°C, is characterized by intense energy production from the breakdown of stored body fuels. In the nonshivering phase, which occurs below about 30°C, the metabolism slows dramatically, resulting at times in multiple organ failure. Individual variation in this progression from catabolism to hypometabolism typically relates not to the overall pattern of metabolic change but to individual differences in the temperature thresholds that trigger the onset or cessation of shivering.

Shivering involves an increase in muscle tone and the powerful rhythmic contraction of both small and large muscle groups. It is therefore not surprising that the metabolic changes during the shivering phase parallel those seen during muscular exercise. In different patient populations with different measurement techniques, heat production has been shown to increase by four times the normal amount [81], oxygen consumption by two to five times [40], and metabolic rate by six times [82]. Central pooling of blood resulting from peripheral vasoconstriction may raise central venous pressure and slightly elevate cardiac output. Because cardiac output remains relatively close to normal and oxygen demand increases dramatically, mixed venous oxygen saturation typically decreases [83]. Although hepatic and muscular glycogenolysis may cause blood sugar to rise, this rise may not be seen in starved or exhausted patients or those with prolonged hypothermia [47,50,84]. The catabolism of fat increases the serum levels of glycerol, nonesterified fatty acids, and ketones. Anaerobic metabolism causes a rise in lactate levels; levels as high as 25.2 mM per liter have been reported [85]. The metabolic acidosis induced by this intense catabolism is compensated for the most part by the increased metabolism of lactate in the liver and increased minute ventilation [84]. As in any severe stress, cortisol levels typically rise [29]. Most of these metabolic changes peak near 34 or 35°C and become much less pronounced near a temperature of 30°C.

As core temperature falls toward 30°C, the body appears to shift from attempts to increase the production of heat to a more hibernationlike state. Below 30°C, shivering nearly ceases and metabolism slows dramatically. Near 30°C, metabolic rate approaches basal levels [86], and it may be half basal value by

Table 72-3. Common Effects of Hypothermia

Metabolic depletion	Anemia/hemoconcentration
Cardiac dysrhythmia	Thrombocytopenia
Hypotension	Ileus
Hypopnea	Pancreatitis
Dehydration	Hyperglycemia
Coma	Pneumonia
Granulocytopenia	Sepsis
	Altered drug clearance

28°C [82]. As shivering and metabolism slow, oxygen consumption declines. At 30°C, oxygen consumption decreases to about 75 percent of basal value [86]; at 26°C to 35 to 53 percent [40]; and by 20°C to only 25 percent of basal value. This profound decrease in metabolism is reflected by changes in every organ system (Table 72-3).

Cardiovascular Function. Increasing degrees of hypothermia produce a tendency for malignant dysrhythmias, depressed cardiac function, and hypotension. A decrease in cardiac conductivity and automaticity [87,88,89] and an increase in refractory period [90,91] begin during the shivering phase and progress as core temperature decreases. The electrocardiogram (ECG) in mild hypothermia may show bradycardia with prolongation of the P–R, QRS, and Q–T intervals. Below 30°C first-degree block is not unusual, and at 20°C third-degree block may be seen [50,92]. Below 33°C, the ECG commonly shows a J point elevation that is characteristic in appearance (Fig. 72-1). As temperature drops, the J wave increases in prominence and is almost always clearly present at core temperatures below 25°C [93,94]. Vectorcardiography reveals that the spatial orientation of the J wave is anterior and leftward, explaining its prominence in the midprecordial and lateral precordial leads [95]. Physio-

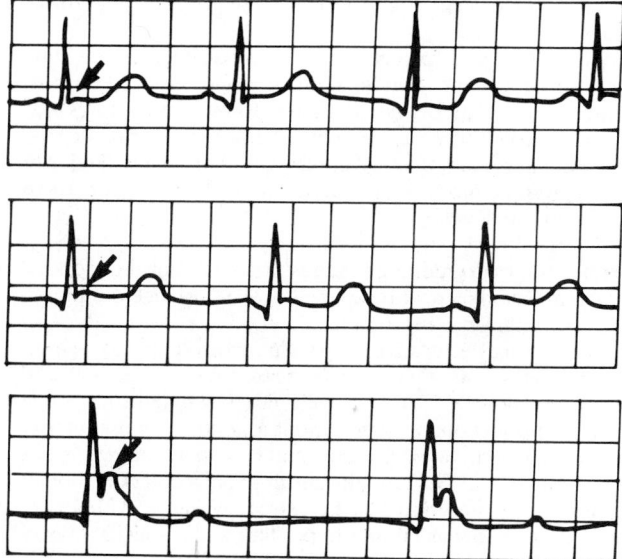

Fig. 72-1. The ECG changes of hypothermia. As temperature decreases (top to bottom), the rate slows and the P–R and Q–T intervals become prolonged. J waves (*arrows*) appear at a temperature less than 35°C and become prominent by a temperature near 25°C. The J wave initially is seen (top) as a widened QRS with a slight S–T elevation at the J point.

logically, this corresponds to delayed depolarization along the inferior surface of the heart. Although the electrophysiologic cause of the J wave remains unclear, reports of J waves occurring in euthermic patients with cerebrovascular accidents suggest that it may be mediated by hypothalamic regulation of autonomic tone [96,97].

Atrial fibrillation is extremely common at temperatures of 34 to 25°C, and ventricular fibrillation frequently occurs below 28°C. The incidence of ventricular fibrillation increases with physical stimulation of the heart and is associated with intracardiac temperature gradients of greater than 2°C [98]. Purkinje cells show marked decreases in excitability in the range of 14 to 15°C [89], and asystole is common when core temperatures drop below 20°C. Recovery of spontaneous electrical activity after hypothermic asystole may be related to protection from the "calcium paradox" afforded by hypothermia [99].

These changes act in concert to produce a gradual decrease in cardiac output. Systole may become extremely prolonged [100], greatly decreasing ejection fraction and aortic pressures. Descriptions of the hearts of hypothermic patients who underwent open-chest resuscitation as being as "hard as stone" [101] suggest a severe decrease in ventricular compliance. Output decreases to about 90 percent of normal at 30°C and may decrease rapidly at lower temperatures, with increasing bradycardia or dysrhythmia. In dogs with induced hypothermia regional blood flow was altered to preserve myocardial and cerebral perfusion [102]. Although cardiac output was reduced to 18 percent of control values in these animals, flow to their hearts and brains was reduced to only 52 and 41 percent of control, respectively.

Although blood pressure appears to be initially maintained by an increase in systemic vascular resistance [103], systemic resistance decreases and hypotension is common [50] below temperatures of 25°C. Oxygen demand usually decreases more rapidly than does cardiac output, causing mixed venous oxygen content to increase as the nonshivering phase begins.

Pulmonary Function. Pulmonary mechanics and gas exchange appear to change little with hypothermia. Compliance, airway resistance, lung volumes, and alveolar-arterial oxygen tension gradient, or $P(A-a)O_2$, are similar to those of euthermic patients [50,104,105,106]. Although the ventilatory response to an elevation in carbon dioxide tension (PCO_2) may be blunted [104], there is no clear decrease in hypoxic drive [50].

As the increased oxygen demand and acidosis of the shivering phase decline, minute ventilation decreases. Both tidal volume and respiratory rate decline at lower temperatures [40]. At 25°C, respirations may be only three or four per minute [50]; at temperatures less than 24°C, respiration may cease [82]. Apnea is presumed to be secondary to failure of respiratory drive at a brainstem level.

Renal Function. Although little is known about the kidneys' role in maintaining acid-base or electrolyte balance during hypothermia, they are instrumental in altering water balance. As blood pressure decreases during the nonshivering phase, glomerular filtration rate (GFR) may decrease by 85 percent [50] and renal blood flow by 75 percent [40], without a significant change in urine production. Maintenance of a good urine output, despite decreases in blood pressure and GFR in hypothermia, has been termed *cold diuresis*. This results from a defect in tubular reabsorption. The urine may be extremely dilute, with an osmolarity of as low as 60 mOsm per liter and a specific gravity of 1.002 [107]. The stimulus for this dilute diuresis may be the triggering of volume receptors as central volume increases with

peripheral vasoconstriction [100]. An alternative explanation is that hypothermia might produce a relative insensitivity to antidiuretic hormone [97] or a direct suppression of antidiuretic hormone release [38]. Although kaliuresis and glycosuria may accompany the dilute diuresis, the net result for the patient is dehydration and a relatively hyperosmolar serum.

Neurologic Function. Hypothermic patients present with profound coma. The brain tolerates hypothermia extremely well: Complete neurologic recovery has been described in hypothermic adults after 20 minutes of complete cardiac arrest [37] and after up to 3.5 hours of cardiopulmonary resuscitation [107]. The mechanism by which hypothermia produces a seemingly protective effect is far from clearly understood; it probably relates to a significant decrease in cerebral metabolism and to the production of a smaller injury by the no-reflow phenomenon [108], a putative mechanism whereby the brain is protected from injury until reperfusion.

Although the cerebral metabolic pathways appear unchanged during hypothermia [109], the level of metabolism is depressed. Cerebral oxygen consumption decreases by about 55 percent for each 10°C decrease in temperature [109]. Cerebral blood flow decreases from 75 percent of normal at 30°C to only 20 percent of normal at 20°C [50]. The fact that the supply of nutrients and removal of wastes is adequate at these extremes is attested to not only by patient recovery but also by experimental evidence that the intracellular pH of brain tissue cooled to 20°C is unchanged even after 20 minutes of anoxia [110].

Visual [111,112] and auditory [113,114] evoked potentials demonstrate delayed latencies; latency increases as temperature decreases. The spectrum of electroencephalographic frequencies also changes with hypothermia. In healthy men cooled to 33°C by immersion, theta and beta activity increased by 17 percent and alpha activity decreased by 34 percent compared with control values [112]. Electromyography during hypothermia has been reported to be normal [115].

Hematologic Function. Hypothermia affects white blood cells (WBCs), red cells, platelets, and perhaps coagulation mechanisms. Although the WBC count in mild hypothermia remains normal to slightly elevated, it may drop severely at temperatures lower than 28°C [116]. Patients show a 35 percent decrease in the number of polymorphonuclear leukocytes (PMNs) by 29°C, and WBC counts may be less than 1000 per ml in some [117]. The hematocrit usually rises in hypothermic patients at a temperature of 30°C. Although this may reflect hemoconcentration from the dehydration caused by cold diuresis, careful studies in dogs rendered hypothermic by packing in ice suggest that the elevation in hematocrit is due primarily to splenic contraction [118]. The increase in blood viscosity in hypothermic patients appears to be due to decreased deformability of the red cell membrane [119]. After intravascular volume and euthermia have been restored, a mild anemia may last up to 6 weeks. Bone marrow aspirates performed on these patients show erythroid hypoplasia and increased ringed sideroblasts, suggesting the anemia may be due to a maturation arrest [120]. Platelet counts drop as temperature decreases, and prolongation of the bleeding time has been noted at 20°C [116]; normal levels and function return on rewarming [121]. The decrease in platelet count is thought to be secondary to hepatic sequestration.

No clear evidence indicates that a coagulopathy is associated with hypothermia. Deep venous thrombosis and disseminated intravascular coagulopathy have been reported in hypothermic patients [55,122], but because they occur frequently in almost every group of severely ill patients this may not reflect a specific effect of hypothermia.

Gastrointestinal Function. Ileus, pancreatitis, and hepatic dysfunction commonly accompany hypothermia. Ileus is frequently present at temperatures above 30°C and is almost always present at lower temperatures. Subclinical pancreatitis appears to be common. Although patients usually lack symptoms of acute pancreatitis, more than half have amylase elevations above 550 Somogyi units. Moreover, up to 80 percent of patients who die of hypothermia have evidence of pancreatitis at autopsy [123]. The relationship between alcohol use and pancreatitis in these patients is unclear. Hepatic dysfunction occurs commonly and involves both synthetic and detoxification abilities [40]. Profoundly hypothermic patients in whom an acidosis develops are less able to clear lactate. Postmortem studies of patients who died from exposure-induced hypothermia have emphasized that gastric submucosal hemorrhage is common [124]. Duodenal ulceration and perforation may also be seen [125].

Endocrine. Although it is generally assumed that acute hypothermia blunts endocrine function, only the effect on insulin metabolism has been clearly described. Hypothermia directly suppresses the release of insulin from the pancreas and increases resistance to insulin's action in the periphery [126,127]. The blood glucose level rises in early hypothermia, due to glycogenolysis and increased corticosteroid levels, and remains elevated because of a decreased concentration and the action of insulin. Elevations in blood glucose, however, are usually mild; only 9 percent of patients in one series had blood glucose levels higher than 200 mg per deciliter [47]. Changes in thyroid and adrenal function occur, but they are less well defined. The responses to TSH and adrenocorticotrophic hormone appear blunted [50]. In hypothyroid patients, TSH increases in response to cold [128]. Although corticosteroid levels vary a great deal among patients, they rarely appear to be severely depressed [84,129,130]. In hypothermic rats, inhibition of adrenocorticotrophic hormone release appears to result from decreased hypothalamic secretion of vasopressin and oxytocin and a subsequent decreased pituitary responsiveness to corticotropin-releasing factors [131]. Urinary catecholamine levels are increased threefold to sevenfold on average in hypothermic deaths, compared with death due to other causes [124].

Immune Function. Infection is a major cause of death in hypothermic patients. Although the cause of the increased susceptibility to infection is not clear, it probably is multifactorial. A number of potential factors can be identified:

1. Hypoperfusion renders the patient more liable to bacterial invasion in ischemic regions of the skin and intestine.
2. Central nervous system depression reduces both gag and cough reflexes, leaving the patient more susceptible to aspiration pneumonia.
3. A decrease in tidal volume and minute ventilation in profound hypothermia increases the risk of atelectasis, making subsequent infection possible.
4. Survival in hypothermia varies directly with the severity of cold-induced granulocytopenia [117,132].
5. Evidence from hypothermic animals with induced sepsis indicates an impaired release of PMNs from the marrow [117,133], as well as delayed clearance of staphylococcal [134] and gram-negative organisms [133] from the blood.
6. Ineffective clearance of organisms may permit a continued low-grade bacteremia [134]. Ineffective clearance probably relates to impaired phagocytosis, migration [135], and a decrease in the half-life of circulating PMNs in hypothermia [132].
7. Impaired killing of bacteria by pulmonary alveolar macrophages exposed to cold in vitro has been reported and presumably increases susceptibility to pneumonia. The role of changes in antigen-antibody interactions, known to be impaired by cold in vitro, has not been clearly defined in hypothermic patients. Thus, the hypothermic host is more susceptible to invasion by pathogens and less equipped to defend itself if invasion occurs.

Drug Clearance. Little is known about the clearance of drugs in hypothermic adults. Complex interactions of reduced cardiac output, dehydration, slowed hepatic metabolism, decreased GFR, abnormal renal tubular filtration and reabsorption, and altered protein-drug dissociation constant (pK) must dramatically alter the volume of distribution and total body clearance of many common drugs. In hypothermic piglets, the clearance of gentamicin was significantly prolonged because of a decrease in GFR [136]. The half-life of thiopental has been shown to increase 4 to 11 times at 24°C [40]. Because bile flow may be reduced by up to 75 percent at similar temperatures, excretion of toxins in the bile is also decreased [40].

DIAGNOSIS. The diagnosis of hypothermia may be suggested by a history of exposure or immersion, clinical examination, and laboratory abnormalities. Elderly, alcoholic, diabetic, quadriparetic, or severely debilitated patients are at high risk of hypothermia and should be evaluated quickly. Signs of hypothermia vary with the patient's temperature. Cool skin, muscle rigidity, some degree of shivering or muscle tremor, and acrocyanosis are present in most noncomatose patients. In more obtunded patients, myxedema-type facies have been reported [123,137]. Although mental status changes vary widely among patients, they follow a typical pattern: between 35 and 32°C the patient may be stuporous or confused; between 32 and 27°C the patient may be verbally responsive but incoherent; at temperatures less than 27°C, 83 percent of patients are comatose but able to respond purposefully to noxious stimuli [138]. Muscle tone remains increased to rigid after shivering stops. Reflexes remain normal until body temperature is lower than 27°C, when they become depressed and frequently are absent. Plantar reflexes may be upgoing. The pupillary reflex may be difficult to detect and sluggish below 30°C and may become fixed at temperatures below 27°C. Electrocardiographic changes are almost always present.

In the absence of an accurate temperature, the ECG may be used to gauge the degree of hypothermia [93,95]. J waves become more prominent as temperature decreases and in the absence of a cerebrovascular accident appear to be pathognomonic for hypothermia. Prolonged P–R or Q–T intervals in the presence of muscle tremor artifact and bradycardia strongly suggest the diagnosis. Because of the increased solubility of carbon dioxide and oxygen, blood gases reported at 37°C may show a value of $PO_2 + PCO_2 > 150$ mm Hg on room air, a biochemical impossibility at euthermia. An elevated hematocrit, a good output of dilute urine with hypotension, ileus, and an elevated amylase are helpful but nonspecific indicators of hypothermia.

Because the symptoms of hypothermia frequently mimic those of other disorders, the diagnosis may be missed unless there is a clear history of exposure or an accurate temperature is taken. Thermometers calibrated to record temperatures below 35°C must be used. Unfortunately, unless mercury thermometers are shaken down below 35°C before use, hypothermia may be missed. Electronic temperature probes, available at most hospitals, are excellent for evaluating and following body temperature because they are accurate at low temperatures, may be used in several body sites, have a rapid response time, and can be left indwelling to provide on-line temperature readings during treatment. The lower temperature limit on individual probes must always be checked.

Where the temperature is taken is also important (see Chap. 29). Oral or nasopharyngeal temperatures may not reflect core temperature because of the influence of surrounding airflow; axillary temperatures may be lower than core temperatures because of decreased axillary perfusion and distance from the core. Bladder, rectal, tympanic, esophageal, or great vessel temperatures are preferable. Bladder temperatures have proved both accurate and convenient for initial measurements [139,140]. Tympanic temperature reflects core temperature, but most physicians have little experience measuring it safely and accurately. Great vessel temperature may be measured using the thermistor on a Swan-Ganz catheter. During rewarming, the choice of where temperature measurement is taken must again be considered because the rewarming technique used may affect the measurement. Esophageal temperature is most influenced by the inhalation of warmed air; great vessel temperature is highly influenced by the inhalation of warm air or the infusion of heated fluids; and rectal temperature is greatly influenced by warmed peritoneal dialysis. During extracorporeal rewarming, bladder and pulmonary artery temperatures may increase faster than esophageal and rectal temperatures [140]. It may be helpful to monitor at least two core sites.

DIFFERENTIAL DIAGNOSIS

Causes of Hypothermia. Once hypothermia is diagnosed, the cause is frequently easy to determine. Exposure, hypoglycemia, and alcohol abuse probably account for more than 80 percent of reported cases. The diagnosis of exposure is usually determined by patient history. Hypoglycemia should be suspected more frequently in diabetic and alcoholic patients and is easily evaluated by a glucose test strip or a blood glucose test. Alcohol abuse can usually be determined by history and physical examination and confirmed by measuring a blood ethanol level. Debility, severe congestive heart failure, renal or hepatic failure, quadriplegia, and severe skin diseases or burns are usually apparent on physical examination. A diagnosis of Wernicke's encephalopathy may be difficult to establish in the hypothermic patient, but it should be suspected in anyone with a history of alcohol abuse, ataxia, or abnormal ocular findings, especially bilateral sixth-nerve palsies and paralysis of conjugate gaze. Ocular movement abnormalities are otherwise unusual in hypothermia [138]. Although hypothyroidism and panhypopituitarism are rare causes of hypothermia, the diagnosis may be difficult to make because the clinical presentations are similar [51]. If the patient is male, the disorder presents during a season other than winter, the cholesterol level is low or normal and myxedema facies is absent, hypothyroidism is unlikely as a cause.

Deep coma is an uncommon complication of hypothermia [138], but when present it may be difficult to distinguish from death. Coma with no response to pain from hypothermia alone has not been reported at temperatures above 27°C. In these cases, patients appear motionless, with rigor of all extremities. Blood pressure may be low and difficult to detect because of peripheral vasoconstriction. The pulse is frequently slow and nonpalpable. The EEG at temperatures below 25°C may show only a flat line. J waves on ECG and the presence of tears or saliva have, in difficult cases, suggested that the patient was actually alive [141]. Clearly, criteria for death cannot be applied in patients with these findings until temperature has been restored to near 37°C. Patients have survived without significant sequelae even after 30 minutes of complete arrest [37,89,122].

Hypothermia versus Other Conditions. Clinical changes produced by hypothermia can both mask and mimic other diseases. Rigidity of the cervical musculature may indicate meningitis. The abdomen is frequently boardlike; absent bowel sounds simulate a state of intraabdominal catastrophe. Because shock and coma have broad differential diagnoses, clinical judgment must guide the work-up of these disorders.

Despite wide interpatient variation, deviation from the temperature-symptom relationship should suggest that the cause of a symptom may be other than hypothermia. For example, ventricular fibrillation or coma with a temperature higher than 30°C or shock with a low hematocrit or heme-positive stools should alert the physician to suspect another diagnosis and pursue further diagnostic evaluations. In a patient with hypothermia, especially after vigorous resuscitation attempts, establishing a diagnosis of myocardial infarction can be difficult. Creatine kinase, lactate dehydrogenase, and serum glutamic oxaloacetic acid-transaminase values may be elevated because of hepatic hypoperfusion and presumed skeletal muscle damage. Elevations in both MB and BB fractions of the creatine kinase have been reported in hypothermic patients with no evidence of myocardial or cerebral infarct [86,142]. The ECG changes in hypothermia do not mimic those seen in myocardial infarction. An ECG is therefore a more reliable indicator of myocardial damage than are enzyme elevations in hypothermic patients.

TREATMENT. With immediate appropriate treatment, mortality should be low. Although exact mortality rates have been difficult to determine because of the large number of techniques used to treat hypothermia, accumulated statistics suggest that mortality varies with both the severity of the underlying disease and the temperature at initial examination. The overall mortality rate in a series of city-dwelling hypothermic patients was 12 percent, but this increased to nearly 50 percent if a serious underlying disease was present [29]. In the same series of patients, mortality increased 1.8 percent for each 1°C decrease in temperature on admission. In healthy young mountain climbers, mortality was also found to vary with body core temperature on admission: Mortality was 25 percent for temperatures higher than 32°C versus 66 percent for temperatures lower than 27°C [82]. In patients in Ireland with hypothermia due to exposure there was an overall mortality of 33 percent, and each 5°C drop in ambient temperature was estimated to double the mortality [31]. Multivariate analysis of the risk factors for death in outpatient hypothermia indicates that the strongest predictors of mortality were prehospital cardiac arrest, low or absent blood pressure, elevated BUN, and the need for tracheal intubation or NG tube placement in the emergency department [143]. The Mount Hood tragedy suggests that serum potassium levels above 10 mEq per liter, fibrinogen less than 50 mg per deciliter, and ammonia above 250 mM per liter at the time of diagnosis makes survival unlikely [139]. The higher survival rates in city-dwelling patients are believed to represent the benefits of immediately accessible care. Many experts believe that without treatment mortality in profound hypothermia may approach 100 percent.

Treatment should be aggressive. Functional survival in adults has been reported even after 6.5 hours of CPR [144]. Treatment should always systematically address initial field care and transport, stabilizing cardiopulmonary status, treating the cause of hypothermia, preventing the common complications of hypothermia, and rewarming.

Initial Field Care and Transport. The field management of hypothermia from exposure or immersion is clearly limited but important. Wet clothes should be removed and replaced with dry ones, if available. The victim should be insulated from cold and wind as much as possible with blankets or a sleeping bag. Sharing heat generated by a companion's body in a sleeping bag may slow the drop in the victim's temperature. Drinking hot drinks is no longer encouraged because it may increase hypothermia by producing peripheral vasodilatation through a pharyngeal reflex [145]. Glucose drinks have been advocated, but recent work has shown that glycogen depletion does not impair shivering or rewarming [146]. Because of vasodilation and depression of consciousness, alcohol should never be given.

The decision of when and how to transport the victim requires careful judgment. A number of precautions should be taken. First, patients should not be transported in the upright position because seizures may result, presumably from orthostatic hypotension [33]. Second, rough handling must be avoided because even minor manipulations can induce ventricular fibrillation [101,145,146]. Third, in profound hypothermia, the victim's clothing should be cut off, and a team of many rescuers should carry the victim as gently as possible. Some investigators have argued against performing CPR on these patients because of concern that vital signs that are difficult to obtain may be misinterpreted and that performing unnecessary CPR may induce fibrillation. However, a patient without a blood pressure or palpable pulse may already be fibrillating. We agree with the American Heart Association [147] that patients without pulses or blood pressures should be resuscitated in the usual fashion until adequate ECG and pressure monitoring are available (see Chap. 32).

Stablizing Cardiopulmonary Status. Because early death from hypothermia is due to hypotension and dysrhythmia, the goal of initial in-hospital management of hypothermic patients should be to achieve a safe, stable cardiopulmonary status.

Shock in mild hypothermia is usually due to the dehydration that results from cold diuresis; in more profound hypothermia, it may be cardiogenic. Fluid resuscitation should be attempted in all patients in hypothermic shock. Delivery of fluids through a central, rather than a peripheral, catheter is preferable for several reasons. First, vasoconstriction makes insertion of peripheral intravenous (IV) catheters difficult. Second, vasoconstriction may impair delivery of peripherally injected medications. Third, peripheral IV catheters may cause unnecessary damage to frostbitten extremities. Fourth, central catheter placement permits monitoring of central venous pressure and helps guide fluid management. Because most patients are hemoconcentrated and hyperosmolar, slightly hypotonic crystalloid fluids should be given. Whenever possible, all IV fluids should be warmed to at least room temperature before infusion. If fluid resuscitation fails, pressor agents should be administered. Although pressor agents increase the risk of ventricular fibrillation, they have been used safely in patients with hypothermia [147,148]. The use of arterial and central venous pressure monitors may help guide treatment. Swan-Ganz catheter monitoring may be performed safely and may aid evaluation and treatment [149]. A low systemic vascular resistance in mild to moderate hypothermia strongly suggests infection or sepsis [103]. Although the older literature emphasized that procedures such as intubation or catheter placement may induce ventricular fibrillation, these procedures have been performed safely in numerous hypothermic patients and should not be withheld because of a fear of dysrhythmia. The increased risk of hemorrhage from hypothermia-induced thrombocytopenia and prolongation of bleeding times must, however, be considered when undertaking invasive procedures such as central venous catheter placement or intubation.

The management of dysrhythmias must be approached in a nontraditional manner, because many pharmacologic agents, pacing efforts, and defibrillation attempts do not work in the hypothermic patient [150–152]. Because atrial dysrhythmias and heart block generally resolve spontaneously on rewarming [94,106], therapy is usually unnecessary. For supraventricular tachydysrhythmias, digitalis should be avoided because the efficacy of the drug is unclear in hypothermia and toxicity increases as the patient is warmed [90]. Although calcium channel blockers are frequently used in treating supraventricular tachydysrhythmias in euthermic patients, little is known about their efficacy in hypothermia.

In hypothermic patients experiencing ventricular fibrillation, procainamide has been of little help [40], and lidocaine has been of only modest benefit [148]. Bretylium appears to be the drug of choice [147,153,154]. Experiments in hypothermic dogs indicate that bretylium not only decreases the incidence of ventricular fibrillation but also increases the likelihood of successful cardioversion [155]. Electrical defibrillation should probably be attempted at least once, but it is unlikely to succeed until core temperatures surpass 30°C [37,98,156]. The role of pacing in patients with fibrillation is unclear; because insertion of pacemakers has been associated with the onset of fibrillation, however, they should not be inserted prophylactically in otherwise stable patients. Pacing theoretically may be helpful in asystole, because conductivity in Purkinje fibers has been shown to continue at temperatures as low as 10°C [89]. Although hearts in digitalized dogs have been successfully paced out of hypothermic asystole [90], attempts at pacing human hearts during asystole have failed [157]. If other avenues of support are unavailable, however, pacing should be tried.

Acid-base status and oxygenation should be assessed immediately. This can be done adequately only by obtaining an arterial blood gas measurement (see Chap. 15). Accurate assessment of acid-base status in hypothermic patients is complicated by several issues. First, blood gases measured at 37°C produce different values of pH and PCO_2 than exist in a patient at a lower temperature. Second, normal values for pH and PCO_2 also change with temperature. Third, body buffer systems respond differently at colder temperatures.

When blood is drawn from a hypothermic patient and then rewarmed to and measured at 37°C, the solubility of carbon dioxide decreases, resulting in higher PCO_2 and lower pH values than actually exist [158].

Normal values for pH and PCO_2 also change with temperature. At a temperature of 20°C, a pH of approximately 7.65 permits continued cellular function and this value, not a pH of 7.40, should be regarded as normal. Normal values for arterial carbon dioxide tension ($PaCO_2$) are altered because of the higher content of carbon dioxide in cooled blood, decreased rate of production of carbon dioxide, and slower rate of carbon dioxide elimination from relative alveolar hypoventilation. R values as low as 0.32 have been reported. On balance, these changes result in lower $PaCO_2$ values at colder temperatures.

Temperature changes the pK of chemical reactions and reduces the ionization level of buffer proteins [158]. This produces a smaller effective protein buffer pool and places a greater reliance for buffering on the less efficient carbonic acid system. Because of this less effective buffering, acid-base disturbances that would be well tolerated at 37°C might be poorly tolerated at lower temperatures.

Despite these complex considerations, $PaCO_2$ and pH values uncorrected for temperature may be accurately used to assess the hypothermic patient's acid-base status. Moreover, they enhance the ease of interpretation. Severinghaus [159], Rahn and colleagues [160], and Blayo and associates [161] argued that there is no loss of accuracy because the changes that take place in anaerobically warmed blood parallel and are almost identical to those that occur in the acid-base system in hypothermic patients. On the basis of their analysis, we recommend that blood obtained from a hypothermic patient be evaluated using the values measured at 37°C and interpreted in the usual fashion, and that the traditional values for normal pH and PCO_2 be used for comparison. The use of nomograms to "correct" pH and PCO_2 values to the patient's temperature may be cumbersome and inaccurate. Moreover, once patient temperature-corrected values are obtained, they must be interpreted in comparison with normal values corrected for the patient's temperature. The use of uncorrected blood gases in hypothermic patients intraoperatively has not resulted in any altered morbidity or mortality [162,163,164].

Because of a decrease in the solubility of oxygen on warming the blood to 37°C, arterial oxygen tension (PaO_2) values reported at 37°C may be substantially higher than the actual value in colder patients. Therefore, PO_2 values must be corrected for temperature, or the presence of significant hypoxemia may be overlooked. Several nomograms to permit correction exist [159,165,166,167]. For clinical purposes, the following formula may be used to correct PO_2 for temperature: decrease the PO_2 measured at 37°C by 7.2 percent for each degree that the patient's temperature is below 37°C.

Because the acute respiratory distress syndrome may and pneumonia [47,125] frequently does accompany hypothermia, a chest radiograph should be obtained. Ninety to 100 percent oxygen should be administered until adequate oxygenation has been demonstrated. Oxygen saturation, after correction for temperature, should be maintained at greater than 90 percent to help prevent hypoxic damage. To avoid the prolonged use of high fractional concentrations of oxygen, positive end-expiratory pressure (PEEP) may be necessary [101]. Stuporous or comatose patients should be prophylactically intubated to decrease the risk of aspiration pneumonitis. Blind nasotracheal intubation may be required; orotracheal intubation may be difficult because the mandible may be unmovable as a result of muscle rigidity [150]. If respiratory failure is evident on blood gas analysis, the patient should be intubated and mechanically ventilated. Experiences during hypothermic surgery and in the treatment of unintentional hypothermia indicate that the initial ventilator settings should be similar to those normally used at temperatures of 37°C [159,160] (see Chap. 66).

Treating the Cause of Hypothermia. Diseases known to predispose to hypothermia should be diagnosed and treated early. Hypoglycemia is easily and rapidly detected by a glucose test strip and confirmed by blood glucose value. As a result of the ineffective action of insulin at low temperatures and the relatively high serum osmolarity from water diuresis, serious and difficult to treat hyperosmolarity may result from boluses of high concentrations of glucose [84,106]. Therefore, treatment with highly concentrated glucose solutions should be delayed until some measure of the blood glucose has been obtained. Once hypoglycemia has been documented, the patient should be given 25 to 50 mg of glucose as a 50 percent dextrose solution. Some patients have been reported to shiver on correction of hypoglycemia and to correct their hypothermia rapidly.

The possibility of alcohol or sedative drug use or overdose is usually indicated by history and confirmed by toxicologic screening. No reports indicate adverse effects of naloxone in hypothermia; it should routinely be given if coma is present.

A thorough neurologic examination may suggest CNS or peripheral nervous system disease. If there is a history of trauma, the neck should be stabilized until a cervical spine radiograph has been obtained. Flaccid extremities suggest a cord or peripheral nerve injury. Cerebral edema secondary to tumor may

be seen on funduscopic examination. Treatment with thiamine is benign and should be given routinely in stuporous hypothermic patients until Wernicke's syndrome can be ruled out. Thiamine should be given with glucose if hyperglycemia is absent to decrease the chance of cerebral dysfunction. If the patient has Wernicke's encephalopathy, response to thiamine treatment may be seen within hours; if thiamine is not given, efforts to increase temperature may be futile [57,61]. Cyclic hypothermia responds to ephedrine and naloxone [168,169].

Thyroid hormone should not be given routinely to every patient with hypothermia, because such treatment is potentially harmful and hypothyroid coma is rare. In all cases of suspected myxedema, however, treatment with thyroid hormone is mandatory because it may be lifesaving. Conventional treatment of myxedema hypothermic coma begins with immediate IV administration of 0.2 to 0.5 mg of thyroxine. If the patient has not clearly responded in 24 hours, this dose is repeated and the patient is maintained on 0.05 to 0.1 mg of thyroxine IV daily until clinically stable (see Chap. 112).

Debilitating diseases such as congestive heart failure, sepsis, or hepatic or renal failure should be treated in a conventional manner. Because of the abnormal physiology of hypothermia, aggressive evaluation of these conditions (e.g., with Swan-Ganz catheter monitoring) should always be considered. In diabetic patients, insulin resistance increases rapidly below 30°C; insulin administration should be delayed when possible until the patient's temperature is above 30°C. If insulin is given during hypothermia, it must be administered IV because subcutaneous absorption is impaired by hypoperfusion. Also, insulin should be given in small doses, because its degradation may be delayed at low temperature and cumulative doses may produce hypoglycemia and rebound hypothermia as the patient is warmed.

Preventing Common Complications. Early attention to the prevention, diagnosis, and treatment of diseases commonly associated with hypothermia may significantly reduce morbidity and mortality [170].

Diabetic patients who have both hypothermia and infection have a particularly grave prognosis. In patients with diabetic ketoacidosis, the prevalence of hypothermia was four times higher in those with underlying infection and mortality was three times higher [171]. The possibility of infection should be carefully evaluated in diabetic persons with hypothermia, and early intervention with antibiotics should be considered.

Pneumonia remains a common complication in hypothermic patients who survive the rewarming period. The incidence of pneumonia can probably be reduced by early intubation in stuporous or comatose patients to protect the airway and thereby minimize aspiration. In addition, periodic hyperinflation [105] and attention to pulmonary toilet decrease the incidence of pneumonia in hypothermic patients. Some investigators [47,172] have advocated giving antibiotics prophylactically because pneumonia develops in nearly all patients. The efficacy of this approach has not been demonstrated, however, and the suggestion should be challenged for several reasons. First, the incidence of pneumonia is as low as 13 percent in some series [170]. Second, host defense mechanisms appear to return to normal soon after euthermia is reached. Third, adequate culturing and proper antibiotic selection may be impaired if infection or superinfection subsequently occurs. We recommend giving antibiotics only when infection is likely already to be present. A study demonstrated that a low systemic vascular resistance (SVR) in patients with mild to moderate hypothermia strongly indicates the presence of infection [103]. In these patients, with a mean temperature of 31.7°C, the average SVR was 486 dyne/sec/cm^{-5} and the average cardiac index 2.2 liters per minute. When SVR is low or diabetic ketoacidosis is present, we believe it is reasonable to give broad-spectrum antibiotic coverage for 24 to 48 hours pending results of the culture.

Because pancreatitis and ileus are both commonly associated with hypothermia, a nasogastric tube should be passed, a baseline amylase level should be obtained, and the patient should not be allowed to eat or drink until fully stable.

Prophylaxis of DVT in patients with hypothermia is a difficult issue. Subcutaneous heparin should not be used because it may be poorly absorbed for several days until skin function returns to normal. Pneumatic boots should not be placed on frostbitten extremities. Because of these concerns and because it is not clear that the risk of DVT from hypothermia outweighs that of systemic anticoagulation, we do not routinely recommend prophylaxis for DVT.

Because disseminated intravascular coagulation (DIC) has been reported, baseline clotting studies may be of value. DIC has occurred even in heparinized patients [173]. Electrolyte levels must be carefully followed, because serum potassium levels vary greatly during treatment. Hypermagnesemia reduces temperatures in hypothermic patients with renal failure and should be avoided [174]. Hypophosphatemia must be observed for because it may result from treatment [175].

Acute tubular necrosis has been reported in hypothermia [92], but it is infrequent and probably results from shock and hypoxia, not as a direct action of hypothermia itself. Renal damage may be minimized by careful cardiovascular support.

In cases of exposure, frostbite frequently occurs on the ears, nose, face, penis, scrotum, and extremities. It may be painless and go unrecognized by the victim until he or she is rewarmed. Frostbite is detectable on physical examination because recently frozen tissue usually appears gray, white, or waxy. Soon after warming, the skin may become edematous, blister, or turn red or black because of hemorrhage or necrosis. The extent of damage and eschar formation is usually demarcated within 10 days. Limbs should be handled gently. Thawing frostbitten areas is best postponed until core temperatures have risen to normal and the patient is otherwise stable. It is best accomplished by immersion for 30 to 60 minutes in water heated to 38 to 43°C. After thawing, whirlpool debridement, intraarterial reserpine, and anticoagulation with heparin or dextran may be helpful. Amputation may be necessary but should always be delayed as long as possible to allow a clear demarcation of viable tissue [145].

Because of the risk of relapse, hypothermic patients require prolonged monitoring. Elderly patients who have had one episode of hypothermia may experience relapse and, in addition, may be at greater risk for future hypothermic episodes [176]. Any patient who has sustained severe hypothermia under conditions other than extreme exposure should be monitored closely for recurrent episodes.

Rewarming. Rewarming methods may be divided into three categories: passive external rewarming, active external rewarming, and active central rewarming. These methods vary in level of invasiveness and the usual speed with which they provide rewarming.

PASSIVE EXTERNAL REWARMING. Passive external rewarming is the least invasive and slowest rewarming technique. It requires only that the patient be dry, sheltered from wind, and covered with blankets to decrease heat loss and thereby allow thermogenesis to restore normal temperature. Temperature increase varies inversely with patient age; the average rate of temperature increase with this method is only 0.38°C per hour [86]. Passive rewarming is, therefore, appropriate only when hypothermia is not profound (i.e., when the patient's core temperature is above 30°C).

ACTIVE EXTERNAL REWARMING. Active external rewarming is by far the most controversial method. It involves raising the core temperature by heating the skin with hot blankets, electric heating pads, and hot water bottles, circulating warmed air immediately adjacent to the skin [177,178], or immersion in a tub of warm water. This method works [37,82,145,176,179] and has been successful in patients with temperatures as low as 17°C [180]. Initial reports [177,178] suggest that rewarming by covering the patient with a plastic blanket which contains tubes of circulating heated air is helpful for the mild hypothermia seen in the perioperative setting. Further studies of the efficacy of this technology need to be conducted before it can be advocated for routine use in more severely hypothermic patients. Mortality with active external rewarming, however, appears to be higher than with passive or central rewarming methods [29]. This possible increase in mortality may be due to a number of factors: (1) less accurate control over the rate of temperature increase; (2) increased risk of peripheral vasodilatation and shock from warming the skin before the core; and (3) increased incidence of acidosis resulting from abrupt return of blood to the core from relatively hypoperfused areas. Treatment by immersion is extremely inconvenient and sometimes impossible in patients who require continuous ECG and temperature monitoring, central venous access, and artificial ventilation and who are in imminent danger of shock or arrest. Experience with patients undergoing external rewarming suggests that aggressive hydration and Swan-Ganz catheter monitoring are helpful [152]. Several studies have shown that the further drop in temperature experienced during the initial phase of active external rewarming is mostly independent of circulatory factors and merely reflects the natural physical laws of heat loss [181,182].

ACTIVE CENTRAL REWARMING. The fastest and most invasive warming methods are those designed to permit active central rewarming. Oxygen that has been humidified and heated to 40 to 46°C is a safe [29,183] and effective [180] rewarming technique; it can be delivered by face mask or an endotracheal tube. In the hospital, heated oxygen can be provided with a cascade humidifier, available in many ventilator systems. In other settings, portable systems that involve heat production by carbon dioxide and soda lime have been useful [184]. Temperature must be monitored orally to ensure that inspired air does not exceed 46°C, or mucosal damage or burns might occur. Temperature increase with heated oxygen is usually less than 1°C per hour.

Lavage by gastric or esophageal balloons also produces a slow temperature increase and has been shown to be effective [185]; however, this method involves risk of aspiration and ventricular fibrillation during balloon insertion.

Peritoneal lavage can be performed conveniently at most hospitals, and it safely raises temperatures at a rate of up to 4°C per hour [107,122,141,186,187]. Average warming rates, however, are closer to 2°C per hour. Saline or dialysate fluid is heated to 38 to 43°C and exchanged every 15 to 20 minutes. Alternatively, two peritoneal trochars may be placed and a continuous infusion and drainage circuit established. Pleural lavage with two chest tubes has also been reported and appears effective [188].

Rewarming by radiofrequency heating has been successful in dogs and was found to be faster than peritoneal lavage or inhalational rewarming, but it has yet to be used in humans [189,190]. Even if radio wave rewarming were shown to be safe and effective in humans, because of the cumbersome nature of the equipment it is unlikely to displace other methods of rewarming.

Insertion of femoral artery and vein catheters allows blood to be removed, heated, and returned to the body. This is usually performed with a hemodialysis machine [171] or pump oxygenator such as that used during cardiopulmonary bypass. Rewarming at a rate of 1 to 2°C per hour has been reported by passing the blood from a surgically created arteriovenous fistula through a countercurrent fluid warmer with [191] or without [192,193] a roller pump. In patients with severe cardiopulmonary collapse, a pump oxygenator offers the advantage of hemodynamic support, rapid elevation of temperature, and nearly complete regulation of acid-base and oxygen disorders [92,101,139,146,154,194,195]. In cases of profound hypothermia, a median sternotomy approach may be preferable because of the possibilities of direct cardiac massage, improved blood flow, and easy access [139].

The desired rate of rewarming varies according to the patient's cardiopulmonary status and underlying disease. Results of experiments performed on hypothermic dogs suggest that if intramyocardial temperature gradients can be maintained at less than 2°C, the risk of fibrillation decreases [98]. This research argues that safe warming should be either slow enough to allow uniformity in tissue temperatures or fast enough to minimize the period of risk. Slower warming techniques allow a prolonged period of hypothermia and presumably should produce a higher risk of infection because of prolonged immune suppression and a higher incidence of acid-base and intravascular volume problems. A diagnosis of diabetes or myxedema may also influence the desired rate of rewarming. In diabetic ketoacidosis, for example, insulin resistance and the severity of the acidosis could be substantially improved by rapid rewarming, and a more active rewarming technique might therefore be preferred [123].

Iatrogenic and Intentional Hypothermia

Both iatrogenic and intentional types of hypothermia occur frequently in surgical recovery rooms and intensive care units [196–201]. Iatrogenic hypothermia results from the infusion of blood products or fluids at lower than body core temperatures [196,202] and from anesthesia and surgery performed in cool operating rooms [42,43,198,203]. Intentional hypothermia has been induced by partial immersion or surface or central cooling techniques to treat cancer [204], limit the toxicity of sepsis [205,206], help prevent the alopecia of chemotherapy [207], retard surgical and posttraumatic brain injury [208], reduce carbon dioxide production in refractory status asthmaticus [209], assist in the amputation of limbs, and minimize the hypoperfusion injury associated with cardiothoracic surgery; it is now commonly used only to assist in cardiothoracic surgery. A detailed review of the evolution of anesthetic practices for hypothermic surgery or the management of specific classes of postoperative patients is beyond the scope of this chapter. Discussion is limited to those problems that are most pertinent to the intensive care physician.

CAUSES AND PATHOGENESIS. Perioperative hypothermia results from increased heat loss, decreased heat production, and compromised thermoregulation. Heat loss may be increased by loss of behavioral control mechanisms, decreased insulation because of exposure of larger skin surfaces, cutaneous vasodilatation resulting from anesthetics, increased evaporative losses from serosal surfaces and volatile antiseptics applied to skin, and exposure to air-conditioned environments. Decreased heat production results from muscular paralysis. Impaired thermoregulation results from slowed or compromised

afferent and efferent nerve impulses and hypothermic reflexes due to sedative anesthetics.

The frequency and severity of heat loss increases with patient age [196,198,200], open chest or abdominal surgery [196,198,210], low operating room temperature [42,43], length of surgery [197], infusion of cool IV solutions, and certain types of anesthetics. Elderly patients experience a decrease in temperature, shiver less frequently, and take longer to rewarm than younger patients [196,200]. Temperature decrease during surgery involving open body cavities may result in almost twice the decrease in temperature seen in extremity surgery [198]. Lightly anesthetized, paralyzed, draped patients provided with no active warming experience a temperature decrease of 0.3°C per hour at ambient temperatures less than 21°C [43]. Surgery involving muscle paralysis with curare-type agents produces twice the temperature decrease of nonparalyzing procedures [198]. Although halothane and epidural anesthesia may increase heat loss because of vasodilatation [211], no major differences have been detected in the heat loss from most inhalational agents [198,200].

Massive infusion of chilled solutions can induce hypothermia, as heat loss from infusion of room temperature solutions approximates 16 kcal per liter [200]. Blood infused at its stored temperature of 4°C produces a heat loss of 32 kcal per liter [202]. In an average human, infusion of 1 liter of 4°C blood produces a 0.5°C decrease in temperature [196]. The mean temperature of patients given more than 20 units of blood in 24 hours has been reported to be 32.9 ± 1.7°C [80]. Although most of these patients had multiple reasons to develop hypothermia, the rapid transfusion of blood not warmed to body temperature must be considered a risk factor for the development of mild hypothermia. The mean temperature of survivors and nonsurvivors after massive transfusion was no different.

Although subnormal temperatures occur frequently during the postoperative period, frank hypothermia (temperature less than 35°C) is uncommon. In one series of 101 patients undergoing elective surgery under general anesthesia, 78 percent had temperatures below 36°C. The average temperature decrease was 0.77°C and maximal decrease was 2.5°C [198]. In a similar series of 195 patients who underwent noncardiothoracic surgery, 60 percent had temperatures below 36°C, 29 percent below 35.5°C, and 13 percent below 35°C [202]. Alternatively, postoperative cardiac surgery patients are more likely to fall into the true hypothermic classification. Intentional hypothermia on cardiopulmonary bypass produces intraoperative temperatures in the range of 24°C. Despite rewarming to 37°C or higher before terminating bypass, patients experience an average temperature decrease of 2.6°C during the next 80 minutes [212].

PATHOPHYSIOLOGY. Perioperative complications from mild hypothermia arise from the hypermetabolism triggered by the patient's efforts to restore body temperature. From the preceding in-depth discussion of patients with noniatrogenic, unintentional hypothermia, it is reasonable to suspect that an otherwise healthy individual with a temperature ranging from 34 to 36°C should do well and should have (1) a slightly increased cardiac output, (2) an oxygen consumption up to five times basal levels, (3) an elevated systemic vascular resistance because of peripheral vasoconstriction, (4) a decrease in mixed venous oxygen saturation because of increased oxygen extraction, (5) shivering or muscle rigidity, and (6) a slightly depressed mental status. The $P(A-a)O_2$ gradient and even arteriovenous oxygen difference [103] may be in the normal range [152]. Therefore, deviations from this pattern in the perioperative period and subsequent morbidity must reflect the additive effects of surgery and anesthesia on metabolism.

Alternatively, in critically ill postoperative patients with cardiac depression, one must be most concerned about the potential effects of mild hypothermia, because an increase in oxygen consumption could easily lead to acidosis and hypoxemia. Although acidosis results from an increase in anaerobic metabolism as metabolic demand outstrips oxygen delivery, minute ventilation is usually maintained to the degree necessary to preserve acid-base balance [212]. Hypoxemia may result from the combination of increased pulmonary parenchymal shunt (venous admixture) after surgery and lower mixed venous PO_2. In one study, shivering appeared to be accompanied by a drop in PO_2; arterial oxygen saturation fell below 90 percent in 53 percent of shivering patients and remained above 90 percent in all nonshivering patients [212]. However, the authors provided little information about inspired oxygen concentrations, raising the possibility that PO_2 may have been significantly improved by merely increasing the concentration of inspired oxygen. Although decreased temperature and shivering can elevate oxygen consumption and in some patients lower PO_2 [200,213], the clinical consequences of these physiologic changes remain obscure. One might speculate that the acidosis and hypoxemia from shivering in mild hypothermia might lead to an increased incidence of dysrhythmia, hypoxic cerebral damage, or myocardial infarction, but no study to date has demonstrated a clear increase in mortality or morbidity in this hypothermic patient group.

PREVENTION AND TREATMENT. Patients with prolonged postoperative hypothermia have a higher mortality than those who return to normal temperatures in the first postoperative hour [214]. It is unclear whether this is due to severe underlying metabolic derangements that slowed rewarming or the consequences of the hypothermia. In either case, efforts to prevent hypothermia and speed rewarming appear indicated.

Numerous interventions have been attempted to minimize perioperative temperature decrease and shivering. The use of warming blankets alone does not prevent significant temperature loss because the body surface area exposed to heat is small [201,203,204,215]. The use of warming blankets plus heating of all infused liquids can maintain average temperature on arrival in the recovery room above 36°C [215]. Heating the carbon dioxide used for laparoscopic insufflation to 30 to 30.5°C decreases the heat loss associated with laparoscopic procedures [216]. Crystalloids can be easily warmed in a microwave oven to 39°C in 2 minutes [217]. For surgery on extremities or neurosurgery, a G-suit apparatus, which circulates warm water over most of the skin surface, has also been effective [218]. The inhalation of heated, humidified air can be safely applied to most intubated patients and is effective in preventing temperature loss [201,213,219–222] and shivering [213]. Although nitroprusside started intraoperatively during cardiopulmonary bypass may limit postbypass temperature decrease by distributing body heat more favorably [223], it must be used cautiously and titrated carefully because hypothermia may increase the toxicity of nitroprusside [224]. In already hypothermic patients, sedation with morphine decreases oxygen consumption and shivering but lengthens the rewarming period [225,226,227]. When started during bypass, the infusion of dopamine and lidocaine has reversed hypothalamic cardiovascular depression in animals. This improvement was equivalent to rewarming by as much as 5°C [151].

All patients undergoing surgery should be observed closely for the development of hypothermia. Simple measures, such as minimizing preoperative and postoperative time in chilled rooms, covering the patient with drapes or blankets whenever possible, and infusing all solutions at least at room temperature, should be taken in all patients. Special measures should be taken in high-risk patients. Groups of patients at high risk of hypothermia include those undergoing major abdominal or cardiothoracic surgery, surgery involving intentional hypothermia, or surgery with anesthesia times in excess of 4 hours; patients older than 60 years of age undergoing surgery; patients with known or expected cardiac depression who are undergoing surgery. In these high-risk patients, preventive measures, including the use of warming blankets, heating of infused solutions to 37.5°C, and inhalation of heated humidified oxygen, should be beneficial. In any patient undergoing any type of extracorporeal bypass, the addition of a heat exchanger to the bypass circuit is simple and effective [228]. Blood and colloid solutions may be safely heated to 37.5°C [229,230]. These measures have been shown to be safe and effective in numerous clinical series and can provide the patient potential benefit at little cost or change in perioperative routine. Esophageal heat exchangers have been ineffective in preventing perioperative hypothermia [231]. The routine use of morphine, nitroprusside, or dopamine solely to regulate temperatures cannot be advocated, however, until further clinical experience is gained in their use for temperature regulation and until the clinical significance of mild temperature decreases in the postoperative patient is clarified.

References

1. Dinarello CA, Wolff SM: Pathogenesis of fever in man. *N Engl J Med* 298:607, 1978.
2. Iampietro PF, Vaughn JA, Goldman RF, et al: Heat production from shivering. *J Appl Physiol* 15:632, 1960.
3. Hensel H: *Thermoreception and Temperature Regulation*. New York, Academic, 1981.
4. Himms-Hagen J: Thermogenesis in adipose tissue as an energy buffer. *N Engl J Med* 311:1549, 1984.
5. Hardy JD, Bard P: Body temperature regulation, in Mountcastle VB (ed): *Medical Physiology*. St Louis, CV Mosby, 1974, p 1305.
6. Hammel HT: Regulation of internal body temperature. *Annu Rev Physiol* 30:641, 1968.
7. Cabanac M: Temperature regulation. *Annu Rev Physiol* 37:415, 1975.
8. Myers RD: The role of hypothalamic transmitter factors in the control of body temperature, in Hardy JD, Gagge AP, Stolwijk JAJ (eds): *Physiological and Behavioral Temperature Regulation*. Springfield, IL, Thomas Books, 1970, p 648.
9. Feldberg W, Myers RD: A new concept of temperature regulation by amines in the hypothalamus. *Nature* 200:1325, 1963.
10. Lomax P, Schonbaum E, Jacob J (eds): *Temperature Regulation and Drug Action*. New York, Karger, 1975.
11. Hardy JD, Gagge AP, Stolwijk JAJ (eds): *Physiological and Behavioral Temperature Regulation*. Springfield, IL, Thomas Books, 1970.
12. Cox B, Kerwin R, Lee TF: Dopamine receptors in central thermoregulatory pathways of the rat. *J Physiol* 282:471, 1978.
13. Burke RE, Fahn S, Mayeaux R, et al: Neuroleptic malignant syndrome caused by dopamine-depleting drugs in a patient with Huntington's disease. *Neurology (NY)* 31:1022, 1981.
14. Henderson VW, Wooten GF: Neuroleptic malignant syndrome: A pathogenetic role for dopamine receptor blockade? *Neurology (NY)* 31:132, 1981.
15. Tollefson GD, Garvey MJ: The neuroleptic syndrome and central dopamine metabolites. *J Clin Psychopharmacol* 4:150, 1984.
16. Sechi GP, Tanda F, Mutani R: Fatal hyperpyrexia after withdrawal of levodopa. *Neurology (NY)* 34:249, 1984.
17. Gale CG: Neuroendocrine aspects of thermoregulation. *Annu Rev Physiol* 35:391, 1973.

18. Wagner JA, Robinson S, Marino RP: Age and temperature regulation of humans in neutral and cold environments. *J Appl Physiol* 37:562, 1974.
19. Collins KJ, Dore C, Exton-Smith AN, et al: Accidental hypothermia and impaired temperature homeostasis in the elderly. *Br Med J* 1:353, 1977.
20. Ellis FP, Exton-Smith AN, Foster KG, et al: Eccrine sweating and mortality during heat waves in very young and very old persons. *Isr J Med Sci* 12:815, 1976.
21. Whittle JL, Bates JH: Thermoregulatory failure secondary to acute illness: Complications and treatment. *Arch Intern Med* 139:418, 1979.
22. Wilson MM, Curley FJ, Larrivee GK, Irwin RS. Hypothermia in critical care units. *Am Rev Respir Dis* 143:A475, 1991.
23. Goldman A, Exton-Smith AN, Francis G, et al: A pilot study of low body temperatures in old people admitted to hospital. *J R Coll Physicians Lond* 11:291, 1977.
24. Fox RH, Woodward PM, Exton-Smith AN, et al: Body temperature in the elderly: A national study of physiological, social, and environmental conditions. *Br Med J* 1:200, 1983.
25. Keilson L, Lambert D, Fabian D, et al: Screening for hypothermia in the ambulatory elderly: The Maine experience. *JAMA* 254:1781, 1985.
26. Hypothermia. *MMWR* 32:46, 1983.
27. Rango N: Exposure-related hypothermia mortality in the United States, 1970–1979. *Am J Public Health* 74:1159, 1984.
28. Kurtz KJ: Hypothermia in the elderly: The cold facts. *Geriatrics* 37:85, 1982.
29. Miller JW, Danzl DF, Thomas DM: Urban accidental hypothermia: 135 cases. *Ann Emerg Med* 9:456, 1980.
30. Mathews JA: Accidental hypothermia. *Postgrad Med* 43:662, 1967.
31. Herity B, Daly L, Bourke GJ, et al: Hypothermia and mortality and morbidity: A epidemiological analysis. *J Epidemiol Community Health* 45:19, 1991.
32. Pugh LGCE: Accidental hypothermia in walkers, climbers and campers: Reports to the medical commission on accident prevention. *Br Med J* 1:123, 1966.
33. Milner JE: Hypothermia. *Ann Intern Med* 89:565, 1978.
34. Hayward JS, Eckerson JD, Collis ML: Thermal balance and survival time prediction of man in cold water. *Can J Physiol Pharmacol* 53:21, 1974.
35. Davidson M, Grant E: Accidental hypothermia: A community hospital perspective. *Postgrad Med* 70:42, 1981.
36. Fitzgerald FT: Hypoglycemia and accidental hypothermia in an alcoholic population. *West J Med* 133:105, 1980.
37. Jessen K, Hagelsten JO: Search and rescue service in Denmark with special reference to accidental hypothermia. *Aerospace Med* 43:787, 1972.
38. Raheja R, Puri BK, Schaeffer RC: Shock due to profound hypothermia and alcohol ingestion. *Crit Care Med* 9:644, 1984.
39. Myers RD: Alcohol's effect on body temperature: Hypothermia, hyperthermia or poikilothermia? *Brain Res Bull* 7:209, 1981.
40. Vandam LD, Burnap TK: Hypothermia. *N Engl J Med* 261:546, 1959.
41. Duff RS, Farrant PC, Leveaux VM, et al: Spontaneous periodic hypothermia. *Q J Med* 30:329, 1961.
42. Morris RH: Operating room temperature and the anesthetized, paralyzed patient. *Arch Surg* 102:95, 1971.
43. Morris RH, Wilkey BR: The effects of ambient temperature on patient temperature during surgery not involving body cavities. *Anesthesiology* 32:102, 1972.
44. Hassel B: Acute hypothermia due to penicillin. *Br Med J* 304:882, 1992.
45. Hassel B: Hypothermia from erythromycin. *Ann Intern Med* 115:69, 1991.
46. Pfeiffer RF: Bromocriptine induced hypothermia. *Neurology* 40:383, 1990
47. Fitzgerald FT, Jessop C: Accidental hypothermia: A report of 23 cases and review of the literature. *Adv Intern Med* 27:128, 1982.
48. Freinkel N, Metzger BE, Harris E, et al: The hypothermia of hypoglycemia: Studies with 2-deoxy-d-glucose in normal human subjects and mice. *N Engl J Med* 287:841, 1972.
49. Gale EAM, Bennett T, Green JH, et al: Hypoglycemia, hypothermia and shivering in man. *Clin Sci* 61:463, 1981.
50. Hardy JD, Bard P: *Body Temperature Regulation in Medical Physiology.* St Louis, CV Mosby, 1974, p 1305.
51. Forrester CF: Coma in myxedema. *Arch Intern Med* 111:100, 1963.
52. Hamburger S, Collier RE: Myxedema coma. *Ann Emerg Med* 11:156, 1982.
53. Branch EF, Burger PC, Brewer DL: Hypothermia in a case of hypothalamic infarction and sarcoidosis. *Arch Neurol* 25:245, 1971.
54. Kearsley JH, Musso AF: Hypothermia and coma in the Wernicke-Korsakoff syndrome. *Med J Aust* 2:504, 1980.
55. Koeppen AH, Daniels JC, Baroron KD: Subnormal body temperatures in Wernicke's encephalopathy. *Arch Neurol* 21:493, 1969.
56. Hansen B, Larsson C, Wiren J, et al: Hypothermia and infection in Wernicke's encephalopathy. *Acta Med Scand* 215:185, 1984.
57. Ackerman WJ: Stupor, bradycardia, hypotension and hypothermia: A presentation of Wernicke's encephalopathy with rapid response to thiamine. *West J Med* 121:428, 1974.
58. Philip G, Smith JF: Hypothermia and Wernicke's encephalopathy. *Lancet* 2:122, 1973.
59. Donnan GA, Seeman E: Coma and hypothermia in Wernicke's encephalopathy. *Aust NZ J Med* 10:438, 1980.
60. Mechlenburg RS, Loriaux DL, Thompson RH, et al: Hypothalamic dysfunction in patients with anorexia nervosa. *Medicine* 53:147, 1974.
61. Shapir WR, Williams GH, Plum F: Spontaneous recurrent hypothermia accompany agenesis of the corpus callosum. *Brain* 92:423, 1969.
62. Summers GD, Young AC, Little RA, et al: Spontaneous periodic hypothermia with lipoma of the corpus callosum. *J Neurol Neurosurg Psychiatry* 44:1094, 1981.
63. Lammens M, Lissoir F, Carton H: Hypothermia in three patients with multiple sclerosis. *Clin Neurol Neurosurg* 91:117, 1989.
64. Sullivan F, Hutchinson M, Bahandeka S, et al: Chronic hypothermia in multiple sclerosis. *J Neurol Neurosurg Psychiatry* 50:813, 1987.
65. Randall WC, Wurster RD, Lewin RJ: Responses of patients with high spinal transection to high ambient temperatures. *J Appl Physiol* 21:985, 1966.
66. Pledger HG: Disorders of temperature regulation in acute traumatic tetraplegia. *J Bone Joint Surg* 44B:110, 1962.
67. Altus P, Hickman JW, Nord J: Accidental hypothermia in a healthy quadriplegic patient. *Neurology* 35:427, 1985.
68. Krook G: Hypothermia in patients with exfoliative dermatitis. *Acta Derm Venereol* 40:142, 1960.
69. Grice KA, Bettley FR: Skin water loss and accidental hypothermia in psoriasis, ichthyosis, and erythroderma. *Br Med J* 2:195, 1967.
70. Moncrief JA: Burns. *N Engl J Med* 288:444, 1973.
71. Roe CF, Kinney JM, Blair C: Water and heat exchange in third-degree burns. *Surgery* 56:212, 1964.
72. Stoner HB: Mechanism of body temperature changes after burns and other injuries. *Ann NY Acad Sci* 150:722, 1968.
73. Buggini RV: Hypothermia in Hodgkin's disease. *N Engl J Med* 312:244, 1985.
74. Weens JH, Hernandez B: Hypothermia following chemotherapy for Hodgkin's disease. *Cancer Treat Rep* 70:313, 1986.
75. Csuka ME, McCarty DJ: Transient hypothermia after corticosteroid treatment of subacute cutaneous lupus erythematosus. *J Rheumatol* 11:112, 1984.
76. Kugler SL, Costakos DT, Aron AM, et al: Hypothermia and systemic lupus erythematosus. *J Rheumatol* 17:680, 1990.
77. Doherty N, Ades A, Shah PK, et al: Hypothermia with acute myocardial infarction. *Ann Intern Med* 101:797, 1984.
78. Luna GK, Maier RV, Pavlin EG, et al: Incidence and effect of hypothermia in seriously injured patients. *J Trauma* 27:1014, 1987.
79. Jurkovich GJ, Greiser WB, Luterman A: Hypothermia in trauma victims: An ominous predictor of survival. *J Trauma* 27:1019, 1987.
80. Wilson RF, Dulchavsky SA, Soullier G, et al: Problems with 20 or more blood transfusions in 24 hours. *Am Surg* 53:410, 1987.
81. Iampietro PF, Faughn JA, Goldman RF, et al: Heat production from shivering. *J Appl Physiol* 15:632, 1960.
82. Martyn JW: Diagnosing and treating hypothermia. *Can Med Assoc J* 125:1089, 1981.
83. Michenfelder JD, Uihlein A, Daw EF, Theye RA: Moderate hypothermia in man: Hemodynamic and metabolic effects. *Br J Anaesth* 37:738, 1965.

84. Stoner HB, Frayn KN, Little RA, et al: Metabolic aspects of hypothermia in the elderly. *Clin Sci* 59:19, 1980.

85. Cohen DJ, Cline JR, Lepinski SM, et al: Resuscitation of the hypothermic patient. *Am J Emerg Med* 6:475, 1988.

86. MacLean D, Griffiths PD, Browning MCK, et al: Metabolic aspects of spontaneous rewarming in accidental hypothermia and hypothermic myxoedema. *Q J Med* 43:371, 1974.

87. Cooper KE: The circulation in hypothermia. *Br Med Bull* 17:48, 1961.

88. Trevino A, Rasi B, Beller BM: The characteristic electrocardiogram of accidental hypothermia. *Arch Intern Med* 127:470, 1971.

89. Southwick FS, Dalglish PH: Recovery after prolonged asystolic cardiac arrest in profound hypothermia. *JAMA* 243:1250, 1980.

90. Angelakos ET, Torres J, Driscoll R: Ouabain on the hypothermic dog heart. *Am Heart J* 56:458, 1958.

91. Bjornstad H, Tande PM, Refsum H: Cardiac electrophysiology during hypothermia and implications for medical treatment. *Arct Med Res* 50(suppl):71, 1991.

92. Kugelberg J, Schuller H, Berg B, et al: Treatment of accidental hypothermia. *Scand J Thorac Cardiovasc Surg* 1:142, 1967.

93. Thompson R, Rich J, Chmelik F, et al: Evolutionary changes in the electrocardiogram of severe progressive hypothermia. *J Electrocardiol* 10:67, 1977.

94. Rankin AC, Rae AP: Cardiac arrhythmias during rewarming of patients with accidental hypothermia. *Br Med J* 289:874, 1984.

95. Clements SD, Hurst JW: Diagnostic value of electrocardiographic abnormalities observed in subjects accidentally exposed to cold. *Am J Cardiol* 29:729, 1972.

96. Abbott JA, Cheitlin MD: The non-specific camel hump sign. *JAMA* 235:413, 1976.

97. DeSweit J: Changes simulating hypothermia in the electrocardiogram in subarachnoid hemorrhage. *J Electrocardiol* 5:193, 1972.

98. Mouritzen CV, Andersen MN: Myocardial temperature gradients and ventricular fibrillation during hypothermia. *J Thorac Cardiovasc Surg* 49:937, 1965.

99. Lomsky M, Ekroth R, Poupa O: The calcium paradox and its protection by hypothermia in human myocardium. *Eur Heart J* 4(suppl):139, 1983.

100. Hervey GR: Hypothermia. *Proc R Soc Med* 66:1055, 1973.

101. Althaus U, Aeberhard T, Schupbach P, et al: Management of profound accidental hypothermia with cardiorespiratory arrest. *Ann Surg* 195:492, 1982.

102. Zarins CK, Skinner DB: Circulation in profound hypothermia. *J Surg Res* 14:97, 1973.

103. Morris DL, Chambers HF, Morris MG, et al: Hemodynamic characteristics of patients with hypothermia due to occult infection and other causes. *Ann Intern Med* 102:153, 1985.

104. Blair E, Esmond WG, Attar S, et al: The effect of hypothermia on lung function. *Ann Surg* 160:814, 1964.

105. Hedley-Whyte J, Pontoppidan H, Laver MB, et al: Arterial oxygenation during hypothermia. *Anesthesiology* 26:595, 1965.

106. Rosenfeld JB: Acid-base and electrolyte disturbances in hypothermia. *Am J Cardiol* 12:678, 1963.

107. Pickering BG, Bristow GK, Craig DB: Core rewarming by peritoneal irrigation in accidental hypothermia with cardiac arrest. *Anesth Analg* 56:574, 1977.

108. Norwood WI, Norwood CR: Influence of hypothermia on intracellular pH during anoxia. *Am J Physiol* 243:C62, 1982.

109. Michenfelder JD, Theye RA: Hypothermia: Effect on canine brain and whole-body metabolism. *Anesthesiology* 29:1107, 1965.

110. Norwood WI, Norwood CR, Castaneda AR: Cerebral anoxia: Effect of deep hypothermia and pH. *Surgery* 86:203, 1979.

111. Russ W, Kling D, Lofsevitz A, et al: Effect of hypothermia on visual evoked potentials (VEP) in humans. *Anesthesiology* 61:207, 1984.

112. FitzGibbon T, Hayward JS, Walker D: EEG and visual evoked potentials of conscious man during moderate hypothermia. *Encephalogr Clin Neurophysiol* 58:48, 1984.

113. Stockard JJ, Sharbrough FW, Tinker JA: Effects of hypothermia on the human brainstem auditory response. *Ann Neurol* 3:368, 1978.

114. Marshall NK, Donchin E: Circadian variation in the latency of brainstem responses and its relation to body temperature. *Science* 212:356, 1981.

115. Maclean D, Griffiths PD, Emslie-Smith D: Serum-enzymes in relation to electrocardiographic changes in accidental hypothermia. *Lancet* 2:1266, 1968.

116. Blair E: A physiologic classification of clinical hypothermia. *Surgery* 58:607, 1965.

117. Doherty P, Bohn D, Bigger D: Hyperthermia and neutrophil dysfunction: Clinical and experimental observations. *Crit Care Med* 12:233, 1984.

118. Kanter GS: Hypothermic hemoconcentration. *Am J Physiol* 214:856, 1968.

119. Poulos ND, Mollitt DL: The nature and reversibility of hypothermia-induced alterations in blood viscosity. *J Trauma* 31:996, 1991.

120. O'Brien H, Ames JAL, Mollin LD: Recurrent thrombocytopenia, erythroid hypoplasia and sideroblastic anaemia associated with hypothermia. *Br J Haematol* 51:451, 1982.

121. Thomas RT, Hessel EA, Harker LA, et al: Platelet function during and after deep surface hypothermia. *J Surg Res* 31:314, 1981.

122. Schissler P, Parker MA, Scott SJ: Profound hypothermia: Value of prolonged cardiopulmonary resuscitation. *South Med J* 74:474, 1981.

123. Maclean D, Murison J, Griffiths PD: Acute pancreatitis and diabetic keto-acidosis in accidental hypothermia and hypothermic myxoedema. *Br Med J* 4:757, 1973.

124. Hirvonen J, Huttunen P: Increased urinary concentration of catecholamines in hypothermia deaths. *J Forensic Sci* 27:264, 1982.

125. Mant AK: Autopsy diagnosis of accidental hypothermia. *J Forensic Med* 16:126, 1969.

126. Baum D, Dillard DH, Porte D: Inhibition of insulin release in infants undergoing deep hypothermic cardiovascular surgery. *N Engl J Med* 279:1309, 1968.

127. Curry DL, Curry KP: Hypothermia and insulin secretion. *Endocrinology* 87:750, 1970.

128. O'Malley BP, Davies TJ, Rosenthal FD: TSH responses to temperature in primary hypothyroidism. *Clin Endocrinol* 13:87, 1980.

129. Maclean D, Browning MC: Plasma 11-hydroxycorticosteroid concentrations and prognosis in accidental hypothermia. *Resuscitation* 52:249, 1974.

130. Woolff PD, Hollander CS, Mitsuma T, et al: Accidental hypothermia: Endocrine function during recovery. *J Clin Endocrinol Metab* 34:460, 1972.

131. Gibbs DM: Inhibition of corticotropin release during hypothermia: The role of corticotropin-releasing factor, vasopressin, and oxytocin. *Endocrinology* 116:723, 1985.

132. Bohn D, Baker C, Kent G, et al: Accidental and induced hypothermia: Effects on neutrophil migration in vivo. *Crit Care Med* 129:A112, 1984.

133. Fedor EJ, Fisher ER, Lee SH, et al: Effect of hypothermia upon induced bacteremia. *Proc Soc Exp Biol Med* 93:510, 1956.

134. deGuzman VC, Webb WR, Grogan JB: The effect of hypothermia on clearance of staphylococcal bacteremia. *Clin Res* 10:58, 1962.

135. Biggar WD, Bohn DJ, Kent G, et al: Neutrophil migration in vitro and in vivo during hypothermia. *Infect Immun* 46:857, 1984.

136. Koren G, Barker C, Bohn D, et al: Influence of hypothermia on the pharmacokinetics of gentamicin and theophylline in piglets. *Crit Care Med* 13:844, 1985.

137. Rosin AJ, Exton-Smith AN: Clinical features of accidental hypothermia, with some observations on thyroid function. *Br Med J* 1:16, 1964.

138. Fischbeck KH, Simon RP: Neurological manifestations of accidental hypothermia. *Ann Neurol* 10:384, 1981.

139. Hauty MG, Esrig BC, Hill JG, et al: Prognostic factors in severe accidental hypothermia: Experience from the Mt. Hood tragedy. *J Trauma* 27:1107, 1987.

140. Lilly JK, Boland JP, Zekan S: Urinary bladder temperature monitoring: A new index of body core temperature. *Crit Care Med* 8:742, 1980.

141. Edwards HA, Benstead JG, Brown K, et al: Apparent death with accidental hypothermia. *Br J Anaesth* 42:906, 1970.

142. Buris L, Debreczeni L: The elevation of serum creatine phosphokinase (CPK) at induced hypothermia. *Forensic Sci Int* 20:35, 1982.

143. Danzl DF, Hedges JR, Pozos RS: Hypothermia outcome score: development and implications. *Crit Care Med* 17:227, 1989.

144. Lexow K: Severe accidental hypothermia: Survival after 6 hours 30 minutes of cardiopulmonary resuscitation. *Arct Med Res* 50(suppl):112, 1991.

145. Bangs C, Hamelt M: Out in the cold: Management of hypothermia, immersion and frostbite. *Top Emerg Med* 2:19, 1980.
146. Neufer PD, Young AJ, Sawka MN, et al: Influence of skeletal muscle glycogen on passive rewarming after hypothermia. *J Appl Physiol* 65:805, 1988.
147. Carden D, Doan L, Sweeney PJ, et al: Hypothermia. *Ann Emerg Med* 11:497, 1982.
148. Towne WD, Geiss WP, Yanes HO, et al: Intractable ventricular fibrillation associated with profound accidental hypothermia: Successful treatment with partial cardiopulmonary bypass. *N Engl J Med* 287:1135, 1972.
149. Steinman AM: Cardiopulmonary resuscitation and hypothermia. *Circulation* 74:IV-29, 1986.
150. DaVee TS, Reineberg EJ: Extreme hypothermia and ventricular fibrillation. *Ann Emerg Med* 9:100, 1980.
151. Nicodemus HF, Chaney RD, Herold R: Hemodynamic effects of inotropes during hypothermia and rapid rewarming. *Crit Care Med* 9:325, 1981.
152. Harari A, Regnier B, Rapin M, et al: Haemodynamic study of prolonged deep accidental hypothermia. *Eur J Intens Care Med* 1:65, 1975.
153. Danzl DF, Sowers MB, Vicario SJ, et al: Chemical ventricular defibrillation in severe accidental hypothermia. *Ann Emerg Med* 11:698, 1982.
154. Dronen S, Nowak RM, Tomlanovich MC: Bretylium tosylate and hypothermic ventricular fibrillation. *Ann Emerg Med* 9:335, 1980.
155. Buckley JJ, Bosch OK, Bacaner MB: Prevention of ventricular fibrillation during hypothermia with bretylium tosylate. *Anesth Analg* 50:587, 1971.
156. Alexander L: *The Treatment of Shock from Prolonged Exposure to Cold, Especially in Water.* London, Combined Intelligence Objectives Subcommittee, APO 413, CIOS Item 24, HMSO, 1945.
157. Truscott DG, Frior WB, Clein LJ: Accidental profound hypothermia: Successful resuscitation by core rewarming and assisted circulation. *Arch Surg* 106:216, 1973.
158. Reeves RB: Temperature-induced changes in blood acid-base status: pH and PCO_2 in a binary buffer. *J Appl Physiol* 40:752, 1976.
159. Severinghaus JW: Respiration and hypothermia. *Ann NY Acad Sci* 80:384, 1959.
160. Rhan H, Reeves RB, Howell BJ: Hydrogen ion regulation, temperature, and evolution. *Am Rev Respir Dis* 112:165, 1975.
161. Blayo MC, Lecompte Y, Pocidalo JJ: Control of acid-base status during hypothermia in man. *Respir Physiol* 42:287, 1980.
162. Ream AK, Reitz BA, Silverberg G: Temperature correction of PCO_2 and pH in estimating acid-base status: An example of the emperor's new clothes? *Anesthesiology* 56:41, 1982.
163. Kroncke GM, Nichols RD, Mendenhall JT, et al: Ectothermic philosophy of acid-base balance to prevent fibrillation during hypothermia. *Arch Surg* 121:303, 1986.
164. Swain JA: Hypothermia and blood pH. *Arch Intern Med* 148:1643, 1988.
165. Malan A: Blood acid-base state at a variable temperature: A graphical representation. *Respir Physiol* 31:259, 1977.
166. Kelman GR, Nunn JF: Nomograms for correction of blood pO_2, pCO_2, pH, and base excess for time and temperature. *J Appl Physiol* 21:1484, 1966.
167. Brooks DK: The meaning of pH at low temperatures during extracorporeal circulation. *Anaesthesia* 19:337, 1964.
168. Flynn MD, Mawson DM, Tooke JE, et al: Cyclical hypothermia: Successful treatment with ephedrine. *J Royal Soc Med* 84:753, 1991.
169. Dunger DB, Leonard JV, Wolff OH, et al: Effect of naloxone in a previously undescribed hypothalamic syndrome: A disorder of the endogenous opiod system? *Lancet* 1:1277, 1980.
170. Hudson LD, Conn RD: Accidental hypothermia: Associated diagnoses and prognosis in a common problem. *JAMA* 227:37, 1974.
171. Guerin JM, Meyer P, Segrestaa JM: Hypothermia in diabetic ketoacidosis. *Diabetes Care* 10:801, 1987.
172. Lewis S, Brettman LR, Holzman RS: Infections in hypothermic patients. *Arch Intern Med* 141:920, 1981.
173. Carr ME Jr, Wolfert AI: Rewarming by hemodialysis for hypothermia: Failure of heparin to prevent DIC. *J Emerg Med* 6:277, 1988.
174. Freeman RM: The role of magnesium in the pathogenesis of azotemic hypothermia. *Proc Soc Exp Biol Med* 137:1069, 1971.
175. Levy LA: Severe hypophosphatemia as a complication of the treatment of hypothermia. *Arch Intern Med* 140:128, 1980.
176. Ledingham IM, Mone JG: Treatment of accidental hypothermia: A prospective clinical study. *Br Med J* 280:1102, 1980.
177. Sessler DI, Moayeri A: Skin surface warming: Heat flux and central temperature. *Anesthesiology* 73:218, 1990.
178. Evaluation of the Bair Hugger warming device. *Anaesth Intensive Care* 20:122, 1992.
179. Myers RA, Britten JS, Cowley RA: Quantitative aspects of therapy. *JACEP* 8:523, 1979.
180. Anderson S, Herbring BG, Widman B: Accidental profound hypothermia. *Br J Anaesth* 42:653, 1970.
181. Mittleman KD, Mekjavic IB: Effect of occluded venous return on core temperature during cold water immersion. *J Appl Physiol* 65:2709, 1988.
182. Hoskin RW, Melinyshyn MJ, Romet TT, et al: Bath rewarming from immersion hypothermia. *J Appl Physiol* 61:1518, 1986.
183. Hayward JS, Steinman AM: Accidental hypothermia: An experimental study of inhalation rewarming. *Aviat Space Environ Med* 46:1236, 1975.
184. Lloyd EL, Conliffe NA, Orgel H, et al: Accidental hypothermia: An apparatus for central rewarming as a first aid measure. *Scott Med J* 17:83, 1972.
185. Ledingham IM, Douglas IHS, Rauth GS, et al: Central rewarming system for treatment of hypothermia. *Lancet* 1:1168, 1980.
186. Johnson LA: Accidental hypothermia: Peritoneal dialysis. *JACEP* 6:556, 1977.
187. Troelsen S, Rybro L, Knudsen F: Profound accidental hypothermia treated with periotoneal dialysis. *Scand J Urol Nephrol* 20:221, 1986.
188. Brunette DD, Sterner S, Robinson EP, et al: Comparison of gastric lavage and thoracic cavity lavage in the treatment of severe hypothermia in dogs. *Ann Emerg Med* 16:1222, 1987.
189. White JD, Butterfield AB, Nucci RC, et al: Rewarming in accidental hypothermia: Radio wave versus inhalation therapy. *Ann Emerg Med* 16:50, 1987.
190. White JD, Butterfield AB, Greer KA, et al: Controlled comparison of radio wave regional hyperthermia and peritoneal lavage rewarming after immersion hypothermia. *J Trauma* 25:989, 1985.
191. Gregory JS, Bergstein JM, Aprahamian C, et al: Comparison of three methods of rewarming from hypothermia: Advantages of extracorporeal blood warming. *J Trauma* 31:1247, 1991.
192. Gentilello LM, Cobean RA, Offner PJ, et al: Continuous arteriovenous reversal of hypothermia in critically ill patients. *J Trauma* 32:316, 1992.
193. Gentillello LM, Rifley WJ: Continuous arteriovenous rewarming: Report of a new technique for treating hypothermia. *J Trauma* 31:1151, 1991
194. Maresda L, Vasko JS: Treatment of hypothermia by extracorporeal circulation and internal rewarming. *J Trauma* 27:89, 1987.
195. Wickstrom E, Ruiz E, Lilja GP, et al: Accidental hypothermia: Core rewarming with partial bypass. *Am J Surg* 131:622, 1976.
196. Roe CF, Goldberg MJ, Blair CS, et al: The influence of body temperature on early postoperative oxygen consumption. *Surgery* 60:85, 1966.
197. Jones HD, McLaren CAB: Postoperative shivering and hypoxaemia after halothane, nitrous oxide and oxygen anesthesia. *Br J Anaesth* 37:35, 1965.
198. Goldberg MJ, Roe CF: Temperature changes during anesthesia and operations. *Arch Surg* 93:365, 1966.
199. Ozuna JM: A study of surgical patients' temperatures: Effects of preoperative procedures on patients' body temperatures. *AORN J* 28:240, 1978.
200. Vaughn MS, Vaughn RW, Cork RC: Postoperative hypothermia in adults: Relationship of age, anesthesia, and shivering to rewarming. *Anesth Analg* 60:746, 1981.
201. Tollofsrud SG, Gundersen Y, Andersen R: Preoperative hypothermia. *Acta Anaesthesiol Scand* 28:511, 1984.
202. Flacke JW, Flacke WE: Inadvertent hypothermia: Frequent, insidious, and often serious. *Anesthesia* 3:183, 1983.
203. Morris RH, Kumar A: The effect of warming blankets on maintenance of body temperature of the anesthetized, paralyzed adult patient. *Anesthesiology* 36:408, 1972.
204. Smith LW, Fay T: Observations on human beings with cancer

maintained at reduced temperature of 75–90° Fahrenheit. *Am J Clin Pathol* 10:1, 1940.

205. Blair E, Henning G, Hornick R, et al: Hypothermia in bacteremic shock. *Arch Surg* 89:619, 1964.
206. Frank ED, Davidoff D, Freidman G, et al: Host resistance to bacteria in hemorrhagic shock. IV. Effect of hypothermia on clearance of intravenously injected bacteria. *Proc Soc Exp Biol Med* 91:188, 1956.
207. Wheelock JB: Ineffectiveness of scalp hypothermia in the prevention of alopecia in patients treated with doxorubicin and cisplatin combinations. *Cancer Treat Rep* 68:1387, 1984.
208. McDowall DG: The current usage of hypothermia in British neurosurgery. *Br J Anaesth* 43:10, 1971.
209. Browning D, Goodrum DT: Treatment of acute severe asthma assisted by hypothermia. *Anaesthesia* 47:223, 1992.
210. Roe CF: Effect of bowel exposure on body temperature during surgical operations. *Am J Surg* 122:13, 1971.
211. Vale RJ: Normothermia: Its place in operative and postoperative care. *Anaesthesia* 29:241, 1973.
212. Bay J, Nunn JF, Prys-Roberts C: Factors influencing arterial PO_2 during recovery from anesthesia. *Br J Anaesth* 40:398, 1968.
213. Pflug AE, Aasheim GM, Foster C, et al: Prevention of post-anaesthesia shivering. *Can Anaesth Soc J* 25:43, 1978.
214. Slotman GJ, Jed EH, Burchard KW: Adverse effects of hypothermia in postoperative patients. *Am J Surg* 149:495, 1985.
215. Roizen MF, Sohn YJ, L'Hommedieu CS, et al: Operating room temperature prior to surgical draping: Effect on patient temperature in recovery room. *Anesth Analg* 59:852, 1980.
216. Ott DE: Correction of laparoscopic insufflation hypothermia. *J Laparoendoscopic Surg* 1:183, 1991.
217. Leaman PL, Martyak GG: Microwave warming of resuscitation fluids. *Ann Emerg Med* 14:876, 1985.
218. Godblat A, Miller R: Prevention of incidental hypothermia in neurosurgical patients. *Anesth Analg* 51:536, 1972.
219. Shanks CA: The effects of inspiration of gases saturated with water vapour on heat and moisture exchange during endotracheal intubation. *Br J Anaesth* 45:887, 1973.
220. Newton DEF: The effect of anaesthetic gas humidification on body temperature. *Br J Anaesth* 47:1026, 1975.
221. Stone DR, Downs JB, Paul WL, et al: Adult body temperature and heated humidification of anesthetic gases during general anesthesia. *Anesth Analg* 60:736, 1981.
222. Caldwell C, Crawford R, Sinclair I: Hypothermia after cardiopulmonary bypass in man. *Anesthesiology* 55:86, 1981.
223. Noback CR, Tinker JH: Hypothermia after cardiopulmonary bypass in man: Amelioration by nitroprusside-induced vasodilation during rewarming. *Anesthesiology* 53:277, 1980.
224. Geller EA, Moore RA, Forsythe M, et al: Cyanide release by nitroprusside during hypothermic CPB. *Anesthesiology* 55(suppl):A20, 1981.
225. Rodriguez JL, Weissman C, Damask MC, et al: Morphine and postoperative rewarming in critically ill patients. *Circulation* 68:1238, 1983.
226. Rouby JJ, Glaser P, Simmoneau G, et al: Cardiovascular response to the IV administration of morphine in critically ill patients undergoing IPPV. *Br J Anaesth* 51:1071, 1979.
227. Rouby JJ, Eurin B, Glaser P, et al: Hemodynamic and metabolic effects of morphine in the critically ill. *Circulation* 64:53, 1981.
228. Ireland KW, Follette DM, Iguidbashian J, et al: Use of a heat exchanger to prevent hypothermia during thoracic and thoracoabdominal aneurysm repairs. *Ann Thorac Surg* 55:534, 1993.
229. Dalili H, Andriani J: Effects of various blood warmers on the components of bank blood. *Anesth Analg* 53:125, 1974.
230. Thornton JA: Blood loss, colloid infusion and blood transfusion, in Gary TC, Nunn F, Utting JE (eds): *General Anesthesia*. 4th ed. Boston, Butterworth, 1980, pp 1037–1059.
231. Kulkarni P, Matson A, Bright J, et al: Clinical evaluation of the oesophageal heat exchanger in the prevention of perioperative hypothermia. *Br J Anaesth* 70:216, 1993.

73. Disorders of Temperature Control: Hyperthermia

Frederick J. Curley and Richard S. Irwin

This chapter reviews the four major hyperthermic syndromes—heat stroke, malignant hyperthermia, neuroleptic malignant syndrome, and drug-induced hyperthermia—with respect to their pathogenesis, pathophysiology, diagnosis, differential diagnosis, and treatment. Because therapy may vary greatly depending on which syndrome produces the hyperthermia and because mortality rises with any delay in treatment, establishing the correct diagnosis and promptly instituting specific therapy are essential to management.

The discussion of these hyperthermic syndromes draws extensively on the analysis of the normal physiology of temperature regulation presented in Chapter 72. Heat stroke is reviewed in greater detail than the other three hyperthermic syndromes, for several reasons: (1) much of our understanding of the pathophysiology of malignant hyperthermia, the neuroleptic malignant syndrome, and drug-induced hyperthermia is derived from our knowledge of the metabolic consequences of the more common and better understood syndrome of heat stroke; (2) all four syndromes share to some degree a common

pathogenesis, clinical presentation, types of clinical sequelae, and methods of treatment; and (3) most deaths from hyperthermic syndromes result from heat stroke.

Heat Stroke

Heat stroke is a syndrome of acute thermoregulatory failure in warm environments characterized by central nervous system (CNS) depression, core temperatures usually above 40°C, and typical biochemical and physiologic abnormalities. Most cases of heat stroke occur in youths exercising in the sun, especially military recruits and athletes, or in elderly or ill patients during severe heat waves. Mortality in some series is as high as 70 percent [1]. During a warm summer in the United States, approximately 4000 deaths may occur as a direct result of heat stroke [2,3,4].

CAUSES AND PATHOGENESIS. Heat stroke may be subclassified by its two distinct clinical presentations: exertional and nonexertional, or classic, heat stroke. Exertional heat stroke is more typically seen in younger individuals exercising at higher than normal ambient temperatures. Although thermoregulatory mechanisms are typically intact, they are overwhelmed by the thermal challenge of the environment and the great increase in endogenous heat production. Nonexertional heat stroke affects predominantly elderly or sick individuals and occurs almost exclusively during a heat wave. Patients frequently have some impairment of thermoregulatory control, and temperatures rise easily with increased thermal challenge.

The causes of heat stroke fall into two pathogenetic categories (Table 73-1): increased heat production and impaired heat loss.

Increased Heat Production. Endogenous heat production during exertion ranges from 300 to 900 kcal per hour. Even in conditions favoring the maximal evaporation of sweat, only 500 to 600 kcal per hour of heat may be lost. Endogenous heat production may also be increased by fever, thyrotoxicosis, or the hyperactivity associated with amphetamine and hallucinogen use. In these conditions of increased thermogenesis, especially during maximal exercise, even a healthy individual with intact regulatory mechanisms may be overwhelmed, and hyperthermia may develop.

Impaired Heat Loss. Schizophrenic, comatose, senile, or mentally deficient patients are at higher risk of heat stroke when ambient temperatures are high, due to impaired voluntary control [5,6]. These patients may fail to perceive a temperature rise, to move to a cooler location, or to change to lighter clothes. Individuals who wear impermeable clothing in hot environments have a great reduction in evaporative heat loss and may suffer heat stroke [7,8].

Acclimatization greatly increases heat tolerance. Acclimatization increases cardiac output, decreases peak heart rate, in-

Table 73-1. Causes of Heat Stroke

Increased heat production
  Exercise
  Fever
  Thyrotoxicosis
  Amphetamines
  Hallucinogens
Impaired heat loss
  High ambient temperature or humidity
  Ineffective voluntary control
  Lack of acclimatization
  Dehydration
  Cardiovascular disease
  Hypokalemia
  Drugs
    Anticholinergics
    Phenothiazines
    Butyrophenones
    Thiothixenes
    Barbiturates
    Anti-Parkinson agents
    Diuretics
    Beta-blockers
    Alcohol
  Debilitating conditions
  Skin diseases
  Cystic fibrosis
  Central nervous system lesions
  Older age

creases stroke volume, lowers the threshold necessary to induce sweating, increases the volume of sweating, and, via an increase in aldosterone, expands extracellular volume and minimizes sweat sodium loss [9,10]. However, unacclimatized individuals who do not have these adaptive increases in cardiovascular and sweating efficiency clearly have an increased chance of suffering exertional heat stroke [11].

Dehydration and impaired cardiovascular performance also predispose to heat stroke because they may decrease skin or muscle blood flow and jeopardize any movement of heat from the core to the environment [10,12]. Adequate fluid intake and maintenance of a normal vascular volume clearly help prevent heat stroke. Heat load places a tremendous stress on the cardiovascular system and may easily produce hyperthermia in patients with cardiovascular dysfunction. In one report, percent of patients with compensated cardiac failure developed overt heart failure and temperatures up to 38°C after as little as 4 hours' exposure to temperatures of 32.2°C. Respiratory rate, blood pressure, and central venous pressure also tended to rise [13].

Hypokalemia poses an increased risk by decreasing muscle blood flow, impairing cardiovascular performance, and possibly decreasing sweat gland function [9,10]. Many drugs are known to predispose to heat stroke. Hypohydrosis may be produced by drugs with anticholinergic properties (e.g., phenothiazines, butyrophenones, thiothixenes, and anti-Parkinson medications [14]). Barbiturate overdose may produce sweat gland necrosis [10]. Diuretics promote dehydration and hypokalemia. Beta-blockers may increase the risk of heat stroke because of cardiodepression. Alcohol use may increase the risk of heat stroke 15 times because of dehydration secondary to antidiuretic hormone inhibition and inappropriate vasodilatation, which may cause a net heat gain [6].

Debilitating conditions are believed to predispose to heat stroke by causing inefficient metabolism, autonomic dysfunction, or circulatory compromise. Although fatigue or exhaustion clearly increase the risk of exertional heat stroke [11,15], physical conditioning prior to exertion decreases the risk [16]. Mortality from heat stroke may be higher for individuals suffering from diabetes, obesity, and chronic obstructive pulmonary disease, but it has not been clearly demonstrated that they are predisposed to heat stroke [6].

Skin disorders that impair sweat gland function, such as cystic fibrosis and chronic idiopathic anhydrosis [17], and CNS lesions (e.g., hypothalamic lesions) that impair thermoregulation may also predispose to heat stroke. During the early stages of heat stroke, hypothalamic regulation appears intact in that appropriate autonomic responses to limit hyperthermia occur. In the later stages, after thermal toxicity has occurred, hypothalamic regulation may be clearly abnormal [18]. Anhidrosis has been reported in up to 100 percent of heat stroke victims in some series [19]. This has been interpreted as an indication of elevated hypothalamic setpoint. The exact cause of hypohidrosis remains unclear and may reflect hypothalamic dysfunction or only the secondary effects of dehydration and cardiovascular collapse. Electron microscopic studies of eccrine sweat glands in a patient with fatal exertional heat stroke show changes suggestive of sweat gland fatigue [20]. Heat stroke can, however, occur in individuals who perspire profusely, indicating that sweat gland malfunction is not inherent to pathogenesis of the syndrome (see Diagnosis).

The increased risk of heat stroke in the elderly results from several impairments of thermoregulation. Although elderly patients normally demonstrate a decreased ability to sweat and a compromised cardiovascular response to heat exposure when compared with younger individuals, their inability to sweat effectively is probably the most important etiologic factor [8,21].

In one report percent of elderly patients showed no evidence of sweating at the time heat stroke was diagnosed [22]. Elderly patients are more likely to have deficient voluntary control and poor acclimatization and to take drugs that adversely affect thermoregulation.

PATHOPHYSIOLOGY. The primary injury in heat stroke is due to the direct cellular toxicity of temperatures above 42°C. Above this temperature, referred to as the critical thermal maximum [23], cell function deteriorates due to cessation of mitochondrial activity, alterations in chemical bonds involved in enzymatic reactions, and cell membrane instability. This toxic effect of temperature accounts for the widespread organ damage seen in all three of the major hyperthermic syndromes. Studies of patients undergoing therapeutic total body hyperthermia reveal that similar patterns of organ toxicity occur [24].

Factors such as dehydration, metabolic acidosis, and local hypoxia potentiate the damage, altering slightly the pathophysiologic consequences and clinical presentation of each of the hyperthermic syndromes. For example, classic heat stroke may occur with relatively little metabolic acidosis because no exertion was involved in its onset; however, it may be associated with more pronounced dehydration due to the gradual rise in temperature and prolonged sweating. Exertional heat stroke, alternatively, may be accompanied by a severe metabolic acidosis and hypoxia due to muscular exercise. It is typically associated with a more normal volume status because the onset of temperature elevation is abrupt.

Muscle Effects. Muscle degeneration and necrosis occur as a direct result of extremely elevated temperature. Muscle damage is more severe in exertional heat stroke due to the local increases in heat, hypoxia, and metabolic acidosis associated with exertion. Significant muscle enzyme elevation and severe rhabdomyolysis are extremely common in exertional heat stroke [12,25,26] but rare in classic heat stroke [27].

Cardiac Effects. Cardiac output is usually high [28] due to increased demands, low peripheral vascular resistance secondary to vasodilatation, and dehydration. Dehydration frequently results from sweat rates that may easily reach 1.5 to 2 liters per hour during episodes of heat stroke [29].

Hypotension occurs commonly as a result of either high output failure or temperature-induced myocardial hemorrhage and necrosis with subsequent cardiac depression and failure [9,12,30]. Tachyarrhythmias are frequent. Postmortem specimens show focal myocytolysis and myocyte necrosis and hemorrhage in subepicardial, intramuscular, subendocardial, or intravalvular tissues [31].

Central Nervous System Effects. Direct thermal toxicity to brain and spinal cord rapidly produces cell death, cerebral edema, and local hemorrhage. These may lead to profound stupor or coma, almost universal features of all the hyperthermic syndromes. Seizures secondary to edema and hemorrhage are not uncommon. Because the Purkinje cells of the cerebellum are particularly sensitive to the toxic effects of high temperatures, ataxia, dysmetria, and dysarthria may be seen acutely and in survivors of hyperthermia [10,32]. Lumbar punctures in both classic and exertional heat stroke may show increased protein levels, xanthochromia, and a slight lymphocytic pleocytosis [12,22]. Survivors of severe heat stroke may show premature cataract formation, considered to be secondary to dehydration [33].

Renal Effects. Some renal damage occurs in nearly all hyperthermic patients; it is potentiated by dehydration, cardiovascular collapse, and rhabdomyolysis. Acute renal failure occurs in an average of 5 percent of patients with classic heat stroke and is considered secondary to dehydration [9]; not unexpectedly, these patients have an elevated blood urea nitrogen (BUN) level. In exertional heat stroke, acute renal failure may occur in up to 35 percent of cases [9,30]. Dehydration, pigment load, hypoperfusion, and urate nephropathy are thought to contribute to a clinical picture of acute tubular necrosis [30]. Low serum osmolarity, moderate proteinuria, active sediment, and characteristic machine oil appearance of the urine are typical of exertional heat stroke. In one series, the incidence of acute tubular necrosis increased with survival time [31]. Hypocalcemia and CPK values above 10,000 U/per liter increase the risk of acute renal failure [34].

Gastrointestinal Effects. The combination of direct thermotoxicity and relative hypoperfusion of the intestines during hyperthermia frequently leads to ischemic intestinal ulcerations that may result in frank bleeding [9]. The liver appears particularly sensitive to temperature damage; it is affected in nearly every case. Hepatic necrosis and cholestasis frequently peak 2 to 3 days after hyperthermic insult and in 5 to 10 percent of cases may be severe enough to cause death [10,35].

Hematologic Effects. White blood cell counts are typically elevated due to catecholamine release and hemoconcentration. Anemia and a bleeding diathesis are frequently present and may result from several factors [29]: (1) direct inactivation of platelets and bleeding factors by the heat, (2) a decrease in coagulation factor synthesis due to liver failure, (3) an as yet unexplained decrease in platelet and megakaryocyte counts, (4) platelet aggregation due directly to heat [36], and (5) disseminated intravascular coagulation (DIC) that may range from mild to severe. Bone marrow specimens indicate that there may be a selective effect of hyperthermia on megakaryocytes. Megakaryocyte counts are reduced in up to 50 percent of specimens, and surviving megakaryocytes are morphologically abnormal [31]. Disseminated intravascular coagulation is present in most cases of fatal hyperthermia [31,37], most frequently appearing on the second or third day following hyperthermic insult. It is thought to be due to the previously mentioned abnormalities coupled with activation of the clotting cascade by vascular endothelial damage and generalized cell necrosis. There is now some evidence that vascular endothelium itself may be heat-sensitive [24]. In cases of DIC, cardiac, CNS, pulmonary, gastrointestinal (GI), and renal complications are exacerbated. An increase in blood viscosity of up to 24 percent to facilitate thromboses has been postulated [38].

Endocrine Effects. Hypoglycemia may occur in severe exertional heat stroke due to metabolic exhaustion [15,26]. In milder heat stroke, hyperglycemia and elevations of serum cortisol have been reported [39]. Although in autopsies the adrenal glands frequently show pericortical hemorrhages, survivors show little evidence of adrenal dysfunction [24,30]. Growth hormone and aldosterone levels actually increase abruptly during severe acute heat exposure and are thought to act to preserve volume.

Electrolyte Effects. Hyperthermia produces frequent imbalances in potassium, sodium, phosphate, and calcium levels [29,40]. In heat stroke, sweating involves the active excretion of potassium from the body, producing normal to low serum potassium levels and slightly decreased total body potassium concentrations. In cases of exertional heat stroke with severe cell injury, potassium may be extremely elevated due to cell lysis. Although mild hypophosphatemia occurs frequently as a result of intracellular trapping and possible parathyroid hormone resistance, phosphate levels may decrease to less than 1 mg per 100 ml in cases of hyperthermia with severe rhabdomyolysis [40]. Calcium values may fall 2 to 3 days after cellular injury owing to intracellular precipitation. In patients with severe tissue injury rebound hypercalcemia may occur 2 to 3 weeks after hyperthermia as a result of parathyroid hormone activation [40].

Pulmonary Effects. Direct thermal injury to the pulmonary vascular endothelium may lead to cor pulmonale or acute respiratory distress syndrome (ARDS). This and the tendency toward myocardial dysfunction make pulmonary edema common. Increased oxygen demands and acidosis frequently produce a respiratory alkalosis. Metabolic acidosis is, however, the most common acid-base disorder [41].

DIAGNOSIS. Heat stroke is usually readily suggested by history and physical examination and the diagnosis confirmed by recording a rectal temperature above 40°C. The temperature of any individual found comatose during a heat wave should be taken. Any laborer or athlete displaying incoordination followed by stupor and collapse while exercising in the heat should be assumed to have heat stroke until proved otherwise. Because more than 6 million workers in the United States experience occupational heat stress [8], a history of the exact events precipitating collapse may be helpful.

Heat stroke should be expected in any patient exercising in hot weather or in susceptible individuals during heat waves (Table 73-1). Coma or profound stupor is nearly always present, but the other traditional criteria of anhidrosis and core temperature above 41°>C may be absent. Although anhidrosis occurs in 84 percent of elderly patients with classic heat stroke [22], profuse sweating is typically present in exertional heat stroke [10]. Thus, the presence of anhidrosis is helpful, but its absence is not. Likewise, by the time the patient receives medical care, the temperature may have fallen significantly owing to cessation of exertion, removal from a hot environment, or cooling measures undertaken during transport. However, most patients do have a temperature above 40°C. Because serum creatine kinase is almost always elevated, we believe diagnostic criteria for heat stroke should include (1) a core temperature above 40°C, (2) severely depressed mental status or coma, (3) elevated serum creatine kinase, and (4) compatible historical setting.

Classic heat stroke occurs more frequently when ambient peak temperatures exceed 32°C and minimum temperatures do not fall below 27°C. The risk is greater in urban areas, where minimum temperatures may exceed that in surrounding communities by more than 5°C [3]. Death rates during these heat waves may exceed twice the normal rates, and heat stroke deaths usually lag behind peak temperatures by approximately 24 hours. More than 80 percent of heat stroke victims are older than 65 years of age [22,37]. Other major high-risk groups are schizophrenics, patients with parkinsonism, alcoholics, and paraplegics or quadriplegics [42,43,44].

Exertional heat stroke may be seen when ambient temperatures are in the 25°C range but more frequently it occurs at higher temperatures. Exertional heat stroke is frequently seen in military recruits during basic training [11,26], amateur football players [10,45], and marathon runners [15,16,46,47]. Miners and others who labor in hot local environments are also at high risk [30]. Heat stroke remains the second leading cause of death in athletes, second only to injuries of the head and spinal cord [9].

DIFFERENTIAL DIAGNOSIS. Table 73-2 lists the causes of hyperthermia. Hyperthermia and coma may occur with hypothalamic injury, severe infection, or endocrinopathy [48]. Hypothalamic tumors or hemorrhage may produce hyperthermia by elevating the regulated temperature setpoint and may be distinguished from heat stroke by the constancy of the temperature and associated defects, such as diabetes insipidus and anhidrosis, which may be unilateral [49]. Meningitis and encephalitis usually lack the characteristic enzyme elevations and may be distinguished by lumbar puncture.

TREATMENT

Primary Therapy of Hyperthermia. Primary therapy includes cooling and decreasing thermogenesis. Some cooling may be achieved in the field by moving the victim to a shaded, cooler area; removing the clothes; and constantly wetting the skin. Fanning or transport in an open vehicle to create a breeze should enhance evaporative cooling. In military installations, helicopter transport to higher, cooler altitudes has also been advocated [10]. Once the victim reaches the hospital, cooling and subsequent supportive care is best provided in an intensive care setting.

Cooling by either evaporative or direct external methods has proved effective. Evaporative cooling methods involve placing a nude patient in a cool room, wetting the skin with water, and encouraging evaporation by the use of fans. In one specially designed evaporative cooling unit, patients were sprayed with 15°C water and their skin fanned at 30 per minute with air heated to 45 to 48°C. Temperature reduction was rapid and mortality was 11 percent [50]. There was no mortality in 25 patients with nonexertional heat stroke treated with cooling by covering with a cool, wet 20°C sheet and fanned with two 35-cm electric fans. Fanning was adjusted to maintain skin temperature at 30 to 32°C; skin temperature fell 1°C every 11 minutes [51]. In 14 patients with nonexertional heat stroke, there was only one death when evaporative/convective cooling was employed. The median time to return to temperature less than 39.4°C was 60 minutes. Direct external cooling involves immersing the patient in ice water or packing the patient in ice. However, because cold skin temperatures produce vasoconstriction, constant massage may be necessary to allow circulation to carry heat from the core. Direct external cooling is highly effective but make patient monitoring and management extremely inconvenient. Therefore, some authors advocate evaporative cooling as a safer cooling method in patients at high risk of cardiovascular collapse [47]. In rare instances when evaporative and direct external cooling methods fail to reduce the temperature, peritoneal lavage with iced saline cooled to 20 or 9°C, gastric lavage, or hemodialysis or cardiopulmonary bypass with external cooling of the blood may be necessary to reduce the temperature. Temperature should be continuously monitored and cooling stopped as it approaches 39°C. Although chlorpromazine in an intravenous dose of 10 to 25 mg has been advocated to prevent shivering during cooling, it is usually unnecessary.

Therapy of the Complications of Hyperthermia. Arrhythmias, metabolic acidosis, and cardiogenic failure complicate the early management of hyperthermic crises. Supraventricular tachyarrhythmias usually require no treatment because they respond to restoration of normal temperature and metabolism. Digitalis should be avoided due to the likelihood of hyperkalemia.

Hypotension should be treated initially with normal saline and, if necessary, with isoproterenol. Dopaminergic and alpha-

Table 73-2. Differential Diagnosis of Hyperthermia

Hyperthermic syndromes
   Exertional heat stroke
   Nonexertional heat stroke
   Malignant hyperthermia
   Neuroleptic malignant syndrome
   Drug-induced hyperthermia
Infection
   Meningitis
   Encephalitis
   Sepsis
Endocrinopathy
   Thyroid storm
   Pheochromocytoma
Central nervous system
   Hypothalamic bleed
   Acute hydrocephalus

agonists, should be avoided because they tend to produce peripheral vasoconstriction. Volume expansion with dextran is contraindicated due to its anticoagulating effect. Swan-Ganz and arterial catheter monitoring may be helpful in the management of hypotension because patients frequently have low peripheral resistance, suffer from dehydration, have impaired cardiac function, and are at a high risk for congestive heart and renal failure. As 64 percent of patients may have a normal central venous pressure prior to resuscitation, volume expansion in most cases should be guided by intravascular pressure monitoring where available [52]. Seizures, quite common in heat stroke, usually respond to diazepam.

Blood gas status should be determined early in treatment. Blood gases drawn at temperatures above 39°C should probably be corrected for temperature, although to our knowledge no studies have demonstrated that this is clinically necessary. The solubility of oxygen and carbon dioxide increases as blood drawn from the patient is cooled to 37°C for analysis. This lowers the carbon dioxide and oxygen tensions and elevates the pH when compared with values present in the patient. The patient is therefore more acidotic and less hypoxic than the uncorrected values indicate. Normal values of intracellular pH and changes on the body's buffering system in hyperthermia have been poorly described. Because normal values for blood gases in hyperthermic patients are unavailable, by convention the blood gas values are corrected for temperature, using any reliable nomogram, and clinical decisions are made as if the patient were euthermic [53,54,55]. Only if the acid-base changes in vivo parallel the acid-base changes of blood in vitro (as in hypothermia) is it unnecessary to correct for temperature. For clinical purposes, the following formulas may be applied to give approximate corrections of arterial blood gas values measured at 37°C for elevations in the patient's temperature. For each 1°C that the patient's temperature is above 37°C, increase the oxygen tension 7.2 percent, increase the carbon dioxide (CO_2) tension 4.4 percent, and lower the pH 0.015 units. More research is needed before definite conclusions can be made. Nevertheless, 100 percent oxygen should be delivered until adequate oxygenation is ensured. Bicarbonate should be administered, guided by frequently obtained arterial blood gases. The base deficit is frequently large, and up to 30 gm of bicarbonate has been required for correction. Comatose patients should be prophylactically intubated to protect their airways from aspiration.

Urine output should be closely monitored with an indwelling bladder catheter. Patients should be routinely given 1 to 2 mg per kilogram of mannitol over 15 to 20 minutes to promote continued urine flow and possibly decrease cerebral edema. Continuous urine output should then be maintained with intermittent doses of furosemide. In all cases of hyperthermia, serum potassium levels should be closely followed. In cases of oliguria or potential renal failure, polystyrene sulfonate should be given early because hyperkalemia frequently increases.

Moderate to severe liver failure is common, may prolong illness, and, in combination with renal failure, may make administration of several drugs difficult or impossible. Although no clinical data are yet available, H_2-blocking drugs given prophylactically may decrease the incidence of GI bleeding.

The occurrence of DIC greatly affects mortality: Most patients who die of heat stroke have evidence of DIC [56]. Coagulation parameters such as prothrombin time, partial thromboplastin time, platelet count, and fibrinogen should be carefully followed. Should DIC occur, traditional recommendations for treatment should be followed (see Chap. 118).

Since steroids are of no benefit in heat stroke, infection has not been reported as a major cause of morbidity and mortality in hyperthermia, and antibiotics are associated with superinfections, the use of steroids and prophylactic antibiotics is not recommended [22,26].

PROGNOSIS. Morbidity and mortality are directly related to the peak temperature reached and time spent at elevated temperatures. A delay in treatment of only 2 hours may result in likelihood of death up to 70 percent [11,47]. When heat stroke is swiftly recognized and aggressively treated, mortality should be minimal. For example, in one series of 15 patients with exertional heat stroke, all were successfully treated with no mortality and little morbidity [11]. Another study predicts mortality of only 5 percent when heat stroke patients are managed properly [10]. A recent review of 34 elderly patients with classic heat stroke revealed an 18 percent mortality. Seventy-three percent recovered without sequelae and 9 percent had some residual neurologic deficit.

Although patients with temperatures as high as 46.5°C have survived without sequelae [57], mortality is increased with premorbid debility and higher maximal temperatures [41]. When ventricular fibrillation, DIC, coma lasting more than 6 to 8 hours, or high lactate levels complicate hyperthermia, mortality is predictably increased.

With respect to morbidity, neurologic function usually rapidly returns to normal after restoration of euthermia; however, some patients may be left with a mild cerebellar disorder [58,59]. Hepatic and renal failure in mild and moderate cases is usually completely resolved. Moderate muscle weakness may persist for several months in patients with severe muscle damage.

Although it has not been proved, patients who have experienced hyperthermic crises should be considered at high risk to develop a recurrence on exposure to similar heat stresses and should be advised accordingly.

Malignant Hyperthermia

Malignant hyperthermia is a drug- or stress-induced hypermetabolic syndrome characterized by vigorous muscle contractions, abrupt increase in temperature, and subsequent cardiovascular collapse. Malignant hyperthermia occurs, on average, in 1 of every 15,000 patients given anesthesia [60]. With treatment, mortality is approximately 30 percent [61].

Table 73-3. Drugs and Malignant Hyperthermia

Drugs known to trigger malignant hyperthermia
    Halothane
    Methoxyflurane
    Enflurane
    Succinylcholine (Anectine)
    Decamethonium
    Gallamine
    Diethyl ether
    Ethylene
    Ethyl chloride
    Trichloroethylene
    Ketamine
    Phencyclidine
    Cyclopropane
Drugs generally considered safe for patients with malignant hyper-
    thermia
    Nitrous oxide
    Barbiturates
    Diazepam (Valium)
    Tubocurarine
    Pancuronium (Pavulon), Vecuronium
    Opiates

CAUSE AND PATHOGENESIS. The cause of the temperature increase in malignant hyperthermia is similar to that of exertional heat stroke: increased thermogenesis overwhelms the patient's ability to dissipate heat. When exposed to various drugs these muscles may develop sustained or repeated contractions (Table 73-3). Current evidence indicates that patients with malignant hyperthermia have a defect in calcium metabolism in skeletal muscles. Postulated abnormalities in calcium metabolism that might underlie this condition include (1) impaired reuptake of calcium into the sarcoplasmic reticulum from the myoplasm, (2) increased release of calcium into the myoplasm with stimulation, and (3) a defect in the calcium-mediated coupling contraction mechanism [61,62]. The most recent evidence from families with an autosomal dominant pattern of inheritance and from swine models of malignant hyperthermia implicate a defect in the ryanodine receptor, which is known to be involved in sarcoplasmic reticulum transverse tubule communication [63]. In humans the gene for the ryanodine receptor and the gene noted to correlate with increased susceptibility to malignant hyperthermia map to the same region of chromosome 19 [64,65].

Sustained or repetitive muscular contractions produce an increase in temperature because of the hydrolysis of adenosine triphosphate (ATP) by muscle and the activation of catabolic pathways involved in the support of muscular exercise. Hepatic and muscular glycogenolysis and catecholamine-induced accelerated turnover of substrates contribute to heat production. Heat is also released during the metabolism of lactate, which reaches high concentrations because of anaerobic metabolism.

Although halothane and succinylcholine are involved in over 80 percent of cases, malignant hyperthermia has developed after the use of many other agents as well (Table 73-3). Stress, excitement, anoxia, viral infections, and lymphoma have also been reported to trigger malignant hyperthermia [66,67]; however, the mechanism is unclear. It is generally assumed that the causes of heat stroke would also increase the likelihood of malignant hyperthermia in susceptible individuals (Table 73-1).

The hyperthermic reaction to anesthetics is not allergic in nature; patients may have received the same anesthetic previously or may be exposed later without developing a reaction. There is little evidence that impaired heat dissipation or altered hypothalamic regulation is instrumental in producing acute hy-

perthermia in these patients. However, sympathetic activity and heat dissipation may be abnormal during exercise [68].

PATHOPHYSIOLOGY. Direct thermal injury is the predominant cause of toxicity in malignant hyperthermia. Damage results from the metabolic consequences of a sudden increase in temperature to levels frequently above 42°C, the critical thermal maximum. Physiologic and pathologic changes parallel those described for patients with exertional heat stroke [69].

Vigorous muscle contracture at the onset of malignant hyperthermia almost immediately precipitates a severe metabolic acidosis, with increased carbon dioxide (CO_2) production and compensatory hyperventilation. High elevations of creatine kinase, lactate dehydrogenase, and aldolase are almost universal in full-blown episodes [62]. All reflect considerable ongoing rhabdomyolysis. Hyperkalemia follows within minutes to hours [62].

Initially, volume status is normal because little volume has been lost in sweat. Cardiac output increases to meet metabolic demands and in response to the vasodilatation of muscle beds. Sinus tachycardia, supraventricular tachyarrhythmias, and ventricular fibrillation occur soon after temperature exceeds 40°C. Tissue hypoxia, acidosis, and hyperkalemia make ventricular arrhythmias common.

Direct thermal injury producing cerebral edema and cerebral hemorrhage results in coma. Seizures occur in most uncontrolled cases.

Renal failure frequently occurs in malignant hyperthermia, most likely secondary to pigment load. Dehydration and low cardiac output do not contribute until later, as the syndrome progresses.

Because higher maximal temperatures are usually seen in malignant hyperthermia, hepatic failure and GI bleeding are more prominent than in heat stroke [70]. In survivors, hepatic necrosis and cholestasis peak in 2 to 3 days and may be severe.

Hematologic abnormalities of elevated white blood cell count and thrombocytopenia are similar in cause and degree to those of heat stroke [70]. A nearly universal finding is DIC.

The degree of hypocalcemia, hypophosphatemia, and hyperkalemia varies with the duration and peak of hyperthermia and degree of secondary myonecrosis. All three disorders are usually more severe in malignant hyperthermia than in heat stroke.

DIAGNOSIS. The metabolic predisposition to malignant hyperthermia appears in general to be inherited in an autosomal dominant fashion, with variable penetrance and expressivity. Although certain pedigrees and myopathies have been described that appear to follow simple mendelian genetics, most investigators now believe several genes and alleles are involved in producing the metabolic defects [62,71]. Human lymphocyte antigen (HLA) typing has not proved helpful in identifying patients at risk [72]. Creatine kinase levels may be elevated in 50 to 70 percent of individuals at risk, but more typically these levels are elevated in those family clusters associated with a myopathy [62]. Tests using caffeine or halothane stimulation of excised muscle are the standard screening tests recommended by the Malignant Hyperthermia Association of the United States [73]. Their false-positive rate is near 10 percent, and their false-negative rate near zero [74]. Studies of muscle ultrastructure, spin labeling of red blood cells, and platelet purine bioassay may also be useful in screening high-risk individuals [61,75,76]. Since there is no one noninvasive test suitable for screening the general population, screening of family members of proved cases remains the best method of identifying susceptible individuals before hyperthermic crisis.

Although malignant hyperthermia may occur under any severe stress, it most commonly follows administration of an anesthetic agent. Malignant hyperthermia occurs at any age but is most frequent in young patients [77]; the mean age is 22 years [78]. Early signs of hyperthermic crisis vary with the anesthetic agent administered but include masseter muscle contracture after the administration of succinylcholine, muscle rigidity, sinus tachycardia, supraventricular tachyarrhythmias, mottling or cyanosis of the skin, increased CO_2 production, and hypertension. Hyperthermia is typically a late sign in an acute crisis, but it may be rapidly followed by hypotension, acidosis, peaked T waves on the electrocardiogram (ECG) due to hyperkalemia, and malignant ventricular arrhythmias [70].

Malignant hyperthermia is not difficult to diagnose late in a full-blown crisis; however, early recognition may be difficult. Mild tachycardia or other arrhythmias early in the anesthetic induction stage are neither infrequent nor specific. In one case report desaturation measured by oximetry preceded temperature elevation by 40 minutes [79]. Two signs may be helpful in making a prehyperthermic diagnosis: increased end-tidal CO_2 and masseter spasm [80–86]. Patients maintained on fixed minute ventilation by mechanical ventilators expel CO_2 at a constant rate. When CO_2 production rises because of increased muscle metabolism, end-tidal, or transcutaneous, CO_2 increases. Monitoring of end-tidal CO_2 is now recommended for virtually all anesthetic procedures and is mandatory for patients at risk of malignant hyperthermia [80,81,82].

Although severe masseter spasm after succinylcholine has been recognized as an early warning sign of malignant hyperthermia, the decision to discontinue anesthesia in patients with succinylcholine-induced spasm remains controversial [83]. Only approximately 1 percent of patients receiving succinylcholine develop masseter spasm [84]. Only 48 to 61 percent of children with masseter spasm had muscle biopsy stimulation tests compatible with a diagnosis of malignant hyperthermia [85,87]. Only 36 percent of patients with malignant hyperthermia had masseter spasm [86]. Nevertheless, because of the increased incidence of masseter spasm in patients who develop malignant hyperthermia, many believe that if masseter spasm occurs, elective surgery should be canceled and the patient referred for diagnostic muscle testing. If surgery must be continued, dangerous triggering anesthetics should be avoided, dantrolene should be given or at least be immediately accessible, and temperature and end-tidal CO_2 should be monitored on-line. Fortunately, 75 percent of patients with succinylcholine-induced masseter spasm who develop hyperthermia have other signs of malignant hyperthermia simultaneously [86].

DIFFERENTIAL DIAGNOSIS. Because malignant hyperthermia occurs almost exclusively in the perioperative setting, the differential diagnosis is more limited than that for heat stroke (Table 73-2). Endocrinopathies and drug reactions, not infection, are the most frequent diseases in the differential diagnosis. Thyroid storm and pheochromocytoma may be very difficult to distinguish from malignant hyperthermia in the anesthetized patient [88]. Thyroid storm is now infrequent, due to ease and extent of preoperative thyroid function test screening and prophylaxis of patients at risk. Dantrolene in doses used for malignant hyperthermia has been shown to decrease temperature in perioperative thyroid storm [89]. The use of dantrolene, therefore, may not distinguish between malignant hyperthermia and thyroid storm but may be therapeutic in both cases. The temperature rise in pheochromocytoma is typically much slower than that in malignant hyperthermia [90]. Hyperthermia due to

narcotic administration in patients taking monoamine oxidase inhibitors also must be considered. Other causes of perianesthesia hyperthermia, such as infection, may be identified by reviewing the patient's history.

TREATMENT. Direct pharmacologic intervention to decrease thermogenesis is mandatory. Dantrolene, a hydantoin derivative, acts by uncoupling the excitation-contraction mechanism in skeletal muscle and lowering myoplasmic calcium. Dantrolene used for fewer than 3 weeks rarely causes toxicity [91]; therefore, patients suspected of having malignant hyperthermia should be given dantrolene as soon as possible. In an acute crisis, 1 to 2.5 mg per kilogram of fresh dantrolene should be administered intravenously every 5 to 10 minutes, not to exceed 10 mg per kilogram [61,62,92,93]. The half-life of action is approximately 5 hours [62], and because relapse may occur, oral or intravenous dosages of 1 to 2 mg per kilogram every 6 hours should continue for at least 24 to 48 hours [62]. Oral dantrolene provides excellent blood levels and may be substituted once the patient is alert [94]. With dantrolene, temperatures often rapidly decrease; without it, they may increase 1 to 2°C every 15 minutes [78,80,92]. The cost of dantrolene is currently approximately $35 per 20-mg IV dose vial. Because even minute quantities of the triggering agent may continue to produce the syndrome, anesthesia should be immediately stopped, and the anesthesia apparatus, tubing, and ventilation equipment should be immediately changed.

Direct external cooling by submersion in ice water is helpful, but management of associated problems such as arrhythmia, arrest, and renal failure then becomes almost impossible. As with heat stroke, iced saline, gastric or peritoneal lavage, evaporative cooling, and infusion of chilled electrolyte solutions may be helpful [93]. Aggressive management with cardiopulmonary bypass with external cooling of the blood may be necessary when dantrolene fails to slow thermogenesis promptly [95].

When patients respond to therapy quickly, before severe temperature elevation occurs, only minimal supportive measures may be necessary. Once temperature exceeds 41°C, complications are widespread and patients frequently require long-term intensive care unit (ICU) support.

Ventricular fibrillation with subsequent cardiac collapse is the most common cause of death in the early stages of the syndrome. Procainamide should be given to all patients prophylactically as soon as malignant hyperthermia is diagnosed [62]. Procainamide acts to increase the uptake of calcium from the myoplasm directly and in early stages may help reduce hyperthermia. Administration of digitalis should be avoided because of the increased likelihood of hyperkalemia.

As with heat stroke, hypotension should be treated with saline infusion and isoproterenol. Dopaminergic and alpha-agonists reduce heat dissipation resulting from peripheral vasoconstriction.

Seizures occur nearly-universally in malignant hyperthermia. Prophylactic treatment with phenobarbital is strongly recommended because seizures may increase heat production, metabolic acidosis, and hypoxia. Arterial blood gas values should be adjusted for temperature, as noted for heat stroke.

Mannitol and furosemide may be needed to promote continued urine output and may reduce the likelihood of cerebral edema and acute tubular necrosis. The serum potassium level usually increases over several hours; the elevation should be treated with polystyrene sulfonates.

Hepatic failure and DIC require supportive treatment. With prolonged supportive care, hepatic, renal, and neurologic functions typically normalize. Muscle weakness may, however, last for months.

PROGNOSIS. With current management techniques, mortality resulting from malignant hyperthermia should be below 30 percent. In one review, prompt dantrolene therapy in cases of confirmed malignant hyperthermia resulted in a 100 percent survival rate [25].

Neuroleptic Malignant Syndrome

Neuroleptic malignant syndrome results primarily from an imbalance of central neurotransmitters, usually due to neuroleptic drug use, and is characterized by hyperthermia, muscular rigidity, and altered consciousness. Most current knowledge is derived from case reports rather than systematic study. Since the syndrome was first described in 1968 [96], fewer than 2000 cases have appeared in the world's literature and most are from the past decade. Early case reports of neuroleptic malignant syndrome frequently centered on psychiatric or neurologic findings, and details such as ECG changes, arterial blood gas abnormalities, and electrolyte changes were inadequately described or not mentioned. An explosion of case reports and analyses of the literature published in the past few years has provided, much better information on incidence, mortality, pathogenesis, and treatment [97,98,99].

Although older, more retrospective studies estimated the incidence of neuroleptic malignant syndrome to be as high as 1 percent of all patients taking neuroleptic agents [100], more recent long-term, prospective studies conducted in inpatient psychiatric hospitals have found incidences as low as 0 percent [101], 0.07 percent [102], 0.2 percent [103], and 0.9 percent [104]. The highest recent estimate of incidence was 2.2 percent [105]. Early estimates of mortality were as high as 30 percent [106]. Incidence also appears to be declining [107]. Recent reviews of all case reports have indicated that the mortality since 1986 has fallen to below 12 percent [108]. Two recent prospective series reported 24 cases and 68 cases with mortality rates of 0 percent [109] and 5 percent [110], respectively.

As data on the syndrome have evolved, controversy regarding its definition has grown [111,112]. The syndrome may be diagnosed in any patient with (1) an unexplained elevation in temperature, (2) muscular rigidity and characteristic extrapyramidal signs, and (3) a history of recent neuroleptic drug use. Mental status changes, coma, and catatonia are common. This definition highlights the cardinal features of the syndrome and is qualified below.

CAUSE AND PATHOGENESIS. In all reports of neuroleptic malignant syndrome, either patients were receiving agents believed to decrease dopaminergic hypothalamic tone or the syndrome appeared after withdrawal of dopaminergic agents (Table 73-4). Butyrophenones [113–127], phenothiazines [113,115,118,121,128,129], thioxanthenes [130,131,132], and dibenzoxazepines [133,134] are believed to act as dopamine receptor-blocking agents. Atypical antipsychotics such as molindone [135], clozepine [136], and fluoxetine [137], and dopamine blockers used to treat GI disease, such as metoclopramide and domperidone [138], have also caused the syndrome. Drugs acting at the D2 dopamine binding sites appear to have the greatest potential for causing the syndrome. Most cases occur in patients taking butyrophenones or piperazines, agents with a high incidence of extrapyramidal reactions. The rate of increase in dose appears more important than the maximal dose achieved [108]. Dopamine-depleting agents such as tetrabenazene and alpha-methyltyrosine produced neuroleptic malignant

Table 73-4. Drugs Associated with the Onset of Neuroleptic Malignant Syndrome

Butyrophenones
  Haloperidol
  Bromperidol
Phenothiazines
  Chlorpromazine
  Levomepromazine
  Trifluoperazine
  Fluphenazine
Thioxanthenes
  Thiothixene
Dibenzoxazepines
  Loxapine
Dihydroindolones
  Molindone
Flurooxypropylamines
  Fluoxetine
Tricyclic-dibenzodiazepines
  Clozapine
Dopamine-depleting agents
  Tetrabenazine
  Alpha-methyltyrosine
  Withdrawal of levodopa, carbidopa, amantadine
  Domperidone
  Metoclopramide

syndrome in a patient with Huntington's disease [106]. Abrupt withdrawal of levodopa (L-dopa), dopa-carbidopa, or amantadine produced the syndrome in patients suspected of having Parkinson's disease [139,140,141]. Tollefson and Garvey [128] reported a patient with neuroleptic malignant syndrome in whom dopamine metabolites were increased in the cerebrospinal fluid (CSF) and postulated that neuroleptics increase dopamine neural firing and dopamine turnover. Initiation of metoclopramide therapy has produced the syndrome, presumably due to alteration in central dopaminergic tone [142,143,144].

The increase in muscular rigidity, akinesia, mutism, and tremor are considered to be due to hypothalamic dopaminergic imbalance. Motor abnormalities vary, but in general they are typical of the parkinsonian-type extrapyramidal reactions commonly seen as side effects of neuroleptic therapy. Unlike typical neuroleptic-induced side effects, however, the muscular effects are frequently seen at low therapeutic doses soon after treatment begins. The central origin of the muscle spasm is further suggested by its resolution with the use of centrally acting dopaminergic agents such as bromocriptine, amantadine, and L-dopa. A role for peripheral muscle abnormality has, however, been suggested, in that sarcoplasmic calcium concentration is higher in patients who have had the syndrome [110], hypocalcemia accompanies 54 percent of cases [109], the syndrome may resolve with nifedipine use [145], and the syndrome has been reported to be triggered by hypoparathyroidism [146].

Hyperthermia results from an increase in endogenous heat production, impaired heat dissipation, loss of voluntary temperature regulation, and possibly an elevation of the hypothalamic setpoint. The fact that the degree of temperature increase varies directly with the severity of rigidity evident on examination strongly suggests that muscle contracture is responsible for increased thermogenesis [113]. A decrease in muscle rigidity by uncoupling contraction with dantrolene or by paralysis with succinylcholine results in a decrease in temperature [147]. Impaired heat dissipation from the anticholinergic-induced hypohydrosis of neuroleptics may also occur. The high prevalence of diaphoresis and presumed dehydration in patients with neuroleptic malignant syndrome suggests, however, that this effect may be minimal. Loss of voluntary control of temperature regulation from akinesis and coma likewise may play a role, but the lack of reports describing neuroleptic malignant syndrome during high ambient temperatures suggests that this has little clinical significance [148]. Although experiments with animals have clearly established that a change in hypothalamic dopamine concentrations affects temperature regulation, the mechanism by which this is accomplished remains obscure. Setpoint is unlikely to be elevated; the increase in diaphoresis seen in neuroleptic malignant syndrome suggests that regulatory mechanisms to dissipate heat have been activated. A likely hypothesis is that regulatory reflexes remain intact, but muscle rigidity from hypothalamic influences and subsequent increased thermogenesis exceed dissipative capacity. In this sense, the syndrome is similar to malignant hyperthermia, in which regulatory mechanisms appear intact but muscle contracture initiated at the level of the muscle, not the hypothalamus, overwhelms dissipative capacity.

Although the development of neuroleptic malignant syndrome is usually described as idiosyncratic, age, sex, and systemic factors appear to be important predisposing factors. The mean and median age at the onset of the syndrome is 40 years [149]. This is surprising, because impairment in temperature regulation and the prevalence of parkinsonian side effects of neuroleptics both increase with age. Onset at an early age suggests that either neuroleptic drugs are more frequently used in this age group or young persons are unusually sensitive to dopaminergic agents. Neuroleptic malignant syndrome develops 1.8 times more frequently in men than in women [149,150]. The larger muscle mass in men may predispose to the development of hyperthermia. There is, however, no difference in mean maximal temperature between men and women. Itoh and co-workers [113] noted that all 14 Japanese patients with neuroleptic malignant syndrome in their review suffered from exhaustion and dehydration. As mentioned previously, debility and dehydration may impair effective heat loss and predispose to hyperthermia.

It is now clear that neuroleptic malignant syndrome is neither an allergic reaction to neuroleptics nor a variant of malignant hyperthermia. An allergic cause is unlikely because onset does not appear to be related to duration of exposure, and neuroleptic malignant syndrome does not typically recur when patients are rechallenged with the offending agent. The fact that patients with muscle biopsy tests both positive and negative for malignant hyperthermia have been reported and that patients with neuroleptic malignant syndrome have had a decrease in temperature with dantrolene has led to confusion [129,130]. The syndromes, however, are clearly different: (1) The causative agents are dissimilar (compare Table 73-3 with Table 73-4); (2) in neuroleptic malignant syndrome the driving force to increased temperature is a change in dopaminergic hypothalamic tone, and in malignant hyperthermia the driving force is a calcium transport defect in skeletal muscle metabolism; and (3) in malignant hyperthermia there is a lack of prominent extrapyramidal symptoms, and in neuroleptic malignant syndrome there is a lack of hereditary predispositions.

PATHOPHYSIOLOGY. Because of the relatively low maximal temperatures—39.9°C, on average [149,150]—in patients with neuroleptic malignant syndrome compared with those of patients with heat stroke and malignant hyperthermia, it is not surprising that direct thermal injury occurs less often. Only 40 percent of patients have temperatures above 40°C [97]. The complications of neuroleptic malignant syndrome are summarized in Table 73-5.

Rhabdomyolysis, most probably secondary to both hyperthermia and muscle rigidity, is frequently seen, with typical

Table 73-5. Complications of Neuroleptic Malignant Syndrome

Rhabdomyolysis
Renal failure
Seizure
Cardiovascular collapse
Disseminated intravascular coagulation
Hepatic failure
Aspiration-pneumonia
Respiratory failure
Death

creatine kinase elevations in the range of 1000 to 5000 IU. Although rhabdomyolysis is usually mild, creatine kinase elevations to greater than 10,000 IU have been reported [132,151,152] and may occur in up to one-third of patients [109]. In cases of severe rhabdomyolysis, muscle biopsies have shown sarcolemmal vacuolization and denervation fiber atrophy, and electromyography has demonstrated a mild neuropathic pattern with prolonged distal latencies and diminished motor nerve conduction velocities [116]. Prolonged muscle weakness or dysfunction in survivors is not described.

Renal failure occurs in 9 to 30 percent of patients [109,149]. Proteinuria occurs in up to 91 percent of patients [109]. Renal failure is due to myoglobin-induced acute tubular necrosis and the dehydration that results from diaphoresis. Renal dysfunction in most patients is transient and mild and, even in cases of acute tubular necrosis, may return to premorbid values after brief periods of dialysis support [116]. Mortality in renal failure patients may, however, be as high as 56 percent [108].

Neuroleptic malignant syndrome does not appear to be associated with any long-term neurologic sequelae other than those usually associated with the patient's underlying neuropsychiatric disease. Coma is not uncommon in severe cases. Grand mal seizure has rarely been reported [116,131]. The electroencephalogram (EEG) typically is normal or shows nonspecific diffuse slowing [109]. Computed tomographic (CT) scans are normal in 95 percent of patients. Cerebrospinal fluid analysis after lumbar puncture is normal in 97 percent of patients, showing an elevated protein in the other 3 percent [111,149]. In one case a magnetic resonance imaging (MRI) scan revealed hyperintensity of the occipitoparietal white matter [153]. Pathologic examinations of patients at autopsy revealed no specific lesions [140].

Although death from cardiovascular collapse has been reported [113], specific cardiac abnormalities have been poorly described. There is no evidence that severe atrophy, heart block, or congestive heart failure occurs frequently in the syndrome.

Hematologic alterations are mild. The white blood cell count is elevated in 78 percent of cases [109,149], usually less than 20,000 mm^3 and rarely exceeding 25,000 mm^3. Elevation may be due to hemoconcentration and catecholamine release. Platelet count is elevated in 56 percent of patients [109]. A hemolytic coagulopathy, possibly DIC, has been reported rarely [119]. Deep venous thrombosis or antemortem embolic phenomena are not reported in the English literature. Thrombotic events, when they do occur, are more likely a result of the patient's immobility due to coma and muscle rigidity than to any temperature-mediated change.

Lactate dehydrogenase, serum glutamic oxaloacetic-acid-transaminase, serum glutamic pyruvic transaminase, and alkaline phosphatase frequently show mild elevations compatible with rhabdomyolysis and mild hepatic dysfunction. Other significant GI abnormalities have not been reported.

Pulmonary complications occur frequently but appear to be

related not to hyperthermia but to the extrapyramidal actions of the neuroleptics. Muscle dysfunction produces frequent dysphagia [113]. Sialorrhea can be copious and necessitate intubation [127]. It is reported that several patients have clearly aspirated, presumably due to muscle dysfunction, and subsequent pneumonias were most likely due to this aspiration. Pneumonia and respiratory distress [118,119,121,127,132,139,147, 150,151] requiring intubation occur in 13 to 21 percent of patients [109,149] and are probably the most serious frequent sequelae of the neuroleptic malignant syndrome.

DIAGNOSIS. The neuroleptic malignant syndrome may occur after any one of the commonly prescribed neuroleptic agents is used and in any age group. Onset of symptoms may occur within hours after the initial neuroleptic treatment or up to 4 weeks later [149]. In the majority of cases, onset occurs within 1 week from initial neuroleptic drug use, and 88 percent occur within 2 weeks of a dosage increase of an already prescribed neuroleptic agent [149]. Most reported cases have occurred in patients with underlying neuropsychiatric disorders.

Early symptoms usually include dysphagia or dysarthria due to diffuse muscular rigidity, pseudoparkinsonism, dystonia, or catatonic behavior. In one series 96 percent of patients demonstrated rigidity, 92 percent tremor, and 96 percent muteness or hypophonia in the 48 hours prior to diagnosis [109]. Rigidity precedes hyperthermia in 59 percent of patients, is concurrent in 23 percent, and is subsequent in only 8 percent [149]. Autonomic signs of hypermetabolism usually suggest the onset of hyperthermia. Diaphoresis, tachycardia, changes in blood pressure, and tachypnea reflect efforts to dissipate the thermogenesis of muscle contracture and to expel CO_2 effectively. Peak temperatures are reached within 48 hours after the onset of symptoms in 88 percent of patients [109]. Temperatures may reach as high as 42.2°C [119] but are typically lower: 53 percent are more than 40°C and 13 percent are higher than 41°C [109]. Because many patients may be tachypneic, rectal or core, rather than oral, temperatures may need to be followed to ensure accuracy (see Chap. 19). Elevations in creatine kinase and transaminase levels and leukocytosis parallel the body temperature. Creatine kinase is elevated in 97 to 100 percent of patients, is typically all MM isoenzyme, exceeds 10,000 IU in 33 percent of patients, and peaks 2 to 3 days after diagnosis in 64 percent and by 1 week in 93 percent [109,149].

DIFFERENTIAL DIAGNOSIS. A thorough examination and diagnostic evaluation for other causes of hyperthermia should be conducted (Table 73-2). In one series all patients referred to an ICU with a suspicion of neuroleptic malignant syndrome had another diagnosis that would explain the fever [104]. Because many patients taking neuroleptic agents develop extrapyramidal side effects and relatively few cases of hyperthermia are a result of neuroleptic malignant syndrome, other, more common causes of hyperthermia (e.g., meningitis or streptococcal pharyngitis) could easily be missed if a hasty diagnosis of neuroleptic malignant syndrome is made. Appropriate cultures, a chest radiographic, lumbar puncture, and thorough physical examination are mandatory. Patients without classic symptoms are more likely to have another cause of hyperthermia [154].

Other causes of catatonia, heat stroke, malignant hyperthermia, and hyperthermic reactions to other drugs may occasionally be confused with the neuroleptic malignant syndrome. However, "lethal catatonia" with rigidity and fatal hyperthermia rarely occurs in patients not taking neuroleptic agents. The treatment and prognosis of these patients remain unclear [150,155,156,157]. However, if rigidity and hyperthermia sub-

sequently develop in a catatonic patient, the development of neuroleptic malignant syndrome should be presumed and all neuroleptic agents should be stopped. If catatonia has been induced or exacerbated by neurolepsis, withdrawal of the neuroleptic drug should aid in clarifying the diagnosis.

Heat stroke must be considered when temperature elevation develops in a patient taking neuroleptics during periods of high ambient temperature or after vigorous exercise. Unlike neuroleptic malignant syndrome, however, heat stroke is usually accompanied by flaccid obtundation and muscle rigidity is rare.

Malignant hyperthermia resembles neuroleptic malignant syndrome in that both conditions have increased thermogenesis secondary to muscular rigidity as well as similar laboratory findings, and both respond to dantrolene. In most cases an adequate history should clearly separate the two syndromes; hyperthermia results from the use of entirely different agents (compare Tables 73-3 and 73-4). Moreover, the symptoms of malignant hyperthermia are much more rapid in onset and more severe. Extrapyramidal symptoms are also very unusual in malignant hyperthermia. In the rare circumstance in which the two syndromes cannot be distinguished, attempts at paralysis with curare or pancuronium may aid diagnosis. These agents produce a flaccid paralysis in neuroleptic malignant syndrome but should have no effect on the postsynaptically medicated muscle contracture of malignant hyperthermia.

Idiosyncratic drug reactions and anaphylaxis accompanying severe hyperthermia may usually be diagnosed by their distinct clinical presentations. Monoamine oxidase inhibitors may produce hyperthermia, especially when administered with meperidine or dextromethorphan [158,159,160]. In patients with neuropsychiatric disorders who are receiving both neuroleptic agents and monoamine oxidase inhibitors, malignant hyperpyrexia may result from either agent. In these cases both agents should be stopped. Therapies for neuroleptic malignant syndrome, such as bromocriptine or L-dopa, are, however, contraindicated in these patients because of their recent use of monoamine oxidase inhibitors.

TREATMENT. The goal of treatment for neuroleptic malignant syndrome is to reduce the temperature, reverse extrapyramidal side effects, and prevent sequelae such as renal failure and pneumonia.

Specific agents used to decrease thermogenesis by reducing muscle contracture include dantrolene, curare, pancuronium, amantadine, bromocriptine, and L-dopa (Table 73-6). Dantrolene reduces thermogenesis by uncoupling muscle contracture at the membrane level and in doses as small as 1 mg per kilogram may result in a temperature decrease of 1 to 2°C within hours [122,123,127,161]. Dantrolene may also favorably alter CNS dopaminergic metabolism [162]. Although doses of up to 10 mg per kilogram have been used, current practice would recommend doses of 1 to 2.5 mg per kilogram IV every 6 hours until a dose of 100 to 300 mg per day by mouth can be given [163,164]. Paralysis with curare or pancuronium should produce a similar prompt decrease in temperature, but this treatment necessitates mechanical ventilation and extensive support [147]. Bromocriptine, amantadine, and dopamine increase central dopaminergic tone; this decreases the central drive, reducing muscular rigidity and thermogenesis. These agents also are beneficial in that they act directly to reduce extrapyramidal side effects. Prompt decreases in temperature have been reported after the use of 2.5 mg of bromocriptine three times per day [121,125,152,165], 100 of 200 mg of amantadine twice per day [126,166], or 10 to 100 mg of carbidopa/-L-dopa three times per day [114,141].

Failures of these therapies, however, have also been pub-

Table 73-6. Treatments for Neuroleptic Malignant Syndrome

Dantrolene
Paralysis (curare, pancuronium)
Bromocriptine
Amantadine
Levodopa
Electroconvulsive therapy
? Nifedepine

lished [128,130,139,165]. The appropriate dosing remains an important question. Some have advocated bromocriptine doses as high as 60 mg per day [163]. Use of a centrally acting dopamine agonist is clearly warranted when the neuroleptic malignant syndrome is believed to occur because of the withdrawal of anti-Parkinson agents. The use of dantrolene, bromocriptine, and amantadine have yet to be shown to reduce mortality significantly [108]. Although nifedepine produced dramatic results with prompt lowering of temperature in one patient [145], further study is necessary to confirm its efficacy. Electroconvulsive therapy has been successful in several patients [118,119,167,168] and is the only therapeutic modality that may be used successfully to treat simultaneously hyperthermia, the extrapyramidal side effects, and the underlying neuropsychiatric disorder for which the neuroleptic drug was prescribed. Because of several reports of cardiovascular collapse in patients undergoing electroconvulsive therapy, this therapy should be given only to patients at low risk of cardiovascular disease who have failed other therapy.

Less specific agents, such as diphenhydramine, benzotropine, valium, and trihexyphenidyl, have been used successfully [114,117,121,124,126,133] but more typically have not been substantially helpful [106,121,127,128,147,165,166]. Little has been published on the use or efficacy of nonspecific measures, such as acetaminophen [169], cooling blankets, iced saline gastric lavage, and cooled peritoneal dialysis. The usefulness of these methods, however, would be restricted simply to lowering body temperature; they would not be expected to inhibit the underlying ongoing drive to thermogenesis or extrapyramidal reactions.

Reduction of core temperature and muscle rigidity should decrease the risk of renal failure and pneumonia. Decreases in temperature are accompanied by a decrease in creatine kinase levels [113]. By minimizing rhabdomyolysis and by aggressive hydration and diuresis, acute tubular necrosis and renal failure might be avoided. Early reversal of coma, dysphagia, and sialorrhea when present should minimize the risk of aspiration and subsequent pneumonia. Prophylactic intubation should be strongly considered for patients with excessive sialorrhea, swallowing dysfunction, or coma. All obtunded patients or those with swallowing difficulty should take nothing by mouth.

The best treatment regimen for neuroleptic malignant syndrome remains to be determined [109,149,170–176]. Because many patients respond to symptomatic treatment after withdrawal of neuroleptic therapy [177] and because all current knowledge is derived from case reports, not clinical trials, treatment recommendations are difficult to make. The average time to recovery with supportive care only is 9.6 days [97]. Treatment should be guided by clinical judgment. Because of the frequency of coma, renal failure, respiratory insufficiency, and cardiovascular collapse, patients with temperatures over 39°C should be initially evaluated and observed in the ICU. Treatment and close observation should be continued for at least 1 week, longer when necessary. The duration of symptoms varies with the rate of excretion of neuroleptic metabolites. In patients receiving long-acting neuroleptic agents such as fluphenazine,

symptoms may last for weeks. When therapy is withdrawn, symptoms may recur up to and after 11 days of drug abstinence [165]. The duration of treatment, therefore, must be adjusted according to the metabolism of the inciting agent, but in most cases it can be tapered over 1 to 2 weeks. Acetaminophen and cooling of intravenous solutions during the acute period produce few side effects and may be beneficial. Bromocriptine therapy appears safe and effective in reducing temperature and minimizing extrapyramidal reactions. Dantrolene therapy does carry a risk of hepatotoxicity, but in patients with temperatures greater than 40°C its use is specific and should be beneficial. Electroconvulsive therapy should be considered only for patients who do not respond properly to bromocriptine, dantrolene, and supportive therapy. More aggressive interventions, such as paralysis, use of cooled dialysate, or cardiopulmonary bypass cooling, should be reserved for refractory life-threatening cases.

PROGNOSIS. Although mortality rates as high as 20 to 30 percent have been reported [100], this rate can probably be reduced to less than 10 percent with appropriate support and treatment. Age and sex do not appear to influence mortality greatly. Mortality rate does appear to be influenced by peak temperature, inciting neuroleptic drug, and renal failure. No deaths among patients with maximal temperatures lower than 40°C have been reported. Haloperidol is statistically less likely to result in death than other neuroleptics [108]. Death has been reported as a result of "cardiovascular collapse" [113], pneumonia [118,147], renal failure [116,132], and hepatic failure [132]. The development of renal failure is particularly ominous; in some series 46 percent of patients with myoglobinuria and 56 percent of those with renal failure died [108].

Typically ICU stay is prolonged due to frequency of complications and slow response to therapy. Although dopaminergic therapy lowers the mean time to response from 6.8 to 1.1 days [178], the mean time to recovery is long—13 days when the syndrome results from nondepot neuroleptics and 26 days for depot neuroleptics [149]. One patient receiving haloperidol decanoate was symptomatic for months [179]. Rechallenge with neuroleptics may cause the syndrome to recur but this occurs much more frequently during the first 2 weeks [180,181]. The prognosis among survivors appears to be excellent, and sequelae other than mild extrapyramidal symptoms compatible with prior neuroleptic treatment appear unusual [182].

Drug-Induced Hyperthermia

Most of our knowledge about drug-induced hyperthermia is anecdotal, having been derived from case reports. Numerous drugs have been suggested to cause hyperthermia. Drugs that blunt cardiovascular performance, such as beta-blockers, or alter heat dissipation, such as chlorpromazine, are widely used and clearly can contribute to temperature elevation. These drugs rarely result in clinically significant hyperthermia without some other precipitant. Patients on such agents typically present with heat stroke. This section focuses on those drugs that independently produce significant elevations of temperature (Table 73-7).

Commonly abused street drugs may result in severe hyperthermia without other pharmacologic or environmental stimuli. Although these drugs all have a low incidence of producing severe hyperthermia, due to the prevalence of their use they may account for a large percentage of cases of hyperthermia presenting to an emergency room. Temperature elevation ac-

Table 73-7. Drugs That Produce Hyperthermia

Cocaine and similar agents
Phencyclidine
Amphetamine
Lysergic acid diethylamine and similar hallucinogens
Monoamine oxidase inhibitors
Tricyclics
Aspirin

companies phencyclidine (PCP) use in 2.6 percent of cases [183]. Temperatures as high as 41.9°C have been reported [183]. Amphetamine use may result in temperature higher than 43°C [184,185] and lysergic acid diethylamine (LSD), a serotonin analog, over 41°C [186]. Monoamine oxidase inhibitors may produce hyperthermia, especially when administered with meperidine or dextromethorphan [158,159,160]. Combination therapy of a monoamine oxidase inhibitor with a tricyclic has also resulted in hyperthermia, although this appears to be rare [158,187]. Aspirin receives mention as a cause of hyperthermia secondary to increased metabolism, but little hard data are available [188].

PATHOGENESIS. These drugs are assumed to cause hyperthermia as a result of muscular contracture or hypermetabolism. Virtually all cases of drug-induced hyperthermia mention increased muscle tone, rigidity, or tremor. Cocaine, amphetamine, PCP, and hallucinogens appear to produce hyperthermia by centrally and perhaps peripherally inducing vigorous muscle contractions [189,190]. Repeated cocaine use may elevate temperature by depletion of postsynaptic dopamine [189]. Tricyclics, amphetamines, and monoamine oxidase inhibitors may elevate CNS serotonin, resulting in hyperthermia [158,159,160,190]. Dextromethorphan and meperidine are believed to inhibit serotonin reuptake and in susceptible patients may increase already high serotonin levels and trigger a hyperthermic crisis [159]. Some patients may have a component of exertional heat stroke, in that they are frequently found running in an agitated or confused manner. Almost all suffer loss of voluntary control of temperature. Status epilepticus frequently accompanies drug-induced hyperthermia but is unlikely to contribute greatly to hyperthermia, in that status is rarely associated with significant temperature elevation in the absence of drug use [191]. Reactions appear mostly idiosyncratic; they are infrequent in comparison to the total number of persons using the drug; occur by IV, enteral, and nasal insufflation usage; and occur after low dose use and massive overdose [192].

PATHOPHYSIOLOGY. The pathophysiology of drug-induced hyperthermia is most similar to that of exertional heat stroke or malignant hyperthermia. Rise in temperature is frequently rapid, and multiple organ failure may rapidly ensue with prolonged elevation of temperature. Patients, however, may also be affected by the direct toxic action of the drug, and it may be difficult to separate the sequelae of hyperthermia from those of direct drug toxicity. Amphetamine overdose, for example, may result in severe rhabdomyolysis, DIC, and renal failure at temperatures of less than 40°C. Hyperthermia can be assumed to have the same physiologic sequelae in these patients as others, but prompt correction of temperature may not be adequate to ensure survival.

DIAGNOSIS. In most case reports patients are described as agitated, hyperexcited, and diaphoretic and have increased muscle tone. The diagnosis of drug-induced hyperthermia should be considered mostly when the patient is young, is an outpatient, has not engaged in recent heavy exertion, or has a history of drug abuse. Because nonexertional heat stroke is uncommon in youth, hyperthermia at a young age always suggests possible drug intoxication. Diagnosis may be confirmed by toxicologic screen or history.

TREATMENT. In all cases treatment should be directed at minimizing the toxicity of the causative drug. Treatment of hyperthermia should be both symptomatic and directed at the underlying physiology. Treatment in general parallels that for exertional heat stroke and is extensively outlined in that section. Evaporative cooling is the preferred method of cooling and should be instituted in any patient with a temperature above 39°C. Many patients may be dehydrated from diaphoresis and require volume replacement. As in malignant hyperthermia and exertional heat stroke, hyperkalemia, acidosis, and myoglobinuria demand careful attention. Because the temperature appears to be generated from muscular contraction, paralysis or use of dantrolene would appear to be useful therapy. Paralysis has been effective in several cases. Paralysis and support with mechanical ventilation should be considered in any patient with a temperature above 40°C not responding promptly to symptomatic cooling. If therapeutic drug levels persist, rebound hyperthermia may occur as paralysis resolves. Use of dopaminergic agents has been advocated, but clinical experience is minimal [189].

PROGNOSIS. Hyperthermia due to amphetamine overdose appears to be well tolerated, with 10 of 11 patients reported in the literature surviving [184,185,193,194]. Hyperthermia in cocaine overdose is frequently accompanied by renal failure [192,195,196], DIC [196,197], and seizure [196,197], and several fatalities [192,196,197,198] have been reported. Survival despite high temperature has been recorded as well [192,195,199]. *Pneumocystis carinii* pneumonia with hyperthermia has resulted in renal failure [200], respiratory and liver failure with coma, and subsequent death [201]. Death and significant morbidity appear to be rare when tricyclics and monoamine oxidase inhibitors are used concurrently [187]. The prognosis when monoamine oxidase inhibitors are combined with meperidine is unclear: no large series have been reported, and both death and cure with appropriate treatment have been reported [160].

References

1. Gauss H, Meyer KA: Heat stroke: A report of 158 cases from Cook County Hospital, Chicago. *Am J Med Sci* 154:554, 1917.
2. Clowes GHA, O'Donnell TF: Heat stroke. *N Engl J Med* 291:564, 1974.
3. Ellis EP: Mortality from heat illness and heat-aggravated illness in the United States. *Environ Res* 5:1, 1972.
4. Heat stroke: United States, 1980. *MMWR* 30:277, 1981.
5. Wise TN: Heat stroke in three chronic schizophrenics: Case reports and clinical considerations. *Compr Psychiatry* 14:263, 1973.
6. Kilbourne EM, Choi K, Jones S, Thacker SB: Risk factors for heat ske: A case control study. *JAMA* 247:3332, 1982.
7. Cole RD: Heat stroke during training with nuclear, biological, and chemical protective clothing: Case report. *Mil Med* 148:624, 1983.
8. Fatalities from occupational heat exposure. *MMWR* 33:410, 1984.
9. Stine FJ: Heat illness. *JACEP* 8:154, 1979.

10. Knochel JP: Environmental heat illness: An eclectic review. *Arch Intern Med* 133:841, 1974.
11. O'Donnell TF: Acute heat stroke: Epidemiologic, biochemical, renal, and coagulation studies. *JAMA* 234:824, 1975.
12. Shibolet S, Coll R, Gilat T, Sohar E: Heat stroke: Its clinical picture and mechanism in 36 cases. *Q J Med* 36:525, 1967.
13. Ansari A, Burch GE: Influence of hot environments on the cardiovascular system. *Arch Intern Med* 123:371, 1969.
14. Adams BE, Manoguerra AS, Lilja GP, et al: Heat stroke: Associated with medications having anticholinergic effects. *Minn Med* 60:103, 1977.
15. Hanson PG, Zimmerman SW: Exertional heat stroke in novice runners. *JAMA* 242:154, 1979.
16. Rose RC, Hughes RD, Yarbrough DR, Dewees SP: Heat injuries among recreational runners. *South Med J* 73:1038, 1980.
17. Dann EJ, Berkman N: Chronic idiopathic anhydrosis: A rare cause of heat stroke. *Postgrad Med J* 68:750, 1992.
18. Chun-Jen S, Mao-Tsun L, Shih-Han T: Experimental study on the pathogenesis of heat stroke. *J Neurosurg* 60:1246, 1984.
19. Attia M, Khogali M, El-Khatib G: Heat stroke: An upward shift of temperature regulation set point at an elevated body temperature. *Int Arch Occup Environ Health* 53:9, 1983.
20. Baba N, Ruppert RD: Alteration of eccrine sweat gland in fatal heat stroke. *Arch Pathol* 85:669, 1968.
21. Sprung CL: Hemodynamic alterations of heat stroke in the elderly. *Chest* 75:361, 1979.
22. Levine JA: Heat stroke in the aged. *Am J Med* 47:251, 1969.
23. McElroy CR: Update on heat illness. *Top Emerg Med* 2:1, 1980.
24. Fajardo LF: Pathologic effects of hyperthermia in normal tissues. *Cancer Res* 44 (suppl):4826S, 1984.
25. Vertel RM, Knochel JP: Acute renal failure due to heat injury: An analysis of 10 cases associated with the high incidence of myoglobinuria. *Am J Med* 43:435, 1967.
26. Costrini AM, Pitt HA, Gustafson AB, Uddin DE: Cardiovascular and metabolic manifestations of heat stroke and severe heat exhaustion. *Am J Med* 66:296, 1979.
27. Hart GR, Anderson RJ, Crumpler CP, et al: Epidemic classical heat stroke: Clinical characteristics and course of 28 patients. *Medicine* 61:189, 1982.
28. Dahmash NS, Al Harthi SS, Akhtar J: Invasive evaluation of patients with heat stroke. *Chest* 103:1210, 1993.
29. Knochel JP: Heat stroke and related heat disorders. *Dis Mon* 35:306, 1989.
30. Kew MC, Abrahams C, Levin NW, et al: The effects of heat stroke on the function and structure of the kidney. *Q J Med* 36:277, 1967.
31. Malamud N, Haymaker W, Custer RP: Heat stroke: A clinico-pathologic study of 125 fatal cases. *Mil Surg* 97:397, 1946.
32. Graham BS, Lichtenstein MJ, Hinson JM, et al: Nonexertional heat-stroke physiologic management and cooling in 14 patients. *Arch Intern Med* 146:87, 1986.
33. Minassian DC, Mehra V, Jones BR: Dehydrational crises from severe diarrhea or heat stroke and risk of cataract. *Lancet* 1:751, 1984.
34. Shieh SD, Lin YF, Lu KC, et al: Role of creatine phosphokinase in predicting acute renal failure in hypocalcemic exertional heat stroke. *Am J Nephrol* 12:252, 1992.
35. Rubel LR: Hepatic injury associated with heat stroke. *Ann Clin Lab Sci* 14:130, 1984.
36. Gader AMA, Al-Mashhadani SA, Al-Harthy SS: Direct activation of platelets by heat is the possible trigger of coagulopathy of heat stroke. *Br J Haematol* 74:86, 1990.
37. Jones TS, Liang AP, Kilbourne EM, et al: Morbidity and mortality associated with the July 1980 heat wave in St. Louis and Kansas City, MO. *JAMA* 247:3328, 1982.
38. Keatinge WR, Coleshaw SRK, Easton JC, et al: Increased platelet and red cell counts, blood viscosity, and plasma cholesterol levels during heat stress, and mortality from coronary and cerebral thrombosis. *Am J Med* 81:795, 1986.
39. Al-Harthi SS, Karrar O, Al-Mashhadani SA: Metabolite and hormonal profiles in heat stroke patients at Mecca pilgrimage. *J Intern Med* 228:343, 1990.
40. Knochel JP, Caskey JH: The mechanism of hypophosphatemia in acute heat stroke. *JAMA* 238:425, 1977.
41. Tucker CE, Stanford J, Graves B, et al: Classic heat stroke: Clinical and laboratory assessment. *South Med J* 78:20, 1985.
42. Buck CW, Carscallen HB, Hobbs GE: Temperature regulation in schizophrenia. *Arch Neurol Psych* 64:828, 1950.
43. Litman RE: Heat stroke in parkinsonism. *Arch Intern Med* 89:562, 1952.
44. Randall WC, Wurster RD, Lewin RJ: Responses of patients with high spinal transection to high ambient temperatures. *J Appl Physiol* 21:985, 1966.
45. McLeod RN: Heat illness in early season football practice. *J Ky Med Assoc* 70:613, 1972.
46. Whitworth JAG, Wolfman MJ: Fatal heat stroke in a long distance runner. *Lancet* 1:545, 1984.
47. Wyndham CH: Heat stroke and hyperthermia in marathon runners. *Ann NY Acad Sci* 301:128, 1977.
48. Talman WT, Florek G, Bullard DE: A hyperthermic syndrome in two subjects with acute hydrocephalus. *Arch Neurol* 45:1037, 1988.
49. Chesanow RL: A 65-year-old woman with heat stroke. *Am J Med* 41:415, 1961.
50. Khogali M, Weiner JS: Heat stroke: Report on 18 cases. *Lancet* 2:276, 1980.
51. Al-Aska AK, Abu-Aisha H, Yaqub B, et al: Simplified cooling bed for heatstroke. *Lancet* 1:381, 1987.
52. Seraj MA, Channa AB, Al Harthi SS, et al: Are heat stroke patients volume depleted? Importance of monitoring central venous pressure as a simple guideline to therapy. *Resuscitation* 21:33, 1991.
53. Severinghaus JW: Respiration and hypothermia. *Ann NY Acad Sci* 80:384, 1959.
54. Malan A: Blood acid base state at variable temperature, a graphical representation. *Respir Physiol* 31:259, 1977.
55. Kelman GR, Nunn JF: Nomograms for correction of blood pO_2, pCO_2, pH, and base excess for time and temperature. *J Appl Physiol* 21:1484, 1966.
56. Chao TC, Simniah R, Pakiam JE: Acute heat stroke deaths. *Pathology* 13:145, 1981.
57. Slovis CM, Anderson GF, Casolaro A: Survival in a heat stroke victim with a core temperature in excess of 46.5°C. *Ann Emerg Med* 11:269, 1982.
58. Lee S, Merriam A, Skim TS, et al: Cerebellar degeneration in neuroleptic malignant syndrome: Neuropathologic findings and review of the literature concerning heat-related nervous system injury. *J Neurol Neurosurg Psychiatry* 52:387, 1989.
59. Yaqub BA, Daif AK, Panayiotopoulos CP: Pancerebellar syndrome in heat stroke: Clinical course and CT scan findings. *Neuroradiology* 29:294, 1987.
60. Slovis CM, Anderson GF, Casolaro A: Survival in a heat stroke victim with a core temperature in excess of 46.5°C. *Ann Emerg Med* 1:269, 1982.
61. Aldrete JA: Advances in the diagnosis and treatment of malignant hyperthermia. *Acta Anaesthesiol Scand* 25:477, 1981.
62. Gronert GA: Malignant hyperthermia. *Anesthesiology* 53:395, 1980.
63. Michelson JR, Gallant EM, Litterer LA, et al: Abnormal sarcoplasmic reticulum ryanodine receptor in malignant hyperthermia. *J Biol Chem* 263:9310, 1988.
64. MacLennan DH, Duff C, Zorzato F, et al: Ryanodine receptor gene is a candidate for predisposition to hyperthermia. *Nature* 343:559, 1990.
65. McCarthy TV, Healy JMS, Heffron JJA, et al: Localization of the malignant hyperthermia susceptibility locus to human chromosome 19q12-13.2. *Nature* 343:562, 1990
66. Schiller HH: Chronic viral myopathy and malignant hyperthermia. *N Engl J Med* 292:1409, 1975.
67. Tsueda K, Dubick MN, Wright BD, et al: Intraoperative hyperthermic crisis in two children with undifferentiated lymphoma. *Anesth Analg* 57:511, 1978.
68. Campbell IT, Ellis FR, Evans RT, Mortimer MG: Studies of body temperatures, blood lactate, cortisol and free fatty acid levels during exercise in human subjects susceptible to malignant hyperpyrexia. *Acta Anaesthesiol Scand* 27:349, 1983.
69. Denborough MA: Etiology and pathophysiology of malignant hyperthermia. *Int Anesthesiol Clin* 7:11, 1979.
70. Steward DJ: Malignant hyperthermia: The acute crisis. *Int Anesthiol* 17:1, 1979.

71. Kalow W, Britt BA, Chan F-Y: Epidemiology and inheritance of malignant hyperthermia. *Int Anesthesiol Clin* 17:119, 1979.
72. Lutsky I, Witkowski J, Henschel EO: HLA typing in a family prone to malignant hyperthermia. *Anesthesiology* 56:224, 1982.
73. Britt BA: Preanesthetic diagnosis of malignant hyperthermia. *Int Anesthesiol Clin* 17:63, 1979.
74. Glisson SN: Malignant hyperthermia. *Compr Ther* 14:33, 1988.
75. Harriman DGF: Preanesthetic investigations of malignant hypothermia: Microscopy. *Int Anesthesiol Clin* 17:97, 1979.
76. Ohnishi ST, Katagi H, Ohnishi T, et al: Detection of malignant hyperthermia susceptibility using a spin label technique on red blood cells. *Br J Anaesth* 61:565, 1988.
77. Britt BA, Kalow W: Malignant hyperthermia: A statistical review. *Can Anaesth Soc J* 17:293, 1970.
78. Felice-Johnson J, Sudds T, Bennett G: Malignant hyperthermia: Current perspectives. *Am J Hosp Pharm* 38:646, 1981.
79. Bacon AK: Pulse oximetry in malignant hyperthermia. *Anaesth Intensive Care* 17:208, 1989.
80. Baudendistel L, Goudsouzian N, Cote C, Strafford M: End tidal CO_2 monitoring: Its use in the diagnosis and management of malignant hyperthermia. *Anesthesia* 39:1000, 1984.
81. Liebenschutz F, Mai C, Pickerodt VWA: Increased carbon dioxide production in two patients with malignant hyperpyrexia and its control by dantrolene. *Br J Anaesth* 51:899, 1979.
82. Triner L, Sherman J: Potential value of expiratory carbon dioxide measurement in patients considered to be susceptible to malignant hyperthermia. *Anesthesiology* 55:482, 1981.
83. Badgwell JM, Heaver JE: Masseter spasm heralds malignant hyperthermia or merely academia gone mad? *Anesthesiology* 61:230, 1984.
84. Schwartz L, Rockoff MA, Koka BV: Masseter spasm with anesthesia: Incidence and implications. *Anesthesiology* 61:772, 1984.
85. Flewellen E, Nelson TE: Halothane-succinylcholine induced masseter spasm: Indicative of malignant hyperthermia susceptibility? *Anesth Analg* 63:693, 1984.
86. Ellis FR, Halsall PJ: Suxamethonium spasm: A differential diagnostic conundrum. *Br J Anaesth* 56:381, 1984.
87. Larach MG, Rosenberg H, Larach DR, Broennle AM: Prediction of malignant hyperthermia susceptibility by clinical signs. *Anesthesiology* 66:547, 1987.
88. Peters KR, Nance P, Wingard DW: Malignant hyperthyroidism or malignant hyperthermia? *Anesth Analg* 60:613, 1981.
89. Bennett MH, Wainwright AP: Acute thyroid crisis on induction of anaesthesia. *Anaesthesia* 44:28, 1989.
90. Crowley KG, Cunningham AJ, Conroy B, et al: Phaeochromocytoma: A presentation mimicking malignant hyperthermia. *Anaesthesia* 43:1031, 1988.
91. Gallant EM, Ahern CP: Malignant hyperthermia: Responses of skeletal muscles to general anesthetics. *Mayo Clin Proc* 58:758, 1983.
92. Kolb ME, Horne ML, Martz R: Dantrolene in human malignant hyperthermia: A multicenter study. *Anesthesiology* 56:254, 1982.
93. Gjessing J, Barsa J, Tomlin PJ: A possible means of rapid cooling in the emergency treatment of malignant hyperpyrexia. *Br J Anaesth* 48:469, 1976.
94. Allen GC, Cattran CB, Peterson RG, et al: Plasma levels of dantrolene following oral administration in malignant hyperthermia-susceptible patients. *Anesthesiology* 69:900, 1988.
95. Ryan JF, Donlon JV, Malt RA, et al: Cardiopulmonary bypass in the treatment of malignant hyperthermia. *N Engl J Med* 290:1121, 1974.
96. Delay J, Deniker P: Drug-induced extrapyramidal syndromes, in Vinken PJ, Bruyn GW (eds): *Diseases of the Basal Ganglia*. Amsterdam, North Holland, 1968, pp 248–266.
97. Caroff SN, Mann SC: Neuroleptic malignant syndrome. *Med Clin North Am* 77:185,1993.
98. Ebadi M, Pfeiffer RF, Murrin LC: Pathogenesis and treatment of the neuroleptic malignant sysndrome. *Gen Pharmacol* 21:367, 1990.
99. Rodnitzky RL, Keyser DL: Neurologic complications of drugs. *Psychiatr Clin North Am* 15:491, 1992.
100. Caroff SN: The neuroleptic malignant syndrome. *J Clin Psychiatry* 41:79, 1980.
101. Modestin J, Toffler G, Drescher JP: Neuroleptic malignant syndrome: Results of a prospective study. *Psychiatry Res* 44:251, 1992.
102. Gelenberg AJ, Bellinghausen B, Wojcik JD, et al: A prospective survey of neuroleptic malignant syndrome in a short-term psychiatric hosptial. *Am J Psychiatry* 145:517, 1988.
103. Friedman JH, Davis R, Wagner RL: Neuroleptic malignant syndrome: The results of a 6-month prospective study of incidence in a state psychiatric hospital. *Clin Neuropharmacol* 11:373, 1988.
104. Keck PE Jr, Pope HG Jr, McElroy SL: Frequency and presentation of neuroleptic malignant syndrome: A prospective study. *Am J Psychiatry* 144:1344, 1987.
105. Hermesh H, Aizenber D, Weizman A, et al: Risk for definite neuroleptic malignant syndrome: A prospective study of 223 consecutive inpatients. *Br J Psychiatry* 161:254, 1992.
106. Burke RE, Fahn S, Mayeaux R, et al: Neuroleptic malignant syndrome caused by dopamine-depleting drugs in a patient with Huntington's disease. *Neurology (NY)* 31:1022, 1981.
107. Keck PE, Pope HG, McElroy SL: Declining frequency of neuroleptic malignant syndrome in a hospital population. *Am J Psychiatry* 148:880, 1991.
108. Shalev A, Hermesh H, Munitz H: Mortality from neuroleptic malignant syndrome. *J Clin Psychiatry* 50:18, 1989.
109. Rosebush PI, Stewart TD: A prospective analysis of 24 episodes of neuroleptic malignant syndrome. *Am J Psychiatry* 146:717, 1989.
110. Lopez JR, Sanchez V, Lopez MJ: Sarcoplasmic ionic calcium concentration in neuroleptic malignant syndrome. *Cell Calcium* 10:223, 1989.
111. Caroff SN, Mann SC: Neuroleptic malignant syndrome. *Psychopharmacol Bull* 24:25, 1988.
112. Guerrera RJ, Chang SS, Romero JA: A comparison of diagnostic criteria for neuroleptic malignant syndrome. *J Clin Psychiatry* 53:56, 1992.
113. Itoh H, Ohtsuka N, Ogita K, et al: Malignant neuroleptic syndrome: Its present status in Japan and clinical problems. *Folia Psychiatr Neurol Jpn* 31:565, 1977.
114. Stoudemire A, Luther JS: Neuroleptic malignant syndrome and neuroleptic induced catatonia: Differential diagnosis and treatment. *Int J Psychiatry Med* 14:57, 1984.
115. Oppenheim G: Mutism and hyperthermia in a patient treated with neuroleptics. *Med J Aust* 2:228, 1973.
116. Eiser AR, Neff MS, Slifkin RF: Acute myoglobinuric renal failure: A consequence of the neuroleptic malignant syndrome. *Arch Intern Med* 142:601, 1982.
117. Geller B, Greydanus DE: Haloperidol induced comatose state with hyperthermia and rigidity in adolescence: Two case reports with a literature review. *J Clin Psychiatry* 40:102, 1979.
118. Jesse SS, Anderson GF: ECT in the neuroleptic malignant syndrome: Case report. *J Clin Psychiatry* 44:186, 1983.
119. Eles GR, Songer JE, DiPette DJ: Neuroleptic malignant syndrome complicated by disseminated intravascular coagulation. *Arch Intern Med* 144:1296, 1984.
120. Liskow BI: Relationship between neuroleptic malignant syndrome and malignant hyperthermia. *Am J Psychiatry* 142:390, 1985.
121. Mueller PS, Vester JW, Fermaglich J: Neuroleptic malignant syndrome: Successful treatment with bromocriptine. *JAMA* 249:386, 1983.
122. May DC, Morns SW, Stewart RM, et al: Neuroleptic malignant syndrome: Response to dantrolene sodium. *Ann Intern Med* 98:183, 1983.
123. Coons DJ, Hillman FJ, Marshall RW: Treatment of neuroleptic malignant syndrome with dantrolene sodium: A case report. *Am J Psychiatry* 139:944, 1982.
124. Feibel JM, Schiffer RB: Sympathoadrenal medullary hyperactivity in the neuroleptic malignant syndrome: A case report. *Am J Psychiatry* 138:1115, 1981.
125. Dhib-Jalbut S, Messelbrock R, Brott T, et al: Treatment of the neuroleptic malignant syndrome with bromocriptine. *JAMA* 250:484, 1983.
126. Amdurski S, Radwan M, Levi A, et al: A therapeutic trial of amantadine in haloperidol-induced malignant neuroleptic syndrome. *Curr Ther Res* 33:225, 1983.
127. Goulon M, deRohan-Chabot P, Elkharrat D, et al: Beneficial effects of dantrolene in the treatment of neuroleptic malignant syndrome: A report of two cases. *Neurology* 33:516, 1983.
128. Tollefson GD, Garvey MJ: The neuroleptic syndrome and central dopamine metabolites. *J Clin Psychopharmacol* 4:150, 1984.
129. Lew T, Tollefson G: Chlorpromazine-induced neuroleptic malig-

nant syndrome and its response to diazepam. *Biol Psychiatry* 18:1441, 1983.

130. Downey GP, Rosenberg M, Caroff S, et al: Neuroleptic malignant syndrome patient with unique clinical and physiologic features. *Am J Med* 77:338, 1984.

131. McAllister RG: Fever, tachycardia and hypertension with acute catatonic schizophrenia. *Arch Intern Med* 138:1154, 1978.

132. Weinberg S, Twersky RS: Neuroleptic malignant syndrome. *Anesth Analg* 62:848, 1983.

133. Tollefson G: A case of neuroleptic malignant syndrome: In vitro muscle comparison with malignant hyperthermia. *J Clin Psychopharmacol* 2:266, 1982.

134. Ewart AL, Klock J, Wells B, Phelps S: Neuroleptic malignant syndrome associated with loxapine. *J Clin Psychiatry* 44:37, 1983.

135. Gradon JD: Neuroleptic malignant syndrome possibly caused by molindone hydrochloride. *Ann Pharmacother* 25:1071, 1991.

136. Anderson ES, Powers PS: Neuroleptic malignant syndrome associated with clozapine use. *J Clin Psychiatry* 52:102, 1991.

137. Halman M, Goldbloom DS: Fluoxetine and neuroleptic malignant syndrome. *Biol Psychiatry* 28: 518, 1990.

138. Spirt MJ, Chan W, Thieberg M, et al: Neuroleptic malignant syndrome induced by domperidone. *Dig Dis Sci* 37:946, 1992.

139. Henderson VW, Wooten GF: Neuroleptic malignant syndrome: A pathogenetic role for dopamine receptor blockade? *Neurology (NY)* 31:132, 1981.

140. Sechi GP, Tanda F, Mutani R: Fatal hyperpyrexia after withdrawal of levodopa. *Neurology* 34:249, 1984.

141. Toru M, Matsuda O, Makiguchi K, et al: Neuroleptic malignant syndrome-like state following withdrawal of anti-parkinsonian drugs. *J Nerv Ment Dis* 1969:324, 1981.

141. Patterson JF: Neuroleptic malignant syndrome associated with metoclopramide. *South Med J* 81:674, 1988.

143. Samie MR: Neuroleptic malignant-like syndrome induced by metoclopramide. *Mov Disord* 2:57, 1987.

144. Friedman LS, Weinrauch LA, D'Elia JA: Metoclopramide-induced neuroleptic malignant syndrome. *Arch Intern Med* 147:1495, 1987.

145. Hermesh H, Molcho A, Aizenberg D, et al: The calcium antagonist nifedipine in recurrent neuroleptic malignant syndrome. *Clin Neuropharmacol* 11:552, 1988.

146. Lim R: Idiopathic hypoparathyroidism presenting as the neuroleptic malignant syndrome. *Br J Hosp Med* 41:182, 1989.

147. Morris HH, McCormick WF, Reinarz JA: Neuroleptic malignant syndrome. *Arch Neurol* 37:462, 1980.

148. Shalev A, Hermesh H, Munitz H: The role of external heat load in triggering the neuroleptic malignant syndrome. *Am J Psychiatry* 145:110, 1988.

149. Addonizio G, Susman VL, Roth SD: Neuroleptic malignant syndrome: Review and analysis of 115 cases. *Biol Psychiatry* 22:1004, 1987.

150. Curley FJ, Irwin RS: Disorders of temperature control, part I. *J Intensive Care Med* 1:5, 1986.

151. Denborough MA, Collins SP, Hopkinson KC: Rhabdomyolysis and malignant hyperpyrexia. *Br Med J* 288:1878, 1984.

152. Granato JE, Stern BJ, Ringel A, et al: Neuroleptic malignant syndrome: Successful treatment with dantrolene and bromocriptine. *Ann Neurol* 4:89, 1983.

153. Becker T, Kornhuber J, Hofmann E, et al: MRI white matter hyperintensity in neuroleptic malignant syndrome (NMS): A clue to pathogenesis? *J Neural Transm* 90:151, 1992

154. Sewell DD, Jeste DV: Distinguishing neuroleptic malignant syndrome (NMS) from NMS-like acute medical illnesses: A study of 34 cases. *J Neuropsychiatry Clin Neurosci* 4:265, 1992.

155. Castillo E, Rubin RT, Holsboer-Trachsler E: Clinical differentiation between lethal catatonia and neuroleptic malignant syndrome. *Am J Psychiatry* 146:324, 1989.

156. Anderson WH: Lethal catatonia and the neuroleptic malignant syndrome. *Crit Care Med* 19:1333, 1991.

157. Chiang WK, Herschman Z: Lethal catatonia and the neuroleptic malignant syndrome. *Crit Care Med* 20:1622, 1992.

158. Gong SNC, Rogers KJ: Role of brain monoamines in the fatal hyperthermia induced by pethidine or imipramine in rabbits pretreated with a monoamine oxidase inhibitor. *Br J Pharmacol* 48:12, 1978.

159. Browne B, Linter S: Monoamine oxidase inhibitors and narcotic analgesics: A critical review of the implications for treatment. *Br J Psychiatry* 151:210, 1987.

160. Meyer D, Halfin V: Toxicity secondary to meperidine in patients on monoamine oxidase inhibitors: A case report and critical review. *J Clin Psychopharmacol* 1:319, 1981.

161. Goekoop JG, Carboat PA: Treatment of neuroleptic malignant syndrome with dantrolene. *Lancet* 2:49, 1982.

162. Nisijima K, Ishiguro T: Does dantrolene influence central dopamine and serotonin metabolism in the neuroleptic malignant syndrome? A retrospective study. *Biol Psychiatry* 33:45, 1993.

163. Olmsted TR: Neuroleptic malignant syndrome: Guidelines for treatment and reinstitution of neuroleptics. *South Med J* 81:888, 1988.

164. Harpe C, Stondemire A: Aetiology and treatment of neuroleptic malignant syndrome. *Med Toxicol* 2:166, 1987.

165. Zubenko G, Pope MG: Management of a case of neuroleptic malignant syndrome with bromocriptine. *Am J Psychiatry* 40:1619, 1983.

166. McCarron MM, Boettger ML, Peck JJ: A case of neuroleptic malignant syndrome successfully treated with amantadine. *J Clin Psychiatry* 43:381, 1982.

167. Hermesh H, Aizenberg D, Weizman A: A successful electroconvulsive treatment of neuroleptic malignant syndrome. *Acta Psychiatr Scand* 75:237, 1987.

168. Addonizio G, Susman VL: ECT as a treatment alternative for patients with symptoms of neuroleptic malignant syndrome. *J Clin Psychiatry* 48:102, 1987.

169. Lotstra F, Linkowski P, Mendlewicz J: General anesthesia after neuroleptic malignant syndrome. *Biol Psychiatry* 18:243, 1983.

170. Maling TJB, MacDonald AD, Davis M, Hawkins T: Neuroleptic malignant syndrome: A review of the Wellington experience. *N Z Med J* 101:193, 1988.

171. Smego RA, Durack DT: The neuroleptic malignant syndrome. *Arch Intern Med* 142:1183, 1982.

172. Birkhimer LJ, DeVane CL: The neuroleptic malignant syndrome: Presentation and treatment. *Drug Intell Clin Pharm* 18:462, 1984.

173. Conner CS: Therapy of syndrome malin. *Drug Intell Clin Pharm* 17:639, 1983.

174. Neuroleptic malignant syndrome. *Lancet* 1:545, 1984.

175. Dallman JH: Neuroleptic malignant syndrome: A review. *Mil Med* 149:471, 1984.

176. Guze BM, Baxter LR: Neuroleptic malignant syndrome. *N Engl J Med* 313:163, 1985.

177. Rosebush PI, Sttewart T, Mazurek MF: The treatment of neuroleptic malignant syndrome: Are dantrolene and bromocriptine useful adjuncts to supportive care? *Br J Psychiatry* 159:709, 1991.

178. Rosenberg MR, Green M: Neuroleptic malignant syndrome. *Arch Intern Med* 149:1927, 1989.

179. Legras A, Hurel D, Dabrowski G, et al: Protracted neuroleptic malignant syndrome complicating long-acting neuroleptic administration. *Am J Med* 85:875, 1988.

180. Wells AJ, Sommi RW, Crismon ML: Neuroleptic rechallenge after neuroleptic malignant syndrome: Case report and literature review. *Drug Intell Clin Pharm* 22:475, 1988.

181. Rosebush PI, Stewart TD, Gelenberg AJ: Twenty neuroleptic rechallenges after neuroleptic malignant syndrome in 15 patients. *J Clin Psychiatry* 50:295, 1989.

182. Koponen H, Repo E, Lepola U: Long-term outcome after neuroleptic malignant syndrome. *Acta Psychiatr Scand* 84:550, 1991.

183. McCarron MM, Schulze BW, Thompson GA, et al: Acute Phencyclidine intoxication: Incidence of clinical findings in 1,000 cases. *Ann Emerg Med* 10:237, 1981.

184. Ginsberg MD, Hertzman M, Schmidt-Nowara WW: Amphetamine intoxication with coagulopathy, hyperthermia, and reversible renal failure: A syndrome resembling heatstroke. *Ann Intern Med* 73:81, 1970.

185. Krisko I, Lewis E, Johnson JE: Severe hyperpyrexia due to tranylcypromine-amphetamine toxicity. *Ann Intern Med* 70:559, 1969.

186. Friedman SA, Hirsch SE: Extreme hyperthermia after LSD ingestion. *JAMA* 217:1549, 1971.

187. Schuckit M, Robins E, Feighner J: Tricyclic antidepressants and monoamine oxidase inhibitors. *Arch Gen Psychiatry* 24:509, 1971.

188. Temple AR: Acute and chronic effects of aspirin toxicity and their treatment. *Arch Intern Med* 141:364, 1981.

189. Kosten TR, Kleber HD: Rapid death during cocaine abuse: A variant of the neuroleptic malignant syndrome? *Am J Drug Alcohol Abuse* 14:335, 1988.
190. Kline SS, Mauro LS, Scala-Barnett DM, Zick D: Serotonin syndrome versus neuroleptic malignant syndrome as a cause of death. *Clin Pharm* 8:510, 1989.
191. Rosenberg J, Pentel P, Pond S, et al: Hyperthermia associated with drug intoxication. *Crit Care Med* 14:964, 1986.
192. Merigian KS, Roberts JR: Cocaine intoxication: Hyperpyrexia, rhabdomyolysis and acute renal failure. *Clin Toxicol* 25:135, 1987.
193. Kendrick WC, Hull AR, Knochel JP: Rhabdomyolysis and shock after intravenous amphetamine administration. *Ann Intern Med* 86:381, 1977.
194. Zalis E, Parmley L JR: Fatal amphetamine poisoning. *Arch Intern Med* 112:822, 1963.
195. Menashe PI, Gottlieb JE: Hyperthermia, rhabdomyolysis, and myoglobinuric renal failure after recreational use of cocaine. *South Med J* 81:379, 1988.

196. Campbell BG: Cocaine abuse with hyperthermia, seizures and fatal complications. *Med J Aust* 149:387, 1988.
197. Bauwens JE, Boggs JM, Hartwell PS: Fatal hyperthermia associated with cocaine use. *West J Med* 150:210, 1989.
198. Loghmanee F, Tobak M: Fatal malignant hyperthermia associated with recreational cocaine and ethanol abuse. *Am J Forens Med Pathol* 7:246, 1986.
199. Bettinger J: Cocaine intoxication: Massive oral overdose. *Ann Emerg Med* 9:429, 1980.
200. Patel R, Das M, Palazzolo M, et al: Myoglobinuric acute renal failure in phencyclidine overdose: Report of observations in eight cases. *Ann Emerg Med* 9:549, 1980.
201. Armen R, Kanel G, Reynolds T: Phencyclidine-induced malignant hyperthermia causing submassive liver necrosis. *Am J Med* 77:167, 1984.

74. Acquired Immunodeficiency Syndrome: Pulmonary Complications and Intensive Care

Mark J. Rosen

Overview

In 1981, a group of patients with *Pneumocystis carinii* pneumonia (PCP), but without a previously recognized cause of immunosuppression, was reported [1]. These were among the first cases of the acquired immunodeficiency syndrome (AIDS), the most important global public health problem of the twentieth century. Now in its second decade, there is little hope that the AIDS epidemic will ever end. By January 1995, 441,528 cases of AIDS were reported in the United States, and 270,870 patients died; 41,085 new cases were reported in 1994 alone [2].

Until effective therapy directed against the underlying immunodeficient state is available, AIDS must be considered virtually uniformly fatal. Decisions regarding the appropriateness of intensive care are inevitable for each individual. While physicians providing intensive care are encountering rapidly increasing numbers of patients with life-threatening complications of AIDS, intensive care resources and health care expenditures are progressively constrained. The AIDS epidemic will undoubtedly present enormous challenges to the field of critical care medicine.

Since the epidemic began, clinical experience and advances in diagnosis and treatment have changed our concept of the spectrum of human immunodeficiency virus (HIV)-related illness. Since the first reports of AIDS, the epidemiology of HIV infection in the United States has shifted from homosexual and bisexual men toward injection drug users and their sexual partners. These trends have influenced the types of infections that occur in the setting of immunosuppression. Furthermore, disorders not previously considered to be complications of HIV infection are now AIDS-defining surveillance diagnoses in HIV-infected persons [3]. These include pulmonary tuberculosis, recurrent bacterial pneumonia, and invasive carcinoma of the cervix. The increased use of antiretroviral therapies has reduced or at least forestalled the development of AIDS-defining events in many patients who choose to use them, and prophylactic strategies aimed at opportunistic infections have changed the spectrum of diseases that people with HIV infection develop [4,5].

Patients with AIDS are usually admitted to intensive care units (ICUs) because of respiratory failure. A variety of infectious, neoplastic, and idiopathic disorders may culminate in severe hypoxemia and the need for mechanical ventilation (Table 74-1), and the literature concerning critical care of patients with HIV infection focuses on this group. However, other life-threatening physiologic derangements may occur in HIV-infected patients, including hypotension, gastrointestinal hemorrhage, and seizures. The basic principles of treatment of these disorders are similar to those in immunocompetent individuals. Patients with HIV infection may also be admitted to ICUs for reasons unrelated to the underlying immunodeficiency state, such as trauma, status asthmaticus, cirrhosis, and drug overdose. Treatment of these conditions is no different than for HIV-negative patients.

Pulmonary Complications of HIV Infection

BACTERIAL PNEUMONIA. The first reported cases of AIDS indicated that pulmonary diseases accounted for a very large share of morbidity and mortality. In 1983, the National Institutes

Table 74-1. Pulmonary Complications of HIV Infection

Bacteria
  Streptococcus pneumoniae
  Hemophilus influenzae
  Staphylococcus aureus
  Moraxella catarrhalis
  Mycobacterium tuberculosis
  Mycobacterium avium-intracellulare
  Other nontuberculous *Mycobacteria*
  Rhodococcus equi
  Nocardia asteroides
Protozoa
  Pneumocystis carinii
  Strongyloides stercoralis
  Toxoplasma gondii
Viruses
  Cytomegalovirus
  Adenovirus
  Herpes simplex
Other pulmonary disorders
  Lymphocytic interstitial pneumonitis
  Nonspecific interstitial pneumonitis
  Bronchiolitis obliterans organizing pneumonia
  Primary pulmonary hypertension
Fungi
  Cryptococcus neoformans
  Histoplasma capsulatum
  Aspergillus fumigatus
  Blastomyces dermatitides
Malignancies
  Kaposi's sarcoma
  Non-Hodgkin's lymphoma
  Lung carcinoma

of Health convened a workshop on the pulmonary complications of AIDS, where investigators from centers across the United States shared their collected experience in the diagnosis and outcomes of pulmonary disorders seen in patients classified as having AIDS using criteria established by the Centers for Disease Control (CDC) [6]. *Pneumocystis carinii* pneumonia occurred in 373 of 441 patients (85%), either alone or together with another pathogen, and it is widely perceived that PCP represents the most common pulmonary disease seen in patients with HIV infection. However, more recent studies suggest that bacterial pneumonia, not previously considered an HIV-related infection, is more common. Surveillance data compiled by the CDC during the 1980s document that mortality rates for pneumonia among persons 25 to 44 years of age more than doubled in cities with a high incidence of injection drug users and AIDS [7]. Selwyn et al. found that the incidence of bacterial pneumonia in injection drug users with HIV infection was five times that of uninfected drug users [8]. In two retrospective analyses of patients with HIV infection hospitalized with respiratory illnesses, bacterial pneumonia was the most common diagnosis, followed by PCP and mycobacterial infections [9,10]. In both of these studies, injection drug users comprised the majority of HIV-infected patients. In a multicenter prospective study of 1353 subjects in six medical centers across the United States, bacterial pneumonia was the most common pulmonary disease diagnosed within 18 months of enrollment, and the incidence among HIV-positive subjects was significantly higher than among a control group of HIV-negative homosexual men and injection drug users [11]. Thus, bacterial pneumonia occurs with increased frequency in HIV-positive individuals, and injection drug users are probably at the highest risk. Although bacterial pneumonia may occur in patients with relatively normal CD4 lymphocyte counts and no other HIV-related symp-

toms, more advanced immunosuppression, as assessed by lower CD4 cell counts, further increases the risk [11a].

Although HIV targets the cell-mediated immune system, qualitative and functional defects in T helper (CD4) lymphocytes impair humoral immunity as well [12]. Defective humoral immunity, in turn, predisposes to pneumonias caused by encapsulated organisms, especially *Streptococcus pneumoniae* and *Hemophilus influenzae* [13,14]. Pneumonia due to *Pseudomonas aeruginosa* may also develop in patients with very low CD4 lymphocyte counts [14a]. Bacterial pneumonias usually present in a typical fashion, with high fever, shaking chills, cough productive of purulent sputum, and localized areas of consolidation on chest radiograph. However, many patients have diffuse pulmonary infiltrates similar to those seen with PCP [9]. Patients may become bacteremic and critically ill, but overall mortality from bacterial pneumonia is similar among HIV-infected and HIV-uninfected persons [15,16]. The approach to diagnosis and treatment of bacterial pneumonia is similar to that for HIV-negative patients.

PNEUMOCYSTIS CARINII PNEUMONIA

Diagnosis. *P. carinii* pneumonia still represents an important cause of respiratory illness and death among HIV-infected persons and is still the most common AIDS indicator disease in surveillance studies [2]. Respiratory failure due to PCP is the most common reason for admission of patients with AIDS to ICUs [17]. Occasionally PCP presents as an acute illness with rapid deterioration over a few days. More often, it progresses insidiously, with gradually increasing cough and dyspnea over weeks or even months. The chest radiograph typically reveals bilateral alveolar and interstitial infiltrates, but unusual manifestations may occur, including nodular densities, cystic lesions, pneumothorax, lobar consolidation, or normal radiographs [18]. Furthermore, the typical radiographic pattern for PCP is not specific, occurring with other infections and neoplastic disorders.

The diagnosis of PCP depends on identification of the organism from specimens derived from the lung. The least invasive diagnostic modality is induction of sputum with 3 percent saline delivered by ultrasonic nebulization. When performed by experienced staff, *P. carinii* can be identified by modified Giemsa, methenamine silver, or immunofluorescent staining in 50 to 80 percent of cases [19,20,21]. Occasionally, other pathogens, particularly *Mycobacterium tuberculosis,* may also be found using appropriate staining and culture techniques.

If sputum induction is not diagnostic, the next step to establish a diagnosis should be fiberoptic bronchoscopy and bronchoalveolar lavage. In the diagnosis of PCP, some have recommended that transbronchial biopsy be omitted initially and performed as part of a second bronchoscopy if the lavage is nondiagnostic [22]. However, biopsy is occasionally diagnostic when lavage is negative in PCP and is the least invasive means of diagnosing other pulmonary conditions that require histologic interpretation. Therefore, the advisability of performing transbronchial biopsy routinely during the evaluation of a patient suspected of having PCP is controversial. It is contraindicated in the presence of bleeding disorders, and the high risk of pneumothorax generally precludes biopsy in patients undergoing mechanical ventilation.

In patients with respiratory failure who have an endotracheal tube in place, bronchoalveolar lavage can be accomplished without the use of the fiberoptic bronchoscope. A diagnosis of PCP was established in 19 of 20 (95%) intubated patients by infusing six 10-ml aliquots of sterile saline into the endotracheal tube, removing the fluid using standard suctioning techniques, and performing appropriate microbiologic analyses on the fluid sediment [23]. Similar high diagnostic yields can be achieved by placing a 12 Fr. nasogastric tube blindly through the endotracheal tube until slight resistance is met and obtaining bronchoalveolar lavage fluid exactly as if a bronchoscope were used. When lavage yields no diagnosis in an intubated patient, open lung biopsy should be considered to establish the diagnosis.

Adjunctive testing is also useful in the diagnosis of PCP. Most patients with PCP have an elevation of serum lactic dehydrogenase (LDH); a normal level is compelling evidence against this infection [24,25]. However, an elevated LDH level may occur in other pulmonary diseases. Similarly, the ^{67}Ga lung scan is almost always positive in cases of PCP but is nonspecific [18]. This test should be reserved for patients with a normal chest radiograph in whom an opportunistic infection is suspected because of symptoms. If there is abnormal gallium uptake in the lungs, further diagnostic studies aimed at demonstrating an opportunistic infection are appropriate. Most patients with a negative scan can be observed.

The CD4 lymphocyte count may also be of value in formulating diagnostic approach. Masur et al., in a retrospective analysis of 100 patients with suspected pulmonary complications of HIV infection, found that 80 of 85 episodes of PCP and other opportunistic infections were associated with a CD4 count below 200×10^6 per liter in the preceding 2 months [26]. In contrast, patients with pulmonary Kaposi's sarcoma or nonspecific interstitial pneumonitis had CD4 counts greater than 200×10^6 per liter. If the CD4 count was greater than 300×10^6 per liter within the prior 2 months the likelihood that pneumonia was due to PCP was less than 10 percent, but if the count was less than 100×10^6 per liter the likelihood was 67.2 percent.

Similarly, Phair et al. found that PCP is very unusual in individuals with CD4 counts greater than 200×10^6 per liter and that when it occurs patients commonly have thrush and antecedent fever [27]. Therefore, HIV-infected individuals known to have CD4 lymphocyte counts greater than 300×10^6 per liter within the past 2 months who have respiratory symptoms but no chronic manifestations of HIV infection (fatigue, fever, thrush, unintentional weight loss) or radiographic abnormalities are unlikely to have PCP.

Treatment. The two most commonly used therapies for PCP are trimethoprim-sulfamethoxazole (TMP-SMX), 15 to 20 mg/kg/day, TMP, 75 to 100 mg/kg/day SMX, or pentamidine isoethionate, 4 mg/kg/day administered intravenously. The optimal duration of treatment is unknown, but a consensus has emerged that 14 to 21 days is necessary. Both regimens have approximately equal efficacy and carry substantial risk of toxicity [28,29]. Trimetrexate, a potent antifolate agent, is an alternative for the treatment of moderate-to-severe PCP. It is less efficacious than TMP-SMX but is also associated with significantly fewer treatment-limiting side effects [29a].

Because TMP-SMX is generally well tolerated, inexpensive, and available in oral and intravenous preparations, it is the preferred agent in patients who have not has a previous adverse reaction [30]. Alternative therapies may be effective and less toxic in mild to moderate episodes, defined as PaO$_2$ breathing room air greater than 70 mm Hg. Intravenous medications may not be necessary in these patients. These alternatives appear promising for outpatient treatment, but definitive studies are still needed before they are applied widely. Regimens include oral TMP-SMX, trimethoprim-dapsone [31], clindamycin-primaquine [32], and aerosolized pentamidine [33,34]. Atovaquone was recently approved as second-line treatment for mild to moderate PCP, defined as PaO$_2$ greater than 60 mm Hg and alveolar-arterial O$_2$ difference less than 45 mm Hg, in patients

intolerant to TMP-SMX [35]. This drug has the advantage of oral administration and is usually well tolerated.

Several studies demonstrate that corticosteroids administered with antimicrobial therapy can lead to more rapid improvement in symptoms and gas exchange and increase survival in patients with PCP. A report by a National Institutes of Health-University of California panel reviewed five randomized, placebo-controlled trials and concluded that adjunctive corticosteroid therapy given at the start of anti-PCP treatment reduces the likelihood of respiratory failure, deterioration of oxygenation, and death in patients with moderate to severe pneumonia [36]. Patients likely to benefit had a PaO$_2$ less than 70 mm Hg or an arterial-alveolar oxygen gradient greater than 35 mm Hg. No benefits were proved with less severe abnormalities in gas exchange at the start of therapy or for patients in whom corticosteroids were administered more than 72 hours after antimicrobial treatment was begun.

The optimal dosage and duration of corticosteroid treatment is unknown. The largest controlled study that demonstrated benefit used oral prednisone in the following regimen: on days 1 through 5, 40 mg was given twice daily; on days 6 through 10, 40 mg was given daily; on days 11 through 21, 20 mg was given daily [37]. Adverse reactions to adjunctive corticosteroid therapy are infrequent, but life-threatening superinfection with opportunistic pathogens may occur [37a,37b,38].

The mechanism by which corticosteroids benefit patients with PCP is unknown. Gas exchange typically deteriorates during the first few days of therapy when corticosteroids are not given [39]. This may be caused by an accelerated inflammatory response to killed organisms, and corticosteroids may attenuate this worsening of gas exchange by reducing inflammation.

Respiratory Failure due to PCP. When treatment of PCP is postponed or ineffective, patients develop hypoxemic respiratory failure. The clinical features and chest radiographs in cases of severe PCP appear similar to those in the acute respiratory distress syndrome (ARDS), with hypoxemia, intrapulmonary shunting, reduced pulmonary compliance, and the radiographic appearance of diffuse alveolar infiltrates [40]. Pathologically, PCP is characterized by foamy intraalveolar exudates; as the disease progresses interstitial inflammation and fibrosis may become prominent. In contrast, the primary site of damage in ARDS is the alveolar capillary membrane, resulting in increased permeability. Alveolar exudates in patients with PCP are not hemorrhagic, and there are no hyaline membranes [40].

Just as severe PCP clinically resembles ARDS, the supportive treatment, including intubation, mechanical ventilation, and application of positive end-expiratory pressure, is similar (see Chaps. 55 and 66). As the disease progresses and pulmonary compliance diminishes, pneumothorax is common. Pulmonary arterial catheterization may be used to optimize intravascular pressures and cardiac output during positive-pressure ventilation.

Continuous positive airway pressure (CPAP) delivered by face mask to patients with PCP may improve gas exchange without endotracheal intubation [41,42]. In one study, 5 of 12 patients treated with CPAP up to 10 cm H$_2$0 improved and did not require intubation, but only 3 were eventually discharged from the hospital [42]. This technique may also afford the patient and physician more time to consider whether mechanical ventilation is desirable. In the same series, five of the seven who did not improve with CPAP decided to forego intubation, opting for supportive care only. The remaining two patients had mechanical ventilatory support and died in the hospital.

Prophylaxis against PCP is very effective and may lead to a decrease in the number of patients with AIDS who require intensive care for this infection [43]. These therapies are discussed in Chapter 93.

TUBERCULOSIS. Coinfection with HIV and *M. tuberculosis* has fueled the resurgence of tuberculosis worldwide [44]. Even modest reductions in cell-mediated immunity increase the likelihood of reactivation of latent tuberculosis. The risk increases as CD4 cell counts decline. Furthermore, impaired T lymphocytic function increases the risk of progressive disease from new infection. In the United States, the association of tuberculosis and HIV infection is particularly striking in groups with a higher prevalence of latent tuberculosis, such as injection drug users, Haitian immigrants, and the homeless. However, tuberculosis is transmissible to the entire community.

In HIV-infected individuals tuberculosis often occurs prior to the development of opportunistic infections that define AIDS, presumably because *M. tuberculosis* is a virulent organism. In patients with relatively intact immune function, the clinical presentation is similar to that of tuberculosis in HIV-negative patients, with the lungs as the most common site of disease [45]. In patients with greater immunosuppression, atypical pulmonary presentations, including diffuse infiltrates, miliary patterns, or normal chest radiographs occur commonly [46]. These patients also have a high incidence of extrapulmonary infection, involving pleura, lymph nodes, gastrointestinal tract, bone marrow, and blood [47].

The diagnosis of tuberculosis may be difficult in HIV-infected patients. Cutaneous anergy becomes more prevalent as CD4 cell counts decline, making tuberculin skin tests relatively insensitive [47a]. Valuable radiographic clues to the diagnosis include the presence of cavitation, hilar and mediastinal lymphadenopathy, and pleural effusions [45,46,47].

When cavitation is present, acid-fast smears and cultures of sputum are usually positive. In patients not expectorating spontaneously, sputum production may be induced with hypertonic saline. Fiberoptic bronchoscopy with bronchoalveolar lavage and transbronchial biopsy, and postbronchoscopy sputum are often diagnostic. Transbronchial biopsy enhances the immediate diagnostic yield of fiberoptic bronchoscopy in the diagnosis of pulmonary tuberculosis, compared with bronchoalveolar lavage alone [48,49]. Despite an appropriate diagnostic evaluation, acid-fast smears of sputum and bronchoscopic specimens may be negative in many patients with pulmonary tuberculosis. Therefore, empiric therapy should be given to patients with radiographic abnormalities consistent with tuberculosis who do not have another plausible disorder identified.

Treatment for tuberculosis due to drug-sensitive organisms is highly successful in patients who adhere to their medical regimen [45]. Because of the recent increased incidence of drug-resistant tuberculosis, the initial regimen recommended includes four drugs: isoniazid, rifampin, pyrazinamide, and either ethambutol or streptomycin [50]. When drug susceptibility results are available, the regimen may be altered. Treatment is continued for at least 9 months and for 6 months after cultures are reported negative.

The factors that fuel the increase in tuberculosis, namely injection drug use, homelessness, and poor social support and public health systems, are also partly responsible for patient noncompliance with medical regimens. This, in turn, has led to a dramatic increase in tuberculosis resistant to conventional drugs [51,52,53]. Outbreaks of multidrug-resistant tuberculosis are reported in hospitals, prisons, and shelters for the homeless. Treatment of pulmonary tuberculosis resistant to isoniazid and rifampin is often unsuccessful and carries a high mortality rate, and failure to control these infections can represent a great threat to public health [52–55].

Mycobacterium avium-intracellulare (MAI). This is another important pathogen in patients with AIDS, often causing devastating complications in patients with advanced immunosuppression. Patients usually suffer from persistent fever, wasting, and diarrhea. However, MAI rarely represents an important pulmonary pathogen in patients with AIDS. Its isolation in patients with overt pulmonary disease usually occurs in association with another pathogen, such as PCP. Patients with HIV infection who have acid-fast bacilli identified from sputum or bronchoscopic specimens should be treated presumptively for *M. tuberculosis* until culture results are known, mainly because tuberculosis is more common and responds better to treatment and because patients represent a potential public health hazard.

CYTOMEGALOVIRUS PNEUMONITIS. Most patients with HIV infection have either latent or overt cytomegalovirus (CMV) infection [56]. In advanced HIV infection, characterized by very low CD4 lymphocyte counts, CMV may cause a host of disorders, ranging from retinitis to esophagitis, gastritis, colitis, hepatitis, encephalitis, pneumonia, and death. Although CMV can often be isolated from the lung, patients with HIV infection rarely develop clinically significant pneumonitis [56,57]. Cultures of bronchoalveolar lavage fluid of patients with AIDS who have pneumonia due to various pathogens are positive for CMV in up to 50 percent of cases; viral inclusion bodies may be seen within lavage cells, and cytopathic changes may be found in pulmonary parenchymal specimens [56–60]. When treatment is directed at coexisting pathogens, such as *P. carinii*, without agents active against CMV, the presence of CMV does not appear to alter the prognosis.

Typically, CMV pneumonitis presents with dyspnea, nonproductive cough, fever, and diffuse pulmonary infiltrates, a presentation similar to that of PCP. The diagnosis of CMV pneumonia in patients with AIDS depends on demonstration of characteristic intranuclear or cytoplasmic inclusion bodies within lung cells, including alveolar macrophages; preferably when no other pulmonary pathogen is identified [56]. Intravenous gancyclovir is the treatment of choice for patients with established CMV pneumonitis and AIDS (see Chap. 93).

FUNGAL PNEUMONIAS. Although not as common as bacterial infections and PCP, serious fungal infections may occur in the setting of immunocompromise, both as new infections and as reactivation of latent disease. The types of fungal infections seen in patients with AIDS depend on the severity of immunodeficiency and whether the patient has lived in endemic areas. Fungal pulmonary infections often precede the appearance of other opportunistic infections but frequently coexist with other pathogens, such as *M. tuberculosis* and *P. carinii*. Treatment of fungal infections is discussed in detail in Chapter 93.

Cryptococcosis. *Cryptococcus neoformans* is distributed throughout the world and is the most common fungus causing life-threatening illness in patients with AIDS. The meninges are the most common site of infection, and meningitis is often the first manifestation of AIDS [61]. Cryptococcal pneumonia typically presents with fever, cough and dyspnea. The chest radiograph usually shows diffuse infiltrates similar to those seen in PCP, but localized infiltrates, nodules, cavitation, pleural effusions, miliary pattern, and lymphadenopathy are also encountered [62,63]. Almost all patients with cryptococcal pneumonia have meningitis and disseminated disease, and CD4 lymphocyte counts are typically below 100×10^6 per liter.

The diagnosis is established by identification of the organism from sputum, bronchoalveolar lavage fluid, pleural fluid, or lung biopsy. A high titer of cryptococcal antigen in serum is strongly suggestive, and an antigen titer of 1:8 or greater in bronchoalveolar lavage fluid is diagnostic of cryptococcal pneumonia [64].

Histoplasmosis. *Histoplasma capsulatum* is endemic in the Ohio and Mississippi river valleys, Central and South America, and the Caribbean islands. Patients with HIV infection who come from endemic areas may develop disseminated disease when immunodeficiency permits reactivation of latent infection [65,66,67]. The clinical presentation is usually subacute and the chest radiograph typically shows a diffuse or miliary pattern, although localized infiltrates may occur. The diagnosis is established by identification or culture of the organism from lung-derived specimens, bone marrow, blood, or liver.

Aspergillosis. Patients with advanced immunosuppression may develop life-threatening pulmonary aspergillosis. Two types of disease have been identified: an invasive parenchymal infection with consolidation or cavitation, favoring the upper lobes, and a predominantly bronchial disease presenting with dyspnea and airway obstruction [68]. Patients generally have CD4 counts below 30×10^6 per liter; prior use of corticosteroids and neutrophil counts less than 500×10^6 per liter appear to increase the risk. As with other fungal infections in patients with AIDS, disseminated disease is common.

Other Fungal Infections. In endemic areas, disseminated coccidioidomycosis and blastomycosis may occur in patients with AIDS. These infections may involve the lung, presenting with cough, fever, dyspnea, and nodular, cavitary, or diffuse disease. [69,70]

NEOPLASTIC DISEASES OF THE LUNG

Kaposi's Sarcoma. Kaposi's sarcoma (KS) is the most common malignancy in individuals with HIV infection, and the skin is the major site of involvement. The etiology of KS is unknown, but epidemiologic data and reports of this tumor in HIV-negative homosexual men suggest that the disease is caused by a sexually transmitted agent other than HIV [71]. Kaposi's sarcoma is much more common among HIV-infected homosexual men; it is distinctly unusual in other HIV transmission groups. The incidence of KS appears to be decreasing.

Disseminated KS may involve virtually any organ, including the lung. Patients with pulmonary KS almost always have obvious cutaneous lesions, but the lung may be the only site of disease. Kaposi's sarcoma can involve the parenchyma, airways, pleura, and intrathoracic lymph nodes, leading to a diverse range of symptoms and radiographic findings [72].

Patients with parenchymal disease usually have dry cough and dyspnea; fever is common, even in the absence of concurrent infection. Airway involvement can cause hemoptysis or wheezing. Pleural disease is unlikely to cause symptoms, but pleural effusions are common. Parenchymal disease is manifested radiographically by focal or diffuse infiltrates, which may resemble opportunistic infections such as PCP. However, nodular infiltrates suggest the diagnosis of KS, especially in patients with cutaneous disease.

The histologic diagnosis of thoracic involvement with KS may be difficult to establish. The finding of typical lesions on inspection of the airways is usually regarded as diagnostic, since the diagnostic yield of forceps biopsy is low and the procedure may cause significant hemorrhage. Transbronchial biopsy of parenchymal KS also has a low diagnostic yield, and even open biopsy of radiographically diffuse disease is often nondiagnostic because of the focality of the pathologic process [73,74]. Clinical clues that suggest pulmonary KS in a patient with respiratory symptoms and an abnormal chest radiograph include the presence of cutaneous involvement, absence of fever and absence of pulmonary uptake on gallium scan, and nodular densities [75].

Pleural fluid, when present, is usually exudative and sanguinous, but cytologic examination is characteristically nondiagnostic [76]. Closed pleural biopsy is rarely positive due to the focality of KS pleural lesions and predominant involvement of the visceral, rather than parietal, pleura. Treatment regimens include chemotherapy and radiotherapy, but response is variable.

Other Malignancies. Non-Hodgkin's lymphoma also occurs with increased frequency in patients with HIV infection. Lymphoma may involve the intrathoracic lymph nodes, pleura, and pulmonary parenchyma, the latter revealing multiple nodules or interstitial infiltrates on chest radiograph [77]. However, severe pulmonary symptoms and impairment are rare.

Solid tumors, including primary lung cancers, are now believed to occur with increased frequency in HIV-infected persons. In two retrospective case-control studies, HIV-positive patients with lung cancer were younger then their HIV-negative counterparts and had a shorter median survival [78,79]. Smoking histories and histologic features of cancer were similar in the two groups.

OTHER PULMONARY DISORDERS. As the AIDS epidemic progresses, more patients are encountered who have pulmonary disorders without a defined infectious or neoplastic etiology. These include lymphocytic interstitial pneumonitis (LIP), nonspecific interstitial pneumonitis (NIP), bronchitis obliterans organizing pneumonia (BOOP), and primary pulmonary hypertension [72,80–83]. With the exception of primary pulmonary hypertension, these disorders generally present with milder symptoms and radiographic abnormalities. The etiology of these disorders is unknown.

Intensive Care of Patients with Pneumocystis carinii *Pneumonia*

Historically, most patients with AIDS admitted to ICUs had respiratory failure due to PCP, and most reports of outcome of intensive care focus on this condition. Respiratory failure is usually defined as the need for intubation and mechanical ventilation, and outcome is defined as survival to discharge from the hospital.

The prognosis of patients with PCP who develop respiratory failure has changed over time, and three distinct periods of differing outcomes have been identified [83a]. Early in the epidemic, the prognosis was uniformly grim, with survival rates of around 15 percent [6,84–88].

Because of these studies, it was widely accepted that endotracheal intubation and mechanical ventilation were unlikely to improve the prognosis of AIDS patients meaningfully and that intensive care admission should not be encouraged, especially when respiratory failure was present or imminent. Between 1984 and 1985, ICU admissions at San Francisco General Hospital declined, while the number of patients with PCP admitted to the hospital increased [85]. It appeared that physicians' awareness of a poor prognosis made them less likely to recommend aggressive interventions. Another study in San Francisco revealed that although patients with AIDS tended to overestimate the likelihood of survival after respiratory failure, 45 percent said they would decline mechanical ventilation, indicating that many patients chose not to be admitted to the ICU [89].

Reports of ICU outcomes after 1986 disputed the notion that intensive care for patients with AIDS has a dismal prognosis. A review of patients at the New York Veterans Administration Medical Center who had mechanical ventilation during a first episode of PCP showed that 8 of 19 (42%) survived [90]. Of the eight survivors, seven deteriorated rapidly after diagnostic fiberoptic bronchoscopy, suggesting that the procedure was largely responsible for the need for mechanical ventilation. In another series, a striking reduction in mortality associated with ventilatory support in PCP was attributed to adjunctive high-dose corticosteroid therapy and early diagnosis [91]. Five of 6 patients who did not receive corticosteroids died, compared with 7 deaths among 18 patients (30%) who were treated.

Wachter et al. compared the course of patients with PCP and respiratory failure admitted to the San Francisco General Hospital ICU from 1986 to 1988 with those hospitalized before 1986 [94]. Mortality in the later period was 60 percent, compared with 87 percent in the earlier period. Only 5 percent of the earlier patients were treated with corticosteroids, compared with 74 percent of the later patients, and the overall survival rate was 22 percent among those who did not receive corticosteroids, compared with 46 percent among those who did. However, when patients in the later period were stratified according to whether they received corticosteroid therapy, there was no statistically significant improvement in survival. Other centers confirmed that the prognosis was not as bleak as previously believed, with mortality rates reported as low as 50 percent [92–100b]. Besides the application of adjunctive corticosteroid therapy, increased survival was associated with higher serum albumin [94] and serum LDH [98,100], and a lower APACHE II score [98,100a] and multisystem organ failure score [100].

Higher mortality rates reported after 1993 tempered optimism for survival in respiratory failure due to PCP. It is likely that the types of patients who require mechanical ventilation for PCP and their severity of illness differ in recent years. In San Francisco General Hospital, mortality increased from 61 percent in the period from 1986 through 1988, to 76 percent in the next two years [83a]. In the latter period, more patients were injection drug users, and there were more episodes of recurrent PCP. Mortality was strongly associated with a CD4 lymphocyte count <50/mm³ (94%), and with the development of a pneumothorax (no survivors).

Furthermore, patients who required mechanical ventilation in recent years are more likely to represent failures of prophylaxis, antipneumocystis treatment and adjunctive corticosteroids. These patients would be expected to have a poor prognosis. In Vancouver, the proportion of patients who received mechanical ventilation for PCP decreased from 1981 through 1991, but mortality rates increased from 50 percent in 1981–1987, to 89 percent in 1987–1991 [100c]. Simultaneously, corticosteroid use before intubation increased from almost never to 50 percent. In another retrospective analysis, Staikowsky et al found an overall mortality rate of 82 percent among patients who required mechanical ventilation for the treatment of PCP between 1987 and 1992 [100d]. Only one of the 22 patients (5%) who started mechanical ventilation after five days of treatment with TMP-SMX and corticosteroids survived, compared with 5 of the 14 (36%) who received a shorter course of therapy. Similarly, 13 of 16 (81%) patients who required mechanical

ventilation for PCP over one year (July 1991–June 1992) died, despite the routine use of adjunctive corticosteroids [100e]. Taken together, these studies show that when respiratory failure follows several days of appropriate therapy for PCP, the probability of survival is only 10 to 20 percent.

Some patients with PCP are admitted to ICUs, but do not undergo mechanical ventilation. The reasons for admission may include performance of fiberoptic bronchoscopy, application of continuous positive airway pressure, pneumothorax, a condition unrelated to PCP, or monitoring that cannot be achieved with routine floor care. These patients can be expected to have a better outcome than those who have more severe respiratory impairment, but published data are scarce and inconclusive.

INTENSIVE CARE FOR REASONS OTHER THAN *PNEUMOCYSTIS CARINII* PNEUMONIA. There is very little information available on the outcome of intensive care for reasons other than respiratory failure due to PCP in patients with AIDS. Admission rates to ICUs for these conditions are unknown, since most studies report exclusively on outcomes for patients with PCP, with no comment on the proportion of patients with HIV infection admitted for other reasons. These patients represent a widely varied group. Depending on local practice patterns, patients may be admitted to ICUs for reasons other than the need for mechanical ventilation, including perioperative monitoring and invasive procedures. Patients may also be admitted for critical illnesses entirely unrelated to HIV infection.

Most data concerning outcome of intensive care for patients who do not have PCP focus on respiratory failure. While PCP is the most common diagnosis leading to admission of patients with HIV into intensive care units, it is not the preponderant cause of critical illness [84,85,86,92,97,100e,100f]. In a multicenter prospective study of 1137 HIV-infected subjects who did not have AIDS at the time of enrollment, only seven of the 50 ICU admissions (14%) in the follow-up period had PCP [100f]. Current data on the incidence and outcomes of disorders other than PCP are meager. The reasons for intubation and mechanical ventilation in these patients are quite diverse, including infection, ARDS, sedative drug overdose, primary neurologic disease, cardiovascular disorder, severe metabolic derangement, and gastrointestinal hemorrhage.

In early reports, respiratory failure necessitating mechanical ventilation due to causes other than PCP appeared to be uniformly fatal [85,86,87]. Later studies reported survival rates of approximately 75 percent, but this estimate was based on a total of 32 patients in different centers, with different illnesses and diverse criteria for ventilatory support [88,92,97].

The spectrum of diseases necessitating ICU management for patients with AIDS is likely to change. The application of antiretroviral therapies and prophylaxis for PCP will probably forestall or reduce the incidence of this infection in those who use them. Moreover, the epidemiologic shift toward patients who acquired HIV infection through injection drug use and heterosexual contact of infected partners may lead to an increase in other life-threatening diseases, such as bacterial infections and tuberculosis. The survival rates for these populations, who are likely to have a high incidence of diseases other than PCP, remain unknown.

INFECTION CONTROL. Human immunodeficiency virus infection may be transmitted by parenteral exposure to blood and body fluids, and ICU staff must be scrupulous in adhering to precautionary measures. Since it is usually not known with certainty whether any patient has HIV infection or other transmissible pathogens, such as hepatitis B, universal infection control measures are recommended for all hospitalized patients [101]. These include the appropriate use of handwashing, gloves, gowns, masks, and protective eyewear when contact with blood or body fluids is possible. To avoid accidental injury, needles should not be recapped but rather disposed of promptly in secure containers.

The risk of transmission of tuberculosis from HIV-infected patients to health care workers is often present, and special precautions are recommended [102]. Effective control of the spread of tuberculosis requires early identification and treatment of infected individuals. Patients suspected of having active pulmonary tuberculosis should be isolated, and the spread of infectious droplet nuclei can be reduced by maintaining adequate exhaust ventilation from patient rooms, supplemented by germicidal ultraviolet irradiation and high-efficiency filtration in areas using recirculated air. Caregivers in close contact with patients with suspected tuberculosis should use protective respiratory masks, because standard paper masks are inadequate to impede transmission of droplet nuclei. Fiberoptic bronchoscopy and endotracheal suctioning must be performed in rooms with adequate ventilation and preferably equipped with ultraviolet irradiation. Although unproved, the use of closed-system suction catheters may reduce the ambient concentration of infectious particles substantially.

References

1. Centers for Disease Control: Pneumocystis pneumonia: Los Angeles. *MMWR* 30:250, 1980.
2. Centers for Disease Control and Prevention. *HIV/AIDS Surveillance Report* 6:1, 1994.
3. Centers for Disease Control: 1993 revised classification system for HIV infection and expanded surveillance case definition for AIDS among adolescents and adults. *MMWR* 41:1, 1992.
4. Hoover RD, Saah AJ, Bacellar H, et al: Clinical manifestations of AIDS in the era of *Pneumocystis* prophylaxis. *N Engl J Med* 329:1922, 1993.
5. Jacobson LP, Kirby AJ, Polk S, et al: Changes in survival after acquired immunodeficiency syndrome (AIDS). *Am J Epidemiol* 138:952, 1993.
6. Murray JF, Felton CP, Garay SM, et al: Pulmonary complications of the acquired immunodeficiency syndrome: Report of National Heart, Lung and Blood Institute Workshop. *N Engl J Med* 310:1682, 1984.
7. Centers for Disease Control: Increase in pneumonia mortality among young adults and the HIV epidemic: New York City, United States. *MMWR* 37:593, 1988.
8. Selwyn PA, Feingold AR, Hartel, et al: Increased risk of bacterial pneumonia in HIV-infected intravenous drug users without AIDS. *AIDS* 2:267, 1988.
9. Magnenat J-L, Nicod L, Aukenthaler R, et al: Mode of presentation and diagnosis of bacterial pneumonia in human immunodeficiency virus-infected patients. *Am Rev Respir Dis* 144:917, 1991.
10. Ruzi JD, Rosen MJ: The changing spectrum of pulmonary complications of HIV infection. *Am Rev Respir Dis* 145:A820, 1992.
11. Wallace JM, Rao AV, Glassroth J, et al: Respiratory illness in persons with acquired immunodeficiency virus infection. *Am Rev Respir Dis* 148:1523, 1993.
11a. Hirschtick R, Glassroth J, Jordan M, Pulmonary Complications of HIV Infection Study Group: Bacterial pneumonia in patients infected with human immunodeficiency virus. *Am Rev Respir Dis* 147:A1003, 1993.
12. Lane HC, Masur H, Edgar LC, et al: Abnormalities of B-cell activation and immunoregulation in patients with the acquired immunodeficiency syndrome. *N Engl J Med* 109:453-8, 1983.
13. Chaisson RE: Bacterial pneumonia in patients with human immunodeficiency virus infection. *Semin Respir Infect* 4:133, 1989.
14. Polsky B, Gold JWM, Whimby E, et al: Bacterial pneumonia in patients with the acquired immunodeficiency syndrome. *Ann Intern Med* 104:38, 1986.
14a. Baron AD, Hollander H: *Pseudomonas aeruginosa* bronchopulmonary infection in late immunodeficiency virus disease. *Am Rev Respir Dis* 148:992, 1993.
15. Pesola GR, Charles A: Pneumococcal bacteremia with pneumonia: Mortality in acquired immunodeficiency syndrome. *Chest* 101:150, 1992.
16. Janoff EN, Breiman RE, Daley CL, et al: Pneumococcal disease during HIV infection: Epidemiologic, clinical and immunologic perspectives. *Ann Intern Med* 117:314, 1992.
17. Wachter RM, Luce JM, Hopewell PC: Critical care of patients with AIDS. *JAMA* 267:541, 1992.
18. Golden JA, Sollitto RA: The radiology of pulmonary disease: Chest roentgenography, computed tomography and gallium scanning. *Clin Chest Med* 9:481, 1988.
19. Pitchenik AE, Ganjei P, Torres A, et al: The usefulness of induced sputum in the diagnosis of *Pneumocystis carinii* pneumonia in patients with the acquired immunodeficiency syndrome. *Am Rev Respir Dis* 133:226, 1987.
20. Bigby TD, Margolskee D, Curtis JL, et al: The usefulness of induced sputum in the diagnosis of *Pneumocystis carinii* pneumonia in patients with the acquired immunodeficiency syndrome. *Am Rev Respir Dis* 133:515, 1986.
21. Kovacs JA, Ng V, Masur H, et al: Diagnosis of *Pneumocystis carinii* pneumonia: Improved detection in sputum with use of monoclonal antibodies. *N Engl J Med* 318:589, 1988.
22. Clement MJ, Luce JM, Hopewell PC: Diagnosis of pulmonary disease. *Clin Chest Med* 9:497, 1988.
23. Karpel JP, Prezant D, Appel D, et al: Endotracheal lavage for the diagnosis of *Pneumocystis carinii* pneumonia in intubated patients with acquired immune deficiency syndrome. *Crit Care Med* 14:741, 1986.
24. Zaman MK, White DA.: Serum lactate dehydrogenase levels and *Pneumocystis carinii* pneumonia. *Am Rev Respir Dis* 137:796, 1988.
25. Kagawa FT, Kirsch CM, Yenokida GG, et al: Serum lactate dehydrogenase activity in patients with AIDS and *Pneumocystis carinii* pneumonia. An adjunct to diagnosis. *Chest* 94:1031, 1988.
26. Masur H, Ognibene FP, Yarchoan R, et al: CD4 counts as predictors of opportunistic pneumonia in human immunodeficiency virus (HIV) infection. *Ann Intern Med* 111:223, 1989.
27. Phair J, Munoz A, Detels R, et al: The risk of *Pneumocystis carinii* pneumonia among men infected with human immunodeficiency virus type I. *N Engl J Med* 322:161, 1990.
28. Wharton JM, Coleman DI, Wofsy CB, et al: Trimethoprim-sulfamethozazole or pentamidine for *Pneumocystis carinii* pneumonia in the acquired immunodeficiency syndrome: A prospective randomized trial. *Ann Intern Med* 105:37, 1986.
29. Sattler FR, Cowan RM, Nielsen DM, et al: Trimethoprim-sulfamethoxazole compared with pentamidine for treatment of *Pneumocystis carinii* pneumonia in the acquired immunodeficiency syndrome: A prospective, noncrossover study. *Ann Intern Med* 109:280, 1988.
29a. Sattler FR, Frame P, Davis R, et al: Trimetrexate with leucovorin versus trimethoprim-sulfamethoxazole for moderate to severe episodes of *Pneumocystis carinii* pneumonia in patients with AIDS: A prospective, controlled multicenter investigation of the AIDS Clinical Trials Group Protocol 029/031. *J Inf Dis* 170:165, 1994.
30. Masur H: Prevention and treatment of *Pneumocystis* pneumonia. *N Engl J Med* 327:1853, 1992.
31. Medina I, Mills J, Leoung G, et al: Oral therapy in the acquired immunodeficiency syndrome: A controlled trial of trimethoprim-sulfamethoxazole versus trimethoprim-dapsone. *N Engl J Med* 323:776, 1990.
32. Black JR, Feinberg J, Murphy R, et al: Clindamycin and primaquine as primary treatment for mild and moderately severe *Pneumocystis carinii* pneumonia in patients with AIDS. *Eur J Clin Microbiol Infect Dis* 10:204, 1991.
33. Montgomery AB, Debs RJ, Luce JM, et al: Aerosolized pentamidine as sole therapy for *Pneumocystis carinii* pneumonia in patients with acquired immunodeficiency syndrome. *Lancet* 2:480, 1987.

34. Conte JE, Hollander H, Golden JA: Inhaled or reduced-dose, intravenous pentamidine for *Pneumocystis carinii* pneumonia. *Ann Intern Med* 107:495, 1987.

35. Falloon J, Kovacs J, Hughes W, et al: A preliminary evaluation of 566C80 for the treatment of *Pneumocystis* pneumonia in patients with the acquired immunodeficiency syndrome. *N Engl J Med* 325:1534, 1991.

36. The National Institutes of Health-University of California Expert Panel for Corticosteroid as Adjunctive Therapy for *Pneumocystis* Pneumonia: Consensus statement on the use of corticosteroid as adjunctive therapy for *Pneumocystis* pneumonia in the acquired immunodeficiency syndrome. *N Engl J Med* 323:1500, 1990.

37. Bozzette SA, Sattler FR, Chin J, et al: Corticosteroids as adjunctive therapy in severe *Pneumocystis carinii* pneumonia in the acquired immunodeficiency syndrome. *N. Engl J Med* 323:1451, 1990.

37a. Jones BE, Taikwel EK, Mercado AL, et al: Tuberculosis in patients with HIV infection who receive corticosteroids for presumed *Pneumocystis carinii* pneumonia. *Am J Respir Crit Care Med* 149:1686, 1994.

37b. Weinberg BJ, DiCostanzo D, Rosen MJ: Cytomegalovirus pneumonitis following adjunctive corticosteroid therapy of AIDS-associated *Pneumocystis carinii* pneumonia. *AIDS Pat Care* 9:4, 1995.

38. Bernstein B, Flomenberg P, Letzer D: Disseminated cryptococcal disease complicating steroid therapy for *Pneumocystis carinii* pneumonia in a patient with AIDS. *So Med J* 87:537, 1994.

39. Montaner JSG, Lawson LM, Levitt N, et al: Corticosteroids prevent early deterioration in patients with moderately severe *Pneumocystis carinii* pneumonia and the acquired immunodeficiency syndrome (AIDS). *Ann Intern Med* 133:14, 1990.

40. Maxfield RA, Sorkin B, Fazzini EP, et al: Respiratory failure in patients with acquired immunodeficiency syndrome and *Pneumocystis carinii* pneumonia. *Crit Care Med* 14:443, 1986.

41. DeVita MA, Greenbaum DM: The critically ill patient with the acquired immunodeficiency syndrome, in Shoemaker WC, Ayres S, Grenvik A, et al (eds): *Textbook of Critical Care Medicine.* Philadelphia, WB Saunders, 1989, pp 862–869.

42. Gregg RW, Friedman BC, Williams JF, et al: Continuous positive pressure by face mask in *Pneumocystis carinii* pneumonia. *Crit Care Med* 18:21, 1990.

43. Centers for Disease Control: Recommendations for prophylaxis against *Pneumocystis carinii* pneumonia for adults and adolescents infected with human immunodeficiency virus. *MMWR* 41:1, 1992.

44. Barnes PF, Bloch AB, Davidson PT, et al: Tuberculosis in patients with human immunodeficiency virus infection. *N Engl J Med* 324:1644, 1991.

45. Chaisson RE, Schecter GF, Theuer CP, et al: Tuberculosis in patients with the acquired immunodeficiency syndrome: Clinical features, response to therapy, and survival. *Am Rev Respir Dis* 136:570, 1987.

46. Pitchenik AE, Rubinson HA: The radiographic appearance of tuberculosis in patients with the acquired immune deficiency syndrome (AIDS) and pre-AIDS. *Am Rev Respir Dis* 131:393, 1985.

47. Shafer RW, Kim DS, Weiss JP, et al: Extrapulmonary tuberculosis in patients with human immunodeficiency virus infection. *Medicine (Baltimore)* 70:384, 1991.

47a. Markowitz N, Hansen NI, Wilcosky TC, et al: Tuberculosis and anergy testing in a cohort of HIV seropositive and HIV-seronegative individuals. *Ann Intern Med* 119:185, 1993.

48. Salzman SH, Schindel ML, Aranda CP, et al: The role of bronchoscopy in the diagnosis of pulmonary tuberculosis in patients at risk for HIV infection. *Chest* 102:143, 1992.

49. Kennedy DJ, Lewis WP, Barnes PF: Yield of bronchoscopy of the diagnosis for tuberculosis in patients with human immunodeficiency virus infection. *Chest* 102:1040, 1992.

50. Centers for Disease Control: Initial therapy for tuberculosis in the era of multidrug resistance: Recommendations of the advisory council for the elimination of tuberculosis. *MMWR* 42:1, 1993.

51. Fischl, MA, Uttamchandani RB, Daikos, GL, et al: An outbreak of tuberculosis caused by multiple drug-resistant tubercle bacilli among patients with HIV infection. *Ann Intern Med* 117:177, 1992.

52. Fischl MA, Daikos GL, Uttachandani RB, et al: Clinical presentation and outcome of patients with HIV infection and tuberculosis caused by multiple drug-resistant bacilli. *Ann Intern Med* 117:184, 1992.

53. Dooley SW, Jarrs WR, Martone WJ, et al: Multidrug-resistant tuberculosis. *Ann Intern Med* 117:184, 1992.

54. Goble M, Iseman MD, Madsen LA, et al: Treatment of 171 patients with pulmonary tuberculosis resistant to isoniazid and rifampin. *N Engl J Med* 323:527, 1993.

55. Small PM, Schechter GF, Goodman PC, et al: Treatment of tuberculosis in patients with advanced human immunodeficiency virus infection. *N Engl J Med* 324:289, 1991.

56. Drew WL: Cytomegalovirus infection in patients with AIDS. *Clin Infect Dis* 14:608, 1992.

57. Millar AB, Patou G, Miller RF, et al: Cytomegalovirus in the lungs of patients with AIDS: Respiratory pathogen or passenger? *Am Rev Respir Dis* 141:1474, 1990.

58. Miles PR, Baugham RP, Linnemann CC: Cytomegalovirus in the bronchoalveolar lavage fluid of patients with AIDS. *Chest* 97:1072, 1990.

59. Klatt EC, Shibata D: Cytomegalovirus infection in the acquired immunodeficiency syndrome. *Arch Pathol Lab Med* 112:540, 1988.

60. Wallace JM, Hannah J: Cytomegalovirus pneumonitis in patients with AIDS. *Chest* 92:198, 1987.

61. Chuck SL, Sande MA: Infectious with *Cryptococcus neoformans* in the acquired immunodeficiency syndrome. *N Engl J Med* 321:794, 1989.

62. Clark RA, Greer DL, Valainis GT, et al: *Cryptococcus neoformans* pulmonary infection in HIV-1-infected patients. *J AIDS* 3:480, 1990.

63. Chechani V, Kamholz SL: Pulmonary manifestations of disseminated cryptococcoses in patients with AIDS. *Chest* 98:1060, 1990.

64. Baugham RP, Rhodes JC, Dohn MN, et al: Detection of cryptococcal antigen in bronchoalveolar lavage fluid: A prospective study of diagnostic utility. *Am Rev Respir Dis* 145:1226, 1992.

65. Johnson PC, Hamill RJ, Sarosi GA: Clinical review: Progressive disseminated histoplasmosis in the AIDS patients. *Semin Respir Infect* 4:139, 1989.

66. Salzman SH, Smith RL, Aranda CP: Histoplasmosis in patients at risk for the acquired immunodeficiency syndrome in a nonendemic setting. *Chest* 93:916, 1988.

67. Wheat LJ, Connoly-Stringfield PA, Baker RL, et al: Disseminated histoplasmosis in the acquired immune deficiency syndrome: Clinical findings, diagnosis and treatment and review of the literature. *Medicine (Baltimore)* 69:361, 1990.

68. Denning DW, Follansbee SE, Scolaro M, et al: Pulmonary aspergillosis in the acquired immunodeficiency syndrome. *N Engl J Med* 324:654, 1991.

69. Pappas PG, Pottage JC, Powderly WG, et al: Blastomycosis in patients with the acquired immunodeficiency syndrome. *Ann Intern Med* 116:847, 1992.

70. Fish DG, Ampel NM, Gagliani JN, et al: Coccidioidomycosis during human immunodeficiency virus infection. *Medicine (Baltimore)* 69:384, 1990.

71. Rutherford GW, Schiowitz SK, Lange GF, et al: The epidemiology of AIDS-related Kaposi's sarcoma in San Francisco. *Infect Dis* 159:569, 1989.

72. White DA, Matthay RA: Noninfectious pulmonary complication of infection with the human immunodeficiency virus. *Am Rev Respir Dis* 140:1763, 1989.

73. Garay SM, Belenko M, Fazzini E, et al: Pulmonary manifestations of Kaposi's sarcoma. *Chest* 91:39, 1987.

74. Ognibene FP, Steis RG, Macher AM, et al: Kaposi's sarcoma causing pulmonary infiltrates and respiratory failure in the acquired immunodeficiency syndrome. *Ann Intern Med* 102:471, 1985.

75. Kaplan LD, Hopewell PC, Jaffe H, et al: Kaposi's sarcoma involving the lung in patients with acquired immunodeficiency syndrome. *J Acquir Immune Defic Syndr* 1:23, 1988.

76. O'Brien RF, Cohn D: Serosanguinous pleural effusions in AIDS-associated Kaposi's sarcoma. *Chest* 96:460, 1989.

77. Polish LB, Cohn DL, Ryder JW, et al: Pulmonary non-Hodgkin's lymphoma in AIDS. *Chest* 96:132, 1989.

78. Karp J, Profeta G, Marantz PR, et al: Lung cancer in patients with immunodeficiency syndrome. *Chest* 103:410, 1993.

79. Sridhar KS, Flores MR, Raub WA, et al: Lung cancer in patients with human immunodeficiency virus infection compared with historic control subjects. *Chest* 102:1704, 1992.

80. Teirstein AS, Rosen MJ: Lymphocytic interstitial pneumonia. *Clin Chest Med* 9:467, 1988.

81. Ognibene FP, Masur H, Rogers P, et al: Nonspecific interstitial pneumonitis without evidence of *Pneumocystis carinii* in asymptomatic patients infected with human immunodeficiency virus (HIV). *Ann Intern Med* 109:874, 1988.

82. Allen JN, Wewers MD: HIV-associated bronchiolitis obliterans organizing pneumonia. *Chest* 96:197, 1989.

83. Coplan NL, Shimony RY, Ioachim HL, et al: Primary pulmonary hypertension associated with human immunodeficiency viral infection. *Am J Med* 89:96, 1990.

83a. Wachter RM, Luce JM, Safrin S, et al: Cost and outcome of intensive care for patients with AIDS, *Pneumocystis carinii* pneumonia, and severe respiratory failure. *JAMA* 273:230, 1995.

84. Rosen MJ, Cucco RA, Teirstein AS: Outcome of intensive care in patients with the acquired immunodeficiency syndrome. *J Intensive Care Med* 1:55, 1986.

85. Wachter RM, Luce JM, Turner J, et al: Intensive care of patients with the acquired immunodeficiency syndrome: Outcome and changing patterns of utilization. *Am Rev Respir Dis* 134:891, 1986.

86. Schein RMH, Fischl MA, Pitchenik AE, et al: ICU survival of patients with the acquired immunodeficiency syndrome. *Crit Care Med* 14:1026, 1986.

87. Baggot LA, Baggot BB: *Pneumocystis carinii* pneumonia (PCP) in AIDS patients in intensive care. *Chest* 92:132S, 1987.

88. Deam R, Kimberley APS, Anderson M, et al: AIDS in ICU's: Outcome. *Anaesthesia* 45:150, 1988.

89. Steinbrook R, Lo B, Moulton J, et al: Preferences of homosexual men with AIDS for life-sustaining treatment. *N Engl J Med* 314:457, 1986.

90. El-Sadr W, Simberkoff MS: Survival and prognostic factors in severe *Pneumocystis carinii* pneumonia following mechanical ventilation. *Am Rev Respir Dis* 137:1264, 1988.

91. Montaner JSG, Russel JA, Lawson L, et al: Acute respiratory failure secondary to *Pneumocystis carinii* pneumonia in the acquired immunodeficiency syndrome: A potential role for systemic corticosteroids. *Chest* 95:881, 1989.

92. Rogers PL, Lane C, Henderson DK, et al: Admission of AIDS patients to a medical intensive care unit: Causes and outcome. *Crit Care Med* 17:113, 1989.

93. DeVita MA, Greenbaum DM: The critically ill patient with the acquired immunodeficiency syndrome, in Shoemaker WC, Ayres S, Grenvik A (eds): *Textbook of Critical Care Medicine*. Philadelphia, WB Saunders, 1989, p 862.

94. Wachter RM, Russi MB, Bloch DA, et al: *Pneumocystis carinii*

pneumonia and respiratory failure in AIDS: Improved outcomes and increased used of intensive care units. *Am Rev Respir Dis* 143:251, 1991.

95. Efferen LS, Nadarajah D, Palat DS: Survival following mechanical ventilation of *Pneumocystis carinii* pneumonia in patients with the acquired immunodeficiency syndrome: A different perspective. *Am J Med* 87:401, 1989.

96. Peruzzi WT, Skoutelis A, Shapiro BA, et al: Intensive care unit patients with immunodeficiency syndrome and *Pneumocystis carinii* pneumonia: Suggested predictors of hospital outcome. *Crit Care Med* 19:892, 1991.

97. Smith RL, Levine S, Lewis ML: Prognosis of patients with AIDS requiring intensive care. *Chest* 96:857, 1989.

98. Benson CA, Spear J, Hines D, et al: Combined APACHE II score and serum lactate dehydrogenase as predictors of in-hospital mortality caused by first episode *Pneumocystis carinii* pneumonia in patients with acquired immunodeficiency syndrome. *Am Rev Respir Dis* 144:319, 1991.

99. Friedman Y, Franklin C, Freels S, et al: Long term survival of patients with AIDS, *Pneumocystis carinii* pneumonia, and respiratory failure. *JAMA* 266:89, 1991.

100. Montaner JSG, Hawley PH, Ronco JJ, et al: Multisystem organ failure predicts mortality of ICU patients with acute respiratory failure secondary to AIDS-related PCP. *Chest* 102:1823, 1992.

100a. Tucker KJ, Anton B, Tucker HJ: The effect of human immunodeficiency virus infection on the distribution and outcome of pneumonia in intensive care units. *West J Med* 157:637, 1992.

100b. Bennett RL, Gilman SC, George L, et al: Improved outcomes in intensive care units for AIDS-related *Pneumocystis carinii* pneumonia: 1987–1991. *J Acquir Immune Defic Syndr* 6:1319, 1993.

100c. Hawley PH, Ronco JJ, Guillemi SA, et al: Decreasing frequency but worsening mortality of acute respiratory failure secondary to AIDS-related *Pneumocystis carinii* pneumonia. *Chest* 106:1456, 1994.

100d. Staikowsky F, Lafon B, Guidet B, et al: Mechanical ventilation for *Pneumocystis carinii* pneumonia in patients with the acquired immunodeficiency syndrome: Is the prognosis really improved? *Chest* 104:756, 1993.

100e. De Palo VA, Millstein BH, Mayo PH, et al: Outcome of intensive care in patients with HIV infection. *Chest* 107:506, 1995.

100f. Rosen MJ, Clayton KJ, Fulkerson WJ, et al: Intensive care of patients with HIV infection. *Chest* 106:51S, 1994.

101. Centers for Disease Control: Recommendations for preventing transmission of human immunodeficiency virus and hepatitis B virus to patients during exposure: Prone invasive procedures. *MMWR* 40:1, 1991.

102. Centers for Disease Control: Guidelines for preventing the transmission of tuberculosis in health care settings, with special focus on HIV-related issues. *MMWR* 39:1, 1990.

75. Severe Upper Airway Infections

Teresa E. Jacobs, Richard S. Irwin,
and Vassilios Raptopoulos

Introduction

The upper airway consists of the nose, mouth, nasopharynx, oropharynx, and hypopharynx; it communicates with the paranasal sinuses. Although minor infections in these areas are common outpatient entities, they may infrequently become severe and life-threatening. This class of disease requires intensive observation and aggressive treatment; it is the focus of this chapter.

Supraglottitis (Epiglottitis)

Acute supraglottitis is an uncommon infection of the epiglottis and other supralaryngeal structures that may progress to abrupt and fatal airway obstruction. The condition is well recognized in children, in whom the presentation and course are usually fulminant. In pediatric age groups, increased awareness and prophylactic airway control have reduced the overall mortality to less than 1 percent [1]. In adults, however, the course is often more indolent and mortality approximates 7 percent, largely because of misdiagnosis and unexpected airway obstruction [2].

PATHOGENESIS AND PATHOPHYSIOLOGY. Supraglottitis, the term preferred to epiglottitis because it is more anatomically correct, is an acute, usually bacterial inflammation of the supraglottic structures, including the epiglottis, aryepiglottic folds, and arytenoids. The true vocal cords are seldom involved. Because the lingual aspect of the epiglottis in children has a looser mucosa than in adults, providing an easy space for edema to collect [3], swelling in this area tends to curl the epiglottis posteriorly and inferiorly, accentuating the juvenile omega shape characteristically seen in children. This swelling reduces the airway aperture [4]. The obstruction increases, and respiratory distress occurs when edema spreads and involves the aryepiglottic folds [5]. Inspiration draws these swollen structures downward, exacerbating the obstruction and producing stridor [6]. The larynx is larger and the epiglottis is shaped less like an omega and more like a spatula in adults [7], and these anatomic differences seem to provide some protection to adults from the rapidly progressive airway narrowing seen in children.

Histologic examination of an acutely infected epiglottis shows three characteristic features [6,7]: edema, polymorphonuclear infiltration, and microabscesses. These processes can also be seen to involve adjacent structures. The changes appear to be the same regardless of the causative agent.

ETIOLOGY. Although a variety of bacteria, viruses, and *Candida* species have been incriminated as the cause of acute supraglottitis (Table 75-1), *Haemophilus influenzae* type B has been identified most often in both pediatric and adult cases [14,21]. About 60 percent of children have documented bacteremia, nearly always due to *H. influenzae* [14,21]. Blood cultures in adults are positive in only 30 percent of cases, and *H. influenzae* is the isolate in one-third of these [2,14,22]. Most of the more severe and rapidly progressive infections have also been associated with this organism [2,14,21,22].

DIAGNOSIS

History and Physical Examination. The classic presentation is of a 3-year-old child who initially complains of a sore throat, then dysphagia, followed within hours by stridor [23]. The child prefers to sit, leaning forward, and is usually pale and frightened. Breathing is slow and quiet, and drooling is characteristic [21]. The progression to respiratory depression and arrest may be sudden. The progression of symptoms is easily remembered as the "four Ds": *d*ysphagia, *d*ysphonia, *d*rooling, *d*istress [24].

In adults, this scenario is more often the exception than the rule. The frequency of misdiagnosis has been reported as high as 60 to 75 percent [25,26,27]. Many patients give histories of preceding upper respiratory tract infections [21,28]. Over 90 percent of adult patients who present to a physician complain of sore throat with or without dysphagia [2,6,10,14]. Other signs and symptoms that occur less often are respiratory difficulty, muffled voice, drooling, fever, and stridor [2,14]. Hoarseness or true dysphonia is not observed because the process spares the true vocal cords [17]. As with children, a preference for an upright posture with the neck extended and mouth slightly open can be observed [17].

The duration of symptoms is highly variable, ranging from hours to almost a week [22,29]. Deeb et al. [8] found that patients who presented within 8 hours of the onset of symptoms were more likely to have signs of upper airway obstruction. This group was also noted to have a higher average white blood cell (WBC) count. In general, patients with more severe symptoms, short times to presentation, fever, and leukocytosis were more likely to be infected with *H. influenzae* [22] and were at increased risk of needing artificial airways or of dying [2].

Evaluation of patients with suspected supraglottitis depends in part on their age and the severity of their symptoms. In young children with a classic presentation, pharyngeal examination should not be attempted. The patient should have an artificial airway established in the controlled setting of an operating room and can be examined at that time without risk of airway

Table 75-1. Organisms Implicated in Acute Epiglottis

Haemophilus influenzae [8]
Streptococcus pneumoniae [9,10]
Beta-hemolytic streptococci [11,12,13]
Staphylococcus aureus [12,14]
Klebsiella pneumoniae [14,15]
Bacteroides species [16]
Hemophilus parainfluenzae [8,17]
Candida albicans* [18,19]
Pasteurella multocida [20]

*Cultured only from epiglottic swab; all others recovered from blood.

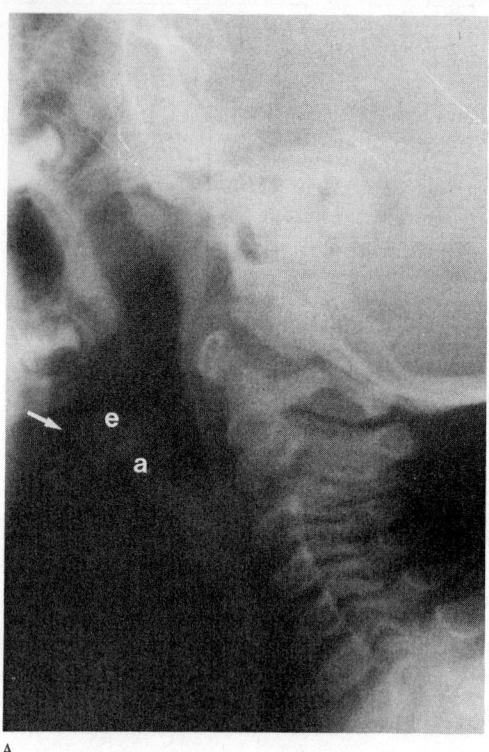

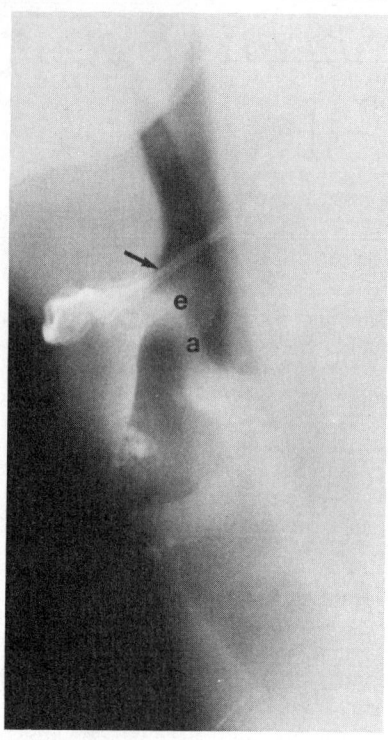

A

B

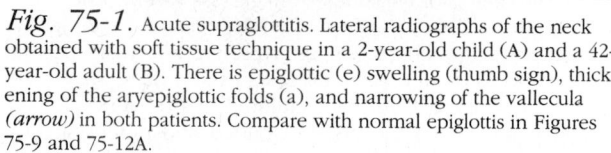

Fig. 75-1. Acute supraglottitis. Lateral radiographs of the neck obtained with soft tissue technique in a 2-year-old child (A) and a 42-year-old adult (B). There is epiglottic (e) swelling (thumb sign), thickening of the aryepiglottic folds (a), and narrowing of the vallecula *(arrow)* in both patients. Compare with normal epiglottis in Figures 75-9 and 75-12A.

obstruction. When there is doubt about the diagnosis in a stable child, a lateral neck radiograph to look for the "thumb" sign of a swollen epiglottis is the proper first step (Fig. 75-1) [23].

In older children and adults, supraglottitis should be considered when sore throat and dysphagia seem to be out of proportion to visible signs of pharyngitis [6]. In this situation, if the patient has no respiratory distress, examination of the larynx and supralaryngeal structures is recommended to diagnose supraglottitis conclusively. The epiglottis may be cherry red but more commonly is pale and edematous. Other supraglottic structures may be swollen as well, so much so that the vocal cords may not be seen [17]. We are not aware of any reported cases of adult airway obstruction precipitated by indirect laryngoscopy [2,10]. Other physical findings, such as pain on laryngeal palpation [30] and cervical adenopathy [31,32], are described, but they are infrequent and not specific.

Diagnostic Tests. Although a lateral soft tissue radiograph of the neck has frequently been used to diagnose or rule out acute supraglottitis, recent reviews question the reliability of this test [2,11,33]. Characteristic changes (Fig. 75-1), however, have been detected in most endoscopically proved infections [2,27]. These include epiglottic thickening of more than 8 mm (producing the thumb sign) [34], swelling of the aryepiglottic folds of more than 7 mm [34], ballooning of the hypopharynx [27], and narrowing of the vallecula [27]. One preliminary, retrospective study [35] suggests that the radiographic ratios of (1) aryepiglottic width to the width of the third cervical vertebra

(AEW/C3W), (2) epiglottic width to the width of the third cervical vertebra (EW/C3W), and (3) epiglottic width to epiglottic height (EW/EH) are very good predictors of both adult and pediatric supraglottitis. Ratios greater than 0.35, 0.5, and 0.6, respectively, were 100 percent sensitive and 87 to 100 percent specific in their 31 patients. However, it is important to remember that if suspicion for supraglottitis is high a normal radiograph is inadequate to exclude the diagnosis and direct visualization of the structures should be pursued. The radiograph should be made in the upright position, since secretions may pool posteriorly when the patient is supine and may increase the obstruction [5]. Given the unpredictable course of the disease, the patient should be observed at all times by someone skilled in airway management.

Few laboratory tests are helpful at the time of initial evaluation. As mentioned, an elevated WBC count may help identify a patient at higher risk. Throat cultures are of no value at presentation and correlate poorly with blood culture results and clinical outcome [2]. Direct swab culture of the epiglottis may reflect more closely the causative agent, but it has not been well studied in adults [2]. Blood cultures and the antibiotic sensitivity pattern are essential to identify the organism and, particularly in cases of *H. influenzae* infection, to guide antibiotic selection [29].

DIFFERENTIAL DIAGNOSIS. The diagnosis of supraglottitis in children is a clinical one. Because immediate airway control is a priority, recognition of other pediatric illnesses that present with a sore throat and that do not require this intervention is important. The most commonly encountered infection is croup, a predominantly viral laryngotracheobronchitis, that occurs up to 40 times more frequently than epiglottitis [23]. Unlike epiglottitis, croup usually presents in a child younger than 3 years of age who has had an upper respiratory tract infection of at least 48 hours' duration. The initial symptom is hoarseness, followed by a distinctive barking cough. Although respiratory distress is common, with inspiratory stridor and expiratory wheezing, intubation is rarely needed; this is in sharp contrast to epiglottitis [23]. Anteroposterior and lateral views of the neck may show the "steeple" sign (Fig. 75-2), a gradual narrowing of the tracheal air column secondary to subglottic edema, with the apex pointed toward the vocal cords. Other less common infectious considerations in children include pseudomembranous croup (bacterial laryngotracheobronchitis), retropharyngeal abscess, lingual tonsillitis, and, rarely, diphtheria [23,36].

One of the above conditions merits special mention. More frequently reported cases of pseudomembranous croup due to bacterial infection, or bacterial tracheitis (BT), are calling attention to this potentially life-threatening illness with features similar to those of both supraglottitis and viral croup. Although more often seen in the pediatric age group, several adult cases have been described [37,38,39]. The clinical presentation is characterized by a brief, progressive upper respiratory prodrome, brassy cough, and stridor, with high fever and toxicity but without dysphagia or drooling [40,41]. Airway obstruction is due to subglottic mucosal edema and thick, inspissated, mucopurulent tracheal secretions [37–41]. The likely etiology is bacterial superinfection, mostly *Staphylococcus aureus* and *H. influenzae*, of a preceding viral tracheitis, with *parainfluenza* the most common viral isolate [40]. Rare cases of membranous tracheobronchitis due to fungus have been described in immunocompromised hosts [42–45], but these infections have involved primarily the lower respiratory tract. Lateral neck radiographs in the bacterial disease demonstrate subglottic narrowing and may show mucosal irregularities or membranes in the tracheal air column [46]. Management is similar to that for supraglottitis, and direct laryngoscopy should be performed for diagnosis [40]. Intubation or tracheostomy is usually necessary to relieve obstruction and provide adequate tracheal suctioning [39,40,41,46]. Antibiotic therapy should be directed against *S. aureus* and other usual respiratory pathogens [38–41].

In adults, the more common illnesses of infectious mononucleosis, often with massive tonsillar hypertrophy leading to stridor, and unilateral pharyngeal mass should be considered when complaints of sore throat and dysphagia are elicited. Pharyngitis may present a picture indistinguishable from that of mild or early supraglottitis [2,8].

Another diagnostic consideration is *Klebsiella rhinoscleromatis* infection [46a]. *Klebsiella rhinoscleromatis* is the etiologic agent of the chronic granulomatous disorder known as rhinoscleroma, the features of which have been reviewed by Colt and colleagues [46a]. The nasal and oral mucous membrane are the most common sites of infection, but laryngotracheal and bronchial infection have also been described. This disease is endemic in areas of Eastern Europe, Asia, the Middle East, Central and South America, and Africa and may be seen in immigrants to the United States from these areas. Chronic rhinorrhea, which may be mucopurulent, and nasal congestion may persist for months. The disease may spread from an initial focus in the nose to the septum, sinuses, palate, vocal cords, and bronchus. Eventually, the indurated tissue takes on a woody consistency. The nasopharyngeal mucosa appears nodular. Radiography may reveal exuberant soft tissue in the nasal cavity, thickening of the nasal septum, sinusitis, and bony destruction. The endoscopic appearance is similar to that of papillomatosis, sarcoidosis, Wegener's granulomatosis, tuberculosis, fungal infections, and carcinoma. Diagnosis is made by culture and histologic examination of multiple biopsies. Prolonged, oral antibiotic treatment is usually effective for *Kleb-*

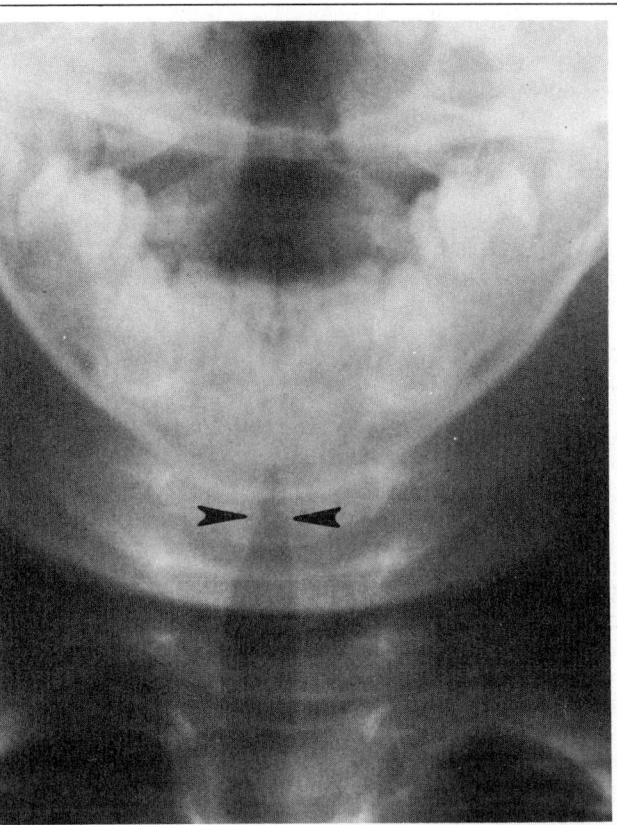

Fig. 75-2. Croup. Anteroposterior radiograph of the neck in a 19-month-old child. Subglottic edema produces smooth tapering *(arrowheads)* of the tracheal air column (the steeple sign).

siella rhinoscleroma [46a]. Antibiotics that have proven effective include ampicillin, streptomycin, tetracycline, chloramphenicol, and trimethaprim-sulfamethoxazole. The antibiotic needs to be continued until complete resolution has occurred. Repeated cultures of biopsy specimens may be needed to ascertain whether bacteriologic cure has been effected [46a].

Noninfectious causes of acute upper airway obstruction are usually suggested by history and the patient's nontoxic appearance [4,36,47]. These include foreign body aspiration, allergic edema, chemical laryngitis from gastroesophageal reflux of stomach acid, and necrotizing tracheobronchitis as a complication of mechanical ventilation. Paraquat poisoning can cause a pharyngeal membrane similar to diphtheria that is accompanied by signs of shock and sepsis [23].

TREATMENT. The treatment of supraglottitis has two major components: airway management and medical therapy. Maintaining airway patency is of utmost importance. The early placement of an artificial airway in children has significantly reduced mortality. Moreover, because airway obstruction is the most common cause of death in adults in whom airways are not secured when the diagnosis of supraglottitis is made [2], some authors favor establishing an artificial airway prophylactically as is done in children [2,5,48,49]. We and others tend to reserve intubation for adult patients with early signs of airway obstruction [8,10,21,22,28,29,31,50,51]. All agree on the need for an intensive care setting and immediate availability of equipment and personnel for emergent intubation.

With respect to the type of artificial airway established, tracheostomy or endotracheal intubation, usually secured orally and changed to a nasal tube, have been used. Although no difference in mortality has been noted in comparisons of the two modalities for this disease [1,52], important differences have been seen in duration of airway control and length of hospitalization: both are significantly reduced in endotracheally intubated patients [52]. Another potential benefit of endotracheal intubation is a decreased rate of upper airway complications [36,52,53]. In general, the mortality of intubation is less than that of tracheostomy: less than 1 percent versus 3 percent [53]. The acute complications of tracheostomy, including pneumothorax, hemorrhage, and subcutaneous or mediastinal emphysema, occur with increased frequency in patients younger than 12 years of age [1]. Accidental extubation, particularly in children, and failure to intubate are the greatest risks of endotracheal intubation [1,54]. Much of the morbidity, including complications of subglottic stenosis, laryngeal ulcers, and tracheal stenosis, is associated with prolonged maintenance of the artificial airway, which is unlikely to occur in supraglottitis. Ninety percent of nasotracheally intubated children in one large series were extubated in less than 24 hours [55]. The choice of airway maintenance should be determined by the skill of available personnel in placing and maintaining the airway. If both modalities are equally available, endotracheal intubation is preferred, with surgical backup should the attempt fail.

Several different criteria have been used to determine the appropriate time to extubate a patient recovering from acute supraglottitis. Some remove the artificial airway when the patient's general toxic appearance and fever have subsided [55]. Others wait until repeat laryngoscopy or lateral neck radiographs show decreased edema of the involved structures [17,28]. A third method to assess readiness for extubation is to test for an air leak around the tube or the patient's ability to breathe with the tube plugged for a few brief moments and the balloon deflated for these maneuvers [54,56]. It is important to understand the limitations of this latter method. Obviously, if the tube is large enough to fill the trachea, the patient is not able to breathe even if supraglottitis has completely resolved.

Medical therapy is crucial for the rapid recovery from supraglottitis. All patients require close observation, humidification [31,57], and, often, mild sedation [3]. Some discussion surrounds the selection of antibiotics, but all regimens are designed to cover *H. influenzae* infection. With the emergence of beta-lactamase-producing strains of the organism, ampicillin is no longer adequate as an initial single agent. The initial drug of choice is a second- or third-generation cephalosporin that covers ampicillin-resistant *H. influenzae* as well as the other possible pathogens in adults: *S. aureus, Streptococcus pneumoniae,* and other streptococcal species [2,7,56]. Ampicillin with chloramphenicol has also been used, primarily in children, in whom the overwhelmingly predominant organism is *H. influenzae* [11,54]. When the organism and its antibiotic sensitivities are known, the regimen should be changed to minimize the toxicity and expense of different antibiotics [11]. The antibiotics should be given intravenously at least for several days, depending on the response, and continued by mouth for 10 or 14 days [50]. When *H. influenzae* is the confirmed or putative causative agent, antibiotic prophylaxis with rifampin, 20 mg per kilogram of body weight (600 mg/day maximum) for 4 days, is recommended for close contacts, especially children younger than 4 years of age [28].

Corticosteroid therapy is controversial in patients with infectious supraglottitis, since no conclusive study has been done. However, their use is suggested based on the premises that any reduction of the inflammatory edema contributes to recovery and a tracheostomy may be averted if the diagnosis proves to be angioneurotic edema [5]. In one study, observation with steroids resulted in an approximate 50 percent decrease in length of hospitalization when compared to observation without steroids and nasotracheal intubation, both with and without steroids [58]. These data were discounted because of small numbers of subjects but may suggest some efficacy in patients who are observed, as are most adults. Many authors, finding no contraindications, use them empirically [1,9,10,26,57]. Racemic epinephrine has not been thought to be effective in this disease [28,57,59].

Complications of the disease differ between the pediatric and adult populations. The former has a higher incidence of pneumonia and accidental extubation [14]. Several cases of pulmonary edema immediately following intubation for severe stridor have been described in children [60]. In adults, an epiglottic abscess may be suggested by a persistent or deteriorating clinical condition [21,28,51]. Both groups face risks and complications associated with intubation and tracheostomy, including tracheal or subglottic stenosis, hoarseness, atelectasis, pneumothorax, and hemorrhage [53,61].

In summary, the most effective management of supraglottitis in any age group is by protocol. The goal is to eliminate death by anticipating unexpected airway obstruction, minimizing complications by optimizing the selection of procedures, and supporting the patient with antibiotics and perhaps antiinflammatory medication (e.g., corticosteroids) through this uniformly self-limiting infection. Our treatment recommendations are outlined in Figure 75-3.

Infections of the Deep Spaces of the Neck

Deep neck infections can be fatal extensions of upper airway infections. Because of prompt treatment of pharyngitis, tonsillitis, and odontogenic infections with antibiotics, these potentially catastrophic infections are a rare occurrence. Early diagnosis and timely intervention of these conditions require an understanding of the complex interconnections between anatomic spaces.

GENERAL PATHOGENESIS AND ANATOMY. Some knowledge of the cervical fasciae is a prerequisite to understanding the etiology, manifestations, complications, and treatment of deep neck infections. The fascial planes both separate and connect distant areas, thereby limiting and directing the spread of infection (Figs. 75-4 and 75-5). Suppurative processes in three cervical spaces (i.e., submandibular, lateral pharyngeal, and retropharyngeal) are considered life-threatening, so emphasis is focused on these areas.

The submandibular space (SMS) (Fig. 75-6) consists of the sublingual and submylohyoid spaces, which communicate around the free posterior border of the mylohyoid muscle. It extends from the mucous membrane of the floor of the mouth above to the superficial layer of the deep cervical fascia below. Anteriorly and laterally, it is bounded by the mandible. Superolaterally is the buccopharyngeal gap, an important opening behind the styloglossus muscle, which connects the SMS to the lateral pharyngeal space (LPS).

The LPS (Fig. 75-7), also called the pharyngomaxillary or parapharyngeal space, is an inverted cone with its apex at the hyoid bone and its base at the base of the skull. The styloid

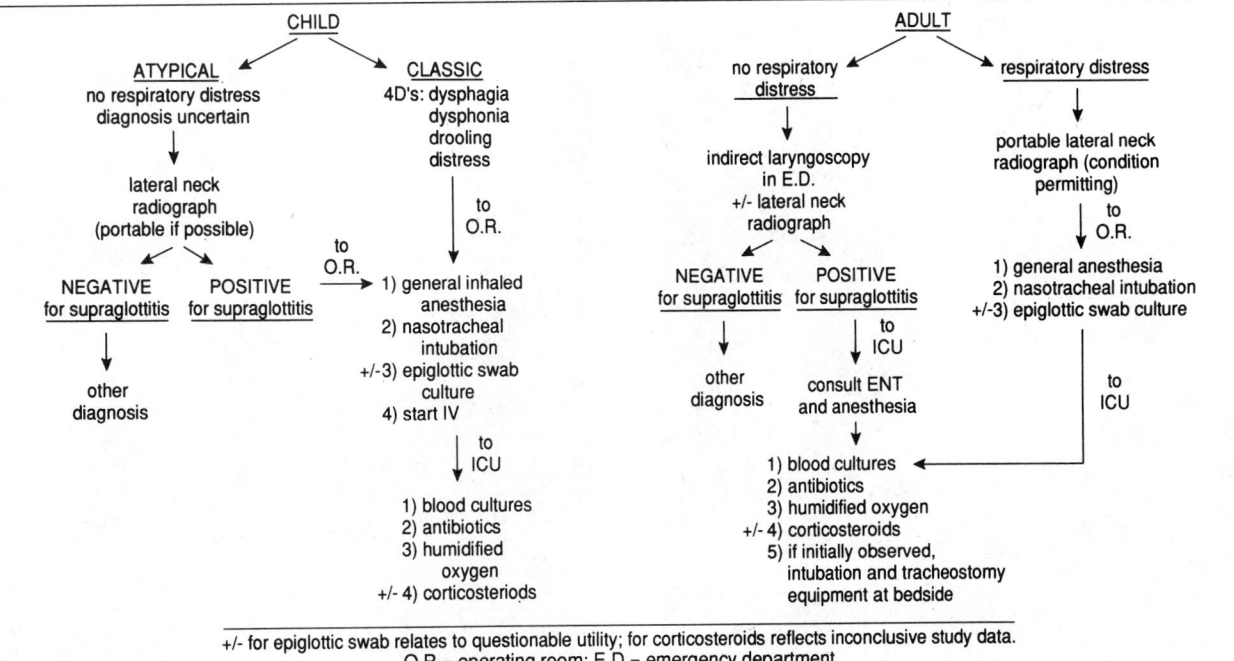

CHILD

ATYPICAL
no respiratory distress
diagnosis uncertain

↓

lateral neck
radiograph
(portable if possible)

NEGATIVE
for supraglottitis

↓

other
diagnosis

POSITIVE
for supraglottitis

CLASSIC
4D's: dysphagia
dysphonia
drooling
distress

↓
to
O.R.

to
O.R. →

1) general inhaled
anesthesia
2) nasotracheal
intubation
+/-3) epiglottic swab
culture
4) start IV

↓ to
ICU

1) blood cultures
2) antibiotics
3) humidified
oxygen
+/- 4) corticosteriods

ADULT

no respiratory
distress

↓

indirect laryngoscopy
in E.D.
+/- lateral neck
radiograph

NEGATIVE
for supraglottitis

↓

other
diagnosis

POSITIVE
for supraglottitis

↓ to
ICU

consult ENT
and anesthesia

↓

respiratory distress

↓

portable lateral neck
radiograph (condition
permitting)

↓ to
O.R.

1) general anesthesia
2) nasotracheal intubation
+/-3) epiglottic swab culture

to
ICU

1) blood cultures
2) antibiotics
3) humidified oxygen
+/- 4) corticosteroids
5) if initially observed,
intubation and tracheostomy
equipment at bedside

+/- for epiglottic swab relates to questionable utility; for corticosteroids reflects inconclusive study data.
O.R.= operating room; E.D.= emergency department.

Fig. 75-3. Management algorithm for acute supraglottitis.

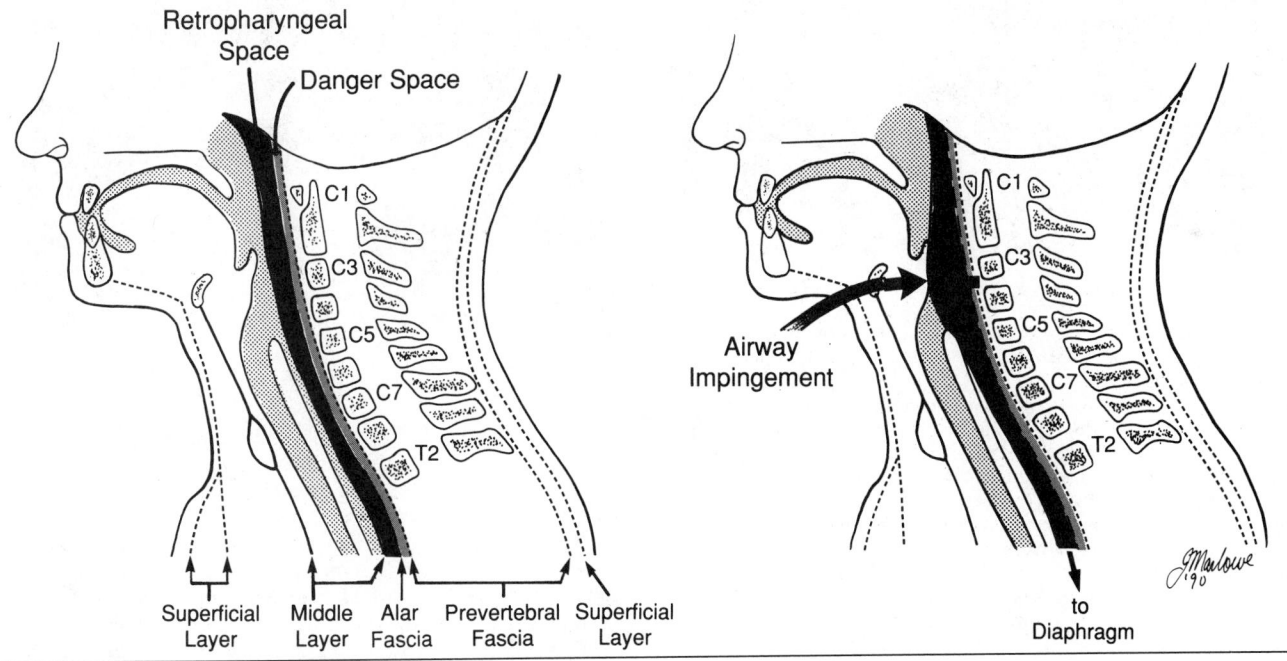

Fig. 75-4. Schematic representation of cervical fascial planes and spaces. Left. Normal. Right. Retropharyngeal space abscess. (Adapted from Netter FH: *Atlas of Human Anatomy.* Summit, NJ, Ciba-Geigy, 1989. With permission.)

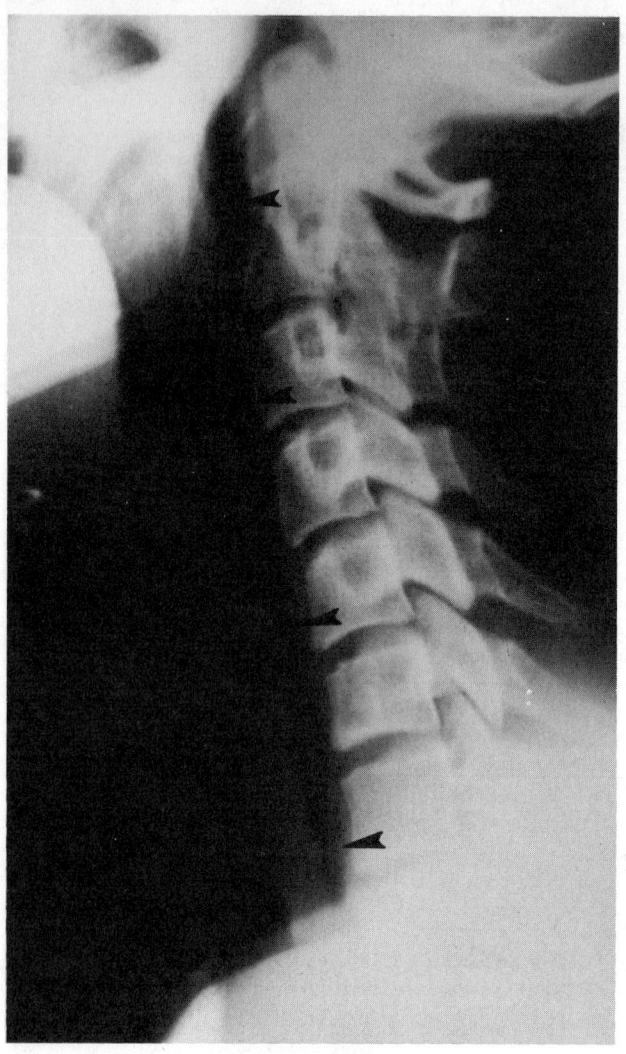

A

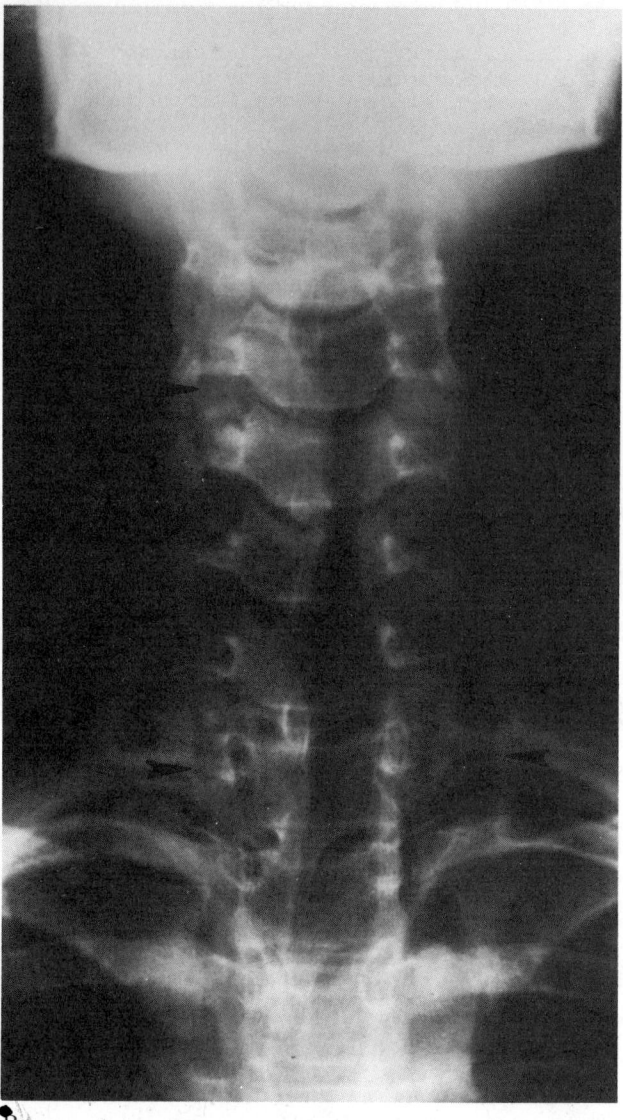

B

Fig. 75-5. Dissection of air along fascial planes of the neck corresponding to common pathways of spread of infections within the soft tissues of the neck. Radiographs (A, B) and computed tomograms (C–E) of the neck of a 16-year-old patient with ruptured pyriform sinus. Air *(arrowheads)* dissects along the posterior (A) and lateral (B) fascial planes of the neck from the base of the skull to the superior mediastinum. Computed tomogram above the level of the hyoid bone (C) shows air in the retropharyngeal space *(arrow)* extending laterally into the posterior (neurovascular) compartment of the lateral pharyngeal space (LPS). p = pharynx; s = styloid process; v = vessels in the posterior compartment of the LPS: internal carotid artery, medially, and internal jugular vein, laterally. Below the hyoid bone (D), the air is again distributed along the prevertebral fascia, posterior to the larynx (l) and along the great vessels (v) (common carotid artery and jugular vein) to the superior mediastinum (E), posterior to the esophagus (e), and along the great neck vessels (v). The prevertebral, retropharyngeal air is in the distribution of the danger space.

process penetrates the space and divides it into two functional units: the anterior (muscular) and posterior (neurovascular) compartments. The former lies lateral to the tonsillar fossa and connects inferomedially to the SMS. The latter contains the carotid sheath and its contents (i.e., internal carotid artery, internal jugular vein, vagus nerve, and lymph nodes), cranial nerves IX through XII, and the cervical sympathetic trunks. Both compartments abut the retropharyngeal space (RPS).

Also called the posterior visceral space, the RPS (Fig. 75-4) lies between the middle layer of the deep cervical fascia, which surrounds the pharynx and esophagus anteriorly and the alar layer of the deep cervical facia posteriorly. It extends from the base of the skull to the level of T_1 or T_2 in the superior mediastinum. Laterally, it abuts the LPS. Two chains of lymph nodes that drain many structures of the head are located on either side of midline.

Immediately posterior to the RPS is the "danger" space (Fig. 75-4), so named because it is the pathway into the chest for all neck infections. It extends from the base of the skull to the diaphragms and is bounded posteriorly by the prevertebral layer of the deep cervical fascia. Involvement of this space by

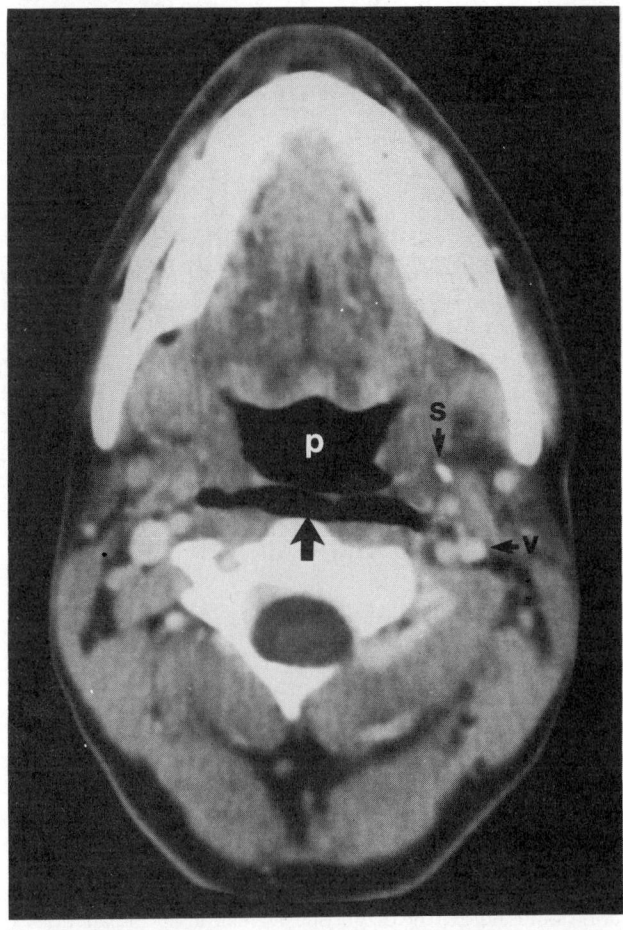

C

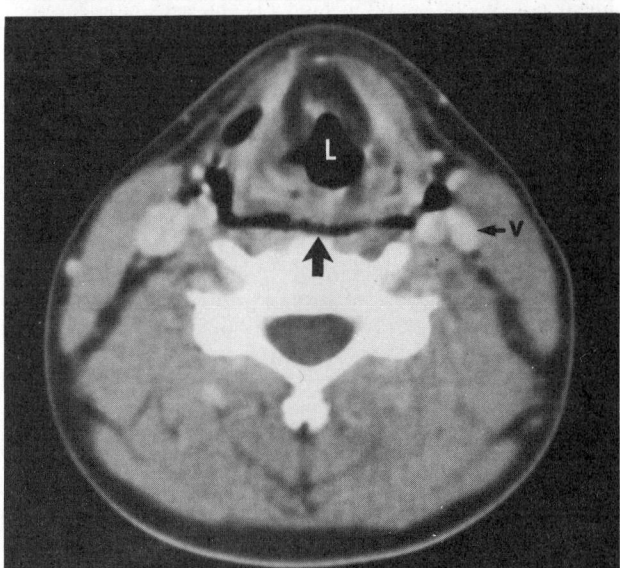

D

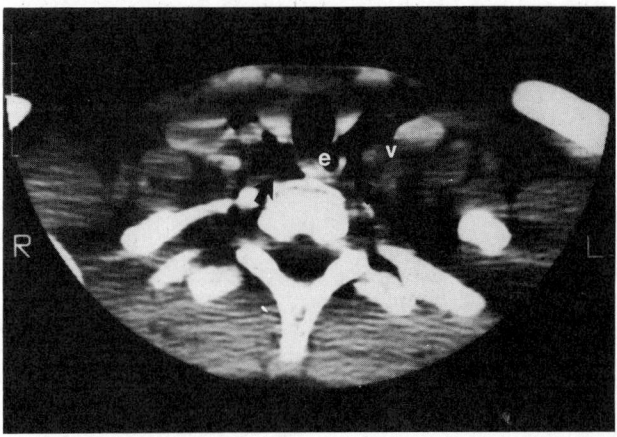

E

infection is a result of extension from the RPS or prevertebral space and gives rise to many life-threatening complications associated with neck infections.

The prevertebral space (PVS) (Fig. 75-4) lies between the vertebral bodies and the prevertebral layer of the deep cervical fascia. Infections here most often represent chronic processes arising from cervical spine injuries or infections. The usual pathogens in this space are different, but the extension to the danger space allows for similar clinical manifestations.

ETIOLOGY. Although fungi and mycobacteria have been occasionally recovered, the bacteria that are normal components of oral flora are chiefly responsible for deep cervical infections. They become pathogenic when mucosal barriers are interrupted, such as during pharyngitis, and they can penetrate into the deeper spaces. These infections usually are due to a mixture of anaerobic and aerobic organisms (e.g., 88% are polymicrobial), anaerobes predominating in a ratio of 3:1 to 6:1 [62,63].

Careful culture technique is crucial to correct identification of the causative bacteria. The major difficulties in obtaining meaningful bacteriologic data are that (1) most patients receive antibiotics before hospitalization, (2) many deep infections resolve with empiric antibiotic therapy without the need for aspiration procedures, and (3) cultures obtained perorally are suspected of contamination by noninfecting oropharyngeal organisms [64]. Several studies using proper anaerobic collection and transport techniques have most frequently identified three anaerobic isolates: *Peptostreptococcus, Fusobacterium* (mostly *nucleatum),* and *Bacteroides* (mostly *melaninogenicus)* [62,63]. Although obligate anaerobes as a class are recovered most often, aerobic streptococci are the most frequent individual isolates [65].

Facultative gram-negative bacilli are less common causes of deep neck infections, but they do colonize the oropharynx of 6 to 18 percent of healthy adults [66,67]. This number can increase to 60 percent in hospitalized patients, diabetic persons, alcoholic persons, and institutionalized patients [66]. *Escherichia coli, Pseudomonas aeruginosa, Klebsiella pneumoniae, H. influenzae, Enterobacter, Proteus mirabilis, Citrobacter freundii,* and *Actinomyces* have been isolated from deep cervical infections [68–71]. One gram-negative rod, a facultative anaerobe, is of particular concern: *Eikenella corrodens.* It is an emerging pathogen in head and neck infections, and it is uniformly resistant to clindamycin, an antibiotic of potential use in cervical infections [72,73,74].

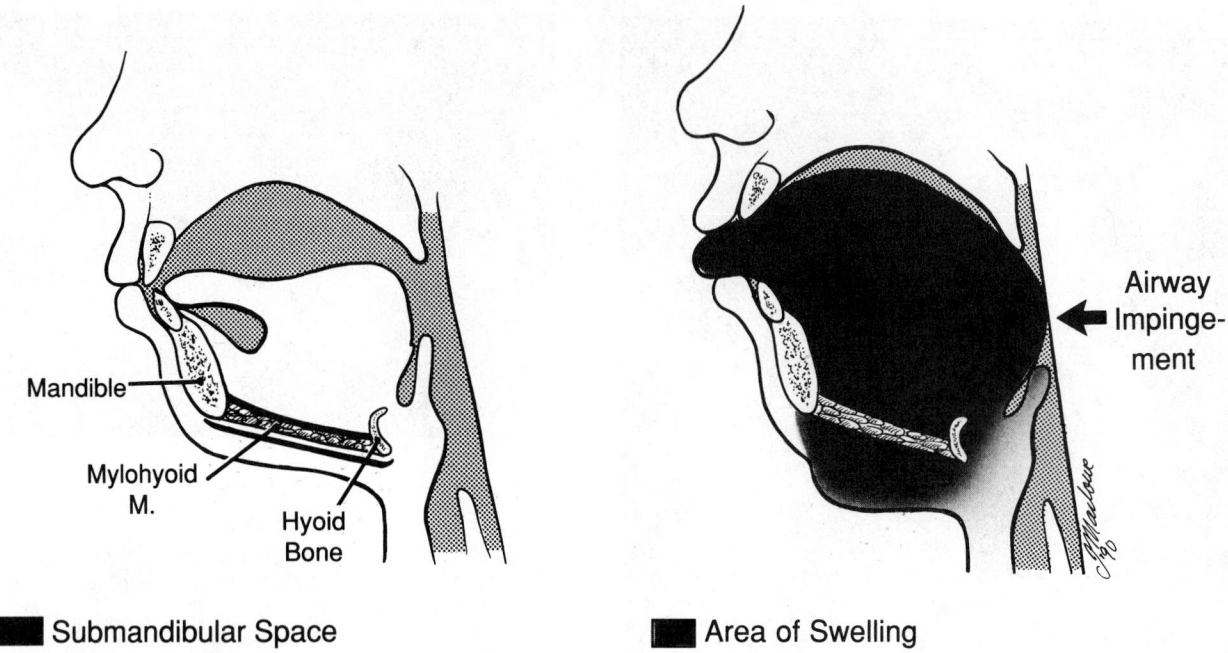

Submandibular Space   **Area of Swelling**

Fig. 75-6. Schematic representation of submandibular space. Left. Normal. Right. Ludwig's angina.

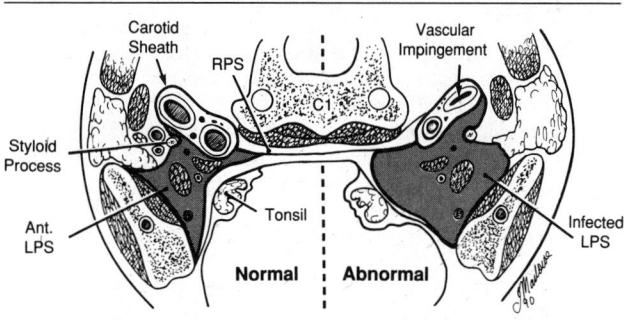

Fig. 75-7. Cross-sectional view of lateral pharyngeal space, showing normal anatomic landmarks and effects of space infection on them.

Staphylococci are rare isolates in deep neck infections but should be considered in certain circumstances, such as penetrating trauma, as in cervical IV drug use [75], and deep infections that originate from osteomyelitis of the cervical spine [65,76].

When cultural confirmation of anaerobic infection is lacking, certain clinical clues may be helpful in suggesting the presence of anaerobes [63]. A foul-smelling discharge is considered diagnostic but may be absent in half of confirmed cases. Gas production, tissue necrosis, and abscess formation are also suggestive. Gram stain of the exudate may reveal anaerobic organisms of specific morphologic characteristics, such as clostridia and fusobacteria. Because anaerobes are more fastidious, failure to discover a likely pathogen from the more rapidly available aerobic cultures can suggest an anaerobic pathogen.

DIAGNOSIS. It is important to distinguish the space or spaces involved in deep neck infections so the potentially devastating

complications can be prevented or recognized early and treated surgically if necessary. The clinical picture may be confusing because of involvement of multiple spaces and interference with the examination by trismus. Because fever and systemic toxicity are common to most processes beyond the early stages, other signs and symptoms may be helpful to localize the primary site of infection (Table 75-2) [77]. Laboratory blood testing contributes little to the diagnostic evaluation (most patients with cervical deep space infections exhibit leukocytosis [71]), but initial assessment should include a lateral neck radiograph.

Submandibular Space Infection. Infection in the SMS is exemplified by Ludwig's angina, a bilateral, brawny cellulitis spread by continuity, not lymphatics, sparing glandular structures, and producing gangrene with putrid serosanguineous infiltration, with little or no pus and no abscess formation (Fig. 75-6) [78]. Most patients are young, healthy adults, with a two or three times greater incidence in males [65,71]. The presenting symptoms are neck pain and swelling, tooth pain or recent extraction, and dysphagia [71,79]. Odontogenic infections are implicated in 70 to 90 percent of cases of Ludwig's angina [64,71,77,79]. Respiratory complaints of dyspnea, tachypnea, and stridor have been reported in as many as 27 percent of cases [71]. Other symptoms have included a muffled voice [80], drooling [75], and tongue swelling [79].

Ludwig's angina is essentially a clinical diagnosis. Physical examination (Fig. 75-8) reveals bilateral, woody submandibular swelling [62,71,79]; mouth distortion secondary to enlargement of the tongue, which is elevated and often protruding [65,71,81]; fever; and general toxicity [71,80]. Trismus, seen in up to 51 percent of patients, indicates that infection has spread to the LPS [71,77]. Airway obstruction is a much feared and frequent complication of Ludwig's angina. Before 1945, the mortality of this infection approached 60 percent, airway problems contributing in 80 percent of fatalities [71,79]. Current mortality rates are much lower—zero in some series [64]—because of improved antibiotic therapy and early airway control [65]. Respiratory compromise may result from obstruction by the swollen, displaced tongue, edema of the neck and glottis, extension of

Table 75-2. Comparative Features of Infections of the Deep Cervical Spaces

Space infections	Usual site of origin	Clinical features				
		Pain	Trismus	Swelling	Dysphagia	Dyspnea
Submandibular	Second and third mandibular molars	Present	Minimal	Submandibular	Absent	Absent
Sublingual	Mandibular incisors	Present	Minimal	Floor of mouth (tender)	Present if involvement is bilateral	Present if involvement is bilateral
Lateral pharyngeal						
Anterior	Masticator spaces	Intense	Prominent	Angle of jaw	Present	Occasional
Posterior	Masticator spaces	Minimal	Minimal	Posterior pharynx (unilateral)	Present	Severe
Retropharyngeal (and danger)	Lateral pharyngeal space; distant via lymphatics	Present	Minimal	Posterior pharynx (often unilateral)	Present	Present
Prevertebral	Cervical vertebrae	Present	None	Posterior pharynx (usually midline)	Occasional	Occasional

Modified from Megran DW, Scheifele DW, Chow AW: Odontogenic infections. *Pediatr Infect Dis* 3:257, 1984. With permission, © by Williams and Wilkins.

edema to involve the epiglottis, and poor control of pharyngeal secretions [62,65]. Most patients with SMS involvement show soft tissue swelling (Fig. 75-9) [71], a finding that should prompt radiographic examination of the mandible in patients without a clear odontogenic source [64].

Lateral Pharyngeal Space Infections. The signs and symptoms of LPS infections are determined by which of the two compartments is affected (Fig. 75-7). There are four major clinical signs of anterior compartment involvement [62,81]. Unilateral trismus is due to irritation of the internal pterygoid muscle. Induration and swelling along the angle of the jaw may be prominent. Systemic toxicity with high fever and rigors may be evidence of the formation of an abscess. The lateral pharyngeal wall may be seen to bulge medially, with the palatine tonsil

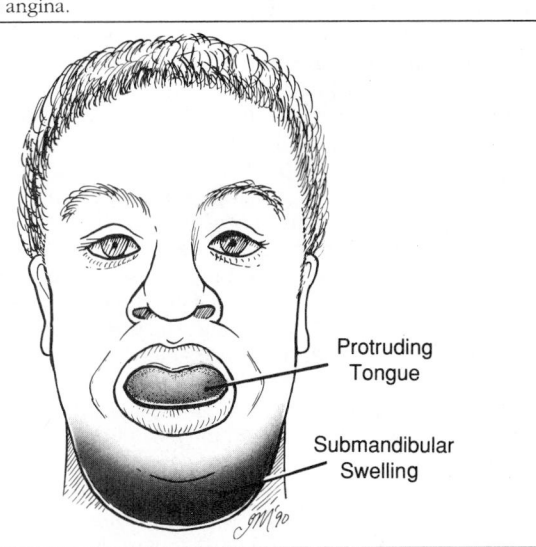

Fig. 75-8. Schematic representation of salient clinical findings of Ludwig's angina.

Protruding Tongue

Submandibular Swelling

bulging into the airway (Fig. 75-10). Other findings may include dysphagia and pain involving the jaw or side of the neck. This pain may be referred to the ipsilateral ear and may worsen with turning the head to the unaffected side, which compresses the inflamed space by contraction of the sternocleidomastoid muscle. A history of recent upper respiratory infection, pharyngitis, or tonsillitis is often elicited [82]. Other sites of initial infection, especially in children, include teeth, adenoids, parotid gland, middle ear with associated mastoiditis, and lymph nodes draining the nose and pharynx [81]. The SMS and RPS have also been implicated.

In infection of the posterior compartment, signs of sepsis consisting of fever, leukocytosis, and often hypotension and respiratory alkalosis are the cardinal features. Trismus and tonsillar prolapse are notably absent [77,81]. Dyspnea may be present as edema descends to involve the larynx and epiglottis [65]. External swelling may be visible when it spreads to the parotid space (Fig. 75-10), but most patients have no localizing signs.

Many symptoms and signs relate to the complications of involvement of the neurovascular structures. Suppurative jugular venous thrombosis is most common. The most frequent consequences of this entity are bacteremia and septic emboli, each of which occurs in half of cases [83,84]. Also reported are suppurative subclavian thrombosis [83], lateral sinus thrombosis [83], cavernous sinus thrombosis [85], and metastatic infections [86].

Involvement of the carotid artery has the highest morbidity and mortality [65,84,87] of any vascular complication in the LPS. Carotid artery rupture carries a mortality of 20 to 40 percent, regardless of treatment [87]. The internal carotid is the most likely to rupture (62%), followed by the external carotid and its branches (25%) and then the common carotid (13%) [88]. Arteritis develops from the contiguous inflammation, which results in false aneurysm formation [89]. Because the carotid sheath is so dense and not easily invaded, 1 or 2 weeks of illness usually precedes arterial erosion [87]. Signs suggestive of carotid sheath involvement include persistent tonsillar swelling after resolution of a peritonsillar abscess, ipsilateral Horner's syndrome, and cranial nerve palsies [89,90,91]. Impending rupture of a carotid aneurysm may be signalled by recurrent "her-

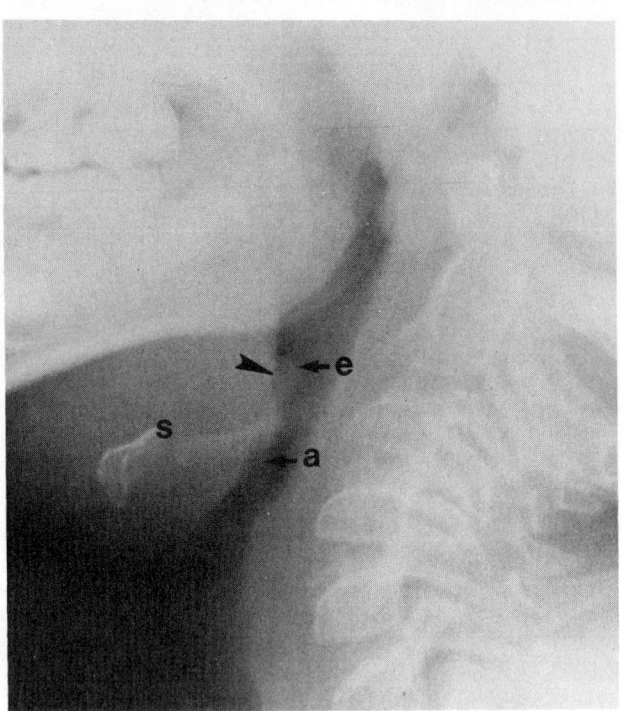

Fig. 75-9. Ludwig's angina. Lateral radiographs of the neck obtained with soft tissue technique in a 7-year-old child. There is soft tissue swelling of the submandibular space (s), producing a smooth impression on the airway anteriorly, compressing and practically ablating the vallecula *(arrowhead)*; the epiglottis (e) and aryepiglottic folds (a) are normal.

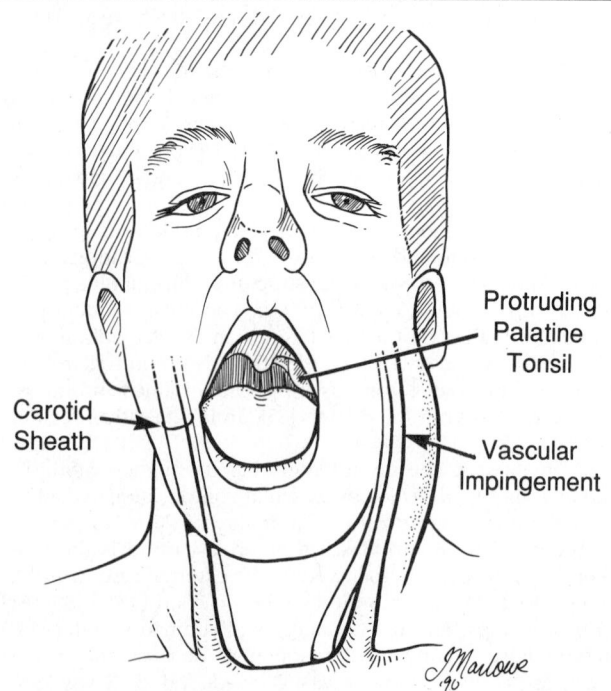

Fig. 75-10. Schematic representation of salient clinical findings of lateral pharyngeal space abscess.

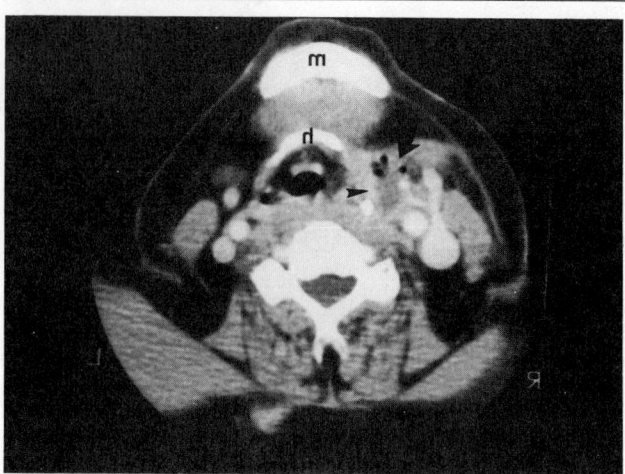

Fig. 75-11. Abscess in the lateral pharyngeal space. Computed tomography at the level of the hyoid bone (h), at the apex of the inverted LPS cone. m = base of mandible. There is a cystic mass *(arrow)* with floating air bubbles and enhancing rim *(arrowhead)*, findings virtually pathognomonic of abscess caused by gas-forming organisms.

ald bleeds" from the nose, mouth, or ears; hematoma in the surrounding tissue; a protracted clinical course; and the onset of shock [87]. Death after carotid hemorrhage is more likely from asphyxiation by aspiration of blood than from exsanguination [87].

Computed tomography (CT) has been used to define neck masses, particularly in the LPS, with excellent results (Fig. 75-11) [92]. One study of contrast-enhanced scans yielded an accuracy of 100 percent in separating abscess, cellulitis, and neoplastic lymphadenopathy [93]. Additional CT findings suggestive of abscess are cystic or multiloculated masses with central air or fluid, soft tissue air, and surrounding edema [65]. Because the complications of deep neck abscesses are potentially fatal, CT scan of the neck is indicated in all cases, especially when surgical intervention is contemplated. Based on clinical information or routine tests, the scan can be extended inferiorly to include the mediastinum and chest. Intravenous contrast is helpful to enhance the abscess capsule and better evaluate the vascular structures of the LPS, but it may not specifically identify thrombosis of the internal jugular vein [72].

Ultrasonography of the neck has been evaluated for its ability to identify fluid-filled masses and guide needle aspiration for culture material and surgical drainage techniques. Several studies show a 95 percent sensitivity of ultrasound in identifying neck abscesses [94,95]. Specificity is probably not as high as that of neck CT scan. An unpublished study in children found that ultrasonography could not distinguish abscess and lymphadenitis, identifying abscesses in less than half of cases and at the same time underestimating their size when compared with CT scans [92]. Therefore, CT is preferable to ultrasonography. Magnetic resonance imaging (MRI) offers little advantage over CT except its multiplanar capability, particularly sagittal sections in the evaluation of RPS infections [96].

Studies used to identify vascular complications in the LPS are plagued by false negatives, with the exception of carotid angiography. If arterial involvement is suggested and time permits, carotid artery angiography is recommended to locate the aneurysm before surgery [87,89]. Doppler venous flow studies [72,97], gallium scans [65], and retrograde venography [65] have been used to diagnose internal jugular vein thrombosis, with mixed results. They cannot be recommended at this time.

Retropharyngeal Space Infections. Retropharyngeal space abscesses are uncommon but potentially fatal infections, most often seen in children younger than 6 years of age [98]. The clinical presentation differs between children and adults. The two chains of lymph nodes in this space are the source of most RPS abscesses and, since they regress by about the age of 4 years, explain the higher frequency of this process in young children [81,99,100]. These nodes drain adjacent muscles, nose, nasopharynx, pharynx, middle ear, eustachian tubes, and paranasal sinuses. In pediatric patients, the initial symptoms may be vague, including fever, irritability, and refusal to eat [99]. The neck is often held stiffly, sometimes tilted away from the involved side [81]; interference with breathing and swallowing occurs as the swelling increases. Respiratory embarrassment can occur secondary to the abscess as it protrudes anteriorly (Fig. 75-4), spontaneous rupture into the airway, or inability to handle secretions [65].

In children, spontaneous rupture of a retropharyngeal abscess, with aspiration and asphyxiation, and upper airway obstruction from a combination of a high larynx (compared with adults) and anterior displacement of the pharyngeal wall, are of most immediate concern [99,100]. These events occur in adults as well, but the larger airway offers some protection from rapid airway occlusion. Severe uncommon complications include meningitis and epiglottitis [101].

Adults generally exhibit signs and symptoms directly referable to the pharynx. There may be a history of trauma to the posterior pharynx as in intubation [102] or by foreign bodies such as chicken bones [99] and external penetrating injuries [99]. Fever, sore throat, dysphagia, nasal obstruction, noisy breathing, stiff neck, and dyspnea are most common [65,81,99]. One suggestive symptom may be pain originating in or radiating to the posterior neck that increases with swallowing [98]. Severe respiratory distress, particularly if accompanied by chest pain or pleurisy, suggests mediastinal extension.

With the possibility of extension to or primary infection in the RPS, the lateral neck radiograph is particularly helpful because of the ability to evaluate prevertebral soft tissue dimensions for swelling (Fig. 75-12) [103,104]. Wholey et al. identified normal dimensions as less than 7 mm in all age groups at the C_2 (retropharyngeal) level and less than 14 mm in children or 22 mm in adults at the C_6 (retrotracheal) level [103]. The radiograph should be a true lateral, with the neck in full extension, and should be taken during inspiration. Exhalation, crying, and swallowing, especially in children, may cause thickening of the upper cervical soft tissues and imitate a mass [99]. Another radiographic finding with involvement of the RPS is loss or reversal of the normal cervical lordosis secondary to inflammation-induced muscle spasm. A PVS source of the symptoms can be inferred by evidence of vertebral abnormalities (e.g., fracture, osteomyelitis).

Descending Infections. Any deep neck infection can have access to the posterior mediastinum and diaphragms by the common pathways of the RPS and danger space [65,74,81,105–108]. Descending necrotizing mediastinitis carries a mortality greater than 40 percent, primarily because of the difficulty in making an early diagnosis [107]. The process can develop within 12 hours to as long as 2 weeks from the onset of the primary infection. The patient usually complains of severe dyspnea and pleuritic or retrosternal chest pain concomitant with or subsequent to the onset of symptoms referable to an oropharyngeal infection. The suppurative process manifests in one of three ways: (1) a widespread necrotizing process ex-

tending to the diaphragms and occasionally into the retroperitoneal space, (2) a mediastinal abscess that may rupture into the pleural cavity, or (3) purulent pleural and pericardial effusions [107]. Suggestive physical findings include diffuse brawny induration of the neck and upper chest associated with pitting edema or crepitation [107].

Cervical necrotizing fasciitis, fascial infection with muscle necrosis and often without pus or abscess formation, can progress superficially along the fascial planes of the neck and chest wall [109,110,111]. Early in the course of disease, the physical appearance may be deceptively benign. Skin erythema occurs initially, progressing to dusky skin discoloration, blisters, or bullae and eventually to visible skin necrosis [109]. Crepitations may be absent, but gas in the tissues can readily be seen using CT. Surgical exploration and wide excision, however, are still essential to determine the full extent of necrosis and improve prognosis [109,110,111].

Because there is the potential for pus in the oral cavity in all of these deep space infections, aspiration pneumonia and lung abscess are possible complications [64,69,99].

DIFFERENTIAL DIAGNOSIS. Few clinical entities must be distinguished from deep cervical infections. Patterns of local swelling should suggest certain conditions. Common causes of submandibular swelling to consider include cervical adenitis and submandibular sialoadenitis [65]. Severe rare entities should also be evaluated in the proper settings and include anticoagulant overdose with sublingual hematoma, tumor of the floor of the mouth, superior vena cava syndrome, and angioedema [112]. However, none of these entities presents with the classic physical findings or respiratory symptoms of SMS infection due to Ludwig's angina.

The major entities from which LPS infection must be differentiated are peritonsillar abscess, anaerobic tonsillitis, and masticator space infections. In the last, the patient presents with fever, trismus, pain, and swelling over the mandible, and oropharyngeal examination is normal [65]. Peritonsillar abscess presents with fever and tonsillar prolapse but without extreme toxicity, trismus, or parotid swelling [113]. Vincent's angina is an anaerobic tonsillitis due to *Fusobacterium necrophorum*, which produces a foul discharge that forms a pseudomembrane [114]. This tonsillitis can be associated with bacteremia and metastatic abscesses [86].

The septic complications of LPS infection can mimic right-sided bacterial endocarditis [65] and be misdiagnosed as community-acquired pneumonia [72], pancreatic abscess [72], periorbital cellulitis [97], temporomandibular joint pain [85], and impending delirium tremens [83].

Retropharyngeal swelling might be due to tumor (e.g., thyroid) [100], hematoma (e.g., posttraumatic) [114], lymphadenopathy (e.g., lymphoma) [99], enlargement of the prevertebral space, as in edema secondary to a cervical spine fracture [99], or tendinitis of the prevertebral muscles [100].

In children with combinations of fever, sore throat, nuchal rigidity, drooling, and respiratory distress, which are components of RPS abscess, severe croup, epiglottitis, and meningitis must also be considered [65].

TREATMENT. All deep neck infections require hospitalization for proper treatment, even if detected early. Therapy has three components: airway management, IV antibiotics, and timely surgical exploration [65].

Airway Management. Establishment of an artificial airway is not universally required but should be done when evidence of

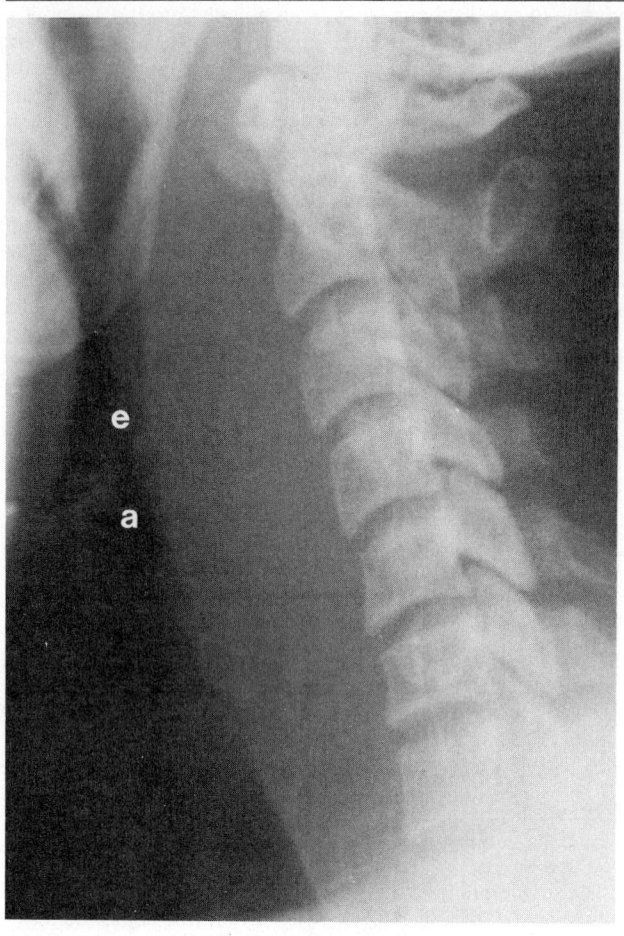

A

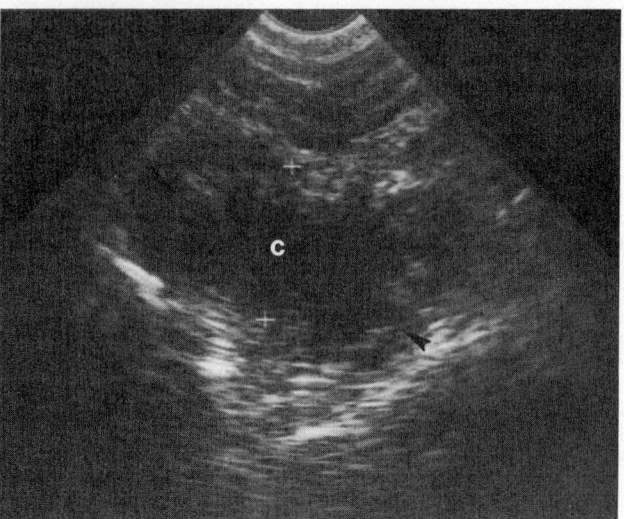

B

Fig. 75-12. Retropharyngeal abscess. Lateral neck radiograph (A) and ultrasound scan of the neck (B). There is marked swelling of the prevertebral soft tissues extending from the base of the skull to the base of the neck, with bulging and anterior displacement of the airway. There is mild reversal of the normal lordosis of the neck secondary to muscle spasm. The epiglottis (e) and aryepiglottic folds (a) are normal. Sonography of the area (B) shows a 7 × 3.5-cm cystic mass (c) with thick irregular wall *(arrowheads)* compatible with abscess.

airway obstruction exists, such as dyspnea and stridor or inability to handle secretions [71]. Upper airway obstruction is most often a complication of infections involving the SMS, for which the standard method of airway control has been tracheostomy [64,80,115,116]. However, there is not uniform agreement that tracheostomy is always the preferred method. Some authors express concern about the risk of aspiration pneumonia and anterior mediastinitis, because of the proximity of the tracheostomy to submandibular wounds created for drainage [116]. Moreover, the surgical risks of tracheotomy may be increased by the distortion of the neck with edema, and there is the known risk of tracheal stenosis [117]. Due to these concerns, cricothyroidotomy has been recommended as an alternative, particularly in emergent situations [118], because of the low immediate and delayed complication rates and because it can be performed rapidly [119]. Distortion of neck landmarks may equally complicate this procedure, but fewer critical structures are in proximity, which may reduce some procedure-related risks.

Another alternative, endotracheal intubation, is often difficult to perform because of trismus and intraoral swelling. Trismus is a more significant problem when infection has spread to the LPS. Blind intubation is unsafe because of potential trauma to the posterior pharyngeal wall, potential rupture of abscesses in the lateral pharyngeal or retropharyngeal spaces [120], and possible laryngospasm precipitating airway obstruction [69]. Intubation over a fiberoptic laryngoscope requires a cooperative, stable patient and may therefore be useful in only certain cases [65]. There has been some success with intubation under direct vision in patients pretreated with an antisialogogue and given inhaled anesthesia to relieve trismus [120]. If this is attempted, the neck should be marked and skilled personnel should be available to establish an emergent surgical airway if needed.

For all of these reasons, the method chosen for establishing an airway in patients with deep cervical infections must be individualized for the patient and to the expertise of the available personnel.

Antimicrobial Therapy. Antibiotic therapy should be given intravenously for all neck infections. Although most oral pathogens are exquisitely sensitive to penicillin, there have been reports of increasing penicillin resistance among oral anaerobes, notably 20 to 40 percent of cases of *B. melaninogenicus* [83]. Therefore, to cover streptococci and oral anaerobes, the combination of high-dose penicillin G (12–20 × 10^6 units per day in divided doses) and metronidazole is recommended. Metronidazole is preferred over clindamycin because it is often less expensive and is more active against most oral flora, particularly *Eikenella* [62,72,73] and the peptostreptococci [121]. An alternate choice, particularly in a seriously ill, penicillin-allergic patient, is chloramphenicol [65,121]. Clindamycin alone and cefoxitin or erythromycin with metronidazole have also been used, but they have drawbacks: clindamycin has a somewhat restricted activity, cefoxitin may cross-react with a penicillin allergy; and erthromycin may not achieve adequate tissue levels [121]. Agents active against facultative gram-negative bacilli are used in patients at increased risk or if they are identified in culture.

Coagulase-positive staphylococci should be covered in the choice of empiric antibiotics when circumstances such as penetrating trauma and vertebral disease exist [76]; an IV beta-lactamase-resistant penicillin is recommended. Vancomycin is recommended for infections in patients with intravenous drug use, as there is a high incidence of methicillin-resistant *S. aureus* (MRSA) [122]. Reports of unusual organisms such as *Mycobacterium tuberculosis* [123] and *Coccidioides immitis* [99] emphasize the importance of careful culture techniques.

Anticoagulation with heparin, then warfarin, for septic internal jugular thrombosis has been used and recommended [87], but the efficacy of this adjuvant therapy to antibiotics has not been conclusively demonstrated [97]. Resection of a thrombosed vein is not widely recommended but may be unavoidable in a patient deteriorating despite prior drainage of the LPS or in one whose vein is frankly suppurative [72].

Surgery. Surgical intervention is most important when infections involve the RPS and LPS; the traditional teaching is that drainage is avoidable almost never in the former and in only 10 to 15 percent of cases of the latter [82]. There has been some recent advocacy for conservative therapy using antibiotics and selective needle aspirates [124,125], but others believe this approach is risky and unnecessarily prolongs hospitalization [126]. In contrast, up to half of cases of Ludwig's angina are cured without surgical drainage procedures [64,71,118] and up to 43 percent require tooth extraction [79].

In general, the surgical approaches to drainage are intraoral or extraoral, depending on the space involved, and should be guided by results of imaging techniques. The specific surgical approaches are not delineated here since they are well described in the surgical literature [115,116,127].

Sinusitis

Sinusitis usually presents in the ICU in two situations: (1) as an uncommon, potentially fatal complication of a community-acquired sinus infection such as meningitis, osteomyelitis, orbital infection, or brain abscess; and (2) as a hospital-acquired sinus infection that may be a frequent cause of occult fever in a critically ill, often nasally intubated or previously intubated, patient. In the nosocomial setting in patients on mechanical ventilatory support sinusitis has been shown to be one of the four most common causes of fever, along with pneumonia, catheter-related infection, and urinary tract infection [127a]. In this study, sinusitis alone or in combination with another infection(s) had a prevalence of 34 percent.

This section covers acute and chronic community-acquired sinusitis and nosocomial sinusitis in a general way and then sphenoid sinusitis specifically.

PATHOGENESIS. The normal paranasal sinuses are air-filled cavities lined with nasal mucosa. They communicate with the upper airway by openings called ostia. Although several hypotheses have been proposed, there does not seem to be a clear function for ostias in humans. They may serve to provide resonance to the voice or reduce the transmission of one's voice to the ears. They may also help humidify and warm inspired air. Lastly, they may help protect the orbit in trauma and reduce the weight of the skull.

The key primary factors that contribute to the development of sinusitis are decreased sinus ostial patency and impaired sinus mucociliary clearance. Inflammation and edema of the nasal mucosa associated with a viral upper respiratory infection or allergic rhinitis can obstruct the ostia [128,129,130], as do other intranasal anatomic abnormalities (e.g., nasal polyps) or foreign bodies (e.g., nasotracheal tube). Any impingement on

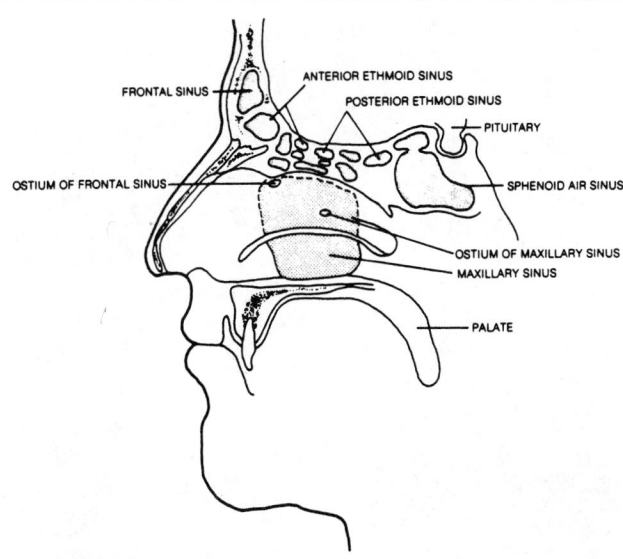

Fig. 75-13. Sagittal section of paranasal sinuses showing anatomic relationships of the ostia and the sinuses as they drain. (From Thadepalli H, Mandal AK: Air sinuses and sinusitis, in *Anatomical Basis of Infectious Disease*. 1984. Courtesy of Charles C. Thomas, Springfield, Illinois.)

ostial size is of potential pathogenetic significance, since they are tenuous protective structures. The diameter of the ostia, normally as small as 1 or 2 mm, has been shown to decrease with recumbency as much as 23 percent because of venous hydrostatic pressures [131]. In addition, many sinus ostia (e.g., maxillary) are poorly located for gravitational drainage (Fig. 75-13) [131,132].

Viral infections may set the stage for sinusitis because they can disrupt the mucociliary action that normally clears the sinuses of bacteria. (Viruses may cause sinusitis by themselves [132a].) The degree of this effect varies among viral agents: whereas influenza produces widespread mucosal destruction, rhinoviruses produce little damage except for ciliary dysfunction [132]. Repeated infections can lead to irreversible mucosal damage that results in chronic sinusitis [133]. In this setting, the normal ciliated epithelium becomes replaced by stratified squamous epithelium, so the sterile environment can no longer be maintained [133]. Other factors shown to impair mucociliary clearance are cold, dry air [134], cigarette smoking [130], topical drugs (e.g., cocaine, decongestants) [134], metal vapors [134], qualitative mucous abnormalities (e.g., cystic fibrosis) [134], and dysmotile cilia (e.g., Kartagener's syndrome) [134].

Secondary changes occur in the nondraining sinus that promote and maintain infection. Without ventilation through the ostia, local oxygen tension decreases and carbon dioxide tension increases; thus, an environment that favors bacterial growth, especially of anaerobic and facultative organisms, is created [131,135,136]. These changes also impair granulocyte function [135]. The accumulation of purulent secretions reduces local immunoglobulin levels [131], and proteolytic enzymes released by granulocytes directly damage the mucosa, which adversely affects clearance [135,136].

A special situation seems to exist in patients infected with human immunodeficiency virus (HIV). The incidence of sinusitis in patients with HIV has been reported to be as high as 68 percent, higher than that of the general population [137]. Some of this increased incidence may be explained by an observed

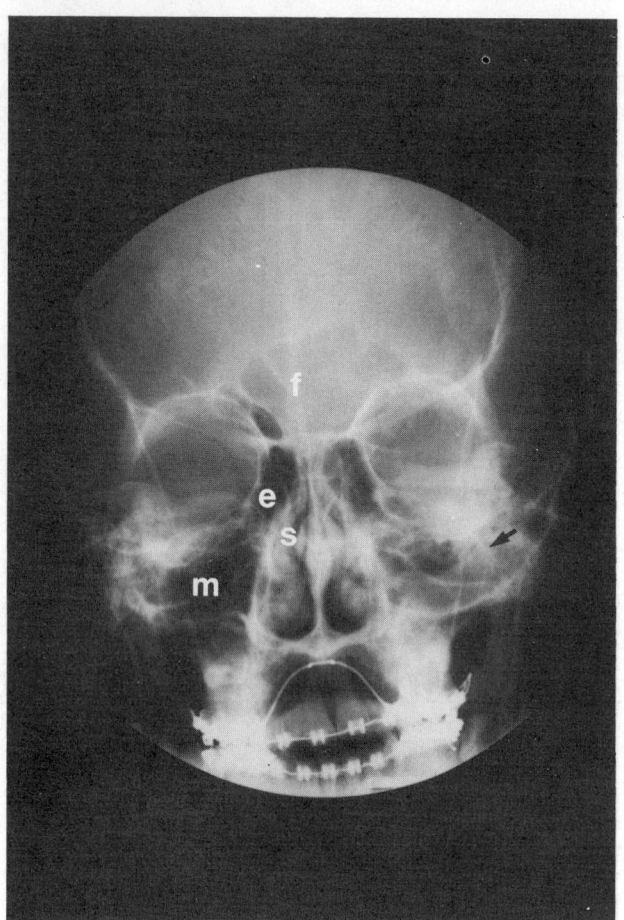

A

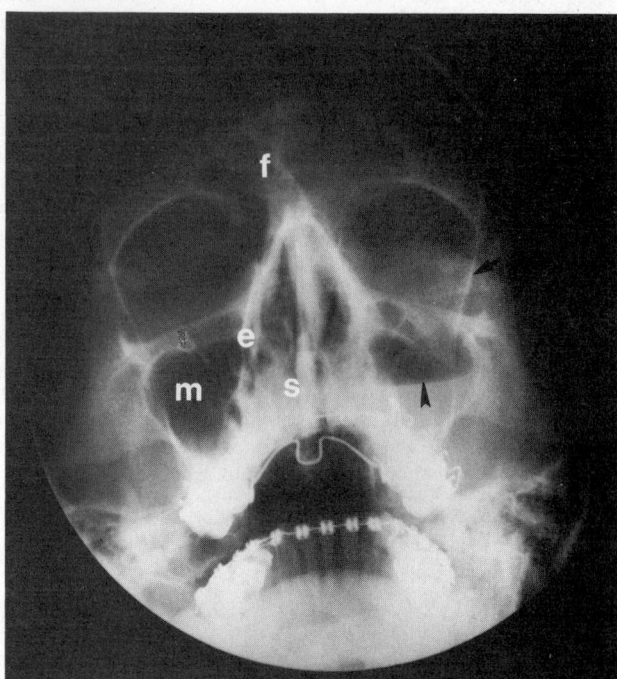

B

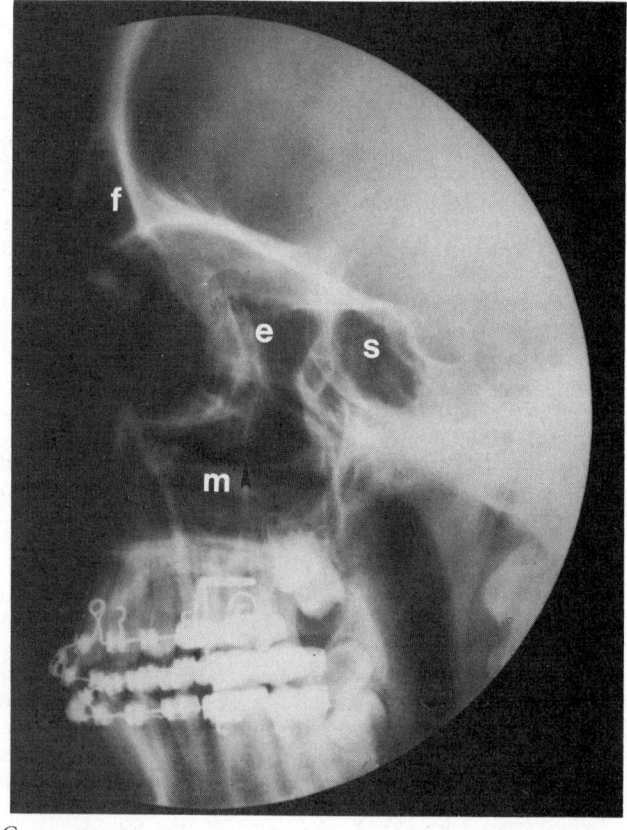

C

Fig. 75-14. Maxillary sinusitis. Standard radiographic examination of the paranasal sinuses in a 17-year-old patient with maxillary sinusitis and periorbital cellulitis. X-ray projections: Caldwell's (A), Water's (B), lateral (C), and axial (D). Computed tomography scan (E) was obtained to evaluate the extent of periorbital cellulitis. f = frontal sinus; m = maxillary sinus; e = ethmoid sinuses; s = sphenoid sinus. There is an air-fluid level in the left maxillary sinus *(arrowhead)* as well as infraorbital soft tissue swelling *(arrow)*.

acquired atopic state. Total serum IgE levels are elevated and increase with progression of HIV disease [138]. The high IgE level is associated with functional allergic reactivity revealed by skin testing with common environmental allergens such as ragweed and dust mite [138]. The role of the T cell deficiency in the risk of sinusitis is unclear. While a decreasing CD4 to CD8 ratio was not an independent risk factor for developing sinusitis [138], it has been observed that the most severe infections occur in patients with the most severe immunodeficiency [138]. An absolute CD_4 count of less than 200 per mm^3 has correlated with chronic or recurrent sinusitis [139].

ETIOLOGY. Most investigators agree that the normal sinus is a sterile environment [140,141]. Although one study demonstrated normal flora, primarily anaerobes, in 12 preoperative patients with no symptoms [128], these patients were undergoing corrective surgery for nasal septal deviation, which could have predisposed them to chronic sinusitis.

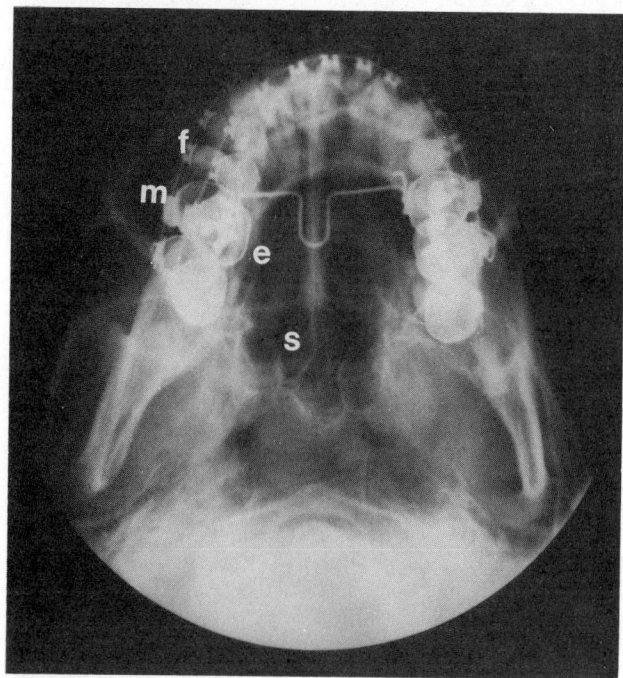

D

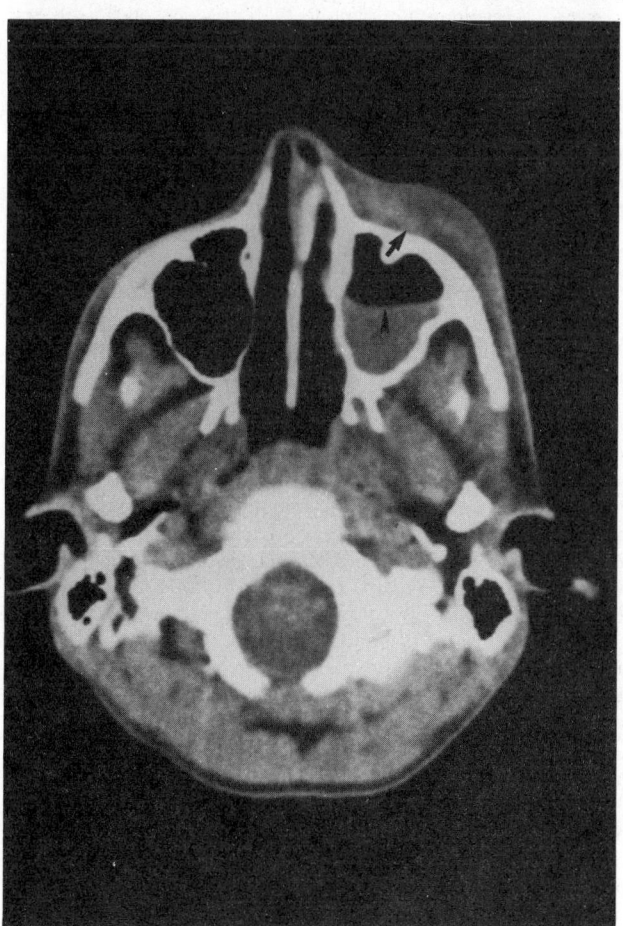

E

In community-acquired acute sinusitis, the most common causes are *H. influenzae, S. pneumoniae,* viruses, and, in children, *Moraxella catarrhalis.* Multiple reports of culture data obtained from maxillary antra by needle aspiration of patients with acute (i.e., < 3 weeks) outpatient sinusitis have identified *H. influenzae* and *S. pneumoniae* as pathogens in more than half of cases [134,136,142,143,144]. Viruses, including rhinovirus, parainfluenza, adenovirus, and influenza, have been recovered in 15 percent of acute maxillary infections either alone or with bacteria [143]. *M. catarrhalis* is seen nearly as frequently as *H. influenzae* in children [134].

In adult community-acquired chronic sinusitis, over 90 percent of surgically obtained specimens were culture-positive; nearly 90 percent of these grew anaerobes [145]. The most common organisms isolated were anaerobic streptococci, *Bacteroides* (mostly *melaninogenicus*), *Propionibacterium* (mostly *acnes*), alpha-hemolytic streptococci, and *S. aureus* [145]. Similar evaluation in children has shown a striking preponderance for anaerobes [146]. Of note in both population groups is the significant number of beta-lactamase-producing organisms, which is important in antibiotic selection [135,145].

The organisms implicated in nosocomial sinusitis are those that frequently cause other types of hospital-acquired infections. Facultative gram-negative bacilli, especially *Pseudomonas aeruginosa,* are most frequently recovered, but *S. aureus, S. epidermidis,* and yeast are also common [147,148, 149,149a]. Twenty-five to over 50 percent of hospital-acquired sinusitis is polymicrobial in origin [147,149a,150]. Anaerobes are relatively uncommon in this setting [147,148,150].

Several special circumstances give rise to infection with more unusual pathogens. Rhinocerebral mucormycosis, an invasive infection usually caused by *Rhizopus* fungi of the class Zygomycetes and order Mucorales, is seen most often in association with diabetes mellitus with acidosis, burns, chronic renal disease, cirrhosis, and immunosuppression [151]. Other fungal infections, primarily with *Aspergillus* species, can be seen in normal hosts but are usually invasive diseases of immunocompromised patients [136,152,153]. Several fungi, especially *Aspergillus* sp. and those of the Dematiaceous (darkly pigmented) family, have been seen to produce a noninvasive sinusitis in immunocompetent, often atopic, hosts [154–157]. This form has been called allergic fungal sinusitis (AFS) because of histologic findings of fungal hyphae scattered within thick "allergic" mucin also containing abundant eosinophils and Charcot-Leyden crystals [154–157]. Intracranial complications can occur as a result of expansile disease or pressure necrosis. *Cryptococcus neoformans* can cause sinusitis with a high relapse rate and significant mortality in both immunocompetent and immunocompromised patients [158]. *Actinomycosis* [151], *Candida* [159], *Pseudallescheria boydii* in patients with acquired immunodeficiency syndrome [136], and other unusual organisms have also been isolated.

DIAGNOSIS

History. The symptoms of acute sinusitis are often nonspecific. Nevertheless, the most important clinical clue to the diagnosis is the failure of nasal symptoms to resolve after a typical cold [160]. Facial pain and a change in nasal discharge from clear to purulent are the most common complaints in adults [133,136]. The location of the pain can vary according to the sinus involved [132]. Other complaints include postnasal drip, nasal obstruction, cough, loss of vocal resonance, and decreased sense of smell [132,133,135,136,161]. A recent prospective study identified five clinical elements—maxillary toothache, poor response to decongestants, abnormal transillumination, report of colored nasal discharge, and the physical finding of purulent nasal mucus—as independent predictors of sinusitis [162]. When none were present, there was a 9 percent predicted probability of sinusitis; when all were present there was a 92 percent probability. Symptoms in children differ by age. Before 5 years, when the maxillary and frontal sinuses are incompletely pneumatacized, ethmoid sinusitis predominates, with symptoms of rhinorrhea and cough; older children may complain of more focal symptoms, such as pain consistent with increased incidence of maxillary and frontal involvement [134,140,161]. Fever is present in only half of all patients [132,134]. In addition, patients may present with complications of acute sinusitis that have specific associated signs and symptoms (see later discussion).

Symptoms of chronic sinusitis are also nonspecific and by definition exist for more than 3 weeks. Patients in general complain of nasal stuffiness, purulent nasal discharge, and postnasal drip. Cough, sore throat, and fetid breath are frequent, whereas headache and facial pain are frequently absent [130]. Patients with chronic sinusitis can also be devoid of nasal symptoms and pain.

Nosocomial sinusitis, which occurs in 5 to 8 percent of ICU admissions [147,163], is usually diagnosed after routine evaluation for a source of fever is unrevealing [147,148,150, 163,164]. It is not easily, definitively diagnosed without sinus CT scans and antral punctures (see Other Modalities section). It can be the cause of the sepsis syndrome [149a]. Maxillary sinusitis in the critically ill is associated with air fluid levels and/or opacification of ethmoid and sphenoid sinuses in more than 90 percent of patients [149a] Of the predisposing factors, the most important is nasopharyngeal instrumentation with nasotracheal airways, nasogastric tubes, or nasal packing [147, 148,149a,150,165]. Other contributing factors observed primarily in head trauma patients are history of corticosteroid therapy, obtundation (secondary to injury or sedation), immobility, supine positioning, and blood in the sinuses on admission [147,148,149a,150,166].

Physical Examination. In adults, although a normal nasal examination is unusual, the physical examination is not often reliable to make the diagnosis of sinusitis [140]. One study of antral aspirates showed negative cultures in 40 percent of patients suspected of having acute sinusitis on the basis of history and examination by an otolaryngologist [143]. Findings in acute infection usually include engorgement of the turbinates, mucosal edema, generalized erythema, and often purulent nasal discharge [128,132,162,165]. When clinical signs, symptoms, and history are considered together, however, the diagnosis of acute sinusitis may be made accurately [167]. Chronic sinusitis has an even less specific examination in which only edematous nasal mucosa and purulent secretions are seen [130]. In nosocomial sinusitis, a purulent nasal discharge may be observed in nearly 30 percent [147,168] of cases. Transillumination is too often inaccurate, even in the most proficient hands, to be a useful screening test [132,140,169].

Radiology. There are four standard x-ray projections of the paranasal sinuses (Fig. 75-14): occipitofrontal (Caldwell's), occipitomental (Water's), lateral, and submental vertex (axial). Studies to evaluate the accuracy of radiographs to identify infection documented by needle aspiration of the maxillary antra have been primarily of the occipitomental view. As the maxillary sinuses are the most commonly involved, some authors have suggested it is reasonable to substitute a single Water's view for a four-view series in some situations [170].

Sinus radiographs are predictive of culture-positive antral aspirates in 70 to 80 percent of acute and more than 90 percent of chronic cases [135,140,143,145]. Positive radiographic findings include an air-fluid level (Fig. 75-14), opacification and mucosal thickening of more than 5 mm in adults [132,135,140,171]. Portable sinus radiographs, including supine horizontal beam lateral, a supine submental-vertex, and horizontal-beam affected side down occipitomental views have been recommended to look for sinus infection in critically ill patients who cannot travel for standard sinus films or a CT scan [147,163,164,172,173]. Others have advocated simpler radiographic series, such as portable anteroposterior and lateral [174] or "reverse Water's" (supine occipitomental) [165] views. We have frequently found portable sinus films in the critically ill to be of poor quality (see section on other modalities).

Ultrasonography. Because of the expense of sinus radiographs and the exposure to ionizing radiation, many studies have examined the utility of ultrasound in diagnosing sinusitis. Whereas some investigators have found excellent correlation between maxillary ultrasound and radiographic findings, especially in sinuses that are normal or contain air-fluid levels [175,176], others have determined that it is not more accurate and may even be less accurate than radiographs [177,178]. Another limitation of ultrasound examination of the sinuses is poor differentiation of mucosal abnormalities (e.g., thickening, polyps, cysts) [176,179]. Because this technique requires special instrumentation and personnel and since its accuracy is no better than that of radiography, we reserve its use for special circumstances (e.g., pregnant patients avoiding x-ray exposure, uncooperative children). To our knowledge, ultrasonography has yet to be evaluated in patients with nosocomial sinusitis as a portable technique.

Rhinoscopy. Although data are limited, the flexible fiberoptic rhinoscope can provide an easy and direct way to evaluate the sinus ostia for purulent drainage in patients without nasopharyngeal catheters or tubes. It is usually well tolerated. A study of patients with headache and evidence of sinusitis by rhinoscopy with and without radiographic findings showed good response to antibiotic therapy, with resolution of the purulence and headache [180].

Antral Aspirate/Antroscopy. Aspiration or washout of the maxillary antrum is considered the gold standard technique by which to diagnose infectious maxillary sinusitis. As an outpatient invasive technique, it should be reserved for patients with poor responses to initial therapy or severe illness [181]. Antral aspiration in hospitalized, critically ill patients can help distinguish between infectious and noninfectious sinus involvement as well as direct the most appropriate antibiotic therapy for nosocomial infections [147,168]. Direct visualization of the sinus mucosa by antroscopy can complement radiographic evaluation of a chronically opacified sinus [135]: it distinguishes fluid from extreme mucosal thickening and allergic from infective mucosa and identifies sinus tumors [182]. This may be useful before surgical treatment of chronic maxillary sinus symptoms [182].

Other Modalities. Computed tomography and MRI (Fig. 75-15) are sensitive techniques to evaluate soft tissue changes in the sinuses [135]. Computed tomography of the sinuses using contrast, high resolution, and thin sections is particularly useful for evaluating possible bony or soft tissue complications of sinusitis (Fig. 75-14E) [183], for evaluating for changes consistent with sinusitis in the critically ill, and when surgical intervention is contemplated [184]. Based on microbiological analysis of antral punctures, it has been determined that air fluid levels and/or opacification of maxillary sinuses on CT scan of

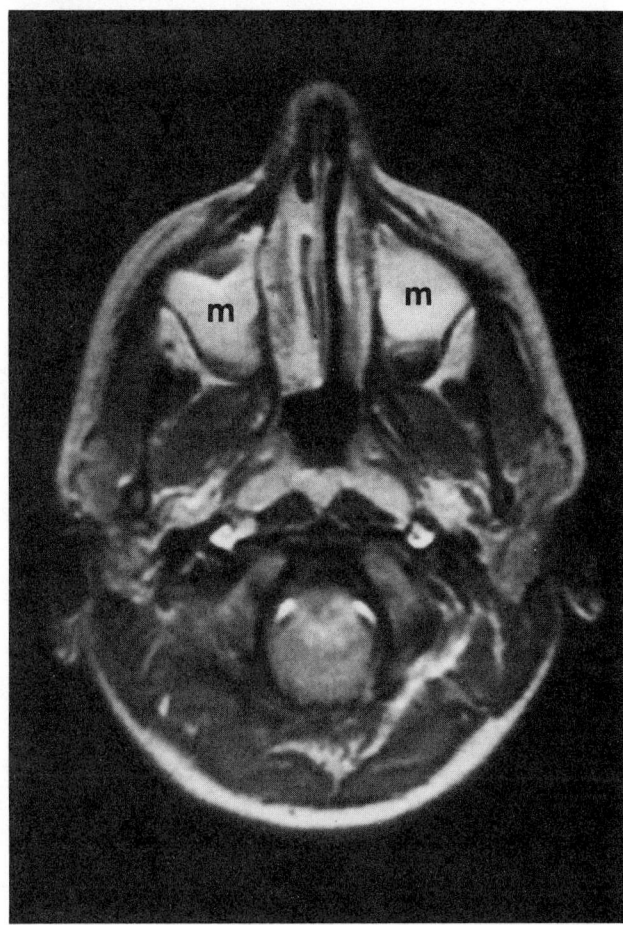

A

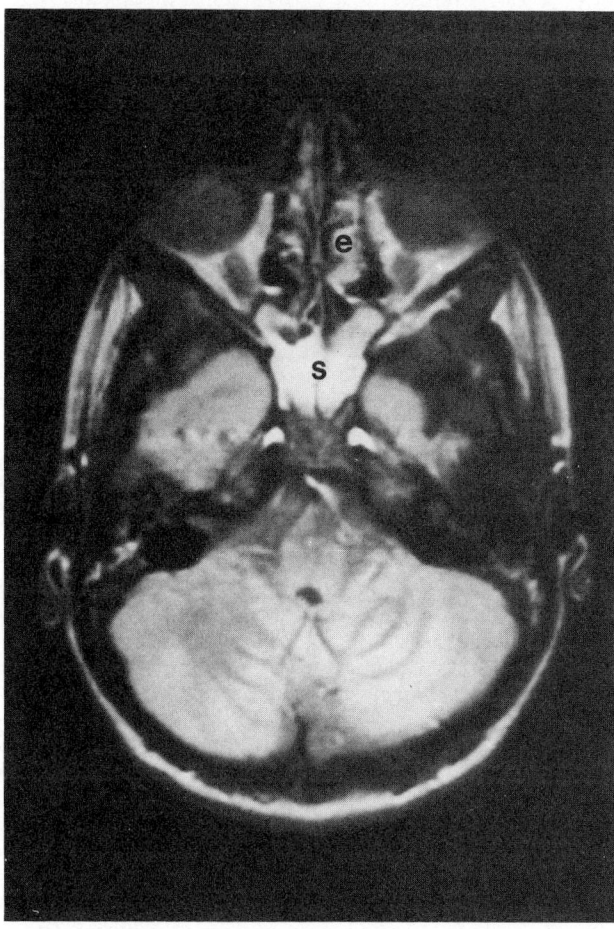

B

Fig. 75-15. Pansinusitis. Magnetic resonance images (T_2-weighted long TR and TE-) at the level of the maxillary (A) and sphenoid (B) sinuses. There is a high signal intensity material (indicating fluid) in the visualized maxillary (m), sphenoid (s), and ethmoid (e) sinuses.

sinuses is due to an infectious cause 38 percent of the time and a noninfectious cause 62 percent of the time [149a].

TREATMENT. The therapy for uncomplicated sinusitis includes antibiotics and decongestants. Initial antibiotic selection depends on whether the infection is acute, chronic, or nosocomial.

In acute community-acquired sinusitis, the choice must be effective against *H. influenzae* and *Streptococcus* species and also *M. catarrhalis* in children. Ampicillin, amoxicillin, trimethoprim-sulfamethoxazole, and cefaclor have all been used successfully [132,134,135,136,160]. Empiric treatment is appropriate, reserving sinus aspiration for complicated or refractory cases [136]. Effective bacterial eradication can be achieved with 3 to 10 days of antibiotics [144,184a]. A recent randomized, double-blind controlled trial showed that 3 days of trimethoprim-sulfamethoxazole was as effective as 10 days [184a].

In chronic community-acquired sinusitis, with the preponderance of anaerobes and increasing numbers of beta-lactamase-producing organisms, the antibiotics of choice are those that are effective against these organisms [145]. Recommendations for the duration of therapy have varied, but at least 3

weeks is preferred to ensure eradication of infection [130,160]. Concomitant use of topical vasoconstrictors and oral decongestants is important to facilitate sinus drainage [132,136,181]. Because reduction of mucosal swelling is important, antihistamines and often topical steroids are suggested, particularly in patients with an allergic component [130].

Nosocomial sinusitis is most often related to the presence of nasopharyngeal catheters and tubes [165]; therefore, in addition to decongestants [147] and antibiotics, treatment includes removing all nasal tubes on the affected side to eliminate the source of obstruction and irritation [164,165]. Whereas some have suggested that topical decongesting agents be used prophylactically in the presence of nasal tubes [163], we reserve their use for cases with evidence of sinusitis. If empiric antibiotics are given, they should be effective against facultative gram-negative rods and *S. aureus* and be given intravenously for 2 weeks. Response should be rapid, within 48 to 96 hours [147,168]. Despite some advocacy for early surgical drainage, it seems that invasive procedures other than a needle aspirate for Gram stain and culture can be reserved for those patients who do not respond to medical therapy or those with the sepsis syndrome who do not respond to needle aspiration [149a].

COMPLICATIONS. The complications of acute sinusitis are rare but often rapidly fatal [185,186]. They fall primarily into two groups: orbital and intracranial [183]. The former is divided into five categories: (1) reactionary edema, predominantly of the eyelids, (2) orbital cellulitis, (3) orbital abscess, (4) subperiosteal abscess, and (5) cavernous sinus thrombosis [187,188]. The last of these is the most severe, with a greater than 20 percent mortality and 50 percent morbidity [151,186]. The intracranial complications, with an overall mortality of 40 percent, include osteomyelitis, meningitis and epidural abscess, subdural empyema, and brain abscess [135,183,189,190]. When evaluating for these entities, it is important to consider the sinuses as a source of the infection; for instance, up to 80 percent of subdural empyemas are secondary to sinusitis [151,191]. In these cases, sinus drainage is imperative and antibiotic choices should be culture-specific.

SPHENOID SINUSITIS. Sphenoid sinusitis merits separate mention because of its potentially fulminant nature and diagnostic difficulty. Delay in diagnosis has been associated with serious morbidity and mortality [192]. The typical presentation primarily in acute infection is of severe headache that interferes with sleep, often accompanied by fever and nasal discharge [167,192]. Neurologic deficits can be prominent features, trigeminal hyperesthesia or hypoesthesia occurring in one-third of cases [192]. Gram-positive organisms have been isolated from sphenoid sinus cultures of most patients with acute sinusitis, whereas equal numbers of gram-positive and facultative gram-negative pathogens have been cultured from those with chronic sphenoid sinusitis [192]. Treatment should include high-dose IV penicillinase-resistant penicillin or appropriate alternative. Spread to nearby structures (e.g., cavernous sinus, pituitary gland, optic chiasm) explains the seriousness of reported sequelae; 8 of 15 patients in one series either died or had permanent neurologic deficits [192]. Early CT scan of the sinuses is essential to evaluate the possibility of extension in patients with suggestive findings. Surgical drainage may be necessary if symptoms persist or neurologic signs develop while the patient is on appropriate antibiotic therapy.

References

1. Cantrell RW, Bell RA, Morioka WT: Acute epiglottitis: Intubation versus tracheostomy. *Laryngoscope* 88:994, 1978.
2. MayoSmith MF, Hirsch PJ, Wodzinski SF, et al: Acute epiglottitis in adults: An eight-year experience in the state of Rhode Island. *N Engl J Med* 314:1133, 1986.
3. Fearon B, Cinnamond M: Tracheotomy in acute supraglottitis (epiglottitis): The treatment of choice. *Laryngoscope* 87:879, 1977.
4. Vetto RR: Epiglottitis: Report of thirty-seven cases. *JAMA* 173:990, 1960.
5. Morgenstein KM, Abramson AL: Acute epiglottitis in adults. *Laryngoscope* 81:1066, 1971.
6. Gorefinkel HJ, Brown R, Kabins SA: Acute infectious epiglottitis in adults. *Ann Intern Med* 70:289, 1969.
7. Black MJ, Harbour J, Remsen KA, et al: Acute epiglottitis in adults. *J Otolaryngol* 10:23, 1981.
8. Deeb ZE, Yenson YC, DeFries HO: Acute epiglottitis in the adult. *Laryngoscope* 95:289, 1985.
9. Lederman MM, Lowder J, Lerner PI: Bacteremic pneumococcal epiglottitis in adults with malignancy. *Am Rev Respir Dis* 125:117, 1982.
10. Stair TO, Hirsch BE: Adult supraglottitis. *Am J Emerg Med* 3:512, 1985.
11. Sendi K, Crysdale WS: Acute epiglottitis: Decade of change—A 10-year experience with 242 children. *J Otolaryngol* 16:196, 1987.
12. Bass JW, Steel RW, Wiebe RA: Acute epiglottitis: A surgical emergency. *JAMA* 229:671, 1974.
13. Schwartz RH, Knerr RJ, Hermansen K: Acute epiglottitis caused by beta-hemolytic group C streptococci. *Am J Dis Child* 136:558, 1982.
14. Murrage KJ, Janzen VD, Ruby RR: Epiglottitis: Adult and pediatric comparisons. *J Otolaryngol* 17:194, 1988.
15. Stanley RE, Liang TS: Acute epiglottitis in adults (the Singapore experience). *J Laryngol Otol* 102:1017, 1988.
16. Devita MA, Wagner IJ: Acute epiglottitis in the adult. *Crit Care Med* 14:1082, 1986.
17. Warner JA, Finlay WEI: Fulminating epiglottitis in adults: Report of three cases and review of the literature. *Anaesthesia* 40:348, 1985.
18. Cole S, Zawin M, Lundberg B, et al: *Candida* epiglottitis in an adult with acute nonlymphocytic leukemia. *Am J Med* 82:662, 1987.
19. Walsh TJ, Gray WC: *Candida* epiglottitis in immunocompromised patients. *Chest* 91:482, 1987.
20. Johnson RH, Rumans LW: Unusual infections caused by *Pasteurella multocida. JAMA* 237:146, 1977.
21. Hawkins DB, Miller AH, Sachs GB, et al: Acute epiglottitis in adults. *Laryngoscope* 1211:83, 1973.
22. Mustoe T, Strome M: Adult epiglottitis. *Am J Otolaryngol* 4:393, 1983.
23. Freeland AP: Acute laryngeal infections in childhood, in Kerry AG (ed): *Scott-Brown's Otolaryngology.* 5th ed. Boston, Butterworth, 1987, p 449.
24. Diaz JH: Croup and epiglottis in children: The anesthesiologist as diagnostician. *Anesth Analg* 64:621, 1985.
25. Sheikh KH, Nostow SR: Epiglottitis: An increasing problem for adults. *West J Med* 151:520, 1989.
26. Procino ND: Acute epiglottitis in adults. *Ear Nose Throat J* 57:30, 1978.
27. Schabel SI, Katzberg RW, Burgener FA: Acute inflammation of epiglottitis and supraglottic structures in adults. *Radiology* 122:601, 1977.
28. Warshawski J, Havas TE, McShane DP, et al: Adult epiglottitis. *J Otolaryngol* 15:362, 1986.
29. Shih L, Hawkins DB, Stanley RB Jr: Acute epiglottitis in adults: A review of forty-eight cases. *Ann Otol Rhinol Laryngol* 97:527, 1988.
30. Andreassen UK, Husum B, Tos M, et al: Acute epiglottitis in adults: A management protocol based on a 17-year material. *Acta Anaesthesiol Scand* 28:155, 1984.
31. Ossoff RH, Wolff AP, Ballenger JJ: Acute epiglottitis in adults: Experience with fifteen cases. *Laryngoscope* 90:1155, 1980.
32. Cohen EL: Epiglottitis in adults. *Ann Emerg Med* 13:620, 1984.
33. Stankiewicz JA, Bowes AK: Croup and epiglottitis: A radiologic study. *Laryngoscope* 95:1159, 1985.
34. Schumaker HM, Doris PE, Birnbaum G: Radiographic parameters in adult epiglottitis. *Ann Emerg Med* 13:588, 1984.
35. Rothrock SG, Pignatiello GA, Howard RM: Radiologic diagnosis of epiglottitis: Objective criteria for all ages. *Ann Emerg Med* 19:978, 1990.
36. Burns JE, Hendley JO: Epiglottitis, in Mandell GL, Douglas RG, Bennett JE (eds): *Principles and Practice of Infectious Disease.* 3rd ed. New York, Wiley, 1990, p 514.
37. Campbell TP, Paris PM, Stewart RD: Tracheitis: The 'other' cause of upper airway obstruction. *Ann Emerg Med* 17:66, 1987.
38. Ruddy J: Bacterial tracheitis in a young adult. *J Laryngol Otol* 102:656, 1988.
39. Valor RR, Polnitsky CA, Tanis DJ, et al: Bacterial tracheitis with upper airway obstruction in a patient with the acquired immunodeficiency syndrome. *Am Rev Respir Dis* 146:1598, 1992.
40. Donnelly BW, McMillan JA, Weiner LB: Bacterial tracheitis: Report of eight new cases and review. *Rev Infect Dis* 12:729, 1990.
41. Jones R, Santos JI, Overall JC Jr: Bacterial tracheitis. *JAMA* 242:721, 1979.
42. Edmonds LC, Prakash UBS: Lymphoma, neutropenia, and wheezing in a 70-year-old man. *Chest* 103:585, 1993.
43. Kramer MR, Denning DW, Marshall SE, et al: Ulcerative tracheobronchitis after lung transplantation: A new form of invasive aspergillosis. *Am Rev Respir Dis* 144:552, 1991.
44. Hines DW, Haber MH, Yaremko L, et al: Pseudomembranous tracheobronchitis caused by *Aspergillus. Am Rev Respir Dis* 143:1408, 1991.

45. Pervez NK, Kleinerman J, Kattan M, et al: Pseudomembranous necrotizing bronchial aspergillosis: A variant of invasive aspergillosis in a patient with hemophilia and acquired immune deficiency syndrome. *Am Rev Respir Dis* 131:961, 1985.

46. Han BK, Dunbar JS, Striker TW: Membranous laryngotracheobronchitis (membranous croup). *AJR* 133:53, 1979.

146a. Colt HG, Gumpert BC, Harrell JH: Tracheobronchial obstruction caused by *Klesiella rhinoscleromatis:* Diagnosis, pathological features, and treatment. *J Bronchology* 1:34, 1994.

47. Chechani V, Vasudevan VP, Kamholz SL: Necrotizing tracheobronchitis: Complication of mechanical ventilation in an adult. *South Med J* 84:271, 1991.

48. Robbins JP, Fitz-Hugh GS: Epiglottitis in the adult. *Laryngoscope* 81:700, 1971.

49. Bishop MJ: Epiglottitis in the adult. *Anesthesiology* 55:701, 1981.

50. Baker AS, Eavey RD: Adult supraglottitis (epiglottitis). *N Engl J Med* 314:1185, 1986.

51. Wolf M, Strauss B, Kronenberg J, et al: Conservative management of adult epiglottitis. *Laryngoscope* 100:183, 1990.

52. Oh TH, Motoyama EK: Comparison of nasotracheal intubation and tracheostomy in management of acute epiglottitis. *Anesthesiology* 46:214, 1977.

53. McGovern FH, Fitz-Hugh GS, Edgemon LJ: The hazards of endotracheal intubation. *Ann Otol* 80:556, 1971.

54. Crockett DM, McGill TJ, Healy GB, et al: Airway management of acute supraglottitis at the Children's Hospital, Boston: 1980–1985. *Ann Otol Rhinol Laryngol* 97:114, 1988.

55. Butt W, Shann F, Walker C, et al: Acute epiglottitis: A different approach to management. *Crit Care Med* 16:43, 1988.

56. Baxter FJ, Dunn GL: Acute epiglottitis in adults. *Can J Anaesth* 35:428, 1988.

57. Strome M, Jaffe B: Epiglottitis: Individualized management with steroids. *Laryngoscope* 84:921, 1974.

58. DiTirro FR, Silver MH, Hengerer AS: Acute epiglottitis: Evolution of management in the community hospital. *Int J Pediatr Otorhinolaryngol* 7:145, 1984.

59. Adair JC, Ring WH: Management of epiglottitis in children. *Anesth Analg* 54:622, 1975.

60. Bonadio WA, Losek JD: The characteristics of children with epiglottitis who develop the complication of pulmonary edema. *Arch Otolaryngol Head Neck Surg* 117:205,1991.

61. Aass AS: Complications to tracheostomy and long-term intubation: A follow-up study. *Acta Anaesth Scand* 19:127, 1975.

62. Chow AW, Roser SM, Brady FA: Orofacial odontogenic infections. *Ann Intern Med* 88:392, 1978.

63. Bartlett JG, Gorbach SL: Anaerobic infections of the head and neck. *Otolaryngol Clin North Am* 9:655, 1976.

64. Patterson HC, Kelly JH, Strome M: Ludwig's angina: An update. *Laryngoscope* 92:370, 1982.

65. Blomquist IK, Bayer AS: Life-threatening deep fascial space infections of the head and neck. *Infect Dis Clin North Am* 2:237, 1988.

66. Greenberg RN, James RB, Marier RL, et al: Microbiologic and antibiotic aspects of infections in the oral and maxillofacial region. *J Oral Surg* 37:873, 1979.

67. Rosenthal S, Tager IB: Prevalence of gram-negative rods in the normal pharyngeal flora. *Ann Intern Med* 83:355, 1975.

68. Tovi F, Fliss DM, Zirkin HJ: Necrotizing soft-tissue infections in the head and neck: A clinicopathological study. *Laryngoscope* 101:619, 1991.

69. Meyers BR, Lawson W, Hirschman SZ: Ludwig's angina: Case report with review of bacteriology and current therapy. *Am J Med* 53:257, 1972.

70. Murray PM, Finegold SM: Anaerobic mediastinitis. *Rev Infect Dis* 6:S123, 1984.

71. Moreland LW, Corey J, McKenzie R: Ludwig's angina: Report of a case and review of the literature. *Arch Intern Med* 148:461, 1988.

72. Celikel TH, Muthuswamy PP: Septic pulmonary emboli secondary to internal jugular vein phlebitis (postanginal sepsis) caused by *Eikenella corrodens. Am Rev Respir Dis* 130:510, 1984.

73. Tami TA, Parker GS: *Eikenella corrodens:* An emerging pathogen in head and neck infections. *Arch Otolaryngol Head Neck Surg* 110:752, 1984.

74. Strauss HR, Tilghman DM, Hankins J: Ludwig's angina, empyema, pulmonary infiltration, and pericarditis secondary to extraction of a tooth. *J Oral Surg* 38:223, 1980.

75. Myers EM, Kirkland LS, Mickey R: The head and neck sequelae of cervical intravenous drug abuse. *Laryngoscope* 98:213, 1988.

76. Bryan CS, King BG, Bryant RE: Retropharyngeal infection in adults. *Arch Intern Med* 134:127, 1974.

77. Megran DW, Scheifele DW, Chow AW: Odontogenic infections. *Pediatr Infect Dis* 3:257, 1984.

78. Grodinsky M: Ludwig's angina: An anatomical and clinical study with review of the literature. *Surgery* 5:678, 1939.

79. Juang YC, Cheng DL, Wang LS, et al: Ludwig's angina: An analysis of 14 cases. *Scand J Infect Dis* 21:121, 1989.

80. Finch RG, Snider GE, Sprinkle PM: Ludwig's angina. *JAMA* 243:1171, 1980.

81. Levitt GW: Cervical fascia and deep neck infections. *Laryngoscope* 80:409, 1970.

82. Dzyak WR, Zide MF: Diagnosis and treatment of lateral pharyngeal space infections. *J Oral Maxillofac Surg* 42:243, 1984.

83. Wills PI, Vernon RP: Complications of space infections of the head and neck. *Laryngoscope* 91:1129, 1981.

84. Scully RF, Galdabini TJ, McNeely BU: Case records of the Massachusetts General Hospital: Weekly clinicopathological exercises. *N Engl J Med* 298:894, 1978.

85. Harbour RC, Trobe JD, Ballinger WE: Septic cavernous sinus thrombosis associated with gingivitis and parapharyngeal abscess. *Arch Ophthalmol* 102:94, 1984.

86. Vogel CC, Boyer KM: Metastatic complications of *Fusobacterium necrophorum* sepsis: Two cases of Lemierre's postanginal septicemia. *Am J Dis Child* 134:356, 1980.

87. Alexander DW, Leonard JR, Trail ML: Vascular complications of deep neck abscesses. *Laryngoscope* 78:361, 1968.

88. Salinger S, Pearlman SJ: Hemorrhage from pharyngeal and peritonsilar abscesses. *Arch Otolaryngol* 18:464, 1933.

89. Blum DJ, McCaffrey TV: Septic necrosis of the internal carotid artery: A complication of peritonsillar abscess. *Otolaryngol Head Neck Surg* 91:114, 1983.

90. Johnson JT, Tucker HM: Recognizing and treating deep neck infection. *Postgrad Med* 59:95, 1976.

91. Eneroth C-M, Tham R: Pseudoaneurysm of the internal carotid artery: A warning of a septic erosion. *Acta Otolaryngol* 72:445, 1971.

92. Healy GB: Inflammatory neck masses in children: A comparison of computed tomography, ultrasound, and magnetic resonance imaging. *Arch Otolaryngol* 115:1027, 1989.

93. Holt GR, McManus K, Newman RK, et al: Computed tomography in the diagnosis of deep-neck infections. *Arch Otolaryngol* 108:693, 1982.

94. Kreutzer EW, Jafek BW, Johnson ML, et al: Ultrasonography in the preoperative evaluation of neck abscesses. *Head Neck Surg* 4:290, 1982.

95. Siegert R: Ultrasonography of inflammatory soft tissue swellings of the head and neck. *J Oral Maxillofac Surg* 45:842, 1987.

96. Weber AL, Baker AS, Montgomery WW: Inflammatory lesions of the neck, including fascial spaces: Evaluation by computed tomography and magnetic resonance imaging. *Isr J Med Sci* 28:241, 1992.

97. Yau PC, Norante JD: Thrombophlebitis of the internal jugular vein secondary to pharyngitis. *Arch Otolaryngol Head Neck Surg* 106:507, 1980.

98. Greene JS, Asher IM: Retropharyngeal abscess: A previously unreported symptom. *Ann Emerg Med* 13:615, 1984.

99. Barratt GE, Koopman CF, Coulthard SW: Retropharyngeal abscess: A ten-year experience. *Laryngoscope* 94:455, 1984.

100. Husaru AD, Nedzelski JM: Retropharyngeal abscess and upper airway obstruction. *J Otolaryngol* 8:443, 1979.

101. Ramsey PG, Weymuller EA: Complications of bacterial infections of the ears, paranasal sinuses, and oropharynx in adults. *Emerg Med Clin North Am* 3:143, 1985.

102. Heath LK, Pierce TH: Retropharyngeal abscess following endotracheal intubation. *Chest* 72:776, 1977.

103. Wholey MH, Bruwer AJ, Baker HL: The lateral roentgenogram of the neck. *Radiology* 71:350, 1958.

104. Haug RH, Wible RT, Lieberman J: Measurement standards for the

prevertebral region in the lateral soft-tissue radiograph of the neck. *J Oral Maxillofac Surg* 49:1149, 1991.

105. Brondbo K, Rubin A, Chapnik JS, et al: Ludwig's angina following dental extraction as a cause of necrotizing mediastinitis. *J Otolaryngol* 12:50, 1983.

106. Moncada R, Warpeha R, Pickleman J, et al: Mediastinitis from odontogenic and deep cervical infection. *Chest* 73:497, 1978.

107. Estrera AS, Landay MJ, Grisham JM, et al: Descending necrotizing mediastinitis. *Surg Gynecol Obstet* 157:545, 1983.

108. Young JN, Samson PC: Extrapleural empyema thoracis as a direct extension of Ludwig's angina: Case report. *J Thorac Cardiovasc Surg* 80:25, 1980.

109. Stoykesych AA, Beecroft WA, Cogan AG: Fatal necrotizing fasciitis of dental origin. *J Can Dent Assoc* 58:59, 1992.

110. Rapoport Y, Himelfarb MZ, Zikk D, et al: Cervical necrotizing fasciitis of odontogenic origin. *Oral Surg Oral Med Oral Pathol* 72:15, 1991.

111. Legreid RJ II, Hendrix RA. Cervical necrotizing fasciitis: Two case reports and review of the literature. *Trans Pa Acad Ophthalmol Otolaryngol* 41:864, 1989.

112. Smith RG, Parker TJ, Anderson TA: Noninfectious acute upper airway obstruction (pseudo-Ludwig phenomenon): Report of a case. *J Oral Maxillofac Surg* 45:701, 1987.

113. Hora JF: Deep neck infections. *Arch Otolaryngol* 77:25, 1963.

114. Owens DE, Calcaterra TC, Aarstad RA: Retropharyngeal hematoma: A complication of therapy with anticoagulants. *Arch Otolaryngol* 101:565, 1975.

115. Gross BD, Roark DT, Meador RC, et al: Ludwig's angina due to bacteroides. *J Oral Surg* 34:456, 1976.

116. Holland CS: The management of Ludwig's angina. *Br J Oral Surg* 13:153, 1975.

117. Andrews MJ, Pearson FG: Incidence and pathogenesis of tracheal injury following cuffed tube tracheostomy and assisted ventilation: Analysis of a two-year prospective study. *Ann Surg* 173:249, 1971.

118. Hought RT, Fitzgerald BE, Latta JE, et al: Ludwig's angina: Report of two cases and review of the literature from 1945 to January, 1979. *J Oral Surg* 38:849, 1980.

119. Brantigan CD, Grow JB: Cricothyroidotomy: Elective use in respiratory problems requiring tracheotomy. *J Thorac Cardiovasc Surg* 71:72, 1976.

120. Allen D, Loughnan TE, Ord RA: A re-evaluation of the role of tracheostomy in Ludwig's angina. *J Oral Maxillofac Surg* 43:436, 1985.

121. Finegold SM, George WL, Mulligan ME: Anaerobic infections: Part I. *Dis Mon* 31:8, 1985.

122. Lee KC, Tami TA, Echavez M, et al: Deep neck infections in patients at risk for acquired immunodeficiency syndrome. *Laryngoscope* 100:915, 1990.

123. Carroll N, Jibain R, Tseung MH, et al: Tuberculous retropharyngeal abscess producing respiratory obstruction. *Thorax* 44:599, 1989.

124. de Marie S, Tjon A, Tham RTO, et al: Clinical infections and nonsurgical treatment of parapharyngeal space infections complicating throat infection. *Rev Infect Dis* 11:975,1989.

125. Gradon JD, Lutwick LI: Retropharyngeal space infections in a community hospital. *Am J Emerg Med* 9:77, 1991.

126. Sethi DS, Stanley RE: Parapharyngeal abscesses. *J Laryngol Otol* 105:1025, 1991.

127. Levitt GW: The surgical treatment of deep neck infections. *Laryngoscope* 81:403, 1970.

127a. Meduri GU, Mauldin GL, Wunderink RG, et al: Causes of fever and pulmonary densities in patients with clinical manifestations of ventilator-associated pneumonia. *Chest* 106:221, 1994.

128. Brook I: Aerobic and anaerobic bacterial flora of normal maxillary sinuses. *Laryngoscope* 91:372, 1981.

129. Frederick J, Braude AI: Anaerobic infection of the paranasal sinuses. *N Engl J Med* 290:135, 1974.

130. Slavin RG: Sinusitis in adults and its relation to allergic rhinitis, asthma, and nasal polyps. *J Allergy Clin Immunol* 82:950, 1988.

131. Rohr AS, Spector SL: Paranasal sinus anatomy and pathophysiology. *Clin Rev Allergy* 2:387, 1984.

132. Johnson CM III, Gwaltney JM Jr: Sinusitis, in Schlossberg D (ed):

Infections of the Head and Neck. New York, Springer-Verlag, 1987, p 81.

132a. Gwaltney JM Jr, Phillips CD, Miller RD, et al: Computed tomographic study of the common cold. *N Engl J Med* 330:25, 1994.

133. Gwaltney JM Jr: Sinusitis, in Mandell GL, Douglas RG, Bennett JE (eds): *Principles and Practice of Infectious Disease.* 3rd ed. New York, Wiley, 1990, p 510.

134. Rachelefsky GS: Sinusitis in children: Diagnosis and management. *Clin Rev Allergy* 2:397, 1984.

135. Daley CL, Sande M: The runny nose: Infection of the paranasal sinuses. *Infect Dis Clin North Am* 2:131, 1988.

136. Malow JB, Creticos CM: Nonsurgical treatment of sinusitis. *Otolaryngol Clin North Am* 22:809, 1989.

137. Rubin JS, Honigberg R: Sinusitis in patients with the acquired immunodeficiency syndrome. *Ear Nose Throat J* 69:460, 1990.

138. Small CB, Kaufman A, Armenaka M, et al: Sinusitis and atopy in human immunodeficiency virus infection. *J Infect Dis* 167:283, 1993.

139. Godofsky EW, Zinreich J, Armstrong M, et al: Sinusitis in HIV-infected patients: A clinical and radiographic review. *Am J Med* 93:163, 1992.

140. Evans FO, Sydnor JB, Moore WEC, et al: Sinusitis of the maxillary antrum. *N Engl J Med* 293:735, 1975.

141. Goldman JL: Infectious rhinitis and sinusitis, in Goldman JL (ed): *The Principles and Practice of Rhinology.* New York, Wiley, 1987, p 249.

142. Jousimies-Somer HR, Savolainen S, Ylikoski JS: Bacteriological findings of acute maxillary sinusitis in young adults. *J Clin Microbiol* 26:1919, 1988.

143. Hamory BH, Sande MA, Sydnor A Jr: Etiology and antimicrobial therapy of acute maxillary sinusitis. *J Infect Dis* 139:197, 1979.

144. Gwaltney JM Jr, Scheld WM, Sande MA, et al: The microbial etiology and antimicrobial therapy of adults with acute communtiy-acquired sinusitis: A fifteen-year experience at the University of Virginia and review of other selected studies. *J Allergy Clin Immunol* 90:457, 1992.

145. Brook I: Bacteriology of chronic maxillary sinusitis in adults. *Ann Otol Rhinol Laryngol* 98:426, 1989.

146. Brook I: Bacteriologic features of chronic sinusitis in children. *JAMA* 244:967, 1981.

147. Caplan ES, Hoyt NJ: Nosocomial sinusitis. *JAMA* 247:639, 1982.

148. Humphrey MA, Simpson GT, Gindlinger GA: Clinical characteristics of nosocomial sinusitis. *Ann Otol Rhinol Laryngol* 96:687, 1987.

149. Guerin JM, Meyer P, Reizine D, et al: Search for purulent rhinosinusitis in intensive care unit patients with nosocomial pulmonary infections (letter). *Crit Care Med* 16:914, 1988.

149a. Rouby J-J, Laurent P, Gosnach M, et al: Risk factors and clinical relevance of nosocomial maxillary sinusitis in the critically ill. *Am J Respir Crit Care Med* 150:776, 1994.

150. Gindlinger GA, Niehoft J, Hughes L, et al: Acute paranasal sinusitis related to nasotracheal intubation of head-injured patients. *Crit Care Med* 15:214, 1987.

151. Kaplan RJ: Neurologic complications of infections of the head and neck. *Otolaryngol Clin North Am* 9:729, 1976.

152. Morgan MA, Wilson WR, Neel HB III: Fungal sinusitis in healthy and immunocompromised individuals. *Am J Clin Pathol* 82:597, 1984.

153. Parnes LS, Brown DH, Garcia B: Mycotic sinusitis: A management protocol. *J Otolaryngol* 18:176, 1989.

154. Goldstein MF, Dvorin DJ, Dunsky EH, et al: Allergic Rhizomucor sinusitis. *J Allergy Clin Immunol* 90:394, 1992.

155. Friedman GC, Hartwick RWJ, Ro JY, et al: Allergic fungal sinusitis: Report of three cases associated with dematiaceous fungi. *Am J Clin Pathol* 96: 368, 1991.

156. Manning SC, Schaefer SD, Close LG, et al: Culture-positive allergic fungal sinusitis. *Arch Otolaryngol Head Neck Surg* 117:174, 1991.

157. Alluphin AL, Strauss M, Abdul-Karim FW: Allergic fungal sinusitis: problems in diagnosis and treatment. *Laryngoscope* 101:815, 1991.

158. Choi SS, Lawson W, Bottone EJ, et al: Cryptococcal sinusitis: A case report and review of the literature. *Otolaryngol Head Neck Surg* 99:414, 1988.

159. Dooley DP, McAllister CK: Candidal sinusitis and diabetic ketoacidosis: A brief report. *Arch Intern Med* 149:962, 1989.

160. Friedman WH, Slavin RG: Diagnosis and medical and surgical treatment of sinusitis in adults. *Clin Rev Allergy* 2:409, 1984.

161. Riding KG, Irvine R: Sinusitis in children. *J Otolaryngol* 16:239, 1987.

162. Williams JW Jr, Simel DL, Roberts L, et al: Clinical evaluation for sinusitis: Making the diagnosis by history and physical examination. *Ann Intern Med* 117:705, 1992.

163. O'Reilly MJ, Reddick EJ, Black W, et al: Sepsis from sinusitis in nasotracheally intubated patients: A diagnostic dilemma. *Am J Surg* 147:601, 1984.

164. Linden BE, Aguilar EA, Allen SJ: Sinusitis in the nasotracheally intubated patient. *Arch Otolaryngol Head Neck Surg* 114:860, 1988.

165. Salord F, Gaussorgues P, Marti-Flich J, et al: Nosocomial maxillary sinusitis during mechanical ventilation: A prospective comparison of orotracheal versus the nasotracheal route for intubation. *Intensive Care Med* 16:390,1990.

166. Hansen M, Pulsen MR, Bendixen DK, et al: Incidence of sinusitis in patient with nasotracheal intubation. *Br J Anaesth* 61:231, 1988.

167. Williams JW Jr, Simel DL: Does this patient have sinusitis? Diagnosing acute sinusitis by history and physical examination. *JAMA* 270:1242, 1993.

168. Deutschman CS, Wilton P, Sinow J, et al: Paranasal sinusitis associated with nasotracheal intubation: A frequently unrecognized and treatable source of sepsis. *Crit Care Med* 14:111, 1986.

169. Spector SL, Lotan A, English G, et al: Comparison between transillumination and the roentgenogram in diagnosing paranasal sinus disease. *J Allergy Clin Immunol* 67:22, 1981.

170. Williams JW Jr, Roberts L Jr, Distell B, et al: Diagnosing sinusitis by X-ray: Is a single Waters view adequate? *Gen Intern Med* 7:481,1992.

171. Salit IE: Diagnostic approaches to head and neck infections. *Infect Dis Clin North Am* 2:35, 1988.

172. Chidekez N, Jensen C, Axelsson A, et al: Diagnosis of fluid in the maxillary sinus. *Acta Radiol Diagn (Stockh)* 10:433, 1970.

173. Aebert H, Hunefeld G, Regel G: Paranasal sinusitis and sepsis in ICU patients with nasotracheal intubation. *Intensive Care Med* 15:27, 1988.

174. Kulber DA, Santora TA, Shabot MM, et al: Early diagnosis and treatment of sinusitis in the critically ill trauma patient. *Am Surg* 57:775, 1991.

175. Landman MD: Ultrasound screening for sinus disease. *Otolaryngol Head Neck Surg* 94:157, 1986.

176. Revonta M, Kunliala I: The diagnosis and follow-up of pediatric sinusitis: Water's view radiography versus ultrasonography. *Laryngoscope* 99:321, 1989.

177. Pfleiderer AG, Drake-Lee AB, Lowe D: Ultrasound of the sinuses: A worthwhile procedure? A comparison of ultrasound and radiography in predicting the findings of proof puncture on the maxillary sinuses. *Clin Otolaryngol* 9:335, 1984.

178. Shapiro GG, Furukawa CT, Pierson WE, et al: Blinded comparison of maxillary sinus radiography and ultrasound for diagnosis of sinusitis. *J Allergy Clin Immunol* 77:59, 1986.

179. Jensen C, von Sydow C: Radiology and ultrasonography in paranasal sinuses. *Acta Radiol* 28:31, 1987.

180. Castellanos J, Axelrod D: Flexible fiberoptic rhinoscopy in the diagnosis of sinusitis. *J Allergy Clin Immunol* 83:91, 1989.

181. Kern EG: Sinusitis. *J Allergy Clin Immunol* 73:25, 1984.

182. Pfleiderer AG, Croft CB, Lloyd AS: Antroscopy: Its place in clinical practice—A comparison of antroscopic findings with radiographic appearances of the maxillary sinus. *Clin Otolaryngol* 11:455, 1986.

183. Carter BL, Bankoff MS, Fisk JD: Computed tomographic detection of sinusitis responsible for intracranial and extracranial infections. *Radiology* 147:739, 1983.

184. Zinreich SJ: Imaging of chronic sinusitis in adults: X-ray, computed tomography, and magnetic resonance imaging. *J Allergy Clin Immunol* 90:445, 1992.

184a. Williams JW Jr, Holleman DR Jr, Samsa GP, et al: Radomized controlled trial of 3 vs 10 days of trimethoprim/sufamethoxasole for acute maxillary sinusitis. *JAMA* 273:1015, 1995.

185. Quick CA, Payne E: Complicated acute sinusitis. *Laryngoscope* 82:1248, 1972.

186. Yarington CT Jr: Sinusitis as an emergency. *Otolaryngol Clin North Am* 12:447, 1979.

187. Chandler J, Langenbrunner DT, Steven ER: The pathogenesis of orbital complications in acute sinusitis. *Laryngoscope* 80:1414, 1970.

188. Shahin J, Gullane PJ, Dayal VS: Orbital complications of acute sinusitis. *J Otolaryngol* 16:23, 1987.

189. Parker GS, Tami TA, Wilson JF, et al: Intracranial complications of sinusitis. *South Med J* 82:563, 1989.

190. Clayman GL, Adams GL, Paugh DR, et al: Intracranial complications of paranasal sinusitis: A combined institutional review. *Laryngoscope* 101:234, 1991.

191. Kaufman DM, Miller MH, Steigbigel NH: Subdural empyema: Analysis of 17 recent cases and review of the literature. *Medicine* 54:485, 1975.

192. Lew D, Southwick FS, Montgomery WW, et al: Sphenoid sinusitis: A review of 30 cases. *N Engl J Med* 309:1149, 1983.

76. *Acute Infectious Pneumonia*

Michael S. Niederman and Alan M. Fein

Overview

Pneumonia is a common infection, in both the community and the hospital, that comes to the attention of the critical care physician when it leads to acute respiratory failure or complicates the course of an otherwise serious illness. Modern medical technology has not been able to eliminate this infection. Rather, it has promoted its emergence by the application of novel, life-sustaining therapies that lead to groups of patients with specific impairments in respiratory tract host defenses [1]. This chapter reviews the scope of the problem of pneumonia in the seriously ill patient, along with a discussion of its pathogenesis, clinical features, diagnostic dilemmas, therapeutic approaches, and possible preventive strategies. Emphasis is on the concept that pneumonia occurs in specific hosts for specific reasons. Thus, a thorough understanding of the patient and any host defense impairment that he or she might harbor can help identify the high-risk individual and the most likely etiologic pathogens.

Pneumonia is common, occurring in up to 6 million patients annually, with up to 1 million of these individuals requiring hospitalization [2,3]. Pneumonia commonly develops in the hospital, particularly in those patients with serious illness, in whom over 275,000 cases are identified each year [4]. In the hospital, the incidence of pneumonia is directly related to the degree of underlying systemic illness in a given patient, which is in turn a reflection of the underlying integrity of the patient's host defense system. Thus, nosocomial pneumonia has been observed in 10 percent of patients who have general surgery and require mechanical ventilation in an intensive care unit (ICU); in 20 percent of a general medical ICU population treated with mechanical ventilation; and in 70 percent of patients with the acute respiratory distress syndrome (ARDS) [5,6,7].

Certain patient populations are at increased risk for pneumonia, primarily as a result of disease-associated impairments in lung host defenses. These include the elderly and those with cardiac disease, alcoholism, chronic obstructive lung disease, malnutrition, head injury, cystic fibrosis, bronchiectasis, malignancy, splenic dysfunction, renal failure, diabetes mellitus, and any immunosuppressive illness or therapy [8,9]. In addition, many hospitalized individuals receive therapeutic interventions that predispose them to pneumonia. These interventions include antibiotic therapy, gastric acid neutralization (in the form of enteral feeding or medications to prevent stress ulceration), endotracheal intubation and tracheostomy, use of an enteral feeding tube, and use of medications such as corticosteroids, aspirin, digitalis, morphine, and pentobarbital [6,9].

Mortality related to pneumonia is staggering; it currently ranks as the sixth leading cause of death in the United States, at a rate of 24.1 per 100,000 population, and is the number one cause of death from infectious diseases [3]. Certain patient populations are particularly susceptible to an adverse outcome from this infection. Among the elderly, pneumonia is the fourth leading cause of death, with a mortality rate of 169.7 per 100,000 [8]. Although community- acquired pneumonia (CAP) can vary from a mild to a severe illness, those who enter the ICU with this infection have a mortality rate that can vary from 20 percent to greater than 50 percent [10–14].

Among patients who acquire life-threatening nosocomial infections pneumonia is most common, being seen in 60 percent of those who die as a direct result of a hospital-acquired infection [15,16] (see Chap. 86). In the ICU, the mortality of nosocomial pneumonia in those requiring mechanical ventilation is at least 50 percent [7]. In those with ARDS, the mortality of pneumonia is high, with only 12 percent of patients with pneumonia surviving, in contrast to 67 percent in the absence of infection [17]. For many years it was unclear whether patients with nosocomial pneumonia in the ICU died because of this infection or simply with this infection. Recently, Fagon and colleagues observed that ventilator-associated pneumonia has its own attributable mortality. This conclusion was reached by comparing the mortality of ICU patients with pneumonia to matched patients without pneumonia. Using this methodology, pneumonia had a 27 percent attributable mortality, but this rate rose to 43 percent if the infection was due to *Pseudomonas* sp. or *Acinetobacter* sp. [18].

Types of Pneumonia Encountered in the Intensive Care Unit

Critical care physicians treat pneumonias that arise in both the community and the hospital. Certain community-acquired infections are so virulent, or the host so impaired, that overwhelming infection and respiratory failure follow. Conversely, a patient who is already critically ill and in the hospital or ICU may have an illness that is complicated by pneumonia and, as stated above, a fatal outcome may follow.

COMMUNITY-ACQUIRED PNEUMONIAS. Although less than 20 percent of all cases of community-acquired pneumonia require hospitalization, patients ill enough to enter the hospital may have a substantial mortality rate. Austrian and Gold reported that penicillin did not eliminate mortality from pneumococcal pneumonia; this prompted the development of a vaccine for this illness [19]. More recently, Hook et al. observed that pneumococcal bacteremia had a 76 percent mortality rate in those admitted to an ICU, despite the use of modern antimicrobial therapy [20]. When community-acquired pneumonia of all types leads to ARDS, which occurs in less than 5 percent of cases, the mortality rate exceeds 70 percent [21]. Pneumonia caused by bacteria, viruses, fungi, and protozoa can occasionally be severe enough to prompt admission to the ICU. Pathogens described as causing ARDS include pneumococcus, *Legionella pneumophila*, enteric gram-negative bacteria, *Staphylococcus aureus, Pneumocystis carinii, Mycobacterium tuberculosis,* influenza, respiratory syncytial virus, varicella, and the bacteria associated with aspiration pneumonia [22,23,24].

Recently, "severe" community-acquired pneumonia has been described [10–14]. Although there is not a uniform definition, the term has been used to refer to all patients with CAP who are admitted to an ICU. Torres et al. estimated that this illness accounted for 10 percent of all admissions to an ICU over a 4-year period; patients with severe CAP were admitted directly to the ICU 42 percent of the time, after admission to another ward 37 percent of the time, and in transfer from another hospital 21 percent of the time [10]. In recently reported series of severe CAP, the mortality rates have varied from 21 to 54 percent, with the lower mortality rates in case series where not all patients were mechanically ventilated and the higher rates seen when nearly 90 percent were being ventilated [10–14]. These studies contrast with the high mortality rate (76%) of pneumococcal pneumonia in the ICU reported by Hook and colleagues, which led these authors to conclude that ICU care could not reduce the mortality rate of this infection [20]. It is quite likely that the lower mortality rates of severe CAP in more recent studies reflects a better understanding of when to use the ICU for CAP. Unlike years past, when the ICU was used only in extreme circumstances and usually only when mechanical ventilation was needed, patients with CAP are now admitted to the ICU before the onset of overt respiratory failure. With this expectant use of critical care for high-risk patients, it does seem that outcome can be favorably affected.

Several investigators have attempted to define the clinical features of CAP that predict a poor outcome or need for admission to the ICU. In one study, the factors predicting a poor prognosis were bronchopneumonia, lobar pneumonia involving more than two lobes, respiratory rate greater than 30 per minute, severe hypoxemia, abnormal liver function, low serum albumin, and signs of clinical sepsis [12]. Those ill enough to require intensive care and mechanical ventilation had a mortality rate of 47 percent, in contrast to a mortality rate of 5 percent in those not requiring intubation. In another study the most important predictor of mortality was bacteremia, present in 63 percent of patients admitted to the ICU because of pneumonia, which was associated with a 70 percent mortality rate, in contrast to a 26 percent mortality rate in those without bacteremia [13]. The degree of underlying illness, as estimated by the Simplified Acute Physiology Score System, was similar in those with and without bacteremia; thus, the presence of a positive blood culture itself was a predictor of a rapidly fatal outcome, independent of the extent of coexisting illness [13].

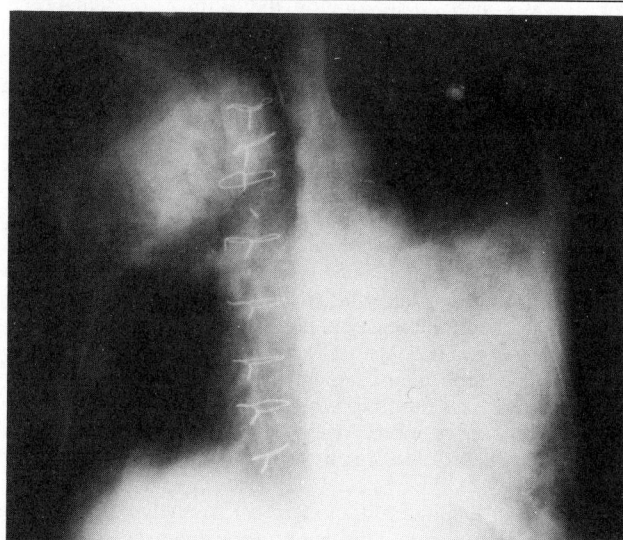

Fig. 76-1. This 68-year-old man who had previous cardiac bypass surgery and chronic congestive heart failure presented with fever, dyspnea, cough, and yellow sputum. The patient required mechanical ventilation for hypoxemic respiratory failure and died within 6 hours of admission. Blood cultures were positive for *S. pneumoniae.* The radiograph shows multilobar consolidation.

Table 76-1. Risk Factors for Pneumonia Mortality

Physical findings
  Abnormal vital signs
    Respiratory rate > 30/min
    Hemodynamic compromise: systolic or diastolic hypotension
    Tachycardia (>120/min)
    Afebrile or high fever (>38°C)
  Altered mental status or coma
Laboratory findings
  Respiratory failure: hypoxemic or hypercarbic
  Multilobar infiltrates
  Rapidly progressive infiltrates
  Positive blood culture
  Multiple organ failure
  Hypoalbuminemia
  Renal insufficiency
  Polymicrobial infection
Historical information
  Serious comorbidity or advanced age
  Recent hospitalization
  Nosocomial onset of infection
  Immunosuppression (including systemic corticosteroids)
  Nonrespiratory clinical presentation
  Delayed or inappropriate therapy
  Prolonged mechanical ventilation

Bacteremia as a pneumonic complication may be an important predictor of mortality for specific bacterial pathogens such as pneumococcus, *Haemophilus influenzae,* and multiple enteric gram-negative bacteria. Data such as these demonstrate that pneumonia can be such a virulent infection that survival may already be determined in certain patients by the time of admission and aggressive intensive care may be unable to save an individual who is already "too far gone" (Fig. 76-1).

A number of studies that have attempted to define prognostic features for CAP were recently summarized by Farr and colleagues [25]. In general, these risk factors fall into several categories (Table 76-1): severe physiologic abnormalities (respiratory rate > 30/min, diastolic blood pressure < 60 mm Hg, need for mechanical ventilation); serious underlying illness (recent hospitalization, hypoalbuminemia, underlying malignancy, immunosuppression) or advanced age; and atypical clinical presentations (lack of fever or clear-cut respiratory symptoms). Among patients with severe CAP, the most important prognostic finding is radiographic progression during therapy [10]. These adverse prognostic factors are particularly evident among the elderly. In one series, the mortality of pneumonia was 30 percent in those 65 years or older, compared to 10 percent in those who were younger [26]. One factor that may explain this finding is that older patients often have atypical clinical presentations of pneumonia, indicating an inappropriate inflammatory response to infection, which may lead to diagnosis at a later, more advanced stage of illness. Starczewski et al. found that elderly patients who died of CAP had chills, sweats, and rigors less often and confusion and tachycardia more often than those who survived [27].

All of these outcome studies were put into perspective by Farr and colleagues when they used stepwise logistic regression analysis to evaluate 245 patients with CAP to define predictors of survival [25]. Although 42 prognostic factors were examined, only 3 emerged as relevant in a multivariate analysis: respiratory rate of 30 per minute or greater, diastolic blood pressure of 60 mm Hg or less, and a serum BUN greater than 19.6 mg per deciliter. When a patient had any two of these three factors present, mortality rose nine fold when compared to patients who had no or one factor present. Because these three important prognostic factors are easily measured and readily available when first evaluating a patient with CAP, accurate identification of patients likely to fare poorly may become quite simple.

NOSOCOMIAL PNEUMONIA. Pneumonia is the nosocomial infection most likely to causally contribute to death, particularly in patients treated with mechanical ventilation. Risk factors for this infection can be conceptually grouped into four categories: underlying acute illnesses that predispose to secondary pneumonia; coexisting medical illness, commonly seen in the critically ill; factors associated with therapy frequently used in the ICU; and malnutrition. Thus, some of the conditions commonly associated with nosocomical pneumonia are general surgery, ARDS, head injury, advanced age, obesity, chronic cardiac or pulmonary disease, renal failure, malignancy, diabetes mellitus, mechanical ventilation, tracheostomy, nasogastric tube use, corticosteroid use, antibiotic therapy, and cimetidine use [6,7,28,29,30].

Among ICU patients, those with the highest risk of pneumonia are individuals treated with mechanical ventilation [30]. Several studies have concluded that intubation increases the risk of pneumonia 7- to 21-fold [29,31,32]. One study estimated the risk of nosocomial pneumonia at 1 percent per day of mechanical ventilation. Thus, a patient treated for 30 days with a ventilator would have approximately a 30 percent risk of developing pneumonia [33]. Fatality rates are also high, particularly in mechanically ventilated patients. Cross and Roup found a mortality rate of 39 percent among 107 patients with pneumonia that developed during the use of respiratory assistance devices [29]. Craven et al. observed a 55 percent mortality rate in 49 patients with nosocomial pneumonia treated with mechanical ventilation [7]. Bryan and Reynolds examined the influence of bacteremia on the outcome of nosocomial pneumonia and found a 58 percent mortality rate in patients with this illness [28]. Seidenfeld et al. studied 129 patients with ARDS and found that pneumonia in this setting was associated with an 88 percent rate of death [17].

The risk factors for nosocomial pneumonia in a combined medical and surgical ICU were examined by Joshi and colleagues [34]. This population had a 12.8 percent incidence of pneumonia, a rate that was not unexpected since 58 percent of these patients were intubated. Risk factors for pneumonia included: use of H-2 blocker therapy, altered mental status, endotracheal intubation, nasogastric tube use, underlying fatal illness, recent upper abdominal or thoracic surgery, and recent bronchoscopy. During the first 4 days of exposure, the greatest risk factors were endotracheal intubation, altered consciousness, and nasogastric tube use. Other investigators have focused primarily on surgical ICU patients and have identified risk factors including: duration of mechanical ventilation, emergency intubation, head injury, shock on admission, blunt trauma, and coma [35,36]. In all ICU populations, common risk factors for nosocomial pneumonia include serious illness of any type, prolonged intubation and mechanical ventilation, and systemic antibiotic use. Antibiotics increase the risk of all pneumonias as well as bacteriologically virulent infections, such as those caused by *P. aeruginosa* and *Acinetobacter,* and therefore must be used carefully among the critically ill [18,33].

The relation between pneumonia and ARDS is particularly interesting. As many as one-third of all cases of ARDS may be the result of pneumonia, and in some series pneumonia is the most common cause of acute lung injury [37,38]. Not only can a variety of CAPs serve as a cause of ARDS, but secondary pneumonia is the most common nosocomial infection acquired by patients with established ARDS [6,17]. In Seidenfeld's study of 129 patients with ARDS, pneumonia was the inciting cause in 21 percent but a complication in 38 percent [17]. In that study, only 21 patients remained free of any infection; these individuals had a mortality rate of 33 percent, in contrast to the 108 patients who had infection of any type and a mortality rate of 79 percent [17]. Those with pneumonia had a high incidence of multiple organ failure (MOF). Often when nosocomial pneumonia complicates ARDS, it is the start of a progressive downhill course characterized by MOF [17,39]. In one study, when a site of nosocomial infection complicating ARDS could be determined, the lung was identified in 56 of 82 patients. Montgomery et al. studied 47 patients with ARDS and reached similar conclusions [40]. Among 20 patients who developed sepsis after the onset of ARDS, pneumonia was present in 15 [40]. In the European collaborative study of 583 patients with ARDS, pneumonia was the cause in 33 percent of cases and a complication in 34 percent [41]. There is ongoing debate about how best to diagnose nosocomial pneumonia, and many of the conclusions about the high rate of this infection among patients with ARDS are based on clinical, not bacteriologic, definitions of pneumonia (see Chap. 55).

Pathogenesis of Pneumonia

NORMAL HOST DEFENSES. When an organism enters the respiratory tract, it encounters a host defense system designed to repel and remove it from every anatomic site in the airway [9]. Pneumonia develops when the size of the organism inoculum overcomes the host defense system, when the organism is so virulent that it cannot be repelled, or when the patient is too impaired to resist an organism type or inoculum size that could ordinarily be handled by a fully functioning host defense system. This system consists of anatomic, mechanical, humoral, secretory, and cellular factors, which can be either nonspecific

or organism-directed. In addition, the nature of presentation of the organism to the lung may be important. It appears that aerosol challenges of bacteria are more easily repelled than bolus liquid challenges (as occurs with aspiration), and a larger number of organisms is required to cause infection by the aerosol route.

The oropharynx is ordinarily free of enteric gram-negative bacilli because salivary proteases, secretions, and local IgA antibody prevent these bacteria from establishing a foothold on the mucosal surface. In addition, the oropharyngeal epithelium is regularly regenerated as cells are desquamated, thereby removing any bound bacteria. Healthy individuals have a poor intrinsic ability of the oral epithelium to bind or adhere to gram-negative bacteria [42]. With a variety of acute illnesses, such as malnutrition, uremia, and general surgery, however, gram-negative bacteria can bind more avidly to the oral epithelium, as these cells expose more "receptors" for binding by bacterial "adhesins" present on organisms such as *Pseudomonas aeruginosa* [30,43,44,45].

The lower respiratory tract has an extremely complex host defense system that keeps this site sterile in normal individuals [46,47]. For this area to become infected, organisms must first pass through the vocal cords and then overcome the physical barriers of the tracheobronchial tree, which include cough, bronchoconstriction, airway angulation, and upward transport of the mucociliary blanket [9]. As in the oropharynx, bacterial adherence is necessary for gram-negative bacteria to colonize the tracheobronchial tree [45]. Organisms must also overcome secretory and cellular defenses in the lower respiratory tract, which function in an immune fashion, and can be organism-specific or nonspecific. Protective materials in respiratory secretions include IgA, the predominant immunoglobulin of the upper airway; IgG, which dominates in the lower respiratory tract; complement; lysozymes; surfactant; and fibronectin [9,48,49]. Cellular defenses in the lower respiratory tract include the alveolar macrophage, neutrophil, and bronchus-associated lymphoid tissue. The resident phagocytic cell of the lower respiratory tract is the alveolar macrophage, but its function can be augmented by systemic host responses, such as recruitment of blood neutrophils and development of cell-mediated and humoral immunity. The alveolar macrophage has intrinsic microbial killing activity, but it can also respond to lymphokines and secrete inflammatory peptides, such as tumor necrosis factor and interleukin-1, thereby serving as an important modulator of the integrated pulmonary and systemic immune response to invading pathogens [9].

The lower airway handles individual pathogens in specific ways that demonstrate the complex integration of the host defense system. For example, *S. aureus* is removed by resident alveolar macrophages, whereas certain enteric gram-negative bacteria require the recruitment of neutrophils to be cleared [9]. Other bacteria, such as *Listeria monocytogenes,* require additional alveolar macrophages to be recruited to the lung to be eliminated [9]. Cell-mediated immunity is required to resist infection with *L. pneumophila* and *M. tuberculosis*. Viruses are handled somewhat differently than bacteria. Important factors in defense against these agents include the alveolar macrophage, neutralizing antibodies (IgG, IgA, IgM), cytotoxic T lymphocytes, and cytokines, such as interferon [50].

HOW MICROORGANISMS REACH THE LUNG. Traditionally, bacteria and other infectious agents reach the lung by one of four routes: inhalation from ambient air, hematogenously from distal sites of infection, by direct extension or exogenous penetration, and by aspiration from a colonized oropharynx and nasopharynx [9]. Inhalation is an uncommon route of or-

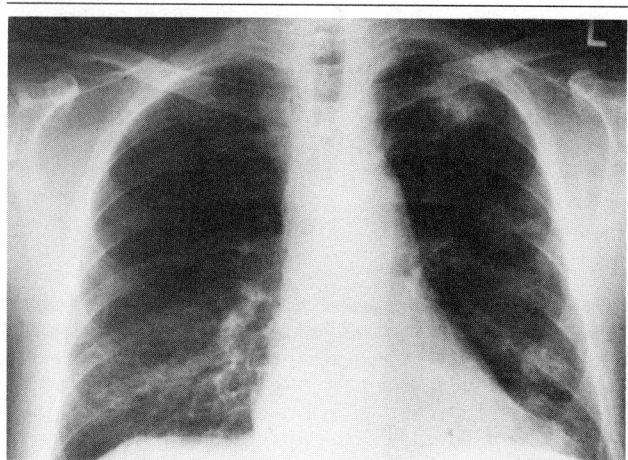

Fig. 76-2. This 25-year-old intravenous drug user came to the hospital with complaints of fever, cough, and blood-tinged sputum. Physical examination showed a systolic and diastolic murmur over the right sternal border along with V waves in the jugular veins. Blood cultures showed *S. aureus* and the chest radiograph showed multiple nodular infiltrates, particularly in the left lung, some of which were cavitary. This radiograph is characteristic of septic emboli from endocarditis of the tricuspid valve.

ganism entry except for agents such as *L. pneumophila* and *M. tuberculosis*. Hematogenous spread can occur with septic emboli from such sites as the valves of the right cardiac chambers (Fig. 76-2). Exogenous penetration is an unlikely route of bacterial entry but can occur, for example, with a stab wound to the chest. Most pneumonias result when microorganisms are aspirated to the lung from a previously colonized oropharynx [9]. Nosocomial pneumonia is frequently preceded by gram-negative bacillary colonization of the upper airway [51,52]. The source of bacteria that colonize the upper airway is most likely the patient's own intestinal flora, but staff members can transmit their flora to patients, particularly when nonsterile techniques are used to handle the airway mucosa.

In the critically ill patient two other routes of organism entry exist, both related to prosthetic devices commonly used in the ICU: the endotracheal tube and the nasogastric tube. Insertion of an endotracheal tube allows organisms direct access from the ICU staff and environment to the tracheobronchial tree, thereby avoiding all the defense mechanisms present above the vocal cords. The endotracheal tube can traumatize the mucosa of the airway and can itself become colonized, serving as a nidus from which bacteria can be disseminated to the distal portions of the lung [53,54]. Any organisms that reach the inside of the endotracheal tube can proliferate to large numbers, because this site is free from host defenses. Sottile et al. observed that 84 percent of endotracheal tubes studied had an amorphous matrix on the inside, and this matrix contained bacteria [55]. Inglis et al. quantitated this biofilm and found as many as 1×10^6 organisms per centimeter of endotracheal tube [56]. The importance of this site of bacteria is the large number of organisms present and the fact that these organisms can reach the lung every time an intubated patient is suctioned.

In addition, contamination of the ventilator's tubing circuit can expose the lung to large numbers of bacteria. Craven et al. showed that patients can contaminate ventilator tubing circuits and bacteria can proliferate in the water condensate in the tubing [57]. If this condensate is inadvertently washed back to the patient, pneumonia can follow [57]. Studies by Schwartz et al. and Niederman et al. showed that when an endotracheal

tube is present some bacteria, particularly *P. aeruginosa,* can colonize the lower airway directly, without first colonizing the oropharynx [58,59].

The gastrointestinal tract, particularly the stomach, can serve as a reservoir for bacteria. Several investigators have shown that gram-negative bacilli can move retrograde from the stomach to the oropharynx and then antegrade into the lung [60,61,62]. The stomach can be the source of 20 to 40 percent of the enteric gram-negative bacteria that colonize the trachea of intubated patients [60,61,62], but it is difficult to determine whether these colonizing gastric bacteria also lead to pneumonia. In one study of 40 neurosurgical patients, gram-negative tracheal colonization often began in the stomach, but only 1 of 15 cases of nosocomial pneumonia had a gastric origin [63]. One way the stomach can be an important source of pneumonic organisms is through the mechanism of reflux and aspiration. When a nasogastric tube is used for feeding, it can promote aspiration, especially if a large-bore tube is used with a bolus feeding method rather than with a continuous infusion of enteral nutrients and if the patient is kept in a supine position [60,64].

When a nasogastric tube is present, it may be important to consider both the pH and the volume of the gastric contents. It has been shown that when gastric pH rises above 4 to 6, as can occur with the use of antacids, H-2 blockers, and enteral feeding, the number of gram-negative bacteria in the stomach increases to as many as 1 to 100 million per milliliter of gastric juice [61]. This may be related to the finding that elevation of gastric pH and the use of cimetidine therapy have been reported as risk factors for nosocomial pneumonia [7,65,66,67]. Driks et al.'s prospective study showed that the use of sucralfate for intestinal bleeding prophylaxis, which does not cause a rise in gastric pH, was associated with a lower rate of nosocomial pneumonia and mortality than if H-2 blockers, antacids, or both were used for this purpose [67]. A number of subsequent studies of this issue have reached differing conclusions, and two meta-analyses have been published [68,69]. In both of these, sucralfate was associated with a reduced risk of pneumonia when compared to antacids or H-2 blockers. However, in one evaluation, H-2 blockers were not associated with a higher pneumonia risk than a placebo-treated group [69]. One recent study of critically ill patients also found that cimetidine did not increase the risk of pneumonia when compared to placebo [70]. It is possible that antacids are more of a risk factor for pneumonia than H-2 antagonists, because the former increase both gastric pH and gastric volume, while the latter increase pH but reduce volume. Interventions that increase both gastric volume and pH may be the greatest risk for pneumonia, because the size of the gastric reservoir is expanded at the same time aspiration is facilitated by the large volume of stomach contents. If this analysis is correct, then it may explain the observation that when continuous enteral feeding led to an elevation of gastric pH (and, presumably, an elevation of gastric volume), the incidence of pneumonia was higher than when continuous feeding was used and did not raise pH [71]. One alternative to elevation of gastric pH and volume by continuous feeding of the stomach is to place enteral feedings into the jejunum, although in one study this strategy did not reduce the risk of pneumonia [72].

AIRWAY COLONIZATION AND NOSOCOMIAL PNEUMONIA. When bacteria encounter the respiratory tract host defense system, they may be repelled entirely, lead to invasive infection, or colonize the airway epithelium. Colonization can be defined as the persistence of organisms at a particular body site, in the absence of a host response and without evidence of an adverse effect to the host. For many patients, colonization of the respiratory tract by enteric gram-negative bacilli is the first step toward invasive infection and serves as both a "marker" of a seriously ill individual and as a harbinger of subsequent nosocomial pneumonia [45].

The rate of colonization of the oropharynx by gram-negative bacilli parallels the extent of systemic illness in a given patient. Thus, although only 6 percent of normals have these bacteria in their oropharynx, up to three-fourths of the sickest patients in the hospital have them in the upper airway. In a study of 213 ICU patients, colonization of the oropharynx preceded and predicted the occurrence of nosocomial pneumonia in 22 of 26 individuals who developed this infection [52]. The close association of colonization and pneumonia may result from the possibility that when a colonized patient aspirates oropharyngeal secretions, gram-negative bacteria enter the lung. Aspiration alone does not always lead to pneumonia, however, and it is likely that patients ill enough to become colonized also have impairments in lower respiratory tract host defenses as a result of their underlying systemic illness, and these impairments add to the risk of pneumonia [9].

Risk factors for gram-negative colonization of the upper and lower respiratory tract are similar and include antibiotic therapy, endotracheal intubation, smoking, malnutrition, general surgery, and therapies that raise gastric pH [45]. Additional factors for oropharyngeal colonization include azotemia, diabetes, coma, hypotension, advanced age, and underlying lung disease [30,45]. Factors that increase the risk of tracheobronchial colonization include chronic bronchitis, cystic fibrosis, ciliary dysfunction, tracheostomy, bronchiectasis, acute lung injury, and viral infection [45].

One pathogenetic mechanism that links many of the clinical risk factors for upper and lower airway colonization is a cell-cell interaction termed bacterial mucosal adherence. Many clinical disease states can alter the oropharyngeal or tracheal epithelium, making the cell surface more receptive for binding by such bacteria as *P. aeruginosa* [45]. At multiple mucosal sites throughout the body, including the oropharynx and tracheobronchial tree, epithelial cells possess receptors that can bind to bacteria. This binding interaction may be the first step in allowing organisms to gain a foothold on the epithelial surface, from which they can proliferate and lead to colonization. Colonization of both the upper and lower airway is more likely to occur in patients who have an increased number of epithelial cell receptors for gram-negative bacteria than in patients with a normal number of such receptors [42–45]. Diseases that can result in an increased number of oropharyngeal bacterial receptors include azotemia, malnutrition, general surgery, endotracheal intubation, smoking, and other serious illness [42,43,45]. Tracheal cell adherence can be increased by endotracheal intubation, malnutrition, tracheostomy, viral infection, and general surgery [44,45,53]. How systemic illnesses lead to an increase in cell surface receptors is unknown, but the nature of a given patient's sputum may be an important factor. The quantity of proteases in the sputum, the pH of the airway secretions, and the nature of sputum mucins all may be affected by a variety of acute illnesses and may in turn influence how avidly bacteria adhere to the epithelial cell surface [45,73,74,75]. Thus, many acute illnesses may act to increase the number of respiratory epithelial cell receptors for gram-negative bacilli and thereby predispose to both colonization and pneumonia by similar pathogenetic mechanisms.

HOST DEFENSE IMPAIRMENTS IN ACUTE AND CHRONIC ILLNESS THAT PREDISPOSE TO PNEUMONIA. Many systemic diseases are associated with an increased

incidence of pneumonia; this may be the result of multiple disease-associated malfunctions in the respiratory host defense system. Such diseases include ARDS, congestive heart failure, malnutrition, renal failure, diabetes mellitus, chronic liver disease, alcoholism, cancer, and collagen vascular disease. For example, ARDS may lead to increased tracheal and buccal cell adherence, as coexisting serious illness and the presence of high levels of neutrophilic proteases in the airway alter the number of epithelial cell receptors for bacteria. Ciliary dysfunction can also occur as a result of high levels of neutrophil elastase [6]. The presence of alveolar edema, hypoxia, overwhelming infection, or shock can lead to dysfunction of polymorphonuclear cells and alveolar macrophages [6,48]. Sepsis, a common cause of ARDS, can lead to a number of inflammatory events that interfere with respiratory tract immune defenses. With endotoxemia, neutrophils can be sequestered in the pulmonary vascular bed but be unable to reach the alveoli in response to a pulmonary bacterial challenge [76]. In addition, the use of endotracheal intubation can lead to a bypassing of upper airway defenses and injury of the tracheal mucosa. Finally, alveolar edema can reduce the amount of surfactant and eliminate its beneficial antibacterial activity. In addition, many of the illnesses that are complicated by pneumonia may develop this complication because they require therapy with medications that increase the risk of infection [9].

Similarly, malnutrition has multiple effects on the respiratory host defense system (Table 76-2), and this common illness in hospitalized patients may add to the risk of pneumonia. Several studies have shown that acute and chronic malnutrition can increase the risk of bacterial and viral infections both in and out of the hospital [9,77]. Malnutrition can increase both oropharyngeal and tracheal cell bacterial adherence; it can reduce alveolar macrophage function, reduce levels of airway IgA, impair cell-mediated immunity by lymphocytes, cause defective neutrophil migration, and impair recruitment of alveolar macrophages to the lung in times of need [43,44,77].

Etiology of Pneumonia

COMMUNITY-ACQUIRED PNEUMONIA. Even with extensive diagnostic testing, a specific etiologic agent can be identified in only approximately 50 percent of pneumonias that develop outside of the hospital [78]. Although the exact incidence of viral pneumonias is unknown, these agents may account for up to one-third of all cases of CAP. The most common pathogen identified in pneumonias arising out of the hospital is pneumococcus, followed by *Mycoplasma pneumoniae, L. pneumophila, H. influenzae, Chlamydia pneumoniae* (TWAR strain), anaerobes, *S. aureus,* and enteric gram-negatives. The exact incidence of each pathogen varies depending on a number of factors, including the severity of the acute illness, the patient's age, and the types of comorbidity present in a given patient population [79]. In the elderly, although pneumococcus is still the most common pathogen, enteric gram-negatives may be

Table 76-2. Lung Host Defense Impairments with Malnutrition

Increased tracheal and buccal cell adherence
Altered macrophage function and migration
Reduced recruitment of neutrophils
Impaired cell mediated immunity and T cell depletion
Diminished secretory IgA
Complement deficiency

responsible for 20 to 40 percent of all cases of pneumonia, and anaerobes and *H. influenzae* are other common agents [80,81]. As mentioned previously, the community-acquired infections most likely to lead to respiratory failure or ICU admission (severe pneumonia) include pneumococcus, *L. pneumophila* and enteric gram-negatives (Fig. 76-3). Other pathogens that can lead to respiratory failure include *H. influenzae, S. aureus,* pathogens associated with aspiration such as anaerobes, *Pneumocystis carinii* (PCP), tuberculosis, influenza, varicella, respiratory syncytial virus, and the recently described Hantavirus.

When evaluating a patient with pneumonia, it is important to understand the status of the respiratory host defense system so as better to evaluate which possible pathogen is most likely (Table 76-3). Thus, if a previously healthy person has pneumonia, it is probably due to a pathogen of such intrinsic virulence that it can overcome even an intact host defense system. These pathogens include pneumococcus, *Legionella* sp., *S. aureus,* and *M. pneumoniae.* Certain agents should be suspected in specific clinical settings. If the patient has some underlying illness, then organisms of less intrinsic virulence that would ordinarily be eliminated by a normal host can be responsible. When an alcoholic has pneumonia, *Klebsiella pneumoniae* becomes more likely; those with chronic bronchitis may be infected with *H. influenzae* and *M. catarrhalis* ; cardiac patients commonly have pneumococcal infection; those with cystic fibrosis are infected by *S. aureus* and *P. aeruginosa*; those with risk factors for or a history of aspiration can have anaerobic lung infection; splenectomized patients are infected by encapsulated organisms; postinfluenza patients may be infected by *S. aureus,* pneumococcus, enteric gram-negatives, or *H. influenzae*; leukemics have fungal and gram-negative pneumonias; and AIDS patients have infections with *P. carinii* and other organisms that require cell-mediated immunity to be repelled. In patients with an appropriate travel or exposure history, unusual pathogens should be considered, including tularemia (hunters), plague (exposure to small animals), anthrax (wool sorters and tanners), cryptococcosis (southwestern United States), histoplasmosis (bat droppings), or psittacosis (infected birds).

NOSOCOMIAL PNEUMONIA.

When pneumonia develops in the hospital, the predominant pathogens are the enteric gram-negative bacilli. Other common agents include *S. aureus, H. influenzae,* pneumococcus, and anaerobes (in the presence of aspiration). One recent study observed that *S. aureus* is a common pathogen when pneumonia begins shortly after intubation and in patients with impaired consciousness, while enteric gram-negatives are more common with later onset pneumonias in patients who are alert on admission [82]. However, later onset pneumonias can involve Methicillin-resistant *S. aureus.* Certain hospitals have foci of *Legionella* in the water system, and viral pneumonia can be transmitted from infected staff members who come to work when their illness is incubating. Among patients who are hospitalized with serious illnesses, such as those who have received corticosteroids or antibiotics, those requiring long-term mechanical ventilation, and those with ARDS, the pathogen most likely to cause pneumonia is *P. aeruginosa.* In one study, this organism was recovered from 40 percent of all tracheobronchial samples collected from patients undergoing long-term mechanical ventilation, for a variety of reasons [59]. Another pathogen to consider when nosocomial pneumonia arises in the setting of corticosteroid therapy for chronic obstructive lung disease is *Aspergillus* sp. [83]. Recently, methicillin-resistant *S. aureus* has emerged as a common pathogen in the ventilated patient, especially in the presence of acute lung injury. In addition, the mechanically ventilated pa-

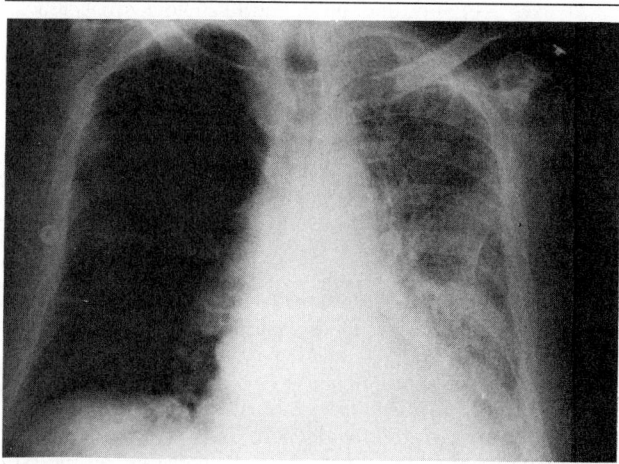

Fig. 76-3. This 57-year-old alcoholic with confusion, cough, and fever came to the hospital because of dyspnea noted by his family. Sputum culture revealed *K. pneumoniae* and the chest radiograph shows a multilobar infiltrate in the left lung.

tient may develop pneumonia from not just one organism; a polymicrobial infection may be present in up to 40 percent of the pneumonias that develop in intubated patients [33].

Clinical Features of Pneumonia

GENERAL FEATURES OF COMMUNITY-ACQUIRED PNEUMONIA. The signs and symptoms of pneumonia depend on both host and bacterial factors, but from a clinical perspective the presentation is often classified as typical or atypical. Although it has been suggested that making the distinction between these clinical patterns can help define the likely etiologic pathogen for a given patient with CAP, this approach is often unsuccessful. In several studies, the clinical presentations

Table 76-3. Likely Pathogens for Pneumonia in the Critically Ill

Patient characteristics/risk factors	Suspected pathogen
Alcoholism—acute or chronic	Pneumococcus, *S. aureus, H. influenzae, K. pneumoniae,* Tuberculosis
Chronic obstructive pulmonary disease	Pneumococcus, *H. influenzae, M. catarrhalis*
Recent viral infection	Pneumococcus, *S. aureus, H. influenzae,* gram-negative bacilli
Nursing home, age > 75 yr	Gram-negative bacilli, pneumococcus, *H. influenzae,* aspiration (anaerobes)
AIDS (risk groups: IV drug abuser, hemophilia, homosexual)	Pneumococcus, *Salmonella,* cytomegalovirus, *H. influenzae, Cryptococcus, P. carinii*
Hospital-acquired	Gram-negative bacilli (incl. *P. aeruginosa*), *S. aureus*
High-risk aspiration	Anaerobes, gram-negative bacilli
Cardiac disease	Pneumococcus, gram-negative bacilli
Neutropenia	*P. aeruginosa, Aspergillus,* gram-negative bacilli

of CAP have overlaped enough among all etiologies that clinical features could not be used to identify the likely pathogen [84,85,86]. Classic typical pneumonia is characterized by the sudden onset of high fever, chills, pleuritic chest pain, and cough along with the findings of a lobar infiltrate, leukocytosis, purulent sputum, and a toxic appearance. Although bacterial pathogens such as pneumococcus, *H. influenzae, K. pneumoniae, S. aureus,* anaerobes, and gram-negative bacilli can present in this manner, these same pathogens can present in a more subtle fashion, particularly if the patient is elderly or has an altered immune system. Atypical pneumonia is described as an illness of more insidious onset, with preceding upper respiratory symptoms, moderate fever without chills, nonproductive cough, headache, myalgia, mild leukocytosis, and the absence of organisms on a sputum Gram's stain. The chest radiograph may demonstrate a bronchopneumonia (patchy distribution adjacent to bronchi, not filling an entire lobe) or a diffuse interstitial pattern and may be more severely affected than the patient appears to be. This pattern is often attributed to viral agents, *M. pneumoniae, C. pneumoniae* (TWAR), and unusual agents such as those causing psittacosis and Q fever. Some agents, particularly *Legionella* sp., can present a mixed picture, with high fever, chills, and leukocytosis, but a dry cough can be present along with prodromal symptoms.

To the extent that the symptoms of pneumonia result from the host inflammatory response, patients with altered immune function will have less dramatic symptoms. Thus, those with advanced age, chronic lung disease, cardiac disease, renal failure, diabetes, immunosuppressive therapy, and other chronic illnesses have not only an increased incidence of pneumonia but a less distinct and more subtle clinical presentation. In those older than 65 years, chills, rigors, and fever may be absent and pneumonia may present as confusion or deterioration of an underlying chronic illness [26,27]. In this patient population, fever has been absent in up to 10 percent of those with bacteremic pneumonia [87]. Given that the elderly and those with multiple comorbidities enter into the case mix of patients with CAP, it is not surprising that it is often difficult to determine the identity of the etiologic pathogen simply by looking at patterns of clinical presentation [85,86]. The failure of clinical features to predict the identity of an etiologic pathogen has been observed for all patients with CAP, including those with severe forms [10].

GENERAL FEATURES OF NOSOCOMIAL PNEUMONIA. One of the major controversies in critical care medicine is how to determine when hospital-acquired pneumonia is present. On clinical grounds alone, the diagnosis is imprecise, and patients with ARDS may be both overdiagnosed and underdiagnosed for nosocomial pneumonia [6]. Fagon et al., using the protected specimen brush to define this infection (see below) in mechanically ventilated patients, reported that up to two-thirds of cases diagnosed based on clinical criteria alone are not truly pneumonia [88]. Most clinical definitions of nosocomial pneumonia require the patient to be hospitalized 48 to 72 hours before the onset of purulent sputum, leukocytosis, fever, and a new and persistent infiltrate. If these features exist along with isolation of a potential pathogen from the sputum, then the organism is deemed responsible for the infection. The findings of a positive blood culture or radiographic cavitation add to the likelihood of pneumonia. One approach to the clinical definition of ventilator-associated pneumonia, developed by Pugin and associates, is to use a scoring system that weights the likelihood of pneumonia using six clinical variables: fever, white blood cell count and differential, the presence of pathogens in the sputum, sputum purulence, radiographic patterns, and oxygenation

changes [89]. When such a clinical scoring system has been compared to invasive diagnostic methods, the clinical and bacteriologic definitions of pneumonia have correlated very well [89]. These observations suggest that there may still be a role for careful clinical judgment in the diagnosis of this confusing infection.

In the presence of diseases such as ARDS, atelectasis, pulmonary embolism, and congestive heart failure, all of which may be associated with lung infiltrates, pneumonia can be overlooked or these processes may be incorrectly called pneumonia. In addition, the elderly and immunosuppressed may have few clinical findings when pneumonia develops in the hospital. Limited sputum production due to impaired immunologic status and mobilization of leukocytes compound the difficulties in diagnosis. Conversely, those on a mechanical ventilator with infectious tracheobronchitis may have purulent sputum, fever, and pathogens colonizing the sputum but not have invasive parenchymal lung infection. Significant alterations in alveolar to arterial oxygen tension gradients can be due to a new or extending infection, although arterial blood gases may be significantly disturbed due to underlying illness. In the mechanically ventilated patient, the development of new diagnostic methods to confirm the presence of pneumonia to supplement traditional bedside criteria has been proposed because of all the attendant problems associated with a clinical approach (see below).

Approach to the Patient with Overwhelming Pneumonia

Three groups of patients are likely to confront the critical care physician evaluating the patient with possible pneumonia: the community patient with a life-threatening pulmonary infection; the compromised host, either in the hospital already or coming from the community or a nursing home; or the patient already in the ICU, often on mechanical ventilation, who clinically deteriorates in a way that raises the possibility of acute pulmonary infection. Historical, physical, and laboratory findings pertinent to diagnoses are helpful in determining whether lung infection is present and, if so, how severely ill the patient is, which etiologic agent is responsible, and what specific therapy should be instituted (see Tables 76-3 and 76-4).

HISTORICAL INFORMATION. Initially, the history is needed to determine whether the patient does have pneumonia as the cause of acute illness. Elderly, immunocompromised, and mechanically ventilated patients may have an altered presentation of pneumonia, and this diagnosis may easily be overlooked or confused with another diagnosis. The systemic response to respiratory infection, which includes fever and tachypnea, occurs early and, in the case of pneumococcal infection in the normal host, usually several days after the onset of an upper respiratory infection. This response is determined cellularly, possibly by mediators released from monocytes and macrophages in response to bacterial cell wall products [9]. These findings, along with chest pain and purulent sputum production, are common in the normal host, but such "typical" symptoms of bacterial pneumonia are likely to be muted in the elderly and compromised host, in whom the infection may be heralded only by lethargy and altered mental activity [80]. In the compromised host with malignancy or immunosuppressive therapy, the presentation may be so stunted that pneumonia may be discovered only serendipitously at autopsy.

Table 76-4. Historical Features Useful in Pneumonia Diagnosis

	Organisms
Environmental contact	
Birds	*Chlamydia psittaci*
Bird droppings	*C. psittaci*
	H. capsulatum
Ungulates	*Coxiella burnetii* (Q fever)
Hunting: animal and insect bites	*Yersinia pestis*
	F. tularensis
Travel or location	
Southeast Asia	*Pseudomonas pseudomallei*
Southwestern U.S.	*Coccidioides immitis*
Midwest	*H. capsulatum*
Prison environment	*M. tuberculosis*

Table 76-5. Extrapulmonary Findings in Pneumonia

Dermatologic findings	Organism
Herpes labialis	Pneumococcus
Erythema multiforme	*Mycoplasma*
	Chlamydia psittaci
Erythema nodosum	*Mycobacterium tuberculosis*
	C. immitis
	H. capsulatum
Skin nodules	*Nocardia*
	Aspergillus
	C. immitis
	Blastomyces
Pharyngitis, bullous myringitis	*Mycoplasma*
Splenomegaly	*F. tularensis*
	C. psittaci
	Coxiella burnetii (Q fever)
Pleural effusion	*H. Influenzae*
	Pneumococcus
	Pyogenic *Streptococcus*
	Aspergillus
	F. tularensis

Historical information can be extremely helpful in the normal host, while more reliance must be placed on laboratory and radiographic information in ICU or ventilator-treated patients. Initially, patients should be classified by whether the pneumonia began in the community or in the hospital and by whether there is a known secondary illness or medication that could increase the risk of infection. An understanding of immune status can help narrow the etiologic considerations. Next, a careful history, including information about contact with animals, especially birds, rats, and rabbits, can suggest the diagnosis of psitticosis, tularemia, and plague. Fungal pneumonia should be considered in appropriate endemic areas, since the acute presentation of endemic fungi can be confused with bacterial pneumonia. Q fever and anthrax are more common in specific occupations, such as contact with infected ungulates in the former and with infected hides and wool in the latter.

Hemoptysis implies tissue necrosis and is more common with pyogenic streptococcal pneumonia (groups A–D), anaerobic lung abscess, *S. aureus*, necrotizing gram-negative organisms, and invasive aspergillosis. Microaspiration of anaerobic organisms leading to pneumonia is more likely when preexisting severe periodontal disease is present along with a history of seizure disorder, altered consciousness, or esophageal obstructive disease. Extrapulmonary symptoms may give clues to specific etiologic agents, with diarrhea and abdominal discomfort being seen in the case of *Legionella* and otitis media and pharyngitis with *M. pneumoniae* (Table 76-5).

PHYSICAL EXAMINATION. The physical examination is of the most value in suggesting the presence of pneumonia and grading its severity. Signs of consolidation suggest pneumonia, whereas rales are less specific, especially in the ICU. Tachypnea (>20 breaths/min) may be the earliest sign of pneumonia in the elderly [90]. In patients with CAP, an admission respiratory rate greater than 30 per minute is an important negative prognostic feature; in some studies mortality increased dramatically when respiratory rate exceeded this level [25]. Signs of pleural effusion are particularly common in *H. influenzae* and pneumococcal, streptococcal, and *Aspergillus* pneumonia, where pleural friction rubs may be detected. Pleural involvement can be seen, although less often, in *Legionella*, and *Mycoplasma* pneumoniae, and is strong evidence against *P. carinii* pneumonia in the compromised host. Relative bradycardia is a frequent finding in pneumonias, caused by *Mycoplasma, Legionella,* and *Chlamydia* organisms. Dermatologic manifestations (erythema nodosum, erythema multiforme, and skin nodules) may be observed in *Mycoplasma,* fungal, nocardia, and tuberculous infections. Horder's spots (pale macular rash), long considered part of the presentation of psittacosis, should lead to a

search for other evidence of this infection. Ecthyma gangrenosum, an indurated, round skin lesion with a central dark area surrounded by erythema, is characteristic of gram-negative septicemia, especially with *P. aeruginosa*. Central nervous system abnormalities can be found with pneumococcus, tuberculosis, *H. influenzae,* gram-negatives, cryptococcus, *Aspergillus* sp., *Legionella,* toxoplasma, varicella zoster, and cytomegalovirus. Other physical findings that narrow the differential diagnosis include splenomegaly in the case of psittacosis and tularemia, herpes labialis in pneumococcal infection, bullous myringitis with *M. pneumoniae,* and lymphadenopathy with tularemia. The predictive value of many of these observations has not been evaluated rigorously (Table 76-5).

ROUTINE DIAGNOSTIC TESTING

Routine Laboratory Testing. A white blood cell count greater than 20,000 cells per cubic centimeter with the presence of immature forms (left shift) suggests infection, particularly in the normal host. Elderly patients and those with acute and chronic alcoholism may be unable to mobilize neutrophils from the bone marrow. Leukopenia can be associated with viral infection but may also result from chemotherapy for malignancy, immunosuppressive therapy, and overwhelming sepsis and may itself be a poor prognostic finding in patients with severe CAP [14]. The majority of patients with *Mycoplasma* infection do not have a white blood cell count above 10,000 [91]. Elevated liver function tests are not a specific finding but can be seen in a variety of viral and bacterial pneumonias, including *Legionella,* tuberculosis, *Mycoplasma,* Q fever, tularemia, and psittacosis as well as pneumococcal infection. Similarly, electrolyte disturbance, including hypophosphatemia and hyponatremia, is not predictive of a specific pathogen [85]. Arterial blood gases are abnormal in patients with severe pneumonia, and the findings from this test can help to guide supportive therapy measures.

Serology. Because even the normal host needs time to mount a humoral response, such examinations are not available for decision-making during the first 24 to 48 hours of critical illness. The nonspecific IgM autoantibody against the I antigen on the red blood cell causes cold agglutination of the erythrocyte and is present in up to 75 percent of patients with *Mycoplasma* infection, becoming evident during the first 7 to 14 days [91].

This response is not uniform, however, and may also be seen in *Legionella* and viral infections. Serologic responses are useful for confirmation of clinical suspicion of many atypical and viral pneumonias. This technique is useful to diagnose a specific viral agent retrospectively, but is not useful if a specific virus is not suspected and targeted for testing. Genetic probes for specific viral DNA and RNA are becoming available for cytomegalovirus, varicella zoster, *H. simplex,* and adenovirus. The direct immunofluorescent stain of sputum for *Legionella* has a sensitivity of 25 to 50 percent and specificity above 90 percent. This methodology is also available for *Chlamydia* and influenza virus but is rarely applied. Counterimmunoelectrophoresis can detect pneumococcal antigen in sputum and less frequently in urine when the diagnosis is in doubt, and occasionally can provide information on an emergent basis.

In general, serologic studies are useful for epidemiologic evaluations and retrospective confirmation of diagnosis but have little value in the routine care of patients with CAP. In one study, even with extensive serologic and bacteriologic testing, an etiologic pathogen could not be defined for 50 percent of patients with CAP, and serology provided useful information in only 25 percent of all cases [78]. Given the cost of these methods and the fact that the necessary convalescent titers are often not collected, serologic testing should not be routinely ordered for patients with CAP [79]. However, if epidemiologic evaluation is needed or if the patient is not responding to appropriate empiric therapy (below), then serologic testing may provide useful information.

Chest Radiographs. The use of the chest radiograph in the diagnosis of pneumonia in the critically ill is of paramount importance (Table 76-6). Although it is not infallible, the application of pattern reading can narrow the differential diagnosis, particularly when used in concert with other available information (see Chap. 70). For example, the rapid development of a diffuse alveolar pattern frequently implies a hematogenously disseminated infection such as varicella or cytomegalovirus or the development of ARDS as a pneumonic complication. Hyperinflation is characteristic of respiratory syncytial virus pneumonia [92]. A more subacute presentation of diffuse alveolar infiltrates may represent hematogenous dissemination of tuberculosis. With the increasing incidence of HIV infection, *P.*

carinii must be considered in the setting of a diffuse alveolar or reticulonodular pattern in groups at risk for AIDS [93]. Noninfectious causes of pulmonary infiltrates, such as heart failure, drug toxicity, and lymphangitic carcinomatosis, frequently present in this fashion.

Focal infiltrates, confined to single segments or lobes, are most likely to represent bacterial pneumonia related to microaspiration into a particular area of the lung. Severe CAPs such as pneumococcus, *S. aureus,* and *Legionella* can present in this manner, although multilobar involvement can occur and carries a worse prognosis. In addition, the systemic inflammatory response to these infections may lead to diffuse acute lung injury (ARDS), and the distinction between focal pneumonia complicated by acute lung injury versus a diffuse pneumonia may be blurred [94].

The acute bacterial pneumonias generally progress more rapidly (hours to days) than fungal or mycobacterial infections (days to weeks). Pleural effusions occur commonly in *H. influenzae* pneumonia (>50%) and pneumococcal infection (25%). Hilar adenopathy and pleural effusion make the diagnosis of PCP extremely unlikely [93], whereas cavitation can occur in both infectious and noninfectious lung disease. Necrosis occurs in staphylococcal pneumonia, and multiple cavitary nodules suggest septic embolization from right-sided endocarditis (Figs. 76-2 and 76-4). Rapid cavitation is also common in gram-negative pneumonias, while a subacute course with cavitation suggests anaerobic or mycobacterial infection. Occasionally, ventilator-associated bacterial pneumonia can progress rapidly and fatally, emphasizing the need for timely recognition and therapy (Fig. 76-5). Chronic cavitation (weeks to months) is more likely due to a noninfectious problem, such as carcinoma, lymphoma, or Wegener's granulomatosis, especially in the absence of the systemic signs of acute infection.

The limitation of the chest radiograph must be stressed, however. In the ICU, coexisting and preexisting lung disease may obscure the findings of pneumonia. In addition, the radiographic patterns that develop with community-acquired infection may not always be specific in determining the pathogen. One study of 196 patients with CAP found that multilobar dis-

Table 76-6. Radiographic Patterns in Diagnosis of Pneumonia

Acute	Chronic	Cavitation
Diffuse infiltrate		
P. carinii pneumonia	TB (typical or atypical)	—
Viral	Fungi	—
Cardiogenic edema	Radiation injury	—
Drug reaction	Drug reaction	—
Alveolar hemorrhage	Lymphangitic cancer	—
Focal infiltrate		
Pneumococcus	TB	Fungi/nocardia
S. aureus	Fungi	Anaerobes
Legionella sp.	Malignancy	Gram-negatives
Gram-negative bacilli		*S. aureus*
Lung infarction		TB
Bronchiolitis obliterans and organizing pneumonia (BOOP)		Malignancy
		Wegener's granulomatosis

Fig. 76-4. One week after recovering from "the flu," this 48-year-old man noted fever and cough. The symptoms persisted for several days before he saw his physician. At the time of evaluation, the chest radiograph showed multiple large cavities with air-fluid levels in the left lung. Sputum culture showed *S. aureus.* The necrotizing cavities of staphylococcal pneumonia are larger and arise in a different setting than the cavities caused by the same organism in the case of septic emboli to the lung (see Fig. 76-2).

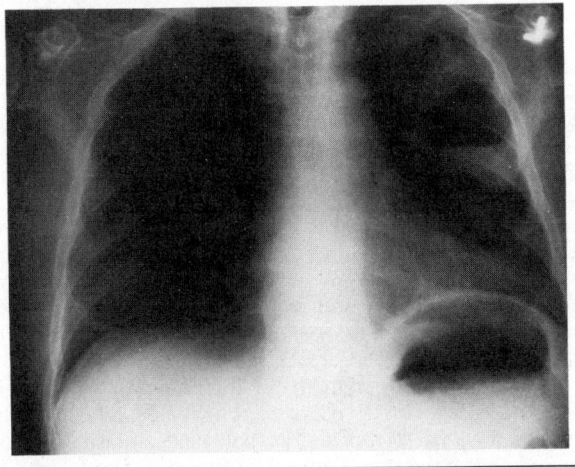

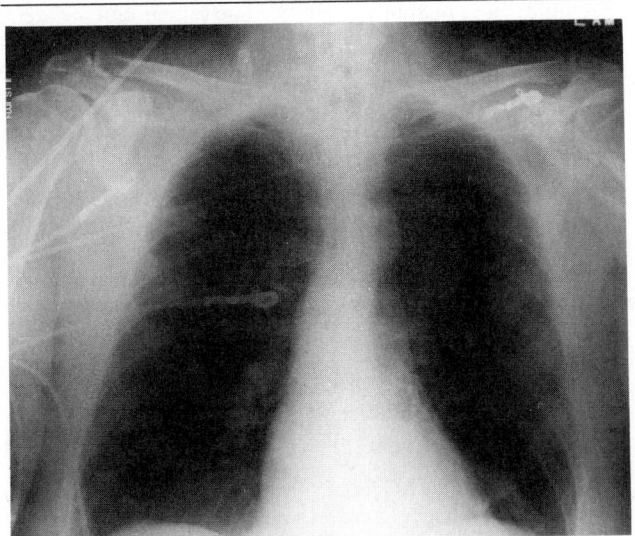

A

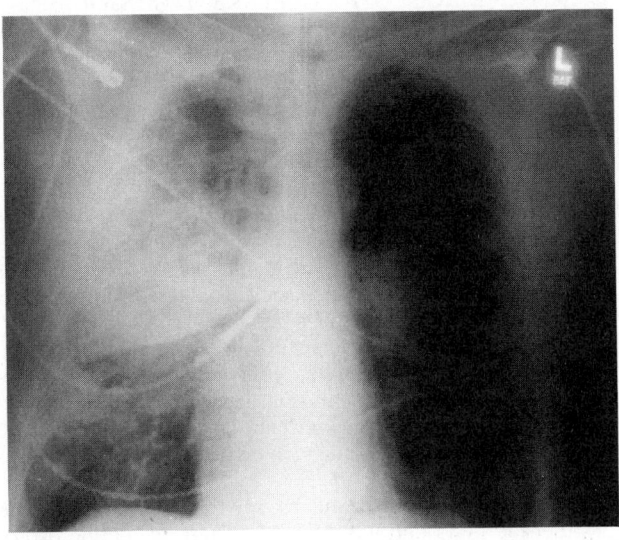

B

Fig. 76-5. This 71-year-old man with chronic obstructive lung disease was being treated with mechanical ventilation, bronchodilators, and corticosteroids for 2 weeks when he developed a fever to 38.2°C, purulent sputum, and a new right upper lobe infiltrate (A). In spite of appropriate antibiotic therapy, 24 hours later his infiltrate had rapidly progressed (B) to involve the entire right lung and the patient died from overwhelming infection. Sputum cultures revealed *P. aeruginosa*.

ease, pleural effusion, lung collapse, and cavitation were common enough in those with pneumococcal infection, Legionnaire's disease, and *Mycoplasma* infection that the radiograph could not be used to determine the responsible pathogen [84].

Sputum Examination. An in-depth discussion on methods of sampling the lower respiratory tract can be found in Chapter 13. Although Gram stain of the sputum has been the traditional first step in evaluation of patients with suspected pneumonia, this is problematic in the critically ill. A specimen may be unavailable if the patient is too weak to generate the pressure necessary to expectorate. When a specimen is obtained, interpretation is dependent on the quality of the sample and the criteria used to define a "positive" sample. In fact, the ability of a sputum Gram stain to predict the recovery of pneumococcus from sputum culture varies widely depending on the criteria [95]. Although no studies correlate Gram stain findings to alveolar cultures in patients with pneumonia, the goal is to evaluate respiratory secretions from deep in the lower airway, and the specimen should have more than 25 polymorphonuclear cells and less than 10 epithelial cells per low-power field. When such criteria are met and intracellular organisms are identified, a bacterial density above 10^5 colony forming units per milliliter of secretions is present [96]. These findings suggest the presence of pneumonia, but the Gram stain may be positive in the presence of bronchitis or with airway colonization. The presence of elastin fibers on potassium hydroxide staining along with positive Gram stain is more suggestive of pneumonia than airway infection or colonization [97]. In addition to not always distinguishing airway colonization from pneumonia, the sputum Gram stain may be falsely negative in up to 50 percent of cases when compared with blood cultures [98,99]. Despite these limitations, sputum may be the only material available to provide rapid information in a critically ill patient, but the interpretation should be cautious. Some findings in sputum may be useful. For example, an inflammatory Gram stain (PMNs) without organisms in a patient with pneumonia suggests evidence of a *Legionella* or *Mycoplasma* infection or viral cause [100]. The use of special stains for tuberculosis and silver or Giemsa staining for PCP may provide definitive evidence of these organisms. Monoclonal antibodies and genetic probes may improve both the sensitivity and specificity of sputum analysis in the near future, but the clinical utility of these methods must be verified.

Culture. Definitive diagnosis that pneumonia is the result of a specific pathogen can be obtained only if cultures of blood, pleural fluid, or spinal fluid are positive in the presence of a lung infiltrate and a compatible clinical picture. Bacteremia is uncommon in most pneumonias, however, usually occurring in less than 20 percent of pneumococcal infections and in only 8 to 15 percent of nosocomial pneumonias [28]. Expectorated or suctioned sputum can be cultured, but results are difficult to interpret because of the problem in separating infection from colonization in the critically ill. In one study of bacteremic nosocomial pneumonia, sputum culture yielded both false positive and false negative findings when compared with blood cultures, with only 49 percent of cases having the same organism recovered from both blood and sputum. In 23 percent of cases no pathogen was found in the sputum and in 28 percent of cases organisms not present in the blood were isolated from sputum [28]. The false positive findings in sputum cultures relate to the high rates of colonization in patients with many acute and chronic diseases, such as general surgery, intubation, alcoholism, diabetes, chronic bronchitis, and advanced age [45]. Oropharyngeal colonization with potential pathogens may be expected in approximately 50 percent of critically ill patients within 4 days of hospitalization [51].

Viruses may be cultured from respiratory secretions, but this procedure may take up to 20 days depending on the virus. Thus, cytologic evidence of viral infection, which can be recognized sooner, may provide helpful information. For example, inclusion bodies and multinucleated giant cells are suggestive of cytomegalovirus (CMV) or herpesvirus infection. Culture of *M. tuberculosis* (TB) or nocardia from respiratory secretions is unlikely to represent colonization, but results are frequently obtained long after clinical decisions have been made.

INVASIVE DIAGNOSTIC CULTURE TECHNIQUES. Because of the inherent problems with expectorated sputum, techniques that bypass the upper airway have been devised. Transtracheal aspiration involves the aspiration of secretions via cricothyroid puncture through a catheter. While the technique has few false negatives, false positives exceed 20 percent; therefore it has limited value in patients with preexisting colonization and is not widely employed (see Chap. 13) [74].

The use of percutaneous needle aspiration of the lung in an area of infiltrate permits direct collection of respiratory secretions from the radiologically identified site of infection. This technique is limited by a high incidence of false negative results in some series and an unacceptable complication rate in debilitated patients. These include pneumothorax in up to 30 percent of patients and a 10 percent rate of hemoptysis [98]. This procedure is particularly dangerous in patients with bullous lung disease and those receiving mechanical ventilation and is most useful in a pediatric population where less invasive techniques cannot be used.

The role of fiberoptic bronchoscopy has expanded over the past decade. Although we do not recommend routine use of this semi-invasive procedure, it is the technique of choice in perplexing infection in the critically ill, particularly in those who are immunosuppressed or who already have an endotracheal tube in place [33,88,101,102,103]. There has been a resurgence of interest in using the bronchoscopically directed protected specimen brush and bronchoalveolar lavage to aid in the diagnosis of nosocomial pneumonia in the mechanically ventilated patient, where clinical criteria of infection have proved oversensitive and inaccurate. Chastre et al. showed that the protected specimen brush (PSB), when cultured quantitatively, can give an accurate estimate of the numbers and types of bacteria present in lung tissue [101]. They suggested that by using this technique, patients with pneumonia will have greater than 10^3 organisms per milliliter of respiratory secretions The accuracy of bronchoscopic diagnosis of bacterial pneumonia using the PSB has not been firmly established (see Chaps. 12 and 13). Other investigators have advocated the use of quantitative culture applied to bronchoalveolar lavage to determine whether pneumonia is present, but this method has not proved useful in the hands of all investigators [103,104]. In some studies, lower airway cells recovered by lavage have been examined for the presence of intracellular organisms; the finding of more than 25 percent of cells with intracellular bacteria has been proposed as a rapid, accurate method to predict the results of PSB culture and to diagnose pneumonia [104]. Whether this method will prove useful is unclear, but most investigators agree that the technique of bronchoalveolar lavage is of greatest value in establishing a nonbacterial cause of infection, especially in the immunocompromised host or the patient with AIDS, where it can reliably diagnose PCP pneumonia, and CMV infection [105].

Although there is no question that clinical diagnosis of pneumonia is fraught with problems, there are few data to suggest that invasive methods for diagnosis of pneumonia can solve these problems [106]. There is no agreement as to which invasive method is most accurate or what criteria should define a "positive" test. The technique of PSB cannot reliably distinguish airway infection from parenchymal lung infection, and all invasive methods have a high rate of false negative findings if the patient is receiving antibiotics at the time of testing [103,106]. Most important, no data exist to show that patient outcome is improved if invasive methods are used in place of clinical diagnosis when managing patients. Data from PSB studies show that antibiotics rapidly sterilize the lung of patients with ventilator-associated pneumonia; these methods may help define the appropriate duration of therapy for this infection [107]. For example, these methods might be especially useful for identifying patients with infection and a small burden of organisms (i.e., early infection), and possibly this population, once identified, could be successfully treated with a shortened duration of antibiotic therapy.

The use of open lung biopsy is the unequivocal standard for the diagnosis of infection; it has been applied primarily in the immunocompromised host. This technique may be expected to provide a diagnosis of infection in those with rapidly advancing, life-threatening infections. *Aspergillus*, CMV, *H. simplex*, and toxoplasmosis are more readily diagnosed by open lung biopsy than by other described techniques. Several studies have suggested that the potential for demonstrating a treatable infection that will alter outcome is low [108]; therefore we recommend extremely judicious use in selected patients (Table 76-7). (See Chap. 77 on lung biopsy for further discussion.)

DIFFERENTIAL DIAGNOSIS. In the differential diagnosis of pneumonia two major questions must be answered: (1) Is pneumonia responsible for the constellation of symptoms and signs being evaluated? (2) What is the etiologic nature of the pneumonia? The decision about whether pneumonia is present is often complicated by the nonspecificity of many of the signs and symptoms of pneumonia. Fever, respiratory distress, pleuritic chest pain, and radiologic infiltrates may accompany acute pulmonary embolism or atelectasis, as well as infectious pneumonia. Bilateral lung infiltrates can be seen with cardiogenic pulmonary edema as well as with viral or *Legionella* and *Chlamydia* pneumonia. Because cardiogenic pulmonary edema is often overdiagnosed in the critically ill, we recommend measurement of pulmonary capillary wedge pressure using a flow-directed pulmonary artery catheter when there is uncertainty [109].

Table 76-7. Diagnostic Techniques in Pneumonia

Test	Advantages	Disadvantages
Expectorated sputum Gram stain	Easy to perform, rapidly available, inexpensive	High false positive and false negative rates
Expectorated sputum culture	Easy to obtain	High false positive and false negative rates
Blood culture	High specificity	Low sensitivity
Transtracheal aspiration	Less contamination than expectorated sputum	High false positive rates in colonized patient, bleeding
Needle aspiration (percutaneous)	High specificity, useful for children and malignancy	High risk of pneumothorax, especially in COPD and ventilated patients
Bronchoscopy (protected brush, BAL)	Low morbidity and mortality, useful in ventilated patients and for nonbacteriologic diagnosis, useful in compromised host	Invasive, requires special training, less useful in patient already on antibiotics, unproven sensitivity, unproven to improve outcome
Open lung biopsy	Excellent for nonbacterial diagnosis and in compromised host	Most invasive, critically ill may not be able to undergo procedure, may not change prognosis

An increasingly common problem is the differentiation of acute infectious pneumonia from drug-induced pneumonitis. This is particularly difficult in the immunocompromised host receiving chemotherapy. While no clear guidelines exist, the use of agents commonly known to produce lung toxicity (e.g., bleomycin, busulfan, and methotrexate in the appropriate dosage range) should raise this possibility; and bronchoscopic or open lung biopsy is sometimes necessary to make such a diagnosis. Eosinophilia is an important clue to the diagnosis of methotrexate toxicity. Amiodarone, increasingly used for refractory arrhythmias, may produce a syndrome indistinguishable from acute infectious pneumonia. Unlike the diffuse infiltrates seen with chemotherapeutic agents, amiodarone frequently produces focal changes on chest radiographs and occasionally pleural effusion [110]. This diagnosis should be suspected in patients who have received more than 400 mg per day and who have a history of a subacute pneumonia. While there are no characteristic laboratory findings, patients tend to have low or declining diffusing capacity, and lipid-laden cells may be present in bronchoalveolar lavage, although this finding is a nonspecific consequence of amiodarone use.

The likely etiologic agent is suggested by historical information, physical findings, and chest radiograph. In addition, culture material can be evaluated to confirm the epidemiologic impression of the likely pathogen. For patients with nosocomial pneumonia, the sputum culture, especially in an intubated patient, is likely to contain the likely etiologic pathogen(s), and antibiotic therapy should be modified to account for these data. Identifying the etiologic pathogen in nonintubated patients, especially those with CAP, is more problematic. Given the difficulties associated with using clinical features to predict microbial etiology and the limitations of extensive diagnostic testing in patients with CAP, one proposed approach is to select an empiric therapy regimen based on three simple clinical assessments: whether the patient will be treated in or out of the hospital; whether the patient has mild, moderate, or severe pneumonia; and whether the patient is elderly (> age 65) or whether comorbidity is present [79]. These assessments can lead to a list of likely etiologic pathogens and which can be used to select appropriate antimicrobial therapy.

In addition to the immune abnormalities associated with common medical illnesses, there are specific immune impairments related to an underlying disease (usually malignancy) or as a result of medical therapy (typically chemotherapy); these patients are identified as immunocompromised hosts (ICH). This category includes AIDS. When these patients are in the ICU, a new lung infiltrate may represent infection, progression of the underlying primary disease, or drug-induced lung disease. As in all patients, the nature of the immune impairment determines which pathogens are most likely. Those with neutropenia from chemotherapy may be infected with gram-negative bacilli or *Aspergillus* sp. Patients with abnormal T cell function (lymphoma or AIDS) may be infected with intracellular bacteria, such as *Listeria monocytogenes, Legionella, Mycobacterium avium,* and tuberculosis; fungi, such as *Cryptococcus neoformans* or *Coccidioides immitis*; viruses, such as cytomegalovirus; and parasites, such as *Toxoplasma gondii* or *P. carinii* [111,112]. While *P. carinii* is a frequent cause of rapidly progressive hypoxic respiratory failure in the patient with AIDS, a similar picture may be seen with tuberculosis (TB). Recent data suggest that TB is poorly recognized in the ICU [113] and should be considered in patients with a history of inadequately treated TB or radiographic evidence of previous infection. Corticosteroid therapy in doses above 20 mg per day also increases the likelihood of *P. carinii* infection (especially during dosage reduction) as well as opportunistic fungi. Recent reports have stressed the occurrence of invasive *Aspergillus* in chronic obstructive pulmonary disease (COPD) patients receiving high-dose steroid therapy for exacerbations of COPD [83,114]. Patients with B cell-specific problems, such as multiple myeloma, are particularly prone to pneumonia with encapsulated organisms, including pneumococcus and *H. influenzae*. A similar organism profile can be seen in the splenectomized patient and in those with complement defects.

Therapy

SUPPORTIVE THERAPY. Supportive therapy for pneumonia in the critically ill is crucial, since antibiotics may not alter outcome during the first 24 hours of treatment. Many of the commonly applied measures are based on traditional practice, with little documentation of efficacy.

Nutritional Therapy. Evidence implicating malnutrition as a cofactor in pneumonia is substantial [9,43,44,77]; the specific host defense impairments related to malnutrition have been discussed (Table 76-2). Evidence that nutritional intervention alters the outcome of severe pneumonia is lacking. Catabolic stress may be expected in septic syndrome and has been related to progressive multiorgan failure if the patient survives the acute phase of critical illness [115]. We recommend nutritional evaluation and support early in the course of pneumonia. Enteral nutrition is preferred, if it can be practically accomplished, as recent data have suggested better preservation of immune function using this route compared with total parenteral nutrition [116]. When enteral feedings are given, a small-bore tube, preferably placed in the jejunum, and a continuous infusion method should be used. Large-bore tubes placed in the stomach with bolus feeding have been associated with an increased risk of aspiration [117]. If gastric feeding is chosen, several issues should be considered. In one study, patient positioning played a vital role in allowing gastric organisms to reflux into the oropharynx and be aspirated into the lung; thus patients getting gastric feeding should be kept semierect, and not supine, as much as possible [64]. In addition, if continuous feeding is being used the gastric pH should be monitored, because patients with high morning pH (>3.5) may have an enhanced risk of pneumonia [71]. If continuous feeding leads to an elevated gastric pH, the feedings should be turned off overnight to allow the stomach to restore a normal pH. Another recently described appoach to this problem uses acidified enteral feedings, but the efficacy of this approach has not been established [118].

Chest Physiotherapy. This modality, long a mainstay of therapy in the management of pneumonia, is based on the assumption that physiotherapy techniques can enhance removal of excessively viscid secretions from the bronchial tree and that such removal will positively affect the outcome of acute pneumonia. However, there is little support for the routine application of these techniques in patients who have an effective cough and scant amounts of respiratory secretions. Such maneuvers have the potential to worsen hypoxemia and mucociliary clearance when applied to routine pneumonia and have not been demonstrated to affect duration of hospitalization [119,120]. Because of the labor-intensive nature of this intervention, techniques such as percussion, vibration, and postural drainage should be specifically targeted at patients with large volumes of purulent secretions (> 30 ml/day) and an ineffective cough. Candidates for this therapy include those with pneumonia along with chronic bronchitis, bronchiectasis, cystic fibrosis, and diseases associated with respiratory muscle weakness or neurologic impairment. In patients at bed rest in the

ICU, the use of positioning and rotation may be helpful in clearing secretions [121,122,123]. In several studies, particularly in surgical trauma patients, the use of beds that rotate patients from side to side, and presumably accelerate mucus clearance, led to a reduced incidence of pneumonia [121,122].

Aerosols and Humidification. Humidification has traditionally been used in respiratory therapy to reduce sputum viscosity and promote mucociliary clearance [124]. Because the deposition of water vapor is dependent on particle size and degree of airway obstruction, however, it is likely that most such aerosols are deposited above the glottis and act only to stimulate cough. Although mucolytic agents such as acetylcysteine offer the theoretic benefit of reducing the viscosity of purulent secretions, they may act as irritants that can provoke bronchospasm and thus must be used selectively. Bronchodilator therapy with beta$_2$ agents can enhance mucociliary clearance and ciliary beat frequency [125], but no controlled trials have demonstrated improved outcome with their use in pneumonia in the absence of underlying bronchospasm. The greatest benefit of bronchodilator therapy may be expected in the patient with COPD who develops pneumonia. Intermittent positive pressure breathing (IPPB) offers no advantage for delivery of aerosolized medication, but it may be used to reduce atelectasis in patients with neuromuscular disease.

ANTIBIOTIC THERAPY. When a specific etiologic pathogen has been identified, antibiotic therapy with a narrow and focused regimen can be employed. Because of the many problems associated with the diagnosis of pneumonia, however, this is an unusual circumstance, occurring in less than 20 percent of patients who have a definitive culture result from material such as blood or pleural fluid. In most patients, the clinical history, chest radiograph, and epidemiologic assessment narrow the etiologic possibilities, but still a broad and "empiric" antibiotic regimen must be applied. Such a therapeutic approach necessarily requires more drugs, some of which may have a risk of toxicity, than if a specific organism is identified. Nonetheless, a broad-spectrum single antibiotic or combination antibiotic regimen may be necessary because of the uncertain cause and the possibility that the pneumonia may be caused by multiple organisms simultaneously. Such polymicrobial infections are common in the case of nosocomial pneumonia in patients treated with mechanical ventilation.

Community-Acquired Pneumonia. When pneumonia leads to admission to the hospital or the ICU, initial therapy should be empiric and broad-spectrum, with the choice of agents guided by the severity of the illness (which, as mentioned, can have a relationship to the etiologic pathogen), the type and extent of comorbidity present, and patient age [79]. The use of clinical syndromes to guide therapy is often inaccurate and not recommended.

If the patient has a severe pneumonia requiring hospitalization but not intensive care, then the infection is likely due to pneumococcus, *H. influenzae,* anaerobic organisms, aerobic gram-negative bacilli, and possibly *Legionella.* Other pathogens, including respiratory viruses and *S. aureus,* are possible but less likely. This type of patient should be treated with either a second-generation cephalosporin (e.g., cefuroxime), a nonpseudomonal third-generation cephalosporin (e.g., cefotaxime or ceftriaxone), or a beta lactam–beta lactamase inhibitor combination (e.g., ampicillin-sulbactam). If atypical pathogens or *Legionella* are a real concern, then a macrolide should be added to this regimen. If the patient is ill enough for admission to the ICU, then, in addition to targeting the previously mentioned

pathogens, therapy should be directed at *Legionella,* a common cause of severe CAP. If the patient has structural lung disease (bronchiectasis), has received antibiotics recently, or is taking corticosteroids, then *P. aeruginosa* should be empirically treated. Thus, therapy should include a macrolide (initially 4 gm/day of erythromycin) plus an agent that is active against *H. influenzae* and enteric gram-negative bacteria, with some anaerobic coverage. If *Legionella* is documented, rifampin (600 mg daily) can be added. In certain situations, an antipseudomonal agent is required. Effective antimicrobials for this type of patient with severe CAP, in combination with a macrolide, include the third-generation cephalosporins ceftazidime or cefoperazone; other beta-lacatams, such as aztreonam or imipenem; the aminoglycosides; and the quinolone ciprofloxacin.

Occasionally these broad empiric approaches should be modified , particularly if culture data lead to the diagnosis of a specific organism or if deep respiratory tract secretion culture reveals an organism not included in the initial regimen (e.g., *S. aureus*). In addition, certain comorbidities predispose to specific pathogens, and these should be covered by any empiric regimen (Table 76-3). Thus, those with recent influenza should be treated for pneumococcus, *S. aureus,* and *H. influenzae,* whereas those with chronic obstructive lung disease should be treated for *H. influenzae* and·*Moraxella catarrhalis* (*Branhamella catarrhalis*).

Antimicrobial resistance to traditional antibiotics has become a problem with some of the common CAP pathogens. Pneumococcus resistant to penicillin (> 0.1 µg/ml) may account for up to 5 percent of clinical isolates in the United States and is more common in immunocompromised patients and those who have previously received beta-lactam antibiotics [126]. If resistant pneumococcus is present, therapy should be initiated with vancomycin, cefotaxime, ceftriaxone, or imipenem. Erythromycin, tetracyclines, quinolones, and clindamycin are not always reliable in the setting of resistant pneumococcus. *H. influenzae* is also becoming increasingly resistant to common antimicrobials because of the production of beta-lactamases; these organisms can be treated with second- or third-generation cephalosporins, trimethoprim-sulfamethoxazole, or ampicillin-sulbactam. *M. catarrhalis* can also produce beta lactamases; the previously mentioned antimicrobials are active against this organism as well.

Pneumonia in the Hospitalized Patient. Although gram-negative bacterial infection is the most common cause of nosocomial pneumonia, in the impaired host opportunistic fungi and mycobacterial infections are also possible. Defining the underlying disease that predisposed to pneumonia helps narrow the likely possibilities. In addition, the patterns of bacteria found in the hospital and the recent history of antibiotic use in the patient should be considered.

Frequently no specific diagnosis can be made during the earliest phases of illness and empiric therapy is initiated. A variety of antibiotic regimens have been advocated, but several general principles apply. First, antibiotic coverage in the critically ill must include enteric gram-negative organisms, including highly resistant organisms such as *P. aeruginosa, Serratia marcesens,* acinetobacter, and *S. aureus.* In some hospitals with high rates of methicillin-resistant *S. aureus,* vancomycin must be added. When the patient is seriously ill or bacteremic due to *K. pneumoniae* or *P. aeruginosa,* the regimen should contain at least two antibiotics that are active against these organisms. A beta-lactam antibiotic (third-generation cephalosporin such as ceftazidime or cefoperazone; or semisynthetic penicillin such as piperacillin or mezlocillin), along with an aminoglycoside, has been considered the standard regimen for these bacteria. Combination therapy reduces the possibility of emerging resistance during treatment, and many studies have demonstrated that combination therapy with an aminoglycoside-containing regimen is superior to single drug therapy, especially when *P. aeruginosa* is a potential pathogen or when bacteremia with this organism is present [127,128]. In vitro data suggest that two antipseudomonal antibiotics provide better intrapulmonary killing than a regimen including one effective drug only. In nonbacteremic, nonneutropenic patients the second agent can be dropped only in the absence of *P. aeruginosa* and after a clinical response has occurred. Therapy is usually continued for 2 to 3 weeks, longer if the course has been complicated by abscess or empyema.

Several newly available antibiotics hold promise in the treatment of nosocomial pneumonia. The monobactam aztreonam has a spectrum similar to that of the aminoglycosides and has proved effective in the therapy of gram-negative lower respiratory tract infections, with much less toxicity [129]. Despite limited experience with this agent in the critically ill, it may be considered an alternative to aminoglycosides in combination regimens aimed at gram-negative bacteria, especially in patients at high risk for aminoglycoside toxicity. Imipenem-cilastatin, the first of a new class of carbapenem antibiotics, has the broadest activity of any single agent, including most gram-positive and gram-negative aerobes as well as anaerobic bacteria. Although imipenem may be useful in the initial empiric therapy of pneumonia in the ICU, recent reports have shown that *P. aeruginosa* may be initially sensitive to this drug but then develop resistance during therapy if this agent is used alone [130]. Fluoroquinolones (ciprofloxacin, ofloxacin) provide effective therapy in community- and hospital-acquired lower respiratory infections, although activity against pneumococcus is only moderate and treatment failures with this organism have been reported [131]. Although experience is limited, ciprofloxacin appears to be useful against most gram-negative bacteria in the ICU and penetrates well into respiratory secretions.

While combination therapy has been considered the standard approach to nosocomial pneumonia, there is increasing evidence that in some situations monotherapy with a broad-spectrum antimicrobial is safe and effective. Monotherapy has been successful with regimens of aztreonam, cefoperazone, ceftazidime, imipenem, and ciprofloxacin [132,133]. In spite of these encouraging data, there are circumstances when monotherapy should not be used and combination therapy is required. These include situations where infection with both *S. aureus* and *P. aeruginosa* is suspected (no single agent covers both organisms adequately) and suspected infection (bacteremic and nonbacteremic) with *P. aeruginosa*.

The traditional combination regimen for therapy of *P. aeruginosa* involves a beta-lactam and an aminoglycoside, but other alternatives are possible. Dual beta-lactam coverage could be used, but there would be no anti-bacterial synergy and there is the possibility of one beta-lactam inducing resistance to both agents. Another alternative is to use a beta-lactam with an antipseudomonal quinolone (e.g., ciprofloxacin). Although this regimen may not be synergistic, the two antibiotics would have different mechanisms of inducing resistance. In addition, one of the potential limitations of aminoglycosides is poor penetration into respiratory secretions; quinolones avoid this problem by providing excellent levels in respiratory secretions. When anti-pseudomonal therapy is chosen, it can include the penicillins (piperacillin, azlocillin, mezlocillin, ticarcillin, carbenicillin), which should not be used as monotherapy; the third-generation cephalosporins ceftazidime and cefoperazone; aztreonam and imipenem, which are beta-lactams; the quinolone ciprofloxacin; and the aminoglycosides, which include gentamicin, tobramycin, and amikacin.

The role of aminoglycosides remains problematic because

they achieve only 40 percent of the serum concentration in respiratory secretions. In addition, there is concern about the high incidence of complicating renal dysfunction (especially in the elderly) and concern about these drugs being less active at the low pH levels that may predominate in areas of pneumonia. Because of these factors and the finding that aminoglycosides lead to a better outcome from pneumonia if serum levels are at least 6 µg per milliliter (gentamicin or tobramycin), it is often necessary to use doses that border on toxicity [134]. To overcome this problem, two approaches have emerged. One involves the use of these agents intravenously in a once daily dosing regimen. This approach takes advantage of the postantibiotic effect of aminoglycosides in an effort to enhance efficacy, while reducing the need for monitoring serum levels and possibly reducing the incidence of toxicity [135]. This interesting approach requires validation of its putative benefits. Another approach is direct instillation of aminoglycosides into the airway, which can achieve high levels of antibiotic at the site of infection with little risk of systemic absorption and toxicity. The aminoglycosides have been either directly instilled or aerosolized into the lower respiratory tract. When this route of administration is used, pretreatment with bronchodilators may be necessary to avoid therapy-associated bronchospasm. Clinical studies have shown this approach to be effective in cystic fibrosis and severe gram-negative pneumonia [136,137]. We believe this therapy should be used as an adjunct to systemic antibiotics in patients with severe gram-negative pneumonias who do not respond to intravenous therapy or those infected by a relatively resistant organism that might be eliminated with high local concentrations of drug.

When antibiotics are used in the critically ill, certain precautions are necessary. Since most drugs are eliminated by the liver or kidney, dosage adjustment may be needed when these organs malfunction. Renally excreted drugs include the aminoglycosides, certain cephalosporins, and penicillins. Drugs removed by the liver include erythromycin, cefoperazone, and nafcillin. In patients with a reduction in lean body mass and an increase in fat (e.g., the elderly), drug levels may rise if chosen on a per kilogram basis. In those with reduced serum albumin, free drug concentrations may rise if the antibiotic is normally highly bound to proteins. The sodium content of many drugs, especially the penicillins, may be important in patients with renal or cardiac failure.

Passive immunization using either antibodies to the lipopolysaccharide (endotoxin) of the gram-negative bacterial cell wall or hyperimmune globulin against *P. aeruginosa* cell wall antigens could theoretically be used for therapy of gram-negative pneumonia, but clinical trials in patients with sepsis have shown no mortality benefit, in spite of initially encouraging reports [138,139,140]. Further clinical studies are necessary to evaluate whether immunologic adjuncts can improve the outcome of patients with severe nosocomial respiratory tract infections.

Strategies for Prevention of Pneumonia

COMMUNITY-ACQUIRED PNEUMONIA. Preventive strategies aimed at reducing either the incidence or the severity of pneumonia can be divided into those applied in the outpatient (prehospital) setting and those applied in the hospital and critical care unit. Outpatient measures proved to reduce the incidence of severe lower respiratory tract infection are immunization against pneumococcal and influenza infection in susceptible populations [141]. These measures, although effective and relatively safe, are out of the usual realm of the ICU. In the case of pneumococcal vaccine, a randomized study demonstrated no significant efficacy in a group of patients with serious coexisting chronic illnesses [142]. Other studies have shown efficacy of the vaccine in less ill populations, however, and in the absence of any proven side effects we still recommend the vaccine to all patients at risk [143]. In fact, one recent study suggested that the vaccine is most effective, and its protection lasts longest, if it is given to patients younger than age 55, particularly when these patients are compared to patients who are vaccinated after age 85 [144]. Hospital-based immunization programs represent one strategy for prevention of pneumonia that can be applied to inpatients. This approach capitalizes on the observation that many hospitalized patients have indications for pneumococcal vaccine and that most patients who ultimately develop pneumonia have been hospitalized in the preceding 4 years [145].

Annual influenza vaccination has reduced the frequency and severity of influenza in the elderly and chronically ill, although there are numerous reports of institutional outbreaks in spite of vaccination [146]. Vaccination of medical personnel may reduce nosocomial transmission of influenza from staff to patients, and annual influenza vaccination is recommended for ICU staff. Antibiotic prophylaxis may be an adjunct to immunization. Amantadine chemoprophylaxis is 70 to 90 percent effective in avoiding infections with influenza A and can be initiated in high-risk individuals at the earliest recognition of an outbreak. A controlled trial of amantadine prophylaxis demonstrated substantial reduction in nosocomial attack rates [146]. The dosage recommended for prophylaxis is 100 to 200 mg per day, not to exceed 100 mg per day in those older than 65 years.

The patient with chronic obstructive lung disease is at high risk for complicated pneumonia, and it has been suggested that antibiotic therapy of bronchitic exacerbations could minimize this complication. Although prophylactic use of antibiotics is of unproved value, therapy of exacerbations may be useful, particularly because these exacerbations are accompanied by a high bacterial burden in the lung [147,148]. Although Nicotra et al. were unable to show improvement in hospitalized COPD patients treated with antibiotics for acute exacerbation [149], antibiotic therapy is recommended for exacerbations of obstructive lung disease requiring admission to the ICU. Choices of therapy are based on local practice and usually include trimethoprim-sulfamethoxazole, tetracycline, or amoxicillin.

NOSOCOMIAL PNEUMONIA. In the ICU, several general strategies may be employed to reduce the incidence of pneumonia (Table 76-8).

Environmental Control. The SENIC study suggested that effective infection control and surveillance programs could potentially reduce the rate of nosocomial pneumonia by 20 percent [150]. Emphasis has been placed on measures designed to reduce colonization in the patient's environment, many of them common-sense measures that do not require specific documentation of efficacy. Handwashing, although simple and effective in reducing the spread of resistant organisms, is frequently neglected in the ICU. Attention should also be directed at respiratory therapy equipment, as it may frequently be colonized with pathogenic bacteria. Proper disinfection of nebulization equipment after each use, as well as the use of cascade humidifiers that do not generate significant contaminated aerosols, has reduced the formerly important role of these devices as a source of nosocomial pneumonia. The use of a heat moisture exchanger in the ventilator circuit, which eliminates the

Table 76-8. Preventive Strategies Available in ICU Pneumonia

Colonization
  Environmental control
    (hand washing, respiratory therapy equipment)
Aspiration avoidance
  Reduce use of nasogastric tubes
  Avoid CNS depressants
  Aspiration of secretions that collect above intratracheal balloon of endotracheal tube
Host defense fortification
  Nutritional support
  Avoid immunosuppressants
  Influenza and pneumococcal vaccine
  Amantadine prophylaxis (influenza A)
  Antibiotic prophylaxis in COPD
Potentially useful measures
  Topical antibiotics
  "Selective decontamination"—oropharynx and GI tract
  Preserve normal gastric pH
  Active and passive immunization against groups of potential pathogens
  Measures to reduce bacterial adherence by altering microenvironment by
    Altering airway pH
    Receptor or adhesin analogues
    Alter secretion of mucins and proteases

need for cascade humidification, may also be effective. Ventilator circuit changes should be made no more often than every 48 hours; more frequent changes and manipulations may actually add to the risk of infection [7,57]. One recent study found no increased risk of infection if tubing was never changed [151]. Trauma to the airways during suctioning may predispose to infection; thus careful sterile suctioning techniques should be employed. The role of the closed suctioning system in either preventing or promoting pneumonia is unclear.

Prophylactic Antibiotics. Numerous studies have documented the efficacy of topical antibiotics applied to the lower airway in preventing nosocomial pneumonia in the ICU. However, these studies, done in the early 1970s, showed that this approach was associated with the emergence of resistant bacteria that could themselves cause fatal pneumonia; thus the strategy was deemed unsafe and abandoned [152]. The studies used either polymyxin B or aminoglycosides, but several methodologic problems existed and this type of prophylaxis is being reconsidered [141]. In the future, this strategy might be applied selectively to high-risk patients, particularly those on mechanical ventilation, and the therapy could be given with aerosol delivery systems that were unavailable in the past.

More recently, intense interest has been focused on "selective digestive decontamination" (SDD) as a means of preventing nosocomial pneumonia and sepsis [153–157]. This approach attempts to sterilize the intestine and oral cavity of all gram-negatives, under the assumption that the gastrointestinal tract is the source of the organisms that cause pneumonia. Such regimens have included the application of an oral paste containing nonabsorbable antibiotics aimed at gram-negative organisms (polymyxin, tobramycin). An antifungal agent (amphotericin) is included to prevent mycotic overgrowth, and some regimens also include a systemic antibiotic to eliminate any incubating infections present at the time of entry in the ICU. Similar agents are also instilled through a nasogastric tube into the stomach to decontaminate the gastrointestinal tract. Most studies have demonstrated reduced rates of respiratory infection, but not all have shown a reduction of in-hospital mortality. Some of the published studies are unblinded, but one large blinded study involved 445 patients randomized to SDD or placebo [156]. Not only was no reduction in mortality observed, but there was a trend toward the emergence of pneumonia with organisms resistant to the SDD regimen. An American study of SDD also observed the possibility of emergent antibiotic-resistant organisms and no reduction in mortality, despite a reduced incidence in tracheobronchitis (but not pneumonia) [157]. Wide application of this technique does not yet appear to be justified, and questions about efficacy in reducing mortality and avoiding emergence of resistant organisms must be answered. In addition, most series have been weighted toward postoperative and trauma patients, and the efficacy in a general medical population needs further study [153–157].

Immunizations. Early studies suggested some efficacy of active immunization with the lipopolysaccharide antigen of *P. aeruginosa* in lowering the incidence of pneumonia and mortality secondary to this organism [158]; however, side effects and the prolonged time necessary for active immunity to develop have limited its application. In addition, many patients develop pneumonia as a result of host defense failure, and it would be optimistic to think they could effectively respond to a vaccine. In these patients, the use of hyperimmune, preformed antibody against *P. aeruginosa* offers an approach that circumvents these objections [159,160]. Another approach to immunotherapy would encompass protection against a larger number of gram-negative organisms by using antibodies against the core gram-negative antigen lipid A, which is common to most species. Although antibody to the J5 mutant of *Escherichia coli* fits this description, its use for prophylaxis has not been established.

Control of Respiratory Secretions. Stagnation of respiratory secretions can lead to pneumonia and atelectasis, and efforts to remove these secretions could theoretically reduce the incidence of pneumonia. One way to achieve this objective is through the use of continuous lateral rotation delivered by a rotating bed used in place of a traditional hospital bed. This type of therapy could theoretically improve mucociliary clearance, improve ventilation/perfusion balance in the lung, and help mobilize patients. Several studies of trauma and medical patients have shown a reduced incidence of pneumonia (especially early onset infection) when high-risk patients receive this type of therapy [121,122,123]. Another way to control respiratory secretions is to remove oropharyngeal contents before they can be aspirated into the lung. In one study, an endotracheal tube was adapted with a suction port above the endotracheal tube cuff and was designed to remove aspirated secretions [161]. This approach reduced the incidence of pneumonia and delayed the time of onset of infection.

Intestinal Bleeding Prophylaxis. Several clinical studies have documented that neutralization of gastric pH with antacids or histamine type 2 (H-2) blockers can add to the risk of nosocomial pneumonia in patients treated with mechanical ventilation [7,30,65,66,67]. One prospective randomized study showed that when sucralfate was used in place of acid-neutralizing therapy, the rate of bleeding was comparable but the incidence of pneumonia was reduced [67]. As mentioned, these findings may arise from the observation that the stomach can serve as a source of gram-negative bacteria that enter the lung and the number of organisms in this gastric reservoir can increase when gastric pH rises [61,62]. In addition, in vitro data have shown that sucralfate may have direct antibacterial activity against gram-negative bacteria [66]. Based on these data, sucralfate has been used by some institutions in place of antacids or H-2 blocking agents for intestinal bleeding prophylaxis in patients treated with me-

chanical ventilation. We agree that the use of sucralfate should be considered in this setting, but we believe the issue is complex, involving consideration of not only gastric pH but also gastric volume. For this reason, antacids, which increase both gastric pH and volume, may present more of a risk than H-2 blockers, which raise pH but reduce volume. In two meta-analyses of this subject, findings have differed. The two studies agree that antacids are more of a risk for pneumonia than sucralfate, but one study found H-2 blockers to pose no more risk than placebo while the other found these agents to pose a risk themselves [68,69]. The choice of intestinal bleeding prophylaxis should also be made in the context of how enteral feeding is delivered. If enteral feedings are placed in the stomach, they too can raise pH and overcome the influence of any intestinal bleeding prophylaxis on gastric pH [71]. To avoid this problem, feedings can be placed into the jejunum, but then a decision must be made about whether to place a second feeding tube in the stomach to give sucralfate or whether to use H-2 blockers, which may be relatively safe in an otherwise empty stomach. In addition to these considerations, it is important to realize that the need for routine stress bleeding prophylaxis may not be as ubiquitous as once believed, and this type of therapy is not indicated in all ICU patients. Finally, since the stomach is not the source for all gram-negative bacteria that reach the lung, the use of any specific strategy directed only at the gastrointestinal tract cannot be expected to prevent all cases of gram-negative pneumonia.

References

1. Niederman MS: Elimination or propagation of pneumonia in the intensive care unit? A challenge for critical care technology. *J Intensive Care Med* 7:1, 1992.
2. Dixon RE: Economic costs of respiratory tract infections in the United States. *Am J Med* 78:45, 1985.
3. Garibaldi RA: Epidemiology of community-acquired respiratory tract infections in adults: Incidence, etiology, impact. *Am J Med* 78:32, 1985.
4. Garibaldi RA, Britt MR, Coleman ML, et al: Risk factors for postoperative pneumonia. *Am J Med* 70:677, 1981.
5. Bell RC, Coalson JJ, Smith JD, et al: Multi-organ system failure and infection in adult respiratory disease syndrome. *Ann Intern Med* 99:293, 1983.
6. Niederman M, Fein A: The interaction of infection and the adult respiratory distress syndrome. *Crit Care Clin* 2:471, 1986.
7. Craven DE, Kunches LM, Kilinsky V, et al: Risk factors for pneumonia and fatality in patients receiving continuous mechanical ventilation. *Am Rev Respir Dis* 133:792, 1986.
8. Schneider EL: Infectious diseases in the elderly. *Ann Intern Med* 98:395, 1983.
9. Skerrett SJ, Niederman MS, Fein AF: Respiratory infections and acute lung injury in systemic illness. *Clin Chest Med* 10:469, 1989.
10. Torres A, Serra-Batlles J, Ferrer A, et al: Severe community-acquired pneumonia: Epidemiology and prognostic factors. *Am Rev Respir Dis* 144:312, 1991.
11. Pachon J, Prados MD, Capote F, et al: Severe community-acquired pneumonia: Etiology, prognosis, and treatment. *Am Rev Respir Dis* 142:369,1990.
12. Van Eeden SF, Coetzee AR, Joubert JR: Community-acquired pneumonia: Factors influencing intensive care admission. *S Afr Med J* 73:77, 1988.
13. Feldman C, Kallenbach JM, Reinach SG, et al: Community-acquired pneumonia of diverse aetiology: Prognostic features in patients admitted to an intensive care unit and a "severity of illness" score. *Intensive Care Med* 15:302, 1989.
14. Ortqvist A, Sterner G, Nilsson JA: Severe community-acquired pneumonia: Factors influencing need of intensive care treatment and prognosis. *Scand J Infect Dis* 17:377, 1985.

15. Gross PA, Neu HC, Aswapokee P, et al: Deaths from nosocomial infection: Experience in a university hospital and a community hospital. *Am J Med* 68:219, 1980.

16. Gross PA, Van Antwerpen C: Nosocomial infections and hospital deaths: A case-control study. *Am J Med* 75:658, 1983.

17. Seidenfeld JJ, Pohl DF, Bell RD, et al: Incidence, site, and outcome of infections in patients with the adult respiratory distress syndrome. *Am Rev Respir Dis* 134:12, 1986.

18. Fagon JY, Chastre J, Hance A, et al: Nosocomial pneumonia in ventilated patients: A cohort study evaluating attributable mortality and hospital stay. *Am J Med* 94:281, 1993.

19. Austrian R, Gold J: Pneumococcal bacteremia with especial reference to bacteremic pneumococcal pneumonia. *Ann Intern Med* 60:759, 1964.

20. Hook EW, Horton CA, Schaberg DR: Failure of intensive care unit support to influence mortality from pneumococcal bacteremia. *JAMA* 249:1055, 1983.

21. Baumann WR, Jung RC, Koss M, et al: Incidence and mortality of adult respiratory distress syndrome: A prospective analysis from a large metropolitan hospital. *Crit Care Med* 14:1, 1986.

22. Maxfield RA, Sorkin B, Fazzini EP, et al: Respiratory failure in patients with acquired immune deficiency syndrome and *Pneumocystis carinii* pneumonia. *Crit Care Med* 14:443, 1986.

23. Zaroukian MH, Kashyap GH, Wentworth BB: Case report: Respiratory syncytial virus infection—A cause of respiratory distress syndrome and pneumonia in adults. *Am J Med Sci* 295:218, 1988.

24. Fruchtman SM, Gombert ME, Lyons HA: Adult respiratory distress syndrome as a cause of death in pneumococcal pneumonia: Report of ten cases. *Chest* 83:598, 1983.

25. Farr BM, Sloman AJ, Fisch MJ: Predicting death in patients hospitalized for community-acquired pneumonia. *Ann Intern Med* 115:428, 1991.

26. Marrie TJ, Haldane EV, Faulkner RS, et al: Community-acquired pneumonia requiring hospitalization: Is it different in the elderly? *J Am Geriatr Soc* 33:671, 1985.

27. Starczewski AR, Allen SC, Vargas E, et al: Clinical prognostic indices of fatality in elderly patients admitted to hospital with acute pneumonia. *Age Ageing* 17:181, 1988.

28. Bryan CS, Reynolds KL: Bacteremic nosocomial pneumonia: Analysis of 172 episodes from a single metropolitan area. *Am Rev Respir Dis* 129:668, 1984.

29. Cross AS, Roup B: Role of respiratory assistance devices in endemic nosocomial pneumonia. *Am J Med* 70:681, 1981.

30. Niederman MS, Craven DE, Fein AM, et al: Pneumonia in the critically ill hospitalized patient. *Chest* 97:170, 1990.

31. Celis R, Torres A, Gatell JM, et al: Nosocomial pneumonia: A multivariate analysis of risk and prognosis. *Chest* 93:318, 1988.

32. Haley RW, Hooton TM, Culver DH, et al: Nosocomial infections in U.S. hospitals, 1975–1976: Estimated frequency by selected characteristics of patients. *Am J Med* 70:947, 1981.

33. Fagon JY, Chastre J, Domart Y, et al: Nosocomial pneumonia in patients receiving continuous mechanical ventilation: Prospective analysis of 52 episodes with use of a protected specimen brush and quantitative culture techniques. *Am Rev Respir Dis* 139:877, 1989.

34. Joshi N, Localio AR, Hamory B: A predictive risk index for nosocomial pneumonia in the intensive care unit. *Am J Med* 93:135, 1992.

35. Rodriguez JL, Gibbons KJ, Bitzer LG, et al: Pneumonia: incidence, risk factors, and outcome in injured patients. *J Trauma* 31:907, 1991.

36. Rello J, Quintana E, Ausina V, et al: Incidence, etiology, and outcome of nosocomial pneumonia in mechanically ventilated patients. *Chest* 100:439, 1991.

37. Suchyta M, Clemmer T, Elliot G: Adult respiratory distress syndrome: A report of survival and modifying factors. *Chest* 101:1074, 1992.

38. Sloane PJ, Gee MH, Gottlieb JE, et al: A multicenter registry of patients with acute respiratory distress syndrome. *Am Rev Respir Dis* 146:419, 1992.

39. DeCamp MM, Demling RH: Posttraumatic multisystem organ failure. *JAMA* 260:530, 1988.

40. Montgomery AB, Stager MA, Carrico C, et al: Causes of mortality in patients with the adult respiratory distress syndrome. *Am Rev Respir Dis* 132:485, 1985.

41. Carlet J, Hemmer M, Flandre P, et al: Infection and ARDS: A complex interaction: A prospective study of 583 patients. *Am Rev Respir Dis* 139:A270, 1989.

42. Johanson WG, Higuchi JH, Chaudhuri TR, et al: Bacterial adherence to epithelial cells in bacillary colonization of the respiratory tract. *Am Rev Respir Dis* 121:55, 1980.

43. Higuchi JH, Johanson WG: The relationship between adherence of *Pseudomonas aeruginosa* to upper respiratory cells in vitro and susceptibility to colonization in vivo. *J Lab Clin Med* 95:698, 1980.

44. Niederman MS, Merrill WW, Ferranti RD, et al: Nutritional status and bacterial binding in the lower respiratory tract in patients with chronic tracheostomy. *Ann Intern Med* 100:795, 1984.

45. Niederman MS: Gram negative colonization of the respiratory tract: Pathogenesis and clinical consequences. *Semin Respir Infect* 5:173, 1990.

46. Laurenzi GA, Potter RT, Kass EH: Bacteriologic flora of the lower respiratory tract. *N Engl J Med* 265:1273, 1961.

47. Lees AW, McNaught W: Bacteriology of the lower respiratory tract secretions, sputum, and upper respiratory tract secretions in "normals" and chronic bronchitics. *Lancet* 2:1112, 1959.

48. LaForce FM, Mullane JF, Boehme RF, et al: The effect of pulmonary edema on antibacterial defenses of the lung. *J Lab Clin Med* 82:634, 1973.

49. Juers J, Rogers RM, McCurdy JB: Enhancement of bactericidal capacity of alveolar macrophages by human "alveolar lining material." *Clin Res* 23:348, 1975.

50. Rose RM, Pinkston P, O'Donnell C, et al: Viral infection of the lower respiratory tract. *Clin Chest Med* 8:405, 1987.

51. Johanson WG, Pierce AK, Sanford JP: Changing pharyngeal flora of hospitalized patients: Emergence of gram-negative bacilli. *N Engl J Med* 281:1137, 1969.

52. Johanson WG, Pierce AK, Sanford JP, et al: Nosocomial respiratory infections with gram-negative bacilli: The significance of colonization of the respiratory tract. *Ann Intern Med* 77:701, 1972.

53. Ramphal R, Small PM, Shands JW Jr, et al: Adherence of *Pseudomonas aeruginosa* to tracheal cells injured by influenza infection or endo-tracheal intubation. *Infect Immunol* 27:614, 1980.

54. Levine SA, Niederman MS: The impact of tracheal intubation on host defenses and risks for nosocomial pneumonia. *Clin Chest Med* 12:523, 1991.

55. Sottile FD, Marrie TJ, Prough DS, et al: Nosocomial pulmonary infection: Possible etiologic significance of bacterial adhesion to endotracheal tubes. *Crit Care Med* 14:265, 1986.

56. Inglis TJ, Millar MR, Jones G, Robinson DA: Trachel tube biofilm as a source of bacterial colonization of the lung. *J Clin Microbiol* 27:2014, 1989.

57. Craven DE, Goularte TA, Make BJ: Contaminated condensate in mechanical ventilator circuits: A risk factor for nosocomial pneumonia. *Am Rev Respir Dis* 129:625, 1984.

58. Schwartz SN, Dowling JN, Benkovic C, et al: Sources of gram-negative bacilli colonizing the tracheae of intubated patients. *J Infect Dis* 138:227, 1978.

59. Niederman MS, Mantovani R, Schoch P, et al: Patterns and routes of tracheobronchial colonization in mechanically ventilated patients: The role of nutritional status in colonization of the lower airway by *Pseudomonas* species. *Chest* 95:155, 1989.

60. Pingleton SK, Hinthorn DR, Liu C: Enteral nutrition in patients receiving mechanical ventilation: Multiple sources of tracheal colonization include the stomach. *Am J Med* 80:827, 1986.

61. du Moulin GC, Paterson DG, Hedley-Whyte J, et al: Aspiration of gastric bacteria in antacid-treated patients: A frequent cause of post-operative colonization of the airway. *Lancet* 1:242, 1982.

62. Atherton ST, White DJ: Stomach as source of bacteria colonizing respiratory tract during artificial ventilation. *Lancet* 2:968, 1978.

63. Reusser P, Zimmerli W, Scheidegger D, et al: Role of gastric colonization in nosocomial infections and endotoxemia: A prospective study in neurosurgical patients on mechanical ventilation. *J Infect Dis* 160:414, 1989.

64. Torres A, Serra-Batlles J, Ros E, et al: Pulmonary aspiration of gastric contents in patients receiving mechanical ventilation: The effect of body position. *Ann Intern Med* 116:540, 1992.

65. Donowitz GL, Page MC, Mileur BL, et al: Alteration of normal gastric flora in critical care patients receiving antacid and cimetidine therapy. *Infect Control* 7:23, 1986.

66. Tryba M: Risk of acute stress bleeding and nosocomial pneumonia in ventilated intensive care unit patients: Sucralfate versus antacids. *Am J Med* 83(suppl 3B):117, 1987.

67. Driks MR, Craven DE, Celli BR, et al: Nosocomial pneumonia in intubated patients given sucralfate as compared with antacids or histamine type 2 blockers. *N Engl J Med* 317:1376, 1987.

68. Tryba M: Sucralfate versus antacids or H2-antagonists for stress ulcer prophylaxis: A meta-analysis on efficacy and pneumonia rate. *Crit Care Med* 19:942, 1991.

69. Cook DJ, Laine LA, Guyatt GH, Raffin TA: Nosocomial pneumonia and the role of gastric pH: A meta-analysis. *Chest* 100:7, 1991.

70. Martin LF, Booth FV, Karlstadt RG, et al: Continuous intravenous cimetidine decreases stress-related upper gastrointestinal hemorrhage without promoting pneumonia. *Crit Care Med* 21:19, 1993.

71. Jacobs S, Chang R, Lee B, Bartlett FW: Continuous enteral feeding: A major cause of pneumonia among ventilated intensive care unit patients. *J Parenter Enter Nutr* 14:353, 1990.

72. Montecalvo MA, Steger KA, Farber HW, et al: Nutritional outcome and pneumonia in critical care patients randomized to gastric versus jejunal tube feedings. *Crit Care Med* 20:1377, 1992.

73. Palmer LB, Merrill WW, Niederman MS, et al: Bacterial adherence to respiratory tract cells: Relationships between in vivo and in vitro pH and bacterial attachment. *Am Rev Respir Dis* 133:784, 1986.

74. Doig P, Smith NR, Todd T, et al: Characterization of the binding of *Pseudomonas aeruginosa* alginate to human epithelial cells. *Infect Immun* 55:1517, 1987.

75. Grant MM, Niederman MS, Poehlman MA, et al: Mucins in human sputum affect the binding of *Pseudomonas aeruginosa* to cultured tracheal epithelial cells. *Am Rev Respir Dis* 139:A33, 1989.

76. Nelson S, Bagby GJ, Bainton BG, et al: Compartmentalization of intraalveolar and systemic lipopolysaccharide-induced tumor necrosis factor and the pulmonary inflammatory response. *J Infect Dis* 159:189, 1989.

77. Martin TR: The relationship between malnutrition and lung infections. *Clin Chest Med* 8:359, 1987.

78. Bates JH, Campbell GD, Barron AL, et al: Microbial etiology of acute pneumonia in hospitalized patients. *Chest* 101:1005, 1992.

79. Mandell LA, Niederman MS, The Canadian Community Acquired Pneumonia Consensus Group: Antimicrobial treatment of community acquired pneumonia in adults: A conference report. *Can J Infect Dis* 4:25, 1993.

80. Niederman MS, Fein AM: Pneumonia in the elderly. *Geriatr Clin North Am* 2:241, 1986.

81. Verghese A, Berk SL: Bacterial pneumonia in the elderly. *Medicine* 62:271, 1983.

82. Rello J, Ausina V, Castella J, et al: Nosocomial respiratory tract infections in multiple trauma patients: Influence of level of consciousness with implications for therapy. *Chest* 102:525, 1992.

83. Rodrigues, JM, Niederman MS, Fein AM, Pai P: Nonresolving pneumonia in steroid treated patients with obstructive lung disease. *Am J Med* 93:29, 1992.

84. MacFarlane JT, Miller AC, Smith WH, et al: Comparative radiographic features of community acquired Legionnaires' disease, pneumococcal pneumonia, *Mycoplasma* pneumonia, and psittacosis. *Thorax* 39:28, 1984.

85. Fang GD, Fine M, Orloff J, et al: New and emerging etiologies for community-acquired pneumonia with implications for therapy: A prospective multicenter study of 359 cases. *Medicine* 69:307, 1990.

86. Farr BM, Kaiser DL, Harrison BDW, Connolly CK: Prediction of microbial aetiology at admission to hospital for pneumonia from the presenting clinical features. *Thorax* 44:1031, 1989.

87. Gleckman RA, Hibert D: Afebrile bacteremia: A phenomenon in geriatric patients. *JAMA* 248:1478, 1982.

88. Fagon JY, Chastre Y, Hance AJ, et al: Detection of nosocomial lung infection in ventilated patients: Use of a protected specimen brush and quantitative culture technique in 147 patients. *Am Rev Respir Dis* 138:110, 1988.

89. Pugin J, Auckenthaler R, Mili N, et al: Diagnosis of ventilator-associated pneumonia by bacteriology analysis of bronchoscopic and nonbronchoscopic "blind" bronchoalveolar lavage fluid. *Am Rev Respir Dis* 143:1121, 1991.

90. McFadden JP, Price RC, Eastwood HD, et al: Raised respiratory rate in elderly patients: A valuable physical sign. *Br Med J* 1:626, 1982.

91. Atmar RL, Greenberg SB: Pneumonia caused by *Mycoplasma pneumoniae* and TWAR agent. *Semin Respir Infect* 4:19, 1989.

92. Osborne D: Radiologic appearance of viral disease of the lower respiratory tract in infants and children. *Am J Roentgenol* 130:29, 1978.

93. Levine SJ, White DA: *Pneumocystis carinii. Clin Chest Med* 9:395, 1988.

94. Wollschlager CM, Jhan FA, Khan A: Utility of radiography and clinical features in the diagnosis of community acquired pneumonia. *Clin Chest Med* 8:393, 1987.

95. Rein MF, Gwaltney JM Jr, O'Brien WM, et al: Accuracy of Gram's stain in identifying pneumococci in sputum. *JAMA* 239:2671, 1978.

96. Winterbauer RH, Dreis DF: New diagnostic approaches to the hospitalized patient with pneumonia. *Semin Respir Infect* 2:57, 1987.

97. Salata RA, Lederman MM, Shlaes DM, et al: Diagnosis of nosocomial pneumonia in intubated, intensive care unit patients. *Am Rev Respir Dis* 135:426, 1987.

98. Tobin MJ: Diagnosis of pneumonia: Techniques and problems. *Clin Chest Med* 8:513, 1987.

99. Barret-Connor E: The nonvalue of sputum culture in the diagnosis of pneumococcal pneumonia. *Am Rev Respir Dis* 103:845, 1971.

100. Edelstein PH, Meyer RD, Finegold SM: Laboratory diagnosis of Legionnaire's disease. *Am Rev Respir Dis* 121:37, 1980.

101. Chastre J, Viau F, Brun P, et al: Prospective evaluation of the protected specimen brush for the diagnosis of pulmonary infections in ventilated patients. *Am Rev Respir Dis* 130:924, 1984.

102. Torres A, Gonzalez J, Ferrer M: Evaluation of the available invasive and non-invasive techniques for diagnosing nosocomial pneumonia in mechanically ventilated patients. *Intensive Care Med* 17:439, 1991.

103. Meduri GU: Diagnosis of ventilator-associated pneumonia. *Infect Dis Clin North Am* 7:295, 1993.

104. Chastre J, Fagon JY, Soler P, et al: Diagnosis of nosocomial bacterial pneumonia in intubated patients undergoing ventilation: Comparison of the usefulness of bronchoalveolar lavage and the protected specimen brush. *Am J Med* 85:499, 1988.

105. Stover DE, Zaman MB, Hajdu SI, et al: Bronchoalveolar lavage in the diagnosis of diffuse pulmonary infiltrates in the immunosuppressed host. *Ann Intern Med* 101:1, 1984.

106. Niederman MS: Diagnosing nosocomial pneumonia: To brush or not to brush. *J Intensive Care Med* 6:151, 1991.

107. Montravers P, Fagon JY, Chastre J, et al: Follow-up protected specimen brushes to assess treatment in nosocomial pneumonia. *Am Rev Respir Dis* 147:38, 1993.

108. Potter D, Poss HI, Brower S, et al: Prospective randomized study of open lung biopsy versus empirical antibiotic therapy for acute pneumonitis in non-neutropenic cancer patients. *Ann Thorac Surg* 40:422, 1985.

109. Niederman MS, Fein AM, Sklarek H, et al: Pulmonary edema with low pulmonary capillary wedge pressure after acute myocardial infarction: Clinical features and prognostic implications. *J Crit Illness* 4:194, 1989.

110. Vrobel TR, Miller PE, Mostow ND, et al: A general overview of amiodarone toxicity: Its prevention, detection, and management. *Prog Cardiovasc Dis* 6:343, 1989.

111. Rosenow EC, Wilson WR, Cockerill FR: Pulmonary disease in the immunocompromised host. *Mayo Clin Proc* 60:473, 610, 1985.

112. Shelhammer JH, Toews GB, Masur H, et al: Respiratory disease in the immunosuppressed patient. *Ann Intern Med* 117:415, 1992.

113. Heffner JE, Strange C, Sahn SA: Impact of respiratory failure on the diagnosis of tuberculosis. *Arch Intern Med* 148:1103, 1988.

114. Wiest P, Flanigan T, Salata RA: Serious infectious complications of corticosteroid therapy for COPD. *Chest* 95:1180, 1989.

115. Barton R, Cerra F: The hypermetabolism multiple organ failure syndrome. *Chest* 96:1153, 1989.

116. Moore FA, Moore EE, Jones TN, et al: TEN versus TPN following

major abdominal trauma: Reduced septic mortality. *J Trauma* 29:916, 1989.

117. Pingleton SK: Enteral nutrition as a risk factor for nosocomial pneumonia. *Eur J Clin Microbiol Infect Dis* 8:51, 1989.

118. Heyland D, Bradley C, Mandell LA: Effect of acidifed enteral feedings on gastric colonization in the critically ill patient. *Crit Care Med* 20:1388, 1992.

119. Graham WB, Bradley DA: Efficacy of chest physiotherapy and intermittent positive pressure breathing in the resolution of pneumonia. *N Engl J Med* 299:624, 1978.

120. Britton S, Bejstedt M, Vedin L: Chest physiotherapy in primary pneumonia. *Br Med J* 290:1703, 1985.

121. Sahn SA: Continuous lateral rotational therapy and nosocomial pneumonia. *Chest* 99:1263, 1991.

122. Fink MP, Helsmoortel CM, Stein KL, et al: The efficacy of an oscillating bed in the prevention of lower respiratory tract infection in critically ill victims of blunt trauma: A prospective study. *Chest* 97:132, 1990.

123. deBoisblanc BP, Castro M, Everret B, et al: Effect of air-supported, continuous postural oscillation on the risk of early ICU pneumonia in nontraumatic critical illness. *Chest* 103:1543, 1993.

124. Wanner A, Rao A: Clinical indications for and effects of bland, mucolytic and antimicrobial aerosols. *Am Rev Respir Dis* 122:79, 1980.

125. Iravani J, Melville GN: Mucociliary function of the respiratory tract as influenced by drugs. *Respiration* 31:350, 1974.

126. Pallares R, Gudiol F, Linare SJ: Risk factors and response to antibiotic therapy in adults with bacteremic pneumonia caused by penicillin resistant pneumococci. *N Engl J Med* 317:18, 1987.

127. Pennington J: New therapeutic approach to hospital acquired pneumonia. *Semin Respir Infect* 2:67, 1987.

128. Hilf M, Yu VL, Sharp J, et al: Antibiotic therapy for *Pseudomonas aeruginosa* bacteremia: Outcome correlations in a prospective study of 200 patients. *Am J Med* 87:540, 1989.

129. Sobel JD: Imipenem and aztreonam infectious disease. *Med Clin North Am* 3:613, 1989.

130. Acar JF: Therapy for lower respiratory tract infections with Imipenem/Cilastatin: A review of worldwide experience. *Rev Infect Dis* 7(suppl 3):S513, 1985.

131. Nolan PE, Bass JB: New drugs for treating lung infection. *Chest* 94:1076, 1988.

132. Mangi RJ, Ryan J, Thornton G, et al: Cefoperazone vs combination antibiotic therapy of hospital acquired pneumonia. *Am J Med* 84:68, 1988.

133. Salacata A, Chow JW: Cephalosporin therapeutics for intensive care infections. *New Horizons* 1:181, 1993.

134. Moore RD, Smith CR, Lietman PS: Association of aminoglycoside plasma levels with therapeutic outcome in gram negative pneumonia. *Am J Med* 77:657, 1984.

135. Miyagawa CI: Aminoglycosides in the intensive care unit: An old drug in a dynamic environment. *New Horizons* 1:172, 1993.

136. Klastersky J, Hsysman E, Weerts D, et al: Endotracheally administered gentamicin for the prevention of infections of the respiratory tract in patients with tracheostomy: A double-blind study. *Chest* 65:650, 1974.

137. Ilowite JS, Niederman MS: Problems and opportunities in the topical treatment of infectious diseases of the respiratory tract. *Adv Drug Delivery Rev* 5:93, 1990.

138. Ziegler EJ, McCutchan L, Fierer J, et al: Treatment of gram-negative bacteremia and shock with human antiserum to a mutant *Escherichia coli*. *N Engl J Med* 307:1225, 1982.

139. Ziegler EJ, Fisher CJ Jr, Sprung CL, et al: Treatment of gram-negative bacteremia and septic shock with HA-1A human monoclonal antibody against endotoxin. *N Engl J Med* 324:429, 1991.

140. Ackerman S, Bone R, Wenzel R, et al, and the Xoma Sepsis Study Group: The use of E5, an anti-endotoxin monoclonal antibody, in gram-negative sepsis. Presented at the French Society of Microbiology annual meeting, December 1991.

141. Niederman MS: Strategies for the prevention of pneumonia. *Clin Chest Med* 8:543, 1987.

142. Simberkoff MS, Cross AP, Al Ibrahim M: Efficacy of pneumococcal vaccine in high risk patients: Results of a Veterans Administration cooperative study. *N Engl J Med* 315:1318, 1986.

143. LaForce FM, Eickhoff TC: Pneumococcal vaccine: An emerging consensus. *Ann Intern Med* 108:757, 1988.

144. Shapiro E, Berg AT, Austrian R, et al: The protective efficacy of polyvalent pneumococcal polysaccharide vaccine. *N Engl J Med* 325:1453, 1991.

145. Fedson DS, Harward MP, Reid RA, Kaiser DL: Hospital-based pneumococcal immunization: Epidemiologic rationale from the Shenandoah study. *JAMA* 264:1117, 1990.

146. Arden NH, Patriarca PA, Fasano MB, et al: The roles of vaccination and amantadine prophylaxis in controlling an outbreak of influenza A (H3N2) in a nursing home. *Arch Intern Med* 148:865, 1988.

147. Ruben FL: The prevention of severe lower respiratory infections in chronic bronchitis. *Semin Respir Infect* 4:261, 1989.

148. Fagon JY, Chastre J, Trouillet JL, et al: Characterization of distal bronchial microflora during acute exacerbation of chronic bronchitis: Use of the protected specimen brush technique in 54 mechanically ventilated patients. *Am Rev Respir Dis* 142:1004, 1990.

149. Nicotra MB, Rivera M, Awe RJ: Antibiotic therapy of acute exacerbations of chronic bronchitis. *Ann Intern Med* 97:18, 1982.

150. Italey RW, Culber DH, White JW, et al: The nationwide nosocomial infection rate: Need for new vital statistics. *Am J Epidemiol* 21:159, 1985.

151. Dreyfuss D, Djedaini K, Weber P, et al: Prospective study of nosocomial pneumonia and of patient and circuit colonization during mechanical ventilation with circuit changes every 48 hours versus no change. *Am Rev Respir Dis* 143:738, 1991.

152. Feely TW, DuMoulin GC, Hedley-Whyte J, et al: Aerosol polymyxin and pneumonia in seriously ill patients. *N Engl J Med* 293:471, 1975.

153. Stoutenbeek CP, van Saene HKF, Miranda DR, et al: The effect of selective decontamination of the digestive tract on colonization and infection rate in multiple trauma patients. *Intensive Care Med* 10:185, 1984.

154. Unertl K, Ruckdeschel G, Selbmann HK, et al: Prevention of colonization and respiratory infections in long-term ventilated patients by local antimicrobial prophylaxis. *Intensive Care Med* 13:106, 1987.

155. Ledingham IM, Alcock SR, Eastaway AT, et al: Triple regimen of selective decontamination of the digestive tract, systemic cefotaxime, and microbiological surveillance for prevention of acquired infection in intensive care. *Lancet* 1:785, 1988.

156. Gastinne H, Wolff M, Delatour F, et al, and the French Study Group on Selective Decontamination of the Digestive Tract: A controlled trial in intensive care units of selective decontamination of the digestive tract with nonabsorbable antibiotics. *N Engl J Med* 326:594, 1992.

157. Cockerill FR, Muller SR, Anhalt JP, et al: Prevention of infection in critically ill patients by selective decontamination of the digestive tract. *Ann Intern Med* 117:545, 1992.

158. Young LS, Meyer RD, Armstrong D: *Pseudomonas aeruginosa* vaccine in cancer patients. *Ann Intern Med* 79:518, 1973.

159. Pennington JE: Properties and characteristics of a new immunoglobulin G intravenous preparation. *Rev Infect Dis* 8(suppl):S371, 1986.

160. Collins MS, Roby RE: Protective activity of intravenous immune globulin (human) enriched antibody against lipopolysaccharide antigens of *Pseudomonas aeruginosa*. *Am J Med* 76:168, 1984.

161. Mahul P, Auboyer C, Jospe R, et al: Prevention of nosocomial pneumonia in intubated patients: Respective role of mechanical subglottic secretions drainage and stress ulcer prophylaxis. *Intensive Care Med* 18:20, 1992.

77. Lung Biopsy

Richard S. Irwin and Gerald Nash

Overview

Lung biopsy is an invasive, diagnostic procedure that allows for histologic, cytologic, microbiologic, and chemical analyses of lung tissue. In general, it is indicated whenever it is necessary to obtain a definitive diagnosis of a localized or diffuse pulmonary disease, usually after noninvasive diagnostic modalities have been employed unsuccessfully.

There are currently available multiple lung biopsy techniques that have been well characterized with regard to tissue yield, diagnostic yield, complications, contraindications, and mortality rate (Table 77-1). The relative usefulness of a particular biopsy technique depends not only on the availability of local expertise but also on the clinical situation (e.g., diffuse pulmonary infiltrates vs. intrapulmonary mass, stable vs. unstable patient). Each biopsy procedure is briefly described and an approach to the lung biopsy procedure in the critically ill patient that focuses on the following questions is outlined: (1) When should a lung biopsy be considered in the critically ill patient? (2) Which biopsy technique should be chosen? (3) How should the specimens be handled?

Biopsy Procedures

GENERAL CONSIDERATIONS. Lung biopsy procedures can be grouped in two broad categories: open (i.e., surgical) or closed (i.e., nonsurgical). The major distinction between the two is that closed procedures avoid major surgical intervention and general anesthesia at the expense of a lower likelihood of obtaining a definitive diagnosis. Open procedures are contraindicated in any patient who is too ill to undergo thoracotomy and general anesthesia. Contraindications to closed procedures may be either absolute or relative [1–9]. Absolute contraindications to closed biopsy include (1) coagulopathy (including uremia) that cannot be corrected prior to the procedure, (2) pulmonary hypertension, (3) poor cardiopulmonary reserve, (4) emphysematous lung disease in the area to be biopsied by percutaneous transthoracic procedures, (5) poor patient cooperation, (6) suspected echinococcal lung disease, and (7) uncontrollable cough. Relative contraindications include (1) recent myocardial infarction and/or unstable angina, (2) nearby vascular abnormalities, (3) positive-pressure ventilation (transbronchial methods have been safely performed in this setting), (4) cavitating lesions (especially with air fluid levels or lesions

Table 77-1. Methods of Sampling Lung Tissue

1. Open thoracotomy biopsy
2. Percutaneous transthoracic needle aspiration biopsy
3. Percutaneous transthoracic cutting biopsy
4. Percutaneous transthoracic trephine drill biopsy
5. Transbronchial forceps biopsy
6. Bronchial brush biopsy
7. Transbronchial needle aspiration biopsy
8. Bronchoalveolar lavage
9. Thoracoscopic lung biopsy

>10 cm in diameter), and (5) hypoxemia that cannot be improved with supplemental oxygen to 60 to 70 mm Hg prior to the procedure.

OPEN THORACOTOMY LUNG BIOPSY. Since thoracotomy allows the surgeon to obtain relatively large specimen(s) of lung tissue under direct observation, open lung biopsy is the most consistently accurate lung biopsy technique (Table 77-2, Fig. 77-1). The procedure requires endotracheal intubation, general anesthesia, and pleural catheter drainage for at least 24 hours following the biopsy. A "conventional" open thoracotomy, utilizing a posterolateral incision, is used when hilar adenopathy is present and/or uneven parenchymal infiltrates exist [10]. A more limited or "modified" open thoracotomy is preferred in other situations [10]. Although the modified procedure limits the area from which the biopsy can be obtained, it does not require rib resection and utilizes a small anterior incision. Several precautions will maximize diagnostic yield [1]. (1) Biopsies of the tip of the lingula or right middle lobe should be avoided, since these are common sites of prior scarring, inflammation, and passive congestion. (2) Average, rather than normal or markedly abnormal, lung tissue should be preferentially biopsied, since it is more likely to show an active and recognizable process. (3) In cases of diffuse pulmonary disease, more than one site should be sampled, if possible.

CLOSED BIOPSY PROCEDURES

Percutaneous Transthoracic Needle Aspiration Biopsy. This procedure involves the insertion, under guidance of fluoroscopy or computed tomography (CT), of a sterile needle through the chest wall into the area of the lung to be biopsied [11]. Needles of varying sizes (18, 20, 22, and 24–25 gauge) can be used. In general, the thinner the needle, the fewer the complications [12]. A specimen is obtained by aspiration; it usually consists of cells (neoplastic, parenchymal, inflammatory), tissue fluids, and/or small tissue fragments (Fig. 77-2). The major advantage of this procedure is that it can be easily performed with local anesthesia. The major disadvantage is that lung architectural integrity is usually not maintained in the specimen.

Percutaneous Transthoracic Cutting Needle Biopsy. This procedure involves the insertion—blindly, in the case of diffuse disease or under fluoroscopic guidance when the process to be biopsied is more localized—of a sterile, large cutting needle (14–16 gauge) through the chest wall into the area of lung to be biopsied [13]. When successfully performed, this procedure can extract a core of tissue with well-maintained lung architecture. Although this procedure can be easily performed with local anesthesia, it can be associated with excessive morbidity and mortality and may not yield tissue. To maximize the risk-benefit ratio of this procedure, we perform it only under fluoroscopic guidance and restrict its use to biopsy of large masses that are in contact with the chest wall.

Percutaneous Transthoracic Trephine Drill Biopsy. This procedure is performed by percutaneous insertion of a large, sterile trephine (7.5 cm long, 3 mm outer diameter, 2.1 mm

Table 77-2. Results of Four Lung Biopsy Procedures in Diffuse Lung Disease

Procedure	Cases (no.)	Mortality (%)	Complications (%)	Tissue obtained (%)	Diagnosis made (%)
Open	2290	1.8	7[a]	100	94
Transbronchial					
forceps biopsy	1289	0.2	13[b]	82	72
Trephine drill	551	0.5	44[c]	84	72
Cutting needle	789	1.1	42[d]	74	63

[a]Pneumothorax, empyema, bleeding into pleural space, pain and subsequent respiratory failure due to analgesics.
[b]Pneumothorax, hemorrhage in uremic or thrombocytopenic patients.
[c]Pneumothorax, bleeding, cardiac arrest.
[d]Pneumothorax, air embolism, pulmonary hemorrhage.
Modified from Berquist TH, Bailey PB, Cortese DA, et al: Transthoracic needle biopsy. *Mayo Clin Proc* 55:475, 1980. With permission.

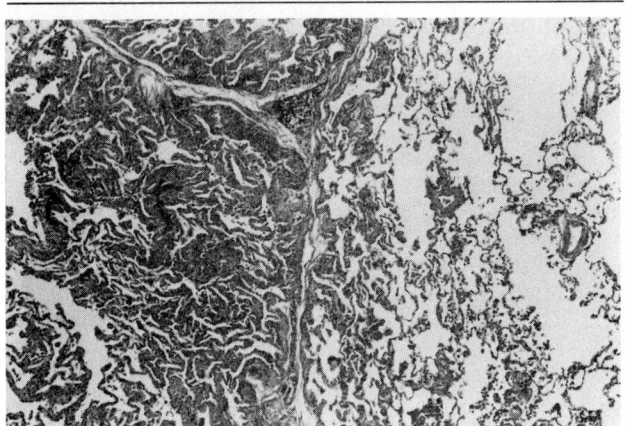

Fig. 77-1. Open lung biopsy of a case of usual interstitial pneumonia with interstitial fibrosis, showing the patchy distribution of the process. An interlobular septum traverses the center of the photomicrograph. Portions of lobules to the left of the septum exhibit interstitial disease, whereas the portion of the lobule to the right shows mostly normal lung. In this situation a smaller sample, such as a transbronchial biopsy, might not be representative of the pathologic process. (Hematoxylin-eosin stain; × 10)

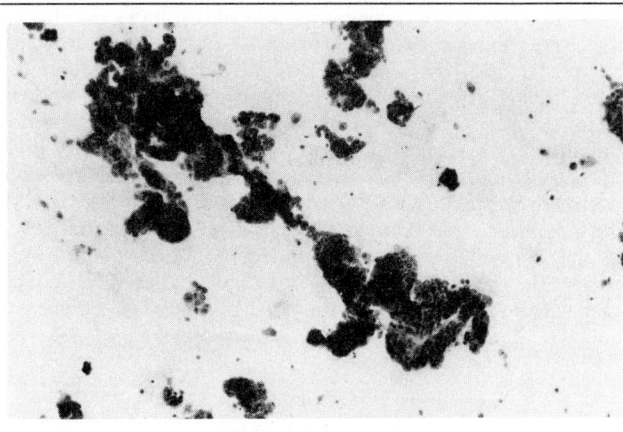

A

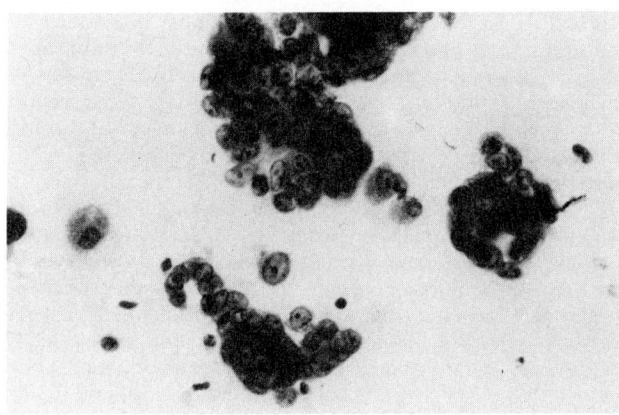

B

Fig. 77-2. Percutaneous transthoracic needle aspiration biopsy of an adenocarcinoma, bronchoalveolar type. A. Low-power view of tiny fragments of tumor present in the aspirate. (Papanicolaou's stain; × 25) B. Higher-power view of clusters of tumor cells showing large cells with macronucleoli characteristic of adenocarcinoma. (× 100)

inner diameter) with a sharp cutting edge with internal rifling into the area of lung to be biopsied [14]. A specimen is obtained when the trephine is attached to and driven by compressed air. The trephine rotates at an estimated 12,000 to 15,000 rotations per minute. With proper technique, the operator can obtain a core of tissue 2 to 4 cm long (approximately 1.5 mm in diameter) that adequately represents the disease process. Since the trephine air drill is short, blunt, and clumsy, it is unsuitable, even with fluoroscopic guidance, for reaching lesions distant from the pleura [15]. Another disadvantage of this technique is the frightening noise generated by the turbine drill [16].

Bronchoscopic Procedures. A variety of techniques, including bronchial and transbronchial forceps biopsy, bronchial brushing, transbronchial needle aspiration, and bronchoalveolar lavage, can be easily and safely performed with the flexible fiberoptic bronchoscope. A detailed discussion of flexible fiberoptic bronchoscopy is presented in Chapter 12.

TRANSBRONCHIAL FORCEPS LUNG BIOPSY. This procedure is performed by passing the endoscope to the segmental level, instilling a dilute solution of epinephrine, and then advancing flexible biopsy forceps into the radiographically abnormal area [17]. Generally, the forceps are advanced under fluoroscopic

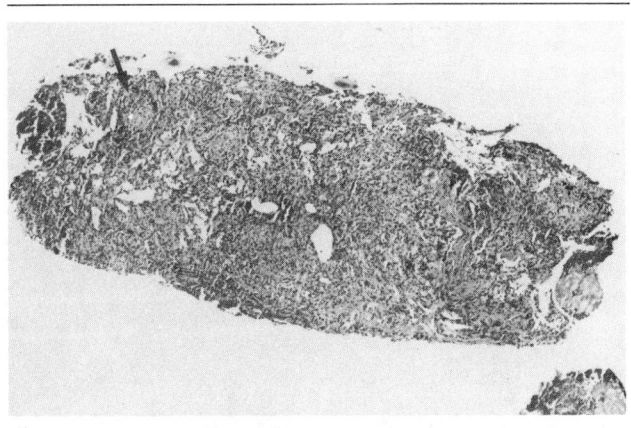

A

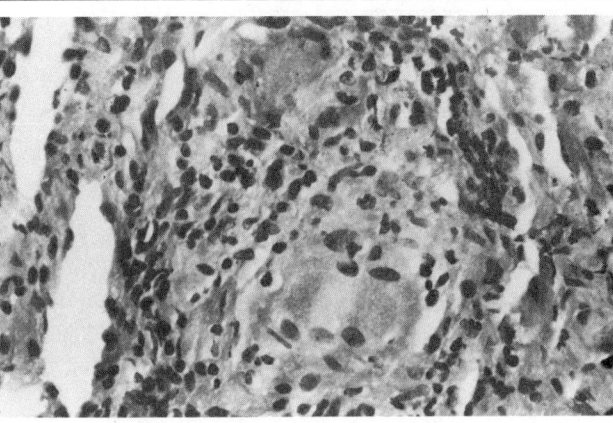

B

Fig. 77-3. Transbronchial forceps biopsy of a case of sarcoidosis. A. Low-power view of one of multiple pieces of lung showing alveolar tissue with a cellular infiltrate. The arrow denotes a nodular focus suggestive of a granuloma. (Hematoxylin-eosin stain; × 10) B. Higher-power view of the nodular area reveals a noncaseating granuloma consistent with sarcoidosis. (× 100)

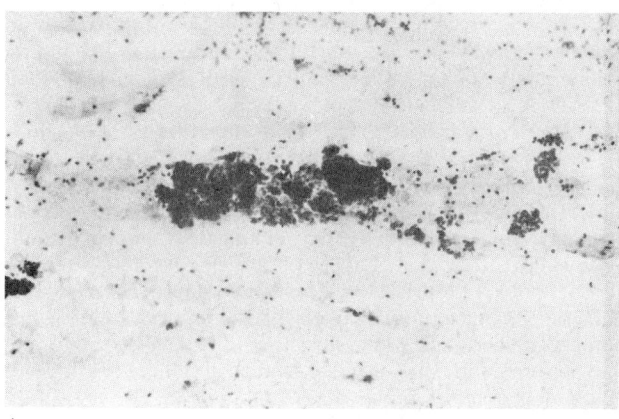

A

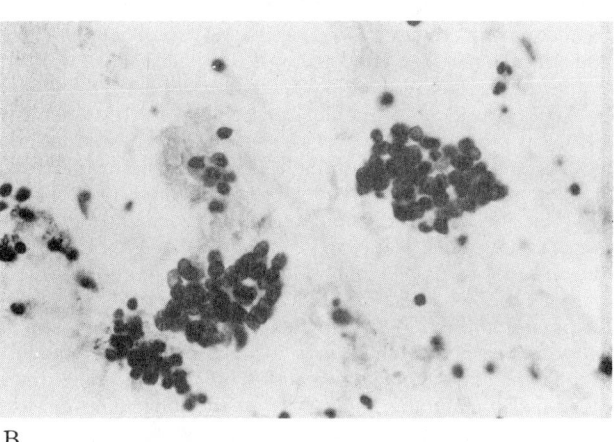

B

Fig. 77-4. Bronchial brush biopsy of a bronchogenic small cell carcinoma. A. Low-power view, showing fragments of neoplasm removed by the brush. (Papanicolaou's stain; × 25) B. Higher-power view of nests of tumor cells with small hyperchromatic nuclei, absent nucleoli, and scanty cytoplasm characteristic of small cell carcinoma. (× 100)

guidance. They are passed in the closed position until resistance is met and/or the patient signals that he or she has chest (pleural) pain. If pain is felt, the forceps are withdrawn in 1-cm increments until pain is no longer perceived. If no pain is felt, the forceps are opened, pressure is gently applied, and the forceps are closed. If no chest pain is felt, the forceps are then removed. As soon as the biopsy is taken, the endoscope is wedged into the airway from which the biopsy was taken to tampónade any potential bleeding and to prevent any blood from spilling out into other airways. A recent study found that synchronization of the biopsy to the respiratory phase affected neither the amount of alveolar tissue obtained nor the integrity of the specimen [18]. Since specimens are small (not >3.9 mm² on average [18]), multiple specimens should be obtained to maximize the yield of this technique (Fig. 77-3).

BRONCHIAL BRUSH BIOPSY. Using a flexible wire brush, the operator performs this procedure in a manner similar to forceps biopsy [19,20,21]. Generally, under fluoroscopic guidance, the brush is passed as far as possible into the radiographically abnormal area. The usefulness of this method is limited by the fact that only cellular material can be obtained and generally only endobronchial processes are sampled (Fig. 77-4). A nodule

not in communication with the bronchial tree cannot be entered with the brush, even though the nodule could be readily biopsied with a needle passed transthoracically.

TRANSBRONCHIAL NEEDLE ASPIRATION. This technique allows one to pierce the walls of airways and aspirate cellular contents and tissue fluid or processes not in communication with the tracheobronchial tree. Specially designed catheters with attached needles are passed through the suction channel of the bronchoscope to the abnormal area [4,22,23,24]. As long as the vascularity of the area to be aspirated is appreciated and/or has been defined, transbronchial puncture with aspiration can be safely performed. This was demonstrated in a report on the aspiration of carinal and peritracheal nodes [24]. This procedure appears to have a role in the diagnosis and staging of lung cancer and in the diagnosis of some benign mediastinal diseases, such as bronchogenic cysts. When appropriately applied and with good cytopathologic support, this procedure can eliminate the need for surgical staging in a substantial number of patients with inoperable lung cancer.

BRONCHOALVEOLAR LAVAGE. This procedure is a quick, safe diagnostic extension of routine flexible fiberoptic bronchoscopy [25]. The tip of the bronchoscope is wedged into a segmental or smaller airway, and physiologic saline is instilled and withdrawn through the suction channel. Using this technique, it is possible to sample cellular and soluble components from the distal airways and alveoli. Although bronchoalveolar lavage has a number of limitations, it can be useful in diagnosing some infectious or other diffuse parenchymal diseases (e.g., *Pneumocystis carinii* pneumonitis [26], intraalveolar hemorrhage [27], alveolar cell carcinoma [28], exogenous lipoid pneumonia [29], alveolar proteinosis [30], and pulmonary histiocytosis X [31]) (Fig. 77-5). A detailed discussion of the use of bronchoalveolar lavage analysis in a variety of lung diseases can be found elsewhere [32]. The usefulness of bronchoalveolar lavage and bronchoscopy protected brush catheter cultures is reviewed in Chapter 12. Since bronchoalveolar lavage is not really a biopsy procedure and little or no associated bleeding occurs, it may be performed in patients with bleeding abnormalities and pulmonary hypertension.

THORACOSCOPIC LUNG BIOPSY. Thoracoscopy is a percutaneous procedure that involves the endoscopic exploration and sampling of the contents of the thoracic cavity [33,34]. Unlike the other closed biopsy procedures, thoracoscopic lung biopsy is considered a surgical procedure. First described in 1910, this procedure has been the subject of renewed interest in the past 10 to 15 years, primarily because of new optical and video imaging technology and improved methods of providing local anesthesia and sedation that avoid general anesthesia in many cases. While there are a variety of potential uses for thoracoscopy (e.g., pleural and lung biopsy, pleurodesis, pleurectomy, wedge resection of peripheral nodules, bullectomy for pneumothorax, mediastinal exploration, laser bullectomy, and lung resection), lung biopsy is highlighted here. Thoracoscopic lung biopsy involves multiple chest wall incisions and a controlled pneumothorax to collapse the lung. One incision allows the insertion of a sterile fiberoptic endoscope (e.g., thoracoscope, arthroscope, laryngoscope, bronchoscope) to visualize the lung and pleural surfaces. A biopsy device is inserted through another incision and guided by direct endoscopic vision/video monitoring. Multiple points of entry may be necessary to determine the ideal endoscopic approach.

With the resurgence of interest in thoracoscopy, the role of this procedure in performing lung biopsies in a variety of settings should be sorted out in the next few years. At this point, although prospective studies are needed to compare the yield, morbidity, mortality, and cost of this procedure with the other techniques, an intuitive advantage of thoracoscopy is that it can obtain a larger piece of lung tissue than bronchoscopy techniques, equal in size to that obtained at open lung biopsy.

Expected Results from Lung Biopsy

GENERAL CONSIDERATIONS. To determine when and what type of lung biopsy procedure should be performed, it is important to appreciate the expected results in any individual patient. The yield of positive diagnoses and the complications incurred depend on the procedure performed, the disease process, and the clinical stability of the patient.

DIFFUSE PARENCHYMAL DISEASE IN CLINICALLY STABLE PATIENTS. To maximize the diagnostic yield, the ideal biopsy procedure would be one that maintains the architectural lung integrity in the specimen. The procedures that best meet this requirement are (1) open lung biopsy, (2) transbroncho-

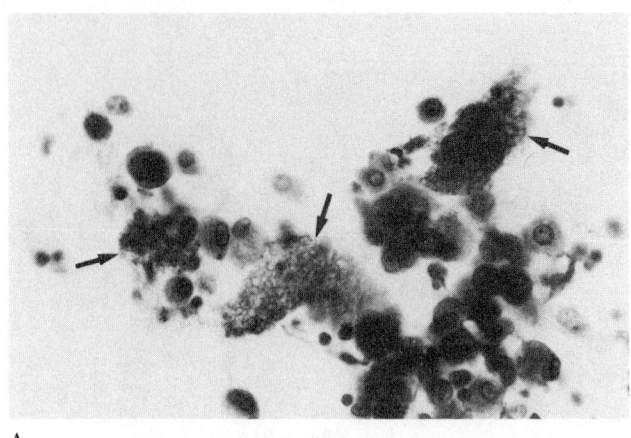

A

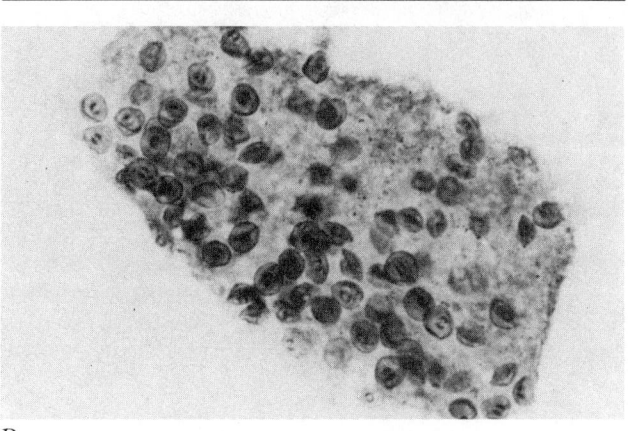

B

Fig. 77-5. Smear of bronchoalveolar lavage sediment in *Pneumocystis carinii* pneumonia in a patient with AIDS. A. Most of the cells in the preparation are macrophages, indicating that alveolar contents were sampled. Three clumps of foamy material (*arrows*) characteristic of *P. carinii* are present in the field. (Papanicolaou's stain; × 100) B. Methenamine silver stain of one of the foamy masses showing numerous cysts of *P. carinii.* Many of the cysts exhibit paired comma-shaped densities characteristic of the organism. (× 250)

scopic forceps lung biopsy, (3) trephine drill biopsy, (4) cutting needle biopsy, and (5) thoracoscopic biopsy. A number of reports on stable patients with diffuse lung disease have documented average rates of mortality, complications, tissue yield, and diagnostic yield for the first four of these procedures (Table 77-2). In four relatively small studies, sensitivities of thoracoscopic lung biopsy approached 100 percent [35–38]; complications have included pneumothorax in up to 11 percent and fever in up to 15 percent [35]; intraoperative hemorrhage requiring conversion to open lung biopsy occurred in one patient [38]. In a recent study, thoracoscopy-guided lung biopsy results correlated directly with the pathologic and microbiologic results of open lung biopsy obtained from the same patients [37].

These data demonstrate that open lung biopsy and transbronchoscopic forceps and perhaps thoracoscopy lung biopsy are preferred for evaluating diffuse pulmonary disease in immunocompetent patients. The highest tissue and diagnostic yields with low morbidity and very low mortality are obtained with open and thoracoscopic lung biopsies. Transbronchoscopic forceps lung biopsy has equivalent tissue and diagnostic yields when compared to other closed techniques, but carries the lowest morbidity and mortality of any of the biopsy procedures.

Although open and thoracoscopic lung biopsies more consistently yield adequate tissue and an increased likelihood of definitive diagnosis than transbronchoscopic forceps lung biopsy, the latter may be preferred as an initial procedure to avoid the morbidity of general anesthesia, postoperative chest tube drainage, residual parenchymal and pleural scarring, postoperative pain, and increased length of hospital stay. The potential morbidity of empyema that may complicate an open or thoracoscopic lung biopsy procedure is also avoided with transbronchoscopic forceps lung biopsy. This closed procedure requires no or a shorter hospital stay, is much less expensive and less painful, and carries less mortality than open lung biopsy.

The overall complication rate for transbronchoscopic forceps lung biopsy is 13 percent. The most common complication is pneumothorax, which may require chest tube drainage in up to 50 percent of cases [8,39]. Although the definitive diagnostic accuracy of transbronchoscopic forceps lung biopsy is less than that of open lung biopsy (the tissue is smaller in quantity, often crushed, usually only peribronchiolar in origin, and not obtained under direct vision), its diagnostic yield is sufficiently high under certain conditions to justify its use as the initial biopsy procedure. For instance, in diffuse diseases such as carcinomatosis, sarcoidosis, and *Pneumocystis carinii* infection, transbronchoscopic forceps lung biopsy yields a specific diagnosis in 67 to 90 percent of individuals [20,40–47].

Percutaneous needle aspiration (lung tap) also has a role in individuals with diffuse parenchymal disease due to infectious disease. The diagnostic yield in this setting varies from 50 to 90 percent [48,49]. Although percutaneous needle aspiration rarely causes mortality or air embolism, pneumothorax is common, occurring in 8 to 49 percent of cases (5–21% of these pneumothoraces may require chest tube drainage). Hemoptysis occurs in 1 to 11 percent of individuals [12,50,51,52].

LUNG MASS IN CLINICALLY STABLE PATIENTS. Since solid or cavitary masses are most often due to malignant and/or infectious causes, and since these diagnoses can often be readily confirmed by analyzing cellular material and fluid, open lung biopsy is usually not the preferred initial procedure. However, when open biopsy is performed, tissue and diagnostic yields should consistently approach 100 percent. Since nodules are usually resected in their entirety, surgical mortality depends on the severity of illness and extent of the resection [53]. The operative mortality associated with wedge resections of benign nodules in otherwise healthy young patients is less than 1 percent, while it may vary from 5 to 10 percent in older patients with bronchogenic carcinomas who undergo pneumonectomy. Complications of thoracotomy for lung masses in clinically stable patients are similar to those in such patients with diffuse lung disease.

Percutaneous needle aspiration is extremely useful in evaluating lung masses. Of the closed biopsy techniques, it carries the highest diagnostic yield. A definite diagnosis is obtained in 80 to 97 percent of all masses [12,50,51,52,54,55], and adequate samples are obtained in 82 to 98 percent of cases [12,50,51,52,54,55]. If the lesion is less than 2 cm in diameter, the likelihood of obtaining adequate material is significantly decreased [50,55]. The diagnostic yield in solid malignant nodules is approximately 86 percent [12,55], in malignant and infectious cavitary lesions 90 to 100 percent [12,50], and in "benign" inflammatory disease, such as granulomatous nodules, only 19 percent [56]. Although percutaneous needle aspiration is rarely associated with fatalities (a review of the literature up

to 1974 revealed only 7 deaths in 9000 patients [57]), complications such as pneumothorax, hemoptysis, and intraparenchymal hemorrhage or hemothorax are not uncommon [12,50,52, 55,57]. The frequency and type of complication are related to the location of the lesion and whether the nodule is solid or cavitary (Table 77-3). Hemorrhage and pneumothorax occur much more frequently in cavitary lesions. It has been demonstrated that aspiration biopsy utilizing smaller, ultrathin 24- to 25-gauge needles should result in a significant decrease in complications without loss of excellent diagnostic yield [12]. The risk of needle track implantation of cancer is a rare complication and should not be considered a contraindication to the procedure [57].

Peripheral lung nodules and masses can also be biopsied using the transbronchoscopic brush and forceps techniques. Complication rates are less than those for percutaneous needle aspiration biopsy. While the diagnostic yield is also diminished and the procedures are more difficult and time-consuming than percutaneous needle biopsy, transbronchial forceps biopsies more frequently yield tissue with architectural integrity. This may allow the pathologist a better opportunity to diagnose benign conditions. In peripheral malignant lesions, the diagnostic yield of transbronchial biopsy relates directly to the number of biopsies obtained under fluoroscopic guidance. With brushing alone, the diagnostic yield is approximately 40 percent; with brushing plus one transbronchoscopic forceps lung biopsy, diagnostic accuracy improves to 55 percent; with brushing plus four transbronchoscopic forceps lung biopsies, accuracy reaches 60 percent; and with brushing plus five transbronchoscopic forceps lung biopsies, diagnostic accuracy improves to 75 percent [58].

Based on scant data, the sensitivity of thoracoscopy in diagnosing the etiology of localized parenchymal lesions approaches 70 percent [35]. Theoretically, only the most peripheral lesions are accessible to this procedure.

DIFFUSE AND LOCALIZED DISEASE IN CLINICALLY UNSTABLE PATIENTS. Some type of lung biopsy procedure in critically ill, clinically unstable patients is most commonly considered in individuals who are immunocompromised hosts or who have the acute respiratory distress syndrome (ARDS).

Numerous studies have considered the merits of various lung biopsy procedures in the non-acquired immunodeficiency syndrome (AIDS) immunocompromised host. We are unaware of results of thoracoscopic biopsy in this setting. A comparison of results of a variety of other lung biopsy techniques in these patients (Table 77-4) reveals that there is no consensus about which biopsy technique is best and under which clinical circumstances. A wide range of expected diagnostic yields exists for all procedures, and the etiology of lung disease in these patients may remain unknown in 19 to 45 percent of patients, even when adequate tissue is obtained by open lung biopsy. Deciding who, when, and how to biopsy is further complicated by the occasionally excessive mortality rates associated with lung biopsy procedures and by the knowledge that even with adequate biopsy material and appropriate therapy, the high mortality rates (25–75%) seen in these patients may not be altered [64,66]. Since the existing data do not allow generalizations concerning consistent diagnosis, one must adopt a practical approach to management that combines empirical therapy with available biopsy procedures.

In patients with AIDS, open lung biopsy is the most sensitive and specific procedure. However, because (1) diffuse pulmonary infiltrates are most likely due to opportunistic infections, (2) these patients have multiple problems that present in this way, and (3) overall, bronchoscopic procedures accurately di-

Table 77-3. Complications of Percutaneous Needle Aspiration of the Lung

Tissue obtained	Cases (No.)	Pneumothorax (%)	Hemoptysis (%)	Parenchymal hemorrhage or hemothorax (%)
Type				
Solid nodule	400	49	10	24
Cavity	12	75	17	67
Location				
Central	100	51	19	70
Peripheral	297	49	9	14
Mediastinal	24	66	4	0
Pleural	9	11	0	0

Modified from Berquist TH, Bailey PB, Cortese DA, et al: Transthoracic needle biopsy. *Mayo Clin Proc* 55:475, 1980. With permission.

Table 77-4. Results of Lung Biopsy Procedures in Clinically Unstable Patients

Procedure	Mortality (%)	Complications (%)	Diagnostic yield (%)
Open lung biopsy [45,59–66]	Up to 38	8–30	55–81
Bronchial brush biopsy [20,44,67–74]	—	—	28–63
Transbronchial forceps biopsy [20,44,65–71]	Up to 51	9	32–74
Transbronchial brush plus forceps biopsy [20,44,65–71]	—	0–26	30–84
Cutting needle [57]	—	15–46	46–75
Needle aspiration [13,48,49,52,60]	—	8–30	35–76
Trephine drill [62,64]	Up to 20	Up to 60	20–65

Table 77-5. Management of the Compromised Host with Pulmonary Disease

1. Identify the patient as a compromised host.
2. Construct a list of differential possibilities that remains constant from patient to patient.
3. Integrate the history, physical examination, and laboratory data with the chest radiographic pattern to narrow the diagnostic possibilities.
4. Assess the urgency of the situation and the need for invasive diagnostic studies, including lung biopsy.

Indications for Lung Biopsy in Critically Ill Patients

GENERAL CONSIDERATIONS. A lung biopsy is indicated in critically ill patients when (1) the pulmonary disease process progresses and its etiology remains unknown, (2) an initial evaluation short of lung biopsy has failed to reveal the etiology and logical empirical therapy has failed to reverse the process, (3) no contraindications exist to performing the procedure(s), (4) the prognosis of the patient's underlying disease is good, and (5) the potential benefit from performing the procedure outweighs associated morbidity and mortality [64,66].

MANAGEMENT OF CRITICALLY ILL PATIENTS WITH PULMONARY DISEASE. The lung biopsy is part of an extensive evaluation of a pulmonary abnormality, yet in critically ill patients it is never the initial step. Any critically ill patient is, for clinical purposes, a compromised host and should be managed as such (Table 77-5).

Because of their altered defense mechanisms, critically ill patients are particularly susceptible to infection by opportunistic as well as pathogenic organisms. Nonimmunologic defenses (altered physical barriers, altered indigenous microbiologic flora) as well as immunologic defenses (altered humoral and/or cellular immunity) may be impaired. These impairments may be partial or transient (alcoholism, diabetes mellitus, sickle cell anemia, uremia, malnutrition) as well as prolonged or permanent (Hodgkin's disease, chronic lymphatic leukemia, acute myelogenous leukemia, multiple myeloma, inherited immune deficiency diseases, cytotoxic chemotherapy, corticosteroids, irradiation).

Four major differential diagnostic possibilities should be considered in every critically ill (compromised) patient with pulmonary disease (Table 77-6). After general diagnostic considerations, the diagnostic possibilities are narrowed by integrating

agnose infections in 90 percent of cases or more [75], open lung biopsy should not be the first procedure contemplated or attempted. Open lung biopsy is (and perhaps thoracoscopic biopsy will be determined to be) appropriate when at least one bronchoscopic examination with bronchoalveolar lavage and transbronchial biopsy (unless contraindicated) has been nondiagnostic [76]. It is rarely useful in patients who worsen after treatment for a diagnosis established by bronchoscopy [75], and it should not be repeated often.

Bronchoalveolar lavage has assumed a most important role in diagnosing opportunistic infections in immunocompromised hosts with diffuse parenchymal disease. In non-AIDS patients, bronchoalveolar lavage in combination with forceps and brush biopsies has a high yield for identifying *P. carinii, Legionella* species, and cytomegalovirus infections [20,77]. In patients with AIDS, the sensitivity of lavage alone for diagnosing *Pneumocystis* can be as high as 97 percent [78]. Bronchoalveolar lavage does not increase the already low complication rate of routine diagnostic fiberoptic bronchoscopy (see Chap. 12).

In patients with ARDS, lung biopsy may be considered to ensure that no treatable disease process is overlooked. In 42 patients with ARDS due to trauma, pneumonia, systemic sepsis, and paraquat intoxication, open lung biopsy added additional diagnostic information in only 4 percent [79]. In these few patients, lung cultures revealed *Aspergillus* and cytomegalovirus infections that had not been identified by other methods. The morbidity and mortality of performing open lung biopsy in these patients remained low (4% and 0%, respectively).

the history, physical examination, and laboratory data (routine blood work; serologic studies; and smears and cultures of blood, urine, sputum, cerebrospinal fluid [CSF], ascites, and pleural effusion) with the chest radiographic pattern. A previous recent or remote chest radiograph may confirm or rule out the presence of another stable process. While unilateral or focal infiltrates suggest bacterial infection, the presence of bilateral disease does not rule out infectious processes [79]. Unusual and opportunistic organisms such as *P. carinii* often present as bilateral infiltrates after administration of immunosuppressive drugs or chemotherapy [80].

The final step involves assessing clinical urgency to evaluate the need for invasive diagnostic studies such as lung biopsy. For example, in the spontaneously breathing, acutely ill patient undergoing treatment for acute myelogenous leukemia who has a focal unilateral infiltrate and cannot expectorate sputum, quantitative cultures obtained by bronchoscopy with plugged telescoping catheters should be the first diagnostic procedure considered. If this is contraindicated, broad-spectrum antibiotics should be started empirically [65]. In an intubated, elderly patient with diffuse pulmonary infiltrates associated with pancreatitis, the first diagnostic procedure might be pulmonary artery catheterization. If the pulmonary capillary wedge pressure (PCWP) is normal, the patient is likely to have developed ARDS.

As noted previously, lung biopsy in nonimmunocompromised patients who have developed ARDS infrequently (approximately 4% of cases [79]) adds useful information. In the thrombocytopenic, immunocompromised host who has diffuse pulmonary infiltrates and who is clinically stable with supplemental oxygen, platelet transfusions and observation may be adequate therapy. As many as 70 percent of infiltrates in these patients may be due to intrapulmonary bleeding [27]. If this conservative management fails and the patient continues to deteriorate, and if the patient's underlying disease is under control (e.g., acute myelogenous leukemia is in remission), erythromycin and trimethoprim/sulfamethoxasole should be started and a lung biopsy seriously contemplated. In a patient who has metastatic carcinomatosis unresponsive to chemotherapy and who develops diffuse pulmonary disease, empirical therapy for any possible reversible disease is appropriate.

Selection of Lung Biopsy Procedure

Three factors should be considered in choosing a particular lung biopsy procedure: (1) local expertise, (2) the patient's condition, and (3) the potential yield of the procedure.

LOCAL EXPERTISE. This factor includes the availability of both individuals skilled in performing the procedure and laboratory personnel skilled in specimen processing and analysis. If local expertise is limited (e.g., a skilled cytopathologist is not available to read bronchial brush or percutaneous needle aspiration specimens, or the microbiology laboratory is not equipped to process reliably specimens for the variety of organisms seen in immunocompromised hosts) the patient should be transferred to another institution with expanded resources.

PATIENT CONDITION. Once it has been decided that the patient's prognosis is potentially good enough to justify a lung biopsy technique, the next decision is the choice of biopsy

Table 77-6. Differential Diagnosis of Pulmonary Disease in the Compromised Host

1. Manifestations of basic disease
2. Complications of management
   a. Lipid embolization
   b. Pulmonary edema
   c. Pulmonary hemorrhage
   d. Leukoagglutinin reaction
   e. Radiation pneumonitis
   f. Drug-induced pneumonitis
3. Presence of another unrelated basic disease
4. Infection
   a. Bacterial
   b. Viral
   c. Fungal
   d. Parasitic

procedure. If it is determined that the patient's condition allows time for only one diagnostic procedure (i.e., the patient is rapidly deteriorating), then an open lung biopsy (or, depending on local expertise, perhaps thoracoscopy biopsy) should be performed. Immediate morbidity and mortality of open lung biopsy in critically ill, immunocompromised patients on ventilators appear to be minimal except in patients with a poor prognosis from their underlying disease [64,65,66]. Data on thoracoscopic biopsy are not yet available in this regard. If there are no contraindications to any of the closed procedures and the patient's condition is such that there will be time for another diagnostic procedure if necessary, then one of the closed procedures may be preferable. Although mechanical ventilation has been considered by some to be a contraindication to transbronchial biopsy, two retrospective studies [81,82] indicate this should be reconsidered. These studies revealed that useful information can be obtained with transbronchial lung biopsy with acceptable morbidity (e.g., pneumothorax, hemorrhage) in a limited number of hemodynamically stable, mechanically ventilated patients.

POTENTIAL YIELD. The potential yield of a particular biopsy procedure depends on both local expertise and the individual clinical setting. For example, in the elderly patient with a solitary pulmonary nodule and clinically obvious disseminated carcinomatosis, percutaneous needle aspiration biopsy, which has a high diagnostic yield and relatively low complication rate, should be the initial procedure of choice to document whether the nodule is malignant. When a patient with a solitary pulmonary nodule has a clinical picture of vasculitis, however, open lung biopsy (or thoracoscopy biopsy if the lesion is peripheral) might be considered first or performed after bronchial brushing and forceps biopsies and percutaneous needle aspirations yield nonspecific findings without evidence of malignancy or infection.

In patients with diffuse pulmonary disease, the clinical setting influences the choice of procedure. When a biopsy is performed to document the presence and type of inorganic pneumoconiosis, open lung biopsy and thoracoscopic biopsy [38] are the only procedures that will yield a sufficient amount of tissue for all the requisite analyses (chemical analysis must be included). When diffuse pulmonary infiltrates suggesting sarcoidosis or carcinomatosis occur in the appropriate clinical setting, transbronchoscopic forceps lung biopsy should be initially considered, since it has an extremely high yield in these situations [20,40,41,42,47]. In the non-HIV immunocompromised host with diffuse pulmonary infiltrates, transbronchoscopic forceps lung biopsy and transbronchoscopic brush biopsy may yield a diagnosis overall up to 71 percent of the time [43–46,69–74]. Open lung biopsy should be used selectively in the immunocompromised host. Those individuals whose diseases are characterized by brief survival (acute leukemia unresponsive to chemotherapy) benefit the least from open lung biopsy, since potentially treatable results may not alter the outcome. Moreover, open lung biopsy can miss second treatable diseases in a significant number of these patients (6–44%), as noted at autopsy [64,65,66]. The most likely explanation for a nondiagnostic open lung biopsy is the selection of an inadequate biopsy site. Gaensler and Carrington pointed out the fallacy of selecting the most radiologically involved areas, since they inevitably demonstrate end-stage lung disease [10]. Average and/or least involved areas in advanced diffuse lung disease are more likely to yield a recognizable process [10]. In chronic interstitial pneumonias (e.g., idiopathic usual interstitial pneumonitis [UIP]), open lung biopsy is diagnostically superior to transbronchoscopic forceps lung biopsy [1,10,47]. However, if chronic eosinophilic pneumonia, desquamative interstitial pneumonitis, or bronchiolitis obliterans organizing pneumonia (BOOP) can be ruled in by transbronchoscopic forceps lung biopsy, open lung biopsy may not be necessary. If infection and malignancy can be ruled out by transbronchoscopic forceps lung biopsy and other nonbiopsy laboratory techniques, it also may be unnecessary to perform an open lung biopsy. If the diffuse process worsens, corticosteroids can be empirically initiated and the response to therapy can be assessed by noninvasive means (e.g., chest radiograph, gallium scan, pulmonary function studies).

Handling of Specimens

To maximize the diagnostic yield from any lung biopsy procedure, specimens must be rapidly transported to the appropriate laboratories by an individual directly involved in the patient's management. All analyses should be planned in advance by the team involved in the case (pathologists, microbiologists, pulmonologists, infectious disease specialist).

Since large samples of tissue are obtained from an open lung biopsy and thoracoscopy biopsy, multiple pieces should be processed for a variety of analyses. First, under sterile conditions, a piece of fresh tissue should be kept moist with physiologic saline and transported immediately to the microbiology laboratory to be minced, ground, and cultured for aerobic and anaerobic bacteria, fungi, and *Mycobacterium* and *Legionella* species. A second piece should be snap-frozen and stored at −60°C to ensure that immunofluorescent studies (immunoglobulin deposition as well as T and B lymphocyte markers; direct fluorescent antibody staining for *Legionella* species), oil-red-O staining, and viral cultures can be performed if necessary. A third small piece should be cut into 2-mm cubes and placed in electron microscopy fixative. If a pneumoconiosis is suspected, special studies can be performed on formalin-fixed, paraffin-embedded tissue. At this juncture, touch preps of a freshly cut surface of the tissue can be made for cytologic analysis and special stains can be used for rapid diagnosis of microorganisms. The pathologist should perform a frozen section to (1) advise the surgeon whether or not an adequate biopsy has been obtained (i.e., the tissue does or does not exhibit a pathologic lesion), (2) obtain information that could focus the work-up of the specimen (e.g., order a lymphoma work-up or specific viral culture, and (3) attempt to obtain a rapid definitive diagnosis. The remainder of the tissue should be placed in 10% formalin for routine histology and special stains.

Unlimited analysis on specimens from transbronchoscopic forceps lung biopsies cannot be performed, because of the relatively small amount of tissue obtained. (This is less of a problem with cutting needle and trephine drill biopsies.) To maximize the diagnostic yield, 4 to 10 pieces should be obtained [42,58]. In immunocompromised patients, touch preps of transbronchial biopsies should be obtained and stained for microorganisms. If an exogenous lipoid pneumonia, immunologic disease, or *Legionella* infection is suspected, one piece should be snap-frozen for fat stains and immunofluorescent studies. One piece can be submitted to microbiology and the remaining pieces processed for routine and special pathologic stains. Once the slides have been made from bronchial brush biopsies, they can be stained in a manner similar to the filters and slides made from needle aspiration specimens.

A specimen obtained by percutaneous, transthoracic needle aspiration should be sent for microbiologic as well as cytologic analyses unless infection is not even a remote possibility. A portion for cytologic analysis can be injected into a test tube with physiologic saline so that it can be processed using the Millipore filter and/or cytocentrifuge technique, or a few drops of the aspirate can first be smeared onto frosted glass slides that are immediately placed in 95% alcohol. Filters and slides can be stained routinely by the Papanicolaou technique and specifically by Gomori-methenamine silver (for fungi and *Pneumocystis*), periodic acid (PAS) (for fungi), and Ziehl-Neelsen stains (for acid-fast organisms). The portion for microbiology should be immediately injected into prereduced anaerobic transport media and transported to the microbiology laboratory. In the laboratory, drops of the specimen are placed on several sterile slides and allowed to air dry for Gram, Ziehl-Neelsen, and direct fluorescent antibody stains for *Legionella* organisms. The remaining specimen can be cultured for anaerobic and aerobic bacteria, fungi, and *Mycobacterium* and *Legionella* species.

After submitting an aliquot of bronchoalveolar lavage fluid for microbiologic analysis, the specimen should be handled in the cytology laboratory in a manner similar to that of percutaneous aspiration specimens.

References

1. Gaensler EA: Open and closed lung biopsy, in Sackner MA (ed): *The Human Lung in Biology: Techniques in Pulmonary Disease*, part 2. New York, Marcel Dekker, 1980, p 579.
2. Landa JF: Bronchoscopy: General considerations, in Sackner MA (ed): *The Human Lung in Biology: Techniques in Pulmonary Disease*, part 2. New York, Marcel Dekker, 1980, p. 655.
3. Sinner WN: Indications and contraindications for needle biopsy, in Sinner WN (ed): *Needle Biopsy and Transbronchial Biopsy*. New York, Thieme-Stratton, 1982, p 118.
4. Haitor IS, Horai T: Transbronchial needle aspiration biopsy (TBAB), in Sinner WN (ed): *Needle Biopsy and Transbronchial Biopsy*. New York, Thieme-Stratton, 1982, p 118.
5. Oho K: Transbronchial lung biopsy (TBLB), in Sinner WN (ed): *Needle Biopsy and Transbronchial Biopsy*. New York, Thieme-Stratton, 1982, p 123.
6. Hanson RR, Zavala DC, Rhodes ML, et al: Transbronchial biopsy via flexible fiberoptic bronchoscope: Results in 164 patients. *Am Rev Respir Dis* 114:67, 1976.
7. Zavala DC: Diagnostic fiberoptic bronchoscopy: Techniques and results in 600 patients. *Chest* 68:12, 1975.
8. Andersen NA: Transbronchoscopic lung biopsy for diffuse pulmonary disease: Results in 939 patients. *Chest* 73 (suppl):734, 1978.
9. Berquist TH, Bailey PB, Cortese DA, et al: Transthoracic needle biopsy: Accuracy and complications in relation to location and type of lesion. *Mayo Clin Proc* 55:475, 1980.

10. Gaensler EA, Carrington CB: Open lung biopsy for chronic diffuse infiltrative lung disease: Clinical, roentgenographic, and physiologic correlations in 502 patients. *Ann Thorac Surg* 30:411, 1980.
11. Sinner WN: Technique of needle aspiration biopsy, in Sinner WN (ed): *Needle Biopsy and Transbronchial Biopsy.* New York, Thieme-Stratton, 1982, p 35.
12. Zavala DC, Schoell JE: Ultrathin needle aspiration of the lung in infections and malignant diseases. *Am Rev Respir Dis* 123:125, 1981.
13. Zavala DC, Bedell GH: Percutaneous lung biopsy with a cutting needle. *Am Rev Respir Dis* 106:186, 1972.
14. Steel SJ, Winstanley DP: Trephine biopsy of the lung and pleura. *Thorax* 24:576, 1969.
15. King EJ, Baychynski JE, Mielke B: Percutaneous trephine drill biopsy: Evolving role. *Chest* 70:212, 1976.
16. Jones FL Jr: A comparison of trephine and Franklin-Silverman needles for percutaneous lung biopsy. *Am Rev Respir Dis* 109:625, 1974.
17. Zavala DC: Transbronchial biopsy in diffuse lung disease. *Chest* 73(suppl):727, 1978.
18. Schure D, Abraham JL, Konopka R: How should transbronchial biopsies be performed and processed? *Am Rev Respir Dis* 126:342, 1982.
19. Kovnat DM, Rath GS, Anderson WM, et al: Bronchial brushing through the flexible fiberoptic bronchoscope in the diagnosis of peripheral pulmonary lesions. *Chest* 67:179, 1975.
20. Ellis JH: Transbronchial lung biopsy via the fiberoptic bronchoscope. *Chest* 68:524, 1975.
21. Cortese DA, McDougall JC: Biopsy and brushing of peripheral lung cancer with fluoroscopic guidance. *Chest* 75:141, 1979.
22. Wang KP, Terry P, Marsh BR: Bronchoscopic needle aspiration biopsy of paratracheal tumors. *Am Rev Respir Dis* 118:17, 1978.
23. Wang KP, March BR, Summer WR, et al: Transbronchial needle aspiration for diagnosis of lung cancer. *Chest* 80:48, 1981.
24. Wang KP, Terry PB: Transbronchial needle aspiration in the diagnosis and staging of bronchogenic carcinoma. *Am Rev Respir Dis* 127:344, 1983.
25. Strumpf IJ, Feld MK, Cornelius MJ, et al: Safety of fiberoptic bronchoalveolar lavage in evaluation of interstitial lung disease. *Chest* 80:268, 1982.
26. Drew WL, Finley TN, Mintz L, et al: Diagnosis of *Pneumocystis carinii* pneumonia by bronchoalveolar lavage. *JAMA* 230:713, 1974.
27. Drew WL, Finley TH, Golde DW: Diagnostic lavage and occult pulmonary hemorrhage in thrombocytopenic immunocompromised patients. *Am Rev Respir Dis* 116:215, 1977.
28. Springmeger SC, Hackman R, Carlson JJ, et al: Bronchoalveolar cell carcinoma diagnosed by bronchoalveolar lavage. *Chest* 83:278, 1983.
29. Corwin RW, Irwin RS: Sensitivity and specificity of the lipid-laden macrophage in diagnosing exogenous lipoid pneumonia. *Am Rev Respir Dis* 127(suppl):94, 1983.
30. Martin RJ, Coalson JJ, Rogers RM, et al: Pulmonary alveolar proteinosis: The diagnosis by segmental lavage. *Am Rev Respir Dis* 121:819, 1980.
31. Basset F, Soler P, Jaurand ML, et al: Ultrastructural examination of bronchoalveolar lavage for diagnosis of pulmonary histiocytosis X: Preliminary report of 4 cases. *Thorax* 32:303, 1977.
32. Reynolds HY: Bronchoalveolar lavage. *Am Rev Respir Dis* 135:250, 1987.
33. Colt HG: Thoracoscopy: New Frontiers. *Pul Perspect* 9:1, 1992.
34. Mathur P, Marin WJ II: Clinical utility of thoracoscopy. *Chest* 102:2, 1992.
35. Boutin C, Viallat JR, Cargnino P, et al: Thoracoscopic lung biopsy: Experimental and clinical preliminary study. *Chest* 82:44, 1982.
36. Dijkman JH, van der Meer JWM, Bakker W, et al: Transpleural lung biopsy by the thoracoscopic route in patients with diffuse interstitial pulmonary disease. *Chest* 82:76, 1982.
37. Hartman DL, Mylet D, Gaither JG, et al: Comparison of thoracoscopic lung biopsy with open lung biopsy in diffuse interstitial lung disorders. *Am Rev Respir Dis* 145:A750, 1992.
38. Bensard DD, McIntyre RC Jr, Waring BJ, et al: Comparison of video thoracoscopic lung biopsy to open lung biopsy in the diagnosis of interstitial lung disease. *Chest* 103:765, 1993.
39. Herf SM, Suratt PM, Arora NS: Deaths and complications associated with transbronchial lung biopsy. *Am Rev Respir Dis* 111:853, 1975.
40. Koerner SK, Sakowitz AJ, Appleman RI, et al: Transbronchial lung biopsy for the diagnosis of sarcoidosis. *N Engl J Med* 293:268, 1975.
41. Koontz CH, Joyner LR, Nelson RA: Transbronchial lung biopsy via the fiberoptic bronchoscope in sarcoidosis. *Ann Intern Med* 85:64, 1976.
42. Poe RH, Israel RH, Utell MJ, et al: Possibility of a positive transbronchial lung biopsy result in sarcoidosis. *Arch Intern Med* 139:761, 1979.
43. Mathay RA, Farmer WC, Odero D: Diagnostic fiberoptic bronchoscopy in the immunocompromised host with pulmonary infiltrates. *Thorax* 32:539, 1977.
44. Repsher LH, Schroter G, Hammond WS: Diagnosis of *Pneumocystis carinii* pneumonitis by means of endobronchial brush biopsy. *N Engl J Med* 287:340, 1972.
45. Scheinhorn DI, Joyner LR, Whitcomb ME: Transbronchial forceps lung biopsy through the fiberoptic bronchoscope in *Pneumocystis carinii* pneumonia. *Chest* 66:294, 1974.
46. Mathay RS, Moritz ED: Invasive procedures for diagnosing pulmonary infections, in Reynolds HY (ed): *Clinics in Chest Medicine: Pulmonary Infections.* Philadelphia, WB Saunders, 1981, p 3.
47. Wall CP, Gaensler EA, Carrington CB, et al: Comparison of transbronchial and open biopsies in chronic infiltrative lung disease. *Am Rev Respir Dis* 123:280, 1981.
48. Bandt DB, Blank N, Castellino RA: Needle diagnosis of pneumonitis: Value in high risk patients. *JAMA* 220:1578, 1972.
49. Palmer DL, Davidson M, Lusk R: Needle aspiration of the lung in complex pneumonias. *Chest* 78:16, 1980.
50. Berquist TH, Bailey PB, Cortese DA, et al: Transthoracic needle biopsy. *Mayo Clin Proc* 55:475, 1980.
51. Gibney RTN, Man GCW, King EG, et al: Aspiration biopsy in the diagnosis of pulmonary disease. *Chest* 80:300, 1981.
52. Sagel SS, Ferguson TB, Forrest JV, et al: Percutaneous transthoracic aspiration needle biopsy. *Ann Thorac Surg* 26:399, 1978.
53. Lillington GA: The solitary pulmonary nodule 1974. *Am Rev Respir Dis* 110:699, 1974.
54. Wallace JM, Deutsch L: Flexible fiberoptic bronchoscopy and percutaneous needle lung aspiration for evaluating the solitary pulmonary nodule. *Chest* 81:665, 1982.
55. Poe RH, Robin RE: Sensitivity and specificity of needle biopsy in lung malignancy. *Am Rev Respir Dis* 122:755, 1980.
56. Sinner WN: Material and results, in Sinner WN (ed): *Needle Biopsy and Transbronchial Biopsy.* New York, Thieme-Stratton, 1982, p 18.
57. Sinner WN: Complications, in Sinner WN (ed): *Needle Biopsy and Transbronchial Biopsy.* New York, Thieme-Stratton, 1982, p 44.
58. Popovich J, Koace PA, Eichenhorn MS, et al: Diagnostic accuracy of multiple biopsies from flexible fiberoptic bronchoscopy. *Am Rev Respir Dis* 125:521, 1982.
59. Rosen PP, Martini N, Armstrong D: *Pneumocystis carinii* pneumonia: Diagnosis by lung biopsy. *Am J Med* 58:794, 1975.
60. Greenman RL, Goodall PT, King D: Lung biopsy in immunocompromised hosts. *Am J Med* 59:488, 1975.
61. Wolff LJ, Bartlett MS, Baehner RL, et al: The causes of interstitial pneumonitis in immunocompromised children: An aggressive systematic approach to diagnosis. *Pediatrics* 60:41, 1977.
62. Leight GS, Michaelis LL: Open lung biopsy for the diagnosis of acute, diffuse, pulmonary infiltrates in the compromised host. *Chest* 73:477, 1978.
63. Singer L, Armstrong D, Rosen PD, et al: Diffuse pulmonary infiltrates in immunosuppressed patients. *Am J Med* 66:110, 1979.
64. Rossiter SJ, Miller DC, Churg AM, et al: Open lung biopsy in the immunosuppressed patient: Is it really beneficial? *J Thorac Cardiovasc Surg* 77:338, 1979.
65. Jaffe JJ, Maki DG: Lung biopsy in immunocompromised patients: One institution's experience and an approach to management of pulmonary disease in the compromised host. *Cancer* 48:1144, 1981.
66. Hiatt JR, Gong H, Mulder DG, et al: The value of open lung biopsy in the immunosuppressed patient. *Surgery* 92:285, 1982.
67. Repsher LH, Schroter G, Hammond WS: Diagnosis of *Pneumocystis carinii* pneumonitis by means of endobronchial brush biopsy. *N Engl J Med* 287:340, 1972.
68. Pennington JD, Feldman NT: Pulmonary infiltrates and fever in patients with hematologic malignancy. *Am J Med* 62:581, 1977.
69. Cunningham JH, Zavala DC, Corry RJ, et al: Trephine air drill, bron-

chial brush, and fiberoptic transbronchial biopsy in immunosuppressed patients. *Am Rev Respir Dis* 115:213, 1977.

70. Poe RH, Utell MJ, Israel RH, et al: Sensitivity and specificity of the non-specific transbronchial biopsy. *Am Rev Respir Dis* 119:25, 1979.

71. Lauver GL, Husan FM, Morgan RB, et al: The usefulness of fiberoptic bronchoscopy in evaluations of new pulmonary lesions in the compromised host. *Am J Med* 66:580, 1979.

72. Phillips MJ, Knight RR, Green M: Fiberoptic bronchoscopy and diagnosis of pulmonary lesions in lymphoma and leukemia. *Thorax* 35:19, 1980.

73. Nisho JH, Lynch JP: Fiberoptic bronchoscopy in the immunocompromised host: The significance of a "non-specific" transbronchial biopsy. *Am Rev Respir Dis* 121:307, 1980.

74. Hedemark LL, Kronenberg RS, Rasp FL, et al: The value of bronchoscopy in establishing the etiology of pneumonia in renal transplant recipients. *Am Rev Respir Dis* 126:981, 1982.

75. Fitzgerald W, Bevelaqua FA, Garay SM, et al: The role of open lung biopsy in patients with the acquired immunodeficiency syndrome. *Chest* 91:659, 1987.

76. Rankin JA, Collman R, Daniele RP: Acquired immune deficiency syndrome and the lung. *Chest* 94:155, 1988.

77. Springmeyer SC, Silvestri RC, Sale GE, et al: The role of transbronchial biopsy for the diagnosis of diffuse pneumonias in immunocompromised marrow transplant recipients. *Am Rev Respir Dis* 126:763, 1982.

78. Hopewell PC: *Pneumocystis carinii* pneumonia: Diagnosis. *J Infect Dis* 157:1115, 1988.

79. Hill JD, Ratliff JL, Parrott JCW, et al: Pulmonary pathology in acute respiratory insufficiency: Lung biopsy as a diagnostic tool. *J Thorac Cardiovasc Surg* 71:64, 1976.

80. Tenholder MF, Hooper RG: Pulmonary infiltrates in leukemia. *Chest* 78:468, 1980.

81. Pincus PS, Kallenbach JM, Hurwitz MD, et al: Transbronchial biopsy during mechanical ventilation. *Crit Care Med* 15:1136, 1987.

82. Papin TA, Grum CM, Weg JG: Transbronchial biopsy during mechanical ventilation. *Chest* 89:168, 1986.

V. Renal Problems in the Intensive Care Unit

Section Editor
Andrew J. Cohen

78. Physiologic Concepts in the Management of Renal, Fluid, and Electrolyte Disorders in the Intensive Care Unit

Andrew J. Cohen

Overview of Renal Physiology— Key Concepts

The kidneys maintain water and solute homeostasis, guarding the body's "internal milieu" [1]. They are provided with 20 to 25% of cardiac output (at rest) and filter approximately 180 liters of fluid per day (Table 78-1). The enormous filtration rate is permitted by the specialized nature of the glomerular capillary network, which provides a large, porous surface area for filtration and a sufficiently high hydraulic driving force (see below). Despite the impressive filtered load of water and solutes, however, only a tiny fraction of these substances are excreted. Moreover, their excretion rate is normally equal to the rate of intake for each substance. This marvelous feat, separately regulating water and individual solute excretion, is due to the exquisite processing of glomerular filtrate by the nephron. An elaborate system of local physical forces and circulating hormones participate in tubular solute and water transport activities.

GLOMERULAR FUNCTION

Glomerular Blood Flow and Glomerular Filtration. The kidneys receive approximately 25% of cardiac output (Table 78-2) and consume more oxygen per gram of tissue weight than any other visceral organ. Over 90% of renal blood flow is directed to the renal cortex and courses through glomeruli. The predominant driving force for glomerular filtration, however, is the hydrostatic pressure in glomerular capillaries.

As shown in Figure 78-1, there is a large step-down in hydrostatic pressure at the level of the *afferent* glomerular arteriole. Hence, the pressure in the glomerular capillary (approximately 45 mm Hg) is less than half of systemic blood pressure; however, this pressure is considerably greater than the average

hydrostatic pressure of peripheral blood capillaries (approximately 24 mm Hg) and is one of the reasons for the high filtration rate.

The forces that govern the filtration rate through a single nephron (SNGFR) are characterized by the Starling equation and are the net effect of the forces favoring filtration minus the forces that oppose filtration.

Forces favoring filtration = $P_{GC} + \pi_{BS}$

where P_{GC} is the glomerular capillary hydrostatic pressure and π_{BS} is the colloid osmotic pressure in Bowman's space

Forces opposing filtration = $P_T + \pi_{GC}$

where P_T is the proximal tubular (or Bowman's space) hydrostatic pressure and π_{GC} is the colloid osmotic pressure in glomerular capillaries

$$SNGFR = \{(P_{GC} + \pi_{BS}) - (P_T + \pi_{GC})\} \times K_f$$

where K_f is a constant, the *ultrafiltration coefficient*, which represents glomerular capillary *surface area* and *hydraulic conductivity* (i.e., permeability to small solutes like water, Na, Cl, and glucose).

If the hydrostatic pressures are combined into a pressure gradient, $\Delta P = P_{GC} - P_T$ and it is assumed that π_{BS} is negligible (since glomerular capillaries are normally relatively impermeant to macromolecules), the equation can be simplified as follows:

$$SNGFR = K_f (\Delta P - \pi_{GC})$$

Hence, the glomerular filtration rate in a single nephron represents the balance between the hydrostatic pressure gradient, P, the predominant force driving filtration, and glomerular capillary colloid osmotic pressure, π_{GC}.

Although it is a "constant," the ultrafiltration coefficient K_f can be altered by changes in glomerular capillary surface area or permeability. It is believed that capillary surface area is under dynamic control by glomerular mesangial cells. These are functionally and histologically similar to vascular smooth muscle

Table 78-1. Filtration and Excretion Rates of Water and Solutes

Substance	Plasma concentration (mM)	Filtered load (mmoles/ day)	Excreted (mmoles/day)	Percent substance resorbed
Sodium	140	27,000	~100	>99
Chloride	105	19,000	~100	>99
Bicarbonate	25	4,500	~2	>99
Potassium	4	720	~100	>86
Glucose	5	900	0–trace	>99
Urea	5	900	360	60
Water	—	180	1–1.5	>99

Table 78-2. Common Values for Whole-Kidney Hemodynamics

Measurement	Value
Renal blood flow (RBF)	1200 ml/min (20–25% of cardiac output)
Renal plasma flow (RPF)	RBF × (1-HCT) = 660 ml/min
Glomerular filtration rate (GFR)	125 ml/min
Filtration fraction	GFR/RPF = 0.18–0.20

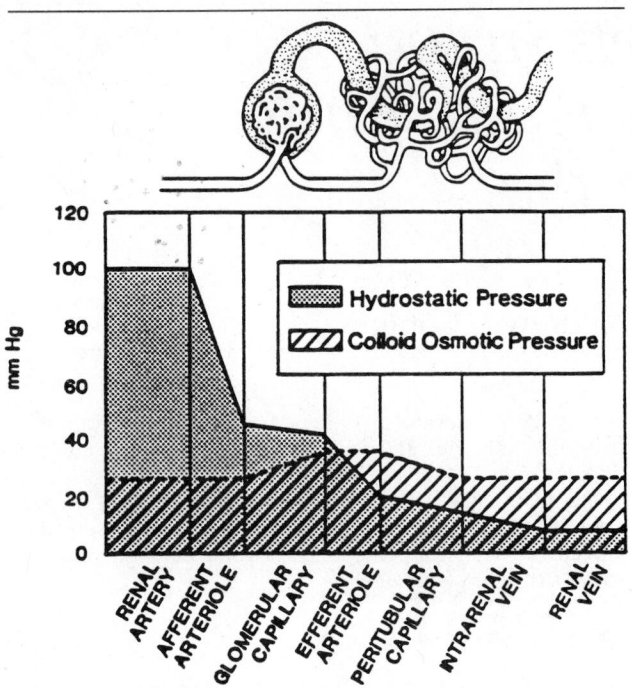

Fig. 78-1. Hydrostatic and colloid osmotic pressures at various levels of the renal vasculature, (From Sullivan & Grantham, *Physiology of the Kidney*. Reproduced with permission).

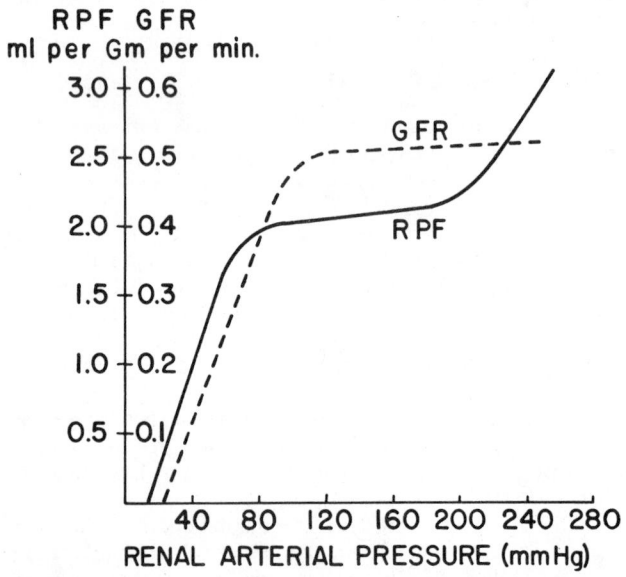

Fig. 78-2. The effect of changes in mean arterial pressure on both RBF and GFR.

cells, expressing membrane receptors for and contracting in response to angiotensin II, vasopressin, and possibly other hormonal stimuli [2].

Autoregulation. The term *autoregulation* encompasses the maintenance of renal blood flow (RBF) and glomerular filtration over a wide range of arterial pressures. As can be seen in Figure 78-2, between mean arterial pressures of 80 mm Hg and 200 mm Hg, both RBF and glomerular filtration rate (GFR) are relatively constant. Separate mechanisms regulate the autoregulation of blood flow and filtration, but both appear to be intrinsic to the kidney, i.e., they are observed in the isolated, perfused organ, free of extrarenal neural or humoral inputs. RBF autoregulation may be controlled by local factors that govern cytosolic calcium in vascular smooth muscle. Increasing hydrostatic pressure in the renal artery (perhaps by directly enhancing membrane calcium permeability) leads to heightened contractility of the afferent arteriole, thus maintaining constancy of glomerular blood flow (GBF). Contrariwise, diminished arterial pressure causes relaxation of the afferent arteriole and maintenance of GBF. This is referred to as the *myogenic reflex*.

Filtration autoregulation, a more complex process, requires the coordination of afferent and efferent glomerular capillary sphincters to maintain constancy of glomerular capillary pressure. Figure 78-3 shows that lowering systemic blood pressure or renal artery pressure within the autoregulatory range results in dilation of the afferent arteriole, possibly mediated by the synthesis of vasodilatory prostaglandins. Coupled with the constriction of the efferent arteriole, mediated by local formation of angiotensin II, this leads to an elevation of P_{GC} and maintenance of GFR.

The proposed mechanism of filtration autoregulation is depicted in Figure 78-3. Capillary hydrostatic pressure P_{GC} (and GFR) is maintained by a combination of afferent arteriolar dilation and efferent constriction. The latter is mediated by a selective effect of intrarenal angiotensin (ANG II), the former presumably is mediated by vasodilatory prostaglandins or nitric oxide [3].

Angiotensin II appears to selectively operate at the efferent sphincter [4] when locally produced. At higher circulating levels, sufficient to raise blood pressure, angiotensin II also causes afferent vasoconstriction, perhaps due to a myogenic reflex.

Fig. 78-3. Mechanism of autoregulation of GFR.

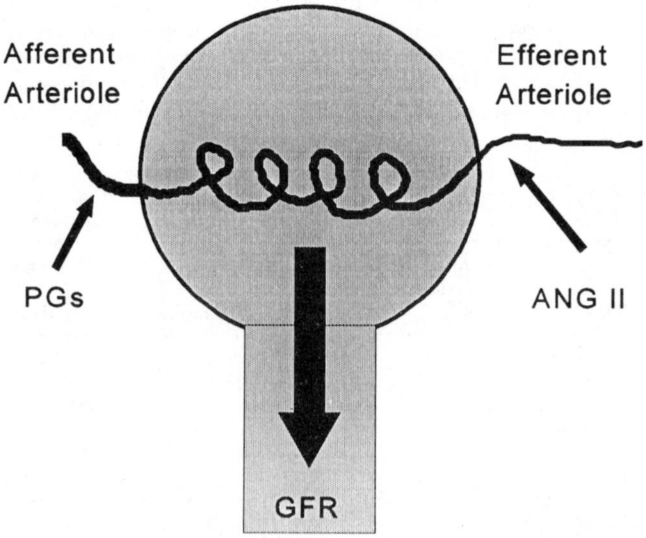

Afferent Arteriole   Efferent Arteriole

PGs   ANG II

GFR

Alternatively, offsetting vasodilatory hormones or autocoids, such as prostacylin or nitric oxide, might compensate for the vasoconstrictor action of the angiotensin II at the afferent but not the efferent arteriole.

Filtration autoregulation is central to maintenance of renal function during conditions when renal perfusion pressure is low, such as in renal artery stenosis [5] and in severe congestive heart failure [6]. The elevation of postglomerular arteriolar tone not only preserves GFR but also leads to reduced pressure in postglomerular, peritubular capillaries. The attendant changes in the physical forces mediated by hydrostatic factors in the postglomerular capillaries that lie in series with glomerular capillaries serve to enhance sodium reabsorption in the proximal tubule, thus contributing to so-called glomerulotubular balance, which is described below.

Macromolecular Sieving. The glomerular capillary wall is composed of endothelial cell, basement membrane, and epithelial cell podocyte. It is freely permeable to water and small solutes, as described earlier. Molecules of larger size, allosteric configuration, and molecular weight (macromolecules, MW > 5000 daltons) are normally restricted from passage into the urinary space, however. The major limitations are size (molecular radius) and electrostatic charge. Regarding electrostatic charge, it should be recalled that the glomerular capillary basement membrane is rich in sialoproteins that confer upon it a negative electrostatic charge. Hence, albumin (MW ~69,000 daltons, negatively charged) largely is withheld from crossing the glomerular capillary; consequently, less than 60 mg is normally excreted in 24 hours.

In certain glomerular disease, to be described later, changes in the glomerular barrier result in the abnormal appearance of albumin in the urine.

TUBULAR SODIUM REABSORPTION

Proximal Tubule. Of the 27,000 mmoles of sodium filtered by the glomeruli each day, only 10 to 250 mmoles (<1%), equivalent to dietary sodium intake, are excreted in the urine. Sodium is reabsorbed along the entire nephron, as shown in Figure 78-4. Approximately two-thirds of the delivered load of sodium is reabsorbed by each major nephron segment.

Figure 78-5 depicts the close relationship between glomerular filtration and proximal tubular reabsorption. On the left, in the normal subject, Figure 78-5A shows that along the length of the glomerular capillary the colloid osmotic pressure ($\Delta\pi$) rises until it meets the level of the capillary hydrostatic pressure gradient (ΔP). Since the area *between* the two lines represents net ultrafiltration pressure, filtration equilibrium exists at the efferent end of the capillary, and no further filtration takes place. In the peritubular (postglomerular) capillary, the forces are reversed, $\Delta\pi > \Delta P$, and *reabsorption* of fluid takes place. This is reflected by the arrow (for $\Delta\pi$) pointing into the peritubular capillary in Figure 78-5B.

The right side of Figures 78-5A and 78-5B depict the situation of filtration autoregulation (as occurs in congestive heart failure [CHF]). As can be seen, the resultant elevation of P_{GC} and ΔP lead to a steeper incline of $\Delta\pi$ and a larger *step-down* of ΔP in the peritubular capillary. The attendant increase in the area between $\Delta\pi$ and ΔP in the peritubular capillary signifies enhancement of forces favoring reabsorption. This is depicted by the broader arrow into the peritubular capillary on the right of Figure 78-5B. The impact of this process on edema formation in CHF will be described below.

Distal Nephron. The proximal tubule reclaims the bulk of filtered sodium, and the remaining 30 to 40% is reabsorbed in

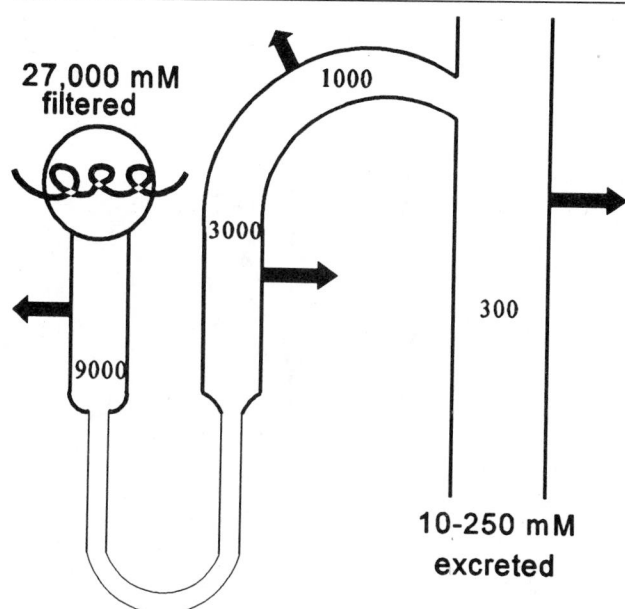

Fig. 78-4. Reabsorption of sodium along the nephron. Numbers beside each nephron segment represent millimoles of sodium remaining in the tubule.

the thick ascending limb of Henle's loop, distal tubule, and collecting duct. In these segments, "fine tuning" adjustments are made for the regulation of sodium reabsorption.

The mineralocorticoid aldosterone, under the influence of the renin-angiotensin system, stimulates sodium absorption in the distal tubule and collecting duct. In addition, circulating catecholamines (predominantly epinephrine) and angiotensin II may directly stimulate sodium reabsorption. Furthermore, increased renal sympathetic neuronal tone contributes to sodium reabsorption by inducing renal vasoconstriction, local renin release, and the release of local catecholamines.

Locally produced autacoids and circulating hormones also appear to regulate sodium metabolism by *increasing* sodium excretion. Prostaglandin E_2, produced in glomeruli and medullary interstitial cells, promotes renal vasodilation and inhibits sodium chloride uptake in the cortical thick ascending limb, thereby increasing sodium excretion.

A series of peptides, known collectively as atrial natriuretic peptide (ANP, atriopeptin, auriculun, and cardionatrin), isolated from cardiac myocytes have been fully purified and sequenced. When given intravenously or directly into the renal artery, ANP promotes mild renal vasodilation, an increase in GFR, and a substantial increase in urinary sodium excretion. This substance is measurable in the circulation and appears to be released by atrial stretch or increase in plasma volume (e.g., with saline infusion). Its importance in volume homeostasis in normal and pathologic states (e.g., CHF) remains to be determined [7].

BODY WATER HOMEOSTASIS. The regulation of renal water excretion is segregated from that of sodium excretion, as can be demonstrated by the classic experiment depicted in Figure 78-6 [8]. In this experiment, a normal subject, given either 1000 ml of water or 1% sodium chloride by mouth, excretes most of the water after 3 hours but only a fraction of the saline solution. This experiment demonstrates that the water-excre-

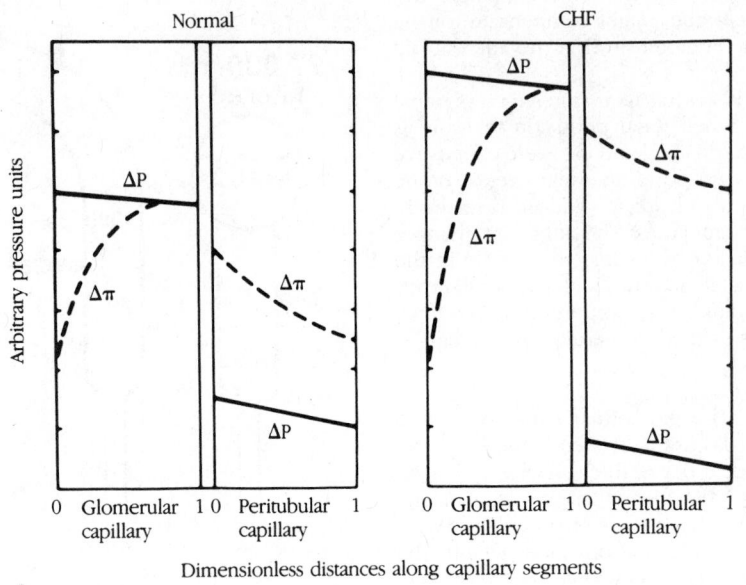

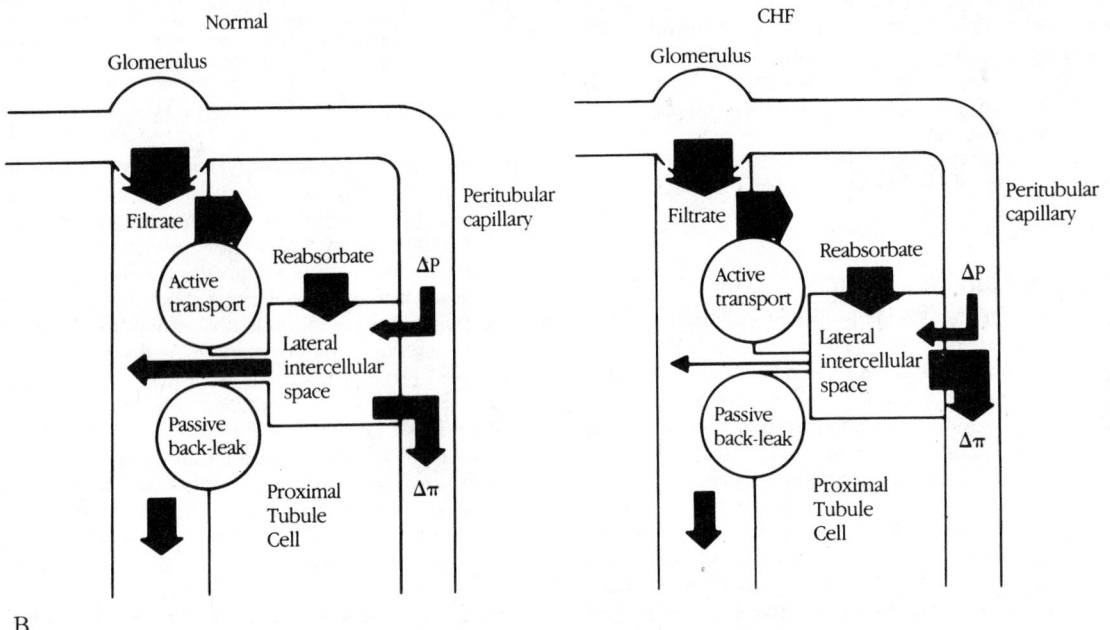

Fig. 78-5. Comparison of hydraulic forces in glomerular and peritubular capillaries in the normal state and in congestive heart failure (CHF). *A.* Demonstration of hydraulic pressure profiles in glomerular and peritubular capillaries in normal (*left*) and CHF (*right*). *B.* Proximal nephron in normal subject (*left*) and patient with CHF (*right*) undergoing filtration autoregulation. The enhanced proximal tubular reabsorption in CHF stems from more favorable hydrostatic forces for reuptake by the peritubular capillaries.

tory response is both exceedingly rapid (more rapid than the response to saline, which requires more than a full day) and separately controlled.

The mechanism responsible for this almost instantaneous response to water intake (or deprivation) is the hypothalamo-pituitary regulation of antidiuretic hormone (ADH, also known as vasopressin or arginine vasopressin [AVP]) secretion. ADH release by the supraoptic and paraventricular hypothalamic nuclei tightly guards body fluid osmolarity around a range of no more than 4%, as shown below:

> 2% decrease in body water → ADH secretion → renal water retention
> 2% increase in body water → ADH suppression → renal water excretion

The centrality of ADH in the regulation of renal water excretion hinges on its instantaneous and sensitive response to very

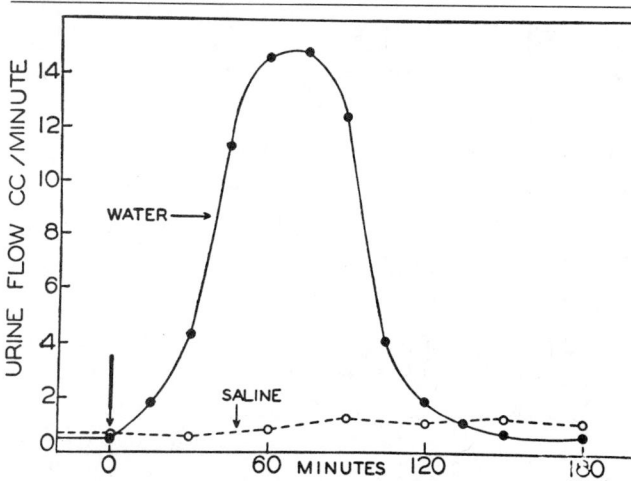

Fig. 78-6. Effect of ingestion of 1 liter of either water (solid line) or isotonic saline (dashed line) on urine flow in a normal subject (From Smith HW: Excretion of sodium and other strong electrolytes, in Smith HW (ed).: *The Kidney: Structure and Function in Health and Disease.* New York, Oxford University Press, 1951. Reproduced with permission).

minor changes in body fluid tonicity and to the unique properties of the renal medulla and collecting duct. The renal medullary interstitium displays an increasing level of tonicity from the outer medulla to the papillary tip. In normal human subjects, the osmolarity at the papillary tip may approach 1200 mOsm/kg H_2O. Interstitial hyperosmolarity is produced and maintained by the countercurrent multiplier depicted in Figure 78-7 [9].

As shown in Figure 78-7, the process of generating a hypertonic medullary interstitium is established by countercurrent flow in the ascending and descending limbs and their differences in water permeability. Although the descending limb is water-permeable, the ascending limb is not, as signified by the darkened lines. Active reabsorption of chloride and sodium in the thick ascending limb (process 1) dilutes the tubular fluid but makes the outer medulla slightly hypertonic. In the distal tubule and cortical collecting duct, water is reabsorbed because of the established osmotic gradient (process 2). This takes place only if ADH is present, rendering the collecting duct permeable to water. Otherwise, in its native state, this segment is not water-permeable. Because of the outflow of water, the urea concentration in the collecting duct lumen rises, as depicted by the increasing letter-size. Because of the rise in the intraluminal urea concentration, at the inner medullary collecting duct, urea diffuses into the interstitium following its concentration gradient (process 3). This accumulation of urea in the inner medullary interstitium contributes to its tonicity and leads to the abstraction of water from the descending limb (process 4). The resultant increase in luminal sodium chloride concentration causes it to diffuse outward at the inner medullary ascending limb (process 5), thus adding to the interstitial osmolar gradient. Thus, ADH is required to establish a maximal interstitial gradient and for the final concentration of the urine.

The process of urinary dilution is *not* the mirror image of urinary concentration. Maximal urinary dilution, like urinary concentration, requires active removal of NaCl by the thick ascending limb. This process establishes a dilute tubular fluid. Inadequate sodium chloride delivery to the thick ascending limb or inhibition of the thick ascending limb function (e.g.,

with a diuretic) impairs urinary dilution. With adequate function of the thick ascending limb (also known as the diluting segment) and suppression of ADH secretion urinary, however, osmolarity can fall to below 50 mOsm/kg H_2O. Hence, ingestion of water results in prompt excretion of the water load.

Renal Mechanisms in the Pathophysiology of Edema Formation

The kidney controls sodium and water homeostasis with exquisite precision, depending on the perceived extracellular fluid (ECF) volume. When ECF is decreased by extrarenal losses (e.g., hemorrhage, GI losses), the kidney attempts to restore this compartment by intensely reclaiming most of the filtered sodium and water. This complex system involves the stimulation of both intrarenal (juxtaglomerular apparatus) and extrarenal (atrial volume receptors, carotid and aortic baroreceptors) sensor elements, which thereby trigger renal sodium retention. Edema formation results when the kidney is signaled by some or all of these mechanisms to conserve sodium due to a reduction in "effective circulating volume." The concept of *effective circulating volume* means that the volume *perceived* by the kidney is reduced, although the absolute plasma volume may actually be normal or even elevated.

EFFECTOR MECHANISMS. The effector limb of sodium retention in edema-forming states involves several elements that increase sodium reabsorption at different sites along the nephron. The process of edema formation can be explored using CHF as a model.

Glomerular Filtration, Renal Blood Flow, and Peritubular Physical Factors. If a reduction in cardiac output produces a parallel decrease in the GFR, it should effect a similar change in sodium excretion. Unless cardiac output is severely reduced, however, GFR usually remains near normal. GFR is protected from reduced cardiac output and arterial pressure by filtration autoregulation. The mechanism by which glomerular filtration is autoregulated is uncertain, but it appears to involve local activation of the renin-angiotensin system, as described above [10]. As perfusion pressure decreases, local mechanisms promote renin secretion and angiotensin formation. Angiotensin II is a potent vasoconstrictor and apparently constricts the efferent glomerular arteriole selectively [4]. The resultant increase in efferent arteriolar resistance maintains hydrostatic pressure within glomerular capillaries and GFR.

Figure 78-5 plots transcapillary hydraulic pressure, ΔP, and colloid osmotic pressure π along the glomerular and peritubular capillaries in both normal subjects and patients with CHF. Note that at the efferent end of glomerular capillaries, both ΔP and π are considerably higher in patients with CHF. Because of elevated efferent resistance, however (presumably a result of the effect of angiotensin II), there is a larger step-down of ΔP in CHF. The reduced ΔP and larger increment in π in peritubular capillaries provides more favorable Starling forces for uptake of reabsorbate, as shown in Fig. 78-5 [11].

When RBF is reduced, blood flow to the deep cortex is relatively spared. Perfusion is preferentially shunted to juxtaglomerular nephrons with long loops of Henle. Since these present a greater reabsorptive surface area, this mechanism theoretically contributes to sodium retention; however, shunting of renal perfusion to deep cortical nephrons has not been found

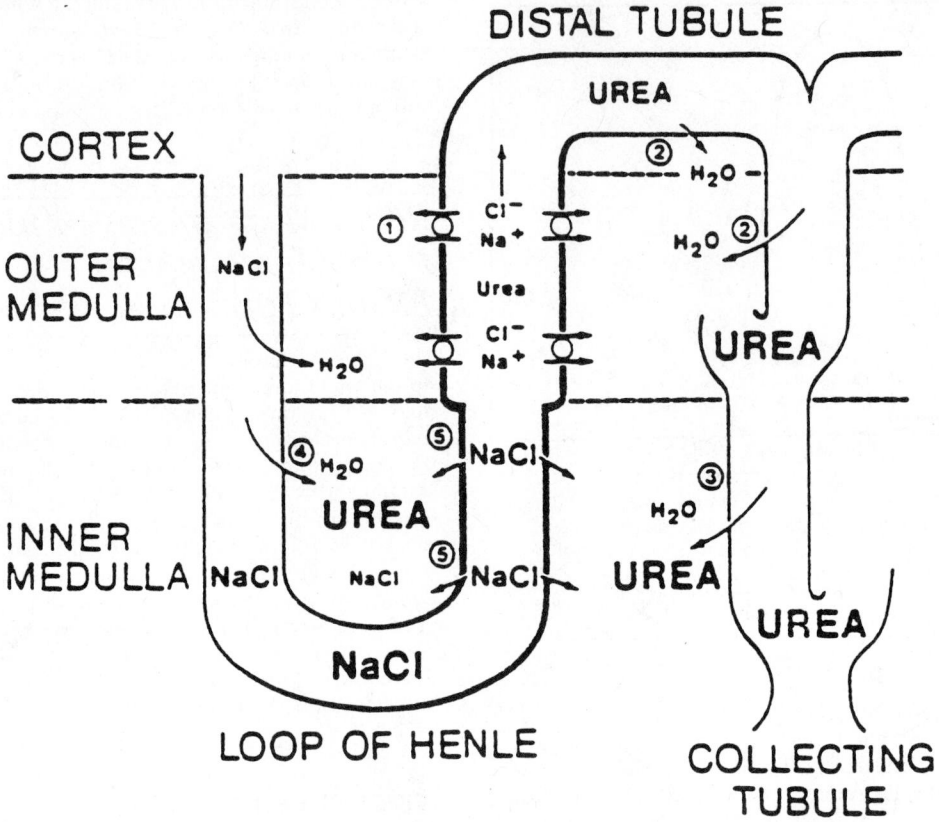

Fig. 78-7. Countercurrent multiplier with resultant interstitial osmotic gradient. (Reproduced from Jamison RL, Maffly RH: Mechanism of urinary concentration. *N Engl J Med* 295:1062, 1976.)

uniformly in experimental heart failure, and its importance is debated [12].

Renin-Angiotensin-Aldosterone. The changes in filtration fraction and peritubular physical forces that accompany heart failure promote equiproportional increases in filtered sodium load and proximal tubular sodium uptake; however, the net increase in renal sodium retention probably rests on distal nephron mechanisms. Although there is aldosterone-independent sodium reabsorption in the distal tubule, much attention has focused on aldosterone because its release is controlled partly by angiotensin II. Hence, in edema-forming states in which there are elevations of plasma renin and angiotensin levels, aldosterone also is high. Aldosterone exerts its effects at the cortical collecting duct [13].

Doubt, however, has arisen concerning the importance of secondary hyperaldosteronism in the sodium retention of edema-forming states, because some patients with CHF do not have elevated plasma aldosterone levels [14]. Nonetheless, experimental cardiac failure in dogs is invariably accompanied by acute hyperreninemia, hyperaldosteronism, and sodium retention, later followed by normalization of renin and aldosterone values [15]. Chronic angiotensin-converting enzyme inhibition, which prevents secondary hyperaldosteronism in these animals, also reduces the degree of sodium retention [15]. These studies suggest that activation of the renin-angiotensin-aldosterone system may be critical in the acute generation of sodium retention. Once positive sodium balance and extracellular vol-

ume expansion have occurred, however, the stimuli to this system are no longer operative, and a new steady-state level of sodium balance is achieved. In experimental models, inhibition of angiotensin and aldosterone formation before induction of heart failure reduces but does not completely abolish renal sodium avidity in cardiac failure. Presumably, therefore, other forces also contribute to the control of sodium excretion in heart failure.

Atrial Natriuretic Peptide and Other Humoral Substances. In addition to the renin-angiotensin-aldosterone system, the presence or absence of other humoral factors also may contribute to renal salt conservation in heart failure. The relative contribution of these agents to edema formation has yet to be determined.

Both increased renal sympathetic neural tone [16] and increased circulating catecholamines [17] are typically found in patients with heart failure. These mechanisms may contribute to renal vasoconstriction and redirect blood flow to the inner cortex. They also appear to stimulate tubular sodium reabsorption directly, as shown by in vitro studies in the isolated perfused kidney [18]. Beta-adrenergic catecholamines also stimulate juxtaglomerular cell renin secretion, as does renal nerve stimulation [19]. Hence, both circulating and neuronal catecholamines may enhance sodium retention and edema formation.

Substantial evidence has accrued for the existence of a so-called natriuretic hormone [20]. Extracted samples of plasma or urine from subjects given volume expansion with saline and placed in water up to the neck (which increases central venous blood volume), or from patients with chronic renal failure, induce increased sodium excretion in isolated nephron segments [21] and intact animals [22]. Identification of the source of this hormone and the importance of its deficiency in sodium-retaining states such as heart failure has been hampered by the lack of a reliable assay.

In 1981, deBold and others [23] described a vasodilatory substance, released from mammalian cardiac atria, which had potent natriuretic properties [24]. The so-called atrial natriuretic peptide (ANP) has since been fully characterized as a peptide hormone with a known amino acid sequence. It participates in the homeostatic control of sodium excretion during volume expansion. Isoncotic extracellular expansion with normal saline increases the radioimmunoassayable levels of ANP [25]. It is stored in cardiac myocytes as a prohormone and released, presumably in response to stretch, into the circulation. Analysis of ANP action reveals that it increases renal sodium excretion by a combination of increasing GFR and the filtered load of sodium and by inhibition of distal nephron sodium reabsorption [26]. Chronic heart failure may be characterized by a loss of ANP release or a reduced renal response to ANP [27].

Renal prostaglandins may be more noted in edema formation in their absence than for their presence. These substances are potent renal vasodilators and thus enhance sodium excretion [28]. There is evidence that they inhibit sodium chloride transport by the cortical collecting duct, thereby also increasing sodium excretion [29]. Induction of prostaglandin E_2 (PGE_2) may also be responsible for the action of loop diuretics such as furosemide, since the inhibition of prostaglandin synthesis blunts the natriuretic effect of these agents [30]. Although there is no evidence to date that the absence of renal prostaglandins is important in edema formation in CHF, *inhibition of prostaglandin synthesis* with NSAIDS such as indomethacin may act synergistically with other factors and add to positive sodium balance and edema formation in patients with cardiac failure [31,32] as well as liver disease [33,34]. Moreover, concomitant use of NSAIDS may blunt the efficacy of some diuretics.

Pharmacology and Uses of Diuretics

Diuretics promote the excretion of solute and water by acting along distinct nephron sites. Although agents that enhance glomerular filtration (e.g., digoxin, dopamine, glucocorticoids) increase urine flow, they are pharmacologically distinct from diuretics and are not considered here.

In general, a diuretic causes the loss of either *solute* or *water* predominantly. A solute diuresis ensues when nephron solute reabsorption is blocked and a larger fraction of filtered solute is excreted in the urine. This can occur when an impermeant substance like mannitol, once filtered by the glomerulus, subsequently impedes the reabsorption of water. This is known as an *osmotic* diuresis. A solute diuresis will also develop when reabsorption is blocked at specific sites along the nephron by agents that selectively impair transepithelial transport. Although these types of diuretic agents have been identified with specific nephron segments, their intracellular mechanisms of action remain obscure. In water diuresis, on the other hand, urinary water loss exceeds solute excretion. Agents that cause this type of diuresis work in the collecting ducts and tubules by impairing vasopressin-induced water reabsorption.

The efficacy of a given diuretic to reduce plasma volume by inhibiting transport in one nephron segment is limited by the capacity of other portions of the nephron to compensate for the induced loss of salt and water. Hence, if sodium reabsorption is inhibited, in the loop of Henle for example, sites proximal and distal to this nephron segment will reclaim proportion-

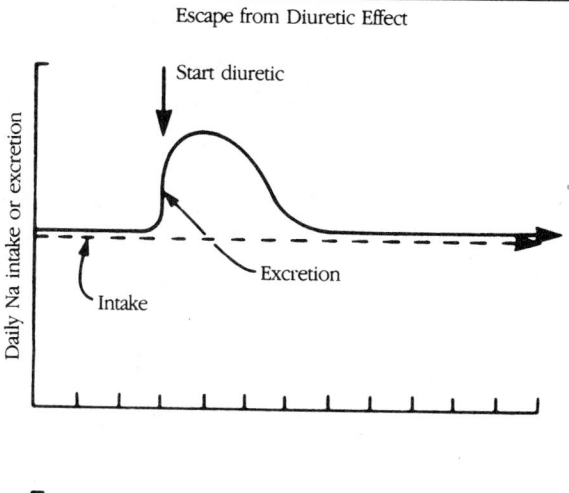

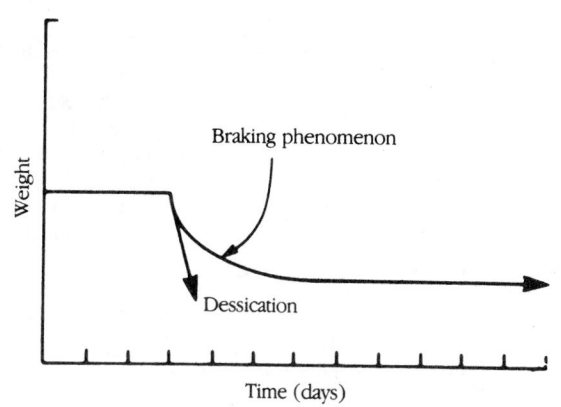

Fig. 78-8. The "braking phenomenon" in subjects placed on limited salt intake and a loop diuretic. There is an initial negative salt balance and weight loss. By 3 days a new steady state is achieved and no additional weight loss occurs. (From Grantham JJ, Chonko AM: The physiological basis and clinical use of diuretics, in Brenner BM, Stein JH [eds]: *Sodium and Water Homeostasis:* New York, Churchill Livingstone, 1978, p 178, with permission.)

ately more glomerular filtrate, thereby attenuating the effect of the diuretic. Ultimately, this mechanism will restore sodium homeostasis after a brief period of negative salt balance. This is known as the *braking phenomenon* (Fig. 78-8) [35]. The braking phenomenon explains why certain agents are ineffective diuretics. Since the loop of Henle and the distal nephron can compensate for a decrease in proximal reabsorption, agents that act primarily in the proximal tubule (e.g., acetazolamide) are weak diuretics. Conversely, a loop diuretic (e.g., furosemide) and a thiazide (which acts in the distal tubule) make a potent combination, since simultaneous administration of those agents prevents the compensating response.

SITES OF DIURETIC ACTION. Diuretics generally are classified according to their site of action along the nephron. Much information regarding their mechanisms of inhibiting solute transport emanates from studies in which tubules were micropunctured in vivo or nephron segments were perfused in vitro. The site of action for each agent is summarized in Table 78-3.

Proximal Tubule. In the proximal nephron, in which the bulk (70%) of glomerular filtrate is reabsorbed without any alteration

Table 78-3. Summary of Diuretic Site of Action, Diuresis, and Complications

Diuretic	Site of action	Type of diuresis	Frequent complications
Mannitol	Proximal tubule	Hypotonic	Hypernatremia, volume depletion
Acetazolamide	Proximal tubule	Bicarbonaturia, potassium wasting	Metabolic acidosis
Loop diuretics	Thick ascending limb (± proximal tubule)	Potassium wasting, large natriuresis, hypo- or isoosmotic	Hypokalemia, metabolic alkalosis, volume depletion, azotemia
Thiazide-type	Distal tubule (± proximal tubule)	Moderate natriuresis, potassium wasting	Hypokalemia, metabolic alkalosis, volume depletion
Spironolactone, triamterene, amiloride	Collecting duct	Potassium sparing	Hyperkalemia, metabolic acidosis
Lithium, demeclocycline	Collecting duct	Water diuretic	Nephrogenic diabetes insipidus

of total solute concentration (osmolarity), agents such as mannitol and acetazolamide are known to produce a diuresis.

MANNITOL. Mannitol is a polysaccharide, freely filtrable by the glomerulus, but unlike glucose, it is not reabsorbable. Its osmotic activity thus constrains fluid absorption by the proximal nephron and presents an overwhelming solute and fluid load to the distal tubules and collecting ducts. Although all diuretics increase solute excretion and therefore might be considered "osmotic," the characteristics of a mannitol diuresis are manifestations of increased fluid flow along the length of the nephron, thereby producing a urine that is generally isoosmotic with plasma. Under conditions in which the urine is concentrated, it produces a relative water diuresis. Mannitol is useful in the treatment of hypoosmolar (hyponatremic) conditions in which both the total body water and the plasma volume are expanded, such as heart failure. Since mannitol generally is given intravenously and remains confined to the extracellular space, however, its role in the management of congestive heart failure is limited: The osmotic gradient it creates may temporarily draw more fluid into the vascular compartment, increasing plasma volume and vascular congestion.

ACETAZOLAMIDE. Unlike mannitol, acetazolamide is secreted into the proximal nephron from the peritubular capillaries by a potent organic acid transport pathway [36], which is similar to the mechanism of secretion for thiazides and for the loop diuretics ethacrynic acid and furosemide. Acetazolamide inactivates the enzyme carbonic anhydrase, which catalyzes the conversion of CO_2 and water into bicarbonate. This inhibition causes a loss of tubular hydrogen ion secretion and consequent decrement in bicarbonate absorption. In the distal tubule, bicarbonate behaves as a nonreabsorbable anion and promotes a sodium and water diuresis. By reducing urinary hydrogen ion secretion, acetazolamide induces a metabolic acidosis. It is, however, a relatively weak diuretic because the resultant acidemia reduces its efficacy. In those with CHF, it may be used either to correct a metabolic alkalosis or in combination with a loop diuretic for the treatment of refractory edema.

Loop of Henle

LOOP DIURETICS. In the thick portion of the ascending limb of the loop of Henle, sodium and potassium cross the luminal cell membrane together with two chlorides. The energy for this carrier-mediated uptake is provided by the action of sodium-potassium ATPase on the basolateral membrane. The loop diuretics inhibit this apical cotransport system, thereby enhancing sodium and chloride secretion.

The entire thick ascending limb is the site of action for the potent loop diuretics ethacrynic acid, furosemide, and butme-

tanide. These drugs are secreted by the organic acid transport route into the proximal tubule, where they demonstrate carbonic anhydrase inhibition and a weak blockade of solute reabsorption. The predominant effect of loop diuretics is exerted at the luminal surface of the ascending limb [37], however. Although 70% of glomerular filtrate NaCl is reabsorbed proximally, nearly 20% is reclaimed by the ascending limb. Hence, complete blockade of chloride, and consequently sodium, transport in this segment presents an overwhelming solute and fluid load to the distal tubule and collecting system. Therefore, all of the loop agents are potent diuretics. They are all effective at GFRs below 25 ml per minute. This gives them some advantages over thiazide diuretics, which generally are ineffective at low GFRs.

The loop diuretics stimulate renal prostaglandin synthesis, thereby increasing RBF [30]. Since PGE_2 may impair solute transport in the ascending limb, this prostaglandin has been proposed as an intermediary of the diuretic action of furosemide and ethacrynic acid; however, this hypothesis requires additional substantiation.

The efficacy of ethacrynic acid, furosemide, and bumetanide in reducing vascular congestion may stem partly from a nondiuretic action. These agents increase systemic venous capacitance, reduce cardiac preload, and lower left ventricular end-diastolic pressure (LVEDP) within 5 minutes of intravenous administration [38]. This effect precedes their diuretic effect and can occur in anephric patients. These observations suggest that the venodilator effect of the loop diuretics is probably responsible for their acute amelioration of pulmonary congestion.

Although head-to-head comparisons of the loop diuretics have not been definitive, it is sometimes found in intensive care patients that failure to respond to one loop diuretic is not predictive of a response to another. Hence, a trial of a second or third agent may be warranted. In addition, since these agents are all tightly protein-bound, hypoalbuminemia (often a complication of severe illness) may be associated with a diminished diuretic response as a consequence of decreased delivery and secretory transport of the agent. Coadministration of an albumin solution mixed with furosemide appears to augment the diuretic response in such cases [39].

The newest agent, bumetanide, may offer some advantages in the intensive care setting. Its onset of action after an intravenous injection (5–10 minutes) and its peak effect after an oral dose (30 minutes) occur twice as fast as with furosemide. In addition, its side-effect profile reveals a much lower incidence of either ototoxicity or glucose intolerance compared with the other two agents.

Distal Tubule and Collecting Duct

THIAZIDE-TYPE DIURETICS. This group includes thiazides, chlorthalidone, and metolazone. The major sites of action of the thiazide diuretics have been clearly established at the early distal tubule [40]. These agents may also exert a modest inhibition of solute reabsorption in the proximal nephron. Compared with loop diuretics, their effect on salt and water excretion is more modest, reflecting the proportionately smaller role of the distal tubule in sodium chloride reabsorption. Nonetheless, they can raise the fractional excretion of sodium to as much as 5% of the filtered load, more than a fivefold increase over normal. Like the loop diuretics, these agents also promote potassium wasting and a metabolic alkalosis. Like other diuretics, they are primarily secreted and not filtered into the proximal tubule, but they are less effective than the loop diuretics in patients with renal failure. Chlorthalidone and metolazone are thiazide-like in effect but more potent and with more prolonged action.

SPIRONOLACTONE, TRIAMTERENE, AND AMILORIDE. In the cortical collecting duct, three drugs—spironolactone, triamterene, and amiloride—inhibit sodium reabsorption by blocking the exchange of this cation for potassium and hydrogen ion. Thus, they are said to be "potassium sparing" and may also induce a metabolic acidosis. Spironolactone inhibits tubular cation exchange as a competitive antagonist of aldosterone and so is ineffective in conditions in which aldosterone is not present. Amiloride and triamterene act independently of aldosterone to inhibit sodium-potassium and sodium-hydrogen exchange. All these agents are weak diuretics. Both the utility and the potential hazard of their use lie in their potassium-sparing effect. In conjunction with kaliuretic diuretics, they provide normalization of the serum potassium. This feature makes them useful in patients taking digitalis, since the toxicity of the cardiac glycoside is potentiated by hypokalemia. They are relatively contraindicated in patients with renal insufficiency and oliguria because of the hyperkalemia that may result from their use in these situations.

VASOPRESSIN ANTAGONISTS. Agents in this group of drugs have different mechanisms of action but share the common characteristic of promoting a water diuresis by blocking the action of vasopressin (antidiuretic hormone) at the collecting duct level. These agents are thus useful adjuncts in the treatment of water-intoxication states (hyponatremia) (see Chap. 79).

Lithium, which is often used in the treatment of bipolar affective disorders (manic depression), causes a water diuresis, sometimes leading to polyuria and nephrogenic diabetes insipidus [41]. It impairs the action of vasopressin, presumably by blocking the formation of the "second messenger," cyclic AMP [41]. Because of its CNS toxicity, however, lithium generally is not recommended for use as a diuretic.

The tetracycline derivative demeclocycline (demethylchlortetracycline) impairs vasopressin-induced water reabsorption by an unknown mechanism [42]. Its toxicity is usually mild (photosensitivity), but it occasionally causes azotemia when given to cirrhotic patients [43].

Although primarily known as natriuretics, the loop diuretics may also induce a mild water diuresis. Several explanations have been offered for this phenomenon: (1) stimulation of prostaglandin biosynthesis causing locally produced PGE_2 to antagonize vasopressin action [30], (2) medullary vasodilation and "washout" of the medullary concentration gradient [44], and (3) direct antagonism of vasopressin (ADH) action at the collecting duct [45]. The loop diuretics do not promote sufficient water excretion to be used as the sole agents for water overload conditions, but they can be used as adjunctive therapy, particularly in patients with edematous conditions who require hypertonic saline.

A new group of synthetic vasopressin analogs has recently been developed that selectively and competitively inhibits vasopressin-induced water reabsorption [47]. Although not yet available for clinical use, these agents may offer considerable advantages as diagnostic as well as therapeutic tools.

CLINICAL APPLICATIONS OF DIURETIC THERAPY. An appropriate choice of a diuretic requires that the clinician be familiar with its pharmacology and the predicted pattern of solute excretion. For example, a thiazide diuretic would be a poor candidate for the treatment of water intoxication, since drugs of this class typically impair urinary dilution and exacerbate hyponatremia. The clinical situations for which diuretics are indicated in the intensive care unit, as well as the recommended drug and dosage range, are shown in Table 78-4.

Edematous Conditions

CONGESTIVE HEART FAILURE. Any inotropic drug, by improving cardiac output and renal perfusion, attenuates the forces for renal sodium retention and thereby promotes a diuresis. In this context, digoxin and dopamine can be considered diuretic agents. However, the intensive care physician often uses a diuretic agent selective for the treatment of pulmonary edema.

Since their introduction in the 1960s, the loop diuretics have been most frequently used for this purpose. The acute reduction in pulmonary capillary wedge (PCW) pressure often seen within minutes of drug administration is due to the venodilatory effects of these agents and usually precedes the diuretic response by several hours [38]. Thiazides may have a similar, although less potent, effect and are less potent diuretic agents. Both produce a considerable kaliuresis, often resulting in hypokalemia (see Chap. 79). For cardiac patients taking digoxin or those with atrial or ventricular arrhythmias, this side effect may be particularly hazardous. The serum potassium level should be carefully monitored and sufficient potassium should be administered to maintain the concentration above 4 mEq per hour. Alternatively, a potassium-sparing diuretic such as spironolactone or triamterene can be added to the regimen.

The edematous patient "resistant" to the diuretic effects of a single agent may be demonstrating the braking phenomenon (see Pharmacology of Diuretics section, and Fig. 78-8). In such cases, the synergy of two drugs that operate at different nephron sites (e.g., a loop diuretic and a thiazide) may be useful. The combination of furosemide and a potassium-sparing diuretic may be less potent, but it carries less risk of severe hypokalemia.

The use of diuretics in patients with severe left ventricular dysfunction poses a dilemma. As illustrated in Fig. 78-9, if the patient's left ventricular end-diastolic pressure cardiac index curve is "flat," diuretic-induced preload reduction will lower the cardiac index further, and tissue perfusion may be compromised. Renal hypoperfusion will result in prerenal azotemia. In such cases, it may be useful to combine diuretics with an inotropic agent or vasodilator. These will move the patient up to a new Starling curve (see Fig. 78-9) and permit the use of diuretics without resultant hypoperfusion. The potential benefits of this approach are depicted in Fig. 78-10. When only furosemide is used in patients with severe CHF, renal hypoperfusion develops, as signified by a rising serum creatinine. In contrast, combined use of furosemide with the vasodilator captopril (an angiotensin-converting enzyme inhibitor) results in forced renal circulation and glomerular filtration and a lower serum creatinine level [48].

HEPATIC CIRRHOSIS. Diuretics may provide relief from edema and ascites in patients with cirrhosis, but they must be used cautiously. Diuretics mobilize fluid directly from the intravas-

Table 78-4. Indications for Diuretic Use in the Intensive Care Unit

Clinical setting	Diuretic type	Drug (daily dose range)	Comment
Edematous condition			
Heart failure	Thiazide or loop	Hydrochlorothiazide (25–100 mg) Furosemide (40–200 mg)	May worsen renal hypoperfusion and azotemia
Hepatic cirrhosis	Thiazide or potassium sparing	Hydrochlorothiazide (25–100 mg) Spironolactone (25–100 mg)[a]	May cause hyperkalemia and metabolic acidosis
Hypertension	Loop or thiazide	Furosemide (40–200 mg) Hydrochlorothiazide (25–100 mg)	May exacerbate hypokalemia
Electrolyte-acid base disturbance			
Hyponatremia	ADH antagonist or loop	Demeclocycline (150–600 mg)[a] Furosemide (40–200 mg)	May cause azotemia, may also require hypertonic saline
Nephrogenic diabetes insipidus	Thiazide	Hydrochlorothiazide (25–100 mg)	
Hyperkalemia	Loop	Furosemide (40–200 mg)	May produce hypovolemia
Hypercalcemia	Loop	Furosemide (40–200 mg)	May produce hypovolemia and should be given together with saline
Metabolic alkalosis	Carbonic anhydrase inhibitor	Acetazolamide (250–1000 mg)	Limited efficacy in volume-depleted condition
Acute tubular necrosis	Loop or osmotic agent	Furosemide (40–480 mg)	May exacerbate hypovolemia and renal hypoperfusion
		Mannitol (12.5[b]–100[c] gm)	May produce pulmonary edema if not excreted
Drug intoxication			
Aspirin	Carbonic anhydrase inhibitor	Acetazolamide (250–1000 mg)	Other modalities may be more effective for drug removal
Phenobarbitol	Carbonic anhydrase inhibitor	Acetazolamide (250–1000 mg)	

[a] Drug may be given only by mouth.
[b] Initial intravenous bolus.
[c] Infused intravenously over 24 hr.

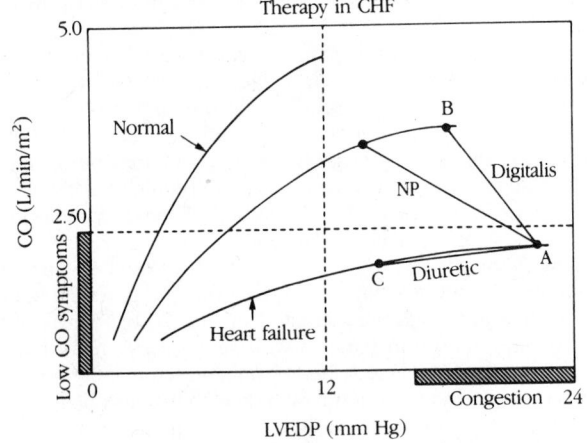

Fig. 78-9. Relation of cardiac output (CO) to left ventricular end-diastolic pressure (LVEDP) in normal versus failing hearts. In the failing heart, a large increase in LVEDP may precipitate pulmonary edema with a persistent reduction in CO (point A). Diuretics reduce LVEDP along the same curve, out of the range of congestive symptoms, and modestly reduce CO. Inotropes such as digitalis shift the curve toward normal (point A to point B). Vasodilators such as nitroprusside (NP) increase cardiac output by reducing afterload impedance, thus also shifting the curve upward. By virtue of venodilation, however, they also may reduce ventricular filling, thus reducing CO along the new curve. (From Grantham JJ, Chonko AM: The physiological basis and clinical use of diuretics, in Brenner BM, Stein JH [eds]: *Sodium and Water Homeostasis.* New York, Churchill-Livingstone, 1978, pp 178–211, with permission.)

cular compartment. When the intravascular volume is reduced, fluid is recruited into the plasma compartment from the interstitial space [49]. This process may be delayed in cirrhotic patients because of hypoalbuminemia, exposing them to the risk of severe hypovolemia and azotemia [50].

It is best to attempt sodium restriction alone first. If the patient's edema and ascites are so disabling that additional intervention is required, spironolactone may be beneficial. Spironolactone ameliorates the secondary hyperaldosteronism of liver disease, and the potassium-sparing effect of this agent prevents the untoward consequences of hypokalemia (such as exacerbation of hepatic encephalopathy). Although spironolactone is a weak diuretic, this feature may be an advantage in patients with liver disease, in whom a brisk diuresis may induce hepatorenal syndrome (see Chap. 81) [50,51]. Spironolactone may also pose some danger in severely cirrhotic patients with prerenal azotemia, however. In this setting, secondary hyperaldosteronism compensates for low urinary flow and a marginal capacity to excrete a potassium and hydrogen ion load: An aldosterone antagonist may, therefore, lead to hyperkalemia and metabolic acidosis (see Chap. 80) [52]. Thiazide-type diuretics should be employed with caution to avoid the potential complications of hypovolemia and hypokalemia.

Patients with cirrhosis and portal hypertension characteristically have a reduced "effective circulating volume" and thus are at risk for renal hypoperfusion. Seemingly small changes in plasma volume can produce dire consequences, such as the hepatorenal syndrome (see Chap. 81) [50,51]. Hence, more potent diuretic agents such as furosemide should be used only in exceptional cases.

Hypertension. Dietary sodium restriction and diuretics are primary antihypertensive modalities. Moderate sodium depletion is beneficial in treating most forms of hypertension. For the treatment of severe or malignant hypertension, however, diu-

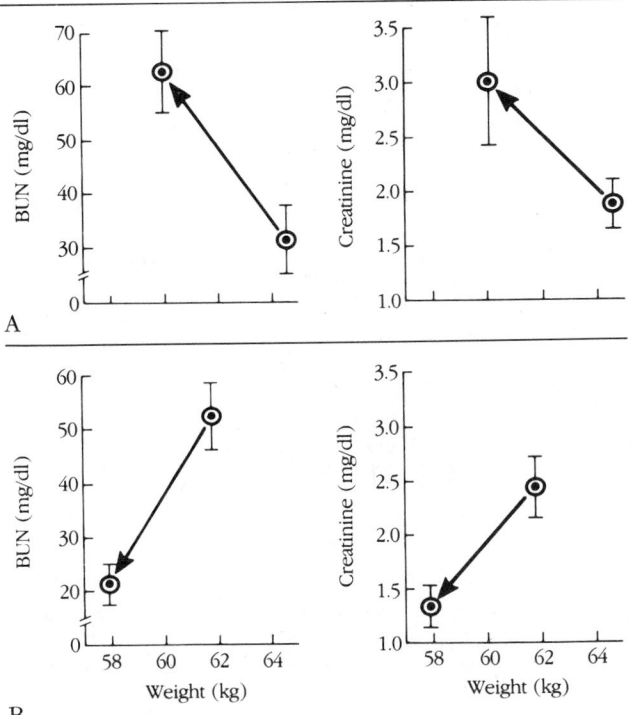

Fig. 78-10. Effect of diuretic therapy on blood urea nitrogen (BUN) and serum creatinine levels in patients with severe congestive heart failure. A. Before captopril treatment, diuresis resulted in both weight loss and azotemia. B. With combined captopril and diuretic therapy, however, BUN and serum creatinine fell despite weight loss equivalent to that which occurred before captopril treatment. (From Dzau VJ, Colucci WS, Williams GH, et al: Sustained effectiveness of converting enzyme inhibition in patients with severe congestive heart failure. *N Engl J Med* 302:1373, 1980. Reprinted by permission of *The New England Journal of Medicine.*)

retics are often used as adjunctive therapy in conjunction with a more potent agent (see Chap. 52). The venodilatory properties of furosemide may also account for its acute antihypertensive effect [38]. Arterial vasodilators typically promote renal sodium retention, which can be avoided with diuretic administration. Thiazide-type or loop diuretics are usually recommended for this purpose. Since hypokalemia may coexist with some forms of secondary hypertension, diuretics may exacerbate this problem and necessitate potassium supplementation.

Disorders of Water Metabolism. Mild water overload can be treated with water restriction. More severe cases of hyponatremia may require induction of a water diuresis (see Chap. 79). We recommend demeclocycline for this purpose, although other nondiuretic modalities are available (see Chap. 79). Synthetic vasopressin antagonists may be available in the future for use in these circumstances.

Water intoxication with mental obtundation or seizures requires rapid correction with hypertonic saline (see Chap. 79). In patients with CHF or other edema-forming states, concurrent administration of furosemide with hypertonic saline causes a relatively hypotonic diuresis while preventing excessive volume expansion [46].

Nephrogenic diabetes insipidus is characterized by polyuria and an impaired nephronal response to vasopressin. The impaired renal response distinguishes this form of diabetes insipidus from central diabetes insipidus, which is vasopressin-responsive. The use of a diuretic for the nephrogenic disease may seem paradoxical; however, thiazide diuretics comprise one of the few available treatments. Thiazides impair urinary dilution but do not disturb urinary concentration by virtue of their site of action in the early distal tubule. The resultant modest volume depletion enhances urinary concentrating ability and limits water excretion.

Hyperkalemia. The causes of hyperkalemia are fully discussed in Chapter 79. With the exception of the potassium-sparing drugs and water diuretics, most agents promote a kaliuresis. Other nondiuretic therapies also may be necessary (sodium polystyrene-Kayexalate, dialysis), particularly in patients with oliguric renal failure. Loop diuretics produce considerable potassium loss. Saline administration may be necessary to prevent the complication of volume depletion.

Hypercalcemia. Furosemide and other loop diuretics promote urinary calcium excretion by blocking absorption of this ion in the loop of Henle [53]. In addition, the incremental sodium delivery to the distal nephron competes with calcium for reabsorption at this site. Hence, furosemide is a first-line therapy for severe hypercalcemia [54]. Volume expansion with simultaneous saline administration maintains the calciuresis by continued delivery of sodium to the distal nephron [54].

In contrast to furosemide, the thiazide diuretics reduce urinary calcium excretion and may provoke or exacerbate hypercalcemia [55]; however, they may be useful in hypercalciuric states leading to stone formation.

Metabolic Alkalosis. Treatment of metabolic alkalosis is best accomplished by removal of factors that initiate hydrogen ion loss (e.g., discontinuing nasogastric suction) or those that maintain renal bicarbonate reclamation (e.g., volume depletion). Carbonic anhydrase inhibitors (e.g., acetazolamide) block bicarbonate reabsorption in the proximal nephron and thereby may correct a metabolic alkalosis. They are useful only when the primary factors involved in the pathogenesis of this disorder cannot be ameliorated. For example, a patient with diuretic-induced metabolic alkalosis may continue to require use of a thiazide or loop diuretic for the underlying condition. The efficacy of carbonic anhydrase inhibitors is limited by both volume depletion and acidemia [56].

Acute Tubular Necrosis. The role of diuretics in the treatment of acute tubular necrosis (ATN) is still controversial (see Chap. 78). Several studies employing either furosemide or mannitol suggest that these agents may help protect against ATN developing when given as prophylaxis against a potential ischemic or nephrotoxic insult [57]. Furosemide in particular has been shown to be effective in preventing radiocontrast-induced acute renal failure [58]. There has been accruing evidence that loop diuretics ameliorate cellular ischemia by reducing tubular transport work and its associated oxygen consumption [59]. Little advantage is afforded by these agents once ATN is established, however. Moreover, the use of diuretics in clinically established ATN appears to improve urine flow but has no effect on mortality [60]. Furosemide, combined with low-dose dopamine, has been shown to be protective in an ischemic model of ATN [61]. Recently, this combination of agents has been shown to improve urine flow and to stabilize or improve glomerular filtration in patients with ATN [62]. These early results require confirmation in a controlled study with larger numbers of patients. The ameliorative effect of dopamine may be due to renal vasodilation and enhanced nephron delivery of furosemide.

Both furosemide and hypertonic mannitol are frequently recommended as diagnostic and therapeutic agents in patients with oliguric renal failure. Even in patients who convert to nonoliguria, however, improvement in survival has not been demonstrated (see Chap. 81).

Caution should be exercised when administering diuretics for the treatment of ATN. Since volume depletion may aggravate this disorder, diuretics should be withheld from hypovolemic patients. Conversely, hypertonic mannitol may lead to pulmonary congestion if renal failure delays its urinary excretion.

Drug Intoxications. Diuretics play a limited role in the treatment of drug overdoses, particularly since dialysis and hemoperfusion are more efficient means of drug removal (see Chap. 83). In specific circumstances such as phenobarbital overdose [63] and salicylate poisoning [64], a carbonic anhydrase inhibitor enhances the urinary excretion and renal clearance of the drug. In both instances, the effect of alkalinizing the urine brings the urine pH up to a range close to the pK of these drugs. For phenobarbital, a sevenfold increase in renal excretion can be anticipated, and renal clearance can increase by five- to sixfold (see Chap. 155) [65].

Assessment of Renal Function

THE CLEARANCE OF INULIN AND MEASUREMENT OF GFR.
Although there are many renal functions, none is more important than excretory capacity. Water and many (but not all) substances enter the nephron "from above" via glomerular filtration. Hence, measurement of GFR is generally equated with determination of "renal function." Since the days of Homer Smith, a patriarch of renal physiology, clearance techniques have been used to measure GFR. Clearance describes the rate at which a volume of plasma is cleared of a substance. Clearance is expressed as units of volume per unit time (ml/min or l/day.) The volume of plasma "cleared" of a substance is a virtual rather than an actual volume. When renal excretion is the mode of clearance, the formula is expressed as:

$$C_x = U_x \times V / P_x$$

where C_x is the clearance of substance, "x", U_x is the urinary concentration of "x," and P_x is the plasma concentration.

Inulin, a 5,200 dalton polymer of fructose, is ideal for measuring glomerular filtration because it is freely filtrable by the glomerular capillaries and undergoes no tubular reabsorption or secretion. The clearance of inulin, as will be demonstrated, is therefore equivalent to the GFR. Since there is no tubular processing of inulin, the filtered load of inulin that enters the proximal tubule is equivalent to the excreted inulin:

Filtered load of inulin = excreted inulin

$$GFR \times P_{inulin} = U_{inulin} \times V$$

where GFR is glomerular filtration rate (ml/min), P_{inulin} is plasma inulin concentration (mg/dl) and U_{inulin} is urinary inulin (mg/dl). Rearranging terms, we get:

$$GFR = U_{inulin} \times V / P_{inulin}$$

Since the clearance of inulin C_{inulin} is equivalent to $U_{inulin} \times V / P_{inulin}$,

$$GFR = C_{inulin}$$

The clearance of inulin remains the "gold standard" for measurement of GFR; however, the measurement of inulin in plasma and urine is cumbersome and requires reagents to measure fructose. Plasma must first be deproteinated. Reactions using indoleacetic acid [66] or anthrone are commonly used [67]. An infusion of inulin is required to produce a steady-state plasma concentration. Alternatively, a bolus method can be employed, although this method may produce considerable variability in results [68].

Alternative clearance techniques have employed radiolabled substances, including ^{99m}Tc-DTPA (diethylenetriaminepenta-acetic acid) and ^{51}Cr-EDTA (ethylenediaminetetra-acetic acid). A description of these methods is beyond the scope of this chapter.

It should be remembered that the clearance of inulin or other GFR markers may not correlate with the loss of renal mass. This is because as nephrons are lost, the remaining functional nephrons may undergo hypertrophy and hyperfiltration, thereby providing normal or near-normal total kidney GFR [69].

CREATININE CLEARANCE AND THE PLASMA CREATININE.
Creatinine is an endogenous compound generated by the nonenzymatic hepatic conversion of creatine. Virtually all creatine is released from skeletal muscle, and creatine production (as well as creatinine synthesis) is proportional to skeletal muscle mass. This is important in interpretation of plasma creatinine levels, as will be discussed below.

Unlike inulin, creatinine is filtered by the glomerulus *and* secreted by the proximal tubule. Hence, the urinary excretion of creatinine represents both the filtered load as well as the secreted creatinine,

$$U_{cr}V = GFR \times P_{cr} + TS_{cr}$$

where $U_{cr}V$ is the urinary excretion, $GFR \cdot P_{cr}$ is the filtered load, and TS_{cr} is the tubular secretion of creatinine, respectively. By dividing by P_{cr}, we get:

$$U_{cr}V / P_{cr} = GFR + TS_{cr} / P_{cr}$$

or,

$$C_{cr} = GFR + TS_{cr} / P_{cr}$$

where C_{cr} is the creatinine clearance and TS_{cr} / P_{cr} represents creatinine clearance due to tubular secretion. At normal GFRs, the TS_{cr} / P_{cr} is considerably smaller than the GFR, hence $C_{cr} \approx$ GFR. In renal failure with low GFRs, however, TS_{cr} / P_{cr} assumes a larger proportion of the total C_{cr}, hence $C_{cr} <$ GFR.

The creatinine clearance requires a timed collection of urine. Clearance determinations may be altered by low urine flow or by poor bladder emptying. In addition, measurement of creatinine, a colorimetric assay known as the Jaffe method, may be altered by compounds in the urine or plasma that react with the alkaline picrate reagent. These compounds include acetoacetate, glucose, pyruvate, proteins, and exogenous agents such as cephalosporin antibiotics. Newer automated methods now measure true creatinine and therefore circumvent these confounding agents.

Creatinine clearance also may be estimated by one of several nomograms that derive C_{cr} from the plasma creatinine value. The formula by Cockcroft and Gault [70] uses the patient's age and body weight and is based on data from hospitalized patients:

$$C_{cr} = (140 - age) \times weight / (P_{cr} \cdot 72)$$

where weight is expressed in kilograms and P_{cr} is expressed as mg/dl.

This formula factors both patient's weight and age, both of which affect the generation of creatinine. Since muscle mass declines in older patients, age is a negative term. Creatinine synthesis is directly proportional to weight. C_{cr} may be overestimated if body weight exceeds lean body mass by a large proportion, as may occur in obese or edematous patients. In women, since the muscle mass is lower, the resultant number is multiplied by 0.85 to determine the C_{cr}.

By far the most common method of estimating GFR is the use of P_{cr}. As indicated by the Cockcroft-Gault formula, however, muscle mass as determined by age, sex, and body weight must be considered. For example, consider that a P_{cr} of 1.2 mg/dl, the upper limit of normal in many laboratories, represents a C_{cr} of only 22 ml/min in an 85-year-old woman weighing 40 kg. In a 25-year-old male weighing 70 kg, however, the C_{cr} would be 93 ml/min.

Furthermore, because the relationship between the P_{cr} and GFR is asymptotic (Fig. 78-11) the P_{cr} can remain "normal" despite a reduced GFR. Note that because of the mathematical relationship between the two, as GFR falls below 25 ml/min, P_{cr} rises sharply. Hence, at marginal GFRs, small decrements in renal function will result in steep increases in P_{cr}. The clinician should bear this in mind when assessing a patient with chronic renal failure. A small reduction in renal blood flow that might result from hypovolemia might effect a large jump in the P_{cr}.

In patients with acute renal failure, it is useful to assess slope of the change of P_{cr}. As demonstrated in Figure 78-12, recovery of renal function in acute renal failure may be heralded by an increase in urine flow. In addition, however, the *change in the slope of the rise in* P_{cr} can be predictive of recovery of renal function. Plotting the P_{cr} in this way permits the physician to prognosticate about recovery of renal function and the need for dialysis.

MEASUREMENT OF URINARY ELECTROLYTES

Sodium and Chloride. The measurement of urinary sodium excretion is an extremely useful adjunct to diagnosis and also

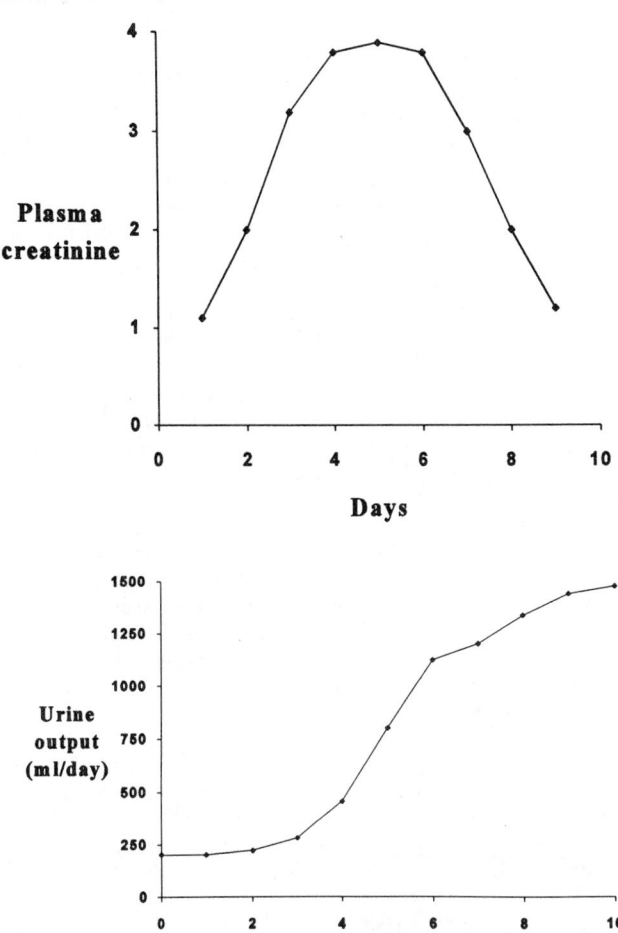

Fig. 78-12. Course of patient with acute renal failure. *A.* Plasma creatinine, which peaks by day 4. *B.* Urine flow: increases herald recovery of renal function.

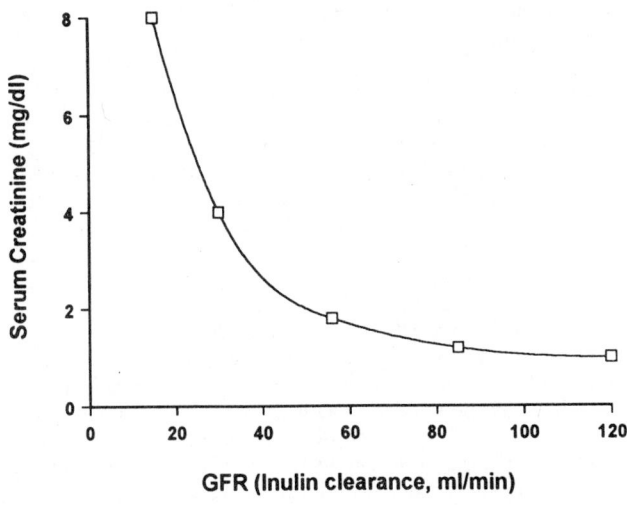

Fig. 78-11. Relationship of GFR, as determined by inulin clearance, and the serum creatinine. As is demonstrated, a considerable decrease in GFR can occur before any increment in serum creatinine is observed.

is of use for guiding therapy in the intensive care unit. With certain caveats, sodium and chloride excretion reflect the state of the renal circulation. When renal perfusion is reduced due to absolute or effective arteriolar volume depletion, urinary sodium and chloride excretion diminish for the reasons described above.

Urinary sodium or chloride *concentration* in a spot aliquot of urine is usually below 10 to 20 mM in patients with renal hypoperfusion. Exceptions to this principle include salt-wasting renal diseases, adrenal insufficiency, and the use of diuretics. If any of these coexists with renal hypoperfusion, the capacity to maximally reabsorb sodium and chloride will be impaired, thus causing inappropriately high levels in the final urine.

The concentration of sodium or chloride in the urine reflects the ratio of these ions to water. Under some conditions of either oliguric or nonoliguric acute renal failure, this ratio may be affected so that water reabsorption remains intact while sodium reabsorption is attenuated. In such cases, the urinary sodium or chloride concentration will be spuriously elevated. To compensate for this, the *fractional excretion of sodium* (FE_{Na}) can be calculated.

The FE_{Na} is the proportion of the filtered load of sodium excreted:

$$FE_{Na}(\%) = \text{urinary sodium excreted} / \text{Filtered load of sodium} \times 100$$
$$= U_{Na}V / GFR \times P_{Na} \times 100$$

Substituting C_{cr} for GFR and rearranging terms, we get:

$$FE_{Na} = U_{Na} / P_{Na} \times P_{cr} / U_{cr} \times 100$$

where U_{Na} and P_{Na} are expressed as mM and U_{cr} and P_{cr} are expressed as mg/dl. Substituting the C_{cr} allows for cancelling of the urinary volume (V) terms. Hence, no timed collection of urine is required. Instead, simultaneous aliquots of plasma and urine are analyzed for sodium and creatinine.

The FE_{Na} is a marker of renal perfusion. Under normal circumstances, the FE_{Na} is <1%. This indicates that >99% of the filtered sodium is reabsorbed by the nephrons. As in normal conditions, when renal hypoperfusion creates "prerenal azotemia," the FE_{Na} is <1%. As described in Chapter 81, in acute renal failure patients, a value of >1% suggests nephronal damage and an inability to reabsorb sodium indicative of acute tubular necrosis.

In general, the urinary sodium concentration and the FE_{Na} suffice for estimates of renal perfusion. Under circumstances where anions are nonreabsorbable, however, the increased sodium excretion necessitated by presentation of the anion to the distal nephron will mask hypovolemia or a decrease in effective arteriolar blood volume and thus require the use of the urinary chloride. Table 78-5 lists those conditions in which the urinary chloride is preferred.

The finding of low FE_{Na} in azotemic or oliguric patients obligates the physician to identify the underlying cause of renal hypoperfusion. This may prove difficult, particularly in patients with CHF in whom renal hypoperfusion may be the result of either overdiuresis or worsening left ventricular dysfunction. Empiric trials of more vigorous diuresis or "volume loading" with intravenous normal saline may be hazardous. In such cases, measurement of pulmonary capillary wedge pressure is warranted.

Potassium. Determination of urinary potassium excretion is most useful in establishing the cause of hypokalemia due either to renal or extrarenal losses. The urinary potassium concentration in a spot sample is usually less than 20 in patients in whom potassium wastage is extrarenal (e.g., diarrhea) and usually >20 with those with urinary potassium wastage. It should be remembered that the *volume* of urine may influence urinary potassium concentration. A urinary potassium concentration of 30 mM in a patient with only 500 ml of urine output suggests extrarenal potassium losses, since the total urinary excretion of potassium is low. In such cases, a 24-hour collection for urinary potassium excretion may be desirable (see Chap. 79).

URINANALYSIS AND THE MEASUREMENT OF URINARY CONCENTRATION.
Urine represents the final product of a process initiated by glomerular filtration and completed by tu-

Table 78-5. Conditions in Which Urinary Chloride is Preferred Over Urinary Sodium

Condition	Reason
Recent vomiting	HCO_3^- obligates augmented Na excretion despite hypovolemia
Ketoacidosis	Excretion of ketones obligates augmented Na excretion despite hypovolemia
Drugs	Excretion of anionically charged drugs (e.g. carbenicillin) obligates augmented Na excretion

bular processing. The examination of the urine and its constituents provides valuable clues for the diagnosis of ICU patients with renal, electrolyte, and acid-base disturbances. Therefore, it is essential that clinicians become familiar with the tools available in the laboratory and develop the skills to perform reliable urine microscopy.

If possible, urine should be obtained by spontaneous voiding, since catheterization may traumatize the bladder and cause iatrogenic hematuria. If this is not possible (as is often the case in the ICU), however, a catheterized specimen should be viewed with the knowledge that hematuria may not represent intrinsic urinary tract disease. The urine should be examined promptly to avoid contamination of formed elements and loss of bicarbonate, thereby changing the pH.

Urine Dipstick. Examination of the urine usually commences with a "dipstick" semiquantitative evaluation of several components:

PROTEIN. Usually, less than 60 mg of albumin are excreted in 24 hours. The appearance of a positive dipstick test for protein connotes albuminuria, which is usually of glomerular origin. If heavy albuminuria is found by dipstick (3+ to 4+), quantitation with a 24-hour urine collection is advisable. Other, low molecular weight proteins, such as Tamm-Horsfall protein, may be present in the urine, but these are not detected by the dipstick (but they *can* be detected with other reagents, such as sulfosalicylic acid.) Urinary proteins in paraproteinemias, usually made up of light chains of immunoglobulins, will also be eluded by dipstick but will give a positive result with sulfosalicylic acid or other reagents. The dipstick reagent, tetra-bromophenol, is buffered at pH 3. False positive results may occur with urine of very high pH.

URINE PH. The physiologic range for urinary pH is 4.5 and 8. Since an ash diet and metabolic processes obligate the excretion of titratable acid, the usual urinary pH is between 5 and 6. Indicator dyes on the dipstick (methyl red and bromthymol blue) respond by release or absorption of hydrogen ions. Urine pH is useful in assessing patients with metabolic acidosis in whom an alkaline urine may connote renal tubular acidosis and in those with certain stone-forming disorders. Although the dipstick reagents generally are accurate, a more precise pH may require the use of a pH meter.

GLUCOSE. Glucose is converted by the reagent glucose oxidase to gluconic acid with subsequent production of peroxide, which turns orthotolidine to a blue color. The appearance of glucose in the urine may connote diabetes mellitus, but proximal tubular disorders ("renal glycosuria") may be manifest by a positive test.

HEMOGLOBIN AND OCCULT BLOOD. The dipstick reagent here is also orthotolidine, which is oxidized by hemoglobin in the presence of cumene hydroperoxide. Both free hemoglobin (as well as myoglobin) and red blood cells may be detected with this reagent. If the urine osmolality is low and the red cells lyse, hemoglobin may be detected even if there are no visible red cells (due to lysis.) The reducing agent ascorbate may prevent this reaction. Hence, patients taking vitamin C in large doses may have falsely negative results. Ideally, the urine should be examined under the microscope not only to confirm the presence of red blood cells but also to examine their morphology as well as the appearance of red cell casts to determine whether the cells are of glomerular or nonglomerular origin.

LEUCOCYTES. The reagent leucocyte esterase on the dipstick can be used to screen for the presence of white cells (more than 4 per high-power field.) As is the case for red cells, urine microscopy should be used for confirmation.

BACTERIA. The nitrite test reflects the capacity of bacteria to reduce nitrates to nitrites. The Greiss reagent produces a red dye in the presence of nitrites. This test is not recommended for the diagnosis of urinary tract infection. Rather, a clean catch (or midstream) urine sample should be sent for culture.

Urine Microscopy. The urine dipstick tests may be performed in any laboratory, but urine microscopy should be performed by a physician familiar with the clinical presentation of the patient. Care should be given to the collection of a *fresh, clean* specimen, preferably at a low urinary pH and high specific gravity. A midstream sample collected after retraction of the foreskin in males or the labia in females is best.

Formed elements in the urine may include free cells, casts, lipid droplets, and crystals. Casts are usually made up a matrix, presumed to be Tamm-Horsfall protein, a low molecular weight molecule secreted by the proximal nephron. Red or white blood cells, tubular epithelial cells, or other cellular components may appear in these casts. A description of the casts likely to be seen in acute renal failure appears in Chapter 81.

Measurement of Urinary Concentration. Measurement of urinary concentrating ability is necessary to assess hyponatremic and polyuric conditions. In these circumstances, urinary osmolality (measured by either freezing point or vapor pressure determination) will be necessary. Urine specific gravity (the relative density of urine to water) is not satisfactory, since the *mass* of particles as well as their number affect the test. Therefore, the relationship between specific gravity and osmolality is not uniform and will be exaggerated by heavy particles in the urine. For example, iodine (as found in radiocontrast agents) by virtue of its heavier mass, will raise the specific gravity disproportionately to the increment in urinary osmolality.

As described in detail in Chapter 79, highly concentrated urine in the face of hypoosmolar hyponatremia suggests the presence of antidiuretic hormone. By careful clinical examination and determination of the urinary sodium concentration to establish whether there is renal hypoperfusion, the clinician can establish whether the hyponatremia is due to nonosmotic stimulation of ADH or to the syndrome of inappropriate ADH secretion. A dilute urine ($U_{osm} < 100$ mOsm/kg) in a hyponatremic subject suggests primary polydipsia.

Polyuric conditions such as diabetes insipidus also require assessment of urinary and plasma osmolality, as discussed in Chapter 79.

References

1. Smith HW: The evolution of the kidney, in Smith HW (ed): *Lectures on the Kidney*. Lawrence, KS, University of Kansas, 1943, pp 3–23.
2. Schlondorff D: The glomerular mesangial cell: An expanding role for a specialized pericyte. *FASEB J* 1:272, 1987.
3. Kon V, Harris RC, Ichikawa I: A regulatory role for large vessels in organ circulation. Endothelial cells of the main renal artery modulate intrarenal hemodynamics in the rat. *J Clin Invest* 85:1728, 1990.
4. Edwards RM: Segmental effects of norepinephrine and angiotensin II on isolated renal microvessels. *Am J Physiol (Renal Fluid Electrolyte Physiol)* 244:F526, 1983.
5. Hricik DE, Browning PJ, Kopelman R, et al: Captopril-induced functional renal insufficiency in patients with bilateral renal-artery stenoses or renal-artery stenosis in a solitary kidney. *N Engl J Med* 308:373, 1983.
6. Hricik DE, Dunn MJ: Angiotensin-converting enzyme inhibitor-induced renal failure: Causes, consequences, and diagnostic uses. *J Am Soc Nephrol* 1:845, 1990.
7. Ballermann BJ, Zeidel ML, Gunning ME, et al: Vasoactive peptides and the kidney, in Brenner BM, Rector FC Jr (eds): *The Kidney*. 4th ed. Philadelphia, WB Saunders, 1991, p 584.
8. Smith HW: Excretion of sodium and other strong electrolytes, in Smith HW (ed): *The Kidney: Structure and Function in Health and Disease*. New York, Oxford University Press, 1951, p 295.
9. Jamison RL, Maffly RH: Mechanism of urinary concentration. *N Engl J Med* 295:1062, 1976.
10. Hall JE, Guyton AC, Jackson TE, et al: Control of glomerular filtration rate by renin-angiotensin system. *Am J Physiol* 233:F366, 1977.
11. Myers BD, Deen WM, Brenner BM: Effects of norepinephrine and angiotensin II on the determinants of glomerular ultrafiltration and proximal tubule fluid reabsorption in the rat. *Circ Res* 37:101, 1975.
12. Boudreau R, Mandin H: Cardiac edema in dogs II. Distribution of glomerular filtrate and renal blood flow. *Kidney Int* 10:578, 1976.
13. Hierholzer K, Lange S: The effect of adrenal steroids on renal function, in Thurau K (ed): *Kidney and Urinary Tract Physiology*. London, Butterworths, 1974, p 273.
14. Chonko AM, Bay WH, Stein JH: The role of renin and aldosterone in the salt retention of edema. *Am J Med* 63:881, 1977.
15. Watkins L, Burton JA, Haber E, et al: The renin-angiotensin-aldosterone system in congestive failure in conscious dogs. *Am J Physiol* 1970.
16. Schrier RW, Humphreys MH, Ufferman RC: Role of cardiac output and the autonomic nervous system in the antinatriuretic effect response to acute constriction of the thoracic superior vena cava. *Circ Res* 29:490, 1971.
17. Johnson MD, Barger AC: Circulating catecholamines in control of renal electrolyte and water excretion. *Am J Physiol* 250:F192, 1981.
18. Besarab A, Silva P, Landsberg L, et al: Effect of catecholamines on tubular function in the isolated perfused rat kidney. *Am J Physiol* 233:F39, 1977.
19. Fray JCS: Stimulus secretion coupling of renin. Role of hemodynamic factors. *Circ Res* 47(4):485, 1980.
20. DeWardener HE: Kidney, salt intake, and Na$^+$,K$^+$-ATPase inhibitors in hypertension: 1990 Corcoran Lecture. *Hypertension* 17:830, 1991.
21. Fine LG, Bourgoignie JJ, Hwang KH, et al: On the influence of the natriuretic factor from patients with chronic uremia on the bioelectric properties and sodium transport of the isolated mammalian collecting tubule. *J Clin Invest* 58:590, 1976.
22. Bricker NS, Schmidt RW, Favre H, et al: On the biology of sodium excretion: The search for a natriuretic hormone. *Yale J Biol Med* 48:293, 1975.
23. deBold AJ, Borenstein AJ, Veress AT: A rapid and potent natriuretic response to intravenous injection of atrial myocardial extracts in rats. *Life Sci* 33:297, 1981.
24. Currie MG, Geiler DM, Cole BR, et al: Bioactive cardiac substances: Potent vasorelaxant activity in mammalian atria. *Science* 221:171, 1983.
25. Lattion AL, Aubert JF, Fluckiger JP, et al: Effect of sodium intake on gene expression and plasma levels of ANF in rats. *Am J Physiol* 255:H245, 1988.
26. Biollaz J, Bidiville J, Diezi J, et al: Site of the action of a synthetic atrial natriuretic peptide evaluated in humans. *Kidney Int* 32:537, 1987.
27. Goy JJ, Waeber B, Nussberger J, et al: Infusion of atrial natriuretic peptide to patients with congestive heart failure. *J Cardiovasc Pharmacol* 12:562, 1988.
28. Morrison AR: Prostaglandin and the kidney. *Am J Med* 69:171, 1980.
29. Stokes JB, Kokko JP: Inhibition of sodium transport by prostaglandin E2 across the isolated, perfused rabbit collecting tubule. *J Clin Invest* 59:1099, 1977.
30. Abe K, Yasuima M, Cherba L, et al: Effect of furosemide on urinary excretion of prostaglandin E in normal volunteers and patients with essential hypertension. *Prostaglandins* 14:513, 1977.
31. Walshe JJ, Venuto RC: Acute oliguric renal failure induced by indomethacin: Possible mechanism. *Ann Intern Med* 91:47, 1979.
32. Clive DM, Stoff JS: Renal syndromes associated with nonsteroidal anti-inflammatory drugs. *N Engl J Med* 310:563, 1984.
33. Boyer TD, Zia P, Reynolds TB: Effect of indomethacin and prostaglandin A1 on renal function and plasma renin activity in alcoholic liver disease. *Gastroenterology* 77:215, 1979.
34. Levy M, Wexler MJ, Fechner C: Renal perfusion in dogs with experimental hepatic cirrhosis: Role of prostaglandins. *Am J Physiol* 245:F521, 1983.
35. Grantham JJ, Chonko AM: The physiological basis and clinical use

of diuretics, in Brenner BM, Stein JH (eds): *Sodium and Water Homeostasis*. 178th ed. New York, Churchill Livingstone, 1978.

36. Weiner IM, Washington JA, Mudge GH: Studies on the renal excretion of salicylate in the dog. *Bull Johns Hopkins Hosp* 105:284, 1959.

37. Burg M, Stoner L, Cardinal J, et al: Furosemide effect on isolated perfused tubules. *Am J Physiol* 225:119, 1973.

38. Dikshit K, Vyden JK, Forrester JS, et al: Renal and extrarenal hemodynamic effects of furosemide in congestive heart failure after myocardial infarction. *N Engl J Med* 288:1087, 1973.

39. Inoue M, Okajima K, Itoh K, et al: Mechanism of furosemide resistance in analbuminemic rats and hypoalbuminemic patients. *Kidney Int* 32:198, 1987.

40. Kunan RT, Weller DR, Webb HL: Clarification of site of action of chlorothiazide in the rat nephron. *J Clin Invest* 56:401, 1975.

41. Cox M, Singer I: Lithium and water metabolism. *Am J Med* 59:153, 1975.

42. Singer I, Rotenberg D: Demeclocycline-induced nephrogenic diabetes insipidus. *Ann Intern Med* 79:679, 1973.

43. deTroyer A, Pillow W, Broeckaert I, et al: Demeclocycline treatment of water retention cirrhosis. *Ann Intern Med* 85:336, 1976.

44. Hook JB, Williamson HE: Effect of furosemide on renal medullary sodium gradient. *Proc Soc Exp Biol Med* 118:372, 1965.

45. Schrier RW, Lehman D, Zacherle B, et al: Effect of furosemide on free water excretion in edematous patients with hyponatremia. *Kidney Int* 3:30, 1973.

46. Hautman D, Rossier B, Zohlman R, et al: Rapid correction of hyponatremia in the syndrome of inappropriate antidiuretic hormone: An alternative treatment to hypertonic saline. *Ann Intern Med* 78:870, 1973.

47. Sawyer WH, Pang PKT, Seto J, et al: Vasopressin analogs that antagonize antidiuretic responses by rats to the antidiuretic hormone. *Science* 212:49, 1981.

48. Dzau VJ, Colucci WS, Williams GH, et al: Sustained effectiveness of converting enzyme inhibition in patients with severe congestive heart failure. *N Engl J Med* 302:1373, 1980.

49. Levy M, Richard C: Mobilization of ascites in cirrhotic dogs following furosemide or mannitol. *Am J Physiol* 235:F12, 1978.

50. Levy M: The kidney in liver disease, in Brenner BM, Stein JH (eds): *Sodium and Water Homeostasis*. New York, Churchill Livingstone, 1978, p 73.

51. Papper S: Hepatorenal syndrome. *Contrib Nephrol* 23:55, 1980.

52. Gabow PA, Moore S, Schrier RW: Spironolactone-induced hyperchloremic metabolic acidosis in cirrhosis. *Ann Intern Med* 90:338, 1979.

53. Edwards BR, Baer PG, Sutton RAC, et al: Micropuncture study of diuretic effects on sodium and calcium reabsorption in the dog nephron. *J Clin Invest* 52:2418, 1973.

54. Suki WN, Yium JJ, Von Minden M, et al: Acute treatment of hypercalcemia with furosemide. *N Engl J Med* 283:836, 1970.

55. Costanzo LS, Weiner IM: On the hypocalciuric effect of chlorothiazide. *J Clin Invest* 54:628, 1974.

56. Chew S, Parish JG, Slater A, et al: Effects of acetazolamide on proximal tubule Cl, Na, HCO_3 transport in normal and acidotic dogs during distal blockade. *J Clin Invest* 60:162, 1977.

57. Levinsky NG, Bernard DB, Johnston PA: Mannitol and loop diuretics in acute renal failure, in Brenner BM, Lazarus JM (eds): *Acute Renal Failure*. Philadelphia, WB Saunders, 1983, p 712.

58. Heyman SN, Brezis M, Greenfeld Z, et al: Protective role of furosemide and saline in radiocontrast-induced acute renal failure in the rat. *Am J Kidney Dis* 14:377, 1989.

59. Brezis M, Rosen S, Silva P, et al: Transport activity modifies thick ascending limb damage in the isolated perfused kidney. *Kidney Int* 25:65, 1984.

60. Minuth AN, Terrell JB, Suki WN: Acute renal failure: A study of the course and prognosis of 104 patients and of the role of furosemide. *Am J Med Sci* 271:317, 1976.

61. Lindner A, Cutler RL, Goodman WG: Synergism of dopamine plus furosemide in preventing acute renal failure in the dog. *Kidney Int* 16:158, 1979.

62. Lindner A: Synergism of dopamine and furosemide in diuretic-resistant oliguric acute renal failure. *Nephron* 33:121, 1983.

63. Bloomer HA: A critical evaluation of diuresis in the treatment of barbiturate intoxication. *J Lab Clin Med* 64:898, 1966.

64. Lawson AA, Proudfoot AT, Brown SS, et al: Forced diuresis in the treatment of acute salicylate poisoning in adults. *Q J Med* 30:31, 1969.

65. Reineck HJ, Stein JH: Mechanisms of action and clinical uses of diuretics, in Brenner BM, Rector FC (eds): *The Kidney*. Philadelphia, WB Saunders, 1981, p 1097.

66. Heyrovsky A: A new method for determination of inulin in plasma and urine. *Clin Chim Acta* 1:470, 1956.

67. White HK, Gann D: An automatic anthrone method for the determination of inulin in plasma and urine. *J Lab Clin Medj* 67:689, 1966.

68. Levey AS, Madaio MP, Perrone RD: Laboratory assessment of renal disease: Clearance, urinanalysis, and renal biopsy, in Brenner BM, Rector FC (eds): *The Kidney*. 4th ed. Philadelphia, WB Saunders, 1991, p 919.

69. Dunn BR, Anderson S, Brenner M: The hemodynamic basis of progressive renal disease. *Semin Nephrol* 6:122, 1986.

70. Cockcroft DW, Gault MH: Prediction of creatinine clearance from serum creatinine. *Nephron* 16:31, 1976.

79. Disorders of Plasma Sodium and Plasma Potassium

Robert M. Black

Disorders of Plasma Sodium

Hyponatremia and hypernatremia are conditions commonly observed in the intensive care unit. They occur when the plasma Na^+ concentration falls below 135 mEq per liter or increases above 145 mEq per liter, respectively. The correct management of individuals with these disorders depends on an understanding of normal salt and water physiology.

It is important to appreciate that hyponatremia represents a disorder of water balance; this is in contrast to true volume depletion (due to gastrointestinal or renal losses) or to edematous states, which are disorders of sodium balance.

This distinction can be illustrated by a review of the difference between osmoregulation and volume regulation (Table 79-1). The former involves maintenance of the plasma osmolality, which is usually composed primarily of sodium salts. Hypothalamic osmoreceptors influence thirst and the release of antidiuretic hormone. The latter increases the urine osmolality and causes water retention by enhancing the permeability of the collecting tubules to water.

Volume regulation, on the other hand, attempts to maintain tissue perfusion. The effectors of this process (see Table 79-1) regulate volume balance by affecting urinary sodium excretion rather than the urine osmolality. Antidiuretic hormone does play a small role, since its release is enhanced by hypovolemia. The associated increase in water reabsorption tends to cause some extracellular volume expansion, although about two-thirds of the water enters the cells. This volume-mediated antidiuretic hormone release occurs even in states of hyponatremia (see below).

RELATIONSHIP BETWEEN PLASMA Na$^+$ AND PLASMA OSMOLALITY. The osmolality of plasma (P_{Osm}) is determined by the sum of the individual osmotically active substances. In plasma, Na$^+$ salts, glucose, and urea (blood urea nitrogen [BUN]) are the major determinants of osmolality. Therefore, the P_{Osm} can be estimated by the following formula:

$$P_{Osm} \approx 2 \times \text{plasma Na}^+ + \text{glucose}/20 + \text{BUN}/3$$

Using this equation [1],* it is evident that the major determinant of the P_{Osm} in normal individuals is the plasma Na$^+$ concentration. In contrast, knowledge of the plasma Na$^+$ alone provides no information about the total content of sodium in the body. For example, an individual with severe gastroenteritis who becomes volume-depleted from vomiting and diarrhea loses a significant quantity of sodium and water through the gastrointestinal tract. If only a portion of these losses were replaced, and if the replacement solution contained only water and no Na$^+$, the plasma Na$^+$ concentration would fall. At that time, the patient would be hyponatremic and, if the BUN and glucose concentrations remained normal, hypoosmolar. Total body Na$^+$ would be reduced more than total body water. In comparison, body water and Na$^+$ are increased in the edematous, hyponatremic patient with congestive heart failure.

The ability of a solute to promote shifts of H$_2$O between the intracellular and extracellular compartments depends not only on its capacity to increase the P_{Osm} but also on its exclusion from one of these compartments. Urea, which can cross almost all cell membranes rapidly, cannot promote the movement of H$_2$O out of cells [2]. As such, urea is referred to as an *ineffective osmole*. A rise in the plasma BUN concentration is detected as an increase in the measured (by the laboratory) and calculated P_{Osm}, but there is no change in the plasma Na$^+$ concentration, because urea does not obligate H$_2$O movement from the intracellular to the extracellular space. Furthermore, because the glucose concentration is normally much lower than that of Na$^+$, the effective P_{Osm} usually correlates best with the plasma Na$^+$. Thus, effective P_{Osm} can be described as follows:

$$P_{Osm} \text{ (effective)} \approx 2 \times \text{plasma Na}^+ \text{ concentration}$$

Sodium is confined primarily to the extracellular fluid by the Na-K antiporter (Na-K ATPase) present in most cells. This pump also maintains a high (about 130 mEq/L) intracellular K$^+$ concentration; as a result, potassium is the principal effective osmole inside cells. The ability of water to cross almost all cell membranes indicates that the P_{Osm} must be in equilibrium with

Table 79-1. Difference Between Osmoregulation and Volume Regulation

	Osmoregulation	Volume regulation
What is being sensed	Plasma osmolality	Effective circulating volume
Sensors	Hypothalamic osmoreceptors	Carotid sinus Afferent arteriole Atria
Effectors	Antidiuretic hormone Thirst	Sympathetic nervous system Renin-angiotensin-aldosterone system Atrial natriuretic peptide Intrarenal hemodynamics Antidiuretic hormone
What is affected	Urine osmolality and, via thirst, water intake	Urinary sodium excretion

the intracellular osmolality. This concept permits the effective P_{Osm} to be calculated as follows:

$$P_{Osm} \text{ effective} =$$
$$\frac{\text{Effective extracellular osmoles} + \text{effective intracellular osmoles}}{\text{Total body water}}$$

$$P_{Osm} \text{ (effective)} \approx \frac{\text{Na}^+ \text{ (exchangeable)} + \text{K}^+ \text{ (exchangeable)}}{\text{Total body water}}$$

$$2 \times (\text{Plasma Na}^+) \approx \frac{\text{Na}^+ \text{ (exchangeable)} + \text{K}^+ \text{ (exchangeable)}}{\text{Total body water}}$$

This equation is important because it helps to explain two important concepts. First, calculation of water deficits or excesses, when dealing with a hyponatremic or hypernatremic individual, respectively, must be performed using total body water, not the extracellular fluid volume. Second, loss of potassium from the body, as might occur with diuretic administration, will affect the plasma Na$^+$ concentration [3,4].

Two processes apparently are operative in the reduction in plasma Na$^+$ concentration induced by hypokalemia: sodium movement into cells to maintain electroneutrality, thus lowering the plasma Na$^+$; and H$^+$ movement into cells in exchange for K$^+$. Since H$^+$ entering the cell becomes bound, it loses its osmotic effect, leading to a relative decrease in effective intracellular osmolality followed by H$_2$O movement out of cells.

Finally, although plasma hypoosmolality is always associated with hyponatremia, a high P_{Osm} may not be evidenced by hypernatremia. Other ineffective osmoles (in addition to urea) have the ability to raise the P_{Osm} without affecting water shifts. The most important of these are the alcohols: ethanol, ethylene glycol, and methanol. As discussed in Chapter 80, the presence of an osmolal gap (a P_{Osm} measured by the clinical laboratory that is more than 10 to 15 mOsm/kg higher than calculated) suggests that one or more of these substances has been ingested. By comparison, these alcohols readily move between fluid compartments without obviating water shifts. Consequently, they do not cause hyponatremia.

REGULATION OF PLASMA OSMOLALITY. Maintenance of the plasma Na$^+$ concentration within narrow limits (285–292

---

* The molecular weights of glucose and nitrogen are 180 and 14, respectively. As a result, the osmotic effect of glucose is determined by dividing by 18 (since the concentration is in 100 ml of plasma and not 1 liter), whereas that of BUN is obtained by dividing by 2.8 (there are two nitrogens on each molecule of urea).

mOsm/kg) depends on the ability of the kidneys to excrete water (thus preventing hypoosmolality) and on a normal thirst mechanism with access to water (defending against hypernatremia). Under normal conditions, the quantity of water that can be excreted in the urine far exceeds the amount ingested.

Renal water excretion is determined by two factors: urinary solute excretion and the ability to generate a maximally dilute urine (urine osmolality <100 mOsm/kg) [5]. In a typical American diet, solute intake equals between 600 and 1200 mOsm per day. Assuming an output that approximates intake, daily urinary solute excretion in a 70-kg man might average 900 mOsm. Dietary NaCl, KCl, and protein (which is broken down to urea) make up most of this solute load. Consequently, the individual who excretes 900 mOsm of solute per day and who can dilute the urine maximally (down to 50 mOsm/kg) has the capacity to excrete about 18 liters of water in a 24-hour period:

$$\frac{900 \text{ mOsm}}{50 \text{ mOsm/kg}} = 18 \text{ L}$$

Anything that impairs maximal diluting ability limits the quantity of water that can be excreted.

The capacity to dilute the urine maximally begins in the loop of Henle and continues to the collecting tubule. This portion of the nephron therefore is often referred to as the diluting segment (Fig. 79-1). As filtrate passes through the loop of Henle, solute is removed by the Na-K-2Cl transporter located in the cells of thick ascending limb [6], and by the NaCl carrier in the distal tubule [7]. Filtrate leaving the diluting segment characteristically has a urinary osmolality (U_{Osm}) below 100 mOsm per

kilogram because this nephron segment is impermeable to water.

A dilute urine cannot be produced if the removal of NaCl by the pumps and carriers in the diluting segment is impaired or if there is permeability of the collecting tubule to water due to the presence of antidiuretic hormone (see below). If, for example, the urine cannot be diluted below 300 mOsm per kilogram, the amount of water that can be excreted is reduced to 3 liters:

$$\frac{900 \text{ mOsm}}{300 \text{ mOsm/kg}} = 3 \text{ L}$$

Similarly, tubular damage (as in chronic interstitial nephritis) or dysfunction (when diuretics are administered) has the same effect. The inability to remove solute limits the ability to dilute the urine in the diluting segment. The minimum U_{Osm} that can be generated in this setting is about 250 to 300 mOsm/kg.

In normal individuals, solute excretion is determined by solute intake [5]. A reduction in dietary solute (as in the patient subsisting on only tea and toast, which contains little protein or salt) limits the capacity to excrete water. If solute intake falls to 150 mOsm per day, for instance, water excretion is limited to about 3 liters even when urinary dilution is normal:

$$\frac{150 \text{ mOsm}}{50 \text{ mOsm/kg}} = 3 \text{ L}$$

It is easy to see that the combination of impaired diluting ability with a concomitant reduction in solute intake is more likely to limit H_2O excretion and cause hyponatremia than either disturbance alone.

REGULATION OF ANTIDIURETIC HORMONE. In contrast to individuals who are unable to excrete a water load, normal adults can excrete very large or very small volumes of urine, the concentration of which varies according to the P_{Osm}. The

Fig. 79-1. Excretion of a dilute urine. Solute entering the early proximal tubule has an osmolality identical to plasma; fluid is isotonically reabsorbed in this nephron segment. Separation of solute from water within the tubule begins in the thick ascending limb of Henle, which is impermeable to water. Excretion of a urine with a minimum osmolality of 50 to 100 mOsm per liter requires intact function of this nephron segment as well as suppression of ADH release. (Adapted from Black RM: Diagnosis and management of hyponatremia. *J Intensive Care Med* 4:205, 1989, with permission.)

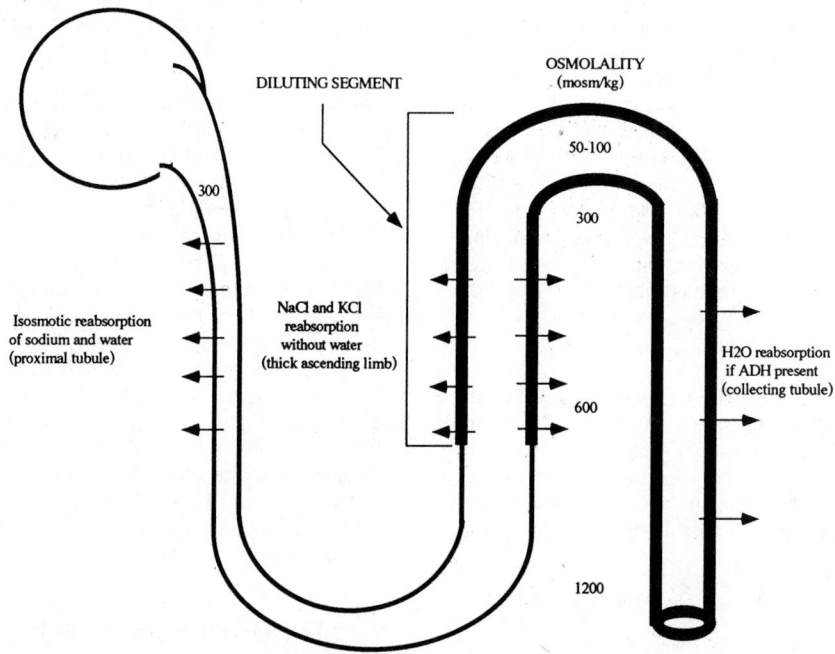

primary hormone regulating water excretion in health is antidiuretic hormone (ADH). ADH (called arginine vasopressin in humans) is synthesized in the supraoptic and paraventricular nuclei of the hypothalamus. Hypothalamic osmoreceptors for ADH release are stimulated by hyperosmolality and inhibited by hypoosmolality. A change in osmoreceptor volume is probably the factor that modifies ADH secretion in response to changes in the P_{Osm}, because urea, which is an ineffective osmole that cannot alter cell volume, does not promote or inhibit ADH release [8].

A 1 to 2% reduction in P_{Osm} (P_{Osm} <280 mOsm/kg) maximally inhibits ADH release, leading to a U_{Osm} that is normally less than 100 mOsm per kilogram [8]. By contrast, a 1% to 2% increase in P_{Osm} above normal or a 7% to 10% decrease in blood pressure or volume (even in the presence of plasma hypoosmolality) normally stimulates ADH release [8,9]. In the presence of ADH, the luminal membranes of the cortical and medullary collecting tubules become permeable as water channels are inserted [10]. This change permits reabsorption and an increase in the final urine osmolality.

HYPONATREMIA.
In most settings, the development of hyponatremia with hypoosmolality represents the retention of ingested or administered water. As a result, causes of this disorder can be divided into those in which water excretion is abnormal and those in which water excretion is normal (but water ingestion is considerably increased).

Hypoosmolar Disorders with Impaired Water Excretion.
The U_{Osm} is typically greater than 100 mOsm per kilogram in patients with reduced water excretion (Table 79-2). An exception to this rule occurs when solute intake is markedly reduced, as may occur with a tea-and-toast diet (see Reduced solute intake, following).

Table 79-2. Causes of Hyponatremia

Impaired water excretion (U_{Osm} >100 mOsm/kg and usually >300 mOsm/kg)
  Hypovolemic states
    True volume depletion (by gastrointestinal, skin, or renal losses)
    Edematous states with reduced effective arterial blood volume (advanced liver and heart disease)
  Diuretics (particularly thiazides)
  Advanced renal failure
  Endocrine deficiencies (hypothyroidism and hypoadrenalism)
  SIADH
  Cerebral salt-wasting
  Reduced solute intake (tea and toast diet; beer drinkers' hyponatremia)*
Normal water excretion (U_{Osm} >100 mOsm/kg)
  Primary polydipsia
    Psychiatric disorders (particularly with phenothiazines)
    Hypothalamic disorders
Hyponatremia without hypoosmolality
  Normal P_{Osm}
    Pseudohyponatremia (hypertriglyceridemia, hyperproteinemia, genitourinary tract irrigation)
  Increased P_{Osm}
    Hyperosmolar hyponatremia (hyperglycemia, mannitol infusion in renal failure)
    Azotemia (effective osmolality is reduced)

*U_{Osm} < 100 mOsm/kg, but normal water excretion is impaired by the reduced solute load; see text for details. (Adapted from Black RM: Diagnosis and management of hyponatremia. *J Intensive Care Med* 4:205, 1989; and Rose BD, Black RM: *Manual of Clinical Problems in Nephrology.* Boston, Little, Brown, 1988, pp 3-10, with permission.)

HYPOVOLEMIC HYPONATREMIA. A fall in effective perfusion pressure stimulates release of the three hypovolemic hormones: norepinephrine (which redirects blood flow away from the kidneys toward the brain and heart), angiotensin II (which enhances renal Na^+ retention directly and by promoting aldosterone release), and ADH [11]. Hypovolemic hyponatremia can occur in states of dehydration or in edematous individuals with congestive heart failure or advanced liver disease, since each of these conditions is associated with a reduced effective arterial blood volume. As discussed previously, the resulting increase in the U_{Osm} (e.g., to 600 mOsm/kg) would limit renal water excretion on a 900 mOsm per day diet to 1.5 liters, assuming all of the ingested solute were excreted (900 mOsm/kg 600). Furthermore, enhanced renal tubular sodium reabsorption limits solute excretion, and most stimuli that activate angiotensin II release also stimulate thirst, despite concurrent hypoosmolality.

DIURETIC-INDUCED HYPONATREMIA. The ability to excrete a dilute urine is impaired by diuretics, whether they act in the thick ascending limb of Henle (loop diuretics) or in the distal tubule (thiazide-type diuretics) (Fig. 79-2). Each class reduces NaCl transport out of the diluting segment, thus raising the minimum U_{Osm} that can be generated from 50 to about 250 mOsm per kilogram, even in the absence of ADH [5]. Reducing the minimum U_{Osm} to this level, however, does not usually lead to hypoosmolality, because a large volume of urine can still be excreted in most patients. For example, if urinary solute excretion is 900 mOsm and the U_{Osm} is 250 mOsm per kilogram, 3.6 liters of water can be eliminated (900 mOsm/kg 250). Despite these similarities, almost all cases of diuretic-induced hyponatremia in otherwise normal individuals have been caused by thiazide-type diuretics, not by agents that act in the thick ascending limb of Henle's loop [12].

This distinction may be due to different sites of the action within the renal tubule (see Fig. 79-2). Loop diuretics, which act in the outer medulla, reduce the solute concentration in the renal medullary interstitium. Since medullary osmolality is the principal determinant of urinary concentrating ability when

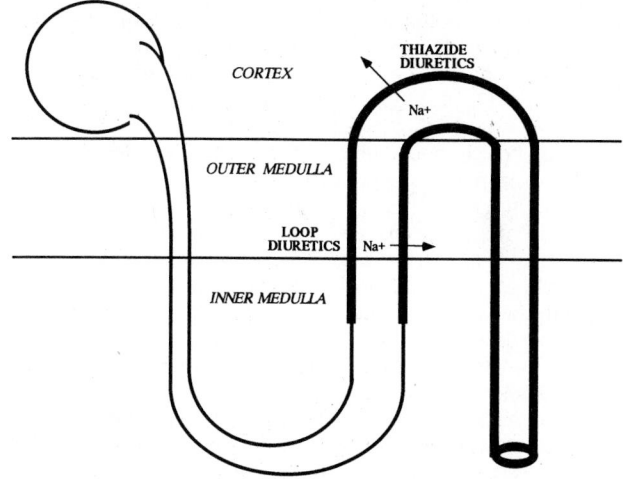

Fig. 79-2. Site of action of loop and thiazide diuretics. Loop diuretics inhibit the Na-K-2Cl cotransporter in the medullary portion of the thick ascending limb of Henle, whereas thiazides block a simple NaCl carrier in the cortical portion of the distal tubule. These differences explain, in part, the susceptibility of individuals treated with thiazide-type diuretics to develop hyponatremia; see text for details. (Adapted from Black RM: Diagnosis and management of hyponatremia. *J Intensive Care Med* 4:205, 1989, with permission.)

ADH is present, a fall in the interstitial osmolality (from 1200 to 300 mOsm/kg, for instance) limits the maximum U_{Osm} that can be generated from 1200 to 300 mOsm per kilogram. By comparison, thiazide diuretics (which act in the cortex) impair diluting capacity but do not greatly limit concentrating ability. Thus, the U_{Osm} may be 600 mOsm per kilogram in the thiazide-treated individual; if the urinary osmoles are primarily NaCl and KCl, urinary electrolyte losses can exceed those contained in an equal volume of plasma. In these patients, therefore, the plasma Na^+ may fall without any water intake. For reasons that are not well understood, however, individuals with thiazide-induced hyponatremia gain weight, indicating that the hyponatremia is at least in part a result of increased water intake [13]. This disorder occurs more frequently in women, typically occurs early in therapy (within 1 to 4 weeks). As discussed previously, accompanying hypokalemia also may contribute to the fall in plasma osmolality.

ADVANCED RENAL FAILURE. The normal glomerular filtration rate (GFR) is approximately 180 liters per day. As renal function decreases, the ability to excrete water also falls. The limitation in H_2O excretion occurs for two reasons: tubular dysfunction leads to an inability to dilute the urine maximally, even in the absence of ADH; and the drop in GFR, particularly when severe, may reduce daily solute excretion.

ENDOCRINE DEFICIENCY. Hypothyroidism and hypocortisolism can impair water excretion [14,15]. Both may reduce cardiac output or stroke volume, leading to increased ADH release. The resulting fall in GFR directly diminishes free water excretion by diminishing water delivery to the diluting segments. Decreased delivery may be particularly important in patients with myxedema in whom hyponatremia develops despite appropriate suppression of ADH release [16]. Another factor appears to be important is hypocortisolism, since corticotropin-releasing factor appears to promote the co-release of adrenocorticotrophic hormone (ACTH) and ADH, although the reason for the concomitant release of these hormones is not known [17]. It is important to note that panadrenal hypofunction (as in Addison's disease) leads to reduced cortisol and aldosterone levels, the latter predisposing to hyperkalemia. The presence of low cortisol levels due to pituitary or hypothalamic disease, on the other hand, may cause hyponatremia but should not alter potassium homeostasis, because aldosterone release is relatively normal [18].

SYNDROME OF INAPPROPRIATE ANTIDIURETIC HORMONE SECRETION. The syndrome of inappropriate ADH secretion (SIADH) is characterized by plasma hypoosmolality; U_{Osm} above 100 to 150 mOsm per kilogram; urinary Na^+ concentration above 20 mEq per liter; normal adrenal, renal, and thyroid function; and normal potassium and acid-base balance [5]. SIADH may be caused by enhanced hypothalamic ADH secretion, ectopic hormone production (usually by cancer), potentiation of ADH effect (as with chlorpropamide), or by administration of medications with ADH activity (Table 79-3).

In about one-third of patients, the SIADH is associated with resetting of the hypothalamic osmostat. This disorder has been described in patients with hypovolemia, psychosis, chronic malnutrition, and in normal pregnancy (in which the plasma Na^+ concentration decreases by the second month from 140 to 135 mEq/L) [19]. ADH release is not suppressed until the P_{Osm} falls well below normal in this disorder. As a result, the P_{Osm} may vary between 240 and 250 mOsm per kilogram (plasma Na^+ about 120 to 125 mEq/L) compared with the normal value of approximately 285 to 292 mOsm per kilogram. In contrast to the classic form of the SIADH, in which nonsuppressible ADH release is seen, ADH secretion stops when the P_{Osm} falls below this new, reset level. Since suppression of ADH prevents

Table 79-3. Major Causes of SIADH

Disorders	Comments
Pulmonary diseases	Acute asthma, atelectasis, empyema, pneumothorax, acute respiratory failure, tuberculosis, carcinoma, pneumonia
Neurologic disorders	Meningitis, tumors, psychiatric disorders, subarachnoid hemorrhage, herpes zoster, Wernicke's encephalopathy
Ectopic production	Cancer (particularly oat-cell carcinoma of lung)
Drugs	Intravenous cyclophosphamide, carbamazepine, chlorpropamide, nonsteroidal antiinflammatory drugs (since prostaglandins block ADH effect), cisplatin*
Following major surgery	Pain afferents stimulate hypothalamic ADH release (lasts for 2 to 5 days), after mitral commissurotomy for mitral stenosis (acute decrease in left atrial pressure releases ADH)
Administration of exogenous ADH or oxytocin	Oxytocin can reduce plasma Na^+ concentration in mother and fetus
Symptomatic HIV infection	See text for details
Idiopathic	Important to continue periodic monitoring for an underlying disorder, particularly carcinoma; vasculitis (such as temporal arteritis) should be considered in elderly patients when no other etiology is apparent
Cerebral salt wasting	See text for details

*Hyponatremia induced by cisplatin may be due to renal salt wasting.

a further fall in the plasma Na^+ concentration, less progressive hyponatremia occurs in this condition.

An increasingly common cause of hyponatremia is symptomatic HIV infection, either the acquired immune deficiency syndrome (AIDS) or AIDS-related complex [20,21]. Although volume deficiency (due, for example, to gastrointestinal losses) or adrenal insufficiency may be responsible, many patients have SIADH. Pneumonia due to *Pneumocystis carinii* or other organisms, CNS infections, and malignant disease are most often responsible in this setting (see Chap. 93).

CEREBRAL SALT WASTING. This rare disorder is characterized by a low P_{Osm}, a U_{Osm} above 100 to 150 mOsm per kilogram, and a urine Na^+ concentration greater than 20 mEq per liter [22]. Unlike SIADH, however, evidence of volume depletion (including low central filling pressures) is present. In affected individuals, therefore, the high urinary Na^+ represents inappropriate salt wasting rather than a response to normal tissue perfusion (as in SIADH patients).

The cause of this putative syndrome is unclear. It has been proposed that there may be increased release of atrial natriuretic peptide (or perhaps the recently described brain natriuretic peptide) from hormone-producing neurons in the brain that are activated by CNS dysfunction [23]. Both hypouricemia and tubular dysfunction have been reported. Mineralocorticoid replacement therapy with fludrocortisone acetate has been effective in some people [24].

REDUCED SOLUTE INTAKE. A reduction in salt and protein intake can lead to hypoosmolality if water intake exceeds output. Severely reduced solute intake, as occurs with a tea-and-toast diet, can cause hyponatremia even with normal degrees of water intake. "Beer drinker's hyponatremia" occurs for a similar reason; the ingestion of the limited quantity of NaCl in beer may be inadequate to permit the water (ingested in beer) to be excreted. In both conditions, the U_{Osm} should be maximally dilute (U_{Osm} 100 mOsm/kg). The absence of polyuria and the development of hyponatremia with normal or slightly above normal fluid intake distinguishes these individuals from those with primary polydipsia (see following).

Hypoosmolar Disorders with Normal Water Excretion.

Psychiatric patients, particularly those with schizophrenia, often have abnormalities in water balance [25,26]. Evaluation of psychotic patients has revealed that a variety of defects in water handling can occur that affect thirst, the release of antidiuretic hormone (ADH), and the renal response to ADH. Depending upon the abnormality that is present, the patient may present with polydipsia and polyuria and/or hyponatremia.

PRIMARY POLYDIPSIA. Many chronically psychotic patients have a moderate to marked increase in water intake [25–28]. This may be manifested clinically by exaggerated weight gain during the day [27] associated with a transient reduction in the plasma sodium concentration [29].

Presumably, a central defect in thirst regulation plays an important role in the pathogenesis of polydipsia [25,28]. In some patients, for example, the osmotic threshold for thirst is reduced below the threshold for the release of antidiuretic hormone (ADH) [30]. These patients continue to drink until the plasma osmolality is less than the threshold level. This may be difficult to achieve, however, since ADH secretion is suppressed by the fall in plasma osmolality, resulting in rapid excretion of the excess water and continued stimulation of thirst. The osmotic regulation of thirst differs from that of normal subjects, in whom the thirst threshold is roughly equal to or a few mOsmol/kg higher than the threshold for ADH [31].

The mechanism responsible for abnormal thirst regulation in this setting is unclear [32]. Drug therapy may contribute to the increase in water intake in schizophrenic patients. Many antipsychotic drugs induce the sensation of a dry mouth, which will enhance the sensation of thirst [33].

Normal subjects can excrete more than 10 to 15 liters of urine per day, a response that is mediated by suppression of ADH secretion and the subsequent formation of a dilute urine with a minimum osmolality between 40 and 100 mOsmol/kg. Thus, if ADH regulation were intact, primary polydipsia should not lead to clinically important disturbances in the plasma sodium concentration unless intake is massively increased. There are, for example, rare patients in whom severe and potentially fatal hyponatremia has developed even though the urine osmolality was appropriately below 100 mOsmol/kg [34]. More commonly, however, the development of hyponatremia is associated with a higher urine osmolality, indicating a concurrent increase in ADH release and or response [28,35,36].

Several abnormalities in ADH regulation have been identified in psychotic patients, each of which can impair water excretion: (1) Transient stimulation of ADH release during acute psychotic episodes can produce SIADH [36]. (2) The net renal response to ADH may increase so that psychotic patients have a higher urine osmolality and therefore a lower rate of free water excretion than healthy controls [28]. (3) The osmostat regulating ADH release may be reset downward.

The effect is that most modestly hyponatremic patients with primary polydipsia do not have a maximally dilute urine, as would be expected if ADH were appropriately suppressed by the fall in plasma osmolality and if there were not increased sensitivity to ADH [28]. The likelihood of developing hyponatremia increases further if there is some other cause for enhanced ADH release. Concurrent thiazide diuretic therapy for systemic hypertension can lead to a marked and symptomatic reduction in the plasma sodium concentration in these patients [37].

There is no proven specific therapy for primary polydipsia with or without hyponatremia in psychotic patients. Limiting water intake will rapidly raise the plasma sodium concentration, as the excess water is readily excreted in a dilute urine. The risk of inducing osmotic demyelination in this setting is unclear; it has been suggested that patients with primary polydipsia and repeated episodes of acute hyponatremia are generally resistant to neurologic injury induced by rapid correction (see below).

Over time, limiting the use of drugs that cause dry mouth, restricting fluid intake, and frequent weighing (to detect water retention) may be helpful. Some physicians have tried the tetracycline derivative demeclocycline, which induces reversible ADH resistance; however, this agent generally has not been effective [38]. Anecdotal observations suggest that the novel antipsychotic agent clozapine may be beneficial, at least in some patients [39].

Hyponatremia Without Hypoosmolality.

Hyponatremia may occur without plasma hypoosmolality. An increase in the plasma concentration of proteins (as immunoglobulins in multiple myeloma) or lipids (primarily triglycerides in lipemic plasma) can reduce the plasma Na^+ concentration. Lipids and proteins displace H_2O from each liter of plasma but do not affect the Na^+ concentration in the water phase of plasma [40]. As a result, the measured P_{Osm} is normal in this condition, which is called *pseudohyponatremia*.

An unusual form of hyponatremia, sometimes associated with a normal P_{Osm}, can be observed after transurethral prostatectomy (TURP) and with uterine irrigation after endometrial ablation. Transurethral resection of the prostate or bladder often requires the use of as much as 20 to 30 liters of nonconductive flushing solutions containing glycine, sorbitol, or mannitol [41–43]. Some patients absorb 3 liters or more of fluids, leading to a dilutional reduction in the plasma sodium concentration that may fall below 100 mEq/L. In one prospective study of 100 patients, the incidence of hyponatremia following TURP was 7%; there was one death [44].

Confusion, disorientation, twitching, seizures, and hypotension may occur in this setting, for obscure reasons [41–47]. Several methods have been devised to attempt to monitor the amount of fluid absorbed so that patients at risk of severe hyponatremia can be detected [42]. The most promising is adding small amounts of ethanol to the irrigant fluid and monitoring breath samples [48]. The presence of ethanol in the breath sample indicates significant irrigant absorption.

Hyponatremia also may be identified in patients with plasma hyperosmolality (hyperosmolar hyponatremia). This disorder, most commonly due to hyperglycemia or the infusion of mannitol in patients with renal failure, results in an osmotic shift of water from cells into the extracellular fluid, thus diluting the plasma Na^+ concentration. In contrast to hypoosmolar individuals, treatment is directed at correcting the high glucose concentration with insulin and giving water, since cellular dehydration is present. For every 100 mg per deciliter rise in the blood sugar, the plasma Na^+ concentration falls by about 1.6 mEq per liter [49].

Symptoms of Hypoosmolality.

The neurologic symptoms of hyponatremia appear to be entirely due to the consequences of plasma hypoosmolality. A fall in P_{Osm} causes water movement from the extracellular space into cells. The resulting increase in cell water, which is of particular importance in the CNS, can lead to brain swelling [50,51]. A variety of symptoms may be found, including lethargy, confusion, nausea, vomiting, and, in severe cases, seizures and coma. Focal neurologic symptoms are uncommon. Hyponatremic encephalopathy may be reversible, although permanent neurologic damage or death can occur, particularly in premenopausal women [52]. The reason for the higher incidence of residual neurologic injury from acute hyponatremia in this patient population is not well understood [52]. Hyponatremic women must be watched carefully, because they may progress rapidly from minimal symptoms (such as headache and nausea) to respiratory arrest. Cerebral edema and herniation have been found in those women who died, suggesting a possible hormonally mediated decrease in the efficiency of the osmotic adaptation.

The likelihood that symptoms will develop is related to the level of hyponatremia and the rapidity with which it develops [53]. For example, a rapid decline in the plasma Na^+ concentration over several hours or days (from 140 to 115 mEq/L, for example) may be associated with severe neurologic findings. In comparison, a similar fall in plasma sodium occurring over a week or more may not cause any changes. In the latter, the degree of cerebral edema is much less than with acute hyponatremia [53a]. This protective response, which begins on the first day and is complete within several days, occurs in two major steps:

1. The initial cerebral edema elevates the interstitial hydraulic pressure, creating a gradient for extracellular fluid movement out of the brain into the cerebrospinal fluid [54].
2. The brain cells lose solutes, leading to the osmotic movement of water out of the cells and less brain swelling [51,55,56]. Most of this volume regulatory response initially consists of the loss of potassium and sodium salts; this is followed by the loss of organic solutes, particularly the amino acids glutamine, glutamate, and taurine, and, to a lesser degree, the carbohydrate inositol. Electrolyte movement occurs quickly because it is mediated by the activation of quiescent cation channels in the cell membrane; organic solute loss occurs later because it requires synthesis of new transporters.

The organic solutes (called *osmolytes*) account for approximately one-third of the solute loss in chronic hyponatremia [56]. Changes in the concentration of these solutes have the advantage of restoring cell volume without interfering with protein function; in comparison, a potentially deleterious effect on protein function would occur if the volume adaptation were mediated entirely by changes in the cell cation (potassium plus sodium) concentration.

This adaptation is so efficient that it is not uncommon to see patients with heart failure or SIADH who are asymptomatic despite a plasma sodium concentration that is persistently between 115 and 120 mEq/L. When symptoms do occur in chronic hyponatremia, there is almost always severe disease, with plasma sodium concentrations usually below 110 to 115 mEq/L.

Diagnosis. Three laboratory findings provide important information in the differential diagnosis of hyponatremia: plasma osmolality, urine osmolality, and urine sodium concentration.

PLASMA OSMOLALITY. Plasma osmolality is reduced in most hyponatremic patients because it is primarily determined by the plasma sodium concentration. In some cases, however, the plasma osmolality is either normal or elevated. The former may be due to hyperlipidemia, hyperproteinemia, or absorption of isotonic glycine during transurethral resection of the bladder or

prostate (see above). High plasma osmolality, on the other hand, may be seen with hyperglycemia or the administration of hypertonic mannitol, both of which induce osmotic water movement out of the cells and lower the plasma sodium concentration by dilution. Since there is no hypoosmolality and therefore no risk of cerebral edema due to water movement into the brain, therapy directed at the hyponatremia, with the exception of glycine administration, is not indicated in any of these disorders. In this setting, plasma osmolality may fall with time as the glycine is metabolized.

URINE OSMOLALITY. In patients with hyponatremia and a low plasma osmolality, the urine osmolality can be used to distinguish between patients with impaired water excretion (which is present in almost all cases) and primary polydipsia, in which water excretion is normal but intake is so high that it exceeds excretory capacity. The normal response to hyponatremia (which is maintained in primary polydipsia) is to completely suppress ADH secretion, resulting in the excretion of a maximally dilute urine with an osmolality below 100 mOsmol/kg and a specific gravity less than 1.003. Values above this level indicate an inability to normally excrete free water, which is generally due to continued secretion of ADH. Most hyponatremic patients have a relatively marked impairment in urinary dilution that is sufficient to maintain the urine osmolality at 300 mOsmol/kg or greater.

URINE SODIUM CONCENTRATION. In the absence of adrenal insufficiency or hypothyroidism, the two major causes of hyponatremia, hypoosmolality, and an inappropriately concentrated urine are one of the causes of effective volume depletion or of the SIADH. These disorders can usually be distinguished by measuring the urine sodium concentration, which is typically below 25 mEq/L with hypovolemia (unless there is renal salt-wasting, due most often to diuretic therapy) and above 40 mEq/L in patients with SIADH who are normovolemic and whose rate of sodium excretion is determined by dietary or intravenous sodium intake [57,58].

In addition to the initial value, serial monitoring of the urine sodium concentration may be helpful in selected cases in which the correct diagnosis may not be apparent. Suppose, for example, that urine sodium concentration falls from 50 to 10 mEq per liter following the administration of 1 to 2 liters of isotonic saline. Surreptitious thiazide diuretic ingestion should be suspected in this setting. The urine sodium concentration was elevated on the first measurement because of the action of the diuretic. Once this wore off, the true state of volume depletion was unmasked even though the patient had been partially rehydrated.

As another example, suppose that the initial urine sodium concentration is 5 mEq per liter, suggesting hyponatremia due to effective volume depletion. If this were the only problem, then fluid repletion should lead to the excretion of a dilute urine (due to elimination of hypovolemic stimulus to ADH release) and rapid correction of the hyponatremia. If, however, the urine sodium concentration rises to above 40 mEq per liter and the urine osmolality remains above 100 mOsmol/kg, then the patient also has SIADH.

To summarize, hyponatremia caused by SIADH is characterized by (1) a reduction in the plasma osmolality; (2) an inappropriately elevated urine osmolality (above 100 mOsmol/kg and usually above 300 mOsmol/kg); (3) a urine sodium concentration usually above 40 mEq per liter; (4) a relatively normal plasma creatinine concentration; (5) normal adrenal and thyroid function; and (6) normal acid-base and potassium balance.

Evaluation of acid-base and potassium balance may help determine a diagnosis in selected hyponatremic patients. As examples, metabolic alkalosis and hypokalemia suggest diuretic use or vomiting, metabolic acidosis and hypokalemia suggest diarrhea or laxative abuse, and metabolic acidosis and hyperkalemia suggest adrenal insufficiency. On the other hand, plasma bicarbonate and potassium concentrations are typically normal in patients with SIADH [58]. Although water retention tends to lower these values by dilution (as it does the plasma sodium and chloride concentrations), normal levels are restored by the factors that normally regulate acid-base and potassium balance. The release of potassium from cells in an attempt to minimize cell swelling induced by hypoosmolality also raises the plasma potassium concentration to normal.

The initial water retention and volume expansion in patients with SIADH leads to another frequent finding that is the opposite of that typically seen with volume depletion: hypouricemia (plasma uric acid concentration less than 4 mg/dL) due to increased uric acid excretion in the urine [58,59]. Presumably, early volume expansion diminishes proximal sodium reabsorption, leading to a secondary decline in the net reabsorption of uric acid. A similar sequence of urinary wasting can occur with urea, as the BUN may fall to below 5 mg/dL, in contrast to the elevation in BUN and in the BUN/plasma creatinine ratio often seen with volume depletion.

All of these findings seen in SIADH also have been described in the putative syndrome of cerebral salt-wasting, a disorder in which the high urine sodium concentration occurs as a result of defective tubular reabsorption, and the elevation in ADH and subsequent development of hyponatremia are due to the associated volume depletion. Hypouricemia also may be present which presumably is another manifestation of impaired renal tubular function (see above).

FRACTIONAL EXCRETION OF SODIUM. The fractional excretion of sodium (FENa) is a more accurate assessment of volume status than the urine sodium concentration in patients with acute renal failure; a FENa below 1% suggests effective volume depletion. This observation has led many physicians to use the FENa in any situation in which the urine sodium concentration might be helpful. FENa may be misleading in patients with relatively normal renal function, however, since the expected value to differentiate volume depletion from euvolemia varies with the glomerular filtration rate. A value of 1% is not the correct dividing line in this setting, since this value may occur in euvolemic patients (such as those with SIADH) who have a urine sodium concentration above 50 mEq per liter and who excrete more than 100 mEq of sodium per day. As a result, random urine sodium concentration is more accurate for assessing the volume status in patients with hyponatremia with a normal plasma creatinine concentration.

Treatment of Hyponatremia.
A variety of therapeutic issues that need to be addressed in the treatment of hyponatremia are discussed below.

SALINE OR WATER RESTRICTION. In general, plasma sodium concentration can be raised either by giving salt (either as saline or salt tablets) or by restricting water intake to below the level of excretion. The choice of therapy is primarily governed by the cause of the hyponatremia.

Salt administration, usually as isotonic saline, is appropriate in those with true volume depletion, diuretic therapy, or adrenal insufficiency (in which cortisol replacement is also indicated). Water restriction is used with edematous states (such as heart failure and hepatic cirrhosis), SIADH, primary polydipsia, and advanced renal failure.

In states of true volume depletion, isotonic saline corrects the hyponatremia by two mechanisms. It slowly raises the plasma sodium by 1 to 2 mEq per liter for every liter of fluid infused, since saline has a higher sodium concentration (154 mEq/L) than the hyponatremic plasma. By eventually causing volume repletion, it removes the stimulus to ADH release,

thereby allowing the excess water to be excreted. At this time, the plasma sodium concentration may return rapidly toward normal.

Isotonic saline should be considered in patients with mild to moderate or asymptomatic hyponatremia. In contrast, symptomatic patients or those with a plasma sodium below 110 to 115 mEq per liter usually require initial therapy with hypertonic saline. It must be emphasized, however, that careful monitoring is essential, since overly rapid correction carries the risk of possibly inducing central demyelinating lesions [60,61].

In primary polydipsia, the initiation of water restriction may result in a dramatic rise in the plasma sodium concentration. There is, however, some evidence suggesting that these patients may be at less risk of developing pontine myelinolysis, since the hyponatremia often is of rapid onset, with less adaptation occurring [62]. As described above, removal of the hypovolemic stimulus to ADH release by the administration of isotonic saline in the volume-depleted patient may also promote prompt correction of hyponatremia. Thus, careful monitoring of the plasma sodium concentration is required.

SODIUM DEFICIT AND RATE OF CORRECTION. The optimal rate of correction of hyponatremia varies with the clinical state of the patient. The following represents a reasonable approach given the information currently available [53,63–65]. In asymptomatic patients (who are more likely to have chronic hyponatremia), the plasma sodium concentration should be raised at a maximum rate averaging 0.5 mEq per liter per hour and, perhaps more importantly, less than 12 mEq per liter per day; a more rapid elevation can increase the risk of osmotic demyelination [53,63–66].

More rapid correction is indicated in patients with symptomatic hyponatremia who present with seizures or other severe neurologic manifestations, which primarily result from cerebral edema induced by acute (developing over 2 to 3 days) hyponatremia [53,63,65]. In this circumstance, the plasma sodium concentration can be raised at an initial rate of 1.5 to 2 mEq per liter per hour for the first 3 to 4 hours (or longer if the patient remains symptomatic), since the risk of persistent severe hyponatremia is greater than the possible danger of overly rapid correction. This appears to be particularly true in premenopausal women, who may progress from minimal symptoms (headache and nausea) to coma and respiratory arrest; furthermore, irreversible neurologic damage or death is relatively common in younger women with symptomatic hyponatremia, even if the hyponatremia is corrected at an appropriate rate. In comparison, men are at much less risk of symptomatic hyponatremia and of permanent neurologic injury.

The quantity of sodium required to achieve the desired elevation in the plasma sodium concentration can be estimated from the product of the plasma sodium deficit per liter and the total body water (TBW), which represents the osmotic space of distribution of the plasma sodium concentration. Normal values for the TBW are 0.5 and 0.6 times the lean body weight in women and men, respectively. Thus, if the initial aim in an asymptomatic hyponatremic 60-kg woman is to raise the plasma sodium concentration from 110 to 120 mEq per liter, then:

Sodium deficit for initial therapy

$$= 0.5 \times 60 \times (120 - 110)$$
$$= 300 \text{ mEq}$$

Thus, 600 ml of hypertonic saline (which contains roughly a mEq of sodium per 2 ml) should be given over 20 hours at a rate of 30 ml per hour; this regimen should raise the plasma sodium concentration at the desired rate of 0.5 mEq/L per hour.

It must be emphasized, however, that this formula is only an estimate and that serial monitoring of the plasma sodium concentration (beginning at 2 to 3 hours) is still required.

The above formula assumes that sodium is being given in excess of water (as with hypertonic saline); isotonic saline, in which sodium and water are given in proportion, will have a relatively minor direct effect on the hyponatremia. Isotonic saline will, however, eventually correct hyponatremia due to true volume depletion. In this setting, restoration of normovolemia will eliminate the hypovolemic stimulus to ADH release, thereby allowing the excess water to be excreted in a maximally dilute urine. Careful monitoring is required, since there is the potential risk of overly rapid correction of the hyponatremia [60,61].

A loop diuretic, such as furosemide, can be added if there is a concern about fluid overload or if the urine is very concentrated (above 500 mOsmol/kg) in a patient with SIADH [1] (see below).

EFFECT OF POTASSIUM. Potassium is as osmotically active as sodium, and giving potassium can raise the plasma sodium concentration and osmolality in a hyponatremic subject [4,61,67]. As most of the excess potassium goes into the cells, electroneutrality is maintained in one of three ways, each of which will raise the plasma sodium concentration. (1) Intracellular sodium moves into the extracellular fluid. (2) Extracellular chloride moves into the cells with potassium; the increase in cell osmolality promotes free water entry into the cells. (3) Intracellular hydrogen moves into the extracellular fluid. These hydrogen ions are buffered by extracellular bicarbonate and, to a much lesser degree, by plasma proteins. This buffering renders the hydrogen ions osmotically inactive; the ensuing fall in extracellular osmolality leads to water movement into the cells.

Thus, any administration of potassium must be taken into account when calculating the sodium deficit. This relationship becomes clinically important in the patient with severe diuretic or vomiting-induced hyponatremia who is also hypokalemic. Suppose, for example, that the plasma potassium concentration is 2 mEq per liter and it is decided to give 400 mEq of potassium during the first day. If the patient is a 70-kg man, the total body water will be approximately 40 liters (60% of body weight). In this setting, 800 mEq of osmotically active potassium chloride (400 mEq of each) distributed through 40 liters will raise the plasma osmolality by 20 mOsmol/kg and the plasma sodium concentration by roughly 10 mEq per liter, which is near the desired rate of maximum correction. Thus, giving potassium chloride alone will correct both the hyponatremia and the hypokalemia [61]. Giving additional sodium may lead to an overly rapid elevation in the plasma sodium concentration.

RISK OF OSMOTIC DEMYELINATION. Severe hyponatremia, especially if acute in onset, can lead to cerebral edema (due to osmotic water movement into the brain), potentially irreversible neurologic damage, and death [52,68]. This most often occurs when large volumes of hypotonic fluids are given to postoperative patients (who have pain-induced ADH release that impairs the ability of the kidney to excrete water) or to those with acute thiazide-induced hyponatremia. Within 24 hours, however, the brain begins to lose extracellular water into the cerebrospinal fluid and loses intracellular water by extruding sodium and potassium salts and certain organic solutes (called osmolytes), thereby lowering the brain volume toward normal (see above) [51,55].

The effect is that hyponatremia that develops slowly (over more than 2 to 3 days) is associated with a lesser likelihood of neurologic symptoms [53,63]. In this setting, in which brain volume has fallen toward normal, rapid correction of severe hyponatremia (plasma sodium concentration usually less than 110 to 115 mEq/L) may lead within 1 to several days to the development of a neurologic disorder called osmotic demyelination or central pontine myelinolysis (although more diffuse demyelination that does not necessarily involve the pons can occur) [53,63–65]. These lesions (which are not seen with slow correction) can be detected by CT scanning or MRI [69]. Results of these diagnostic tests may not become positive for as long as 4 weeks, however [65,69]. Thus, negative radiologic study in a patient who develops neurologic symptoms after the treatment of hyponatremia does not exclude osmotic demyelination.

The mechanisms responsible for osmotic demyelination are not completely understood. Rapid elevation in the plasma sodium concentration leads to water movement out of the brain, which can lower the brain volume below normal [51]. This osmotic shrinkage in the axons could sever their connections with the surrounding myelin sheaths [70]. An alternative mechanism involves the initial brain cell response to brain shrinkage, which is the uptake of potassium and sodium from the extracellular fluid; this elevation in cell cation concentration could be toxic to the cells [51,55].

It has been suggested that there are differences in individual susceptibility to osmotic demyelination. For example, observations indicate that psychiatric patients with primary polydipsia are relatively resistant to osmotic demyelination despite having repeated episodes of hyponatremia and, due to normal water excretory capacity, rapid correction of the plasma sodium concentration [62]. The reasons for this are not known, but this resistance to demyelination may not apply to polydipsia in chronic alcoholics [71].

The manifestations of osmotic demyelination, which may be irreversible, include mental status changes, dysarthria, dysphagia, paraparesis or quadriparesis, and coma; seizures may occur but are less common [63,65,68]. Patients in whom the plasma sodium concentration is raised more than 20 mEq/L in the first 24 h or is overcorrected to greater than 140 mEq/L are at greatest risk [53,63–65]. On the other hand, late neurologic deterioration is rare if the hyponatremia is corrected at an average rate equal to or less than 0.5 mEq per liter per hour [64,65].

Studies in experimental animals indicate that the total rate of correction over the first 24 hours is more important than the maximum rate in any given hour [66,72]. Demyelinating lesions are most common when the plasma sodium concentration in severe hyponatremia is raised more than 20 mEq per liter per day and are rare at a rate below 10 to 12 mEq per liter per day [66]. This is similar to the safe average rate of correction of 0.5 mEq per liter per hour observed in humans.

RECOMMENDATIONS. The preferred rate at which the plasma sodium concentration should be elevated varies with the clinical presentation. Patients and animals with chronic asymptomatic hyponatremia are generally at little risk for neurologic symptoms due to the cerebral adaptation described above. In this setting, rapid correction is not indicated and may be harmful. Although the optimal rate of correction is not clearly proven [63], the current recommendation in asymptomatic patients is that the plasma sodium concentration be raised at a maximum rate of 12 mEq per liter per day (which represents an average correction of 0.5 mEq/L per hour) [53,64,65]. Although it may be safe to increase the plasma sodium concentration at a rate above 12 mEq/day [66], there is no reason to correct more rapidly in the absence of symptoms.

The potential benefit of administering water to lower the plasma sodium concentration in hyponatremic patients who have been corrected much too rapidly is unresolved. Preliminary studies in rats noted a marked reduction in the incidence and severity of brain lesions if overly rapid correction (30 mEq/L or more over several hours) was partially reversed so that the net daily elevation in the plasma sodium concentration was less than 20 mEq per liter [72]. This improvement was seen if therapy was begun before the onset of neurologic symptoms; benefit was much less likely in animals with symptomatic demyelination. The applicability of these findings to humans is uncertain.

More aggressive initial correction, at a rate of 1.5 to 2 mEq per liter per hour, is indicated for the first 3 to 4 hours (or until the symptoms resolve) in patients who present with seizures or other severe neurologic abnormalities due to untreated and usually acute hyponatremia [53,63,65]. The primary problem in these patients is cerebral edema, and the risk of delayed therapy is greater than the potential risk of too rapid correction. Even in this setting, however, the plasma sodium concentration should probably not be raised by more than 12 mEq per liter in the first 24 hours [65], since partial cerebral adaptation has already occurred [51].

Patients with acute symptomatic hyponatremia generally require treatment with hypertonic saline; this solution also has been used initially in symptomatic patients with primary polydipsia in whom cessation of water intake alone results in an often rapid elevation in the plasma sodium concentration as a result of urinary excretion of the excess water [62]. Overly rapid correction of the plasma sodium concentration may occur in this setting.

Rapid correction of hyponatremia also can occur when patients with end-stage renal disease are hemodialyzed against a dialysate with a higher sodium concentration. It has been estimated, for example, that dialysis against a dialysate sodium concentration of 145 mEq per liter can raise the plasma sodium concentration from 110 to 130 mEq per liter in 4 hours [73]. These patients may be partially protected against osmotic demyelination by the fact that the concurrent removal of urea tends to lower the plasma osmolality, thereby promoting water movement into the brain and minimizing the degree of cerebral contraction induced by the elevation in the plasma sodium concentration. Nevertheless, there probably is some risk in asymptomatic patients, and it has been recommended that the sodium concentration in the dialysate should not be more than 15 to 20 mEq per liter higher than that in the plasma [73].

TREATMENT OF HYPONATREMIA IN SIADH AND WITH A RESET OSMOSTAT. Hyponatremia in SIADH results primarily from ADH-induced retention of ingested water. Appropriate therapy in this disorder depends on the severity of the hyponatremia and on the fact that, although water excretion is impaired, sodium handling is intact since there is no abnormality in volume-regulating mechanisms such as the renin-angiotensin-aldosterone system or atrial natriuretic peptide.

Correction of the hyponatremia may include water restriction, which is the mainstay of therapy in asymptomatic hyponatremia and in chronic SIADH due, for example, to an oat cell carcinoma of the lung. The associated negative water balance raises the plasma sodium concentration toward normal.

Severe, symptomatic, or resistant hyponatremia often requires the administration of salt. If the plasma sodium concentration is to be elevated, the osmolality of the fluid given must exceed that of the urine. This can be illustrated by a simple example (Table 79-4). Suppose a patient with SIADH and hyponatremia has a urine osmolality that is relatively fixed (cannot be below) at 616 mOsm/kg. If 1000 ml of isotonic saline is given (containing 154 mEq each of Na and Cl or 308 mOsmol), all of the NaCl will be excreted (because sodium handling is intact) but in only 500 ml of water (308 mOsmol in 500 ml of water equals 616 mOsm/kg). The retention of one-half of the administered water will lead to a further reduction in the plasma sodium concentration. As a result, correction of the hyponatremia in these cases requires the administration of hypertonic saline (or salt tablets), preferably with a drug that lowers the urine osmolality and increases water excretion by impairing the

Table 79-4. Mechanism of Normal Saline-induced Worsening of Hyponatremia in the SIADH*

	Solute (mOsm)	Water (ml)
Input	308	1000
Output	308	500
Net gain	0	+500

*This calculation assumes that the individual cannot dilute the urine below a U_{Osm} of 616 mOsm/kg and that all the administered solute is excreted in the urine.

renal responsiveness to ADH. A loop diuretic (such as 20 mg of furosemide once or twice a day) is most often used in this setting, since it directly interferes with the countercurrent concentrating mechanism by decreasing NaCl reabsorption in the medullary aspect of the loop of Henle [74].

Demeclocycline and lithium act on the collecting tubule cell to diminish its responsiveness to ADH, thereby increasing water excretion [1D,3D–5D]. These drugs should be considered only for use in the rare patient with persistent marked hyponatremia who is unresponsive to or cannot tolerate water restriction, a high salt intake, and a loop diuretic. Demeclocycline (300–600 mg twice a day) is more predictably effective and less toxic than lithium [75].

Dietary manipulation is another method to treat persistent SIADH. In normal subjects, the urine volume is primarily determined by water intake via changes in ADH release. When ADH levels are relatively fixed, as in SIADH, however, the main determinant of the urine output is the rate of solute excretion. If, for example, the urine osmolality were 600 mOsmol/kg in the SIADH, then the urine volume would be 1000 ml/day if solute excretion (sodium and potassium salts and urea) were 600 mOsmol/day and 1500 ml/day if solute excretion were increased to 900 mOsmol/day with a higher-salt, higher-protein diet. Thus, the elevation in the plasma sodium concentration induced by salt occurs in two stages: the direct effect of the ingestion of salt without water, followed by the excretion of the excess salt with water leading to net negative water balance. Unfortunately, many patients with chronic SIADH have a major debilitating underlying illness (such as an oat cell carcinoma) that limits compliance with increased dietary intake.

Another way to use solute excretion to enhance water excretion is the direct administration of 30 g of urea per day [76,77]. This regimen is generally well tolerated, although it should be considered only in patients with marked hyponatremia that does not respond to the above modalities.

The necessity for chronic therapy is limited to patients with persistent hyponatremia. Many causes of SIADH (e.g., meningitis, pneumonia, and tuberculosis) are transient, however, and resolve as the underlying condition is corrected [78].

RESET OSMOSTAT. Hyponatremia due to a reset osmostat can be seen with any of the causes of SIADH and accounts for between 25 and 30% of cases overall [79]. In addition, downward resetting of the osmostat can occur in hypovolemic states (in which the baroreceptor stimulus to ADH release is superimposed on osmoreceptor function), quadriplegia (in which effective volume depletion may result from venous pooling in the legs), psychosis, tuberculosis, and chronic malnutrition [78,79]. The plasma sodium concentration also falls by about 5 mEq per liter in normal pregnancy; how this occurs is incompletely understood, but human chorionic gonadotropin may play an important role [79a].

The presence of a reset osmostat should be suspected in any patient with apparent SIADH who has mild hyponatremia (usually between 125 and 135 mEq/L) that is stable over many days despite variations in sodium and water intake. The diagnosis can be confirmed clinically by observing the response to a water load (10–15 ml/kg given orally or intravenously). Normal subjects and those with a reset osmostat should excrete more than 80% within 4 hours, whereas excretion will be impaired in SIADH [74].

Identification of a reset osmostat is important, because the above therapeutic recommendations for SIADH do not apply in this setting. These patients have mild, asymptomatic hyponatremia in which there is downward resetting of the threshold for both ADH release and thirst. Since osmoreceptor function is normal around the new baseline, attempting to raise the plasma sodium concentration will increase ADH levels and make the patient very thirsty, a response that is similar to that seen with water restriction in normal subjects. Thus, efforts to raise the plasma sodium concentration are both unnecessary (given the lack of symptoms and lack of risk of more severe hyponatremia) and likely to be ineffective (due to increased thirst). Treatment should be primarily directed at the underlying disease (e.g., tuberculosis) [78].

TREATMENT OF HYPONATREMIA IN EDEMATOUS STATES. Raising the plasma sodium concentration in patients with edema may be more difficult than in those conditions described earlier. Most of these individuals have advanced congestive heart failure or liver disease. Consequently, sodium administration is generally contraindicated.

Congestive heart failure. Restricting water intake is the mainstay of therapy in hyponatremic patients with heart failure [80], although this is often not tolerable because of the intense stimulation of thirst. In refractory cases, the combination of an angiotensin converting enzyme (ACE) inhibitor and a loop diuretic may induce an elevation in the plasma sodium concentration [81,82].

These agents may act in three ways: (1) the increase in cardiac output following ACE inhibition can lower the levels of ADH, angiotensin II, and norepinephrine [82]; (2) ACE inhibitors (via the local generation of prostaglandins) appear to antagonize the effect of ADH on the collecting tubules, thereby decreasing water reabsorption at this site [83]; and (3) the loop diuretic increases water delivery to the collecting tubules, which (due to the decrease in ADH secretion) are now less permeable to water. The increment in cardiac output and fall in angiotensin II levels may be beneficial because they reduce the sensation of thirst, thus making the patient more comfortable.

Despite these benefits, ACE inhibitors may be poorly tolerated in patients with advanced CHF and may lead to symptomatic hypotension, worsening azotemia, or hyperkalemia. When this occurs, the addition of drugs that directly increase cardiac contractility, such as digitalis and perhaps newer inotropic agents, may be considered.

One final modality that has been evaluated in the patient with heart failure and hyponatremia is the administration of demeclocycline, a tetracycline derivative that increases free water excretion by partially antagonizing the action of ADH [75]. Use of this drug has been limited by the common development of nephrotoxicity, which is due to high circulating drug levels that result from diminished hepatic drug metabolism [84].

Liver disease. Hyponatremia in patients with hepatic cirrhosis usually develops slowly and produces no cerebral edema or symptoms. It is possible, however, that a low plasma sodium concentration can exacerbate hepatic encephalopathy [85]. In view of the marked sodium and water retention, the mainstay of therapy in this setting is restricting water intake to a level sufficient to induce negative water balance and partial correction of the hyponatremia. Hypertonic saline or salt tablets are indicated only in patients with symptomatic hyponatremia. Diuretics can be given concurrently to prevent worsening of the edema, but overly rapid correction must be avoided to minimize the risk of central demyelinating lesions.

As in hyponatremic patients with CHF, the administration of demeclocycline has been evaluated in this setting, but use of this drug has been limited because of its nephrotoxicity [84].

HYPERNATREMIA. Hypernatremia is a relatively common problem that can be produced either by the administration of hypertonic sodium solutions or, in almost all cases, by the loss of free water [86]. It should be emphasized that persistent hypernatremia does not occur in normal subjects, because the ensuing rise in plasma osmolality stimulates both the release of ADH (thereby minimizing further water loss) and, more importantly, thirst [86,87]. The associated increase in water intake then lowers the plasma sodium concentration back to normal. This regulatory system is so efficient that the plasma osmolality is maintained within a range of 1 to 2% despite wide variations in sodium and water intake. Even patients with diabetes insipidus, who often have marked polyuria due to diminished ADH effect, maintain a near-normal plasma sodium concentration by appropriately increasing water intake.

The result is that hypernatremia primarily occurs in those patients who cannot express thirst normally: infants and adults with impaired mental status most often, in the elderly [88], who also appear to have diminished osmotic stimulation of thirst via an unknown mechanism [89]. A patient with a plasma sodium concentration of 150 mEq per liter or more who is alert but not thirsty has, by definition, a hypothalamic lesion affecting the thirst center.

Etiology of Hypernatremia. The major causes of hypernatremia are listed in Table 79-5.

UNREPLACED WATER LOSS. The loss of solute-free water that is not replaced will lead to an elevation in the plasma sodium concentration. It is important to recognize in this regard that the plasma sodium concentration and plasma osmolality are determined by the ratio between total body solutes (primarily sodium and potassium salts) and the total body water. Thus, sodium plus potassium content determine the effect of loss of a given fluid [67]. The composition of diarrheal fluid can be used to illustrate this point. Patients with secretory diarrheas (cholera, VIP oma) have a sodium plus potassium concentration in the diarrheal fluid that is similar to that in the plasma [90]. Loss of this fluid will lead to volume and potassium depletion but will not directly affect the plasma sodium concentration.

In comparison, many viral enteritides and the osmotic diarrhea induced by lactulose (to treat hepatic encephalopathy) or charcoal-sorbitol (to treat a drug overdose) are associated with an isosmotic diarrheal fluid that has a sodium plus potassium concentration between 40 and 100 mEq per liter [90–92]; or-

Table 79-5. Major Causes of Hypernatremia

Unreplaced water loss
  Insensible and sweat losses
  Gastrointestinal losses
  Central or nephrogenic diabetes insipidus
  Hypothalamic lesions affecting thirst or osmoreceptor function
    Primary hypodipsia
    Essential hypernatremia
    Reset osmostat in mineralocorticoid excess
Water loss into cells
  Severe exercise or seizures
Sodium overload
  Intake of hypertonic sodium solutions

ganic solutes, which do not affect the plasma sodium concentration, make up the remaining osmoles. Loss of this fluid tends to induce hypernatremia, because water is being lost in excess of sodium plus potassium [67,91]. Similar considerations apply to urinary losses during an osmotic diuresis induced by glucose, mannitol, or urea (see below) [93,94].

With these considerations in mind, the sources of free water loss that can lead to hypernatremia if intake is not increased include [1]:

Insensible and sweat losses. Insensible water losses from the skin by evaporation and sweat are dilute. The loss of this fluid is increased by fever, exercise, and by exposure to high temperatures.

Gastrointestinal losses. As mentioned earlier, some gastrointestinal losses, particularly osmotic diarrheas, promote the development of hypernatremia, because the sodium plus potassium concentration is less than that in the plasma. An elevation in the plasma sodium concentration with a diarrheal illness is particularly common in infants even though fluid replacement with a relatively dilute solution (sodium plus potassium concentration of 95 mEq/L) can minimize this risk [95].

Central or nephrogenic diabetes insipidus. Decreased release of ADH or renal resistance to its effect cause the excretion of a relatively dilute urine (see below). Most affected patients have a normal thirst mechanism [96] and therefore typically present with polyuria and polydipsia, and, at most, a high-normal plasma sodium concentration. Marked and symptomatic hypernatremia can occur if a central lesion impairs both ADH release and thirst, however, thereby preventing replacement of the urinary water losses [97].

Osmotic diuresis. An osmotic diuresis due to glucose, mannitol, or urea causes an increase in urine output in which the sodium plus potassium concentration is well below that in the plasma because of the presence of the nonreabsorbed organic solute [93,94]. Thus, patients with diabetic ketoacidosis or nonketotic hyperglycemia typically present with marked hyperosmolality, although the plasma sodium concentration may not be elevated due to hyperglycemia-induced water movement out of the cells.

Hypothalamic lesions affecting thirst or osmoreceptor function. Hypernatremia can occur in the absence of increased water losses if there is primary hypothalamic disease impairing thirst (called hypodipsia). Two syndromes have been described that are most often due to tumors, granulomatous diseases (such as sarcoidosis), or vascular disease [86,87]. One disorder involves a defect in thirst, with or without concomitant diabetes insipidus [87,98]. In this disorder, forced water intake is usually sufficient to maintain a normal plasma sodium concentration, although central diabetes insipidus, if present, should be treated.

Other hypodipsic patients will not respond to water loading, as the excess water is excreted in the urine with little change in the plasma sodium concentration. These patients have selective injury to the hypothalamic osmoreceptors, with ADH secretion being primarily governed by changes in volume. Thus, the suppression of ADH release by water loading in such patients is due to the associated mild volume expansion rather than to a fall in plasma osmolality [86,99,100]. This disorder is termed *essential hypernatremia.*

True resetting of the osmostat upwards has been described only in patients with primary mineralocorticoid excess (such as primary hyperaldosteronism). Presumably, suppressive effect of chronic mild volume expansion on ADH release is responsible for the resetting; the plasma sodium concentration in these patients is usually between 143 and 147 mEq per liter [79].

The best therapy for essential hypernatremia is uncertain. Affected patients are generally asymptomatic because the hypernatremia is chronic. There is some evidence that chlorpropamide, which increases the renal effect of ADH, may lead to a modest lowering of the plasma sodium concentration [86]. In addition, a careful neurologic and radiologic evaluation may demonstrate a treatable disease (such as a benign tumor) that, if corrected, can restore osmoreceptor function.

WATER LOSS INTO CELLS. Transient hypernatremia (in which the plasma sodium concentration can rise by 10 to 15 mEq/L within a few minutes) can be induced by severe exercise or seizures, which are also associated with the development of lactic acidosis. In this setting, the breakdown of glycogen into smaller, more osmotically active molecules (such as lactate) can increase the cell osmolality, thereby causing the osmotic movement of water into the cells [1,33]. The plasma sodium concentration returns to normal within 5 to 15 minutes after the cessation of exertion [33].

SODIUM OVERLOAD. Acute and often marked hypernatremia (in which the plasma sodium concentration can exceed 175 to 200 mEq/L) can be induced by administration of hypertonic sodium-containing solutions. Examples include accidental or nonaccidental salt poisoning in infants and young children, infusion of hypertonic sodium bicarbonate to treat metabolic acidosis, and massive salt ingestion, as can occur when a highly concentrated saline emetic or gargle is swallowed [101–104].

This type of hypernatremia will correct spontaneously if renal function is normal, since the excess sodium will be rapidly excreted in the urine. This process can be facilitated by inducing a sodium and water diuresis with a loop diuretic and then replacing the urine output solely with water [86]. Too rapid correction should be avoided if the patient is asymptomatic; these patients are, however, less likely to develop cerebral edema during correction, since the hypernatremia is generally very acute with little time for cerebral adaptation (see below). Even with optimal therapy, however, the mortality rate is extremely high in adults with a plasma sodium concentration that has suddenly risen to above 180 mEq per liter [104]; for reasons that are not well understood, severe hypernatremia is often better tolerated in young children [102].

Patients with concurrent renal failure or infants can be treated with peritoneal dialysis. An electrolyte-free, hypertonic (8%) dextrose and water solution can be used to remove the excess sodium [101]. The high osmolality of the dialysate will minimize water movement from the dialysate into the patient, thereby minimizing further volume expansion.

Symptoms of Hypernatremia. Hypernatremia is basically a mirror image of hyponatremia [51,105,106]. The rise in the plasma sodium concentration and osmolality causes acute water movement out of the brain; this decrease in brain volume can cause rupture of the cerebral veins, leading to focal intracerebral and subarachnoid hemorrhages and possible irreversible neurologic damage [105,106]. The clinical manifestations of this disorder begin with lethargy, weakness, and irritability and can progress to twitching, seizures, and coma. Severe symptoms usually require an acute elevation in the plasma sodium concentration to above 158 mEq per liter. Values above 180 mEq per liter are associated with a high mortality rate, particularly in adults [104].

Beginning on the first day, however, brain volume is largely restored due both to water movement from the cerebrospinal fluid into the brain (thereby increasing the interstitial volume)

[51,107] and to the uptake of solutes by the cells (thereby pulling water into the cells and restoring the cell volume) [51,108,109]. The latter response involves an initial uptake of sodium and potassium salts, followed by the later accumulation of osmolytes, such as inositol and the amino acids glutamine and glutamate [108,109]. Inositol is taken up from the extracellular fluid via an increase in the number of sodium-inositol cotransporters in the cell membrane [110], whereas the source (uptake from the extracellular fluid or production within the cells) of glutamine and glutamate is unknown. The effect is that these osmolytes, which do not interfere with protein function [111], account for about 35% of the new cell solute [109].

As in hyponatremia, the cerebral adaptation in hypernatremia has two important clinical consequences:

1. Chronic hypernatremia is much less likely to induce neurologic symptoms. Assessment of symptoms attributable to hypernatremia is often difficult because most affected adults have underlying neurologic disease, which is required to diminish the protective thirst mechanism that normally prevents the development of hypernatremia, even in patients with diabetes insipidus.

2. Correction of chronic hypernatremia must occur slowly to prevent rapid fluid movement into the brain and cerebral edema, which can lead to seizures and coma [106,112]. Although the brain cells can rapidly lose potassium and sodium in response to this cell swelling, the loss of accumulated osmolytes occurs more slowly, a phenomenon that acts to hold water within the cells [51,109]. The loss of inositol, for example, requires both a reduction in synthesis of new sodium-inositol cotransporters [110] and the activation of a specific inositol efflux mechanism in the cell membrane [113]. The delayed clearance of osmolytes from the cell can predispose to cerebral edema if the plasma sodium concentration is lowered too rapidly.

Diagnosis of Hypernatremia and Polyuric Disorders. The cause of the hypernatremia is usually evident from the history. If, however, the etiology is unclear, the correct diagnosis can usually be established by evaluation of the integrity of ADH-renal axis via measurement of the urine osmolality [114]. A rise in the plasma sodium concentration is a potent stimulus to ADH release as well as to thirst; furthermore, a plasma osmolality above 295 mOsmol/kg (which represents a plasma sodium concentration above 145–147 mEq/L) generally leads to sufficient ADH secretion to maximally stimulate urinary concentration.

Thus, if both hypothalamic and renal function are intact, the urine osmolality in the presence of hypernatremia will be above 700 to 800 mOsmol/kg. Exogenous ADH will not produce a further rise in the urine osmolality. In this setting, unreplaced insensible or gastrointestinal losses, sodium overload, or, rarely, a primary defect in thirst is likely to be responsible for the hypernatremia [114]. Measurement of the urine sodium concentration may help to distinguish between these disorders: it should be less than 25 mEq per liter when water loss and volume depletion are the primary problems, but it is typically well above 100 mEq per liter following the ingestion or infusion or a hypertonic sodium solution [102].

If, on the other hand, the urine osmolality is lower than that of the plasma, then either central (ADH-deficient) or nephrogenic (ADH-resistant) diabetes insipidus is present.

DIAGNOSIS OF POLYURIC STATES AND DIABETES INSIPIDUS. Polyuria can be arbitrarily defined as a urine output exceeding 3 liter/day. It must be differentiated from the more common complaints of frequency and nocturia, which are not associated with an increase in the total urine output. In the absence of a glucose-induced osmotic diuresis in uncontrolled diabetes mellitus, there are three major causes of polyuria in the outpatient setting. Each is due to a defect in water balance leading to the excretion of large volumes of dilute urine (urine osmolality usually below 250 mOsmol/kg) [115].

Primary polydipsia. Primary polydipsia (also called psychogenic polydipsia) is characterized by a primary increase in water intake (see Hyponatremia above). This disorder is most often seen in anxious, middle-aged women and in patients with psychiatric illnesses, including those taking a phenothiazine, which can lead to the sensation of a dry mouth. Primary polydipsia can also be induced by hypothalamic lesions that directly affect the thirst center, as may occur with an infiltrative disease such as sarcoidosis [115].

Central diabetes insipidus. Central diabetes insipidus (CDI) is associated with deficient secretion of ADH. This condition is most often idiopathic (possibly due to autoimmune injury to the ADH-producing cells) or induced by trauma, pituitary surgery, or hypoxic or ischemic encephalopathy.

Nephrogenic diabetes insipidus. Nephrogenic diabetes insipidus (NDI) is characterized by normal ADH secretion but varying degrees of renal resistance to its water-retaining effect. In its mild form, this problem is relatively common, since most patients who are elderly or who have underlying renal disease have a reduction in maximum concentrating ability. This defect, however, is not severe enough to produce a symptomatic increase in urine output. True polyuria due to ADH-resistance primarily occurs in four settings: X-linked hereditary NDI in children, in which there is an abnormality in the V2, antidiuretic receptors for ADH [116]; chronic lithium use, which can lead to polyuria in about 20 percent of patients [117,118]; hypercalcemia [119]; and severe hypokalemia.

Each of these conditions is associated with an increase in water output and the excretion of a relatively dilute urine. With primary polydipsia, the polyuria is an appropriate response to enhanced water intake; in comparison, the water loss is inappropriate with either form of diabetes insipidus. Thus, a low plasma sodium concentration at presentation (less than 137 mEq/L due to water overload) is usually indicative of primary polydipsia, whereas a high-normal plasma sodium concentration (greater than 142 mEq/L due to water loss) points toward diabetes insipidus [115]. Marked hypernatremia is uncommon in diabetes insipidus, because the initial loss of water stimulates the thirst mechanism, resulting in an increase in intake to match the urinary losses. An exception to this general rule occurs in patients with a central lesion that impairs both ADH release and thirst; in such patients, the plasma sodium concentration can exceed 160 mEq per liter [97].

The correct diagnosis is often suggested from the plasma sodium concentration and from the history. The patient should be questioned about one of the causes of central or nephrogenic diabetes insipidus and about the rate of onset of the polyuria: the latter is usually abrupt in CDI ("I suddenly began urinating excessively 2 days ago"), but gradual in NDI or primary polydipsia.

Even if the history or plasma sodium concentration appears to be helpful, the diagnosis should be confirmed by raising the plasma osmolality either by water restriction or, less commonly, by the administration of hypertonic saline (0.05 ml/kg per minute for no more than 2 hours).

The water restriction test for the evaluation of polyuria involves measurement of the urine volume and osmolality every hour and plasma sodium concentration osmolality every 2 hours. We generally recommend that the patient stop drinking 2 to 3 hours before coming to the office or clinic; overnight fluid restriction should be avoided, since potentially severe volume depletion and hypernatremia can be induced in patients with marked polyuria.

Interpretation of the water restriction test (or the administration of hypertonic saline) is based upon the following observations [115,120,121]: (1) Raising the plasma osmolality leads to a progressive elevation in ADH release and therefore the urine osmolality in normal individuals. (2) Once the plasma osmolality reaches 295 to 300 mOsmol/kg (normal 275–290 mOsmol/kg), endogenous ADH effect on the kidney is maximal. At this point, administering ADH will not elevate the urine osmolality unless endogenous ADH release is impaired (i.e., unless the patient has CDI).

Thus, the water restriction test is continued until the urine osmolality reaches a clearly normal level (about 600 mOsmol/kg, indicating that both ADH release and effect are intact), the urine osmolality is stable on two or three successive measurements despite a rising plasma osmolality, or the plasma osmolality exceeds 295 to 300 mOsmol/kg. In the last two cases, exogenous ADH is then given (5 units of aqueous vasopressin subcutaneously or 10 mg of dDAVP by nasal insufflation) and the urine osmolality and volume are monitored. Each of the causes of polyuria produces a distinct pattern [115,120,121]:

1. CDI may be partial and therefore associated with a rise in the urine osmolality as the plasma osmolality rises. The degree of urinary concentration is clearly submaximal, however, and, since ADH release is inadequate, exogenous ADH will lead to a rise in the urine osmolality of 15% to 50% and an equivalent fall in urine output.
2. NDI also is associated with a submaximal rise in urine osmolality, but there is no urinary response to exogenous ADH. It must be emphasized that NDI is a rare cause of true polyuria in adults in the absence of lithium use, hypercalcemia, hypokalemia or, rarely, tubular damage in patients with amyloidosis or Sjögren's syndrome [115].
3. Primary polydipsia is associated with a rise in urine osmolality, usually to above 500 mOsmol/kg, and no response to exogenous ADH, since endogenous release is intact. The chronic polyuria in this disorder can partially wash out the medullary interstitial solute gradient; as a result, maximal concentrating ability is impaired and the urine osmolality may reach 500 to 600 mOsmol/kg, as compared to 800 mOsmol/kg or more in normal subjects.

A properly performed test in which ADH is not given until the plasma osmolality exceeds 295 mOsmol/kg will usually establish the correct diagnosis. The different patterns of response are depicted in Figure 79-3. There is, however, one major potential source of error. Patients with partial CDI may be hyperresponsive to the submaximal rise in ADH induced by water restriction, perhaps because of receptor upregulation. As a result, they may be polyuric at the normal plasma osmolality of 285 to 290 mOsmol/kg when ADH levels are very low, but they may have a maximally concentrated urine at a plasma osmolality above 295 mOsmol/kg when ADH levels are somewhat higher. In such patients, exogenous ADH will be without effect, resulting in a pattern suggestive of primary polydipsia [12]. Therefore, measurement of plasma ADH levels may be useful.

The above discussion has emphasized the diagnostic approach to a water diuresis. In some polyuric patients, however, the increase in urine output is due to a solute or osmotic diuresis in which decreased solute reabsorption is the primary abnormality. Although glucosuria is the major cause of an osmotic diuresis in outpatients, other conditions are often responsible

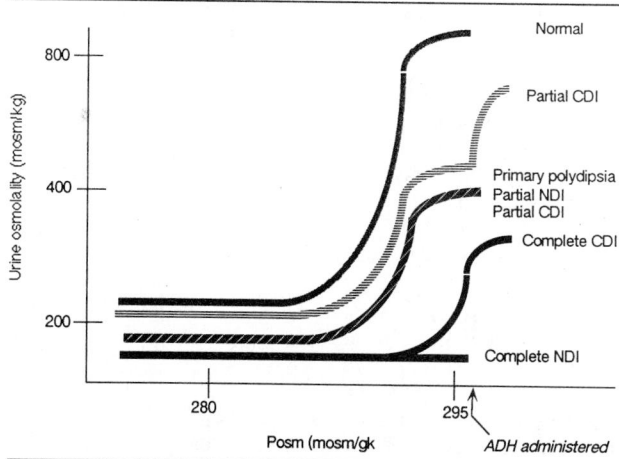

Fig. 79-3. Response to ADH after a water restriction text. ADH is given when the P_{Osm} reaches 295 mOsm per kilogram, the level at which maximal ADH release and response should be present. This test will identify the cause of polyuria in about 80 percent of patients. Confusion may arise, however, with partial central diabetes insipidus. In this disorder, some individuals have lower than normal ADH levels at a normal P_{Osm}, but the increase in ADH (although still subnormal) generates a maximum urine response, presumably due to increased sensitivity. Consequently, these patients exhibit polyuria at a normal P_{Osm}, but the curve during the water restriction test may mimic partial NDI or primary polydipsia. Measurement of plasma ADH levels may be needed to distinguish these possibilities. (Zerbe RL, Robertson GL: A comparison of plasma vasopressin measurements with a standard indirect test in the differential diagnosis of polyuria. *N Engl J Med* 305:1539, 1981).

when polyuria develops in the hospital. These include high-protein feedings (in which urea acts as the osmotic agent) and volume expansion due to saline loading or the administration of mannitol. The urine osmolality in these disorders is usually above 300 mOsmol/kg, in contrast to the dilute urine typically found with a water diuresis. Furthermore, total solute excretion (calculated on a 24-hour urine collection from the product of the urine osmolality and the urine output) is normal with a water diuresis (600 to 900 mOsmol per day) but markedly increased with an osmotic diuresis.

As a general rule, underlying renal disease can impair sodium conservation in the presence of volume depletion but does not cause sufficient sodium wasting to induce true polyuria. Thus, polyuria in which there is a marked increase in sodium excretion is almost always appropriate, resulting from volume expansion induced either by saline loading or following relief of urinary obstruction by fluid retained during the period of obstruction [92,122,123].

The cause of the polyuria in a postobstructive diuresis is often misunderstood. Many physicians faced with a urine output that may initially exceed 1000 ml per hour feel compelled to replace the urine output with intravenous fluids. This will only prolong the polyuria, since the volume expansion persists. Optimal therapy of a postobstructive diuresis consists of fluid infusion at a maintenance level, such as 75 ml of one-half isotonic saline per hour. The development of volume depletion, as evidenced by hypotension or a rise in the BUN, is unusual with this regimen [122,123].

One exception to the usually appropriate nature of a marked natriuresis is the polyuria that can occur when dopamine is given to treat hypotension in a septic patient. In these patients, infection seems to enhance (via an uncertain mechanism) the normal natriuretic action of dopamine [124].

Treatment of Hypernatremia. The water deficit in the hypernatremic patient can be estimated from the following considerations. The quantity of osmoles in the body is equal to the osmolal space [the total body water (TBW)] times the osmolality of the body fluids:

Total body osmoles = TBW × POsm

Since the P_{Osm} is primarily determined by two times the plasma sodium concentration (to account for the accompanying anions)

Total body osmoles = TBW × 2 × plasma Na$^+$
If hypernatremia results only from water loss, then
Current body osmoles = Normal body osmoles
or, if the normal plasma sodium concentration is 140 mEq per liter,
Current body water (CBW) × plasma Na$^+$ = Normal body water (NBW) × 140
(The multiple 2 cancels out, since it is present on both sides of the above equation.) If this equation is solved for NBW:

$$NBW = CBW \times \frac{plasma\ Na^+}{140}$$

The water deficit can now be estimated from:
Water deficit = NBW − CBW
or by substituting from the equation for NBW:

$$Water\ deficit = \left(CBW \times \frac{plasma\ Na^+}{140}\right) - CBW$$

$$Water\ deficit = CBW \left(\frac{plasma\ Na^+}{140} - 1\right)$$

The TBW is normally above 60 and 50% of lean body weight in men and women, respectively, but it is probably reasonable to use values about 10% lower in hypernatremic patients who are water-depleted, since loss of muscle mass in debilitated individuals lowers the percent of body weight that is water. Thus, in a 60-kg woman with a plasma sodium concentration of 168 mEq per liter, the water deficit can be approximated from:

Water deficit = 0.4 × 60 (168/140 − 1)
= 4.8 liters

This formula estimates the amount of positive water balance required to return the plasma sodium concentration to 140 mEq per liter. It does not include any additional isosmotic fluid deficit, which is frequently present when both sodium and water have been lost, as occurs with an osmotic diuresis or with diarrhea. In addition, hypernatremia itself may cause mild urinary sodium-wasting in hypovolemic subjects, largely as a result of reduced aldosterone release [125]. Both hypernatremia and concurrent hypokalemia (due to gastrointestinal or renal losses) may act directly on the adrenal gland, and it has been suggested that the loss of sodium might be appropriate from an osmotic viewpoint by tending to reduce the plasma sodium concentration [125].

RATE OF CORRECTION. Overly rapid correction is potentially dangerous in hypernatremia (as it is in hyponatremia) [109]. Hypernatremia initially causes fluid movement out of the brain and cerebral contraction that is primarily responsible for the associated symptoms. Within 1 to 3 days, however, brain volume is largely restored due both to water movement from the cerebrospinal fluid into the brain (thereby increasing the interstitial volume) and to the uptake of solutes by the cells (thereby pulling water into the cells and restoring the cell volume) [109].

Rapidly lowering the plasma sodium concentration once this adaptation has occurred causes osmotic water movement into the brain, increasing brain size above normal. This cerebral edema can lead to seizures, permanent neurologic damage, or death [106].

This sequence of an adverse response to therapy primarily has been described in children in whom the hypernatremia was corrected at a rate exceeding 0.7 mEq per liter per hour [126]. In comparison, no neurologic sequelae were induced when the plasma sodium concentration was lowered at 0.5 mEq per liter per hour [127].

These principles can be applied to the above patient with a plasma sodium concentration of 168 mEq per liter and an estimated water deficit of 4.8 liters. The 28 mEq per liter rise in the plasma sodium concentration should be corrected over 56 hours, which involves the administration of 4.8 liters of free water at a rate of approximately 80 ml per hour. It should be emphasized, however, that water deficit estimates the positive water balance that must be achieved; thus, continuing free water losses must also be replaced, such as insensible losses (about 40 ml/h) and any continued dilute urinary or gastrointestinal losses. "Dilute" in this context refers to a sodium plus potassium concentration in the fluid lost that is lower than that in the plasma. Simply comparing osmolalities is not sufficient; both urine and intestinal fluids contain urea and other organic solutes that contribute to the total osmolality but, since they are ineffective solutes, do not contribute to regulation of the plasma sodium concentration [67]. Thus, the excretion of 100 ml per hour of urine with a sodium plus potassium concentration half that of the plasma is equivalent to losing 50 ml per hour of free water.

In summary, appropriate therapy in this patient requires the administration of about 120 ml of free water per hour, with careful monitoring of the plasma sodium concentration to confirm that there is the desired rate of correction. This fluid can be administered orally or intravenously as dextrose in water. Sodium or potassium can be added if there are concurrent losses of these solutes, but the addition of these solutes decreases the amount of free water that is being given. If, for example, one-quarter isotonic saline is infused, then only three-quarters of the solution is free water. As a result, 160 ml must be given to provide 120 ml of free water. If potassium is also added, then even less free water is present, and a further adjustment to the rate must be made.

This discussion primarily applies to the majority of patients in whom hypernatremia is induced by water loss. Other factors must be considered in patients with diabetes insipidus (in whom the plasma sodium concentration is usually near normal and the primary aim of therapy is to decrease the urine output; see below), in patients with hypothalamic lesions impairing the thirst mechanism, and in patients with primary sodium overload. It should be emphasized that an isotonic saline solution should be used as initial therapy in the volume-depleted, hypotensive patient since restoration of tissue perfusion is of primary importance in these patients.

Treatment of Diabetes Insipidus. The major symptoms of diabetes insipidus are polyuria and polydipsia due to the concentrating defect (see above). Treatment in this disorder is aimed at decreasing the urine output.

CENTRAL DIABETES INSIPIDUS. Since the primary problem is deficient secretion of ADH, control of the polyuria can be achieved by hormone replacement with dDAVP, a two amino acid substitute of ADH. dDAVP is administered by nasal spray in a usual dose of 5 to 20 mg once or twice a day. In addition to its long duration of action, dDAVP has the advantage of having no vasopressor activity [128].

There is an important potential risk to the administration of dDAVP in CDI: water retention and the development of hyponatremia. Patients with this disorder are polyuric but are not in danger of marked fluid loss and hypernatremia as long as their thirst mechanism is intact. Once dDAVP is given, however, the patient has nonsuppressible ADH activity and may be unable to excrete ingested water normally. This problem can be avoided by giving the minimum dose that is required to control the polyuria. The first dose (5 to 10 mg) is usually given in the late evening to control the most troubling symptom of nocturia. The size and necessity for a daytime dose can be determined by the effectiveness of the evening dose. If, for example, polyuria does not recur until noon, then one-half the evening dose may be sufficient at that time.

Some patients have an incomplete response to dDAVP. Coupled with the fact that dDAVP is very expensive, it may be necessary or desirable to add other (cheaper) drugs that either increase ADH release, enhance ADH effect on the kidney (both of which require at least some endogenous ADH secretion), or directly decrease the urine output independent of ADH.

Chlorpropamide, an oral hypoglycemic agent, has been the most widely used antidiuretic [129,130]; it apparently acts by promoting the renal response to ADH or to dDAVP. Studies in animals suggest that this response may be mediated by enhanced sodium chloride reabsorption in the thick ascending limb (thereby increasing the degree of medullary hypertonicity) or by augmented collecting tubule permeability to water; how these changes occur is unclear [131,132]. The usual dose is 125 to 250 mg, once or twice a day; higher doses may produce a somewhat greater response but increase the risk of hypoglycemia [130].

Carbamazepine (used to treat seizures and tic douloureux) in a dose of 100 to 300 mg twice daily and clofibrate (used in the treatment of hyperlipidemia) in a dose of 500 mg every 6 hours can ameliorate the polyuria in patients with CDI [130,133, 134]. Carbamazepine appears to enhance the response to ADH [135], whereas clofibrate may increase ADH release [134]. These drugs, as well as chlorpropamide, can lower the urine output by as much as 50% [129].

NEPHROGENIC DIABETES INSIPIDUS. Nephrogenic diabetes insipidus results from partial or complete resistance of the kidney to the effects of antidiuretic hormone. As a result, patients with this disorder are not likely to respond to either hormone administration (as dDAVP) or to drugs such as chlorpropamide and carbamazepine that either increase the renal response to ADH or ADH secretion.

In adults, a concentrating defect severe enough to produce polyuria due to NDI is most often due to chronic lithium use or hypercalcemia. Less frequently, it is caused by other conditions that impair tubular function, such as Sjögren's syndrome (see above). Therapy is usually aimed at correcting the underlying disorder or discontinuing an offending drug. In hypercalcemic patients, for example, normalization of the plasma calcium concentration usually leads to amelioration of polyuria. In contrast, lithium-induced NDI may be irreversible if the patient already has severe tubular injury and a marked concentrating defect [117].

Thiazide diuretics can diminish the degree of polyuria in patients with persistent and symptomatic NDI [136–140]. The potassium-sparing diuretic amiloride may be helpful because of its additive effect with a thiazide diuretic [141] and, with reversible lithium-induced disease, its allowing the lithium to be continued (see below) [142].

The combination of a low-sodium diet with a thiazide diuretic (such as hydrochlorothiazide, 25 mg once or twice daily) acts by inducing mild volume depletion. As little as a 1- to 1.5-kg weight loss can reduce the urine output by more than 50%,

from 10 liters per day to below 3.5 liters per day in one study of patients with NDI [137]. This effect is presumably mediated by a hypovolemia-induced increase in proximal sodium and water reabsorption, thereby diminishing water delivery to the ADH-sensitive sites in the collecting tubules and reducing the urine output. The initial natriuresis and therefore the antipolyuric response can be enhanced by combination therapy with amiloride (or other potassium-sparing diuretic) [142]. This regimen has an additional benefit in that amiloride partially blocks the potassium wasting induced by the thiazide.

Thiazide diuretics limit the ability to maximally dilute the urine. As a result, the hypotonic urine in an individual with NDI will typically rise, even in the absence of ADH. If solute excretion (NaCl, KCl, and urea) remains constant, the urine volume will fall. As a example, in a patient with a normal solute excretion rate of 900 mOsm/kg per day and a maximum UOsm of 150 mOsm/kg due to NDI, urine output will be at least 6 liters per day (900/150). In contrast, if a thiazide diuretic limits the minimum UOsm to 300 mOsm/day, daily urine output will decrease to about 3 liters each day (900/300).

The efficacy of amiloride in patients with reversible lithium nephrotoxicity is directly related to its site and mechanism of action. This drug closes the sodium channels in the luminal membrane of the collecting tubule cells. These channels constitute the mechanism by which filtered lithium normally enters these cells and then interferes with their response to ADH [141]. Compared to amiloride, thiazide diuretics should be used cautiously, if at all, in patients with lithium-induced NDI (who are still taking lithium), since volume depletion can lead to increased reabsorption and potentially toxic plasma lithium levels.

The efficacy of nonsteroidal antiinflammatory drugs (NSAID) depends on the inhibition of renal prostaglandin synthesis. This has the effect of increasing concentrating ability, since prostaglandins normally antagonize the action of ADH [143,144]. If, for example, normal subjects are given a submaximal dose of ADH, the ensuing rise in urine osmolality can be increased by more than 200 mOsmol/kg if the patient has been pretreated with a NSAID [143]. The result in patients with NDI may be a 25 to 50% reduction in urine output [138–140], a response that is partially additive to that of a thiazide diuretic [139–142]. Not all NSAIDs are equally effective in a given patient; for example, some patients have a good response to indomethacin but derive little if any benefit from ibuprofen [138].

Dietary modification via the use of a low-sodium, low-protein diet can diminish the urine output in patients with NDI [136]. The ensuing decrease in net solute excretion (as sodium salts and urea) will, at a given urine osmolality, reduce the urine output. Suppose that the maximum urine osmolality is 200 mOsmol/kg. In this case, the daily urine volume will be 4.5 liters if solute excretion is in the normal range at 900 mOsmol/ day, but will only be 2.5 liters if solute excretion is lowered to 500 mOsmol/day by dietary modification.

Most patients with NDI have partial rather than complete resistance to ADH. It is therefore possible that attaining supraphysiologic hormone levels can increase the renal effect of ADH to a clinically important degree. One case report of a patient with lithium-induced NDI suggested that this benefit is more likely to be achieved if dDAVP is combined with an NSAID [145].

Disorders of Plasma Potassium

Potassium is the major intracellular cation. Only about 2% of body potassium is located in the extracellular space, where the concentration (3.5–5.0 mEq/L) is much lower than inside cells (125–140 mEq/L). This concentration difference is preserved by the Na^+/K^+ ATPase pump that actively transports sodium out of and potassium into most cells. Despite the relatively small quantity of K^+ in the extracellular space, slight changes in plasma potassium can have dramatic effects on muscle contraction and nerve conduction, since the concentration difference between K^+ inside and outside the cell is the major determinant of membrane excitability.

NORMAL POTASSIUM HOMEOSTASIS. Daily dietary potassium intake in this country varies between 40 and 120 mEq. Most of this (about 90%) is eliminated by the kidney; the rest is excreted in stool. Gastrointestinal potassium excretion can increase in renal failure, a process that depends, in part, on aldosterone [146].

Only about 50% of potassium ingested in the diet or administered parenterally appears in the urine during the first 4 hours [146]. As a result, over half of an acute potassium load must be transported into cells before excretion to prevent life-threatening hyperkalemia.

Transcellular Potassium Shifts. The most important factors that are involved in translocating K^+ intracellularly are insulin

and beta-adrenergic stimulation. Insulin stimulates the Na^+/K^+ ATPase pump present in most cells, leading to a more rapid rate of transfer [147]. By comparison, the effect of insulin is permissive; whereas an insulin infusion increases the rate of K^+ transport, the administration of K^+ does not stimulate insulin secretion.

Activation of beta-adrenergic receptors (specifically the beta2 receptor) also stimulates K^+ movement from the plasma into cells. The pathophysiology is due in part to direct stimulation of the Na^+/K^+ ATPase pump [147]. The observation that the hypokalemic effect of the beta-adrenergic agonist, terbutaline, can be limited by somatostatin indicates a possible role for insulin in the hypokalemic response to beta-adrenergic stimulation [148].

Aldosterone is the principal hormone stimulating K^+ secretion by the renal tubule (see following). This effect is important in all epithelial cell surfaces, whereas the importance of aldosterone on translocation of K^+ into cells is less clear [146].

Renal Regulation of Potassium Excretion. Potassium is freely filtered at the glomerulus so that the concentration of K^+ entering the early proximal tubule is approximately 4 mEq liter. Ninety percent of the filtered potassium load is reabsorbed by the time the glomerular filtrate reaches the distal tubule. As a result, renal K^+ excretion normally occurs almost exclusively by secretion in the distal nephron [149].

Potassium secretion occurs in the principal cells of the cortical collecting tubule (Fig. 79-4). Movement of potassium from the tubular cell into the lumen is controlled by dietary potassium intake, the rate of sodium reabsorption (a process driven by aldosterone) that generates a lumen-negative electrical gradient down which K^+ can move, and the rate of distal urine flow that maintains a high tubular cell to tubule lumen potassium gradient by washing away secreted K^+

Aldosterone enters the principal cell from the basolateral (antiluminal) side. Once inside, it binds to receptors, which increase the number of open luminal sodium channels and increase the number and activity of the Na^+/K^+ ATPase pumps in the basolateral membrane. The ensuing rise in cell potassium favors the secretion of K^+ into the lumen down the electrochemical gradient provided by Na^+ reabsorption [150].

In states of potassium depletion, potassium secretion in the cortical collecting tubule is reduced, whereas potassium reabsorption is stimulated. Reabsorption takes place in the intercalated cells of this nephron segment (see Fig. 79-5).

Fig. 79-4. Schematic representation of sodium and potassium transport mechanisms in the sodium reabsorbing cells in the collecting tubules. The entry of filtered sodium into the cells is mediated by selective sodium channels in the apical (luminal) membrane; the energy for this process is provided by the favorable electrochemical gradient for sodium (cell interior electronegative and low cell sodium concentration). Reabsorbed sodium is pumped out of the cell by the Na/K ATPase pump in the basolateral (peritubular) membrane. The reabsorption of cationic sodium makes the lumen electronegative, thereby creating a favorable gradient for the secretion of potassium into the lumen via potassium channels in the apical membrane. Aldosterone, after combining with the cytosolic mineralocorticoid receptor (Aldo-R), leads to enhanced sodium reabsorption and potassium secretion in the cortical collecting tubule by increasing both the number of open sodium channels and the number of Na/K ATPase pumps. Atrial natriuretic peptide, on the other hand, acts primarily in the inner medullary collecting duct by combining with its basolateral membrane receptor (ANP-R) and activating guanylate cyclase. ANP inhibits sodium reabsorption by closing the sodium channels. The potassium-sparing diuretics act by closing sodium channels, amiloride and triamterene directly and spironolactone by competing with aldosterone for binding to the mineralocorticoid receptor.

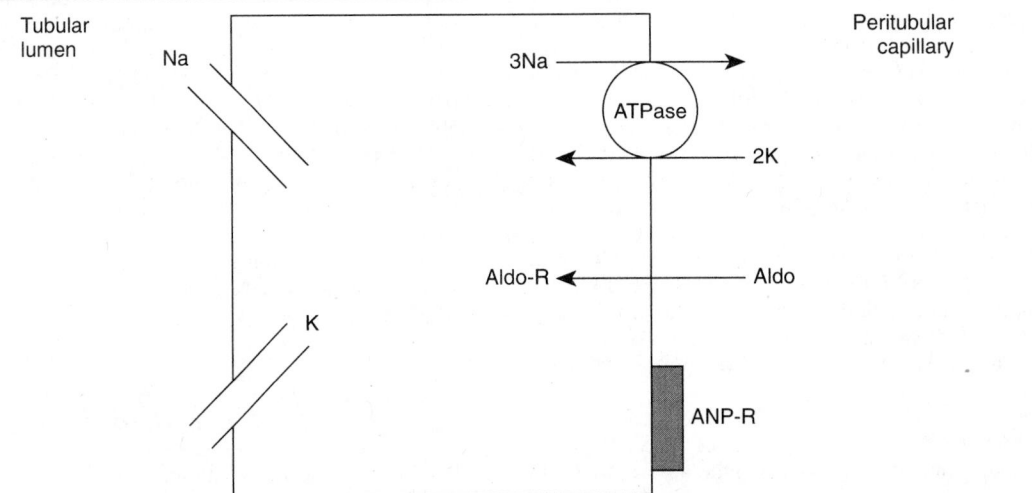

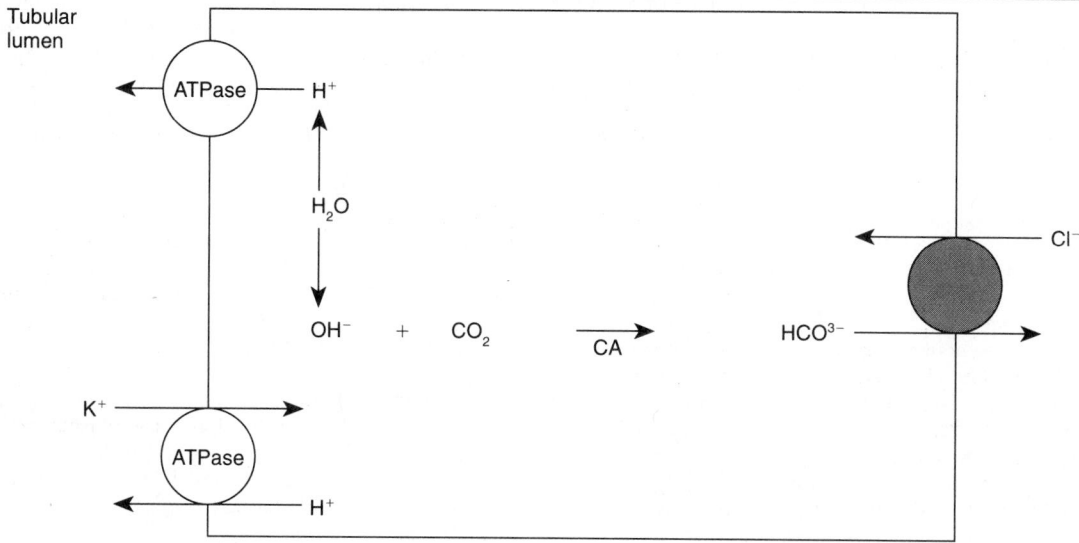

Fig. 79-5. Transport mechanisms involved in hydrogen secretion and bicarbonate and potassium reabsorption in type A intercalated cells in the cortical collecting tubule and in the outer medullary collecting tubule cells. Water within the cell dissociates into hydrogen and hydroxyl anions. The former are secreted into the lumen by H-ATPase pumps in the luminal membrane; chloride may be cosecreted with hydrogen to maintain electroneutrality. The hydroxyl anions in the cell combine with carbon dioxide to form bicarbonate in a reaction catalyzed by carbonic anhydrase (CA). Bicarbonate is then returned to the systemic circulation via chloride-bicarbonate exchangers in the basolateral membrane. The favorable inward concentration gradient for chloride (plasma and interstitial concentration greater than that in the cell) provides the energy for bicarbonate reabsorption. H-K-ATPase pumps, which lead to both hydrogen secretion and potassium reabsorption, may also be present in the luminal membrane. The number of these pumps increases with potassium depletion, suggesting that their main function is to promote potassium conservation.

HYPOKALEMIA.

Hypokalemia is a common clinical problem. Potassium enters the body via oral intake or intravenous infusion, is largely stored in the cells, and then excreted in the urine. Thus, decreased intake, increased translocation into the cells, or, most often, increased losses in the urine (or gastrointestinal tract or sweat) can lead to potassium depletion and a reduction in the plasma potassium concentration.

Causes of Hypokalemia (Table 79-6)

DECREASED POTASSIUM INTAKE. The normal range of potassium intake is 40 to 120 mEq per day. Most is excreted in the urine. The kidney can lower potassium excretion to a minimum of 5 to 25 mEq per day when potassium depletion is occurring [151]. Thus, decreased intake alone rarely causes hypokalemia, but it can contribute to the severity of potassium depletion when another problem is superimposed, such as diuretic therapy or the used of hypocaloric, liquid protein diets for rapid weight loss [152].

INCREASED ENTRY INTO CELLS. The normal distribution of potassium between the cells (which contains approximately 98% of exchangeable potassium) and the extracellular fluid is maintained by the Na^+/K^+ ATPase pump in the cell membrane. In some cases, however, there is increased potassium entry into cells, resulting in transient hypokalemia.

Elevation in extracellular pH. Metabolic or respiratory alkalosis can promote potassium entry into cells. When this occurs, hydrogen ions leave the cells to minimize the change in extracellular pH; the necessity to maintain electroneutrality then requires the entry of some potassium (and sodium) into the cells. In general, this direct effect is relatively small, as the plasma potassium concentration falls less than 0.4 mEq per liter for every 0.1 unit rise in pH [153]. (A similar change can be induced by the administration of sodium bicarbonate to treat metabolic acidosis; under this circumstance, however, a direct effect of bicarbonate may also contribute, independent of the elevation in pH [154].)

Although the direct effect of alkalemia is relatively small, hypokalemia is common in metabolic alkalosis. The major reason for this association probably is that the underlying disorder (diuretics, vomiting, or hyperaldosteronism) causes both hydrogen and potassium loss (see below).

Increased availability of insulin. Insulin apparently promotes the entry of potassium into skeletal muscle and hepatic cells by increasing the activity of the Na^+/K^+ ATPase pump [147,154,155]. This effect is most prominent after the adminis-

Table 79-6. Major Causes of Hypokalemia

Decreased potassium intake
Increased entry into cells
  An elevation in extracellular pH
  Increased availability of insulin
  Elevated β-adrenergic activity
  Hypokalemic periodic paralysis
  Marked increase in blood cell production
  Hypokalemia
Increased gastrointestinal losses
Increased urinary losses
  Diuretics
  Primary mineralocorticoid excess
  Loss of gastric secretions
  Nonreabsorbable anions
  Metabolic acidosis
  Hypomagnesemia
  Amphotericin B
  Salt-wasting nephropathies—including Bartter's syndrome
  Polyuria
Increased sweat losses
Dialysis

tration of insulin to patients with diabetic ketoacidosis or severe nonketotic hyperglycemia [156].

The plasma potassium concentration can also be reduced by a carbohydrate load. Thus, intravenous administration of potassium chloride in a dextrose-containing solution in an effort to correct hypokalemia can transiently further reduce the plasma potassium concentration and possibly lead to cardiac arrhythmias [157].

Elevated β-adrenergic activity. Catecholamines, acting via the β2-adrenergic receptors [158], can promote potassium entry into the cells, primarily by increasing Na$^+$/K$^+$ ATPase activity [147]. As a result, transient hypokalemia can occur whenever there is stress-induced release of epinephrine, as with acute illness, coronary ischemia, or theophylline intoxication [159,160]. A similar effect, in which the plasma potassium concentration can fall acutely by more than 0.5 to 1 mEq per liter, can be achieved by the administration of a β-adrenergic agonist (such as albuterol, terbutaline, or dopamine) to treat asthma or heart failure or to prevent premature labor [161–163]. This effect must be considered when diuretic therapy is considered for the treatment of hypertension in a patient with asthma or chronic lung disease. The hypokalemic response to epinephrine can be blocked by a nonselective β-blocker (such as propranolol), but a β1-selective agent (such as atenolol) offers no protection [164].

Hypokalemic periodic paralysis. Hypokalemic periodic paralysis is a rare disorder of uncertain cause characterized by potentially fatal episodes of muscle weakness or paralysis that can affect the respiratory muscles [165]. Acute attacks, in which the sudden movement of potassium into the cells can lower the plasma potassium concentration to as low as 1.5 to 2.5 mEq per liter, are often precipitated by rest after exercise, stress, or a carbohydrate meal, events that are often associated with increased release of epinephrine or insulin.

Hypokalemic periodic paralysis may be familial with autosomal dominant inheritance, or may be acquired in patients (particularly Asian males) with thyrotoxicosis [165,166]. Thyroid hormone increase Na$^+$/K$^+$ ATPase activity (thereby tending to drive potassium into cells), and thyrotoxic patients with periodic paralysis have higher sodium pump activity than those without paralytic episodes [167]. Excess thyroid hormone may therefore predispose to paralytic episodes by increasing the susceptibility to the hypokalemic action of epinephrine or insulin [166]. Recent studies indicate that the abnormal gene in this disorder appears to code for part of a calcium channel in skeletal muscle [167a]. How this predisposes to hypokalemia is unclear.

Oral administration of 60 to 120 mEq of potassium chloride usually aborts acute attacks within 15 to 20 minutes. Another 60 mEq can be given if no improvement is noted. The presence of hypokalemia must be confirmed prior to therapy, however, since potassium can worsen episodes caused by the normokalemic or hyperkalemic forms of periodic paralysis [165]. Furthermore, excess potassium administration during an acute episode may lead to posttreatment hyperkalemia as potassium moves back out of the cells [166].

Prevention of hypokalemic episodes consists of the restoration of euthyroidism in thyrotoxic patients and the administration of a β-adrenergic blocker in either form of periodic paralysis. β-blockers can minimize the number and severity of attacks and, in most cases, the fall in the plasma potassium concentration [166]. A nonselective β-blocker (such as propranolol) should be given; β1-selective agents are less likely to inhibit the β2 receptor-mediated hypokalemic effect of epinephrine and so may be less likely to prevent paralytic episodes [166].

Marked increase in blood cell production. An acute increase in hematopoietic cell production is associated with potassium uptake by the new cells and possible hypokalemia. This most often occurs after the administration of vitamin B12 or folic acid to treat a megaloblastic anemia or of granulocyte-macrophage colony-stimulating factor (GM-CSF) to treat neutropenia [168,169].

Metabolically active cells can also take up potassium after blood has been drawn. This in vitro phenomenon has been described in patients with acute myeloid leukemia and a high white blood cell count [170]. In these patients, the measured plasma potassium concentration may be below 1 mEq per liter (without symptoms) if the blood is allowed to stand at room temperature for a prolonged period before separation of the plasma from the cells.

Hypothermia. Accidental or induced hypothermia can drive potassium into the cells and lower the plasma potassium concentration to below 3.0 to 3.5 mEq per liter [171]. In contrast, hyperkalemia in an individual with severe hypothermia is usually due to irreversible tissue necrosis and is associated with a high mortality rate [171].

INCREASED GASTROINTESTINAL LOSSES. Loss of gastric or intestinal secretions from any cause (vomiting, diarrhea, laxatives, or tube drainage) is associated with potassium wasting and, possibly, hypokalemia. It should be emphasized, however, that the concentration of potassium in gastric secretions is relatively low (5 to 10 mEq/L) and that the potassium depletion is primarily due to increased urinary losses [172].

The associated metabolic alkalosis seen with loss of gastric secretions raises the plasma bicarbonate concentration and therefore the filtered bicarbonate load above its readsorptive threshold. As a result, more sodium bicarbonate and water are delivered to the distal potassium secretory site in combination with a hypovolemia-induced increase in aldosterone release. The result is increased potassium secretion and potentially large urinary potassium losses.

The urinary potassium wasting seen with loss of gastric secretions is typically most prominent in the first few days; thereafter, bicarbonate reabsorptive capacity increases, leading to a marked reduction in urinary sodium, bicarbonate, and potassium losses [172]. At this time, the urine pH falls from above 7.0 (due to bicarbonate wasting) to acid (below 6.0); see Chap. 69.

INCREASED URINARY LOSSES. Urinary potassium excretion is mostly derived from potassium secretion in the distal nephron, particularly by the principal cells in the cortical collecting tubule [173,174]. This process is primarily influenced by two factors: aldosterone and the distal delivery of sodium and water [173,175]. Aldosterone acts partly by stimulating sodium reabsorption; the removal of cationic sodium makes the lumen relatively electronegative, thereby promoting passive potassium secretion from the tubular cell into the lumen through specific potassium channels in the luminal membrane. Thus, urinary potassium wasting generally requires increases in either aldosterone or distal flow; the other parameter is at least normal or increased [173,175]. On the other hand, hypovolemia-induced hyperaldosteronism does not usually lead to hypokalemia, since the associated decline in distal flow (caused by enhanced proximal reabsorption, in part under the influence of angiotensin II) and urine volume (due to increased ADH release) counterbalances the stimulatory effect of aldosterone [175].

Diuretics. Any diuretic that acts proximal to the potassium secretory site, such as carbonic anhydrase inhibitors, loop diuretics, and thiazide-type diuretics, both increases distal delivery and, via the induction of volume depletion, activates the renin-angiotensin-aldosterone system. As a result, urinary potassium excretion increases, leading to hypokalemia if these losses are greater than intake.

Primary mineralocorticoid excess. Urinary potassium wasting is characteristic of any condition associated with primary hypersecretion of a mineralocorticoid, such as an aldosterone-producing adrenal adenoma. Affected patients are almost always hypertensive, and the differential diagnosis includes diuretic therapy (which may be surreptitious) in a patient with underlying hypertension, and renovascular disease, in which increased secretion of renin leads to enhanced aldosterone release.

Loss of gastric secretions. The mechanism by which loss of gastric secretions leads to urinary potassium wasting is described above. This problem is usually suggested from the history. If the history is not helpful, the differential diagnosis of a normotensive patient with hypokalemia, urinary potassium wasting, and metabolic alkalosis includes surreptitious vomiting or diuretic use and Bartter's syndrome (see Chap. 80).

Nonreabsorbable anions. The lumen-negative electrical gradient created by sodium reabsorption in the cortical collecting tubule is partially attenuated by chloride reabsorption. There are, however, a number of clinical situations in which sodium is presented to the distal nephron with relatively large quantities of a nonreabsorbable anion, including bicarbonate with vomiting or type 2 (proximal) renal tubular acidosis, β-hydroxybutyrate in diabetic ketoacidosis, hippurate following toluene use (glue-sniffing), or a penicillin derivative in patients receiving high-dose penicillin therapy. In these settings, more of the delivered sodium is reabsorbed in exchange for potassium, leading to a potentially marked increase in potassium excretion [176,177]. As an example, the plasma potassium concentration has been reported to be below 2 mEq per liter in approximately one-fourth of patients with toluene-induced metabolic acidosis [177].

The effect of nonreabsorbable anions is likely to be most prominent when there is concurrent volume depletion. When this occurs, the decrease in distal chloride delivery (thereby limiting the ability of chloride reabsorption to dissipate the lumen-negative gradient) and the enhanced secretion of aldosterone both promote potassium secretion [178].

Metabolic acidosis. Increased urinary potassium losses can occur in several forms of metabolic acidosis by mechanisms similar to those already described. In diabetic ketoacidosis, for example, increased distal sodium and water delivery (due to the glucose-induced osmotic diuresis), hypovolemia-induced hyperaldosteronism, and β-hydroxybutyrate acting as a nonreabsorbable anion all can contribute to potassium wasting [156]. Potassium wasting can also occur in both type 1 (distal) and type 2 (proximal) renal tubular acidosis (see Chapter 80).

In each of these disorders, however, the degree of potassium depletion is masked by the tendency of acidemia to promote potassium movement out of the cells. Thus, the plasma potassium concentration is higher than it should be given the presence of potassium depletion. In some patients, the plasma potassium concentration may be normal or even elevated, although correction of the acidemia will uncover the true state of potassium balance. An important exception can occur in patients with organic acidoses (lactic and ketoacidosis) in whom potassium shifts due to acidemia may not occur (see Chap. 110).

Hypomagnesemia. Hypomagnesemia is present in up to 40 percent of patients with hypokalemia [179]. In many cases, as with diuretic therapy, vomiting, or diarrhea, there are concurrent potassium and magnesium losses. In addition, hypomagnesemia of any cause can lead to increased urinary potassium losses possibly by depleting ATP and opening potassium chan-

nels in the tubular cells. This would lead to a loss of intracellular K^+ into the tubule lumen [179a]. Documenting the presence of hypomagnesemia is particularly important because the hypokalemia often cannot be corrected until the magnesium deficit is repaired [179]. The concurrent presence of hypocalcemia (due both to decreased release of parathyroid hormone and resistance to its calcemic effect) is often a clue to underlying magnesium depletion.

Amphotericin B. Hypokalemia occurs in up to one-half of patients treated with amphotericin B [180]. Amphotericin interacts with membrane sterols, leading to an increase in membrane permeability that can promote potassium secretion from intracellular stores across the luminal membrane and into the tubule lumen. Concurrent type 1 (proximal) renal tubular acidosis also may play a contributory role.

Salt-wasting nephropathies. Occasionally, renal diseases associated with decreased proximal, loop, or distal sodium reabsorption can lead to hypokalemia via a mechanism similar to that induced by diuretics. This problem can be seen in patients with Bartter's syndrome, tubulointerstitial diseases (such as interstitial nephritis due to Sjögren's syndrome or lupus), hypercalcemia, and tubular injury that may be induced by lysozyme in patients with leukemia, particularly acute monocytic or myelomonocytic leukemia [181–184]. Increased potassium uptake by the leukemic cells may contribute to the fall in the plasma potassium concentration [170].

Polyuria. In the presence of potassium depletion, normal subjects can lower the urine potassium concentration to a minimum of 5 to 10 mEq per liter [151]. If, however, the urine output is greater than 5 to 10 liters per day, obligatory potassium losses can exceed 50 to 100 mEq in this period. This problem is most likely to occur in primary polydipsia, in which the urine output may be elevated over a prolonged period [35]. An equivalent degree of polyuria can also occur in central diabetes insipidus, but patients with this disorder typically seek medical care soon after the polyuria has begun.

INCREASED SWEAT LOSSES. Daily sweat losses are normally negligible, since the volume is low and the potassium concentration is only 5 to 10 mEq per liter; however, subjects exercising in a hot climate can produce 10 liters or more of sweat per day, leading to potassium depletion if these losses are not replaced [185]. Urinary potassium excretion also may contribute, since aldosterone release is enhanced both by exercise (via catecholamine-induced renin secretion) and volume loss [185,186].

Extensive burns are another situation in which potassium losses through the skin may cause hypokalemia. Despite the low potassium concentration in sweat, the potassium concentration of fluid lost through the skin after burns may greatly exceed the plasma level because of local tissue breakdown, which leads to the release of potassium from cells.

DIALYSIS. Although patients with end-stage renal disease typically retain potassium and tend to be mildly hyperkalemic, hypokalemia can be induced in some patients by maintenance dialysis. Dialysis potassium losses can reach 30 mEq per day in patients on chronic peritoneal dialysis. This can become clinically important if intake is reduced or if there are concurrent gastrointestinal losses [187].

A different mechanism may be operative in patients treated with hemodialysis who have underlying potassium depletion. In these patients, the metabolic acidosis induced by renal failure can result in a relatively normal predialysis plasma potassium concentration owing to potassium movement out of the cells. The high flows attained during hemodialysis can rapidly correct the acidemia, however, leading to potassium entry into cells and a potentially large, although transient, reduction in the plasma potassium concentration [188]. As a result, care must be exercised in treating hypokalemia based on an early post-dialysis potassium level.

Clinical Manifestations. Most individuals with mild hypokalemia exhibit no symptoms relative to the low plasma K^+ concentration. The major disturbances seen with more severe K^+ deficiency are due to changes in cardiovascular, neuromuscular, and renal function. Cardiac toxicity may be manifested by serious arrhythmias due to hyperpolarization of the myocardial cell membrane, leading to a prolonged refractory period and increased susceptibility to reentrant arrhythmias [189]. Earlier electrocardiographic changes of hypokalemia include T-wave depression with prominent U waves (Fig. 79-6).

Hyperpolarization also slows nerve conduction and muscle contractions, which may contribute to symptoms such as muscle weakness, cramps, and paresthesias, although these are usually not observed until the plasma K^+ concentration is below 2.5 mEq per liter. Severe hypokalemia may cause rhabdomyolysis, since K^+ permits vasodilation in response to muscle contraction, such as occurs during extreme physical exercise [190]. When severe, hypokalemia can impair respiratory muscle function, leading to hypoventilation [191].

Polyuria due to stimulation of thirst as well as resistance to the action of antidiuretic hormone are the primary renal manifestations of hypokalemia. Increased thirst results from direct stimulation of the hypothalamic thirst center as well as to an appropriate response to polyuria [192].

Diagnosis. The cause of hypokalemia can usually be determined from the history (as with diuretic use, vomiting, or diarrhea). In some cases, however, the diagnosis is not readily apparent. Measurement of blood pressure and urinary potassium excretion and assessment of acid-base balance are often helpful in such cases.

URINARY RESPONSE. In the presence of potassium depletion, a normal subject can lower urinary potassium excretion below 25 to 30 mEq per day [151]; values above this level reflect at least a contribution from urinary potassium wasting. Random measurement of the urine potassium concentration can be used but may be less accurate than a 24-hour collection. Extrarenal losses probably are present if the urine potassium concentration is less than 15 mEq per liter (unless the patient is markedly polyuric). Higher values, however, do not necessarily indicate potassium wasting if the urine volume is reduced. For example, a urine potassium concentration of 40 mEq per liter represents seemingly appropriate potassium conservation of 20 mEq per day if the urine volume is only 500 ml.

Most of the filtered potassium is reabsorbed in the proximal tubule and loop of Henle, whereas the majority of potassium that is excreted in the urine is derived from tubular secretion by the principal cells in the cortical and outer medullary collecting tubules (see Fig. 79-4) [175]. The response to potassium depletion is twofold: decreased potassium secretion by the

principal cells (mediated in part by a reduction in the cell potassium concentration), and increased active potassium reabsorption by H/K ATPase pumps in the luminal membrane of the adjacent type A intercalated cells in the cortical collecting tubule (see Fig. 79-5) [174,193,194]. These pumps, which are activated by hypokalemia, reabsorb potassium and secrete hydrogen. Hypokalemia-induced reductions in aldosterone release and in the tubular cell potassium concentration mediate at least part of these tubular adaptations [174,175,193–195].

The minimum urine potassium concentration that can be achieved with hypokalemia is 5 to 15 mEq per liter; this value is higher than the ability to virtually eliminate sodium from the urine in the presence of volume depletion [151]. This minimal degree of potassium wasting with potassium depletion may reflect passive potassium leakage out of the inner medullary collecting cells down a favorable concentration gradient through a nonselective cation channel in the luminal membrane [196].

Once urinary potassium excretion is measured, the following diagnostic possibilities should be considered in the patient with hypokalemia of uncertain origin:

Metabolic acidosis with a low rate of potassium excretion is, in an asymptomatic patient, suggestive of lower gastrointestinal losses due to laxative abuse or a villous adenoma [197].

Metabolic acidosis with potassium wasting is most often caused by diabetic ketoacidosis or to type 1 (distal) or type 2 (proximal) renal tubular acidosis. A salt-wasting nephropathy can produce similar findings, as the associated renal insufficiency is responsible for the acidemia.

Metabolic alkalosis with a low rate of potassium excretion is due to surreptitious vomiting or diuretic use (in which the urinary collection is obtained after the diuretic effect has worn off).

Metabolic alkalosis with potassium wasting and a normal blood pressure most often results from surreptitious vomiting or diuretic use or from Bartter's syndrome. In this situation, measurement of the urine chloride concentration is often helpful, as the concentration is low in vomiting patients at a time when urinary sodium and potassium excretion may be relatively high due to the need to maintain electroneutrality as some of the excess bicarbonate is being excreted. This possibility can be determined at the bedside from the urine pH, which should be above 7.0 if significant bicarbonaturia is present (see Chap. 80).

Metabolic alkalosis with potassium wasting and hypertension suggests surreptitious diuretic therapy in patients with underlying hypertension, renovascular disease, or one of the causes of primary mineralocorticoid excess.

The possible presence of primary mineralocorticoid excess (with aldosterone and, to a lesser degree, deoxycorticosterone [DOC] being the major endogenous mineralocorticoids) should be suspected in any patient with hypertension and unexplained hypokalemia and metabolic alkalosis [198–200]. Although occasional patients with this disorder are normokalemic [199], it is not realistic to screen every hypertensive patient for hyperaldosteronism. Even less common are patients with hypokalemia but a normal systemic blood pressure [201]. Surreptitious vomiting or diuretic therapy or Bartter's syndrome should be excluded in this setting, but some patients have findings diagnostic of primary hyperaldosteronism: low plasma renin activity and nonsuppressible hypersecretion of aldosterone.

The two other major causes of hypertension and hypokalemia are renovascular disease (in which the hypersecretion of renin leads sequentially to increased secretion of angiotensin II

Fig. 79-6. Both hypokalemia and hyperkalemia can cause changes in the patient's electrocardiogram. The ECG from a patient with moderate hypokalemia shows prominent U waves.

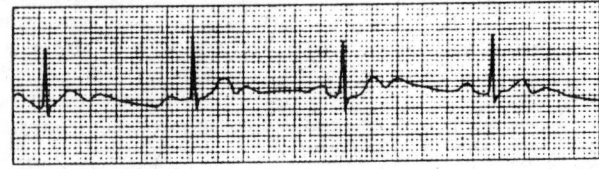

and then aldosterone) and diuretic therapy, which may be surreptitious. The development of new hypokalemia in a patient on diuretic therapy is relatively common and is not an indication for further evaluation for adrenal disease unless there is an unusually marked reduction in the plasma potassium concentration.

Diagnosis in the patient with hypokalemia and hypertension (including primary hyperaldosteronism). The sequential evaluation of a patient with hypertension and hypokalemia should include the following tests:

24-hour urine collection. The low plasma potassium concentration induced by mineralocorticoid excess is a result of increased urinary potassium losses. Thus, a 24-hour urine collection should be obtained (in the absence of known diuretic therapy) to document the presence of inappropriate potassium wasting (defined as more than 25 mEq/day in a patient with hypokalemia). An appropriately low rate of potassium excretion suggests either extrarenal losses (vomiting, diarrhea) or the use of diuretics, with the urine being collected after the diuretic effect has worn off.

Attention must be paid to the patient's volume status and rate of sodium excretion. The patient must not be hypovolemic (as evidenced by less than 20 mEq of sodium being excreted per day), since the associated decrease in sodium and water delivery to the distal potassium secretory site can diminish potassium excretion even in patients with hyperaldosteronism. On the other hand, the degree of potassium wasting and therefore the diagnostic accuracy can be enhanced by a high-sodium diet, as the combination of increased distal flow and hypersecretion of aldosterone will maximize potassium losses [175,199].

A high-sodium diet can be used as a provocative test in patients with an initial plasma potassium concentration in the low-normal range. Sodium-induced hypokalemia is strongly suggestive of nonsuppressible hyperaldosteronism [199]. Normal subjects do not waste potassium in this setting because the increase in distal flow is offset by reduced secretion of aldosterone.

Plasma renin activity. The plasma renin activity should be measured once urinary potassium wasting has been documented [199,201]. An elevated value is most often due to renovascular or malignant hypertension or to diuretic usage; rarely, renin-secreting tumors can produce this pattern [202]. On the other hand, plasma renin activity is typically very low (due in part to the associated mild volume expansion) with primary mineralocorticoid excess [199].

Cushing's syndrome can lead to hypokalemia, in part as a result of ACTH-dependent compounds such as deoxycorticosterone, corticosterone, and, in some cases, cortisol (see below). The hypertension in this disorder, however, is usually not related to mineralocorticoid excess or sodium retention, and the plasma renin activity is typically normal [203]. The presence of cortisol excess is usually suspected from the classic cushingoid appearance (central obesity, ecchymoses, abdominal striae, and hirsutism).

Estimation of aldosterone secretion. The combination of urinary potassium wasting and low plasma renin activity strongly suggests increased mineralocorticoid activity. The different causes of this problem can be differentiated by measuring the plasma aldosterone concentration or the urinary excretion of aldosterone metabolites.

A low plasma or urinary level of aldosterone indicates the presence of some nonaldosterone mineralocorticoid. A complete review of this relatively rare problem is beyond the scope of this discussion. Among the settings in which it can occur are:

Some types of congenital adrenal hyperplasia, including familial cortisol resistance, which has a similar presentation

Settings in which cortisol acts as the primary mineralocorticoid, as with chronic licorice or licorice-like compounds (such as carbenoxolone) ingestion. Although intitial studies suggested that the excess mineralocorticoid activity in such patients was derived from a steroid in licorice (glycyrrhetinic acid), it now appears that the major action of glycyrrhetinic acid is to inhibit the enzyme 11β-hydroxysteroid dehydrogenase. Inhibition of this enzyme permits cortisol to act as the major endogenous mineralocorticoid [204]

A DOC-producing tumor, which can usually be detected by CT scanning or magnetic resonance imaging (MRI) [200]

Liddle's syndrome, a rare condition in which there is a possibly humorally-mediated increase in collecting tubule sodium reabsorption and potassium secretion [205]

On the other hand, a clearly high plasma aldosterone concentration ($>$30 mg/dl) or elevated 24-hour urinary aldosterone excretion points toward one of the causes of hyperaldosteronism. The diagnostic accuracy of these measurements can be enhanced by attempting to suppress endogenous aldosterone production via the administration of 2 liters of isotonic saline intravenously over 4 hours (while the patient is recumbent) [199,200,206]. The plasma aldosterone concentration will fall to 6 mg/dl or below in normal subjects, whereas values above 10 mg/dl are consistent with primary hyperaldosteronism [206]. Levels between 6 and 10 mg/dl are nondiagnostic; in this setting, a more prolonged suppression test can be performed by inducing volume expansion with the combination of a high sodium diet plus 0.6 to 1.2 mg/day of fludrocortisone (a synthetic mineralocorticoid) for 3 days [199,206]. The plasma aldosterone concentration should fall to less than 6 mg/dl with this regimen in subjects without adrenal disease.

Potentially confounding variables should be eliminated to prevent possible misinterpretation of these tests. Thus, the plasma aldosterone concentration should be measured when the patient is relatively normokalemic and off potassium supplements, since hypokalemia can inhibit and potassium loading can enhance aldosterone release in normal subjects [207]. The patient should be recumbent; standing causes venous pooling with a subsequent increase in the activity of the renin-angiotensin-aldosterone system.

The presence of high plasma aldosterone levels and low plasma renin activity (PRA) in primary hyperaldosteronism has led to the suggestion that the plasma aldosterone/PRA ratio can be used as an effective screening test for this disorder. Patients in whom antihypertensive medications could be discontinued for 2 weeks had blood drawn at 8 A.M. after 2 hours of ambulation. The combination of a plasma aldosterone/PRA above 30 and a plasma aldosterone concentration above 20 mg/dl had a sensitivity and specificity of 90% for the diagnosis of primary hyperaldosteronism [208]. In a selected population in which the incidence of primary hyperaldosteronism was 20%, the positive and negative predictive values for these findings were 70 and 98%, respectively.

ADENOMA VS ADRENAL HYPERPLASIA. Once the diagnosis of nonsuppressible primary hyperaldosteronism has been established, a unilateral adenoma (or rarely carcinoma) must be distinguished from bilateral hyperplasia because of their differing therapy requirements: surgery for an adenoma or carcinoma versus medical therapy with a potassium-sparing diuretic for idiopathic hyperplasia [199,200]. Hyperplasia is generally a milder disease with less hypersecretion of aldosterone and less hypokalemia; there is, however, substantial overlap.

The mechanism responsible for idiopathic adrenal hyperplasia is not well understood. Aldosterone secretion can be markedly reduced in some patients by the administration of cyproheptadine, a serotonin antagonist [209]. This finding suggests that central serotoninergic pathways may mediate the release of a hypothalamic secretagogue for aldosterone, such as β-lipotropin or an as yet unidentified aldosterone-stimulating factor [200,210].

Increased sensitivity of the adrenal zona glomerulosa to angiotensin II is another mechanism by which hypersecretion of aldosterone might occur [200]. This phenomenon could explain the characteristic rise in the plasma aldosterone concentration between an 8 A.M. supine sample and an upright noon sample [200,211]. Assumption of the upright posture leads sequentially to pooling of blood in the lower extremities, mild effective volume depletion, and activation of the renin-angiotensin system. This response is diagnostically useful, since there is no change or even a slight decrease in aldosterone levels during the day in patients with an adrenal adenoma in whom there is autonomous hypersecretion of aldosterone.

Adrenal vein aldosterone levels can help to establish the correct diagnosis. Unilateral disease is associated with a marked (usually greater than ten-fold) increase in aldosterone concentration on the side of the tumor, whereas there is little difference between the two sides with bilateral hyperplasia [200]. To ensure that the samples are from the adrenal veins, an ACTH-stimulated cortisol level should be measured on the same sample; the cortisol concentration should be roughly the same in both adrenal veins, but much higher than that in a peripheral vein [199,200].

In another form of adrenal hyperplasia with hyperaldosteronism, ACTH, which does not normally play an important role in mineralocorticoid regulation, is responsible for the hypersecretion of aldosterone. This form of the disease may be corrected by glucocorticoid administration [212].

RADIOLOGIC TESTS. The diagnosis of an adrenal adenoma or carcinoma can usually be confirmed by demonstrating a unilateral adrenal mass by CT scan or MRI [200,213,214]. These radiologic tests have an overall sensitivity of 67 to 85% in patients with primary hyperaldosteronism. They are most accurate when a unilateral mass is seen. Bilateral lesions are not diagnostic of hyperplasia, however, since some patients with a functioning aldosteronoma in one adrenal gland have a nonfunctioning adrenal nodule in the other [213,214]. As an example, one study of 24 patients with primary hyperaldosteronism determined that 22 had a unilateral adenoma by adrenal vein sampling and subsequent surgery [214]. Only 17 of these 22 patients were diagnosed correctly by CT; the other 5 appeared to have bilateral lesions. Thus, adrenal vein sampling should be performed to confirm a CT-suggested diagnosis of bilateral hyperplasia or to distinguish between an adenoma and hyperplasia when no mass is seen [213,214]. Although not widely available, scintillation scanning with 131-I-iodocholesterol (a precursor of aldosterone) may be even more accurate in detecting a unilateral lesion [215].

Treatment. Although hypokalemia can be transiently induced by the entry of potassium into the cells, most cases are caused by unreplaced gastrointestinal or urinary losses. Optimal therapy depends on the severity of the potassium deficit; somewhat different considerations are required to minimize continued urinary losses due to diuretic therapy or, less often, to one of the causes of primary hyperaldosteronism.

POTASSIUM DEFICIT. The total potassium deficit can only be approximated, since there is no strict correlation between the plasma potassium concentration and total body potassium stores. In general, the loss of 200 to 400 mEq of potassium is required to lower the plasma potassium concentration from 4.0 to 3.0 mEq per liter; the loss of an additional 200 to 400 mEq will lower the plasma potassium concentration to approxi-

mately 2.0 mEq per liter [216]. Continued potassium losses will not produce much more hypokalemia owing to release of potassium from the cell stores.

These estimates assume that there is a normal distribution of potassium between the cells and the extracellular fluid. The most common setting in which this does not apply is diabetic ketoacidosis, a disorder in which hyperosmolality, insulin deficiency, and, perhaps, acidemia favor the movement of potassium out of the cells. As a result, patients with this disorder may have a normal or even elevated plasma potassium concentration at presentation, despite having a marked potassium deficit due to urinary and gastrointestinal losses [156]. In these patients, potassium supplementation is usually begun once the plasma potassium concentration is 4.5 mEq per liter or below (assuming the patient is making urine), since the administration of insulin and fluids often leads to a rapid reduction in the plasma potassium concentration.

POTASSIUM PREPARATION. Intravenous or oral potassium chloride preparation generally is the preferred treatment for hypokalemia. Use of the chloride salt has two important advantages. First, potassium chloride will more rapidly raise the plasma potassium concentration than will potassium bicarbonate (or potassium citrate, with the citrate being rapidly metabolized to bicarbonate) [217]. This difference is probably attributable to the fact that bicarbonate has a greater ability to enter the cells than does chloride. The persistence of chloride in the extracellular fluid will, because of the need to maintain electroneutrality, limit the initial entry of potassium into the cells, thereby maximizing the rise in the plasma potassium concentration.

Second, most patients with hypokalemia also have metabolic alkalosis. For example, with diuretic therapy, vomiting, and hyperaldosteronism, hydrogen loss accompanies that of potassium. In such patients, potassium must be given with chloride to optimally correct both the hypokalemia and the alkalosis. Other anions act as nonreabsorbable anions in the kidney. As a result, sodium reabsorption in the collecting tubules cannot be accompanied by the nonreabsorbable anion; electroneutrality can be maintained only by the increased secretion of potassium and hydrogen [218]. With potassium chloride, on the other hand, chloride reabsorption follows that of sodium without an inappropriate rise in potassium and hydrogen excretion [218].

In comparison, potassium bicarbonate or citrate can be given to patients with hypokalemia and metabolic acidosis. This most often occurs in renal tubular acidosis and chronic diarrheal states.

Oral potassium chloride can be given in crystalline form (salt substitutes), as a liquid, or in a slow-release tablet or capsule. Salt substitutes contain 50 to 65 mEq per level teaspoon; they may be the ideal form of oral therapy, as they are safe, well tolerated, and much cheaper than the other preparations [219]. Potassium chloride solutions, on the other hand, are often unpalatable, and the slow-release preparations can in rare cases cause ulcerative or stenotic lesions in the gastrointestinal tract as a result of the local accumulation of high concentrations of potassium [220].

Increasing the intake of potassium-rich foods (such as oranges and bananas) is generally less effective. These foods contain phosphate and citrate rather than chloride and are therefore less likely to correct the hypokalemia and metabolic alkalosis [221].

Potassium chloride can be given intravenously to patients who are unable to eat or who have severe hypokalemia (see below). In general, 20 to 40 mEq of potassium is added to each liter of fluid, since concentrations over 60 mEq per liter can lead to pain and sclerosis of the peripheral vein. A saline solution is preferred to a dextrose solution for initial therapy, since the administration of dextrose can lead to a transient 0.2 to 1.4 mEq per liter reduction in the plasma potassium concentration, particularly if only 20 mEq per liter of potassium chloride is present [157]. This effect, which can induce arrhythmias in susceptible patients (such as those taking digitalis), is thought to be mediated by dextrose-stimulated release of insulin, which then drives potassium into the cells by enhancing the activity of the cellular Na/K ATPase pump [222].

MILD TO MODERATE POTASSIUM DEPLETION. The majority of patients have a plasma potassium concentration between 3 and 3.5 mEq per liter; this degree of potassium depletion usually produces no symptoms, except in patients with heart disease (particularly if they are taking digitalis) or advanced hepatic cirrhosis [223]. Treatment in this setting is directed toward replacing the lost potassium (usually beginning with 60–80 mEq of potassium chloride per day) and toward treating the underlying disorder (such as vomiting or diarrhea).

Another problem occurs in patients with continued urinary losses due to diuretic therapy (in hypertension or heart failure, for example) or to primary hyperaldosteronism. Potassium replacement alone is often only partially corrective in these conditions, perhaps in part as a result of concurrent hypomagnesemia, which also promotes potassium wasting.

The use of a potassium-sparing diuretic (amiloride, triamterene, or spironolactone) in these patients is generally more effective than other agents because it limits the further urinary losses of both potassium and magnesium [224]. It is frequently underappreciated, however, that, in the presence of high levels of aldosterone, greater than usual doses (up to 20–40 mg of amiloride, and 150–300 mg of spironolactone) are required to block potassium secretion [225,226]. Amiloride is preferred because it lacks the gastrointestinal or hormonal (amenorrhea, gynecomastia) side effects of spironolactone. Potassium-sparing diuretic in combination with potassium supplements should be used only with careful monitoring to prevent possible overcorrection and the development of hyperkalemia.

Severe hypokalemia. Potassium must be given more rapidly to patients with severe or symptomatic (arrhythmias, marked muscle weakness) hypokalemia. This is most easily done orally, as the plasma potassium concentration will rise by as much as 1 to 1.5 mEq per liter after 40 to 60 mEq and by 2.5 to 3.5 mEq per liter after 135 to 160 mEq [227,228]. These effects, however, are transient, as most of the exogenous potassium will be taken up by the cells [229]. Thus, careful monitoring is required, and more potassium should be given as necessary. A patient with a plasma potassium concentration of 2 mEq per liter, for example, may have a 400 to 800 mEq potassium deficit [216].

Some patients with severe hypokalemia must be treated intravenously because of a life-threatening disease or an inability to take medication orally. There are, however, two potential constraints to intravenous therapy: a maximum of 60 mEq per liter can be given into a peripheral vein; and, since saline solutions are preferable, volume overload is a potential risk in susceptible subjects.

The necessity for aggressive intravenous therapy has been reported primarily in patients with diabetic ketoacidosis or nonketotic hyperglycemia who present with hypokalemia due to marked potassium losses [230]. As described above, treatment with insulin and fluids will exacerbate the hypokalemia. Fortunately, these patients are also quite volume-depleted. Thus, the addition of 40 to 60 mEq of potassium chloride to each liter of half-isotonic saline can supply large quantities of potassium without the risk of pulmonary congestion. (Although isotonic saline is generally the initial replacement fluid of choice in patients with uncontrolled diabetes mellitus, the addition of

potassium will make this a hypertonic fluid, thereby delaying reversal of the hyperosmolality that is primary responsible for neurologic symptoms in this disorder. On the other hand, the combination of potassium in half-isotonic saline is almost the osmotic equivalent of isotonic saline, since potassium is as osmotically active as sodium).

In general, the maximum rate of intravenous potassium administration is 10 to 20 mEq/hour, although as much as 40 to 100 mEq/hour have been given to selected patients with paralysis or life-threatening arrhythmias [230]. In these patients, solutions containing as much as 200 mEq of potassium per liter (20 mEq in 100 ml of isotonic saline) have been used [231]. These solutions should be infused into a large vein, such as the femoral vein; a central venous line has also been used, but a local increase in the potassium concentration possibly could have a deleterious effect on cardiac conduction [231].

It must be emphasized that rapid intravenous administration of potassium is potentially dangerous, even in potassium-depleted patients. Thus, careful monitoring of the physiologic effects of hypokalemia (ECG abnormalities, muscle weakness or paralysis) is essential. Once these problems are no longer severe, the rate of potassium repletion should be slowed (to 10–20 mEq/h) even though there is persistent hypokalemia.

HYPERKALEMIA. Hyperkalemia is a relatively common laboratory abnormality in critically ill patients, particularly in those with oliguric acute or chronic renal failure.

Etiology. Hyperkalemia is rare in normal subjects, because the cellular and urinary adaptations prevent significant potassium accumulation in the extracellular fluid. Furthermore, the efficiency of potassium handling is increased if potassium intake is slowly enhanced, thereby allowing what might be a fatal potassium load to be tolerated. This phenomenon, called *potassium adaptation,* is mostly due to more rapid potassium excretion in the urine. Studies in rats indicate that early adaptation begins after a single potassium-containing meal. Compared to rats given a potassium-free meal, rats fed a meal with potassium were better able to excrete a potassium load several hours later, leading to a lesser rise in the plasma potassium concentration [232]. The result is that adapted animals excrete more potassium at a given plasma potassium concentration than normal animals.

The effect of potassium adaptation in humans can be illustrated by a recent study evaluating the response of normal subjects to increasing potassium intake from 100 up to 400 mEq/day [233]. Urinary potassium excretion rose to equal intake by the end of the second day; this effect was mediated by an elevation in both aldosterone release and the plasma potassium concentration (from 3.8 to 4.8 mEq/L). At day 20, urinary potassium excretion remained high, but aldosterone levels had returned to near baseline, and the plasma potassium concentration had fallen to 4.2 mEq per liter. The increased efficiency of potassium excretion at this time was presumably mediated by increased Na/K ATPase activity in the collecting tubule cells [233,234], thereby enhancing potassium uptake and therefore the size of the secretory pool.

These observations led to the following conclusions concerning the development of hyperkalemia:

Increasing potassium is not a cause, unless very acute or occurring in a patient with impaired potassium excretion. As examples, acute hyperkalemia can be induced (primarily in infants because of their small size) by the administration of intravenous potassium penicillin as an intravenous bolus, the accidental ingestion of a potassium-containing salt substitute, or the use of stored blood for exchange transfusion.

The net release of potassium from the cells (due either to enhanced release or decreased entry) can cause a transient elevation in the plasma potassium concentration.

Persistent hyperkalemia requires an impairment in urinary potassium excretion; in view of the above discussion, this is generally associated with a reduction in either aldosterone effect or in the delivery of sodium and water to the distal secretory site.

The causes of hyperkalemia are listed in Table 79-7.

INCREASED POTASSIUM RELEASE FROM CELLS. *Pseudohyperkalemia*. Pseudohyperkalemia refers to conditions in which the elevation in the measured plasma potassium concentration is due to potassium movement out of the cells during or after the blood specimen has been drawn. The major cause of this problem is mechanical trauma during venipuncture, resulting in the release of potassium from red cells and a characteristic reddish tint of the serum due to the concomitant release of hemoglobin.

Potassium also moves out of white cells and platelets after clotting has occurred. Thus, the serum potassium concentration normally exceeds the true value in the plasma by 0.1 to as much as 0.5 mEq per liter [235]. Although this difference in normal levels is not clinically important, the measured serum potassium concentration may be as high as 9 mEq per liter in patients with marked leukocytosis or thrombocytosis (white cell or platelet count greater than 100,000 per mm^3 or 400,000 mm^3, respectively), as may occur with leukemia or a myeloproliferative disease [235,236]. With thrombocytosis, for example, the measured serum potassium concentration rises by approximately 0.15 mEq per liter for every 100,000 per mm^3 elevation in the platelet count [235].

Pseudohyperkalemia should be suspected whenever there is no apparent cause for the elevation in the plasma concentration in an asymptomatic patient. Careful venipuncture to avoid hemolysis and measurement of the plasma potassium concentration (with a heparinized specimen tube) usually establishes the correct diagnosis.

Metabolic acidosis. The buffering of excess hydrogen ions in the cells can lead to potassium movement into the extracellular fluid; this transcellular shift is obligated, in part, by the need to maintain electroneutrality. This phenomenon is less likely to occur in the organic acidoses, ketoacidosis and lactic acidosis.

Insulin deficiency, hyperglycemia, and hyperosmolality. Insulin promotes potassium entry into cells; thus, the ingestion of

Table 79-7. Major Causes of Hyperkalemia

Increased potassium release from cells
 Pseudohyperkalemia
 Metabolic acidosis
 Insulin deficiency, hyperglycemia, and hyperosmolality
 Increased tissue catabolism
 β-adrenergic blockade
 Exercise
 Other
  Digitalis overdose
  Hyperkalemic periodic paralysis
  Succinylcholine
  Arginine hydrochloride
Reduced urinary potassium excretion
 Hypoaldosteronism
 Renal failure
 Effective circulating volume depletion
 Selective impairment of potassium excretion
Dapsone

glucose (which stimulates endogenous insulin secretion) minimizes the rise in the plasma potassium concentration induced by concurrent potassium intake. On the other hand, the combination of insulin deficiency and the hyperosmolality induced by hyperglycemia frequently leads to hyperkalemia in patients with uncontrolled diabetes mellitus, even though a patient may be markedly potassium depleted due primarily to potassium losses in the urine [156].

An elevation in plasma osmolality results in osmotic water movement from the cells into the extracellular fluid. This is accompanied by potassium movement out of the cells by two mechanisms. First, the loss of water raises the cell potassium concentration, thereby creating a favorable gradient for passive potassium exit through potassium channels in the cell membrane. Second, the friction forces between solvent (water) and solute can result in potassium being carried along with water through the water pores in the cell membrane. This phenomenon of solvent drag is independent of the electrochemical gradient for potassium diffusion. In addition to hyperglycemia, hyperosmolality-induced hyperkalemia can occur with the administration of hypertonic mannitol or the development of hypernatremia, particularly in patients with renal failure [237].

In one other setting, insulin deficiency can raise the plasma potassium concentration: following the administration of somatostatin (which is now available) to treat disorders such as postprandial hypotension. Somatostatin can raise the plasma potassium concentration by an average of 0.6 mEq per liter in normal subjects, but by more than 1.5 mEq per liter to potentially dangerous levels in selected patients with end-stage renal disease [238].

Increased tissue catabolism. Any cause of increased tissue breakdown can result in the release of potassium into the extracellular fluid, and can result in hyperkalemia, particularly if renal failure is also present. Clinical examples include trauma, the administration of cytotoxic or radiation therapy to patients with lymphoma or leukemia (the tumor-lysis syndrome), and patients who are terminally ill following severe accidental hypothermia [171].

β-adrenergic blockade. β-adrenergic blockers interfere with the β2-adrenergic facilitation of potassium uptake by the cells (see Fig. 79-4). This effect is associated with only a minor elevation in the plasma potassium concentration in normal subjects (less than 0.5 mEq/L), since the excess potassium can be easily excreted in the urine [216]. True hyperkalemia is rare except in conjunction with an additional defect in potassium handling, such as a large potassium load, marked exercise, hypoaldosteronism, or renal failure [239].

Exercise. Potassium is normally released from muscle cells during exercise. This response may reflect both a delay between potassium exit during depolarization and subsequent reuptake by the Na/K ATPase pump and, with severe exercise, an increased number of open potassium channels in the cell membrane due to a decline in ATP levels [240]. The release of potassium may have a physiologic function, since the local increase in the plasma potassium concentration has a vasodilator effect, increasing blood flow and energy delivery to the exercising muscle.

The degree of elevation in the systemic plasma potassium concentration is less pronounced and is related to the degree of exercise: 0.3 to 0.4 mEq per liter with slow walking; 0.7 to 1.2 mEq per liter with moderate exertion (including prolonged aerobic exercise with marathon running); and as much as 2 mEq per liter following exercise to exhaustion [241–243]. Both lactic acidosis [243] and ECG changes may be seen in the last example [242].

The rise in the plasma potassium concentration is reversed after several minutes of rest, and is typically associated with a mild rebound hypokalemia (averaging 0.4 to 0.5 mEq/L below the baseline level) [242,243] that may be arrhythmogenic in susceptible subjects [242]. The degree of potassium release is attenuated by prior physical conditioning (perhaps due to increased Na/K ATPase activity) [244], but may be exacerbated by the administration of β-blockers.

Exercise can interfere with accurate measurement of the plasma potassium concentration. Repeated fist clenching during blood drawing can acutely raise the plasma potassium concentration by more than 1 mEq per liter in that forearm, thereby representing another form of pseudohyperkalemia [245].

Other. Other rare causes of hyperkalemia due to translocation of potassium from the cells into the extracellular fluid include digitalis overdose, due to dose-dependent inhibition of the Na/K ATPase pump [246]; and the hyperkalemic form of periodic paralysis, an autosomal dominant disorder in which episodes of weakness or paralysis are usually precipitated by cold exposure, rest after exercise, or the ingestion of small amounts of potassium [247]. These attacks are also associated with a fall in the plasma sodium concentration and a rise in the plasma protein concentration, suggesting that sodium and water enter the cell as potassium leaves [247].

The primary abnormality in at least some families with hyperkalemic periodic paralysis appears to be a point mutation in the gene for the a-subunit of the skeletal muscle cell sodium channel [248]. How this abnormality accounts for episodic muscle weakness is not clear; one possibility is that the activity of the sodium channel is inappropriately increased by a slight elevation in the plasma potassium concentration. The ensuing entry of sodium into the cell down a very favorable concentration gradient depolarizes the cell membrane, thereby favoring potassium diffusion out of the cells (because the cell potassium concentration is so much higher than that in the extracellular fluid) and the development of hyperkalemia.

Administration of succinylcholine to patients with burns, extensive trauma, or neuromuscular disease can also cause hyperkalemia.

Administration of arginine hydrochloride, which partly metabolizes in hydrochloric acid and has been used to treat refractory metabolic alkalosis. The entry of cationic arginine into the cells presumably obligates potassium exit to maintain electroneutrality [249].

REDUCED URINARY POTASSIUM EXCRETION. Impaired urinary potassium excretion generally requires an abnormality in one or both of the two major factors required for adequate renal potassium handling: aldosterone and distal sodium and water delivery.

Hypoaldosteronism. Any cause of decreased aldosterone release or effect can diminish the efficiency of potassium secretion and lead to hyperkalemia (Table 79-8). The ensuing rise

Table 79-8. Major Causes of Hypoaldosteronism

Hyporeninemic hypoaldosteronism
  Renal disease, most often diabetic nephropathy
  Nonsteroidal antiinflammatory drugs
  Angiotensin converting enzyme inhibitors
  Cyclosporine
  HIV infection, including trimethoprim administration
Primary adrenal insufficiency
Potassium-sparing diuretics (trimethoprim may act similarly)
Heparin
Congenital adrenal hyperplasia, with 21-hydroxylase deficiency being
  most common
Isolated impairment in aldosterone synthesis
Pseudohypoaldosteronism (end-organ resistance)
Severe illness

in the plasma potassium concentration directly stimulates potassium secretion, partially overcoming the relative absence of aldosterone. The result is that the rise in the plasma potassium concentration is generally small in patients with normal renal function, but it can be clinically important in the presence of underlying renal insufficiency.

Hyperkalemia in this disorder is usually associated with a mild metabolic acidosis. This condition has been called *type 4 renal tubular acidosis* and appears to be due primarily to decreased urinary ammonium excretion. A transcellular cation exchange has been thought to play an important role [250]. Some of the excess potassium enters the cells. Electroneutrality is maintained, in part, by the movement of cellular sodium and hydrogen ions into the extracellular fluid. The ensuing intracellular alkalosis in the kidney would then diminish proximal ammonium production. More recent studies suggest that the primary defect may be in the thick ascending limb, however, where ammonium delivered out of the proximal tubule normally recycles within the medullary interstitium and is resecreted into the medullary collecting tubule [251]. Hyperkalemia decreases medullary recycling by inhibiting ammonium reabsorption in the thick ascending limb. Potassium and ammonium compete for a common transporter in the luminal membrane, which can function as a Na-K-2Cl or a Na-NH4-2Cl transporter.

Although aldosterone also promotes sodium retention, decreased availability of aldosterone is not typically associated with prominent sodium wasting (except in young children) because of the ability of other sodium-retaining factors (such as angiotensin II and norepinephrine) to compensate [252]. Hyponatremia is also uncommon, since there is no hypovolemia-induced stimulation of ADH release [252]. When hyponatremia is present, primary adrenal insufficiency should be suspected. In this disorder, the concurrent lack of cortisol is a potent stimulus to ADH secretion, leading to water retention and a fall in the plasma sodium concentration.

The causes of hypoaldosteronism include disorders that affect adrenal aldosterone synthesis, the renal response to aldosterone, or renal (and perhaps adrenal) renin release (Table 79-8) [250]. The plasma renin activity is generally increased in those disorders in which there is diminished aldosterone effect; the exception is different forms of hyporeninemic hypoaldosteronism.

Hyporeninemic hypoaldosteronism. The syndrome of hyporeninemic hypoaldosteronism is characterized by decreased angiotensin II production (due to diminished renin release) and an intraadrenal defect, both of which may contribute to the decline in aldosterone secretion [250,252]. The adrenal dysfunction may involve a local renin-angiotensin system, since there is evidence that angiotensin II produced within the adrenal gland may stimulate the release of aldosterone [253].

This relatively common disorder most often occurs in patients with mild to moderate renal insufficiency due to diabetic nephropathy or chronic interstitial nephritis. Low plasma renin levels are common in diabetics due, in part, to a defect in the conversion of the precursor prorenin into active renin [254]. Volume expansion induced by diabetic and other chronic renal diseases may play a contributory role; the increase in atrial natriuretic peptide release in this setting can suppress both the release of renin and the hyperkalemia-induced secretion of aldosterone [255].

Similar hemodynamic and humoral changes occur in acute glomerulonephritis (such as postinfectious glomerulonephritis): volume expansion, leading to appropriate suppression of renin release and enhanced secretion of atrial natriuretic peptide [256]. In some patients, these changes can lead to hyperkalemia that responds to mineralocorticoid replacement [257]. Recovery of renal function within 1 to 2 weeks is associated with restoration of normal potassium balance [257].

Low renin and aldosterone levels also may be seen in several other settings:

Nonsteroidal antiinflammatory drugs. Nonsteroidal antiinflammatory drugs lower renal renin secretion, which is normally partially mediated by locally produced prostaglandins. The result is that the plasma potassium rises about 0.2 mEq per liter in subjects with normal renal function, but can rise by more than 1 mEq per liter when renal insufficiency is superimposed [258,259]. This observation illustrates an important point in hypoaldosteronism: the degree of hyperkalemia is generally mild unless an additional factor, such as renal insufficiency or a high potassium diet, is also present.

Angiotensin converting enzyme inhibitors. Similar considerations apply to angiotensin converting enzyme (ACE) inhibitors, which diminish aldosterone release by impairing the conversion of angiotensin I to angiotensin II, both systemically and perhaps within the adrenal zona glomerulosa. In addition, the normal stimulatory effect of an elevation in the plasma potassium concentration on aldosterone release may be partially mediated by the adrenal generation of angiotensin II [253]. Thus, an ACE inhibitor may decrease both angiotensin II- and potassium-mediated aldosterone release [253,260].

ACE inhibitors generally raise the plasma potassium concentration by less than 0.5 mEq per liter in patients with relatively normal renal function. More prominent hyperkalemia may be seen in patients with renal insufficiency or concurrent use of a potassium-sparing diuretic [261].

Other. Other causes of hyporeninemic hypoaldosteronism include the use of cyclosporine, which can lead to hyperkalemia in 15 to 25 percent of renal transplant recipients (due in part to diminished secretion of, as well as responsiveness to, aldosterone; see below) [262,263], and human immunodeficiency virus (HIV) infection [21,264]. An adrenalitis is frequently present in the latter disorder; this abnormality may be infectious in origin, perhaps being induced by cytomegalovirus or *Mycobacterium avium intracellulare* [21]. The administration of trimethoprim-sulfamethoxazole is another common cause of hyperkalemia in HIV-infected patients; in this setting, trimethoprim given in much higher than usual doses appears to act as a potassium-sparing diuretic, directly diminishing collecting tubule potassium secretion in the manner described below [265].

Primary adrenal insufficiency. Primary adrenal disease is associated with lack of cortisol as well as aldosterone. Pituitary disease, in comparison, does not lead to hypoaldosteronism, since ACTH does not have a major role in the regulation of aldosterone release.

Primary adrenal insufficiency is frequently due to autoimmune destruction of the steroid-producing cells in the adrenal cortex. One major antigen against which the autoantibodies are directed appears to be the enzyme 21-hydroxylase [266]. This enzyme converts progesterone into deoxycorticosterone in the zona glomerulosa and 17-hydroxyprogesterone into deoxycortisol in the zona fasciculata.

Potassium-sparing diuretics. Potassium-sparing diuretics are probably the most common cause of hyperkalemia due to hypoaldosteronism. These drugs antagonize the action of aldosterone on the collecting tubule cells: spironolactone by competing for the aldosterone receptor, and amiloride and, probably, triamterene by closing the sodium channels in the luminal membrane [250].

Heparin. Heparin (or perhaps its preservative chlorbutol) has a direct toxic effect on the adrenal zona glomerulosa cells [250,267]. Even low-dose heparin can lead to a 75% reduction in plasma aldosterone levels [268]; once again, hyperkalemia is only seen if renal insufficiency is also present [267].

Adrenal enzyme deficiency. In children, hypoaldosteronism can result from a deficiency of enzymes required for aldosterone synthesis, which may be associated with concurrent abnormalities in cortisol and androgen production [250,269,270].

Pseudohypoaldosteronism. Decreased aldosterone activity also occurs in the syndrome of pseudohypoaldosteronism. This disorder is associated with generalized resistance to the actions of aldosterone due to a marked reduction in the number of mineralocorticoid receptors in the kidney and in other target organs such as the colon and sweat glands [271,272].

A second, rare, form of pseudohypoaldosteronism has been described in which patients present with hyperkalemia, hypertension, normal renal function, and low or low-normal levels of renin and aldosterone [273–275]. It has been proposed that the primary defect in this disorder is enhanced distal chloride reabsorption [273,275]. As a result, sodium is reabsorbed distally with chloride, not in exchange for potassium and hydrogen. The result is hyperkalemia, volume expansion and hypertension, which has the secondary effect of suppressing renin secretion. This mechanism may contribute to the hyperkalemia associated with cyclosporine therapy [263].

Two findings are compatible with this chloride hypothesis [275]. First, the administration of sodium chloride is associated with impairments in both sodium and potassium excretion in affected patients. These defects are not seen with sodium sulfate or sodium bicarbonate, indicating a central role for chloride transport. Second, many of the abnormalities can be corrected by a thiazide diuretic, suggesting that the primary defect in this condition may be increased activity of the thiazide-sensitive sodium-chloride cotransporter in the luminal membrane of the cells in the distal tubule and adjacent connecting segment. Increased sodium chloride reabsorption at this site will lead to volume expansion and to diminished sodium and water delivery to the potassium-secreting cells in the cortical collecting tubule, thereby reducing potassium excretion.

Severe illness. Hypoaldosteronism due to decreased adrenal production is common in critically ill patients. The stress-induced hypersecretion of ACTH in these patients may be responsible for this defect by inducing activity of 17a-hydroxylase in the zone glomerulosa [276]. This enzyme enhances the synthesis of cortisol and is normally restricted to the zona fasciculata. Its expression in the zona glomerulosa may promote the production of cortisol (which is beneficial in the presence of severe illness) at the expense of aldosterone.

Renal failure. The ability to maintain potassium excretion at near normal levels is generally maintained in patients with renal disease as long as both aldosterone secretion and distal flow are maintained [277]. Thus, hyperkalemia generally develops in patients who are oliguric or who have an additional problem such as a high potassium diet, increased tissue breakdown, hypoaldosteronism, or fasting in dialysis patients (which may both lower insulin levels and cause resistance to β-adrenergic stimulation of potassium uptake) [278,279]. The last effect may be important in patients who are fasted prior to surgery; the administration of insulin and glucose or, to a lesser degree, glucose alone in nondiabetics can minimize the elevation in the plasma potassium concentration [279].

Impaired cell uptake of potassium also contributes to the development of hyperkalemia in patients with advanced renal failure. Diminished Na/K ATPase activity may be particularly important in these patients; how this occurs is not clear, but retained uremic toxins may decrease the transcription of mRNA for the a1 isoform of the Na/K ATPase pump in skeletal muscle [278, 280].

Effective circulating volume depletion. Decreased distal flow due to marked effective volume depletion (as in heart failure, hepatic cirrhosis, or a salt-wasting nephropathy) can lead to hyperkalemia [281,282].

Hyperkalemic type 1 renal tubular acidosis. In some patients with type 1 (distal) renal tubular acidosis (RTA), the primary defect is impaired sodium reabsorption in the cortical collecting tubule. The movement of sodium from the lumen into the cell at this site makes the lumen electronegative, thereby promoting both hydrogen and potassium secretion. Inhibiting the transport of sodium therefore reduces both hydrogen and potassium secretion, leading to metabolic acidosis and hyperkalemia. This form of type 1 RTA is most often seen in patients with urinary tract obstruction or sickle cell disease. In comparison to hypoaldosteronism, patients with type 1 RTA have normal or even high aldosterone levels and are unable to normally acidify the urine (urine pH above 5.5).

Selective impairment of potassium secretion. Some patients have hyperkalemia and impaired potassium excretion despite normal aldosterone release and normal sodium handling. This seemingly selective impairment in potassium handling, which does not respond to exogenous mineralocorticoid, has been described in those with acute transplant rejection and those with lupus nephritis [283,284]. It may also occur in cyclosporine-treated patients, perhaps partly as a result of a toxic effect on the potassium-secreting cells in the cortical and outer medullary collecting tubules.

Other hyperkalemic patients have volume expansion, hypertension, and otherwise normal renal function [273,274]. It has been proposed that enhanced distal chloride reabsorption may be the primary problem in these individuals. Such a defect would lead to sodium being reabsorbed with chloride, rather than in exchange for potassium and hydrogen, thereby accounting for all the abnormalities that are seen.

The diagnosis of these disorders is made by exclusion. Plasma aldosterone levels are normal and the administration of a mineralocorticoid leads to an appropriate reduction in sodium excretion, but does not appreciably increase that of potassium. Therapy consists of a high sodium-low potassium diet and, if necessary, a loop or, perhaps preferably, a thiazide diuretic [274,283].

Clinical Manifestations. The symptoms induced by hyperkalemia are related to impaired neuromuscular transmission [285,286]. The ease of generating an action potential (called *membrane excitability*) is related both to the magnitude of the resting membrane potential and to the activation state of membrane sodium channels. Opening up of these sodium channels, leading to the passive diffusion of extracellular sodium into the cells, is the primary step in this process. According to the Nernst equation, the resting membrane potential is related to the ratio of the intracellular to the extracellular potassium concentration. An elevation in the plasma (extracellular) potassium concentration will decrease this ratio and therefore partially depolarize the cell membrane (that is, make the resting potential less electronegative). This change initially increases membrane excitability, since less of a depolarizing stimulus is required to generate an action potential. The later effect seen in patients is different. Persistent depolarization inactivates sodium channels in the cell membrane, thereby producing a net decrease in membrane excitability that may be manifested clinically by impaired cardiac conduction and/or muscle weakness or paralysis [286].

In general, severe symptoms of hyperkalemia do not occur until the plasma potassium concentration is above 7.5 mEq per liter. There is, however, substantial interpatient variability, since factors such as hypocalcemia and metabolic acidosis can increase the toxicity of excess potassium. Thus, careful monitoring of the ECG and muscle strength are indicated to assess the functional consequences of the hyperkalemia. A plasma potassium concentration above 7.5 to 8 mEq per liter, severe muscle weakness, or marked electrocardiographic changes are potentially life-threatening and require immediate treatment with almost all of the modalities described below.

The earliest electrocardiogram (ECG) abnormality is symmetric peaking of T waves. This is followed by reduced P wave voltage and widening of the QRS complexes (Fig. 79-7). If untreated, severe hyperkalemia may ultimately cause a sinusoidal ECG pattern, with one oscillation representing a wide QRS complex and the complementary oscillation an abnormal T wave. ECG changes are not usually present until the plasma K^+ concentration exceeds 6.5 mEq per liter and are more likely to develop when the rise in K^+ occurs rapidly [287]. There is, however, no absolute predictive relationship between the severity of the electrolyte disturbance and the ECG; in rare cases, the ECG can remain unchanged even with a plasma potassium concentration above 9 mEq per liter [288].

The neuromuscular manifestations of hyperkalemia are nonspecific. The earliest findings are paresthesias and weakness, which can progress to paralysis affecting the respiratory muscles. These symptoms are similar to those seen with hypokalemia; cranial nerve function remains unaffected.

Diagnosis. Pseudohyperkalemia should be considered when there is evidence of hemolysis in the sample or when the platelet or white blood cell counts are markedly increased. Discontinuation of all medications that adversely affect potassium handling, and removal of any exogenous sources of potassium are mandatory. When hyperkalemia is sustained, renal excretion is almost always impaired. The plasma cortisol concentration should be measured when hypoaldosteronism is documented to exclude the presence of primary adrenal insufficiency.

Treatment. An asymptomatic patient with a plasma potassium concentration of 6.5 mEq per liter can be treated only with a cation exchange resin (Kayexalate), whereas patients with a value below 6 mEq per liter can often be treated with a low potassium diet and diuretics. In addition, any extra source of potassium intake (such as salt substitutes or potassium supplements) should be eliminated, and any potentiating drugs (such as nonsteroidal antiinflammatory drugs or angiotensin converting enzyme inhibitors) should be discontinued.

Specific treatment of severe or symptomatic hyperkalemia is directed at antagonizing the membrane effects of potassium, driving extracellular potassium into the cells, or removing excess potassium from the body. The following modalities, which are listed according to their rapidity of action, all may be beneficial.

Calcium. Calcium directly antagonizes the membrane actions

Fig. 79-7. Marked hyperkalemia results in peaked T waves and widened QRS complexes in this ECG.

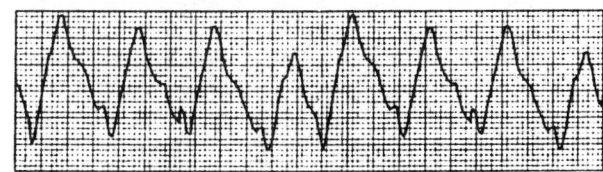

of hyperkalemia. As mentioned above, hyperkalemia-induced depolarization of the resting membrane potential leads to inactivation of sodium channels and decreased membrane excitability. Calcium antagonizes this membrane effect of hyperkalemia, although how this is achieved is not well understood [286].

The protective effect of calcium begins within minutes but is relatively short-lived. As a result, calcium infusions are indicated only for severe hyperkalemia, when it is potentially dangerous to wait the 30 to 60 minutes for insulin and glucose or sodium bicarbonate to act. The usual dose is 10 mL (1 ampul) of a 10% calcium gluconate solution infused slowly over 2 to 3 minutes with constant cardiac monitoring. This dose can be repeated after 5 minutes if the ECG changes persist.

Calcium should not be given in bicarbonate-containing solutions, since this can lead to the precipitation of calcium carbonate. Calcium should be administered only when absolutely necessary (as with loss of P waves or widening of the QRS complex) in patients taking digitalis, since hypercalcemia can induce digitalis toxicity.

Insulin and glucose. Increasing the availability of insulin lowers the plasma potassium concentration by driving potassium into the cells, apparently by enhancing the activity of the Na/K ATPase pump in skeletal muscle [155]. Hyperinsulinemia can be induced in either by giving insulin (with glucose to prevent hypoglycemia) or by the intravenous administration of glucose (50 mL of a 50% glucose solution), which will rapidly enhance endogenous insulin secretion. Glucose alone may produce a smaller rise in the plasma insulin concentration and a lesser reduction in plasma potassium concentration than the insulin plus glucose regimen [279]. Effective therapy usually leads to a 0.5 to 1.5 mEq per liter fall in the plasma potassium concentration. This effect begins in 15 minutes, peaks at 60 minutes, and lasts for several hours [289,290]. Although patients with renal failure are resistant to the glycemic effect of insulin, they are not resistant to the hypokalemic effect, as Na/K ATPase activity is still enhanced [291,292].

Exogenous insulin can induce symptomatic hypoglycemia unless adequate glucose is given concurrently [289]. If, for example, 10 units of regular insulin is given with 25 g of glucose, the plasma glucose concentration may fall below 55 mg/dL in as many as 75% of initially normoglycemic patients [289]. Increasing the initial glucose dose to 40 g followed by a continuous dextrose infusion generally prevents this problem [278,289].

Proper therapy in diabetic patients varies with the plasma glucose concentration. Both insulin and glucose should be given when the plasma glucose concentration is normal or mildly elevated, since endogenous insulin release is impaired. Insulin in this case both reduces the plasma potassium concentration directly and prevents a rise in the plasma glucose concentration that can exacerbate the hyperkalemia by solvent drag (the rise in plasma osmolality pulls water and secondarily potassium out of the cells) [228]. In comparison, insulin alone is sufficient if the patient is already hyperglycemic.

Sodium bicarbonate. Raising the systemic pH with sodium bicarbonate results in hydrogen ion release from the cells (as part of the buffering reaction); this change is accompanied by potassium movement into the cells to maintain electroneutrality. In addition, the elevation in the plasma bicarbonate concentration appears to have a direct effect on lowering the plasma potassium concentration (via an unknown mechanism) that is independent of pH [154].

The potassium-lowering action of sodium bicarbonate is most prominent in patients with metabolic acidosis and begins within 30 to 60 minutes and persists for several hours. Sodium bicarbonate should not be used as the only therapy in patients with advanced renal failure, since it generally produces little acute reduction in the plasma potassium concentration (other than that due to dilution by the associated volume expansion) [290,293]. Insulin plus glucose and a β2 agonist are more predictably effective in this setting [278].

The usual dose is 45 mEq (1 ampul of a 7.5% sodium bicarbonate solution) infused slowly over 5 minutes; this dose can be repeated in 30 minutes if necessary. Alternatively, sodium bicarbonate can be added to a glucose and saline solution. This regimen may have an additional advantage in hyponatremic patients, since raising the plasma sodium concentration with this hypertonic solution can also reverse the electrocardiographic effects of hyperkalemia. Both an increase in the rate of membrane depolarization and a fall in the plasma potassium concentration by dilution may contribute to this effect [294]. These sodium containing solutions should be used with extreme caution in edematous patients with advanced heart failure or renal failure. In these patients, 50 mL of a 50% glucose solution (and insulin if necessary) plus small doses of sodium bicarbonate (45 to 90 mEq) can be infused slowly.

β2-adrenergic agonists. Like insulin, the β2-adrenergic agonists drive potassium into the cells by increasing Na/K ATPase activity [222]. As a result, these drugs can be effectively used in the acute treatment of hyperkalemia. Albuterol (20 mg in 4 mL of saline by nasal inhalation over 10 minutes or 0.5 mg by intravenous infusion) or epinephrine (0.05 mg/kg per minute by intraveous infusion) can lower the plasma potassium concentration by 0.5 to 1.5 mEq per liter within 30 to 60 minutes [278,289,290]. Furthermore, the effect of these agents is additive to that of insulin plus glucose [289].

Patients with end-stage renal disease generally show a blunted hypokalemic response to epinephrine but not albuterol [290,295]. This difference appears to be related to the α-adrenergic (as well as β2-adrenergic) activity of epinephrine. The α-receptors tend to cause potassium movement out of, not into, the cells; for reasons that are unclear, patients with renal failure show increased response to the alpha effect, thereby limiting or even preventing any fall in the plasma potassium concentration [295].

The only side effects of the β2 agonists are mild tachycardia and the possible induction of angina in susceptible subjects. Thus, these agents should probably be avoided in patients with known active coronary disease.

Loop or thiazide diuretics. The above modalities only transiently lower the plasma potassium concentration; therefore, additional therapy is required to remove potassium from the body. Although this can easily be achieved in normal subjects with loop and thiazide diuretics, patients with persistent hyperkalemia typically have an abnormality in renal potassium secretion and are unlikely to have a good response to diuretic therapy.

Cation exchange resin. The major cation exchange resin available is sodium polystyrene sulfonate (Kayexalate), prepared in the sodium phase. In the gut, this resin takes up potassium (and calcium and magnesium to lesser degrees) and releases sodium. Each gram of resin may bind as much as 1 mEq of potassium and release 1 to 2 mEq of sodium [285]. Thus, a potential side effect is exacerbation of edema due to sodium retention.

The resin can be given either orally or as a retention enema. The oral dose is usually 20 g given with 100 mL of a 20% sorbitol solution to prevent constipation. This can be repeated every 4 to 6 hours as necessary. Lower doses (5 to 10 g with meals) are generally well tolerated (no nausea or constipation) and can be used to control chronic mild hyperkalemia in patients with renal insufficiency.

When given as an enema, 50 g of resin is mixed with 50 mL

of 70% sorbitol plus 100 to 150 mL of tap water. This solution should be kept in the colon for at least 30 to 60 minutes and preferably for 2 to 3 hours. Each enema can lower the plasma potassium concentration by as much as 0.5 to 1 mEq per liter and can be repeated every 2 to 4 hours.

Intestinal necrosis is an occasional occurrence, particularly when Kayexalate is given orally with sorbitol within the first week after surgery [296,297]. Why this occurs is not clear; it is possible that postoperative ileus plays an important role by increasing the duration of drug contact with the intestinal mucosa [296]. Cleansing enemas given before and after Kayexalate enemas may be protective by preventing drug retention in the intestinal lumen [297].

Dialysis. Dialysis can be used if the conservative measures listed above are ineffective, if the hyperkalemia is severe, or if the patient has marked tissue breakdown and is releasing large amounts of potassium from the injured cells [290]. Hemodialysis is preferred in the last two settings, since the rate of potassium removal is many times faster than with peritoneal dialysis [298].

References

1. Gabow P: Ethylene glycol intoxication. *Am J Kidney Dis* 11:277, 1988.
2. Rose B: Hypoosmolal states—hyponatremia, in *Clinical Physiology of Acid-Base and Electrolyte Disorders*. New York, McGraw-Hill, 1989, p 601.
3. Laragh J: The effect of potassium chloride on hyponatremia. *J Clin Invest* 33:807, 1954.
4. Fichman M, Vorherr H, Kleeman C, et al: Diuretic-induced hyponatremia. *Ann Intern Med* 75:853, 1971.
5. Black R: Diagnosis and management of hyponatremia. *J Intensive Care Med* 4:205, 1989.
6. Herbert S, Reeves W, Molony D, et al: The medullary thick limb: Function and modulation of the single effect multiplier. *Kidney Int* 31:580, 1987.
7. Ellison D, Velazquez H, Wright F: Thiazide-sensitive sodium chloride cotransport in early distal tubule. *Am J Physiol* 253, 1987.
8. Robertson G: Thirst and vasopressin function in normal and disordered states of water balance. *J Lab Clin Med* 101:351, 1983.
9. Schrier R: Pathogenesis of sodium and water retention in high-output and low-output cardiac failure, nephrotic syndrome, cirrhosis, and pregnancy. *N Engl J Med* 319:1065, 1988.
10. Brown D: Membrane recycling and epithelial cell function. *Am J Physiol* 256:F1, 1989.
11. Schrier R: An odyssey into the milieu intérieur. Pondering enigmas. *J Am Soc Nephrol* 2:1549, 1992.
12. Ashouri O: Severe diuretic-induced hyponatremia in the elderly. *Arch Intern Med* 146:1355, 1986.
13. Friedman E, Shadel M, Halkin H, et al: Thiazide-induced hyponatremia. Reproducibility by a single dose rechallenge and an analysis of pathogenesis. *Ann Intern Med* 110:24, 1989.
14. Skowsky W, Kikuchi T: The role of vasopressin in the impaired water excretion of myxedema. *Am J Med* 64:613, 1978.
15. Linas S, Berl T, Robertson G, et al: Role of vasopressin in impaired water excretion of glucocorticoid deficiency. *Kidney Int* 18:58, 1980.
16. Iwasaki Y, Oiso Y, Yamauchi K, et al: Osmoregulation of plasma vasopressin in myxedema. *J Clin Endocrinol Metab* 70:534, 1990.
17. Klingbeil C, Keil L, Chang D, et al: Effects of CRF and ANG II on ACTH and vasopressin release in conscious dogs. *Am J Physiol* 255:E46, 1988.
18. Oelkers W: Hyponatremia and inappropriate secretion of vasopressin (antidiuretic hormone) in patients with hypopituitarism. *N Engl J Med* 321:492, 1989.
19. Davison J, Shiells E, Philips P, et al: Serial evaluation of vasopressin release in human pregnancy. Role of human chorionic gonadotropin in the osmoregulatory changes of gestation. *J Clin Invest* 81:798, 1988.
20. Vitting K, Gardenswartz M, Zabatekis P, et al: Frequency of hyponatremia and nonosmolar vasopressin release in the acquired immune deficiency syndrome. *JAMA* 263:973, 1990.
21. Glassock R, Cohen A, Danovitch G, et al: Human immunodeficiency virus (HIV) infection and the kidney. *Ann Intern Med* 112:35, 1990.
22. Tanneau R, Pennec Y, Jouquan J, et al: Cerebral salt-wasting in elderly patients. *Ann Intern Med* 107:120, 1987.
23. Ganong C, Kappy M: Cerebral salt wasting in children. The need for recognition and treatment. *Am J Dis Child* 147:167, 1993.
24. Ishikawa S, Saito T, Kaneko K, et al: Hyponatremia responsive to fludrocortisone acetate in elderly patients after head injury. *Ann Intern Med* 106:187, 1987.
25. Illowsky B, Kirch D: Polydipsia and hyponatremia in psychotic patients. *Am J Psychiatr* 145:675, 1988.
26. Jose C, Perez-Cruet J: Incidence and morbidity of self-induced water intoxication in state mental hospital patients. *Am J Psychiatry* 136:221, 1979.
27. Vieweg W, Godleski L, Graham P, et al: Abnormal diurnal weight gain among long-term patients with schizophrenic disorders. *Schizophrenia Res* 1:67, 1988.
28. Goldman M, Luchins D, Robertson G: Mechanisms of altered water metabolism in psychotic patients with polydipsia and hyponatremia. *N Engl J Med* 318:397, 1988.
29. Vieweg W, Hundley P, Godelski L, et al: Diurnal weight gain as a predictor of serum sodium concentration among patients with psychosis, intermittent hyponatremia, and polydipsia. *Psychiatr Res* 26:305, 1988.
30. Thompson C, Edwards C, Baylis P: Osmotic and non-osmotic regulation of thirst and vasopressin secretion in patients with compulsive water drinking. *Clin Endocrinol (Oxford)* 35:221, 1991.
31. Thompson C, Selby P, Baylis P: Reproducibility of osmotic and nonosmotic tests of vasopressin secretion in men. *Am J Physiol* 260:R533, 1991.
32. Goldman M, Blake L, Marks R, et al: Association of nonsuppression of cortisol on the DST with primary polydipsia in chronic schizophrenia. *Am J Psychiatr* 150:653, 1993.
33. Rao K, Miller M, Moses A: Water intoxication and thioridazine. *Ann Intern Med* 82:61, 1975.
34. Gillum D, Linas S: Water intoxication in a psychotic patient with normal water excretion. *Am J Med* 77:773, 1984.
35. Hariprasad M, Eisinger R, Nadler I, et al: Hyponatremia in psychogenic polydipsia. *Arch Intern Med* 140:1639, 1980.
36. Dubovsky S, Grabon S, Berl T, et al: Syndrome of inappropriate secretion of antidiuretic hormone with exacerbated psychosis. *Ann Intern Med* 79:551, 1973.
37. Levine S, McManus B, Blackbourne B, et al: Fatal water intoxication, schizophrenia, and diuretic therapy for systemic hypertension. *Am J Med* 82:153, 1987.
38. Alexander R, Karp B, Thompson S, et al: A double blind, placebo-controlled trial of demeclocycline treatment of polydipsia-hyponatremia in chronically psychotic patients. *Biol Psychiatr* 30:417, 1991.
39. Lee H, Kwon K, Alphs L, et al: Effect of clozapine on psychogenic polydipsia in chronic schizophrenia (letter). *J Clin Psychopharmocol* 11:222, 1991.
40. Weisberg L: Pseudohyponatremia: A reappraisal. *Am J Med* 86:315, 1984.
41. Sunderrajan S, Bauer J, Vopat R, et al: Posttransurethral prostatic resection hyponatremic syndrome: Case report and review of the literature. *Ann J Kidney Dis* 4:80, 1984.
42. Editorial: Monitoring TURP. *Lancet* 338:606, 1991.
43. Campbell H, Fincher M, Sklar A: Severe hyponatremia without severe hypoosmolality following transurethral resection of the prostate (TURP) in end-stage renal disease. *Am J Kidney Dis* 12:152, 1988.
44. Hahn R: Relations between irrigant absorption rate and hyponatremia during transurethral resection of the prostate. *Acta Anesthesiol Scand* 32:53, 1988.
45. Beirne G, Madsen P, Burns R: Serum electrolyte and osmolality changes following transurethral resection of the prostate. *J Urol* 93:83, 1965.
46. Ryder K, Olson J, Kahnoski R, et al: Hyperammonemia after trans-

urethral resection of the prostate: A report of 2 cases. *J Urol* 132:995, 1984.

47. Bernstein G, Loughlin K, Gittes R: The physiologic basis of the TUR syndrome. *J Surg Res* 46:135, 1989.

48. Hahn R: Prevention of TUR syndrome by detection of trace ethanol in expired breath. *Anaesthesia* 45:577, 1990.

49. Katz M: Hyperglycemia-induced hyponatremia: Calculation of expected serum sodium depression. *N Engl J Med* 289:843, 1973.

50. Rose B, Black R: *Manual of Clinical Problems in Nephrology.* Boston, Little, Brown, 1988, p 3.

51. Strange K: Regulation of solute and water balance and cell volume in the central nervous system. *J Am Soc Nephrol* 3:12, 1992.

52. Ayus J, Wheeler J, Arieff A: Postoperative hyponatremic encephalopathy in menstruant woman. *Ann Intern Med* 117:891, 1992.

53. Cluitmans F, Meinders A: Management of severe hyponatremia: Rapid or slow correction. *Am J Med* 88:161, 1990.

53a. Berl T: Treating hyponatremia: Damned if we do and damned if we don't. *Kidney Int* 37:1006, 1990.

54. Melton J, Patlak C, Pettigrew D, et al: Volume regulatory loss of Na, Cl, and K from rat brain during acute hyponatremia. *Am J Physiol* 252:F661, 1987.

55. Lien V, Shapiro, J, Chan L: Study of brain electrolytes and osmolytes during correction of chronic hyponatremia. Implications for the pathogenesis of central pontine myelinolysis. *J Clin Invest* 88:303, 1991.

56. Verbalis J, Gullans S: Hyponatremia causes sustained reductions in brain content of multiple organic osmolytes in rats. *Brain Res* 567:274, 1991.

57. Chung H-M, Lluge R, Schier R, et al: Clinical assessment of extracellular fluid volume in hyponatremia. *Am J Med* 83:905, 1987.

58. Graber M, Corish D: The electrolytes in hyponatremia. *Am J Kidney Dis* 18:527, 1991.

59. Beck L: Hypouricemia in the syndrome of inappropriate secretion of antidiuretic hormone. *N Engl J Med* 301:528, 1979.

60. Oh M, Uribarri J, Barrido D, et al: Danger of central pontine myelinolysis in hypotonic dehydration and recommendation for treatment. *Am J Med Sci* 298:41, 1989.

61. Kamel K, Bear R: Treatment of hyponatremia: A quantitative analysis. *Am J Kidney Dis* 21:439, 1993.

62. Cheng J, Zikos D, Skopicki H, et al: Long-term neurologic outcome in psychogenic water drinkers with severe symptomatic hyponatremia: The effect of rapid correction. *Am J Med* 88:561, 1990.

63. Berl T: Treating hyponatremia: Damned if we do and damned if we don't *Kidney Int* 37:1006, 1990.

64. Sterns R: Severe symptomatic hyponatremia: Treatment and outcome. A study of 64 cases. *Ann Intern Med* 107:656, 1987.

65. Sterns R: The treatment of hyponatremia: First, do no harm. *Am J Med* 88:557, 1990.

66. Soupart A, Penninckx R, Stenuit A, et al: Treatment of chronic hyponatremia in rats by intravenous saline: Comparison of rate versus magnitude of correction. *Kidney Int* 41:1662, 1992.

67. Rose B: New approach to disturbances in the plasma sodium concentration. *Am J Med* 81:1033, 1986.

68. Rose B: *Clinical Physiology of Acid-Base and Electrolyte Disorders.* 4th ed. New York, McGraw-Hill, 1994, p 669.

69. Brunner J, Redmond J, Haggar A, et al: Central pontine myelinolysis and pontine lesions after rapid correction of hyponatremia: A prospective magnetic resonance imaging study. *Ann Neurol* 27:61, 1990.

70. Sterns R, Thomas D, Herndon R: Brain dehydration and neurologic deterioration after correction of hyponatremia. *Kidney Int* 35:69, 1989.

71. Tanneau R, Bourbigot B, Rouhart F, et al: High incidence of neurologic complications following rapid correction of severe hyponatremia in psychogenic water drinkers (abstract). *Kidney Int* 44:471, 1993.

72. Soupart A, Penninckx R, Stenuit A, et al: Prevention of brain demyelination after excessive correction of chronic hyponatremia in rats by excessive serum sodium lowering (abstract). *J Am Soc Nephrol* 3:329, 1992.

73. Sterns R, Silver S: Hemodialysis in hyponatremia: Is there a risk? *Semin Dial* 3:3, 1990.

74. Rose B: *Clinical Physiology of Acid-Base and Electrolyte Disorders.* 4th ed. New York, McGraw-Hill, 1994, p 681.

75. Forrest J Jr, Cox M, Hong C, et al: Superiority of demeclocycline over lithium in the treatment of chronic syndrome of inappropriate secretion of antidiuretic hormone. *N Engl J Med* 298:173, 1978.

76. Decaux G, Brimioulle S, Genette F, et al: Treatment of the syndrome of inappropriate secretion of antidiuretic hormone by urea. *Am J Med* 69:99, 1980.

77. Decaux G, Prospert F, Penninckx R, et al: 5-year treatment of the chronic syndrome of inappropriate secretion of antidiuretic hormone with oral urea. *Nephron* 63:468, 1993.

78. Hill A, Uribarri J, Mann J, et al: Altered water metabolism in tuberculosis. Role of vasopressin. *Am J Med* 88:357, 1990.

79. Robertson G, Aycinena P, Zerbe R: Neurogenic disorders of osmoregulation. *Am J Med* 72:339, 1982.

79a. Lindheimer MD, Barron WM, Davison JM: Osmoregulation of thirst and vasopressin release in pregnancy. *Am J Physiol* 257:F503, 1989.

80. Oster J, Materson B: Renal and electrolyte complications of congestive heart failure and effects of treatment with angiotensin-converting enzyme inhibitors. *Arch Intern Med* 152:704, 1992.

81. Dzau V, Hollenberg N: Renal response to captopril in severe heart failure: Role of furosemide in natriuresis and reversal of hyponatremia. *Ann Intern Med* 100:777, 1984.

82. Riegger G, Kochsiek K: Vasopressin, renin and norepinephrine levels before and after captopril administration in patients with congestive heart failure due to dilated cardiomyopathy. *Am J Cardiol* 58:300, 1986.

83. Rouse D, Dalmeida W, Williamson F, et al: Captopril inhibits the hydroosmotic effect of ADH in the cortical collecting tubule. *Kidney Int* 32:845, 1987.

84. Miller P, Linas S, Schrier R: Plasma demeclocycline levels and nephrotoxicity: Correlation in hyponatremic cirrhotic patient. *JAMA* 243:2513, 1980.

85. Papadakis M, Fraser C, Arieff A: Hyponatraemia in patients with cirrhosis. *Q J Med* 76:675, 1990.

86. Rose B: *Clinical Physiology of Acid-Base and Electrolyte Disorders.* 4th ed. New York, McGraw-Hill, 1994, p 698.

87. Robertson G: Abnormalities of thirst regulation. *Kidney Int* 25:460, 1984.

88. Snyder N, Feigal D, Arieff A: Hypernatremia in elderly patients. A heterogeneous, morbid, and iatrogenic entity. *Ann Intern Med* 107:309, 1987.

89. Phillips P, Bretherton M, Johnston C, et al: Reduced osmotic thirst in healthy elderly men. *Am J Physiol* 261:R166, 1991.

90. Shiau Y, Feldman G, Resnick M, et al: Stool electrolyte and osmolality measurements in the evaluation of diarrheal disorders. *Ann Intern Med* 102:773, 1985.

91. Nelson D, McGrew W, Hoyumpa A: Hypernatremia and lactulose therapy. *JAMA* 249:1295, 1983.

92. Allerton J, Strom J: Hypernatremia due to repeated doses of charcoal sorbitol. *Am J Kidney Dis* 17:581, 1991.

93. Gipstein R, Boyle J: Hypernatremia complicating prolonged mannitol diuresis. *N Engl J Med* 272:1116, 1965.

94. Gault M, Dixon M, Doyle M, et al: Hypernatremia, azotemia, and dehydration due to high-protein tube feeding. *Ann Intern Med* 68:778, 1968.

95. Pizzarro D, Castillo B, Posada G, et al: Efficacy comparison of oral rehydration solutions containing 90 or 75 millimoles of sodium per liter. *Pediatrics* 79:190, 1987.

96. Thompson C, Baylis P: Thirst in diabetes insipidus: Clinical relevance of quantitative assessment. *Q J Med* 65:853, 1987.

97. McIver B, Connacher A, Whittle I, et al: Adipsic hypothalamic diabetes insipidus after clipping of anterior communicating artery aneurysm. *BJM* 303:1465, 1991.

98. Hammond D, Moll G, Robertson F, et al: Hypodipsic hypernatremia with normal osmoregulation of vasopressin. *N Engl J Med* 315:433, 1986.

99. DeRubertis F, Michelis M, Beck N, et al: Essential hypernatremia due to ineffective osmotic and intact volume regulation of vasopressin secretion. *J Clin Invest* 50:97, 1971.

100. DeRubertis F, Michelis M, Davis B: Essential hypernatremia. *Arch Intern Med* 134:889, 1974.

101. Miller N, Finberg L: Peritoneal dialysis for salt poisoning. *N Engl J Med* 263:1347, 1960.

102. Meadow R: Non-accidental salt poisoning. *Arch Dis Child* 68:448, 1993.
103. Mattar J, Weil M, Shubin H, et al: Cardiac arrest in the critically ill. II. Hyperosmolal states following cardiac arrest. *Am J Med* 56:162, 1974.
104. Moder K, Hurley D: Fatal hypernatremia from exogenous salt intake: Report of a case and review of the literature. *Mayo Clin Proc* 65:1587, 1990.
105. Rose B: *Clinical Physiology of Acid-Base and Electrolyte Disorders.* 4th ed. New York, McGraw-Hill, 1994, p 669.
106. Pollack A, Arieff A: Abnormalities of cell volume regulation and their functional consequences. *Am J Physiol* 239:F195, 1980.
107. Pullen R, DePasquale M, Cserr H: Bulk flow of cerebrospinal fluid into brain in response to acute hyperosmolality. *Am J Physiol* 253:F538, 1987.
108. Heilig C, Stromski M, Blumenfeld J, et al: Characterization of the major brain osmolytes that accumulate in salt-loaded rats. *Am J Physiol* 257:F1108, 1989.
109. Lien Y, Shapiro J, Chan L: Effect of hypernatremia on organic brain osmoles. *J Clin Invest* 85:1427, 1990.
110. Paredes A, McManus M, Kwon H, et al: Osmoregulation of Na$^+$-inositol cotransporter activity and mRNA levels in brain glial cells. *Am J Physiol* 263:C1282, 1992.
111. Somero G: Protons, osmolytes, and fitness of internal milieu for protein function. *Am J Physiol* 251:R197, 1986.
112. Hogan G, Dodge P, Gill S, et al: Pathogenesis of seizures occurring during restoration of plasma tonicity to normal in animals previously chronically hypernatremic. *Pediatrics* 43:54, 1969.
113. Morrison R, Strange K: Mechanism of osmoregulatory inositol loss in brain glial cells (abstract). *J Am Soc Nephrol* 3:832, 1992.
114. Rose B: *Clinical Physiology of Acid-Base and Electrolyte disorders.* 4th ed. New York, McGraw-Hill, 1994, p 712.
115. Rose B: *Clinical Physiology of Acid-Base and Electrolyte Disorders.* 4th ed. New York, McGraw-Hill, 1994, p 698.
116. Holzman E, Harris H Jr, Kolakowski L Jr, et al: Brief report: A molecular defect in the vasopressin V2-receptor gene causing nephrogenic diabetes insipidus. *N Engl J Med* 328:1534, 1993.
117. Boton R, Gaviria, M, Batlle D: Prevalence pathogenesis, and treatment of renal dysfunction associated with chronic lithium therapy. *Am J Kidney Dis* 10:329, 1987.
118. Cogan E, Svoboda M, Abramow M: Mechanisms of lithium-vasopressin interaction in rabbit cortical collecting tubule. *Ann J Physiol* 252:F1080, 1987.
119. Berl T: The cyclic AMP system in vasopressin-sensitive nephron segments of the vitamin D-treated rat. *Kidney Int* 31:1065, 1987.
120. Miller M, Kalkos T, Moses A, et al: Recognition of partial defects in antidiuretic hormone secretion. *Ann Intern Med* 73:721, 1970.
121. Zerbe R, Robertson G: A comparison of plasma vasopressin measurements with a standard indirect test in the differential diagnosis of polyuria. *N Engl J Med* 305:1539, 1981.
122. Howards S: Post-obstructive diuresis: A misunderstood phenomenon. *J Urol* 110:537, 1973.
123. Bishop M: Diuresis and renal functional recovery in chronic retention. *Br J Urol* 57:1, 1985.
124. Flis R, Scoblionco D, Bastl C, et al: Dopamine-related polyuria in patients with gram-negative infection. *Arch Intern Med* 137:1547, 1977.
125. Merrill D, Skelton M, Cowley A Jr: Humoral control of water and electrolyte excretion during water restriction. *Kidney Int* 29:1152, 1986.
126. Kahn A, Brachet E, Blum D: Controlled fall in natremia and risk of seizures in hypertonic dehydration. *Intensive Care Med* 5:27, 1979.
127. Blum D, Brasseur D, Kahn A, et al: Safe oral rehydration of hypertonic dehydration. *J Pediatr Gastroenterol Nutrition* 5:232, 1986.
128. Richardson D, Robinson A: Desmopressin. *Ann Intern Med* 103:228, 1985.
129. Webster B, Bain J: Antidiuretic effect and complications of chlorpropamide therapy in diabetes insipidus. *J Clin Endocrinol Metab* 30:215, 1970.
130. Rado J: Combination of carbamazepine and chlorpropamide in the treatment of "hyporesponder" pituitary diabetes insipidus. *J Clin Endocrinol Metab* 38:1, 1974.
131. Welch W, Ott C, Lorenz J, et al: Effects of chlorpropamide on loop of Henle function and plasma renin. *Kidney Int* 30:712, 1986.
132. Rocha A, Ping W, Kudo L: Effect of chlorpropamide on water and urea transport in the inner medullary collecting duct. *Kidney Int* 39:79, 1991.
133. Wales J: Treatment of diabetes insipidus with carbamazepine. *Lancet* 2:948, 1975.
134. Moses A, Howanitz J, van Gemmert M, et al: Clofibrate-induced antidiuresis. *J Clin Invest* 52:535, 1973.
135. Gold P, Robertson G, Ballenger J, et al: Carbamazepine diminishes the sensitivity of the plasma arginine vasopressin response to osmotic stimulation. *J Clin Endocrinol Metab* 57:952, 1983.
136. Rose B: *Clinical Physiology of Acid-Base and Electrolyte Disorders.* 4th ed. New York, McGraw-Hill, 1994, p 702.
137. Earley L, Orloff J: The mechanism of antidiuresis associated with the administration of hydrochlorothiazide to patients with vasopressin-resistant diabetes insipidus. *J Clin Invest* 41:1988, 1952.
138. Libber S, Harrison H, Spector D: Treatment of nephrogenic diabetes insipidus with prostaglandin synthesis inhibitors. *J Pediatr* 108:305, 1986.
139. Monnens L, Jonkman A, Thomas C: Response to indomethacin and hydrochlorothiazide in nephrogenic diabetes insipidus. *Clin Sci* 66:709, 1984.
140. Allen H, Jackson R, Winchester M: Indomethacin in the treatment of lithium-induced nephrogenic diabetes insipidus. *Arch Intern Med* 149:1123, 1989.
141. Batlle D, von Riotte A, Gaviria M, et al: Amelioration of polyuria by amiloride in patients receiving long-term lithium therapy. *N Engl J Med* 312:408, 1985.
142. Knores N, Monnens L: Amiloride-hydrochlorothiazide versus indomethacin-hydrochlorothiazide in the treatment of nephrogenic diabetes insipidus. *J Pediatr* 117:499, 1990.
143. Berl T, Raz A, Wald H, et al: Prostaglandin synthesis inhibition and the action of vasopressin: Studies in man and rat. *Am J Physiol* 232:F529, 1977.
144. Stokes J: Integrated actions of renal medullary prostaglandins in the control of water excretion. *Am J Physiol* 240:F471, 1981.
145. Stasior D, Kikeri D, Duel B, et al: Nephrogenic diabetes insipidus responsive to indomethacin plus dDAVP (letter). *N Engl J Med* 324:850, 1991.
146. Brown R: Extrarenal potassium homeostasis. *Kidney Int* 30:116, 1986.
147. Clausen T, Flatman J: Effect of insulin and epinephrine on Na$^+$-K$^+$-ATPase and glucose transport in soleus muscle. *Am J Physiol* 252:F492, 1987.
148. Schnack C, Podolsky A, Watzke H, et al: Effects of somatostatin and oral potassium administration on terbutaline-induced hypokalemia. *Am Rev Respir Dis* 139:176, 1989.
149. Wright F: Renal potassium handling. *Semin Nephrol* 7:174, 1987.
150. Stanton B: Regulation of Na$^+$ and K$^+$ transport by mineralocorticoids. *Semin Nephrol* 7:82, 1987.
151. Squires R, Huth E: Experimental potassium depletion in normal human subjects: I. Relation of ionic intakes to the renal conservation of potassium. *J Clin Invest* 38:1134, 1959.
152. Amatruda J, Biddle T, Patton M, et al: Vigorous supplementation of a hypocaloric diet prevents cardiac arrhythmias and mineral depletion. *Am J Med* 74:1016, 1983.
153. Adrogu H, Madias N: Changes in plasma potassium concentration during acute acid-base disturbances. *Am J Med* 71:456, 1981.
154. Fraley D, Adler S: Correction of hyperkalemia by bicarbonate despite constant blood pH. *Kidney Int* 12:354, 1977.
155. Ferrannini E, Taddei S, Santoro D, et al: Independent stimulation of glucose metabolism and Na$^+$-K$^+$ exchange by insulin in the human forearm. *Am J Physiol* 255:E953, 1988.
156. Adrogu H, Lederer E, Suki W, et al: Determinants of plasma potassium levels in diabetic ketoacidosis. *Medicine (Baltimore)* 65:163, 1986.
157. Kunin A, Surawicz B, Sims E: Decrease in serum potassium concentration and appearance of cardiac arrhythmias during infusion of potassium with glucose in potassium-depleted patients. *N Engl J Med* 266:228, 1962.
158. Brown M, Brown D, Murphy M: Hypokalemia from beta 2-receptor stimulation by circulating epinephrine. *N Engl J Med* 309:1414, 1983.

159. Morgan D, Young R: Acute transient hypokalemia: New interpretation of a common event. *Lancet* 2:751, 1982.

160. Shannon M, Lovejoy F Jr: Hypokalemia after theophylline intoxication. The effects of acute vs chronic poisoning. *Arch Intern Med* 149:2725, 1989.

161. Lipworth B, McDevitt D, Struthers A: Prior treatment with diuretic augments the hypokalemic and electrocardiographic effects of inhaled albuterol. *Am J Med* 86:653, 1989.

162. Wong C, Pavord I, Williams J, et al: Bronchodilator, cardiovascular, and hypokalaemic effects of fenoterol, salbutamol, and terbutaline in asthma. *Lancet* 336:1396, 1990.

163. Goldenberg I, Olivari M, Levine T, et al: Effect of dobutamine on plasma potassium in congestive heart failure secondary to idiopathic or ischemic cardiomyopathy. *Am J Cardiol* 63:843, 1989.

164. Reid J, Whyte K, Struthers A: Epinephrine-induced hypokalemia: The role of beta adrenoceptors. *Ann J Cardiol* 57:23F, 1986.

165. Pearson C, Kalyanaraman K: Periodic paralysis, In Stanbury J, Wyngaarden J (eds): *The Metabolic Basis of Inherited Disease.* 3rd ed. New York, McGraw-Hill, 1972.

166. Ober K: Thyrotoxic periodic paralysis in the United States. Report of seven cases and review of the literature. *Medicine (Baltimore)* 71:109, 1992.

167. Chan A, Shinde R, Cockram C, et al: In vivo and in vitro sodium pump activity in subjects with thyrotoxic periodic paralysis. *Br Med J* 303:1096, 1991.

167a. Ptacek LJ, Tawil R, Griggs RC, et al: Dihydropyridine receptor mutations cause hypokalemic periodic paralysis. *Cell* 77:863, 1994.

168. Lawson D, Murray R, Parker J: Early mortality in the megaloblastic anaemias. *Q J Med* 41:1, 1972.

169. Viens P, Thyss A, Garnier G, et al: GM-CSF treatment of hypokalemia (letter). *Ann Intern Med* 111:236, 1989.

170. Adams P, Woodhouse K, Adela M, et al: Exaggerated hypokalemia in acute myeloid leukaemia. *Br Med J* 282:1034, 1981.

171. Schaller M, Fischer A, Perret C: Hyperkalemia: A Prognostic factor during acute severe hypothermia. *JAMA* 264:1842, 1990.

172. Kassirer J, Schwartz W: The response of normal man to selective depletion of hydrochloric acid: Factors in the genesis of persistent gastric alkalosis. *Am J Med* 40:10, 1966.

173. Rose B: *Clinical Physiology of Acid-Base and Electrolyte Disorders.* 4th ed. New York, McGraw-Hill, 1994, p 333.

174. Stanton B: Renal potassium transport: Morphological and functional adaptations. *Am J Physiol* 257:R989, 1989.

175. Young D: Quantitative analysis of aldosterone's role in potassium regulation. *Am J Physiol* 255:F811, 1988.

176. Mohr J, Clark R, Waack T, et al: Nafcillin-associated hypokalemia. *JAMA* 242:544, 1979.

177. Carlisle E, Donnelly S, Vasuvattakul S, et al: Glue-sniffing and distal renal tubular acidosis: Sticking to the facts. *J Am Soc Nephrol* 1:1019, 1991.

178. Carlisle E, Donnelly S, Ethier J, et al: Modulation of the secretion of potassium by accompanying anions in humans. *Kidney Int* 39:1206, 1991.

179. Whang R, Whang D, Ryan M: Refractory potassium depletion. A consequence of magnesium deficiency. *Arch Intern Med* 152:40, 1992.

179a. Nichols CG, Ho K, Hebert S: $Mg^{(2+)}$-dependent inward rectification of ROMK 1 potassium channels expressed in Xenopus oocytes. *J Physiol* 476:399, 1994.

180. Douglas J, Healy J: Nephrotoxic effects of amphotericin B, including renal tubular acidosis. *Am J Med* 46:154, 1969.

181. Aldinger K, Samann N: Hypokalemia with hypercalcemia: Prevalence and significance in treatment. *Ann Intern Med* 87:571, 1977.

182. Mir M, Brabin B, Tang O, et al: Hypokalaemia in acute myeloid leukaemia. *Ann Intern Med* 82:54, 1975.

183. Perazella M, Eisen R, Frederick W, et al: Renal failure and severe hypokalemia associated with acute myelomonocytic leukemia. *Am J Kidney Dis* 22:462, 1993.

184. Wrong W, Feest T, MacIver A: Immune-related potassium-losing interstitial nephritis: A comparison with distal renal tubular acidosis. *Q J Med* 86:513, 1993.

185. Knochel J, Cotin L, Hamburger R: Pathophysiology of intense physical conditioning in hot climate: I. Mechanism of potassium depletion. *J Clin Invest* 51:242, 1972.

186. Kosunen K, Pakarinen A: Plasma renin, angiotensin II, and plasma and urinary aldosterone in running exercise. *J Appl Physiol* 41:26, 1976.

187. Rostand S: Profound hypokalemia in continuous ambulatory peritoneal dialysis. *Arch Intern Med* 143:377, 1983.

188. Wiegand C, Davin T, Raij L, et al: Severe hypokalemia induced by hemodialysis. *Arch Intern Med* 141:167, 1981.

189. Helfant R: Hypokalemia and arrhythmias. *Am J Med* 80(suppl 4A):13, 1986.

190. Knochel J: Neuromuscular manifestations of electrolyte disorders. *Am J Med* 72:521, 1982.

191. Tillman C: Hypokalemic hypoventilation complicating severe diabetic ketoacidosis. *South Med J* 73:231, 1980.

192. Berl T, Linas S, Aisenbrey G, et al: On the mechanism of polyuria in potassium depletion. *J Clin Invest* 60:620, 1977.

193. Cheval L, Barlet-Bas C, Khadouri C, et al: K^+-ATPase-mediated Rb^+ transport in rat collecting tubule: Modulation during K^+ deprivation. *Am J Physiol* 260:F800, 1991.

194. Okuso M, Unwin R, Velazquez H, et al: Active potassium absorption by the renal distal tubule. *Am J Physiol* 262:F488, 1992.

195. Linas S, Peterson L, Anderson R, et al: Mechanism of renal potassium conservation in the rat. *Kidney Int* 15:601, 1979.

196. Light D, McCann F, Keller T, et al: Amiloride-sensitive cation channel in apical membrane of inner medullary collecting duct. *Am J Physiol* 255:F278, 1988.

197. Schwartz W, Relman A: Metabolic and renal studies in chronic potassium depletion resulting from overuse of laxatives. *J Clin Invest* 32:258, 1953.

198. Rose R: *Clinical Physiology of Acid-Base and Electrolyte Disorders.* New York, McGraw-Hill, 1989, p 722.

199. Bravo E, Tarazi R, Dustan H, et al: The changing clinical spectrum of primary aldosteronism. *Am J Med* 74:641, 1983.

200. Biglieri E: Spectrum of mineralocorticoid hypertension. *Hypertension* 17:251, 1991.

201. Kono T, Ikeda F, Oseko F, et al: Normotensive primary aldosteronism: Report of a case. *J Clin Endocrinol Metab* 52:1009, 1981.

202. Baruch D, Corvol P, Alhenc-Gelas F, et al: Diagnosis and treatment of renin-secreting tumors. Report of three cases. *Hypertension* 6:760, 1984.

203. Whitworth J: Mechanisms of glucocorticoid-induced hypertension. *Kidney Int* 31:1213, 1987.

204. Whorwood C, Sheppard M, Steward P: Licorice inhibits 11β-hydroxysteroid dehydrogenase message ribonucleic acid levels and potentiates glucocorticoid hormone action. *Endocrinology* 132:2287, 1993.

205. Nakada T, Koike H, Akiya T, et al: Liddle's syndrome, an uncommon form of hyporeninemic hypoaldosteronism: Functional and histopathological studies. *J Urol* 137:636, 1987.

206. Holland O, Brown H, Kuhnert L, et al: Further evaluation of saline infusion for the diagnosis of primary aldosteronism. *Hypertension* 6:717, 1984.

207. Kaplan N: Hypokalemia in the hypertensive patient, with observations on the incidence of primary aldosteronism. *Ann Intern Med* 66:1079, 1967.

208. Weinberger M, Fineberg N: The diagnosis of primary aldosteronism and separation of two major subtypes. *Arch Intern Med* 153:2125, 1993.

209. Gross M, Grekin R, Gniadek T, et al: Suppression of aldosterone by cyproheptadine in idiopathic aldosteronism. *N Engl J Med* 305:181, 1981.

210. Matsuoka H, Mulrow P, Franco-Saenz T, et al: Effects of β-lipotropin and β-lipotropin-derived peptides on aldosterone production in the rat adrenal gland. *J Clin Invest* 68:752, 1981.

211. Weinberger M: Primary aldosteronism: Diagnosis and differentiation of subtypes. *Ann Intern Med* 100:300, 1984.

212. Rich G, Ulick S, Cook S, et al: Glucocorticoid-remediable aldosteronism in a large kindred: Clinical spectrum and diagnosis using a characteristic biochemical phenotype. *Ann Intern Med* 116:813, 1992.

213. Radin D, Manoogian C, Nadler J: Diagnosis of primary hyperaldosteronism: Importance of correlating CT findings with endocrinologic studies. *Am J Roentgenol* 158:553, 1992.

214. Doppman J, McGill J, Miller D, et al: Distinction between hyperaldosteronism due to bilateral hyperplasia and unilateral aldosteronoma: Reliability of CT. *Radiology* 184:677, 1992.

215. Gross M, Shapiro B, Grekin R, et al: Scintigraphic localization of adrenal lesions in primary aldosteroinism. *Am J Med* 77:839, 1984.

216. Sterns R, Cox M, Feig P, et al: Internal potassium balance and the control of the plasma potassium concentration. *Medicine (Baltimore)* 60:339, 1981.

217. Villamil M, DeLand E, Henney R, et al: Anion effects on cation movements during correction of potassium depletion. *Am J Physiol* 229:161, 1975.

218. Schwartz W, van Ypersele de Strihou C, Kassirer J: Role of anions in metabolic alkalosis and potassium deficiency. *N Engl J Med* 279:630, 1968.

219. Sopko J, Freeman R: Salt substitutes as a source of potassium. *JAMA* 238:608, 1977.

220. Aselton P, Jick H: Short-term follow-up study of wax matrix potassium chloride in relation to gastrointestinal bleeding. *Lancet* 1:184, 1983.

221. Kopyt N, Dalal F, Narins R: Renal retention of potassium in fruit (letter). *N Engl J Med* 313:582, 1985.

222. Clausen T, Everts M: Regulation of the Na, K-pump in skeletal muscle. *Kidney Int* 35:1, 1989.

223. Shapiro W, Taubert K: Hypokalaemia and digoxin-induced arrhythmias. *Lancet* 2:604, 1975.

224. Dyckner T, Wester P-O, Widman L: Amiloride prevents thiazide-induced intracellular potassium and magnesium losses. *Acta Med Scand* 224:25, 1988.

225. Griffing G, Cole A, Aurecchia S, et al: Amiloride in primary hyperaldosteronism. *Clin Pharmacol Ther* 31:57, 1982.

226. Brown J, Davies D, Ferriss J, et al: Comparison of surgery and prolonged spironolactone therapy in patients with hypertension, aldosterone excess, and low plasma renin. *Br Med J* 2:729, 1972.

227. Keith N, Osterberg A, Burchell H: Some effects of potassium salts in man. *Ann Intern Med* 16:879, 1942.

228. Nicolis G, Kahn T, Sanchez A, et al: Glucose-induced hyperkalemia in diabetic subjects. *Arch Intern Med* 141:49, 1981.

229. Sterns R, Feig P, Pring M, et al: Disposition of intravenous potassium in anuric man: A Kinetic analysis. *Kidney Int* 15:651, 1979.

230. Abramson E, Arky R: Diabetic acidosis with initial hypokalemia. *JAMA* 196:401, 1966.

231. Kruse J, Carlson R: Rapid correction of hypokalemia using concentration intravenous potassium chloride infusions. *Arch Intern Med* 150:613, 1990.

232. Jackson C: Rapid renal potassium adaptation in rats. *Am J Physiol* 263:F1098, 1992.

233. Rabelink TJ, Koomans HA, Hene RJ, Dorhout Meese EJ: Early and late adjustment to potassium loading in humans. *Kidney Int* 38:942, 1990.

234. Garg L, Narang N: Renal adaptation to potassium in the adrenalectomized rabbit. Role of distal tubular sodium-potassium adenosine triphosphatase. *J Clin Invest* 76:1065, 1985.

235. Graber M, Subramani K, Copish D: Thrombocytosis elevates serum potassium. *Am J Kidney Dis* 12:116, 1988.

236. Chumbley L: Pseudohyperkalemia in acute myelocytic leukemia. *JAMA* 211:1007, 1970.

237. Conte G, Dal Canton A, Imperatore P, et al: Acute increase in plasma osmolality as a cause of hyperkalemia in patients with renal failure. *Kidney Int* 38:301, 1990.

238. Sharma A, Thiede H, Keller F: Somatostatin-induced hyperkalemia in a patient on maintenance hemodialysis. *Nephron* 59:445, 1991.

239. Arthur S, Greenberg A: Hyperkalemia associated with intravenous labetalol therapy for acute hypertension in renal transplant recipients. *Clin Nephrol* 33:269, 1990.

240. Daut J, Maiser-Rudolph W, von Beckerath N, et al: Hypoxic dilation of coronary arteries is mediated by ATP-sensitive potassium channels. *Science* 247:1341, 1990.

241. Struthers A, Quigley C, Brown M: Rapid changes in plasma potassium during a game of squash. *Clin Sci* 74:397, 1988.

242. Thomson A, Kelly D: Exercise stress-induced changes in systemic arterial potassium in angina pectoris. *Am J Cardiol* 63:1435, 1989.

243. Lindinger M, Heigenhauser G, McKelvie R: Blood ion regulation during repeated maximal exercise and recovery in humans. *Am J Physiol* 262:R126, 1992.

244. Knochel J, Blachley J, Johnson J, et al: Muscle cell electrical hyperpolarization and reduced exercise hyperkalemia in physically conditioned dogs. *J Clin Invest* 75:740, 1985.

245. Don B, Sebastian A, Cheitlin M, et al: Pseudohyperkalemia caused by fist clenching during phlebotomy. *N Engl J Med* (322), 1990.

246. Reza M, Kovick R, Shine K, et al: Massive intravenous digoxin overdosage. *N Engl J Med* 291:777, 1974.

247. Clausen T, Wang P, Orskov H, et al: Hyperkalemic periodic paralysis: relationship between changes in plasma water, electrolytes, insulin, and catecholamines during attacks. *J Clin Lab Invest* 40:211, 1980.

248. Rojas C, Wang J, Schwartz L, et al: A met-to-val mutation in the skeletal muscle Na$^+$ channel alpha-subunit in hyperkalemic periodic paralysis. *Nature* 354:387, 1991.

249. Bushinsky D, Gennari F: Life-threatening hyperkalemia induced by arginine. *Ann Intern Med* 89:632, 1978.

250. Rose B: *Clinical Physiology of Acid-Base and Electrolyte Disorders.* 4th ed. New York, McGraw-Hill, 1994, p 834.

251. Dubose T Jr, Good D: Chronic hyperkalemia impairs ammonium transport and accumulation in the inner medulla of the rat. *J Clin Invest* 90:1443, 1992.

252. DeFronzo R: Hyperkalemia in hyporeninemic hypoaldosteronism. *Kidney Int* 17:118, 1980.

253. Kifor I, Moore T, Fallo F, et al: Potassium-stimulated angiotensin release from superfused adrenal capsules and enzymatically digested cells of the zona glomerulosa. *Endocrinology* 129:823, 1991.

254. Lush D, King J, Fray J: Pathophysiology of low renin syndromes: Sites of renal secretory impairment and prorenin over expression. *Kidney Int* 43:983, 1993.

255. Clark B, Brown R, Epstein F: Effect of atrial natriuretic peptide on potassium-stimulated aldosterone secretion: Potential relevance to hypoaldosteronism in man. *J Clin Endocrinol Metab* 75:399, 1992.

256. Rodriguez-Iturbe B, Colic D, Parra G, et al: Atrial natriuetic factor in the acute nephritic and nephrotic syndromes. *Kidney Int* 38:512, 1990.

257. Don B, Schambelan M: Hyperkalemia in acute glomerulonephritis due to transient hyporeninemic hypoaldosteronism. *Kidney Int* 38:1159, 1990.

258. Zimran A, Kramer M, Plaskin M, et al: Incidence of hyperkalaemia induced by indomethacin in a hospitalized population. *Br Med J* 291:107, 1985.

259. Oates J, FitzGerald G, Branch R, et al: Clinical implications of prostaglandin and thromboxane A2 formation. *N Engl J Med* 319:761, 1988.

260. Pratt J: Role of angiotensin II in potassium-mediated aldosterone secretion in the dog. *J Clin Invest* 70:667, 1982.

261. Textor S, Bravo E, Fouad F, et al: Hyperkalemia in azotemic patients during angiotensin-converting enzyme inhibition and aldosterone reduction with captopril. *Am J Med* 73:719, 1982.

262. Bantle J, Nath K, Sutherland D, et al: Effect of cyclosporine on the renin-angiotensin system and potassium excretion in renal transplant recipients. *Arch Intern Med* 145:505, 1985.

263. Kamel K, Ethier J, Quaggin S, et al: Studies to determine the basis for hyperkalemia in recipients of a renal transplant who are treated with cyclosporine. *J Am Soc Nephrol* 2:1279, 1991.

264. Kalin M, Poretsky L, Seres D, et al: Hyporeninemic hypoaldosteronism associated with AIDS. *Am J Med* 82:1035, 1987.

265. Choi M, Fernancez P, Patnaik A, et al: Brief report: trimethoprim-induced hyperkalemia in a patient with AIDS. *N Engl J Med* 328:703, 1993.

266. Winqvist O, Karlsson F, Kampe O: 21-hydroxylase, a major autoantigen in idiopathic Addison's disease. *Lancet* 339:1559, 1992.

267. O'Kelly R, Magee F, McKenna T: Routine heparin therapy inhibits adrenal aldosterone production. *J Clin Endocrinol Metab* 56:108, 1983.

268. Sherman R, Ruddy M: Suppression of aldosterone production by low-dose heparin. *Am J Nephrol* 6:165, 1986.

269. White P, New M, Dupont B: Congenital adrenal hyperplasia. *N Engl J Med* 316:1519, 1987.

270. Ulick S, Wang J, Morton D: The biochemical phenotypes of two inborn errors in the biosynthesis of aldosterone. *J Clin Endocrinol Metab* 74:1415, 1992.

271. Armanini D, Kuhnle U, Strasser T, et al: Aldosterone-receptor de-

ficiency in pseudohypoaldosteronism. *N Engl J Med* 313:1178, 1985.

272. Kuhnle U, Nielsen M, Teitze H-U, et al: Pseudohypoaldosteronism in eight families: Different forms in inheritance are evidence for various genetic defects. *J Clin Endocrinol Metab* 70:638, 1990.

273. Schambelan M, Sebastian A, Rector F Jr: Mineralocorticoid-resistant renal hyperkalemia without salt-wasting (type II pseudohypoaldosteronism): Role of increased renal chloride reabsorption. *Kidney Int* 19:716, 1981.

274. Gordon R: Syndrome of hypertension and hyperkalemia with normal gomerular filtration rate. *Hypertension* 8:93, 1986.

275. Take C, Ikeda K, Kurasawa T, et al: Increased chloride reabsorption as an inherited renal tubular defect in familial type II pseudohypoaldosteronism. *N Engl J Med* 324:472, 1991.

276. Braley L, Adler G, Mortensen R: Dose effect of adrenocorticotropin on aldosterone and cortisol biosynthesis in cultured bovine adrenal glomerulosa cells. In vitro correlate of hyperreninemic hypoaldosteronism. *Endocrinology* 131:187, 1992.

277. Gonick H, Kleeman C, Rubini M, et al: Functional impairment in chronic renal disease: III. Studies of potassium excretion. *Am J Med Sci* 261:281, 1971.

278. Allon M: Treatment and prevention of hyperkalemia in end-stage renal disease. *Kidney Int* 43:1197, 1993.

279. Allon M, Takeshian A, Shanklin N: Effect of insulin-plus-glucose infusion with or without epinephrine on fasting hyperkalemia. *Kidney Int* 43:212, 1993.

280. Bonilla S, Goecke A, Bozzo S, et al: Effect of chronic renal failure on Na,K,-ATPase a1 and a2 mRNA transcription in rat skeletal muscle. *J Clin Invest* 88, 1991.

281. Chakko S, Frutchey J, Gheorghiade M: Life-threatening hyperkalemia in severe heart failure. *Am Heart J* 117:1083, 1989.

282. Popovtzer M, Katz F, Pinggera W, et al: Hyperkalemia in salt-wasting nephropathy: Study of the mechanism. *Arch Intern Med* 132:203, 1973.

283. DeFronzo R, Goldberg M, Cooke C, et al: Investigations into mechanisms of hyperkalemia following renal transplantation. *Kidney Int* 11:357, 1977.

284. DeFronzo R, Cooke C, Goldberg M, et al: Impaired renal tubular potassium secretion in systemic lupus erythematosus. *Ann Intern Med* 86:268, 1977.

285. Rose D: *Clinical Physiology of Acid-Base and Electrolyte Disorders*. New York, McGraw-Hill, 1994, p 848.

286. Berne R, Levy M: Cardiovascular Physiology. 4th ed. St. Louis, Mosby, 1981, p 7.

287. Surawicz B, Chlebus H, Mussoleni A: Hemodynamic and electrocardiographic effects of hyperpotassemia. Differences in response to slow and rapid increases in concentration of plasma K. *Am Heart* 73:647, 1967.

288. Szerlip H, Weiss J, Singer I: Profound hyperkalemia without electrocardiographic manifestations. *Am J Kidney Dis* 7:461, 1986.

289. Allon M, Copkney C: Albuterol and insulin for treatment of hyperkalemia in hemodialysis patients. *Kidney Int* 38:869, 1990.

290. Blumberg A, Weidmann P, Shaw S, et al: Effect of various therapeutic approaches on plasma potassium and major regulating factors in terminal renal failure. *Am J Med* 85:507, 1988.

291. Alvestrand A, Wahren J, Smith D, et al: Insulin-mediated potassium uptake is normal in uremic and healthy subjects. *Am J Physiol* 246:E174, 1984.

292. Goecke I, Bonilla S, Marusic E, et al: Enhanced insulin sensitivity in extrarenal potassium handling in uremic rats. *Kidney Int* 39:39, 1991.

293. Blumberg A, Weidmann P, Ferrari P: Effect of prolonged bicarbonate administration on plasma potassium in terminal renal failure. *Kidney Int* 41:369, 1992.

294. Ballantyne F III, Davis L, Reynolds E Jr: Cellular basis for reversal of hyperkalemic electrocardiographic changes by sodium. *Am J Physiol* 229:935, 1975.

295. Allon M, Shankin N: Adrenergic modulation of extrarenal potassium disposal in men with end-stage renal disease. *Kidney Int* 40:1103, 1991.

296. Gerstman B, Kirkman R, Platt R: Intestinal necrosis associated with postoperative orally administered sodium polystyrene sulfonate in sorbitol. *Am J Kidney Dis* 20:159, 1992.

297. Shepard K: Cleansing enemas after sodium polystyrene sulfonate enemas (letter). *Ann Intern Med* 112:711, 1990.

298. Nolph K, Popovich R, Ghods A, et al: Determinants of low clearances of small solutes during peritoneal dialysis. *Kidney Int* 13:117, 1978.

80. Metabolic Acidosis and Metabolic Alkalosis

Robert M. Black

Normal Acid-Base Physiology

The blood pH is normally maintained between 7.35 and 7.45. *Acidemia* and *alkalemia* define decreases or increases in blood pH, respectively. A simple (single) acid-base disturbance always causes the blood pH to change. For example, an infusion of hydrochloric acid decreases the blood pH below 7.35 (acidemia). In comparison, the presence of two opposing primary acid-base disturbances, such as a metabolic acidosis due to diarrhea and metabolic alkalosis due to vomiting, may result in little or no deviation of the blood pH from normal. As a result, a thorough understanding of the normal compensatory processes that protect against changes in body pH are important in the assessment of acid-base abnormalities.

RENAL REGULATION OF H$^+$ SECRETION. Maintenance of a normal plasma bicarbonate (HCO_3^-) concentration depends on reclamation of the 4500 mEq of HCO_3^- filtered by the kidneys each day (normal HCO_3^- concentration is 25 mEq/L $\times$ glomerular filtration rate, which equals 180 L/day = 4500 mEq/day). Reabsorption of filtered bicarbonate takes place primarily in the proximal tubule (Fig. 80-1). In this process, luminal HCO_3^- is free to combine with H$^+$ secreted into the proximal tubular lumen by an Na-H antiporter [1]. The formation and

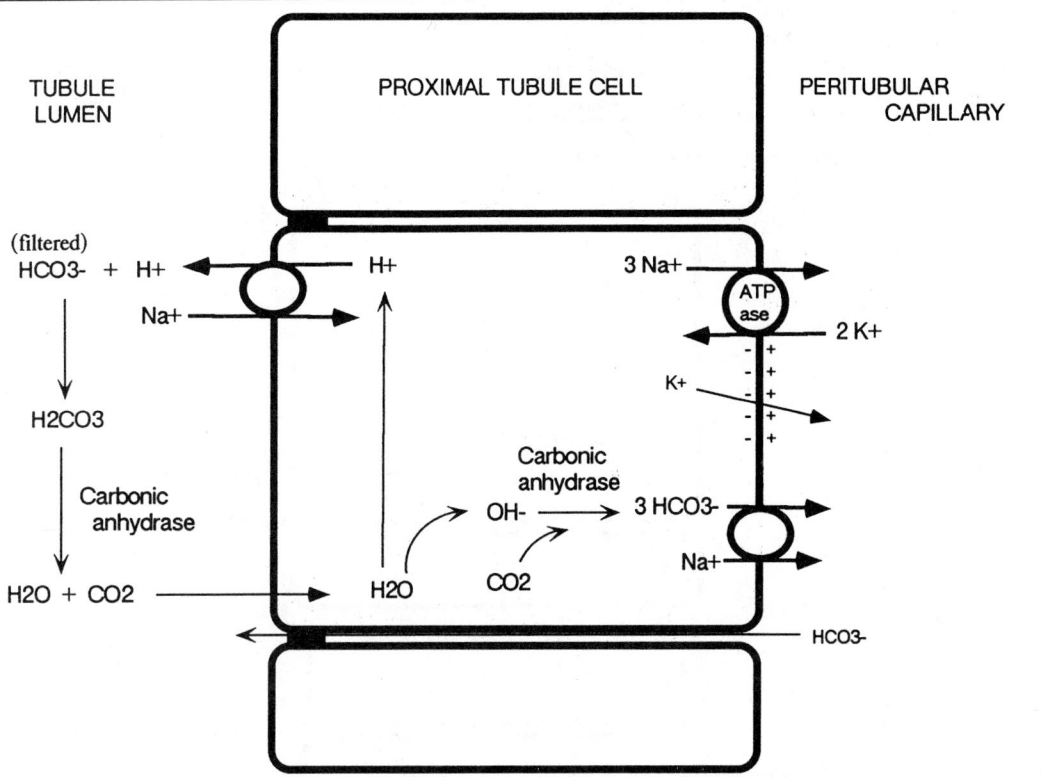

Fig. 80-1. Proximal tubular reclamation of filtered bicarbonate. The first step in maintaining normal acid-base balance is the reabsorption of all filtered bicarbonate. Inability to accomplish this results in metabolic acidosis (proximal, type 2, RTA). See text for details.

subsequent dissociation of carbonic acid (H_2CO_3) to CO_2 and H_2O (catalyzed by carbonic anhydrase) permit CO_2 to enter the luminal membrane of the proximal tubular cell. Once inside the cell, CO_2 combines with OH^- to form HCO_3^-. A Na-3HCO_3 cotransporter then carries HCO_3^- across the peritubular membrane into the blood. As a result, filtered bicarbonate is returned to the circulation without any net loss of H^+.

Any insult that limits H^+ secretion into the proximal tubule lumen results in urinary bicarbonate losses, which may lead to a fall in plasma HCO_3^- concentration and to metabolic acidosis. The carbonic anhydrase inhibitor acetazolamide, for example, reduces the activity of luminal carbonic anhydrase, thereby decreasing the entry of water and CO_2 across the luminal membrane, which decreases bicarbonate reabsorption by the tubular cell. As a result, less CO_2 enters the cell across the luminal membrane. This limits the quantity of H^+ that is available for secretion in exchange for Na^+ (see Fig. 80-1). It is not surprising, therefore, that these agents generate a metabolic acidosis while concomitantly increasing urinary sodium (and HCO_3^-) excretion.

Reclamation of all filtered HCO_3^- is not sufficient to maintain a normal blood pH. The kidney must also excrete the 1 to 3 mEq per kg of H^+ generated each day from the metabolism of dietary proteins, particularly sulfur-containing amino acids (methionine, cystine), which are converted to sulfuric acid. This acid load is initially buffered in the body to minimize changes in blood pH and is reflected by a decrease in the plasma HCO_3^- concentration. The kidney must excrete the daily acid load to replete the HCO_3^- used in this process.

The ability of the kidney to excrete H^+ ions is limited by

urinary pH. Below a urine pH of 4.5, the gradient between the H^+ inside of the tubule cell and the tubule lumen exceeds the energy capacity of the H^+ pumps throughout the nephron. As a consequence, buffers are added to the urine to raise the urine pH above this limiting value. This permits excretion of the daily acid load, thereby regenerating plasma HCO_3^-.

Two distinct buffering processes are used in the regeneration of buffer. *Titratable acids* (primarily HPO_4)* are freely filtered through the glomerulus and can combine with H^+.

$$HPO_4^- + H^+ \rightarrow H_2PO_4^-$$

Approximately 40 to 50% of the daily acid load is excreted in this way. For each H^+ secreted, a HCO_3^- is regenerated (Fig. 80-2), thus replenishing the HCO_3^- used to buffer the net daily surplus of dietary acid. By comparison, the most important urinary buffer is ammonia (which is secreted as ammonium, NH_4^+), since this buffer can be varied according to physiologic needs. The quantity of titratable acid is limited by the plasma concentration of the buffer and by the glomerular filtration rate [2].

Ammonia synthesis takes place in the proximal tubule. Synthesis occurs principally from the breakdown of glutamine to alpha-ketoglutarate (Fig. 80-2) [3]. This process is stimulated by intracellular acidosis and by *hypokalemia*, which may act by decreasing the intracellular pH (see following). Ammonia thus generated can combine with intracellular H^+, forming NH_4^+. NH_4^+ is then secreted into the proximal tubule lumen by substituting for H^+ on the Na-H antiporter. Ammonia (NH_3) that forms by the dissociation of H^+ from NH_4^+ is largely reabsorbed, recycled, and then secreted. It is primarily secreted by the collecting tubule, where it is trapped in the tubule lumen

*Titratable acidity is determined by adding HCO_3^- to the daily urine volume. It is equal to the quantity of HCO_3^- required to return the urine pH to 7.4.

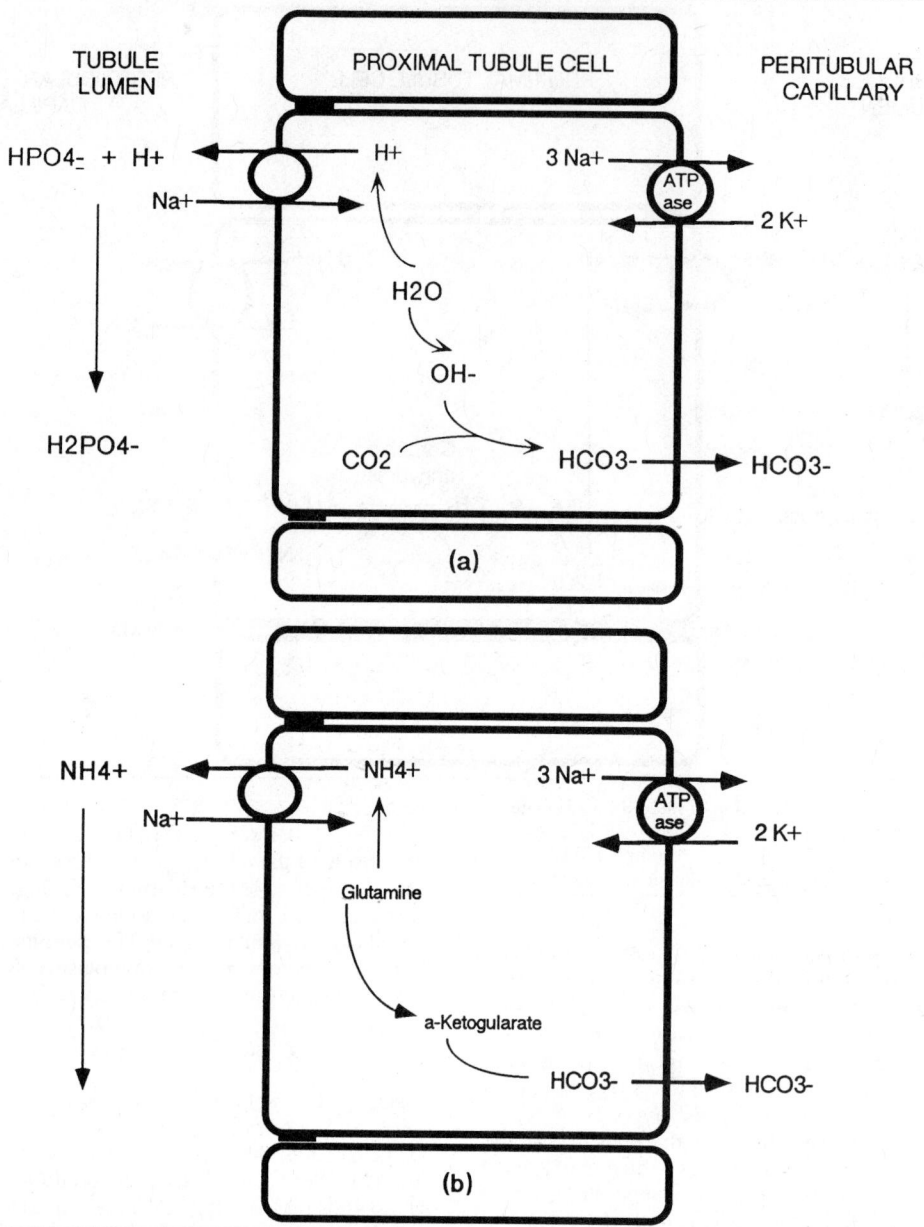

Fig. 80-2. Excretion of the daily acid load permits the regeneration of bicarbonate that was used as a buffer. Two processes are involved: (A) the excretion of titratable acid; and (B) the excretion of ammonium. The latter is particularly important since acidosis stimulates the breakdown of glutamine to NH_3. By comparison, hyperkalemia impairs the capacity of the proximal tubule to make ammonia, thus contributing to the metabolic acidosis observed in hyperkalemic disorders.

as NH_4^+ and excreted (since the urine pH is lowest in this nephron segment). As will be seen, limited secretion of NH_4^+ is a common cause of impaired H^+ secretion and metabolic acidosis.

Metabolic Acidosis

Metabolic acidosis is defined as an increase in the blood H^+ concentration. The H^+ concentration can be derived from the plasma HCO_3^- and PCO_2 using the nonlogarithmic form of the Henderson-Hasselbalch equation:

$$H^+ = 24 \, PCO_2/HCO_3^-$$

This relationship shows that a fall in the HCO_3^- concentration will also cause a metabolic acidosis, since it leads to an increase in H^+ concentration.

Metabolic acidosis can be categorized by the presence or absence of an increased anion gap. The *anion gap* (AG) refers to the difference between measured cations (Na$^+$) and measured anions (Cl$^-$ and HCO$_3^-$).*

$$AG = Na^+ - (Cl^- + HCO_3^-)$$

The normal AG had been considered to range between 7 and 13 mEq/per liter. The AG may be as low as 3 to 11 mEq/per liter, however, due to a higher chloride concentration measured with the newer autoanalyzers [4,4a]. As a result, knowing the normal range in a particular laboratory is often essential for proper interpretation of AG, particularly if the rise in AG is to be compared to the fall in plasma HCO$_3^-$ concentration.

These unmeasured anions consist of proteins (primarily albumin), sulfates, phosphates, and circulating organic acids. Uric acid is a large molecule and therefore does not contribute significantly to the AG even when hyperuricemia is present.

A reduction in the plasma albumin concentration can reduce the baseline AG (approximately 2.5 mEq for every 1 g/dl fall in the albumin concentration) [5]. Thus, the hypoalbuminemic patient may not have a high AG even in the presence of a disorder that typically causes an elevation (e.g., lactic acidosis).

ANION GAP METABOLIC ACIDOSIS. The causes of metabolic acidosis associated with an increased anion gap are listed in Table 80-1. Lactic acidosis is the most frequent cause in hospitalized patients, whereas chronic renal failure is the principal cause of an increased AG in ambulatory individuals.

Renal Failure. Renal failure presents an interesting example of the potential overlap between normal and elevated AG acidosis. The high AG in patients with renal failure is usually a late finding and reflects a severe reduction in glomerular filtration rate. Early in renal failure, metabolic acidosis appears because H$^+$ secretion is reduced.

As discussed previously, the daily acid load, generated primarily by the metabolism of sulfur-containing amino acids to sulfuric acid, is about 50 to 100 mEq per day in someone consuming a typical American diet. This acid is immediately buffered by NaHCO$_3^-$

$$H_2SO_4 + 2\ NaHCO_3^- \rightarrow Na_2SO_4 + 2\ CO_2 + 2\ H_2O$$

The excess sulfate is excreted in the urine. The rate of excretion is determined by the difference between glomerular filtration and tubular reabsorption; in comparison, the excess H$^+$ enters the tubule lumen by secretion. If glomerular and tubular function decline in parallel, then both the H$^+$ and the SO$_4^=$ will be retained, producing metabolic acidosis with a high AG. If, however, there is more prominent tubular dysfunction, the excretion of acid will be diminished, but excretion of sulfate may be maintained due to reduced reabsorption. The result is that sulfate is excreted as Na$_2$SO$_4$, and metabolic acidosis occurs without a rise in AG [6].

As the glomerular filtration rate falls below 20 to 30 ml per minute (plasma creatinine >3–4 mg/dl), however, anionic substances that are normally filtered (including phosphates and sulfates) are retained [7]. Therefore, the ability of the tubules to secrete hydrogen ions does not necessarily correlate quantitatively with the retention of unmeasured anions. Thus, the decrease in plasma bicarbonate and the severity of acidemia do

Table 80-1. Causes of Metabolic Acidosis with an Increased Anion Gap

Renal failure*
Lactic acidosis
Ketoacidosis (diabetic, alcoholic, starvation)*
Rhabdomyolysis
Ingestions
    Salicylates
    Methanol
    Ethylene glycol
    Paraldehyde†
    Toluene‡

*May be associated with normal AG early in course (renal failure) or during therapy (ketoacidosis); see text for details.
†Earlier cases of paraldehyde-induced metabolic acidosis may have been caused by alcoholic ketoacidosis.
‡Toluene also may cause a non-AG acidosis (see Table 80-3).

not predict the degree to which the AG will increase. Although the AG may be normal or increased, it is rarely greater than 23 mEq per liter, and the plasma bicarbonate is typically above 12 mEq per liter in patients with uncomplicated renal failure. A search for a second acid-base disorder is indicated when a higher gap or lower bicarbonate concentration is identified.

Lactic Acidosis. Lactic acidosis is probably the most common cause of severe metabolic acidosis encountered in the ICU. The AG is always increased above baseline (normal lactate level is below 1.0 mM/L)*; lactate does not appear in the urine until a higher plasma concentration is achieved because the renal threshold is 6 to 8 mM per liter [8]. Lactate levels greater than 5 mM per liter are considered diagnostic of lactic acidosis [9], although levels between 2 and 5 mM per liter may be representative in the appropriate clinical circumstances. This disorder is discussed in detail in Chapter 115.

Ketoacidosis. Ketoacidosis occurs when acetoacetic acid and beta-hydroxybutyric acid (beta-HBA) are overproduced by the liver (see Chap. 110 for a complete discussion). Acetone, which forms as a breakdown product of acetoacetic acid, is not an acid; as such, it does not contribute to the acidemia or to the AG.†

Although ketoacidosis is generally associated with an elevated AG, loss of ketone anions in the urine, particularly during intravenous fluid therapy, may attenuate the expansion of the AG. During fluid repletion therapy, the blood level of ketoacids diminishes as acetoacetic acid and beta-HBA are excreted in the urine since the renal threshold for ketones (in contrast to lactic acid; see preceding) is only 1 to 2 mM per liter. As a result, ketones generated may be lost through the kidneys before they can be metabolized back to bicarbonate by the liver in the presence of insulin. Since the production of ketoacids titrates the plasma bicarbonate concentration downward, the loss of urinary ketone anions is tantamount to the renal loss of bicarbonate. The net effect is that the AG metabolic acidosis present

---

* Potassium is usually not included in the calculation of the AG, since changes large enough to alter the gap significantly are uncommon or incompatible with life.

* The more recently described condition of D-lactic acidosis requires a specific search for D-lactic acid, which is not routinely measured (see Chap. 115 for details). This acid may be present in patients with short bowel syndrome and is formed by intestinal bacteria. Diagnosis requires a specific enzymatic assay since human lactic dehydrogenase metabolizes only L-lactate.
† Isopropyl alcohol is metabolized to acetone and can cause renal failure. In this setting, ketonemia and ketonuria are characteristically present, whereas any increase in the AG is typically not due to ketoacidosis since acetoacetic acid and beta-hydroxybutyric acid are not usually produced.

before therapy may be converted to a non-AG metabolic acidosis during recovery [10].

Rhabdomyolysis. Massive muscle breakdown is an important cause of metabolic acidosis with an increased AG (see Chap. 81). Acute renal failure may develop with the retention of metabolic acids and anions (such as phosphate) that have been released from damaged myocytes.

Ingestions. The most common acid-base abnormality observed with *salicylate* intoxication (see Chap. 154) is a respiratory alkalosis caused by direct stimulation of the medullary respiratory center. In fact, the presence of respiratory alkalosis appears to be necessary for the development of metabolic acidosis [11]. Consequently, a pure metabolic acidosis due to aspirin toxicity is uncommon. In contrast, moderate-to-severe salicylate intoxication causes the AG to increase as salicylic acid (as well as other metabolic acids) is retained, leading to a mixed respiratory alkalosis with a high AG metabolic acidosis [12].

Methanol and ethylene glycol ingestions require early diagnosis, since removal by hemodialysis may be lifesaving. Ingestion is suggested by the appropriate history and physical findings (see Chap. 132) in the presence of a concomitant AG metabolic acidosis. The turnaround time for measurement of these toxins may delay treatment; in comparison, the detection of an osmolal gap (see following) can support the suspected diagnosis, thereby permitting earlier intervention. Mannitol, which may be given to enhance diuresis if oliguria is present, does not only elevate the measured plasma osmolality (Posm; see following), but also can cause a false-positive ethylene glycol reaction with some assays [13].

The *osmolal gap* refers to the difference between the Posm measured by the laboratory and that calculated using the following formula (see Chap. 79) [14]:

$$\text{Calculated Posm (mOsm/kg)} = 2 \times \text{Na}^+ + \frac{\text{glucose}}{20} + \frac{\text{BUN}}{3}$$

Normally, the measured Posm is less than 10 mOsm per kg higher than the calculated value [15]. A larger osmolal gap indicates the presence of osmotically active substances not normally present. The most frequent causes of an increased osmolal gap are ethyl alcohol, isopropyl alcohol, ketones, lactate, mannitol, ethylene glycol, and methanol. If the presence of ethanol, lactate, and ketones cannot be identified in a patient with an AG metabolic acidosis, the diagnosis of ethylene glycol or methanol intoxication should be strongly suspected [15a].

Paraldehyde (metabolized to acetic acid) and *toluene* (metabolized to hippuric acid) are rare causes of an increased AG. Earlier cases of "paraldehyde-induced" metabolic acidosis possibly may have been due to the concomitant presence of alcoholic ketoacidosis.

NORMAL ANION GAP (HYPERCHLOREMIC) METABOLIC ACIDOSIS.

Metabolic acidosis with a normal AG may be observed in the conditions listed in Table 80-2. The decrement in the plasma bicarbonate concentration is replaced by a rise in the plasma chloride level to maintain electroneutrality.

Acid and Chloride Administration. The infusion of amino acid solutions during hyperalimentation is a common source of hydrochloric acid (HCl). The generation of a metabolic acidosis is more common in patients with renal insufficiency.

Oral administration of cholestyramine chloride reportedly occasionally also causes acidemia. This resin, which is used in

Table 80-2. Causes of Metabolic Acidosis with a Normal Anion Gap

Acid administration
  Hyperalimentation with HCl-containing amino acid solutions
  Cholestyramine chloride
  Hydrochloric acid administration during treatment of severe metabolic alkalosis
Bicarbonate losses
  Gastrointestinal
    Diarrhea
    Pancreatic or biliary drainage
    Urinary diversions (ureterosigmoidostomy)
  Renal
    Proximal (type 2) renal tubular acidosis
    Ketoacidosis (particularly during therapy)
    Postchronic hypocapnia
Impaired renal acid excretion
  With hypokalemia
    Classic distal (type 1) renal tubular acidosis
  With hyperkalemia
    Hyperkalemic distal renal tubular acidosis
    Hypoaldosteronism (type 4 renal tubular acidosis)
Reduced renal perfusion

the management of hypercholesterolemia, is nonreabsorbable and can act as an anion-exchange resin, exchanging its Cl^- for endogenous HCO_3^- and producing a metabolic acidosis [16].

Bicarbonate Losses. Bicarbonate that is lost from the gastrointestinal tract or kidneys can lead to a reduction in the plasma HCO_3^- level. Bowel contents are alkaline compared to blood because bicarbonate is added by pancreatic and biliary secretions. Bicarbonate is later exchanged for chloride in the ileum and colon. The result is that most alkali secreted into the gut lumen is reclaimed by the colon. Gastrointestinal losses of bicarbonate (or bicarbonate precursors such as lactate and acetate) are most commonly observed in patients with severe diarrhea in whom there is inadequate time for alkali reabsorption in the colon. At times, the resulting stool bicarbonate losses can approach 40 mEq per liter [17]. Less frequently, metabolic acidosis due to bicarbonate depletion results from pancreatic fistulae, biliary drainage, or a ureterosigmoidostomy. In the last circumstance, the excretion of acid (as NH_4Cl) urine directly into the colon permits the exchange of HCl for bicarbonate, since the colon is permeable to H^+ and Cl^-, unlike the urinary bladder [18].

Renal bicarbonate losses can cause or contribute to acidemia in type 2 (proximal) renal tubular acidosis (RTA; see Table 80-2)*, during recovery from ketoacidosis (see preceding), and in patients who are postchronic hypocapnia. In patients with proximal RTA (Table 80-3), the normal reabsorptive threshold for bicarbonate is reduced [19]. As a result, bicarbonate can no longer be reabsorbed at a rate adequate to maintain the normal plasma level of approximately 25 mEq per liter. If the new plasma threshold is now 18 mEq per liter, bicarbonate is lost in the urine. As a consequence, the urine pH is alkaline (>5.3), and the fractional excretion of bicarbonate is elevated (above 15% of the filtered load).[†] Normally, this value is less than 3%,

---

*The RTAs can be classified as type 1 (distal), type 2 (proximal), and type 4 (hypoaldosteronism). Type 3 refers to what is now considered to be an infantile variant of type 1 and therefore type 3 RTA is a term not generally used in adults.
[†] The fractional excretion of bicarbonate is equal to the amount of HCO_3^- excreted divided by the filtered load:

$$\text{Fractional excretion } [\text{HCO}_3] = \frac{\text{urine HCO}_3^- \times \text{plasma creat}}{\text{urine creat} \times \text{plasma HCO}_3^-} \times 100$$

Table 80-3. Causes of Types 1 and 2 Renal Tubular Acidosis

Distal (type 1) RTA	Proximal (type 2) RTA
Idiopathic	Hereditary disorders
Genetic	Cystinosis
Familial	Tyrosinemia
Marfan's syndrome	Wilson's disease[b]
Ehler-Danlos syndrome	Glycogen storage disease,
Disorders of calcium metabo-	type 1
lism	Pyruvate carboxylase defi-
Idiopathic hypercalciuria	ciency
Hypervitaminosis D	Galactosemia
Hyperparathyroidism	Acquired disorders
Hypergammaglobulinemic	Multiple myeloma[b]
states	Vitamin D deficiency
Amyloidosis[a]	Nephrotic syndrome
Cryoglobulinemia	Toxins and drugs
Drugs and toxins	Lead
Amphotericin B	Cadmium
Lithium carbonate	Mercury
Toluene[c]	Uranium
Autoimmune diseases	Copper (Wilson's disease)[b]
Sjögren's syndrome[a]	Carbonic anhydrase inhibi-
Thyroiditis	tors
Chronic active hepatitis	Outdated tetracycline
Primary biliary cirrhosis	Streptozotocin
Miscellaneous	
Cirrhosis	
Medullary sponge kidney	
Associated with hyperkale-	
mia	
Urinary tract obstruction	
Sickle cell anemia	
Systemic lupus erythemato-	
sus	
Renal transplant rejection[a]	

[a]Also may cause proximal RTA.
[b]Also may cause distal RTA.
[c]Metabolism to hippuric acid may cause AG to increase.

since over 97% of bicarbonate filtered through the glomerulus is reabsorbed, primarily in the proximal tubule (see Fig. 80-1). Bicarbonate wasting ceases, however, and the urine becomes acidic (pH <5.3) once the plasma bicarbonate concentration has stabilized at the new (lower) level. This process explains why the urine pH may be high or low in proximal RTA.

Renal bicarbonate losses also occur as compensation for chronic respiratory alkalosis (chronic hypocapnia) [20]. During chronic hyperventilation, the blood pH increases as the PCO_2 decreases. As can be seen in Figure 80-1, an increase in intracellular pH diminishes H^+ excretion, leading to a concomitant decrease in bicarbonate reabsorption. These changes cause the plasma HCO_3^- concentration to fall, partially compensating for the rise in blood pH. If the stimulus for hyperventilation (e.g., hypoxemia) is suddenly corrected, the PCO_2 rapidly returns to normal. Renal compensation, by comparison, continues for 1 to 2 more days, causing a persistent reduction in the plasma bicarbonate concentration. The resulting *posthypocapneic metabolic acidosis* normally resolves spontaneously.

Reduced Renal H^+ Excretion. Reduced renal acid excretion can be observed in four conditions: renal failure; type 1 (distal) RTA (see Table 80-3); type 4 (hypoaldosteronism) RTA; and states of reduced renal perfusion [19]. The *acidosis of renal failure* is due primarily to a reduction in ammonia production.

In contrast to individuals with RTA (types 1 and 4), in whom ammonia synthesis per nephron is reduced, patients with chronic renal failure have a substantial drop in the number of functioning nephrons. Nephrons that continue to filter, however, characteristically have filtration rates and acid excretion rates per nephron that are above normal. Impaired acid excretion in these patients occurs because the number of hyperfiltering nephrons is inadequate to compensate for those that are nonfunctioning.

The classic form of type 1 (distal) RTA (see Table 80-3) occurs when H^+ cannot be pumped into the tubule lumen by the intercalated cells of the collecting tubule (see Chap. 79) [21]. The result is urine that cannot be maximally acidified (urine pH always >5.3). In addition to the generation of a metabolic acidosis, hypokalemia is typically present [22]. The potassium deficit is caused by enhanced distal nephron Na-K exchange, a process that is necessary to maintain sodium balance since H^+ cannot be secreted in response to Na^+ reabsorption.

The most important clinical complication of distal RTA is the formation and deposition of calcium salts throughout the kidney (nephrocalcinosis). This process begins in the collecting tubules, where the urine is most concentrated, and is commonly accompanied by the formation of calcium phosphate calculi. The factors that may contribute to the renal stone disease in this disorder include hypercalciuria (due to metabolic acidosis, which releases bone calcium that can then be filtered and excreted); the alkaline urine pH, which predisposes to the precipitation of calcium phosphate crystals; and, most importantly, hypocitraturia. The reduction in urinary citrate is a direct result of the metabolic acidosis, which increases proximal tubular citrate reabsorption [23]. Since calcium citrate is significantly more soluble than calcium phosphate, hypocitraturia facilitates the precipitation of calcium phosphate crystals in the tubule lumen.*

It is possible that the lack of a tendency toward stone formation in most patients with proximal RTA is due to the concomitant presence of Fanconi's syndrome, in which proximal tubular reabsorption of bicarbonate and many other substances, including citrate, is impaired.

In addition to the classic form of type 1 (distal) RTA, in which hypokalemia is characteristic, a hyperkalemic variety has been recently described. This disorder, as well as type 4 (hypoaldosteronism) RTA, is discussed in Chapter 79.

CLINICAL SIGNS AND SYMPTOMS OF METABOLIC ACIDOSIS. Results of the physical examination can suggest the presence of metabolic acidosis when Kussmaul respirations are present. These ventilatory changes are due to an increase in tidal volume rather than to respiratory rate, which results from stimulation of the respiratory center in the brainstem by the low blood pH. As acidemia becomes more severe, nausea and vomiting or mental status changes, including coma, may occur.

Secondary hypotension also may occur in severely acidemic patients [24]. The reduced blood pressure in such patients is the result of depressed myocardial contractility and arterial vasodilation, both induced by the fall in blood pH. Initially, the cardiovascular effects of acidemia are antagonized by elevated levels of circulating catecholamines; however, the effect of acidemia may predominate below a blood pH of 7.15 to 7.20.

The plasma potassium concentration may be altered by the degree of metabolic acidosis. Infusion of a mineral acid such as arginine HCl, for example, causes a prompt rise in the plasma

* Most renal calculi are composed of calcium oxalate. In comparison, the presence of a persistently alkaline urine pH presdisposes to calcium phosphate stone formation.

potassium concentration as K^+ moves out of cells in exchange for H^+. By comparison, a shift of potassium is less likely to occur in those with metabolic acidosis caused by organic acids, such as lactic and ketoacidosis [24a]. The reason for this apparent difference is uncertain, but it may be due to the release of insulin by organic substrates (such as lactate and beta-hydroxybutyrate), which would drive potassium into cells (see Chap. 79). On the other hand, the applicability of these findings to humans remains to be proved.

DIAGNOSIS. The diagnosis of a simple metabolic acidosis is made relatively easily in the presence of a low blood pH and plasma bicarbonate concentration. The detection of an AG can then be used to identify a specific cause for the disorder. The likelihood of identifying a specific acid(s) in a patient with an AG acidosis increases as the size of the AG increases [25].

In comparison with patients with a simple metabolic acidosis, many individuals have a concomitant respiratory or second metabolic acid-base disorder. Consequently, knowledge of the appropriate respiratory compensation as well as an understanding of the ratio of the increment in AG to decrement in plasma bicarbonate concentration is needed to evaluate these patients properly.

Respiratory Compensation. Stimulation of the brainstem respiratory center by acidemia causes a fall in the PCO_2 that, in uncomplicated metabolic acidosis, can be estimated from the following equation [26]:

$$\text{Expected } PCO_2 \text{ (mm Hg)} = [(1.5 \times HCO_3^-) + 8] \pm 2$$

A PCO_2 that is substantially different from the expected value indicates a superimposed respiratory acidosis or alkalosis. For example, if the plasma bicarbonate concentration were 10 mEq per liter, the expected PCO_2 would be approximately 23 mm Hg $\{(1.5 \times 10) + 8\} = 23$. A lower PCO_2 indicates the presence of a concomitant respiratory alkalosis (as might be seen with a salicylate overdose), whereas a higher PCO_2 signifies a simultaneous respiratory acidosis. It should be emphasized that this calculation is useful only in the evaluation of the respiratory response to metabolic acidosis and that it is inaccurate when the plasma bicarbonate concentration is above 20 mEq per liter.

Identification of a Second (Nonanion Gap) Metabolic Acidosis or a Metabolic Alkalosis. The identification of a second *metabolic* acid-base disorder can be made by comparing the *change* in the AG with the *change* in the plasma HCO_3^- concentration.

The AG is elevated in those forms of metabolic acidosis in which there is buffering of excess acid by extracellular HCO_3. If hydrogen is retained with an unmeasured anion such as lactate (L), for example, then

$$HL + NaHCO_3 \rightarrow NaL + H_2CO_3 \rightarrow CO_2 + H_2O$$

The ensuing increase in the unmeasured anion lactate will raise the AG. From this equation, it might be assumed that there is a 1:1 relationship between the increase in AG (ΔAG) and the decrease in plasma bicarbonate (ΔHCO_3). The Δ/Δ ratio is typically greater than 1 in lactic acidosis, however, since the space of distribution of the hydrogen ion and the lactate anion are different [27]. Most of the lactate anions remain in the extracellular fluid, thereby raising the AG. In comparison, more than 50% of the excess hydrogen ions is buffered in the cells and in bone in mild metabolic acidosis, a process that does not lower the plasma bicarbonate concentration.

Thus, the rise in anion gap tends to exceed the reduction in the plasma bicarbonate concentration lactic acidosis [12,27]. This disparity increases in proportion to the severity of the acidosis. As the plasma bicarbonate concentration falls, there is a progressive reduction in extracellular buffering capacity (which almost entirely consists of bicarbonate) [27a]. As a result, buffering of newly produced acid occurs primarily in the cells and bone, minimizing a further fall in the plasma bicarbonate concentration (which is rarely below 5 mEq/L) while the AG continues to rise.

The result is that the Δ/Δ ratio averages about 1.6:1 in lactic acidosis [23]. Thus, a patient with a plasma bicarbonate concentration of 14 mEq per liter (10 mEq/L below normal) should have an AG that is approximately 25 mEq per liter (16 mEq/L above normal, assuming that a mean of 9 mEq/L is normal).

Urinary Losses of Unmeasured Anions. Although the same principles apply to ketoacidosis, the Δ/Δ ratio averages about 1:1 [23,27b]. In this disorder, the loss of ketoacid anions in the urine (as the sodium and potassium salts of beta-hydroxybutyrate and acetoacetate) lowers the AG without affecting the plasma bicarbonate concentration, therefore tending to balance the effect of intracellular buffering of hydrogen. In contrast, urinary anion loss is minimal in lactic acidosis, because shock is typically associated with the virtual cessation of renal function, and most of the lactate that is filtered can be reabsorbed by a specific sodium-L-lactate cotransporter in the luminal membrane of the proximal tubular cells.

The amount of ketoacid anions excreted in ketoacidosis depends on the degree to which glomerular filtration is maintained. Patients with impaired renal function (due to underlying diabetic nephropathy or volume depletion) retain the ketoacid anions and have a relatively high anion gap in relation to the fall in the plasma bicarbonate concentration, similar to that in lactic acidosis [27b]. In comparison, patients with relatively normal renal function (including those with alcoholic or fasting ketoacidosis) can lose large quantities of ketoacids in the urine and may have a Δ/Δ below 1.

The loss of ketoacid anions in the urine has another effect: the common development of a hyperchloremic (normal AG) metabolic acidosis during the treatment of diabetic ketoacidosis [23]. Suppose, for example, that a patient has a Δ/Δ ratio of 1, with a plasma HCO_3 of 8 mEq per liter ($\Delta HCO_3 = 16$ mEq/L) and an AG of 24 mEq per liter ($\Delta AG = 16$ mEq/L, assuming that the plasma albumin concentration is normal). Administration of insulin will convert all 16 mEq per liter of ketoacid anion back into HCO_3; the plasma HCO_3, however, may only rise by about 8 mEq per liter (to 16 mEq/L), with the rest of the HCO_3 replenishing the cell and bone buffer stores. At this point, the patient will have metabolic acidosis with a normal AG, due to the combination of the previous production of the intact ketoacid and the subsequent loss of the anion in the urine [23].

The ability to calculate the Δ/Δ is dependent on two assumptions: (1) That the baseline AG can be estimated accurately, an issue that is particularly important in view of the lower normal AG now often measured with newer autoanalyzers [4a,27c]. Evaluation of recent previous blood test results, if available, provides the best way of determining the normal AG for that patient. (2) That accumulating anions are derived from acids that are responsible for the acidemia. In some cases, for example, unmeasured anions accumulate in the plasma that may be unrelated to the genesis of the metabolic acidosis. As an example, severe diarrhea may induce both hyperproteinemia due to hemoconcentration and hyperphosphatemia due to acidosis-induced movement of phosphate from the cells into the extracellular fluid [27d]. The result is an elevation in AG even though diarrhea alone produces a normal AG acidosis (unless the volume losses are so large that lactic acidosis is superimposed). Hyperphosphatemia also may contribute to a high AG in some patients with nonketotic hyperglycemia even though the plasma bicarbonate concentration is normal or only slightly reduced [27c].

Changes in the concentration of other unmeasured cations or anions in the plasma can also lead to misestimation of the AG [27c]. As an example, both hypoalbuminemia (decreased unmeasured anions) and hyperkalemia (increased unmeasured cations) can lower the AG. Thus, a patient with one or both of these disorders may have a baseline AG of 4 rather than 8 mEq per liter. In this setting, an AG of 13 mEq per liter, which is mildly above "normal," represents a true elevation in the AG of 9 mEq per liter. As a result, calculation of the Δ/Δ is most accurate when the pre-acidosis anion gap is known.

Summary. In summary, strict recommendations that apply to all patients cannot easily be made. Assuming that the baseline AG is known or can be estimated accurately, the Δ/Δ ratio in an uncomplicated high AG metabolic acidosis should be between 1 and 2. A lower value (in which the ΔAG is less than expected from the ΔHCO$_3$) reflects either urinary ketone losses (as in diabetic ketoacidosis), some cases of chronic renal failure (in which tubular damage allows filtered anions to be excreted but limits the degree of hydrogen secretion) [27e], or a combined high and normal AG acidosis, as might occur if diarrhea were superimposed upon chronic renal failure. On the other hand, a Δ/Δ ratio above 2 indicates the plasma HCO$_3$ is higher than expected from the rise in the AG; this usually reflects a concurrent metabolic alkalosis, as with vomiting.

URINARY ANION GAP. Another useful tool in the evaluation of a metabolic acidosis is the urinary AG (UAG). The UAG is the difference between the sum of the urinary Na$^+$ and K$^+$ and the urinary Cl$^-$:

$$UAG = (Na^+ + K^+) - Cl^-$$

The most frequent use of the UAG is to identify the cause of a non-AG acidosis [29]. Normally, extrarenal causes of metabolic acidosis with a normal AG (e.g., diarrhea) are associated with a concomitant increase in renal H$^+$ secretion. This higher rate of renal acid secretion is lost in the urine primarily as NH$_4$Cl. Since NH$_4^+$ is not measured in the calculation of the UAG, but Cl$^-$ is, an increased rate of renal H$^+$ secretion causes the UAG to become a negative number. Conversely, the presence of a positive UAG in an individual with a non-AG metabolic acidosis suggests that the disorder is due to impaired renal H$^+$ excretion (renal tubular acidosis or renal failure) and not to extrarenal bicarbonate losses (as in diarrhea).

TREATMENT OF METABOLIC ACIDOSIS.
Treatment of metabolic acidosis must be directed at correction of acidemia as well as the cause of the acid-base disturbance. The likelihood that alkali administration is necessary and that it will be effective depends on the blood pH, compensatory mechanisms, and the underlying cause.

The degree of acidemia and hypobicarbonatemia should be evaluated before administering alkali. Until the blood pH falls below 7.15 to 7.20, the adverse effects of acidemia are usually compensated for by elevated plasma catecholamines, thus avoiding a decrease in cardiac output and hypotension [24]. As a result, alkali therapy generally is not needed until the arterial blood pH drops below this level.

An exception to this rule may occur when the plasma HCO$_3^-$ concentration falls to less than 10 to 12 mEq per liter, despite a blood pH above 7.15. As can be seen using equation 1, as the plasma levels of bicarbonate and PCO$_2$ fall, the effect of a minor change in either has a greater impact on the H$^+$ concentration (and blood pH). For example, an individual with a PCO$_2$ of 21 mm Hg and a plasma HCO$_3^-$ concentration of 8 mEq per liter has a H$^+$ concentration of 63 mEq per liter (pH = 7.20):

$$H^+ = 24 \times \frac{21}{8} = 63$$

Although the arterial blood pH is in a range not normally associated with hypotension or cardiac arrhythmias, the total body buffer reserve (reflected in the HCO$_3^-$ concentration) is depleted. As a result, a further fall in the plasma HCO$_3^-$ concentration to 4 mEq per liter, as might be seen if septic shock developed, would be associated with a profound fall in the blood pH to a potentially life-threatening level of 6.87:

$$H^+ \text{ concentration} = 24 \times \frac{PCO_2}{HCO_3^-}$$

$$H = 24 \times \frac{21}{4} = 126 \text{ mEq/L}$$

$$pH = 6.87$$

It has therefore been recommended that the plasma bicarbonate concentration be maintained above 10 to 12 mEq per liter with alkali therapy. Alkali administration is usually unnecessary if the acidosis is likely to resolve spontaneously (e.g., lactic acidosis following a grand mal seizure).

Alkali Administration. Bicarbonate therapy should be considered in patients with moderate-to-severe metabolic acidosis, depending on the etiology (see following). The initial goal of alkali therapy is to raise the arterial blood pH to 7.20, a typically safe level at which the patient is at less risk of cardiovascular compromise. The pH does not need to be corrected back to normal, since the potential risks of bicarbonate therapy (hypernatremia, hypercapnia, cerebrospinal fluid acidosis, and overshoot alkalosis) are likely to outweigh the benefits, as long as renal function (and therefore acid-excretory ability) is relatively intact.

Calculation of the bicarbonate deficit is useful in estimating the quantity of bicarbonate required. In a patient with an arterial pH of 7.10, for example, a plasma HCO$_3^-$ concentration of 6 mEq per liter, and a PCO$_2$ of 20 mm Hg, the amount of sodium bicarbonate required to increase the blood pH to 7.20 can be calculated using equation 1:

$$H^+ \text{ concentration} = 24 \times \frac{PCO_2}{HCO_3^-}$$

The H$^+$ concentration at a pH of 7.20 is 63 mEq per liter. Since the administration of bicarbonate is likely to suppress ventilation to some extent, a rise in the PCO$_2$ by 4 to 5 mm Hg is likely. Thus:

$$63 = 24 \times \frac{25}{HCO_3^-}$$

$$HCO_3^- = 10 \text{ mEq/L}$$

Therefore, a 4 mEq per liter increase in the plasma HCO$_3^-$ concentration from 6 to 10 mEq per liter is all that is required to raise the blood pH to 7.20.

The quantity of bicarbonate required to produce this change in pH is determined by estimating the total body bicarbonate deficit. The apparent bicarbonate space is about 50% of lean body weight in normal subjects. By comparison, in patients with moderate-to-severe metabolic acidosis (plasma HCO_3^- concentration below 10 mEq/L), cellular and bone buffering become more prominent due to the marked reduction in the quantity of available extracellular buffer (primarily bicarbonate) [30]. This preferential entry of H^+ into cells causes the bicarbonate space to expand to approximately 70% of lean body weight.

In the preceding example, the quantity of bicarbonate required to raise the plasma HCO_3^- concentration from 6 to 10 mEq per liter in a 70-kg subject can be estimated using these calculations:

$$HCO_3^- \text{ deficit} = (\text{volume of distribution}) \times \left(\frac{\text{deficit}}{2}\right)$$
$$= (0.7 \times 70) \times (10 - 6) = 196 \text{ mEq}$$

Approximately 196 mEq of $NaHCO_3$ given over the first few hours should increase the arterial blood pH to about 7.20. More bicarbonate is usually unnecessary if the pH remains at or above this level, since the kidney will eventually excrete the excess acid, assuming renal function is normal. It must be emphasized that these are only rough guidelines and cannot replace serial measurements of the extracellular pH. One potential problem is that the above formula assumes that the patient is in a steady state. If, for example, there is continuing acid loss from diarrhea, then the alkali requirements may be substantially increased.

Treatment of Specific Causes of Metabolic Acidosis

RENAL FAILURE. Treatment of the metabolic acidosis of renal failure depends both on the clinical manifestations and the severity of the acidosis (see Chap. 81). Most individuals with acute renal failure can be managed with dialysis or using the guidelines for alkali administration in metabolic acidosis listed previously. Although many patients with chronic renal failure might benefit from alkali therapy, there are insufficient data to recommend the level of acidemia at which such treatment should be started.

Symptomatic hypocalcemia with tetany is a potential risk of alkali therapy in patients with renal failure, since it diminishes the ionized fraction of total serum calcium. Failure to mobilize calcium may acutely exacerbate this problem. The common use of calcium carbonate as a phosphate-binding antacid has the advantages of increasing the plasma HCO_3^- level while protecting against hypocalcemia.

Treatment of hyperkalemia (see Chap. 79) also may improve acid excretion and raise the plasma HCO_3^- concentration. A high plasma potassium suppresses ammonia production from glutamine in the proximal tubular cells (see preceding), thereby limiting H^+ secretion [31].

KETOACIDOSIS. The plasma glucose concentration does not correlate with the degree of acidemia in ketoacidosis. This may result from reduced glycogen stores, impaired gluconeogenesis, or, rarely, renal glycosuria [32]. Moreover, the blood glucose level may normalize before ketoacid production has ceased; as a result, alleviation of hyperglycemia should not be the only measure that determines a reduction of the insulin infusion rate. Although some patients with ketoacidosis can be treated in the emergency ward and released after the episode resolves [33], most patients are admitted to the hospital for close observation as well as to investigate for a precipitating event.

The initial management of patients with diabetic ketoacidosis with very large fluid volumes has recently been challenged [10]. The advantages of intensive fluid administration may be limited after the intravascular volume has been restored, because volume expansion then leads to the excretion of ketone anions in the urine. Moreover, excessive expansion of the plasma volume

reduces proximal tubular bicarbonate reabsorption, in part by reducing Na-H exchange. The net effect is normalization of the AG without a significant increase in the plasma HCO_3^- concentration. In this setting, correction of the metabolic acidosis requires regeneration of "new" bicarbonate by the kidney (a process that may take several days), in contrast to the rapid increase in bicarbonate that occurs when ketone anions are metabolized back to HCO_3^- in the liver as insulin is given. As a result, vigorous fluid administration may delay recovery of acidosis and should be slowed after intravascular volume compromise manifested by a reduction in blood pressure or a rise in the plasma creatinine and blood urea nitrogen (BUN) concentrations has been corrected. A rise in the plasma creatinine in ketoacidosis does not always indicate renal insufficiency, since acetoacetic acid is a noncreatinine chromogen that is measured as creatinine in the standard colorimetric assay [34].

Alkali administration is not usually necessary in patients with ketoacidosis, since there appears to be no difference in mortality between patients treated with $NaHCO_3$ and controls [35]. Insulin therapy should normalize the plasma HCO_3^- concentration as ketone anions are metabolized. Furthermore, there is evidence that alkali administration can increase the rate of ketoacid production [36].

Selected patients may benefit from cautious alkali therapy, however, including patients with severe acidemia (in whom cardiovascular compromise may ensue) [37] and those with a normal AG acidosis [10,38]. As discussed previously, the latter setting is associated with a reduced quantity of organic anion from which HCO_3^- can be generated. The goal of therapy should be to raise the arterial blood pH to a relatively safe level of 7.15 to 7.20.

Bicarbonate administration is indicated in patients with severe hyperkalemia, which is due primarily to insulin deficiency (see Chap. 79) and to hyperglycemia. The latter can increase the plasma K^+ concentration by solvent drag, in which the osmotic effect of hyperglycemia causes water (and potassium) to leave the intracellular space.

Hypophosphatemia may occur with insulin administration during treatment of ketoacidosis. Observations have not shown that phosphate replacement alters the course of this disorder [39].

LACTIC ACIDOSIS. Correction of the underlying disorder is the primary therapy for lactic acidosis. Reversal of circulatory failure, hypoxemia, or sepsis reduces the rate of lactate production and enhances its removal (see Chap. 115).

The use of $NaHCO_3$ in the treatment of lactic acidosis is controversial [37,40]. The potential benefits of alkali administration principally involve the maintenance of normal cardiovascular homeostasis [43]. This potential benefit must be weighed against possible deleterious effects such as volume overload, hypernatremia, and overshoot alkalosis after restoration of tissue perfusion. Recent data also suggest that HCO_3^- therapy may not improve the blood pH or survival in lactic acidosis.

Both in experimental models [40,41] and in patients with lactic acidosis [40,42], alkali therapy has been relatively ineffective, since the increment in the plasma HCO_3^- concentration is transient. Furthermore, the administration of HCO_3^- has been observed to reduce cardiac performance in patients with cardiac arrest, congestive heart failure, and acute myocardial infarction [43,44].* Experimental studies suggest that this lack of efficacy is due to an associated increase in net lactate production, a process that leads to a rise in the AG. The mechanism underlying this increased lactic acid production is probably complex, but may include alterations in intracellular pH, a left-

* By comparison, dialysis with a solution containing HCO_3^- may improve cardiac function in patients with renal failure.

ward shift of the hemoglobin-oxygen dissociation curve, as well as altered cardiac function.

As the lactic acid production rate increases, administered bicarbonate is titrated and forms carbon dioxide. In the presence of fixed or impaired ventilation, respiratory excretion of carbon dioxide becomes limited at this extremely high production rate [45].

$$HCO_3^+ + H^+ \rightarrow H_2CO_3 \rightarrow CO_2 + H_2O$$

The problem of CO_2 accumulation may be masked clinically by reduction in pulmonary blood flow, as occurs, for example, during cardiopulmonary resuscitation [46]. Blood entering the pulmonary circulation may be normally cleared of CO_2, leading to a relatively normal *arterial* PCO_2. In this setting, the *mixed venous* PCO_2, representing blood that has not yet entered the pulmonary circulation, may be markedly elevated because of both the increased rate of CO_2 production at the tissue level and the low cardiac output that slows the return of CO_2-carrying venous blood from the tissues to the lungs. If the mixed venous results more closely reflect the pH at a cellular level, then the arterial values may lead to the mistaken assumption that the pH is being well controlled.

It is possible that alkali therapy may have a direct negative effect on cardiac function by reducing coronary perfusion pressure. This could explain the fall in cardiac output observed in some patients treated with bicarbonate in this setting [46a].

As a result of these findings, no definite recommendations can be made regarding alkali therapy in lactic acidosis. A reasonable approach might be to administer HCO_3^- to maintain the arterial blood pH above 7.15 to 7.20 and the plasma HCO_3^- concentration above 10 to 12 mEq per liter, as determined previously (see section on alkali administration in this chapter). In contrast, if the lactate level increases or the arterial or mixed venous PCO_2 rises without a significant improvement in clinical status or blood pH, the benefit of continuing alkali administration should be questioned.

There are two potential alternatives to the administration of $NaHCO_3$ in lactic acidosis: sodium carbonate and dichloroacetate (DCA). Sodium carbonate (Na_2CO_3) has been observed to improve the acid-base and circulatory status in individuals with experimental lactic acidosis when compared with sodium bicarbonate [47]. This difference appears to be due to the generation of CO_2 with HCO_3^- therapy; in comparison, sodium carbonate is metabolized to bicarbonate and so does not directly cause a rise in the PCO_2.

$$Na_2CO_3 + H^+ \text{ lactate} \rightarrow Na^+HCO_3^- + Na^+ \text{ lactate}$$

Dichloroacetate, by contrast, stimulates pyruvate dehydrogenase (PDH) activity in many tissues, thereby limiting lactate production from pyruvate (catalyzed by lactate dehydrogenase, LDH) by increasing the oxidation of pyruvate to acetyl CoA.

$$\text{Lactate} \overset{\text{LDH}}{\leftarrow} \text{pyruvate} \overset{\text{PDH}}{\rightarrow} \text{acetyl CoA} \rightarrow CO_2 + H_2O$$

Early studies with this investigational drug had shown promise experimentally and in some patients with lactic acidosis [48,49]. A more recent large clinical trial, however, failed to show a difference in mortality in patients treated with this agent [49a]. This lack of improvement in outcome occurred despite a fall in plasma lactate concentration and a rise in bicarbonate level with therapy. These findings are consistent with the hypothesis that the high mortality in lactic acidosis results from the underlying disorder causing the acidosis, not from the acidemia per se.

DRUG AND TOXIN INGESTIONS. The treatment of salicylate intox-

ication is discussed in Chapter 154, and the therapy of methanol and ethylene glycol ingestions is considered in Chapter 132.

RENAL TUBULAR ACIDOSIS. The acidemia in type 1 (distal) RTA can be corrected with HCO_3^- or a bicarbonate precursor such as citrate. The usual requirement is 1 to 3 mEq per kg per day, which should be sufficient to buffer that fraction of the daily acid load (50–100 mEq/day) that is not being excreted. Generally, a potassium salt is administered (such as potassium citrate), since this will repair the potassium deficit as well.* Large doses of oral $NaHCO_3$ can cause gastrointestinal symptoms due to gas formation as gastric acid is titrated to form carbonic acid and then CO_2 and water. This problem can be minimized by the use of citrate, which is ultimately metabolized in the body to bicarbonate. Solutions are available that contain 1 to 2 mEq per ml of sodium, potassium, or sodium and potassium citrate.

The initial step in the management of type 2 (proximal) RTA is to determine the presence of treatable underlying disorder, such as vitamin D deficiency, multiple myeloma, or the use of a carbonic anhydrase inhibitor. Even if no specific therapy is available, correction of the acidemia may not be required in adults if the patient is asymptomatic and if there is only a mild-to-moderate reduction in the plasma HCO_3^- concentration. In comparison, treatment is always indicated in children, since restoring acid-base balance can permit normal growth to resume [50].

The evaluation and treatment of the hyperkalemic form of distal renal tubular acidosis and of type 4 (hypoaldosteronism) RTA, in which hyperkalemia is also present, can be found in Chapter 79.

Metabolic Alkalosis

Primary metabolic alkalosis is characterized by an elevated plasma HCO_3^- concentration in the presence of an arterial pH above 7.40. When there is a concomitant metabolic acidosis, however, the blood pH may be increased, decreased, or normal. Furthermore, hyperbicarbonatemia alone is not diagnostic of this disorder, since it may also represent the appropriate response to chronic respiratory acidosis.† These conditions can be easily distinguished by measurement of the arterial blood pH, which is reduced in respiratory acidosis.

PATHOPHYSIOLOGY AND ETIOLOGY. There are two steps involved in the development of metabolic alkalosis; the alkalosis must first be generated, and then it must be maintained [51]. The factors that mediate the generation phase may differ from those that maintain it. As a result, the evaluation and treatment of this disorder are made easier by first reviewing the pathophysiology of these changes.

A primary rise in the plasma HCO_3^- concentration can be induced by one or more of three mechanisms: (1) loss of acid from the gastrointestinal tract or in the urine; (2) administration of HCO_3^- or a bicarbonate precursor such as citrate; or (3) loss of fluid with a chloride-bicarbonate concentration ratio that is higher than that contained in an equal volume of plasma. The latter condition is sometimes referred to as "contraction alka-

---

* The response of the kidney in respiratory acidosis is to retain HCO_3^- and excrete H^+. The change in the plasma HCO_4^- concentration is typically less than 3 mEq per liter when this occurs acutely. Consequently, an increase in the plasma concentration of HCO_4^- that is greater than this amount (e.g., a rise from 25 to 32 mEq/L) indicates that the respiratory disturbance is chronic.
† Rarely, potassium deficiency may be severe enough to cause respiratory muscle dysfunction, leading to a superimposed respiratory acidosis.

losis," since the total bicarbonate content remains normal while the extracellular fluid volume contracts around it, thereby elevating the plasma HCO_3^- concentration [52]. In contrast to the rise in HCO_3^- that may be observed in (1) and (2), contraction alkalosis contributes to metabolic alkalosis, but it is rarely responsible for more than a mild increase in the plasma HCO_3^- concentration. The reason for this limitation can be seen by the following example: Suppose a patient with a normal plasma HCO_3^- level loses 3 liters of extracellular fluid through vomiting but that all H^+ losses are replaced. The normal HCO_3^- space is equal to approximately 50% of lean body weight (see Metabolic Acidosis, preceding). Thus, a 70-kg man has an HCO_3^- volume of distribution of about 35 liters. Assuming a baseline plasma HCO_3^- concentration of 25 mEq per liter, the estimated bicarbonate stores are 875 mEq. The removal of 3 liters of chloride-containing extracellular fluid without bicarbonate would cause the plasma HCO_3^- concentration to rise to only 27.3 mEq per liter [875/(35 − 3) = 27.3].

Loss of fluid with an electrolyte composition similar to plasma, as occurs with gastrointestinal bleeding, produces contraction of the extracellular fluid volume that may lead to hypotension. By comparison, it does not result in a contraction alkalosis because there is no direct change in the plasma HCO_3^- concentration.

Under normal circumstances, the excess in bicarbonate generated by any of these processes is rapidly excreted in the urine [52]. Consequently, *the maintenance of a metabolic alkalosis requires an impairment in renal bicarbonate excretion* [53]. This is most commonly due to volume and chloride depletion.

A fall in effective arterial blood volume* reduces the ability of the kidney to excrete HCO_3^-, an alteration that is particularly important in the proximal tubule [54]. This nephron segment is responsible for reabsorption of over 80% of the bicarbonate load filtered through the kidneys each day (see Fig. 80-1). Under ordinary conditions, bicarbonate appears in the urine when the plasma level increases above the normal value of about 25 mEq per liter. In the presence of volume depletion, however, the capacity of the proximal tubule to reabsorb bicarbonate increases, thereby permitting the plasma level to rise without bicarbonaturia. Several mechanisms account for these changes; two of the most important may be stimulation of the luminal Na-H antiporter by angiotensin II (AII) (AII is usually generated in response to volume contraction) and enhanced bicarbonate transport out of the proximal tubular cell (see Fig. 80-1) [55,56]. In addition, most hypovolemic states are associated with chloride depletion. Since luminal chloride appears to be important in chloride-bicarbonate exchange, it is not surprising that correction of the metabolic alkalosis usually requires chloride repletion as well [56a]. In comparison, giving chloride is ineffective when hyperaldosteronism, marked hypokalemia, renal failure, or an edematous state is responsible for the defect in bicarbonate excretion. The cause of metabolic alkalosis can usually be identified by this ability of chloride to repair only some types of metabolic alkalosis (see Diagnosis, following).

Alkali Administration. Since administered bicarbonate is normally excreted rapidly in the urine, alkali administration must be massive or renal impairment must limit the excretion of bicarbonate if metabolic alkalosis is to develop. The administration of large quantities of $NaHCO_3$ or a bicarbonate precursor (such as citrate with multiple blood transfusions) can cause metabolic alkalosis [57]. By comparison, if renal impairment is significant, lesser amounts may raise the blood pH.

Milk-alkali syndrome is an uncommon cause of hypercal-

cemia and metabolic alkalosis, probably because nonabsorbable antacids and H_2-blockers have largely supplanted the use of large quantities of baking soda and milk as treatment of gastritis and peptic ulcer disease [58]. The chronic ingestion of milk and calcium carbonate-containing antacids leads to the development of metabolic alkalosis because the increased HCO_3^- load cannot be excreted as a result of renal impairment from chronic hypercalcemia [59].

Chloride-Responsive Metabolic Alkalosis

GENERATION OF CHLORIDE-RESPONSIVE METABOLIC ALKALOSIS. The two most common causes of metabolic alkalosis are diuretic therapy and loss of gastric secretions (resulting from nasogastric suction or vomiting) (Table 80-4) [60]. Both *thiazide* and *loop diuretics* can generate a metabolic alkalosis, regardless of whether they are given to treat hypertension or states of volume overload such as congestive heart failure. H^+ loss results from increased distal sodium presentation in the presence of elevated aldosterone levels; this causes enhanced distal nephron Na-H exchange (see Chap. 79 for a description of the tubular mechanisms involved in distal H^+ secretion) [52]. Hydrogen secretion in this, as in other nephron segments, is associated with increased HCO_3^- reabsorption. The proximal tubule may also play an important role, since stimulation of the renin-angiotensin system by volume depletion enhances the activity of the Na-H antiporter, thereby increasing H^+ secretion and HCO_3^- reabsorption. To the degree that the urinary anion losses are primarily chloride, a component of contraction alkalosis can contribute as well.

Contraction can also play a role in the metabolic alkalosis observed with vomiting and nasogastric suction (even in patients with achlorhydria in whom NaCl replaces HCl in the gastric secretions), and, less commonly, with some forms of diarrhea in which chloride is the predominant anion that is lost [60a]. In contrast, gastric H^+ losses are primarily responsible for the generation of metabolic alkalosis in this setting.

Secretion of gastric acid results in the retention of 1 mEq of HCO_3^- for each milliequivalent of H^+ that is secreted, because

---

Table 80-4. Major Causes of Metabolic Alkalosis

Hydrogen loss
  Gastrointestinal
    Removal of gastric secretions (vomiting or nasogastric suction)[a]
    Chloride-losing diarrheal states
  Renal
    Loop or thiazide-type diuretics[a]
    Mineralocorticoid excess[a]
    Postchronic hypercapnia
    Hypercalcemia[b]
    High dose intravenous penicillins
    Bartter's syndrome
Bicarbonate retention
  Massive blood transfusion
  Administration of large amounts of $NaHCO_3$
  Milk alkali syndrome
Contraction alkalosis
  Diuretics[a]
  Loss of high chloride/low bicarbonate gastrointestinal secretions[a]
    (vomiting and some diarrheal states)
Hydrogen movement into cells
  Hypokalemia
  Refeeding

[a]Most common causes.
[b]Primary hyperparathyroidism is frequently associated with a mild metabolic acidosis (see text for details).

---

* The effective arterial blood volume refers to that portion of the blood volume perfusing tissues, particularly the kidney.

both of the ions are derived from the intracellular dissociation of carbonic acid.

$$H_2CO_3 \rightarrow HCO_2^- + H^+$$

This process does not normally lead to metabolic alkalosis, since the 80 to 200 mEq of HCl secreted by the stomach each day enters the duodenum, where it stimulates an equivalent amount of bicarbonate secretion from the pancreas. By comparison, the H^+ secreted by the stomach cannot enhance pancreatic HCO_3^- secretion when vomiting or nasogastric suctioning is present, thereby leading to net retention of HCO_3^-. As in diuretic use, distal nephron Na-H exchange usually contributes to the development of this disorder because aldosterone levels are stimulated by the loss of extracellular volume.

Renal H^+ and K^+ losses also contribute to the metabolic alkalosis and potassium depletion observed in *hypercalcemic* states [61]. Malignancy-induced hypercalcemia is frequently severe. Calcium may impair tubular function and cause nausea and vomiting, leading to volume depletion and increased H^+ and K^+ losses. As a result, humoral hypercalcemia of malignancy, caused by a parathyroid-like hormone, may cause metabolic alkalosis. On the other hand, primary hyperparathyroidism is commonly associated with a mild metabolic *acidosis,* probably due to the inhibitory action of parathyroid hormone on the Na-H antiporter in the proximal tubule. This difference may result from a lack of inhibitory effect of tumor-induced parathyroid hormone-like protein on this transporter [62].

Metabolic alkalosis also may be observed after the rapid correction of chronic respiratory acidosis. This *posthypercapneic metabolic alkalosis* occurs because chronic respiratory acidosis activates compensatory renal mechanisms that induce HCl loss in the urine; the ensuing rise in the plasma HCO_3^- concentration is appropriate in that it returns the arterial pH toward normal [63]. Generally, the plasma HCO_3^- increases by about 3.5 mEq per liter for every 10 mm Hg rise in the arterial PCO_2. If hypercapnia is rapidly reversed, however (most frequently by artificial ventilation), the excess HCO_3^- that has been generated persists, and the pH may rise to alkalemic levels.

MAINTENANCE OF CHLORIDE-RESPONSIVE METABOLIC ALKALOSIS. As reviewed previously, renal excretion of bicarbonate typically begins when the plasma level rises above 25 mEq per liter, and the normal kidney can excrete large quantities (>1000 mEq/L) without a substantial increase in the plasma HCO_3^- concentration [57]. As a result, maintenance of a chloride-responsive alkalosis depends on a reduction in renal bicarbonate excretion. Both reduced glomerular filtration rate and, more importantly, enhanced proximal tubular NaHCO$_3$ reabsorption limit HCO_3^- excretion, thus allowing the increase in plasma bicarbonate to persist [64]. Normally, Cl^- is the major anion reabsorbed with Na^+. In states of chloride depletion (as occurs in chloride-responsive metabolic alkalosis), however, sodium must be reabsorbed with the next most abundant anion, bicarbonate. Thus, the need to preserve volume prevents correction of the alkalosis.

Hypokalemia also can enhance renal HCO_3^- reabsorption and contribute to the maintenance of metabolic alkalosis. Potassium losses frequently occur when diuretic administration or gastric acid losses cause the acid-base disturbance (see Diagnosis, following) [65]. If the plasma HCO_3^- concentration exceeds the capacity of the proximal renal tubule to reabsorb it, bicarbonaturia obligates excretion of a cation (such as Na^+) so that electrical charge is not altered. Some of the Na^+ that leaves the proximal tubule with bicarbonate is then reabsorbed distally in exchange for potassium. These urinary K^+ losses are primarily responsible for the hypokalemia seen with vomiting;

gastric losses are usually less important, since these secretions have a potassium concentration below 10 mEq per liter. As a result of potassium depletion, intracellular acidosis occurs as H^+ shifts into cells to maintain electroneutrality as K^+ moves extracellularly to defend against hypokalemia [66].* Ultimately, proximal tubular Na-H exchange is stimulated, which further reduces renal HCO_3^- excretion (see Fig. 80-1).

In the presence of effective volume depletion, high-dose penicillins (including ticarcillin and carbenicillin) act as nonreabsorbable anions [67]. The negative charge in the tubular lumen facilitates secretion of both H^+ and K^+ and may contribute to the maintenance of metabolic alkalosis.

Chloride-Resistant Metabolic Alkalosis. Metabolic alkalosis in some individuals is not responsive to the administration of chloride-containing solutions. In these disorders, hypokalemia, a primary increase in mineralocorticoid activity, or renal tubular chloride wasting (Bartter's syndrome) is usually responsible for the generation and maintenance of the alkalosis. In all of these disorders, there is enhanced renal H^+ excretion and HCO_3^- reabsorption. There is no chloride depletion or an inability to reabsorb chloride, which explains why NaCl and KCl will not correct the metabolic alkalosis in these individuals. Edematous states also are generally unresponsive to volume (and chloride) replacement, despite the reduction in effective arterial blood volume.

MINERALOCORTICOID EXCESS. Mineralocorticoids, such as aldosterone, act in the cortical collecting tubule (see Chap. 79), where they enhance Na-K exchange as well as H^+ secretion [68]. As a result, overproduction of an endogenous mineralocorticoid (as occurs in primary aldosteronism) or administration of an exogenous substance with mineralocorticoid activity (such as glycyrrhizic acid in licorice) leads to hypokalemia and metabolic alkalosis. Hypertension is characteristically present in these disorders. In contrast to patients with secondary increases in mineralocorticoid activity (e.g., as in congestive heart failure), edema does not occur. This phenomenon, called "aldosterone escape," results from the high renal interstitial pressures generated by the hypertension that limits further NaCl reabsorption; it is also possible that atrial natriuretic peptide, released in response to volume expansion, contributes to this phenomenon [69].

In addition to the direct effect of aldosterone on H^+ secretion, hypokalemia also appears to be necessary for the development of a significant metabolic alkalosis in patients with primary mineralocorticoid excess [70]. The mechanism of this effect involves the development of intracellular acidosis with increased H^+ secretion and HCO_3^- reabsorption by the proximal tubule and enhanced distal nephron Na-H exchange [70].

SEVERE HYPOKALEMIA. The effect of mild-to-moderate hypokalemia on the generation and maintenance of metabolic alkalosis has been discussed. In contrast, severe hypokalemia (plasma K^+ <2 mEq/L) can impair distal chloride reabsorption by an unknown mechanism [71]. In this setting, some of the Na^+ that is normally reabsorbed with Cl^- must be reabsorbed in exchange for H^+.

BARTTER'S SYNDROME. Bartter's syndrome is a rare cause of

---

* The pathophysiology of this event is more complex and probably depends on a change in the membrane potential induced by hypokalemia. As can be seen in Figure 80-1, the interior of the tubular cell is electronegative compared with the outside. This potential difference is determined primarily by the difference between K^+ intracellular and K^+ extracellular. Because there is substantially more potassium inside the cell (about 130 mEq/L) than in plasma (about 4 mEq/L), a fall in the plasma K^+ concentration causes the inside of the cell to become more electronegative as the membrane potential increases. It appears that this negative intracellular charge on the basolateral membrane is the driving force for Na-3HCO$_3$ reabsorption. Thus, the cell interior may become more acid in hypokalemic states because more HCO_3^- leaves the cell.

metabolic alkalosis typically seen in women under 30 years old who are typically normotensive or slightly hypotensive. It is due to impaired NaCl reabsorption in the loop of Henle or distal tubule [72]. The ensuing volume depletion activates the renin-angiotensin-aldosterone system, increasing distal nephron K^+ and H^+ secretion, similar to a loop diuretic.

Renal prostaglandin production is increased in this disorder, although the reason this occurs is not completely understood. The increase in renal prostaglandin synthesis enhances renin (and subsequently aldosterone) release, further contributing to the hypokalemia and metabolic alkalosis. The fact that inhibitors of prostaglandin synthesis improve the electrolyte abnormalities, but do not normalize them, indicates that the increase in prostaglandin synthesis is not the primary abnormality (see Treatment of Metabolic Alkalosis, following).

EDEMATOUS STATES. Congestive heart failure and advanced liver disease may be associated with metabolic alkalosis in patients treated with loop or thiazide diuretics or in whom vomiting occurs. Although the pathogenesis of the alkalosis is similar to that in normal individuals, Cl^- replacement may be ineffective in correcting the disorder. Chloride resistance persists because the effective arterial blood volume cannot be normally expanded by NaCl or KCl in edematous states. Consequently, there is continued stimulation of proximal tubular HCO_3^- reabsorption and distal nephron K^+ and H^+ secretion.

Intracellular Shift of H^+ Causing Metabolic Alkalosis.
The effect of hypokalemia on metabolic alkalosis has been discussed previously. *Refeeding* with carbohydrate after a prolonged fast can cause a metabolic alkalosis, possibly through a shift of H^+ into cells, since neither volume depletion nor increased renal H^+ excretion is present [73]. The maintenance of the alkalosis in this condition may result from renal Na^+ (and HCO_3^-) retention, possibly due to increased insulin secretion.

CLINICAL MANIFESTATIONS.
Most patients with metabolic alkalosis do not suffer clinically from the adverse effects of alkalemia. When symptoms are present, they are typically those associated with volume depletion (weakness, muscle cramps, postural dizziness) or hypokalemia (muscle weakness, polyuria, polydipsia). The usual symptoms of alkalemia are due to increased neuromuscular excitability and are exhibited as paresthesias, carpopedal spasm, or lightheadedness. These findings are much more likely to be seen in patients with acute respiratory alkalosis, since the fall in plasma PCO_2 causes the intracellular CO_2 tension to fall [51]. This intracellular alkalosis occurs more slowly in those with metabolic alkalosis, since HCO_3^-, in contrast to CO_2, is not lipid soluble and crosses the cell membrane less rapidly.

DIAGNOSIS.
The cause of metabolic alkalosis can usually be elicited from the history and physical examination. One of the most important aspects of the physical examination in identifying a cause is the determination of blood pressure. Except for the hypertensive individual taking a diuretic, hypokalemia in the presence of metabolic alkalosis and hypertension should suggest the presence of a primary mineralocorticoid-induced disease.

Normotensive individuals in whom there is no obvious cause almost always have surreptitious vomiting or diuretic ingestion as the cause of the metabolic alkalosis. Some individuals with self-induced vomiting may have dental erosions (due to re-

Table 80-5. Urine Chloride Concentration in Metabolic Alkalosis

Less than 15 mEq/L	Greater than 20 mEq/L
Vomiting	Mineralocorticoid excess
Nasogastric suction	Alkali loading
Postdiuretic administration	During diuretic administration
Posthypercapnia	Severe hypokalemia
High dose penicillin therapy	Bartter's syndrome
Alkali loading*	

*Since the maintenance of metabolic alkalosis requires impairment of renal bicarbonate excretion, the pathophysiology of the renal limitation will determine the urinary chloride concentration. If, for example, there is underlying hypovolemia, the urinary chloride concentration will be low (<15 mEg/L); in comparison, the urinary chloride concentration will be >20 mEq/L when the cause of renal bicarbonate retention is due to a reduction in glomerular filtration rate, as in the milk-alkali syndrome or in patients with acute tubular necrosis who receive large alkali loads.

peated exposure to gastric acid), calluses, and scarring on the dorsum of the hand [74].

Measurement of the urinary chloride concentration is useful in differentiating these disorders (Table 80-5). The urinary chloride concentration is typically less than 15 mEq per liter with hypovolemia due to vomiting or diuretic therapy (if the effect of the diuretic has worn off). Higher values are found if the diuretic is still active, if Bartter's syndrome or severe hypokalemia is present, or if there is primary mineralocorticoid excess. Diuretic abuse may be distinguished from Bartter's syndrome in some individuals by screening the urine for diuretics.

The urinary chloride concentration is important because urinary Na^+ wasting may occur in the presence of a high plasma bicarbonate concentration even if volume depletion is present. $NaHCO_3$ losses develop when the plasma HCO_3^- level exceeds the renal reabsorptive threshold, a condition that obligates the excretion of HCO_3^- with a cation to maintain electroneutrality. The most abundant extracellular fluid cation is Na^+, even in low perfusion states. As a result, the urine Na^+ concentration should not be used to suggest the volume status of an individual with an increased plasma HCO_3^- concentration unless it is less than 20 mEq per liter. By comparison, the urinary chloride concentration characteristically is low in hypoperfusion states, since Cl^- is not affected by bicarbonaturia.

Mixed Acid-Base Disturbances with Metabolic Alkalosis

RESPIRATORY COMPENSATION. The increased arterial pH in metabolic alkalosis leads to a compensatory rise in the PCO_2. This decrease in respiration is due to direct suppression of the medullary respiratory center by alkalemia. In general, *the PCO_2 rises about 0.7 mm Hg for every 1 mEq per liter elevation in the plasma HCO_3^-* concentration [75]. This compensatory mechanism holds true until the PCO_2 rises to about 60 mm Hg (plasma HCO_3^- concentration = 53 mEq/L); values above this level are unusual because further hypoventilation is limited by the development of hypoxemia. The identification of a PCO_2 greater or less than predicted suggests the presence of a second primary acid-base disturbance, respiratory acidosis, or respiratory alkalosis, respectively.

METABOLIC ALKALOSIS WITH METABOLIC ACIDOSIS. The ratio of the increment in AG to decrement in the plasma HCO_3^- concentration (Δ/Δ) can be used to identify the presence of a metabolic alkalosis in a patient with metabolic acidosis. This concept is demonstrated by the following example:

A 47-year-old man with a history of alcohol abuse and vomiting is admitted to the hospital with the following laboratory studies:

Na^+ = 140 mEq/L	BUN = 23 mg/dl
K^+ = 3.6 mEq/L	Creatinine = 1.3 mg/dl
Cl^- = 92 mEq/L	Plasma ketones = 4^+
HCO_3^- = 16 mEq/L	Plasma lactate <1 mEq/L
AG = 32 mEq/L	PCO_2 = 32 mm Hg pH = 7.31

The diagnosis of alcoholic ketoacidosis with appropriate respiratory compensation was made based on the clinical history and positive blood ketones. On closer inspection, however, it can be seen that the increment in the AG (above the normal value of about 10 mEq/L) is 22. If all of the circulating anions were metabolized back to HCO_3^-, the final plasma HCO_3^- concentration would be 38 mEq per liter (22 + 16). Consequently, the presence of a second primary acid-base disturbance, a metabolic alkalosis caused by vomiting, was suggested by the admission laboratory studies. This was confirmed as the plasma HCO_3^- concentration rose above normal as ketones were metabolized during insulin administration.

TREATMENT OF METABOLIC ALKALOSIS. Rapid correction of metabolic alkalosis is usually not necessary owing to the general lack of adverse effects directly related to the rise in pH. As a result, there is ordinarily time to identify the cause of the disorder and to institute specific therapy. Exogenous sources of alkali (such as HCO_3^-, acetate, lactate, and citrate) can exacerbate the alkalemia and should be discontinued.

Chloride-Responsive Metabolic Alkalosis. Chloride replacement (as NaCl, KCl, or both) is appropriate for management of individuals with a low urinary chloride concentration. Administration of chloride-containing fluid with potassium ameliorates the alkalosis by permitting renal excretion of the excess HCO_3^-. It allows more sodium to be reabsorbed with Cl^-, rather than in exchange for H^+; it reduces the volume stimulus for Na^+ retention, permitting HCO_3^- excretion in the urine; and it increases the plasma K^+ concentration, which raises the tubular cell pH and reduces renal H^+ secretion. Replacement of the volume deficit with nonchloride-containing solutions of Na^+ or K^+ will not correct the alkalosis or hypokalemia, since nonchloride anions obligate further K^+ and H^+ excretion [76].

Patients with vomiting or nasogastric suction also may benefit from H_2-blockers or other medications that impair gastric acid secretion [77]. They are not, however, substitutes for Cl^- replacement, which is still necessary to correct the already present chloride deficit.

The therapy of metabolic alkalosis in edematous patients (such as those with congestive heart failure and advanced liver disease) is more difficult. Although renal perfusion is characteristically reduced, leading to a low urinary chloride concentration, chloride administration (as 0.9% saline, for instance) will not enhance HCO_3^- excretion, since the reduced effective arterial blood volume will not be corrected by this therapy. In this setting, the carbonic anhydrase inhibitor, acetazolamide (at a dose of 250 to 375 mg once or twice daily orally or intravenously), can be useful since it permits fluid mobilization while decreasing HCO_3^- reabsorption in the proximal tubule. An adverse consequence of acetazolamide administration is the tendency for more K^+ wasting. Thus, careful monitoring of the plasma potassium concentration is necessary. When the plasma K^+ level is low, the use of a distally acting potassium-sparing diuretic (such as amiloride or spironolactone) should be considered.

In rare instances, these recommendations may be ineffective or the metabolic alkalosis may be so severe that adverse neurologic symptoms of alkalemia are present. When this occurs, HCl can be given intravenously to lower the plasma HCO_3^- concentration. HCl is usually given as a solution isotonic to plasma (150 mEq H^+ and 150 mEq Cl^- in each liter of distilled water). The volume needed to reduce the plasma HCO_3^- concentration can be estimated from the HCO_3^- deficit. Since the volume of distribution of bicarbonate is approximately 50% of lean body weight, the amount of HCl needed to lower the plasma HCO_3^- concentration from 45 to 35 mEq per liter in a 70-kg man can be calculated as follows (assuming there are no ongoing HCO_3^- losses):

$$HCO_3^- \text{ excess} = 0.5 \times 70 \times (45 - 35) = 350 \text{ mEq}$$

This would require administration of slightly over 2 liters of an isotonic HCl solution. The very low pH of this solution can injure small veins, particularly if extravasation occurs; thus, administration should generally occur over at least 24 hours using a large (central) vein. A peripheral vein can be safely used if the HCl is buffered in an amino acid solution and infused with a fat emulsion [78]. Ammonium chloride and arginine hydrochloride have metabolic side effects (encephalopathy [79] and hyperkalemia [80], respectively) that preclude their use in this setting.

Dialytic therapy may be useful in the rare patient with metabolic alkalosis, volume overload, and renal failure. Peritoneal dialysis typically contains lactate as the HCO_3^- precursor at a concentration of about 40 mEq per liter, an amount that may worsen the alkalosis. It is possible, however, to constitute a solution containing more chloride in place of lactate. In contrast, newer volumetric hemodialysis machines use HCO_3^-, the concentration of which can be adjusted. In the uncommon patient in whom dialytic therapy is considered for treatment of metabolic alkalosis, when both techniques are available, hemodialysis or continuous arteriovenous hemofiltration may be preferable to peritoneal dialysis depending on the vascular stability of the individual [81,82].

Chloride-Resistant Metabolic Alkalosis. Individuals with a urinary chloride concentration greater than 15 mEq per liter are unlikely to respond to chloride-containing solutions such as physiologic saline, with correction of the metabolic alkalosis. Since the effective perfusion volume is already normal, the administered Cl^- is rapidly excreted in the urine. Moreover, enhanced distal Na^+ presentation increases Na-K exchange, leading to a rise in urinary K^+ excretion with more severe hypokalemia in states of primary mineralocorticoid excess.

In a hypertensive individual, primary aldosterone should be considered. Removing the source of aldosterone (by adrenalectomy when an aldosterone-secreting adenoma is present) or blocking its action (with a potassium-sparing diuretic, such as amiloride [83]) is usually sufficient to correct the hypokalemia and metabolic alkalosis and to control hypertension in this disorder.

The abnormality in Bartter's syndrome, impaired Cl^- reabsorption, cannot be corrected with treatment. Therapy is, therefore, directed at improving the laboratory abnormalities, particularly hypokalemia and metabolic alkalosis. Nonsteroidal antiinflammatory drugs reduce renin secretion (a prostaglandin-dependent process) and may be effective in reducing the plasma HCO_3^- and K^+ levels to or near normal, although potassium supplementation also may be required [84]. Angiotensin-converting enzyme inhibitors [85] or potassium-sparing diuretics [86] may be useful either alone or in combination, but they have the potential risk of causing the already slightly low blood pressure to fall. It is important to exclude surreptitious diuretic use or forced vomiting in these individuals before assigning a diagnostic or therapeutic regimen used for Bartter's syndrome, since the former are far more common disorders.

The associated chloride reabsorptive defect in severe hypokalemia is corrected with KCl supplementation [71]. Potassium treatment will convert the chloride-resistant alkalosis to one that is responsive to NaCl.

The treatment of edematous patients has been discussed. These individuals are typically not chloride-responsive despite the usual finding of a low urinary chloride concentration.

References

1. Seifter J, Aronson P: Properties and physiologic roles of the plasma membrane sodium-hydrogen exchanger. *J Clin Invest* 78:859, 1986.
2. Clark E, Evans B, MacIntyre I: Acidosis in experimental electrolyte depletion. *Clin Sci* 14:421, 1955.
3. Schoolwerth AC: Regulation of renal ammoniagenesis in metabolic acidosis. *Kidney Int* 40:961, 1991.
4. Nasraway S, Black R, Sottile F: The anion gap in patients admitted to the medical intensive care unit (abstract). *Chest* 96:287S, 1989.
4a. Winter SD, Pearson R, Gabow PA, et al: The fall of the serum anion gap. *Arch Intern Med* 150:311, 1990.
5. Emmett M, Narins R: Clinical use of the anion gap. *Medicine* 56:38, 1977.
6. Wallia R, Greenberg A, Piraino B, et al: Serum electrolyte patterns in end-stage renal disease. *Am J Kidney Dis* 8:98, 1986.
7. Widmer B, Gerhardt R, Harrington J, et al: Serum electrolyte and acid-base composition: The influence of graded degrees of chronic renal failure. *Arch Intern Med* 139:1099, 1979.
8. Yudkin J, Cohen R: The contribution of the kidney to removal of lactic acid load under normal and acidotic conditions in the conscious rat. *Clin Sci Molec Med* 48:121, 1975.
9. Oliva P: Lactic acidosis. *Am J Med* 48:209, 1970.
10. Adrogue H, Barrero J, Eknoyan G: Salutary effects of modest fluid replacement in the treatment of adults with diabetic ketoacidosis. *JAMA* 262:2108, 1989.
11. Gabow P, Anderson R, Potts D, et al: Acid-base disturbances in the salicylate intoxicated adult. *Arch Intern Med* 138:1481, 1978.
12. Gabow P: Disorders associated with an altered anion gap. *Kidney Int* 27:472, 1985.
13. Gilmour I, Blanchard R, Perry W: Mannitol gives false positive biochemical estimation of ethylene glycol. *N Engl J Med* 291:51, 1974.
14. Gabow P: Ethylene glycol intoxication. *Am J Kidney Dis* 11:277, 1988.
15. Schelling J, Howard R, Goldberg C, et al: Utility of osmolar gap in anion gap metabolic acidosis (abstract). *Kidney Int* 37:268, 1990.
15a. Schelling JR, Howard RL, Winter SO, Linas SL: Increased osmolal gap in alcoholic ketoacidosis and lactic acidosis. *Ann Intern Med* 113:580, 1990.
16. Kleinman P: Cholestyramine and metabolic acidosis. *N Engl J Med* 290:861, 1974.
17. Walter R, Morgan F, Songkhla Y, et al: Water and electrolyte studies in cholera. *J Clin Invest* 38:1879, 1959.
18. Stamy T: The pathogenesis and implications of the electrolyte imbalance in ureterosigmoidostome. *Surg Gynecol Obstet* 103:736, 1959.
19. Kurtzman N: Renal tubular acidosis: A constellation of syndromes. *Hosp Pract* 22:131, 1987.
20. Gougoux A, Kaenhy W, Cohen J: Renal adaptation to chronic hypocapnia. *Am J Physiol* 229:1330, 1975.
21. Rose B: *Clinical Physiology of Acid-Base and Electrolyte Disorders*. New York, McGraw-Hill, 1989, p 527.
22. Gill J Jr, Bell N, Bartter F: Impaired conservation of sodium and potassium in renal tubular acidosis and its correction by buffer anions. *Clin Sci* 33:577, 1967.
23. Simpson D: Citrate excretion: A window on renal metabolism. *Am J Physiol* 244:F223, 1983.
24. Mitchell J, Wildenthal K, Johnson R Jr: The effect of acid-base disturbances on cardiovascular and pulmonary function. *Kidney Int* 1:375, 1973.
24a. Adrogue HJ, Madias NE: Changes in plasma potassium concentration during acute acid-base disturbances. *Am J Med* 71:456, 1981.
25. Gabow P, Kaehay W, Fernessey P, et al: Diagnostic importance of an increased serum anion gap. *N Engl J Med* 303:854, 1980.
26. Bushinsky D, Coe F, Katzenberg C, et al: Arterial PCO_2 in chronic metabolic acidosis. *Kidney Int* 22:311, 1982.
27. Oh M, Carroll H, Goldstein D, et al: Hyperchloremic acidosis during the recovery phase of diabetic ketoacidosis. *Ann Intern Med* 89:925, 1978.
27a. Fernandez PC, Cohen RM, Feldman GM: The concept of bicarbonate distribution space: The crucial role of body buffers. *Kidney Int* 36:747, 1989.
27b. Androgue HJ, Eknoyan G, Suki WN: Diabetic ketoacidosis: Role of the kidney in the acid-base homeostasis re-evaluated. *Kidney Int* 25:591, 1984.
27c. Salem MM, Mujais SK: Gaps in the anion gap. *Arch Intern Med* 152:1625, 1992.
27d. Wang F, Butler T, Rabbari GH, et al: The acidosis of cholera. Contributions of hyperproteinemia, lactic acidemia, and hyperphosphatemia to an increased anion gap. *N Engl J Med* 315:1591, 1986.
27e. Walka R, Greenberg AS, Piraino B, et al: Serum electrolyte patterns in end-stage renal disease. *Am J Kidney Dis* 8:98, 1986.
28. Rose B, Black R: *Manual of Clinical Problems in Nephrology*. Boston, Little, Brown, 1988, p 39.
29. Batle D, Hizon M, Cohen E, et al: The use of the urinary anion gap in the diagnosis of hyperchloremic metabolic acidosis. *N Engl J Med* 318:594, 1988.
30. Adrogue H, Brensilver J, Cohen J: Influence of steady-state alterations in acid-base equilibrium on the fate of administered bicarbonate in the dog. *J Clin Invest* 71:867, 1983.
31. Warnock D: Uremic acidosis. *Kidney Int* 34:278, 1988.
32. Brandt K, Miles J: Relationship between severity of hyperglycemia and metabolic acidosis in diabetic ketoacidosis. *Mayo Clin Proc* 63:1071, 1988.
33. Bonadio WA, Gutzeit MS, Losek JD, et al: Outpatient management of diabetic ketoacidosis. *Am J Dis Child* 142:448, 1988.
34. Molitch M, Roidman E, Hirsch C, et al: Spurious serum creatinine elevations in ketoacidosis. *Ann Intern Med* 93:280, 1980.
35. Morris L, Murphy M, Kitabachi A: Bicarbonate therapy in severe diabetic ketoacidosis. *Ann Intern Med* 105:836, 1986.
36. Hood V, Danforth E Jr, Horton E, et al: Impact of hydrogen ion on fasting ketogenesis: Feedback regulation of acid production. *Am J Physiol* 11:F238, 1982.
37. Narins R, Cohen J: Bicarbonate therapy for organic acidosis: The case for its continued use. *Ann Intern Med* 106:615, 1987.
38. Adrogue H, Eknoyan G, Suki W: Diabetic ketoacidosis: Role of the kidney in the acid-base homeostasis revisited. *Kidney Int* 25:591, 1984.
39. Wilson H, Kener S, Lea A, et al: Phosphate therapy in DKA. *Arch Intern Med* 142:517, 1982.
40. Stacpoole P: Lactic acidosis: The case against bicarbonate therapy. *Ann Intern Med* 105:276, 1986.
41. Graf H, Leach W, Arieff A: Evidence for detrimental effect of bicarbonate therapy in hypoxic lactic acidosis. *Science* 227:754, 1985.
42. Fields A, Wolman S, Halperin M: Chronic lactic acidosis in a patient with cancer: Therapy and metabolic consequences. *Cancer* 47:2026, 1981.
43. Ayus J: Effect of bicarbonate administration on cardiac function. *Am J Med* 87:5, 1989.
44. Bersin R, Chatterjee K, Arieff A: Metabolic and hemodynamic consequences of sodium bicarbonate administration in patients with heart disease. *Am J Med* 87:7, 1989.
45. Bishop R, Weisfeldt M: Sodium bicarbonate administration dur-

ing cardiac arrest: Effect on arterial pH, PCO_2, and osmolality. *JAMA* 235:506, 1976.

46. Weil M, Rackow E, Trevino R, et al: Differences in acid-base state between venous and arterial blood during cardiopulmonary resuscitation. *N Engl J Med* 315:153, 1986.

46a. Kette F, Weil MH, Gazmuri RJ: Buffer solutions may compromise cardiac resuscitation by reducing coronary perfusion pressure. *JAMA* 266:2121, 1991.

47. Bersin R, Arieff A: Improved hemodynamic function during hypoxia with carbicarb, a new agent for the management of acidosis. *Circulation* 77:227, 1988.

48. Stacpoole P, Harman E, Curry H, et al: Treatment of lactic acidosis with dichloroacetate. *N Engl J Med* 309:390, 1983.

49. Graf H, Leach W, Arieff A: Effects of dichloroacetate in the treatment of hypoxic lactic acidosis in dogs. *J Clin Invest* 76:919, 1985.

49a. Stacpoole PW, Wright EC, Baumgartner TG, et al: A controlled clinical trial of dichloroacetate for treatment of lactic acidosis in adults. *N Engl J Med* 327:1564, 1992.

50. Rose B, Black R: *Manual of Clinical Problems in Nephrology.* Boston, Little, Brown, 1988, p 49.

51. Rose B, Black R: *Manual of Clinical Problems in Nephrology.* Boston, Little, Brown, 1988, p 57.

52. Garella S, Chang B, Kahn S: Dilution acidosis and contraction alkalosis: Reviews of a concept. *Kidney Int* 8:279, 1975.

53. Jacobson H, Seldin S: On the generation, maintenance, and correction of metabolic alkalosis. *Am J Physiol* 245:F425, 1983.

54. Sabatini S, Kurtzman NA: The maintenance of metabolic alkalosis: Factors which decrease bicarbonate excretion. *Kidney Int* 25:357, 1984.

55. Liu F-Y, Cogan MG: Angiotensin II stimulates early proximal bicarbonate absorption in the rat by decreasing cAMP. *J Clin Invest* 84:83, 1989.

56. Pastoriza E, Harrington R, Graber M: PTH inhibits base exit in rat proximal tubule (abstract). *Kidney Int* 37:211, 1990.

56a. Wesson DE, Dolson GM: Enhanced HCO_3 secretion by distal tubule contributes to NaCl induced correction of chronic alkalosis. *Am J Physiol* 264:F899, 1993.

57. Van Goidsenhoven G, Gray O, Price A, et al: The effect of prolonged administration of large doses of sodium bicarbonate in man. *Clin Sci* 13:383, 1954.

58. Orwoll E: The milk-alkali syndrome: Current concepts. *Ann Intern Med* 97:241, 1982.

59. Kapsner P, Langsdorf L, Marcus R, et al: Milk-alkali syndrome in patients treated with calcium carbonate after cardiac transplantation. *Arch Intern Med* 146:1965, 1986.

60. Rose B: *Clinical Physiology of Acid-Base and Electrolyte Disorders.* New York, McGraw-Hill, 1989, p 478.

60a. Perez GO, Oster JR, Rogers TJ: Acid-base disturbances in gastrointestinal disease. *Dig Dis Sci* 32:1033, 1987.

61. Heinemann H: Metabolic alkalosis in patients with hypercalcemia. *Metabolism* 14:1137, 1965.

62. Jaeger P, Tellier M, Fowler N, et al: Effect of parathyroid hormone related peptides on proximal tubular handling of HCO_3 (abstract). *Kidney Int* 37:467, 1990.

63. Polak A, Haynie G, Hays G, et al: Effects of chronic hypercapnia on electrolyte and acid-base equilibrium: I. Adaptation. *J Clin Invest* 40:1223, 1961.

64. Berger B, Cogan M, Sebastian A: Reduced glomerular filtration and enhanced bicarbonate reabsorption maintain metabolic alkalosis in humans. *Kidney Int* 26:105, 1984.

65. Hernandez R, Schambelan M, Cogan M, et al: Dietary NaCl determines the severity of potassium depletion-induced metabolic alkalosis. *Kidney Int* 31:1356, 1987.

66. Cooke R, Segar W, Cheek D, et al: The extrarenal correction of alkalosis associated with potassium deficiency. *J Clin Invest* 31:798, 1952.

67. Lipner H, Ruzany F, Dasgupta M, et al: The behavior of carbenicillin as a nonreabsorbable anion. *J Lab Clin Med* 86:183, 1975.

68. Young D: Quantitative analysis of aldosterone's role in potassium regulation. *Am J Physiol* 255:F811, 1988.

69. Capuccio F, Markandu N, Buckley M, et al: Changes in the plasma levels of atrial natriuretic peptides during mineralocorticoid escape in man. *Clin Sci* 72:531, 1987.

70. Hulter H, Sigala J, Sebastian A: K deprivation potentiates the renal alkalosis-producing effect of mineralocorticoid. *Am J Physiol* 235:F298, 1978.

71. Garella S, Chazan J, Cohen J: Saline-resistant metabolic alkalosis or "chloride-wasting nephropathy." *Ann Intern Med* 73:31, 1970.

72. Stein J: The pathogenetic spectrum of Bartter's syndrome. *Kidney Int* 28:85, 1985.

73. Stinebaugh B, Schloeder F: Glucose-induced alkalosis in fasting subjects: Relationship to renal bicarbonate reabsorption during fasting and refeeding. *J Clin Invest* 51:1326, 1972.

74. Mitchell J, Seim H, Colon E, et al: Medical complications and medical management of bulimia. *Ann Intern Med* 107:71, 1987.

75. Javaheri S, Shore N, Rose B, et al: Compensatory hypoventilation in metabolic alkalosis. *Chest* 81:296, 1982.

76. Schwartz W, Jenson R, Relman A: Role of anions in metabolic alkalosis and potassium deficiency. *N Engl J Med* 279:630, 1968.

77. Barton C, Vaziri N, Ness R, et al: Cimetidine in the management of metabolic alkalosis induced by nasogastric drainage. *Arch Surg* 114:70, 1979.

78. Knutsen O: New method for administration of hydrochloric acid in metabolic alkalosis. *Lancet* 1:953, 1983.

79. Warren S, Swerdlin A, Steinberg S: Treatment of alkalosis with ammonium chloride: A case report. *Clin Pharmacol Ther* 25:624, 1979.

80. Bushinsky D, Gennari F: Life-threatening hyperkalemia induced by arginine. *Ann Intern Med* 89:632, 1978.

81. Swartz R, Jabobs J: Modified dialysis for metabolic alkalosis. *Ann Intern Med,* 88:432, 1978.

82. Kaplan A, Longnecker R, Folkert V: Continuous arteriovenous hemofiltration. *Ann Intern Med* 100:358, 1984.

83. Griffing G, Cole A, Aurecchia S, et al: Amiloride in primary hyperaldosteronism. *Clin Pharmacol* 31:56, 1982.

84. Chan J: Bartter's syndrome. *Nephron* 26:155, 1980.

85. Morales J, Ruilope L, Praga M, et al: Long-term enalapril therapy in Bartter's syndrome. *Nephron* 48:327, 1988.

86. Griffing G, Komanicky P, Aurecchia S, et al: Amiloride in Bartter's syndrome. *Clin Pharmacol Ther* 31:713, 1982.

81. Acute Renal Failure in the Intensive Care Unit

Andrew J. Cohen and David M. Clive

Overview of Acute Renal Failure

The sudden disruption of previously normal or stable kidney function is termed *acute renal failure* (ARF). The precipitous decline in the glomerular filtration rate (GFR) usually takes place over hours or days. This decline may be accompanied by either *oliguria* (urine output < 400 ml per day) or *anuria* (urine output < 50 ml per day), but it may also occur with more copious urine flow (nonoliguric ARF.) Both the etiology and the pathophysiology of ARF differ from those of chronic renal failure, in which nephron loss is more gradual; however, ARF can occur in the setting of antecedent chronic renal insufficiency.

ARF is a common complication of many forms of serious illness, hemodynamic perturbation, or metabolic stress. A patient with severe left ventricular dysfunction and poor cardiac output may develop acute (prerenal) renal failure as a result of reduced blood flow to the kidneys. Septic or hemorrhagic shock may lead to the syndrome of acute tubular necrosis, as may exposure to nephrotoxic antibiotics or angiographic contrast agents. ARF also may result from a primary renal parenchymal disease or from obstruction of the urinary tract.

Most commonly, ARF is diagnosed when a patient has both oliguria and azotemia. Oliguria, however, need not be present. If tubular reabsorption of glomerular filtrate is reduced as a result of either tubular dysfunction or diuretic-administration, urine flow rates may be high even in conjunction with a markedly reduced GFR.

Azotemia (the retention of nitrogenous wastes such as urea and creatinine in the blood) is invariably present, since the glomerular filtration rate is diminished in all forms of ARF. Compromise of the renal clearance and excretion of metabolic waste lead to an accumulation of these substances in the blood. Elevations of either BUN or serum creatinine may also result from oversynthesis of nitrogenous wastes or interference with their renal clearance without any decline in GFR, as indicated in Table 81-1. Elevation of one laboratory value without a concomitant increase in the other value may indicate the presence of one of these conditions. In addition, increased ureagenesis may be established by an increased fractional clearance of urea, as detailed in the section on Prerenal Azotemia and Autoregulatory Failure.

ARF may stem from any of three general conditions: impaired renal perfusion, injury to the renal parenchyma itself, or obstruction of the urinary tract. Thus, renal failure is referred to as *prerenal, renal,* or *postrenal* on the basis of etiology. The general causes of ARF are summarized in Table 81-2. Although it is helpful to consider the complete array of renal diseases when evaluating new-onset ARF in an inpatient setting, two-thirds of patients are likely to have either acute tubular necrosis or prerenal azotemia [1]. Hence, an extensive search for other forms of renal disease is indicated in the ICU setting only when suggested by clinical signs such as urinary abnormalities indicative of glomerular disease. Obstructive uropathy should be considered in searching for causes for ARF, particularly in middle-aged or older men, since prostatic obstruction is a common cause in this group.

PRERENAL AZOTEMIA AND AUTOREGULATORY FAILURE. Prerenal azotemia is a functional condition in which renal hypoperfusion leads to retention of nitrogenous wastes. Prerenal azotemia can exist in the absence of intrinsic renal disease, or it may be superimposed on preexisting renal disease. The causes of prerenal azotemia are listed in Table 81-3. Prerenal azotemia is not caused by renal injury but rather, it results from extrarenal factors responsible for glomerular hypoperfusion; therefore, correction of these factors, if possible, promptly restores renal function.

Patients with hypovolemia from gastrointestinal losses, hemorrhage, venous pooling, or sequestering of fluid in "third spaces" are particularly vulnerable to prerenal azotemia. Similarly, urinary or skin losses of sodium and water result in extracellular volume depletion. In all such cases of true extracellular volume depletion, the patient usually exhibits signs of hypovolemia, including thirst, diminished skin turgor and mucous membrane moistness, and postural hypotension.

In addition, patients whose vascular volume is functionally reduced by the hemodynamic alterations of congestive heart failure, cirrhosis, or hypoalbuminemia may develop prerenal azotemia. This group of patients may actually have an expanded extracellular fluid volume space and peripheral edema. As a result of the reduced effective circulatory volume, however, renal perfusion is impaired just as it is in true hypovolemia.

Glomerular hypoperfusion may lead to decreased GFR, but autoregulatory mechanisms (see Chap. 78) usually preserve

Table 81-1. Causes of BUN or Serum Creatinine Elevation Without Reduction of GFR

Increased biosynthesis of urea
  Gastrointestinal bleeding
  Drug administration
    Corticosteroids
    Tetracycline
  Increased protein intake
  Amino acid administration
  Hypercatabolism and febrile illness

Increased biosynthesis of creatinine
  Increased release of creatine from muscle (rhabdomyolysis)

Drug-interference with tubular creatinine secretion
  Cimetidine
  Trimethoprim

Spuriously elevated creatinine colorimetric assay
  Ketoacids (DKA)
  Cephalosporins

Table 81-2. Causes of Acute Renal Failure

Prerenal azotemia
    Hypovolemia
    Reduced effective circulating volume
    Autoregulatory failure

Intrinsic renal disease
    Glomerular diseases
    Vascular diseases (main renal artery and microcirculation)
    Tubulointerstitial disease
    Acute tubular necrosis
    Acute cortical necrosis

Postrenal failure
    Ureteric obstruction (bilateral or solitary kidney)
    Lower tract obstruction (bladder neck or urethra)

Table 81-3. Causes of Prerenal Azotemia

Hypovolemia
    Gastrointestinal losses
        Vomiting
        Diarrhea
        Surgical drainage
    Renal losses
        Osmotic agents
        Diuretics
        Renal salt wasting disease
        Adrenal insufficiency
    Skin losses
        Burns
        Excessive diaphoresis
    Hemorrhage
    Translocation of fluid ("third-spacing")
        Postoperative
        Pancreatitis
Reduced effective circulating volume
    Hypoalbuminemia
    Hepatic cirrhosis
    Left ventricular cardiac failure
    Peripheral blood pooling (vasodilator therapy, anesthetics, anaphylaxis, sepsis, toxic-shock syndrome)
    Renal artery occlusion
    Small vessel disease (malignant hypertension, toxemia, scleroderma)
    Renal vasoconstriction (hypercalcemia, hepatorenal syndrome, cyclosporine, pressor agents)
Autoregulatory failure
    NSAIDs (Preglomerular vasoconstriction)
    CEIs (Postglomerular vasodilation)

NSAIDs = nonsteroidal antiinflammatory drugs; CEIs = converting enzyme inhibitors.

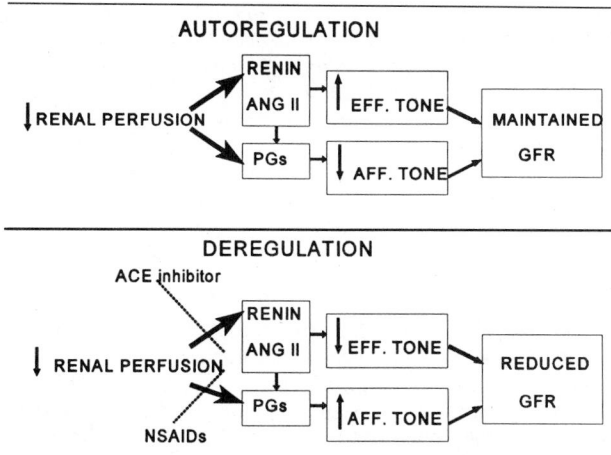

Fig. 81-1. Diagrammatic representation of autoregulation and deregulation caused by use of either NSAIDs which lead to afferent vasoconstriction or angiotensin converting enzyme inhibitors (ACE inhibitors), which produce efferent vasodilation.

glomerular capillary pressure and offset the reduction in glomerular blood flow. Hence, the GFR tends to be preserved with relatively little change in the creatinine clearance or serum creatinine. Impairment of autoregulatory mechanisms may create a sharp decline in GFR, however. The mechanisms of these processes are shown in Figure 81-1. Use of nonsteroidal antiinflammatory drugs (NSAIDs) in patients with renal hypoperfusion, for example, can lead to severe ARF [2-4]. Likewise, administration of ACE inhibitors in patients with bilateral renovascular disease causes severe azotemia [5].

Reduced renal perfusion also results in a low tubular flow rate, allowing for increased reabsorption and diminished clearance of urea. Since creatinine is not reabsorbed in the renal tubules, its clearance is unaffected by these nephronal factors and more nearly approximates the GRF. This disparity between urea and creatinine clearances is the basis for the unusually high blood urea nitrogen (BUN)-to-creatinine ratio often seen in prerenal states. In such situations, the BUN:creatinine ratio may rise from the normal 10:1 to *greater* than 20:1.

A high urea-to-creatinine ratio, however, is not pathognomonic of reduced renal perfusion. When the body's "urea pool" is augmented by accelerated catabolism (as is seen in tetracycline and corticosteroid therapy) or reabsorption of blood from the gastrointestinal tract, BUN levels will rise, sometimes beyond normal limits, even though urea clearance may be normal or even high. Such increases may be quite high in patients with antecedent renal insufficiency who cannot adequately raise urea clearance to meet the increased load. To establish whether a high BUN:creatinine ratio is due to increased urea production or reduced excretion, calculation of the fractional urea clearance may be useful.

The hallmark of prerenal conditions is the intense renal conservation of salt and water as reflected in the urine composition, which generally shows a low sodium concentration (U_{Na} <10 mEq/L) and a high osmolality (U_{Osm} >500 mOsm/kg). Several aspects of this phenomenon merit special attention. Renal tubular conservation of NaCl involves the entire length of the nephron. Both enhanced proximal and distal nephronal sodium transport apparently occur in prerenal conditions like congestive heart failure (see Chap. 42). A low urinary sodium concentration generally reflects renal hypoperfusion with resultant sodium conservation, but there are circumstances in which this may not occur. The presence of a nonreabsorbable anion (e.g., bicarbonate in patients with metabolic alkalosis, or penicillin) will obligate excretion of accompanying cations such as sodium, thereby elevating the urinary sodium concentration. In addition, patients with chronic renal failure, particularly those with salt-wasting diseases, suffer an obligatory natriuresis. Under these conditions, the U_{Na} may be elevated despite renal hypoperfusion.

INTRINSIC RENAL DISEASE. Reduced renal function may also result from diseases of, or insults to, the renal parenchyma.

The pathogenesis of renal parenchymal disease includes glomerular, vascular, and tubulo-interstitial conditions (see Table 81-2). Such processes may reflect primary kidney disease or may be part of an underlying systemic illness (e.g., systemic lupus erythematosus). ARF may result from direct parenchymal involvement by systemic disease, such as lupus, vasculitis, and malignant hypertension. Some systemic processes (e.g., sepsis, shock, or toxin exposure) can produce ARF in a nonspecific fashion by inducing ATN or acute cortical necrosis. These are the most common causes of ARF in the intensive care unit and are discussed in detail below.

Glomerular and Vascular Diseases. The GFR may be abruptly reduced in severe glomerulonephritis. With poststreptococcal glomerulonephritis, the prototypic nephritic disorder, the patient may present with ARF and oliguria. Hypertension probably reflects salt and water retention in these patients. The history of a previous sore throat or streptococcal strain infection often provides clues. The key findings are in the urine sediment, however. In nephritic disease, the urine sediment contains many free red blood cells and may be grossly bloody or, more often, "tea-colored." The microscopic examination often reveals red blood cell casts (Fig. 81-2). Similar findings are likely in patients with other nephritic disorders such as systemic lupus, vasculitis, and bacterial endocarditis. The appearance of oliguric renal failure in a patient with a nephritic disorder requires that a rapid diagnosis be made so that appropriate therapy may be initiated.

Vascular diseases of either the main renal arteries or their branches may precipitate ARF. Renal artery occlusion by acute thrombosis or thromboembolism typically only causes ARF if it is bilateral or involves a solitary functioning kidney. The disease may be silent or may produce both flank pain and hematuria. Fever, moderate leukocytosis, and an elevated lactate dehydrogenase (LDH) suggest renal infarction.

Acute renal vein thrombosis seldom causes renal failure unless both kidneys are simultaneously occluded. Once again, acute flank pain and hematuria are the clinical hallmarks. Renal venous obstruction may accompany other conditions such as nephrotic syndrome and renal cell carcinoma with carcinomatous involvement of the renal venous system.

Microscopic occlusion of smaller vessels occurs in a variety of disorders, including atheroembolic renal disease (see Atheroembolic Renal Disease below). Other vascular diseases, such as thrombotic thrombocytopenic purpura, hemolytic-uremic syndrome, scleroderma, postpartum renal failure, and malignant hypertension, occlude the microvasculature by a process involving intimal hypertrophy and fibrin deposition. Scleroderma or malignant hypertension may appear as ARF with severe blood pressure elevation due to activation of the renin-angiotensin system. These vascular disorders produce renal failure by reducing glomerular blood flow. Since the lesion is proximal to the glomerulus, the urine sediment in these disorders is usually acellular and bland.

Acute vasculitides can cause ARF. Typically, microscopic polyarteritis or Wegener's granulomatosis may present with evident renal parenchymal disease, as suggested by urinary abnormalities such as microscopic hematuria, red blood cell casts, and proteinuria. These patients may present to the ICU when there is multiorgan involvement, such as with the pulmonary disease that occurs in Wegener's granulomatosis. Fulminant presentations with severe hypoxemia and pulmonary hemorrhage may be accompanied by rapidly progressive renal failure. In these cases, glomerular involvement may range from focal and segmental necrotizing glomerulitis to severe crescenteric glomerulonephritis.

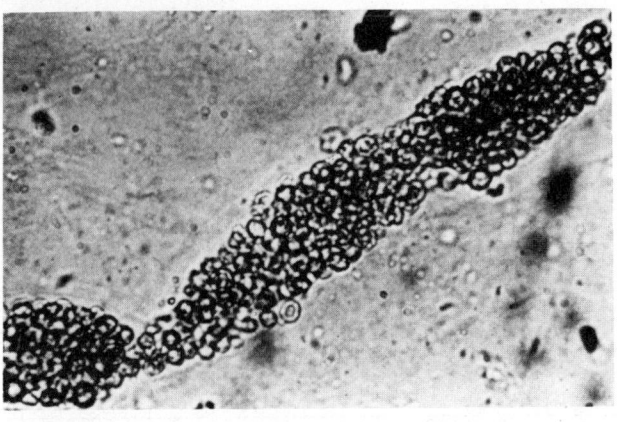

A

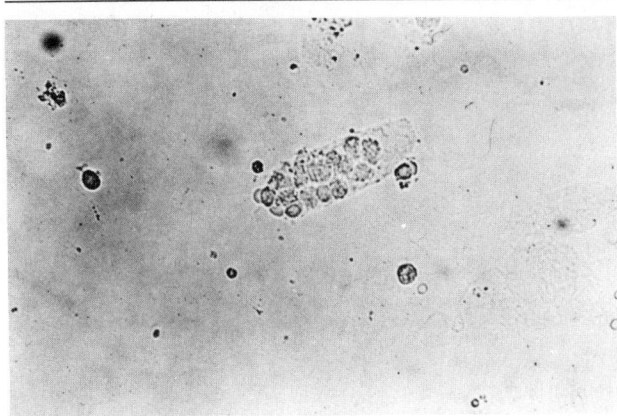

B

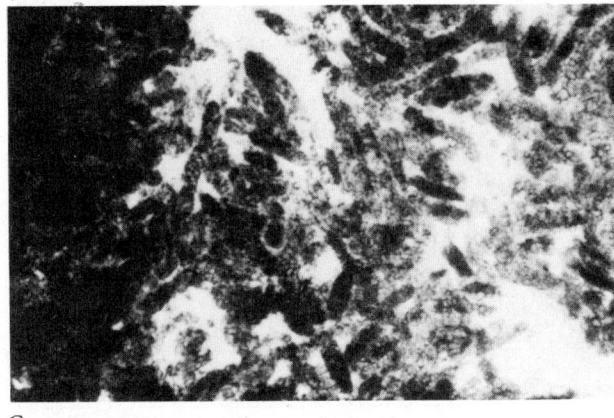

C

Fig. 81-2. Typical urinary sediments from patients with parenchymal renal diseases. A. Sediment from patient with acute glomerulonephritis showing free red blood cells and red blood cell casts. B. Sediment from patient with acute interstitial nephritis demonstrating pyuria and white blood cell cast. C. Typical muddy brown coarse granular casts in a patient with acute tubular necrosis.

Tubulointerstitial Diseases. In hospitalized patients, two parenchymal disease syndromes are likely: acute interstitial nephritis (AIN) or acute tubular necrosis (ATN).

ACUTE TUBULAR NECROSIS (ATN). ATN is a term frequently applied to acutely disordered renal function developing in the context of renal ischemia or exposure to certain nephrotoxins (aminoglycoside antibiotics, radiocontrast agents, heavy metals, myoglobin). Although many other names have been applied (*vasomotor nephropathy, postischemic renal failure, lower nephron nephrosis*), the term "ATN" prevails even though frank tubular cell necrosis does not appear in all cases [6–8]. The earliest pathophysiologic theory suggested that necrotic tubular cell debris caused nephronal impaction, which led to a reduction of GFR [9]. Other hypotheses have arisen, partly because of the disparity between the degree of renal failure and severity of histopathologic findings. *Back-leak* refers to the abnormal transmigration of filtered solutes across the disrupted tubular epithelium, which are then returned to the circulation. Since these substances (e.g., inulin) are ordinarily filtered and excreted with reabsorption, their return to the circulation represents a reduction in the effective GFR. This phenomenon apparently occurs in experimental postischemic renal failure [10] and in some subjects with ATN following cardiac surgery [11].

Considerable attention has focused on the hemodynamic abnormalities of the renal microcirculation in patients with ATN. Severe vasoconstriction, particularly in the outer cortex, has been noted early in the course of ATN [12]. This has led to speculation that preglomerular vasospasm and reduced glomerular blood flow predominate in the pathogenesis of this form of renal failure. The so-called "no-reflow" phenomenon [13] has been advanced as a potential mechanism of glomerular hypoperfusion whereby an initial reduction in renal blood flow leads to prolonged vasoconstriction, mediated by either endothelial swelling or the release of locally acting vasoconstrictors, such as the newly described peptide, endothelin [14]. A variety of animal models of ARF have failed to identify a central role for renal vasoconstriction, however, because restoring renal blood flow with vasodilators fails to restore GFR [15]. Nonetheless, this factor may be important in the initiation of certain forms of ATN such as radiocontrast toxicity (see below). Furthermore, agents that attenuate renal vasoconstriction, such as dopamine [16] and atrial natriuretic peptide [17], appear to have ameliorative affects in experimental forms of ATN.

In addition to the hydrostatic forces that drive glomerular filtration, a critical determinant of GFR is the ultrafiltration coefficient (K_f), which encompasses both the available glomerular capillary surface area and the hydraulic permeability of the capillary. Reduction in K_f may account for the glomerular hypofiltration in certain forms of ATN, particularly aminoglycoside nephrotoxicity and myoglobinuria [18]. A central role for the renin-angiotensin system has been suggested by the finding that the abnormalities of both K_f and GFR can be reversed by blocking angiotensin II formation. Whether this maneuver has any therapeutic value remains to be determined.

ATN is part of a larger spectrum of injuries related to renal hypoperfusion. The renal hypoperfusion syndromes constitute a range of injuries [19] (listed in Table 81-4) related to the severity, duration, and underlying cause of the circulatory insult. Patients may present with features characteristic of one syndrome or with an "intermediate" picture, having the attributes of more than one entity. *Cortical hypoperfusion,* which leads to prerenal azotemia, is characterized by a modest reduction of urine output and GFR, preservation of tubular function as evidenced by intact urinary concentration, and sodium reabsorption. It is rapidly reversible. Patients with cortical hypoperfusion or prerenal azotemia can expect complete recovery of renal function so long as the underlying factors (e.g., hypovolemia) are reversible. In patients with renal hypoperfusion due to protracted and severe reduction in blood flow to the kidneys, such as in cardiogenic shock or hepatic failure, reversibility would not be anticipated, however [20]. More critical decreases in renal perfusion lead to *medullary hypoperfusion and ischemia.* Ischemia eventuates in the syndromes of ATN associated with histologic evidence of injury, more severe reductions in GFR, abnormalities of tubular function, and prolonged time to recovery of renal function. The most extreme form of hypoperfusion injury is *cortical ischemia* associated with either patchy or diffuse cortical necrosis. The lesions of cortical (and glomerular) necrosis correspond with the most severe reductions in GFR and either partial or no recovery of renal function.

Recent attention has focused on the cellular and metabolic correlates of renal ischemia. An analogy can be made to coronary ischemia, as shown in Table 81-5, so that kidney ischemia can be seen as a kind of "renal angina." The medullary thick ascending limb (MTAL) segment of the loop of Henle is particularly vulnerable to ischemic and nephrotoxic insults because of a combination of low ambient PO_2 and intense, transport-driven oxygen consumption [21–23]. This is similar to the area at risk in coronary ischemia: the subendocardium. Therefore, maneuvers that diminish oxygen consumption or improve oxygen delivery prevent ischemic damage to the MTAL [8,24–26]. Furosemide, which inhibits sodium chloride transport and reduces oxygen consumption by the thick ascending limb, preserves tubular cell integrity during ischemia in the isolated per-

Table 81-4. The Spectrum of Renal Hypoperfusion

Pathogenesis	Syndrome	Urine output ml/day	U_{osm} mOsm/kg	FE_{Na} %	GFR ml/min	Reversibility
Cortical hypoperfusion	Prerenal azotemia	~500	>500	<1	40–100	Immediate
Medullary hypoperfusion	Intermediate syndrome	Variable	Variable	<1	20–60	1–3 days
Medullary ischemia	Nonoliguric "ATN"	>400	~300	varies	2–25	1–2 weeks
	Oliguric "ATN"	<400	~300	>1	0–20	Usually 2–3 weeks
Cortical ischemia	Incomplete cortical necrosis	Oligoanuria	~300	>1	0–5	Not predictable
	Complete cortical necrosis	Anuria	No urine	No urine	0	Little or no recovery

U = clearance of urea; C = clearance of creatinine.

Table 81-5. Comparison of Coronary and Renal Ischemia

	Coronary	Renal
Area at risk	subendocardium	outer medulla
O$_2$-consumption	contractile work	transport work
Remedy	↑ contraction (β-blockers)	↑ sodium transport (? loop diuretics)

fused kidney. Likewise, radiocontrast-mediated injury can be prevented by furosemide administration in the perfused kidney [25]. In addition, other factors such as ATP depletion [27], activation of phospholipases, cytosolic and mitochondrial calcium overload [28], and release of free radicals [29–32] may contribute to cellular damage.

A suggestive history (e.g., nephrotoxin exposure or renal ischemia) can be elicited in about 80% of patients with ATN. Most patients with this disease have the classic findings of sloughed renal tubular epithelial cells, epithelial cell casts, and/or muddy brown granular casts in the urinary sediment (see Fig. 81-2).

The fractional excretion of filtered sodium (FE$_{Na}$) may be useful. FE$_{Na}$ is very low in prerenal azotemia, as a result of active sodium reabsorption by the renal tubules. When frank tubular damage has occurred, as in ATN, the tubules can no longer reclaim sodium efficiently, and the FE$_{Na}$ is generally high (>1%). (See Chap. 78 for a discussion of how to calculate and interpret FE$_{Na}$.) Urinary concentration is also impaired in tubular necrosis; as a result, urinary osmolality approximates that of plasma, and the U:P creatinine ratio is less than 20 (see Fig. 81-3).

ACUTE INTERSTITIAL NEPHRITIS. This term encompasses a collection of disorders that lead to progressive renal failure accompanied by an acute inflammatory reaction of the renal interstitium. Depending on the nature of the condition, the inflammatory infiltrate may consist of a combination of neutrophils, eosinophils, and lymphocytes or plasma cells. Acute pyelonephritis is a form of interstitial disease usually associated with enteric gram-negative rods. Interstitial disease can occur as a result of other infectious agents, including brucellosis, leptospirosis, legionella, toxoplasmosis, and Epstein-Barr virus. Acute interstitial nephritis occurring in the setting of an allergic reaction with eosinophilia and skin eruption is usually a drug-induced phenomenon and is discussed in detail below.

POSTRENAL AZOTEMIA. This term refers to azotemia caused by obstruction of urine flow from the kidneys. There are many causes of renal outflow obstruction, but the most common causes are prostatic enlargement and stones, infections, and tumors in the urinary tract. For obstruction to produce azotemia, both kidneys must be involved (since one normally functioning kidney is sufficient to maintain a normal glomerular filtration rate). Renal failure may occur with unilateral obstruction in a patient who has one functioning kidney or in whom unilateral obstruction is superimposed on an underlying decrease in renal reserve.

The clinical history may be very helpful in establishing an obstructive cause. A previous history of renal stones should raise the index of suspicion for a recurrent obstruction, particularly with symptoms of renal colic. Acute renal failure in an elderly man who has been experiencing urinary hesitancy most likely represents obstruction of the bladder outlet by an en-

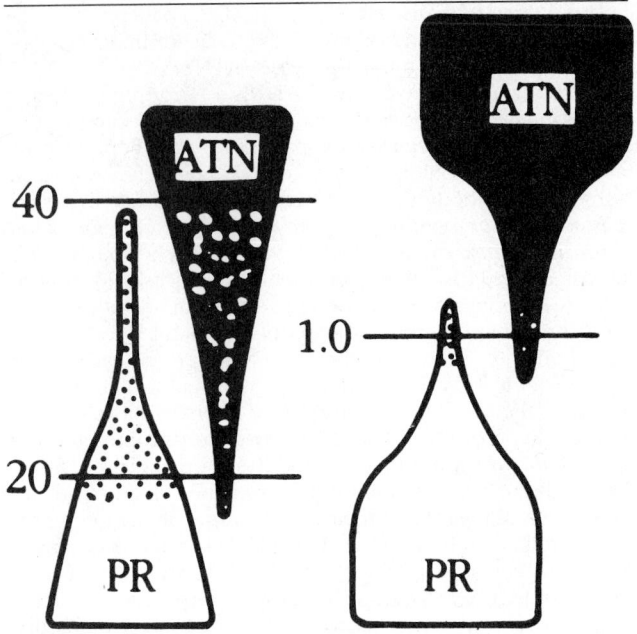

Fig. 81-3. Diagnostic parameters in acute renal failure. Two laboratory tests used to distinguish prerenal (PR) azotemia from acute tubular necrosis (ATN) are shown. *Left:* urinary sodium concentration (U$_{Na}$, mEq/L). *Right:* fractional excretion of sodium (FE$_{Na}$,%). Area within each symbol denotes the proportion of patients with each condition correlated with the laboratory parameter. Note that while considerable numbers of patients with both PR and ATN fall in an intermediate zone of U$_{Na}$ (20–40 mEq/L), the FE$_{Na}$ almost completely differentiates the two groups. (Adapted from Bastl CP, Rudnick MR, Narins RG: Diagnostic approaches to acute renal failure, in Brenner BM, Stein JH: *Acute Renal Failure.* New York, Churchill Livingstone, 1980, with permission.)

larged prostate. A history of genitourinary malignancy in an azotemic patient also makes obstruction the most likely diagnosis. Finally, renal failure in a newborn infant is likely to be due to congenital anatomic ureteral obstruction.

When urine output declines precipitously or when cessation of urine flow occurs (anuria), complete obstruction of the urinary tract must be considered. Such an obstruction is likely to be located at the bladder outlet, since the probability of simultaneous obstruction in both ureters from any cause is remote. If the patient has only one kidney (e.g., previous nephrectomy, unilateral renal disease, or congenital solitary kidney), however, anuria may occur with unilateral ureteral obstruction. Even though obstruction is the most common cause of anuria, such lesions are not always associated with a decline in urine output. In partial obstruction anywhere in the urinary tract, the kidney may lose the ability to concentrate urine, resulting in a polyuric state (acquired nephrogenic diabetes insipidus) [33,34]. In patients with complete unilateral obstruction of a ureter, the contralateral kidney often sustains a normal urine output.

As discussed later, urologic causes of ARF are best diagnosed by renal imaging techniques. The urine chemistry is generally of little help in diagnosing obstructive uropathy. Likewise, the urinalysis provides only indirect evidence of a possible cause of ARF. Hematuria may suggest an irritative, obstructing lesion. Crystals (calcium oxalate or uric acid) in the urine sediment may suggest an impacting stone.

Clinical Syndromes Associated with ARF in the Intensive Care Setting

Advances in antibiotics and cancer therapy, the increasing use of cardiac surgery, and invasive radiologic techniques make ARF more common in the modern hospital. As with other areas of clinical medicine, patterns of presentation often can be recognized and can lead the physician to the most likely diagnoses. The section below describes the common intensive care syndromes of ARF (listed in Table 81-6) and appropriate therapeutic measures.

ISCHEMIC ARF. The most common causes of ARF in the ICU are associated with renal hypoperfusion. Since frank hypotension is present in fewer than half of these cases, the causal events may often be overlooked or obscured by multiple factors. Frequently, more than one causal factor is necessary to provoke ARF. For example, sepsis-induced ARF often occurs in the setting of extracellular volume depletion.

Extracellular Volume Depletion. This accounted for approximately 17% of cases of ARF in a prospective study of ARF in a major hospital [20]. In most instances, renal losses are the cause of hypovolemia. Injudicious use of diuretics and the osmotic diuresis that accompanies diabetic ketoacidosis are the most common causes. Cessation of diuretic therapy and volume repletion lead to rapid recovery; consequently, the mortality rate is quite low [20].

In rare instances, GI losses of substantial magnitude may lead

Table 81-6. Intensive Care Syndromes Associated with ARF

Ischemic ARF
  Extracellular volume depletion
  Postoperative (particularly cardiac surgery)
  Severe ventricular dysfunction or cardiogenic shock
  Sepsis
  Pancreatitis
  Trauma
  Burns
Acute bilateral cortical necrosis
Nephrotoxicity and drug-induced ARF
  Myoglobinuric ARF
  Radiocontrast nephropathy
  Drugs (See Table 81-9)
Renal vascular disease
  Major vessel disease
    Renal artery embolism or thrombosis
    Renal vein thrombosis
  Microvascular disease
    Atheroembolism
    Vasculitis
    Scleroderma
Cancer-related
  Obstructive uropathy
  Hypercalcemia
  Tumor-lysis syndrome
  ATN secondary to chemotherapy
Renal dysfunction with liver disease
  Prerenal azotemia
  ATN
  Hepatorenal syndrome

to ARF. (Worldwide, however, this is one of the most common causes of ARF, as it is the major cause of morbidity and mortality in epidemic cholera.) In such cases, the source of the GI losses, either gastric or intestinal, may lead to disparate electrolyte abnormalities. In the former, metabolic alkalosis dictates repletion with chloride-containing replacement solutions (normal saline, usually with potassium chloride, as most patients are also hypokalemic). With intestinal losses of fluid, metabolic acidosis often ensues, and appropriate replacement may consist of a buffer solution of either isotonic bicarbonate or lactate-containing (Ringer's) in combination with saline. (This is more fully discussed in Chap. 80.)

Dermal losses of fluid usually occur in the setting of major *burns* in which the extent of thermal injury (body surface area involvement) corresponds to the degree of hypovolemia and the severity of ARF. The ARF that accompanies burns is probably the result of both hypovolemia and increased sympathetic outflow with resultant renal vasoconstriction. In some instances the severity of renal vasoconstriction, superimposed on hypovolemia, leads to ATN. In addition, deeper thermal injury with skeletal muscle involvement may induce myoglobinuric ARF. Dermal losses of fluid are also seen in the setting of heat stroke. The evaporative loss of sweat, which is hypotonic, leads to a hypertonic dehydration in these cases. Replacement fluid in hypertonic dehydration should therefore consist of hypotonic saline. The ARF is usually the result of volume depletion and accompanying hyperpyrexia and rhabdomyolysis (see below). The prognosis of patients with heat stroke depends on age and the presence of underlying medical conditions.

Postoperative. This form of ARF has long been recognized as a complication of major vascular, abdominal, and open-heart surgery. The pathogenesis of postoperative renal failure varies with the nature of the surgery and the preoperative condition of the patient. Acute renal failure following abdominal surgery is often the result of translocation of fluid into the peritoneal cavity. In this phenomenon, "third spacing" causes hypovolemia and subsequent renal underperfusion. ATN is uncommon in patients undergoing routine abdominal surgery, but the risk of ATN is substantial in surgery for obstructive jaundice; approximately 10% of patients may develop this complication [35]. Major vascular surgery, particularly aortic repairs, is associated with ARF. ATN occurs mainly after a ruptured aortic aneurysm, however, [36] with subsequent emergent surgery. Elective repair of an aortic aneurysm is seldom associated with ARF unless cross-clamping is placed above the renal arteries.

Cardiac surgery generates most of the cases of postoperative ARF in an acute care hospital. In a prospective study, ARF following cardiac surgery accounted for nearly two-thirds of the postoperative renal failure with a 15% incidence of ARF [20]. In a case-control study of 572 patients undergoing open heart surgery, 42 patients developed ARF (7% incidence) [37]. Preoperative risk factors included age, preexisting renal insufficiency, and combined bypass and valvular surgery. Analysis of these three variables correctly identified 77 percent of the patients destined to develop ARF.

Identification of intraoperative risk factors does not improve predictive ability. Nearly 40 percent of patients do not have frank hypotension prior to ARF, thereby confirming the principle that renal hypoperfusion occurs without evident shock (see above). Prolonged cardiopulmonary bypass and poor postoperative left ventricular function are likely contributory factors.

Several factors have been identified with a poor prognosis. Repeated episodes of ARF and sepsis complicating ARF are associated with substantially higher mortality (85%). Myers and colleagues [12] have described three distinct patterns of ARF following open heart surgery (Fig. 81-4). The "abbreviated" pattern, observed in 80 to 90 percent of patients, usually has an abrupt onset following surgery followed by a brief and mild rise in the serum creatinine, peaking by 3 to 4 days and followed by a rapid recovery. We have found that this form of ARF frequently is associated with the use of renal vasoconstrictors, such as norepinephrine and epinephrine, in the immediate postoperative period. The "overt" form is associated with a more severe reduction in GFR and rise in serum creatinine, which peaks 1 to 2 weeks after surgery. This is generally associated with poor cardiac performance following surgery, whereas recovery is associated with improved ventricular function. The "protracted" form of ARF generally follows a second insult following surgery, such as sepsis, and is associated with prolonged ARF and a poor prognosis.

Prevention of postoperative renal failure hinges upon adequate volume expansion prior to and during surgery. In postcardiac surgery cases, weaning of renal vasoconstrictors coupled with doses of dopamine sufficient for renal vasodilation (1–3 μg/kg/min) may promote more rapid recovery of GFR. Mannitol or furosemide should be used only in those patients in whom volume overload has been determined.

Severe Ventricular Dysfunction or Cardiogenic Shock. These are relatively rare causes of ARF. In the prospective analysis of ARF by Hou et al, these two causes combined to account for only 14 of 129 cases (11%) [20]. The mortality rate in these conditions is quite high: all four patients with cardiogenic shock and ARF died, and four of 10 patients with severe heart failure died. It is likely that the incidence of ARF in cardiogenic shock is low because patients expire for other reasons before renal failure has developed. It has been theorized that the kidney might be "protected" in cardiogenic shock. Acute atrial enlargement might evoke renal vasodilation via release of atrial natriuretic peptide [38,39].

Sepsis. Sepsis is among the most common medical causes of ARF. In one series of 276 patients with ATN, sepsis was believed to be the cause in 15% and with a mortality rate of 40% [40]. The association between septicemia and ATN is confounded by the experience that ATN due to other causes may be complicated by infection. The incidence of sepsis has been reported as high as 75% [41]. At the outset of ARF, however, only one third of patients have clinically apparent septicemia [42]

The mechanism whereby sepsis provokes ARF and ATN is unclear. It is likely that endotoxin causes a reduction in GFR by hemodynamic mechanisms, including vascular pooling and renal vasoconstriction. The latter phenomenon may be mediated by local vasoconstrictors such as thromboxane and endothelin. Although cardiac output is usually elevated in patients with sepsis, the extreme systemic vasodilation coupled with renal vasoconstriction theoretically shunts perfusion away from the renal circulation. The vascular pooling or leakage leads to intravascular hypovolemia (usually indicated by low pulmonary capillary wedge pressures). This usually necessitates volume expansion with isotonic saline, a prospect viewed squeamishly by the ICU physician who may be dealing with an oliguric patient. Careful monitoring of the pulmonary capillary wedge or pulmonary artery diastolic pressures will permit judicious use of appropriate crystalloid solutions.

Pancreatitis. Pancreatitis may occur in association with other etiologies of ARF but can itself induce ATN. This is a rare phenomenon and is generally seen in patients with severe or hemorrhagic pancreatitis with serum amylase values above 1000 U/l. A 1976 report of pancreatitis-associated ATN described five

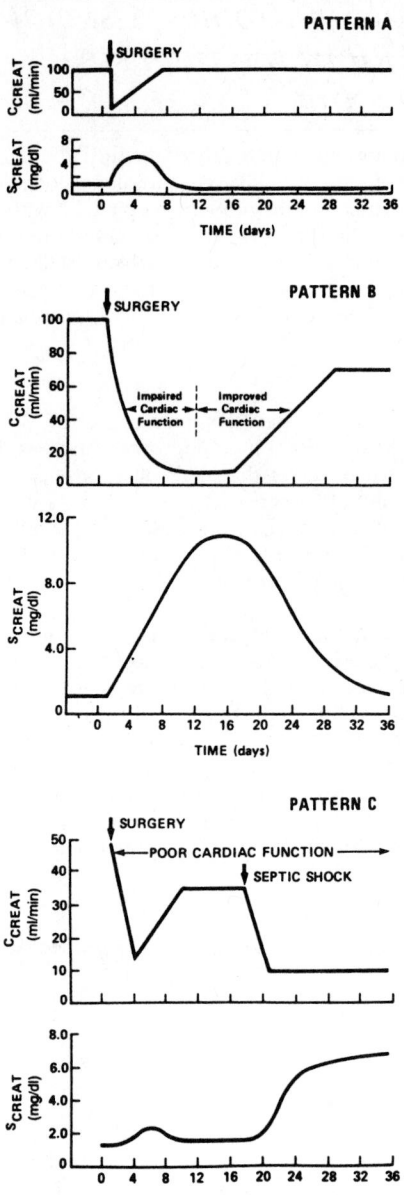

Fig. 81-4. Three typical courses of acute renal failure after cardiac surgery, illustrated by creatinine clearance (C_{creat}) and serum creatinine (S_{creat}) levels in representative patients without impact of dialysis. *Panel A* displays a step decrement that is followed immediately by a ramp increment in creatinine clearance typical of abbreviated acute renal failure. *Panel B* displays an exponential decrement of clearance that is accompanied by a linear increase in the serum level of creatinine (days 1–12). Recovery, which follows improved cardiac performance from day 12, is manifested during days 16–30 by a ramp increment in clearance that is accompanied by a sigmoidal decline in serum creatinine. In *Panel C,* successive ramp decrements in clearance (days 1–4 and 18–21) are accompanied by sigmoid elevation of the serum creatinine level. Recovery of creatinine clearance (ramp increment, days 4–7) is seen only after the first episode. A persistent low cardiac output state prevents recovery from the second insult. (From Myers BD, Moran SM: Hemodynamically mediated acute renal failure. *N Engl J Med* 314:97, 1986.)

patients with the condition, all of whom survived. [42a] More recent collections of cases have reported mortality rates of 70% to 80%. Deaths are more likely to occur in those with multiple organ system involvement, such as acute respiratory distress syndrome (ARDS) and hepatic failure.

Trauma. ARF associated with severe *trauma* is generally due to a combination of acute volume depletion, hemorrhage, and myoglobinuria (see below). Survival after trauma is markedly reduced when complicated by ARF.

ACUTE BILATERAL CORTICAL NECROSIS. Acute bilateral cortical necrosis is rare. Unlike ATN, in which only tubular elements are involved, in acute cortical necrosis both glomeruli and tubules are destroyed by a process in which cortical vessels may be occluded with fibrin thrombi. Cortical necrosis usually occurs following profound hypotension. Approximately two-thirds of cases are related to obstetric complications, including abruptio placentae, pre-eclampsia and eclampsia, septic abortion, and amniotic fluid embolism [43]. Nonobstetric cortical necrosis is most common in shock, sepsis, and disseminated intravascular coagulopathy (DIC), but isolated cases have been reported with snakebites [44], arsenic ingestion [45], and hyperacute renal allograft rejection [46]. The pathogenesis of ARF in these conditions involves both the hemodynamic insults of hypoperfusion and renal vasoconstriction and an intravascular coagulopathy suggested by the appearance of the fibrin thrombi.

Typically, patients with bilateral cortical necrosis have anuric ARF and, although the diagnosis may be suspected early in the course of renal failure, ATN is a far more likely condition. If urine is available, the urinalysis may show moderate proteinuria and hematuria, occasionally with red blood cell casts. When renal function fails to recover after several weeks, cortical necrosis may be confirmed by a renal biopsy. Other diagnostic tests are less specific. Intravenous urography generally shows absence of a nephrogram; however, a "cortical rim sign" occasionally is seen, indicating continued viability of the subcapsular cortex. Renal angiography shows patency of the main renal arteries and either a complete absence of cortical filling or a mottled nephrogram. Computed tomography with contrast enhancement may demonstrate similar findings, indicating absence of perfusion to the renal cortex. Renal scintigraphy most often demonstrates complete absence of isotope in the region of the kidneys.

Because of the nature of the underlying disease, the mortality rate is high in those with acute cortical necrosis; fewer than 20 percent of patients with this condition survive. Twenty-five percent of survivors eventually require maintenance dialysis [43]. The remainder of patients may recover sufficient renal function to obviate the need for dialysis but may later undergo progressive nephron loss and ultimately require endstage renal care.

NEPHROTOXICITY AND DRUG-INDUCED ARF. In the general categories of ARF in the ICU, a large proportion of patients can be identified with toxicity from a variety of endogenous and exogenous agents.

Myoglobinuria and Hemoglobinuria. Rhabdomyolysis is often associated with leakage into the plasma of myocyte contents, including the pigment protein myoglobin. Myoglobin has a molecular weight of approximately 17,000. It is freely filtered by the glomerulus. On entering the distal nephron, myoglobin participates in the formation of proteinaceous casts that obstruct nephronal flow; it may also exert direct cytotoxic effects on tubular epithelium. Myoglobinuric acute renal failure is a consequence of massive skeletal muscle injury of diverse causes.

Traumatic rhabdomyolysis occurs in the setting of direct mechanical injury ("crush syndrome"), burns, or prolonged pressure. Myoglobinuric renal failure is an important cause of morbidity in virtually all widescale human catastrophes. Indeed, much of what is known about the syndrome was derived from experiences during the bombing of London in World War II and in the Vietnam War. Crush injuries during the Arménian earthquake of 1988 necessitated emergent mobilization of dialysis resources on a massive scale [47].

Nontraumatic rhabdomyolysis has been reported in association with the use of heroin, amphetamines, and cocaine as well as during therapy with the lipid-lowering agent lovastatin [48,49]. Toxic, metabolic, and inflammatory myopathies, vigorous exercise, severe potassium and phosphate depletion, and hyperthermic states such as the neuroleptic malignant syndrome and malignant hyperthermia may also provide a setting for rhabdomyolysis.

As with other forms of ARF, the prognosis depends largely on the gravity of the predisposing condition; ARF following massive trauma can be expected to run a longer course than that associated with nontraumatic causes, such as drugs. In particularly severe cases, oliguria and dialysis dependence may persist for weeks.

The risk of myoglobinuric renal failure is present whenever extensive skeletal muscle injury has occurred. Patients with rhabdomyolysis due to trauma are usually easily recognized. Clinical signs and symptoms of muscle injury, such as muscle tenderness, are absent in at least half of cases of significant nontraumatic rhabdomyolysis, however. The diagnosis is suggested by markedly elevated serum levels of muscle enzymes; serum creatine kinase levels are usually higher than 5000.

The serum phosphate level is usually elevated in rhabdomyolysis, since lysis of muscle cells causes release of intracellular phosphate stores into the blood. A reciprocal fall in the serum calcium is quite common. Rebound hypercalcemia often occurs during the recovery phase.

The therapy of myoglobinuria is similar to that of other forms of ARF, but there are several particular considerations. The tubular toxicity of myoglobin is enhanced when nephronal flow rates are low, urine is concentrated, and urinary acidification is maximal. It is therefore important in the early phases of the illness to ensure that the patient is in a volume-replete state and maintaining a rapid diuresis (i.e., urine output of at least 150 ml per hour). To this end, isotonic fluids may be administered. Most experts recommend the administration of bicarbonate-rich fluids to alkalinize the urine. Diuresis may be enhanced with concurrent administration of diuretics. Some have argued that loop diuretics may introduce the potentially adverse effect of encouraging urinary acid excretion, and they have advocated the use of osmotic diuretic agents such as mannitol [50]. Mannitol, however, offers the potential drawback of causing intravascular volume overload in patients whose kidneys may already be unable to diurese in response to it. For this reason, it is our practice to administer loop diuretics to patients at risk for myoglobinuric renal failure.

Hemoglobinuria can also result in ARF. The pathophysiologic mechanisms are similar to those involved in myoglobinuric acute renal failure. Hemoglobinuric renal failure is relatively rare. Hemoglobin, with a molecular weight almost four times that of myoglobin, is less readily filtered. Furthermore, when hemoglobin is released into the plasma, it binds to haptoglobin, forming a bulky, nonfilterable molecular complex. Only when the haptoglobin binding capacity is saturated (at hemoglobin concentrations greater than 100 mg/dl of plasma) can free hemoglobin gain entrance into the renal tubules. Thus, only massive intravascular hemolysis might conceivably induce acute renal failure (e.g., fulminant transfusion reactions, auto-immune hemolytic crises, and the mechanical hemolysis that may accompany prosthetic heart valve dysfunction ["Waring blender syndrome"]) [51].

Radiocontrast-induced Nephropathy. The administration of intravascular radiocontrast agents leads to a syndrome of rapidly developing ARF. The typical patient suffers a brief episode of oliguric ARF. The serum creatinine level peaks around 4 days after the procedure [52]. Most patients do not require dialysis.

Prospective studies report that the incidence of radiocontrast-induced renal failure varies between 3.7 and 70% [52–54]. This large variance in frequency is a result of the disparity in definitions of ARF. In addition, reporting institutions may vary widely in the proportion of patients with risk factors for radiocontrast nephropathy (see Table 81-7). Disagreement remains about the significance of some risk factors for contrast-induced nephropathy. Preexisting renal insufficiency, however, particularly in patients with diabetes (which confers a 6- to 10-fold increased likelihood of radiocontrast-induced ARF), appears to be an irrefutable risk.

A mechanistic understanding of how radiocontrast induces renal injury has not evolved owing to the lack of a suitable animal model. One theory has advanced the role of hemodynamic factors. Following injection of contrast, the renal circulation undergoes initial vasodilation followed by prolonged vasoconstriction. The finding of a low FE_{Na} in some patients with contrast-induced renal failure [55] and the tendency toward rapid recovery suggest a role for reversible vasoconstriction. The intensity and duration of the vasoconstriction may be influenced by the underlying characteristics of the renal microcirculation. Endothelial factors which promote vasoconstriction of preglomerular vessels such as the newly discovered peptide, endothelin, may participate in the pathogenesis of radiocontrast-induced nephropathy [14,56].

Since there is no specific treatment for radiocontrast-induced nephropathy other than supportive measures, attention has focused on methods of prevention. Obviously, the best preventive measure is avoidance of radiocontrast and use of an alternative noncontrast imaging procedure. This is clearly not feasible, however, if, for example, the patient requires definitive coronary angiography in preparation for angioplasty or coronary bypass surgery.

A number of prophylactic measures (listed in Table 81-8) have been promoted. There are few, if any, clinical data to support these measures. Nonetheless, experimental data and retrospective clinical studies suggest that radiocontrast injury is augmented by preexisting hypovolemia, particularly in the presence of prostaglandin inhibitors [25,57,58]. Therefore, modest hydration prior to the procedure (0.45% saline, 0.5–2.0 ml/kg/hr to start 6 hours before contrast administration and to continue for 6 hours following contrast administration) and avoidance of NSAIDs is justifiable. The use of diuretics, furosemide or mannitol, has been supported by experimental stud-

Table 81-7. Risk Factors Associated with Radiocontrast Nephropathy

Preexisting renal insufficiency
Diabetic nephropathy, with renal insufficiency
Volume depletion
Large contrast dose (>2 ml/kg)
Age > 60
Hyperuricemia
Hepatic failure
Multiple myeloma

Table 81-8. Preventive Measures for Radiocontrast Nephropathy

Volume expansion with half-normal saline (0.5–1.0 ml/kg/hr for 8–12 hr)
Limit radiocontrast load to ≤1 ml/kg in high-risk patients
Discontinue NSAIDs in high-risk patients
? Dopamine
? Diuretics (mannitol, furosemide)

ies that suggest that these agents protect the nephron against ischemic injury. Mannitol may prevent the "no-reflow" phenomenon by decreasing endothelial swelling. By reducing cellular oxygen consumption, furosemide may reduce damage to the MTAL, which appears to be a nephron segment targeted in radiocontrast nephropathy. There is no evidence in randomly controlled prospective trials to support the use of either furosemide or mannitol. On the contrary, evidence suggests that these agents might aggravate renal injury, particularly in patients with preexisting risk factors [59].

Considerable attention has been given to the newer nonionic, low osmolality radiocontrast media. Although earlier studies failed to provide convincing evidence that the use of these very expensive agents reduces the incidence of radiocontrast nephropathy [60], a more recent metaanalysis indicates a small benefit, particularly in patients at high risk [61].

Drug-induced Syndromes. Hospitalized patients, particularly those in ICUs, are exposed to numerous diagnostic agents. Since many drugs are capable of inducing abnormalities in renal function, the appearance of ARF in any patient should prompt the clinician to investigate a possible drug-related cause. There are four major syndromes of drug-induced ARF (Table 81-9).

ACUTE TUBULAR INJURY. This syndrome is caused by drugs exerting direct toxic effects; the proximal tubular epithelium is most often affected. Such agents include aminoglycoside antibiotics, heavy metals, certain cephalosporins, and amphotericin B [62]. The incidence of tubular injury varies among these drugs and ranges from 10 to 15% for tobramycin, to 20 to 30% for gentamicin, to as high as 50% for *cis*-platin. The new antiviral agent, foscarnet, has been found to have an incidence of nephrotoxicity of up to 65% [63]. Volume contraction, preexisting renal insufficiency, and liver disease enhance the risk of drug-induced tubular injury. Logically, the risk of nephrotoxicity is reduced by ensuring that patients are well hydrated prior to therapy. If possible, nonnephrotoxic therapeutic alternatives

Table 81-9. Syndromes of Drug-Induced Renal Failure

Acute tubular injury
    Aminoglycoside antibiotics
    Cephalosporin antibiotics
    Antifungal agents (amphotericin)
    Antiviral agents (foscarnet)
    Heavy metals (*cis*-platin)

Intratubular micro-obstruction
    Methotrexate
    Acyclovir
    Sulfamethoxazole
    Dextran

Acute interstitial nephritis
    (see list in Table 81-10)

Autoregulatory failure
    Angiotensin converting enzyme (ACE) inhibitors
    Nonsteroidal antiinflammatory drugs (NSAIDs)

should be sought in patients with underlying renal and hepatic disease.

Tubular injury is almost always reversible following withdrawal of the inciting agent, although recovery may take several days to 2 weeks. Occasionally, specific renal tubular functional abnormalities may persist indefinitely; these include magnesium and potassium wasting, renal tubular acidosis, and mild impairment of renal concentrating ability.

INTRATUBULAR MICRO-OBSTRUCTION. A second form of acute nephrotoxicity is caused by drugs that precipitate in and impact the nephrons. Such agents are generally poorly soluble at low pH, as is found in distal nephronal fluid. This syndrome has been reported in patients receiving relatively high doses of intravenous methotrexate, acyclovir, low-molecular-weight dextran, and sulfamethoxazole. It has also been described in the setting of oral therapy with NSAIDs such as sulindac. Other NSAIDs, presumably because of their uricosuric properties, can precipitate tubular blockade with uric acid crystals.

Prevention of micro-obstructive ARF necessitates optimal hydration of the patient and maintenance of a high urine flow rate. Adjunctive use of urinary alkalinization has not been well studied. There is no evidence to suggest that these measures may shorten the course of established nephrotoxicity. The syndrome is usually readily reversible and short-lived.

ACUTE INTERSTITIAL NEPHRITIS (AIN). An ever-enlarging list of drugs has been associated with the syndrome of ARF accompanied by signs of allergy as evidenced by the frequent findings of skin rash and eosinophilia (Table 81-10). Since the disorder is nearly always an allergic response to a drug, it behaves more idiosyncratically than the other disorders, varying widely in the time of onset following exposure to the allergenic agent (days to years), the severity of the renal failure, and the time required for reversal following withdrawal of the drug (days to months). In addition to hematuria and pyuria, the urine sediment may show a preponderance of eosinophils [64,65]. White blood cell casts are a common finding (see Fig. 81-2). The pathogenesis of ARF in this disorder is poorly understood. The renal histopathology early in the course of the disease shows mainly interstitial infiltration with inflammatory cells, often (but not always) eosinophils.

Although steroids have never been shown to reduce morbidity in a controlled trial, most experts employ them in severe cases of acute interstitial nephritis (i.e., those in which supportive dialysis may become necessary). In these instances, our choice is to offer a 2-week course of prednisone or methylprednisolone (1 mg/kg BW/day), followed by a rapid taper.

A variant form of acute interstitial nephritis is occasionally encountered in patients taking NSAIDs, particularly fenoprofen, meclofenamate, tolmetin, and indomethacin. The hallmarks of allergy (i.e., drug rash, eosinophilia and eosinophiluria) are absent. The urinalysis is nonspecific; some patients may experience nephrotic-range proteinuria. The renal pathology shows interstitial inflammation and normal-appearing glomeruli. As with classic allergic interstitial nephritis, this disorder regresses following cessation of therapy with the offending agent. Patients who have had this disorder should probably be considered at risk for recurrence with other NSAIDs.

AUTOREGULATORY FAILURE. The final form of drug-related ARF pertains to drugs that cause abnormalities of glomerular blood flow. In this disorder, the pharmacologic effect is not to engender any cytotoxic or inflammatory effect, but rather to disturb the renal microcirculation sufficiently to cause ARF. With underperfusion of the kidneys, modern pharmacotherapeutics may upset the precarious balance between reduced renal blood flow and maintenance of GFR.

Two pathophysiologic subsets of hemodynamically mediated ARF may be identified, depending on whether the main action of the drug is on the afferent or efferent glomerular arteriole. When the action of the drug is to cause or permit afferent vasoconstriction, failure to autoregulate renal blood flow ensues, and the patient develops prerenal azotemia. This effect may be seen in association with NSAIDs, which reduce the synthesis of vasodilatory prostaglandins [66], or drugs that directly constrict the preglomerular vessels (i.e., vasopressors, and possibly radiocontrast agents). When preglomerular vasoconstriction is severe and prolonged, frank ischemic tubular necrosis may result. More often, a rapidly reversible, prerenal form of ARF occurs.

The other subset of hemodynamically mediated, drug-induced renal failure is seen in association with angiotensin-converting enzyme inhibitors (CEIs; captopril, enalapril, fosinopril, etc.), which block the formation of angiotensin II from angiotensin I. These agents are potent antihypertensives and are increasingly used for the treatment of congestive heart failure. In most instances, their use is associated with improvement of renal perfusion (since reduced peripheral vascular resistance leads to reduced left ventricular impedance). Under conditions of attenuated and fixed renal blood flow, however (as would occur with bilateral renal artery stenoses), CEIs may cause a sharp reduction in GFR [5,67].

These syndromes are encountered almost exclusively in patients with significant underlying cardiovascular or renal dysfunction. Unless severe renal ischemia has occurred, renal function should rapidly return to baseline levels after withdrawal of the responsible drug.

RENAL VASCULAR DISEASE

Major Renal Vascular Disease. Renal vascular disease is divisible into major vascular and microvascular syndromes. *Major renal vascular disease* is an unusual cause of ARF. In a prospective series from a major teaching hospital, renal artery occlusion accounted for only one of 129 reported cases of ARF [20]. Renal artery occlusion does not produce ARF unless it is

Table 81-10. Drugs Most Often Implicated in Acute Interstitial Nephritis

1. Antibiotics
   a. Penicillinase-resistant penicillins
   b. Cephalosporins
   c. Ampicillin
   d. Amoxicillin
   e. Penicillin G
   f. Sulfonamides and sulfa-trimethoprim
   g. Rifampin
   h. Ethambutol
   i. Tetracycline
2. Diuretics
   a. Furosemide
   b. Thiazides and related compounds
3. Nonsteroidal antiinflammatory drugs
   a. Ibuprofen
   b. Indomethacin
   c. Fenoprofen
   d. Naproxen
   e. Phenylbutazone
   f. Mefenamic acid
   g. Tolmetin
4. Miscellaneous drugs
   a. Diphenylhydantoin
   b. Cimetidine
   c. Alpha-methyldopa
   d. Allopurinol
   e. Captopril

bilateral or occurs in a solitary functioning kidney. The sudden appearance of flank pain and a rising serum creatinine should lead the physician to consider acute renal artery embolism or thrombosis. The differential diagnoses in this scenario include nephrolithiasis, pyelonephritis (with or without urinary obstruction), and renal vein thrombosis. Pain, however, is not a *sine qua non* of renal artery occlusion. In a series of cases of renal artery embolism, 5 of 17 patients experienced no flank or abdominal pain [68].

Renal artery embolus occurs most frequently in the setting of cardiac disease, particularly in patients with arrhythmias and/or mural cardiac thrombi. Frequently, multiple organs are involved, including brain, lung, and spleen. Renal failure is more likely to occur with a distribution of emboli to both kidneys, although azotemia has been reported with a unilateral embolus [68].

If the thrombus or embolus involves a solitary functioning kidney, oligoanuria and a rising level of azotemia can be expected. In a series of 17 cases of renal embolism, 15 patients experienced a rising serum creatinine. Seven of nine patients in whom urine volumes were recorded were either anuric or oliguric [68]. In addition to flank pain and diminished urine volume, at least 50% of patients experience nausea and/or fever. The urinalysis is not specific. Leucocyturia, hematuria, and low-grade proteinuria have been found, as has a bland urine sediment.

Diagnosis of renal arterial disease requires radiologic or nuclear imaging studies. Intravenous urography is nonspecific, demonstrating only a nonfunctional kidney. Arteriography demonstrates the occlusive process and gives the most detailed anatomic information. Radionuclide scanning with newer agents of DPTA, DMSA, or MAG 3 often demonstrates patchy uptake of isotope or, in the case of total occlusion, no isotopic uptake. Computed tomography may demonstrate similar findings of diminished contrast uptake either by the whole kidney or localized "wedge-shaped" areas of nonperfusion.

Occlusion of the renal artery does not inevitably lead to infarction. Particularly in patients with slowly developing atherosclerotic disease, collateral circulation via capsular or ureteric vessels may protect the kidney from infarction even though renal arterial blood flow is inadequate to provide function. Surgery may be preferable in patients with renal artery thrombosis although supportive care with anticoagulation has been the preferred treatment for renal arterial embolism. Recent reports of successful treatment with fibrinolytic agents (either urokinase or streptokinase) has led some to consider this the preferred treatment for renal artery occlusive disease, particularly in patients for whom surgery represents too great a risk.

Renal Vein Thrombosis (RVT). This is a particularly rare cause of ARF. Bilateral renal vein occlusion may occur in children with severe dehydration. In adults, it usually accompanies nephrotic syndrome or may occur in patients with renal cell carcinoma. Occasionally, extension of caval thrombosis, sickle cell disease, pregnancy, use of oral contraceptives, or trauma may cause RVT. RVT generally does not cause ARF unless it is acute and bilateral or occurs in a solitary kidney. Flank pain and microscopic hematuria are the usual clinical manifestations in acute RVT. Diagnosis depends on renal venography. With intravenous urography, however, "notching" of the ureter caused by venous collaterals may suggest RVT. Treatment usually consists of anticoagulation, although fibrinolytic therapy might be more desirable in patients with ARF and RVT.

Atheroembolic Renal Disease (Cholesterol Emboli). This condition has only recently been recognized as a cause of ARF; consequently, it is seldom listed among the etiologic diagnoses.

In the prospective study by Hou et al [20], none of the 129 episodes of ARF were identified with this diagnosis. These findings may be explained by the recognition that the diagnosis is frequently missed or found only during postmortem examination.

Showers of cholesterol emboli occur only in patients with severe aortic atherosclerosis. They may occur spontaneously but more often follow a specific event that usually is associated with increased shearing forces on the wall of the aorta. These precipitating factors include aortography, repair of an aortic aneurysm, or blunt trauma to the abdomen [69,70]. The result may either be a subtle series of small vessel occlusions or a more dramatic illness. Patients may suffer from minor abnormalities such as infarction of the tip of a single toe. Renal involvement is particularly common when a massive shower accompanies major arteriography or aortic surgery. There may also be involvement of other visceral organs, including the pancreas, bowel, spleen, retina, and brain. Typically, the cholesterol emboli form needlelike occlusions in small vessels, which then develop a chronic inflammatory response that can include the formation of a granulomatous reaction [69,70]. Extensive infarction of bowel or sudden neurologic abnormalities may bring the patient to the ICU where, in addition to the presenting findings, ARF is noted. In the kidney, occlusion of a sufficient proportion of the microvasculature results in varying degrees of azotemia. The azotemia may be sudden, following the precipitating event, or may develop more slowly. The latter course helps to distinguish this diagnosis from radiocontrast nephropathy, which typically occurs within 24 to 48 hours after arteriography.

The diagnosis is often missed unless there are peripheral signs of involvement. Typically, manifestations in the skin such as blue distal digits or a mottled appearance of the lower extremities known as *livido reticularis* provide the necessary clue. A more subtle and less frequently observed physical manifestation is the finding of cholesterol emboli on examination of the retina. Less specific manifestations include eosinophilia and hypocomplementemia. The urine sediment is usually not helpful; there usually either are no findings or only a few red blood cells. Red blood cell casts have been reported occasionally.

Patients with atheroembolic renal disease suffer the full spectrum of renal failure, from minor degrees of azotemia to full-blown, irreversible renal failure. After an initial rise in serum creatinine, there may be an improvement in GFR over several weeks, probably owing to nephron adaptation with hyperfiltration in remnant glomeruli.

There is no specific management for atheroembolic renal disease. Management of renal failure, including dialytic therapy, may be indicated. Use of anticoagulatants may worsen the course of this condition.

ACUTE RENAL FAILURE IN THE CANCER PATIENT. Acute renal failure occasionally complicates the course of neoplastic diseases. Many malignancies cause *hypercalcemia*, a well-defined cause of ARF. Hypercalcemia may induce ARF both through alterations in renal hemodynamics (afferent arteriolar vasoconstriction and diminished GRF) and by causing volume depletion. The pathogenesis and therapy of hypercalcemia of malignancy are described in greater detail in Chapters 114 and 127.

The term *tumor lysis syndrome* refers to the sudden release of tumor cell contents in response to induction chemotherapy. These intracellular products include phosphates, uric acid, and other purine metabolites. They may cause diffuse nephronal microbstruction once they are filtered by the kidney, with sudden onset of ARF. The syndrome occurs almost exclusively in patients with hematologic and lymphoproliferative malignancies, especially when the tumor cell mass is large. Patients at risk for this syndrome should routinely receive prophylaxis prior to the initiation of chemotherapy, including volume expansion and maintenance of a diuresis, alkalinization of the urine, and pretreatment with allopurinol. Once established, the syndrome is difficult to treat and usually requires a period of 1 to 2 weeks to run its course. During this time, dialytic support is required for oliguric patients. In nonoliguric patients, it may be possible to attenuate the illness with an alkaline diuresis, although care must be taken not to cause systemic alkalinization or fluid overload.

A number of the commonly employed *antineoplastic agents* have renal side effects and can cause ARF. Prinicipal among these is *cis*-platin, which, like other heavy metals, can engender acute tubular necrosis [71]. The incidence of this complication is less with the newer analog, carbiplatinum. Saline loading of patients about to receive platinum-containing chemotherapeutic agents helps reduce the risk of ARF. High dose (> 2 g/day) methotrexate therapy can cause ARF; the mechanism is felt to represent tubular micro-obstruction from intraluminal crystallization of methotrexate metabolites. As is usually the case with renal failure syndromes arising through this mechanism, maintenance of a forced diuresis is usually effective prophylaxis.

Many neoplasms metastasize to the ureteric bed or periureteric lymph nodes. *Obstructive uropathy* must be considered in any case of unexplained ARF in an oncologic patient, particularly those with lymphoma or with prostatic, colorectal, or cervical carcinoma. Such obstructions are usually readily detectable by ultrasonographic examination; if the ultrasonogram fails to detect hydronephrosis but obstruction is felt to remain a strong possibility, the clinician should proceed to retrograde cysto-ureterography. Immediate treatment involves the placement of ureteral stents or establishment of nephrostomy drainage. Such drainage measures may only be needed temporarily in tumors that respond sufficiently to radiation or chemotherapy [72].

Tumor infiltration of the renal parenchyma is an unusual cause of ARF, despite the frequency of metastases to the kidneys. Imaging studies frequently reveal kidney enlargement. Successful reversal with radiation or chemotherapy is unusual. The use of dialysis in patients with widespread metastatic disease should be weighed carefully and in the light of the prognosis of the underlying disease.

RENAL DYSFUNCTION IN PATIENTS WITH LIVER DISEASE.

Renal dysfunction is extremely common in patients with advanced liver disease. The most common renal syndrome associated with liver disease is prerenal azotemia (i.e., a reduction in the glomerular filtration rate attributable to hypoperfusion of the kidney). The systemic hemodynamic abnormalities associated with portal hypertension, the hypoalbuminemia of hepatocellular failure, and probably other neurohumoral influences that are active even in the incipient stages of liver disease cause a reduction in renal perfusion. There is evidence that the increase in intraabdominal pressure due to ascites may exert an adverse effect on blood flow to the kidneys.

Although reversible, prerenal azotemia in the liver disease patient makes salt and water balance more difficult to maintain, predisposes to encephalopathy, and may render the patient susceptible to the more severe *hepatorenal syndrome*.

Endless debate has centered around the proper definition of the hepatorenal syndrome and its specific relationship to prerenal azotemia. A good working definition of the syndrome describes it as progressive oliguria and azotemia with severe sodium retention that is unresponsive to volume loading or diuretics and occurs in patients with liver disease. Much of the literature concerning hepatorenal syndrome is weakened by the great difficulty in distinguishing severely prerenal cirrhotic patients from those who truly meet the criteria above. Indeed, in the clinical setting, it is often impossible to establish which of the two states a given patient may have.

The hepatorenal syndrome is usually seen in advanced cirrhosis, but it has also been reported in patients with acute hepatitis [73] or hepatic neoplasm [74,75]. Onset of the syndrome may be sudden or insidious. Most commonly, it appears in patients with cirrhosis following a major physiologic insult, such as hypotensive GI hemorrhage, sepsis, or surgery. Overzealous diuresis has also been implicated, although its importance in the etiology of hepatorenal syndrome has been questioned [76,77].

The pathogenesis of the hepatorenal syndrome remains obscure. The kidneys' tendency to retain salt and water suggests a hemodynamic alteration rather than parenchymal injury. Postmortem angiography of hepatorenal kidneys has demonstrated severe vasoconstriction with cortical ischemia (Fig. 81-5). This process appears to reverse when the involved kidney is transplanted into a hepatically intact host. Factors that may contribute to vasomotor instability of the kidney in those with the hepatorenal syndrome include endotoxin, increased sympathetic neural activity, hyperbilirubinemia, circulating catecholamines, and other humoral imbalances related to hepatocellular dysfunction. The renin-angiotensin system is probably activated [78], but its causal relationship to the pathophysiology of the syndrome is arguable. The kidneys of cirrhotic patients appear to excrete large amounts of prostaglandins, which dilate the renal vasculature. When these patients receive NSAIDs, renal blood flow and GFR fall in parallel with the reduction in prostaglandin excretion [79,80]. A role for disordered prostaglandin metabolism in the pathogenesis of the hepatorenal syndrome is unproved but seems plausible [81]. Other vasoactive mediators, such as endothelin, merit further study in this regard.

Cirrhotic patients are in a tenuous physiologic state; they have little tolerance for small deviations, either positive or negative, from their optimal state of fluid balance. The degree of azotemia in cirrhotic patients often underestimates the true severity of their renal failure. A serum creatinine of 1.5 mg/dl may correspond to a glomerular filtration rate of under 30 ml/minute [82]. This is generally because of the reduction in muscle mass, creatine release, and consequent creatinine biosynthesis in patients with advanced cirrhosis.

Management of cirrhotic patients with sodium retention and azotemia is, at the very least, challenging. In the prerenal and hepatorenal states, urinary sodium excretion is reduced (usually less than 20 mEq/day). Sodium balance must be regulated with dietary restriction and/or diuretics if ascites and edema are to be controlled. When oliguria develops in patients with advanced cirrhosis, conventional therapy may be ineffective in promoting a diuresis. High doses of intravenous diuretics, perhaps in combination, may be tried, and strict bed rest instituted. Because aldosterone appears to play a role in the sodium retention of cirrhosis, spironolactone may be a useful adjunct in diuretic therapy. Infusing salt poor albumin may be attempted to raise plasma oncotic pressure and consequently renal blood flow. Infusions of fresh frozen plasma may be more effective in stimulating a diuresis than albumin or stored plasma, perhaps due to its ability to provide plasma renin substrate or other vasoactive principles [83]. It is important to recall that this is merely a temporizing measure.

Hyponatremia is most common in patients with cirrhosis, since this state is often complicated by a diminished capacity to excrete free water. The more advanced the disease, the greater the likelihood of hyponatremia; such patients should

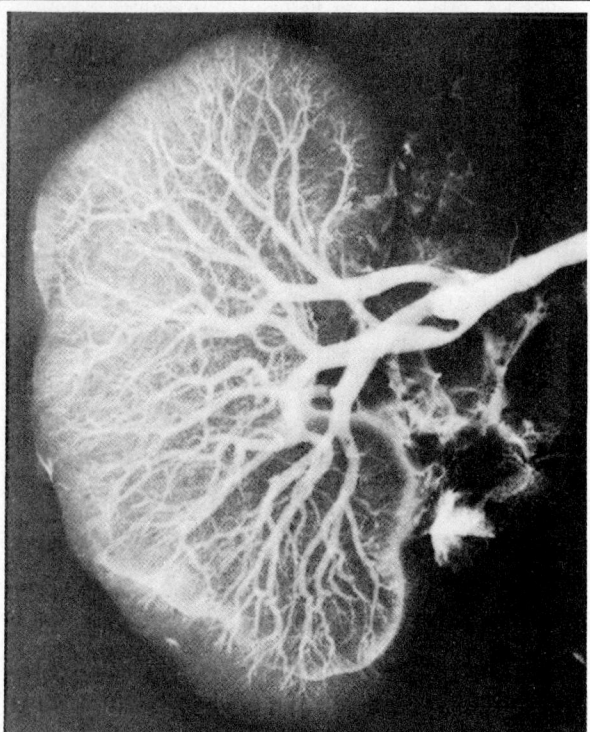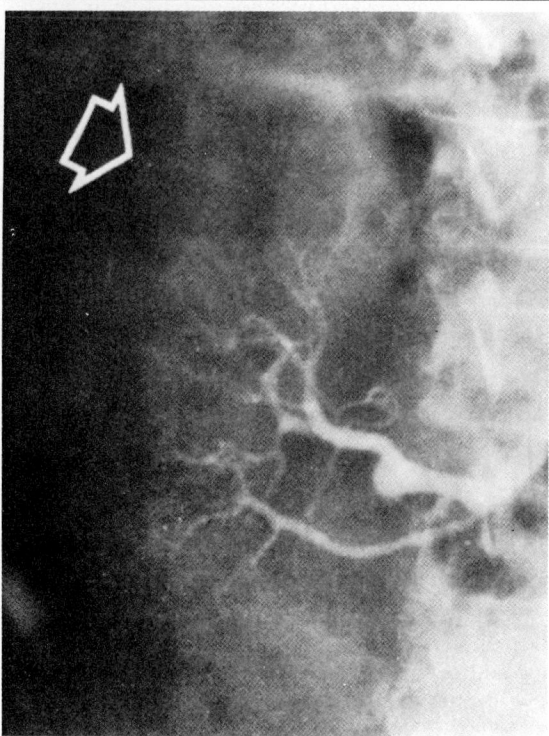

Fig. 81-5. Angiographic pattern in hepatorenal syndrome with severe renal cortical vasoconstriction. Premortem (left) and postmortem (right) angiograms of a representative patient are shown. Arrow points to severe cortical vasoconstriction; it is a process that appears to reverse when the involved kidney is transplanted into a hepatically intact host. (From Epstein M, Berk DP, Hollenberg NK, et al: Renal failure in the patient with cirrhosis. *Am J Med* 49:175, 1970, with permission.)

have their water intake restricted (less than 1500 ml per day). Fluid challenges should be undertaken with great caution, particularly in patients with existing edema and ascites. Volume removal should be approached gingerly. Although the danger of precipitating hepatorenal syndrome with aggressive diuretic therapy has historically been exaggerated, we generally advise clinicians to limit *net* negative fluid balance to under 3 liters per day in any cirrhotic patient with ascites.

Paracentesis represents a more aggressive technique of fluid removal. Recent studies have shown that removal of greater than 4 liters at a time of peritoneal fluid may be undertaken safely and with salutory results [84–87]. Albumin infusion should be performed simultaneously with paracentesis. Since ascitic fluid forms at least partially at the expense of the plasma volume in patients with portal hypertension, there is a rationale for collecting ascites fluid and reinfusing it intravenously, several liters at a time. The technique can be useful for palliating ascites in hospitalized patients provided they have sufficient renal function to diurese in response to this expansion of the vascular space.

Peritoneovenous shunts (of which the Denver and LeVeen shunts are the most familiar) represent a novel extension of the concept of ascitic reinfusion. These shunts comprise a plastic catheter linking the peritoneal cavity with the venous system, generally the internal jugular vein, with a valve in the catheter permitting one-way conduction of fluid from the peritoneum to the venous system when ascites pressure reaches a predetermined point.

Peritoneovenous shunting has been used effectively in am-

bulatory patients for long-term control of ascites. The procedure should be reserved for patients without a history of variceal hemorrhage, a limited expected survival, or insufficient renal reserve to handle the steady reinfusion of ascites. A patient's ability to meet the latter eligibility criterion may be tested by subjecting them to several days' trial of ascites reinfusion. Diuretics may be used to maximize the patient's renal response both pre- and postoperatively. There have been reports of spontaneous reversal of the hepatorenal syndrome [88] and recovery following portosystemic [89–91] or peritoneovenous [83,91–97] shunting procedures. Although such reports may represent hope for the hepatorenal patient, they must be interpreted with caution. Experience along these lines is still limited and has not been uniformly favorable [98], and only a small percentage of patients may be considered candidates for surgical therapy.

In hepatorenal syndrome, as in other causes of irreversible renal failure, dialysis is ultimately needed to sustain life (see Chap. 83). Unfortunately, most patients have associated medical problems that preclude long-term survival on dialytic therapy.

Hepatic disease predisposes patients to acute tubular necrosis of the usual causes (i.e., nephrotoxic drug exposure, radiographic contrast material exposure, hypotension, and sepsis). Patients with severe hepatic disease often have one or more of these risk factors. Furthermore, hyperbilirubinemia may predispose to ARF through the actions of bile on renal tubules [98,99]. Although the urinary sediment in most cases of acute tubular necrosis is distinctive, showing renal tubular epithelial cells and muddy brown granular casts, jaundiced patients without tubular necrosis may manifest pigmented granular casts simply as a result the interaction of bilirubin with tubular cells [99].

Azotemic patients with hepatic failure have increased metabolic substrate for ammonia production, and therefore are at heightened risk for encephalopathy. Potassium depletion, a common electrolyte imbalance in cirrhosis, further enhances ammonia synthesis.

Acid-base disturbances are extremely common in patients with advanced hepatocellular disease. Primary respiratory alkalosis is common in cirrhotics, but the mechanism is poorly understood. Metabolic acidosis occurs in patients developing renal failure (Chap. 80). Lactic acidosis has several causes (Chap. 115), and may be particularly severe in patients with liver disease, since extraction and metabolism of lactic acid from the blood depend largely on hepatic reserve.

A mixed acid-base disturbance, respiratory alkalosis and metabolic acidosis, often develops in cirrhotic patients. Typically, patients with a primary respiratory alkalosis subsequently suffer an additional insult (such as sepsis) with an attendant metabolic acidosis. This is a particularly treacherous combined acid-base disturbance, since a near-normal serum pH may belie the true extent of the acidosis. As the acidotic component worsens, pH may plummet due to depletion of the bicarbonate buffer system, deficiencies of protein buffers, and inability to maintain adequate respiratory compensation. Bicarbonate supplementation may be unavoidable.

Metabolic alkalosis usually reflects vomiting or severe secondary hyperaldosteronism. The importance of metabolic alkalosis resides in its tendency to aggravate hepatic encephalopathy. As plasma pH rises, ammonium ions lose protons to the plasma; the resulting ammonia penetrates the blood-brain barrier more readily. Metabolic alkalosis may be treated with chloride salts (potassium or sodium), or, if indicated, spironolactone.

Patients with combined hepatic and renal dysfunction have lost both major physiologic means for metabolizing and detoxifying drugs. Consequently, drug doses should be adjusted to compensate for the loss of both excretory routes when appropriate.

Diagnosis of Acute Renal Failure

Since the symptoms of renal failure are nonspecific, if present at all, the history provided by the patient may not always be of diagnostic help. The history may be useful in establishing whether renal failure is truly acute or a progressive, long-standing problem. If the patient has been known to have pallor, anemia, or anorexia for several months or more, it is likely that renal failure is chronic. Occasionally, a history of previous renal or urinary abnormalities may be elicited, such as hypertension, proteinuria, or diabetes mellitus.

A thirsty patient or one in whom daily weight loss has been documented may have dehydration causing prerenal azotemia. If avenues of fluid loss are identifiable (e.g., vigorous diuretic therapy, surgical blood loss), a prerenal cause is substantiated. Exposure to nephrotoxic agents or a recent episode of hypotension should suggest the possibility of ATN. Symptoms of renal colic, abnormal voiding pattern, or a history of genitourinary malignancy make an obstructive cause likely.

The physical examination occasionally furnishes some diagnostic information. Diminished skin turgor, sunken eyes, dry mucous membranes, the absence of axillary sweat, or orthostatic hypotension supports a diagnosis of prerenal azotemia. In disorders characterized by an "ineffective circulatory volume," however, such as congestive heart failure and nephrotic syndrome, prerenal azotemia may exist in the setting of severe edema.

Hypertension in patients with ARF raises suspicion of intrinsic renal disease. The clinician must be alert for signs of systemic disease that can cause acute renal injury, including vasculitis, endocarditis, and sepsis. Bladder distention and prostatic enlargement point to an obstructive cause.

The laboratory work-up should commence with a urinalysis. The measurements of urine osmolality, electrolytes, and creatinine concentration are simple and useful, particularly in differentiating between ATN and prerenal renal failure. Urine specific gravity can be measured at the bedside while the results of the more accurate urine chemistry tests are pending. A high urine specific gravity generally correlates with a concentrated urine and suggests a prerenal form of renal failure.

The familiar dipstick tests provide a readily available method for determining whether the urine contains protein or heme pigments. When positive, they should raise the suspicion of intrinsic renal pathology. A patient with multiple myeloma may have ARF resulting from intratubular deposition of immunoglobulin light chains. These Bence Jones proteins do not interact with dipstick reagents. Light chains can be made to precipitate in urine by adding sulfosalicylic acid to the specimen and heating it to 60°C.

Formed elements in the urine sediment yield invaluable information about the nature of ARF, particularly in intrinsic renal disease. The significance of hematuria, pyuria, renal tubular epithelial cells, and casts in the urine has already been discussed. The presence of red blood cell casts distinguishes the hematuria associated with glomerulonephritis from that of "postrenal" or urologic causes. Broad and waxy casts suggest that renal disease is chronic. Virtually any lesion that can cause obstruction in the genitourinary tract can produce hematuria. Crystalluria often occurs in association with obstruction due to renal calculi.

In anemic patients the likelihood of a chronic form of renal disease is high. Eosinophilia frequently accompanies AIN. The most important blood tests are routine chemistries, which should be monitored closely to aid in the management of the critical acid-base and electrolyte abnormalities that may characterize the course of ARF.

Specialized serologic tests may help answer specific diagnostic questions. The presence of antinuclear antibodies is consistent with autoimmune nephropathy such as lupus nephritis or scleroderma, both of which may cause ARF. The serum protein electrophoresis or immunoelectrophoresis may aid in the diagnosis of multiple myeloma, which has been reported to present as ARF of uncertain cause [100].

Various radiographic techniques may contribute to the evaluation of ARF. The abdominal flat plate (KUB) is an easily obtained study that can help establish the presence and size of both kidneys. If both kidneys are small, azotemia may be of a chronic nature. Radiopaque stones may be identified on an abdominal flat plate.

The intravenous pyelogram (IVP) is rarely indicated in the diagnosis of ARF. The contrast agent administered during the test can itself produce severe impairment of renal function in hypovolemic patients and patients with diabetic nephropathy or multiple myeloma. It should therefore be avoided when any of these conditions is suspected. Furthermore, good imaging cannot be obtained in patients with moderate-to-severe azotemia (creatinine of 4.0 mg/dl or more). The IVP, however, offers the best delineation of renal morphology of any imaging technique. It is particularly useful in the recognition of hydronephrosis (Fig. 81-6), if performed early in the course. In ATN, a dense, persistent nephrogram can be seen (Fig. 81-7).

Renal ultrasonography, a safe, quick, high-yield procedure, is probably the first radiologic test that should be ordered in the evaluation of any azotemic patient. It permits the identification and measurement of both kidneys and is a very sensitive for detecting obstructive uropathy (Fig. 81-8). Ultrasonography provides almost as much information as IVP with none of the risks; it may be used in severely azotemic patients. Computed tomography (CT) offers an additional method of establishing

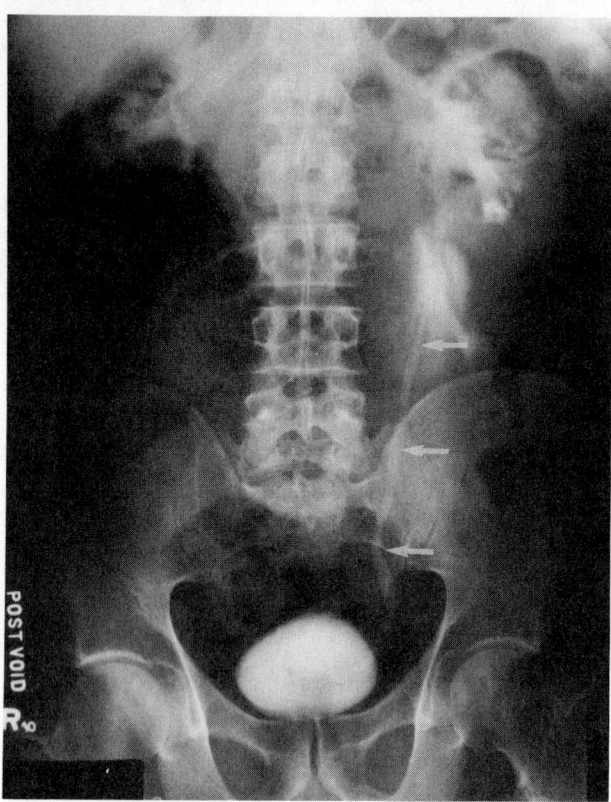

Fig. 81-6. Intravenous pyelogram with unilateral left ureteral obstruction. (Right, nonobstructed ureter is shown for comparison.) Note that left ureter is visible throughout (see arrows) and dilated to the level of the bladder.

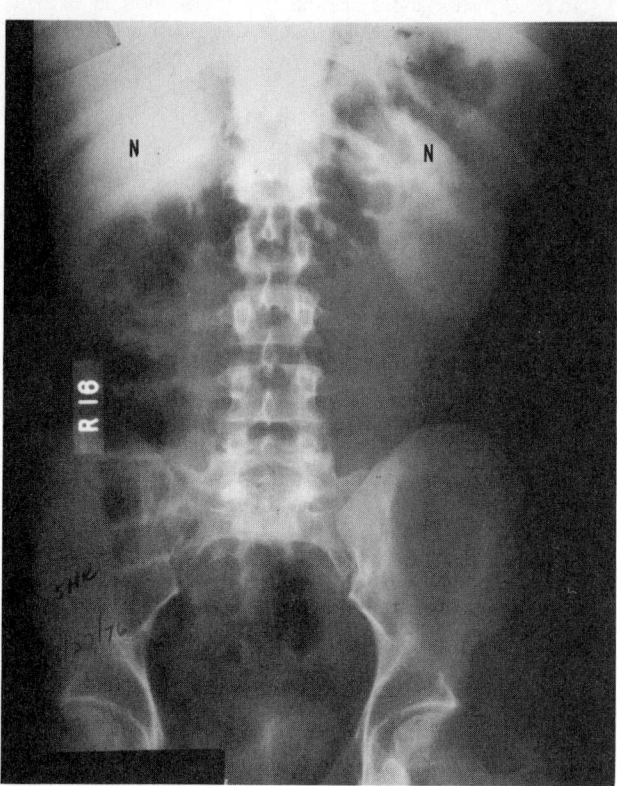

Fig. 81-7. Persistent nephrograms in a patient with acute tubular necrosis. Bilateral renal shadows are each marked with an "N."

the size of the kidneys and recognizing hydronephrosis (Fig. 81-9). The same caveats regarding the administration of radiocontrast agents in IVP apply to CT scanning.

Retrograde pyelography is reserved for patients in whom urinary tract obstruction is strongly suspected. It is generally performed in anticipation of relieving such obstructions as soon as they are identified (usually by placement of ureteral catheters).

Isotopic renal scanning provides a safe means for locating the kidneys and allows estimation of their functional capacity. Radionuclide flow studies may be used to assess the rapidity of uptake of tracer by the kidneys. A delay in uptake helps to substantiate the diagnosis of impaired renal perfusion, whether due to structural renovascular disease or functionally impaired renal blood flow. Prolonged retention of radioisotope by the kidneys is suggestive of outflow obstruction. We have found radioisotopic scanning to be particularly helpful in assessing patients with prolonged ARF for the absence of blood flow and the possible diagnosis of cortical necrosis or renal infarction (Fig. 81-10).

Renal biopsy is reserved for patients who are thought to have parenchymal renal disease. The indications for renal biopsy are a matter of some controversy, but the procedure should be considered when (1) azotemia is of recent onset and unknown cause; (2) there is a possibility that the patient has a renal disease that may require drug treatment (e.g., steroids or cytotoxic drugs)—this applies to patients with probable glomeru-

lonephritis, vasculitis, or AIN; or (3) the biopsy result might be of prognostic importance.

Consequences of Acute Renal Failure

Regardless of the cause, the consequences of severe and abrupt reductions in GFR are similar. Before deciding on specific therapy, the physician should carefully assess the patient for potential complications.

HYPERKALEMIA. This is perhaps the most life-threatening electrolyte imbalance encountered in patients with renal disease (Chap. 79). Hyperkalemia arises from the inability of the kidneys to respond to potassium loads. Sources of potassium should be identified and regulated appropriately. Potassium loads may be endogenous (e.g., tissue breakdown, hematoma reabsorption) or exogenous (e.g., dietary, intravenous, medicational). Even when the GFR is substantially reduced, however, the kidneys can excrete large amounts of potassium provided that tubular secretion is intact. For this reason, hyperkalemia more often occurs in patients with renal or postrenal azotemia in whom damage to tubular cells is likely. Urine flow rate is an important determinant of tubular potassium secretion, so oliguric patients are more prone to potassium imbalance than are nonoliguric patients.

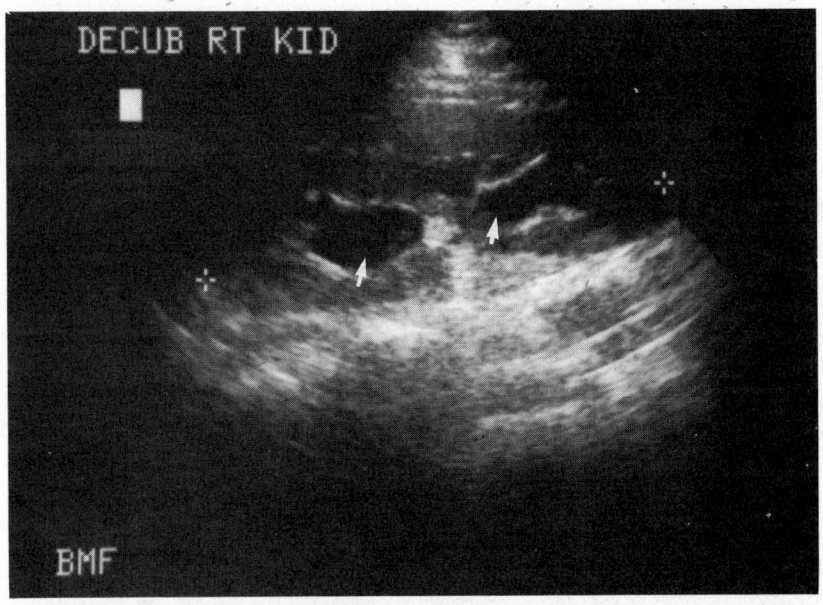

Fig. 81-8. Sonogram with right hydronephrosis. Kidney poles are marked by crosses. Dark, echolucent areas (arrows) in center represent dilated collecting system.

METABOLIC ACIDOSIS. The kidneys' ability to excrete metabolically produced acids may be reduced, particularly in parenchymal and obstructive disease. Since acid excretion is primarily a tubular function, the degree of acidosis may not always correlate with the degree of GFR impairment (and thus, the degree of azotemia). Indeed, pure tubular acid excretion abnormalities may exist independently of azotemia (renal tubular acidosis). Metabolic acidosis that results from failure of the tubules to excrete hydrogen ions normally produces a hyperchloremic or "low anion gap" acidosis (see Chap. 80). When

the GFR is severely impaired, retention of acid wastes in the extracellular fluid may produce a high anion gap acidosis.

ABNORMAL SALT AND WATER METABOLISM. Although most fluids ingested by or administered to patients are hypotonic, plasma osmolality normally remains within tightly fixed limits. The process by which plasma tonicity is preserved depends on the suppression of vasopressin release and the formation of "free water" in the cortical ascending limb of the loop of Henle. This latter function is impeded *whenever GRF is reduced,* which results in water retention and hyponatremia.

Conversely, some renal disorders are characterized by a failure to conserve water. This situation, referred to as *nephrogenic diabetes insipidus,* is most common in tubulointerstitial disease and in partial obstruction of the urinary tract. Patients with these disorders are prone to dehydration and hypernatremia (see Chap. 79).

Fig. 81-9. CT scan with right hydronephrosis. Left, unobstructed kidney is shown for comparison. Note enlarged pelvocalyceal system on right (arrowhead).

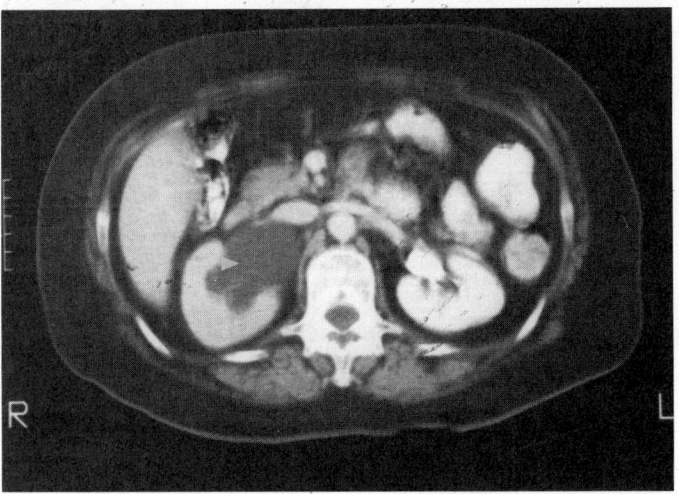

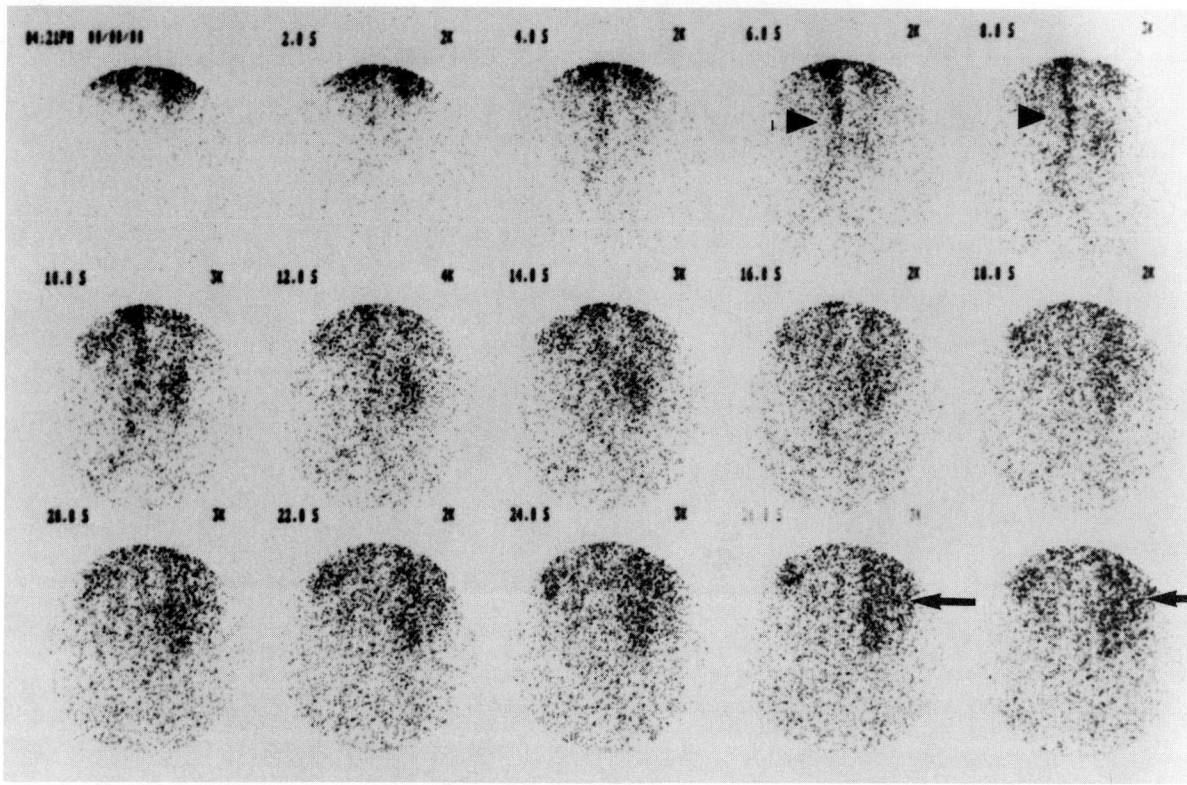

A

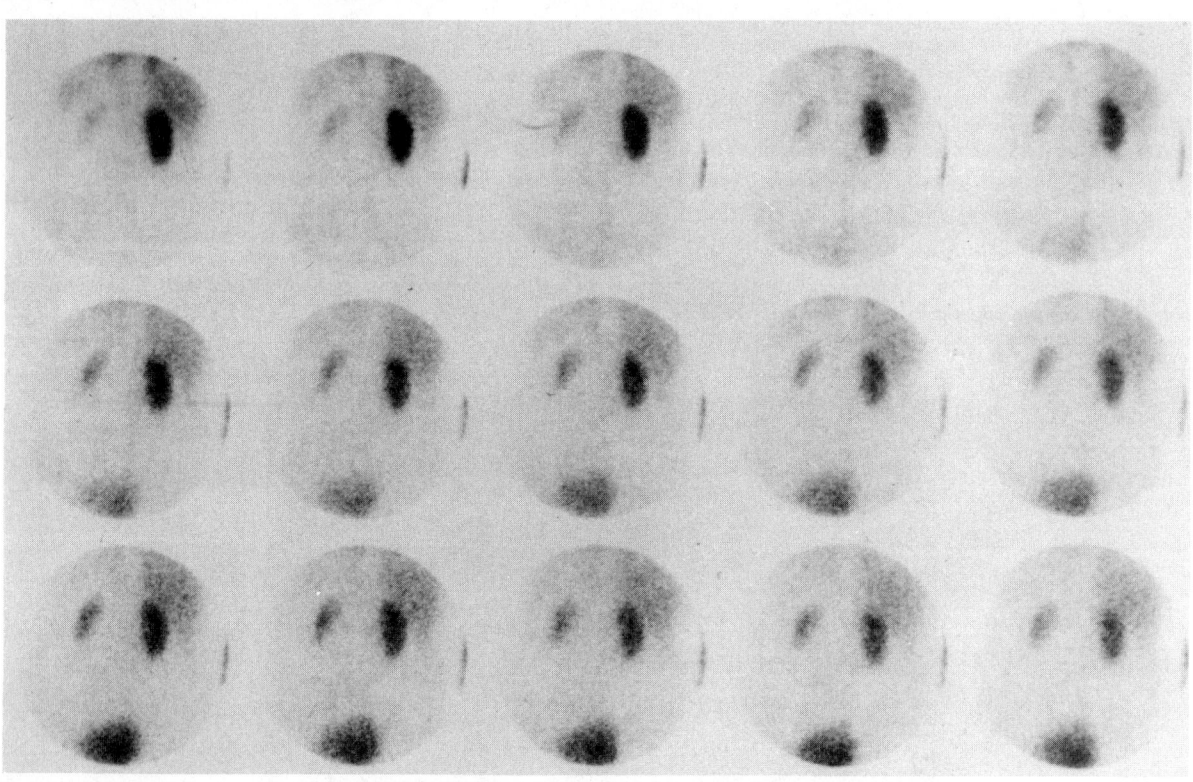

B

Fig. 81-10. Renal radioisotopic scan with MAG 3 demonstrating poor uptake of tracer in patient with left renal artery occlusion. A. Early flow phase in which each panel represents a 2-second interval. Scintigraphic activity is seen in proximal aorta (arrowheads) and right kidney (arrows). Note the absence of scintigraphic activity over the area of left kidney. B. Functional scan (1-minute intervals). Note marked diminution of scintigraphic activity over the area of left kidney.

The situation is similar regarding sodium. Patients with pure prerenal azotemia generally retain sodium avidly. However, it is wise to think of patients with other forms of azotemia as having sodium homeostasis that is "contracted at both ends"—that is, the kidney can neither maximize sodium excretion in response to a sodium load nor conserve sodium with peak efficiency during sodium depletion. Consequently, such patients are constantly at risk for either fluid overload or hypovolemia.

ABNORMAL CALCIUM AND PHOSPHORUS METABOLISM. The ability of the kidney to excrete phosphorus normally is impaired when the GFR falls to about one-third of normal. High serum phosphorus levels lead to formation of insoluble calcium phosphate salts, which may precipitate in soft tissue. If the product of the initial serum calcium and phosphorus concentrations exceeds 70, precipitation in soft tissues becomes more likely. For this reason, administration of calcium to patients in ARF should be reserved for emergent situations, such as the appearance of tetany, seizures, or refractory hypotension. Since untreated hypocalcemia may lead to secondary hypoparathyroidism, however, and eventually to bone disease, phosphate binders such as aluminum hydroxide gels should be used early to prevent these pathophysiologic consequences of hyperphosphatemia. The hypocalcemic tendency may be additionally aggravated by the injured kidney's failure to form 1,25-dihydroxycholecalciferol, although vitamin D therapy is rarely required in cases of ARF.

Occasionally, during the early part of the recovery phase from ARF, a period of "rebound hypercalcemia" may be observed. This phenomenon is more characteristic of myoglobinuria-associated ATN than of other forms of ARF and is thought to represent release of calcium from deposits in injured muscle tissue [101].

UREMIA. Accumulation of endogenous toxins in the body eventually results in uremia. The uremic syndrome comprises a variety of multisystemic disorders. Although uremia is considered an indication to initiate dialytic therapy, the syndrome may be insidious in onset and produce only vague symptoms. Lethargy, anorexia, nausea, and malaise, all of which may herald uremia, may well be attributed to extrarenal disease in the patient with ARF. For this reason, the physician may delay dialysis, especially if there are relative contraindications such as hypotension or problems related to establishing dialytic access. Other, "harder" uremic symptoms constitute stronger indications for prompt initiation of dialysis, including bleeding diathesis, seizures, coma, and the appearance of a pericardial rub.

The exact identities of the so-called uremic toxins are not known, although many possibilities have been suggested. Urea and creatinine are *not* uremic toxins, but rather are markers of renal excretory capacity. One cannot deduce on the basis of urea nitrogen and creatinine levels exactly when a patient will become uremic. In general, the syndrome manifests itself as a GFR of less than 10 ml per minute.

ABNORMAL DRUG METABOLISM. A careful review of all medications is imperative in the care of the patient with ARF. Some drugs (e.g., aminoglycoside antibiotics, digoxin) are excreted almost entirely by the kidneys. If the dose or dosing intervals are unchanged, a reduced GFR will lead to accumulation of the drug in body fluids and eventual drug toxicity.

Other agents are hepatically metabolized, but the active metabolites are renally excreted (e.g., benzodiazepines). Still other agents may have greater toxic potential, since a larger proportion of the administered drug is displaced from albumin-binding sites in uremia (e.g., phenytoin). Drug doses need to be altered in most instances to account for both residual renal function and the effect of dialysis on drug removal. This subject is covered fully in Chapter 83.

Treatment of Acute Renal Failure

GENERAL PRINCIPLES OF TREATMENT. The predialysis management of ARF is outlined in Table 81-11. These steps are applicable for any patient with ARF. Despite the availability of technologic wonders in the modern hospital, the simplest procedures may be critical for the patient's survival. Fluid balance should be measured during each 8-hour nursing shift with input/output recordings, and body weight should be recorded daily. Serum electrolytes and arterial blood gases may need daily or more frequent measurement, depending on the patient's status.

Fluid management is crucial, since sodium and water excretion may be limited, particularly in oliguric patients. In patients with pure prerenal azotemia attributable to hypovolemia, restoration of normal volume is usually sufficient to return BUN and creatinine to their normal levels. A volume-depleted, azotemic patient can receive up to a liter of saline over a 4-hour period with the expectation that renal perfusion and urine flow will improve rapidly. This maneuver is of diagnostic as well as

Table 81-11. Predialysis Management of ARF

Fluid Balance
  Weigh patient daily
  Monitor input and output
  In volume depleted patients, replace ECF with isotonic saline (or bicarbonate).
  In normovolemic or edematous patients, restrict fluid intake (~1500 ml/day) and sodium intake (≤2 gm/day)

Acid/Base and Electrolyte
  Avoid water overload and hyponatremia (restrict free water intake, particularly in oliguric patients)
  Restrict potassium intake (≤2 gm/day) and treat hyperkalemia (see Chap. 79)
  Maintain serum bicarbonate ≥12 and 15 mM
  Use phosphate binders ($CaCO_3$) to maintain PO_4 ≤5.0 mg/dl
  Treat symptomatic hypocalcemia (see text)

Drugs
  Avoid nephrotoxins where possible
  Adjust doses of all renally excreted drugs
  Withhold NSAIDs and ACE inhibitors in patients with prerenal conditions
  Avoid magnesium containing drugs (e.g., antacids, milk of magnesia)

Nutrition
  Restrict protein intake to ≤0.5 gm/kg/day
  Caloric (carbohydrate) intake of ≥400 kCal/day

Reduction of Infectious Risks
  Remove indwelling urinary catheter in oliguric, non-obstructed patients
  Strict aseptic technique and rapid removal, when feasible, of vascular catheters

therapeutic benefit, since rapid response to the fluid challenge will establish that azotemia is due, at least in part, to prerenal factors. Hypovolemia may complicate intrinsic renal disease and urinary tract obstruction, superimposing a prerenal component on the azotemia caused by these conditions.

It is essential not only to have a reasonable estimate of the patient's extracellular fluid volume but also to monitor fluid volumes with daily weights and input/output records. It should not be assumed that because the patient has renal failure, that fluid intake must be restricted. If the patient is clinically hypovolemic as indicated by diminished skin turgor, orthostasis, or dry mucous membranes, fluid replacement should be given with isotonic saline. (Isotonic bicarbonate should be used if the patient is acidotic with a serum bicarbonate of ≤15 mM. Use of saline in an acidotic patient may result in a worsening acidosis due to expansion of the ECF with chloride instead of bicarbonate.) The estimate of isotonic fluid replacement should be based on the clinical findings. With orthostasis, it may be estimated that the patient is suffering from an ECF deficit of at least 10%. Fluid replacement in these circumstances should be administered regardless of the patient's urine output or the presumptive diagnosis of ATN. In either case, recovery of renal function might be hastened by rapid volume repletion.

In normovolemic or edematous patients, fluid restriction is necessary. The physician should aim for a target weight loss of 0.5 lb (~0.25 kg) per day. The following formula can be applied:

Daily Fluid Replacement (ml/day)
= (Urinary + Extrarenal + Insensible losses*) − 250

Treatment of electrolyte and acid-base disorders is covered in Chapters 79 and 80. It should be noted that attention needs to be paid to mineral metabolism in patients with ARF. Hyperphosphatemia is common, particularly in patients with rhabdomyolysis or tumor lysis syndrome. Control of hyperphosphatemia usually requires the use of a phosphate-binding agents. If the patient is hypocalcemic, calcium carbonate can be administered (1–1.5 gm with meals) as the phosphate-binding agent. Hypocalcemia should be treated only if the patient is symptomatic with neuromuscular irritability or if bicarbonate therapy is anticipated in an acidotic, hypocalcemic patient. At least 1 gm of elemental calcium is necessary to raise the serum calcium 1 mg/dl. Calcium gluconate (~10% elemental calcium) should be administered slowly in a large vein.

A complete survey of all of the patient's medications should be taken when renal failure develops. Drugs that may interfere with renal blood flow or GFR-autoregulation, such as NSAIDs or ACE inhibitors, should be discontinued. In addition, the dosage of drugs that require renal metabolism and excretion should be adjusted appropriately (see Chap. 82). It is important to remember that, as the patient recovers renal function, upward adjustment of some renally excreted drugs will be necessary.

Prevention of ATN or worsening of pre-existing renal failure can best be accomplished by averting nephrotoxin exposure in high-risk patients. For example, contrast procedures should be avoided in patients with ARF. If this is not feasible, the risk should be minimized by ensuring that the patient is optimally volume-expanded before the procedure (see above). Similarly, aminoglycoside antibiotics can be replaced with nonnephrotoxic agents (see Chap. 82). When this is not possible, however, the appropriately reduced drug dose should be employed.

Patients suffering from ARF are often catabolic and increase their production of nitrogenous products that require excretion.

At the same time, such patients require caloric replacement to reduce tissue catabolism and prevent ketosis. In the early stages of renal failure, particularly before dialysis is required, minimal caloric replacement (e.g., 400 kCal or 100 gm of carbohydrate) should be sufficient. This should be administered in a concentrated solution such as 1 liter of a 10% glucose solution infused over 24 hours. This permits fluid restriction while the patient is oliguric. Protein (or amino acid) intake should likewise be restricted to prevent increased urea synthesis.

It is not our purpose to describe nutritional therapy here (see Chap. 202). The guidelines for nutritional therapy in ARF are similar to those in other ICU patients. Patients on dialysis, however, allowed a more liberal fluid intake, can receive the necessary caloric, protein, and fat requirements provided that the fluid administration can be matched by dialytic fluid removal (see Chap. 83). The use of nutritional therapy to enhance survival and recovery from ARF is controversial. Early studies suggested that recovery and survival were enhanced [102,103], but these were not confirmed by more recent, controlled trials [104,105].

The physician should try to minimize iatrogenic factors that may contribute to mortality and morbidity. Since infection, particularly of the urinary tract, is a leading cause of mortality, unnecessary indwelling urinary and vascular catheters must be avoided. In an oliguric patient who is too obtunded to void spontaneously, periodic "straight" catheterization suffices to collect urine and carries a lower risk of inducing iatrogenic urosepsis than an indwelling device [106].

SPECIFIC THERAPEUTIC INTERVENTIONS. Few definitive modes of therapy exist for intrinsic renal diseases. If renal damage occurs as a result of exposure to a drug with allergic or nephrotoxic potential, the offending agent should be withdrawn if feasible.

Acute interstitial nephritis usually responds to withdrawal of the culpable drug. Recovery of renal function may, however, be protracted. A short course of corticosteroids (usually oral prednisone at an initial dose of approximately 1 mg/kg/day) has been found to hasten recovery in uncontrolled trials [107].

In rapidly progressive renal diseases, a renal biopsy may be helpful not only to aid in diagnosis but also as a means of predicting response to therapy. Specific treatment may not be required, such as in postinfectious glomerulonephritis or glomerulonephritis associated with bacterial endocarditis. In the former case, spontaneous remission usually occurs; in the latter, antibiotic treatment of the underlying condition may result in clearing of the immune complex-induced renal lesion (see Chap. 88). Renal failure in association with systemic lupus or one of the idiopathic forms of rapidly progressive glomerulonephritis may respond to high-dose intravenous corticosteroids ("pulse therapy" consisting of 1 gm methylprednisolone/day for 3–5 days) or a combination of oral prednisone, a cytotoxic agent (cyclophosphamide or azathioprine), and plasmapheresis [108,109]. The latter therapy is aimed at clearing the plasma of the offending antibody (antiglomerular basement membrane) or immune complexes while simultaneously decreasing their formation [110]. Renal failure associated with necrotizing vasculitis may be treated with corticosteroid alone, cytotoxic agents alone, or a combination of both. Cyclophosphamide is generally accepted as the treatment of choice for Wegener's granulomatosis [111].

Both the loop diuretics and mannitol have been recommended as therapy for ATN. Diuretic therapy should only be administered to oliguric patients who are judged to be either normo- or hypervolemic. In these circumstances, the patient may convert to a nonoliguric state. Unfortunately, evidence that

---

* Insensible losses = 500 ml/day. For febrile patients, add 500 ml/day for every degree Fahrenheit over 101.

this maneuver improves patient survival is lacking [112]. Moreover, diuretic administration may worsen renal perfusion in a patient with antecedent hypovolemia.

Recent attention has focused on two new therapeutic approaches. The use of dopamine in combination with furosemide appears effective in both an experimental model of ischemic ATN [16] and in human patients with newly established ATN [113]. It is thought that dopamine, a renal vasodilator, either directly enhances solute excretion or improves delivery of the diuretic to the peritubular blood and its subsequent secretion into the nephron. Early results in small numbers of patients with this form of combination therapy are promising, but additional randomized trials are needed.

The calcium channel antagonists have recently been proposed for use in the treatment of ATN [112]. The rationale for their use lies not only in their vasodilating properties but also in the accruing evidence that raised intracellular and mitochondrial calcium is the harbinger and possibly a final common pathway of cell death [114]. The studies of these agents have so far been confined to animals, although human investigations are under way.

Relief of urinary obstruction is the object of therapy in this form of ARF. Acute intervention is mandatory in the presence of complete or bilateral urinary tract obstruction, severe azotemia, or any of the metabolic or hemodynamic complications of ARF. Coexisting fever or any other evidence that urinary infection lies proximal to the obstruction requires a rapid decompression procedure to avoid bacteremic shock.

When bladder outlet obstruction is suspected, insertion of a urethral catheter should be attempted. If this is not possible, as is occasionally the case in patients with prostatic enlargement or ureteral stricture, ureteral dilation or percutaneous cystostomy should be performed.

When obstruction is confined to the upper urinary tract, the need for intervention is tempered by the presence or absence of bilateral obstruction (or obstruction of a solitary kidney) sufficient to cause renal failure and symptoms. When indicated, upper tract obstruction can be relieved by either the retrograde insertion of a ureteral catheter or the percutaneous placement (under ultrasonic, fluoroscopic, or CT scan guidance) of a catheter in the renal pelvis.

The metabolic and hemodynamic complications of urinary obstruction need attention regardless of whether the process can be relieved. Obstructive uropathy is associated with defects of the distal nephron, including hydrogen ion and potassium secretion, as well as urinary concentration. Consequently, the patient, particularly if there is prolonged high-grade obstruction, may display hyperkalemia [115], hyperchloremic metabolic acidosis [116], hypernatremia, or a combination of all three. Water and bicarbonate replacement are often required and can be administered as a solution of 5% glucose and water to which sodium bicarbonate has been added. The patient's plasma volume and serum sodium should determine the tonicity of the administered fluid. If the patient is hypovolemic, an isotonic solution should be used. If the patient is primarily hypernatremic, a hypotonic solution is needed. Hyperkalemia may respond to both the institution of a diuresis that relieves the obstruction and correction of the acidosis. In patients with severe hyperkalemia, exchange resins (sodium polystyrene) or dialysis may be required.

A diuresis often ensues following relief of urinary obstruction, particularly when prolonged. This usually reflects both the trapping of urine within the expanded bladder and ureters and the retained extracellular fluid during the period of obstruction. As such, this diuresis is considered "appropriate" to the preexisting volume expansion [117]. In some patients with correction of bilateral obstruction, a large diuresis and natriuresis may ensue, which results in hypovolemia and, sometimes, frank shock. The mechanism for this "inappropriate" diuresis is poorly understood but may involve the synthesis of a natriuretic substance [118]. These patients require fluid replacement, usually with hypotonic saline to repair the deficit and match urinary losses. A useful technique is to measure the urinary sodium and potassium concentrations periodically to determine the composition of the replacement fluid.

PROGNOSIS AND OUTCOME OF ACUTE RENAL FAILURE. Overall, the mortality rate from acute renal failure ranges from 25 percent [20] to 64 percent [119]. The large disparity in mortality rates no doubt reflects the varied intensities of illness and case mixes in the reports. A large retrospective study by McMurray et al demonstrated a 14% mortality rate in patients with nephrotoxic forms of ARF compared with a 35% mortality for all other causes. Similarly, in the prospective study by Hou and colleagues, mortality ranged between a low of 6% in radiocontrast-induced nephropathy to 80% in cases of hepatorenal syndrome. Even within the group of patients with ARF due to renal hypoperfusion, mortality varied between 9% in patients with volume depletion and 100% in patients with cardiogenic shock.

These data explain why dialysis therapy fails to dramatically improve the survival rates in ARF. Patients with multisystem conditions, in particular, fail to show any benefit from dialysis therapy. A recent analysis of survival in ARF in the ICU demonstrated that certain comorbid factors—acute respiratory distress syndrome, requirement for antibiotics, and ventilatory failure—caused lower survival [120]. Ventilatory failure, in particular, was associated with 100% mortality in patients who also required dialysis. The particularly high mortality in ARF complicating multiorgan system failure and the associated increments in hospital costs have led some to call for a reanalysis of the use of dialytic procedures in critically ill patients.

The causal basis for mortality in ARF is seldom due to uremia. As can be seen in Figure 81-11, as reported by Kleinknecht et al [42], most deaths are the result of either sepsis, GI hemorrhage, or cardiac causes. The excessively high mortality from GI bleeding in this study, published in 1971, raises some question about its relevance for current practice. This study also reported improved mortality figures in posttraumatic and postsurgical patients who were dialyzed "prophylactically" to maintain a BUN level of no more than 100 mg/dl.

Nonoliguria accounts for at least half of the current cases of ARF [121]. Nonoliguria is associated with an improved likelihood of recovery of renal function and approximately half the mortality (26%) of oliguric ARF (50%) [121]. Nonoliguric patients are more likely to have suffered ARF as a result of exposure to a nephrotoxin than are oliguric patients [121]. The converse, that is, that these patients are less likely to have multiorgan system failure, is also probably true. Hence, their improved survival may be the result of a less severe insult. It is therefore unclear whether pharmacologic conversion from oliguria to nonoliguria improves survival. Initial studies showed no demonstrable improvement in patient survival when patients became nonoliguric after use of high-dose loop diuretics [122]. More recent uncontrolled studies indicated improved survival in diuretic-responsive patients compared with nonresponsive patients. Shorter duration of oliguria and preservation of tubular function, as indicated by a low U_{Na} or FE_{Na}, were predictive of responsiveness to diuretics.

Recovery of renal function can be expected in most patients who survive ARF. With the exception of those who have acute bilateral cortical necrosis or other irreversible forms of paren-

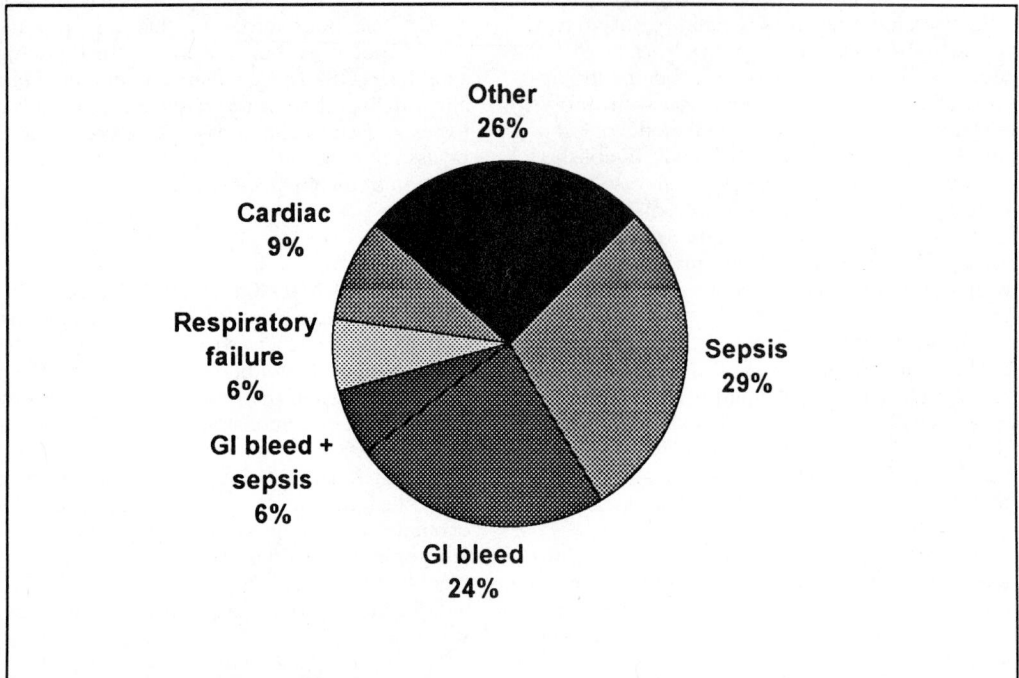

Fig. 81-11. Primary causes of death in patients with ARF. (Data from Kleinknecht et al: Uremic and non-uremic complications of acute renal failure: Evaluation of early and frequent dialysis on prognosis. *Kidney Int* 1:190, 1972.)

chymal renal disease, partial or complete recovery occurs in more than 90%. Prolongation of recovery can be anticipated in those patients with poor cardiac output [123] or in patients with hypovolemia. It is therefore imperative that extracellular fluid volume be assessed, particularly in patients on hemodialysis or peritoneal dialysis in whom volume depletion may occur. Measurement of pulmonary wedge pressure, if available, is helpful. The finding of a low U_{Na} or FE_{Na} in a patient with previously high values for these indices might indicate recovery of tubular function and simultaneous hypovolemia.

References

1. Rose BD: Acute renal failure, in Rose BD (ed): *Pathophysiology of Renal Disease*. New York, McGraw-Hill, 1981, p 55.
2. Stoff JS, Clive DM: Role of arachidonic acid metabolites in acute renal failure, in Brenner BM, Lazarus JM (eds): *Acute Renal Failure*. 2nd ed. New York, Churchill Livingstone, 1988, p 143.
3. Francis GS: Neuroendocrine manifestations of congestive heart failure. *Am J Cardiol* 62:9A, 1988.
4. Clive DM, Stoff JS: Renal syndromes associated with nonsteroidal anti-inflammatory drugs. *N Engl J Med* 310:563, 1984.
5. Hricik DE, Browning PJ, Kopelman R, et al: Captopril-induced functional renal insufficiency in patients with bilateral renal-artery stenoses or renal-artery stenosis in a solitary kidney. *N Engl J Med* 308:373, 1983
6. Bohle A, Jahnecke D, Meyer D, et al: Morphology of acute renal failure: Comparative data from biopsy and autopsy. *Kidney Int* 10(Suppl 1):S9, 1976.
7. Solez K, Morel Maroger L, Sraer JD: The morphology of "acute tubular necrosis" in man: analysis of 57 renal biopsies and a comparison with the glycerol model. *Medicine* 58:362, 1979.
8. Brezis M, Rosen S, Silva P, et al: Renal ischemia: A new perspective. *Kidney Int* 26:375, 1984.
9. Baker SL, Dodds EC: Obstruction of the renal tubules during the excretion of hemoglobins. *Br J Exp Pathol* 6:247, 1925.
10. Donohoe JF, Venkatachalam MA, Bernard DB, et al: Tubular leakage and obstruction after renal ischemia: Structural functional correlations. *Kidney Int* 13:208, 1978.
11. Myers BD, Carrie BJ, Yee RR, et al: Pathophysiology of hemodynamically mediated acute renal failure in man. *Kidney Int* 18:495, 1980.
12. Myers BD, Moran SM: Hemodynamically mediated acute renal failure. *N Engl J Med* 314:97, 1986.
13. Flores J, DiBona DR, Beck CH, et al: The role of cell swelling in ischemic renal damage and the protective effect of hypertonic solute. *J Clin Invest* 51:118, 1972.
14. Tomita K, Ujiie K, Nakanishi T, et al: Plasma endothelin levels in patients with acute renal failure. *N Engl J Med* 321:1127, 1989.
15. Smolens P, Stein JH: Hemodynamic factors in acute renal failure: Pathophysiologic and therapeutic implications, in Brenner BM, Stein JH (eds): *Acute Renal Failure (Contemporary Issues in Nephrology Series)*. New York, Churchill Livingstone, 1980, p 180.
16. Lindner A, Cutler RL, Goodman WG: Synergism of dopamine plus furosemide in preventing acute renal failure in the dog. *Kidney Int* 16:158, 1979.
17. Lieberthal W, Sheridan AM, Valeri CR: Protective effect of atrial natriuretic factor and mannitol following renal ischemia. *Am J Renal Fluid Electrolyte Physiol* 258:F1266, 1990.
18. Hostetter TH, Wilkes BM, Brenner BM: Mechanisms of impaired glomerular filtration in acute renal failure, in Brenner BM, Stein JH (eds): *Acute Renal Failure (Contemporary Issues in Nephrology Series)*. New York, Churchill Livingstone, 1980, p 52.
19. Brezis M, Rosen S, Epstein FH: Acute renal failure, in Brenner BM, Rector FC (eds): *The Kidney*. 4th ed. Philadelphia, WB Saunders, 1991, p 993.
20. Hou S, Bushinsky DA, Wish JB, et al: Hospital-acquired renal insufficiency: A prospective study. *Am J Med* 74:243, 1983.
21. Heyman SN, Brezis M, Reubinoff CA, et al: Acute renal failure with selective medullary injury in the rat. *J Clin Invest* 82:401, 1988.
22. Brezis M, Shanley P, Silva P, et al: Disparate mechanisms for hypoxic cell injury in different nephron segments. Studies in the isolated perfused rat kidney. *J Clin Invest* 76:1796, 1985.

23. Brezis M, Rosen S, Silva P, et al: Selective anoxic injury to thick ascending limb: An anginal syndrome of the renal medulla. *Adv Exp Med Biol* 180:239, 1984.

24. Brezis M, Rosen S, Silva P, et al: Transport activity modifies thick ascending limb damage in the isolated perfused kidney. *Kidney Int* 25:65, 1984.

25. Heyman SN, Brezis M, Greenfeld Z, et al: Protective role of furosemide and saline in radiocontrast-induced acute renal failure in the rat. *Am J Kidney Dis* 14:377, 1989.

26. Brezis M, Rosen SN, Epstein FH: The pathophysiological implications of medullary hypoxia. *Am J Kidney Dis* 13:253, 1989.

27. Farber JL: Membrane injury and calcium homeostasis in the pathogenesis of coagulative necrosis. *Lab Invest* 47:114, 1982.

28. Humes HD: Role of calcium in pathogenesis of acute renal failure. *Am J Physiol* 250:F579, 1986.

29. Paller MS, Hoidal IR, Ferris TF: Oxygen-free radicals in ischemic acute renal failure in the rat. *Kidney Int* 25:519, 1984.

30. Ratych RE, Bulkley GB: Free-radical-mediated postischemic reperfusion injury in the kidney. *J Free Radical Biol Med* 2:311, 1986.

31. Humes HD, Jackson NM, O'Connor RP, et al: Pathogenetic mechanisms of nephrotoxicity: Insights into cyclosporine nephrotoxicity. *Transplant Proc* 17:51, 1985.

32. Brezis M, Epstein FH: Cellular mechanisms of acute ischemic injury in the kidney. *Ann Rev Med* 44:27, 1993.

33. Badr KF, Brenner BM: Renal circulatory and nephron function in experimental obstruction of the urinary tract, in Brenner BM, Lazarus JM (eds): *Acute Renal Failure*. 2nd ed. New York, Churchill Livingstone, 1988, p 91.

34. Early LE: Extreme polyuria in obstructive uropathy. *N Engl J Med* 255:600, 1956.

35. Dawson JL: Acute post-operative renal failure in obstructive jaundice. *Ann R Coll Surg* 42:163, 1968.

36. Berisa F, Beaman M, Adu D, et al: Prognostic factors in acute renal failure following aortic aneurysm surgery. *Q J Med* 76:689, 1990.

37. Corwin HL, Sprague SM, DeLaria GA, et al: Acute renal failure associated with cardiac operations. A case-control study Nutrition in acute renal failure. *J Thorac Cardiovasc Surg Crit Care Clin* 3:155, 1987.

38. Nakamoto M, Shapiro JI, Shanley PF, et al: In vitro and in vivo protective effect of atriopeptin III on ischemic acute renal failure. *J Clin Invest* 80:698, 1987.

39. Burkart F, Kiowski W: Circulatory abnormalities and compensatory mechanisms in heart failure. *Am J Med* 90:19S, 1991.

40. McMurray SD, Luft FC, Maxwell DR, et al: Prevailing patterns and predictor variables in patients with acute tubular necrosis. *Arch Intern Med* 136:950, 1978.

41. Schaefer JH, Jochimsen F, Keller F, et al: Outcome prediction of acute renal failure in medical intensive care. *Intensive Care Medicine* 17:19, 1991.

42. Kleinknecht D, Jungers P, Chanard J, et al: Uremic and non-uremic complications of acute renal failure: Evaluation of early and frequent dialysis on prognosis. *Kidney Int* 1:190, 1972.

42a. Goldstein DA, Llach F, Massry SG: Acute renal failure in patients with acute pancreatitis. *Arch Intern Med* 136:1363, 1976.

43. Kleinknecht D, Grunfeld JP, Cia Gomez P: Diagnostic procedures and longterm prognosis in bilateral renal cortical necrosis. *Kidney Int* 4:390, 1973.

44. Kaplinsky C, Frand M, Rubenstein ZJ: Disseminated intravascular clotting and renal cortical necrosis complicating snake bite. *Clin Pediatr* 19:229, 1980.

45. Gerhardt RE, Hudson JB, Rao RN, et al: Chronic renal insufficiency from cortical necrosis induced by arsenic poisoning. *Arch Intern Med* 138:1267, 1978.

46. Williams GM, Horne DM, Hudson KP Jr: Hyperacute renal homograft rejection in man. *N Engl J Med* 279:611, 1968.

47. Solez K, Bihari D, Collins AJ, et al: International dialysis aid in earthquake and other disasters. *Kidney Int* 44:479, 1993.

48. Honda N, Kurokawa K: Acute renal failure and rhabdomyolysis. *Kidney Int* 23:888, 1983.

49. Roth D, Alarcon FJ, Fernandez JA, et al: Acute rhabdomyolysis associated with cocaine intoxication. *N Engl J Med* 319:673, 1990.

50. Better OS, Stein JH: Early management of shock and prophylaxis of acute renal failure in traumatic rhabdomyolysis. *N Engl J Med* 322:825, 1990.

51. Dubrow A, Flamenbaum W: Acute renal failure associated with myoglobinuria and hemoglobinuria, in Brenner BM, Lazarus JM (eds): *Acute Renal Failure*. 2nd ed. New York, Churchill Livingstone, 1988, p 279.

52. Berns AS: Nephrotoxicity of contrast media [clinical conference]. *Kidney Int* 36:730, 1989.

53. Kumar S, Hull JD, Lathi S, et al: Low incidence of renal failure after angiography. *Arch Intern Med* 141:1268, 1981.

54. Mason RA, Arbeit LA, Giron F: Renal dysfunction after angiography. *JAMA* 253:1001, 1985.

55. Fang LST, Sirota RA, Ebert TH, et al: Low fractional excretion of sodium with contrast media induced acute renal failure. *Arch Intern Med* 140:531, 1980.

56. Margulies KB, Hildebrand FL, Heublein DM, et al: Radiocontrast increases plasma and urinary endothelin. *J Am Soc Nephrol* 2:1041, 1991.

57. Shusterman N, Strom BL, Murray TG, et al: Risk factors and outcome of hospital-acquired acute renal failure Clinical epidemiologic study. *Am J Med* 83:65, 1987.

58. Porter GA: Experimental contrast-associated nephropathy and its clinical implications. *Am J Cardiol* 66:18F, 1990.

59. Margulies K, Schirger J, Burnett J, Jr: Radiocontrast-induced nephropathy: current status and future prospects. *International Angiology* 11:20, 1992.

60. Brezis M, Epstein FH: A closer look at radiocontrast-induced nephropathy [editorial]. *N Engl J Med* 320:179, 1989.

61. Barrett BJ, Carlisle EJ: Metaanalysis of the relative nephrotoxicity of high- and low-osmolality iodinated contrast media. *Radiology* 188:171, 1993.

62. Humes HD: Aminoglycoside toxicity. *Kidney Int* 33:900, 1988.

63. Deray G, Martinez F, Katlama C: Foscarnet nephrotoxicity: mechanism, incidence, and prevention. *Am J Nephrol* 9:316, 1989.

64. Galpin JE, Shinaberger JH, Stanley TM: Acute interstitial nephritis due to methicillin. *Am J Med* 65:756, 1978.

65. van Ypersele de Strihou C: Acute oliguric interstitial nephritis. *Kidney Int* 16:751, 1979.

66. Walshe JJ, Venuto RC: Acute oliguric renal failure induced by indomethacin: possible mechanism. *Ann Intern Med* 91:47, 1979.

67. Hricik DE, Dunn MJ: Angiotensin-converting enzyme inhibitor-induced renal failure: Causes, consequences, and diagnostic uses. *J Am Soc Nephrol* 1:845, 1990.

68. Lessman RK, Johnson SF, Coburn JW, et al: Renal artery embolism. *Ann Intern Med* 89:477, 1978.

69. Fraser I, Ihle B, Kincaid-Smith P: Renal failure due to cholesterol emboli. *Austr N Z J Med* 21:418, 1991.

70. Smith MC, Ghose MK, Henry AR: The clinical spectrum of renal cholesterol embolization. *Am J Med* 71:174, 1981.

71. Blachley JD, Hill JB: Renal and electrolyte disturbances associated with cisplatin. *Ann Intern Med* 95:628, 1981.

72. Garnick MB, Mayer RJ: Management of acute renal failure associated with neoplastic disease, in Yarboro J, Bornstein R (eds): *Oncologic Emergencies*. New York, Grune and Stratton, 1981.

73. Ring Larsen H, Palazzo U: Renal failure in fulminant hepatic failure and terminal cirrhosis: A comparison between incidence, types, and prognosis. *Gut* 22:585, 1981.

74. Mas A, Arroyo V, Rodes J, et al: Ascites and renal failure in primary liver cell carcinoma. *Br Med J* iii:692, 1975.

75. Rosanasky SJ, Mullens CC: The hepatorenal syndrome associated with angiosarcoma of the gall bladder. *Ann Intern Med* 96:191, 1982.

76. Conn HO: Diuresis of ascites: Fraught with or free from hazard? *Gastroenterology* 73:619, 1977.

77. Gregory PB, Broekelschen PH, Hill MD: Complications of diuresis in the alcoholic patient with ascites: A controlled trial. *Gastroenterology* 73:534, 1977.

78. McDonald FD, Brennan LA, Turcotte JG: Severe hypertension and elevated plasma renin activity following transplantation of the "hepatorenal donor" kidneys into anephric recipients. *Am J Med* 54:39, 1973.

79. Boyer TD, Zia P, Reynolds TB: Effect of indomethacin and prostaglandin A1 on renal function and plasma renin activity in alcoholic liver disease. *Gastroenterology* 77:215, 1979.

80. Zipser RD, Hoefs JS, Speckert PF, et al: Prostaglandins: Modulators

of renal function and pressor resistance in chronic liver disease. *J Clin Endocrinol Metab* 48:895, 1979.

81. Kronborg IJ, Radvan G, Zipser RD: Urinary excretion of prostaglandins and thromboxanes in the hepatorenal syndrome, in Samuelsson P, Paoletti R, Ramwell P (eds): *Advances in Prostaglandin, Thromboxane, and Leukotriene Research*. New York, Raven, 1983.

82. Papadakis MA, Arieff AI: Unpredictability of clinical evaluation of renal function in cirrhosis. *Am J Med* 82:945, 1987.

83. Cade R, Wagemaker H, Vogel S, et al: Hepatorenal syndrome. *Am J Med* 82:427, 1987.

84. Kao HW, Ralkov NE, Savage E, et al: The effect of large volume paracentesis on plasma volume: A cause of hypovolemia? *Hepatology* 5(3):403, 1985.

85. Pinto PC, Amerian J, Reynolds TB: Large-volume paracentesis in nonedematous patients with tense ascites. Its effect on intravascular volume. *Hepatology* 8(2):207, 1988.

86. Gines P, Arroyo V, Quintero E, et al: Comparison of paracentesis and diuretics in the treatment of cirrhotics with tense ascites. *Gastroenterology* 93:234, 1987.

87. Kellerman P, Linas S: Large-volume paracentesis in treatment of ascites. *Ann Intern Med* 112(12):889, 1990.

88. Clark F, O'Leary JP: Survival associated with hepatorenal syndrome. *South Med J* 72:87, 1979.

89. Ariyan S, Sweeney T, Kerstein MD: The hepatorenal syndrome: Recovery after portacaval shunt. *Ann Surg* 181:847, 1975.

90. Fischer JE, Foster GS: Survival from acute hepatorenal syndrome following splenorenal shunt. *Ann Surg* 814:22, 1976.

91. Epstein M: Peritoneovenous shunt in the management of ascites and hepatorenal syndrome. *Gastroenterology* 82:790, 1982.

92. Fullen WD: Hepatorenal syndrome: Reversal of peritoneovenous shunt. *Surgery* 82:337, 1977.

93. Kinney MJ, Schneider A, Sapnick S, et al: The hepatorenal syndrome and refractory ascites. *Nephron* 23:228, 1979.

94. Schroeder ET, Anderson GH, Smulyan H: Effects of portacaval or peritoneovenous shunt on renin in the hepatorenal syndrome. *Kidney Int* 15:54, 1979.

95. Schwartz ML, Vogel SG: Treatment of hepatorenal syndrome. *Am J Surg* 139:370, 1980.

96. Wapnick S, Grosberg A, Kinney M, et al: LeVeen continuous peritoneo-jugular shunt. *JAMA* 237:131, 1977.

97. Epstein M: The LeVeen shunt for ascites and hepatorenal syndrome. *N Engl J Med* 302:628, 1980.

98. Linas SL, Schaefer JW, Moore EE, et al: Peritoneovenous shunt in the management of the hepatorenal syndrome. *Kidney Int* 30:736, 1986.

99. Levinsky NG: Pathophysiology of acute renal failure. *N Engl J Med* 296:1453, 1977.

100. Border WA, Cohen AH: Renal biopsy diagnosis of clinically silent multiple myeloma. *Ann Intern Med* 93:43, 1980.

101. Knochel JP: Serum calcium derangements in rhabdomyolysis. *N Engl J Med* 305:161, 1981.

102. Abel RM, Beck CH, Abbott WM, et al: Improved survival from acute renal failure after treatment with intravenous essential L-amino acids and glucose. Results of a prospective, double-blind study. *N Engl J Med* 288:695, 1973.

103. Back SM, Makabali GG, Bryan-Brown CW, et al: The influence of parenteral nutrition on the course of acute renal failure. *Surg Gynecol Obstet* 141:405, 1975.

104. Freund H, Harmian S, Fischer JE: Comparative studies of parenteral nutrition in renal failure using essential and non-essential amino acid containing solutions. *Surg Gynecol Obstet* 151:652, 1980.

105. Feinstein EI, Blumenkrantz MJ, Healy M, et al: Clinical and metabolic responses to parenteral nutrition in acute renal failure. *Medicine* 60:124, 1981.

106. Warren JW, Platt R, Thomas J, et al: Antibiotic irrigation and catheter-associated urinary tract infection. *N Engl J Med* 299:570, 1978.

107. Linton AL, Clark WF, Driedger AA: Acute interstitial nephritis due to drugs. Review of the literature with a report of nine cases. *Ann Intern Med* 93:735, 1980.

108. Kincaid-Smith P, d'Apice AJF: Plasmapheresis in rapidly progressive glomerulonephritis. *Am J Med* 65:564, 1978.

109. Lockwood CM, Pinching AJ, Swemy P, et al: Plama-exchange and immunosuppression in the treatment of fulminating immune complex crecentic glomerulonephritis. *Lancet* 1:63, 1977.

110. Lockwood CM, Pearson TA, Rees AJ, et al: Immunosuppression and plasma-exchange in the treatment of Goodpasture's syndrome. *Lancet* 1:711, 1976.

111. Fauci AS, Haynes BF, Katz P, et al: Wegener's granulomatosis: Prospective clinical and therapeutic experience with 85 patients for 21 years. *Ann Intern Med* 98:76, 1983.

112. Goldfarb D, Iaina A, Serban I, et al: Beneficial effects of verapamil in ischemic acute renal failure in the rat. *Proc Soc Exp Biol Med* 172:389, 1983.

113. Lindner A: Synergism of dopamine and furosemide in diuretic-resistant oliguric acute renal failure. *Nephron* 33:121, 1983.

114. Wilson DR, Arnold PE, Burke TJ, et al: Mitochondrial calcium accumulation and respiration in ischemic acute renal failure in the rat. *Kidney Int* 25:519, 1984.

115. Battle DC, Arruda JAL, Kurtzman NA: Hyperkalemic distal renal tubular acidosis associated with obstructive uropathy. *N Engl J Med* 304:373, 1981.

116. DeFronzo RA: Hyperkalemia and hyporeninemic hypoaldosteronism. *Kidney Int* 17:118, 1980.

117. Rose BD: Urinary tract obstruction, in Rose BD (ed): *Pathophysiology of Renal Disease*. New York, McGraw Hill, 1981, p 347.

118. Wilson DR, Honrath V: Cross circulation of natriuretic factors in post-obstructive diuresis. *J Clin Invest* 57:380, 1976.

119. Lien J, Chan V: Risk factors influencing survival in acute renal failure treated by hemodialysis. *Arch Intern Med* 145:2015, 1985.

120. Spiegel DM, Ullian ME, Zerbe GO, et al: Determinants of survival and recovery in acute renal failure patients dialyzed in intensive-care units. *Am J Nephrol* 11:44 1991.

121. Dixon BS, Anderson RJ: Nonoliguric acute renal failure. *Am J Kidney Dis* 6:71, 1985.

122. Minuth AN, Terrell JB, Suki WN: Acute renal failure: A study of the course and prognosis of 104 patients and of the role of furosemide. *Am J Med Sci* 271:317, 1976.

123. Moran SM, Myers BD: Pathophysiology of protracted acute renal failure in man. *J Clin Invest* 1440:1448, 1985.

82. Drug Dosing in the Intensive Care Unit: The Patient with Renal Failure

Gail Morrison

Very ill hospitalized patients are at risk of having or developing abnormal renal function. Many of these patients may have underlying disease processes such as diabetes mellitus, hypertension, and congestive heart failure that may have directly affected their kidneys and already led to renal insufficiency prior to hospitalization. During hospitalization, the development of intravascular volume depletion, shock due to sepsis or blood loss, myocardial failure, or cardiac arrest makes these acutely ill patients more susceptible to worsening renal function and makes patients with normal renal function more predisposed to developing acute renal failure (ARF). One of the many problems facing physicians caring for such patients is selecting and then adjusting the various drug regimens to provide adequate therapeutics while avoiding adverse drug reactions and toxicity. It is hoped that the discussion and Tables 82-1 to 82-17 that follow will assist physicians in selecting and adjusting a drug regimen for acutely ill patients with varying degrees of renal impairment.

Renal Failure: Effect on Drug Pharmacokinetics

Renal failure (either mild, GFR >50 ml/min; moderate, GFR 10–50 ml/min; or severe, GFR < 10 ml/min) has the potential to affect every aspect of drug disposition by the body, including a drug's bioavailability, protein binding, volume of distribution (Vd), metabolism, and excretion. Knowing the exact method by which renal failure affects these pharmacokinetic parameters for specific drugs can be helpful in deciding if a drug's dosing regimen has to be altered.

BIOAVAILABILITY. Although drugs administered intravenously enter the bloodstream directly and have a rapid onset of action even in patients with renal failure, this is not true for orally administered drugs, in which absorption (bioavailability) may be incomplete and thus decreased. The primary reasons for decreased drug absorption include nausea and vomiting, delayed gastric emptying associated with uremia, and frequent drug–drug interactions that occur in many patients as a result of multiple drug combinations. It has been proposed that patients with renal failure associated with edematous states may have "edema" of their gastrointestinal tract, which prevents complete absorption of drugs. Certainly, as renal function declines, elevated levels of salivary urea are converted to ammonia by urease, resulting in alkalinization of the gastric pH. Specific drugs that need an acid environment for absorption are then incompletely absorbed.

PROTEIN BINDING. In patients with renal failure, drug-protein binding may be altered because of a decreased quantity of plasma proteins (particularly albumin) are available for binding (e.g., nephrotic syndrome and malnourished individuals) or because of a reduction in the affinity of albumin for a drug. Changes in the structural orientation of the albumin molecule or the accumulation of endogenous uremic toxins that compete with these drugs for specific albumin binding sites have been cited as reasons for a reduced affinity of albumin for a drug. Drugs that are structurally organic acids often bind to a single albumin site, whereas drugs that are structurally organic bases probably have several sites of attachments [1]. As a consequence, the binding of many acidic drugs is decreased in patients with renal failure; the binding of many basic drugs is less affected by uremia [1].

Reduced drug-protein binding significantly increases the availability of "unbound" or active drug, which can result in drug toxicity. On the other hand, although decreased drug-protein binding results in greater availability of unbound drug at the site for drug action or toxicity, more unbound drug is also available for metabolism and excretion, which can result in a decreased half-life and reduced therapeutic effect of that drug. Thus, predicting the clinical consequences of decreased drug-protein binding for any drug in uremia is difficult.

VOLUME OF DISTRIBUTION. The apparent Vd reflects the ratio of the amount of drug in the body to its plasma concentration at equilibrium. Vd helps provide an estimate for the initial or loading dose of a drug needed to reach a plasma therapeutic concentration. Highly protein-bound drugs or those that are highly water soluble tend to be confined to the extracellular fluid compartment and have relatively small Vd. In contrast, highly lipid-soluble drugs easily cross the cell membrane into tissues and have large Vd [2]. Renal failure can alter a drug's volume of distribution. Decreased drug-protein binding can increase the Vd of a drug by providing more "unbound" drug for distribution. Edema and ascites can increase the Vd of highly water soluble or protein-bound drugs. Normal or "usual" doses of drugs given to patients with significant edema may result in low or inadequate drug plasma or serum drug levels because the drug disperses into edematous fluids. In contrast, in patients with dehydration or muscle wasting, there is usually a decrease in the Vd of most water-soluble drugs, since total body water is decreased. Therefore, in these patients, a normal or "usual" dose may result in unexpectedly high plasma or serum drug concentrations [2].

METABOLISM. Renal failure can substantially affect drug metabolism or drug biotransformation. Most drugs are metabolized in the liver. Reduction and hydrolysis reaction are generally slowed in patients with uremia, whereas glucuronidation, sulfated conjugation, and microsomal oxidation usually occur at normal rates [3]. Many drugs are metabolized to active metabolites that may be equally or more potent than the parent drug. Many of these metabolites are eliminated via the kidney [4]. Often, failure to recognize this accumulation of active metabolites when using a drug leads to the high incidence of adverse drug reactions reported in patients with renal failure.

EXCRETION. The kidney is responsible for the excretion of many drugs (and drug metabolites). It accomplishes this function by three primary processes: glomerular filtration, active tubular secretion, and passive tubular reabsorption. The prime determinant of whether a drug is eliminated by glomerular filtration is its molecular size and protein-binding capacity. When glomerular filtration is reduced, the elimination of water-soluble drugs of low molecular weight is decreased; consequently, the plasma half-life of these drugs is prolonged.

The renal tubular secretion of drugs eliminated by an active transport system can be affected by renal failure. Drugs dependent on renal tubular secretion for elimination are excreted more slowly as the creatinine clearance decreases, because less drug reaches the tubule sites. Furthermore, because the proximal tubular secretion of some drugs is mediated by the carrier and limited by capacity, concurrent use of several drugs eliminated by renal tubular secretion may saturate the transport system [2]. Therefore, certain drug combinations may result in more adverse drug reactions and drug toxicity (e.g., digoxin-quinidine combination) in patients with renal failure.

Comparing pharmacokinetic data from individuals with normal renal function to data from patients with end-stage renal disease (ESRD) is helpful in determining whether a drug dose has to be altered for patients with renal failure. Extensive guidelines and nomograms [2,5–13] as well as several textbooks [14,15] have been published to facilitate drug dosing in patients with renal failure. Most of the data found in Tables 82-3 to 82-17 come from these cited publications and textbooks. Unfortunately, data are still not available for many commonly used drugs. For those drugs, clinical and laboratory evaluation may be the only means of monitoring patients to determine adequacy of therapy and drug *toxicity.*

Assessment of Renal Function

Since the rate of elimination of drugs excreted by the kidneys is proportional to the glomerular filtration rate (GFR), a measurement of the GFR is often needed. Clinically, the GFR can be approximated from a patient's creatinine clearance, which can be calculated from a timed 24-hour urine collection for creatinine and a mid-point serum creatinine measurement. This type of collection is often not practical in an acutely ill patient who requires institution of an immediate drug regimen. In most acute situations, the equation of Cockroft and Gault [16] can be used to estimate the creatinine clearance (see Chap. 78).

Estimating the GFR from either the timed urine collection or the formulas in Chapter 78 assumes that the patient's renal function is stable, which is indicated by a constant (unchanging) serum creatinine measurement. A fluctuating serum creatinine level is no longer a true representative measurement of the creatinine clearance; if used to calculate the GFR, an erroneous value will result. Of particular importance, whenever a patient is oliguric (< 400 ml/24 hours of urine), regardless of the serum creatinine concentration, the creatinine clearance should be estimated to be less than 10 ml/min.

Since serum creatinine is a function of muscle mass as well as GFR, the serum creatinine measurement alone cannot be used as an indicator of normal renal function unless the patient is a young, relatively healthy, well-nourished individual with a sudden acute illness. Elderly or debilitated (malnourished) patients with diminished muscle mass may have serum creatinine levels in the "normal" range. When the equation of Cockroft and Gault is applied, which takes into account their age and

weight, normal range values for these individuals are indicative of a markedly reduced GFR (see Chap. 78).

Adverse Drug Reactions

Adverse drug reactions are common in patients with renal impairment [17,18]. Some of these adverse reactions could be prevented by avoiding drugs that are nephrotoxic, drugs that are not efficacious in renal insufficiency, or drugs that produce an increased metabolic load that cannot be excreted (Table 82-1). The development of adverse drug reactions only complicates the hospital course of an acutely ill patient, and attempts should be made to minimize such complications by carefully reviewing all drugs prescribed to patients with or without renal impairment. Whenever possible, the drug tables (Tables 82-3 to 82-17) have identified some of the common adverse drug reactions associated with a category of drugs or a specific drug.

Dosing of Drugs in Renal Disease

Before initiating a drug in a patient with renal impairment, it is important to assess whether there is a history of previous drug allergies or adverse drug reactions, any concurrently prescribed medications, and all nonprescription medications. As part of the physical examination, an estimation of the extracellular fluid volume is essential because the presence of dehydration, edema, or ascites often requires alteration of the dose of a drug. For obese and edematous patients, the ideal body weight should be calculated. Liver function studies should be assessed since further drug alterations are frequently needed in patients with both renal and liver impairment.

The initial drug dose or loading dose for a patient with renal impairment is usually the same as that for a patient with normal renal function with two exceptions; a larger initial dose may be

Table 82-1. Drugs to Avoid in Renal Insufficiency

Drug	Reason for avoiding drug
Antibiotics	
Tetracycline	Antianabolic causes rise in BUN
	May potentiate acidosis
	Nephrotoxic
Cardiovascular drugs	
Acetazolamide	Potentiates metabolic acidosis
	Ineffective in renal failure
Spironolactone	Hyperkalemia
Triamterene	Hyperkalemia
Amiloride	Hyperkalemia
Analgesics and narcotics	
Aspirin	Antiplatelet effect
NSAIDs	Antiplatelet effect
	Gastrointestinal irritation
	Nephrotoxic
Sedatives, hypnotics, and tranquilizers	
Lithium carbonate	Nephrogenic diabetes insipidus
	Lithium toxicity
Miscellaneous	
Magnesium compounds	Accumulates in renal insufficiency
	CNS side effects

necessary if substantial edema or ascites is evident, whereas a smaller initial dose may be required in dehydrated or severely debilitated patients. The initial loading dose rapidly produces a therapeutic plasma drug concentration. Without a loading dose, steady-state plasma levels will be achieved giving just a maintenance dose after four to five half-lives of the drug. A loading dose should be considered when the half-life of the drug is particularly prolonged in patients with renal insufficiency or when rapid achievement of therapeutic plasma levels is critical [2], as is often the case in acutely ill patients.

Following the loading dose or initial dose, the subsequent maintenance doses often need adjustment in patients with renal insufficiency. Options include a reduction in the normal maintenance dose, a prolongation of the dosing interval with normal maintenance doses, and both a reduction in the maintenance doses and a prolongation of the dosing interval. The option selected depends on the drug (see Tables 82-3 to 82-17). Guidelines for adjusting normal drug doses in patients with renal impairment are provided in Tables 82-3 to 82-17.

Therapeutic Drug Monitoring

Whenever possible, measuring the plasma drug concentration can help in assessing a particular drug dosing regimen. This is especially true when the relationship between drug levels and efficacy or toxicity has been established [19,20]. Such measurements are important for drugs with a narrow range between their therapeutic and their toxic levels. For some drugs, maximum concentrations measured 30 to 60 minutes after an infusion (peak levels) and minimum concentrations (trough levels) measured immediately before the next dose are relevant. In patients with renal impairment, the trough or minimum levels are more reliable measurements of drug elimination; if elevated, they seem to more closely reflect the potential for drug accumulation and toxicity. Many hospital centers offer formal dosing services that provide advice on drug dose, interval, routes of administration, and timing of plasma levels [19].

Effect of Dialysis

Hospitalized patients who develop renal impairment or those with prior renal impairment may progress to renal failure which may necessitate the initiation of a form of acute dialytic therapy (see Chap. 83). Many patients with ESRD who become acutely ill may need admission to an intensive care setting and will require maintained on dialysis for the duration of their hospitalization. Since most of these patients will be prescribed multiple drug combinations, it is necessary to ascertain for each drug whether the dialytic therapy would alter a drug's clearance and result in subtherapeutic levels. For drugs significantly removed by hemodialysis, supplemental doses are often given prior to or at the conclusion of the 4 to 5 hour hemodialysis treatment. For drugs cleared by chronic ambulatory peritoneal dialysis (CAPD), supplemental doses are added to each peritoneal dialysate bag. For drugs cleared by continuous arteriovenous hemofiltration (CAVH), supplemental doses are added to each hemofiltration dialysate bag. These supplemental doses maintain the therapeutic plasma drug concentration necessary for treatment and prevent the development of subtherapeutic plasma drug levels.

Use of the Tables

Tables 82-3 to 82-17 identify the most common drugs prescribed in clinical medicine. The drugs are listed by generic name by major categories (e.g., antimicrobial, cardiovascular) and are subdivided by pharmacologic action or similarity of structure (e.g., beta blockers, cardiac glycosides). The major route of elimination is noted as either "R," representing renal excretion; "H," representing hepatic metabolism; or "NR," representing nonrenal or other routes of elimination such as bile, feces, and other metabolic pathways. Other abbreviations are defined in Table 82-2.

For each drug, the half-life (t1/2) in individuals with normal renal function and in those with ESRD is given. Since t1/2 represents the time it takes for half of an administered dose of a drug to be eliminated from the body, prolongation of the t1/2 of a drug in ESRD is usual for drugs that are primarily eliminated via the kidney. Drugs eliminated by hepatic metabolism do not exhibit prolonged t1/2 in ESRD. The t1/2 is often used to estimate the appropriate dosing intervals of a drug.

The "normal" drug dose recommendations given in the tables represent reasonable standard doses for an average-sized patient with normal renal and hepatic function. These doses are meant to be used only as a guide for the range of dosing regimens used for a particular drug. These doses are not a recommendation for treating a specific clinical disorder. The eventual selection of a specific drug-dosing regimen must take into account the clinical condition needing treatment and the

Table 82-2. Abbreviations used in Tables 82-3 to 82-17

ESRD	End stage renal disease
GFR	Glomerular filtration rate
HEMO	Hemodialysis
CAPD	Chronic ambulatory peritoneal dialysis
CAVH	Continuous arteriovenous hemofiltration
T½	Biological half life
g	Grams
mg	Milligrams
kg	Kilograms
q	Every
h	Hour
d	Day
hs	At bed time
mg/l	Milligrams per liter
mg/dl	Milligrams per deciliter
μg	Micrograms
NA	Not applicable
QD	Daily
TID	Three times a day
BID	Twice a day
QID	Four times a day
R	Renal
H	Hepatic
NR	Non-renal
Vd	Volume of distribution
mEq/g	Milliequivalent per gram
IV	Intravenous
CNS	Central nervous system
BUN	Blood urea nitrogen
MIN	Minute
GI	Gastrointestinal
NSAIDs	Nonsteroidal anti-inflammatory drugs
IM	Intramuscular
U	Units
SIADH	Syndrome of inappropriate secretion of antidiuretic hormone

patient's age, weight, volume status, nutritional status, and renal and hepatic function. For most drugs, steady-state plasma levels should be achieved after approximately 4 to 5 t1/2 of a drug. If rapid therapeutic drug levels need to be achieved, however, a loading dose of that drug has to be administered.

For each drug, where appropriate, a dosage adjustment is recommended for mild (GFR > 50 ml/min), moderate (GFR 10–50 ml/min), and severe (GFR < 10 ml/min) renal failure. If no dosage adjustment is required, the recommendation is "none." For drugs needing a dose adjustment, two methods are used. If the recommendation is to reduce the dose (dosage reduction method), the percent of the usual dose to be given at the normal dosing interval is reported. If the recommendation is to prolong the dosing interval (interval extension method), the number of hours (or days) between normal doses is given.

For many drugs (e.g., aminoglycosides), a combination of prolonging the dosing interval and reducing the dose is both effective and convenient. For patients on dialysis, supplemental doses of a drug may be necessary if significant quantities of a drug are removed (e.g., cleared) during dialysis. Specific recommendations for supplemental doses, if known, are given for each drug.

Antimicrobial Drugs

Most antimicrobial drugs are eliminated by the kidney (Table 82-3). Therefore, for patients with renal impairment, selection of an antimicrobial drug must be done with care and with concern about a drug's route of elimination. The greatest care is needed when prescribing aminoglycoside antibiotics, because they are almost exclusively eliminated by glomerular filtration; in patients with renal impairment, if an appropriate dose reduction is not made, these antibiotics may result in ototoxicity and nephrotoxicity. Drugs such as metronidazole and cefotaxime that are converted to active metabolites and eliminated by the kidney can be associated with drug toxicity if these metabolites accumulate. Most tetracycline drugs, exept doxycycline, are anti-anabolic and will cause an increase in the BUN concentration potentiating uremic symptoms if used in patients with renal impairment. Certain drugs can produce an increased metabolic load of either sodium (e.g., moxalactam) or potassium (e.g., penicillin G and ticarcillin). The accumulation of these cations can lead to hypernatremia and edema or hyperkalemia in patients with renal impairment who are unable to excrete them.

For patients with renal impairment, unfortunately there are no good controlled clinical trials comparing the relevant efficacy of modifying drug dose either by decreasing the individual maintenance dose or by increasing the dosing interval. For patients with renal impairment, the most frequent recommendation is to modify the dosing regimen by prolonging the dosing interval. Of obvious importance in any dosing regimen is the need to maintain therapeutic drug concentrations at all times. The concern with giving a normal maintenance dose but prolonging the dosing interval is that this regimen may result in a dosing interval as long as 48 to 72 hours or longer for some drugs. Whenever the dosing interval is prolonged to that extent, the possibility of reaching subtherapeutic plasma concentrations during that interval becomes a concern. Therefore it may be prudent to avoid prolonging the dosing interval beyond 24 hours in severely ill patients with renal impairment. Instead, a regimen of both a reduction in the maintenance dose and a prolongation of the dosing interval probably assures the safest therapeutic drug levels over time. Dosing of the aminoglycoside

antibiotics is the perfect example of such a dosing regimen: with these drugs, there is both a decrease in the maintenance dose and an increase in the dosing interval for patients with moderate to severe renal impairment.

For most antimicrobial drugs, there is a direct relationship between plasma levels and antimicrobial efficacy or toxicity. This suggests that whenever possible, drug levels should be measured and monitored. Generally, drug levels should be measured after four to five doses of a drug are given to assure that steady-state concentrations have been reached. For some drugs, both peak levels, drawn 30 to 60 minutes after an intravenous infusion, and trough levels, drawn immediately before the next dose, are necessary to determine the best dosing regimen. As stated previously, for patients with renal impairment the trough levels appear to be more reliable for measuring elimination and seem to reflect drug accumulation more closely. Particularly for patients with unstable renal function, these drug measurements are essential to assess safety and efficacy of the drug regimen adequately.

ANTIHYPERTENSIVE DRUGS. Antihypertensive drugs are frequently prescribed for patients in ICUs (Table 82-4). For these drugs, the patient's response to a blood pressure drug is the most important determinant of drug selection, not the pharmacokinetic characteristics associated with an individual drug (see Chapter 210). Unfortunately, in patients with renal impairment, the pharmacologic response of these drugs is so variable that careful dose titration must be done to prevent hypotension. It is therefore prudent to start patients on the lowest recommended doses and gradually increase the dose. Close monitoring of both the patient's blood pressure and renal function (serum creatinine) should be done during the initiation of any blood pressure medication. The physician should be alert for the significant complication of a transient decrease in renal function, which can occur in hypertensive patients with renal impairment when the blood pressure is initially lowered. Once renal homeostatic mechanisms are restored, renal function should return to baseline. For patients with severe atherosclerosis, however, angiotensin converting enzyme (ACE) inhibitors can significantly affect blood flow across the kidney and worsen underlying renal function. Immediate discontinuation of these drugs should result in return of renal function to baseline levels. Careful monitoring of patients with renal impairment being started on ACE inhibitors is an absolute necessity to prevent irreversible renal failure.

For most patients with renal impairment, both ACE inhibitors and calcium channel blockers appear to be the drugs of choice for treatment of hypertensive events. In general, these drugs have the fewest side effects and maintain renal blood flow even during blood pressure reduction in most patients.

DIURETICS. Most patients with renal impairment require diuretics as part of their drug regimen (Table 82-5). In patients with renal impairment, endogenous organic acids accumulate and compete with diuretics for secretion into the tubular lumen (see Chapter 78). Consequently, as renal function declines, increasing doses of diuretics are required to produce a diuresis. Once the GFR is less than 30 ml/min, all thiazide diuretics are generally ineffective. Metolazone is the only distal tubule diuretic that is effective even in patients with ESRD. Large doses of loop diuretics, furosemide, bumetanide, or ethacrynic acid will continue to produce a diuresis, although maximum doses may be required as renal function declines. Overzealous use of loop diuretics may produce intravascular volume depletion, which may cause a further decline in renal function or pre-renal

(Text continues on page 1043.)

Table 82-3A. Antimicrobial Drugs

Drug	Route of elimination	Normal half life (h) T½	Half life in ESRD (h) T½	Dose: normal Renal function	Renal failure adjustment (GFR ml/min)		Dialysis supplementation	Adverse reactions comments
Aminoglycoside antibiotics Nephrotoxic and ototoxic. Blood levels best guide to therapy.								
Amikacin (Amikin)	R	2-3	30	5 mg/kg q8h	>50 10-50 <10	60-90% q12h 30-70% q12-18h 20-30% q24-48h	HEMO: 2/3 normal dose after dialysis CAPD: 15-20 mg/L·d CAVH: 20 mg/L·d	
Gentamicin (Garamycin)	R	2	24-28	1 mg/kg q8h	>50 10-50 <10	60-90% q8-12h 30-70% q12h 20-30% q24-48h	HEMO: 2/3 normal dose after dialysis CAPD: 3-4 mg/L·d CAVH: 4 mg/L·d	Concurrent penicillins may result in subtherapeutic aminoglycoside levels.
Netilmicin (Netromycin)	R	2-5	40	5 mg/kg q8h	>50 10-50 <10	50-90% q8-12h 20-60% q12h 10-20% q24-48h	HEMO: 2/3 normal dose after dialysis CAPD: 3-4 mg/L·d CAVH: 4 mg/L·d	
Streptomycin	R	2-5	100	1 g/day	>50 10-50 <10	500 mg q24h 300-400 mg q24h 200 mg q24h or 500 mg q48-72h	HEMO: 1/2 normal dose after dialysis CAPD: 20-40 mg/L·d CAVH: 20-40 mg/L·d	Less nephrotoxic
Tobramycin (Nebcin)	R	2-5	56	1 mg/kg q8h	>50 10-50 <10	60-90% q8-12h 30-70% q12h 20-30% q24-48h	HEMO: 2/3 normal dose after dialysis CAPD: 3-4 mg/L·d CAVH: 4 mg/L·d	Concurrent penicillins may result in subtherapeutic aminoglycoside levels.
Cephalosporin antibiotics Rare allergic interstitial nephritis **First generation**								
Cefadroxil (Doricef)	R	1.5	22	0.5-1 g q12h	>50 10-50 <10	none q12-24h 0.5 gm q24-48h	HEMO: 0.5-1 g after dialysis CAPD: 0.5 g/d CAVH: not applicable	
Cephradine (Velosef)	R	1	10	0.5 g q6h	>50 10-50 <10	none q8h q12-24h	HEMO: dose after dialysis CAPD: dose q 12-24 h CAVH: 50-100 mg/L·d	
Cephalexin (Keflex)	R	0.9	20-40	0.25-0.5 g q6h	>50 10-50 <10	none q8-12h q12-24h	HEMO: 250 mg after dialysis CAPD: 250 mg TID CAVH: none	
Cephalothin (Keflin)	R	0.5-0.9	3-18	0.5-2 g q6h	>50 10-50 <10	none q8h q12h	HEMO: dose after dialysis CAPD: 1 g q12h CAVH: 30-50 mg/L·d	
Cephapirin (Cefadyl)	R	0.7	2-5	0.5-2 g q6h	>50 10-50 <10	none q8h q12h	HEMO: dose after dialysis CAPD: 1 g q12h CAVH: 30-50 mg/L·d	
Cefazolin (Ancef, Kefzol)	R	2	18-36	0.5-1.5 g q6h	>50 10-50 <10	q8h q12h q24-48h	HEMO: 0.5-1 g after dialysis CAPD: 0.5 g q12h CAVH: 30 mg/L·d	

Table 82-3A. Antimicrobial Drugs *(Cont.)*

Drug	Route of elimination	Normal half life (h) T½	Half life in ESRD (h) T½	Dose: normal renal function	Renal failure adjustment (GFR ml/min)			Dialysis supplementation	Adverse reactions comments
					>50	10-50	<10		
Second generation									
Cefaclor (Ceclor)	R	1	3	0.25-0.5 g q8h	none	none	none	HEMO: 250 mg after dialysis CAPD: 250 mg q8-12h CAVH: Not applicable	
Cefonicid (Monocid)	R	4	17-59	1-2 g q24h	none	q24-48h	q3-5days	HEMO: none CAPD: none CAVH: none	
Lefotetan (Cefotan)	R	3.5	13-25	1-2 g q12h	none	q24h	q48h	HEMO: 1 g after dialysis CAPD: 1 g/d CAVH: 10-30 mg/L·d	
Cefoxitin (Mefoxine)	R	0.7	13-23	1-2 g q4-6h	q8h	q12h	q24-48h	HEMO: 1 g after dialysis CAPD: 1 g/d CAVH: 50 mg/L·d	
Cefuroxime (Zinacef)	R	1.2	17	.75-1.5 g q8h	none	q8-12h	q24h	HEMO: dose after dialysis CAPD: dose q24h CAVH: 750 mg q12h	
Third generation									
Cefoperazone (Cefobid)	NR	1.6-2.5	2.9	1.2 g q8-12h	none	none	none	HEMO: 1 g after dialysis CAPD: none CAVH: none	
Cefotaxime (Claforan)	R	1	2.6	1-2 g q4-6h	q6h	q8-12h	1 g q12h	HEMO: 1 g after dialysis CAPD: 1 g/d CAVH: 30-50 mg/L·d	Active metabolite with t½ 1.4-1.9 hours
Ceftazidime (Tazicef, Captaz)	R	1.2	13-25	1-2 g q6-8h	q8-12h	q24-48h	q48-72h	HEMO: 1 g after dialysis CAPD: 0.5 g/d CAVH: 30 mg/L·d	Vd increases with infection
Ceftrizoxime (Cefizox)	R	1.4	35	1-2 g q6-8h	q8-12h	q36-48h	q48-72h	HEMO: 1 g after dialysis CAPD: 0.5 – 1 g/d CAVH: 30 mg/L·d	
Ceftriaxone (Rocephin)	R/H	7-9	12-24	1.2 q 12-24h	none	q24h	q24h	HEMO: dose after dialysis CAPD: 750 mg q12h CAVH: 10 mg/L·d	

Carbapenems—combination of imipenem and cilastatin. Cilastatin inhibits renal metabolism in the proximal tubule and prolongs t½ of imipenem.

Drug	Route of elimination	Normal half life (h) T½	Half life in ESRD (h) T½	Dose: normal renal function	Renal failure adjustment (GFR ml/min)			Dialysis supplementation	Adverse reactions comments
					>50	10-50	<10		
Imipenem	R	1	4	250 mg-1 g q6h	q6-8h	q6-12h	q12-24h	HEMO: dose after dialysis CAPD: dose q12-24h CAVH: 20 mg/L·d	Seizures in ESRD.
Cilastatin	R	1	13	Combination with imipenem	none	50%	avoid	HEMO: avoid CAPD: avoid CAVH: avoid	Dose with imipenem. Unnecessary in renal failure.
Monobactams									
Aztreonam	R	1.7-2.9	6-8	0.5-2.0 g q6-12h	q8-12h	q12-24h	q24-36h	HEMO: 0.5 g after dialysis CAPD: dose q24-36h CAVH: 50 mg/L·d	

Drug		$t_{1/2}$ normal	$t_{1/2}$ ESRD	Usual dose	GFR	Dose adjustment	Dialysis	Comments
Moxalactam (Moxam)	R	2.3	18-23	1-2 g q8-12h	>50 10-50 <10	q8-12h q12-24h q24-48h	HEMO: dose after dialysis CAPD: dose q24-48h CAVH: dose 50 mg/L·d	Monitor prothrombin time. Platelet dysfunction at high doses. Sodium 3.8 mEq/g.
Macrolides								
Clindamycin (Cleocin)	H	2-4	3-5	150-300 mg q6h	>50 10-50 <10	none none none	HEMO: none CAPD: none CAVH: none	
Erythromycin	H	1.4	5-6	256-500 mg q6-12h	>50 10-50 <10	none none 50%	HEMO: none CAPD: none CAVH: none	Ototoxicity with high doses in ESRD.
Penicillins								
Penicillin G	R	0.5	6-20	1-3 million units q4-6h	>50 10-50 <10	q6-8h q8-12h q12-24h	HEMO: dose after dialysis CAPD: dose q12-24h CAVH: dose q12-24h	Potassium, 1.7 mEq/million units. Seizures. False-positive urine protein reactions. For ESRD, upper limits, 6 million units/day
Penicillin V	R	0.5	6-20	250-500 mg q6h	>50 10-50 <10	q6-8h q8-12h q12-24h	HEMO: dose after dialysis CAPD: dose q12-24h CAVH: q12-24h	Same as for Pen G.
Penicillinase-resistant penicillins								
Dicloxacillin	R/NR	0.7	1.2	250 mg q6h	>50 10-50 <10	none none none	HEMO: none CAPD: none CAVH: none	
Methicillin (Staphcillin)	R	0.5-1	4	1-2 g q4-6h	>50 10-50 <10	q6h q8h q12h	HEMO: none CAPD: none CAVH: none	Acute interstitial nephritis
Nafcillin (Unipen)	H	0.5	1.2	1-2 g q4-6h	>50 10-50 <10	none none none	HEMO: none CAPD: none CAVH: none	Coagulopathy.
Broad-spectrum penicillins								
Amoxicillin	R	0.8-2.3	10-15	250-500 mg q6h	>50 10-50 <10	none 500 mg q8-12h 500 mg q12h	HEMO: 500 mg after dialysis CAPD: no data CAVH: no data	
Amoxicillin/Clavulanate (Augmentin)	R	1.3 1.0	10-15 unknown	250-500 mg q8h	>50 10-50 <10	q8h q12h q12-24h	HEMO: NA CAPD: NA CAVH: NA	One tablet (250-500 mg amoxicillin/125 mg clavulanate acid)
Ampicillin	R	0.8-1.5	20	250-500 mg q6h	>50 10-50 <10	none q12h 50% q12h	HEMO: dose after dialysis CAPD: 500 mg q8h CAVH: no data	
Ampicillin/Sulbactam (Unasyn)	R	1	9	1.5-3.0 g q6h	>50 10-50 <10	q6-8h q12h q24h	HEMO: dose after dialysis CAPD: no data CAVH: no data	1.5 g (1 g ampicillin/0.5 g sulbactam) 3.0 g (2 g ampicillin/1 g sulbactam)
Azlocillin	R	0.8-1.5	5.6	2-3 g q4-6h	>50 10-50 <10	none q6-8h q12h	HEMO: dose after dialysis CAPD: dose q12h CAVH: 100 mg/L·d	Sodium, 2.7 mEq/g may cause hypokalemic metabolic acidosis.

Table 82-3A. Antimicrobial Drugs *(Cont.)*

Drug	Route of elimination	Normal half life (h) T½	Half life in ESRD (h) T½	Dose: normal renal function	Renal failure adjustment (GFR ml/min)			Dialysis supplementation	Adverse reactions comments
					>50	10-50	<10		
Carbenicillin (Geocillin)	R	1.0	10-20	4-5 g q4-6h	q6-8h	q12-24h	q24-48h	HEMO: 1-2 g after dialysis CAPD: none CAVH: none	
Mezlocillin (Mezlin)	R	0.6-1.2	2.6-5.4	2-4 g q4-6h	none	q6-8h	q8-12h	HEMO: dose after dialysis CAPD: none CAVH: none	
Piperacillin (Pipracil)	R	0.8-1.5	3.3-5.1	3-4 g q4-6h	none	q8-12	q12-16	HEMO: dose after dialysis CAPD: dose q12-16 CAVH: dose q12-16	Measure plasma levels as guide Sodium, 1.9 mEq/g
Ticarcillin (Ticar)	R	1.2	11-16	2-3 g q4-6h	q8-12h	q12-24h	q24-48h	HEMO: 3 g after dialysis CAPD: dose q24-48h CAVH: dose q24-48h	Sodium, 5.2 mEq/g
Tetracyclines Doxycycline	R/NR	15-24	18-25	50-100 mg q12h	none	none	none	HEMO: none CAPD: none CAVH: none	Group drug of choice for decreased renal function. Not anti-anabolic.
Tetracycline	R	6-10	57-108	250-500 mg qid	avoid	avoid	avoid	HEMO: avoid CAPD: avoid CAVH: avoid	
Quinolones Ciprofloxacin (Cipro)	R	3-6	6-9	250-750 mg q12h	none	q12-24h	q24h	HEMO: 250 mg q12h CAPD: 250 mg q12h CAVH: 250 mg q8-12h	
Norfloxacin (Noroxin)	NR/R	3.5-6.5	8	400 mg q12h	none	q 12-24 h	avoid	HEMO: avoid CAPD: avoid CAVH: avoid	
Miscellaneous Chloramphenicol (Chloromycetin)	H	1.6-3.3	3.7	1 g q6h	none	none	none	HEMO: none CAPD: none CAVH: none	Measure plasma levels as guide.
Metronidazole (Flagyl)	H	6-14	7-21	7.5 mg/kg q6h	none	none	50%	HEMO: dose after dialysis CAPD: none CAVH: no data	Active metabolite can accumulate
Trimethoprim/ Sulfamethoxazole (Bactrim)	R R	8-11 9-11	24-30 30-60	2 tablets q12h	none	q18-24h	q24 h-48h	HEMO: dose after dialysis CAPD: no data CAVH: no data	1 tablet = 80 mg trimethoprim and 400 mg sulfamethoxazole.
Vancomycin (Vancolin)	R	6-11	150-250	500 mg-1 g q12-24h	1-2 days	q2-4days	q4-7days	HEMO: 1 g q weekly CAPD: 15-30 mg/L CAVH: no data	

Table 82-3B. Antifungal Drugs

Drug	Route of elimination	Normal half life (h) T½	Half Life in ESRD (h) T½	Dose: normal renal function	Renal failure adjustment (GFR ml/min)		Dialysis supplementation	Adverse reactions comments
Amphotericin B (Fungizone)	H	24	24	0.5-1.0 mg/kg q24h	>50 10-50 <10	none none q24-36h	HEMO: none CAPD: none CAVH: none	Initial test dose: 1 mg IV Nephrotoxic. Renal tubular acidosis. Potassium wasting Nephrogenic diabetes insipidus.
Fluconazole (Diflucan)	R	22	?	100-200 mg q24	>50 10-50 <10	none q24-48h q48-72h	HEMO: 200 mg after dialysis CAPD: dose for GFR <10 CAVH: dose for GFR <10	
Flucytosine (Ancobon)	R	3-6	75-200	500 mg-1 g q6h	>50 10-50 <10	q6-8h q12-24h q24-48h	HEMO: dose after dialysis CAPD: dose q24h CAVH: dose q24h	Hepatic dysfunction. Marrow suppression more common in azotemic patients
Ketoconazole (Nizoral)	H	1.5-3.3	3.3	200 mg q24h	>50 10-50 <10	none none none	HEMO: none CAPD: none CAVH: none	

Table 82-3C. Antituberculous Drugs

Drug	Route of elimination	Normal half life (h) T½	Half life in ESRD (h) T½	Dose: normal renal function	Renal failure adjustment (GFR ml/min)	Dialysis supplementation	Adverse reactions comments
Capreomycin (Capastat)	R	2	Prolonged	1 g q day	>50 q 48 10-50 q 60-96 <10 avoid	HEMO: none CAPD: none CAVH: none	
Cycloserine (Seromycin)	R	0.5	?	250 mg q12h	>50 none 10-50 q12-24h <10 avoid	HEMO: avoid CAPD: avoid CAVH: avoid	CNS toxicity Measure blood levels
Ethambutol (Myambutol)	R	4	7-15	15 mg/kg q24h	>50 none 10-50 q24-36h <10 q48h	HEMO: dose after dialysis CAPD: dose for GFR <10 CAVH: dose q24-36h	Decreases visual acuity. Peripheral neuritis.
Ethionamide (Trecator)	H	2-4	?	250-500 mg q12h	>50 none 10-50 avoid <10 avoid	HEMO: avoid CAPD: avoid CAVH: avoid	
Isoniazid (INH)	H	0.7-4	8-17	5 mg/kg q24h	>50 none 10-50 none <10 q48h	HEMO: dose after dialysis CAPD: dose for GFR <10 CAVH: dose for GFR <10	Dosing is for slow acetylators
PAS	R	1	?	50 mg/kg q8h	>50 none 10-50 q12-18h <10 q24h	HEMO: dose after dialysis CAPD: dose for GFR <10 CAVH: dose for GFR <10	Significant sodium load.
Pyrazinamide	H	9	?	10 mg/kg q8h	>50 none 10-50 avoid <10 avoid	HEMO: avoid CAPD: avoid CAVH: avoid	Impairs urate excretion. Can precipitate gout.
Streptomycin	(see Aminoglycoside Antibiotics)						
Rifampin (Rifadin)	H	1.5-5	1.8-11	600 mg q6h	>50 none 10-50 none <10 none	HEMO: none CAPD: none CAVH: none	Acute interstitial nephritis. Potassium wasting. Renal tubular defects. Biologically active metabolite.

Table 82-3D. Antiviral Drugs

Drug	Route of elimination	Normal half life (h) T½	Half life in ESRD (h) T½	Dose: normal renal function	Renal failure adjustment (GFR ml/min)	Dialysis supplementation	Adverse reactions comments
Acyclovir (Zovirax)	R	2-4	20	5 mg/kg q8h	>50 none 10-50 q12-24h <10 2.5 mg/kg q24h	HEMO: dose after dialysis CAPD: dose for GFR <10 CAVH: 3.5 mg/kg·d	Neurotoxicity in ESRD. Intravenous preparations can cause renal failure if injected rapidly.
Amantadine	R	12	500	100 mg q12h	>50 q12-24h 10-50 q48-72h <10 q168h	HEMO: none CAPD: none CAVH: none	
Ganciclovir (Cytovene)	R	3.6	30	2.5 mg/kg q8h	>50 q12h 10-50 q24h <10 q48-96h	HEMO: dose after dialysis CAPD: dose for GFR <10 CAVH: 2.5 mg/kg·d	Marrow toxicity
Ribavirin (Virazole)	H	30-60	?	200 mg q8h	>50 none 10-50 none <10 50% q8h	HEMO: dose after dialysis CAPD: dose for GFR <10 CAVH: dose for GFR <10	Loading dose required
Vidarabine (Vira)	NR/R	2-6	Prolonged	15 mg/kg infusion q24h	>50 q24-48h 10-50 avoid <10 avoid	HEMO: avoid CAPD: avoid CAVH: avoid	
Zidovudine (AZT)	H	1.1-1.4	1.4-3	200 mg q4h	>50 none 10-50 none <10 100 mg q4h	HEMO: 100 mg after dialysis CAPD: 100 mg q4h CAVH: 100 mg q4h	Marrow suppression

Table 82-4. Antihypertensive Drugs (Blood Pressure is Best Guide to Dose and Intervals)

Drug	Route of elimination	Normal half life (h)	Half life in ESRD (h)	Dose: normal renal function	Renal failure adjustment (GFR ml/min)		Dialysis supplementation	Adverse reactions comments
Anti Adrenergic Drugs								
Peripheral alpha antagonists								
Prazosin (Minipres)	H	2-3	2-3	1-5 mg BID-TID	>50 10-50 <10	none none none	HEMO: none CAPD: none CAVH: none	May produce profound first dose hypotension
Terazosin (Hytrin)	H	9-12	8-12	1-10 mg qd-BID	>50 10-50 <10	none none none	HEMO: no data CAPD: no data CAVH: no data	
Central alpha agonists								All agents may cause sedation, dry mouth, sexual dysfunction.
Alpha-methyldopa (Aldomet)	R	1.5-6	6-16	250-1000 mg BID-TID	>50 10-50 <10	none q8-12h q12-24h	HEMO: dose after dialysis CAPD: none CAVH: no data	Orthostatic hypotension Retroperitoneal fibrosis Active metabolites with long t½
Clonidine (Catapres)	R	6-23	39-42	0.1-0.6 mg BID	>50 10-50 <10	none none none	HEMO: none CAPD: none CAVH: no data	Rebound hypertension if drug is abruptly withdrawn.
Guanabenz (Wytensin)	H	12-14	?	4-32 mg BID	>50 10-50 <10	none none none	HEMO: no data CAPD: no data CAVH: no data	
Other Agents								
Reserpine (Serpasil)	H	46-168	87-323	100-250 mg qd	>50 10-50 <10	none none avoid	HEMO: none CAPD: none CAVH: no data	
Angiotensin-Converting Enzyme (ACE) Inhibitors								
Monitor renal function in patients with congestive heart failure or possible renovascular hypertension. Hypotensive response in patients taking diuretics. May cause hyperkalemia. Dry cough in 5-10%.								
Captopril (Captopen)	H/R	1.9	21-32	12.5-50 mg BID-TID	>50 10-50 <10	100% q 8-12 h 75% q12-18h 50% q24h	HEMO: 25 mg after dialysis CAPD: none CAVH: no data	Rare proteinuria, nephrotic syndrome, dysqeusia and granulocytopenia.
Enalapril (Vasotec)	R	11-24	34-60	2.5-20 mg qd-BID	>50 10-50 <10	none 50-75% 25-50%	HEMO: 20-25% after dialysis CAPD: none CAVH: no data	Enaliprilat, active metabolite formed in the liver.
Lisinopril (Prinivil, Zestril)	R	12.6	40-50	5-40 mg qd	>50 10-50 <10	none 50-75% 25-50%	HEMO: 20% after dialysis CAPD: none CAVH: no data	
Beta-adrenergic Blockers								
Hyperkalemia in ESRD. Hypoglycemia in dialysis patients can occur.								

Drug	Route	t½ Normal (h)	t½ ESRD (h)	Dose	GFR (mL/min)	Adjustment	Dialysis	Comments
Acebutolol (Sectral)	H	7-9	7	200-400 mg qd-BID	>50 / 10-50 / <10	none / 50% / 30-50%	HEMO: none / CAPD: none / CAVH: no data	Active metabolites with long half life.
Atenolol (Tenormin)	R	6.7	15-35	50-100 mg qd	>50 / 10-50 / <10	none / 50% q48h / 30-50% q96h	HEMO: none / CAPD: none / CAVH: no data	Accumulates in ESRD
Labetalol (Normodyne, Trandate)	H	3-9	3-9	100-600 mg BID	>50 / 10-50 / <10	none / none / none	HEMO: none / CAPD: none / CAVH: no data	
Metoprolol (Lopressor)	H	3.5	2.5-4.5	50-100 mg qd-BID	>50 / 10-50 / <10	none / none / none	HEMO: none / CAPD: none / CAVH: no data	
Nadolol (Corgard)	R	19	45	40-320 mg qd	>50 / 10-50 / <10	none / 50% / 25%	HEMO: none / CAPD: none / CAVH: no data	
Penbutolol (Levatol)	H	22	24	20-80 mg qd	>50 / 10-50 / <10	none / none / none	HEMO: none / CAPD: none / CAVH: no data	
Pindolol (Visken)	H	2.5-4	3-4	5-20 mg BID	>50 / 10-50 / <10	none / none / none	HEMO: none / CAPD: none / CAVH: no data	
Propranolol (Inderal)	H	2-6	1-6	40-160 mg BID	>50 / 10-50 / <10	none / none / none	HEMO: none / CAPD: none / CAVH: no data	
Sotalol (Betapace)	R	7.5-15	56	80-160 mg BID	>50 / 10-50 / <10	none / 30% / 15-30%	HEMO: none / CAPD: none / CAVH: no data	
Timolol (Blocadren)	H	2.7	4	10-20 mg BID	>50 / 10-50 / <10	none / none / none	HEMO: none / CAPD: none / CAVH: no data	

Direct Vasodilators

Commonly cause reflex tachycardia, headache and edema. May precipitate angina in patients with coronary artery disease.

Drug	Route	t½ Normal (h)	t½ ESRD (h)	Dose	GFR (mL/min)	Adjustment	Dialysis	Comments
Diazoxide (Hyperstat)	H/R	17-31	30-60	150-300 mg bolus	>50 / 10-50 / <10	none / none / none	HEMO: none / CAPD: none / CAVH: NA	Sodium and water retention
Hydralazine (Apresoline)	H	2-4.5	7-16	25-100 mg BID-TID	>50 / 10-50 / <10	none / none / q8-16h	HEMO: none / CAPD: none / CAVH: no data	Drug induced lupus at high doses
Minoxidil (Loniten)	H	2.8-4.2	2.8-4.2	2.5-20 mg qd-BID	>50 / 10-50 / <10	none / none / none	HEMO: none / CAPD: none / CAVH: no data	
Nitroprusside	H	<10 min	<10 min	0.25-8 µg/kg/min by infusion	>50 / 10-50 / <10	none / none / none	HEMO: none / CAPD: none / CAVH: no data	Toxic metabolite thiocyanate accumulates causing seizures and coma. Measure thiocyanate levels. Thiocyanate is hemodialyzable.

Table 82-4. Antihypertensive Drugs (Blood Pressure is Best Guide to Dose and Intervals) *(Cont.)*

Drug	Route of elimination	Normal half life (h)	Half life in ESRD (h)	Dose: normal renal function	Renal failure adjustment (GFR ml/min)		Dialysis supplementation	Adverse reactions comments
				Calcium Channel Blockers				
				May increase serum digoxin level or cause edema, headache and flushing. Used as antianginal drugs.				
Diltiazem (Cardizem)	H	2-8	3-5	30-90 mg TID-QID	>50 10-50 <10	none none none	HEMO: none CAPD: none CAVH: no data	Active metabolites
Nicardipine (Cardene)	H	5	5-7	20-30 mg TID	>50 10-50 <10	none none none	HEMO: none CAPD: none CAVH: no data	
Nifedipine (Procardia, Adalat)	H	4.5-5	5-7	10-30 mg TID-QID	>50 10-50 <10	none none none	HEMO: none CAPD: none CAVH: no data	Protein binding decreased in ESRD
Verapamil (Calan, Isoptin, Verelan)	H	3-7	2.4-4	80-120 mg TID	>50 10-50 <10	none none none	HEMO: none CAPD: none CAVH: no data	

1037

Table 82-5. Diuretics

Drug	Route of elimination	Normal half life (h)	Half life in ESRD (h)	Dose: normal renal function	Renal failure adjustment (GFR ml/min)		Dialysis supplementation	Adverse reactions comments
Thiazide and related drugs								Associated with photosensitivity, pancreatitis and interstitial nephritis.
Hydrochlorothiazide (Esidrix, Oretic, Hydrodiuril)	R	6-8	12-20	12.5-50 mg qd	>50 / 10-50 / <10	none / none / avoid	HEMO: avoid / CAPD: avoid / CAVH: NA	Ineffective with GFR <30 ml/min
Indapamide (Lozol)	H	14-18	14-18	2.5-5 mg qd	>50 / 10-50 / <10	none / none / avoid	HEMO: avoid / CAPD: avoid / CAVH: NA	Ineffective with GFR <30 ml/min
Metolazone (Zaroxolyn, Diulo)	R	4-20	?	2.5-20 mg qd	>50 / 10-50 / <10	none / none / none	HEMO: avoid / CAPD: avoid / CAVH: NA	High doses effective for ESRD.
Loop Diuretics								Ototoxicity may occur at high doses
Bumetanide (Bumex)	R	1.2-1.5	1.5	1-2 mg q8-12h	>50 / 10-50 / <10	none / none / none	HEMO: none / CAPD: none / CAVH: NA	High doses effective in ESRD, ototoxicity occurs in combination with aminoglycosides.
Ethacrynic Acid (Edecrin)	H/NR	2-4	?	25-100 mg qd-BID	>50 / 10-50 / <10	none / none / avoid	HEMO: none / CAPD: none / CAVH: NA	Ototoxicity in combination with aminoglycosides
Furosemide (Lasix)	R	0.5-1.1	2-4	20-160 mg BID	>50 / 10-50 / <10	none / none / none	HEMO: none / CAPD: none / CAVH: NA	High doses effective in ESRD. Ototoxicity in combination with aminoglycosides.
Potassium sparing diuretics								
Amiloride (Midamor, Moduretic)	R	6-8	10-144	5-10 mg qd	>50 / 10-50 / <10	none / 50% / avoid	HEMO: avoid / CAPD: avoid / CAVH: avoid	Hyperkalemia with GFR <30 ml/min especially in diabetics. Hyperchloremic metabolic acidosis.
Spironolactone (Aldactone, Aldactazide)	H	10-35	10-35	25 mg TID-QID	>50 / 10-50 / <10	q6-12h / q12-24h / avoid	HEMO: avoid / CAPD: avoid / CAVH: avoid	Hyperkalemia with GFR <30 mL/min especially in diabetics. Active metabolites with long half-life.
Triamterene (Dyrenium, Dyazide, Maxide)	H	2-12	10	25-50 mg BID	>50 / 10-50 / <10	none / none / avoid	HEMO: avoid / CAPD: avoid / CAVH: avoid	Hyperkalemia common with GFR <30 mL/min especially in diabetics. Active metabolites with long half-life.
Others								
Acetazolamide (Diamox)	R	1.7-5.8	?	500 mg BID	>50 / 10-50 / <10	none / avoid / avoid	HEMO: avoid / CAPD: avoid / CAVH: avoid	Ineffective in ESRD. May potentiate acidosis.

Table 82-6. Cardiovascular Drugs

Drug	Route of elimination	Normal half life (h)	Half life in ESRD (h)	Dose: normal renal function	Renal failure adjustment (GFR ml/min)		Dialysis supplementation	Adverse reactions comments
Antiarrhythmic drugs								Blood levels most often best guide to therapy.
Class IA								
Quinidine	H	6	4-14	200-400 mg q4-6h	>50 10-50 <10	none none 75%	HEMO: none CAPD: none CAVH: no data	Active metabolite. Increases level of digoxin. Hemodialysis useful in poisoning.
Procainamide (Procan)	R	2.5-4.9	5-6	350-400 mg q3-4h	>50 10-50 <10	none q6-12h avoid	HEMO: Replace depending on blood levels CAPD: none CAVH: Replace, depending on blood levels	Active metabolite. N-acetyl procainamide (NAPA). Lupus-like syndrome. Hemofiltration useful in poisoning.
Disopyramide (Norpace)	R	5-8	10-18	100-200 mg q6h	>50 10-50 <10	q8h q12-24h q24h	HEMO: none CAPD: none CAVH: no data	Vd decreased in ESRD. Urinary retention.
Class IB								
Lidocaine (Xylocaine)	H	2-2.2	1.3-7	50 mg over 2 min, repeat q5 min × 3	>50 10-50 <10	none none none	HEMO: none CAPD: none CAVH: no data	
Tocainide (Tonocard)	H	14	22-27	200-400 mg q4-6h	>50 10-50 <10	none none 50%	HEMO: none CAPD: none CAVH: no data	
Mexiletene (Mexitil)	H	8-13	16	100-300 mg q6-12h	>50 10-50 <10	none none 50-75%	HEMO: none CAPD: none CAVH: none	
Phenytoin	H	24	24	1000 mg loading dose. Then 400-600 mg/day	>50 10-50 <10	none none none	HEMO: none CAPD: none CAVH: none	Protein binding decreased and Vd increased in renal failure.
Class IC								
Flecainide (Tambocor)	H	12-20	19-26	100-200 mg BID	>50 10-50 <10	none none 50-75%	HEMO: none CAPD: none CAVH: no data	
Encainide	R	2-3	6-9	Withdrawn	>50 10-50 <10	none 75% 50%	HEMO: no data CAPD: no data CAVH: no data	Encephalopathy. Converted to active metabolite t½ 6 hours
Propafenone (Rhythmol)	H	5	?	150-300 mg q8h	>50 10-50 <10	none none none	HEMO: none CAPD: none CAVH: no data	
Class III								
Sotalol (Betapace)	R	15-17	30-50	80-160 mg BID	>50 10-50 <10	none 80-120 mg q48-72h 80 mg q48-72h	HEMO: none CAPD: none CAVH: none	
Amiodarone (Cardarone)	H	14-120 days	14-120 days	1200-1600 mg loading dose; then 200-400 mg/day	>50 10-50 <10	none none none	HEMO: none CAPD: none CAVH: no data	Hepatotoxicity. Thyroid dysfunction. Peripheral neuropathy. Pulmonary fibrosis. Increases digoxin plasma levels. Active metabolite.

Drug		Half-life Normal	Half-life ESRD	Dose	GFR (ml/min)	Adjustment	Supplement	Comments
Bretylium (Bretylol)	R	6–14	32	5–30 mg/kg IV loading dose; then 1–2 mg/min IV or 5–10 mg/kg q6-8h	>50 10–50 <10	none q8-12h avoid	HEMO: 5 mg/kg after dialysis CAPD: no data CAVH: no data	Hypotension due to adrenergic blockade.
Cardiac Glycosides								
Digitoxin	H	144–200	210	0.1–0.2 mg/day	>50 10–50 <10	none none 50-75%	HEMO: none CAPD: none CAVH: no data	Measure serum levels Vd decreased in uremia.
Digoxin	R	36–44	80–120	1–1.5 mg loading dose; 0.25–50 mg/day	>50 10–50 <10	none 25-75% q36h 10-25% q48h	HEMO: none CAPD: none CAVH: 0.5 mg q12h	Decrease loading dose by 50% in ESRD. Vd and total body clearance decreased in ESRD.
Ouabain	R	21	60–70	0.25 mg loading dose; 0.1 mg q12h	>50 10–50 <10	q12-24h q24-36h q36-48h	HEMO: none CAPD: none CAVH: no data	
Nitrates								
Isosorbide (Isordil)	H	0.15–0.5	4	10–20 mg TID	>50 10–50 <10	none none none	HEMO: none CAPD: none CAVH: no data	
Nitroglycerin	(See Parenteral Cardiac Drugs)							
Parenteral Drugs for CHF								
Direct-Acting Vasodilators								
Nitroprusside	H	10 min	10 min	0.5–10 µg/kg/min	>50 10–50 <10	none none none	HEMO: none CAPD: none CAVH: no data	Toxic metabolite, thiocyanate accumulates, causing seizures, coma. Thiocyanate is dialyzable. Measure thiocyanate levels.
Nitroglycerin	H	2–4 min	2–4 min	100–200 µg/min	>50 10–50 <10	none none none	HEMO: no data CAPD: no data CAVH: no data	
Sympathomimetic Agents								
Dopamine	H	2–5 min	2–5 min	1–10 µg/kg/min	>50 10–50 <10	none none none	HEMO: none CAPD: none CAVH: none	
Dobutamine	H	2 min	?	2.5–20 µg/kg/min	>50 10–50 <10	none none none	HEMO: no data CAPD: no data CAVH: no data	
Phosphodiesterase Inhibitors								
Bipyridine derivatives								
Amrinone	H	2.5–8	2.5–8	0.5 mg/kg bolus × 2; 40 µg/kg/min infusion	>50 10–50 <10	none none 50-75%	HEMO: no data CAPD: no data CAVH: no data	Thrombocytopenia. GI upset.
Milrinone	R	1	1.5–3	12.5–75 µg/kg (given as 10-mg boluses)	>50 10–50 <10	none none 50-75%	HEMO: no data CAPD: no data CAVH: no data	2.5–15 mg q6h po

Table 82-7A. Non-Narcotic Analgesics

Drug	Route of elimination	Normal half life (h)	Half life in ESRD (h)	Dose: normal renal function	Renal failure adjustment (GFR ml/min)		Dialysis supplementation	Adverse reactions comments
Acetaminophen	H	2	2	325-650 mg q4h	>50 10-50 <10	none none q8h	HEMO: none CAPD: none CAVH: no data	Metabolites may accumulate in ESRD
Salicylates Aspirin	H/R	2-3	2-3	650 mg q4h	>50 10-50 <10	none q4-6h avoid	HEMO: dose after dialysis CAPD: none CAVH: no data	Nephrotoxic in high doses. Protein binding reduced in ESRD.
NSAID-Non-Steroidal Anti-Inflammatory Drugs May decrease renal function. Can cause Nephrotic syndrome and interstitial nephritis. Hyperkalemia and sodium retention. Decreased platelet aggregation.								
Short Acting NSAIDS								
Diclofenac (Voltaren)	H	1-2	1-2	25-75 mg BID/TID	>50 10-50 <10	none none none	HEMO: none CAPD: none CAVH: none	
Fenoprofen Calcium (Nalfon)	H	2-3	2-3	300-600 mg q6h	>50 10-50 <10	none none none	HEMO: none CAPD: none CAVH: none	
Ibuprofen (Motrin)	H	2-2.5	2-2.5	400-600 mg q6h	>50 10-50 <10	none none none	HEMO: none CAPD: none CAVH: none	
Indomethacin (Indocin)	H	4-12	4-12	25-50 mg q8h	>50 10-50 <10	none none none	HEMO: none CAPD: none CAVH: none	High rate of dyspepsia
Ketoprofen (Orudas)	H	1.5	1.5	50-75 mg q6-8h	>50 10-50 <10	none none none	HEMO: none CAPD: none CAVH: none	

Drug		t½ (normal)	t½ (ESRD)	Dose	GFR			Supplement	Comments
					>50	10-50	<10		
Meclofenamate sodium (Meclomen)	H	3	3	50-100 mg TID/QID	none	none	none	HEMO: none CAPD: none CAVH: none	
Mefenamic Acid (Ponstel)	H	3-4	3-4	500 mg, then 250 mg q6h	none	none	none	HEMO: none CAPD: none CAVH: none	High rate of nausea.
Tolmetin Sodium (Tolectin)	H	1-1.5	1-1.5	400 mg q6-8h	none	none	none	HEMO: none CAPD: none CAVH: none	
Intermediate Acting NSAIDs Diflunisal (Dolobid)	H	5-20	5-20	500 mg q12h	none	none	none	HEMO: none CAPD: none CAVH: none	
Flurbiprofen (Ansaid)	H	3-5	3-5	50-100 mg BID/TID	none	none	none	HEMO: none CAPD: none CAVH: none	
Naproxen (Naprosyn)	H	12-15	12-15	250-500 mg q12h	none	none	none	HEMO: none CAPD: none CAVH: none	
Sulindac (Clinoril)	H	8-16	8-16	150-200 mg q12h	none	none	none	HEMO: none CAPD: none CAVH: none	Active sulfide metabolite
Long-Acting NSAID Piroxicam (Feldene)	H	45-55	45-55	10-20 mg q24h	none	none	none	HEMO: none CAPD: none CAVH: none	High rate of gastric upset.
Parenteral NSAID Ketorolac (Toradol)	H	13.6	5.3	30-60 mg initially, then 15-30 mg q6h (Im)	none	none	50%	HEMO: none CAPD: none CAVH: none	

Table 82-7B. Narcotic Analgesics

Drug	Route of elimination	Normal half life (h)	Half life in ESRD (h)	Dose: normal renal function	Renal failure adjustment (GFR ml/min)		Dialysis supplementation	Adverse reactions comments
Butorphanol (Stadol)	H	2-4	?	2-3 mg q3-4h IM	>50 10-50 <10	none 75% 50%	HEMO: no data CAPD: no data CAVH: no data	
Codeine	H	2.5-3.5	2.5-3.5	15-60 mg q4h	>50 10-50 <10	none 75% 50%	HEMO: no data CAPD: no data CAVH: no data	Analgesia enhanced when combined with acetaminophen, aspirin or NSAIDS.
Fentanyl (Sublimaze)	H	2-7	?	0.05-0.10 q1-2h IM	>50 10-50 <10	none 75% 50%	HEMO: NA CAPD: NA CAVH: NA	
Meperidine (Demerol)	H	2-7	7-32	50-125 mg q3-4h IM 50-100 mg q4h	>50 10-50 <10	none 75% avoid	HEMO: none CAPD: none CAVH: no data	Normeperidine, an active metabolite, accumulates in ESRD and may cause seizures.
Methadone (Dolophine)	H	13-58	?	5-10 mg q4-6h	>50 10-50 <10	none none 50-75%	HEMO: none CAPD: none CAVH: no data	Fecal elimination is increased in ESRD.
Morphine Sulfate (Roxanol)	H	1-4	1-4	5-20 mg q4h IM	>50 10-50 <10	none 75% 50%	HEMO: none CAPD: no data CAVH: no data	Increased sensitivity to drug effect in ESRD.
Naloxone (Narcan)	H	1-1.5	?	0.4-2 mg IV up to 10 mg	>50 10-50 <10	none none none	HEMO: NA CAPD: NA CAVH: NA	
Pentazocine (Talwin)	H	2-5	?	30-60 mg q3-4h IM 50-100 mg q4h	>50 10-50 <10	none 75% 50%	HEMO: none CAPD: no data CAVH: no data	
Propoxyphene (Darvon)	H	9-15	12-20	65 mg TID/QID	>50 10-50 <10	none none avoid	HEMO: none CAPD: none CAVH: no data	Active metabolite, norpropoxyphene, accumulates in ESRD.

azotemia. The potassium-sparing diuretics, amiloride, spirono-lactone, and triamterene, produce hyperkalemia in patients with GFR's of less than 30 ml/min, and these drugs should be avoided at all costs. Acetazolamide, a carbonic acid inhibitor, should also be avoided in patients with renal impairment since it potentiates metabolic acidosis.

CARDIOVASCULAR DRUGS. Many patients with renal impairment may need specific cardiovascular drugs to treat congestive heart failure or potentially lethal arrhythmias. All cardiovascular drugs are difficult to prescibe because they have a very narrow therapeutic range and because there is marked individual patient variability in response to any specific drug (see Chaps. 131 and 207). Many of these drugs (Table 82-6) are metabolized to active metabolites (e.g., quinidine, procainamide) that are eliminated by the kidney or have decreased drug-protein binding or Vd, which makes more unbound or free drug available for receptor sites.

The antiarrhythmic drug procainamide is a particular concern. Both the parent drug and its primary active metabolite, n-acetyl procainamide, depend on renal function for elimination. Careful monitoring of patients on this drug is essential to prevent the development of toxic cardiac arrhythmias.

The choice of cardiac glycosides is between digitoxin and digoxin, both of which have narrow therapeutic ranges. Digitoxin is metabolized primarily by non-renal routes, and renal impairment has little effect on digotoxin pharmacokinetics. The digitoxin t1/2 in patients with normal renal function is 6 days; in ESRD patients, it has a t1/2 of 8.5 days. Only minor reductions in dose are necessary in patients with severe renal impairment. If a patient develops digitoxin toxicity, its long t1/2 (8.5 days) means that it would be days before the digitoxin would be effectively metabolized; during that time, lethal arrhythmias could persist. Digoxin is excreted primarily through the kidney. Its dose must be substantially reduced even in patients with moderate renal impairment, but it has a relatively short t1/2 (1.6 days in patients with normal renal function, and 4.4 days in patients with ESRD). In patients with advanced renal impairment, very little digoxin appears in the urine. These patients can achieve therapeutic serum concentrations with a dosage of 0.125 mg given three to five times a week. Digoxin is the drug of choice for patients with renal impairment. Both digitoxin and digoxin appear to have a smaller volume of distribution in patients with renal impairment. For that reason, both a reduction in the loading dose and a reduction in the maintenance dose are necessary for both drugs. The measurement of plasma drug levels is the best guide to assessing the therapeutic drug levels of either of these drugs.

Parenteral cardiovascular drugs are often necessary for the acutely ill patient. Cardiac inotropes can be used in normal dosages but because of their extreme vasoconstrictive effects, the minimum effective dose is recommended. Dobutamine and dopamine are the drugs of choice. Dopamine at low doses (2–5 mg/kg/min) has primarily vasodilatory effects. Intravenous nitrates can be used at a normal dose. Sodium nitroprusside can be administered by constant infusion for hypertensive emergencies or for left ventricular failure. The metabolism of nitroprusside to thiocyanate presents some risk to patients with renal impairment, since thiocyanate is eliminated by the kidneys. Owing to the potential for accumulation of thiocyanate, nitroprusside infusions in patients with renal impairment should be terminated at 48 hours. Symptoms of thiocyanate toxicity, which include nausea, vomiting, myoclonus, and seizures, can be reversed with hemodialysis.

ANALGESICS. The most commonly used analgesics (Table 82-7) (see Chaps. 154 and 215) are eliminated primarily by hepatic metabolism, and patients with renal impairment need little dose reduction. Because patients with renal impairment are more prone to bleeding diathesis, however, aspirin should be avoided in these patients.

Although they are primarily hepatically metabolized, non-steroidal anti-inflammatory drugs (NSAIDs) can produce significant adverse effects in patients with renal impairment. All NSAIDs are potent inhibitors of the synthesis of renal prostaglandins, which are important in maintaining renal vasodilatation and ensuring adequate renal blood flow in the kidney. NSAIDs cause renal arteriolar constriction, decreased renal blood flow, and diminished glomerular filtration rate [2].

Inhibition of prostaglandins causes an increase in tubular chloride reabsorption in the loop of Henle and an increased effect of ADH on the distal tubule, leading to salt and water retention. Diminished prostaglandin synthesis is also associated with decreased renin levels and results in a reduction of plasma aldosterone production. Hypoaldosteronism is associated with potassium retention and elevated plasma potassium levels in patients with renal impairment. Patients with decreased effective circulating blood volume, such as those with congestive heart failure, chronic liver failure, chronic renal failure, dehydration, and hemorrage, are more prone to these adverse effects. NSAIDS can cause a hypersensitivity reaction leading to acute renal failure. Proteinuria or the nephrotic syndrome, hematuria, or pyuria is the clinical presentation. Biopsies show evidence of glomerulonephritis or interstitial nephritis. Discontinuation of NSAIDs is essential if these conditions develop. Renal function usually returns to baseline values.

Narcotic analgesics (Table 82-7B) given at the recommended doses to patients with renal impairment produce sedation that may be more profound than in patients with normal renal function. It is essential that doses of these drugs be carefully titrated. The minimal dose should be used for the shortest period in patients with renal impairment. There is particular concern with the use of meperidine in patients with renal impairment. Although the primary metabolite, normeperidine, has little analgesic effect, it accumulates in patients with renal impairment and may decrease the seizure threshold. Therefore, long-term therapy with meperidine should be avoided in patients with renal impairment.

SEDATIVES AND HYPNOTICS. Psychotherapeutic drugs (Table 82-8) are commonly given to patients with renal impairment to relieve anxiety and depression (see Chaps. 209 and 155). The most important side effect of these drugs is excessive sedation. Since malaise, somnolence and mental status changes are also common symptoms of uremia, this particular adverse drug reaction may be overlooked. Benzodiazepines are often used as anti-anxiety drugs in patients with renal impairment. Many of these drugs are metabolized to active metabolites, which are normally excreted by the kidney. When these accumulate in patients with renal impairment, they produce enhanced and prolonged sedation. (Diazepam, chlordiazepoxide, and flurazepam are examples of such compounds.) Therefore, care must be taken when using certain drugs in this category in patients with renal impairment.

DRUGS USED IN THE AFFECTIVE DISORDERS. Tricyclic anti-depressants (Table 82-9) can be used to treat severe depression in patients with renal impairment. They all produce excessive sedation, even at normal doses. In addition, patients

(Text continues on page 1056.)

Table 82-8. Sedatives and Hypnotics

Drug	Route of elimination	Normal half life (h)	Half life in ESRD (h)	Dose: normal renal function	Renal failure adjustment (GFR ml/min)			Dialysis supplementation	Adverse reactions comments
					>50	10-50	<10		
Barbiturates									
Amobarbital (Amytal)	H	15-48	?	65-200 mg hs	none	none	none	HEMO: none CAPD: no data CAVH: no data	
Pentobarbital (Nembutal)	H	18-48	18-48	100 mg hs	none	none	none	HEMO: none CAPD: no data CAVH: no data	
Secobarbital (Seconal)	H	20-35	?	100 mg hs	none	none	none	HEMO: none CAPD: none CAVH: no data	
Benzodiazepines									
Short Acting									
Oxazepam (Serax)	H	5-10	25-90	15-30 mg TID/QID	none	none	none	HEMO: none CAPD: no data CAVH: no data	Glucoronide metabolite increases in ESRD. Protein binding decreased and volume of distribution increased in ESRD.
Triazolam (Halcion)	H	2-4	2-4	0.25-0.50 mg hs	none	none	none	HEMO: none CAPD: none CAVH: no data	
Intermediate-Acting									
Alprazolam (Xanax)	H	10-20	10-20	0.25-5 mg TID	none	none	none	HEMO: no data CAPD: no data CAVH: no data	
Lorazepam (Ativan)	H	5-10	32-70	1-2 mg BID/TID	none	none	none	HEMO: none CAPD: no data CAVH: no data	
Temazepam (Restoril)	H	4-10	?	30 mg hs	none	none	none	HEMO: none CAPD: none CAVH: no data	

		Half-life (hrs) Normal	Half-life (hrs) ESRD	Dose	GFR >50	GFR 10-50	GFR <10	Dialysis	Notes
Long-Acting									
Chlordiazepoxide (Librium)	H	5-30	5-30	15-100 mg/d	none	none	50%	HEMO: none / CAPD: no data / CAVH: no data	Active metabolite
Chlorazepate (Tranxene)	H/R	30-60	36	15-60 mg/d	none	none	none	HEMO: no data / CAPD: no data / CAVH: no data	Active metabolite
Clonazepam (Klonopin)	H	18-50	?	0.5 mg TID	none	none	none	HEMO: none / CAPD: no data / CAVH: no data	
Diazepam (Valium)	H	20-50	20-50	5-40 mg/d	none	none	none	HEMO: none / CAPD: no data / CAVH: no data	Active metabolite
Flurazepam (Dalmane)	H	47-100	47-100	15-30 mg hs	none	none	none	HEMO: none / CAPD: no data / CAVH: no data	Active metabolite
Prazepam (Centrax)	H/R	30-100	36	20-60 mg hs	none	none	none	HEMO: no data / CAPD: no data / CAVH: no data	Active metabolite
Miscellaneous									
Chloral hydrate (Noctec)	H	7-14	?	250 mg TID	none	avoid	avoid	HEMO: none / CAPD: no data / CAVH: no data	Active metabolite. Excessive sedation
Glutethimide (Doriden)	H	10-16	?	250-500 mg/d	none	none	avoid	HEMO: none / CAPD: no data / CAVH: no data	Active metabolite. Hemoperfusion for overdose.
Meprobamate (Miltown)	H/R	9-11	9-11	1200-1600 mg/d	none	none	none	HEMO: none / CAPD: no data / CAVH: no data	Excessive sedation
Paraldehyde (Paral)	H/NR	7.5	?	4-8 ml q2-4h	none	50%	avoid	HEMO: avoid / CAPD: no data / CAVH: no data	Can develop metabolic acidosis.
Pure Anxiolytic									
Buspirone (Buspar)	H	2-3	5.8	5 mg TID	none	none	none	HEMO: none / CAPD: no data / CAVH: no data	Active metabolite

Table 82-9. Drugs Used in the Affective Disorders

Drug	Route of elimination	Normal half life (h)	Half life in ESRD (h)	Dose: normal renal function	Renal failure adjustment (GFR ml/min)		Dialysis supplementation	Adverse reactions comments
Tricyclic Anti-Depressants (TCAs)					Anticholinergic Urinary Retention. Orthostatic hypotension Excessive sedation.			
Amitriptyline (Elavil)	H	24-40	24-40	25 mg TID	>50 10-50 <10	none none none	HEMO: none CAPD: none CAVH: no data	
Desipramine (Norpramin)	H	12-54	?	75-150 mg/d	>50 10-50 <10	none none none	HEMO: none CAPD: none CAVH: no data	Active metabolites
Doxepin (Sinequan)	H	8-25	10-30	25 mg TID	>50 10-50 <10	none none none	HEMO: none CAPD: none CAVH: no data	
Imipramine (Tofranil)	H	6-20	?	25 mg TID	>50 10-50 <10	none none none	HEMO: none CAPD: none CAVH: no data	Active metabolites
Nortriptyline (Aventyl)	H	25-38	15-66	25 mg TID/Qid	>50 10-50 <10	none none none	HEMO: none CAPD: none CAVH: no data	
Protriptyline (Vivactil)	H	54-98	?	15-60 mg/d	>50 10-50 <10	none none none	HEMO: none CAPD: none CAVH: no data	
Trimipramine (Surmontil)	H	24	?	50-150 mg/d	>50 10-50 <10	none none avoid	HEMO: none CAPD: none CAVH: no data	
Tetracyclic								
Amoxapine (Ascendin)	H	8-30	?	75-200 mg/d	>50 10-50 <10	none none none	HEMO: no data CAPD: no data CAVH: no data	

Drug				Dose	GFR >50	GFR 10-50	GFR <10	Supplement	Comments
Maprotiline (Ludiomil)	H	48	?	75 mg/d	none	none	none	HEMO: no data CAPD: no data CAVH: no data	
Heterocyclic Trazodone (Desyrel)	H	6-9	?	75 mg BID	none	none	50%	HEMO: none CAPD: no data CAVH: no data	
Fluoxetine (Prozac)	H	24-72	24-72	20 mg/d	none	none	none	HEMO: no data CAPD: no data CAVH: no data	Active metabolite with $t^{1/2}$ 7-9 days
MAO inhibitors Phenelzine (Nardil)	H	1.5-4	?	45-75 mg/d	none	none	none	HEMO: no data CAPD: no data CAVH: no data	
Tranylcypromine (Parnate)	H	1.9-3.5	?	15 mg BID	none	50%	avoid	HEMO: no data CAPD: no data CAVH: no data	
Miscellaneous Lithium Carbonate	R	14-28	40	0.9-1.2 g/d	none	50-75%	25-50%	HEMO: dose after dialysis CAPD: none CAVH: no data	Nephrogenic diabetes insipidus. Renal tubular acidosis.
Haloperidol (Haldol)	H	10-36	?	1-2 mg BID/TID	none	none	none	HEMO: none CAPD: none CAVH: no data	
Sertraline (Zoloft)	H	24	?	50-200 mg/d	no data	no data	no data	HEMO: no data CAPD: no data CAVH: no data	Active metabolite
Paroxetine (Paxil)	H	21	?	20-50 mg/d	none	50%	50%	HEMO: no data CAPD: no data CAVH: no data	

Table 82-10. Anticoagulants

Drug	Route of elimination	Normal half life (h)	Half life in ESRD (h)	Dose: normal renal function	Renal failure adjustment (GFR ml/min)		Dialysis supplementation	Adverse reactions comments
Dipyridamole	NR	12	?	50 mg TID	>50 10-50 <10	none none none	HEMO: no data CAPD: no data CAVH: no data	
Heparin	H	0.3-2	0.3-2	Individualized	>50 10-50 <10	none none none	HEMO: none CAPD: none CAVH: none	
Streptokinase	H	1-1.5	1-1.5	250,000 U loading dose, then 100,000 U/h	>50 10-50 <10	none none none	HEMO: NA CAPD: NA CAVH: NA	
Urokinase	?	?	?	4400 U/kg loading dose, then 4400 U/kg·h	>50 10-50 <10	none none none	HEMO: no data CAPD: no data CAVH: no data	
Warfarin	H	35-45	35-45	10-15 mg loading dose, then 2-10 mg/d	>50 10-50 <10	none none none	HEMO: none CAPD: none CAVH: none	Follow prothrombin time

Table 82-11. Anticonvulsants (Monitor Serum Levels)

Drug	Route of elimination	Normal half life (h)	Half life in ESRD (h)	Dose: normal renal function	Renal failure adjustment (GFR ml/min)		Dialysis supplementation	Adverse reactions comments
Carbamazepine (Tegretol)	H	12-17	?	600-1200 mg/d	>50 10-50 <10	none none 50-75%	HEMO: none CAPD: none CAVH: no data	Aplastic anemia Agranulocytosis
Ethosuximide (Zarontin)	H/R	30-50	30-50	750-2000 mg/d	>50 10-50 <10	none none 50%	HEMO: 250 mg after dialysis CAPD: no data CAVH: no data	
Phenobarbital (Luminal)	H/R	90-120	117-160	30-200 mg/d	>50 10-50 <10	none 75% 25-50%	HEMO: 50% after dialysis CAPD: 25% after dialysis CAVH: no data	
Phenytoin (Dilantin)	H	24-72	24-72	300-400 mg/d	>50 10-50 <10	none none none	HEMO: none CAPD: none CAVH: none	Measure free and bound levels Nystagmus indicates toxicity
Primidone (Mysoline)	H	7-14	7-14	500-1500 mg/d	>50 10-50 <10	none 75% avoid	HEMO: 1/3 dose after dialysis CAPD: no data CAVH: no data	Partially converted to phenobarbital. Excessive sedation. Nystagmus. Folate deficiency
Valproic Acid (Depakote)	H	10-12	10-12	1000-3000 mg/d	>50 10-50 <10	none none none	HEMO: none CAPD: none CAVH: none	

Table 82-12. Antiemetics

Drug	Route of elimination	Normal half life (h)	Half life in ESRD (h)	Dose: normal renal function	Renal failure adjustment (GFR ml/min)		Dialysis supplementation	Adverse reactions comments
Histamine (H₁) blocker								
Dimenhydrinate (Dramamine)	?	4-7	?	50-100 mg q4h	>50 10-50 <10	none q9h q12h	HEMO: no data CAPD: no data CAVH: no data	
Diphenhydramine (Benadryl)	H	3.4-9.3	?	25-100 mg q6h	>50 10-50 <10	none none none	HEMO: none CAPD: none CAVH: none	Anticholinergic effects may cause urinary retention. May cause excessive sedation.
Hydroxyzine (Vistaril, Atarax)	H	14-20	?	25-100 mg q6h	>50 10-50 <10	none none none	HEMO: no data CAPD: no data CAVH: no data	Active metabolite excreted by the kidney. May cause excessive sedation.
Meclizine (Antivert)	NR	6	?	12.5-37.5 mg TID	>50 10-50 <10	none none avoid	HEMO: no data CAPD: no data CAVH: no data	Long duration of action (12-24 hours) due to conversion to active metabolites
CTZ Effect—(Chemoreceptor Trigger Zone)								
Trimethobenzamide (Tigan)	?	?	?	250 mg TID/QID	>50 10-50 <10	no data no data no data	HEMO: no data CAPD: no data CAVH: no data	
Metoclopramide (Reglan)	H	2.5-4	14-15	1.25-2.50 mg q4h	>50 10-50 <10	none 75% 50%	HEMO: none CAPD: no data CAVH: no data	Extrapyramidal side effects common in ESRD.
Droperidol (Inapsine)	H	2-2.5	?	2.5-10 mg IM	>50 10-50 <10	none 50% avoid	HEMO: no data CAPD: no data CAVH: no data	
Phenothiazines					Anticholinergic. Urinary retention. Orthostatic hypotension. Confusion. Extrapyramidal symptoms			
Chlorpromazine (Thorazine)	H	11-42	11-42	10-25 mg q4-6h 25-50 mg q3-4h IM	>50 10-50 <10	none none none	HEMO: none CAPD: none CAVH: no data	Plasma levels rebound after oral dose.
Prochlorperazine (Compazine)	H	7	?	5-10 mg q6h	>50 10-50 <10	none none none	HEMO: no data CAPD: no data CAVH: no data	
Promethazine (Phenergan)	H	9-12	?	12.5-25 mg q4-6h	>50 10-50 <10	none none none	HEMO: no data CAPD: no data CAVH: no data	Excessive sedation

Table 82-13. Bronchodilators

Drug	Route of elimination	Normal half life (h)	Half life in ESRD (h)	Dose: normal renal function	Renal failure adjustment (GFR ml/min)		Dialysis supplementation	Adverse reactions comments
Albuterol (Proventil)	H/R	4	?	2-4 mg TID/QID	>50 10-50 <10	none 75% 50%	HEMO: no data CAPD: no data CAVH: no data	
Dyphylline (Dilor, Lufyllin)	R	1.8-2.3	12	1.5 mg/kg·d	>50 10-50 <10	75% 50% 25%	HEMO: no data CAPD: no data CAVH: no data	
Ipratropium (Atrovent)	NR	1.6	?	2 inhalators QID	>50 10-50 <10	none none none	HEMO: none CAPD: none CAVH: none	
Terbutaline (Brethine)	H/R	3	?	2.5-5 mg TID	>50 10-50 <10	none 50% avoid	HEMO: no data CAPD: no data CAVH: no data	Parenteral doses should be avoided in ESRD.
Theophylline (Aminophylline)	H	4-12	4-12	6 mg/kg loading dose, then 9 mg/kg·d	>50 10-50 <10	none none none	HEMO: 50% CAPD: no data CAVH: no data	May exacerbate uremic gastrointestinal symptoms.

Table 82-14. Corticosteroids and Immunosuppressive Drugs (May Aggravate Azotemia. Associated with Sodium Retention, Glucose Intolerance and Hypertension)

Drug	Route of elimination	Normal half life (h)	Half life in ESRD (h)	Dose: normal renal function	Renal failure adjustment (GFR ml/min)		Dialysis supplementation	Adverse reactions comments
Corticosteroids								
Betamethasone	H	5.5	?	0.5-9 mg/d	>50 10-50 <10	none none none	HEMO: no data CAPD: no data CAVH: no data	
Cortisone	H	0.5-2	3.5	25-500 mg/d	>50 10-50 <10	none none none	HEMO: no data CAPD: no data CAVH: no data	
Dexamethasone	H	3-4	?	0.75-9 mg/d	>50 10-50 <10	none none none	HEMO: no data CAPD: no data CAVH: no data	
Hydrocortisone	H	1.5-2	?	20-500 mg/d	>50 10-50 <10	none none none	HEMO: no data CAPD: no data CAVH: no data	
Methylprednisolone	H	1.9-6	1.9-6	4-48 mg/d	>50 10-50 <10	none none none	HEMO: dose after dialysis CAPD: no data CAVH: no data	
Prednisolone	H	2.5-3.5	2.5-3.5	5-60 mg/d	>50 10-50 <10	none none none	HEMO: dose after dialysis CAPD: no data CAVH: no data	
Prednisone	H	2.5-3.5	2.5-3.5	5-60 mg/d	>50 10-50 <10	none none none	HEMO: none CAPD: no data CAVH: no data	
Triamcinolone	?	1.9-6	1.9-6	4-48 mg/d	>50 10-50 <10	none none none	HEMO: no data CAPD: no data CAVH: no data	
Immunosuppressive Drugs								
Azathioprine (Imuran)	H	0.16-1	?	1.5-2.5 mg/kg·d	>50 10-50 <10	none 75% 50%	HEMO: dose after dialysis CAPD: no data CAVH: no data	
Cyclophosphamide (Cytoxan)	H	4-7.5	10	1-5 mg/kg·d	>50 10-50 <10	none none 75%	HEMO: 50% after dialysis CAPD: no data CAVH: no data	Hemorrhagic cystitis. SIADH.
Cyclosporine (Sandimmune)	H	3-16	3-16	3-10 mg/kg·d	>50 10-50 <10	none none none	HEMO: none CAPD: none CAVH: no data	Nephrotoxic. Hypertension, seizures.

Table 82-15. H₂ Antagonists

Drug	Route of elimination	Normal half life (h)	Half life in ESRD (h)	Dose: normal renal function	Renal failure adjustment (GFR ml/min)			Dialysis supplementation	Adverse reactions comments
					>50	10-50	<10		
Cimetidine (Tagamet)	R	1.5-2	2	400 mg BID	none	50%	25%	HEMO: none CAPD: none CAVH: no data	Increases serum creatinine and decreases creatinine clearance by inhibition of tubular creatinine secretion. Mental confusion in ESRD.
Famotidine (Pepcid)	R	2.5-4	12-19	20-40 mg q hs	50%	25%	10%	HEMO: none CAPD: none CAVH: none	
Nizatidine (Axid)	R	1.3-1.6	5.3-8.5	150-300 mg q hs	75%	50%	25%	HEMO: no data CAPD: no data CAVH: no data	
Ranitidine (Zantac)	R	1.5-3	6-9	150-300 mg q hs	75%	50%	25%	HEMO: 50% dose after dialysis CAPD: none CAVH: none	

Table 82-16. Neuromuscular Drugs

Drug	Route of elimination	Normal half life (h)	Half life in ESRD (h)	Dose: normal renal function	Renal failure adjustment (GFR ml/min)			Dialysis supplementation	Adverse reactions comments
					>50	10-50	<10		
Non-Depolarizing d-Tubocurarine	R	0.5-4	5.5	0.1-0.2 mg/kg	75%	50%	avoid	HEMO: no data CAPD: no data CAVH: no data	Recurarization may occur.
Pancuronium	H/R	1.7-2.2	4.3-8.2	0.04-0.1 mg/kg	none	50%	avoid	HEMO: no data CAPD: no data CAVH: no data	Recurarization may occur up to 24 h after a dose.
Gallamine	R	2.3-2.7	6-20	0.5-1.5 mg/kg	75%	avoid	avoid	HEMO: NA CAPD: NA CAVH: NA	Recurarization may occur up to 24 h after a dose.
Polarizing Succinylcholine	H	3	?	0.3-1.1 mg/kg loading dose, then 0.04-0.07 mg/kg PRN	none	none	none	HEMO: no data CAPD: no data CAVH: no data	Hyperkalemia in ESRD.

Table 82-17. Antineoplastic Drugs

Drug	Route of elimination	Normal half life (h)	Half Life in ESRD (h)	Dose: normal renal function	Renal failure adjustment (GFR ml/min)			Dialysis supplementation	Adverse reactions comments
					>50	10-50	<10		
Busulfan	H	2.5	?	4-8 mg/d	none	none	none	HEMO: no data CAPD: no data CAVH: no data	May cause hemorrhagic cystitis
Bleomycin	R	9	20	10-20 u/m²	none	75%	50%	HEMO: none CAPD: no data CAVH: no data	Drug accumulation predisposes to pulmonary fibrosis. Hypertension and dysuria.
Chlorambucil	?	1	?	0.1 mg/kd·d	no data	no data	no data	HEMO: no data CAPD: no data CAVH: no data	
Cisplatin	R	0.3-0.5	?	20-50 mg/m²·d	no data	75%	50%	HEMO: none CAPD: no data CAVH: no data	Nephrotoxic Renal magnesium wasting.
Daunorubicin	H	18-27	?	30-45 mg/m²	none	none	none	HEMO: no data CAPD: no data CAVH: no data	
Etoposide	R	4-8	?	35-100 mg/m²·d	none	75%	50%	HEMO: none CAPD: no data CAVH: no data	
Fluorouracil	NR	0.1	0.1	12 mg/kg·d	none	none	none	HEMO: none CAPD: no data CAVH: no data	
Hydroxyurea	R	?	?	20-30 mg/kg·d	none	50%	20%	HEMO: no data CAPD: no data CAVH: no data	
Melphalan	H	1.1-1.4	4-6	6 mg/d	none	75%	50%	HEMO: no data CAPD: no data CAVH: no data	

Drug		Half-life		Dose	GFR	Adjust	Dialysis	Comments
Methotrexate	R	8-12	increases	5-10 mg/week for RA; 15 mg/d to 12 g/m² for cancer	>50 / 10-50 / <10	none / 50% / avoid	HEMO: none; CAPD: none; CAVH: no data	Nephrotoxicity prevented by urinary alkalinization and forced diuresis.
Mitomycin C	?	0.5-1	?	20 mg/m² 6-8 weeks	>50 / 10-50 / <10	none / none / 75%	HEMO: no data; CAPD: no data; CAVH: no data	Nephrotoxicity. Hemolytic-uremic syndrome.
Nitrosoureas	?	short	?	varies	>50 / 10-50 / <10	none / 75% / 25-50%	HEMO: none; CAPD: no data; CAVH: no data	Prototype: methyl CCNU. Metabolites with variable $T_{1/2}$, irreversible toxicity at dose > 1500 mg/m²
Tamoxifen	?	18	?	10-20 mg BID	>50 / 10-50 / <10	no data / no data / no data	HEMO: no data; CAPD: no data; CAVH: no data	
Teniposide	H	6-10	?	50-250 mg/m²	>50 / 10-50 / <10	none / none / none	HEMO: none; CAPD: none; CAVH: none	
Vinblastine	H	1-1.5	?	3.7 mg/m²	>50 / 10-50 / <10	none / none / none	HEMO: no data; CAPD: no data; CAVH: no data	May cause SIADH.
Vincristine	H	1-2.5	?	1.4 mg/m²	>50 / 10-50 / <10	none / none / none	HEMO: no data; CAPD: no data; CAVH: no data	

taking these drugs may exhibit anticholinergic effects, orthostatic hypotension, confusion and extrapyramidal symptoms. Lithium carbonate is often used for treating manic-depressive conditions. It is excreted primarily by the kidney and has a very narrow therapeutic range. It is therefore important to markedly reduce the dose and to monitor plasma lithium levels in all patients with renal impairment or unstable renal function. (See also Chaps. 140, 147, 221 to 223.)

ANTICOAGULANTS. When needed, both warfarin and heparin can be used in normal dosages for patients with renal impairment (Table 82-10). Following the prothrombin time is the best guide for determining if the warfarin dosage is therapeutic. Both streptokinase and urokinase may be needed in a patient with renal impairment, particularly one who has a vascular access that may need declotting (see Chap. 121).

ANTICONVULSANTS. Phenytoin is one of the most frequently used drugs for seizures in patients with renal impairment (Table 82-11) (see Chaps. 134 and 213). Phenytoin protein binding is decreased and the volume of distribution is increased in renal failure patients. For any given total serum phenytoin level, the concentration of active free drug is higher in patients with renal impairment than in patients with normal renal function. Since most laboratories measure the total serum drug concentration, a low total phenytoin level in patients with renal impairment may not correspond to a subtherapeutic plasma concentration. Since the physical finding of nystagmus is an indication of phenytoin toxicity, its presence should preclude any further dosing with this drug. Whenever possible, free serum phenytoin concentrations should be measured frequently in patients with renal impairment who are receiving this drug. For the long-acting barbiturates, a marked decrease in the drug dosage is necessary for patients with severe renal impairment, and close monitoring of plasma levels and observations for toxic effects is necessary.

ANTIEMETICS. A variety of drugs are used for patients with renal impairment who experience symptoms of nausea and vomiting (Table 82-12). Of these drugs, metoclopramide requires dosage reduction in patients with severe renal impairment to prevent adverse side effects. Since this drug blocks the effects of dopamine, both drowsiness and extrapyramidal reactions are especially common in patients with ESRD. Phenothiazines, which are also used as antiemetic drugs, are primarily hepatically metabolized, and dosage adjustments are not necessary in patients with renal impairment. These drugs all have an anticholinergic effect, however, and therefore can cause urinary retention and orthostatic hypotension (see Chap. 133). They also can cause extrapyramidal symptoms and sedation in patients with ESRD.

BRONCHODILATORS. Beta agonists (Table 82-13) administered by inhalation or parenteral routes usually do not require adjustment in patients with renal impairment. Aminophylline and theophylline can be given in usual doses (see Chaps. 56 and 211). Plasma drug concentrations should be monitored if possible.

CORTICOSTEROIDS AND IMMUNOSUPPRESSIVE DRUGS. Most corticosteroid preparations are eliminated by hepatic metabolism (Table 82-14) and do not have to be re-

duced in patients with renal impairment. Azathioprine does accumulate in patients with renal impairment, and the dose needs to be reduced significantly as renal function decreases. Cyclosporine is primarily metabolized by the liver and only a small amount is excreted as the parent drug into the urine. Renal impairment does not affect its metabolism, and the dose does not have to be reduced. Since cyclosporine is metabolized by the cytochrome P-450 system, the concomitant use of drugs that are also metabolized by the cytochrome can significantly alter plasma concentration of this drug (see Chaps. 193 and 214). Cyclophosphamide is also hepatically metabolized, but its metabolites, which are excreted into the urine, are responsible for producing a chemical hemorrhagic cystitis. For patients on cyclophosphamide, a high urine flow rate is essential when high doses of drug are given.

HISTAMINE H_2 ANTAGONISTS. The H_2 antagonists are often used in patients with renal impairment for treatment of acid dyspepsia (Table 82-15). All of these drugs are primarily eliminated by the kidneys and therefore require significant adjustment in patients with renal impairment. Cimetidine can cause a mild increase in the serum creatinine level because it blocks the tubular secretion of creatinine, thus decreasing creatinine clearance. This drug also can cause an increased risk of confusional states in patients with renal impairment.

NEUROMUSCULAR DRUGS. Paralyzing agents should be used cautiously in patients with renal impairment. (Table 82-16). Drugs identified as nondepolarizing drugs (D-tubocurarine, pancuronium, or gallamine) undergo significant renal elimination, and prolonged neuromuscular blockade may occur when they are administered to patients with renal impairment. Although the depolarizing drug succinylcholine is not significantly eliminated by the kidneys, some of its pharmacologically active metabolites undergo renal excretion. Succinylcholine can result in hyperkalemia in patients with renal impairment. (See Chap. 208.)

ANTINEOPLASTIC DRUGS. A variety of antineoplastic drugs are available for use in patients with renal impairment (Table 82-17). Many depend on renal elimination for the removal of either the parent drug or its active metabolite and therefore require significant reduction in dose and careful monitoring for toxic effects when used in patients with renal impairment.

References

1. Reidenberg MM: The binding of drugs to plasma proteins and the interpretation of measurements of plasma concentration of drugs in patients with poor renal function. *Am J Med* 62:466, 1977.
2. Bennett WM, Aronoff GR, Golper TA, et al: *Drug Prescribing in Renal Failure: Dosing Guidelines for Adults.* Philadelphia, American College of Physicians, 1991.
3. Reidenberg MM: The biotransformation of drugs in renal failure. *Am J Med* 62:482, 1977.
4. Verbeeck RK, Branch RA, Wilkinson GR: Drug metabolites in renal failure: Pharmacokinetic and clinical applications. *Clin Pharmacokinet* 6:329, 1981.
5. Carmichael DJ: Handling of drugs in kidney disease, in Cameron S, Davison AM, Grunfeld JP, et al (eds): *Oxford Textbook of Clinical Nephrology,* Vol 1, Oxford, Oxford University Press, 1992.
6. Bennett WM: Use of drugs in renal failure and dialysis, in Massry SG, Glonich, RJ (eds): *Textbook of Nephrology,* Baltimore, Williams and Wilkins, 1983.

7. Anderson RJ, Bennett WM, Gambertoglio JG, et al: Fate of drugs in renal failure, in Brenner B, Rector F (eds): *The Kidney.* 4th ed. Philadelphia, WB Saunders, 1991.

8. Bennett WM, Aronoff GR, Morrison G, et al: I. Drug prescribing in renal failure: Dosing guidelines for adults. *Am J Kidney Dis* 3:155, 1983.

9. Bennett WM, Aronoff GR, Golper TA, et al: *Drug Prescribing in Renal Failure: Dosing Guidelines for Adults,* Philadelphia, American College of Physicians, 1987.

10. Brater DC: *Handbook of Drug Use in Patients with Renal Disease.* 3rd ed. Dallas, Texas, Improved Therapeutics, 1985.

11. Reed WE, Sabatini S: The use of drugs in renal failure. *Semin Nephrol* 6(3):259, 1986.

12. Stein JH, editor: *Internal Medicine: Diagnosis and Therapy.* 3rd ed. Norwalk, CT, Appleton and Lange, 1992.

13. Ramsey PG, Larson EB, (eds): *Medical Therapeutics,* ed 2, Philadelphia, WB Saunders, 1993.

14. Seyffart, G, editor: *Drug Dosage in Renal Insufficiency,* Boston, Kluwer, 1991.

15. Anderson RJ, Schrier RW, Gambertoglio JG (eds): *Clinical Use of Drugs in Patients with Kidney and Liver Disease.* Philadelphia, WB Saunders, 1981.

16. Cockroft DW, Gault MH: Prediction of creatinine clearance from serum creatinine. *Nephron* 16:31, 1976.

17. Jick H: Adverse drug effects in relation to renal function. *Am J Med* 62:514, 1977.

18. Smith JW, Seidl LG, Cluff LE: Studies on the epidemiology of adverse drug reaction. Clinical factors influencing susceptibility. *Ann Intern Med* 65:629, 1966.

19. Elenbaas RM, Payne VW, Bauman JL: Influence of clinical pharmacist consultants on the use of drug blood level tests. *Am J Hosp Pharm* 37:61, 1980.

20. Aronoff GR, Abel SR: Principles of administering drugs to patients with renal failure, in Brenner BM, Stein JH (eds): *Contemporary Issues in Nephrology.* New York, Churchill-Livingstone, 1986.

83. Dialysis Therapy in the Intensive Care Setting

William F. Owen, Jr.

Historical Perspectives on Dialytic Therapy

Bones can break, muscles can atrophy, glands can loaf, even the brains can go to sleep, without immediately endangering our survival; but should the kidneys fail . . . neither bone, muscle, gland, nor brain could carry on.

Homer W. Smith (1895–1962)

In 1839, Addison reported that stupor, coma, and convulsions were consequences of "diseased kidneys" [1], an illness referred to for much of that century as Bright's disease [2]. Approximately 50 years later, Hughes and Carter accurately defined uremia as:

An intoxication brought about by the accumulation in the blood of substances which it is the function of the kidneys to excrete [3].

Further, Tyson noted that:

Uremic symptoms are dependent on retention of urea and allied substances in the blood, which when they have accumulated to a sufficient quantity act on the nervous system producing delirium and convulsions or coma [4].

These rudimentary observations relevant to the pathobiology of symptomatic renal failure suggested that therapy should be directed at the reversal or attenuation of the retention of nitrogenous products of metabolism. Sweating, bowel evacuation, forced diuresis, bloodletting, and volume expansion were variably successful therapies and were often deleterious to the patient. These therapeutic failures stimulated the development of hemodialysis:

There are numerous toxic states in which the eliminating organs of the body, more especially the kidneys, are incapable of removing from the body, at an adequate rate, the autochthonous or foreign substances whose presence in excessive amounts is detrimental to life processes. In the hope of providing a substitute in such emergencies, which might tide over a dangerous crisis . . . we devised a method by which the blood of a living animal may be submitted to dialysis outside the body and again returned to the natural circulation [5].

The practical application of these principles to humans with renal insufficiency was not realized for another 30 years. In September 1945, Kolff successfully dialyzed a 67-year-old woman with acute oliguric renal failure. At the initiation of hemodialysis, her blood urea nitrogen (BUN) concentration was approximately 400 mg/dl, and she was in a uremic coma. Therapy in Kolff's "kidney room" was so successful that after an initial 11-hour dialysis session, her uremic encephalopathy resolved. Her recovery and spontaneous diuresis occurred after 1 week of dialysis therapy [6]. Initially, it was only used as a research tool applied only at academic health care centers, but the Korean War validated the crucial role of hemodialysis. In this conflict, hemodialysis was applied for acute renal failure (ARF) in previously healthy young men secondary to shock, trauma, and nephrotoxins [7]. Using a Brigham-modified Kolff rotating drum dialyzer configuration, Teschan described that in over 30 such patients:

Dramatic clinical improvement was frequently obtained. . . . A reduction in case fatality has, we think, been achieved through the use of dialysis in these patients (and) has demonstrated the value of dialysis therapy of combat casualties with posttraumatic renal insufficiency.

As acceptance of dialytic therapy for acute renal failure was gained, it was appreciated that regular hemodialysis treatments of chronic (irreversible) terminal renal failure were impractical until a means of safely and reproducibly gaining access to the vascular system was achieved. This was accomplished in March, 1960 with a newly developed arteriovenous cannula system. This device was exteriorized in the arm. Scribner initiated twice-weekly repetitive hemodialysis on a 39-year-old man with end-stage renal failure (ESRD). He survived for 11 years on dialysis. Death finally occurred secondary to a myocardial infarction [8]. By 1965, hemodialysis was being performed on a worldwide basis for the management of ESRD, and the number of patients requiring treatment soon exceeded the number of available facilities, equipment, trained personnel, and available finances. In 1978, Congress mandated federal funding of dialysis and transplantation for therapy of ESRD. One consequence of the elimination of financial barriers to the treatment of chronic renal failure is that the number of patients being treated has increased by approximately 10% annually [9].

Conceptually, peritoneal dialysis is an older technique than hemodialysis, but its practical application was compromised by numerous unsuccessful attempts to treat both acute and chronic renal failure patients.

The author suggests using the peritoneum as a dialysis membrane and to perfuse the peritoneal cavity because this would be more physiological. . . . The peritoneum has indeed a large surface area and dialysis does occur for the non-protein nitrogen in the perfusion fluid is increased, but the clinical results are negative [10].

Despite anecdotal reports of short-term success with peritoneal dialysis for acute renal failure in the 1950s, it was used as an experimental technique and attempted only as a last resort in preterminal cases of uremia. Therapeutic success with peritoneal dialysis required the development of a closed dialysate administration system, the commercial preparation of standardized dialysis fluids and tubing, and the development of reliable peritoneal dialysis catheters. Therefore, it is unsurprising that peritoneal dialysis technically lagged behind hemodialysis and renal transplantation. Because stylet catheters were safe only for short intervals, repeated abdominal perforations were required even for the management of ARF. The development of the dual-cuffed Tenckhoff catheter in 1968 [11] helped improve the status of peritoneal dialysis from that of

. . . a good leaden bullet which . . . should perhaps be more commonly fired [12].

Overview of Dialysis Modalities

Patients undergo dialysis for either chronic renal failure, in which the azotemia is the consequence of preexisting irreversible, structural renal insufficiency, or for ARF, which denotes a wide variety of disorders associated with the acute retention of nitrogenous products of metabolism. Because ARF is potentially reversible, an aggressive pursuit should be undertaken to identify and correct the cause. Within the intensive care unit (ICU) setting, most cases of renal failure that require dialytic support are acute in nature. Therefore, most of the subsequent discussion focuses on dialysis for ARF within the ICU. Except where specifically denoted, all subsequent discussions are applicable to both patients with ARF and those with chronic renal failure.

Despite vastly improved medical, surgical, and nursing care within the ICU, the use of mechanical ventilators, inotrophs, intracardiac pressure monitoring, total parenteral nutrition, an expanded choice of antimicrobial agents, and the ready avail-

ability of multiple dialysis techniques, mortality from ARF greatly exceeds that of chronic renal failure. Whereas the annual gross mortality from ESRD has declined from 50% to approximately 20% over the last 20 years [9], the mortality for ARF has remained relatively stable at approximately 50% since the 1950s [13–18].

Adverse determinants of patient survival that contribute to this excessive mortality include (1) the shifting pattern of clinical characteristics of affected patients, (2) comorbid illness, and (3) the provocative factors that culminate in ARF [18]. As an example of the first issue, the age of the patient base that is affected with acute renal failure has increased; this demographic variable has an adverse influence on disease survival [15,16,18–21]. Nonoliguric acute renal failure, however, which is being recognized with increased frequency as a distinct entity, is associated with a substantially lower mortality than oliguric disease [22,23]. The inclusion or exclusion of these patients skews survival statistics for ARF. Relevant to the second issue are the observations that despite therapeutic advances for comorbid disorders such as infections [16,24,25], cardiovascular conditions [16,21,26], respiratory failure [21,27,28], and hypercatabolism and malnutrition [21,29,30], their presence continues to adversely influence the course of ARF. Lastly, it is unclear if the underlying illness defines the patient's prognosis for ARF. Earlier observations suggested an increased likelihood of death in patients with ARF secondary to "surgical" disorders (trauma, vascular catastrophes, and complicated orthopedic, thoracic, and abdominal procedures) compared to "medical" disorders (nephrotoxic medications, infections/sepsis, cardiovascular events, and intrarenal pathologies) [15,31,32]. More recent multivariate analysis has not supported this assessment, however [33,34]. The percentage and absolute number of patients with medical disorders that require care in the ICU setting have increased [34], and the suggestion of an increased mortality for this group is distressing. In summary, the advent and widespread availability of dialysis have eliminated ARF itself as a direct and significant factor in the prognosis of patients with ARF.

Approximately 90% of the patients with ARF do not require dialytic support [20,35]. Because of the potential for recovery of renal function, the cause of renal insufficiency alone should not be a determinant in deciding the patient's candidacy for dialysis. Other issues such as the patient's educational status, financial resources, social status, ethnicity, and mental competence are likewise of no primary relevance in this situation. If the patient has an active and aggressive neoplastic disease that will significantly abbreviate the subject's lifespan, dialysis should be approached with greater deliberation. If the development of ARF has compromised the capacity of the oncology patient to receive chemotherapy and nutrition, dialysis is indicated. Only the terminally ill patient with such severe medical complications that dialysis cannot be technically performed should be denied this therapy.

Dialysis fulfills two biophysical goals: (1) solute removal, as is the case for potassium and urea, or the addition of solute, as is the case for bicarbonate and calcium ("clearance"); and (2) the elimination of volume from the patient ("ultrafiltration"). These two processes can be performed simultaneously or at different times. The dialysis procedures used are hemodialysis, hemofiltration, and peritoneal dialysis (Table 83-1).

HEMODIALYSIS. Hemodialysis is a diffusion-driven and size discriminatory process for the clearance of small solutes such as electrolytes and urea (<300 daltons). The clearance of larger solutes is typically far less. During hemodialysis, ultrafiltration

Table 83-1. Dialysis Modalities*

Technique	Dialyzer	Physical principle
Hemodialysis		
Conventional	Hemodialyzer	Concurrent diffusive clearance & UF
Sequential UF/ Clearance	Hemodialyzer	UF followed by diffusive clearance
Ultrafiltration	Hemodialyzer	UF alone
Hemofiltration		
SCUF	Hemofilter	Arteriovenous UF without a blood pump
CAVH	Hemofilter	Arteriovenous convective transport without a blood pump
CAVHD	Hemofilter	Arteriovenous hemodialysis without a blood pump
CAVHDF	Hemofilter	Arteriovenous hemofiltration & hemodialysis without a blood pump
CVVH	Hemofilter	Venovenous convective transport with a blood pump
CVVHD	Hemofilter	Venovenous hemodialysis with a blood pump
CVVHDF	Hemofilter	Venovenous hemofiltration & hemodialysis with a blood pump
Peritoneal Dialysis		
Intermittent	None	Exchanges performed for 10-12 hours every 2-3 days
CAPD	None	Manual exchanges performed daily during waking hours
CCPD	None	Automated cycling device performs exchanges nightly

*Abbreviations: CAPD = continuous ambulatory peritoneal dialysis
CAVH = continuous arteriovenous hemofiltration
CAVHD = continuous arteriovenous hemodialysis
CAVHDF = continuous arteriovenous hemodiafiltration
CCPD = continuous cycling peritoneal dialysis
CVVH = continuous venovenous hemofiltration
CVVHD = continuous venovenous hemodialysis
CVVHDF = continuous venovenous hemodiafiltration
SCUF = slow continuous ultrafiltration
UF = ultrafiltration.

is driven by the generation of negative hydraulic pressure on the dialysate side of the dialyzer. The major components of the hemodialytic process are (1) the artificial kidney or dialyzer; (2) the delivery system, which is the mechanical device(s) that pumps the patient's blood and the dialysate through the dialyzer; and (3) the dialysate, which is the fluid having a defined chemical composition used for solute clearance. During the performance of "conventional" hemodialysis, the patient's blood and dialysate are pumped continuously through the dialyzer in opposite (countercurrent) directions at flow rates of approximately 300 and 500 ml per minute, respectively. The dialysate passes through the dialyzer only once (single pass system) and is discarded after interaction with the blood across the dialyzer's semipermeable membrane. The efficiency of hemodialysis can be augmented by the use of dialyzers that are more porous to water and solutes. These kidneys with enhanced performance characteristics are described as *high-efficiency* and *high-flux* dialyzers, depending upon their ultrafiltration capacity. High-efficiency hemodialysis uses a high-

porosity dialyzer that has an ultrafiltration coefficient greater than 10 and less than 20 ml/mm Hg/hour. High-flux hemodialysis uses an even more porous dialyzer with an ultrafiltration coefficient greater than 20 ml/mm Hg/hour. Typically, these enhanced performance dialyzers have greater clearances of solutes of large molecular weight (>300 daltons).

Variables of the hemodialysis procedure that may be manipulated are the type of dialyzer (determine the solute clearance and ultrafiltration capacity), the dialysate composition (influence solute clearance and loading), the blood and dialysate flow (influence solute clearance), and the hydraulic pressure that drives ultrafiltration.

HEMOFILTRATION. Compared with the diffusion-driven solute clearance of hemodialysis, hemofiltration depends on convective transport. Specifically, the patient's blood is conveyed through an extremely high-porosity dialyzer (hemofilter); the result is formation of a protein-free hemofiltrate that resembles plasma water in composition. The driving force for perfusion of the hemofilter is typically the patient's mean arterial pressure, whereas the hydrostatic pressure in the hemofiltrate compartment provides the driving force for the formation of the filtrate. For effective hemofiltration, the mean arterial pressure should be maintained >70 mm Hg. Blood is usually conveyed into the hemofilter from an arterial cannula and is returned into a large-caliber vein. If the hemofiltrate is formed and is not replaced by a replacement solution, the process is described as *slow continuous ultrafiltration* (SCUF). Little solute clearance occurs during SCUF. An alternative technique that enhances solute clearance is to continually replace the lost volume with a solution that lacks the solute being removed. If an arteriovenous blood path is used, the process is called *continuous arteriovenous hemofiltration* (CAVH). If a venovenous path is used (driven by a blood pump at a rate of 100 ml/minute), the procedure is described as *continuous venovenous hemofiltration* (CVVH). Optimal solute clearance is achieved by combining diffusive clearance and convective transport. This is accomplished by circulating a dialysate through the hemofilter with or without a high ultrafiltration rate (continuous arteriovenous hemodialysis [CAVHD] and continuous arteriovenous hemodiafiltration [CAVHDF], respectively). Alternatively, these procedures may be performed using venovenous access with a blood pump to generate adequate flow rates (CVVHD and CVVHDF, respectively). Hemofiltration, which is impractical for maintenance dialysis, is typically performed with arteriovenous access.

PERITONEAL DIALYSIS. Peritoneal dialysis relies on the diffuse clearance of solutes across the peritoneal membrane, whereas ultrafiltration during peritoneal dialysis depends on the instillation of a hyperosmolal solution. Typically, maintenance peritoneal dialysis is performed daily, either by the performance of manual instillation and drainage of the dialysate during waking hours (continuous ambulatory peritoneal dialysis [CAPD]), or while sleeping using an automated dialysate cycling device (*continuous cycling peritoneal dialysis* [CCPD]). The dialysate volume is usually 2 to 3 liters per instillation, and it dwells in the peritoneal cavity for variable intervals depending on the clearance and ultrafiltration goals (described as an "exchange"). In the acute setting, peritoneal dialysis is performed through a straight stylet peritoneal catheter or through a surgically implanted and tunneled, cuffed catheter (such as the Tenckhoff catheter). Chronic peritoneal dialysis is performed through a cuffed catheter.

Indications for Dialysis in Renal Failure

In patients with ARF, the goal of dialytic therapy is to support the patient while awaiting the recovery of adequate renal function to sustain life, whereas in chronic renal failure, the objective is for dialysis to substitute for renal function indefinitely. Because there has been inadequate time for the establishment of compensatory or adaptive alterations, it is mandatory that dialysis be speedily initiated in patients with ARF. Premortal conditions that can be corrected by dialysis are absolute indications for its initiation. These absolute indications for the initiation of dialysis are uremic serositis, uremic encephalopathy, hyperkalemia that is inadequately corrected with conservative therapy, hypervolemia that is inadequately corrected with optimal doses of diuretics, and acidosis that is not adequately corrected with alkali. In addition, selected conditions are not typically life-threatening and can be managed by more conservative means. These conditions are relative indications for the initiation of dialysis. These include azotemia in the absence of uremia, hypercalcemia, hyperuricemia, hypermagnesemia, and uremic bleeding.

ABSOLUTE INDICATIONS

Uremia. Historically, uremic encephalopathy and hyperkalemia were the absolute indications for the initiation of dialysis [36]. The degree of clinical improvement observed with these woefully inadequate quantities of dialysis is rather remarkable. Of the complications of uremia, none are corrected as dramatically as those of the central nervous system. This complication of renal failure improves rapidly with the institution of an adequate dialysis regimen. Tremor, asterixis, diminished cognitive function, neuromuscular irritability, seizures, somnolence, and coma are all reversible manifestations of uremia that merit the initiation of dialysis [37].

Reversible cardiopulmonary complications of uremia, such as uremic pericarditis and uremic lung, respond to the initiation of an adequate dialysis regimen, but clinical resolution is more protracted than for the CNS manifestations of uremia [38,39]. Uremic pericarditis is defined by the presence of sterile inflammation of both layers of the pericardium. It is accompanied by pericardial neovascularization and the development of a serofibrinous exudative effusion. As a consequence of the injudicious use of systemic anticoagulation during dialysis for uremic pericarditis, intrapericardial hemorrhage and cardiac tamponade may occur. In untreated patients, however, spontaneous tamponade will occur. In addition, uremic pericarditis may be associated with systolic dysfunction of the left ventricle as well as serosal inflammation with pleural hemorrhage. Uremic lung is a poorly understood late pulmonary complication of uremia that refers to a roentgenographic pattern of atypical pulmonary edema that is not necessarily associated with elevated pulmonary capillary wedge pressures. It is treated by the initiation of dialysis.

There is a poor correlation between the BUN and the development of uremic signs and symptoms. The BUN is determined by the degree of renal insufficiency, dietary protein intake, hepatocellular function, and protein catabolic rate. Therefore, it is unsurprising that uremic manifestations can occur with a BUN less than 100 mg/dl. In addition to the absolute value, the temporal rate of increase of the BUN seems to influence the development of uremia. Patients with a sudden and rapid decline in renal function, such as those with ARF, typically manifest uremic symptoms at lesser degrees of azotemia than do patients with more gradual declines in renal function, such as those with chronic progressive renal failure. This is especially true in uremic encephalopathy. Lastly, selected patient populations, such as children, the elderly, and individuals with diabetes mellitus, manifest uremic symptoms sooner.

The initiation of dialysis for uremia is associated with only two management issues relevant to the dialysis prescription. The first of these, and an interesting paradox of dialytic therapy for uremia, is that the greater the patient's symptomatic need for dialysis, the less intense can be the initial provision of dialysis. This is because a rapid reduction in the BUN is associated with the sudden development of an admixture of neurologic symptoms ranging from restlessness, headache, nausea, and vomiting to confusion, tremors, myoclonic twitching, seizures, coma, and even death [37,40]. Described as the "dysequilibrium syndrome," it apparently arises as a consequence of delayed equilibration of cerebral osmolality to declining serum osmolality with dialysis. Therapeutic strategies to prevent dysequilibrium are discussed in greater detail in a later section. They involve modifications of the dialysis prescription to limit fluctuations in serum osmolality during solute clearance.

The second issue is that the structurally unstable neovascularization associated with uremic serositis can result in devastating local bleeding into the pericardial sac. Therefore, anticoagulation during dialysis for uremic pericarditis should be "regional" (inclusive of the extracorporeal dialytic circuit) or should be withheld altogether. Typically, this poses no significant problems for the performance of hemodialysis. Because the occurrence of severe platelet dysfunction is associated with untreated, advanced renal insufficiency (uremic thrombocytopathy), anticoagulation is frequently unnecessary during the initiation of dialysis.

Hyperkalemia. During the course of progressive renal insufficiency, the capacity to excrete potassium is compromised, and the adaptive cellular uptake of potassium declines [41]. Although hyperkalemia is a frequent complication during the course of renal failure, its severity and the degree of renal insufficiency at which it is first noted are influenced by the cause of renal failure, comorbid conditions, medications administered, and the exogenous potassium load (see Chap. 79). For example, ARF that complicates the tumor lysis syndrome, crush injuries, rhabdomyolysis, hyperthermia, burns, hemolytic uremic syndrome/thrombotic thrombocytopenic purpura, disseminated intravascular coagulation, sepsis with high fevers, and extensive orthopedic injuries may be associated with severe and rapidly developing hyperkalemia due to hypercatabolism and cytolysis. Although renal insufficiency complicating parenchymal liver disease is not typically associated with early-occurring hyperkalemia, upper gastrointestinal bleeding predisposes the patient to the development of hyperkalemia.

Medications administered during the course of renal failure may contribute to the evolution of hyperkalemia. These drugs interfere with potassium excretion, alter its transcellular distribution, or contain potassium. Drug-induced hyperkalemia may occur with spironolactone, triamterene, angiotensin-converting enzyme inhibitors, beta-blockers, nonsteroidal anti-inflammatory drugs (NSAIDs), digitalis intoxication, potassium-based salt substitutes, and potassium penicillin preparations [42]. The contribution of blood transfusions to the development of hyperkalemia in patients with renal insufficiency is uncertain. During prolonged ex vivo storage, erythrocytes spontaneously release intracellular potassium, and their half-life in vivo is abbreviated [43,44]. The transfusion of senescent erythrocytes and their relatively hyperkalemic preservative may account for the increase in serum potassium reported when dialysis patients are transfused in the interdialytic interval [45]. The reported increment in the serum potassium concentration was a modest 0.4 mEq/l, however.

Conservative measures to treat hyperkalemia include limiting the daily dietary intake of potassium to less than 2 g per day, discontinuing provocative medications, augmenting potassium excretion from the gastrointestinal tract and urine, altering its transcellular distribution, and limiting its cardiotoxicity. For nonemergent hyperkalemia (neither EKG changes nor symptoms), augmenting potassium excretion by the gastrointestinal tract and in the urine may be adequate acute therapy. Enhanced gastrointestinal clearance of potassium can be induced with oral or rectal administration of a cation exchange resin such as sodium polystyrene sulfonate (Kayexalate). Oral polystyrene sulfonate is typically administered every 2 hours as a 15- to 30-gm slurry mixed with a bowel cathartic such as 70% sorbitol. Rectal polystyrene sulfonate is given every 45 minutes as a high retention enema of 60 gm mixed in 200 ml of water. Because rectal administration of sorbitol can cause colonic epithelial necrosis, Kayexalate enemas must not be mixed with sorbitol [46]. In addition, a recent report suggests that the administration of oral Kayexalate with sorbitol within the first postoperative week can induce intestinal necrosis [47]. With optimal cation exchange and bowel evacuation, polystyrene sulfonate can induce the loss of 30 mEq per hour of potassium, in comparison to the maximal 12 mEq per hour that can be eliminated by peritoneal dialysis [48]. This value for potassium elimination rivals the amount eliminated by conventional hemodialysis. Because sodium is the cation exchanged for potassium, however, volume expansion can limit the usefulness of polystyrene sulfonate. In addition, if the patient is responsive to diuretics, the administration of furosemide alone or with metolazone will induce a kaliuresis. Such urinary losses of potassium with sodium must be monitored to prevent hypovolemia.

If hyperkalemia is sufficiently severe to produce electrocardiographic alterations and (or) symptoms, therapy is of greater urgency [49]. Typically, such life-threatening complications of hyperkalemia do not occur until the potassium exceeds 7.5 mEq/l, but significant variability exists between the degree of hyperkalemia and the development of symptoms and signs. Typically, patients with chronic renal failure and prior episodes of hyperkalemia have acclimated to this metabolic disturbance. In contrast, hyperkalemia in the setting of ARF occurs with such rapidity that it is poorly tolerated. Because the response to the therapeutic strategies outlined earlier is delayed, the management for symptomatic hyperkalemia focuses on minimizing cardiotoxicity. This is accomplished acutely by the administration of calcium salts such as calcium gluconate (10 ml of a 10% solution every 1 to 5 minutes up to a maximal volume of 100 ml) that directly antagonize the membrane depolarizing action of hyperkalemia. Because hypercalcemia enhances the pharmacologic effect of cardiac glycosides, extreme care must be exercised by the administration of calcium salts to patients on digoxin. The biologic effect of calcium salts is dramatic and begins within minutes. Unfortunately, its effect is short-lived.

Cardiac toxicity from hyperkalemia can be diminished further by acutely augmenting its cellular uptake and lowering the plasma concentration. Transcellular potassium shifts can be induced by acute systemic alkalization, increasing the systemic level of insulin, and administering beta$_2$-agonists. The conventional mechanism of alkalization for hyperkalemia is the administration of 45 mEq of bicarbonate over 5 minutes, with supplemental dosing after 30 minutes as needed. The clinical effect of bicarbonate is noted within 30 to 60 minutes and persists for several hours. As part of the adaptive mechanism

to acute systemic alkalization, protons move from the cells, and to maintain electrical neutrality, potassium shifts to an intracellular location. In patients with advanced renal insufficiency, alkalization as a solitary therapy for hyperkalemia is not particularly effective, and volume expansion from the sodium limits total dose [50].

Hyperinsulinemia acutely lowers the serum potassium by direct stimulation of the Na^+-K^+ ATPase of skeletal muscle [51]. Plasma insulin levels may be increased acutely by the administration of parenteral glucose (100 ml of 50% dextrose) or the direct administration of intravenous insulin (10 units of regular insulin, with or without dextrose). Glucose infusion alone is less effective than the combination of insulin and glucose and obviously cannot be used in patients with diabetes mellitus. Although the glycemic response in patients with chronic renal failure is attenuated compared to that in healthy individuals, potassium uptake is not altered [52]. Potassium uptake begins approximately 15 minutes after insulin administration. The maximal clinical benefit is noted in approximately 60 minutes and persists for several hours.

Similarly, by augmenting activity of the Na^+-K^+ ATPase, beta-agonists effectively reduce the serum potassium concentration by approximately 1 mEq per liter in 30 to 60 minutes. Specific agonists include albuterol sulfate (0.5 mg intravenously over 10 minutes or 20 mg in 4 ml of saline intranasal) and epinephrine (0.05 μg per kg per minute intravenously) [42,50,53,54]. Interestingly, the alpha-agonist effect of epinephrine attenuates its capacity to induce a transcellular shift of potassium [55].

An improved therapy for hyperkalemic patients with advanced renal failure is the concomitant administration of alkali, insulin, and a beta-agonist [42]. The combination of therapies for life-threatening hyperkalemia is particularly effective and allows adequate time for the institution of a regimen that will diminish the total body potassium load. For those few patients that cannot be treated by more conservative means, dialysis should be performed. As stated earlier, hemodialysis is the most efficient dialytic modality for the elimination of potassium, but it is not much more effective than an optimal response to polystyrene sulfonate.

Hypervolemia. Excessive volume expansion is a common complication of renal insufficiency, both in and out of the hospital settings. For an outpatient with established renal failure, overzealous fluid intake and dietary indiscretion are typical contributors to hypervolemia. For hospitalized patients, the obligatory volume of fluids, medications, and food administered to care for the patient can often exceed the excretory capacity of even patients with nonoliguric renal failure.

Some of the specific medical interventions that incite hypervolemia are worthy of review. In the absence of intravascular volume monitoring, parenteral fluid challenges are typically administered to patients with ARF to correct suspected hypovolemia. In such cases, the therapeutic result often is the development of mild hypervolemia. An excessive sodium load administered as the sodium salt of medications (such as sodium penicillins), hyperalimentation, alkali loads (such as sodium citrate or bicarbonate), and cation exchange resins (such as sodium polystyrene sulfonate) are often unappreciated contributors to the development of hypervolemia. Another scenario is a critically ill patient whose nutritional needs have not been fully met during the hospitalization. Such a patient has a loss of lean mass of up to 0.5 to 1.0 kg per day. The inappropriate matching of sensible and insensible losses in these patients results in the maintenance of a stable weight at the expense of expansion of the patient's body water.

The mainstay of therapy for prevention of hypervolemia and for the urgent and emergent treatment of hypervolemia is the administration of diuretics. Even patients with advanced renal insufficiency (glomerular filtration rate [GFR] <15 ml per min) may respond to optimal doses of loop diuretics. These agents are highly protein-bound and depend upon tubular secretion, not GFR, for entry into the luminal side of the tubular loop. Because their efficacy depends upon the administration of a threshold dose [56], an inadequate response after a single dose should be countered by doubling the dose. It is not unusual to require 400 mg of furosemide or 10 mg of bumetanide intravenously to induce an optimal diuretic response. Because of the greatly increased risk of ototoxicity, ethacrynic acid should be avoided. If an inadequate response occurs, the efficacy of the loop diuretic can be enhanced by administering it as a continuous infusion that maintains the tubular concentration in excess of the threshold [57], combining it with salt poor albumin to diminish the volume of distribution [58], and including a thiazide diuretic to diminish sodium reabsorption at an additional nephron segment. Even in the absence of an adequate diuretic effect, the vasodilatory response to parenteral furosemide can be of therapeutic benefit in cases of emergent hypervolemia [59]. Osmotic cathartics such as sorbitol can be used to induce significant gastrointestinal losses of fluid. Additionally, nitrates and parenteral narcotics can be used to temporize the patient until more definitive therapy is instituted.

The absence of an adequate diuretic response (diuresis that is adequate to meet the volume challenge from obligatory fluids) is an absolute indication for dialysis. Fluid removal can be accomplished by hemodialysis, hemofiltration, or peritoneal dialysis (ultrafiltration). Ultrafiltration rates of more than 3 liters per hour can be achieved during hemodialysis, 1 to 2 liters per hour during hemofiltration, and less than 1 liter per hour during peritoneal dialysis.

Acidosis. As renal function declines, endogenously generated organic acids and exogenously ingested acids are retained, and the capacity to generate and reclaim bicarbonate becomes increasingly compromised [60]. Typically, endogenous acid generation occurs at a rate of 1 mEq/kg/day, resulting in a decline in the serum bicarbonate concentration by ~2 mEq per liter [61]. Therefore, in patients with renal insufficiency, metabolic acidosis is the typical acid-base disturbance. The severity of the acidosis will be influenced by comorbid occurrences such as the loss of gastric acid secondary to vomiting or nasogastric suctioning or the concurrent administration of alkali. In patients with ESRD treated by dialysis, the steady-state serum bicarbonate concentration is influenced by the dialytic modality, type of alkali in the dialysate, frequency of dialysis, and interdialytic weight increase [60]. For hemodialysis patients dialyzed against acetate buffered dialysates, the usual serum bicarbonate is 17 mEq per liter; for hemodialysis patients dialyzed against bicarbonate buffered dialysates, the serum bicarbonate concentration is 21 mEq per liter; and for chronic ambulatory peritoneal dialysis patients dialyzed against lactate buffered dialysates, serum bicarbonate concentration is 26 mEq per liter.

Metabolic acidosis in renal insufficiency is usually well tolerated until the systemic pH declines below 7.2. Less severe acidosis may be corrected by administration of oral alkali in the form of sodium bicarbonate or a metabolized alkali equivalent such as sodium citrate. The usual dose of either of these compounds is 0.5 to 1.0 mEq per day, which is sufficient to match endogenous acid production in nonhypercatabolic patients. Although sodium citrate is more palatable than sodium bicarbonate, acute aluminum intoxication can occur in the setting of the ingestion of citrate and aluminum [62]. The citrate stabilizes enteral aluminum in aqueous solution by forming an aluminum salt and enhances intestinal epithelial absorption [63]. Therefore, patients on sodium citrate must not receive aluminum hydroxide as a dietary phosphate binder.

Both bicarbonate and citrate are administered as sodium salts. Therefore, volume expansion can limit the capacity to correct systemic acidosis. In these circumstances, or if emergent therapy is required, dialysis is indicated. During the performance of hemodialysis, alkali is provided as bicarbonate or acetate. In contrast, lactate is the buffer used for peritoneal dialysis or continuous hemofiltration. Acetate is no longer available in peritoneal dialysates because of their causal relationship to the development of peritoneal fibrosis [64].

RELATIVE INDICATIONS. Nonlife-threatening indications for dialysis can typically be managed by more conservative interventions. All of the absolute indications defined in the previous section may provoke consideration of dialysis when present to a lesser extent. For example, a hypercatabolic trauma patient with acute renal failure manifest by a rapidly increasing serum potassium concentration, declining serum bicarbonate concentration, falling urine output, and a mildly diminished sensorium does not fulfill any of the absolute criteria for the initiation of dialysis. In such a case, however, the need for dialysis is inevitable, and the patient's care is not improved by withholding dialysis until one of the life-threatening complications of renal failure has developed.

Hypercalcemia and hyperuricemia associated with ARF are common in patients with malignancies and tumor lysis syndrome, respectively [65,66]. Hypermagnesemia in renal failure is usually the result of the injudicious use of magnesium containing cathartics or antacids [67]. These metabolic disorders are readily corrected by deletion of the excessive electrolyte from the dialysate. For example, hypercalcemia that is unresponsive to conventional conservative interventions may be corrected by hemodialysis with a reduced calcium dialysate (<2.5 mEq per liter).

Gastrointestinal and dermatologic bleeding are common manifestations of platelet dysfunction in renal insufficiency. The hemostatic defect of renal insufficiency that best illustrates the impairment of platelet aggregation and adherence is the typical three-fold prolongation of the bleeding time [68]. The mechanisms for platelet dysfunction in renal insufficiency include (1) anemia that alters the flow pattern within the vasculature, thereby diminishing the physical interaction between the platelets and the endothelium; (2) decreased binding of Von Willebrand factor to the platelet receptor; and (3) increased endothelial generation of nitric oxide [68–71]. Although either peritoneal or hemodialysis will correct the platelet defect [72,73], more conservative therapies are available. Platelet dysfunction can be rapidly corrected by: (1) erythrocyte transfusion to a hematocrit level above 35% [69], (2) infusion of 10 units of cryoprecipitate, which is rich in von Willebrand factor, every 12 to 24 hours, [74], or (3) intravenous (0.3 μg per kg), or subcutaneous (0.3 μg per kg) administration of deamino-8-D-arginine vasopressin (DDAVP), which induces the endothelial release of factor VIII - von Willebrand multimers [75]. Although not uniformly effective and of diminishing benefit after repeated administration, DDAVP is the safest and most rapid way to correct the platelet defect of renal insufficiency. Interventions that produce a more protracted response that have a delayed onset of action are the administration of erythropoietin [76], conjugated estrogens (0.6 mg per kg for 5 days), or Premarin (25 mg per day for 7 days) [77,78].

Prophylactic Dialysis and Residual Renal Function

In the absence of absolute indications, the decision to initiate dialysis for ARF alone or for acute superimposed upon chronic renal failure is often subjective. This is because there is only a very limited body of data that specifically attempts to address the issue of the timing of dialysis in this setting (i.e., prophylactic dialysis). In a small prospective study of eighteen patients with posttraumatic ARF, the subjects were randomized into one of two clinical treatment groups: low BUN group (frequent and early hemodialysis to maintain predialysis BUNs and serum creatinine concentrations of <70 and 5.0 mg per dl, respectively) and high BUN group (hemodialysis not initiated until predialysis BUN and creatinine of approximately 150 and 10 mg per dl, respectively, were reached, or until uremic complications developed). Because of the inefficiency of the hemodializers and the patients' hypercatabolic states, the low BUN group required daily dialysis to stay within the defined parameters. Within the low BUN group, only 36% of the patients died, whereas 80% of the high BUN patients died [79]. Interestingly, death most often resulted from infections and hemorrhaging. Although the results appear to be plain, the design of this study did not permit the exclusion of patients with milder forms of ARF who would have done well even without dialysis. Further, the sample size was extremely small, and the evaluation of the patients' nutritional status and antibiotic selection were not given.

In an attempt to clarify these issues, a second larger study was instituted that segregated its thirty-four patients by medical and surgical causes of ARF [80]. The study design was altered such that all patients initiated hemodialysis at a serum creatinine concentration above 8.0 mg per dl; this prevented the inclusion of patients with presumably milder forms of ARF. After dialysis was initiated, the patients were dialyzed to target BUN and creatinine values of less than 60 and 5.0 mg per dl (low BUN group) or approximately 100 and 9.0 mg per dl, respectively (high BUN group). Therefore, this study addressed the issue of dialysis intensity in the setting of ARF rather than the timing of initiation of dialytic therapy. No difference in patient mortality was observed between the two groups (41% for the low and 53% for the high BUN groups). On the basis of these data, it appears that early intense dialysis to maintain low BUN and creatinine values is of no proven benefit.

A critical variable in this analysis, however, is the influence of dialysis on residual renal function and the length of recovery from ARF. Numerous observations have suggested an important and potentially deleterious interaction between the initiation of dialysis and residual renal function. Several investigators have observed that patients with posttraumatic ARF who were treated by hemodialysis had pathologically demonstrable fresh, focal areas of tubular necrosis 3 to 4 weeks after the original hemodynamic insult [81,82]. The only recent hemodynamic insult sustained by these patients was short-lived hypotension, characteristic of that hypotension frequently observed during hemodialysis. Further, the institution of hemodialysis is often associated with an acute decline in urine output that is typically ascribed to the intradialytic clearance of sodium, urea, and water [83]. The institution of hemodialysis for acute ischemic renal failure may be associated with a prolongation in recovery [84,85]. Lastly, for patients with advanced chronic renal failure, the institution of hemodialysis results in a progressive decline in glomerular filtration rate over several months [86,87]. Interestingly, peritoneal dialysis does not provoke a similar relentless, and accelerated, decline in residual renal function. As dis-

cussed in greater detail in later sections, these deleterious effects may be a consequence of dialysis-induced hypotension and abnormal compensatory vascular responses [88], and complement activation by the dialysis membrane resulting in complement-mediated immunologic injury [84,89]. In summary, these observations suggest that the dialysis procedure may have significant and potentially deleterious ramifications for the patient with ARF, ARF superimposed on chronic renal failure, or chronic renal failure alone. In view of the questionable benefit of prophylactic dialysis, the physician must avoid the temptation to intervene with dialysis during the course of ARF to simply lower an asymptomatic increase in the BUN and creatinine.

Preserving residual renal function is of significant benefit in the management of patients with advanced renal insufficiency [90]. Even modest preservation of urine output simplifies the management of the patient's volume status and permits liberalization of fluid intake. A residual glomerular filtration rate of approximately 15 ml per minute is equivalent to 5 hours of hemodialysis with a dialyzer having a urea clearance of 160 ml per minute. For the patient on hemodialysis, the effect of residual renal function is disproportionately great for the clearance of larger solutes (>500 daltons) that are minimally cleared by conventional hemodialysis. For patients treated by peritoneal dialysis, which is much less efficient than hemodialysis, preserving residual renal function is even more critical. For some individuals treated by CAPD, adequate dialysis depends upon both solute clearance from dialysis and the patient's endogenous renal function. For example, in comparison to an anuric patient treated with CAPD, who exchanges 8 liters of dialysate per day, a residual glomerular filtration rate of only 3 ml per minute increases the clearance of urea by approximately 50%.

Because it is useful for adjusting drug dosing in renal failure and for evaluating a patient's recovery from ARF, the residual renal clearance of a marker solute in a hemodialysis patient is calculated by:

$$BUN_{avg} = (BUN_{post\ HD} + BUN_{pre\ HD})/2$$
and
$$clearance_{urea} = (V \times urea_u)/(T \times BUN_{avg})$$

in which $BUN_{post\ HD}$ and $BUN_{pre\ HD}$ are the blood urea concentrations at the end and at the beginning of the dialysis session that flank the 48-hour interdialytic interval, V is the urine volume in the 48-hour interdialytic interval, $urea_u$ is the concentration of urea in the collected urine, and T is the duration of the urine collection (typically 48 hours). By substituting the appropriate creatinine concentrations in this formulation, the clearance of creatinine is computed in an identical manner. In comparison to either value alone, the average of the clearance$_{urea}$ and the clearance$_{creatinine}$ may provide a more accurate measurement of the glomerular filtration rate [91]. For nonoliguric patients on peritoneal dialysis, residual renal function can be calculated by the conventional timed urine collection.

Practical Application of Engineering Principles

HEMODIALYSIS AND HEMOFILTRATION

Clearance. During the performance of hemodialysis, solutes such as potassium and urea are moved from the blood into the dialysate by diffusion. Likewise, the translocation of solutes such as bicarbonate or calcium from the dialysate into the blood is also driven by diffusion. Diffusion can be expressed by Fick's Law as:

$$J = -DA \times (dc/dx)$$

where J is the solute flux, D its diffusivity, A the area available for diffusion, and dc the change in the concentration of the solute over the distance, dx. For a particular model dialyzer, the dx is constant, and for an individual solute, D is constant. Expressed in a more practical manner for dialysis:

$$K = Q_{Bi} (C_{Bi} - C_{B0})/C_{Bi}$$

In this expression, K is the diffusive clearance of the solute from the blood, Q_{Bi} the rate of blood flow into the dialyzer that contains the solute, C_{Bi} the concentration of the solute in the blood entering the dialyzer (arterial end), and C_{B0} the remaining concentration of the solute in the egress side of the blood compartment ("venous end") [92]. This mathematical description is accurate for the situation in which the solute is not initially present in the dialysate ($C_{Di} = 0$), the dialysate passes through the dialyzer only once (single-pass dialysate system), and there is no convective transport of the solute during its clearance. Thus, the clearance of a solute during dialysis may be functionally defined as the volumetric removal of the solute from the patient's blood. Within the practical application of this formulation, the clearance of a solute can be modified by altering the patient's blood flow into the dialyzer (Q_{Bi}).

A similar relationship exists for the dialysate and the diffusive clearance of a solute from the blood:

$$K = Q_{Di} (C_{D0} - C_{Di})/C_{Bi}$$

in which Q_{Di} is the flow rate of the dialysate into the dialyzer and C_{D0} and C_{Di} are the concentrations of solute at the dialysate outlet and inlet ends of the hemodialyzer, respectively [92]. Therefore, an additional means of augmenting the diffusive clearance of a solute from blood to the dialysate, or vice versa, is to increase the dialysate flow rate.

Practically, increases in the Q_{Bi} and Q_{Di} increase the clearance of a solute to an asymptote that is defined by the specific dialyzer and the solute. As blood and dialysate flow rates are increased, resistance and turbulence within the dialyzer increase. The result is nonlinear flow and a decline in the clearance per unit flow of blood or dialysate. For conventional dialyzers, this limitation occurs for blood and dialysate flow rates above 300 and 500 ml per minute; for high-flux dialyzers, this limitation is observed at blood and dialysate flow rates above 400 and 800 ml per minute. In choosing a dialyzer for the clearance of a particular solute, such as urea, creatinine, uric acid, dextrose, vitamin B_{12}, inulin, or cytochrome C, it is important to remember that these values are typically determined in vitro in the absence of protein. Therefore, Gibbs-Donnan effects, protein binding, membrane interactions, and solute aggregation are not taken into account, and the "diffusive dialysance" in vivo may be different [93]. Nonetheless, the capacity to compare this aspect of the performance between various dialyzers is important in planning the patient's dialysis prescription.

Solutes that are larger than 300 daltons, such as vitamin B_{12} or β_2-microglobulin, have low K values compared to smaller solutes, such as urea and potassium. The clearance of these larger solutes from blood depends upon ultrafiltration and the passive movement of solute (convective transport). The summary interaction between the diffusive clearance and convective transport of a solute is expressed as:

$$J = (K \times [1 - Q_f/Q_{Bi}] + Q_f) \times C_{Bi} = K'C_{Bi}$$

in which Q_f is the ultrafiltration rate and K' is the sum of the convective and diffuse clearances [92,94]. If the diffusive clearance (K) is large, as is true for urea, the influence of the ultrafiltration rate is not great. As the diffusive clearance for a solute declines because of increasing size (value of K approaches Q_f), the contribution of convective transport to solute movement increases greatly [95].

The practical application of convective transport of solutes is observed during hemofiltration. These techniques are performed by passing the patient's blood through a dialyzer that has great hydraulic permeability but is able to retain protein and cellular elements [96]. During hemofiltration, ultrafiltration is accomplished by either the generation of a positive pressure gradient on the blood side of the hemofilter or a negative pressure on the dialysate side.

Ultrafiltration. An equally important operational component of the dialysis procedure is the "ultrafiltration coefficient" (K_F), defined by:

$$K_F = Q_F/P_B - P_D$$

in which Q_F is the ultrafiltration rate and P_B and P_D the mean pressures in the blood and dialysate compartments, respectively [92,94]. Analogous to the information derived for the clearance of a particular solute for a specific dialyzer, each dialyzer also has an ultrafiltration coefficient. Because these values are typically derived in vitro, similar limitations exist for their application to the in vivo situation. Therefore, it is not unusual for the ultrafiltration coefficient in vitro to be amiss by 10% to 20% in either direction.

The ultrafiltration coefficient for a dialyzer operationally defines the volume of ultrafiltrate formed for a given pressure across the dialysis membrane per unit time (ml/mm Hg/hour). Therefore, it is possible to use the ultrafiltration coefficient to calculate the quantity of pressure that must be exerted across the dialysis membrane (transmembrane pressure) to achieve a given volume of ultrafiltration during a dialysis session. To make this calculation, it is first necessary to quantitate the pressure that is exerted across the dialysis membrane from the blood to the dialysate compartment. During ultrafiltration, the serum oncotic pressure increases in the blood compartment from the arterial to the venous ends, but it is a negligible biophysical factor. Therefore, the net pressure across the dialysis membrane that arises from the flow of blood and dialysate is calculated by:

$$P_{net} = (P_{Bi} - P_{B0})/2 - (P_{Di} + P_{D0})/2$$

in which P_{Bi}, P_{B0}, P_{D0}, and P_{Di} are the pressures measured at the inflow and outflow ports of the blood and dialysate compartments, respectively. If the P_{net} is too low to provide for adequate ultrafiltration during a dialysis session ($P_{net} \times$ ultrafiltration coefficient $\times$ dialysis time <target ultrafiltrate volume), additional pressure can be generated across the dialysis membrane by creating negative pressure in the dialysate compartment or positive pressure in the blood compartment.

For example, a patient with a 2.0-kg interdialytic weight gain who undergoes hemodialysis for 4 hours with a dialyzer that has an ultrafiltration coefficient of 4.0 ml/mm Hg/hr would require a transmembrane dialyzer pressure of 125 mm Hg to achieve the desired 2000 ml weight loss. If the P_{net} is only 75 mm Hg, an additional 50 mm Hg would be required as negative pressure during the dialysis session. If additional volume were to be removed, the negative pressure would have to be increased accordingly. During hemofiltration, added driving pressure for ultrafiltration is produced across the dialysis membrane by generating both positive and negative pressures. The effective pressure required to achieve a particular intradialytic weight loss is described as the transmembrane pressure (TMP) and is calculated by:

$$TMP = desired\ weight\ loss/(ultrafiltration\ coefficient \times dialysis\ time)$$

The performance of ultrafiltration during hemodialysis has been greatly simplified by the development of dialysis machines that possess ultrafiltration control systems (ultrafiltration controller). Ultrafiltration with these devices is remarkably precise, and weight loss is effected in a linear manner [97]. Hemodialysis with high porosity dialyzers, some having massive ultrafiltration coefficients as great as approximately 55 ml/mm Hg/hour ("high flux hemodialysis"), is unsafe without an ultrafiltration controller.

Typically during hemodialysis, ultrafiltration and clearance are performed simultaneously. However, it is possible to temporally segregate the two procedures by a modification of the hemodialysis procedure described as "sequential ultrafiltration-clearance" [98,99]. This modification of the conventional hemodialysis procedure is accomplished by first ultrafiltering the desired volume, followed by the performance of diffusive clearance without ultrafiltration. During the initial ultrafiltration phase, diffusive clearance is prevented by not circulating dialysate through the dialyzer. During the second phase, no negative pressure is instituted, and fluid losses secondary to P_{net} are balanced by the infusion of saline. Sequential ultrafiltration-clearance has distinct hemodynamic advantages over conventional hemodialysis, such that it is a particularly useful technique for large volume fluid removal over a short interval. When ultrafiltration is performed concurrently with diffusive solute clearance, intravascular volume losses may exceed the rate of translocation of fluid from the interstitium. If these losses are not counterbalanced by an appropriate increase in the peripheral vascular resistance and venous refilling, hypotension occurs [98–103]. With sequential ultrafiltration-clearance, these hemodynamic abnormalities are attenuated, such that up to 4 liters per hour may be removed. Unfortunately, unless the total time allotted to dialysis is increased during sequential ultrafiltration-clearance, solute clearance will be compromised and inadequate dialysis will occur.

During hemofiltration, ultrafiltration is governed by different physical principles than those for hemodialysis. Because the driving force for blood flow during arteriovenous hemofiltration is the mean arterial pressure, and the resistance in the blood path that arises from the hemofilter and the lines is low, the hydraulic pressure in the blood compartment of the hemofilter is also low. Therefore, during hemofiltration, the driving force for the formation of an ultrafiltrate is the hydrostatic pressure within the ultrafiltrate compartment of the hemofilter. This effective negative pressure (P_h) that is generated by the weight of the column within the ultrafiltration collection line is calculated by:

$$P_h = height\ difference\ between\ the\ hemofilter\ and\ collection\ bag \times 0.74$$

Therefore, to increase or decrease the rate of fluid formation during hemofiltration, the collection bag is either lowered from, or raised to, the level of the hemofilter, respectively. In contrast to hemodialysis, the increase in oncotic pressure at the venous end of the hemofilter is of sufficient magnitude that little ultrafiltration occurs at this end of the device. Because solute clearance is convective in hemofiltration, little clearance occurs at the venous end of the hemofilter. This situation is most likely to occur when the amount of ultrafiltrate formed is maximal and when the blood flow rate through the hemofilter is low.

The ultrafiltrate that is formed during hemofiltration is free of protein with a solute composition that closely resembles plasma water (94). However, because of the constraints of maintaining Gibbs-Donnan equilibrium, cations such as calcium are less well represented, and anions such as chloride are excessively represented in the ultrafiltrate as compared with plasma. These differences are modest, typically <5 mEq per liter. The quantity of a selected solute that is cleared will be determined by the volume of ultrafiltrate formed, by its concentration in the blood (and therefore in the ultrafiltrate), and by the composition of the replacement solution. For example, if hemofiltration results in the formation of 0.5 liter of ultrafiltrate per hour, and the ultrafiltrate and the replacement solution contain 5 mEq per liter and 0 mEq per liter of potassium, respectively, 30 mEq of potassium will be cleared in 12 hours.

It is not unusual for hemofiltration to result in the formation of >500 ml per hour of ultrafiltrate. Although this rate of ultrafiltration is less than that achieved with hemodialysis, the continuous nature of hemofiltration permits the removal of a greater total volume over an extended interval. Because of the capacity to acutely tailor the rate and volume of replacement, greater prospective fluid management can occur with hemofiltration. For example, if the patient is volume overloaded in the setting of oliguric acute renal failure, hemofiltration is allowed to occur without fluid maintain replacement until euvolemia is achieved. Thereafter, an adequate volume of replacement solution is infused to maintain euvolemia. In contrast, if the patient is already euvolemic and nonoliguric, replacement fluid is infused in an adequate volume to match the losses through the hemofilter. It should not be overlooked that the volume of replacement solution that is required can be diminished by minimizing the vertical distance between the hemofilter and the collection bag. However, because clearance is dependent upon convective transport, clearance will likewise be attenuated.

Because there are no commercial replacement solutions for hemofiltration in the United States, these must be individually prepared. Many centers use Ringer's lactate solution (sodium 130 mEq per liter, potassium 4.0 mEq per liter, chloride 109 mEq per liter, lactate 28 mEq per liter, calcium 3.0 mEq per liter) as a replacement solution, but because of its potassium content, it is not ideal for many patients with renal failure. Also, patients with tissue hypoperfusion, and renal and hepatic insufficiency, may not be able to accommodate the lactate load in Ringer's solution. Therefore, most patients are better managed by custom fluid formulations such as that generated for parenteral hyperalimentation. This is particularly advantageous because it allows caloric obligations to be met, volume constraints controlled, and optimization of the electrolyte solution.

The replacement solution can be administered immediately before ("predilutional hemofiltration") or after the hemofilter ("postdilutional hemofiltration"), simultaneously into both locations ("pre-postdilution hemofiltration), or into the peripheral venous circulation [104,105]. Predilution hemofiltration offers the advantage of diluting plasma proteins that effectively lower the thrombogenicity of the hemofilter and increase the ultrafiltration rate for a given hydrostatic pressure. However, this technique also reduces the concentration of solutes in the blood entering the hemofilter and therefore may compromise their clearance. Alternatively, the replacement solution can be administered incompletely before the hemofilter, with the balance being infused immediately after the hemofilter. This offers the advantages of predilutional hemofiltration and avoids the clearance disadvantages.

PERITONEAL DIALYSIS

Clearance. Clearance during the performance of peritoneal dialysis depends on the anatomic and functional status of the peritoneum. The surface area of the human peritoneum is approximately 21,000 cm^2; the area to weight ratio is 284 cm^2 per kg [106,107]. The simplest practical model of solute transport from the peritoneal cavity is based upon a two-compartment model, in which one pool is the dialysate in the peritoneal cavity and the other pool is the extraperitoneal fluid compartment [108]. The unique transport characteristics of a solute during peritoneal dialysis may be defined by its mass transfer coefficient:

$$m = m_t \times A \times (C_B - C_D)$$

in which m_t is mass transfer rate for the solute, A is the effective surface area of the peritoneum, and C_B and C_D are the concentrations of the solute in the blood and dialysate, respectively. The mass transfer rate is the net solute removal per unit time that has occurred during a dialysis exchange. Variations from these formulations occur in vivo because of the contribution of convective transport and bidirectional movement of solutes. If the solute being examined is not present in the dialysate, such as urea or potassium, its clearance is the product of the dialysate volume and the solute concentration in the dialysate. If the solute is infused with the dialysate, such as sodium, its clearance can be determined by subtracting the original quantity from the amount of solute in the dialysate after an exchange is completed.

A useful index of peritoneal dialysis solute efficiency is the plasma clearance rate, which is calculated by dividing the mass transfer rate by the concentration of the solute in the blood. An important practical consideration derived from this formulation is that the instantaneous clearance of a solute from the blood will be greatest at the beginning of an exchange when the dialysate concentration is at its lowest and the blood concentration at its greatest. As the dwell time increases and the dialysate and blood concentrations approach each other, the instantaneous clearance begins to decline to zero. Therefore, solute clearance is optimized during peritoneal dialysis by frequent exchanges with shortened dwell times. For example, the performance of rapid exchanges can increase the clearance of a small solute such as urea by approximately 25% [109].

Shortened dwell times with an increased number of exchanges increase the time spent infusing and draining the dialysate, and decrease the relative amount of time available for contact between the dialysate and the peritoneum. Therefore, at dialysate flow rates above 3.5 liters per hour, solute clearance may begin to decline [110]. A successful alternative to increasing the number of exchanges per unit time is to increase the volume of dialysate per exchange from 2.0 to 3.0 liters. These volumes are usually well tolerated by adults, especially when recumbent. Because ultrafiltration and clearance occur concurrently during peritoneal dialysis, the use of hyperosmolal dialysates augments the clearance of small solutes. In this situation, convective transport is added to diffusive clearance. The use of the maximal 4.25% dextrose-containing dialysate can increase urea clearance by approximately 50% [111,112]. Surprisingly, if the peritoneal vascular surface area is adequate, urea clearance and ultrafiltration are not limited by peritoneal blood flow [113–115]. In patients in shock, the clearance of urea is depressed only by approximately 30%, whereas intraperitoneal vasodilators augment its clearance by only 20%.

Considering that a typical 2 liter exchange of 1.5% dextrose containing dialysate results in the clearance of urea of approximately 20 ml per minute, peritoneal dialysis is a low-efficiency procedure. Therefore, it is unsurprising that this technique is inappropriate for the management of patients with hypercatabolic acute renal failure. Likewise, an acutely ill, maintenance peritoneal dialysis patient who has been on an adequate and stable dialysis regimen when healthy may not achieve adequate clearance for their increased needs on continued peritoneal dialysis. Further, as discussed earlier, the contribution of residual renal function to dialysis adequacy is critical for successful peritoneal dialysis. In a peritoneal dialysis patient, the loss of residual renal function secondary to a severe comorbid illness often heralds the occurrence of inadequate dialysis. Such patients should have their number of exchanges increased empirically or should be considered for a switch to hemodialysis.

Ultrafiltration. By using dextrose as an active osmotic solute, ultrafiltration occurs during peritoneal dialysis. As is the situation for solute clearance, ultrafiltration is maximal at the beginning of an exchange and declines as the gradient declines during the exchange. Even with optimal exchange frequency and volume, ultrafiltration rates during peritoneal dialysis are usually ~700 ml per hour. The ultrafiltrate formed is hypoosmolal to serum, so hypernatremia is a relatively common complication of excessive ultrafiltration.

Components of the Dialysis Process

HEMODIALYSIS AND HEMOFILTRATION

Dialyzers and Hemofilters. Virtually all of the commercial dialyzers available for hemodialysis in the United States are configured as large cylinders packed with hollow fibers through which the blood flows (hollow fiber dialyzer). The dialysate flows through the dialyzer around these fibers. The membrane within these dialyzers is composed of a variety of modified biologic or synthetic materials such as regenerated cellulose, cuprophane, hemophan, cellulose acetate, polysulfone (PS), polymethylmethacrylate (PMMA), and polyacrilonitrile (PAN). The surface area available for solute transport and the filling volume of the blood and dialysate compartments varies significantly among the different membranes. These materials vary in their characteristics for solute transport and ultrafiltration, capacity to interact with cellular and soluble components of the blood ("biocompatibility"), and costs and reuse capacity. The choices of dialyzer for the management of either acute or chronic renal failure are usually dictated by these three variables in this exact rank order.

The development of a wide array of dialyzers and delivery systems with ultrafiltration controllers has simplified the selection of a dialyzer to fulfill a particular solute or ultrafiltration target. An increasingly important and controversial topic in the acute and chronic management of patients with renal insufficiency is membrane selection based upon biocompatibility [116,117]. The interaction of both soluble and cellular components within the blood with the dialysis membrane may be important in the pathobiology of such varied issues as duration of recovery from acute ischemic renal failure [84,85], adverse intradialytic symptoms and signs such as fever, hypotension, and hypoxemia [118–122], immunologic dysfunction and infectious susceptibility [123–125], and the development of beta$_2$-microglobulin amyloidosis [126]. A plethora of alterations of cellular functions and physiologic responses have been described in association with hemodialysis using selected membranes, including the intradialytic generation of complement-derived anaphylatoxins such as C3a and C5a via the alternate complement pathway in vivo [89], induction of enhanced membrane expression of selected granulocyte adhesion molecules such as MAC-1 and LAM-1 in vivo [127,128], inappropriate production of reactive oxygen species such as superoxide by granulocytes in vivo [129], the enhanced monocyte elaboration of endogenous pyrogens such as interleukin (IL)-1, IL-6, and tumor necrosis factor in vitro and perhaps in vivo [119,130–132], altered monocyte phagocytosis in vitro [124], and altered IL-2 receptor expression in vivo [133]. These issues are discussed in detail in two recent reviews [116,117]. Many of the adverse pathobiologic consequences of hemodialysis that arise from membrane interactions are absent or attenuated by dialysis against synthetic membrane materials such as PS, PMMA, and PAN. In contrast, hemodialysis against cellulosic membranes is associated with the greatest number of acute perturbations, and perhaps long-term complications.

Unfortunately, although the synthetic dialysis membranes are more biocompatible, they are typically far more costly than conventional cellulosic dialyzers. A practical reality of the financial constraints imposed by Medicare's fixed funding of the End Stage Renal Disease Program is that few dialysis providers can afford a single dialysis use of these relatively expensive dialyzers. Therefore, in most maintenance hemodialysis facilities, reuse of disposable dialyzers is performed. Dialyzer reuse is a common practice within the United States. In 1990, 70% of the centers reused their dialyzers, and this number has increased yearly [134]. Dialyzer reuse may be performed manually or with an automated rinsing device. Formaldehyde, glutaraldehyde, or paracetic acid (Renalin) is used as a chemical disinfectant. After reuse, dialyzer adequacy is assessed indirectly by measuring the blood compartment volume. In addition, many hemodialysis centers check the dialysis membrane integrity by pressurizing the dialyzer. The safety, efficacy, cost-effectiveness, and morality of this procedure have been closely scrutinized. Most nephrologists feel that neither the patient nor dialyzer reuse personnel are placed at risk if strict quality assurance and control are implemented [135–137]. The reuse of dialyzers is far less common in the acute hemodialysis setting. An additional putative benefit from the reuse of cuprophane dialyzers is the attenuation of the ill-health, dyspnea, nausea, hypotension, leukopenia, and complement-activation observed during the first use of these membranes (first-use syndrome). Thus, if biocompatibility issues are a significant clinical concern and synthetic membranes are unavailable, a reused cellulosic dialyzer can provide intermediate compatibility. The practice of rinsing the dialyzer with a dilute bleach solution to clarify the membrane will return the dialyzer membrane to its original reactivity.

A putative disadvantage of high-flux dialyzers is that their relatively open pore configuration may permit the transmembrane flux of bacterial derived-lipopolysaccharides from the dialysate into the dialyzer blood compartment (backfiltration) [138]. The resultant patient exposure to the pyrogen results in a febrile illness without bacteremia described as a "pyrogen reaction" and may occur more often with reused high-flux dialyzers. The use of bicarbonate-buffered dialysates, which are permissive for the growth of gram negative bacteria, and ultrafiltration controllers that limit the rate of ultrafiltration contributes to the occurrence of pyrogen reactions [138–140].

Hemofilters are available in two geometric configurations: the hollow fiber configuration and the "parallel plate" geometry. Parallel plate dialyzers are series of parallel plates segregating the device into multiple compartments through which either blood or dialysate traverses [141]. Hemofilters are usually composed of PS, PMMA, or PAN. One single report suggests that both ultrafiltration and diffusive clearance may be greater when CAVHD is performed using a hemofilter of the parallel plate geometry [142]. In contrast, performance differences between hemofilters have not been observed with venovenous hemofiltration [143].

Dialysates for Hemodialysis. The composition of the dialysate is the other major component of the dialysis process that determines the outcome of this procedure. Although sodium and potassium are typically the only components of the dialysate that are altered in response to different clinical situations, the other constituents are equally critical. The dialysate is stored as a liquid or powdered concentrate that is diluted in a fixed ratio to yield the final solute concentration. Dialysate concentrates and water can be appropriately proportioned by using on-line measurements of the conductivity of the dialysate prior to its entry into the hemodialyzer.

GLUCOSE. Before hydraulic-driven ultrafiltration became available, the dialysate glucose concentration was maintained at above 1.8 g per dl to generate an osmotic gradient between the blood and the dialysate [144]. Although this was effective for inducing ultrafiltration, some patients developed the morbid symptoms and signs of hyperosmolality. Currently, dialysates are either glucose-free, normoglycemic (0.20–0.25% dextrose) or modestly hyperglycemic (0.25% dextrose). Hemodialysis with a glucose-free dialysate results in a net glucose loss of approximately 30 g and stimulates ketogenesis and gluconeogenesis [145]. Such alterations in intermediary metabolism may be particularly deleterious in chronically or acutely ill hemodialysis patients who are malnourished or on a medication such as propranolol that is provocative for hypoglycemia [146,147]. These effects are ameliorated by the use of a normoglycemic dialysate. Additional metabolic consequences occurring from the use a glucose-free dialysate include an accelerated loss of free amino acids into the dialysate [148], a decline in serum amino acids [149], and enhanced potassium clearance because of relative hypoinsulinemia [145]. Therefore, the dialysate glucose concentration should be maintained at normoglycemic concentrations.

SODIUM. Historically, the dialysate sodium concentration was maintained at hypoosmolal levels (less than 135 mEq per liter) to prevent interdialytic hypertension, exaggerated thirst, and excessive weight gains. Hyponatremic dialysates increase the likelihood of intradialytic hypotension, cramps, headaches, nausea, and vomiting, and are provocative for the dialysis dysequilibrium syndrome [150–154]. During conventional hemodialysis with a hyponatremic dialysate or during the clearance phase of sequential ultrafiltration-clearance, the decline in extracellular volume exceeds the volume ultrafiltered. As solute is removed from the extracellular compartment, there is a relative increase in intracellular osmolality, which drives transcellular volume movement [155]. These hemodynamic alterations are absent in the setting of equal dialysate and serum sodium concentrations. Thus, there has been an appropriate increase the dialysate sodium to 140 to 145 mEq per liter.

Unfortunately, an increase in the dialysate sodium can result in polydipsia and increased interdialytic weight gains [152]. The enhanced capacity to ultrafilter these patients permits ready management of this problem, however. The pressor response to an increased dialysate sodium varies. In patients who are hypertensive because of hyperreninemia during ultrafiltration, a higher dialysate sodium may be associated with a reduction in blood pressure; however, most patients exhibit no increment in blood pressure with a physiologic dialysate sodium concentration [152]. A minority who is typically hypertensive at baseline have worsened pressor control with a higher sodium dialysate [150,153].

The newer dialysate delivery systems permit the active alteration of the sodium concentration during a session by the use of variable-dilution proportioning systems. The technique of "sodium modeling" to fit a patient's hemodynamic needs has been espoused as a mean of accomplishing optimal blood pressure support without increased thirst at the completion of the treatment. The alteration in the dialysate sodium can occur in two patterns. It may be performed in a "step" in which the dialysate sodium concentration is initially high (>145 mEq per liter) and is promptly reduced (~135 mEq per liter) during the second half of the dialysis session, or it may be reduced as a linear "gradient" from above 145 mEq per liter to approximately 135 mEq per liter [156,157]. Although sodium modeling reduces the frequency of hypotension during ultrafiltration without decreasing time committed to diffusive clearance, as is the case with sequential ultrafiltration-clearance, it is unclear if this technique offers any advantage over a fixed dialysate sodium of 140 to 145 mEq per liter [158,159]. Further, interdialytic weight gains appear unaffected by sodium modeling [156–158]. Therefore, for most hemodialysis patients, the dialysate sodium concentration should be maintained at 140 to 145 mEq per liter.

POTASSIUM. Unlike urea, which usually behaves as a solute distributed in a single pool with a variable volume of distribution [160], only 1 to 2% of the 3000 to 3500 mEq of potassium are present in the extracellular space [161]. The flux of potassium from the intracellular compartment to the extracellular space and subsequently across the dialysis membrane to the dialysate compartment is unequal. Therefore, the efficacy of potassium removal in hemodialysis is highly variable, difficult to predict, and influenced by dialysis specific and patient specific factors [162]. In a study that controlled for dialyzer specific components of the dialysis procedure (blood and dialysate flow, dialyzer type and surface area, duration of dialysis, dialysate composition), potassium removal varied by approximately 70%. Even for the same patient, approximately 20% variability in potassium removal was noted using the same hemodialysis prescription [163].

During hemodialysis, approximately 70% of the potassium removed is derived from the intracellular compartment [145]. As 50 to 80 mEq of potassium are removed in a single dialysis session, and only 15 to 20 mEq of potassium are present in the plasma, life-threatening hypokalemia would be the consequence of dialysis if these were not the case [162]. The volume of distribution of potassium is not constant however; the greater the total body potassium, the lower its volume of distribution [164]. The practical consequence of these observations is that the fractional decline in the plasma potassium during a single dialysis session will be greater if the pre-hemodialysis potassium is higher. Therefore, optimal potassium elimination by hemodialysis is accomplished by daily short hemodialysis treatments instead of protracted sessions every other day. The transfer of potassium from the intracellular compartment to the extracellular compartment usually occurs more slowly than the transfer from the plasma across the dialysis membrane [164,165]. This discrepancy further complicates predicting the quantity of potassium removed during hemodialysis. A practical consequence of these discordant transfer rates is that the plasma potassium measured immediately after the completion of hemodialysis is approximately 30% less than the steady state value measured after 5 hours. Therefore, hypokalemia diagnosed immediately after the completion of hemodialysis should not be treated with potassium supplements.

The transcellular distribution of potassium is influenced by several variables, including the relative degree of hyperinsulinemia (promotes potassium uptake into cells and lowers its intradialytic clearance) [145], catecholamine tone (beta-agonists promote cellular uptake of potassium and alpha-agonists stimulate the cellular egress of potassium — attenuate and increase the intradialytic clearance of potassium, respectively) [161,166], sodium-potassium ATPase activity (pharmacologic inhibition diminishes potassium uptake into cells, which may enhance intradialytic clearance) [167], and systemic pH (alkalemia augments transcellular potassium uptake, which may diminish dialytic clearance of potassium) [161]. Surprisingly, although the degree of systemic alkalization is greater and more rapid in onset with bicarbonate-buffered dialysates than with acetate-buffered dialysates, the choice of buffer does not appear to be critical in determining potassium removal during hemodialysis [145,168]. Paradoxically, it has been observed that as the gradient for potassium clearance from blood into the dialysate is increased by decreasing the dialysate potassium concentration, the uptake of bicarbonate from the dialysate declines [169]. This interaction between alkali and potassium in the dialysate is sizable: a 1 mEq increase in the potassium gradient results in a decline in bicarbonate dialysance of 50 mEq. This interaction should not be overlooked in planning the dialysate prescription for patients being dialyzed for severe acidosis.

As the selection of the dialysate potassium is empirical, most patients are dialyzed with a potassium concentration of 1 to 3 mEq per liter. For patients who have excessive potassium loads from their diet, medications, hemolysis, trauma, or gastrointestinal bleeding, the dialysate potassium concentration should be 0 to 1 mEq per liter. For stable patients who do not have significant cardiac disease or who are not taking cardiac glycosides, a dialysate potassium concentration of 2 to 3 mEq per liter is appropriate. In a patient with a history of cardiac disease, especially with arrhythmias and cardiac glycoside usage, the dialysate potassium should be increased to 3 to 4 mEq per liter [170]. Such patients are at the greatest risk for the development of dysrhythmias associated with the potassium flux of hemodialysis. They are best managed by tolerating a greater degree of interdialytic hyperkalemia so that they may receive a higher dialysate potassium concentration.

Most of the cardiac morbidity that arises from the dialysate potassium concentration occurs during the first half of the dialysis session. The rapidity of the fall in the plasma potassium concentration, rather than the absolute plasma concentration, determines the risk of cardiac arrhythmias [165,170]. For this reason, hyperkalemic patients should be managed by an incremental decline in the dialysate potassium concentration of approximately 1.0 mEq per liter per hour [171]. If the patient has a significant deficit in total body potassium, post-dialysis hypokalemia can occur, even if the dialysate potassium concentration is greater than the serum potassium concentration [172]. This seemingly contradictory situation arises because of the potential for a delayed conductance of potassium from the dialysate into the patient, in comparison to its movement from the extracellular space into the intracellular compartment.

BASES. Initially, bicarbonate was used as the buffer in the dialysate. In the early 1960s, it was superseded by acetate, which is stable in aqueous solution at neutral pH in the presence of divalent cations. Acetate is metabolized in skeletal muscle and, to a lesser extent, in the liver, to acetyl CoA, which is subsequently metabolized further via Krebs cycle to carbon dioxide and water. In the latter process, one proton is consumed and one molecule of bicarbonate is liberated [173]. During conventional hemodialysis with large surface area dialyzers, acetate flux above 300 mmol per hour can occur, resulting in acetate accumulation as the amount translocated exceeds the capacity to metabolize the base. This complication occurs most often in women, elderly patients, and patients who are malnourished [174]. The resultant clinical consequences of acetate accumulation include variable degrees of nausea, vomiting, headache, fatigue, peripheral vasodilatation, decreased myocardial contractility, metabolic acidosis, and arterial hypoxemia [60,175–180]. Therefore, it is unsurprising that vascular instability is much more problematic with acetate-buffered dialysates than bicarbonate-buffered dialysates. The hemodynamic instability with acetate is worsened by hyponatremic dialysates and is lessened with a normonatremic dialysate [177,181,182].

Hemodialysis using a bicarbonate-buffered dialysate prevents these complications. The paradoxical anion gap metabolic acidosis associated with acetate dialysis occurs because the intradialytic loss of bicarbonate from blood into the dialysate exceeds the patient's capacity to generate alkali from metabolized acetate. A raised bicarbonate concentration in the dialysate attenuates the diffusive gradient from blood to dialysate. Likewise, dialysis-induced hypoxemia is attenuated by a bicarbonate dialysate. During hemodialysis with acetate, there is a large diffusive loss of carbon dioxide into the dialysate such that the minute ventilation falls by approximately 25%. Therefore, despite the loss of carbon dioxide across the dialytic circuit, there is little decline in the arterial carbon dioxide tension. During hemodialysis with acetate, hypoxemia is most prominent during the first 60 minutes of hemodialysis and may be associated with an approximately 35 mm Hg decline in arterial oxygen tension [183,184].

Because of the amelioration of many intradialytic symptoms with bicarbonate-buffered dialysate and the increased use of high-efficiency and high-flux hemodialysis, acetate is used for hemodialysis in less than 20% of the dialysis facilities in the United States [134]. Bicarbonate dialysis is now feasible because of the widespread availability of proportioning systems that permit mixing of the separate concentrates containing bicarbonate and divalent cations close to the entry point of the final dialysate into the dialyzer [97]. As mentioned earlier, unlike the more acidic and hyperosmolal acetate-buffered dialysate, liquid bicarbonate concentrates and reconstituted bicarbonate dialysate support the growth of gram-negative bacteria such as *Pseudomonas, Acinetobacter, Flavobacterium,* and *Achromobacter,* filamentous fungi, and yeast [140]. Because of the propensity of the dialysate to support bacterial growth and the morbidity associated with the presence of such growth in the dialysate, strict guidelines exist for the acceptable limit of bacterial growth and for the presence of lipopolysaccharide in the dialysate and dialyzer reuse system [185].

For these reasons, a bicarbonate-buffered dialysate of 30 to 35 mEq per liter should be used, if available. Bicarbonate concentrations above 35 mEq per liter may result in the development of a metabolic alkalosis with secondary hypoventilation, hypercapnia, and hypoxemia. If bicarbonate is unavailable, acetate at an equivalent concentration is suitable, but large-surface-area dialyzers or dialyzers with high-efficiency of high-flux solute clearances cannot be used. The dialysate sodium should be maintained at 140 to 145 mEq per liter.

CALCIUM. Patients with renal failure are prone to develop hypocalcemia, hyperphosphatemia, hypovitaminosis D, and hyperparathyroidism. Therefore, positive calcium balance is useful as an adjunct during hemodialysis for controlling metabolic bone disease [186–188]. In patients with renal failure requiring dialysis, 61% of the calcium is not bound to plasma proteins and is in a diffusible equilibrium during hemodialysis [189]. Assuming free conductance of calcium across the dialysis membrane secondary to diffusive clearance and an additional contribution secondary to convective losses, a dialysate calcium concentration of roughly 3.5 mEq per liter (7.0 mg per dl) is necessary to prevent intradialytic calcium losses [190,191]. Because such elevated calcium dialysates transiently induce hypercalcemia, which temporarily reduces parathyroid hormone secretion [192], they used to be the standard for dialysate calcium concentrations.

Over the last decade, increasing and appropriate concerns arose for the development of aluminum intoxication syndromes secondary to the protracted use of oral aluminum hydroxide as a phosphate binder. The three aluminum intoxication disorders, which arise because of the intestinal absorption and retention of ingested aluminum, are progressive osteomalacia, iron-resistant microcytic anemia, and progressive encephalopathy [193–196]. Instead of using aluminum salts alone, calcium carbonate or calcium acetate have been increasingly employed alone or with small quantities of aluminum hydroxide as oral phosphate binders [197,198]. Because variable amounts of calcium are absorbed from the ingested calcium salt, persistent hypercalcemia is a frequent complication of a dialysate calcium of greater than 3.0 mEq per liter, especially if a vitamin D supplement is also used [186]. To minimize the likelihood of hypercalcemia, there is a trend towards lowered dialysate calcium concentrations. In most outpatient dialysis facilities, a dialysate calcium concentration of 2.5 to 3.0 mEq per liter is used. Despite these reduced dialysate calcium concentrations, some patients are still hypercalcemic between dialysis sessions. The combination of a reduced ingested dose of calcium salt and the inclusion of a small quantity of aluminum hydroxide can minimize the risk of hypercalcemia and treat the hyperphosphatemia.

A reduction in the dialysate calcium may increase vascular instability during hemodialysis [199,200]. Dialysis-induced changes in the serum calcium concentration correlate with the intradialytic systolic and diastolic blood pressures. This interaction is secondary to alterations in left ventricular performance without an accompanying alteration in the peripheral vascular resistance [201].

MAGNESIUM. Like potassium, serum magnesium concentration is a poor determinant of total body magnesium stores. Only approximately 1% of the total body magnesium is present in the extracellular fluid, and only 60% of this amount (approximately 25 mEq) is free and diffusible [202]. Because of scant extrarenal clearance, clearance during hemodialysis is the primary route of elimination for magnesium. The magnesium flux that occurs during a dialysis session is difficult to predict despite knowledge of the serum and dialysate magnesium concentrations. When using a low magnesium dialysate, however, the postdialytic decline in serum magnesium concentration is virtually resolved after 24 hours [203].

Because the "ideal" serum magnesium concentration in patients with ESRD is debatable, the appropriate dialysate magnesium concentration is unresolved. Many centers use a 1.0 mEq per liter dialysate magnesium concentration, and mild interdialytic hypermagnesemia is often observed. Although elevated magnesium concentrations impair bone formation in vitro and in vivo, its clinical significance is unresolved [202,204–206]. The reduction of the dialysate magnesium concentration to less than 0.5 mEq per liter has been reported to improve osteomalacic bone pathology and symptoms.

CHLORIDE. Chloride is the major anion in the dialysate. Because its concentration is defined by the constraints of maintaining electrical neutrality in the dialysate, chloride concentration varies depending upon the concentration of the cations.

Dialysates for Hemofiltration. An advantage of CAVHD, CVVHD, CAVHDF, and CVVHDF over conventional hemodialysis is the lack of need for complex dialysate delivery systems. Therefore, the costs and the nursing personnel required to perform hemofiltration are less. Dialysate flow is relatively compromised, however. Typical dialysate flow rates for hemofiltration or hemodiafiltration are 800 to 1000 ml per hour (versus 500 to 800 ml per minute for hemodialysis), and these flow rates are usually delivered by a continuous infusion pump. Because it is impractical to mix and store conventional hemodialysis dialysate for hemofiltration and hemodiafiltration, and the formation of a custom dialysate in the volumes required for these techniques is not feasible, most centers use conventional peritoneal dialysate for CAVHD, CVVHD, CAVHDF, and CVVHDF. Despite the use of a commercially prepared dialysate formulation, it is this component of the hemofiltration procedure that is responsible for the relatively increased cost in comparison to CAVH [207]. Peritoneal dialysate formulations are discussed in greater detail below.

The need for a custom dialysate for hemofiltration most often arises in situations in which the calcium concentration requires modification or the patient cannot tolerate a lactate-buffered dialysate. Commercial dialysates for peritoneal dialysis are available in only three calcium concentrations: 3.5, 3.0, and 2.5 mEq per liter. Such a limited selection of dialysates significantly compromises the treatment of hypercalcemic patients by CAVHD, CVVHD, CAVHDF, CVVHDF, or peritoneal dialysis. If such circumstances arise, the dialysate formula should be tailored to the individual using an appropriately reduced calcium concentration. The standard lactate-buffering of peritoneal dialysates may become problematic for patients with an impaired capacity to metabolize lactate, such as those with lactic acidosis secondary to impaired hepatic and renal function, and hypotensive patients with ongoing tissue ischemia and tissue lactate generation. In these circumstances, a custom dialysate should be formulated with bicarbonate as the buffer.

Anticoagulation for Hemodialysis. Despite the impaired capacity of platelets to aggregate and adhere in most patients with advanced renal failure, the interaction of plasma with the dialysis membrane results in activation of the clotting cascade, thrombosis in the extracorporeal circuit, and the resultant dysfunction of the dialyzer [208]. Dialyzer thrombogenicity is determined by its composition, surface charge, surface area, and configuration [209]. In addition, the propensity for intradialytic clotting is influenced by the blood flow through the dialyzer, the extent of recirculation in the extracorporeal circuit, the amount of ultrafiltration, and the length, diameter, and composition of the lines between the patient and the dialyzer. Patient-specific variables that influence thrombogenicity and determine the requirements for anticoagulants include the presence of congestive heart failure, malnutrition, neoplasia, blood transfusions, and comorbid coagulopathies such as disseminated intravascular coagulation, warfarin therapy, or hepatic synthetic dysfunction [210].

Because of its low cost, ready availability, ease of administration, simplicity of monitoring, and relatively short biologic half-life, the anionic mucopolysaccharide heparin is the most widely used anticoagulant for dialysis (see Chap. 121). The time constraints of hemodialysis are such that the partial thromboplastin time (PTT) cannot be used to monitor the effectiveness of anticoagulation. Instead, an "activated clotting time" (ACT) is used. In this assay, whole blood is mixed with an activator of the extrinsic clotting cascade such as kaolin, diatomaceous earth, or ground glass, and the time necessary for the blood to first congeal is monitored. The normal range is 90 to 140 seconds.

The precise method of administration of heparin is influenced by the patient's comorbid illness and varies among dialysis providers. The simplest method of heparin administration is "systemic" administration, in which 2000 to 5000 units of heparin are administered at the initiation of dialysis followed by the bolus of 1000 units per hour. The target ACT is approximately 50% above baseline. Another method of systemic anticoagulation is to bolus the patient with heparin (100 units per kilogram of dry weight) at the initiation of dialysis. Because the degree of anticoagulation during systemic anticoagulation is relatively intensive, it is appropriate only for stable patients who are at no risk for bleeding. Therefore, in the ICU, systemic anticoagulation is rarely used.

Less intensive anticoagulation is achieved with "fractional" heparinization, in which the target ACT is maintained at 15% ("tight fractional") or 25% ("fractional") greater than the baseline value. Five hundred to 3000 units of heparin are administered at the initiation of dialysis, followed by a continuous infusion at an initial rate of 500 to 1000 units per hour.

Minimal heparinization occurs with "regional" heparinization. By this method, the extracorporeal circuit alone is anticoagulated [211]. Five hundred units of heparin are given at the beginning of dialysis, and 500 to 750 units per hour are infused into the arterial line. Simultaneously, 3.75 mg per hour of protamine are infused into the venous line. Using frequent checks of the ACT from the arterial and venous lines as a guide, the heparin and protamine infusion rates are adjusted to maintain the ACT for the patient at baseline and for the dialytic circuit at approximately 10 seconds. Because heparin has a longer half-life than protamine, an additional 50 mg of protamine should be given at the end of dialysis [212]. Alternatively, regional anticoagulation may be achieved with sodium citrate as the anticoagulant [213]. Citrate binds to calcium and forms a dialyzable salt, thus depleting the extrinsic and intrinsic clotting cascades of the obligatory cofactor calcium. A 45% solution of sodium citrate is initially infused into the arterial line at 30 ml per hour, and the infusion rate is adjusted after 20 minutes to maintain the ACT of the patient and the machine 10 and 25% over baseline, respectively.

If the nursing personnel are not experienced with regional anticoagulation, this technique can be associated with significant and relatively frequent side effects without significant advantage over low-dose heparin [214]. Therefore, in high-risk situations in which regional anticoagulation may be contraindicated (heparin-induced thrombocytopenia, allergy to protamine, personnel unfamiliar with technique), dialysis may be performed without heparin [215,216]. In this technique, the hemodialyzer is first rinsed with 1 liter of 0.45% saline containing 3000 to 5000 units of heparin. Hemodialysis is immediately initiated using the greatest blood flow that can be tolerated, and the dialyzer is flushed every 15 to 30 minutes with 50 ml of saline. This technique is not conducive to large volume ultrafiltration, compromised blood flows, or the intradialytic administration of blood products.

Anticoagulation must be individualized based on the patient's risk of hemorrhage. Clearly, the risk of thrombosis of the dialytic circuit is a secondary consideration. Guidelines for anticoagulation based upon comorbid conditions are

1. Patients who are bleeding, at significant risk of bleeding, have a baseline major thrombostatic defect, or are within 7 days of a major operative procedure or within 14 days of intracranial surgery should be dialyzed without heparin or by regional anticoagulation.
2. Patients who are within 72 hours of a needle or forceps biopsy of a visceral organ should be dialyzed without heparin or by regional anticoagulation.
3. Patients who are beyond the temporal limits established for items 1 and 2 can be dialyzed by fractional heparinization. If they have previously received fractional heparinization, they can now be considered for systemic anticoagulation.
4. Patients with pericarditis should be dialyzed without heparin or by regional anticoagulation.
5. Patients who have undergone minor surgical procedures within the previous 72 hours should be dialyzed under fractional anticoagulation.
6. Patients anticipated to receive a major surgical procedure within 8 hours of hemodialysis should be dialyzed without heparin or by regional anticoagulation. If they are within 8

hours of a minor procedure, fractional anticoagulation is appropriate.

Anticoagulation for Hemofiltration. As with hemodialysis, anticoagulation is usually necessary with hemofiltration. The slower blood flows (50 to 100 ml per hour) are more conducive to intradialytic clotting. Thus, even by modifying the procedure to minimize thrombogenicity (using relatively short arterial and venous lines, changing to a parallel plate configuration for the hemofilter, performing predilutional hemofiltration), heparin is usually required [96,141,217,218]. On the contrary, the use of aggressive ultrafiltration that results in hemoconcentration, reduced blood flows, and the blood passage through long venous lines is very thrombogenic. During hemofiltration, the required intensity of anticoagulation usually is similar to that associated with systemic heparinization for hemodialysis. After a systemic loading dose of heparin, an initial maintenance infusion of approximately 10 units per kg per hour is administered and titrated to maintain the PTT in the arterial line 50% greater than control. Obviously, such concentrated heparinization limits the use of this technique to patients who are not at risk for bleeding. Anticoagulation guidelines for continuous veno-venous hemofiltration are the same as those given for conventional hemodialysis.

Hemofiltration can be performed without heparin. This involves rinsing the kidney and lines with heparinized saline in the method described for heparin-free hemodialysis [219]. The parallel plate configuration for the hemofilter is less thrombogenic and may preserve its clearance to a greater degree than a hollow fiber geometry [141]. Regional anticoagulation can be performed during hemofiltration [220], but it is labor intensive and greatly compromises the utility of hemofiltration. Thrombosis within the hemofilter is easy to recognize by the characteristic striped clotting of the usually white fibers within the hollow fiber dialyzer. Unfortunately, the parallel plate configuration is assembled in such a manner that the interior of the hemofilter cannot be visualized. In this circumstance, clotting of the hemofilter can only be defined inferentially by the decline in the ultrafiltration rate in the absence of decreased mean arterial pressure.

Angioaccess for Hemodialysis and Hemofiltration. For optimal performance of these vascular-based clearance techniques, adequate angioaccess must be established and maintained. The issues relevant to the permanent angioaccess and temporary angioaccess differ, but a few principles are common and critical to both. For example, the angioaccess should be dedicated to the performance of dialysis alone. In the ICU, where the establishment of angioaccess may be problematic, the temptation to use the dialysis access for vascular cannulation must be avoided. Because of prior compromise of arterial and venous vasculature and the unique requirements of blood flow necessary for the performance of dialysis, establishing adequate dialysis angioaccess may be a formidable task for patients with renal failure. This task is typically much more difficult than achieving access for the infusion of fluids or for arterial monitoring that may be routinely required in the intensive care unit. Therefore, routine care to preserve the angioaccess involves: (1) no catheter cannulation of the angioaccess, (2) no phlebotomy, blood pressure measurements, or intravenous catheters in the extremity with the angioaccess, (3) no constricting bandages or dressings over the vascular access, (4) no medication infusions or hyperalimentation through dialysis catheters, and (5) no use of the dialysis catheter to measure central venous pressures.

For maintenance hemodialysis patients, vascular access is established through either the surgical generation of an anas-

tomosis between an artery and a vein ("fistula"), or by the placement of a catheter in a large-caliber vein. For temporary vascular access in hemodialysis patients with ARF or for maintenance hemodialysis patients who are transiently without a fistula but in need of angioaccess, a catheter placed in a large-diameter vein may be used. Similarly, for hemofiltration, angioaccess is typically provided with catheters. Although the type of catheter and its location should be determined by short-term care issues, it should be remembered that the consequences of these decisions may have major ramifications for the subsequent establishment of a permanent angioaccess. For example, because subclavian vein dialysis catheters are associated with subclavian vein stenosis or thrombosis [221,222], temporary dialysis catheters should not be placed in the subclavian vein on the side of an anticipated fistula. Likewise, patent cephalic and basilic veins in the nondominant upper extremity should be preserved in anticipation of a permanent endogenous arteriovenous fistula.

The vascular access of choice for long-term hemodialysis patients is the endogenous arteriovenous fistula native vein fistula. This is because of its ease of construction, long-term survival, and lower incidence of infection compared to other modalities of vascular access [223]. Preferred sites for the generation of an endogenous fistula are the radial artery and the cephalic vein at the wrist or at the anatomic snuffbox, the radial or brachial artery and the median cubital vein near the antecubital fossa, and the brachial artery and the cephalic vein proximal to the elbow. Infrequently, the saphenous vein may be anastomosed to the femoral artery.

Most older patients and diabetics with ESRD do not have adequate arterial and venous anatomy to allow the generation of an endogenous fistula. In these patients, a prosthetic arteriovenous fistula is generated. The most frequently used material for a "graft fistula" is 6-mm polytetrafluoroethylene (PTFE). Common sites of placement and configurations for prosthetic grafts are as a forearm loop graft in a U-configuration between the radial artery and a convenient vein proximal to the antecubital space (preferred site), as a straight graft between the distal radial artery and a convenient vein at the antecubital fossa, as a loop graft between the radial artery and the basilic vein in the mid upper arm, as a straight graft between the brachial artery at the antecubital space and the proximal brachial vein, and as a straight graft between the brachial artery at the antecubital space and the infraclavicular portion of the axillary vein.

Patency rates for fistulae vary greatly. In our center, the 2-year survival for grafts is roughly 70%, whereas for endogenous fistulae, the comparable survival rate is 50% [224]. Early failure of either an endogenous or prosthetic fistula (<1 month after generation) is usually secondary to anatomic inadequacies, such as poor arterial inflow, or to a surgical variance, such as a technically unsatisfactory anastomosis. Late failure (> 1 month after generation) of an endogenous fistula most often is caused by thrombosis and much less frequently is due to local infection or aneurysmal dilatation and dysfunction. In contrast, late failure of a prosthetic graft most often occurs as a result of infection or thrombosis. Most graft infections are secondary to *Staphylococcus aureus* or *Staphylococcus epidermidis* and require therapy with antibiotics and surgical excision. Late-occurring thrombosis arises most often from neointimal proliferation at the venous anastomotic site and typically requires surgical revision. Relevant to the ICU, it should be appreciated that acute thrombosis of either a native vein or graft fistula may occur from dehydration with modest hypotension secondary to overzealous ultrafiltration, systemic hypotension from a comorbid condition like sepsis, or excessively vigorous local pressure for hemostasis after removal of the dialysis needles.

As a precedent to thrombotic failure of the angioaccess, the "venous pressure" in the dialytic circuit (hydraulic pressure in the venous limb of the extracorporeal circuit) becomes raised. The increased venous pressure is a consequence of the impedance to blood return arising in the fistula. In addition to frank thrombosis of the angioaccess, incipient venous occlusion of the fistula decreases the efficiency of hemodialysis. As the laminar flow of blood is increasingly compromised, turbulent non-laminar blood flow occurs within the fistula. Under these conditions, blood returning to the fistula from the dialyzer may regurgitate back to the arterial side of the fistula. This blood, which has already entered the dialyzer once, reenters the dialytic circuit. The overall effect of this recirculation of blood within the dialysis circuit is that the relative percentage of systemic blood entering the dialyzer per unit time declines. Thus, a small volume of blood gets dialyzed very well, but a significant portion of the blood volume does not undergo solute clearance. The percentage of "blood recirculation" during a dialysis treatment can be calculated by

$$100 \times (P_{BUN} - A_{BUN})/(P_{BUN} - V_{BUN})$$

in which P_{BUN}, A_{BUN}, and V_{BUN} are the BUN concentrations measured in the peripheral blood and the arterial and venous dialysis blood lines, respectively. A well functioning fistula will have less than 15 percent circulation. Values greater than this result in compromised solute clearance, which is manifest by hyperkalemia and worsening azotemia that are unexplained by dietary indiscretion and alterations in the dialysis prescription. An increase in the recirculation percentage should prompt an angiographic evaluation of the fistula for outflow obstruction.

Alternatively, acute angioaccess for hemodialysis or hemofiltration may be achieved with vascular catheters. The oldest and safest means of establishing angioaccess for hemodialysis is to place a single- or double-lumen coaxial catheter in the femoral vein by the Seldinger technique [225]. The incidence of serious complication from femoral vein dialysis catheters is only 0.2% [226,227], and they may be left in position for up to 14 days without significant sequelae. Femoral vein catheters are available in a number of lengths and diameters.

Alternative sites for catheter-based angioaccess are the subclavian or internal jugular veins. These sites have the advantage of fewer local infections, longer local positioning, and enhanced patient mobility [228]. Early-occurring complications such as local bleeding, hemothorax, pneumothorax, hemopericardium, and hemomediastinum are usually related to catheter placement. Late-occurring complications such as arteriovenous fistula formation, local catheter infection or sepsis, central vein thrombosis or stenosis, and catheter malfunction are particularly vexing. Infectious complications are a function of the duration of catheter usage.

If the catheter is left in place for less than 2 weeks, the incidence of infections is less than 5%. Longer periods of catheter placement in situ are associated with an increased incidence of infections (as great as 25%) [229,230]. The usual pathogenesis for catheter infections is from bacteria colonizing the skin adjacent to the catheter entry site that migrate down the catheter sheath [231]. The usual therapy is 10 to 14 days of systemic antibiotics and removal of the dialysis catheter if clinical improvement is not noted after 24 to 48 hours of therapy. Suppurative thrombophlebitis requires discontinuation of the catheter and 4 to 6 weeks of bacteriocidal antibiotics.

Central venous thrombosis is a serious complication of venous cannulation [228,232]. The precise incidence is unknown and varies depending upon how aggressively the diagnosis is established. Most cases are clinically silent until an ipsilateral fistula is created distal to the site of obstruction. At this time,

the classic finding of unilateral arm edema develops. Similarly, anatomic stricture of the central veins may occur as a long-term catheter complication; like central vein thrombosis, it is frequently without clinical signs. Precise pathogenic factors remain undefined for these disorders, but risk factors appear to be the choice of blood vessel cannulated (subclavian vein is riskier than internal jugular vein) and the duration of cannulation (longer has greater risk than shorter). Thrombolytic therapy and percutaneous transluminal angioplasty may be beneficial for central vein thrombosis and for central vein stenosis, respectively [233,234].

Catheter malfunction with inadequate or absent blood flow is most often secondary to intraluminal thrombosis or catheter malposition [228]. Forced irrigation is usually of no benefit and may be detrimental. Instead, inadequate blood flow should be treated by the instillation of 7500 units of urokinase in a volume large enough to fill the catheter. After 15 minutes, the solution should be aspirated out of the catheter and dialysis attempted again. If unsuccessful, the procedure should be repeated. If thrombolytic therapy is of no benefit, catheter malposition should be considered. The catheter can be threaded with a guide wire, removed, and a replacement catheter repositioned.

Catheter complications can be diminished by the use of an implantable, Dacron-cuffed, double-lumen catheter, such as the modified Hickman-Broviac catheter [235]. Usually, these catheters are inserted surgically in a sterile environment. They are most often positioned in the internal jugular vein, but there have been successful installations in the subclavian and femoral veins. For a minority of maintenance hemodialysis patients who lack adequate peripheral arterial vasculature to construct a fistula for long-term angioaccess, these catheters may be used as permanent vascular access [236]. They also are useful for maintenance hemodialysis patients who are awaiting maturation of a fistula, patients with a protracted recovery from ARF and who require hemodialysis, and patients anticipated to have a limited life span with ESRD.

The choice of catheter is usually dictated by the clinical circumstance. For hemodialysis, double-lumen catheters that have virtually no dead space have supplanted the use of single-lumen catheters. For the performance of SCUF, CAVH, CAVHD, and CAVHDF, arterial and venous blood flow is usually achieved through single-lumen femoral artery and vein catheters, respectively. For CVVH, CVVHD, and CVVHDF, femoral vein or central vein double-lumen catheters are used with a blood pump running at 100 ml per minute. For hemofiltration, a 8-Fr catheter is ideal, but smaller catheters may be used successfully, especially with a blood pump.

PERITONEAL DIALYSIS

Dialysates. As discussed earlier, compared to the dialysates used for hemodialysis or hemofiltration, the composition of the dialysates used for peritoneal dialysis is relatively constant. The conventional dialysate sodium concentration is 140 mEq per liter, potassium concentration 0 mEq per liter, and lactate concentration 35 mEq per liter. Hypokalemia in peritoneal dialysis patients is usually managed by increasing the dietary potassium intake. If oral therapy is either ineffective or unfeasible, potassium can be added to the dialysate to attenuate the diffusive gradient. A typical potassium concentration in the dialysate is 1 to 4 mEq per liter. The dialysate calcium concentration varies from 2.5 to 3.5 mEq per liter; the choice of dialysate calcium depends upon the propensity to develop hypercalcemia. Many peritoneal dialysis patients, who ingest calcium salts as phosphate binders, become hypercalcemic using the traditional 3.5 mEq per liter containing calcium dialysate. Therefore, like hemodialysis, the trend has been to lower the calcium concentration in peritoneal dialysates. The only additional electrolyte present in the dialysate is chloride, the concentration of which is determined solely by the requirements to achieve electrical neutrality.

As described earlier, ultrafiltration during peritoneal dialysis is achieved by the infusion of a hyperosmolal dialysate. Dextrose in concentrations of 1.5, 2.5, and 4.25% is used to induce ultrafiltration. Because the osmotic gradient is less with a 1.5% dextrose containing dialysate than with a 4.25% dialysate, the nadir in the ultrafiltration rate occurs sooner using the 1.5% dextrose solution. Likewise, if the osmotic gradient is attenuated by the development of hyperglycemia, the ultrafiltration rate will decline. Therefore, in peritoneal dialysis patients with glucose intolerance, ultrafiltration with dialysates containing high levels of glucose may be compromised if glycemic control is not maintained.

Access into the Peritoneal Cavity.

Access for peritoneal dialysis may be provided acutely by the percutaneous placement of a stylet-guided catheter connected to a closed-gravity, manual instillation drainage system or to an automated cycler. Although simple to install and position in the peritoneal cavity, patients cannot be ambulatory, and the risk of infection is so great that the catheters must be removed after only 48 hours. An alternative means of establishing access to the peritoneal cavity with much greater permanency permits ambulation is to place a soft Silastic catheter with one or two Dacron cuffs. The most frequently used dual-cuffed catheter is the Tenckhoff catheter, which has an open end and multiple holes in the last 15 cm (11). Therefore, Tenckhoff catheters or similar models are the preferred access for peritoneal dialysis in maintenance dialysis patients [237].

Placement of stylet-guided temporary catheters can be difficult and dangerous in patients who have intraabdominal adhesions, which usually are secondary to prior major abdominal surgery. Even if successfully positioned, the resultant compartmentalization of the dialysate in the peritoneal cavity greatly decreases the surface area available for solute clearance and ultrafiltration. Similar limitations exist for the placement of surgically implanted Tenckhoff catheters. For this reason, peritoneal dialysis is not generally offered to renal failure patients with previous major abdominal surgery, but with adequate peripheral vasculature for hemodialysis.

Late-occurring catheter complications include cuff extrusion, dialysate leaks, infection at the percutaneous exit site, catheter tunnel infection, and inadequate catheter function. A well-healed catheter exit site is clean and without redness, crusting, or drainage. Exit site infections are tender, red, and suppurative. These infections usually resolve with oral antibiotics, but if the infectious process extends down the catheter tunnel to the cuff, antibiotic therapy alone is inadequate. Infected catheters typically require removal.

Catheter malfunction, manifest by slow dialysate instillation and (or) drainage, may be caused by catheter malpositioning (tip migration, trapped in adhesions, or kinking) or luminal obstruction (clot, blood, or incarcerated omentum). This problem should be evaluated by a KUB to determine the position of the catheter. If appropriately positioned, urokinase may be instilled into the catheter. After the liquid is aspirated, an exchange may be attempted [238]. If catheter failure continues, the catheter should be replaced. Interestingly, poor catheter function may occur as a consequence of constipation and is easily treated with bowel cathartics. Additional situations in which the peritoneal dialysis catheter should be removed include (1) bowel perforation, (2) noncorrectable catheter dysfunction, (3) tunnel infection, (4) persistent peritonitis despite appropriate antibiotics, (5) persistent catheter-related abdominal pain, and (6) a physical break in the catheter.

Selected Complications of Dialysis

HEMODIALYSIS. The complications of hemodialysis are best managed conceptually in the same manner as those arising from ultrafiltration, solute clearance, and from technical variances (Table 83-2). A common complication is intradialytic hypotension, which is typically ascribed to excessive ultrafiltration (frank intravascular volume depletion resulting in diminished left ventricular filling pressure) or to an excessive rate of ultrafiltration (volume removal from the intravascular space at a rate that exceeds the capacity of interstitial fluid to migrate into this compartment). Common additional contributory factors include left ventricular dysfunction (systolic or diastolic secondary to comorbid illness or medications), autonomic dysfunction (secondary to disease processes or medications), inappropriate vasodilatation (secondary to sepsis, medications), disease of the pericardium or the pericardial space, and bleeding [171,239,240]. It is important to appreciate that there are other critical components of the dialysis procedure that contribute to the development of hypotension. These include the choice of dialysate (buffer, sodium, and calcium concentration) and dialyzer membrane composition and porosity. Specific provocative issues are the (1) vasodilatory and cardiodepressant effects of acetate, (2) impairment of vasoconstriction, exacerbation of autonomic dysfunction, and declining serum osmolality with a hyponatremic dialysate, (3) vasodilatory and cardiodepressant

Table 83-2. Dialysis Complications

Hemodialysis
  Hypotension
  Cramps
  Bleeding
  Leukopenia
  Arrhythmias
  Infections
  Hypoxemia
  Pyrogen reactions
  Dialysis dysequilibrium syndrome
  Angioaccess dysfunction
  Technical mishaps:
    Incorrect dialysate mixture, contaminated dialysate, air embolism, spallation
Hemofiltration
  Bleeding
  Thrombosis of hemofilter
  Technical mishaps:
    Incorrect dialysate mixture, incorrect replacement solution, contaminated dialysate, air embolism
  Hemolysis
  Angioaccess dysfunction
  Hypotension
  Congestive heart failure
Peritoneal Dialysis
  Peritonitis
  Catheter infections
  Catheter dysfunction
  Abdominal pain
  Visceral perforation
  Pleural effusion
  Respiratory failure
  Technical mishaps:
    Inappropriate dialysate composition, contaminated dialysate

effects of a lowered calcium dialysate, (4) cellulosic membrane-induced complement activation, (5) cellulosic membrane-induced and/or acetate-induced hypoxemia, (6) complement and/or pyrogen-induced pyrogenic cytokine production, and (7) dialysis membrane hypersensitivity manifest by kallikrein/bradykinin activation [89,116–120,122,177,180,181,183–185,199,200].

Specific strategies to manage intradialytic hypotension include, but are not limited to, withholding antihypertensive and anti-inotropic medications for 6 hours prior to the dialysis treatment, using a more biocompatible dialysis membrane material such as polysulfone, increasing the dialysate sodium concentration to 140 to 145 mEq per liter and the calcium concentration to 3.5 mEq per liter, switching to a bicarbonate-buffered dialysate, decreasing the blood flow and dialyzer surface area, administering supplemental oxygen during the dialysis session, augmenting impaired intropy by using cardiac glycosides or parenteral inotrophs and removing large volumes by increasing the dialysis time (less volume ultrafiltered per unit time), increasing the frequency of dialysis sessions, ultrafiltering the patient alone, or performing sequential ultrafiltration/clearance. Postdialysis hypotension is typically secondary to hypovolemia and may be managed by the administration of saline or the ingestion of salty foodstuffs such as bouillon or crackers. Other potential causes of hypotension such as occult bleeding or pericardial disease should not be overlooked.

As discussed earlier, dialysis-associated arrhythmias occur most often in patients with comorbid cardiovascular disease and/or cardiac glycoside administration and a concurrent rapid decline in plasma potassium [170]. In high-risk patients, the dialysate potassium concentration should be increased to 3 to 4 mEq per liter. Interdialytic hyperkalemia can be managed by the ingestion of Kayexalate between dialysis treatments.

As mentioned earlier, the dialysis dysequilibrium syndrome is an easily preventable complication of overzealous solute removal at the initiation of hemodialysis, or a dramatic increase in the amount of dialysis delivered to a poorly dialyzed patient. The precise pathobiology of this disorder is undefined, but it appears to arise because of intra- and postdialytic cerebral edema. Although not uniformly supported experimentally [241,242], most evidence suggests that with excessively aggressive solute clearance, urea departure from the cerebrospinal fluid (CSF) is delayed, and the brain becomes hyperosmolal [243]. An additional contributant to the CSF abnormality is the transient, paradoxical development of CSF acidosis, with a resultant increase in osmotic activity. There may be an inappropriate intracerebral accumulation of osmolytes such as inositol, glutamine, and glutamate [244–246]. All of these alterations result in paradoxical intracerebral cell swelling.

The simplest way to prevent dialysis dysequilibrium is to attenuate solute clearance during hemodialysis by using a smaller surface area dialyzer, decreasing blood and dialysate flows, circulating the blood and dialysate in a cocurrent direction, and decreasing the dialysis time. Typically, a urea clearance of 1 to 2 ml per minute per kg is well tolerated; however, such a low urea clearance results in a protracted recovery from uremia. This limitation can be overcome without increasing the risk of the dialysis dysequilibrium syndrome by performing dialysis with low solute clearance for 3 consecutive days [210]. Dialysis can also be initiated by an alternative modality that has less efficient solute clearance, such as peritoneal dialysis. Additional preventive strategies include intradialytic administration of mannitol, dextrose, or dialysis with a hypernatremic dialysate to minimize the decline in serum osmolality. The use of a high-sodium dialysate appears to be the most effective strategy [154,247]. Lastly, in high-risk patients who require aggressive solute clearance, the patient should be loaded

with phenytoin (1 g) prior to the dialysis session, and the dosage should be continued over the subsequent 72 hours as a full dialysis schedule is achieved. Once dialysis dysequilibrium has developed, therapy consists of administration of anti-epileptics and institution of strategies such as hyperventilation and mannitol to reduce intracerebral edema. Neurosurgical patients with stable ESRD treated by hemodialysis may exhibit a similar propensity to develop cerebral edema. Even in the setting of solute clearance not associated with a major change in the dialysis prescription, caution should be undertaken in performing solute clearance that may be associated with a deleterious degree of superimposed cerebral edema [248,249].

The 5- to 35-mm Hg decline in arterial oxygen tension that occurs during dialysis-induced hypoxemia is usually of no clinical significance. In critically ill patients who require supplemental oxygen to maintain an acceptable oxygen tension, this intradialytic decline can result in overt respiratory failure, CNS dysfunction, cardiac arrhythmias, and (or) hypotension. This disorder appears to result from the interaction of the dialysate, dialysis membrane, lungs, and respiratory control center. Specifically, the dialysance of CO_2 across the dialysis membrane results in hypocapnia, which causes a compensatory hypoventilation and hypoxemia (normocapnic hypoventilation); dialysis membrane interactions with plasma complement components result in the intradialytic generation of anaphylatoxins and altered pulmonary regional ventilatory and perfusion patterns; and leukocyte interactions with the dialysis membrane enhance cell membrane expression of leukocyte adhesion molecules, causing pulmonary leukocyte sequestration [120,128,183,184]. Modifications of the hemodialysis procedure that minimize this complication include use of a bicarbonate-buffered dialysate containing 30 to 35 mEq per liter and conversion to a more biocompatible membrane material such as polysulfone. In addition, patients at high risk should have the inspired oxygen concentration empirically increased during the dialysis treatment.

As the monitoring techniques for the performance of hemodialysis have improved, technical errors are now remarkably uncommon. As discussed earlier, pyrogen reactions are a persistent and vexing problem that result from the development of high-porosity dialysis membranes and ultrafiltration controllers, combined with the greatly increased utility of bicarbonate-buffered dialysates. Arguably, strict adherence to prescribed guidelines for water and dialysate purity can minimize this occurrence [250]. In the case of a suspected pyrogen reaction, the patient should be treated with systemic antibiotics until septicemia has been eliminated as the cause of the illness.

HEMOFILTRATION. The most common and significant complication of hemofiltration is bleeding. This is a consequence of the need for intensive anticoagulation in most cases of hemofiltration. Bleeding in this circumstance is managed as for patients with normal renal function, but it should be appreciated that heparin appears to have a prolonged biologic half-life in patients with advanced renal insufficiency [251]. In addition, platelet dysfunction may contribute to the bleeding, and this should be considered in the therapeutic management if the bleeding does not abate [68]. Clotting of the hemofilter is easily managed by replacing the hemofilter and lines if continued dialytic support is required, and by transfusing the patient as is required to replace the lost blood volume.

Because the monitoring associated with hemofiltration is much less than that occurring during hemodialysis, technical errors are more common. A host of metabolic abnormalities may develop as a consequence of variances in the replacement solution or the dialysate. For example, if CAVH is performed in the absence of a bicarbonate-containing replacement solution, severe hyperchloremic metabolic acidosis develops [60]. Excessive solute replacement results in hypernatremia, metabolic alkalosis, hyperkalemia, hypercalcemia, and hypermagnesemia. Inadequate solute replacement causes hyponatremia, hyperchloremic metabolic acidosis, hypokalemia, hypocalcemia, and hypomagnesemia.

Additionally, undetected dysfunction of the hemofilter may occur unless there is active monitoring. Thrombosis of the hemofilter may compromise its performance. For parallel plate dialyzers, this complication cannot be detected early unless hourly monitoring of the ultrafiltration rate occurs. Rupture of the fibers or perforation or tears in the plates in the hemofilter that place the patient at risk of pyrogen contamination or sepsis can be detected early by monitoring the ultrafiltrate for heme moieties with urine dipsticks. Small leaks do not require replacement of the hemofilter. Intradialytic hemolysis is an infrequent complication that is more common when using parallel plate hemofilters than when using the hollow fiber configuration. Adequate patient and technical surveillance can prevent most of these complications.

PERITONEAL DIALYSIS. The most grave complication of peritoneal dialysis is peritonitis, which is reviewed in detail elsewhere [252–254]. Although peritonitis may occur as a consequence of bacteremia, it is usually a complication of introduction of bacteria through the catheter during an exchange. The incidence of peritonitis has declined, predominantly because of improvements in the connectors between the dialysis bag and the intraperitoneal catheter [255]. Current popular systems segregate the lines for instillation and for drainage of the dialysate (Y-set). If the connector sets are the nidus for bacterial entry into this otherwise closed system, limiting the number of times that the system is opened to the environment should be advantageous. This assumption has been validated: CCPD patients, who open their system only once daily, have fewer episodes of peritonitis than CAPD patients, who open their system 4 to 5 times daily [256].

The diagnosis of peritonitis is not difficult. If a particular provocative event can be identified, symptoms and signs begin within 6 to 24 hours. Most patients have low-grade fevers, abdominal pain and tenderness, a cloudy dialysate that contains more than 100 leukocytes per mm^3, and a peripheral blood leukocytosis [253]. After culture of the dialysate and blood have been obtained, the patient should perform two manual exchanges with no dwell to lavage the peritoneum. Because the Gram stain is often negative for bacterial organisms, empiric antibiotic therapy should be initiated immediately. *S. epidermidus* and *S. aureus* account for approximately 50% of the cases of bacterial peritonitis. Although the incidence of polymicrobial peritonitis is increasing, such infections still represent the minority of cases (~10 percent of the cases) [257]. Polymicrobial peritonitis should always raise the differential of ruptured intraabdominal viscera and usually requires removal of the peritoneal dialysis catheter and a course of antibiotics. Well-defined algorithms for antibiotic therapy for bacterial peritonitis are available elsewhere [254]. Most of these protocols suggest initial therapy with intraperitoneal vancomycin (2 g per week) and an aminoglycoside (4 to 8 mg per liter), ceftazidime (125 mg per liter), or ceftriazone (1 g per day). Subsequent therapy should be dictated by the results of cultures. Fungal peritonitis usually requires antifungal therapy and discontinuation of the dialysis catheter.

Metabolic abnormalities associated with peritoneal dialysis are relatively uncommon. This is a result of the relatively inefficient manner in which solute clearance occurs during peritoneal dialysis. Typically, aberrations are detected early in their course, and corrective action is instituted. More common abnormalities include hypernatremia, hypokalemia, and hypercalcemia.

Matching the Dialysis Modality to the Patient

Although typically viewed as an issue only for patients with ARF who have not yet been committed to a particular dialysis modality, the matching of the type of dialysis to a particular patient and his or her comorbid conditions can require an equivalent amount of deliberation for patients on maintenance dialysis. This is especially true for critically ill patients in the ICU. An important principle is that virtually no maintenance dialysis patients are "married" to their dialysis modality. For most patients, the choice of dialysis technique was determined by subjective issues such as patient and physician preference and prejudice, access to transportation, support in the home and community, and the likelihood of medical compliance. Therefore, when the patient is sufficiently ill that choice the maintenance dialysis technique is being reconsidered, the objective medical concerns should be the overwhelming point of convergence for resolving this issue.

As may be appreciated from the previous sections, the decision of the optimal dialysis modality for a particular clinical situation is imprecise. For example, a recent nephrology publication debated (*without* resolution) the choice of hemodialysis versus peritoneal dialysis for patients with cardiovascular instability [258], and hemofiltration versus hemodialysis for patients with ARF [207,259]. Therefore, the following expresses only guidelines that reflect the experiences and the bias of the author (Table 83-3).

1. If the patient is severely hypervolemic or is receiving large obligatory volumes (hyperalimentation, antibiotics, or inotrophs) but is otherwise hemodynamically stable, hemodialysis should be performed with a hemodialyzer having a large ultrafiltration coefficient. If the patient is hemodynamically unstable, SCUF should be performed. If clearance is required as well as ultrafiltration, CAVH or CAVHD (or the equivalent veno-venous technique) is necessary.
2. If the patient is hypercatabolic from a comorbid condition, such as sepsis, burns, or trauma, either hemodialysis or hemofiltration should be performed. If hemodialysis is selected, the surface area of the dialyzer should be large, with maximal blood and dialysate flow. If solute clearance is inadequate despite a long dialysis time, daily hemodialysis may be necessary. If such scheduling is impractical, the patient should undergo CAVHD or CAVHDF (or the equivalent veno-venous technique).
3. If the patient has a poor cardiovascular reserve, does not require large volumes to be ultrafiltered, and clearance requirements are modest, peritoneal dialysis may be substituted for hemofiltration.
4. If the patient cannot be anticoagulated (e.g., postoperative neurosurgical patients), hemodialysis can be performed with no heparin. Alternatively, peritoneal dialysis can be used.
5. If vascular access cannot be established, such as in diabetics with severe peripheral vascular disease, peritoneal dialysis should be used.
6. If attenuated clearances are required, such as in patients who are severely uremic and at great risk for the dysequi-

Table 83-3. Considerations Relevant to the Selection of a Dialysis Modality

Patient Specific
  Residual renal function
  Cardiovascular status
  Pulmonary status
  Volume status
  Volume load
  Medications
  Comorbid conditions:
    Surgery
    Myocardial or coronary disease
    Coagulopathy
    Hemorrhage
    Sepsis
    Arrhythmias
    Malnutrition
    Diabetes mellitus
    Burns
    Vasculopathy
Dialysis Specific
  Membrane composition
  Membrane surface area
  Ultrafiltration coefficient
  Dialysate composition
    Sodium
    Potassium
    Base
    Calcium
    Dextrose
    Magnesium
  Blood and dialysate flow
  Dialysis duration and frequency
  Dialysate volume*
  Angioaccess
  Peritoneal access*
  Anticoagulation

*Applicable to peritoneal dialysis only.

librium syndrome, hemodialysis may be performed with low blood and dialysate flows, cocurrent blood and dialysate flow, short dialysis time, and a small surface area dialyzer. Alternatively, patients may be dialyzed by peritoneal dialysis.

7. In postoperative neurosurgical patients at risk of developing worsening cerebral edema with intermittent hemodialysis, peritoneal dialysis may be used.
8. If patient mobility is an issue, such as the requirement to frequently transport the patient for different investigations or procedures, hemofiltration should not be performed.
9. Hemofiltration cannot be performed where 1:1 nursing is unavailable.
10. Rapid removal of drugs from intoxications, such as aminophylline or lithium, is best accomplished by hemodialysis.

Regardless of the dialysis modality selected, it is critical that the full range of dialysis techniques be used as necessary. For example, if hemodynamic instability compromises fluid removal during hemodialysis, which otherwise would be the best modality for the patient, sequential ultrafiltration/clearance should be tried. If the patient requires a continuous therapy such as CAVHD but cannot tolerate the lactate load in the conventional peritoneal dialysate, pre-post dilutional CAVH may provide adequate clearance. If continuous therapy is required but the patient cannot tolerate heparin, hemofiltration

should be performed using a parallel plate dialyzer, short lines, and a predilutional technique.

References

1. Addison T: On the disorders of the brain connected with diseased kidneys. *Guys Hosp Rep* 4:1, 1839.
2. Bright R: Cases and observations illustrative of renal disease accompanied with the secretion of albuminous urine. *Guys Hosp Rep* 1:338, 1836.
3. Hughes WE, Carter WS: A clinical and experimental study of uraemia. *Am J Med Sci* 108:177, 1894.
4. Tyson J: Acute parenchymatous nephritis. *Boston Med Surg J* 111:193, 1884.
5. Abell JJ, Rowntree LC, Turner BB: On the removal of diffusable substances from the circulating blood of living animals by dialysis. *J Pharmacol Exp Ther* 5:611, 1913.
6. Kolff WJ: The artificial kidney. M.D. thesis, University of Groningen. The Netherlands, Kampen JH, Kok NV, 1946.
7. Teschan PE: Hemodialysis in military casualties. *Trans Am Soc Artif Int Organs* 2:52, 1955.
8. Scribner BH, Buri R, Caner JEZ, Hegstrom R, Burnell JM: The treatment of chronic uremia by means of intermittent dialysis: A preliminary report. *Trans Am Soc Artif Int Organs* 6:114, 1960.
9. Feldman H, Klag MJ, Chiapella AP, Whelton PK: End-stage renal disease in US Minority Groups. *Am J Kidney Dis* 5:397, 1992.
10. Drukker W: Peritoneal dialysis: A historical review, In Maher JF (ed): *Replacement of Renal Function by Dialysis*. Dordrecht, The Netherlands, Kluwer Academic Publishers, 1989, p 475.
11. Tenckhoff H, Schechter H: A bacteriologically safe peritoneal access device. *Trans Am Soc Artif Int Organs* 14:181, 1968.
12. Leading article (anonymous): Intermittent peritoneal ravage. *Lancet* 2:551, 1959.
13. Swan RC, Merrill JP: The clinical course of acute renal failure. *Medicine* 32:215, 1953.
14. Kiley JE, Powers SR, Beebe RT: Acute renal failure: Eighty cases of renal tubular necrosis. *N Engl J Med* 262:481, 1960.
15. Kennedy AC, Burton JA, Luke RG, et al: Factors affecting prognosis in acute renal failure. *Q J Med* 165:73, 1973.
16. McMurray SD, Luft SC, Maxwell DR, et al: Prevailing patterns and predictor variables in patients with acute tubular necrosis. *Arch Int Med* 138:950, 1978.
17. Rasmussen HH, Pitt EA, Ibels LS, McNeil DR: Prediction of outcome in acute renal failure by discriminant-analysis of clinical variables. *Arch Int Med* 154:2015, 1985.
18. Corwin HL, Bonventre JV: Factors influencing survival in acute renal failure. *Semin Dial* 2:220, 1989.
19. Stott RB, Cameron JS, Ogg CS, Bewick M: Why the persistently high mortality in acute renal failure? *Lancet* 2:75, 1972
20. Kjellstrand CM, Ebben J, Davin T: Time of death, recovery of renal function, development of chronic renal failure and need for chronic hemodialysis in patients with acute tubular necrosis. *Trans Am Soc Artif Int Organs* 27:45, 1981.
21. Bullock ML, Umen AJ, Finkelstein M, Keane WF: The assessment of risk factors in 462 patients with acute renal failure. *Am J Kidney Dis* 5:97, 1985.
22. Anderson RJ, Linas SL, Berns AS, et al: Nonoliguric acute renal failure. *N Engl J Med* 296:1134, 1977.
23. Diamond JR: Nonoliguric acute renal failure. *Arch Intern Med* 142:1882, 1982.
24. Montgomerie JZ, Kalmanson GM, Guze LB: Renal failure and infection. *Medicine* 47:1, 1968.
25. Woodrow G, Turney JH: Causes of death in acute renal failure. *Nephrol Dial Transplant* 7:230, 1992.
26. Kumar R, Hill CM, McGeown MG: Acute renal failure in the elderly. *Lancet* 1:90, 1973.
27. Broyer M, Brunner FP, Brygner H, et al: Combined report on regular dialysis and transplantation in Europe. XIII. 1982 Acute (reversible) renal failure. *Proc Eur Dial Transplant Assoc* 20:64, 1983.

28. Cameron JS: Acute renal failure—the continuing challenge. *Q J Med* 228:337, 1986.

29. Feinstein EI, Blumenkrantz MJ, Healy M et al: Clinical and metabolic responses to parenteral nutrition in acute renal failure. *Medicine* 60:124, 1981.

30. Rainford DJ: Nutritional management of acute renal failure. *Acta Chir Scand Suppl* 507:327, 1981.

31. Kleinknecht D, Jungers P, Charnard BJ, et al: Uremic and non-uremic complications in acute renal failure: Evaluation of early and frequent dialysis on prognosis. *Kidney Int* 1:190, 1972.

32. Gillum DM, Dixon BS, Yanover MJ, et al: The role of intensive dialysis in acute renal failure. *Clin Nephrol* 25:249, 1986.

33. Rasmussen HH, Ibels LS: Acute renal failure: Multivariate analysis of causes and risk factors. *Am J Med* 73:211, 1982.

34. Beaman M, Turney JH, Roger RSC, et al: Changing patterns of acute renal failure. *Q J Med* 62:15, 1987.

35. Hou S, Bushinsky DA, Wish H et al: Hospital-acquired renal insufficiency: A prospective study. *Am J Med* 74:243, 1983.

36. Merrill JP: Medical progress: The artificial kidney. *N Engl J Med* 246:17, 1952.

37. Locke S, Merrill JP, Tyler HR: Neurologic complications of acute uremia. *N Engl J Med* 108:75, 1961.

38. Drueke T, Le Pailleur C, Zingraff J, Jungers P: Uremic cardiomyopathy and pericarditis. *Adv Nephrol* 9:33, 1980.

39. DeBroe ME, Lins RR, DeBacker WA: Pulmonary aspects of dialysis patients, in Maher JF (ed): *Replacement of Renal Function by Dialysis*. Dordrecht, The Netherlands, Kluwer Academic Publishers, 1989, p 828.

40. Arieff AI: Dialysis dysequilibrium syndrome: current concepts on pathogenesis. *Controv Nephrol* 4:367, 1982.

41. Allon M, Dansky L, Shonklin N: Glucose modulation of the disposal of an acute potassium load in patients with end-stage renal disease. *Am J Med* 94:475, 1993.

42. Allon M: Treatment and prevention of hyperkalemia in end-stage renal disease. *Kidney Int* 43:1197, 1993.

43. Michael JM, Bruns DD, Ladenson JH, Sherman LA: Potassium load in CPD-preserved whole-blood and two types of packed red blood cells. *Transfusion* 15:144, 1975.

44. Simon GE, Bove JR: The potassium load from blood transfusion. *Postgrad Med* 49:61, 1971.

45. Schlarrman J, Schurek HJ, Neumann KH, Eckert G: Chloride-induced increase of plasma potassium after transfusion of erythrocytes in dialysis patients. *Nephron* 37:240, 1984.

46. Lillemoe KD, Romolo JL, Hamilton SR, et al: Intestinal necrosis due to sodium polystyrene (Kayexalate) in sorbitol enemas. Clinical and experimental support for the hypothesis. *Surgery* 101:267, 1987.

47. Gerstman BB, Kirkman RL, Platt R: Intestinal necrosis associated with postoperative administered sodium polystyrene sulfonate in sorbitol. *Am J Kidney Dis* 20:159, 1992.

48. Brown TS, Ahern DJ, Nolph KD: Potassium removal with peritoneal dialysis. *Kidney Int* 4:67, 1978.

49. Bearne RM, Levy MN: in (ed): *Cardiovascular Physiology*. St. Louis, Mosby, 1981, p 7.

50. Blumberg A, Weidmann P, Shaw S, Gnadinger M: Effect of various therapeutic approaches on plasma potassium and major regulating factors in terminal renal failure. *Am J Med* 85:507, 1988.

51. Ferramnini E, Tuddei S, Santoro D, et al: Independent stimulation of glucose metabolism and sodium potassium exchange by insulin in human forearm. *Am J Physiol* 255:E953, 1988.

52. Alvestrand A, Wahren J, Smith D, Defronzo RA: Insulin-mediated potassium uptake is normal in uremic and healthy subjects. *Am J Physiol* 246:F174, 1984.

53. Montoliu J, Lenz XM, Revert L: Potassium-lowering effect of albuterol for hyperkalemia in acute renal failure. *Arch Int Med* 147:713, 1987.

54. Allon M, Copkney C: Albuterol and insulin for treatment of hyperkalemia in hemodialysis patients. *Kidney Int* 38:869, 1990.

55. Allon M, Shanklin N: Adrenergic modulation of extrarenal potassium disposal in men with end-stage renal disease. *Kidney Int* 40:1103, 1991.

56. Bratre DC, Day B, Burdette A, Anderson S: Bumetaninde and furosemide in heart failure. *Kidney Int* 26:183, 1984.

57. Rudy DW, Voelker JR, Greene PK, et al: Loop diuretics for chronic renal failure: A continuous infusion is more efficacious than bolus therapy. *Ann Int Med* 115:360, 1991.

58. Inoue M, Okajima K, Itoh K, et al: Mechanism of furosemide resistance in analbuminemic rats and hypoalbuminemic patients. *Kidney Int* 32:198, 1987.

59. Anderson CC, Shavari MBG, Zimmerman JE: The treatment of pulmonary edema in the absence of renal function—A role for sorbitol and furosemide. *JAMA* 241:1008, 1979.

60. Gennari FJ, Rimmer JM: Acid-base disorders in end stage renal disease. Part I. *Semin Dial* 3:81, 1990.

61. Van Ypersele de Strihou C, Frans A: The pattern of respiratory compensation in chronic uremic acidosis. *Nephron* 7:37, 1970.

62. Walker JA: Aluminum and citrate: A cautionary note. *Semin Dial* 1:91, 1988.

63. Walker JA, Sherman RA, Cody RF: The effect of oral bases on enteral aluminum absorption. *Arch Int Med* 150:2037, 1990.

64. Slingeneyer A, Mion C, Mourad G, Canaud B, et al: Progressive sclerosing peritonitis. A late and severe complication of maintenance peritoneal dialysis. *Trans Am Soc Artif Int Organs* 29:633, 1983.

65. Benabe JE, Martinez-Maldonado M: Hypercalcemic nephropathy. *Arch Int Med* 138:777, 1978.

66. Kjellstrand CM, Campbell DC, von Hartitzch B, Buselmeier TJ: Hyperuricemic acute renal failure. *Arch Int Med* 133:349, 1974.

67. Randall RE, Cohen MD, Spray CC: Hypermagnesemia in renal failure. *Ann Int Med* 61:73, 1964.

68. Remuzzi G: Bleeding in renal failure. *Lancet* 1:1205, 1988.

69. Livio M, Gotti E, Marchesi D, et al : Uremic bleeding: Role of anemia and beneficial effect of red cell transfusion. *Lancet* 2:1013, 1982.

70. Escolar G, Cases A, Bastida E, et al: Uremic platelets have a functional defect affecting the interaction of von Willebrand factor with glycoprotein IIb–IIIa. *Blood* 76:1336, 1990.

71. Remuzzi G, Perico N, Zoja C, et al: Role of endothelium-derived nitric oxide in the bleeding tendency of uremia. *J Clin Invest* 86:1768, 1990.

72. Lindsay RM, Friesen M, Koens F, et al: Platelet function in patients on long term peritoneal dialysis. *Clin Nephrol* 6:335, 1976.

73. Nenci G, Berrittini M, Agnelli G, et al: The effect of peritoneal dialysis, hemodialysis, and kidney transplantation on blood platelet function. Platelet aggregation to ADP and epinephrine. *Nephron* 23:287, 1979.

74. Janson PA, Jubeliere SJ, Weinstein MJ, Deykin D: Treatment of the bleeding tendency in uremia with cryoprecipitate. *N Engl J Med* 308:8, 1980.

75. Mannuccci PM, Remuzzi G, Pusineri F, et al: Deamino-8-D-arginine vasopressin shortens the bleeding time in uremia. *N Engl J Med* 308:8, 1983.

76. Moia M, Vizzotto L, Cattaneo M, et al: Improvement of the hemostatic defect of uraemia after treatment with recombinant human erythropoietin. *Lancet* 2:1227, 1987.

77. Livio M, Mannucchi PM, Bignano G, et al: Conjugated estrogens for the management of bleeding associated with renal failure. *N Engl J Med* 315:731, 1986.

78. Lohr JW, Schwab SJ: Minimizing hemorrhagic complications in dialysis patients. *J Am Soc Nephrol* 2:961, 1991.

79. Conger JD: A controlled evaluation of prophylactic dialysis in post-traumatic acute renal failure. *J Trauma* 15:1056, 1975.

80. Gillum DM, Dixon BS, Yanover MJ, et al: The role of intensive dialysis in acute renal failure. *Clin Nephrol* 25:249, 1986.

81. Solez L, Morel-Maroger L, Sraer J: The morphology of acute tubular necrosis in man: Analysis of 57 renal biopsies and comparison with the glycerol model. *Medicine (Baltimore)* 58:362, 1979.

82. Conger JD: Does hemodialysis delay recovery from acute renal failure? *Semin Dial* 3:146, 1990.

83. Yeh BPY, Tomki DJ, Stacy WK, et al: Factors influencing sodium and water excretion in uremic man. *Kidney Int* 7:103, 1975.

84. Schulman G, Fogo A, Gung A, et al: Complement activation retards renal failure in the rat. *Kidney Int* 40:1069, 1991.

85. Hakim RM, Wingard RL, Lawrence P, et al: Use of biocompatable membranes improves outcome and recovery from acute renal failure (abstract). *J Am Soc Nephrol* 3:367, 1992.

86. Ogata K: Clinicopathological study of kidneys from patients on chronic dialysis. *Kidney Int* 37:1333, 1990.

87. Rottembourg J: Residual renal function and recovery of renal function in patients treated by CAPD. *Kidney Int* 43(suppl 40):S-106, 1993.

88. Conger JD, Robinette JB, Schrier RW: Smooth muscle calcium and endothelial-derived relaxing factor in abnormal vascular responses of acute renal failure. *J Clin Invest* 82:532, 1988.

89. Hakim RM, Fearon DT, Lazarus JM: Biocompatibility of dialysis membranes: effects of chronic complement activation. *Kidney Int* 26:194, 1984.

90. Lynn RI, Feinfeld DA: Importance of residual renal function in end-stage renal disease. *Semin Dial* 2:1, 1989.

91. Skov PE: GFR in patients with severe and very severe renal insufficiency. *Acta Med Scand* 187:419, 1970.

92. Sargent JA, Gotch FA: Principles and biophysics of dialysis, in Maher JF (ed): *Replacement of Renal Function by Dialysis*. Dordrecht, The Netherlands, Kluwer Academic Publishers, 1989, p 87.

93. Babb AL, Farrell P, Uvelli DA Scribner BH: Hemodialyzer evaluation by examination of solute molecular spectra. *Trans Am Soc Artif Int Organs* 18:98, 1972.

94. Henderson LW: Biophysics of ultrafiltration and hemofiltration, in Maher JF (ed): *Replacement of Renal Function by Dialysis*. Dordrecht, The Netherlands, Kluwer Academic Publishers, 1989, p 300.

95. Nolph KD, Nothum RJ, Maher JF: Ultrafiltration: A mechanism for removal of intermediate molecular weight substances in coil dialyzers. *Kidney Int* 6:55, 1974.

96. Laurer A, Saccaggi A, Ronco C, et al: Continuous arteriovenous hemofiltration in the critically ill patient. *Ann Int Med* 99:255, 1983.

97. Keshaviah PR, Shaldon S: Hemodialysis monitors and monitoring, in Maher JF (ed): *Replacement of Renal Function by Dialysis*. Dordrecht, The Netherlands, Kluwer Academic Publishers, 1989, p 276.

98. Asaba H, Bergstrom J, Furst P, et al: Sequential ultrafiltration and diffusion as alternatives to conventional hemodialysis. *Proc Clin Dial Transplant Forum* 6:29, 1976.

99. Shaldon S: Sequential ultrafiltration and dialysis. *Proc Eur Dial Transplant Assoc* 13:300, 1976.

100. Wehle B, Asaba H, Castenfores J, et al: Hemodynamic changes during sequential ultrafiltration and dialysis. *Kidney Int* 15:411, 1979.

101. Keshaviah P, Ilstrup K, Constantini E, et al: The influence of ultrafiltration and diffusion on cardiovascular parameters. *Trans Am Soc Artif Int Organs* 26:328, 1980.

102. Fleming SJ, Wilkinson JS, Aldridge C, et al: Blood volume change during isolated ultrafiltration and combined ultrafiltration-dialysis. *Nephrol Dial Transplant* 3:272, 1988.

103. Bradley JR, Evans DB, Cowley AJ: Comparison of vascular tone during haemodialysis with ultrafiltration and during ultrafiltration followed by haemodialysis: A possible mechanism for dialysis hypotension. *Br Med J* 19:300, 1990.

104. Geronemus R, von Albertini B, Glabman S, et al: Enhanced molecular clearance in hemofiltration. *Proc Clin Dial Transplant Forum* 8:47, 1985.

105. Kaplan AA: Predilution vs postdilution for continuous arteriovenous hemofiltration. *Trans Am Soc Artif Int Organs* 3:28, 1985.

106. Kallen RJ: A method for approximating the efficacy of peritoneal dialysis for uremia. *Am J Kidney Dis* 3:156, 1966.

107. Esperanca MJ, Collins DL: Peritoneal dialysis efficiency in relation to body weight. *J Ped Surg* 10:162, 1966.

108. Popovich RP, Moncrief JW, Nolph KD, et al: Physiological transport parameters in peritoneal and hemodialysis. 3rd Annual Report No. N01-AM-3-2205, AK-CUP, Bethesda, MD, NIAMDD, National Institutes of Health, 1977

109. Bomar JB, Dechard JF, Hlavinka D, et al: The elucidation of maximum efficiency minimum costs peritoneal dialysis protocols. *Trans Am Soc Artif Int Organs* 20:120, 1974.

110. Penzotti SC, Mattocks AM: Effects of dwell time, volume of dialysis fluid, and added accelerators on peritoneal dialysis of urea. *J Pharm Sci* 60:1520, 1971.

111. Henderson LW: Peritoneal ultrafiltration dialysis. Enhanced urea transfer using hypertonic peritoneal dialysis fluid. *J Clin Invest* 45:950, 1966.

112. Nolph KD, Ghods AJ, Van Stone JC: The effects of intraperitoneal vasodilators on peritoneal clearances. *Trans Am Soc Artif Int Organs* 22:586, 1976.

113. Nolph KD, Ghods AJ, Brown PA: Effects of intraperitoneal nitroprusside on peritoneal clearances with variations in dose, frequency of administration, and dwell times. *Nephron* 24:4, 1979.

114. Miller FN, Nolph KD, Harris PD: Microvascular and clinical effects of altered peritoneal solutions. *Kidney Int* 15:630, 1979.

115. Grzegorzewska AE, Moore HL, Nolph KD, Chen TW: Ultrafiltration and effective peritoneal blood flow during peritoneal dialysis in the rat. *Kidney Int* 39:608, 1991.

116. Lazarus JM, Owen WF: Role of biocompatibility in dialysis morbidity and mortality. *Am J Kidney Dis* 24:1019, 1994.

117. Schulman G, Hakim R: Recent advances in the biocompatibility of haemodialysis membranes. *Nephrol Dial Transplant* 6 (suppl 2): S-10, 1991.

118. Henderson LW, Koch KM, Dinarello CA, Shaldon S: Hemodialysis hypotension: The interleukin hypothesis. *Blood Purif* 1:3-8, 1983.

119. Dinarello CA, Koch KM, Shaldon S: Interleukin-1 and its relevance to patients treated with hemodialysis. *Kidney Int* 33 (suppl 24): S-21, 1988.

120. Ross EA, Nissenson AR: Dialysis-associated hypoxemia: insights into pathophysiology and prevention. *Semin Dial* 1:33, 1988.

121. Tetta C, David S, Biancone L, et al: Role of platelet activating factor in hemodialysis. *Kidney Int* 43 (suppl 39): S-154, 1993

122. Schulman G, Hakim R, Arias R, Silverberg M, et al: Bradykinin generation by dialysis membranes: possible role in anaphylactic reaction. *J Am Soc Nephrol* 3:1563, 1993.

123. Roccatello D, Mazzucco G, Coppo R, et al: Functional changes of monocytes due to dialysis membranes. *Kidney Int* 32:84, 1989.

124. Vanholder R, Ringoir S, Dhondt A, Hakim R: Phagocytosis in uremic and hemodialysis patients: a prospective and cross sectional study. *Kidney Int* 39:320, 1991.

125. Vanholder R, Ringoir S: Polymorphonuclear cell function and infection in dialysis. *Kidney Int* 42 (suppl 38):S-91, 1992.

126. van Ypersele de Strihou C, Jadoul M, Malghem J, Maldague B: Effect of dialysis membrane and patient's age on signs of dialysis-related amyloidosis. The Working Party on Dialysis Amyloidosis. *Kidney Int* 39:1012, 1991.

127. Aranout A, Hakim RM, Todd R, et al: Increased expression of an adhesion-promoting surface glycoprotein in the granulocytopenia of hemodialysis. *N Engl J Med* 312:457, 1985.

128. Himmelfarb J, Zaoui P, Hakim R: Modulation of granulocyte LAM-1 and MAC-1 during dialysis—A prospective, randomized controlled trial. *Kidney Int* 41:388, 1992.

129. Himmelfarb J, Lazarus JM, Hakim R: Reactive oxygen species production by monocytes and polymorphonuclear leukocytes during dialysis. *Am J Kidney Dis* 17:271, 1991.

130. Shaldon S, Lonnemann G, Koch KM: Cytokine relevance in biocompatibility. *Contrib Nephrol* 79:227, 1989.

131. Schindler R, Lonnemann G, Shaldon S, et al: Transcription, not synthesis, of interleukin-1 and tumor necrosis factor by complement. *Kidney Int* 37:85, 1990.

132. Pertosa G, Gesualdo L, Tarantino EA, et al: Influence of hemodialysis on interleukin-6 production and gene expression by peripheral blood mononuclear cells. *Kidney Int* 43(suppl 39):S-149, 1993.

133. Zaoui P, Green W, Hakim RM: Hemodialysis with cuprophane membrane modulates interleukin-2 receptor expression. *Kidney Int* 39:1020, 1991.

134. Tokars JI, Alter MJ, Favero MS, et al: National surveillance of hemodialysis associated diseases in the United States, 1990. *Am Soc Artif Int Organs J* 33:71, 1993.

135. Kaye M, Lella J, Gagnon R, Low G: Consent to dialyzer reuse: Is it ethically necessary? *Am J Nephrol* 5:138, 1985.

136. Garred LJ, Canaud B, Flavier JL, et al: Effect of reuse on dialyzer efficacy. *Artif Organs* 14:80, 1990.

137. Baris E, McGregor M: The reuse of hemodialyzers: An assessment of safety and potential savings. *Can Med Assoc J* 148:175, 1993.

138. Petersen J, Hyver SW, Collins J: Backfiltration during hemodialysis: A critical assessment. *Semin Dial* 5:13, 1992.

139. Ward RA, Luehmann DA, Klein E: Are current standards for the microbiological purity of hemodialysate adequate? *Semin Dial* 2:69, 1989.

140. Klein E, Pass T, Harding GB, et al: Microbial and endotoxin contamination in water and dialysate in the central United States. *Artif Organs* 14:85, 1990.

141. Kovalik EC, Schwab SJ, Quarles LD: Hollow-fiber versus parallel-plate dialyzers in continuous arteriovenous hemodialysis. *Semin Dial* 6:229, 1993.

142. Yohay DA, Butterly DW, Schwab SJ, Quarles LD: Continuous arteriovenous hemodialysis: Effect of dialyzer geometry. *Kidney Int* 42:448, 1992.

143. Ifediora OC, Teehan BP, Sigler MH: Solute clearances in continuous venovenous hemodialysis: A comparison of cuprophane polyacrilonitrile, and polysulfone membranes. *Am Soc Artif Int Organs J* 38:M697, 1992.

144. Mendelssohn S, Swartz CD, Yudis M, et al: High glucose concentration dialysate in chronic hemodialysis. *Trans Am Soc Artif Int Organs* 13:249, 1967.

145. Ward RA, Walthen RL, Williams TE, Harding GB: Hemodialysate composition and intradialytic metabolic, acid-base, and potassium changes. *Kidney Int* 32:129, 1987.

146. Arem R: Hypoglycemia. *Endocrinol Metab Clin North Am* 18:103, 1989.

147. Grajower MM, Walter L, Albin J: Hypoglycemia in chronic hemodialysis patients: Association with propranolol use. *Nephron* 26:126, 1980.

148. Kopple JD, Swendseid ME, Shinaberger JH, Umezawa CY: The free and bound amino acids removed by hemodialysis. *Trans Am Soc Artif Int Organs* 19:309, 1973.

149. Ganda OP, Aoki TT, Soeldner JS, et al: Hormone-fuel concentrations in anephric subjects: Effects of hemodialysis (with special references to amino acids). *J Clin Invest* 57:1403, 1976.

150. Wilkinson R, Barber SG, Robson V: Cramps, thirst, and hypertension in hemodialysis patients—The influence of dialysate sodium concentration. *Clin Nephrol* 7:101, 1977.

151. Ogden D: A double-blind crossover comparison of high and low sodium dialysate. *Proc Clin Dial Transplant Forum* 88:157, 1978.

152. Henrich WL, Woodard TD, McPhaul JJ: The chronic efficacy and safety of high sodium dialysate: Double-blind crossover study. *Am J Kidney Dis* 2:349, 1982.

153. Cybulsky AVE, Materi A, Hollombh DJ: Effects of high sodium dialysate during maintenance hemodialysis. *Nephron* 41:57, 1985.

154. Port FK, Johnson WJ, Klass DW: Prevention of dialysis disequilibrium syndrome by use of high sodium concentration in the dialysate. *Kidney Int* 3:327, 1973.

155. Van Stone JC, Bauer J, Carey J: The effect of dialysate sodium concentration on body fluid distribution during hemodialysis. *Trans Am Soc Artif Int Organs* 26:383, 1980.

156. Dumler F, Grondin G, Levin NW: Sequential high/low sodium hemodialysis: An alternative to ultrafiltration. *Trans Am Soc Artif Int Organs* 25:351, 1979.

157. Daugirdas JT, Al-Kudsi RR, Ing TS, Norusis MJ: A double-blind evaluation of sodium gradient hemodialysis. *Am J Nephrol* 5:163, 1985.

158. Raja R, Kramer M, Barber K, Chin S: Sequential changes in dialysate sodium during hemodialysis. *Trans Am Soc Artif Int Organs* 29:649, 1983.

159. Palmer BF: The effect of dialysate composition on systemic hemodynamics. *Semin Dial* 5:54, 1992.

160. Depner TA: Standards for dialysis adequacy. *Semin Dial* 4:245, 1991.

161. William M, Epstein FH: Internal exchanges of potassium, in Seldin DW, Giebisch G (eds): *The Regulation of Potassium Balance.* New York, Raven Press, 1989, p 3.

162. Ketchersid TL, Van Stone JC: Dialysate potassium. *Semin Dial* 4:46, 1991.

163. Sherman RA, Hwang ER, Bernholc AS, Eisinger RP: Variability in potassium removal by hemodialysis. *Am J Nephrol* 6:284, 1986.

164. Feig PU, Shook A, Sterns RH: Effect of potassium removal during hemodialysis on the plasma potassium concentration. *Nephron* 27:25, 1981.

165. Hou S, McElroy PA, Nootes S, Beach M: Safety and efficacy of low potassium dialysate. *Am J Kidney Dis* 13:137, 1989.

166. Ozuer M, Aksoy, Dortlmez O, Dortlemez H: Effects of cardioselective (β_1) and nonselective (both β_1 and β_2) adrenergic blockade on serum potassium in patients with chronic renal failure undergoing hemodialysis. *Kidney Int* 26:584, 1984.

167. Papadakis MA, Wexman MP, Fraser C, Sedlacek SM: Hyperkalemia complicating digoxin toxicity in a patient with renal failure. *Am J Kidney Dis* 5:64, 1985.

168. Williams AJ, Barnes JN, Cunningham J, et al: Effect of dialysate buffer on potassium removal during haemodialysis. *Proc EDTA-ERA* 21:209, 1985.

169. Redaelli B, Sforzini B, Bonoldi L, et al: Potassium removal as a factor limiting the correction of acidosis during dialysis. *Proc EDTA* 19:366, 1982.

170. Morrison G, Michelson EL, Brown S, Morganroth J: Mechanism and prevention of cardiac arrhythmias in chronic hemodialysis patients. *Kidney Int* 17:811, 1980.

171. Lazarus JM: Complications in hemodialysis. An overview. *Kidney Int* 18:783, 1980.

172. Wiegand CF, Davin TD, Raij L, Kjellstrand CM: Severe hypokalemia induced by hemodialysis. *Arch Int Med* 141:167, 1981.

173. Kveim M, Nesbakken R: Utilization of exogenous acetate during hemodialysis. *Proc Dial Transplant Forum* 5:138, 1975.

174. Vinay P, Prud'homme M, Vinet B, et al: Acetate metabolism and bicarbonate generation during hemodialysis: 10 years of observation. *Kidney Int* 31:1194, 1987.

175. Graefe U, Multinovich J, Follette WC, et al: Less dialysis-induced morbidity and vascular instability with bicarbonate dialysate. *Ann Int Med* 88:332, 1978

176. Mastrangelo F, Rizzelli S, Corliano C: Benefits of bicarbonate dialysis. *Kidney Int* 28(suppl 17):S-188, 1985.

177. Henrich WL: Hemodynamic instability during hemodialysis. *Kidney Int* 30:605, 1986.

178. Wolff J, Pendersen T, Rossen M, Cleeman-Rasmussen K: Effects of acetate and bicarbonate dialysis on cardiac performance, transmural myocardial perfusion and acid-base balance. *Int J Artif Organs* 9:105, 1986

179. Daugirdas JT: Dialysis hypotension: A hemodynamic analysis. *Kidney Int* 39:233, 1991.

180. Palmer BF: The effect of dialysate composition on systemic hemodynamics. *Semin Dial* 5:54, 1992.

181. Wehle B, Asaba H, Castenfors J, et al: The influence of dialysis fluid composition on the blood pressure response during dialysis. *Clin Nephrol* 10:62, 1978.

182. Velez RL, Woodard TD, Henrich WL: Acetate and bicarbonate hemodialysis in patients with and without autonomic dysfunction. *Kidney Int* 26:59, 1984.

183. Garella S, Chang BS: Hemodialysis-associated hypoxemia. *Am J Nephrol* 4:272, 1984.

184. Nissenson AR, Kraut JA, Shinaberger JH: Dialysis-associated hypoxemia: Pathogenesis and prevention. *Am Soc Artif Int Organs J* 7:1, 1984.

185. Ward RA, Luehmann DA, Klein E: Are current standards for the microbiological purity of hemodialysate adequate? *Semin Dial* 2:69, 1989.

186. Sherman RA: On lowering dialysate calcium. *Semin Dial* 1:78, 1988.

187. Goodman WG, Coburn JW: The use of 1,25-dihydroxyvitamin D3 in early renal failure. *Ann Rev Med* 43:27, 1992.

188. Sutton RA, Cameron EC: Renal osteodystrophy: Pathophysiology. *Semin Nephrol* 12:91, 1992.

189. Wing AJ: Optimum calcium concentration of dialysis fluid for hemodialysis. *Br Med J* 4:145, 1968.

190. Mirahmadi KS, Duffy BS, Shinaberger JH, et al: A controlled evaluation of clinical and metabolic effects of dialysate calcium levels during regular hemodialysis. *Trans Am Soc Artif Int Organs* 17:118, 1971.

191. Raman A, Chong YK, Sreenevasan GA: Effects of varying dialysate calcium concentrations on the plasma calcium fractions in patients on dialysis. *Nephron* 16:181, 1976.

192. Bouillon R, Verberckmoes R, Moor PD: Influence of dialysate calcium concentration and vitamin D on serum parathyroid hormone during repetitive dialysis. *Kidney Int* 7:422, 1975.

193. Salusky IB, Foley J, Nelson P, Goodman WG: Aluminum accumulation during treatment with aluminum hydroxide and dialysis in children and young adults with chronic renal failure. *N Engl J Med* 324:527, 1991.

194. Delmez JA, Slatopolsky E: Hyperphosphatemia: Its consequence and treatment in chronic renal failure. *Am J Kidney Dis* 19:303, 1992.

195. Touam M, Martinez F, Lacour B, et al: Aluminum-induced, reversible microcytic anemia in chronic renal failure: Clinical and experimental studies. *Clin Nephrol* 19:295, 1983.

196. Alfrey AC, Le Gendre GR, Kaehny WD: The dialysis encephalopathy syndrome. Possible aluminum intoxication. *N Engl J Med* 294:184, 1976.

197. Slatopolsky E, Weerts C, Lopez-Hilker S, et al: Calcium carbonate as a phosphate binder in patients with chronic renal failure undergoing dialysis. *N Engl J Med* 315:157, 1986.

198. Mai ML, Emmett M, Sheikh MS, et al: Calcium acetate, an effective phosphorus binder in patients with renal failure. *Kidney Int* 36:690, 1989.

199. Sherman RA, Bialy GB, Gazinski B, et al: The effect of dialysate calcium levels on blood pressure during hemodialysis. *Am J Kidney Dis* 8:244, 1986.

200. Maynard JC, Cruz C, Kleerekoper M, Levin NW: Blood pressure response to changes in serum ionized calcium during hemodialysis. *Ann Int Med* 104:358, 1986.

201. Fellner SK, Lang RM, Neumann A, et al: Physiological mechanisms for calcium-induced changes in systemic arterial pressure in stable dialysis patients. *Hypertension* 13:213, 1989.

202. Vaporean ML, Van Stone JC: Dialysate magnesium. *Semin Dial* 6:46, 1993.

203. Breuer J, Moniz C, Baldwin D, Parsons V: The effects of zero magnesium dialysate and magnesium supplements on ionized calcium concentration in patients on regular dialysis treatment. *Nephrol Dial Transplant* 2:347, 1987.

204. Gonella M, Ballanti P, Rocca C, et al: Improved bone morphology by normalizing serum magnesium in chronically hemodialyzed patients. *Miner Electrolyte Metab* 14:240, 1988.

205. Gonella M, Calabrese G: Magnesium status in chronically haemodialyzed patients: The role of dialysate magnesium concentration. *Magnesium Res* 2:259, 1989.

206. Coburn JW, Slatopolsky E: Vitamin D, parathyroid hormone and the renal osteodystrophies, in Brenner BM, Rector FC, Jr (eds): *The Kidney*. Philadelphia, WB Saunders, 1991, p 2036.

207. Mehta RL: Renal replacement therapy for acute renal failure: Matching the method to the patient. *Semin Dial* 6:253, 1993.

208. Cazenave JP, Mulvihill J: Interaction of blood with surfaces: Hemocompatibility and thromboresistance of biomaterials. *Contrib Nephrol* 62:188, 1988.

209. Grant ME, Lovell HB, Wiegmann TB: Current use of anticoagulation in hemodialysis. *Semin Dial* 4:168, 1991.

210. Owen WF, Lazarus JM: Dialytic management of acute renal failure, in Lazarus JM, Brenner BM (eds): *Acute Renal Failure*. New York, Churchill Livingstone, 1993, p 487.

211. Gordon LA, Simon ER, Richards JM: Studies in regional heparinization. II Artificial kidney hemodialysis without systemic heparinization—preliminary report of a method using simultaneous infusion of heparin and protamine. *N Engl J Med* 255:1063, 1956.

212. Hampers CL, Blaufox MD, Merrill JP: Anticoagulation rebound after hemodialysis. *N Engl J Med* 255:1063, 1966.

213. von Brecht J, Flanagan M, Freeman R, Lim V: Regional anticoagulation: hemodialysis with hypertonic trisodium citrate. *Am J Kidney Dis* 8:196, 1986.

214. Swartz R, Port F: Preventing hemorrhage in high risk hemodialysis: Regional versus low-dose heparin. *Kidney Int* 16:513, 1979.

215. Schwab S, Onorato J, Shara L, Dennis P: Hemodialysis without anticoagulation: 1 year prospective trial in hospitalized patients at risk for bleeding. *Am J Med* 83:405, 1987.

216. Caruna R, Raiai R, Bush J, et al: Heparin free dialysis: comparative data and results in high risk patients. *Kidney Int* 31:35, 1987.

217. Ronco C, Brendolan A, Gragantini L, et al: Continuous arteriovenous hemofiltration. *Contrib Nephrol* 48:70, 1985.

218. Golper TA, Ronco C, Kaplan AA: Continuous arteriovenous hemofiltration: Improvements, modifications, and future directions. *Semin Dial* 1:50, 1988.

219. Smith D, Paganini EP, Suhoza K, et al: Non-heparin continuous renal replacement therapy is possible, in J Nose, CM Kjellstrand, P Ivanovich (eds): *Progress in Artificial Internal Organs*. Cleveland, OH, ISAO Press, 1985, p 32.

220. Kaplan AA, Petrillo R: Regional heparinization for continuous arteriovenous hemofiltration. *Trans Am Soc Artif Int Organs* 33:312, 1987.

221. Vanherweghem JL, Yassine T, Goldman M, et al: Subclavian vein thrombosis: A frequent complication of subclavian vein cannulation for hemodialysis. *Clin Nephrol* 26:235, 1986.

222. Cimochowski G, Sartan J, Worley E, et al: Clear superiority of internal jugular access route over the subclavian vein for temporary access: An angiographic study in 52 patients with 102 venograms. *Kidney Int* 31:230, 1987.

223. Whittemore AD: Vascular access for hemodialysis, in Tilney NL, Lazarus JM (eds): *Surgical Care of the Patient with Renal Failure*. Philadelphia, WB Saunders, 1982, p 49.

224. Palder SB, Kirkman RL, Whittemore AD, et al: Tilney NL: Vascular access for hemodialysis. *Ann Surg* 202:235, 1985.

225. Nidus B, Matalon R, Katz C: Hemodialysis using femoral vein cannulation. *Nephron* 13:416, 1974.

226. Kjellstrand CN, Merino GE, Mauer SM, et al: Complications of percutaneous femoral vein catheterization for hemodialysis. *Clin Nephrol* 4:37, 1975.

227. Nidus BD, Neusy AJ: Chronic hemodialysis by repeated femoral vein cannulation. *Nephron* 29:195, 1981.

228. Bander SJ, Schwab SJ: Central venous angioaccess for hemodialysis and its complications. *Semin Dial* 5:121, 1992.

229. Dahlberg RJ, Falk RJ, Huffman KA: Subclavian hemodialysis catheter infections. *Am J Kidney Dis* 5:421, 1986.

230. Vanherweghem JL, Cabolet P, Dheane M, et al: Complications related to subclavian catheters for hemodialysis. *Am J Nephrol* 6:339, 1986.

231. Goldstein MB: Prevention of sepsis from central vein dialysis catheters. *Semin Dial* 5:106, 1992.

232. Schwab SJ: Hemodialysis-associated central vein thrombosis and stenosis: unresolved problems. *Semin Dial* 2:141, 1989.

233. Becker GJ, Holden RW, Rabe FE, et al: Local thrombolytic therapy for subclavian and axillary vein thrombosis. *Radiology* 149:419, 1983.

234. Schwab SJ, Quarles LD, Middleton JP, et al: Hemodialysis-associated subclavian vein stenosis. *Kidney Int* 33:1156, 1988.

235. Reed WP, Light PF, Sadler JH: Access for hemodialysis by means of long-term central venous catheters. *Kidney Int* 25:838, 1984.

236. Schwab SJ, Buller GL, McCann RL, et al: Prospective evaluation of a Dacron cuffed hemodialysis catheter for prolonged use. *Am J Kidney Dis* 11:166, 1988.

237. Khanna R, Twardowski ZJ: Peritoneal dialysis access, in Nolph KD (ed): *Peritoneal Dialysis*. Boston, Kluwer Academic Publishers, 1989, p 319.

238. Strippoli P, Pilolli D, Dimgrone G, et al: A hemostasis study in CAPD patients during fibrinolytic intraperitoneal therapy with urokinase (UK). *Adv Perit Dial* 5:97, 1989.

239. Sherman RA: The pathophysiologic basis for hemodialysis-related hypotension. *Semin Dial* 1:136, 1988.

240. Travis M, Henrich WL: Autonomic nervous system and hemodialysis hypotension. *Semin Dial* 2:158, 1989.

241. Arieff AI, Massry SG, Barrientos A, Kleeman CR: Brain water and electrolyte metabolism in uremia: Effects of slow and rapid hemodialysis. *Kidney Int* 4:177, 1973.

242. Basile C, Miller JD, Koles ZJ, Grace M, Ulan RA: The effects of dialysis on brain water and EEG in stable chronic uremia. *Am J Kidney Dis* 9:462, 1987.

243. Silver SM, DeSimone JA Jr, Smith DA, Sterns RH: Dialysis dysequilibrium syndrome in the rat: Role of the "reverse urea effect." *Kidney Int* 42:161, 1992.

244. Wakim KG: Predominance of hyponatremia or hypo-osmolality in simulation of the dialysis disequilibrium syndrome. *Mayo Clin Proc* 44:433, 1969.

245. Arieff AI, Massry SG: Dialysis dysequilibrium syndrome, in Massry SG, Sellers AL (eds): *Clinical Aspects of Uremia and Dialysis*. Springfield, IL, Charles C Thomas, 1976, p 34.

246. Strange K: Regulation of solute and water balance and cell volume in the central nervous system. *Am Soc Nephrol* 3:12, 1992.

247. Stewart WK, Fleming LW, Manuel MA: Benefits obtained by the use of a high sodium dialysate during maintenance hemodialysis. *Proc Eur Dial Transplant Assoc* 9:111, 1972.

248. Yoshida S, Tajika T, Yamasaki N, et al: Dialysis dysequilibrium syndrome in neurosurgical patients. *Neurosurgery* 20:716, 1987.

249. Intracranial pressure measurement in a patient undergoing hemodialysis and peritoneal dialysis. *Am J Kidney Dis* 13:336, 1989.

250. Bland LA, Favero MS, Arduino MJ: Should hemodialysis fluid be sterile? *Semin Dial* 6:34, 1993.

251. Teien AN, Bjoornson J: Heparin elimination in uraemic patients on haemodialysis. *Scand J Haematol* 17:29, 1976.

252. Vas SI: Peritonitis, in Nolph KD (ed): *Peritoneal Dialysis*. Boston, Kluwer Academic Publishers, 1989, p 261.

253. Traneus A, Heimburger O, Lindholm B: Peritonitis in chronic ambulatory peritoneal dialysis (CAPD): Diagnostic findings, therapeutic outcome and complications. *Perit Dial Int* 9:179, 1989.

254. Keane WF, Everett ED, Golper TA, et al: Peritoneal dialysis-related peritonitis treatment recommendations. 1993 update. *Perit Dial Int* 13:14, 1993.

255. Port FK, Held PJ, Nolph KD, et al: Risk of peritonitis and technique failure by CAPD connection technique: A national study. *Kidney Int* 42:967, 1992.

256. deFijter CWH, Verbrugh HA, Oe LP, et al: Peritonitis defense in continuous ambulatory vs chronic cycling peritoneal dialysis. *Kidney Int* 42:947, 1992.

257. Holley JL, Bernardini J, Piraino B: Polymicrobial peritonitis on continuous peritoneal dialysis. *Am J Kidney Dis* 19:162, 1992.

258. Lazarus JM: Which dialytic therapy is best for the patient with an unstable cardiovascular system? Hemodialysis is the optimal therapy. *Semin Dial* 5:208, 1992.

259. Bellomo R, Boyce N: Does continuous hemodiafiltration improve survival in acute renal failure? *Semin Dial* 6:16, 1993.

VI. Infectious Disease Problems in the Intensive Care Unit

Section Editor
Richard T. Ellison

84. Approach to Fever in the Intensive Care Patient

Marie J. George and Richard H. Glew

Approach to the Febrile Patient

Fever is a common problem in the intensive care unit. This chapter discusses both noninfectious and infectious causes of fever and provides a diagnostic framework for evaluation and treatment.

PATHOPHYSIOLOGY. Fever has been recognized for centuries as a sign of disease. Unlike other types of hyperthermia, fever represents an increase in body temperature in which thermoregulatory mechanisms are functional but acting to produce and sustain an elevated body temperature or set point [1]. Physiologically, fever begins with the production of one or more of a group of endogenous pyrogens in response to exogenous pyrogenic substances, such as microorganisms, toxic agents, or immunologic mediators [2,3]. Endogenous pyrogens are more accurately named cytokines because they are produced by a variety of cells, including lymphocytes, tissue macrophages, circulating monocytes, and endothelial cells. Cytokines produce a wide range of responses in both leukocytes and nonleukocytes. The principal mediator of fever is interleukin-1 (IL-1) [4,5], although others, including tumor necrosis factor (TNF) and interleukin-6 (IL-6), have been shown to be similar effectors of fever [5–8]. Cytokines interact with receptors in the preoptic anterior hypothalamic thermoregulatory area, causing synthesis and release of prostaglandins, chiefly prostaglandin E_2 (PGE_2). PGE_2 in turn initiates local cyclic adenosine monophosphate (AMP) production, which ultimately resets the thermoregulatory set point of the hypothalamus. In addition, prostaglandins coordinate other adaptive responses like shivering and peripheral vasoconstriction, thereby raising body temperature by several mechanisms [9,10].

Because fever results from a new set point of body temperature and is unassociated with impairments of either thermosensory or thermoeffector mechanisms, any attempt to reduce body temperature by simple physical means such as external cooling is resisted physiologically and can be physically distressing to the patient [1]. Moreover, except for a few uncommon states of hyperthermia, such as malignant hyperpyrexia during anesthesia and classic heat stroke, febrile episodes rarely produce body temperatures that are life-threatening [1,2].

TEMPERATURE MEASUREMENT. No single body temperature exists, and temperatures measured at different sites may vary. A person's body temperature varies physiologically; it is lowest in the morning and elevates with marked activity such as exercise or seizures. A recent study among adults 40 years old and younger suggested that 37.2°C (98.9°F) in the early morning and 37.7°C (99.9°F) for the remainder of the day and night represent the upper limits of the normal oral temperature range in individuals in this age group [11]. The febrile response to pyrogenic stimuli may be blunted or even absent in the elderly, in patients with azotemia or congestive heart failure, and in those receiving therapy with antipyretics or corticosteroids [12].

Because fever can be an early sign of common nosocomial complications in the ICU or CCU patient, prompt detection is essential. All ICU or CCU patients should be monitored with regular, reliable temperature determinations [13] (see Chap. 29). Although rectal temperature generally rises more slowly than oral temperature, the time delay in most febrile illnesses is too brief for this differential to be of clinical significance [14]. Moreover, rectal temperature generally is about 0.3° to 0.4°C higher than simultaneous oral temperature [15,16], and a glass-mercury rectal thermometer reaches maximal readings faster than similar oral thermometers—about 2 to 4 minutes compared with about 10 minutes for an oral thermometer [17,18]. Electronic thermometers operate in a predictive manner and complete a temperature reading before thermal equilibrium is reached, thereby providing accurate readings at either site in less than 1 minute [19,20]. Infrared detection tympanic thermometers appear to be equivalent to rectal probes when placed in the external auditory canal in the correct manner to record from the anterior, inferior one-third of the tympanic membrane [21,22]. Notably, oral temperatures obtained with an electronic thermometer in a tachypneic patient may be misleadingly low [16]. In general, axillary and skin temperature recordings are unreliable.

In most patients, a carefully obtained temperature is considered to indicate fever when a reading of 38°C (100.4°F) is obtained. Lesser degrees of temperature elevation warrant investigation in patients likely to manifest blunted pyrogenic responses, such as the elderly and patients with azotemia. Moreover, debilitated patients who exhibit a flattened temperature plot without the normal diurnal variation should be examined for possible underlying pyrogenic processes as well, even if maximal daily temperature is unimpressive (i.e., ≤100°F).

FEVER PATTERNS. Despite medical folklore, fever patterns generally are not helpful in suggesting or establishing specific diagnoses [23]. First, in many hospitalized patients insufficient data exist to establish a pattern of fever, because of brevity of illness, infrequency of temperature recordings, or administration of confounding medications. Moreover, even when there are sufficient recordings to identify a fever pattern, there is generally no relation between specific diagnoses and the occurrence of so-called intermittent, remittent, or hectic fevers [23]. Similarly, although rigors are considered to be suggestive of the presence of severe bacterial infection, shaking chills may also be seen in various nonbacterial disease states, including viral infections, drug reactions, and other inflammatory conditions.

Etiology of Fever in the Intensive Care Unit Patient

NONINFECTIOUS CAUSES OF FEVER. Although acute bacterial infections are among the most common and serious causes of fever in the ICU or CCU patient, fever may be a prominent manifestation of several noninfectious illnesses as well (Table 84-1). For example, fever can be a major presenting symptom in patients admitted critically ill with an acute vasculitis [24,25], subarachnoid hemorrhage, dissection of an aortic aneurysm [26], mesenteric ischemia [27], heat stroke [28], or hyperthyroidism [29]. Fever may appear as a nosocomial complication in the patient in whom the stress of surgery unmasks adrenal insufficiency [29] or in the patient in whom malignant hyperpyrexia develops during surgery or is associated with administration of nonanesthetic agents such as phenothiazines [30]. Fever associated with acute alcohol withdrawal is well described although in this setting it may be difficult to exclude other sequelae of chronic alcoholism such as pulmonary aspiration [31]. Likewise, fever related to generalized or partial seizures must be differentiated from possible underlying causes of seizure, such as meningitis or brain abscess. Fever occurring several days after admission and restriction to bed can signal the development of deep venous thrombosis [32] and/or pulmonary embolism [33,34]. A common cause of nosocomial fever is adverse reaction to medications, including therapeutic and diagnostic agents as well as blood products [35,36]. Notably, drug fever often occurs in the absence of traditionally held common signs and symptoms like eosinophilia and rash [37]. Fever has also been described in a few patients secondary to multiple intramuscular injections of analgesics, particularly hydroxyzine [38].

Table 84-1. Noninfectious Sources of Fever in the ICU or CCU Patient

A. Inflammatory conditions
   1. Reaction to medications
   2. Reaction to blood products
   3. Collagen vascular diseases
      a. Systemic lupus erythematosus
      b. Rheumatoid arthritis
   4. Vasculitis
      a. Hypersensitivity vasculitis
      b. Henoch-Schönlein purpura
      c. Wegener's granulomatosis
      d. Giant cell arteritis
   5. Microcrystalline arthritis
      a. Gout
      b. Pseudogout
   6. Postpericardiotomy syndrome
B. Hemorrhage/thromboembolism
   1. Deep venous thrombophlebitis
   2. Pulmonary embolism
   3. Dissecting aortic aneurysm
   4. Hemorrhage into
      a. CNS
      b. Retroperitoneum
      c. Joint
      d. Lung
   5. Myocardial infarction
C. Metabolic conditions
   1. Heat stroke
   2. Malignant hyperthermia during anesthesia or secondary to medications
   3. Hyperthyroidism
   4. Adrenal insufficiency
   5. Alcohol withdrawal
D. Neoplasia
   1. Lymphoma
   2. Renal cell carcinoma
   3. Hepatoma
   4. Malignancy metastatic to liver
   5. Colon carcinoma

Particular diagnostic and therapeutic difficulties arise with the appearance of fever in patients with malignancy, because it is important to differentiate between fever attributable to the tumor itself (especially common with lymphomas, primary and metastatic liver tumors, and renal cell carcinoma, and occasionally seen with colon carcinoma), fever from a mechanical complication caused by the malignancy (perforation, obstruction, or hemorrhage), and fever caused by superinfection [39,40].

The patient infected with human immunodeficiency virus (HIV-1 or HIV-2) who develops fever poses a formidable diagnostic challenge. Possible acute or chronic infections can elude diagnosis and are discussed in greater detail in Chapter 93. Additionally, HIV-infected persons have a greater incidence of adverse reactions to new or previously administered drugs, including drug-related fever [41]. Febrile episodes attributable to HIV itself are common in these patients, as are intermittent fevers without clear cause.

Conspicuously absent from Table 84-1 is atelectasis. Despite anecdotal belief among physicians in this relationship, there is no clear evidence of such. Rather, in two studies from the rabbit model, atelectasis alone was not sufficient to cause fever. In these same investigations, fever did occur in animals when pulmonary infection existed concurrently [42,43,44].

INFECTIOUS CAUSES OF FEVER. Nosocomial infections are an endemic problem in the ICU, in part because of the numerous invasive devices used to monitor and support critically ill patients, but also because of the acute illnesses and general debility that predispose critically ill patients to the development of acute infections [45,46,47] (see Chap. 86). Although nosocomial infections can arise in many sites, the most common sources of bacterial infection in the ICU or CCU include the urinary tract, respiratory tract, and wounds (Table 84-2). Secondary bacteremia can complicate infection in any of these sites but can also develop as a consequence of vascular invasion through intravenous lines, intraarterial monitors, temporary transvenous pacemakers, and intraaortic assist devices [48,49].

The gastrointestinal tract can serve as the source for severe nosocomial infections as well. Acute acalculous cholecystitis may occur after surgery and severe trauma [50,51]. Mesenteric infarction can be seen in patients with hypotension or atrial fibrillation, or in the setting of advanced age, severe generalized atherosclerosis, or recent myocardial infarction [26,52]. Another cause of fever and abdominal pain in the ICU patient is pseudomembranous colitis, caused by *Clostridium difficile* and related to antibiotic administration [53,54,55].

Diagnostic Considerations

In general, fever in the ICU or CCU patient warrants immediate assessment for several reasons: (1) Patients requiring ICU support are severely ill, often have complex underlying illnesses, and thereby are less likely than other hospitalized patients to survive serious nosocomial infections. (2) The organisms commonly operative in nosocomial infections in seriously ill patients include *Staphylococcus aureus*, gram-negative bacilli, and fungi. Infections caused by these organisms are characterized by necrotizing destruction of tissue and relative resistance of the organisms to antibiotics. (3) Fever may herald exacerbation or progression of the disease that prompted hospitalization (e.g., extension of a recent myocardial infarction, lung abscess or empyema developing in a patient with a necrotizing pneumonia, or persistent bacteremia in a patient with *S. aureus* endocarditis).

Table 84-2. Infectious Sources of Fever in the ICU or CCU
Patient

A. Urinary tract
B. Vascular support
   1. Intravenous access site
      a. Phlebitis
      b. Bacteremia or fungemia
      c. Cellulitis
   2. Intraarterial access site (bacteremia or fungemia)
C. Pulmonary
   1. Tracheobronchitis
   2. Pneumonia
D. Surgery-related
   1. Wound infection (superficial or deep)
   2. Undetected abscess
E. Decubitus ulcers
F. Gastrointestinal
   1. Antibiotic-associated colitis
   2. Ischemic colitis (mesenteric infarction)
   3. Acalculous cholecystitis
   4. Hepatitis (transfusion-related)
      a. Cytomegalovirus
      b. Non-A, non-B hepatitis
      c. Hepatitis B

HISTORY AND PHYSICAL EXAMINATION. If the patient can communicate, he or she should be interviewed concerning localizing complaints. The patient and hospital chart should be reinvestigated for a history of relevant antecedent problems (e.g., allergic reactions to drugs). In the case of an unconscious patient, the chart and paramedical personnel can provide useful information concerning duration of vascular cannulation, quantity and purulence of sputum or wound drainage, changes in skin condition, apparent abdominal or musculoskeletal pain or tenderness, and difficulty in handling respiratory secretions and food.

Physical examination of the febrile ICU patient may be more difficult to carry out with constraints of catheters, ventilator attachments, and monitors, but nonetheless should be thorough. Skin examination may demonstrate a bilateral, symmetric, erythematous, multiforme rash suggestive of drug reaction, or an acral, bilateral but often asymmetric rash of vasculitis. A tender intravenous access site, with or without purulence, can indicate septic phlebitis. Spreading erythema, warmth, and tenderness that appear to indicate cellulitis of an extremity can also be the hallmarks of deep venous phlebitis, pyarthrosis, or gout. After the first 24 hours postoperatively, wound dressings should be taken down and examined. Wound inspection may require fenestrating or changing a cast to allow examination of a fractured extremity if no other source of hectic fever is found. All intravenous and intraarterial line sites should be inspected.

Head and neck examination can provide important signs of systemic as well as localized infection. Funduscopic lesions of disseminated candidiasis may be the first identifiable site of this often elusive pathogen. The lesions of candidal endophthalmitis have a white cotton-wool appearance and are principally located in choroid and retina but may advance to involve the lens, cornea, vitreous humor, and uveal tract [56]. Purulent sinusitis can occur in the nasally or orally intubated patient and may have a paucity of associated symptoms. Oral lesions of recrudescent herpetic stomatitis are common in the ICU setting. These lesions may be more ulcerated and necrotic (i.e., black) and less vesicular in appearance in a seriously ill patient.

Examination of the lungs can be difficult in the ICU patient whose mobility necessarily is restricted, and often is unrewardingly nonlocalizing and nonspecific in the ventilator-dependent patient. More sensitive (though nonspecific) indicators of pneu-

monia include the chest roentgenogram and the finding of unexplained deterioration in arterial oxygenation. Unfortunately, pulmonary infiltrates and arterial hypoxemia also can be seen with congestive heart failure, acute respiratory distress syndrome, and, less commonly, reactions to medications and pulmonary hemorrhage [57,58]. Cardiac examination may demonstrate a pericardial friction rub caused by Dressler's syndrome, or a new or changing murmur possibly attributable to endocarditis.

Abdominal findings can be misleadingly unremarkable in the elderly, in the patient with diminished sensorium, and in the patient receiving potent analgesics. They may be confoundingly positive in the patient with recent abdominal or thoracic surgery. Abdominal pain and tenderness may be localized (cholecystitis, intraabdominal abscess, diverticulitis) or generalized (diffuse peritonitis, ischemic bowel, antibiotic-associated colitis). Examination of the genitals and rectum may demonstrate unsuspected epididymitis, prostatitis, prostatic abscess, or perirectal abscess.

LABORATORY STUDIES. Initial laboratory evaluation of fever in the ICU patient should include urinalysis and culture, two sets of blood cultures (each obtained from a separate venipuncture and/or intravascular catheter with catheter-obtained specimens sent labeled as such when sent to the microbiology laboratory), and chest roentgenogram. Efforts should be made to obtain sputum for Gram stain and culture [59–62]. See Chapters 13 and 76 for in-depth discussions of obtaining lower respiratory tract secretions in pneumonia.

In general, all abnormal fluid collections (pleural effusion, joint effusion, ascites) should be sampled for microscopic, chemical, and cultural evaluation. Microbiologic yield from ascites culture has been shown to be greater when ascitic fluid is placed into blood culture [63] or fungal isolator [64] media. Because small pleural effusions are noted commonly after uncomplicated abdominal surgery, however, pleural fluid need not be sampled in the first several postoperative days unless the volume is large or increasing or there is associated pleuritic chest pain [65]. Except in cases of head trauma, neurosurgery, or high-grade bacteremia with virulent, invasive pathogens such as *S. aureus* or gram-negative bacilli, meningitis is an uncommon nosocomial infection [66,67]; thus, sampling of CSF usually need not be considered in the initial work-up for nosocomial fever. However, lumbar puncture should be considered in the febrile ICU patient with sudden, unexplained change in mental status or in the febrile patient who has undergone recent neurosurgery or head trauma and whose mental status is difficult to evaluate. Symptomatic complaints or physical findings referable to the abdomen dictate the need for determination of liver chemistries and serum amylase and abdominal roentgenogram.

Examination of fluid from an inflamed, effused joint necessarily includes analysis for crystals. Exacerbations of gout and pseudogout often mimic the symptoms and physical examination and even leukocytosis of the septic joint [68]. Identification of crystals expedites treatment for these rheumatologic entities that do not benefit from drainage and antibiotics. Coexistence of gout and joint infection, although uncommon, may occur [69].

If the examinations and studies already mentioned are unrewarding and fever continues, or if impressive, enigmatic local findings are observed in the central nervous system or abdomen, additional laboratory studies such as computed tomography (CT) scan and radionuclide studies may be indicated.

In many instances thorough evaluation of the febrile ICU or CCU patient establishes the cause of fever, thereby guiding selection of antibiotic therapy or, conversely, indicating that no antimicrobial therapy is required. In the acutely ill, unstable patient, however, it may be necessary to begin empiric broad-spectrum antibiotic therapy before an infectious cause is established. If the pretherapeutic work-up has been thorough, re-adjustment, addition of, or even termination of initial antibiotic therapy will be made possible by reevaluation of the clinical situation, including response of the patient to therapy and results of cultures and other laboratory tests. Positive cultures may permit narrowing of the spectrum of antibiotic coverage or may dictate that additional organisms need to be covered by added antimicrobial therapy. Negative cultures in a patient who is unimproved yet stable on broad therapy indicate that antibiotics should be discontinued and the patient reevaluated. Negative cultures in a febrile patient who is unimproved or worsened may be a clue to disseminated fungal infection, and empiric antifungal therapy should be considered.

Approach to Initial Presumptive Antibiotic Therapy

Because little or no microbiologic information usually is forthcoming for the first 24 to 48 hours of management, initial antibiotic therapy in the acutely infected patient often is based on presumptive conclusions derived from initial clinical evaluation (see Chap. 85). Rapid but thorough evaluation of the febrile ICU or CCU patient by means of history, physical examination, and simple laboratory tests as above often identifies a likely primary site of infection, such as pneumonia or pyelonephritis. However, infections even in these sites may be difficult to define with certainty in some patients, because cardiogenic pulmonary edema or the acute respiratory distress syndrome can produce roentgenographic infiltrates and hypoxemia, and instrumentation of the lungs and urinary bladder results in purulent secretions and positive cultures even in the absence of invasive infection [59].

Once efforts have been made to determine the most likely site or sites of infection, one can make a reasonable estimate of infecting pathogens. In an ICU or CCU patient, one should assume that in addition to the usual expected pathogens, infection is likely to involve more opportunistic, hospital-associated pathogens such as S. aureus, coagulase-negative staphylococci, and gram-negative enteric bacilli. Similarly, in light of possible impaired mechanical and immunologic defenses and the presence of intravascular lines, the febrile ICU or CCU patient should be considered to be bacteremic until proved otherwise. Patients with intravascular lines and suspected bacteremia should have blood cultures obtained and their lines removed if at all possible. Lines can be replaced, if necessary, after antibiotic therapy has been initiated.

Once the spectrum of potential infecting organisms has been narrowed to one or a few likely candidates, empiric antibiotic therapy should be initiated according to generally accepted principles [70,71,72] as outlined in Table 84-3 and in Chapter 85. However, such guidelines must be interpreted in light of the types of organisms and patterns of drug resistance prevalent in the specific institution and ICU. Ultimately, definitive antibiotic therapy is determined by review of the final microbiologic data with identification of the isolated infecting microorganism and its antibiotic sensitivities.

DOSAGE AND ROUTE OF ADMINISTRATION. Because infections in the ICU often are severe and fulminant, because

of either the nature of the infecting organism, the site of infection, or impaired defenses and resources of the patient, antimicrobial therapy generally should be administered parenterally and in maximal recommended doses. As a rule, the intravenous route is preferred over intramuscular injections because of the possibility of unreliable absorption from muscle because of impaired hemodynamics.

Antibiotics such as the penicillins and cephalosporins, which exhibit a high therapeutic-toxic ratio, are usually administered to adults according to a standardized dosage regimen (gm/day) independent of the patient's weight. For antibiotics such as the aminoglycosides and vancomycin, which exhibit a narrow toxic-therapeutic ratio and with which likelihood of toxicity is proportional to serum and tissue levels, dosing should be based on the patient's estimated lean body weight and renal function. The creatinine clearance, calculated by using the serum creatinine, age, and patient's lean body weight, is an important first step for antimicrobial dosing determinations, especially for the aminoglycosides [73] (see Chap. 78):

$$\frac{\text{Creatinine clearance (CrCl)}}{\text{(males)}} = \frac{(140 - \text{age (yrs)}) \times \text{weight (kg)}}{\text{serum creatinine} \times 72}$$

$$\text{CrCl (females)} = \text{CrCl} \times 0.85$$

Serum creatinine concentrations should be checked frequently, and serum antibiotic levels (peak and trough) should be monitored at least weekly and more often if renal function or hemodynamics are unstable.

Dosing intervals for most antibiotics are selected so that the drugs are administered every three to four serum half-lives ($T^{1/2}$). Because most of the older parenterally administered beta-lactam antibiotics have a $T^{1/2}$ of approximately 1 hour, intravenous penicillins and cephalosporins traditionally were given every 4 hours. However, the $T^{1/2}$ for cefazolin and newer cephalosporins such as cefotaxime, ceftazidime, and cefoperazone is approximately 1.5 to 2.5 hours, and these agents can be administered less frequently, perhaps every 6 to 8 hours even for serious infections; for ceftriaxone the $T^{1/2}$ is 8 hours, and the administration frequency is every 12 to 24 hours [74,75,76].

ANTIBIOTIC COMBINATIONS. Although infection caused by a single well-characterized organism can be successfully treated with a single antimicrobial agent in most patients, combination antimicrobial therapy is justified in a variety of clinical and microbiologic situations that may be obtained in the ICU or CCU patient [77,78]. Three such indications for use of antibiotic combinations are discussed.

Initial Therapy of Life-Threatening Infection. During the initial management of a seriously ill patient in the ICU in whom the diagnosis remains in question, it may be necessary to administer two or three antibiotics to cover multiple possible sources of fever pending return of microbiologic and other laboratory studies. For example, suspected acute overwhelming infection of unknown or uncertain source in an ICU patient warrants therapy with a penicillinase-resistant penicillin (oxacillin or nafcillin) or a cephalosporin to cover S. aureus, plus an aminoglycoside (gentamicin, tobramycin, or amikacin) to treat gram-negative bacilli. If methicillin-resistant S. aureus is common in the facility, vancomycin should be substituted for a penicillin or cephalosporin. If pneumonia seems more likely than line-associated bacteremia, a third-generation cephalosporin should be substituted for oxacillin to provide better coverage for gram-negative enteric bacilli and Haemophilus influenzae, respectively. If gross aspirational soiling of the lungs is suspected or if lower airway obstruction is present (e.g., lung

Table 84-3. Presumptive Antibiotic Therapy in the ICU or CCU Patient

Site/diagnosis	Potential causes	Definitive therapy	Alternative therapy
Vascular/line-associated bacteremia	*Staphylococcus aureus*, GNR	Oxacillin[a] or nafcillin[a] *plus* an aminoglycoside[b]	Vancomycin or cephalosporin[c] *plus* an aminoglycoside[b]
Vascular/acute endocarditis	*S. aureus*	Oxacillin[a] or nafcillin[a] *plus* an aminoglycoside[b] (if enterococcus is suspected, add penicillin G)	Vancomycin or cephalosporin[c] *plus* an aminoglycoside[b]
Vascular/acute endocarditis	GNR	A third-generation cephalosporin[d] or imipenem or piperacillin *plus* an aminoglycoside[b]	Aztreonam *plus* an aminoglycoside[b]
Pulmonary/pneumonia	Diverse GNR	Third-generation cephalosporin[d] *plus* an aminoglycoside[b]	Imipenem or piperacillin or aztreonam *plus* an aminoglycoside;[b] trimethoprim-sulfamethoxazole
Pulmonary/pneumonia	*S. aureus*	Oxacillin[a] or nafcillin[a]	Cephalosporin[c] or vancomycin
Pulmonary/pneumonia	GNR, mouth anaerobes, *S. aureus*, *Haemophilus influenzae*	Third-generation cephalosporin[d] *plus* an aminoglycoside[b]	Imipenem or piperacillin (*plus* clindamycin) *plus* an aminoglycoside[b]
Urinary tract/pyelonephritis	GNR, enterococcus	Ampicillin or piperacillin *plus* an aminoglycoside[b]	Third-generation cephalosporin[d] or aztreonam (with vancomycin if enterococcus suspected)
Abdomen/peritonitis, abscess, pelvic infection associated with female GU tract	GNR, anaerobes, enterococcus	Ampicillin or penicillin G or piperacillin or mezlocillin *plus* clindamycin or metronidazole *plus* an aminoglycoside[b]	Vancomycin in place of penicillin *plus* clindamycin, or metronidazole *plus* an aminoglycoside[b] or a third-generation cephalosporin[d]; or imipenem
Abdomen/biliary tract	GNR, enterococcus, anaerobes (less often)	Ampicillin or penicillin G or piperacillin or mezlocillin *plus* an aminoglycoside[b]	Add clindamycin or metronidazole if initial therapy is unsuccessful
CNS/meningitis	*Streptococcus pneumoniae*	Penicillin G	Ceftriaxone, cefuroxime or chloramphenicol
CNS/meningitis	*Neisseria meningitidis*	Penicillin G	Ceftriaxone, cefuroxime or chloramphenicol
CNS/meningitis	GNR, *S. aureus*	Oxacillin[a] or nafcillin[a] *plus* ceftriaxone *plus* an aminoglycoside[b]	Vancomycin *plus* ceftriaxone *plus* an aminoglycoside[b]
CNS/acute abscess	*S. aureus*	Oxacillin[a] or nafcillin[a] *plus* an aminoglycoside[b]	Vancomycin
CNS/subacute or chronic abscess	Anaerobes	Penicillin G *plus* metronidazole	Chloramphenicol

[a]Vancomycin if methicillin-resistant *S. aureus* common.
[b]Gentamicin, tobramycin, or amikacin.
[c]First-generation cephalosporin (cephalothin, cefazolin, or cephapirin).
[d]Cefotaxime, ceftriaxone, or ceftazidime.
GNR = gram-negative rods.

tumor), anaerobic coverage can be obtained by the addition of metronidazole or clindamycin to the above regimen, or by substituting imipenem for a third-generation cephalosporin. Similarly, it is common to administer three antibiotics to the septic neutropenic patient with fever—a semisynthetic, penicillinase-resistant penicillin to cover gram-positive organisms like *S. aureus*; a semisynthetic, anti-pseudomonal penicillin (piperacillin or a third-generation cephalosporin (e.g., ceftazidime); and an aminoglycoside to provide a broad, potentially synergistic gram-negative coverage [77–82]. In the seriously ill neutropenic patient with long-term intravascular access in place, vancomycin should replace oxacillin or nafcillin as empiric therapy for gram-positive organisms, because *S. epidermidis* and other sources of line infection are not consistently susceptible to the penicillinase-resistent penicillins [83].

Therapy of Mixed Bacterial Infection. Combination therapy is necessary to provide broad, effective coverage in specific infections expected to involve numerous, diverse microorganisms. For example, intraabdominal and intrapelvic infections frequently exhibit complex infecting flora, involving diverse aerobic and anaerobic pathogens [84–91]. Definitive treatment of such infections often includes an aminoglycoside for members of the *Enterobacteriaceae* family, clindamycin or metronidazole for *Bacteroides fragilis* and other anaerobes, and penicillin G or ampicillin for enterococci [71]. An alternative regimen, particularly in the patient with known or suspected (long-term residence in the ICU or recent receipt of broad-spectrum antibiotic therapy) multiresistant gram-negative bacteria, is imipenem plus an aminoglycoside.

Synergism of Antibiotic Regimens. Therapy with combinations of antibiotics is indicated in several circumstances in which these regimens are or may be synergistic against a single organism, usually when bactericidal effect of therapy is considered optimal (e.g., bacteremic infections caused by enterococcal group D streptococci, especially those involving endocarditis; therapy involves penicillin G or ampicillin plus an aminoglycoside) [78,92–94]. Synergistic antibiotic regimens also are employed against severe, invasive, or blood-borne infections by *Pseudomonas aeruginosa* and other highly resistant gram-negative bacilli (e.g., *Enterobacter, Serratia,* and *Acinetobacter* species) to provide possible improved efficacy (especially in neutropenic patients) and to retard emergence of increasing antibiotic resistance. In this setting, therapy commonly involves a semisynthetic beta-lactam with anti-Pseudomonal activity (ceftazidime, piperacillin, azlocillin, or imipenem) plus an aminoglycoside [95–100]. Bacteremic *S. aureus* infections may warrant initial therapy with a penicillinase-resistant penicillin (oxacillin or nafcillin) plus an aminoglycoside to provide optimal early bactericidal effect [101,102,103]. This treatment combination is associated with earlier sterilization of blood cultures from *S. aureus* than treatment with penicillinase-resistant penicillin alone [104]. The fixed combination of trimethoprim and sulfamethoxazole (cotrimoxazole) provides bactericidal activity against a variety of microorganisms, including members of the Enterobacteriaceae family, *Haemophilus influenzae, Streptococcus pneumoniae,* Salmonella and Shigella species, and the fungi *Pneumocystis carinii* [105,106].

References

1. Stitt JT: Fever versus hyperthermia. *Fed Proc* 138:39, 1979.
2. Bernheim HA, Block LH, Atkins E: Fever: Pathogenesis, pathophysiology, and purpose. *Ann Intern Med* 91:261, 1979.
3. Dinarello CA, Wolff SM: Molecular basis of fever in humans. *Am J Med* 72:799, 1989.
4. Dinarello CA: Interleukin-1 and interleukin-1 antagonism. *Blood* 77:1627, 1991.
5. Cannon JG, Tompkins RG, Gelfand JA, et al: Circulating interleukin-1 and tumor necrosis factor in septic shock and experimental endotoxin fever. *J Infect Dis* 161:79, 1990.
6. Kapas L, Hong L, Cady AB, et al: Somnogenic, pyrogenic and anorectic activities of tumor necrosis factor-α and TNF-α fragments. *Am J Physiol* 263:R708, 1992.
7. Karunaweena ND, Graw GE, Gamage P, et al: Dynamics of fever and serum levels of tumor necrosis factor are closely associated during clinical paroxysms in *Plasmodium vivax* malaria. *Proc Natl Acad Sci U S A* 89:3200, 1992.
8. Heney D, Lewis LJ, Evans SW, et al: Interleukin-6 and its relationship to C-reactive protein and fever in children with febrile neutropenia. *J Infect Dis* 165:886, 1992.
9. Coceani F, Bishai I, Lees J, et al: Prostaglandin E2 in the pathogenesis of pyrogen fever: Validation of an intermediary role. *Adv Prostaglandin Thromboxane Leukotriene Res* 19:394, 1989.
10. Davidson J, Milton AS, Rotondo D: α-Melanocyte stimulating hormone suppresses fever and increases in plasma levels of protstaglandin E_2 in the rabbit. *J Physiol* 451:491, 1992.
11. Mackowiak PA, Wasserman SS, Levine MM: A critical appraisal of 98.6°F, the upper limit of the normal body temperature, and other legacies of Carl Reinhold August Wunderlich. *JAMA* 26:1578, 1992.
12. Gleckman R, Hibert D. Afebrile bacteremia: A phenomenon in geriatric patients. *JAMA* 1248:1478, 1982.
13. Clarke DE, Kimelman J, Raffin TA: The evaluation of fever in the intensive care unit. *Chest* 100:213, 1991.
14. Cranston WI: Temperature regulation. *Br Med J* 5505:69, 1966.
15. Cranston WI, Gerbrandy J, Snell ES: Oral, rectal and oesophageal temperatures and some factors affecting them in man. *J Physiol* 126:347, 1954.
16. Tandberg D, Sklar D: Effect of tachypnea on the estimation of body temperature by an oral thermometer. *N Engl J Med* 308:945, 1983.
17. Nichols GA, Ruskin MM, Glor BAK, et al: Oral, axillary, and rectal temperature determinations and relationships. *Nurs Res* 15:307, 1966.
18. Nichols GA, Kucha DH: Oral measurements. *Am J Nurs* 72:1091, 1972.
19. New thermometers. *Medical Letter* 21:19, 1979.
20. Erickson R: Thermometer placement for oral temperature measurement in febrile adults. *Int J Nurs Stud* 13:199, 1976.
21. Kenny RD, Fortenberry JB, Surratt SS, et al: Evaluation of an infrared tympanic membrane thermometer in pediatric patients. *Pediatrics* 85:854, 1990.
22. Terndrup TE: An appraisal of temperature assessment by infrared emission detection tympanic thermometer. *Ann Emerg Med* 21:1483, 1992.
23. Musher DM, Fainstein V, Young EJ, et al: Fever patterns: Their lack of clinical sigificance. *Arch Intern Med* 139:1225, 1979.
24. Fauci AS, Haynes BF, Katz P: The spectrum of vasculitis: Clinical, pathologic, immunologic, and therapeutic considerations. *Ann Intern Med* 89:660, 1978.
25. Stahl NI, Klippel JH, Decker JL: Fever in systemic lupus erythematosus. *Am J Med* 67:935, 1979.
26. Mackowiak PA, Lipscomb KM, Millis LJ, et al: Dissecting aortic aneurysm manifested as fever of ukhown origin. *JAMA* 236:1725, 1976.
27. Ottinger LW: Acute mesenteric ischemia. *N Engl J Med* 307:535, 1982.
28. Hart GR, Anderson RJ, Crumpler CP, et al: Epidemic classical heat stroke: Clinical characteristics and course of 28 patients. *Medicine* 61:189, 1982.
29. Simon HB, Daniels GH: Hormonal hyperthermia: Endocrinologic causes of fever. *Am J Med* 66:257, 1979.
30. Arens JF, McKinnon WMP: Malignant hyperpyrexia during anesthesia. *JAMA* 215:919, 1971.
31. Bartlett JG, Gorbach SL, Finegold SM: The bacteriology of aspiration pneumonia. *Am J Med* 56:202, 1974.
32. Faris IB, Rosengarten DS, Dudley HAF: Temperature-chart analysis in the diagnosis of postoperative deep-vein thrombosis. *Lancet* 2:775, 1972.
33. Dalen JE, Haffajee CI, Alpert JS, et al: Pulmonary embolism, pulmonary hemorrhage and pulmonary infarction. *N Engl J Med* 296:1431, 1977.
34. Murray HW, Ellis GC, Blumenthal DS, et al: Fever and pulmonary thromboembolism. *Am J Med* 67:232, 1979.
35. Lipsky BA, Hirschmann JV: Drug fever. *JAMA* 245:851, 1981.
36. Young EJ, Fainstein V, Musher DM: Drug-induced fever: Cases seen in the evaluation of unexplained fever in a general hospital population. *Rev Infect Dis* 4:69, 1982.
37. Mackowiak PA, LeMaistre CF: Drug fever: A critical appraisal of conventional concepts. *Ann Intern Med* 106:728, 1987.
38. Semel JD: Fever associated with repeated intramuscular injections of analgesics. *Rev Infect Dis* 8:68, 1986.
39. Young CW: Studies on fever in neoplastic disease, in Lipton JM (ed): *Fever.* New York, Raven Press, 1980.
40. Warshaw AL, Carey RW, Robinson DR: Control of fever associated with visceral cancers by indomethacin. *Surgery* 89:414, 1981.
41. Gordin FM, Simon GL, Wofsy CB, et al: Adverse reactions to trimethoprim-sulfamethoxazole in patients with the acquired immunodeficiency syndrome. *Ann Intern Med* 100:495, 1984.
42. Shlenke JD, Huban CA: The pathogenesis of postoperative atelectasis. *Arch Surg* 107:846, 1973.
43. Lansing AM, Jamieson WG: Mechanisms of fever in pulmonary atelectasis. *Arch Surg* 87:168, 1963.
44. Shields RT: The pathogenesis of postoperative pulmonary atelectasis. *Arch Surg* 48:489, 1949.
45. Britt MR, Schleupner CJ, Matsumiya S: Severity of underlying disease as a predictor of nosocomial infection. *JAMA* 239:1047, 1978.
46. Maki DG: Risk factors for nosocomial infection in intensive care:

devices vs nature and goals for the next decade. *Arch Intern Med* 149:30, 1989.

47. Craven DE, Kunches LM, Lichtenberg DA, et al: Nosocomial infection and fatality in medical and surgical intensive care unit patients. *Arch Intern Med* 148:1168, 1988.

48. McGowan JE Jr: Changing etiology of nosocomial bacteremia and fungemia and other hospital-acquired infections. *Rev Infect Dis* 7(suppl):2357, 1985.

49. Maki DG, Hassemer CA: Endemic rate of fluid contamination and related septicemia in arterial pressure monitoring. *Am J Med* 70:733, 1981.

50. Long TN, Helmbach DM, Carrico CJ: Acalculous cholecystitis in critically ill patients. *Am J Surg* 136:31, 1978.

51. Howard RJ: Acute acalculous cholecystitis. *Am J Surg* 141:194, 1981.

52. Ottinger LW, Austen WG: A study of 136 patients with mesenteric infarction. *Surg Gynecol Obstet* 124:251, 1967.

53. Tedesco FJ, Barton RW, Alpers DH: Clindamycin-associated colitis. *Ann Intern Med* 81:429, 1974.

54. Bartlett JG: Antibiotic-associated diarrhea. *Clin Infect Dis* 15:573, 1992.

55. McFarland LV, Mulligan ME, Kwok RYY, et al: Nosocomial acquisition of *Clostridium difficile* infection. *N Engl J Med* 320:204, 1989.

56. Edwards JE Jr: *Candida* endophthalmitis, in Bodey GP, Fainstein V (eds): *Candidiasis*. New York, Raven Press, 1985, p 211.

57. Rinaldo JE, Rogers RM: Adult respiratory distress syndrome. Changing concepts of lung injury and repair. *N Engl J Med* 306:900, 1982.

58. Divertie MB: The adult respiratory distress syndrome. *Mayo Clin Proc* 57:371, 1982.

59. Glew RH, Moellering RC Jr, Kunz LJ: Infection with *Acinetobacter calcoaceticus (Herellea vaginicola)*: Clinical and laboratory studies. *Medicine* 56:79, 1977.

60. Geckler RW, Gremillion DH, McAllister CK, et al: Microscopic and bacteriological comparison of paired sputa and transtracheal aspirates. *J Clin Microbiol* 6:396, 1977.

61. Murray PR, Washington JA II: Microscopic and bacteriologic analysis of expectorated sputum. *Mayo Clin Proc* 50:339, 1975.

62. Johanson WG Jr, Pierce AK, Sanford JP, et al: Nosocomial respiratory infections with gram-negative bacilli: The significance of colonization of the respiratory tract. *Ann Intern Med* 77:701, 1972.

63. Siersema PD, deMarie S, Van Zeijl JH, et al: Blood culture bottles are superior to lysis centrifugation tubes for bacteriological diagnosis of spontaneous bacterial peritonitis. *J Clin Microbiol* 30:667, 1992.

64. Castellote J, Xiol X, Verdaguer R, et al: Comparison of two ascitic fluid culture methods in cirrhotic patients with spontaneous bacterial peritonitis. *Am J Gastroenterol* 85:1605, 1990.

65. Light RW, George RB: Incidence and significance of pleural effusion after abdominal surgery. *Chest* 69:621, 1976.

66. Hodges GR, Perkins RL: Hospital-associated bacterial meningitis. *Am J Med Sci* 271:335, 1976.

67. National Nosocomial Infection Study Report. US Department of Health and Human Services, Centers for Disease Control, March 1982.

68. Smith JW: Infectious arthritis. *Infect Dis Clin North Am* 4:523, 1990.

69. Baer PA, Tenenbaum J, Fam AG, et al: Coexistent septic and crystal arthritis: Report of 4 cases and literature review. *J Rheumatol* 13:604, 1986.

70. Wilkowske CJ: General principles of antimicrobial therapy. *Mayo Clinic Proc* 66:931, 1991.

71. The choice of antimicrobial drugs. *Medical Letter* 32:41, 1990.

72. Sanford JP: *Guide to Antimicrobial Therapy*. Dallas, Antimicrobial Therapy Inc., 1993.

73. Cockcroft DW, Gault MH: Prediction of creatinine clearance from serum creatinine. *Nephron* 16:31, 1976.

74. Gustaferro CA, Steckelberg JM: Cephalosporin antimicrobial agents and related compounds. *Mayo Clin Proc* 66:1064, 1991.

75. Neu HC: New antibiotics: Areas of appropriate use. *J Infect Dis* 155:403, 1987.

76. Gustaferro CA, Steckelberg JM: Cephalosporin antimicrobial agents and related compounds. *Mayo Clin Proc* 66:1064, 1991.

77. Eliopoulos GM: Synergism and antagonism. *Infect Dis Clin North Am* 3:399, 1989.

78. Rahal JJ Jr: Antibiotic combinations: The clinical relevance of synergy and antagonism. *Medicine* 57:179, 1978.

79. Pizzo PA: Management of fever in patients with cancer and treatment-induced neutropenia. *N Engl J Med* 328:1323, 1993.

80. Schimpff S, Satterlee W, Young VM, et al: Empiric therapy with carbenicillin and gentamicin for febrile patients with cancer and granulocytopenia. *N Engl J Med* 284:1061, 1971.

81. Whimbey E, Kiehn TE, Brannon P, Blevins A, et al: Bacteremia and fungemia in patients with neoplastic disease. *Am J Med* 82:723, 1987.

82. Klastersky J: Empiric treatment of infections in neutropenic patients with cancer. *Rev Infect Dis* 5:S21, 1983.

83. Shapiro ED, Wald ER, Nelson KA, et al: Broviac catheter-related bacteremia in oncology patients. *Am J Dis Child* 8:42, 1986.

84. Styrt B, Gorbach SL: Recent developments in the understanding of the pathogenesis and treatment of anaerobic infections. *N Engl J Med* 321:240, 298, 1989.

85. Rotstein OD, Pruett TL, Simmons RL: Mechanisms of microbial synergy in polymicrobial surgical infections. *Rev Infect Dis* 7:151, 1985.

86. Field TC, Pickleman J: Intra-abdominal abscess unassociated with prior operation. *Arch Surg* 120:821, 1985.

87. Sutter VL: Frequency of occurrence and antimicrobial susceptibility of bacterial isolates from the intestinal and female genital tracts. *Rev Infect Dis* 5:S84, 1985.

88. Peterson HB, Walker CK, Kahn JG, et al: Pelvic inflammatory disease: Key treatment issues and options. *JAMA* 266:2605, 1991.

89. Eschenbach DA, Buchanan TM, Pollock HM, et al: Polymicrobial etiology of acute pelvic inflammatory disease. *N Engl J Med* 293:166, 1975.

90. Dodson MG, Faro S: The polymicrobial etiology of acute pelvic inflammatory disease and treatment regimens. *Rev Infect Dis* 7:S696, 1985.

91. Finegold SM, Wexler HM: Therapeutic implications of bacteriologic findings in mixed aerobic-anaerobic infections. *Antimicrob Agents Chemother* 32:611, 1988.

92. Moellering RC Jr: Antimicrobial synergism: An elusive concept. *J Infect Dis* 140:639, 1979.

93. Mandell GL, Kaye D, Levison ME, et al: Enterococcal endocarditis. *Arch Intern Med* 125:258, 1970.

94. Moellering RC JR, Wennersten C, Weinberg AN: Studies on antibiotic synergism against enterococci: I. Bacteriologic studies. *J Lab Clin Med* 77:821, 1971.

95. Parry MF, Neu HC: Ticarcillin for treatment of serious infections with gram-negative bacteria. *J Infect Dis* 134:476, 1976.

96. Glew RH, Moellering RC Jr, Buettner KR: In vitro synergism between carbenicillin and aminoglycosidic aminocyclitols against Acinetobacter calcoaceticus var. anitratus. *Antimicrob Agent Chemother* 11:1036, 1977.

97. Johnson DG, Thompson B, Calia FW: Comparative activities of piperacillin ceftazidime and amikacur alone and in all possible combinations against experimental *Pseudomonas aeruginosa* infections in neutropenic rats. *Antimicrob Agent Chemother* 27:735, 1985.

98. The EORTC International Antimicrobial Therapy Cooperative Group: Ceftazidime combined with a short or long course of amikacin for empirical therapy of gram-negative bacteremia in cancer patients with granulocytopenia. *N Engl J Med* 317:1092, 1987.

99. Anderson ET, Young IS, Hewitt WL: Antimicrobial synergism in the therapy of gram-negative rod bacteremia. *Chemotherapy* 24:45, 1978.

100. Glew RH, Pavuk RA: Early synergistic interaction between semisynthetic penicillins and aminoglycosidic aminocyclitols against Enterobacteriaceae. *Antimicrob Agent Chemother* 23:902, 1983.

101. Kaye D: The clinical significance of tolerance of *Staphylococcus aureus*. *Ann Intern Med* 93:924, 1980.

102. Mayhall CG, Medoff G, Marr JJ: Variation in the susceptibility of strains of *Staphylococcus aureus* to oxacillin, cephalothin, and gentamicin. *Antimicrob Agent Chemother* 10:707, 1976.

103. Rajashekaraiah KR, Rice T, Rao Vs, et al: Clinical significance of

tolerant strains of *Staphylococcus aureus* in patients with endo-carditis. *Ann Intern Med* 93:796, 1980.

104. Korzeniowski O, Sande MA: Combination antimicrobial therapy for *Staphylococcus aureus* endocarditis in patients addicted to parenteral drugs and nonaddicts: A prospective study. *Ann Intern Med* 97:496, 1982.

105. Rubin RH, Swartz MN: Trimethoprim-sulfamethoxazole. *N Engl J Med* 303:426, 1980.

106. Cockerill FR III, Edson RS: Trimethoprim-sulfamethoxazole. *Mayo Clin Proc* 66:1260, 1991.

85. Use of Antimicrobials in the Treatment of Infection in the Critically Ill

Richard H. Glew and Neil R. Blacklow

This chapter covers the specific agents used in the treatment of viral, fungal, and protozoan infections as well as the therapy of aerobic and anaerobic bacterial infections. Ten groups of antibacterial antimicrobial agents commonly used in the ICU are discussed: the penicillins, cephalosporins, carbapenems, monobactams, beta-lactamase inhibitor/beta-lactam combinations, aminoglycosides, fluoroquinolones, vancomycin, antimicrobials used for therapy of anaerobic infections, and macrolides. (See also Chap. 212.)

Penicillins

Penicillin G continues to be highly active against streptococci, meningococci, pneumococci (high-level resistance to penicillin G occurs commonly among *Streptococcus pneumoniae* in certain locales such as South Africa), and most mouth anaerobes. However, treatment of severe enterococcal infections such as endocarditis mandates the addition of an aminoglycoside. *Staphylococcus aureus* should be presumed to be resistant to penicillin G, and infections caused by this organism should be treated with a penicillinase-resistant penicillin (or, alternatively, a cephalosporin or vancomycin). The activity of penicillin G and ampicillin against most gram-negative bacilli is poor, and various semisynthetic penicillins have been created for use against these organisms [1].

The serum half-life ($t\frac{1}{2}$) of most penicillins is short, and rapid clearance occurs through the kidneys. A few of the semisynthetic penicillins, particularly nafcillin and oxacillin, are metabolized to a large extent by the liver, so adjustment in dosage is not required for these agents in the face of renal insufficiency. For most other penicillins, moderate adjustments should be made in dosage in patients with severe renal insufficiency. Penicillins are relatively nontoxic at usual doses (Table 85-1), and side effects most commonly involve hypersensitivity reactions.

PENICILLIN G. In the ICU, aqueous penicillin G is appropriate in the therapy of severe, overwhelming infections caused by susceptible organisms, including pneumococcal pneumonia, necrotizing fasciitis due to group A streptococci, and clostridial cellulitis and myonecrosis. Aspiration pneumonia, particularly in patients arriving from outside the hospital, commonly involves mouth anaerobes, for which penicillin G usually provides excellent therapy. However, studies have suggested that penicillin-resistant anaerobes can be operative in putrid, cavitary pneumonia, and clindamycin (or penicillin plus metronidazole) is the preferred regimen in such patients [2,3,4]. Patients in the ICU commonly and rapidly develop pharyngeal colonization with gram-negative bacilli [5,6,7], and initial therapy of nosocomial aspiration pneumonia requires the addition of an aminoglycoside and a third-generation cephalosporinlike agent. Optimal therapy for enterococcal endocarditis is penicillin G plus an aminoglycoside [8,9], preferably gentamicin [10].

In most ICU infections for which penicillin G is indicated, high doses at frequent intervals should be administered (see Table 85-1). In patients with marked renal impairment, adjustment in penicillin dosage should be made [11].

PENICILLINASE-RESISTANT SEMISYNTHETIC PENICILLINS. Because most strains of *S. aureus* are resistant to penicillin G by virtue of beta-lactamase production, treatment of severe infections caused by these organisms involves one of the beta-lactamase–resistant semisynthetic penicillins (see Table 85-1). Methicillin no longer is used, in part because it is the least active of these agents on a comparative microgram-per-milliliter basis [12], and in part because it appears to cause interstitial nephritis more frequently than do newer agents [13]. Nafcillin and oxacillin are interchangeable: both exhibit excellent in vitro activity against most isolates of *S. aureus,* are slightly less active (though generally effective) than penicillin G against streptococci, are highly protein bound [12], and are sufficiently metabolized by the hepatic route that no adjustment in dose is necessary in patients with renal insufficiency [14,15,16]. These agents should not be relied on to provide effective therapy of infections caused by enterococci [12] or anaerobes usually sensitive to penicillin G. In patients with suspected overwhelming or disseminated infection caused by *S. aureus,* therapy should be instituted with 9 to 12 gm per day of intravenous oxacillin or nafcillin, in divided 4-hourly doses (see Table 85-1). Over the past decade, staphylococci resistant to the penicillinase-resistant penicillins (and cephalosporins) have become increasingly more common. Resistance to beta-lactams is attributable to chromosomally mediated production of an altered penicillin-binding protein with diminished affinity for these penicillins as well as cephalosporins. In settings where the prevalence of these so-called methicillin-resistant *S. aureus* (MRSA) is high, vancomycin should be used for empiric therapy of suspected staphylococcal infections. Although controversial, the occasional demonstration of tolerance to killing by semisynthetic

Table 85-1. Uses of Parenteral Penicillins

Penicillin	Indications	Dose	Frequency	Total daily dosage
Penicillin G/Ampicillin	Meningitis/*Streptococcus pneumoniae, Neisseria meningitidis*	2×10^6 units	q2h	24×10^6 units
	Endocarditis/enterococci (plus gentamicin), viridans group streptococci	3×10^6 units	q4h	18×10^6 units
	Aspiration pneumonia/anaerobes	2×10^6 units	q4h	12×10^6 units
Nafcillin or oxacillin	Bacteremia, endocarditis, skin-soft tissue infection/*Staphylococcus aureus*	2 gm	q4h	12 gm
Piperacillin	*Pseudomonas aeruginosa* or sensitive Enterobacteriaceae (plus an aminoglycoside)	2 gm	q4h	12 gm
Azlocillin	*Pseudomonas aeruginosa* (plus an aminoglycoside)	2 gm	q4h	12 gm
Mezlocillin	Sensitive enterobacteriaceae (plus an aminoglycoside)	3 gm	q4h	12–18 gm
Ticarcillin *plus* clavulanate	Sensitive enterobacteriaceae (usually plus an aminoglycoside) and anaerobes	3.1 gm	q6h	12.4 gm
Piperacillin *plus* tazobactam	Sensitive enterobacteriaceae or *Pseudomonas aeruginosa* plus an aminoglycoside	3.37 gm	q6h	13.5 gm

penicillins among *S. aureus* isolates [17] has led some investigators to argue for addition of gentamicin to oxacillin or nafcillin in the treatment of suspected *S. aureus* endocarditis pending laboratory characterization of the blood isolate [18].

Untoward Reactions. Untoward reactions (other than typical penicillin hypersensitivity rash or fever) to these agents are relatively uncommon. Bone marrow and hepatic toxicities have been described caused by semisynthetic penicillins, with neutropenia more commonly seen with nafcillin, and hepatitis more likely to occur with oxacillin [19].

ANTI–GRAM-NEGATIVE PENICILLINS. Several semisynthetic penicillins have been developed for use against gram-negative organisms. Ampicillin is active against beta-lactamase-negative *Haemophilus influenzae* and many strains of *Escherichia coli, Proteus mirabilis,* and *Salmonella* and *Shigella* species. Most other Enterobacteriaceae as well as *Pseudomonas* species are highly resistant to ampicillin. In light of its restricted spectrum, ampicillin has limited usefulness in the ICU and should not be relied on for gram-negative coverage.

Broad-spectrum semisynthetic penicillins, including piperazine penicillins (piperacillin) and acylureido penicillins (azlocillin and mezlocillin) have replaced earlier penicillins in the treatment of infections caused by gram-negative bacilli. These drugs exhibit activity against many Enterobacteriaceae usually resistant to carbenicillin and ticarcillin, including many isolates of *Klebsiella, Serratia,* indole-positive *Proteus, Enterobacter,* and *Citrobacter.* Piperacillin is the most active of the three against the Enterobacteriaceae, followed by mezlocillin and then azlocillin [20,21,22]. Against *P. aeruginosa,* the order of potency is piperacillin, then azlocillin, followed by mezlocillin [21,22].

Because of their broader spectrum and greater potency, piperacillin, azlocillin, and mezlocillin generally are administered at lower doses than carbenicillin and ticarcillin (see Table 85-1). Because of greater nonrenal excretion of the three newer agents [23], serum $t^{1/2}$ is only mildly increased in patients with renal failure, necessitating only modest adjustments in dose. For example, in patients with moderate-to-severe renal insufficiency, piperacillin, azlocillin, and mezlocillin should be administered as 2 gm IV every 6 to 8 hours. Because these agents are monosodium salts, the frequency of sodium overload and hypokalemia is less than with the carboxypenicillins. Similarly, piperacillin, azlocillin, and mezlocillin exhibit less binding to

platelets than earlier agents and rarely result in prolonged bleeding time or clinically significant bleeding diathesis [24]. In general, none of these semisynthetic, extended-spectrum penicillins should be used as single-agent therapy in patients with suspected bacteremia or overwhelming infection by gram-negative bacilli. Their gram-negative spectrum is not as broad as that of the aminoglycosides, third-generation cephalosporins, or imipenem, and resistance to these semisynthetic penicillins rapidly arises when they are used alone. Accordingly, whichever of these agents is employed in the ICU patient, an aminoglycoside should be administered concomitantly. In addition to providing broader gram-negative coverage, such combinations provide synergistic killing in vitro against *P. aeruginosa* and many Enterobacteriaceae [25,26].

Cephalosporins

For the past 20 years, cephalosporin antibiotics have enjoyed wide clinical use because of their relative safety and because their antibacterial spectrum includes activity against both gram-positive and gram-negative bacteria. The term *cephalosporin* is used broadly, because some of the newer agents are characterized chemically as cephamycins (cefoxitin, cefotetan, cefmetazole, and moxalactam) or oxa-beta-lactams (moxalactam) [27]. Examples of parenteral cephalosporins currently available are listed in Table 85-2.

FIRST-GENERATION CEPHALOSPORINS. All of the first-generation cephalosporins exhibit a virtually identical spectrum of antibacterial activity, and they differ only in their pharmacokinetic properties. These agents are active against staphylococci (*S. aureus* and often against outpatient-acquired *S. epidermidis*) but are not effective against enterococci, *Listeria monocytogenes,* or methicillin-resistant *S. aureus* and *S. epidermidis.* In addition, they do not exhibit in vivo effectiveness in the therapy of prosthetic valve endocarditis caused by *S. epidermidis* [28]. Community-acquired strains of *E. coli, P. mirabilis,* and (less commonly) *K. pneumoniae* often are sensitive to the first-generation cephalosporins, but nosocomial isolates of Enterobacteriaceae (including indole-positive *Proteus* and *Enterobacter* species and *Serratia marcescens*) frequently are resistant, as are *Pseudomonas* and *Acinetobacter* species. Although these antibiotics exhibit in vitro activity against many

Table 85-2. Examples of Parenteral Cephalosporins and Related Beta-lactams

	Dose (gm)	Frequency	Total daily dosage (gm)
1. First-generation cephalosporins			
a. Cephalothin (Keflin)	1.5–2	q4h	9–12
b. Cefazolin (Ancef, Kefzol)	1–2	q8h	3–6
2. Second-generation cephalosporins			
a. Anti–*H. influenzae*			
1) Cefuroxime (Zinacef, Kefurox)	0.75–1.5	q8h	2.25–4.5
2) Cefonicid (Monocid)	1	q12h	2
b. Anti-anaerobes			
1) Cefoxitin (Mefoxin)	1–2	q6h	4–8
2) Cefotetan (Cefotan)	1–2	q12h	2–4
3) Cefmetazole (Zefazone)	2	q6-8h	6–8
3. Third-generation cephalosporins			
a. Cefotaxime (Claforan)	1–2	q6h	4–8
b. Ceftriaxone (Rocephin)	1–2	q12h	2–4
c. Ceftazidime (Fortaz, Tazidime, Tazicef)	1–2	q8h	3–6
d. Cefoperazone (Cefobid)	1–2	q8	3–6
e. Ceftizoxime (Ceftizox)	1–2	q8h	3–6
f. Investigational			
1) Cefpirome			
2) Cefepime			
4. Third-generation equivalent beta-lactams			
a. Imipenem/cilastatin (Primaxin)	0.5–1	q6h	2–4
b. Aztreonam (Azactam)	1–2	q8h	3–6

anaerobes with the exception of *Bacteroides fragilis* [29,30], more effective or specific agents are available, and the cephalosporins generally are not indicated for therapy of proven anaerobic infections.

Pharmacologically, cefazolin is unique among the first-generation cephalosporins because it exhibits a longer $t\frac{1}{2}$ (1.5–2.5 hr) and results in higher serum levels than the other agents [27]. Thus, cefazolin can be administered at lower doses and less often than other first-generation cephalosporins and is the preferred agent if the intramuscular route must be employed.

SECOND-GENERATION CEPHALOSPORINS. The second-generation cephalosporins are notable for a moderately extended spectrum of activity against some gram-negative bacilli resistant to first-generation cephalosporins. Cefuroxime exhibits activity against gram-positive organisms nearly equivalent to that of cephalothin and is more active against indole-positive *Proteus, Citrobacter,* and *Providencia* species, as well as some strains of *Serratia marcescens* and some isolates of cephalothin-resistant *E. coli* and *Klebsiella.* Cefuroxime and cefonicid are particularly active against *H. influenzae,* including beta-lactamase–producing strains [27,31].

Cefoxitin, a cephamycin, also exhibits a broader spectrum of activity than cephalothin against gram-negative bacilli but is much less potent than the first-generation cephalosporins against gram-positive cocci, including *S. aureus* [27]. Cefoxitin is active against most organisms sensitive to other second-generation cephalosporins, including some indole-positive *Proteus* and *Providencia* species, some strains of *Serratia marcescens,* and many strains of cephalothin-resistant *E. coli* and *Klebsiella.* Moreover, cefoxitin exhibits moderately good activity in vitro against anaerobes, including a majority of *B. fragilis* isolates [30].

THIRD-GENERATION CEPHALOSPORINS. The third-generation cephalosporins exhibit an expanded spectrum and

markedly increased potency against gram-negative infections compared with older cephalosporins [27]. Against the *Enterobacteriaceae,* the in vitro activity of the third-generation cephalosporins is outstanding [27,32]. Moreover, these agents are active against many isolates resistant to first- and second-generation cephalosporins and semisynthetic penicillins. However, some of these agents, particularly ceftazidime and cefoperazone, are substantially less active than first-generation cephalosporins against gram-positive cocci [32,33,34].

The activity of most third-generation cephalosporins against *P. aeruginosa* is variable and unpredictable; ceftazidime is more potent against this organism than all other cephalosporins but is less active than imipenem. Each hospital needs to assess the potency of these drugs and related beta-lactams (piperacillin, imipenem, aztreonam) against its own *Pseudomonas* flora. Each of these anti-*Pseudomonas* beta-lactam antibiotics should be used in combination with an aminoglycoside when infection with *P. aeruginosa* is likely.

Activity against anaerobes is poor with most of these agents. The activity of ceftizoxime is comparable to that of cefoxitin against anaerobes, that is, moderate and less than that of metronidazole and imipenem.

Adverse Reactions. In comparison with other agents (e.g., the aminoglycosides) exhibiting efficacy against gram-negative bacilli, the cephalosporins are a relatively nontoxic group of agents. As with the penicillins, the most commonly noted adverse effects are hypersensitivity reactions, including rashes, drug fever, interstitial nephritis, and anaphylaxis [27]. In patients with documented penicillin allergy, the risk of cross-reactive allergic reactions to the cephalosporins is approximately 5 to 15 percent. Accordingly, it is generally believed that cephalosporins should be avoided in patients with a history of documented anaphylaxis or immediate hypersensitivity (urticaria) reaction to the penicillins, but may be given to patients with a history of other types of reactions to penicillins, including morbilliform rash and fever.

Seemingly unique reactions have been described with the

newer cephalosporins. Hypoprothrombinemia, sometimes associated with clinically significant bleeding, has been described, especially with cefamandole and moxalactam, leading to discontinuation of their use, and less so with cefoperazone [35,36]. Diminished platelet adhesiveness has been noted to occur with moxalactam [36]. In patients receiving cefonicid, ceforanide, or moxalactam, a disulfiramlike effect has been noted after ingestion of alcohol [37]. Enterococcal superinfections occur with any of the extended-spectrum cephalosporins because none of these agents has significant activity against enterococci [27].

Most evidence suggests that the cephalosporins do not potentiate aminoglycoside nephrotoxicity. However, a few studies suggest that the combination of cephalothin and an aminoglycoside is more commonly nephrotoxic than penicillin-aminoglycoside therapy [38,39].

Indications for Cephalosporins. Because the activity of the first- and second-generation cephalosporins is unpredictable against gram-negative bacilli, they should not be employed as empiric, single-drug therapy for the treatment of serious infections by these organisms. If in vitro susceptibility testing demonstrates that an infecting strain of the *Enterobacteriaceae* is sensitive to a cephalosporin, this agent is preferable to an aminoglycoside because of its less frequent toxicity.

The broad spectrum and potency of the third-generation cephalosporins enable these agents to provide effective single-agent therapy of many hospital-acquired infections. However, several gaps or weak points may occur in such single-drug coverage, including (1) enterococcal infections of the urinary tract or gallbladder, as well as enterococcal endocarditis, (2) *P. aeruginosa* infections in neutropenic patients, (3) emergence of broad-spectrum resistance by means of chromosomally mediated inducible beta-lactamases during cephalosporin monotherapy of deep-seated infections by species of *Enterobacter, Providencia, Pseudomonas,* and *Acinetobacter,* (4) intraabdominal or intrapelvic infections likely to involve *B. fragilis,* and (5) *S. aureus* bacteremia, endocarditis, or meningitis. Thus, third-generation cephalosporins should be employed ordinarily as part of combination therapy or as specific single-agent treatment of documented gram-negative bacillary infections involving organisms sensitive to the agent in vitro. Because the most inexpensive cephalosporin with acceptable activity generally should be used, the main indication for use of a third-generation cephalosporin should be in the treatment of infections caused by organisms demonstrated (or suspected) to be resistant to other drugs.

Dosage. When used in the treatment of severe infections in ICU patients, all of the cephalosporins should be employed, at least initially, at maximal doses and frequencies (Table 85-2). Because of high serum levels and prolonged serum half-lives, therapy with cefazolin can be administered as 1 to 2 gm every 8 hours, cefotaxime as 1 to 2 gm IV every 6 hours, ceftazidime as 1 to 2 gm every 8 hours, and ceftriaxone 1 to 2 gm every 12 to 24 hours. In patients with severe impairment of renal function, dosages of all cephalosporins except ceftriaxone and cefoperazone must be adjusted to avoid accumulation [27,40,41].

Carbapenems

IMIPENEM. Imipenem is the first of a class of beta-lactam antibiotics known as carbapenems [42,43]. It is administered in combination with cilastatin, which inhibits metabolism of imipenem by the kidney. Imipenem has the broadest and most potent antibacterial spectrum of any available beta-lactam. Its activity against gram-negative bacilli is at least equal to that of the third-generation cephalosporins (including anti-*Pseudomonas* potency equal to that of ceftazidime), against gram-positive cocci similar to that of semisynthetic penicillins (oxacillin, nafcillin) or first-generation cephalosporins (cephalothin), and against anaerobic bacteria equal to metronidazole or clindamycin [42,43]. Methicillin-resistant strains of *S. aureus* and coagulase-negative staphylococci tend to be resistant to imipenem. Among enterococci, *Enterococcus faecalis* appears sensitive but *E. faecium* usually is resistant, and imipenem should not be regarded as effective therapy for serious infections caused by enterococci. Among nonfermentative gram-negative bacilli associated with nosocomial infections, *Xanthomonas maltophilia, P. cepacia* and *Flavobacterium* species usually are resistant to imipenem. Resistance to imipenem arises infrequently (most commonly with *P. aeruginosa*) during therapy, usually through alteration in porin channels in the cell membrane, resulting in diminished permeability of the organism for the drug, and the organism usually remains susceptible to other beta-lactams if susceptible initially.

Usual dosage of imipenem/cilastatin is 2 gm per day in four divided doses, with up to 4 gm per day in life-threatening infections by less susceptible organisms (e.g., *P. aeruginosa*). Dosage adjustment is necessary for patients with renal dysfunction because serum level–related myoclonus and seizures can occur, particularly when used at higher doses, in elderly patients with impaired renal function, or in patients with a history of seizures [43]. In patients with creatinine clearance <50 ml/mm, usual dosage is 0.5 gm every 12 hours, and for anuric patients 0.5 gm every 24 hours. Treatment of highly resistant gram-negative bacilli (e.g., *P. aeruginosa, Enterobacter cloacae, Acinetobacter* spp.) with imipenem generally should involve coadministration of an aminoglycoside.

Adverse Reactions. Adverse reactions to imipenem include rash and fever (as with other beta-lactams; the frequency of cross-reactivity with other classes of beta-lactams is unknown; although estimated to be about that observed with penicillins and cephalosporins, the rate may be somewhat higher with imipenem). Nausea and vomiting are noted during administration and can be reduced by slowing the rate of infusion. Risk of seizures can be minimized by adjustment of dosing in the elderly and in patients with reduced renal function; usage should be avoided when possible in patients with a history of seizures or CNS lesions.

Monobactams

AZTREONAM. Aztreonam is the only synthetic monocyclic beta-lactam (monobactam) approved for clinical use in the United States [44]. Monobactams differ from penicillins and cephalosporins in that they have a monocyclic rather than a bicyclic nucleus; it is probably this novel structure that grants aztreonam little cross-allergenicity with these other beta-lactams. Although skin rashes occur occasionally with this drug, aztreonam has been given safely to patients with immediate hypersensitivity-type reactions (anaphylaxis, urticaria) to penicillins or cephalosporins [45].

Aztreonam has no antibacterial activity against gram-positive or anaerobic bacteria, thus minimizing its use as a single, empiric agent. Against most facultatively aerobic gram-negative bacilli, aztreonam exhibits a spectrum and potency much like that of the third-generation cephalosporins [44]. Aztreonam is highly active against *H. influenzae* and *N. gonorrhoeae* (including beta-lactamase–producing strains), and against most of the Enterobacteriaceae (including *E. coli, Klebsiella, Proteus, Providencia, Serratia, Shigella,* and *Salmonella* species). Against *P. aeruginosa,* aztreonam is slightly less active than imipenem or ceftazidime but is more active than other third-generation cephalosporins. Some isolates of *P. aeruginosa* and *Enterobacter cloacae* are resistant, as are most non-aeruginosa pseudomonads (*P. cepacia, Xanthomonas maltophilia*) and many *Acinetobacter* and *Flavobacterium* species. Usual dosage of aztreonam is 1 to 2 gm IV every 8 hours. Aztreonam is cleared by the kidneys, and the dosage must be reduced in patients with renal insufficiency.

Beta-Lactamase Inhibitors

Clavulanic acid, sulbactam, and tazobactam are beta-lactamase inhibitors—beta-lactam agents with only weak antibacterial activity (sulbactam and tazobactam are active against *Acinetobacter calcoaceticus*). They bind irreversibly to beta-lactamases derived from *S. aureus* and anaerobes, as well as some beta-lactamases from gram-negative bacilli [46]. Thus, the combination of one of these beta-lactamase inhibitors with ampicillin, ticarcillin, or piperacillin results in a drug combination that is active against beta-lactamase–producing strains of *S. aureus, Bacteroides* species, *H. influenzae, N. gonorrhoeae,* and enteric gram-negative bacilli such as *E. coli, Klebsiella,* and *Proteus* species. However, class I inducible, chromosomally mediated beta-lactamases of other gram-negative bacilli are unaffected by these beta-lactamase inhibitors, so that these combinations are ineffective against many isolates of *P. aeruginosa, Enterobacter cloacae, Citrobacter freundii,* and *Serratia marcescens* [47]. Class 3 and 4 enzymes, produced by *X. maltophilia,* also are unaffected by these combinations.

Three beta-lactamase combination formulations are available parenterally: ampicillin-sulbactam (Unasyn; Roerig, New York), ticarcillin-clavalanate (Timentin; SmithKline Beekman, Philadelphia), and piperacillin-tazobactam (Zosyn; Lederle, Wayne, NJ). These agents can be effective in the treatment of mixed infections, such as nosocomial pneumonia, intraabdominal infections, and severe skin–soft tissue infections. However, the lack of efficacy against multiply resistant gram-negative bacilli commonly found in the ICU warrants limitation of their use in this setting, or the inclusion of an aminoglycoside as part of a combination regimen to ensure broad efficacy against gram-negative bacilli.

The usual suggested dosages of the available combinations are 6 to 12 gm per day (the higher dose in serious or nosocomial infections) ampicillin-sulbactam, 12.4 gm per day ticarcillin-clavulanate, and 13.5 gm/day piperacillin-tazobactam, each in four divided doses. For treatment of *P. aeruginosa* infections, the dosage of ticarcillin-clavulanate should be increased to 3.1 gm IV every four hours, and piperacillin-tazobactam to 3.375 gm IV every four hours. The pharmacology of the beta-lactamases inhibitors is similar to that for other beta-lactams: clearance is by renal mechanisms, and dosage adjustments must be made with these combinations in the setting of renal impairment.

Aminoglycosides

The aminoglycoside antibiotics, more correctly designated aminoglycosidic aminocyclitols, are bactericidal agents of great value in the treatment of gram-negative infections in ICU patients. Aminoglycosides in common clinical use for parenteral therapy in the critically ill patient include gentamicin, tobramycin, and amikacin.

PHARMACOLOGY. All available aminoglycosides exhibit similar pharmacologic properties: (1) absorption from the gastrointestinal tract is negligible, and adequate serum levels are obtained only by the IV or IM routes; (2) volume of distribution is similar to total volume of extracellular fluid (ECF) and therefore can be somewhat unpredictable under conditions of abnormal ECF such as dehydration, congestive heart failure, or ascites; (3) protein binding is negligible; (4) penetration into the cerebrospinal fluid (CSF) is poor even in the presence of meningeal inflammation; (5) drug levels in bronchial secretions are only two-thirds those in serum, and are poor in vitreous fluid, prostate, and bile; (6) excretion is predominantly by glomerular filtration; serum half-life of the aminoglycosides in the presence of normal renal function is approximately 2 to 3 hours (shorter for gentamicin and tobramycin than for amikacin) and is prolonged in patients with renal impairment, approaching 24 hours in patients with end-stage renal failure; (7) all aminoglycosides are dialyzable, greater efficacy of removal occurs with hemodialysis (approximately 60–75% cleared in 6 hr) than with peritoneal dialysis; and (8) aminoglycoside activity is reduced under conditions of reduced pH and oxygen tension (such as in purulent, particularly anaerobic fluids and tissues) [48–51].

SPECTRUM OF ACTION AND INDICATIONS FOR THERAPY. The primary clinical indication for aminoglycoside therapy is serious infection caused by gram-negative bacilli. Although more toxic than penicillins and cephalosporins, the aminoglycosides provide the broadest range of potent, bactericidal antibiotic activity against gram-negative bacilli, particularly when multiply resistant enteric gram-negative bacilli (e.g., *Enterobacter* spp.) or nonfermentative gram-negatives such as *Pseudomonas* and *Acinetobacter* species are considered possible pathogens, such as occurs in severely ill, hospitalized patients.

Resistance to aminoglycosides emerges slowly and infrequently. Because of the narrow toxic-therapeutic relationship of aminoglycosides and their limited activity against gram-positive organisms, these agents commonly are employed in the ICU as part of combination therapy together with an extended spectrum beta-lactam antibiotic, particularly in the therapy of pneumonia (because aminoglycoside levels and activity in infected lung are suboptimal).

Resistance to aminoglycosides has increased dramatically among enterococci, and currently in many hospitals up to one-fourth of isolates are gentamicin resistant [52]. Treatment of infections by these organisms is problematic, especially in light of recent emergence of beta-lactamase–producing and vancomycin-resistant strains.

Gentamicin. Gentamicin continues to exhibit efficacy against a broad range of gram-negative bacilli. The cost advantage of this agent and 20 years of experience with the drug render it the aminoglycoside of choice in many infections involving members of the *Enterobacteriaceae.* However, in many ICUs gentamicin resistance is prevalent among local isolates of gram-negative bacilli, and either amikacin or tobramycin is preferred in the initial management of gram-negative bacillary infections, pending results of microbiologic studies and sensitivity testing. In addition, gentamicin in combination with ampicillin, penicillin, or vancomycin is indicated for treatment of endocarditis due to enterococci or viridans group streptococci, and in combination with vancomycin and rifampin for treatment of prosthetic valve endocarditis caused by *S. epidermidis*.

Tobramycin. The spectrum of antibacterial activity and indications for use of tobramycin are similar to those for gentamicin. However, tobramycin generally is more potent in vitro against *P. aeruginosa*, and along with amikacin, often is effective against gentamicin-resistant strains of this organism. However, the frequency of cross-resistance is unpredictable, and in some institutions it may be alarmingly common [53]. In addition, tobramycin is less active than gentamicin against some organisms, such as *Serratia* and *Acinetobacter* species [53,54].

Amikacin. Amikacin is the semisynthetic aminoglycoside most resistant to aminoglycoside-inactivating enzymes. For most gentamicin-resistant gram-negative bacilli, amikacin is the most active aminoglycoside [55,56] and should be the aminoglycoside of choice in hospitals or ICUs in which gentamicin and tobramycin resistance is prevalent.

Aminoglycosides such as netilmicin and sisomicin have spectra of action similar to gentamicin and have no documented clinical pharmacologic advantage over the aforementioned agents.

ADVERSE REACTIONS. Unlike the beta-lactam antibiotics, the aminoglycosides are characterized by a narrow therapeutic-toxic ratio, and therapy with these agents can be associated with considerable toxicity. Hypersensitivity reactions such as fever and rash are uncommon but have been reported in 1 to 3 percent of patients receiving these drugs [57]. Anaphylaxis has been observed on rare occasions. Neuromuscular blockade has been described uncommonly, and appears to be of concern only in patients with myasthenia gravis or severe hypocalcemia, or who are receiving neuromuscular-blocking agents.

Ototoxicity appears to occur with equal frequency (up to 10% of patients) among the modern aminoglycosides [49,56]. Vestibular damage has been described more commonly with gentamicin and tobramycin, whereas impairment of auditory acuity seems more common with amikacin [49]. Ototoxicity occurs unpredictably (either early or late in therapy), appears to be only partially related to elevated serum levels, most closely correlates with duration of therapy and total dosage administered, and often is irreversible.

Nephrotoxicity has been reported to occur in 2 to 10 percent of all patients receiving aminoglycoside therapy [13] and in up to 10 to 25 percent of critically ill patients when broadly inclusive criteria are employed [56,58]. However, renal damage usually is mild and promptly reversible with cessation of therapy. Aminoglycoside-induced nephrotoxicity appears to be related to dose and duration of therapy as well as to serum levels, especially elevated trough levels. It is seen more commonly in elderly patients, patients with preexisting renal disease, those with diminished tissue perfusion caused by cardiogenic or peripheral vascular factors, and patients receiving other nephrotoxic agents such as vancomycin or potent diuretics. The most useful laboratory tests available to detect aminoglycoside nephrotoxicity are the serum creatinine and determinations of peak and trough serum aminoglycoside levels. Although a few studies have suggested that tobramycin is less nephrotoxic than gentamicin when used at maximal doses [58], most studies have failed to document significant differences in toxicity among the modern aminoglycosides. In critically ill patients, however, especially those with one or more of the aforementioned risk factors and who are to be treated with aggressive aminoglycoside regimens designed to achieve relatively high serum drug

levels, the mildly diminished nephrotoxic potential of tobramycin is an argument for its preference over gentamicin.

THERAPY AND DETERMINATION OF SERUM LEVELS. Recommended dosage schedules and serum concentrations for the aminoglycosides are shown in Table 85-3. In patients with impaired renal function, the interval between doses should be extended to a value (in hours) of approximately eight times the serum creatinine level for gentamicin and tobramycin and nine times that level for amikacin; serum levels (and serum creatinine and blood urea nitrogen [BUN]) should be monitored to ensure safe and effective levels, as shown in Table 85-3 [41]. Serum concentrations of aminoglycosides and creatinine should be monitored frequently (and dosage/frequency adjusted accordingly) in patients with fluctuating cardiovascular function/fluid volumes or renal function and in patients anticipated to receive prolonged therapy. Alternatively, a dose-variable, interval-constant regimen for adjustment of therapy can be employed [41].

Some authorities have suggested that administration of a single large, once-daily dose of aminoglycoside may reduce nephrotoxicity [59]. However, clinical studies are limited, and there is no experience on patients who are critically ill or with impaired renal function.

In patients undergoing hemodialysis, it can be estimated that approximately two-thirds to three-quarters of a dose will need to be given at the end of each hemodialysis session, and serum levels (trough at end of dialysis, peak after supplemental dose given) should be monitored. In patients undergoing peritoneal dialysis, instillation of the aminoglycoside into the dialysate at a therapeutic concentration (i.e., 4 μg/ml = 4 mg/liter for gentamicin and tobramycin, and 20 μg/ml = 20 mg/liter for amikacin) eliminates a serum-dialysis concentration gradient and minimizes loss of drug through dialysis.

Fluoroquinolones

Fluoroquinolones are broad-spectrum agents that extend their antimicrobial activity by binding to and inhibiting DNA gyrase, the enzyme that introduces negative superhelical twists into double-stranded bacterial DNA [60–62]. Although there is variability in potency among the fluoroquinolones in vitro, these agents are highly active and generally bactericidal against enteric gram-negative bacilli (including enteric pathogens such as *Salmonella* and *Shigella* species) and *H. influenzae* and are

Table 85-3. Recommended Dosage Regimens and Serum Concentrations of Aminoglycosides in ICU Patients with Normal Renal Function

Drug	Route	Regimen (mg/kg)	Serum Concentration (μg/ml)*	
			Peak	Trough
Gentamicin	IV,IM	1.3–1.7 (q8h)	4–8	1–1.5
Tobramycin	IV,IM	1.3–1.7 (q8h)	4–8	1–1.5
Amikacin	IV,IM	7.5 (q12h)	20–25	5–10

*Serum for determination of peak aminoglycoside concentration obtained 30 min after completion of intravenous infusion or 1 hr after intramuscular injection. Serum for trough level obtained just before dose.

also active against other gram-negative bacteria such as *P. aeruginosa, Acinetobacter* species, and *Aeromonas hydrophila.* Nonfermenters such as *P. cepacia, P. fluorescens,* and *X. maltophilia* are less susceptible to the quinolones.

Activity of quinolones against aerobic gram-positive cocci is variable, with good activity of ofloxacin, ciprofloxacin, and perfloxacin against methicillin-sensitive *S. aureus* and *S. epidermidis.* In general, streptococci (particularly *S. pneumoniae, S. pyogenes* [Group A streptococcus] and enterococci) exhibit poor susceptibility to quinolones. Against anaerobes, currently available quinolones have little or no activity.

Ciprofloxacin and ofloxacin are the most active of the quinolones against mycobacteria, including *M. tuberculosis, M. kansasii,* and *M. fortuitum.* Ofloxacin, followed by ciprofloxacin, has the lowest minimal inhibitory concentration against *Mycoplasma hominis, Chlamydia trachomatis,* and *Ureaplasma urealyticum.* Most agents demonstrate activity against *Legionella pneumophila. Nocardia* species are resistant to the quinolones.

The half-life of the fluoroquinolones is relatively long (3–4 hours for ciprofloxacin, 6–7 hours for ofloxacin). In general, the quinolones are cleared primarily by renal excretion. Ofloxacin is cleared only by the kidneys, whereas some component of hepatic excretion occurs with ciprofloxacin. Thus, adjustment in ofloxacin dosage must be made in patients with renal insufficiency. The fluoroquinolones are not eliminated by hemodialysis or peritoneal dialysis.

Although several oral fluoroquinolones are available that result in adequate serum and tissue levels to treat infections outside the urinary tract, parenteral therapy is preferred in the acute management of serious infections in hospital patients, particularly in the ICU. Ciprofloxacin and ofloxacin are available in intravenous preparations, and of these, ciprofloxacin has greater potency against *P. aeruginosa.* Gastrointestinal absorption of quinolones can be impaired by concomitant administration of antacids containing magnesium or aluminum and multivitamins containing zinc, iron, or sucralfate.

ADVERSE REACTIONS. In general, the fluoroquinolones are remarkably safe and well-tolerated broad-spectrum (vs. gram-negative bacilli) antibiotics. The most common adverse reactions include gastrointestinal symptoms (nausea, vomiting, dyspepsia, abdominal pain, diarrhea), central nervous system symptoms (insomnia, restlessness, headache, dizziness, confusion, and, rarely, seizures) and occasional hypersensitivity reactions (rash, pruritus, drug fever). Ciprofloxacin increases serum concentrations and potentiates the effects of theophylline, warfarin, and cyclosporine.

INDICATIONS. The fluoroquinolones are indicated in the treatment of (1) complicated urinary tract infections involving multiply resistant gram-negative bacilli, (2) prostatitis, (3) bacterial diarrhea of diverse causes, including traveler's diarrhea, and enteritis due to *Shigella, Salmonella,* and *Campylobacter* species, (4) invasive (malignant) external otitis, usually occurring in elderly diabetic patients, and (5) gram-negative bacterial pneumonia. In treating nosocomial pneumonia, it must be remembered that the quinolones have limited spectrum of activity against gram-positive pathogens and no activity against anaerobes, so that addition of an agent active against these organisms should be considered. In addition, it is important to note that resistance to fluoroquinolones is becoming increasingly common among gram-negative bacilli, especially *P. aeruginosa.*

Vancomycin

Vancomycin was introduced into clinical use in 1958. Although it quickly proved to be highly effective in the treatment of serious infections caused by staphylococci, initially it was replaced by less toxic agents, i.e., antistaphylococcal penicillins and cephalosporins [63]. Recently, use of vancomycin has increased as broadened indications for its use have appeared, including therapy of infections due to *S. aureus* resistant to semisynthetic penicillins, infections due to non-*aureus,* coagulase-negative staphylococci (especially *S. epidermidis*) or Diphtheroides species associated with infection on prosthetic heart valves, and endovascular infections in patients undergoing chronic hemodialysis [64].

Vancomycin is bactericidal at low concentrations against most gram-positive cocci and bacilli, such as *S. aureus* (including MRSA), coagulase-negative staphylococci (e.g., *S. epidermidis*), *S. pneumoniae* (including multidrug-resistant strains), viridans group streptococci, *S. bovis,* and *Clostridium* species [64,65]. Although most enterococci are inhibited by low concentrations of vancomycin, bactericidal killing of these organisms usually requires the addition of an aminoglycoside such as gentamicin [66]. Resistance to vancomycin is an emerging problem, particularly in strains of *E. faecium.*

Because of poor absorption from the gastrointestinal tract and severe pain with IM injection, vancomycin is given IV for the treatment of systemic infections. Oral vancomycin is employed only in patients with antibiotic-associated colitis caused by *Clostridium difficile* [67]. Vancomycin has not been demonstrated to be metabolized and is excreted primarily by the kidneys.

Pharmacokinetics of IV administered vancomycin are unpredictable. In patients with normal renal function, serum $t^{1}/_{2}$ varies from 2.7 to 13.3 hours, and peak and trough serum concentrations are unpredictable [68,69]. The usual recommended dose for adults with normal renal function is 1 gm every 12 hours, or 0.5 gm every 6 hours, administered IV over 60 minutes. Some investigators have recommended that initial dosage regimens be based on body weight, with 6.5 to 8 mg per kg administered every 6 to 12 hours [68]. Whichever regimen is employed, serum levels should be monitored and the administration schedule adjusted to give a peak serum concentration of 25 to 30 μg per ml and a trough concentration of 10 to 15 μg per ml. Although nomograms are available to guide vancomycin dosing in patients with varying degrees of renal insufficiency [70,71], serum vancomycin and creatinine levels need to be monitored closely in these patients.

ADVERSE REACTIONS. Although recent experience suggests that adverse reactions to vancomycin occur less commonly than was noted with earlier crude drug preparations, vancomycin is associated with hypersensitivity reactions such as rash and fever in approximately 3 to 5 percent of patients [72]. Because there is no cross-reaction with other antibiotics, vancomycin is the drug of choice in the therapy of serious gram-positive infections in patients allergic to penicillins and cephalosporins. Rapid IV administration of vancomycin can produce a histamine-associated reaction characterized by flushing, tingling, pruritus, tachycardia, hypotension, and an erythematous rash over the upper trunk and face. This "red-neck syndrome" is not a manifestation of hypersensitivity and can be avoided by slow IV administration of the drug (i.e., at a rate no faster than 15 mg/min, or 0.5 gm over 60 min and 1 gm over 60–90 min) or by pretreatment with antihistamines [73]. Neutropenia occurs occasionally [74].

Ototoxicity appears to occur in approximately 1 percent of

patients receiving vancomycin, usually in association with elevated serum levels (>50 µg/ml), and generally is reversible with discontinuation of therapy [72]. Nephrotoxicity occurs in 25 to 35 percent of patients receiving vancomycin in conjunction with an aminoglycoside, but in only 5 percent of patients receiving vancomycin alone. In the latter group nephrotoxicity usually is associated with elevated serum vancomycin levels [72].

Therapy of Anaerobic Infections

CHLORAMPHENICOL. Chloramphenicol is a bacteriostatic antibiotic used occasionally in the treatment of rickettsial infections and rarely in the treatment of infections due to anaerobes, *Salmonella typhi,* or *H. influenzae.* Hepatic metabolism is the major route of clearance, and chloramphenicol penetrates well into all tissues, including the brain and CSF [75,76].

The most important adverse effect of chloramphenicol therapy is bone marrow suppression, which occurs in two forms. Idiosyncratic aplastic anemia is rare (1 case per 40,000 courses of therapy), not dose related, and usually is irreversible and fatal. Although seen most often with oral therapy, it has occurred with IV and topical therapy as well [77,78]. Dose-related pancytopenia occurs when serum concentrations exceed 25 µg per ml, with prolonged therapy, and with doses greater than 4 gm per day [75,76]. To prevent dose-related marrow toxicity, patients receiving chloramphenicol should be monitored frequently (about every 3 days) with serum chloramphenicol levels and granulocyte and platelet counts [75,76].

Therapy with chloramphenicol should consist of 50 to 100 mg per kg per day, or approximately 1 gm every 6 hours in the severely ill patient. These doses should be adjusted to maintain serum levels in the safe yet therapeutic range (peak of 25 µg/ ml, trough of 5–10 µg/ml). No adjustment in dosage is needed in patients with renal insufficiency, but diminished dosages or frequencies (maximum 2 gm/day) are recommended in patients with severe hepatic dysfunction [76].

Although virtually all species of anaerobes are susceptible to chloramphenicol [29,79,80], many investigators question its efficacy in comparison with alternate agents such as metronidazole, imipenem, clindamycin, and cefoxitin. Chloramphenicol is highly effective against rickettsiae and is used to treat Rocky Mountain spotted fever and typhus group infections in patients unable to receive tetracyclines.

METRONIDAZOLE. Metronidazole is highly active against obligate anaerobes. Although orally administered metronidazole is absorbed nearly completely, critically ill patients should receive therapy by the IV route. In severe anaerobic infections, metronidazole is administered as a loading dose of 15 mg per kg IV followed by 7.5 mg per kg every 6 hours [76,81]. Intravenous metronidazole requires neutralization, and current preparations are prebuffered and ready to use. Metronidazole is metabolized by the liver; no dose adjustment is required in patients with renal insufficiency, but dosages must be reduced in patients with hepatic insufficiency [76,81]. Penetration into CSF is excellent [81].

Metronidazole is active in vitro against anaerobic gram-negative bacilli and is probably the most potent agent for treatment of infections due to *B. fragilis* [29,80]. Like clindamycin, metronidazole must be used in conjunction with an aminoglycoside, extended-spectrum beta-lactam, or fluoroquinolone in the treatment of intraabdominal and intrapelvic infections in which aerobic organisms can be expected to be operative as well.

CLINDAMYCIN. Although clindamycin is well absorbed from the gastrointestinal tract, therapy in critically ill patients should be administered IV. Usual parenteral therapy for severe infections consists of 600 to 900 mg IV every 8 hours (25–40 mg/ kg/day) [76]. Clindamycin is metabolized by the liver and excreted in inactive form in bile, so no adjustment in dosage is required in patients with renal insufficiency [82]. The drug penetrates well into most tissues and fluids, with the exception of CSF and brain [82,83].

The most important side effects of clindamycin are gastrointestinal. The incidence of diarrhea during therapy with clindamycin has been reported to range from 3 percent to 30 percent, with variable severity [76,82]. Pseudomembranous colitis associated with clindamycin administration has been reported to occur in up to 10 percent of patients receiving the drug and appears to be caused by overgrowth of *C. difficile* and elaboration of a toxin by this organism [84,85]. Pseudomembranous colitis can be precipitated by many different antibiotics, particularly penicillins and cephalosporins, but its association with clindamycin is among the most common. The appearance of characteristic symptoms (diarrhea, abdominal pain, cramps, fever, and bloody diarrhea) is an indication for discontinuation of clindamycin therapy, which may result in cessation of symptoms. In cases of severe pseudomembranous colitis, in milder cases that do not spontaneously remit with cessation of clindamycin therapy, or in patients in whom antibiotic therapy cannot be discontinued, treatment should be instituted with oral vancomycin or metronidazole [82,86,87,88].

Clindamycin is active in vitro against a wide variety of anaerobic bacteria [29]. Although clindamycin-resistant strains of *B. fragilis* have been detected, close to 90 percent of isolates remain sensitive [80,89]. Clindamycin has been used with great success in the treatment of anaerobic infections of the head, neck, and lungs/pleural space. Although penicillin G generally is effective in these settings, studies have suggested the possible superiority of clindamycin in patients with necrotizing, cavitary anaerobic pneumonia and lung abscesses [4,6,90].

Macrolides

Erythromycin is the oldest of the macrolide antibiotics in common use; the macrolides are bacteriostatic antibiotics that act on the 50S ribosome subunit [76]. The most common use of erythromycin is to treat community-acquired, non–life-threatening infections in normal hosts: primary atypical pneumonia due to *M. pneumoniae* or *C. pneumoniae,* pharyngitis due to *S. pyogenes, B. pertussis* infections, enteritis due to *Campylobacter* species, and eradication of the carrier state of diphtheria. In addition, erythromycin is the drug of choice at high IV doses for legionellosis.

Erythromycin is well absorbed from the gastrointestinal tract, but concomitant administration with food diminishes absorption. In the ICU, parenteral therapy usually is indicated, dosage ranges from 0.5 gm every 6 hours for mycoplasma and chlamydial pneumonia to 0.75 to 1 gm every 6 hours for pneumonia due to *Legionella* species. Erythromycin is excreted primarily in the bile, so that dosage adjustment is not necessary in patients with renal impairment.

Erythromycin is relatively free of serious effects. Dose-related upper gastrointestinal irritation with epigastric pain, nausea, or vomiting is noted commonly with oral administration, and occasionally with IV administration. Cholestatic hepatitis occurs rarely, most commonly with oral erythromycin in its estolate form. Transient auditory impairment may occur in patients receiving high doses of erythromycin intravenously; recovery of hearing follows discontinuation of treatment and may occur with continued administration of erythromycin at reduced dosages.

Two newer oral macrolides (azithromycin and clarithromycin) have become available [91,92]. In addition to sharing the microbiologic spectrum of activity of erythromycin, azithromycin is active against *Chlamydia trachomatis* but is less active than erythromycin or clarithromycin against staphylococci and streptococci. Although azithromycin is more active in vitro than the other two macrolides against *H. influenzae*, its activity is insignificant compared with the potency of newer cephalosporins or sulfamethoxazole-trimethoprim. Clarithromycin shares the antimicrobial spectrum of erythromycin but is more active against gram-positive cocci and *Legionella* species and also demonstrates activity against *Mycobacterium avium-intracellulare*, an organism that can be problematic in AIDS patients.

Therapy of Fungal Infections

Invasive and disseminated fungal infections are increasingly common in ICU patients, especially among those receiving immunosuppressive therapy or broad-spectrum antibiotics, in patients with lymphoreticular malignancies or transplants, and in individuals with T cell depletion due to HIV-1 infection. During the past several years, newer antifungals of the imidazole (ketoconazole) and triazole (fluconazole, itraconazole) classes have become available for the treatment of systemic mycoses. However, amphotericin B remains the standard agent for most serious fungal infections [93,94,95].

AMPHOTERICIN B. Amphotericin B is a polyene antibiotic, insoluble in water and solubilized by the addition of sodium desoxycholate, forming a colloidal dispersion. Its mechanism of action is due to its binding to ergosterol, a sterol present in the cell membrane of sensitive fungi, resulting in altered membrane permeability and causing leakage of cell components and resultant cell death [93]. Amphotericin B is effective against most species of fungi that are pathogenic in humans and is the drug of choice for deep, invasive, or systemic candidiasis, aspergillosis, mucormycosis, cryptococcosis, histoplasmosis, coccidioidomycosis, and torulopsosis [93,94,95]. It also is effective for blastomycosis and extracutaneous sporotrichosis [93,94,95]. Whereas *Candida albicans* generally is sensitive to amphotericin B, non-albicans species of *Candida* often are less susceptible, and variable activity is evident against species of *Aspergillus* and *Mucor, Pseudallescheria* (*Petriellidium*) *boydii, Fusarium* species, and dematiaceous fungi [93,95]. The combination of amphotericin B plus flucytosine is synergistic against *Candida* species and *Cryptococcus neoformans* [93,95,96].

Amphotericin B for IV administration should be prepared in 5% dextrose because saline solutions result in drug precipitation [95]. The drug is highly protein bound and is distributed into many tissues (liver, spleen, lung, muscle, kidney, skin, adrenals); because penetration into CSF is poor [93,95], intrathecal/intracisternal administration may be necessary for some CNS mycoses, especially coccidioidomycosis. The metabolism of amphotericin B is poorly understood, but renal and hepatic insufficiency have little effect on serum levels of the drug, and hemodialysis does not affect serum levels [93,95].

Amphotericin B usually is given IV by infusion once daily over 2 to 6 hours, at a concentration of 0.1 mg per milliliter. Daily and total dosage are adjusted according to the fungal species, sites and extent of infection, and the individual tolerance of the patient. A test dose of 1 mg (in 25–100 ml 5% dextrose) is infused over 30 minutes; if this dose is well tolerated, therapy can be continued with 0.25 mg per kilogram administered over 2 to 6 hours. For patients who are critically ill with apparently rapidly progressive fungal disease, the second day of therapy can achieve the full daily dose of 0.5 to 1 mg per kilogram. For patients exhibiting intolerance with the test dose or subsequent increased doses as well as patients with subacute fungal infection, amphotericin B dosing can be increased in a gradual fashion, with increase in the dose by 5 to 10 mg daily, until the final daily dose (0.4–0.6 mg/kg for candidiasis) is reached. The usual duration of amphotericin B therapy for systemic mycoses is 4 to 12 weeks, to a total of 1 to 2 gm. For infections due to less susceptible fungi (e.g., *Aspergillus, Zygomycete* species [*Mucor*], and *C. immitis*), treatment warrants daily doses of up to 1 mg per kilogram and a total dose of 2 gm. Candida esophagitis not responding to less toxic drugs and candidemia without apparent dissemination may be treated with a total of 250 to 1000 mg. Candiduria related to an indwelling bladder catheter often responds to bladder irrigation with amphotericin B (50 mg/1000 ml sterile water, instilled intravesicularly continuously at 40 ml/hr through a three-way catheter) [93]. Candiduria in the patient without a catheter may respond to oral fluconazole. Recalcitrant, persistent candiduria in the setting of fever and deteriorating renal function suggests candida pyelonephritis (ascending or hematogenous) and may be an indication for IV therapy with amphotericin B. Cryptococcosis can be treated successfully with reduced (0.3 mg/kg/day) dosages of amphotericin B plus flucytosine (150 mg/kg/day orally) for 6 weeks. Coccidioidal meningitis usually requires concomitant intrathecal administration [93].

Adverse Reactions. Adverse effects of amphotericin B most frequently include infusion-associated constitutional symptoms such as fever, chills, hypotension, and tachypnea, a reaction that is most common and most severe with the first few doses of the drug and during escalation of dosage and can be minimized by increasing daily dosage slowly (if the clinical situation permits) or by pretreatment with acetaminophen, hydrocortisone (25–50 mg IV), and/or meperidine (25 mg IV). Dantrolene (10 mg IU) has been used successfully as an alternative or adjunctive agent in patients with severe rigors. Nephrotoxicity occurs frequently with amphotericin B therapy and results in sodium and potassium wasting, renal tubular acidosis, and azotemia. Potassium levels should be monitored closely and supplementation with potassium begun as soon as serum potassium decreases toward the lower end of normal range. Azotemia is potentiated by sodium depletion and can be reduced by avoidance of diuresis, poor fluid intake, and administration of other nephrotoxic agents [94,95,96]. Sodium supplementation (150 mEq/day above normal sodium intake of 150–200 mEq/day in patients able to tolerate such treatment) also appears protective [97]. Although amphotericin B dosage need not be adjusted for renal insufficiency, an increase of serum creatinine to greater than 2.0 mg per deciliter during therapy warrants reduction in the dosage or interruption of therapy until creatinine starts to decrease; then amphotericin B can be restarted at a lower daily dose or on an alternate-day basis [93]. Mild anemia occurs commonly during amphotericin B therapy, but thrombocytopenia, leukopenia, and severe hepatitis are rare. Reduction in amphotericin B toxicity by use of novel delivery systems, such as liposomal preparations, is under investigation [98].

FLUCYTOSINE. Flucytosine is an orally administered pyrimidine analog with a narrow spectrum of action [95,96]. Most strains of *C. neoformans, Candida* species, and the most common agents of chromomycosis (*Fonsecaea* and *Cladosporium* spp.) are susceptible initially, whereas most other fungi pathogenic for humans are resistant. Except in chromomycosis, flucytosine seldom is used alone because resistance emerges rapidly. The use of combination therapy with flucytosine allows a reduction in dosage and duration (0.3 mg/kg/day for 6 weeks) of amphotericin B in the treatment of cryptococcal meningitis, and improves efficacy in the treatment of candidal meningitis and peritonitis because of its excellent penetration into these sites.

Flucytosine is water soluble, demonstrates nearly complete absorption after oral administration, exhibits little protein binding, and has excellent penetration into most tissues and fluids. The drug is cleared by the kidneys, with a serum t$\frac{1}{2}$ of 3 hours in patients with normal renal function and 85 hours in anuric patients [96]. The usual recommended dosage in patients with normal renal function is 150 mg per kilogram daily in four divided doses; the interval between doses should be doubled (every 12 hours) when the creatinine clearance is 20 to 40 ml per minute and quadrupled (every 24 hours) when creatinine clearance is 10 to 20 ml per minute [96]. The serum level of flucytosine should be monitored, particularly in patients with renal impairment, and the dose should be adjusted to maintain a level of 50 to 100 μg per milliliter.

Leukopenia is the most serious complication of flucytosine therapy and occurs most commonly in patients with renal insufficiency and when serum levels exceed 100 μg per milliliter. Gastrointestinal intolerance (nausea, vomiting, anorexia, diarrhea), hepatitis, and rash occur occasionally.

IMIDAZOLES. Ketoconazole is an orally administered antifungal agent that interferes with the synthesis and permeability of fungal membranes and has activity against *Candida* species, *B. dermatitides, H. capsulatum, C. neoformans, C. immitis,* and most dermatophytes [93,99,100]. The usual dosage of ketoconazole is 400 mg once daily for deep or systemic mycoses and 200 mg once daily for candida esophagitis or vaginitis. Ketoconazole requires an acid environment for absorption and is poorly absorbed in the setting of achlorhydria (e.g., patients with gastrectomy, HIV-induced gastropathy, pernicious anemia, or receiving H$_2$-blocker medications); uncertainty of bioavailability limits the utility of this drug in the ICU. Adverse effects include the relatively common occurrence of gastrointestinal symptoms (nausea, vomiting, anorexia) and suppression of testosterone synthesis (gynecomastia in men, menstrual irregularities in women). Mild, often transient, asymptomatic elevation of serum transaminases occurs in up to 10 percent of patients; severe hepatotoxicity occurs rarely (in approximately 1 in 10,000 patients) and can be fatal if the drug is not discontinued [95]. Ketoconazole can enhance the effect of oral anticoagulants and the toxicity of cyclosporine.

TRIAZOLES

Fluconazole. Fluconazole is a water-soluble bis-triazole available for IV and oral use and exhibits good activity in vitro against *Candida* species and *C. neoformans* [95,101]. As with other azoles, its mode of action is mediated through inhibition of ergosterol synthesis. Oral absorption is excellent, resulting in serum levels nearly as high as with IV administration, and is independent of gastric acidity. Fluconazole penetrates well into bodily fluids, including CSF (50–90% of serum concentrations).

Fluconazole has a long (30 hours) half-life; because of its renal clearance, adjustments must be made in dosing in patients with renal impairment. The usual dosage (oral or IV) of fluconazole is 200 mg on the first day of therapy, followed by 100 mg once daily for patients with oropharyngeal or esophageal candidiasis; therapy is continued until clinical findings resolve and for a total of two to three weeks. The potential role of fluconazole is uncertain in the treatment of systemic or invasive candidiasis [102], for which amphotericin B remains the drug of choice [93]. Despite its high cost, fluconazole likely will prove to be the antifungal of preference for suppressive prophylaxis of candidiasis in immunocompromised patients. Fluconazole is the drug of choice for suppressive maintenance therapy of cryptococcal meningitis in AIDS patients. Side effects of fluconazole are relatively minor and uncommon, with gastrointestinal symptoms (nausea) most frequent. Mild, transient elevation of serum transaminase levels occurs occasionally. Unlike ketoconazole, fluconazole does not affect adrenal function or androgen synthesis, but does inhibit the metabolism and potentiate the effects of warfarin, phenytoin, cyclosporine, and oral hypoglycemics.

Itraconazole. Itraconazole is an orally administered, broad-spectrum triazole antifungal with notable activity against *Aspergillus* species, *H. capsulatum, C. immitis, Sporothrix schenckii,* and the agents of chromomycosis [95,103]. Absorption is unpredictable between individuals and over time, suggesting the need for monitoring of serum levels during the treatment of serious infections. Itraconazole is widely distributed in most tissues, but with poor levels in CSF [103]. Daily dosage is 200 to 400 mg orally, but higher doses are indicated in patients with CNS infection. Clearance is by hepatic metabolism, and no adjustment of dosage is required in patients with renal failure. Limited clinical experience indicates that itraconazole likely has a role in the treatment of sporotrichosis, paracoccidioidomycosis, and chromomycosis and may be of use in treating patients with histoplasmosis, coccidioidomycosis, cryptococcosis, or aspergillosis who have experienced failure of prior therapy with amphotericin B or other azoles [103]. Trials suggest that itraconazole is well tolerated, with occasional gastrointestinal symptoms (abdominal discomfort, nausea, diarrhea) or minor elevation of liver chemistries noted. Unlike ketoconazole, itraconazole has only a minimal effect on the synthesis of androgens or cortisol but appears to be able to produce a picture of mineralocorticoid excess with hypokalemia, edema, and hypertension [95].

Therapy of Viral Infections

As viral infections have become more common, diverse, and severe in an era of expanding populations of immunocompromised hosts, several antiviral agents have become available. Nevertheless, antiviral therapy remains problematic and limited in scope as compared with antibacterial treatments. Anti-retroviral therapy will not be covered in this chapter.

ACYCLOVIR. Acyclovir is a nucleoside analog of guanosine with antiviral activity against herpesviruses, particularly herpes simplex virus (HSV) types 1 and 2 and varicella-zoster virus (VZV) [104,105,106]. Administered as a prodrug, acyclovir requires phosphorylation to a monophosphate form by a virus-generated thymidine kinase and then to a triphosphate form by host cellular enzymes. Because cytomegalovirus (CMV) lacks a thymidine kinase, acyclovir has limited activity against the virus.

Acyclovir is available as 200-mg, 400-mg, and 800-mg capsules for oral administration and as an IV preparation, with the latter route preferred for serious infections in critically ill patients and for milder illnesses in patients unable to take medications by mouth. Dosage varies according to the condition under treatment. After oral administration, absorption is slow and incomplete, with oral bioavailability of only 15 to 30 percent [106].

Serum half-life is 2 to 3 hours in patients with normal renal function. Because 85% of clearance is renal, dosage must be reduced in patients with impaired renal function. In patients with creatinine clearance greater than 50 ml per minute, full unit dosage (generally 10 mg/kg) should be administered every 8 hours; with creatinine clearance of 25 to 50 ml per minute, full dose should be administered every 12 hours; with creatinine clearance 10 to 25 ml per minute, full dose every 24 hours; with creatinine clearance greater than 10 ml per minute, the dose should be reduced by one-half and given every 24 hours [106].

Acyclovir is well tolerated. Reversible renal impairment occurs occasionally, usually in patients receiving high doses by rapid IV infusion or who are elderly, dehydrated, or have antecedent renal insufficiency. At high doses, especially IV, neurologic reactions (confusion, delirium, hallucinations, seizures, tremors) have occurred in approximately 1 percent of patients. Occasionally, patients experience nausea, vomiting, or rash.

Intravenous acyclovir at 10 mg per kilogram every 8 hours is the drug of choice for HSV encephalitis (for a course of 10–14 days), for neonatal HSV infection (10–14 days), and for VZV infections (chicken pox or shingles) in immunocompromised patients (7–10 days). Acyclovir at 5 mg per kilogram IV every 8 hours is effective against mucocutaneous HSV in immunocompromised patients. Topical and particularly oral (200 mg 5 times daily) acyclovir can be of benefit in patients with recurrence of HSV labialis or genitalis. High-dose (800 mg 5 times daily) oral administration of acyclovir accelerates the rate of healing and may reduce somewhat the intensity of acute neuritis in patients with shingles. Acyclovir has been used prophylactically in patients undergoing bone marrow or organ transplantation.

GANCICLOVIR. Ganciclovir (DHPG) is highly active against CMV, in part because of high concentration of the triphosphylated form of the drug in infected cells [107]. The most problematic adverse effect is myelosuppression, particularly neutropenia, which is sufficiently common with coadministration of zidovudine as to preclude simultaneous use of the two drugs in most AIDS patients. Other side effects include nausea/vomiting and CNS abnormalities [104,107]. Ganciclovir alone is effective in the treatment of CMV retinitis, gastrointestinal infection (colitis, esophagitis, gastritis), and pneumonitis in AIDS patients. However, in bone marrow transplant patients the drug must be used in combination with IV CMV hyperimmune globulin for the treatment of CMV pneumonitis [104,107,108].

Treatment with ganciclovir usually involves induction therapy with 5 mg per kilogram IV twice daily for 14 to 21 days, followed by maintenance therapy (5–6 mg/kg once daily 5 days per week) in AIDS patients [105]. Clearance of ganciclovir is by renal elimination; dosage adjustments must be made in patients with renal impairment, especially in light of the relationship between drug serum levels and myelosuppression.

FOSCARNET. Foscarnet (trisodium phosphoneoformate) is an inorganic pyrophosphate analog that acts by inhibiting viral DNA polymerases of most human herpes viruses (particularly CMV) and reverse transcriptases of human retroviruses (particularly HIV-1) [104,105,107,109]. Foscarnet has been demonstrated to be effective in the therapy of CMV retinitis in patients with AIDS and has two potential advantages as compared with ganciclovir, namely, little or no myelosuppression, and inherent antiretroviral activity toward HIV-1 [104]. However, foscarnet is more expensive than ganciclovir and is associated with a significant (25%) incidence of nephrotoxicity. Therapy involves IV administration at a dosage of 60 mg per kilogram 3 times a day for induction and at 90 to 120 mg per kilogram once daily for maintenance therapy. Clearance is by renal excretion, and dosage adjustment is required in patients with renal impairment. Nonrenal adverse effects include nausea, vomiting, anemia, seizures, and metabolic abnormalities (hyperphosphatemia and hypophosphatemia, hypercalcemia and hypocalcemia, hypokalemia, hypomagnesemia).

Therapy of Protozoan Infections

TRIMETHOPRIM-SULFAMETHOXAZOLE. Trimethoprim-sulfamethoxazole (cotrimoxazole) works through sequential, two-stage inhibition of folate synthesis and is the regimen of choice in the treatment of *Pneumocystis carinii* pneumonia (PCP) in patients able to tolerate this antimicrobic combination [110,111,112]. In moderately to severely ill patients, it is administered IV or orally at a dosage of 20 mg per kilogram daily of the trimethoprim component (or 100 mg/kg daily of the sulfa component) in four divided doses for a total course of 14 days in non-AIDS patients and 21 days in patients with AIDS. Failure to obtain satisfactory response in 5 days (7 days in individuals with HIV-1 infection) warrants change to an alternative regimen (e.g., pentamidine isethionate). Adverse reaction to trimethoprim-sulfamethoxazole occurs in approximately 10 to 15 percent of patients uninfected with HIV-1 and in up to two-thirds of patients with AIDS. The most common problems are neutropenia and/or thrombocytopenia (particularly in patients with advanced HIV-1–induced immunodeficiency and/or receiving zidovudine), rash/fever, nausea/vomiting, and abnormalities of hepatic chemistries. In patients with AIDS, therapy may be tolerated better with reduced dosages (i.e., 15 mg/kg of the trimethoprim component, or 75 mg/kg of the sulfa component, daily) without reduction in efficacy.

PYRIMETHAMINE-SULFADIAZINE. For the treatment of systemic and invasive (including encephalitis) toxoplasmosis in the compromised host, the alternate double antifolate combination of pyrimethamine-sulfa usually is employed [112]. Pyrimethamine is administered orally with a loading dose of 200 mg, then as 75 mg daily (with folinic acid 5 mg daily) together with sulfadiazine orally as 6 gm daily in four divided doses. Adverse reactions can be expected to occur in similar frequency and type as with cotrimoxazole. Alternative therapies for CNS toxoplasmosis include clindamycin (900 mg IV every 6 hours) plus pyrimethamine [113].

PENTAMIDINE ISETHIONATE. Equally efficacious but more toxic therapy for PCP can be obtained with pentamidine, administered IV by slow infusion (1–2 hours) at 4 mg per kilogram once daily [112,114]. Generally, intramuscular therapy is avoided because of problems with sterile abscesses. Adverse reactions are common, occurring in up to two-thirds of patients and occasionally serious enough to require change in therapy. Common side effects include nausea, vomiting, and hypotension, and more serious problems include azotemia, pancreatitis (which may become chronic), hypoglycemia followed by hyperglycemia, leukopenia, and thrombocytopenia [111,114]. Dosage adjustment is indicated in patients with renal impairment, e.g., increasing the interval to every 36 hours in patients with creatinine clearance of 10 to 50 ml per minute and to every 48 hours in patients with creatinine clearance less than 10 ml per minute

References

1. Wright AJ, Wilkowske, CJ: The penicillins. *Mayo Clin Proc* 66:1047, 1991.
2. Perline CA: Metronidazole vs. clindamycin treatment of anaerobic pulmonary infection: Failure of metronidazole therapy. *Arch Intern Med* 141:1424, 1981.
3. Sanders CV, Hanna BJ, Lewis AC: Metronidazole in the treatment of anaerobic infections. *Am Rev Respir Dis* 120:337, 1979.
4. Levison ME, Mangura CT, Lorber B, et al: Clindamycin compared with penicillin for the treatment of anaerobic lung abscess. *Ann Intern Med* 98:466, 1983.
5. Johanson WG Jr, Pierce AK, Sanford JP, et al: Nosocomial respiratory infections with gram-negative bacilli: The significance of colonization of the respiratory tract. *Ann Intern Med* 77:701, 1972.
6. Lorber B, Swenson RM: Bacteriology of aspiration pneumonia: A prospective study of community and hospital-acquired cases. *Ann Intern Med* 81:329, 1974.
7. Johanson WG, Pierce AK, Sanford JP, et al: Nosocomial respiratory infections with gram-negative bacilli: The significance of colonization of the respiratory tract. *Ann Intern Med* 77:701, 1972.
8. Mandell GL, Kaye D, Levison ME, et al: Enterococcal endocarditis. *Arch Intern Med* 125:258, 1970.
9. Wilkowske CJ: Enterococcal endocarditis. *Mayo Clin Proc* 57:101, 1982.
10. Moellering RC Jr, Emergence of enterococcus as a significant pathogen. *Clin Infect Dis* 14:1173, 1992.
11. Bryan CS, Stone WJ: "Comparably massive" penicillin G therapy in renal failure. *Ann Intern Med* 82:189, 1975.
12. Glew RH, Moellering RC Jr: Effect of protein binding on the activity of penicillins in combination with gentamicin against Enterococci. *Antimicrob Agents Chemother* 15:87, 1979.
13. Appel GB, Neu HC: The nephrotoxicity of antimicrobial agents (first of three parts). *N Engl J Med* 296:663, 1977.
14. Diaz CR, Kane JG, Parker RH, et al: Pharmacokinetics of nafcillin in patients with renal failure. *Antimicrob Agents Chemother* 12:98, 1977.
15. Bulger RJ, Lindholm DD, Murray JS, et al: Effect of uremia on methicillin and oxacillin blood levels excretion and inactivation in renal failure and hemodialysis. *JAMA* 187:319, 1964.
16. Kind AC, Tupasi TE, Standiford HC, et al: Mechanisms responsible for plasma levels of nafcillin lower than those of oxacillin. *Arch Intern Med* 125:685, 1970.
17. Mayhall CG, Medoff G, Marr Jr JJ: Variation in the susceptibility of strains of *Staphylococcus aureus* to oxacillin, cephalothin, and gentamicin. *Antimicrob Agents Chemother* 10:707, 1976.
18. Rajashekaraiah KR, Rice T, Rao VS, et al: Clinical significance of tolerant strains of *Staphylococcus aureus* in patients with endocarditis. *Ann Intern Med* 93:796, 1980.
19. Bruckstein AH, Attia AA: Oxacillin hepatitis: Two patients with liver biopsy and review of the literature. *Am J Med* 64:519, 1978.
20. Bodey GP, LeBlanc B: Piperacillin: In vitro evaluation. *Antimicrob Agents Chemother* 14:78, 1978.
21. Wise R, Andrews JM, Bedford KA: Comparison of the in vitro activity of Bay k 4999 and piperacillin, two new antipseudomonal broadspectrum penicillins, with other beta-lactam drugs. *Antimicrob Agents Chemother* 14:549, 1978.
22. Eliopoulos GM, Moellering RC Jr: Azlocillin, mezlocillin, and piperacillin: New broad-spectrum penicillins. *Ann Intern Med* 97:755, 1982.
23. Bergan T: Overview of acylureidopenicillin pharmacokinetics. *Scand J Infect Dis* 29:33, 1981.
24. Gentry LO, Jemsek JG, Natelson EA: Effects of sodium piperacillin on platelet function in normal volunteers. *Antimicrob Agents Chemother* 19:532, 1981.
25. Glew RH, Pavuk RA: Early synergistic interaction between semisynthetic penicillins and aminoglycosidic aminocyclitols against Enterobacteriaceae. *Antimicrob Agents Chemother* 23:902, 1983.
26. White GW, Malow JB, Zimelis VM, et al: Comparative in vitro activity of azlocillin, ampicillin, mezlocillin, piperacillin, and ticarcillin, alone and in combination with an aminoglycoside. *Antimicrob Agents Chemother* 15:540, 1979.
27. Gustaferro CA, Steckelberg JM: Cephalosporin antimicrobial agents and related compounds. *Mayo Clin Proc* 66:1064, 1991.
28. Karchmer AW, Archer GL, Dismukes WE: *Staphylococcus epidermidis* causing prosthetic valve endocarditis: Microbiologic and clinical observations as guides to therapy. *Ann Intern Med* 98:447, 1983.
29. Sutter L, Finegold SM: Susceptibility of anaerobic bacteria to 23 antimicrobial agents. *Antimicrob Agents Chemother* 10:736, 1976.
30. Rolfe RD, Finegold SM: Comparative in vitro activity of new beta-lactam antibiotics against anaerobic bacteria. *Antimicrob Agents Chemother* 20:600, 1981.
31. Tantaglione TA, Polk RR: Review of the new second-generation cephalosporins: Cefonicid, cefonamide and cefuroxime. *Drug Intell Clin Pharm* 19:188, 1985.
32. Neu HC: The new beta-lactamase-stable cephalosporins. *Med Clin North Am* 66:283, 1982.
33. Moellering RC Jr: Ceftazidime: A new broad spectrum cephalosporin. *Pediatr Infect Dis* 4:390, 1985.
34. Salzer W, Pegram PS Jr, McCall CE: Clinical evaluation of moxalactam: Evidence of decreased efficacy of gram-positive aerobic infections. *Antimicrob Agents Chemother* 23:565, 1983.
35. Clancy CM, Glew RH: Hypoprothrombinaemia and bleeding associated with cephamandole. *Lancet* 1:250, 1983.
36. Bang NU, Tessler SS, Heidenrich RO, et al: Effect of moxalactam on blood coagulation and platelet function. *Rev Infect Dis* 4:S546, 1982.
37. Buening MK, Wold JS: Ethanol-moxalactam interactions in vivo. *Rev Infect Dis* 4:S555, 1982.
38. Wade JC, Petty BG, Conrad G, et al: Cephalothin plus an aminoglycoside is more nephrotoxic than methicillin plus an aminoglycoside. *Lancet* 2:604, 1978.
39. Klastersky J, Hensgens C, Debusscher L: Empiric therapy for cancer patients: Comparative study of ticarcillin/tobramycin, ticarcillin/cephalothin, and cephalothin/tobramycin. *Antimicrob Agents Chemother* 7:640, 1975.
40. Balant L, Dayer P, Aukenthaler R: Clinical pharmacokinetics of the third generation cephalosporins. *Clin Pharmacokinet* 10:101, 1985.
41. Van Scoy RE, Wilson WR: Antimicrobial agents in patients with renal insufficiency. *Mayo Clin Proc* 58:246, 1983.
42. Wise R: In vitro and pharmacokinetic properties of the carbapenems. *Antimicrob Agents Chemother* 30:343, 1986.
43. Bellinger WC, Brewer NS: Imipenem. *Mayo Clin Proc* 66:1074, 1991.
44. Brewer NS, Hellinger WC: The monobactams. *Mayo Clin Proc* 66:1152, 1991.
45. Saxon A, Hassuen A, Swabb EA, Wheelen B, et al: Lack of cross-reactivity between aztreonam, a monobactam antibiotic, and penicillin in penicillin-allergic subjects. *J Infect Dis* 149:16, 1984.
46. Bush K: β-lactamase inhibitors from laboratory to clinic. *Clin Microbiol Rev* 1:109, 1988.
47. Jacoby GA, Medeiros AA: More extended-spectrum beta-lactamases. *Antimicrob Agents Chemother* 35:1897, 1991.
48. Riff LJ, Jackson GG: Pharmacology of gentamicin in man. *J Infect Dis* 124:S98, 1971.
49. Edson RS, Terrell CL: The aminoglycosides. *Mayo Clin Proc* 66:1158, 1991.
50. Sarubbi FA Jr, Hull JH: Amikacin serum concentrations: Prediction of levels and dosage guidelines. *Ann Intern Med* 89:612, 1978.
51. Briedis DJ, Robson HG: Cerebrospinal fluid penetration of amikacin. *Antimicrob Agents Chemother* 13:1042, 1978.
52. Wells VD, Wong ES, Murray BE, et al: Infections due to beta-lactamase-producing, high-level gentamicin-resistant *Enterococcus faecalis*. *Ann Intern Med* 116:285, 1992.

53. John JF Fr, Rubens CE, Farrar WE Jr: Characteristics of gentamicin resistance in nosocomial infections. *Am J Med Sci* 279:25, 1980.

54. Glew RH, Moellering RC Jr, Buettner KR: In vitro synergism between carbenicillin and aminoglycosidic aminocyclitols against *Acinetobacter calcoaceticus* var. *anitratus. Antimicrob Agents Chemother* 11:1036, 1977.

55. Price KE, DeFuria MD, Pursiano TA: Amikacin, an aminoglycoside with marked activity against antibiotic-resistant clinical isolates. *J Infect Dis* 134:S249, 1976.

56. Smith CR, Baughman KL, Edwards CQ, et al: Controlled comparison of amikacin and gentamicin. *N Engl J Med* 296:351, 1977.

57. Anderson JA, Adkinson NF Jr: Allergic reactions to drugs and biologic agents. *JAMA* 258:2891, 1987.

58. Smith CR, Lipsky JJ, Laskin OL, et al: Double-blind comparison of the nephrotoxicity and auditory toxicity of gentamicin and tobramycin. *N Engl J Med* 302:1106, 1980.

59. Gilbert DN: Once-daily aminoglycoside therapy. *Antimicrob Agents Chemother* 35:399, 1991.

60. Wolfson JS, Hooper DL: The fluoroquinolones: Structures, mechanisms of action and resistance, and spectra of activity in vitro. *Antimicrob Agents Chemother* 28:581, 1985.

61. Hooper DC, Wolfers JS: The fluoroquinolones: Pharmacology clinical uses and toxicity in humans. *Antimicrob Agents Chemother* 28:718, 1985.

62. Walker RC, Wright AJ: The fluoroquinolones. *Mayo Clin Proc* 66:1249, 1991.

63. Cook V, Farrar WE Jr: Vancomycin revisited. *Ann Intern Med* 88:813, 1978.

64. Wilhelim MP: Vancomycin. *Mayo Clin Proc* 66:1165, 1991.

65. Geraci JE, Heilman FR, Nichols DR, et al: Antibiotic therapy of bacterial endocarditis: VII. Vancomycin for acute micrococcal endocarditis. *Mayo Clin Proc* 33:172, 1958.

66. Harwick HJ, Kalmanson GM, Guze LB: In vitro activity of ampicillin or vancomycin combined with gentamicin or streptomycin against enterococci. *Antimicrob Agents Chemother* 4:383, 1973.

67. Silva J Jr, Fekety R: *Clostridia* and antimicrobial enterocolitis. *Annu Rev Med* 32:327, 1981.

68. Rotschafer JC, Crossley K, Zaske DE, et al: Pharmacokinetics of vancomycin: Observations in 28 patients and dosage recommendations. *Antimicrob Agents Chemother* 22:391, 1982.

69. Blouin RA, Bauer LA, Miller DD, et al: Vancomycin pharmacokinetics in normal and morbidly obese subjects. *Antimicrob Agents Chemother* 21:575, 1982.

70. Moellering RC Jr, Krogstad DJ, Greenblatt DJ: Vancomycin therapy in patients with impaired renal function: A nomogram for dosage. *Ann Intern Med* 94:343, 1981.

71. Krogstad DJ, Moellering RC Jr, Greenblatt DJ: Single-dose kinetics of intravenous vancomycin. *J Clin Pharmacol* 20:197, 1980.

72. Farber BF, Moellering RC Jr: Retrospective study of the toxicity of preparations of vancomycin from 1974 to 1981. *Antimicrob Agents Chemother* 23:138, 1983.

73. Polk RE, Healy DP, Schwartz LB, et al: Influence of antihistamine pretreatment on vancomycin-induced red-man syndrome. *J Infect Dis* 160:876, 1989.

74. Farwell AP, Kendall LG, Vakil RD, et al: Delayed appearance of vancomycin-induced neutropenia in a patient with chronic renal failure. *South Med J* 77:664, 1984.

75. Smith AL, Weber A: Pharmacology of chloramphenicol. *Pediatr Clin North Am* 30:209, 1983.

76. Smilack JD, Wilson WR, Cockerill FR III: Tetracyclines, chloramphenicol, erythromycin, clindamycin and metronidazole. *Mayo Clin Proc* 66:1270, 1991.

77. Daum RS, Cohen DL, Smith AL: Fatal aplastic anemia following apparent "dose-related" chloramphenicol toxicity. *J Pediatr* 94:403, 1979.

78. Matthews SJ, Shawver-Matthews S: Chloramphenicol toxicity: Oral vs. intravenous administration. *J Pediatr* 97:869, 1980.

79. Bartlett JG, Joiner KA, Dezfulian M, et al: Efficacy of moxalactam in an animal model of subcutaneous abscesses: Penetration into infected sites and in vivo activity against *Bacteroides fragilis. Rev Infect Dis* 4:S664, 1982.

80. Cuchural GJ Jr, Tally FP, Jacobus NV, et al: Susceptibility of the *Bacteroides fragilis* group in the United States: Analysis by site of isolation. *Antimicrob Agents Chemother* 32:717, 1988.

81. Molavi A, LeFrock JL, Prince RA: Metronidazole. *Med Clin North Am* 66:121, 1982.

82. Dhawan VK, Thadepalli H: Clindamycin: A review of fifteen years of experience. *Rev Infect Dis* 4:1133, 1982.

83. Picardi JL, Lewis HP, Tan JS, et al: Clindamycin concentrations in the central nervous system of primates before and after head trauma. *J Neurosurg* 43:717, 1975.

84. Larson HE, Price AB: Pseudomembranous colitis: Presence of clostridial toxin. *Lancet* 2:1312, 1977.

85. Bartlett JG, Onderdonk AB, Cismeros RL, et al: Clindamycin-associated colitis due to a toxin-producing species of *Clostridium* in hamsters. *J Infect Dis* 136:701, 1977.

86. Tedesco F, Markham R, Gurwith M, et al: Oral vancomycin for antibiotic-associated pseudomembranous colitis. *Lancet* 2:226, 1978.

87. Keighley MRB, Burdon DW, Arabi Y, et al: Randomized controlled trial of vancomycin for pseudomembranous colitis and postoperative diarrhea. *Br Med J* 2:1667, 1978.

88. Trinh DH, Kernbaum S, Frottier J: Treatment of antibiotic-induced colitis by metronidazole. *Lancet* 1:338, 1978.

89. Musial CE, Rosenblutt JE: Antimicrobial susceptibilities of anaerobic bacteria isolated at the Mayo Clinic during 1982 through 1987: Comparison with results from 1977 through 1981. *Mayo Clin Proc* 64:392, 1989.

90. LeFrock JL, Molavi A, Prince RA: Clindamycin. *Med Clin North Am* 66:103, 1982.

91. Neu HC: New macrolide antibiotics: Azithromycin and clarithromycin. *Ann Intern Med* 116:517, 1992.

92. Clarithromycin and azithromycin. *The Medical Letter* 34:45, 1992.

93. Gallis HA, Drew RH, Pickard WW: Amphotericin B: 30 years of clinical experience. *Rev Infect Dis* 12:308, 1990.

94. Hoeprich PD: Clinical use of amphotericin B and derivatives: Lore, mystique, and fact. *Clin Infect Dis* 14(suppl):S114, 1992.

95. Terrell CL, Hughes CE: Antifungal agents for deep-seated mycotic infections. *Mayo Clin Proc* 67:69, 1992.

96. Bennett JE: Flucytosine. *Ann Intern Med* 86:319, 1977.

97. Branch RA: Prevention of amphotericin B-induced renal impairment: A review on the use of sodium supplementation. *Arch Intern Med* 148:2389, 1988.

98. Brajtburg J, Powerdly WG, Kobayashi GS, Medoff G: Amphotericin B: Delivery systems. *Antimicrob Agents Chemother* 34:381, 1990.

99. Craven PC, Graybill JR, Jorgensen JH, Dismukes WE, Levine BE: High-dose ketaconazole for treatment of fungal infections of the central nervous system. *Ann Intern Med* 98:160, 1983.

100. Hansen RM, Reinerio N, Sohnle PG, et al: Ketoconazole in the prevention of candidiasis in patients with cancer: A prospective, randomized, controlled, double-blind study. *Arch Intern Med* 147:710, 1987.

101. Galgiani JN: Fluconazole, a new antifungal agent. *Ann Intern Med* 113:177, 1990.

102. Evans TG, Mayer J, Cohen S, et al: Fluconazole failure in the treatment of invasive mycoses. *J Infect Dis* 164:1232, 1991.

103. Sharkey PK, Rinaldi MG, Dunn JF, et al: High-dose itraconazole in the treatment of severe mycoses. *Antimicrob Agents Chemother* 34:707, 1991.

104. Keating MMR: Antiviral agents. *Mayo Clin Proc* 67:160, 1992.

105. Drugs for viral infections. *The Medical Letter* 34:31, 1992.

106. Whitley RJ, Gnann JW Jr: Acyclovir: A decade later. *N Engl J Med* 327:782, 1992.

107. Balfour HH Jr: Managment of cytomegalovirus disease with antiviral drugs. *Rev Infect Dis* 12:S849, 1990.

108. Reed EC, Bowden RA, Bandliker PS, et al: Treatment of cytomegalovirus pneumonia with ganciclovir and intravenous immunoglobulin in patients with bone marrow transplants. *Ann Intern Med* 109:783, 1988.

109. Studies of Ocular Complications of AIDS Research Group, in collaboation with the AIDS Clinical Trials Group: Mortality in patients with the acquired immunodeficiency synndrome treated with either foscarnet or ganciclovir for cytomegalovirus retinitis. *N Engl J Med* 326:213, 1992.

110. Cockerill FR III, Edson RS: Trimethoprim sulfamethoxazole. *Mayo Clin Proc* 66:12680, 1991.

111. Davey RT Jr, Masur H: Recent advances in the diagnosis, treatment

and prevention of *Pneumocystis carinii* pneumonia. *Antimicrob Agents Chemother* 34:499, 1990.
112. Rosenblatt JE: Antiparasitic drugs. *Mayo Clin Proc* 67:276, 1992.
113. Dannemann BR, Israelski DM, Remington JS: Treatment of toxo-

plasmic encephalitis with intravenous clindamycin. *Arch Intern Med* 148:2477, 1988.
114. Sands M, Kron MA, Brown RB: Pentamidine: A review. *Rev Infect Dis* 7:625, 1985.

86. *Prevention and Control of Nosocomial Infection in the Intensive Care Unit*

Gary L. Dudek, Carlos R. Ortiz,
and F. Marc LaForce

Nosocomial infections have been defined by the Centers for Disease Control and Prevention (CDC) as those infections that occur in hospitalized patients that were not present or incubating at the time of admission [1]. Hence, nosocomial infections are potentially preventable complications of hospitalization that result in excess health care costs estimated at between 5 and 10 billion dollars annually in the United States [2]. These costs are attributable to extended lengths of hospital stay and additional antibiotic utilization [2,3]. Nosocomial infections are morbid events, and excess mortality associated with these infections [2–5] have been well described. These complications become especially prominent in the intensive care unit where the rate of nosocomial infections is 2 to 5 times that of the general inpatient population [6–9]. The intensivist, therefore, can play an important role in minimizing the financial and human costs associated with hospital-acquired infections. This requires a thorough knowledge of the epidemiology of nosocomial infections in the critical care unit, some familiarity with general preventive and control strategies, and an appreciation of the controversies surrounding some of the newer control measures that are being proposed.

Prevalence of Intensive Care Unit–Associated Nosocomial Infection

CDC's National Nosocomial Infection Surveillance (NNIS) System defines intensive care unit (ICU)-associated infections as those occurring after ICU admission or within 48 hours after transfer from an ICU [10]. Using these definitions, as well as the CDC criteria for documentation of infection at specific sites [1], nosocomial infections occurring in ICUs of various types have been characterized.

Table 86-1 summarizes ten recent reports on the prevalence of nosocomial infections in critical care units. Although the largest study [11] describes a mean prevalence of 9.2 nosocomial infections per 100 admissions to adult and pediatric ICUs, review of infection rates by specific ICU type demonstrates considerable variability, ranging from 0.8% in a cardiac surgery ICU [12] to 78% in a pediatric ICU [13]. In general, coronary care units have the lowest rates of nosocomial infections, and burn and surgical ICUs suffer the highest rates.

The reasons for the variability in nosocomial infection rates include, but are not limited to, the following: size of the unit, severity of illness, and variability in management practices, particularly with regard to use of invasive devices such as urinary catheters, endotracheal tubes, and vascular catheters. Not unexpectedly, the most important risk factor is length of stay. Review of NNIS data by Jarvis et al. [11] showed a strong correlation between nosocomial infection rate and length of ICU stay. A strong correlation between device utilization and site-specific infection (e.g., urinary tract infection and the presence of a urinary catheter) was also noted even after controlling for length of ICU stay. ICUs could be grouped according to site-specific nosocomial infection rates (Table 86-2). Coronary care and medical ICUs had similar infection profiles; surgical ICUs had a second type, and pediatric ICUs exhibited a third nosocomial infection profile. The medical-surgical and surgical ICUs have the highest prevalence of ventilator-associated pneumonias. Rates of catheter-related urinary tract infection were greatest in the coronary care unit (CCU) and medical intensive care unit (MICU) patient populations, and vascular catheter infections were most frequent in pediatric ICUs. The incidence of vascular catheter infections [14] among neonates was inversely related to a birth weight of less than 1500 gm (14.6 versus 5.1 infections/1000 central line days).

Proper comparisons of ICU-associated nosocomial infection rates, therefore, should include both measures of general nosocomial infection rates and device-specific infection rates. Such an analysis can serve as the basis for the identification of infection control problems such as an increase in device-associated infection rates.

Distribution and Microbiology of Nosocomial Infections

Critical care units provide an environment where the most immunologically compromised individuals by virtue of their underlying diseases (diabetes, renal insufficiency, shock, pharmacologic immunosuppression, malnutrition) are treated with intensive supportive efforts using invasive devices that bypass host defense mechanisms (e.g., endotracheal tubes, urinary catheters, and intravascular catheters). It should come as no surprise that ICU-acquired infections are strongly correlated with device utilization [6,7,11] and

Table 86-1. Prevalence of ICU-Acquired Infection

Reference	ICU Type	Nosocomial Infections (infections/100 patients)	No. of Patients
Craven et al. [7]	SICU	62	799
	MICU	35	526
Chandrasekar et al. [8]	SICU	35.2	88
	MICU	13.9	101
	BCU	29.8	47
	CCU	6.6	106
Jarvis et al. [11]	Adult and pediatric	9.2	164,572
Gaynes et al. [14]	NICU	13.5	24,480
Brown et al. [12]	MSICU	11.2	5,189
	CCU	1.8	5,017
	PICU	6.2	965
	NICU	5.9	1,848
	CSICU	0.8	1,341
Pories et al. [9]	Trauma	9.2	2,496
Goldman et al. [17]	NICU	4.4	911
Bjerke et al. [32]	SICU	4.1	2,122
Klein et al. [13]	PICU	78	70
Aavitsland et al. [15]	MSICU	22	67
	MICU	8.7	126
	SICU	17	178

MICU = medical ICU; SICU = surgical ICU; NICU = neonatal ICU; MSICU = medical/surgical ICU; PICU = pediatric ICU; CCU = coronary care unit; BCU = burn care unit; CSICU = cardiac surgery ICU.

Table 86-2. Device-Associated Infection Rates [11]

Infection Type	CCU/MICU	MSICU/SICU	PICU
Central line infections/ 1000 catheter days	6.9	5.3	11.4
Pneumonias*/ 1000 ventilator days	12.8	17.6	4.7
Urinary tract infection†/ 1000 catheter days	10.7	7.6	5.8

* Ventilator-associated pneumonia.
† Catheter-associated urinary tract infection.

that the sites of these infections reflect the host defense barrier that has been breached.

Table 86-3 is a summary of site-specific nosocomial infection rates among a wide variety of ICUs taken from several studies [7,9,12,15]. Although there is variability in infection rates, all studies are consistent in showing a relative preponderance of nosocomial pneumonias and urinary tract infections (UTIs). UTIs are particularly common among SICU patients [7,9], a difference that may be attributable to a longer duration of urinary catheterization among surgical intensive care unit (SICU) patients. Others [11] have demonstrated a greater incidence of nosocomial UTI in the MICU rather than the SICU when length of catheterization was controlled as a confounding variable (see Table 86-2). Device utilization, therefore, is only one of many determinants for the observed variability in sites of infection.

The microbiology of ICU-acquired infection varies among institutions (Table 86-4). As a rule, gram-negative organisms are responsible for most isolates. Among the gram-negative organisms, *Escherichia coli* and the *Klebsiella-Enterobacter-Serratia* group are the most common, followed by *Pseudomonas* spe-

cies. *Pseudomonas* isolates are less common in the coronary, pediatric, and neonatal settings. *Haemophilus influenzae* is a predominant organism in the pediatric ICU.

Gram-positive organisms constitute approximately 20% of nosocomial isolates [8]; *Staphylococcus aureus* remains the predominant pathogen. It is followed rather closely by streptococcal species and enterococci. Some institutions have higher infection rates from *Staphylococcus epidermidis* [16]. Methicillin-resistant *Staphylococcus aureus* (MRSA) is a common problem in all ICU settings. These variations underscore the importance of a regular, systematic review of ICU isolates and the antimicrobial susceptibilities of these isolates.

Among fungal isolates, *Candida* species are the most important pathogens, and they have increased in importance over the past decade. Whether the emergence of these yeasts is related to selection because of antibiotic pressure or because of cross-infection is unclear [6].

In summary, the urinary and respiratory tracts are the major sites of nosocomial infection in the ICU. Aerobic gram-negative rods are the most common isolates, although resistant gram-positive organisms, such as methicillin-resistant *Staphylococcus aureus* and aminoglycoside-resistant enterococci, may colonize units, thus altering the choices for empiric antibiotic therapy.

Risk Factors and Mortality

The identification of risk factors for nosocomial infections in critical care unit patients is complicated by the interdependence of several potential risk factors such as length of ICU stay, device utilization, and severity of illness. It is important that statistical analysis, usually in the form of logistic regression stratification, be used to analyze these risks [11,14].

Craven and associates investigated nosocomial infections among 1300 patients admitted to the SICU or MICU at Boston City Hospital [7]. Univariate analysis showed a significant association between 23 variables and the development of nosocomial infection. These variables included demographic data (age, race), markers for severity of illness (shock, coma, acute physiologic score >20, blood urea nitrogen [BUN] >20 mg per deciliter, creatinine >1.5 mg per deciliter, bicarbonate <20 mEq per liter, steroids/chemotherapy), admission diagnosis (head/multiple trauma, neurologic disease, cardiopulmonary arrest, respiratory failure, acute myocardial infarction), ICU stay >10 days, and device utilization (urinary catheters, ventilator, central line, arterial line, Swan-Ganz catheter). Stepwise logistic regression analysis was used to eliminate codependent variables. This analysis demonstrated statistical association with only five variables: urinary catheter days >10, arterial line days >3, intracranial pressure monitoring, shock on admission, and ICU stay >10 days. Because invasive devices could be considered as markers of severity of illness, they were eliminated from a second logistic regression analysis. Results of this more refined analysis reinforced the association of nosocomial infection with shock on admission and days in the ICU. Surgical ICU admission, use of steroids or chemotherapy, and a creatinine >1.5 mg per deciliter replaced devices as risk factors for infection. In summary, this important study has shown a significant and independent association between host factors (shock, immunosuppression, and renal insufficiency) and nosocomial infection rates.

Mortality in the ICU is significantly higher than that seen on a general medical ward. Whether this difference is partially caused by ICU-acquired infections or explained by the severity of underlying disease is a key question that has not been an-

Table 86-3. Site-Specific Nosocomial Infection Rates*

ICU Type	Pulmonary	Urinary	Blood	Wound	Abdomen	CNS
			(Craven et al. [7])			
SICU	7.8	15.1	7.5	9.5	1.5	1.3
MICU	9.9	9.9	4.8	2.3	0.2	0
			(Brown et al. [12])			
MSICU	8.8	5.8	0.2	1.2	3.2	0.4
CCU	1.4	2.4	0.2	<0.1	0.1	<0.1
PICU	5.5	4.9	0.3	0.5	0.1	5.8
NICU	4.4	0.2	1.2	0	0.1	0.2
			(Pories et al. [9])			
SICU	1.3	5.6	0.7	0.6		
			(Aavitsland et al. [15])			
All	7.3	2.2	2.4	1.1		

* Rates are no. of infections per 100 patients.
SICU = surgical ICU; MICU = medical ICU; MSICU = medical/surgical ICU; CCU = coronary care unit; NICU = neonatal ICU.

Table 86-4. Bacterial Isolates in ICU-Associated Infections*

Species	Craven et al. [7]	Chandrasekar et al. [8]	Brown et al. [12]			
			MS	C	P	N
GRAM-NEGATIVES						
E. coli	13	18	12	26	10	5
K-E-S	24	17	17	11	6	3
Pseudomonas	13	21	10	6	4	8
Other	15					
Haemophilus sp.	2				18	
GRAM-POSITIVES						
S. aureus	9	11	9	10	12	8
Enterococci	5	6	7	6	1	4
Streptococci	7					
Other	5					
FUNGI						
Candida sp.	7	5	11	6	3	7
Other (gram-negative and -positive)			15	13	27	31

* Expressed as percentage of total isolates to the nearest 1%.
E. coli = *Escherichia coli*; K-E-S = *Klebsiella, Enterobacter, Serratia* species; *S. Aureus* = *Staphylococcus aureus*; MS = medical/surgical ICU; C = coronary care unit; P = pediatric ICU; N = neonatal ICU.

swered. Chandrasekar et al. [8] documented a mortality rate among ICU patients with nosocomial infection that was statistically greater (p < 0.0005) than that of unmatched patients from their medical, surgical, burn, and coronary care units. Smith and associates [4] documented an increased mortality (82.4% versus 52.9%) among critically ill patients with nosocomial bloodstream infections relative to noninfected controls chosen by matching APACHE II scores. In a neonatal ICU, Goldmann and others [17] noted an increased mortality rate among infants with nosocomial infection (relative risk = 1.96) but found the greatest impact on mortality in patients without a patent ductus arteriosus (PDA) and an acquired infection (relative risk = 3.42). This suggested that the increased mortality seen in the group with a PDA was more dependent on their underlying disease. Craven and colleagues [7] measured the effect of 30 variables on ICU mortality, and when submitted to stepwise logistic regression analysis, nosocomial intraabdominal infection or peritonitis remained the only nosocomial infection associated with increased mortality. Although certain subgroups of critically ill patients appear to die as a direct result of an acquired infection, most ICU deaths are determined by the severity of underlying disease in which nosocomial infection serves as a surrogate for disease severity.

General Preventive and Control Measures

MODES OF TRANSMISSION. Prevention and control of nosocomial infections in the critical care unit requires a clear understanding of the reservoir of pathogenic bacteria and the mode of spread of these pathogens within a critical care unit. For example, in a recent *Xanthomonas maltophilia* outbreak in a surgical ICU [18], patients with surgical wounds colonized or infected with *X. maltophilia* were identified as reservoirs from which further colonization/infection was disseminated. The hands of ICU staff members were similarly colonized, as were respirometers, which were shared among all patients and were believed to be the mode of transmission. Institution of strict handwashing practices, secretion/drainage precautions, use of gloves for endotracheal suctioning, and high-level decontamination of respirometers resulted in a marked reduction in the prevalence of *Xanthomonas* colonization/infection (17.7/1000 patient days to 2.6/1000 patient days).

In contrast to contact spread of pathogens, airborne transmission appears to play a minor role in the ICU setting. Evidence for this assertion comes from a prospective microbiologic and epidemiologic study in a medical ICU specifically designed to evaluate modes of transmission of nosocomial pathogens in the ICU [19]. In this study, 15% of air samples were culture positive for pathogenic bacteria. However, the spectrum of organisms so obtained bore no relation to the organisms cultured from patients. In contrast, cultures of the hands of care-givers were indistinguishable from patient isolates, supporting the primacy of contact over airborne nosocomial transmission.

These findings must be interpreted in light of colonization rates in patients before their transfer to an ICU. This distinction is especially problematic in medical ICUs. Of the 100 patients colonized by *Pseudomonas aeruginosa* in an MICU over a 6-month period, Olson and co-workers [20] found that 63% were colonized on admission. Furthermore, of the 37 remaining cases, only 12 cases were unequivocally attributable to cross-infection. Of these 12 cases, only five were believed to have been preventable through institution of barrier isolation.

ARCHITECTURAL FEATURES.

Concerns about ICU design and its impact on nosocomial infection rates have prompted many recommendations aimed at limiting the environmental transmission of microbes [21]. These recommendations include standards of room ventilation (8–20 air exchanges/hour, use of HEPA filters, positive- and negative-pressure patient rooms, laminar flow environments), individual room temperature/humidity control, space per bed (11 m²/bed), and the design of sinks that minimize aerosolization of potentially contaminated water. Despite all of this effort, such interventions have resulted an variable impact on nosocomial infection rates [6].

Shirani and associates [22] described a reduction in nosocomial infection rate from 28.9 percent to 19.2 percent (p < 0.05) after they moved from a burn unit with multiple beds in a ward setting with regional sinks to a renovated unit with individual patient cubicles, each with its own sink. Similarly, Goldmann et al. [23] described the impact of moving from a ward-style neonatal ICU with unknown ventilation to a renovated unit with one isolation room and the ability to separate neonates by a chest-high barrier in an otherwise open environment. Ventilation of 12 air exchanges per hour was assured, and a separate sink was provided for each incubator. A reduction in the number of nosocomially infected infants was seen (5.8% to 1.8%). The authors postulated that increased space and availability of sinks together with increased staffing resulted in improved compliance with basic infection control procedures, especially handwashing. Handwashing compliance, however, was not measured.

In contrast, Huebner and others [24] describe the consequences of moving an open anesthesiology ICU to a new facility comprising a four-bed open area, a two-bed room, and three single-bed isolation rooms having independent environmental controls. Ventilation was maintained at 20 changes per hour in a positive-pressure mode. No difference in nosocomial infection rate (34.2% versus 33%) was observed in the new unit environment.

Improvement in nosocomial infection rates with alterations in the ICU environment is probably more related to facilitating compliance with basic infection control procedures such as handwashing. Any potential effect is, in turn, influenced by the fraction of endogenous vs. exogenous infections among the patient population studied, because environmental changes are likely to affect only those infections acquired exogenously.

HANDWASHING.

Handwashing as a means of preventing transmission of microorganisms from patient to patient by health care personnel seems deceptively simple. Villarino and colleagues [18] documented a significant reduction in infection and colonization rates with institution of basic control measures in which strict handwashing was a prominent component. Unfortunately, several studies have documented an embarrassingly low compliance rate for handwashing among ICU personnel, ranging from 22 percent to 32 percent of observed encounters [25–28]. Educational activities directed at improving handwashing practices have in some cases shown no improvement [27], whereas others report significant improvements in compliance [26,29].

This improved compliance has also been shown to correlate with a reduction in nosocomial infection rates. Conly et al. [26] studied handwashing compliance in an MICU at a time when the nosocomial infection rate was 32.8 percent. At the beginning of the study, handwashing by ICU personnel was documented to have occurred 14 percent before patient contact and 28 percent after patient contact. An educational program that used posters and direct feedback to personnel on their handwashing practices resulted in significant improvements in pre-patient- and postpatient-contact handwashing rates (38% and 60%). This change was associated with a decrease in nosocomial infection rates to 12 percent. However, over the course of several years, both handwashing compliance and nosocomial infection rates returned to pre-educational levels, requiring reinstitution of educational activities followed by a second decrease in nosocomial infection rates.

The effectiveness of various handwashing agents has also been investigated in the critical care setting. Doebbeling et al. [30] evaluated the relative efficacies of 4% chlorhexidine and 60% isopropyl alcohol among 1894 adult ICU patients in a multiple cross-over study. Chlorhexidine was associated with a lower rate of nosocomial infection (3.4/100 patient days versus 5.1/100 patient days). However, the compliance rates with handwashing despite the intense activity surrounding this study was only 42 percent in the chlorhexidine group and 38 percent in the isopropyl alcohol group. Although the choice of agent used in handwashing may influence the effectiveness of this strategy, its significance pales in comparison with the problem of ensuring general compliance with handwashing guidelines among ICU personnel [25].

BARRIER PRECAUTIONS.

Barrier precautions, in the form of disposable gloves and gowns, may also prevent contact transmission of microbes among ICU patients and thus reduce nosocomial infection rates. Like handwashing, barrier methods suffer from poor compliance among the ICU staff. Furthermore, compliance was lowest when use of barrier precautions required the health care worker to interpret its necessity for a given encounter (e.g., wound/skin precautions or excretion/secretion isolation) and best when required for all encounters. Pettinger and Nettleman [31] measured compliance with isolation precautions in a surgical ICU. Compliance with wound/skin isolation and excretion/secretion isolation was 40 percent and 36 percent, respectively, whereas compliance with strict isolation was 65 percent. Overall health care worker compliance with any form of isolation precautions was only 41 percent.

Barrier methods have been shown to be effective in reducing nosocomial infections in surgical and pediatric ICU populations

[18,32]. Klein et al. [13] evaluated the impact of isolation precautions (nonsterile latex gloves and disposable, nonwoven polypropylene gowns) in a pediatric ICU in which patients needed mechanical ventilation for longer than 3 days. Patients were randomized to receive standard care (n = 38) or strict isolation precautions (n = 32). Nosocomial colonization by *S. aureus*, MRSA, gram-negative bacilli, or fungi was similar among those in isolation (31%) and the group receiving standard care (42%). Nosocomial infection rates, however, were significantly reduced in the cohort receiving strict isolation (8.6 infections/100 patient days—standard care, versus 4.4 infections/100 patient days—isolation). Moreover, patients in isolation remained uninfected for a much longer period (median 20 days) compared with those receiving standard care (median 8 days). Strict enforcement of barrier precautions did not adversely interfere with the delivery of health care or the social interaction of patients with relatives [13]. Further studies are required to prove the efficacy of strictly enforced barrier precautions in ICUs of all types. In addition, studies to determine if barrier precautions are cost-effective by a direct comparison with handwashing have not been published.

The issue of barrier precautions to prevent transmission of organisms from patient to patient (isolation precautions) should not be confused with universal precautions, which seek to protect the health care worker from bloodborne pathogens. Although "isolation precautions" also protect the health care worker, universal precautions do not afford the patient a similar degree of protection. The use of the same gloves or gown when caring for more than one patient fulfills the mandates of universal precautions but results in transmission of pathogens between patients. This potential was demonstrated by Patterson and others [33], who recently reported an outbreak of *Acinetobacter calcoaceticus* among Yale University surgical and medical ICU patients, which was traced to nonsterile latex gloves that were used for universal precautions and that were not changed between patients.

EXTERNAL DEVICES. Contamination of medical devices in contact with the patient from endogenous or exogenous organisms is another aspect of intensive care that is amenable to preventive measures. Pressure transducers and ventilator circuits, because of the frequency of their use in the ICU setting, deserve special emphasis.

Reusable pressure transducers have been associated with nosocomial bacteremias because of inadequate sterilization. This problem has continued despite the development of disposable domes because of the presence of a saline interface between the dome and the transducer. Such colonization at the transducer head was refractory to alcohol sterilization and was directly traced to epidemics of bacteremia [34,35]. High-level sterilization of the transducer heads and replacement of transducer heads every 48 hours were recommended [34,35,36]. The introduction of completely disposable transducers has considerably reduced this problem while permitting their use for up to 96 hours without an increased incidence of colonization [37].

Microbiologic studies of ventilator circuits have shown that colonization begins at the endotracheal tube, which is colonized by oropharyngeal bacteria [38,39]. Because of this phenomenon, frequent ventilator circuit changes are not helpful; tubing colonization is the same at 24 and 48 hours [40]. In fact, tubing changes every 24 hours has been found to be an independent risk factor for development of nosocomial pneumonia, perhaps as a result of patient inoculation with contaminated condensate at the time of the circuit change [39,41]. Data supporting the indefinite use of a ventilator circuit for a given patient without increasing the incidence of nosocomial pneu-

monia are becoming available despite the use of cascade humidifiers, which increase tubing condensate [42]. Use of heated-wire circuits and condensation traps to reduce the volume of condensate in the tubing may improve the longevity of ventilator circuits beyond the 24 hours currently recommended by the CDC [43]. Such a change has the potential to save millions of dollars in equipment costs annually.

Infections of Special Interest

Detailed discussion of all sites of nosocomial infection is beyond the scope of this chapter. Further information on nosocomial pneumonia, central nervous system infections, catheter-related bacteremia, and urinary tract infections can be found in Chapters 76, 87, 89, and 90, respectively. The special problems posed by MRSA and *Clostridium difficile* are discussed below.

METHICILLIN-RESISTANT *STAPHYLOCOCCUS AUREUS*. Methicillin-resistant staphylococci (MRSA) are now common isolates in acute care hospital ICUs [44]. Once these organisms are established within a unit they are difficult to eradicate and can account for up to 50 percent of nosocomial staphylococcal infections. In such units an important, but expensive, rule is the need to presumptively treat all staphylococcal infections with vancomycin, an agent that is more toxic than beta-lactam antibiotics, until sensitivity results are available. MRSA produce a low-affinity penicillin-binding protein (PBP-2a or PBP-2′), which appears to be the major determinant of antibacterial resistance [45]. MRSA strains are resistant to methicillin, oxacillin, and the cephalosporins. Epidemiologically these resistant strains behave like methicillin-sensitive strains. They colonize the anterior nares, the skin, open wounds, and the urinary bladder in patients with catheters [46]. Once introduced into ICUs, these organisms tend to spread among patients within the unit.

The in-hospital spread of MRSA has been well studied. The major reservoir for MRSA in hospitals is colonized and infected patients. Transmission of resistant staphylococci to other hospitalized patients is through contact spread, from one patient to another, or through the hands of hospital personnel. Colonized employees with dermatitis or paronychiae are especially likely to transmit the organism to patients [47]. Approximately 5 percent of ICU personnel involved in the care of patients have positive anterior nares cultures for MRSA. Longitudinal study of these employees has shown that their carriage occurs transiently and asymptomatically. Therefore, positive nasal cultures with MRSA in ICU personnel do not require that these persons be removed from work in the ICU setting.

Control Measures. Nonspecific but important measures for managing MRSA in the ICU setting include prospective surveillance of infections in the ICU and review of microbiologic data. Because of the important role of contact spread of MRSA, handwashing is considered to be the most effective way to limit spread of this organism. The role of specific isolation practices in limiting the spread of MRSA has been studied in a controlled manner. Ribner compared strict isolation (masks, gowns, gloves and private room) with modified isolation (masks, gloves and handwashing) to control MRSA in an intensive and intermediate care unit [48]. The frequency of acquisition of MRSA was the same for both isolation practices, but compliance was better with the less stringent form of isolation. In general, we favor modified isolation for the care of MRSA-colonized patients in the ICU except for patients with colonized burn surfaces or patients with pneumonia when strict isolation is recommended. Because of the tendency for MRSA to spread in the immediate environment, MRSA-colonized patients should be placed in private rooms. Cohorting of colonized patients is a reasonable strategy if it is logistically feasible.

Attempts at eradicating MRSA colonization with antibiotics have met with variable success. Approximately half of nasally colonized patients are cleared after a regimen of trimethoprim-sulfamethoxazole, rifampin, and intranasal bacitracin. Local instillation of mucopirin, an antistaphylococcal ointment, has also been shown to reduce colonization with MRSA [49]. This approach, however, is of limited use in ICU patients, who are usually colonized at wound sites or at sites with foreign bodies, clinical conditions usually associated with antibiotic failure. Vancomycin therapy does not result in eradication of carriage. Some studies have shown that eradication of the carrier state in personnel has helped end hospital outbreaks [50,51].

Environmental cultures to test for the presence of MRSA are unnecessary. Similarly, routine culturing of ICU personnel is unnecessary unless there is epidemiologic evidence linking cases of MRSA with contact with a specific employee.

CLOSTRIDIUM DIFFICILE COLITIS. Nosocomial *C. difficile* colitis is an all too familiar disease to hospital personnel. A typical case begins with a hospitalized patient who is being given antibiotics to prevent or to treat an infection. Two to 5 days later the patient complains of loose stools and lower abdominal cramps. If untreated the loose stools progress to frank diarrhea, the abdominal pain worsens, and the patient becomes febrile and develops leukocytosis. Polymorphonuclear leukocytes are invariably present in stool samples, which are sometimes bloody and test positively for the presence of the *C. difficile toxin*. The disease can progress to colonic perforation, and fatal cases have been reported. Pseudomembranous plaques are easily seen in the rectum and sigmoid colon. With oral vancomycin or metronidazole the patient gradually improves over a week to 10 days. The morbidity and extra costs associated with nosocomial cases of *C. difficile* colitis are excessive.

The disease is caused by the proliferation of toxin producing *C. difficile*, a phenomenon that is greatly facilitated by antibiotic perturbation of colonic flora. The pathogenesis of the colitis is related to the production of two exotoxins, Toxins A and B. Toxin A causes mucosal damage, and Toxin B is a cytotoxin that causes the cytopathic effect in tissue culture and forms the basis for the laboratory diagnosis of colitis attributable to *C. difficile* [52]. Virtually all antibiotics, but particularly clindamycin, have been associated with the development of *C. difficile* colitis. Groups at high risk include the elderly, the debilitated, postoperative patients, and those bedded in ICUs [52].

Oral vancomycin or oral metronidazole are both effective treatments; however, relapses occur in approximately one fourth of cases. Cessation of systemic antibiotics to allow for normalization of bowel flora is an important curative maneuver. Most ICU patients are treated with antibiotics, and for most patients it is not possible to discontinue systemic antibiotics despite the suspicion or the proof that diarrhea is caused by *C. difficile*. In such situations simultaneous treatment using systemic antibiotics and oral metronidazole or vancomycin is appropriate.

Hospitalized patients frequently become colonized with *C. difficile*. McFarland and co-workers followed 399 patients who had negative stool cultures on admission; 83 patients became colonized, and 26 of these patients developed antibiotic-associated diarrhea [53]. Gerding has shown that the ratio of colonized to clinical cases can be as high as 6 to 1 [54]. Patient-to-

patient transmission has been shown to occur through careful studies of clusters of cases and the identification of identical immunoblot isolates among such cases [55]. Spread by the hands of health care workers is also common. Approximately 60 percent of hospital personnel who care for patients with *C. difficile* colitis have positive hand cultures. Furthermore, routine handwashing is not effective in removing *C. difficile* because 88 percent of hand cultures are still positive after handwashing [55]. Electronic thermometers that go from patient to patient can become contaminated with *C. difficile*, and in one study replacement of electronic thermometers with single-use disposable devices significantly reduced the incidence of *C. difficile*-associated diarrhea in an acute care facility [56]. The message from these studies is quite clear: *C. difficile* is a hardy, ubiquitous pathogen that can circulate widely throughout a hospital.

Control Measures. The use of gloves is the only proven way of limiting spread of *C. difficile*. There are no controlled studies that have been done in an ICU setting, but in a prospective trial on a general medical ward the use of vinyl gloves by hospital personnel for all body substance contact was associated with a significant decrease in the incidence of *C. difficile* diarrhea [57]. Prophylactically treating carriers of *C. difficile* with vancomycin or metronidazole has not been successful [58]. Johnson and co-workers identified fecal carriers of *C. difficile* on admission and randomly assigned patients to placebo, metronidazole, or vancomycin therapy. Treatment with metronidazole was not effective, and vancomycin therapy was associated with a higher rate of *C. difficile* carriage 2 months after treatment [58].

References

1. Garner JS, Jarvis WR, Emori TG, et al: CDC definitions for nosocomial infections, 1988. *J Infect Control* 16:128, 1988.
2. Wenzel RP, Pfaller MA: Feasible and desirable targets for reducing the costs of hospital infections. *J Hosp Infect* 18(suppl A):94, 1991.
3. French GL, Cheng AFB: Measurement of the costs of hospital infections by prevalence surveys. *J Hosp Infect* 18(suppl A):65, 1991.
4. Smith RL, Meixler SM, Simberkoff MS: Excess mortality in critically ill patients with nosocomial bloodstream infections. *Chest* 100:164, 1991.
5. Davey P, Hernanz C, Lynch W, et al: Human and non-financial costs of hospital-acquired infection. *J Hosp Infect* 18(suppl A):79, 1991.
6. Weinstein RA: Epidemiology and control of nosocomial infections in adult intensive care units. *Am J Med* (suppl 3B):179s, 1991.
7. Craven DE, Kunches LM, Lichtenberg DA, et al: Nosocomial infection and fatality in medical and surgical intensive care unit patients. *Arch Intern Med* 148:1161, 1988.
8. Chandrasekar PH, Kruse JA, Mathews MF: Nosocomial infection among patients in different types of intensive care units at a city hospital. *Crit Care Med* 14(15):508, 1986.
9. Pories SE, Gamelli RL, Mead PB, et al: The epidemiologic features of nosocomial infections in patients with trauma. *Arch Surg* 126:97, 1991.
10. Emori TG, Culver DH, Horan TC, et al: National nosocomial infections surveillance system (NNIS): Description of surveillance methods. *Am J Infect Control* 19:19, 1991.
11. Jarvis WR, Edwards JR, Culver DH, et al: Nosocomial infection rates in adult and pediatric intensive care units in the United States. *Am J Med* 91(suppl 3B):185s, 1991.
12. Brown RB, Hosmer D, Chen HC, et al: A comparison of infections in different ICUs within the same hospital. *Crit Care Med* 13(6):472, 1985.
13. Klein BS, Perloff WH, Maki GD: Reduction of nosocomial infection during pediatric intensive care by protective isolation. *N Engl J Med* 320:1714, 1989.
14. Gaynes RP, Martone WJ, Culver DH, et al: Comparison of rates of

nosocomial infections in neonatal intensive care units in the United States. *Am J Med* 91(suppl 3B):192s, 1991.

15. Aavitsland P, Stormark M, Lystad A: Hospital-acquired infections in Norway: A national prevalence survey in 1991. *Scand J Infect Dis* 24:477, 1992.

16. Massanari RM: Nosocomial infections in critical care units: Causation and prevention. *Crit Care Nurs Q* 11(4):45, 1989.

17. Goldman DA, Freeman J, Durbin WA: Nosocomial infection and death in a neonatal intensive care unit. *J Infect Dis* 147(4):635, 1983.

18. Villarino ME, Stevens LE, Schable B, et al: Risk factors for epidemic Xanthomonas maltophilia infection/colonization in intensive care unit patients. *Infect Control Hosp Epidemiol* 13:201, 1992.

19. Bauer TM, Ofner E, Just HM, et al: An epidemiologic study assessing the relative importance of airborne and direct contact transmission of microorganisms in a medical intensive care unit. *J Hosp Infect* 15(4):301, 1990.

20. Olson B, Weinstein RA, Nathan C: Epidemiology of endemic Pseudomonas aeruginosa: Why infection control efforts have failed. *J Infect Dis* 150(6):808, 1984.

21. du Moulin G: Minimizing the potential for nosocomial pneumonia: Architectural, engineering, and environmental considerations for the intensive care unit. *Eur J Clin Microbiol Infect Dis* 8(1):69, 1989.

22. Shirani KZ, McManus AT, Vaughan GM, et al: Effects of environment on infection in burn patients. *Arch Surg* 121:31, 1986.

23. Goldman DA, Durbin WA, Freeman J: Nosocomial infections in a neonatal intensive care unit. *J Infect Dis* 144(5):449, 1981.

24. Huebner J, Frank U, Kappstein I: Influence of architectural design on nosocomial infections in intensive care units: A prospective 2 year analysis. *Intensive Care Med* 15:179, 1989.

25. Goldman DA, Larson E: Hand-washing and nosocomial infections. *N Engl J Med* 327(2):120, 1992.

26. Conly JM, Hill S, Ross J, et al: Handwashing practices in an intensive care unit: The effects of an educational program and its relationship to infection rates. *Am J Infect Control* 17:330, 1989.

27. Simmons B, Bryant J, Neiman K, et al: The role of handwashing in prevention of endemic intensive care unit infections. *Infect Control Hosp Epidemiol* 11(11):589, 1990.

28. Graham M: Frequency and duration of handwashing in an intensive care unit. *Am J Infect Control* 18:77, 1990.

29. Dubbert PM, Dolce J, Richter W, et al: Increasing ICU handwashing: Effects of education and group feedback. *Infect Control Hosp Epidemiol* 11:191, 1990.

30. Doebbeling BN, Stanley GL, Sheetz CT, et al: Comparative efficacy of alternative hand-washing agents in reducing nosocomial infections in intensive care units. *N Engl J Med* 327:88, 1992.

31. Pettinger A, Nettleman MD: Epidemiology of isolation precautions. *Infect Control Hosp Epidemiol* 12:303, 1991.

32. Bjerke HS, Leyerle B, Shabot MM: Impact of ICU nosocomial infections on outcome from surgical care. *Am Surg* 57(12):798, 1991.

33. Patterson JE, Vechio J, Pantelick EL: Association of contaminated gloves with transmission of Acinetobacter calcoaceticus var. anitratus in an intensive care unit. *Am J Med* 91:479, 1991.

34. Beck-Sague CM, Jarvis WR, Brook JH, et al: Epidemic bacteremia due to Acinetobacter baumanii in five intensive care units. *Am J Epidemiol* 132(4):723, 1990.

35. Villarino ME, Jarvis WR, O'Hara C, et al: Epidemic Serratia marcescens bacteremia in a cardiac intensive care unit. *J Clin Microbiol* 27(11):2433, 1989.

36. Simmons BP: Guidelines for prevention of infections related to intravascular pressure monitoring systems. *J Infect Control* 3:68, 1982.

37. Luskin RL, Weinstein RA, Nathan C, et al: Extended use of disposable pressure transducers. *JAMA* 255:916, 1986.

38. Craven DE, Steger KA, Barber TW: Preventing nosocomial pneumonia: State of the art and perspectives for the 1990's. *Am J Med* 91(suppl 3B):44s, 1991.

39. Craven DE, Goularte TA, Make BJ: Contaminated condensate in mechanical ventilator circuits. *Am Rev Respir Dis* 129:625, 1984.

40. Craven DE, Connolly MG, Lichtenberg DA, et al: Contamination of mechanical ventilators with tubing changes every 24 or 48 hours. *N Engl J Med* 306:1505, 1982.

41. Craven DE, Kunches LM, Kilinsky V, et al: Risk factors for pneumonia and fatality in patients receiving continuous mechanical ventilation. *Am Rev Respir Dis* 133:792, 1986.

42. Dreyfuss D, Djedaini K, Weber P, et al: Prospective study of nosocomial pneumonia and of patient and circuit colonization during mechanical ventilation with every 48 hours versus no change. *Am Rev Respir Dis* 143:738, 1991.

43. Simmons BP, Wong ES: Guideline for prevention of nosocomial pneumonia. *J Infect Control* 3:327, 1982.

44. Boyce JM: Methicillin resistant Staphylococcus aureus. *Infect Clin North* 3:901, 1989.

45. Chambers HF: Methicillin-resistant staphylococci. *Clin Microbiol Rev* 1:173, 1988.

46. Thompson RL, Cabezudo I, Wenzel RP: Epidemiology of nosocomial infections caused by methicillin-resistant Staphylococcus aureus. *Ann Intern Med* 97:309, 1982.

47. Craven DE, Reed C, Kollisch N, et al: A large outbreak of infections caused by a strain of Staphylococcus aureus resistant to oxacillin and aminoglycosides. II. Epidemiologic studies. *Am J Med* 71:53, 1981.

48. Ribner BS, Landry MN, Gholson GL: Strict versus modified isolation for prevention of nosocomial transmission of methicillin-resistant Staphylococcus aureus. *Infect Control* 7:313, 1986.

49. Reagan DR, Doebbeling BN, Pfaller MA, et al: Elimination of coincident Staphylococcus aureus nasal and hand carriage with intranasal application of mucopirin calcium ointment. *Ann Intern Med* 114:101, 1991.

50. Reboli AC, John JF, Platt CB, et al: Methicillin-resistant Staphylococcus aureus outbreak at a Veterans' Affairs Medical Center: Importance of carriage of the organism by hospital personnel. *Infect Control Hosp Epidemiol* 11:291, 1990.

51. Hill RL, Duckworth GJ, Casewell MW: Elimination of nasal carriage of methicillin-resistant Staphylococcus aureus and therapy of colonized personnel during a hospital-wide outbreak. *J Antimicrob Chemother* 22:377, 1988.

52. Bartlett JG: Clostridium difficile: Clinical considerations. *Rev Infect Dis* 12(Supp l2):S243, 1990.

53. McFarland LV, Surawicz CM, Stamm WE: Risk factors for Clostridium difficile carriage and C. difficile-associated diarrhea in a cohort of hospitalized patients. *J Infect Dis* 162:678, 1990.

54. Gerding DN: Disease associated with Clostridium difficile infection. *Ann Intern Med* 110:255, 1989.

55. McFarland LV, Mulligan ME, Kwork RYY, et al: Nosocomial acquisition of Clostridium difficile infection. *N Engl J Med* 320:204, 1989.

56. Brooks SE, Veal RO, Kramer M, et al: Reduction in the incidence of Clostridium difficile-associated diarrhea in an acute care hospital and a skilled nursing facility following replacement of electronic thermometers with single use disposables. *Infect Control Hosp Epidemiol* 13:98, 1992.

57. Johnson S, Gerding DN, Olson MM, et al: Prospective, controlled study of vinyl gloves use to interrupt Clostridium difficile nosocomial transmission. *Am J Med* 88:137, 1990.

58. Johnson S, Homann SR, Bettin KM, et al: Treatment of asymptomatic Clostridium difficile carriers (fecal excretors) with vancomycin or metronidazole. *Ann Intern Med* 117:297, 1992.

87. Central Nervous System Infections

Sarah H. Cheeseman and
Alan L. Rothman

The central nervous system (CNS) infections of major interest in the ICU are bacterial meningitis, encephalitis, brain abscess, and other parameningeal foci of infection. These quite discrete disease entities may overlap considerably in their presentation as clinical syndromes. *Meningitis* means inflammation of the leptomeninges, and its hallmark is stiff neck. Headache and photophobia are the usual symptoms. These are usually the only findings in viral meningitis, but they may also occur as part of other illnesses such as Rocky Mountain spotted fever and leptospirosis. When there is no inflammatory response in the spinal fluid, these symptoms are called *meningismus*. *Encephalitis* is a syndrome that consists of disturbance of cerebral function accompanied by cerebrospinal fluid pleocytosis. Many cases of bacterial meningitis would certainly fit within this definition because of the occurrence of seizures or coma.

The terms *purulent* and *aseptic* describe contrasting spinal fluid formulas, although again overlap exists. The typical purulent spinal fluid has a white cell count in excess of 1000 cells per cubic millimeter, most of which are polymorphonuclear leukocytes; a depressed glucose concentration (<40 mg/dl); and an elevated protein level (>100 mg/dl). An aseptic formula would have a lower total leukocyte count with a predominance of mononuclear cells, a glucose concentration greater than 40 to 50 percent of the blood level, and less marked elevation of protein content.

In general, the purulent picture represents bacterial meningitis, although it may occasionally arise from brain abscess or acute bacterial endocarditis, whereas the aseptic picture characterizes most other forms of central nervous system infection. One must be particularly careful not to interpret aseptic as equivalent to viral, because parameningeal foci, subacute bacterial endocarditis, spirochetal infection, and noninfectious diseases can give rise to a similar spinal fluid picture. An intermediate formula in which a moderate pleocytosis, usually lymphocytic, is accompanied by depressed glucose and elevated protein suggests granulomatous disease.

General Clinical Approach

Evaluation of the patient with suggested central nervous system infection should focus on defining the syndrome on three levels:

1. Nature of the symptoms—meningitic versus encephalitic
2. Presence and pattern of neurologic involvement—focal versus diffuse
3. Character of the cerebrospinal fluid—purulent versus aseptic

If the neurologic examination suggests a focal lesion, the possibility that localized edema and mass will produce a pressure cone after lumbar puncture should dissuade one from obtaining cerebrospinal fluid (CSF) until computed tomographic scanning has excluded this possibility. The other circumstance in which lumbar puncture should not be performed is when lumbar spinal epidural abscess is suspected. Because speed is so important in diagnosing and treating bacterial meningitis, it is fortu-

nate that brain abscess is a much rarer disease, and only half of the cases have an infectious disease presentation at all; the others present like tumors, without fever. Spinal epidural abscess is also uncommon, and the presence of radicular symptoms tends to distinguish it from meningitis. Thus most patients clinically suspected of having meningitis should have lumbar puncture performed as soon as that suspicion arises.

If lumbar puncture proves difficult, the expertise of a senior person, particularly a neurologist, neurosurgeon, or anesthesiologist, should be requested promptly. Occasionally, distorted anatomy makes the lumbar puncture impossible unless performed by a neuroradiologist under fluoroscopic control. In these situations of unavoidable delay, antibiotics should be begun while efforts to obtain CSF continue; however, blood cultures should be drawn before instituting therapy.

In the normal situation, when the lumbar puncture has been performed expeditiously, the return of purulent fluid should lead to immediate institution of antibiotics. Even if the fluid appears clear, Gram stain should be performed. The finding of many organisms and few cells implies rapidly progressive disease and a need for haste if there is to be any hope that therapy will affect the outcome. Patients who have an aseptic formula can then be evaluated with respect to the question of meningitis versus encephalitis, and if the latter is the case, the search for the focus can begin.

Virtually all patients with the diagnoses reviewed here require initial admission to an ICU. Specific therapies are of no avail if a lapse in the vigor of supportive care causes irreversible damage.

Bacterial Meningitis

Bacterial meningitis is perhaps the most clear-cut emergency in the field of infectious diseases. Therapy promptly initiated may restore life and health, but delay or inadequate treatment increases the risk of death and of significant neurologic impairment for those who survive. Bacterial meningitis is more common at the extremes of age and among the immunosuppressed, but cases occur in all age groups.

ETIOLOGY. Three organisms, *Haemophilus influenzae*, *Neisseria meningitidis* (the meningococcus), and *Streptococcus pneumoniae* (the pneumococcus), have accounted for 70 to 85 percent of cases of bacterial meningitis, although the fraction of meningitis cases caused by other bacteria has increased in recent years [1–4]. The predominant organisms can be predicted on the basis of the age and underlying condition of the host (Table 87-1).

H. influenzae type B was for many years the most common cause of meningitis in patients between 3 months and 6 years of age. Infection is frequently accompanied by pharyngitis (20%–60%) or otitis (20%–50%) [1,2,5]. Recently, the incidence of *H. influenzae* type B meningitis in infants has declined by almost 90 percent after the introduction of new *H. influenzae* type B conjugate vaccines [6]. *H. influenzae* is a much less

Table 87-1. Antibiotic Therapy for Meningitis of Known Cause in Adults

Organism	Preferred Therapy		Alternative Therapy	
	Antibiotic	Dosage/24 hr	Antibiotic	Dosage/24 hr
Pneumococcus	Penicillin G	24 million units IV	Ceftriaxone[a] or chloramphenicol or erythromycin	4 gm IV 4 gm IV 4 gm IV
Streptococcus groups A and B	Penicillin G	24 million units IV	Ceftriaxone[a] or erythromycin	4 gm IV 4 gm IV
Enterococcus	Penicillin G + gentamicin[b]	24 million units IV 5 mg/kg IV + ? IT	Vancomycin + gentamicin[b]	2 gm IV 5 mg/kg IV + ? IT
Staphylococcus aureus	Nafcillin[c]	12 gm IV	Vancomycin	2 gm IV
Listeria monocytogenes	Penicillin G or ampicillin + gentamicin[b]	24 million units IV 12 gm IV 5 mg/kg IV	Trimethoprim-sulfamethoxazole	10 mg/kg trimethoprim IV
Meningococcus	Penicillin G	24 million units IV	Ceftriaxone[a] or chloramphenicol	4 gm IV 4 gm IV
Haemophilus influenzae	Ceftriaxone[a,d]	4 gm IV	Chloramphenicol	4 gm IV
Pseudomonas	Ceftazidime + tobramycin	6 gm IV 5 mg/kg IV + ? IT	Piperacillin + tobramycin	24–30 gm IV 5 mg/kg IV + 10 mg IT
Others (e.g., *Escherichia coli, Klebsiella, Proteus*)[e]	Ceftriaxone[a] + gentamicin[b]	4 gm IV 5 mg/kg IV	Trimethoprim-sulfamethoxazole or gentamicin[b]	10 mg/kg trimethoprim IV 5 mg/kg IV + 10 mg IT

[a] Or other third-generation cephalosporin.
[b] Tobramycin may be used in place of gentamicin.
[c] Unless organism known or suspected to be methicillin-resistant.
[d] If organism is ampicillin-sensitive, use ampicillin 12 gm IV.
[e] Final choice of specific antibiotic therapy depends on antibiotic susceptibility studies of the organism.
IT = intralumbar or intraventricular.

frequent cause of meningitis in adults, and is usually associated with predisposing factors, such as anatomic defects (head trauma, CSF leaks) or defects in humoral immunity [7]. Otitis or sinusitis is seen in 25 to 30 percent of these cases. The predominance of type B strains seen in childhood does not carry over to meningitis in adulthood.

N. meningitidis is the most common cause in older children and young adults, but is uncommon after age 45. It is the one form of bacterial meningitis associated with epidemic spread. Serogroup B, for which there is currently no vaccine, is responsible for most sporadic cases in the United States, whereas serogroups A and C are more often associated with outbreaks [3,8].

S. pneumoniae is the predominant cause of meningitis in adults, and is seen in all age groups. Pneumococcal meningitis is particularly common after head trauma or in the presence of a CSF leak, hypogammaglobulinemia, asplenism, or alcoholism [9–12]. Pneumonia, otitis, or sinusitis accompanies meningitis in up to 50 percent of cases [1,2,5].

Listeria monocytogenes is a common cause of meningitis in the neonatal period or in the setting of malignancy, organ transplantation, immunosuppression, or debilitation, particularly alcoholism [13–17]. Up to 30 percent of patients have no apparent immunocompromising condition [13]. Most of these patients are older than age 50. This organism accounted for 10 percent of community-acquired meningitis among adults in one recent series [18].

Gram-negative bacillary meningitis occurs in the neonatal period or after neurosurgery or trauma [3,14,18–22]. Community-acquired gram-negative bacillary meningitis is rare in adults (fewer than 4% of cases [18]). When it occurs, it is usually a complication of bacteremia from a distant site, often the urinary tract, with a predilection for patients with cancer or alcohol-induced liver disease [14,15,18,21,22,23]. *Staphylococcus aureus* meningitis is also associated with neurosurgery or trauma.

Community-acquired cases occur in the presence of a focus of infection outside the CNS, such as endocarditis or soft-tissue infections [24,25,26]. Both *S. aureus* and *Staphylococcus epidermidis* are associated with meningitis in patients with CSF shunts [27] or congenital dermal sinus tracts, as are other skin flora, such as *Propionibacterium acnes* and gram-negative bacilli. Group B streptococcus is the most common cause of neonatal meningitis [4]. Anaerobic bacteria and streptococci other than *S. pneumoniae* are otherwise uncommon causes of meningitis that are usually related to spread from brain abscess or parameningeal foci such as chronic otitis or sinusitis [2,28].

PATHOGENESIS. The meninges become infected by either hematogenous spread or contiguous extension of infection. The former route is by far the more common. Bacteremia does not require an established focus of infection but apparently can arise from simple colonization of the nasopharynx. It is presumed that respiratory spread of the organism carries it to the nasopharynx, and that this is followed by bacteremia in a proportion of patients lacking specific antibody. The opsonic role of antibody is a major defense against *S. pneumoniae* and *H. influenzae*, as evidenced by the increased incidence and the fulminant course of meningitis in patients with primary hypogammaglobulinemia, poor production of specific antibody (as in multiple myeloma), splenectomy (especially combined with radiation and chemotherapy for the treatment of lymphoma), or a functional asplenic state [10,11,12].

Spread from contiguous foci of infection is more often a cause of intracranial abscess than of acute purulent meningitis, except when abnormal connections exist. Occult or obvious CSF leaks after fractures of the skull predispose to pneumococcal [1,2] and, less commonly, *H. influenzae* [7] meningitis and should always be searched for in patients who have recurrent disease. Fractures through the cribriform plate and the ethmoid and frontal sinuses are most frequently involved, but the injury that gave rise to the defect may have occurred in the remote past. An abnormal connection is much more obvious in post-traumatic and postneurosurgical cases, particularly with use of intracranial pressure-monitoring devices [29,30].

Lumbar puncture itself may serve as a portal of entry of bacteria to the subarachnoid space. This may result from a breach of aseptic technique, introducing skin flora. This should be a rare complication and is avoided by careful attention to proper technique, especially during long and difficult procedures. A theoretic concern is the possibility that lumbar puncture in bacteremic patients may facilitate the subsequent occurrence of meningitis. Several clinical studies failed to show a significant increase in the occurrence of meningitis after lumbar puncture [31,32]. One study did find such an association in children younger than 1 year of age, but a bias favoring the performance of lumbar puncture in children already developing meningitis could not be excluded [33]. Therefore, the possibility of lumbar puncture-induced meningitis during bacteremia remains unproved, and should not deter one from performing the procedure whenever indicated.

Once bacteria have reached the CSF, both bacterial and host factors contribute to the pathophysiologic responses. In the initial phase, bacterial products stimulate endothelial and astroglial cells of the CNS to produce endogenous mediators of inflammation such as tumor necrosis factor (TNF), interleukin 1 (IL-1), and arachidonic acid metabolites [34]. These in turn stimulate the adherence of neutrophils to the local endothelium and neutrophil diapedesis into the CNS. Neutrophil activation by cytokines leads to the release of toxic intermediates, which disrupt the integrity of the tight junctions between endothelial cells. This incites CSF inflammation and impairs the blood-brain barrier. Elevated cytokine levels in CSF distinguish bacterial meningitis from nonpyogenic meningitis [35] and have been associated with poor outcome [36]. Antibiotics that rapidly lyse bacteria, such as certain beta-lactam antibiotics, actually generate a transient increase in inflammation as a response to the release of bacteria cell wall products [37].

Intracranial pressure (ICP) increases as a consequence of the disruption of the blood-brain barrier. Other factors, such as obstruction to CSF outflow, may also contribute to increased ICP. Together with a loss of the normal mechanisms of cerebrovascular autoregulation, this causes global and regional fluctuation in cerebral blood flow [38]. Inflammation in the Virchow-Robin spaces may progress to involve the vessels and produce cortical venous thrombophlebitis with resultant cortical necrosis [39,40]. Occasionally major dural sinuses become involved, and arterial obliteration may also occur [41] with corresponding neurologic signs. The exudate pools in the basilar cisterns, where it may damage cranial nerves and produce sufficient adhesions to lead to hydrocephalus, usually of the communicating type.

The clinical consequence of these pathologic processes is a generalized disturbance of cerebral function. An early phase of agitation or mania may be noted, particularly in meningococcal disease. Lethargy progresses to obtundation and sometimes coma. Seizures occur early in 20 to 30 percent of adults with meningitis [2,18,20,39]. Focal neurologic deficits may be observed, either as transient postictal effects or because of the vascular phenomena previously enumerated. Hyponatremia, caused by the syndrome of inappropriate antidiuretic hormone (SIADH) excretion, may contribute to obtundation and seizures.

Given the multiple forms of parenchymal damage possible, it is not surprising that nearly any neurologic disorder may be a sequela of meningitis, but sensorineural deafness is particularly characteristic [42,43,44]. In cases in which profound mental

retardation, hydrocephalus, or significant paralysis occurs, seizures may also persist. In most patients, however, seizures resolve after the period of acute infection [44,45]. The frequency of significant neurologic impairment after meningitis is greatest when the infection occurs in infancy, and most studies of the sequelae have been in pediatric patient populations [42–46]. Limited data suggest that neurologic impairment persists in approximately 30 percent of survivors of meningitis in adulthood [20,39].

DIAGNOSIS

History. History may be of little help in the patient with meningitis, because there may be none. In fact, the patient's inability to give a coherent history should lead one to consider the diagnosis. Patients found unresponsive alone in their homes or with hypothermia from exposure should be highly suspect for meningitis. Patients with fever and derangement of cerebral function, even if there is another cause for the latter, must have meningitis excluded. Persons with coexistent alcoholism, general debility, head trauma, or neurosurgery are at higher risk for meningitis.

When patients can describe their symptoms, headache, photophobia, and stiff neck suggest meningitis. Headache may be the only complaint in some immunosuppressed patients. The symptoms of a primary focus of infection such as otitis or pneumonia may also be present. It is very important to inquire about head trauma, skull fracture, and presence or recent history of clear nasal or ear discharges, because the possibility of a CSF leak in an adult alters the probable causes. It is also important to discover whether the patient has been taking any antibiotics, which could interfere with obtaining cultures of the responsible organism. A history of exposure to a patient with known meningococcal disease is usually forthcoming if present. In children one should inquire about close contacts with others (such as in a day-care setting), with respect to both origin and spread of *H. influenzae* and meningococcal disease.

Physical Examination. Nuchal rigidity suggests meningitis when present, but it may be absent, especially in infants. In the elderly, limitation of motion caused by degenerative cervical arthritis may be a confounding variable. The Kernig sign may help, because extending the knee on the flexed hip stretches the meninges but not the neck. Resistance to this maneuver represents either meningeal irritation or flexion contractures of the knees. The initial neurologic examination should be directed toward evaluating the mental status and presence of focal deficits. Papilledema is rarely present in meningitis and when observed should suggest other diagnoses as well as alter the approach to lumbar puncture [39,47]. Serial examinations document the presence or absence of functional improvement and define sequelae.

The systemic examination may give clues to the cause of meningitis, particularly the skin findings. Any patient with meningitis and petechiae should be placed on respiratory precautions immediately to limit the number of people potentially exposed to meningococcus, although petechiae can also occur in aseptic meningitis caused by enterovirus, Rocky Mountain spotted fever, and other forms of bacterial meningitis. Purpuric lesions with irregular but well-defined margins and skin infarcts (often gunmetal gray in color) strongly suggest meningococcal disease, although the same lesions have been seen in bacteremic meningitis caused by *S. pneumoniae* and *H. influenzae*. Bilateral symmetric peripheral gangrene, affecting the fingers and toes, has been described in pneumococcal disease, and multiple pustular skin lesions have been noted with *S. aureus*.

*Whenever skin lesions occur, an effort should be made to ob*tain material from them for a Gram stain. Even the tiniest pustule or petechia can be opened with a very small needle and a touch preparation made of the drop of fluid that exudes.

Laboratory Tests. Evaluation of the CSF is essential for the diagnosis of meningitis [47]. The typical features of purulent CSF have already been discussed. A few cases may demonstrate minimal pleocytosis, and this is a bad prognostic sign if it occurs in the presence of many organisms on Gram stain [48]. Polymorphs constitute more than 50 percent of the cells in nearly all cases and more than 85 percent in the majority [2,49,50]. Instances of lymphocytic predominance have been reported more frequently in recent series [51,52] and may be associated with spread from contiguous foci, unusual organisms (including *H. influenzae* in the adult), or previous antibiotic therapy [2,7,46,49,50]. Despite its species name, *L. monocytogenes* usually gives a polymorphonuclear pleocytosis [14]. Elevated protein is also almost always present and, when marked, tends to differentiate bacterial from aseptic meningitis [49]. Severe depression of the CSF glucose (<20 mg/dl) is strong evidence for a pyogenic process [49,53,54]. The definition of decreased CSF glucose is variably given as less than 40 or 50 percent of the blood level, but this point becomes less important when one considers that whatever definition one takes, CSF glucose is normal in 13 to 40 percent of patients with bacterial meningitis [46,49,53,54]. In patients with abnormally high blood sugars, such as diabetics, a cutoff of 30 percent of the simultaneous blood glucose provides better specificity for bacterial meningitis, but the same caveat applies [55]. The CSF sugar is thus useful when it is unequivocally low, but a normal value cannot be used to exclude bacterial meningitis.

Blood and CSF cultures remain the mainstays of diagnosis. Gram stain of CSF or skin lesions can identify the causative organism rapidly in at least 75 percent of cases [1,2,46,50] but should be reviewed by an experienced person to prevent errors of technique or interpretation. Antigen detection by the latex agglutination method has a similar yield for those bacteria tested and may be useful when Gram stain is negative and antimicrobial therapy has been given before CSF is obtained [56,57]. It should not be regarded as any more definitive than the Gram stain, because false negatives, false positives, and cross-reactions may occur. Newer techniques, including polymerase chain reaction (PCR) detection of bacterial DNA, may eventually prove useful for rapid diagnosis in patients with negative Gram stain of CSF [58]. Ultimately at least 90 percent of patients with unequivocally purulent CSF have an organism isolated in culture [1,2]. Antibiotic administration is much more likely to render cultures negative than it is to alter the CSF formula [2,46,50].

The laboratory should perform formal susceptibility testing on all isolates from CSF and blood in cases of meningitis, including penicillin susceptibility for pneumococci (using an oxacillin disc and a zone diameter ≥20 mm [59]) and determine both beta-lactamase production and ampicillin susceptibility for *H. influenzae*. Susceptibility testing of meningococci is not routinely indicated in the United States; however, resistance to penicillin among clinical isolates of *N. meningitidis* has recently been observed in areas of Spain, South Africa, and the United Kingdom and should be considered in the appropriate epidemiologic setting [60].

Radiologic studies are of secondary importance in the diagnosis of meningitis. Radiographs of the chest and paranasal sinuses may identify other foci of infection. Computed tomography (CT) and magnetic resonance imaging (MRI) are most useful for excluding focal intracranial processes such as brain abscess or subdural empyema.

DIFFERENTIAL DIAGNOSIS. The most common conditions to be differentiated from pyogenic meningitis are aseptic and tuberculous meningitis, because there may be overlap in the spinal fluid formulas in these conditions. Very high CSF white blood cell counts and a high proportion of polymorphonuclear leukocytes occur in a few cases of enteroviral meningitis. Mumps and lymphocytic choriomeningitis are the viruses most often responsible for low glucose levels. Early in viral meningitis there may be a polymorphonuclear predominance, with a shift to lymphocytes taking place with time, so repeating the lumbar puncture after 8 to 12 hours may be helpful [61]. Clinical features such as young adult age and onset of illness during the summer months can be helpful clues to a viral rather than bacterial origin [51]. Viral cultures, which may yield an enterovirus within 48 to 72 hours, can also provide useful clarification, although coexistent viral and bacterial meningitis has been reported. PCR-based assays for diagnosis of enteroviral meningitis may also prove useful [62]. In the few instances in which there is real doubt as to the bacterial or viral nature of the process, it is always safer to continue therapy for the possibility of a bacterial cause.

Tuberculous meningitis may have a total leukocyte count in the range of purulent meningitis and may be predominantly polymorphonuclear (≥80% in 3 of 11 cases in one series [49]). The first phase of tuberculous meningitis is described as a nonspecific illness, so that by the time headache or other central nervous system signs occur, the patient is in the second stage, and there may be a period of only 10 days or 2 weeks to act before permanent damage is done [63,64,65]. A history of previous tuberculosis, of exposure to active disease or belonging to a group in which that is likely, or the presence of an immunocompromising condition such as infection with human immunodeficiency virus (HIV) [66] must raise the physician's suspicion. If an initial diagnosis of purulent meningitis is not confirmed by culture and the patient does not improve, repeat lumbar puncture with studies for acid-fast bacilli and a tuberculin test should be performed. A switch to lymphocytic predominance, additional decrease in CSF glucose and increase in protein, positive chest radiograph or tuberculin reaction, or well-founded clinical suspicion would mandate institution of antituberculous therapy. Acid-fast bacilli are rarely observed on microscopic examination of CSF [64,65], although the yield may be improved by repeated spinal tap [64]. Newer techniques, such as the PCR, hold hope for facilitating earlier diagnosis [67].

Two other nonbacterial processes in which the CSF mimics pyogenic meningitis are eastern equine encephalitis and amebic (*Naegleria*) meningitis. The latter is acquired through freshwater swimming and may be diagnosed on wet mount of CSF. In the appropriate epidemiologic setting, the assistance of public health authorities should be requested in making these diagnoses.

Mollaret's meningitis is recurrent culture-negative purulent meningitis [1] and can be diagnosed only after observation of several episodes. Medications, such as sulfonamides or nonsteroidal antiinflammatory agents, may cause meningitis indistinguishable from pyogenic infection [68]. Acute bacterial endocarditis, especially that caused by *S. aureus,* can also mimic bacterial meningitis (see Chap. 88) [69].

Parameningeal foci of infection, such as subdural empyema or phlebitis of major dural sinuses, can sometimes present a purulent picture, usually with a normal glucose concentration, and brain abscess that has ruptured into the ventricles may duplicate the clinical picture of bacterial meningitis. Isolation of an anaerobe or more than one organism from the CSF should strongly suggest one of these diagnoses. Persistent, localizing neurologic findings should make one think about them [39].

Hypoglycorrhachia may be seen in carcinomatous meningitis or fungal meningitis. An indolent course and lymphocytic pleocytosis in the CSF usually distinguishes these from pyogenic infection. *Cryptococcus neoformans* is a major cause of meningitis in patients with acquired immunodeficiency syndrome (AIDS) or other immunosuppressive conditions [15,16,70], although it can also occur in normal hosts. Meningismus is uncommon, and there is typically only mild to moderate lymphocytic pleocytosis [71,72]. The HIV-infected patient also may have lymphocytic meningitis with normal CSF glucose due to either syphilis or HIV itself [73].

THERAPY. The appropriate management of patients with bacterial meningitis involves prompt initiation of antimicrobial therapy, aggressive control of the potential complications of the disease, and prevention of spread of disease. Mortality from bacterial meningitis ranges from 3 to 6 percent for childhood *H. influenzae* meningitis to over 50 percent for pneumococcal or gram-negative bacillary meningitis in the elderly [2,3,4], with 70 percent of deaths occurring in the first 48 hours [2]. This fact underlies the recommendation that most if not all such patients be treated in an intensive care setting.

The principal consideration in choosing an antibiotic regimen for bacterial meningitis is that the agent or agents reach the CSF in concentrations that are bactericidal for the likely pathogens. The presence of inflammation assists the penetration of many drugs, such as the penicillins and cephalosporins, into the CSF. It is important to continue high-dose antibiotic therapy throughout the course of treatment, because antibiotic levels in the CSF are likely to diminish as inflammation subsides [34]. Table 87-1 lists current recommendations for therapy of bacterial meningitis of known cause.

When initial examination of CSF does not indicate a specific pathogen, or when lumbar puncture is delayed, antibiotic therapy should be directed against the likely pathogens based on the age and underlying condition of the patient. Recommendations for empiric antimicrobial therapy of bacterial meningitis are listed in Table 87-1.

Penicillin or ampicillin has long been the mainstay of therapy for community-acquired meningitis in immunocompetent older children and adults, in whom *S. pneumoniae* and *N. meningitidis* predominate. Therapeutic failures or early relapses occur, however, in patients infected with penicillin-resistant pneumococci (PR-Sp). These organisms are commonly encountered outside the United States [74]. In the United States, surveillance data through 1987 demonstrated a low prevalence of PR-Sp, approximately 5 percent of isolates [75]. More recent data published in abstract form only have shown a rapid increase in PR-Sp in areas of the United States [76–79]. Where local conditions dictate, the choice of empiric antimicrobial therapy should reflect the risk of PR-Sp. Vancomycin or the third-generation cephalosporins are most active for such infections; most PR-Sp have also been resistant to chloramphenicol, tetracycline, and trimethoprim-sulfamethoxazole [76–81].

Combination therapy with penicillin plus a third-generation cephalosporin should be used in immunosuppressed or debilitated patients who have a higher incidence of *H. influenzae* or gram-negative bacillary meningitis; the penicillin is necessary because the cephalosporins are inactive against *L. monocytogenes*. An alternative is the combination of trimethoprim and sulfamethoxazole, which is active against *L. monocytogenes* as well as many gram-negative bacilli other than *Pseudomonas aeruginosa* [82]. Many authorities recommend using the broader-spectrum antimicrobial regimens in all elderly patients with meningitis. For patients with meningitis after neurosurgery

or trauma, in whom staphylococci and resistant gram-negative bacilli are more common, initial therapy with nafcillin or vancomycin, a third-generation cephalosporin, and an aminoglycoside would provide reasonable coverage while culture data are pending.

Indiscriminate use of multiple antibiotics or reliance on newer antibacterial agents should be avoided. In vitro antagonism between penicillin and tetracycline is associated with an increase in mortality in patients with meningitis receiving both drugs [83]. Similarly, some studies have suggested that mortality or the frequency of neurologic sequelae may be higher in patients receiving ampicillin plus chloramphenicol than in patients receiving either drug alone [84,85]. Some newer antibiotics, such as imipenem, aztreonam, and ciprofloxacin, have been shown to achieve bactericidal concentrations in the presence of inflamed meninges; however, the clinical experience with these agents in the treatment of meningitis is very limited. The use of imipenem carries the risk of drug-induced seizures [86]. Aztreonam and ciprofloxacin are notable for their absent or minimal activity against *S. pneumoniae*. These drugs should not be used for empiric treatment of meningitis but should be reserved for treatment of meningitis caused by organisms resistant to other agents.

The recommended duration of antimicrobial therapy for meningitis depends on the specific organism and the clinical response [87]. Seven to 10 days of therapy are adequate for infection with *H. influenzae* or the meningococcus [88,89]; 10 to 14 days are preferred for pneumococcal meningitis. Gram-negative bacillary meningitis is typically treated for 3 weeks; staphylococcal disease, when accompanied by bacteremia, for 4 to 6 weeks. Repeat lumbar punctures are not useful in determining when to discontinue therapy as long as the patient has responded clinically; the CSF cell count, glucose, or protein remains abnormal in at least 30 percent of cases after curative therapy [90,91].

The pathophysiologic role of endogenous mediators of inflammation, such as IL-1 and TNF, has provided a strong theoretical rationale for the use of antiinflammatory agents in the therapy of bacterial meningitis. Several studies have demonstrated that dexamethasone, 0.15 mg/kg four times daily for 4 days, accelerates the normalization of CSF glucose, improves cerebral perfusion pressure, and reduces the incidence of hearing loss and other neurologic abnormalities in children with meningitis [92–96]. Shorter courses of dexamethasone may also be effective [97]. Initiation of dexamethasone therapy before the first antimicrobial dose has been recommended [96,97], and there seem to be no adverse effects of this approach for children ultimately shown to have aseptic meningitis [98].

The routine use of steroids in adults with bacterial meningitis remains controversial. One study from Egypt found a reduction in mortality and in subsequent hearing loss in patients of all ages with pneumococcal meningitis treated with dexamethasone, 8 to 12 mg IM every 12 hours for 3 days [99]. However, the antibiotic regimen used in that study, IM ampicillin plus chloramphenicol, would be considered suboptimal by U.S. standards, and many of the patients presented with coma (64%) and had symptoms for more than 2 days (87%), indicating more severe illness. A similar benefit might not be seen in the patient population typically seen in the United States. Dexamethasone therapy for meningitis has been associated with GI bleeding and secondary fever [92,97]. Older studies on steroid therapy for sepsis had shown a higher incidence of secondary infection or an increase in mortality attributed to secondary infections [100,101]. A prudent approach in adult patients would be to reserve steroid therapy for those patients with more severe illness, as indicated by markedly elevated CSF pressure or floridly positive Gram stain of CSF, especially if there is minimal CSF pleocytosis. If steroids are administered, dexamethasone is the preferred agent and should be begun as early as possible.

In animal models of bacterial meningitis beneficial effects on the CSF profile and development of cerebral edema have been seen with other agents directed at a variety of steps in the inflammatory cascade, including antibodies to bacterial cell wall or cytokines, cyclooxygenase inhibitors, inhibitors of leukocyte adhesion, and pentoxyfylline [102]. Some of these agents have reduced mortality in these experimental systems. However, there is little clinical information on the use of these agents in patients with meningitis, and their therapeutic value is not currently known.

Treatment of meningitis also requires attention to the problems of seizures and increased intracranial pressure as a result of cerebral edema. Seizures should be controlled by anticonvulsants as necessary (see Chap. 213), and aspiration and hypoxia must be prevented. Severe cerebral edema, with evidence of uncal or cerebellar herniation, may be managed with mannitol and steroids. To minimize cerebral edema, fluid intake should be carefully balanced with expected maintenance requirements. The traditional practice of routine fluid restriction may be counterproductive [103,104]. Nevertheless, excessive fluid administration may cause further elevation of intracerebral pressure, and hyponatremia secondary to SIADH may develop, and should be managed by fluid restriction. Systemic complications such as hypotension, disseminated intravascular coagulation (DIC), hypoxemia, or metastatic infection arising during the course of meningitis require additional therapeutic interventions.

Patients with CSF shunts or intracranial pressure monitoring devices who develop bacterial meningitis present additional considerations. Cure of infection is unlikely without removal of the device, having been achieved in only 3 of 10 patients in one randomized study [105]. Best results are obtained with complete removal of the shunt [27,105,106]. Hydrocephalus can be managed by temporary external drainage or periodic ventricular or spinal taps until a clinical response and sterilization of CSF is achieved, followed by reinsertion of a new shunt. Generally favorable results have also been obtained with immediate replacement of the shunt [27,105,106]. If removal and reinsertion will be difficult, a trial of nonoperative management may be given.

To prevent spread of infection, respiratory isolation until 24 hours after initiation of antibiotics is recommended for patients with meningococcal or *H. influenzae* meningitis. Household and day care contacts of patients with meningococcal disease and intimately exposed hospital personnel (e.g., those who have performed cardiopulmonary resuscitation (CPR), intubation, or suctioning) should receive chemoprophylaxis with rifampin, 10 mg per kilogram (maximum dose, 600 mg) PO bid for 2 days, or sulfisoxazole, 1 g (500 mg for children 1–12 years of age) PO bid for 2 days, if the organism is known to be sulfa sensitive [107]. Chemoprophylaxis with rifampin, 20 mg per kilogram (maximum dose, 600 mg) PO daily for 4 days, is recommended for household contacts of patients with *H. influenzae* disease only in families with children younger than 4 years of age [108]. The risk of secondary disease in day care contacts is probably lower than the risk in household contacts but may justify the use of chemoprophylaxis [109]. If two or more cases have occurred in the same day care group within 60 days, chemoprophylaxis is recommended. Of equal importance to chemoprophylaxis is the thorough evaluation of any contact who becomes ill, with the institution of antibiotic therapy if bacteremia seems likely [110]. Quadrivalent (serogroups A, C, Y, and W-135) meningococcal polysaccharide vaccine is recommended as an adjunct to chemoprophylaxis to prevent late secondary cases in contacts or to control outbreaks of disease [111].

Encephalitis

Encephalitis is a rarer infection than meningitis and a far less uniform one. Both actual viral replication in the CNS and an inflammatory response to systemic viral infection or immunization may produce the syndrome. Only autopsy or brain biopsy, with viral isolation attempts, can definitely distinguish between these two situations. Although important prognostic and epidemiologic information may derive from a specific diagnosis, the only forms of viral encephalitis for which specific treatment is currently available are those due to herpes simplex and varicella-zoster viruses. Infections of the brain that do not present as acute encephalitis but rather as subacute-to-chronic processes include subacute sclerosing panencephalitis caused by rubeola (measles) virus; the subacute spongiform encephalitides such as kuru and Creutzfeldt-Jakob disease; progressive multifocal leukoencephalopathy caused by JK papovavirus; and dementia caused by HIV, none of which are discussed further in this chapter. We also do not discuss important causes of encephalitis in the tropics, beyond mentioning that cerebral malaria (which may not give CSF abnormalities) and trypanosomiasis (acute Chagas' disease and African sleeping sickness) should be considered in travelers and recent immigrants from endemic areas.

ETIOLOGY. The causes of encephalitis endemic to the United States are predominantly viruses, although rickettsiae, *Mycoplasma pneumoniae*, spirochetes, amoebae, *L. monocytogenes*, and *Toxoplasma gondii* have all been associated with the syndrome. *T. gondii* encephalitis occurs only in patients with acquired immune deficiency syndrome (AIDS) or other conditions associated with cellular immunodeficiency (see Chap. 93). In contrast, the acute viral encephalitides exhibit no particular predilection for the immunosuppressed host. The relative frequency of various viruses in the cause of encephalitis is not well established. In recent years, pressure to diagnose herpes simplex because of the potential for therapy has led to its documentation more frequently than any other form [112,113]. However, most cases of encephalitis elude a causative diagnosis [112,114,115,116]. Table 87-2 lists the causes of encephalitis indigenous to the United States in general prognostic categories. Despite the favorable prognosis, encephalitis caused by organisms listed in group 1 may be extremely severe with prolonged unresponsiveness followed by gradual but eventually complete clearing.

PATHOGENESIS. Arboviruses are transmitted by the bite of their insect vector. The mosquito-borne infections have seasonal prevalence in late summer and early fall, and their prominence in any year depends on the climatic conditions affecting the vector [117,118]. In each case except the California group viruses, there is a bird reservoir from which mosquitoes carry the virus to humans and horses. Surveillance of bird populations and deaths of horses is used to track the localities at risk for human disease and to define the magnitude of the problem to guide mosquito control efforts [118]. The various arboviruses differ in their likelihood of producing overt disease and in the proportion of patients with nonspecific illness as opposed to

Table 87-2. Prognostic Categorization of Encephalitides Indigenous to the United States

1. Causes of encephalitis that tend to resolve spontaneously and rarely leave neurologic residua

	Comment
a. Epstein-Barr virus	
b. Enterovirus	
c. Mumps	
d. Lymphocytic choriomeningitis	
e. California encephalitis	Arbovirus
f. St. Louis encephalitis	Arbovirus
g. Colorado tick fever	Arbovirus
h. Herpes zoster	
i. Cat scratch disease	Especially acute cerebellar ataxia
j. *Mycoplasma pneumoniae*	Especially acute cerebellar ataxia
k. Rocky Mountain spotted fever	Contingent on recovery from the systemic illness
l. Leptospirosis	Contingent on recovery from the systemic illness

2. Causes of encephalitis that carry a small but definite risk of death and a sizable risk of sequelae

	Comment
a. Measles	
b. Powassan virus	Arbovirus
c. Western equine encephalitis	Arbovirus
d. Venezuelan equine encephalitis	Arbovirus
e. Smallpox vaccine	

3. Causes of encephalitis with a large risk of death; most survivors have significant residua

	Comment
a. Herpes simplex	
b. Eastern equine encephalitis	Arbovirus
c. Rabies	3 reported survivors

clinically manifest encephalitis, but they all attack young children particularly severely. Eastern equine encephalitis is the most virulent, causing death or severe neurologic sequelae in more than 60% of cases [119]. The prognosis in St. Louis encephalitis is worse in the older age group [120,121]. The insect vector inoculates the virus into the bloodstream, so viremia is the earliest event in pathogenesis. The organism replicates in reticuloendothelial tissues, where a secondary viremia arises and infects the CNS. By the time encephalitic symptoms develop, the virus has usually been cleared from the circulation and specific antibody is present, facilitating diagnosis [122].

Rabies virus, however, reaches the brain by spread up neural pathways from its site of inoculation, a process that may take a period of weeks to over a year. The saliva of infected animals contains the virus, which is usually introduced by a bite or salivary contamination of an open wound. Human-to-human transmission has occurred by corneal transplantation from donors with undiagnosed rabies [123,124]. Human-to-human transmission through saliva is feasible but has not been documented.

The pathogenesis of herpes simplex encephalitis (HSE) is not clear. The same virus causes this devastating infection and the common cold sore or fever blister. In the latter case the virus is thought to persist in the trigeminal ganglion and travel down the nerve route at the time of reactivation. Encephalitis may occur in patients with or without preexisting antibody [125] and may be caused by a virus identical to or different from that isolated from a typical lip lesion in the same patient [126]. The characteristic feature of HSE is its focal nature. It is an acute hemorrhagic necrotizing process with a predilection for the temporal lobe. A few cases resolve spontaneously, but without

antiviral therapy more than 70 percent progress to death with extensive brain destruction and cerebral edema [127,128].

DIAGNOSIS. The diagnostic process is directed primarily at determining the likelihood of HSE or a treatable nonviral cause of encephalitis.

History. The epidemiologic features reviewed in the section on pathogenesis are major contributors to the diagnosis. There are a few cases of rabies in which no apparent source can be determined, but often the appropriate history was not sought until the patient was unable to answer questions. One should always inquire about travel, which may widen the differential diagnosis beyond the considerations reviewed here.

Fever is nearly universal in encephalitis, and headache is also common. The presence of systemic complaints does not assist in the distinction between herpes simplex and other forms of viral encephalitis [129]. A neurologic presentation may occur, with seizures, mania, personality change, or other neuropsychiatric disorder as the first sign. Aphasia, or a disturbance of taste or smell, may favor a diagnosis of HSE [129,130]. The aversion to water, refusal to swallow, and delirious behavior from which the terms *hydrophobia* and *rabid* derive have not been present in some cases of rabies [131]. These have presented as coma with flaccid paralysis [132].

Physical Examination. The critical component of the physical examination, as with subsequent laboratory studies, is the attempt to determine whether an anatomic focus of abnormality is present, increasing the likelihood of HSE. Typical skin findings may suggest alternative diagnoses, such as Rocky Mountain spotted fever, measles, or herpes zoster.

Laboratory Tests. The spinal fluid usually has an aseptic character in encephalitis, with the exceptions already mentioned. It may be normal at the outset in 10 to 20 percent of patients subsequently proved to have HSE [129,133]. The presence of red cells may indicate a hemorrhagic type of encephalitis rather than a traumatic tap, so the count in the first and last tubes should be compared before disregarding this abnormality.

The neurodiagnostic procedures used in the effort to demonstrate focality are electroencephalography (EEG), technetium brain scan, and CT or MRI. In the largest series of patients with biopsy-proven HSE, a focal EEG abnormality was seen in 81 percent of patients, whereas technetium brain scan localization and CT scan localization were seen in 50 percent and 59 percent, respectively [129]. The specificity of EEG was substantially lower than brain scan or CT, however. Characteristic abnormalities may not be seen until late in the course. In one older series, four of six CT scans performed within 5 days of onset of HSE were normal [134]. MRI appears to be more sensitive than CT in demonstrating temporal lobe involvement [135]. Angiography is rarely used now but may be the procedure of choice when the differential diagnosis includes vasculitis or cerebral infarct in culture-negative endocarditis. No one procedure should be relied on to exclude a focus. EEG and CT scanning, which are widely available, are useful first-line studies. If the clinical suspicion is high and these studies fail to identify a focal abnormality, MRI or technetium brain scan should be performed. The initial studies should also be repeated after several days if a suspicion of HSE remains.

Serologic testing is unreliable for the diagnosis of HSE, because seropositivity to HSV at onset of disease is equally high (70%) in biopsy-proven and biopsy-negative cases, and false positive increases in antibody titer occur in 40 percent of seropositive biopsy-negative patients [125]. The situation is different for the arboviruses, because antibody is usually present at the onset of neurologic signs and sufficiently rare in the general population to permit presumptive diagnosis. Similarly, a single serum specimen may suffice to document primary Epstein-Barr virus infection, and a rare patient may even have a positive heterophil [136]. A distinctive preceding or accompanying illness, such as mumps or herpes zoster [137], may permit clinical diagnosis with fair certainty in a few cases, but in general the demonstration of a significant increase in antibody titer between acute and convalescent phase serum samples will be required. This is, of course, not useful for acute management of patients with encephalitis.

Other noninvasive diagnostic tests for HSE have been studied. The detection of antibodies to herpes simplex virus in CSF is specific but is insensitive during the first 7 days of illness [138]. Methods for PCR detection of HSV DNA in CSF have shown promise for the early and specific diagnosis of HSE [138], but these tests are not yet widely available.

The most reliable and definitive way to prove HSE is the demonstration of viral antigen or recovery of virus in brain tissue obtained at biopsy. This procedure can be performed safely by experienced neurosurgeons [139]. Few false negatives have been reported, and many of these appear related to biopsy at sites other than the affected one [139,140]. This may, of course, be appropriate in some cases, when the focus is in a critical neurologic region.

Given the relative safety and effectiveness of acyclovir therapy for HSE, considerable attention has been directed at the merits of empiric antiviral therapy without brain biopsy. The relative value of different management strategies depends on the likelihood of HSE and other treatable diseases, the risk of acyclovir therapy, and also on characteristics of the medical center, such as the skill of the neurosurgeons and pathologists and the availability of a viral diagnostic laboratory [141,142]. Most specialists recommend empiric acyclovir therapy when the likelihood of HSE is increased as demonstrated by focal findings on neurologic examination or neurodiagnostic testing. If no clinical response is seen after several days of acyclovir therapy, a biopsy should be performed to exclude other treatable lesions. Patients who have no focal findings on repeated examination and testing have a very low likelihood of HSE [142]. Empiric antiviral therapy is therefore unlikely to be of benefit. Little information is available on the yield of brain biopsy for treatable diseases in this patient group. If initial serologic tests fail to identify a cause, and repeated neurodiagnostic testing shows no focal lesion, brain biopsy should be considered.

The premortem noninvasive diagnosis of rabies is difficult. In one series, virus isolation from saliva or throat washings was the most sensitive test early in the disease [131]. Fluorescent antibody staining of a skin biopsy specimen from the nape of the neck [143] or a corneal impression [144,145] were less sensitive, but others have found skin biopsy to be very sensitive for rabies encephalitis [146]. The detection of antibody in serum or CSF of unvaccinated subjects is specific but insensitive early in disease [131].

T. gondii must be strongly suspected when multiple abscess-like areas are seen on CT scan of an immunosuppressed host, although solitary lesions also occur [147,148]. In patients with AIDS the presence of IgG to toxoplasma is sufficient indication to begin empiric therapy, and a presumptive diagnosis is made based on the therapeutic response [148]. Biopsy is reserved for those who fail to respond quickly.

DIFFERENTIAL DIAGNOSIS. A focal lesion appears to be a relatively sensitive but not very specific finding for HSE. Only

about one-half of focal abnormalities examined through biopsy for suspicion of HSE have yielded that diagnosis [149]. Nearly every other form of encephalitis as well as granulomatous meningitis and tumor have been found on such biopsy specimens. Treatable lesions were found in 16 percent of patients with brain biopsy specimens negative for HSE [149].

THERAPY. Treatment for most cases of encephalitis is supportive, with particular attention to the management of cerebral edema, hyponatremia due to SIADH, and seizures. Status epilepticus (see Chap. 186) without tonic-clonic activity, or seizures so frequent that the patient is in a postictal state when not convulsing, may lead to a false clinical assessment of the depth of coma and may produce additional neurologic damage as well. Intubation may frequently be necessary to prevent aspiration and to provide ventilatory assistance when respiratory drive is depressed because of either anticonvulsant medication or the disease itself. The risks of nosocomial infection, particularly pneumonia, are very high for patients with prolonged periods of unconsciousness.

Specific therapy is available for most nonviral causes of encephalitis. Early institution of chloramphenicol (50–75 mg/kg/d, maximum 4 g/d) or a tetracycline (e.g., doxycycline 100 mg bid) is associated with reduced mortality in Rocky Mountain spotted fever [150]. Therapy should be given for 6 to 10 days until the patient has been afebrile for at least 2 to 3 days [151]. Neurosyphilis should be treated with 10 days of high-dose penicillin G [152]. Meningoencephalitis caused by the Lyme disease spirochete can be treated with high-dose penicillin or with a third-generation cephalosporin (ceftriaxone or cefotaxime) for 14 to 21 days [153]. Treatment for toxoplasmic encephalitis consists of pyrimethamine plus either sulfadiazine or clindamycin [148].

Among the viral encephalitides, specific therapy is available only for herpes simplex and varicella-zoster infection. Acyclovir (10 mg/kg every 8 hours in adults) is the agent of choice for both diseases [128,154]. Vidarabine can reduce mortality in HSE, but is less effective than acyclovir [127,128,139,154]. The likelihood and quality of survival are strongly related to the neurologic condition of the patient at the time treatment is started and his or her age. Patients younger than 30 years who are only lethargic or semicomatose can be expected to have a good outcome with therapy [128,139]. Although herpes zoster–associated encephalitis is usually self-limited [137], it has been reported that patients improve more rapidly and have better outcome when treated with acyclovir [155,156].

Brain Abscess

ETIOLOGY AND PATHOGENESIS. Brain abscesses most commonly arise from chronic infections of the paranasal sinuses, middle ear, or mastoid [157–161]. Streptococci and anaerobes are the major organisms, with *Staphylococcus aureus* involved less frequently. Enteric gram-negative bacilli are commonly found in otogenic brain abscess [160]. Contiguous spread is also the mechanism of brain abscess after penetrating trauma or surgery, where staphylococci and gram-negative bacilli are important pathogens [158].

Metastatic hematogenous spread occurs in patients with cyanotic congenital heart disease and anaerobic pleuropulmonary infections as well as some normal hosts, with microaerophilic streptococci and anaerobes the likely organisms [160]. *S. aureus* endocarditis and nocardial infections are additional causes of hematogenous brain abscess.

Brain abscesses caused by fungi or mycobacteria are occasionally seen in immunosuppressed patients [16,73]. In patients infected with HIV, mass lesions are most often caused by *Toxoplasma gondii* [73,148].

DIAGNOSIS. Brain abscess usually presents more as a focal mass lesion—with headache, seizures, or neurologic deficit—than as an infectious disease [157,158]. Low-grade fever is present in approximately half of patients. Cranial CT scanning is important for diagnosis and localization of brain abscesses and is also useful for staging the disease and evaluating the underlying cause [162]. Magnetic resonance imaging has not demonstrated a clinical advantage over CT scanning but may provide better definition of brainstem lesions or extraparenchymal spread [163]. Abnormalities identified by either modality can also be seen with tumor and infarct [163,164].

THERAPY. Brain abscess is best treated with a combination of antibiotics and surgery. Initial antimicrobial therapy should be based on the likely pathogens as predicted by the probable underlying source. Penicillin plus either metronidazole or chloramphenicol has been a successful approach [157,158,160]. For otogenic brain abscesses, either cefotaxime or ceftriaxone should be added to cover aerobic gram-negative bacilli [158,160]. Antistaphylococcal therapy may also be required.

Prolonged antimicrobial therapy alone is curative in some patients, especially when the lesions are small (<2.5 cm) and do not have a well-defined capsule by CT criteria [165]. However, in the absence of a medical contraindication, most specialists would recommend prompt aspiration of the abscess contents using CT-guided stereotactic techniques [165,166]. This provides confirmation of the diagnosis and material for culture and may suffice for drainage. In patients with multiple abscesses, the largest lesions are usually aspirated. Total excision of the abscess capsule has been favored by some neurosurgeons [166]. The hospital stay and need for second surgical procedures is reduced by excision [165], but deep or multiple abscesses, abscesses in the early (cerebritis) stage, or abscesses in vital regions are poor candidates for this approach.

Parameningeal Foci

SUBDURAL EMPYEMA. Subdural empyema arises from the same foci as brain abscess and has the same microbiology, except in infancy when bacterial meningitis is the predominant cause [167–170]. The route of spread from sinus or mastoid infections is through venous drainage into intracranial vessels, which course through the subdural space. The clinical features of subdural empyema relate to local inflammation and cerebral edema, leading to increased ICP and herniation. Patients demonstrate depression of consciousness, hemiplegia, focal seizures, papilledema, and meningitic signs. MRI is the most sensitive diagnostic modality [171]; cranial CT is also useful, but occasional false negative scans occur [169]. Surgical decompression and drainage are urgent adjuncts to antibiotic therapy.

DURAL SINUS THROMBOPHLEBITIS. Major dural sinus occlusion caused by inflammation may occur in pyogenic meningitis but more often arises from spread of contiguous infection [172]. The site of origin may be sinusitis, mastoiditis, otitis, or cranial skin and soft tissue infection. The microbiology reflects

that of acute infection at these sites: *Staphylococcus aureus,* streptococci of all kinds, pneumococci, and anaerobes. Sagittal sinus thrombosis may result in seizures and hemiplegia, and its source is usually the meninges or the frontal sinuses. Cavernous sinus thrombosis presents with proptosis, marked chemosis, and ophthalmoplegia. Because of the connection between the two cavernous sinuses, the syndrome frequently becomes bilateral. One pathogenetic sequence is ethmoid (and often maxillary) sinusitis eroding the lamina papyracea to enter the orbit, with infection then spreading retrograde along ophthalmic veins. Direct extension can occur from sphenoid sinusitis. It may also arise from midface erysipelas or furuncle by direct spread through penetrating diploic veins. Sigmoid sinus thrombophlebitis may give no neurologic signs but produce persistent fever in a case of chronic otitis media and mastoiditis. Angiography has been the diagnostic procedure of choice, but CT and MRI often can demonstrate dural sinus thrombosis [173,174]. Antibiotics and drainage or excision of the focus from which the problem originates are the mainstays of therapy. The role of heparin and surgical attack on the dural sinus must be decided on the basis of their merits for each case.

SPINAL EPIDURAL ABSCESS. This infection may be a metastatic focus seeded during bacteremia or a complication of vertebral osteomyelitis or surgery [170,175–179]. More than half of the cases are caused by *Staphylococcus aureus.*

The classic description is a sequence of events from back pain to root pain, weakness, and then paralysis. Frank meningitic signs develop in up to one-third of cases [175,176,177], but the presence of percussion tenderness over the vertebral spinous processes should raise the suspicion of spinal epidural abscess. Early recognition of this entity is critical, because neurologic progression may be rapid, even if symptoms have been chronic, and patients may not recover from paralysis. MRI should be performed quickly to distinguish the nature and extent of spinal involvement to evaluate adjacent structures [177–181]. False negative scans have been reported [177,178], and if the suspicion of disease is high or MRI is unavailable, myelography with or without CT scanning should be performed quickly.

Immediate neurosurgical consultation is mandatory. Almost all patients should have prompt surgical intervention to prevent or relieve paraplegia. A nonoperative approach may be considered initially in patients with poor medical condition or if the neurologic condition is stable (without weakness or with paralysis of >3 days' duration) and a microbial cause is identified quickly from blood cultures or culture of aspirated material [182,183]. There is risk in this approach that neurologic progression may proceed rapidly even after several weeks of antimicrobial therapy [178], so MRI scanning and neurosurgical facilities must be available on an emergent basis. Antistaphylococcal antibiotics should be begun and the therapy adjusted after Gram stains and cultures of the material obtained at surgery. Therapy should be administered for 4 weeks unless vertebral osteomyelitis is also present, in which case it should be continued for 6 weeks or longer.

References

1. Swartz MN, Dodge PR: Bacterial meningitis: A review of selected aspects. I. General clinical features, special problems and unusual meningeal reactions mimicking bacterial meningitis. *N Engl J Med* 272:725, 1965.
2. Geiseler PJ, Nelson KE, Levin S, et al: Community-acquired puru-

lent meningitis: A review of 1316 cases during the antibiotic era, 1954–1976. *Rev Infect Dis* 2:725, 1980.

3. Schlech WF, Ward JI, Band JD, et al: Bacterial meningitis in the United States, 1978 through 1981: The national bacterial meningitis surveillance study. *JAMA* 253:1749, 1985.

4. Wenger JD, Hightower AW, Facklam RR, et al: Bacterial meningitis in the United States, 1986: Report of a multistate surveillance study. *J Infect Dis* 162:1316, 1990.

5. Carpenter RR, Petersdorf RG: The clinical spectrum of bacterial meningitis. *Am J Med* 33:262, 1962.

6. Adams WG, Deaver KA, Cochi SL, et al: Decline of childhood *Haemophilus influenzae* type B disease in the Hib vaccine era. *JAMA* 269:221, 1993.

7. Spagnuolo PJ, Ellner JJ, Lerner PI, et al: *Haemophilus influenzae* meningitis: The spectrum of disease in adults. *Medicine* 61:74, 1982.

8. Feigin RD, Baker CJ, Herwoldt LA, et al: Epidemic meningococcal disease in an elementary-school classroom. *N Engl J Med* 307:1255, 1982.

9. Hand WL, Sanford JP: Posttraumatic bacterial meningitis. *Ann Intern Med* 72:869, 1970.

10. Eraklis AJ, Kevy SV, Diamond LK, et al: Hazard of overwhelming infection after splenectomy in childhood. *N Engl J Med* 276:1225, 1967.

11. Zarrabi MH, Rosner F: Serious infections in adults following splenectomy for trauma. *Arch Intern Med* 144:1421, 1984.

12. Baccarani M, Fiacchini M, Galieni P, et al: Meningitis and septicaemia in adults splenectomized for Hodgkin's disease. *Scand J Haematol* 36:492, 1986.

13. Nieman RE, Lorber B: Listeriosis in adults: A changing pattern. Report of eight cases and review of the literature, 1968–1978. *Rev Infect Dis* 2:207, 1980.

14. Cherubin CE, Marr JS, Sierra MF, et al: Listeria and gram-negative bacillary meningitis in New York City, 1972–1979: Frequent causes of meningitis in adults. *Am J Med* 71:199, 1981.

15. Chernik NL, Armstrong D, Posner JB: Central nervous system infections in patients with cancer: Changing patterns. *Cancer* 40:268, 1977.

16. Hooper DC, Pruitt AA, Rubin RH: Central nervous system infection in the chronically immunosuppressed. *Medicine* 61:166, 1982.

17. Jurado RL, Farley MM, Pereira E, et al: Increased risk of meningitis and bacteremia due to *Listeria monocytogenes* in patients with human immunodeficiency virus infection. *Clin Infect Dis* 17:224, 1993.

18. Durand ML, Calderwood SB, Weber DJ, et al: Acute bacterial meningitis in adults: A review of 493 episodes. *N Engl J Med* 328:21, 1993.

19. Mangi RJ, Quintiliani R, Andriole VT: Gram-negative bacillary meningitis. *Am J Med* 59:829, 1975.

20. Gorse GJ, Thrupp LD, Nudleman KL, et al: Bacterial meningitis in the elderly. *Arch Intern Med* 144:1603, 1984.

21. Berk SL, McCabe WR: Meningitis caused by gram-negative bacilli. *Ann Intern Med* 93:253, 1980.

22. Gower DJ, Barrows AA, Kelly DL, et al: Gram-negative bacillary meningitis in the adult: Review of 39 cases. *South Med J* 79:1499, 1986.

23. Crane LR, Lerner AM: Non-traumatic gram-negative bacillary meningitis in the Detroit Medical Center, 1964–1974. *Medicine* 57:197, 1978.

24. Gordon JJ, Harter DH, Phair JP: Meningitis due to *Staphylococcus aureus*. *Am J Med* 78:965, 1985.

25. Schlesinger LS, Ross SC, Schaberg DR: *Staphylococcus aureus* meningitis: A broad-based epidemiologic study. *Medicine* 66:148, 1987.

26. Kim JH, Horst CVD, Mulrow CD, et al: *Staphylococcus aureus* meningitis: Review of 28 cases. *Rev Infect Dis* 11:698, 1989.

27. Walters BC, Hoffman HJ, Hendrick EB, et al: Cerebrospinal fluid shunt infection: Influences on initial management and subsequent outcome. *J Neurosurg* 60:1014, 1984.

28. Heerema MS, Ein ME, Musher DM, et al: Anaerobic bacterial meningitis. *Am J Med* 67:219, 1979.

29. Mayhall CG, Archer NH, Lamb VA, et al: Ventriculostomy-related infections: A prospective epidemiologic study. *N Engl J Med* 310:553, 1984.

30. Aucoin PJ, Rosen Kotilainen H, Gantz NM, et al: Intracranial pressure monitors: Epidemiologic study of risk factors and infections. *Am J Med* 80:369, 1986.

31. Pray LG: Lumbar puncture as a factor in the pathogenesis of meningitis. *Am J Dis Child* 62:295, 1941.

32. Eng RHK, Seligman SJ: Lumbar puncture-induced meningitis. *JAMA* 245:1456, 1981.

33. Teele DW, Dashefsky B, Rakusan T, et al: Meningitis after lumbar puncture in children with bacteremia. *N Engl J Med* 305:1079, 1981.

34. Tunkel AR, Wispelwey B, Scheld WM: Bacterial meningitis: Recent advances in pathophysiology and treatment. *Ann Intern Med* 112:610, 1990.

35. Lopez-Cortes LF, Cruz-Ruiz M, Gomez-Mateos J, et al: Measurement of levels of tumor necrosis factor-alpha and interleukin-1beta in the CSF of patients with meningitis of different etiologies: Utility in the differential diagnosis. *Clin Infect Dis* 16:534, 1993.

36. Mustafa MM, Lebel MH, Ramilo O, et al: Correlation of interleukin-1beta and cachectin concentrations in cerebrospinal fluid and outcome from bacterial meningitis. *J Pediatr* 115:208, 1989.

37. Arditi M, Ables L, Yogev R: Cerebrospinal fluid endotoxin levels in children with *H. influenzae* meningitis before and after administration of intravenous ceftriaxone. *J Infect Dis* 160:1005, 1989.

38. Ashwal S, Stringer W, Tomasi L, et al: Cerebral blood flow and carbon dioxide reactivity in children with bacterial meningitis. *J Pediatr* 117:523, 1990.

39. Dodge PR, Swartz MN: Bacterial meningitis: A review of selected aspects: II. Special neurologic problems, postmeningitic complications and clinicopathologic correlations. *N Engl J Med* 272:954, 1965.

40. Gilles F: Bacterial meningitis: A symposium. III. Morbid anatomical changes. *Pediatrics* 52:592, 1973.

41. Thomas VH, Hopkins IJ: Arteriographic demonstration of vascular lesions in the study of neurologic deficit in advanced *Haemophilus influenzae* meningitis. *Dev Med Child Neurol* 14:783, 1972.

42. Kabani A, Jadavji T: Sequelae of acute bacterial meningitis in children. *Antibiot Chemother* 45:209, 1992.

43. Taylor HG, Mills EL, Ciampi A, et al: The sequelae of *Haemophilus influenzae* meningitis in school-age children. *N Engl J Med* 323:1657, 1990.

44. Pomeroy SL, Holmes SJ, Dodge PR, et al: Seizures and other neurologic sequelae of bacterial meningitis in children. *N Engl J Med* 323:1651, 1990.

45. Annegers JF, Hauser WA, Beghi E, et al: The risk of unprovoked seizures after encephalitis and meningitis. *Neurology* 38:1407, 1988.

46. Feigin RD, Dodge PR: Bacterial meningitis: Newer concepts of pathophysiology and neurologic sequelae. *Pediatr Clin North Am* 23:541, 1976.

47. Marton KI, Gean AD: The spinal tap: A new look at an old test. *Ann Intern Med* 104:840, 1986.

48. Weiss W, Figueroa W, Shapiro WH, et al: Prognostic factors in pneumococcal meningitis. *Arch Intern Med* 120:517, 1967.

49. Karandanis D, Shulman JA: Recent survey of infectious meningitis in adults: Review of laboratory findings in bacterial, tuberculous, and aseptic meningitis. *South Med J* 69:449, 1976.

50. Bohr V, Rasmussen N, Hansen B, et al: 875 cases of bacterial meningitis: Diagnostic procedures and the impact of preadmission antibiotic therapy. Part III of a three-part series. *J Infect* 7:193, 1983.

51. Spanos A, Harrell FE, Durack DT: Differential diagnosis of acute meningitis. An analysis of the predictive value of initial observations. *JAMA* 262:2700, 1989.

52. Powers WJ: Cerebrospinal fluid lymphocytosis in acute bacterial meningitis. *Am J Med* 79:216, 1985.

53. Donald PR, Malan C, vanderWalt A: Simultaneous determination of cerebrospinal fluid glucose and blood glucose concentrations in the diagnosis of bacterial meningitis. *J Pediatr* 103:413, 1983.

54. Lindquist L, Linne T, Hansson LO, et al: Value of cerebrospinal fluid analysis in the differential diagnosis of meningitis: A study in 710 patients with suspected central nervous system infection. *Eur J Clin Microbiol Infect Dis* 7:374, 1988.

55. Powers WJ: Cerebrospinal fluid to serum glucose ratios in diabetes mellitus and bacterial meningitis. *Am J Med* 71:217, 1981.

56. Ringelmann R, Heym B, Kniehl E: Role of immunological tests in

diagnosis of bacterial meningitis. *Antibiot Chemother* 45:68, 1992.

57. Tilton RC, Dias F, Ryan RW: Comparative evaluation of three commercial products and counterimmunoelectrophoresis for the detection of antigens in cerebrospinal fluid. *J Clin Microbiol* 20:231, 1984.

58. Ni H, Knight AI, Cartwright K, et al: Polymerase chain reaction for diagnosis of meningococcal meningitis. *Lancet* 340:1432, 1992.

59. Swenson JM, Hill BC, Thornsberry C: Screening pneumococci for penicillin resistance. *J Clin Microbiol* 24:749, 1986.

60. Saez-Nieto JA, Lujan R, Berron S, et al: Epidemiology and molecular basis of penicillin-resistant *Neisseria meningitidis* in Spain: A 5-year history (1985–1989). *Clin Infect Dis* 14:394, 1992.

61. Varki AP, Puthuran P: Value of second lumbar puncture in confirming a diagnosis of aseptic meningitis: A prospective study. *Arch Neurol* 36:581, 1979.

62. Rotbart HA: Diagnosis of enteroviral meningitis with the polymerase chain reaction. *J Pediatr* 117:85, 1990.

63. Lincoln EM, Sordillo SVR, Davies PA: Tuberculous meningitis in children: A review of 167 untreated and 74 treated patients with special reference to early diagnosis. *J Pediatr* 57:807, 1960.

64. Kennedy DH, Fallon RJ: Tuberculous meningitis. *JAMA* 241:264, 1979.

65. Klein NC, Camsker B, Hirschman SZ: Mycobacterial meningitis: Retrospective analysis from 1970 to 1983. *Am J Med* 79:29, 1985.

66. Berenguer J, Moreno S, Laguna F, et al: Tuberculous meningitis in patients infected with the human immunodeficiency virus. *N Engl J Med* 326:668, 1992.

67. Shankar P, Manjunath N, Mohan KK, et al: Rapid diagnosis of tuberculous meningitis by polymerase chain reaction. *Lancet* 337:5, 1991.

68. Joffe AM, Farley JD, Linden D, et al: Trimethoprim-sulfamethoxazole-associated aseptic meningitis: Case reports and review of the literature. *Am J Med* 87:332, 1989.

69. Pruitt AA, Rubin RH, Karchmer AW, et al: Neurologic complications of bacterial endocarditis. *Medicine* 57:329, 1978.

70. Levy RM, Bredesen DE, Rosenblum ML: Neurological manifestations of the acquired immunodeficiency syndrome (AIDS): Experience at UCSF and review of the literature. *J Neurosurg* 62:475, 1985.

71. Kovacs JA, Kovacs AA, Polis M, et al: Cryptococcosis in the acquired immunodeficiency syndrome. *Ann Intern Med* 103:533, 1985.

72. Lewis JL, Rabinovich S: The wide spectrum of cryptococcal infections. *Am J Med* 53:315, 1972.

73. McArthur JC: Neurologic manifestations of AIDS. *Medicine* 66:407, 1987.

74. Appelbaum PC: Antimicrobial resistance in *Streptococcus pneumoniae*: An overview. *Clin Infect Dis* 15:77, 1992.

75. Spika JS, Facklam RR, Plikaytis BD, et al: Antimicrobial resistance of *Streptococcus pneumoniae* in the United States, 1979–1987. *J Infect Dis* 163:1273, 1991.

76. Thornsberry C, Marler JK, Rich TJ: Increased penicillin resistance in recent U.S. isolates of *Streptococcus pneumoniae*. *Abstracts of the 92nd general meeting of the American Society for Microbiology* (C-268), 1992, p. 465.

77. Barnett ED, Pelton SI, Bolduc G, et al: Antimicrobial resistance of respiratory isolates of *Streptococcus pneumoniae* in pediatric patients in Boston. *Abstracts of the 33rd Interscience Conference on Antimicrobial Agents and Chemotherapy* (#1045), 1993, p. 310.

78. Block S, Hedrick J, Harrison C, et al: Penicillin-resistant *S. pneumoniae* In acute otitis media: *In vitro* study of alternative antimicrobials. *Abstracts of the 33rd Interscience Conference on Antimicrobial Agents and Chemotherapy* (#1046), 1993, p. 311.

79. Duchin J, Diamond A, Block S, et al: Community-wide spread of drug-resistant *Streptococcus pneumoniae* among children in rural Kentucky. *Abstracts of the 33rd Interscience Conference on Antimicrobial Agents and Chemotherapy* (#1183), 1993, p. 336.

80. Viladrich PF, Gudiol F, Linares J, et al: Characteristics and antibiotic therapy of adult meningitis due to penicillin-resistant pneumococci. *Am J Med* 84:839-846, 1988.

81. Jacobs MR: Treatment and diagnosis of infections caused by drug-resistant *Streptococcus pneumoniae*. *Clin Infect Dis* 15:119, 1992.

82. Levitz RE, Quintiliani R: Trimethoprim-sulfamethoxazole for bacterial meningitis. *Ann Intern Med* 100:881, 1984.

83. Lepper NH, Dowling HF: Treatment of pneumococcic meningitis with penicillin compared with penicillin plus aureomycin: Studies including observations on apparent antagonism between penicillin and aureomycin. *Arch Intern Med* 88:489, 1951.

84. Wehrle PF, Mathies AW, Leedom JM, et al: Bacterial meningitis. *Ann NY Acad Sci* 145:488, 1967.

85. Lindberg J, Rosenthall U, Nylen O, et al: Long term outcome of *Haemophilus influenzae* meningitis related to antibiotic treatment. *Pediatrics* 60:1, 1977.

86. Eng RHK, Munsif AN, Yangco BG, et al: Seizure propensity with imipenem. *Arch Intern Med* 149:1881, 1989.

87. Radetsky M: Duration of treatment in bacterial meningitis: A historical inquiry. *Pediatr Infect Dis J* 9:2, 1990.

88. Peltola H, Antilla M, Renkonen OV, et al: Randomised comparison of chloramphenicol, ampicillin, cefotaxime, and ceftriaxone for childhood bacterial meningitis. *Lancet* 1:1281, 1989.

89. Jadavji T, Biggar WD, Gold R, et al: Sequelae of acute bacterial meningitis treated for seven days. *Pediatrics* 78:21, 1986.

90. Chartrand SA, Cho CT: Persistent pleocytosis in bacterial meningitis. *J Pediatr* 88:424, 1976.

91. Durack DT, Spanos A: End-of-treatment spinal tap in bacterial meningitis: Is it worthwhile? *JAMA* 248:75, 1982.

92. Lebel MH, Freij BJ, Syrogiannopoulos GA, et al: Dexamethasone therapy for bacterial meningitis: Results of two double-blind, placebo-controlled trials. *N Engl J Med* 319:964, 1988.

93. Lebel MH, Hoyt MJ, Waagner DC, et al: Magnetic resonance imaging and dexamethasone therapy for bacterial meningitis. *Am J Dis Child* 143:301, 1989.

94. Havens PL, Wendelberger KJ, Hoffman GM, et al: Corticosteroids as adjunctive therapy in bacterial meningitis: A meta-analysis of clinical trials. *Am J Dis Child* 143:1051, 1989.

95. Kennedy WA, Hoyt MJ, McCracken GH: The role of corticosteroid therapy in children with pneumococcal meningitis. *Am J Dis Child* 145:1374, 1991.

96. Odio CM, Faingezicht I, Paris M, et al: The beneficial effects of early dexamethasone administration in infants and children with bacterial meningitis. *N Engl J Med* 324:1525, 1991.

97. Schaad UB, Lips U, Gnehm HE, et al: Dexamethasone therapy for bacterial meningitis in children. *Lancet* 342:457, 1993.

98. Waagner DC, Kennedy WA, Hoyt MJ, et al: Lack of adverse effects of dexamethasone therapy in aseptic meningitis. *Pediatr Infect Dis J* 9:922, 1990.

99. Girgis NI, Farid Z, Mikhail IA, et al: Dexamethasone treatment for bacterial meningitis in children and adults. *Pediatr Infect Dis J* 8:848, 1989.

100. Sprung CL, Caralis PV, Marcial EH, et al: The effects of high-dose corticosteroids in patients with septic shock: A prospective, controlled study. *N Engl J Med* 311:1137, 1984.

101. Bone RC, Fisher CJ, Clemmer TP, et al: A controlled clinical trial of high-dose methylprednisolone in the treatment of severe sepsis and septic shock. *N Engl J Med* 317:653, 1987.

102. Tuomanen E: Adjunctive therapy of experimental meningitis: Agents other than steroids. *Antibiot Chemother* 45:184, 1992.

103. Tureen JH, Tauber MG, Sande MA: Effect of hydration status on cerebral blood flow and cerebrospinal fluid lactic acidosis in rabbits with experimental meningitis. *J Clin Invest* 89:947, 1992.

104. Powell KR, Sugarman LI, Eskenazi AE, et al: Normalization of plasma arginine vasopressin concentrations when children with meningitis are given maintenance plus replacement fluid therapy. *J Pediatr* 117:515, 1990.

105. James HE, Walsh JW, Wilson HD, et al: Prospective randomized study of therapy in cerebrospinal fluid shunt infection. *Neurosurgery* 7:459, 1980.

106. Forward KR, Fewer HD, Stiver HG: Cerebrospinal fluid shunt infections: A review of 35 infections in 32 patients. *J Neurosurg* 59:389, 1983.

107. *Report of the Committee on Infectious Diseases.* 22nd ed. Elk Grove Village, IL, American Academy of Pediatrics, 1991, p 325.

108. *Report of the Committee on Infectious Diseases.* 22nd ed. Elk Grove Village, IL, 1991, p 224.

109. Broome CV, Mortimer EA, Katz SL, et al: Use of chemoprophylaxis

to prevent the spread of *Hemophilus influenzae* B in day-care facilities. *N Engl J Med* 316:1226, 1987.

110. Artenstein MS: Prophylaxis for meningococcal disease. *JAMA* 231:1035, 1975.

111. Lepow ML, Gold R: Meningococcal A and other polysaccharide vaccines: A five-year progress report. *N Engl J Med* 308:1158, 1983.

112. Koskiniemi M, Manninen V, Vaheri A, et al: Acute encephalitis: A survey of epidemiological, clinical and microbiological features covering a twelve-year period. *Acta Med Scand* 209:115, 1981.

113. Koskiniemi MJ, Vaheri A: Acute encephalitis of viral origin. *Scand J Infect Dis* 14:181, 1982.

114. Centers for Disease Control: Encephalitis surveillance. Annual Summary 1978. U.S. Department of Health and Human Services, Public Health Service, 1981.

115. Beghi E, Nicolosi A, Kurland LT, et al: Encephalitis and aseptic meningitis, Olmstead County, Minnesota, 1950–1981: I. Epidemiology. *Ann Neurol* 16:283, 1984.

116. Koskiniemi M, Rautonen J, Lehtokoski-Lehtiniemi E, et al: Epidemiology of encephalitis in children: A 20-year survey. *Ann Neurol* 29:492, 1991.

117. Grady GF, Maxfield HK, Hildreth SW: Eastern equine encephalitis in Massachusetts, 1957–1976: A prospective study centered upon analyses of mosquitoes. *Am J Epidemiol* 107:170, 1978.

118. Centers for Disease Control: Arboviral surveillance—United States, 1990. *MMWR* 39:593, 1990.

119. Przelomski MM, O'Rourke E, Grady GF, et al: Eastern equine encephalitis in Massachusetts: A report of 16 cases, 1970–1984. *Neurology* 38:736, 1988.

120. Powell KE, Kappus KD: Epidemiology of St. Louis encephalitis and other acute encephalitides. *Adv Neurol* 19:197, 1978.

121. Tsai TF, Canfield MA, Reed CM, et al: Epidemiological aspects of a St. Louis encephalitis outbreak in Harris County, Texas, 1986. *J Infect Dis* 157:351, 1988.

122. Johnson RT, Mims CA: Pathogenesis of viral infections of the nervous system. *N Engl J Med* 278:23, 1968.

123. Houff SA, Burton RC, Wilson RW, et al: Human to human transmission of rabies virus by a corneal transplant. *N Engl J Med* 300:603, 1979.

124. Centers for Disease Control: Human to human transmission of rabies via a corneal transplant—France. *MMWR* 29:25, 1980.

125. Nahmias AJ, Whitley RJ, Visintine AN, et al: Herpes simplex virus encephalitis: Laboratory evaluations and their diagnostic significance. *J Infect Dis* 145:829, 1982.

126. Whitley R, Lakeman AD, Nahmias AJ, et al: DNA restriction-enzyme analysis of herpes simplex virus isolates obtained from patients with encephalitis. *N Engl J Med* 307:1060, 1982.

127. Whitley RJ, Soong SJ, Dolin R, et al: Adenine arabinoside therapy of biopsy-proved herpes simplex encephalitis. *N Engl J Med* 297:289, 1977.

128. Whitley RJ, Alford CA, Hirsch MS, et al: Vidarabine versus acyclovir therapy in herpes simplex encephalitis. *N Engl J Med* 314:144, 1986.

129. Whitley RJ, Soong SJ, Linneman C Jr, et al: Herpes simplex encephalitis: Clinical assessment. *JAMA* 247:317, 1982.

130. Drachman DA, Adams RD: Herpes simplex and acute inclusion-body encephalitis. *Arch Neurol* 7:45, 1962.

131. Anderson LJ, Nicholson KG, Tauxe RV, et al: Human rabies in the United States, 1960 to 1979: Epidemiology, diagnosis, and prevention. *Ann Intern Med* 100:728, 1984.

132. Chopra JS, Banerjee AK, Murthy MK, et al: Paralytic rabies: A clinico-pathological study. *Brain* 103:789, 1980.

133. Koskiniemi M, Vaheri A, Taskinen E: Cerebrospinal fluid alterations in herpes simplex virus encephalitis. *Rev Infect Dis* 6:608, 1984.

134. Davis JM, Davis KR, Kleinman GM, et al: Computed tomography of herpes simplex encephalitis, with clinicopathological correlation. *Radiology* 129:409, 1978.

135. Neils EW, Lukin R, Tomsick TA, et al: Magnetic resonance imaging and computerized tomography scanning of herpes simplex encephalitis: Report of two cases. *J Neurosurg* 67:592, 1987.

136. Grose C, Henle W, Henle G, et al: Primary Epstein-Barr virus infections in acute neurologic diseases. *N Engl J Med* 292:392, 1975.

137. Jemsek J, Greenberg SB, Taber L, et al: Herpes zoster-associated encephalitis: Clinicopathologic report of 12 cases and review of the literature. *Medicine* 62:81, 1983.

138. Aurelius E, Johansson B, Skoldenberg B, et al: Rapid diagnosis of herpes simplex encephalitis by nested polymerase chain reaction assay of cerebrospinal fluid. *Lancet* 337:189, 1991.

139. Whitley RJ, Soong SJ, Hirsch MS, et al: Herpes simplex encephalitis: Vidarabine therapy and diagnostic problems. *N Engl J Med* 304:313, 1981.

140. Landry ML, Booss J, Hsiung GD: Duration of vidarabine therapy in biopsy-negative herpes simplex encephalitis. *JAMA* 247:332, 1982.

141. Barza M, Pauker SG: The decision to biopsy, treat, or wait in suspected herpes encephalitis. *Ann Intern Med* 92:641, 1980.

142. Soong SJ, Watson NE, Caddell GR, et al: Use of brain biopsy for diagnostic evaluation of patients with suspected herpes simplex encephalitis: A statistical model and its clinical implications. *J Infect Dis* 163:17, 1991.

143. Blenden DC, Creech W, Torres-Anjel MJ: Use of immunofluorescence examination to detect rabies virus antigen in the skin of humans with clinical encephalitis. *J Infect Dis* 154:698, 1986.

144. Schneider LG: The cornea test: A new method for the intra-vitam diagnosis of rabies. *Zentralbl Veterinarmed* [B] 16:24, 1969.

145. Cifuentes E, Calderon E, Bijlenga G: Rabies in a child diagnosed by a new intra-vitam method: The cornea test. *J Trop Med Hyg* 74:23, 1971.

146. Warrell MJ, Looareesuwan S, Manatsathit S, et al: Rapid diagnosis of rabies and post-vaccinal encephalitides. *Clin Exp Immunol* 71:229, 1988.

147. Townsend JJ, Wolinsky JJ, Baringer JR, et al: Acquired toxoplasmosis, a neglected cause of treatable central nervous system disease. *Arch Neurol* 32:335, 1975.

148. Luft BJ, Remington JS: Toxoplasmic encephalitis in AIDS. *Clin Infect Dis* 15:211, 1992.

149. Whitley RJ, Cobbs CG, Alford CA, et al: Diseases that mimic herpes simplex encephalitis: Diagnosis, presentation, and outcome. *JAMA* 262:234, 1989.

150. Helmick CG, Bernard KW, D'Angelo LJ: Rocky mountain spotted fever: Clinical, laboratory, and epidemiological features of 262 cases. *J Infect Dis* 150:480, 1984.

151. *Report of the Committee on Infectious Diseases*. 22nd ed. Elk Grove Village, IL, 1991, p 407.

152. Hook EW: Treatment of syphilis: Current recommendations, alternatives, and continuing problems. *Rev Infect Dis* 11:S1511, 1989.

153. Steere AC: Lyme disease. *N Engl J Med* 321:586, 1989.

154. Skoldenberg B, Forsgren M, Alestig K, et al: Acyclovir versus vidarabine in herpes simplex encephalitis: Randomised multicentre study in consecutive Swedish patients. *Lancet* 2:707, 1984.

155. Johns DR, Gress DR: Rapid response to acyclovir in herpes zoster-associated encephalitis. *Am J Med* 82:560, 1987.

156. Peterslund NA: Herpes zoster associated encephalitis: Clinical findings and acyclovir treatment. *Scand J Infect Dis* 20:583, 1988.

157. Nielsen H, Gyldensted C, Harmsen A: Cerebral abscess: Aetiology and pathogenesis, symptoms, diagnosis, and treatment: A review of 200 cases from 1935–1976. *Acta Neurol Scand* 65:609, 1982.

158. Chun CH, Johnson JD, Hofstetter M, et al: Brain abscess: A study of 45 consecutive cases. *Medicine* 65:415, 1986.

159. Nicolosi A, Hauser WA, Musicco M, et al: Incidence and prognosis of brain abscess in a defined population: Olmsted County, Minnesota, 1935–1981. *Neuroepidemiology* 10:122, 1991.

160. Richards J, Sisson PR, Hickman JE, et al: Microbiology, chemotherapy, and mortality of brain abscess in Newcastle-upon-Tyne between 1979 and 1988. *Scand J Infect Dis* 22:511, 1990.

161. Seydoux C, Francioli P: Bacterial brain abscesses: Factors influencing mortality and sequelae. *Clin Infect Dis* 15:394, 1992.

162. Britt RH, Enzmann DR: Clinical stages of human brain abscesses on serial CT scans after contrast infusion. Computerized tomographic, neuropathological, and clinical correlations. *J Neurosurg* 59:972, 1983.

163. Haimes AB, Zimmerman RD, Morgello S, et al: MR imaging of brain abscesses. *AJR* 152:1073, 1989.

164. New PFJ, Davis KR: The role of CT scanning in diagnosis of infections of the central nervous system, in Remington JS, Swartz MN

(eds): *Current Clinical Topics in Infectious Diseases*. New York, McGraw-Hill, 1980, vol 1, p 1.

165. Mampalam TJ, Rosenblum ML: Trends in the management of bacterial brain abscesses: A review of 102 cases over 17 years. *Neurosurgery* 23:451, 1988.

166. Stephanov S: Surgical treatment of brain abscess. *Neurosurgery* 22:724, 1988.

167. Farmer TW, Wise GR: Subdural empyema in infants, children and adults. *Neurology* 23:254, 1973.

168. Miller ES, Dias PS, Uttley D: Management of subdural empyema: A series of 24 cases. *J Neurol Neurosurg Psychiatry* 50:1415, 1987.

169. Feuerman T, Wackym PA, Gade GF, et al: Craniotomy improves outcome in subdural empyema. *Surg Neurol* 32:105, 1989.

170. Krauss WE, McCormack PC: Infections of the dural spaces. *Neurosurg Clin North Am* 3:421, 1992.

171. Weingarten K, Zimmerman RD, Becker RD, et al: Subdural and epidural empyemas: MR imaging. *AJR* 152:615, 1989.

172. Southwick FS, Richardson EP, Swartz MN: Septic thrombosis of the dural venous sinuses. *Medicine* 65:82, 1986.

173. Goldberg AL, Rosenbaum AE, Wang H, et al: Computed tomography of dural sinus thrombosis. *J Comput Assist Tomogr* 10:16, 1986.

174. Macchi PJ, Grossman RI, Gomori JM, et al: High field MR imaging of cerebral venous thrombosis. *J Comput Assist Tomogr* 10:10, 1986.

175. Baker AS, Ojemann RG, Swartz MN, et al: Spinal epidural abscess. *N Engl J Med* 293:463, 1975.

176. Curling OD, Gower DJ, McWhorter JM: Changing concepts in spinal epidural abscess: A report of 29 cases. *Neurosurgery* 27:185, 1990.

177. Darouiche RO, Hamill RJ, Greenberg SB, et al: Bacterial spinal epidural abscess: Review of 43 cases and literature survey. *Medicine* 71:369, 1992.

178. Hlavin ML, Kaminski HJ, Ross JS, et al: Spinal epidural abscess: A ten-year perspective. *Neurosurgery* 27:177, 1990.

179. Nussbaum ES, Rigamonti D, Standiford H, et al: Spinal epidural abscess: A report of 40 cases and review. *Surg Neurol* 38:225, 1992.

180. Post MJD, Quencer RM, Montalvo BM, et al: Spinal infection: Evaluation with MR imaging and intraoperative US. *Radiology* 169:765, 1988.

181. Sandhu FS, Dillon WP: Spinal epidural abscess: Evaluation with contrast-enhanced MR imaging. *AJNR* 12:1087, 1991.

182. Leys D, Lesoin F, Viaud C, et al: Decreased morbidity from acute bacterial spinal epidural abscesses using computed tomography and nonsurgical treatment in selected patients. *Ann Neurol* 17:350, 1985.

183. Hanigan WC, Asner NG, Elwood PW: Magnetic resonance imaging and the nonoperative treatment of spinal epidural abscess. *Surg Neurol* 34:408, 1990.

88. Infective Endocarditis

Sarah H. Cheeseman and Karen Carroll

Overview

Infective endocarditis is infection of the endothelial lining of the heart, characterized pathologically by vegetations. The infected site is usually a valve, but endocarditis may be situated on mural thrombi (rare) or the endothelial surface on which the jet stream from a stenotic lesion (patent ductus, ventricular septal defect, or stenotic valve) impinges. With a slight extension of this concept the term encompasses infection of the endothelial surface of any blood vessel, which most frequently occurs on hemodynamically or structurally abnormal ones such as abdominal aortic aneurysms, arteriovenous fistulas (either natural or created to provide access for hemodialysis), and prosthetic grafts. The peculiarities of these infections are beyond the scope of this chapter, but the general principles of diagnosis and treatment are the same.

Infective endocarditis has challenged physicians diagnostically and therapeutically for many years. In the preantibiotic era, the challenge was predominantly therapeutic. The diagnosis became abundantly clear as a symptom complex of fever, changing murmurs, characteristic skin lesions, anemia, splenomegaly, and major organ emboli evolved over time and progressed relentlessly to death. Today, it has become possible to cure many patients, although not all, and the pressure for early recognition and institution of therapy, which clearly correlate with improved prognosis, is therefore greater. The therapeutic modalities that have improved the outcome are long-term, high-dose antibiotics and, in selected cases, cardiac surgery. These interventions are not without risk, so accuracy in diagnosis is critical. A new dilemma has now arisen, particularly keen in coronary and intensive care unit patients. Which patients with bacteremia actually have endocarditis? This question is particularly difficult in patients with prosthetic valves, intravascular foreign bodies, and staphylococcal or enterococcal bacteremia.

Table 88-1 reviews the mortality rate of endocarditis over time and points out that therapy for this infection is still not wholly satisfactory [1–9]. The introduction of penicillin abruptly decreased the hitherto inevitable fatality of the disease. From the late 1940s up to 1970, reported mortality ranged from 25 to 60 percent of treated patients. This plateau over nearly 30 years appears to represent a stalemate between our improving antibiotic armamentarium and increasingly difficult-to-treat organisms and hosts. Possible progress in the past decade [7,9] may relate to the use of cardiac surgery as a mode of treatment.

Review of experience at a number of centers suggests that the decline in mortality has occurred predominantly among young patients. Mortality remains high in the elderly, diabetics, and patients with other predisposing underlying diseases [9–12] as well as in those infected with staphylococci [11,12].

Traditionally two clinical forms of endocarditis have been delineated, and a high proportion of all cases can still be placed in one of the two categories: acute and subacute. Subacute disease denotes a form, often of insidious onset, with slow development of the characteristic lesions and absence of marked toxicity for a long period. A high proportion of these cases occur on valves previously damaged by either congenital, rheumatic, or degenerative cardiovascular disease, and many are caused by organisms of relatively low virulence, such as alpha-hemolytic streptococci (viridans streptococci). In contrast, acute bacterial endocarditis presents as a fulminant infection, with abrupt onset, high fever, more frequent leukocytosis, and rapid downhill course with respect to both valve destruction and systemic toxicity. This is most frequently secondary to

Table 88-1. Mortality of Endocarditis Over 50 Years

Series [reference]	Overall Mortality %	Comments	
University of Iowa [1]			
1924–1939	100		
1940–1944	96.5	SBE only	
1944–1949	25.5	Sulfa	
1950–1963[a]		Penicillin	
Massachusetts General Hospital [2]		*ABE*	*SBE*
1944–1958	40.4	85	32
1958–1964	29	60	13
New England Medical Center [3]			
1956–1964	25		10[b]
University of Washington [4]			
1963–1972	36.8		
Columbia-Presbyterian [5]			
1968–1973	32.5		
Collaborative Study [6]			
1972	25.5		
Beth Israel Hospital [7]			
1970–1977	15		
Mayo Clinic [8]			
1950–1959[c]	60		
1960–1969	33		
1970–1981	32		
Louisiana Statewide Prospective Study [9]			
1985–1986	12		

[a] Mortality of treated cases only.
[b] Mortality for cases of SBE treated within 2 weeks of onset.
[c] Mortality in first 60 days.
ABE = acute bacterial endocarditis; SBE = subacute bacterial endocarditis.

Staphylococcus aureus and may occur on previously normal valves.

The value of the clinical differentiation into these two types does not rest predominantly on prediction of cause. Rather, the clinical grouping has great importance in predicting the pace of the disease and hence the haste to institute therapy. In the subacute form of endocarditis, the slower rate of progression of the disease permits careful and vigorous culturing for a few days before institution of antimicrobial therapy. In the acute form, valvular destruction may proceed so rapidly that appropriate antibiotics must be begun urgently, even at the cost of excess toxicity engendered by the use of multiple drug combinations and before the causative agent is isolated. In recent series of endocarditis, the acute form of the infection has come to predominate [2,3,4], and among patients who require intensive care, this certainly will be the more frequent problem.

All observers of infective endocarditis have noted a decrease in the frequency of rheumatic heart disease as a predisposing lesion and an increase in degenerative disease [5,13]. Infants younger than age 2 very rarely have endocarditis, nor do children of any age in the absence of preexisting heart disease [3,14]. Those with congenital heart disease are distinctly at risk for endocarditis [5,6,14] and are more often surviving into adulthood as a result of cardiac surgery. Taking these trends together, the universal observation of an increasing proportion of cases in older age-groups is not surprising. Less explicable is the predilection of the disease for men, who account for two to three times as many cases as women [1,3,5,13]. Women predominate only in the subgroup with isolated mitral valve involvement [1,4,13].

Other populations particularly at risk for endocarditis are

intravenous drug addicts, who respond unusually well to therapy, and patients with prosthetic valves. Prosthetic valve endocarditis is usually subdivided into "early" (<60 days after implantation) and "late" varieties, with the former having a particularly bleak prognosis. Problems in endocarditis particularly relevant to patients in cardiac or intensive care units include

1. Acute bacterial endocarditis
2. Prosthetic valve endocarditis
3. The diagnosis of endocarditis in patients with intravascular foreign bodies, such as pacemakers and indwelling catheters (Broviac and Hickman lines)
4. Indications for surgery in endocarditis

Etiology

The term *infective endocarditis*, rather than the more commonly used term *bacterial endocarditis*, properly includes the whole world of microorganisms that can cause the disease. Fungi, rickettsiae (*Coxiella burnetii*, which causes Q fever), chlamydia, and perhaps even viruses have been implicated in endocarditis [13,15], although bacteria are still the predominant cause. Osler's description of "malignant endocarditis" mentioned staphylococci, streptococci (particularly beta-hemolytic, if we are to judge by his association of endocarditis with erysipelas), the pneumococcus, and the gonococcus as causative organisms [16]. These organisms, the same ones noted at Boston City Hospital in 1933 to 1935 [17], suggest a large proportion of cases of the acute type, because *Streptococcus viridans* is recorded as the cause of nearly all cases of subacute bacterial endocarditis in that era [1].

Table 88-2 presents trends in the bacterial etiology of endocarditis compiled from a number of series [1–7,17–20]. Note that since 1950, one third to one half of all cases are still caused by viridans streptococci (non–beta-hemolytic, nonenterococcal; thus, microaerophilic, anaerobic, or nonhemolytic). With improved microbiologic techniques, it is now possible to identify to species level the viridans group of organisms. The taxonomy still requires standardization; nevertheless, some investigators believe that species identification may have important therapeutic and prognostic implications. For example, *Streptococcus milleri* tends to cause more severe infection with a higher incidence of suppurative extracardiac complications, such as septic arthritis, splenic abscess, and disseminated intravascular coagulation [21,22]. Nutritionally deficient streptococci constitute 5 to 6 percent of cases of endocarditis caused by viridans streptococci [23,24]. These organisms require pyridoxal, the active form of vitamin B_6, for growth and were probably responsible for a significant proportion of culture-negative cases of endocarditis in the 1950s and 1960s. Unlike other species of viridans streptococci, these organisms are tolerant to penicillin and thus are associated with a high relapse rate [23]. Most cases of viridans streptococcal endocarditis (80%) are caused by *S. sanguis*, *S. mitis*, and *S. mutans*, which are associated with dental plaque [25]. There do not appear to be any statistically significant differences in the symptoms, demographics, or complications among patients with infections caused by this group of organisms [21].

Among the non–viridans streptococci, pneumococci are still relatively uncommon causes of endocarditis, and enterococci continue to rank third after staphylococci. Although the proportion of cases caused by beta-hemolytic streptococci has not increased since 1950, it appears that infections with group G and group B are being seen more frequently [26,27,28]. Patients

Table 88-2. Etiology of Endocarditis in the Past 60 Years[a]

Cause	1930–1950			1950–1965			1965–1980			1980 +		
	[1]	[17]	[18][b]	[1]	[2]	[3]	[5]	[7]	[6]	[9]	[19]	[20]
Streptococci												
Viridans	72.4	30.6	65	33.3	40	27	30.9	34	38.6	25.3	48.5	21
Pneumococci	NS	26.4	NS		2	0	0	1	2.8	1.3	0.9	4
Beta-hemolytic	NS	13.9	NS		7	3	0	3.8	23	5.3	3.1	4
Enterococci	NS	1.4	4	1.4	6	8	5.5	6	65	9.3	6.1	9
Not speciated	5.2	[c]	NS	8.5	3	18	13.9	9.6	1.9	6.7	5.1	3
Staphylococci												
S. aureus	9.4	4.2	8	18.4	23	20	13.9	25	19	34.7	11	30
Coagulase negative		2.8	0	5	2	3	6.1	3	4.2	5.3	7.9	4
Gram-negative bacilli	NS	2.8	NS	3.5	2	4	5.4	3.8	11.2	2.7	8	3.2
Enteric							3.0			NS	2	1.6
HACEK							0.6	3.8		1.3	4	0.9
Other							1.8			NS	2	0.7
												2
Gram-positive bacilli						2	0.6			2.7	1.3	8
Yeast		0	NS		0	0	6.7	2	4.7	2.7	NS	0
Other	9.4	17.9	14	9							2.8	0
Culture negative	3.4	NS	9	25.5	14	14	16.4[d]	4.8	12.1	2.7	9.7	9

[a] All figures are the percentages of episodes reported [reference].
[b] Estimated from bar graphs.
[c] Included under viridans streptococci.
[d] Includes seven with organism isolated from valve at surgery or autopsy; and tabulated above.
NS = not stated.

with these infections usually have underlying valvular disease, numerous predisposing factors, and acute onset of their infection [26,27,28]. Finally, *S. bovis* deserves mention because of its association with benign and malignant disorders of the gastrointestinal tract. When this organism is isolated, the patient should be carefully evaluated for gastrointestinal malignancy, although it may occur months to years after the bacteremic episode [29].

S. aureus may be increasing in frequency and accounts for up to 50 percent of cases in more recent series. Coagulase-negative staphylococci are recognized pathogens on prosthetic valves, but they also seem to be accounting for more cases on native valves in recent series [3,10,19,20,30,31].

Before 1950, endocarditis caused by gram-negative organisms composed less than 3 percent of cases. More recent reports indicate that gram-negative organisms may now constitute 5 to 10 percent of all native valve endocarditis and an even higher proportion of prosthetic valve endocarditis [11,20,24,32]. Of particular interest is the emergence of the HACEK group (*Haemophilus* spp., *Actinobacillus actinomycetemcomitans, Cardiobacterium hominis, Eikenella corrodens, Kingella kingae*), which may cause up to 50 percent of cases of gram-negative endocarditis [32]. These organisms are fastidious, nonmotile, slow-growing coccobacilli that require up to 4 weeks of incubation. The HACEK organisms rarely cause endocarditis in patients without preexisting valvular disease or in the absence of predisposing factors.

Also of note is the decline in culture-negative endocarditis (8%–12% of cases). This is most likely the result of improved microbiologic techniques. Causes of culture negativity include prior antibiotic administration, fungal endocarditis, uremia, and advanced disease [13,33].

S. aureus is by far the most common cause of endocarditis in IV drug users, but gram-negative bacilli, *Candida,* and other yeasts are also important [3,4,5,18,34,35]. Since 1976, the incidence of polymicrobial endocarditis has increased among IV drug users [36,37,38]. Methicillin-resistant *S. aureus* and meth-

icillin-tolerant staphylococci as single pathogens have also become more prevalent [38].

On prosthetic valves, the common causes of early-onset endocarditis are *S. aureus, S. epidermidis,* gram-negative bacilli, and fungi, whereas late-onset disease is caused mainly by the organisms usually associated with the subacute picture and by *S. epidermidis* and diphtheroids [39–42]. This difference is thought to be explained by intraoperative or early postoperative contamination of the prosthesis with resistant hospital flora in the early type. Late cases represent either smoldering infection with relatively avirulent organisms seeded at the original surgery or subsequent transient bacteremias, such as those that induce endocarditis on native valves [4,5,41–45].

Pathophysiology

The laboratory model of endocarditis is a rabbit in which a catheter passed through a valve produces mild trauma with the elaboration of a fibrin-platelet thrombus, and a subsequent injection of bacteria either through the catheter or at a distant vascular site leads to infection of the traumatized valve [46]. It appears that the fibrin-platelet thrombus acts as both a trap to catch the bacteria and a barrier to protect them from phagocytosis and other host defenses. This model conforms with the propensity of damaged human valves toward endocarditis and even accounts for the distribution of organisms.

One would anticipate that the organisms that cause frequent transient bacteremia would be the most common causes of endocarditis. The fact that chewing, toothbrushing, and the like cause transient bacteremia with mouth flora, predominantly viridans streptococci [47], certainly explains the pattern observed in subacute bacterial endocarditis. More virulent organisms such as *S. aureus* seem to be able to invade even normal hearts. Bacteremia with this organism may result from trivial points of entry as well as manipulation of furuncles [48], biting nails down to paronychia, and excoriation of the skin to the point of secondary infection. Again it is clear that bacteremia occurs far more often than valvular attachment, but in any disease of hematogenous origin *Staphylococcus* is the most common pathogen. Intravenous drug users combine the injection of contaminated materials with particulate and often irritant matter, probably accounting for the frequency of endocarditis in this setting. The use of intravascular central lines reaching near the tricuspid valve or even crossing tricuspid and pulmonic valves reproduces the rabbit model of endocarditis in humans. With the inadvertent but all too frequent introduction of bacteria, especially staphylococci, through these lines comes the specter of iatrogenic endocarditis.

Once the fibrin-platelet thrombus has become infected, the pathologic process is the enlargement of this mass into a vegetation and invasion of tissue by the infection with eventual disruption. In addition to the more or less bulky mass of the vegetation, there are perforations or total erosions of valve cusps, rupture of chordae tendinae, fistulas from the sinus of Valsalva to atrium or pericardium, and burrowing myocardial abscesses.

Depending on the valve involved, the physiologic consequences may be predicted. Rarely, a vegetation will be so large as to function as an occlusive or stenotic lesion [13,49]. More often the tissue destruction process predominates and valvular incompetence results. New regurgitant murmurs of mitral, tricuspid, or aortic origin may acutely stress the heart with resultant congestive failure. Aortic valve disease carries the worst prognosis [1,4,5,13,49] for several reasons: (1) The heart tolerates acute aortic insufficiency least well; (2) pericardial tamponade or massive left-to-right shunt may develop if a sinus of Valsalva aneurysm erodes into pericardium or right atrium, respectively; (3) heart block may occur if a myocardial abscess invades the conducting system; and (4) aortic valve ring vegetations are most likely to be flipped into the coronary arteries, infarcting already overworked muscle. These catastrophes are all even more likely in the presence of a prosthetic aortic valve, in which case the infection has its seat at the annulus. By analogy, tricuspid valve endocarditis is the most benign. Even total tricuspid insufficiency can be tolerated for a time, and acute right-sided heart failure is not as life-threatening as is the pulmonary edema of left-sided failure.

The vegetations themselves may break off in whole or part as emboli to the brain, viscera (spleen and kidney are particularly common targets), coronary arteries, and—notably in fungal endocarditis—large arteries of the extremities. Right-sided cardiac lesions produce septic emboli to the lungs, resulting in pulmonary infiltrates, often nodular and sometimes cavitating in nature. Similarly, emboli to other organs produce infarction, which is usually bland, although microscopic brain abscess and even purulent meningitis may occur in staphylococcal endocarditis. The most common cerebral lesion, however, is embolic infarct with the clinical appearance of a stroke [49]. Splenic emboli produce acute left upper quadrant pain, sometimes pleuritic in nature. The smaller vascular lesions of endocarditis may be of an immunologic, "vasculitic" nature or truly embolic and suppurative in character. Emboli to the vasa vasorum or vasculitis of the arteries leads to mycotic aneurysms of both cerebral and peripheral vessels. The cerebral emboli are generally asymptomatic until they rupture and present as subarachnoid or intracerebral hemorrhage, whereas peripheral mycotic aneurysms may come to attention because of their obvious enlargement and frequent overlying inflammation. Other phenomena that fall into this category are the cutaneous stigmata of endocarditis—Osler's nodes, Janeway lesions, splinter hemorrhages, and petechiae—as well as the frequent renal involvement. Kidney pathology may take at least four forms: microscopic renal infarcts, focal embolic glomerulonephritis, chronic glomerulonephritis, and acute diffuse glomerulonephritis [13]. The last is thought to represent immune complex disease, and circulating immune complexes have been detected in endocarditis, as might be expected from a prolonged illness in which a foreign antigen (the causative organism) exists intravascularly.

The pathophysiology of endocarditis also includes the poorly understood effects of chronic illness, particularly anemia and weight loss. There may be a nonspecific effect on cerebral function, so-called toxic-metabolic encephalopathy, producing confusion, lethargy, or near coma. It should be noted that even after successful treatment and eradication of the infection, valvular damage may progress and emboli continue. Worsening valve function is attributed to the process of cicatrization with resultant distortion of the leaflet [3]. Emboli have occurred as late as 8 to 20 months after the end of therapy without signaling relapse or reinfection [3]; they do of course cause concern in physician and patient and warrant evaluation.

Diagnosis

Before or in the absence of autopsy or surgical confirmation of vegetations [50], endocarditis is diagnosed on the basis of signs and symptoms that reflect the pathology: fever, embolic phenomena, and evidence of valvular dysfunction. A continuous bacteremia is characteristic and, indeed, highly suggestive of endovascular infection, although the entity of culture-negative endocarditis also exists.

CRITERIA. The following criteria for the certainty of the diagnosis of infective endocarditis (IE) have been used in many studies [7]:

Definite IE: Histologic evidence of infected endocardial vegetation(s) from examination of tissue obtained from cardiac surgery, embolectomy, or autopsy.
Probable IE: (a) Persistently* positive blood cultures and either new regurgitant murmur or known underlying heart disease and evidence of emboli to the skin or viscera, or (b) negative blood cultures with fever (>38°C), new regurgitant valvular heart murmurs, and embolic phenomena.
Possible IE: (a) Persistently* positive blood cultures and either predisposing heart disease or embolic phenomena, or (b) negative blood cultures with fever, known underlying heart disease, and embolic episodes.

Revised criteria proposed by investigators at Duke University provide for classification of the diagnosis as definite infective endocarditis in the absence of histologic confirmation [51]. The Duke criteria incorporate certain echocardiographic findings, give greater weight to the type of organisms recovered from blood, and add intravenous drug use as a predisposition to endocarditis.

Classification of a case on the basis of criteria such as these is the end of a process that must begin with a clinical suspicion based on data from history, physical examination, and laboratory studies. The frequency of various findings in infective endocarditis is tabulated in Table 88-3 [1,3,4,5,7,52,53].

*At least two blood cultures obtained, with two of two positive, three of three positive, or at least 70 percent of cultures positive, if four or more were obtained.

Table 88-3. Clinical Features of Endocarditis[a]

Feature	Iowa[1] 1924–1939 (SBE only)	Iowa[1] 1950–1963	NEMC 1956–1972[3]	UW 1963–1972[4]	CPMC 1968–1973[5]	BI 1970–1977[7]	Chicago 1972–1980[28]	Belgium 1980–1986[52]
History								
Fever	41.2[b]	100[c]	97[c]	84	63	86	80	91
Malaise/weakness	29			} 24	12	94	30	74
Anorexia	3.8					75		30
Weight loss	8.8			24	15	50	20	30
Arthralgias	12.5	25		12			33	11
Back pain	2.5			7		37	18	2
Mental status change or obvious neurologic event	7.5		20	34	15	16	20	4
Previous heart disease	83.7	91.5	61	72	52[d]	77	31	53
Physical examination								
Fever	97.5	100[c]	97[c]	77	80	73,90[c,e]	93	91
Murmur		96.4	85	89			83,93[c,e]	96
Change in murmur		9.9	10		11,25[e]			
Splenomegaly	58	43.2	23	28	27	21,31[e]	20	30
Petechiae	59	47.5	26	34	19	13,20[e]		—
Osler's nodes		11.3		12		10,16[e]		4
	} 36.3						} 18	
Janeway lesions		4.9				3,5[e]		—
Splinters	1.2			12.8		14,28[e]		6
Fundus abnormalities	20	17	2	9		2,8[e]	5	—
Clubbing	10	15	13	12		NS	—	4
Without other known cause	6.3	10		8	3			
Laboratory tests								
Hematuria	75	28.3	26	55		25	72.5	
Elevated ESR			90		70.8	93	95	
Rheumatoid factor			SBE:50		47	24	33	

[a] All figures are percentages.
[b] Presenting complaint.
[c] Fever by history not distinguished from fever recorded in hospital.
[d] Excludes patients with history of a murmur but no formal cardiac diagnosis.
[e] The first number is the percentage of patients who had the findings on admission, and the second number is the cumulative percentage who developed it over the course of observation.
NEMC = New England Medical Center; UW = University of Washington; CPMC = Columbia Presbyterian Medical Center; BI = Beth Israel; SBE = subacute bacterial endocarditis; ESR = erythrocyte sedimentation rate; NS = not stated.

HISTORY. The most frequent symptoms reported by patients with endocarditis are fever and malaise, but some present with acute musculoskeletal (most frequently lower back) pain [54] and others because of an embolus, without complaining of or perhaps even noticing fever [53]. A common feature of endocarditis is loss of appetite, and its return may be the first clinical sign of response to treatment.

Any febrile illness in a patient with known valvular heart disease must bring to mind the question of endocarditis. Hence determining whether a patient has ever been told of a murmur or is likely to have had rheumatic carditis is of prime importance. Similarly, a history of recent dental cleaning or extraction or genitourinary manipulation may indicate an opportunity for bacteremia and seeding of the valve, and should be sought, as should suggestions of intravenous drug abuse. The history of appropriate antibiotic prophylaxis for these procedures is, unfortunately, not enough to exclude the possibility of endocarditis, because failures occasionally occur with currently recommended regimens.

It is important to establish the duration and tempo of the illness by history. Abrupt onset of symptoms, shaking chills, and fever greater than 38.9°C (102°F) strongly suggest acute endocarditis. A symptom pattern that provides a useful clue to the diagnosis of subacute bacterial endocarditis is that of vague illness over a period of several weeks or months that responds transiently to courses of outpatient antibiotics but recurs shortly after they are discontinued [4,13]. This phenomenon should be sought in the history of all patients with "fever of unknown origin" and those with stroke as well.

PHYSICAL EXAMINATION. In contrast to the vagueness of the symptoms of endocarditis, many findings on physical examination are characteristic, although not pathognomonic. Most pertinent to the diagnosis are cardiac murmurs and mucocutaneous "embolic" phenomena. *Any* heart murmur is compatible with a diagnosis of endocarditis, because it is evidence of the turbulent flow that provides the proper nidus for infection. The fact that a murmur has been documented for a long time and is unchanged is encouraging because it suggests that significant hemodynamic alteration has not yet taken place, but it in no way excludes the possibility of active endocarditis. Similarly, a stenotic murmur, although rarely the result of endocarditis, provides evidence of a damaged valve that is susceptible to endocarditis. Changing murmurs, and particularly new regurgitant murmurs, are much less commonly observed but are highly significant with respect to both certainty of the diagnosis and functional consequences. Thus patients must be examined both supine and sitting up leaning forward, so that an aortic regurgitant murmur is not missed acutely or interpreted as "new" the first day the patient is well enough to be out of bed and in a chair during rounds. In addicts, careful listening on both sides of the sternum during inspiration must similarly be a routine to detect the murmur of tricuspid insufficiency. Signs of congestive heart failure are not early findings in endocarditis, but must be watched for because the onset of failure signals a need to consider cardiac surgical intervention.

The most commonly observed mucocutaneous lesions of endocarditis are petechiae. They are distinguished from the ordinary petechiae of thrombocytopenia by their distribution. They do not favor dependent areas (such as the ankles and dorsum of the feet) but appear on the plantar surface of the toes and fingertips, as well as the conjunctival and buccal mucosa. They may be larger and more irregular in outline than conventional petechiae (see Plate I-1) but are not the skin infarcts or large purpuric areas or ecchymoses seen in disseminated intravascular coagulation or meningococcemia. They may sometimes have a white or even pustular center. Conjunctival petechiae commonly occur in patients on cardiopulmonary bypass [55], so it is necessary to record their presence or absence on first encounter with a patient after cardiac surgery and to interpret only those that develop under observation. The same necessity applies to subungual splinter hemorrhages, which are so commonly a result of trauma that many patients will have one or two on admission; only those that appear subsequently, while the patient is at rest in the hospital, have diagnostic usefulness [56].

The famed Osler's nodes and Janeway lesions of endocarditis also favor the plantar and palmar surfaces. Janeway lesions are uncommon; very few have been studied histologically [57]. In terms of clinical importance, it is not necessary to distinguish between Osler's nodes and Janeway lesions, because both strongly support a diagnosis of endocarditis. The Osler's node is a painful, tender, bluish-purple nodular lesion located on the pads of the fingers or toes. The Janeway lesion is a painless, pink, nontender macular lesion that is located commonly on the palms or soles [58].

Funduscopic examination may show evidence of endocarditis only slightly less often than does the skin. In fact, "showering" of emboli often occurs, as in the patient whose findings are illustrated in Plate I-1: the fingertip, subungual, conjunctival, and retinal lesions all developed the day after admission for what proved to be acute staphylococcal endocarditis. The retinal lesions are mainly hemorrhages whose shape is dependent on the layer of the retina in which the bleeding occurs rather than on its cause. Those with a central white or pale area are designated *Roth spots*.

Clubbing is mentioned in almost all discussions of endocarditis, even though nearly every author finds it unusual and not helpful; approximately one third of the patients in whom it is noted have had it on some other basis, predating the endocarditis. Splenomegaly is found in nearly half of patients with subacute bacterial endocarditis and in very few of those with the acute variety.

Other findings on physical examination may include evidence of intravenous drug injection; likely sources for bacteremia such as periodontal disease, severely carious teeth, or chronic furunculosis; and the consequences of embolic disease, such as hemiplegia.

LABORATORY TESTS. The key to the diagnosis of endocarditis is blood cultures. Two to three separate blood cultures within a 24-hour interval are recommended based on studies [59,60] that showed that 99.3 percent of all septic episodes will be detected by the first two blood cultures. In adults, 20 to 30 ml blood per culture is optimal [61]. Resin devices used to

neutralize antibiotics are no longer recommended. Although the detection of *S. aureus* has reportedly been increased with these devices, adverse or no effects on the recovery of most other organisms have been demonstrated [61]. Their effectiveness in culture-negative endocarditis has not been established. In cases that appear to be culture negative [62], the advice of a clinical microbiologist should be sought regarding the need for special media, such as those adequate for the propagation of nutritionally deficient streptococci, *Brucella* species, and cell-wall defective forms. Prolonged incubation may be necessary for some fastidious organisms, but routine subculture to plates may speed recognition of an isolate. Broths should not be discarded until the organism has been successfully propagated in subculture. Nor should "diphtheroids" and non–*aureus* staphylococci be disregarded as skin contaminants if isolated repeatedly; they are well reported as causes of endocarditis. A particularly troublesome problem is the recovery of *S. epidermidis* of different colony types or susceptibility patterns from different blood cultures. This is not evidence for multiple "contaminated" cultures because the pattern can be observed in true *S. epidermidis* endocarditis.

One form of endocarditis that may be persistently culture negative is fungal endocarditis [5,13]. Only 50 percent of blood cultures have been found to be positive in patients with *Candida* endocarditis, and the rate is even lower for filamentous fungi such as *Aspergillus* [62]. Premortem microbiologic diagnosis has often been made by culture and special histologic stains of large arterial emboli retrieved at surgery to save an extremity [3]. The diagnosis of Q-fever endocarditis can be made by serologic study [63].

Other laboratory tests are not nearly as useful in the diagnosis of endocarditis. The findings of elevated erythrocyte sedimentation rate (ESR), high titer of rheumatoid factor (RF), and hematuria help to demonstrate the existence of chronic illness and antigen-antibody complex phenomena in these patients, and certainly raise one's level of suspicion. They may weigh heavily in a decision to call an illness "culture-negative endocarditis" or to treat as endocarditis a bacteremia that was only documented in a single blood culture before antibiotics were started. ESR and RF may also be used to follow the response of a patient to therapy.

The hematologic pattern expected with endocarditis is an anemia of chronic disease (which may be combined with hemolysis in patients with prosthetic valvular leaks or certain artificial valves known to cause a "Waring blender syndrome") with a mild leukocytosis. Marked leukocytosis and pronounced shift-to-the-left strongly suggest either staphylococcal disease or sepsis other than endocarditis.

OTHER DIAGNOSTIC TESTS. Diagnostic modalities that may be used to assess the impact of infection on the heart are listed in Table 88-4. The electrocardiogram (ECG) is the simplest test for evaluation of perivalvular extension of infection in endocarditis [54,64–67]. In aortic valve disease, especially on prosthetic valves, serial ECGs should be used to monitor for abscess development. Persistent (> 2–3 days) prolongation of the P-R interval in the absence of digitalis toxicity, new persistent bundle branch block, or complete heart block is quite specific for predicting extension into myocardial or aortic root tissue and the subsequent need for surgery [67,68].

Echocardiography is a valuable adjunct in the patient with endocarditis. Detection of a vegetation by echocardiography is not required for the diagnosis of IE. Current roles for echocardiography include: (1) characterization of underlying valvular disease; (2) clarification of destructive nature of endocarditis; (3) assessment of the persistently febrile patient for evidence

Table 88-4. Diagnostic Modalities Available to Evaluate
Complications of Infective Endocarditis

Electrocardiography
M-mode echocardiography
Transthoracic 2D echocardiography
Transesophageal echocardiography
Doppler techniques
Magnetic resonance imaging
Computer tomography
Indium-111 leukocyte scan
Cardiac catheterization

of perivalvular extension of infection; and (4) assessment of valvular function in prosthetic valve endocarditis.

M-mode echocardiography was the first echocardiographic technique to be used clinically. Although it is still applied in the assessment of patients with IE, anatomic information is limited [69]. The overall sensitivity for detecting vegetations is reported to be 57 percent [70]. It is too insensitive to be used for the detection of perivalvular abscess [67]. Transthoracic two-dimensional (2D) images (TTE) of the heart have improved the sensitivity of vegetation detection to 70% [70]. The literature is less clear, however, on the ability of TTE to detect abscess extension, with sensitivities for abscess detection reported from 0% to 100%, and overall accuracy approximating 70 percent [67].

Although TTE is a valuable tool in the management of patients with endocarditis, it is of limited value in as many as 30% of patients because of obesity, chronic lung disease, and thoracic deformity, which preclude obtaining the high-quality images needed to detect vegetations [71,72]. In addition, equivocal results due to thickening or myxomatous degeneration of native valves and artifact from prosthetic valves are problems with TTE [70,73].

Transesophageal echocardiography (TEE) is the latest advance in the evaluation of the patient with IE [74,75]. The procedure consists of the insertion of a modified endoscope equipped with a biplane transducer capable of high-resolution imaging into the esophagus of the patient [75]. Despite the somewhat invasive nature of TEE, the procedure is quite safe when performed by a skilled physician, with interruption of the procedure or complications occurring less than 1 percent of the time [76]. Contraindictions to the procedure include esophageal diseases, severe atlantoaxial joint disease (preventing neck flexion), prior irradiation to the chest, and perforated viscus [75].

Image quality of the TEE is much improved because of the high-resolution transducer and unobstructed view of cardiac structures [67–75]. The TEE is much more sensitive than TTE for the detection of valvular vegetations; sensitivity with current biplane TEE is >90%, with vegetations as small as 1 mm being seen [70,71,73,77]. TEE is also superior to TTE for detection of perivalvular abscess with approximately 87% sensitivity [78]. Finally, TEE also appears to be superior to TTE in the assessment of prosthetic valve dysfunction and in the intraoperative assessment of cardiac structure and hemodynamics [73]. However, at this time, investigators do not routinely recommend TEE in all patients with IE. TEE may be useful when the diagnostic quality of TTE is inadequate or inconclusive. TEE also appears to be indicated when there is an abnormality on TTE requiring further evaluation and to assess prosthetic valve dysfunction [72].

The prognostic implications of vegetations identified by echocardiagraphic studies remain controversial. Some recent studies have indicated an increased risk of embolization in patients with vegetations > 10 mm in size [79], particularly in patients with left-sided endocarditis [70,80]. Still others have found that the predictive value of size for embolization depended on the organism [81]. Most investigators agree that the presence of a vegetation alone is not an independent indication for valve replacement [69,82,83]. However, patients with echocardiographic evidence of valvular destruction, such as chordal rupture or torn aortic cusps, do have more complicated courses [83].

Doppler studies employ ultrasound to measure blood flow and pressure gradients through intracardiac and extracardiac vascular structures. Blood flow can be displayed as a color map that enables the examiner to estimate valvular regurgitation. When combined with TTE or TEE, Doppler studies permit more accurate assessment of the functional significance of any identified anatomic lesion [69,73].

Magnetic resonance imaging (MRI) has been used successfully to diagnose aortic root abscess, but its exact role in evaluating patients with endocarditis remains to be clarified [67]. Data on the indium-111 leukocyte scan indicate difficulties in interpretation, no role in the detection of vegetations, and an uncertain role in the diagnosis of abscess [67].

Finally, cardiac catheterization is reserved for patients in whom prior studies have failed to detect a highly suspected complication and for patients who require surgery. In the latter instance, the anatomic information to be gained allows the surgeon to be better prepared because significant unanticipated lesions are often discovered [84]. The potential risk of dislodging a fragment of vegetation may be lessened by low-pressure injection and the fact that regurgitant lesions often obviate the need to cross the valve bearing the vegetation [85]. In aortic insufficiency, for instance, a supravalvular injection, via retrograde filling, may demonstrate the degree of regurgitation as well as left ventricular contractility, mitral valve function, and abnormalities of the aortic root such as aneurysm of the sinus of Valsalva.

Differential Diagnosis

Three issues in differential diagnosis will be considered:

1. Syndromes for which infective endocarditis is a possible cause
2. Syndromes that may mimic infective endocarditis
3. The distinction between endocarditis and simple bacteremia

The first category represents the situation in which one of the features of endocarditis is the cardinal symptom; the others may need to be searched for or may only evolve later in the clinical course. Syndromes of this nature are stroke, particularly in a young person, fever of unknown origin, and new-onset congestive heart failure or sudden worsening of preexisting failure. Any fever in a person with a heart murmur must raise the question of endocarditis, and the suspicion must be stronger in the presence of known valvular disease and stronger yet with a prosthetic valve in place. Fever in addicts always calls for ruling out endocarditis. Sudden onset of renal failure is not a common presentation of endocarditis, but does occur, and should be an indication for blood cultures even in the afebrile patient. Endocarditis may not come to mind readily in the patient with low back pain, but enough patients present in this fashion to warrant looking for fever and other physical findings of endocarditis and checking for leukocytosis, anemia, and elevated sedimentation rate when there is no definite orthopedic diagnosis.

Diseases that actually mimic many of the features of infective endocarditis are limited in number, but the distinction from culture-negative endocarditis may be extremely difficult. Such is the case with marantic endocarditis in the debilitated or chronically ill host, in whom the presence of sterile vegetations clearly can duplicate the clinical hallmarks of infective endocarditis, although progression to valve destruction and heart failure is rare in this condition. Failure of the fever to respond to antibiotics may be the tip-off to this diagnosis, which may be made definitively only postmortem. Atrial myxoma can also present all of the features of endocarditis, including congestive heart failure, but a clue sometimes may be found in failure that comes and goes, because that caused by the destructive process of infective endocarditis rarely remits spontaneously . Echocardiographic or angiographic visualization of the tumor makes this diagnosis. The older literature refers to difficulties in distinguishing between some cases of acute rheumatic fever and infective endocarditis and notes that the presence of pericarditis strongly favors the former, although it does not absolutely exclude the latter [3].

By far the most common difficulty confronting the present-day practitioner is deciding which episodes of bacteremia represent endocarditis. The question becomes particularly acute in patients with intravascular foreign bodies, such as pacemakers, valves, and patches, and when the organism is *S. aureus*. The approach to this problem must take into account the propensity for the foreign body to become infected and of the organism to cause endocarditis. An additional major consideration in the analysis is the duration of bacteremia. Because sustained bacteremia characterizes infection of endovascular sites, the longer bacteremia lasts, the more suspicious one becomes of its endothelial origin. In addition, even if the origin is distant and known, the longer the organisms circulate the greater is the risk that they *have* settled out and seeded the intravascular foreign body secondarily.

Prosthetic valves, both mechanical and of biologic origin, have a very high risk of becoming infected, whereas permanent pacemakers, once endothelialized, appear to carry a relatively low risk. In one study, distancing the pacemaker wire skin entrance site from the venous insertion site markedly reduced the rate of infection associated with these systems [86]. This supports the concept that infection usually occurs at the skin-catheter junction and is thus most likely to invade the circulation when the vessel is in close proximity to the skin wound. There seems to be agreement in published discussions that sustained bacteremia implies infection of the pacemaker electrode, which should be removed in its entirety [86–89], whereas transient bacteremia from another focus, treated in a fashion appropriate to the primary infection, has generally not resulted in complications related to the heart [89].

As mentioned, organisms differ in their propensity to cause endothelial infection. Enteric gram-negative bacilli are among the most common blood culture isolates at most hospitals but are less common as a cause of endocarditis (see Table 88-2). For example, many elderly men sustain *Escherichia coli* bacteremia from pyelonephritis without infecting their sclerotic aortic valves, even though such valves are quite susceptible to attack by enterococci or other streptococci. Notable exceptions to this characterization of enteric gram-negative bacilli are salmonellae, particularly *S. typhimurium* and *S. choleraesuis,* which seem to have an affinity for damaged vascular endothelium and to have infected aortic aneurysms [90] as well as pacemaker tracts [91].

Even in patients with highly susceptible prosthetic valves, gram-negative bacteremia does not always constitute endocarditis. It has been claimed that early-onset (<60 days post–cardiac surgery) gram-negative bacteremia with an obvious source rarely indicates involvement of the valve [92]. These patients have done better in terms of valve function and survival with

antibiotic treatment alone than have patients with prosthetic valve endocarditis caused by other organisms. Others have argued that gram-negative endocarditis on prosthetic valves seems to respond better to antibiotics than does gram-positive infection [39,40,41], although the numbers in any series are too small for statistical significance. A working solution to the management of gram-negative bacteremia in the setting of a prosthetic valve without obvious endocarditis lies in choosing antibiotic therapy adequate for both the primary focus of infection and possible endocarditis.

In contrast, a classic study reported that 64 percent of *all* bacteremias with *S. aureus* in the period 1940 to 1954 represented endocarditis, proved by autopsy in 38 percent [93]. A subsequent report from the same center defined 16 percent of 134 patients with *S. aureus* bacteremia in the years 1975 to 1977 as having definite or probable endocarditis by the criteria listed above [94]. Although others have claimed that *S. aureus* bacteremia associated with a clear-cut focus of infection or a removable intravenous catheter is not likely to represent endocarditis [95,96], this series found the risk of endocarditis in patients with catheter-associated bacteremia (18%) not different from that of the group as a whole. These and other studies have amply demonstrated the ability of *S. aureus* to produce endocarditis on a valve previously presumed normal and have shown that established endocarditis may be found at postmortem examination in patients in whom no murmur was ever heard during life [1,3,4,6,17,93,97].

Thus, *S. aureus* bacteremia always raises the question of whether treatment as endocarditis is warranted. The absence of a primary focus appears to be the most powerful predictor of endocarditis in community-acquired staphylococcal bacteremia [98,99]. Intravenous drug users are also at high risk for endocarditis and metastatic abscesses, and staphylococcal bacteremia should be treated in a fashion appropriate to endocarditis whenever it occurs in this group. In contrast, many currently believe a 2-week course of antibiotic therapy is adequate for catheter-associated *S. aureus* bacteremia in patients at low risk for endocarditis, that is, without valvular heart disease (or prosthetic valves) and in whom the catheter has been removed promptly and subsequent blood cultures are negative [95,96,98,100,101]. Failures may still occur in as many as 5 percent to 24 percent of patients with catheter-associated bacteremia, usually within 10 weeks of discontinuing therapy [100,102]. Clearly, patients who have prolonged fever or bacteremia after catheter removal should receive the longer course of antibiotic therapy, because catheter-associated *S. aureus* endocarditis can be fatal [101,103–106].

The overall mortality rate for staphylococcal endocarditis in one collaborative study was 20 percent [104]. In contrast, parenteral drug users have only a 2 percent mortality, although considerable morbidity, including congestive heart failure, occurs in 23 percent. The more favorable outcome of addicts is generally attributed to their younger age and absence of underlying systemic illness, as well as the location of their valve involvement.

Even less clear than the literature on *S. aureus* bacteremia and endocarditis is the significance of enterococcal bacteremia in the hospitalized patient. The incidence of enterococcal bacteremia has increased over the last decade, especially in the surgical patient [107–110]. Predisposing risk factors include: (1) immunosuppression related to cancer, alcoholism, and diabetes mellitus; (2) breakdown in local skin barriers from decubitus ulcers, burns, or central lines; (3) instrumentation of the gastrointestinal and genitourinary tracts; (4) long-term hospitalization (>3 weeks); and (5) treatment with cephalosporins and other broad-spectrum agents that have no anti-enterococcal activity [110,111]. Frequently, the enterococcus occurs in polymicrobial bacteremic infections along with enteric gram-negative bacilli [111]. Mortality is high, ranging from 34 percent to 68 percent, and seems to correlate directly with the severity of underlying illness [110].

Nosocomial enterococcal bacteremia is much less likely to represent endocarditis than is community-acquired disease [108–111], and polymicrobial enterococcal bacteremia almost never does [109,110,111]. Suspicion for endocarditis is heightened by the absence of an identifiable source of infection and the presence of a heart murmur [109,110,111].

It is important to make the distinction between endocarditis and enterococcal bacteremia without cardiac involvement, because the treatment approaches are different. Short course (<2 weeks), single-drug therapy and drainage or removal of a focus is adequate in the absence of endocarditis [110,111,112]. The treatment of enterococcal endocarditis, however, requires prolonged and potentially toxic therapy [113].

Infections of Prosthetic Devices: Pacemakers, Automatic Implantable Cardioverter Defibrillators (AICDS)

Infections involving permanent pacemakers present diagnostic and management dilemmas. The incidence of such infections has declined over the last several decades to approximately 6 percent [114]. Predisposing factors include diabetes mellitus, corticosteroid and anticoagulant therapy, remanipulation of the electrode after implantation, hematoma of the generator pocket, skin erosion over the generator, and infection at sites elsewhere in the body such as pneumonia and skin ulcers [88,115,116,117]. Infections of pacemakers can be divided into several distinct syndromes:

1. Generator pocket infections, which tend to occur within 2 months of surgery, are usually caused by *S. aureus.*
2. Infections associated with the lead wire and electrode generally present months later and more typically are caused by *Staphylococcus epidermidis.*
3. Endocarditis usually follows contiguous spread of infection along the pacer system.

Local erythema, erosion over the generator site, or drainage characterize pocket infections, whereas electrode infections and endocarditis present more typically with sepsis and sustained bacteremia.

Early literature suggested that pocket infections could be treated with local surgery and antibiotics, but more recent articles report failure with such a conservative approach [88,115]. Infections that involve pacemaker wires and electrodes are almost never cured with antibiotics alone, and the entire system should be removed [87,88,115,118,119,120]. This usually can be accomplished in a one-stage procedure in which the old system is removed and the new system placed at a site remote from the infection [88,115,116], followed by a course of antibiotics of 4 to 6 weeks' duration [120].

Removal of the old system may not always be easy to accomplish. Sometimes defective or infected electrodes become firmly enclosed by fibrous tissue and are adherent to the vessel endothelium, precluding easy extraction through the venous system [115,117,118]. In some instances, the wire has been severed and sutured into place in the venous system. Although this practice is safe with noninfected electrodes, 23.5 percent of patients died of sepsis when infected electrodes were retained, despite appropriate antibiotic therapy [117]. Removal of a retained wire using traction devices has been successful in some instances, but serious complications such as avulsion of the tricuspid valve and creation of atrioventricular fistulae have been reported [118]. Cardiopulmonary bypass surgery with dissection of the electrode is recommended for those patients who can tolerate surgery [115,117,118].

Infection is one of the most serious complications of automatic implantable cardioverter defibrillators (AICDS). These devices consist of a pulse generator, a bipolar sensing device, and two defibrillating electrodes. The sensing electrode is either a right ventricular endocardial lead or an epicardial electrode pair. The defibrillating electrodes are usually mesh patches that are applied to the epicardium or one epicardial patch coupled with a spring lead positioned at the superior vena caval–right atrial junction.

Infection rates of AICDS range from 0 percent to 7 percent [121,122]. Early infections typically involve the generator pocket and are caused by *S. aureus* [122,123]. Late infections involving the patch and associated purulent pericarditis, usually caused by coagulase-negative staphylococci and corynebacteria, have also been described [122,124]. There is now agreement that these infections, whether early or late, require removal of the entire system [121,122,124]. Radical debridement of the pericardium is necessary if infection extends beyond the electrode patch capsule [124]. Prolonged antibiotic therapy, i.e., 6 weeks, follows these procedures. After appropriate gas sterilization, the generator may be reimplanted using new electrodes and wires [122].

Treatment

The traditional treatment of endocarditis has been 4 to 6 weeks of intravenous administration of a drug that is bactericidal for the infecting organism. Tables 88-5 to 88-8 present the current recommendations for antimicrobial therapy from the American Heart Association Committee on Rheumatic Fever, Endocarditis, and Kawasaki Disease [125]. Shorter courses of therapy, oral antimicrobial regimens, and outpatient management are currently under investigation [126].

USE OF COMBINATION THERAPY. For many years it has been known that certain organisms, such as the enterococcus, cannot be killed in vitro by a single antibiotic at achievable serum levels. For this organism both laboratory and clinical data support the greater efficacy of a combination of two antibiotics, a cell-wall active agent (penicillin, ampicillin, or vancomycin—a cephalosporin) plus an aminoglycoside, in the therapy of endocarditis [127]. However, recent trends in antimicrobial resistance, namely, the increasing prevalence of enterococci with high-level aminoglycoside resistance, have compromised our ability to use combination therapy. These isolates are characteristically resistant to the synergistic bactericidal action of cell-wall active agents and aminoglycosides [112,113,128,129]. Endocarditis due to enterococci that are highly resistant to gentamicin has been reported [130,131]. Approximately 30 percent to 50 percent of these isolates are susceptible to streptomycin, which then may be used for combination therapy [128]. If the enterococcal isolate is resistant to both aminoglycosides, one is left with single-drug therapy with cell-wall active agents, which are not bactericidal for this organism. Nonetheless, there

Table 88-5. Therapy for Endocarditis Due to Strains of Viridans Streptococci and Streptococcus Bovis Relatively Resistant to Penicillin (Minimum Inhibitory Concentration >0.1 μg/ml and <0.5 μg/ml[a])

Antibiotic	Adult dose and route	Pediatric dose and route	Duration (wk)
Aqueous crystalline penicillin G	20 million units/24 hr IV either continuously or in 6 equal divided doses	200,000 to 300,000 units/kg per 24 hr IV (not to exceed 20 million units/24 hr) given continuously or in 6 equally divided doses	4
With streptomycin[b]	7.5 mg/kg IM (not to exceed 500 mg) every 12 hr	15 mg/kg IM (not to exceed 500 mg) every 12 hr	2
Or with gentamicin[b]	1 mg/kg IM or IV (not to exceed 80 mg) every 8 hr	2.0 to 2.5 mg/kg IM or IV (not to exceed 80 mg) every 8 hr	2

[a] Cephalothin or cefazolin (with an aminoglycoside for the first 2 weeks) or vancomycin alone can be used in patients whose penicillin hypersensitivity is not of the immediate type. Vancomycin also can be used in patients with immediate penicillin allergy. Antibiotic doses should be modified appropriately for patients with impaired renal function.

[b] Streptomycin or gentamicin should be given in addition to penicillin for the first 2 weeks. Peak streptomycin levels of approximately 20 μg/ml and peak gentamicin levels of about 3 μg/ml are desirable. For the rare viridans streptococcus with minimum inhibitory concentration greater than or equal to 0.5 μg/ml penicillin G, aminoglycoside therapy should be continued for 4 weeks with appropriate monitoring of serum levels of streptomycin or gentamicin. Aminoglycosides given on a milligram per kilogram basis will produce higher serum concentrations in obese than in lean patients.

Source: Bisno AL, Dismukes WE, Durack, et al: Antimicrobial treatment of infective endocarditis due to viridans streptococci, enterococci and staphylococci. *JAMA* 261:1471, 1989.

IV = intravenously; IM = intramuscularly.

Table 88-6. Therapy for Endocarditis Due to Enterococci (or to Viridans Streptococci with a Minimum Inhibitory Concentration >0.5 μg/ml)[a]

Antibiotic	Adult dose and route	Pediatric dose and route	Duration (wk)
Regimen for non-penicillin-allergic patients			
1. Aqueous crystalline penicillin G	20–30 million units/24 hr IV given continuously or in 6 equally divided doses	200,000 to 300,000 units/kg per 24 hr IV (not to exceed 30 million units/24 hr) given continuously or in 6 equally divided doses	4–6
With gentamicin[b,c,d]	1 mg/kg IM or IV (not to exceed 80 mg) every 8 hr	2.0–2.5 mg/kg IM or IV (not to exceed 80 mg) every 8 hr	4–6
Or with streptomycin[b,d,e]	7.5 mg/kg IM (not to exceed 500 mg) every 12 hr	15 mg/kg IM (not to exceed 500 mg) every 12 hr	4–6
2. Ampicillin	12g/24 hr IV given continuously or in 6 equally divided doses	300 mg/kg per 24 hr IV (not to exceed 12 g/24 hr) in 4 to 6 equally divided doses	4–6
With gentamicin[b,c,d]	1 mg/kg IM or IV (not to exceed 80 mg) every 8 hr	2.0 to 2.5 mg/kg IM or IV (not to exceed 80 mg) every 8 hr	4–6
Or with streptomycin[b,d,e]	7.5 mg/kg IM (not to exceed 500 mg) every 12 hr	15 mg/kg IM (not to exceed 50 mg) every 12 hr	4–6
Regimen for penicillin-allergic patients (desensitization should be considered; cephalosporins are not satisfactory alternatives)			
Vancomycin[f]	30 mg/kg per 24 hr IV in 2 or 4 equally divided doses, not to exceed 2 g/24 hr unless serum levels are monitored	40 mg/kg per 24 hr IV in 2 or 4 equally divided doses, not to exceed 2 gm/24 hr unless serum levels are monitored	4–6
With gentamicin[b,c,d]	1 mg/kg IM or IV (not to exceed 80 mg) every 8 hr	2.0 to 2.5 mg/kg IM or IV (not to exceed 80 mg) every 8 hr	4–6
Or with streptomycin[b,d,e]	7.5 mg/kg IM (not to exceed 500 mg) every 12 hr	15 mg/kg IM (not to exceed 500 mg) every 12 hr	4–6

[a] Antibiotic doses should be modified appropriately in patients with impaired renal function.

[b] Choice of aminoglycoside depends on resistance level of infecting strain (see text). Enterococci should be tested for high-level resistance (minimum inhibitory concentration, ≥2000 μg/ml).

[c] Serum concentration of gentamicin should be monitored and dose adjusted to obtain a peak level of approximately 3 μg/ml.

[d] Dosing of aminoglycosides and vancomycin on a milligram per kilogram basis will give higher serum concentrations in obese than in lean patients.

[e] Serum concentration of streptomycin should be monitored if possible and dose adjusted to obtain a peak level of approximately 20 μg/ml.

[f] Peak serum concentrations of vancomycin should be obtained 1 hour after infusion and should be in the range of 30 to 45 μg/ml for twice-daily dosing and 20 to 35 μg/ml for four times daily dosing. Each dose should be infused over 1 hour.

Source: Bisno AL, Dismukes WE, Durack DT, et al: Antimicrobial treatment of infective endocarditis due to viridans streptococci, enterococci and staphylococci. *JAMA* 261:1471, 1989.

IV = intravenously; IM = intramuscularly.

Table 88-7. Therapy for Endocarditis Due to *Staphylococcus* in the Absence of Prosthetic Material[a]

Antibiotic	Adult dose and route	Pediatric dose and route	Duration
Methicillin-susceptible staphylococci Regimen for nonpenicillin-allergic patients			
Nafcillin	2 gm IV every 4 hr	150–200 mg/kg per 24 hr IV (not to exceed 12 gm/24 hr) in 4–6 equally divided doses	4–6 wk
Or oxacillin	2 gm IV every 4 hr	150–200 mg/kg per 24 hr (not to exceed 12 gm/24 hr) in 4–6 equally divided doses	4–6 wk
With optional addition of gentamicin[b,c]	1 mg/kg IM or IV (not to exceed 80 mg) every 8 hr	2.0–2.5 mg/kg IV (not to exceed 80 mg) every 8 hr	3–5 days
Regimen for penicillin-allergic patients 1. Cephalothin[d]	2 gm IV every 4 hr	100–150 mg/kg per 24 hr IV (not to exceed 12 gm/24 hr) in equally divided doses every 4–6 hr	4–6 wk
Or cefazolin[d]	2 gm IV every 8 hr	80–100 mg/kg per 24 hr IV (not to exceed 6 gm/24 hr) in equally divided doses every 8 hr	4–6 wk
With optional addition of gentamicin[b]	Same as for non–penicillin-allergic patient	Same as for non–penicillin-allergic patient	—
2. Vancomycin[b,e]	30 mg/kg per 24 hr IV in 2 or 4 equally divided doses, not to exceed 2 gm/24 hr unless serum levels are monitored	40 mg/kg per 24 hr IV in 2 of 4 equally divided doses, not to exceed 2 gm/24 hr unless serum levels are monitored	4–6 wk
Methicillin-resistant staphylococci Vancomycin[b,e]	30 mg/kg per 24 hr IV or in 2 or 4 equally divided doses, not to exceed 2 gm/24 hr unless serum levels are monitored	40 mg/kg per 24 hr IV in 2 or 4 equally divided doses, not to exceed 2 gm/24 hr unless serum levels are monitored	4–6 wk

[a] Antibiotic doses should be modified appropriately for patients with impaired renal function. For treatment of endocarditis due to penicillin-susceptible staphylococci (minimum inhibitory concentration, ≤0.1 μg/ml), aqueous crystalline penicillin G should be used for 4 to 6 weeks instead of nafcillin or oxacillin. Shorter antibiotic courses have been effective in some drug addicts with right-sided endocarditis due to *Staphylococcus aureus*. See text for comments on use of rifampin.
[b] Dosing of aminoglycosides and vancomycin on a milligram per kilogram basis will give higher serum concentrations in obese than in lean patients.
[c] Benefit of additional aminoglycosides has not been established. Risk of toxic reactions due to these agents is increased in patients who are older than age 65 years or who have renal or eighth nerve impairment.
[d] There is potential cross-allergenicity between penicillins and cephalosporins. Cephalosporins should be avoided in patients with immediate type hypersensitivity to penicillin.
[e] Peak serum concentration of vancomycin should be obtained 1 hour after infusion and should be in the range of 30–45 μg/ml for twice-daily dosing and 20–35 μg/ml for four times daily dosing. Each dose of vancomycin should be infused over 1 hour. See text for consideration of optional addition of gentamicin.
Source: Bisno AL, Dismukes WE, Durack DT, et al: Antimicrobial treatment of infective endocarditis due to viridans streptococci, enterococci and staphylococci. *JAMA* 261:1471, 1989.
IV = intravenously; IM = intramuscularly.

are reports of success using beta-lactams alone in divided doses or by continuous infusion [128,129]. The latter regimen has shown promise for the treatment of experimental endocarditis in the rat model, but there is minimal clinical experience to date [132,133]. Current recommendations are ≥6 weeks of therapy with ampicillin for strains demonstrating high-level resistance to all aminoglycosides, along with strong consideration of early surgery [113,130].

Some enterococci with high-level gentamicin resistance also produce beta-lactamase. Animal studies suggest that ampicillin-sulbactam or a glycopeptide such as vancomycin may be successful. Finally, vancomycin-resistant enterococci are becoming a problem, and these isolates are also resistant to beta-lactams [134]. Cases of entercoccal endocarditis involving resistant organisms require a cooperative effort between the consultant in infectious diseases, the microbiology laboratory, and a cardiac surgeon.

In several other clinical situations, combination antimicrobial therapy may also be considered. In endocarditis caused by nonenterococcal, non–beta-hemolytic streptococci, results with either 4 weeks of penicillin alone or 2 weeks of penicillin plus an aminoglycoside followed by 2 more weeks of penicillin have been excellent, and a preference may be largely a matter of local tradition, except when the organism is demonstrated to

be relatively resistant to penicillin (minimal inhibitory concentration [MIC] >0.1 and <0.5 μg/ml) [135]. Patients who develop streptococcal endocarditis while on chronic penicillin prophylaxis for rheumatic fever are particularly likely to have such strains. Some authors have used 2 weeks of combination parenteral therapy to shorten the period of hospitalization [136]. This is not recommended for relatively resistant organisms, prosthetic valve endocarditis, or otherwise complicated cases [135].

In staphylococcal endocarditis, there is clearly room for improvement in therapeutic results, and there is some suggestion of impaired in vitro killing of a large proportion of strains by the semisynthetic penicillins alone (tolerance), which is ameliorated by the addition of an aminoglycoside [137,138,139]. In two clinical trials, however, the addition of gentamicin to oxacillin or nafcillin did not improve the outcome [140,141]. In one, however, combination-treated patients cleared their bacteremia more rapidly, but at the expense of greater nephrotoxicity [140]. This has led to the recommendation for addition of an aminoglycoside to the semisynthetic penicillin for the first 3 to 5 days of therapy. The goal of short-term use is to minimize damage to the heart valve while avoiding the nephrotoxicity associated with prolonged courses of aminoglycosides [125].

Patients infected with penicillin-susceptible *S. aureus* should

Table 88-8. Treatment of Staphylococcal Endocarditis in the Presence of a Prosthetic Valve or Other Prosthetic Material[a]

Antibiotic	Adult dose and route	Pediatric dose and route	Duration
Regimen for methicillin-resistant staphylococci			
Vancomycin[b,c]	30 mg/kg per 24 hr IV in 2 or 4 equally divided doses, not to exceed 2 gm/24 hr unless serum levels are monitored	40 mg/kg per 24 hr IV in 2 or 4 equally divided doses, not to exceed 2 gm/24 hr unless serum levels are monitored	≥6
With rifampin[d]	300 mg PO every 8 hr	20 mg/kg per 24 hr PO (not to exceed 900 mg/24 hr) in 2 equally divided doses	≥6
And with gentamicin[c,e,f]	1.0 mg/kg IM or IV (not to exceed 80 mg) every 8 hr	2.0–2.5 mg/kg per 24 hr IV (not to exceed 80 mg) every 8 hr	2
Regimen for methicillin-susceptible staphylococci			
Nafcillin or oxacillin[g]	2 gm IV every 4 hr	150–200 mg/kg per 24 hr IV (not to exceed 12 gm/24 hr) in 4 to 6 equally divided doses	≥6
With rifampin[d]	300 mg PO every 8 hr	20 mg/kg per 24 hr PO (not to exceed 900 mg/24 hr) in 2 equally divided doses	≥6
And with gentamicin[c,e,f]	1.0 mg/kg IM or IV (not to exceed 80 mg) every 8 hr	2.0–2.5 mg/kg IV (not to exceed 80 mg) every 8 hr	2

[a] Vancomycin and gentamicin doses must be modified appropriately in patients with renal failure.
[b] Peak serum concentrations of vancomycin should be obtained 1 hour after infusion and should be in the range of 30–45 μg/ml for twice-daily dosing and 20–35 μg/ml for four times daily dosing. Each dose should be infused over 1 hour.
[c] Aminoglycosides or vancomycin given on a milligram per kilogram basis will produce higher serum concentrations in obese than in lean patients.
[d] Rifampin is recommended for therapy of infections due to coagulase-negative staphylococci. Its use in coagulase-positive staphylococcal infections is controversial. Rifampin increases the amount of warfarin sodium required for antithrombotic therapy.
[e] Serum concentration of gentamicin should be monitored and dose should be adjusted to obtain a peak level of approximately 3 μg/ml.
[f] Use during initial 2 weeks. See text on alternative aminoglycoside therapy for organisms resistant to gentamicin.
[g] First-generation cephalosporins or vancomycin should be used in penicillin-allergic patients. Cephalosporins should be avoided in patients with immediate type hypersensitivity to penicillin and in patients infected with methicillin-resistant staphylococci.
Source: Bisno AL, Dismukes WE, Durack DT, et al: Antimicrobial treatment of infective endocarditis due to viridans streptococci, enterococci and staphylococci. *JAMA* 261:1471, 1989.
IV = intravenously; IM = intramuscularly.

receive penicillin with or without an aminoglycoside in a manner similar to treatment of viridans streptococci. For those patients whose isolates are resistant to methicillin, vancomycin is the treatment of choice (see Table 88-7); these strains are also resistant to cephalosporins, although they may appear susceptible by in vitro tests [125].

Staphylococcus epidermidis, a frequent cause of endocarditis on prosthetic valves, presents a situation not unlike that of the enterococcus. Poor therapeutic results in both patients and the animal model have led to careful examination of conventional susceptibility data and the finding that a large proportion of these isolates have a property called heteroresistance. Among the progeny of a single colony are a proportion with high-level resistance to the beta-lactam agents [142]. In disc susceptibility testing, this phenomenon may give rise to a few colonies within the zone of inhibition or it may not be recognized unless a heavy inoculum of the organism is plated on agar containing 100 μg per milliliter of methicillin and growth occurs [143]. *S. epidermidis* strains exhibiting resistance to methicillin but susceptibility to cephalothin by disc usually fall in this class. Vancomycin is the cornerstone of therapy for these infections, as it is for methicillin-resistant *S. aureus,* but is not sufficient by itself. The addition of rifampin or gentamicin improves therapeutic results (see Table 88-8). Rifampin is currently recommended because of the greater nephrotoxicity of the vancomycin-aminoglycoside combination, but emergence of rifampin resistance on therapy has been documented, and adverse effects of rifampin are common as well [143]. Ongoing studies address the efficacy and toxicity of using all three drugs in combination, compared with two-drug regimens.

Ampicillin and gentamicin in combination have traditionally been the recommended therapy for endocarditis caused by the HACEK group of organisms. Therapeutic failures with this combination in the treatment of *Actinobacillus actinomycetemcomitans* endocarditis and a nearly 30% mortality in one series of patients indicate the need for therapeutic improvement [144,145]. In addition, in vitro susceptibility to ampicillin and penicillin may be quite variable, and synergy between ampicillin or penicillin and gentamicin has not been demonstrated for this particular organism [144,146,147].

A number of recent reports indicate excellent in vitro activity of ceftriaxone and other third-generation cephalosporins against this group of organisms [143,146–150]. Successful monotherapy of endocarditis caused by *Haemophilus* spp. in eight patients treated with ceftriaxone has been reported [150]. Reports of beta-lactamase production by *Eikenella corrodens* have led to the suggestion that third-generation cephalosporins should become the agents of choice for the treatment of *E. corrodens* infections [148], perhaps in combination with gentamicin for the first 2 weeks of therapy [148,149].

Gram-negative-rod (other than HACEK organisms) endocarditis on native valves has had a very poor response rate, and the use of antibiotic combinations, usually an aminoglycoside plus a beta-lactam or cephalosporin to which the organism is susceptible, is accepted practice [127,148]. When possible one would like to demonstrate that the combination chosen is synergistic against the patient's organism in vitro.

ROLE OF LABORATORY STUDIES TO ASSESS TREATMENT EFFICACY. Because host defenses appear to be ineffective in eradicating endocarditis, the concept has developed that the antibiotic regimen must be bactericidal, parenteral, and usually prolonged [151]. How best to monitor in vivo antibiotic efficacy has been controversial, but it is generally agreed that tests that measure only inhibition of the organism do not provide enough information to guide therapy [152]. Hence, the serum bactericidal test has traditionally been recommended for this purpose [153]. This test determines the greatest dilution of the patient's serum that kills 99.9 percent or more of an inoculum of the infecting pathogen [151].

Many factors influence serum bactericidal levels, including inoculum size, type of media, and the time that the samples are obtained in relation to antibiotic therapy (reviewed in references 151, 152, 154, and 155). In the last decade, standardization of the methodology for the test has eliminated laboratory variability of results noted in earlier studies [154]. The peak level is obtained 30 to 60 minutes after completion of a 30-minute parenteral infusion, 1 hour after an IM dose, and $1\frac{1}{2}$ hours after oral therapy. If more than one antibiotic is used, the peak should be obtained 30 to 60 minutes after completion of the second antibiotic. The trough is obtained within 15 minutes before the next dose.

The advantages of the serum bactericidal titer (SBT) are:

1. It correlates well with the minimum bactericidal concentration of the infecting microorganism.
2. It is a convenient test for evaluating the efficacy of combination therapy. For example, gentamicin can be removed by treating the patient's serum with cellulose phosphate; the SBT can then be measured with and without the contribution of the aminoglycoside. If the bactericidal activity of the serum does not decrease appreciably, combination therapy may not be needed.
3. The test can be modified easily for fastidious bacteria.

Two major disadvantages are:

1. Studies in rabbits have failed to demonstrate a correlation between SBT and sterilization of experimentally induced vegetations [156].
2. Retrospective studies in humans have shown no evidence that the SBT is of prognostic value [152,157,158].

In the only prospective study performed to date using a standardized method, the SBT predicted cure in patients with infective endocarditis at peak titers of 1:64 or greater and trough titers of 1:32 or greater. The predictive values for cure at a titer of 1:8 or greater were 93 percent at peak and 97.5 percent at trough [159]. However, there were many patients with lower titers who were also cured of their infections. Therefore, the serum bactericidal titer alone did not predict who would fail. Because of the limitations of this study and its conclusion that SBTs alone are inadequate to predict the outcome of infective endocarditis, many investigators discourage routine use of SBT in uncomplicated patients who are doing well on recommended conventional therapy (e.g., viridans streptococcal endocarditis due to penicillin-susceptible isolates) [152,157]. The greatest utility of the test appears to be in demonstrating bactericidal activity in patients with unusual organisms and to assess the need for potentially toxic drug combinations.

ROLE OF CARDIAC SURGERY. Although it may at first seem folly to replace a native valve with a prosthetic one in the face of active infection, at times failure of antibiotics to sterilize the blood necessitates surgical debridement and removal of the infected focus—the valve. Similarly, even if bacteriologic cure is achieved, the patient may die of hemodynamic compromise

unless a valve is replaced. The surprisingly favorable outcomes of a number of patients operated on in these desperate circumstances [50,160–164] has led to an examination of the role of cardiac surgery at an earlier point in the course of endocarditis [68,165,166,167].

If the need for surgery could be predicted, it could be performed before severe congestive failure greatly increases its risk. No study has randomly selected patients for operation, and the bias has always been toward reserving surgery for those patients who clearly need it. Thus when the survival of surgically treated patients, who are the sicker ones, exceeds that of patients treated medically, superior therapeutic efficacy can be assumed. The urge to "go the last measure" for the young, previously healthy, or heart-rendingly tragic patient may of course weaken the premise on which this conclusion is based. Whatever guidelines for the probable need for cardiac surgery are devised, it must be remembered that the patient who can do well without valve replacement is spared both the immediate operative mortality and the additional lifelong risks associated with a prosthetic valve. There is an unusually high incidence of paraprosthetic leaks on a mechanical basis, often requiring repeat replacement, in patients whose valve replacements are performed during endocarditis [50,160,165], as well as a roughly 6 percent risk of recurrence of the initial episode of endocarditis [50,163,167].

The indications for surgery already mentioned—microbiologic failure and congestive failure—are now well accepted. Conventional blood cultures should become sterile within 3 to 5 days after the institution of appropriate antibiotic therapy, and patients should defervesce within 9 days [20,50,104,163]. In patients with isolated right-sided lesions, most often addicts, tricuspid valvulectomy without immediate replacement has permitted cure of resistant *Pseudomonas* endocarditis, and not all patients have required subsequent prosthetic valves [38]. In left-sided endocarditis, valve replacement must be performed in the same operation and is followed by a minimum of 4 and more often 6 weeks of potent antibiotics directed at the infecting organism. Fungal endocarditis carries such a certainty of failure of medical therapy that surgery should be undertaken when the diagnosis is established. There is not general agreement as to whether any other organisms fall into this category. Although early surgery has been proposed in all cases of left-sided staphylococcal endocarditis [165], too many patients do well with medical therapy to justify this approach without additional refinement of the indications [104,166]. It would seem desirable, whenever possible, to define the optimal antibiotic regimen for the infecting organism before the new valve is inserted.

Many patients with endocarditis have preexisting congestive failure as a result of their underlying valvular disease, but new onset or worsening heart failure carries an ominous prognosis—a mortality of 49 percent in one series [4]. Significant failure presaging a poor course includes cases that require any therapy other than digitalis. Urgent surgery is indicated for these patients, and a number of authors have noted that medical stabilization may be impossible once severe progressive failure begins [50,68,162,168]. Pathologic studies suggest that coronary artery emboli are a frequent contribution to the sudden catastrophic decompensations that occur in patients with aortic endocarditis and cardiac failure [3,4,5,169]. It cannot be overemphasized that once surgery is clearly indicated, it should not be delayed, because of the unpredictability of the clinical course and the increasing risk of the operation as failure progresses.

The definite visualization of vegetations has been proposed as a criterion for surgery before the onset of hemodynamic decompensation. As previously discussed, vegetations on echocardiography are not in themselves an indication for surgery.

However, echocardiography may be very helpful in defining the presence of complications that do require surgery, including destruction of the valve or extension of infection beyond the valve ring as a myocardial abscess [83]. Myocardial abscess may be the reason for prolonged fever [170], be present as conduction defects [50,65,66,171], or cavitate into the pericardium with resultant purulent pericarditis [171].

Table 88-9, adapted from the review by DiNubile, summarizes indications for surgery in active endocarditis [68]. One of the "major criteria" or three of the "minor criteria" are indicative of a very high likelihood of medical failure and a need for urgent surgery at a later date if not performed early. Individual patient situations may modify the readiness to resort to surgery. For instance, in a patient with another condition that made the risk of general anesthesia prohibitive, such as severe restrictive lung disease, one might elect to operate only for uncontrollable congestive heart failure. The guidelines for surgical intervention are not absolute predictors of failure of medical management but overall can predict a low success rate.

There is surprisingly little difference in the clinical indications for surgery in native and prosthetic valve endocarditis, but the proportion of patients requiring surgery is higher in those with prosthetic valves, approximately 50 percent [68,142,172,173,174]. Early surgical intervention reduces the mortality of prosthetic valve endocarditis [44,175]. It should be stressed that in any patient who displays any of the characteristics enumerated, as well as all patients with staphylococcal or prosthetic valve endocarditis, it is wise early in the course to mention the possibility of a need for surgery to the patient and family, to consult with the cardiac surgical team, and to make provisions to facilitate scheduling of urgent surgery should that become necessary. This may require transfer to a cardiac surgical center of some patients who subsequently do not require an operation, but this is preferable to transporting a patient who has become seriously unstable.

In summary, therapy for endocarditis requires skillful manipulation of antibiotics and careful day-to-day judgment of the relative risks of expectant versus surgical management. We lack rigorously derived answers to many questions because of the relatively low incidence of the disease and the great variability among individual cases when it does occur. Only multicenter collaborative trials can accumulate enough patients to provide valid statistical comparisons of treatment options, and these, extending over several years, can be initiated only to answer the most major questions, using relatively gross but objective end points, such as mortality. Hence we rely heavily on tradition and adhere to conservative approaches to therapy, even while continuously reviewing our experience with this changing disease.

Table 88-9. Criteria for Surgical Intervention in Active Endocarditis

1. Major criteria (Any single criterion necessitates early operation)
   a. Progressive heart failure
   b. Significant heart failure[a]
   c. Multiple embolic episodes
   d. Persistent bacteremia despite appropriate antibiotics
   e. Fungal endocarditis
   f. Extravalvular foreign body
   g. Development of heart block, bundle-branch block, or purulent pericarditis[b]
   h. Prosthetic valve dehiscence or obstruction
   i. Relapse after "adequate" trial[c]
2. Minor criteria (Any three criteria predict a high rate of antibiotic failure with resultant [often sudden and major] complications; surgery should be considered in certain patients even if only two criteria are met)
   a. Congestive heart failure resolved with medical therapy
   b. Single embolus
   c. Definite left-sided vegetations seen on M-mode echocardiography
   d. Early mitral valve closure or flail valve leaflets
   e. Early prosthetic endocarditis caused by other than highly penicillin-sensitive streptococci
   f. Gram-negative rod tricuspid endocarditis
   g. Persistent fever without other identifiable cause
   h. New regurgitant murmur in aortic prosthetic endocarditis
   i. Lack of appropriate cell wall antibiotic

[a] Failure of symptoms and signs of heart failure to resolve after "simple" medical therapy. If heart failure predated endocarditis, "resolution" would imply a return to baseline.
[b] Conduction defects should be persistent and unrelated to drug therapy or ischemic cardiac disease; these should occur in the setting of aortic valve involvement.
[c] "Adequate" here implies the use of the best available antibiotics in the maximum tolerated dosage for a minimum of 6–8 wk.
Source: Adapted from DiNubile MJ: Surgery in active endocarditis. *Ann Intern Med* 96:656, 1982, with permission.

References

1. Rabinovich S, Evans J, Smith IM, et al: A long-term view of bacterial endocarditis, 337 cases 1924 to 1963. *Ann Intern Med* 63:185, 1965.
2. Uwaydah MM, Weinberg AN: Bacterial endocarditis: A changing pattern. *N Engl J Med* 273:1231, 1965.
3. Lerner PI, Weinstein L: Infective endocarditis in the antibiotic era. Parts I-IV. *N Engl J Med* 274:199, 259, 323, 388, 1966.
4. Pelletier LL Jr, Petersdorf RG: Infective endocarditis: A review of 125 cases from the University of Washington Hospitals, 1963–72. *Medicine* 56:287, 1977.
5. Garvey GJ, Neu HC: Infective endocarditis: An evolving disease: A review of endocarditis at the Columbia-Presbyterian Medical Center 1968–1973. *Medicine* 57:105, 1978.
6. Kaplan EL, Rich H, Gersony W, et al: A collaborative study of infective endocarditis in the 1970s: Emphasis on infections in patients who have undergone cardiovascular surgery. *Circulation* 59:327, 1979.
7. Von Reyn CF, Levy BS, Arbeit RD, et al: Infective endocarditis: An analysis based on strict case definitions. *Ann Intern Med* 94:505, 1981.
8. Griffin MR, Wilson WR, Williams ED, et al: Infective endocarditis, Olmsted County, Minnesota, 1950 through 1981. *JAMA* 254:1199, 1985.
9. King JW, Nguyen VQ, Conrad SR: Results of a prospective state-wide reporting system for infectious endocarditis. *Am J Med Sci* 295:517, 1988.
10. King JW, Shehane RR, Lierl J: Infectious endocarditis at three hospitals in the same city: Two studies a decade apart. *South Med J* 79:151, 1986
11. Ernst AL, Claus OS, Tore K: Infective endocarditis 1973–1984. The Bergen University Hospital: Clinical features, treatment and prognosis. *Scand J Infect Dis* 20:239, 1988.
12. Terpenning M, Buggy B, Kauffman C: Infective endocarditis: Clinical features in young and elderly patients. *Am J Med* 83:626, 1987.
13. Weinstein L, Rubin RH: Infective endocarditis—1973. *Prog Cardiovasc Dis* 16:239, 1973.
14. Johnson CM, Rhodes KH: Pediatric endocarditis. *Mayo Clin Proc* 57:86, 1982.
15. Shapiro DS, Kenney SC, Johnson M, et al: *Chlamydia psittaci* endocarditis diagnosed by blood culture. *N Engl J Med* 326:1192, 1992.
16. Osler W: *The Principles and Practice of Medicine* (1892), reprinted. Birmingham, AL, Classics of Medicine Library, 1978, p 592.
17. Finland M, Barnes MW: Changing etiology of bacterial endocarditis in the antibacterial era. *Ann Intern Med* 72:341, 1970.
18. Cherubin CE, Neu HC: Infective endocarditis at the Presbyterian Hospital in New York City from 1938–1967. *Am J Med* 51:83, 1971.

19. Bayliss R, Clarke C, Oakley CM, et al: The microbiology and pathogenesis of infective endocarditis. *Heart* 50:513, 1983.
20. McKinsey DS, Ratts TE, Bisno AL: Underlying cardiac lesions in adults with infective endocarditis, the changing spectrum. *Am J Med* 82:681, 1987.
21. Sussman JI, Baron EJ, Tenenbaum MJ, et al: Viridans streptococcal endocarditis: Clinical, microbiological and echocardiographic correlations. *J Infect Dis* 154:597, 1986.
22. Gossling J: Occurrence and pathogenicity of the *Streptococcus milleri* group. *Rev Infect Dis* 10:257, 1988.
23. Stein D, Kenrad N: Endocarditis due to nutritionally deficient streptococci: Therapeutic dilemma. *Rev Infect Dis* 9:908, 1987.
24. Bouvet A, Acar GF: New bacteriological aspects of infective endocarditis. *Eur Heart J* 5(suppl C):45, 1984.
25. Haroud T, Delbas F: Viridans streptococci in infective endocarditis, species distribution and susceptibility to antibiotics. *Eur Heart J* 5(suppl C):39, 1984.
26. Venezio FR, Gullberg RM, Westenfelder GO, et al: Group G streptococcal endocarditis and bacteremia. *Am J Med* 81:29, 1986.
27. Gallagher P, Watanakunakorn C: Group B streptococcal endocarditis: Report of seven cases and review of the literature 1962–1985. *Rev Infect Dis* 8:175, 1986.
28. Venezio FR, Westenfelder GO, Cook FV, et al: Infective endocarditis in a community hospital. *Arch Intern Med* 142:789, 1982.
29. Panwalker AP: Unusual infections associated with colorectal carcinoma. *Rev Infect Dis* 10:347, 1988.
30. Caputo GM, Archer GL, Calderwood SB, et al: Native valve endocarditis due to coagulase negative staphylococci: Clinical and microbiologic features. *Am J Med* 83:619, 1987.
31. Sanabria TJ, Alpert JS, Goldberg R, et al: Increasing frequency of staphylococcal infective endocarditis: Experience at a university hospital, 1981–1988. *Arch Intern Med* 150:1305, 1990.
32. Geraci JR, Wilson WR: Endocarditis due to gram-negative bacteria. *Mayo Clin Proc* 57:145, 1982.
33. Pesanti E, Smith I: Infective endocarditis with negative blood cultures: An analysis of 52 cases. *Am J Med* 66:43, 1979.
34. Reisberg BE: Infective endocarditis in the narcotics addict. *Prog Cardiovasc Dis* 22:193, 1979.
35. Reyes MP, Lerner AM: Current problems in the treatment of infective endocarditis due to *Pseudomonas aeruginosa*. *Rev Infect Dis* 5:314, 1982.
36. Baddour LM, Meyer J, Henry B: Polymicrobial infective endocarditis in the 1980's. *Rev Infect Dis* 13:963, 1991.
37. Raucher B, Dobkin J, Mandel L, et al: Occult polymicrobial endocarditis with *Haemophilus parainfluenzae* in intravenous drug abusers. *Am J Med* 86:169, 1989.
38. Szabo S, Lieberman JP, Lue YA: Unusual pathogens in narcotic-associated endocarditis. *Rev Infect Dis* 12:412, 1990.
39. Block PC, DeSanctis RW, Weinberg AN, et al: Prosthetic valve endocarditis. *J Thorac Cardiovasc Surg* 60:540, 1970.
40. Slaughter L, Morris JE, Starr A: Prosthetic valve endocarditis: A 12 year review. *Circulation* 47:1319, 1973.
41. Dismukes WE, Karchmer AW, Buckley MJ, et al: Prosthetic valve endocarditis; analysis of 38 cases. *Circulation* 48:365, 1973.
42. Wilson WR, Jaumin PM, Danielson GK, et al: Prosthetic valve endocarditis. *Ann Intern Med* 82:751, 1975.
43. Karchmer AW, Dismukes WE, Buckley MJ, et al: Late prosthetic valve endocarditis. *Am J Med* 64:199, 1978.
44. Saffle JR, Gardner P, Schoenbaum SC, et al: Prosthetic valve endocarditis. *J Thorac Cardiovasc Surg* 73:416, 1977.
45. Watanakunakorn C: Prosthetic valve infective endocarditis. *Prog Cardiovasc Dis* 22:181, 1979.
46. Wright AJ, Wilson WR: Experimental animal endocarditis. *Mayo Clin Proc* 57:10, 1982.
47. Lowy F, Steigbigel NH: Infective endocarditis: III. Prevention of bacterial endocarditis. *Am Heart J* 96:689, 1978.
48. Richards JH: Bacteremia following irritation of foci of infection. *JAMA* 99:1496, 1932.
49. Pruitt AA, Rubin RH, Karchmer AW, et al: Neurologic complication of bacterial endocarditis. *Medicine* 57:329, 1978.
50. Stinson EB: Surgical treatment of active endocarditis. *Prog Cardiovasc Dis* 22:145, 1979.
51. Durack DT, Lukes AS, Bright DK, and the Duke Endocarditis Service: New criteria for the diagnosis of infective endocarditis: Utilization of specific echocardiographic findings. *Am J Med* 96:200, 1994.
52. Hollander G, DeScheerder M, De Buyzere GI, et al: Six years review on 53 cases of infective endocarditis: Clinical, microbiological and therapeutical features. *Acta Cardiol* 43:121, 1988.
53. Hardin RC: The variability of embolic phenomena in subacute bacterial endocarditis. *J Iowa State Med Soc* 31:95, 1941.
54. Holler JW, Pecora JS: Backache in bacterial endocarditis. *NY State J Med* 70:1903, 1970.
55. Willerson JT, Moellering RC Jr, Buckley MJ, et al: Conjunctival petechiae after open-heart surgery. *N Engl J Med* 284:539, 1971.
56. Dowling RH: Sub-ungual splinter haemorrhages. *Postgrad Med J* 40:595, 1964.
57. Kerr A Jr, Tan JS: Biopsies of the Janeway lesion of infective endocarditis. *J Cutan Pathol* 6:124, 1979.
58. Farrior JB, Silverman ME: Consideration of the differences between Janeway's lesion and an Osler's node in infective endocarditis. *Chest* 70:239, 1976.
59. Belli J, Waisbren BA: Number of blood cultures necessary to diagnose most cases of bacterial endocarditis. *Am J Med Sci* 232:284, 1956.
60. Werner AS, Cobbs CG, Kaye D, et al: Studies on the bacteremia of bacterial endocarditis. *JAMA* 202:199, 1967.
61. Washington JA, Ilstrup DM: Blood cultures, issues and controversies. *Rev Infect Dis* 8:792, 1986.
62. Washington JA: The microbiological diagnosis of infective endocarditis. *Antimicrobial Chemotherapy* 20(suppl A):29, 1987.
63. Robin MJ, Cahill N, Gearty G, et al: Q fever endocarditis. *Am J Med* 72:396, 1983.
64. Davis RS, Strom JA, Frishman W, et al: The demonstration of vegetations by echocardiography in bacterial endocarditis: An indication for early surgical intervention. *Am J Med* 69:57, 1980.
65. Wang K, Gobel F, Gleason DF, et al: Complete heart block complicating bacterial endocarditis. *Circulation* 46:939, 1972.
66. Roberts NK, Somerville J: Pathologic significance of electrocardiographic changes in aortic valve endocarditis, abstract. *Br Heart J* 31:395, 1969.
67. Carpenter JL: Perivalvular extension of infection in patients with infective endocarditis. *Rev Infect Dis* 13:127, 1991.
68. DiNubile MJ: Surgery in active endocarditis. *Ann Intern Med* 96:650, 1982.
69. Parker JD, St. John Sutton MG, Martin G, et al, in Remington and Swartz (eds): *Current Clinical Topics in Infectious Diseases,* vol II, Boston, Blackwell Scientific Publications, 246, 1991.
70. Mügge A, Daniel WG, Frank G, et al: Echocardiography in infective endocarditis: Reassessment of prognostic implications of vegetation size determined by the transthoracic and the transesophageal approach. *J Am Coll Cardiol* 14:631, 1989.
71. Erbel R, Rohmann S, Drexler M, et al: Improved diagnostic value of echocardiography in patients with infective endocarditis by transesophageal approach: A prospective study. *Eur Heart J* 9:43, 1988.
72. Birmingham GD, Rahko PS, Ballantyne F: Improved detection of infective endocarditis with transesophageal echocardiography. *Am Heart J* 123:774, 1992.
73. Shapiro SM, Bayer AS: Transesophageal and Doppler echocardiography in the diagnosis and management of infective endocarditis. *Chest* 100:1125, 1991.
74. Seward JB, Khandheria BK, Edwards WD, et al: Biplanar transesophageal echocardigraphy: Anatomic correlations, image orientation, and clinical applications. *Mayo Clin Proc* 65:1193, 1990.
75. Khandheria BK, Oh J: Transesophageal echocardiography state of the art and future directions. *Am J Cardiol* 69:61H, 1992.
76. Werner DG, Erbel R, Kasper W, et al: Safety of transesophageal echocardiography: A multicenter survey of 10,419 examinations. *Circulation* 83:817, 1991.
77. Shively BK, Gurule FT, Roldan CA: Diagnostic value of transesophageal compared with transthoracic echocardiography in infective endocarditis. *J Am Coll Cardiol* 18:391, 1991.
78. Daniel WG, Mügge A, Martin RP, et al: Improvement in the diagnosis of abscesses associated with endocarditis by transesophageal echocardioography. *N Engl J Med* 324:795, 1991.
79. Jaffe WM, Morgan DE, Pearlman AS, et al: Infective endocarditis,

1983–1988: Echocardiographic findings and factors influencing morbidity and mortality. *J Am Coll Cardiol* 15:1227, 1990.

80. Sanfilippo AJ, Picard MH, Newell JB, et al: Echocardiographic assessment of patients with infectious endocarditis: Prediction of risk for complications. *J Am Coll Cardiol* 18:1191, 1991.

81. Steckelberg JM, Murphy JG, Ballard D, et al: Emboli in infective endocarditis: The prognostic value of echocardiography. *Ann Intern Med* 114:635, 1991.

82. Manolis AS, Melita H: Echocardiographic and clinical correlates in drug addicts with infective endocarditis. *Arch Intern Med* 148:2461, 1988.

83. Lutas EM, Roberts RB, Deveraux RB, et al: Relation between the presence of echocardiographic vegetations and the complication rate in infective endocarditis. *Am Heart J* 112:107, 1986.

84. Welton DE, Young JB, Raizner AE, et al: Value and safety of cardiac catheterization during active infective endocarditis. *Am J Cardiol* 44:1306, 1979.

85. Mills J, Abbott J, Utley JR, et al: Role of cardiac catheterization in infective endocarditis. *Chest* 72:576, 1977.

86. Morgan G, Ginks W, Siddons H, et al: Septicemia in patients with an endocardial pacemaker. *Am J Cardiol* 44:221, 1979.

87. Lemire GG, Morin JE, Dobell ARC: Pacemaker infections: A 12 year review. *Can J Surg* 18:181, 1975.

88. Choo MH, Holmes DR, Gersh BJ, et al: Permanent pacemaker infections: Characterization and management. *Am J Cardiol* 48:559, 1981.

89. Case 36—1980: Case records of the Massachusetts General Hospital. *N Engl J Med* 303:628, 1980.

90. Rubin RH, Weinstein L: *Salmonellosis: Microbiologic, Pathologic, and Clinical Features*. New York, Stratton Intercontinental, 1977, p 60.

91. Svanborn M, Gastrin B, Rodriguez L: Transvenous cardiac pacemaker as a focus of *Salmonella* infection in a patient with heart block. *Acta Med Scand* 196:218, 1974.

92. Sande MA, Johnson WD, Hook EW, et al: Sustained bacteremia in patients with prosthetic cardiac valves. *N Engl J Med* 286:1067, 1972.

93. Wilson R, Hamburger M: Fifteen years' experience with *Staphylococcus* septicemia in a large city hospital: Analysis of fifty-five cases in the Cincinnati General hospital 1940–1954. *Am J Med Sci* 22:437, 1957.

94. Shah M, Watanakunakorn C: Changing patterns of *Staphylococcus aureus* bacteremia. *Am J Med Sci* 278:115, 1979.

95. Nolan CM, Beaty HN: *Staphylococcus aureus* bacteremia. *Am J Med* 60:495, 1976.

96. Iannini PB, Crossley D: Therapy of *Staphylococcus aureus* bacteremia associated with a removable focus of infection. *Ann Intern Med* 84:558, 1976.

97. Watanakunakorn C, Tan JS, Phair JP: Some salient features of *Staphylococcus aureus* endocarditis. *Am J Med* 54:473, 1973.

98. Mylotte JM, McDermott C, Spoone JA: Prospective study of 114 consecutive episodes of *Staphylococcus aureus* bacteremia. *Rev Infect Dis* 90:891, 1987.

99. Bayer A, Lam K, Ginzton L, et al: *Staphylococcus aureus* bacteremia: Clinical, serologic and echocardiographic findings in patients with and without endocarditis. *Arch Intern Med* 147:457, 1987.

100. Ehni WF, Reller LB: Short-course therapy for catheter associated *Staphylococcus aureus* bacteremia. *Arch Intern Med* 149:533, 1989.

101. Jernigan JA, Farr BM: Short-course therapy of catheter-related *Staphylococcus aureus* bacteremia: A meta-analysis. *Ann Intern Med* 119:304, 1993.

102. Rahal JJ, Chan YK, Johnson G: Relationship of staphylococcal tolerance, teichoic acid antibody, and serum bactericidal activity to therapeutic outcome in *Staphylococcus aureus* bacteremia. *Am J Med* 81:43, 1986.

103. Raad II, Sabbagh MF: Optimal duration of therapy for catheter-related *Staphylococcus aureus* bacteremia: A study of 55 cases and review. *Clin Infect Dis* 14:75, 1992.

104. Chambers HF, Korzeniowski OM, Sande MA, et al: *Staphylococcus aureus* endocarditis: Clinical manifestations in addicts and non-addicts. *Medicine* 62:170, 1983.

105. Powell DC, Bivins B, Bell RM, et al: Bacterial endocarditis in the critically ill surgical patient. *Arch Surg* 116:311, 1981.

106. Watanakunakorn C, Baird IM: *Staphylococcus aureus* bacteremia and endocarditis associated with a removable infected intravenous device. *Am J Med* 63:253, 1977.

107. Shlaes DM, Levy J, Wolinsky E. Enterococcal bacteremia without endocarditis. *Arch Intern Med* 141:578, 1981.

108. Malone DA, Wagner RA, Myers JP, et al: Enterococcal bacteremia in two large community teaching hospitals. *Am J Med* 81:601, 1986.

109. Bryan CS, Reynolds KL, Brown JJ: Mortality associated with enterococcal bacteremia. *Surg Gynecol Obstet* 160:557, 1985.

110. Maki DG, Agger WA: Enterococcal bacteremia: Clinical features, the risk of endocarditis, and management. *Medicine* 67:248, 1988.

111. Gullberg RM, Homann SR, Phair JP: Enterococcal bacteremia: Analysis of 75 episodes. *Rev Infect Dis* 11:74, 1989.

112. Graninger W, Ragette R: Nosocomial bacteremia due to *Enterococcus faecalis* without endocarditis. *Clin Infect Dis* 15:49, 1992.

113. Megran DW: Enterococcal endocarditis. *Clin Infect Dis* 15:63, 1992.

114. Heimberger TS, Duma RJ: Infections of prosthetic heart valves and cardiac pacemakers. *Infect Dis Clin North Am* 3:221, 1989.

115. Lewis AB, Hayes DL, Holmes DR, et al: Update on infections involving permanent pacemakers: Characterization and management. *J Thorac Cardiovasc Surg* 89:758, 1985.

116. Kennelly BM, Peller LW: Management of infected transvenous permanent pacemakers. *Br Heart J* 36:1133, 1974.

117. Rettig G, Doenecke P, Sen S: Complications with retained transvenous pacemaker electrodes. *Am Heart J* 98:587, 1979.

118. Beeler B: Infections of permanent transvenous and epicardial pacemakers in adults. *Heart Lung* 11:152, 1982.

119. Wohl B, Peters R, Carliner N, et al: Pacemaker pocket infection due to *Staphylococcus epidermidis*: A new clinical entity. *PACE* 5:190, 1982.

120. Morgan G, Ginks W, Siddons H, et al: Septicemia in patients with an endocardial pacemaker. *Am J Cardiol* 44:221, 1979.

121. Kelly PA, Wallace S, Tucker B, et al: Post-operative infection with the automatic implantable cardioverter defibrillator: Clinical presentation and use of the Gallium scan in diagnosis. *PACE* 11:1220, 1988.

122. Wunderly D, Maloney J, Edel T, et al: Infections in implantable cardioverter defibrillator patients. *PACE* 13:1360, 1990.

123. Minowski M, Reid PR, Mower MM, et al: Clinical performance of the implantable cardioverter defibrillator. *PACE* 7:1345, 1984.

124. Alamassi GH, Oinger GN, Troup OJ, et al: Delayed infection of the automatic implantable cardioverter defibrillator: Current recognition and management. *J Thorac Cardiovasc Surg* 95:908, 1988.

125. Bisno AL, Dismukes WE, Durack DT, et al: Antimicrobial treatment of infective endocarditis due to viridans streptococci, enterococci and staphylococci. *JAMA* 261:1471, 1989.

126. Chambers HC: Short-course combination and oral therapies of *Staphylococcus aureus* endocarditis. *Infect Dis Clin North Am* 7:69, 1993.

127. Sande MA, Scheld WM: Combination antibiotic therapy of bacterial endocarditis. *Ann Intern Med* 92:390, 1980.

128. Eliopoulos GH: Aminoglycoside resistant enterococcal endocarditis. *Infect Dis Clin North Am* 7:117, 1993.

129. Rice LB, Calderwood SB, Eliopoulos GM, et al: Enterococcal endocarditis: A comparison of prosthetic and native valve disease. *Rev Infect Dis* 13:1, 1991.

130. Fernandez-Guerro ML, Barros C, Rodriguez Tudela JL, et al: Aortic endocarditis caused by gentamicin-resistant *Enterococcus faecalis*. *Eur J Clin Microbiol Infect Dis* 7:525, 1988.

131. Lipman ML, Silva J Jr.: Endocarditis due to *Streptococcus faecalis* with high-level resistance to gentamicin. *Rev Infect Dis* 11:325, 1989.

132. Eliopoulos GM, Thauvin-Eliopoulos C, Moellering RC: Contribution of animal models in the search for effective therapy for endocarditis due to enterococci with high-level resistance to gentamicin. *Clin Infect Dis* 15:58, 1992.

133. Thauvin C, Eliopoulos GM, Willey S, et al: Continuous-infusion ampicillin therapy of enterococcal endocarditis in rats. *Antimicrob Agents Chemother* 31:139, 1987.

134. Frieden TR, Munsiff SS, Low DE, et al: Emergence of vancomycin-resistant enterococci in New York City. *Lancet* 342:76, 1993.

135. Bisno AL, Dismukes WE, Durack DT, et al: Treatment of infective endocarditis due to viridans streptococci. *Circulation* 63:730, 1981.

136. Wilson WR, Thompson RL, Wilkowske CJ, et al: Short-term therapy for streptococcal infective endocarditis: Combined intramuscular administration of penicillin and streptomycin. *JAMA* 245:360, 1981.

137. Best GK, Koval AV, Best NH: Susceptibility of clinical isolates of *Staphylococcus aureus* to killing by oxacillin. *Can J Microbiol* 21:1692, 1975.

138. Mayhall CG, Medoff G, Marr JJ: Variation in the susceptibility of strains of *Staphylococcus aureus* to oxacillin, cephalothin, and gentamicin. *Antimicrob Agents Chemother* 10:707, 1976.

139. Sabath LD, Wheeler N, Laverdiere M, et al: A new type of penicillin resistance of *Staphylococcus aureus*. *Lancet* 1:443, 1977.

140. Korzeniowski O, Sande MA, National Collaborative Endocarditis Study Group: combination antimicrobial therapy for *Staphylococcus aureus* endocarditis in patients addicted to parenteral drugs and in nonaddicts. *Ann Intern Med* 97:496, 1982.

141. Abrams B, Sklaver A, Hoffman T, et al: Single or combination therapy of staphylococcal endocarditis in intravenous drug abusers. *Ann Intern Med* 90:789, 1979.

142. Archer GL: Antimicrobial susceptibility and selection of resistance among *Staphylococcus epidermidis* isolates recovered from patients with infections of indwelling foreign devices. *Antimicrob Agents Chemother* 14:353, 1978.

143. Karchmer AW, Archer G, Dismukes WE: *Staphylococcus epidermidis* causing prosthetic valve endocarditis: Microbiologic and clinical observations as guides to therapy. *Ann Intern Med* 98:447, 1983.

144. Kaplan AH, Weber DJ, Oddone EZ, et al: Infection due to *Actinobacillus actinomycetemcomitans*. 15 cases and review. *Rev Infect Dis* 11:46, 1989.

145. Schack SH, Smith PW, Penn RG, et al: Endocarditis caused by *Actinobacillus actinomycetemcomitans*. *J Clin Microbiol* 20:579, 1986.

146. Yogev R, Shulman D, Shulman S, et al: In vitro activity of antibiotics alone and in combination against *Actinobacillus actinomycetemcomitans*. *Antimicrob Agents Chemother* 29:179, 1986.

147. Chen Y-C, Chang SC, Luh KT, et al: *Actinobacillus actinomycetemcomitans* endocarditis: A report of four cases and review of the literature. *Q J Med* 81:871, 1991.

148. Francioli PB: Ceftriaxone and outpatient treatment of infective endocarditis. *Infect Dis Clin North Am* 7:97, 1993.

149. Patrick WD, Brown WD, Bowmer MI, et al: Infective endocarditis due to *Eikenella corrodens*: Case report and review of the literature. *Can J Infect Dis* 1:139, 1990.

150. Reller LB, Baines RD, Brandt D, et al: Activity of ceftriaxone against HACEK bacteria and efficacy in treatment of *Haemophilus spp.* endocarditis, in *Programs and Abstracts of the 27th Interscience Conference on Antimicrobial Agents and Chemotherapy*, 1987, abstr 120.

151. Wolfson JS, Swartz MN: Serum bactericidal activity as a monitor of antibiotic therapy. *N Engl J Med* 312:968, 1985.

152. Reller LB: The serum bactericidal test. *Rev Infect Dis* 8:803, 1986.

153. Schlichter JG, MacLean H, Milzer A: Effective penicillin therapy in subacute bacterial endocarditis and other chronic infections. *Am J Med Sci* 217:600, 1949.

154. Stratton CW: Standardization of the serum bactericidal test and its relationship to levels of antimicrobial agents. *Eur J Clin Microbiol* 5:61, 1986.

155. Standiford HC, Tatem BA: Technical aspects and clinical correlations of the serum bactericidal test. *Eur J Clin Microbiol* 5:79, 1986.

156. Hackbarth CJ, Chambers HF, Sande MA: Serum bactericidal titer as a predictor of outcome in endocarditis. *Eur J Clin Microbiol* 5:93, 1986.

157. Mellors JW, Coleman DL, Andriole VT: Value of the serum bactericidal test in management of patients with bacterial endocarditis. *Eur J Clin Microbiol* 5:67, 1986.

158. Jordan GW, Kawachi MM: Analysis of serum bactericidal activity in endocarditis, osteomyelitis and other bacterial infections. *Medicine* 60:49, 1981.

159. Weinstein MP, Stratton CW, Ackley A, et al: Multicenter collaborative evaluation of a standardized serum bactericidal test as a prognostic indicator in infective endocarditis. *Am J Med* 78:262, 1985.

160. Stason WB, DeSanctis RW, Weinberg AN, et al: Cardiac surgery in bacterial endocarditis. *Circulation* 38:514, 1968.

161. Jung JY, Saab SB, Almond CH: The case for early surgical treatment of left-sided primary infective endocarditis: A collective review. *J Thorac Cardiovasc Surg* 70:509, 1975.

162. Stinson EB, Griepp RB, Vosti K, et al: Operative treatment of active endocarditis. *J Thorac Cardiovasc Surg* 71:659, 1976.

163. Boyd AD, Spencer FC, Isom OW, et al: Infective endocarditis: Analysis of 54 surgically treated patients. *J Thorac Cardiovasc Surg* 73:23, 1977.

164. Wilson WR, Danielson GK, Giuliani ER, et al: Valve replacement in patients with active infective endocarditis. *Circulation* 58:585, 1978.

165. Richardson JV, Karp RB, Kirklin JW, et al: Treatment of infective endocarditis: A 10-year comparative analysis. *Circulation* 58:589, 1978.

166. Rapaport E: The changing role of surgery in the management of infective endocarditis. *Circulation* 58:598, 1978.

167. Cukingnan RA Jr, Carey JS, Wittig JH, et al: Early valve replacement in active infective endocarditis: Results and survival. *J Thorac Cardiovasc Surg* 85:163, 1983.

168. Griffin FM Jr, Jones G, Cobbs CG: Aortic insufficiency in bacterial endocarditis. *Ann Intern Med* 76:23, 1972.

169. Brunson JG: Coronary embolism in bacterial endocarditis. *Am J Pathol* 29:689, 1953.

170. Mildvan D, Goldberg E, Berger M, et al: Diagnosis and successful management of septal myocardial abscess: A complication of bacterial endocarditis. *Am J Med Sci* 274:311, 1977.

171. Arnett EN, Roberts WC: Valve ring abscess in active infective endocarditis: Frequency, location, and clues to clinical diagnosis from the study of 95 necropsy patients. *Circulation* 54:140, 1976.

172. Nunez L, de la Llana R, Aguado M, et al: Bioprosthetic valve endocarditis: Indicator for surgical intervention. *Ann Thorac Surg* 35:262, 1983.

173. Rossiter SJ, Stinson EB, Oyer PE, et al: Prosthetic valve endocarditis comparison of heterograft tissue valves and mechanical valves. *J Thorac Cardiovasc Surg* 176:795, 1978.

174. Baumgartner WA, Miller DC, Reitz BA, et al: Surgical treatment of prosthetic valve endocarditis. *Ann Thorac Surg* 35:89, 1983.

175. Calderwood SB, Swinski LA, Waternaux CM, et al: Risk factors for the develpment of prosthetic valve endocarditis. *Ann Thorac Surg* 35:87, 1983.

89. Infections Associated with Vascular Catheters

Suzanne F. Bradley and
Carol A. Kauffman

Medical technology has led to the creation of many intravascular devices for the purpose of fluid and drug administration, hemodynamic monitoring, hemodialysis, and other functions that have greatly improved our ability to deliver care to critically ill patients. With improvements in life-saving technology have come life-threatening complications, including infection. Nosocomial infection as a consequence of medical devices was not perceived as a problem until the latter half of this century [1,2]. It has been estimated that 50% of the 40 million persons hospitalized each year require a vascular catheter [3]. Most patients that develop bacteremia as a serious complication of their hospitalization do so as a consequence of an intravascular device [3–6]. Intensive care unit patients are at great risk of acquiring nosocomial bacteremia as a complication of an intravascular device [5,7]. As many as 35 percent to 45 percent of nosocomial bacteremias occur in intensive care unit patients, who constitute only 10% of the inpatient population [5]. No doubt the percentage of patients requiring intravenous catheters and subsequent problems associated with these catheters will increase as the acuity of the hospital population increases.

Catheter-related infection is common, and most physicians must deal with it frequently. Approaches to catheter-related infection vary widely from institution to institution; many accepted practices may in fact have little scientific basis. Great strides have been made in understanding how catheter-related infection is acquired and how it might be prevented, but many "gray areas" concerning optimum diagnostic methods and treatment still exist. In this chapter, we provide some historical perspective, discuss current areas of controversy, and when appropriate, give some practical recommendations for the management of catheter-related infection.

Pathophysiology

GENERAL. Foreign bodies that penetrate the cutaneous barriers of the host induce a chronic inflammatory response and are coated with proteins such as fibronectin, fibrin, and collagen, as well as immunoglobulins [6,8,9,10]. The coated catheter can then provide a niche for microorganisms that can adhere to it through structures such as fimbriae, adhesins that bind to surface receptors present on some of the coating proteins, or by electromagnetic interactions. Fibronectin in particular provides a binding surface for *Staphylococcus aureus*. Bacteria such as *S. epidermidis* can also "hide" from host phagocytes by lying in catheter crevices, coating themselves with their own slimy glycocalyx, or hiding under the excrescences of other microbes or host cells (biofilm) [9,10]. Catheters that bear thrombus on either their outside or inside surfaces are significantly more likely to yield positive cultures for microorganisms than catheters that have no thrombus formation [11]. The likelihood that a catheter will stimulate thrombus formation increases with the duration of insertion [11].

It has been hypothesized that microorganisms colonizing the skin gain entry primarily along the insertion site. There is a strong correlation between the infecting organism isolated from the catheter and results of microbial cultures obtained from the insertion site [12–19]. In addition, most catheter-related infections are caused by skin flora [12–19]. Additional studies suggest that contamination of the catheter hub and ultimately the internal lumen of the catheter may have a role in the development of catheter-related infection as well [20–24]. Catheter-related infections occur less often as a result of hematogenous seeding from a distant focus of infection [14,18,19].

DIAGNOSIS. Various diagnostic techniques have increased our understanding of how catheter-related infections occur and have improved our ability to identify these important iatrogenic complications as well.

Insertion Site Culture. Various methods have been used in an attempt to differentiate catheter-associated infection from colonization of the catheter. In one study, cultures of the insertion site that grew more than 15 colonies of a microorganism predicted catheter-related infection 66 percent of the time, whereas negative surface cultures correlated with negative catheter cultures 97 percent of the time [21]. Although this method is effective in ruling out catheter-related infection, it is overly sensitive in that all patients with insertion site colonization will not necessarily have catheter-related infections [8,18,21].

Quantitative Blood Culture. Positive blood cultures in a patient without another obvious source of infection are more specific for catheter-related infection than insertion site cultures. Differential quantitation of numbers of microorganisms in blood taken simultaneously from the catheter and from peripheral blood have been used in experimental studies to determine if catheter-associated infection is present [25–31]. Although quantitative blood culture systems, such as the lysis centrifugation system, are commercially available, most clinical laboratories do not routinely perform quantitative blood cultures.

Culturing the Catheter: Which Segment? Documentation of catheter-related infection has been attempted by culturing various segments of the catheter. The optimum choice of segment to be cultured is controversial. Catheters found to have distal thrombus are more likely to be associated with infection than catheters with clean sheaths [9]. On this basis, some investigators suggest culturing the distal tip of the catheter [32]. However, recent studies suggest that the hub and lumen of the catheter may be important in the pathophysiology of catheter-related infection as well [20,32,33]. Cultures from intradermal and intravascular segments yield identical organisms most of the time [34,35], but positive proximal cultures are more predictive of colonization and positive distal cultures more sensitive and specific for infection [34]. The choice of method to culture catheters is often dependent on one's laboratory resources.

Catheter Culture: Quantitative Methods. Catheter segments have been cultured by incubating them in broth overnite. This method is very sensitive in the identification of microorganisms that might colonize or infect a catheter. Because any number of microorganisms can multiply in broth cultures, this method is not effective for determining how many microorganisms are present on a catheter at the time of removal or how those numbers might correlate with the patient's clinical condition [35]. Agitation of the catheter in broth followed by serial dilution and quantitation of microbial growth by pour plate methods can accurately determine the numbers of microorganisms present on a catheter or within the lumen at the time of removal [35,36,37]. Even though accurate, these methods are not practical.

Catheter Culture: Semiquantitative Methods. Rolling a segment of catheter on agar is a less time consuming and effective semiquantitative method to determine numbers of microbes present on a catheter. In studies by Maki et al., the results of this method were comparable to those of a quantitative broth method [38]. The presence of 15 or more colonies on an agar plate correlated significantly with the presence of local inflammation or signs and symptoms of septicemia [38–41]. These guidelines are still empiric because patients with a clinical course compatible with catheter-related infection may have fewer colonies, and cultures from asymptomatic patients may yield more than 15 colonies. Although this method is simpler than broth methods, some infections might be missed because only the external portion of the catheter is cultured, not the hub or lumen [32,33,41].

Direct Examination of Catheter Segments. The diagnosis of catheter-related infection might be achieved more rapidly by direct microscopic examination. In experimental studies, catheter segments have been placed on a slide, stained with Gram's stain or acridine orange, and the number of microbes assessed under oil immersion [42,43,44]. Such a rapid method potentially could allow early diagnosis of catheter-related infection, but although direct staining appears to be simple and inexpensive, a trained observer is required. Although all of these methods have been devised to improve our detection of catheter-related infections, one study has shown that only positive blood cultures had a significant impact on decision-making by physicians [45].

Summary. Although multiple laboratory methods have been used to try to definitively differentiate catheter-related contamination, colonization, and infection, each has its shortcomings, and no "gold standard" exists. Catheter tip cultures by the "roll-plate method" have gained the greatest acceptance by microbiology personnel because of the simplicity, low cost, and ease of interpretation. Catheter-related infection is still primarily a clinical diagnosis based on the presence of signs and symptoms of infection in a patient with an intravascular device in place from which pathogenic organisms have been isolated.

DEFINITIONS. The development of a warm, tender, erythematous, sometimes purulent site of current or recent venous or arterial catheter placement is commonly assumed to be caused by infection. In fact, the likelihood of infection is much greater in patients with phlebitis, but other causes such as a localized host response to the catheter itself or to the infusate are more common. In turn, many catheters yield microorganisms on culture, but their presence does not necessarily correlate with the presence of clinical signs and symptoms. Adherence to stan-dardized definitions of catheter-related infection by authors is critical if the reader is to make informed comparisons between the myriad of studies that have been performed in this area. Although definitions may vary slightly from investigator to investigator, some consensus has been reached in recent years [46–49].

Colonization. The patient has no signs and symptoms of infection, i.e., pain, erythema, swelling, warmth, or discharge from the catheter site, but a routine surveillance culture is found to have fewer than 15 colonies of an organism present by semiquantitative culture.

Catheter-Related Infection. The patient has a clinical syndrome compatible with local or systemic infection and semiquantitative cultures with 15 or more colonies present. Although suggestive, a positive culture from the catheter is not definitive evidence that a catheter-related infection is causing the patient's symptoms.

Catheter-Related Bacteremia or Fungemia. Microorganisms found in the blood of a patient are also present on the catheter as measured by semiquantitative cultures. There is no other clinical evidence that the organism may emanate from a focus of infection other than the catheter.

Infusate-Related Bacteremia or Fungemia. The infusate and the patient's blood are positive for the same organism. The catheter may or may not be positive.

Contamination. The inadvertent introduction of microorganisms while obtaining a catheter segment for culture.

THE ROLE OF THE CATHETER

Catheter Materials. Catheter-related factors that may be important in the development of thrombophlebitis and infection include material, length, and diameter [46,47]. After World War II, plastic (polyethylene) catheters were introduced for the administration of fluids and blood [50,51,52]. Rates of thrombophlebitis with these early plastic catheters were very high [50,51]. Plastic catheters were temporarily supplanted by steel scalp-vein needles introduced in the 1950s; these devices were less often associated with phlebitis, local infection, or bacteremia [53,54,55]. Newer small Teflon catheters eventually supplanted steel scalp vein needles even though there was a somewhat greater risk of phlebitis [56]. Studies have shown that bacteria have the least affinity for steel needles, followed by Teflon catheters, polyvinylchloride, and polyethylene plastic catheters [57,58]. More recently, polyetherurethane and silicone elastomer (polytetrafluoroethylene) catheters, which are smoother, more flexible, more hydrophilic, and less thrombogenic than Teflon, have been made available [59,60,61].

Investigators have also attempted to further reduce the likelihood of infection by bonding disinfectants and antibiotics directly to the catheter. Penicillins, cephalosporins, silver nitrate, iodine, chlorhexidine-silver sulfadiazine, and sodium bisulfite have been bonded to catheters with or without the presence of carrier substances such as benzalkonium, polyvinylpyrrolidone, tridodecylmethylammonium (TDMAC), heparin, or graphite [62–66]. Because most of the antimicrobial activity of these catheters dissipates within the first 48 hours, the maximum benefit from the use of these catheters is seen shortly after insertion. Significant reductions in catheter colonization and bacteremia by gram-positive cocci and gram-negative rods have been demonstrated in in vitro studies and in animal models [62–66].

Semipermanent Catheters. In the 1970s, Broviac et al. introduced a cuffed, silicone rubber central venous catheter for the purpose of hyperalimentation, and Hickman devised a similar catheter of larger gauge that would allow the administration and withdrawal of more viscous blood products [67–77]. The double-lumen catheter resulted when both Hickman and Broviac catheters were combined for the purpose of infusing total parenteral nutrition solutions as well as other drugs [73,74]. Although the risk of infection with a semipermanent catheter appears to be low, its routine use in the intensive care setting is not practical [76,78].

Pulmonary Artery Catheters. The percutaneously inserted pulmonary artery catheter allows both drawing of blood and measuring of cardiac output by thermodilution of fluids administered at the proximal port, pressure monitoring at the distal port, and the simultaneous administration of hyperalimentation, drugs, or fluids at the medial port. The risk of infection appears to be low in those patients in whom the catheter requires little manipulation and is left in place for less than 72 hours [79–85]. However, the risk of pulmonary artery catheter colonization, infection, and associated sepsis increases significantly when the catheter is left in longer than 72 hours [80–85]. Rates of catheter-related sepsis vary widely from study to study [80–85]. Determination of prior colonization of the insertion site, the catheter hub, the catheter tip, or the proximal extravascular portion of the catheter was helpful in differentiating infection from colonization in two studies, but cultures of the catheter tip were not useful in another study [83,84,85]. Autopsy evidence of right-sided endocardial damage has been noted in 36 percent to 53 percent of patients with pulmonary artery catheters, and subsequent endocarditis has developed in 7 percent to 10 percent of these patients [82,86,87].

Multi-Lumen Catheters. In patients who do not require hemodynamic monitoring, triple-lumen catheters may be used for total parenteral nutrition, drugs, and fluids. As with pulmonary artery catheters, there appears to be little risk of catheter-related infection if the catheter is removed by 72 hours [88–92]. Multi-lumen catheters instead of single-lumen catheters may be required by patients with more severe illness, medication needs, and poor venous access [89]. In some studies, multi-lumen catheters have been associated more often with colonization [88,89,92,95], infection [93,94], and sepsis [81,85] than single-lumen catheters. There is a trend for increased rates of multi-lumen catheter-associated sepsis with prolonged duration of catheterization [90,95]. A few studies have suggested that patients receiving total parenteral nutrition through multi-lumen catheters are at greater risk of colonization or infectious complications [89,93,95], but this hypothesis has not been confirmed by others [94,96]. No significant differences in catheter materials or the gauge of the catheter used have been noted that might account for differences seen between single- and multi-lumen catheters [89]. Although these studies yield conflicting results, it would appear that the greatest risk of the multi-lumen catheter is not the catheter itself but the frequent manipulations that are required in the care of critically ill patients. In one study only one of three lumens was used in most of the multi-lumen catheters that were inserted [94]. We recommend limiting the care of these multi-lumen lines to a few well-trained personnel (the intensive care unit staff or TPN [total parenteral nutrition] team), especially if hyperalimentation is required, to change to a single-lumen line if all the ports are no longer needed, and to use these types of catheters predominantly in patients in the intensive care setting.

Arterial Catheters. Contrary to early reports, as indwelling arterial catheters have been used more frequently, they appear to have rates of complications similar to those for venous catheters [97–107]. It has been estimated that thrombosis complicates as many as 19 percent to 38 percent of arterial catheterizations, whereas infection may occur in as many as 4 percent to 23 percent of patients with arterial catheters in place [97–100]. Signs and symptoms of infection in arterial catheters are similar to those for venous catheters except that the presence of distal embolic lesions and hemorrhage are highly predictive of arterial catheter-related sepsis [98,99,100]. Band and Maki have warned that the absence of local signs of inflammation does not preclude arterial catheter-related infection [100]. Late complications such as pseudoaneurysm and even rupture of the artery may occur [104].

It has been suggested that limiting the duration of catheterization to less than 4 days may be an important factor in reducing arterial catheter thrombosis, colonization, local infection, and septicemia [100,101,102]. Although some studies have found no increase in the rate of septicemia when catheterization is extended beyond 4 days, several have noted significant local colonization and infection of the catheter [103,105,106]. As with pulmonary artery and multi-lumen catheters, it is difficult to assess whether the arterial catheter itself, or more likely the increased use of in-line devices, infusates, and other manipulations needed in the critically ill patient, increase the risk of infection.

THE ROLE OF THE INSERTION SITE

Local Skin Flora. Regardless of the type of catheter inserted, the major risk factor for the development of catheter-related infection is the breach of a major host defense against infection, the skin. Catheter-related infections are usually due to normal skin flora, particularly aerobic gram-positive cocci such as *S. epidermidis* and *S. aureus* [108,109]. However, it should be recognized that the distribution of microorganisms on the skin of even healthy hosts varies. *S. aureus* may be found in the axillae and perineums of carriers, and aerobic gram-negative bacilli, *Candida* species, and anaerobes are increased in the groin area and on the lower extremities [108,109,110].

The ecology of normal human flora is further altered by illness, hospitalization, and the presence of foreign bodies [110,111,112]. Hospitalized patients are at increased risk of oropharyngeal colonization with gram-negative bacilli [113]. The use of antimicrobial agents may inhibit the growth of normal flora and allow the emergence of gram-negative bacilli, *S. aureus*, and yeasts [110]. Patients with productive coughs or tracheostomies may contaminate their skin with organisms from their respiratory tract [111]. The presence of a foreign body (the catheter) may predispose the patient to become colonized with *S. aureus* [112,114].

Choice of Insertion Site. The site of catheter insertion may influence the patient's risk of infection [36,46,59,115–119]. Central venous catheters inserted in the internal jugular vein may become infected more often than catheters inserted in the subclavian vein, perhaps because of difficulties in dressing the area and contamination with respiratory secretions [85,115,116,119,120]. Catheter insertion in the lower extremities has generally been avoided because of its intrinsic "dirtiness" and because of difficulties in keeping the site clean [111]. In addition, peripheral vascular occlusive disease is greatest in the lower extremities where poor blood supply might also increase the patient's risk of infection [46,108,109]. Although it has not been shown conclusively that femoral lines are at greater risk of infection than lines in upper extremities, their placement should be a last resort in emergent situations where no other means of vascular access is available [95,116]. These lines should be used temporarily and removed as soon as possible.

Insertion Techniques. How the catheter is inserted may also be an important determining factor in the development of infection. Catheter-related phlebitis and infection are more likely to occur when inserted by inexperienced personnel than by an intravenous therapy team or trained personnel [1,49,117,121,122]. In early studies, arterial and venous catheters were inserted by cutdown, until it was determined that catheters that were placed percutaneously were less likely to become infected [100,123,124,125].

To limit the tracking of bacteria from the skin insertion site along the catheter, other surgical procedures such as tunneling or subcutaneous ports were developed for semipermanent central venous indwelling catheters [76,125–128]. Central venous catheters inserted percutaneously are probably no more likely to become infected than surgically implanted catheters if strict attention is paid to aseptic technique [126]. Infection of subcutaneous implantable devices occurs infrequently (0.01–0.1 infections per 100 patient-days), but mechanical complications are frequent, occurring in 10 percent to 25 percent of catheters inserted [76,127].

Dacron cuffs have been used as an additive method to impede the entry of skin flora along the insertion site of Hickman and Broviac catheters [127]. More recently, attachable biodegradable collagen cuffs impregnated with silver ions have been used in the percutaneous insertion of central venous catheters. In two studies, these cuffs significantly reduced the likelihood of catheter-related colonization (8%–9% vs. 29%–35%) and septicemia (0%–1% vs. 4%–14%) [129,130]. The silver-impregnated cuffs are expensive, but their antimicrobial activity appears to be efficacious. Catheter-related infection rates may also be reduced by ensheathing the catheter in a protective sterile sleeve [131]. Although sheathing devices and silver-impregnated cuffs may ultimately prove to be cost-effective, we have little information on which to base a strong recommendation for or against these items at this time.

PREPARATION OF THE INSERTION SITE

Disinfection of the Insertion Site. Many different methods have been used in an attempt to reduce microbial contamination at the insertion site of the catheter. The effect of disinfection of the skin by 70% alcohol, 2% aqueous chlorhexidine, or 10% povodine-iodine solution before catheter insertion has been assessed. In one study, catheter-associated infection and bacteremia occurred least often in the group treated with chlorhexidine (2.3 and 0.5 per 100 catheters) as compared with alcohol (7.1 and 2.3 per 100 catheters) and povidone-iodine (9.3 and 2.6 per 100 catheters) [132]. The success of chlorhexidine might be attributable to antimicrobial activity that persists longer than that for the other two agents. Other methods of insertion site preparation such as "defatting" the skin with acetone have been shown to be of little benefit in preventing infection [133]. Although the chlorhexidine data are interesting, further studies should clarify whether it will become the disinfectant of choice.

Prophylactic Use of Systemic Antibiotics. The use of systemic antibiotics as prophylaxis before the placement of central venous devices has been suggested. However, it has been shown that many patients develop infection despite being on appropriate antimicrobial therapy [100]. In cancer patients, the use of antimicrobial agents was shown to be effective in preventing exit site infection after Hickman catheter placement in one study, but it did not prevent catheter-related sepsis in bone marrow transplant patients after the insertion of central venous catheters or in cancer patients requiring hepatic artery catheterization [107,134,135]. In light of these studies, we do not advocate the routine use of prophylactic systemic antibiotics.

LOCAL CARE OF THE INSERTION SITE AND CATHETER

Antimicrobial Ointments. Protection of the catheter site by antimicrobial ointments has been advocated. Infection and bacteremia associated with venous cutdowns appear to be reduced with the use of an ointment containing polymyxin B, neomycin, and bacitracin [124]. Some, but not all, studies of percutaneous catheters suggest that the use of this ointment might decrease colonization, and in some instances infection, especially against *S. aureus,* when compared with a placebo group [136–139]. Polymyxin B, neomycin, and bacitracin ointment also appear to be more effective against staphylococci than povidone-iodine ointment [134]. Emergence of *Candida* colonization after the use of bacitracin, neomycin, and polymyxin B has been noted in all studies [129,136–139]. Povidone-iodine ointment has been used primarily with hyperalimentation and arterial catheters, although there is little evidence that it is effective [118,139]. Mupirocin ointment has excellent activity against staphylococci, but its usefulness will probably be limited by the rapid development of resistance [140]. Although the use of an ointment at the insertion site has become an accepted practice, no specific recommendation regarding the choice of ointment can be made at this time.

Local Care of the Catheter and Hub. If catheter-related infection begins at the catheter hub, then alternative methods to prevent infection might be necessary. In one study, the interiors of catheter hubs, contaminated in vitro with *S. epidermidis, P. aeruginosa,* or *C. parapsilosis,* were routinely swabbed with chlorhexidine alone, chlorhexidine plus 70% ethanol, 70% or 95% ethanol alone, or saline [141]. The ethanol-containing solutions were the most effective means of disinfecting the catheters. In addition, the in situ decontamination of catheters has been attempted by the local irrigation of the catheter with a combination of chlorine dioxide and cefazolin or vancomycin and heparin [24,142,143]. These concepts have not been sufficiently explored, and we do not currently recommend that they be done.

Dressing the Insertion Site. Traditional gauze and tape bandages may be uncomfortable and limit the ability of health care personnel to monitor the insertion site without frequent manipulation and the inherent risk of possibly contaminating the site in the process. Transparent semipermeable polyurethane dressings eliminate the problems seen with gauze, but have been associated with trapping of moisture and body fluids underneath the bandage. In several studies of peripheral and central venous catheters, increases in insertion site colonization, local infection, and bacteremia were seen when transparent dressings were compared with gauze dressings [144–147]. However, in other studies of peripheral and central venous catheters, no significant differences in colonization were seen when either gauze or transparent dressings were used [148,149]. The benefits of improved monitoring of the insertion site and decreased manipulation of the catheter with the use of transparent dressings must be weighed against the potential for increased infection for individual patients. Such decisions should be made in conjunction with intravenous therapy teams and nursing staff.

THE ROLE OF THE INFUSION SET. Although early recommendations were to change the infusion set every 24 hours, subsequent studies found that changing the infusion set every 48 hours and ultimately every 72 hours resulted in no significant increase in infection but led to a significant decrease in cost [150–153]. Exceptions to these recommendations include lines used in the administration of blood products, lipid emulsions, arterial pressure monitoring, or if an outbreak related to the use of an infusate is suspected. Under these circumstances, sets should be changed every 24 hours [150,153]. Because the catheter hub may be a significant site for the introduction of infection, future emphasis on changing the design of infusion sets to reduce the possibility of contamination by the hands of personnel may be of great benefit to the patient.

THE ROLE OF IN-LINE DEVICES. In-line devices may also be a significant source of catheter-related infection. Pressure transducers have been implicated as sources of outbreaks of catheter-related bacteremia, particularly caused by water-associated gram-negative bacilli, including *Pseudomonas, Serratia, Enterobacter, Citrobacter,* and *Acinetobacter* [154–162]. Reusable transducer domes could not be sterilized effectively despite various recommendations including the use of glutaraldehyde or ethylene oxide, and infection developed even with the use of disposable domes when other components of the transducer were improperly cleaned [157,159]. Stopcocks are easily contaminated by the constant manipulation by hands of personnel or by injection with contaminated syringes [97,102,159,163]. Disposable transducer domes, stopcocks, and other in-line devices should be changed with the rest of the infusion set as just outlined.

THE ROLE OF THE INFUSATE

Infusates: Local Effects. Intravenous solutions and drugs that are acidic, hypertonic (>600 mOsm/l) (hypertonic glucose, amino acids, lipids), or directly irritative to vascular endothelium (potassium chloride, antibiotics, chemotherapeutic agents, and others) may lead to a local inflammatory response, thrombosis, and phlebitis, with an increased risk of infection, particularly in small-caliber peripheral veins [59,61]. If such solutions are necessary, the risk of complications may be reduced by infusion through large-caliber vessels, or possibly with the addition of heparin or hydrocortisone to the solution [59,61]. In addition, some investigators have suggested the use of vasodilators, such as a glyceryl trinitrate patch [61].

Contamination of Infusates. In addition, infection may occur by the direct contamination of intravenous solutions. In the 1970s, epidemics of bacteremia and sepsis occurred primarily related to defects in the design of elastomer screw tops on glass bottles, which allowed the introduction of microorganisms into intravenous solutions [164–168]. Some aerobic gram-negative bacilli, such as *Enterobacter, Klebsiella, Serratia, Citrobacter,* and *Erwinia* species, are particularly adept at proliferating in the acid environment of intravenous fluids containing minimal nutrients such as dextrose [164–169]. Other organisms, such as *Candida* species, have a propensity to grow in hypertonic TPN solutions [170–175]. The addition of albumin directly to TPN solutions increases the growth of bacteria and fungi, and the addition of fat emulsions has been associated with the growth of corynebacteria, gram-positive cocci, and *Malasezzia furfur* [171–176]. Although contamination with microorganisms during manufacture now occurs rarely, breaks in sterile technique by hospital personnel continue to be an important factor in causing

sporadic outbreaks of infusion-related bacteremia, particularly with gram-positive cocci and other skin flora [163,166].

In-Line Filters. In-line millipore filters to remove microorganisms and other particulate debris that might contribute to the development of phlebitis and infection have been tried [177–180]. Although the use of in-line filters reduced the incidence of phlebitis, the filters clogged frequently, impeded the infusate flow, and required changing every 24 hours [177,178,179]. Although these filters led to a decline in the rate of phlebitis, few studies showed a decline in the rate of infection, and their use is not recommended [180].

CATHETER REPLACEMENT

General Guidelines. Phlebitis is a well-recognized harbinger of infection [1]. Although the presence of phlebitis at a catheter insertion site is not an absolute indication of the presence of catheter-related infection, the consequences of misdiagnosing catheter-related infection are severe enough to make removal of a catheter mandatory when patients have alternative access sites [47,59]. Some exception may be made for the patient with poor access who is dependent on the surgically implanted central catheter. Under those circumstances, a trial of antimicrobial therapy with or without the use of thrombolytics to dissolve associated thrombus in an attempt to save the catheter is reasonable [6,49,68,69–74,77,78,181]. It should be recognized that tunnel infections and infection with some microorganisms, particularly *Candida, Pseudomonas,* and *S. aureus,* may be very difficult, if not impossible, to treat [48,71,72]. If the patient's clinical condition deteriorates despite therapy, significant drug toxicity develops, or bacteremia/fungemia persists, then salvage therapy of the semipermanent catheter should be abandoned [48,77].

After 72 hours, complications of peripheral venous catheter insertion such as thrombus formation (15%–20%), phlebitis (30%–70%), catheter colonization (27%–50%), catheter-related infection (5%–17%), and bacteremia (0%–4%) increase [1,8,11, 50,51,56,59,122,182]. Pulmonary artery catheter insertion sites become colonized or local infection develops in as many as 16 percent to 30 percent of patients, but septicemia occurs in only 1 percent to 5 percent of patients. However, the risk of infection is greatest for patients in whom catheters are left in place for more than 72 hours [48,80,82,83,85,119,131]. Overall, rates of local infection for arterial catheter insertion sites range from 4 percent to 18 percent, and bacteremia may result in 4 percent of patients, but the overall likelihood of infection increases markedly in adult patients with arterial catheters left in place for more than 96 hours [47,48,97,100,119].

Recommendations for routine replacement of these catheters are based on these studies [183]. Peripheral venous catheters and pulmonary artery catheters should be changed every 72 hours, and arterial lines should be changed every 96 hours. For percutaneous central venous catheters, which are not used for blood draws or pressure monitoring, the maximum duration of catheterization that can be attained without a significant increase in risk to the patient is unknown [47,118,125]. Under these circumstances the routine rotation of a central catheter to a different site is not warranted because the increased risks of pneumothorax, laceration of the vessel with hemothorax, and cardiac arrhythmias are well known [184,185].

The Role of the Guidewire. Considerable controversy exists as to whether central catheter-related infection might be prevented by changing the catheter over a guidewire at regular intervals [93,184–191]. Bozzetti et al. found a significant decline in colonization rates, local infection, and sepsis compared with historical controls if central venous catheters were changed weekly [186]. In a comparison between guidewire replacement and changing the catheter site every 3 days, two groups of investigators found an increased risk of bloodstream infection in the guidewire group and an increased risk of insertion complications in the site change group [184,185]. In burn patients, catheters that were changed over a guidewire at 3 days became colonized more often than catheters that remained in place for the 7-day duration of the study [190]. A large study assessing the effect of not changing catheters, changing every 7 days over a guidewire, or changing the site every 7 days showed no difference in the risk of infection among these three methods [191]. If culture of the catheter after guidewire change demonstrates organisms, the newly placed catheter is almost assuredly infected and must be removed [188]. Given the lack of benefit of guidewire changes in preventing infection, we recommend leaving a central venous catheter in place unless signs and symptoms of infection develop. Under those circumstances, the catheter should be removed and a new catheter inserted at another site.

Microbiology of Catheter-Related Infection

Coagulase-negative staphylococci (including *S. epidermidis* and other species) are most commonly implicated in catheter-related infections, followed by *S. aureus,* a variety of aerobic gram-negative bacilli, other gram-positive cocci and bacilli, and *Candida* and other yeasts [34,48,120,192,193]. In some series, coagulase-negative staphlyococci have been found twice as often as *S.aureus* [34,120], but in others they have been implicated with equal frequency [192].

The type of catheter (central versus peripheral) influences the organism found as the cause of infection. *Candida* are found most often in infections related to central venous catheters, and *S. aureus* and coagulase-negative staphylococci cause infection in association with both peripheral and central venous catheters [48,193]. *Candida* and *Malasezzia* infections most often occur in patients receiving TPN [175,176,194]. Infections with gram-negative bacilli have been associated with contaminated infusate but also occur after infection of the catheter insertion site for both peripheral and central venous catheters [164–169,192,193].

Although most common, coagulase-negative staphylococci are associated with less severe disease than *S. aureus* and *Candida*. The latter two organisms are most likely to cause complications, such as suppurative thrombophlebitis, endocarditis, metastatic infections, and sustained sepsis.

Complications of Catheter-Related Infection

Despite improvements in catheter care, it has been estimated that approximately 30,000 cases of catheter-related sepsis occur each year in the United States, at a cost of $4000 to $6000 in additional cost per patient [192,195–198]. In one study, major complications included septic shock (12%), sustained septicemia (12%), suppurative thrombophlebitis (7%), metastatic infection (5%), endocarditis (2%) and arteritis (2%) (192). Com-

plicated catheter-related septicemia may require aggressive management combining appropriate antimicrobial therapy as well as surgical intervention.

SUPPURATIVE PHLEBITIS. Catheter-associated infection is the most common cause of suppurative thrombophlebitis in the modern era [199–213]. Patients with burns or those who have required cutdowns or hyperalimentation are at the greatest risk of developing suppurative phlebitis [202,205,208,210]. Patients usually present with fever, positive blood cultures, and a history of catheter placement, but signs of phlebitis—pain, redness, and swelling—may be absent [202–205,207,208].

In a febrile patient in whom suppurative phlebitis is suspected, healed insertion sites require exploration by needle aspiration or incision; purulent material may occasionally be expressed if the vein is "milked" [203,205,207]. If gross purulence is present or sepsis persists despite adequate antibiotic therapy, excision of the vein has been advocated instead of venous interruption or excision of the thrombus alone because those procedures probably do not treat proximal infection [201,204–208]. Suppurative complications of central veins, particularly of the subclavian veins and superior vena cava, have increased with the use of central venous catheters [210,211]. Because any of the surgical procedures recommended in the management of peripheral suppurative thrombophlebitis are technically difficult in the treatment of central venous infection, therapy of this infection is controversial.

ENDOCARDITIS. Endocarditis is one of the most dreaded complications of catheter-related infection, occurring after the use of peripheral as well as central catheters (see Chap. 88). The aortic and mitral valves are involved most often; presumably "normal" valves as well as those damaged from congenital, rheumatic, and degenerative diseases may be infected [214]. Right atrial catheters that cross the tricuspid valve may cause endothelial damage and turbulence, predisposing the patient to the development of right-sided endocarditis if transient bacteremia or fungemia occurs [215,216,217]. Persistent or intermittent bacteremia or fungemia despite catheter removal along with evidence of pulmonary, cutaneous, central nervous system, or visceral emboli by physical or laboratory examination suggests the possible diagnosis of endocarditis. If complications of endocarditis are suggested, echocardiography may be useful in determining the valves involved and their function, the size of the vegetation, and the presence of myocardial abscesses, information that is necessary if surgical intervention is anticipated [218]. Although transesophageal echocardiography has greatly improved the detection of vegetations, especially on right-sided lesions, endocarditis remains a diagnosis established by persistently positive blood cultures. Even if endocarditis is not present, metastatic foci to bone and visceral organs may occur as a consequence of *S. aureus* bacteremia with significant morbidity and mortality [192,219,220].

Treatment of Catheter-Related Infection

Treatment depends on the infecting microorganism, the type of catheter, and the patient. In general, the catheter should be removed because it serves as a persistent nidus of infection [1,18]. In the case of semipermanent central catheters in febrile patients with limited vascular access, treatment of some forms of catheter-associated infection, predominantly exit site infection, with antibiotics alone and without the removal of the catheter has been accomplished [181]. Success has most always been with coagulase-negative staphylococcal infections, whereas infections due to *S. aureus, Candida,* and gram-negative bacilli almost always require catheter removal [72]. If the patient continues to have persistent fever, bacteremia, and evidence of local infection despite 48 hours of appropriate antibiotic therapy, then the catheter should be removed [181]. If the patient responds to therapy, most investigators recommend treating bacteremia with a course of intravenous therapy for 2 weeks. Even with coagulase-negative staphylococci, recurrence of infection is common after treatment unless the catheter is removed [221].

In the febrile patient in whom catheter-related septicemia is suspected, one should treat with antimicrobial agents, such as vancomycin and gentamicin, that cover both gram-positive cocci and gram-negative bacilli. Vancomycin is chosen most frequently because not only does it have excellent anti-staphylococcal and anti-streptococcal activity; it is the only agent consistently active against methicillin-resistant strains of *S. aureus* and coagulase-negative staphylococci, which predominate in many tertiary care centers. Aminoglycosides have been shown to be highly effective therapy, when compared with beta-lactam antibiotics used as monotherapy, in the treatment of gram-negative bacillary septicemia and should be used as a component of initial empiric therapy of catheter-related sepsis while awaiting the results of cultures [222].

In the setting of catheter-associated coagulase-negative staphylococcal bacteremia, it is unclear how long a patient must be treated if the catheter is promptly removed. In contrast to *S. aureus* and *Candida,* coagulase-negative staphylococci have a rare propensity to cause metastatic foci of infection unless prosthetic devices or other foreign bodies are in place. Although some authorities recommend no treatment once the catheter is removed [15], many physicians prefer to treat with a brief course (usually 10–14 days) of an appropriate anti-staphylococcal antibiotic based on antimicrobial susceptibilities. Persistently positive blood cultures despite catheter removal, especially in susceptible hosts, would mandate longer treatment and a search for a focus of infection [216,217,223,224].

There is considerable debate concerning the appropriate length of therapy for catheter-associated *S. aureus* bacteremia. If the catheter is promptly removed, *S. aureus* infection is often treated with a minimum of 2 weeks of a penicillinase-resistant beta-lactam antibiotic, first-generation cephalosporin, or vancomycin, if the patient is allergic to penicillins or cephalosporins or if the organism is methicillin resistant. The recommendation of "short-course" (2-week) therapy was made recognizing that some persons with transient *S. aureus* bacteremia and prompt removal of the catheter source might be at less risk of complications of endocarditis and metastatic foci than persons with prolonged bacteremia and sources of infection that could not be removed [225,226]. However, it should be recognized that even if persons with catheter-associated *S. aureus* bacteremia appear to be candidates for short-course therapy and receive 2 weeks of treatment, they may still develop metastatic foci or endocarditis [219,220,227]. Raad and Sabbagh, in a retrospective review, found that patients with bacteremia or fever persisting greater than 3 days after catheter removal and initiation of antibiotic therapy were at high risk for complications and required a longer course (4–6 weeks) of anti-staphylococcal therapy [228]. In fact, several authorities question whether short-course therapy of *S. aureus* bacteremia is safe [227,229,230]. We recommend short course (2 weeks) of intravenous anti-staphylococcal therapy only if the catheter is

removed immediately, the patient defervesces promptly, resolution of bacteremia is documented by repeatedly negative blood cultures, and no metastatic foci are found.

Catheter-related sepsis due to gram-negative bacilli requires treatment with antibiotics to which the microorganisms have been shown to be susceptible. Organisms such as *Pseudomonas* and *Xanthomonas* may be especially difficult to treat, particularly in the immunocompromised host [28,231]. Most times, an aminoglycoside, third-generation cephalosporin, or extended spectrum penicillin will be required, and on some occasions combination therapy is appropriate. Those organisms likely to develop resistance on monotherapy (*P. aeruginosa, Enterobacter,* or *Serratia*) should also be treated with both an aminoglycoside and a beta-lactam antibiotic.

The appropriate treatment of catheter-associated infections caused by *C. albicans* and other yeasts has been debated extensively in the literature [232–237]. Removal of the catheter is the first step in effective treatment. Although early studies implied that catheter removal alone was effective therapy for fungemia [232], recent data question this concept. The possibility that the organism has seeded to distant sites, especially retina, bones, and other organs, is high and the consequences of infection in those sites may be catastrophic [233,234,237]. Current recommendations from several authorities are to treat all patients with *Candida* catheter-associated infections [235,236]. Amphotericin B remains the standard of therapy, although studies comparing fluconazole to amphotericin, when reported, may show a role for this drug as well. The length of therapy and total dose of amphotericin B are not known [235]. We currently use between 300 and 500 mg amphotericin B if the catheter tip grows yeast or if fungemia occurs and no evidence of metastatic foci has been documented. For patients with persistent fungemia or evidence of metastatic disease, 1000 mg, and sometimes as much as 2000 mg, may be required. In patients who continue to do poorly in spite of therapy of amphotericin B, the addition of 5-flucytosine should be considered.

References

1. Bentley DW, Lepper MH: Septicemia related to indwelling venous catheter. *JAMA* 206:1749, 1968.
2. Darrell JH, Garrod LP: Secondary septicaemia from intravenous cannulas. *BMJ* 2:481, 1969.
3. Maki DG: Nosocomial bacteremia: An epidemiologic overview. *Am J Med* 70:719, 1981.
4. Yagupsky P, Nolte FS: Quantitative aspects of septicemia. *Clin Microbiol Rev* 3:269, 1990.
5. Smith RL, Meixler SM, Simberkoff MS: Excess mortality in critically ill patients with nosocomial blood stream infections. *Chest* 100:164, 1991.
6. Dickinson GM, Bisno AL: Infections associated with indwelling devices: Concepts of pathogenesis; infections associated with intravascular devices. *Antimicrob Agents Chemother* 33:597, 1989.
7. Jarvis WR, Edwards JR, Culver DH, et al: Nosocomial infection in adult and pediatric intensive care units in the United States. *Am J Med* 91(3B):185S, 1991.
8. Goldmann DA, Pier GB: Pathogenesis of infections related to intravascular catheterization. *Clin Microbiol Rev* 6:176, 1993.
9. Franson TR, Sheth NK, Rose HD, et al: Scanning electron microscopy of bacteria adherent to intravascular catheters. *J Clin Microbiol* 20:500, 1984.
10. Marrie TJ, Costerton JW: Scanning and transmission electron microscopy of *in situ* bacterial colonization of intravenous and intra-arterial catheters. *J Clin Microbiol* 19:687, 1984.
11. Stillman RM, Soliman F, Garcia L, et al: Etiology of catheter-associated sepsis. *Arch Surg* 112:1497, 1977.
12. Snydman DR, Pober BR, Murray SA, et al: Predictive value of

surveillance skin cultures in total-parenteral-nutrition-related infection. *Lancet* 2:1385, 1982.

13. Armstrong CW, Mayhall CG, Miller KB, et al: Clinical predictors of infection of central venous catheters used for total parenteral nutrition. *Infect Control Hosp Epidemiol* 11:71, 1990.

14. Bjornson HS, Colley R, Bower RH, et al: Association between microorganism growth at the catheter insertion site and colonization of the catheter in patients receiving total parenteral nutrition. *Surgery* 92:720, 1982.

15. Sitges-Serra A, Puig P, Jaurrieta E, et al: Catheter sepsis due to *Staphylococcus epidermidis* during parenteral nutrition. *Surg Gynecol Obstet* 151:481, 1980.

16. Tenney JH, Moody MR, Newman KA, et al: Adherent microorganisms on lumenal surfaces of long-term intravenous catheters: Importance of *Staphylococcus epidermidis* in patient with cancer. *Arch Intern Med* 146:1949, 1986.

17. Hansell DT, Park R, Jensen R, et al: Clinical significance and etiology of infected catheters used for total parenteral nutrition. *Surg Gynecol Obstet* 163:469, 1986.

18. Bozzetti F, Terno G, Camerini E, et al: Pathogenesis and predictability of central venous catheter sepsis. *Surgery* 91:383, 1982.

19. Morgensen JV, Frederiksen W, Jensen JK: Subclavian vein catheterization and infection: A bacteriological study of 130 catheter insertions. *Scand J Infect Dis* 4:31, 1972.

20. Sitges-Serra A, Linares J, Garau J: Catheter sepsis: The clue is the hub. *Surgery* 97:355, 1985.

21. Cercenado E, Ena J, Rodriguez-Creixems M, et al: A conservative procedure for the diagnosis of catheter-related infections. Arch Intern Med 150:1417, 1990.

22. Segura M, Alia C, Valverde J, et al: Assessment of a new hub design and the semiquantitative catheter culture method using an *in vivo* experimental model of catheter sepsis. *J Clin Microbiol* 28:2551, 1990.

23. Rello J, Coll P, Net A, et al: Evaluation of different catheter parts for identification of pulmonary artery catheter colonization. *Scand J Infect Dis* 23:655, 1991.

24. Salzman MB, Isenberg HD, Shapiro JF, et al: A prospective study of the catheter hub as the portal of entry for microorgansims causing catheter-related sepsis in neonates. *J Infect Dis* 167:487, 1993.

25. Wing EJ, Norden CW, Shadduck RK, et al: Use of quantitative bacteriologic techniques to diagnose catheter-related sepsis. *Arch Intern Med* 139:482, 1979.

26. Andremont A, Paulet R, Nitenberg G, et al: Value of semiquantitative cultures of blood drawn through catheter hubs for estimating the risk of catheter tip colonization in cancer patients. *J Clin Microbiol* 26:2297, 1988.

27. Capedevila JA, Planes AM, Palomar M, et al: Value of differential quantitative blood cultures in the diagnosis of catheter-related sepsis. *Eur J Clin Microbiol Infect Dis* 11:403, 1992.

28. Benezra D, Kiehn TE, Gold JWM, et al: Prospective study of infections in indwelling central venous catheters using quantitative blood cultures. *Am J Med* 85:495, 1988.

29. Ascher DP, Shoupe BA, Robb M, et al: Comparison of standard and quantitative blood cultures in the evaluation of children with suspected central venous line sepsis. *Diagn Microbiol Infect Dis* 15:499, 1992.

30. Flynn PM, Shenep JL, Barrett FF: Differential quantitation with a commercial blood culture tube for diagnosis of catheter-related infection. *J Clin Microbiol* 26:1045, 1988.

31. Moyer MA, Edwards LD, Farley L: Comparative culture methods on 101 intravenous catheters: Routine, semiquantitative, and blood cultures. *Arch Intern Med* 143:66, 1983.

32. Linares J, Sitges-Serra A, Garau J, et al: Pathogenesis of catheter sepsis: A prospective study with quantitative and semiquantitative cultures of catheter hub and segments. *J Clin Microbiol* 21:357, 1985.

33. Raad I, Costerton W, Sabharwal U, et al: Ultrastructural analysis of indwelling vascular catheters: A quantitative relationship between luminal colonization and duration of placement. *J Infect Dis* 168:400, 1993.

34. Haslett TM, Isenberg HD, Hilton E, et al: Microbiology of indwelling central intravascular catheters. *J Clin Microbiol* 26:696, 1988.

35. Cleri DJ, Corrado ML, Seligman SJ: Quantitative culture of intravenous catheters and other intravascular inserts. *J Infect Dis* 141:781, 1980.

36. Brun-Buisson C, Abrouk F, Legrand P, et al: Diagnosis of central venous catheter-related sepsis: Critical level of quantitative tip cultures. *Arch Intern Med* 147:873, 1987.

37. Sherertz RJ, Raad II, Belani A, et al: Three-year experience with sonicated vascular catheter cultures in a clinical microbiology laboratory. *J Clin Microbiol* 28:76, 1990.

38. Maki DG, Weise CE, Sarafin HW: A semiquantitative culture method for identifying intravenous-catheter-related infection. *N Engl J Med* 296:1305, 1977.

39. Jones PG, Hopfer RL, Elting L, et al: Semiquantitative cultures of intravascular catheters from cancer patients. *Diagn Microbiol Infect Dis* 4:299, 1986.

40. Rello J, Coll P, Prats G: Laboratory diagnosis of catheter-related bacteremia. *Scand J Infect Dis* 23:583, 1991.

41. Raad II, Sabbagh MF, Rand KH, et al: Quantitative tip culture methods and the diagnosis of central venous catheter-related infections. *Diagn Microbiol Infect Dis* 15:13, 1992.

42. Cooper GL, Hopkins CC: Rapid diagnosis of intravascular catheter-associated infection by direct gram staining of catheter segments. *N Engl J Med* 312:1142, 1985.

43. Collignon P, Chan R, Munro R: Rapid diagnosis of intravascular catheter-related sepsis. *Arch Intern Med* 147:1609, 1987.

44. Coutlee F, Lemieux C, Paradis J-F: Value of direct catheter staining in the diagnosis of intravascular-catheter-related infection. *J Clin Microbiol* 26:1088, 1988.

45. Widmer AF, Nettleman M, Flint K, et al: The clinical impact of culturing central venous catheters: A prospective study. *Arch Intern Med* 152:1299, 1992.

46. Norwood S, Ruby A, Civetta J, et al: Catheter-related infections and associated septicemia. *Chest* 99:968, 1991.

47. Plit ML, Lipman J, Eidelman J, et al: Catheter related infection: A plea for consensus with review and guidelines. *Intensive Care Med* 14:503, 1988.

48. Raad II, Bodey GP: Infectious complications of indwelling vascular catheters. *Clin Infect Dis* 15:197, 1992.

49. Hampton AA, Sherertz RJ: Vascular-access infections in hospitalized patients. *Surg Clin North Am* 68:57, 1988.

50. Druskin MS, Siegel PD: Bacterial contamination of indwelling intravenous polyethylene catheters. *JAMA* 185:966, 1963.

51. Collins RN, Braun PA, Zinner SH, et al: Risk of local and systemic infection with polyethylene intravenous catheters: A prospective study of 213 catheterizations. *N Engl J Med* 279:340, 1968.

52. Frederick GR, Guze LB: Infectious complications of intravenous polyethylene catheters. *California Medicine* 114:50, 1971.

53. Crossley K, Matsen JM: The scalp vein needle: A prospective study. *JAMA* 220:985, 1972.

54. Harbin RL, Schaffner W: Septicemia associated with scalp-vein needles. *South Med J* 66:638, 1973.

55. Band JD, Maki DG: Steel needles used for intravenous therapy: Morbidity in patients with hematologic malignancy. *Arch Intern Med* 140:31, 1980.

56. Tully JL, Friedland GH, Baldini LM, et al: Complications of intravenous therapy with steel needles and teflon catheters: A comparative study. *Am J Med* 70:702, 1981.

57. Ashkenazi S, Weiss E, Drucker MM: Bacterial adherence to intravenous catheters and needles and its influence by cannula type and bacterial surface hydrophobicity. *J Lab Clin Med* 107:136, 1986.

58. Sheth NK, Franson TR, Rose HD, et al: Colonization of bacteria on polyvinyl chloride and Teflon intravascular catheters in hospitalized patients. *J Clin Microbiol* 18:1061, 1983.

59. Maki DG, Ringer M: Risk factors for infusion-related phlebitis with small peripheral venous catheters: A randomized controlled trial. *Ann Intern Med* 114:845, 1991.

60. Legha SS, Haq M, Rabinowitz M, et al: Evaluation of silicone elastomer catheters for long-term intravenous chemotherapy. *Arch Intern Med* 145:1208, 1985.

61. Madan M, Alexander DJ, McMahon MJ: Influence of catheter type on occurrence of thrombophlebitis during peripheral intravenous nutrition. *Lancet* 339:101, 1992.

62. Illner H, Hsia WC, Rikert SL, et al: Use of topical antiseptic in prophylaxis of catheter-related septic complications. *Surg Gynecol Obstet* 168;481, 1989.

63. Trooskin SZ, Donetz AP, Harvey RA, et al: Prevention of catheter sepsis by antibiotic bonding. *Surgery* 97:547, 1985.

64. Jansen B, Kristinsson KG, Jansen S, et al: *In-vitro* efficacy of a central venous catheter complexed with iodine to prevent bacterial colonization. *J Antimicrob Chemother* 30:135, 1992.

65. Kropec A, Huebner J, Frank U, et al: *In vitro* activity of sodium bisulfite and heparin against staphylococci: New strategies in the treatment of catheter-related infection. *J Infect Dis* 168:235, 1993.

66. Mermel LA, Stolz SM, Maki DG: Surface antimicrobial activity of heparin-bonded and antiseptic-impregnated vascular catheters. *J Infect Dis* 167:920, 1993.

67. Editorial. Indwelling venous catheters. *Lancet* 1:499, 1985.

68. Lazarus HM, Lowder JN, Herzig RH: Occlusion and infection in Broviac catheters during intensive cancer therapy. *Cancer* 52:2342, 1983.

69. Shapiro ED, Wald ER, Nelson KA, et al: Broviac catheter-related bacteremia in oncology patients. *Am J Dis Child* 136:679, 1982.

70. Fuchs PC, Gustafson ME, King JT, et al: Assessment of catheter-associated infection risk with the Hickman right atrial catheter. *Infect Control* 5:226, 1984.

71. Prince A, Heller B, Levy J, et al: Management of fever in patients with central vein catheters. *Pediatr Infect Dis J* 5:20, 1986.

72. Dugdale DC, Ramsey PG: *Staphylococcus aureus* bacteremia in patients with Hickman catheters. *Am J Med* 89:137, 1990.

73. Wurzel CL, Halom K, Feldman JG, et al: Infection rates of Broviac-Hickman catheters and implantable venous devices. *Am J Dis Child* 142:536, 1988.

74. Schropp KP, Ginn-Pease ME, King DR: Catheter-related sepsis: A review of the experience with Broviac and Hickman catheters. *Nutrition* 4:195, 1988.

75. Pasquale MD, Campbell JM, Magnant CM: Groshong versus Hickman catheters. *Surg Gynecol Obstet* 174:408, 1992.

76. Sariego J, Bootorabi B, Matsumoto T, et al: Major long-term complications in 1,422 permanent venous access devices. *Am J Surg* 165:249, 1993.

77. Wang EEL, Prober CG, Ford-Jones L, et al: The management of central intravenous catheter infections. *Pediatr Infect Dis J* 3:110, 1984.

78. Moosa HH, Julian TB, Rosenfeld CS, et al: Complications of indwelling central venous catheters in bone marrow transplant recipients. *Surg Gynecol Obstet* 172:275, 1991.

79. Pracher H, Dittel M, Jobst Ch, et al: Bacterial contamination of pulmonary artery catheters. *Intensive Care Med* 4:79, 1978.

80. Applefeld JJ, Caruthers TE, Reno DJ, et al: Assessment of the sterility of long-term cardiac catheterization using the thermodilution Swan-Ganz catheter. *Chest* 74:377, 1978.

81. Hudson-Civetta JA, Civetta JM, Martinez OV, et al: Risk and detection of pulmonary artery catheter-related infection in septic surgical patients. *Crit Care Med* 15:29, 1987.

82. Becker RC, Martin RG, Underwood DA: Right-sided endocardial lesions and flow-directed pulmonary artery catheters. *Cleve Clin J Med* 54:384, 1987.

83. Michel L, Marsh M, McMichan JC, et al: Infection of pulmonary artery catheters in critically ill patients. *JAMA* 245:1032, 1981.

84. Myers ML, Austin TW, Sibbald WJ: Pulmonary artery catheter infections: A prospective study. *Ann Surg* 201:237, 1985.

85. Mermel LA, McCormick RD, Springman SR, et al: The pathogenesis and epidemiology of catheter-related infection with pulmonary artery Swan-Ganz catheters: A prospective study utilizing molecular subtyping. *Am J Med* 91(3B):197S, 1991.

86. Greene JF, Fitzwater JE, Clemmer TP: Septic endocarditis and indwelling pulmonary artery catheters. *JAMA* 233:891, 1975.

87. Rowley KM, Clubb KS, Walker Smith GJ, et al: Right-sided infective endocarditis as a consequence of flow-directed pulmonary-artery catheterization: A clinicopathological study of 55 autopsied patients. *N Engl J Med* 311:1152, 1984.

88. Miller JJ, Venus B, Mathru M: Comparison of the sterility of long-term central venous catheterization using single lumen, triple lumen, and pulmonary artery catheters. *Crit Care Med* 12:634, 1984.

89. Pemberton LB, Lyman B, Lander V, et al: Sepsis from triple- vs single-lumen catheters during total parenteral nutrition in surgical or critically ill patients. *Arch Surg* 121:591, 1986.

90. Kelly CS, Ligas JR, Smith CA, et al: Sepsis due to triple lumen central venous catheters. *Surg Gynecol Obstet* 163:14, 1986.

91. Mantese VA, German DS, Kaminski DL, et al: Colonization and sepsis from triple-lumen catheters in critically ill patients. *Am J Surg* 154:597, 1987.

92. Yeung C, May J, Hughes R: Infection rate for single lumen v triple lumen subclavian catheters. *Infect Control Hosp Epidemiol* 9:154, 1988.

93. Hilton E, Haslett TM, Borenstein MT, et al: Central catheter infections: Single- versus triple-lumen catheters: Influence of guide wires on infection rates when used for replacement of catheters. *Am J Med* 84:667, 1988.

94. Gil RT, Kruse JA, Thill-Baharozian MC, et al: Triple-vs single-lumen central venous catheters: A prospective study in a critically ill population. *Arch Intern Med* 149:1139, 1989.

95. Frawley LW: Multi-lumen lines. *Infect Control* 7:34, 1986.

96. Farkas J-C, Liu N, Bleriot J-P, et al: Single-versus triple-lumen central catheter-related sepsis: A prospective randomized study in a critically ill population. *Am J Med* 93:277, 1992.

97. Stamm WE, Colella JJ, Anderson RL, et al: Indwelling arterial catheters as a source of nosocomial bacteremia: An outbreak caused by *Flavobacterium* species. *N Engl J Med* 292:1099, 1975.

98. Fanning WL, Aronson M: Osler node, Janeway lesions, and splinter hemorrhages. *Arch Dermatol* 113:648, 1977.

99. Maki DG, McCormick RD, Uman SJ, et al: Septic endarteritis due to intra-arterial catheters for cancer chemotherapy: I. Evaluation of an outbreak. II. Risk factors, clinical features and management. III. Guidelines for prevention. *Cancer* 44:1228, 1979.

100. Band JD, Maki DG: Infections caused by arterial catheters used for hemodynamic monitoring. *Am J Med* 67:735, 1979.

101. Adams JM, Speer ME, Rudolph AJ: Bacterial colonization of radial artery catheters. *Pediatrics* 65:94, 1980.

102. Spaccavento LJ, Hawley HB: Infections associated with intra-arterial lines. *Heart Lung* 11:118, 1982.

103. Shinozaki T, Deane RS, Mazuzan JE, et al: Bacterial contamination of arterial lines: A prospective study. *JAMA* 249:223, 1983.

104. Arnow PM, Costas CO: Delayed rupture of the radial artery caused by catheter-related sepsis. *Rev Infect Dis* 10:1035, 1988.

105. Leroy O, Billiau V, Beuscart C, et al: Nosocomial infections associated with long-term radial artery cannulation. *Intensive Care Med* 15:241, 1989.

106. Furfaro S, Gauthier M, Lacroix J, et al: Arterial catheter-related infections in children: A 1-year cohort analysis. *Am J Dis Child* 145:1037, 1991.

107. Wong E, Khardori N, Carrasco CH, et al: Infectious complications of hepatic artery catheterization procedures in patients with cancer. *Rev Infect Dis* 13:583, 1991.

108. File TM, Tan JS: Treatment of bacterial skin and soft tissue infections. *Surg Gynecol Obstet* 172:17S, 1991.

109. Bisno AL: Cutaneous infections: Microbiologic and epidemiologic considerations. *Am J Med* 76(5A):172, 1984.

110. Larson EL, McGinley KJ, Foglia AR, et al: Composition and antimicrobic resistance of skin flora in hospitalized and healthy adults. *J Clin Microbiol* 23:604, 1986.

111. Brook I, Frazier EH: Aerobic and anaerobic bacteriology of wounds and cutaneous abscesses. *Arch Surg* 125:1445, 1990.

112. Sheagren JN: Treatment of skin and skin structure infections in the patient at risk. *Am J Med* 76(5A):180, 1984.

113. Scheld WM, Mandell GL: Nosocomial pneumonia: Pathogenesis and recent advances in diagnosis and therapy. *Rev Infect Dis* 13:S743, 1991.

114. Tuazon CU: Skin and skin structure infections in the patient at risk: Carrier state of *Staphylococcus aureus*. *Am J Med* 76(5A):166, 1984.

115. Gertner J, Herman B, Pescio M, et al: Risk of infection in prolonged central venous catheterization. *Surg Gynecol Obstet* 149:567, 1979.

116. Collignon P, Soni N, Pearson I, et al: Sepsis associated with central vein catheters in critically ill patients. *Intensive Care Med* 14:227, 1988.

117. Tomford JW, Hershey CO, McLaren CE, et al: Intravenous therapy team and peripheral venous catheter-associated complications: A prospective controlled study. *Arch Intern Med* 144:1191, 1984.

118. Prager RL, Silva J: Colonization of central venous catheters. *South Med J* 77:458, 1984.

119. Pinilla JC, Ross DF, Martin T, et al: Study of the incidence of intravascular catheter infection and associated septicemia in critically ill patients. *Crit Care Med* 11:21, 1983.

120. Richet H, Hubert B, Nitemberg G, et al: Prospective multicenter study of vascular-catheter-related complications and risk factors for positive central-catheter cultures in intensive care unit patients. *J Clin Microbiol* 28:2520, 1990.

121. Bernard RW, Stahl WM, Chase RM: Subclavian vein catheterization: A prospective study. II. Infectious complications. *Ann Surg* 173:191, 1971.

122. Hershey CO, Tomford JW, McLaren CE, et al: The natural history of intravenous catheter-associated phlebitis. *Arch Intern Med* 144:1373, 1984.

123. Bogen JE: Local complications in 167 patients with indwelling venous catheters. *Surg Gynecol Obstet* 110:112, 1960.

124. Moran JM, Atwood RP, Rowe MI: A clinical and bacteriologic study of infections associated with venous cutdowns. *N Engl J Med* 272:554, 1965.

125. Lindblad B, Wolff T: Infectious complications of percutaneously inserted central venous catheters. *Acta Anaesthesiol Scand* 29:587, 1985.

126. Keohane PP, Attrill H, Northover J, et al: Effect of catheter tunneling and a nutrition nurse on catheter sepsis during parenteral nutrition: A controlled trial. *Lancet* 2:1388, 1983.

127. Toltzis P, Goldmann DA: Current issues in central venous catheter infection. *Annu Rev Med* 41:169, 1990.

128. De Cicco M, Chiaradia V, Veronesi A, et al: Source and route of microbial colonization of parenteral nutrition catheters. *Lancet* 2:1258, 1989.

129. Flowers RH, Schwenzer KJ, Kopel RF, et al: Efficacy of an attachable subcutaneous cuff for the prevention of intravascular catheter-related infection: A randomized, controlled trial. *JAMA* 261:878, 1989.

130. Maki DG, Cobb L, Garman JK, et al: An attachable silver-impregnated cuff for prevention of infection with central venous catheters: A prospective randomized multicenter trial. *Am J Med* 85:307, 1988.

131. Heard SO, Davis RF, Sherertz RJ, et al: Influence of sterile protective sleeves on the sterility of pulmonary artery catheters. *Crit Care Med* 15:499, 1987.

132. Maki DG, Ringer M, Alvarado CJ: Prospective randomized trial of povidone-iodine, alcohol, and chlorhexidine for prevention of infection associated with central venous and arterial catheters. *Lancet* 338:339, 1991.

133. Maki DG, McCormack KN: Defatting catheter insertion sites in total parenteral nutrition is of no value as an infection control measure: Controlled clinical trial. *Am J Med* 83:833, 1987.

134. Al-Sibai MB, Harder EJ, Faskin RW, et al: The value of prophylactic antibiotics during the insertion of long-term indwelling silastic right atrial catheters in cancer patients. *Cancer* 60:1891, 1987.

135. Ranson MR, Oppenheim BA, Jackson A, et al: Double-blind placebo controlled study of vancomycin prophylaxis for central venous catheter insertion in cancer patients. *J Hosp Infect* 15:95, 1990.

136. Levy RS, Goldstein J, Pressman RS: Value of a topical antibiotic ointment in reducing bacterial colonization of percutaneous catheters. *J Albert Einstein Medical Center* 18:67, 1970.

137. Zinner SH, Denny-Brown BC, Braun P, et al: Risk of infection with intravenous indwelling catheters: Effect of application of antibiotic ointment. *J Infect Dis* 120:616, 1969.

138. Norden CW: Application of antibiotic ointment to the site of venous catheterization: A controlled trial. *J Infect Dis* 120:611, 1969.

139. Maki DG, Band JD: A comparative study of polyantibiotic and iodophor ointments in prevention of vascular catheter-related infection. *Am J Med* 70:739, 1981.

140. Bradley SF: Efficacy of mupirocin ointment in the control of methicillin-resistant *Staphylococcus aureus*. *Infections in Medicine* 10:23, 1993.

141. Salzman MB, Isenberg HD, Rubin LG: Use of disinfectants to reduce microbial contamination of hubs of vascular catheters. *J Clin Microbiol* 31:475, 1993.

142. Dennis MB, LeCaptain L, Cole JJ, et al: Septic implanted vascular catheters: Models and *in situ* disinfection, in Hall CW (ed): *Sur-*

gical Research, Recent Developments. New York, Pergamon Press, 1985.

143. Schwartz C, Henrickson KJ, Roghmann K, et al: Prevention of bacteremia attributed to luminal colonization of tunneled central venous catheters and vancomycin-susceptible organisms. *J Clin Oncol* 8:1591, 1990.

144. Conly JM, Grieves K, Peters B: A prospective randomized study comparing transparent and dry gauze dressings for central venous catheters. *J Infect Dis* 159:310, 1989.

145. Kelsey MC, Gosling M: A comparison of the morbidity associated with occlusive and non-occlusive dressings applied to peripheral intravenous devices. *J Hosp Infect* 5:313, 1984.

146. Anderson PT, Herlevsen P, Schaumburg H: A comparative study of "Op-site" and "Nobecutan gauze" dressings for central venous line care. *J Hosp Infect* 7:161, 1986.

147. Craven DE, Lichtenberg DA, Kunches LM, et al: A randomized study comparing a transparant polyurethane dressing to a dry gauze dressing for peripheral intravenous catheter sites. *Infect Control* 6:361, 1985.

148. Maki DG, Ringer M: Evaluation of dressing regimens for prevention of infection with peripheral intravenous catheters: Gauze, a transparent polyurethane dressing, and an iodophor-transparent dressing. *JAMA* 258:2396, 1987.

149. Schwartz-Fulton J, Colley R, Valanis B, et al: Hyperalimentation dressings and skin flora. *National Intravenous Therapy Association* 4:354, 1981.

150. Band JD, Maki DG: Safety of changing intravenous delivery systems at longer than 24-hour intervals. *Ann Intern Med* 91:173, 1979.

151. Buxton AE, Highsmith AK, Garner JS, et al: Contamination of intravenous infusion fluid: Effects of changing administration sets. *Ann Intern Med* 90:764, 1979.

152. Birnbaum DW: Safety of maintaining intravenous sites for longer than 48 H. *J Clin Microbiol* 13:833, 1981.

153. Maki DG, Botticelli JT, LeRoy ML, et al: Prospective study of replacing administration sets for intravenous therapy at 48- vs 72-hour intervals: 72 hours is safe and cost-effective. *JAMA* 258:1777, 1987.

154. Centers for Disease Control: Nosocomial *Pseudomonas cepacia* bacteremia caused by contaminated pressure transducers. *MMWR* 23:423, 1974.

155. Centers for Disease Control: Transducer-associated bacteremia—North Carolina. *MMWR* 24:295, 1975.

156. Weinstein RA: The design of pressure monitoring devices: Infection control considerations. *Medical Instrumentation* 10:287, 1976.

157. Buxton AE, Anderson RL, Klimek J, et al: Failure of disposable domes to prevent septicemia acquired from contaminated pressure transducers. *Chest* 74:508, 1978.

158. Weinstein RA, Stamm WE, Kramer L, et al: Pressure monitoring devices: Overlooked source of nosocomial infection. *JAMA* 236:936, 1976.

159. Maki DG, Band JD: Septicemia from disposable pressure-monitoring chamber domes. *Chest* 74:486, 1978.

160. Donowitz LG, Marsik FJ, Hoyt JW, et al: *Serratia marcescens* bacteremia from contaminated pressure transducers. *JAMA* 242:1749, 1979.

161. Aduan RP, Iannini PB, Salaki J: Nosocomial bacteremia associated with contaminated blood pressure transducers: Report of an outbreak and a review of the literature. *Am J Infect Control* 8:33, 1980.

162. Abbott N, Walrath JM, Scanlon-Trump E: Infection related to physiologic monitoring: Venous and arterial catheters. *Heart Lung* 12:28, 1983.

163. Duma RJ, Warner JF, Dalton HP: Septicemia from intravenous infusions. *N Engl J Med* 284:257, 1971.

164. Felts SK, Schaffner W, Melly A, et al: Sepsis caused by contaminated intravenous fluids: Epidemiologic, clinical, and laboratory investigation of an outbreak in one hospital. *Ann Intern Med* 77:881, 1972.

165. Centers for Disease Control: Septicemias associated with contaminated intravenous fluids—Wisconsin, Ohio. *MMWR* 22:99, 1973.

166. Maki DG, Anderson RL, Shulman JA: In-use contamination of intravenous infusion fluid. *Appl Microbiol* 28:778, 1974.

167. Maki DG, Martin WT: Nationwide epidemic of septicemia caused by contaminated infusion products. IV. Growth of microbial path-

ogens in fluids for intravenous infusion. *J Infect Dis* 131:267, 1975.

168. Maki DG, Rhame FS, Mackel DC, et al: Nationwide epidemic of septicemia caused by contaminated intravenous products. I. Epidemiologic and clinical features. *Am J Med* 60:471, 1976.

169. Crichton EP: Infusion fluids as culture media. *Am J Clin Pathol* 59:199, 1973.

170. Goldmann DA, Martin WT, Worthington JW: Growth of bacteria and fungi in total parenteral nutrition solutions. *Am J Surg* 126:314, 1973.

171. Mirtallo JM, Caryer K, Schneider PJ, et al: Growth of bacteria and fungi in parenteral nutrition solutions containing albumin. *Am J Hosp Pharm* 38:1907, 1981.

172. Scheckelhoff DJ, Miratallo JM, Ayers LW, et al: Growth of bacteria and fungi in total nutrient admixtures. *Am J Hosp Pharm* 43:73, 1986.

173. Solomon SL, Khabbaz RF, Parker RH, et al: An outbreak of *Candida parapsilosis* bloodstream infections in patients receiving parenteral nutrition. *J Infect Dis* 149:98, 1984.

174. Brennan MF, Goldman MH, O'Connell RC, et al: Prolonged parenteral alimentation: *Candida* growth and the prevention of candidemia by amphotericin instillation. *Ann Surg* 176:265, 1972.

175. Curry CR, Quie PG: Fungal septicemia in patients receiving parenteral hyperalimentation. *N Engl J Med* 285:1221, 1971.

176. Dankner WM, Spector SA, Fierer J, et al: Malassezia fungemia in neonates and adults: Complication of hyperalimentation. *Rev Infect Dis* 4:743, 1987.

177. Collin J, Tweedle DEF, Venables CW, et al: Effect of a millipore filter on complications of intravenous infusions: A prospective clinical trial. *BMJ* 4:456, 1973

178. Friedland G: Infusion-related phlebitis: Is the in-line filter the solution? *N Engl J Med* 312:113, 1984.

179. Falchuk KH, Peterson L, McNeil BJ: Microparticulate-induced phlebitis: Its prevention by in-line filtration. *N Engl J Med* 312:78, 1985.

180. Quercia RA, Hills SW, Klimek JJ, et aL: Bacteriologic contamination of intravenous infusion delivery systems in an intensive care unit. *Am J Med* 80:364, 1986.

181. Press OW, Ramsey PG, Larson EB, et al: Hickman catheter infections in patients with malignancies. *Medicine* 63:189, 1984.

182. Tager IB, Ginsberg MB, Ellis SE, et al: An epidemiologic study of the risks associated with peripheral intravenous catheters. *Am J Epidemiol* 118:839, 1983.

183. Simmons BP, Hooton TM, Wong ES, et al: Guideline for prevention of intravenous therapy-related infections. *Hosp Infect Control* 9:28K, 1982.

184. Snyder RH, Archer FJ, Endy T, et al: Catheter infection: A comparison of two catheter maintenance techniques. *Ann Surg* 208:651, 1988.

185. Cobb DK, High KP, Sawyer RG, et al: A controlled trial of scheduled replacement of central venous and pulmonary-artery catheters. *N Engl J Med* 327:1062, 1992.

186. Bozzetti F, Terno G, Bonfanti G, et al: Prevention and treatment of central venous catheter sepsis by exchange via a guidewire: A prospective controlled trial. *Ann Surg* 198:48, 1983.

187. Sitzmann JV, Townsend TR, Siler MC, et al: Septic and technical complications of central venous catheterization. *Ann Surg* 202:766, 1985.

188. Armstrong CW, Mayhall CG, Miller KB, et al: Prospective study of catheter replacement and other risk factors for infection of hyperalimentation catheters. *J Infect Dis* 154:808, 1986.

189. Pettigrew RA, Lang SDR, Haydock DA, et al: Catheter-related sepsis in patients on intravenous nutrition: A prospective study of quantitative catheter cultures and guidewire changes for suspected sepsis. *Br J Surg* 72:52, 1985.

190. Kowalewska-Grochowska K, Richards R, Moysa GL, et al: Guidewire catheter change in central venous catheter biofilm formation in a burn population. *Chest* 100:1090, 1991.

191. Eyer S, Brummitt C, Crossley K, et al: Catheter-related sepsis: Prospective, randomized study of three methods of long-term catheter maintenance. *Crit Care Med* 18:1073, 1990.

192. Arnow PM, Quimosing EM, Beach M: Consequences of intravascular catheter sepsis. *Clin Infect Dis* 16:778, 1993

193. Henderson DK: Intravascular device-associated infection: Current concepts and controversies. *Infections in Surgery* 7:365, 1988.

194. Montgomerie JZ, Edwards JE: Association of infection due to *Candida albicans* with intravenous hyperalimentation. *J Infect Dis* 137:197, 1978.

195. Stamm WE: Infections related to medical devices. *Ann Intern Med* 89(Part 2):764, 1978.

196. Smits H, Freedman LR: Prolonged venous catheterization as a cause of sepsis. *N Engl J Med* 276:1229, 1967.

197. Harris LF, Alford RH, Dan BB, et al: Bacteremia related to IV cannulation: Variability of underlying venous infection. *South Med J* 73:719, 1980.

198. Thomas MG, Lang SDR: Intravascular cannula-related sepsis: Two years experience. *N Z Med J* 98:804, 1985.

199. Neuhof H: Excision of vein for suppurative thrombophlebitis. *Ann Surg* 106:311, 1937.

200. Phillips RW, Eyre JD: Septic thrombophlebitis with septicemia: Report of three cases due to *Staphylococcus aureus* infection after the intravenous use of polyethylene catheters for parenteral therapy. *N Engl J Med* 259:729, 1958.

201. Crane C: Venous interruption for septic thrombophlebitis. *N Engl J Med* 262:947, 1960.

202. O'Neill JA, Pruitt BA, Foley FD, et al: Suppurative thrombophlebitis: A lethal complication of intravenous therapy. *J Trauma* 8:256, 1968.

203. Stein JM, Pruitt BA: Suppurative thrombophlebitis: A lethal iatrogenic disease. *N Engl J Med* 282:1452, 1970.

204. Barenholtz L, Kaminsky NI, Palmer DL: Venous intramural microabscess: A cause of protracted sepsis with intravenous cannulas. *Am J Med Sci* 265:335, 1973.

205. Munster AM: Septic thrombophlebitis: A surgical disorder. *JAMA* 230:1010, 1974.

206. Zinner MJ, Zuidema GD, Lowery BD: Septic nonsuppurative thrombophlebitis. *Arch Surg* 111:122, 1976.

207. Baker CC, Petersen SR, Sheldon GF: Septic phlebitis: A neglected disease. *Am J Surg* 138:97, 1979.

208. Pruitt BA, McManus WF, Kim SH, et al: Diagnosis and treatment of cannula-related intravenous sepsis in burn patients. *Ann Surg* 191:546, 1980.

209. Sears N, Grosfeld JL, Weber TR, et al: Suppurative thrombophlebitis in childhood. *Pediatrics* 68:630, 1981.

210. Winn RE, Tuttle KL, Gilbert DN: Surgical approach to extensive suppurative thrombophlebitis of the central veins of the chest. *J Thorac Cardiovasc Surg* 81:564, 1981.

211. Verghese A, Widrich WC, Arbeit RD: Central venous septic thrombophlebitis: The role of medical therapy. *Medicine* 64:394, 1985.

212. Johnson RA, Zajac RA, Evans ME: Suppurative thrombophlebitis: Correlation between pathogen and underlying disease. *Infect Control* 7:582, 1986.

213. Walsh TJ, Bustamente CI, Vlahov D, et al: Candidal suppurative peripheral thrombophlebitis: Recognition, prevention, and management. *Infect Control* 7:16, 1986.

214. Terpenning MS, Buggy BP, Kauffman CA: Hospital-acquired infective endocarditis. *Arch Intern Med* 148:1601, 1988.

215. Tsao MMP, Katz D: Central venous catheter-induced endocarditis: Human correlate of the animal experimental model of endocarditis. *Rev Infect Dis* 6:783, 1984.

216. Liepman MK, Jones PG, Kauffman CA: Endocarditis as a complication of indwelling right atrial catheters in leukemic patients. *Cancer* 54:804, 1984.

217. Martino P, Micozzi A, Venditti M, et al: Catheter-related right-sided endocarditis in bone-marrow transplant recipients. *Rev Infect Dis* 12:250, 1990.

218. Sochowski RA, Chan K-L: Implication of negative results on a monoplane transesophageal echocardiographic study in patients with suspected infective endocarditis. *J Am Coll Cardiol* 21:216, 1993.

219. Libman H, Arbeit RD: Complications associated with *Staphylococcus aureus* bacteremia. *Arch Intern Med* 144:541, 1984.

220. Mylotte JM, McDermott, Spooner JA: Prospective study of 114 consecutive episodes of *Staphylococcus aureus* bacteremia. *Rev Infect Dis* 9:891, 1987.

221. Raad I, Davis S, Khan A, et al: Impact of central venous catheter removal on the recurrence of catheter-related coagulase negative staphylococcal bacteremia. *Infect Control Hosp Epidemiol* 13:215, 1992.

222. Hilf M, Yu VL, Sharp J, et al: Antibiotic therapy for *Pseudomonas aeruginosa* bacteremia: Outcome correlations in a prospective study of 200 patients. *Am J Med* 87:540, 1989.

223. Power J, Wing EJ, Talamo TS, et al: Fatal bacterial endocarditis as a complication of permanent indwelling catheters: Report of two cases. *Am J Med* 81:166, 1986.

224. Sattler FR, Foderaro JB, Aber RC: *Staphylococcus epidermidis* bacteremia associated with vascular catheters: An important cause of febrile morbidity in hospitalized patients. *Infect Control* 5:279, 1984.

225. Iannini PB, Crossley K: Therapy of *Staphylococcus aureus* bacteremia associated with a removable focus of infection. *Ann Intern Med* 84:558, 1976.

226. Ehni WF, Reller LB: Short-course therapy for catheter-associated *Staphylococcus aureus* bacteremia. *Arch Intern Med* 149:533, 1989.

227. Watanakunakorn C, Baird IM: *Staphylococcus aureus* bacteremia and endocarditis associated with a removable device. *Am J Med* 63:253, 1977.

228. Raad II, Sabbagh MF: Optimal duration of therapy for catheter-related *Staphylococcus aureus* bacteremia: A study of 55 cases and review. *Clin Infect Dis* 14:75, 1992.

229. Rahal JJ: Preventing second-generation complications due to *Staphylococcus aureus* [Editorial]. *Arch Intern Med* 149:503, 1989.

230. Jernigan JA, Farr BM: Short-course therapy of catheter-related *Staphylococcus aureus* bacteremia: A meta-analysis. *Ann Intern Med* 119:304, 1993.

231. Elting LS, Bodey GP: Septicemia due to *Xanthomonas* species and non-*aeruginosa Pseudomonas* species: Increasing incidence of catheter-related infections. *Medicine* 69:296, 1990.

232. Ellis CA, Spivak ML: The significance of candidemia. *Ann Intern Med* 67:511, 1967.

233. Lecciones JA, Lee JW, Navarro EE, et al: Vascular catheter-associated fungemia in patients with cancer: Analysis of 155 episodes. *Clin Infect Dis* 14:875, 1992.

234. Fraser VJ, Jones M, Dunkel J, et al: Candidemia in a tertiary care hospital: Epidemiology, risk factors, and predictors of mortality. *Clin Infect Dis* 15:414, 1992.

235. Edwards JE: Editorial response: Should all patients with candidemia be treated with antifungal agents? *Clin Infect Dis* 15:422, 1992.

236. Edwards JE, Filler SG: Current strategies for treating invasive candidiasis: Emphasis on infections in nonneutropenic patients. *Clin Infect Dis* 14:106S, 1992.

237. Komshian SV, Uwaydah AK, Sobel JD, et al: Fungemia caused by Candida species and *Torulopsis glabrata* in the hospitalized patient: Frequency, characteristics, and evaluation of factors influencing outcome. *Rev Infect Dis* 11:379, 1989.

90. Urinary Tract Infections

Steven M. Opal

Introduction

Urinary tract infection (UTI) remains the most common nosocomially acquired infectious disease, accounting for approximately 40 percent of all infectious complications in the hospitalized patient population in the United States [1,2]. Furthermore, the urinary tract is the most frequently recognized source of gram-negative rod bacteremia, which constitutes a major cause of infectious morbidity and mortality in the critically ill patient [1,3]. Approximately 100,000 annual admissions to acute care hospitals in the United States are attributable to severe infections of the urinary tract [4]. The progressive development of resistance to antimicrobial agents by urinary pathogens and the difficulties attendant to the management of patients with indwelling urinary catheters remain major challenges in current critical care practice. Those urinary tract infections of sufficient severity to require intensive care management and the omnipresent risk of infectious complications with urinary catheters are the principal focus of this review of urinary tract infections.

Microbiology and Pathophysiology of UTI

Urinary tract infections are primarily caused by enteric gram-negative bacilli and occasionally by gram-positive cocci including staphylococci and enterococci. *Escherichia coli* is by far the most common cause of community-acquired and nosocomially acquired UTI. Most UTIs arise from ascending infection by enteric organisms that colonize the perineum and distal urethra. Because *E. coli* is the most common enteric gram-negative aerobic bacterium in the human colon, it most frequently contaminates the lower urinary tract and results in infection. *E. coli* also has the ability to adhere to and persist on the vaginal epithelial cells, which facilitates its capacity to cause recurrent UTI in women.

Specific clones of *E. coli* have evolved the potential to colonize uroepithelium and cause UTI. A restricted number of serotypes make up the uropathogenic clones of *E. coli* that cause most urinary tract infections. This is particularly striking in upper urinary tract infections, where only eight of the more than 170 O antigen serotypes of *E. coli* account for up to 80 percent of community-acquired episodes of pyelonephritis. Serotypes O1, O2, O4, O6, O7, O16, O18, and O75 are the major uropathogenic strains in human infections. These somatic antigen types are often associated with capsular serotypes K1, K2, K5, K12, K13, and K51 antigens [5–17]. Uropathogenic strains of *E. coli* possess a number of other features that may enhance the organism's capacity to cause UTI. These potential virulence factors include an iron assimilation system [18,19,20] and hemolysin production [21,22,23]. Invasive strains of *E. coli* frequently possess an iron-sequestering system known as aerobactin, which allows the organism to acquire iron from the human host and disseminate from extraintestinal sites. Hemolysin may increase iron availability to the infecting organism [24], interfere with leukocyte function [25], or damage uroepithelial cell membranes [26]. These factors potentiate the invasive capacity of uropathogenic strains of *E. coli*.

An additional virulence property that potentiates colonization by uropathogenic *E. coli* is its adhesive capacity to uroepithelial membranes. Urinary isolates of *E. coli* possess numerous adhesins including type I or common pili and P pili, which facilitate attachment to epithelial surfaces. Type I pili bind to mannose-containing polysaccharides on the cell surface of epithelial membranes. This allows the organism to attach and persist within the urinary tract and thereby avoid elimination during micturation [27,28].

Another important adherence property of uropathogenic *E. coli* is the expression of P pili on the bacteria's outer membrane [29,30,31]. P pili bind to alpha-D-Galactose 1 → 4 beta-D-Galactose (Gal-Gal) containing disaccharides of the globoseries of glycolipids. The globoseries of glycolipids are found primarily on the epithelial surfaces of the urinary tract and kidney as well as the large intestinal epithelial cells and erythrocytes. The ability of *E. coli* to express P pili is particularly important in the establishment of upper UTIs where Gal-Gal disaccharide-containing glycolipids are found in large concentration. *E. coli* strains that lack P pili also lack the ability to produce UTI in experimental animals. Genetically engineered transformants that have regained the ability to express P pili also reacquire the ability to cause pyelonephritis in experimental models of UTI [32]. Clinical surveys of *E. coli* isolates from patients with UTI support the relevance of P pili in the pathogenesis of UTI [33].

Other aerobic gram-negative bacterial organisms of the Enterobacteriaceae may also cause UTI. *Klebsiella, Enterobacter, Serratia, Proteus,* and *Providencia* species become increasingly common urinary pathogens in patients who have recently received antibiotics for UTI and in patients with anatomic or functional abnormalities in urine flow [34]. The microbiology of UTI after short-term urinary catheterization is similar to that observed in the non-catheterized patient. However, long-term (>30 days) urinary catheterization generates an environment that supports a complex and often polymicrobial microflora. The microbiology of the chronic catheterized patient with UTI differs considerably from microbiology of the noncatheterized or short-term catheterized patient. Strains from *Proteus, Providencia, Morganella,* and *Pseudomonas* species become more common whereas *E. coli* and *Klebsiella* species become less common (Fig. 90-1) [35]. The unique attributes of *Proteus* and *Providencia* strains that contribute to their ability to cause UTIs in catheterized patients will be considered in a later section of this chapter on catheter-related UTI.

Proteus species, as well as some other gram-negative enteric organisms and *Staphylococcus saprophyticus,* synthesize the enzyme urease, a known bacterial virulence factor in the urinary tract. The generation of ammonia from urea changes regional pH, favoring the generation of the "triple-phosphate crystals" struvite and apatite in an alkaline environment. Struvite crystals participate in obstruction of urinary flow in urinary catheters and promote the generation of renal calculi, which may complicate the management of UTI [36].

Gram-positive bacterial species occasionally cause UTIs. Coagulase-negative staphylococci such as *S. saprophyticus* are a common cause of lower UTI in sexually active women [37]. The isolation of *Staphylococcus aureus* in the urine is important in that it is frequently seen in patients who have staphylococcal bacteremia. *S. aureus* isolation in urine cultures should prompt a search for extrarenal sources of staphylococcal infection. *S. aureus* is also associated with suppurative complications in the genitourinary tract, with severe consequences [38,39]. *S. aureus* may also colonize chronically catheterized patients. This is particularly true for methicillin-resistant *S. aureus* strain, which may thrive in hospital settings with many elderly, catheterized patients [40].

Enterococci have become increasingly prevalent urinary pathogens in elderly populations and in patients with long-term

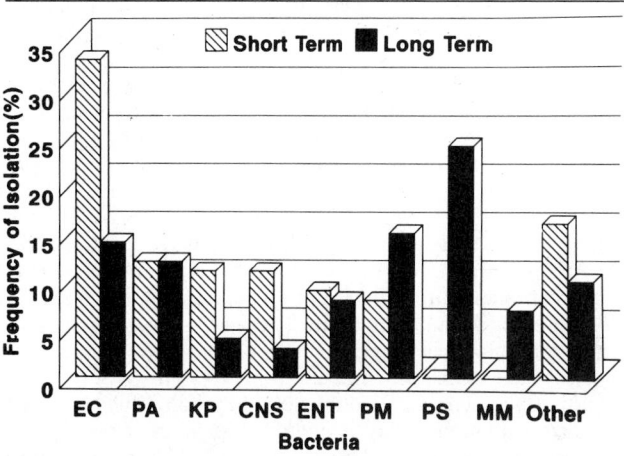

Fig. 90-1. Distribution of bacterial isolation associated with catheter-related UTI. EC = *Escherichia coli;* PA = *pseudomones aeruginosa;* KP = *klebsiella pneumoniae;* CNS = coagulase-negative staphylococci; ENT = Enterococci; PM = *Proteus mirabilis;* PS = *Providencia stuartii;* and MM = *morganella morganii.*

urinary catheters in place. The remarkable ability of this organism to resist antimicrobial agents, including beta-lactam antibiotics, aminoglycosides, and vancomycin, has made this organism a formidable pathogen in the urinary tracts of hospitalized patients [41]. *Candida* species and other fungal organisms may also necessitate special consideration. *Candida* species are particularly common and recalcitrant urinary pathogens that often complicate urinary catheterization. Candiduria may be associated with hematogenous dissemination or ascending UTIs [42]. The unique problems associated with the isolation of *Candida* species of the urinary tract are considered in the final section of this chapter.

Host Defense Mechanisms Against UTI

The human genitourinary tract is remarkably resistant to colonization and infection of the urinary tract because of a series of mechanical, mucosal, and immunologic mechanisms. Certainly, the establishment and maintenance of normal urinary flow is the most important defense against UTI. The frequent occurrence of UTI after obstruction or incomplete bladder emptying attests to the importance of mechanical clearance of bacteria during micturition as an important defense against UTI. Patients with a neurogenic bladder and those with vesicoureteral reflux are highly susceptible to UTI and renal scarring as a consequence of such infections. Although urinary pathogens must possess a full complement of virulence factors to cause infection in anatomically normal urinary tract, patients with mechanical obstruction to urine flow may become infected with bacterial species devoid of special urinary virulence [43,44].

Urinary osmolarity, urea concentration, pH, and oxygen concentration limit the growth of multiple potential bacterial pathogens such as the anaerobic microflora [45]. It has been postulated that the continuous sloughing of uroepithelial cells, urinary mucosal glycocalyx (slime), and secretion of the Tamm-Horsfall protein may assist in the mechanical removal of adherent bacteria that have entered the urinary tract [46].

The mucosal surface of uroepithelial cells may vary in its ability to prevent the attachment of bacteria on entrance to the urinary tract. The mucopolysaccharide content and chemical composition of this epithelial surface determines its adherence properties. A genetic susceptibility to UTIs has been ascribed to individuals who possess the P1 blood group antigen [47]. This blood group antigen consists of surface antigens that contain the Gal-Gal disaccharide. These are similar to glycolipids, which promote bacterial adherence of p-piliated *E. coli* to uroepithelial cells. It has also been observed that patients who are nonsecretors of blood group antigens have an increased risk of UTI [48,49]. Blood group antigens coat the surface of the uroepithelial cells when secreted onto the mucosal surface. This interferes with the binding of bacteria to adhesin-receptor oligosaccharides on the surface of epithelial cells and results in inhibition of colonization of the bladder by urinary pathogens. Individuals who fail to secrete these blood group antigens lack this defense mechanism and are prone to UTI.

Although secretory immunoglobulin, neutrophils, and cell-mediated immunity play a limited role in the host defense against UTI, their role is largely overshadowed by mechanical and physical barriers to UTI. Recent evidence suggests that uroepithelial cells produce the proinflammatory cytokine interleukin-8 in response to *E. coli* infection. Interleukin-8 serves as a chemoattractant for neutrophils that then migrate to the bladder mucosa. Neutrophils may limit the infection to the urinary bladder and prevent disseminated infection [50].

Males are generally spared from UTI when compared with their female counterparts except at the extremes of age where obstruction to urinary flow is frequently problematic in males. The increased anatomic distance from the urethral orifice to the urinary bladder, the infrequent presence of gram-negative bacteria around the male urethra, and the production of inhibitory secretions from the prostate protect the male from UTI throughout most of adult life. However, the prostate becomes a liability to men as they age. Bladder neck obstruction from benign prostatic hypertrophy is a frequent occurrence and contributes to urinary obstruction and UTI in elderly men [51].

Severe UTI in the ICU Setting

ACUTE PYELONEPHRITIS. Pyelonephritis is generally not of sufficient severity to warrant ICU admission unless complicated by bacteremia and septic shock, urinary obstruction, papillary necrosis, or other local suppurative complications. Patients who become bacteremic and develop septic shock from a urinary tract source should respond rapidly to supportive measures and appropriate antimicrobial therapy. Patients with gram-negative sepsis originating from the urinary tract have a more favorable prognosis when compared with those with sepsis from other sources [52]. Failure to respond within 48 to 72 hours to appropriate therapy should prompt a search for complications of UTI. Functional or mechanical obstruction to urinary flow is the principal underlying cause of treatment failure in the management of UTI. Obstruction may arise from extrarenal causes such as retroperitoneal or pelvic masses or abnormalities intrinsic to the genitourinary (GU) tract such as renal calculi or bladder outlet obstruction. Alleviation of obstruction facilitates antimicrobial treatment and is often essential to successfully eradicate infections in the upper urinary tract system [53].

SUPPURATIVE COMPLICATIONS OF UTI. Suppurative complications of the GU tract should be considered in those patients who fail to respond to conventional therapy for UTI. Abscess formation within the GU tract may take several forms and may present a diagnostic and therapeutic challenge. It is important to distinguish between these entities because the clinical implications and medical management of each process differ substantially. The principal complications of infection of the upper urinary tract are described in Table 90-1. Radiographic findings in a typical case of emphysematous pyelonephritis are seen in Fig. 90-2A and B. The presence of suppurative complications of UTI indicate the need for consultation with an invasive radiologist or urologist to assist in the management of these patients.

DIAGNOSTIC METHODS IN UTI. The clinical diagnosis of acute UTI is usually straightforward, with a history of urinary frequency and dysuria often accompanied with costovertebral angle (CVA) tenderness and signs of systemic toxicity. The urinalysis often shows positive "dipstick" results for leukocyte esterase and nitrite, which suggest leukocytes and enteric bacteremia are present. An examination of the urinary sediment is generally sufficient for a presumptive diagnosis of UTI. The presence of excess numbers of urinary leukocytes and bacteria in the absence of evidence of vaginal contamination by epithelial cells in women is indicative of a UTI.

The urinary Gram stain of unspun urine is helpful in determining the most likely agent causing the UTI. The presence of gram-negative rods in the urine is frequently found and confirms the presence of excess numbers of bacteria in the urine. The consistent finding of greater than 1 organism per high-powered field in unspun urine is indicative of $>10^5$ colony-forming units (CFU) per milliliter [54]. Urinary Gram stain also provides an opportunity to detect gram-positive microorganisms with a reasonable degree of accuracy. Enterococci and staphylococci are readily distinguished by microscopic examination of the urinary Gram stain and permit early intervention with appropriate antimicrobial therapy. Fungal elements are also easily identified by the urinary Gram stain. Polymicrobial bacteriuria is often apparent by urinary Gram stain and may be seen in UTI from long-standing urinary catheterization, enterovesical fistula, or complicated UTI associated with obstruction or foreign bodies [55].

UTIs of sufficient severity to require critical care management should have a quantitative urinary culture performed, preferably before the initiation of antimicrobial therapy. The urine culture serves to confirm the diagnostic impression and to direct the most appropriate antimicrobial agent for use in the management of UTI. The progressive increase in antimicrobial resistance in common urinary tract bacterial pathogens now makes it imperative to carefully select antimicrobial agents based on susceptibility patterns of the infecting microorganism. Greater than 10^5 CFU per milliliter of urine is diagnostic of a UTI in the appropriate clinical situation. This quantitative level of bacteriuria and its association with acute UTI was developed from a laboratory-based study of hospitalized adult, primarily female, patients [56]. It has become apparent from clinical surveys that symptomatic women may have acute UTI with as little as 10^2 pathogenic microorganisms per milliliter [57]. Catheterized patients may also have significant symptomatic UTI with fewer than 10^5 CFU per milliliter. The presence of a Foley catheter may not permit ongoing replication of microorganisms in the urinary bladder to generate greater than 10^5 CFU per milliliter. Moreover, urinary cultures from noninstrumented men are significant with as little as 10^3 CFU per milliliter [58].

The absence of pyuria and significant bacteriuria does not exclude the possibility of a potentially serious UTI. Patients with severe neutropenia may not have significant levels of pyuria associated with UTI. Urine cultures may be negative in more than 40 percent of patients with perinephric abscess [59], and most patients with renal cortical abscesses have urinalyses that

Table 90-1. Suppurative Complications of UTI

Disease Process	Pathogenesis	Predisposing Factors	Common Pathogens	Radiographic Features	Standard Treatment
Papillary necrosis	Ischemia, necrosis, infection	Analgesics, diabetes, obstruction	Gram-negative enterics	Sloughed papilla, in calyx	Antibiotics alone
Pyonephrosis	Infection with hydronephrosis	Ureteral obstruction, calculi	Gram-negative enterics	Hydronephrosis with gas, debris in collecting system	Nephrostomy tube, antibiotics
Focal bacterial nephritis	Ascending UTI with focal renal inflammation	UTI with upper tract involvement	Gram-negative enterics	Focal defect on contrast-enhanced CT scan	Antibiotics alone
Corticomedullary abscess	Ascending UTI with focal renal liquification	UTI with obstruction, diabetes	Gram-negative enterics	Focal fluid-filled defect on CT or US	Antibiotics alone or percutaneous drainage
Xanthgranulomatous pyelonephritis	Enlarging granulomatous process with cholesterol-laden macrophages	Chronic obstruction with infection	*Proteus sp. Klebsiella sp.*	Large heterogenous mass	Partial or complete nephrectomy
Emphysematous pyelonephritis	Ischemic necrosis with infection from gas-forming organisms	Elderly diabetic	Gram-negative enterics, rarely anaerobes	Gas on plain film, CT	Closed or open drainage or nephrectomy, antibiotics
Cortical abscess (renal carbuncle)	Hematogenous seeding of kidney	Extrarenal infection with *S. aureus*	*S. aureus*	Semi-solid intrarenal mass with caliceal distortion	Antibiotics alone or with percutaneous drainage.
Perinephric abscess	Rupture of intrarenal abscess	Obstruction, diabetes, renal transplants	*E. coli, Proteus sp., S. aureus*, others	Displaced renal tissue, perinepheric mass	Closed or open surgical drainage, antibiotics

do not show significant bacteriuria [60]. Complete urinary obstruction associated with pyonephrosis may also fail to show the primary pathogen within voided urine. Complicated UTIs often require radiologic methods to establish the correct diagnosis.

Blood cultures should be obtained on all patients who are septic as a result of a UTI. The acquisition of adequate volumes of blood before the initiation of antimicrobial therapy is crucial in the establishment of a diagnosis of bacteremic UTI. Urine cultures should also be performed from nephrostomy tube drainage in patients with prior urinary diversion procedures. It is generally unnecessary to change a urinary catheter before the acquisition of urine cultures in patients with acute UTI.

Radiographic Procedures in the Diagnosis of UTI

Routine abdominal radiographs are a useful diagnostic tool in some patients with complicated UTI. The presence of radiopaque renal calculi can be readily detected and their position determined on abdominal radiography. Emphysematous pyelonephritis appears as an abnormal collection of gas within the renal parenchyma [61]. Gas may also be detected in the urinary collecting system in patients with pyonephrosis. Abnormal renal shadows and loss of psoas margins may suggest the presence of a perinephric abscess. Renal ultrasonography and computed tomography (CT) have replaced the intravenous pyelogram (or excretory urogram) as the principal radiographic technique in the detection of complicated UTI. The anatomic definition of the kidney and perirenal tissues is superior with

abdominal CT scan. Nonetheless, the renal ultrasound may be a rapid method of detecting hydronephrosis and gives reasonably detailed anatomic information of the renal parenchyma as well. Ultrasonography also assists in the determination of the solid or cystic nature of a renal mass detected on abdominal CT. The ultrasound has the additional advantage of studying the kidney on any plane and may also be performed on an urgent basis in the absence of intravenous contrast media. CT of the kidney, particularly with intravenous contrast media, supplies excellent anatomic detail of the kidney and perirenal structures and has become the imaging study of choice for complicated UTI. Sufficient anatomic detail of renal parenchyma with CT scanning allows the differentiation of acute focal bacterial nephritis and corticomedullary abscess, cortical abscess, and perinephric abscess (see Table 90-1) [62]. The CT scan or renal ultrasound are indispensable in the localization of inflammatory processes during diagnostic aspiration or percutaneous drainage procedures. Magnetic resonance imaging (MRI) provides detailed information about the renal structures and retroperitoneal space, but MRI does not exceed the CT in resolving power for most renal inflammatory diseases [63].

The gallium-67– scan or indium-111–labeled leukocyte studies may occasionally be useful in the diagnosis of complicated UTI. These nuclear medicine studies may assist in the differentiation between renal neoplasms and focal inflammatory processes of the kidney. These studies may occasionally be useful in the evaluation of patients with fever of unknown origin who are subsequently found to harbor a small perinephric abscess or renal cortical abscess [64].

Intravenous pyelography (IVP) continues to provide the most detailed information of the calyces and ureters and may assist in the radiographic evaluation of UTIs associated with obstruction of the collecting system. This radiographic method remains

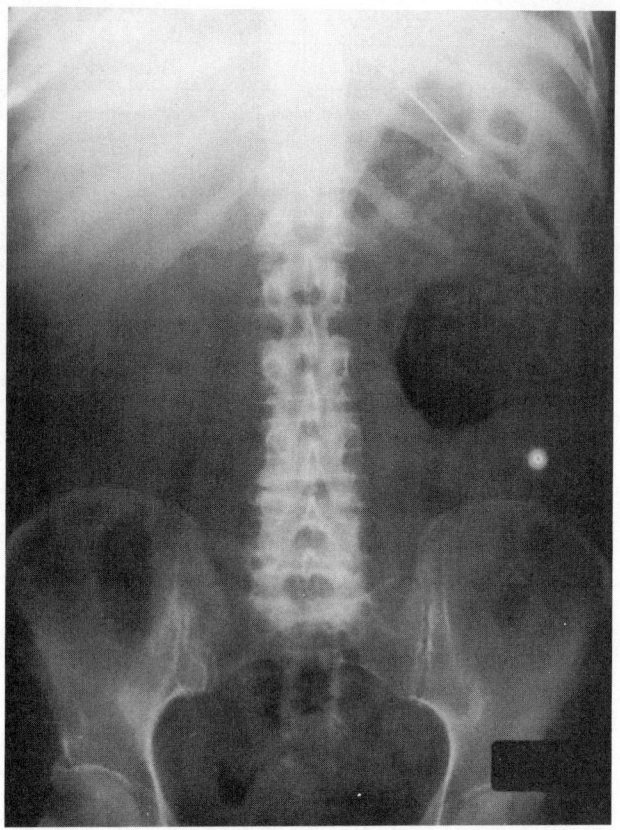

A

B

Fig. 90-2. Radiographic findings in a 73-year-old diabetic woman with emphysematous pyelonephritis caused by *E. coli;* A. Plain abdominal radiograph demonstrating the presence of gas in the right renal fossa. B. Computed tomography confirming the presence of gas in the right kidney. This patient was successfully treated with emergency nephrectomy and antimicrobial therapy.

the preferred method for the diagnosis of papillary necrosis and the detection of radiolucent urinary calculi. The need for intravenous contrast media carries with it the attendant risks of radiocontrast-induced renal failure. The potential for toxicity and lack of detailed resolution within the renal parenchyma has relegated the IVP to an infrequently performed procedure in the work-up of UTI [65].

Medical Management of UTI

Patients admitted to the intensive care unit as the result of UTI usually suffer from severe infections complicated by a systemic inflammatory response (sepsis) or complicated UTI with suppurative complications of the GU tract. Medical management initially consists of stabilization of the patient's hemodynamic parameters and intensive care support measures in the management of septic shock. Another priority is the rapid assessment of patients for possible suppurative or obstructive complications of UTI that necessitate urgent surgical management. After the completion of appropriate diagnostic studies, empiric antimicrobial therapy is then initiated and directed toward the most likely infecting urinary pathogen(s). A urinary Gram stain usually provides evidence of either a gram-negative or a gram-positive bacterial pathogen. If this is unavailable, as may be the case with urinary obstruction, then broad-spectrum, empiric antimicrobial therapy is indicated. The use of an extended spectrum bactericidal beta-lactam antibiotic in combination with an aminoglycoside has become the standard therapeutic regimen in UTIs associated with septic shock caused by gram-negative bacilli. The beta-lactam/aminoglycoside combination supplies optimal therapy for systemic infections with enterococci, *Pseudomonas*, and other multiresistant gram-negative urinary pathogens. This regimen remains the mainstay of therapy in septic patients who have nosocomially acquired urinary infections, catheter-related UTIs, or complicated UTIs with obstruction. Severely ill patients who are immunocompromised also warrant combination antimicrobial therapy [66,67].

Community-acquired UTIs in nonimmunocompromised patients who have not received antimicrobial agents infrequently harbor multiresistant gram-negative bacilli or *Pseudomonas* species. Should the urinary Gram stain exclude enterococci as a potential pathogen, then single therapy with a third-generation cephalosporin, extended-spectrum penicillin, trimethoprim-sulfamethoxazole, or a quinolone is acceptable therapy while awaiting culture results. Local susceptibility patterns of urinary pathogens should be used as a guide to the selection of antimicrobial therapy until susceptibility data of the specific urinary pathogen are available. There is no evidence that combination antimicrobial therapy is necessary for UTIs caused by gram-negative bacilli in the absence of neutropenia or complicated by infections caused by *Pseudomonas aeruginosa*. A single antimicrobial agent known to be active against the infecting uropathogen should be employed throughout the remainder of the patient's treatment once the causative organism is known. Parenteral therapy is generally administered until the patient has been rendered nontoxic and afebrile for 24 to 48 hours. Therapy may then be administered orally and should be given for a total of approximately 2 weeks [67,68]. Patients with obstructive lesions and complicated UTIs not amenable to corrective surgery may require prolonged courses of antimicrobial therapy as indicated by their underlying urologic disorder. Common antimicrobial agents useful in the treatment of severe UTIs are listed in Table 90-2.

Antimicrobial therapy for severe enterococcal UTIs has traditionally included ampicillin and an aminoglycoside. Although this regimen remains active against most enterococcal isolates, progressive antimicrobial resistance to aminoglycosides [69], ampicillin and other beta-lactams [41], and vancomycin [70] has complicated the antimicrobial therapy for enterococcal infections. High-level beta-lactam resistance may be the result of aberrant penicillin-binding proteins with low affinity to beta-lactam antibiotics [41]. These isolates require vancomycin or another class of antimicrobial agents to eradicate these infections. Beta-lactamase–producing enterococci are susceptible to beta-lactam inhibitor combinations such as ampicillin/sulbactam or ticarcillin/clavulanic acid [71]. High-level aminoglycoside-resistant strains of enterococci are increasing in frequency and pose a therapeutic dilemma in that the addition of aminoglycoside no longer contributes to synergistic clearance of these infections [69]. Aminoglycosides should not be used in the treatment of these enterococcal isolates in that the aminoglycoside only adds to toxicity and does not contribute to the antimicrobial activity against the organism. Glycopeptide-resistant strains of enterococci that express resistance to vancomycin and in some cases teicoplanin pose a serious threat to the antimicrobial management of enterococcal infections. Some of these isolates remain susceptible to beta-lactam agents. The quinolones have moderate activity against enterococci and may be useful in the treatment of glycopeptide- and beta-lactam–resistant strains of enterococci [70,71].

Anti-staphylococcal penicillins such as nafcillin or oxacillin are indicated in the empiric therapy of renal cortical abscesses (renal carbuncle). Vancomycin should be instituted if there is a suspicion of the presence of methicillin-resistant staphylococcal isolates in a patient with a cortical abscess or perinephric abscess. Treatment of *Candida* infections and other fungal infections of the urinary tract are considered in a subsequent section of this chapter.

Preventive Measures Against Urinary Tract Infection

Suppressive therapy with antimicrobial agents has been shown to be a useful strategy in infection-prone women with recurrent UTI. Continuous antimicrobial prophylaxis, postcoital prophylaxis, and self-initiated therapy for symptomatic UTIs have all been shown to be beneficial in infection-prone women [72]. Other behavior modifications such as avoidance of the use of diaphragms and spermicidal agents may also be useful in the prevention of recurrent UTIs [73]. The most efficacious method of prevention of UTIs in patients with uncorrectable structural abnormalities is less clear. Patients with structural or functional obstruction to urinary flow should be advised of the symptoms of UTIs and should seek medical attention at the early phases of symptomatic urinary infection. Asymptomatic bacteriuria in pregnant women and immunocompromised patients should be treated with specific antimicrobial agents in that the risk of ascending UTI is considerable and may be avoided by early medical intervention.

It is hoped that a detailed understanding of the molecular pathogenesis of UTIs will lead to innovative strategies against UTI. The recognition of specific virulence factors in uropathogens and the finding that a limited number of clones of bacteria are adapted to the urinary tract make it plausible that a polyvalent vaccine against UTI may be developed. Although progress toward this goal is being made, treatment with urinary receptor analogs [74], vaccine strategies [75], and alteration of

Table 90-2. Common Antimicrobial Agents in the Treatment of Severe UTI*

Agent	Dose	Frequency	Comments
Ampicillin/ sulbactam	3.0 gm IV	q6–8h	Other beta-lactam/inhibitor combinations also effective
Cefazolin	1.0 gm IV	q8h	
Cefotaxime	1 gm IV	q8h	Other second and third generation cephalosporins also effective
Ciprofloxacin	400 mg IV	q12h	IV ofloxacin also available
Gentamicin**	1.5 mg/kg IV	q8–12h	Dosing interval dependent on renal function
TMP-SMX	160/800 mg IV	q12h	Watch for sulfa allergies
Mezlocillin	3.0 gm IV	q8h	Other extended spectrum penicillins also effective

* Adult dosing in patients with normal renal function; follow susceptibility test results and treat parenterally until systemic toxicity resolves.
** Gentamicin or other aminoglycosides often given with a beta-lactam agent in gram-negative septic shock or severe enterococcal infections.

host factors that promote adherence of urinary pathogens to the mucosal surfaces remain experimental approaches that may prove to be useful in the prevention of UTI in the future.

The Management of Catheter-Related UTI

The ubiquitous presence of the indwelling urinary catheter in hospitalized patients provides perineal bacterial populations ready access to the urinary tract with subsequent development of UTI. It is estimated that 10 percent of all hospitalized patients in the United States will have a urinary catheter inserted during their hospitalization [76]. The prevalence of catheterized patients in the intensive care unit (ICU) is undoubtedly much higher and contributes to the high frequency of bacteriuria in the ICU setting. The risk of bacteriuria after urinary tract catheterization is approximately 5 percent for each day of catheterization. Chronically catheterized (>30 days) patients almost invariably have bacteriuria, and their admission to the ICU poses a threat of cross-contamination of urinary pathogens to other ICU patients. Despite considerable efforts to decrease the frequency of UTI associated with catheterization, UTI remains the major complication of the use of the urinary catheter.

PATHOGENESIS. The presence of a urinary catheter interferes with physiologic host defense mechanisms against UTI. Trauma produced by an indwelling catheter may damage the bladder mucosa and the mucous layer that coats uroepithelial cells [77]. This exposes the cell surface of epithelial cells to bacterial adhesins and increases the risk of UTI. Indwelling catheters prevent complete bladder emptying. Residual urine serves as culture media for bacteria in an inadequately drained urinary bladder. Additionally, temporary obstruction of urine flow caused by kinking or clamping of the urinary catheter leads to bladder distension, vesicoureteral reflux, and upper UTI.

Bacteria may gain access to the urinary tract in catheterized patients by one of three mechanisms: (1) introduction of bacteria during the insertion of the urinary catheter; (2) entrance of bacteria along the external mucous sheath between the urethra and urinary catheter; and (3) influx of urinary pathogens through the lumen of the urinary catheter. Implantation of bacteria into the bladder during catheter placement occurs at a frequency of approximately 0.5 percent to 8 percent [78]. This risk varies with the experience of the health care worker placing the catheter and with the level of periurethral colonization by potential uropathogens. Ascending UTI with the inner lumen as the portal of entry accounts for approximately 20 percent of catheter-related UTIs [79]. The use of sterile, closed urinary collecting devices that have a sterile vent to avoid a standing column of urine from the bladder to the collecting bag has decreased the frequency of UTI from the catheter lumen. Catheter design should include a sampling port that can be maintained in a sterile condition and avoid the need to open the system to collect urine samples. The urinary collecting bag should have a large reservoir with a device to measure urine output with minimal manipulation of the catheter system.

Most catheter-related UTIs are derived from bacterial organisms that enter the urinary bladder along the external surface of the urinary catheter [79,80]. The periurethral space becomes colonized with enteric organisms, which then migrate along the periurethral mucous sheath that surrounds the surface of the catheter. It is difficult to anchor the urinary catheter in place. Continued movement of the catheter in and out of the urinary bladder occurs on repositioning of the patient or other catheter manipulations. This process provides ample opportunity for bacteria that coat the catheter surface to gain access to the urinary bladder and cause infection.

Numerous enteric organisms avidly adhere to the mucosal surface of the urinary bladder. Some organisms, such as *Providencia stuartii* and *Pseudomonas aeruginosa,* also possess surface adhesins that bind directly to the urinary catheter itself. The urinary catheter becomes an ecologic niche for these organisms, resulting in prolonged infections that may persist for months in the catheterized patient [81]. The urease produced by *Proteus* sp. affects the local pH surrounding the catheter, which facilitates the deposition of struvite microcrystals on the surface of the catheter. These encrustations serve as a nidus for persistent colonization with urinary pathogens. The continued buildup of this biofilm within the lumen of the urinary catheter eventually leads to obstruction of urinary flow [82]. The presence of a foreign body within the urinary bladder may also interfere with the antimicrobial action of antibiotics. Bactericidal antimicrobial agents may inhibit but often fail to kill microorganisms that are adherent to catheter materials. Furthermore, the presence of the catheter functions as a foreign body, which leads to early degranulation and loss of bactericidal activity of neutrophils. These factors contribute to the difficulties inherent in the therapeutic efforts to eradicate urinary pathogens in the catheterized patient.

DIAGNOSIS. The presence of bacteriuria in the catheterized patient documents colonization of the urinary tract but does not necessarily confirm the presence of an actual UTI. UTI indicates that a host response has occurred to the presence of microbial pathogens in the urine. As many as 70 percent of patients who develop catheter-related bacteriuria remain symptom free and resolve spontaneously with the catheter removal [83]. It is generally acknowledged that the treatment of asymptomatic bacteriuria in the catheterized patient is not warranted,

except in some specific circumstances [84]. The severely neutropenic patient with asymptomatic bacteriuria should be treated because of the risk of systemic infection in this patient population. Additionally, the treatment of asymptomatic bacteriuria in the catheterized patient may be warranted in an outbreak setting of nosocomially acquired infection in an ICU if the patient has been epidemiologically linked to the spread of specific urinary pathogens [85].

It is often difficult to recognize that a symptomatic UTI is present in the catheterized patient. Altered levels of consciousness may interfere with the patient's awareness of the UTI. Furthermore, the presence of a urinary catheter removes the symptoms of urinary frequency and the perception of dysuria. Hematuria and pyuria may be found in the catheterized patient in the absence of urinary colonization with bacteria. This is presumably related to sterile inflammation and trauma induced by the catheter itself. Nonetheless, the presence of high-grade pyuria (>50 WBC/HPF) has been associated with fever and supports the diagnosis of a UTI in the catheterized patient [86]. Quantitative urine culture is valuable in the confirmation of catheter-related UTI. Clearly the presence of more than 10^5 CFU per milliliter indicates that the urinary bladder is colonized with a significant number of microorganisms. The presence of lower numbers of bacteria in catheterized urine may also suggest infection in catheterized patients [87]. Quantitative counts as low as 10^2 CFU per milliliter may be significant in the catheterized patient [87,88]. It has been shown that low colony counts in catheterized urine progress to high-grade bacteriuria in most patients who do not receive suppressive antimicrobial therapy. Clinical laboratories should isolate and characterize urinary isolates from catheterized patients even if the quantitative counts are below 10^5 CFU per milliliter. The high flow rate of catheterized urine, presence of inhibitors to bacterial growth, and significance of slow-growing organisms such as enterococci and *Candida* make it incumbent on the laboratory to characterize even low numbers of uropathogens in these patients. Moreover, polymicrobial bacteriuria occurs in more than 15 percent of patients with catheter-related UTI [89]. Multiple organisms must be isolated, characterized, and subjected to susceptibility testing to ensure adequate treatment of catheter-related UTIs.

Most patients who have symptomatic UTIs associated with urinary catheters have lower urinary tract involvement. Upper tract involvement occurs in up to one third of catheter-related UTIs and may have serious consequences [90]. The clinical and laboratory recognition of upper urinary tract involvement in persons with UTI (with or without a catheter) remains imprecise and unsatisfactory. ICU patients with UTIs may have altered levels of consciousness and may not be able to relate the symptoms of upper tract involvement. Antibody-coated bacteria have not proved to be sufficiently reproducible and reliable to distinguish upper from lower UTI [91]. Bladder washout techniques may be effective [92] but are cumbersome and infrequently used in the ICU setting. Radiographic indicators of upper tract involvement with evidence of enlarged kidneys on ultrasound or CT are expensive, impractical, and inconvenient methods of diagnosis in ICU patients. The patient is generally assumed to have upper tract disease if evidence of systemic toxicity is present and treated accordingly. Bacteria confined to the urinary bladder, in contrast, should clear with removal of the urinary catheter followed by a short course of antimicrobial therapy if necessary.

TREATMENT. Perhaps the most important therapeutic modality in the treatment of catheter-related UTIs is the removal of the urinary catheter itself. Up to two thirds of patients with bacteriuria associated with urinary catheterization spontaneously resolve within 1 week after catheter removal [83]. Patients with persistent bacteriuria after catheter removal should be treated with a short course (3 days) of an appropriate antimicrobial agent, which should be sufficient to eradicate bladder bacteriuria. If patients have persistent bacteriuria after short-course therapy, then a 14-day course of an active antimicrobial agent would be appropriate to treat a presumed upper UTI [93].

Should a patient become systemically ill from a UTI, treatment is warranted even if the catheter must remain in place. It is possible to successfully treat UTIs in patients with indwelling catheters, although treatment failures and reinfection occur at a greater frequency than in noncatheterized patients [94]. Antimicrobial agents useful in the treatment of catheter-related UTI are described in Table 90-2.

Routine replacement of indwelling urinary catheters complicated by UTI is generally unnecessary. Although some organisms such as *Proteus, Providencia, Morganella,* and *Pseudomonas* species and the enterococci may colonize the urinary catheter in greater quantities than the actual urinary bladder, the microbiology of urine samples from indwelling catheters and replacement catheters does not differ markedly in the presence of a UTI [95]. Catheters should be replaced if they are malfunctioning, obstructed, or leak around urethral orifice. Leaking urinary catheters generally indicate luminal obstruction and require replacement.

It is important to recognize that long-term urinary catheterization may be associated with other local suppurative complications, particularly in adult men. These include prostatitis, prostatic abscess, epididymitis, scrotal abscess, and other urethral complications [96,97]. These local complications require urologic management and necessitate the removal of the urethral catheter.

PREVENTION

Alternatives to Urethral Catheterization. The recognition of the high frequency of catheter-related UTIs has led to concerted efforts to find alternative methods to manage the incontinent patient and patients with urinary outflow obstruction. Bladder training, meticulous nursing care, and special linens and diapers may assist some incontinent patients and avoid long-term catheterization. Avoidance of sedative-hypnotic drugs, maintenance of physical activity, and regular socialization may assist in the preservation of continence in elderly populations without resorting to indwelling catheters. Should these methods fail to maintain dryness in the perineal area, other alternatives have been attempted with limited success.

Condom catheterization has been used for men with urinary incontinence and consists of the application of an external collector about the penis with a collection tube and drainage bag. Condom catheterization may be a reasonable alternative in selected patients who are cooperative and highly motivated. However, leakage of the catheter, kinking and disruption of the collecting system, and maceration and ulceration of the epithelium of the penis are frequent complications of condom drainage [98]. The incidence of UTIs may not be significantly lowered by the use of a condom catheter when compared with an indwelling catheter in many patients [98,99]. This has limited the utility of this alternative approach to urinary drainage.

Intermittent catheterization has been used for many years in centers for spinal cord injury patients. This strategy may be more efficacious if combined with a urinary antiseptic such as oral methenamine or systemic antimicrobial prophylaxis [100]. This method of urinary drainage is infrequently appropriate for the ICU patient. Similarly, suprapubic catheterization is not often an option available in the critical care unit. Some evidence

suggests that this may be an appropriate alternative to long-term urethral catheterization in selected patient populations [101].

Catheter Design, Maintenance, and Care. Because most catheter-related infections are derived from endogenous perineal organisms adherent to the exterior surface of the catheter itself, daily urethral meatal care with the application of antimicrobial materials at the urethral orifice would seem to be a logical preventive measure. However, randomized, controlled, clinical trials with meatal care and application of povidone-iodine solution or topical polyantimicrobic applications have failed to convincingly demonstrate a reduction in catheter-related infections [102,103,104]. This procedure cannot be recommended as a means of prevention of catheter-associated UTI.

Considerable effort has been undertaken by manufacturers to develop a urinary catheter that interferes with the binding of bacteria, inhibits biofilm formation, or possesses antibacterial properties. The value of siliconized catheters [105,106], antibacterial-coated catheters, and other catheter innovations designed to decrease the risk of UTI remains to be demonstrated in carefully controlled, clinical trials [107,108]. Closed drainage with latex catheters with sterile portals for urine sampling remain the standard of care for indwelling urethral catheters.

Exogenous contamination of the urethral catheter and the urine within the collection bag remains an infrequent but significant problem associated with indwelling urethral catheters. The instillation of antiseptic agents within the drainage bag as a means of prevention of catheter-related UTIs has met with conflicting results [109,110]. The procedure appears to increase the risk of acquisition of multiple drug-resistant gram-negative bacilli. Urinary irrigation with antimicrobial agents or the instillation of antiseptic in the urinary drainage drainage bag is not recommended.

Antimicrobial Prophylaxis for Catheter-Related UTI. A number of reports indicate the potential utility of systemic antimicrobial prophylaxis in the prevention of UTIs in catheterized patients [111,112]. The clinical benefits of this preventive measure appear to be limited to short-term catheterization. This method fails to prevent the development of bacteriuria in chronically catheterized patients and predisposes to the acquisition of multi–drug-resistant gram-negative bacilli. A recent report illustrates the potential benefits and hidden risks of this approach to antimicrobial prophylaxis [113]. Patients with acute spinal cord injury were randomized to trimethoprim-sulfamethoxazole (TMP-SMX) or placebo in a double-blind fashion in an effort to decrease the frequency of UTIs after intermittent catheterization. Symptomatic bacteriuria occurred in 7 percent of TMP-SMX–treated patients and 35% in the placebo-treated patients (p < 0.0003). However, TMP-SMX–resistant organisms were found to be increasingly prevalent over the following 3 years at this special care unit. TMP-SMX–resistant bacteria were found in 49 percent of treated patients and 42 percent of placebo-treated patients. The prevalence of antibiotic resistance limits the utility of this preventive approach. Systemic antimicrobial prophylaxis must be considered an experimental approach to prevention of catheter-related UTI.

The Problem of Candiduria

The clinical interpretation of the isolation of *Candida* species from the urine is problematic in that this organism's presence in the urine may occur in a spectrum of illnesses ranging from simple contamination to life-threatening systemic candidiasis. *Candida* species are normal inhabitants of the vaginal tract of women and may contaminate inadequately collected urine specimens. This is particularly true in older women, diabetics, and patients receiving antibacterial therapy. Additionally, *Candida* species frequently colonize the urinary tract in catheterized patients. These organisms are of marginal clinical significance and frequently disappear on removal of the urinary catheter without any specific antifungal therapy [114]. However, tissue invasive infection of the urinary bladder has been documented cystoscopically in patients with genitourinary candidiasis. Candida cystitis may produce a friable white pseudomembrane on the bladder mucosa similar to the findings of oral thrush. Furthermore, ascending urinary infection of the kidney and renal pelvis may follow genitourinary candidiasis [115,116]. Papillary necrosis, fungus ball formation, urinary obstruction, and perinephric abscess have all been described from ascending infection with *Candida* species. Moreover, *Candida* infection of the upper urinary tract may arise from hematogenous dissemination of *Candida* organisms from extrarenal sites. Microabscesses of the renal parenchyma with subsequent candiduria is a frequent finding in disseminated candidiasis. Therefore, the isolation of *Candida* in the urine poses a diagnostic dilemma as to its clinical significance.

Quantitative culture of the urine has been used in an attempt to determine the clinical ramifications of candiduria. Unfortunately, the quantitative colony counts of *Candida* species in the urine do not have the same diagnostic and prognostic implications as quantitative bacteriology of the urine [117]. The finding of urinary casts made up of *Candida* elements is of diagnostic significance and indicates invasive upper tract candidiasis. Candiduria associated with a fungus ball in the urinary collecting system dictates the need for antifungal therapy, as does papillary necrosis or abscess formation within the renal parenchyma. Recurrent isolation of *Candida* species in urine cultures in immunocompromised patients, or patients with unexplained fever and pyuria, suggests UTI with *Candida* species. Evidence of concomitant infection with *Candida* organisms in other organ systems increase the likelihood of the significance of *Candida* isolates in the urine. Disseminated candidiasis should be considered in patients with repeated and unexplained *Candida* isolates in the urinary tract [118].

The Treatment of Genitourinary Candidiasis

There are several treatment options available in the management of candiduria, depending on the clinical circumstances in each patient. The discontinuation of antibacterial agents, removal of immunosuppression, or removal of urinary catheters may be sufficient for the spontaneous eradication of candiduria and remains an acceptable treatment strategy in medically stable patients.

Bladder instillation of amphotericin B or other antifungal agents has become the mainstay of therapy for catheter-related UTI with *Candida* species. Recent evidence suggests that the conventional bladder irrigation with 50 mg amphotericin B and 1000 ml sterile water is potentially toxic to uroepithelial cells and is not necessary for eradication of *Candida* infections of the bladder [119]. Amphotericin at a dose of 5 to 10 mg per liter sterile water instilled in the bladder for 60 to 90 minutes twice daily for 2 days is the current recommendation for the treatment of *Candida* cystitis. Systemic amphotericin B is indicated in patients with candiduria and suspected systemic candidiasis,

renal abscess formation, and fungus balls within the urinary collecting system.

The triazole compound, fluconazole, is a water-soluble antifungal agent and is excreted in the urine in high concentration as the active compound [120]. Although this is not yet an approved indication for its use, *Candida* UTI may be readily treated with oral or intravenous fluconazole. A short course of fluconazole at 200 mg orally followed by 100 mg daily for 3 days is generally effective in the treatment of *Candida* cystitis. Fluconazole has yet to be shown to be an acceptable alternative to amphotericin B in systemic candidiasis resulting in candiduria. Until clinical trials demonstrate the efficacy of fluconazole in this setting, amphotericin B remains the treatment of choice in disseminated candidal infections.

References

1. Centers for Disease Control. Nosocomial infection surveillance. 33:9SS, 1983.
2. Haley RW, Colver DH, White JW, et al: The nationwide nosocomial infection rate: A need for vital statistics. *Am J Epidemiol* 121:159, 1985.
3. Krieger JN, Kaiser DL, Wenzel RP: Nosocomial urinary tract infections: Secular trends, treatment and economics in a university hospital. *J Urol* 130:102, 1983.
4. McCarty E: Inpatient utilization of short-stay hospitals, by diagnosis: United States, 1980, in *Vital and Health Statistics.* Data From the National Health Survey, Series 13. Hyattsville, MD, National Center for Health Statistics, No. 74, 1983.
5. Zachtman M, Mercer A, Kusecek B, et al: Six widespread bacterial clones among Escherichia coli K1 isolates. Infect Immun 39:315, 1983.
6. Enerbäck S, Larsson AC, Jodal U, et al: Binding of galactose alpha 1 → 4 galactose beta-containing receptors as a potential diagnostic tool in urinary tract infection. *J Clin Microbiol* 25:407, 1987.
7. Kaijser B, Hanson LA, Jodal U, et al: Frequency of E. coli K antigens in urinary tract infections in children. *Lancet* 1:663, 1977.
8. Källenius G, Svensson SB, Hultburg H: Occurrence of P-fimbriated Escherichia coli in urinary tract infections. *Lancet* 2:1369, 1981.
9. Leffler H, Svanborg Edén C: Glycolipid receptors for uropathogenic Escherichia coli binding to human erythrocytes in uroepithelial cells: Globoseries of glycolipids vs other receptors. *Infect Immun* 34:920, 1981.
10. Lidin-Janson G, Hanson LA, Kaijser B, et al: Comparison of Escherichia coli from bacteriuric patients with those from faeces of healthy school children. *J Infect Dis* 136:346, 1977.
11. Olling S, Hanson LA, Holmgren J, et al: The bactericidal effect of normal human serum on E. coli strains from normals and from patients with urinary tract infections. *Infection* 1:24, 1973.
12. Sandberg T, Stenquist K, Svanborg Edén C, et al: Host-parasite relationship in urinary tract infections during pregnancy. *Prog Allergy* 33:223, 1983.
13. Stenqvist K, Sandberg T, Lindin-Janson G, et al: Virulence factors in Escherichia coli urinary isolates from pregnant women. *J Infect Dis* 156:870, 1987.
14. Ørskov I, Ørskov F, Birch-Andersen A, et al: O,K,H, and fimbrial antigens in Escherichia coli serotypes associated with pyelonephritis and cystitis. *Scand J Infect Dis* 33:18, 1982.
15. Svanborg Edén C, Bjursten LM, Hull R, et al: Influence of adhesins on the interaction of Escherichia coli with human phagocytes. *Infect Immun* 44:407, 1984.
16. Väisänen-Rhen V, Elo J, Väisänen E, et al: P-fimbriated clones among uropathogenic Escherichia coli strains. *Infect Immun* 43:149, 1984.
17. Ørskov I, Ørskov F: Escherichia coli in extra-intestinal infections. *J Hyg Camb* 95:551, 1985.
18. Opal SM, Cross AS, Gemski P, et al: Aerobactin in alpha-hemolysin as virulence determinants in Escherichia coli isolated from human blood, urine, and stool. *J Infect Dis* 161:994, 1990.

19. Arthur M, Johnson CE, Rubin RH, et al: Molecular epidemiology of adhesin and hemolysin virulence factors among uropathogenic Escherichia coli. *Infect Immun* 57:301, 1989.
20. Brun V: Escherichia coli cells containing the plasmid Col V produce the iron ionophore aerobactin. *FEMS Microbiol Lett* 11:225, 1981.
21. Maslow JN, Mulligan ME, Adams KS, et al: Bacterial adhesins and host factors: Role in the development and outcome of Escherichia coli bacteremia. *Clin Infect Dis* 17:89, 1993.
22. Welch RA, Dillinger AP, Minshew B, et al: Haemolysin contributes to virulence of extra-intestinal E. coli infections. *Nature* 297:665, 1981.
23. O'Hanley P, Lalonde G, Ji G: Alpha-hemolysin contributes to the pathogenicity of piliated digalactoside-binding Escherichia coli in the kidney: Efficacy of an alpha-hemolysin vaccine in preventing renal injury in the BALB/c mouse model of pyelonephritis. *Infect Immun* 59:1153, 1991.
24. Payne SM: Iron and virulence in the family Enterobacteriaceae. *CRC Crit Rev Microbiol* 16:81, 1988.
25. Cavalieri SJ, Snyder JS: Effect of Escherichia coli alpha-hemolysin on human peripheral leukocyte function in vitro. *Infect Immun* 37:966, 1982.
26. Keane WF, Welch R, Gakker G, et al: Mechanism of Escherichia coli alpha-hemolysin-induced injury to isolated renal tubular cells. *Am J Pathol* 126:350, 1987.
27. Hagberg L, Jodal U, Korhonen TK, et al: Adhesion hemagglutination and virulence in Escherichia coli causing urinary tract infections. *Infect Immun* 31:564, 1981.
28. Reid G, Sobel JD: Bacterial adherence in the pathogenesis of urinary tract infection: A review. *Rev Infect Dis* 9:470, 1987.
29. de Man P, Jodal U, Lincoln K, et al: Bacterial attachment and inflammation in the urinary tract. *J Infect Dis* 158:29, 1988.
30. O'Hanley P, Low D, Romero I, et al: Gal-Gal binding and hemolysin phenotypes and genotypes associated with uropathogenic Escherichia coli. *N Engl J Med* 313:414, 1985.
31. KSllenius G, Mollby R, Svensson SB et al: The PKantigen as receptor for the haemagglutination of pyelonephritic E. coli. *FEMS Microbiol Lett* 7:297, 1980.
32. Hagberg L, Hull R, Hull S, et al: Contribution of adhesion to bacterial persistence in the mouse urinary tract. *Infect Immun* 40:265, 1983.
33. Dominque GJ, Roberts JA, Laucirica R, et al: Pathogenic significance of P fimbriated Escherichia coli in urinary tract infections. *J Urol* 133:983, 1985.
34. Asher EF, Oliver BG, Fry DE: Urinary tract infections in the surgical patient. *Am Surg* 54:466, 1988.
35. Warren JW, Tenney JH, Woopes JM, et al: A prospective microbiologic study of bacteriuria in patients with chronic indwelling urethral catheters. *J Infect Dis* 146:719, 1982.
36. McLean R, Nickel JC, Noakes VC, et al: An in vitro ultrastructural study of infectious kidney stone genesis. *Infect Immun* 49:805, 1985.
37. Hovelius B, Mardh P: Staphylococcus saprophyticus as a common cause of urinary tract infections. *Rev Infect Dis* 6:328, 1984.
38. Cluff LE, Reynolds RC, Page DL, et al: Staphylococcal bacteremia in altered host resistance. *Ann Intern Med* 69:856, 1968.
39. Lee BK, Crossley K, Gerding DN: The association between Staphylococcus aureus bacteremia and bacteriuria. *Am J Med* 65:301, 1978.
40. Hsu CCS, Macaluso CP, Special L, et al: High rate of methicillin resistance of Staphylococcus aureus isolated from hospitalized nursing home patients. *Arch Intern Med* 148:569, 1988.
41. Spera RV, Farber BF: Multiply-resistant Enterococcus faecium: The nosocomial pathogen of the 1990s. *JAMA* 268:2563, 1992.
42. Fisher JF, Chew WH, Shadomy S, et al: Urinary tract infections due to Candida albicans. *Rev Infect Dis* 4:1107, 1982.
43. Stamm WE: Catheter-associated urinary tract infections: Epidemiology, pathogenicity and prevention. *Am J Med* 91(S3B):865, 1991.
44. Lomberg H, Hellstrom M, Jodal U, et al: Virulence-associated traits in Escherichia coli causing first and recurrent urinary tract infection in children with or without vesicoureteral reflux. *J Infect Dis* 150:561, 1984.
45. Kaye D: Antibacterial activity of human urine. *J Clin Invest* 47:2374, 1968.
46. Sobel JD, Kaye D: Reduced uromucoid excretion in the elderly. *J Infect Dis* 152:653, 1985.
47. Lomberg H, Hanson LA, Jacobsson B, et al: Correlation of P blood group, vesicoureteral reflux, and bacterial attachment in patients with recurrent pyelonephritis. *N Engl J Med* 308:1189, 1983.
48. Lomberg H, Cedergren B, Leffler H, et al: Influence of blood groups on the availability of receptors for attachments of uropathogenic Escherichia coli. *Infect Immun* 51:919, 1986.
49. Sheinfeld J, Schaeffer AJ, Cordon-Cardo C, et al: Association of Lewis blood group phenotype with recurrent urinary tract infections in women. *N Engl J Med* 320:773, 1989.
50. Agace WW, Hedges SR, Ceska M, et al: Interleukin-8 and the neutrophil response to mucosal gram-negative infection. *J Clin Invest* 92:780, 1993.
51. Stamey TA, Fair WR, Timothy MM: Antibacterial nature of prostatic fluid. *Nature* 218:444, 1968.
52. Knaus WA, Harrell FE, Fisher CJ, Jr., et al: The clinical evaluation of new drugs for sepsis: A prospective study design based on survival analysis. *JAMA* 270:1233, 1993.
53. Silverman DE, Stamey TA: Management of infection stone: The Stanford experience. *Medicine* 62:44, 1983.
54. Jenkins RD, Fenn JP, Matsen JM: Review of urine microscopy for bacteriuria. *JAMA* 255:3397, 1986.
55. New HC: Urinary tract infections. *Am J Med* 92(4A):63S, 1992.
56. Stamm WE: Quantitative urine cultures revisited. *Eur J Microbiol* 3:279, 1984.
57. Stamm WE, Counts GW, Running KR, et al: Diagnosis of coliform infection in acutely dysuric women. *N Engl J Med* 207:463, 1982.
58. Lipsky BA: Urinary tract infection in men: Epidemiology, pathophysiology, diagnosis and treatment. *Ann Intern Med* 110:138, 1989.
59. Thorley JD, Jones SR, Sanford JP: Perinephric abscess. *Medicine* 53:41, 1974.
60. Schiff M, Glickman M, Weiss RM, et al: Antibiotic treatment for renal carbuncle. *Ann Intern Med* 87:305, 1977.
61. Allen HA, Walsh JW, Brewer WH, et al: Sonography of emphysematous pyelonephritis. *J Ultrasound Med* 3:533, 1984.
62. Mendez G, Isikoff MB, Morillo G: The role of computerized tomography in the diagnosis of renal and perirenal abscesses. *J Urol* 122:582, 1979.
63. Baumgartner BR, Chezmar JL: Magnetic resonance imaging of kidneys and adrenal glands. *Semin Ultrasound CT MR* 10:43, 1989.
64. Piccirillo M, Rigsby C, Rosenfield AT: Contemporary imaging of renal inflammatory disease. *Infect Dis Clin North Am* 1:927, 1987.
65. Kanel KT, Kroboth FJ, Schwentker FN, et al: The intravenous pyelogram in acute pyelonephritis. *Arch Intern Med* 148:2144, 1988.
66. Kunin CM: Use of antimicrobial agents in treating urinary tract infection. *Adv Nephrol* 14:39, 1985.
67. Klein LA, Koyle M, Berg S: The emergency management of patients with urethral calculi and fever. *J Urol* 129:938, 1983.
68. Stamm WE, McKevitt M, Counts GW: Acute renal infection in women: Treatment with trimethoprim-sulfamethoxazole or ampicillin for two or six weeks. A randomized trial. *Ann Intern Med* 104:341, 1987.
69. Rhinehart E, Smith NE, Wennersten C: Rapid dissemination of beta-lactamase-producing aminoglycoside-resistant Enterococcus faecalis among patients and staff of an infant-toddler surgical ward. *N Engl J Med* 323:1814, 1990.
70. Fraimow HS, Venuti E: Inconsistent bactericidal activity of triple-combination therapy with vancomycin, ampicillin and gentamicin against vancomycin-resistant, highly ampicillin-resistant Enterococcus faecium. *Antimicrob Agents Chemother* 36:1563, 1992.
71. Murray BE: The life and times of the enterococcus. *Clin Microbiol Rev* 3:46, 1990.
72. Stapleton A, Latham RH, Johnson C, et al: Postcoital antimicrobial prophylaxis for recurrent urinary tract infection. *JAMA* 264:703, 1990.
73. Strom BL, Collins M, West SL, et al: Sexual activity, contraceptive use, and other risk factors for symptomatic and asymptomatic bacteriuria: A case-controlled study. *Ann Intern Med* 107:816, 1987.
74. Svanborg EdQn C, Freter R, Hagberg L, et al: Inhibition of experimental ascending urinary tract infection by an epithelial cell-surface receptor analogue. *Nature* 298:560, 1982.

75. O'Hanley P, Lark D, Falkow S, et al: Molecular basis for Escherichia coli colonization of the upper urinary tract in BALB/c mice. *J Clin Invest* 75:347, 1985.
76. Garibaldi RA, Burke JP, Dickman ML, et al: Factors predisposing to bacteriuria during indwelling urethral catheterization. *N Engl J Med* 291:215, 1974.
77. Vardi Y, Meshulam T, Obedeanu H, et al: In vivo adherance of Pseudomonas aeruginosa to rat bladder epithelium. *Proc Soc Exp Biol Med* 172:449, 1983.
78. Kunin CM: Care of the urinary catheter, in Kunin CM (ed): *Detection, Prevention, and Management of Urinary Tract Infections*. Philadelphia, Lea and Febiger, 1987, p 245.
79. Schaberg DR, Haley RW, Highsmith AK, et al: Nosocomial bacteriuria: A prospective study of case clustering and antimicrobial resistance. *Ann Intern Med* 93:420, 1980.
80. Garibaldi RA, Burke JP, Britt MR, et al: Meatal colonization and catheter-associated bacteriuria. *N Engl J Med* 303:316, 1980.
81. Mobley HL, Chippendale GR, Tenney JH, et al: MR/K hemagglutination of Providencia stuartii correlates with adherence to catheters and with persistence in catheter-associated bacteriuria. *J Infect Dis* 157:264, 1988.
82. Mobley HL, Warren JW: Urease-positive bacteriuria in obstruction of long-term indwelling urinary catheters. *Arch Phys Med Rehabil* 69:25, 1988.
83. Harding GKM, Nicolle LE, Ronald AR, et al: How long should catheter-acquired urinary tract infection in women be treated. *Ann Intern Med* 114:713, 1991.
84. Warren JW: Catheter-associated urinary tract infections. *Infect Dis Clin North Am* 1:823, 1987.
85. Okuda T, Endo N, Osada Y, et al: Outbreak of nosocomial urinary tract infections caused by Serratia marcescens. *J Clin Microbiol* 20:691, 1984.
86. Peterson JR, Roth EJ: Fever, bacteriuria and pyuria in spinal cord injured patients with indwelling urethral catheters. *Arch Phys Med Rehabil* 70:839, 1989.
87. Garibaldi RA, Mooney BR, Epstein BJ, et al: An evaluation of daily bacteriologic monitoring to identify to preventable episodes of catheter-associated urianry tract infection. *Infect Control* 3:466, 1982.
88. Stark RP, Maki D: Bacteriuria in the catheterized patient: What quantitative level of bacteriuria is relevant? *N Engl J Med* 311:560, 1984.
89. Warren JW, Tenney JH, Hoopes JM, et al: A prospective microbiologic study of bacteriuria in patients with chronic indwelling urethral catheters. *J Infect Dis* 146:719, 1982.
90. Warren JW, Damron D, Tenney JH, et al: Fever, bacteremia, and death as complications of bacteriuria in women with long-term urethral catheters. *J Infect Dis* 155:1151, 1987.
91. Thomas VL, Forland M: Antibody-coated bacteria in urinary tract infections. *Kidney Int* 21:1, 1982.
92. Fairley KF, Bond AG, Brown RB, et al: Simple test to determine the site of urinary tract infection. *Lancet* 2:427, 1967.
93. Stamm WE, Hooten TM, Johnson C Jr., et al: Urinary tract infections: From pathogenesis to treatment. *J Infect Dis* 159:400, 1989.
94. Butler HJ, Kunin CM: Evaluation of specific antimicrobial therapy in patients while on closed catheter drainage. *J Urol* 100:567, 1968.
95. Grahn D, Norman DC, White ML, et al: Validity of urinary catheter specimens for the diagnosis of urinary tract infection in the elderly. *Arch Intern Med* 145:1858, 1985.
96. Weinberger M, Cytron S, Servadio C, et al: Prostatic abscess in the antibiotic era. *Rev Infect Dis* 10:239, 1988.
97. Corrado ML, Cierra MF, Eng R, et al: Anaerobic prostatic abscess. *NY State J Med* 80:652, 1980.
98. Hirsh DD, Fainstein V, Musher DM: Do condom catheter collecting systems cause urinary tract infection? *JAMA* 242:340, 1979.
99. Ouslander JG, Greengold B, Chen S: External catheter use in urinary tract infections among incontinent male nursing home patients. *J Am Geriatr Soc* 35:1063, 1987.
100. Krebs M, Halvorsen RB, Fishman IJ, et al: Prevention of urinary tract infection during intermittent catheterization. *J Urol* 131:82, 1984.
101. Sethia KK, Selkon JB, Barry AR, et al: Prospective randomized controlled trial of urethral versus suprapublic catheterization. *Br J Surg* 74:624, 1987.
102. Burke JP, Garibaldi RA, Britt MR, et al: Prevention of catheter-associated urinary tract infections: Efficacy of daily meatal care regimens. *Am J Med* 70:655, 1981.
103. Burke JP, Jacobson JA, Garibaldi RA, et al: Evaluation of daily meatal care with polyantimicrobic ointment in the prevention of urinary catheter-associated bacteriuria. *J Urol* 129:331, 1983.
104. Classen DC, Larsen RA, Burke JP, et al: Daily meatal care for prevention of catheter-associated bacteriuria: Results following frequent applications of polyantibiotic cream. *Infect Control Hosp Epidemiol* 12:157, 1991.
105. Cox AJ, Millington RS, Hukins DW, et al: Resistance of catheters coated with a modified hydrogel to encrustation during an in vitro test. *Urol Res* 17:353, 1989.
106. Lopez G, Pascual A, Martinez L, et al: Effect of a siliconized latex urinary catheter on bacterial adherence in human neutrophil activity. *Diagn Microbiol Infect Dis* 14:1, 1991.
107. Leidbeig H, Lundeberg T: Silver alloy coated catheters reduce catheter-associated bacteriuria. *Br J Urol* 65:379, 1990.
108. Johnson JR, Roberts PL, Olsen RJ, et al: Prevention of catheter-associated urinary tract infection with a silver oxide-coated urinary catheter: Clinical and microbiologic correlates. *J Infect Dis* 162:1145, 1990.
109. Thompson RL, Haley CE, Searcey MA, et al: Catheter-associated bacteriuria: Failure to reduce attack rates using periodic instillations of a disinfectant into urinary drainage systems. *JAMA* 251:747, 1984.
110. Holliman RC, Seal DV, Archer H, et al: Controlled trial of chemical disinfection of urinary drainage bags: Reduction in hospital-acquired, catheter-associated infection. *Br J Urol* 60:419, 1987.
111. Vollaard EJ, Clasener HAL, Zambon JV, et al: Prevention of catheter-associated, gram-negative bacilluria with norfloxacin by selective decontamination of the bowel and high urinary concentration. *J Antimicrob Chemother* 23:915, 1989.
112. Kuhlemeier KV, Stover SL, Lloyd LK: Prophylactic antibacterial therapy for preventing urinary tract infections in spinal cord injury patients. *J Urol* 134:514, 1985.
113. Gribble MJ, Puterman ML: Prophylaxis of urinary tract infection in patients with recent spinal cord injury: A prospective, randomized, double-blind, placebo-controlled study of trimethoprim-sulfamethoxazole. *Am J Med* 95:141, 1993.
114. Thornton GF, Lytton B, Andriole VT: Bacteriuria during indwelling catheter drainage. *JAMA* 195:179, 1966.
115. Frye KR, Donovan JM, Drach GW: Torulopsis glabrata urinary infections: A review. *J Urol* 139:1245, 1988.
116. Roy JB, Gejer JR, Ohr JA: Urinary tract candidiasis. An update. *Urology* 79:455, 1986.
117. Gregory MC, Schumann GB, Schumann JL, et al: The clinical significance of Candida casts. *Am J Kidney Dis* 4:179, 1984.
118. Martino P, Girmania C, Vanditti M, et al: Candida colonization and systemic infection in neutropenic patients. *Cancer* 464:2030, 1989.
119. Sanford JP: The enigma of Candiduria: Evolution of bladder irrigation with amphotericin B for management: from anecdote to dogma with a lesson from Machiavelli. *Clin Infect Dis* 16:145, 1993.
120. Body GP: Azole antifungal agents. *Clin Infect Dis* 14:S161, 1992.

91. Life-Threatening Community-Acquired Infections

Debra D. Poutsiaka

Several infectious disease entities exist that arise in the community and are rapid in onset, fulminant in course, and possess a relatively high rate of mortality. Their presentation, typically in an emergency room and often nonspecific, should prompt suspicion and frequently admission to an intensive care unit. Several selected entities are discussed here. For additional information, referral to a standard infectious disease text is recommended.

Many of the diseases discussed here have a similar initial presentation, despite vastly different causes, clinical courses, and treatment. Therefore, it is sensible to adopt a thorough and uniform evaluation and initial management of the patient who may have a severe and unusual infectious disease. Below is a general approach, which should assist but not supersede clinical judgment.

History taking, whether from the patient or others, is extremely important and may be the only source of clues to the correct diagnosis. A complete history should be obtained, including travel, exposure to children or pets, past surgeries or trauma, human immunodeficiency virus (HIV) risk factors, and occupation. Although this takes time, it should not delay the initiation of other aspects of care, particularly cardiopulmonary and fluid resuscitation.

A complete physical examination, with particular attention to the skin, mucous membranes, nervous system, and, in women, the pelvic examination, should be undertaken. Specimens for the following initial laboratory and other examinations should be obtained: complete blood count with platelet and differential counts; prothrombin and partial thromboplastin times; electrolytes, including calcium and magnesium; blood glucose; renal and liver functions; at least two blood cultures, obtained at least 30 minutes apart; a serum sample to be stored for acute serologic analysis; urine for culture and urinalysis; chest radiograph; and an electrocardiogram. Depending on the clinical situation, it may be desirable to obtain other tests, including the following: an arterial blood gas, a disseminated intravascular coagulation (DIC) screen; blood and urine toxicology screens; thick and thin peripheral blood smears to rule out malaria or babesiosis; cerebrospinal fluid for cell count with differential count, glucose, protein, bacterial, fungal, and viral cultures, and Gram stain; Gram stain of the buffy coat of peripheral blood; and cervical and vaginal bacterial cultures.

The initiation of empiric or specific therapy should proceed without delay. The choice of appropriate agents should be guided by the information gained through the history and physical and laboratory examinations. However, it is prudent to involve a specialist in infectious diseases early in the patient's course because of the wide array of infectious agents that may be involved and the equally wide array of unfamiliar therapeutic agents that may be required.

Toxic Shock Syndrome

Toxic shock syndrome is a toxin-mediated multisystem disease characterized by the rapid onset of high fever, hypotension,

diffuse macular erythroderma, mucous membrane inflammation, severe myalgia, vomiting, diarrhea, headache, and nonfocal neurologic abnormalities [1–5]. Toxic shock syndrome as initially defined is clearly associated with infection or colonization with *Staphylococcus aureus* strains that elaborate one or more toxins [6,7]. Although first formally described in children in 1978 [6], the syndrome has gained notoriety in subsequent years because of its association with menstruating women who use tampons [1,7–11]. In addition, increasing numbers of nonmenstrual cases have been recognized in men and women [11]. In the late 1980s, a similar syndrome caused by group A *Streptococcus* was described [12] and is discussed further.

ETIOLOGY. Toxic shock syndrome occurs when toxin-producing strains of *S. aureus* infect or colonize persons who possess risk factors for developing the illness. Nearly all menstrually related and half of nonmenstrually related toxic shock syndrome cases are closely associated with a staphylococcal toxin, now called toxic shock syndrome toxin-1 (TSST-1), originally described as pyrogenic exotoxin C and enterotoxin F [13–19]. However, nearly 40 percent of staphylococcal strains causing nonmenstrual toxic shock syndrome do not produce TSST-1. Most of these strains produce other staphylococcal enterotoxins [14,19] and current concepts are that these staphylococcal enterotoxins are involved in the induction of toxic shock syndrome [13,20–23].

Toxic shock syndrome occurred in 1981 and 1982 with a rate of about 10 per 100,000 menstruating women per year [11] and has had only a moderate decline in incidence since removal of implicated tampons from the market. Several risk factors for the development of toxic shock syndrome in menstruating women have been identified. They include tampon use, particularly superabsorbent tampons [1, 8–11]; vaginal colonization with toxin-producing *S. aureus* [24], although the vaginal colonization rate in healthy women is approximately 9 percent [25]; and the lack of serum antibody to staphylococcal toxins at the onset of disease, in contrast to its presence in the sera of a great majority of healthy women and men [17,18]. Interestingly, most women convalescing from the syndrome develop a serum antibody response to these toxins [20], suggesting that antibody to the toxin(s) may play a role in recovery and protection from subsequent episodes.

PATHOGENESIS. The precise pathogenesis of toxic shock syndrome is unproved. Colonization or infection with certain strains of *S. aureus* is likely followed by the production of one or more toxins that are absorbed systemically because of certain underlying conditions such as a high growth titer of organism in a closed environment containing blood or devitalized tissue. When superabsorbant tampons are present in the vagina, physiologic conditions, including the tension of O_2 and CO_2 and low magnesium concentrations, favor the production of TSST-1. The toxin or toxins then produce the systemic manifestations of the syndrome in persons who lack protective antitoxin antibody. Possible mediators of the effects of the toxins to produce the clinical syndrome of toxic shock are cytokines because TSST-1 and other toxic shock syndrome toxins induce the production of cytokines such as interleukin-1 and tumor necrosis factor (TNF) [13,19,26,27]. Additionally, there is increasing evidence to support the possibility that the toxins are superantigens; that is, they stimulate nonspecific T cell proliferation, resulting in the release of large amounts of cytokines (reviewed in [23]).

Support for toxin-induced injury came from postmortem pathologic studies of the vagina, cervix, lung, liver, and kidney [28,29]. Findings included ulceration with mucosal separation and desquamation of vaginal tissue, hyaline membrane formation characteristic of shock lung, periportal hepatic inflammation and fatty changes, acute tubular necrosis of the kidney, and subacute vasculitis and interstitial edema in various organs. These pathologic changes are not specific for toxic shock syndrome but are consistent with changes produced by a toxin.

DIAGNOSIS. Toxic shock syndrome has a rapid, dramatic, fulminant onset. It is important to recognize the syndrome quickly to institute treatment promptly in the intensive care unit.

Clinical Features. The syndrome occurs most commonly in women, most of whom are using tampons, usually within 5 days after the onset of menstruation [1]. However, toxic shock syndrome occurs over a wide range of clinical settings associated with *S. aureus* infections at a variety of sites. These include surgical wound infections, postpartum infections, focal cutaneous and subcutaneous lesions, deep abscesses, adenitis, bursitis, empyema, fasciitis, peritonsillar abscess, sinusitis, and osteomyelitis [30,31,32].

The possibility of toxic shock syndrome should be entertained in anyone who presents with the sudden onset of fever, rash, orthostatic signs, and systemic evidence of toxicity, although it is likely that the syndrome occurs in a milder form [33]. The case definition employed by the Centers for Disease Control (CDC) is shown in Table 91-1 [34]. Five categories of clinical features are needed for diagnosis: (1) fever, (2) rash, typically a diffuse macular erythroderma, although other dermatologic findings may be observed such as a localized erythematous, papulopustular, or petechial eruption, and Nikolsky's sign (rupture and separation of the upper portion of the epidermis after light stroking of bullae) (see Chap. 218) [1–5], (3) desquamation 1 to 2 weeks after onset of illness [1–5], (4) hypotension, and (5) evidence of multisystem involvement in three or more of the following areas: (a) gastrointestinal [1–5], (b) muscular, (c) mucous membrane involvement [1–5], (d) renal [35], (e) hepatic [36], (f) hematologic, and (g) central nervous system. In addition, there should be reasonable evidence for the absence of other potential causes of the illness. Particularly prominent and noteworthy clinical signs of the syndrome are depicted in the series of photographs shown in Plate I-2.

Complications. Severe complications include prolonged and refractory hypovolemic shock, adult respiratory distress syndrome, acute renal failure, electrolyte and acid-base imbalances, cardiac dysrhythmia, and DIC with thrombocytopenia [1–5,37]. As currently defined, toxic shock syndrome carries a mortality rate of 3 percent [9,38,39,40], which is particularly striking because the syndrome affects predominantly healthy young adults.

Clinical Sequelae. Clinical sequelae occur in a minority of patients. These include a pruritic, total-body, maculopapular rash 9 to 13 days after the onset of symptoms [37] which may represent a drug reaction to penicillin compounds or a delayed

Table 91-1. Centers for Disease Control Case Definition of Toxic Shock Syndrome

1. Fever: temperature ≥38.9°C (102°F)
2. Rash: diffuse macular erythroderma
3. Desquamation 1 to 2 weeks after onset of illness, particularly of palms and soles
4. Hypotension: systolic blood pressure ≥90 mm Hg for adults or below fifth percentile by age for children younger than 16 years of age; orthostatic drop in diastolic blood pressure ≥15 mm Hg for lying-to-sitting, orthostatic syncope, or orthostatic dizziness
5. Multisystem involvement—three or more of the following:
   a. Gastrointestinal: vomiting or diarrhea at onset of illness
   b. Muscular: severe myalgia or creatine phosphokinase level at least twice the upper limit of laboratory normal
   c. Mucous membrane: vaginal, oropharyngeal, or conjunctival hyperemia
   d. Renal: blood urea nitrogen or creatinine at least twice the upper limit of laboratory normal, or urinary sediment with pyuria (≥5 leukocytes/high power-field) in the absence of urinary tract infection
   e. Hepatic: total bilirubin, serum glutamic-oxaloacetic transaminase, serum glutamic pyruvic transaminase at least twice the upper limit of laboratory normal
   f. Hematologic: platelet 100,000/mm³
   g. Central nervous system: disorientation or alterations in consciousness without focal neurologic signs when fever and hypotension are absent
6. Negative results on the following tests, if obtained:
   a. Blood, throat, or cerebrospinal fluid cultures (blood cultures may be positive for *Staphylococcus aureus*)
   b. Rise in titer to Rocky Mountain spotted fever, leptospirosis, or rubeola

Source: Adapted from Reingold AL, Hargrett NT, Shands KN, et al: Toxic shock syndrome surveillance in the United States, 1980 to 1981. *Ann Intern Med* 96:879, 1982, with permission.

effect of or reaction to a staphylococcal toxin (see Chap. 218); chronic renal failure [10, 37]; asymptomatic cyanotic extremities [37]; and prolonged neuromuscular abnormalities such as myopathy with muscle weakness and paresthesia [37]. Neuropsychological sequelae may occur 2 to 12 months after recovery and include difficulty concentrating, headache, recent memory lapses, irritability, inability to compute, and loss of other higher integrative functions, and are usually accompanied by electroencephalographic abnormalities [41]. It is not known if these findings are caused by a direct effect of a staphylococcal toxin on the central nervous system.

Toxic shock syndrome may recur in up to 60 percent of patients who are not treated with β-lactamase–resistant antimicrobial drugs [11,42]. Clinical recurrences typically occur within 1 to 2 months and are usually milder than the initial episode [7,42]. They are uncommon in patients who have been treated with appropriate antibiotics [42].

Laboratory Features. There is no one laboratory test that is diagnostic of toxic shock syndrome or abnormal in all patients. However, more than 50 percent of affected persons show the following abnormalities [5]: leukocytosis with a polymorphonuclear shift to the left; sterile pyuria; prolonged prothrombin and partial thromboplastin times; hypocalcemia; low serum protein and albumin concentrations; and elevated blood urea nitrogen, transaminase, bilirubin, and creatine phosphokinase levels. Other laboratory abnormalities may include thrombocytopenia, hypophosphatemia, elevated serum creatinine, and a mild normochromic normocytic, nonhemolytic anemia [5].

S. aureus is easily identified by Gram stain and cultured from patients with a well-defined focus of infection such as an abscess or wound infection. Of cases associated with menstruation, more than 90 percent demonstrate the organism in cultures from the cervix or vagina [1,24]. Of particular importance is the fact that *S. aureus* bacteremia is very uncommon in patients with the toxic shock syndrome [1–5]. Tests for production of staphylococcal toxins are limited to a few research laboratories.

DIFFERENTIAL DIAGNOSIS. Toxic shock syndrome is a rather distinct clinical entity that need not be confused with more than a few other diseases. The differential diagnosis includes infectious conditions such as leptospirosis, rubeola, Rocky Mountain spotted fever, rash-associated viral infections, meningococcemia, and streptococcal or staphylococcal scarlet fever. Noninfectious entities that enter the differential diagnosis include drug reactions, Kawasaki disease, and toxic epidermal necrolysis (Lyell's disease). Toxic shock syndrome has also been mistaken for a number of conditions not listed above [3]. These include acute pyelonephritis, septic shock, acute rheumatic fever, legionnaires' disease, acute pelvic inflammatory disease, hemolytic uremic syndrome, systemic lupus erythematosus, tick typhus, and gastroenteritis. This last group of conditions should not be seriously confused with toxic shock syndrome in an individual patient.

TREATMENT. It is crucially important to diagnose toxic shock syndrome rapidly and to institute therapy immediately. Usually the most urgent need is to correct hypovolemic shock, which necessitates the administration of between 2 and 20 liters of crystalloid during the first 24 hours of hospitalization [37]. Severely ill patients have required vasopressors, fresh frozen plasma, plasma protein fraction, or normal serum albumin.

After obtaining samples of blood for culture, large doses of a beta-lactamase–resistant antistaphylococcal antimicrobial agent should be given intravenously, such as 1.5 to 2.0 gm nafcillin or oxacillin every 4 hours. Additionally, because it is difficult to differentiate between staphylococcal and streptococcal toxic shock syndrome on clinical grounds alone (see below), intravenous penicillin should be administered until a bacteriologic diagnosis is confirmed by culture. Alternatively, a first-generation cephalosporin or, for those who cannot tolerate β-lactams, vancomycin can be used. A reasonable length of therapy is 10 days, but the patient's condition may dictate modification [2,3,33]. The efficacy of this therapy for correction of the toxin-induced toxic shock syndrome has not been conclusively proved, but it is known to reduce the likelihood of recurrent toxic shock syndrome in a given patient [7,42]. Any infected area should be surgically drained, and foreign bodies, such as tampons or sutures, must be removed. The administration of intravenous human immunoglobulin has been useful in the amelioration of the toxicity observed in toxic shock syndrome [43] and should be considered in severe cases [44].

Therapy for complications, such as deranged electrolyte and acid-base status, adult respiratory distress syndrome, myocardial irritability, hypocalcemia, acute renal failure, thrombocytopenia, and DIC [1–5,35,37,45] should be administered, as discussed elsewhere in this volume.

Because patients who recover are at risk for recurrent episodes of toxic shock syndrome [7,42], it seems reasonable to consider or recommend forms of preventive therapy such as discontinuation of tampon usage and administration of oral antistaphylococcal antibiotics before and during each menstrual period for several months.

Future possibilities for therapy include the development of an antitoxin, and for prevention, the development of a toxoid vaccine.

STREPTOCOCCAL TOXIC SHOCK SYNDROME. In the late 1980s, a toxic shock–like syndrome caused by group A *Streptococcus* was described in 20 adults [12]. As with staphylococcal toxic shock syndrome, bacterial toxins are thought to mediate the toxicity [12,46]. Prominent features are fever, shock, renal or respiratory failure, mental status changes, and a mortality rate of 30 percent. Skin manifestations are varied and include bullae, scarlet fever–like rash, petechial or maculopapular rashes, and desquamation [12]. In comparison with staphylococcal toxic shock syndrome, blood cultures are usually positive. Underlying infections are varied and include cellulitis, pharyngitis, necrotizing fasciitis, postpartum myometritis, and surgical wound infection. Diagnosis is made by culture of blood and other bodily fluids. Treatment is similar to that for staphylococcal toxic shock syndrome in that supportive care such as fluids, vasopressors, ventilatory assistance, etc., should be administered, and surgical drainage of pyogenic sites is imperative. The antibiotic of choice is intravenous penicillin. For those intolerant to penicillin, other suitable agents are cephalosporins, vancomycin, and clindamycin. Until the bacteriologic diagnosis is confirmed by culture, staphylococcal coverage should be included in the antibiotic regimen.

Rocky Mountain Spotted Fever

Rocky Mountain spotted fever (RMSF) is a potentially severe illness classically characterized by the triad of fever, rash, and tick bite (see [47] for a recent review). The causative agent is endemic in most if not all of the continental United States [48]. Particular areas of recent high endemicity are the southeastern states, primarily North Carolina, and mountainous regions of Oklahoma and Arkansas [48]. However, foci of RMSF have occurred previously in northeastern urban centers such as New York City and Long Island, and the New England States [49,50,51]. RMSF is a seasonal disease, with most cases occurring during the late spring, summer, and early fall. Occasionally, cases occur in endemic areas during the winter months [52]. The disease most commonly involves those younger than 20 years of age, but all age-groups are affected [48,53]. It is essential to recognize or consider RMSF early in the course of the illness, because the prompt institution of proper therapy is correlated with a better outcome [54].

ETIOLOGY. RMSF, caused by the obligate intracellular bacterium *Rickettsia rickettsii,* is an arthropod-borne infection. It is transmitted by the tick vectors, *Dermacentor virabilis,* the dog tick, found in eastern and southern states, and *Dermacentor andersoni,* the wood tick, found in the Rocky Mountain states [53]. However, a sizable proportion of those with confirmed RMSF have no history of a tick bite [53,55,56,57]. Other risk factors for RMSF include exposure to dogs and living in a wooded area [56,57]. There are rare reports of RMSF infection occurring through occupational exposure [53].

PATHOGENESIS. RMSF is a multisystem disease. Once *R. rickettsii* is inoculated into the host through the saliva of the tick, it is widely disseminated to various organs in the body, including the central nervous system, lungs, liver, spleen, and kidneys [58]. The organisms enter endothelial cells, where they multiply [58]. Immunofluorescence studies have demonstrated the rickettsia within smooth muscle cells of the walls of blood vessels [59]. In vitro studies have elucidated several possible mechanisms whereby infection causes the vasculitislike events that occur during the course of RMSF. They include the release of von Willebrand factor from *R. rickettsii*–infected endothelial cells, which may contribute to the observed thrombosis [51]; the adherence of platelets to infected endothelial cells, which may partially explain the thrombocytopenia commonly found in RMSF [60]; and the release of peroxides from infected endothelial cells, which may explain the widespread endothelial damage observed in RMSF [61]. In vivo studies of experimentally infected human volunteers have suggested that early in the course of infection, there is activation of the fibrinolytic and coagulation systems, as well as perturbation of endothelial cells [62]. In the most severe cases, multisystem organ failure ensues, with coma, respiratory failure, and renal failure.

DIAGNOSIS

Clinical Features. A most important component of correct diagnosis is the history. The onset of illness may be abrupt or gradual [55], usually appearing within 2 weeks of tick exposure [56]. Because tick exposure is not always noticed, determining the presence of other risk factors, such as dog exposure or length of time spent in wooded areas, may aid in diagnosis. The classical triad of fever, rash, and tick bite is present in two-thirds of confirmed cases [55,57] (see Chap. 218). In general, symptoms include fever and malaise, seen in almost 100 percent of cases, headache in most cases, and rash [49,53,55,57]. Other common symptoms include myalgia, nausea or vomiting, abdominal pain, and diarrhea [49,53,55,57].

The classic rash occurs within 3 days of onset of illness, is petechial, originates on the distal extremities and spreads centripetally to the trunk, and involves the palms and soles but spares the face [49,55,56,57] (see Chap. 218). Atypical presentations are not rare and include a maculopapular or evanescent rash, an atypical distribution, and appearance late in the disease [63]. Survey of several large series demonstrates that rash appeared in 84 to 100 percent of confirmed cases [53,56]. Therefore, it is important to note that rash might not occur in RMSF, leading some to call it "Rocky Mountain spotless fever" [63]. Spotless fever is more likely to occur in males and in African-Americans [63].

The clinical findings of RMSF are varied. As discussed above, fever and rash are important clues, as is the finding of tick infestation, which may occur in obscure sites, such as the perineum. Neurologic involvement, ranging from irritability and confusion to meningismus, seizures, stupor, and coma, has been described. Pneumonitis, at times leading to respiratory failure, has been described in 2 to 13 percent of cases [49,53,55]. Lymphadenopathy, hepatomegaly, and splenomegaly also occur. Other less common findings include shock, cardiac dysrhythmia, peripheral edema, jaundice, conjunctivitis, and decreased hearing [53,55].

Laboratory Features. The laboratory findings in RMSF are varied and nonspecific. There is leukocytosis, frequently with a significant proportion of immature neutrophils present, and anemia [55,57]. Thrombocytopenia is frequent [53,55], as is hyponatremia, present in approximately 90 percent of cases [57]. Rhabdomyolysis, elevation in hepatic transaminases, and elevated clotting indices (prothrombin time, partial thromboplastin time, and fibrin degradation products) have also been observed

in half or more cases. Acute renal failure has been observed in up to 5 percent of patients [57]. Results of cerebrospinal fluid (CSF) examination are also nonspecific. In one study of 32 patients who underwent lumbar puncture, one-third had normal CSF profiles. The remaining two-thirds had abnormal CSF profiles with a mononuclear pleocytosis [57]. Less common were elevated CSF protein and low CSF glucose levels.

The diagnosis of RMSF is often made on clinical grounds. However, because a number of other diseases may be easily confused with RMSF, specific diagnosis is important (see [47] for a more complete discussion). Currently, the only rapid diagnostic approach is the demonstration through immunofluorescence of *R. rickettsii* in skin biopsy specimens [59,64]. In the future, the polymerase chain reaction may prove a rapid, sensitive, and specific test [65]. Serologic assays can definitively confirm the diagnosis of RMSF. Specific serologic tests have supplanted the nonspecific Weil-Felix OX 19 agglutination test. A fourfold rise in titers in the indirect immunofluorescent antibody assay, the indirect hemagglutination assay, or the latex agglutination assay is considered diagnostic [47]. Although these tests are very specific (96–100%), they vary in sensitivity, with the first two being the most sensitive (91–100% vs. 71–94% for latex agglutination) [47].

DIFFERENTIAL DIAGNOSIS. Given the varied clinical presentations of RMSF, the differential diagnosis is broad. It includes meningococcal disease, infectious mononucleosis, hepatitis, pneumonia, acute abdominal illness, exanthemous viral infections such as rubella or measles, meningitis, viral encephalitis, rheumatic fever, ehrlichiosis, typhoid fever, leptospirosis, idiopathic thrombocytopenic purpura, thrombotic thrombocytopenic purpura, drug reaction, and vasculitis [47,55,57,66].

TREATMENT. The mortality from RMSF has declined from almost 60 percent in the preantibiotic era, to 5 to 10 percent or less in recent years [49,53,55,57]. It is essential that therapy be instituted early for best outcome [54]. Because the most specific serologic assays do not become positive until several days into the illness, treatment must be started before the diagnosis is confirmed. Specific treatment is with tetracycline or doxycyline (25–50 mg/kg/day or 100 mg every 12 hours, respectively) for 7 days or until the patient has been afebrile for 2 days [58]. For those who cannot or should not be treated with a drug in the tetracycline class, chloramphenicol (50–75 mg/kg/day) is the drug of choice [58]. Persons in this group include pregnant women, children younger than 8 years of age, and persons with hypersensitivity to tetracycline. In addition to specific therapy, attention should be paid to supports such as the maintenance of fluid and electrolyte balance, ventilatory support, and other measures. The use of corticosteroids has not been studied. However, it is recommended by some for the adjunctive care of the patient with severe RMSF [54].

Meningococcal Sepsis

Meningococcal infection is a serious and frequently life-threatening event. Primary concerns are meningococcal meningitis and acute meningococcemia, which are discussed here. Other types of meningococcal infections include chronic meningococcemia, pneumonia, and otitis. For a more detailed discussion on bacterial meningitis, refer to Chapter 87.

A recent study on the epidemiology of meningococcal disease in the United States estimated there were 2600 cases annually, yielding an attack rate of 1.1:100,00 [67]. The highest and lowest attack rates were during February to March and September, respectively. The highest age-specific attack rate was in those younger than 1 year of age. Additionally, African-American and Latino groups had a higher attack rate than Caucasians [67,68]. However, race and age did not influence outcome [69].

Meningitis and primary bacteremia accounted for 57 to 65 percent and 35 to 49 percent of cases, respectively [67,68]. Other syndromes, including when more than one syndrome presented in a single patient, were pneumonia (3%), otitis (2%), and arthritis (2%). The observed case fatality rate was 12 to 14.2 percent. However, the fatality rate if blood cultures were positive, regardless of the culture result of the CSF, was 18.5 percent, compared with 9.9 percent when only CSF cultures were positive [68].

ETIOLOGY. Meningococcal disease is caused by infection with *Neisseria meningitidis,* a gram-negative coccus. There are several serogroups of *N. meningitidis* that are clinically relevant, groups A, B, C, W135, and Y. Serogroup A is important in epidemics worldwide but is less of a concern in the United States. In a study of isolates from the United States, 46 percent were group B, 45 percent were group C, 3 percent were due to group W135, and 2 percent were due to group Y [67]. There was no difference between serogroups in the clinical syndrome or case fatality rate.

PATHOGENESIS. It is estimated that 2 to 18 percent of individuals are colonized with *N. meningitidis* at any one time [70]. Infection is transmitted through aerosolization of or direct contact with infected respiratory secretions [71]. The portal of entry appears to be the nasopharyngeal epithelium (reviewed in [72]). The initial phase of invasion is the passage of the meningococcus through the mucus layer lining the epithelium. During the invasion process, host cellular damage, particularly to ciliated cells, includes disruption of intercellular tight junctions, ciliostasis, and sloughing of ciliated cells. This occurs without attachment of the organism to ciliated cells and suggests a soluble bacterial or host-derived toxin as the mediator [72]. Attachment of meningococci to nonciliated nasopharyngeal cells occurs through pili. After attachment, there is "parasite-directed" endocytosis of the organism. The bacteria traverse the host cell undamaged within membrane-bound vesicles and are deposited to the subepithelium within 24 hours [72]. Presumably, there the bacteria gain access to blood vessels.

The major host defense against invasive meningococci lies in the complement system (reviewed in [73]). Fragments of C3 provide opsonophagocytic activity through fixation to the organism, and the formation of the membrane attack complex (MAC) by the terminal complement components, C5 to C9, provides direct serum bactericidal activity. The importance of the complement system in protection from serious meningococcal infection is demonstrated by (1) the 7000- to 10,000-fold increased incidence of such infection in persons with a deficiency in a single late complement component compared with persons with an intact complement system [73] and (2) the fact that congenital or acquired complement deficiencies are common in persons with meningococcal disease [73–78].

At the tissue level, damage appears to occur through thrombosis and ischemia [79,80,81].

DIAGNOSIS

Clinical Features. Patients with acute meningococcal sepsis may present with or without meningitis. Those in the former group may exhibit the classic signs and symptoms of acute bacterial meningitis: fever, headache, and signs of meningeal irritation. A frequently encountered presentation of meningococcal sepsis is septic shock, with hypotension, poor peripheral perfusion, impaired mentation, and anuria or oliguria [69,82–85]. Other signs and syndromes present on admission include fever, cutaneous purpura, hemorrhage, cardiac failure, acute renal failure, and thrombocytopenia with or without DIC [69,82–85]. Other less common complications of meningococcal sepsis include adrenal hemorrhage and failure, chronic renal failure necessitating hemodialysis, cutaneous necrosis with sloughing requiring skin grafting, extremity gangrene requiring subsequent amputation and often several surgical revisions, septic arthritis, endopthalmitis, and pericarditis [69,79,80,81,86].

Death can occur within hours of admission [82,87,88]. Case fatality rates ranged from 0 to 29 percent [67,68,69,82,84,85,87]. However, crude case fatality rates can be misleading because patients with low-severity disease had one-tenth the mortality rate of those with high-severity illness (2.7% vs. 29.7%, respectively, with a crude case fatality rate of 10%) [69] based on the prognostic factors of peripheral and CSF leukocyte count, heart rate, and mental status. Other studies have shown that unfavorable prognostic indicators of meningococcal disease include rapid onset of petechiae, absence of meningitis, shock, and the absence of leukocytosis [89].

Laboratory Features. Numerous laboratory abnormalities are noted in patients with severe meningococcal disease. These include an abnormal CSF profile in patients with meningitis, such as polymorphonuclear pleocytosis, low CSF glucose, elevated CSF protein, and CSF Gram stain demonstrating intracellular and extracellular gram-negative diplococci. Abnormal hematologic indices include leukocytosis or leukopenia, both with the presence of immature polymorphonuclear leukocytes, and thrombocytopenia with or without other laboratory evidence of DIC. Findings of abnormal blood chemistries include acidemia, hypoglycemia, decreased cortisol levels, and elevated blood urea nitrogen and creatinine [85].

The cornerstone to the microbiologic diagnosis of meningococcal disease is the isolation of *N. meningitidis* from the blood, CSF, or other sterile fluids such as synovial or pericardial fluid. Approximately 50 percent of patients with severe meningococcal disease have positive blood cultures [90,91]. The yield from CSF cultures is higher, ranging from 46 to 96 percent [90,91,92]. Also, approximately two-thirds of cases of primary meningococcemia have positive CSF cultures [91].

Other and more rapid means to specific diagnosis can be achieved through immunoassay, such as latex agglutination of bodily fluids. However, false-positive latex agglutination tests attributable to povidone-iodine contamination of CSF have been reported [93]. Finally, the polymerase chain reaction may be used as a diagnostic method in the future [94].

DIFFERENTIAL DIAGNOSIS. The differential diagnosis of severe meningococcal disease is that of acute bacterial meningitis and severe illnesses presenting with fever and rash. Etiologic agents to consider in the former case include *S. pneumoniae* and *H. influenzae* (see Chap. 87). Severe illnesses presenting with fever and a petechial or purpuric rash include Rocky Mountain spotted fever, gram-negative sepsis, fulminant staphylococcal sepsis, overwhelming postsplenectomy infection, and malaria [95]. Additionally, viral illnesses such as coxsackievirus, Epstein-Barr virus, cytomegalovirus, measles, and echovirus infections may present with a petechial rash [95]. Finally, other causes of fever and rash include vasculitis, thrombotic thrombocytopenic purpura, and thrombocytopenia coexisting with fever, such as in a person with acute leukemia or DIC.

TREATMENT

Antibiotics. The drug of choice in the United States for the treatment of severe meningococcal infection is penicillin G, 24 million units intravenously per day for adults, and 300,000 units per kilogram body weight per day for children [96], for 7 to 14 days [91,97]. An alternative is a third-generation cephalosporin such as ceftriaxone, 2 gm intravenously every 12 hours in adults and, in children, 100 mg/kg body weight in one or divided into two doses per day [98]. Finally, for those who cannot tolerate β-lactam antibiotics, chloramphenicol, 100 mg per kilogram body weight per day intravenously up to a maximum of 4 gm per day, is recommended [96].

Resistance of *N. meningitidis* to penicillin has been documented in Spain, the United Kingdom, and South Africa [99]. Resistant strains remain sensitive to third-generation cephalosporins [99]. Therefore, in areas where penicillin resistance is suspected, a third-generation cephalosporin is the drug of choice.

Additional Management. Additional management includes admission into an intensive care unit, attention to fluid and electrolyte balance, respiratory isolation until after 24 hours of appropriate antibiotic therapy, and, if needed, the use of vasopressors, hemodialysis, and respiratory ventilation. Also, necrotic skin lesions and gangrenous limbs require surgical care. In the presence of hypotension, after obtaining a blood sample for a cortisol level, corticosteroids should be administered pending cortisol level results in the event of bilateral adrenal necrosis. In severe meningococcal infection, plasmapheresis has been shown to be of benefit in a limited number of patients [100,101]. A possible explanation for its efficacy is the removal of cytokines from the circulation [100].

In cases of meningococcal meningitis in children, steroids should be administered. A suggested dosing regimen is dexamethasone, 0.6 mg/kg/day in four divided doses for 4 days, starting before or at the time of antibiotic administration [98,102]. In adults with meningitis, the use of steroids should be given strong consideration, although the data supporting it are less compelling.

Consideration should be given to testing for complement deficiency after the patient has recovered from the acute illness.

Prophylaxis. Chemoprophylaxis after exposure to persons with *N. meningitidis* infection is recommended for household, daycare and other intimate contacts; for persons in close contact with infected respiratory secretions, such as those performing mouth-to-mouth resuscitation; and closed populations such as those in college dormitories and military barracks [96,98]. The agent currently recommended for chemoprophylaxis is rifampin, 600 mg orally (adults) or 10 mg per kilogram orally (children) every 12 hours for four doses [67]. Ciprofloxacin and ceftriaxone have also been successful in eliminating carriage [103,104]. Routine chemoprophylaxis is not required for medical personnel unless they have had prolonged close contact before the institution of antibiotic therapy.

Immunization with the tetravalent (serogroups A, C, W135, and Y) meningococcal polysaccharide vaccine is indicated for the following populations: populations at risk during an outbreak (such as school or dormitory mates), those with complement deficiencies, although this view is not universally held [105]; travelers to endemic areas; and persons with asplenia [73,106,107]. Serogroup B is not included in the vaccine because it is poorly immunogenic [96].

Postsplenectomy Infection

Increased incidence and severity of infection after splenectomy has been recognized for decades. In its most fulminant form, it is known as overwhelming postsplenectomy infection (OPSI), defined as a rapidly progressive bacterial infection, initially manifested by nonspecific symptoms, and frequently accompanied by DIC, multiple organ failure, and death (see [108,109] for recent reviews). Since initial descriptions, similar infections have been described in functionally asplenic individuals.

In a compilation of series reviewed by Francke and Neu [110], the incidence of sepsis in 4846 children splenectomized for a variety of reasons was 5 percent, with a mortality of 2.4 percent within the total population. For 1416 adults, 3.9 percent experienced sepsis, with a mortality of 2.6 percent, leading the authors to conclude that sepsis in the splenectomized host carries with it a mortality of greater than 50 percent. This is supported by a series of case reports, which demonstrate a mortality of 60 to 88 percent [111,112]. However, other studies demonstrated a much lower mortality rate (1% or less) for postsplenectomy infections [113,114,115].

In summary, although it is difficult to draw unifying conclusions from the literature, infection after splenectomy has the potential to be relatively common and frequently fatal.

ETIOLOGY. Serious postsplenectomy infections are generally bacterial in nature. Classically, *Streptococcus pneumoniae* is the most common organism involved [111,116]. However, several studies demonstrate significant involvement by other organisms, perhaps because of the advent of the polyvalent pneumococcal polysaccharide vaccine. Other organisms involved include other encapsulated organisms such as *Haemophilus influenzae* and *Neisseria meningitidis;* and to a lesser extent, *Escherichia coli, Pseudomonas aeruginosa, Staphylococcus aureus,* and other streptococcal, staphylococcal, and gram-negative species [110–115,117]. There are also accounts of serious postsplenectomy infections with unusual agents such as *Neisseria gonorrhoeae, Capnocytophagia canimorsus* (see below), *Babesia microti,* a protozoal parasite resembling malaria (see below), and viruses in the herpes group [109,118].

PATHOGENESIS. The spleen is a site of intense immune activity, most notably antibody production and phagocytosis. In the immune response to encapsulated organisms, the spleen is thought to play a critical role in protecting the host from pneumococcus through the production of type-specific antibodies. However, the production of specific antibody to encapsulated organisms, specifically pneumococcus, was defective in persons with asplenia compared with normal individuals [119, 120,121]. In contrast, several studies have shown no difference in antibody response to pneumococcal polysaccharide challenge in splenectomized patients compared with healthy controls [122,123,124].

The clearance of pneumococci from the bloodstream is adversely affected by splenectomy [125], thought to be attributable in part to the loss of the phagocytosing function of the spleen in the absence of specific antibody [110]. The alternative complement pathway can be viewed as additional protection against bacterial invasion because its activation and subsequent formation of the bactericidal membrane attack complex does not require specific antibody. However, splenectomized persons have an acquired deficit in alternative complement function [110]. Thus, splenectomy impairs at least three protective mechanisms: production of specific antibacterial antibody, splenic phagocytosis in the absence of specific antibody, and normal activation of the alternative complement pathway [108,110].

Age is a risk factor for infection in the splenectomized host because most patients with overwhelming infection are younger than 2 years of age [110]. Also, the presence of underlying disease in the splenectomized host may be a risk factor for the occurrence and severity of OPSI [110,114,126,127]. Those persons who were splenectomized because of trauma generally fared the best, with a lower risk of infection and death from infection. The groups with a higher incidence of infection or death included those with hematologic or other malignancies, immunocompromised persons, and those who underwent abdominal surgery for reasons other than splenectomy.

DIAGNOSIS

Clinical Features. Serious postsplenectomy infections can present in several manners. The most typical is sepsis without an obvious focus, occurring in more than half to three-quarters of individuals [110,111,112]. Other common presentations include meningitis and pneumonia [110,111,112]. Postsplenectomy infections should be considered in any person presenting with signs of sepsis with a history or a scar suggestive of splenectomy or in those with conditions associated with functional asplenia, such as sickle cell disease, advanced age, Felty's syndrome, splenic irradiation, inflammatory bowel disease, or systemic lupus erythematosus [128–133]. Overwhelming infection has occurred more than 40 years after splenectomy, although the risk is thought by some to be greatest within the first 2 to 3 years [109,110,112,115].

The classic presentation of OPSI is heralded by a prodrome consisting of fever, chills with rigors, pharyngitis, myalgias, nausea, and vomiting. It rapidly progresses to hypotension, DIC, purpura, and respiratory distress with additional complications such as adrenal hemorrhage, gangrene, and coma [109, 115,127]. Death can ensue in less than 24 hours [109,111, 115]. Reported long-term sequelae include amputation caused by gangrene, deafness, chronic pyoderma, and aortic insufficiency attributable to endocarditis [109,111].

Laboratory Features. Laboratory features are varied and include leukocytosis with the presence of immature forms, leukopenia, thrombocytopenia, and other laboratory evidence of DIC, hyponatremia, and acidemia. Evidence of bacterial meningitis may also be present.

The appearance of bacteria, particularly pneumococci, on peripheral blood smears in patients with OPSI has been noted [116,134,135]. Additionally, the peripheral smear shows erythrocyte Howell-Jolly bodies, erythrocyte Heinz bodies, and target or burr cells characteristic of the asplenic state. The offending bacteria are often grown in blood culture, as well as in cultures of CSF.

DIFFERENTIAL DIAGNOSIS. Overwhelming sepsis in the setting of anatomic or functional asplenia is not a subtle diag-

nosis. It might be confused with fulminant sepsis in the setting of other immunocompromised states such as neutropenia or acute leukemia if the asplenic state is not noted historically. In addition, noninfectious disorders, such as thrombotic thrombocytopenic purpura, should be considered.

TREATMENT. After obtaining blood and other specimens for culture, the expedient initiation of broad-spectrum antibiotic therapy, particularly with an agent with activity against encapsulated organisms and with CSF penetration, is essential. A suitable choice is a third-generation cephalosporin, such as ceftriaxone, 2 gm intravenously every 12 hours in adults and, in children, 100 mg per kilogram per day in one dose or divided into two doses [98]. Antibiotic therapy can be further tailored after identification of the infecting organism.

Supportive therapy, such as intravenous fluids, ventilatory support, and vasopressors, may be necessary. In the presence of hypotension, corticosteroids should be administered until the integrity of adrenal function can be verified. If meningitis is present, corticosteroids should be administered (see section on meningococcemia in this chapter).

PREVENTION. There are three approaches to the prevention of subsequent episodes of severe postsplenectomy infection. The first is vaccination against encapsulated organisms. The efficacy of pneumococcal vaccine in preventing infection in asplenic individuals, including those with sickle cell disease, has been demonstrated [136,137,138] despite the occurrence of vaccine failures [139] and varied specific antibody responses to capsular polysaccharide [119,121,122,124,136]. Given the relative safety of vaccination and the potential morbidity and mortality from postsplenectomy infection, vaccination against encapsulated organisms is recommended [106,108,110,123, 137,138,140]. Additionally, revaccination of asplenic persons with pneumococcal vaccine after 6 years is also recommended [141].

Another approach is the administration of prophylactic antibiotics, such as penicillin or a similar agent. This approach is controversial because the optimal duration of prophylaxis is undefined, adverse antibiotic reactions might occur, and infection with agents insensitive to penicillin is not uncommon [109,111]. A number of authors recommend the use of prophylactic antibiotics on an individual basis, for instance, in those within the first 2 to 3 years of splenectomy, younger than 5 years of age, with hematologic and other malignancies undergoing chemotherapy or with high risk of exposure [60,110].

A final approach is the early use of amoxicillin or a similar agent for any febrile or flu-like illness in splenectomized individuals, along with seeking prompt medical attention [108–112].

Malaria

Malaria is a major health problem worldwide, particularly in developing countries. It is estimated that there are 100 million cases, with one million deaths, annually [142]. In the United States, foci of endemicity have long since been eradicated, and therefore, malaria cannot be considered a "community-acquired infection." However, from 1972 to 1988, there were 2697 cases of malaria in U.S. civilians older than 18 years of age reported to the national surveillance system [143]. Approximately half of those cases were falciparum malaria. Because the sensitivity of reporting is estimated to be 50 percent, and

U.S. military personnel and non-U.S. citizens were excluded from the survey, the actual number of cases of malaria in the United States during that period was likely much higher. Approximately 80 percent of imported falciparum malaria in developed countries was acquired in Africa [144,145].

There were 68 deaths from falciparum malaria in U.S. travelers from 1959 to 1987 [144], 50 percent of whom were tourists. This yielded a case fatality rate of 3.8 percent. However, mortality was age related because those in the 70- to 79-year age range experienced a 30 percent mortality. Of note, the number of deaths from falciparum malaria has increased annually [144].

Given the increase in travel to developing countries, as well as the deployment of U.S. military troops to endemic areas, malaria will continue to be seen in the United States. For a detailed discussion of malaria, refer to the review by Wyler [142].

ETIOLOGY. Malaria is caused by the intracellular parasite *Plasmodium.* There are four species that cause disease in humans: *P. falciparum, P. malariae, P. ovale,* and *P. vivax. Plasmodium* is transmitted to human hosts by its vector, the female anopheles mosquito (Fig. 91-1). Other, much less common routes of transmission include congenital transmission, intravenous drug use, and blood transfusion [143]. During a blood meal, an infected mosquito injects saliva containing sporozoites, the infectious form of the parasite [142]. The sporozoites travel hematogenously to the liver, invading hepatocytes (the exoerythrocytic or hepatic phase). Within hepatocytes, schizonts form from sporozoites and eventually rupture their contents, merozoites, into the bloodstream. For *P. falciparum* and *P. malariae,* this heralds the end of the exoerythrocytic phase. However, *P. vivax* and *P. ovale* can maintain chronic hepatocyte infection and merozoite release. This has implications for disease course and therapy, as discussed below.

Merozoites invade erythrocytes, where their morphology is similar to signet rings, hence the designation of "ring forms" for their light microscopic appearance. The merozoites enlarge into trophozoites, which asexually divide into clusters of merozoites termed schizonts. The schizonts rupture, releasing merozoites into the bloodstream. Subsequently, the erythrocytic stage of infection is repeated.

PATHOGENESIS. This discussion is restricted to falciparum malaria, which accounts overwhelmingly for the morbidity and mortality from malaria. The effects of falciparum alaria, especially the feared complication of cerebral malaria, are largely attributable to vents within the capillaries (reviewed in [146]). The membranes of parasitized erythrocytes contain electron-dense knobs that are associated with malarial proteins. These sites are thought to be involved in the binding of parasitized erythrocytes to capillary endothelial cells. In addition, nonparasitized erythrocytes adhere to parasitized erythrocytes attached to endothelium, causing further blockage of the capillary lumen. Data are not conclusive, however, in that parasitized erythrocytes without knobs adhere to endothelium, and not all investigators have found the proteins thought to be the binding sites on cerebral endothelium [146].

Metabolic derangements, specifically hypoglycemia and increased levels of lactate in the blood and CSF [146], also likely are involved in the development of cerebral malaria. Hypoglycemia is associated with seizures, an altered mental status, and decerebrate signs in some patients with malaria. However, the administration of intravenous dextrose does not always reverse these effects [146]. The packing of erythrocytes into capillaries in the absence of inflammation suggest that tissue damage is

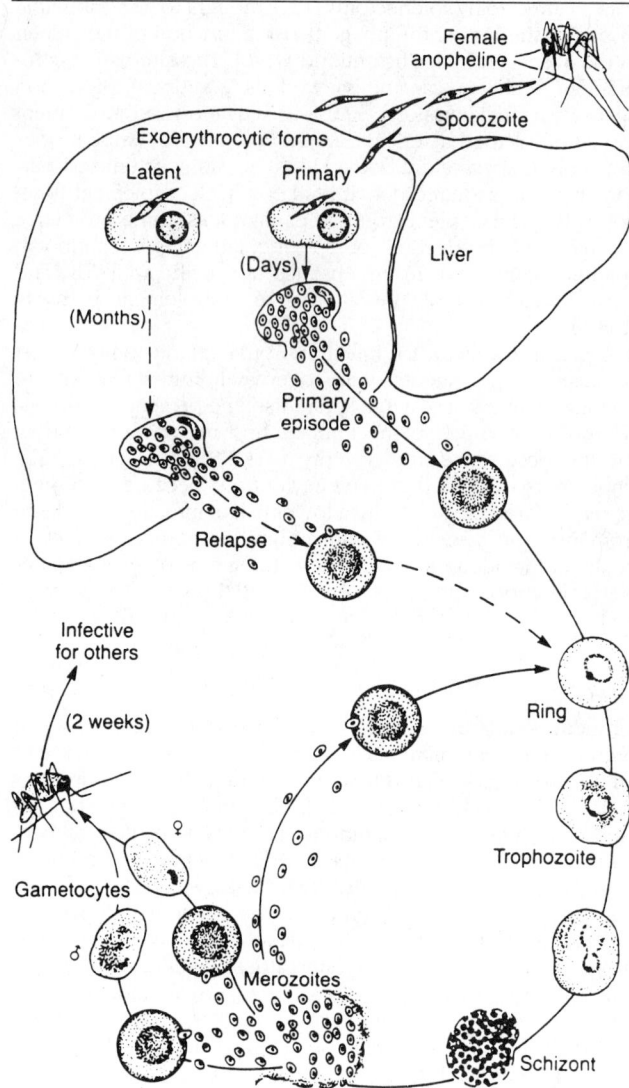

Fig. 91-1. From Wyler DJ: Plasmodium and babesia, in Gorbach SL, Bartlett JG, Blacklow NR (eds): *Infectious Disease.* Philadelphia, Saunders, 1992: pp 1967–1978. Reproduced by permission.

caused by anoxia [147]. Finally, the cytokine tumor necrosis factor (TNF) is thought by some to play a role in the pathogenesis of cerebral malaria as suggested by in vitro and in vivo studies [146].

DIAGNOSIS

Clinical Features. Imported malaria occurs at varying intervals after leaving a malarious area [143,145]. Almost all cases of falciparum malaria occur within 5 months, with 75 percent occurring within 3 months of return from travel. However, malaria due to *P. malariae, P. ovale,* and *P. vivax* can occur more than a year after return. Therefore, in any patient with a fever of unknown origin, a detailed travel history should be obtained.

The classic presenting features of malaria are fever and chills, seen in 80 percent or more of individuals with imported malaria in developed countries [144,145,148]. Other symptoms include malaise or weakness, neurologic complaints, gastrointestinal symptoms, headache, myalgia, shortness of breath or cough, and to a lesser extent, lower back pain, pharyngitis, and neck stiffness [144,145,148].

Malaria in pregnancy presents as a more severe disease [149,150]. In addition to the usual presenting features and complications of malaria, especially hypoglycemia, acute pulmonary edema, and anemia, other features are maternal mortality, premature labor with preterm birth, miscarriage, and congenital malaria.

Physical findings include fever (in 54–73% of patients on admission), orthostatic hypotension, splenomegaly, hepatomegaly, abdominal tenderness, neurologic findings, jaundice, and, rarely, purpura [145,148].

Complications. The most common and feared complication of malaria is cerebral malaria. It has been variably defined as fever, seizure, and coma for more than 30 minutes after a seizure [151]; impaired consciousness in the presence of parasites in the blood [146]; or nonlocalizing or absent motor response to noxious stimuli in the presence of parasites in the blood and in the absence of other causes of encephalopathy [152]. The incidence of cerebral malaria in three series of imported severe falciparum malaria ranged from 6 to 59 percent of cases [146,151,152]. Although it is thought that recovery from cerebral malaria is the rule, 6 to 50 percent of children suffer from sequelae such as hemiparesis, seizure disorder, blindness, or spasticity [146,151]. In contrast, Ethiopian adults who survived cerebral malaria experienced no sequelae [152].

Other complications of malaria include severe anemia, presumably caused by hemolysis, DIC, acute renal failure, adult respiratory distress syndrome, shock, and bacterial sepsis [145,153,154]. Death from imported falciparum malaria in developed countries occurred in up to 19 percent of cases [144,145,148,154].

Laboratory Features. A number of abnormalities are evident on laboratory examination. The total white blood cell count is generally normal, although up to 30 percent exhibit leukopenia, whereas leukocytosis is rare. An increased percentage of band forms is frequently present. Anemia is observed in one-third of patients and can be profound in those with severe falciparum malaria. Other manifestations include thrombocytopenia, renal impairment, hyperbilirubinemia, hyponatremia, elevated liver function tests, hypoalbuminemia, microscopic hematuria, and, rarely, hypoglycemia [145,148].

Laboratory Diagnosis

The most efficient and reliable diagnostic test for malaria is the examination of peripheral blood thick or thin smears by light microscopy (reviewed in [155]). The test is sensitive in that one parasitized erythrocyte in one million can be detected. Over 90 percent of patients with imported malaria have been diagnosed by examination of the thick or thin smear [145,148]. Because up to 10 percent of patients with malaria have negative microscopic studies, malaria should be presumed when history of travel to an endemic area is accompanied by the typical clinical scenario in the absence of positive smears and another explanation for the illness.

The utility of the thick smear is its greater sensitivity in detecting parasites. Because erythrocytes are lysed in this test, the parasites are more easily seen, but an estimation of the percentage of erythrocytes parasitized (% parasitemia) is impossible. This and speciation are accomplished by review of a thin smear, where erythrocytes remain intact. After the diagnosis of

malaria is made, thin smears are repeated at intervals to assess the efficacy of therapy. For a discussion of the thick-and-thin smear method, refer to Makler and Gibbins [155].

Other methods of diagnosis that are not used routinely or are research tools include fluorescence microscopy, polymerase chain reaction and immunologic testing, such as serology, for use in epidemiologic studies, blood banking, and screening.

DIFFERENTIAL DIAGNOSIS. Because of the nonspecific signs and symptoms of malaria, the differential diagnosis is extensive and encompasses several febrile illnesses endemic to developing countries. These include dengue fever and other viral hemorrhagic fevers, yellow fever, typhoid fever, rickettsioses (particularly before the development or in the absence of rash), acute visceral leishmaniasis, and acute American or African trypanosomiasis. Babesiosis, a disease caused by *Babesia microti,* a protozoan similar to *Plasmodium,* may cause a clinical syndrome similar to malaria (see below). Additionally, the diagnosis of babesiosis is made by thick or thin smear. The morphology is varied and includes ring forms. However, the geographic distribution, mode of transmission, and specific morphologic characteristics of *Babesia* differ from those of *Plasmodium.* Finally, bacterial sepsis should be considered in the differential diagnosis of malaria.

TREATMENT. The treatment of malaria is complex because of the different regimens for falciparum and nonfalciparum malaria, unfamiliarity of physicians in developed countries with antimalarial agents and drug resistance. For a complete review, refer to Panisko and Keystone (156).

Drug Resistance. The development of single and multiple drug resistance has become a difficult problem in the treatment of malaria, particularly in Southeast Asia [156]. Thus, it is important in the management of patients with malaria to know where travel occurred and what resistance patterns occur in that geographic area.

Resistance of *P. falciparum* to several antimalarial agents is well documented. Chloroquine resistance is widespread such that areas without significant resistance are primarily the Middle East and Central America. Readers are referred to the resource *Health Advice for International Travel,* published annually by the CDC, for more detailed information. It should be noted that chloroquine resistance is independent of resistance to quinine or mefloquine [156]. Quinine and mefloquine resistance have been documented in Southeast Asia, the latter particularly along the Thai-Burmese border [157]. Pyrimethamine-sulfadoxine (Fansidar) resistance of *P. falciparum* is not uncommon. It is found in Southeast Asia, Bangladesh, Oceania, the Amazon basin, and East Africa. *P. vivax* is frequently resistant to pyrimethamine-sulfadoxine.

Primaquine resistance is a serious problem in the eradication of the exoerythrocytic phase of infection with *P. ovale* or *P. vivax,* because no other agent for this purpose exists [156]. Resistance is found in Southeast Asia and New Guinea. Additionally, there are case reports of resistance in India, South America, and Africa.

Nonfalciparum Malaria. The treatment for nonfalciparum malaria is chloroquine phosphate, the oral form of chloroquine (Table 91-2). An alternative is quinine sulfate. In the event oral dosing is not possible, intravenous quinidine gluconate infusion is recommended because parenteral quinine is no longer available in the United States from the CDC [158]. The patient should be switched to oral chloroquine as soon as feasible. Addition-

Table 91-2. Drug Treatment of Nonfalciparum and Chloroquine-Sensitive Falciparum Malaria

Agent	Adults	Children	Comments
Chloroquine phosphate[a] (oral)	1 gm then 500 mg q.o.d. for 2 days	16.7 mg/kg then 8.3 mg/kg in 6 hr then 8.3 mg/kg for 2 days	Safe in pregnancy
Quinine sulfate[b] (oral)	600 mg q 8 hr for 5 to 7 d	19 mg/kg q 8 hr for 5 to 7 d	
Quinidine gluconate[b] (intravenous infusion)	10 mg/kg over 1 to 2 hr then 0.02 mg/kg/min for up to 72 hr	Same as for adults	Change to oral chloroquine when possible.
Primaquine sulfate[c] (oral)	15 mg q.o.d. for 14 d OR 45 mg q week for 8 weeks	0.3 mg/kg/d for 14 d	Treatment for the exoerythrocytic phase of *P. ovale* and *P. vivax.* Use in pregnancy?

[a]Toxicities: gastrointestinal distress, headache, fatigue, dyskinesia, hearing loss, neuromuscular disorders, hemolytic anemia in glucose-6-phosphate dehydrogenase (G-6-PD) deficiency.
[b]Toxicities: cinchonism, diarrhea, constipation, drug fever, pruritus, urticaria, bronchospasm, angioedema, hemolysis, agranulocytosis, hypoglycemia, hemolytic anemia in G-6-PD deficiency. Also seen with parenteral administration: hypotension, increased QTc interval, seizures, blindness, deafness, death.
[c]Toxicities: gastrointestinal distress, methemoglobinemia, agranulocytosis, hemolytic anemia in G-6-PD deficiency.

ally, infection with *Plasmodium* forms definitely or possibly identified as *P. vivax* or *P. ovale* merits treatment with primaquine to eradicate the exoerythrocytic phase of disease.

Chloroquine-Sensitive Falciparum Malaria. Persons with falciparum malaria (1) which was contracted in an area that has no documented chloroquine resistance, (2) who have mild disease without complications, and (3) who were not taking chloroquine prophylaxis [159] should be treated as for nonfalciparum malaria with oral chloroquine.

Chloroquine-Resistant Falciparum Malaria. The recommended treatment for mild chloroquine-resistant falciparum malaria is oral quinine (Table 91-3) [156]. Consideration should be given to the addition of pyrimethamine-sulfadoxine, tetracycline, or clindamycin on completion of quinine. The latter two are useful in patients with a history of hypersensitivity to sulfonamides or if malaria was contracted in an area with pyrimethamine-sulfadoxine resistance.

Quinidine gluconate administration by intravenous infusion is the recommended treatment for chloroquine-resistant falciparum malaria (or other forms of malaria) if (1) oral intake is impossible, (2) neurologic dysfunction is present, or (3) greater than 5 percent of erythrocytes are infected (Table 91-2) [154,158]. Thin smears to assess the degree of parasitemia and hence therapeutic efficacy should be performed every 12 to 24 hours. Because of the possibility of adverse cardiac effects and hypoglycemia attributable to quinidine, it should be administered in an intensive care unit, and blood glucose, quinidine levels, and cardiac monitoring, specifically the QTc interval, is recommended. A change to oral quinine should occur once oral intake is possible, parasitemia is less than 1 percent, and mental status is normal [154]. Improvement usually occurs within 28 to 72 hours [154]. If not, drug resistance or poor drug delivery is to be suspected [158]. A total treatment duration of 72 hours is recommended, followed by treatment with pyrimethamine-sulfadoxine, tetracycline, or clindamycin.

Other agents have been used in the treatment of malaria in countries with endemic disease. The use of mefloquine in the treatment of falciparum malaria, including chloroquine-resistant falciparum malaria, has been studied recently [160,161,162]. It was equal to or more effective than chloroquine and relatively well tolerated in both adults and children. Additionally, artemisinine, also known as *qinghaosu,* and related compounds de-

rived from the plant, *Artemisia annua,* have been promising in the treatment of falciparum malaria [156,163]. Originally used as a Chinese herbal remedy for fever, the agent is not presently available in the United States. Its major advantage is the rapid reduction in parasitemia in severe *P. falciparum* infection. It is unlikely that artemisinine will be used as a single agent because of high rates of recrudescence when used alone [156].

Treatment During Pregnancy. Treatment of malaria during pregnancy presents additional challenges (reviewed in [149,150]). Chloroquine is safe for use in pregnant women for the treatment of nonfalciparum or chloroquine-sensitive falciparum malaria. In chloroquine-resistant falciparum malaria, quinine has been used safely, despite its abortifacient properties [164]. Because intravenous forms of quinine are no longer available in the United States, a pregnant women with severe falciparum malaria would ideally be treated with intravenous quinidine, although the efficacy and safety of quinidine under these circumstances have not been studied. Obviously, the serious consequences of severe falciparum malaria in a pregnant woman must be considered when choosing therapy. Clindamycin is an acceptable second agent, after completion of quinidine or oral quinine treatment. Exchange transfusion (see below) has been used in pregnant women as adjunctive treatment for malaria [165]. In addition to the usual supportive care and monitoring, fetal monitoring should be performed. Emergency cesarean delivery may be necessary [150].

Adjunctive Therapy. Exchange transfusion for complicated malaria, particularly in the presence of a high degree of parasitemia, has been shown to be beneficial [154,166,167]. It has been recommended by some experts to use exchange transfusion when the following exist: parasitemia of at least 5 to 10 percent, cerebral malaria, DIC, or acute renal failure. Exchange transfusion should continue until parasitemia is less than 1 to 5 percent [154,166,167]. This is usually accomplished by exchanging 8 to 10 units [154]. Exchanges can be accomplished manually or mechanically with a cell sorter. Blood banking practices that assure proper cross-matching and a blood supply free from human immunodeficiency virus, hepatitis B, hepatitis C, and parasites are essential.

Persons with severe malaria should be cared for in an intensive care unit. Fluids, electrolytes, blood glucose, drug concen-

Table 91-3. Drug Treatment of Chloroquine-Resistant Falciparum Malaria

Agent	Adults	Children	Comments
Quinine sulfate	As in Table 91-2	As in Table 91-2	Consider adding second agent after quinine.*
Quinidine sulfate (intravenous)	As in Table 91-2	As in Table 91-2	Change to oral quinine as soon as possible. Add second agent after quinidine.

*Pyrimethamine-sulfadoxine, 75 mg of pyrimethamine and 1500 mg of sulfadoxine in adults (1.25 mg/kg pyrimethamine and 25 mg/kg sulfadoxine in children) in one dose on day 3 of quinine. Avoid in late pregnancy, premature infants or infants younger than 1 month of age because of kernicterus. Other toxicities: hypersensitivity, including severe cutaneous reactions, hepatitis, agranulocytosis, serum sickness, hemolytic anemia in glucose-6-phosphate dehydrogenase deficiency. **OR** Tetracycline, 250 mg p.o. q 6 hr for 7 days starting several days after discontinuation of quinine. Doxycycline, 100 mg p.o. q 12 hr, is an alternative. Both are contraindicated in pregnancy and children younger than 8 years of age. Toxicities: hypersensitivity, especially in sunlight, rash, gastrointestinal upset. **OR** Clindamycin, 10 mg/kg p.o. q 8 hr in children and adults, for 5 days starting several days after discontinuation of quinine. May be used during pregnancy. Toxicities: rash and pseudomembranous colitis.

trations, and cardiac and neurologic function should be closely monitored. In addition, renal function and the integrity of the clotting system should be assessed. Respiratory ventilation may be necessary.

In the past, steroids were used in the treatment of cerebral malaria. However, they have been shown not to be beneficial and may be harmful in this instance [153,168,169]. Therefore, steroids are not indicated for the treatment of cerebral malaria.

Miscellaneous Infectious Diseases

It is beyond the scope of this chapter to include all unusual infectious diseases that might require admission to an intensive care unit. However, several diseases merit brief discussions.

BABESIOSIS. Babesiosis is caused by the protozoan *Babesia microti* [170]. It is transmitted by the tick vector, *Ixodes dammini,* the deer tick that transmits *Borrelia burgdorferi,* the agent of Lyme disease, or by transfusion of infected blood [171]. *B. microti* is endemic to the northeastern United States, particularly the coastal regions. It causes a self-limited disease characterized by fever, rigors, headache, generalized myalgias and arthralgias, and hemolytic anemia [172,173]. However, in certain high-risk groups, including persons with asplenia, the disease can pursue a fulminant and frequently fatal course [174]. Diagnosis is made through epidemiologic associations in combination with examination of the thick and thin peripheral blood smears (see Malaria in this chapter), which show protozoa parasitizing erythrocytes. Treatment is quinine and clindamycin in combination for 7 to 10 days [170]. Severe cases benefit from exchange transfusion [171,175]

PLAGUE. Plague, caused by *Yersinia pestis,* is a potentially fatal illness that exists in several forms (reviewed in [176]). The disease is primarily transmitted by fleas harbored by rodents. Other modes of transmission include direct inoculation into wounds, inhalation, and mechanical introduction. Enzootic foci of infection exist in the southwestern United States, especially New Mexico. Plague exists in several forms. Bubonic plague is the form involving buboes, enlarged lymph nodes draining the site of a flea bite. In the absence of treatment, the infection can disseminate to cause septicemic plague (secondary septicemic plague). Alternatively, septicemia can exist without the presence of buboes (primary septicemic plague). Septicemic plague can involve any organ system and be fulminant and rapidly

fatal [176,177]. In one recent study, one-third of cases of primary septicemic plague were fatal, as compared with 12 percent of bubonic plague cases [177]. Its presenting signs and symptoms include fever, chills, malaise, gastrointestinal symptoms, and gangrene of the skin and digits [176,177]. Pneumonic plague can occur secondary to septicemia or through inhalation and thus has implications concerning person-to-person spread. However, not since 1925 has pneumonic plague occurred caused by human-to-human spread [176].

The diagnosis of plague is by the isolation of *Y. pestis* from blood or other bodily fluids; the identification of the organism, with its characteristic bipolar appearance, in Wayson's or Giemsa-stained samples of fluid from buboes or sputum; and immunofluorescence. Treatment is with the aminoglycoside streptomycin (30 mg/kg body weight intramuscularly in two divided doses per day for 10 days) [178]. The dosage should be adjusted in the presence of renal failure. Tetracycline or sulfadiazine is also effective. The former is particularly useful for the prophylaxis of persons exposed to patients with plague [176]. For meningitis or endophthalmitis, chloramphenicol is recommended because of its superior penetration [176,178]. The drug is administered intravenously as a loading dose of 25 mg/kg body weight, then 60 mg/kg/day in four divided doses until there is clinical improvement, whereby the dose can be reduced to 30 mg/kg/day and administered by the oral route for a total of 10 days [178]. Respiratory isolation is necessary for persons suspected of having pneumonic plague.

CAPNOCYTOPHAGIA CANIMORSUS. *C. canimorsus,* also known as CDC group DF-2, is a thin gram-negative rod that causes septicemia and meningitis [179–182]. Most severe cases occur in individuals with underlying diseases such as asplenia or alcoholism (180,181,182), although fatal septicemia has occurred in healthy individuals [183]. The source of the organism is most often dog bites, although cat bites have been implicated [184]. Presentations include sepsis, meningitis, cellulitis, and endocarditis [185] and can be fulminant [183]. Diagnosis is through culture and identification of the organism on peripheral smear [179]. Antibiotic treatment is usually with penicillin or amoxicillin-clavulanic acid, although the organism is sensitive to a variety of antibiotics such as other β-lactams (excepting aztreonam), vancomycin, clindamycin, ciprofloxacin, and erythromycin [179,186]. In immunocompromised persons, parenteral therapy with ticarcillin-clavulanate or ampicillin sulbactam should be instituted [179].

TULAREMIA. Tularemia, caused by the organism *Francisella tularensis,* is typically associated with human contact with infected game, notably rabbits, where the skin is the portal of entry (reviewed in [176]). Other modes of transmission are through the bites of infected animals or insects, inhalation of infectious aerosols, inoculation onto mucous membranes, and ingestion. Of the several forms, pneumonic tularemia is the most severe, with the highest mortality [(187]. The disease is associated with high fever, headache, rigors, meningitis, rhabdomyolysis, DIC, and hypotension [176,187,188]. Diagnosis is by measurement of serum agglutinins or culture. If the organism is suspected, the microbiogy laboratory should be notified because of the hazard of aerosolization [176,187]. The drug of choice for treatment is an aminoglycoside, such as streptomycin or gentamicin, for 10 days [176,187]. Effective oral alternatives are tetracycline and chloramphenicol, although treatment failures occur [176].

AMERICAN HANTAVIRUS INFECTION. In May 1993, an acute illness characterized by a prodrome of fever, myalgia, headache, and cough with rapid progression to respiratory failure was described [189,190]. The illness occurred most commonly in members of the Navajo Nation in the Four Corners region of the southwestern United States, although cases outside that area have been described [189,191]. The causative agent is hantavirus or a related virus [189]. The reservoir is the deer mouse and possibly other rodents, with transmission through contact with infected rodent excreta, after the bite of an infected rodent or possibly through ingestion of contaminated food or water [192]. A confirmed case is described as unexplained acute respiratory distress syndrome or acute bilateral pulmonary interstitial infiltrates with or without prodromal symptoms, with the onset in 1993, and with laboratory evidence of recent hantavirus infection [189]. The treatment suggested by the CDC is ribavirin because of its efficacy in the treatment of Hantaan virus infection [189], although its efficacy in treating American hantavirus infection is unknown.

References

1. Shands KN, Schmid GP, Dan BB, et al: Toxic-shock syndrome in menstruating women: Association with tampon use and *Staphylococcus aureus* and clinical features in 52 cases. *N Engl J Med* 303:1436, 1980.
2. Tofte RW, Williams DN: Toxic shock syndrome: Clinical and laboratory features in 15 patients. *Ann Intern Med* 94:149, 1981.
3. Chesney PJ, Davis JP, Purdy WK, et al: Clinical manifestations of toxic shock syndrome. *JAMA* 246:741, 1981.
4. Fisher RF, Goodpasture HC, Peterie JD, et al: Toxic shock syndrome in menstruating women. *Ann Intern Med* 94:156, 1981.
5. Tofte RW, Williams DM: Clinical and laboratory manifestations of toxic shock syndrome. *Ann Intern Med* 96:843, 1982.
6. Todd J, Fishaut M: Toxic-shock syndrome associated with phage-group-1 staphylococci. *Lancet* 2:1116, 1978.
7. Davis JP, Chesney PJ, Wand PJ, et al: Toxic-shock syndrome: Epidemiologic features, recurrence, risk factors, and prevention. *N Engl J Med* 303:1429, 1980.
8. Kehrberg MW, Latham RH, Haslam BT, et al: Risk factors for staphylococcal toxic-shock syndrome. *Am J Epidemiol* 114:873, 1981.
9. Osterholm MT, Davis JP, Gibson RW, et al: Tri-state toxic-shock syndrome study. I. Epidemiologic findings. *J Infect Dis* 145:431, 1982.
10. Schlech WF, Shands KN, Reingold AL, et al: Risk factors for development of toxic shock syndrome. *JAMA* 248:835, 1982.
11. Kass EH: Toxic shock syndrome: A reprise. *Ann Intern Med* 97:608, 1982.
12. Stevens DL, Tanner MH, Winship J, et al: Severe group A streptococcal infections associated with a toxic shock-like syndrome and scarlet fever toxin A. *N Engl J Med* 321:1, 1989.
13. Parsonnet J, Hickman RK, Eardley DD, et al: Induction of human interleukin-1 by toxic-shock-syndrome toxin-1. *J Infect Dis* 151:514, 1985.
14. Stone RL, Schlievert PM: Evidence for the involvement of endotoxin in toxic shock syndrome. *J Infect Dis* 155:682, 1987.
15. Schlievert PM, Shands KN, Dan BB, et al: Identification and characterization of an exotoxin from *Staphylococcus aureus* associated with toxic-shock syndrome. *J Infect Dis* 143:509, 1981.
16. Schlievert RM, Kelly JA: Staphylococcal pyrogenic exotoxin type C: Further characterization. *Ann Intern Med* 96:982, 1982.
17. Bergdoll MS, Crass BA, Reiser RF, et al: A new staphylococcal enterotoxin, enterotoxin F associated with toxic-shock-syndrome *Staphylococcus aureus* isolates. *Lancet* 1:1017, 1981.
18. Bergdoll MS, Crass BA, Reiser RF: An enterotoxin-like protein in *Staphylococcus aureus* strains from patients with toxic shock syndrome. *Ann Intern Med* 96:969, 1982.
19. Parsonnet J, Gillis JA, Pier GB: Induction of interleukin-1 by strains of *Staphylococcus aureus* from patients with nonmenstrual toxic shock syndrome. *J Infect Dis* 154:55, 1986.
20. Whiting JL, Rosten PM, Chow AW: Determination by Western blot (immunoblot) of seroconversions to toxic shock syndrome (TSS) toxin 1 and enterotoxin A, B, or C during infection with TSS- and non-TSS-associated *Staphylococcus aureus*. *Infect Immun* 57:231, 1989.
21. Crass BA, Bergdoll MS: Involvement of staphylococcal enterotoxins in nonmenstrual toxic shock syndrome. *J Clin Microbiol* 23:1138, 1986.
22. Garbe PL, Arko RJ, Reingold AL, et al: *Staphylococcus aureus* isolates from patients with nonmenstrual toxic shock syndrome. *JAMA* 253:2538, 1985.
23. Schlievert PM: Role of superantigens in human disease. *J Infect Dis* 167:997, 1993.
24. Wannamaker LW: Toxic shock: Problems in definition and diagnosis. *Ann Intern Med* 96:775, 1982.
25. Guinan ME, Dan BB, Guidotti RJ: Vaginal colonization with *Staphylococcus aureus* in healthy women: A review of four studies. *Ann Intern Med* 96:944, 1982.
26. Parsonnet J, Gillis ZA: Production of tumor necrosis factor by human monocytes in response to toxic-shock-syndrome toxin-1. *J Infect Dis* 158:1026, 1988.
27. Ikejima T, Okusawa S, van der Meer JWM, et al: Induction by toxic-shock-syndrome toxin-1 of a circulating tumor necrosis factor-like substance in rabbits and of immunoreactive tumor necrosis factor and interleukin-1 from human mononuclear cells. *J Infect Dis* 158:1017, 1988.
28. Paris AL, Herwaldt LA, Blum D: Pathologic findings in twelve fatal cases of toxic shock syndrome. *Ann Intern Med* 96:852, 1982.
29. Larkin SM, Williams DN, Osterholm MT: Toxic shock syndrome: Clinical laboratory and pathologic findings in nine fatal cases. *Ann Intern Med* 96:858, 1982.
30. Reingold AL, Hargrett NT, Dan BB: Nonmenstrual toxic shock syndrome: A. *Ann Intern Med* 96:871, 1982.
31. Bartlett P, Reingold AL, Graham DR, et al: Toxic shock syndrome associated with surgical wound infections. *JAMA* 247:1448, 1982.
32. Reingold AL, Dan BB, Shands KN, et al: Toxic-shock syndrome not associated with menstruation: A review of 54 cases. *Lancet* 1:1, 1982.
33. Tofte RW, Williams DN: Toxic shock syndrome: Evidence of a broad clinical spectrum. *JAMA* 246:2163, 1981.
34. Reingold AL, Hargrett NT, Shands KN: Toxic shock syndrome surveillance in the United States. *Ann Intern Med* 96:875, 1982.
35. Chesney RW, Chesney PJ, Davis JP, et al: Renal manifestations of the staphylococcal toxic-shock syndrome. *Am J Med* 71:583, 1981.
36. Gourley GR, Chesney PJ, Davis JP, et al: Acute cholestasis in patients with toxic-shock syndrome. *Gastroenterology* 81:928, 1981.
37. Chesney JP, Crass BA, Polyak MD: Toxic shock syndrome: Management and long-term sequelae. *Ann Intern Med* 96:847, 1982.
38. Glasgow LA: Staphylococcal infection in the toxic-shock syndrome. *N Engl J Med* 303:1473, 1980.
39. Shands KN, Dan BB, Schmid GP: Toxic shock syndrome: The emerging picture. *Ann Intern Med* 94:264, 1981.
40. Wolff SM: Introduction to volume on the toxic shock syndrome. *Ann Intern Med* 96:835, 1982.
41. Rosene DA, Copass MK, Kastner LS: Persistent neuropsychological

sequelae of toxic shock syndrome. *Ann Intern Med* 96:865, 1982.

42. Davis JP, Osterholm MT, Helms CM, et al: Tri-state toxic-shock syndrome study. II. Clinical and laboratory findings. *J Infect Dis* 145:441, 1982.
43. Barry W, Hudgins L, Donta ST, et al: Intravenous immunoglobulin therapy for toxic shock syndrome. *JAMA* 267:3315, 1992.
44. Todd JK: Therapy of toxic shock syndrome. *Drugs* 39:856, 1990.
45. Burns JR, Menapace FJ: Acute reversible cardiomyopathy complicating toxic shock syndrome. *Arch Intern Med* 142:1032, 1982.
46. Bisno AL: Group A streptococcal infections and acute rheumatic fever. *N Engl J Med* 325:783, 1991.
47. Weber DJ, Walker DH: Rocky Mountain spotted fever. *Infect Dis Clin North Am* 5:19, 1991.
48. Centers for Disease Control: Summary of notifiable diseases, United States 1991. *MMWR* 40:1, 1992.
49. Vianna NJ, Hinman AR: Rocky Mountain spotted fever on Long Island. *Am J Med* 51:725, 1971.
50. Massachusetts Department of Public Health: On the alert for Rocky Mountain spotted fever. *N Engl J Med* 292:1127, 1975.
51. Sporn LA, Shi RJ, Lawrence SO, et al: *Rickettsia rickettsii* infection of cultured endothelial cells induces release of large von Willebrand factor multimers from Weibel-Palade bodies. *Blood* 78:2595, 1991.
52. Lange JV, Walker DH, Wester TB: Documented Rocky Mountain spotted fever in wintertime. *JAMA* 247:2403, 1982.
53. Hattwick MA, O'Brien RJ, Hanson BF: Rocky Mountain spotted fever: Epidemiology of an increasing problem. *Ann Intern Med* 84:732, 1976.
54. Woodward RE: Rocky Mountain spotted fever: Epidemiological and early clinical signs are keys to treatment and reduced mortality. *J Infect Dis* 150:465, 1984.
55. Helmick CG, Bernard KW, D'Angelo LJ: Rocky Mountain spotted fever: Clinical, laboratory, and epidemiological features of 262 cases. *J Infect Dis* 150:480, 1984.
56. Wilfert CM, MacCormack JN, Kleeman K, et al: Epidemiology of Rocky Mountain spotted fever as determined by active surveillance. *J Infect Dis* 150:469, 1984.
57. Kirk JL, Fine DP, Sexton DJ, et al: Rocky Mountain spotted fever: A clinical review based on 48 confirmed cases, 1943. *Medicine* 69:35, 1990.
58. Raoult D, Walker DH: *Rickettsia rickettsii* and other spotted fever group rickettsiae (Rocky Mountain spotted fever and other spotted fevers), in Mandell GL, Douglas RG, Bennett JE (ed): *Principles and Practice of Infectious Diseases*. 3rd ed. New York, Churchill Livingstone, 1990, pp 1465-1471.
59. Walker DH, Cain BG, Olmstead PM: Laboratory diagnosis of Rocky Mountain spotted fever by immunofluorescent demonstration of *Rickettsia rickettsii* in cutaneous lesions. Am J Clin Pathol 69:619, 1978.
60. Silverman DJ: Adherence of platelets to human endothelial cells infected by *Rickettsia rickettsii*. *J Infect Dis* 153:694, 1986.
61. Silverman DJ, Santucci LA: Potential for free radical-induced lipid peroxidation as a cause of endothelial cell injury in Rocky Mountain spotted fever. *Infect Immun* 56:3110, 1988.
62. Rao AK, Schapira M, Clements ML, et al: A prospective study of platelets and plasma proteolytic systems during the early stages of Rocky Mountain spotted fever. N Engl J Med 318:1021, 1988.
63. Sexton DJ, Corey GR: Rocky Mountain "spotless" and "almost spotless" fever: A wolf in sheep's clothing. *Clin Infect Dis* 15:439, 1992.
64. Woodward TE, Pedersen CE Jr., Oster CN, et al: Prompt confirmation of Rocky Mountain spotted fever: Identification of rickettsiae in skin tissues. *J Infect Dis* 134:297, 1976.
65. Tzianabos T, Anderson BE, McDade JE: Detection of *Rickettsia rickettsii* DNA in clinical specimens by using polymerase chain reaction technology. *J Clin Microbiol* 27:2866, 1989.
66. Walker DH: Rocky Mountain spotted fever: A disease in need of microbiological concern. *Clin Microbiol Rev* 2:227, 1989.
67. Centers for Disease Control: Laboratory-based surveillance for meningococcal disease in selected areas—United States, 1989-1991. *MMWR* 42:21, 1993.
68. Pinner RW, Gellin BG, Bibb WF, et al: Meningococcal disease in

the United States—1986. Meningococcal Disease Study Group. *J Infect Dis* 164:368, 1991.
69. Havens PL, Garland JS, Brook MM, et al: Trends in mortality in children hospitalized with meningococcal infections, 1957 to 1987. *Pediatr Infect Dis J* 8:8, 1989.
70. Greenfield S, Sheehe PR, Feldman HA: Meningococcal carriage in a population of "normal" families. *J Infect Dis* 123:67, 1971.
71. Schwartz B, Moore PS, Broome CV: Global epidemiology of meningococcal disease. *Clin Microbiol Rev* 2:S118, 1989.
72. Stephens DS, Farley MM: Pathogenic events during infection of the human nasopharynx with *Neisseria meningitidis* and *Haemophilus influenzae*. *Rev Infect Dis* 13:22, 1991.
73. Figueroa JE, Densen P: Infectious diseases associated with complement deficiencies. *Clin Microbiol Rev* 4:359, 1991.
74. Merino J, Rodriguez-Valverde V, Lamelas JA, et al: Prevalence of deficits of complement components in patients with recurrent meningococcal infections. *J Infect Dis* 148:331, 1983.
75. Nagata M, Hara T, Aoki T, et al: Inherited deficiency of ninth component of complement: An increased risk of meningococcal meningitis. *J Pediatr* 114:260, 1989.
76. Rasmussen JM, Brandslund I, Teisner B, et al: Screening for complement deficiencies in unselected patients with meningitis. *Clin Exp Immunol* 68:437, 1987.
77. Ellison RT, Mason SR, Kohler PF, et al: Meningococcemia and acquired complement deficiency: association in patients with hepatic failure. *Arch Intern Med* 146:1539, 1986.
78. Ellison RT, Kohler PF, Curd JG, et al: Prevalence of congenital or acquired complement deficiency in patients with sporadic meningococcal disease. *N Engl J Med* 308:913, 1983.
79. Grogan DP, Love SM, Ogden JA, et al: Chondro-osseous growth abnormalities after meningococcemia: A clinical and histopathological study. *Am J Bone Joint Surg* 71:920, 1989.
80. Chervu I, Koss M, Campese VM: Bilateral renal cortical necrosis in two patients with *Neisseria meningitidis* sepsis. *Am J Nephrol* 11:411, 1991.
81. Genoff MC, Hoffer MM, Achauer B, et al: Extremity amputations in meningococcemia-induced purpura fulminans. *Plast Reconstr Surg* 89:878, 1992.
82. Tuncer AM, Gur I, Ertem U, et al: Once daily ceftriaxone for meningococcemia and meningococcal meningitis. *Pediatr Infect Dis J* 7:711, 1988.
83. Girardin E, Grau GE, Dayer JM, et al: Tumor necrosis factor and interleukin-1 in the serum of children with severe infectious purpura. *N Engl J Med* 319:397, 1988.
84. Jacobs RF, Sowell MK, Moss MM, et al: Septic shock in children: Bacterial etiologies and temporal relationships. *Pediatr Infect Dis J* 9:196, 1990.
85. Fourrier F, Lestavel P, Chopin C, et al: Meningococcemia and purpura fulminans in adults: Acute deficiencies of proteins C and S and early treatment with antithrombin III concentrates. *Intensive Care Med* 16:121, 1990.
86. Morse JR, Oretsky MI, Hudson JA: Pericarditis as a complication of meningococcal meningitis. *Ann Intern Med* 74:212, 1971.
87. Emparanza JI, Aldamiz EL, Perez YE, et al: Prognostic score in acute meningococcemia. *Crit Care Med* 16:168, 1988.
88. Romijn JA, Godfried MH, Wortel C, et al: Hypoglycemia, hormones and cytokines in fatal meningococcal septicemia. *J Endocrinol Invest* 13:743, 1990.
89. Stiehm ER, Damrosch DS: Factors in the prognosis of meningococcal infections. *J Pediatr* 68:457, 1966.
90. Hoyne AL, Brown RH: 727 meningococcic cases, an analysis. *Ann Intern Med* 28:248, 1948.
91. Levin S, Painter MB: The treatment of acute meningococcal infection in adults. *Ann Intern Med* 64:1049, 1966.
92. Carpenter RR, Petersdorf RG: The clinical spectrum of bacterial meningitis. *Am J Med* 33:262, 1962.
93. D'Amato RF, Hochstein L, Fay EA: False-positive latex agglutination test for *Neisseria meningitidis* groups A and Y caused by povidone-iodine antiseptic contamination of cerebrospinal fluid. *J Clin Microbiol* 28:2134, 1990.
94. Kristiansen BE, Ask E, Jenkins A, et al: Rapid diagnosis of meningococcal meningitis by polymerase chain reaction. *Lancet* 337:1568, 1991.
95. Weber DJ, Gammon WR, Cohen MS: The acutely ill patient with

fever and rash, in Mandell GL, Douglas RG, Bennett JE (ed): *Principles and Practice of Infectious Diseases*. 3rd ed. New York, Churchill Livingstone, 1990, pp 479–488.

96. Apicella MA: *Neisseria meningitidis,* in Mandell GL, Douglas RG, Bennett JE (ed): *Principles and Practice of Infectious Diseases*. 3rd ed. New York, Churchill Livingstone, 1990, pp 1600–1613.

97. Wispelway B, Tunkel AR, Scheld WM: Bacterial meningitis in adults. *Infect Dis Clin North Am* 4:645, 1990.

98. Saez-Llorens X, McCracken GH: Bacterial meningitis in neonates and children. *Infect Dis Clin North Am* 4:623, 1990.

99. Saez-Nieto JA, Lujan R, Berron S, et al: Epidemiology and molecular basis of penicillin-resistant *Neisseria meningitidis* in Spain: A 5-year history (1985-1989). *Clin Infect Dis* 14:394, 1992.

100. Drapkin MS, Wisch JS, Gelfand JA, et al: Plasmapheresis for fulminant meningococcemia. *Pediatr Infect Dis J* 8:399, 1989.

101. Brandtzaeg P, Sirnes K, Folsland B: Plasmapheresis in the treatment of severe meningococcal or pneumococcal septicaemia with DIC and fibrinolysis: Preliminary data on eight patients. *Scand J Clin Lab Invest* 45(suppl 178):53, 1985.

102. Tauber MG, Sande MA: General principles of therapy of pyogenic meningitis. *Infect Dis Clin North Am* 4:661, 1990.

103. Pugsley MP, Dworzack DL, Roccaforte JS, et al: An open study of the efficacy of a single dose of ciprofloxacin in eliminating the chronic nasopharyngeal carriage of *Neisseria meningitidis. J Infect Dis* 157:852, 1988.

104. Schwartz B: Chemoprophylaxis for bacterial infections: Principles of and application to meningococcal infections. *Rev Infect Dis* 13(suppl 2):S170, 1991.

105. Potter PC, van Frasch CE, et al: Prophylaxis against *Neisseria meningitidis* infections and antibody responses in patients with deficiency of the sixth component of complement. *J Infect Dis* 161:932, 1990.

106. Centers for Disease Control: Recommendations of the Advisory Committee on Immunization Practices (ACIP): Use of vaccines and immune globulins in person with altered immunocompetence. *MMWR* 42:1, 1993.

107. Centers for Disease Control: Meningococcal vaccines. *MMWR* 34:255, 1985.

108. Shaw JH, Print CG: Postsplenectomy sepsis. *Br J Surg* 76:1074, 1989.

109. Styrt B: Infection associated with asplenia: risks, mechanisms, and prevention. *Am J Med* 88:1990.

110. Francke EL, Neu HC: Postplenectomy infection. *Surg Clin North Am* 61:135, 1981.

111. Zarrabi MH, Rosner F: Serious infections in adults following splenectomy for trauma. *Arch Intern Med* 144:1421, 1984.

112. Van Wyck DB: Overwhelming postsplenectomy infection (OPSI): The clinical syndrome. *Lymphology* 16:107, 1983.

113. Hays DM, Ternberg JL, Chen TT, et al: Postsplenectomy sepsis and other complications following staging laparotomy for Hodgkin's disease in childhood. *J Pediatr Surg* 21:628, 1986.

114. Schwartz PE, Sterioff S, Mucha P, et al: Postsplenectomy sepsis and mortality in adults. *JAMA* 248:2279, 1982.

115. Green JB, Shackford SR, Sise MJ, et al: Late septic complications in adults following splenectomy for trauma: A prospective analysis in 144 patients. *J Trauma* 26:999, 1986.

116. Gopal V, Bisno AL: Fulminant pneumococcal infections in "normal" asplenic hosts. *Arch Intern Med* 137:1526, 1977.

117. Holmes FF, Weyandt T, Glazier J, et al: Fulminant meningococcemia after splenectomy. *JAMA* 246:1119, 1981.

118. Austin TW, Sargeant HL, Warwick OH: Fulminant gonococcemia after splenectomy. *Can Med Assoc J* 123:195, 1980.

119. Hosea SW, Burch CG, Brown EJ, et al: Impaired immune response of splenectomised patients to polyvalent pneumococcal vaccine. *Lancet* 1:804, 1981.

120. Di Padova F, Durig M, Wadstrom J, et al: Role of spleen in immune response to polyvalent pneumococcal vaccine. *Br Med J* 287:1829, 1983.

121. Siber GR, Gorham C, Martin P, et al: Antibody response to pretreatment immunization and post-treatment boosting with bacterial polysaccharide vaccines in patients with Hodgkin's disease. *Ann Intern Med* 104:467, 1986.

122. Giebink GS, Foker JE, Kim Y, et al: Serum antibody and opsonic responses to vaccination with pneumococcal capsular polysaccha-

ride in normal and splenectomized children. *J Infect Dis* 141:404, 1980.

123. Caplan ES, Boltansky H, Snyder MJ, et al: Response of traumatized splenectomized patients to immediate vaccination with polyvalent pneumococcal vaccine. *J Trauma* 23:801, 1983.

124. Oldfield S, Jenkins S, Yeoman H, et al: Class and subclass antipneumococcal antibody response in splenectomized patients. *Clin Exp Immunol* 61:664, 1985.

125. Hosea SW, Brown EJ, Hamburger MI, et al: Opsonic requirements for intravascular clearance after splenectomy. *N Engl J Med* 304:245, 1981.

126. O'Neal BJ, McDonald JC: The risk of sepsis in the asplenic adult. *Ann Surg* 194:775, 1981.

127. Chaikof EL, McCabe CJ: Fatal overwhelming postsplenectomy infection. *Am J Surg* 149:534, 1985.

128. Barrett-Connor E: Bacterial infection and sickle cell anemia: An analysis of 250 infections in 166 patients and a review of the literature. *Medicine* 50:97, 1971.

129. Coleman CN, McDougall IR, Dailey MO, et al: Functional hyposplenia after splenic irradiation for Hodgkin's disease. *Ann Intern Med* 96:44, 1982.

130. Dillon AM, Stein HB, English RA: Splenic atrophy in systemic lupus erythematosus. *Ann Intern Med* 96:40, 1982.

131. Corrigan JJ, Wyck DBV, Crosby WH: Clinical disorders of splenic function: The spectrum from asplenism to hypersplenism. *Lymphology* 16:101, 1983.

132. Markus HS, Toghill PJ: Impaired splenic function in elderly people. *Age & Aging* 20:287, 1991.

133. Brzeski M, Smart L, Baird D, et al: Felty's syndrome. *Ann Rheum Dis* 50:724, 1991.

134. Torres J, Bisno AL: Hyposplenism and pneumococcemia. *Am J Med* 55:851, 1973.

135. Scott SD, Lowes JA, McGinn FP, et al: Overwhelming post-splenectomy infection. *Br J Clin Practice* 44:110, 1990.

136. Ammann AJ, Addiego J, Wara DW, et al: Polyvalent pneumococcal-polysaccharide immunization of patients with sickle-cell anemia and patients with splenectomy. *N Engl J Med* 297:897, 1977.

137. Bolan G, Broome CV, Facklam RR, et al: Pneumococcal vaccine efficacy in selected populations in the United States. *Ann Intern Med* 104:1, 1986.

138. Konradsen HB, Henrichsen J: Pneumococcal infections in splenectomized children are preventable. *Acta Paediatr Scand* 80:423, 1991.

139. Schlaeffer F, Rosenheck S, Baumgarten-Kleiner A, et al: Pneumococcal infections among immunized and splenectomized patients in Israel. *J Infect* 10:38, 1985.

140. Lucas CE: Splenic trauma. Choice of management. *Ann Surg* 213:98, 1991.

141. Centers for Disease Control: Immunization Practices Advisory Committee: pneumococcal polysaccharide vaccine. *MMWR* 38:64, 1989.

142. Wyler DJ: *Plasmodium* species (malaria), in Mandell GL, Douglas RG, Bennett JE (ed): *Principles and Practice of Infectious Diseases*. 3rd ed. New York, Churchill Livingstone, 1990, pp 2056–2066.

143. Nahlen BL, Lobel HO, Cannon SE, et al: Reassessment of blood donor selection criteria for United States travelers to malarious areas. *Transfusion* 31:798, 1991.

144. Greenberg AE, Lobel HO: Mortality from *Plasmodium falciparum* malaria in travelers from the United States, 1959 to 1987. *Ann Intern Med* 113:326, 1990.

145. Wiselka MJ, Kent J, Nicholson KG: Malaria in Leicester 1983-1988: A review of 114 cases. *J Infect* 20:103, 1990.

146. Phillips RE, Solomon T: Cerebral malaria in children. *Lancet* 336:1355, 1990.

147. MacPherson GG, Warrell MJ, White NJ, et al: Human cerebral malaria: A quantitative ultrastructural analysis of parasitized erythrocyte sequestration. *Am J Pathol* 119:385, 1985.

148. Wiest PM, Opal SM, Romulo RL, et al: Malaria in travelers in Rhode Island: A review of 26 cases. *Am J Med* 91:30, 1991.

149. Subramananian D, Moise KJ, White AC: Imported malaria during pregnancy: Report of four cases and review of management. *Clin Infect Dis* 15:408, 1992.

150. Nathwani D, Currie PF, Douglas JG, et al: *Plasmodium falciparum* malaria in pregnancy: A review. *Br J Obstet Gynaecol* 99:118, 1992.

151. Brewster DR, Kwiatkowski D, White NJ: Neurological sequelae of cerebral malaria in children. *Lancet* 336:1039, 1990.

152. Endeshaw Y, Assefa D: Cerebral malaria: Factors affecting outcome of treatment in a suboptimal clinical setting. *J Trop Med Hyg* 93:44, 1990.

153. Hoffman SL, Rustama D, Punjabi NH, et al: High-dose dexamethasone in quinine-treated patients with cerebral malaria: A double-blind, placebo-controlled trial. *J Infect Dis* 158:325, 1988.

154. Miller KD, Greenberg AE, Campbell CC: Treatment of severe malaria in the United States with a continuous infusion of quinidine gluconate and exchange transfusion. *N Engl J Med* 321:65, 1989.

155. Makler MT, Gibbins B: Laboratory diagnosis of malaria. *Clin Lab Med* 11:941, 1991.

156. Panisko DM, Keystone JS: Treatment of malaria—1990. *Drugs* 39:160, 1990.

157. Nosten F, ter Kuile F, Chongsuphajaisiddhi T, et al: Mefloquine-resistant falciparum malaria on the Thai-Burmese border [see comments]. *Lancet* 337:1140, 1991.

158. Centers for Disease Control: Treatment of severe *Plasmodium falciparum* malaria with quinidine gluconate: Discontinuation of parenteral quinine from CDC drug service. *MMWR* 40:21, 1991.

159. Pithie AD, Ellis CJ: Falciparum malaria: The current status of antimalarials in therapy and prophylaxis. *J Antimicrob Chemother* 25:5, 1990.

160. Anh TK, Kim NV, Arnold K, et al: Double-blind studies with mefloquine alone and in combination with sulfadoxine-pyrimethamine in 120 adults and 120 children with falciparum malaria in Vietnam. *Trans R Soc Trop Med Hyg* 84:50, 1990.

161. Sowunmi A, Salako LA, Walker O, et al: Clinical efficacy of mefloquine in children suffering from chloroquine-resistant *Plasmodium falciparum* malaria in Nigeria. *Trans R Soc Trop Med Hyg* 84:76761, 1990.

162. Hellgren U, Kihamia CM, Bergqvist Y, et al: Standard and reduced doses of mefloquine for treatment of *Plasmodium falciparum* in Tanzania: Whole blood concentrations in relation to adverse reactions, in vivo response, and in vitro susceptibility. *Am J Trop Med Hyg* 45:254, 1991.

163. Arnold K, Tran TH, Nguyen TC, et al: A randomized comparative study of artemisinine *(qinghaosu)* suppositories and oral quinine in acute falciparum malaria. *Trans R Soc Trop Med Hyg* 84:499, 1990.

164. Looareesuwan S, Phillips RE, White NJ: Quinine and falciparum malaria in late pregnancy. *Lancet* 2:4, 1985.

165. Malin AS, Cass PL, Hudson CN: Exchange transfusion for severe falciparum malaria in pregnancy. *Br Med J* 300:1240, 1990.

166. Lancet Editor: Exchange transfusion in falciparum malaria. *Lancet* 335:324, 1990.

167. Phillips P, Nantel S, Benny WB: Exchange transfusion as an adjunct to the treatment of severe falciparum malaria: Case report and review. *Rev Infect Dis* 12:1100, 1990.

168. Warrell DA, Looareesuwan S, Warrell MJ, et al: Dexamethasone proves deleterious in cerebral malaria: A double blind trial in 100 comatose patients. *N Engl J Med* 306:313, 1982.

169. Wyler DJ: Steroids are out in the treatment of cerebral malaria: What's next? *J Infect Dis* 158:320, 1988.

170. Gelfand JA: Babesia, in Mandell GL, R G Douglas J, Bennett JE (eds): *Principles and Practice of Infectious Diseases*. 3rd ed. New York, Churchill Livingstone, 1990, pp 2119–2122.

171. Jacoby GA, Hunt JV, Kosinski KS: Treatment of transfusion-transmitted babesiosis by exchange transfusion. *N Engl J Med* 303:1098, 1980.

172. Ruebush TK, Cassaday PB, Marsh HJ, et al: Human babesiosis on Nantucket Island: Clinical features. *Ann Intern Med* 86:6, 1977.

173. Ruebush TK, Juranek DD, Chisholm ES, et al: Human babesiosis on Nantucket Island: Evidence for self-limited and subclinical infections. *N Engl J Med* 297:825, 1977.

174. Rosner F, Zarrabi MH, Benach JL, et al: Babesiosis in splenectomized adults: Review of 22 reported cases. *Am J Med* 76:696, 1984.

175. Iacopino V, Earnhart T: Life-threatening babesiosis in a woman from Wisconsin. *Arch Intern Med* 150:1527, 1990.

176. Craven RB, Barnes AM: Plague and tularemia. *Infect Dis Clin North Am* 5:165, 1991.

177. Hull HF, Montes JM, Mann JM: Septicemic plague in New Mexico. *J Infect Dis* 155:113, 1987.

178. Butler T: Yersinia species (including plague), in Mandell GL, Douglas RG, Bennett JE (eds): *Principles and Practice of Infectious Diseases*. 3rd ed. New York, Churchill Livingstone, 1990, pp 1748–1756.

179. Job L, Horman JT, Grigor JK, et al: Dysgonic fermenter-2: A clinico-epidemiologic review. *J Emerg Med* 7:185, 1989.

180. Bobo RA, Newton EJ: A previously undescribed gram-negative bacillus causing septicemia and meningitis. *Am J Clin Pathol* 65:564, 1976.

181. Hicklin H, Verghese A, Alvarez S: Dysgonic fermenter 2 septicemia. *Rev Infect Dis* 9:884, 1987.

182. Brenner DJ, Hollis DG, Fanning GR, et al: *Capnocytophaga canimorsus* sp. nov. (formerly CDC group DF-2), a cause of septicemia following dog bite, and *C. cynodegmi* sp. nov., a cause of localized wound infection following dog bite. *J Clin Microbiol* 27:231, 1989.

183. Hantson P, Gautier PE, Vekemans MC, et al: Fatal Capnocytophaga canimorsus septicemia in a previously healthy woman. *Ann Emerg Med* 20:93, 1991.

184. Carpenter PD, Heppner BT, Gnann JW: DF-2 bacteremia following cat bites. *Am J Med* 82:621, 1987.

185. Butler T, Weaver RE, Ramani TKV, et al: Unidentified gram-negative rod infection, a new disease of man. *Ann Intern Med* 86:1, 1977.

186. McGowan JE, Rio CD: Other Gram-negative bacilli, in Mandell GL, Douglas RG, Bennett JE (eds): *Principles and Practice of Infectious Diseases*. 3rd ed. New York, Churchill Livingstone, 1990, pp 1782–1793.

187. Sanford JP: Tularemia. *JAMA* 250:3225, 1983.

188. Kaiser AB, Rieves D, Price AH, et al: Tularemia and rhabdomyolysis. *JAMA* 253:241, 1985.

189. Centers for Disease Control: Update: Outbreak of Hantavirus infection—Southwestern United States, 1993. *MMWR* 42:441, 1993.

190. Centers for Disease Control: Outbreak of acute illness—Southwestern United States, 1993. *MMWR* 42:421, 1993.

191. Centers for Disease Control: Update: Hantavirus Disease—United States, 1993. *MMWR* 42:612, 1993.

192. Centers for Disease Control: Hantavirus infection—Southwestern United States: Interim recommendations for risk reduction. *MMWR* 42:1, 1993.

92. Acute Infection in the Immunocompromised Host

Mark A. Keroack and Richard H. Glew

Overview

Advances in the management of leukemia, lymphoma, and solid tumors have resulted in marked improvement in the prognosis of patients with these neoplasms. Similarly, developments in transplant immunology have produced improved survival of patients with various transplanted organs, with a resultant expansion in programs for transplantation of kidney, heart, liver, bone marrow, endocrine organs, and other tissues and organs. However, patients with either neoplasia or transplants are rendered highly susceptible to infection by virtue of both their basic diseases and their associated therapies, including chemotherapy, radiation therapy, and surgery. Infection remains the leading cause of death in patients with leukemia and lymphoma and a major cause of morbidity and mortality in patients with solid tumors or transplants [1–11]. Traditionally, infection has accounted for up to 75 percent of deaths in patients with acute leukemia [1,4,8] or transplant recipients [2,3,9,11]. Infection was found at autopsy in about 50 to 70 percent of patients with Hodgkin's disease [6]. The epidemic of human immunodeficiency virus (HIV-1) infection has added to the numbers of immunocompromised hosts, by virtue of the central event of the virus' pathogenesis: a progressive, irreversible weakening of cell-mediated immunity [12].

Although a great variety of microorganisms have been noted to cause severe, life-threatening infections in immunocompromised hosts, one can formulate a diagnostic plan and decide on empiric therapy by giving careful consideration to the nature and severity of the immunosuppression predisposing the patient to infection.

Epidemiology and Pathophysiology of Defective Immunity

In the compromised patient, infection can arise as a consequence of derangements in host defenses that result from the primary disease, the medical and surgical treatment of the condition, or a combination of these factors.

DEFECTS RELATED TO AN UNDERLYING DISEASE

Anatomic Barriers. The skin and mucosal surfaces serve a primary role in the defense of the host against invasion by both endogenous and exogenous microorganisms. Mucous membrane ulceration in the mouth and gastrointestinal (GI) tract can occur spontaneously in patients with acute leukemia, although this complication more commonly arises after chemotherapy. In patients with solid tumors, disruption of mucocutaneous barriers can result from invasion, obstruction, or perforation by the malignancy. Patients with esophageal obstruction secondary to tumor frequently aspirate oropharyngeal secretions, which may result in repeated pneumonias, including nec-

rotizing pneumonia caused by anaerobes or gram-negative bacilli. Obstruction of a major bronchus by bronchogenic carcinoma may also present as recurrent pneumonia in the related lung area, often poorly responsive to appropriate antibiotic therapy. Obstructing tumors involving the genitourinary tract may result in pyelonephritis and necessitate ureteral stents or nephrostomy drainage to obtain satisfactory clinical response. Tumors involving the GI or female genital tracts can lead to intestinal perforation with development of peritonitis, intraabdominal abscesses, or bowel obstruction. Bacteremia may result from any of the above derangements.

Defective Phagocytosis. Defense against infection by bacteria and many fungi is provided by neutrophils and macrophages. Patients with leukemia, particularly the acute leukemias, commonly have a reduction in their absolute number of circulating neutrophils; qualitative defects of neutrophil function have also been described in these patients [13]. Aplastic anemia, as well as extensive bone marrow involvement caused by lymphoma or metastatic solid tumors, may result in neutropenia [14]. By far the most common cause of neutropenia, however, is cytotoxic chemotherapy. Patients whose neutrophils are reduced in number by malignancy or chemotherapy are at risk to develop spontaneous bacteremia. This becomes a notable risk at absolute neutrophil counts that are persistently below $500/mm^3$ (or below $1000/mm^3$ and falling). The risks for infection increase dramatically at counts below $100/mm^3$ [15–18].

Invasive and disseminated fungal infections also may be a consequence of neutropenia and become more common after the neutropenic patient has received broad-spectrum antibiotic therapy [11,14,16,17,19,20]. *Candida* and *Aspergillus* species are the most common fungal pathogens observed in compromised hosts, but unusual genera such as *Fusarium, Trichosporon, Pseudallescheria,* and *Cunninghamella* have been described with increasing frequency [21,22,23].

Altered Humoral Immunity. B-cell lymphocytic function and antibody production may be impaired in untreated patients with chronic lymphocytic leukemia, multiple myeloma, and certain lymphomas [24,25]. Acquired deficits in antibody production may also be encountered in otherwise healthy patients (e.g., IgA deficiency, common variable immunodeficiency). Hypogammaglobulinemia or impaired antibody response (as in patients with splenectomy) predispose patients to infections attributable to encapsulated bacteria, such as *Streptococcus pneumoniae, Haemophilus influenzae,* and *Neisseria meningitidis;* moreover, these infections are likely to be severe and associated with fulminant bacteremia. Infections caused by enteric gram-negative bacilli and *Pseudomonas aeruginosa* also may be seen in previously untreated patients with defective humoral immunity secondary to B-cell malignancies [26].

Impaired Cell-Mediated Immunity. T-cell–mediated immunity includes cytotoxic (killer) T cells, activated macrophages, and antibody-dependent cellular cytotoxicity. These critical components of immunity are impaired in patients with Hodgkin's disease and other lymphomas [27] and in those taking antirejection drugs (cyclosporine, azathioprine) or corticosteroids [7,28]. A progressive and devastating loss of T-cell–mediated immunity is suffered by patients infected with HIV-1. This virus selectively infects and lyses CD4 + lymphocytes (also called T4 lymphocytes or helper T-cells), which play a central role in governing both humoral and cellular immune responses [12].

Defects in cell-mediated immunity commonly are associated with infections by viruses (varicella-zoster virus [VZV]), cytomegalovirus (CMV), herpes simplex virus (HSV)), protozoa (*Pneumocystis carinii, Toxoplasma gondii,* and *Cryptosporidium* species), fungi (*Cryptococcus neoformans, Histoplasma capsulatum, Coccidioides immitis,* and *Candida* species), helminths (*Strongyloides stercoralis*), mycobacteria (*Mycobacterium tuberculosis, Mycobacterium avium-intracellulare*), and intracellular bacteria (*Listeria monocytogenes, Salmonella* and *Legionella* species) [2,3,5,11,29,30,31].

DEFECTS RELATED TO TREATMENT

Immunosuppressive Medications. Cytotoxic chemotherapy, corticosteroids, and other immunosuppressive therapeutic regimens can alter host defenses in several ways. Immunosuppressive effects depend on the class of drug, dose and duration of therapy, and timing relative to other therapeutic modalities (e.g., radiation). All arms of the host defense mechanisms can be impaired as a result of immunosuppressive agents, but the most common defects include neutropenia caused by cytotoxic agents or, alternatively, impaired phagocyte function, immunoglobulin synthesis, and cell-mediated immunity related to corticosteroid administration. Intermittent chemotherapy with drug-free grace periods tends to be less immunosuppressive than continuous chemotherapy.

Nosocomial Infections. Immunocompromised patients are prone especially to nosocomial infections complicating the medical and surgical support efforts common to the intensive care unit (ICU), including intravenous and intraarterial catheters and urinary catheters [32] (see Chaps. 86 and 89). Organisms most frequently causing infection of intravenous catheter include *Staphylococcus epidermidis, Staphylococcus aureus, Corynebacterium* species (including *C. jeikeium*), and *Candida* species. The risk of infection with vascular catheters can be reduced, though not eliminated, through the use of permanent, subcutaneously tunneled cannulae (e.g., Hickman, Broviac, Groshung, or Portacath systems) [33,34].

Antibiotic therapy frequently is employed in the management of documented infections and febrile episodes in the compromised host. These agents are double-edged swords, however, and promote a shift toward increasing frequency of infections caused by progressively more resistant organisms, including *Pseudomonas aeruginosa, Enterobacter* species, enterococci, methicillin-resistant staphylococci (MRSA), and *Candida albicans.* Unusual, intrinsically resistant bacteria (e.g., *Capnocytophaga* and *Corynebacterium* species) and fungi (e.g., *Pseudallescheria* and *Fusarium* species) are being seen with increasing frequency in oncology centers [16–20,35–38].

Splenectomy. Splenectomy has been employed in the therapeutic staging of patients with Hodgkin's disease, and this procedure predisposes patients to fulminant, overwhelming bacteremia caused by encapsulated bacteria (*S. pneumoniae, H. influenzae, N. meningitidis*) as well as *S. aureus* [39]. Although the syndrome of overwhelming postsplenectomy infection (OPSI) is most common in patients whose splenectomy was for malignancy or reticuloendothelial disease, OPSI can occur in any splenectomized patient regardless of underlying disease or interval since surgery [40,41,42] (see Chap. 91). Accordingly, fever over 38°C in the splenectomized patient warrants immediate investigation for possible bacteremia or focal bacterial infection. Consideration of ICU admission and presumptive antibiotic therapy is appropriate if the patient appears systemically toxic. A third-generation cephalosporin (e.g., ceftriaxone or cefotaxime) is reasonable empiric therapy. Many of these patients manifest the full systemic inflammatory response syndrome with hypotension, disseminated intravascular coagulopathy, and multiple organ dysfunction with its attendant high mortality.

Organisms and Infections

SITES OF INFECTION. In general the most common sites of serious, definable infection in the compromised host are the bloodstream and lung and mucosal surfaces (including oral and perirectal areas) [4,18,43]. Bacteremia or fungemia may be associated with an obvious focus of infection but commonly occurs without a documented source. The gastrointestinal tract is the likely source of many of these occult infections; chemotherapy and neutropenia cause a breakdown in normal mucosal defenses of the gut, facilitating entry of bacteria or yeast into the bloodstream [18,44]. Attempts to control this potential reservoir of infection with oral antimicrobials are discussed later in the chapter. Clinically apparent intestinal problems seen in neutropenic patients include typhlitis, anorectal cellulitis/fasciitis/abscess, necrotizing colitis, and pseudomembranous colitis caused by chemotherapy [45–49]. Typhlitis, an inflammatory disease of the cecum, may lead to toxic megacolon and perforation and requires a high index of suspicion, prompt diagnosis, and urgent surgical intervention [46,47]. Unusually severe and prolonged viral gastroenteritis caused by adenovirus, rotavirus, and coxsackievirus has been observed in marrow transplant recipients [49].

Herpes simplex virus should be suspected as a possible cause for any lesion of mucous membranes in an immunocompromised host. These lesions often are crusted and hemorrhagic and may be difficult to distinguish from mucositis caused by neutropenia, chemotherapy, or trauma [50,51]. Necrotizing gingivostomatitis (noma) caused by oral anaerobes as well as severe periodontal infection may also complicate neutropenia [52]. Genitourinary tract infections are relatively uncommon except in the elderly, those requiring urinary catheter drainage, or patients with pelvic tumors causing ureteral obstruction. Infections of the central nervous system (CNS) are unusual, with the exception of meningitis caused by *Cryptococcus* or *Listeria* species in patients with impaired cell-mediated immunity (e.g., lymphoma, HIV-1 infection, corticosteroid therapy) or as part of a disseminated infection (especially by *S. aureus* or fungi) [31] or in the setting of recent head trauma or neurosurgery.

Organisms. The diverse organisms frequently or uniquely associated with infections in the compromised host are listed in Table 92-1. Although virtually any organism can cause infection in a severely immunosuppressed patient, the predominant organisms in most hospitals are gram-negative bacilli such as *P. aeruginosa, E. coli,* and *Enterobacter,* followed by common gram-positive cocci such as *S. aureus* (including MRSA), coagulase-negative staphylococci, and various streptococci. Fungal infections increase in frequency with increasing duration of granulocytopenia and therapy with broad-spectrum antibiotics. Infections caused by *P. carinii* and CMV are seen predomi-

Table 92-1. Organisms Commonly or Uniquely Associated with
Acute Infection in the Compromised Host

A. Bacteria
 1. Enteric gram-negative bacilli
  a. *Escherichia coli*
  b. *Klebsiella* species
  c. *Enterobacter* species
  d. *Proteus* species
 2. *Staphylococcus aureus*
 3. *Pseudomonas aeruginosa*
 4. *Listeria monocytogenes*
 5. *Legionella pneumophila* and related organisms
 6. Skin/mucous membrane saprophytes
  a. *Corynebacterium jeikeium*
  b. *Capnocytophaga* species
  c. *Eikenella corrodens*
  d. Coagulase-negative staphylococci
 7. *Nocardia* species
 8. Mycobacteria
 9. Organisms involved in immunoglobulin deficiencies or hyposplenism
  a. *Streptococcus pneumoniae*
  b. *Haemophilus influenzae*
  c. *Neisseria meningitidis*
B. Fungi and Yeasts
 1. Saprophytic fungi and yeasts
  a. *Candida albicans* and other *Candida* species
  b. *Torulopsis glabrata*
  c. *Aspergillus* species
  d. *Zygomycete* species
  e. *Trichosporon* species
  f. *Fusarium* species
 2. Endemic fungi and yeasts
  a. *Cryptococcus neoformans*
  b. *Histoplasma capsulatum*
  c. *Coccidioides immitis*
C. Protozoa
 1. *Pneumocystis carinii*
 2. *Toxoplasma gondii*
D. Parasites
 1. *Strongyloides stercoralis*
E. Viruses
 1. Cytomegalovirus
 2. Varicella-zoster virus
 3. Herpes simplex virus

nantly in patients with defects in cell-mediated immunity (e.g., lymphoma, AIDS, corticosteroid therapy or transplant recipients).

DIAGNOSTIC APPROACH TO FEVER. Patients with neutropenia and infection exhibit fewer and less striking physical findings of infection (e.g., local warmth, swelling, adenopathy, exudate, or fluctuance) than ordinarily encountered in normal patients with similar infections of skin, pharynx, urinary tract, lung, or anorectal areas [53]. Moreover, the types of organisms and sites of infection in the immunocompromised host are diverse and occasionally unique compared with those seen in most ICU patients. In evaluating the acutely ill, immunocompromised patient with fever in the ICU, therefore, a meticulous and thorough history and physical examination must be performed initially and repeated daily. Particular attention should be directed to sites of high risk, such as oropharynx, anorectal region, lungs, skin, optic fundi, and vascular catheter sites [53–56]. Patients with focal abnormalities such as solid tumors, organ transplants, or recent surgery need to have these specific sites investigated with special care.

Initial laboratory studies that should be performed in the evaluation of the acutely ill, febrile compromised host include (1) cultures of blood and urine, (2) culture of sputum (see Chap. 13), if obtainable, in patients with symptoms or signs of pulmonary disease (including those who have only shortness of breath, mild cough, or tachypnea); (3) swab, aspiration or biopsy of suspicious skin, mucous membrane, or other lesions for smears (Gram's stain, fungal preparation), cultures (routine, fungal, and viral), and pathologic examination; (4) semiquantitative culture of intravenous catheters in place when fever develops, if possible (if the cannula is a critical lifeline or a subcutaneously tunneled device showing no local signs of infection, removal can be deferred pending results of routine blood cultures; blood should be obtained by catheter for blood culture as well [32,33,34]); (5) chest roentgenography; and (6) serum chemistries (electrolytes, liver chemistries, creatinine), in part to detect possible visceral involvement or multiorgan failure caused by disseminated infection and also to serve as baselines for monitoring possible adverse reactions to subsequent antimicrobic therapy.

Patients with defects in cell-mediated immunity (e.g., AIDS, lymphoma, transplant recipient) often harbor organisms best diagnosed by histologic examination (e.g., *Pneumocystis, Toxoplasma*) or special culture techniques (e.g., mycobacteria, viruses). In instances when such organisms are high in the differential diagnosis, initial evaluation often entails immediate biopsy of the pathologic process by gastrointestinal endoscopy, bronchoscopy, or surgery. Localizing symptoms and signs may indicate the need for other studies, such as computed tomography, magnetic resonance imaging, or nuclear medicine scans (e.g., gallium[67] scan to detect *Pneumocystis carinii* pneumonia [PCP]). Tachypnea warrants arterial blood gas studies because progressive hypoxemia in the absence of radiographic findings can be an early indicator of pulmonary infection, especially as a result of PCP, and may indicate a need for bronchoscopy [57,58,59].

In patients with fever and neutropenia, septic shock may be an early complication of bacteremia. Although only one-third of these patients have documented infection [16,17,60], empiric broad-spectrum antibiotic therapy is indicated for all patients with fever greater than 38°C and absolute neutrophil counts less than 500/mm³ (or <1000/mm³ and falling). The immediate institution of such therapy in these patients (even in the absence of documentation of bacterial infection) dramatically reduces morbidity and mortality [61,62,63].

APPROACH TO SPECIFIC INFECTIOUS DISEASE PRESENTATIONS

Fever Without Obvious Source—Neutropenia. The most rapidly fatal infectious agents documented to cause acute fever in the critically ill neutropenic cancer patient are enteric gram-negative bacilli (*E. coli, Klebsiella* species, *Proteus* species, *P. aeruginosa,* and *S. aureus*[6,16,17,64,65]. In the patient without an obvious site of infection, initial empiric antibiotic therapy should be directed against these pathogens. Such therapy should (1) provide bactericidal coverage against the aforementioned organisms; (2) be administered parenterally (usually intravenously) and at maximal recommended dosages; (3) provide synergism, if possible, against gram-negative bacilli [66,67]; and (4) take into consideration idiosyncrasies of the antimicrobial susceptibility patterns of organisms in the institutions where the patient has resided in the months before infection. (For example, the emergence of *Enterobacter* species resistant to third-generation cephalosporins has been a major concern in some cancer centers [35]).

In most hospitals, a two-drug regimen is employed, such as

Table 92-2. Empiric Regimens for Initial Therapy of the Febrile Adult Neutropenic Cancer Patient

1. Piperacillin or azlocillin, 12–18 gm/day IV (divided q4h), plus tobramycin, 4–5 mg/kg/day IV or amikacin 20–25 mg/kg/day (divided q8h)
2. Ceftazidime, 3–6 gm/day IV (divided q8h) plus tobramycin 4–5 mg/kg/day IV or amikacin 20–25 mg/kg/day (divided q8h)
3. Imipenem/cilastatin, 2–4 gm/day IV (divided q6h)
4. Aztreonam, 3–6 gm/day IV (divided q8h), plus vancomycin, 2 gm/day (divided q6–12 hr), plus tobramycin, 4–5 mg/kg/day IV or amikacin 20–25 mg/kg/day (divided q8h)

those indicated in Table 92-2. An anti-pseudomonal beta-lactam such as piperacillin or azlocillin (either at 2–3 gm IV q4h) or reftazidine (1–2 gm IV q8h) often is coupled with tobramycin (4–5 mg/kg/d IV divided q8h) or amikacin (20–25 mg/kg/d IV divided q8h) to provide a highly effective synergistic regimen with superior coverage of gram-negative bacilli [16,17,68–71]. In critically ill patients, an initial loading dose of aminoglycoside is advisable (2 mg/kg tobramycin or 10 mg/kg amikacin). Aztreonam has activity equivalent to other beta-lactam drugs against gram-negative bacilli and may be used with an aminoglycoside in patients with immediate hypersensitivity reactions to cephalosporins and penicillins; vancomycin typically is added to this regimen because aztreonam has no gram-positive activity [72].

Some authors have questioned the need for specific antistaphylococcal therapy, because aminoglycosides exhibit activity against *S. aureus*, and studies have failed to show increased rates of staphylococcal infections in patients treated with empiric regimens that lacked specific antistaphylococcal activity. In contrast, other investigators have recommended routine inclusion of vancomycin in empiric regimens, particularly in patients with indwelling plastic venous access catheters [73]. However, two recent studies demonstrated no increased morbidity when the vancomycin was added to initial empiric therapy only after patients demonstrated bacteremia with a gram-positive isolate [74,75].

The conventional wisdom of beta-lactam/aminoglycoside combinations has been challenged in several recent studies. When ceftazidime monotherapy was compared with traditional combination therapy, no increase in mortality was seen in the monotherapy group [60], although it was more often necessary to modify monotherapy when the results of cultures became known. Extensive use of ceftazidime also has led to the emergence of resistant isolates in some units [35], and an extensive European trial supported the continued use of aminoglycoside therapy in the empiric regimen [76]. Numerous trials of imipenem, a more broad-spectrum agent, as sole therapy for the febrile neutropenic patient have been more encouraging [77–80]. One study of 750 febrile episodes in 567 patients showed equivalent response rates between imipenem monotherapy and ceftazidime with amikacin [78]. The addition of amikacin to imipenem failed to improve the outcome. The propensity for imipenem to promote fungal colonization is cause for some concern, but this agent now should be considered an acceptable alternative to combination regimens in empiric therapy.

After initial evaluation of the patient and institution of empiric antibiotic therapy, subsequent management is based on (1) identification of a focus of infection, (2) isolation of an etiologic agent, (3) defervescence versus continued fever, and (4) duration of neutropenia [16,17,81]. In the patient for whom an infection has been documented clinically or by culture and who has defervesced on broad-spectrum therapy, antibiotics should be continued until all of the following conditions have been met: (1) 3 days or more without fever, (2) 10 days or more total

duration of antibiotic therapy, (3) clearance of clinical and laboratory signs of infection, and (4) reversal of neutropenia with a total neutrophil count at least 500 cells per cubic mullimeter. If a specific pathogen is identified by culture, changes in the initial regimen may be necessary based on susceptibility testing; in all cases, however, a broad-spectrum regimen should be maintained for the duration of neutropenia [16,17,82].

If an infection cannot be documented but the patient has defervesced, empiric antibiotic therapy should be continued until (1) the patient has been afebrile for 3 days or more *and* (2) the total neutrophil count is at least 500 per cubic millimeter. In patients likely to suffer permanent or extremely prolonged granulocytopenia, attempts to stop therapy are reasonable but should be made with continuing close clinical observation [17,83].

If fever has not been eliminated by the third day of treatment, efforts should be directed toward optimizing aminoglycoside levels. In many patients with hematologic malignancies, enhanced aminoglycoside clearance may necessitate administration of high doses (up to 6 mg/kg/d of tobramycin or 30 mg/kg/d of amikacin) to achieve effective levels [84]. The search should continue for potential sites of focal infection (optic fundi, oropharynx, chest, abdomen, and perirectal area). Consideration should be given to empiric addition of vancomycin, particularly in patients with permanent intravenous catheters.

Should fevers persist for 7 days of neutropenia, it is customary to begin empiric antifungal therapy with amphotericin B [16,17]. The rationale for such therapy is based on a number of considerations: (1) *Candida* species are the most common fungal pathogens in neutropenic hosts [19,20]; (2) blood cultures in autopsy-proved cases of disseminated candidiasis are positive in only 50 percent of cases during life [16,19]; (3) funduscopic and cutaneous findings usually appear only when disease is far advanced [85]; (4) rapid serum antigen detection assays often fail to detect non-albicans species of *Candida* [86,87]; and (5) effective therapy for candidiasis may be achieved with lower doses of amphotericin B than used traditionally for other fungi (e.g., 500 mg vs. 1000–2000 mg total dose), thus reducing toxicity [17,88]. Amphotericin also is the drug of choice for infections caused by *Aspergillus* and many other filamentous fungi. Patients who had low-dose amphotericin B instituted empirically for persistent fever and advanced to high-dose therapy (1 mg/kg/d) when *Aspergillus* was isolated had an improved survival over those in whom therapy was instituted only after definitive diagnosis [89]. Prognosis remains poor, however, for patients treated for documented invasive fungal infection in the setting of persistent neutropenia [14,85]. Patients at particularly high risk of disseminated fungal disease include those with (1) anticipated prolonged granulocytopenia; (2) parenteral nutrition; (3) *Candida* colonization in oropharynx or urine; (4) corticosteroid therapy; and (5) advancing multiple organ dysfunction (renal, hepatic, pulmonary), which often is a reflection of disseminated candidiasis [85]. Hepatosplenic (also called chronic disseminated) candidiasis presents with fevers and elevation of serum alkaline phosphatase that continue through the return of neutrophils to >1000/cells per cubic millimeter [90]. Multiple embolic lesions are present in liver and spleen. Responses to amphotericin have been poor with this condition, although fluconazole (400 mg/d) has shown promising results [91].

Pneumonia in the Compromised Host. The lung is one of the most common identifiable sites of infection in immunocompromised patients [3,57,92]. Pulmonary disease can be caused by a wide variety of agents, including bacteria, protozoa, helminths, viruses, fungi, and mycobacteria (Table 92-3) (see Chap. 76). The differential diagnosis is made even more difficult

Table 92-3. Common Causes of Acute Pulmonary Disease in Immunocompromised Patients

I. Infectious causes
  A. Bacteria
    1. Common organisms
      a. *Streptococcus pneumoniae*
      b. *Haemophilus influenzae*
    2. *Pseudomonas aeruginosa*
    3. Enteric gram-negative bacilli
    4. *Staphylococcus aureus*
    5. *Legionella* species
    6. *Nocardia* species
    7. Mycobacteria
  B. Protozoa: *Pneumocystis carinii*
             Toxoplasma gondii
  C. Viruses
    1. Cytomegalovirus
    2. Herpes simplex virus
  D. Fungi
    1. *Aspergillus* species
    2. *Candida* species
    3. *Zygomycete* species
    4. *Cryptococcus neoformans*
  E. Parasites: *Strongyloides stercoralis*
II. Noninfectious causes
  A. Primary disease
    1. Malignancy
      a. Primary
      b. Metastatic
    2. Vasculitis
  B. Drug toxicity
    1. Bleomycin
    2. Busulfan
    3. Cyclophosphamide (Cytoxan)
  C. Hemorrhage
  D. Congestive heart failure
  E. Radiation

by the various noninfectious pulmonary complications that can present abruptly with acute respiratory symptoms and fever: involvement by an underlying malignancy or vasculitis, drug toxicity, pulmonary hemorrhage, radiation pneumonitis, cardiogenic pulmonary edema, and pulmonary embolism [57,92–95].

The clinical picture of pneumonia in the compromised patient generally is nonspecific. Regardless of cause, fever and progressive shortness of breath (and concomitant tachypnea and arterial hypoxemia) tend to be common symptoms, and in the neutropenic patient, cough, sputum production, and physical examination (as well as roentgenographic findings) are likely to be unimpressive or absent [96]. Chest roentgenograms should be obtained promptly in the compromised patient with fever or dyspnea and should be repeated every few days in the acutely ill compromised host with unexplained fever, particularly those with pulmonary symptoms or signs.

DIFFERENTIAL DIAGNOSIS. Developing an appropriate differential diagnosis for the causative agents of pneumonia in the immunocompromised host rests first on an appreciation of the nature, severity, and duration of the immune suppression. Neutropenic patients are most prone to gram-negative bacillary pneumonias [96]; those with prolonged (>7 days) or profound (<100 neutrophils/mm³) neutropenia may develop infection with *Aspergillus* or *Zygomycete* species [57,92]. T-cell–deficient hosts (e.g., patients with HIV infection, transplant, or lymphoma) are more likely to acquire infection with PCP [58], CMV, HSV, [97,98], fungi (*Cryptococcus, Histoplasma*) [99,100], or in-

tracellular bacteria (mycobacteria, *Legionella*) [101,102]. Patients who have resided in tropical countries may reactivate latent infection by *Strongyloides stercoralis* in the setting of altered cell-mediated immunity. Pulmonary infiltrates, polymicrobial bacteremia, and bacterial meningitis are the hallmarks of this syndrome [103,104]. Patients with both deficient neutrophil and T cell function (e.g., bone marrow transplant recipients) may be at risk for all of these pathogens [105].

Chest radiographs may provide useful clues: focal or multifocal infiltrates tend to favor infections by bacteria and those caused by *Aspergillus* or *Zygomycete* species. Diffuse disease is more characteristic of viral causes (HSV, CMV, PCP, or noninfectious processes (drug toxicity, lymphangitic carcinomatosis, and radiation pneumonitis) [57,92]. Cavitary disease can be seen with certain of the necrotizing gram-negative bacilli such as *Pseudomonas* as well as *S. aureus* and anaerobes (e.g., postaspiration or postobstructive) and can also be a late finding with pneumonia due to *Aspergillus, Mucor,* and *Nocardia* species. It is impossible, however, to make firm rules with regard to radiographic patterns. Gram-negative bacilli or *Legionella* may progress to diffuse disease or incite the adult respiratory distress syndrome (ARDS). Patients with severe defects in cell-mediated immunity may manifest a miliary pattern because of disseminated tuberculosis or histoplasmosis. Conversely, radiation pneumonitis may present as focal, sharply demarcated infiltrates confined to the irradiated portion of the lung [92]. The timing of immune suppression is particularly important in transplant recipients, in whom the incidence of CMV disease tends to peak within the first 1 to 6 months after transplantation [106].

DIAGNOSTIC APPROACH/EMPIRIC THERAPY. The diagnostic approach to pulmonary disease in the immunocompromised host also depends on the nature of the immune deficit. As a general rule, all accessible sites (blood, urine, sputum) should be cultured, although sputum of high quality is rarely obtained in these circumstances (see Chap. 12). In *neutropenic hosts,* empiric antibacterial therapy is begun at the outset regardless of radiographic pattern, using one of the regimens discussed previously for fever and neutropenia [16,17,57]. The use of a synergistic beta-lactam (piperacillin, azlocillin, or ceftazidime) with aminoglycoside (tobramycin or amikacin) combination is encouraged because of the common isolation of gram-negative bacilli in these settings. If a clinical response occurs, then therapy is continued until neutropenia resolves. In the setting of advancing pulmonary disease despite antibiotic therapy, saprophytic fungi are the principal concern (especially *Aspergillus,* but also *Mucor, Fusarium,* and *Trichosporon*) [20,21,57]. Expectorated sputum or bronchial lavage fluid may provide presumptive evidence of these pathogens, but prompt definitive diagnosis usually requires open lung biopsy. Typically, pneumonia caused by *Aspergillus* or *Mucor* causes large areas of lung infarction that may be missed by transbronchial biopsy [57,92,107]. Standard therapy for confirmed pulmonary disease caused by *Aspergillus* involves intravenous amphotericin B, usually at a dosage of 0.7 to 1.0 mg/kg/day and for a total course of 1.5 to 2 gm over 6 to 8 weeks [19,20,108]. Unfortunately there is no established therapy for some emerging fungal pathogens such as *Trichosporon* or *Fusarium;* surgical resection of grossly infected tissues together with amphotericin therapy is often necessary for cure [19,21]. Diffuse pulmonary infiltrates may occur in the setting of disseminated candidiasis, but this pathogen rarely is associated with primary pneumonia.

In patients with compromised T-cell immunity, the list of diagnostic possibilities is longer and more diverse, making satisfactory empiric therapy a virtual impossibility [57,106]. Expectorated or induced sputum may demonstrate the organism by special stains in a minority of cases (*P. carinii, M. tuberculosis, N. asteroides*), but fiberoptic bronchoscopy with lavage or biopsy remains a valuable technique for these patients [57,109,110]. It is particularly helpful for diffuse or interstitial disease, where it provides not only lavage fluid with reasonable diagnostic accuracy for infectious agents such as PCP and bacteria, but also pathologic specimens that may allow diagnosis of CMV, drug pneumonitis, hemorrhage, or lymphangitic carcinomatosis. In patients with focal or nodular disease, alternative techniques such as needle aspiration or open-lung biopsy may be useful [94,95].

In the immunodeficient host with T cell impairment not caused by HIV infection, the authors often employ trimethoprim-sulfamethoxazole (5 mg/kg of the trimethoprim component IV q6h) plus erythromycin (1 gm IV q6h) as empiric therapy for the pathogens most likely to progress rapidly as diagnostic efforts proceed (e.g., PCP, *Legionella*, *Mycoplasma*, encapsulated bacteria). Serum drug level monitoring, if available, should be used to adjust therapy to obtain a peak serum sulfamethoxazole level of 100 μg/ml or TMP levels of 5 to 8 μg/ml [111]. Non-AIDS patients with suspected PCP require bronchoscopy with bronchoalveolar lavage and/or biopsy as soon as possible after starting therapy, because organisms may no longer be demonstrable after only a few days of treatment [112]. The establishment of histologic or microbiologic diagnosis by invasive techniques will allow institution of specific therapy, such as acyclovir for HSV pneumonia [97], ganciclovir with CMV-immune globulin for CMV pneumonia [113], TMP/SMX for nocardiosis, or corticosteroids for radiation pneumonitis [92].

PNEUMONIA IN THE PATIENT WITH HIV-I INFECTION. The patient with known or suspected HIV infection and pneumonia presents special challenges. Chapters 74 and 93 discuss AIDS and the pulmonary complications of AIDS.

Prevention of Infection

In recent years there has been increased emphasis on the prevention of opportunistic infections in immunocompromised hosts. These strategies have taken many different forms. Early efforts were directed at modifications of the environment of neutropenic patients through laminar air flow, nonabsorbable antibiotics, and elaborate efforts at disinfecting the inanimate environment. These approaches have proven expensive and laborious and have been abandoned by most centers for all but the most profoundly immunocompromised hosts (e.g., bone marrow transplant recipients) [114].

Oral fluoroquinolone administration has been studied in patients with prolonged neutropenia [115,116,117]. These agents reduce levels of aerobic gram-negative bacilli within the gut lumen, the major reservoir for dissemination of infection in the neutropenic host [18,44]. Although the incidence of gram-negative bacillary infections is favorably affected by these regimens, there has been no proven effect on morbidity or mortality. Potential disadvantages include the development of resistant bacterial strains caused by widespread use and a possible increase in infections caused by gram-positive species [118].

Antifungal prophylaxis with oral fluconazole (400 mg po qd or 200 mg IV q12hr) has proven effective in reducing infection by *Candida* species in bone marrow transplant recipients [119]. In patients with leukemia, superficial fungal infections were reduced by fluconazole, whereas invasive disease was unaffected [120]. One center noted an increase in fluconazole-resistant *Candida krusei* infections because of this practice [121]. Infections caused by saprophytic fungi (e.g., *Aspergillus*) would not be expected to be affected by fluconazole.

Antiviral prophylaxis with acyclovir has been shown to reduce mucocutaneous infections by HSV both in transplant recipients and in patients with leukemia [122,123,124]. Studies on the prevention of CMV infection in transplant recipients have focused on the avoidance of CMV-positive blood transfusion to CMV-negative patients and the prophylactic use of acyclovir, ganciclovir, or hyperimmune globulin [125,126]. No clear consensus has emerged.

Finally, there is increasing interest in the routine use of hematopoietic growth factors such as granulocyte colony-stimulating factor (G-CSF) and granulocyte-monocyte colony-stimulating factor (GM-CSF) for patients with neutropenia [127]. The use of G-CSF in patients undergoing chemotherapy for small-cell carcinoma of the lung reduced the days of neutropenia, episodes of fever, use of antibiotics, and days in hospital when compared with controls [128]. Clinical practice guidelines for the use of colony-stimulating factors have been published recently [129].

References

1. Hersh EM, Bodey GP, Nies BA, et al: Causes of death in acute leukemia. *JAMA* 193:105, 1965.
2. Kusne S, Dummer JS, Singh N, et al: Infections after liver transplantation: An analysis of 101 consecutive cases. *Medicine* 67:132, 1988.
3. Peterson PK, Ferguson R, Fryd DS, et al: Infectious diseases in hospitalized renal transplant recipients: A prospective study of a complex and evolving problem. *Medicine* 61:360, 1982.
4. Chang HY, Rodriguez V, Narboni G, et al: Causes of death in adults with acute leukemia. *Medicine* 55:259, 1976.
5. Winston DJ, Gale RP, Meyer DV, et al: Infectious complications of human bone marrow transplantation. *Medicine* 58:1, 1979.
6. Notter DT, Grossman PL, Rosenberg SA, et al: Infections in patients with Hodgkin's disease: A clinical study of 300 consecutive adult patients. *Rev Infect Dis* 2:761, 1980.
7. Masur H, Cheigh JS, Stubenbord WT: Infection following renal transplantation: A changing pattern. *Rev Infect Dis* 4:1208, 1982.
8. Bodey GP, Bolivar R, Fainstein V: Infectious complications in leukemic patients. *Semin Hematol* 19:193, 1982.
9. Hofflin JM, Potasman I, Baldwin JC, et al: Infectious complications in heart transplant recipients receiving cyclosporine and corticosteroids. *Ann Intern Med* 106:209, 1987.
10. Elting LS, Bodey GP, Fainstein V: Polymicrobial septicemia in the cancer patient. *Medicine* 65:218, 1986.
11. Pirsch JD, Maki DG: Infectious complications in adults with bone marrow transplantation and T-cell depletion of donor marrow. *Ann Intern Med* 104:619, 1986.
12. Pantaleo G, Graziosi C, Fauci AS: The immunopathogenesis of human immunodeficiency virus infection. *N Engl J Med* 328:327, 1993.
13. Pickering LK, Anderson DC, Choi S, et al: Leukocyte function in children with malignancies. *Cancer* 35:1365, 1975.
14. Weinberger M, Elattar I, Marshall D, et al: Patterns of infection in patients with aplastic anemia and the emergence of *Aspergillus* as a major cause of death. *Medicine* 71:24, 1992.
15. Bodey GP, Buckley M, Sathe YS, Freireich EJ: Quantitative relationships between circulating leukocytes and infections in patients with acute leukemia. *Ann Intern Med* 64:328, 1966.
16. Pizzo PA: Management of fever in patients with cancer and treatment induced neutropenia. *N Engl J Med* 328:1323, 1993.
17. Hughes WT, Bodey GP, Meyers JD, et al: Guidelines for the use of antimicrobial agents in neutropenic patients with unexplained fever. *J Infect Dis* 161:381, 1990.
18. Schimpff SC, Young VM, Greene WH, et al: Origin of infection in acute nonlymphocytic leukemia: Significance of hospital acquisition of potential pathogens. *Ann Intern Med* 77:707, 1972.
19. Sugar AM: Empiric treatment of fungal infections in the neutropenic host. *Arch Intern Med* 150:2258, 1990.

20. Armstrong D: Treatment of opportunistic fungal infections. *Clin Infect Dis* 16:1, 1993.

21. Anaissie E, Bodey GP, Kantarjian H, et al: New spectrum of fungal infections in patients with cancer. *Rev Infect Dis* 11:369, 1989.

22. Walsh TJ, Newman KR, Moody M, et al: Trichosporonosis in patients with neoplastic disease. *Medicine* 65:268, 1986.

23. Bodey GP: Fungal infection and fever of unknown origin in neutropenic patients. *Am J Med* 80:112, 1986.

24. Stiehm RE, Ashida E, Sik K, et al: Intravenous immunoglobulins as therapeutic agents. *Ann Intern Med* 107:367, 1987.

25. Cooperative Group: Intravenous immunoglobulin for the prevention of infection in chronic lymphocytic leukemia: A randomized, controlled clinical trial. *N Engl J Med* 319:902, 1988.

26. Savage DG, Lindenbaum J, Garrett TJ: Biphasic pattern of bacterial infection in multiple myeloma. *Ann Intern Med* 96:47, 1982.

27. Fisher RI, DeVita VT Jr, Bostick F, et al: Persistent immunologic abnormalities in long-term survivors of advanced Hodgkin's disease. *Ann Intern Med* 92:595, 1980.

28. Hellmann DB, Petri M, Whiting-O'Keefe Q: Fatal infections in systemic lupus erythematosus: The role of opportunistic organisms. *Medicine* 66:341, 1987.

29. Wheat LJ, Smith EJ, Sathapatayavongs B, et al: Histoplasmosis in renal allograft recipients: Two large urban outbreaks. *Arch Intern Med* 143:703, 1983.

30. Rubin RH, Wolfson JS, Cosimi AB, et al: Infection in the renal transplant recipient. *Am J Med* 70:405, 1981.

31. Hooper DC, Pruitt AA, Rubin RH: Central nervous system infection in the chronically immunosuppressed. *Medicine* 61:166, 1982.

32. Raad II, Bodey GP: Infectious complications of indwelling vascular catheters. *Clin Infect Dis* 15:197, 1992.

33. Press OW, Ramsey PG, Larson EB, et al: Hickman catheter infections in patients with malignancies. *Medicine* 63:189, 1984.

34. Groeger JS, Lucas AB, Thaler HT et al: Infectious morbidity associated with long term use of venous access devices in patients with cancer. *Ann Intern Med* 119:1168, 1993.

35. Johnson MP, Ramphal R: β-Lactam-resistant *Enterobacter* in febrile neutropenic patients receiving monotherapy. *J Infect Dis* 162:981, 1990.

36. Forlenza SW: *Capnocytophaga* sepsis: A newly recognized clinical entity in granulocytopenic patients. *Lancet* 1:567, 1980.

37. Young VM, Meyers WF, Moody MR, et al: The emergence of coryneform bacteria as a cause of nosocomial infections in compromised hosts. *Am J Med* 70:646, 1981.

38. Van Elta LL, Filice GA, Ferguson RM, et al: *Corynebacterium equi:* A review of 12 cases of human infection. *Rev Infect Dis* 5:1012, 1983.

39. Coker DD, Morris DM, Coleman J, et al: Infection among 210 patients with surgically staged Hodgkin's disease. *Am J Med* 75:97, 1983.

40. Gopal V, Bisno AL: Fulminant pneumococcal infections in "normal" asplenic hosts. *Arch Intern Med* 137:1526, 1977.

41. Zarrabi HM, Rosner F: Serious infections in adults following splenectomy for trauma. *Arch Intern Med* 144:1421, 1984.

42. Bohnsack JF, Brown EJ: The role of the spleen in resistance to infection. *Annu Rev Med* 37:49, 1986.

43. Pizzo PA, Robichaud KJ, Wesley R, et al: Fever in the pediatric and young adult patient with cancer. *Medicine* 61:153, 1982.

44. Fainstein V, Rodriguez V, Turek M, et al: Patterns of oropharyngeal and fecal flora in patients with acute leukemia. *J Infect Dis* 144:10, 1981.

45. Barnes SG, Sattler FR, Ballard JO: Perirectal infections in acute leukemia: Improved survival after incision and debridement. *Ann Intern Med* 100:515, 1984.

46. Pokorney BH, Jones JM, Shaikh BS, et al: Typhlitis: A treatable cause of recurrent septicemia. *JAMA* 243:682, 1980.

47. Weinberger M, Hollingsworth H, Feuerstein IM, et al: Successful surgical management of neutropenic enterocolitis in two patients with severe aplastic anemia. *Arch Intern Med* 153:107, 1993.

48. Cudmore MA, Silva J, Fekety R, et al: *Clostridium difficile* colitis associated with cancer chemotherapy. *Arch Intern Med* 142:333, 1982.

49. Yolken RH, Bishop CA, Townsend TR, et al: Infectious gastroenteritis in bone-marrow-transplant recipients. *N Engl J Med* 306:1009, 1982.

50. Muller SA, Hermann EC Jr, Winklemann RK: Herpes simplex infectious in hematologic malignancies. *Am J Med* 52:102, 1972.

51. Pass RF, Whitley RJ, Whelchel JD, et al: Identification of patients with increased risk of infection with herpes simplex after renal transplantation. *J Infect Dis* 140:487, 1979.

52. Overholser DC, Peterson DE, Williams LT, et al: Periodontal infection in patients with acute nonlymphocytic leukemia. *Arch Intern Med* 142:551, 1982.

53. Sickles EA, Greene WH, Wiernik PH: Clinical presentation of infection in granulocytopenic patients. *Arch Intern Med* 135:715, 1975.

54. Fishman LS, Griffin JR, Sapico FL, et al: Hematogenous candida endophthalmitis: A complication of candidemia. *N Engl J Med* 286:675, 1972.

55. Wolfson JS, Sober AJ, Rubin RH: Dermatologic manifestations of infections in immunocompromised patients. *Medicine* 64:115, 1985.

56. Allo MD, Miller J, Townsend T, et al: Primary cutaneous aspergillosis associated with Hickman intravenous catheters. *N Engl J Med* 317:1105, 1987.

57. Shelhammer JH, Toews GB, Masur H, et al: Respiratory disease in the immunosuppressed patient. *Ann Intern Med* 117:415, 1992.

58. Sepkowitz KA, Brown AE, Telzak EE, et al: *Pneumocystis carinii* pneumonia among patients without AIDS at a cancer hospital. *JAMA* 267:832, 1992.

59. Kovacs JA, Hiemenz JW, Macher AM, et al: *Pneumocystis carinii* pneumonia: A comparison between patients with the acquired immunodeficiency syndrome and patients with other immunodeficiencies. *Ann Intern Med* 100:663, 1984.

60. Pizzo PA, Hathorn JW, Hiemenz J, et al: A randomized trial comparing ceftazidime alone with combination antibiotic therapy in cancer patients with fever and neutropenia. *N Engl J Med* 315:552, 1986.

61. Love LJ, Schimpff SC, Schiffer CA, et al: Improved prognosis for granulocytopenic patients with gram-negative bacteremia. *Am J Med* 68:643, 1980.

62. Pizzo PA, Robichaud KJ, Gill FA, et al: Empiric antibiotic and antifungal therapy for cancer patients with prolonged fever and granulocytopenia. *Am J Med* 72:101, 1982.

63. Schimpff S, Satterlee W, Young VM, et al: Empiric therapy with carbenicillin and gentamicin for febrile patients with cancer and granulocytopenia. *N Engl J Med* 284:1061, 1971.

64. EORTC International Antimicrobial Therapy Project Group: Three antibiotic regimens in the treatment of infection in febrile granulocytopenic patients with cancer. *J Infect Dis* 137:14, 1978.

65. Singer C, Kaplan MH, Armstrong D: Bacteremia and fungemia complicating neoplastic disease: A study of 364 cases. *Am J Med* 62:731, 1977.

66. Scott RE, Robson HG: Synergistic activity of carbenicillin and gentamicin in experimental *Pseudomonas* bacteremia in neutropenic rats. *Antimicrob Agents Chemother* 10:646, 1976.

67. Glew RH, Pavuk RA: Early synergistic interaction between semisynthetic penicillins and aminoglycosidic aminocytitols against *Enterobacteriaceae. Antimicrob Agents Chemother* 23:902, 1983.

68. Eliopoulos GM, Moellering RC Jr: Azlocillin, mezlocillin, and piperacillin: New broad-spectrum penicillins. *Ann Intern Med* 97:755, 1982.

69. Feliu J, Artal A, Gonzales M, et al: Comparison of two antibiotic regimens (piperacillin plus amikacin versus ceftazidime plus amikacin) as empiric therapy for febrile neutropenic patients with cancer. *Antimicrob Agents Chemother* 36:2816, 1992.

70. Klastersky J, Glauser MP, Schimpff SC, et al: Prospective randomized comparison of three antibiotic regimens for empirical therapy of suspected bacteremic infection in febrile granulocytopenic patients. *Antimicrob Agents Chemother* 29:263, 1986.

71. Viscoli C, Moroni C, Boni L, et al: Ceftazidime plus amikacin versus ceftazidime plus vancomycin as empiric therapy in febrile neutropenic children with cancer. *Rev Infect Dis* 13:387, 1991.

72. Jones PG, Rolston KVI, Fainstein V, et al: Aztreonam therapy in neutropenic patients with cancer. *Am J Med* 81:243, 1986.

73. Karp JE, Dick JD, Angelopulos C, et al: Empiric use of vancomycin during prolonged treatment-induced granulocytopenia: Randomized, double-blind, placebo-controlled clinical trial in patients with acute leukemia. *Am J Med* 81:237, 1986.

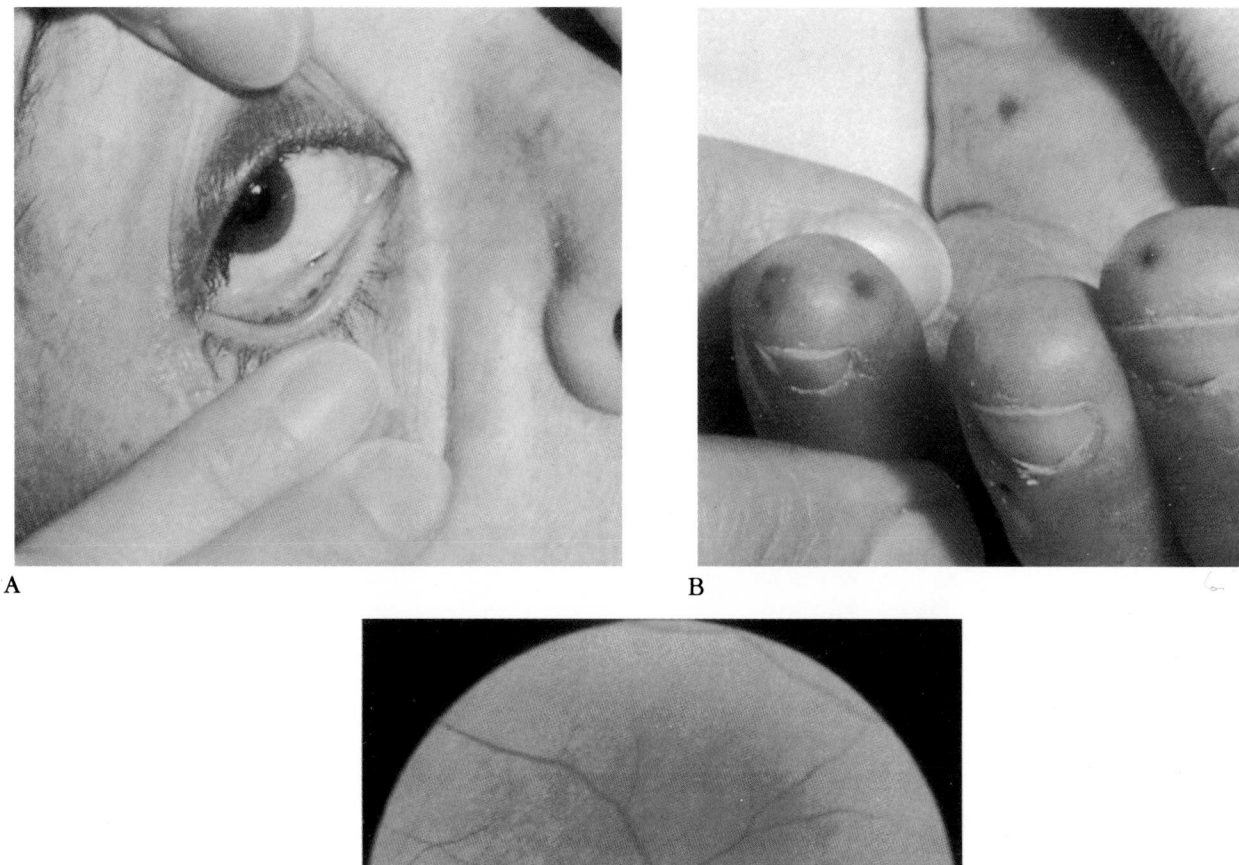

A

B

C

Plate I-1. Embolic phenomena in a single patient with *Staphylococcus aureus* endocarditis. A. Conjunctival petechiae. B. Petechiae on fingertips; note irregular margins. (A and B courtesy of Biomedical Media, University of Massachusetts Medical Center.) C. Fundus hemorrhage with white center, known as *Roth spot*. (Courtesy of Harry Kachadoorian, Ophthalmology Clinic, University of Massachusetts Medical Center.)

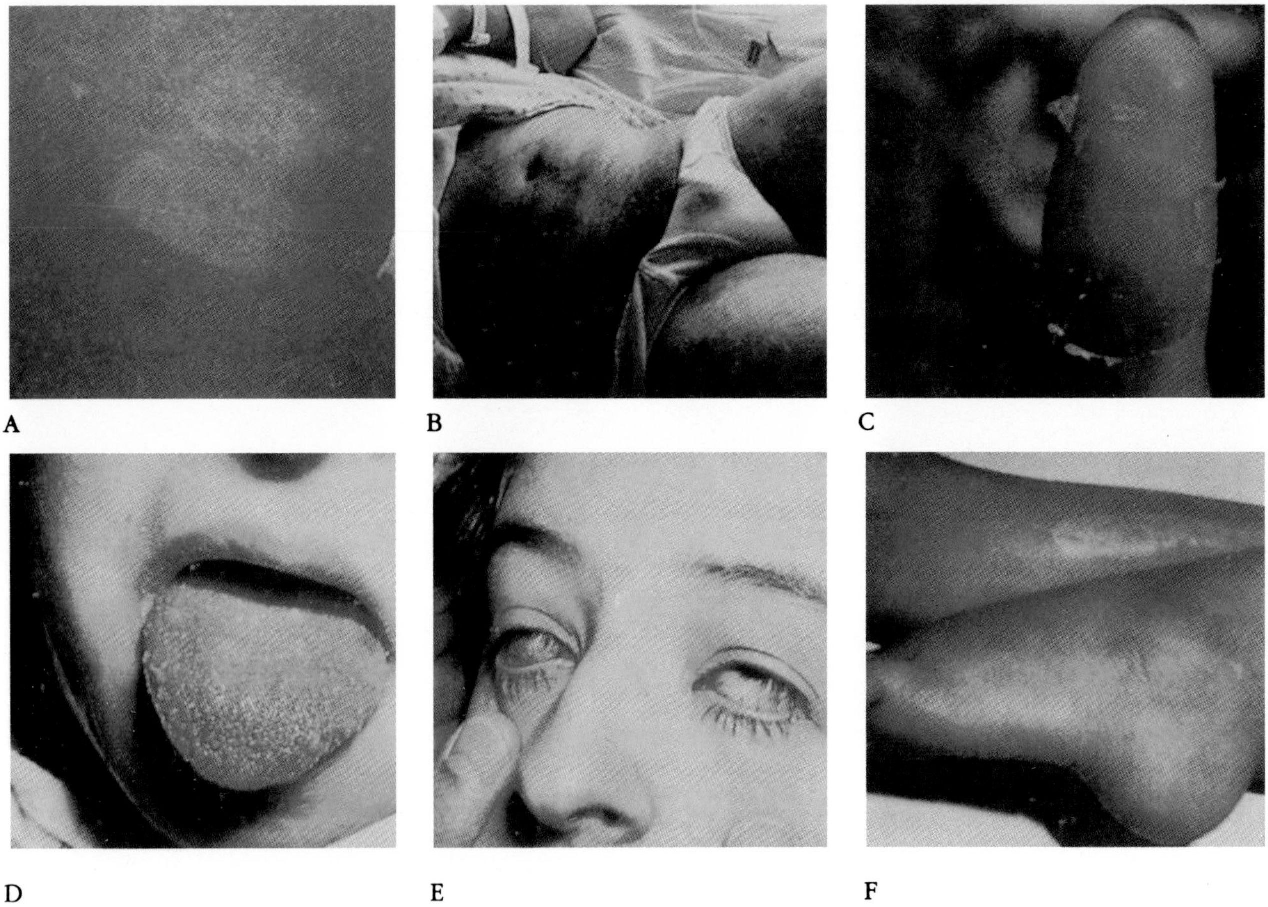

A   B   C

D   E   F

Plate I-2. Clinical signs of toxic shock syndrome. A. Diffuse, blanching macular erythroderma. B. Localized erythematous, papulopustular rash with zones of sparing at the waist and over both thighs corresponding to usual location of elastic in the underwear. C. Full-thickness desquamation involving the tip of the thumb. D. Strawberry tongue with denuded lingual mucosa and hyperplastic papillae. E. Bilateral nonpurulent bulbar and palpebral conjunctivitis. F. Diffuse pedal edema with accentuation around the metatarsophalangeal and ankle joints. (From Tofte RW, Williams DM: Clinical and laboratory manifestations of toxic shock syndrome. *Ann Intern Med* 96:843, 1982, with permission.)

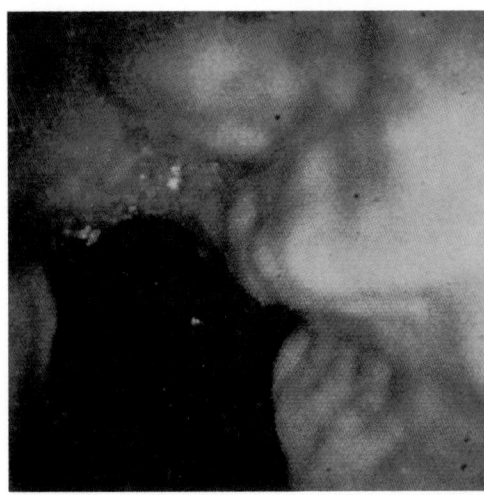

Plate I-3. Endoscopic appearance of esophageal varices. Because varices are distended submucosal veins, they appear as bluish, raised, irregular ridges.

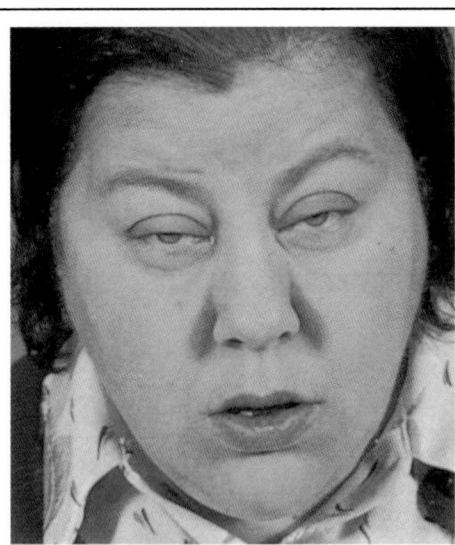

Plate I-4. Characteristic facies of severe hypothyroidism. Note the facial and periorbital puffiness and the dull, lethargic expression.

74. Rubin M, Hathorn JW, Marshall D, et al: Gram-positive infections and the use of vancomycin in 550 episodes of fever and neutropenia. *Ann Intern Med* 108:30, 1988.

75. EORTC and National Cancer Institute of Canada: Vancomycin added to empirical combination antibiotic therapy for fever in granulocytopenic cancer patients. *J Infect Dis* 163:951, 1991.

76. EORTC International Antimicrobial Therapy Cooperative Group: Ceftazidime combined with a short or long course of amikacin for empirical therapy of gram-negative bacteremia in cancer patients with granulocytopenia. *N Engl J Med* 317:1692, 1987.

77. Norrby SR, Vandercam B, Louie T, et al: Imipenem/cilastatin versus amikacin plus piperacillin in the treatment of infections in neutropenic patients: A prospective, randomized multi-clinic study. *Scand J Infect Dis* 52:65, 1987.

78. Rolston KVI, Berkey G, Bodey P, et al: A comparison of imipenem to ceftazidime with or without amikacin as empiric therapy in febrile neutropenic patients. *Arch Intern Med* 152:283, 1992.

79. Riikonen P: Imipenem compared with ceftazidime plus vancomycin as initial therapy for fever in neutropenic children with cancer. *Pediatr Infect Dis J* 10:918, 1991.

80. Winston DJ, Ho WG, Bruckner DA, et al: Beta-lactam antibiotic therapy in febrile granulocytopenic patients. *Ann Intern Med* 115:849, 1991.

81. Pizzo PA, Robichaud KJ, Gill FA, et al: Duration of empiric antibiotic therapy in granulocytopenic patients with cancer. *Am J Med* 67:194, 1979.

82. Pizzo PA, Ladisch S, Robichaud K: Treatment of gram-positive septicemia in cancer patients. *Cancer* 45:206, 1980.

83. Dinubile MJ: Stopping antibiotic therapy in neutropenic patients. *Ann Intern Med* 108:289, 1988.

84. Zeitany RG, Saghir NE, Santhosh-Kumar CR, et al: Increased aminoglycoside dosage requirements in hematologic malignancy. *Antimicrob Agents Chemother* 34:702, 1990.

85. Maksymiuk AW, Thongprasert S, Hopfer R, et al: Systemic candidiasis in cancer patients. *Am J Med* 77:20, 1984.

86. Platenkamp GP, Van Duin AM, Porsius JC, et al: Diagnosis of invasive candidiasis in patients with and without signs of immune deficiency: A comparison of six detection methods in human serum. *J Clin Pathol* 40:1162, 1987.

87. Fisher JF, Trincher RC, Agel JF, et al: Disseminated candidiasis: A comparison of two immunologic techniques in the diagnosis. *Am J Med Sci* 290:135, 1985.

88. Medoff G, Dismukes WE, Meade RH, et al: A new therapeutic approach to *Candida* infections. *Arch Intern Med* 130:241, 1972.

89. Karp JE, Merz WG, Charache P: Response to empiric amphotericin B during antileukemic therapy-induced granulocytopenia. *Rev Infect Dis* 13:592, 1991.

90. Thaler M, Pastakia B, Shawker TH, et al: Hepatic candidiasis in cancer patients: The evolving picture of the syndrome. *Ann Intern Med* 108:88, 1988.

91. Anaissie E, Bodey GP, Kantarjian H, et al: Fluconazole therapy for chronic disseminated candidiasis in patients with leukemia and prior amphotericin B therapy. *Am J Med* 91:142, 1991.

92. Rosenow EC III, Wilson WR, Cockerill FR III: Pulmonary disease in the immunocompromised host (two parts). *Mayo Clin Proc* 60:473, 610, 1985.

93. Singer C, Armstrong D, Rosen PP, et al: Diffuse pulmonary infiltrates in immunocompromised patients. Prospective study of 80 cases. *Am J Med* 66:110, 1979.

94. Cockerill FR III, Wilson WR, Carpenter HA, et al: Open lung biopsy in immunocompromised patients. *Arch Intern Med* 145:1398, 1985.

95. Cheson BD, Samlowski WE, Tang TT, Spruance SL: Value of open-lung biopsy in 87 immunocompromised patients with pulmonary infiltrates. *Cancer* 55:453, 1985.

96. Valdivieso M, Gil-Extremera B, Zornoza J, et al: Gram-negative bacillary pneumonia in the compromised host. *Medicine* 56:241, 1977.

97. Graham BS, Snell JD: Herpes simplex virus infection of the adult lower respiratory tract. *Medicine* 62:384, 1983.

98. Crawford SW, Bowden RA, Hackman RC, et al: Rapid detection of cytomegalovirus pulmonary infection by bronchoalveolar lavage and centrifugation culture. *Ann Intern Med* 108:80, 1988.

99. Kerkering TM, Duma RJ, Shadomy S: The evolution of pulmonary cryptococcosis. *Ann Intern Med* 94:611, 1981.

100. Wheat LJ, Slama TG, Norton JA, et al: Risk factors for disseminated or fatal histoplasmosis. *Ann Intern Med* 96:159, 1982.

101. Slavin RE, Walsh TJ, Pollack AD: Late generalized tuberculosis: A clinical pathologic analysis and comparison of 100 cases in the preantibiotic and antibiotic eras. *Medicine* 59:352, 1980.

102. Dowling JN, Pasculle WA, Frola FN, et al: Infections caused by *Legionella micdadei* and *Legionella pneumophila* among renal transplant patients. *J Infect Dis* 149:703, 1984.

103. Scowden EB, Schaffner W, Stone WJ: Overwhelming strongyloidiasis: An unappreciated opportunistic infection. *Medicine* 57:527, 1978.

104. Davidson RA, Fletcher RH, Chapman LE: Risk factors for strongyloidiasis: A case-control study. *Arch Intern Med* 144:321, 1984.

105. Meyers D, Flournoy N, Thomas ED: Nonbacterial pneumonia after allogeneic marrow transplantation: A review of ten years' experience. *Rev Infect Dis* 4:1119, 1982.

106. Ramsey PG, Rubin RH, Tolkoff-Rubin NE, et al: The renal transplant patient with fever and pulmonary infiltrates: Etiology, clinical manifestations, and management. *Medicine* 59:206, 1980.

107. Rinaldi MG: Invasive aspergillosis. *Rev Infect Dis* 5:1061, 1983.

108. Denning DW, Stevens DA: Antifungal and surgical treatment of invasive aspergillosis: Review of 2,121 published cases. *Rev Infect Dis* 12:1147, 1990.

109. Pisani RJ, Wright AJ: Clinical utility of bronchoalveolar lavage in immunocompromised hosts. *Mayo Clin Proc* 67:221, 1992.

110. Springmeyer SC, Silvestri RC, Sale GE, et al: The role of transbronchial biopsy for the diagnosis of diffuse pneumonias in immunocompromised marrow transplant recipients. *Am Rev Respir Dis* 126:763, 1982.

111. Sattler FR, Cowan R, Nielsen DM, et al: Trimethoprim-sulfamethoxazole compared with pentamidine for treatment of *Pneumocystis carinii* pneumonia in the acquired immunodeficiency syndrome: A prospective, noncrossover study. *Ann Intern Med* 109:280, 1988.

112. Sattler FR, Remington JS: Intravenous trimethoprim-sulfamethoxazole therapy for *Pneumocystis carinii* pneumonia. *Am J Med* 70:1215, 1981.

113. Emanuel D, Cunningham I, Jules-Elysee K, et al: Cytomegalovirus pneumonia after bone marrow transplantation successfully treated with the combination of ganciclovir and high-dose intravenous immune globulin. *Ann Intern Med* 15:777, 1988.

114. Pizzo PA: Considerations for the prevention of infectious complications in patients with cancer. *Rev Infect Dis* 11(suppl 7):S1551, 1989.

115. The GIMEMA Infection Program: Prevention of bacterial infection in neutropenic patients with hematologic malignancies: A randomized, multicenter trial comparing norfloxacin with ciprofloxacin. *Ann Intern Med* 115:7, 1991.

116. Karp JE, Merz WG, Hendricksen C, et al: Oral norfloxacin for prevention of gram-negative bacterial infections in patients with acute leukemia and granulocytopenia. *Ann Intern Med* 106:1, 1987.

117. Dikker AW, Rozenberg-Arska M, Verhoef J: Infection prophylaxis in acute leukeima: A comparison of ciprofloxacin with trimethoprim-sulfamethoxazole and colistin. *Ann Intern Med* 106:7, 1987.

118. Muder RR, Brennen C, Goetz AM, et al: Association with prior fluoroquinolone therapy of widespread ciprofloxacin resistance among gram-negative isolates in a Veterans Affairs medical center. *Antimicrob Agents and Chemother* 35:256, 1991.

119. Goodman JL, Winston DJ, Greenfield RA, et al: A controlled trial of fluconazole to prevent fungal infections in patients undergoing bone marrow transplantation. *N Engl J Med* 326:845, 1992.

120. Winston DJ, Chandrasekar PH, Lazarus HM, et al: Fluconazole prophylaxis of fungal infections in patients with acute leukemia. *Ann Intern Med* 118:495, 1993.

121. Wingard JR, Merz WG, Rinaldi MG, et al: Increase in *Candida krusei* infection among patients with bone marrow transplantation and neutropenia treated prophylactically with fluconazole. *N Engl J Med* 325:1274, 1991.

122. Saral R, Burns WH, Laskin OL, et al: Acyclovir prophylaxis of herpes-simplex virus infections: A randomized, double-blind, controlled trial in bone-marrow transplant recipients. *N Engl J Med* 305:63, 1981.

123. Wade JC, Newton B, Flournoy N, et al: Oral acyclovir for prevention of herpes simplex virus reactivation after marrow transplantation. *Ann Intern Med* 100:823, 1984.
124. Seale L, Jones CJ, Kathpalia S, et al: Prevention of herpes virus infections in renal allograft recipients by low-dose oral acyclovir. *JAMA* 254:3435, 1985.
125. Meyers JD, Leszczynski J, Zaia JA, et al: Prevention of cytomegalovirus infection by cytomegalovirus immune globulin after marrow transplantation. *Ann Intern Med* 98:442, 1983.
126. Balfour HH, Chace BA, Stapleton JT, et al: A randomized, placebo-controlled trial of oral acyclovir for the prevention of cytomegalovirus disease in recipients of renal allografts. *N Engl J Med* 320:1381, 1989.

127. Lieschke GJ, Burgess AW: Granulocyte colony-stimulating factor and granulocyte-macrophage colony-stimulating factor. *N Engl J Med* 327:28, 1992.
128. Crawford J, Ozer H, Stoller R, et al: Reduction by granulocyte colony-stimulating factor of fever and neutropenia induced by chemotherapy in patients with small-cell lung cancer. *N Engl J Med* 325:164, 1991.
129. American Society for Clinical Oncology: American Society for Clinical Oncology recommendations for the use of hematopoietic colony-stimulating factors: Evidence-based, clinical practice guidelines. *J Clin Oncol* 12:2471, 1994.

93. Acquired Immunodeficiency Syndrome

Patrick G. Fairchild

AIDS is an acronym for the acquired immunodeficiency syndrome, a condition that represents the end stage of infection with the human immunodeficiency virus (HIV). First recognized in the early 1980s, AIDS is a clinical state of immunosuppression with multisystem manifestations that usually results in death. Severe impairment of the immune system leads to the development of unusual and life-threatening opportunistic infections and malignancies.

Because of the severity of these illnesses and the involvement of critical organ systems, many patients are admitted to the intensive care unit. Although in some cases decisions concerning the extent of aggressiveness and support remain difficult, prompt diagnosis and appropriate therapy can lead to a successful outcome for many patients [1]. Recent advances in the areas of antiviral therapy and prophylaxis of opportunistic infection have improved the outlook for longer patient survival [2–5]. Such intervention is changing the natural history of this disease from one of rapid demise to that of a chronic illness.

Etiology

During 1983 and 1984, a human lentivirus, now referred to as the human immunodeficiency virus type one (HIV-1), was identified by researchers in the United States and France as the infectious agent responsible for AIDS [6,7,8]. HIV-1 is classified as a retrovirus because it uses reverse transcriptase, a DNA polymerase, which transcribes RNA into DNA. Another human retrovirus, designated HIV-2, has been identified in persons from West Africa and Western Europe and appears to cause a syndrome indistinguishable from AIDS [9]. No cases of HIV-2 infection definitely acquired in the United States have been documented; however, HIV-2–associated disease has been found in patients who have immigrated to the United States.

Pathogenesis

HIV appears to preferentially infect a specific subset of lymphocytes referred to as T-4 helper cells or CD4 lymphocytes [10,11]. The first step in infection involves the attachment of HIV to the CD4 antigen on the lymphocyte surface. After binding to the CD4 receptor, HIV enters the cell and ultimately is incorporated into the cell genome. HIV infection of gastrointestinal cells, monocytes, macrophages, and neurons can also occur independent of this specific CD4 receptor binding site interaction [12,13]. After genomic integration, HIV replicates by using host cellular machinery. Infection appears to be lifelong [14,15].

After infection with HIV, many of the CD4 lymphocytes die or become dysfunctional, which probably accounts for the decrease in the absolute CD4 lymphocyte population associated with HIV disease. How HIV kills CD4 cells is unknown, but the destruction of the helper T4 cell ultimately leads to significant defects in cell-mediated immunity. The impairment of the immune response interferes with tumor surveillance as well as response to antigens and the effective clearance of viruses, fungi, protozoa, mycobacteria, and certain bacteria. Several weeks after acute HIV infection, there is a rapid rise in plasma viremia, which is followed by the appearance of HIV-specific cytotoxic lymphocyte (CTL) activity (Fig. 93-1). Although this CTL activity does not completely clear HIV from the body, there is a sharp drop in detectable virus in the plasma. Antibodies to HIV envelope (ENV) and core proteins (p24) appear soon thereafter. This CTL and antibody response is sustained in most individuals for many years, and the loss of these antiviral immune responses correlates closely with the recurrence of plasma viremia and the onset of clinical symptomatology because of immunodeficiency.

HIV is directly neurotropic and can cause a variety of both central nervous system (CNS) and peripheral nervous system disorders [16]. Neurologic disease directly attributable to HIV infection alone may have a varied and frequently insidious presentation. Dementia, chronic meningitis, spinal cord myelopathy, and cranial and peripheral neuropathy have been described. Because HIV can infect brain cells directly, any effective antiviral agent must be able to penetrate the blood-brain barrier.

Epidemiology

By the end of 1993, more than 300,000 cases of AIDS in the United States had been reported to the Centers for Disease

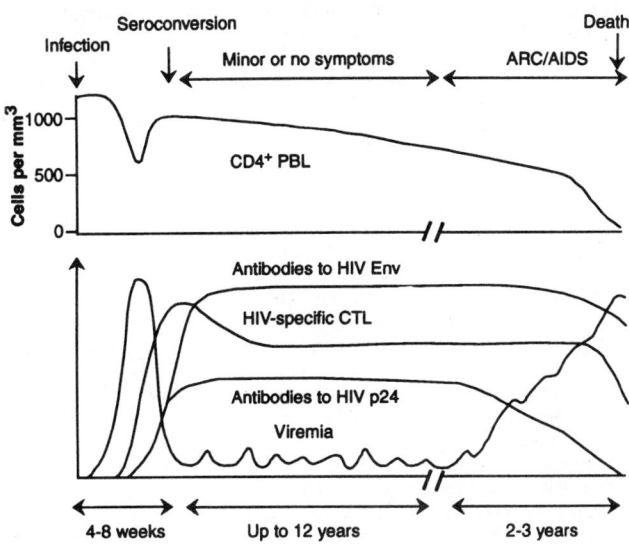

Fig. 93-1. Schematic course of HIV infection. Reproduced with permission from *Science* 260: 1273, 1993.

Control (CDC) [17]. At least one million individuals in the United States are thought to be infected with HIV [18]. AIDS has been reported from all 50 states, but major urban centers account for most cases. AIDS has been reported in more than 100 countries throughout the world, and millions worldwide are known to be seropositive for HIV.

Minorities are overrepresented in the AIDS epidemic. Current reporting indicates that 30 percent of persons with AIDS are black, and 17 percent are Hispanic [17]. Whites account for 52 percent of the cases, and 1 percent are of unknown or other racial background.

Several important risk factors have been identified for the acquisition of HIV infection. In the United States, these include homosexual or bisexual activity (57%), intravenous (IV) drug use (23%), homosexual activity or IV drug use (6%), heterosexual contact with a member of a high-risk group (7%), hemophilia (1%), and receipt of blood or blood products (2%) [17,19]. In approximately 4 percent of AIDS patients no identifiable risk factor has been ascertained.

Transmission of HIV occurs almost exclusively through contact with blood, semen, or vaginal secretions. HIV does not appear to be spread by casual contact. The most efficient mode of transmission is probably inoculation by transfusion with a significant quantity of infected blood. Fortunately, in the United States, routine screening of all blood and plasma donors for HIV-1 antibody has substantially reduced HIV-1–infected blood or plasma products from the nation's blood supply.

Needle sharing by IV drug users also appears to be a relatively efficient means of transmitting HIV from one person to another. IV drug users are now thought to account for most newly acquired cases of HIV infection in the United States and are the most important route of HIV transmission into the heterosexual and pediatric populations.

In the United States, transmission by sexual contact first occurred primarily among homosexual men. The number of new cases of HIV infection in the homosexual population has been steadily decreasing, presumably secondary to safer sex practices. In central Africa, where heterosexual transmission is the primary route of spread, HIV infection is equally distributed between men and women. Heterosexual transmission occurs from men to women and from women to men. The risk of HIV infection after a single unprotected sexual contact with an infected person is unknown but has been estimated to be 1 in 300 [20]. Use of latex condoms and spermicidal compounds containing nonoxynol-9, which also has anti-HIV activity, has been advocated to decrease the risk of transmission.

Diagnosis of HIV Infection

The diagnosis of HIV infection is usually made by demonstrating the presence of antibody to the virus. HIV-antibody tests use inactivated HIV antigen in an enzyme-linked immunoabsorbent assay (ELISA)[21]. Because the ELISA is a very sensitive test that may yield false-positive results, further confirmation is performed by another serologic assay called the Western blot analysis, which is highly specific. The sensitivity and specificity of serotesting in a high-risk population is well over 99 percent under optimal laboratory conditions [22].

Persons who have recently experienced acute primary HIV infection may have a negative ELISA test because insufficient time may have elapsed to produce levels of HIV antibody adequate to permit detection [23]. This may account for the rare instances of HIV transmission through blood products even though the blood donor had been appropriately screened. Although HIV-2 shares many similarities with HIV-1, routine serologic tests used to screen blood donors and other individuals for HIV-1 antibody do not detect the presence of HIV-2 envelope proteins [24].

Recently, rapid diagnostic assays have been developed that directly detect HIV antigens instead of HIV antibody. The polymerase chain reaction is one such exciting new modality [25,26]. This procedure permits detection of very small quantities of HIV by amplifying the viral gene products to detectable levels. Although widespread availablity of these assays is still several years away, it is hoped that they will prove to be a quick and reliable means to screen individuals at risk for HIV infection and help to identify those infected with HIV who have undetectable antibody levels.

HIV testing should be performed only for legitimate medical reasons and then only with permission of the patient or appropriate guardian [27]. In some states, HIV testing can be performed only with written informed consent. HIV test results should remain confidential.

Clinical Manifestations of HIV Infection

Acute primary infection with HIV is characterized by a mononucleosislike syndrome that develops 3 to 6 weeks after exposure [28,29,30]. Clinical illness typically consists of fever, rigors, arthralgias, myalgias, lymphadenopathy, headache, diarrhea, and rash. Acute symptoms usually last 2 to 3 weeks before resolving. Some patients may develop progressive symptoms after acute HIV infection and quickly develop more advanced stages of disease. Persistent high fever for a 10- to 14-day period during acute HIV infection may herald a rapidly progressive course [31].

After resolution of acute primary infection, most patients appear to recover fully and remain asymptomatic. This asymptomatic group represents the vast majority of those infected with HIV. They usually demonstrate serologic evidence of an antibody response to HIV 8 to 12 weeks after exposure but are without complaints or findings indicative of HIV infection. A period of clinical latency subsequently ensues, which may last from months to years in different individuals. Although HIV may be undetectable in the peripheral blood during this period, it has recently been shown that HIV is present and actively replicating in the lymphoid tissue of the body [32]. Therefore, a true state of microbiologic latency does not coincide with the period of clinical latency.

Early in the course of HIV infection, some patients develop the syndrome of persistent generalized lymphadenopathy, which is characterized by a greater than 1-cm enlargement of lymph nodes for at least a 3-month duration at two or more extrainguinal sites that cannot be explained by other reasons [33,34]. A quantitative T cell deficiency may not be present, and there are usually no defects in delayed hypersensitivity. Many patients with this syndrome do not feel ill.

In the later stages of HIV disease, effective immune containment of the large resevoir of latently infected cells in the lymphoid tissue is lost. This spillover of virus leads to a rapid rise in plasma viremia and may be followed by signs of clinical symptomology.

As the immune system becomes further impaired, many patients develop a syndrome called AIDS-related complex (ARC) [35]. This condition is characterized by a constellation of signs and symptoms that include intermittent fever, fatigue, weight loss, diarrhea, and lymphadenopathy (Table 93-1). As HIV continues to ravage the immune system, and host defenses become profoundly deranged, severe or total suppression of immune function develops that results in increased susceptibility to a variety of opportunistic infections, malignancies, and neurologic abnormalities, many of which establish the diagnosis of AIDS.

Definition of AIDS

The case definition of AIDS was created by the CDC in 1982 for epidemiologic surveillance, but was recognized to work well for clinical purposes [36]. AIDS was defined as the occurrence of a reliably diagnosed disease at least moderately indicative of underlying cellular immunodeficiency in a person without a condition known to be associated with an increased incidence of disease related to cellular immunodeficiency [37]. The CDC added several refinements to the case definition in 1985, when HIV-antibody testing became available [38]. Further revisions to the case definition were subsequently made in 1987 and 1993 as the expanded clinical spectrum of HIV-associated diseases became apparent [39,40]. Classification of HIV disease is dependent on the results of laboratory testing for HIV anti-

Table 93-1. AIDS-Related Complex

Any Two Clinical Findings	*Plus* Any Two Laboratory Abnormalities
Lymphadenopathy >3 mo	Helper T cells <400/mm³
Fever over 100° F >3 mo	T helper/T suppressor ratio <1.0
Weight loss >10%	Leukopenia
	Thrombocytopenia
Fatigue	Anemia
Persistent diarrhea	Elevated serum globulins
Night sweats	Reduced blastogenesis
	Anergy to skin tests
	Positive HIV antibody test

Table 93-2. Diseases That Indicate AIDS When HIV Antibody Testing Is Negative or Unknown and the Patient Has No Other Reasons for Immunodeficiency

Candidiasis of the esophagus, trachea, bronchi, or lungs
Cryptococcosis, extrapulmonary
Cryptosporidiosis, with diarrhea persisting >1 mo
Cytomegalovirus disease of an organ other than liver, spleen, or lymph nodes in a patient >1 mo of age
Herpes simplex virus infection causing a mucocutaneous ulcer that persists longer than 1 mo; or bronchitis, pneumonitis, or esophagitis for any duration affecting a patient >1 mo of age
Kaposi's sarcoma affecting a patient <60 yr of age
Lymphoma of the brain (primary) affecting a patient <60 yr of age
Lymphoid interstitial pneumonia and/or pulmonary lymphoid hyperplasia affecting a child <13 yr of age
Mycobacterium avium complex or *M. kansasii* disease, disseminated (at a site other than or in addition to lungs, skin, or cervical or hilar lymph nodes)
Pneumocystis carinii pneumonia
Progressive multifocal leukoencephalopathy
Toxoplasmosis of the brain affecting a patient >1 mo of age

Table 93-3. Diseases That Indicate AIDS When HIV-Antibody Test Results Are Positive

Bacterial infections, multiple or recurrent in child <13 yr of age
Coccidiodomycosis, disseminated
HIV encephalopathy
Histoplasmosis, disseminated
Isosporiasis with diarrhea persisting >1 mo
Kaposi's sarcoma at any age
Lymphoma of the brain (primary) at any age
Non-Hodgkin's lymphoma of B-cell type or unknown immunologic phenotype
Any mycobacterial disease caused by mycobacteria other than *M. tuberculosis,* disseminated
Diseases caused by *M. tuberculosis,* extrapulmonary
Salmonella septicemia, recurrent
HIV wasting syndrome
Pulmonary tuberculosis
Recurrent pneumonia within a 12-mo period
Invasive cervical carcinoma

body, the patients' CD4 count, and certain clinical conditions. If the results of HIV-antibody testing are unknown or are negative and the patient has no other recognized reason for underlying immunodeficiency, the presence of any of the indicator diseases listed in Table 93-2 is considered presumptive evidence of AIDS. If the HIV-antibody test results are positive and the patient has evidence of any of the indicator diseases listed in Table 93-3, the patient is considered to have AIDS. This is independent of other factors that may cause the patient to be immunodeficient, such as cytotoxic or immunosuppressive drugs. Additionally, the expanded 1993 definition of AIDS includes all HIV-infected individuals with less than 200 CD4 T lymphocytes or less than 14 percent CD4 T lymphocytes compared with the total lymphocyte count.

Opportunistic infections by a variety of organisms account for most AIDS-defining conditions. Some pathogens may cause multisystem disease, whereas others mainly affect one organ system (Table 93-4). Several non-AIDS defining conditions, such as oral candidiasis, Epstein-Barr virus–induced oral hairy leukoplakia, and multidermatomal zoster, are associated with

Table 93-4. Opportunistic Infections Associated With AIDS

Clinical diseases	Etiologic agents
Pneumonia	*Pneumocystis carinii, Aspergillus fumigatus, Legionella, Nocardia,* cytomegalovirus, *Cryptococcus neoformans, Mycobacterium avium* complex, and *M. tuberculosis*
Persistent gastroenteritis	*Cryptosporidium,* Microsporidia, *Isospora belli*
Mucous membrane disease	Herpes simplex virus, varicella zoster virus, *Candida,* Epstein-Barr virus
Meningitis, encephalitis, CNS abnormalities	*Toxoplasma gondii, Cryptococcus neoformans,* cytomegalovirus, papovavirus
Disseminated infections with multiple findings	*Mycobacterium avium* complex, *M. tuberculosis, Cryptococcus neoformans, Histoplasma capsulatum, Aspergillus fumigatus, Candida, Zygomycoses, Toxoplasma gondii, Strongyloides,* cytomegalovirus, herpes simplex virus

an increased risk of developing AIDS in subsequent years [41–44].

Several types of malignancy are recognized to be associated with advanced HIV infection. Kaposi's sarcoma [45,46], non-Hodgkin's lymphoma [47,48,49], and primary central nervous system (CNS) lymphoma [50,51] are AIDS-defining conditions. Although not diagnostic of AIDS, Hodgkin's lymphoma [52,53], squamous cell carcinoma [54,55], testicular carcinoma [56,57], and basal cell carcinoma [58,59] have been reported to occur with increased frequency in HIV-infected individuals.

The natural history of HIV infection is still unclear. Years of follow-up will be required before it can be fully understood. There appears to be remarkable variation among individuals with regard to clinical manifestations and the rate of disease progression. However, once AIDS develops, it appears to be a universally fatal disease. The use of prophylactic agents against such life-threatening illnesses as *Pneumocystis carinii* pneumonia (PCP) and the early use of antiviral therapy directed against HIV appear to have favorably affected the natural course of HIV disease [2,3,4].

Antiviral Therapy Against HIV

There is no cure for HIV infection. Azidothymidine (AZT), now called zidovudine (ZDV), was the first agent shown to improve the clinical and laboratory status of patients with HIV infection. Zidovudine is a thymidine analog that blocks the replication of HIV by inhibiting reverse transcriptase activity [60,61]. Early studies demonstrated that zidovudine, 250 mg taken by mouth every 4 hours, was beneficial for AIDS patients with a history of PCP [62]. Similar benefit was shown for patients with severe ARC whose CD4 counts were less than 200 cells per cubic millimeter. In both of these groups, patients lived longer and had fewer serious clinical events. Subsequent clinical trials have shown that zidovudine can also slow the rate of disease progression in both asymptomatic and symptomatic patients

whose CD4 counts are 500 cells per cubic millimeter or less [63,64].

Based on these results, the current FDA recommendation is to begin zidovudine, 200 mg po tid, in any HIV-infected person with a CD4 count less than 500. Unfortunately, long-term use of zidovudine has been associated with an apparent loss of efficacy over time. Several factors have been postulated to be responsible, including the appearance of syncytium-inducing virus [65–68] and viral resistance to zidovudine [69–72].

The major toxicity of zidovudine is bone marrow suppression [73]. During early studies that used dosages of 200 to 250 mg every 4 hours, anemia and leukopenia were common side effects, and a reduction in dosage was often required. Approximately one-third of patients on long-term zidovudine therapy required blood transfusions. Later studies have demonstrated that zidovudine, 100 mg every 4 hours, is as efficacious in its antiviral effect and improvement in clinical status as 200 mg every 4 hours but with significantly less hematologic toxicity [74]. Exogenous recombinant erythropoietin has also been successfully used to treat anemia in patients on zidovudine who have low endogenous erythropoietin levels [75], as has granulocyte-macrophage colony stimulating factor (GM-CSF) for zidovudine-associated leukopenia [76].

An important characteristic of zidovudine is its ability to penetrate the blood-brain barrier. Concentrations in the CNS are approximately 30 to 50 percent of serum concentrations [61]. Recently, an intravenous preparation of zidovudine has become available. Its exact role in adults remains to be ascertained, but it probably will be used in patients who are unable to take oral medication because of gastrointestinal (GI) problems or altered sensorium.

Didanosine (dideoxyinosine or ddI), another nucleoside analog that interferes with reverse transcriptase, initially was shown to have benefit in patients with advanced HIV infection who were intolerant of or unresponsive to zidovudine [77,78]. Subsequent studies demonstrated that patients receiving ddI had a significant delay in progression to AIDS compared with those who had received prior zidovudine therapy [79]. The major side effects of ddI are peripheral neuropathy and pancreatitis [77,78]. Neuropathy is more common in patients with a history of neuropathy or prior or concomitant neurotoxic drug therapy. Didanosine-associated pancreatitis can vary in presentation from asymptomatic elevated serum amylase levels to a fulminant rapidly fatal process. Renal insufficiency or a previous history of pancreatitis appears to increase the risk. Like zidovudine, viral resistance to ddI may develop after prolonged therapy [80,81].

Zalcitabine (dideoxycytidine or ddC), like zidovudine and ddI, is a reverse transcriptase inhibitor [82,83]. However, it is approved by the FDA only for use in combination with zidovudine in patients with CD4 counts less than 300 with evidence of clinical progression on zidovudine alone. Rash and stomatitis are the two major side effects, but individuals usually can be treated symptomatically without interruption in ddC therapy. Pancreatitis may also occur.

Combination therapy with zidovudine and ddI or ddC has been under intense study [84,85,86]. Their different toxicity profiles and in vitro synergism make combination therapy an attractive approach. It is still too early to tell if combination therapy will prove to be superior to monotherapy or decrease the emergence of resistance in a clinically meaningful way.

Multiple other antiviral agents that act at different sites in the life cycle of HIV are being evaluated [61,87]. Ultimately, successful treatment of HIV infection may involve the combination of antiviral agents with immunopotentiating drugs that effectively reconstitute the immune system.

Clinical Spectrum of HIV-Associated Disease by Organ System

DERMATOLOGIC MANIFESTATIONS. Skin disease is very common in the course of HIV disease (see Chap. 218). Multiple manifestations of infection, malignancy, and autoimmunity may be evident. Of greatest concern is Kaposi's sarcoma (KS). The emergence of an aggressive form of KS in the early 1980s was one of the first clues to the existence of AIDS [88,89]. For reasons that are not clear, KS disproportionately affects HIV-infected male homosexuals but is exceptionally rare in other risk groups [90–93]. The incidence of KS, a cause of great morbidity and mortality, is fortunately, but inexplicably, decreasing in the United States [94,95].

An endothelial neoplasm of the capillaries or lymphatics, KS may involve any part of the body. The characteristic lesion is an erythematous or violaceous nodule or papule. Lesions may be isolated or multiple in distribution. Although the lesion is fairly characteristic, a punch biopsy of a suspicious skin lesion should be done to confirm the diagnosis. Significant hemorrhage after skin biopsy is infrequent. Visceral involvement is common, and any organ can be involved. The GI tract is the most common site of extracutaneous involvement [96–99]. Pulmonary involvement when it occurs can be quite extensive and is often rapidly fatal [100,101,102].

Several therapeutic modalities are available to treat KS. In a small number of patients, the use of zidovudine has been associated with regression of the lesions. Recombinant interferon-alpha, 18 to 36 million units subcutaneously each day, has been reported to achieve partial or complete remissions [103,104]. Unfortunately, therapy may be limited by high fever, arthralgias, myalgias, and other flulike symptoms. The vinca alkaloids, vinblastine and vincristine, are two chemotherapeutic agents that can effectively control or cause regression of lesions in most cases [105,106]. The use of vinblastine may be restricted by its tendency to cause myelosuppression. Likewise, the neurotoxic side effect of peripheral neuropathy can complicate the use of vincristine. Alternating these agents often permits continuation of therapy by sparing the susceptible end organ. Bleomycin and etoposide (VP-16) have also been employed with success. Adriamycin, which is cardiotoxic, is generally reserved for very severe cases but usually provides only limited benefit [107]. Radiation therapy can be helpful for isolated lesions [108,109].

Herpes simplex virus (HSV) can cause recurring mucocutaneous lesions of the perioral and genital areas. The more advanced the state of immunosuppression, the more frequent and chronic these recurrences may become. Chronic mucocutaneous HSV disease for longer than 1 month is an AIDS-defining condition. Lesions characteristically begin as painful erythematous papules that undergo vesiculation and eventually ulcerate. Many patients experience a prodrome of tingling and pain before the appearance of painful vesicles and ulcers. Giant perirectal ulcers and proctitis can be associated with severe rectal pain and obstipation. Anoscopy may be required for diagnosis.

Treatment with oral or intravenous acyclovir usually promotes healing and decreases the pain of HSV lesions. In profoundly immunocompromised patients, the usual dose of acyclovir for mucocutaneous disease is 5 mg per kilogram IV every 8 hours for 7 days [110]. Rapid infusion may lead to renal dysfunction, and care should be taken to infuse this medication slowly over 1 hour. Patients with less severe immunosuppression may respond to acyclovir 200 mg by mouth five times a day for 5 to 7 days. The recent identification of acyclovir-resistant isolates has been a cause for concern, and alternate agents like vidarabine and foscarnet are under investigation [111,112].

Latent varicella zoster virus (VZV) infection frequently reactivates during the course of HIV disease and may be a marker of HIV disease progression [42]. Pruritus and pain in a dermatomal distribution often heralds the development of the characteristic erythematous vesiculopapular eruption. Single dermatomal outbreaks are most common, but a significant number of patients have multidermatomal disease. Cutaneous and visceral dissemination may occur. Postherpetic neuralgia is common and may be unresponsive to medical intervention. High-dose acyclovir, 10 mg per kilogram IV every 8 hours for 7 days, is usually effective if begun within 72 hours of onset [113].

Molluscum contagiosum lesions are painless, pearly white papules with central umbilication that are usually spread by sexual transmission. In HIV-infected patients, these lesions may be multiple, and the distribution may be varied [114]. Giant lesions have been described. Cutaneous cryptococcal infection may mimic molluscum contagiosum, and biopsy may be necessary to differentiate between these two conditions [115].

Drug eruptions are extremely common in HIV-infected patients [116]. Most cutaneous reactions are related to sulfa compounds [117]. The reason for the frequency of these reactions is unknown but is probably related to derangement of the immune system.

PULMONARY DISEASE. The multiple causes of pulmonary disease in patients with HIV infection can be broadly categorized as infectious, neoplastic, or immunologic (Table 93-5). Numerous treatable infectious agents, including organisms such as *Pneumocystis carinii (PCP)*, cytomegalovirus (CMV), fungi, mycobacteria, and encapsulated bacteria, have been described to cause pneumonitis in patients with HIV infection [118]. Pneumonia secondary to pyogenic bacteria occurs frequently in patients with HIV disease and is especially common in IV drug users [119]. Encapsulated bacteria, such as *Streptococcus pneumoniae* and *Haemophilus influenzae*, are the most common pathogens [120]. In contrast to patients with PCP, most of these patients have a productive cough and complain of pleuritic chest pain. Bacterial pneumonia in HIV-infected patients is often associated with bacteremia and tends to have a more abrupt onset than other opportunistic pulmonary pathogens [121]. Noninfectious causes include the malignancies, KS and non-Hodgkin's lymphoma, as well as nonspecific interstitial pneumonitis. A more comprehensive discussion of these pulmonary processes can be found in Chapter 74.

Table 93-5. Pulmonary Involvement in HIV Diseases

Infectious
    Bacteria—*Streptococcus pneumoniae, Haemophilus influenzae, Legionella, Nocardia*
    Mycobacteria—*M. tuberculosis, M. avium* complex
    Fungus—*Cryptococcus neoformans, Coccidiodes immitis, Histoplasma capsulatum, Candidia*
    Viral—CMV, HSV, VZV
    Protozoa—*Pneumocystis carinii*
Neoplastic
    Kaposi's sarcoma
    Non-Hodgkin's lymphoma
Immunologic
    Lymphoid interstitial pneumonitis

CMV = cytomegalovirus, HSV = herpes simplex virus, VZV = varicella zoster virus.

TUBERCULOSIS. Tuberculosis (TB) may present either early or late in the course of HIV infection. The clinical picture varies with the degree of immunosuppression [122,123,124]. TB in the AIDS patient may be the result of reactivation of earlier infection or the result of recent acquisition. The reversal of the downward trend of TB cases in the United States noted in 1985 is primarily the result of TB cases in HIV-infected individuals [125,126]. More common among the black and Hispanic minorities, TB occurs with especially high frequency in the IV drug user population [127].

Tuberculosis most commonly involves the respiratory tract. Pulmonary tuberculosis is an AIDS-defining condition under the revised 1993 case definition. Extrapulmonary TB may occur in 20 to 40 percent of patients and is an AIDS-defining condition [123,124]. The purified protein derivative (PPD) test may be negative if the patient has severe immunosuppression, and a 5-mm reaction should be considered positive [128]. The diagnosis of TB should always be entertained in any HIV-infected patient with pneumonia, and appropriate infection control procedures should be employed until TB is ruled out. Sputum specimens should be stained for acid-fast organisms and cultured for mycobacteria.

AIDS patients usually have an excellent response to antituberculous chemotherapy if the organism has a routine sensitivity pattern. Because of an increase in multidrug–resistant TB in the United States, the CDC now recommends the use of four agents until sensitivity data are available [129]. Once-daily oral administration of isoniazid, 300 mg, rifampin, 600 mg, pyrazinamide, 15 to 30 mg/kg/day, and either ethambutol, 15 mg/kg/day, or streptomycin, 15 mg per kilogram IM (1 gm maximum), should be administered for the first 2 months. The regimen can be altered if sensitivity testing demonstrates a susceptible isolate. The standard duration of therapy is 9 months or for at least 6 months after sputum conversion [130]. Pyridoxine, 50 mg, is given once daily by mouth to prevent the neurotoxicity associated with isoniazid. Isoniazid, rifampin, and pyrazinamide can all cause hepatitis. They should be used judiciously in patients with elevated transaminases. (See Chap. 95 for discussion of how to manage this complication.) Ethambutol can cause optic neuritis. This side effect appears to be dose related, and the first manifestation is usually loss of color vision. Streptomycin is both vestibulo-ototoxic and nephrotoxic.

MYCOBACTERIUM AVIUM **COMPLEX DISEASE.** Nontuberculous mycobacterial disease tends to occur late in the course of HIV infection when patients are more severely immunosuppressed and CD4 counts are less than 100 [131,132,133]. Most of these cases are caused by *M. avium* complex (MAC), ubiquitous environmental saprophytes that usually gain entry through the GI or respiratory tract. In addition to the lungs, infection often involves multiple other organs, including the liver, spleen, lymph nodes, bone marrow, GI tract, and adrenal glands. Because these strains often colonize the respiratory tract in AIDS patients, it may be difficult to ascertain if MAC is actually causing pulmonary disease. For this reason, patients should be thoroughly evaluated for other pulmonary pathogens before attributing respiratory illness to MAC.

The treatment of nontuberculous mycobacterial disease is controversial. As many as 70 percent of selected patients experienced improvement in their constitutional symptoms in one early study involving combination therapy with rifampin, ethambutol, clofazimine, and amikacin (with or without ciprofloxacin) [134]. More recently, a retrospective analysis indicated that patients with MAC infection receiving multidrug therapy had a prolonged life span [135]. However, this has not yet been confirmed in prospective studies, and an optimal therapeutic approach has not been defined. Two newly developed macrolide antibiotics, azithromycin and clarithromycin, have been shown to have activity against MAC [136,137]. The CDC has published recommendations for the treatment of disseminated MAC infection. These interim recommendations suggest that treatment regimens should contain either azithromycin or clarithromycin with at least one of the following agents: ethambutol, clofazamine, rifabutin, rifampin, ciprofloxacin, or amikacin [138,139]. Lifetime treatment is warranted if the patient demonstrates clinical or microbiologic improvement without significant toxicity.

Because of the devastating impact of disseminated MAC disease, patients with CD4 counts less than 100 should receive lifelong prophylaxis against MAC. Although azithromycin and clarithromycin have shown laboratory and clinical activity against MAC, only rifabutin, 300 mg po daily, has been demonstrated to prevent or delay serious MAC disease [140].

CARDIOVASCULAR MANIFESTATIONS. Most cardiac abnormalities associated with AIDS are secondary to neoplasms and opportunistic infections [141]. The asymptomatic incidence of cardiac involvement in AIDS is high. Echocardiograms commonly show fractional shortening, pericardial effusions, and other findings not appreciated clinically [142,143]. Endocarditis is a frequent occurrence in IV drug users and may involve unusual organisms. Nonbacterial thrombotic endocarditis has also been reported. Pericardial disease with effusion is most often secondary to *M. tuberculosis, M. avium* complex, *Cryptococcus neoformans,* and cytomegalovirus [144,145]. Fibrinous pericarditis of uncertain origin has also been reported. Occasionally pericardial effusions are associated with tamponade [146]. The myocardium may be involved with KS, lymphoma, or toxoplasmosis [147,148]. Cardiac dysfunction related to the use of interferon-alpha has been described [149,150]. *Torsades de pointes* during IV pentamidine infusion has been reported [151,152,153]. Ventricular tachycardia has been reported in AIDS patients receiving ganciclovir [154].

Cardiomyopathy is another severe manifestation and is associated with a high overall mortality [155,156,157]. Although direct HIV infection of myocytes has been suggested [158,159], the exact cause has not been defined. It is possible that HIV has a direct toxic effect on myocytes. Alternatively, cardiotoxic cytokines like tumor necrosis factor may have an indirect effect. Antiretroviral cardiac toxicity has also been implicated [160–163]. The recognition that HIV-infected individuals with other risk factors for heart disease have an increased likelihood of having cardiac abnormalities at autopsy [164] makes it important to search for other factors that may possibly contribute to cardiac dysfunction.

RENAL DISEASE. The existence of HIV-related renal dysfunction has been difficult to prove because most patients in whom the condition has been implicated have multiple other risk factors for kidney disease. Blacks appear to be more susceptible to this condition than Hispanics or whites, and it appears to occur more frequently in IV drug users than in other risk groups [165]. Although HIV has been demonstrated in the renal epithelium of patients with HIV-associated nephropathy, the exact pathophysiologic mechanism remains unclear [166,167]. In terms of laboratory findings, most patients with AIDS-associated nephropathy demonstrate proteinuria and an elevated serum creatinine level [168]. Autopsy or biopsy specimens show focal or segmental sclerosis similar to heroin nephropathy [169,170]. Some patients may unexpectedly develop rapidly progressive renal failure that requires hemodialysis [171,172]. The prognosis for AIDS patients requiring maintenance hemodialysis is very poor, with most patients dying within a few months after its initiation. However, asymptomatic HIV seropositive and ARC patients may have prolonged survival on dialysis [173].

Interestingly, recent reports suggest that antiretroviral therapy with zidovudine may have a favorable impact on proteinuria and renal function in some patients with HIV-associated nephropathy [174,175].

Other causes of renal disease in HIV patients include the nephrotoxic drugs used to treat opportunistic infection, such as amphotericin B, pentamidine, foscarnet, and the aminoglycosides. Involvement of the kidneys with fungal or mycobacterial infections may also occur as a result of systemic disease.

ENDOCRINE MANIFESTATIONS. Although endocrine abnormalities are not a salient feature of AIDS, opportunistic infection, malignancy, and medications may all affect the endocrine system [177].

The adrenal gland appears to be the most commonly affected endocrine gland in AIDS [178,179,180]. Although postmortem examination frequently shows involvement of the adrenal gland, clinical adrenal insufficiency is uncommon [181,182,183]. KS, cytomegalovirus, MAC, and *Cryptococcus neoformans* have all been reported to involve the adrenals [180]. Despite extensive involvement by tumor or infection, clinical adrenal insufficiency is distinctly uncommon in most HIV-infected individuals. Several studies have demonstrated a normal cortisol response after adrenocorticotropic hormone (ACTH) stimulation in patients with early HIV disease or ARC but a subnormal response in those with AIDS [181,182]. These findings may indicate that the adrenal glands of AIDS patients have a limited ability to respond to stress. The neurotropic tendency of HIV may account for the necrosis of the adrenal medulla seen in some AIDS patients [184]. Ketoconazole, an antifungal agent that interferes with cytochrome P-450 enzyme activity, may produce adrenal insufficiency [185,186]. The degree of adrenal insufficiency is usually dose related and reversible after drug cessation [187]. Rifampin can increase hepatic cytochrome P-450 activity and alter cortisol metabolism and may result in a decrease in cortisol bioavailability [188,189].

Hyponatremia occurs frequently in patients with AIDS and has multiple causes [180]. The syndrome of inappropriate antidiuretic hormone (SIADH) may occur as a result of CNS or pulmonary involvement as well as medication effect. Adrenal insufficiency can also contribute to the development of hyponatremia.

Hypoglycemia secondary to IV pentamidine therapy is a well-recognized complication associated with the use of this drug [190,191]. The mechanism of hypoglycemia appears to be secondary to a direct lytic effect of pentamidine on the pancreatic beta islet cell resulting in a nonphysiologic release of insulin. Sustained glucose intolerance or diabetes mellitus may ensue as a consequence of islet cell damage. All patients undergoing therapy with pentamidine should be monitored for the development of hypoglycemia. In some cases, seizures may occur. The periods of hypoglycemia may be brief or prolonged and may occur during or after the course of therapy. Renal insufficiency may promote the development of hypoglycemia.

Calcium metabolism may be affected by the use of aminoglycosides and amphotericin B, both of which can cause magnesium wasting and result in hypocalcemia [192,193]. Significant renal losses of potassium may also occur with the use of amphotericin. Hyperkalemia has been reported in 16 to 21 percent of hospitalized AIDS patients [194,195,196]. Hyperkalemia may also occur in AIDS patients receiving high doses of

trimethoprim in combination with sulfamethoxazole or dapsone during therapy for PCP [197]. The structural similarity of trimethoprim to the potassium-sparing diuretics amiloride and triamterene may account for this effect [198]. Foscarnet has also been associated with significant derangement of calcium, magnesium, and phosphate homeostasis. The euthyroid sick syndrome may occur, but clinical hypothyroidism is rare.

GASTROINTESTINAL DISEASE. The oral cavity may demonstrate a variety of abnormalities throughout the course of HIV infection [199]. Most common of these is oral candidiasis, which is also referred to as thrush. Characteristic white plaques that can be easily removed by scraping with a tongue blade may be seen on the dorsum of the tongue, soft palate, and buccal mucosa. An atrophic form of candidiasis may produce flat, red plaques without overlying white exudate in the same areas. Angular cheilitis, the result of infection with *Candida* at the corners of the mouth, can present as painful fissures, which in some cases may impair oral intake.

Thrush usually responds well to oral antifungal agents. Clotrimazole troches five times a day, ketoconazole, 200 mg twice a day, and fluconazole, 100 mg once daily, are all effective. Angular cheilitis often responds to topical antifungal therapy with either clotrimazole 1% or ketoconazole 2% cream.

Oral hairy leukoplakia (OHL) is observed during more advanced stages of HIV infection [200]. Its name is derived from the furry or hairy appearance of the lesions. OHL is characterized by asymptomatic fine, white, vertical striations on the lateral aspects or undersurface of the tongue. There is evidence that OHL is the result of Epstein-Barr virus (EBV) infection of the epithelium of the buccal mucosa and tongue [201]. Although the natural history of OHL is to wax and wane, some patients appear to have regression of their lesions on high-dose acyclovir. The major significance of OHL is as a prognostic indicator of rapid progression to AIDS within subsequent years [43].

Severe, necrotizing gingivitis and periodontitis can occur in HIV disease. Patients may complain of severe dental pain, bleeding gums, loose teeth, and halitosis. The cause of the gingivitis and periodontal disease has not been clearly established, but both aerobic and anaerobic flora have been implicated. Chlorhexidine rinses (Peridex), oral penicillin or metronidazole, and meticulous dental hygiene often have a favorable impact.

Aphthous ulcers of the oral cavity can also be seen in HIV disease. In some cases, the ulcers are large and painful enough to interfere with oral intake. The cause is uncertain, but HIV itself is thought to be responsible. Topical therapy with steroid creams such as Kenalog in Orabase three or four times a day usually results in improvement. Infrequently, systemic treatment with prednisone, 1 mg/kg/day, may be required.

Esophageal disease is common in patients with HIV infection. Both infectious and malignant involvement can occur, with most of these processes being AIDS-defining conditions. Patients usually present with odynophagia and dysphagia. Decreased oral intake and weight loss are often seen. In the infectious category, *Candida*, HSV, cytomegalovirus, and HIV itself are the most common causative agents [202,203]. Involvement of the esophagus with either lymphoma or KS may also occur. A number of patients have been described with idiopathic steroid-responsive esophageal ulcerations.

An empiric trial of antifungal therapy with an imidazole or amphotericin B may be warranted if the patient has extensive thrush [204]. Ketoconazole, 200 mg twice a day, and fluconazole, 100 mg once a day for 2 to 3 weeks, are both effective. Optimal absorption of ketoconazole requires an acid stomach pH. The use of H2 blockers or antacids may impair absorption. Amphotericin B, 0.3 mg/kg/day IV for 7 to 10 days, can be used in patients unable to tolerate oral medication or who have triazole-resistant isolates such as *Candida krusei*. Because some patients may have coexistent disease with one or more of the causative agents listed above, the most reliable approach is upper endoscopy, which usually provides the diagnosis by direct observation, culture, and biopsy data. Endoscopy should be performed if the condition fails to respond to empiric antifungal therapy within 3 to 5 days. If HSV is identified, acyclovir, 200 mg po five times daily, is usually effective. A patient with the finding of CMV on biopsy should initially be treated with ganciclovir, 5 mg/kg IV bid daily. In patients with esophageal ulcerations in whom no pathogen or malignancy can be indentified, an empiric trial of prednisone, 40 to 60 mg po qd, may be effective [205,206].

Gastritis secondary to cytomegalovirus can produce extensive ulceration throughout the stomach. Patients present with complaints of nausea, vomiting, abdominal pain, and occasionally hematemesis. Barium studies are usually abnormal but not specific. Definitive diagnosis can usually be made by an endoscopic procedure. KS of the stomach is usually asymptomatic but can be associated with nausea, abdominal pain, and occasionally obstruction or hemorrhage [207]. Gastric lymphoma may present with symptoms similar to those of KS, and evidence of lymphoma is usually present elsewhere. Endoscopic evaluation is usually necessary for diagnosis.

Acalculous cholecystitis has been reported in AIDS patients who present with fever, right upper quadrant pain, and an elevated alkaline phosphatase. Ultrasound or computed tomography (CT) scanning usually shows the findings typically associated with cholecystitis. Both cryptosporidium and CMV have been implicated as responsible pathogens [208,209].

Sclerosing cholangitis and papillary stenosis have also been described in AIDS patients [210,211]. The presentation is similar to cholecystitis, with the findings of fever, right upper quadrant tenderness, and an elevated alkaline phosphatase. Cryptosporidium, microsporidium, and CMV are often found to be associated with both of these conditions [212,213,214]. Ultrasonography usually shows dilatation of the intrahepatic and extrahepatic ducts. Endoscopic retrograde cholangiopancreatography usually demonstrates irregularity of the ducts or stenosis at the papilla of Vater. Sphincterotomy usually results in a reduction in pain and a decrease in the alkaline phosphatase.

Liver disease occurs frequently in the HIV-infected patients [215–218]. Although alcohol and hepatotoxic drugs can cause elevated transaminases, viral injury secondary to hepatitis A, B, C, and D as well as CMV probably accounts for most cases of liver abnormalities. Involvement of the liver with MAC, TB, fungi, KS, and lymphoma can all cause hepatic disease in patients with HIV infection. Liver biopsy may be necessary to make a definitive diagnosis.

Pancreatitis secondary to ddI and ddC has been reported [77,78]. Although most patients have only asymptomatic amylase elevation, some patients develop symptoms consistent with clinical pancreatitis. A small but significant number of patients have had fulminant fatal pancreatitis with little or no warning. Some of these patients have died despite aggressive intervention.

Small and large bowel disease as a result of infection or malignancy frequently causes GI distress for patients with AIDS [219,220,221]. Infectious causes include *Salmonella, Shigella, Campylobacter, Cryptosporidium,* Microsporidia, and *Isospora* species. Novel enteric viruses such as astrovirus and picobirvirus have also been associated with diarrhea in HIV-infected patients [222]. Although some patients are asymptomatic, many complain of diarrhea and abdominal cramping with or without fever. In some patients, the diarrhea is associated with massive volume depletion, weight loss, and electrolyte imbalance requiring aggressive repletion.

There is no effective treatment for cryptosporidial or microsporidial enteritis. Some patients may improve on zidovudine. Both oral and IV spiramycin have been used, but the results have been disappointing. The use of a somatostatin analog has been reported to decrease diarrheal output in some patients [223,224,225]. *Isospora* infection usually responds well to TMP-SMZ (trimethoprim, 160 mg, sulfamethoxazole, 800 mg) four times a day for 2 weeks, but relapse is common. In sulfa-intolerant patients, pyrimethamine or metronidazole may be effective.

Colitis and proctitis are often associated with tenesmus and crampy lower abdominal pain. *Entamoeba histolytica, Giardia lamblia,* HSV, CMV, and *Clostridium difficile* should be considered as possible pathogens in patients with lower bowel symptoms. Stool studies usually show the responsible pathogen in most symptomatic patients. In patients in whom the cause cannot be ascertained from examination of the stool, colonoscopy with biopsy may be required to establish the diagnosis.

NERVOUS SYSTEM INVOLVEMENT. Ninety percent of AIDS patients demonstrate some type of affective, cognitive, or psychomotor abnormalities; measurable impairment appears to develop early in the course of overall HIV disease [226]. Aseptic meningitis secondary to HIV may occur during acute retroviral infection but also can occur in a more chronic form [227,228,229]. In both situations, meningeal signs may be minimal or absent, and the cerebrospinal fluid (CSF) may show only a mild pleocytosis and a slight elevation of the CSF protein.

HIV encephalopathy is a progressive neurologic syndrome that is the direct result of HIV infection of the CNS white matter. Memory loss, difficulty with concentration, and slowed mentation are typical of early HIV encephalopathy. At this stage of illness, head CT scans show generalized atrophy advanced for the patient's age [230]. Magnetic resonance imaging (MRI) also demonstrates cerebral atrophy as well as increased signal intensity in the subcortical white matter. CSF analysis is usually not helpful and often shows only a slight CSF pleocytosis with a normal glucose and modestly elevated protein. Late HIV encephalopathy is characterized by more dramatic changes. Patients display serious cognitive impairment with behavioral changes and severe memory loss [231,232,233]. Profound weakness, psychomotor retardation, and seizures may occur. Cranial CT and MRI scans demonstrate even more severe cerebral atrophy and changes in the white matter. The diagnosis of HIV encephalopathy is made clinically by excluding other causes of encephalopathy, malignancy, and opportunistic infection. Routine biopsy of the brain is not usually required. In some patients with early HIV encephalitis, therapy with zidovudine has resulted in significant improvement.

Symptomatic peripheral nerve disease occurs frequently in AIDS patients [234,235]. The most common HIV-associated peripheral neuropathy is a sensory polyneuropathy characterized by chronic, bilateral painful dysesthesias in a stocking glove distribution [236]. Pain with light touch and numbness are the most common complaints. Ankle reflexes may be decreased or absent, and motor weakness may be observed because of the lack of any effective therapy. Many patients require narcotics to control their chronic pain.

Acute or chronic inflammatory demyelinating polyneuropathy can occur secondary to HIV or CMV [237,238,239]. These patients predominantly have findings of motor weakness but only minimal sensory abnormalities. Prolonged therapy with ganciclovir may improve CMV polyradiculopathy. Guillain-Barré syndrome, vacuolar myelopathy, and transverse myelitis have also been reported [240].

Central nervous system toxoplasmosis is responsible for the majority of intracranial mass lesions observed in AIDS patients [241,242]. Approximately 75 percent of patients with CNS toxoplasmosis have altered mental status. Approximately half complain of headache. Focal neurologic findings such as hemiparesis or ataxia are common. Fever occurs in fewer than half of the patients. Although the onset may be subacute, some patients may have a fulminant presentation with seizures. CT scanning with contrast typically shows ring-enhancing lesions. If the head CT is negative, and the clinical suspicion is high, an MRI scan should be performed. MRI will often show multiple lesions, particularly in the basal ganglia, if the patient has CNS toxoplasmosis. *Toxoplasma* serology is neither sensitive nor specific and is not a reliable test on which to base treatment decisions [243].

Patients with a consistent clinical presentation and typical ring-enhancing lesions on head CT often receive empiric therapy for presumptive CNS toxoplasmosis with pyrimethamine, 50 to 100 mg PO once daily, sulfadiazine, 1.5 to 2.0 gm PO every 6 to 8 hours, and folinic acid, 10 to 20 mg per day. Although not FDA approved for this indication, clindamycin, 600 to 900 mg IV three times per day or 600 mg po four times per day, has been used as an alternative agent in patients who are intolerant of sulfa [242,244]. Azithromycin and atovaquone are also under investigation for the treatment of CNS toxoplasmosis [245,246]. Response to therapy is usually quite rapid, with more than half of patients displaying a response within 3 days and 86 percent showing a response by day 7 [242]. If the patient displays signs of further clinical deterioration or a lack of a clinical or radiographic response after 10 to 14 days of empiric therapy, a brain biopsy should be strongly considered to establish a diagnosis. Primary CNS lymphoma, which has an extremely poor prognosis even with aggressive intervention, may mimic CNS toxoplasmosis. Because of its high relapse rate, patients with CNS toxoplasmosis require chronic suppressive therapy with one or more of the above agents to prevent recrudescence [247].

Progressive multifocal leukoencephalopathy (PML) is a disease of the cerebral white matter characterized by multiple discrete areas of demyelination [248]. Papovavirus is thought to be the causative agent of this disorder. Usual symptoms of PML include headache, confusion, hemiparesis, and ataxia. Contrast CT scan of the head may show low-density, nonenhancing lesions involving the periventricular white matter. MRI scans demonstrate nonenhancing lesions with high signal intensity. CSF analysis is usually nonspecific, and the diagnosis can be established only by brain biopsy. There is no definite therapy, although some patients may manifest improvement while on antiretroviral therapy [249]. Progressive deterioration over time is the usual course.

Other causes of encephalitis in the AIDS patient include VZV and CMV [250,251]. If recognized early, both of these conditions may respond to appropiate antiviral therapy.

Cryptococcal meningitis usually has a subtle presentation with nonspecific complaints of headache and photophobia as the only symptoms [252,253,254]. Meningeal signs are usually absent, and focal neurologic deficits are rare [254]. The diagnosis of cryptococcal meningitis can be made by serum cryptococcal antigen assays (sensitivity 90–95%) and by lumbar puncture [255,256]. The CSF cellular and chemical findings are usually not helpful and typically disclose a mild pleocytosis with a slightly elevated protein. Although India ink examination may show the organism in more than half of cases, it has been supplanted by the cryptococcal antigen test, which is positive in more than 95 percent of cases. Most patients have a positive CSF fungal culture.

The most important predictor of early mortality for cryptococcal meningitis is abnormal mental status at the time of initial presentation. Other factors predictive of a poor outcome include a high opening pressure, a low CSF white blood cell count (WBC) (less than 20), a CSF cryptococcal antigen titer greater than 1:1024, hyponatremia, and age younger than 35 years [254,256]. A patient with these risk factors should initially receive IV amphotericin rather than fluconazole. If there is clinical and laboratory improvement after 2 to 3 weeks of IV amphotericin, the patient can usually be switched cautiously to fluconazole to complete another 8 to 10 weeks of therapy. Patients who do not respond to IV amphotericin should be reevaluated for other causes of CNS compromise.

Standard therapy for severe acute HIV-associated cryptococcal meningitis involves the use of amphotericin B, 0.7 mg/kg/day IV [255,257]. Patients may require as much as 15 mg per kilogram total dose to clear the CSF. Although many AIDS patients do not tolerate 5-flucytosine because of its myelosuppressive effects, it may be of benefit when used in combination with amphotericin in patients with severe disease [254]. Fluconazole, 200 to 400 mg daily, has been shown to be effective alone in the treatment of acute cryptococcal meningitis [258,259]. Serial lumbar punctures should be performed to demonstrate a decrease in the cryptococcal antigen and conversion of the CSF cultures.

Because of the serious adverse effects and quality of life issues associated with IV amphotericin, liposomal amphotericin, high-dose fluconazole 600 to 2,000 mg/day, and combination therapy with fluconazole plus flucytosine are under investigation.

Because cryptococcal meningitis has a very high recurrence rate, prophylactic therapy is required to prevent relapse. Amphotericin, 1 mg per kilogram administered once per week intravenously, or fluconazole, 200 mg PO per day, have both been shown to be effective [255,260,261]. Recent evidence suggests that fluconazole is more efficacious and better tolerated than amphotericin B for maintenance therapy [262].

Other less common causes of meningitis in patients with HIV infection include *M. tuberculosis, Histoplasma capsulatum,* and *Candida albicans.*

OCULAR COMPLICATIONS. Several causative agents have been associated with retinitis in the AIDS patient [263]. These include CMV, toxoplasmosis, and syphilis. Cottonwool spots are very common in patients with AIDS and are thought to be secondary to HIV [264,265]. These fluffy exudates tend to wax and wane but usually do not affect vision. CMV is by far the most common cause and is an AIDS-defining condition [266,267,268]. The onset may be rapid but is more often insidious. Patients with CMV retinitis usually give a history of blurred vision, scotoma, or decreased visual acuity. Unilateral presentation accounts for most cases, but the opposite eye often eventually becomes involved. On funduscopic examination, areas of white exudate with surrounding hemorrhage and edema are seen. Blood and urine cultures for CMV are usually positive.

Intravenous ganciclovir was the first agent shown to be effective in the treatment of CMV retinitis [269]. Acute treatment consists of twice-daily IV administration of ganciclovir, 5 mg per kilogram, for 2 weeks followed by lifetime suppressive IV maintenance therapy with 5 mg per kilogram 7 days per week. The major adverse effect of ganciclovir is neutropenia, which often necessitates the discontinuation of AZT. The coadministration of colony-stimulating factors with ganciclovir shows promise [270,271].

Foscarnet, which is active against both HIV and CMV, has also been shown to be effective in the treatment of CMV retinitis [272,273,274]. In a recent study, foscarnet and ganciclovir showed comparable efficacy for CMV retinitis, but patients receiving foscarnet had a more prolonged survival, possibly because of its antiretroviral activity [275]. Standard induction dosing of foscarnet for acute retinitis is 60 mg per kilogram IV q8h for 14 days followed by daily IV maintenance therapy with 90 to 120 mg per kilogram for life to prevent recurrence. The major toxicities of foscarnet are renal impairment, hypokalemia, and ionic fluxes of calcium and magnesium that may lead to seizures. Combination therapy with ganciclovir and foscarnet may be more effective than either agent alone in treating CMV in AIDS patients [276].

HEMATOLOGIC MANIFESTATIONS. The cytopenias, anemia, leukopenia, and thrombocytopenia, are frequently seen in HIV-infected patients [277]. In general, anemia and leukopenia appear to be related to primary HIV infection of hematopoietic precursors. Thrombocytopenia may also relate to such infection or to immune-mediated processes [278]. Infiltration of the bone marrow by opportunistic pathogens, especially MAC, *Histoplasma,* and *Cryptococcus,* or by neoplasms like B cell lymphoma, can interfere with effective hematopoiesis. Certain therapeutic agents such as sulfa, dapsone, pyrimethamine, amphotericin, and ZDV can also impair bone marrow function.

Multiple factors may account for the normochromic, normocytic anemia commonly seen in patients with HIV disease. Infection of erythroid precursors by HIV itself may inhibit the production of red cells [279]. Parvovirus B19 infection can cause profound anemia in HIV-positive patients that may respond to treatment with high-dose IV gamma globulin [280]. Splenic sequestration can also contribute to anemia. Depressed erythropoietin elaboration by an undefined mechanism also may result in decreased red cell production. Exogenous administration of recombinant erythropoietin may raise the hematocrit in some patients with endogenous erythropoietin levels less than 500 μg per milliliter [281,282]. Infiltration of the bone marrow by opportunistic pathogens or malignancy can impair erythropoiesis. Some of the medications given to HIV patients may result in red cell suppression or destruction. Drugs such as zidovudine and sulfa compounds can cause macrocytic anemia.

Leukopenia is common in HIV disease. Although lymphopenia is characteristic, neutropenia may also occur [277]. In some patients, antineutrophil antibodies may be an important mechanism for granulocytopenia. Based on the response of patients with other types of autoimmune neutropenia, treatment with high doses of IV gamma globulin may increase circulating levels of granulocytes in these HIV-infected patients [283,284]. Multiple drugs can lead to impairment of white cell production. Zidovudine, ganciclovir, TMP-SMZ, pyrimethamine, sulfadiazine, dapsone, amphotericin, and some chemotherapeutic agents are all associated with myelosuppression. Recombinant human colony-stimulating factors have been shown to effectively increase white cell production in severely leukopenic AIDS patients with impaired hematopoiesis [281, 285]. The co-administration of colony-stimulating factors with myelosuppressive agents like zidovudine and ganciclovir often allows continuation of therapy.

Thrombocytopenia has been reported to occur in as many as 5 to 15 percent of HIV-seropositive individuals. Peripheral destruction of platelets on an immune basis clearly contributes to HIV-related cases of thrombocytopenia. Many of these patients have specific platelet membrane antigens against which antibodies are directed [278]. Although bone marrow examination usually shows normal or increased production of megakaryocytes, recent kinetic studies have shown that a decreased rate of platelet production makes a major contribution to the thrombocytopenic state. Although petechiae, easy bruisability, and prolonged bleeding may be early manifestations of thrombocytopenia, most patients are asymptomatic and are incidentally found to have low platelet levels during routine laboratory investigation. Spontaneous severe bleeding occurs infrequently and is usually related to underlying mucosal damage. Splenomegaly is often detected by physical examination or abdominal CT scanning [286]. Drug-induced thrombocytopenia also occurs, particularly in alcoholics or IV drug users whose street drugs are cut with such compounds as quinine.

The administration of zidovudine is often associated with a reversal of the immune thrombocytopenia seen in many HIV-seropositive patients, and increased platelet counts may occur while on therapy [287]. Danazol and vincristine have also been used with limited success. High doses of intravenous immunoglobulin infused intermittently have also been used successfully in some patients. In general, the chronic use of steroids is not routinely recommended because of the potential for further immunosuppression, but glucocorticoids are often quite effective when the previous modalities fail. Splenectomy or splenic irradiation may be necessary for patients with severe thrombocytopenia or significant episodes of bleeding [288–291].

PSYCHIATRIC MANIFESTATIONS. The psychiatric aspects of HIV disease are diverse and complex. Anxiety, depression, dysthymia, and substance abuse are common and may interfere with treatment [292,293]. There is an increased risk of suicide for HIV-infected persons. Several early studies reported the relative risk of suicide for AIDS patients to be 7 to 36 times that of demographically similar groups [294,295]. Times of greatest risk appear to coincide with time of initial HIV diagnosis, guilt related to infecting another person, loss of a job or loved one, drop in CD4 count, first illness or hospitalization, diagnosis of AIDS, termination of aggressive treatment, painful or debilitating disease, and impending death. Overdose secondary to illicit drugs or prescription antidepressants and benzodiazepines is a common method that often results in the need for intensive care. Although mild depression may be the baseline for these patients, suicidal or homicidal ideation is not. Therapeutic support in a controlled environment is often effective in maintaining patients through periods of severe depression until the suicidal/homicidal ideation resolves. See Chapter 227 for a complete discussion of the neuropsychiatric aspects of AIDS.

Fever of Unknown Origin

The approach to fever of unknown origin in the AIDS patient is a challenging task because of the myriad possible causes. Often clues to the source of fever can be ascertained from the history, physical examination, or routine laboratory tests. Despite intensive evaluation, some patients continue to have unexplained fever. In many of these patients, fever is ultimately attributable to mycobacterial, viral (CMV), or fungal disease [296]. Although easily obtainable, mycobacterial and fungal blood cultures are a relatively slow and nonspecific method to establish a diagnosis [297]. Liver biopsy in patients with unexplained fever and liver abnormalities appears to be a rapid and reliable method for detecting occult mycobacterial or fungal infection [298]. The presence of organisms or granulomas may suggest the diagnosis in up to 75 percent of such cases. Bone marrow biopsy has a lower yield (25%) but is associated with less morbidity and mortality. Although a recent study indicates that urine and blood cultures for CMV are neither sensitive nor specific, positive cultures may provide an important clue to look for clinically significant disease [299]. Intravenous drug users pose a special problem because of their risk for infective endocarditis [300]. Finally, drugs and tumor should always be considered as possible causes of fever.

Advice for Health Care Workers

There is a small but definite risk of infection with HIV for individuals working in the laboratory or hospital setting. To date, at least 36 health care workers have become infected with HIV after occupational exposure [301]. Thirty-one sustained percutaneous injury by a needle contaminated with body fluids from an HIV-infected patient; four had mucocutaneous injuries; and one had both. Still, the risk of HIV infection by needlestick is quite low, estimated to be approximately 0.4 percent [302]. Although a small number of health care workers have become infected after mucocutaneous exposure to blood from an HIV-infected individual, the risk of such exposure is so low it cannot be quantified in prospective studies.

Because most individuals infected with HIV do not display signs or symptoms of infection, the CDC has recommended that health care workers should treat blood and body fluids from all patients as if they are potentially infectious. This concept has been referred to as universal precautions [303]. One should always use gloves when drawing blood or handling any body fluid. A gown and eye goggles or eye shields should be worn whenever blood or body fluid splattering is anticipated. When spills occur, surfaces contaminated with HIV-infected material can be disinfected with 1:10 dilution of sodium hypochlorite (household bleach). All mucocutaneous exposures or needlestick punctures that involve contaminated blood or body fluids should be reported to the Infection Control or Employee Health Department.

Although routinely advocated at some centers, the CDC has not recommended the use of zidovudine after a critical exposure because of the lack of supportive data [304]. A prophylactic trial with zidovudine after massive exposure to HIV in health care or laboratory workers was discontinued because of low enrollment. Because of the low toxicity with short-course therapy, the psychological trauma associated with high-risk HIV exposure, and the possible small therapeutic benefit, zidovudine prophylaxis is offered in many institutions to individuals with known high-risk HIV exposures. The failure of zidovudine prophylaxis to prevent HIV infection despite rapid IV administration immediately after exposure has been reported [305]. Thus, the role of zidovudine for prophylaxis in various types of exposures is still undefined.

References

1. Dobkin JF: AIDS, ethics, and ICU's. *Infections in Medicine* 10(6):16, 1993.
2. Lemp GF, Payne SF, Neal D, et al: Survival trends for patients with AIDS. *JAMA* 263:402, 1990.
3. Chaisson RE: Editorial: Living with AIDS. *JAMA* 263:434, 1990.
4. Gail MH, Rosenberg PS, Goedert JJ: Therapy may explain recent deficits in AIDS incidence. *J Acquir Immune Defic Syndr* 3:296, 1990.
5. Graham et al: Survival of early treatment of human immunodeficiency virus infection. *N Engl J Med* 326:1037, 1992.
6. Barre-Sinoussi F, Chermann JC, Rey F, et al: Isolation of T-lymphotropic retrovirus from a patient at risk for acquired immunodeficiency syndrome (AIDS). *Science* 220:868, 1983.
7. Gallo RC, Salahudin SZ, Popovic M, et al: Frequent detection and isolation of cytopathic retroviruses (HTLV-III) from patients with AIDS and at risk for AIDS. *Science* 224:500, 1984.
8. Levy JA, Hoffman AD, Kramer SD, et al: Isolation of lymphocytopathic retrovirus from San Francisco patients with AIDS. *Science* 225:840, 1984.
9. Clavel F, et al: Isolation of a new human retrovirus from West African patients with AIDS. *Science* 233:343, 1986.
10. Dalgleish A et al: The CD4 (T4) antigen is an essential component of the reception for the AIDS virus. *Nature* 312:763, 1984.
11. Klatzman D, Champagne E, Chamaret S, et al: T-Lymphocyte T4 molecule behaves as receptor for human retrovirus LAV. *Nature* 312:767, 1984.
12. Cheng-Mayer C, Rutha JT, Rosenblum ML, et al: The human immunodeficiency virus (HIV) can productively infect cultured human glial cells. *Proc Natl Acad Sci USA* 84:3526, 1987.
13. Tateno M, Gonzalez-Scarano F, Levy JA: The human immunodeficiency virus can infect CD4-negative human fibroblastoid cells. *Proc Natl Acad Sci USA* 86:4287, 1989.
14. Fauci AS, Schnittman SM, Poli G, et al: Immunopathogenetic mechanisms in human immunodeficiency virus infection. *Ann Intern Med* 114:678, 1991.
15. Pantaleo G, Graziosi C, Fauci AS: The immunopathogenesis of human immunodeficiency virus infection. *N Engl J Med* 328:327, 1993.
16. Brew BJ: Medical management of AIDS patients: Central and peripheral nervous system abnormalities. *Med Clin North Am* 76(1):63, 1992.
17. Centers for Disease Control and Prevention. HIV/AIDS Surveillance Report. *MMWR* 5(No. 3):7, 1993.
18. World Health Organization: Current and future dimensions of the HIV/AIDS pandemic: A capsule summary. *Who/GPA/SFI/90* 2 September:1990.
19. Summary of notifiable diseases, United States 1992. *MMWR* 41:18, 1992.
20. Marcus Rand, CDC Cooperative Needlestick Surveillance Group: Surveillance of health care workers exposed to blood from patients with the human immunodeficiency virus. *N Engl J Med* 319:1118, 1988.
21. Centers for Disease Control: Update: Serologic testing for antibody to human immunodeficiency virus. *MMWR* 36:833, 1988.
22. Meyer RB, Pauker SG: Sounding Board: Screening for HIV: Can we afford the false positive rate? *N Engl J Med* 317(4):238, 1987.
23. Horsburgh CR Jr, Ou Cy, Jason J, et al: Duration of human immunodeficiency virus infection before detection of antibody. *Lancet* 2:637, 1989.
24. Guyader M, Emerman M, Sonigo P, et al: Genome organization and transactivation of the human immunodeficiency virus type 2. *Nature* 326:662, 1987.
25. Ou CY, Kwok S, Mitchell SW, et al: DNA amplification for direct detection of HIV-1 DNA of peripheral blood mononuclear cells. *Science* 239:295, 1988.
26. Saiki RK, Gelfand DH, Stoffel S, et al: Primer-directed enzymatic amplification of DNA with a thermostable DNA polymerase. *Science* 239:487, 1988.
27. Gostin LO: Public health strategies for confronting AIDS: Legislative and regulatory policy in the United States. *JAMA* 261:1621, 1989.
28. Cooper DA, Gold J, MacLean P, et al: Acute AIDS retrovirus infection: Definition of a clinical illness associated with seroconversion. *Lancet* 1:1376, 1985.
29. Needlestick transmission of HTLV-III from a patient infected in Africa. *Lancet* 2:1376, 1984.
30. Tindall B, Lindhardt BO, Jensen BL, et al: Characteristics of the acute clinical illness associated with human immunodeficiency virus infection. *Arch Intern Med* 148(4):945, 1988.

31. Pedersen C, Lindhardt BO, Jensen BL et al: Clinical course of primary HIV infection: Consequences for the subsequent course of infection. Abstract presented at the 5th International AIDS Conference. 5th International AIDS Conference 1989. (Abstract)

32. Pantaleo G, Graziosi C, Demarest JF, et al: HIV infection is active and progressive in lymphoid tissue during the clinically latent stage of disease. *Nature* 362:355, 1993.

33. Abrams DI, Lewis BJ, Beckstead JP, et al: Persistent diffuse lymphadenopathy in homosexual men: Endpoint or prodrome? *Ann Intern Med* 100:801, 1984.

34. Abrams DI: Lymphadenopathy syndrome in male homosexuals, in Gallin JI, Fauci AS (eds): *Acquired Immunodefiency Syndrome. Advances in Host Defense Mechanisms.* Vol 5. New York, Raven Press, 1985, pp 75–97.

35. Abrams DI: AIDS-related conditions. *Clin Immun Allergy* 6:581, 1986.

36. Centers for Disease Control: Opportunistic infections and Kaposi's sarcoma among Haitians in the United States. *MMWR* 31:353, 1982.

37. Centers for Disease Control: Update on acquired immunodeficiency syndrome (AIDS)—United States. *MMWR* 31:507, 1982.

38. Center for Disease Control: Update: Acquired immunodeficiency syndrome—United States. *MMWR* 34:245, 1985.

39. Centers for Disease Control: Revision classification system for HIV infection and expanded surveillance case definition for AIDS among adolescents and adults. *MMWR* 44:1992.

40. Centers for Disease Control: Revision of the CDC surveillance case definition for acquired immunodeficiency syndrome. *MMWR* 36(suppl):I, 1987.

41. Klein RS, Harris CA, Small CB, et al: Oral candidiasis in high-risk patients as the initial manifestation of the acquired immunodeficiency syndrome. *N Engl J Med* 311(6):354, 1984.

42. Friedman-Kien AE, Lafleur FL, Gendler E, et al: Herpes zoster: A possible early clinical sign for development of acquired immunodeficiency syndrome in high-risk individuals. *J Am Acad Dermatol* 14:1023, 1986.

43. Greenspan D, Greenspan JS, Hearst NG, et al: Relation of oral hairy leukoplakia to infection with the human immunodeficiency virus and the risk of developing AIDS. *J Infect Dis* 155:475, 1987.

44. Melbye M, Grossman RJ, Goedert JJ, et al: Risk of AIDS after herpes zoster. Lancet 1:728, 1987.

45. Haverkos HW, Drotman DP: Prevalence of Kaposi's sarcoma among patients with AIDS. *N Engl J Med* 312:1518, 1985.

46. Rogers MF, Morens DM, Stewart JA, et al: National case-control study of Kaposi's sarcoma and *Pneumocystis carinii* pneumonia in homosexual men: Part 2, laboratory results. *Ann Intern Med* 99:151, 1983.

47. Ziegler JL, Beckstead JA, Volberding PA, et al: Non-Hodgkin's lymphoma in 90 homosexual men. *N Engl J Med* 311:565, 1984.

48. Ioachim HL, Cooper MC, Hellman GC: Lymphomas in men at high risk for acquired immune deficiency syndrome (AIDS). *Cancer* 56:2831, 1985.

49. Levine AM: Non-Hodgkin's lymphomas and other malignancies in the acquired immune deficiency syndrome. *Semin Oncol* 14:34, 1987.

50. Loeffler JS, Ervin TJ, Mauch P, et al: Primary lymphomas of the central nervous system: Patterns of failure and factors that influence survival. *J Clin Oncol* 3:490, 1985.

51. Elkin CM, Leon E, Grenell SL, et al: Intracranial lesions in the acquired immunodeficiency syndrome. *JAMA* 253:393, 1985.

52. Robert J, Schneiderman H: Hodgkins disease and the acquired immunodeficiency syndrome. *Ann Intern Med* 100:142, 1984.

53. Ioachim HL, Cooper MC, Hellman GC: Hodgkin's disease and the acquired immunodeficiency syndrome. *Ann Intern Med* 101:876, 1984.

54. Frager DH, Wolf EL, Competiello LS, et al: Squamous cell carcinoma of the esophagus in patients with acquired immunodeficiency syndrome. *Gastrointest Radiol* 13:358, 1988.

55. Enck RE: Squamous cell cancers and the acquired immunodeficiency syndrome. *Ann Intern Med* 106:773, 1987.

56. Tessler AN, Catanese A: AIDS and germinal cell tumors of testis. *Urology* 203:203, 1987.

57. Logothetis CJ, Newell GR, Samuels ML: Testicular cancer in homosexual men with cellular immune deficiency: Report of 2 cases. *J Urol* 133:484, 1985.

58. Slazinski L, Staff JR, Matthews CR: Basal cell carcinoma in a man with acquired immunodeficiency syndrome. *J Am Acad Dermatol* 11:140, 1984.

59. Sitz KV, Keppen M, Fohnson DF: Metastatic basal cell carcinoma in acquired immunodeficiency syndrome-related complex. *JAMA* 257:340, 1987.

60. Hirsch MS: AIDS Commentary: Azidothymidine. *J Infect Dis* 157:427, 1988.

61. Hirsch MD, Martin S, D'Aquila MD, et al: Therapy for human immunodeficiency virus infection. *N Engl J Med* 328(23):1686, 1993.

62. Fischl MA, et al: The efficacy of azidothymidine (AZT) in the treatment of patients with AIDS and AIDS-related complex: A double-blind, placebo-controlled trial. *N Engl J Med* 317:185, 1987.

63. Volberding PA, Lagakos SW, Koch MA, et al: Zidovudine in asymptomatic human immunodeficiency virus infection. *N Engl J Med* 322:941, 1990.

64. Fischl MA, Richman DD, Hansen N, et al: The safety and efficacy of zidovudine (AZT) in the treatment of subjects with mildly symptomatic human immunodeficiency virus type 1 (HIV) infection. *Ann Intern Med* 112:727, 1990.

65. Cheng-Mayer C, Quiroga M, Tung JW, et al: Viral determinants of human immunodeficiency virus type 1 T-cell or macrophage tropism, cytopathogenicity, and CD4 antigen modulation. *J Virol* 64:4390, 1990.

66. Boucher CAB, Lange JMA, Miedema FF, et al: HIV-1 biological phenotype and the developement of zidovudine resistance in relation to disease progression in asymptomatic individuals during treatment. *AIDS* 6:1259, 1992.

67. Cann AJ, Churcher MJ, Boyd M, et al: The region of the envelope gene of human immunodeficiency virus type 1 responsible for determination of cell tropism. *J Virol* 66:305, 1992.

68. Schuitemaker H, Koot M, Kootstra NA, et al: Biological phenotype of human immunodeficiency virus type 1 clones at different stages of infection: Progression of disease is asociated with a shift from monocytotropic to T-cell tropic virus population. *J Virol* 66:1354, 1992.

69. Larder BA, Darby G, Richman DD: HIV with reduced sensitivity to zidovudine (AZT) isolated during prolonged therapy. *Science* 243:1731, 1989.

70. Rooke R, Tremblay M, Soudeyns H, et al: Isolation of drug-resistant variants of HIV-1 from patients on long-term zidovudine therapy: Canadian Zidovudine Multi-Centre Study Group. *AIDS* 3:411, 1989.

71. Land S, Terloar G, McPhee D, et al: Decreased in vitro susceptibility to zidovudine of HIV isolates obtained from patients with AIDS. *J Infect Dis* 161:326, 1990.

72. Richman DD: Zidovudine resistance of human immunodeficiency virus. *Rev Infect Dis* 12(suppl 5):S507, 1990.

73. Richman DD et al: The toxicity of azidothymidine (AZT) in the patients with AIDS and AIDS-related complex. *N Engl J Med* 317:192, 1987.

74. Fischl MA, Parker CB, Pettinelli C, et al: A randomized controlled trial of a reduced daily dose of zidovudine in patients with the acquired immunodeficiency syndrome. *N Engl J Med* 323:1009, 1990.

75. Fischl M, Galpin JE, Levine JD, et al: Recombinant human erythropoietin for patients with AIDS treated with zidovudine. *N Engl J Med* 322:1488, 1990.

76. Pluda JM, Yarchoan R, Smith PD, et al: Subcutaneous recombinant granulocyte-macrophage colony-stimulating factor used as a single agent and in an alternating regimen with azidothymidine in leukopenic patients with severe human immunodeficiency virus infection. *Blood* 76(3):463, 1990.

77. Lambert JS, Seidlin M, Reichman RC, et al: 2',3'-Dideoxyinosine (ddI) in patients with the acquired immunodeficiency syndrome or AIDS-related complex. *N Engl J Med* 322:1333, 1990.

78. Cooley TP, Kunches LM, Saunders CA, et al: Once-daily administration of 2',3'-dideoxyinosine (ddI) in patients with the acquired immunodeficiency syndrome or AIDS-related complex. *N Engl J Med* 322:1340, 1990.

79. Kahn JO, Lagakos SW, Richman DD, et al: A controlled trial comparing continued zidovudine with didanosine in human immunodeficiency virus infection. *N Engl J Med* 327:581, 1992.

80. St Clair MH, Martin JL, Tudor-Williams G, et al: Resistance to ddI

and sensitivity to AZT induced by a mutation in HIV-1 reverse transcriptase. *Science* 253:1557, 1991.

81. Gu Z, Gao Q, Li X, et al: Novel mutation in the human immunodeficiency virus type 1 reverse transcriptase gene that encodes cross-resistance to 2',3'-dideoxyinosine and 2',3'-dideoxycytidine. *J Virol* 66:7128, 1992.

82. Yarchoan R, Perno CF, Thomas RV, et al: Phase I studies of 2',3'-dideoxycytidine in severe human immunodeficiency virus infection as a single agent and alternating with zidovudine (AZT). *Lancet* 1:76, 1988.

83. Merigan TC, Skowron G, Bozzette SA, et al: Circulating antigen levels and responses to dideoxycytidine in human immunodeficiency virus (HIV) infections: A phase I and II study. *Ann Intern Med* 110:189, 1989.

84. Meng TC, Fischl MA, Boota AM, et al: Combination therapy with zidovudine and dideoxycytidine in patients with advanced human immunodeficiency virus infection: A phase I/II study. *Ann Intern Med* 116:13, 1992.

85. Skowron G, Bozzette SA, Lim L, et al: Alternating and intermittent regimens of zidovudine and dideoxycytidine in patients with AIDS or AIDS-related complex. *Ann Intern Med* 118:321, 1993.

86. Yarchoan R, Mitsuya H, Broder S: Strategies for the combination therapy of HIV infection. *J AIDS* 3(suppl)2:S99, 1990.

87. Johnston Margaret I, Hoth Daniel F: Present status and future prospects for HIV therapies. *Science* 260:1286, 1993.

88. Urmacher C, Myskowski P, Ochoa M, et al: Outbreak of Kaposi's sarcoma with cytomegalovirus infection in young homosexual men. *Am J Med* 72:569, 1990.

89. Friedman-Kien AE, Laubenstein LJ, Rubinstein P, et al: Disseminated Kaposi's sarcoma in homosexual men. *Ann Intern Med* 96:693, 1982.

90. Jaffe HW, Keewhan C, Thomas P, et al: National case-control study of Kaposi's sarcoma and *Pneumocystis carinii* pneumonia in homosexual men: Part I, epidemiologic results. *Ann Intern Med* 99:145, 1983.

91. DeJarlais DC, Marmor M, Thomas P, et al: Kaposi's sarcoma among four different AIDS risk groups. *Lancet* 1:1119, 1988.

92. Jaffe HW, Bregman D, Selik RM: Acquired immune deficiency syndrome in the United States: The first 1,000 cases. *J Infect Dis* 148:339, 1983.

93. Garrett TJ, Lange M, Ashford A, et al: Kaposi's sarcoma in heterosexual intravenous drug users. *Cancer* 55:1146, 1985.

94. Haverkos HW, Amsel Z, Drotman DP, et al: Kaposi's sarcoma in homosexual men with AIDS, by race. *Lancet* 2:1075, 1988.

95. Drew WL, Mills J, Hauer LB, et al: Declining prevalence of Kaposi's sarcoma in homosexual AIDS patients paralleled by fall in cytomegalovirus transmission. *Lancet* 1:66, 1988.

96. Scott LF, Wright TL, Altman DF: Gastrointestinal Kaposi's sarcoma in patients with acquired immunodeficiency syndrome. *Gastroenterology* 89:102, 1988.

97. Dworkin B, Wormser GP, Rosenthal WS, et al: Gastrointestinal manifestations of the acquired immunodeficiency syndrome: A review of 22 cases. *Am J Gastroenterol* 80:774, 1985.

98. Friedman SL, Wright TL, Altman DF: Gastrointestinal Kaposi's sarcoma in patients with acquired immunodeficiency syndrome. *Gastroenterology* 89:102, 1985.

99. Lustbader I, Sherman A: Primary gastrointestinal Kaposi's sarcoma in a patient with acquired immune deficiency syndrome. *Am J Gastroenterol* 82:894, 1987.

100. Ognibene FP, Steis RG, Macher AM, et al: Kaposi's sarcoma causing pulmonary infiltrates and respiratory failure in the acquired immunodeficiency syndrome. *Ann Intern Med* 102:471, 1985.

101. Caray SM, Belenko M, Fazzini E, et al: Pulmonary manifestations of Kaposi's sarcoma. *Chest* 91:39, 1987.

102. Kaplan LD, Hopewell PC, Jaffe HW, et al: Kaposi's sarcoma involving the lung in patients with the acquired immunodeficiency syndrome. *J AIDS* 1:23, 1988.

103. Flepp M, Tauber MG, Luthy R, et al: Kaposi's sarcoma in AIDS patients: Long-term treatment with recombinant interferon alpha-2A and chemotherapy. *Klin Wochenschr* 66:437, 1988.

104. Gelmann EP, Preble OT, Steis R, et al: Human lymphoblastoid interferon treatment of Kaposi's sarcoma in the acquired immune deficiency syndrome. *Am J Med* 78:737, 1985.

105. Volberding PA, Abrams DI, Conant MA, et al: Vinblastine therapy for Kaposi's sarcoma in the acquired immunodeficiency syndrome. *Ann Intern Med* 103:335, 1985.

106. Kaplan LD, Abrams DI, Volberding PA: Treatment of Kaposi's sarcoma and thrombocytopenia with vincristine in patients with the acquired immunodeficiency syndrome. *Ann Intern Med* 102:200, 1985.

107. Laubenstein LJ, Krigel RL, Odajnyk CM, et al: Treatment of epidemic Kaposi's sarcoma with etoposide or a combination of doxorubicin, bleomycin, and vinblastine. *J Clin Oncol* 2:1115, 1984.

108. Hill DR: The role of radiotherapy for epidemic Kaposi's sarcoma. *Semin Oncol* 14:19, 1987.

109. Nobler MP, Leddy ME, Huh SH: The impact of palliative irradiation on the management of patients with acquired immune deficiency syndrome. *J Clin Oncol* 5:107, 1987.

110. Balfour HH, Bean B, Laskin OL, et al: Acyclovir halts progression of herpes zoster in immunocompromised patients. *N Engl J Med* 308:1448, 1983.

111. Erlich KS, Jacobson MA, Koehler JE, et al: Foscarnet therapy for severe acyclovir-resistant herpes simplex virus type-2 infections in patients with the acquired immunodeficiency syndrome (AIDS): An uncontrolled trial. *Ann Intern Med* 110:710, 1989.

112. Safrin S, Crumpacker C, Chatis P, et al: A controlled trial comparing foscarnet with vidarabine for acyclovir-resistant mucocutaneous herpes simplex in the acquired immunodeficiency syndrome. *N Engl J Med* 325:551, 1991.

113. Shepp DH, Dandliker PS, Meyers JD: Treatment of varicella zoster virus infection in severely immunocompromised patients. *N Engl J Med* 314:208, 1986.

114. Dover JS, Johnson RA: Cutaneous manifestations of human immunodeficiency virus infection. *Arch Dermatol* 127:1383, 1991.

115. Concus AP, Helfand RF, Imber MJ, et al: Cutaneous cryptococcosis mimicking molluscum contagiosum in a patient with AIDS. *J Infect Dis* 158:897, 1988.

116. Coopman MD, Serge A, Johnson MD, et al: Cutaneous disease and drug reactions in HIV infection. *N Engl J Med* 328(23):1670, 1993.

117. Gordin FM, Simon GL, Wofsy CB, et al: Adverse reactions to trimethoprim-sulfamethoxazole in patients with the acquired immunodeficiency syndrome. *Ann Intern Med* 100:49, 1984.

118. Menduri G, Stein D: Pulmonary manifestations of acquired immunodeficiency syndrome. *Clin Infect Dis* 14:98, 1992.

119. Selwyn PA, Feingold AR, Hartel D, et al: Increased risk of bacterial pneumonia in HIV-infected intravenous drug abusers without AIDS. *AIDS* 2:267, 1988.

120. Schlamm HT, Yancovitz SR: Haemophilus influenzae pneumonia in young adults with AIDS/ARC or risk of AIDS. *Am J Med* 86:11, 1989.

121. Polsky B, Gold JWM, Whimbey E, et al: Bacterial pneumonia in patients with acquired immunodeficiency syndrome. *Ann Intern Med* 104:38, 1986.

122. Sunderam G, McDonald RJ, Maniatis T, et al: Tuberculosis as a manifestation of the acquired immunodeficiency syndrome. *JAMA* 256:762, 1986.

123. Chaisson RE, Schecter GF, Theuer CP, et al: Tuberculosis in patients with the acquired immunodeficiency syndrome: Clinical features, response to therapy, and survival. *Am Rev Respir Dis* 136:570, 1987.

124. Chaisson RE, Slutkin G: Tuberculosis in patients with human immunodeficiency virus infection. *J Infect Dis* 159:96, 1989.

125. Jereb JA, Kelly GD, Dooley SW, et al: Tuberculosis morbidity in the United States: Final data. *MMWR* 40(SS-3):23, 1991.

126. Ellner JJ, Hinman AR, Dooley SW, et al: Tuberculosis symposium: emerging problems and promise. *J Infect Dis* 168:537, 1993.

127. Selwyn PA, Hartel D, Lewis VA, et al: A prospective study of the risk of tuberculosis among intravenous drug users with human immunodeficiency virus infection. *N Engl J Med* 320:545, 1989.

128. Tuberculosis and human immunodeficiency virus infection: Recommendations of the Advisory Committee for the Elimination of Tuberculosis (ACET). *MMWR* 38:236, 1989.

129. Initial therapy for tuberculosis in the era of multidrug resistance: Recommendations of the Advisory Council for the Elimination of Tuberculosis. *MMWR* 42(RR-7):1, 1993.

130. Small PM, Schecter GF, Goodman PC, et al: Treatment of tuberculosis in patients with advanced human immunodeficiency virus infection. *N Engl J Med* 324:289, 1991.

131. Horsburgh CR, Selik RM: The epidemiology of disseminated non-tuberculosous mycobacterial infection in AIDS. *Am Rev Respir Dis* 139:4, 1989.

132. Ellner JJ, Goldberger MJ, Parenti DM: Mycobacterium avium infection and AIDS: A therapeutic dilemma in rapid evolution. *J Infect Dis* 163:1326, 1991.

133. Benson CA, Ellner JJ: Mycobacterium avium complex infection and AIDS: Advances in theory and practice. *Clin Infect Dis* 17:7, 1993.

134. Young LS: Mycobacterium avium complex infection. *J Infect Dis* 157:863, 1988.

135. Horsburgh CR Jr., Havlik JA, Ellis EA, et al: Survival of patients with acquired immune deficiency syndrome and disseminated Mycobacterium avium complex infection with and without antimycobacterial chemotherapy. *Am Rev Respir Dis* 144:557, 1991.

136. Young LS, Wiviott L, Wu M, et al: Azithromycin for treatment of Mycobacterium avium-intracellulare complex infection in patients with AIDS. *Lancet* 338:1107, 1991.

137. Dautzenberg B, Truffot C, Legris S, et al: Activity of clarithromycin against Mycobacterium avium infection in patients with the acquired immune deficiency syndrome. *Am Rev Respir Dis* 144:564, 1991.

138. Recommendations on prophylaxis and therapy for disseminated Mycobacterium avium complex disease in patients infected with the human immunodeficiency virus. *N Engl J Med* 329:898, 1993.

139. Recommendations for counseling persons infected with human T-lymphotrophic virus, types I and II. *MMWR* 42(RR-9):1993.

140. Nightingale SD, Cameron WD, Gordin FM, et al: Two controlled trials of rifabutin prophylaxis against Mycobacterium avium complex infection in AIDS. *N Engl J Med* 329:828, 1993.

141. Acierno LJ: Cardiac complications in acquired immunodeficiency syndrome (AIDS): A review. *J Am Coll Cardiol* 13:1144, 1989.

142. Hecht SR, Berger M, Van Tosh A, et al: Unsuspected cardiac abnormalities in the acquired immunedeficiency syndrome: An echocardiographic study. *Chest* 96:805, 1989.

143. Himelman RB, Chng WS, Chernoff DN, et al: Cardiac manifestations of human immunodeficiency virus infection: A two-dimensional echocardiographic study. *J Am Coll Cardiol* 13:1030, 1989.

144. Kinney EL, Monsuez JJ, Kitzis M, et al: Treatment of AIDS-associated heart disease. *Angiology* 40:970, 1989.

145. Horn DL, Hewlett D Jr., Alfalla C, et al: Fatal hospital-acquired multidrug-resistant tuberculous pericarditis in two patients with AIDS. *N Engl J Med* 327:1816, 1992.

146. Stotka JL, Good CB, Downer WR, et al: Pericardial effusion and tamponade due to Kaposi's sarcoma in acquired immunodeficiency syndrome. *Chest* 95:1359, 1989.

147. Adair OV, Randive N, Krasnow N: Isolated toxoplasma myocarditis in acquired immune deficiency syndrome. *Am Heart J* 118:856, 1989.

148. Kelsey RC, Saker A, Morgan M: Cardiac lymphoma in a patient with AIDS. *Ann Intern Med* 115(5):370, 1991.

149. Cohen MC, Huberman MS, Nesto RW: Interferon alfa-induced cardiac dysfunction. *N Engl J Med* 322:1469, 1989.

150. Deyton LR, Walker RE, Kovacs JA, et al: Reversible cardiac dysfunction associated with interferon alpha therapy in AIDS patients with Kaposi's sarcoma. *N Engl J Med* 321:1246, 1989.

151. Mitchell P, Dodek P, Lawson L, et al: *Torsades de pointes* during intravenous drug pentamidine isethionate therapy. *Can Med Assoc J* 140:173, 1989.

152. Wharton JM, Demopulos PA, Goldschlager N: *Torsades de pointes* during administration of pentamidine isethionate. *Am J Med* 83:571, 1987.

153. Stein KM, Fenton C, Lehany AM, Incidence of QT interval prolongation during pentamidine therapy of Pneumocystis carinii pneumonia. *Am J Cardiol* 68:1091, 1991.

154. Cohen AJ, Weiser B, Afzal Q, et al: Ventricular tachycardia in two patients with AIDS receiving ganciclovir (DHPG). *AIDS* 4:807 1990.

155. Francis CK: Cardiac involvement in AIDS. *Curr Probl Cardiol* 15:569, 1990.

156. Jacob AJ, Boon NA: HIV cardiomyopathy: A dark cloud with a silver lining? *Br Heart J* 66:1, 1991.

157. Kaul S, Fishbein MC, Siegel RJ: Cardiac manifestations of acquired immune deficiency syndrome: A 1991 update. *Am Heart J* 122:535, 1991.

158. Grody WW, Cheng L, Lewis W: Infection of the heart by the human immunodeficiency virus. *Am J Cardiol* 66:203, 1990.

159. Lipshultz SE, Fox CH, Perez-Atayde AR, et al: Identification of human immunodeficiency virus-1 RNA and DNA in the heart of a child with cardiovascular abnormalities and congenital acquired immune deficiency syndrome. *Am J Cardiol* 66:246, 1990.

160. Lipshultz SE, Orav EJ, Sanders SP, et al: Cardiac structure and function in children with human immunodeficiency virus infection treated with Zidovudine. *N Engl J Med* 327 (18):1260, 1992.

161. Herskowitz A, Willoughby SB, Baughman KL, et al: Cardiomyopathy associated with antiretroviral therapy in patients with HIV infection: A report of six cases. *Ann Intern Med* 116:311, 1992.

162. Walter EB, Drucker RP, McKinney RE, et al: Myopathy in human immunodeficiency virus-infected children receiving long-term zidovudine therapy. *J Pediatr* 119:152, 1991.

163. Lewis W, Grody WW: AIDS and the heart: Review and consideration of pathogenic mechanisms. *Cardiovasc Pathol* 1:53, 1992.

164. Van Hoeven KH, Segal B, Factor SM: AIDS cardiomyopathy: First rule out other myocardial risk factors. *Int J Cardiol* 29:35, 1990.

165. Pardo V, Meneses R, Ossa L, et al: AIDS-related glomerulopathy: Occurrence in specific risk groups. *Kidney Int* 31:1167, 1987.

166. Cohen AH, Sun NCJ, Shapshak P, et al: Demonstration of human immunodeficiency virus in renal epithelium in HIV-associated nephropathy. *Mod Pathol* 2:125, 1989.

167. Rao TKS, Friedman EA: AIDS (HIV) associated nephropathy: Does it exist? An in-depth review. *Am J Nephrol* 9:441, 1989.

168. Seney FD Jr, Berns DK, Silva FG: Acquired immunodeficiency syndrome and the kidney. *Am J Kidney Dis* 16:1, 1990.

169. Rao TKS, Friedman EA, Nicastri AD: The types of renal disease in the acquired immunodeficiency syndrome. *N Engl J Med* 316:1062, 1987.

170. Bourgoignie JJ, Meneses R, Ortiz C, et al: The clinical spectrum of renal disease associated with human immunodeficiency virus. *Am J Kidney Dis* 12:131, 1988.

171. Ortiz C, Meneses R, Jaffe D, et al: Outcome of patients with human immunodeficiency virus on maintenance hemodialysis. *Kidney Int* 34:248, 1988.

172. Langes C, Galle GR, Schacht RG, et al: Rapid renal failure in AIDS-associated fecal glomerulosclerosis. *Arch Intern Med* 150:287, 1990.

173. Schoenfeld P, Feduska N: Acquired immunodeficiency syndrome and renal disease: Report of the National Kidney Foundation—National Institutes of Health Task Force on AIDS and Kidney Disease. *Am J Kidney Dis* 16(1):14, 1990.

174. Babut-Gay ML, Mechard M, Kleiknecht D, et al: Zidovudine and nephropathy with human immunodeficiency virus (HIV) infection. *Ann Intern Med* 111:856, 1989.

175. Lam M, Park MC: HIV-associated nephropathy: Beneficial effect of zidovudine therapy. *N Engl J Med* 323:1775, 1990.

176. Cook PP, Appel RG: Prolonged clinical improvement in HIV-associated nephropathy with zidovudine therapy. *J Am Soc Nephrol* 1:842, 1990.

177. Aron DC: Endocrine complications of the acquired immunodeficiency syndrome. *Arch Intern Med* 149:330, 1989.

178. Reichert CM, O'Leary TJ, Levens DL, et al: Autopsy pathology in the acquired immune deficiency syndrome. *Am J Pathol* 112:357, 1983.

179. Mobley K, Rotterdam HZ, Lerner CW, et al: Autopsy findings in the acquired immunodeficiency syndrome. *Pathol Annu* 20:45, 1985.

180. Glasgow BJ, Steinsapir KD, Anders K, et al: Adrenal pathology in the acquired immune deficiency syndrome. *Am J Clin Pathol* 84:594, 1985.

181. Dobs AS, Dempsey MA, Ladenson PW, et al: Endocrine disorders in men infected with human immunodeficiency virus. *Am J Med* 84:611, 1988.

182. Membreno L, Irony I, Dere W, et al: Adrenocortical function in acquired immunodeficiency syndrome. *J Clin Endocrinol Metab* 65:482, 1987.

183. Greene LW, Cole W, Green JB, et al: Adrenal insufficiency as a complication of the acquired immune deficiency syndrome. *Ann Intern Med* 101:497, 1984.

184. Weiss CD: The human immunodeficiency virus and the adrenal medulla. *Ann Intern Med* 105:300, 1986.

185. Sonio N: The use of ketoconazole as an inhibitor of steroid production. *N Engl J Med* 317:812, 1987.

186. Best TR, Jenkins JK, Murphy FY, et al: Persistent adrenal insufficiency secondary to low-dose ketoconazole therapy. *Am J Med* 82:676, 1987.

187. Tucker WS Jr., Snell BB, Island DP, et al: Reversible adrenal insufficiency induced by ketoconazole. *JAMA* 253:2413, 1985.

188. Kyriazopoulou V, Parparousi O, Vagenaskis AG: Rifampin-induced adrenal crisis in Addisonian patients receiving corticosteroid replacement therapy. *J Clin Endocrinol Metab* 59:1204, 1984.

189. Elansary EH, Earis JE: Rifampin and adrenal crisis. *Br Med J* 286:1861, 1983.

190. Stahl-Bayliss CM: Pentamidine-induced hypoglycemia in patients with the acquired immune deficiency syndrome. *Clin Pharmacol Ther* 39:271, 1986.

191. Ganda OP: Pentamidine and hypoglycemia. *Ann Intern Med* 39:271, 1984.

192. Davis SV, Murray JA: Amphotericin B, aminoglycosides, and hypomagnesemic tetany. *Br Med J* 292:1395, 1986.

193. Clements JS Jr., Peacock JE Jr.: Amphotericin B revisited: Reassessment of toxicity. *Am J Med* 88:5, 1990.

194. Seney FD Jr., Burns DK, Silva FG: Acquired immunodeficiency syndrome and the kidney. *Am J Kidney Dis* 16:1 1990.

195. Vaziri ND, Barbari A, Licorish K, et al: Spectrum of renal abnormalities in acquired immune-deficiency syndrome. *J Natl Med Assoc* 77:369, 1985.

196. Kalin MF, Poretsky L, Seres DS, et al: Hyporeninemic hypoaldosteronism associated with acquired immune deficiency syndrome. *Am J Med* 82:1035, 1987.

197. Medina I, Mills J, Leoung G, et al: Oral therapy for Pneumocystis carinii pneumonia in the acquired immunodeficiency syndrome: A controlled trial of trimethoprim-sulfamethoxazole versus trimethoprim-dapsone. *N Engl J Med* 323:776, 1990.

198. Choi MJ, Fernandez PC, Patnaik A, et al: Brief report: Trimethoprim-induced hyperkalemia in a patient with AIDS. *N Engl J Med* 328:703, 1993.

199. Greenspan JS, Greenspan D, Winkler JR: Diagnosis and management of the oral manifestations of HIV infection and AIDS. *Infect Dis Clin North Am* 2:373, 1988.

200. Greenspan D, Greenspan JS, Conant M, et al: Oral "hairy" leukoplakia in male homosexuals: Evidence of association with both papillomavirus and a herpes-group virus. *Lancet* 2:831, 1984.

201. Greenspan JS, Greenspan D, Lennette ET, et al: Replication of Epstein-Barr virus within the epithelial cells of oral "hairy" leukoplakia and AIDS-associated lesion. *N Engl J Med* 313:1564, 1985.

202. Connolly GM, Hawkins D, Harcourt-Webster JN, et al: Oesophageal symptoms, their causes, treatment, and prognosis in patients with the acquired immunodeficiency syndrome. *Gut* 30:1033, 1989.

203. Wilcox CM, et al: Esophageal disease in the acquired immunodeficiency syndrome: Etiology, diagnosis, and management. *Am J Med* 92:412, 1992.

204. Tavitian A, Raufman JP, Rosenthal LE: Oral candidiasis as a marker for esophageal candidiasis in the acquired immunodeficiency syndrome. *Ann Intern Med* 104:54, 1986.

205. Bach MC, Valenti AJ, Howell DA, et al: Odynophagia from aphthous ulcers of the pharynx and esophagus in the acquired immunodeficiency syndrome (AIDS). *Ann Intern Med* 113:338, 1988.

206. Bach MC, Howell DA, Valenti AJ, et al: Aphthous ulceration of the gastrointestinal tract in patients with the acquired immunodeficiency syndrome (AIDS). *Ann Intern Med* 112:465, 1990.

207. Friedman SL, Wright TL, Altman DF: Gastrointestinal KS in patients with acquired immunodeficiency syndrome: Endoscopic and autopsy findings. *Gastroenterology* 89:102, 1985.

208. Blumberg RS, Kelsey P, Perrone I, et al: Cytomegalovirus- and cryptosporidium-associated acalculous gangrenous cholecystitis. *Am J Med* 76:1118, 1984.

209. Kavin H, Jonas RB, Chowdhury L, et al: Acalculous cholesystitis and cytomegalovirus infection in the acquired immunodeficiency syndrome. *Ann Intern Med* 104:53, 1986.

210. Margulis SJ, Honig CL, Soave R, et al: Biliary tract obstruction in the acquired immunodeficiency syndrome. *Ann Intern Med* 105:207, 1986.

211. Schneiderman DJ, Cello JP, Laing FC: Papillary stenosis and sclerosing cholangitis in the acquired immunodeficiency syndrome. *Ann Intern Med* 106:546, 1987.

212. Jacobson MA, Cello JP, Sande MA: Cholestasis and disseminated cytomegalovirus disease in patients with acquired immunodeficiency syndrome. *Am J Med* 84:218, 1987.

213. Cello JP: Gastrointestinal manifestations of HIV infection. *Infect Dis Clin North Am* 2:387, 1988.

214. Rabeneck L, Fyorkey F, Genta RM, et al: The role of microsporidia in the pathogenesis of HIV-related chronic diarrhea. *Ann Intern Med* 119:895, 1993.

215. Glasgow BJ, Anders K, Layfield LJ, et al: Clinical and pathologic finding of the liver in the acquired immunodeficiency syndrome. *Am J Clin Pathol* 83:582, 1985.

216. Lebovics E, Thung SN, Schaffner F, et al: The liver in the acquired immunodeficiency syndrome: A clinical and histologic study. *Hepatology* 5:293, 1985.

217. Schneiderman DJ, Arenson DM, Cello JP, et al: Hepatic disease in patients with acquired immunodeficiency syndrome (AIDS). *Hepatology* 7:925, 1987.

218. Bonacini M: Hepatobiliary complications in patients with human immunodeficiency virus infection. *Am J Med* 92:404, 1992.

219. Laughon BE, Druckman DA, Vernon A, et al: Prevalence of enteric pathogens in homosexual men with and without AIDS. *Gastroenterology* 94:984, 1988.

220. Soave R, Johnson WD: Cryptosporidum and Isospora belli infections. *J Infect Dis* 157:225, 1988.

221. Bartlett JG, Belitsos PC, Sears CL: AIDS enteropathy. *Clin Infect Dis* 15:726, 1992.

222. Grohmann GS, Glass RI, Pereira HG, et al: Enteric viruses and diarrhea in HIV-infected patients. *N Engl J Med* 329: 14, 1993.

223. Robinson EN Jr, Fogel R: SMS 201-995, a somatostatin analogue, and diarrhea in the acquired immunodeficiency syndrome (AIDS). *Ann Intern Med* 109(8):680, 1988.

224. Cook DJ, Kelton JG, Stanisz AM, et al: Somatostatin treatment for cryptosporidial diarrhea in a patient with the acquired immunodeficiency syndrome (AIDS). *Ann Intern Med* 108(5):708, 1988.

225. Katz MD, Erstad C, Rose C: Treatment of severe cryptosporidium-related diarrhea with octreotide in a patient with AIDS. *Drug Intell Clin Pharm* 22(2):134, 1988.

226. Koralnik IJ, Beaumanoir A, Hausler R, et al: A controlled study of early neurologic abnormalities in men with asymptomatic human immunodefieiency virus infection. *N Engl J Med* 323(13):864, 1990.

227. Hollander H, Stringari S: Human immunodeficiency virus-associated meningitis: Clinical course and correlations. *Am J Med* 83:813, 1987.

228. Hollander H, Levy JA: Neurologic abnormalities and recovery of human immunodeficiency virus from cerebrospinal fluid. *Ann Intern Med* 106:692, 1987.

229. Chalmers MC, Antoino C, Aprill MC, et al: Cerebrospinal fluid and human immunodeficiency virus findings in healthy, asymptomatic, seropositive men. *Arch Intern Med* 150:1538, 1990.

230. De La Paz R, Enzmann D: Neuroradiology of the acquired immunodeficiency syndrome, in Rosenblum ML, Levy RM, Bredesen DE (eds): *AIDS and the Nervous System.* New York, Raven Press, 1988.

231. Navia BA, Jordan BD, Price RW: The AIDS dementia complex: I. Clinical features. *Ann Neurol* 19:517, 1986.

232. Navia BA, Co Eun-Sook, Petito CK, et al: The AIDS dementia complex: II. Neuropathology. *Ann Neurol* 19:525, 1986.

233. Ho DD, Bredesen DE, Vinters HV: The acquired immunodeficiency syndrome (AIDS) dementia complex. *Ann Intern Med* 111:400, 1989.

234. Levy RM, Bredesen DE, Rosenblum ML: Neurological manifestations of the acquired immunodeficiency syndrome (AIDS): Experience of UCSF and review of the literature. *J Neurosurg* 62:75, 1985.

235. McArthur JC: Neurologic manifestations of AIDS. *Medicine* 66:407, 1985.

236. Cornblath DR, McArthur JC: Predominantly sensory neuropathy in patients with AIDS and AIDS-related complex. *Neurology* 38:794, 1988.

237. Cornblath DR, McArthur JC, Kennedy PG, et al: Inflammatory demyelinating peripheral neuropathies associated with human T-cell lymphotrophic virus type III infection. *Ann Neurol* 21:32, 1987.

238. Lipkin WI, Perry G, Kiprov D, et al: Inflammatory neuropathy in homosexual men with lymphadenopathy. *Neurology* 35:1479, 1985.

239. Young Kim S, Hollander H: Polyradiculopathy due to cytomegalovirus: Report of two cases in which improvement occurred after prolonged therapy and review of the literature. *Clin Infect Dis* 17:32, 1993.

240. Gabuzda DH, Hirsch MS: Neurolgic manifestations of infection with human immunodeficiency virus. *Ann Intern Med* 107:383, 1987.

241. Luft BJ, Remington JS: Toxoplasmic encephalitis. *J Infect Dis* 157:1, 1988.

242. Luft BJ, Hafner R, Korzun AH, et al: Toxoplasmic encephalitis in patients with the acquired immunodeficiency syndrome. *N Engl J Med* 329(14):995, 1993.

243. Potasman I, Resnick L, Luft BJ, et al: Intrathecal production of antibodies against *T. gondii* in patients with toxoplasmic encephalitis and AIDS. *Ann Intern Med* 108:49, 1988.

244. Danneman BR, et al: Treatment of toxoplasmic encephalitis with intravenous clindamycin. *Arch Intern Med* 148:2477, 1988.

245. Araujo FG, Guptil DR, Remington JS: Azithromycin, a macrolide antibiotic with potent activity against Toxoplasma gondii. *Antimicrob Agents Chemother* 32:755, 1988.

246. Araujo FG, Shepard RM, Remington JS: In vivo activity of the macrolide antibiotics azithromycin, roxithromycin and spiramycin against Toxoplasma gondii. *Eur J Clin Microbiol Infect Dis* 10:519, 1991.

247. Israelski DM, Remington JS: AIDS-associated toxoplasmosis, in Sande MA, Volberding PA (eds): *The Medical Management of AIDS*. 3rd ed. Philadelphia, Saunders, 1992, p 319.

248. Berger JR, Kaszovitz B, Post MJ, et al: Progressive multifocal leukoencephalopathy associated with human immunodeficency virus infection. *Ann Intern Med* 107:78, 1987.

249. Berger JR, Mucke L: Prolonged survival and partial recovery in AIDS-associated progressive multifocal leukoencephalopathy. *Neurology* 38:1060, 1988.

250. Kalayjian RC, Cohen ML, Bonomo RA, et al: Cytomegalovirus ventriculoencephalitis in AIDS: A syndrome with distinct clinical and pathologic features. *Medicine* 72:67, 1993.

251. Ryder JW, Croen K, Kleinschmidt BK, et al: Progressive encephalitis three months after resolution of cutaneous zoster in a patient with AIDS. *Ann Neurol* 19:182, 1986.

252. Kovacs JA, Kovacs AA, Polis M, et al: Cryptococcosis in the acquired immunodeficiency syndrome. *Ann Intern Med* 103:533, 1985.

253. Dismukes WE: Cryptococcal meningitis in patients with AIDS. *J Infect Dis* 157:624, 1988.

254. Chuck SL, Sande MA: Infections with cryptoccocus neoformans in the acquired immunodeficiency syndrome. *N Engl J Med* 321:794, 1989.

255. Zuger A, et al: Maintenance amphotericin B for cryptococcal meningtis in the acquired immunodeficiency syndrome (AIDS). *Ann Intern Med* 109:592, 1988.

256. Saag MS, et al: Comparison of amphotericin B with fluconazole in the treatment of acute AIDS-associated cryptococcal meningitis. *N Engl J Med* 326:83, 1992.

257. Larsen RA, Leal ME, Chan LS: Fluconazole compared with amphotericin B plus flucytosine for cryptococcal meningitis in AIDS. *Ann Intern Med* 113:183, 1990.

258. Byrne WR, Wajszczuk CP: Cryptococcal meningitis in the acquired immunodeficiency syndrome: Successful treatment with fluconazole after failure with amphotericin B. *Ann Intern Med* 108:384, 1988.

259. Robinson PA, Knirsch AK, Joseph JA: Fluconazole for life-threatening fungal infections in patients who cannot be treated with conventional antifungal agents. *Rev Infect Dis* 12(suppl 3):S349, 1990.

260. Stern JJ, et al: Oral fluconazole therapy for patients with acquired immunodeficiency syndrome and cryptococcosis: Experience with 22 patients. *Am J Med* 85:477, 1988.

261. Sugar AM, Sanders C: Oral fluconazole as suppressive therapy of disseminated cryptococcosis in patients with acquired immunodeficiency syndrome. *Am J Med* 85:481, 1988.

262. Powderly WG, et al: A controlled trial of fluconazole or amphotericin B to prevent relapse of cryptococcal meningitis in patients with the acquired immunodeficiency syndrome. *N Engl J Med* 326:793, 1992.

263. DeSmet MD: Differential diagnosis of retinitis and choroiditis in patients with acquired Immunodeficiency syndrome. *Am J Med* 92(suppl 2A):17S, 1992.

264. Shulman JS, Orellana J, Friedman AH, et al: Acquired immunodeficiency syndrome (AIDS). *Surv Ophthalmol* 31:384, 1987.

265. Culbertson WW: Infections of the retina in AIDS. *Int Ophthalmol Clin* 29:108, 1989.

266. Jacobson MA, Mills J: Serious cytomegalovirus disease in acquired immunodeficiency syndrome (AIDS): Clinical findings, diagnoses, and treatment. *Ann Intern Med* 108:585, 1988.

267. Bloom JN, Palestine AG: The diagnosis of cytomegalovirus retinitis. *Ann Intern Med* 109:963, 1988.

268. Jabs DA, Enger C, Bartlett JG: Cytomegalovirus retinitis and acquired immunodeficiency syndrome. *Arch Ophthalmol* 109:963, 1988.

269. Henderly DE, Freeman WR, Causey DM, et al: Cytomegalovirus retinitis and response to therapy with ganciclovir. *Ophthalmology* 94:425, 1987.

270. Grossberg HS, et al: GM-CSF with ganciclovir for the treatment of CMV retinitis in AIDS. *N Engl J Med* 320:1560, 1989.

271. Jacobson MA, Stanley HD, Heard SE: Ganciclovir with recombinant methionyl human granulocyte colony stimulating factor for treatment of cytomegalovirus disease in AIDS patients. *AIDS* 6:515, 1992.

272. LeHoang P, Girard B, Robinet M, et al: Foscarnet in the treatment of cytomegalovirus retinitis in acquired immune deficiency syndrome. *Ophthalmology* 96:865, 1989.

273. Jacobson MA, O'Donnell JJ, Mills J: Foscarnet treatment of cytomegalovirus retinitis in patients with the acquired immunodeficiency syndrome. *Antimicrob Agents Chemother* 33:736, 1989.

274. Fanning MM, Read SE, Benson M, et al: Foscarnet therapy of cytomegalovirus retinitis in AIDS. *AIDS* 3:472, 1990.

275. Studies of Ocular Complications of AIDS Research Group, in collaboration with the AIDS Clinical Trials Group: Mortality in patients with the acquired immunodeficiency syndrome treated with either foscarnet or ganciclovir for cytomegalovirus retinitis. *N Engl J Med* 326:213, 1992.

276. Dieterich DT, Poles MA, Lew EA, et al: Concurrent use of ganciclovir and foscarnet to treat cytomegalovirus infection in AIDS patients. *J Infect Dis* 167:1184, 1993.

277. Zon LI, Groopman JE: Hematological manifestations of the human immune deficiency virus (HIV). *Semin Hematol* 25:208, 1988.

278. Stricker RB, Abrams DI, Corash L, et al: Target platelet antigen in homosexual men with immune thrombocytopenia. *N Engl J Med* 313:1375, 1985.

279. Folks TM, Kessler SW, Orenstein JM, et al: Infections and replication of HIV-1 in purified progenitor cells of normal human bone marrow. *Science* 242:919, 1988.

280. Frickhofen N, et al: Persistence of B19 parvovirus infection in patients infected with HIV type I. *Ann Intern Med* 113:926, 1990.

281. Groopman JE, et al: Effect of recombinant human GM-CSF on myelopoiesis in AIDS. *N Engl J Med* 317:593, 1987.

282. Phair JP, Abels RI, NcNeill MV, et al: Recombinant human erythropoietin treatment: Investigational new drug protocol for the anemia of the acquired immunodeficiency syndrome. *Arch Intern Med* 153:2669, 1993.

283. Dwyer JM: Manipulating the immune system with immune globulin. *N Engl J Med* 326(2):107, 1992.

284. Dietriach G, Kaveri SV, Kazatchkine MD: Modulation of autoimmunity by intravenous immune globulin through interaction with the function of the immune/idiotypic network. *Clin Immunol Immunopathol* 62(1):S73, 1992.

285. Miles SA, Mitsuyasu RT, Moreno J, et al: Combined therapy with recombinant granulocyte colony-stimulating factor and erythropoietin decreases hematologic toxicity from zidovudine. *Blood* 77:2109, 1991.

286. Jeffrey RB Jr, Nyberg DA, Bottles W, et al: Review: Abdominal CT in acquired immunodeficiency syndrome. *AJR* 146:7, 1986.

287. The Swiss Group for Clinical Studies on AIDS, Luthy R, Chairman: Zidovudine for the treatment of thrombocytopenia associated with

human immunodeficiency virus (HIV): A prospective study. *Ann Intern Med* 109:718, 1988.

288. Ravikumar TS, Allen JD, Bothe A Jr., et al: Splenectomy: The treatment of choice for human immunodeficiency virus-related immune thrombocytopenia. *Arch Surg* 124(5):625, 1989.

289. Tyler DS, Shaunak S, Bartlett JA, et al: HIV-1-associated thrombocytopenia: The role of splenectomy. *Ann Surg* 211(2):211, 1990.

290. Calverley DC, Jones GW, Kelton JG: Splenic radiation for corticosteroid-resistant immune thrombocytopenia. *Ann Intern Med* 116(12 pt1):977, 1992.

291. Needleman SW, Sorace J, Poussin-Rossillo H: Low-dose splenic irradiation in the treatment of autoimmune thrombocytopenia in HIV-infected patients. *Ann Intern Med* 116(4):310, 1992.

292. Atkinson JH Jr., Grant I, Kennedy CJ, et al: Prevalence of psychiatric disorders among men infected with human immunodeficiency virus: A controlled study. *Arch Gen Psychiatry* 45:859, 1988.

293. Brooner RK, Greenfield L, Schmidt C, et al: Antisocial personality disorder and HIV infection among intravenous drug abusers. *Am J Psychiatry* 150(1):53, 1993.

294. Marzuk PM, Tierney H, Tardiff K, et al: Increased risk of suicide in persons with AIDS. *JAMA* (259):1333, 1988.

295. McKegney FP, O'Dowd MA: Suicidality and HIV status. *Am J Psychiatry* 149(3):396, 1992.

296. Sepkowitz KA, Telzak EE, Carrow M, et al: Fever among outpatients with advanced human immunodeficiency virus infection. *Arch Intern Med* 153:1909, 1993.

297. Katz SJ, Wenger NS, Shapiro MF: Diagnostic value of bacterial and fungal blood cultures in patients with the acquired immunodeficiency syndrome. *Am J Med* 88:5, 1990.

298. Prego V, Glatt AE, Roy V, et al: Comparative yield of blood culture for fungi and mycobacteria, liver biopsy, and bone marrow biopsy in the diagnosis of fever of undetermined origin in human immunodeficiency virus-infected patients. *Arch Intern Med* 150:333, 1990.

299. Zurlo JJ, O'Neill D, Polis MA, et al: Lack of clinical utility of cytomegalovirus blood and urine cultures in patients with HIV infection. *Ann Intern Med* 118 (1):12, 1993.

300. Weisse AB, Heller DR, Schimenti RJ, et al: The febrile parenteral drug user: A prospective study in 121 patients. *Am J Med* 94:274, 1993.

301. Ciesielski C, Metler R, Hammett T, et al: Occupationally acquired HIV infection in health care workers. Abstracts of the 33rd ICAAC Session 57:231, 1993 (Abstract).

302. Tokars JI, Marcus R, Culver, et al: Surveillance of HIV infection and zidovudine use among health care workers after occupational exposure to HIV-infected blood. *Ann Intern Med* 118(12):913, 1993.

303. Centers for Disease Control: Recommendations for prevention of HIV transmission in health-care settings. *MMWR* 36(suppl 2S):1S, 1987.

304. Center for Disease Control: Public health service statement on management of occupational exposure to human immunodeficiency virus, including considerations regarding zidovudine postexposure use. *MMWR* 39:1, 1990.

305. Lange JMA, Boucher CAB, Hollak CEM, et al: Failure of zidovudine prophylaxis after accidental exposure to HIV-1. *N Engl J Med* 322:1375, 1990.

94. Infectious Complications of Drug Abuse

Neil M. Ampel

Drug abuse is a growing and pervasive problem in our society. Since the 1980s, there has been a marked increase in the amount of illicit drug use in the United States [1,2]. A working definition of drug abuse is the taking of any drug beyond medical need [3]. A variety of drugs are abused, including opiates, depressants, stimulants, and hallucinogens. Although two licit substances, alcohol and tobacco, are associated with significant health problems, this chapter focuses on either drugs that are explicitly illegal or those that are legal but are used by the patient for purposes other than for which they were prescribed. Abused drugs can be administered by a variety of means, including "snorting" through the nasal mucosa, inhalation through smoking, and by a parenteral route, including injection into the soft tissues or directly into the vascular system.

Individuals who abuse drugs are at risk for a variety of problems. They are more likely to be involved in crime, to sustain trauma, and to develop psychiatric illness [1]. Drug abuse also is attended by an increased risk in a number of infections, some of which may lead patients to be admitted to the intensive care unit. Most of these infections are associated with parenteral injection [4]. Illicit drug injection occurs under unsanitary conditions, using a drug that is usually not sterile and by injection equipment that has generally been used more than once, often by someone other than the patient. Such practices provide a

mechanism for passage of a variety of infectious agents. Although in some instances, particularly for the hepatitis viruses and HIV, the infectious agent is passed directly from blood-contaminated drug paraphernalia to the patient, the mode of spread is less clear for other agents. Tuazon and colleagues cultured 100 samples of heroin and injection equipment. The most frequent organisms cultured were *Bacillus* species, coagulase-negative staphylococci, *Clostridium perfringens,* and gram-negative bacilli. However, *Staphylococcus aureus,* the most frequent cause of infection in their population, was not isolated. Hence, it seems probable that the skin of the injecting drug user, and not the drug or injection paraphernalia, is the most likely source of infection for many bacterial infections [5].

Infections associated with parenteral drug abuse include skin and soft tissue infection, endocarditis, bone and joint infections, pneumonia, ophthalmologic infections, and hepatitis [2,3,6]. Parenteral drug abusers are also now recognized as a major group at risk for infection with the human immunodeficiency virus (HIV), the cause of the acquired immunodeficiency syndrome (AIDS) [7,8]. Finally, many patients with substance-abuse problems are homeless, have poor nutrition, and live under crowded conditions, placing them at increased risk for tuberculosis. This problem has recently been compounded by the epidemic of HIV among these patients [9,10,11].

Fever

Fever is one of the most common complaints of parenteral drug users presenting to the hospital. It may be attributable to a variety of causes, some life threatening, others benign. Based on recent studies [12,13], the most common cause of fever is a variety of self-limited syndromes, including viral upper respiratory tract infections, pharyngitis, and acute pyrogenic reactions [14,15]. Other common causes include pneumonia, cellulitis, and soft tissue abscesses. Of note, endocarditis accounts for fewer than 15 percent of all cases of fever [12,13].

All febrile parenteral drug users should undergo a thorough history and physical examination, and have routine blood laboratories and chest radiographs taken. Particular attention should be paid to abnormalities of the skin and soft tissues, to any cardiac valvular abnormalities, to any bony tenderness, and to any pulmonary abnormalities, because these are among the commonest sites of major illness. However, clinical evaluation alone often does not differentiate major disease from trivial illness in these patients. In particular, specific signs and symptoms of bacterial endocarditis are frequently lacking [12,13,16]. Because of this, febrile parenteral drug users should be admitted to the hospital for further observation.

Weisse and co-workers [16] have developed an algorithm for febrile parenteral drug abusers with no apparent source of infection. In this approach, blood cultures are obtained on all patients, and empiric antibiotic therapy is started. If blood cultures are positive or if the patient has clinical stigmata indicative of endocarditis, an echocardiogram is performed. If valvular vegetations are seen, the diagnosis of endocarditis is considered established. Conversely, if blood cultures are negative and the patient is clinically well, antibiotic therapy may be stopped. However, it is important to realize that parenteral drug users commonly self-administer antibiotics [17,18]. This practice may substantially reduce the likelihood of positive blood cultures. Hence, careful clinical evaluation is advised when making antibiotic decisions in these patients.

Bacteremia

Bacteremia is a frequent occurrence in the febrile parenteral drug user [19,20]. In most instances, it is a reflection of an underlying infection. Approximately 60 percent of bacteremias in parenteral drug abusers are attributable to causes other than endocarditis [20]. Among these nonendocarditis infections, most are secondary to either skin or soft tissue infections or to mycotic aneurysms of peripheral arteries. A smaller number are due to miscellaneous causes, such as septic arthritis, septic thrombophlebitis, or pneumonia. In about 3 percent of cases, the source of the bacteremia is undiscovered.

Although it is well recognized that the organisms associated with bacteremias in the parenteral drug user may vary based on geographic location [20] and the type of drug abused [21], some basic generalizations can be made. Staphylococci remain the most common organisms isolated. Drug users have an increased incidence of staphylococcal carriage of the skin, nose, and throat when compared with the general population [22], and there is a high frequency of such carriage among parenteral drug users with endocarditis [23]. Because, as already mentioned, bacterial infection appears to derive principally from the user's own flora and not from the drug or its paraphernalia [5], it is not surprising that *S. aureus* constitutes the majority of bacteremias in these patients [19]. One issue of concern is the frequency of isolation of methicillin-resistant *S. aureus*. In one

study from Detroit [19], such isolates accounted for more than 40 percent of all bacteremic isolates of *S. aureus*. Prior antibiotic therapy, including that self-administered by the drug user [17,18], appears to increase the incidence of methicillin-resistant staphylococcal infections [20]. The second most frequent causes of bacteremia are streptococci. In a recent report, a marked increase in Group A beta-hemolytic streptococcal bacteremia was associated with intravenous drug use in inner-city Philadelphia. These organisms appeared to be community acquired and were most often associated with skin and soft tissue infections [24]. Gram-negative aerobic bacilli are the third most frequently isolated bacteria in single-organism bacteremias. Of these, *Pseudomonas aeruginosa* has been most commonly cultured. Finally, polymicrobial bacteremias occur in about 10 percent of cases. Although a large range of organisms may be involved, in about two-thirds of the cases at least one of the organisms isolated is a staphylococcus [19].

The approach toward the bacteremic parenteral drug user should be to search for an underlying cause and to begin empiric antibiotic treatment, if this has not already been done. Eliciting an appropriate history with careful physical examination of the patient, especially looking for soft-tissue swelling and tenderness, peripheral pulsatile masses, skeletal tenderness, or peripheral emboli suggestive of endocarditis, along with careful review of the chest radiograph for either pneumonia or pulmonary emboli, should establish the cause of the bacteremia in the majority of patients. The isolation of a group A beta-hemolytic streptococci from the blood should prompt a search for a cutaneous or soft tissue focus of infection [24]. Empiric antibiotic therapy may vary based on local experience, but should generally include agents directed against staphylococci and streptococci as well as aerobic gram-negative bacilli. If methicillin-resistant *S. aureus* has previously occurred as a bacteremia in parenteral drug users in the community, empiric use of vancomycin should be considered.

Skin and Soft Tissue Infections

Skin and soft tissue infections are extremely frequent occurrences in the parenteral drug user. Conditions range from local cellulitis or skin abscess at the site of injection to necrotizing fasciitis and gangrene [25–32].

The microbiology of these soft tissue infections is complex and often polymicrobial. The most common pathogens are *S. aureus,* streptococci, and oral anaerobes [25,29,32]. However, it is not uncommon to isolate any number of aerobic gram-negative bacilli, such as *Klebsiella* and *Serratia* species, and even *P. aeruginosa.*

Cutaneous infection in the parenteral drug user occurs at the site of injection. This is usually in the antecubital fossa, forearm, and hand in the intravenous drug user, because these are the most accessible veins. However, because intravenous injection results in thrombosis and sclerosis of veins, intravenous drug users may avail themselves of other, less accessible sites when these first areas are no longer usable. In this case, sites of infection commonly include the feet, legs, anterior neck, groin, and even axilla [26,30]. In addition, subcutaneous injection or skin-popping may be performed in all accessible parts of the body, leading to subcutaneous abscesses and chronic scarring [31,33]. Moreover, inadvertent or purposeful injection into arteries may result in localized gangrene [26,30].

The most common skin infections in the injecting drug user are simple cellulitis or localized skin abscess [28]. The patient may appear generally toxic and have localized redness, tenderness, and swelling. However, it is imperative to exclude the possibility of a deep subcutaneous infection at the earliest possible moment. Deep soft tissue infections may be indistinguishable from simple cellulitis in their early stages. The presence of vesicles or bullae, an area of central necrosis within a larger area of erythema, and the presence of subcutaneous crepitation in a patient with systemic toxicity are suggestive of necrotizing fasciitis [27]. Gas seen in the soft tissues on radiographs is also indicative of deep infection [34]. If there is any question of a deep, soft tissue infection, immediate local surgical exploration at the bedside should be performed. The diagnosis is established if serosanguinous fluid exudes or gray or frankly necrotic fascia or muscle is observed after incision [27]. Direct visualization of the soft tissues not only provides immediate diagnosis, it allows initial debridement. As well, any abnormal material from this exploration should be immediately examined using Gram stain to provide the basis for empiric antimicrobial therapy. Examination of a sample of tissue using frozen-section biopsy may also be useful [35].

Simple cellulitis usually requires only antibiotic therapy directed against staphylococci and streptococci. A penicillinase-resistant penicillin, such as nafcillin or oxacillin, or a first-generation cephalosporin, such as cefazolin, is an appropriate choice. Localized soft tissue abscesses that do not penetrate into the deep subcutaneous tissue should be drained. Antibiotic therapy may be given and should be directed by Gram stain of the drained material. However, antibiotic therapy is not always necessary in the treatment of cutaneous abscesses [36].

Necrotizing fasciitis, pyomyositis, or gangrene require immediate, aggressive debridement in the operating room in association with parenteral antibiotics [25]. Gram stain and culture are imperative to guide antimicrobial therapy because the number of potential pathogens is large. Empiric therapy should be directed against staphylococci, streptococci, anaerobes, and aerobic gram-negative bacilli. Morbidity is significant, and surgical debridement may be required on multiple occasions before infection is controlled [37].

Peripheral Vascular Infections

Because parenteral drug use so often involves vascular injection of material under nonsterile conditions, it is not surprising that a wide range of vascular complications may result from these practices. The most frequent manifestations of such infections are fever associated with pain, redness, and swelling over the involved area. Bacteremia with septic thromboembolism is a common association [20] and may be mistaken for endocarditis. When the injecting site is into the deep tissues of the groin or neck, it may be difficult to distinguish involvement of vascular structures from simple cellulitis, soft tissue abscess, or fasciitis. If there is any question, angiography should be performed to determine if vascular tissue is involved.

Mycotic aneurysms are one of the most frequent complications of intravenous drug use and result when the user injects directly into the artery [20,38,39]. Aneurysms most frequently occur in the femoral arteries, but carotid aneurysms are not uncommon, and are often due to attempts at injection into the internal jugular vein between the two heads of the sternocleidomastoid muscle above the clavicle [26,40]. Brachial artery aneuryms occasionally occur [19]. The classic presentation of this syndrome is a febrile patient with a tender, pulsatile mass, usually in the groin or the neck. Sometimes, there is a small amount of bleeding at the site. If there is any question of an aneurysm, a vascular surgical consultation should be obtained

before any exploration of the lesion. Angiography confirms the site and the extent of the aneurysm. *S. aureus* and streptococci are the most frequent microbiologic agents involved with aerobic gram-negative bacilli occasionally occurring [19]. Empiric antibiotic therapy should be directed against these organisms. Of note, ligation and excision of the involved arterial segment is usually successful and generally does not result in loss of limb or paralysis [39].

Another frequent vascular complication is septic thrombophlebitis. The usual clinical syndrome is fever, bacteremia, and swelling over the involved vein. Again, when the infection involves veins in the groin or neck, it may be impossible to distinguish septic thrombophlebitis from infection of other tissues without surgical exploration. Septic thrombophlebitis can often be treated with antibiotics alone, although incision, drainage and removal of the vein is sometimes necessary. Anticoagulation is generally not needed [20,38].

Endocarditis

Endocarditis in the parenteral drug abuser differs in several respects from endocarditis in the nonaddict [20,41–46] (see Chap. 88). It is more likely occur in persons without underlying valvular heart disease, to involve the tricuspid valve, to be due to *S. aureus,* and to have a more benign outcome [42,46]. Certain types of intravenous drug abuse may predispose to the development of endocarditis. Heroin use has long been associated with this complication [47], and an association between intravenous cocaine abuse and endocarditis has been recently noted [48].

There is a prototypical presentation of tricuspid-valve endocarditis in the parenteral drug user [45,46,49,50]. The patient complains of fever, usually for less than 1 week. There may also be a history of chills and pleuritic chest pain, and occasionally hemoptysis. On physical examination, fever is a nearly universal finding. A systolic murmur may or may not be present on admission but often develops during the course of therapy. Signs of peripheral embolization, such as Osler's nodes, Janeway lesions, or Roth spots, are uncommon. On chest radiograph, multiple patchy infiltrates indicative of pulmonary emboli are strongly suggestive of the diagnosis of tricuspid endocarditis. Blood cultures are almost invariably positive and, in the majority of instances, *S. aureus* is isolated. When blood cultures are negative in the face of the appropriate clinical syndrome, one should suspect that the patient has recently taken antibiotics.

Endocarditis involving the valves of the left side of the heart may also occur in the parenteral drug user and may be increasing in incidence [20,51]. Tricuspid valve endocarditis may be concomitantly present in these patients. Compared with patients with tricuspid-valve endocarditis alone, there is more likely to be a history of underlying heart disease, although this is not universal [20,51]. On examination, a heart murmur is usually evident on presentation, and peripheral emboli are frequent. Streptococci are more likely to be isolated from the blood, but *S. aureus* is still frequently isolated [20,46,51].

In addition to staphylococci and streptococci, a variety of other organisms have been associated with endocarditis in the parenteral drug user, including aerobic gram-negative bacilli, particularly *P. aeruginosa* [21], and fungi, notably *Candida* species [52]. Moreover, polymicrobial bacteremia is a well-recognized complication of endocarditis in this population [53] and is usually indistinguishable on clinical grounds from that caused by a single organism [54].

Echocardiography has been used for both establishing the

diagnosis and determining the prognosis of endocarditis in the parenteral drug user. Dubois and Ginzton [55] found that bacteremia and pulmonary emboli on chest radiograph were highly predictive of tricuspid-valve endocarditis in this group of patients. Echocardiography added no further information regarding the diagnosis. The newer technique of transesophageal echocardiography does not appear to be more sensitive in detecting vegetations than the transthoracic method among this group of patients but is able to more precisely characterize the vegetations [56]. Because it adds little to the diagnosis of endocarditis and because some individuals who do not have active endocarditis by clinical criteria may demonstrate valvular vegetations [55], echocardiography should be obtained only in those patients with bacteremia or who have clinical stigmata of endocarditis [16]. Echocardiography may be more useful for determining prognosis. Hecht and Berger [49] found that patients with valvular vegetations of greater than 2.0 cm had a significantly higher mortality when compared with those with vegetations smaller than this.

Empiric therapy for endocarditis in parenteral drug users should be directed against staphylococci, streptococci, and aerobic gram-negative bacilli. Nafcillin, oxacillin, or cefazolin are reasonable choices if methicillin resistance among staphylococci has not been encountered. Vancomycin is the current alternative for the treatment of methicillin-resistant staphylococcal infections as well as for the penicillin-allergic patient. Empirically, an aminoglycoside, such as gentamicin or tobramycin, should also be added to the regimen, both for initial therapy of aerobic gram-negative bacilli and for potential synergism against the staphylococcus [57,58].

The prognosis for tricuspid-valve endocarditis in the parenteral drug user is good, with mortality below 10 percent [49]. Staphylococcal endocarditis in the parenteral drug user in general appears to have a better prognosis compared with that in non–drug users. In two studies [42,59], mortality was less than 10 percent among drug abusers compared with 20 percent or more among others with native valve endocarditis. A variety of therapies have been used to treat staphylococcal endocarditis in the parenteral drug user. Abrams and colleagues [60] cured 25 consecutive cases using a beta-lactam antibiotic either alone or in combination with an aminoglycoside for 4 weeks, with no difference in either regimen. Chambers and colleagues [57] found that intravenous nafcillin plus tobramycin for 2 weeks led to a cure in 94 percent of patients treated. Parker and Fossieck [61] successfully treated 33 patients with staphylococcal endocarditis, 29 of whom were parenteral drug users, by using approximately 2 weeks of intravenous therapy followed by approximately 1 month of treatment with an oral antistaphylococcal agent.

Nonstaphylococcal endocarditis, particularly involving the aortic and mitral valves, has a significantly worse prognosis. Left-sided endocarditis secondary to *P. aeruginosa* has a particularly poor outcome, with a mortality rate of nearly 70 percent [21]. To achieve cure, an antipseudomonal beta-lactam antibiotic plus an aminoglycoside, both at high doses, administered for 6 weeks intravenously and combined with early surgical removal of the involved valve is usually required [21,62]. Candidal endocarditis also has an extremely high mortality rate [52] even with prompt valve replacement and systemic antifungal therapy.

The role of surgery in endocarditis in the parenteral drug user is no different from endocarditis in the general population. Hemodynamic decompensation, persistently positive blood cultures in the face of appropriate antimicrobial therapy, multiple embolic episodes after therapy is initiated, fungal endocarditis, and evidence of extravalvular extension of infection constitute major criteria for valve replacement [63]. For patients with isolated tricuspid-valve involvement and intractable infection, tricuspid valvulotomy is successful in the majority of cases. Only about 10 percent of patients require a subsequent prosthetic valve to control congestive right-heart failure [64].

Skeletal Infections

Infections of the bones and joints represent a distinct clinical syndrome in the drug abuser. Most cases have been reported among intravenous heroin users [65–68]. Bacterial osteomyelitis of the vertebral column is the most frequent skeletal infection reported among this group of patients. The lumbar, cervical, and thoracic spine are involved, in that order. Patients generally present with weeks to months of pain in the involved area. There may be an antecedent history of nonpenetrating trauma. High fevers are unusual, and many patients are afebrile. On examination, there is usually tenderness over the involved vertebral bodies, and there is often radiographic evidence of osteomyelitis. Laboratory values are generally normal, although the peripheral white blood cell count may be modestly elevated [66]. Because of the chronicity of symptoms and the general lack of toxicity of these patients, it is not unusual for the diagnosis to be missed for weeks or even months. The complaint of low back or neck pain in an intravenous drug user should always suggest the diagnosis of vertebral osteomyelitis.

Septic arthritis among this group of patients often involves the sacroiliac and sternoarticular joints and the symphysis pubis, relatively unusual sites in non–drug users. Symptoms and signs are similar to those seen in osteomyelitis, with weeks to months of pain at the site and tenderness to palpation at the site of involvement. Radiographs are usually normal at presentation.

The bacteriology of skeletal infections among drug users is quite different from that seen in other patients. Aerobic gram-negative bacilli, particularly *P. aeruginosa,* have been most frequently isolated [67,68], with gram-positive cocci, such as staphylococci and streptococci, less commonly noted [65]. In addition, skeletal infections due to *Candida* species may occur alone [69] or as part of a dissemination syndrome [70,71,72]. Because of this, it is imperative that a bacteriologic diagnosis be established in such patients. In most cases, this can be achieved by needle aspirate of the involved bone or joint. For sternoarticular infections, open surgical exploration is often required [67]. Therapy involves long-term antibiotic therapy and, in some cases, surgical debridement.

HIV Infection

Intravenous drug use represents the second most common risk behavior for infection with HIV in the United States, accounting for 17 percent of cases of AIDS [73,74]. It is estimated that between 61,000 and 398,000 intravenous drug users are infected with HIV in this country [8]. Studies that have examined the prevalence of HIV infection have found great variability based on geographic location. The highest rates are in the northeastern United States and Puerto Rico, and are as high as 60 percent in areas of New York City and northern New Jersey. Some metropolitan regions, notably Atlanta, Detroit and San Francisco, have rates approximating 10 percent. Outside of these areas, rates of infection with HIV among intravenous drug users are generally less than 5 percent [8]. Most surveys have been performed using drug abuse treatment centers involving predominantly chronic heroin abusers. Hence, data may not be entirely representative [73]. In addition to geographic variation, black and Hispanic ethnic groups are disproportionately represented among those with HIV infection and intravenous drug use [8,75,76].

Certain practices increase the risk for an intravenous drug user to acquire HIV infection. These include frequent injections, injection in "shooting galleries," places where users rent the injecting paraphernalia and return it after use, injection with used needles, and sharing needles with others during injection. Additional factors associated with an increased risk include use of cocaine and having sex partners who use intravenous drugs. The latter is significantly associated with HIV infection in women [76].

HIV infection in intravenous drug users differs in several respects from other risk groups. Intravenous drug users are more likely to develop infections not directly related to HIV infection before reaching an AIDS-defining diagnosis [7,77]. In particular, they have a high risk of developing bacterial pneumonia and bacterial sepsis, especially due to encapsulated organisms such as *Streptococcus pneumoniae* or *Haemophilus influenzae* [7]. In addition, they are at significant risk for developing pulmonary tuberculosis [7,78]. These early complications appear to lead to an earlier morbidity and mortality than seen in patients with HIV from other causes [77]. However, progression to severe immunodeficiency occurs at the same rate in intravenous drug users as in other patient groups. Moreover, zidovudine therapy prolongs the time to the development of AIDS in these patients [7].

Any intravenous drug user should be considered at risk for HIV infection, and such patients should be offered testing for such infection [79]. In areas of high prevalence, the clinician should be aware that HIV-related immunodeficiency may be complicating the clinical course in an intravenous drug abuser. In such cases, diseases specifically related to HIV infection, such as *Pneumocystis carinii* pneumonia, *Mycobacterium avium* infection, toxoplasmosis, or cytomegalovirus disease, should be also considered in the differential diagnosis.

Viral Hepatitis

Acute and chronic hepatitis have long been recognized as among the most common reasons for hospital admission among drug users [4,28,80,81]. Of the infectious causes, hepatitis B remains the principal pathogen. It is estimated that from 60 to 80 percent of parenteral drug users in the United States are infected with hepatitis B and that nearly 10 percent are chronic carriers [2]. Intravenous drug use has become the major risk factor for acquiring hepatitis B infection in the United States and the risk appears to be increasing [82]. Moreover, co-infection with the delta virus, a hepatotrophic agent that requires hepatitis B for replication, is relatively common among parenteral drug users in this country, occurring in up to 40 percent of those infected with hepatitis B [83,84,85]. Individuals who are co-infected with hepatitis B and the delta agent may have a more fulminant acute course [86] and are more likely to develop chronic active hepatitis [83].

Hepatitis A has also long been suspected as a cause for acute hepatitis among intravenous drug users [80]. This has recently been confirmed in studies of recent outbreaks [87]. Moreover, parenteral drug abusers are at increased risk for acquiring non-A, non-B hepatitis, most cases of which are now recognized as being due to hepatitis C [88,89]. Although hepatitis C infection is less commonly associated with acute fulminant hepatitis than

hepatitis B infection, it often leads to chronic liver disease. In one recent survey of emergency departments, infection with hepatitis C was identified in 83 percent of intravenous drug users and was the most common risk factor for this infection [88]. Other studies have confirmed that intravenous drug use is highly associated with hepatitis C infection [89,90].

Parenteral drug abusers may suffer multiple attacks of acute hepatitis and are also likely to have significant structural and functional abnormalities of their liver, even if they are asymptomatic [91]. Noninfectious factors, particularly the use of alcohol and other drugs, may act synergistically with the hepatitis viruses to lead to a poorer outcome [2]. Moreover, concomitant infection with HIV also has the potential to cause increased activity of these viruses and promote more liver damage [92].

Patients with acute hepatitis present with fever, anorexia, and malaise. On examination, scleral icterus and an enlarged and tender liver are often found. Stigmata of chronic liver disease may also be present. Severe disease is associated with an elevated prothrombin time and encephalopathy, both of which suggest significant hepatic destruction.

Disseminated Candidiasis

A distinctive form of disseminated candidiasis has been described in intravenous drug abusers. This syndrome occurs virtually exclusively in individuals who abuse brown heroin. This form of heroin, because of its poor solubility, is often dissolved in an acidic solution, such as lemon juice [72]. *Candida albicans* has been the only candidal species implicated in these cases [70,71,72]. The source of infection is unclear but appears to be derived from the drug user's own flora [70,72].

The syndrome is characterized by an episode of fever within hours after injection, followed days to weeks later by skin, eye, and osteoarticular lesions. The skin lesions consist of deep subcutaneous nodules, confined to the scalp or other hairy areas, and painful pustules on an erythematous base found in all areas of the body [70]. Direct examination of expressed material from these pustules demonstrates budding yeast and culture that is usually positive for *C. albicans*. Ocular involvement, which generally occurs soon after the skin involvement, is manifested by eye pain, photophobia, and decreased visual acuity. White or yellow exudates either confined to the retina or with vitreal involvement are seen on ophthalmologic examination [70,72]. Costochondritis, osteomyelitis, and arthritis, if they occur, tend to occur later than the skin and eye involvement. The skin lesions may have disappeared by the time of appearance of skeletal symptoms [70]. Costochondral tumors are a unique part of the syndrome and present as pain and swelling over the involved ribs. Biopsy of such lesions is often diagnostic, demonstrating both pseudohyphae and yeast forms [72].

Optimal therapy is not established. Azole antifungals, such as ketoconazole, have been used successfully in many cases of skin involvement alone [70,72]. For ocular involvement, both oral azoles and intravenous amphotericin B have been used. Vitrectomy has been necessary in some cases. Costochondral tumors have required surgical removal in some instances [72].

Ocular Infections

Parenteral drug users are well recognized as having an increased risk of eye infections. In general, these are due to hematogenous spread from another site. Most cases are secondary to *Candida* species, either as part of the disseminated candidiasis syndrome described above or with eye involvement alone [93]. Candida endophthalmitis may involve parts of the eye in addition to the retina and vitreous. Uveitis with an intense anterior chamber reaction is well described [93].

In addition to *Candida*, *Aspergillus* species have been frequently associated with endophthalmitis in the parenteral drug user [94]. Again, ocular involvement is presumed to result from hematogenous spread, although usually only one eye is involved and there are no other sites of infection [93]. Treatment usually requires vitrectomy combined with systemic amphotericin B.

Endophthalmitis due to bacteria is far less common than that due to fungi [93,95]. Unlike fungal endophthalmitis, which often presents indolently, bacterial endophthalmitis is usually explosive with acute pain, redness, and decreased visual acuity. It may be mistaken initially for conjunctivitis [93]. Progressive destruction of the eye may occur rapidly and immediate ophthalmologic consultation is requisite. Unusual organisms have been frequently isolated in this disease, such as *Bacillus* species and *Staphylococcus epidermidis* [93,95].

Central Nervous System Infections

Epidural abscess is probably the most frequent central nervous system infection and is increasing in frequency [96]. Pain associated with radicular symptoms is the most common presentation, and symptoms are often indolent. These infections are usually secondary to an underlying vertebral osteomyelitis. Imaging studies, such as myelography, CT scan, or MRI, are useful in defining the extent of the infectious process. Needle aspiration under radiographic visualization can be used to establish the microbiologic etiology, but care must be taken not to enter the subarachnoid space, which can spread the infection into the cerebrospinal fluid, if this has not already occurred. Staphylococci are the most frequent cause, but *P. aeruginosa* and *M. tuberculosis* have also been isolated. Antibiotics alone may be curative in some cases, but surgery is often required [96]. Hence, neurosurgical consultation should be obtained at the time the diagnosis is first suspected.

Brain abscesses may occur in the parenteral drug user, usually as a result of embolization from either endocarditis or a mycotic aneurysm [28]. They are usually multiple and generally due to *S. aureus*. Antibiotic therapy alone has led to cure in some cases [97]. In addition, it is believed parenteral drug users are at increased risk for both bacterial and aseptic meningitis [2]. The finding of a pleocytosis or frank meningitis on examination of the cerebrospinal fluid should prompt a search for an underlying etiology, such as vertebral osteomyelitis, epidural abscess, or brain abscess.

Bacterial Pneumonia

Pneumonia has long been recognized as a frequent event among parenteral drug abusers [28,80,81] (see Chap. 76). Louria and Hensle [28] have described three acute pulmonary complications in the intravenous drug user. The first is an acute pulmonary edema secondary to drug injection. This is not associated with infection and usually clears in 1 to 2 days. The second is a unilateral bacterial pneumonia, usually due to community-acquired pathogens, and generally responds well to antibiotic

therapy. The third manifestation is septic pulmonary embolism, usually due to tricuspid valve endocarditis but sometimes secondary to peripheral mycotic aneurysms. In a more recent study [98], a similar pattern of pulmonary disease among intravenous drug abusers was found, with septic pulmonary embolism and community-acquired pneumonia the most likely causes. Tuberculosis occurred in about 10 percent of patients. Although HIV infection was present in more than half of the patients, AIDS-related pulmonary infections were not common.

A unilateral infiltrate on chest radiograph in a drug abuser should suggest a bacterial pneumonia. See Chapter 13 for an in-depth discussion on obtaining lower respiratory tract secretions for diagnosing the cause of pneumonia. Antibiotic therapy should be directed against community-acquired pathogens, such as *S. pneumoniae*, *S. aureus* and non-pseudomonal gram-negative bacilli, such as *H. influenzae* and *Klebsiella pneumoniae*. If there is a recent history of unconsciousness suggesting aspiration of oropharyngeal contents, antimicrobial therapy directed against anaerobes should be considered.

Tuberculosis

From 1953 to 1984, the incidence of active tuberculosis steadily declined in the United States (see Chap. 95). Since that time, it has increased by about 7% each year. The catalyst for this increase is infection with HIV, which dramatically increases both the risk of reactivation of previously acquired tuberculosis and the rate of progressive disease from new infection. The marked increase in tuberculosis has occurred particularly in the urban regions of the northeastern United States, an area of high prevalence for both HIV infection and intravenous drug use. Moreover, the predominant ethnic groups involved have been black and Hispanic [99]. In essence, the new tuberculosis epidemic is closely linked to the HIV epidemic among intravenous drug users [9].

Parenteral drug users in general have a high rate of infection with *Mycobacterium tuberculosis*, as indicated by a 20 percent rate of dermal reactivity to tuberculin [10,100,101]. The risk of developing active tuberculosis among these patients is significant, particularly if they are co-infected with HIV and homeless [10,11]. Moreover, many drug users with HIV infection may not demonstrate cutaneous tuberculin reactivity and yet be infected with *M. tuberculosis* [101]. These patients have been shown to be at even greater risk for developing active tuberculosis [78]. Because of this, some have advocated preventive isoniazid therapy for all intravenous drug users who are HIV infected and live in areas of high prevalence of tuberculosis, regardless of their tuberculin skin test reaction [102,103].

Two patterns of tuberculosis have been recognized in the recent epidemic among HIV-infected patients. Those patients with positive tuberculin reactions and relatively high CD4 lymphocyte counts tend to present with reactivation tuberculosis, often manifested by an upper lobe pulmonary infiltrate with cavitation and hilar adenopathy. However, those with cutaneous anergy and low CD4 counts often present with primary tuberculosis, indicated by hilar adenopathy, pleural effusions, or a miliary chest radiograph pattern. These patients often have extrapulmonary tuberculosis, including meningitis. In such patients, there is a high rate of positive blood cultures for *M. tuberculosis* [99].

Because tuberculosis may present atypically, the clinician must maintain a high index of suspicion for this disease in any drug user with pulmonary disease, particularly if they are infected with HIV. If there is any question of the possibility of pulmonary tuberculosis, patients should be placed in appropriate respiratory isolation. Acid-fast smears should be performed on at least three respiratory specimens before active pulmonary tuberculosis is ruled out. If smears are positive, antituberculous therapy should be immediately started and should include isoniazid, rifampin, pyrazinamide, and either ethambutol or streptomycin. To further complicate the management of tuberculosis in these patients, outbreaks of infection due to *M. tuberculosis* strains that are resistant to multiple antibiotics have occurred, chiefly in New York and Florida. Because of this, patients with sputa containing acid-fast bacilli should be treated and kept in respiratory isolation until there is evidence of decreasing mycobacterial numbers. If multidrug resistance is strongly suspected, drugs in addition to those mentioned may be required [104]. See Chapter 95 for further discussion of this disease.

Tetanus

Older reviews have recognized tetanus as a significant medical complication of parenteral drug users (see Chap. 97). A long history of narcotic abuse, subcutaneous injection, and the use of heroin adulterated with quinine were associated with these cases [28,81]. Although tetanus now appears to be a rare infection in the injecting drug user [4], it remains a possible complication in this group of patients. Abdominal and back pain, stiffness, and pain and inability to open the jaw are common presenting symptoms of tetanus. There are no diagnostic laboratory tests. Any patient suspected of having tetanus should be admitted to the intensive care unit and carefully monitored for airway patency, cardiac arrhythmias, and blood pressure [6]. To reduce the risk of tetanus among drug-abusing patients, tetanus toxoid should be administered if no booster or primary series has been given for 10 years. A primary series should be given to any adult who has not received three previous injections [105]. See Chapter 97 for further discussion of this disease.

References

1. Hoffman RS, Goldfrank LR: The impact of drug abuse and addiction on society. *Emerg Med Clin North Am* 8:467, 1990.
2. Haverkos HW, Lange WR: Serious infections other than human immunodeficiency virus among intravenous drug abusers. *J Infect Dis* 161:894, 1990.
3. Michelson JB, Robin HS, Nozik RA: Nonocular manifestations of parenteral drug abuse. *Surv Ophthalmol* 30:314, 1986.
4. Brettle RP: Infection and injection drug use. *J Infect* 25:121, 1992.
5. Tuazon CU, Hill R, Sheagren JN: Microbiologic study of street heroin and injection paraphernalia. *J Infect Dis* 129:327, 1974.
6. Shepherd SM, Druckenbrod GG, Haywood YC: Other infectious complications in intravenous drug users: The compromised host. *Emerg Med Clin North Am* 8:683, 1990.
7. Selwyn PA, Alcabes P, Hartel D, et al: Clinical manifestations and predictors of disease progression in drug users with human immunodeficiency virus infection. *N Engl J Med* 27:1697, 1992.
8. Hahn RA, Onorato IM, Jones TS, et al: Prevalence of HIV infection among intravenous drug users in the United States. *JAMA* 261:2677, 1989.
9. Brudney K, Dobkin J: Resurgent tuberculosis in New York City: Human immunodeficiency virus, homelessness, and the decline of tuberculosis control programs. *Am Rev Respir Dis* 144:745, 1991.
10. Selwyn PA, Hartel D, Lewis VA, et al: A prospective study of the risk of tuberculosis among intravenous drug users with human immunodeficiency virus infection. *N Engl J Med* 320:545, 1989.

11. Torres RA, Mani S, Altholz J, et al: Human immunodeficiency virus infection among homeless men in a New York City shelter: Association with *Mycobacterium tuberculosis* infection. *Arch Intern Med* 150:2030, 1990.
12. Samet JH, Shevitz A, Fowle J, et al: Hospitalization decision in febrile intravenous drug users. *Am J Med* 89:53, 1990.
13. Marantz PR, Linzer M, Feiner CJ, et al: Inability to predict diagnosis in febrile intravenous drug abusers. *Ann Intern Med* 106:823, 1987.
14. Tuazon CU, Elin RJ: Endotoxin content of street heroin [letter]. *Arch Intern Med* 141:1385, 1981.
15. Shragg T: "Cotton fever" in narcotic addicts. *JACEP* 7:279, 1978.
16. Weisse AB, Heller DR, Schimenti RJ, et al: The febrile parenteral drug user: a prospective study in 121 patients. *Am J Med* 94:274, 1993.
17. Schaffer SR: Use of prophylactic antibiotics by drug abusers [letter]. *MA* 252:1410, 1984.
18. Novick DM, Ness FL: Abuse of antibiotics by abusers of parenteral heroin or cocaine. *South Med J* 77:302, 1984.
19. Crane LR, Levine DP, Zervos MJ, et al: Bacteremia in narcotic addicts at the Detroit Medical Center. I. Microbiology, epidemiology, risk factors, and empiric therapy. *Rev Infect Dis* 8:364, 1986.
20. Levine DP, Crane LR, Zervos MJ: Bacteremia in narcotic addicts at the Detroit Medical Center. II. Infectious endocarditis: A prospective comparative study. *Rev Infect Dis* 8:374, 1986.
21. Wieland M, Lederman MM, Kline-King C, et al: Left-sided endocarditis due to *Pseudomonas aeruginosa. Medicine* [Baltimore] 65:180, 1986.
22. Tuazon CU, Sheagren JN: Increased rate of carriage of *Staphylococcus aureus* among narcotic addicts. *J Infect Dis* 129:725, 1974.
23. Tuazon CU, Sheagren JN: Staphylococcal endocarditis in parenteral drug abusers: Source of the organism. *Ann Intern Med* 82:788, 1975.
24. Lentnek AL, Giger O, O'Rourke E: Group A beta-hemolytic streptococcal bacteremia and intravenous substance abuse: A growing clinical problem? *Arch Intern Med* 150:89, 1990.
25. Biderman P, Hiatt JR: Management of soft-tissue infections of the upper extremity in parenteral drug abusers. *Am J Surg* 154:526, 1987.
26. Espiritu MB, Medina JE: Complications of heroin injections of the neck. *Laryngoscope* 90:1111, 1980.
27. Jacobson JM, Hirschman SZ: Necrotizing fasciitis complicating intravenous drug abuse. *Arch Intern Med* 142:634, 1982.
28. Louria DB, Hensle T: The major medical complications of heroin addiction. *Ann Intern Med* 67:1, 1967.
29. Orangio GR, Pitlick SD, Della Latta P, et al: Soft tissue infections in parenteral drug abusers. *Ann Surg* 199:97, 1984.
30. Somers WJ, Lowe FC: Localized gangrene of the scrotum and penis: a complication of heroin injection into the femoral vessels. *J Urol* 136:111, 1986.
31. Vollum DI: Skin lesions in drug addicts. *Br Med J* 2:647, 1970.
32. Webb D, Thadepalli H: Skin and soft tissue polymicrobial infections from intravenous abuse of drugs. *West J Med* 130:200, 1979.
33. Schiff BL, Kern AB: Unusual cutaneous manifestations of pentazocine addiction. *JAMA* 238:1542, 1977.
34. Fisher JR, Conway MJ, Takeshita RT, et al: Necrotizing fasciitis: The importance of roentgenographic studies for soft-tissue gas. *JAMA* 241:803-6, 1979.
35. Stamenkovic I, Lew PD: Early recognition of potentially fatal necrotizing fasciitis: The use of frozen-section biopsy. *N Engl J Med* 310:1689, 1984.
36. Meislin HW, Lerner SA, Graves MH, et al: Cutaneous abscesses: Anaerobic and aerobic bacteriology and outpatient management. *Ann Intern Med* 87:145, 1977.
37. Sudarsky LA, Laschinger JC, Coppa GF, et al: Improved results from a standardized approach in treating patients with necrotizing fasciitis. *Ann Surg* 206:661-65, 1987.
38. Yeager RA, Hobson RW II, Padberg FT, et al: Vascular complications related to drug abuse. *J Trauma* 27:305, 1987.
39. Johnson JR, Ledgerwood AM, Lucas CE: Mycotic aneurysm: New concepts in therapy. *Arch Surg* 118:577, 1983.
40. Lewis JW Jr., Groux N, Elliott JP Jr., et al: Complications of attempted central venous injections performed by drug abusers. *Chest* 78:612, 1980.

41. Anand A: Complications of infective endocarditis in the 1980s [letter]. *Arch Intern Med* 153:1017, 1993.

42. Chambers HF, Korzeniowski OM, Sande MA: *Staphylococcus aureus* endocarditis: Clinical manifestations in addicts and nonaddicts. *Medicine* [Baltimore] 62:170, 1983.

43. Cherubin CE, Sapira JD: Endocarditis in drug abusers [letter]. *South Med J* 85:1036, 1992.

44. Hubbell G, Cheitlin MD, Rapaport E: Presentation, management, and follow-up evaluation of infective endocarditis in drug addicts. *Am Heart J* 102:85, 1981.

45. Reisberg BE: Infective endocarditis in the narcotic addict. *Prog Cardiovasc Dis* 22:193, 1979.

46. Sheagren JN: Endocarditis complicating parenteral drug abuse, in Remington JS, Swartz MN (Eds): *Current Clinical Topics in Infectious Diseases,* Vol. 2. New York, McGraw-Hill Book Company, 1981, pp 211-233.

47. Lange M, Salaki JS, Middleton JR, et al: Infective endocarditis in heroin addicts: Epidemiological observations and some unusual cases. *Am Heart J* 96:144, 1978.

48. Chambers HF, Morris DL, Taüber MG, et al: Cocaine use and the risk for endocarditis in intravenous drug users. *Ann Intern Med* 106:833, 1987.

49. Hecht SR, Berger M: Right-sided endocarditis in intravenous drug users: Prognostic features in 102 episodes. *Ann Intern Med* 117:560, 1992.

50. Tuazon CU, Cardella TA, Sheagren JN: Staphylococcal endocarditis in drug users: Clinical and microbiologic aspects. *Arch Intern Med* 135:1555, 1975.

51. Graves MK, Soto L: Left-sided endocarditis in parenteral drug abusers: Recent experience at a large community hospital. *South Med J* 85:378, 1992.

52. Rubinstein E, Noriega ER, Simberkoff MS, et al: Fungal endocarditis: Analysis of 24 cases and review of the literature. *Medicine [Baltimore]* 54:331, 1975.

53. Baddour LM, Meyer J, Henry B: Polymicrobial infective endocarditis in the 1980s. *Rev Infect Dis* 13:963, 1991.

54. Saravolatz LD, Burch KH, Quinn EL, et al: Polymicrobial infective endocarditis: An increasing clinical entity. *Am Heart J* 95:163, 1978.

55. Dubois RW, Ginzton LW: Role of echocardiography in suspected infective endocarditis in intravenous drug abusers. *Am J Cardiol* 58:649, 1986.

56. San Román JA, Vilacosta I, Zamorano JL, et al: Transesophageal echocardiography in right-sided endocarditis. *J Am Coll Cardiol* 21:1226, 1993.

57. Chambers HF, Miller RT, Newman MD: Right-sided *Staphylococcus aureus* endocarditis in intravenous drug abusers: Two-week combination therapy. *Ann Intern Med* 109:619, 1988.

58. Korzeniowski O, Sande MA: Combination antimicrobial therapy for *Staphylococcus aureus* endocarditis in patients addicted to parenteral drugs and in nonaddicts. *Ann Intern Med* 97:496, 1982.

59. Sanabria TJ, Alpert JS, Goldberg R, et al: Increasing frequency of staphylococcal infective endocarditis: Experience at a university hospital, 1981 through 1988. *Arch Intern Med* 150:1305, 1990.

60. Abrams B, Sklaver A, Hoffman T, et al: Single or combination therapy of staphylococcal endocarditis in intravenous drug abusers. *Ann Intern Med* 90:789, 1979.

61. Parker RH, Fossieck BE: Intravenous followed by oral antimicrobial therapy for staphylococcal endocarditis. *Ann Intern Med* 93:832, 1980.

62. Komshian SV, Tablan OC, Palutke W, et al: Characteristics of left-sided endocarditis due to *Pseudomonas aeruginosa* in the Detroit Medical Center. *Rev Infect Dis* 12:693, 1990.

63. Dinubile MJ: Surgery in active endocarditis. *Ann Intern Med* 96:650, 1982.

64. Arbula A, Holmes RJ, Asfaw I: Tricuspid valvulectomy without replacement. *J Thorac Cardiovasc Surg* 102:917, 1991.

65. Chandrasekar PH, Narula AP: Bone and joint infections in intravenous drug abusers. *Rev Infect Dis* 8:904, 1986.

66. Lohr KM: Rheumatic manifestations of diseases associated with substance abuse. *Semin Arthritis Rheum* 17:90, 1987.

67. Roca RP, Yoshikawa TT: Primary skeletal infections in heroin users: a clinical characterization, diagnosis and therapy. *Clin Orthop* 144:238, 1979.

68. Sapico FL, Montgomerie JZ: Vertebral osteomyelitis in intravenous drug abusers: Report of three cases and review of the literature. *Rev Infect Dis* 2:196, 1980.

69. Rowe IF, Wright ED, Higgens CS, et al: Intervertebral infection due to *Candida albicans* in an intravenous heroin abuser. *Ann Rheum Dis* 47:522, 1988.

70. Dupont B, Drouhet E: Cutaneous, ocular, and osteoarticular candidiasis in heroin addicts: New clinical and therapeutic aspects in 38 patients. *J Infect Dis* 152:577, 1985.

71. Collignon PJ, Sorrell TC: Disseminated candidiasis: Evidence of a distinctive syndrome in heroin abusers. *Br Med J* 287:861, 1983.

72. Bisbe J, Miro JM, Latorre X, et al: Disseminated candidiasis in addicts who use brown heroin: Report of 83 cases and review. *Clin Infect Dis* 15:910, 1992.

73. Curran JW, Jaffe HW, Hardy AM, et al: Epidemiology of HIV infection and AIDS in the United States. *Science* 239:610, 1988.

74. CDC: Update: Acquired immunodeficiency syndrome—United States, 1981–1988. *MMWR* 38:229, 1989.

75. CDC: Human immunodeficiency virus infection in the United States. *MMWR* 36(49):801, 1987.

76. Schoenbaum EE, Hartel D, Selwyn PA, et al: Risk factors for human immunodeficiency virus infection in intravenous drug users. *N Engl J Med* 321:874, 1989.

77. Stoneburner RL, Des Jarlais DC, Benezra D, et al: A larger spectrum of severe HIV-1-related disease in intravenous drug users in New York City. *Science* 242:916, 1988.

78. Selwyn PA, Sckell BM, Alcabes P, et al: High risk of active tuberculosis in HIV-infected drug users with cutaneous anergy. *JAMA* 268:504, 1992.

79. Brickner PW, Torres RA, Barnes M, et al: Recommendations for control and prevention of human immunodeficiency virus (HIV) infection in intravenous drug users. *Ann Intern Med* 110:833, 1989.

80. White AG: Medical disorders in drug addicts. 200 consecutive admissions. *JAMA* 223:1469, 1973.

81. Cherubin CE: Infectious disease problems of narcotic addicts. *Arch Intern Med* 128:309, 1971.

82. CDC: Changing patterns of groups at high risk for hepatitis B in the United States. *MMWR* 37:429, 1988.

83. Ponzetto A, Seeff LB, Buskell-Bales Z, et al: Hepatitis B markers in United States drug addicts with special emphasis on the delta hepatitis virus. *Hepatology* 4:1111, 1984.

84. Barry MA, Gleavy D, Herd K, et al: Prevalence of markers for hepatitis B and hepatitis D in a municipal house of correction. *Am J Public Health* 80:471, 1990.

85. Lange WR, Cone EJ, Snyder FR: The association of hepatitis delta virus and hepatitis B virus in parenteral drug users. *Arch Intern Med* 150:365, 1990.

86. Lettau LA, McCarthy JG, Smith MH, et al: Outbreak of severe hepatitis due to delta and hepatitis B viruses in parenteral drug users and their contacts. *N Engl J Med* 317:1256, 1987.

87. CDC: Hepatitis A among drug abusers. *MMWR* 37:297, 1988.

88. Kelen GD, Green GB, Purcell RH, et al: Hepatitis B and hepatitis C in emergency department patients. *N Engl J Med* 326:1399, 1992.

89. Weinstock HS, Bolan G, Reingold AL, et al: Hepatitis C virus infection among patients attending a clinic for sexually transmitted diseases. *JAMA* 269:392, 1993.

90. van den Hoek JA, van Haastrecht HJ, Goudsmit J, et al: Prevalence, incidence, and risk factors of hepatitis C virus infection among drug users in Amsterdam. *J Infect Dis* 162:823, 1990.

91. Gelb AM, Mildvan D, Stenger RJ: The spectrum and causes of liver disease in narcotic addicts. *Am J Gastroenterol* 67:314, 1977.

92. Kreek MJ, Des Jarlais DC, Trepo CL, et al: Contrasting prevalence of delta hepatitis markers in parenteral drug abusers with and without AIDS. *J Infect Dis* 162:538, 1990.

93. McLane NJ, Carroll DM: Ocular manifestations of drug abuse. *Surv Ophthalmol* 30:298, 1986.

94. CDC: *Aspergillus* endophthalmitis in intravenous-drug users—Kentucky. *MMWR* 39:48, 1990.

95. Kreeger R, Pearson PA, Bullock JD, et al: Endophthalmitis associated with intravenous drug abuse. *Ann Emerg Med* 16:585. 1987.

96. Koppel BS, Tuchman AJ, Mangiardi JR, et al: Epidural spinal infection in intravenous drug abusers. *Arch Neurol* 45:1330, 1988.

97. Boom WH, Tuazon CU: Successful treatment of multiple brain abscesses with antibiotics alone. *Rev Infect Dis* 7:189, 1985.

98. O'Donnell AE, Pappas LS: Pulmonary complications of intravenous drug abuse. *Chest* 94:251, 1988.

99. Barnes PF, Bloch AB, Davidson PT, et al: Tuberculosis in patients with human immunodeficiency virus infection. *N Engl J Med* 324:1644, 1991.

100. Markowitz N, Hansen NI, Wilcosky TC, et al: Tuberculin and anergy testing in HIV-seropositive and HIV-seronegative persons. *Ann Intern Med* 119:185, 1993.

101. Graham NMH, Nelson KE, Soloman L, et al: Prevalence of tuberculin positivity and skin test anergy in HIV-1-seropositive and -seronegative intravenous drug users. *JAMA* 267:369, 1992.

102. Moreno S, Baraia-Etxaburu J, Bouza E, et al: Risk for developing tuberculosis among anergic patients infected with HIV. *Ann Intern Med* 119:194, 1993.

103. Jordan TJ, Lewit EM, Montgomery RL, et al: Isoniazid as preventive therapy in HIV-infected intravenous drug abusers. *JAMA* 265:2987, 1991.

104. Dooley SW, Jarvis WR, Martone WJ, et al: Multidrug resistant tuberculosis [editorial]. *Ann Intern Med* 117:257, 1992.

105. Fedson DS, Dismukes WE, Gardner P, et al: *Guide for Adult Immunization.* 2nd ed. Philadelphia, American College of Physicians, 1990.

95. *Tuberculosis*

Randall R. Reves

Historical Overview

Tuberculosis has made the transition from a disease thought to be destined for elimination from the United States in the 1980s to a disease of increasing importance to physicians and other health care providers in the 1990s. When the annual collection of death statistics in the United States began, the annual death rate attributable to tuberculosis was nearly 200 per 100,000 population [1] and among young, urban adults tuberculosis was the leading cause of death. Tuberculosis mortality rates were steadily declining but the rate of change accelerated in 1950s [2] with the beginning of the chemotherapy era. Streptomycin and para-aminosalicylic acid (PAS) were introduced in the mid-1940s, isoniazid in 1952, and ethambutol in the 1960s [3]. However, despite multidrug treatment with these drugs for 18 to 24 months, late relapses continued to occur in about 10 percent [4]. The introduction of rifampin in the 1970s allowed the development of highly effective 6- and 9-month regimens [5]. The major advance in tuberculosis control in the early 1980s was the development of effective, short-course therapy in twice or thrice weekly, directly observed protocols to ensure compliance [6,7]. In 1989 a national plan of tuberculosis elimination was announced [8].

The observed decline in tuberculosis morbidity in the United States ended in 1984 with 22,255 reported cases. The 26,283 cases reported in 1991 represented an increase of 18 percent over the number in 1984 and an increase in the annual rate from 9.4 to 10.4 cases per 100,000 population [9]. This increase has resulted in an estimated excess of 39,000 cases over the number expected. The three factors known to be associated with the increase in tuberculosis morbidity are the increased immigration of foreign-born individuals to the United States, the impact of the epidemic of human immunodeficiency virus (HIV), and the deterioration in the health care infrastructure [9]. Decreased funding of tuberculosis control programs over the past decade in some urban areas has led to low rates of completion of therapy and to the emergence of multidrug-resistant tuberculosis [10,11].

IMPORTANCE OF TUBERCULOSIS IN INTENSIVE CARE UNITS. The changing epidemiologic features of tuberculosis in the United States have important implications for all health care providers, with particular importance for those in the intensive care settings [12,13]. The rising incidence of tuberculosis in recent years, particularly of HIV-associated tuberculosis and of multidrug-resistant tuberculosis, have increased the likelihood of tuberculosis cases being admitted to intensive care units in many geographic areas. Prompt recognition of tuberculosis and early institution of effective therapy with multiple-drug therapy along with appropriate supportive measures are required to achieve the dual goals of the successful treatment of the patient and the prevention of tuberculosis transmission [14]. In situations where multidrug-resistant tuberculosis is suspected, effective empiric therapy may require treatment with four to six antituberculous drugs in an individual already receiving numerous medications for complications of the acquired immunodeficiency syndrome (AIDS) [15].

Microbiology

The genus *Mycobacterium* is composed of more than 50 species of mycobacteria distinguished by their ability to withstand decolorization by acid alcohol when stained with Ziehl-Neelsen or auramine-O methods; hence their designation as acid-fast bacilli (AFB) [16,17]. Tuberculosis is defined as disease caused by one of the three species of *Mycobacterium tuberculosis* complex. In addition to *M. tuberculosis,* the members of the complex are *M. bovis,* a rare cause of tuberculosis in foreign-born U.S. residents, and *M. africanum,* rarely seen even in Africa. *M. tuberculosis* is a nonpigmented, slow-growing organism measuring 0.2 to 0.5 μ wide and 2 to 4 μ in length. Typical buff-colored colonies can be detected after 2 to 6 weeks' incubation on potato- or egg-based media. Identification of *M. tuberculosis* is done by biochemical tests, including niacin production, nitrate reduction, and catalase production. Drug susceptibility is defined by the proportional method because of the heterogeneity of mycobacterial populations. When the number of colonies growing on agar containing a drug equals at least 1 percent of the number growing on control media, the strain is considered resistant to that drug [17].

SPUTUM MICROSCOPY. Examination of sputum or other lower respiratory specimens for AFB remains an important diagnostic tool in providing a presumptive diagnosis [17]. The accuracy of acid-fast smears is dependent on the collection of appropriate specimens and proper preparation by decontamination and liquefaction followed by centrifugation for concentration. The preparation of smears should be done in a biologic safety cabinet because of the potential of generating infectious aerosols. With the Ziehl-Neelsen stain this involves the examination of 300 fields at 1000× magnification, a process requiring 15 minutes per slide. Auramine-stained smears can be more rapidly screened at lower power with fluorescence microscopy. A skilled technologist is able to detect AFB with concentrations of 5 to 10 thousand bacilli per milliliter of sputum. The examination of a direct sputum smear for AFB by an on-call physician or inexperienced technologist not only is inadequate to exclude the diagnosis of infectious tuberculosis but could also result in laboratory transmission of tuberculosis. Mycobacteria are not reliably detected on routine sputum Gram stains, although they may occasionally be seen as gram-positive bacilli or as unstained ghost bacilli.

CULTURE AND DRUG SUSCEPTIBILITY TESTING. Because of the slow growth of mycobacterial pathogens, delays of several weeks or months for results of cultures and drug susceptibility tests were unavoidable until the 1980s, when the use of liquid media and radiometric detection was introduced. Incubation on selective agar (Middlebrook 7H10 or 7H11) or egg-based (Lowenstein-Jensen) media and speciation by biochemical testing requires 3 to 6 weeks for completion. Direct susceptibility testing with plating of concentrated sputum specimens onto control and drug-containing solid agar may provide results within 2 to 4 weeks if growth is sufficient [17,18]. When only a few colonies are isolated, direct susceptibility testing cannot be done, and several additional weeks are required for susceptibility testing of subcultures. Further delay before the clinician receives final laboratory results frequently occurs if the initial laboratory performs only primary isolation, using a reference laboratory for further studies. The BACTEC system (Becton Dickinson Diagnostic Instrument System) using a liquid Middlebrook 7H9 medium containing [14C]-labeled palmitic acid has been a major advance in the diagnosis and treatment of mycobacterial diseases. Growth of mycobacteria is often detected within 2 to 6 days by the release of [14C], and the time required for detection, speciation, and the results of drug susceptibility testing can be reduced to a total of 2 to 4 weeks [17,19]. Presumptive identification can be made in a matter of days because of the selective inhibition of *M. tuberculosis* complex by para-nitro-α-acetyl-amino-betahydroxypropiophenone (NAP). Identification of *M. tuberculosis* and speciation of most mycobacterial isolates can be done rapidly by the application of genetic mycobacterial probes. The importance of using rapid diagnostic techniques in clinical mycobacteriology has been tragically illustrated in recent outbreaks of drug-resistant tuberculosis among immunocompromised hosts whose median survival with standard, ineffective therapy was 8 weeks [20].

INVESTIGATIONAL DIAGNOSTIC TECHNIQUES. A variety of other techniques have been investigated, with the aims of increasing the rapidity of diagnosis of tuberculosis or providing methods more suitable in developing country settings [21]. These include serologic assays for antigen or antibody, tuberculostearic acid, polymerase chain reaction, and luciferase assay. The diagnostic yield of serologic techniques appears no better than that of standard AFB smears and cultures. Analysis of cerebrospinal fluid for tuberculostearic acid, done through the Centers for Disease Control (CDC), appears to have some

utility in supporting the diagnosis of tuberculous meningitis. Detection of *M. tuberculosis* by the polymerase chain reaction also appears promising as a method to increase diagnostic yield from spinal fluid and may have a role in direct identification from sputum specimens. Results from some studies have found lower sensitivity from specimens that are negative by AFB smear. The application of the luciferase assay is in early stages of development [22]. Although a number of these investigational techniques are commercially available, none are currently recommended for routine use [23].

Pathogenesis

The pathogenesis of tuberculosis is a two-stage process [1,24], the first being the development of tuberculous infection. Most infected individuals with intact cell-mediated immunity remain in this first stage, never progressing to the second stage of disease. Tuberculous infection, with rare exceptions, results from the airborne transmission of tubercle bacilli from an infectious case of pulmonary tuberculosis to a susceptible host. The transmissible particles are tubercle bacilli within droplet nuclei 1 to 5 μ in diameter, particles small enough to reach the alveolus without being trapped in the mucociliary blanket [25]. In the susceptible host the tubercle bacilli multiply to produce a localized pneumonia and spread to involve the hilar lymph nodes. The tubercle bacilli then enter the bloodstream through the thoracic duct and disseminate. This initial period of the primary infection is usually clinically inapparent but may be recognized as primary tuberculosis, particularly in children. The development of cell-mediated immunity to *M. tuberculosis* brings the infection under control in most individuals over a period of weeks. About 1 percent of immunocompetent individuals progress directly to miliary or progressive primary disease; this risk is higher among individuals with defects in cell-mediated immunity such as those with AIDS. The tuberculin skin test usually becomes positive 2 to 10 weeks after the onset of tuberculous infection. Despite the initial immunologic control of tuberculous infection in most individuals, viable tubercle bacilli remain in scattered foci with high tissue oxygen tension [24].

The second stage, the development of active tuberculosis, occurs in about 10 percent of immunocompetent individuals with tuberculous infection. About half the tuberculosis cases develop within the first 1 to 2 years after initial infection [1,24]. Among individuals with intact cell-mediated immunity, tuberculosis is characterized by the development of an intense, destructive, granulomatous inflammatory process [26]. The mechanism for disseminated disease during the second stage of tuberculosis is believed to be the direct entry of tubercle bacilli into the bloodstream because of the erosion of a tuberculous focus into a blood vessel [27]. Such a source for dissemination may be chronic pulmonary tuberculosis or an occult extrapulmonary focus.

There are significant clinical and pathologic differences noted in individuals with abnormalities of cell-mediated immunity, such as that resulting from HIV infection, that are characterized by accelerated pathogenesis. The risk of progressive primary or disseminated disease at the time of the initial tuberculous infection increases with the degree of impairment of cell-mediated immunity. Paralleling the decline in cell-mediated immunity is a decrease in the extent of granulomatous inflammation histologically and an increase in the numbers of AFB seen in tissues [28]. For instance, AFB are readily detected in lymph node aspirates in HIV-associated lymphatic tuberculosis compared with the detection of a few AFB in only a third of lymph node biopsy specimens in immunocompetent individuals. Reinfection tuberculosis, although rare in normal hosts, has been well documented [29].

Epidemiology

Determining the likelihood of tuberculosis in a critically ill patient should include an assessment of risk factors for the two stages of its pathogenesis (Table 95-1).

RISK FACTORS FOR TUBERCULOUS INFECTION. The first stage, tuberculous infection, is associated with various risk factors reflecting the likelihood of prior exposure to tuberculosis [1,30]. Tuberculosis case rates per 100,000 population in the United States in 1987 [12] were twice as high among men as among women. Compared with white non-Hispanics, the rates were higher by a factor of 4.3 for Hispanics, by 6.4 for blacks, by 4.7 for Native Americans, and by 11.2 for Pacific Islanders. Rates in all population groups were highest among the elderly because of prior exposure in childhood and transmission in long-term care facilities [31]. Foreign-born cases composed 23 percent of reported cases in the United States in 1987, but the proportion of foreign-born cases was 44 percent in Hispanics and 93 percent among Pacific Islanders [12]. Higher rates among United States–born minorities reflect the association of tuberculosis exposure with poverty and perhaps a greater risk of infection among blacks compared with whites [32].

RISK FACTORS FOR PROGRESSION TO TUBERCULOSIS. After tuberculous infection, a different set of risk factors are

Table 95-1. Factors That Should Prompt Consideration of Tuberculosis in the Differential Diagnosis

History of tuberculous infection (positive tuberculin test)
History of tuberculosis, particularly if never or inadequately treated
Risk factors for tuberculous infection but tuberculin status unknown
    Contact with known or suspected tuberculosis
    Presence of fibrotic lung lesions compatible with inactive tuberculosis
    Immigration from countries with high risk for tuberculosis
    Advanced age
    Medically underserved populations
    Alcohol or other drug use
    Institutional exposure
        Homeless shelters
        Correctional facilities
        Nursing homes
        Some hospitals and mental institutions
Higher risk for progression to disease, if tuberculin status positive or unknown
    Known or suspected HIV infection
    Other immunosuppressed states
        Lymphatic and reticuloendothelial disorders
        High-dose corticosteroids and other immunosuppressive therapy
    Recent tuberculous infection
    Presence of upper lobe scars compatible with inactive tuberculosis
    Certain medical conditions
        Silicosis
        Chronic renal failure
        Diabetes mellitus
        Intravenous drug use
        Gastrectomy or other conditions associated with weight loss

associated with progression to active tuberculosis [1,30]. The duration of tuberculous infection is an important factor because approximately half the tuberculosis cases will develop during the first 2 years after infection. The risk of progression from tuberculous infection to disease also varies with age, with the highest risk periods during infancy, during the early 20s, and after 70 years of age [33]. Individuals with pulmonary parenchymal scars of healed, untreated tuberculosis are also at increased risk of disease recurrence, ranging up to 1.4 percent per year in some studies [34]. In the critically ill individual, the presence of these and other factors associated with risk for progression to active disease (Table 95-1) should prompt consideration of tuberculosis in the differential diagnosis. The tuberculin status in such individuals is often unknown and cannot be determined because of anergy [17]. The 7 percent annual risk of tuberculosis reported by Selwyn among HIV-infected and tuberculin-positive individuals indicates that HIV infection is the greatest risk factor yet identified for progression to tuberculosis [35].

Accelerated progression from exposure to disease has been noted in several nosocomial outbreaks of multidrug-resistant tuberculosis. In one housing facility 37 percent of individuals with AIDS developed active tuberculosis within 5 months of exposure to residents with smear-positive tuberculosis [36]. The impact of HIV on the epidemiology of tuberculosis is reflected in the rising case rates since 1984 among minority groups, particularly among Hispanics and blacks in the 20- to 44-year age-group [12]. This increase has been particularly marked in locations with high morbidity due to HIV infection associated with injection drug use. New York City has experienced the greatest increase in tuberculosis morbidity among U.S. cities since 1984 [13,37].

EPIDEMIOLOGY OF DRUG-RESISTANT TUBERCULOSIS. A CDC survey of drug susceptibility tests of tubercle bacilli from newly diagnosed cases of tuberculosis in the first quarter of 1991 showed another disturbing statistic. Tuberculosis caused by strains resistant to at least one first-line drug constituted 13.3 percent of cases, and 3 percent of isolates were resistant to both isoniazid and rifampin [38]. In New York City 19 percent of cases were attributable to strains resistant to isoniazid and rifampin [11]. Acquired or secondary drug resistance is a preventable complication of treatment; it results from prescribing an inadequate treatment regimen, from failure on the part of the patient to adhere to an appropriate regimen, or frequently from a combination of the two [39]. Primary drug resistance, with resistant strains isolated from previously untreated cases, results from the transmission of drug-resistant strains. During the early decades of the antimicrobial era, drug-resistant strains of tuberculosis were believed to be less pathogenic, and potential for transmission of such strains relatively unimportant. However, two outbreaks of tuberculosis in the 1970s with primary resistance to isonicotinoylhydrazine (INH), streptomycin, and PAS dispelled the notion of benign drug-resistant tuberculosis [40,41]. Numerous additional outbreaks of multidrug-resistant tuberculosis have now been reported [38].

Clinical Manifestations and Diagnostic Features

PRESENTATIONS IN THE INTENSIVE CARE UNIT. The two likely presentations of tuberculosis in the intensive care unit include severe forms of tuberculosis as the primary disease or active tuberculosis presenting as a coincidental illness in patients being treated for another condition (Table 95-2). This latter presentation may be the result of active tuberculosis developing during a prolonged hospitalization as well as coexisting tuberculosis on admission. Respiratory failure is the most likely reason for this disease to precipitate admission to the intensive care unit. Other presentations one might expect in the intensive care unit include massive hemoptysis, pericardial tamponade, neurologic deterioration, and rarely an acute abdomen attributable to obstruction or perforation.

The symptoms and signs of tuberculosis are variable, depending on the site and extent of disease. A history of a chronic, progressive illness with fever, night sweats, and weight loss is most suggestive of tuberculosis, along with a chronic cough in pulmonary disease [42]. Associated yet nonspecific laboratory abnormalities include anemia of chronic disease, mild hypoalbuminemia, increased alkaline phosphatase, and hyponatremia caused by inappropriate secretion of antidiuretic hormone or from the occasional association with Addison's disease [43].

The most common form of tuberculosis is pulmonary, accounting for 82 percent of the 25,701 cases reported in 1990 [44]. An additional 5 percent of cases are both pulmonary and extrapulmonary, with only 18 percent of cases involving only extrapulmonary sites. The distribution of total cases by extrapulmonary sites was 5 percent for lymphatic, 4 percent for pleural, and 2 percent each for skeletal and genitourinary. Miliary, meningeal, and peritoneal each accounted for about 1 percent of cases and all other sites for only 2 percent. Even with the greater frequency of extrapulmonary tuberculosis among cases associated with AIDS, the lungs are involved in more than 70 percent of cases reviewed by Pitchenik and Fertel [45]. Fertel patients with tuberculosis admitted to the intensive care unit represent an obvious selection of the most severely ill cases. Acute respiratory failure, which occurs at a frequency of less than 2 percent of hospitalized cases [46,47], is the most common reason for admission to an intensive care unit. Acute respiratory failure may present with features of the acute respiratory distress syndrome (ARDS), as has been documented in some instances, but may also be due to fulminant tuberculous pneumonia.

PULMONARY TUBERCULOSIS. Chronic cough and chest discomfort, particularly when associated with systemic symptoms, should suggest the diagnosis of pulmonary tuberculosis. Cough is present in about two-thirds of cases and is typically productive of mucoid sputum. Dyspnea may be minimal despite fairly extensive lung destruction. Hemoptysis is reported

in about 20 percent of cases but is usually self-limited. Massive hemoptysis, classically described as caused by a Rasmussen's aneurysm of a pulmonary artery within a large cavity [48], as well as less severe forms of hemoptysis, may precipitate admission to the intensive care unit.

Routine chest radiography is an invaluable initial diagnostic test and screening test for patients at risk for tuberculosis because it is possible to detect most active cases that involve the lungs, to detect nearly all cases likely to be contagious (i.e., parenchymal disease, often with cavitation) and to identify fibrotic residuals of previously active tuberculosis. Primary tuberculosis, developing weeks to months after infection, typically presents as a lower lobe infiltrate, often with ipsilateral hilar adenopathy in children. Primary tuberculosis can be seen at any age, including the elderly, as described among recently infected nursing home residents [31]. The classic pattern of fibrotic and cavitary infiltrates in the apical segment of the upper lobe and superior segment of the lower lobes generally develops as a result of reactivation of latent infection in foci with high tissue oxygen tension (Fig. 95-1). There is considerable variation in the pattern of disease that includes focal infiltrates of alveolar or nodular patterns, with or without cavitation, as well as diffuse infiltrates of disseminated or miliary tuberculosis. The frequency of atypical presentations of pulmonary tuberculosis ranges from 34 to 45 percent in series of HIV-negative individuals [42,49,50]. An example of a delayed diagnosis of pulmonary tuberculosis in an alcoholic without HIV infection is shown in Fig. 95-2. The development of acute respiratory failure during the first 2 weeks of effective antituberculous therapy for pulmonary nondisseminated tuberculosis has been described [51].

In the presence of HIV infection, particularly with more advanced immunodeficiency, there is greater variation in the radiographic patterns of tuberculosis with a greater frequency of lower lobe involvement, diffuse infiltrates, hilar or mediastinal

Table 95-2. Presentations of Tuberculosis in the Intensive Care Unit

Tuberculosis as the primary diagnosis
  Respiratory failure
    Fulminant tuberculous pneumonia
    Disseminated tuberculosis
    Acute respiratory distress syndrome
  Hemoptysis
  Pericardial tamponade
  Neurologic deterioration from central nervous system disease
  Complications of gastrointestinal tract involvement
    Bowel obstruction or perforation
    Tuberculous peritonitis
Tuberculosis as a secondary diagnosis
  Coincidental tuberculosis
  Progression of prior infection to active disease
  Rapid progression to disease in immunocompromised hosts

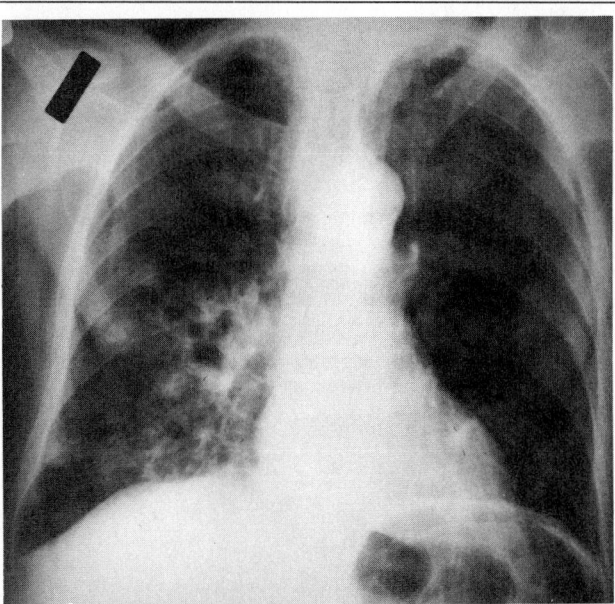

Fig. 95-1. Radiograph of 85-year-old man with cavitary tuberculosis involving the superior segment of the right lower lobe that developed 1 week after resection of the sigmoid colon for diverticular disease. The bilateral apical scars were radiographically stable and are typical of previously active tuberculosis.

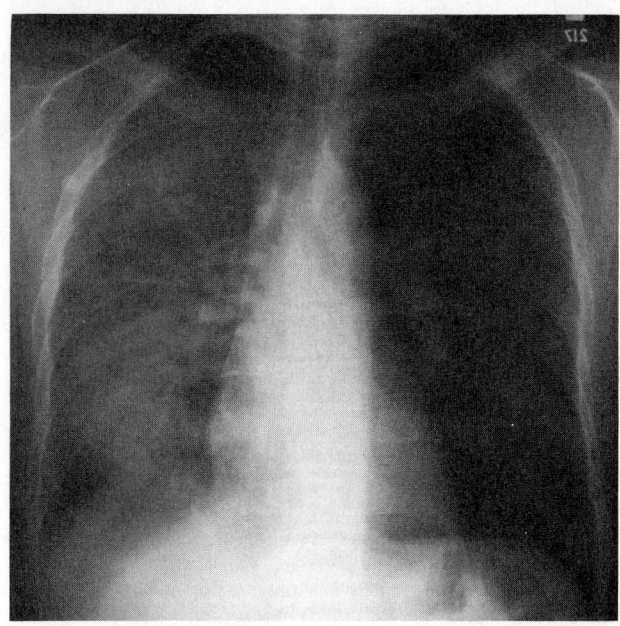

A

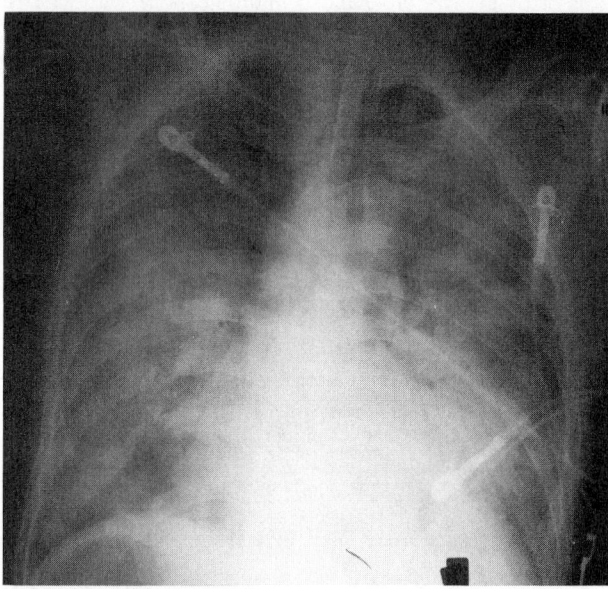

B

Fig. 95-2. Chest radiographs of a 40-year-old HIV-negative man with rapidly progressive tuberculous pneumonia. The admission radiograph (A) shows extensive right alveolar infiltrates with respiratory failure due to bilateral pneumonia on day 4 (B). He died on day 6 after receiving 2 days of antituberculous therapy. Five-lobe tuberculous pneumonia and diffuse alveolar damage was found post mortem. Tuberculosis subsequently developed in two immunocompromised hospital roommates (strains were identical on DNA fingerprinting).

adenopathy, and pleural effusions. Unfortunate delays in the diagnosis of tuberculosis have been noted in more than half of patients admitted to community hospitals, with nearly a third of those with the classic presentation not suspected on admission [42]. The diagnosis of pulmonary tuberculosis among HIV-infected individuals is frequently delayed or missed because of the more atypical radiographic patterns, as illustrated in Figs. 95-3 and 95-4, and high frequency of other pulmonary disorders [52,53].

It is important to recognize the radiographic patterns of upper lobe parenchymal scars or calcified granulomas representing residual fibrotic foci of healed, inactive tuberculosis (see Fig. 95-1). Some radiographically stable parenchymal lung scars may represent indolent active disease that may be diagnosed by the growth of tubercle bacilli from screening sputum cultures. A careful review of chest radiographs for evidence of active or inactive pulmonary tuberculosis may provide a valuable diagnostic clue to the cause of disease at other sites such as the central nervous system [54] or pericardium [55].

PLEURAL TUBERCULOSIS. Pleural tuberculosis may present as an isolated pleural process from the rupture of a granuloma into the pleural space [56] or in conjunction with pulmonary disease [57]. Symptoms may be minimal or the presentation may be more acute, suggesting a viral or bacterial cause [58]. Isolated pleural disease often resolves without treatment but is associated with a high risk of recurrent pulmonary disease [56]. Pleural effusions are associated with pulmonary tuberculosis among 20 percent of cases with AIDS and among 23 percent of age-matched control cases [59]. The pleural fluid characteristics in tuberculous pleurisy are typically those of a serous exudate with elevated protein and lactic dehydrogenase levels, glucose levels of 30 to 60 mg/dl, and pH range of 7.05 to 7.45 [60]. Early in the process there is a predominance of polymorphonuclear leukocytes in pleural fluid that is replaced by a lymphocytic predominance within days. Specimens of sputum as well as pleural fluid and pleural biopsy should be collected in cases of suspected pleural tuberculosis. The earliest presumptive diagnosis is likely to be obtained by pleural biopsy because granulomas with or without caseation are seen histologically in 60 percent of biopsy specimens. AFB are detected in 20 percent or less of pleural fluid or biopsy specimens. The frequency of culture positivity ranges from 20 to 30 percent for pleural fluid or sputum specimens to 55 to 80 percent for pleural biopsy specimens.

DISSEMINATED TUBERCULOSIS. Disseminated tuberculosis may occur early during the initial stage of tuberculous infection, or later as a complication of chronic tuberculosis. It is increasingly being seen in association with AIDS. Historically the term *miliary tuberculosis* was used to describe the pathologic lesions occurring among small children who develop progressive dissemination during their primary tuberculous infection [61]. Disseminated tuberculosis during primary infection may also occur among adults, although less commonly than among the very young [62–67]. Among adults with disseminated tuberculosis, a focus of chronic pulmonary or extrapulmonary disease is found in 23 to 32 percent of cases. More recently the term *late generalized tuberculosis* has been used to describe a more chronic, cryptic form of tuberculosis usually seen in the elderly or those with other underlying illnesses [27]. In this cryptic form of disseminated tuberculosis, miliary infiltrates are the exception, and a diagnosis is often made post mortem.

The duration of symptoms before diagnosis may vary from 1 week to over a year. Fever and other constitutional symptoms

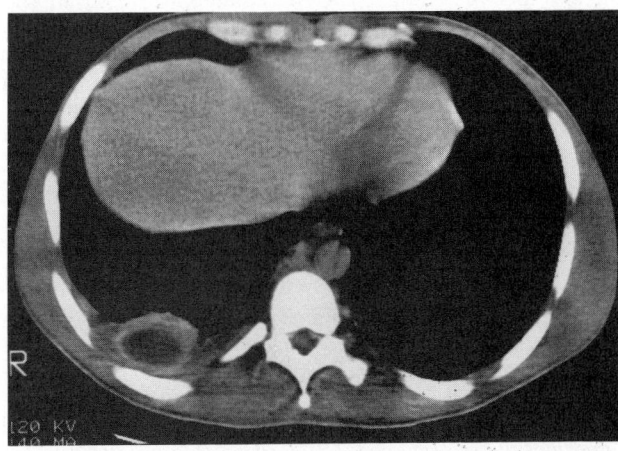

Fig. 95-3. Computerized tomographic scan showing a right lower lung pleural-based tuberculous abscess in a 25-year-old man with AIDS and bowel obstruction due to abdominal tuberculosis. The chest radiographic appearance was of a small effusion. Sputum was smear negative but culture positive for *M. tuberculosis.*

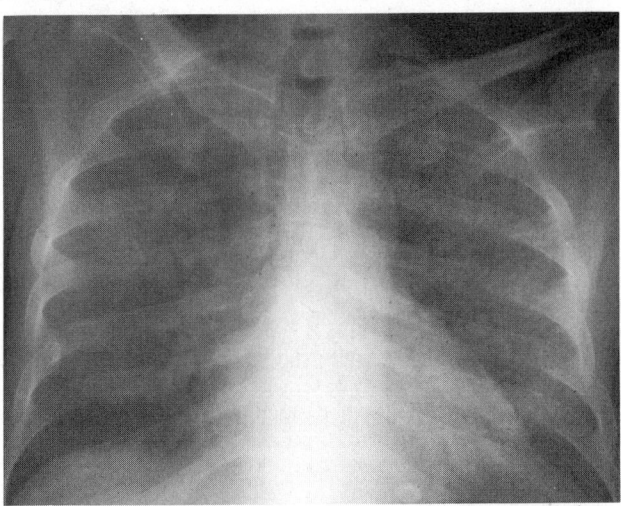

Fig. 95-4. Chest radiograph showing diffuse bilateral reticulonodular infiltrates in a 51-year-old man with AIDS, schizophrenia, and noncompliance with prior treatment for tuberculosis. Sputum smears were AFB positive. The patient survived with parenteral amikacin, ciprofloxacn, rifampin, and isoniazid plus oral ethambutol and pyrazinamide. High-dose corticosteroids were also used. The amikacin and ciprofloxacin were discontinued when drug-susceptible *M. tuberculosis* was identified, and full recovery resulted.

are seen in over 90 percent, respiratory symptoms in 75 percent, abdominal symptoms in 25 percent, and central nervous system symptoms in 20 percent. The physical findings include fever in over 90 percent, auscultatory crackles on chest examination in 75 percent, hepatomegaly in 50 percent, and lymphadenopathy in about 20 percent. Choroidal tubercles were reported in about 10 to 20 percent in earlier series [62,68] but rarely seen more recently [67]. Laboratory abnormalities are nonspecific and include anemia and levels of leukocytes and platelets ranging from markedly elevated to severely depressed [69,70,71]. Alkaline phosphatase levels are frequently elevated, suggesting a

granulomatous hepatitis. Chest radiographs may be normal or show no evidence of dissemination in about 10 percent, particularly early in the illness or if not carefully examined. In addition to miliary nodules of 1 to 3 mm diameter, larger nodules of 5 to 7 mm may be seen, as shown in Fig. 95-4. Acute respiratory failure, as illustrated in Figs. 95-2 and 95-4, is an atypical but well-characterized complication [46,47,73–76]. ARDS is occasionally seen during the initial 2 weeks of therapy of advanced pulmonary tuberculosis in the absence of dissemination [51]. Presentations of acute respiratory failure in individuals may be caused by ARDS or extensive tuberculous pneumonia. In some reports the presentation has been similar to that of gram-negative septicemia [73].

Sputum smears should be examined for AFB but are positive in fewer than a third of cases of miliary tuberculosis. Histology and cultures of transbronchial, thoracoscopic, or traditional open lung biopsy usually confirm the diagnosis, but a careful search for chronic skin lesions [77,78], scrotal involvement, or lymphadenopathy may disclose other sites amenable to diagnostic biopsy. Other potentially useful diagnostic tests include culture of urine or spinal fluid and biopsy of liver or bone marrow. Granulomas are seen in about 90 percent of liver biopsies; the yield is lower from bone marrow biopsy unless pancytopenia is present [79]. Lumbar puncture of patients with headache or other central nervous system symptoms may be diagnostic because meningitis is found in 17 to 19 percent of cases of disseminated tuberculosis.

The frequency of disseminated tuberculosis has increased in recent years as a result of the epidemic of tuberculosis among HIV-infected individuals [28]. Clinical evidence of dissemination is seen in up to 10 percent of HIV-associated tuberculosis cases, with presentations ranging from generalized lymphadenopathy to fulminant respiratory failure [76]. In most cases it appears that dissemination arises from a prior previously latent focus because of declining cell-mediated immunity associated with HIV infection, rather than early dissemination of a new infection.

Among immunocompetent individuals, mycobacteremia is uncommon [80]. A study from 1917 reported positive blood cultures in 67 percent of miliary tuberculosis cases, but only 7 percent of other forms [82]. However, there are now numerous reports of bacteremia due to *M. tuberculosis* in recent years with the increasing use of mycobacterial blood cultures [80,83–86]. Tuberculosis in HIV-infected individuals may be confirmed by culture of blood in about 26 to 42 percent of cases, with blood being the only culture-positive specimen in some cases. Urine cultures are positive in about 40 percent and stool in about 40 percent of such cases.

CENTRAL NERVOUS SYSTEM TUBERCULOSIS. Tuberculosis involving the central nervous system presents as a chronic meningitis, as one or more parenchymal tuberculomas, or as a combination of both conditions [54,86a,87]. The clinical presentation varies from an indolent illness with headache and subtle changes in mental status to more acute presentations. Focal neurologic symptoms and signs may result from involvement of cranial nerves with the inflammatory basilar meningitis, from infarction due to involvement of intracranial arteries or from tuberculomas. Evidence of active or inactive tuberculosis at another site is noted in about three-fourths of cases, most often miliary infiltrates on chest radiographs. The key to the diagnosis rests on examination of spinal fluid. The findings of a lymphocytic pleocytosis, low glucose, and elevated protein have been classically described in tuberculous meningitis. However, the absence of these findings should not be used to completely exclude the diagnosis of tuberculous meningitis because the white cell count may range from 0 to 1500, a polymorphonuclear predominance may be seen in 27 percent of cases, the protein may be under 100 in 25 percent, and the glucose greater than 45 mg per 100 ml in 83 percent [54]. AFB are detected in cerebrospinal fluid sediment of 10 to 37 percent of cases with a yield of up to 87 percent with four spinal taps. Tuberculomas of the central nervous system are readily detected by computed tomography or magnetic resonance imaging [88,89]. Antituberculous therapy is usually curative for tuberculomas, and surgical intervention is required only if necessary for diagnosis. The survival and neurologic sequelae of tuberculous meningitis are correlated with delays in therapy and severity of neurologic symptoms before treatment. Tuberculous meningitis in HIV-infected individuals presents with signs, symptoms, and laboratory findings that are similar to those found in individuals who are uninfected with HIV [90,91,92]. Intracerebral lesions are more commonly found among cases associated with HIV infection (60% vs. 14%) [92].

LYMPHATIC TUBERCULOSIS. The typical presentation of lymphatic tuberculosis is that of an enlarging cervical, supraclavicular, or axillary mass that may become fluctuant and drain spontaneously. Systemic symptoms are usually relatively minor, and an intensive care unit presentation of this form of tuberculosis would be considered unlikely before the AIDS era. Among individuals with AIDS, lymphatic tuberculosis often presents as one manifestation of disseminated disease with more marked systemic symptoms [28,53,81,93]. Enlarging peripheral, mediastinal, or intraabdominal adenopathy, particularly when associated with fever in an individual with documented or possible HIV infection, should raise the clinical suspicion for tuberculosis. In AIDS-associated lymphatic tuberculosis sputum cultures and even smears may be AFB positive despite chest radiographs that are normal or that show only hilar adenopathy [94,95]. In individuals with AIDS a percutaneous needle aspirate of an involved lymph node, with computed tomographic guidance if necessary, is a useful diagnostic step because the AFB smear is frequently positive in such cases [53]. Culture results confirm the diagnosis or provide the alternative diagnosis of disease due to *M. avium* complex, *M. kansasii*, or other nontuberculous mycobacteria that cause disseminated disease among individuals with AIDS.

OTHER EXTRAPULMONARY FORMS OF TUBERCULOSIS. Other forms such as cutaneous, skeletal, or genitourinary tuberculosis may be either coincidental findings or may provide clues to the diagnosis of disseminated tuberculosis or disease at other sites. This is particularly true for individuals with AIDS, among whom reported sites of extrapulmonary tuberculosis are innumerable [45].

Diagnosis

The most important step in making a timely diagnosis of tuberculosis is to include tuberculosis in the differential diagnosis of a variety of pulmonary and extrapulmonary disorders. Delayed or missed diagnoses of tuberculosis are all too frequent with hospitalized cases of tuberculosis, both with the typical adult form of pulmonary disease [42] and with the more atypical forms seen in association with HIV infection [53]. Tuberculosis should be reconsidered when a disease presumed to be caused by standard bacterial pathogens fails to respond to empiric therapy and when routine bacterial cultures are nondiagnostic. One should be aware that initial or empiric antibacterial therapy with some commonly used antimicrobial agents may result in a misleading initial or partial clinical response because of their activity against *M. tuberculosis*. Such agents include the fluoroquinolones such as ciprofloxacin and ofloxacin, gentamicin, amikacin, streptomycin, and rifampin [15,96].

TUBERCULIN SKIN TESTING. The tuberculin skin test is the only test available for detecting tuberculous infection [17]. Documentation of a previously positive or of a currently positive tuberculin test indicates the presence of tuberculous infection or may reflect a false-positive test caused by sensitivity to similar antigens from nontuberculous mycobacteria, but it cannot be used to confirm the diagnosis of active tuberculosis. Similarly, the tuberculin test that is negative, even with positive delayed hypersensitivity reactions to other antigens, does not rule out the diagnosis of tuberculosis. Selective anergy to tuberculin from the sequestration of sensitized lymphocytes at the site of the disease process has been demonstrated in pleural tuberculosis [97].

COLLECTION OF CLINICAL SPECIMENS. Empiric therapy for tuberculosis based on a strong clinical suspicion may be critical to the survival of the critically ill patient, but culture confirmation should be pursued aggressively because of the increasing importance of determining drug susceptibility results of *M. tuberculosis* strains. A minimum of three sputum or other lower respiratory tract specimens should be collected initially and may be useful in the absence of pulmonary infiltrates. Positive cultures of sputum in the absence of radiographic abnormalities, though relatively rare, have been reported in the pre-AIDS era [98] and among tuberculosis cases associated with AIDS [99]. If AFB smears are negative on sputum or secretions obtained by endotracheal tube suctioning, additional specimens that may yield a diagnostic smear or culture include pleural fluid, pleural biopsy, bronchoalveolar lavage, or transbronchial biopsy [28,53,67]. More invasive procedures such as transthoracic needle biopsy of lung or mediastinal lymph nodes or open lung biopsy may occasionally be indicated if the diagnosis is uncertain. Culture confirmation may be achieved with specimens from a variety of extrapulmonary sites. Virtually any body fluid, tissue, or organ may yield a diagnosis, particularly with clinical or laboratory abnormalities that suggest an extrapulmonary site of disease. Because AFB stains of involved extrapulmonary tissues are frequently negative because of the lower burden of organisms compared with that in pulmonary disease, the greatest diagnostic yield for many forms of extrapulmonary tuberculosis is from histologic examination and culture of biopsy specimens. The finding of granulomas, even noncaseating, may provide sufficient basis for a diagnosis even in the absence of AFB, as is often the case with pleural tuberculosis. Collection of a variety of appropriate specimens for confirmation may be done before and even during the initial days of empiric therapy because tubercle bacilli are not rapidly cleared from involved sites.

Treatment

PRINCIPLES OF THERAPY FOR TUBERCULOSIS. The two characteristics of *M. tuberculosis* that form the theoretical basis for current therapy of tuberculosis are their high frequency of spontaneous mutations and their slow and intermittent growth

Table 95-3. Recommended Dosage, Routes of Administration, and Major Adverse Reactions of Antituberculosis Drugs

Drug	Daily dosage (route)	Adverse effects
Isoniazid	300 mg (PO) 300 mg (IM)	Hepatitis rash, neuropathy, mood changes
Rifampin	10–20 mg/kg up to 600 mg (PO or IV)	Abdominal distress, rash, increased bilirubin & ALT, hepatitis, thrombocytopenia, renal failure, drug interactions
Pyrazinamide	15–30 mg/kg (PO) usually 2 gm/day	Rash, nausea, hepatitis, hyperuricemia, arthralgias
Ethambutol	15–25 mg/kg (PO) usually 1 to 1.6 gm/day	Nausea, optic neuritis
Streptomycin, Kanamycin, Amikacin, Capreomycin	15 mg/kg (IM or IV) (IM only for streptomycin)	Auditory & vestibular toxicity, renal toxicity, rash, transient oral paresthesias
Ofloxcin	400 mg bid (PO) 400 mg bid (IV)	Nausea, emessis, rash, headache, anxiety
Ciprofloxacin	500–750 mg bid (PO) 300–400 mg bid (IV)	Nausea, emesis, rash, headache, anxiety, drug interactions
Ethionamide	250 mg bid or tid (PO)	Nausea, emesis, rash hepatitis, neuropathy, goiter, arthralgias
Cycloserine	250 mg bid or tid (PO)	Headache, depression, psychosis, insomnia, seizures
Aminosalicylic acid	3 gm QID (PO)	Nausea, emesis, diarrhea, rash, edema, hepatitis

Adapted from information appearing in *The New England Journal of Medicine* with permission [15].

characteristics [3]. Because of these two characteristics, successful therapy of tuberculosis requires multidrug therapy for extended periods. Resistance caused by mutation occurs at a frequency of 1 of 10^5 bacilli for streptomycin, 1 of 10^6 for ethambutol and isoniazid (INH), and $1/10^8$ for rifampin [100]. A single cavitary lesion may contain up to 10^9 bacilli, so it is not surprising that individuals receiving single-drug therapy for active disease experience high failure rates because of acquired drug resistance. The theoretical probability of a spontaneous mutation resulting in a tubercle bacillus with resistance to the combination of INH plus rifampin would be reduced to $1/10^{14.}$ A combination of three drugs would reduce the likelihood of a strain resistant to the regimen to $1/10^{19-20.}$ The use of four drugs during the initial 2 months of treatment provides an additional margin of safety when the bacillary burden is high and when the results of drug susceptibility testing are not available.

Extended durations of therapy are required to ensure killing and prevent relapse of the slow-growing and intermittently dormant tubercle bacilli. To reduce the frequency of relapse, treatment for 18 to 24 months was required with the early regimens of INH plus para-aminosalicylic acid or ethambutol [4]. The addition of rifampin to INH-containing regimens was a major advance, allowing successful treatment in 9 months in nearly 100 percent of drug-susceptible cases with relapse rates of less than 5 percent [5]. Similar results have been achieved with the combination of INH, rifampin, and pyrazinamide for the initial 2 months, followed by 4 months of INH and rifampin [101].

RECOMMENDATIONS FOR INITIAL THERAPY. Table 95-3 lists the drugs used in the treatment of tuberculosis with dosages, routes of administration, and common adverse effects. The two 6- and 9-month regimens were considered the standard by the American Thoracic Society and Centers for Disease Control from 1983 to 1993, when they were revised in light of the increased prevalence of tuberculosis due to drug-resistant strains (Table 95-4) [11,102]. The new recommendations consider the four-drug combinations of INH, rifampin, and pyrazinamide with either ethambutol or streptomycin as the standard initial therapy of cases of tuberculosis, unless drug susceptibility results are known or unless initial drug resistance is improbable. The goal of these recommendations is to avoid the inadvertent treatment of drug-resistant cases with inadequate regimens [9]. Equally important as the choice of several recommended regimens is the issue of compliance with therapy [103]. Compliance should be less an issue in the intensive care setting, but the goal of eventual discharge planning should be to ensure compliance with outpatient therapy.

DRUG-RESISTANT TUBERCULOSIS. Treatment of tuberculosis caused by documented drug-resistant strains requires an individualized approach based on the results of several important sources of information. The results of recent cultures and drug susceptibility testing are important but may not be completely reliable in previously treated cases [15]. Other invaluable information includes the results of previous drug susceptibility studies and details of previous antituberculous treatment received. Resources that should be used in documenting previous treatment and susceptibility results include local and state health departments as well as prior health care providers. Results of drug susceptibility studies may vary during long courses of ineffective therapy, and previous findings of resistance to a drug should not be ignored even with subsequent results indicating susceptibility. Even in the absence of in vitro resistance, previous use of a drug may render that agent less effective in cases being retreated [104].

In designing a regimen for the treatment of drug-resistant tuberculosis, the goal is to ensure that initial treatment includes a minimum of three and preferably four drugs to which the organism is susceptible and that have not previously been used. Table 95-5 lists the regimens often used for therapy of tuberculosis caused bacilli with various patterns of drug resistance. Treatment of tuberculosis due to bacilli resistant to INH alone

Table 95-4. Recommended Initial Regimens for the Therapy of Tuberculosis in 1993 [a]

Option	Regimen	Comments
Standard (susceptibilities unknown)	INH, RIF, & PZA, plus EMB or SM	Reduces infectiousness most rapidly Effective for most 1–2 drug-resistant strains Amenable to early intermittent use [b]
Alternate option (proven susceptible strains)	INH, RIF, PZA	Inadequate for INH- or RIF-resistant strains May be adopted once susceptibilities known Sputum cleared less rapidly

[a] American Thoracic Society, Centers for Disease Control 1993, revised recommendations for initial 2 months' treatment. If INH- & RIF-susceptible, INH and RIF alone continued for 4 additional months (7 additional months for HIV-positive individuals). INH and RIF alone no longer considered a standard regimen.
[b] Initial use of this regimen permits an early change (2 weeks or less) to twice or thrice weekly, directly observed therapy (DOT) with altered dosage to ensure outpatient compliance.

Table 95-5. Suggested Regimens [a] for Patients with Drug-Resistant Tuberculosis

Resistance	Regimen	Comments
INH	RIF, EMB, PZA, AG	Highly effective
INH & EMB	RIF, PZA, AG, OFL	Highly effective
INH & RIF	EMB, PZA, AG, OFL	Consider surgery
INH, RIF & EMB	PZA, OFL, AG, plus 2 [b]	Consider surgery
INH, RIF, PZA	EMB, OFL, AG, plus 2 [b]	Consider surgery
INH, RIF, EMB, & PZA	OFL, AG, plus 2 [b]	Consider surgery

[a] Abbreviations as follows: INH = isoniazid, RIF = rifampin, EMB = ethambutol, PZA = pyrazinamide, OFL = ofloxacin (ciprofloxacin may be substituted), AG = aminogloycoside. With resistance to streptomycin, amikacin or kanamycin may be used; capreomycin is used with resistance to the latter.
[b] Potential agents from which to choose include ethionamide, cycloserine, or para-aminosalicylic acid.
Adapted from Iseman [15], with permission.

or in combination with streptomycin is 95 to 100 percent effective with regimens that include rifampin, ethambutol, and pyrazinamide [15]. The addition of streptomycin or amikacin, if resistance to streptomycin is present, should be strongly considered initially. The combination of resistance to INH plus ethambutol is more troublesome, but treatment with an aminoglycoside, rifampin, pyrazinamide, and ofloxacin (or ciprofloxacin) is quite effective. The fluoroquinolones exhibit good in vitro activity against *M. tuberculosis* [105], and limited clinical experience with ofloxacin appears promising [106,107]. Because of their lower frequency of treatment-limiting adverse effects, these agents are often used before the older second-line drugs ethionamide, cycloserine, and PAS [15].

Treatment of disease due to tubercle bacilli resistant to INH and rifampin, often accompanied with resistance to other drugs, is much more difficult. Treatment failures occur in 35 percent of such cases, with later relapse in 20 percent [104]. These discouraging results have been obtained despite the occasional use of resectional surgery, hospital stays of 7 months, and durations of therapy extended to 18 to 24 months. The poorly tolerated second line drugs with known activity (cycloserine, ethionamide, and para-aminosalicylic acid) are often required in the treatment of such cases. Other unproven agents that may be used as a last resort are clofazamine or amoxacillin/clavulanate.

Given the relatively poor antituberculosis activity of the alternative drugs used in the treatment of drug-resistant tuberculosis, some experts have recommended the measurement of serum drug levels to push levels of the agents well above the minimal inhibitory concentrations [15]. Although not ex-

amined in a comparative trial, surgical resection appears to be a useful adjunct in the therapy of multidrug-resistant tuberculosis [108].

OTHER SPECIAL TREATMENT CONSIDERATIONS. Several situations requiring special considerations in the treatment of tuberculosis are listed in Table 95-6.

Empiric Therapy for Suspected Drug Resistance. The need to initiate treatment for suspected rather than documented drug-resistant tuberculosis is more likely in the intensive care unit because of more fulminant presentations in that setting. In a number of situations the standard four-drug regimens may be inadequate and result in treatment failures with the loss of activity of additional antituberculous drugs. Table 95-7 lists several situations in which drug-resistant tuberculosis is more likely and in which modifications of the standard recommendations should be considered. Recognition of exposure to an infectious case of drug-resistant tuberculosis, or knowledge of epidemic or high-level endemic transmission of a particular drug-resistant strain can be invaluable. In the settings of some institutional and community outbreaks, initial treatment with up to five or six drugs has been recommended [11,15]. Treatment failures or relapses require additional consideration because of the uncertainty they engender. Not surprisingly, the frequency of drug-resistant bacilli is higher among previously treated than among untreated cases. Clinical judgment concerning the likelihood of drug resistance dictates whether one should continue a standard but failing regimen pending susceptibility results or

Table 95-6. Treatment Recommendations for Tuberculosis in Special Situations

Situation	Recommendation	Comments
Possible primary drug resistance	Ascertain resistance patterns of epidemic, or endemic strains	Initiate standard therapy, including at least 3 drugs likely to be active against the suspected strain.
Treatment failure[a]	Repeat culture and susceptibility testing. Continue current drugs or add 2–3 new[b] drugs.	Add 2–3 new drugs pending results if prior regimen was suboptimal or if resistance is likely.
Treatment relapse	Obtained records of prior treatment & susceptibilities. Repeat susceptibilities.	Standard 4-drug regiment is still susceptible. Consider 2–3 new agents pending results. Alter regimen based on susceptibility.
Pregnancy	INH, RIF, PZA, and EMB	Avoid aminoglycosides, fluoroquinolones; ethionamide only late in pregnancy; limited data on PZA.
Questionable oral absorption	Use parenteral drugs initially. Consider testing drug levels.	Malabsorption reported in AIDS. Use parenteral aminoglocosides, rifampin, fluoroquionolones, and INH.

[a] Failure occurs during treatment and is defined as persistence of positive sputum smears or cultures beyond 3 months, poor clinical response, or deterioration (clinical or microbiologic) during treatment despite an initial response.
[b] New drugs are ones not previously received by the patients and to which the organism is likely to be susceptible.

Table 95-7. Risk Factors for Tuberculosis Caused by Drug-Resistant Organisms

Tuberculin conversion after exposure to a documented resistant case
Exposure to known epidemic or endemic foci or drug resistance
Birth and residence in a high-risk developing country
Treatment failure or relapse, particularly if poorly compliant

whether it is better to add two or three new drugs; the latter should generally be done in the critically ill patient.

Pregnancy. The treatment of tuberculosis in pregnancy is not particularly difficult if it is attributable to drug-susceptible organisms. INH, rifampin, and ethambutol have been used most extensively without apparent adverse effects on the fetus [96,102,109]. No evidence of fetal risk has been reported with the limited experience in pregnancy with pyrazinamide, and some experts recommend its use. The use of the aminoglycosides during pregnancy may result in fetal deafness and malformation and should be avoided. The fluoroquinolones are contraindicated during pregnancy and childhood based on animal studies showing skeletal abnormalities. Ethionamide may be teratogenic and should not be used in early pregnancy. As with any life-threatening maternal disease during pregnancy, multidrug-resistant tuberculosis presents ethical dilemmas.

Parenteral Therapy. Poor absorption of antituberculous drugs has been associated with clinical failure in the treatment of drug-resistant tuberculosis in individuals with AIDS. Malabsorption of rifampin, ciprofloxacin and ethambutol has also been noted among individuals with disseminated *M. avium* complex infection associated with AIDS [110]. Drugs that can be given by the parenteral route should be used initially in the treatment of fulminant cases of tuberculosis, particularly when malabsorption is a consideration (Table 95-6). In addition to the aminoglycosides, rifampin and the fluoroquinolones may be administered intravenously. INH may be given by the intramuscular route.

MANAGEMENT OF ADVERSE DRUG EFFECTS. During the treatment of tuberculosis, serious mistakes can result from the failure to appropriately recognize and manage adverse drug effects [96]. These mistakes may result from the failure to permanently interrupt therapy in the face of a serious adverse effect as well as from abandoning valuable drugs because of minor adverse effects. Minor side effects such as gastrointestinal problems can often be managed symptomatically or by alteration in dosing schedules. Transient rashes are often associated with pyrazinamide and may be managed with antihistamines. Increased transaminase levels are more common with the combination of INH, rifampin, and pyrazinamide than when these drugs are used alone. When aspartate transaminase (AST) levels exceed 5 times the upper limit of normal, the drugs are usually discontinued, and the offending drug is identified by cautiously rechallenging with one drug at a time. With a rapid rise in AST to levels of 10 to 20 times normal, a rechallenge with INH should probably be avoided. Isolated bilirubin elevations caused by rifampin-associated cholestasis may occur but resolve despite continued therapy. Rifampin-associated renal failure, hemolysis, or thrombocytopenia should result in its permanent discontinuation.

THE ROLE OF CORTICOSTEROIDS. In certain circumstances, corticosteroids play a useful role in the therapy of tuberculosis by reducing the intensity of the inflammatory response [102,111,112]. The addition of corticosteroids to effective chemotherapy may serve a useful function in controlling disabling local and systemic effects of tuberculosis, and in selected circumstances may reduce morbidity and mortality. In early comparative studies of pulmonary or pleural tuberculosis, corticosteroid use was associated with a more rapid resolution of the symptoms of fever and anorexia and a more rapid improvement in radiographic abnormalities. However, no long-term benefit in reducing lung destruction was seen. In meningitis and pericarditis, where the inflammatory response may cause irreversible damage, corticosteroids may play a significant, even life-saving role. In randomized, placebo-controlled trials, corticosteroids were shown to lower the mortality and morbidity of patients being treated for tuberculous meningitis [113] and to reduce the need for pericardiocentesis in patients being treated for tuberculous pericarditis [114,115]. There appears to be no long-term benefit of corticosteroids in reducing the late complication of constrictive pericarditis. In most studies showing a benefit of corticosteroids, initial daily doses of 40 to 80 mg prednisone were used, followed by tapering doses over several weeks. The role of corticosteroids in acute respiratory failure caused by tuberculosis is undefined but may be helpful [51].

In summary, the use of corticosteroids should be considered in patients for whom fever, anorexia, and other systemic symptoms are disabling or interfere with nutrition and ingestion of oral medications. Corticosteroids should be used in most cases of tuberculous meningitis and pericarditis. Studies of corticosteroids in HIV-associated tuberculosis have not been published, but given their demonstrated benefit in the therapy of severe AIDS-associated pneumocystosis, they may be of benefit in individuals with AIDS-associated tuberculosis who otherwise meet the indications for corticosteroid use.

Infection Control and Respiratory Isolation

Nosocomial transmission of tuberculosis was considered an unavoidable occupational hazard for health care professional in the 1920s when up to 80 percent of nursing students became infected per year [116]. In the past few decades in the United States, annual infection rates in hospital personnel were expected to be less than 1 percent and by the 1980s, questions were raised concerning the utility of routine tuberculin testing of hospital personnel [117]. The nosocomial outbreaks of multidrug-resistant tuberculosis in the 1990s, with annual infection rates in hospital personnel similar to those early in this century, have banished all controversy over the necessity for highly effective infection control measures for tuberculosis.

NOSOCOMIAL TRANSMISSION OF MULTIDRUG-RESISTANT TUBERCULOSIS. During 1990 to 1992, there were eight reported outbreaks of nosocomial multidrug-resistant tuberculosis involving more than 200 cases among individuals in hospitals or prisons [38]. One third of exposed health care workers had documented tuberculin skin test conversion in two hospitals, and disease attributable to the epidemic strain occurred in 17 personnel. The high rates of nosocomial transmission in these and other outbreaks were associated with the failure to initiate and maintain recommended respiratory isolation, and with the rapid development of infectious tuberculosis after infection in HIV-infected individuals [118–122]. Subsequent reports from several of the institutions indicate that rigorous application of respiratory isolation procedures has interrupted nosocomial transmission [118,119] (see Chap. 86).

FACTORS ASSOCIATED WITH TRANSMISSION. As discussed earlier in this chapter, tuberculosis is transmitted by the airborne route by droplet nuclei. Because of their size, droplet nuclei remain suspended for hours, settling slowly to the floor, where they becoming noninfectious or disperse through the air by diffusion. These characteristics of droplet nuclei permit the transmission of tuberculosis at some distance through air handling systems as shown experimentally in guinea pigs [123] and as illustrated during a tuberculosis epidemic aboard a naval vessel [124]. Other less common modes of transmission of tuberculosis include the generation of infectious aerosols in laboratories or during debridement of tuberculous infected wounds [125], direct inoculation [126], and rarely from congenital transmission [127]. Individuals with active, cavitary pulmonary or laryngeal tuberculosis who have frequent, productive coughs are most likely to be contagious [14,17]. Cough-inducing

measures such as sputum induction, bronchoscopy, and administration of inhaled medications such as pentamidine have the potential to increase infectiousness. Reflecting the greater concentration of bacilli, cases with AFB-positive sputum smears are more infectious. Infection is more likely to result when exposure to such infectious cases occurs in settings where droplet nuclei remain suspended in the air in high concentrations. Rooms with smaller air volume and with poor ventilation or with recirculated ventilation present the highest risk for transmission of tuberculosis. Compared with most communicable diseases, tuberculosis cases are generally of low infectiousness. An average of a third of household contacts of smear-positive cases become infected, yet an occasional highly infectious case results in outbreaks with high attack rates of tuberculosis infection and disease in a variety of settings, including hospitals.

PREVENTING NOSOCOMIAL TRANSMISSION. Measures to prevent the transmission of tuberculosis in health care settings were updated by the Centers for Disease Control in 1990 [14]. Table 95-8 represents an adaptation of these recommendations to the intensive care unit setting. Early recognition of tuberculosis is the most important step in preventing the transmission of tuberculosis, because this allows the appropriate use of respiratory isolation and because it allows the prompt initiation of treatment. The infectiousness of tuberculosis begins to decrease within days of the initiation of effective therapy, probably by decreasing the cough as well as by reducing the number of tubercle bacilli. Timely examination of AFB smears and rapid diagnostic techniques for culture, identification, and drug susceptibility testing of mycobacteria are required to ensure prompt, effective therapy. Decisions about respiratory isolation need to be made carefully because most institutions have limited numbers of rooms designed for respiratory isolation. Decisions about discontinuing isolation should be carefully individualized, avoiding a decision based only on the number of days on therapy. The criteria that should be used in determining infectiousness are listed in Table 95-8. The safest approach in a patient receiving treatment in the hospital is to isolate until three sputum smears are negative, particularly when drug susceptibilities are unknown.

Environmental controls are important in preventing nosocomial transmission of tuberculosis, both in preventing the spread of droplet nuclei within the institution and in clearing them from the air in the isolation room. The major focus for removing droplet nuclei in isolation rooms has been on dilution of room air with exhaust directly to the outside. Most state or local hospital regulations require 10 or 12 air exchanges per hour, well in excess of the six recommended for isolation rooms. In most hospitals these high levels of air are achieved by recirculation of air after filtration through high-efficiency particulate (HEPA) filters, a practice not recommended for tuberculosis isolation rooms. Some institutions have relied on ultraviolet [128] light, and others have used the recirculation of air filtered through high-efficiency particulate filters (HEPA), although complete reliance on either method has not been recommended by the Centers for Disease Control. Additional measures that are likely to be of benefit in the intubated patient with tuberculosis include the use of closed suctioning systems to avoid generation of infectious aerosols and the use of submicron filters for air exhausted from ventilated patients [129]. Regardless of the methods used, periodic maintenance and monitoring of effectiveness must be done.

The method to be used as an adjunct to the measures above is that of personal protective devices. Properly fitted disposable particulate respirators designed to remove particles of 1- to 5-μ size are recommended, particularly in those settings where

Table 95-8. Methods of Preventing Tuberculosis Transmission in the Intensive Care Unit

I. Decrease the generation of droplet nuclei
  A. Early identification and effective treatment of active tuberculosis
  B. Maintain a clinical suspicion for tuberculosis
  C. Ensure the use of timely, reliable sputum AFB bacteriology examintaions
  D. Ensure the use of rapid diagnostics in mycobacteriology
  E. Assess the infectiousness of tuberculosis
    1. Infectious—isolation required
      a. Positive sputum smear
      b. Untreated, early in treatment or not clinically responding
    2. Probably not infectious—isolation usually continued while hospitalized
      a. Effectively treated for 2–3 weeks
      b. Definite clinical and bacteriologic improvement
    3. Not infectious—respiratory isolation not required
      a. Clinically responding to effective chemotherapy
      b. Sputum smears negative on 3 consecutive days.
II. Prevent the transmission of droplet nuclei
  A. Removal of droplet nuclei from the air
    1. Negative pressure rooms with air exhausted on the outside
    2. Ensure at least 6 air exchanges per hour
    3. Consider the use of supplemental measures
      a. Submicron filters on air exhausted from ventilators of suspected cases
      b. Closed system for endotracheal tube suctioning to avoid aerosol generation
      c. Germicidal ultraviolet irradiation with safety precautions
      d. High-efficiency particulate air filtration in general areas
III. Protection for exposed personnel
  A. Disposable particulate respirator masks (dust-mist-fume)
    a. Must exclude 1–5 μ particles
    b. Must be tight fitting

there is high-level generation of droplet nuclei. Standard surgical masks probably provide no protection because of the large pore sizes but may be placed on patients with contagious tuberculosis as a method of covering the mouth to reduce the generation of droplet nuclei. Periodic tuberculin testing of hospital personnel should be continued as a means of monitoring the effectiveness of other measures and of evaluating tuberculin converters and providing preventive therapy when appropriate [130,131]. Health care workers with documented tuberculin skin test using the Mantoux method should be evaluated for active tuberculosis by a history and physical examination and by chest radiograph. Those without evidence of active tuberculosis should be evaluated for preventive therapy with isoniazid [102] or with alternative regimens if infection with a tubercle bacillus resistant to isoniazid or to multiple drugs is likely [130]. The possibility of HIV infection in the health care worker should be considered and anergy testing included if tuberculin tests are negative [131]. See previous discussion concerning tuberculin skin testing in the Diagnosis section.

PUBLIC HEALTH ASPECTS. Presumptive and confirmed cases of tuberculosis should be promptly reported to the local public health department as required by law in every state. The function of this reporting is to provide the opportunity to conduct timely contact investigations, which may be critical to preventing life-threatening complications of tuberculosis among small children or immunocompromised household members.

In addition, many health departments can assist in ensuring completion of outpatient therapy and thus prevent a hospital readmission for treatment failure or relapse with drug-resistant tuberculosis.

References

1. Comstock GW: Epidemiology of tuberculosis. *Am Rev Respir Dis* 125(No. 3, Pt 2):8, 1982.
2. Comstock GW: Advances toward the conquest of tuberculosis. *Public Health Reports* 95:444, 1980.
3. Grosset JH: Present status of chemotherapy for tuberculosis. *Rev Infect Dis* 11:347, 1989.
4. Medical Research Council—Tuberculosis Chemotherapy Trials Committee: Long-term chemotherapy in the treatment of chronic pulmonary tuberculosis with cavitation. *Tubercle* 43:201, 1962.
5. British Thoracic and Tuberculosis Association: Short-course chemotherapy in pulmonary tuberculosis: A controlled trial. *Lancet* 2:1102, 1976.
6. Hong Kong Chest Service/British Medical Research Council: Five-year follow-up of a controlled trial of five 6-month regimens of chemotherapy for pulmonary tuberculosis. *Am Rev Respir Dis* 136:1339, 1987.
7. Hong Kong Chest Service/British Medical Research Council: Controlled trial of 2, 4, and 6 months of pyrazinamide in 6-month, three-times-weekly regimens for smear-positive pulmonary tuberculosis, including an assessment of a combined preparation of isoniazid, rifampin, and pyrazinamide: Results at 30 months. *Am Rev Respir Dis* 143:700, 1991.
8. Advisory Committee for the Elimination of Tuberculosis: A strategic plan for the elimination of tuberculosis in the United States. *MMWR* 38(suppl 3):1, 1989.
9. Centers for Disease Control: Initial therapy for tuberculosis in the era of multidrug resistance: Recommendations of the Advisory Council for the Elimination of Tuberculosis. *MMWR* 42(RR-7):1, 1993.
10. Brudney K, Dobkin J: Resurgent tuberculosis in New York City. *Am Rev Respir Dis* 144:745, 1991.
11. Frieden TR, Sterling T, Pablos-Mendez A, et al: The emergence of drug-resistant tuberculosis in New York City. *N Engl J Med* 328(8):521, 1993.
12. Rieder HL, Cauthen GM, Kelly GD, et al: Tuberculosis in the United States. *JAMA* 262:385, 1989.
13. Barnes PF, Bloch AB, Davidson PT, et al: Tuberculosis in patients with human immunodeficiency virus infection. *N Engl J Med* 324:1644, 1991.
14. Guidelines for preventing tuberculosis transmission in health-care settings, with special focus on HIV-related issues. *MMWR* 39(RR-17):1, 1990.
15. Iseman MD: Treatment of multidrug-resistant tuberculosis. *N Engl J Med* 329:784, 1993.
16. Wayne LG: Microbiology of tubercle bacilli. *Am Rev Respir Dis* 25(No. 3,Pt 2):31, 1982.
17. American Thoracic Society/Centers for Disease Control: Diagnostic standards and classification of tuberculosis. *Am Rev Respir Dis* 142(No. 3):725, 1990.
18. Heifets LB: Rapid automated methods (BACTEC System) in clinical mycobacteriology. *Semin Respir Infect* 1(No. 4):242, 1986.
19. Snider DE, Good RC, Kilburn JO, et al: Rapid susceptibility testing of *Mycobacterium tuberculosis*. *Am Rev Respir Dis* 123:422, 1981.
20. Fischl MA, Daikos GL, Uttamchandani RB, et al: Clinical presentation and outcome of patients with HIV infection and tuberculosis caused by multiple-drug-resistant bacilli. *Ann Intern Med* 117:184, 1992.
21. Daniel TM: The rapid diagnosis of tuberculosis: A selective review. *J Lab Clin Med* 116(3):277, 1990.
22. Cooksey RC, Crawford JT, Jacobs WR, et al: A rapid method for screening antimicrobial agents for activity against a strain of *Mycobacterium tuberculosis* expressing firely luciferase. *Antimicrob Agents Chemother* 37:1348, 1993.
23. Centers for Disease Control: Diagnosis of tuberculosis by nucleic

acid amplification methods applied to clinical specimens. *MMWR* 42(No. 35):686, 1993.

24. Stead WW: Pathogenesis of a first episode of chronic pulmonary tuberculosis in man: Recrudescence of residuals of the primary infection or exogenous reinfection? *Am Rev Respir Dis* 95:729, 1967.

25. Riley RL: Disease transmission and contagion control. *Am Rev Respir Dis* 125:16, 1982.

26. Pratt PC: Pathology of tuberculosis. *Semin Roentgenol* 14:196, 1979.

27. Slavin RE, Walsh TJ, Pollack AD: Late generalized tuberculosis: A clinical pathologic analysis and comparison of 100 cases in the preantibiotic and antibiotic eras. *Medicine* 59:352, 1980.

28. Hill AR, Premkumar S, Brustein S, et al. Disseminated tuberculosis in the acquired immunodeficiency era. *Am Rev Respir Dis* 144:1164, 1991.

29. Small PM, Shafer RW, Hopewell PC, et al: Exogenous reinfection with multidrug-resistant *Mycobacterium tuberculosis* in patients with advanced HIV infection. *N Engl J Med* 328:1137, 1993.

30. Rieder HL, Cauthen GM, Comstock GW, et al: Epidemiology of tuberculosis in the United States. *Epidemiol Rev* 11:79, 1989.

31. Stead WW, Lofgren JP, Warren E, et al: Tuberculosis as an endemic and nosocomial infection among the elderly in nursing homes. *N Engl J Med* 312:1483, 1985.

32. Stead WW, Senner JW, Lofgren JP, et al: Racial differences in susceptibility to infection by *Mycobacterium tuberculosis. N Engl J Med* 322:422, 1990.

33. Stead WW, Lofgren JP: Does the risk of tuberculosis increase in old age? *J Infect Dis* 147:371, 1983.

34. Edwards LB, Doster B, Livesay VT, et al: Risk of tuberculosis among persons with "not active—not treated" lesions. *Bull Int Union Tuberc* 47:151, 1972.

35. Selwyn PA, Hartel D, Lewis VA, et al: A prospective study of the risk of tuberculosis among intravenous drug users with human immunodeficiency virus infection. *N Engl J Med* 320:545, 1989.

36. Daley CL, Small PM, Schecter GF, et al: An outbreak of tuberculosis with accelerated progression among persons infected with the human immunodeficiency virus: An analysis using restriction-fragment-length polymorphisms. *N Engl J Med* 326:231, 1992.

37. Barnes PF, Barrows SA: Tuberculosis in the 1990's. *Ann Intern Med* 119:400, 1993.

38. Villarino ME, Geiter LJ, Simone PM: The multidrug-resistant tuberculosis challenge to public health efforts to control tuberculosis. *Public Health Reports* 107(6):616, 1992.

39. Mahmoudi A, Iseman, MD: Pitfalls in the care of patients with tuberculosis. *JAMA* 270:65, 1993.

40. Steiner, M: Common errors and their association with the acquisition of drug resistance: Primary drug-resistant tuberculosis: Report of an outbreak. *N Engl J Med* 283:1353, 1970.

41. Reves R, Blakey D, Snider D, et al: Transmission of multiple drug-resistant tuberculosis: Report of a school and community outbreak. *Am J Epidemiol* 113: 423, 1981.

42. Counsell SR, Tan JS, Dittus RS: Unsuspected pulmonary tuberculosis is a community teaching hospital. *Arch Intern Med* 149:1274, 1989.

43. Braidy J, Pothel C, Amra S: Miliary tuberculosis presenting as adrenal failure. *Can Med Assoc J* 124:748, 1981.

44. Centers for Disease Control: Tuberculosis statistics in the United States, 1990. U.S. Department of Health and Human Services, National Center for Prevention Services, pp 6-7, 1992.

45. Pitchenik AE, Fertel D: Tuberculosis and nontuberculosis mycobacterial disease. *Med Clin North Am* 76(1):121, 1992.

46. Levy H, Kallenbach JM, Feldman C, et al: Acute respiratory failure in active tuberculosis. *Crit Care Med* 15(3):221, 1987.

47. Dyer RA, Chappell WA, Potgieter PD: Adult respiratory distress syndrome associated with miliary tuberculosis. *Crit Care Med* 13:12, 1985.

48. Plessinger VA, Jolly PN: Rasmussen's aneurysms and fatal hemorrhage in pulmonary tuberculosis. *Am Rev Tuberc* 60:589, 1949.

49. Kahn MA, Koynat DM, Bachus B, et al: Clinical and roentgenographic spectrum of pulmonary tuberculosis in the adult. *Am J Med* 62:31, 1977.

50. Miller WT, MacGregor RR: Tuberculosis: Frequency of unusual radiographic findings. *AJR* 130:867, 1978.

51. Onwubalili JK, Scott GM, Smith H: Acute respiratory distress related to chemotherapy of advanced pulmonary tuberculosis: A study of two cases and review of the literature. *Q J Med* 50(230):599, 1986.

52. Flora GS, Modilevsky T, Antoniskis D, et al: Undiagnosed tuberculosis in patients with human immunodeficiency virus infection. *Chest* 98:1056, 1990.

53. Kramer F, Modilevsky T, Waliany AR, et al: Delayed diagnosis of tuberculosis in patients with human immunodeficiency virus infection. *Am J Med* 89:451, 1990.

54. Kennedy DH, Fallon RJ: Tuberculosis meningitis. *JAMA* 241:264, 1979.

55. Rooney JJ, Crocco JA, Lyons HA: Tuberculosis pericarditis. *Ann Intern Med* 72:72, 1970.

56. Roper WH, Waring JJ: Primary serofibrinous pleural effusion in military personnel. *Am Rev Tuberc* 71:616, 1955.

57. Berger HW, Mejia E: Tuberculosis pleurisy. *Chest* 63:88, 1973.

58. Levine H, Szanto PB, Cugell DW: Tuberculous pleurisy. An acute illness. *Arch Intern Med* 122:329, 1968.

59. Chaisson RE, Schecter GF, Theuer CP, et al: Tuberculosis in patients with the acquired immunodeficiency syndrome: Clinical features, response to therapy, and survival. *Am Rev Respir Dis* 136:570, 1987.

60. Epstein DM, Kline LR, Albelda SM, et al: Tuberculous pleural effusions. *Chest* 91:106, 1987.

61. Auerbach O: Acute generalized miliary tuberculosis. *Am J Pathol* 20:121, 1944.

62. Munt PW: Miliary tuberculosis in the chemotherapy era: With a clinical review in 69 American adults. *Medicine* 51:139, 1971.

63. Biehl JP: Miliary tuberculosis: A review of sixty-eight adult patients admitted to a municipal general hospital. *Am Rev Respir Dis* 77:605, 1958.

64. Gelb AF, Leffler C, Brewin A, et al: Miliary tuberculosis. *Am Rev Respir Dis* 108:1327, 1973.

65. Sahn SA, Neff TA: Miliary tuberculosis. *Am J Med* 56:495, 1974.

66. Proudfoot AT, Akhtar AJ, Douglas AC, et al: Miliary tuberculosis in adults. *Br Med J* 2:273, 1969.

67. Martens G, Willcox PA, Benatar SR: Miliary tuberculosis: Rapid diagnosis, hematologic abnormalities, and outcome in 109 treated adults. *Am J Med* 89:291, 1990.

68. Massaro D, Katz S, Sachs M: Choroidal tubercles: A clue to hematogenous tuberculosis. *Ann Intern Med* 60:231, 1964.

69. Twomey JJ, Leavell BS: Leukemoid reactions to tuberculosis. *Arch Intern Med* 116:21, 1965.

70. Krauss JS, Walker DH: Miliary tuberculosis and comsumption of clotting factors by multifocal vasculopathic coagulation. *South Med J* 72:1479, 1979.

71. Cockcroft DW, Donevan RE, Copland GM, et al: Miliary tuberculosis presenting with hyponatremia and thrombocytopenia. *Can Med Assoc J* 115:871, 1976.

72. Huseby JS, Hudson LD: Miliary tuberculosis and adult respiratory distress syndrome. *Ann Intern Med* 85:609, 1976.

73. Ahuja SS, Ahuja SK, Phelps KR, et al: Hemodynamic confirmation of septic shock in disseminated tuberculosis. *Crit Care Med* 20(6):901, 1992.

74. Heap MJ, Bion JF, Hunter KR: Miliary tuberculosis and the adult respiratory distress syndrome. *Respir Med* 83:153, 1989.

75. Piqueras AR, Marruecos L, Artigas A, et al: Miliary tuberculosis and adult respiratory distress syndrome: *Intensive Care Med* 13:175, 1987.

76. Gachot B, Wolff B, Regnier C, et al: Severe tuberculosis in patients with human immunodeficiency vrus infection. *Intensive Care Med* 16:491, 1990.

77. Kennedy C, Knowles GK: Miliary tuberculosis presenting with skin lesions. *Br Med J* 2:356, 1975.

78. Fisher JR: Miliary tuberculosis with unusual cutaneous manifestations. *JAMA* 238;241, 1977.

79. Cucin RL, Coleman M, Eckardt JJ, et al: The diagnosis of miliary tuberculosis: Utility of peripheral blood abnormalities, bone marrow and liver needle biopsy. *J Chronic Dis* 26:355, 1973.

80. Bouza E, Diaz-Lopez MD, Moreno S, et al: *Mycobacterium tuber-*

culosis bacteremia in patients with and without human immunodeficiency virus infection. *Arch Intern Med* 153:496, 1993.

81. Hill AR, Premkumar S, Brustein S, et al: Disseminated tuberculosis in the acquired immunodeficiency era. *Am Rev Respir Dis* 144:1164, 1991.

82. Clough MC: The cultivation of tubercle bacille from the circulation blood in milary tuberculosis. *Am Rev Tuberc* 1:598, 1917.

83. Barnes PF, Arevalo C: Six cases of *Mycobacterium tuberculosis* bacteremia. *J Infect Dis* 156:377, 1987.

84. Saltzman BA, Motyl MR, Friendland GH, et al: *Mycobacterium tuberculosis* bacteremia in the acquired immunodeficiency syndrome. *JAMA* 256:390, 1986.

85. Shafer RW, Goldberg R, Sierra M, et al: Frequency of Mycobacterium tuberculosis bacteremia in patients with tuberculosis in an area endemic for AIDS. *Am Rev Respir Dis* 140:1611, 1989.

86. Barber TW, Craven DE, McCabe WR: Bacteremia due to *Mycobacterium tuberculosis* in patients with human immunodeficency virus infection. *Medicine* 69:375, 1990.

86a. Haas EJ, Mahavan T, Quinn EL, et al: Tuberculosis meningitis in an urban general hospital. *Arch Intern Med* 137:1518, 1977.

87. Falk A, U.S. Veterans Administration Armed Forces cooperative study on the chemotherapy of tuberculosis. 13. Tuberculosis meningitis in adults, with special reference to survival, neurologic residents, and work status. *Am Rev Respir Dis* 91:823, 1965.

88. Witham RR, Johnson RH, Roberts DL: Diagnosis of miliary tuberculosis by cerebral computerized tomography. *Arch Intern Med* 139:479, 1979.

89. Harder E, Al-Kawi MZ, Carney P: Intracranial tuberculoma: Conservative management. *Am J Med* 74:570, 1983.

90. Bishburg E, Sunderam G, Reichman LB: Central nervous system tuberculosis with acquired immunodeficiency syndrome and its related complex. *Ann Intern Med* 105:210, 1986.

91. Berenguer J, Moreno S, Laguna F, et al. Tuberculous meningitis in patients infected with the human immunodeficiency virus. *N Engl J Med* 326:668, 1992.

92. Dube MP, Holtom PD, Larsen RA: Tuberculosis meningitis in patients with and without human immunodeficiency virus infection. *Am J Med* 93:520, 1992.

93. Shafer RW, Kim DS, Weiss JP, et al: Extrapulmonary tuberculosis in patients with human immunodeficiency virus infection. *Medicine* 70:384, 1991.

94. Pitchenik AE, Burr J, Suarez M, et al: Human T-cell lymphotrophic virus-III (HTLV-III) seropositivity and related disease among 71 consecutive patients in whom tuberculosis was diagnosed. *Am Rev Respir Dis* 135:875, 1987.

95. Pitchenik AE, Rubinson HA: The radiographic appearance of tuberculosis in patients with the acquired immune deficiency syndrome (AIDS) and pre-AIDS. *Am Rev Respir Dis* 131:393, 1985.

96. Davidson PT, Le QH: Drug treatment of tuberculosis—1992. *Drugs* 43(5):651, 1992.

97. Rossi GA, Balbi B, Manca F: Tuberculous pleural effusions, evidence for selective presence of PPD-specific T-lymphocytes at site of inflammation in the early phase of the infection. *Am Rev Respir Dis* 138:575, 1987.

98. Husen L, Fulkerson LL, Del Vecchio E, et al: Pulmonary tuberculosis with negative findings on chest x-ray films: A study of 40 cases. *Chest* 60:540, 1971.

99. Pedro-Botet J, Gutierrez J, Miralles R, et al: Pulmonary tuberculosis in HIV-infected patients with normal chest radiographs. *AIDS* 6:91, 1992.

100. David HL: Drug-resistance in M. Tuberculosis and other mycobacteria. *Clin Chest Med* 1:227, 1980.

101. British Thoracic Society: A controlled trial of 6 months chemotherapy in pulmonary tuberculosis. Final report: Results during the 36 months after the end of chemotherapy and beyond. *Br J Dis Chest* 78:330, 1984.

102. American Thoracic Society, Centers for Disease Control: Treatment of tuberculosis and tuberculosis infection in adults and children. *Am Rev Respir Dis* 134:355, 1986.

103. Iseman MD, Cohn DL, Sbarbaro JA: Directly observed treatment of tuberculosis. *N Engl J Med* 328:576, 1993.

104. Goble M, Iseman MD, Madsen LA, et al: Treatment of 171 patients with pulmonary tuberculosis resistance to isoniazid and rifampin. *N Engl J Med* 328:527, 1993.

105. Chen C-H, Shih J-F, Lindholm-Levy PJ, et al: Minimal inhibitory concentrations of rifabutin, ciprofloxacin against Mycobacterium tuberculosis isolated before treatment of patients in Taiwan. *Am Rev Respir Dis* 140:987, 1989.

106. Hong Kong Chest Service/British Medical Research Council: A controlled study of rifabutin and an uncontrolled study of ofloxacin in the retreatment of patients with pulmonary tuberculosis resistant to isoniazid, streptomycin, and rifampicin. *Tuber Lung Dis* 73:59, 1992.

107. Tsukanura M, Nakamura E, Yoshii S, et al: Therapeutic effect of a new antibacterial substance ofloxacin (DL82880) on pulmonary tuberculosis. *Am Rev Respir Dis* 131:353, 1985.

108. Mahoudi A, Iseman MD: Surgical intervention in the treatment of drug-resistant tuberculosis: Update and extended follow-up. *Am Rev Respir Dis* 145(suppl):A816, 1992.

109. Hamadeh MA, Glassroth J: Tuberculosis in pregnancy. *Chest* 101:1114, 1992.

110. Berning SE, Huitt GA, Iseman MD, et al: Malabsorption of antituberculosis medications by a patient with AIDS. *N Engl J Med* 327:1817, 1992.

111. Lee CH, Wang WJ, Lan RS, et al: Corticosteroids in the treatment of tuberculosis pleurisy: A double-blind, placebo controlled, randomised study. *Chest* 94:1256, 1988.

112. Committee on Tuberculosis Treatment: Adrenal corticosteroids and tuberculosis. *Am Rev Respir Dis* 97:484, 1968.

113. O'Toole RD, Thornton GF, Mukherjee MK, et al: Dexamethasone in tuberculosis meningitis: Relationship of cerebrospinal fluid effects of therapeutic efficacy. *Ann Intern Med* 70:39, 1969.

114. Strang JIG, Kakaza HHS, Gibson DG, et al: Controlled clinical trial of complete open surgical drainage and of prednisolone effusion in Transkei. *Lancet* 2:759, 1988.

115. Fowler NO: Tuberculous pericarditis. *JAMA* 266(1):99, 1991.

116. Heimbeck J: Incidence of tuberculosis in young adult women with special reference to employment. *Br J Tuberc* 32:154, 1938.

117. Aitken ML, Anderson KM, Albert RK: Is the tuberculosis screening program of hospital employees still required? *Am Rev Respir Dis* 136:805, 1987.

118. Edlin BR, Tokars JL, Grieco MH, et al: Nosocomial transmission of multidrug-resistant tuberculosis among AIDS patients: Epidemiologic studies and restriction fragment length polymorphism analysis. *N Engl J Med* 326:1514, 1992.

119. Pearson ML, Jereb JA, Frieden TR, et al: Nosocomial transmission of multidrug-resistant Mycobacterium tuberculosis: A risk to patients and healthcare workers. *Ann Intern Med* 117:191, 1992.

120. Dooley SW, Villarino ME, Lawrence M, et al: Nosocomial transmission of tuberculosis in a hospital unit for HIV-infected patients. *JAMA* 267:2632, 1992.

121. Edlin BR, Tokars JL, Grieco MH, et al: Nosocomial transmission of multidrug-resistant tuberculosis among AIDS patients: Epidemiologic studies and restriction fragment length polymorphism analysis. *N Engl J Med* 326:1514, 1992.

122. Beck-Sagué C, Dooley SW, Hutton MD, et al: Hospital outbreak of multidrug-resistant Mycobacterium tuberculosis infections: Factors in transmission to staff and HIV-infected patients. *JAMA* 268:1280, 1992.

123. Riley RL, Mills CC, O'Grady F, et al: Infectiousness of air from a tuberculosis ward: Ultraviolet irradiation of infected air: Comparative infectiousness of different patients. *Am Rev Respir Dis* 84:511, 1962.

124. Houk VN, Kent DC, Baker JH: The epidemiology of tuberculosis infection in a closed environment. *Arch Environ Health* 16:26, 1968.

125. Frampton MW: An outbreak of tuberculosis among hospital personnel caring for a patient with a skin ulcer. *Ann Intern Med* 117:312, 1992.

126. Kramer F, Sasse SA, Simms JC: Primary cutaneous tuberculosis after a needlestick injury from a patient with AIDS and undiagnosed tuberculosis. *Ann Intern Med* 119:594, 1993.

127. Morens DM, Baublis JV, Heidelberger KP: Congenital tuberculosis and associated hypoadrenocorticism. *South Med J* 72(2):160, 1979.

128. Iseman MD: A leap of faith: What can we do to curtail intrainstitutional transmission of tuberculosis? *Ann Intern Med* 117:251, 1992.

129. Suzukawa M, Usuda Y, Numata K: The effects on sputum characteristics of combining an unheated humidifier with a heat-moisture exchanging filter. *Res Care* 34(11):976, 1989.

130. Centers for Disease Control: Management of persons exposed to multidrug-resistant tuberculosis. *MMWR* 41 (No. RR-11):61, 1992.

131. Centers for Disease Control: Purfied protein derivative (PPD): For anergy testing and management of anergic testing and management of anergic persons at risk of tuberculosis. *MMWR* 40:27, 1991.

96. Botulism

Nelson M. Gantz

Botulism is a rare disease requiring prompt diagnosis and early treatment to decrease the case fatality rate. The term *botulism* comes from the Latin word *botulus,* which means "sausage," an important source of infection in the past. Today sausage is rarely implicated in a food-borne outbreak, and most infections are associated with plant sources. Disease results from the action of a potent neurotoxin produced by *Clostridium botulinum* and is classified into four types: (1) food-borne, (2) wound, (3) infant botulism, and (4) an undetermined type in which no vehicle has been incriminated. Patients should be closely monitored in an intensive care unit during the early stages of the illness, because pulmonary complications are the major cause of death. The insidious development of respiratory failure and pneumonia are the two principal complications. Elective intubation is often indicated to prevent the development of unrecognized respiratory failure and death. This chapter focuses on the diagnosis and treatment of patients with food-borne and wound botulism. Infant botulism is not discussed in detail.

Etiology

The causative agent of botulism is *Clostridium botulinum,* an anaerobic gram-positive bacillus that produces spores. The property that distinguishes *C. botulinum* from other clostridial species is its ability to produce a potent neurotoxin, which causes paralysis by acting on the peripheral nervous system. There are at least eight antigenically distinct toxin types designated as A, B, C_1, C_2, D, E, F, and G. Disease in humans is caused by strains that produce toxin types A, B, E, and rarely F and G. Both the vegetative form of the organism and the toxins are heat labile and destroyed in 10 to 15 minutes at 80°C. The spores, in contrast, are highly heat resistant and can survive boiling for hours. However, spores do not germinate and grow unless conditions are favorable; these include an anaerobic environment, adequate water and nutrients, low acidity (pH > 4.6), a suitable temperature (which may be as low as 4°C), and lack of inhibitory substances. Highly acidic fruits and vegetables such as tomatoes are usually safe, because the low pH prevents spore germination and growth [1].

Epidemiology

The organism and its spores are ubiquitous in nature so that foods are often contaminated. Under suitable conditions, such as improperly preserved food, toxin production can occur. Most of the cases of botulism are food-borne and involve home-canned or home-processed foods. The foods that have been implicated most often are home-canned green beans or peppers. The diagnosis should not, however, be excluded if there is no history of eating home-canned food, because an outbreak occurred at a restaurant in Clovis, New Mexico, involving 34 persons who acquired the disease after eating bean or potato salad [2]. Of the food-borne outbreaks in which toxin type is identified, 58 percent are attributable to type A, 25 percent to type B, and 17 percent to type E [3]. Type E outbreaks have usually involved fish or seafood and have been reported primarily from Alaska [4]. Foods contaminated with toxin, especially type E, may appear and taste normal. Sometimes disease associated with toxin types A or B spoils the food, resulting in gas production and swollen cans. Wound botulism should be considered in parenteral drug abusers who present with neurologic symptoms such as dysphagia, dysphonia, and a wound infection [5]. Intranasal cocaine abuse has also been associated with *Clostridium botulinum* maxillary sinusitis [6]. In 1994 approximately 20 cases of food-borne botulism were reported [6a]. In the 17 previous years there were an average of 32 cases per year [7]. This contrasts with the 72 cases reported to the Centers for Disease Control (CDC) in 1978 as a result of the large outbreak in New Mexico. In 1991 in Cairo, Egypt, there was a massive outbreak of type E botulism associated with eating salted fish. In this outbreak, 91 patients were hospitalized, and 20 percent of patients died. Wound-associated botulism is uncommon, with an average of one to two reported cases each year. Infant botulism was first described as an entity in 1976. In 1991, 93 cases of infant botulism were reported to the CDC. In 1989, there were only 25 cases of infant botulism reported, which is the fewest number of the past decade.

Pathogenesis

In food-borne botulism, the preformed toxin in the food is ingested and is absorbed from the small intestine. The toxin is distributed by the lymphatic and circulatory systems to the peripheral nervous system. The toxin acts at the neuromuscular junctions, where it inhibits the release of acetylcholine at the cholinergic synapses. The toxin does not affect the central nervous system or the adrenergic nerve endings. Once the toxin is bound to the presynaptic membrane, it is not inactivated by antitoxin. Wound botulism is the rarest of the types of botulism and occurs when *C. botulinum* infects a wound and produces toxin, which then is carried to the peripheral nervous system by the circulatory and lymphatic systems. Infant botulism occurs when the organism or its spores are swallowed and colonize the intestinal tract, resulting in in vivo toxin production. Recently, there is evidence that adults may develop botulism by eating foods contaminated with the production of toxin in vivo [8]. This illness in adults resembles infant botulism and has occurred in patients with predisposing factors including intestinal surgery, gastric achlorhydria, and antibiotic therapy. Infant botulism occurs in infants between 3 and 26 weeks of age and has been associated with the ingestion of honey contaminated with *C. botulinum* [9]. Thus, honey should not be fed to infants younger than 1 year of age. Death from botulism results from respiratory paralysis. The findings on postmortem examination are nondiagnostic.

Clinical Manifestations

The onset of symptoms and signs after the ingestion of the contaminated food may be as soon as 6 hours or as long as 8 days, with the usual interval being 18 to 36 hours [1,3]. A shorter incubation period is usually associated with more severe disease [1]. Botulism should be suspected in a patient who develops bilateral cranial nerve impairment with descending paralysis or weakness [10]. The diagnosis is usually not difficult when many persons are ill simultaneously, but most outbreaks involve only one or two persons [1]. Gastrointestinal complaints, which include nausea, vomiting, and abdominal cramps, often precede the neurologic manifestations. However, in one-third of patients gastrointestinal complaints are absent [11]. Frequent neurologic symptoms include dysphagia, diplopia, dysarthria, upper- and lower- extremity weakness, and blurred vision. Dizziness, dyspnea, and fatigue also occur commonly. Impaired autonomic nerve function results in a patient complaining of a dry mouth, tongue, and throat because of the decreased saliva production. Table 96-1 lists the frequency of symptoms of types A and B food-borne botulism from a review of 55 cases reported

to the CDC [6]. The physical findings are listed in Table 96-2 and typically show an alert afebrile patient with ptosis, upper- and lower-extremity weakness, and a hypoactive gag reflex [11]. Ocular findings are common, and, in addition to ptosis, include extraocular palsies, nystagmus, and dilated, poorly reactive, or fixed pupils. One study noted sixth cranial nerve dysfunction in 98 percent of patients [10]. In summary, clues to the diagnosis include the absence of fever, a normal mental status although the patient may be anxious or drowsy, symmetric neurologic findings, and no sensory deficits [1].

The symptoms and signs in wound botulism are identical to those seen with food-borne botulism except that fever secondary to the wound infection may be present, and there is no epidemiologic evidence to implicate a food. Gastrointestinal complaints usually do not occur [12]. The incubation period in wound botulism varies from 4 to 14 days. Prominent manifestations seen in infant botulism include constipation, impaired sucking and swallowing, and a flaccid paralysis.

Diagnosis

The diagnosis of botulism, suspected on the clinical presentation, can be confirmed by demonstrating the presence of the botulinal toxin in the patient's serum or feces or incriminated food. The toxin can be identified using a mouse toxin neutralization test. The test requires 24 to 96 hours to complete and is available at selected state health department laboratories as well as from the laboratory at the CDC in Atlanta, Georgia.*

Suitable materials to be collected and sent for examination for botulinal toxin assay include serum, stool, vomitus, gastric contents, and the suspected food. Because the toxins are lethal for humans, the suspected specimens should be handled with gloves in a safety cabinet. Ten to 15 ml of serum and 25 to 50 gm of stool should be sent under refrigeration in a leakproof container to the laboratory [1]. The CDC should be notified

* Telephone number during weekdays is 404-639-2206; number during night, holiday, or weekend is 404-639-2888.

Table 96-1. Frequency of Symptoms in Patients with Food-borne Botulism

Symptoms	Cases (%)
Neurologic	
Dysphagia	96
Dry mouth	93
Diplopia	91
Dysarthria	84
Upper extremity weakness	73
Lower extremity weakness	69
Blurred vision	65
Dyspnea	60
Paresthesias	14
Gastrointestinal	
Constipation	73
Nausea	64
Vomiting	59
Abdominal cramps	42
Diarrhea	19
Miscellaneous	
Fatigue	77
Sore throat	54
Dizziness	51

Source: Modified from Hughes JM, Blumenthal JR, Merson MH, et al: Clinical features of type A and B food-borne botulism. *Ann Intern Med* 95:442, 1981, with permission.

Table 96-2. Frequency of Physical Findings in Patients with Food-borne Botulism

Physical findings	Cases (%)
Upper extremity weakness	75
Ptosis	73
Lower extremity weakness	69
Hypoactive gag reflex	65
Extraocular muscle weakness	65
Facial nerve dysfunction	63
Tongue weakness	58
Pupils fixed or dilated	44
Nystagmus	22
Ataxia	17
Initial mental status	
Alert	90
Lethargic	4
Obtunded	6
Deep tendon reflexes	
Normal	54
Hypoactive or absent	40
Hyperactive	6

Source: Modified from Hughes JM, Blumenthal JR, Merson MH, et al: Clinical features of type A and B food-borne botulism. *Ann Intern Med* 95:442, 1981, with permission.

before sending the samples. The diagnosis can also be established by isolating the organism, *C. botulinum,* from the stool, wound, or suspected food. The organism must be cultured using strict anaerobic techniques. The finding of the organism in a patient's feces strongly supports the diagnosis, because it is not part of the normal fecal flora [13,14]. In one large outbreak of food-borne botulism, toxin was identified in half the serum specimens and in one-third of the stool samples; the organism was cultured from 79 percent of the stool specimens [2]. Overall, laboratory confirmation occurred in 76 percent of cases. In a review of 309 patients, the laboratory failed to confirm the diagnosis in about one-third of the cases [14]. In general, specimens should be obtained early to increase the yield. Toxin is much more likely to be found in samples obtained less than 1 day after the onset of symptoms [2]. In cases of infant botulism, toxin and the organism can be found in the feces, but toxin is rarely identified in the serum. Another test that can be used to establish the diagnosis of botulism is the performance of repetitive nerve stimulation. Stimuli of low frequency evoke a decrease in the amplitude of the muscle action potential, whereas repetitive stimuli at a higher frequency (50/sec) produces a marked incremental response [15]. The findings on repetitive nerve stimulation with botulism are the opposite of those seen in patients with myasthenia gravis [15]. Routine laboratory findings, including the complete blood count (CBC), electrolytes, serum enzymes, and cerebrospinal fluid, are normal unless there are secondary complications.

Differential Diagnosis

Some of the disorders that are most often confused with botulism include Guillain-Barré syndrome, myasthenia gravis, cerebrovascular accidents, other cases of food poisoning, carbon monoxide poisoning, drug reactions, tick paralysis, poliomyelitis, diphtheria, and Eaton-Lambert syndrome. Guillain-Barré syndrome (see Chap. 189) usually causes an ascending motor paralysis, but it can produce a descending pattern of paralysis and can be confined to the cranial nerves occasionally. The presence of paresthesias and an elevated concentration of cerebrospinal fluid (CSF) protein help distinguish this disease from botulism. Myasthenia gravis (see Chap. 190) may also mimic botulism. However, a positive response to edrophonium (Tensilon) and a characteristic response to repetitive nerve stimulation are helpful. Sometimes a positive response to edrophonium can occur in patients with botulism. Cerebrovascular accidents usually produce sensory defects as well as asymmetric changes in the deep tendon reflexes. Other causes of food poisoning usually have a more rapid onset, paresthesias, as seen with shellfish poisoning, and other signs. Because drugs such as phenothiazines may simulate botulism, a history of their use should be obtained. Fever, which is absent in food-borne botulism unless a secondary complication has occurred, is present in the other infectious disorders that can be confused with botulism. In cases of tick paralysis, paresthesias occur. The Eaton-Lambert syndrome, usually associated with bronchogenic lung carcinoma, can mimic certain features of botulism.

Treatment

The diagnosis and institution of specific therapy for botulism must be based on the clinical evidence, because laboratory confirmation is often delayed. One goal of therapy is to remove unabsorbed toxin from the gastrointestinal tract using a nasogastric tube for lavage and a cathartic or a tap water enema. A second goal is to administer trivalent antitoxin (A, B, E) to neutralize any circulating antitoxin in the serum. Because the toxin binds irreversibly to the nerve endings, antitoxin must be given as soon as possible [16,17]. The toxin is of equine origin, and the patients should be skin tested for hypersensitivity to the product. Reactions to the antitoxin occur in 10 to 20 percent of patients. If the patient tolerates the antitoxin, then one vial is given intravenously, and one vial is given intramuscularly. The same dose is repeated in 4 hours [1]. The third goal and the mainstay of therapy is meticulous nursing and medical supportive care. Pulmonary complications are the principal cause of death. Elective intubation should be performed when the vital capacity approaches 30 percent of the predicted value [18]. The vital capacity is a more sensitive indicator than the arterial blood gas measurements [18]. Pneumonia secondary to aspiration also occurs and requires therapy based on the etiology. Wound botulism is treated with debridement and high-dose intravenous penicillin G (3 million units IV q4h) as well as antitoxin. Infant botulism is managed with good supportive care without the use of antitoxin or antibiotics. A clinical trial involving human-derived botulism immune globulin is underway for infant botulism. The role of guanidine, a substance that acts to release acetylcholine from the serum terminals, is uncertain, and most authorities do not advocate its use.

Prognosis

The case fatality rate of food-borne botulism is about 15 percent. More severe disease occurs in patients with an early onset of neurologic signs. Patients may be hospitalized for several months and require meticulous care to prevent complications. Infant botulism is rarely fatal, but the hospital course may be prolonged [9].

References

1. Centers for Disease Control: *Botulism in the United States 1899–1977: Handbook for Epidemiologists, Clinicians, and Laboratory Workers.* Atlanta, GA, Centers for Disease Control, 1979.
2. Mann JM, Hathaway CL, Gardiner TM: Laboratory diagnosis in a large outbreak of type A botulism. *Am J Epidemiol* 115:598, 1982.
3. MacDonald KL, Cohen ML, Blake PA: The changing epidemiology of adult botulism in the United States. *Am J Epidemiol* 124:794, 1986.
4. Wainwright RB, Heyward WL, Middaugh JP, et al: Food-borne botulism in Alaska, 1947-1985: Epidemiology and clinical findings. *J Infect Dis* 157:1158, 1988.
5. MacDonald KL, Rutherford GW, Friedman SM, et al: Botulism and botulism-like illness in chronic drug abusers. *Ann Intern Med* 102:616, 1985.
6. Kudrow DB, Henry DA, Haake DA, et al: Botulism associated with *Clostridium botulinum* sinusitis after intranasal cocaine abuse. *Ann Intern Med* 109:984, 1988.
6a. Centers for Disease Control: unpublished data.
7. Weber JT, Hibbs RG, Darwish A, et al: A massive outbreak of type E botulism associated with traditional salted fish in Cairo. *J Infect Dis* 167:451, 1993.
8. Chia JK, Clark JB, Ryan CA, et al: Botulism in an adult associated with food-borne intestinal infection with *Clostridium botulinum*. *N Engl J Med* 315:239, 1986.
9. Arnon SS: Infant botulism, in Finegold SM, George WL (eds): *Anaerobic Infections in Humans*. San Diego, CA, Academic Press, 1989.

10. Terranova W, Palumbo JN, Breman JG: Ocular findings in botulism type B. *JAMA* 241:475, 1979.
11. Hughes JM, Blumenthal JR, Merson MH, et al: Clinical features of type A and B food-borne botulism. *Ann Intern Med* 95:442, 1981.
12. Merson MH, Dowell VR Jr: Epidemiologic, clinical and laboratory aspects of wound botulism. *N Engl J Med* 289:1105, 1973.
13. Dowell VR Jr, McCroskey LM, Hathaway CL, et al: Coproexamination for botulinal toxin and *Clostridium botulinum*. *JAMA* 238:18292, 1977.
14. Woodruff BA, Griffin PM, McCroskey LM, et al: Clinical and laboratory comparison of botulism for toxin types A, B, and E in the United States, 1975-1988. *J Infect Dis* 166:1281, 1992.

15. Cherington M: Botulism: Ten-year experience. *Arch Neurol* 30:432, 1974.
16. Sugiyama H: *Clostridium botulinum* neurotoxin. *Microbiol Rev* 44:420, 1980.
17. Tacket CO, Shandera WX, Mann JM, et al: Equine antitoxin use and other factors that predict outcome in type A foodborne botulism. *Am J Med* 76:794, 1984.
18. Schmidt-Nowara WW, Samet JM, Rosario PA: Early and late pulmonary complications. *Arch Intern Med* 143:451, 1983.

97. Tetanus

Sam T. Donta

Tetanus is a prime example of a toxigenic disease, i.e., one in which the organism produces the disease with little or no multiplication or spread, where cell-free toxin mimics the disease, and immunization against the toxin is effective in preventing the disease. The clinical picture is the result of the action of a neurotoxin produced by most strains of *Clostridium tetani*. The toxin, sometimes referred to as tetanospasmin, is one of the most poisonous substances known, with as little as 10 pg of toxin capable of killing a mouse [1,2]. The organism is ubiquitous in soil, and commonly colonizes the intestinal tract of humans and other vertebrates. Because of its requirement of anaerobic conditions for growth or toxin production, clinical disease is seen in conditions where the organism gains access to deep tissue and the redox potential is low, such as could occur after puncture wounds or deep lacerations when there has been inadequate debridement or premature closure of wounds. Neonatal tetanus results when the umbilical cord stump is contaminated in an infant whose mother lacks toxin immunity. Tetanus may result in narcotic addicts after intramuscular injection of quinine-containing preparations, creating conditions favorable for toxin production. Local tetanus results when there is minimal toxin production.

Pathogenesis

Toxin is produced once the spores of *Clostridium tetani* have germinated and are in stationary phase. The toxin then migrates to neural tissue, where it binds to membrane gangliosides GD1b and GT1b [2,3,4]. After membrane binding, the toxin is internalized and transported to the central nervous system by retrograde intraaxonal movement [5]. Although the exact mechanisms of action remain to be defined, the toxin is thought to act primarily on inhibitory (Renshaw) neurons, inhibiting the release of acetylcholine, and perhaps other neurotransmitters, from synaptic nerve endings [6,7]. Probably because of similar relationships between the ganglioside receptors for tetanus toxin on neural cells and those for thyrotropin on thyroid cells [8,9], tetanus is frequently accompanied by increased sympathetic nervous system activity, as is often seen in hyperthyroidism [10,11]. There are no means to reverse the effects of the toxin, once bound; instead, one must wait until the toxin is eventually degraded and eliminated.

Clinical Manifestations

After an incubation period of 3 to 10 days (range 1–54), clinical symptoms begin. In the generalized form of tetanus, including neonatal tetanus, the patient becomes restless and suffers from headaches, muscle pains, and muscular rigidity. The jaws and neck are affected early, causing trismus (lockjaw) and difficulty in swallowing. Dysphagia may be the only presenting symptom. All muscle groups may be affected, including the muscles of respiration. Generalized seizures are common, and minor sensory stimuli (e.g., sounds) may evoke seizures. The patient remains mentally lucid; thus, tetanus can be a very painful disorder.

In localized tetanus, the symptoms of muscle pain and rigidity are limited to the involved area. Cephalic tetanus may be viewed as a form of localized tetanus, which can occur as a rare complication of dental caries or dental procedures (e.g., root canal). Facial pain may be the first sign of cephalic tetanus.

The major complications of tetanus are the results of respiratory paralysis and excess sympathetic activity, including cardiac arrhythmias. The most common electrocardiogram (ECG) finding is sinus tachycardia, and supraventricular tachycardias are not uncommon. Nonspecific ST-T wave and P wave changes are also common, as are prolonged QT intervals [12]. Infections of the respiratory and urinary tracts also add to the morbidity and mortality of the disease. Improvements in the management of tetanus have led to decreased mortality rates in recent years [13,14]. Case-fatality rates generally increase with age, ranging from 15 to 20 percent in middle-aged individuals to 50 percent in the elderly.

Diagnosis

The diagnosis of tetanus is based on the clinical picture, even in the absence of an identifiable portal of entry for the organism.

Few conditions mimic the sustained muscle rigidity and sympathetic hyperreactivity. In strychnine poisoning, the muscles are relaxed between seizures. Hypocalcemic tetany and phenothiazine reactions can be diagnosed by an appropriate history and testing of blood and urine. Stiff-man syndrome is characterized by its slower progression. Meningitis and intracranial hemorrhage may rarely confuse the diagnosis of neonatal tetanus.

The laboratory is of little value in the diagnosis of tetanus. The amount of toxin capable of causing disease is too small to be detected and does not result in any consistent immunologic response. Immunization, therefore, is essential if second attacks of tetanus are to be avoided.

Treatment

The successful management of generalized tetanus depends most on the provision of adequate respiratory support. Early tracheostomy, especially in elderly patients, muscle paralysis with curarelike agents, and ventilatory support for periods up to 2 months may be needed to ensure a successful outcome.

The patient should be placed in a quiet room and stimuli kept to a minimum. Diazepam should be administered intravenously (5 mg q4h for adults, increased to 20 mg q4h if needed) to further sedate the patient and to prevent seizures. Meperidine, 75 to 100 mg, should be given as needed to reduce pain.

The excess sympathetic activity is probably best managed with the use of propranolol, beginning with 1 mg/kg/day divided into four doses, and increasing until a mild bradycardia occurs. The patient should be continuously monitored for the occurrence of arrhythmias and other ECG abnormalities. Anecdotally, baclofen has been used intrathecally to reduce the muscle contractures [15].

As soon as the diagnosis of tetanus is made, the patient should be given 500 units human tetanus immune globulin (TIG) intramuscularly. Repeated or greater doses do not appear to be any more efficacious. In the absence of TIG, commercially available immune globulin (IVIG) preparations usually contain adequate amounts of antitoxin and may be useful [16]. Immunization with tetanus toxoid should be initiated concomitantly, using another muscle site. A second and third toxoid injection should be given 1 and 2 months later, with booster injections 1 year later and then at 10-year intervals.

Penicillin is probably of little value in the management of tetanus, unless there is no obvious portal of entry. In that case, 600,000 units of procaine penicillin twice daily for 2 weeks should be used. In cases in which there is a site of injury, the involved area should be exposed, thoroughly debrided, and cleansed.

Because of the duration of convalescence, special care must be taken to avoid secondary infections of the respiratory and urinary tracts and complications such as decubitus ulcers. Adequate nutrition may require parenteral hyperalimentation. There is no evidence that hyperbaric oxygenation is of value.

Prevention

To prevent tetanus, all individuals should be immunized early in life with alum-precipitated tetanus toxoid (in combination with pertussis vaccine and diphtheria toxoid). A series of three injections at monthly intervals, with booster immunizations 1 year later and at 10-year intervals thereafter ensures adequate protection. Further booster immunizations are not needed for individuals who have received boosters within the previous 10 years [17]. Even in individuals who have not received toxoid boosters for up to 30 years, antitoxic immunity is restored by a single booster immunization [18]. Special attention should be given to pregnant women to ensure that they have been properly immunized before parturition [19]. Immunization with toxoid may be given in any trimester. If a neonate is born of a nonimmune mother, the infant should be given 250 units TIG in the first day. Special attention should also be given to individuals older than age 50, because measured levels of antitoxin in this group of people were below what are generally considered as protective levels [20].

Because tetanus is not contagious, no special measures are needed for contacts or personnel.

References

1. Bizzini B: Tetanus toxin. *Microbiol Rev* 43:224, 1979.
2. Matsuda M, Lei DL, Sugimoto N, et al: Isolation, purification, and characterization of Fragment B, the NH2-terminal half of the heavy chain of tetanus toxin. *Infect Immun* 57:3588, 1989.
3. van Heyningen S: Binding of gangliosides by the chains of tetanus toxin. *FEBS Lett* 68:5, 1976.
4. Simpson L: Pharmacological experiments on the binding and internalization of the 50,000 dalton carboxyterminus of tetanus toxin at the cholinergic neuromuscular junction. *J Pharm Exp Ther* 234:100, 1985.
5. Price D, Griffin J, Young A, et al: Tetanus toxin: Direct evidence for retrograde intraaxonal transport. *Science* 188:945, 1975.
6. Bigalke H, Ahnert-Hilger G, Habermann E: Tetanus toxin and botulinum A toxin inhibit acetylcholine release from but not calcium uptake into brain tissue. *Arch Pharm* 316:143, 1981.
7. Habermann E, Dryer F: Clostridial neurotoxins: handling and action at the cellular and molecular level. *Curr Top Microbiol Immunol* 129:93, 1986.
8. Lee G, Grollman EF, Dyer S, et al: Tetanus toxin and thyrotropin interactions with rat brain membrane preparations. *J Biol Chem* 254:3826, 1979.
9. Pierce EJ, Davison MD, Parton RG, et al: Characterization of tetanus toxin binding to rat brain membranes. *Biochem J* 236:845, 1986.
10. Kanarek DJ, Kaufman B, Zwi S: Severe sympathetic hyperactivity associated with tetanus. *Arch Intern Med* 132:602, 1973.
11. Domenighetti GM, Savary G, Stricker H: Hyperadrenergic syndrome in severe tetanus: extreme rise in catecholamines responsive to labetalol. *B Med J* 288:1483, 1984.
12. Mitra RC, Gupta RD, Sack SRB: Electrocardiographic changes in tetanus: A serial study. *J Indian Med Ass* 89:164, 1991.
13. Prevots R, Sutter RW, Strebel PM, et al: Tetanus surveillance—United States, 1989–1990. *MMWR CDC Surveill Summ* 41:19, 1992.
14. Nolla-Salas M, Garces-Bruses J: Severity of tetanus in patients older than 80 years: Comparative study with younger patients. *Clin Infect Dis* 16:591, 1993.
15. Demaziere J, Saissy JM, Vitris M, et al: Intermittent intrathecal baclofen for severe tetanus. *Lancet* 337:427, 1991.
16. Bleck TP: Intravenous immune globulin for passive tetanus prophylaxis. *J Infect Dis* 167:498, 1993.
17. Bizzini B: Tetanus, in Germainier R (ed): *Bacterial Vaccines*. New York, Academic Press, 1984, pp 37–67.
18. Simonsen O, Kjeldsen K, Heron I: Immunity against tetanus and effect of revaccination 2530 years after primary vaccination. *Lancet* 332:1240, 1984.
19. Varela LR, Black FL, Mendizabal-Morris CA: Tetanus antitoxin titers in women of childbearing age from nine diverse populations. *J Infect Dis* 151:850, 1985.
20. Hilton E, Singer C, Kozarsky P, et al: Status of immunity to tetanus, measles, mumps, rubella, and polio among US travelers. *Ann Intern Med* 115:32, 1991.

VII. Gastrointestinal and Hepatobiliary Problems in the Intensive Care Unit

Section Editor
Ray E. Clouse

98. Gastrointestinal Bleeding: Principles of Diagnosis and Management

Gary R. Zuckerman

Acute massive or subacute gastrointestinal (GI) bleeding is a common clinical emergency that often necessitates admission to the intensive care unit (ICU) or represents a superimposed morbidity on a patient already residing in the ICU. Data looking at epidemiologic trends would suggest that although hospital admissions for uncomplicated peptic ulcer disease declined in the early 1980s, possibly related to the introduction of histamine H-2-receptor antagonists, admissions for GI bleeding increased [1]. The mortality rate from GI bleeding has remained steady at 6 to 12 percent but it is hoped that recently introduced non-surgical therapies will result in improved survival rates [2]. Other advances in the recognition of clinical and endoscopic prognostic signs should improve our ability to triage patients who need urgent ICU admission and to recognize earlier those patients who can be transferred safely from the ICU to the hospital floor. The following reviews key elements in the diagnosis and management of GI bleeding. Special emphasis is placed on newer endoscopic therapies and criteria for assessing prognosis.

Initial Evaluation and Resuscitation

Hemorrhagic shock and its management are discussed in more specific detail in Chapter 172. The issue of resuscitation is brought up early in this chapter because it must be addressed immediately in the actively bleeding patient. At this point in the patient's clinical course the source or bleeding level (within the GI tract) is not as important as is stabilizing the condition of the hemorrhaging patient. In most cases, the diagnostic evaluation will proceed after the patient's condition has been stabilized. In the patient with exsanguinating hemorrhage, proceeding immediately to the operating room or having a limited endoscopy to help direct the surgical approach may be necessary. The priority is to recognize and replete intravascular volume and prevent irreversible shock. A physical examination that includes serial vital signs and evaluation of the volume and character of the bleeding is important at this point to establish the degree of hemodynamic instability. Repeating this examination periodically to establish adequacy of intravascular volume repletion or ongoing or recurrent bleeding is imperative. Primary resuscitation may have taken place in the emergency room, but volume expansion must continue until the patient's bleeding slows or stops, and continued observation is necessary to detect recurrent bleeding.

The urgency and degree of resuscitation depend on the presence of various clinical factors noted on the physical examination, e.g., hypovolemic shock versus orthostatic hypotension. The patient's general appearance should be noted for signs that may accompany hemorrhagic shock. These include mental confusion, agitation, diaphoresis, mottled skin (livedo reticularis), and cold extremities. A quantitative estimate of the amount of blood lost, by looking at volume of blood being passed per

rectum or by hematemesis, is also helpful in determining the urgency and degree of resuscitation. Although blood testing should be performed to obtain baseline values and to type and cross-match blood for possible transfusion, the initial hemoglobin and hematocrit values frequently will not reflect the degree of acute blood lost (both plasma and red cells) until the intravascular space equilibrates with extravascular or intravenous fluids. This may take as long as 72 hours [3]. The initial history and physical examination may be necessarily brief, but inquiring early for critical information can influence management. GI bleeding is not associated generally with abdominal pain, and such a complaint should alert the interviewer to include hematobilia, intestinal infarction, and intestinal perforation in the differential diagnoses. Chest pain may imply a superimposed myocardial infarction or dissecting aneurysm, whereas a history of abdominal vascular surgery will add aortoenteric fistula to the differential diagnoses.

Resuscitation of the unstable patient must take precedence over other treatment, but frequently many activities are occurring simultaneously. If the bleeding is massive with hematemesis, endotracheal intubation may be necessary to provide airway protection and facilitate endoscopic evaluation and therapy. Intravenous access with one or two large-bore catheters in large peripheral veins will usually suffice for aggressive administration of fluids and blood products. Normal saline or lactated Ringer's solution should be administered promptly to replete volume and may obviate the need for blood products when bleeding is mild to moderate or subacute in character. Moderate to massive GI hemorrhage will necessitate transfusion with blood products to replete red blood cell mass and improve tissue oxygenation. The blood bank should be notified of the anticipated transfusion need.

Further Evaluation and Management

Once the initial volume deficit has been corrected, the need for further crystalloid or colloid replacement can be best followed by monitoring vital signs and evidence of ongoing or renewed gross bleeding. Because of the laxative properties of fresh blood in the GI tract, repeated passage of liquid blood per rectum implies ongoing or recurrent bleeding. As bleeding stops, the stool will go from liquid to formed stool and from red or maroon blood to darker stool and eventually to brown guaiac-positive stool. The stool may remain guaiac positive for as long as two weeks after GI bleeding has ceased. During the initial period the gastroenterologist and surgeon should be consulted for further diagnostic evaluation.

In patients without hematemesis or melena the passage of a nasogastric tube may be helpful if the return is positive for gross blood, thus determining that the bleeding is upper GI in origin. The value of a nasogastric tube for gastric lavage to stop

GI bleeding has not been substantiated, however. In fact, in the experimental model, gastric lavage with iced saline prolonged the bleeding time and increased the clotting time [4], prolonging ulcer bleeding, compared with no gastric lavage [5]. Thus, although gastric lavage is used frequently to clear clots from the stomach, no evidence exists that it stops clinical bleeding. Many gastroenterologists, including the author, do not believe that gastric lavage is necessary for endoscopic visualization in most cases and sense that the tube produces mucosal suction artifacts, which often confuse the endoscopic evaluation.

Histamine H-2-receptor antagonists (H2RA) are prescribed frequently for patients with GI bleeding. Although the reasons for administering these medications may vary, prescribing patterns during GI bleeding would suggest that H2RAs are administered primarily to stop bleeding rather than to treat peptic ulcer disease [6]. The rationale for the use of H2RAs in upper GI bleeding is implied by studies that show clotting abnormalities associated with an acid milieu [7]. The largest U.S. randomized controlled study comparing an H2RA with placebo in patients with acute upper GI bleeding did not show a statistical advantage for H2RA in stopping bleeding [8]. H2RAs also were not useful in preventing rebleeding. A meta-analysis of a number of randomized trials suggests that H2RAs can decrease the frequency of surgery and death, but this conclusion is difficult to interpret because the analysis did not find a concomitant decrease in persistent or recurrent upper GI bleeding [9]. The potent parietal cell proton pump inhibitor omeprazole, which can bring gastric acid pH into a neutral range, has also been examined for its potential to prevent rebleeding from an upper GI source. The largest randomized controlled study did not show a significant difference in rebleeding, transfusion requirements, operative rates, or mortality when omeprazole was compared with a placebo [10]. Thus, although therapy directed toward decreasing gastric acidity for patients bleeding from peptic ulcer disease may be helpful in ulcer healing, there is no firm evidence that this therapy can stop bleeding or prevent rebleeding.

Risk Factors for Rebleeding, Surgery, and Mortality

Although the great majority (at least 80%) of patients with acute GI bleeding will stop bleeding [8], it is important to recognize factors that can identify those patients at higher risk for morbidity and mortality. It is this group of high-risk patients that will likely necessitate urgent ICU admission, require specific invasive therapeutic efforts, and remain longer in the ICU. The patient's record should be reviewed for details about the clinical presentation to the paramedics or to the emergency room personnel, as these data can offer early prognostic information (Table 98-1). Other prognostic information can be obtained from the upper endoscopy report, and it should detail ulcer location and whether stigmata of recent bleeding or no stigmata (clean ulcer base) were found in association with a gastric or duodenal ulcer (Table 98-2). These endoscopic criteria can be used to predict rebleeding and the need for therapeutic intervention [14,15,16]. Endoscopic descriptors have also been used to characterize stigmata of recent bleeding in patients with lower GI bleeding, but their usefulness for prognostication has not been evaluated. A separate terminology is used to describe the endoscopic appearance of esophageal varices that may continue to bleed (e.g., hemocytic spots, red wale sign).

Table 98-1. Clinical Risk Factors for Mortality in Acute Upper Gastrointestinal Bleeding

Clinical Feature	Mortality (%)
Age >60	11
Age < 60	1
Shock on admission	23
No shock	4
Rebleeding in 72 hours	30
No rebleeding	3
Failure to clear red nasogastric aspirate	50
Red to clear nasogastric return	8

Data derived from references 11, 12, and 13.

Table 98-2. Endoscopic Risk Factors for Continued Bleeding or Rebleeding from Gastric or Duodenal Ulcers

Endoscopic Finding	Percent of Patients Who Continue to Bleed or Rebleed
Arterial bleeding	90
Nonbleeding visible vessel	40–50
Adherent clot	10–25
Oozing	<20
Flat pigmented spot	<10
Clean ulcer base	<5
Ulcer of posterior inferior duodenal bulb (gastroduodenal artery)	*
Ulcer of lesser-curve gastric body (left gastric artery)	*

* Percent unknown but frequent finding at surgery for ongoing bleeding
Data from references 14, 16, and 18.

Diagnostic Evaluation

Upper Versus Lower Gastrointestinal Bleeding. Although textbook chapters commonly divide the management of GI bleeding into upper and lower bleeding, it is sometimes, if not frequently, difficult to predict the bleeding level at the initial bedside evaluation. When the nasogastric aspirate is "positive," the bleeding source is not always determined to be upper GI in origin. When patients have hematochezia associated with hemodynamically significant bleeding, even when the nasogastric aspirate is negative, a number of authors recommend upper endoscopy for most if not all such patients [17,18]. This recommendation is based on the evidence that about 15 percent of patients with hematochezia and a negative nasogastric aspirate will turn out to have an upper GI bleeding source determined by endoscopy [17]. Thus, there will be patients requiring diagnostic evaluations of both the upper and lower GI tracts.

Upper Endoscopy. With the suspicion of a bleeding source above the level of the jejunum, esophagogastroduodenoscopy (EGD) is the diagnostic procedure of choice. It should identify the bleeding source in 80 to 90 percent of cases and offers a significantly higher diagnostic yield than upper GI x-ray series [19]. This high diagnostic yield drops when the procedure is delayed beyond 12 hours. Barium studies are not helpful in detecting small mucosal lesions such as gastric erosions, angiodysplasia, and Mallory-Weiss tears, whereas endoscopy has the added advantage of detecting prognostic risk factors and the ability to deliver thermal or injection therapy through the endoscope. Patients should have the endoscope placed as they are approaching or after they have achieved hemodynamic stability, but frequently resuscitation is ongoing at the time of endoscopy. Endoscopy may rarely be necessary in the unstable patient being transferred to the operating room for torrential bleeding in the hope of identifying the bleeding location and guiding the surgical approach. Even when an exact diagnosis cannot be made by EGD, localizing the bleeding to a region, e.g., proximal stomach, can be helpful to the surgeon or interventional radiologist. Complications related to endoscopy are higher when the procedure is performed on an emergency basis for GI bleeding.

Sigmoidoscopy/Colonoscopy. When a lower GI bleeding source is suspected, sigmoidoscopy may be helpful if the bleeding is distal and not of a magnitude that would prevent adequate visualization. For the patient with subacute bleeding or hemorrhage that has ceased, colonoscopy, after adequate bowel preparations, can detect lower bleeding sources and offer the added benefit of endoscopic therapy [17]. Even when the exact cause of bleeding cannot be determined, colonoscopy can localize the fresh blood to a segment of colon or anorectal area and thus direct other therapeutic endeavors.

Radionuclide Bleeding Scan. The technetium-99m (^{99m}Tc)-labeled red blood cell scan offers a reasonable noninvasive early diagnostic approach to patients suspected of having GI bleeding originating below the second duodenum beyond the reach of upper endoscopy. Although bleeding rates as low as 0.1 ml per minute can be detected by this method, the patient should have signs of gross bleeding at test time. If the test reveals a positive bleeding site, angiography or colonoscopy will be needed for confirmation, to further define the cause, and to offer therapy for ongoing bleeding. If the test is negative, colonoscopy usually is employed to evaluate potential colonic bleeding sources.

Mesenteric Arteriography. Because a more rapid bleeding rate is necessary for a positive arteriogram (0.5 ml/min) the radiologist will usually decline to perform a mesenteric arteriogram if the radionuclide bleeding scan is negative [20]. However, because of the intermittent nature of bleeding and the variable timing of mesenteric arteriography, a positive red blood cell scan does not always result in a diagnostic arteriogram.

Therapy for Gastrointestinal Bleeding

Endoscopic Therapy (Endotherapy). Endotherapy offers a convenient and expedient method for treatment of GI bleeding via the endoscope. It has been used primarily for the treatment of upper GI and peptic ulcer bleeding. This therapeutic approach can be applied to patients with lower GI bleeding, but the experience with endotherapy for colonic bleeding is scant [17]. Endoscopic therapy for bleeding esophageal varices is discussed in a separate chapter. An NIH Consensus Conference on Therapeutic Endoscopy and Bleeding Ulcers concluded that endotherapy for hemostasis is indicated for patients at high risk

for persistent or recurrent upper GI bleeding and death [14]. The previously mentioned prognostic criteria will be helpful in categorizing this therapeutic subgroup. Patients with evidence of significant blood loss or other clinical risk factors and patients with endoscopic evidence of ongoing bleeding or a nonbleeding visible vessel would be typical candidates for endotherapy. The most common modalities used are thermal therapy (heater probe, electrocoagulation, laser) and injection therapy (epinephrine, hypertonic saline, sclerosing solutions, etc.). In a number of studies, randomized trials of various thermal and injection modalities have shown that these treatments can decrease further bleeding, shorten hospital stay, decrease transfusions, decrease emergency surgery, and lower costs [18,21]. Most reports have not shown a benefit in terms of decreased mortality, but meta-analysis has shown a significant improvement in mortality with endotherapy [22,23]. The literature would also suggest that these various treatment modalities are comparable with respect to efficacy and safety, and sometimes they are used in combination. Laser therapy has not been as popular in the United States because of its cost and relative lack of portability.

Angiotherapy. The interventional radiologist can be very helpful in the management of patients with GI bleeding, from both diagnostic and therapeutic standpoints. Intraarterial vasopressin has been used for angiographic control of various bleeding lesions from anatomic sites such as the esophagus (esophagitis, Mallory-Weiss tear), stomach (stress ulcer), duodenum, and colon [24]. The results of intraarterial vasopressin for bleeding duodenal ulcers have been disappointing, with control of this form of bleeding in less than 50 percent of cases. Vasopressin also has the potential disadvantage of cardiovascular complications. Gelfoam or metal coil emboli are effective because they can be delivered close to the terminal vessel and result in localized thrombosis with vessel occlusion. The timing for the use of angiography and angiotherapy must be individualized and will usually be a consensus decision made by the involved physicians. Angiotherapy may be a first-line treatment for lower GI bleeding from lesions such as diverticula and angiodysplasia, whereas its use in patients with bleeding peptic ulcers is reserved for those who fail to respond to endotherapy and have a prohibitive surgical risk.

Surgical Therapy. Once clinical or endoscopic risk factors suggesting high morbidity and mortality are identified, surgical consultation should be obtained. The indications for surgery should not be cookbook or rigid but be based on the overall assessment of the patient and an inability to maintain hemodynamic stability. Patients falling into this category are usually those who have failed to respond to medical and/or endoscopic therapy. For the patient with massive hemorrhage that overwhelms the resuscitation effort, proceeding directly to the surgical suite during ongoing resuscitation may be necessary. When the patient is a high-risk surgical candidate, angiotherapy (arterial vasopressin, arterial embolization) or percutaneously placed shunts for variceal bleeding are alternatives.

Specific Bleeding Lesions

Mallary-Weiss Tear. Mallory-Weiss tears represents bleeding from a rent or tear at the area of the esophagogastric junction and are an uncommon cause of upper GI bleeding (5–15%). The classic history describes a patient who has had vomiting of nonbloody gastric contents just prior to hematemesis, although this presentation is variably present (29–86%) [25]. The great majority of patients with bleeding from a Mallory-Weiss tear stop bleeding (80–90%) without any therapeutic intervention, and the rebleeding rate is low (≤5%). Endoscopy will offer both diagnosis and prognosis.

Angiodysplasia. These small (3–15 mm) vascular lesions can be responsible for GI bleeding from the stomach, small bowel, or colon. The character of the bleeding is usually subacute and recurrent rather than massive. The bleeding lesions in the stomach and duodenum are diagnosed with EGD, and the colonic lesions can be detected with angiography or colonoscopy. Bleeding upper GI lesions have been found frequently in patients with chronic renal failure [26,27], whereas vascular heart disease has been associated with colonic lesions [28]. Endotherapy, angiotherapy, and surgery have been used in treating these bleeding vascular lesions.

Aortoenteric Fistula. The key to recognizing an aortoenteric fistula is to remember to escalate it in the differential diagnosis of every patient with GI bleeding and a history of aortic surgery. Although fistulas can occur rarely between a native aortic aneurysm and the intestinal lumen, they more commonly occur in patients who have undergone abdominal aortic graft surgery (0.5–2.4%) [29]. This communication with resultant GI bleeding presents, on average, 4 years after the surgery. The point of intestinal breach can be anywhere from the esophagus to the colon but occurs most often in the third duodenum (75%). Commonly, the massive bleeding episode is preceded by a small "herald bleed" that stops spontaneously. The interval between the first event and the exsanguinating hemorrhage can be hours, weeks, or months (average 1–3 weeks). Making the diagnosis is difficult, and EGD is most useful in excluding the diagnosis by identifying another lesion that is actively bleeding or has stigmata of recent bleeding. Endoscopic visualization of the graft eroding through the intestinal wall is diagnostic but uncommon. In some cases, computed tomography of the abdomen has identified graft abnormalities that indicate an enteric communication [30]. Angiography has not been helpful in the diagnosis. If available, a vascular surgeon should be part of the evaluating team because definitive surgery is required for a confirmed diagnosis and exploratory surgery likely will be necessary for a presumed diagnosis.

Dieulafoy's Lesion. This unusual cause of massive GI bleeding represents a mucosal defect, not an ulcer, that exposes an end artery of the same caliber as its feeding submucosal artery [31]. The lesions have been located typically in the gastric cardia/proximal stomach but have been found rarely in the duodenum and other parts of the GI tract [32]. Bleeding often is massive and recurrent but difficult to diagnose. The site is minute, innocent looking, and frequently not appreciated at endoscopy once bleeding has stopped. EGD can offer diagnosis and therapy for a lesion that was previously considered amenable only to surgical resection [33].

Colonic Diverticula. Bleeding colonic diverticula have been considered the major cause of lower GI bleeding, but their preeminence has been challenged by the high prevalence of bleeding colonic angiodysplasia in more recent studies of bleeding patients [17]. Problems related to determining the prevalence of the various causes for lower GI bleeding relate to many factors, including difficulty in confirming bleeding from a diverticulum. Diverticular bleeding confirmed by angiography is usually found in the right colon [34], whereas the left colon is the more common location (descending colon 21%, rectosigmoid 35%) when colonoscopy has been used to arrive at the diagnosis [34]. Nevertheless, even though the majority of diverticular bleeding found by colonoscopy was located in the left colon, colonoscopy also determined that 32 percent of cases were bleeding from diverticula in the right colon [35]. The character of diverticular bleeding is invariably bright red or maroon blood per rectum associated with orthostasis or hypotension. The majority of patients stop bleeding spontaneously, but approximately 20 to 30 percent rebleed. The diagnostic approach depends on whether the patient is actually bleeding at the time of presentation. For those patients with ongoing bleeding, a radionuclide bleeding scan can be the initial test. If positive, angiography can be used to localize the bleeding site and for angiotherapy. An alternative approach is colonoscopy after colonic purge, but adequate cleaning of the colon may take 4 to 6 hours [17]. Colonoscopy can also be performed when bleeding has stopped and is preferable to barium studies. Angiotherapy and surgery have been the primary therapeutic approaches for continued or recurrent diverticular bleeding.

Other uncommon causes of lower GI bleeding include intestinal infarction, ischemic colitis, and radiation proctitis, but the character of such bleeding usually is mild to moderate and self-limited. Profuse bleeding related to inflammatory bowel disease also is uncommon.

References

1. Kurota JH, Corboy ED: Current peptic ulcer time trends: An epidemiological profile. *J Clin Gastroenterol* 10:259, 1988.
2. Pitcher JL: Therapeutic endoscopy and bleeding ulcers: Historical overview. *Gastrointest Endosc* 36(Suppl 5):2, 1990.
3. Ebert RV, Stead EA, Gibson JA: Response of normal subjects to acute blood loss. *Arch Intern Med* 68:578, 1941.
4. Waterman NG, Walker JL: The effect of gastric cooling on hemostasis. *Surg Gynecol Obstet* 137:80, 1973.
5. Ponsky J, Hoffman M, Swaynigim D: Saline irrigation in gastric hemorrhage: The effect of temperature. *J Surg Res* 28:204, 1980.
6. Bhatt BD, Meriano FV, Phipps TL, et al: Survey of H2RA usage in acute upper gastrointestinal hemorrhage. *J Clin Gastroenterol* 12:14, 1990.
7. Green FW, Kaplan MM, Curtis LE, et al: Effects of acid and pepsin on blood coagulation and platelet aggregation. *Gastroenterology* 74:38, 1978.
8. Zuckerman G, Welch R, Douglas A, et al: Controlled trial of medical therapy for active gastrointestinal bleeding and prevention of rebleeding. *Am J Med* 76:361, 1984.
9. Collins R, Langman M: Treatment with histamine H2RA in acute upper gastrointestinal hemorrhage: Implications of randomized trials. *N Engl J Med* 313:660, 1985.
10. Daneshmen TK, Hawkey CJ, Langmann MJ, et al: Omeprazole vs. placebo for acute upper gastrointestinal bleeding: A randomized controlled trial in 1154 patients. *Gut* 31:A1206, 1990.
11. Branicki FJ, Boey J, Fok PJ, et al: Bleeding duodenal ulcer: A prospective evaluation of risk factors for rebleeding and death. *Ann Surg* 211:411, 1989.
12. Hunt PS: Bleeding gastroduodenal ulcers: Selection of patients for surgery. *World J Surg* 11:289, 1987.
13. MacLeod IA, Mills PR: Factors predicting the probability of further hemorrhage after upper gastrointestinal hemorrhage. *Br J Surg* 69:256, 1982.
14. NIH Consensus Conference: Therapeutic endoscopy and bleeding ulcers. *JAMA* 262:1369, 1989.

15. Lane L, Cohen H, Brodhead J, et al: Prospective evaluation of immediate versus delayed refeeding and prognostic value of endoscopic findings in patients with upper gastrointestinal hemorrhage. *Gastroenterology* 102:314, 1992.

16. Swain CP: Pathology of bleeding lesions, in Sugawa C, Schuman B, Lucas C (eds): *Gastrointestinal Bleeding*. New York, Igaku-Shoin, 1992, chap 3, pp 26–41.

17. Jensen DM, Machicado GA: Diagnosis and treatment of severe hematochezia: The role of urgent colonoscopy after purge. *Gastroenterology* 95:1567, 1988.

18. Lane L: Rolling review: Upper gastrointestinal bleeding. *Aliment Pharmacol Ther* 7:207, 1993.

19. Dronfield MW, Langman MJ, Atkinson J, et al: Outcome of endoscopy and barium radiography for acute upper gastrointestinal bleeding: Controlled trial in 1037 patients. *BMJ* 284:545, 1982.

20. McKusick KA, Froelich J, Callahan RJ, et al: Tc-99 red blood cells for detection of gastrointestinal bleeding: Experiences with 80 patients. *AJR* 137:1113, 1981.

21. Fleisher DE: Endoscopic control of upper gastrointestinal bleeding. *J Clin Gastroenterol* 12(Suppl 2):S41, 1990.

22. Sacks HS, Chalmers TC, Blum AL, et al: Endoscopic hemostasis: An effective therapy for bleeding peptic ulcers. *JAMA* 264:494, 1990.

23. Ring EJ: Angiographic management, in Sugawa C, Shuman B, Lucas C (eds): *Gastrointestinal Bleeding*. New York, Igaku-Shoin, 1992, pp 365–390.

24. Cook DJ, Guyatt GH, Salena BJ, Laine L: Endoscopic therapy for acute non-variceal hemorrhage—a meta-analysis. *Gastroenterology* 102(1):139, 1992.

25. Graham DY, Schwartz JT: The spectrum of the Mallory-Weiss tear. *Medicine* 57:302, 1977.

26. Zuckerman GR, Cornette GL, Clouse RE, Harter HR: Upper gastrointestinal bleeding in patients with chronic renal failure. *Ann Intern Med* 102:588, 1985.

27. Clouse RE, Costigan DJ, Mills BA, et al: Angiodysplasia as a cause of upper gastrointestinal bleeding. *Arch Intern Med* 145:458, 1985.

28. Boley SJ, Sammartano R, Adams A, et al: On the nature and etiology of vascular ectasias of the colon. *Gastroenterology* 72:650, 1977.

29. Champion MC, Sullivan S, Coles JC, et al: Aortoenteric fistula: Incidence, presentation, recognition and management. *Ann Surg* 195:314, 1982.

30. Low RN, Wall SD, Jeffrey RB Jr, et al: Aortoenteric fistula and perigraft infection: Evaluation with CT. *Radiology* 175:157, 1990.

31. Eidus LB, Rasuli P, Manion D, Heringer R: Caliber-persistent artery of the stomach (Dieulafoy's vascular malformation). *Gastroenterology* 99:1507, 1990.

32. McClave SA, Goldschmid S, Cunningham JT, Boyd WP: Dieulafoy's cirsoid aneurysm of the duodenum. *Dig Dis Sci* 33:801, 1988.

33. Lin HJ, Lee FY, Tsai YT, et al: Therapeutic endoscopy for Dieulafoy's disease. *J Clin Gastroenterol* 11:507, 1989.

34. Casarella WJ, Kanter IE, Seaman WB: Right sided colonic diverticula as a cause of acute rectal hemorrhage. *N Engl J Med* 286:450, 1972.

35. Hurwich DB, Gostout CJ, Balm RK: Acute lower GI bleeding from diverticulosis: Prevalence, clinical features and outcome. *Gastrointest Endosc* 39:297, 1993 (Abstract).

99. *Stress Ulcer Syndrome*

Thomas M. Sherman and
Gary R. Zuckerman

The term *stress ulcer* has been inconsistently used to define erosive or ulcerative mucosal abnormalities of the upper gastrointestinal (GI) tract in the face of extreme stress, ranging from physiologic to psychological trauma. In this broad context, it lacks clinical significance and applicability. A more concise definition has been advocated to describe the gastric mucosal process encountered under conditions of severe physiologic stress. Animal studies using endoscopic and pathologic analyses have demonstrated a characteristic progressive gastric mucosal response to the physiologic stress of induced shock [1]. The clearly documented progression from normal mucosa to ulcer has been reproduced in humans under similar conditions [1,2,3]. The earliest changes occur in the gastric fundus, the most proximal part of the stomach. The mucosa initially becomes mottled, progressing to an overall appearance of ischemia, marked by pallor and enhancement of the submucosal vessels. These changes are followed by development of submucosal petechiae, which may then coalesce to form superficial linear erosions and ulcers along the crests of the rugal folds of the fundus. Eventually this process may involve antrum and small bowel if intervention or prophylaxis is inadequate. The result is a diffuse area of involvement that may ooze blood but can, in a small number of cases, result in massive, acute hemorrhage or perforation [4,5]. The mucosal lesion and associated clinical bleeding or perforation have been termed *stress ulcer syndrome*.

Clinical Characteristics and Presentation

Documentation of gastric mucosal ulceration as a complication of surgery, thermal injury, or neurologic damage has existed in autopsy and surgical specimens for over 150 years [6–10]. Stress ulcer is somewhat of a misnomer in that most of the lesions appear to be shallow mucosal erosions without the submucosal depth of an ulcer (Table 99-1). These mucosal lesions can be found prior to any bleeding, and, in fact, most will not progress to bleeding. These lesions have been found with endoscopy as early as 5 hours after ICU admission, and most will be evident within 72 hours. Stress ulcers/erosions are usually multiple and occur in the proximal stomach (cardia, fundus, body). It has been observed that when patients bleed, there are usually ten or more stress ulcers/erosions found at endoscopy [11]. Within 24 hours of ICU admission they have the appearance of small (1–2 mm) round shallow erosions, and by 48 hours the lesions can be larger (2–25 mm), deeper, and associated with minimal

Table 99-1. Characteristics of Stress Ulcer

- Endoscopic evidence of gastric mucosal disease may be noted within 72 hours of ICU admission.
- Multiple ulcers are located in the proximal stomach. (Peptic ulcer is typically found in the distal stomach.)
- Duodenal ulcers are uncommon. When present, they are usually associated with proximal gastric ulcers and are more common in patients with intracranial disease and thermal injury.
- Progression to overt upper GI bleeding occurs in 5–22% of patients.
- Onset of hemorrhage is within 14 days of ICU admission.
- Abdominal pain is unusual except in setting of perforation.
- Gastroduodenal perforation is infrequent (but may be more common with intracranial injury/disease).

clot. They differ from chronic peptic ulcers in that stress ulcers appear punched out with little or no surrounding inflammation, induration, or edema. Their typical proximal location in the stomach also differs from the usual antral location for gastric ulcers. They also differ in histology as they have minimal acute inflammatory cell reaction and none of the fibrin reaction found with chronic peptic ulcer disease [3]. Duodenal stress ulcers do not usually occur unless they are associated with proximal gastric stress ulcers. Simultaneous stress ulcers in the stomach and duodenum have been noted in 15 percent of burn patients [12]. Stress ulcers confined to the duodenum without associated proximal gastric ulcers would appear to be very rare but have been reported at autopsy.

The advent of upper endoscopy has allowed direct visualization of gastric mucosa in vivo and a more reliable assessment of the prevalence of stress ulcers. However, the bulk of clinical reports over the last 20 years have not always used endoscopy to substantiate that upper GI bleeding in the ICU is related to stress ulcer. Thus, studies failing to document endoscopically that stress ulcer is the cause of the upper GI bleeding may have led to an inaccurate estimate of the prevalence of stress ulcer syndrome [13]. The available endoscopy data indicate that gastric mucosal changes (erythema, erosions, or ulcers) are visualized in 73 to 82 percent of patients admitted to the ICU and given no prophylactic treatment for stress ulcer syndrome [11,14,15]. The finding at preemptory endoscopy of small amounts of blood on the ulcers without associated clinical signs of bleeding has been noted in 22 to 36 percent of cases [14,15].

Although stress-related mucosal lesions are frequently found in the asymptomatic patient at endoscopy, the progression to stress ulcer syndrome (clinical bleeding, intestinal perforation) is much less common. Abdominal pain is rarely reported except in association with perforation, and gastroduodenal perforation is the least common clinical presentation of stress ulcer syndrome. Intestinal perforation has been described more often in critically ill patients with intracranial injury [5]. GI bleeding usually presents within 14 days of the onset of physiologic stress or ICU admission. Hematemesis, gross blood from the nasogastric tube, or melena is the unusual presentation, with massive bleeding occurring in up to 10 percent of bleeding patients. The true incidence of GI bleeding resulting from stress ulcer is difficult to ascertain and will vary depending on the definition of bleeding and the category of ICU patients. There is even some consideration that the incidence of stress ulcer bleeding is decreasing, related to the common use of prophylaxis and improved patient care. The overall occurrence of bleeding ranges from 5 to 22 percent [4,15]. Overt GI bleeding has been noted in 6 percent of patients in a medical ICU [4], and bleeding requiring transfusions was noted in 22 percent of patients with extensive burns [15].

Pathophysiology

The common denominator in the pathogenesis of stress ulcer appears to be mucosal ischemia resulting from splanchnic hypoperfusion in the setting of physiologic stress and an acid milieu [16,17]. While Cushing's ulcers (ulcers related to intracranial injury) are associated with increased acid and pepsin secretion, the classic stress ulcer is marked by a normal or even decreased intraluminal gastric acid concentration [16,17,18]. The failure of the gastric mucosal barrier to provide a normal level of acid protection in the face of stress-related hypoperfusion leads to the mucosal damage of stress ulcer, suggesting the predominant importance of intramural acid concentration over intraluminal pH in the pathogenesis of stress ulcer syndrome [19].

The most superficial gastric mucosal defense against stress ulcer is the mucus and mucus-bound bicarbonate that provides a physical barrier and buffering of intraluminal hydrogen ions [20]. This bicarbonate is derived mostly from basilateral parietal cell secretion. Hydrogen ions that reach the mucous cell layer are handled by a process of back-diffusion, allowing access to the blood-vessel–rich gastric interstitium [16,17,21,22]. It is in this environment that back-diffused acid is buffered by bicarbonate supplied principally by the systemic circulation via the interstitial microvasculature. Mucosal cell restitution allows for rapid restoration of the mucous cell layer integrity by the lateral migration of existing mucosal cells to areas of damaged epithelium [22].

While classic stress ulcer is not associated with an increased intraluminal acid content, ischemia may decrease secretion of bicarbonate to the surface mucus layer from mucosal cells, resulting in a diminished buffering capacity [23]. The systemic acidosis and sympathetically mediated splanchnic vasoconstriction with hypoperfusion that accompany physiologic stress impair the ability of the gastric intramucosal blood supply to buffer and remove the back-diffused acid [16,24]. In the face of mucosal ischemia, gastric intramural pH falls as back-diffusing H^+ ions accumulate [16,24,25]. Hypoperfusion may be transient, resulting in mucosal ischemia and subsequent reperfusion with production of oxygen-derived free radicals and superoxides [18,26]. The resulting lipid peroxidation and destruction of both cellular and lysosomal membranes lead to cell death and further local damage from the ensuing inflammatory response [27]. A recent human study demonstrated the efficacy of therapeutic doses of free-radical scavengers in preventing stress ulcer syndrome [28]. The role of a diminished cellular energy supply in the pathogenesis of stress ulcer is controversial [16,23,29]. A reduction in available ATP in the hypoperfused mucous cell layer coupled with the relatively higher energy requirements of parietal cells may explain the typical fundic location of stress ulcer [16,29]. Factors such as elevated gastrin and pepsin levels, increased intraluminal bile and urea concentrations, decreased gastric motility from enhanced vagal stimulation, and a diminished supply of prostaglandin also appear to be contributory to the development of a stress ulcer but inadequate by themselves to induce the lesion [16,23]. The impact, if any, of *Helicobacter pylori* on the risk and development of stress ulcer is unknown.

Risk Factors for Stress Ulcer

Experimental studies have utilized septic shock, hypotension, restraint, and hypoxia to produce stress-related mucosal disease

[1,30–36]. These animal models demonstrate the key elements required for the development of stress ulcer: physiologic stress and gastric acid. Clinical risk factors commonly associated with stress ulcer syndrome include major surgery, hemorrhagic shock, hypotension, long-term mechanical ventilation, coagulopathy, trauma, and sepsis [5]. While these conditions reflect the severity of illness among ICU patients, they may not constitute independent individual risk factors for the development of stress ulcer syndrome (Table 99-2). Few well-designed endoscopy-based studies exist to validate these risk factors. A statistically significant predisposition to stress ulcer syndrome has been demonstrated in medical ICU patients with a coagulopathy or a requirement for prolonged mechanical ventilation [4]. Hypotension and shock were more common among patients with bleeding attributed to stress ulcer syndrome, but they failed to achieve statistical significance as independent risk factors [4]. The surgical literature suggests multiple organ system failure, trauma, surgery, shock, hypotension, and sepsis as risk factors for stress ulcer syndrome, but the statistical significance of these factors has not always been demonstrated [2,3,11,37]. Patients with thermal injury from burns and those with acute intracranial disease, including head trauma and coma, are also at an increased risk of having stress ulcers (Curling's and Cushing's ulcers, respectively) [16,38,39].

Several studies have demonstrated a worse prognosis and risk for bleeding in patients who have a combination of "accepted" risk factors as opposed to a single risk factor. A clinical syndrome of respiratory failure, hypotension, sepsis, and jaundice has been described in association with a high mortality rate from stress ulcer hemorrhage [2]. The concept of risk factors in combination as predicting stress ulcer syndrome and subsequent outcome has been adapted for ICU application in scoring systems [40,41]. Modified forms of the Glasgow Coma Scale and Apache II Score have been utilized in determining severity of illness, but their usefulness in predicting patients at risk for stress ulcer syndrome has yet to be demonstrated [42]. Elucidating more fully the specific individual and combined risk factors should help identify those patients most likely to incur bleeding complications and, therefore, to benefit from prophylactic therapy [13]. Conditions that appear to present a low risk for stress ulcer syndrome include myocardial infarction, renal failure on dialysis, chronic obstructive pulmonary disease, and malignancy [5].

Prophylaxis

The logic of prophylaxis therapy lies in the assumptions that the formation of stress ulcers can be prevented or that, once formed, the progression from ulcer to bleeding or perforation can be halted. Because the great majority of critically ill patients develop evidence of gastroduodenal injury very soon after their ICU admission, it may be that the latter assumption is more applicable. If those patients at risk can be identified sufficiently early in their ICU stays, then mucosal integrity can be enhanced by three different pharmacologic approaches. The most common therapy involves decreasing or neutralizing gastric acid. Antacids and histamine-2 (H-2) receptor antagonists (H2RA) have fulfilled this role and have long been a mainstay in the prevention of bleeding and perforation. A second pharmacologic approach involves the use of sucralfate, the aluminum salt of sulfated sucrose. While this agent coats the early shallow mucosal ulcers and protects them from further acid and pepsin damage, the primary mechanism of action is probably related

to its intestinal mucosal cytoprotection effect and the ability to preserve microvascular integrity. Sucralfate does not affect gastric acidity. Prostaglandins also have been utilized in stress ulcer prophylaxis for their mucosal protection properties. A third approach to prophylaxis, still in the experimental phase, involves the use of free radical scavengers such as dimethyl sulfoxide (DMSO). This approach is based on the concept that oxygen-derived free radicals are cytotoxic and mediate tissue damage in the critically ill patient. An initial clinical trial suggests that the free radical scavengers DMSO and allopurinol protect against stress-induced mucosal injury and its complications [28].

The difficulties of evaluating and interpreting studies of prophylaxis therapy in stress ulcer syndrome include the variability in patient populations, severity of disease, definition of bleeding, and the type and method of drug delivery. Several studies that have evaluated the use of acid-reducing or -neutralizing therapies have strived to maintain the gastric pH at 3.5 to 4.0 or greater by titrating antacids or H2RA. Although it has been assumed that gastric pH should be 3.5 to 4.0 or greater to prevent bleeding, the ideal pH threshold and duration of pH elevation are unknown. Certainly, studies that have used intermittent fixed IV doses of H2RA appear to have achieved the goal of bleeding prophylaxis equally well as studies utilizing titrated dosing [43]. In fact, stress ulcer bleeding is not always pH dependent, as bleeding has occurred in patients with a mean gastric pH greater than 4.0 [44]. There are now several meta-analyses that have looked at the combined outcomes of studies using titrated antacids or H2RA for prophylaxis [45–48]. The initial review pointed out the flaw of using occult bleeding as an endpoint [45]. This reappraisal of 16 studies involving 2,133 patients found that prophylaxis with either antacids (overt bleeding 3.3%) or H2RA (overt bleeding 2.7%) was superior to placebo (overt bleeding 15%), but there was no advantage of one active therapy over another [45]. More recent meta-analyses have all shown a significant advantage of antacids or H2RA (intermittent and continuous infusion dosage) in preventing overt bleeding when compared to no prophylaxis, and H2RA was superior to antacids. One meta-analysis looked at a subgroup of patients with "clinically important bleeding" (defined as overt bleeding associated with hemodynamic changes or the need for transfusion) and found that only H2RA significantly reduced (by 50%) the incidence of clinically important bleeding [48].

Sucralfate, usually delivered in the form of a slurry through a nasogastric tube at a dose of 4 to 6 gm per day, also has been studied as a prophylactic agent. With regard to the ability of sucralfate to prevent stress ulcer bleeding, the data are conflicting. One meta-analysis concluded that sucralfate was significantly superior to H2RA and as effective as antacids in preventing stress ulcer bleeding, but noted that the results should be interpreted with caution because of the small number of patients involved in the studies [47]. In another meta-analysis reviewing many of the same studies, there were insufficient data to compare H2RA to sucralfate [48]. These somewhat divergent conclusions may just reflect the small number of studies that have utilized sucralfate for stress ulcer prophylaxis.

Complications of Prophylaxis

Although almost every therapeutic agent studied has been successful in reducing stress ulcer bleeding compared with no prophylaxis, there is growing concern about the potential complications, such as nosocomial pneumonia, associated with the use of certain therapies. The incidence of nosocomial pneumonia in long-term mechanically ventilated patients is up to 20 times higher than in patients not on mechanical ventilation, and the mortality rate in these ventilated patients can be as high as 60 percent. Drugs that decrease or neutralize gastric acidity may promote the growth of gram-negative bacteria in previously sterile gastric fluid, predisposing the upper and lower respiratory tracts to bacterial colonization. Thus, there is the potential problem that pH-altering drugs can have their advantages in preventing stress ulcer bleeding offset by the development of nosocomial pneumonia. Sucralfate, a drug that does not alter gastric pH and appears to have bactericidal properties, may offer a clinical advantage. One statistical review of prophylaxis studies came to the conclusion that the subgroup of critically ill patients on long-term mechanical ventilation receiving sucralfate had a significantly lower risk for the development of pneumonia than patients receiving pH-altering drugs [47]. However, another meta-analysis found the incidence of pneumonia in critically ill patients receiving antacids or H2RAs to be lower than in patients receiving no prophylaxis, but statistical significance was not reached [49]. A number of questions have been raised about the study designs of prophylaxis trials, including the often retrospective look at pneumonia and the indirect clinical criteria used to diagnose pneumonia. Thus, the relationship of stress ulcer prophylaxis to nosocomial pneumonia needs further clarification before one prophylactic agent can be recommended over another.

Therapy for Established Bleeding

Once clinically significant bleeding commences it should be evaluated and diagnosed as with any other upper GI bleed. Upper GI endoscopy should be performed as soon as possible to establish the diagnosis and to determine the need for endoscopic thermal or injection therapy. Although multiple stress ulcers or erosions have the potential to bleed at the same time, it is not unusual for only one or two ulcers to be actively bleeding and to respond to endoscopic therapy. For treatment of multiple diffuse bleeding sites, continuous gastric lavage with 5 to 10 liters of ice-cold lactated Ringer's solution has been advocated [50]. The lavage is administered over a 1- to 2-hour period or until bleeding stops. Surgical therapy should be reserved for patients with continuing life-threatening hemorrhage that is unresponsive to endoscopic therapy. Because of the proximal gastric locations and multiplicity of the bleeding lesions, surgical procedures that leave significant amounts of gastric mucosa intact are associated with a recurrent bleeding rate that approaches 50 percent [51]. However, the mortality rate associated with total gastrectomy in these critically ill patients approaches 100 percent. The addition of vagotomy may decrease the high rebleeding rate and has prompted the use of subtotal gastrectomy with vagotomy and oversewing of any ulcers in the remaining stomach [52].

Outcome

The mortality rate for critically ill patients with or without stress ulcer bleeding varies in large part with the type and severity of the underlying disease. Studies evaluating patients with extensive thermal injury have found mortality rates approaching 75 percent [15]. Although mortality can be very high in ICU patients, the relationship of stress ulcer bleeding to mortality is

not well characterized. A natural history study from a medical ICU that did not use prophylaxis found that the overall mortality rate for patients who bled was 90 percent, whereas the mortality rate was 13 percent for nonbleeders [4]. Nevertheless, meta-analyses of studies performed to evaluate stress ulcer prophylaxis came to the conclusion that antacids or H-2 antagonists had no effect on mortality [47,48]. One analysis found that the mortality rate for a subgroup of critically ill patients (long-term ventilated patients) was lower in those given sucralfate prophylactically [47], whereas another meta-analysis did not find any overall mortality advantage for sucralfate-treated patients [48].

Summary: Regimens for Prophylaxis

The prevalence of stress ulcer syndrome may be decreasing, and this decrease may be related largely to the administration of prophylactic agents for those ICU patients at high risk for the development of mucosal disease and subsequent bleeding [53]. There also may be a hierarchy of risk among critically ill patients, burn and neurologic ICU patients being more susceptible to such complications. It is evident that once patients at risk are identified, the administration of any standard prophylactic agent (H2RA, antacids, sucralfate) shortly after the patient is admitted to the ICU will decrease the rate of stress ulcer bleeding. Various high-potency antacids are administered through a nasogastric tube every 1 or 2 hours. H2RAs are administered intravenously either as a standard intermittent bolus or by continuous infusion. Both antacids and H2RAs have been administered without checking pH, although most antacid trials have titrated the frequency and dose of the antacid against a gastric pH level. There is no evidence that one method of administration has any advantage over another. In fact, the

Table 99-2. Risk Factors for Gastrointestinal Bleeding and Perforation in Stress Ulcer Syndrome

Patient Categories Presumed at High Risk

- Burns on more than 50% of body surface area
- Intracranial lesions associated with coma
- Fulminant hepatic failure
- Sepsis, especially pulmonary and intraperitoneal sources
- Major trauma
- Postoperatively, especially following abdominal, cardiovascular, or thoracic surgery
- Intensive care patients with superimposed complications: shock, prolonged mechanical ventilation, acute renal failure, jaundice, coagulopathy
- Multi-organ system failure

Patient Categories Presumed Not at High Risk

- Burns on less than 35% of body surface area (unless shock or sepsis superimposed)
- Intracranial lesions without coma
- Chronic obstructive pulmonary disease or other respiratory illnesses that are transient
- Dialyzed chronic renal failure
- Cardiac disease, including myocardial infarction, arrhythmias, and congestive heart failure

(Adapted from Zuckerman GR, Cort D, Shuman RB: Stress ulcer syndrome. *J Intensive Care Med* 3(1):21, 1988.)

optimal gastric pH level is unknown, the need for 24-hour pH control does not appear to be critical, and the practice of titrating gastric pH is not of proven necessity for adequate prophylaxis. Sucralfate, incorporated into a liquid slurry and administered through a nasogastric tube at the standard dose for treatment of peptic ulcer disease (1 gm four times a day), has also been shown to decrease the rate of stress ulcer bleeding. Although all of these agents would appear effective, only certain specified H2RAs and antacids have received FDA approval for the prevention of upper GI bleeding in critically ill patients. The approved adult dosing regimen for cimetidine is continuous IV infusion of 50 mg per hour. Patients with a creatinine clearance of less than 30 ml per minute should receive half the recommended dose. Treatment beyond 7 days has not been evaluated. Maalox TC (therapeutic concentrate) suspension (Rhone-Poulenc Rorer) and double-strength Mylanta (Mylanta DS liquid, Johnson & Johnson, Merck) are FDA-approved antacids when administered in accord with the following directions:

1. Aspirate nasogastric tube and check pH.
2. Instill 10 ml of Maalox TC or Mylanta DS followed by 30 ml of water via nasogastric tube; clamp tube.
3. Wait 1 hour, then aspirate and record pH.
4a. If pH equals or exceeds 4.0, apply drainage or intermittent suction for 1 hour, then repeat cycle.
4b. If pH is less than 4.0, instill a double dose (20 ml) of Maalox TC or Mylanta DS followed by 30 ml of water; clamp tube.
5. Wait 1 hour; if pH equals or exceeds 4.0, see number 7. If pH is still less than 4.0, instill another double dose (40 ml) of Maalox TC followed by 30 ml water; clamp tube.
6. Wait 1 hour. If pH is still less than 4.0, instill a double amount (80 ml) of antacid.
7. Drain for 1 hour and repeat cycle with the effective dosage.

The advantage, if any, of one prophylactic agent over another or of a non–pH-altering drug over one that does affect pH has not been clarified at this time. The choice of a prophylactic agent will be influenced not only by one's interpretation of the scientific literature but also by the willingness of the ICU staff to adhere to a particular protocol for stress ulcer prophylaxis.

References

1. Goodman AA, Osborne MP: An experimental model and clinical definition of stress ulceration. *Surg Gynecol Obstet* 134(4):563, 1972.
2. Skillman JJ, Bushnell LS, Goldman H, Silen W: Respiratory failure, hypotension, sepsis, and jaundice. *Am J Surg* 117:523, 1969.
3. Lucas CE, Sugawa C, Riddle J, et al: Natural history and surgical dilemma of "stress" gastric bleeding. *Arch Surg* 102:266, 1971.
4. Schuster DP, Rowley H, Feinstein S, et al: Prospective evaluation of the risk of upper gastrointestinal bleeding after admission to a medical intensive care unit. *Am J Med* 76:623, 1984.
5. Zuckerman GR, Cort D, Shuman RB: Stress ulcer syndrome. *J Intensive Care Med* 3(1):21, 1988.
6. Cushing H: Peptic ulcers and the interbrain. *Surg Gynecol Obstet* 55(1):1, 1932.
7. Selye H: Gastrointestinal system, in *The Physiology and Pathology of Exposure to Stress: A Treatise Based on the Concepts of the General Adaptation Syndrome and the Diseases of Adaptations*. Montreal, ACTA, 1950, pp 688–707.
8. Curling TB: On acute ulceration of the duodenum in cases of burns. *Medico-Chirurgal Transactions* 25:260, 1842.
9. Beil AR Jr, Mannix H Jr, Beal JM: Massive upper gastrointestinal hemorrhage after operation. *Am J Surg* 108:324, 1964.
10. Goodman AA, Frey CF: Massive upper gastrointestinal hemorrhage following surgical operations. *Ann Surg* 167:180, 1968.
11. Martin LF, Booth FV, Reines D, et al: Stress ulcers and organ failure in intubated patients in surgical intensive care units. *Ann Surg* 215:332, 1991.
12. Pruitt BA Jr, Goodwin CW Jr: Stress ulcer disease in the burned patient. *World J Surg* 5:209, 1981.
13. Schuster DP. Stress ulcer prophylaxis: In whom? With what? *Crit Care Med* 21:4, 1993.
14. Peura DA, Johnson LF. Cimetidine for prevention and treatment of gastroduodenal mucosal lesions in patients in an intensive care unit. *Ann Intern Med* 103:173, 1985.
15. Czaja AJ, McAlhany JC, Pruitt BA: Acute gastroduodenal disease after thermal injury: An endoscopic evaluation of incidence and natural history. *N Engl J Med* 291(18):925, 1974.
16. Marrone GC, Silen W: Pathogenesis, diagnosis and treatment of acute gastric mucosal lesions. *Clinics in Gastroenterology* 3(2):635, 1984.
17. Hase T, Moss BJ: Microvascular changes of gastric mucosa in the development of stress ulcer in rats. *Gastroenterology* 65:224, 1973.
18. Yabana T, Yachi A: Stress-induced vascular damage and ulcer. *Dig Dis Sci* 33:751, 1988.
19. Fiddian-Green RG, McGough E, Pittenger G, Rothman E: Predictive value of intramural pH and other risk factors for massive bleeding from stress ulceration. *Gastroenterology* 85:613, 1983.
20. Pilchman J, Lefton HB, Braden GL: Cytoprotection and stress ulceration. *Med Clin North Am* 75:853, 1991.
21. Kilvaasko EG, Silen W: Pathogenesis of experimental gastric mucosal injury. *N Engl J Med* 301:364, 1979.
22. Silen W: Pathogenetic factors in erosive gastritis. *Am J Med* 79(Suppl 2C):45, 1985.
23. Bresalier RS: The clinical significance and pathophysiology of stress-related gastric mucosal hemorrhage. *J Clin Gastroenterol* 13(Suppl 2):S35, 1991.
24. Cheung LY: Gastric mucosal blood flow: Its measurement and importance in mucosal defense mechanisms. *J Surg Res* 36:282, 1984.
25. Skillman JJ, Gould SA, Chung RSK, Silen W: The gastric mucosal barrier: clinical and experimental studies in critically ill and normal man, and in the rabbit. *Ann Surg* 172:564, 1970.
26. Mantor PC, Tuggle DW, Perkins TA, et al: Stress-induced gastric ulcers. *Current Surgery* 46:388, 1989.
27. Itoh M, Guth PH: Role of oxygen-derived free radicals in hemorrhagic shock-induced gastric lesions in the cat stomach. *Gastroenterology* 90:362, 1986.
28. Salim AS: Protection against stress-induced acute gastric mucosal injury by free radical scavengers. *Intensive Care Med* 17:455, 1991.
29. Menguy R, Masters YF: Mechanism of stress ulcer. *Gastroenterology* 66:509, 1974.
30. Harjola PT, Sivula A: Gastric ulceration following experimentally induced hypoxia and hemorrhagic shock. *Ann Surg* 163:21, 1966.
31. Zinner MJ, Turtinen L, Gurll NJ: The role of acid and ischemia in production of stress ulcers during canine hemorrhagic shock. *Surgery* 77:807, 1975.
32. Arvidsson S, Haglund V: Acute gastric ulceration in septic shock: An experimental model. *Scand J Gastroenterol* 105:46, 1984.
33. Kuroiwa M, Sugiyama S, Goto H, et al: The role of mucosal prostaglandin levels in healing water-immersion-induced gastric ulcers in rats. *Scand J Gastroenterol* 25:59, 1990.
34. Robert A, Northam JI, Wezomis JE: Exertion ulcers in the rat. *Am J Dig Dis* 15:497, 1970.
35. Kawarada Y, Lambeck J, Matsumoto T: Pathophysiology of stress ulcer and its prevention. II. Prostaglandin E1 and microcirculatory responses in stress ulcer. *Am J Surg* 129:217, 1975.
36. Hanson HM, Brodie DA: Use of the restrained rat technique for study of anti-ulcer drugs. *J Appl Physiol* 15:291, 1960.
37. LeGall JR, Mignon FC, Rapin M, et al: Acute gastroduodenal lesions related to severe sepsis. *Surg Gynecol Obstet* 142:377, 1976.
38. Haglund U: Stress ulcers. *Scand J Gastroenterol* 25(Suppl 175):27, 1990.
39. Fitts C, Cathcart R, Artz C, et al: Acute gastrointestinal tract ulceration: Cushing's ulcer, steroid ulcer, Curling's ulcer, and stress ulcer. *Am J Surg* 37:218, 1971.
40. Tryba M, Zevounow F, Torok M, Zenz M: Prevention of acute stress bleeding with sucralfate, antacids or cimetidine: A controlled study with pirenzepine as a basic medicine. *Am J Med* 79(Suppl 2C):55, 1985.
41. Zinner MJ, Zuidema GD, Smith PL, Miguosa M: The prevention of

upper gastrointestinal tract bleeding in patients in an intensive care unit. *Surg Gynecol Obstet* 153:214, 1981.

42. Driks MR, Craven DE, Celli BR, et al: Nosocomial pneumonia in intubated patients given sucralfate as compared with antacids or histamine type 2 blockers. *N Engl J Med* 317:1376, 1987.

43. Zuckerman GR, Shuman R: Therapeutic goals and treatment options for prevention of stress ulcer syndrome. *Am J Med* 83(Suppl 6A):29, 1987.

44. Martin L, Booth F, Karlstadt R, et al: Continuous intravenous cimetidine decreased stress-related upper gastrointestinal hemorrhage without promoting pneumonia. *Crit Care Med* 21:19, 1993.

45. Shuman R, Zuckerman G, Schuster D: Prophylactic therapy for stress ulcer bleeding: A reappraisal. *Ann Intern Med* 106:562, 1987.

46. Lacroix J, Infante-Rivard C, Jenicek M, Gauthier M: Prophylaxis of upper gastrointestinal bleeding in intensive care units: A meta-analysis. *Crit Care Med* 17:862, 1989.

47. Tryba M: Prophylaxis of stress ulcer bleeding: A meta-analysis. *J Clin Gastroenterol* 13(Suppl 2):544, 1991.

48. Cook DJ, Witt LG, Cook RJ, Guyatt GH: Stress ulcer prophylaxis in the critically ill: A meta-analysis. *Am J Med* 91:519, 1991.

49. Cook DJ, Laine LA, Guyatt GH, Raffin TA: Nosocomial pneumonia and the role of gastric pH: A meta-analysis. *Chest* 100:7, 1991.

50. Tryba M, May B: Conservative treatment of stress ulcer bleeding: A new approach. *Scand J Gastroenterol* 27(Suppl 191):16, 1992.

51. Hubert JP, Kiernan PD, Welch JS, et al: The surgical management of bleeding stress ulcers. *Ann Surg* 191:672, 1980.

52. Ritchie WP: Stress ulceration, in Nyhus LM, Wastell C (eds): *Surgery of the Stomach and Duodenum*. 4th ed. Boston, Little, Brown & Co, 1986, p 663.

53. Sherman TM, Zuckerman GR: Significant stress ulcer bleeding in the intensive care unit: A rare entity. *Gastrointest Endosc* 40:88, 1994.

100. Variceal Bleeding

Paul E. Buse and
Gary R. Zuckerman

Upper gastrointestinal (GI) variceal bleeding is one of the most feared complications of portal hypertension. In western countries the most frequent cause of portal hypertension is cirrhosis related to alcohol abuse and viral etiologies. Gastroesophageal varices are the source of bleeding in only 10 percent of patients who present with acute upper GI hemorrhage [1], although the 30 to 50 percent mortality associated with acute variceal bleeding is much greater than that typically associated with bleeding from acid-peptic disease (9%). Disappointingly, no specific therapy has been found to reproducibly decrease mortality in this patient population. The reason for this is multifactorial, related to the typically brisk rate of bleeding, the high incidence of rebleeding, and the poor functional status and comorbid medical problems associated with chronic liver disease. This creates tremendous challenges for the intensivist responsible for the management of these patients and requires a team approach involving critical care physicians, gastroenterologists, surgeons, and radiologists.

Pathophysiology of Variceal Hemorrhage

The development of portal hypertension in the cirrhotic patient is a complex pathophysiologic event. Hemodynamic manifestations of cirrhosis include peripheral vasodilatation with decreased systemic vascular resistance, increased cardiac output, splanchnic hyperemia, and resultant increased portal venous blood flow [2]. Increases in portal blood flow alone do not produce portal hypertension except in extreme situations such as arteriovenous fistula and splenomegaly (unrelated to liver disease). This results from the very low resistance encountered at the level of the hepatic sinusoid in the normal liver. But with chronic liver disease there appears to be increased resistance of hepatic flow at the sinusoidal level; to compensate for this

one witnesses the development of the portosystemic collateral circulation. This merely represents the body's attempts to decompress the portal venous system. Numerous vascular collaterals exist between the portal and systemic circulations, the most clinically significant sites being at the juncture of squamous and columnar mucosa (gastroesophageal, rectal, and peristomal). With increasing levels of portal hypertension these channels progressively enlarge to form varices. Risk factors associated with variceal rupture include a portal pressure greater than 12 mm Hg [3], increasing variceal size, and progressive hepatic dysfunction.

Diagnosis. These patients typically present with hematemesis, melena, or hematochezia coupled with hemodynamic instability. Although the diagnosis of variceal hemorrhage rests on endoscopic documentation, appropriate resuscitative efforts should be undertaken prior to proceeding with endoscopy. The use of blood and colloid will usually be necessary to expand intravascular volume and to maintain an adequate hemoglobin. Excessive amounts of saline and glucose can lead to progressive ascites, edema, and hyponatremia. When titrating volume expansion and transfusion it is important to remember that the hemodynamic alterations associated with the cirrhosis frequently result in lower basal peripheral blood pressures. It is best to titrate transfusions to maintain an adequate blood pressure (systolic pressure greater than 90 mm Hg), correct orthostatic changes, and maintain an adequate urine output and stable hemoglobin. A nasogastric tube may document the level of bleeding in patients in whom it is not clinically obvious. Although there is a theoretical concern that a nasogastric tube could traumatize a varix and induce more bleeding, this has not been found to be the case in clinical practice. Once the patient is stable or on the positive side of the resuscitation phase, endoscopy should be performed for both diagnostic and therapeutic purposes. Approximately 50 percent of patients with cirrhosis and peripheral stigmata of chronic liver disease who present with acute bleeding will have other sources of hemmorrhage documented at the time of endoscopy. A thorough examination of the stomach and duodenum is performed to exclude alternative bleeding sources. There are several endoscopic scenarios that can confirm that bleeding originates from esophageal or gastric varices. The least common is the endoscopist visualizing a rent in a varix with blood pouring out. The typical clinical setting will be the documentation of upper GI bleeding (hematemesis, gross blood per nasogastric tube, esophageal or gastric blood noted at endoscopy) and endoscopic evidence of only one potential bleeding source, varices. This evidence for a variceal "smoking gun" will be all the impetus needed to plan therapeutic options. Occasionally, a fresh or fibrinous clot will be seen protruding from the variceal wall. For patients with varices that have not as yet bled, the appearance and color of the vessels appear to be predictive of the subsequent bleeding risk and include such signs as cherry red spots, hemocytic spots, and red wale marks (whiplash-like markings).

Table 100-1. Complications of Endoscopic Sclerotherapy and Band Ligation

Esophageal complications
   Ulceration
   Stricture formation
   Perforation (early or delayed)
   Dysmotility
Pulmonary complications
   Pleural effusions
   Pulmonary infiltrates
   Aspiration
   Mediastinitis
   Adult respiratory distress syndrome
Septic complications
   Bacteremia
   Sepsis
   Subacute bacterial peritonitis

Endoscopic Therapy

Endoscopic sclerotherapy was initially described 50 years ago but only recently has gained universal acceptance as a useful modality in the acute management of esophageal variceal hemorrhage. The technique involves injection of a sclerosing solution into the lumen of a varix in the distal 5 cm of the esophagus. Randomized trials comparing sclerotherapy to medical management of variceal bleeding (balloon tamponade and pharmacologic manipulation of portal hypertension) have revealed somewhat conflicting results, but of the eight studies, only three showed no statistically significant benefit to sclerotherapy [4,5,6]. The other five studies showed an advantage to sclerotherapy in terms of control of acute hemorrhage [7,8,9], control of early rebleeding [7,8,10], and long-term, but not short-term, survival [11]. In these studies sclerotherapy was nearly uniformly successful in controlling acute bleeding, and, thus, it has evolved as the therapy of choice in the initial management of acute bleeding. Nonetheless, the incidence of early rebleeding is high (17–37%) [4–11]. Repeat endoscopy after sclerotherapy may be indicated within the first 24 hours in cases of persistent or recurrent hemorrhage. If this is unsuccessful in controlling bleeding, alternative therapeutic options will become necessary. In addition to controlling the acute bleeding episode, sclerotherapy has proven value in preventing rebleeding when used on a chronic basis to eradicate varices [12].

Esophageal sclerotherapy is associated with a high incidence of complications (20–40%) [13] (Table 100-1). Esophageal ulcers develop in the vast majority of patients and should be considered an expected side effect of therapy. Deep ulceration can develop and can be complicated by bleeding, stricture formation (10%), and occasionally necrosis and perforation. Transient bacteremia occurs in a significant portion of patients who have emergency sclerotherapy performed for acute bleeding [14]. Transient chest pain, fever, effusions, and fleeting pulmonary infiltrates also occur in a significant number of patients. The majority of these latter complications are not clinically significant and resolve spontaneously, but there is a procedure-associated mortality of 2 to 12 percent.

Endoscopic band ligation of esophageal varices is an alternative to sclerotherapy for controlling acute hemorrhage. This technique involves the endoscopic placement of multiple elastic "O" rings around varices in the distal esophagus. A recent study showed sclerotherapy and band ligation of varices to be equally effective in controlling acute bleeding [15]. The inci-

dence of complications was 22 percent in the sclerotherapy group and only 2 percent in the ligated group. This lower complication rate may be related to the shallow nature of the esophageal ulcerations compared to sclerotherapy ulcers, the lower incidence of bacteremia, and protection against aspiration through the use of an overtube that is required with the ligating device.

Gastric varices are detected in approximately 20 percent of patients with portal hypertension. Endoscopic visualization of acute gastric variceal hemorrhage can be difficult because of blood pooling over varices in the gastric fundus. Gastric variceal hemorrhage has a tendency to be more severe than the esophageal counterpart. A recent study suggests that gastric varices bleed less frequently than esophageal varices, but the mean transfusion requirement per bleeding episode was significantly higher for gastric varices [16]. The endoscopic control of gastric variceal hemorrhage has not been well characterized, but past experience has shown it to be refractory to endoscopic sclerotherapy with a high rate of rebleeding and sclerotherapy-associated complications [17]. Thus, gastric variceal hemorrhage may dictate an earlier nonendoscopic approach to bleeding control. Isolated gastric varices may result from left-sided portal hypertension (splenic vein thrombosis or hypersplenism). The treatment of choice for gastric varices related to left-sided portal hypertension is splenectomy.

Pharmocotherapy for Variceal Bleeding

Vasopressin. Attempts at pharmacologic manipulation of portal hemodynamics to control acute variceal hemorrhage have been by and large unsuccessful. Vasopressin is a hormone produced by the posterior pituitary that serves to regulate water balance. At high blood levels it acts as a potent vasoconstrictor, thus reducing portal venous blood flow (as well as flow to other crucial organs such as the heart and brain). Controlled clinical data are limited in supporting the utility of vasopressin to control acute variceal bleeding [18]. The typically small studies vary with regard to the dosage and route of administration (continuous intravenous, bolus intravenous, and continuous intraarterial infusions), management of the control group, and documentation of the source of bleeding. A minority of the studies documented significant benefit. Toxicity associated with vasopressin is high, and in an attempt to minimize end-organ damage from vasoconstrictive side effects, investigators have advocated using it in conjunction with nitroglycerin. In addition to the theoretical effect of reducing toxicity, nitroglycerin also has unique beneficial effects on portal hemodynamics. A few controlled studies have compared combination therapy of vasopressin and nitroglycerin to vasopressin alone. Most revealed less toxicity and better control of hemorrhage in the nitroglycerin-treated group. Nitroglycerin has been administered orally, sublingually, and intravenously.

For patients with documented variceal bleeding unresponsive to sclerotherapy, vasopressin in conjunction with sublingual or intravenous nitroglycerin can be considered. There is no definite evidence that vasopressin impacts beneficially on variceal hemorrhage, and, for this reason, at the earliest signs of any toxicity one should discontinue the medication. Coronary artery disease and severe peripheral vascular disease are contraindications for its use. Vasopressin is typically started at 0.3 unit per minute and titrated to control bleeding. Dosage should not generally exceed 0.9 unit per minute. Once bleeding is controlled, the drug should be tapered off. Nitroglycerin may be administered sublingually (0.6 mg every 30 minutes) or intravenously (40 mg/min) titrated to keep systolic blood pressure greater than 90 mm Hg. Though apparently as effective, topical nitrates are not typically recommended due to variable absorption, particularly in the critically ill patient.

Somatostatin, Beta-Blockers. Somatostatin is a hormone that decreases splanchnic blood flow in normal individuals and possibly in patients with portal hypertension. Two randomized trials comparing continuous infusion of somatostatin (250–500 mg/hour) to a placebo revealed contradictory results [19,20]. Somatostatin was more effective than vasopressin in 3 of 4 randomized trials [21–24]. Somatostatin is as efficacious as balloon tamponade with less associated toxicity in the control of acutely bleeding varices [25,26]. A recent study compared somatostatin to sclerotherapy and found similar rates of hemostasis with less toxicity in the somatostatin group [6]. Somatostatin is currently not available in the United States; octreotide acetate (Sandostatin ®Sandoz) is a long-acting analog of somatostatin that is available. One small randomized study comparing octreotide to balloon tamponade revealed similar rates of hemostasis between the two groups, although there was a trend toward higher rebleeding rates in the octreotide-treated group [27]. The analog may offer control of bleeding at least comparable to that of vasopressin but without the systemic toxicity. One study showed octreotide to be equal to sclerotherapy for control of variceal bleeding during the first 48 hours [27a].

Beta-blockers appear to be efficacious in the long-term prevention of recurrent variceal hemorrhage, although they have no role in the management of active variceal bleeding [18].

In summary, the scientific data concerning the efficacy of using pharmacologic agents such as vasopressin to manipulate portal blood flow and control acute variceal bleeding are not convincing. The available somatostatin/octreotide data appear promising but are still preliminary.

Balloon Tamponade

The vast majority of patients with esophageal varices will stop bleeding spontaneously or in response to endoscopic therapy. For those patients with persistent or recurrent variceal bleeding, the use of esophageal and gastric balloon devices for direct tamponade of the bleeding is appropriate. These devices function to apply direct pressure on the bleeding varix and to decrease flow through the portosystemic collaterals. There are two basic types of balloons available: those consisting of a large-volume gastric balloon alone (Linton-Nachlas) and those with both gastric and esophageal balloons (Sengstaken-Blakemore and Minnesota tubes). Tamponade is an effective technique to control acute hemorrhage with initial success in approximately 90 percent of the cases. The incidence of rebleeding is high, occurring in 35 to 50 percent of patients. These data reflect the fact that balloon tamponade is effective only while mechanical pressure is applied. For this reason, one should be making appropriate plans for more definitive interventional therapy once the balloon is decompressed.

Complications associated with the use of these devices are variable though typically high (15–30%) [28,29]. Balloon-related deaths occur in up to 6 percent of patients. The most frequent major complications include aspiration, balloon migration with occlusion of the airway, inadvertent inflation of the balloon in the esophagus with subsequent mucosal tear or perforation, and gastric or esophageal pressure necrosis. See Table 100-2 regarding issues concerning tube management. The Sengstaken-Blakemore and Minnesota tubes are used more frequently than the Linton-Nachlas tube, as they have both esophageal and gastric balloons. The Linton-Nachlas tube is thought to be more effective for patients with actively bleeding gastric varices [30]. For a more thorough overview of techniques involved in the placement of these balloon devices, refer to the package insert provided with the tube and to a recent review [31].

Surgical Therapy

For patients with severe, recurrent, or persistent bleeding, surgical treatment may become necessary. Surgically created shunts have the definite advantage of being the most reliable means to control acute bleeding (greater than 90%) and prevent recurrent bleeding (9%) [32,33]. The main limitation to emergent surgical intervention in the acutely bleeding cirrhotic patient is the high associated operative mortality. Improvements in patient selection, medical management, surgical techniques, and anesthesia are likely responsible for the decreased mortal-

Table 100-2. Important Points in Using Balloon Tamponade for Acute Variceal Hemorrhage

1. Temporizing measure only. Make arrangements while the balloon is inflated for more definitive therapy (chronic sclerotherapy, shunt surgery, TIPS, transplantation).
2. Refer to package insert for details concerning specific tube insertion and usage.
3. Endotracheal intubation will be necessary in patients with a high risk for aspiration.
4. Document (x-ray) the position of the gastric balloon prior to inflating to full volume.
5. Ensure drainage of the proximal esophagus either with an accessory nasogastric tube placed above the esophageal balloon or use a balloon with proximal aspiration ports (Minnesota tube, Linton tube).
6. Label all ports.
7. Limit balloon use to periods of 24 hours.
8. Have scissors readily available for emergent transection and removal of device.
9. Monitor closely for complications.

ity in series reported since 1980. The operative mortality before 1980 was 52 percent as compared with 21 percent since that time [33]. Operative mortality is best predicted by the severity of liver disease, with Childs C patients having poorer outcomes. Nonetheless, these patients are likewise at a higher risk to continue bleeding and succumb to complications related to continued medical therapies. A frequent complication related to surgical shunting is encephalopathy. This likely results from the diversion of a hyperemic, low-resistance portal system into the systemic circulation. Subsequent enhanced absorption of nitrogenous intestinal products that bypass the hepatic circulation results in altered mental status. Selective shunt procedures such as the distal splenorenal shunt are designed to separate the gastrosplenic and portomesenteric circulations, thus partially preserving portal venous pressure and offering the potential for lower encephalopathy rates. The selective shunts are more challenging technically than a portacaval shunt. Nonshunting operations such as the Sugiura procedure (transection and devascularization of the esophagus) have shown promising results in Japan. Limitations of the procedure are related primarily to the redevelopment of varices and recurrent bleeding in upward of 20 percent of patients. The operative mortality in cirrhotic patients undergoing the procedure on an emergent basis was similar to that of standard shunt procedures (23%) [34]. The associated incidence of encephalopathy is low.

A randomized trial comparing surgical portosystemic shunts to sclerotherapy revealed shorter hospital stays and fewer transfusions in those treated endoscopically without any difference in mortality. In long-term follow-up, bleeding recurred in 75 percent of the sclerotherapy group and in none of the surgically treated patients [35]. Warren and his associates from Emory University found that utilizing sclerotherapy for acute bleeding, while reserving shunt surgery for sclerotherapy failures, provided the best overall chance for survival in comparison with shunt surgery alone [36].

Transjugular Intrahepatic Portosystemic Shunt

A transjugular intrahepatic portosystemic shunt (TIPS) is an interventional radiologic procedure whereby a fistula is created between the hepatic vein and the portal vein. This technique involves passing a catheter, under fluoroscopy guidance, through the internal jugular vein to the level of the hepatic vein. A needle is subsequently passed through the hepatic vein until a branch of the portal vein is cannulated. This track is dilated, and a metallic expandable stent is placed in the liver to create a shunt between the portal and hepatic veins. A report of the first 94 patients treated for variceal bleeding at the University of California San Francisco was recently published; TIPS resulted in control of variceal bleeding in all except one patient [37]. Long-term follow-up (a mean of 4.7 months) revealed recurrent variceal bleeding in 10 patients (11%). All of these patients had documented stent stenosis or occlusions, and 90 percent were successfully retreated with stent revision. Seventeen patients developed new or worsening encephalopathy, and 14 were successfully managed with lactulose. The 30-day mortality associated with this procedure was 13 percent. At follow-up, 26 percent of patients had died, 22 percent were transplanted, and 48 percent were alive without transplant. The main issues that remain unresolved regarding this therapy are long-term shunt patency and risk of significant encephalopathy. It may prove to be an invaluable tool in the acute management of variceal bleeding.

Liver Transplantation

Liver transplantation is the only available therapy that treats both the underlying liver disease and portal hypertension. Indications for liver transplantation in patients with variceal bleeding are identical to those in nonbleeding patients (i.e., liver failure). If a patient has advanced liver disease and refractory bleeding and is considered a candidate for liver transplantation a referral to an appropriate center is warranted. If he or she has relatively preserved liver function, a shunt procedure may potentially provide better quality of life, reserving transplantation until absolutely necessary. Shunt procedures that avoid the hepatic hilum (mesocaval, splenorenal, or TIPS) or esophageal transection will interfere less with subsequent efforts at hepatic transplantation. The 1-year survival for patient undergoing transplantation for variceal bleeding is on the order of 70 to 80 percent [38]. An important issue in the management of variceal bleeding is to consider liver transplantation as one of the management options.

Summary

Management of acute variceal bleeding requires a coordinated team approach. Aggressive resuscitation followed by early endoscopy is mandatory for the diagnosis and initial management of variceal hemorrhage. Endoscopic therapy will stop variceal bleeding in the majority of patients. If the patient experiences recurrent or persistent bleeding, repeat endoscopy may prove helpful, but this may be the point in management to move on to other definitive therapies. Balloon tamponade can be used successfully to temporize ongoing bleeding while arrangements are made for more definitive interventional therapy. Pharmacotherapy to alter portal hemodynamics is of unproved benefit. If used, vasopressin should be combined with nitroglycerin to decrease toxicity. Somatostatin is currently unavailable in the United States, although the preliminary data and the low toxicity profile of its long-acting analog, octreotide, are very promising. Early surgical and/or interventional radiologic consultation is necessary so that therapeutic intervention can be arranged if medical management proves fruitless. Transjugular intrahepatic portosystemic shunting is a technique that shows great promise for nonoperative decompression of the portal circulation. Patients with advanced liver disease who are considered to be transplant candidates should be referred early to a center experienced in hepatic transplantation.

References

1. Elta GH: Approach to the patient with gross gastrointestinal bleeding, in Yamada T (ed): *Textbook of Gastroenterology.* Philadelphia, JB Lippincott, 1991.
2. MacMathuna P: The pathogenesis of varice rupture. *Gastrointest Endoscopy Clin North Am* 2:1, 1992.
3. Groszman RJ, Basch J, Grace ND, et al: Hemodynamic events in a prospective randomized trial of propranolol versus placebo in the prevention of a first variceal hemorrhage. *Gastroenterology* 99:1401, 1991.
4. Sorensen T, Anderson B, Backer O, et al: Sclerotherapy after first variceal hemorrhage in cirrhosis. *N Engl J Med* 311:1594, 1984.
5. Soderlund C, Ihre C: Endoscopic sclerotherapy vs. conservative management of bleeding oesophageal varices: A 5-year prospective trial of emergency and long term treatment. *Acta Chir Scand* 151:449, 1985.

6. Shields R, Jenkins SA, Baxter JN: A prospective randomized controlled trial comparing the efficacy of somatostatin with injection sclerotherapy in the control of bleeding oesophageal varices. *J Hepatol* 16:128, 1992.
7. Barsoum MS, Bolous FI, EL-Rooby AA, et al: Tamponade and injection sclerotherapy in the management of bleeding oesophageal varices. *Br J Surg* 69:76, 1982.
8. Moreto D, Zaballa M, Bernal A, et al: A randomized trial of tamponade or sclerotherapy as immediate treatment of bleeding esophageal varices. *Surg Gynecol Obstet* 167:331, 1988.
9. Westaby D, Hayes PC, Gimson AE et al: Controlled clinical trial of injection sclerotherapy for active variceal bleeding. *Hepatology* 9:274, 1989.
10. Larson AW, Cohen H, Zweiban B, et al: Acute esophageal variceal sclerotherapy. Results of a prospective randomized controlled trial. *JAMA* 255:497, 1986.
11. Paquet KJ, Feussner H: Endoscopic sclerosis esophageal balloon tamponade in acute hemorrhage from esophagogastric varices: A prospective controlled randomized trial. *Hepatology* 5:580, 1985.
12. Pagliaro L, Burroughs AK, Sorensen TIA, et al: Therapeutic controversies and randomized clinical trials (RCTs). Prevention of bleeding and rebleeding in cirrhosis. *Gastroenterol Int* 2:71, 1989.
13. Shuman BM, Bekman JW, Tedesco FJ, et al: Complications of endoscopic sclerotherapy: A review. *Am J Gastroenterol* 82:823, 1987.
14. Ho H, Zuckerman MJ, Wassem C: A prospective controlled study of the risk of bacteremia in emergency sclerotherapy of esophageal varices. *Gastroenterology* 101:1642, 1991.
15. Stiegmann GV, Goff JS, Michaletz-Onody PA, et al: Endoscopic sclerotherapy as compared with endoscopic ligation for bleeding esophageal varices. *N Engl J Med* 326:1527, 1992.
16. Sarin SK, Lahoti D, Saxena SP, et al: Prevalence, classification and natural history of gastric varices: A long-term follow-up study in 568 portal hypertension patients. *Hepatology* 16:1343, 1992.
17. Sarin SK, Lahoti D: Management of gastric varices. *Baillieres Clin Gastroenterol* 6(3):527, 1992.
18. Zuckerman GR, Buse PE: Pharmacologic approach to the control of acute GI bleeding, in Lewis JR (ed): *A Pharmacologic Approach to Gastrointestinal Disorders.* Baltimore, Williams & Wilkins, 1994.
19. Valenzuela JE, Schubert T, Fogel MR, et al: A multicenter, randomized, double-blind trial of somatostatin in the management of acute hemorrhage from esophageal varices. *Hepatology* 10:958, 1989.
20. Burroughs AK, McCormick PA, Hughes MD, et al: Randomized, double-blind, placebo-controlled trial of somatostatin for variceal bleeding. *Gastroenterology* 99:1388, 1990.
21. Kravetz D, Bosch J, Teres J, et al: Comparison of continuous somatostatin and vasopressin infusions in the treatment of acute variceal hemorrhage. *Hepatology* 4:442, 1984.
22. Saari A, Livilaakso E, Inberg M, et al: Comparison of somatostatin and vasopressin in bleeding esophageal varices. *Am J Gastroenterol* 85:804, 1900.
23. Jenkins SA, Baxter JN, Corbet W, et al: A prospective randomized, controlled, clinical trial comparing somatostatin and vasopressin in controlling acute variceal hemorrhage. *BMJ* 290:275, 1985.
24. Bagarini M, Albertini M, Anza M, et al: Effect of somatostatin in controlling bleeding from esophageal varices. *Ital J Surg Sci* 17:21, 1987.
25. Jamarillo JL, Mata M, Mino G, et al: Somatostatin versus Sengstaken balloon tamponade for primary hemostasis of bleeding esophageal varices: A randomized pilot study. *J Hepatol* 12:100, 1991.
26. Avgeromps A, Klonis C, Rekoumis G, et al: A prospective randomized trial comparing somatostatin, balloon tamponade, and the combination of both methods in the management of acute variceal hemorrhage. *J Hepatol* 13:78, 1991.
27. McKee RF, Garden OJ, Anderson JR, et al: A comparison of SMS 201-995 and oesophageal tamponade in the control of acute variceal hemorrhage. *HBP Surgery* 6:7, 1992.
27a. Sung JJ, Chung SC, Lai CW, et al: Octreotide infusion or emergency sclerotherapy for variceal hemorrhage. *Lancet* 342:637, 1993.
28. Panes J, Teres J, Bosch J, et al: Efficacy of balloon tamponade in treatment of bleeding gastric and esophageal varices: Results in 151 consecutive episodes. *Dig Dis Sci* 33:454, 1988.
29. Haddock G, Garden OJ, McKee RF, et al: Esophageal tamponade in the management of acute variceal hemorrhage. *Dig Dis Sci* 34:913, 1989.
30. Teres J, Cecilia A, Bordas J, et al: Esophageal tamponade for bleeding varices. Controlled trial between the Sengstaken-Blakemore tube and the Linton-Nachlas tube. *Gastroenterology* 75:566, 1978.
31. Pasquale MD, Cerr FB: Sengstaken-Blakemore tube replacement. Use of balloon tamponade to control bleeding varices. *Crit Care Clin* 8:743, 1992.
32. Cavallari A, DeRaffele E, Bellusci R: Bleeding esophageal varices: Today's role of portosystemic shunts. *Dig Dis* 10:74, 1992.
33. Spina G, Santambrogio R: The role of portosystemic shunting in the management of portal hypertension. *Baillieres Clin Gastroenterol* 6:497, 1992.
34. Idezuki Y: Transection and devascularization procedures for bleeding from oesophagogastric varices. *Baillieres Clin Gastroenterol* 6:549, 1992.
35. Villeneuve JP, Pomier-Layrarques G, Duguay L, et al: Emergency portacaval shunt for variceal hemorrhage. *Ann Surg* 206:48, 1987.
36. Warren WD, Henderson JM, Millikan WJ, et al: Distal splenorenal shunt versus endoscopic sclerotherapy for long-term management of variceal bleeding. *Ann Surg* 203:454, 1986.
37. LaBerge JM, Ring EJ, Gordon RL, et al: Creation of transjugular intrahepatic portosystemic shunts with the Wallstend endoprosthesis: Results in 100 patients. *Radiology* 187:413, 1993.
38. Iwatsuki S, Starzl TE, Todo S, et al: Liver transplantation in the treatment of bleeding esophageal varices. *Surgery* 104:697, 1988.

101. Intestinal Pseudo-obstruction (Ileus)

John R. Mathias and Thomas E. Ducker

The clinical presentation suggesting intestinal obstruction in the intensive care patient is often a diagnostic and therapeutic challenge. Symptoms may include acute onset of nausea, vomiting, abdominal pain, and/or abdominal distention, suggesting a catastrophic, life-threatening condition. Yet the patient's only clinical problem may be that of marked abdominal distention [1,2,3]. The obstruction presentation can be secondary to either a mechanical factor or a neuromuscular dysfunction of known or unknown cause [4–15], commonly referred to as pseudo-obstruction or ileus [1]. Pseudo-obstruction may be either acute (new onset) [4–7] or chronic (intermittent or continuous) [8–15]. Recent technological developments are available to help diagnose intestinal pseudo-obstruction. Thus, the intensivist must be aware of the differential diagnosis and the diagnostic and therapeutic approaches to these hollow-organ disorders.

Acute intestinal pseudo-obstruction was first described in 1948 by Ogilvie [2]. The syndrome of predominantly large-bowel dilatation in the absence of mechanical obstruction subsequently was given his name, but the descriptive term *acute intestinal pseudo-obstruction* is now preferred. Ogilvie described two older patients who had abdominal distention and gastrointestinal (GI) symptoms without apparent cause. The patients underwent surgery despite normal barium studies; exploratory laparotomy showed that the small intestine and large intestine were normal, but both patients had unexpected cancer of the celiac plexus. Ogilvie concluded that the ileus was due to interference of sympathetic innervation. Other cases in elderly and chronically ill patients without cancer have been described [16–20]; typically, the patients were older, often with chronic medical problems, and had had procedures performed for urologic disorders, orthopedic problems, or fractures from accidents. Today, we appreciate that acute intestinal pseudo-obstruction can occur from any medical insult. Certainly patients in the intensive care unit are prime candidates for GI tract dysfunction from such causes as life-threatening systemic diseases, drugs, vascular insufficiency, and electrolyte abnormalities.

The first cases termed chronic intestinal pseudo-obstruction were described by Dudley et al. in 1958 [3]. More reports of this problem in children as well as in adults and in both sexes followed [18–24]. In 1969 Dyer, Dawson, Smith and colleagues [20] used a silver staining technique developed by Smith to describe histologic changes of the myenteric plexus. In 1977 Schuffler et al. [25,26] defined specific histologic abnormalities of longitudinal and circular muscle of the intestine, suggesting that visceral myopathies were responsible for the syndromes. However, in 1985, Smout et al. [27] reported intestinal pseudo-obstruction as a combined myopathy and neuropathy that involved myenteric plexus neurons of the enteric nervous system within the wall of the intestine. Current information suggests that most cases of chronic pseudo-obstruction involve neural degeneration or neural receptor dysfunction of the enteric nervous system. Strategic areas of the central nervous system may be involved as well, resulting in a complex interaction between both nervous systems [28,29].

A more extensive form of pseudo-obstruction involves additional hollow viscera such as the urinary tract, reproductive system, and/or biliary tract. In 1938 Weiss et al. [30] described hollow visceral disease as a myopathy; in 1979 Schuffler et al. [25,26] described the first histologic findings as a degeneration of the longitudinal muscle layer of the intestine. Today, we recognize that most patients with hollow visceral disease have dysfunction or degeneration of nerves in the enteric nervous system [31,32]. In our experience, cases of myopathy are usually familial and rare [10,33]; most cases are neuropathies or neuroreceptor dysfunctional disorders that are idiopathic and acquired [8,9]. Recognizing that alterations in nerve and muscle function may cause significant and life-threatening disease has advanced the understanding that not all cases presenting with severe or recurrent obstruction symptoms are mechanical and require surgical intervention.

Etiology

The list of known causes of chronic intestinal pseudo-obstruction is rapidly growing and includes collagen vascular disorders; endocrine abnormalities, such as diabetes mellitus; neurologic disorders, such as Parkinson's disease; and drugs [8–11,33]. In the intensive care setting, recognizing these disorders as known causes of ileus is important because the patient may have chronic GI symptoms that have gone undiagnosed by conventional testing. However, after a major medical insult like myocardial infarction, vascular accident, or surgery, the

patient may have life-threatening problems not only from the acute condition, but also from distended, nonfunctioning bowel. This situation can cause a diagnostic dilemma for the intensivist and consultants, leading to difficult decisions about whether the patient can withstand certain tests and what therapeutic approach to consider. The outcome can be critical for survival of the patient.

Acute intestinal pseudo-obstruction may also have no history of chronic underlying disease. Common known causes are listed in Table 101-1. Frequently encountered are electrolyte abnormalities, infections, inflammation, vascular abnormalities, drugs, and postoperative ileus.

Pathophysiology

PATHOGENESIS. In the intensive care setting the pathogenesis of acute intestinal pseudo-obstruction usually remains undefined, most patients being severely ill from different disease processes. However, electrolyte abnormalities (such as low potassium, calcium, or magnesium), hypotension, hypovolemia, or hypoxemia from any cause; inflammation from any source; and drugs used to treat the underlying problems are the most commonly associated abnormalities. Viral infection causing an inflammatory neuropathy is a rapidly growing concept as a common factor in neural dysfunction [34–42]. Acute ileus has been described in Guillain-Barré syndrome [35,36], herpes zoster [37], Epstein-Barr virus [38,39], cytomegalovirus [40,41], and botulism B [42]. Retroviruses such as human foamy virus [43] have recently been implicated as causative factors in inflammation of nerves in the gastrointestinal tract as well as in the central nervous system. Neurotropic viruses utilize intracellular machinery for their own purposes at the expense of normal end-organ response.

Ileus occurs postoperatively to a variable extent, especially after the abdomen is actually opened [44]. Although the mechanism of ileus remains unknown, opening the peritoneal cavity or (especially) handling the intestine causes sudden cessation of contractile activity. The slow wave (pacemaker rhythm) remains unchanged, but enteric nerves and circular smooth muscles fail to function for several days. It is now appreciated, however, that ileus predominantly involves the stomach and large intestine, with small bowel function quickly returning to normal [45]. As a result, enteral feedings may be possible in some cases of acute ileus if stomach and colon decompression is maintained by nasogastric suction.

Especially in postoperative ileus, there is evidence that catecholamines, particularly norepinephrine, are released within the wall of the intestine and act on alpha$_1$-adrenergic receptors to interfere with motor function [46]. Pharmacologic treatment with the ganglionic blocker guanethidine followed by cholinergic stimulation with neostigmine has provided immediate and effective relief for some patients, supporting the concept of excessive sympathetic stimulation and/or release [47,48].

Ileus associated with pregnancy or cesarean section occurs in another large group of patients [49,50,51]. Trauma to the sacral nerve roots [52,53] or compression by the postpartum uterus [54] has been suggested as the underlying factor.

Although, in general, we do not understand the cellular pathophysiology, the common theme in most causes of acute ileus is neural insult, either by direct trauma or disruption of intracellular function. Prolonged ileus (> 8–10 days) associated with surgery should suggest either an unsuspected cause (as listed in Table 101-1) or an associated cause of chronic intestinal pseudo-obstruction [55]. The key factor is that any insult to the

Table 101-1. Common Causes of Acute Intestinal Pseudo-obstruction

Electrolyte abnormalities
   Hypocalcemia
   Hypokalemia
   Hyperkalemia
   Hypomagnesemia
   Hypomanganesia
Infections
   Sepsis (bacterial)
   Pneumonia
   Viral hepatitis
   Viral pancreatitis
   Gastroenteritis (viral or bacterial)
   Pelvic inflammatory disease
   Peritonitis
   Pseudomembranous enterocolitis secondary to *C. difficile*
Inflammation
   Pancreatitis
   Cholecystitis
   Crohn's ileitis or colitis
   Ulcerative colitis
   Appendicitis
Vascular disease
   Superior or inferior mesenteric or celiac artery obstruction
   Hypotension with hypoperfusion of mesenteric vessels
   Hypovolemia from decreased intravascular volume
   Hypoxemia
Drugs
   Opiates
   Phenothiazines
   Tricyclic antidepressants
   Antiparkinsonian medications
   Alpha$_1$-adrenergic agonists (e.g., ephedrine sulfate, phenylpropanolamine HCl)
   Alpha$_2$-adrenergic agonists (e.g., clonidine HCl)
   Calcium channel antagonists
   Anticholinergics
   Interleukin-2
Trauma
   Abdominal insult
   Trauma to the head (cerebrovascular accident or subarachnoid hemorrhage)
   Back injury (pelvic or spinal fractures)
Postoperative ileus
   Abdominal
   Urologic
   Orthopedic
   Other
Toxic
   Organophosphate poisoning
   Mushroom poisoning (*Amanita*)
   Radiation sickness
   Heavy metal poisoning (lead, arsenic, mercury)
Metabolic
   Acute intermittent porphyria
   Sickle cell crises
   Hypothyroidism (myxedema)
   Renal failure
   Diabetes mellitus (ketoacidosis, nonketotic hyperosmolar coma, hypoglycemia, "akee poisoning" or "Jamaican vomiting illness")
Pregnancy
   Premature labor
   Placenta previa
   "Postdelivery" ileus
   Cesarean section

GI tract may cause ileus. The puzzle then evolves to identifying the underlying insult.

PATHOLOGIC CHANGES. The changes associated with acute ileus are often disclosed by a plain x-ray film of the abdomen and may be as subtle as an area of localized ileus, or "sentinel loop," as shown in Figure 101-1. Because localized areas of ileus are usually associated with neighboring inflammation, the disease process most commonly considered is unsuspected pancreatitis.

Figure 101-2 shows multiple air–fluid levels, which indicate the pattern of small bowel obstruction. This type of finding on a plain x-ray film can reflect mechanical obstruction, making surgery a serious consideration. However, acute intestinal pseudo-obstruction may also produce the same radiographic pattern. Differentiating between the two is discussed under Diagnosis, following.

The typical pattern of large bowel pseudo-obstruction (Ogilvie's syndrome) is massive dilatation of the large intestine (Fig. 101-3). The degree of dilatation influences the physician's deciding between conservative or invasive diagnosis and therapy. When the cecum approaches 9 to 10 cm (one can read newsprint through the wall of the cecum when it is dilated at ≥10 cm), the possibility of perforation begins to increase rapidly.

Free air in the peritoneal cavity visualized on a plain film of

Fig. 101-1. Radiograph of the abdomen shows an area of localized ileus (*arrow*) in the left upper quadrant. The patient had unsuspected pancreatitis causing the local ileus.

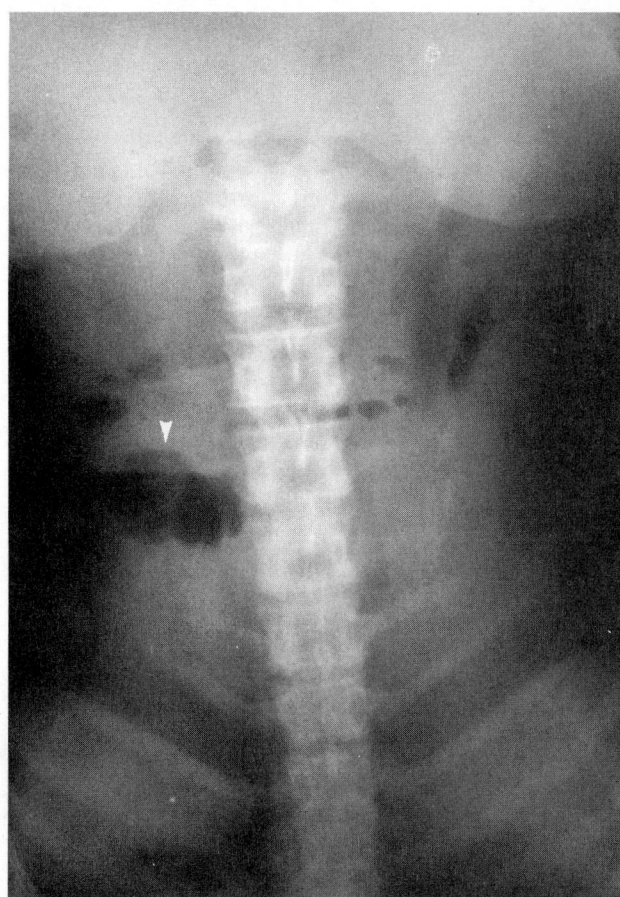

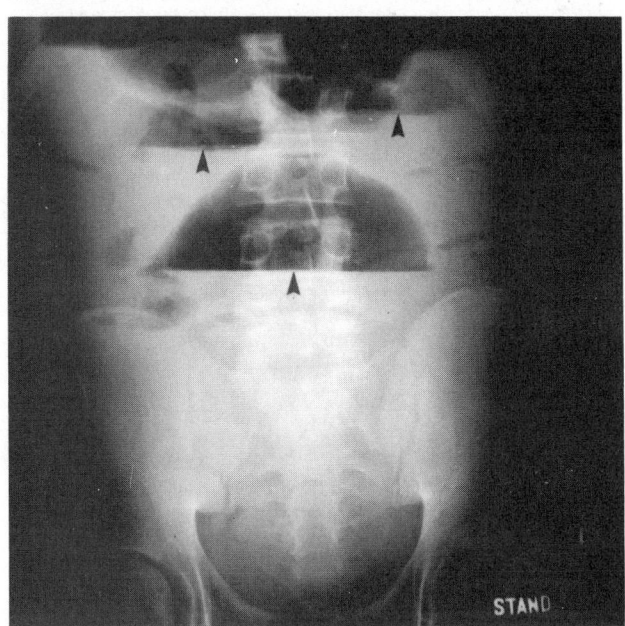

Fig. 101-2. Radiograph of the abdomen shows multiple air–fluid levels (*arrows*) suggestive of small bowel obstruction. Although the initial diagnosis was mechanical obstruction, no lesions were found on exploratory laparotomy and the diagnosis of chronic intermittent pseudo-obstruction was established.

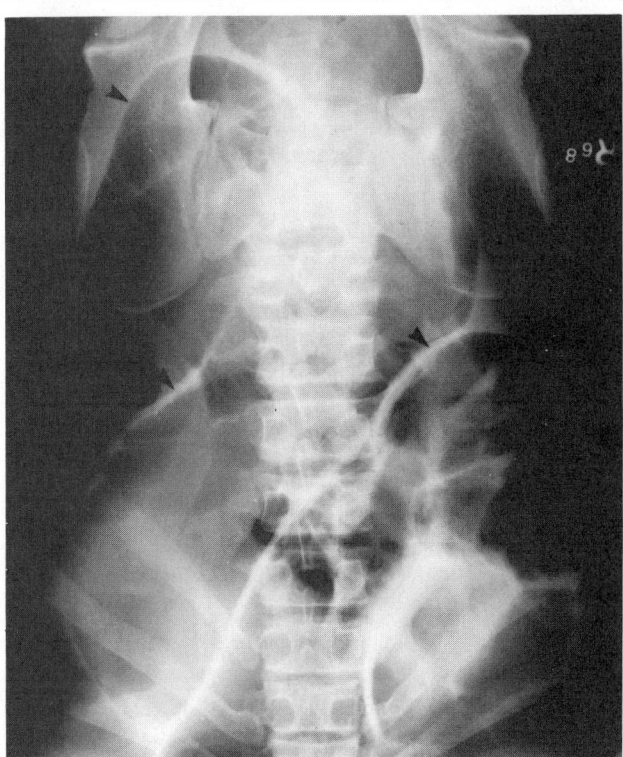

Fig. 101-3. Radiograph of the abdomen shows markedly dilated loops of large bowel (*arrows*), suggestive of large bowel obstruction. Mechanical obstruction was suspected, but colonic pseudo-obstruction (Oglivie's syndrome) was established by diagnostic and decompressive colonoscopy and later by air-contrast barium enema.

the abdomen is also alarming (Fig. 101-4). Although surgical consultation is always required, there are some situations in which free air in the peritoneal cavity may be handled conservatively. For instance, in pneumatosis intestinalis, a condition of mucoid cysts in the wall of the intestine, the cysts may rupture and produce free air in the peritoneal cavity (Fig. 101-5). Although this condition has been commonly reported to accompany idiopathic motility disease, it has been our experience that connective tissue diseases are almost always the associated underlying factors.

Fig. 101-4. Radiograph of the abdomen shows free air under both the right and left hemidiaphragm (*arrows*). Perforation was suspected and exploratory surgery was considered, but computed tomography showed pneumatosis intestinalis of the colon and the patient was treated successfully with supportive therapy.

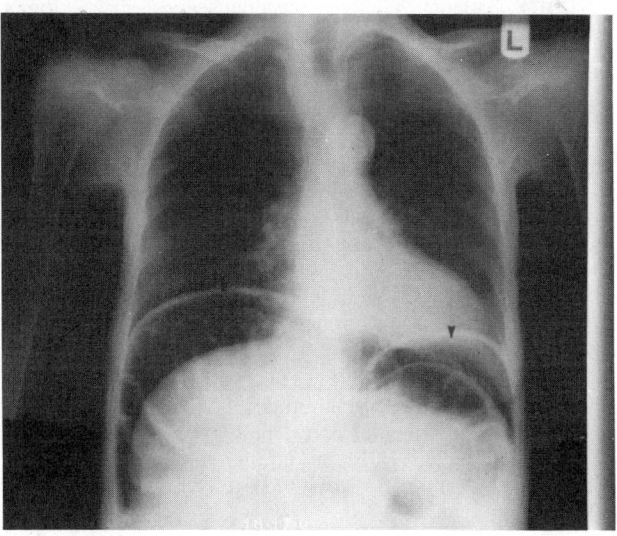

Fig. 101-5. Example of pneumatosis intestinalis by computed tomography of the abdomen, showing free air in cystic lesions in the large bowel wall (*arrows*). Free air is also visible in the anterior portion of the peritoneal cavity (*large dark space*).

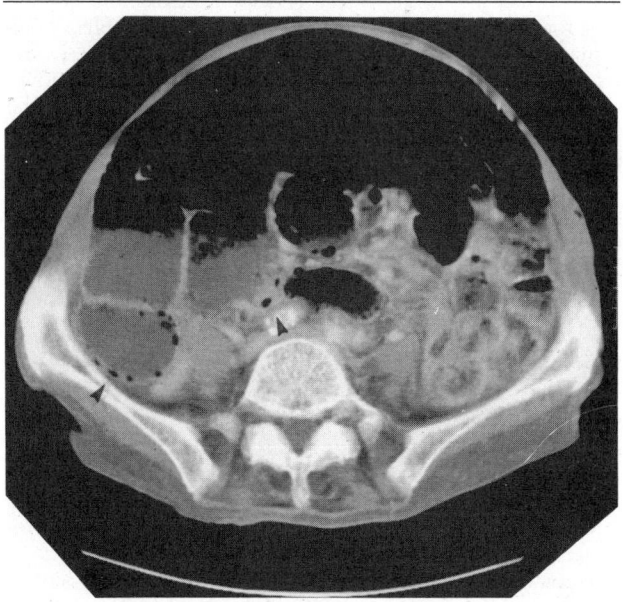

Flexible sigmoidoscopy or therapeutic colonoscopy may disclose other pathologic changes. Pseudomembranous enterocolitis may cause ileus, and inflammation and pseudomembranes are present in the rectosigmoid area. Because antibiotics are commonly used in intensive care, pseudomembranous enterocolitis should always be considered. Other causes of intestinal inflammation such as ulcerative colitis, Crohn's colitis, or ischemic disease will show ulceration and inflammation; rectal inflammation is usually suggestive of ulcerative colitis. The rectum is characteristically spared in both Crohn's colitis and ischemic disease.

Diagnosis

HISTORY. Patients with acute intestinal pseudo-obstruction or ileus often have had no past episodes or problems with the disease. Therefore it is most important to begin with the *history of the present illness* and the *past medical history.* Table 101-2 provides questions that help differentiate between mechanical obstruction and pseudo-obstruction.

Because hollow visceral disease is common but poorly recognized, inquiry into the integrity of the patient's other hollow viscera—urinary, biliary, and reproductive tracts—is important. The single most useful question that will provide a clue to hollow visceral disease concerns the patient's usual frequency of urination during a 24-hour period. The mean urinary frequency of persons in the United States is 5 to 6 times per day. An abnormal response to the question may be either once or twice a day or more than 12 to 15 times a day. A low frequency implies a hypotonic or atonic urinary bladder, and increased frequency implies bladder or urethral spasticity. In addition, eye problems such as ptosis or ophthalmoplegia can be associated with visceral myopathies; the eye problems may be the only clue.

PHYSICAL FINDINGS. In classic acute intestinal pseudo-obstruction, the abdomen is markedly distended, with prominent tympany by percussion, absence of bowel sounds, and relatively little, if any, abdominal pain. The lack of abdominal pain does not always indicate an innocent cause, as similar findings may be associated with vascular ischemia. The examiner should look for other evidence of recent or ongoing peripheral ischemic injury as well as physical findings that might accompany the other disorders listed in Table 101-1. The search for a Virchow's lymph node, a left axillary lymph node, or prominence of the posterior cul-de-sac (Blumer's shelf) on rectal examination may provide the diagnostic information for cancer of the celiac plexus. Abdominal pain on percussion or palpation and rebound tenderness should alert the physician to an intraabdominal inflammatory process involving the GI tract or other abdominal organs. Immediate appropriate tests are necessary to define the cause of this process.

DIAGNOSTIC TESTS. We emphasize that the evaluation and decision to use one of the tests mentioned below *always* begins with a careful history and physical examination. Conventional laboratory tests will then guide and assist in establishing a more objective assessment of the patient's problem. The task is to define the problem and effectively resolve it in the simplest and safest possible manner. The diagnosis of acute obstruction requires all the skills learned as a physician.

All patients should first have supine and upright abdominal and chest x-ray films to assess for the presence of abdominal

Table 101-2. Characteristics that May Help Differentiate Mechanical Obstruction from Acute Intestinal Pseudo-obstruction

Mechanical Obstruction	Acute Intestinal Pseudo-obstruction
1. No previous episode.	1. May have had a prior history or chronic intermittent symptoms of GI distress.
2. No history of GI symptoms.	2. History of dysphagia, early satiety, constipation, and/or diarrhea.
3. Symptom-free between attacks.	3. Chronic abdominal pain, nausea, intermittent vomiting.
4. No history of urinary tract symptoms.	4. History of recurrent urinary tract infections, markedly infrequent or frequent urination.
5. No family history.	5. May have a family history of similar problems.
6. Esophageal manometry is normal.	6. Esophageal manometry may show aperistalsis, lower esophageal sphincter abnormalities, or both.
7. Gastric emptying is normal.	7. May show delayed gastric emptying.
8. Upper GI x-ray series may show obstructing lesion.	8. Upper GI x-ray series may show hypotonic or atonic segments of small intestine.
9. Barium enema may show obstructing lesion.	9. Barium enema may show redundant colon.
10. Plain x-ray film of the abdomen may not show air in the rectum.	10. Plain x-ray film of the abdomen usually shows air in the rectum.
11. Enteroclysis may show obstructing lesion.	11. Enteroclysis may show hypotonic or atonic segments of small intestine.
12. Intravenous pyelogram gives normal findings.	12. Intravenous pyelogram may show dilated bladder or ureters.
13. Jejunal manometry may show peristaltic rushes. Migrating motor complexes are present.	13. Jejunal manometry may show few or no migrating motor complexes.
14. No history of causes of chronic intestinal pseudo-obstruction [8,15,33].	14. May have history of causes of chronic intestinal pseudo-obstruction [8,15,33].
15. No current surgical procedure.	15. Postoperative or a current orthopedic or urologic procedure.
16. No history of toxin exposure.	16. May have been exposed to environmental toxins.
17. No eye abnormalities.	17. Ptosis or external ophthalmoplegia may be present.
18. Obstructing lesion found on exploratory laparotomy.	18. No obstructing lesion found on exploratory laparotomy.

air and its distribution. The decision of which test to perform next is based largely on the history, physical examination, and laboratory data. Figure 101-6 shows an algorithm for proceeding to further tests. For example, if the plain film shows predominantly dilated large intestine, the classic approach is to consider examining the large bowel with a barium enema using a thin solution of barium. If the barium findings are normal, a small-bowel series with thin-contrast barium given orally may be performed. An alternative approach, colonoscopy, can be both diagnostic and therapeutic, defining through biopsy the

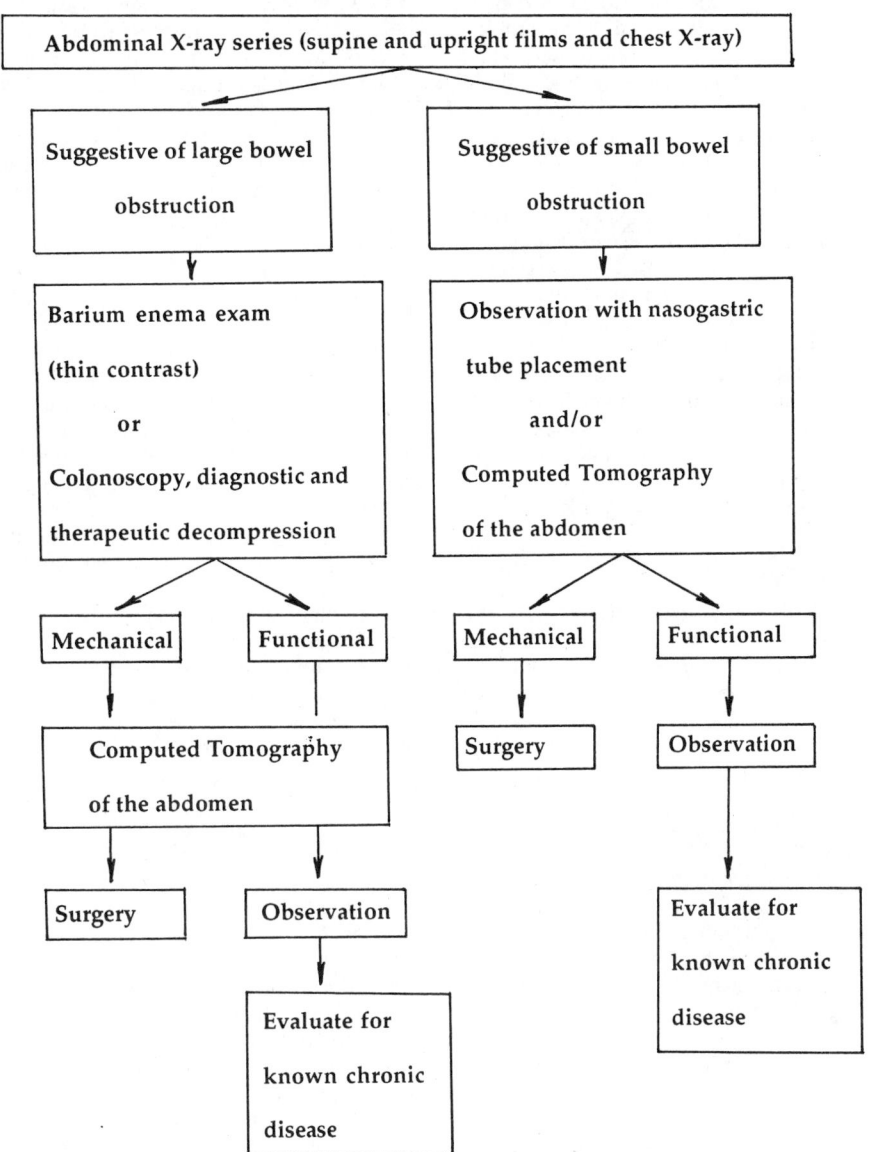

Fig. 101-6. Algorithm of acute intestinal pseudo-obstruction.

presence and histology of a lesion such as a colonic cancer, and it may also be therapeutic, as with a sigmoid volvulus or through decompression of a massively dilated bowel. Deciding what approach to take depends largely on the personnel who have been trained to perform these procedures. When the air–fluid distribution seen on the x-ray film suggests small bowel disease, one may wish to observe the patient if he or she is not ill and conventional tests suggest a cause such as pancreatitis. If the patient is ill, ultrasound or computed tomography of the abdomen should follow; these tests may be focused, especially if the radiologic findings suggest a specific problem, such as acute pancreatitis with a sentinel loop.

A complete blood count is important for assessing the white blood cell count and the cell differential. Serum electrolyte levels, including calcium and magnesium, are important. A biochemical profile that includes amylase and lipase may provide clues to metabolic abnormalities. If "sickle crisis" is considered, a sickle preparation or hemoglobin electrophoresis is indicated.

DIFFERENTIAL DIAGNOSIS. The differential diagnosis for known causes is shown in Table 101-1. Many cases of acute intestinal pseudo-obstruction are idiopathic.

Treatment

OBSERVATION. Many causes of acute intestinal pseudo-obstruction respond only to supportive care and time. The history, repeated physical examination, and laboratory testing will help guide the physician in determining when to be conservative or aggressive in therapy.

SUPPORTIVE MEASURES. The patient with acute obstruction requires basic supportive care. Fluid replacement and correction of electrolytes are essential. If inflammation is a factor, correct selection of antibiotic therapy is crucial. For example, pneumococcal pneumonia responds dramatically to penicillin, but a bacterial infection of the abdomen involving enteric flora may not respond to it at all—such an abdominal infection requires an antibiotic effective in killing enteric pathogens.

EVALUATION OF DRUGS.

Assessing the patient's current medication is essential. Persons in the intensive care setting are often taking multiple medications. Although many drugs alter motility of the GI tract to some extent, others in common use can induce intestinal pseudo-obstruction. For example, adrenergic agonists used to treat hypertension (the alpha$_2$-agonist clonidine) are powerful inhibitors of neuromuscular function of the GI tract. Antidepressant medication, especially the tricyclic antidepressants, can also induce acute intestinal pseudo-obstruction. Finally, opiates of any type inhibit motor function. Assessment of drugs and of their transmitter effect on the GI tract requires careful thought when they are prescribed to debilitated and ill patients.

NUTRITIONAL SUPPORT.

Although nutritional support often is not thought of early in the course of a pseudo-obstruction illness, adequate calories and nutrition are essential for a bedridden patient. If fever and inflammation are present, the number of calories needed for healing is even greater. Total parenteral nutrition may be necessary as a temporary measure until the intestine can function again.

Over the past ten years, experimentation in postoperative or posttrauma animals and humans has shown that the small intestine can be used successfully to provide adequate fluid, electrolytes, and nutrition under those conditions because it retains motor function that allows the perfusion of basic nutrient meals [45,56]. The postoperative or posttrauma stomach and colon, however, remain atonic or hypotonic for 1 to 2 days and 3 to 5 days, respectively [45]. Using enteral nutrition has been shown to be effective in patients undergoing laparotomy for trauma [57]. The intestine has also been employed with excellent success for nutritional support after aortic aneurysm repair with associated acute ileus [58] and has been suggested for use in pseudo-obstruction in general [59]. In addition, enteral feeding has been applied successfully in patients with acute intestinal pseudo-obstruction associated with Guillain-Barré syndrome. This form of nutritional support obviously needs more investigation before it is considered the approach of choice for either acute or chronic intestinal pseudo-obstruction.

NASOGASTRIC SUCTION.

The key to controlling intestinal accumulation of air is to prevent swallowed air from being passed through the GI tract. A 16-Fr. nasogastric tube attached to suction should be placed. If the patient has chronic disease and the nasogastric tube is required for longer than 10 days, a percutaneous endoscopic gastrostomy (PEG) tube should be seriously considered for decompression. Prolonged use of nasogastric tubes causes inflammation of the esophagus, incompetence of the lower esophageal sphincter with chronic gastroesophageal reflux, and potential stricture formation. Obviously, these are complications to be prevented.

RECTAL SUCTION.

Decompression of the rectosigmoid colon may be assisted with a rectal tube attached to intermittent suction [60,61]. This technique is often used in conjunction with decompressive colonoscopy and nasogastric suction.

COLONOSCOPY.

The successful use of colonoscopy for acute large bowel ileus was first described by Kukora and Dent in 1977 [62]. This therapeutic choice is widely favored by gastroenterologists for acute large bowel ileus because it can be both therapeutic and diagnostic [4,63-67] (see Table 101-2). Colonoscopy should be considered early in the course of large bowel ileus [7]. Conservative management consisting of a repeated physical examination (preferably by the same examiner), assessment of cecal dilatation by plain films of the abdomen every 12 to 24 hours, fluid and electrolyte replacement, nasogastric suction, and *repeated* white blood cell counts should be implemented during the first 48 to 72 hours. If the condition does not change or even progresses, decompression should be carried out immediately. The colonoscope may be passed safely by an accomplished endoscopist, even in the presence of retained stool; if stool interferes with decompression, repeated gentle saline enemas may be administered before colonoscopy to improve visibility. The administration of air to distend the bowel should be kept at a minimum to avoid additional pressures within the bowel lumen. If signs of ischemic bowel disease are present (erythematous or friable mucosa, or the presence of blood-stained fluid within the lumen), the procedure should be immediately terminated and surgery becomes the treatment of choice. In addition, if there are signs of peritoneal inflammation (tender right lower quadrant, guarding, or rebound tenderness), fever, or an elevated white count, or a combination of these findings, surgical intervention is clearly indicated. Successful decompression may be expected in approximately 80 percent of patients with one procedure [68]. If dilatation recurs, repeat colonoscopy is usually successful. Successful decompression may be accomplished even when only the hepatic flexure is reached, without visualization of the cecum [62,68]. The use of a fenestrated tube placed in the cecum or transverse colon during decompressive colonoscopy has also been successful [69-72]. This retained tube may be attached to suction to maintain decompression until full recovery. One should understand that decompressive colonoscopy is not indicated for small bowel ileus.

If a diagnostic barium study is considered, a *limited* enema involving only the rectosigmoid region is recommended. Gastrografin enemas are also discouraged because they are hyperosmolar substances that draw water from the intravascular space. The colonoscopic examination then becomes very difficult because of the enormous volume of fluid, and the intravascular space may be compromised, resulting in hypovolemia. Decompressive colonoscopy may need to be repeated until the intestine can recover sufficiently.

When the pattern of colonic obstruction is present, colonoscopy is often used as the initial procedure because of its dual diagnostic and therapeutic capabilities. A barium enema examination using a thin solution of barium may be used later in the evaluation, if at all. Colonoscopy and limited barium enema for chronic or recurrent disease should be viewed as complementary tests. If lesions observed by colonoscopy explain the underlying symptoms, biopsies can be taken to help the surgeon better prepare for a definitive procedure. If lesions noted during colonoscopy do not explain the obstructive symptoms, they should be left alone and removed later, when the colon can be properly cleansed before therapeutic colonoscopy. Decompression of the colon without laparotomy is the primary objective of colonoscopy in critically ill patients.

SURGICAL INTERVENTION.

Surgery may be needed to assess the acute problem effectively and to treat the underlying problem. In the absence of perforation or ischemic bowel changes, either tube cecostomy or formal cecostomy is the treatment of choice [53,73,74]. If clinical signs suggest perforation, ischemia, or mechanical obstruction such as a volvulus, laparotomy should be performed immediately through a midline abdominal incision. Surgical colleagues should be involved in the initial evaluation and decision-making and *should not be asked to consult on an emergency basis when all else has failed.* Acute intestinal pseudo-obstruction is a difficult problem and requires a number of different medical disciplines for effective patient care. The well-being of the patient is the common goal. If exploratory surgery is performed and no obstructive lesion is found, full-thickness biopsies should *always* be obtained for histologic assessment of nerve and muscle. If repeated explorations can be prevented because the biopsies define chronic nerve or muscle disease, then preventing intraabdominal adhesions is a significant gain. Chronic mechanical obstruction superimposed on neuromuscular disease becomes a therapeutic nightmare.

OTHER SPECIFIC MEDICAL TREATMENTS. Using medication to speed the recovery of ileus is always tempting, especially after surgery [6]. In acute intestinal pseudo-obstruction from surgery [44,55,75], the intestine is shut down because of an underlying insult. The nerve and muscle can be expected to respond when the recovery phase is complete; it is best not to hurry this defense mechanism of the body. In general, the intestine will recover and be functional 5 to 7 days postoperatively. If the ileus persists longer than 10 days, evaluation for known causes of chronic intestinal pseudo-obstruction should be pursued [8–11,33].

Recently, the use of intravenous erythromycin, a macrolide antibiotic that acts as a motilin agonist [76,77,78], has been reported to stimulate motor activity in the stomach and small intestine. This drug has been effective in refractory cases of postoperative ileus [79,80]. It should be used carefully, however, and only after the patient has been appropriately examined. Promising results have also been shown recently in animals with the kappa-opioid agonist fedotozamine [81]. Trials in humans are pending.

Several different pharmacologic agents have been used to treat acute ileus medically. Guanethidine, an adrenergic neuronal blocker associated with the pseudocholine esterase inhibitor neostigmine [48,82], produced excellent results in eight patients. This combination was used because one of the theories of acute ileus, especially of postoperative ileus, is that it involves excessive sympathetic discharge. This approach was repeated in a double-blind study using bethanidine, an analog of guanethidine, and showed no significant difference from saline controls [48]. Other drugs such as the cholinergic agonist bethanechol (Urecholine) and metoclopramide (Reglan) have also been used, with mixed results [83]. Extreme caution should be taken when considering use of these prokinetic agents because they may stimulate the upper GI tract but have little effect on the lower tract, thereby increasing the possibility of perforation. Cisapride has been used favorably in a patient with acute ileus [84] and in chronic intestinal pseudo-obstruction [85], but formal double-blind, placebo-controlled studies are lacking and caution should be exercised until such information is available [46]. Another study that used conservative therapy exclusively resulted in 23 of 24 patients recovering successfully from acute ileus [86]. These subjects all had cancer, and their main causes of acute ileus were the results of either chemotherapy or radiation therapy, opiates for pain, or sepsis—all potentially treatable or correctable etiologies.

The use of suppositories or laxative agents is strongly discouraged. If the patient is able to ambulate, the time-honored remedy of short walks should be encouraged; however, we do not know if this exercise helps or how it may contribute to improved gut function. We again suggest that although it is tempting to hurry the recovery phase of the intestine along, especially in postoperative ileus, patience and careful attention to the details of care usually result in a recovered and well patient.

Summary

Intestinal pseudo-obstruction is a commonly encountered problem in the intensive care setting. The disorder results from dysfunction of the enteric nervous system and the circular smooth muscle layer within the wall of the intestine. Typical presenting symptoms include marked distention with a minimum of abdominal pain. Dilatation with air–fluid levels of the large intestine (Ogilvie's syndrome) or small intestine, or both, may be seen by radiography. To determine the therapeutic approach, assessment of the underlying cause is important. Intestinal pseudo-obstruction, if appropriately recognized early and effectively evaluated, need not result in significant morbidity or mortality.

References

1. Cantor MO: Ileus. *Am J Gastroenterol* 47:461, 1967.
2. Ogilvie H: Large-intestine colic due to sympathetic deprivation: New clinical syndrome. *BJM* 2:671, 1948.
3. Dudley HAF, Sinclair ISR, McLaren IF, et al: Intestinal pseudo-obstruction. *J R Coll Surg Edinb* 3:206, 1958.
4. Dorudi S, Berry AR, Kettlewell MGW: Acute colonic pseudo-obstruction. *Br J Surg* 79:99, 1992.
5. VanTrappen G: Acute colonic pseudo-obstruction (Commentary). *Lancet* 341:152, 1993.
6. Camilleri M, Phillips S: Acute and chronic intestinal pseudo-obstruction. *Adv Intern Med* 36:287, 1991.
7. Krige JEJ, Hudson DA, Kottler RE: Acute colonic pseudo-obstruction: Current diagnosis and management. *S Afr Med J* 75:271, 1989.
8. Mathias JR, Finelli DS: Functional disorders of the small intestine, in Cohen S, Soloway RD (eds): *Functional Disorders of the Gastrointestinal Tract (Contemporary Issues in Gastroenterology, vol 6)*. New York, Churchill Livingstone, 1987, pp 39–58.
9. Reeves-Darby VG, Mathias JR: Motility disorders of the small intestine. *Contemp Int Med* 3(10):92, 1991.
10. Anuras S: Intestinal pseudo-obstruction syndrome. *Annu Rev Med* 39:1, 1988.
11. Anuras S: Clinical presentation: Chronic intestinal pseudo-obstruction. *Prac Gastroenterol* 15(3):13, 1991.
12. Colemont LJ, Camilleri M: Chronic intestinal pseudo-obstruction: Diagnosis and treatment. *Mayo Clin Proc* 64:60, 1989.
13. Schuffler MD: Chronic intestinal pseudo-obstruction syndromes. *Med Clin North Am* 65(6):1331, 1981.
14. Faulk DL, Anuras S, Christensen J: Chronic intestinal pseudo-obstruction. *Gastroenterology* 74:922, 1978.
15. Anuras S, Crane SA, Faulk DL, et al: Intestinal pseudo-obstruction. *Gastroenterology* 74:1318, 1978.
16. Melamed M, Kubian E: Relationship of the autonomic nervous system to "functional" obstruction of the intestinal tract: Report of four cases, one with perforation. *Radiology* 80:22, 1963.
17. Caves PK, Crockard HA: Pseudo-obstruction of the large bowel. *BMJ* 1:583, 1970.
18. Chaimoff C, Dintsman M: The pseudo-obstruction of bowel syndrome: A suggestion of a simple surgical remedy. *Am J Proctol* 25(1):39, 1974.
19. Bardsley D: Pseudo-obstruction of the large bowel. *Br J Surg* 61:963, 1974.

20. Dyer HH, Dawson AM, Smith BF, et al: Obstruction of bowel due to lesion in the myenteric plexus. *BMJ* 1:686, 1969.
21. Vargas JH, Sachs P, Ament ME: Chronic intestinal pseudo-obstruction syndrome in pediatrics (Review). *J Pediatr Gastroenterol Nutr* 7(3):323, 1988.
22. Byrne WJ, Cipel L, Euler AR, et al: Chronic idiopathic intestinal pseudo-obstruction syndrome in children: Clinical characteristics and prognosis. *J Pediatr* 90:585, 1977.
23. Kapila L, Haberkorn S, Nixon HH: Chronic adynamic bowel simulating Hirschsprung's disease. *J Pediatr Surg* 10:885, 1975.
24. Piñeiro-Carrero VM, Andres JM, Davis RH, et al: Abnormal gastrointestinal motility in children and adolescents with recurrent functional abdominal pain. *J Pediatr* 113:820, 1988.
25. Schuffler MD, Lowe MC, Bill AH: Studies of idiopathic intestinal pseudo-obstruction. I. Hereditary hollow visceral myopathy: Clinical and pathological studies. *Gastroenterology* 73:327, 1977.
26. Schuffler MD, Pope CE II: Studies of idiopathic intestinal pseudo-obstruction. II. Hereditary hollow visceral myopathy: Family studies. *Gastroenterology* 73:339, 1977.
27. Smout AJPN, DeWilde K, Kooyman CD, et al: Chronic idiopathic intestinal pseudo-obstruction, coexistence of smooth muscle and neuronal abnormalities. *Dig Dis Sci* 30:282, 1985.
28. Gue M, Junien JL, Bueno L: Conditioned emotional response in rats enhances colonic motility through the central release of corticotropin-releasing factor. *Gastroenterology* 100:964, 1991.
29. Koch KL, Stern RM, Vasey MW, et al: Neuroendocrine and gastric myoelectrical responses to illusory self-motion in humans. *Am J Physiol* 258:E304, 1990.
30. Weiss W: Zur Atiologie des Megaduodenums. *Dtsch Z Chir* 25:317, 1938.
31. Krishnamurthy S, Schuffler MD, Rohrmann CA, et al: Severe idiopathic constipation is associated with a distinctive abnormality of the colonic myenteric plexus. *Gastroenterology* 88:26, 1985.
32. Krishnamurthy S, Schuffler MD: Pathology of neuromuscular disorders of the small intestine and colon. *Gastroenterology* 93:610, 1987.
33. Chokhavatia S, Anuras S: Neuromuscular disease of the gastrointestinal tract. *Am J Med Sci* 301:201, 1991.
34. Oh JJ, Kim CH: Gastroparesis after a presumed viral illness: Clinical and laboratory features and natural history. *Mayo Clin Proc* 65:636, 1990.
35. Susman E, Maddox K: The Guillain-Barré syndrome. *Med J Aust* 1:158, 1940.
36. Lichtenfeld P: Autonomic dysfunction in the Guillain-Barré syndrome. *Am J Med* 50:772, 1971.
37. Wyburn-Mason R: Visceral lesions in herpes zoster. *BMJ* 1:678, 1957.
38. Yahr MD, Frontera AT: Acute autonomic neuropathy: Its occurrence in infectious mononucleosis. *Arch Neurol* 32:132, 1975.
39. Vassallo M, Camilleri M, Caron BL, et al: Gastro-intestinal motor dysfunction in acquired selective cholinergic dysautonomia associated with infectious mononucleosis. *Gastroenterology* 100:252, 1991.
40. Sonsino E, Mouy R, Foucaud P, et al: Intestinal pseudo-obstruction related to cytomegalovirus infection of the myenteric plexus (Letter to the Editor). *N Engl J Med* 311:196, 1984.
41. Mathias JR, Baskin GS, Reeves-Darby VG, et al: Chronic intestinal pseudoobstruction in a patient with heart-lung transplant: Therapeutic effect of leuprolide acetate. *Dig Dis Sci* 37:1761, 1992.
42. Jenzer G, Mumenthaler M, Ludin HP, et al: Autonomic dysfunction in botulism B: A clinical report. *Neurology* 25:150, 1975.
43. Bothe K, Aguzzi A, Lassmann H, et al: Progressive encephalopathy and myopathy in transgenic mice expressing human foamy virus genes. *Science* 253:555, 1991.
44. Waldhausen JHT, Shaffrey ME, Skenderis BS II, et al: Gastrointestinal myoelectric and clinical patterns of recovery after laparotomy. *Ann Surg* 211(6):777, 1990.
45. Ryan JA Jr, Page CP: Intrajejunal feeding: development and current status. *Ann J Parenter Enteral Nutr* 8:187, 1984.
46. Vantrappen G: Commentary: Acute colonic pseudo-obstruction. *Lancet* 341:152, 1993.
47. Hutchinson R, Griffiths C: Acute colonic pseudo-obstruction: A pharmacological approach. *J R Coll Surg Engl* 74:364, 1992.
48. Heimbach DM, Crout JR: Treatment of paralytic ileus with adrenergic neuronal blocking drugs. *Surgery* 69:582, 1971.

49. Reece EA, Petrie RH: Ogilvie's syndrome in the postcaesarean patient. *Am J Obstet Gynecol* 144:849, 1948.
50. Morre JG, Gladstone NS, Lucas GW, et al: Successful management of post-Caesarean-section acute pseudo-obstruction of the colon (Ogilvie's syndrome) with colonoscopic decompression: A case report. *J Reprod Med* 31:1001, 1986.
51. Rodriguez-Ballesteros R, Torres-Bautista A, Torres-Valadez F, et al: Ogilvie's syndrome in the postcaesarean section patient. *Int J Gynaecol Obstet* 28:185, 1989.
52. Spira IA, Rodrigues R, Wolff WI: Pseudo-obstruction of the colon. *Am J Gastroenterol* 65:397, 1976.
53. Bachulis BL, Smith PE: Pseudo-obstruction of the colon. *Am J Surg* 136:66, 1978.
54. Monro A, Jones PF: Abdominal surgical emergencies in the puerperium. *BMJ* 4:691, 1975.
55. Livingston EH, Pasaro EP: Postoperative ileus. *Dig Dis Sci* 35:121, 1990.
56. Clifton GL, Robertson CS, Contant CF: Enteral hyperalimentation in head injury. *J Neurosurg* 62:186, 1985.
57. Adams S, Dellinger EP, Wertz MJ, et al: Enteral versus parenteral nutrition support following laparotomy for trauma: A randomized prospective trial. *J Trauma* 26:882, 1986.
58. Barker SGE, Dodds RDA, Middlemiss A, et al: Small bowel function after aortic repair. *Postgrad Med J* 67:757, 1991.
59. Randall HT: Enteral nutrition: Tube feeding in acute and chronic illness. *J Parenter Enteral Nutr* 8:113, 1984.
60. Caves PK, Crockard HA: Pseudo-obstruction of the large bowel. *BMJ* 2:583, 1970.
61. Layman RV, Reddy P, Nivatvongs S: Acute pseudo-obstruction in the colon: A serious complication of urological surgery. *J Urol* 126:415, 1981.
62. Kukora JS, Dent T: Colonoscopic decompression of massive nonobstructive cecal dilatation. *Arch Surg* 112:512, 1977.
63. Nivatvongs S, Vermeulen FD, Fang DT: Colonoscopic decompression of acute pseudo-obstruction of the colon. *Ann Surg* 196:598, 1982.
64. Nakhgevany KB: Colonoscopic decompression of the colon in patients with Ogilvie's syndrome. *Am J Surg* 148:317, 1984.
65. Bode WE, Beart RW, Spencer RJ, et al: Colonoscopic decompression for acute pseudo-obstruction of the colon (Ogilvie's syndrome). *Am J Surg* 147:243, 1984.
66. Freilech HS, Chopra S, Gilliam JI: Acute colonic pseudo-obstruction or Ogilvie's syndrome. *J Clin Gastroenterol* 8:457, 1986.
67. Gosche JR, Sharpe JN, Larson GM: Colonoscopic decompression for pseudo-obstruction of the colon. *Am Surg* 55:111, 1989.
68. Stroder WE, Nostrant TT, Eckhauser FE, et al: Therapeutic and diagnostic colonoscopy in nonobstructive colonic dilatation. *Ann Surg* 197:416, 1983.
69. Bernton E, Myers R, Reyne T: Pseudo-obstruction of the colon: Case report including a new endoscopic treatment. *Gastrointest Endosc* 28:90, 1982.
70. Messmer JM, Wolper JC, Loewe CJ: Endoscopic assisted tube placement for decompression of acute colonic pseudo-obstruction. *Endoscopy* 16:135, 1984.
71. Groff W: Colonoscopic decompression and intubation of the cecum for Ogilvie's syndrome. *Dis Colon Rectum* 26:503, 1983.
72. Burke G, Shellito PC: Treatment of recurrent colonic pseudo-obstruction by endoscopic placement of a fenestrated overtube. *Dis Colon Rectum* 30:615, 1987.
73. Adams JT: Adynamic ileus of the colon: An indication for caecostomy. *Arch Surg* 109:503, 1974.
74. Dudley HAF, Patterson-Brown S. Pseudo-obstruction. *BMJ* 292:1157, 1986.
75. Kraft RO, Fry WJ, DeWeese MS: Post-vagotomy gastric atony. *Arch Surg* 88:865, 1964.
76. Tomomasa T, Kuroume T, Wakabayashi K, et al: Erythromycin induces migrating motor complex in human gastrointestinal tract. *Dig Dis Sci* 31:157, 1986. ♦
77. Itoh Z, Nakaya M, Suzuke T, et al: Erythromycin mimics exogenous motilin in gastrointestinal contractile activity in the dog. *Am J Physiol* 247:G688, 1984.
78. Tack J, Janssens J, Vantrappen G, et al: Effect of erythromycin on gastric motility in controls and in diabetic gastroparesis. *Gastroenterology* 103:72, 1992.

79. Mozwecz H, Paval D, Pitrak D, et al: Erythromycin stearate as prokinetic agent in postgastrectomy gastroparesis. *Dig Dis Sci* 35:902, 1990.

80. Bonacini M, Smith OJ, Pritchard T: Erythromycin as therapy for acute colonic pseudo-obstruction (Ogilvie's syndrome). *J Clin Gastroenterol* 13:475, 1991.

81. Rivière PJM, Pascaud X, Chevalier E, et al: Fedotozine reverses ileus induced by surgery or peritonitis: Action at peripheral κ-opioid receptors. *Gastroenterology* 104:724, 1993.

82. Catchpole BN: Ileus: Use of sympathetic blocking agents in its treatment. *Surgery* 66:811, 1969.

83. Vanek VW, Al-Salti M: Acute pseudo-obstruction of the colon (Ogil-

vie's syndrome): An analysis of 400 cases. *Dis Colon Rectum* 29:203, 1986.

84. MacColl C, MacCannell KL, Baylis B, et al: Treatment of acute colonic pseudoobstruction (Ogilvie's syndrome) with cisapride. *Gastroenterology* 98:773, 1990.

85. Camilleri M, Malagelada JR, Abell TL, et al: Effect of six weeks of treatment with cisapride in gastroparesis and intestinal pseudoobstruction. *Gastroenterology* 96:704, 1989.

86. Sloyer AF, Panella VS, Demas BE, et al: Ogilvie's syndrome: Successful management without colonoscopy. *Dig Dis Sci* 33:1391, 1988.

102. Fulminant Colitis and Toxic Megacolon

Ira M. Hanan and Stephen B. Hanauer

Ulcerative colitis is characterized by a diffuse, continuous inflammatory process that usually is limited to the superficial mucosa of the colon. Fulminant colitis implies progression of mucosal inflammation to involvement of deeper layers of the colon wall. It is generally associated with severe bloody diarrhea, fever, tachycardia, and abdominal tenderness. These toxic manifestations are due to the transmural nature of this advanced form of colitis. The transmural extension of inflammation may result in muscle paralysis, precipitating dilatation. Once dilatation is recognized, the term *toxic megacolon* applies.

Toxic megacolon refers to the acute dilatation of the colon, generally as a complication of ulcerative colitis, but it may occur with any severe inflammatory bowel disease. This condition has been described with both idiopathic and infectious colitis, including ulcerative colitis, Crohn's disease [1,2,3], amebic colitis [4], pseudomembranous colitis [5], and other infections [6].

Toxic megacolon has been reported to complicate from 1 to 13 percent of all ulcerative colitis cases [7,8]. Its frequency has been estimated to be 2 to 3 percent in patients with Crohn's colitis [7]. Although mortality has been as high as 25 percent, it may reach 50 percent if colonic perforation occurs before surgical intervention. More recently, early recognition and management of toxic megacolon have substantially lowered mortality to below 15 percent [7,9]. Factors associated with increased mortality include age over 40 years, the presence of colonic perforation, and the delay of surgery [7]. Colonic perforation, whether free or localized, is the greatest risk factor leading to death in these patients.

cerative colitis, with most cases developing within the first 5 years of disease, and 25 to 40 percent of cases present with the initial attack [8,12]. The onset of toxic megacolon has been linked to patients who have recently undergone diagnostic examinations (Table 102-1). Numerous cases have been reported in which a barium enema was performed within 72 hours of the onset of toxic megacolon, raising suspicion that manipulation of the inflamed bowel or vigorous laxative preparation may exacerbate electrolyte imbalance [8,10].

Certain drug therapies have been implicated in the development of toxic megacolon. Diphenoxylate hydrochloride–atropine sulfate (Lomotil) and loperamide, potent antidiarrheal compounds, and other inhibitors of colonic motility such as opiates and narcotics have been suspected as contributors to the development of toxic megacolon by inhibiting colon muscle function in severe, transmural disease.

Electrolyte and pH disturbances contribute to the development of toxic megacolon. Severe potassium depletion is known to inhibit colonic motility by producing smooth muscle atony. Hypokalemia (serum potassium <3.0) was a pronounced finding in more than half of the patients with toxic megacolon in one series [12]. In addition, severe hypokalemia has been associated with a higher mortality in patients in whom toxic megacolon developed [13]. Potassium requirements of patients with colitis may be massive, and restoration of serum potassium may not be adequate to replenish sufficient body stores to prevent toxic megacolon [12].

Early reports speculated that corticosteroid therapy may precipitate toxic megacolon [14,15]. Despite these earlier concerns,

Predisposing Factors

The severity of disease activity is the most important predictor of toxic megacolon, which is more common in extensive colitis than in disease limited to the left colon [10]. However, limited right- or left-sided segmental colitis [7,8] and even rectosigmoiditis, generally considered milder forms of colitis, have been associated with toxic megacolon [10,11].

Toxic megacolon typically occurs early in the course of ul-

Table 102-1. Potential Precipitants of Toxic Megacolon

Concurrent pathogens

Narcotics

Anticholinergics

Antidiarrheal agents (diphenoxylate with atropine, loperamide)

Barium enema

Colonoscopy

most experienced clinicians do not accept the implication that corticosteroids or adrenocorticotropic hormone (ACTH) are precipitating factors in the development of toxic megacolon [12,16,17]. Concern remains, however, that corticosteroids may suppress signs of perforation, thereby delaying surgical therapy.

Clinical Features

Toxic megacolon sometimes occurs during the first attack of ulcerative or Crohn's colitis; however, in most cases chronic ulcerative colitis will have been present for years (in some patients, for more than 30 years) before the onset of toxic megacolon [12,18]. The usual presentation develops with progressive symptoms of diarrhea, bloody stool, and crampy abdominal pain, although, paradoxically, in chronically (steroid) treated or bedridden patients, a decrease in stool frequency with passage of only bloody discharge or bloody membranes may be an ominous sign (Table 102-2). Thereafter, clinical signs of toxemia, including pyrexia (temperature >101.5°F), tachycardia, and leukocytosis (total white blood cell count >10.5), develop as abdominal pain and distention become progressive and bowel sounds diminish or cease completely. Signs of peritoneal irritation, including rebound tenderness and abdominal guarding, represent transmural inflammation to the serosa, despite the absence of free perforation. Conversely, peritoneal signs may be minimal or absent in an elderly patient or those receiving high-dose or prolonged corticosteroid therapy. In such a patient, loss of hepatic dullness may be the first clinical indication of colonic perforation. Mental status changes, including confusion, agitation, and apathy, are occasionally noted [12]. Leukocytosis with a left shift generally is present. The total leukocyte count may approach 40,000, especially if perforation has occurred. Anemia, hypokalemia, and hypoalbuminemia are common.

Radiographic studies should be limited to plain films of the abdomen and reveal loss of haustration with segmental or total colonic dilatation. The magnitude of dilatation may not be severe, averaging 8 to 9 cm (normal is <5–6 cm), although it may be as high as 15 cm before rupture. Maximal dilatation may

Table 102-2. Clinical Features of Toxic Megacolon

Symptoms and signs
  Increased diarrhea and bleeding
  Fever >101.5°F
  Abdominal distention
  Decreased or absent bowel sounds
  Peritoneal signs (potentially masked by corticosteroids)
  Hemodynamic instability
  Mental status changes
Radiographic findings
  Progressive segmental or pancolonic dilatation (may not correlate
    with physical findings)
Laboratory test findings
  White blood cell count >10,000, with pronounced left shift
  Anemia (may not be reflected in initial measurement if dehydrated)
  Hypernatremia (if dehydrated)
  Hypokalemia
  Metabolic alkalosis (diarrhea)/acidosis (sepsis)
  Hypomagnesemia
  Hypophosphatemia
  Hypoalbuminemia

occur in any part of the colon. Accompanying mucosal thumb-printing or pneumatosis cystoides coli reflects severe, transmural disease. Free peritoneal air should serve as an immediate indication for surgery [8,12]. Infrequently, retroperitoneal tracking of air from a colonic perforation may produce subcutaneous emphysema and pneumomediastinum without pneumoperitoneum [19]. In patients with severe colitis, small bowel ileus may signal toxic megacolon [20,21]. Discrepancies may exist between physical and radiographic findings. Abdominal distention by physical examination may be minimal despite massive colonic dilatation. Conversely, physical findings may dominate the presentation, and peritoneal signs in the absence of free air or dilatation should not be ignored.

A limited proctoscopic examination generally shows extensive ulceration with friable, bleeding mucosa. However, the rectum may be normal in rare instances, especially if Crohn's colitis is the underlying abnormality. An abdominal radiograph after minimal proctoscopic insufflation of air can provide a partial contrast study to define the proximal extent of disease. There is no correlation between proctoscopic findings of severe rectal disease and the clinical course and eventual outcome of toxic megacolon. More extensive endoscopic examinations are contraindicated, and the examining physician should be careful to avoid excessive air insufflation.

Management

Few gastrointestinal emergencies require as close cooperation between medical and surgical personnel as fulminant colitis and toxic megacolon. A team approach with early management by both groups is vital not only to determine whether surgery is indicated but to support critically ill patients preoperatively and postoperatively. Early recognition and institution of therapy by an experienced team can alter the outcome of this life-threatening illness (Table 102-3) [20].

MEDICAL TREATMENT. Despite the absence of bowel rest as a primary therapy for severe colitis, oral intake of fluids should be discontinued in fulminant colitis or once colonic dilatation is recognized [22]. A nasogastric tube is indicated for patients with associated small bowel ileus. Rolling the less toxic patient from front to back may redistribute colonic air and assist in decompression. Rarely, patients with dilatation in the absence of toxic signs or symptoms may benefit by rectal tube

Table 102-3. Management of Toxic Megacolon

1. Team approach toward management, including medical and surgical personnel
2. Resuscitation and stabilization—electrolyte and fluid repletion, central venous pressure measurements, blood transfusions to maintain hematocrit greater than 30%, nasogastric suctioning, broad-spectrum antibiotics, administration of intravenous corticosteroids (e.g., methylprednisolone 40 mg/day, hydrocortisone 400 mg/day)
3. Evaluate status—abdominal exam every 6 hours, radiographs of abdomen every 12 to 24 hours
4. Surgical intervention required for clinical deterioration at any time, failure of medical management to improve status within 48 hours, evidence of perforation, shock, persistent hemorrhage

decompression or gentle oral feeding. Anticholinergic and narcotic agents should be discontinued immediately. Resuscitative measures, including vigorous fluid, electrolyte, and blood replacement, are paramount. Extracellular fluid loss may be severe, and when combined with a low oncotic pressure secondary to the hypoalbuminemia that is frequent in these patients, the hemodynamic state is often unstable. The goal of fluid replacement should be to restore previous losses and to continue replenishing ongoing losses from diarrhea, fever, and third spacing of fluids. Transfusion of packed red blood cells should be instituted to maintain the serum hematocrit above 30 percent.

Although severe hyokalemia may not be present, total body potassium depletion is common, and resuscitative measures should include adequate potassium replacement. Phosphate, calcium, and magnesium depletion should be corrected.

Broad-spectrum antibiotics, with adequate gram-negative and anaerobic coverage, are considered standard therapy and should be administered without delay once transmural inflammation or toxic megacolon is suspected. Antibiotics should be continued until the patient stabilizes over several days to a week, or through the initial postoperative period. Whether antibiotics help avert progression of toxic megacolon is not known.

Corticosteroids have long been used in the management of ulcerative colitis as well as in Crohn's colitis. However, the efficacy of parenteral corticosteroids or ACTH to abort progression of dilatation in patients with toxic megacolon has been controversial. Generally, parenteral corticosteroids are essential to patients with toxic megacolon because they were most likely receiving the drugs before the toxic megacolon developed. Augmented doses of corticosteroids should be administered in view of the additional stress of the toxic state. There is no general agreement regarding which corticosteroid preparation or dose should be given [23]. Prednisone 25 mg intravenously every 6 hours, hydrocortisone sodium succinate 100 mg intravenously every 4 to 6 hours, and prednisolone sodium phosphate have been used successfully [9,17]. In the United States, hydrocortisone, 100 mg every 6 hours, and methylprednisolone, 6 to 15 mg every 6 hours, are available for intravenous administration. A continuous infusion of corticosteroids may be beneficial to maintain steady plasma levels. While ACTH has not been shown to be superior to corticosteroids [6], it may be preferred in patients not previously exposed to corticosteroids (100–150 units/day).

Most physicians include corticosteroids or ACTH in the treatment of severe colitis despite limited data regarding their efficacy in toxic megacolon. In the absence of randomized controlled trials, empirical evidence exists that supports the benefit of steroid therapy. Norland and Kirsner [12] noted that while many of their 36 patients eventually required surgical therapy, 25 (70%) had a dramatic and prompt response to medical management that included corticosteroids. This response included 6 patients in whom corticosteroids had not previously been used. Further experience supports the contention that corticosteroids may induce remission and thereby obviate the need for surgical intervention [8]. Conversely, patients managed without corticosteroids had a higher mortality than those managed with corticosteroids, regardless of the need for surgery. We favor the introduction of parenteral steroids for all patients with severe idiopathic inflammatory colitis with the expectation that potential medical benefit will outweigh rare surgical complications attributed solely to steroid therapy. A recent trial has demonstrated the benefit of intravenous cyclosporin A in severe ulcerative colitis for patients failing to improve after 7 to 10 days of intensive intravenous hydrocortisone therapy [22]. Whether or not any long-term benefit will be achieved awaits further follow-up [24].

Resuscitative measures for fulminant infectious colitis resulting in toxic megacolon should be initiated in the same manner as for idiopathic ulcerative colitis. Broad-spectrum antibiotic coverage should be followed by pathogen-specific therapy after the causative organism has been identified. Vancomycin or metronidazole hydrochloride should be used if *Clostridium difficile* is considered likely because of prior antibiotic exposure or the presence of pseudomembranes. The same criteria for surgical treatment should be employed.

SURGICAL INTERVENTION. When no improvement or deterioration occurs, despite 12 to 24 hours of intensive medical management, surgical intervention is required for toxic megacolon. Some physicians actually view surgical management of toxic megacolon as the conservative approach, noting that delay of operative therapy may promote higher mortality.

Evidence of colonic perforation is an unequivocal indication for emergent surgery. If physical signs of perforation are absent, 12- to 24-hour radiographic surveillance is necessary. Perforation is associated with severe complications, including peritonitis, extreme fluid and electrolyte imbalance, and hemodynamic instability. Early recognition of perforation should lessen morbidity and mortality. Other indications for emergent surgery precluding protracted medical management include signs of septic shock and imminent transverse colon rupture (diameter >12 cm). Soyer and Aldrete [25] noted that the presence of severe malnutrition or pregnancy in a patient with toxic megacolon should be factors that indicate emergent surgery.

While the medical management of fulminant colitis is similar to that of toxic megacolon, the absence of acute colonic dilatation may permit delay of surgical intervention. However, the timing of surgical intervention in these less urgent cases requires experienced clinical judgment. Early intervention to reduce mortality must be balanced against the potential for intensive medical management to control the inflammatory process and complications, thereby potentially preventing the psychosocial and medical stigmata of colectomy. Generally, in the absence of colonic dilatation, medical management may be continued for 5 to 7 days, in a further attempt to reverse transmural inflammation, as long as the patient is stable and improving. Should the additional days of medical therapy not dramatically improve the clinical course, fulminant colitis should be treated surgically.

The type of operation that should be performed for treatment of fulminant colitis or toxic megacolon depends on the clinical status of the patient and the experience of the surgeon [25]. A one-stage procedure that cures ulcerative colitis without the need for a second operation is appropriate for older patients or those not desiring restorative ileal pouch–anal anastomosis. Most surgeons prefer a limited abdominal colectomy with ileostomy, leaving the rectosigmoid as a mucous fistula or the rectum alone, using a Hartmann procedure [9,26]. This approach has the advantages of limiting the lengthy pelvic dissection in acutely ill patients while allowing for the option of a subsequent restorative, sphincter-saving procedure (ileoanal anastomosis) [27]. In patients with indeterminant colitis or Crohn's disease, preservation of the rectum may provide the opportunity for an eventual ileorectal or ileoanal anastomosis to preserve anal continence after temporary diversion and pathologic review of the colectomy specimen [27].

The surgical management of toxic megacolon must be individualized for each patient. The type of operation selected will depend on the clinical condition of the patient and the experience of the surgeon.

References

1. Greenstein AJ, Kark AE, Dreiling DA: Crohn's disease of the colon. III. Toxic dilatation of the colon in Crohn's colitis. *Am J Gastroenterol* 63:117, 1975.
2. Grieco MB, Bordan DL, Greiss AC, et al: Toxic megacolon complicating Crohn's colitis. *Ann Surg* 191:75, 1980.
3. Whorwell PJ, Isaacson P: Toxic dilatation of colon in Crohn's disease. *Lancet* 2:1334, 1981.
4. Stein D, Bank S, Louw JH: Fulminating amoebic colitis. *Surgery* 85:349, 1979.
5. Brown CH, Ferrante WA, Davis WD: Toxic dilatation of the colon complicating pseudomembranous enterocolitis. *Am J Dig Dis* 13:813, 1968.
6. Schofield PF, Mandal BK, Ironside AG: Toxic dilatation of the colon in salmonella colitis and inflammatory bowel disease. *Br J Surg* 66:5, 1979.
7. Greenstein AJ, Sachar DB, Gribas A, et al: Outcome of toxic dilatation in ulcerative and Crohn's colitis. *J Clin Gastroenterol* 7:137, 1985.
8. Jalan KN, Sirues W, Card WI, et al: An experience of ulcerative colitis. I. Toxic dilatation in 55 cases. *Gastroenterology* 57:68, 1969.
9. Mungas JE, Mooja AR, Block GE: Treatment of toxic megacolon. *Surg Clin North Am* 56:95, 1976.
10. Farmer RG, Easley KA, Rankin GB: Clinical patterns, natural history, and progression of ulcerative colitis: A long-term follow-up of 1116 patients. *Dig Dis Sci* 38:1137, 1993.
11. Kisloff B, Adkins JC: Toxic megacolon developing in a patient with longstanding distal ulcerative colitis. *Am J Gastroenterol* 75:451, 1981.
12. Norland CC, Kirsner JB: Toxic dilatation of colon (toxic megacolon): Etiology, treatment and prognosis in 42 patients. *Medicine* 48:229, 1969.
13. Caprilli R, Vernia P, Colaneir O, et al: Risk factors in toxic megacolon. *Dig Dis Sci* 25:817, 1980.
14. Marshak RH, Lester LJ, Friedman AI: Megacolon, a complication of ulcerative colitis. *Gastroenterology* 16:768, 1950.
15. Binder HJ: Steroids and toxic megacolon. *Gastroenterology* 76:888, 1979.
16. Meyers S, Janowitz HD: The place of steroids in the therapy of toxic megacolon. *Gastroenterology* 75:729, 1978.
17. Truelove SC, Marks CG: Toxic megacolon. I: Pathogenesis, diagnosis and treatment. *J Clin Gastroenterol* 10:107, 1981.
18. Binder SC, Miller HH, Deterling RA: Emergent and urgent operations for ulcerative colitis. *Arch Surg* 110:284, 1975.
19. Mogan GR, Sachar DB, Bauer J, et al: Toxic megacolon in ulcerative colitis complicated by pneumomediastinum: Report of two cases. *Gastroenterology* 79:559, 1980.
20. Caprilli R, Vernia P, Latella G, et al: Early recognition of toxic megacolon. *J Clin Gastroenterol* 9:160, 1987.
21. Chew CN, Noland DJ, Jewell DP: Small bowel gas in severe ulcerative colitis. *Gut* 32:1535, 1991.
22. McIntyre PB, Powell-Tuck J, Wood SR, et al: Controlled trial of bowel rest in the treatment of severe acute colitis. *Gut* 27:481, 1986.
23. Rosenberg WMC, Ireland A, Jewell DP: High-dose methylprednisolone in the treatment of active ulcerative colitis. *J Clin Gastroenterol* 12:40, 1990.
24. Lichtiger S, Present DH, Kornbluth A, Hanauer S: Cyclosporin A in the treatment of severe, refractory ulcerative colitis: A double-blinded placebo controlled trial. *Gastroenterology* 104(4) (Suppl):A732, 1993 (Abstract).
25. Soyer MT, Aldrete JS: Surgical treatment of toxic megacolon and proposal for a program of therapy. *Am J Surg* 140:421, 1980.
26. Ritchie JK, Ritchie SM, McIntyre PB, et al: Management of severe acute colitis in district hospitals. *J R Soc Med* 77:465, 1984.
27. Mowschenson PM: New surgical approaches. *Semin Colon Rect Surg* 4:25, 1993.

103. Evaluation and Management of Liver Failure

Heather M. White

Liver abnormalities are seen very commonly in clinical practice. Fortunately, overt liver failure is uncommon because of the tremendous reserve capacity of the liver and its resiliency to changes in hepatic blood flow and nutrient deprivation. Two major subgroups of liver failure include fulminant hepatic failure and chronic end-stage liver disease. In either of these situations, patients may present to the intensive care unit for evaluation and management. This chapter focuses on the complications of hepatic failure that are encountered in the intensive care unit (ICU).

Fulminant Hepatic Failure

Fulminant hepatic failure (FHF) occurs when a patient without prior evidence of liver disease develops evidence of encephalopathy and severe synthetic dysfunction. The time period for the development of abnormalities that define FHF has varied over the years. Clinicians initially required 8 weeks [1,2], but more recent definitions require a diagnosis of encephalopathy within 2 weeks of the onset of jaundice [3]. Both prolongation of the prothrombin time and mental status changes in the setting of acute hepatic dysfunction are needed for the diagnosis.

A number of causes may be responsible for FHF, the most common being viral hepatitis and drugs or toxins (Table 103-1). Identification of the etiology is important. First, certain causes (e.g., acetaminophen) have specific treatments. If a toxin or drug is identified, local poison control authorities can help determine if the administration of an antidote will be helpful. Second, the etiology may have important public health implications. If a patient is determined to have acute viral hepatitis, public health departments must be notified and contacts of the patient should be made aware of appropriate postexposure prophylaxis if available. Third, the prognosis may have a variable outcome dependent on the etiology. Despite having ex-

Table 103-1. Etiologies of Fulminant Hepatic Failure

Viral Hepatitis
  Hepatitis A
  Hepatitis B
  Hepatitis C
  Hepatitis D
  Hepatitis E
  Hepatitis non-A, non-B
Common drugs/toxins
  Acetaminophen
  Alcohol
  Cotrimazole
  Gold
  Halothane
  Isoniazid
  Ketoconazole
  Nonsteroidal antiinflamatory drugs
  Phenytoin
  Sodium valproate
  Sulfonamides
Vascular
  Portal vein thrombosis
  Hepatic vein thrombosis (Budd-Chiari)
  Veno-occlusive disease
  Ischemic hepatitis
Other
  Wilson's disease
  Reye's syndrome
  Acute fatty liver of pregnancy

Adapted from references 3, 4, and 5.

cellent medical management, patients with FHF generally do poorly without liver transplantation, the average survival rate being less than 20 percent [6,7,8]. Low survival rates are particularly common when FHF is due to idiosyncratic drug reactions, acute Wilson's disease, halothane hepatitis, and non-A, non-B hepatitis [6,9,10,11]. Higher survival rates have been quoted for fulminant failure secondary to hepatitis A, hepatitis B, and acetaminophen [9].

For patients with acute liver failure, liver transplantation has emerged as an important treatment modality, with reported survival rates greater than 50 percent in most series [5,6,7,12–18]. Diminished posttransplant survival in FHF patients is attributed to early postoperative deaths from sepsis and neurologic complications [19]. A number of studies have been performed to identify prognostic criteria for patients being evaluated and managed for fulminant hepatic failure. The single most important predictor of outcome is the degree of encephalopathy [20]. Predictors of adverse outcome have best been addressed by

Table 103-2. Prognostic Indicators in Fulminant Hepatic Failure

Variable	Prognostic Indicator
Acetaminophen-related FHF	
Arterial pH	<7.3
Prothrombin time	>100 seconds
Serum creatinine	>3.4 mg/dl
Non-acetaminophen-related FHF	
Disease etiology	Non-A, non-B hepatitis *or* drug/toxin
Age	<10 or >40 years
Duration of jaundice	>1 week prior to encephalopathy
Serum bilirubin concentration	>18 mg/dl
Prothrombin time	>50 seconds

Modified from reference 21.

the King's College Group [21] (Table 103-2). These factors should be considered early, and, if appropriate, patients should be referred to a facility capable of performing transplantation.

Because of the devastating consequences of FHF, attempts have been made to develop other supportive therapies. Prostaglandin E1 has been used with some success in an uncontrolled study but has not been evaluated in controlled studies [22]. Two modalities presently under investigation are hepatocyte transplantation and filtration devices [19].

Specific Complications of Fulminant Hepatic Failure

ENCEPHALOPATHY AND CEREBRAL EDEMA. Hepatic encephalopathy and cerebral edema are two distinct but related conditions that affect patients with FHF. By definition, all patients with FHF have encephalopathy, but not all patients will have cerebral edema. Hepatic encephalopathy is graded on a scale of 0 to 4, but may fluctuate during the course of disease [4] (Table 103-3). Cerebral edema is an increase in the content of brain tissue water and appears to be the initial event that results in increased intracranial pressure (ICP). There are two primary theories regarding the mechanisms of brain edema. The first theory suggests that cerebral edema is "vasogenic," with a breakdown in the blood-brain barrier. The second theory states that the edema is "cellular," due to impaired cellular osmoregulation [24,25]. While there is some evidence to support each of these theories, the exact mechanisms of hepatic encephalopathy and cerebral edema are not well understood and are beyond the scope of this text.

Patients with cerebral edema and encephalopathy are best managed with close observation, frequent monitoring, and rapid institution of appropriate therapy. Transfer of the patient to a center capable of performing liver transplantation should

Table 103-3. Hepatic Encephalopathy Grading System

Grade	Level of Consciousness	Neurologic Abnormalities	EEG Abnormalities
0	Normal	None	None
1	Personality changes; day-night reversal; short attention span	Tremor; asterixis	Symmetric slowing; triphasic waves
2	Lethargic; loss of orientation; inappropriate behavior	Asterixis; abnormal reflexes	Symmetric slowing; triphasic waves
3	Drowsy but arousable; confused when awake	Asterixis; abnormal reflexes	Triphasic waves
4	Comatose; no meaningful intellectual function	Babinski response; decerebrate posturing; pupillary responses preserved	Delta waves

Modified from reference 23.

be strongly considered. Optimally, transfer should occur before the patient develops hemodynamic or neurologic instability. Hepatic encephalopathy is managed importantly by the identification and correction of precipitants. In FHF, the primary precipitant is loss of functional liver tissue. Because no extracorporeal hepatic systems are clinically available, patients are managed with supportive care until transplantation can be performed. Some patients will benefit from the institution of standard therapies for chronic portosystemic encephalopathy, including neomycin and lactulose (see Complications of Chronic Liver Disease, following). However, 50 to 85 percent of patients with FHF develop cerebral edema despite this therapy [26–30], and death due to cerebral herniation occurs in 30 to 50 percent of untransplanted patients [9,26–30].

Neurologic checks for mental status should be evaluated frequently, sometimes hourly, with attention to increased muscle tone, hyperreflexia, and abnormal pupillary relexes [28]. Unfortunately, typical clinical manifestations of increased intracranial pressure are noticeably absent in FHF; these include papilledema, bradycardia, vomiting, and headache [28,29,31,32]. Many of these patients are either comatose or intubated for airway protection, which may make a standard neurologic examination unreliable. An uncooperative patient or a patient who has received sedatives or neuromuscular blocking agents while mechanically ventilated cannot receive an accurate neurologic assessment.

Computed tomography of the brain in FHF has been found to be neither sensitive nor specific for diagnosing increased ICP [33,34]. Cerebral edema may occur prior to the development of increased ICP [35]. However, an initial computed tomography scan should be considered in patients with abnormal mental status to evaluate for structural lesions that would alter clinical management [19]. Obviously, patients with structural lesions or intracranial hemorrhage would not be candidates for liver transplantation. This is particularly important in FHF since either cerebral herniation from edema or intracranial bleeding from coagulopathy may occur. Thus, while the information obtained from an initial computed tomography scan of the head is beneficial, serial scanning in FHF is neither practical nor useful to assess for cerebral edema or increased ICP.

In FHF the most sensitive method for detecting increased ICP is ICP monitoring [29,33,35,36]. Patients with grade 1 or grade 2 encephalopathy do not require placement of an ICP monitor but should be electively transferred to a facility where monitors can be placed and transplantation can be performed [28]. ICP monitoring is recommended for patients who present with grade 3 encephalopathy [30] or for any patient with grade 4 encephalopathy [37]. Rapid changes in neurologic function as well as increases in ICP have been observed over periods as brief as 5 minutes [19,28].

ICP monitoring should be performed by individuals familiar with the technique. The monitors are most frequently placed by neurosurgical colleagues. Coagulopathy is normalized as much as possible to minimize the risk of epidural or intracranial bleeding during the procedure. Volume challenge associated with the administration of blood products to correct coagulopathy, infection, and intracranial or epidural bleeding are the major risks of ICP monitor placement. The incidence of intracranial hemorrhage varies from center to center and with the type of transducer, but ranges from 5 to 15 percent [34,38]. Epidural transducers are most frequently associated with inaccurate readings but have the lowest rate of complications. Intraventricular transducers have the highest rate of complications but are the most accurate. Subarachnoid transducers have intermediate levels of both complications and fidelity [19]. Generally, attempts are made to maintain ICP below 15 mm Hg with a cerebral perfusion pressure greater than 50 mm Hg (the

difference between the mean arterial pressure and the ICP) [28]. In the acute setting, hyperventilation to maintain an arterial PCO_2 of 25 to 30 mm Hg may decrease ICP [19]. Patients should be maintained in a quiet, nonstimulated environment with minimal physical movement. A 30-degree elevation of the head is optimal. If this is not possible, positioning of the bed to prevent the head-down position is essential [28].

A variety of pharmacologic agents have been tried in the management of intracranial hypertension. Mannitol, at 0.5 to 1.0 gm per kilogram intravenously, has been used with a success rate of around 60 percent; however, the use of mannitol requires intact renal function [29]. Thiopental, at 30 to 40 mg per kilogram intravenously as a loading dose, then 5 mg per kilogram intravenously as needed, is similarly effective but may result in hypotension requiring vasopressors. Barbiturates may alter objective neurologic findings [39]. Studies evaluating corticosteroids have shown no benefits for the management of increased ICP [29].

Intraoperative intracranial hypertension is common and may occur throughout the period of liver transplant [33,40]. In patients with elevated ICP, it is essential to attempt to determine those who will recover neurologic function. ICP monitoring may help to determine whether comatose patients have a potential for neurologic recovery or if irreversible neurologic injury has occurred. Refractory and sustained intracranial hypertension, as determined by a cerebral perfusion pressure below 40 mm Hg, has been associated with a high frequency of postoperative neurologic deaths [15]. Therefore, some transplant centers use this level as a contraindication to liver tranplantation, a criterion that appears to prevent postoperative neurologic deaths [33,41].

CARDIORESPIRATORY COMPLICATIONS. Patients with FHF may have impaired cardiopulmonary status. Hemodynamics in FHF mimic septic shock: high cardiac output and low systemic vascular resistance [4]. Patients will have relative intravascular hypovolemia resulting from this vasodilation. Treatment of hypovolemia should be preferentially with blood products that stay in the intravascular space but also may involve colloid (albumin, plasma, or dextran) or crystalloid [4]. Persistent need for inotropic agents such as dobutamine or dopamine is associated with a poor outcome [4]. Although arrhythmias may be seen, they are related typically to metabolic (e.g., hypokalemia, acidosis, hypoxia) or mechanical events (e.g., cardiac irritation from a Swan-Ganz catheter). Paroxysmal hypertension may herald bouts of increased ICP.

Patients with FHF frequently have respiratory abnormalities or complications. Approximately 40 percent of patients with FHF have pulmonary edema, cardiogenic or noncardiogenic [42]. Arterial hypoxemia may occur from a variety of factors, including bacterial infection, intrapulmonary hemorrhage, atelectasis, intrapulmonary vascular shunting (from liver disease), and noncardiogenic pulmonary edema. Hypoxemia can exacerbate cerebral edema as well as precipitate multiorgan failure. Hypoxemia is managed with supplemental oxygen or by intubation, if needed. Positive-pressure ventilation may be helpful in some patients but also can increase ICP by decreasing vascular return. Hyperventilation and resultant hypocapnea are typical of patients with FHF. This results from rising ICP and metabolic acidosis. Unfortunately, as hyperventilation persists, patients may either become fatigued or the hypocapnea may actually decrease central respiratory drive. Both may lead to respiratory depression or failure.

Besides being used for management of hypoxemia, intubation is done for airway protection to prevent aspiration or to assist in the management of cerebral edema [28]. The administration of lidocaine at 1 mg per kilogram intravenously prior to intubation will diminish or eliminate the rise in ICP associated with intubation [28]. Ultimately, inability to maintain cardiopulmonary status generally contributes to multiorgan failure. This accounts for about 20 percent of FHF patients who become ineligible for liver transplantation [42]. Swan-Ganz catheter placement may be necessary for optimization of hemodynamics and is essential in any patient with coexistent renal failure [19].

COAGULOPATHY. Hemostatic disturbances result from defects in any of the following components: vascular endothelium; platelet aggregation, activation, or number; formation of the fibrin clot; or synthesis, consumption, or containment of coagulation factors [43]. Typically, patients with FHF have reduced synthesis of coagulation factors as the primary reason for disordered coagulation. Except for factor VIII, all clotting factors are synthesized exclusively in the liver. Although the half-lives are variable, certain factors are very sensitive to hepatic injury. Factor V has the shortest half-life [4]. Prothrombin time is prolonged in liver disease and also in vitamin K deficiency, because vitamin K–dependent carboxylase is required for production of factors II, VII, IX, and X, as well as protein C and protein S [44]. To differentiate hepatic failure from vitamin K deficiency, patients should be given parenteral vitamin K, 10 mg subcutaneously for 3 days. A picture consistent with disseminated intravascular coagulation (DIC) also can be seen, resulting from decreased levels of antithrombin III and other clotting factor inhibitors. Although overt DIC is unusual, tests for fibrin degradation products (FDPs) often will be positive [45]. Both qualitative and quantitative defects in platelet function have been described [4,44].

Gross hemorrhage is uncommon and usually occurs in the setting of combined platelet and clotting factor deficiency. Gastrointestinal hemorrhage is the most common site wherein bleeding usually results from superficial mucosal lesions. Prophylactic use of H-2 receptor antagonists is recommended to keep the gastric pH above 4 [4,19]. Other bleeding sites include skin puncture wounds, kidneys, retroperitoneum, lungs, nasopharynx, and endometrium. Packed red cell replacement is recommended for clinically significant bleeding. Clotting factors in the form of fresh-frozen plasma may be needed for active bleeding. Studies have demonstrated that neither morbidity nor mortality was affected by the prophylactic administration of fresh-frozen plasma in the absence of overt bleeding [46]. Platelet transfusions should be reserved for patients with active bleeding, and levels should be maintained at above 50,000 per cubic millimeter for any invasive procedures such as Swan-Ganz catheter placement [4].

METABOLIC DISORDERS. A variety of metabolic disorders occur in patients who have FHF, the most important being lactic acidosis. Acidosis occurs for a number of reasons, including excess lactate production from tissue hypoxia (this occurs primarily with hypotension or multiorgan failure), impaired hepatic uptake of lactate, or impaired metabolism of lactate by the liver. Lactic acidosis may be difficult to correct and requires intravenous bicarbonate or dialysis for control [19]. Associated renal dysfunction (see following) may contribute to the acidosis while producing a host of other metabolic abnormalities (e.g., hypocalcemia, hyperphosphatemia, and hypermagnesemia).

Hypoglycemia is the other major metabolic derangement in severe FHF. The liver is essential to normal glucose metabolism as it is the primary site for gluconeogenesis as well as glycogen storage. Blood glucose is generally preserved until massive hepatic parenchymal damage has occurred. Maintenance of nor-

mal serum glucose is essential to preservation of neurologic and cellular function. Serum glucose should be checked frequently, and dextrose solutions with concentrations ranging from 5 to 50 percent may be required to maintain normal levels [19].

RENAL FAILURE. Renal failure is an ominous complication of FHF. Impairment of renal function is usually multifactorial, with the most common causes being intravascular volume depletion, acute tubular necrosis, and hepatorenal syndrome. Oliguric renal failure has been variously defined, but the definition most commonly used in FHF is a urine output of less than 300 ml per 24 hours [4]. Renal failure occurs in up to 75 percent of patients with acetaminophen toxicity and has been used as a marker for poor prognosis [4,9,19,21]. The renal failure associated with acetaminophen is partially a consequence of direct toxicity to the kidney and is frequently present prior to the development of advanced encephalopathy; however, cases with isolated renal failure and little encephalopathy have been reported [4]. Although renal failure is less common with other types of FHF, it occurs in about 30 percent [9,21]. Diagnosis includes assessment of urine output (<300 ml/24 hr), volume status (may require a Swan-Ganz catheter), and determination of urine sodium and creatinine (to distinguish acute tubular necrosis from either prerenal azotemia or hepatorenal syndrome). Patients are initially managed by the institution of dopamine infusions at 2 to 4 µg/kg/hr, which increases renal blood flow and thus hopefully reverses or delays progressive failure [4]. Placement of a Swan-Ganz catheter is often required for fluid management because of total body volume overload in the setting of hypotension and oliguria [19]. Great care should be taken in the use of nephrotoxic agents, especially antibiotics, and patients with renal impairment may not tolerate mannitol [4]. Some patients will require dialysis for management; the technique of continuous hemodiafiltration has some advantages [4,19].

SEPSIS. A number of factors play a role in the increased risk of infection, including impaired neutrophil cell function, altered Kupffer cell function, and a deficiency of opsonins. Sepsis in FHF jeopardizes the suitability of the patient for transplantation and can contribute to metabolic derangements, cardiopulmonary complications, and renal failure. The recognition of sepsis is challenging because the hemodynamics and hematologic picture of all patients with FHF mimic septic shock [19]. Urinary and respiratory sources are responsible for the vast majority of bacterial infections. While the prevalence of bacterial infection may be as high as 80 percent [47], bacteremia is much less common, occurring in 20 to 25 percent of patients [47,48]. The most common organisms include *Staphylococcus* sp., *Streptococcus* sp., gram-negative organisms, and fungi, especially *Candida* sp. Patients should have surveillance cultures of blood, sputum, and urine with a very low clinical threshold for the institution of antibiotics. Given the spectrum of infection and likely coexistent renal dysfunction, the best antibiotic selections include vancomycin in combination with a third-generation cephalosporin [19]. Aminoglycosides should be avoided if at all possible. The use of prophylactic antibiotics in FHF remains an unresolved issue.

Chronic Liver Disease

Chronic liver disease may be complicated by a variety of conditions that result in an admission to the intensive care unit or may complicate an admission for other types of medical illness. The identification and management of the most common of these complications are delineated below.

Consideration of liver transplantation may be appropriate in selected patients with chronic liver disease. Although criteria for inclusion and exclusion vary from center to center, the ICU physician should be cognizant of features in patients with chronic liver disease that may warrant a referral to a transplantation center. Patients who experience an episode of spontaneous bacterial peritonitis, medically intractable ascites, encephalopathy, or variceal bleeding should undergo at least the initial stages of consideration for transplantation. Liver transplantation has evolved as an effective treatment for chronic liver disease and affords an 85 percent 1-year survival in better transplant programs [49].

Specific Complications of Chronic Liver Disease

ENCEPHALOPATHY. Chronic portosystemic encephalopathy is a condition that may wax and wane in severity through the course of a patient's life. The grading system and manifestations are described in Table 103-3. Interestingly, patients with chronic portosystemic encephalopathy do not generally experience either the cerebral edema or increased ICP encountered in FHF. It also has been demonstrated that brain histology differs between the acute and chronic conditions [23]. No single test is reliable for establishing the diagnosis of chronic portosystemic encephalopathy. Although frequently considered a marker indicating a hepatic etiology for depressed mental status, serum ammonia may be normal in individuals with hepatic encephalopathy and abnormal in those without clinical manifestations. Several studies demonstrate poor correlation between ammonia levels and clinical disease [50,51,52]. In chronic liver disease, encephalopathy is usually precipitated by an event or condition. These commonly include increased nitrogen load (gastrointestinal bleeding, excess dietary protein, azotemia, constipation), electrolyte imbalance (hypokalemia, alkalosis, hypoxia, hypovolemia), drugs (narcotics, tranquilizers, sedatives, diuretics), infection, surgery, superimposed acute liver disease, and progressive liver disease.

Clinicians must be vigilant for the causes of encephalopathy so that appropriate diagnostic tests are performed and specific treatments that correct the precipitant may be instituted. The first step is to identify any metabolic abnormalities (e.g., hypo- or hyperglycemia, electrolyte imbalance, hypophosphatemia, hypoxemia). Of particular concern is chronic hyponatremia, which frequently accompanies liver disease; too rapid a correction may result in central pontine myelinolysis and an abnormal mental status [53]. Accurate assessment of volume status is important, because some patients with encephalopathy are simply dehydrated. Patients may appear volume overloaded, yet intravascular volume is usually depleted, most commonly by diuretic therapy. In addition to metabolic abnormalities, a search for sources of infection must be made. Fever is an atypical feature of hepatic encephalopathy, and its presence increases the likelihood of sepsis. Particular attention should be given to obtaining cultures of blood, urine, sputum, and ascites. The issue of pursuing a lumbar puncture must be individualized; coagulopathy may increase the risk of this procedure. Either constipation or gastrointestinal bleeding may produce encephalopathy, and their presence should be determined. Certain medications or toxins including alcohol, antihistamines, anti-

emetics, sedatives, hypnotics, anxiolytics, and narcotics may precipitate encephalopathy. A toxicology screen may be helpful.

Therapies aimed directly at reversing encephalopathy include dietary adjustments, medications, and, for intractable disease, transplantation. Patients presenting to the ICU likely will have significantly depressed mental status and initially will not be fed. For prolonged ICU stays, preservation of nitrogen balance requires some form of nutritional support. The most commonly prescribed diets for patients who remain encephalopathic on modest protein reductions [40–60 g/day] utilize commercial products rich in branched-chain amino acids. These diets have shown some promise in correcting encephalopathy [54–57]. Other dietary supplements, such as multivitamins and zinc [58], also have been used. The major medications employed for hepatic encephalopathy are a group of agents that work by decreasing nitrogen delivery to the liver. Lactulose is an artificial, nonabsorbable disaccharide that is metabolized to small organic acids in the colon. The metabolized and nonmetabolized lactulose creates both an osmotic diarrhea and an acidic environment in the colon [23]. The dose required varies from patient to patient and should be titrated to achieve at least 3 stools per day. In the ICU setting, patients are typically given 30 ml orally every 4 to 6 hours until bowel movements are initiated, and then the dose is titrated to 3 stools per day. To prevent aspiration of the lactulose in comatose patients, it may be given as an enema, 300 ml lactulose plus 700 ml of water or saline every 4 to 6 hours. Lactilol, a compound used in Europe, is similar to lactulose but is dispensed as a powder. Lactilol is as effective as lactulose [59] but is less sweet than lactulose and may be better tolerated. Antibiotics also have been used to destroy colonic bacteria that produce ammonia. The most popular antibiotic currently used in practice is neomycin, a minimally absorbed aminoglycoside, given orally in doses of 500 to 1000 mg every 6 to 12 hours. Potential toxicities center around ototoxicity, nephrotoxicity, and secondary colonic infections [60]. Although metronidazole has been used as an effective agent in bowel decontamination, the irreversible neurotoxicity associated with long-term use limits its clinical utility. For patients with recurrent, uncontrolled encephalopathy, hepatic transplantation is the treatment of choice [61].

HEPATORENAL SYNDROME. Renal abnormalities in chronic liver disease are common. The following have been described in chronic liver disease patients: increased renal sodium retention; impaired renal water excretion, concentrating ability, and renal acidification; and altered potassium metabolism. Clinically, these may manifest as acute renal failure, glomerulonephropathies, chronic renal insufficiency, or hepatorenal syndrome. For the purposes of this discussion, comments will be limited to hepatorenal syndrome. This disorder is a progressive oliguric renal failure occurring in patients with advanced hepatic disease, most often cirrhosis. It has occasionally been described in acute hepatitis [62] and hepatic malignancy [63]. Renal failure occurs in the absence of anatomic, laboratory, or clinical evidence of other recognized causes. The renal failure may develop over hours to days. Generally, the phenomenon has been observed in patients with preexisting ascites and portal hypertension. Interestingly, hepatorenal syndrome almost always develops while patients are in the hospital [64]. Diagnosis is made by determination of urine sodium, creatinine, and osmolarity, with a calculation of urine creatinine to plasma creatinine ratio, and evaluation of urinary sediment [63] (Table 103-4). However, prerenal azotemia and hepatorenal syndrome cannot be distinguished on the basis of these tests, and accurate diagnosis usually requires an assessment of intravascular vol-

Table 103-4. Findings in Oliguric Renal Failure

	Hepatorenal Syndrome	Prerenal Azotemia	Acute Renal Failure
Urine osmolality	Urine >100 mOsm than plasma osmolality	Urine >100 mOsm than plasma osmolality	Equal to plasma
Urine sodium concentration	<10 mEq/liter	<10 mEq/liter	>30 mEq/liter
Urine-to-plasma-creatinine ratio	>30:1	>30:1	<20:1
Urine sediment	Usually normal	Normal	Casts

Modified from reference 63.

ume (e.g., with a Swan-Ganz catheter). Patients with hepatorenal syndrome may be managed acutely by dialysis or hemofiltration, but ultimately require liver transplantation for long-term survival [63]. Renal abnormalities of hepatorenal syndrome are corrected by liver transplantation, and most patients require little if any dialysis after transplant unless underlying renal disease antedated the onset of hepatorenal syndrome. Other modalities attempted for hepatorenal syndrome include portacaval shunting [65], peritoneovenous shunts [66,67,68], and more recently transjugular intrahepatic portosystemic shunts (TIPS) [69]. Experience with all of these modalities is limited.

ASCITES AND SPONTANEOUS BACTERIAL PERITONITIS.
Ascites is the accumulation of fluid in the peritoneal space. Ascites may occur in a number of settings, including cardiac failure, renal failure, intraabdominal malignancy, intraabdominal infections, pancreatitis, and liver disease [70]. Liver disease is the most common cause. The pathogenesis involves alterations in hepatic outflow that result in intrahepatic portal hypertension. These events lead to primary renal sodium retention, diminished effective circulating volume with secondary renal sodium retention, and increased production of hepatic lymph [71]. Spontaneous bacterial peritonitis (SBP) occurs when the ascitic fluid becomes "spontaneously" infected with bacterial organisms, and is diagnosed when the polymorphonuclear (PMN) leukocyte count is greater than 250 PMNs/per cubic millimeter and/or organisms are cultured [72]. The most recent data suggest SBP occurs when spontaneous bacteremia seeds susceptible ascites [73]. Susceptible ascites results from immune defects in patients with liver disease, including complement deficiencies, defects in neutrophil function, and deficiencies in reticuloendothelial system function [74–77]. Another important feature of susceptible ascites is the demonstration of low protein ascites (<1 gm/dl), with depressed opsonic activity [78–82]. SBP is very common. Studies show that between 10 and 27 percent of patients with ascites have SBP on admission [82,83,84].

Clinical examination may reveal a distended abdomen (with or without an umbilical or ventral hernia), a fluid wave, shifting dullness, or normal findings. Patients admitted to the ICU may appear to "blossom" ascites overnight, as they are repleted with sodium-laden crystalloid or blood products. Other patients may exhibit respiratory compromise from intraabdominal pressure or have sympathetic pleural effusions (ascites equivalents), especially on the right side. Unfortunately, clinical examination for small amounts of ascites has poor results, and patients may require ultrasound for localization. The clinical presentation of SBP may be very subtle, with vague mental status changes, a feeling of discomfort in the abdomen, or frank abdominal pain [70]. One third of patients will have no specific abdominal symptoms [70].

The management of ascites in the ICU should focus on determining the etiology of ascitic fluid (if unknown), excluding SBP, and controlling volume. The two most serious complications of ascites are SBP and umbilical hernia rupture; less serious complications include respiratory compromise as a result of compression of the diaphragm or pleural effusions, anorexia, development of umbilical and ventral hernias, and abdominal discomfort from distention. Patients are rarely admitted to the ICU with ascites as the primary indication. More often, ascites develops during the course of the ICU admission. The most important aspect of management is restriction of sodium intake. If the patient is able to eat, dietary sodium should be restricted to 500 mg per day; more liberal diets may be acceptable if ascites is minimal. The largest sodium intake comes from the administration of intravenous fluid, crystalloid solutions, and medications. Restriction of free water intake is not usually necessary, unless patients develop hyponatremia (<125 mEq/L). If so, free water should be restricted to 1 to 1.5 liters per day.

The two groups of drugs most commonly used to manage sodium fluid overload in cirrhotic patients are the distal tubular diuretics (spironolactone, amiloride, triamterene) and the loop of Henle diuretics (furosemide, bumetanide). Spironolactone is particularly effective in cirrhotic patients because it inhibits sodium reabsorption in the distal tubules and collecting ducts by blocking the effects of aldosterone. Major side effects include hyperchloremic acidosis and hyperkalemia. In the ICU setting, loop diuretics are more commonly used. These drugs inhibit sodium transport in the ascending limb of the loop of Henle. Major side effects include hypokalemia, metabolic alkalosis, and hypovolemia. Loop of Henle diuretics tend to produce a greater natriuresis diuresis than do the distal tubule diuretics. Optimal weight loss through diuretics to prevent intravascular volume depletion is 0.3 to 0.5 kg per day [85]. In the presence of peripheral edema, intravascular volume appears to be conserved, so diuresis of more than 1 kg per day is possible without impairment of renal function [85,86]. However, it is important to remember that ascitic fluid is resorbed at only a rate of 300 to 500 ml per day [87]. In the ICU, large-volume paracentesis (5 L) is usually only necessary as a therapeutic measure if there is respiratory compromise. Large-volume paracentesis is well tolerated generally by cirrhotic patients, especially if peripheral edema is present [86,87,88]. The use of albumin infusions with large-volume paracentesis goes in and out of fashion. Major disadvantages of albumin infusions are sodium load and cost, as well as limited "staying power" in the intravascular space. However, albumin may have a role in selected patients with very low serum albumin and intravascular volume depletion.

Refractory ascites occurs when patients who are adhering to a sodium- and fluid-restricted diet can no longer tolerate diuretic therapy due to intravascular volume depletion or electrolyte imbalance, or when patients no longer respond even to maximal doses of diuretics. Patients with truly refractory ascites are rare, but they may require consideration of a peritoneovenous shunt, transjugular intrahepatic portosystemic shunt, or transplantation. Peritoneovenous shunts were very popular prior to the advent of transplantation and are still used in patients who are either not yet ready for transplantation or are ineligible. The principle is to return ascitic fluids and proteins back into the systemic circulation. Peritoneovenous shunts have no effect on survival, and potential complications have dampened the enthusiasm for their use. Complications include disseminated intravascular coagulopathy, central venous thrombosis, infection, variceal hemorrhage, shunt malfunction/dislodgement, fluid overload, air embolism, pulmonary edema, and bowel obstructions/perforations [70]. These shunts are contraindicated in patients with SBP, hyperbilirubinemia (>3–4 mg/dl), or a pleural effusion [70]. The only portosystemic surgical shunt that has any effect on ascites is a side-to-side portacaval shunt [89]; unfortunately, mortality rates in this setting exceed 30 percent [89]. Recent interest in TIPS for refractory ascites has surfaced. Preliminary data suggest that because TIPS is a side-to-side shunt, it is effective [90,91,92]. Finally, transplantation is successful for refractory ascites and is among the indications for the procedure.

Diagnostic paracentesis is an essential skill for intensivists and crucial to the evaluation of ascites and SBP. Paracentesis is a safe procedure, even in the setting of severe coagulopathy. A midline lower abdominal approach is favored by most clinicians because of its avascular tissue [93], although the left lower quadrant also may be used. The major concerns regarding the procedure are the risk of causing an infection and bleeding. Infection resulting from the needle entering bowel is a rare occurrence (approximately 0.6% risk) and seldom results in clinical peritonitis [94]. Bleeding from coagulopathy is also uncommon, occurring in approximately 1 percent of paracenteses [95]. The procedure should be performed in any patient with new-onset ascites, in any patient with cirrhosis admitted to the hospital, and in any cirrhotic patient with clinical deterioration [73,96]. Fluid should be sent for cell count, protein, and cytology; cultures for acid-fast organisms and fungus should be obtained, but the culture may be positive in only half of cases. Bacterial culture should be performed by the inoculation of 10 ml of ascitic fluid into each of two blood culture bottles at the bedside. This technique is far superior to conventional laboratory microbiologic culture techniques for detecting SBP (91% vs. 42% positive cultures) [97]. Tests that may be helpful in selected cases include triglycerides (for chylous ascites), carcinoembryonic antigen (for malignant ascites), and amylase (for pancreatic ascites) [70]. Tests that are not helpful include ascitic pH, glucose, and LDH [98].

SBP is diagnosed when more than 250 PMNs per cubic millimeter are present. Generally cultures will be positive when obtained appropriately [97]. Blood cultures will also be positive in 54 percent of patients with SBP [73]. The most common organisms include gram-negative enterics with *E. coli* and *Klebsiella* responsible for the majority, 46 percent and 10 percent, respectively; gram-positive cocci, with *Streptococcus sp.* and *Staphylococcus aureus* responsible for 19 percent and 1 percent, respectively; anaerobic bacteria, 6 percent; and miscellaneous organisms responsible for the remainder [98–101]. There is an increase in the percentage of *Staphylococcus* infections after placement of a LeVeen shunt, with the incidence of *S. aureus* peritonitis equal to that caused by gram-negative enterics (38 percent) [102]. The older literature on SBP suggests mortality rates of 100 percent [103,104]; more recent data suggest that despite awareness of SBP, the hospital mortality from SBP is as high as 70 percent even with appropriate antibiotics [98]. Although SBP has been reported to resolve spontaneously [98] this course is presumably very rare.

Given the high mortality rate even with treatment, clinicians should always search for and treat SBP. When selecting therapy for SBP, the clinician should consider several important points: (1) the organisms most commonly found in SBP, (2) the adequacy of antibiotic tissue penetration to the peritoneum and concentration in ascitic fluid [105,106], and (3) the consideration of nephrotoxicity. Patients with cirrhosis appear to be particularly susceptible to aminoglycoside nephrotoxicity [107]. When initiating therapy without bacteriologic identification, the drug of choice is a third-generation cephalosporin [70]. Cefotaxime in a dose of 2 gm intravenously every 8 hours adjusted for renal function has been evaluated and has been shown to be less toxic and to have greater efficacy than ampicillin with an aminoglycoside [108]. Aztreonam has also been shown to be effective, but a high incidence of superinfection (21%) makes it a second-line choice to cefotaxime [108]. Duration of therapy has not been standardized completely. A recent study demonstrated no difference in infection-related mortality, hospitalization mortality, bacteriologic cure, and recurrence of ascitic fluid infection between groups treated with cefotaxime 2 gm intravenously every 8 hours for 5 days or 10 days [109]. Repeat paracentesis should be performed after 48 hours of therapy and should demonstrate a 50 percent drop in the PMN count; cultures should be sterile [70]. If the patient did not grow an organism (so that selective antimicrobials could be administered) or if the patient does not show evidence of clinical improvement, additional paracenteses may be necessary. In patients surviving the initial episode, recurrent SBP at 1 year is estimated at 69 percent [110]. In a controlled study evaluating recurrent SBP, patients treated with norfloxacin at 400 mg orally daily were found to have a 1-year recurrence rate of 20 percent, whereas those in the placebo group had a 1-year recurrence rate of 68 percent [111]. Patients who develop SBP on norfloxacin have a higher incidence of gram-positive infections [111], an observation that should be taken into account when selecting antimicrobial regimens.

PORTAL HYPERTENSION. Portal hypertension contributes to the development of encephalopathy by shunting portal blood systemically, induces the development of collateral blood flow in the form of varices, participates in the production of ascites, and produces hypersplenism. Bleeding from esophageal varices is the most common cause for ICU admissions related to liver disease. A discussion of variceal bleeding is covered in Chapter 100. The management of a variety of ICU complications of liver disease may be difficult because of thrombocytopenia from splenic sequestration. In chronic liver disease, the platelets are usually functional unless uremia has developed. Transfusion of platelets should be reserved for active bleeding.

SYNTHETIC DYSFUNCTION. Synthetic dysfunction is a gradually progressive indicator of chronic liver disease. Generally, synthetic function is preserved until large portions of hepatic parenchyma have been replaced by fibrosis. Serum albumin and prothrombin time (uncorrected by vitamin K administration) are two easily measured determinants of synthetic function that have long been used to establish the prognosis and severity of liver disease [112,113]. Patients with synthetic dysfunction often will have severe muscle wasting and other apparent nutritional deficiencies despite adequate oral intake. In contrast to FHF, hypoglycemia in chronic liver disease is rare. However, hypoglycemia may be seen in association with specific challenges to the chronic liver disease patient, particularly alcohol ingestion or congestive heart failure [114]. In the absence of these conditions, the occurrence of hypoglycemia in chronic liver disease patients is a preterminal event.

References

1. Trey C, Davidson CS: The management of fulminant hepatic failure, in Popper H, Schaffner F (eds): *Progress in Liver Disease,* vol 3, New York, Grune & Stratton, 1970.
2. Gimson AES, White YS, Eddleston ALWF, et al: Clinical and prognostic differences in fulminant hepatitis type A, B, and non-A, non-B. *Gut* 24:1194, 1983.
3. Bernuau J, Rueff B, Benhamou J-P: Fulminant and subfulminant liver failure: Definitions and causes. *Semin Liver Dis* 6:97, 1986.
4. Williams R, Gimson AES: Intensive liver care and management of acute hepatic failure. *Dig Dis Sci* 36(6):820, 1991.
5. Iwatsuki S, Stieber AC, Marsh JW, et al: Liver transplantation for fulminant hepatic failure. *Trans Proc* 21(1):2431, 1989.
6. Bismuth H, Samuel D, Gugenheim J, et al: Emergency liver transplantation for fulminant hepatitis. *Ann Intern Med* 107:337, 1987.
7. Peleman RR, Gavaler JS, Van Thiel D, et al: Orthotopic liver transplantation for acute and subacute hepatic failure in adults. *Hepatology* 7:484, 1987.
8. Edmond J, Aran P, Thistlethwaite J, et al: Liver transplantation and the management of fulminant hepatic failure. *Gastroenterology* 94:A537, 1988 (Abstract).
9. O'Grady JG, Gimson AES, O'Brien CJ, et al: Controlled trials of charcoal hemoperfusion and prognostic factors in fulminant hepatic failure. *Gastroenterology* 94:1186, 1988.
10. Rakela J: Etiology and prognosis in fulminant hepatitis: Acute hepatic failure study group. *Gastroenterology* 77:A33, 1979 (Abstract).
11. Papaevangelou G, Tassopoulos N, Roumeliotou-Karayannis A, et al: Etiology of fulminant viral hepatitis in Greece. *Hepatology* 4:15S, 1984.
12. Gimson AES, O'Grady J, Ede R, et al: Late-onset hepatic failure: Clinical, serological and histological features. *Hepatology* 6:288, 1988.
13. Iwatsuki S, Esquivel CO, Gordon RD, et al: Liver transplantation for fulminant hepatic failure. *Semin Liver Dis* 5:325, 1985.
14. Edmond JC, Aran PP, Whitington PF, et al: Liver transplantation in the management of fulminant hepatic failure. *Gastroenterology* 96:1583, 1989.
15. Schafer DF, Shaw BW. Fulminant hepatic failure and orthotopic liver transplantation. *Semin Liver Dis* 9:189, 1989.
16. Munoz SJ, Moritz M, Martin P, et al: Liver transplantation for fulminant hepatic failure and orthotopic liver transplantation. *Hepatology* 12:1019, 1990.
17. Rakela J, Perkins JD, Gross JB, et al: Acute hepatic failure: The emerging role of orthotopic liver transplantation. *Mayo Clin Proc* 64:424, 1989.
18. Castells A, Salmeron JM, Navasa M, et al: Liver transplantation for acute liver failure: Analysis of applicability. *Gastroenterology* 105:532, 1993.
19. Lidofsky SD: Liver transplantation for fulminant hepatic failure. *Gastroenterol Clin North Am* 22(2):257, 1993.
20. Tygstrup N, Ranek L: Assessment of prognosis in fulminant hepatic failure. *Semin Liver Dis* 6:129, 1986.
21. O'Grady JG, Alexander GJM, Hayallar KM, et al: Early indicators of prognosis in fulminant hepatic failure. *Gastroenterology* 97:439, 1989.
22. Sinclair SB, Greig PD, Blendis LM, et al: Biochemical and clinical response of fulminant viral hepatitis to administration of prostaglandin E. *J Clin Invest* 84:1063, 1989.
23. Schafer DF, Jones EA: Hepatic encephalopathy, in Zakim D, Boyer TD (eds): *Hepatology: A Textbook of Liver Disease.* 2nd ed. Philadelphia, WB Saunders, 1990.
24. Klatzo I: Neuropathological aspects of brain edema. *J Neuropathol Exp Neurol* 26:1, 1967.
25. Joo F: A unifying concept on the pathogenesis of brain oedemas. *Neuropathol Appl Neurobiol* 13:161, 1987.
26. Ware AJ, D'Agostino A, Combes B: Cerebral edema: A major complication of massive hepatic necrosis. *Gastroenterology* 61:877, 1971.
27. Bismuth H, Didier S: Liver transplantation in fulminant and subfulminant hepatitis, in Morris PJ, Tilney NL (eds): *Transplantation Reviews.* Vol 2. Philadelphia, WB Saunders, 1988.
28. Nora LM, Bleck TP: Increased intracranial pressure complicating hepatic failure. *J Crit Illness* 4:87, 1989.
29. Canalese J, Gimson AES, Davies C, et al: Controlled trial of dexamethasone and mannitol for the cerebral edema of fulminant hepatic failure. *Gut* 23:625, 1982.
30. Silk DBA, Hanid MA, Trewby PN, et al: Treatment of fulminant hepatic failure by polyacrylonitrile membrane hemodialysis. *Lancet* 2:1, 1977.
31. Ede RJ, Gimson AES, Bihari D, Williams R: Controlled hyperventilation in the prevention of cerebral edema in fulminant hepatic failure. *J Hepatol* 2:43, 1986.
32. Ede JE, Williams R: Hepatic encephalopathy and cerebral edema. *Semin Liver Dis* 6:107, 1986.
33. Munoz SJ, Robinson M, Northrup B, et al: Elevated intracranial pressure and computed tomography of the brain in fulminant hepatocellular failure. *Hepatology* 13:209, 1991.
34. Lidofsky SD, Bass NM, Prager MC, et al: Intracranial pressure monitoring and liver transplantation for fulminant hepatic failure. *Hepatology* 16:1, 1992.
35. Blei AT: Cerebral edema and intracranial hypertension in acute liver failure: Distinct aspects of the same problem. *Hepatology* 13:376, 1991.
36. Hanid MA, Davies M, Mellon PJ: Clinical monitoring of intracranial pressure in fulminant hepatic failure. *Gut* 21:866, 1980.
37. Hetzel D: Fulminant hepatic failure. *Anaesth Intensive Care* 13:272, 1985.
38. Donovan JP, Shaw B, Langnas AN, et al: Brain water and acute liver failure: The emerging role of intracranial pressure monitoring. *Hepatology* 16:267, 1992.
39. Forbes A, Alexander GJM, O'Grady JG, et al: Thiopental infusion in the treatment of intracranial hypertension complicating fulminant hepatic failure. *Hepatology* 10:306, 1989.
40. Keays R, Potter D, O'Grady J, et al. Intracranial and cerebral perfusion pressure changes before, during and immediately after liver transplantation for fulminant hepatic failure. *Q J Med* 79:425, 1991.
41. Inagaki M, Shaw B, Schafer D, et al: Advantages of intracranial pressure monitoring in patients with fulminant hepatic failure. *Gastroenterology* 102:A826, 1992 (Abstract).
42. Bihari DJ, Gimson AES, Williams R: Cardiovascular, pulmonary, and renal complications of fulminant hepatic filure. *Semin Liver Dis* 6:119, 1986
43. Porte RJ, Knot EAR, Bontempo FA: Hemostasis in liver transplantation. *Gastroenterology* 97:488, 1989
44. Fiore L, Levine J, Deykin D: Alterations of hemostasis in patients with liver disease, in Zakim D, Boyer TD (eds): *Hepatology: A Textbook of Liver Disease.* 2nd ed. Philadelphia, WB Saunders, 1990.
45. O'Grady JG, Langley PG, Isola LM, et al: Coagulopathy of fulminant hepatic failure. *Semin Liver Dis* 6:159, 1986.
46. Gazzard BG, Henderson JM, William R: Early changes in coagulation following a paracetamol overdose and a controlled trial of fresh frozen plasma therapy. *Gut* 16:617, 1975.
47. Rolando N, Harvey F, Brahm J, et al: Prospective study of bacterial infection in acute liver failure: An analysis of fifty patients. *Hepatology* 11:49, 1990.
48. Wyke RJ, Canalese JC, Gimson AES, et al: Bacteraemia in patients with fulminant hepatic failure. *Liver* 2:45, 1982.
49. Health Resources and Services Administration, Bureau of Health Resources Development: *1991 Report of Center-Specific Graft and Patient Survival Rates.* Rockville, MD, US Department of Health and Human Services, 1992.
50. Sullivan JF, Linder H, Holdener P, et al: Blood ammonia in cerebral dysfunction. *Am J Med* 30:893, 1961.
51. Phear EA, Sherlock S, Summerskill WHJ: Blood ammonium levels in liver disease and hepatic coma. *Lancet* 1:836, 1955.

52. Phillips GB, Schwartz R, Gabuzda GJ, et al: The syndrome of impending hepatic coma in patients with cirrhosis of the liver given certain nitrogenous substances. *N Engl J Med* 247:239, 1952.

53. Sterns RH: Severe symptomatic hyponatremia: Treatment and outcome. *Ann Intern Med* 107:656, 1987.

54. Cerra FB, Cheung NK, Fischer JE, et al: Disease-specific amino acid infusion (F080) in hepatic encephalopathy: A prospective, randomized, double-blind, controlled trial. *J Parenter Enteral Nutr* 9:288, 1985.

55. Michel H, Bories P, Aubin JP, et al: Treatment of acute hepatic encephalopathy in cirrhosis with a branched-chain amino acids versus a conventional amino acids mixture. A controlled study of 70 patients. *Liver* 5:282, 1985.

56. Egbers EH, Schomerus H, Hamster W, et al: Branched-chain amino acids in the treatment of latent portosystemic encephalopathy: A double-blind placebo-controlled crossover study. *Gastroenterology* 88:887, 1985.

57. Mendenhall C, Bongiovanni G, Goldberg S, et al: VA cooperative study on alcoholic hepatitis III. Changes in protein-calorie malnutrition associated with 30 days of hospitalization with and without enteral nutritional therapy. *J Parenter Enteral Nutr* 9:590, 1985.

58. Reding P, Duchateau J, Bataille C: Oral zinc supplementation improves hepatic encephalopathy. *Lancet* 2:493, 1984.

59. Morgan MY, Hawley KE: Lactilol vs. lactulose in the treatment of acute hepatic encephalopathy in cirrhotic patients: A double-blind randomized trial. *Hepatology* 7:1278, 1987.

60. Berk PD, Chalmers T: Deafness complicating antibiotic therapy of hepatic encephalopathy. *Ann Intern Med* 73:393, 1970.

61. Parkes JD, Murray-Lyon IM, Williams R: Neuropsychiatric and electroencephalographic changes after transplantation of the liver. *Q J Med* 39:515, 1970.

62. Ritt DJ, Whelan G, Werner DJ, et al: Acute hepatic necrosis with stupor or coma. *Medicine* 48:151, 1969.

63. Epstein M: Functional renal abnormalities in cirrhosis: Pathophysiology and management, in Zakim D, Boyer TD (eds): *Hepatology: A Textbook of Liver Disease*. 2nd ed. Philadelphia, WB Saunders, 1990.

64. Epstein M: Hepatorenal syndrome, in Epstein M (ed): *The Kidney in Liver Disease*. 3rd ed. Baltimore, Williams & Wilkins, 1988.

65. Schroeder ET, Numann PJ, Chamberlain BE: Functional renal failure in cirrhosis: Recovery after portacaval shunt. *Ann Intern Med* 72:923, 1970.

66. Kinney MJ, Wapnick S, Ahmed N, et al: Cirrhosis, ascites, and impaired renal function: Treatment with the LeVeen-type chronic peritoneal-venous shunt, in Epstein M (ed): *The Kidney in Liver Disease*. New York, Elsevier-North Holland, 1978.

67. Kinney MJ, Schneider A, Wapnick S, et al: The "hepatorenal" syndrome and refractory ascites: Successful therapy with the LeVeen-type peritoneal-venous shunt and valve. *Nephron* 23:228, 1979.

68. Epstein M: The role of peritoneovenous shunt in the management of ascites and the hepatorenal syndrome, in Epstein M (ed): *The Kidney in Liver Disease*. New York, Elsevier-North Holland, 1978.

69. Conn HO: Transjugular intrahepatic portal-systemic shunts: The state of the art. *Hepatology* 17:148, 1993.

70. Wright TL, Boyer TD: Diagnosis and management of cirrhotic ascites, in Zakim D, Boyer TD (eds): *Hepatology: A Textbook of Liver Disease*. 2nd ed. Philadelphia, WB Saunders, 1990.

71. Rocco VK, Ware AJ: Cirrhotic ascites. *Ann Intern Med* 105:573, 1986.

72. Runyon BA: Spontaneous bacterial peritonitis: An explosion of information. *Hepatology* 8:171, 1988.

73. Hoefs JC, Runyon BA: Spontaneous bacterial peritonitis. *Dis Mon* 31:1, 1985.

74. Fox RA, Dudley FS, Sherlock S: The serum concentrations of the third component of complement in liver disease. *Gut* 12:574, 1971.

75. Kourilsky O, LeRoy C, Peltier AP: Complement and liver cell function in 53 patients with liver disease. *Am J Med* 55:783, 1973.

76. Rajkovic IA, William R: Abnormalities of neutrophil phagocytosis, intracellular killing, and metabolic activity in alcoholic cirrhosis and hepatitis. *Hepatology* 6:252, 1986.

77. Rimola A, Soto R, Bory F, et al: Reticuloendothelial system phagocytic activity in cirrhosis and its relation to bacterial infections and prognosis. *Hepatology* 4:53, 1984.

78. Kurtz RC, Bronzo RL: Does spontaneous bacterial peritonitis occur in malignant ascites? *Am J Gastroenterol* 77:146, 1982

79. Runyon BA: Spontaneous bacterial peritonitis associated with cardiac ascites. *Am J Gastroenterol* 79:796, 1984.

80. Runyon BA, Hoefs JC: Ascitic fluid analysis before, during, and after spontaneous bacterial peritonitis. *Hepatology* 5:257, 1985.

81. Runyon BA, Morrissey R, Hoefs JC, et al: Opsonic activity of human ascitic fluid: A potentially important protective mechanism against spontaneous bacterial peritonitis. *Hepatology* 5:634, 1985.

82. Runyon BA: Low-protein-concentration ascitic fluid is predisposed to spontaneous bacterial peritonitis. *Gastroenterology* 91:1343, 1986.

83. Almdal TP Skinhoj P: Spontaneous bacterial peritonitis in cirrhosis: Incidence, diagnosis, and prognosis. *Scand J Gastroenterol* 22:295, 1987.

84. Pinzello G, Simonetti RG, Craxi A, et al: Spontaneous bacterial peritonitis: A prospective investigation in predominantly nonalcoholic cirrhotic patients. *Hepatology* 3:545, 1983.

85. Boyer TD, Warnock D: Use of diuretics in the treatment of cirrhotic ascites. *Gastroenterology* 84:1051, 1983.

86. Pockros PJ, Reynolds TB: Rapid diuresis in patients with ascites from chronic liver disease: The importance of peripheral edema. *Gastroenterology* 90:1827, 1986.

87. Shear L, Ching S, Gabuzda GJ: Compartmentalization of ascites and edema in patients with hepatic cirrhosis. *N Engl J. Med* 282:1391, 1970.

88. Simon DM, McCain JR, Bonkovsky HL, et al: Effects of therapeutic paracentesis on systemic and hepatic hemodynamics and on renal and hormonal function. *Hepatology* 7:432, 1987.

89. Welch HF, Welch CS, Carter JH: Prognosis after surgical treatment of ascites: Results of side-to-side shunt in 40 patients. *Surgery* 56:75, 1964.

90. Sanyal AJ, Freedman AM, Shiffman ML: Transjugular intrahepatic porto-systemic shunt for ascites: A preliminary report. *Am J Gastroenterol* 87:1305, 1992 (Abstract).

91. Ochs A, Sellinger M, Haag K: Transjugular intrahepatic portosystemic stent-shunt (TIPS) for the treatment of refractory ascites and hepatorenal syndrome: Results of a pilot study. *Gastroenterology* 102:A862, 1992 (Abstract).

92. Garcia-Villarreal L, Zozaya MJM, Quiroga J, et al: Transjugular intrahepatic portosystemic shunt (TIPS) for intractable ascites (IA): Preliminary results. *J Hepatol* 16:S36, 1992 (Abstract).

93. Hoefs JC: Diagnostic paracentesis: A potent clinical tool. *Gastroenterology* 98:230, 1990.

94. Runyon BA, Hoefs JC, Canawati HN: Polymicrobial bacterascites: A unique entity in the spectrum of infected ascitic fluid. *Arch Intern Med* 146:2173, 1986.

95. Runyon BA: Paracentesis of ascitic fluid: A safe procedure. *Arch Intern Med* 146:2259, 1986.

96. Hoefs JC, Runyon BA: Spontaneous bacterial peritonitis. *Dis Mon* 31:3, 1985.

97. Macrae F: Spontaneous bacterial peritonitis: Reversible cause of clinical deterioration in patients with cirrhosis. *Med J Aust* 2:201, 1980.

98. Runyon BA, Umland ET, Merlin T: Inoculation of blood culture bottles with ascitic fluid: Improved detection of spontaneous bacterial peritonitis. *Arch Intern Med* 147:73, 1987.

99. Garcia Tsao G, Conn HO, Lerner E: The diagnosis of bacterial peritonitis: Comparison of pH, lactate concentration and leukocyte count. *Hepatology* 5:91, 1985.

100. Stassen WN, McCullough AJ, Bacon BR, et al: Immediate diagnostic criteria for bacterial infection of ascitic fluid: Evaluation of ascitic fluid polymorphonuclear leukocyte count, pH, and lactate concentration alone and in combination. *Gastroenterology* 90:1247, 1986.

101. Targan SR, Chow AW, Guze LB: Role of anaerobic bacteria in spontaneous peritonitis: A report of two cases and review of the literature. *Am J Med* 62:397, 1977.

102. Prokesch RC, Rimland D: Infectious complications of the peritoneovenous shunt. *Am J Gastroenterol* 78:235, 1983.

103. Conn HO, Fessel JM: Spontaneous bacterial peritonitis in cirrhosis: Variations on a theme. *Medicine* 50:161, 1971.

104. Correia JP, Conn HC: Spontaneous bacterial peritonitis in cirrhosis: Endemic or epidemic? *Med Clin North Am* 59:963, 1975.

105. Gerding DN, Hall WH, Schierl EA: Antibiotic concentrations in ascitic fluid of patients with ascites and bacterial peritonitis. *Ann Intern Med* 86:708, 1977.
106. Ariza J, Gudio F, Dolz C, et al: Evaluation of aztreonam in the treatment of spontaneous bacterial peritonitis in patients with cirrhosis. *Hepatology* 6:906, 1986.
107. Cabrera J, Arroyo V, Ballesta AM, et al: Aminoglycoside nephrotoxicity in cirrhosis. Value of urinary B2–microglobulin to discriminate functional renal failure from acute tubular damage. *Gastroenterology* 82:97, 1982.
108. Felisart J, Rimola A, Arroyo V, et al: Cefotaxime is more effective than is ampicillin-tobramycin in cirrhotics with severe infections. *Hepatology* 5:457, 1985.
109. Runyon BA, McHutchison JG, Antillon MR, et al: Short-course versus long-course antibiotic treatment of spontaneous bacterial peritonitis: A randomized controlled study of 100 patients. *Gastroenterology* 100:1737, 1991.
110. Tito L, Rimola A, Gines P, et al: Recurrence of spontaneous bacterial peritonitis in cirrhosis: Frequency and predictive factors. *Hepatology* 8:27, 1988.
111. Gines P, Rimola A, Planas R, et al: Norfloxacin prevents spontaneous bacterial peritonitis recurrence in cirrhosis: Results of a double-blind, placebo-controlled trial. *Hepatology* 12:716, 1990.
112. Child CG III, Turcotte J: Surgery and portal hypertension. In Child CG III (ed): *The Liver and Portal Hypertension*. Philadelphia, WB Saunders, 1965.
113. Stolz A, Kaplowitz N: Biochemical tests for liver disease, in Zakim D, Boyer TD (eds): *Hepatology: A Textbook of Liver Disease*, 2nd ed. Philadelphia, WB Saunders, 1990.
114. Zakim D: Metabolism of glucose and fatty acids by the liver, in Zakim D, Boyer TD (eds): *Hepatology: A Textbook of Liver Disease*. 2nd ed. Philadelphia, WB Saunders, 1990.

104. Diarrhea

George Stathopoulos
and Eugene B. Chang

Diarrhea frequently complicates the course of the critically ill patient, occurring in 40 to 50 percent of intensive care unit (ICU) patients, making it the most common nonhemorrhagic gastrointestinal (GI) complication in this population [1,2,3]. Despite its prevalence, diarrhea is frequently overlooked by the physician and the ICU team, especially when more emergent cardiovascular, respiratory, and infectious complications are present. Inattention to excessive stool output, however, can often result in serious perturbations of fluid and electrolyte balance, promote skin breakdown and infection, and create difficulty in the administration of proper nutritional support. In these instances, proper and immediate evaluation and management are essential in preventing further compromise of the already stressed patient. An alternative approach to these patients is often mandated by the patient's tenuous state and the practical limitations in performing many diagnostic studies in the ICU setting. The patient care team must also be aware that the differential diagnosis differs considerably from that of diarrhea in the general population.

The term *diarrhea* surprisingly carries a different meaning for the patient, physician, and nursing staff. Increases in stool frequency, changes in consistency, and increased volume all have been used as criteria to define diarrhea; however, increases in stool frequency or fluidity do not necessarily indicate the presence of diarrhea. In the general patient population, an increase in daily stool weight or volume (exceeding 250 gm/ml) has been used as a more objective defining criterion [4]. In the critically ill patient, however, accurate quantitation of stool output may be difficult, if not impossible. The physician, therefore, must use his or her best judgment to decide whether diarrhea is present and to determine whether it represents a clinical problem requiring immediate attention. In this chapter, we provide helpful insights for making these decisions, present guidelines for rapid and directed evaluation, and suggest effective approaches for the management of diarrhea in this setting.

Etiology

The numerous causes of diarrhea in the ICU setting can be broadly divided into iatrogenic causes, causes secondarily related to an underlying disease, and diarrhea as a primary manifestation of specific diseases. Careful review of historical and laboratory data will allow the physician to narrow the diagnostic possibilities and avoid overlooking the simple and perhaps most common causes (Table 104-1). In some patients, however, diarrhea may be the result of a combination of these factors. It is therefore incumbent on the physician to review the available data carefully to determine the cause or causes of the patient's diarrheal syndrome.

IATROGENIC CAUSES. Iatrogenic causes of diarrhea in the critically ill patient must be first and foremost in the physician's differential diagnosis because they are both the most common and the most frequently overlooked factors. In addition, in most situations, rapid and successful treatment can be achieved simply by eliminating the offending agent or process.

Drugs. Medication is perhaps the most frequent cause of iatrogenic diarrhea in this patient population. Many of the drugs commonly used in the ICU cause diarrhea (Table 104-2). However, any medication or combination of medications should be suspect, and uncertainty on the part of the physician warrants consultation with the pharmacist or drug company.

Antibiotics head the list of agents implicated in diarrhea. Some studies show a definite correlation between antibiotic usage and the incidence of diarrhea [5]. Although any antibiotic may cause diarrhea, ampicillin, the tetracyclines, erythromycin, and clindamycin are most frequently implicated. Certain cephalosporins, such as cefoperazone, are excreted in bile, which

Table 104-1. Differential Diagnosis of Diarrhea in the Intensive Care Unit Setting

Iatrogenic causes
  Medications
  Enteral feeding
  Pseudomembranous colitis
Diarrhea secondarily related to underlying disease
  Infections in immunosuppressed patients
  Neoplastic disease in immunosuppressed patients
  Gastrointestinal bleeding
  Neutropenic enteropathy
  Ischemic bowel disease
  Postsurgical diarrhea (postcholecystectomy, following gastric surgery)
  Surgically induced short bowel syndrome or pancreatic insufficiency
  Fecal impaction
  Opiate withdrawal
Diarrhea as a primary manifestation of disease
  Diabetic diarrhea
  Renal failure
  Sepsis
  Cirrhosis?
  Adrenal insufficiency
  Graft versus host disease
  Vasculitis
  Diarrhea-causing pathogens
  Inflammatory bowel disease
  Celiac sprue

Table 104-2. Medications Associated with Diarrhea*

Antibiotics (especially erythromycin, ampicillin, clindamycin, cephalosporins)
Antacids (magnesium containing)
Magnesium and phosphorus supplements
Lactulose
Colchicine
Digitalis
Quinidine
Theophylline
Levothyroxine
Aspirin
Nonsteroidal antiinflammatory agents
Cimetidine
Misoprostol
Diuretics
Beta-blocking agents
Chemotherapeutic agents

* Additives in the physical formulation of medications (e.g., sorbitol, lactose) may produce diarrhea independent of the primary medication.

may make gastrointestinal side effects more common. Antibiotic agents most frequently cause a nonspecific noninflammatory diarrhea associated with other abdominal complaints such as nausea, vomiting, abdominal cramping, and bloating. Diagnostic studies, including stool examination, are generally negative. Fluid and electrolyte losses are minimal and, in most cases, symptoms abate on withdrawal or change of the medication. Alterations in intestinal flora, breakdown of dietary carbohydrate products, and prokinetic effects (erythromycin) are all postulated mechanisms.

Antibiotic-associated (pseudomembranous) colitis (AAC) resulting from infection with *Clostridium difficile* is a less frequent but serious and sometimes life-threatening complication in the ICU. The incidence of this complication varies depending on the study and patient population, with infection rates as high

as 45 percent occurring in patients with diarrhea in a Seattle burn unit [6]. Other studies have shown a much lower prevalence, but the possibility of AAC causing diarrhea must always be considered in ICU patients because of its potentially devastating sequelae. AAC may be caused by any antibiotic, including the agents that are used to treat the infection (metronidazole and vancomycin). Clindamycin, ampicillin, and broad-spectrum cephalosporins have been especially implicated. Infection may occur in single patients or spread among patients within the hospital setting. Patients who are elderly; who have insulin-dependent diabetes, hepatic failure, renal failure, or malnutrition; or who have undergone upper GI surgery or cytotoxic chemotherapy (i.e., methotrexate, cytoxan) especially may be at risk. Colitis can be induced by administration of only one or two antibiotic doses by the intravenous, oral, or even topical routes.

C. difficile produces multiple toxins, two of which have been well characterized [7]. Toxin-induced changes in brush border function, intestinal fluid transport, and GI peristalsis appear important in disease pathogenesis and symptom manifestations. Prompt recognition and treatment are essential, in that severe cases may result in profound colitis that may progress to a toxic megacolon or colonic perforation requiring surgical intervention.

Agents that increase the osmotic load of the gut lumen frequently cause diarrhea. Magnesium-containing antacids (e.g., Maalox and Mylanta) are probably the most common example of this group. Aggressive enteral repletion of nutrients such as magnesium and phosphorus will also result in diarrhea by this mechanism. The semisynthetic disaccharide lactulose, useful in treating portal systemic encephalopathy, remains unhydrolyzed in the gut lumen, increasing the osmotic gradient, fluid secretion, and stool output. Degradation in the terminal ileum may also lower pH, which may have a negative effect on intestinal absorption. In addition, many medications contain, as inert additives, sorbitol or lactose, which may cause an osmotic diarrhea. Of 29 tube-fed patients with diarrhea in a recent study, 48 percent had diarrhea that was caused by sorbitol-containing elixirs [8].

Other agents capable of causing a nonspecific and rarely severe diarrhea include agents such as colchicine, quinidine, digitalis, metoclopramide, theophylline, levothyroxine, aspirin, nonsteroidal antiinflammatory drugs, misoprostol, cimetidine, diuretics, cholinergic agents (e.g., bethanechol), beta-blockers, and various chemotherapeutic agents. The pathophysiology in most instances remains unclear; however, it is presumed that these agents act as irritants, affecting gut motility, nerve conduction, secretion, and absorption. Symptoms can frequently be lessened by dose reduction or eliminated by discontinuance.

Enteral Feedings. Numerous studies have investigated the role of enteral feeding in causing diarrhea in the previously fasted critically ill patient. Certain aspects, such as administration of antibiotics, osmolality of solution, type of solution, and serum albumin, have been assessed to determine their contributing roles in the occurrence and severity of diarrhea in these patients [9].

In most instances, diarrhea in enterally fed patients has been shown to be associated with concurrent antibiotic administration [5,10]. Changes in intestinal function caused by antibiotics, coupled with the intestinal effects of enteral feeding administration, have an additive role in causing changes in gut function that result in diarrhea. Osmolality of solution may play a role in feeding-induced diarrhea, especially when elemental-type diets are used and when feedings are rapidly administered directly into the small bowel. Bolus feeding may be more physiologic, especially with regard to glucose homeostasis; however, feedings administered in this manner (especially tbe feedings distal to the pylorus) may result in rapid, uncontrolled emptying of high caloric contents into the small bowel with rapid transit and a higher incidence of diarrhea [11]. Bacterial contamination of enteral feedings is a rare cause of diarrhea due to intestinal bacterial overgrowth.

Enteral formulas high in lactose or fat content may also be a factor in susceptible patients. Starved or parenterally fed patients who have developed small bowel villus atrophy and a decrease in mucosal disaccharidase enzyme activities may experience diarrhea when enteral feedings are initiated. In these patients, initial management with elemental diets that require less digestion and are low in fat and residue may be indicated. Elemental dietary supplementation may also be considered in patients with short bowel syndrome, pancreatic insufficiency, radiation enteritis, fistulas, and inflammatory bowel disease. Their major disadvantages are high cost and increased osmolality [12]. The use of peptide-based and fiber-rich formulas has not consistently been shown to reduce the incidence of diarrhea but may be useful in individual patients.

The role of hypoalbuminemia is controversial. Brinson found that when ICU patients with and without diarrhea were compared, the albumin level was statistically different between the groups (1.90 gm/dl vs. 3.40 gm/dl in the groups with and without diarrhea, respectively). Patients with an albumin level below 2.6 gm per deciliter developed diarrhea, whereas those with a level above 2.6 gm per deciliter did not [2]. Hypoalbuminemia, which decreases colloid osmotic pressure, may cause diarrhea by causing mucosal edema and changes in the Starling forces sufficient to inhibit intestinal fluid absorption. Some authors claim that concurrent nutritional intake and correction of the albumin deficit with intravenous salt-poor albumin may result in normalization and maintenance of albumin levels with an improved tolerance of enteral feedings and resolution of diarrhea [13]. Conversely, however, patients with severe hypoalbuminemia secondary to cirrhosis or the nephrotic syndrome do not uniformly have diarrhea. Until further studies show efficacy, the aggressive use of intravenous albumin repletion cannot be routinely recommended.

DIARRHEA SECONDARILY RELATED TO UNDERLYING DISEASE.
Diarrhea may result from various processes or pathogens associated with disease states commonly seen in the critically ill patient. Diarrhea may occur more frequently in patients with drug-induced or disease-induced immunosuppression, alterations in cardiac output and blood flow, and various primary GI diseases.

In immunosuppressed patients, such as posttransplant patients, diarrhea may be caused by several infectious agents, most commonly cytomegalovirus (CMV). Patients may also be infected with herpes simplex; *Giardia, Salmonella, Shigella, Cryptosporidium, Isospora,* and *Campylobacter* species; and fungi (*Candida* and *Aspergillus* species). Posttransplantation patients receiving long-term immunosuppression may also develop intestinal lymphoma manifesting as diarrhea.

Diarrhea is perhaps the most common symptom found in patients with the acquired immunodeficiency syndrome (AIDS). These patients can develop diarrhea from a single pathogen or simultaneous infection with several pathogens. CMV, *Mycobacterium avium intracellulare* (MAI), and *Cryptosporidium* are the most common organisms, with *Cryptosporidium* being the agent most likely to cause a severe large-volume secretory diarrhea (often in excess of 1 liter/day) [14]. *Isospora belli, Giardia lamblia, Salmonella, Shigella, Campylobacter* species, *Entamoeba histolytica, Microsporidium* species, and various viruses (i.e., adenoviruses) are also capable of causing diarrhea

in patients with AIDS [15]. Infections such as salmonellosis or from *Campylobacter* may become chronic and relapsing, posing difficult treatment problems. The herpes simplex virus may cause perianal ulceration, urgency, and frequent mucopurulent discharge, which may be interpreted as diarrhea [16]. In many patients, extensive investigation of diarrhea will not yield a causative pathogen, suggesting a primary enteropathy associated with the disease, possibly due to the causative virus itself [17]. However, as our knowledge of the disease and of other potential opportunistic infections increases, most if not all cases of diarrhea will probably be shown to be caused by specific pathogens and not by an associated enteropathy. Patients with AIDS may also develop high-grade intestinal lymphomas predominantly of B-cell origin, which may present as diarrhea. Kaposi's sarcoma may cause GI bleeding but rarely, if ever, causes diarrhea [18].

GI bleeding is a particularly common cause of increased stool output and diarrhea. Common etiologies include stress ulceration, peptic ulcer disease, Mallory-Weiss tears, esophagitis, esophageal varices, and hemorrhagic gastropathy. The presence of intraluminal blood will increase stool output by virtue of its effect as a gut irritant and to some extent as an osmotic agent.

Neutropenic patients receiving chemotherapy for malignancy or posttransplant immunosuppressed patients can experience diarrhea, with or without abdominal pain, as a result of bowel pathology ranging from bowel edema to frank infarction. The cause of these changes is unclear; however, infection, chemotherapeutic agents, neutropenia itself, and a primary intestinal injury have been postulated as initiating factors [19].

Intestinal ischemia, especially involving the colon, may result in abdominal pain and, occasionally, diarrhea in the ICU patient. Postsurgical patients, especially those who have undergone resection of an abdominal aortic aneurysm, may have as high as a 6 percent incidence of colonoscopically documented ischemia [20]. Patients who have undergone an abdominoperineal resection or therapeutic angiography are also at risk. Compromise of the inferior mesenteric artery with left-sided colonic involvement is the primary etiologic factor. Occurrence is generally a few days following the procedure but can be delayed for weeks. Patients in shock with depressed cardiac output may be more likely to present with right-sided colonic involvement [21]. Severity can range from mild, transient ischemic changes, to mucosal ulceration or bowel necrosis. Sympathomimetic drugs, vasopressin, ergot preparations, and perhaps digitalis may further place susceptible patients at risk [22]. Likewise, small intestinal ischemia may initially present with bloody or nonbloody diarrhea.

Other problems that may occur in the postsurgical patient include intestinal fistulas with a blind loop syndrome, small bowel bacterial overgrowth, abscesses, and the well-described diarrhea in the patient following cholecystectomy, gastric surgery, or massive intestinal or pancreatic resection. Fecal impaction in both medical and surgical patients may paradoxically cause diarrhea. Drugs such as analgesics, sedatives, aluminum-containing antacids, and sucralfate, combined with ileus, may decrease intestinal motility and fecal fluidity, resulting in the formation of a partially obstructing fecal mass and diarrhea. Diverticulitis may also present with accompanying diarrhea.

Patients who are active drug abusers may suffer from the opiate withdrawal syndrome, which involves a constellation of symptoms, including nausea, vomiting, and severe diarrhea.

DIARRHEA AS A PRIMARY MANIFESTATION OF DISEASE.
Several common diseases may occasionally be characterized by diarrhea during their courses. Patients with diabetes,

uremia, or sepsis can experience severe bouts of diarrhea. Although the mechanisms of the latter two remain unclear, the diarrhea of diabetes is thought to result from an autonomic neuropathy and its effect on intestinal fluid absorption [23]. Abnormalities in motility, with intestinal stasis and bacterial overgrowth, may play a role, as may incontinence (misinterpreted as diarrhea). These patients invariably have other signs of autonomic neuropathy, including orthostatic hypotension, gastroparesis, anhidrosis, abnormalities in R-R wave variation on electrocardiogram (ECG), and neurogenic bladder [24].

Cirrhosis with portal hypertension has been hypothesized to be a possible cause of diarrhea. Increases in intestinal lymphatic pressure and hypoalbuminemia theoretically may result in diarrhea. Most patients with cirrhosis and portal hypertension, however, do not present with diarrhea, leaving cirrhosis-induced diarrhea as a diagnosis made with reservation.

Several unusual causes of diarrhea may occur in patients with certain disease states. Patients with primary adrenal insufficiency (e.g. secondary to sepsis or anticoagulants) or patients on long-term steroid replacement who develop adrenal crisis may present with diarrhea. This etiology may be overlooked in the patient with hemodynamic compromise or may be attributed to infection in the patient who, as part of the syndrome, presents with fever and abdominal pain.

Graft-versus-host disease (GVHD) may complicate both the acute and the long-term course of the posttransplant (usually of the bone marrow) immunosuppressed patient [25,26]. Acute (less than 3 months posttransplant) GVHD may present with severe diarrhea. Significant intestinal protein losses are common. Bowel changes are most common in the distal ileum and proximal colon and consist of villus atrophy, with a lymphocyte and plasma cell infiltrate, and necrosis of colonic epithelial cells with enterochromaffin cell sparing, respectively. Chronic GVHD is characterized by a less severe form of diarrhea. Intestinal strictures and a scleroderma-type picture with intestinal stasis, bacterial overgrowth, and malabsorption may occur. Concurrent esophageal involvement is common. Therapy generally consists of increased immunosuppression.

Vasculitic diseases, such as systemic lupus erythematosus, dermatomyositis, polyarteritis, the rheumatic diseases, and Wegener's granulomatosis, can involve the medium-sized and small-sized vessels supplying the gut. Abdominal pain, fever, bleeding, and diarrhea are common resulting symptoms.

Finally, one must always consider causes of diarrheal disease that are not unique to the critically ill patient. Infectious causes of diarrhea in the immunocompetent hospitalized patient are mentioned for completeness, but they are unusual in clinical practice unless the onset of diarrhea is within the first few days of hospitalization or a nosocomial outbreak of infection is present [27]. Infectious causes include *Salmonella, Shigella, Campylobacter, Giardia,* or *Entamoeba histolytica.* Nonenteric infectious causes of diarrhea include toxic shock syndrome and Legionnaires' disease. For a more complete review of infectious causes of diarrhea, see reference 28. Other causes to be considered include lactose intolerance, inflammatory bowel disease, and celiac sprue.

Diagnosis

HISTORY AND PHYSICAL EXAMINATION. Historical data are very important in the diagnosis of diarrhea but may be difficult to obtain in the ICU patient. Depressed neurologic function as the result of the disease state or iatrogenic sedation and intubation may make it impossible to obtain a history. Attention

to the onset, duration, character, relation to enteral intake, and associated symptoms of diarrhea may be helpful etiologic clues. Information on prior episodes of diarrhea, the patient's underlying medical conditions (which may be associated with diarrhea), or prior use of antibiotics can also be helpful. Not uncommonly, pseudomembranous colitis may occur up to 6 weeks after the offending antibiotic has been discontinued.

Next, a careful review of the patient's current medications and their administration relative to the onset of diarrhea should be performed. Any suspected agent should be discontinued if at all possible or changed to an alternative medication. Every effort should be made at decreasing the number of medications and continuing only those that are absolutely necessary. The physician should also determine whether the institution of enteral feedings may correlate with the onset of symptoms. Important patient symptoms include abdominal pain, which may suggest ischemia, infection, or various inflammatory conditions such as vasculitis or GVHD. Bloody diarrhea may suggest primary GI bleeding, ischemia, or, occasionally, pseudomembranous colitis. Passage of frequent small-volume stools with urgency and tenesmus suggests distal, left-sided intestinal involvement, whereas passage of less frequent, large-volume stools suggests more proximal involvement (small bowel or right colon). These historical clues, however, are not mutually exclusive and in disease states with extensive bowel involvement the distinction may not be appreciable.

The physical examination may provide further clues as to etiology but usually is nonspecific. More importantly, the physical examination is essential in assessing the clinical severity of diarrhea. Profound postural hypotension suggests severe volume loss, adrenal insufficiency, or autonomic neuropathy (e.g., of diabetes). Fever may signify infection, vasculitis, or adrenal insufficiency. Abdominal tenderness may suggest infectious or ischemic causes. Skin rashes or mucosal ulcerations in the appropriate patient may suggest inflammatory bowel disease or vasculitis. Cutaneous manifestations of AIDS and lymphadenopathy should be sought. Abdominal distention, palpable bowel loops, or abnormal rectal examination may suggest a partially obstructing fecal impaction.

LABORATORY STUDIES. Serum electrolytes, especially sodium, potassium, magnesium, and phosphorus, should be obtained and carefully monitored in patients with diarrhea. Severe diarrhea may result in a hyperchloremic metabolic acidosis and prerenal azotemia if not adequately treated. The serum sodium may be normal, elevated, or depressed, depending on severity of diarrhea, the patient's access to water, type of intravenous fluid administered, and other disease states (e.g., hepatic or renal dysfunction). The serum potassium, magnesium, and phosphorus may be normal or depressed, whereas elevations (e.g., in potassium) may suggest adrenal insufficiency or uremia. Leukocytosis may suggest infection or ischemia, whereas neutropenia may suggest resultant changes of the intestinal mucosa.

Examination of the stool may be the single most important and most overlooked laboratory investigation in this patient population. The presence of occult blood should be checked and a methylene blue stain performed to look for fecal leukocytes. The presence of fecal leukocytes suggests infection, ischemia, or mucosal inflammation such as GVHD or vasculitis. A culture and toxin assay for *C. difficile* should be obtained. A positive assay for the toxin of *C. difficile* is highly suggestive but not specific for pseudomembranous colitis. It is positive in 95 to 100 percent of patients with the disease, 15 to 25 percent of patients with antibiotic-associated diarrhea without pseudomembranes, and 2 to 8 percent of patients receiving antibiotics without diarrhea [29,30].

Fresh stool specimens should also be sent for culture and ova and parasite examination, which may yield a treatable diagnosis. Immunosuppressed patients, such as patients with AIDS, require more extensive examination of the stool. Sugar flotation techniques to concentrate the stool may be necessary for isolation of *Cryptosporidium* species or *Isospora belli*. Other pathogens such as CMV or MAI isolated from stool do not necessarily represent infection and require evidence of tissue invasion on biopsy for diagnosis. As is discussed subsequently, the diagnosis of certain other infections such as *Microsporidium, Cryptosporidium,* or *Giardia* may be aided by small bowel biopsy.

A Sudan stain for fecal fat may be helpful if a malabsorptive state is suspected. Osmotic diarrhea secondary to carbohydrate malabsorption will decrease stool pH (to approximately 5 from a normal of 7) due to short-chain fatty acid production from bacterial action on carbohydrate. Objective measurements of stool composition and weight may be difficult to perform in the ICU setting. Quantitation of stool weight is important not only in assessing volume loss, but also in monitoring effectiveness of antidiarrheal therapy. Determination of the stool osmolar gap (the difference between expected stool osmolality ($[Na^+]$ + $[K^+]$) × 2) and measured osmolality) may help distinguish between osmotic and secretory causes. High-volume stool output that persists with fasting suggests a secretory etiology, whereas an elevated stool osmolar gap (generally greater than 70 mOsm) suggests osmotic causes.

SPECIAL DIAGNOSTIC INVESTIGATIONS. Abdominal radiographs are sometimes helpful and may show signs of ischemia, partial obstruction, perforation, or a toxic megacolon associated with colitis. Contrast studies better define GI pathology that may result in diarrhea but often cannot be performed in the critically ill patient.

Flexible or rigid proctosigmoidoscopy can be extremely useful in the diagnosis of antibiotic-associated colitis, distal ischemic colitis, GVHD, or vasculitis, to name a few, but may be difficult to perform in the severely traumatized or burned patient. Classic findings in antibiotic-associated colitis include distinct, adherent, raised plaques (pseudomembranes), 2 to 5 mm in size, that can, on occasion, be confluent. Normal mucosal appearance, however, should not rule out the diagnosis. Mucosal biopsy can be useful in some cases with negative endoscopic findings and may reveal pseudomembranes, composed of polymorphonuclear leukocytes, chronic inflammatory cells, fibrin, and epithelial debris. In addition, it must be remembered that up to one-third of patients with antibiotic-associated colitis will have findings confined to the right colon beyond the reach of the sigmoidoscope [31]. Patients with suspected CMV colitis or herpes proctitis should undergo proctosigmoidoscopic examination with biopsy. CMV colitis may manifest as discrete ulcerations or widespread mucosal edema, erythema, and erosion. The characteristic vesicles of herpes may or may not be present and may be replaced by extensive ulceration. MAI should also be a diagnosis made at biopsy. Small bowel biopsy may reveal PAS-positive macrophages simulating a Whipple's type picture. Closer inspection will reveal acid-fast bacilli. In addition, the dilated lacteals and clinical evidence of arthralgias in true Whipple's disease will be absent in MAI infection. The diagnosis of *Cryptosporidium* and *Giardia* will be enhanced by small bowel biopsy, whereas the identification of *Microsporidium* requires electron microscopic examination of mucosal biopsies.

Management

Initial Management. The first and most important step in the management of patients with diarrhea, regardless of etiology, is the correction of fluid and electrolyte imbalance (Fig. 104-1). Careful monitoring of the patient's physical examination and laboratory parameters will help to guide replacement therapy. Most likely, free water, sodium, potassium, phosphorus, magnesium, and possibly bicarbonate replacement will be needed. If fluid losses are particularly severe or the patient's circulatory status is tenuous or compromised, central venous access and monitoring are essential. The physician and nursing staff should ensure that proper patient hygiene and skin care are maintained. Suspected infectious causes of diarrhea warrant patient isolation and enteric precautions until the diagnosis is made and proper treatment instituted.

Therapy of Iatrogenic Causes. Iatrogenic causes of diarrhea are among the most readily diagnosed and easily treated etiologies. Suspect medications, especially antibiotics, should be withdrawn or changed to those less likely to cause diarrhea.

If the diagnosis of pseudomembranous colitis is suspected or made, the offending agent should be discontinued immediately, especially in severe cases (Table 104-3). In some patients, antibiotic discontinuance alone, without definitive treatment, may result in spontaneous improvement or resolution of symptoms. In milder cases, the antibiotic may be continued concurrently with therapy for *C. difficile* or changed to an agent with a lower associated incidence. Vancomycin administered by the enteral route has been a time-honored and highly efficacious therapy, resulting in improvement in over 95 percent of patients [32]. High intestinal concentrations, uniform susceptibility of the organism, and lack of systemic absorption make this agent attractive. Expense, however, is a major drawback, and with trials showing equal efficacy of oral metronidazole [33] and bacitracin [34], vancomycin should probably be reserved for treatment failures, relapses, or severe cases. Patients will generally respond within 24 to 48 hours with improvement in diarrhea, pain, fever, and leukocytosis. Relapse rates may be high, occurring in as many as 24 percent of patients [35]. Anion exchange resins, such as cholestyramine or colestipol, may be useful as adjunctive therapy in mild cases or in relapses but, based on existing data, should not be used exclusively, especially in moderate to severe diarrhea. These agents can bind vancomycin, making this combination less desirable. Treatment should be continued for 7 to 14 days. Antimotility agents should not be used because they may lengthen the course of illness [36].

Enteral feedings suspected of causing diarrhea should be reduced in volume, diluted, given by continuous infusion, or temporarily discontinued. The intravenous administration of albumin to the hypoalbuminemic patient or the use of elemental diets or peptide-based or fiber-rich formulas cannot be routinely recommended, but they may be of benefit in individual patients.

Treatment of Diarrhea Secondarily Related to Disease. Efforts should always be made to treat the underlying disease, which may or may not have an effect on the course of diarrhea. The diarrhea of sepsis will resolve as the source of sepsis is treated, whereas the diarrhea of diabetes or uremia generally will not respond to treatment of the primary disease.

Diarrhea-causing pathogens in both immunocompetent and immunocompromised hosts should be aggressively treated. Certain infections in patients with AIDS, such as CMV, *Isospora*

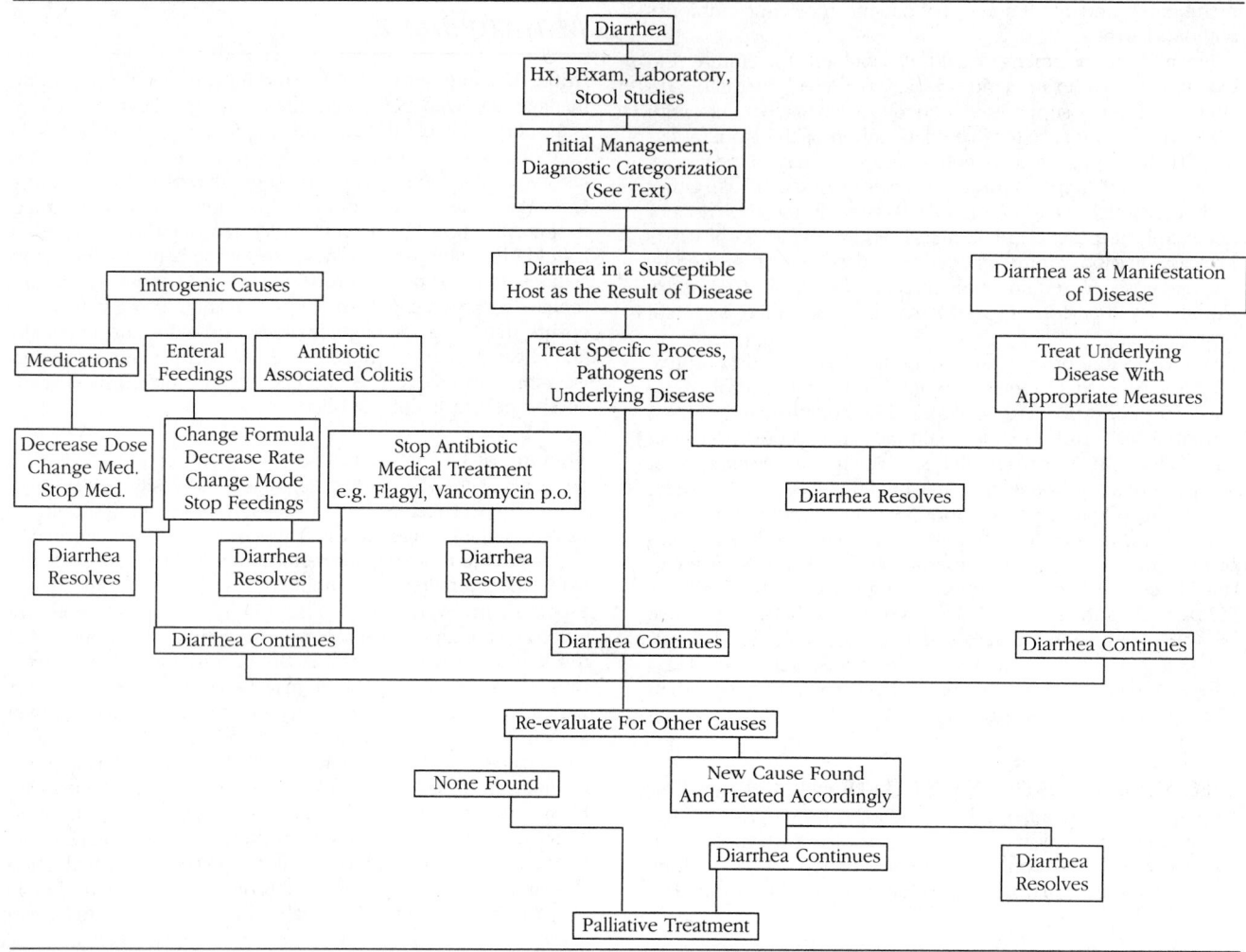

Fig. 104-1. Algorithm for management of diarrhea in the intensive care unit.

belli, *Salmonella, Shigella, Campylobacter, Giardia,* and *Entamoeba histolytica,* may be amenable to current therapy (see reference 14 for review), whereas effective treatments for MAI, *Cryptosporidium,* and *Microsporidium* are not yet available.

Patients with ischemic bowel disease without clinical signs of bowel necrosis may be managed conservatively with close observation, bowel rest, and antibiotics. Drugs that may exacerbate ischemia should be discontinued if possible. Aggressive efforts at maintaining circulatory blood volume and maximizing oxygen delivery should be emphasized. Signs of infarction or perforation warrant operative management.

Fistulas should be managed by bowel rest or surgery, depending on the clinical circumstances. Somatostatin analog may also be useful as adjunctive therapy. Postcholecystectomy diarrhea may respond to bile acid sequestrants such as cholestyramine. Surgically induced cases of short bowel syndrome or malabsorption may be aided by enteral nutrition in the form of elemental diets or, if unsuccessful, parenteral nutrition. Fecal impactions should be removed by manual disimpaction, followed by cleansing enemas consisting of tap water, Fleet's solution, water-soluble contrast medium (Gastrografin), or docusate sodium. More proximal and firm impactions can be broken up using a sigmoidoscope and a dental irrigating device (Water-

Pik), by directing the water jet into the fecal mass under direct vision. Prevention following treatment with appropriate stool wetting agents, laxatives, or enemas is paramount.

Treatment of Diarrhea as a Primary Manifestation of Disease. Every effort should be made to treat the disease responsible for the diarrheal syndrome. The general supportive measures previously discussed should be employed in all patients. Diseases such as vasculitis should be managed with corticosteroid or immunosuppressive therapy. Adrenal insufficiency will respond promptly to the administration of corticosteroids. GVHD should be managed with corticosteroids and immunosuppressive agents. The chronic form of the disease may be more effectively treated, whereas the acute variety may be less responsive, with a substantial mortality rate. The intricacies of the treatment of inflammatory bowel disease are beyond the scope of this chapter but include the aminosalicylates (e.g., sulfasalazine), corticosteroids, immunosuppressives, nutritional therapy, and surgery. Celiac sprue will respond to supportive measures and a gluten-free diet.

Palliative Measures. The aforementioned diagnostic and treatment regimen will result in proper diagnosis and directed treatment in the majority of patients with diarrhea in this setting. In a modest number of patients, however, a cause for diarrhea will not be found or a specific treatment will not be readily

Table 104-3. Treatment of Pseudomembranous Colitis

General
    Discontinue offending antibiotic if possible
    Avoid antimotility agents
    Isolation and enteric precautions
Antimicrobial
    Metronidazole 250 mg PO tid for 7–14 days
    Vancomycin 125–500 mg PO qid for 7–14 days
    Bacitracin 25,000 units PO qid for 7–14 days
Anion exchange resins (in combination with metronidazole in mild cases)
    Cholestyramine 4 gm PO tid
    Colestipol 5 gm PO tid

available. For this category of patients, palliative therapies are available to lessen fluid losses, patient discomfort, and morbidity (Table 104-4). Antimotility agents such as loperamide, diphenoxylate with atropine, and deodorized tincture of opium (DTO) may decrease frequency and severity of diarrhea in patients with diarrhea of unclear etiology or diarrhea due to enteral feeding or other noninfectious causes. Advantages of loperamide include the absence of central nervous system activity and resultant side effects, whereas DTO is administered in drop form, enhancing dosing flexibility. The availability and increased half-life of the long-acting somatostatin analog SMS 201995 (Sandostatin) allow the intermittent subcutaneous use of this drug for palliation of diarrhea in patients with AIDS, GVHD, hormone-producing tumors, and other causes of secretory diarrhea [37]. Several agents such as clonidine and the phenothiazines are under investigation as possible palliative treatment, but until further studies determine efficacy, they cannot be routinely recommended.

Conclusion

Diarrhea is a frequently occurring complication in the ICU setting. It is a symptom that tends to be overshadowed by other processes in the ICU but in and of itself may result in significant

Table 104-4. Antidiarrheal Agents and Dosages

Loperamide (Imodium)
    Available forms: capsules (2 mg) and liquid (5 ml [1 teasp] = 1 mg)
    Dosage: 4 mg initially, followed by 2 mg after each diarrheal stool
    Maximum daily recommended dose: 16 mg per day
Diphenoxylate with atropine (Lomotil)
    Available forms: 1 tablet or 5 ml liquid = 2.5 mg diphenoxylate and .025 atropine
    Dosage: 2 tablets or 10 ml four times a day (20 mg of diphenoxylate) initially, then decrease and titrate to symptoms
    Maximum daily recommended dose: 20 mg per day (based on diphenoxylate)
Deodorized opium tincture
    Available form: 10 mg morphine per milliliter
    Dosage: 0.6 ml four times a day (range: 0.3 to 1 ml four to six times a day)
    Maximum daily recommended dose: 6 ml per day
Camphorated opium tincture (Paregoric)
    Available form: 0.4 mg morphine per milliliter
    Dosage: 5–10 ml one to four times a day
    Maximum daily recommended dose: 40 ml per day

morbidity. In most instances, however, it can be managed with the institution of proper diagnostic, treatment, or palliative measures.

References

1. Kelly TWJ, Patrick MR, Hillman KM, et al: Study of diarrhea in critically ill patients. *Crit Care Med* 11:7, 1983.
2. Brinson RR, Kolts BE: Hypoalbuminemia as an indicator of diarrheal incidence in critically ill patients. *Crit Care Med* 15:506, 1987.
3. Dark DS, Pingleton SK: Nonhemorrhagic gastrointestinal complications in acute respiratory failure. *Crit Care Med* 17:755, 1989.
4. Fine KD, Krejs GJ, Fordtran JS: Diarrhea-definitions, in Sleisenger MH, Fordtran JS (eds): *Gastrointestinal Disease.* 4th ed. Philadelphia: WB Saunders, 1989, pp 290–316.
5. Keohane PP, Attrill H, Love M, et al: Relation between osmolality of diet and gastrointestinal side effects in enteral nutrition. *BMJ* 288:678, 1984.
6. Grube BJ, Heimbach DM, Marvin JA: *Clostridium difficile* diarrhea in critically ill burned patients. *Arch Surg* 122:655, 1987.
7. Lyerly DM, Krivan HC, Wilkins TD: *Clostridium difficile*: Its diseases and toxins. *Clin Microbiol Rev* 1:1, 1988.
8. Edes TE, Walk BE, Austin JL: Diarrhea in tube fed patients: Feeding formula not necessarily the cause. *Am J Med* 88:91, 1990.
9. Cataldi-Betcher EL, Seltzer MH, Slocum BA, Jones KW: Complications occurring during enteral nutritional support: A prospective study. *JPEN* 7:546, 1983.
10. Keohane PP, Attril H, Jones BJM, et al: Roles of lactose and *Clostridium difficile* in the pathogenesis of enteral feeding associated diarrhoea. *Clin Nutrition* 1:259, 1983.
11. McHugh P, Moran T: Calories and gastric emptying: A regulatory capacity with implications for feeding. *Am J Physiol* 236:254, 1979.
12. Randall HT: Enteral nutrition: Tube feeding in acute and chronic illness. *JPEN* 8:113, 1984.
13. Ford EG, Jennings LM, Andrassy RJ: Serum albumin (oncotic pressure) correlates with enteral feeding tolerance in the pediatric surgical patient. *J Pediatr Surg* 22:7, 1987.
14. Rodgers VD, Kagnoff MF: Gastrointestinal manifestations of the acquired immunodeficiency syndrome. *West J Med* 146:57, 1987.
15. Santangelo WC, Krejs GJ: Southwestern Internal Medicine Conference. The gastrointestinal manifestations of the acquired immunodeficiency syndrome. *Am J Med Sci* 292:328, 1986.
16. Baker RW, Peppercorn MA: Gastrointestinal ailments of homosexual men. *Medicine* 61:390, 1982.
17. Kotler DP, Gaetz HP, Lange M, et al: Enteropathy associated with the acquired immunodeficiency syndrome. *Ann Intern Med* 101:421, 1984.
18. Weber JN, Carmichael DJ, Boylston A, et al: Kaposi's sarcoma of the bowel presenting as apparent ulcerative colitis. *Gut* 26:295, 1985.
19. Starnes HF, Moore FD, Mentzer S, et al: Abdominal pain in neutropenic cancer patients. *Cancer* 57:616, 1986.
20. Ernst CB, Hagihara PF, Daugherty ME, et al: Ischemic colitis incidence following aortic reconstruction: A prospective study. *Surgery* 80:417, 1976.
21. Sakai L, Keltner R, Kaminski D: Spontaneous and shock-associated ischemic colitis. *Am J Surg* 140:755, 1980.
22. Mueller PD, Benowitz NL: Toxicologic causes of acute abdominal disorders. *Emerg Med Clin North Am* 7:667, 1989.
23. Chang EB, Bergenstal RM, Field M: Diarrhea in streptozocin treated rats. *J Clin Invest* 75:1666, 1985.
24. Whalen GE, Soergel KH, Geenen JE: Diabetic diarrhea. *Gastroenterology* 56:1021, 1969.
25. McDonald GB, Shulman HM, Sullivan KM, Spencer GD: Intestinal and hepatic complications of human bone marrow transplantation. Part I. *Gastroenterology* 90:460, 1986.
26. McDonald GB, Shulman HM, Sullivan KM, Spencer GD: Intestinal and hepatic complications of human bone marrow transplantation. Part II. *Gastroenterology* 90:770, 1986.
27. Siegel DL, Edelstein PH, Nachamkin I: Inappropriate testing for diarrheal diseases in the hospital. *JAMA* 263:979, 1990.

28. Fine KD, Krejs GJ, Fordtran JS: Diarrhea, and Gorbach SL: Infectious diarrhea, in Sleisenger MH, Fordtran JS (eds): *Gastrointestinal Disease*. 4th ed. Philadelphia, WB Saunders, 1989, pp 290–316 and pp 1191–1232.
29. Bartlett JG, Taylor NW, Chang TW, et al: Clinical and laboratory observations in *Clostridium difficile* colitis. *Am J Clin Nutr* 33:2521, 1981.
30. Viscidi R, Willey S, Bartlett JG: Isolation rates and toxigenic potential for *Clostridium difficile* isolates from various patient populations. *Gastroenterology* 81:5, 1981.
31. Tedesco FJ, Corless JK, Brownstein RE: Rectal sparing in antibiotic-associated pseudomembranous colitis: A prospective study. *Gastroenterology* 83:1259, 1982.
32. Bartlett JG: Treatment of *Clostridium difficile* colitis. *Gastroenterology* 89:1192, 1985.
33. Teasley DG, Gerding DN, Olson M, et al: Prospective randomized trial of metronidazole versus vancomycin for *Clostridium difficile* associated diarrhea and colitis. *Lancet* 2:1043, 1983.
34. Young GP, Ward PB, Bayley N: Antibiotic-associated colitis due to *Clostridium difficile*: Double blind comparison of vancomycin with bacitracin. *Gastroenterology* 89:1038, 1985.
35. Bartlett JG, Tedesco FJ, Schull S, et al: Relapse following oral vancomycin therapy of antibiotic-associated pseudomembranous colitis. *Gastroenterology* 78:431, 1979.
36. Tedesco FJ, Napier J, Gamble W, et al: Therapy of antibiotic-associated pseudomembranous colitis. *J Clin Gastroenterol* 1:51, 1979.
37. Gorden P, Comi RJ, Maton PN, Go VLW: Somatostatin and somatostatin analogue (SMS 201995) in treatment of hormone-secreting tumors of the pituitary and gastrointestinal tract and non-neoplastic diseases of the gut. *Ann Intern Med* 110:35, 1989.

105. Severe and Complicated Biliary Tract Disease

Steven A. Edmundowicz
and Daniel Picus

A wide spectrum of biliary tract diseases may be seen in the intensive care unit (ICU). Presentations vary from mildly abnormal blood chemistries to life-threatening septic shock. Unrecognized biliary disease can lead to significant morbidity. Awareness of the different biliary disorders commonly encountered in the ICU, in conjunction with a logical approach to invasive and noninvasive patient evaluation, will allow the clinician to diagnose and treat these conditions appropriately.

Approximately 500 ml per day of bile are secreted into the biliary tree at the level of the canaliculus in the hepatic lobule. Bile flows through progressively larger ductules until reaching the main intrahepatic duct system. Flow into the duodenum and gallbladder is regulated by the sphincter of Oddi. Tonic contraction of the sphincter increases pressure in the common bile duct and allows the gallbladder to fill from the cystic duct. Relaxation of the sphincter of Oddi in the postprandial state is thought to be mediated by cholecystokinin, a hormone well known to stimulate gallbladder contraction. The anatomy of the biliary tree is demonstrated in Figure 105-1. Access to the biliary tree for diagnostic and therapeutic purposes may be obtained percutaneously, operatively through the peritoneal cavity, and endoscopically by cannulation of the ampulla in the second duodenum.

Diagnostic Evaluation

PHYSICAL EXAMINATION. Physical signs in patients with biliary tract disease may encompass a spectrum from the acute abdomen with localized right upper quadrant pain to less impressive or nonspecific findings, such as fever or ileus. When biliary tract disease is suspected, careful inspection and examination for findings of icterus, hepatomegaly, ascites, and focal tenderness over the liver should be undertaken.

LABORATORY EVALUATION. In the obtunded or otherwise compromised ICU patient, abnormal laboratory values are often the first clue to biliary tract disease. All ICU patients should have appropriate laboratory testing on admission, including serum bilirubin, alkaline phosphatase, and aspartate aminotransferase (AST, SGOT) or alanine aminotransferase (ALT, SGPT). In acutely ill patients, bilirubin elevation is common and may be due to sepsis, drug effects, hemolysis, or other non-biliary etiologies (see Chap. 107). Biliary tract causes of bilirubin elevation should be included in the differential diagnosis if fractionation yields an elevated direct (conjugated) level that is associated with abnormalities of other liver enzymes.

Alkaline phosphatase elevation is often seen in patients with biliary tract disease. Alkaline phosphatase may be released from other tissues in the body (e.g., bone, placenta), and, therefore, it is not a specific test for hepatobiliary disease. Hepatobiliary origin for an elevated serum level of this enzyme can be confirmed by isoenzyme analysis or by detection of concomitantly elevated 5' nucleotidase or gamma-glutamyltransferase.

Serum transaminase elevations are the hallmark of hepatocellular injury. AST (SGOT) and ALT (SGPT) elevation can also be seen in patients with biliary tract disease, especially when an inflammatory or infectious etiology is present. Occasionally, a patient with significant biliary tract disease may present with a normal laboratory evaluation, as in cholecystitis without involvement of the common bile duct and without substantial pericholecystic hepatitis.

NONINVASIVE IMAGING STUDIES. Noninvasive radiologic imaging is essential in the evaluation of patients with suspected biliary tract disease.

Plain Abdominal Radiograph. The plain radiographic features of biliary tract disease usually are nonspecific. The most common bowel gas finding seen in patients with acute biliary

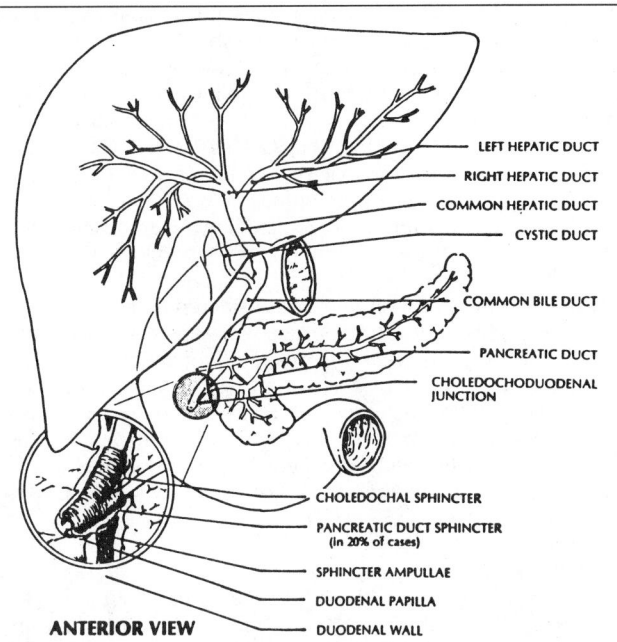

LEFT HEPATIC DUCT
RIGHT HEPATIC DUCT
COMMON HEPATIC DUCT
CYSTIC DUCT
COMMON BILE DUCT
PANCREATIC DUCT
CHOLEDOCHODUODENAL JUNCTION
CHOLEDOCHAL SPHINCTER
PANCREATIC DUCT SPHINCTER (In 20% of cases)
SPHINCTER AMPULLAE
DUODENAL PAPILLA
ANTERIOR VIEW
DUODENAL WALL

Fig. 105-1. Normal anatomy of the biliary tract. (From Turner MA, Cho S-R, Messmer JM: Pitfalls in cholangiographic interpretation. *Radiographics* 7:1067, 1987, with permission.)

disease is a generalized ileus. Gallstones are rarely detected on plain radiographs, since only 10 to 15 percent of stones will have a sufficient calcium concentration to make them radiopaque. Air in the biliary tree, in the absence of a known biliary enteric fistula, prior sphincterotomy, or surgical anastomosis, is strongly suggestive of biliary tract infection with gas-producing organisms.

Ultrasonography. Ultrasonography of the biliary tree is an extremely useful technique in the ICU setting and can be performed at the bedside with good results. It is a sensitive test for determining biliary duct dilatation, and the accuracy of ultrasonography in detecting cholelithiasis exceeds 95 percent. Findings on ultrasonography that indicate acute gallbladder disease include focal tenderness over the gallbladder, thickening of the gallbladder wall, and pericholecystic fluid collections. The technique may also detect other abnormalities, including choledocholithiasis, liver lesions, pancreatic masses, and ascites.

Hepatobiliary Scanning. Scanning the abdomen following an intravenous injection of technetium 99m (^{99m}Tc) iminodiacetic acid (HIDA) yields both physiologic and structural information regarding the biliary tract. Filling of the gallbladder with radionuclide confirms the patency of the cystic duct and virtually excludes the diagnosis of acute cholecystitis. False-positive examinations can be seen in patients with chronic cholecystitis, on long-term parenteral hyperalimentation, or following prolonged fasting. However, delayed views and routine pretreatment with cholecystokinin increase the accuracy of HIDA scanning for acute cholecystitis to greater than 95 percent [1].

Hepatobiliary scanning is also useful in identifying structural abnormalities of the biliary tree. Significant bile duct leaks can be identified in almost all patients with this entity. Scanning has a limited role in patients with poor hepatocellular function,

complete biliary obstruction, and cholangitis because these defects often prevent adequate uptake or excretion of the radiopharmaceutical into the biliary tree.

Computed Tomography. Computed tomography (CT) is highly accurate for the detection of biliary tract disease. Unfortunately, unlike ultrasonography or radionuclide scanning, CT cannot be used portably in the ICU. Findings on CT for gallbladder disease include thickening of the gallbladder wall, pericholecystic fluid, and adjacent abscesses. Additionally, CT is highly accurate for the detection of biliary tract obstruction, both the level and the cause. Frequently, the area of the head of the pancreas will be obscured on ultrasonographic studies because of overlying bowel gas. CT generally provides better images of the bile duct in the region of the head of the pancreas, especially in acutely ill patients.

Summary. When evaluating the ICU patient with suspected biliary tract disease, ultrasonography and hepatobiliary scanning should be the initial procedures of choice. Both are portable and noninvasive. Ultrasonography is highly accurate for the detection of calculi as well as structural pathology. Hepatobiliary scanning, on the other hand, provides physiologic information, primarily regarding patency of the cystic duct. Such physiologic data are especially important for patients with suspected calculous or acalculous cholecystitis. CT should be reserved for those patients in whom sonographic or radionuclide findings are equivocal or in whom ductal dilatation is seen without a clearly defined etiology.

INVASIVE DIAGNOSTIC TESTS

Endoscopic Retrograde Cholangiopancreatography. The technique of endoscopic retrograde cholangiopancreatography (ERCP) is described in some detail in Chapter 19. A side-viewing endoscope is passed through the mouth into the second duodenum, where the ampulla of Vater is identified and cannulated. The biliary tree is then opacified with contrast medium injected through a plastic cannula, allowing a retrograde cholangiogram to be obtained. Fluoroscopy and standard radiographs are used to examine the biliary tree and define such abnormalities as stones, strictures, leaks, and obstruction. ERCP can be used in the evaluation and therapy of the ICU patient as long as the patient can be stabilized for endoscopy and transported to a fluoroscopy room. Rarely, it is necessary to perform emergent biliary decompression at the bedside using portable fluoroscopy. Patients usually require some form of intravenous conscious sedation with benzodiazepines or narcotics, but in the critically ill this can be omitted. Reversible coagulopathies should be corrected prior to the procedure, especially if an endoscopic sphincterotomy (incision of the sphincter of Oddi in the duodenal wall for stone removal or drainage) is anticipated. Major morbidity from the diagnostic procedure includes pancreatitis, cholangitis, perforation, and hemorrhage. These complications occur in less than 10 percent of patients under standard conditions. ERCP can be highly successful in the delineation and treatment of biliary disease in the ICU patient.

Percutaneous Transhepatic Cholangiography. Percutaneous transhepatic cholangiography (PTC) may also be used in evaluating the ICU patient. The technique requires high-quality fluoroscopic guidance and transport of the patient to the interventional radiology suite. The use of PTC for the diagnosis of biliary tract pathology has been supplanted primarily by less invasive examinations, such as ultrasonography and CT, as well as ERCP. Currently, PTC is used primarily as an initial step in percutaneous transhepatic biliary drainage. Decompression of the biliary tree via a percutaneous catheter is a highly effective method for rapid nonoperative biliary decompression. Indications for the procedure in the ICU patient include sepsis from cholangitis, postoperative bile leak, and the treatment of biliary tract calculi. The technique involves initial PTC followed by puncture of an appropriate intrahepatic bile duct with an 18-gauge needle. A guide wire is then passed into the biliary tree. The tract is dilated and a drainage catheter placed. This catheter can be left either to external drainage or passed through the obstruction into the duodenum and capped to internal drainage. Successful drainage can be established in almost all patients. Percutaneous biliary drainage is an invasive procedure, and major acute complications occur in 5 to 10 percent of patients. These complications include hemorrhage, sepsis, and bile leakage. Sepsis most commonly occurs in patients who have been obstructed chronically. Extreme care must be taken to avoid extensive manipulations in these patients before establishing drainage.

Percutaneous Liver Biopsy. Liver biopsy is an important technique in the evaluation of selected patients with hepatobiliary abnormalities. A rapid pathologic diagnosis can be made in the patient with intrinsic liver disease, and tissue can be cultured for bacterial, viral, and fungal organisms. Microscopic analysis of the specimen may also provide information regarding unexpected diagnoses, response to therapy, and prognosis. The biopsy is performed at the bedside. Ultrasonographic localization may be needed in patients in whom ascites is suspected or in those with small livers or right-sided pleural effusions. Risks of the procedure primarily include hemorrhage and inadvertent damage to surrounding organs such as lung, kidney, or bowel. Liver biopsy should be employed only in those patients who would benefit from the procedure and in whom the results of biopsy are likely to dictate a change in management. Any coagulopathy must be corrected prior to standard percutaneous biopsy. In some patients with prolonged bleeding times or uncorrectable prothrombin times, a biopsy may be obtained by way of the hepatic vein using a transjugular approach [2] or percutaneously using a sheath, embolizing the tract with Gelfoam following completion of the biopsy [3].

Biliary Tract Disorders Encountered in the Intensive Care Unit

CHOLANGITIS. Acute cholangitis occurs when bacterial infection of the biliary tree is associated with an elevated intraductal pressure that allows reflux of bacteria or endotoxins into the bloodstream. The presentation of patients with cholangitis may range from intermittent low-grade fevers to fulminant septic shock. This diagnosis must be considered and excluded in all patients who present to the ICU with shock and sepsis of unknown origin because it is associated with an extremely high mortality in such patients if urgent biliary decompression is not accomplished. Because partial or complete biliary obstruction is thought to be a prerequisite, the occurrence of cholangitis is restricted to those patients with biliary stasis secondary to stones, strictures, or recent manipulations of the biliary tree [4].

The clinical manifestations of cholangitis include fever or chills, abdominal pain, and jaundice. The classic triad of fever, right upper quadrant pain, and jaundice was described by Char-

cot [5] in 1877, and is seen in a small percentage of patients presenting with cholangitis today [4]. Laboratory abnormalities are present in the overwhelming majority of patients, with more than 90 percent having elevation of bilirubin, alkaline phosphatase, or transaminases. Blood cultures are positive in the minority of patients in most series (44–47%) [6,7]. When bacteremia is documented, solitary isolates of *Escherichia coli, Klebsiella pneumoniae,* or enterococcus are found most commonly. Polymicrobial infections including anaerobes are identified frequently if bile is cultured at operation [6,8]. Often it is difficult to prospectively diagnose cholangitis in the ICU population, and this entity should be considered in the differential diagnosis of all patients who present with sepsis. Although most patients with cholangitis will respond to antibiotic therapy alone, those with biliary obstruction may progress to a more fulminant state despite general resuscitative measures and broad-spectrum antibiotics. These patients must be identified rapidly and treated with emergent biliary decompression by endoscopic, percutaneous, or surgical means if therapy is to be successful.

Treatment. Once cholangitis is suspected, the patient should be treated empirically with broad-spectrum antibiotics [7]. Recent controlled trials have demonstrated the utility of the extended-spectrum penicillins in this setting. In the septic patient it is reasonable to begin with broad-spectrum antibiotic coverage for both aerobic and anaerobic organisms until a clear response is seen. The regimen can then be tapered to a more specific therapy pending the results of cultures.

Patients who do not respond rapidly to resuscitative efforts and who have evidence of complete obstruction by laboratory or imaging studies should undergo emergent biliary decompression. This can be accomplished by endoscopic, percutaneous, or surgical means. Selection of a particular approach should be tailored to the patient's condition as well as local expertise and the rapid availability of the procedure. Initial efforts in decompensated patients should concentrate solely on decompression of the biliary tree. Definitive therapy may be completed at a later time even if this requires a second laparotomy. It must be recognized that even with modern support, biliary decompressive techniques, and broad-spectrum antibiotics, the mortality for acute fulminant cholangitis approaches 50 percent [8,9].

BILIARY OBSTRUCTION. Biliary obstruction may present in the ICU patient without cholangitis. The multiple causes of biliary obstruction are listed in Table 105-1, the most common being stone disease, benign stricture, and malignancy. The patient with physical findings and laboratory studies suggesting obstruction should be evaluated with noninvasive imaging to verify and define the level of obstruction. In the noninfected patient an elective direct cholangiogram by ERCP or PTC should be obtained when the patient's condition allows. This provides anatomic details of the biliary tree and allows one to plan definitive therapy. Care must be taken to ensure that the entire biliary tree is visualized at cholangiography and that adequate prophylactic antibiotics are administered. In addition, adequate drainage following the procedure is essential to prevent the development of cholangitis.

Treatment. Biliary obstruction without cholangitis is seen more often with malignancy than with stone disease or inflammatory strictures. The diagnosis can usually be made prior to laparotomy with ERCP or PTC. Definitive therapy for stone disease and palliative therapy for benign and malignant strictures may also be accomplished during either procedure. Re-

Table 105-1. Causes of Biliary Obstruction

I. Intrinsic lesions
    Stones
    Cholangiocarcinoma
    Benign stricture
    Sclerosing cholangitis
    Periarteritis nodosa
    Ampullary stenosis
    Parasites
II. Extrinsic lesions
    Pancreatic carcinoma
    Metastatic carcinoma
    Pancreatitis
    Pancreatic pseudocyst
    Visceral artery aneurysm
    Lymphadenopathy
    Choledochal cyst
    Hepatic cyst or cysts
    Duodenal diverticulum
III. Iatrogenic lesions
    Postoperative stricture
    Hepatic artery infusion chemotherapy

cent reviews of endoscopic or transhepatic stenting of malignancies demonstrate the utility of these approaches when compared with surgical decompression for unresectable disease [10,11]. Surgical approaches are preferred in those patients who are good operative candidates and who may have resectable malignancy, symptomatic cholelithiasis requiring therapy, or duodenal or gastric outlet obstruction in the setting of unresectable malignancy.

BILIARY FISTULA. Leakage of bile into the peritoneal cavity or pleural space is an uncommon complication of biliary disease. Biliary-enteric fistulas occur in association with stone disease of the biliary tract but are usually not a significant management problem. Iatrogenic bile duct fistulas can be seen after open or laparoscopic cholecystectomy. The resultant bile peritonitis usually is associated with abdominal pain, ascites, leukocytosis, and fever. The occasional patient may present with only new-onset ascites and an elevated serum bilirubin level. Diagnosis of a biliary fistula can usually be made with hepatobiliary scanning. This can be followed by ERCP or PTC to determine the exact location of the leak.

Treatment. Patients with suspected biliary fistulas should be placed on broad-spectrum antibiotics, and the presence of a bile leak should be confirmed with hepatobiliary scanning followed by direct cholangiography. ERCP or PTC should be performed as soon as possible after a bile leak is identified in order to limit the degree of bile leakage and patient symptoms. Postoperative cystic duct leak or premature removal of a T-tube can often be managed definitively with endoscopic decompression at the same setting as ERCP. Larger bile duct leaks or those associated with ischemia, trauma, or surgical anastomosis are more complicated and eventually may require surgical repair or bypass.

ACUTE CHOLECYSTITIS. Although the diagnosis can be suspected on clinical grounds alone, the use of noninvasive testing, including ultrasonography and hepatobiliary scanning, is essential before embarking on a potentially hazardous therapeutic course. Acalculous cholecystitis deserves special mention as it can result in significant morbidity and mortality in the ICU pa-

tient [12]. Although the signs and symptoms may be similar to those seen with calculous cholecystitis, the presentation in the postoperative or acutely ill ICU patient may be masked by the complicated underlying situation. In this setting an aggressive diagnostic and therapeutic approach is essential, because mortality from complicated acalculous cholecystitis may approach 50 percent.

Treatment. Supportive measures should be undertaken while the patient is evaluated with noninvasive testing. Antibiotic therapy with broad-spectrum coverage should be initiated in patients with clinical evidence of sepsis, leukocytosis, or fever. Percutaneous cholecystostomy has become the therapy of choice for those patients with acute calculous or acalculous cholecystitis who do not respond to conservative therapy and are too unstable for operative cholecystectomy. Percutaneous cholecystostomy is performed at the bedside using ultrasonographic guidance. A 22-gauge needle is inserted into the gallbladder, and bile is aspirated. A guide wire is passed through this needle and the tract is dilated, allowing placement of a drainage catheter. Success rates exceeding 95 percent are generally reported. Complications are few and include local wound infection, bleeding, and rarely bile peritonitis.

The primary advantage of percutaneous cholecystostomy is that it can be done at the bedside without general anesthesia. Percutaneous cholecystostomy is often helpful in patients with suspected gallbladder disease, even if cholecystitis is not found, by excluding the diagnosis. Therefore, percutaneous cholecystostomy should be performed early if gallbladder disease is suspected. Unfortunately, simple aspiration of bile from the gallbladder for Gram stain and culture has not been shown to be sensitive for the diagnosis of acute cholecystitis. Therefore, once the diagnosis is suspected a drainage catheter should be placed in the gallbladder.

A cholecystostomy drainage catheter is left in place until the patient's symptoms resolve, at which time an elective cholecystectomy may be performed. Alternatively, in patients with acute acalculous cholecystitis, percutaneous cholecystostomy may be the sole method of treatment. Frequently, in these patients, the cholecystostomy tube can eventually be removed when the cystic duct becomes patent without the need for a cholecystectomy. In patients with acute calculous cholecystitis and severe underlying medical problems, the gallstones can be removed through the percutaneous tract using various techniques [13]. Such percutaneous gallstone removal is an effective alternate therapy to cholecystectomy for patients with other significant medical conditions.

GALLSTONE PANCREATITIS. Acute pancreatitis often results from biliary stone disease. Although most cases are self-limited and respond to conservative management, fulminant pancreatitis may occur with a mortality in excess of 10 percent. There are several theories regarding the pathogenesis of gallstone pancreatitis. The evidence suggests that stone passage or impaction in the ampulla is likely responsible for this entity. Gallstone pancreatitis should be considered and excluded in the evaluation of all patients with acute pancreatitis because it is a recurrent and treatable cause of this presentation. Standard abdominal ultrasonography in combination with laboratory screening for biliary obstruction can be used to exclude gallstones as the cause for the pancreatitis in most patients [14]. Patients with acute pancreatitis should be classified into risk groups based on one of the accepted prognostic scales [15,16]. These prognostic scales allow physicians to identify those patients who are at risk for developing severe pancreatitis and a complicated hospital course. A scale derived for use in patients with gallstone pancreatitis has been described by Osborn and co-workers [17]. Any patient who has more than two of the following criteria at any time during the first 48 hours of hospitalization would be classified as having severe pancreatitis:

1. WBC greater than 15,000 cells per cubic millimeter[3]
2. Blood glucose greater than 180 mg per milliliter
3. BUN greater than 45 mg per deciliter
4. Arterial pO_2 less than 60 mm Hg
5. Serum calcium less than 8.0 mg per deciliter
6. Serum albumin less than 3.2 gm per deciliter
7. Serum LDH greater than 600 units per liter
8. AST or ALT greater than 200 units per liter

Treatment. Patients with acute pancreatitis from biliary stone disease should be managed initially as detailed in Chapter 160. Although most patients will improve with conservative therapy alone, those patients with severe pancreatitis appear to benefit from early intervention with ERCP and endoscopic sphincterotomy [18,19]. Early ERCP as advocated by some authors allows removal of impacted or retained common bile duct stones, limiting further pancreatic inflammation and preventing cholangitis. Consultation with a skilled biliary endoscopist should be obtained early in the course of all patients with severe gallstone pancreatitis. ERCP should be considered in those patients who do not improve with 24 hours of conservative therapy. It generally is accepted that patients with gallstone pancreatitis require definitive therapy to prevent recurrent bouts of pancreatitis. This may be accomplished by cholecystectomy or endoscopic sphincterotomy in nonoperative candidates. Although debate continues regarding the timing of surgery, generally it is accepted that all patients who are operative candidates should undergo cholecystectomy during the initial hospital admission after the pancreatitis has subsided [20]. Early operative intervention in patients with gallstone pancreatitis has been associated with unacceptably high morbidity [20].

References

1. Weissman HS, Badia J, Sugarman LA, et al: Spectrum of cholescintographic patterns in acute cholecystitis. *Radiology* 138:167, 1981.
2. Gamble P, Colapinto RF, Stronell RD, et al: Transjugular liver biopsy: A review of 461 biopsies. *Radiology* 157:589, 1985.
3. Chuang VP, Alspaugh JP: Sheath needle for liver biopsy in high-risk patients. *Radiology* 166:261, 1988.
4. Pitt HA, Couse WF: Biliary sepsis and toxic cholangitis, in Moody FG (ed): *Surgical Treatment of Digestive Disease.* Chicago, Year Book Medical Publishers, 1990, p 332.
5. Charcot JM: Lecons sur les maladies du foie des voiesbiliaires et des viens. Paris, Faculte de Medecine de Paris. Recueilles et publiees par Bourneville et Sevestre, 1877.
6. Pitt HA, Postier RG, Cameron JL: Consequences of preoperative cholangitis and its treatment on the outcome of surgery for choledocholithiasis. *Surgery* 94:447, 1983.
7. Sinanan MN: Acute cholangitis. *Infect Dis Clin North Am* 6(3):571, 1992.
8. Boey JH, Way LU: Acute cholangitis. *Ann Surg* 191:264, 1980.
9. Thompson JE, Tompkins RK, Longwire WP Jr: Factors in the management of acute cholangitis. *Ann Surg* 195:137, 1982.
10. Brandabur JJ, Kozarek RA, Ball TJ, et al: Non-operative versus operative treatment of obstructive jaundice in pancreatic cancer: Cost and survival analysis. *Am J Gastroenterol* 83:1132, 1988.
11. Shepherd HA, Royle G, Ross APR, et al: Endoscopic biliary endoprosthesis in the palliation of malignant obstruction of the distal common bile duct: A randomized trial. *Br J Surg* 75:1166, 1988.
12. Babb RR: Acute acalculous cholecystitis. *J Clin Gastroenterol* 15(3):238, 1992.
13. Picus D, Hicks ME, Darcy MD, et al: Percutaneous cholecystolithotomy: Analysis of results and complications in 58 consecutive patients. *Radiology* 183(3):799, 1992.
14. Wang SS, Lin XZ, Tsai YT, et al: Clinical significance of ultrasonography, computed tomography, and biochemical tests in the rapid diagnosis of gallstone-related pancreatitis: A prospective study. *Pancreas* 3:153, 1988.
15. Ranson JHC: Etiological and prognostic factors in human acute pancreatitis: A review. *Am J Gastroenterol* 77:623, 1982.
16. Leese T, Shaw D: Comparison of the Glasgow Multifactor Prognostic Scoring Systems in acute pancreatitis. *Br J Surg* 75:460, 1988.
17. Osborne DH, Imrie CW, Carter DC: Biliary surgery in the same admission for gallstone-associated pancreatitis. *Br J Surg* 68:751, 1981.
18. Carr-Locke DL: Role of endoscopy in gallstone pancreatitis. *Am J Surg* 165(4):519, 1993.
19. Fan ST, Edward CS, Lai EC, et al: Early treatment of acute biliary pancreatitis by endoscopic papillotomy. *N Engl J Med* 328(4):228, 1993.
20. Kelly TR, Wagner DS: Gallstone pancreatitis: A prospective randomized trial of the timing of surgery. *Surgery* 104:600, 1988.

106. Complications of Gastrointestinal Procedures

Nadim G. Haddad and
Stanley B. Benjamin

A wide array of gastroenterologic procedures have become a part of the diagnostic and therapeutic armamentarium. Despite the frequent use of these procedures, complications remain remarkably uncommon (Table 106-1). Complications are a part of any procedural specialty and must be anticipated and appropriately treated. Complications associated with endoscopic procedures vary from those related to medications used for conscious sedation to those specific to the type of procedure performed. In this chapter the potential complications of gastrointestinal (GI) procedures and their management are reviewed, the primary focus being on endoscopic procedures.

Complications Related to Medications Used for Conscious Sedation

The success of many GI procedures depends on the use of conscious sedation, i.e., the production of sedation and amnesia to provide a relaxed patient who remains capable of responding and maintaining protective reflexes. Conscious sedation differs from anesthesia, whereby protective reflexes are lost. Surveys from the United States and the United Kingdom indicate that conscious sedation has become the standard for GI endoscopy and that both endoscopists and patients prefer that some form of premedication is employed [8,9]. The spectrum of untoward effects related to medications includes cardiopulmonary, allergic, paradoxical, and local reactions, and reactions to agents used to reverse conscious sedation (see Chap. 155).

CARDIOPULMONARY COMPLICATIONS. Changes in the patient's cardiopulmonary status are common during endoscopy. Arrhythmias related to anxiety or vagal effects are often detected. Serious cardiopulmonary events are uncommon and have hypoxemia as their most common cause. Although several factors can contribute to the hypoxemia seen during upper endoscopy (topical anesthesia, placement of the endoscope in the hypopharynx), premedications make the largest contribution [10–16]. Benzodiazepines, often used in combination with narcotic analgesics, represent the most common medications administerd prior to GI endoscopy. Both types of medications are known to cause some degree of respiratory depression, but the degree and significance of respiratory depression and hypoxemia seen during endoscopic examinations are extremely variable principally because of variability in patient response. Patients with chronic obstructive lung disease or those 65 years of age or older are more likely to have respiratory depression [15].

These observations are of particular relevance in patients with coronary artery disease in whom hypoxemia may produce life-threatening complications. Thorough evaluation prior to the procedure, careful administration of the medications at reduced doses, and pulse oximetry at least in high-risk patients may help prevent hypoxemic complications. Oxygen administration via nasal cannula during endoscopy reduces the likelihood of hypoxemia in patients at risk of respiratory complications [17], but this practice is not uniformly recommended.

Midazolam, a water-soluble benzodiazepine, was initially commonly believed to cause significant respiratory depression. In a recent publication analyzing data from 21,011 patients, midazolam did not place patients at greater risk of cardiopulmonary complications than did diazepam, even in the population over age 65 [18].

ALLERGIC AND LOCAL REACTIONS. True allergy to sedative/narcotic premedication used for conscious sedation is extremely rare and does not represent a significant risk to the patient. The real risk for anaphylaxis exists in those situations wherein antibiotics and IV contrast must be used (see Chap. 217). Antibiotics are currently administered in patients at risk for endocarditis, as discussed in the following. Although water-soluble contrast agents are used during endoscopic retrograde cholangiopancreatography (ERCP), anaphylaxis has not been reported. The reason is not clear, as water-soluble contrast administered during ERCP enters the vascular compartment (evidenced by the presence of nephrograms during or after the study) [19]. If a decision is made to pretreat for dye allergy, corticosteroids given 12 and 2 hours prior to procedure will effectively prevent anaphylaxis [20]. Erythema and phlebitis are common when diazepam is administered through a peripheral line. One advantage of the water-soluble benzodiazepine midazolam is the low incidence of venous irritation.

PARADOXICAL REACTIONS. Some patients develop emotional lability, restlessness, agitation, and even rage as opposed to a calming effect following intravenous administration of sedative medications [21,22]. Paradoxical reactions have been reported in up to 29 percent of patients, 7 percent of the reactions being pronounced. In these situations, the physician must decide if the patient is insufficiently sedated, oversedated, or having a paradoxical reaction. The same clinical features can be a reflection of hypoxemia, making the administration of further medication extremely dangerous. Pulse oximetry is employed to help make this distinction.

ADDITIONAL COMPLICATIONS OF MEDICATIONS THAT REVERSE SEDATION. Flumazenil, a benzodiazepine-receptor antagonist, blocks the actions of benzodiazepines at initial nervous system receptor sites and is effective for complete or partial reversal of the sedative effects of benzodiazepines [23]. Although flumazenil universally reverses sedation, it may not reverse hypoventilation and hypoxemia induced by the medications [24,25]. Seizures may be precipitated when this reversal agent is administered to patients who take benzodi-

Table 106-1. Incidence of Procedure-Related Complications During Gastrointestinal Endoscopy [1–7]

Type	Mortality	Cardiopulmonary	Perforation	Bleeding	Infection
EGD	0.001–0.005%	0.06–0.073%	0.008–0.1%	0.03%	0.008%
Colonoscopy	0.008–0.1%	(D) 0.04–0.13% (T) 0.03–0.32%	(D) 0.08–0.2% (T) 0.11–3%	(D) 0.02–0.045% (T) 1.9–2.7%	(D) 0.01% (T) 0.06%
ERCP	0.1–2%	0.12%	0.03–1%	0.06–3%	Pancreatitis 0.07–7.5%

D = diagnostic; t = therapeutic.

azepines chronically (11% of patients undergoing endoscopy in our institution). Naloxone, a narcotic antagonist, reverses the central nervous system and respiratory effects of narcotics (e.g., meperidine, fentanyl). Its use in patients with clinical narcotic dependence may induce withdrawal and rarely sudden death [26].

Procedure-Related Complications of Endoscopy

An overall low complication rate of gastrointestinal endoscopy has been maintained as noted in large retrospective studies. Complications and their rates vary with the procedure (e.g., a higher incidence of complications from therapeutic vs. diagnostic procedures) (see Chap. 19).

CARDIAC EVENTS. The overall cardiopulmonary complication rate in patients undergoing upper endoscopy is 0.06 percent. Serious cardiorespiratory complications are uncommon, having occurred in 5 per 1000 procedures in a collaborative study on complication rates and drug use during endoscopy [18]. Cardiac arrhythmias occur in patients undergoing upper or lower gastrointestinal endoscopy. Sinus tachycardia from the sympathomimetic stimulation related to endoscope insertion is the most common abnormality [10]. Other acute cardiac abnormalities include premature ventricular contractions and ST segment changes that usually resolve on termination of the procedure [27–32].

COMPLICATIONS OF UPPER ENDOSCOPY

Perforation. The reported incidence of perforation during diagnostic upper endoscopy varies from 0.008 to 0.1 percent of procedures [1,5,10,33]. The esophagus is perforated more commonly than the stomach. Certain predisposing factors have been noted: (1) blind passage of the endoscope through the pharynx and upper esophagus; (2) spurs in the cervical spine; (3) strictures; and (4) diverticula, especially Zenker's.

The incidence of perforation is increased with therapeutic endoscopic intervention [5,6,7,34]. Perforation is the most common serious complication of esophageal dilation and has been reported to occur in 1 to 10 percent of patients undergoing certain therapeutic or diagnostic endoscopic procedures that involve dilation. Balloon dilation of narrowings at other sites of the upper GI tract has become more widely available. The incidence of perforation from such procedures varies from 0.5 percent in patients with pyloric stenosis to 2.2 percent in patients with anastomotic strictures following gastroenterostomy [34].

Endoscopic treatment of nonvariceal bleeding sites in the

upper GI tract using laser, heat-generating probes, or injection therapy is relatively safe but can be complicated by perforation in 0.7 to 0.9 percent of cases [35]. Palliative, endoscopic management of patients with advanced esophageal carcinoma is becoming more widely used. Laser or coagulation probes are used to destroy tumor and widen the esophageal lumen. Esophageal perforation is one of the major complications and reportedly occurs in about 5 percent of patients [36,37,38].

Patients with esophageal perforation usually present with chest pain, subcutaneous emphysema, fever, and tachycardia. Most patients are diagnosed within 6 hours of the procedure, but diagnosis can be delayed up to 24 hours. Diagnosis is suspected by radiographic abnormalities on chest x-ray (pneumomediastinum, pneumoperitoneum). Esophagrams using water-soluble nonionic contrast should be obtained immediately to confirm the diagnosis and may demonstrate a contained or florid leak at the site of perforation. Management of contained esophageal perforation consists of a nonsurgical conservative approach: broad-spectrum IV antibiotics, nasoesophageal or nasogastric suction, close observation, and surgical backup [39].

Retroperitoneal, mediastinal, and subcutaneous emphysema without organ perforation as a complication of diagnostic upper endoscopy is rare [40]. This complication appears to be a benign clinical condition that resolves with conservative nonsurgical management.

Bleeding. Bleeding in patients undergoing diagnostic upper endoscopy is rare (~0.03%) [1]. Patients with underlying coagulopathy occasionally develop major bleeding after biopsy. Iatrogenic Mallory-Weiss tears occur in approximately 0.25 percent of cases [41], rarely requiring blood transfusion.

COMPLICATIONS FOLLOWING ENDOSCOPIC MANAGEMENT OF ESOPHAGEAL VARICES. Complications from endoscopic sclerotherapy occur in up to 78 percent of patients if minor complications are included [7,42,43]. Dysphagia, chest pain, and fever are common and usually transient, but perforation can occur in up to 6 percent of cases [42,43]. Other uncommon complications of sclerotherapy include pericarditis [44], disseminated intravascular coagulopathy [45], and rare but usually fatal cases of portal or mesenteric vein thrombosis [46]. The method of endoscopic variceal ligation, introduced in 1986, is based on principles similar to those of ligation of internal hemorrhoids. Because no sclerosant is used, fewer complications are expected. In a recent study comparing sclerotherapy to band ligation, esophageal strictures were more common with sclerotherapy than with ligation (33% vs. 0%) [47].

COMPLICATIONS OF FLEXIBLE SIGMOIDOSCOPY AND COLONOSCOPY

Perforation. Colonic perforation remains an important complication of colonoscopy. The reported incidence varies from

0.1 to 0.8 percent following diagnostic procedures to 0.5 to 3 percent following therapeutic colonoscopies [1–7]. Colonic perforation during a diagnostic procedure results from mechanical or pneumatic pressures [48,49,50]. Mechanical perforation, most commonly in the sigmoid colon, is usually the result of forceful insertion of the colonoscope. Colonic wall weakness (e.g., from diverticula, inflammation, radiation injury, or ischemia) may be a predisposing factor [48]. Enough intraluminal pneumatic pressure also can be generated to rupture the colon. The cecum is most susceptible to pneumatic rupture, followed in descending order by the transverse colon, sigmoid colon, and rectum [51]. The incidence of perforation is increased with therapeutic colonoscopy. Wadas and co-workers reported an incidence of perforation of 0.31 percent with the coagulation biopsy forceps [52]. Through-the-scope balloon dilations of colonic strictures are accompanied by perforation in approximately 5 percent of cases [34].

Patients with localized colonic perforation usually present within 6 to 24 hours of the procedure with localized pain and tenderness without signs of diffuse peritonitis. These "microperforations" have been well described by Christie [53] and are intermediate in the spectrum between frank perforation with peritonitis and the postpolypectomy coagulation syndrome. Pneumoperitoneum is commonly seen on x-ray films, confirming the suspicion of perforation. Conservative treatment for 48 to 72 hours is sufficient in most cases and consists of intravenous antibiotics, bowel rest, and close observation [51,54].

Patients with postpolypectomy coagulation syndrome [55] usually present within several hours of colonoscopy. Symptoms include localized pain, tenderness, guarding, and rigidity, associated with fever, tachycardia, and leukocytosis. This complication is also referred to as "serositis" or "transmucosal burn." The clinical picture is similar to that seen with localized perforation with peritonitis, except that the abdominal radiographs do not show free air. Conservative management, including antibiotics and bowel rest, is adequate; complete recovery is usually expected in 48 to 72 hours.

Free perforation into the peritoneal cavity may be recognized during the procedure if abdominal viscera and peritoneum are seen; in these situations, immediate surgery is indicated. Nonsurgical conservative management, if even appropriate, is recommended only for those with small perforations and without signs of generalized peritonitis or sepsis [55]. Surgical consultation is imperative and the clinical course must be closely monitored for signs of deterioration necessitating operative treatment.

Bleeding. Hemorrhage following diagnostic colonoscopy is rare and usually is the result of the coagulation biopsy technique. Bleeding that commonly is self-limited occurs in 0.4% of cases when this technique is used. The incidence of postpolypectomy bleeding varies from 0.5 to 2.5 percent [57,58]. Although bleeding usually occurs immediately following polypectomy, it may be delayed up to two weeks in 30 to 50 percent of cases, especially in patients on chronic anticoagulation therapy. Immediate bleeding is usually controlled during endoscopy; occasionally angiography with vasopressin infusion or embolization may be needed. In patients with persistent delayed post-polypectomy bleeding, successful hemostasis is achieved with repeat therapeutic colonoscopy [57]. Blood transfusions are rarely required.

COMPLICATIONS OF ENDOSCOPIC RETROGRADE CHOLANGIOPANCREATOGRAPHY. The most frequent complications of diagnostic ERCP are pancreatitis and cholangitis [33]. Pancreatitis occurs with an average frequency of 1

percent, requires surgical intervention in 0.03 percent of the cases, and has a mortality of 0.02 percent [6]. The etiology of post-ERCP pancreatitis is multifactorial [59]. Septic complications and cholangitis occur almost exclusively in cases of biliary obstruction if adequate drainage is not obtained post-ERCP. The complication rate increases to 5 percent when sphincterotomy is performed; hemorrhage accounts for 45 percent of the complications, and pancreatitis for 20 percent. Hemorrhage is the result of direct vascular injury or partial digestion of the vascular wall by pancreatic enzymes. Immediate bleeding can be stopped endoscopically in most cases. The presentation can be delayed up to 21 days.

In cases of benign or malignant obstruction of the pancreaticobiliary ducts, insertion of an endoprosthesis during ERCP helps ensure drainage. Possible complications of this technique include prosthesis occlusion, cholangitis, and pancreatic sepsis. Treatment consists of intravenous antibiotics and stent replacement to ensure adequate drainage.

Procedure-Related Infections

The number of infections transmitted as a direct consequence of GI procedures is exceedingly small. This is true despite the fact that the human GI tract is heavily populated by many different organisms from the oral cavity to the colon. An estimated 40 million endoscopies were performed in the United States from 1988 to 1992, with only 28 cases of endoscopy-related infection reported [60]. Therefore, the likelihood of infection transmission may be well less than 1 in 1 million. Reported cases are restricted to infections with *Salmonella* sp. and *Pseudomonas* sp. The emergence of the AIDS virus has changed the level of concern related to the potential for endoscopy-related infection. HIV can be found on endoscopes removed from HIV-infected patients, but no case of HIV transmission by endoscopy has been reported.

Factors important in the transmission of organisms during GI endoscopy include the concentration and type of microorganism, the efficacy and compliance with cleaning and disinfection procedures, and equipment design. Most episodes of infection can be traced to procedural errors in cleaning and disinfecting the endoscope or its accessories, underlining the importance of the disinfection process.

GI procedures can cause bacteremia, placing patients with preexisting heart conditions at risk for endocarditis. The rate of bacteremia after endoscopy varies from 4 to 50 percent, depending on the specific procedure performed [61,62]. The bacteremia is usually transient, lasting 10 to 15 minutes. In selected high-risk settings, such as in patients with prior endocarditis or prosthetic valves, prophylactic antibiotics are often used to prevent endocarditis [63,64]. Because of the variability in occurrence of bacteremia, guidelines for best use of antibiotics for GI procedures are still being developed.

References

1. Shahmir M, Schuman BM: Complications of fiberoptic endoscopy. *Gastrointest Endosc* 26(3):86, 1980.
2. Macrae FA, Tan KG, William CB: Towards safer colonoscopy: A report on the complications of 5000 diagnostic or therapeutic colonoscopies. *Gut* 24:376, 1983.
3. Rogers BH, Silvis SE, Nebel OT, et al: Complications of flexible fiberoptic colonoscopy and polypectomy. *Gastrointest Endosc* 22:73, 1975.

4. Hart R, Classen M: Complications of diagnostic gastrointestinal endoscopy. *Endoscopy* 22:229, 1990.
5. Silvis SE, Nebel O, Rogers G, et al: Endoscopic complications: Results of the 1974 American Society for Gastrointestinal Endoscopy Survey. *JAMA* 235:928, 1976.
6. Eimiller A: Complication in endoscopy. *Endoscopy* 24:176, 1992.
7. Muhldorfer SM, Kekos G, Hahn EG, Ell C: Complications of therapeutic gastrointestinal endoscopy. *Endoscopy* 24:276, 1992.
8. Bianchi-Porro G, Lazzaroni M: Premedication for upper gastrointestinal endoscopy: Still a matter for debate? *Endoscopy* 23:32, 1991.
9. Bell GD: Review article: Premedications and intravenous sedation for upper gastrointestinal endoscopy. *Aliment Pharmacol Ther* 4:103, 1990.
10. Miller G: Komplikationen der Endoskopie des oberen Gastrointestinaltraktes. *Leber Magen Darm* 17;299, 1987.
11. Whorwell PJ, Smith CL, Foster KJ: Arterial blood gas tensions during upper gastrointestinal endoscopy. *Gut* 17:797, 1976.
12. Rozen P, Oppenheim D, Ratan J, et al: Arterial oxygen tension changes in elderly patients undergoing upper gastrointestinal endoscopy. I. Possible causes. *Scand J Gastroenterol* 14:577, 1979.
13. Rostykus PS, McDonald GB, Albert RK: Upper intestinal endoscopy induces hypoxemia in patients with obstructive pulmonary disease. *Gastroenterology* 78:488, 1980.
14. Hayward SR, Sugawa C, Wilson RF: Changes in oxygenation and pulse rate during endoscopy. *Am Surg* 55:198, 1989.
15. Bell GD, Morden A, Coady T, et al: A comparison of diazepam and midazolam as endoscopy premedication assessing changes in ventilation and oxygen saturation. *Br J Clin Pharmacol* 26:595, 1988.
16. Bell GD, Reeve PA, Moshiri M, et al: Intravenous midazolam: A study of the degree of oxygen desaturation occurring during upper gastrointestinal endoscopy. *Br J Clin Pharmacol* 23:703, 1987.
17. Bell GD, Morden A, Bown S, Coady T: Prevention of hypoxemia during upper gastrointestinal endoscopy by means of oxygen via nasal cannulae. *Lancet* 1:1022, 1987.
18. Arrowsmith JB, Gerstman BB, Fleischer DE, Benjamin SB: Results from the American Society for Gastrointestinal Endoscopy/U.S. Food and Drug Administration collaborative study on complication rates and drug use during gastrointestinal endoscopy. *Gastrointest Endosc* 37:421, 1991.
19. Lorenz R: Allergic reaction to contrast medium after endoscopic retrograde pancreatography. *Endoscopy* 22:196, 1990.
20. Lasser EC, Berry CC, Talner LB, et al: Pretreatment with corticosteroids to alleviate reactions to intravenous contrast material. *N Engl J Med* 317:845, 1987.
21. Kaplan DS: Paradoxical reaction to midazolam during upper endoscopy. *Gastrointest Endosc* 37:235, 1991 (Abstract).
22. Short TG, Forrest P, Galletly DC: Paradoxical reactions to benzodiazepines—A genetically determined phenomenon. *Anaesth Intensive Care* 15:333, 1987.
23. Roche Laboratories, 340 Kingsland St., Nutley, NJ, 1994.
24. Flumazenil and hypoxic ventilatory response. *Anesth Analg* 70:122, 1990.
25. Gross JB, Weller RS, Conard P: Flumazenil antagonism of midazolam-induced ventilatory depression. *Anesthesiology* 75:179, 1991.
26. Bailey PL, Pace NL, Ashburn MA, et al: Frequent hypoxemia and apnea after sedation with midazolam and fentanyl. *Anesthesiology* 73:826, 1990.
27. Dorta G, Hammer B: Langzeit-EKG bei der Koloskopie. *Schweiz Med Wochenschr* 116:1640, 1986.
28. Pyörälä K, Salmi J, Fussila J, Heikkila J: Electrocardiographic changes during gastroscopy. *Endoscopy* 5:186, 1973.
29. Van Durme JP, Elewaut A, Rosseel MT, et al: Electrocardiographic changes during oesophago-gastro-duodenoscopy. *Endoscopy* 6:134, 1974.
30. Fujita R, Kamura F: Arrhythmias and ischaemic changes of the heart induced by gastric endoscopic procedures. *Am J Gastroenterol* 64:44, 1975.
31. Fletcher GF, Earnest DL, Shuford WF, Wenger NK: Electrocardiographic changes during routine sigmoidoscopy. *Arch Intern Med* 122:483, 1968.
32. Vawter M, Ruiz R, Alaama A, et al: Electrocardiographic monitoring during coloscopy. *Am J Gastroenterol* 63:155, 1975.
33. Bilbao MK, Potter CT, Le TG, Katon M: Complications of endoscopy retrograde cholangiopancreatography (ERCP): A study of 10,000 cases. *Gastroenterology* 70:314, 1976.
34. Kozarek R: Hydrostatic balloon dilation of gastrointestinal stenoses: A national survey. *Gastrointest Endosc* 32(1):15, 1986.
35. Gibert DA, Silverstein FE, Tedesco FJ: National ASGE survey on upper gastrointestinal bleeding: Complications of endoscopy. *Dig Dis Sci* 26(7 Suppl):55s, 1981.
36. Fleischer D, Sivak MV, Jr: Endoscopic Nd:YAG laser therapy as palliation for esophagogastric cancer: Parameters affecting initial outcome. *Gastroenterology* 89:827, 1985.
37. Tytgat GN: Endoscopic therapy of esophageal cancer: Possibilities and limitations. *Endoscopy* 22:263, 1990.
38. Fleischer D: Endoscopic laser therapy for esophageal cancer. *Las Surg Med* 9:6, 1989.
39. Haddad N, Al-Kawas FH, Benjamin SB, et al: Conservative management of instrumental esophageal perforation. *Am J Gastroenterol* 87:A27, 1992.
40. Girardi A, Piazza I, Giunta G, Pappagallo G: Retroperitoneal, mediastinal and subcutaneous emphysema as a complication of routine upper gastrointestinal endoscopy. *Endoscopy* 22:83, 1990.
41. Haddad NG, Al-Kawas FH, Benjamin SB, et al: Incidence and natural history of iatrogenic Mallory-Weiss tear during upper gastrointestinal endoscopy. *Am J Gastroenterol (in press)* (Abstract).
42. Baillie J, Yudelman P: Complications of endoscopic sclerotherapy of esophageal varices. *Endoscopy* 24:284, 1992.
43. Schuman BM, Beckman JW, Tedesco FJ, et al: Complications of endoscopic injection sclerotherapy: A review. *Am J Gastroenterol* 82(9):823, 1987.
44. Caletti GC, Brocchi E, Labriola E, et al: Pericarditis: A probably overlooked complication of endoscopic variceal sclerotherapy. *Endoscopy* 22:144, 1990.
45. Bellary SV, Isaacs P: Letters to the Editor: Disseminated intravascular coagulation (DIC) after endoscopic injection sclerotherapy with ethanolamine oleate. *Endoscopy* 22:151, 1990.
46. Ashida H, Kotoura Y, Nishioka A, et al: Portal and mesenteric venous thrombosis as a complication of endoscopic sclerotherapy. *Am J Gastroenterol* 84(3):306, 1989.
47. Laine L, el-Newihi HM, Migikovsky B, et al: Endoscopic ligation compared with sclerotherapy for the treatment of bleeding esophageal varices. *Ann Intern Med* 119(1):1, 1993.
48. Katon RM, Keeffe EB, Melnyk CS: *Flexible Sigmoidoscopy.* Orlando, Grune & Stratton, 1985.
49. Kozarek RA, Earnest DL, Silverstein ME, Smith RG: Air-pressure-induced colon injury during diagnostic colonoscopy. *Gastroenterology* 78:7, 1980.
50. Razzak IA, Millan J, Schuster MM: Pneumatic ileal perforation: An unusual complication of colonoscopy. *Gastroenterology* 70:268, 1976.
51. Kavin H, Sinicrope F, Esker AH: Management of perforation of the colon at colonoscopy. *Am J Gastroenterol* 87(2):161, 1992.
52. Wadas DD, Sanowski RA: Complications of hot biopsy forceps technique. *Gastrointest Endosc* 34:32, 1988.
53. Christie JP, Marrazzo J 3rd: "Mini-perforation" of the colon: Not all postpolypectomy perforations require laparotomy. *Dis Colon Rectum* 34:132, 1991.
54. Carpio G, Albu E, Gumbs MA, Gerst PH: Management of colonic perforation after colonoscopy: Report of three cases. *Dis Colon Rectum* 32:624, 1989.
55. Waye JD: The postpolypectomy coagulation syndrome. *Gastrointest Endosc* 27:184, 1981.
56. Hall C, Dorricott NJ, Donovan IA, Neoptolemos JP: Colon perforation during colonoscopy: Surgical versus conservative management. *Br J Surg* 78:542, 1991.
57. Rex DK, Lewis BS, Waye JD: Colonoscopy and endoscopic therapy for delayed post-polypectomy hemorrhage. *Gastrointest Endosc* 38:127, 1992.
58. Waye JD, Lewis BS, Yessayan S: Colonoscopy: A prospective report of complications. *J Clin Gastroenterol* 15(4):347, 1992.
59. Sherman S, Lehman GA: ERCP and endoscopic sphincterotomy-induced pancreatitis. *Pancreas* 6:350, 1991.
60. American Society for Gastrointestinal Endoscopy: Technology Assessment Position Paper. Transmission of infection by gastrointestinal endoscopy. April 1993.

61. Botoman VA, Surawicz CM: Bacteremia with gastrointestinal endoscopic procedures. *Gastrointest Endosc* 32:342, 1986.
62. Sontheimer J, Salm R, Friedrich G, et al: Bacteremia following operative endoscopy of the upper gastrointestinal tract. *Endoscopy* 23:67, 1991.
63. Schulman ST, Amren DP, Bisno AL, et al: Prevention of bacterial endocarditis: A statement for health professionals by the Committee on Rheumatic Fever and Infective Endocarditis of the Council on Cardiovascular Disease in the Young. *Circulation* 70:1123A, 1984.
64. Infection control during gastrointestinal endoscopy. Guidelines for clinical application. *Gastrointest Endosc* 34(3 Suppl):375, 1988.

107. Hepatic Dysfunction

Ajay Kumar, and
Caroline A. Riely

Abnormalities of liver function tests occur commonly in patients admitted to a general critical or intensive care unit (ICU) [1]. Even though these abnormalities are common, they should not be discounted, as liver dysfunction in the ICU setting can have important prognostic implications. In patients with multiple organ failure, the mortality rate has been shown to rise progressively in proportion to increasing severity of hepatic dysfunction [2]. In addition, patients in the ICU with a variety of disorders, including adult respiratory distress syndrome (ARDS) [3], trauma [4], or intraabdominal sepsis [4,5] and after cardiopulmonary bypass surgery [6], who also have biochemical liver dysfunction, have been shown to have a higher mortality than those without liver involvement.

It would appear, therefore, that the occurrence of liver disease in patients with critical illnesses is associated with adverse consequences, which worsen as a function of increasing degree of hepatic dysfunction. Many aspects of this dysfunction continue to be poorly understood. The syndrome commonly encountered in the ICU is multifactorial, and this will be covered in the following paragraphs. In some patients, however, specific disorders can be identified (Table 107-1), and these will be discussed in more detail.

Common Scenario

The conditions of patients in the ICU are often complicated, with a variety of medical and surgical problems, and represent a challenge to the consulting internist or gastroenterologist. The typical patient develops abnormal liver tests several days to weeks after the event that resulted in admission to the ICU. Initial findings may include jaundice with dark urine and pale stools, but pruritus, symptoms of hepatitis, complications of portal hypertension, and evidence of true hepatocellular failure are usually absent. Features related to sepsis or concurrent other organ involvement may not only be present but often overshadow the liver dysfunction. The liver is not enlarged in most of the patients, and peripheral stigmata of liver disease are not present. The hemodynamic profile typical of sepsis is common and is difficult to distinguish from that of acute hepatic failure or chronic liver disease complicated by portal hypertension. All of these states can be associated with an increase in cardiac output and oxygen consumption and a decrease in systemic vascular resistance and peripheral oxygen extraction.

Biochemical tests reveal a progressive rise in bilirubin, which usually peaks between 8 to 15 mg per deciliter but can go much higher. Most (70–80%) of the bilirubin is conjugated [1]. Serum aminotransferase concentrations are normal or minimally increased unless there has been a concurrent episode of hepatic ischemia. Serum alkaline phosphatase (ALP) is either normal or mildly to moderately elevated. Marked rise in serum ALP levels with minimal increase in serum bilirubin has also been reported in systemic infections [7]. Serum concentrations of gamma glutamyl transpeptidase (GGT) usually rise to several times normal at about the time of the peak of bilirubin level [8]. Prothrombin time and serum albumin and ammonia levels are minimally abnormal. The serum albumin may be low due to underlying disorder, and major clotting abnormalities may occur due to disseminated intravascular coagulation. There are many reports documenting a return to normal liver function in critically ill patients with jaundice who survive [9,10,11].

The differential diagnosis of such a patient includes a variety of possibilities, ranging from biliary obstruction, drug-induced liver disease, and ischemic hepatitis to multisystem organ failure. In addition, there are a number of possible contributing factors. Within 24 hours of transfusion, 10 percent of the erythrocytes in 500 ml of blood are hemolyzed and produce 250 mg of bilirubin. The normal liver can cope easily with this load, but multiple transfusions in a seriously ill patient may generate a bilirubin quantity that may exceed the hepatic excretory capacity. This could promote development of jaundice by presenting an increased bilirubin load to a depressed transporter system. Drug-induced cholestasis should be ruled out but does not seem to be of major etiologic importance in this setting, and there is usually no clear relationship between the occurrence

Table 107-1. Etiologic Considerations of Hepatic Dysfunction in the Critically Ill

Ischemic hepatitis
Parenteral nutrition
Sepsis
Multiple organ failure
Drugs
    Asymptomatic GGT elevation
    Hepatocellular dysfunction
    Cholestasis
    Vascular injury

of jaundice and the administration of any specific anesthetic agents or drugs in patients with trauma [9,12] or sepsis [4,13]. The role of parenteral nutrition is unclear. This therapy is used almost universally in these critically ill patients, but none of the studies describing the incidence of jaundice in sepsis, trauma, or multiple organ failure has included an evaluation of the nutritional regimen used.

Specific Entities

ISCHEMIC HEPATITIS. The dual blood supply to the liver, from the portal vein and hepatic artery, preserves blood flow under most circumstances. But occasionally even this mechanism fails to protect the liver from the effects of acute circulatory impairment. The resultant hepatic injury is popularly termed *ischemic hepatitis* because it is accompanied by biochemical changes similar to those of acute hepatitis.

This syndrome, equally correctly described as *shock liver syndrome* or *acute hepatic infarction,* occurs in a specific clinical setting. It is due to a reduction in perfusion of the liver. Most but not all patients have an acute event associated with a fall in cardiac output. This fall can be subtle. Systemic hypotension or right heart failure may be detectable in just over half of the patients [14]. This syndrome is not rare and is most likely to occur in patients with chronic elevation in right-sided pressures, such as those that occur with either congenital heart disease or pulmonary hypertension.

The most striking abnormality is a pronounced rise in aminotransferases, both serum aspartate aminotransferase (AST) and alanine aminotransferase (ALT), often in parallel, to forty or more times normal. Thus, these levels are commonly over 1000 IU per liter and sometimes greater than 10,000 IU per liter. Peak elevations usually occur within 24 to 48 hours of the ischemic episode [14]. Serum bilirubin and ALP concentrations are normal or only modestly elevated [15]. Prolongation of prothrombin time occurs early and corrects promptly with recovery. Hypoglycemia has been reported in children [16]. Hepatomegaly occurs in up to 50 percent of patients [16,17,18]. There is a parallel rise in serum of the hepatic isoenzyme of lactate dehydrogenase, which does not occur in uncomplicated viral hepatitis. The elevated aminotransferase levels fall more rapidly than viral hepatitis and return to normal in 3 to 11 days [14].

The characteristic histologic feature is centrilobular hepatic necrosis with little or no inflammatory response. Liver biopsy is not necessary for diagnosis as the syndrome can easily be recognized on clinical grounds. Ischemic hepatitis is usually benign and self-limiting when it affects normal liver, subject to reversal of the precipitating event. More serious damage may be anticipated when the liver is already damaged, for example, by chronic hepatic congestion. Fulminant hepatic failure following acute circulatory disorders has been reported in patients with chronic congestive heart failure [19].

HEPATIC DYSFUNCTION FROM PARENTERAL NUTRITION. Studies evaluating parenteral nutrition in adults have documented abnormalities in liver function tests in 68 to 93 percent of patients receiving total parenteral nutrition (TPN) for two weeks or longer [20,21]. Frequently seen is two- to threefold elevation in ALT, more than that of AST, both of which often improve despite continued therapy. Serum bilirubin and ALP show variable changes. These patients have fatty infiltration or no significant abnormalities on liver biopsy. Cholestatic hepatitis and triaditis can be found in infants [22]. Similar

changes can be seen in adults, and progression to cirrhosis has been reported uncommonly. Steatohepatitis indistinguishable from alcoholic liver disease also has occurred. After six or more weeks of TPN, biliary sludge can form and cause acalculous cholecystitis or cholelithiasis [23].

The pathophysiologic mechanisms underlying the adverse effects of TPN are unclear, but recent interest has been focused on the effect of gut rest on hormone secretion and bacterial overgrowth, linked with bacterial translocation and cytokine-mediated liver injury. The exact contribution of TPN to the hepatic dysfunction seen in the critical care setting is difficult to judge, as the nutritional regimens used have not been reported or evaluated in studies of liver dysfunction in multiple organ failure, trauma, or sepsis.

Steps that may assist in preventing liver dysfunction include using the gut for nutrition whenever possible, even with small feeds; avoidance of overfeeding; balancing nutritional intake and using supplements if indicated; decontaminating the bowel with oral antibiotics; and anticipating and effectively treating sepsis [24]. Observing the patient after discontinuing the TPN is probably the best treatment but, unfortunately, often not an option in these extremely ill patients.

HEPATIC DYSFUNCTION FROM SEPSIS. Sepsis and multiple organ failure are the two most common causes of hepatic dysfunction in the ICU. Up to 54 percent of patients with bacteremia have abnormalities of liver function tests [25,26]. These occur during infections with either gram-positive or gram-negative organisms and sometimes can precede the development of bacteremia [13]. The jaundice usually develops 2 to 3 days after onset of bacteremia. Hepatomegaly is absent in up to half of affected patients [27].

The response of the liver to sepsis is variable, but data obtained from retrospective studies show that moderate elevation of serum bilirubin is common with concentrations in the range of 5 to 10 mg per deciliter [10,27,28]. Enzyme abnormalities, with up to a threefold elevation in ALT, AST and ALP, have been reported in a prospective study [26]. No difference in outcome, site of infection, or bacteria isolated was noted between patients with and without abnormalities. In a study of 9 adults with jaundice complicating severe extrahepatic infection, derangement of organic anion transport (BSP clearance) was demonstrated while synthetic (clotting), cytosolic (galactose elimination capacity), and microsomal (caffeine clearance) functions were preserved [10]. In patients with no serious underlying disease, elevated values return to normal in 1 to 2 weeks, although the clinical course can be more prolonged in severe infections. Common histologic findings are intrahepatic cholestasis, dilatation of bile canaliculi, and some ballooning of hepatocytes with little evidence of hepatocyte necrosis. Electron microscopy reveals swollen mitochondria and endoplasmic reticulum. There is accumulating evidence from animal studies that endotoxin, a lipopolysaccharide derived from the outer walls of all enterobacteria, induces dose-dependent decrease in bile flow and inhibition of sodium–potassium ATPase activity [27]. Endotoxin-mediated cholestasis is unlikely the sole mechanism for hepatic dysfunction during sepsis, however, since jaundice is also seen in patients infected with gram-positive organisms, which do not have endotoxins. Activation of inflammatory mediators and Kupffer cell phagocytic depression may contribute.

DRUG-INDUCED HEPATIC DYSFUNCTION. Drug-induced hepatic dysfunction is common; 2 percent of hospital admissions for jaundice are related to drug-induced liver disease. This figure is substantially higher in the elderly. Up to 25 percent of fulminant hepatic failure may be accounted for by drugs [29]. Drugs can affect the liver in numerous ways. Mild or subclinical hepatic dysfunction appears to be far more common than is overt disease. Drugs like acetaminophen can cause hepatotoxicity that is dose-dependent and predictable, whereas reactions from other drugs like isoniazid and phenytoin are idiosyncratic, dose-independent, and unpredictable. Chronic forms of drug-induced liver injury usually depend on continued or repeated exposure to the agent and do not result from a self-perpetuating process set in motion by a single acute insult. Recovery after withdrawal can sometimes take 5 months or longer [30].

Asymptomatic GGT Elevation. As an isolated serum abnormality, this is caused by induction of hepatic microsomal oxidase enzyme systems, including cytochrome P-450 enzymes. Several drugs act as inducers, most notably phenytoin and alcohol, but also phenobarbital, carbamazepine, rifampicin, and griseofulvin (Table 107-2). The rise is commonly less than five times normal, although higher levels can be seen [32]. This GGT elevation does not represent true cholestasis; more specific tests, such as 5' nucleotidase or serum bile acid levels, are normal or nearly so.

Elevation of Serum Aminotransferases. This occurs with a very large number of drugs, some of which are listed in Table 107-2. Most of these agents cause minor asymptomatic increases in serum aminotransferase levels or mild hepatic dysfunction. In the majority of cases, liver abnormalities develop within a few weeks of commencement of therapy [29]. Submassive or massive hepatic necrosis, which may cause fulminant hepatic failure and death, is occasionally seen. Fulminant hepatic failure associated with isoniazid, methyldopa, phenytoin, sulfonamides, and valproic acid therapy carries a mortality in excess of 10 percent. Chronic active hepatitis clinically or histologically resembling the autoimmune variety can occur with some drugs. Also, drugs will at times produce a granulomatous reaction in the liver.

Cholestasis. Two distinct patterns are associated with drug-induced cholestasis. In the first variety, cholestasis is accompanied by inflammation and hepatocellular necrosis along with systemic manifestations such as fever, rash, arthralgia, and eosinophilia. Phenothiazine tranquilizers, antithyroid medications, oral hypoglycemic agents, and erythromycin may result in this form of cholestatic hepatitis. In the second type of cholestasis, inflammation and systemic symptoms as described above are minor or absent, and the picture is of bland cholestasis. This can be caused by estrogens, androgens, and anabolic steroids (see Table 107-2). After 1 to 5 weeks of drug ingestion, patients who develop cholestasis have onset of jaundice and pruritus, which can be severe, similar to that caused by bile duct obstruction. Biochemical abnormalities consist of elevation of serum bilirubin, ALP, GGT, and cholesterol with only slight increase in aminotransferase activities. Drug-induced cholestasis does not progress to massive necrosis or a fatal outcome, and recovery after cessation of drug therapy is the rule. Recovery often takes several weeks to months, and chlorpromazine reactions may rarely be quite prolonged.

Vascular Injury. Congestive liver injury secondary to venoocclusive disease may result from radiation injury or treatment with certain antineoplastic agents and occurs frequently in bone marrow transplant patients (see Table 107-2). The major site of injury is the subendothelium of small hepatic venules, with clinical features similar to those of hepatic vein thrombosis,

Table 107-2. Hepatotoxicity of Drugs Used in the Intensive Care Unit [1,29,30,31]*

GGT elevation: phenytoin, alcohol, phenobarbital, carbamazepine, and rifampicin

ALT/AST elevation and hepatic necrosis: allopurinol†, amiodarone, amitriptyline, carbamazepine, chlordiazepoxide, captopril, cimetidine, dantrolene, flucytosine, furosemide, fusidic acid, halothane†, heparin, hydralazine, indomethacin, isoniazid†, methoxyflurane, methyldopa†, phenelzine, phenobarbital, phenytoin†, prochlorperazine, oxacillin, sulfonamides, valproic acid†

Chronic hepatitis: acetaminophen, alcohol, amiodarone, aspirin, dantrolene, isoniazid, methyldopa, nitrofurantoin, oxyphenisatin, propylthiouracil, sulfonamides

Granulomas: allopurinol, carbamazepine, erythromycin, hydralazine, methyldopa, procainamide, quinidine

Cholestasis: anabolic steroids, androgens, amitriptyline, captopril, carbamazepine, cephalosporins, chlorpromazine (phenothiazines), cimetidine, cyclosporine, dantrolene, diazepam, fluphenazine, flurazepam, haloperidol, iodipamide, phenytoin, rifampicin, sulfonamides, thiazides, valproic acid

Vascular injury: azathioprine, Adriamycin, cytosine, daunorubicin, mitomycin, 6-thioguanine, valproic acid

* List not complete. Check drug information.
† Can cause submassive or massive necrosis.

including abdominal pain, hepatomegaly, and ascites. This vascular injury may or may not be reversible.

MULTIPLE ORGAN FAILURE. A dreaded disorder encountered in the ICU is multiple organ failure. This multisystem disorder can be difficult to recognize clinically. Most patients have signs of sepsis, including fever, leukocytosis, hypotension, and decreased systemic vascular resistance. Liver dysfunction may occur at any point in the course of the disorder and is characterized by an elevation in serum bilirubin out of proportion to changes in aminotransferases, ALP, and GGT. Serum levels of bile acids may be increased [10,33].

The predominant finding on biopsy is intrahepatic cholestasis with dilated canaliculi containing bile casts. Bile pigment is present in cytoplasm of adjacent hepatocytes and in Kupffer cells near the center of the lobules. A distinctive pattern of marked dilation with bile plugging of periportal cholangioles, called *cholangiolar cholestasis,* has been noted in some patients [34,35]. However, intrahepatic cholestasis is not seen in all patients [4]. The sinusoids are often narrowed by hepatocyte swelling in centrilobular areas [9]. Hepatocyte necrosis is variable.

Hypotheses about the pathogenic mechanisms underlying this disorder abound. Infection clearly plays a central, although undefined, role. Bacteria and endotoxins derived from gut microorganisms may translocate across the bowel wall in circumstances associated with critical illness. They are largely transported in the portal vein to the liver. When exposed to endotoxin, Kupffer cells (fixed hepatic macrophages), which line the vascular sinusoids and are responsible for removal of endotoxin, bacteria, and particulate matter, become activated and release a variety of mediators, including leukotrienes, arachidonic acid metabolites, interleukin-1, tumor necrosis factor, and toxic oxygen radicals [36,37]. Furthermore, the phagocytic capacity of Kupffer cells is depressed by hepatic ischemia, hypoxemia, large loads of material for phagocytosis, and fibronectin deficiency [38]. Various forms of liver disease have also been shown per se to depress Kupffer cell function in experimental models [39,40]. Hepatocytes may therefore become exposed to noxious effects of endotoxin and inflammatory mediators, which can affect hepatocellular function. Many features of the liver dysfunction of multiple organ failure can be explained by the actions of endotoxin derived from the gut or a septic focus.

There is also increasing circumstantial evidence that liver dysfunction predisposes to failure of other organ systems. In the presence of depressed Kupffer cell function, gut-derived bacteria or endotoxin and inflammatory mediators generated during Kupffer cell activation may "spill over" into systemic circulation and lead to remote organ failure [1]. Indeed, it is claimed that changes in hepatocyte metabolism are essential for the definition of multiple organ failure [41].

The first step is thought to be hypermetabolism accompanied by absolute or relative tissue perfusion deficit. This is followed 48 to 72 hours later by development of injury causing multiple organ failure. Evolution of hepatic dysfunction is believed to define multiple organ failure and determine its attendant mortality [42]. A variety of insults including severe hemorrhage, sepsis, tissue injury, and inflammation as in severe pancreatitis, can initiate a hypermetabolic phase of illness in critically ill patients. This phase has a mortality of 25 to 40 percent but resolves or partially resolves in 9 to 14 days in patients who respond to treatment. In nonresponders, illness progresses to multiple organ failure and eventually hyperbilirubinemia disproportionately higher than elevation in aminotransferases and ALP. Reduced hepatic protein synthesis and amino acid clearance, increased ureagenesis, and falling hepatic redox potential ensue, signifying the development of clinical hepatic dysfunction. It is reported that a serum bilirubin level greater than 8 mg/per deciliter, in the absence of biliary obstruction or sequestrated blood, is associated with a mortality approaching 95 percent [42]. Signs and symptoms of liver disease are often overshadowed by the underlying illness. In patients who survive, liver function returns to normal.

Hepatic dysfunction occurs with gram-negative as well as gram-positive infections, and factors as yet not clearly identified must be invoked. Even in gram-negative infections, multiple organ failure can progress despite the absence of endotoxemia [43]. Hence, it has been hypothesized that cell wall–deficient forms (L-form) of gram-negative bacteria, rather than endotoxin, may be responsible for organ failure in compromised patients [44].

Approach to Management

When the clinician is confronted with the problem of hepatic dysfunction in a critically ill patient, clinical features remain quite helpful in leading to a correct diagnosis and appropriate course of action. Such features as antecedent symptoms of liver disease, history of heavy alcohol ingestion, risk factors for various types of hepatitis, and recent medication exposure may all suggest a possible cause of the liver disease. It should be remembered that chronic liver disease is often asymptomatic.

A tenfold or higher elevation of aminotransferase levels is suggestive of hepatocellular necrosis, such as that caused by ischemic hepatitis, viral hepatitis, or reaction to a drug, for example, halothane hepatitis. Serology for hepatitis viruses should be performed and serum acetaminophen levels checked. If the rise in the serum bilirubin or ALP is predominant, then serum amylase and lipase levels should be measured to exclude pancreatitis and abdominal ultrasound, or CT scan should be performed to exclude extrahepatic biliary obstruction.

No comprehensive or specific therapy exists for hepatic dysfunction in the critically ill patient. Therapeutic advances are possible in the future if inflammatory mediators can be manipulated. The primary elements of management are preventative and consist principally of prompt resuscitation, treatment of sepsis, and intensive support [1]. Use of drugs with a propensity to hepatotoxicity should be eliminated or minimized.

RESUSCITATION. Prompt resuscitation from shock is important. Shock can adversely affect hepatic function by promoting translocation of gut bacteria and endotoxin, by predisposing to hepatocyte necrosis, and by impairing Kupffer cell phagocytic ability. Conventional reversal of uncompensated shock by correcting oliguria and hypotension may not be enough. It is now being suggested that oxygen delivery and extraction in tissues should also be optimized. Gastric intramucosal acidosis as measured by gastric tonometry has been shown to represent and correlate well with splanchnic ischemia. Countering this ischemia may diminish translocation. Preliminary data are available on dopexamine, a splanchnic vasodilator that also increases hepatic blood flow, showing improved survival in multiple organ failure [45]. After full replacement of volume dobutamine infusion to reverse low cardiac output was shown to reduce markers of ischemic hepatitis in a patient [46]. A small but significant increase in estimated effective hepatic blood flow beyond the increase in cardiac output has been seen in patients treated with low-dose dopamine (6 μg/kg/min) soon after open heart surgery [47].

TREATMENT OF SEPSIS. In view of the close association of liver dysfunction with sepsis, it is not surprising that studies have demonstrated reversal of hepatic abnormalities with adequate therapy of sepsis [10,26]. Collection of pus should be drained aggressively and appropriate antibiotic therapy instituted. Measures addressing reduction of the incidence of infections in the ICU may also be important. Selective decontamination of the digestive tract has improved outcome in critically ill patients with trauma but not in patients with other diagnoses [48]. Serum level of fibronectin, an opsonizing glycoprotein required for optimal Kupffer cell phagocytic function, is low in critical illness, but replacement has not improved survival in patients with trauma or abdominal sepsis [49,50].

NUTRITIONAL SUPPORT. Control of the malnutrition that is a covariable of morbidity and mortality has been suggested to benefit survival in sepsis and multiple organ failure [41], although no particular nutritional regimen has been shown to improve outcome in this setting [1]. Parenteral nutrition should be balanced. Fat as the source of 25 to 40 percent of nonprotein calories reduces the incidence of fatty liver and maintains microsomal enzyme function. The value of using formulas that are enriched in branched-chain amino acids and glutamine is not clear.

The enteral route for nutrition has several advantages. Fewer septic complications were noted in patients wth trauma on enteral feeding than in those receiving parenteral nutrition [51]. Early initiation of enteral nutrition, which also provides direct luminal nutrition to the gut itself, has been incorporated into the package of measures used to improve survival in organ failure [45]. Enteral feeding causes a fall in serum bilirubin in healthy volunteers [52], reverses parenteral nutrition–related cholestasis in infants [53], and reduces bacterial translocation from the gut in rats [54]. (See Chap. 201.)

OTHER TREATMENT ASPECTS. Gut mucosal injury is increasingly suspected of having a central role in the causation of multiple organ failure [55]. Gastric intramucosal acidosis persisting at 12 hours after admission has been noticed to be a very powerful predictor of outcome [56]. Therefore, therapy should not only be aimed at markers of global hypoxia, such as base excess and blood lactate, but should also include measures designed to protect gut and liver, consisting of early initiation of enteral nutrition and possibly the use of splanchnic vasodilators such as dopexamine. This type of regimen will improve intramucosal acidosis and liver blood flow and has been shown to favorably alter mortality and duration of multiple organ failure [45].

The precise role of immunotherapy using monoclonal antibodies to endotoxin [44,57] or antioxidant therapy [58] is not established in critical care medicine and hence its place in prevention or treatment of hepatic dysfunction is uncertain.

In conclusion, many aspects of the hepatic dysfunction common in critically ill patients are not well understood. Some specific entities can be identified. Liver dysfunction is less directly life threatening than failure of other organ systems but is an indicator of poor outcome. No specific therapy is available. Research is in progress to determine if the inflammatory mediator response can be manipulated, reversed, or protected by various therapeutic agents.

References

1. Hawker F: Liver dysfunction in critical illness. *Anaesth Intensive Care* 19:165, 1991.
2. Marshall JC, Christou NV, Horn R, et al: The microbiology of multiple organ failure: The proximal gastrointestinal tract as an occult reservoir of pathogens. *Arch Surg* 123:309, 1988.
3. Schwartz DB, Bone RC, Balk RA, et al: Hepatic dysfunction in the adult respiratory distress syndrome. *Chest* 95:871, 1989.
4. Te Boekhorst T, Urlus M, Doesburg W, et al: Etiologic factors of jaundice in severely ill patients. *J Hepatol* 7:111, 1988.
5. Pine RW, Wertz MJ, Lennard E, et al: Determinants of organ malfunction or death in patients with intra-abdominal sepsis. *Arch Surg* 118:242, 1983.
6. Collins JD, Bassendine MF, Ferner R, et al: Incidence and prognostic importance of jaundice after cardiopulmonary bypass surgery. *Lancet* 1:1119, 1983.
7. Neale G, Caughey DE, Mollins DL, et al: Effects of intrahepatic and extrahepatic infection on liver function. *BMJ* 1:382, 1966.
8. Champion HR, Jones RT, Trump BF, et al: A clinicopathologic study of hepatic dysfunction following shock. *Surg Gynecol Obstet* 142:657, 1976.
9. Nunes G, Blaisdell FW, Margaretten W: Mechanism of hepatic dysfunction following shock and trauma. *Arch Surg* 100:546, 1970.
10. Pirovino M, Meister F, Rubli E, et al: Preserved cytosolic and synthetic liver function in jaundice of severe extrahepatic infection. *Gastroenterology* 96:1589, 1989.
11. Champion HR, Jones RT, Trump BF, et al: Post-traumatic hepatic dysfunction as a major etiology in post-traumatic jaundice. *J Trauma* 16:650, 1976.
12. Sarfeh IJ, Balint JA: The clinical significance of hyperbilirubinemia following trauma. *J Trauma* 18:58, 1978.
13. Vermillion SE, Gregg JA, Baggenstoss AH: Jaundice associated with bacteremia. *Arch Intern Med* 124:611, 1969.
14. Gibson PR, Dudley FJ: Ischemic hepatitis: Clinical features, diagnosis and prognosis. *Aust NZ J Med* 14:822, 1984.
15. Anonymous [editorial]: Ischemic hepatitis. *Lancet* 1:1019, 1985.
16. Garland JS, Werlin SL, Rice TB: Ischemic hepatitis in children: Diagnosis and clinical course. *Crit Care Med* 16:1209, 1988.
17. Bynum TE, Boitnott JK, Maddrey WC: Ischemic hepatitis. *Dig Dis Sci* 24:129, 1979.
18. Cohen JA, Kaplan MM: Left-sided heart failure presenting as hepatitis. *Gastroenterology* 74:583, 1978.
19. Novel O, Henrion J, Bernau J, et al: Fulminant hepatic failure due to transient circulatory failure in patients with chronic heart disease. *Dig Dis Sci* 25:49, 1980.
20. Lindor KD, Fleming CR, Abrams A, et al: Liver function variables in adults receiving total parental nutrition. *JAMA* 241:2398, 1979.
21. Grant JP, Cox CE, Kleinman LM, et al: Serum hepatic enzyme and bilirubin elevations during parenteral nutrition. *Surg Gynecol Obstet* 145:573, 1977.
22. Whitington PF: Cholestasis associated with total parenteral nutrition in infants. *Hepatology* 4:693, 1985.
23. Messing B, Bories C, Kunstlinger F, et al: Does total parenteral nutrition induce gall bladder sludge formation and lithiasis. *Gastroenterology* 84:1012, 1983.
24. Paynes-James JJ, Silk DBA: Hepatobiliary dysfunction associated with total parenteral nutrition. *Dig Dis* 9:106, 1991.
25. Franson TR, Hierholzer WJ, LaBrecque DR: Frequency and characteristics of hyperbilirubinemia associated with bacteremia. *Rev Infect Dis* 7:1, 1985.
26. Sikuler E, Guetta V, Keynan A, et al: Abnormalities in bilirubin and liver enzyme levels in adult patients with bacteremia: A prospective study. *Arch Intern Med* 149:2246, 1989.
27. Gimson AES: Hepatic dysfunction during bacterial sepsis. *Intensive Care Med* 13:162, 1987.
28. Miller DJ, Keeton GR, Webber BL, et al: Jaundice in severe bacterial infection. *Gastroenterology* 71:94, 1976.
29. Bass NM, Ockner RK: Drug induced liver disease, in Zakim D, Boyer TD (eds): *Hepatology: A Textbook of Liver Disease.* Philadelphia, WB Saunders, 1990, pp 754–791.
30. Lee MG, Hanchard B, Williams NP: Drug-induced acute liver disease. *Postgrad Med J* 65:367, 1989.
31. Ludwig J, Axelsen R: Drug effects on the liver. An updated tabular compilation of drugs and drug-related hepatic diseases. *Dig Dis Sci* 28:651, 1983.
32. Keefee EB, Sunderland MC, Gabourel JD: Serum gamma-glutamyl transpeptidase activity in patients receiving chronic phenytoin therapy. *Dig Dis Sci* 31:1056, 1986.
33. Howarth DM, Sanpson DC, Hawker FH, et al: Digoxin-like immunoreactive substance in the plasma of intensive care unit patients: Relationship to organ dysfunction. *Anaesth Intensive Care* 18:45, 1990.
34. Lefkowitch JH: Bile ductular cholestasis: An ominous histopathologic sign related to sepsis and "cholangitis lenta." *Hum Pathol* 13:19, 1982.
35. Riely CA, Dean PJ, Park AL, et al: A distinct syndrome of liver disease with multisystem organ failure associated with bile ductular cholestasis. *Hepatology* 10:739, 1989.
36. Beutler B, Greenwald D, Hulmes JD, et al: Identity of tumor necrosis factor and the macrophage secreted factor cachetin. *Nature* 316:552, 1985.
37. Keppler D, Hagmann W, Rapp S, et al: The relation of leukotrienes to liver injury. *Hepatology* 5:883, 1985.
38. Jones EA, Summerfield JA: Kupffer cells, in Arias IM, Jakoby WB, Popper H, et al (eds): *The Liver: Biology and Pathobiology.* New York, Raven Press, 1988, pp. 683–704.
39. Holman JM, Rikkers LF: Biliary obstruction and host defense failure. *J Surg Res* 32:208, 1982.
40. Wardle EN, Anderson A, James O: Kupffer cell phagocytosis in relation to BSP clearance in liver and inflammatory bowel disease. *Dig Dis Sci* 24:414, 1980.
41. Steinberg S, Flynn W, Kelley K, et al: Development of a bacteria-independent model of the multiple organ failure. *Arch Surg* 124:1390, 1989.
42. Barton R, Cerra FB: The hypermetabolism: Multiple organ failure syndrome. *Chest* 96:1153, 1989.
43. Danner RL, Elin RJ, Hosseini JM, et al: Endotoxaemia in human septic shock. *Chest* 99:169, 1991.
44. Hurley JC: Reappraisal of the role of endotoxin in the sepsis syndrome. *Lancet* 341:1133, 1993.
45. Beale R, Bihari DJ: Multiple organ failure: The pilgrim's progress. *Crit Care Med* 21:S1, 1993.
46. Kram HB, Evans T, Bundage B, et al: Use of dobutamine for treatment of shock liver syndrome. *Crit Care Med* 16:644, 1988.

47. Schmid E, Angehrn W, Althaus F, et al: The effect of dopamine on hepatic-splanchnic blood flow after open heart surgery. *Intensive Care Med* 5:183, 1979.

48. Ledingham IM, Alcock SR, Eastaway AT, et al: Triple regimen of selective decontamination of the digestive tract, systemic cefotaxime and microbiological surveillance for prevention of acquired infection in intensive care. *Lancet* 1:785, 1988.

49. Saba TM, Jaffe E: Plasma fibronectin [opsonic glycoprotein]: Its synthesis by vascular endothelial cells and role in cardiopulmonary integrity after trauma as related to reticuloendothelial function. *Am J Med* 68:577, 1980.

50. Mansberger AR, Doran JE, Treat R, et al: The influence of fibronectin administration on the incidence of sepsis and septic morbidity in severely injured patients. *Ann Surg* 210:297, 1989.

51. Moore FA, Moore EE, Jones TN, et al: TEN versus TPN following major abdominal trauma-reduced septic morbidity. *J Trauma* 29:916, 1989.

52. Roongpisuthipong C, Heymsfield SB, Casper K, et al: Continuous nasoenteral feeding: Inverse relation between infusion rate and serum levels of bilirubin. *JPEN J Parenter Enteral Nutr* 11:544, 1987.

53. Whitington PF: Cholestasis associated with total parenteral nutrition in infants. *Hepatology* 5:693, 1985.

54. Alverdy JC, Aoys E, Moss GS: Total parenteral nutrition promotes bacterial translocation from the gut. *Surgery* 104:185, 1988.

55. Fiddian-Green RG, Haglund U, Gutierrez G, et al: Goals for the resuscitation of shock. *Crit Care Med* 21:S25, 1993.

56. Doglio GR, Pusajo JF, Egurrola MA, et al: Gastric mucosal pH as a prognostic index of mortality in critically ill patients. *Crit Care Med* 19:1037, 1991.

57. Fink MP: Adoptive immunotherapy of gram-negative sepsis: Use of monoclonal antibodies to liposaccharide. *Crit Care Med* 21:S32, 1993.

58. Schiller HJ, Reilly PM, Bulkley GB: Antioxidant therapy. *Crit Care Med* 21:S92, 1993.

VIII. Endocrine Problems in the Intensive Care Unit

Section Editors
Lewis E. Braverman and Aldo A. Rossini

108. Approach to the Acutely Ill Patient on Chronic Steroid Therapy

Neil Aronin

Introduction

Because glucocorticoids affect the function of multiple organ systems in normal homeostasis (see Chap. 113), it is no surprise that the long-term use of pharmacologic amounts of glucocorticoids is associated with numerous side effects and complications. The following discussion focuses on the management of the acutely ill patient or surgical candidate on long-term glucocorticoid treatment whose response to stress may be abnormal.

Glucocorticoids and Stress

RESPONSE IN NORMAL SUBJECTS. During surgical stress, the plasma concentrations of adrenal glucocorticoids increase 5-fold to 10-fold. High circulating levels of cortisol may persist for 24 hours. The adrenal response is probably maximal, since administration of additional exogenous adrenocorticotropic hormone (ACTH) generally does not produce greater adrenal release of corticosteroids [1]. The cortisol-deoxycortisol ratio in these patients is increased in surgery and after ACTH injection compared with the basal secretion in normal subjects [2]. In operative trauma, there is evidence that both the frequency and the rate of secretion in the episodic release of cortisol are increased [3]. Anesthesia reversal is associated with an especially profound increase in ACTH and cortisol plasma concentrations [4]. Furthermore, in surgical stress there is a larger volume of distribution and an enhanced metabolic clearance rate of injected, labeled cortisol [5]. Available data indicate that cortisol secretion is favored and is maximal during surgical stress and that the extent of increased cortisol is similar to that following adrenal stimulation by ACTH injection or insulin-induced hypoglycemia.

RESPONSE DURING LONG-TERM STEROID TREATMENT. Following the introduction of glucocorticoid therapy, several case reports linked withdrawal of steroids, adrenal suppression, and shock in patients on long-term steroid treatment [6,7]. A causal role for adrenal suppression was based on restoration of normal blood pressure with corticosteroid treatment. These reports indicated that adrenal suppression may be an important complication of corticosteroid administration, but biochemical confirmation that coupled hypotension to adrenal atrophy was lacking. Several years later, such data were obtained in patients on long-term steroid therapy in whom the plasma cortisol remained subnormal after surgical stress and corticotropin administration [8]. It is evident that some patients who have used steroids may be unable to respond adequately to the stress of an acute illness.

How frequent is hypotension in steroid-treated patients who undergo acute stress without glucocorticoid supplementation? The few studies available suggest that hypotension from inadequate adrenal function is uncommon. In one study, 8 of 104 patients who were receiving replacement doses of steroids developed unexplained hypotension during surgery [9]. Only one of these patients had a correspondingly low plasma cortisol concentration. In another series, 117 patients on replacement doses of cortisol (20 mg hydrocortisone or daily equivalent) who were not receiving supplemental cortisol encountered no episodes of hypotension or increased morbidity during 80 occasions of diagnostic or surgical procedures [10]. In this study, 42 patients on replacement or low-dose steroid treatment whose adrenals were unresponsive to metyrapone had no difficulties during surgery, even though supplemental steroids were withheld. More recently, observations in adrenalectomized nonhuman primates undergoing cholecystectomy showed that subphysiologic replacement (one-tenth physiologic value) of cortisol resulted in significantly increased mortality and operative hypotension compared with replacement with physiologic or supraphysiologic dosages (10 times physiologic value) [11]. It is interesting that no difference in subject outcome was found between the physiologic and supraphysiologic amounts.

These studies were not designed to determine the extent of morbidity of patients who receive suppressive doses of steroids. However, the findings suggest that hypotension from adrenal suppression is uncommon. Thus, the development of shock in the acutely ill or surgical patient on steroid therapy (or following withdrawal within 1 year) should not be attributed solely to diminished adrenal responsiveness. Adrenal steroids can and should be administered, but other contributing causes of the hypotension should be sought.

Clinical Presentations

HYPERCORTISOL STATE. Long-term administration of glucocorticoids shares many of the complications found in Cushing's syndrome, such as obesity, psychiatric disturbances, edema (with cortisone), and impaired wound healing. Problems attributable to administration of synthetic corticosteroids that are not associated with natural Cushing's syndrome include benign intracranial hypertension, glaucoma, pancreatitis, aseptic necrosis of bone, panniculitis, and posterior subcapsular cataracts. In contrast, striae, purpura, plethora, hypertension, acne, hirsutism, and menstrual irregularities and impotence are more commonly associated with endogenous hypercortisolism. When present, these features aid in distinguishing the etiology of a hypercortisol state. It should be emphasized that patients on long-term steroid therapy may lack many or all of these complications [12,13,14].

WITHDRAWAL OF STEROID THERAPY. Withdrawal of glucocorticoids can be associated with symptoms of Addison's disease, including anorexia, fever, nausea, lethargy, myalgias, arthralgias, weakness, and weight loss [15]. These symptoms can occur despite a gradual decrease in dosage and in the presence of normal baseline plasma cortisol and satisfactory cortisol response to corticotropin. Moreover, at least some patients with withdrawal symptoms have an intact hypothalamic-anterior pituitary-adrenal axis, as tested by either insulin-induced hypoglycemia or metyrapone administration [16]. These findings are consistent with a widespread and differential action of glucocorticoids in selected patients; the adrenal axis may be less affected than other systems during long-term steroid therapy.

Adrenal suppression may also occur in patients who manifest no obvious signs of hypercortisolism and who lack symptoms of steroid excess or steroid withdrawal. In certain individuals, the hypothalamic-anterior pituitary-adrenal axis is rapidly suppressed in as few as 5 days after prednisone treatment (20–30 mg daily) [17]. Impaired adrenal function may occur up to 5 days after cessation of short-term administration of the steroid. Following more long-term administration of corticosteroids, the adrenal axis may respond poorly to appropriate stimuli up to 1 year after steroid withdrawal [18]. A detailed study of patients treated with glucocorticoids revealed that adrenal suppression cannot be predicted based on glucocorticoid dosage and duration or a normal basal cortisol [19].

In general, the anterior pituitary regains its ability to respond to stress (e.g., hypoglycemia) before normal adrenal function is restored. Consequently, an adequate increase in plasma cortisol that follows corticotropin administration is interpreted to indicate the presence of an intact hypothalamic-anterior pituitary-adrenal axis [1,18,20]. Furthermore, it has been shown that patients receiving long-term glucocorticoid therapy who have a subnormal response to corticotropin or its analog, ACTH 1-24, also have a subnormal cortisol response to stress or surgery, whereas those who have an adequate response to corticotropin respond normally to stress or surgery [21]. Use of corticotropin releasing hormone (CRH) may replace insulin-induced hypoglycemia or metyrapone administration to study the integrity of the hypothalamic-pituitary-adrenal axis [19,22]. To date, CRH is available for investigational use only.

Treatment

MINIMIZING STEROID SUPPRESSION. The alternate-day schedule for steroid administration reduces side effects and complications of long-term glucocorticoid therapy, including suppression of the adrenal gland [23,24]. Patients who receive alternate-day prednisone or cortisone therapy can usually discontinue steroids without experiencing withdrawal symptoms. Complications of steroids (peptic ulcers, psychotic reactions, infections) are also reduced. Of note, the increase in cortisol or 17-hydroxycortisol following ACTH injection in patients on an alternate-day regimen is similar to that observed in normal subjects and significantly greater than in patients on daily steroid therapy. Continued adrenal suppression has been found when dexamethasone is used despite alternate-day treatment [25]. In addition, administration of a single dose in the morning rather than at night is associated with less adrenal suppression [26].

Long-term daily injection of corticotropin has not been found to result in suppression of the hypothalamic-anterior pituitary-adrenal axis and does not retard linear growth in children [11,27]. This form of treatment has limitations, however: intramuscular injection, difficulty in adjusting dosages, possibility of irregular absorption, dependence on adrenal function, and complications similar to those of Cushing's syndrome. For these reasons, alternate-day steroid maintenance is preferred to corticotropin. It should be emphasized that alternate-day therapy is not useful in giant cell arteritis and may be unsatisfactory in the initial management of other generalized disorders (e.g., ulcerative colitis, pemphigus vulgaris) [28].

ANTICIPATING STEROID SUPPRESSION. Patients on glucocorticoid therapy for least 4 weeks at either pharmacologic or replacement levels and those who have stopped glucocorticoids within the past year are generally considered to be at highest risk for adrenal suppression. Time permitting, a corticotropin or (when available) CRH stimulation test provides information on the adequacy of the adrenal response to stress; however, clinical situations do not always abide this opportunity. These patients are prudently treated with hydrocortisone hemisuccinate (or equivalent cortisol ester), 100 mg intravenously every 8 hours, until the critical illness or event has subsided. The subsequent decrease in steroids to pretreatment doses is completed within 2 weeks when the stress lasts less than 10 days. For less stressful procedures (e.g., dental or outpatient surgery), a 2-day replacement with 100 mg hydrocortisone or equivalent in divided doses should suffice.

Summary

1. Normal subjects increase cortisol secretion during surgical procedures and anesthesia reversal.
2. Patients with adrenal hypofunction, including those on long-term glucocorticoid therapy, are at increased risk for morbidity associated with surgical stress.
3. An absolute replacement requirement for cortisol remains unsettled in the acutely ill patient with adrenal hypofunction. In addition, there is a wide range of responses by the hypothalamic-pituitary-adrenal axis to long-term steroid therapy.
4. Because in the acutely ill patient testing the intactness of the adrenal axis may not be practical, replacement with cortisol or equivalents at stress doses is prudent.
5. Available evidence from patient and primate studies indicates that hypotension or shock in patients on physiologic amounts of glucocorticoid replacement is uncommon. Thus, in acutely ill patients on long-term steroid therapy, causes of hypotension or persistent morbidity other than glucocorticoid insufficiency should be determined after appropriate cortisol replacement.

References

1. Kehlet H, Binder C: Value of an ACTH test in assessing hypothalamic-pituitary-adrenocortical function in glucocorticoid-treated patients. *Br Med J* 1:147, 1973.
2. Hume DM, Bell CC, Bartter F: Direct measurement of adrenal secretion during operative trauma and convalescence. *Surgery* 52:174, 1962.
3. Wise L, Margraf HW, Ballinger WF: A new concept on the pre- and postoperative regulation of cortisol secretion. *Surgery* 72:290, 1972.
4. Udelsman R, Ramp J, Gallucci WT, et al: Adaptation during surgical stress: A reevaluation of the role of glucocorticoids. *J Clin Invest* 77:1377, 1986.
5. Kehlet H, Binder C: Alteration in distribution volume and biological half-life of cortisol during major surgery. *J Clin Endocrinol Metab* 36:330, 1973.
6. Fraser CG, Preuss PS, Bigfor WD: Adrenal atrophy and irreversible shock associated with cortisone therapy. *JAMA* 149:1542, 1952.
7. Lewis L, Robinson RF, Yee J, et al: Fatal adrenal cortical insufficiency

precipitated by surgery during prolonged continuous cortisone treatment. *Ann Intern Med* 116:195, 1953.

8. Sampson PA, Brooke BN, Winstone NE: Biochemical confirmation of collapse due to adrenal failure. *Lancet* 1:1377, 1961.
9. Kehlet H, Binder C: Adrenocortical function and clinical course during and after surgery in supplemented glucocorticoid-treated patients. *Br J Anaesth* 45:1043, 1973.
10. Danowski TS, Bonessi JV, Sabeh G, et al: Probabilities of pituitary-adrenal responsiveness after steroid therapy. *Ann Intern Med* 61:11, 1964.
11. Udelsman R, Norton JA, Jelenich SE, et al: Responses of the hypothalamic-pituitary-adrenal and renin-angiotensin axes and the sympathetic system during controlled surgical and anesthetic stress. *J Clin Endocrinol Metab* 64:986, 1987.
12. Axelrod L: Glucocorticoid therapy. *Medicine* 55:39, 1976.
13. Dixon RB, Christy NP: On the various forms of corticosteroid withdrawal syndrome. *Am J Med* 68:224, 1980.
14. Christy NP: Corticosteroid withdrawal, in Krieger DT, Bardin CW (eds): *Current Therapy in Endocrinology*. St. Louis, CV Mosby, 1983, p 318.
15. Amatruda TT Jr, Hurst MM, D'Espo ND: Certain endocrine and metabolic facets of the steroid withdrawal syndrome. *J Clin Endocrinol Metab* 25:1207, 1965.
16. Amatruda TT Jr, Hollingsworth DR, D'Espo ND, et al: A study of the mechanisms of the steroid withdrawal syndrome: Evidence for integrity of the hypothalamic-pituitary-adrenal system. *J Clin Endocrinol Metab* 20:339, 1960.
17. Streck WF, Lockwood DH: Pituitary-adrenal recovery following short-term suppression with corticosteroids. *Am J Med* 66:910, 1979.
18. Graber AI, Ney RL, Nicholson WE, et al: Natural history of pituitary-adrenal recovery following long-term suppression with corticosteroids. *J Clin Endocrinol Metab* 25:11, 1965.
19. Schlaghecke R, Kornely E, Santen RTh, Ridderskamp P: The effect of long-term glucocorticoid therapy on pituitary-adrenal responses to exogenous corticotropin-releasing hormone. *N Engl J Med* 326:226, 1992.
20. Sampson PA, Winston NE, Brooks BN: Adrenal function in surgical patients after steroid therapy. *Lancet* 2:332, 1962.
21. Jasani MK, Freeman PA, Boyle JA, et al: Studies of the rise in plasma 11-hydroxycorticosteroids (11-OHCS) in corticosteroid-treated patients with rheumatoid arthritis during surgery: Correlations with the functional integrity of the hypothalamo-pituitary-adrenal axis. *Q J Med* 37:407, 1968.
22. Christy NP: Pituitary-adrenal function during corticosteroid therapy: Learning to live with uncertainty. *N Engl J Med* 326:266, 1992.
23. Harter JG, Reddy WJ, Thorn GW: Studies on an intermittent corticosteroid dosage regimen. *N Engl J Med* 269:591, 1963.
24. Thorn GW: Clinical considerations in the use of corticosteroids. *N Engl J Med* 274:775, 1966.
25. Rabhan NB: Pituitary-adrenal suppression and Cushing's syndrome after intermittent dexamethasone therapy. *Ann Intern Med* 69:1141, 1968.
26. Nichols T, Nugent CA, Tyler FH: Diurnal variation in suppression of adrenal function by glucocorticoids. *J Clin Endocrinol Metab* 25:344, 1965.
27. Carter ME, James VHT: Pituitary-adrenal response to surgical stress in patients receiving corticotropin treatment. *Lancet* 1:328, 1970.
28. Hunder GG, Sheps SG, Allen GL, et al: Daily and alternate day corticosteroid regimens in treatment of giant cell arteritis: Comparison in a prospective study. *Ann Intern Med* 82:613, 1975.

109. Management of Diabetes in the Critically Ill Patient

Aldo A. Rossini, Peter A. Gottlieb, and John P. Mordes

Introduction

Diabetes mellitus is a common problem that complicates the delivery of intensive care. It afflicts more than 5 percent of Americans, and nearly 80 percent of individuals with the disorder are older than 40 years. In 1990, 7 million people knew they had diabetes, but an equal number with the disease remained undiagnosed. Among certain minorities the disease is epidemic [1,2,3]. Poorly controlled [4] diabetes predisposes to cardiovascular [5,6], renal [7], and infectious [8] complications that often require intensive surgical and medical care. In addition, diabetic patients in the intensive care unit (ICU) are particularly vulnerable to the adverse metabolic consequences of stress.

This chapter describes the management of intercurrent diabetes in the critically ill patient. Whatever the primary problem, diabetes amplifies the difficulty of intensive care. Often diabetes itself is the primary problem, as in ketoacidosis and hyperosmolar coma. These conditions are described in Chapter 110. Whether diabetes is the primary or secondary disorder in an ICU patient, the effects of insulin deficiency and stress on metabolic homeostasis are the same.

Etiology and Pathophysiology

METABOLIC HOMEOSTASIS. Normal individuals always maintain their blood glucose concentration between 60 and 120 mg per deciliter. Maintenance of glucose within this narrow range depends on a complex interaction between metabolites and hormones. This interaction is controlled by the degree of tissue "insulinization" (Fig. 109-1) [9], a function of the amount of insulin available and the responsiveness of target tissues. After eating, blood glucose concentration rises but remains within the normal range as a result of increased insulin secretion. The insulin first promotes the transport of glucose into cells and the repletion of glycogen and protein stores. It then mediates the storage of excess glucose as triglyceride. When absorption of nutrients is complete, the concentrations of all metabolites and hormones return to basal levels.

In the fasting state, two mechanisms keep blood glucose concentration in the normal range, glycogenolysis and gluconeogenesis. Initially, hepatic glycogen is mobilized. If fasting persists longer than 12 to 18 hours, peripheral tissues begin to use free fatty acid for fuel, thereby sparing glucose. A low level of circulating insulin is permissive to the lipolytic release of

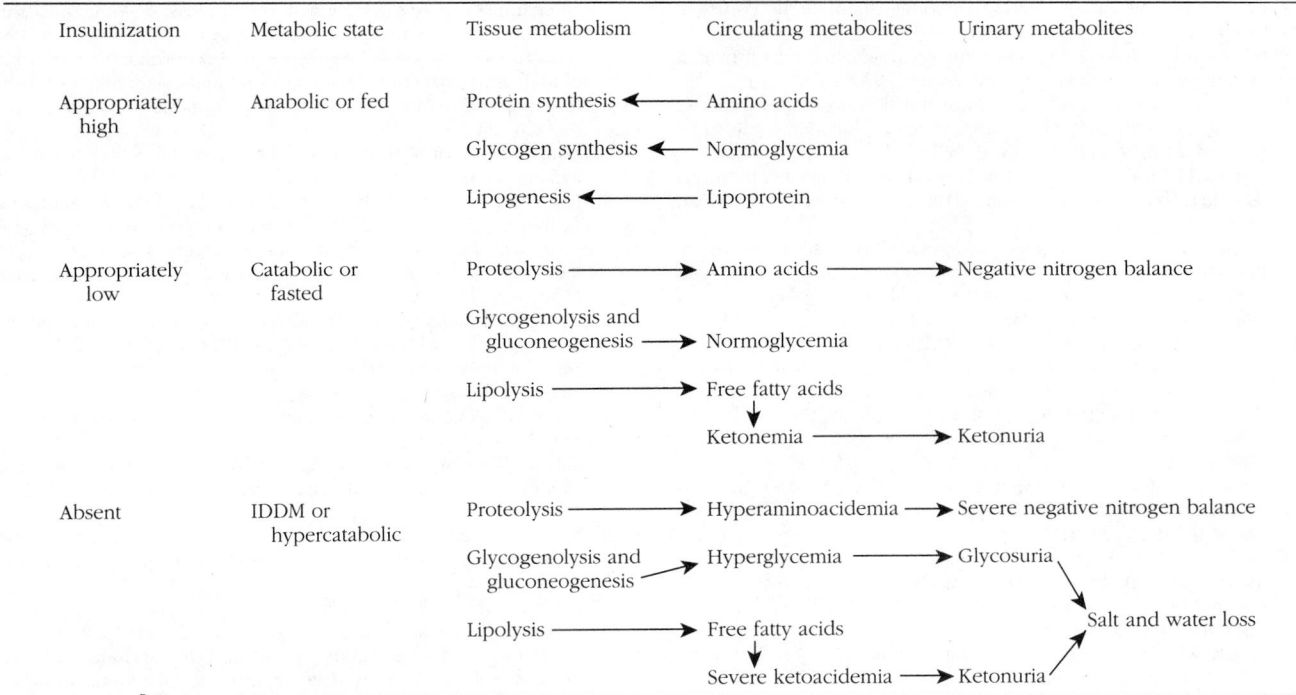

Insulinization	Metabolic state	Tissue metabolism	Circulating metabolites	Urinary metabolites

Fig. 109-1. Metabolic effects of insulin in normal and diabetic states. Upper entries illustrate the anabolic, storage-promoting effects of insulin that occur with eating. Middle entries illustrate the controlled catabolic effects that occur during fasting. Bottom entries illustrate the uncontrolled catabolism that ensues from the absence of insulin in insulin-dependent diabetes mellitus (IDDM).

these fatty acids. At the same time, gluconeogenesis supplies glucose for obligate glycolytic tissues, most notably the central nervous system (CNS).

If starvation persists for more than 72 hours, the brain begins to utilize ketone bodies as an alternative fuel, further sparing glucose utilization [10]. At this stage, a progressive decrease in hepatic gluconeogenesis occurs as a consequence of decreased amino acid release in the periphery. As starvation continues, lactate, pyruvate, and glycerol become the main gluconeogenic precursors in place of amino acids. At all times a low level of circulating insulin regulates the rate of lipolysis, glucose transport, and gluconeogenesis. Normal humans are always "insulinized" to an appropriate degree.

METABOLIC STRESS. Major surgery and critical illness are physiologically stressful events that provoke complex metabolic responses. Tissue hypoxia and hypoxemia adversely affect normal oxidative phosphorylation (see Chap. 115), and counterregulatory "antiinsulin" hormones are secreted. These hormones include epinephrine, norepinephrine, cortisol, growth hormone, and glucagon. They raise blood glucose concentration, mobilize alternative fuels, and increase peripheral resistance to the effects of insulin. In the ICU, their effects may be further amplified by the concurrent administration of exogenous pressors, glucocorticoids, and other drugs that can affect intermediary metabolism.

Normally, stress-induced changes in metabolism lead to increased insulin release. This, in turn, enhances peripheral glucose utilization and inhibits alternative fuel mobilization. The body thus resists stress without losing control of the biochem-

ical machinery. In patients with poor insulinization, failure of this feedback loop produces diverse metabolic complications. Overt diabetes may occur in a previously undiagnosed patient. Severe ketosis and shock may occur in a previously well-controlled patient with insulin-dependent diabetes mellitus (IDDM).

To preclude these complications, careful management of insulin, fluid, and electrolytes is necessary. It should go without saying that every patient admitted to an ICU must have at least one blood glucose determination at the time of admission.

CLASSIFICATION OF DIABETES. In the diabetic state, inadequate insulinization disrupts normal regulatory mechanisms. This can come about in many ways. Diabetes is not one disease, but rather a family of syndromes with hyperglycemia in common (Table 109-1) [9,11].

Diabetes Mellitus

INSULIN-DEPENDENT DIABETES MELLITUS. In IDDM (or type I diabetes mellitus), the insulin-producing beta cells in the pancreatic islets are destroyed by an autoimmune process and an absolute deficiency of insulin ensues [12]. Insulin-dependent diabetes mellitus develops abruptly in individuals of normal weight. Onset is typically during childhood and adolescence but may occur in older adults.

Patients with untreated IDDM can neither store nor utilize glucose. As a result, sustained gluconeogenesis and lipolysis occur (Fig. 109-1). In this hypercatabolic state, accelerating amino acid and fat mobilization produce hyperglycemia, hyperlipidemia, and ketosis. The glucose is the product of uncontrolled gluconeogenesis and remains in the circulation because there is no insulin to stimulate transport into cells. Secondary fluid and electrolyte shifts are produced by the osmotic diuresis of glucose and buffering of ketoacids. Management of IDDM and prevention of ketoacidosis are common ICU problems. The treatment of ketoacidosis is described in Chapter 110.

NON-INSULIN-DEPENDENT DIABETES MELLITUS. Non-insulin-de-

Table 109-1. Classification of Hyperglycemia

I. Diabetes mellitus
   A. Type I—Insulin-dependent (IDDM); ketosis-prone
   B. Type II—Non-insulin-dependent (NIDDM); resistant to ketosis
   C. Associated with certain conditions or syndromes (see Table 109-2)
II. Impaired glucose tolerance (IGT); abnormality in glucose concentrations intermediate between normal and overt diabetes
III. Gestational diabetes mellitus (GDM); glucose intolerance with onset during pregnancy

Source: National Diabetes Data Group: Classification and diagnosis of diabetes mellitus and other categories of glucose intolerance. *Diabetes* 28:1039, 1979.

Table 109-2. Most Common Types of Diabetes Mellitus

Variable	IDDM	NIDDM
Age at onset	Usually <25 years	Usually >40 years
Prevalence in U.S.	0.2–0.5%	3–4%
Sex ratio	♂ = ♀	♀ > ♂
Body habitus	Normal weight	Obesity in 80%
Clinical onset	Subacute to acute; ketosis present	Often insidious; nonketotic
Insulin treatment	Necessary for survival	Not always needed; diet and oral agents often effective
Inheritance	Frequently familial but only ≈50% concordance in monozygotic twins	Strongly familial with ≈100% concordance in monozygotic twins
Associations with autoimmune diseases and the MHC	Yes	No
Other terminology	Juvenile diabetes; ketosis-prone diabetes	Adult or maturity onset diabetes; ketosis-resistant diabetes

IDDM = insulin-dependent diabetes mellitus; NIDDM = non-insulin-dependent diabetes mellitus.

Table 109-3. Secondary Diabetes

Type	Examples
Drug-induced [32]	Thiazides, isoniazid, phenytoin, glucocorticoids, niacin, furosemide, calcium channel blockers, beta-adrenergic blockers, sympathomimetic drugs, phenothiazines, oral contraceptives, lithium
Pancreatic diseases	Hemochromatosis, pancreatic cancer, pancreatitis
Other endocrine disorders	Cushing's syndrome, pheochromocytoma, acromegaly

Source: Podolsky S, Viswanathan M (eds): *Secondary Diabetes: The Spectrum of the Diabetic Syndromes.* New York, Raven, 1980.

[14,32]. The condition is often described as secondary diabetes. Many of the offending drugs and diseases are common in the ICU.

Impaired Glucose Tolerance. Persons with impaired glucose tolerance have either a mildly elevated fasting blood glucose concentration or a borderline abnormal glucose tolerance test [11]. Most progress to overt diabetes, at the rate of 1 to 5 percent per year, but some may remain glucose-intolerant indefinitely or even revert to normal.

Epidemiologic studies suggest that they are at higher risk of atherosclerotic cardiovascular disease and neuropathy than is the general population [15]. They tend, however, to be free of microangiopathic retinal and renal disease. Patients with impaired glucose tolerance often become frankly diabetic when stressed.

Gestational Diabetes. Gestational diabetes typically appears during the last trimester of pregnancy in women who were not previously diabetic [16]. It occurs when maternal insulin reserves prove inadequate to the increased metabolic demands of pregnancy. When gestational diabetes is diagnosed, it always requires insulin therapy for the duration of the pregnancy, but only 2 percent of women will remain diabetic after delivery.

Diagnosis of Diabetes in the Critically Ill

DIAGNOSTIC CRITERIA. Among hyperglycemic patients who are seriously ill, the majority are previously diagnosed diabetics. Others are unable to provide a history, are unaware of preexisting diabetes, experience new onset of IDDM, or develop secondary diabetes in response to their primary illness. The diagnosis of diabetes is based on the observation of hyperglycemia; specific criteria applicable in an ICU are given in Table 109-4 [11]. Diabetes diagnosed in the ICU may or may not persist after the patient recovers. Impaired glucose tolerance should not be diagnosed in the critically ill because diagnosis is not valid in patients under stress. Individuals with minimal abnormality of glucose tolerance must be reassessed after recovery.

ASSESSMENT OF SEVERITY. As soon as diabetes is diagnosed in a critically ill patient, two critical questions must be answered immediately: Is the patient ketoacidotic? Is the patient hyperosmolar? The first question can usually be answered

pendent diabetes mellitus (NIDDM; type II) is characterized by a relative lack of insulin. In this disorder, insulin is ineffective, not absent [13]. Even when NIDDM is untreated, there is usually enough insulin to control lipid mobilization and prevent ketosis. In the ICU, however, intercurrent stress can cause hyperosmolar coma or lactic acidosis in patients with NIDDM. These disorders are discussed in Chapters 110 and 115.

Non-insulin-dependent diabetes mellitus develops insidiously, usually in obese individuals older than 40 years. It may go undetected for years only to be discovered serendipitously or during the stress of surgery or other illness. Patients with NIDDM account for more than 80 percent of the diabetic population.

Insulin is not required for *survival* of individuals with NIDDM; they are not ketosis-prone. They may, however, be given insulin to control the symptoms (e.g., polyuria) and prevent the complications of hyperglycemia. Many patients with NIDDM fare well with diet, exercise, and oral hypoglycemic agents. The small group of lean patients with NIDDM often requires insulin therapy. Characteristics that distinguish IDDM from NIDDM are summarized in Table 109-2.

OTHER TYPES OF DIABETES MELLITUS. Diabetes is associated with many drugs and diseases, some of them listed in Table 109-3

Table 109-4. Diagnosis of Diabetes in an Intensive Care Setting

Fasting glucose concentration greater than any of the following limits on more than one occasion:

1. Venous plasma ≥ 140 mg/dl (7.8 mM)
2. Venous whole blood ≥ 120 mg/dl (6.7 mM)
3. Capillary blood ≥ 120 mg/dl (6.7 mM)

Table 109-5. Diabetes Treatment Goals in Critically Ill and Surgical Patients

Zone	Blood glucose concentration
Hypoglycemia	<100
Safe but low margin for error	100–150
Critical care, surgical	150–250
Hyperglycemia	250–350
Severe hyperglycemia	>350

quickly on the basis of history, physical findings, and the presence of an anion gap acidosis and ketonemia. Osmolarity can be measured by the laboratory or calculated from the serum concentrations of glucose, blood urea nitrogen (BUN), sodium, and potassium (see Table 110-1 in Chap. 110). Hyperosmolar states in the setting of diabetes are associated with severe dehydration, obtundation, and extreme hyperglycemia. Diabetic ketoacidosis and hyperosmolar coma require urgent treatment (see Chap. 110). The remainder of this chapter describes the goals, methods, and pitfalls of treating intercurrent diabetes mellitus in the ICU when neither ketoacidosis nor hyperosmolar coma is the primary disease process.

Treatment of Critically Ill Patients with Intercurrent Diabetes

GOALS. We recommend that the blood glucose concentration in the critically ill or surgical diabetic patient be maintained between 150 and 250 mg per deciliter (Table 109-5). Which extreme of this range is more appropriate for a given patient is a matter of clinical judgment and depends on age and severity of illness, among other factors. Blood glucose concentrations less than 100 mg per deciliter pose the hazard of hypoglycemia. Values between 100 and 150 mg per deciliter in the ICU are not dangerous but offer little margin for error in management. Glucose concentrations in excess of 250 mg per deciliter require intervention. Glycemia between 150 and 250 mg per deciliter constitutes a safe "critical care zone." Although this concentration would not be desirable at other times, it avoids the pitfall of hypoglycemia as well as the short-term consequences of severe hyperglycemia.

WHY CONTROL DIABETES IN THE INTENSIVE CARE UNIT? Control of diabetes in the ICU is important for many reasons [17,18,19]. Patients with IDDM are very susceptible to the development of ketosis when stressed. Ketoacidotic patients develop dehydration and shock, and hyperglycemia predisposes to multiple electrolyte imbalances. Through its osmotic effect, each 100 mg per deciliter increase in glucose causes the serum sodium to fall 1.6 mEq per liter [20]. Since uncontrolled diabetes also provokes an osmotic diuresis, symptomatic hyponatremia can result. Hypokalemia predisposes to arrhythmia, and hypophosphatemia may interfere with platelet function and white cell motility. It may also decrease red cell 2,3-diphosphoglycerate levels, resulting in reduced O_2 delivery to tissues [21]. Control of glycemia prevents these problems and the need for compensatory correction.

The susceptibility of patients with diabetes to infection is well recognized [8]. Uncontrolled glycemia per se impairs leukocyte function and may also impair lymphocyte function and antibody formation [22,23,24]. Another short-term advantage of reasonable glycemic control concerns wound healing. Animal studies indicate that wounds develop less tensile strength in the presence of chronic severe hyperglycemia [25].

ASSESSMENT OF THE CRITICALLY ILL DIABETIC PATIENT. Assessment of diabetes in the ICU requires ascertaining the type of diabetes present, the duration of diabetes, and the degree of previous diabetes control. Patients with IDDM require exogenous insulin at all times; those with NIDDM may not. Patients with secondary diabetes require careful assessment of the precipitating factors.

Long-standing diabetes is also associated with complications that tend to be worse in poorly controlled patients [4]. These sequelae of diabetes complicate the management of critical illness. Diabetes is a leading cause of cardiovascular and peripheral vascular disease. Assessments of both cardiac function and peripheral circulation are obviously necessary for all diabetic patients. Diabetic neuropathy can affect the autonomic nervous system, with implications for management of blood pressure, heart rate, and voiding. Occult infections to which diabetic individuals are particularly susceptible include osteomyelitis, cellulitis, tuberculosis, cholecystitis, gingivitis, sinusitis, cystitis, and pyelonephritis. Because diabetes is a major cause of renal failure, BUN and creatinine should also be monitored. Diabetic eye disease is not a contraindication to anticoagulation, but its severity should be documented before instituting therapy. Patients with NIDDM are frequently hyperlipidemic and may develop pancreatitis on this basis.

A history of poorly controlled diabetes often implies poor nutrition. This has important implications for resistance to infection and wound healing; nutritional assessment and vitamin repletion may be required. Thiamine in particular is a critical cofactor in carbohydrate metabolism (see Chap. 115), and patients with uncontrolled diabetes may be thiamine-deficient.

In addition to this retrospective assessment of diabetes in the critically ill, prospective assessment requires continuously updated information on glycemia. Accurate fingerstick blood glucose monitoring systems for obtaining genuinely "stat" glucose determinations should be available in all ICUs, operating rooms, and recovery rooms [26].

TREATMENT OF HYPERGLYCEMIA IN THE CRITICALLY ILL

Insulin Infusion. All ICU patients known to have IDDM and all patients with blood glucose concentrations above the critical care zone of 150 to 250 mg per deciliter should be treated with a continuous intravenous infusion of regular insulin. This applies to all patients, without regard to previous history of diabetes or treatment modalities. Insulin may also be indicated for some patients with blood glucose concentrations of 200 to 250 mg per deciliter, depending on individual clinical circumstances. Continuous insulin infusion obviates concerns with the patient's state of perfusion, permits fine-tuning of insulinization, and simplifies maintaining stable plasma glucose within the critical care zone. This treatment method can obviously lead to hypoglycemia, but the continuous monitoring available in an ICU minimizes that risk and enables safe exploitation of this technology. Continuous insulin infusion requires frequent (at least every 1–2 hours) determinations of fingerstick blood glucose concentration.

Figure 109-2 indicates appropriate initial insulin infusion rates. Insulin infusions for glucose concentrations of 75 to 150 mg per deciliter are not needed initially unless the patient has IDDM. These patients require exogenous insulin at all times to prevent catabolism and ketoacidosis. Blood glucose concentrations less than 175 mg per deciliter should be covered with infusions of D_5W or $D_{10}W$ as indicated in Figure 109-2.

"Sliding scale" prescriptions for boluses of insulin should be avoided. They offer none of the benefits of continuous infusion while amplifying the risks of hypo- and hyperglycemia. Oral hypoglycemic agents (see Chap. 116) should not be used in the ICU.

In some centers, it is the practice to infuse insulin continuously in a glucose rather than a saline solution. We do not advocate this procedure simply because there is too much variation among individuals to rely on a fixed ratio of insulin to glucose. Either hyperglycemia or hypoglycemia could result. In addition, as the patient's condition changes, resistance to insulin may change, rendering the selected ratio inappropriate. Separate insulin and (when needed) glucose infusions are preferable.

Adjustments to Insulin Infusions. The amount of insulin required by ICU patients depends on (1) the degree of insulin resistance induced by the primary illness and its treatment; (2) insulin resistance due to other factors, such as obesity; and (3) the type and amount of nutritional support being given. An escalating insulin infusion requirement is a sensitive indicator of increasing insulin resistance and requires careful reevaluation of the patient's overall metabolic status.

Stressors that increase insulin resistance include sepsis, occult infections, heart disease, tissue ischemia, hypoxemia, and medications. The most common offending medications are glucocorticoids and pressors.

In otherwise stable patients, increasing insulin requirements sometimes reflect the institution or augmentation of enteral or parenteral nutrition. Insulin-mediated glucose disposal is impaired in stressed patients with diabetes, and even heroic insulin infusion rates cannot prevent hyperglycemia due to unmanageable carbohydrate loads. To control hyperglycemia in the ICU, a choice must sometimes be made between increasing insulin infusion rates or reducing carbohydrate feeding. We suggest that insulin infusion rates not be increased beyond 20 units per hour (480 units/day) without first decreasing any exogenous carbohydrate loads. This suggestion is based on the fact that maximal insulin effects are achieved when only some of the available insulin receptors are occupied [27,28]. High concentrations of insulin, such as those achieved during continuous intravenous infusions at high rates, desensitize target tissues at both the receptor and postreceptor levels, paradoxically enhancing insulin resistance [27,28].

Factors that increase insulin sensitivity in the ICU include improvement in the primary illness, changes in medication, and reductions in enteral or parenteral feeding. Occasionally, hepatic failure, renal failure, and adrenal insufficiency lead to decreased insulin requirements.

When blood glucose concentrations fall to less than 150 mg per deciliter, a common reaction is to discontinue insulin com-

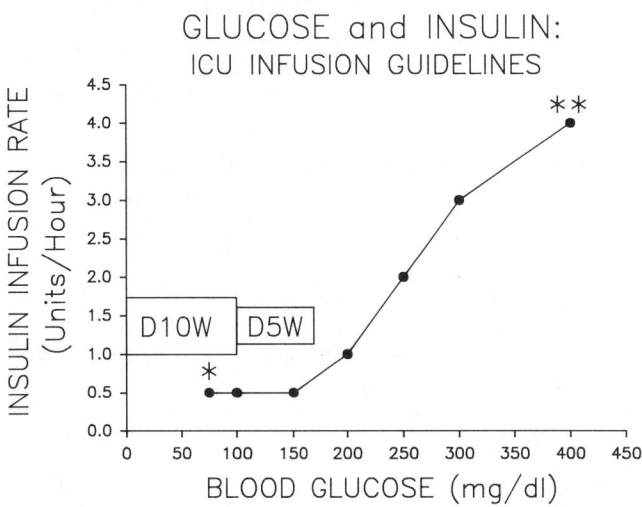

Fig. 109-2. Initial insulin and glucose infusion recommendations. Patients with blood glucose concentrations greater than 150 mg/dl in the ICU should be treated with a continuous insulin infusion. Patients with insulin-dependent diabetes mellitus (IDDM) should receive insulin at all times. ICU patients with glucose concentrations less than 175 mg/dl should receive infusions of glucose as indicated. * ICU patients who do not have IDDM generally require no insulin for glucose concentrations that are consistently less than 100 mg/dl. Patients with IDDM with values this low should be maintained on an insulin infusion of 0.5 units/hr together with a glucose infusion at all times. ** The infusion rate needed to control extreme hyperglycemia cannot be predicted. We counsel starting with conservative infusion rates that can then be adjusted hourly as needed. If a blood glucose concentration greater than 400 mg/dl fails to respond to 4 units/hr within 2 hours, the infusion rate should be doubled.

pletely. For patients with IDDM this is always incorrect: discontinuation of insulin can precipitate hyperglycemia and ketosis within hours. The proper response is to reduce the insulin infusion rate to 1 or even 0.5 unit per hour and, if necessary, to coinfuse glucose in the form of D_5W. We recommend the same strategy for most other ICU patients as well. Unless their primary disease problem has improved dramatically, they frequently experience recurrent hyperglycemia. Diabetic patients in the ICU should receive continuous intravenous insulin until they have demonstrated clear improvement in overall clinical status and stability of glycemic control that extends over several blood glucose determinations.

Transition to Other Forms of Therapy. When the condition of a diabetic patient in the ICU has improved to the point that continuous insulin infusion is no longer needed, additional therapy for diabetes depends largely on the type of diabetes. Patients with drug-induced (e.g., catecholamine- or steroid-induced) diabetes may need no further treatment for diabetes after the offending drug is stopped. In contrast, all patients with IDDM and the majority with NIDDM still require insulin. In these patients, subcutaneous injections of an intermediate-acting insulin should be started as the infusion is being discontinued. We recommend that the intravenous infusion of regular insulin continue for 2 to 3 hours after the first subcutaneous injection of intermediate-acting insulin is given. Some stable patients with NIDDM can be managed with oral hypoglycemic agents or diet alone, but these therapeutic decisions are best made after discharge from the ICU on a regimen of subcutaneous injections of an intermediate-acting insulin.

SURGERY IN THE CRITICALLY ILL PATIENT WITH DI-ABETES. Critically ill patients frequently require urgent invasive procedures, surgery, and intensive postoperative care. In such situations, the treatment of intercurrent diabetes is obviously of great concern.

Transfers from the ICU to the Operating Room. The ICU patient who requires surgery should be sent to the operating room or procedure suite with infusions of both insulin and 5% dextrose in half-normal saline.

Emergency Surgery. The possibility of diabetes must be considered in all surgical emergencies, and both glucose and electrolytes must be measured immediately. A critically ill patient with diabetes, even if previously undiagnosed, can rapidly develop profound metabolic derangements. Unless the diagnosis of diabetes is considered, the proper course of action may not be taken.

Abdominal pain accompanied by guarding and rebound tenderness is a common symptom of diabetic ketoacidosis. The diagnosis of diabetic ketoacidosis has on occasion been made at laparotomy, and this disorder must be excluded in every patient being evaluated for an acute abdomen. The patient with trauma being prepared for surgery should also be evaluated for diabetes, regardless of mental status. The stress of major trauma and shock is not likely to be survived if ketoacidosis or hyperosmolarity is present or allowed to develop. Severe trauma causes the release of contrainsulin hormones and other unidentified factors that can rapidly induce a state of severe insulin resistance.

Treatment of hyperglycemia in diabetic patients being prepared for urgent surgery can be initiated with either 16 to 20 units of subcutaneous intermediate-acting insulin or a continuous insulin infusion, as described above. Frequent monitoring of blood glucose is essential. Proper fluid and electrolyte balance must accompany the proper degree of insulinization; the amount and the type of fluid administered must be assessed on an individual basis.

Surgical Diabetes Management. In general, premedication in diabetic patients should be kept to a minimum. With respect to the type and the route of anesthesia, the first choices are always regional and local. Inhalant and parenteral anesthetics affect carbohydrate metabolism either directly through impairment of insulin secretion or indirectly through interference with the peripheral action of insulin on glucose utilization. Halothane inhibits insulin release, and nitrous oxide, trichloroethylene, and cyclopropane promote sympathetic stimulation and catecholamine release. Barbiturates share some of these effects and also block the removal of glucose and perhaps free fatty acids from the circulation.

Obviously, intraoperative blood glucose concentrations must be measured, particularly during prolonged surgery. The goal is to keep blood glucose in the critical care surgical zone (Table 109-5). In critically ill diabetic patients, insulin infusion as described above should be used during surgery [29].

Management after Emergency Procedures. Patients managed with an insulin infusion must either be maintained on the infusion or switched to a subcutaneous intermediate-acting insulin. Those kept on the infusion must have frequent blood glucose testing. The most important point is that insulin not be abruptly discontinued, since severe hyperglycemia and ketosis may ensue. Patients no longer critically ill and able to resume oral feedings can also generally resume their usual insulin regimen at that time. Patients who remain critically ill should remain on a continuous intravenous insulin infusion.

Postoperative convalescence in the ICU may be accompanied by reduced levels of contrainsulin hormones and may require reduced insulin doses. An increase in insulin requirements in the postoperative period may signify the opposite and should prompt the search for infectious or other postoperative complications.

PERITONEAL DIALYSIS AND DIABETES. Efforts to control glycemia in diabetic patients undergoing peritoneal dialysis commonly rely on the admixture of glucose and insulin in the dialysate. The relative concentrations of both must be determined empirically and are a continuously variable function of the metabolic and fluid status of the patient [30]. It is commonly necessary to administer additional regular insulin to diabetic patients to control hyperglycemia associated with high dialysate glucose concentrations. We recommend that most critically ill diabetic patients being treated with peritoneal dialysis be maintained on a continuous, low-dose insulin infusion at all times to ensure insulinization.

HYPERALIMENTATION AND DIABETES. If blood glucose rises above 250 mg per deciliter in a severely ill patient on hyperalimentation, an insulin infusion should be administered. The hyperalimentation should be continuous. The admixture of insulin with parenteral nutrition formulations, although a common practice, is not recommended. There is too much variability among severely ill patients to rely on a fixed ratio of insulin to carbohydrate. In addition, as is true of combined insulin and glucose infusions, changes in the patient's status can render the fixed ratio inappropriately high or low.

PITFALLS IN THE CARE OF THE CRITICALLY ILL DIABETIC PATIENT

Sliding Scales. We have repeatedly stressed the need to obtain frequent blood glucose specimens for evaluating glucose control. In an ICU these should be used to guide frequent adjustments of the rate of insulin infusion. There is no role for intermittent insulin boluses in the ICU.

Intermittent Insulin Administration. A patient begun on insulin should remain on it daily until the need has unequivocally disappeared. A previously normoglycemic patient who develops diabetes in the course of a severe illness should be treated continuously with insulin until the stress of the illness has been reduced to the point at which an independent assessment of the need for insulin can be made.

Unfortunately, some patients are treated with regular insulin injections on an intermittent schedule whenever a very high blood glucose concentration is noticed. This leads to erratic glycemic control and potentially serious shifts in fluids and electrolytes. When the insulin is given very intermittently, it is possible inadvertently to immunize the patient and generate high titers of antiinsulin antibodies. When this occurs, severe hyperglycemia in the face of ever-increasing insulin requirements results. The best way to avoid these problems is to maintain diabetic patients in the ICU on a continuous infusion of regular insulin.

Hypoglycemia Due to Sensitivity to Regular Insulin. Patients who have had IDDM for 15 years or more often develop extreme sensitivity to the effects of regular insulin. The reason is unclear, but this sensitivity frequently contributes to increased brittleness in these patients.

The use of regular insulin is an important component of the

care of critically ill and postsurgical diabetics. However, in the insulin-dependent patient with long-standing diabetes, the initial use of regular insulin must be approached with caution. Profound hypoglycemia can result from the use of as little as 5 to 10 units given either subcutaneously or intravenously. Because intermediate-acting insulins do not produce this effect, their use is preferred outside the ICU when the situation permits. When regular insulins are needed for patients who might be sensitive, the initial doses should be small (2–4 units) and the response monitored by fingerstick blood glucose determinations.

The Diabetic Kidney and Radiographic Contrast Agents. The risk of angiography in patients with both diabetes and nephropathy has been reassessed. Nephropathy was commonly thought to render patients with long-standing diabetes particularly susceptible to acute renal failure after angiographic procedures. With newer reagents and techniques, however, the risk of angiography may be no higher than in patients without diabetes [31]. A prudent course of action is to alert radiologists to the presence of diabetes, to hydrate such patients before study, and to minimize dye loads.

Conclusions

The key to successful care of the very ill diabetic patient is careful monitoring of glycemia and infused insulin. These patients all have a defect in normal metabolic regulation, and during the amplified metabolic stress of critical illness or surgery only treatment can compensate for the diabetes. Careful monitoring of blood glucose, followed by prudent adjustment of the insulin infusion rate, minimizes swings to either hyperglycemic or hypoglycemic states. Fingerstick blood glucose determination makes this intensive metabolic care possible not only in the ICU but also in the operating room, recovery room, emergency room, and procedure suite. The guidelines presented here have proved workable in our hands. Although they demand time and attention, they should enable physicians to minimize the special risks faced by diabetic patients who experience the stress of severe illness or surgery.

References

1. National Diabetes Data Group: *Diabetes in America. Diabetes Data Compiled 1984.* Bethesda, U.S. Department of Health and Human Services, 1985.
2. Kovar MG, Harris ML, Hadden WC: The scope of diabetes in the United States. *Am J Public Health* 77:1549, 1987.
3. Bransome ED Jr: Financing the care of diabetes mellitus in the U.S. *Diabetes Care* 15(suppl 1):1, 1992.
4. The Diabetes Control and Complications Trial Research Group: The effect of intensive treatment of diabetes on the development and progression of long-term complications in insulin-dependent diabetes mellitus. *N Engl J Med* 329:977, 1993.
5. Kannel WB, McGee DL: Diabetes and cardiovascular disease. The Framingham study. *JAMA* 241:2035, 1979.
6. Keen H, Ashton CE: Mechanisms of excess cardiovascular mortality in diabetes. *Postgrad Med J* 65(suppl 1):S26, 1989.
7. Selby JV, FitzSimmons SC, Newman JM, et al: The natural history and epidemiology of diabetic nephropathy: Implications for prevention and control. *JAMA* 263:1954, 1990.
8. Moutschen MP, Scheen AJ, Lefebvre PJ: Impaired immune responses in diabetes mellitus: Analysis of the factors and mechanisms involved—Relevance to the increased susceptibility of diabetic patients to specific infections. *Diabète Metab* 18:187, 1992.
9. Felig P: The endocrine pancreas: Diabetes mellitus, in Felig P, Baxter JD, Broadus AE, et al (eds): *Endocrinology and Metabolism.* New York, McGraw-Hill, 1981, pp 761–868.
10. Cahill GF Jr: Starvation in man. *N Engl J Med* 282:668, 1970.
11. National Diabetes Data Group: Classification and diagnosis of diabetes mellitus and other categories of glucose intolerance. *Diabetes* 28:1039, 1979.
12. Mordes JP, Greiner DL, Friedman HP, et al: Immunopathogenesis of diabetes mellitus. *Diabet Rev* 1:43, 1993.
13. Martin BC, Warram JH, Krolewski AS, et al: Role of glucose and insulin resistance in development of type 2 diabetes mellitus: Results of a 25-year follow-up study. *Lancet* 340:925, 1992.
14. Podolsky S, Viswanathan M: *Secondary Diabetes: The Spectrum of the Diabetic Syndromes.* New York, Raven, 1980, pp 1–602.
15. Kannel WB, McGee DL: Diabetes and glucose tolerance as risk factors for cardiovascular disease: The Framingham study. *Diabetes Care* 2:120, 1979.
16. Landon MB, Gabbe SG: Diabetes mellitus and pregnancy. *Obstet Gynecol Clin North Am* 19:633, 1992.
17. Santiago JV: Clinical review 38: Intensive management of insulin dependent diabetes—Risks, benefits, and unanswered questions. *J Clin Endocrinol Metab* 75:977, 1992.
18. Robertson RP, Klein DJ: Treatment of diabetes mellitus. *Diabetologia* 35(suppl 2):S8, 1992.
19. Unger RH: Meticulous control of diabetes: Benefits, risks, and precautions. *Diabetes* 31:479, 1982.
20. Katz MA: Hyperglycemia-induced hyponatremia: Calculation of expected serum sodium depression. *N Engl J Med* 289:843, 1973.
21. Alberti KG, Emerson PM, Darley JH, et al: 2,3-Diphosphoglycerate and tissue oxygenation in uncontrolled diabetes mellitus. *Lancet* 2:391, 1972.
22. Bagdade JD, Root RK, Bulger RJ: Impaired leukocyte function in patients with poorly controlled diabetes. *Diabetes* 23:9, 1974.
23. Strom TB, Bear RA, Carpenter CB: Insulin-induced augmentation of lymphocyte-mediated cytotoxicity. *Science* 187:1206, 1975.
24. Bates G, Weiss C: Delayed development of antibody to *Staphylococcus* toxin in diabetic children. *Am J Dis Child* 62:346, 1941.
25. Yue DK, McLennan S, Marsh M, et al: Effects of experimental diabetes, uremia, and malnutrition on wound healing. *Diabetes* 36:295, 1987.
26. North DS, Steiner JF, Woodhouse KM, et al: Home monitors of blood glucose: Comparison of precision and accuracy. *Diabetes Care* 10:360, 1987.
27. Olefsky JM, Kolterman OG, Scarlett JA: Insulin action and resistance in obesity and noninsulin-dependent (type II) diabetes. *Am J Physiol* 243:E15, 1982.
28. Olefsky JM, Garvey WT, Henry RR, et al: Cellular mechanisms of insulin resistance in non-insulin-dependent (type II) diabetes. *Am J Med* 85(suppl 5A):86, 1988.
29. Taitelman U, Reece EA, Bessman AN: Insulin in the management of the diabetic surgical patient: Continuous intravenous infusion vs subcutaneous administration. *JAMA* 237:658, 1977.
30. Berisa F, McGonigle R, Beaman M, et al: The treatment of diabetic renal failure by continuous ambulatory peritoneal dialysis. *Diabet Med* 6:67, 1989.
31. Parfrey PS, Griffiths SM, Barrett BJ, et al: Contrast material-induced renal failure in patients with diabetes mellitus, renal insufficiency, or both: A prospective controlled study. *N Engl J Med* 320:143, 1989.
32. Koffler M, Ramirez LC, Raskin P: The effects of many commonly used drugs on diabetic control. *Diabetes Nutr Metab* 2:75, 1989.

110. The Diabetic Comas

Aldo A. Rossini and John P. Mordes

Introduction

Diabetes mellitus is not one disease but a group of syndromes, all characterized by hyperglycemia. Its major clinical manifestations are due to relative or absolute deficiency of insulin [1]. About 5 percent of the U.S. population is diabetic, and the intensivist must regularly care for patients with the disease and its complications. The most important metabolic complications are the four diabetic comas: (1) hypoglycemia, (2) alcoholic ketoacidosis, (3) diabetic ketoacidosis (DKA), and (4) hyperosmolar hyperglycemic nonketotic coma (HHNKC). These four diagnostic possibilities must be considered in any lethargic or comatose patient. Hypoglycemia in the intensive care setting is discussed briefly here and in detail in Chapter 116.

Blood glucose concentration should be measured in all critically ill patients, even when mental status is normal or another primary diagnosis is evident. Diabetic ketoacidosis alone may cause abdominal pain and tenderness [2]. What appears to be simple alcohol intoxication may be alcoholic ketoacidosis with hypoglycemia. Head trauma may be the consequence of diabetic coma and may not be the patient's primary disease process.

Every emergency room should now have the capacity to perform fingerstick blood glucose determinations. Current chemistries and electronics make determinations of whole blood glucose concentration both rapid and accurate [3,4].

If the whole blood glucose concentration in a comatose patient is less than 50 mg per deciliter, or if for any reason the blood glucose cannot be measured rapidly, the first diagnostic and therapeutic step should be the infusion of 50 ml of a 50% dextrose solution. The hypoglycemic patient who awakens is cured; coma of any other origin is not adversely affected.

There are many causes of stupor and coma, but the diabetic comas are particularly important conditions because they are reversible. Frank coma as a result of diabetes has grown relatively less common [5], but untreated diabetic stupor will inevitably progress to coma. We use *diabetic coma* as a generic term that encompasses the milder metabolic abnormalities that precede loss of consciousness.

Hypoglycemic Coma

Hypoglycemia due to inadvertent insulin overdosage is the most common cause of diabetic coma [6]. It typically affects diabetic patients who have skipped a meal or exercised strenuously. Other causes of hypoglycemia include intentional misuse of insulin [7], liver or kidney failure [8,9], other endocrine deficiency states [10] (e.g., Addison's disease), and drug interactions (e.g., beta-blockers). Patients who take oral hypoglycemic agents rarely become hypoglycemic unless they fail to eat. Another cause of hypoglycemic coma, alcohol [8], is discussed in Alcoholic Ketoacidosis, below.

Successful treatment of hypoglycemia is gratifying; a bolus of concentrated glucose solution reverses the coma. The typical patient with type 1, or insulin-dependent, diabetes (IDDM) and insulin-induced hypoglycemia can be treated in the emergency room and sent home. If the cause of the hypoglycemia is excessive exercise, dietary omission, or a mistake in insulin administration, education must be provided. If the episode represents attempted suicide, psychosocial intervention must be arranged. If there is no immediate explanation for hypoglycemia, the patient should be admitted for evaluation.

When hypoglycemia is due to oral hypoglycemic agents, the patient must be admitted to the hospital (see Chap. 116). The half-life of many oral agents is quite long and the therapeutic administration of glucose further stimulates endogenous insulin secretion. Frequent feedings and continuous intravenous glucose should be given until levels of the oral agent fall. The process generally takes 1 to 2 days.

Alcoholic Ketoacidosis

Alcoholic ketoacidosis is not restricted to individuals with diabetes but is generally included among the diabetic comas. Recognition of the syndrome is important because it is potentially fatal but easily reversed. Ethanol is metabolized by alcohol dehydrogenase to acetaldehyde, which in turn is metabolized to acetyl-CoA. This process generates hydrogen ions and reduced nicotinamide adenine dinucleotide (NADH):

$$CH_3CH_2OH + NAD^+ \rightarrow CH_3CHO + NADH + H^+ \qquad (1)$$
Ethanol Acetaldehyde

The accumulation of reduced NADH leads to a reduction in oxidized NAD^+. Ethanol intoxication impairs the generation of glucose because gluconeogenesis depends on the availability of NAD^+ When glycogen stores are exhausted, hypoglycemia ensues [10]. The resultant low insulin state [11] promotes the breakdown of fatty acids, which are then metabolized to ketone bodies.

Patients with alcoholic ketoacidosis usually have very low blood glucose concentrations, elevated free fatty acid concentrations, and detectable ketone bodies [8]. They typically are stuporous, have not eaten for days, and are prone to nausea, vomiting, and aspiration. Hypothermia and neurologic abnormalities, including trismus, seizures, hemiparesis, and abnormal tendon reflexes, may be observed. By the time patients with this disorder are seen by a physician, the ethanol has often been metabolized and is no longer detectable. These patients are usually quite acidotic, with an arterial pH less than 7.2. Both ketoacids and lactic acid contribute to the acidosis.

The condition may occur in nonalcoholics who have binged and in children after accidental ingestion. Younger individuals are more susceptible than adults. Exercise, Addison's disease, hypopituitarism, hyperthyroidism, and diabetes treated with insulin or oral agents all predispose to alcoholic ketoacidosis. The transition from alcoholic stupor to alcoholic hypoglycemia may be imperceptible. It can be lethal if not recognized.

Management consists of rehydration with intravenous fluids and glucose to correct hypoglycemia. Parenteral thiamine (100 mg) should be given to prevent Wernicke's encephalopathy. Sodium bicarbonate should not be administered in alcoholic ketoacidosis uncomplicated by lactic acidosis (Chap. 115).

Diabetic Ketoacidosis

Any diabetic can develop ketoacidosis, but it most often occurs in those with IDDM (type I, ketosis-prone, or juvenile). Before the discovery of insulin, most patients with IDDM died of DKA [12]. Insulin revolutionized treatment and made recovery possible. As the treatment of DKA has improved steadily, the associated mortality has fallen to approximately 5 percent [13,14]. Most deaths are associated with intercurrent heart disease or infection in older patients, but some deaths still result from therapeutic error. Diabetic ketoacidosis is a medical emergency, requiring treatment that is not only immediate but also appropriate, thorough, and fastidious.

PATHOPHYSIOLOGY AND ETIOLOGY

Normal Glucose Homeostasis. After a meal, pancreatic islet beta cells release insulin into the circulation. The insulin enables fuels to enter cells and activates enzymes for their storage or metabolism. Glucose enters most tissues only in the presence of insulin; erythrocytes, heart, and brain are exceptions. Glucose is stored in the liver as glycogen. Some glucose is metabolized; any excess is converted into triglyceride.

In adipose tissue, insulin activates lipoprotein lipase, clearing lipoproteins from the circulation and storing them intracellularly. Insulin also inhibits the breakdown and release of previously stored fat [15,16,17]. Insulin has similar effects on skeletal muscle, permitting both amino acids and glucose to enter cells for oxidation or storage.

During starvation, insulin concentrations decrease and catabolic processes are activated to meet energy needs [18]. Stored fuels (glucose, amino acids, and fats) are all mobilized. Liver glycogen provides glucose for only several hours. After glycogen stores are exhausted, glucose is synthesized by the liver from muscle-derived amino acids by the process of gluconeogenesis. To conserve muscle mass during starvation, glucose consumption is reduced and fatty acids released from adipose tissue become the principal fuel source. Some fatty acids are transformed by the liver into ketoacids [19].

The rate of catabolism is regulated by insulin. Glucose utilization decreases circulating glucose concentration, leading to decreased insulin concentration. Low insulin levels permit lipolysis and proteolysis, stimulate gluconeogenesis, and restore the glucose concentration toward normal. This increase in glucose concentration stimulates insulin secretion, which in turn reduces or halts catabolism. Precise adjustment of insulin secretion, even in the absence of food intake, achieves continuous control of carbohydrate metabolism.

Abnormal Glucose Homeostasis. Diabetic ketoacidosis can be viewed as the "superfasted" state [16] that occurs when there is no insulin available to regulate carbohydrate metabolism. In the absence of insulin, glucose no longer enters most cells and is neither stored nor metabolized. Glucagon secretion is increased and hepatic glucose production increases without restraint. When the renal threshold for glucose is exceeded ($\approx$180–200 mg/dl), an osmotic diuresis ensues and water and electrolytes are lost.

If insulin deficiency persists, the stress-responsive hormones cortisol, epinephrine, norepinephrine, glucagon, and growth hormone are released and accelerate catabolism [20]. In these circumstances, lipolysis accelerates and large quantities of free fatty acids are circulated to the liver, where they are metabolized to ketone bodies [17,21,22,23]. Once this has happened, diabetic ketoacidosis is present. Most threatening to the patient with ketoacidosis are the accumulation of hydrogen ions, loss of free water, and depletion of electrolytes.

The cause of ketoacidosis is insulin deficiency. Previously undiagnosed IDDM commonly presents as ketoacidosis. Many more cases occur in individuals known to have diabetes. Dietary indiscretion in a treated diabetic may produce classic hyperglycemia, polydipsia, and polyuria, but it never causes ketosis. Ketonuria in any hyperglycemic diabetic patient should suggest the presence of frank DKA. Such patients must be carefully evaluated for the presence of acidemia [24,25]. Ketoacidosis occurs most often in patients who have omitted their insulin or who have an intercurrent infection. Other precipitating factors include acute myocardial infarction, emotional stress, cancer, drugs that interfere with insulin release or action, pregnancy, menstruation, and various endocrinopathies. Occasionally, no precipitating factor can be identified [12].

CLINICAL MANIFESTATIONS. Most patients in DKA are lethargic and about 10 percent are comatose [5]. They have lost large quantities of fluid; their skin, lips, and tongue are dry; and their eyes are soft to palpation. Patients with severe hyperglycemia and DKA have facial rubor in the malar area. Postural hypotension is common, but shock is rare [26].

Patients in DKA have rapid, deep (Kussmaul) respiration, and their breath has a sweet fruity odor. Some patients with new onset DKA have been misdiagnosed as having psychologic hyperventilation [27]. If a patient in DKA is not tachypneic, depressed respiratory drive due to severe acidosis (pH <7.1) should be suspected [28].

It is important to measure temperature accurately. Since the patient is hyperventilating, rectal or tympanic temperature should be measured. Patients in DKA do not have fever unless an intercurrent process, usually infection, is present. Similarly, the rare cases of hypothermia in DKA are associated with sepsis [29].

Abdominal pain is common and may be accompanied by a tender, guarded abdomen with diminished or absent bowel sounds [12]. The physician must always exclude the diagnosis of DKA when evaluating abdominal pain [2]. What may appear to be a surgical condition will resolve with correction of the acidosis.

Patients with DKA may be nauseous and vomit guaiac-positive, coffee grounds-like material. This is probably due to gastric atony, distention, and rupture of mucosal blood vessels. Pleuritic chest pain may also be present. The cause is unknown, but it resolves with treatment of the DKA.

The nose and sinuses of all patients with DKA should be examined. Acute sinusitis and a black intranasal eschar should suggest mucormycosis. This opportunistic fungal infection disseminates rapidly in acidotic patients. Mucormycosis is often fatal; survival depends on prompt diagnosis [30].

Diabetic ketoacidosis can complicate pregnancy. When it represents new onset of diabetes, is complicated by infection, or is due to noncompliance, rates of fetal loss are high [31].

DIAGNOSIS. Hyperglycemia, acidemia, and ketosis in the appropriate clinical setting are the criteria for the diagnosis of DKA. Additional laboratory abnormalities occur commonly but not always.

Blood Glucose. Blood glucose concentration in the range of 400 to 800 mg per deciliter is typical in DKA. Occasionally younger patients with high glomerular filtration rates (GFR) have blood glucose concentrations less than 300 mg per deciliter. More often, the solute diuresis causes dehydration, decreases the GFR, and further increases circulating blood glucose concentration [32].

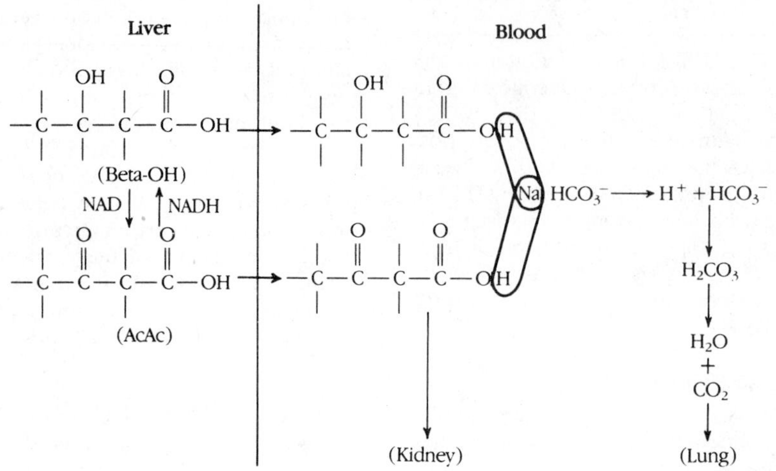

Liver | Blood

(Beta-OH)

NAD ↓ ↑ NADH

(AcAc)

(Kidney)   (Lung)

$HCO_3^- \longrightarrow H^+ + HCO_3^-$

H_2CO_3

H_2O
$+$
CO_2

Fig. 110-1. Neutralization of ketoacids. Hydrogen ion from ketoacids is neutralized by bicarbonate, producing carbonic acid that then decomposes to H_2O and CO_2. The latter is expelled by the lungs. The neutralized salts of ketone bodies are excreted in the urine. NAD = nicotinamide adenine dinucleotide; NADH = reduced form of NAD; AcAc = acetoacetate.

Electrolytes

SODIUM. Serum sodium concentration is quite variable in DKA and is usually not helpful in management unless it is extremely abnormal. Large amounts of sodium are lost during the osmotic diuresis of DKA, and the serum concentration does not necessarily reflect this loss [33]. Since sodium resides principally in the extracellular fluid space, elevated sodium concentration may simply reflect the degree of dehydration and free water loss.

Abnormally low sodium concentrations may be due to the osmotic effect of large amounts of extracellular glucose. The osmotic activity of glucose, drawing free water from the intracellular to the extracellular space, produces a fall of 1.6 mEq per liter of sodium for every increase of 100 mg per deciliter in blood glucose level over 100 mg per deciliter [34]. The "corrected" serum sodium in a patient with a measured concentration of 135 mEq per liter and a glucose concentration of 600 mg per deciliter is $1.6 \times (6 - 1) + 135$, or 143 mEq per liter.

It is important to verify that abnormally low serum sodium concentrations in DKA are not factitious. A common cause of factitiously low sodium concentration is hypertriglyceridemia. Sodium resides only in the aqueous phase of plasma but is measured as sodium per 100 ml of fluid in a sample [35]. When substantial hypertriglyceridemia is present in DKA, the measured concentration of sodium is spuriously low.

CHLORIDE. Chloride concentrations are usually not helpful in the diagnosis of DKA, though they may provide clinically useful information. Hyperchloremia may sometimes represent a more chronic ketoacidotic state [36] and is associated with slower recovery [24]. Extremely low levels of chloride may result from vomiting. Hyperchloremic acidosis can also occur during recovery from DKA as a consequence of the loss of neutralized ketone body salts [37].

POTASSIUM. Potassium is the electrolyte that must be watched most carefully and often during therapy. All patients with DKA risk the development of life-threatening hypokalemia during treatment, despite the fact that the serum potassium concentration is usually elevated initially [38]. This elevation is due to

catabolism of tissue, dehydration, and shifts of potassium from the intracellular to the extracellular space as hydrogen ions are buffered [24,39]. An initially elevated serum potassium concentration should never obscure the fact that total body potassium loss (200–700 mEq) always occurs in ketoacidosis [33]. The greatest loss accompanies the osmotic diuresis of glucose [40]. Additional losses are due to the excretion of ketone bodies as potassium salts, dehydration-induced secondary hyperaldosteronism, and vomiting. Potassium replacement early in the course of therapy for DKA is always necessary. Normal or low concentrations of potassium early in ketoacidosis reflect a very severe potassium deficit.

MAGNESIUM. Like potassium, serum magnesium concentrations in untreated DKA tend to be elevated initially, but they fall with subsequent hydration.

BICARBONATE. Serum bicarbonate concentration is low in ketoacidosis [28] due to neutralization of ketone bodies, which are strong acids. Bicarbonate buffer in the extracellular compartment represents the first-line defense in acid-base homeostasis. The process is summarized in Figure 110-1. The H^+ from ketoacids is neutralized by bicarbonate, producing carbonic acid, water, and CO_2. As CO_2 is expelled through the lungs, the neutralized salts of the ketone bodies are excreted in the urine.

PHOSPHORUS. Elevated serum phosphate concentrations are common in untreated DKA; the mechanism is not clear. After therapy, there is a precipitous decline to subnormal levels [33]. It has been estimated that as much as 1 mM per kilogram of phosphate is lost during DKA. Hypophosphatemia of less than 0.5 mM per liter has been described in both DKA and hyperosmolar hyperglycemic nonketotic coma [33].

Acidosis. Arterial blood gas and pH measurements are essential in the management of severe DKA. If they are unobtainable, venous or capillary gases may be of some use [41]. Diabetic ketoacidosis classically presents as an anion gap acidosis. The anion gap should be calculated for all acidemic patients (Table 110-1). In addition to confirming the diagnosis of DKA, the anion gap can be used together with plasma ketone measurements to obtain important additional insight into the nature and severity of a given case [42]. More chronic ketoacidotic states may be associated with hyperchloremic rather than anion gap acidosis [24,36], probably as a consequence of the loss of neutralized ketone body salts [37]. Rare cases of DKA are complicated by intercurrent metabolic alkalosis, most often from severe vomiting [43].

Table 110-1. Anion Gap and Osmolality Calculation

1. Anion gap

$$(Na^+ + K^+) - (Cl^- + HCO_3^-) + 17 = 0$$
$$\text{or}$$
$$Na^+ - (Cl^- + HCO_3^-) + 12 = 0$$

2. Osmolality*

$$2(Na^+ + K^+) + Glucose/18 + BUN/2.8$$

* Normal osmolality = 285–295 mOsm/kg.

Plasma Ketones. Plasma ketones must be measured in all comatose diabetics initially and then every 12 hours.* Results are usually expressed as the highest dilution of serum that gives a positive reaction. By definition, the test is always positive in DKA, but the result does not necessarily reflect the full extent of ketogenesis. The test measures only ketones. Acetocetone and acetone are ketones, whereas the beta-hydroxybutyrate (BOHB) produced from AcAc, although a "ketone body," is a hydroxyacid, not a ketone (Fig. 110-2). Normally, the BOHB/AcAc ratio is 3:1, but acidosis increases the ratio to 6:1 or even 12:1 as pH decreases. The BOHB/AcAc ratio at a pH of 7.1 is at least 6:1.

With this background information, the results of ketone body, anion gap, and arterial pH measurements can be used to determine whether a pure or mixed anion gap acidosis is present. The highest positive ketone dilution is multiplied by 0.1 mM per liter to obtain an estimate of AcAc concentration. If the serum ketones are positive at 1:32 but negative at 1:64, then multiplying 0.1 mM by 32 estimates the AcAc concentration as 3.2 mM. Multiplying the AcAc by 3 or 6 (depending on the pH) estimates the concurrent BOHB concentration. Acetoacetone (3.2 mM) plus BOHB (9.6 or 19.2) equals 12.8 to 22.4 mM per liter of ketone bodies. This approach roughly quantifies the contribution of ketoacids to the overall acidosis and the anion gap. If a patient's anion gap as calculated in Table 110-1 is greater than the estimated contribution of ketone bodies, the presence of an additional unmeasured anion should be considered (e.g., lactate, salicylate, uremic compounds, methanol, or ethylene glycol; see Chap. 115).

* Any laboratory can provide this service, but the clinician can also perform this test. First, place 5 ml of blood in a green-topped (heparin-containing) tube. Centrifuge the tube until clear plasma is obtained. Decant the undiluted plasma into a clean test tube and place two drops on a crushed Acetest nitroprusside tablet. (Uncrushed tablets have a waterproof coating.) After placing the sample on the powder, wait 60 seconds, then read the color. Do not wait longer. The depth of the purple color indicates the concentration of ketones. Then take 0.5 ml of the plasma, place it in a second test tube, and add 0.5 ml of water to make a 1:2 dilution. After mixing the tube well, test two drops of this sample. Then take 0.5 ml of the 1:2 dilution and again add 0.5 ml of water to produce a 1:4 dilution for testing. Repeat the procedure until a dilution is found that gives a negative (pale yellow) reaction.

Fig. 110-2. Biochemical interrelationships of the ketone bodies. Acetoacetate and acetone are ketones, whereas beta-hydroxybutyrate, although a "ketone body," is beta-hydroxycarboxylic acid and not a ketone. NAD^+ = nicotine adenine dinucleotide; NADH = reduced form of NAD.

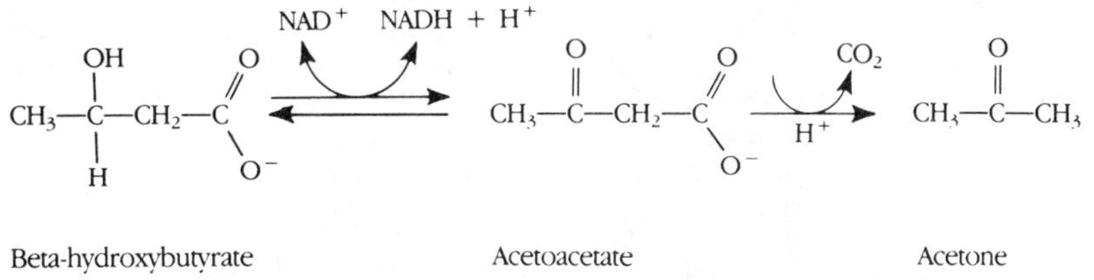

Ketone body measurements are also useful for monitoring the resolution of DKA. In cases of severe acidosis, ketone body measurements initially rise, not fall, as the acidosis improves. This is due to conversion of BOHB back to AcAc. Clearance of ketone bodies occurs slowly; measurement more often than every 12 hours is unnecessary.

Blood Urea Nitrogen and Creatinine. The blood urea nitrogen (BUN) of patients with DKA is typically elevated to values between 25 and 50 mg per deciliter [12,44], due not only to prerenal azotemia from volume depletion but also to increased ureagenesis. Patients in DKA are in a state of uncontrolled gluconeogenesis; the large quantities of amino acids released from muscle for conversion to glucose produce hyperaminoacidemia. These amino acids increase substrate availability for ureagenesis. Although the serum creatinine concentration usually reflects the degree of dehydration and prerenal azotemia in DKA accurately [45], spurious elevations occasionally occur because AcAc interferes with some creatinine assays [44].

Complete Blood Count. Hematocrit and hemoglobin in DKA are usually high and in proportion to the degree of dehydration [12]. Low values suggest preexisting anemia or acute blood loss. A characteristic hematologic finding in DKA is leukocytosis. White blood cell counts in the range of 15,000 to 90,000 per cubic millimeter with a significant left shift often occur in the absence of intercurrent illness [5,12,46]. Leukocytosis and a left shift in DKA do *not* necessarily imply concurrent infection. The absence of leukocytosis should prompt a search for folic acid or vitamin B_{12} deficiency.

Triglycerides. Insulin deficiency impairs clearance of lipid from the circulation and accelerates hepatic production of very low-density lipids (VLDL). In DKA there is marked elevation of serum triglyceride concentrations [25] that may be clinically obvious in the form of lactescent serum. With insulin therapy, this biochemical derangement reverses. If a patient can eat during the onset of DKA, hyperchylomicronemia may also be present. This condition can be distinguished from simple VLDL elevation by lipoprotein electrophoresis. Alternatively, a serum specimen can be refrigerated overnight and observed for a low-density "cream" layer of chylomicrons that has separated and risen to the top of the tube.

Urine. Urinary glucose and acetone should be measured and recorded. If pyuria is present, a urine specimen should be sent for culture and sensitivity. To avoid iatrogenic infection, catheterization should be avoided unless the patient is comatose or anuric.

Serum Amylase and Lipase. Serum amylase and lipase concentrations are sometimes elevated in acute ketoacidosis, but they do not necessarily imply exocrine pancreatic disease [47,48]. In some cases, the amylase may be of salivary gland origin.

Other Laboratory Findings. Uric acid concentrations may be elevated during acute DKA [49,50] as a result of impaired renal function or competition from ketone bodies at sites of tubular secretion. Hepatic enlargement with fatty infiltration of parenchymal cells may occur during acute DKA [12]. Liver function studies may appear transiently abnormal because of interference by ketone bodies with transaminase assays.

TREATMENT. Patients in severe DKA should immediately be hospitalized, preferably in an intensive care unit (ICU). It is unfortunate that some patients remain in the emergency room for hours awaiting laboratory studies other than those needed to establish the diagnosis. Delaying intensive care greatly increases morbidity. Treatment should be directed at three main problems—fluid, electrolytes, and insulin—in that order.

Recording of Data. A comprehensive flowsheet of vital signs, laboratory data, and treatment is essential to follow the response to therapy. An example is shown in Figure 110-3.

Fluid Replacement. Fluid and electrolyte therapy always takes precedence over insulin therapy in the treatment of DKA. As described below in Complications, insulin administration before volume and potassium repletion can cause arrhythmias and shock [51].

The free water deficit in DKA generally ranges between 5 and 11 liters and is due primarily to the osmotic diuresis of glucose [33,52]. Vomiting and hyperventilation may also contribute to water loss. Initial fluid resuscitation should be an infusion of 0.9% saline [53]. Approximately 2 liters should be given during the first hour to restore blood volume, stabilize blood pressure, and establish urine flow. Another liter of 0.9% saline is given during the next 2 hours. The subsequent rate of fluid replacement depends on individual clinical circumstances. During the first 24 hours, 75 percent of the estimated total water deficit should be replaced. Urine flow should be maintained at approximately 30 to 60 ml per hour. A simple method for judging the efficacy of fluid therapy is frequent determination of body weight. Fluid replacement after the first 2 liters may be changed to hypotonic 0.45% saline if hypernatremia is present [54].

Electrolytes. Sodium and chloride are replaced in conjunction with free water as just described. Potassium must be added as a supplement to the saline. Because serum potassium concentration does not accurately reflect total body potassium, replacement should be initiated early in treatment. Until the serum potassium concentration is known, replacement should be carried out cautiously. The recommended initial repletion rate is 20 mEq per hour as KCl or K_3PO_4. When the serum value is known, the rate of potassium administration can be adjusted. If a nasogastric tube is in place, electrolyte losses due to gastric suctioning must also be considered.

Potassium concentration often falls precipitously after starting therapy. K^+ shifts from the extracellular to the intracellular space in the presence of glucose and insulin. As acidemia resolves, buffered intracellular H^+ is exchanged for additional extracellular K^+, further lowering the serum potassium concentration. The electrocardiogram can be helpful in monitoring potassium treatment but cannot substitute for serum potassium determinations. Sudden reduction in serum potassium concentration can cause flaccid paralysis, respiratory failure, and life-threatening cardiac arrhythmias. If a patient in mild DKA is alert and able to tolerate liquids, potassium should be given orally.

Phosphate. Depletion of phosphate occurs in DKA. Initially the concentration of phosphate is elevated, but levels may decrease to less than 1 mM per liter with insulin treatment. Persistent severe hypophosphatemia can cause neurologic disturbances, arthralgias, muscle weakness, rhabdomyolysis, and liver dysfunction. Another important consideration in phosphate metabolism is 2,3-diphosphoglycerate (DPG) deficiency [55]. Deficiency of 2,3-DPG shifts the oxygen dissociation curve to the left, may result in tissue hypoxia, and has the potential to initiate lactic acidosis [56].

Potassium salt is recommended for phosphate replacement therapy. Each vial contains 93 mg phosphorus and 4 mEq potassium per milliliter. It is rarely necessary to administer more than one 5-ml ampule of potassium phosphate to a patient in DKA. Thereafter, potassium should be replaced as KCl. The hazards of parenteral phosphate administration include hypocalcemia and metastatic calcification. Except when hypophosphatemia is severe and persistent, the need for phosphate replacement in DKA may be more theoretic than actual. No studies have demonstrated that replacement of phosphate affects the course or outcome of ketoacidosis [57,58,59].

Bicarbonate. Most authorities suggest that bicarbonate replacement in DKA should be used only in patients with an arterial pH less than 7.1 [12,53,54,60]. Acidosis may impair myocardial contractility and decreases ventricular function, sensitivity of fat and muscle to insulin, and respiratory drive. Neutralization is intuitively appealing, but fluid and electrolyte replacement alone often ameliorate acidosis, and bicarbonate therapy may produce adverse effects. These include severe acute hypokalemia [61], late alkalosis due to paradoxical cerebrospinal fluid acidosis [62,63], and a shift of the oxygen dissociation curve to the left that results in tissue hypoxia and lactic acidosis [56]. At least three studies have questioned the efficacy of sodium bicarbonate therapy in DKA [64,65,66], but most clinicians would probably endorse its continued use in appropriate cases [60,67].

We recommend bicarbonate therapy in DKA (1) when the pH is persistently less than 7.1 after 2 to 3 hours of treatment; (2) when the initial pH is less than 7.0; (3) in cases complicated by depressed respiratory drive; and (4) when hypotensive shock is unresponsive to rapid fluid replacement [68]. To administer sodium bicarbonate, 2 ampules equivalent to 88 mEq should be given over 1 hour. As soon as the pH is greater than 7.2, bicarbonate treatment should be stopped.

Magnesium. Hypermagnesemia may occur early in the course of DKA [69], but serum Mg^{++} concentrations will generally return to normal without specific treatment. In some patients, Mg^{2+} stores may be depleted and may rarely lead to cardiac arrest [70]. Dysrhythmia should alert the physician to the possible need for magnesium supplementation.

Insulin. Insulin therapy in DKA is essential but should be instituted only after fluid and electrolyte resuscitation is underway. Continuous low dose infusion after a single intravenous loading dose is the preferred method [67]. We recommend a bolus of 10 units of regular insulin followed by a continuous intravenous infusion starting at 5 units per hour.* Some authorities recommend higher doses [53]. In children the recom-

---

* If continuous infusion cannot be given, the older bolus method can still be used. For adults, initially 10 to 25 units of regular insulin intravenously plus 10 to 25 units subcutaneously should be given. Subsequent doses of intravenous and subcutaneous regular insulin can be given every 1 to 2 hours, with the dose dependent on the results of glucose, potassium, and pH determinations.

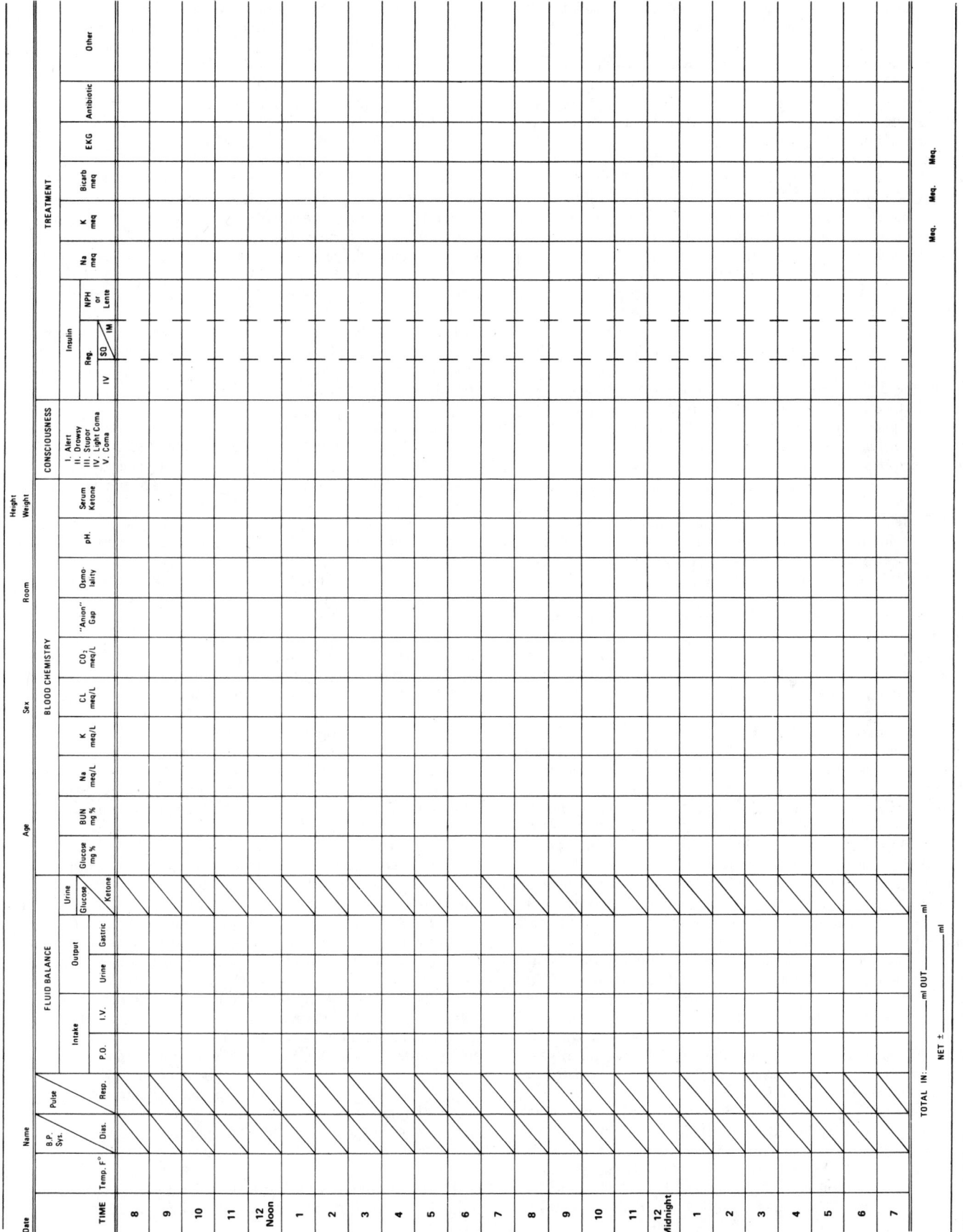

Fig. 110-3. Comprehensive flowsheet for charting vital signs, laboratory data, and treatment in diabetic ketoacidosis.

mended initial bolus is 0.1 unit per kilogram body weight and the infusion rate is 0.1 unit/kg/hr [65].

The insulin for infusion should be added to 0.45% saline (100 units/100 ml) and the bottle swirled before use. Blood glucose concentration should be measured every 1 to 2 hours after starting the infusion. If the glucose concentration has not decreased by 100 mg per deciliter, the insulin infusion rate should be doubled. When glucose has fallen by more than 150 mg per deciliter the infusion rate should be decreased by 50 percent, but it should never be stopped.

The blood glucose concentration during the first 24 hours of treatment should be kept at ≈200 mg per deciliter. If it falls below 200 mg per deciliter, glucose infusion (D₅W) should be started and the insulin infusion rate adjusted to 1.0 unit per hour to maintain insulinization and inhibit ketogenesis. Insulin should never be stopped entirely during DKA treatment, even if the infusion rate is reduced to only 0.5 units per hour.

Resolving DKA is often accompanied by increasing plasma ketones (principally AcAc) as BOHB is reoxidized. Total ketone bodies (AcAc plus BOHB) slowly fall throughout treatment, and the increase in measured ketones is transient. With further resolution of the acidosis, ketones fall. An increase in total ketones during the early hours of DKA treatment should not automatically lead to the conclusion that treatment is inadequate and more insulin is needed. The entire clinical picture must be assessed; if the acidosis and hyperglycemia are resolving, the rise in ketones can be interpreted as a sign of improvement.

COMPLICATIONS.

The morbidity and mortality associated with DKA are proportional to the severity of coma and acidemia at the time of presentation. Many complications can occur despite initiation of appropriate therapy.

Hypotension and Shock. Hypotension is an important complication of DKA [12]. It is usually caused by volume depletion, and normally fluid replacement alone will reverse it [71]. Persistent hypotension should prompt consideration of fluid shifts, bleeding, severe acidosis, hypokalemia, arrhythmia, myocardial infarction, sepsis, and adrenal insufficiency.

When insulin is administered to a patient with DKA, both glucose and water move to the intracellular space. Blood pressure may then fall as extracellular and intravascular volumes decrease. This can usually be reversed by increasing the rate of fluid replacement. Occasionally, hypertonic saline or an osmotically active solute, such as mannitol, may be necessary [72].

If shock persists despite fluid replacement, occult blood loss should be considered. Patients with gastric ulcer, colitis, or hemorrhagic pancreatitis can bleed into the gut lumen or peritoneum. Physical examination and an inappropriately low hematocrit in the face of dehydration are clues that lead to recognition of this complication.

Severe acidemia may impair the pressor effect of catecholamines. Patients with refractory shock and severe (pH < 7.0) acidosis may require bicarbonate to reverse the acidosis before the hypotension can be reversed.

A shift in K⁺ from the extracellular to the intracellular fluid space following insulin administration can lower serum potassium concentration. This common cause of cardiac arrhythmia may compromise blood pressure.

Patients with hypotension and increased central venous pressure should be investigated for heart disease. Myocardial infarction is the most common finding, but other conditions, such as cardiac tamponade, can be found [12]. Myocardial infarction is a common complication in long-standing diabetes, and its classic symptoms may be less obvious in the diabetic popula-

tion. Patients in DKA who have had a myocardial infarction have an ominous prognosis [14,73].

Gram-negative sepsis is another cause of shock in ketoacidosis [68]. Pyelonephritis and pneumonia are common in such cases and must be treated appropriately when encountered. Ketoacidosis per se does not cause fever.

It is not uncommon for insulin-dependent diabetic patients to have other autoimmune diseases, and adrenal insufficiency should be considered in cases of ketoacidosis with refractory shock. The stress of DKA may uncover a state of partial adrenal insufficiency requiring glucocorticoid replacement.

The most logical initial approach to the patient in shock is additional fluid replacement. (See Chaps. 171 and 172 for a detailed discussion of the subsequent management of this problem.) Thereafter, further diagnostic procedures will be necessary. Occasionally, patients who have persistent shock may respond to blood transfusion [54], but this is disputed [74]. Cardiovascular monitoring systems should be used as needed.

Thrombosis. The dehydration and intravascular volume contraction common in DKA may activate coagulation factors [75]. Thrombosis of the cerebral vessels and stroke are recognized complications of DKA.

Cerebral Edema. Subclinical brain edema may be common in DKA [76], but clinically important cerebral edema is a rare complication in adults. In children it usually occurs a few hours after the initiation of therapy. The exact mechanism is unknown, but it may involve a combination of fluid shifts, thrombosis of intracerebral vessels, and effects on ion exchange mechanisms [77,78,79]. The most effective treatment for cerebral edema is probably mannitol [79]. Steroids may also be useful. Unfortunately, even when diagnosed early, this complication may cause permanent neurologic damage or death.

Renal Failure. Hyperglycemic patients given intravenous fluids should have brisk urine flow. Patients in DKA who do not void within a few hours of therapy should be considered oliguric. One of the commonest causes of oliguria is postrenal obstruction. A dilated, atonic bladder is common in comatose patients and even more common in diabetic patients with severe neuropathy and DKA. Occasionally patients in DKA precipitated by pyelonephritis develop acute tubular necrosis [12]. Acute renal failure in the absence of infection is an uncommon complication of DKA [80].

Recurrent Diabetic Ketoacidosis. If ketoacidosis reappears in a patient who has received adequate amounts of insulin, infection or a severe contrainsulin state (e.g., Cushing's syndrome) should be suspected. More commonly the problem is iatrogenic: The physician treating DKA notes that the blood glucose concentration has fallen, mistakenly assumes the condition has been cured, and discontinues insulin treatment. Because the half-life of infused insulin is 20 minutes, and by definition these patients make no insulin, ketone production soon resumes and ketosis recurs [81]. Insulin infusions should be continued, if only at 0.5 to 1 unit per hour, until the patient is well enough to be switched to subcutaneous injections of longer-acting insulin. We recommend that the intravenous infusion of regular insulin continue for 2 to 3 hours after the first subcutaneous injection of intermediate-acting insulin is given.

Low Blood Glucose Concentration. The blood glucose concentration in DKA usually decreases rapidly as soon as fluid is administered and urine flow is established [71]. After insulin is given, glucose is metabolized as well. The physician must be alert to the possibility of precipitous reductions in glycemia. The goal of the first 24 hours of DKA treatment is a blood glucose concentration not less than 200 mg per deciliter to avoid cerebral edema.

Children with ketoacidosis have a high glomerular filtration rate, and their increased renal clearance of glucose following hydration may mask persistent ketone production. When the blood glucose concentration falls to 200 mg per deciliter, intravenous glucose as D_5W should be administered together with insulin. Use of $D_{10}W$ is unnecessary [82]. Dual therapy inhibits ketone production while precluding hypoglycemia. For the first 24 hours of treatment, continuous intravenous infusion of insulin is recommended.

FOLLOW-UP CARE OF DIABETIC KETOACIDOSIS. After a patient has recovered from DKA, the goal should be prevention of further episodes [83]. This requires identification of any precipitating factors. Lack of education regarding diabetes should be remedied. Full recovery from diabetic coma may take several days, during which any necessary investigations can be performed.

Hyperosmolar Hyperglycemic Nonketotic Coma

Severe hyperglycemia, dehydration, and coma frequently occur in older patients with mild or moderate diabetes in the absence of significant acidosis or ketonemia. This syndrome, now designated hyperosmolar hyperglycemic nonketotic coma (HHNKC), was described by Sament and Schwartz in 1957 [84]. Mortality in HHNKC has historically been high, on the order of ≈50 percent [85,86,87]. Increasing recognition and improved ICU-based treatment have substantially improved this figure; 15 percent mortality was reported in one recent series [14]. With optimal care, HHNKC managed in an ICU setting can carry a relatively favorable prognosis.

PATHOPHYSIOLOGY AND ETIOLOGY. The pathophysiology that gives rise to HHNKC requires that three interrelated elements be present: insulin deficiency, renal impairment, and cognitive impairment.

Insulin Deficiency. Relative lack of insulin is the fundamental defect in HHNKC. Patients have sufficient insulin to inhibit ketone body formation but not enough to prevent hyperglucagonemia, glycogenolysis, and gluconeogenesis [88]. The resulting hyperglycemia induces an osmotic diuresis, with resultant fluid and electrolyte losses.

Paradoxically, venous insulin concentration levels in patients with HHNKC are comparable to those sometimes observed in DKA [89]. Animal studies may explain the apparent paradox. Animals with experimentally induced HHNKC have *portal* insulin concentrations higher than those of animals with experimental ketoacidosis [90]. The data suggest that partial insulinization of the liver in HHNKC enables affected patients to metabolize free fatty acids and thereby avoid ketogenesis in the face of severe hyperglycemia.

Additional data indicate, however, that hepatic insulinization alone cannot account for the absence of ketosis in HHNKC.

Ketone bodies can be induced when medium-chain triglycerides (precursors of fatty acids) are administered to animals with an experimental HHNKC syndrome [91]. The result suggests that patients with HHNKC would produce ketones despite hepatic insulinization if enough substrate in the form of free fatty acids were present. Their resistance to ketosis must therefore depend on limited availability of circulating free fatty acids [86].

The low concentrations of free fatty acids in HHNKC may be due to relatively low concentrations of lipolytic hormones [92], including growth hormone and cortisol. Concentrations of these hormones are lower in HHNKC than in DKA [77]. Another explanation is that hyperosmolality itself inhibits the release of free fatty acids [93]. Still other factors may play a role.

Renal Impairment. Some degree of renal impairment accompanies all cases of HHNKC. Younger patients with diabetes have a normal glomerular filtration rate and, even in the event of DKA, filter enough glucose into the urine to prevent extreme hyperglycemia. In contrast, typical patients with the HHNKC syndrome are older. Their renal blood flow and GFR are reduced, and they cannot readily excrete a glucose load. When they become hyperglycemic, the glucose is neither metabolized nor excreted. It remains in the extracellular fluid space. The resulting increase in osmolality, together with the decreased GFR, causes excretion of still less glucose (Fig. 110-4).

The underlying renal abnormality in the HHNKC syndrome may be prerenal, renal, or postrenal. The common result is that affected patients are unable to compensate for the hyperglycemia with an osmotic diuresis. The result is extremely severe hyperglycemia.

Cerebral Impairment. Hyperglycemia leading to hyperosmolality normally activates thirst. The combination of mild diabetes and azotemia does not lead to the HHNKC syndrome unless the affected individual cannot drink sufficient water to prevent hyperosmolality. Invariably, HHNKC involves acute or chronic impairment of cerebral function. The most common history involves an elderly patient with impaired cognitive function due to cerebrovascular disease, dementia, or CNS-depressant medications. This impairment may involve either concurrent impairment of the normal thirst mechanism or an inability to respond to thirst due to speech or motor deficits. Patients with trauma or burns have large insensible water losses, are often unable to drink, and are also susceptible to HHNKC in the absence of adequate parenteral fluids.

Animal studies confirm that fluid restriction is necessary to produce an HHNKC-like disorder. Diabetic rats do not develop HHNKC syndrome unless they are deprived of water [94]. Decreased thirst leads to increased dehydration, increased stupor, and further decreases in fluid intake. Other factors, such as angiotensin, may also be involved [95].

Interrelationships. To summarize, three interrelated factors are required for HHNKC. Insulin deficiency leads to hyperglycemia and glycosuria. Impaired renal function exaggerates the hyperglycemia and leads to hyperosmolality. Decreased water intake precludes dilutional compensation. Together these three factors produce dehydration and the hyperosmolar hyperglycemic state (Fig. 110-5).

The severe dehydration that occurs in this syndrome is due to the osmotic diuresis of glucose in the absence of compensatory free water intake. Dehydration, in turn, leads to hemoconcentration, setting the stage for severe prerenal azotemia, thrombosis, and shock. As glucose and osmolality rise, cerebral function is progressively compromised. Coma ensues when the serum osmolality is 350 mOsm per kilogram or greater [96].

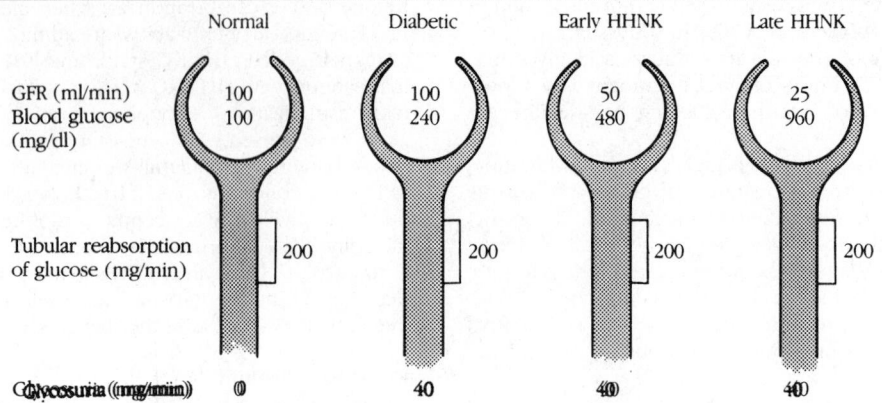

	Normal	Diabetic	Early HHNK	Late HHNK
GFR (ml/min)	100	100	50	25
Blood glucose (mg/dl)	100	240	480	960
Tubular reabsorption of glucose (mg/min)	200	200	200	200
Glycosuria (mg/min)	0	40	40	40

Fig. 110-4. Interrelationship of blood glucose concentration, glomerular filtration rate (GFR), and renal excretion of glucose. This diagram illustrates the importance of dehydration and diminished GFR in the development of extreme hyperglycemia in hyperosmolar hyperglycemic nonketotic coma (HHNC). The normal individual, with normal GFR and normoglycemia, is never glycosuric. A diabetic individual with normal renal function and normal thirst response may become hyperglycemic if glycemic control is poor, but the high GFR leads to glycosuria, and severe hyperglycemia does not usually develop. In a patient with HHNKC, in contrast, osmotic diuresis and impairment of thirst response lead to progressive deterioration in GFR. The kidney's ability to excrete glucose declines and extreme hyperglycemia develops.

CLINICAL FINDINGS IN HYPEROSMOLAR HYPERGLYCEMIC NONKETOTIC COMA. Patients in HHNKC are typically middle-aged or elderly [72,73,85,87,97,98]. The syndrome may occur in younger patients and even infants, but this is unusual [31,99]. Patients often have a history of mild type II diabetes and may have been treated with diet and oral hypoglycemic agents. There may be a prodrome of progressive polyuria and polydipsia and, occasionally, polyphagia lasting days to several weeks.

Most patients have underlying diseases. Renal and cardiovascular disorders are most common. Other intercurrent problems include infection, myocardial infarction, stroke, hemorrhage, and trauma [85,98]. Additional predisposing factors include dialysis [100], hyperalimentation [101], and medications. Thiazide diuretics [102], phenytoin [103], propranolol [104], immunosuppressive agents [105], and cimetidine [106] all impair insulin secretion or action and have been implicated as causes of HHNKC.

Fever is a common finding in HHNKC, even in the absence of infection, but infection must be rigorously excluded in all cases. Patients may have hypotension and tachycardia due to dehydration, and they frequently hyperventilate. Neurologic manifestations include tremors and fasciculations. Mental status may range from mild disorientation to obtundation and coma as a function of the degree of abnormalities in osmolality and perfusion [107]. Up to a third of patients with HHNKC may seize [108], and many in this group are misdiagnosed as having primary intracerebral disease. Once treatment has been instituted, neurologic symptoms may clear rapidly. The hyperventilation may reflect lactic acidosis, a common complication of severe dehydration and hypotension (see Chap. 115). Rapid respirations in hyperglycemic patients do not always imply ketoacidosis.

DIAGNOSIS. The key to the diagnosis of HHNKC is the demonstration of hyperglycemia and hyperosmolality without significant ketosis in the appropriate clinical setting.

Blood Glucose Concentration. Blood glucose concentrations in HHNKC are generally higher than in DKA, usually greater than 600 mg per deciliter. Values as high as 2000 mg per deciliter occur.

Acetone. Most patients in HHNKC are not ketotic. Serum acetone levels are usually normal or only slightly elevated, seldom exceeding 1:2. Occasional patients in HHNKC will develop an intercurrent metabolic acidosis. In these very ill patients, a severe hyperosmolar state may overlap with ketoacidosis. Such cases are uncommon.

Osmolality. Serum osmolality in comatose patients usually exceeds 350 mOsm per kilogram. It can be measured directly in the laboratory but is easily and quickly approximated from other data. The formula for calculating approximate serum osmolality from BUN, sodium, potassium, and glucose concentrations is given in Table 110-1.

Acid-Base Balance. Most patients in HHNKC are only mildly acidotic. Serum bicarbonate concentration and arterial pH are usually close to normal. The average pH is about 7.25 before treatment. The acidemia most often represents either mild lactic acidosis or uremic acidosis. If there is a significant anion gap (see Table 115-4), other causes of acidosis should be considered. These include salicylate, methanol, and ethylene glycol ingestions.

Renal Function. As outlined above, renal function is always impaired in patients with HHNKC. In addition to any preexisting renal disease, dehydration induces prerenal azotemia, and the ratio of BUN to creatinine is usually greater than 30:1. Blood urea nitrogen and creatinine should be repeated after treatment to determine the degree of intrinsic renal impairment.

Electrolytes. The serum sodium concentration in early HHNKC is highly variable, ranging between 100 and 180 mEq per liter. Hyponatremia may result from the dilutional effect of osmotically active glucose in patients with high free water intake in the face of impaired renal function. As mentioned previously, for each 100 mg per deciliter increase in blood glucose in excess of 100 mg per deciliter, serum sodium concentration falls approximately 1.6 mEq per liter. When severe hypotonic fluid losses occur in the later stages of HHNKC, patients may become hypernatremic. Since sodium remains in the extracellular fluid compartment, this electrolyte should be followed to assess the state of hydration.

Serum potassium concentration in HHNKC syndrome is also variable. It may range from 2.2 to 7.8 mEq per liter [85,86,87].

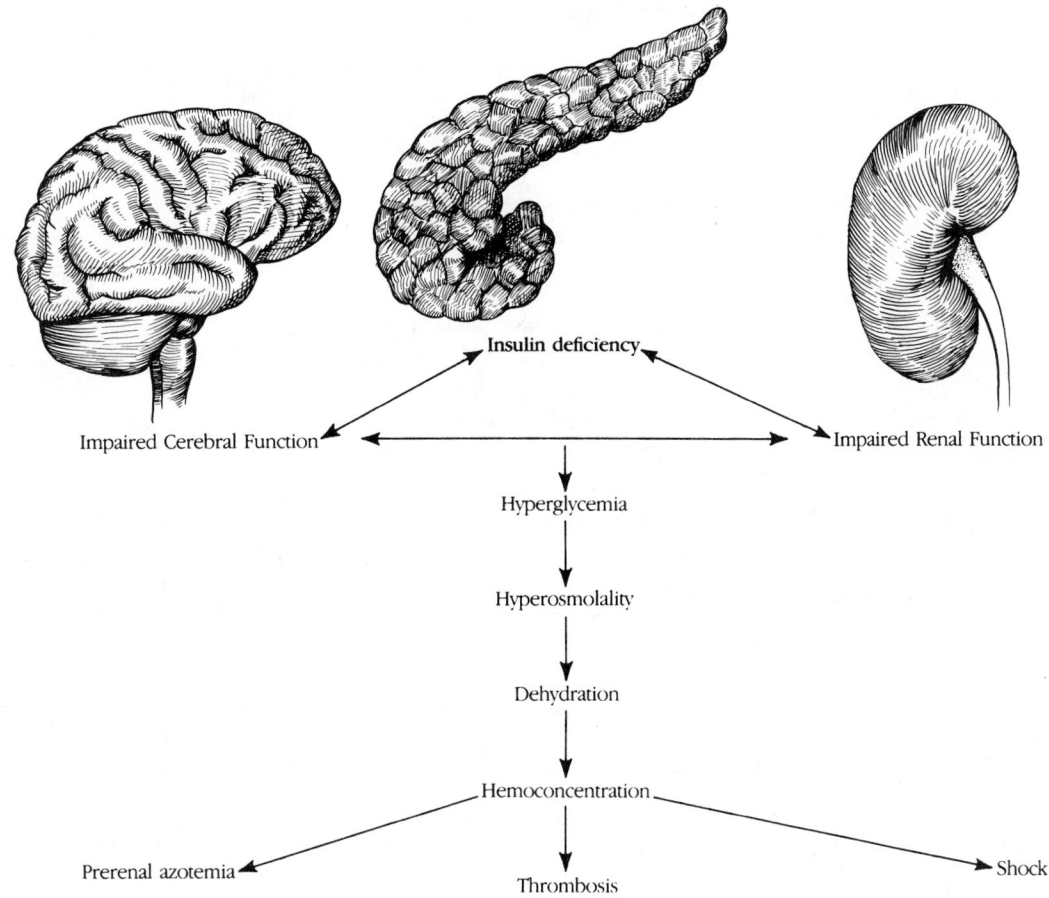

Fig. 110-5. Pathogenesis of hyperosmolar hyperglycemic non-ketotic coma (HHNKC). Three interrelated factors give rise to HHNKC: (1) insufficient insulin leads to hyperglycemia and glycosuria; (2) impaired renal function exaggerates the hyperglycemia and hyperosmolarity; and (3) impaired cognition leads to decreased free water intake. Together, these factors lead to dehydration and the hyperosmolar hyperglycemic state.

Hypokalemia requires immediate potassium replacement. As will be mentioned below, serum potassium concentrations decrease after treatment with insulin is begun. Hyperkalemia often responds to fluid replacement and improvement in urinary output. It must be emphasized that patients with HHNKC, like those with DKA, lose substantial quantities of electrolytes [109].

TREATMENT

Overview. The best treatment for HHNKC is prevention. The condition can easily be avoided by periodic attention to blood glucose control and mental status. Susceptible individuals are those with mildly impaired glucose metabolism. They are often the elderly living alone. They may also be hospitalized inpatients who have experienced trauma, undergone extensive surgery, or been placed on hyperalimentation regimens, or residents of nursing homes, though improvements in care appears to have lessened this classical risk factor [98]. Individuals in all of these settings are at risk for hyperglycemia and hyperosmolality.

Historically, 40 to 70 percent of patients with HHNKC died despite appropriate treatment [85,86,87]. One-third of these pa-

tients succumbed within the first 24 hours. The immediate causes of death included associated illness, shock, electrolyte disturbances, and cerebral edema. With modern ICU-based management of both hyperosmolarity and its precipitants, it is now possible to lower that mortality rate substantially [14]. Continuous vigilance in monitoring the details of the patient's clinical progress at the bedside is the key to achieving a successful outcome.

Fluid Replacement. Patients with HHNKC are without exception profoundly dehydrated. Within the first 2 hours, 1 to 2 liters of 0.9% saline should be given. Normal saline is recommended even if hypernatremia is present, to expand the extracellular fluid compartment rapidly. After initial volume expansion and restoration of normotension, subsequent treatment for dehydration in this syndrome emphasizes free water replacement. The osmotic diuresis of glucose produces free water loss in excess of solute loss. The initial infusion of normal saline must never be overlooked, however. It promptly expands the extracellular compartment and helps reestablish adequate perfusion pressure.

The average patient requires 6 to 8 liters of fluids during the first 12 hours of treatment. The rate of fluid administration must be adjusted as appropriate to the patient's clinical status. Elderly patients with cardiovascular impairment may require less aggressive replacement.

Electrolytes. As soon as adequate urine flow has been established and the degree of hypokalemia estimated, potassium supplementation should be added to the intravenous fluids.

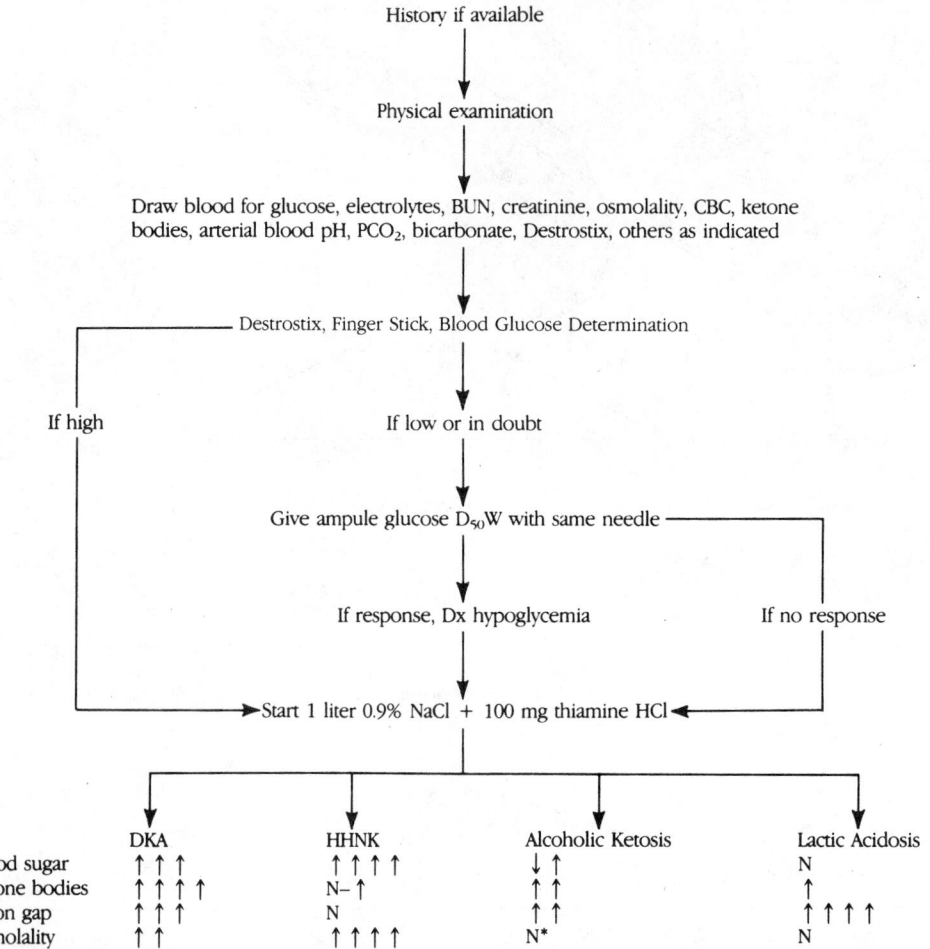

Fig. 110-6. Algorithm for the diagnosis of diabetic coma. Measured osmolality is greater than predicted; result in freezing point depression test is increased by 1 mOsm/5 mg % EtOH. DKA = diabetic ketoacidosis; HHNK = hyperosmolar hyperglycemic nonketotic syndrome; N = normal;   = mildly elevated;   = mildly depressed;   = moderately elevated;   = severely elevated;   = extremely elevated. (Adapted from Hare JW, Rossini AA: Diabetic comas: The overlap concept. *Hosp Pract* 14:95, 1979. With permission. Illustration by Albert Miller.)

During the initial phases of therapy, serum potassium concentration should be checked frequently and the electrocardiogram monitored for changes in morphology and rhythm. A sudden fall in serum potassium concentration frequently accompanies the initiation of insulin therapy [86]. Cardiac arrhythmias induced by hypokalemia may be irreversible, particularly in the elderly. Although total body potassium is invariably decreased in patients with HHNKC, the magnitude of the loss is never as great as that encountered in diabetic ketoacidosis [109].

Insulin. Most patients with HHNKC are more sensitive to insulin than are patients with diabetic ketoacidosis [86]. In addition, blood glucose concentration in HHNKC can fall precipitously when urine output is reestablished after volume expansion with saline. The combination of insulin sensitivity and glucose diuresis puts patients in HHNKC at risk of sudden, unexpected hypoglycemia. Treatment with insulin is essential but should be instituted with careful monitoring and only *after* fluid and electrolyte resuscitation is underway.

Only short-acting regular insulin should be used. Continuous infusion is now standard, but must be used with great caution. We do not recommend an initial intravenous insulin bolus. For the infusion, we recommend a starting dose of only 1 to 5 units per hour, depending on individual circumstances. This dose is sufficient to insulinize the patient and is usually not high enough to cause severe hypoglycemia.*

As emphasized repeatedly, normalization of glucose is not the primary goal of treatment; fluid and electrolyte resuscitation take precedence and often improve glycemia substantially before any insulin is given. An attempt should be made to maintain blood glucose concentration near 250 mg per deciliter for the first 24 hours. Rapid fall in blood glucose concentration correlates with the development of cerebral edema [110,111].

COMPLICATIONS

Hypotension. When insulin is administered to patients with HHNKC syndrome, glucose shifts from the extracellular to the intracellular compartment. Since glucose is osmotically active, the movement of glucose intracellularly draws water from the extracellular compartment. The rapid intracellular movement of free water compromises intravascular volume and may precip-

---

* If continuous infusion therapy is not possible, treatment should be with boluses of intravenous regular insulin. The initial dose should not exceed 10 to 30 units. Boluses should be given every 2 to 4 hours, with dose adjusted on the basis of blood glucose determinations.

itate hypotension and shock [72]. The use of normal (0.9%) saline for initial volume replacement helps prevent hypotension [112]. The higher osmolality of normal (308 mOsm/L) compared with half-normal (154 mOsm/L) saline reduces the osmotic effect of the glucose shifts that follow insulin administration [113].

The magnitude of the fluid shifts that can be induced by insulin was illustrated in a dramatic case report. A patient with congestive heart failure and preexisting renal disease was found to have severe hyperglycemia. Because fluid replacement was contraindicated, he was treated with insulin alone. The insulin treatment resulted in a shift of fluid from the extracellular to the intracellular compartment sufficient to ameliorate the congestive heart failure [114].

Cerebral Edema. Blood glucose concentrations should never be reduced precipitously. Rapid reduction is a major contributor to the development of cerebral edema and a fatal outcome in HHNKC. The exact cause of cerebral edema in HHNKC is unknown, but animal studies suggest that neuronal intracellular osmolality increases in HHNKC. The osmotically active solute has not been identified. The term *idiogenic osmoles* is used to describe these uncharacterized, osmotically active, nondiffusible substances [111]. They draw water into neurons when the extracellular osmolality drops as a result of the intracellular movement of glucose. This is followed by severe edema, increased intracranial pressure, and development of disturbed hypothalamic function.

Conclusions

The diabetic comas are often described as discrete entities, but they frequently present as overlapping disorders [81]. Patients in DKA often have concurrent mild lactic acidosis and may also develop hyperosmolality. Initial treatment of all diabetic comas must always emphasize fluid and electrolytes. Diabetic ketoacidosis and HHNKC also require insulin. Physicians must obtain the relevant history, perform a thorough physical examination, classify the disorder, and treat appropriately. The approach to treatment is summarized in Figure 110-6. With care, nearly all patients with DKA and most with HHNKC can survive.

References

1. Rossini AA, Mordes JP: Diabetes mellitus, in Branch W (ed): *Office Practice of Medicine,* 3rd ed. Philadelphia, WB Saunders, 1994, pp 558–590.
2. Campbell IW, Duncan LJ, Innes JA, et al: Abdominal pain in diabetic metabolic decompensation: Clinical significance. *JAMA* 233:166, 1975.
3. Kubilis P, Rosenbloom AL, Lezotte D, et al: Comparison of blood glucose testing using reagent strips with and without a meter (Chemstrips bG and Dextrostix/Dextrometer). *Diabetes Care* 4:417, 1981.
4. North DS, Steiner JF, Woodhouse KM, et al: Home monitors of blood glucose: Comparison of precision and accuracy. *Diabetes Care* 10:360, 1987.
5. Snorgaard O, Eskildsen PC, Vadstrup S, et al: Diabetic ketoacidosis in Denmark: Epidemiology, incidence rates, precipitating factors and mortality rates. *J Intern Med* 226:223, 1989.
6. Service FJ: Clinical review 42: Hypoglycemias. *J Clin Endocrinol Metab* 76:269, 1993.
7. Horwitz DL: Factitious and artifactual hypoglycemia. *Endocrinol Metab Clin North Am* 18:203, 1989.
8. Arky RA: Hypoglycemia associated with liver disease and ethanol. *Endocrinol Metab Clin North Am* 18:75, 1989.
9. Arem R: Hypoglycemia associated with renal failure. *Endocrinol Metab Clin North Am* 18:103, 1989.
10. Arky RA: Hypoglycemia, in DeGroot LJ, Cahill GF Jr, Martini L, et al (eds): *Endocrinology.* New York, Grune & Stratton, 1979, pp 1099–1123.
11. Turner RC, Oakley NW, Nabarro JDN: Changes in plasma insulin during ethanol-induced hypoglycemia. *Metabolism* 22:111, 1973.
12. Bradley RF: Diabetic ketoacidosis and coma, in Marble A, White P, Bradley RF, et al (eds): *Joslin's Diabetes Mellitus.* Philadelphia, Lea & Febiger, 1971, pp 361–416.
13. Basu A, Close CF, Jenkins D, et al: Persisting mortality in diabetic ketoacidosis. *Diabet Med* 10:282, 1993.
14. Hamblin PS, Topliss DJ, Chosich N, et al: Deaths associated with diabetic ketoacidosis and hyperosmolar coma, 1973–1988. *Med J Aust* 151:439, 1989.
15. Cahill GF Jr: Starvation in man. *N Engl J Med* 282:668, 1970.
16. Cahill GF Jr: The Banting Memorial Lecture 1971: Physiology of insulin in man. *Diabetes* 20:785, 1971.
17. Saudek CD, Felig P: The metabolic events of starvation. *Am J Med* 60:117, 1976.
18. Aoki TT, Muller WA, Brennan MF, et al: Metabolic effects of glucose in brief and prolonged fasted man. *Am J Clin Nutr* 28:507, 1975.
19. McGarry JD, Foster DW: Ketogenesis and its regulation. *Am J Med* 61:9, 1976.
20. Miles JM, Rizza RA, Haymond MW, et al: Effects of acute insulin deficiency on glucose and ketone body turnover in man: Evidence for the primacy of overproduction of glucose and ketone bodies in the genesis of diabetic ketoacidosis. *Diabetes* 29:926, 1980.
21. Alberti KG: Role of glucagon and other hormones in development of diabetic ketoacidosis. *Lancet* 1:1307, 1975.
22. Unger RH, Orci L: Glucagon and the A cell: Physiology and pathophysiology (first of two parts). *N Engl J Med* 304:1518, 1981.
23. Unger RH, Orci L: Glucagon and the A cell: Physiology and pathophysiology (second of two parts). *N Engl J Med* 304:1575, 1981.
24. Adrogu HJ, Wilson H, Boyd AE III, et al: Plasma acid-base patterns in diabetic ketoacidosis. *N Engl J Med* 307:1603, 1982.
25. Fleckman AM: Diabetic ketoacidosis. *Endocrinol Metab Clin North Am* 22:181, 1993.
26. Beigelman PM: Severe diabetic ketoacidosis (diabetic "coma"): 482 episodes in 257 patients—Experience of three years. *Diabetes* 20:490, 1971.
27. Treasure RA, Fowler PB, Millington HT, et al: Misdiagnosis of diabetic ketoacidosis as hyperventilation syndrome. *Br Med J* 294:630, 1987.
28. Verdon F, van Melle G, Perret C: Respiratory response to acute metabolic acidosis. *Bull Eur Physiopathol Respir* 17:223, 1981.
29. Guerin JM, Meyer P, Segrestaa JM: Hypothermia in diabetic ketoacidosis. *Diabetes Care* 10:801, 1987.
30. Sugar AM: Mucormycosis. *Clin Infect Dis* 14(suppl 1):S126, 1992.
31. Montoro MN, Myers VP, Mestman JH, et al: Outcome of pregnancy in diabetic ketoacidosis. *Am J Perinatol* 10:17, 1993.
32. Foster DW: Insulin deficiency and hyperosmolar coma. *Adv Intern Med* 19:159, 1974.
33. Bohannon NJ: Large phosphate shifts with treatment for hyperglycemia. *Arch Intern Med* 149:1423, 1989.
34. Katz MA: Hyperglycemia-induced hyponatremia: Calculation of expected serum sodium depression. *N Engl J Med* 289:843, 1973.
35. Albrink MJ, Hold PM, Man EB, et al: The displacement of serum water by the lipids in hyperlimemic serum: A new method for the rapid determination of serum water. *J Clin Invest* 34:1483, 1955.
36. Halperin ML, Bear RA, Hannaford MC, et al: Selected aspects of the pathophysiology of metabolic acidosis in diabetes mellitus. *Diabetes* 30:781, 1981.
37. Oh MS, Carroll HJ, Uribarri J: Mechanism of normochloremic and hyperchloremic acidosis in diabetic ketoacidosis. *Nephron* 54:1, 1990.
38. Fulop M: Hyperkalemia in diabetic ketoacidosis. *Am J Med Sci* 299:164, 1990.
39. Fulop M: Serum potassium in lactic acidosis and ketoacidosis. *N Engl J Med* 300:1087, 1979.

40. Siperstein MD: Diabetic ketoacidosis and hyperosmolar coma. *Endocrinol Metab Clin North Am* 21:415, 1992.
41. Hale PJ, Nattrass M: A comparison of arterial and non-arterialized capillary blood gases in diabetic ketoacidosis. *Diabet Med* 5:76, 1988.
42. Emmett M, Narins RG: Clinical use of the anion gap. *Medicine* 56:38, 1977.
43. Zonszein J, Baylor P: Diabetic ketoacidosis with alkalemia: A review. *West J Med* 149:217, 1988.
44. Molitch ME, Rodman E, Hirsch CA, et al: Spurious serum creatinine elevations in ketoacidosis. *Ann Intern Med* 93:280, 1980.
45. Owen OE, Licht JH, Sapir DG: Renal function and effects of partial rehydration during diabetic ketoacidosis. *Diabetes* 30:510, 1981.
46. Slovis CM, Mork VG, Slovis RJ, et al: Diabetic ketoacidosis and infection: Leukocyte count and differential as early predictors of serious infection. *Am J Emerg Med* 5:1, 1987.
47. Vinicor F, Lehrner LM, Karn RC, et al: Hyperamylasemia in diabetic ketoacidosis: Sources and significance. *Ann Intern Med* 91:200, 1979.
48. Nsien EE, Steinberg WM, Borum M, et al: Marked hyperlipasemia in diabetic ketoacidosis: A report of three cases. *J Clin Gastroenterol* 15:117, 1992.
49. Leung CB, Li PK, Lui SF, et al: Acute renal failure (ARF) caused by rhabdomyolysis due to diabetic hyperosmolar nonketotic coma: A case report and literature review. *Ren Fail* 14:81, 1992.
50. Goldberg LH: Hyperuricemia, diabetes mellitus, and diabetic ketoacidosis. *Pa Med* 79:40, 1976.
51. Soler NG, Bennet MA, Dixon K, et al: Potassium balance during treatment of diabetic ketoacidosis with special reference to the use of bicarbonate. *Lancet* 2:665, 1972.
52. Gennari FJ, Kassirer JP: Osmotic diuresis. *N Engl J Med* 291:714, 1974.
53. Kreisberg RA: Diabetic ketoacidosis: New concepts and trends in pathogenesis and treatment. *Ann Intern Med* 88:681, 1978.
54. Foster DW, McGarry JD: The metabolic derangements and treatment of diabetic keotacidosis. *N Engl J Med* 309:159, 1983.
55. Kreisberg RA: Phosphorus deficiency and hypophosphatemia. *Hosp Pract* 12:121, 1977.
56. Bellingham AJ, Detter JC, Lenfant C: The role of hemoglobin affinity for oxygen and red-cell 2,3-diphosphoglycerate in the management of diabetic ketoacidosis. *Trans Assoc Am Physicians* 83:113, 1970.
57. Wilson HK, Keuer SP, Lea AS, et al: Phosphate therapy in diabetic ketoacidosis. *Arch Intern Med* 142:517, 1982.
58. Keller U, Berger W: Prevention of hypophosphatemia by phosphate infusion during treatment of diabetic ketoacidosis and hyperosmolar coma. *Diabetes* 29:87, 1980.
59. Fisher JN, Kitabchi AE: A randomized study of phosphate therapy in the treatment of diabetic ketoacidosis. *J Clin Endocrinol Metab* 57:177, 1983.
60. Riley LJ Jr, Cooper M, Narins RG: Alkali therapy of diabetic ketoacidosis: Biochemical, physiologic, and clinical perspectives. *Diabetes Metab Rev* 5:627, 1989.
61. Schade DS, Eaton RP: Dose response to insulin in man: Differential effects on glucose and ketone body regulation. *J Clin Endocrinol Metab* 44:1038, 1977.
62. Posner JB, Plum F: Spinal-fluid pH and neurologic symptoms in systemic acidosis. *N Engl J Med* 277:605, 1967.
63. Bureau MA, Begin R, Berthiaume Y, et al: Cerebral hypoxia from bicarbonate infusion in diabetic acidosis. *J Pediatr* 96:968, 1980.
64. Lever E, Jaspan JB: Sodium bicarbonate therapy in severe diabetic ketoacidosis. *Am J Med* 75:263, 1983.
65. Kecskes SA: Diabetic ketoacidosis. *Pediatr Clin North Am* 40:355, 1993.
66. Gamba G, Oseguera J, Castrejon M, et al: Bicarbonate therapy in severe diabetic ketoacidosis: A double blind, randomized, placebo controlled trial. *Rev Invest Clin* 43:234, 1991.
67. Kitabchi AE: Low-dose insulin therapy in diabetic ketoacidosis: Fact or fiction? *Diabetes Metab Rev* 5:337, 1989.
68. Clements RS Jr, Vourganti B: Fatal diabetic ketoacidosis: Major causes and approaches to their prevention. *Diabetes Care* 1:314, 1978.
69. Mordes JP, Wacker WE: Excess magnesium. *Pharmacol Rev* 29:273, 1977.
70. McMullen JK: Asystole and hypomagnesaemia during recovery from diabetic ketoacidosis. *Br Med J* 1:690, 1977.
71. Waldhausl W, Kleinberger G, Korn A, et al: Severe hyperglycemia: Effects of rehydration on endocrine derangements and blood glucose concentration. *Diabetes* 28:577, 1979.
72. Brown RH, Rossini AA, Callaway CW, et al: Caveat on fluid replacement in hyperglycemic, hyperosmolar, nonketotic coma. *Diabetes Care* 1:305, 1978.
73. Bradley RF, Bryfogle JW: Survival of diabetic patients after myocardial infarction. *Am J Med* 20:207, 1956.
74. deVries HR: Letter. *N Engl J Med* 310:199, 1984.
75. Paton RC: Haemostatic changes in diabetic coma. *Diabetologia* 21:172, 1981.
76. Krane EJ, Rockoff MA, Wallman JK, et al: Subclinical brain swelling in children during treatment of diabetic ketoacidosis. *N Engl J Med* 312:1147, 1985.
77. Van der Meulen JA, Klip A, Grinstein S: Possible mechanism for cerebral oedema in diabetic ketoacidosis. *Lancet* 2:306, 1987.
78. Rosenbloom AL: Intracerebral crises during treatment of diabetic ketoacidosis. *Diabetes Care* 13:22, 1990.
79. Duck SC, Wyatt DT: Factors associated with brain herniation in the treatment of diabetic ketoacidosis. *J Pediatr* 113(1 pt. 1):10, 1988.
80. Murdoch IA, Pryor D, Haycock GB, et al: Acute renal failure complicating diabetic ketoacidosis. *Acta Paediatr* 82:498, 1993.
81. Hare JW, Rossini AA: Diabetic comas: The overlap concept. *Hosp Pract* 14:95, 1979.
82. Krentz AJ, Hale PJ, Singh BM, et al: The effect of glucose and insulin infusion on the fall of ketone bodies during treatment of diabetic ketoacidosis. *Diabet Med* 6:31, 1989.
83. Flexner CW, Weiner JP, Saudek CD, et al: Repeated hospitalization for diabetic ketoacidosis. *Am J Med* 76:691, 1984.
84. Sament S, Schwartz MB: Severe diabetic stupor without ketosis. *South Afr Med J* 31:893, 1957.
85. McCurdy DK: Hyperosmolar hyperglycemic nonketotic diabetic coma. *Med Clin North Am* 54:683, 1977.
86. Gerich JE, Martin MM, Recant L: Clinical and metabolic characteristics of hyperosmolar nonketotic coma. *Diabetes* 20:228, 1971.
87. Arieff AI, Carroll HJ: Nonketotic hyperosmolar coma with hyperglycemia: Clinical features, pathophysiology, renal function, acid-base balance, plasma-cerebrospinal fluid equilibria and the effects of therapy in 37 cases. *Medicine* 51:73, 1972.
88. Lindsey CA, Faloona GR, Unger RH: Plasma glucagon in nonketotic hyperosmolar coma. *JAMA* 229:1771, 1974.
89. Henry DP II, Bressler R: Serum insulin levels in non-ketotic hyperosmotic diabetes mellitus. *Am J Med Sci* 256:150, 1968.
90. Joffe BI, Seftel HC, Goldberg R, et al: Factors in the pathogenesis of experimental nonketotic and ketoacidotic diabetic stupor. *Diabetes* 22:653, 1973.
91. Wilson HK, Keuer SP, Lea AS, et al: Experimental hyperosmolar diabetic syndrome; Ketogenic response to medium-chain triglycerides. *Diabetes* 24:301, 1975.
92. Turpin BP, Duckworth WC, Solomon SS: Simulated hyperglycemic hyperosmolar syndrome: Impaired insulin and epinephrine effects upon lipolysis in the isolated rat fat cell. *J Clin Invest* 63:403, 1979.
93. Gerich J, Penhos JC, Gutman RA, et al: Effect of dehydration and hyperosmolarity on glucose, free fatty acid and ketone body metabolism in the rat. *Diabetes* 22:264, 1973.
94. Bavli S, Gordon EE: Experimental diabetic hyperosmolar syndrome in rats. *Diabetes* 20:92, 1971.
95. Malvin RL, Mouw D, Vander AJ: Angiotensin: physiological role in water-deprivation-induced thirst of rats. *Science* 197:171, 1977.
96. Arieff AI, Carroll HJ: Cerebral edema and depression of sensorium in nonketotic hyperosmolar coma. *Diabetes* 23:525, 1974.
97. Libertino JA, Weiss RM, Lytton B: Pathophysiology and surgical implications of hyperosmolar non-ketotic diabetic coma. *J Urol* 104:642, 1970.
98. Wachtel TJ, Silliman RA, Lamberton P: Predisposing factors for the diabetic hyperosmolar state. *Arch Intern Med* 147:499, 1987.
99. Ginsberg-Fellner F, Primack WA: Recurrent hyperosmolar nonketotic episodes in a young diabetic. *Am J Dis Child* 129:240, 1975.
100. Emder PJ, Howard NJ, Rosenberg AR: Non-ketotic hyperosmolar diabetic pre-coma due to pancreatitis in a boy on continuous ambulatory peritoneal dialysis. *Nephron* 44:355, 1986.
101. Sypniewski E Jr, Mirtallo JM, Schneider PJ: Hyperosmolar, hyper-

glycemic, nonketotic coma in a patient receiving home total parenteral nutrient therapy. *Clin Pharm* 6:69, 1987.

102. Balsam MJ, Baker L, Kaye R: Hyperosmolar nonketotic coma associated with diazoxide therapy for hypoglycemia. *J Pediatr* 78:523, 1971.

103. Gharib H, Munoz JM: Endocrine manifestations of diphenylhydantoin therapy. *Metabolism* 23:515, 1974.

104. Podolsky S, Pattavina CG: Hyperosmolar nonketotic diabetic coma: A complication of propranolol therapy. *Metabolism* 22:685, 1973.

105. Woods JE, Zincke H, Palumbo PJ, et al: Hyperosmolar nonketotic syndrome and steroid diabetes. Occurrence after renal transplantation. *JAMA* 231:1261, 1975.

106. Pomare EW: Hyperosmolar non-ketotic diabetes and cimetidine (letter). *Lancet* 1:1202, 1978.

107. Maccario M: Neurological dysfunction associated with nonketotic hyperglycemia. *Arch Neurol* 19:525, 1968.

108. Daniels JC, Chokroverty S, Barron KD: Anacidotic hyperglycemia and focal seizures. *Arch Intern Med* 124:701, 1969.

109. Walsh CH, Soler NG, James H, et al: Studies on whole-body potassium in non-ketoacidotic diabetics before and after treatment. *Br Med J* 4:738, 1974.

110. Maccario M, Messis CP: Cerebral oedema complicating treated non-ketotic hyperglycaemia. *Lancet* 2:352, 1969.

111. Arieff AI, Kleeman CR: Cerebral edema in diabetic comas. II. Effects of hyperosmolality, hyperglycemia and insulin in diabetic rabbits. *J Clin Endocrinol Metab* 38:1057, 1974.

112. Fulop M, Rosenblatt A, Kreitzer SM, et al: Hyperosmolar nature of diabetic coma. *Diabetes* 24:594, 1975.

113. Feig PU, McCurdy DK: The hypertonic state. *N Engl J Med* 297:1444, 1977.

114. Axelrod L: Response of congestive heart failure to correction of hyperglycemia in the presence of diabetic nephropathy. *N Engl J Med* 293:1243, 1975.

111. Thyroid Storm

Susan L. Abend and
Lewis E. Braverman

Overview

The term *thyroid storm* describes the decompensated clinical presentation of a patient with severe thyrotoxicosis. The syndrome is characterized by hyperpyrexia, tachycardia, and delirium. Thyroid storm generally occurs in patients with severe thyrotoxicosis who then experience stressful events such as trauma, emergency surgery, childbirth, or an intercurrent illness such as pneumonia. The cause of this rapid decompensation is unknown, but it may be due in part to a sudden inhibition in thyroid hormone binding to plasma proteins, which causes a rise in the already elevated free hormone pool [1,2].

In view of the decreasing incidence of thyroid storm, which now accounts for no more than 2 percent of hospital admissions for all forms and complications of thyrotoxicosis, the diagnosis is less readily apparent and often difficult to make because there is such a fine line between severe thyrotoxicosis and thyroid storm. When properly treated, thyroid storm has a mortality rate as low as 7 percent.

Etiology

Prior to the preoperative use of iodides and then the antithyroid propylthiouracil (PTU) and methimazole (MMI; Tapazole), thyroid storm was most frequently seen during and after subtotal thyroidectomy. Because these agents restore euthyroidism it is now rarely seen in this context. Although propranolol has also been used as sole therapy before surgery [3], this is controversial [4,5]. Beta-blocking drugs alone may not prevent thyroid storm [6].

Thyroid storm now occurs most commonly in patients with rather severe underlying thyrotoxicosis, frequently undiagnosed, who become ill for reasons other than thyroid surgery, such as infections or pulmonary and cardiovascular disorders, the latter often aggravated by the thyrotoxicosis (Table 111-1). Thyroid storm may also be precipitated during and after nonthyroid surgery, including orthopaedic surgery for fractures. The widespread use of radioactive iodine (^{131}I; RAI) as the primary treatment of hyperthyroidism, especially in older patients, may also precipitate thyroid storm because of the release of large quantities of thyroxine (T_4) and triiodothyronine (T_3) during radiation destruction of the thyroid.

Thyroid storm may rarely occur approximately 10 to 14 days after the administration of large doses of ^{131}I in patients with very large goiters who have not been recently treated with PTU or MMI. Although propranolol usually reduces the symptoms of this temporary worsening of the thyrotoxicosis, alone it will not necessarily prevent thyroid storm. To avoid this rare but worrisome complication of ^{131}I therapy, it is advisable to use PTU or MMI to deplete thyroid stores of T_4 and T_3 in older patients with severe thyrotoxicosis prior to ^{131}I therapy. The

Table 111-1. Events Associated with the Precipitation of Thyroid Storm

Infection
Surgery
Trauma
Iodinated contrast dyes
Hypoglycemia
Parturition
Vigorous palpation of the thyroid
Emotional stress
Thiourea withdrawal
Radioactive iodine (^{131}I) therapy
Diabetic ketoacidosis
Pulmonary thromboembolism
Cerebrovascular accident

From Wartofsky L: Thyrotoxic storm, in Ingbar SH, Braverman LE (eds): *Werner's, The Thyroid*. Philadelphia, Lippincott, 1986, p 974. With permission.

antithyroid drugs should be stopped for approximately 4 days before ^{131}I treatment. Propranolol should also be employed, unless contraindicated because of bronchospastic lung disease, in which case the selective beta$_1$-blocking or calcium channel blocking drugs may be used [7]. Iodide-induced thyrotoxicosis is not uncommon in areas of endemic iodine-deficient goiter or in areas such as western Europe where iodine intake is marginal. In these regions, iodide-induced thyrotoxicosis not infrequently occurs following the administration of iodine-containing x-ray contrast dyes and drugs, such as amiodarone [8]. Since iodides also block release of T$_4$ and T$_3$ from the thyroid, these patients are at least partially protected while pharmacologic quantities of iodine remain in the circulation. However, a worsening of the thyrotoxicosis and thyroid storm can ensue when the blocking effect of iodide on hormone release has dissipated and large quantities of excess stored hormones are released into the circulation. Although this condition is not common in the United States, where iodine intake is sufficient, this syndrome must still be considered. Finally, overdoses of thyroid hormone (thyrotoxicosis factitia) can lead to thyroid storm [9]. Cardiac deaths that were probably due to ventricular arrhythmias have been reported following the acute ingestion of massive doses of thyroid hormones.

Clinical Manifestations

Patients with thyroid storm are almost always febrile (usually >100° F) and have rapid sinus tachycardia and tachyarrhythmias (especially atrial fibrillation in the elderly) out of proportion to the degree of fever. This condition frequently results in congestive heart failure. Patients are often agitated, delirious and tremulous, with hot, flushed skin due to vasodilatation. The skin may be either moist or dry, depending on the state of hydration. Diarrhea is not infrequent and contributes to the dehydration and hypovolemia. Vascular collapse and shock, which are poor prognostic signs, may occur in these patients. Hepatomegaly with abnormal liver enzymes and splenomegaly are not infrequent; jaundice portends a relatively poor prognosis.

Most patients display the classic signs of thyrotoxic Graves' disease, including ophthalmopathy, or toxic uninodular or multinodular goiter. However, in elderly patients, apathy, severe myopathy, profound weight loss, and congestive heart failure are not uncommon, and thyroid enlargement may be minimal. As thyroid storm progresses, a stupor that leads to coma, hypotension, vascular collapse, and death may ensue within 48 hours unless active therapy is instituted [10,11,12].

Diagnosis and Differential Diagnosis

The diagnosis of thyroid storm is made on clinical grounds. Thyroid function tests do not often differentiate between severe thyrotoxicosis and thyroid storm. Serum T$_4$ concentrations are usually similar, although it has been suggested that the serum-free T$_4$ concentration is significantly higher in patients with thyroid storm [1], which might partially explain their more severe symptoms. On the other hand, the serum T$_3$ concentration is not higher [13] and in fact may be less elevated or even normal in these patients when the precipitating cause is an intercurrent illness or surgery. This phenomenon is not surprising, since a major source of circulating T$_3$ is the peripheral outer-ring monodeiodination (5'-deiodination) of T$_4$, an enzymatic process that is markedly impaired in a wide variety of acute and chronic systemic illnesses [14].

Liver function tests are frequently abnormal, especially in elderly patients in whom congestive heart failure is not uncommon. The mild elevation in total and free serum calcium, which may accompany hyperthyroidism, can be exaggerated. Occasionally, these very ill patients do not have an expected leukocytosis and neutrophilia because the white blood cell count tends to be lower in hyperthyroid patients, with a relative lymphocytosis.

The differential diagnosis for a patient presenting with hyperpyrexia, delirium, and tachycardia includes severe infection, malignant hyperthermia, neuroleptic malignant syndrome, and acute mania with lethal catatonia. Thyroid storm can be distinguished from these disorders clinically by the history of thyroid disease, thyroid hormone, or iodine ingestion and the presence on physical examination of a goiter or stigmata of Graves' disease, including ophthalmopathy, onycholysis, and pretibial myxedema. It must be stressed, however, that the diagnosis of thyroid storm does not rule out the presence of any of the disorders mentioned in the differential diagnosis. Rather, one of the aforementioned illnesses may precipitate thyroid storm in a patient with preexisting hyperthyroidism.

Treatment

UNDERLYING ILLNESS. Since nonthyroidal illness and surgery in previously undiagnosed or only partially treated patients with hyperthyroidism are the most common causes of thyroid storm (Table 111-1), the precipitating disease should be vigorously treated, especially since death in patients treated for thyroid storm is now primarily due to the underlying illness. It should be emphasized that cardiac arrhythmias and congestive heart failure require approximately twice the dose of digoxin needed in euthyroid patients, and refractory arrhythmias should alert the physician to the presence of thyrotoxicosis. Similarly, more insulin may be required to treat diabetic ketoacidosis.

Since diabetes mellitus and Graves' disease occur more frequently in the same patient, due to the autoimmune etiology of both diseases, deterioration in the control of diabetes should suggest the onset of thyrotoxicosis. It is evident that these patients must receive adequate antibiotic therapy; careful fluid, electrolyte, and vitamin supplementation; vigorous pulmonary therapy; and careful pre- and postoperative care. If emergency surgery is required in a thyrotoxic patient, propranolol, PTU or MMI, iodides, and perhaps corticosteroids should be given prior to, during, and after surgery.

SPECIFIC THERAPY

Hyperpyrexia. A cooling blanket should probably be used if the temperature rises above 101° F, but the shivering response should be decreased by using drugs that block the central thermoregulatory centers, such as chlorpromazine or meperidine, 25 to 50 mg every 4 to 6 hours. Antipyretics may also be given. Large doses of salicylate displace the thyroid hormones from the serum-binding proteins and therefore slightly increase the free hormone concentrations [15]. They have also been reported to decrease the peripheral conversion of T$_4$ to the far more biologically active hormone T$_3$ [16]. Thus, it is advisable to use antipyretic drugs other than the salicylates, because the increase in serum-free T_4 induced by salicylates may be detrimental.

Catecholamine Depletion or Blockade. Many of the clinical manifestations of hyperthyroidism can be alleviated by the administration of drugs that deplete or block the peripheral action of the catecholamines (Table 111-2). Prior to the availability of beta-adrenergic blockers, drugs that deplete catecholamine stores—reserpine and guanethidine (which also blocks release)—were used with some success. However, parenteral reserpine has troublesome side effects, including somnolence, diarrhea, flushing, and resistant hypotension. If it must be used, a test dose of 0.25 mg should be administered intramuscularly and blood pressure carefully monitored. Thus, reserpine should be used only in patients in whom the beta-adrenergic blocking agents are contraindicated. Oral guanethidine has also been employed in the treatment of thyroid storm, but its effect is not evident for approximately 12 hours, and, like reserpine, it can cause diarrhea and postural hypotension.

Propranolol and its derivatives (Table 111-2) are potent beta-adrenergic blocking agents; they are now the drugs of choice in alleviating the catecholamine-dependent signs and symptoms of thyrotoxicosis and thyroid storm. The widest experi-

Table 111-2. Treatment of Thyroid Storm

A. Vigorous therapy of underlying intercurrent illness with digoxin, diuretics, antibiotics, intravenous fluid supplemented with complex B vitamins, and insulin for diabetic ketoacidosis
B. Cooling blanket and/or antipyretics (perhaps not aspirin) for hyperpyrexia
C. Beta-adrenergic blocking drugs or, far less commonly, drugs that deplete catecholamines
  1. Propranolol ($beta_1$- and $beta_2$-blocker)
    a. 1 mg IV/min for a total of 2–10 mg
    b. 40–80 mg po q4–6h
  2. Metoprolol ($beta_1$-blocker) 100–400 mg po q12h
  3. Atenolol ($beta_1$-blocker) 50–100 mg po daily
  4. Esmolol ($beta_1$-blocker) 500 mg/kg/min for 1 min, then 50–100 mg/kg/min
  5. Reserpine
    a. Test dose of 0.25 mg IM, then initial dose of 1–5 mg
    b. 1–2.5 mg IM q4–6h
  6. Guanethidine, 1–2 mg/kg po q4–6h
D. Inhibit synthesis of thyroid hormones
  1. Propylthiouracil, approx. 800 mg po stat and 200–300 mg q8h
  2. Methimazole, approx 80 mg po stat and 40 mg po q12h
E. Block release of thyroid hormone from thyroid gland
  1. Iodides
    a. Saturated solution of potassium iodide (SSKI), 5 drops PO q8h
    b. Lugol's solution, 10 drops po q8h
    c. Sodium iodide, 1 gm IV infused over 12 hr q12h
  2. Telepaque or Oragrafin, 1 gm po daily
  3. Lithium (requires careful monitoring)
    a. 800–1200 mg po daily
    b. Serum lithium concentrations range from 0.5 to 1.5 mEq/L
F. Inhibit peripheral 5'monodeiodination of thyroxine (T_4) to triiodothyronine (T_3)
  1. Corticosteroids, equivalent to 300–400 mg hydrocortisone daily, especially dexamethasone, 2 mg q6h
  2. Propranolol, metoprolol, atenolol, and possibly esmolol
  3. Propylthiouracil
  4. X-ray iodine-containing contrast agents
    a. Telepaque, 1 gm daily
    b. Oragrafin, 1 gm daily
G. Remove thyroid hormones from the circulation
  1. Plasmapheresis
  2. Peritoneal dialysis
  3. Cholestyramine, 4 g po q6h

ence has been achieved with propranolol. The cardiac and psychomotor manifestations of thyrotoxicosis are improved within minutes of intravenous administration [17]. While propranolol can also be administered orally, the route of administration depends on the severity of the cardiac symptoms and the urgency of correcting tachycardia or tachyarrhythmias.

In view of the more rapid metabolism of the beta-blocking drugs in patients with severe thyrotoxicosis as well as the variable absorption of the drugs, large doses may be required, with plasma propranolol concentrations greater than 50 ng per milliliter often necessary to maintain a good clinical response [18,19]. Since propranolol may be contraindicated in patients with congestive heart failure, it is frequently debated whether to use the beta-blockers in patients with severe thyrotoxicosis or thyroid storm. However, since tachycardia and tachyarrhythmias are major contributing factors to the congestive failure in many of these patients, propranolol may be used cautiously along with digoxin and other cardiotropic drugs and diuretics [20]. Rarely, hypotension and cardiac arrest may occur following intravenous administration of beta-blockers in patients with severe congestive failure and severe thyrotoxicosis.

In addition to alleviating the catecholamine-dependent signs and symptoms of thyrotoxicosis and thyroid storm, propranolol has the advantage of partially blocking the conversion of T_4 to T_3 [21]. Since propranolol is contraindicated in patients with asthma, the more selective $beta_1$-blocking drugs, such as metoprolol and atenolol, may be used with less risk. Although these drugs were originally reported not to impair the peripheral conversion of T_4 to T_3, another study strongly suggests that there is impairment [22].

A short-acting $beta_1$-blocker, esmolol, was recently used successfully [23]. Diltiazem can also be employed to control the tachyarrhythmias associated with thyrotoxicosis [6]. Thyroid storm has also been treated with dantrolene, which inhibits the effects of high circulating levels of T_4 on calcium flux across the sarcoplasmic reticulum [24].

Inhibition of Thyroid Hormone Synthesis. The sulfonylureas PTU and MMI are potent inhibitors of the synthesis of both T_4 and T_3 (Table 111-2). While the onset of action is rapid, PTU and MMI only partially block thyroid hormone synthesis. Since usually many weeks are required to deplete the thyroid of stored hormones, the clinical effects of these drugs may not be observed for weeks. Since they are not available in a parenteral form in the United States, they must be administered orally, often necessitating the use of a gastric tube in severely ill patients. If a nasogastric tube is not feasible, methimazole, 40 mg every 6 hours, can be dissolved in aqueous solution and given rectally [25]. In Europe, an intravenous preparation of MMI (Thiamazol) is available. Since PTU, but not MMI, has the added advantage of partially blocking the peripheral conversion of T_4 to T_3 [26], PTU may be the drug of choice. It is important to note that these drugs are useful only if thyroid storm is caused by a hyperfunctioning thyroid gland; they are not effective if thyroid storm is due to excess ingestion of thyroid hormone (thyrotoxicosis factitia, see below) or painful or silent thyroiditis, since sulfonylureas affect the synthesis of thyroid hormone and do not affect its release or peripheral activity.

Either drug should be administered at least 1 hour before iodides are given to at least partially prevent the excess thyroid hormone synthesis that occurs in the hyperfunctioning gland treated with iodides. Both PTU and MMI are continued long after iodides have been discontinued, to maintain the euthyroid state so that definitive ablative therapy can be carried out. Thus, ^{131}I therapy cannot be given to patients receiving iodides or for days after iodides have been withdrawn, since the radioactive iodine uptake (RAIU) is suppressed.

Blockade of Thyroid Hormone Release. Iodide administration (Table 111-2) plays a major role in the treatment of thyroid storm, owing to its rapid inhibition of thyroid hormone release from the gland [27]. This effect occurs almost immediately after oral or intravenous administration. Some inhibition of hormone synthesis may also occur in the hyperfunctioning gland. As with PTU and MMI, iodide therapy is not useful in thyroid storm caused by ingestion of excess amounts of thyroid hormone (thyrotoxicosis factitia), since it affects the synthesis and release of endogenously synthesized thyroid hormone.

Lugol's solution or saturated solution of potassium iodide (SSKI) is given orally or sodium iodide intravenously by slow infusion in patients unable to take oral medications. Iodide therapy results in dramatic improvement and should be maintained until the serum T_4 and T_3 concentrations are normal or near normal. Escape from the iodide effect often occurs when PTU or MMI is not concomitantly employed [28]. Lithium, a relatively weak inhibitor of thyroid hormone release, also partially inhibits thyroid hormone synthesis and may also relieve the acute mania occasionally seen in thyroid storm (Table 111-1) [29]. However, its margin of safety in severely ill patients is limited, and its use should be restricted.

Inhibition of Peripheral Generation of Triiodothyronine. It is generally believed that the major bioactive hormone is T_3, that the major source of circulating T_3 is derived from T_4, and that most, if not all, of the metabolic effects of T_4 result from the intracellular generation of T_3 from T_4. A variety of drugs now available to impair the outer-ring monodeiodination of T_4 to T_3 and offer a new dimension to the treatment of thyroid storm by decreasing the peripheral generation of T_3. As noted above, propranolol and some selective beta$_1$-blocking drugs and PTU impair the conversion of T_4 to T_3, although they are relatively weak inhibitors. The corticosteroids, especially dexamethasone, are potent inhibitors when administered in high doses [30] and also have an inhibitory effect on thyroid hypersecretion [31]. Their importance in treating thyroid storm has been well documented; the survival rate in thyroid storm was improved when corticosteroids were added to the treatment regimen. Until studies appeared that demonstrated that dexamethasone inhibited 5'-deiodination of T4, resulting in decreased T_3 generation, it was suggested that the improved survival rate was due to the relative adrenal insufficiency believed to be present in thyroid storm.

Although there is some evidence of impaired conversion of cortisone to the more active corticosteroid hydrocortisone, and plasma cortisol concentrations may not be as elevated as expected, which suggests a degree of decreased adrenal reserve, the major effect of the glucocorticoids, especially dexamethasone, is most likely due to decreased peripheral generation of T_3 from T_4. Indeed, combination therapy of severe hyperthyroidism with PTU, iodides, and dexamethasone has resulted in a reduction of serum T_3 concentration to the euthyroid range within 24 hours [32].

The gallbladder dyes Telepaque and Oragrafin are extremely potent inhibitors of 5'-deiodinase and also partially block the entrance of T_4 into the liver [33,34]. These dyes also have the advantage of containing large quantities of iodide, which is released from the metabolism of the dyes and blocks release of T_4 and T_3 from the thyroid. However, as with the iodides, PTU or MMI should also be used to block the accumulation of excessive thyroid hormone stores associated with iodide administration. These agents, in addition to PTU and propranolol, may be extremely efficacious in the treatment of thyroid storm [35].

The antiarrhythmic and antianginal drug amiodarone inhibits 5'-deiodinase activity [36], is rich in iodine, and may also block entrance of T_4 into the cell. This drug has been employed in the short-term (2 weeks) treatment of thyrotoxicosis, but the decrease in serum T_4 and T_3 concentrations was similar to those induced by an equivalent dose of iodine alone [37]. Moreover, amiodarone has a long half-life (approximately 25–100 days) and is the source of excess iodine for many months, making it difficult to restore euthyroidism in an iodine-rich, hyperfunctioning thyroid. Finally, amiodarone can be associated with iodide-induced thyrotoxicosis, which itself is often difficult to treat. Combined treatment with PTU or MMI, which inhibit thyroid hormone synthesis, and potassium or sodium perchlorate, which block entrance of iodide into the thyroid, has been proposed as the most efficacious therapy of amiodarone-, iodine-induced thyrotoxicosis [38]. Therefore, amiodarone should not be used in the treatment of thyroid storm

Removal of Thyroid Hormone from the Circulation. Direct removal of thyroid hormone from the circulation is occasionally required in patients who do not respond to conventional medical treatment. Plasmapheresis [39], peritoneal dialysis [40], extracorporeal resin perfusion [41], and charcoal plasma perfusion [42] have been used. Cholestyramine, which decreases serum T_3 and T_4 concentrations by increasing the fecal excretion of these hormones [43], was recently reported to lower serum thyroid hormone concentrations in thyrotoxic patients [44], and might also be useful in the management of thyroid storm.

THYROTOXICOSIS FACTITIA. The inadvertent ingestion of excess amounts of thyroid hormone most commonly occurs in children, although adults may also ingest excess hormone for weight reduction or as a suicide attempt [45]. Gastric lavage or emesis induction should be performed as soon as possible after ingestion. Occasionally, oral charcoal administration can be useful. As mentioned above, this form of thyrotoxicosis is not due to endogenous production of thyroid hormone; therefore drugs that inhibit the synthesis of T_4 and T_3 or those that block thyroid hormone release are not helpful. Therapy should focus on preventing the peripheral effects of excessive thyroid hormone with beta-adrenergic blocking drugs and inhibiting the peripheral generation of T_3 from T_4 by employing the gallbladder dyes Oragrafin or Telepaque. As noted above, cholestyramine might be efficacious.

Conclusions

It is evident that each patient must be treated individually and that a set protocol cannot be advised for all patients. Specific therapy should be directed toward inhibiting the synthesis and release of T_4 and T_3 from the thyroid, blocking the peripheral conversion of T_4 to T_3, relieving the catecholamine-mediated effects by beta-adrenergic blockade, and treating the possibility of decreased adrenal reserve with corticosteroids. Associated and precipitating diseases should, of course, be vigorously treated.

References

1. Abend SL, Braverman LE: Acute thyroid disorders, in May HL (ed): *Emergency Medicine.* 2nd ed. Boston, Little, Brown, 1992, p 1274.
2. Brooks MH, Waldstein SS: Free thyroxine concentration in thyroid storm. *Ann Intern Med* 93:694, 1980.
3. Toft AD, Irvine WJ, McIntosh D, et al: Propranolol in the treatment

of thyrotoxicosis by subtotal thyroidectomy. *J Clin Endocrinol Metab* 43:1312, 1976.

4. Feek CM, Sawers JSA, Irvine WJ, et al: Combination of potassium iodide and propranolol in preparation of patients with Graves' disease for thyroid surgery. *N Engl J Med* 302:883, 1980.

5. Unger J, Couturier E, Durez M, et al: Failure to reach euthyroidism with potassium iodide and propranolol in preparation of a patient with Graves' disease for surgery. *J Endocrinol Invest* 4:367, 1981.

6. Eriksson MA, Rubenfeld S, Garber AJ, et al: Propranolol does not prevent thyroid storm. *N Engl J Med* 269:263, 1977.

7. Roti E, Montermini M, Roti S, et al: The effect of diltiazem, a calcium channel-blocking drug, on cardiac rate and rhythm in hyperthyroid patients. *Arch Intern Med* 148:1919, 1988.

8. Fradkin JE, Wolff J: Iodide-induced thyrotoxicosis. *Medicine* 62:1, 1983.

9. Bhasin S, Wallace W, Lawrence JB, et al: Sudden death associated with thyroid hormone abuse. *Am J Med* 71:887, 1981.

10. Mackin JF, Canary JJ, Pittman CS: Thyroid storm and its management. *N Engl J Med* 291:1396, 1974.

11. Menendez CE, Rivlin RS: Thyrotoxic crisis and myxedema coma. *Med Clin North Am* 57:1463, 1973.

12. Urbanic RC, Mazzaferri EL: Thyrotoxic crisis and myxedema coma. *Heart Lung* 7:435, 1978.

13. Brooks MH, Waldstein SS, Bronsky D, et al: Serum triiodothyronine concentrations in thyroid storm. *J Clin Endocrinol Metab* 40:339, 1975.

14. Wartofsky L, Burman KD: Alterations in thyroid function in patients wih systemic illness: The "euthyroid sick syndrome." *Endocr Rev* 3:164, 1982.

15. Larsen PR: Salicylate-induced increases in free triiodothyronine in human serum. *J Clin Invest* 51:1125, 1972.

16. Chopra IJ, Solomon DH, Teco GNC, et al: Inhibition of hepatic outer ring monodeiodination of thyroxine and 3,3′,5′-triiodothyronine by sodium salicylate. *Endocrinology* 106:1728, 1980.

17. Das G, Krieger M: Treatment of thyrotoxic storm with intravenous administration of propranolol. *Ann Intern Med* 70:985, 1969.

18. Hellman R, Kelly KL, Mason WD, et al: Propranolol for thyroid storm. *N Engl J Med* 297:671, 1977.

19. Feely J, Forrest A, Gunn A, et al: Propranolol dosage in thyrotoxicosis. *J Clin Endocrinol Metab* 51:658, 1980.

20. Ikram H: Haemodynamic effects of beta-adrenergic blockade in hyperthyroid patients with and without heart failure. *Br Med J* 1:1505, 1977.

21. Verhoeven RP, Visser TJ, Docter R, et al: Plasma thyroxine, 3,3′5′-triiodothyronine and 3,3′5′-triiodothyronine during beta-adrenergic blockade in hyperthyroidism. *J Clin Endocrinol Metab* 44:1002, 1977.

22. Perrild H, Molholm Hansen J, Skovsted L, et al: Different effects of propranolol, alprenolol, sotalol, atenolol and metoprolol on serum T3 and serum rT3 in hyperthyroidism. *Clin Endocrinol* 18:139, 1983.

23. Vijayakumar HR, Thomas WO, Ferrara JJ: Peri-operative management of severe thyrotoxicosis with esmolol. *Anaesthesia* 44:406, 1989.

24. Bennett MH, Wainwright AP: Acute thyroid crisis on induction of anesthesia. *Anaesthesia* 44:28, 1989.

25. Nabil M, Miner DJ, Amatruda JM: Methimazole: An alternative route of administration. *J Clin Endocrinol Metab* 54:180, 1982.

26. Geffner DL, Azukizawa M, Hershman JM: Propylthiouracil blocks extrathyroidal conversion of thyroxine to triiodothyronine. *J Clin Invest* 55:224, 1975.

27. Wartofsky L, Ransil BJ, Ingbar SH: Inhibition by iodine of the release of thyroxine from the thyroid glands of patients with thyrotoxicosis. *J Clin Invest* 49:78, 1970.

28. Emerson CH, Anderson AJ, Howard WJ, et al: Serum thyroxine and triiodothyronine concentrations during iodide treatment of hyperthyroidism. *J Clin Endocrinol Metab* 40:33, 1975.

29. Lazarus JH, Addison GM, Richards AR, et al: Treatment of thyrotoxicosis with lithium carbonate. *Lancet* 2:1160, 1974.

30. Duick DS, Warren DW, Nicoloff JT, et al: Effect of single dose dexamethasone on the concentration of serum triiodothyronine in man. *J Clin Endocrinol Metab* 39:1151, 1974.

31. Williams DE, Chopra IJ, Orgiazzi J, et al: Acute effects of corticosteroids on thyroid activity in Graves' disease. *J Clin Endocrinol Metab* 45:354, 1975.

32. Croxson MS, Hall TD, Nicoloff JT, et al: Combination drug therapy for treatment of hyperthyroid Graves' disease. *J Clin Endocrinol Metab* 45:623, 1977.

33. Burgi H, Wimpfheimer C, Burger A, et al: Changes of circulating thyroxine, triiodothyronine and reverse triiodothyronine after radiographic contrast agents. *J Clin Endocrinol Metab* 43:1203, 1976.

34. Felicetta JV, Green WL, Nelp WB: Inhibition of hepatic binding of thyroxine by cholecystographic agents. *J Clin Invest* 65:1032, 1980.

35. Sharp B, Reed AW, Tamagna EL, et al: Treatment of hyperthyroidism with sodium ipodate (Oragrafin) in addition to propylthiouracil and propranolol. *J Clin Endocrinol Metab* 53:622, 1981.

36. Burger A, Dinichert D, Nicod P, et al: Effect of amiodarone on serum triiodothyronine, reverse triiodothyronine, thyroxine, and thyrotropin. *J Clin Invest* 58:255, 1976.

37. Sheldon J: Effects of amiodarone in thyrotoxicosis. *Br Med J* 286:267, 1983.

38. Martino E, Aghini-Lombardi F, Mariotti S, et al: Treatment of amiodarone associated thyrotoxicosis by simultaneous administration of potassium perchlorate and methimazole. *J Endocrinol Invest* 9:201, 1986.

39. Herrmann J, Hilger P, Kruskemper HL: Plasmapheresis in the treatment of thyrotoxic crisis (measurement of half-concentration tissues for free and total T_3 and T_4). *Acta Endocrinol* 173(suppl):22, 1973.

40. Herrmann J, Kruskemper HL, Grosser KD, et al: Peritoneal Dialyse in der Behandlung der Thyreotoxischen Krise. *Dtsch Med Wochenschr* 96:742, 1971.

41. Burman KD, Yaeger HC, Briggs WA, et al: Resin hemoperfusion: A method of removing circulating thyroid hormones. *J Clin Endocrinol Metab* 42:70, 1976.

42. Candrina R, DiStefano O, Spandrio S, et al: Treatment of thyrotoxic storm by charcoal plasmaperfusion. *J Endocrinol Invest* 12:133, 1989.

43. Solomon B, Wartofsky L, Burman KD: Cholestyramine treatment of thyrotoxicosis. Presented at the 72nd Annual Meeting of the Endocrine Society, abstract 329, 1990.

44. Shakir KM, Michaels RD, Hays JH, Potter BB: The use of bile acid sequestrants to lower serum thyroid hormones in iatrogenic hyperthyroidism. *Ann Intern Med* 118:112, 1993.

45. Cohen JH III, Ingbar SH, Braverman LE: Thyrotoxicosis due to ingestion of excess thyroid hormone. *Endocr Rev* 10:113, 1989.

112. Myxedema Coma

Charles H. Emerson

Introduction

Myxedema coma is a syndrome that occurs in advanced untreated hypothyroidism [1–8]. It is defined by a group of characteristic clinical features, not by laboratory evidence of severe hypothyroidism (Table 112-1). Myxedema coma is generally preceded by increasingly severe signs and symptoms of thyroid insufficiency. Fortunately, it is quite rare. Hypothyroid patients who are neglectful or whose contact with family and friends is limited are most vulnerable.

Etiology and Pathophysiology

By definition, myxedema coma does not occur in the absence of hypothyroidism. If the hypothyroidism is due to hypothalamic or pituitary insufficiency, the condition is even more serious because it is also accompanied by adrenal failure. Pituitary tumors are the major cause of central hypothyroidism in the United States. In countries with poor access to health care, postpartum pituitary necrosis is quite prevalent and is therefore another important cause of secondary hypothyroidism.

More than 95 percent of patients with hypothyroidism have primary thyroid disease. Most patients with primary hypothyroidism have either autoimmune thyroid failure or hypothyroidism secondary to ablative procedures on the thyroid. These include radioactive iodine and surgery for hyperthyroidism, thyroid resection for thyroid cancer, and external thyroid irradiation for head and neck tumors. Lithium carbonate is a widely used drug with substantial antithyroid properties. Clinical hypothyroidism develops in about 5 percent of patients receiving lithium, and biochemical evidence of hypothyroidism can be found in almost one-third of lithium-treated patients [9]. Amiodarone also affects thyroid function. Its effects are more complex, however, as it has been associated with hypothyroidism, hyperthyroidism, and, most recently, hyperthyroidism followed by hypothyroidism [10]. Myxedema coma has been reported in association with lithium treatment, amiodarone treatment, following deep neck irradiation, in patients with the thyroid-infiltrating disease cystinosis, and even in the syndrome of subacute thyroiditis. The latter is distinctly rare, however, since myxedema coma is usually not a threat without long-standing hypothyroidism.

Table 112-1. Clinical Features of Myxedema Coma

Mental obtundation
Coarse, dry skin
Myxedema facies
Hypothermia
Hypoglycemia
Bradycardia and hypotension
Electrocardiographic changes
Atonic gastrointestinal tract
Atonic bladder
Pleural, pericardial, and peritoneal effusions

Myxedema coma is distinguished from uncomplicated hypothyroidism by a variety of features that relate to central nervous system (CNS) dysfunction. The pathophysiology of myxedema coma will become clearer when there is a better understanding of the effects of thyroid hormone on the brain. Narcotics and hypnotics should be used with caution in hypothyroid patients, since these patients are very sensitive to their sedative effects. These agents, alone or in combination with other factors, may precipitate myxedema coma in hypothyroid patients. Other precipitating factors are trauma, surgery, and severe infection. The most important factor, however, is cold stress. In a recent series, 9 of the 11 patients with myxedema coma were admitted in the late fall or winter [7].

Clinical Manifestations

Patients are partially or completely obtunded. Therefore, the history must often be obtained from other sources. Friends, relatives, and acquaintances might have noted increasing lethargy, complaints of cold intolerance, and changes in the voice. An outdated container of L-thyroxine discovered with the patient's belongings suggests that he or she has been remiss in taking medication. The medical record may also indicate that the patient was taking thyroid hormone or may refer to previous treatment with radioactive iodine. A thyroidectomy scar suggests the possibility of hypothyroidism. Other than coma itself, the cardinal manifestations are hypothermia and hypotension. Hypotonia of the gastrointestinal tract is common and often so severe as to suggest an obstructive lesion. Urinary retention due to a hypotonic bladder is related but less frequent. Most patients have the physical features of severe hypothyroidism, including bradycardia and slow relaxation of the deep tendon reflexes. A myxedematous facies (Plate I-4) results from the dry, puffy skin, pallor, hypercarotinemia, periorbital edema, and patchy hair loss.

Diagnosis

The diagnosis of myxedema coma is based on the presence of the characteristic clinical syndrome in a patient with hypothyroidism. The laboratory's role is to confirm that the patient is hypothyroid and determine whether there are treatable complications of myxedema coma, such as hypoventilation, hypoglycemia, and hyponatremia. Because of the gravity of hypothyroidism, treatment must be instituted before laboratory tests confirm the diagnosis.

The diagnostic laboratory features of primary hypothyroidism are a subnormal serum-free thyroxine index (FTI) and elevated serum thyroid-stimulating hormone (TSH). Serum FTI is calculated by multiplying the serum thyroxine (T_4) concentration by serum triiodothyronine (T_3) uptake, either directly or by first applying a conversion factor to the T_3 uptake test result. The serum T_3 uptake test is not a measure of serum T_3 concentration but an index of the concentration of thyroxine binding globulin (TBG) with unoccupied T_4 binding sites. Other direct or indirect tests measure the free T_4 (FT_4) concentration in serum, which is always low in patients with myxedema coma.

Serum T_3 concentration is a standard laboratory test. It is of no value in the diagnosis of hypothyroidism or myxedema coma, however, because serum T_3 concentrations are reduced in almost all illnesses due to decreased conversion of circulating T_4 to T_3.

Differential Diagnosis

In myxedema coma, the FTI or other tests assessing serum FT_4 are usually less than half the value of the lower limit of normal. The FTI or FT_4 is often in this low range in severely ill patients, where it is associated with the characteristic laboratory profile of the sick euthyroid syndrome. It is obvious that the incidence of sick euthyroid syndrome (see Chap. 117) is far greater than that of myxedema coma. Therefore, the diagnosis of hypothyroidism or myxedema coma cannot be made solely on the basis of a low FTI or FT_4 in an obtunded patient. The markedly elevated serum TSH concentrations in myxedema coma almost always distinguish sick euthyroid syndrome from myxedema coma. Alone, few of the signs and symptoms described in this chapter are unique to myxedema coma. For example, the differential diagnosis of hypothermia (see Chap. 72) includes numerous conditions, such as protein-calorie malnutrition, sepsis, hypoglycemia, and exposure to certain drugs and toxins [11]. Hypotension and hypoventilation, other cardinal features of myxedema coma, occur in other disease states. What distinguishes myxedema coma from other disorders is laboratory evidence of hypothyroidism, characteristic myxedema facies with periorbital puffiness, skin changes, obtundation, and, frequently, a constellation of other physical signs characteristic of severe hypothyroidism.

Treatment

Treatment of myxedema coma (Table 112-2) consists of management of hypoglycemia, respiratory depression, hyponatremia, hypothermia, hypotension, and administration of thyroid hormone. All patients require continuous monitoring of the electrocardiogram and an intravenous line to administer fluids and drugs. Baseline thyroid function tests, serum cortisol, complete blood count (CBC), blood urea nitrogen (BUN), plasma glucose, and electrolytes are mandatory. Pneumonia commonly develops or may be the precipitating factor and must be treated promptly (see Chap. 76). Hypothyroidism and myxedema coma are also associated with hemostatic abnormalities, particularly capillary bleeding and cerebral hemorrhage. Although bleeding should be anticipated in many patients, few strategies have evolved to counter this disorder.

HYPOGLYCEMIA. Since hypoglycemia is not unusual in myxedema coma, 50 ml of 50% glucose should immediately be administered intervenously to avoid any delay in confirming the presence of this complication. Chapter 116 details the management of hypoglycemia.

HYPOVENTILATION. Respiratory center depression is common in severe hypothyroidism and myxedema coma. Arterial blood gases should be routinely obtained, therefore, to rule out

Table 112-2. Treatment of Myxedema Coma

1. Assisted ventilation for hypoventilation
2. Intravenous glucose for hypoglycemia
3. Water restriction or hypertonic saline for severe hyponatremia
4. Passive rewarming for hypothermia
5. Administer T_4 or T_3 IV*
6. Administer hydrocortisone*
7. Treat underlying infection and other illnesses, if present
8. Avoid all sedatives, hypnotics, and narcotics

* Dosage must be individualized (see text).
T_4 = thyroxine, T_3 = triiodothyronine.

hypoventilation. If respiratory center depression is clinically obvious, assisted ventilation with oxygen supplementation must be started without delay, taking care not to correct chronic hypercapnia too rapidly (see Chaps. 66 and 69).

HYPONATREMIA. Hyponatremia is most deleterious to CNS function when it develops rapidly. Although hyponatremia is present in some patients, it is usually not the cause of coma, since its onset is likely to be gradual. A limiting factor is that water intake decreases as myxedema coma develops, offsetting the tendency toward hyponatremia. Treatment consists of restriction of free water. If the serum sodium concentration is less than 110 mEq per liter, hypertonic saline and, in some cases, furosemide should be administered (see Chap. 79).

HYPOTHERMIA. Hypothermia is one of the hallmarks of myxedema coma. It can be overlooked or its severity underestimated, however, if the thermometer is not shaken down or does not register below 30°C. Regardless of the cause, hypothermia is associated with a decrease in the basal metabolic rate, myocardial irritability, and blood pressure alterations. Blood pressure initially rises and then gradually falls. Changes in the cardiovascular status are accompanied by electrocardiographic changes. First there is sinus bradycardia, then T wave inversion, and, finally, the development of a J wave [11]. At core temperatures below 28°C, ventricular fibrillation is a major threat to life. For an in-depth discussion of this complication see Chapter 72.

Despite its gravity, the management of the hypothermia of myxedema coma differs from the treatment of exposure-induced hypothermia in euthyroid subjects. In myxedema coma, the patient should be kept in a warm room and covered with blankets. Active heating should be avoided, since it increases oxygen consumption and promotes peripheral vasodilation and circulatory collapse. Active heating is recommended only for situations of severe hypothermia where ventricular fibrillation is an immediate threat. In these cases, the rate of rewarming should not exceed 0.5°C per hour and core temperature should be raised to approximately 31°C.

HYPOTENSION. Hypotension is another ominous feature of myxedema coma. Hypothermia and thyroid hormone deficiency per se are the two most important causes, but bleeding and, perhaps in some cases, decreased adrenal reserve may play a role. Since hypothermia itself produces hypotension, some improvement in blood pressure can be expected if passive measures to restore body temperature are successful. Anemia is common in hypothyroidism and has a multifactorial basis. In patients in whom anemia is severe or there appears to be active bleeding, a case can be made for transfusion. If this course is chosen it must be done with great caution since patients with myxedema coma are extremely prone to circulatory collapse. Sympathomimetic vasoconstrictors or drugs intended to increase myocardial contractility, such as isoproterenol or digitalis, have very limited use in myxedema coma. The response to these drugs is poor, and myxedematous patients are very sensitive to their toxic effects.

Although there is little evidence that hypotension in myxedema coma results from adrenal insufficiency, there are at least theoretic reasons for considering that these patients have decreased adrenal reserve. Furthermore, it is often unclear whether the myxedema coma is due to primary or pituitary-hypothalamic hypothyroidism. Therefore, one of the immediate measures in treating myxedema coma is to administer 300 mg hydrocortisone intravenously in three divided doses over the first 24 hours. Gradually decreasing doses of hydrocortisone should be administered over the next few days, depending on the patient's response. This protocol is recommended even in the absence of hypotension.

THYROID HORMONE. Administration of thyroid hormone is the definitive treatment of myxedema coma and is essential for reversing hypotension, hypothermia, and depressed consciousness. The sensorium may be improved in a few patients when glucose is given or hypoventilation corrected, but deterioration will recur if thyroid hormone is not given. The gastrointestinal absorption of thyroid hormone is often markedly reduced in myxedema coma. Therefore, thyroid hormone must be given by the intravenous route. To ensure proper dosing, synthetic preparations should be employed.

There are no controlled studies of the optimum form of thyroid hormone for myxedema coma. Both T_4 [4,7] and T_3 [6,7,8] have been employed with varying degrees of success, and each has its theoretic advantages. T_4 is advantageous because most thyroid hormone is secreted in the form of T_4. For this and other reasons, plasma and intracellular T_4 and T_3 profiles are more stable and representative of the normal condition if T_4 rather than T_3 is administered. Conversely, T_3 is advantageous because it has a more rapid onset of action than T_4.

The best doses for treating myxedema coma have not been studied in a rigorous fashion. As is the case when deciding between T_4 and T_3, the choice is not straightforward. In patients with long-standing untreated hypothyroidism, thyroid hormone treatment is usually initiated at low doses. These patients frequently have underlying arteriosclerotic cardiovascular disease, and initial therapy with full replacement doses of thyroid hormone can precipitate angina or myocardial infarction. On the other hand, in near terminal patients with myxedema coma the need for thyroid hormone is urgent. In this setting, the blood pressure and body temperature can increase within hours after thyroid hormone is started.

I prefer to use T_4 in all but the most severe cases of myxedema coma. The initial intravenous dose of T_4 should be between 0.2 and 0.5 mg, with the larger doses employed for more comatose patients, those with more severe hypotension or hypothermia, and those with large body mass. If the patient has received less than 0.5 mg of T_4 and there is no improvement in the state of consciousness, blood pressure, or core temperature during the first 6 to 12 hours after therapy, T_4 should again be administered to bring the total dose during the first 24 hours to 0.5 mg. Thyroid hormone should then be given again 24 hours later and every 24 hours thereafter. After the first 24 hours the dose should range from 0.05 to 0.2 mg daily, depending on the clinical response. If the treatment is not maintained, coma may recur. A smaller dose in comatose patients is justified if they are normotensive and euthermic and have another explanation

for their comatose state, such as CNS trauma or recent sedative ingestion. Another situation that calls for lower doses is the patient who has had an acute myocardial infarction and whose hypotension appears to be secondary to the myocardial infarction, which is a major contributor to the patient's depressed sensorium. In these cases, ventilatory support should be given and intravenous doses of as little as 0.05 to 0.1 mg of T_4 administered in the first 24 hours. Care must be taken in making the diagnosis of myocardial infarction, however, since CK-MB activity is increased in the absence of myocardial infarction in a few patients with myxedema coma [12,13].

Intravenous T_3 may be a better choice as the initial therapy in the most severe cases of myxedema coma. If T_3 is employed, however, greater caution must be exercised to avoid "overstimulation" of the cardiovascular system [7] and too rapid an increase in oxygen consumption. It is clear that T_3 has been lifesaving in some patients, but an inverse correlation between survival and "calculated" plasma T_3 concentrations has actually been reported in myxedema coma [7]. Though doses as high as 0.2 mg of T_3 in the first 24 hours have been used, as little as 0.0025 mg has been reported to increase cardiac output, heart rate, ventricular stroke work, oxygen consumption, and oxygen delivery in myxedema coma [8]. Based on these and other considerations, a good starting dose of T_3 is 0.0125 mg given intravenously [6]. This dose should be repeated every 6 hours for the first 48 hours. If there is no apparent response after 15 to 21 hours as shown by heart rate, blood pressure, and body temperature, the next two doses could be increased to 0.025 mg. If, on the other hand, signs of myocardial ischemia develop, the dose should be reduced. Particularly worrisome would be a decrease in blood pressure in the face of an increase in body temperature, suggesting that cardiovascular decompensation is occurring in the face of increased oxygen demands. If there is gradual improvement of metabolic parameters, the T_3 should be tapered and T_4 treatment introduced, starting with doses of 0.05 mg given intravenously every 24 hours.

Although myxedema coma is associated with a high mortality, many patients can be saved by judicious therapy aimed at correcting the secondary metabolic disturbances and reversing the hypothyroid state. This must be done in a sustained but gradual fashion, however, since an effort to correct hypothyroidism too rapidly may completely negate the beneficial effects of the initial treatment.

References

1. Nickerson JF, Hill SR, McNeil JH, et al: Fatal myxedema, with and without coma. *Ann Intern Med* 53:475, 1960.
2. Catz B, Russell S: Myxedema, shock and coma: Seven survival cases. *Arch Intern Med* 108:407, 1961.
3. Forester CF: Coma in myxedema. *Arch Intern Med* 111:734, 1963.
4. Holvey DN, Goodner CJ, Nicoloff JT: Treatment of myxedema coma with intravenous thyroxine. *Arch Intern Med* 113:89, 1964.
5. Royce PC: Severely impaired consciousness in myxedema: A review. *Am J Med Sci* 261:46, 1971.
6. Pereira VG, Haron ES, Lima-Neto N, Medeiros-Neto GA: Management of myxedema coma: Report on three successfully treated cases with nasogastric or intravenous administration of triiodothyronine. *J Endocrinol Invest* 5:331, 1982.
7. Hylander B, Rosenquist U: Treatment of myxedema coma: Factors associated with fatal outcome. *Acta Endocrinol (Copenh)* 108:65, 1985.
8. McCulloch W, Price P, Hinds CJ, Wass JAH: Effects of low dose oral triiodothyronine in myxedema coma. *Intensive Care Med* 11:259, 1985.
9. Emerson CH, Anderson AJ, Howard WJ, Utiger RD: Serum thyroxine

and triiodothyronine concentrations during iodine treatment of hyperthyroidism. *J Clin Endocrinol Metab* 40:33, 1975.

10. Roti E, Minelli R, Gardini E, et al: Thyrotoxicosis followed by hypothyroidism in patients treated with amiodarone: A possible consequence of a destructive process in the thyroid. *Arch Intern Med* 153:886, 1993.
11. Renler JB: Hypothermia: Pathophysiology, clinical settings and management. *Ann Intern Med* 89:519, 1978.
12. Hickman PE, Sylvester W, Musk AA, et al: Cardiac enzyme changes in myxedema coma. *Clin Chem* 33:622, 1987.
13. Nee PA, Scane AC, Lavelle PH, et al: Hypothermic myxedema coma erroneously diagnosed as myocardial infarction because of increased creatinine kinase MB. *Clin Chem* 33:1083, 1987.

113. Hypoadrenal Crisis

Christopher Longcope

Introduction

The adrenal glands secrete five types of hormones: (1) mineralocorticoids (C-21 steroids, of which aldosterone is the major hormone), which have their major effects on electrolyte balance; (2) glucocorticoids (C-21 steroids, cortisol being the principal hormone), which promote gluconeogenesis but have many other actions; (3) C-19 steroids (primarily dehydroepiandrosterone and its sulfate), which are precursors of potent androgens; (4) C-18 steroids (primarily estrone), which are estrogens secreted in minimal amounts only; and (5) catecholamines, which are secreted by the medulla. The C-21 steroids are life-maintaining and play a critical role in hypoadrenal crises. In contrast, the C-19 and C-18 steroids and the catecholamines do not play a major role in this disorder.

The symptom complex—hypoadrenal crisis—that develops in many individuals with adrenal hypofunction is a true endocrine emergency. However, a moribund patient can be treated and brought back to an essentially normal life, provided the proper diagnosis is made and treated accordingly. Hypoadrenal crisis may be due not only to adrenal disease (i.e., primary adrenal failure) but also to adrenal failure from lack of adrenocorticotropic hormone (ACTH) (i.e., secondary adrenal failure). Hypoadrenal crisis can occur as an acute event not only in an individual with chronic adrenal failure but also in an individual who gives little background history [1,2] of previous adrenal problems. It is in the latter individual, especially, that a high index of suspicion is necessary, because the diagnosis may be easily missed.

Although it can occur as a primary event, hypoadrenal crisis is usually associated with some other stressful situation, such as infection or trauma. Since establishment of the diagnosis by biochemical testing usually requires some time, it may be wise to perform testing procedures immediately prior to the initiation of therapy and not withhold therapy until the results are known.

Addison's disease is now the most common cause [3]. This condition is more common in women than men, the overall sex ratio being 1.25:1.

In idiopathic adrenal cortical insufficiency, the disease appears to be autoimmune in nature; it is frequently associated with antibodies to the adrenal gland and other tissues, such as thyroid, gonads, islet cells, parietal cells, and parathyroid [5–8]. Individuals with idiopathic Addison's disease may also have hypothyroidism, hypogonadism, diabetes mellitus, pernicious anemia, or hypoparathyroidism. The presence of any of these conditions may precede or postdate the appearance of adrenal insufficiency. In idiopathic Addison's disease, the function of the adrenal medulla is usually well preserved.

Tuberculosis of the adrenals has become far less common with the decrease in incidence of tuberculosis. It can be associated with evidence of tuberculosis elsewhere and is often accompanied by calcification in the adrenal areas. In tuberculosis of the adrenals, the medulla is usually also destroyed.

Other causes of Addison's disease include surgery (i.e., bilateral adrenalectomy), fungal disease, amyloidosis, AIDS, hemorrhage that is secondary to overwhelming sepsis, circulating anticoagulants [9], or anticoagulant therapy [10], trauma [2], infarction, irradiation, metastatic disease, and drugs [5]. Adrenal glands stimulated by ACTH are more vulnerable to hemorrhagic lesions than are unstimulated glands [11].

The incidence of acute adrenal insufficiency secondary to bilateral adrenalectomy is of varying frequency, in part reflecting physicians' enthusiasm for the procedure. The once relatively frequent use of adrenalectomy for metastatic disease or hypertension has waned in recent years, however, with the development of other therapeutic regimens for these diseases. Secondary adrenal insufficiency, resulting from a lack of ACTH, can be the result of pituitary tumor or hypothalamic disease, but the most common cause is glucocorticoid suppression of ACTH release.

Etiology

While the incidence appears to be decreasing [3], primary adrenal hypofunction has been estimated to occur in 40 to 60 in 1 million people [4,5]. For many years the most common cause of adrenal hypofunction (Addison's disease) was tuberculosis, which was more common in men than women. With the decrease in the incidence of tuberculosis, however, idiopathic

Pathophysiology

NORMAL ADRENAL FUNCTION. The adrenal glands lie retroperitoneally above the kidneys and are composed of an inner medullary zone and an outer cortex. The cortex is divided into three zones—the outer zona glomerulosa and the inner zonae fasciculata and reticularis. The glomerulosa secretes the mineralocorticoid aldosterone and is stimulated primarily by angiotensin [12,13] but also by ACTH [12,13,14] and high potassium levels [12–15]. The zonae fasciculata and reticularis are stimulated by ACTH to secrete glucocorticoids, primarily cortisol [16,17], and the C-19 steroids, primarily dehydroepiandrosterone sulfate [18].

Adrenocorticotropic hormone, a 39-amino acid product of the parent polypeptide, is secreted by the pituitary in an episodic fashion with a superimposed diurnal rhythm [19]. The secretion of pituitary ACTH is, in turn, controlled by corticotropin-releasing factor (CRF), a hypothalamic polypeptide of 41 amino acids. The release of CRF is controlled in part by higher centers [20,21].

The mineralocorticoid aldosterone is primarily under the control of the renin-angiotensin system [13,22,23]. Renin release can be stimulated by a chloride deficit, a decrease in renal blood pressure, or, to some extent, beta-adrenergic action [24]. Renin is necessary for the conversion of angiotensinogen to the decapeptide angiotensin I, which in turn is cleaved to form the octapeptide angiotensin II, which acts on the zona glomerulosa to increase aldosterone synthesis and secretion [13]. Aldosterone secretion is also stimulated by an increase in the plasma potassium level and by ACTH [12,13]. Although a long-standing lack of ACTH results in a diminution in the increase of aldosterone secretion associated with salt depletion, under normal conditions ACTH plays little role in aldosterone secretion. Aldosterone secretion is also stimulated by sodium deficiency, presumably due to the effects of sodium chloride on the renin-angiotensin system [24,25].

Angiotensin II acts to stimulate aldosterone secretion at an early step of the biosynthetic pathway by increasing the conversion of cholesterol to pregnenolone [13,26]. In addition, it acts at a later step by stimulating the conversion of corticosterone to 18-hydroxycorticosterone and aldosterone [26]. Potassium also seems to affect both the early and late steps in biosynthesis, but ACTH acts primarily at the early step [26], increasing the conversion of cholesterol to pregnenolone [16] in regulating glucocorticoid secretion.

Actions of Aldosterone. The major site of action of the mineralocorticoid aldosterone is the renal tubule, where it promotes the reabsorption of sodium and the secretion of potassium and hydrogen through the classic receptor mechanism [27]. Thus aldosterone enters the cell and binds to a receptor. The aldosterone-receptor complex binds to the genome, stimulating messenger ribonucleic acid (mRNA) synthesis and, in turn, protein synthesis. Aldosterone also affects sodium excretion via the gut, salivary glands, and sweat glands, through the same mechanism.

Actions of Cortisol. Glucocorticoids act on numerous tissues via the classic cytosol-nuclear receptor mechanism [28]; however, the exact process for certain of the receptor mechanism's actions has not been identified. Glucocorticoids affect the sense of well-being, appetite, and mood, but the mechanisms for these effects remain uncertain. Glucocorticoids also directly inhibit the release of ACTH in the central nervous system, probably at the pituitary level, and also through inhibition of hypothalamic release of CRF. Glucocorticoids have a direct effect on the cardiovascular system and help maintain blood pressure, although the means by which they do so is unknown.

One of the major actions of glucocorticoids is their effect on gluconeogenesis and protein wasting. They stimulate hepatic glycogen and glucose production [29] and inhibit insulin action on peripheral tissues via classic steroid receptor mechanisms. In addition, glucocorticoids stimulate protein breakdown and inhibit synthesis in many tissues, thus providing substrate for gluconeogenesis. They also increase the excretion of free water

by the kidney, in part by inhibiting antidiuretic hormone (ADH) release [30], and in large doses they bind to mineralocorticoid receptors, increasing sodium reabsorption and potassium and hydrogen ion excretion.

The effects of glucocorticoids on white cells are manifested as lymphopenia, especially T but also B cells [31], leukocytosis, and eosinopenia. Glucocorticoids suppress the inflammatory and immune responses.

Excess glucocorticoids can lead to osteoporosis and reduction of the hypercalcemia in certain diseases. Although the exact mechanisms whereby glucocorticoids act on bone and calcium metabolism remain uncertain, cortisol administration can inhibit intestinal calcium absorption [32,33], move extracellular calcium into intracellular spaces [34], and increase renal excretion of calcium. In addition, in cell culture studies, cortisol has been reported to inhibit both osteoclast and osteoblast function [32,33].

ADRENAL FAILURE. In primary adrenal failure, the lack of aldosterone results in sodium wasting with concomitant loss of water and an increase in renal reabsorption of potassium. A decrease in plasma volume and dehydration occurs, with subsequent increases in blood urea nitrogen (BUN) and plasma renin activity.

Lack of glucocorticoids results in weakness, fatigue, anorexia, and weight loss, the exact mechanisms of which cannot be clearly related to known actions of glucocorticoids. Because of the withdrawal of feedback inhibition of ACTH synthesis and release, the decrease in circulating levels of cortisol causes a marked increase in circulating levels of ACTH and a corresponding increase in beta-lipotropin [35]. Due to an increase in melanocyte-stimulating hormone (MSH) activity, the skin, especially creases and scars, becomes pigmented.

Hypotension develops, which is initially orthostatic but may progress to frank shock in a crisis. This decrease in blood pressure is due not only to the decrease in plasma volume but also to the direct effect of glucocorticoids on the cardiovascular system. With the decrease in work load, the heart usually becomes smaller. However, in a previously hypertensive patient, the effect on blood pressure and heart size may not be so noticeable in the early stages of hypoadrenalism.

Hypoglycemia develops, and usually the glucose tolerance test is relatively flat with fasting hypoglycemia. Liver glycogen levels fall because of the decrease in gluconeogenesis and glycogen synthesis. There is an increase in sensitivity to insulin as the glucocorticoid peripheral inhibition of insulin action disappears.

Renal excretion of free water is decreased, resulting in a dilutional effect on the already lowered serum sodium level. This effect on free water is manifested, however, as an inability to excrete a free water load. Inappropriate secretion of antidiuretic hormone (ADH) may further contribute to hyponatremia.

There is an increase in circulating eosinophils and lymphocytes and a decrease in red cell mass, with consequent anemia. Lymphoid tissue in the gastrointestinal (GI) tract may be increased and play a role in GI symptoms, which are prominent. The loss of glucocorticoid action results in an increase in calcium, which may be slight but can result in frank hypercalcemia.

Clinical Manifestations

PRIMARY ADRENAL HYPOFUNCTION. When available, there is usually a nonspecific history of increasing weakness, lassitude, fatigue, anorexia, vomiting, and constipation (with the hypoadrenal crisis, there may be diarrhea). In some instances a history of craving for salt or salty foods may also be present.

Patients who present with adrenal hypofunction in crisis are hypotensive or in frank shock, generally have a fever that may be high, show evidence of dehydration, and may be stuporous or comatose [5,36]. However, there may be no pigmentation if the adrenal hypofunction is of recent onset [5]. In individuals whose loss of adrenal function occurs as a precipitous event (i.e., adrenal hemorrhage during the course of an infection or anticoagulant therapy), frequently there is evidence of flank pain.

Patients with chronic adrenal insufficiency may often be able to survive in the basal state, but they will go into crisis in a stress situation, such as infection or trauma [5]. Therefore, signs of these inciting conditions and chronic adrenal hypofunction should be carefully sought. Pigmentation is usually striking in individuals who have an insidious onset of chronic adrenal hypofunction prior to presentation in crisis. The pigmentation is usually dark, present most commonly in the creases of the hands, the soles of the feet, and on any scars incurred after the onset of adrenal hypofunction. In addition, generalized purplish freckling of the skin can be seen. However, only 50 percent of patients presenting in adrenal crisis show evidence of pigmentation [5].

The buccal mucosa may have small, purplish freckles with frank patches of pigmentation. Buccal mucosa pigmentation is usually seen only in those patients who are pigmented elsewhere. When severe, the pigmentation creates a darkish cast to the skin of the entire body, and patients sometimes note that the tan they achieved in August has remained with them through the winter. In some instances there is calcification of the pinnae of the ears.

SECONDARY ADRENAL HYPOFUNCTION. In secondary adrenal failure due to lack of ACTH, the signs and symptoms are primarily those of glucocorticoid deficiency [37]. However, it can be associated with the signs of other endocrine gland dysfunctions if there is a deficit in the pituitary secretion of other tropic hormones. The clinical manifestations of hypoglycemia can be severe, since both cortisol and growth hormone may be lacking; the signs and symptoms of myxedema and/or hypogonadism may also be present. Patients with secondary adrenal failure present with weakness and fatigue, but they often lack the marked weight loss of an addisonian. They are not pigmented, because ACTH and beta-lipotropin are lacking.

Diagnosis

The diagnosis of hypoadrenal function is confirmed by laboratory tests of adrenal function when a patient presents with a compatible clinical picture. Other laboratory tests will likely be abnormal as well.

ADRENAL FUNCTION TESTS. In primary adrenal insufficiency, although plasma levels of cortisol are usually low or in the low-normal range, the levels do not rise after ACTH. This failure to respond to ACTH is the definitive test for primary adrenal hypofunction and should be carried out on anyone in whom the diagnosis is suspected. The ACTH stimulation test may be carried out as follows. Plasma cortisol levels are drawn prior to and 30 and 60 minutes after intravenous administration

of 250 µg of Synacthen (synthetic ACTH 1-24). Normal adrenal function shows cortisol levels rising 7 µg per 100 ml above baseline or reaching a level greater than 18 µg per 100 ml; patients with primary adrenal insufficiency have an absent response. Since the analysis of the plasma for cortisol cannot be done immediately, therapy, if not started before, should be started immediately after the test is completed and before the results are obtained.

Some individuals present with secondary rather than primary adrenal hypofunction; in the secondary form aldosterone secretion is generally preserved. It has been suggested that the measurement of aldosterone and cortisol levels, following the administration of ACTH, provides added information as to whether the adrenal dysfuncton is primary or secondary [38]. In addition, blood should be drawn prior to the ACTH test for ACTH measurement. Elevated levels of ACTH indicate primary dysfunction of the adrenals; normal or decreased levels are seen in normal individuals or those with secondary adrenal hypofunction [39]. Following intravenous administration of 250 µg of ACTH, patients with secondary adrenal insufficiency show an increase in cortisol, although not to the same degree as subjects with normal hypothalamic-pituitary adrenal function.

In primary adrenal insufficiency, urinary levels of free cortisol and cortisol metabolites are decreased and fail to rise with ACTH testing. However, it is usual to administer intravenously 250 µg of ACTH in 8-hour infusions for 3 days, when urinary-free cortisol or 17-hydroxycorticoids are measured. In normal subjects, this causes excretion of urinary 17-OHCS to rise two- to threefold. In secondary adrenal hypofunction the rise is usually delayed and not quite so great; in primary adrenal insufficiency there is no rise.

OTHER LABORATORY TESTS. In individuals who develop acute adrenal insufficiency as a result of adrenal hemorrhage, a computed tomography (CT) scan of the adrenals can be a very useful diagnostic tool [9,40]. Electrolytes in individuals with adrenal hypofunction generally show varying degrees of hyponatremia secondary to the negative sodium balance. Hyperkalemia is usually present, although not always to a major degree. However, the sodium-potassium ratio is almost always less than 30. The blood sugar is generally low, the BUN elevated, and hypercalcemia is often present. Eosinophilia and lymphocytosis are noted, and there is usually a normocytic, normochromic anemia. Urinary sodium and chloride are generally elevated and the urinary potassium decreased. Stool fat may be increased.

Treatment

The management of suspected hypoadrenal crisis depends on the severity of the illness on presentation (Fig. 113-1). The main objective of therapy in the critically ill patient with primary adrenal insufficiency is immediate administration of a glucocorticoid along with saline and glucose. Since large amounts of hydrocortisone are administered intravenously in salt-containing solutions, it is not necessary to administer a mineralocorticoid immediately. It is generally believed that individuals in the hypoadrenal state have a deficit of about 20 percent of their extracellular fluid volume and should receive at least 3 liters of glucose-containing saline in the first 24 hours.

In critically ill patients, the saline and glucose may have to be given in the first few hours. A bolus of 100 mg of hydrocortisone should be administered intravenously immediately and then every 6 hours thereafter for the first 24 hours. If the pa-

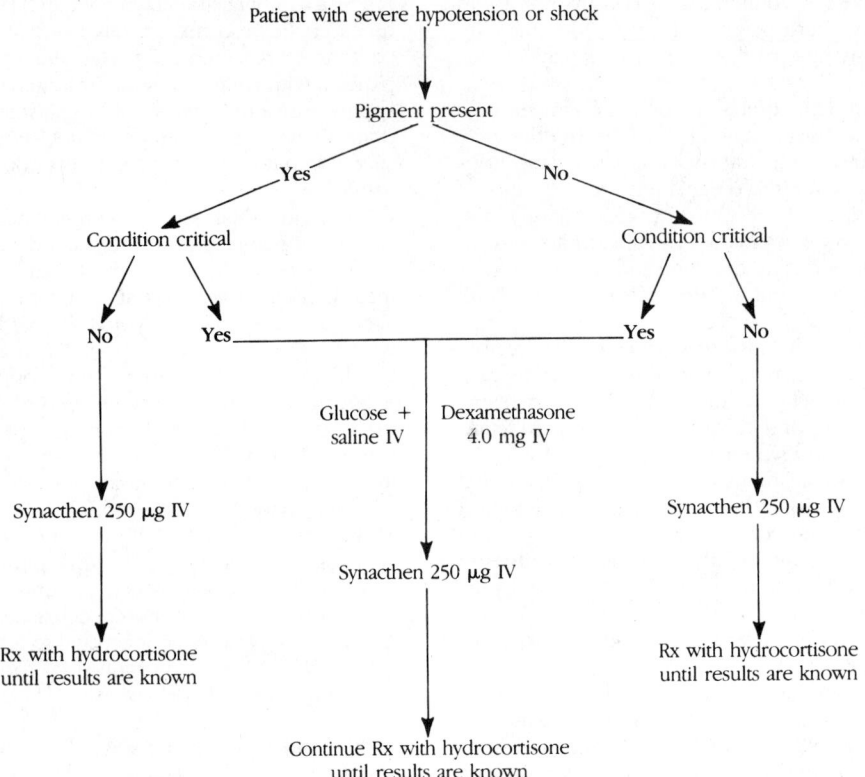

Fig. 113-1. Management of suspected hypoadrenal crisis.

tient's condition is deemed sufficiently grave, 4.0 mg of dexamethasone sodium phosphate may be administered as initial therapy before carrying out the ACTH stimulation [41]. However, since dexamethasone does not have potent salt-retaining activity, hydrocortisone should be used for continuing therapy.

After the initial 24 hours of therapy, generally the hydrocortisone can be decreased by 50 percent per day as the situation improves to reach a standard maintenance dose of 20 to 30 mg per day. As the maintenance dose is achieved, the administration of a mineralocorticoid, 0.1 mg of 9α-fluorocortisol, should be the treatment of choice. This may then be adjusted to achieve a normal blood pressure without excessive salt retention or hypokalemia. Adequate salt intake should be assured, but with a proper dose of mineralocorticoid excessive amounts are not necessary.

In addition to therapy with glucocorticoids and saline and glucose, any underlying infection should be treated vigorously.

Summary

Hypoadrenal crisis can be treated effectively to alleviate the acute signs and symptoms but requires long-term therapy thereafter to maintain a normal life. An individual in crisis is usually febrile, hypotensive, hypoglycemic, and hyponatremic; if the diagnosis is uncertain, the individual should be tested rapidly with intravenous ACTH. Therapy can be begun with saline and glucocorticoids even before the diagnostic test is performed, if the situation warrants, but certainly before the results are known.

References

1. Frederick R, Brown C, Renusch J, et al: Addisonian crisis: Emergency presentation of primary adrenal insufficiency. *Ann Emerg Med* 20:802, 1991.
2. Claussen MS, Landercasper J, Cogbill TH: Acute adrenal insufficiency presenting as shock after trauma and surgery: Three cases and review of the literature. *J Trauma* 32:94, 1992.
3. Dunlop D: Eighty-six cases of Addison's disease. *Br Med J* 2:887, 1963.
4. Nerup J: Addison's disease: A review of some clinical, pathological and immunological features. *Dan Med Bull* 21:201, 1974.
5. Rusnak RA: Adrenal and pituitary emergencies. *Emerg Med Clin North Am* 7:903, 1989.
6. Irvine WJ, Barnes EW: Addison's disease, ovarian failure and hypoparathyroidism. *Clin Endocrinol Metab* 4:379, 1975.
7. Blizzard RM, Chee D, Davis W: The incidence of adrenal and other antibodies in the sera of patients with idiopathic adrenal insufficiency (Addison's disease). *Clin Exp Immunol* 2:119, 1967.
8. Nerup J: Addison's disease: Serological studies. *Acta Endocrinol* 76:142, 1974.
9. Siu SCB, Kitzman DW, Sheedy PF, et al: Adrenal insufficiency from bilateral adrenal hemorrhage. *Mayo Clin Proc* 65:664, 1990.
10. Portnay GI, Vagenakis AG, Braverman LE: Acute adrenal insufficiency associated with anticoagulant therapy. *Ann Intern Med* 81:115, 1974.
11. Xarli VP, Steele AA, Davis PJ: Adrenal hemorrhage in the adult. *Medicine* 57:211, 1978.
12. Fraser R, Mason PA, Buckingham JC: The interaction of sodium and potassium states, of ACTH and of angiotensin II in the control of corticosteroid secretion. *J Steroid Biochem* 11:1039, 1979.
13. Quinn SJ, Williams GH: Regulation of aldosterone secretion. *Annu Rev Physiol* 50:409, 1988.
14. Fakunding JL, Chow R, Cart KJ: The role of calcium in the stimulation of aldosterone production by adrenocorticotropin, angiotensin II, and potassium in isolated glomerulosa cells. *Endocrinology* 105:327, 1979.

15. Williams GH, Bailey LM: Effects of dietary sodium intake and potassium intake and acute stimulation on aldosterone output by isolated human cells. *J Clin Endocrinol Metab* 45:55, 1977.

16. Gill GN: ACTH regulation of the adrenal cortex, in Gill GN (ed): *Pharmacology of Adrenal Cortical Hormones.* New York, Pergamon, 1979, p 35.

17. Jones MT: Control of adrenocortical hormone secretion, in James VHT (ed): *The Adrenal Gland.* New York, Raven, 1979, pp 93–130.

18. Odell W, Parker L: Control of adrenal androgen secretion, in Genazzani AR (ed): *Adrenal Androgens.* New York, Raven, 1980, p 27.

19. Krieger DT: Rhythms of ACTH and corticosteroid secretion in health and disease and their experimental modification. *J Steroid Biochem* 6:785, 1975.

20. Krieger DT: Rhythms in CRF, ACTH, and corticosteroids, in Krieger DT (ed): *Endocrine Rhythms.* New York, Raven, 1979, pp 123–142.

21. Plotsky PM, Cunningham ET, Windmaier EP: Catecholaminergic modulation of corticotropin-releasing factor and adrenocorticotropin secretion. *Endocr Rev* 10:437, 1989.

22. Barrett PQ, Bollag WB, Isales CM, et al: Role of calcium in angiotensin II-mediated aldosterone secretion. *Endocr Rev* 10:496, 1989.

23. Kater CE, Biglieri EG, Brust N, et al: Stimulation and suppression of the mineralocorticoid hormones in normal subjects and adrenocortical disorders. *Endocr Rev* 10:149, 1989.

24. Fray JCS, Park CS, Valentine AND: Calcium and the control of renin secretion. *Endocr Rev* 8:53, 1987.

25. Davis JO, Freeman RH: Mechanisms regulating renin release. *Physiol Rev* 56:1, 1976.

26. Aguilera G, Catt KJ: Loci of action of regulators of aldosterone biosynthesis in isolated glomerulosa cells. *Endocrinology* 104:1046, 1980.

27. Funder JW: Aldosterone action. *Annu Rev Physiol* 55:115, 1993.

28. Baxter JD, Ivarie RD: Regulation of gene expression by glucocorticoid hormones: Studies of receptors and responses in cultured cells, in O'Malley BW, Birnbaumer L (eds): *Receptors and Hormone Action.* New York, Academic, 1978, pp 252–296.

29. Stalmans W, Laloux M: Glucocorticoids and hepatic glycogen metabolism, in Baxter JD, Rousseau GG (ed): *Glucocorticoid Hormone Action,* New York, Springer-Verlag, 1979, pp 518–533.

30. Boykin J, deTorrente A, Erickson A: Role of plasma vasopressin in impaired water excretion of glucocorticoid deficiency. *J Clin Invest* 62:738, 1978.

31. Ilfeld DN, Krakauser RS, Blaese RM: Suppression of the human autologous mixed lymphocyte reaction by physiologic concentrations of hydrocortisone. *J Immunol* 119:428, 1977.

32. Lukert BP, Raisz LG: Glucocorticoid-induced osteoporosis: Pathogenesis and management. *Ann Intern Med* 112:352, 1990.

33. Reid IR: Pathogenesis and treatment of steroid osteoporosis. *Clin Endocrinol* 30:83, 1989.

34. Kimura S, Rasmussen H: Adrenal glucocorticoids, adenine nucleotide translocation, and mitochondrial calcium accumulation. *J Biol Chem* 252:1217, 1977.

35. Krieger DT, Liotta AS, Brownstein MJ: ACTH, beta-lipotropin, and related peptides in brain, pituitary, and blood. *Recent Prog Horm Res* 36:277, 1980.

36. Knowlton AI: Adrenal insufficiency in the intensive care setting. *J Intensive Care Med* 4:35, 1989.

37. Yamamoto T, Fukuyama J, Hasegawa K, et al: Isolated corticotropin deficiency in adults. *Arch Intern Med* 152:1705, 1992.

38. Dluhy RG, Himathongkam T, Greenfield M: Rapid ACTH test with plasma aldosterone levels: Improved diagnostic discrimination. *Ann Intern Med* 80:693, 1974.

39. Besser GM, Cullen DR, Irvine WJ: Immunoreactive corticotrophin levels in adrenocortical insufficiency. *Br Med J* 1:374, 1971.

40. Rao RH, Vagnucci AH, Amico JA: Bilateral massive adrenal hemorrhage: Early recognition and treatment. *Ann Intern Med* 110:227, 1989.

41. Sheridan P, Mattingly D: Simultaneous investigations and treatment of suspected acute adrenal insufficiency. *Lancet* 2:676, 1975.

114. Disorders of Mineral Metabolism

Daniel T. Baran

Introduction

Disorders of mineral metabolism, although common, are rarely the primary cause of admission to an intensive care unit. However, these disorders frequently exacerbate life-threatening medical situations. Calcium ions regulate intracellular enzyme activities, nuclear endonuclease activity, intercellular communication through channels and ion exchange, neurotransmitter release, hormone-receptor interactions, neuromuscular excitation, membrane potentials, and the coagulation cascade. Hypocalcemia can result in laryngospasm and death or can exacerbate neuromuscular irritability and existing seizure disorders. Hypercalcemia can cause asystole or exacerbate peptic ulcer disease and cause a deterioration in mental status.

Magnesium is necessary for parathyroid hormone secretion and maintenance of serum calcium, membrane sodium-potassium ATPase activity, and neuromuscular function. Hypomagnesemia can cause hypocalcemia, with its resultant complications, or enhance digitalis toxicity. Hypermagnesemia is often attended by a loss of deep tendon reflexes and central nervous system (CNS) depression.

Phosphate, the major intracellular anion, is instrumental for normal cellular function. It is a component of nucleic acids, phospholipids, and high-energy nucleotides and is necessary to facilitate oxygen delivery to cells and enhance enzyme activity. Hypophosphatemia can impair oxygen delivery to the body tissues due to decreased 2,3-diphosphoglycerate levels. Rhabdomyolysis, which can occur during severe hypophosphatemia, can result in acute hypercalcemia, hypermagnesemia, and impairment of renal function. Thus, phosphorus metabolism is related to calcium and magnesium homeostasis, and symptoms of abnormal phosphorus metabolism often reflect the abnormalities in circulating calcium and magnesium.

Calcium, magnesium, and phosphate balance are controlled through the interactions of parathyroid hormone, $1\alpha,25$-dihydroxyvitamin D_3, and calcitonin.

Calcium Disorders

CALCIUM PHYSIOLOGY. Ninety-nine percent of total body calcium is stored primarily in bone, whereas less than one percent is located in extracellular fluids. The calcium found in the extracellular fluids is either free (40%) or bound to albumin (50%) or other anions, such as citrate, lactate, and sulfate (10%). It is the free ionized calcium that is biologically active. Acid-base balance affects the binding of calcium to albumin. Hyperventilation, and the resultant respiratory alkalosis, enhances the binding of calcium to albumin, thereby acutely decreasing the ionized calcium and causing symptoms of hypocalcemia despite unchanged levels of total calcium. Similarly, changes in serum protein levels affect total serum calcium. The ionized or free calcium level (normal 4.5–5.5 mg/dl) can be estimated by the following formula:

$$\text{Total serum calcium (mg/dl)} - 0.8 \times \text{serum albumin (mg/dl)}$$
$$= \text{ionized calcium (mg/dl)}$$

Although the formula takes into account changes in serum proteins, it does not consider the impact of alterations in pH, which frequently occur during acute illness. Therefore, when there is suspicion of altered serum calcium levels in the acutely ill patient, it is best to measure the ionized calcium directly.

Calcium balance is a function of absorption from the intestine (primarily the small intestine by active transport and facilitated diffusion), distribution in the body, and excretion. The average diet contains 500 to 1500 mg of calcium per day. In young individuals, the efficiency of intestinal absorption varies inversely with the amount of calcium ingested. The absorbed calcium is in equilibrium with intracellular calcium and calcium in bone and is filtered through the kidney. Approximately 300 mg of calcium is exchanged daily between plasma and bone. Urinary calcium excretion (150–300 mg of calcium per day) depends on glomerular filtration rate and tubular sodium reabsorption. Furosemide diuretics enhance urinary calcium excretion in conjunction with their effect on sodium excretion. It is this property of the furosemide diuretics that serves as a useful adjunct to lower elevated serum calcium levels in the hydrated patient.

HORMONAL REGULATION OF CALCIUM.

Calcium balance depends on (1) bone resorption and formation, (2) gastrointestinal (GI) absorption, and (3) renal excretion. These processes are in large part regulated by three hormones: (1) parathyroid hormone (PTH), (2) $1\alpha,25$-dihydroxyvitamin D_3 [$1,25(OH)_2D_3$], and (3) calcitonin (CT).

Parathyroid Hormone. Parathyroid hormone is an 84-amino acid polypeptide produced and secreted by the chief cells of the parathyroid gland. The cDNA message for PTH has been identified. Secretion of PTH is stimulated by low levels of calcium in the cytoplasm of the parathyroid cells. The target organs for PTH are bone, kidney, and intestine. Parathyroid hormone stimulates bone resorption to release calcium and phosphate from the hydroxyapatite crystals in bone. This effect is augmented in the presence of $1,25(OH)_2D_3$. The renal effects of PTH include decreased proximal tubular reabsorption of phosphate (phosphate wasting), enhanced distal tubular calcium reabsorption (calcium retention), increased renal mitochondrial 1α-hydroxylase activity (enhanced $1,25(OH)_2D_3$ production), and augmented cyclic AMP production. The hormone's effects on the intestine are indirect and mediated through its actions on renal $1,25(OH)_2D_3$ production.

Parathyroid hormone is produced as a large preprohormone of 115 amino acids and undergoes intracellular proteolysis to a prehormone of 90 amino acids and finally the 84-amino acid peptide. The hormone is primarily secreted as the intact 84-amino acid polypeptide. Peripheral metabolism of the intact molecule occurs primarily in the liver, to yield the biologically active 1-34 amino acid fragment (N terminal) and the biologically inactive 35-84 amino acid fragment (C terminal). The N terminal fragment has a short half-life, due in large part to its rapid binding to membrane receptors, whereas the C terminal fragment has a half-life that depends on renal function and the rate of glomerular filtration.

Radioimmunoassays for PTH measure the intact 84-amino acid polypeptide, the N terminal fragment, or various regions of the 50-amino acid C terminal fragment. The intact PTH measurement will play an increasingly important role in the investigation and management of disorders of mineral metabolism. Not only does the intact assay distinguish patients with primary hyperparathyroidism from normals, it also separates those with hypercalcemia due to primary hyperparathyroidism and those with hypercalcemia of malignancy [1].

The N terminal fragment of PTH binds to cell membrane receptors to activate adenylate cyclase and produce cyclic AMP. Measurement of nephrogenous cyclic AMP (cyclic AMP produced by the kidney) is a method of determining PTH bioactivity. The nephrogenous component is determined by measuring total urinary cyclic AMP and plasma cyclic AMP using the following formula:

$$\text{Nephrogenous cyclic AMP/24 hr} =$$
$$\frac{\text{Total urinary cyclic AMP}}{24} - \text{Plasma cyclic AMP (CrCl} \times 1440)$$

The utility of the nephrogenous cyclic AMP determination is limited by the necessity of urine collections and the concomitant measurement of creatinine clearance.

Decrements in parathyroid cell calcium (a reflection of serum ionized calcium) cause the immediate release of preformed PTH. Although catecholamines can modulate PTH secretion, with beta-agonists augmenting and beta-antagonists inhibiting secretion, these effects are rarely apparent in vivo. For example, beta-antagonists are not an effective treatment for hyperparathyroidism. In contrast, magnesium is mandatory for PTH secretion and end-organ response [2]. At magnesium levels below 0.4 mM per liter, the parathyroid glands do not secrete adequate hormone in response to hypocalcemia, and the cyclic AMP response and bone resorption induced by the secreted hormone are reduced. Correction of the hypocalcemia occurs only after correction of the hypomagnesemia.

Parathyroid hormone has both anabolic and catabolic effects on bone. Anabolic effects presumably occur at physiologic levels and may result from PTH-induced production of insulinlike growth factors by osteoblasts [3]. The catabolic, bone resorptive effects of PTH are mediated by enhanced osteoclastic activity, resulting in calcium and phosphate release from the inorganic matrix. The rapid release of PTH in response to the hypocalcemic stimulus is essential for calcium homeostasis.

Vitamin D. Vitamin D is a steroid that is essential for calcium balance. Activation of vitamin D requires 25-hydroxylation in the liver and 1-hydroxylation in the kidney to form the hormone $1,25(OH)_2D_3$. Negative feedback is exerted by $1,25(OH)_2D_3$ on its own production by suppressing 1-hydroxylase activity and stimulating the enzyme 24-hydroxylase to produce the biologically inactive steroid $24,25(OH)_2D_3$.

The effects of $1,25(OH)_2D_3$ are exerted through interaction with nuclear receptors located in a variety of cells, including enterocytes, osteoblasts, and renal tubular cells. The receptor is also located in parathyroid cells. $1,25(OH)_2D_3$ has been shown to suppress PTH gene expression. $1,25(OH)_2D_3$ receptors have also been identified in tissues not associated with calcium balance, such as keratinocytes, hematopoietic lymphoid cells, and islet cells of the pancreas [4]. The steroid hormone has been found to stimulate cell differentiation and suppress cell proliferation in these tissues. It is proving to be useful in patients with psoriasis, a disorder of excessive proliferation of keratinocytes. The hormone also induces differentiation of HL60 cells (a human leukemic cell line) into monocytelike cells [5]. Finally, the steroid acts on cell membranes to cause immediate increments in cellular calcium. These rapid nongenomic actions of 1,25-dihydroxyvitamin D_3 modulate the hormone-induced increments in osteocalcin gene transcription in osteoblasts [6].

Calcitonin. Calcitonin is a 32-amino acid polypeptide produced by the C cells of the thyroid. It is secreted in response to elevations in serum calcium. Gastrointestinal hormones (e.g., gastrin) also stimulate CT secretion. Studies of normal and thyroidectomized dogs given an oral calcium load demonstrated hypercalcemia in the thyroidectomized animals, suggesting that CT may act to buffer the hypercalcemic effects of calcium absorption. Calcitonin is the most potent endogenous inhibitor of bone resorption. It also acts on the kidneys to enhance excretion of calcium, phosphate, magnesium, and sodium. Thus, the hormone is useful in the treatment of hypercalcemia through its inhibitory effects on osteoclastic bone resorption and renal tubular calcium reabsorption.

Extrathyroidal C cells capable of CT production have been identified in multiple organs, including the thymus, lungs, and urinary bladder. Production at these sites contributes to circulating CT levels and may explain the presence of measurable, albeit reduced, levels of CT in patients who have undergone thyroidectomy.

The effect of CT on bone resorption is lost over time due to an "escape phenomenon," which occurs with all forms of CT used clinically (i.e., human, eel, and salmon). This phenomenon, likely due to downregulation of CT receptors, is of clinical importance when treating patients with hypercalcemia due to increased bone resorption with CT. The excellent short-term effects of CT to lower serum calcium (within 12–48 hours) are usually lost after 7 days of treatment. This period of response to CT allows the institution of therapies that require several days to attain maximal effectiveness (e.g., bisphosphonates and gallium nitrate).

The primary physiologic function of CT in humans is unclear. Medullary carcinoma of the thyroid is characterized by elevated CT levels; however, calcium, phosphate, and PTH levels remain normal. Since there are no known syndromes of abnormal calcium balance in humans caused by either excess or deficient CT production, there is no evidence that the diminished CT levels following thyroidectomy are detrimental. Although the role of CT in the development of osteoporosis is controversial, the hormone has been shown to increase bone mass in some women with osteoporosis [7] and to prevent the enhanced bone loss that occurs during the perimenopausal period [8].

HYPERCALCEMIA. Hypercalcemia is an abnormality of balance between different body compartments and can result from increased bone resorption, decreased renal excretion, increased GI absorption, or any combination of these mechanisms.

The signs and symptoms of hypercalcemia are protean and can be divided into four groups: (1) mental, (2) neurologic and skeletal, (3) GI and urologic, and (4) cardiovascular. The mental manifestations of hypercalcemia include stupor, obtundation, apathy, lethargy, confusion, disorientation, and coma. In general, for a given level of hypercalcemia, older patients exhibit more of the mental signs than younger patients. The neurologic and skeletal effects of hypercalcemia are reduced muscle tone and strength, myalgias, and decreased deep tendon reflexes. The GI and urologic signs are vomiting, polyuria and polydipsia, and constipation. The major cardiovascular effect of hypercalcemia, which the intensive care physician must address, is shortening of the Q–T interval. In the presence of ventricular ectopic beats, the calcium-induced shortening of the Q–T interval increases the potential for fatal arrhythmias.

Differential Diagnosis. Elevated serum calcium measurements have been reported in approximately 1 percent of the general population [9]. The elderly, patients with malignancies, and individuals with kidney stones have a higher incidence of hypercalcemia [10]. Primary hyperparathyroidism and malignant disease account for nearly 90 percent of hypercalcemia cases [11]. The remaining causes include granulomatous disease, thyrotoxicosis, immobilization, vitamin D intoxication, Addison's disease, and familial hypocalciuric hypercalcemia. The malignancies most often associated with hypercalcemia include lung, 35 percent; breast, 25 percent; hematologic (myeloma and lymphoma), 14 percent; head and neck, 6 percent; and renal, 3 percent [12]. See Chapter 127 for a complete discussion of the hypercalcemia of malignancy.

Hypercalcemia not associated with malignancy is much less common in the hospitalized patient. Hyperparathyroidism results from inappropriate secretion of PTH despite elevated serum calcium levels. Hypercalcemia develops due to increased bone resorption, increased intestinal calcium absorption secondary to stimulated $1,25(OH)_2D_3$ production, and increased renal tubular calcium reabsorption. The patient is commonly hypophosphatemic due to the phosphaturic effect of PTH. The hormone also induces renal bicarbonate wasting, resulting in a mild hyperchloremic acidosis. A single adenoma is present in 80 to 85 percent of cases, whereas hyperplasia occurs in 10 to 15 percent of cases. Parathyroid cancer is present in less than 5 percent of these patients. Parathyroid cancer occurs in a younger age group, with average serum calcium levels of 15 mg per deciliter.

The routine measurement of serum calcium has altered the clinical presentation of hyperparathyroidism. Whereas bone disease (47–79%) and nephrolithiasis (3–21%) were common signs of hyperparathyroidism in the past, most patients (57%) are now diagnosed before any symptoms occur. In recent reviews, the incidence of nephrolithiasis has decreased to 7 percent, and no patients present with bone disease as their primary symptom [13].

Parathyroid adenomas can also occur as part of the multiple endocrine neoplasia (MEN) syndrome. Type I MEN involves tumors of the pituitary, pancreas, and parathyroid, whereas type II is associated with pheochromocytoma, medullary cancer of the thyroid, and hyperparathyroidism.

Familial hypocalciuric hypercalcemia (FHH) is an autosomal dominant disorder characterized by hypercalcemia with elevated PTH levels [14]. In contrast to hyperparathyroidism, patients have hypocalciuria (mean 24-hour urinary calcium <100 mg), do not develop nephrolithiasis or bone disease, and are not cured by neck surgery.

Calcium balance can be affected by nonparathyroid endocrine conditions. Hyperthyroidism is associated with increased bone turnover resulting in osteoporosis [15] and hypercalciuria. Approximately 20 percent of patients with thyrotoxicosis have mild hypercalcemia (serum calcium 10.8–11.2 mg/dl) despite normal PTH levels. Adrenal insufficiency is occasionally associated with hypercalcemia, presumably due to hemoconcentration and volume depletion. Pheochromocytoma is associated with hyperparathyroidism in type II MEN. Isolated pheochromocytomas have been reported to cause hypercalcemia due to volume contraction and possibly a stimulatory effect of beta-agonists on PTH secretion.

Sarcoidosis is associated with increased intestinal calcium absorption and sensitivity to vitamin D intake. Hypercalcemia occurs in 10 to 20 percent of patients and is the result of autonomous $1,25(OH)_2D_3$ production by the granulomas. Mild hypercalcemia has also been reported in patients with tuberculosis, presumably due to $1,25(OH)_2D_3$ production by the granulomas.

Immobilization causes hypercalcemia as a result of decreased bone formation and persistent bone resorption. Hypercalcemia in the immobilized individual occurs most commonly in patients with high bone turnover—adolescents during the growth spurt or individuals with Paget's disease or thyrotoxicosis. Hypercalcemia is most likely to occur within 4 months of spinal cord injury and to affect one-fourth of children younger than age 16 after paralysis.

Relatively few medications can induce hypercalcemia. Hypercalcemia associated with the use of thiazide diuretics is usually an indicator of underlying primary hyperparathyroidism [16]. Vitamin D and vitamin A intoxication can cause hypercalcemia, as can isotretinoin (13-*cis*-retinoic acid) treatment of acne. Lithium may also affect bone metabolism and is associated with elevated PTH levels, hypercalcemia, and hypocalciuria, similar to patients with FHH [17].

Laboratory Evaluation. Hypercalcemia should always be considered in the patient with altered mental status. An ionized calcium is the most accurate marker of calcium levels. A total serum calcium level alone usually makes the diagnosis; however, altered binding of calcium to proteins, as can occur in hypoalbuminemic states, with abnormal proteins (e.g., myeloma), or in acid-base imbalance, may affect the free calcium level. Because of the interrelationships of calcium, magnesium, and phosphorus, the latter two minerals should be measured in all cases involving altered calcium metabolism. An electrocardiogram to determine the Q–T interval is very important to assess the severity and urgency of the patient's hypercalcemia. If malignancy is suspected, a bone scan usually identifies the metastatic process. Since myeloma is characterized by bone resorption with little bone formation, the bone scan is usually negative and the disease best diagnosed by bone marrow examination, serum protein electrophoresis, and urine immunoelectrophoresis. Intact PTH levels, serum electrolyte and cortisol levels, and thyroid function tests can confirm the diagnosis of primary hyperparathyroidism, Addison's disease, and thyrotoxicosis, respectively. The diagnosis of sarcoidosis is made by fulfilling three criteria: (1) a compatible clinical picture (e.g., symmetric chest radiograph abnormalities); (2) involved tissue that reveals noncaseating granulomata on biopsy; and (3) special stains and cultures that fail to reveal another cause for noncaseating granulomata.

Management of Hypercalcemia. The aim of treatment of hypercalcemia is to minimize its effects on CNS, renal, and cardiovascular function. Appropriate treatment of hypercalcemia depends in part on the etiology. General concepts in the management involve attempts to (1) increase renal calcium clearance, (2) decrease bone resorption, and (3) decrease intestinal calcium absorption. To this end it is critical that the pathophysiology of the disease process be understood. If, for example, the hypercalcemia in a patient with myeloma is due to a combination of increased bone resorption plus decreased renal calcium clearance, successful management of the hypercalcemia requires that both processes be treated (see Chap. 127). Specific measures directed toward the pathophysiology of the hypercalcemia are discussed in the following sections.

HYDRATION AND DIURESIS. Saline hydration creates a diuresis that increases renal calcium excretion by decreasing calcium reabsorption in the proximal tubule. Hydration plays a critical role in the initial management of hypercalcemia because the onset of the therapeutic response is rapid. The aim of therapy is to achieve a urine output of 3 to 5 liters per 24 hours. This requires the administration of 4 to 6 liters of normal saline per 24 hours. Since a potential complication of administration of this amount of saline is congestive heart failure, extreme care must be taken in treating the patient with underlying cardiac disease. The concomitant administration of a diuretic helps prevent fluid overload and further increases renal calcium excretion by inhibiting distal tubular calcium reabsorption. Furosemide (40–80 mg) or ethacrynic acid (50–100 mg) can be administered IV every 1 to 2 hours. Measurement of serum electrolytes, phosphorus, and magnesium is mandatory during saline hydration to replace adequately the quantities lost in the urine. If renal or cardiac failure precludes the use of saline hydration, dialysis with a calcium-free dialysate is an effective alternative.

CALCITONIN. Calcitonin reduces resorption of calcium from bone by inhibiting osteoclasts. It also exerts transient effects to increase excretion of renal calcium, along with sodium, potassium, magnesium, and phosphate. The efficacy of CT was documented in a study of 24 hypercalcemic patients (19 due to malignancy and 5 the result of primary hyperparathyroidism) [18]. All patients remained hypercalcemic despite 48 hours of hydration plus diuresis. At a dose of 4 units per kilogram per 12 hours, there was a 75 percent response by 2 hours and an 80 percent response by 24 hours. Response was defined by a minimum 0.5 mg per deciliter decline in serum calcium. The average decline in calcium after 24 hours was 2 mg per deciliter. Four of the patients with malignancy and two with primary hyperparathyroidism failed to respond. Usually CT is effective for 4 to 7 days [19]. This "escape phenomenon" was initially attributed to the development of antibodies to the CT but is now believed to represent a downregulation of receptors on the osteoclasts. The benefits of CT in the treatment of hypercalcemia include (1) rapid onset (2 hours), (2) maximal effect within 24 hours, (3) analgesic effects, and (4) low toxicity. It can be used safely in patients with renal failure, and its side effects are limited to transient nausea, facial flushing, and occasional hypersensitivity at the injection site.

BISPHOSPHONATES. The bisphosphonates are organic compounds that inhibit osteoclastic activity. They are effective in rehydrated patients with malignancy in whom increased bone resorption is the main cause of hypercalcemia [20]. The bisphosphonates are well tolerated and have few side effects, mainly GI upset. Etidronate disodium (7.5 mg/kg IV every 8 hours) when used along with hydration (3 liters of saline per day) reduces serum calcium in up to 90 percent of patients with hypercalcemia of malignancy [21,22]. Clodronate may be administered orally (1600–3200 mg/day) or IV (300–600 mg over 8 hours). The serum calcium does not usually begin to decline until 48 hours after administration of the bisphosphonate. The decline with clodronate therapy does not appear to differ if the drug is given as one injection or repeated daily injections [20]. In comparison with CT and mithramycin (see following), aminohydroxypropylidene bisphosphonate (APD) given as an infusion of 15 mg in 250 ml normal saline each day had the slowest onset of action but the most sustained effect [23]. Because of the delay in reduction of serum calcium with bisphosphonates, these agents have been used in conjunction with other therapies. The combination of APD and CT [24], clodronate and CT [25], and etidronate and CT [26] have been reported to produce rapid and sustained decrements in calcium levels. The rapid response has been attributed to the skeletal and renal effects of CT, whereas the prolonged response is thought to represent bisphosphonate-induced inhibition of osteoclast activity. At least one recent report suggested that patients whose hypercalcemia is due to production of PTHrP are resistant to multiple infusions of bisphosphonates [27].

MITHRAMYCIN. Mithramycin is an antibiotic used in cancer chemotherapy. At a dose of 25 μg per kilogram IV over 8 hours, it can lower serum calcium levels within 24 to 48 hours as a result of osteoclast inhibition. Its use is limited by bone marrow, renal, and hepatic toxicity [28].

GALLIUM NITRATE. Gallium nitrate causes hypocalcemia as a result of inhibition of bone resorption. In a randomized, double-blind comparison to CT, gallium nitrate therapy (200 mg/m² body surface area for 5 days by continuous IV infusion) resulted in normocalcemia in 75 percent (18 of 24) of patients with hypercalcemia of malignancy [29]. CT (8 IU/kg every 6 hours for 5 days) normalized serum calcium in 31 percent (8 of 26) of patients. Median duration of normocalcemia was 11 days in the gallium nitrate group and 2 days in the CT group. The major side effect of gallium nitrate is nephrotoxicity, and it should not be used until intravascular depletion has been corrected with IV hydration. Use of aminoglycoside antibiotics along with the gallium nitrate may potentiate its nephrotoxic effects. Current recommendations are that patients not receive aminoglycosides within 48 hours before or after treatment with gallium nitrate and that a urine output of 2 liters per day be maintained throughout therapy [29].

HYPOCALCEMIA. Hypocalcemia is frequently encountered in critically ill hospitalized patients [30]. The most frequent cause is low serum albumin, but the ionized, or free, fraction remains normal. The symptoms of hypocalcemia, tingling, paresthesias, tetany, or even seizures are due to decreased serum ionized calcium. Positive Chvostek and Trousseau's signs are suggestive, but not diagnostic, of hypocalcemia. In contrast to the Q–T interval shortening in hypercalcemia, hypocalcemia is attended by an increase in the Q–T interval on electrocardiogram, predisposing patients to cardiac arrhythmias [31]. Chronic hypocalcemia is associated with basal ganglia calcification, cataract formation, and behavioral abnormalities.

Differential Diagnosis. Risk factors for the development of hypocalcemia in hospitalized patients include alkalosis, renal failure, multiple transfusions, and GI bleeding. Although pancreatitis is associated with hypocalcemia, the mechanism is unclear. Recent studies suggest that intracellular magnesium depletion may be responsible for the occurrence of hypocalcemia in patients with pancreatitis [32]. Hyperphosphatemia is the suspected cause of hypocalcemia attending tumor lysis and rhabdomyolysis.

Inadequate, or absent, PTH secretion is a cause of hypocalcemia. Hypoparathyroidism can occur after surgery, after irradiation, as a result of iron deposition in hemochromatosis, or in severe magnesium deficiency. Idiopathic hypoparathyroidism can be familial or sporadic. Autoimmune phenomena may explain the idiopathic variety. Target tissue unresponsiveness, presumably due to a defect in cell membrane G protein, is

characterized by hypocalcemia and hyperphosphatemia in the presence of elevated PTH levels [33]. Somatic abnormalities (short, stocky habitus, round facies, and short metacarpals and/or metatarsals) frequently accompany the chemical manifestations.

Hypocalcemia can also signify vitamin D deficiency. Although nutritional rickets is rare in the United States, liver or renal failure may affect the hydroxylation of the parent compound. Vitamin D deficiency may also be the result of malabsorption and steatorrhea.

Laboratory Evaluation. The most accurate measure of true hypocalcemia is ionized calcium level. Additional studies may include creatinine, phosphate, amylase, magnesium, liver function tests, carotene, 25-hydroxyvitamin D, and PTH levels. In hypoparathyroidism due to the absence of PTH or target tissue unresponsiveness, serum phosphate levels tend to be high as a result of the absent phosphaturic effect of PTH.

Management of Hypocalcemia. Treatment of hypocalcemia depends on its severity and chronicity. Patients with an ionized calcium less than 3 mg per deciliter who are symptomatic should be treated with IV calcium. A 10-ml vial of 10% calcium gluconate provides 93 mg of elemental calcium, whereas 10 ml of calcium chloride (10%) provides 272 mg. Either calcium gluconate or calcium chloride (93–272 mg elemental calcium) should be administered in 50 to 100 ml D_5W over 10 to 15 minutes in the symptomatic patient. After the initial bolus, an infusion of 1 to 2 mg elemental calcium per kilogram per hour can be continued until the ionized calcium is 4.5 mg per deciliter or the total calcium is 7 mg per deciliter. Dietary supplementation should be instituted to provide 1.5 to 2.5 gm of elemental calcium per day. If oral intake is prohibited (e.g., in the comatose patient), a maintenance infusion of 0.3 to 0.5 mg of elemental calcium per kilogram per hour can be administered. Calcium to be administered IV should always be diluted, since concentrated solutions are very irritating to veins. Patients being treated with digitalis must have electrocardiographic monitoring during calcium supplementation, because calcium potentiates the action of digitalis on the heart. Hypocalcemia may mask digitalis toxicity. In these situations, a slower rate of calcium administration is recommended to prevent cardiac arrhythmias.

If calcium supplementation alone cannot maintain serum calcium levels, vitamin D preparations may be administered. Ergocalciferol (vitamin D_2) is the most frequently administered preparation because of its safety margin and low cost. The usual dose is 50,000 to 150,000 units per day. This preparation has a slow onset of action because it must be 25-hydroxylated in the liver and 1-hydroxylated in the kidney. Therefore, significant liver or renal disease limits its utility. The preparation has a long half-life because it is stored in fat. Vitamin D preparations that act more rapidly are also available. Dihydrotachysterol (100–400 μg/day) is an oral synthetic analog of vitamin D that requires 25-hydroxylation in the liver for full activity. $1,25(OH)_2D_3$ (0.25–1.0 μg/day) is also available. These preparations have shorter half-lives than vitamin D but are more potent and more expensive for long-term management. If the patient is unable to take oral medication, vitamin D preparations can be administered parenterally [34].

The goal of treating hypocalcemia is to prevent symptoms attributable to low calcium but to avoid hypercalciuria and hypercalcemia. In the hypoparathyroid patient, total serum calcium should be maintained between 8 and 8.5 mg per deciliter. In the absence of PTH, which acts on the renal tubules to enhance calcium reabsorption, circulating calcium levels greater than 9.0 mg per deciliter are often attended by hypercalciuria and the increased risk of nephrolithiasis.

Magnesium Disorders

MAGNESIUM PHYSIOLOGY. Magnesium is the major intracellular divalent cation. One-half of the total body content of magnesium is found in bone. Muscle and liver are the soft tissues that contain the greatest amount of magnesium. Thirty percent of extracellular magnesium circulates bound to protein. Therefore, as with circulating calcium levels, albumin concentration must be known to interpret total magnesium levels.

Magnesium absorption occurs throughout the small intestine. Absorption is enhanced by $1,25(OH)_2D_3$. Like calcium, magnesium is reabsorbed in the kidney tubules. Therefore, hypomagnesemia may result from decreased intestinal absorption (e.g., steatorrhea), increased renal excretion due to an osmotic diuresis (e.g., hyperglycemia), or drugs (e.g., ethanol, aminoglycosides, or cisplatin).

Magnesium is necessary for normal Na^+/K^+ ATPase activity, PTH secretion, and neuromuscular function. Decreased Na^+/K^+ ATPase activity due to hypomagnesemia can result in intracellular potassium depletion. This, in turn, increases the risk of digitalis toxicity. Magnesium-induced decreases in PTH secretion result in hypocalcemia that can only be corrected by magnesium replacement. Finally, magnesium inhibits the release of acetylcholine by presynaptic fibers and decreases the sensitivity of the motor end plate to the neurotransmitter. Therefore, hypomagnesemia is often attended by CNS hyperexcitability, whereas hypermagnesemia results in CNS depression. Flaccid paralysis, hypotension, confusion, and coma may result from magnesium levels greater than 6 mEq per liter.

HYPERMAGNESEMIA. The most common cause of hypermagnesemia in the hospitalized patient is renal failure. The hypermagnesemia may be aggravated by the administration of magnesium-containing antacids. Diabetic ketoacidosis is usually attended by hypermagnesemia, but this typically reflects dehydration, which masks the total body magnesium depletion resulting from the glucose-induced osmotic diuresis.

Management. The actions of magnesium in neuromuscular function are antagonized by calcium. Emergency treatment of the magnesium-induced CNS depression includes IV administration of 10 ml of 10% calcium gluconate (93 mg elemental calcium) diluted in 50 to 100 ml D_5W to prevent venous irritation. The dose may be repeated as necessary. Total serum calcium must be monitored and not allowed to exceed 11 mg per deciliter.

Definitive treatment of the hypermagnesemia requires increasing renal magnesium excretion. In the presence of normal renal function, increased magnesium excretion can be achieved by IV administration of $D_{5-1/2}NS$ at 150 ml per hour along with bolus furosemide, 40 to 80 mg IV every 1 to 2 hours. Serum electrolytes, particularly potassium, must be closely monitored. Dialysis is the treatment of choice when kidney function is impaired and the patient is symptomatic from the hypermagnesemia.

HYPOMAGNESEMIA. Hypomagnesemia is much more common than hypermagnesemia in the hospitalized patient. Low serum magnesium levels are usually due to combinations of decreased intake and intestinal absorption and increased renal excretion. The increased CNS excitability in the patient with hypomagnesemia is in part due to the accompanying hypocalcemia, which results from impaired PTH secretion and decreased peripheral tissue responsiveness to PTH.

Dietary deficiency alone is rarely the explanation for hypomagnesemia. The exceptions are starvation or prolonged parenteral feeding. Hypomagnesemia has been reported in 40 percent of patients with malabsorption [35]. Steatorrhea is always associated with some degree of magnesium deficiency.

The most common cause of hypomagnesemia is increased renal excretion. Osmotic diuresis resulting from hyperglycemia or hypercalcemia increases magnesium excretion. The hypomagnesemia associated with diabetic ketoacidosis is most commonly encountered once rehydration is begun. Hypercalcemia is associated with hypomagnesemia because of the associated osmotic diuresis and the competition between magnesium and calcium for reabsorption in the renal tubule.

The drugs that most commonly increase renal magnesium excretion are alcohol and diuretics. Hypomagnesemia in the alcohol abuser is also attributable to dietary deficiency. Hypomagnesemia is encountered in 30 percent of severe alcoholics and 80 percent of those with delirium tremens [36]. Serum magnesium levels fall within the first 48 hours of alcohol withdrawal, presumably because of intracellular shifts. The role of magnesium deficiency in alcohol withdrawal syndrome is unknown, but magnesium replacement is indicated in patients admitted for detoxification (see Chap. 158).

Recent studies suggest that patients with acute pancreatitis and hypocalcemia commonly have magnesium deficiency with low intracellular magnesium levels. Normocalcemic patients with pancreatitis have normal intracellular magnesium levels. These results suggest that magnesium deficiency may play a role in the pathogenesis of hypocalcemia in patients with acute pancreatitis [32].

Management. Magnesium may be administered orally or parenterally. If serum magnesium levels are below 1 mEq per liter or the patient is symptomatic, parenteral treatment is indicated. The patient with symptoms usually has a total body magnesium deficit of 1 to 2 mEq per kilogram body weight. Because approximately half of the administered magnesium is lost due to renal excretion, replacement of the deficit requires administration of 2 to 4 mEq per kilogram body weight. Forty-nine milliequivalents of magnesium (6 ampules of 10% $MgSO_4$) can be administered every 12 hours [37]. The magnesium can be added to a liter of IV solution and given over 3 to 6 hours. After each 49-mEq dose, serum magnesium and calcium should be monitored. In the patient with mild magnesium deficiency, oral therapy is satisfactory. Diarrhea is the most common side effect. With all magnesium supplementation, levels must be monitored closely in the patient with renal insufficiency.

Phosphorus Disorders

PHOSPHORUS PHYSIOLOGY. Eighty percent of total body phosphorus is found in bone. Extracellular phosphate accounts for only 0.1 percent of total body phosphorus. Because of shifts in phosphate between intracellular and extracellular compartments, serum phosphate levels do not accurately reflect total body stores. For example, since acidosis causes a shift in phosphate from within cells to the extracellular compartment, serum phosphate levels may be normal in the acidotic patient despite depletion of total body stores.

Phosphorus is a component of nucleic acids and phospholipids and is a cofactor for a number of enzymes. Low phosphate levels increase renal mitochondrial 1α-hydroxylase activity and $1,25(OH)_2D_3$ production. This, in turn, increases intestinal calcium and magnesium absorption. Thus, phosphorus metabolism is closely related to calcium and magnesium metabolism.

HYPERPHOSPHATEMIA. Increased phosphate levels are most often encountered in patients with renal failure or hypoparathyroidism. The loss of tubular function in renal failure results in impaired phosphate excretion. The hyperphosphatemia, along with diminished renal $1,25(OH)_2D_3$ production, results in hypocalcemia. Hyperphosphatemia occurs in the hypoparathyroid patient due to the absent phosphaturic response to PTH. As in the patient with renal failure, symptoms are usually attributable to the accompanying hypocalcemia, not the hyperphosphatemia per se. Therefore, in the symptomatic patient, therapy should be directed at correction of the hypocalcemia.

HYPOPHOSPHATEMIA. Hypophosphatemia results from impaired intestinal phosphate absorption or increased renal phosphate excretion. The cause of hypophosphatemia in alcoholics is multifactorial but most likely reflects malnutrition and the accompanying vomiting. Phosphate-binding antacids impair phosphate absorption. The resulting hypophosphatemia can stimulate $1,25(OH)_2D_3$ production and cause hypercalcemia, which has been confused with hyperparathyroidism.

Renal phosphate excretion is increased in hyperparathyroidism, vitamin D deficiency, and hyperglycemic states. Parathyroid hormone inhibits renal tubular phosphate reabsorption, causing the hypophosphatemia encountered in hyperparathyroidism. Serum phosphate levels are reduced in vitamin D deficiency due to impaired intestinal phosphate absorption (the result of low $1,25(OH)_2D_3$ levels) and increased renal phosphate excretion (the result of secondary hyperparathyroidism in response to the associated hypocalcemia). The patient in diabetic ketoacidosis has a total body phosphorus deficit, despite normal serum phosphorus levels. In the early stages of the illness, the rising serum glucose levels cause an osmotic diuresis with increased renal phosphate loss. This lowers serum phosphorus levels; however, the developing acidosis causes a shift in phosphorus from the intracellular to the extracellular compartment. This shift, along with the accompanying volume depletion, tends to normalize the serum phosphorus levels. Rehydration and insulin treatment cause a rapid fall in serum phosphorus levels.

The potential consequences of severe hypophosphatemia are impaired oxygen delivery to the tissues due to decreased 2,3-diphosphoglycerate levels, muscle weakness, and rhabdomyolysis. The latter is most likely to occur when severe hypophosphatemia occurs after prolonged mild hypophosphatemia, for example in the hospitalized alcoholic in whom phosphate falls precipitously during carbohydrate administration.

Management. Severe hypophosphatemia (<1 mg/dl) requires parenteral therapy. Potassium phosphate for parenteral use contains 3 mM of phosphate per milliliter. The phosphate (0.08–0.16 mM phosphate per kilogram body weight) may be added to $D_{5-1/2}NS$ and given over 6 hours. Initial doses should be 25 to 50 percent higher in the symptomatic patient, lower if the patient is hypercalcemic [38]. Further treatment depends on the serum phosphate levels and clinical condition. Parenteral therapy is contraindicated in the patient with renal failure or hy-

pocalcemia. In the patient with renal failure, IV therapy can cause hyperphosphatemia, worsen hypocalcemia, and cause metastatic calcification, primarily in the kidney. The latter can occur if the patient is hypercalcemic or if the phosphate is administered too rapidly.

The usual oral dose of phosphate is 1 to 4 gm per day in divided doses. The most common side effect is diarrhea.

References

1. Woodhead JS, Silver AC, Aston JP, et al: Measurement of circulating parathyroid hormone. *Horm Res* 32:97, 1989.
2. Chase LR, Slatopolsky E: Secretion and metabolic efficacy of parathyroid hormone in patients with severe hypomagnesemia. *J Clin Endocrinol Metab* 38:363, 1974.
3. McCarthy TL, Centrella M, Canalis E: Parathyroid hormone enhances the transcript and polypeptide levels of insulin-like growth factor I in osteoblast-enriched cultures from fetal rat bone. *Endocrinology* 124:1247, 1989.
4. DeLuca HF: The vitamin D story: A collaborative effort of basic science and clinical medicine. *FASEB J* 2:224, 1988.
5. Desai SS, Appel MC, Baran DT: Differential effects of 1,25-dihydroxyvitamin D_3 on cytosolic calcium in two human cell lines (HL-60 and UJ-937). *J Bone Miner Res* 1:497, 1986.
6. Baran DT, Sorensen AM, Shalhoub V, et al: The rapid nongenomic actions of 1,25-dihydroxyvitamin D_3 modulate the hormone-induced increments in osteocalcin gene transcription in osteoblast-like cells. *J Cell Biochem* 50:124, 1992.
7. Civitelli R, Gonnelli S, Zacchei F, et al: Bone turnover in postmenopausal osteoporosis: Effect of calcitonin treatment. *J Clin Invest* 82:1268, 1988.
8. Reginster JY, Albert A, Lecart MP, et al: 1-year controlled randomized trial of prevention of early postmenopausal bone loss by intranasal calcitonin. *Lancet* 2:1481, 1987.
9. Palmer M, Jakobsson S, Akerstrom G, et al: Prevalence of hypercalcaemia in a health survey: A 14-year follow-up study of serum calcium values. *Eur J Clin Invest* 18:39, 1988.
10. Heath H, Hodgson SF, Kennedy MA: Primary hyperparathyroidism: Incidence, morbidity, and potential economic impact in a community. *N Engl J Med* 302:189, 1980.
11. Mundy GR: Incidence and pathophysiology of hypercalcemia. *Calcif Tissue Int* 46:S3, 1990.
12. Mundy GR, Martin TJ: The hypercalcemia of malignancy: Pathogenesis and management. *Metabolism* 31:1247, 1982.
13. Mundy GR, Cove DH, Fisken R: Primary hyperparathyroidism: Changes in the pattern of clinical presentation. *Lancet* 1:1317, 1980.
14. Marx SJ, Spiegel AM, Levine MA, et al: Familial hypocalciuric hypercalcemia: The relation to primary parathyroid hyperplasia. *N Engl J Med* 307:416, 1982.
15. Paul TL, Kerrigan J, Kelly AM, et al: Long term *l*-thyroxine therapy is associated with decreased hip bone density in premenopausal women. *JAMA* 259:3137, 1988.
16. Christensson T, Hellstrom K, Wengle B: Hypercalcemia and primary hyperparathyroidism: Prevalence in patients receiving thiazides as detected in a health screen. *Arch Intern Med* 137:1138, 1977.
17. Mallette LE, Eichhorn E: Effects of lithium carbonate on human calcium metabolism. *Arch Intern Med* 146:770, 1986.
18. Wisneski LA, Croom WP, Silva OL, et al: Salmon calcitonin in hypercalcemia. *Clin Pharmacol Ther* 24:219, 1978.
19. Wisneski LA: Salmon calcitonin in the acute management of hypercalcemia. *Calcif Tissue Int* 46:S26, 1990.
20. Bonjour J-P, Rizzoli R: Clodronate in hypercalcemia of malignancy. *Calcif Tissue Int* 46:S20, 1990.
21. Hasling C, Charles P, Mosekilde L: Etidronate disodium in the management of malignancy-related hypercalcemia. *Am J Med* 82(suppl 2A):51, 1987.
22. Kanis JA, Urwin GH, Gray RES, et al: Effects of intravenous etidronate disodium on skeletal and calcium metabolism. *Am J Med* 82(suppl 2A):55, 1987.
23. Ralston SH, Gardner MD, Dryburgh FJ, et al: Comparison of ami-

nohydroxypropylidene diphosphonate, mithramycin, and cortico-steroids/calcitonin in treatment of cancer-associated hypercalcae-mia. *Lancet* 2:907, 1985.

24. Ralston SH, Alzaid AA, Gardner MD, et al: Treatment of cancer associated hypercalcaemia with combined aminohydroxypropyli-dene diphosphonate and calcitonin. *Br Med J* 292:1549, 1986.

25. Junghall S, Rastad J, Akerstrom G: Comparative effects of calcitonin and clodronate in hypercalcemia. *Bone* 8:S79, 1987.

26. Fatemi S, Singer FR, Rude RK: Effect of salmon calcitonin and etidronate on hypercalcemia of malignancy. *Calcif Tissue Int* 50:107, 1992.

27. Gallacher SJ, Fraser WD, Logue FC, et al: Factors predicting the acute effect of pamidronate on serum calcium in hypercalcemia of malignancy. *Calcif Tissue Int* 51:419, 1992.

28. Brown JH, Kennedy BJ: Mithramycin in the treatment of disseminated testicular neoplasms. *N Engl J Med* 272:111, 1965.

29. Warrell RP Jr, Israel R, Frisone M, et al: Gallium nitrate for acute treatment of cancer-related hypercalcemia. *Ann Intern Med* 108:669, 1988.

30. Chernow B, Zaloga G, McFadden E, et al: Hypocalcemia in critically ill patients. *Crit Care Med* 10:848, 1982.

31. Connor TB, Rosen BL, Blaustein MP, et al: Hypocalcemia precipitating congestive heart failure. *N Engl J Med* 307:869, 1982.

32. Ryzen E, Rude RK: Low intracellular magnesium in patients with acute pancreatitis and hypocalcemia. *West J Med* 152:145, 1990.

33. Downs RW, Sekura RD, Levine MA, et al: The inhibitory adenylate cyclase coupling protein in pseudohypoparathyroidism. *J Clin Endocrinol Metab* 61:351, 1985.

34. Whyte MP, Haddad JG Jr, Walters DD, et al: Vitamin D bioavailability: Serum 25-hydroxyvitamin D levels in man after oral, subcutaneous, intramuscular, and intravenous vitamin D administration. *J Clin Endocrinol Metab* 48:906, 1979.

35. Booth CC, Hanna S, Babouris N, et al: Incidence of hypomagnesaemia in intestinal malabsorption. *Br Med J* 2:141, 1963.

36. Sullivan JF, Wolpert PW, Williams R, et al: Serum magnesium in chronic alcoholism. *Ann NY Acad Sci* 162:947, 1969.

37. Flink EB: Therapy of magnesium deficiency. *Ann NY Acad Sci* 162:901, 1969.

38. Lentz RD, Brown DM, Kjellstrand CM: Treatment of severe hypophosphatemia. *Ann Intern Med* 89:941, 1978.

115. *Lactic Acidosis*

John P. Mordes, Robert E. Tranquada, and Aldo A. Rossini

Introduction

The lactate anion is a normal product of anaerobic glycolysis. In persons at rest, the venous lactate concentration is ≈ 1 mM per liter. After strenuous exercise it may rise transiently to 20 mM per liter or more [1], but the capacity for lactate disposal is great and perturbations are rapidly corrected. Lactic acidosis is a pathologic state diagnosed when the serum lactate concentration is persistently 5 mM per liter or greater and there is significant acidemia [2]. It is a common disorder, reportedly present in 0.5 to 3.8 percent of consecutive hospital admissions [3].

Lactic acidosis was described in the 1920s [4] but not recognized as a significant clinical problem until the 1960s [5]. It is fatal in the majority of cases [6]. Figure 115-1 illustrates the correlation of mortality with increasing serum lactate concentration in one group of patients [7]. Incidence and fatality rate have changed little in recent decades [6,8].

Pathophysiology

NORMAL LACTATE METABOLISM [9]. Figure 115-2 outlines the place of lactate in carbohydrate metabolism. Catabolism of glucose to pyruvate occurs anaerobically in the cytoplasm of all cells, generating ATP and reduced nicotinamide adenine dinucleotide (NADH). This ATP is the sole energy source in cells like erythrocytes that lack mitochondria. Anaerobic glycolysis depends on the continuing availability of oxidized nicotinamide adenine dinucleotide (NAD^+) as a cofactor.

All tissues containing mitochondria subsequently metabolize

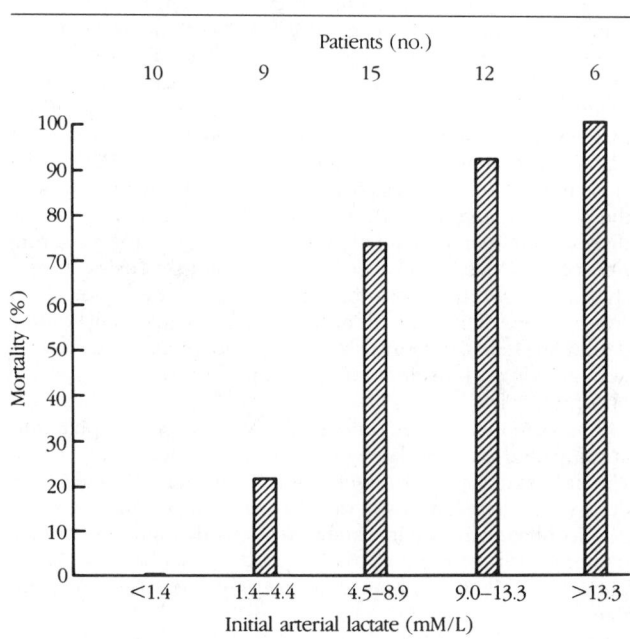

Fig. 115-1. Mortality rate in 52 patients with shock and lactic acidosis as a function of lactate concentration. (From Peretz DI, Scott HM, Duff J, et al: The significance of lacticacidemia in the shock syndrome. *Ann NY Acad Sci* 119:1133, 1965. With permission.)

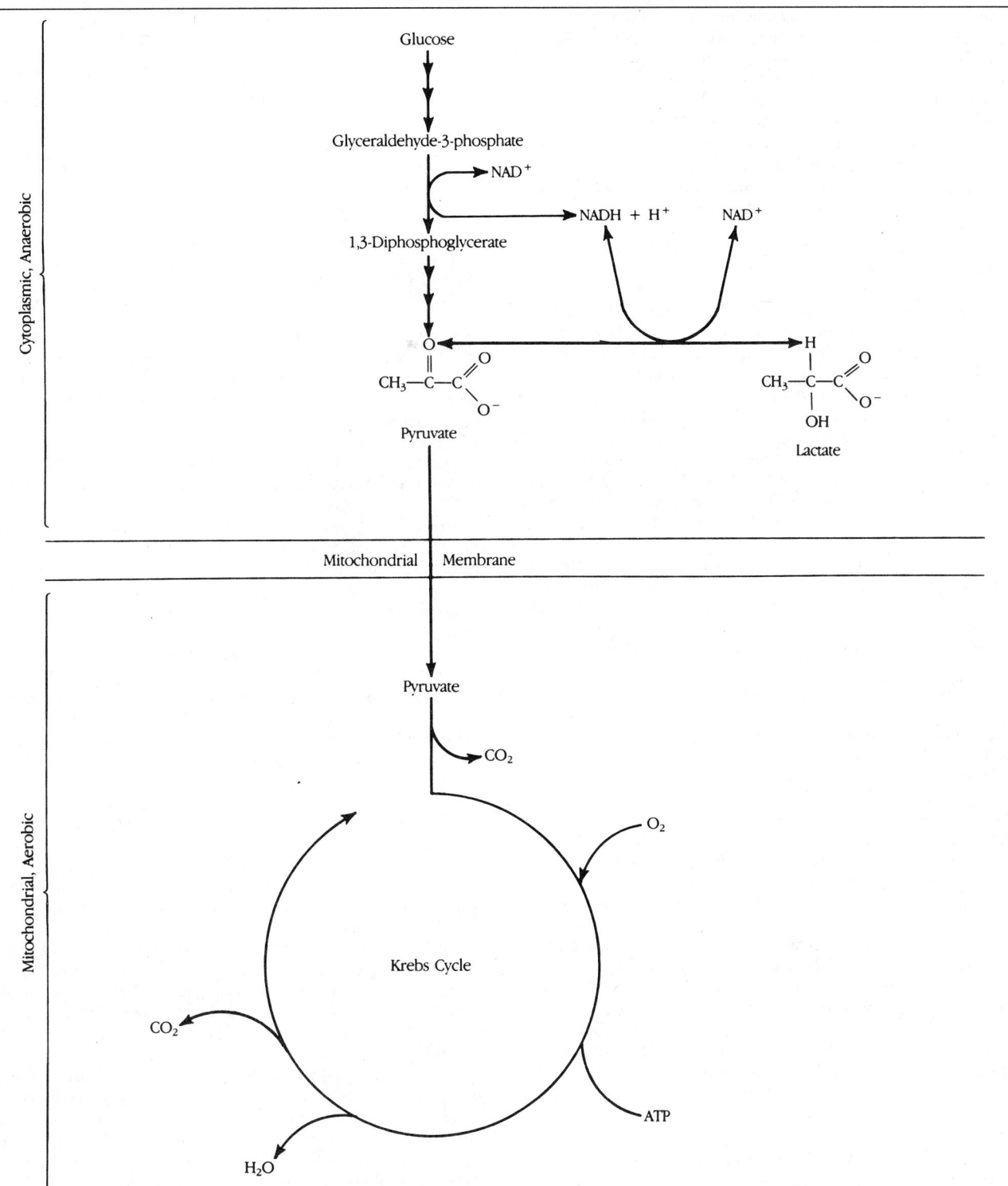

Fig. 115-2. Outline of lactate metabolism. NAD$^+$ = oxidized
nicotinamide adenine dinucleotide (NAD); NADH = reduced NAD;
ATP = adenosine triphosphate.

pyruvate to CO_2 and water. Oxidative phosphorylation generates ATP both from Krebs cycle reactions and from the oxidation of reduced NADH and $FADH_2$ by the cytochrome oxidase complex. Anything that impairs the oxidation of pyruvate results in reduced ATP generation and leads to the accumulation of not only pyruvate but also reduced NADH.

The accumulation of NADH and concomitant depletion of NAD^+ would then fatally halt anaerobic glycolysis (by preventing the generation of 1,3-diphosphoglycerate) were it not for the formation of lactate from pyruvate:

$$CH_3COCOO^- + NADH + H^+ \rightarrow CH_3CHOHCOO^- + NAD^+ \quad (1)$$

Pyruvate   Lactate

Lactate dehydrogenase catalyzes the synthesis of lactate from pyruvate. Using NADH as a cofactor, it regenerates NAD^+. The reaction strongly favors the production of lactate; at equilibrium the ratio of lactate to pyruvate is ≈10:1. Lactate formation is essential to tissues that need NAD^+ to generate energy anaerobically. This is the case in erythrocytes without mitochondria and in exercising skeletal muscle with an "oxygen debt."

Figure 115-3 summarizes the metabolic fates of lactate. The principal route of disposal is via cytosolic reconversion to pyruvate. Most of the pyruvate then either enters the Krebs cycle and is oxidatively phosphorylated or is used for gluconeogenesis. Lactate from erythrocytes is released into the circulation for disposal elsewhere. The same holds true for any other tissue that produces lactate faster than it can be metabolized. The release by skeletal muscle of lactate derived from glycogen is an important response to starvation, comprising a part of the Cori cycle. Disposal of circulating lactate occurs principally in liver (≥50%), kidney, muscle, and the central nervous system. Renal excretion of lactate is quantitatively important only at serum concentrations in excess of 10 mM per liter.

The generation of lactate provides a kind of metabolic buffer for tissues. It permits glycolysis and energy generation to continue despite fluctuations in the rate of oxidative phosphorylation. Lactate itself is a metabolic dead end; it cannot be metabolized unless the process that led to its formation is reversed. Lactate generation "buys time" for tissues that must metabolize glucose anaerobically because oxidative phosphorylation has become impaired. Time eventually runs out, however, because anaerobic glycolysis proceeds at the expense of accumulating a strong (pKa = 3.8) metabolic acid.

Transient increases in lactate concentration are buffered by circulating HCO_3^-. This is what happens during exercise or a seizure. Ultimately, however, all lactate must be oxidized to pyruvate and removed. Persistent failure to oxidize lactic acid to CO_2 and water, thereby removing accumulated free H^+, eventually exhausts the buffering capacity of blood and transforms hyperlactatemia into lactic acidosis.

ABNORMAL LACTATE METABOLISM [10].

Many paths lead to abnormal lactate accumulation; most involve impairment of lactate disposal. Normal daily production of lactate is on the order of only 1.5 M per day. In comparison, the normal capacity for lactate disposal is enormous. The liver alone can clear up to 3.4 M per day, and total body lactate clearance may be as high as 17 M per day [11]. Decreased lactate removal is nearly always present in states of lactic acidosis, whereas increased production may or may not contribute.

Anything that deprives tissues of oxygen (e.g., shock, hypoxemia) impairs oxidative phosphorylation and leads to the accumulation of pyruvate and then lactate. Similarly, drugs, toxins, and metabolites that interfere with oxidative metabolism

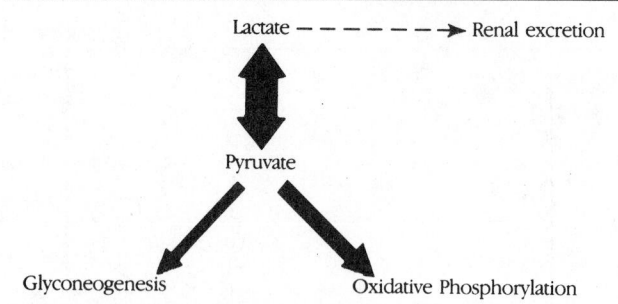

Fig. 115-3. Metabolic fates of the lactate anion.

in general or hepatic metabolism in particular predispose to lactate accumulation. Factors that decrease gluconeogenesis also tend to decrease pyruvate utilization and predispose to lactic acidosis. Deficiencies of vitamins such as thiamine that are cofactors in pyruvate metabolism also predispose to lactic acidosis in states of malnutrition.

Acidosis per se facilitates the accumulation of lactate. Lactate disposal depends on the maintenance of normal tissue pH. At pH 7.40 the liver's capacity for lactate uptake is very great, but that capacity decreases progressively with increasing acidosis. At pH 7.0 or less, the liver produces more lactate than it consumes [12]. The metabolism of lactate by the kidney is similarly affected by acidemia. The more severe the uncompensated acidemia, the more difficult it may be to restore lactate homeostasis [13].

Another factor that influences lactate removal is the availability of oxidized NAD. The ratio of NAD^+ to NADH reflects the cellular redox state. Reduction in the ratio favors lactate accumulation and an increase in the ratio of lactate to pyruvate. As an example, ethanol is metabolized to acetaldehyde using NAD^+ as a cofactor; this reduces the intracellular NAD^+/NADH ratio:

$$CH_3CH_2OH + NAD^+ \rightarrow CH_3CHO + NADH + H^+ \quad (2)$$

Ethanol   Acetaldehyde

The accumulation of NADH favors the generation of lactate from pyruvate (Equation 1), and thus ethanol ingestion favors lactic acid accumulation.

Lactic acidosis due solely to increased pyruvate production is uncommon. Disorders that increase pyruvate production include states of extreme catabolism, such as starvation; insulin deficiency; some parenteral nutrition regimens; grand mal seizures; malaria; and certain hereditary metabolic disorders, such as type I glycogen storage disease.

This sketch of abnormal lactate metabolism indicates only the broad outlines of a complex pathophysiologic process, but two broad themes emerge. First, from a biochemical viewpoint abnormal lactate accumulation is a disorder of pyruvate, not lactate, metabolism. Lactate is a marker of the balance between pyruvate synthesis and disposal. Lactic acidosis is a sign of a disturbance in that balance, and the etiology of lactic acidosis encompasses the disorders that disequilibrate it. Second, the physiologic significance of increased lactate concentration resides less with the lactate anion than with the equimolar amount of dissociated hydrogen ion that challenges acid-base equilibrium. These themes imply that the resolution of lactic acidosis requires, first, restoration of normal pyruvate metabolism, followed by the oxidation of lactate to pyruvate and thence to CO_2 and water, fixing the free hydrogen ion causing the acidemia. More detailed information on normal and abnormal lactate metabolism is available elsewhere [2,8,9,10].

Etiology

Lactic acidosis is commonly divided into two broad categories, types A and B [11]. The former is associated with clinically obvious states of hypoperfusion and/or tissue hypoxia. The latter encompasses all other forms of lactic acidemia (Table 115-1).

This classification is a useful guide in clinical practice, but it oversimplifies the pathophysiology. The A/B distinction is somewhat artificial. Many cases of type B lactic acidosis probably result in part from regional, clinically undetectable tissue hypoperfusion. Furthermore, acidemia per se adversely affects cardiovascular function, and the lactate ion itself may be negatively inotropic. Hence, type A lactic acidosis may become superimposed on type B. Finally, many "causes" of type B lactic acidosis (e.g., hepatic failure) function principally to predispose to the condition in the context of intercurrent hypoperfusion or hypoxia. Types A and B lactic acidosis cannot be distinguished biochemically with respect to the mechanism of lactate production [14].

TYPE A LACTIC ACIDOSIS. Hemorrhagic, cardiogenic, and endotoxic shock are the most common precipitants of lactic acidosis. Many cases occur after trauma, but any cause of severe cardiorespiratory distress or sepsis may lead to the disorder. In most instances, lactic acidosis is only one facet of a critical clinical situation. Its presence in cases associated with shock is ominous. Blair reported 100 percent mortality in patients with septic shock and lactate greater than 3 mM per liter [15]. Peretz et al. reported 73 percent mortality in cases of shock with lactate levels between 4.4 and 8.9 mM per liter (Fig. 115-1) [7]. Lactic acidosis in the context of hypoxemia is often accompanied by an intercurrent perfusion disorder [6]. Control of the underlying disease state and restoration of perfusion are the keys to successful treatment of type A lactic acidosis associated with shock [6].

TYPE B LACTIC ACIDOSIS. Cases of lactic acidosis are categorized as type B if there is no obvious tissue hypoxia or hypoperfusion. The major subcategories include cases associated with intercurrent acquired diseases, drugs and toxins, and congenital diseases. As noted above, overlap with type A states is not uncommon.

Lactic Acidosis Associated with Acquired Diseases. Lactic acidosis associated with seizure disorders is usually self-limiting. Orringer et al. reported a mean lactate concentration of 12.7 mM per liter with a pH of 7.14 immediately after seizures [16]. The acidemia was analogous to that which follows maximal exercise of short duration. In all cases, the acid-base disorder resolved spontaneously and without treatment within 2 hours.

Hepatic [17] and renal [18] disease predispose to lactic acidosis and hypoglycemia. They contribute to lactate accumulation by impairing metabolism and excretion of the anion. Hypoglycemia is commonly associated with lactic acidosis in the context of congenital metabolic defects in glycogenolysis or gluconeogenesis [19,20]. In all such cases, the acidemia may not be correctable unless hypoglycemia is corrected [17,18,21].

The lactic acidosis of acute leukemia has been attributed to unregulated anaerobic glycolysis occurring in packed, poorly perfused, marrow cavities [22,23,24], but some cases may involve other factors, such as intercurrent thiamine deficiency [25,26]. Other neoplasms can also result in the disorder [27–31].

Table 115-1. Clinical Classification of Lactic Acidosis

Type A. States of hypoperfusion and hypoxia [6,8]
    1. Hypoperfusion
        a. Cardiogenic shock
        b. Hemorrhagic shock
        c. Septic shock
        d. Regional (e.g., mesenteric) ischemia
    2. Hypoxia
        a. Carbon monoxide poisoning
        b. Severe asthma
        c. Extreme degrees of anemia [89]
        d. Other causes of severe hypoxemia
Type B. No clinical evidence of hypoperfusion
    1. Associated with acquired diseases
        a. Grand mal seizures [16]
        b. Renal failure [18]
        c. Liver failure [17]
        d. Malignancy [22,23,24,27–31]
        e. Thiamine deficiency [25,26,56]
        f. Infection (sepsis [15,32], AIDS [33,34], cholera [36], malaria [35])
        g. Pheochromocytoma [37]
        h. Diabetes mellitus [38]
    2. Associated with metabolites, drugs, and toxins
        a. Parenteral nutrition (fructose, xylose, sorbitol) [11,39,40,41,90]
        b. Ethanol [42,43,44]
        c. Methanol [42]
        d. Salicylates [45,46]
        e. Acetaminophen [11]
        f. Biguanides (phenformin, metformin) [47,48]
        g. Streptozotocin [11]
        h. Epinephrine, norepinephrine [8]
        i. Terbutaline [6]
        j. Theophylline [91]
        k. Cocaine [92,93]
        l. Cyanide [8]
        m. Nitroprusside [87]
        n. Isoniazid [94]
        o. Propylene glycol [57]
        p. Ethylene glycol [8]
        q. Papaverine [8]
        r. Nalidixic acid [8]
        s. Lactulose [95]
        t. Ritodrine [6]
        u. Diethyl ether [8]
        v. Niacin [96]
        w. Paraldehyde [97]
    3. Associated with hereditary diseases [19]
        a. Glucose-6-phosphatase deficiency (von Gierke's or type 1 glycogen storage disease) [52]
        b. Fructose-1-6-diphosphatase deficiency [98,99]
        c. Pyruvate carboxylase deficiency [51]
        d. Organic acidurias [49]
        e. Leigh's disease [49]
        f. Alper's disease [49]
        g. Kearns-Sayre syndrome [49]
        h. Mitochondrial encephalopathies (MELAS syndrome) [50]
    4. Other
        a. D-lactic acidosis [53–57]
        b. Unexplained [58–61]

MELAS = mitochondrial myopathy, encephalopathy, lactic acidosis, and stroke-like episodes.
Adapted from Cohen RD, Woods HF: Lactic acidosis revisited. *Diabetes* 32:181, 1983.

Bacterial sepsis [15,32], AIDS [33,34], malaria [35], and cholera [36] are the infectious disorders most commonly associated with lactic acidosis. In all of these, tissue hypoperfusion or some other predisposing factor probably plays a major role. In the case of *Plasmodium falciparum*, lactate production by the parasite may also contribute.

Severe lactic acidosis with pulmonary edema and peripheral vasoconstriction has also been reported in pheochromocytoma [37]. Severe lactic acidosis in the setting of diabetes mellitus is not as common as once believed. Alberti and Nattrass note that the decline in biguanide treatment has paralleled the decline in diabetes-associated lactic acidosis [38].

Lactic Acidosis Associated with Metabolites, Drugs, and Toxins.
The list of compounds associated with the development of lactic acidosis grows steadily (Table 115-1), but the pathophysiology in many cases remains poorly understood and the contribution of hypoperfusion is often uncertain.

Infusions of fructose, sorbitol, and other total parenteral nutrition formulations have occasionally led to lactic acidosis [11,39,40,41]. In these cases, infusions were generally performed in fasting patients who required nutritional support and who were consequently in a gluconeogenic state. The pathophysiology is unclear but probably relates to intracellular acidification, consumption of ATP, and net synthesis of lactate from fructose.

Ethanol, as noted in Equation 2, favors the accumulation of lactate and the development of hypoglycemia due to impaired gluconeogenesis. Ethanol also interferes with lactate clearance. Coexisting liver disease, seizures, hyperventilation, thiamine deficiency, and diabetes further predispose to ethanol-induced hypoglycemia, ketosis, and lactic acidosis [42,43,44]. Administration of glucose alone is often sufficient to reverse lactic acidosis in the alcoholic patient.

In cases of salicylate intoxication, salicylate anion accounts for only part of the anion gap (see Chap. 154). Lactate is largely responsible for the ensuing acidosis [45,46]. The mechanism by which this occurs is unknown but may involve both uncoupling of oxidative phosphorylation and an impairment of gluconeogenesis.

Biguanides inhibit absorption of glucose from the gut, enhance glycolysis, and inhibit gluconeogenesis. They probably act by altering the physical-chemical state of mitochondrial membranes. Mild (≤ 2 mM/L) hyperlactatemia is a consequence of the normal action of these drugs. The biguanides phenformin, buformin, and metformin have all been associated with lactic acidosis [47,48]. Why only certain individuals who take the drugs are susceptible to this complication is not clear. The only biguanide made available in the United States, phenformin, was removed from the market. Metformin, now approved for use in the U.S. for diabetes management, appears less likely to cause lactic acidosis but is not free of this side effect [48].

Lactic Acidosis Associated with Hereditary Metabolic Disorders.
Congenital lactic acidosis can be a feature of both classical single enzyme deficiencies [19,49] and more complex disorders of mitochondria [50]. Absence of pyruvate dehydrogenase prevents the oxidation of pyruvate and leads to the accumulation of lactate [51]. Type I glycogen storage disease (glucose-6-phosphatase deficiency) may also lead to fasting lactic acidemia [52]. The inability to form glucose from glycogen in this disease leads to hypoglycemia and enhanced activity of the gluconeogenic and glycolytic pathways. The pyruvate thus generated cannot be disposed of rapidly enough by the glycogen-infiltrated liver and is then shunted to lactate. Fructose-1,6-diphosphatase deficiency also leads to hypoglycemia and lactic acidosis, which may be corrected by glucose administration [21]. Other hereditary syndromes associated to varying degrees with lactic acidosis in childhood are listed in Table 115-1 and reviewed elsewhere [2,19,49,50].

Other Forms of Lactic Acidosis.
Rare cases of lactic acidosis due to d-lactic acid have been reported [53,54,55]. In humans it is the l-stereoisomer of lactate that is normally synthesized from pyruvate. In d-lactic acidosis, most cases have involved preexisting bowel disease, and the d-stereoisomer is thought to be synthesized by gut flora. Clinical and experimental data suggest that other factors, including thiamine deficiency [56] and propylene glycol intoxication [57], could play a role in some cases.

A small number of cases of lactic acidosis in the older literature could not be attributed to any specific underlying process. These cases of "spontaneous" or idiopathic lactic acidosis [58,59,60], including chronic recurrent lactic acidosis [61], may have been due to subclinical regional hypoperfusion or the coexistence of several predisposing conditions, no one of which was severe. A few cases, however, may reflect an as yet undefined intrinsic derangement of the redox state of the tissues. Individual variability in the capacity for oxidative phosphorylation probably affects the severity of lactic acidosis of whatever cause.

Clinical Manifestations

Onset of lactic acidosis generally occurs over a few hours. The typical case is that of unexplained acidemia in a previously ill individual. Symptoms include tachycardia, tachypnea, and Kussmaul's respiration. Mental status may range from mild confusion to deep coma. The tachycardia and tachypnea may be due in part to enhanced sympathetic activity induced by increased lactate concentrations in the cerebrospinal fluid [8].

Patients with lactic acidosis typically exhibit some degree of dehydration and vascular collapse (hypotension, tachycardia, hypothermia, vasoconstriction), as well as manifestations of their underlying disease (Table 115-1). Acute pancreatitis with characteristic symptoms and elevated serum amylase can occur in lactic acidosis, as do elevations of liver transaminases, lactic dehydrogenase, and serum phosphate [62].

Diagnosis

The diagnosis is established by demonstrating significantly elevated serum lactate concentration and anion gap acidemia. There is no agreement on precise numbers, but most authorities concur that lactic acidosis is present when arterial lactate concentration is greater than 5 mM per liter and arterial pH is less than 7.35 [63]. Lactate concentrations of 2 mM per liter or less are probably normal in critically ill patients. The clinical manifestations of lactic acidosis (hyperpnea, tachypnea, and mental status change) usually occur when lactate concentration exceeds 7 mM per liter [64].

Intermediate values of lactic acid (2–5 mM/L) can be worrisome but may not imply impending acidosis. Hyperventilation, for example, produces both hypocapnia and alkalemia; hypocapnia can decrease the activity of pyruvate carboxylase, and alkalemia can increase the activity of the enzyme phosphofructokinase [65]. Together, these may modestly increase rates of glycolysis and lactate production. Poorly controlled diabetes may also lead to enhanced gluconeogenic activity, reduction in pyruvate dehydrogenase activity, and other changes that increase lactate generation [13,38]. Lactate concentration must be interpreted in the context of arterial pH and the patient's clinical state.

Arterial blood is preferred for measuring lactate concentration because it is less susceptible to artifactual elevation and misinterpretation. The normal lactate concentration in arterial blood is 0.4 to 0.8 mM per liter and in venous blood is somewhat higher, 0.45 to 1.30 mM per liter [5]. In resting hospitalized patients without acute illness, the lactate concentration in venous blood reportedly may range up to 3.17 mM per liter [62]. Oliva cautioned, however, that venous stasis distal to a tourniquet and muscle contraction of the extremity can generate misleadingly high venous lactate concentrations [65]. Rules for the interconversion of lactate concentration between metric and SI units are given in Table 115-2. The lactate to pyruvate ratio is not clinically helpful. Accurate blood pyruvate concentrations are difficult to obtain and are of little practical help in determining the cause or prognosis of lactic acidosis.

Differential Diagnosis

Lactic acidosis should be suspected whenever an anion gap is present [66]. The calculation of the anion gap is given in Table 115-3 and the differential diagnosis in Table 115-4. The differential diagnosis also includes primary hyperventilation due to cerebral damage and the tachypnea frequently associated with the onset of gram-negative septicemia. The diagnosis is confirmed by the measurement of circulating lactate concentration. Hyperlactatemia in the absence of significant acidemia may not be detected by measurement of the anion gap [67].

Lactic acidosis may coexist or overlap with other metabolic acidoses. Some degree of lactic acidosis is common in patients with diabetic ketoacidosis. Overlap of diabetic ketoacidosis with lactic acidosis may be suspected when the concentration of acetoacetate plus β-OH butyrate does not fully account for the observed anion gap. Similarly, preexisting alkalosis (e.g., salicylate intoxication and primary respiratory alkalosis) may mask substantial accumulation of lactate before clinical signs of metabolic acidosis appear.

Treatment

At this writing, there is no satisfactory treatment for lactic acidosis per se [6,8]. The primary goal of therapy in lactic acidosis must always focus on correction of the underlying cause. Volume expansion, inotropic agents, vasodilator drugs, and blood transfusion as appropriate for the underlying disease condition are crucial. They comprise the essential therapeutic tools for the majority of adults with lactic acidosis. Thiamine (100 mg) should probably be given empirically in most cases [25,26,56].

Given the high fatality rate, it is not surprising that many other adjunctive therapies for lactic acidosis have been advocated. These include bicarbonate, dialysis, dichloroacetate, methylene blue, *tris*-hydroxymethyl-aminomethane (THAM), nitroprusside, and carbicarb. All have appealing theoretical rationales, but data supporting their use are limited [6,8].

BICARBONATE. Until recently, most authors advocated alkalinization with bicarbonate as a mainstay of therapy in lactic acidosis. Neutralization of acid in lactic acidosis is intuitively

Table 115-2. Concentration of Lactate Expressed in Various Units

1 mM/L = 1 mEq/L
1 mM/L = 9 mg/dl
1 mg/dl = 0.11 mM/L

Standard international (SI) units for lactate are mM/L.

Table 115-3. Calculations of the Anion Gap

$$(Na^+ + K^+) - (Cl^- + HCO_3^-) + 17 = 0$$

or

$$Na^+ - (Cl^- + HCO_3^-) + 12 = 0$$

Table 115-4. Anion Gap Acidoses

1. Lactic acidosis
2. Diabetic ketoacidosis
3. Uremia
4. Salicylate intoxication
5. Methanol intoxication
6. Paraldehyde intoxication
7. Ethylene and propylene glycol intoxication

appealing, but few clinical studies have tested it in controlled studies. The role of bicarbonate therapy is being reevaluated [6,68–72]. Because available data indicate that it may be ineffective and potentially harmful, guidelines for the use of bicarbonate are controversial [8,71,72].

Recognized complications of bicarbonate therapy include inadvertent alkalemia with reduction of cerebrospinal fluid pH and respiratory depression [73,74], severe acute hypokalemia [75], leftward shift of the oxyhemoglobin dissociation curve that might increase tissue hypoxia [76], and substantial sodium loads. In a controlled trial in adults with lactic acidosis, bicarbonate therapy failed to improve hemodynamics [77]. In at least one instance, bicarbonate administration reportedly accelerated neoplastic lactate production [29]. Animal data suggest, in addition, that bicarbonate may paradoxically increase tissue lactate production, lower intracellular pH in muscle and liver, and worsen cardiac output.

Those who advocate bicarbonate therapy generally suggest that it be used in amounts that correct the acidosis only partially (i.e., to pH ≈7.2 with serum HCO_3^- concentration ≈12 mEq/L) [71,72]. Bicarbonate is not generally recommended at all, unless the arterial pH is less than 7.05. In certain circumstances its routine use is particularly discouraged. These include lactic acidosis accompanying pulmonary edema [78], cardiopulmonary arrest [72,79,80], grand mal seizures [16], biguanides [70], ethanol ingestion, and diabetic ketoacidosis.

DIALYSIS. Dialysis is rarely indicated early in the treatment of lactic acidosis except to speed the elimination of drugs. It can be particularly helpful when fluid overload and cardiac or renal insufficiency are present. A few reports have suggested that for severe lactic acidosis, hemodialysis [81] and peritoneal dialysis [82,83] with bicarbonate-based dialysates may be efficacious. Another new approach is hemofiltration combined with bicarbonate infusion [84]. This approach to the management of lactic acidosis is still experimental [8].

OTHER THERAPIES. Dichloroacetate is an activator of pyruvate dehydrogenase. It can lower lactate concentration in acidotic patients, but as a single agent it has no effect on mortality in lactic acidosis [85]. The use of vasodilator drugs such as nitroprusside [86] has been advocated, but there are no convincing data to support their use. Moreover, lactic acidosis is a recognized complication of nitroprusside therapy [87]. Neither THAM nor methylene blue is clinically inefficacious. Carbicarb, a formulation of equimolar amounts of sodium bicarbonate and sodium carbonate [88], has a theoretical advantage as a neutralizing agent in that it does not generate CO_2. Data from animal models are encouraging, but there are as yet no clinical data to support its use in human lactic acidosis.

References

1. Osnes JB, Hermansen L: Acid-base balance after maximal exercise of short duration. *J Appl Physiol* 32:59, 1972.
2. Mizock BA: Lactic acidosis. *Dis Mon* 35:233, 1989.
3. Luft D, Deichsel G, Schmulling RM, et al: Definition of clinically relevant lactic acidosis in patients with internal diseases. *Am J Clin Pathol* 80:484, 1983.
4. Clausen SW: Anhydremic acidosis due to lactic acid. *Am J Dis Child* 29:761, 1925.
5. Huckabee WE: Hyperlactatemia. *Am J Med* 30:833, 1961.
6. Mizock BA, Falk JL: Lactic acidosis in critical illness. *Crit Care Med* 20:80, 1992.
7. Peretz DI, Scott HM, Duff J, et al: The significance of lacticacidemia in the shock syndrome. *Ann N Y Acad Sci* 119:1133, 1965.
8. Stacpoole PW: Lactic acidosis. *Endocrinol Metab Clin North Am* 22:221, 1993.
9. Buchalter SE, Crain MR, Kreisberg R: Regulation of lactate metabolism in vivo. *Diabetes Metab Rev* 4:379, 1989.
10. Arieff AI: Pathogenesis of lactic acidosis. *Diabetes Metab Rev* 5:637, 1989.
11. Cohen RD, Woods HF: Lactic acidosis revisited. *Diabetes* 32:181, 1983.
12. Lloyd MH, Iles RA, Simpson BR, et al: The effect of simulated metabolic acidosis on intracellular pH and lactate metabolism in the isolated perfused rat liver. *Clin Sci Mol Med* 45:543, 1973.
13. Kreisberg RA: Lactate homeostasis and lactic acidosis. *Ann Intern Med* 92:227, 1980.
14. Madias NE: Lactic acidosis. *Kidney Int* 29:752, 1986.
15. Blair E: Acid-base balance in bacteremic shock. *Arch Intern Med* 127:731, 1971.
16. Orringer CE, Eustace JC, Wunsch CD, et al: Natural history of lactic acidosis after grand-mal seizures: A model for the study of an anion-gap acidosis not associated with hyperkalemia. *N Engl J Med* 297:796, 1977.
17. Medalle R, Webb R, Waterhouse C: Lactic acidosis and associated hypoglycemia. *Arch Intern Med* 128:273, 1971.
18. Rutsky EA, McDaniel HG, Tharpe DL, et al: Spontaneous hypoglycemia in chronic renal failure. *Arch Intern Med* 138:1364, 1978.
19. Israels S, Haworth JC, Dunn HG, et al: Lactic acidosis in childhood. *Adv Pediatr* 22:267, 1976.
20. Saudubray JM, Narcy C, Lyonnet L, et al: Clinical approach to inherited metabolic disorders in neonates. *Biol Neonate* 58(Suppl 1):44, 1990.
21. Maguire LC, Sherman BM, Whalen JE: Glucose therapy of recurrent lactic acidosis. *Am J Med Sci* 276:305, 1978.
22. Roth GJ, Porte D Jr.: Chronic lactic acidosis and acute leukemia. *Arch Intern Med* 125:317, 1970.
23. Wainer RA, Wiernik PH, Thompson WL: Metabolic and therapeutic studies of a patient with acute leukemia and severe lactic acidosis of prolonged duration. *Am J Med* 55:255, 1973.
24. Ishibashi M, Kimura N, Kawara T, et al: Lactic acidosis complicating adult T-cell leukemia: Report of two cases. *Eur J Haematol* 50:122, 1993.
25. Rovelli A, Bonomi M, Murano A, et al: Severe lactic acidosis due to

26. Oriot D, Wood C, Gottesman R, et al: Severe lactic acidosis related to acute thiamine deficiency. *J Parenter Enteral Nutr* 15:105, 1991.
27. Stacpoole PW, Lichtenstein MJ, Polk JR, et al: Lactic acidosis associated with metastatic osteogenic sarcoma. *South Med J* 74:868, 1981.
28. Spechler SJ, Esposito AL, Koff RS, et al: Lactic acidosis in oat cell carcinoma with extensive hepatic metastases. *Arch Intern Med* 138:1663, 1978.
29. Fraley DS, Adler S, Bruns FJ, et al: Stimulation of lactate production by administration of bicarbonate in a patient with a solid neoplasm and lactic acidosis. *N Engl J Med* 303:1100, 1980.
30. Nadiminti Y, Wang JC, Chou SY, et al: Lactic acidosis associated with Hodgkin's disease: Response to chemotherapy. *N Engl J Med* 303:15, 1980.
31. Varanasi UR, Carr B, Simpson DP: Lactic acidosis associated with metastatic breast carcinoma. *Cancer Treat Rep* 64:1283, 1980.
32. Hurtado FJ, Gutierrez AM, Silva N, et al: Role of tissue hypoxia as the mechanism of lactic acidosis during *E. coli* endotoxemia. *J Appl Physiol* 72:1895, 1992.
33. Gopinath R, Hutcheon M, Cheema Dhadli S, et al: Chronic lactic acidosis in a patient with acquired immunodeficiency syndrome and mitochondrial myopathy: Biochemical studies. *J Am Soc Nephrol* 3:1212, 1992.
34. Chattha G, Arieff AI, Cummings C, et al: Lactic acidosis complicating the acquired immunodeficiency syndrome. *Ann Intern Med* 118:37, 1993.
35. White NJ, Warrell DA, Chanthavanich P, et al: Severe hypoglycemia and hyperinsulinemia in falciparum malaria. *N Engl J Med* 309:61, 1983.
36. Wang F, Butler T, Rabbani GH, et al: The acidosis of cholera: Contributions of hyperproteinemia, lactic acidemia, and hyperphosphatemia to an increased serum anion gap. *N Engl J Med* 315:1591, 1986.
37. Hollander RG: Lactic acidosis in pheochromocytoma. *Ann Intern Med* 107:259, 1987.
38. Alberti KG, Nattrass M: Lactic acidosis. *Lancet* 2:25, 1977.
39. Woods HF, Alberti KG: Dangers of intravenous fructose. *Lancet* 2:1354, 1972.
40. Batstone GF, Alberti KG, Dewar AK: Reversible lactic acidosis associated with repeated intravenous infusions of sorbitol and ethanol. *Postgrad Med J* 53:567, 1977.
41. Craig GM, Crane CW: Lactic acidosis complicating liver failure after intravenous fructose. *Br Med J* 4:211, 1971.
42. Fulop M: Alcoholism, ketoacidosis, and lactic acidosis. *Diabetes Metab Rev* 5:365, 1989.
43. Kreisberg RA: Lactic acidosis: An update. *J Intensive Care Med* 2:76, 1987.
44. Fulop M, Bock J, Ben Ezra J, et al: Plasma lactate and 3-hydroxybutyrate levels in patients with acute ethanol intoxication. *Am J Med* 80:191, 1986.
45. Gabow PA, Anderson RJ, Potts DE, et al: Acid-base disturbances in the salicylate-intoxicated adult. *Arch Intern Med* 138:1481, 1978.
46. Chapman BJ, Proudfoot AT: Adult salicylate poisoning: Deaths and outcome in patients with high plasma salicylate concentrations. *Q J Med* 72:699, 1989.
47. Luft D, Schmulling RM, Eggstein M: Lactic acidosis in biguanide-treated diabetics: A review of 330 cases. *Diabetologia* 14:75, 1978.
48. Gan SC, Barr J, Arieff AI, et al: Biguanide-associated lactic acidosis: Case report and review of the literature. *Arch Intern Med* 152:2333, 1992.
49. Chaves-Carballo E: Detection of inherited neurometabolic disorders: A practical clinical approach. *Pediatr Clin North Am* 39:801, 1992.
50. Kerr DS: Lactic acidosis and mitochondrial disorders. *Clin Biochem* 24:331, 1991.
51. Farrell DF, Clark AF, Scott CR, et al: Absence of pyruvate decarboxylase activity in man: A cause of congenital lactic acidosis. *Science* 187:1082, 1975.
52. Howell RR, Ashton DM, Wyngaarden JB: Glucose-6-phosphatase deficiency glycogen storage disease. *Pediatrics* 29:553, 1962.
53. Oh MS, Phelps KR, Traube M, et al: D-lactic acidosis in a man with the short-bowel syndrome. *N Engl J Med* 301:249, 1979.

54. Stolberg L, Rolfe R, Gitlin N, et al: d-Lactic acidosis due to abnormal gut flora: Diagnosis and treatment of two cases. *N Engl J Med* 306:1344, 1982.

55. Gurevitch J, Sela B, Jonas A, et al: D-lactic acidosis: A treatable encephalopathy in pediatric patients. *Acta Paediatr* 82:119, 1993.

56. Hudson M, Pocknee R, Mowat NA: D-lactic acidosis in short bowel syndrome: An examination of possible mechanisms. *Q J Med* 74:157, 1990.

57. Christopher MM, Eckfeldt JH, Eaton JW: Propylene glycol ingestion causes D-lactic acidosis. *Lab Invest* 62:114, 1990.

58. Oliva PB: Spontaneous lactic acidosis. *Ann Intern Med* 72:439, 1970.

59. Cederbaum SD, Blass JP, Minkoff N, et al: Sensitivity to carbohydrate in a patient with familial intermittent lactic acidosis and pyruvate dehydrogenase deficiency. *Pediatr Res* 10:713, 1976.

60. Oliva PB, Schwartz HA: Survival of a patient with spontaneous lactic acidosis. *Ann Intern Med* 71:587, 1969.

61. Sussman KE, Alfrey A, Kirsch WM, et al: Chronic lactic acidosis in an adult: A new syndrome associated with an altered redox state of certain NAD-NADH coupled reactions. *Am J Med* 48:104, 1970.

62. Tranquada RE, Grant WJ, Peterson CR: Lactic acidosis. *Arch Intern Med* 117:192, 1966.

63. Mizock BA: Controversies in lactic acidosis. Implications in critically ill patients. *JAMA* 258:497, 1987.

64. Tranquada RE: Lactic acidosis. *California Med* 101:450, 1964.

65. Oliva PB: Lactic acidosis. *Am J Med* 48:209, 1970.

66. Emmett M, Narins RG: Clinical use of the anion gap. *Medicine* 56:38, 1977.

67. Iberti TJ, Leibowitz AB, Papadakos PJ, et al: Low sensitivity of the anion gap as a screen to detect hyperlactatemia in critically ill patients. *Crit Care Med* 18:275, 1990.

68. Stacpoole PW: Lactic acidosis: The case against bicarbonate therapy. *Ann Intern Med* 105:276, 1986.

69. Graf H, Leach W, Arieff AI: Evidence for a detrimental effect of bicarbonate therapy in hypoxic lactic acidosis. *Science* 227:754, 1985.

70. Ryder RE: The danger of high dose sodium bicarbonate in biguanide-induced lactic acidosis: The theory, the practice and alternative therapies. *Br J Clin Pract* 41:730, 1987.

71. Narins RG, Cohen JJ: Bicarbonate therapy for organic acidosis: The case for its continued use. *Ann Intern Med* 106:615, 1987.

72. Hindman BJ: Sodium bicarbonate in the treatment of subtypes of acute lactic acidosis: Physiologic considerations. *Anesthesiology* 72:1064, 1990.

73. Posner JB, Plum F: Spinal-fluid pH and neurologic symptoms in systemic acidosis. *N Engl J Med* 277:605, 1967.

74. Bureau MA, Begin R, Berthiaume Y, et al: Cerebral hypoxia from bicarbonate infusion in diabetic acidosis. *J Pediatr* 96:968, 1980.

75. Schade DS, Eaton RP: Dose response to insulin in man: Differential effects on glucose and ketone body regulation. *J Clin Endocrinol Metab* 44:1038, 1977.

76. Bellingham AJ, Detter JC, Lenfant C: The role of hemoglobin affinity for oxygen and red-cell 2,3-diphosphoglycerate in the management of diabetic ketoacidosis. *Trans Assoc Am Physicians* 83:113, 1970.

77. Cooper DJ, Walley KR, Wiggs BR, et al: Bicarbonate does not improve hemodynamics in critically ill patients who have lactic acidosis: A prospective, controlled clinical study. *Ann Intern Med* 112:492, 1990.

78. Fulop M, Horowitz M, Aberman A, et al: Lactic acidosis in pulmonary edema due to left ventricular failure. *Ann Intern Med* 79:180, 1973.

79. Weil MH, Rackow EC, Trevino R, et al: Difference in acid-base state between venous and arterial blood during cardiopulmonary resuscitation. *N Engl J Med* 315:153, 1986.

80. Adrogue HJ, Rashad MN, Gorin AB, et al: Assessing acid-base status in circulatory failure: Differences between arterial and central venous blood. *N Engl J Med* 320:1312, 1989.

81. Lalau JD, Westeel PF, Debussche X, et al: Bicarbonate haemodialysis: An adequate treatment for lactic acidosis in diabetics treated by metformin. *Intensive Care Med* 13:383, 1987.

82. Foulks CJ, Wright LF: Successful repletion of bicarbonate stores in ongoing lactic acidosis: A role for bicarbonate-buffered peritoneal dialysis. *South Med J* 74:1162, 1981.

83. Vaziri ND, Ness R, Wellikson L, et al: Bicarbonate-buffered peritoneal dialysis: An effective adjunct in the treatment of lactic acidosis. *Am J Med* 67:392, 1979.

84. Barton IK, Streather CP, Hilton PJ, et al: Successful treatment of severe lactic acidosis by haemofiltration using a bicarbonate-based replacement fluid. *Nephrol Dial Transplant* 6:368, 1991.

85. Stacpoole PW, Wright EC, Baumgartner TG, et al: A controlled clinical trial of dichloroacetate for treatment of lactic acidosis in adults. *N Engl J Med* 327:1564, 1992.

86. Taradash MR, Jacobson LB: Vasodilator therapy of idiopathic lactic acidosis. *N Engl J Med* 293:468, 1975.

87. Humphrey SH, Nash DA Jr: Lactic acidosis complicating sodium nitroprusside therapy. *Ann Intern Med* 88:58, 1978.

88. Bersin RM, Arieff AI: Improved hemodynamic function during hypoxia with Carbicarb, a new agent for the management of acidosis. *Circulation* 77:227, 1988.

89. Finch CA, Gollnick PD, Hlastala MP, et al: Lactic acidosis as a result of iron deficiency. *J Clin Invest* 64:129, 1979.

90. Kashner RF: Total parenteral nutrition-associated metabolic acidosis. *J Parenter Enteral Nutr* 10:306, 1986.

91. Leventhal LJ, Kochar G, Feldman NH, et al: Lactic acidosis in theophylline overdose. *Am J Emerg Med* 7:417, 1989.

92. Bethke RA, Gratton M, Watson WA: Severe hyperlactemia and metabolic acidosis following cocaine use and exertion. *Am J Emerg Med* 8:369, 1990.

93. Jonsson S, O'Meara M, Young JB: Acute cocaine poisoning: Importance of treating seizures and acidosis. *Am J Med* 75:1061, 1983.

94. Weil MH, Afifi AA: Experimental and clinical studies on lactate and pyruvate as indicators of the severity of acute circulatory failure (shock). *Circulation* 41:989, 1970.

95. Mann NS, Russman HB, Mann SK, et al: Lactulose and severe lactic acidosis. *Ann Intern Med* 103:637, 1985.

96. Earthman TP, Odom L, Mullins CA: Lactic acidosis associated with high-dose niacin therapy. *South Med J* 84:496, 1991.

97. Beier LS, Pitts WH, Gonick HC: Metabolic acidosis occurring during paraldehyde intoxication. *Ann Intern Med* 58:155, 1963.

98. Rallison ML, Meikle AW, Zigrang WD: Hypoglycemia and lactic acidosis associated with fructose-1,6-diphosphatase deficiency. *J Pediatr* 94:933, 1979.

99. Moses SW, Bashan N, Flasterstein BF, et al: Fructose-1,6-diphosphatase deficiency in Israel. *Isr J Med Sci* 27:1, 1991.

116. Hypoglycemia

John P. Mordes, James Desemone,
Peter A. Gottlieb, and Aldo A. Rossini

Introduction

Hypoglycemia is frequently encountered in emergency departments. Few cases require admission to an intensive care unit (ICU) but severe or prolonged hypoglycemia can lead to permanent neurologic and cardiovascular damage. Because glucose administration makes such sequelae entirely avoidable, every intensivist must be familiar with the symptoms of hypoglycemia, the contexts in which they occur, and the types of hypoglycemia that require intensive care.

Definition of Hypoglycemia

PHYSIOLOGY. No specific blood glucose concentration defines the presence or absence of hypoglycemia. Similarly, there is no one cause to define the context in which hypoglycemia might be expected to appear. For these reasons, we advocate as a physiologic definition of hypoglycemia a blood glucose concentration sufficiently low as to cause the release of counterregulatory hormones and impair the function of the central nervous system. Many disorders lead to blood glucose concentrations low enough to fulfill these criteria.

SYMPTOMS. The physiologic definition of hypoglycemia implies its clinical presentation. The symptoms reflect the relative contributions of neuroglycopenia [1] and elevated concentrations of counterregulatory hormones (e.g., catecholamines) [2]. Whipple recognized this in 1938, and his criteria for the diagnosis of hypoglycemia are an enduring example of clinical acumen, knowledge of physiology, and good sense. "Whipple's triad" [1] defines hypoglycemia as (1) documentation of a low blood glucose concentration, (2) concurrent symptoms of hypoglycemia, and (3) resolution of those symptoms following the administration of glucose. Hypoglycemia should seldom be diagnosed unless all three criteria are fulfilled.

Clinical Manifestations of Hypoglycemia

NEUROLOGIC SIGNS AND SYMPTOMS. Early symptoms and signs of neuroglycopenia include hunger, headache, confusion, slurred speech, and other nonspecific behavioral changes. These mild alterations of perception, affect, and personality can progress to disturbances of integrative function, cognitive deterioration, lethargy, obtundation, seizures, coma, and, occasionally, a permanent vegetative state.

ADDITIONAL SYMPTOMS AND SIGNS. These are caused by counterregulatory hormones released in response to low glucose concentrations. The most prominent symptoms are weakness, palpitations, and anxiety due to the release of catecholamines. Corresponding signs of catecholamine release include diaphoresis, tachycardia, peripheral vasoconstriction, and widening of the pulse pressure.

Normal Glucose Regulatory Physiology

Insulin overdosage is the most common but not the only cause of hypoglycemia. The diagnosis and treatment of many cases of hypoglycemia are challenging problems that require an understanding of normal glucose regulatory physiology.

GLUCOSE UTILIZATION. Plasma glucose concentration is normally maintained in a narrow range (60–120 mg/dl; 3.3–6.7 mM), under a wide range of metabolic circumstances. The narrowness of this range indicates the critical role played by glucose in the maintenance of mammalian homeostasis. The organ most dependent on glucose availability is the brain. The adult brain consumes glucose at the rate of ≈144 gm per day. Unlike adipose tissue and muscle, the central nervous system does not depend on insulin for glucose transport. During periods of starvation the brain uses ketone bodies as a substitute fuel, but acquisition of the capability to use this alternate substrate is a slow process, requiring hours to days. Even during prolonged starvation the brain maintains a minimal obligate glucose requirement of ≈44 gm per day. Other tissues with obligate glucose needs include the circulating erythrocyte mass (≈36 gm/day) and renal medulla (≈25 gm/day) [2].

MAINTENANCE OF PLASMA GLUCOSE CONCENTRATION. There are two sources of glucose: that which is endogenously produced and ingested carbohydrate. In the postprandial state, the concentration of circulating insulin rises in response to increases in glucose concentration. When central nervous system requirements for glucose are met, these levels of insulin promote storage of glucose in the form of liver glycogen by activating glycogen synthase and inhibiting glycogen phosphorylase and glycogenolysis. Glucose is also transported into skeletal muscle for immediate use or storage as muscle glycogen. When all other metabolic demands for glucose are met, any excess is used for de novo synthesis of triglyceride.

During brief periods of starvation, such as a night's sleep, the principal source of circulating glucose is hepatic glycogen. As glycogenolysis occurs, insulin levels are low. During more prolonged starvation the glucose is derived principally from the gluconeogenic conversion of muscle-derived amino acids. Lesser contributions to gluconeogenesis are made by glycerol derived from fat and lactate produced by anaerobic glycolysis from erythrocytes, leukocytes, bone marrow, renal medulla and peripheral nerve.

The liver stores only about 60 to 80 gm of glycogen, a supply that is exhausted by an overnight fast. Muscle glycogen amounts to ≈120 gm, but this store of glycogen is not *directly*

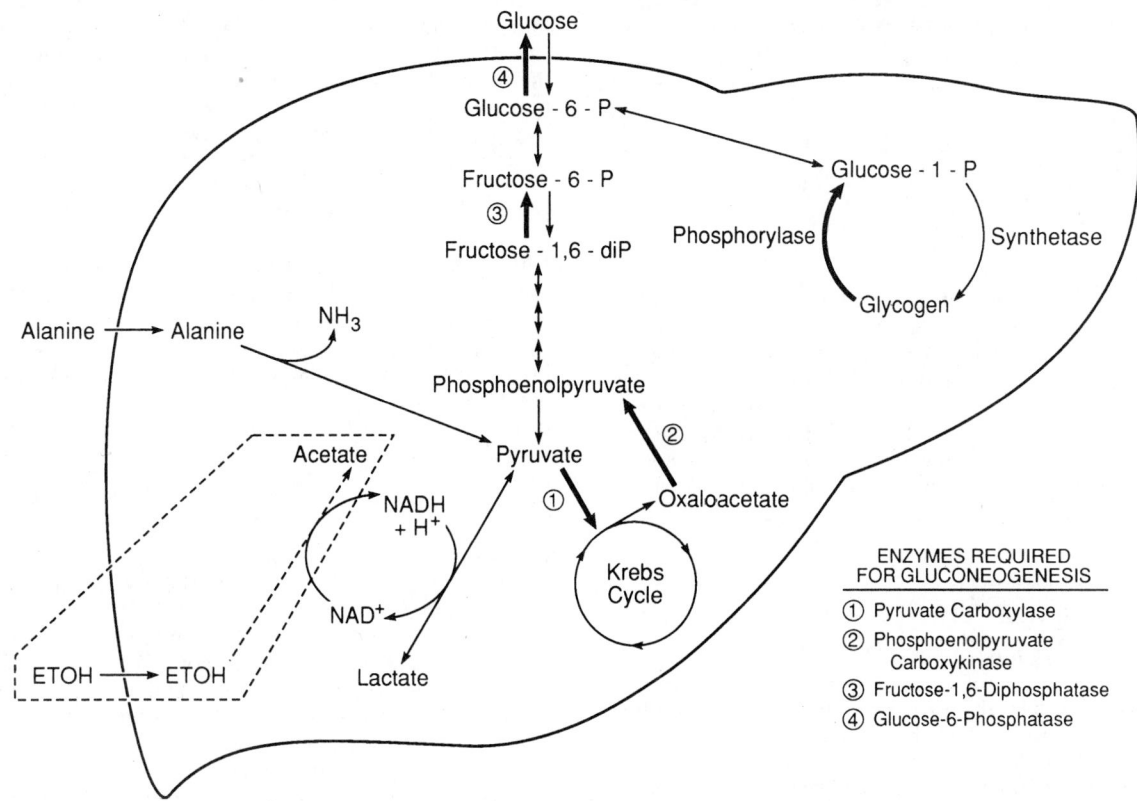

Fig. 116-1. Metabolic pathways important in the response to hypoglycemia. The thick, annotated arrows indicate the key steps in glycogen breakdown and gluconeogenesis. In the presence of low circulating insulin concentrations, phosphorylase activity is increased, leading to the release of glucose-1-phosphate. This moiety is then converted to glucose-6-phosphate and finally to glucose through the action of glucose-6-phosphatase. Glucose is also generated from three carbon precursors by gluconeogenesis. This process essentially reverses glycolysis and is controlled by four enzymes: (1) pyruvate carboxylase, (2) phosphoenolpyruvate carboxykinase, (3) fructose-1,6-diphosphatase, and (4) glucose-6-phosphatase. Within the box delimited by dotted lines, the metabolic effects of ethanol ingestion are indicated. Ethanol is converted to acetaldehyde and then to acetate, producing reduced NADH. The high concentration of NADH favors the generation of lactate from pyruvate, decreasing the concentration of the latter. As the availability of pyruvate as a gluconeogenic precursor declines, glucose production via gluconeogenesis also declines, and hypoglycemia can ensue.

available for the maintenance of systemic glucose concentrations due to the lack of glucose-6-phosphatase in muscle. Muscle glycogen contributes to plasma glucose only via anaerobic glycolysis leading to the production of lactate. The lactate is transported to the liver, where it is converted into glucose. The shuttling of glucose to muscle and lactate to the liver is known as the Cori cycle. In addition to providing lactate as a substrate for gluconeogenesis, muscle can amidate pyruvate to form alanine, which is then exported to the liver.

Gluconeogenesis occurs mainly in the liver and to a lesser extent in the kidney and intestine. The principal substrates are amino acids, glycerol, and lactate. The liver produces the enzymes necessary to convert all three into glucose for release into the systemic circulation. Alanine is quantitatively the most important precursor, providing 50 percent of de novo glucose synthesis in fasted humans. The enzymes required for gluco-

neogenesis are activated by low concentrations of circulating insulin. These enzymes are pyruvate carboxylase, phosphoenolpyruvate carboxykinase (PEP-CK), fructose-1,6-diphosphatase, and glucose-6-phosphatase (Fig. 116-1).

HORMONAL REGULATION OF PLASMA GLUCOSE CONCENTRATION. Insulin is the most important hormone for maintenance of normal levels of glycemia. Elevated concentrations of insulin promote glucose utilization and lower plasma glucose concentrations. Reduced concentrations of insulin enable glycogenolysis, gluconeogenesis, and lipolysis to proceed. Low insulin concentrations also facilitate the provision of substrates needed for the formation of glucose. As glucose concentrations subsequently rise, circulating insulin concentrations increase, suppress gluconeogenesis and lipolysis, and close a classical endocrine feedback loop [2].

Glucagon, glucocorticoids, catecholamines, growth hormone, and, to a lesser degree, thyroxine also contribute to glucose homeostasis. They promote the formation of glucose in the fasted state and, in general, counteract the actions of insulin. Foremost among them is glucagon, which is secreted in response to low glucose concentrations. It promotes both glycogenolysis (an immediate effect) and gluconeogenesis (a delayed but more enduring effect). Glucocorticoids antagonize the action of insulin, stimulating gluconeogenesis and inhibiting extrahepatic glucose utilization. Catecholamines also promote glycogenolysis and gluconeogenesis. The mechanism by which growth hormone promotes blood glucose elevation is not fully understood; it may suppress insulin-mediated glucose uptake and enhance glucose release from the liver. The influence of thyroxine on blood glucose concentration is probably indirect. Fasting blood glucose concentrations tend to be elevated and decreased in hyper- and hypothyroid patients, respectively. Absence of liver glycogen has been observed in hyperthyroid animals [3].

Classification of Hypoglycemia: Fasting versus Nonfasting

For purposes of classification, hypoglycemia is divided into fasting and nonfasting subcategories. The former often implies a major physiologic derangement; hypoglycemia encountered in the intensive care setting generally falls into this category. Nonfasting, "postprandial," and "reactive" hypoglycemic states not associated with surgery of the gastrointestinal tract are poorly defined, controversial entities. Postprandial hypoglycemia is not usually life-threatening. It does not require intensive care management and is not discussed further here.

Differential Diagnosis of Fasting Hypoglycemia

Fasting hypoglycemia always implies a fundamental disturbance in glucose homeostasis. From both clinical and physiologic viewpoints, it can be useful to think of normal glucose homeostasis as dependent on three factors: (1) an appropriate hormonal milieu; (2) ability of organs responsible for glucose production to synthesize at a rate adequate to maintain euglycemia; and (3) availability of substrate for conversion to glucose in these organs.

Disturbance in any of these domains, whether the result of disease, drugs, or toxins, can lead to symptomatic hypoglycemia. The differential diagnosis of fasting hypoglycemia subsumes three corresponding categories: (1) states of hormonal imbalance (principally states of overinsulinization), (2) states of impaired or inadequate endogenous glucose production, and (3) states in which gluconeogenic substrates are unavailable.

Fasting Hypoglycemia Due to an Inappropriate Hormonal Milieu

HYPERGLYCEMIA DUE TO EXCESS OF INSULIN OR INSULIN-MIMETIC AGENTS. Inappropriately elevated concentrations of insulin are most commonly caused by overdosage with exogenous insulin, overdosage with oral sulfonylurea hypoglycemic agents (which enhance endogenous insulin secretion), insulinomas, and tumors that produce peptides with insulinlike activities.

Insulin Overdoses in Diabetic Patients. Overdosage of diabetic patients with insulin is the most common cause of hypoglycemia. In an outpatient/emergency department setting, it is most often encountered among type 1, insulin-dependent diabetics. In most cases, the overdosage is inadvertent. In some cases an apparent overdose is actually the indirect consequence of a missed meal or an increased amount of exercise. Occasionally an overdose is intentional, particularly among adolescents.

In an intensive care setting, changes in the severity of the underlying disease and the presence of a continuous insulin infusion commonly conspire to produce hypoglycemia. Occasionally insulin is administered in the hospital setting either in the wrong dose or to the wrong patient. Total parenteral nutrition solutions containing excessive insulin can also produce hypoglycemia, particularly if improvement in a patient's underlying condition leads to reduced peripheral insulin resistance. The diagnosis is readily made on the basis of the history, clinical setting, and confirmatory response to glucose administration.

Intentional Insulin Overdose in Nondiabetics. "Factitious hypoglycemia" should be suspected in health care workers, relatives of diabetics, or anyone with access to insulin or oral hypoglycemic agents who experiences unexplained fasting hypoglycemia. The diagnosis can be difficult to make. By definition these patients are trying to frustrate rather than facilitate a diagnosis, and they often devise ingenious methods to conceal their abuse. Insulin intended for surreptitious injection has been found hidden in places that range from portable radios to various body orifices.

Insulinoma. Fasting hypoglycemia due to overinsulinization is classically caused by insulinoma. These very rare insulin-secreting tumors are the most common form of pancreatic islet neoplasm. Only a minority (<10%) are malignant. The malignant potential of insulinomas cannot be determined from histologic appearance. Insulinomas are often small and difficult to visualize radiographically. To evaluate a patient with suspected insulinoma, fasting immunoreactive insulin (IRI, measured in μU/ml) and glucose (mg/dl) should be obtained. If the IRI/glucose ratio is greater than 0.3, the insulin concentration may be inappropriately high.

It can be difficult to differentiate among insulinoma, factitious hypoglycemia due to self-administration of insulin, and abuse of oral hypoglycemic agents. If oral agent abuse is suspected, serum and urine should be screened for sulfonylurea compounds. When abusive insulin self-administration is suspected, measurements of circulating insulin concentration are of limited value. Patients with factitious hypoglycemia may have circulating anti-insulin antibodies that interfere with the radioimmunoassay for insulin. This is true even if human insulin is used for self-injection. These patients may therefore appear to have elevated levels of insulin during the period of hypoglycemia just as would patients with an insulinoma. In this circumstance it is best to obtain simultaneous insulin and C-peptide blood concentrations during a hypoglycemic episode. Insulin and C-peptide are normally cosecreted by the pancreas in equimolar quantities, but the latter is not present in commercial insulin preparations. If insulin and C-peptide are not present in equimolar amounts in a patient with unexplained fasting hypoglycemia, the possibility of surreptitious use of insulin is strengthened. C-peptide does not cross-react in the insulin radioimmunoassay. Another useful study is the serum concentration of proinsulin, which is typically elevated (to >30% of the insulin concentration) in cases of insulinoma. Finally, when self-administered insulin is of animal origin, highly specific radioimmunoassays can sometimes establish the species of origin [4].

Nesidioblastosis. This is a form of nonmalignant islet cell adenomatosis that leads to insulin-mediated hypoglycemia. It is a rare condition most commonly diagnosed in children. A very small number of cases have been reported in adults [5,6]. Rapid diagnosis of the childhood form is crucial to avoid hypoglycemic damage to the maturing central nervous system.

Antibody-Mediated ("Autoimmune") Hypoglycemia. An uncommon cause of hypoglycemia is endogenous antibodies that bind to and activate the insulin receptor [7]. Some but not all cases are associated with other autoimmune disorders [8,9,10] and a few have occurred in patients with myeloma [11]. Previous exposure to exogenous insulin is not required, but some patients may have an abnormal insulin molecule [12].

Hypoglycemia Associated with Nonislet Tumors and Nonsuppressible Insulinlike Activity.

Certain tumors not of pancreatic islet origin are associated with fasting hypoglycemia clinically indistinguishable from that caused by islet cell neoplasms. Whereas insulinomas are typically quite small, nonpancreatic tumors associated with hypoglycemia tend to be very large. The large size initially suggested that excessive glucose utilization by the tumor (perhaps in conjunction with tumor-related failure of compensatory mechanisms) was the cause of the hypoglycemia. Another explanation has been provided by the discovery of nonsuppressible insulinlike activity (NSILA) in the serum of some patients with these tumors. Nonsuppressible insulinlike activity comprises a heterogeneous group of substances related to insulinlike growth factors (IGF) 1 and 2, some of which are now well characterized [13,14]. Nonislet cell neoplasms associated with hypoglycemia include mesenchymal tumors, hepatomas, adrenocortical carcinoma, gastrointestinal tumors, lymphoma, and leukemia [15]. Multiple myeloma may also cause hypoglycemia via the antibody-mediated mechanism described above [11]. The diagnosis of NSILA-mediated hypoglycemia due to a nonislet cell tumor requires the exclusion of insulinoma. As noted above, this is most conveniently done by obtaining simultaneous insulin and glucose measurements during hypoglycemia.

Hypoglycemia Due to Oral Hypoglycemic Agents.

After insulin, drugs are the most common cause of hypoglycemia [16] (Table 116-1). Drugs of the sulfonylurea class reduce serum glucose concentrations by increasing insulin secretion, inhibiting glycogenolysis and gluconeogenesis, and enhancing the response of target tissues to the effects of insulin [17]. The prevalence of sulfonylurea-induced hypoglycemia increases with age, but in all age groups the condition is most often observed in the context of decreased carbohydrate intake. Maternal treatment of diabetes with sulfonylureas can lead to postpartum hypoglycemia in neonates. For this reason, and because the teratogenic potential of oral hypoglycemic agents is not known, these drugs should never be used during pregnancy. In patients between the ages of 11 and 30 years, perhaps two-thirds of hypoglycemic comas are due to the accidental or intentional ingestion of sulfonylurea agents. Half of these cases are suicide attempts [16]. In older age categories, sulfonylurea-induced hypoglycemia is a frequent complication of the treatment of type 2 diabetes mellitus. It is the leading cause of hypoglycemia in patients older than 60 years. Liver disease contributes to sulfonylurea-induced hypoglycemia by decreasing the metabolic clearance of tolbutamide (Orinase), acetohexamide (Dymelor), tolazamide (Tolinase), glipizide (Glucotrol), and glyburide (Micronase, Diabeta). Renal failure decreases the clearance of chlorpropamide (Diabinese), acetohexamide, and tolazamide. Sulfonylurea-induced hypoglycemia is classically observed in older individuals in the setting of acute or chronic starvation superimposed on mild to moderate liver or renal failure.

Chlorpropamide and glyburide account for nearly 70 percent of all cases of sulfonylurea-induced hypoglycemia. Chlorpropamide is excreted largely unchanged by the kidney, and its half-life of ≈35 hours is the longest of any sulfonylurea. Glyburide undergoes hepatic transformation to two less active

Table 116-1. Drugs and Toxins Associated with Hypoglycemia

Drugs that increase circulating insulin concentrations
  Direct stimulants of insulin secretion
    Acetohexamide (Dymelor)
    Chloroquine (Aralen)
    Chlorpropamide (Diabinese)
    Disopyramide (Norpace)
    Glipizide (Glucotrol)
    Glyburide, glibenclamide (Micronase, Diabeta)
    Pentamidine (Pentam)
    Quinidine
    Quinine
    Ritodrine (Yutopar)
    Terbutaline (Brethine, Bricanyl)
    Tolazamide (Tolinase)
    Tolbutamide (Orinase)
  Agents that enhance the action of sulfonylureas
    Bishydroxycoumarin (Dicoumarol)
    Imipramine (Tofranil)
    Phenylbutazone (Butazolidin)
Drugs that impair gluconeogenesis
  Ethanol
  Hepatotoxins
    Acetaminophen (Tylenol, Tempra)
    Propoxyphene (Darvon)
  Agents that decrease activity of gluconeogenic enzymes
    Metformin (Glucophage)
    Metoprolol (Lopressor)
    Nadolol (Corgard)
    Phenformin (DBI)
    Pindolol (Visken)
    Propranolol (Inderal)
Unknown mechanism of action
  Acetazolamide-Diamox
  Acetylsalicylic acid (Aspirin)
  Aluminum hydroxide (Dialume)
  Captopril (Capoten)
  Chlorpromazine (Thorazine)
  Cimetidine (Tagamet)
  Diphenhydramine (Benadryl)
  Doxepin (Sinequan, Adapin)
  Enalapril (Vasotec)
  Ethylenediaminetetraacetic acid (EDTA, Versene)
  Haloperidol (Haldol)
  Isoxsuprine
  Lidocaine (Xylocaine)
  Lithium (Eskalith)
  Oxytetracycline (Terramycin)
  Para-aminobenzoic acid (PABA)
  Para-aminosalicylic acid (PASA)
  Ranitidine (Zantac)
  Sulfadiazine
  Sulfamethoxazole (Bactrim, Septra)
  Sulfisoxazole (Gantrisin)
  Warfarin (Coumadin)

A sampling of common trade names is shown in parentheses; the enumeration of trade names is not exhaustive.
Adapted from Seltzer HS: Drug-induced hypoglycemia: A review of 1418 cases. *Endocrinol Metab Clin North Am* 18:163–183, 1989.

metabolites, has a serum half-life of ≈10 hours, and is currently the most frequently prescribed sulfonylurea [16]. Oral hypoglycemic drugs of the biguanide class (phenformin, metformin) probably induce hypoglycemia by inhibiting gluconeogenesis. Phenformin has been associated with the induction of lactic acidosis (see Chap. 115). Only metformin is currently available in the United States.

The long half-life of commonly used oral hypoglycemic agents requires that patients with sulfonylurea-induced hypoglycemia be hospitalized after initial resuscitation with glucose in the emergency department. They require continued treatment with oral and intravenous glucose for a minimum of 18 to 24 hours.

When oral agent overdosage is suspected, serum and urine should be screened for sulfonylurea compounds. These studies are not readily available as part of toxic screens. Testing for sulfonylurea drugs must be requested specifically, and some laboratories require special handling of specimens.

Medication Errors. Severe hypoglycemia can result from inadvertent substitution of an oral hypoglycemic agent for a different medication. These cases can present a diagnostic challenge, because high insulin concentrations may suggest an insulinoma. To make the diagnosis, the physician must be inquisitive and have a high index of suspicion. Medication errors due to phonetic similarity in name are exemplified by cases in which acetazolamide (Diamox) has been prescribed but acetohexamide (Dymelor) inadvertently dispensed [16,18,19]. Illegible prescriptions enhance the possibility of such errors. Examples of hypoglycemic medications that have been substituted for prescribed medications are listed in Table 116-2. As noted above, oral hypoglycemic agents are sometimes ingested intentionally by nondiabetic individuals and produce "factitious" hypoglycemia. Testing of serum and urine specimens as described above may reveal the diagnosis.

Hypoglycemia Associated with Other Drugs that Increase Serum Insulin Levels. In addition to sulfonylureas, a number of other medications can produce hypoglycemia by increasing serum insulin levels (Table 116-1). Pentamidine, used to treat *Pneumocystis carinii* infection in immunocompromised patients, particularly those with AIDS, can be toxic to pancreatic beta cells. It may cause transient hypoglycemia due to the release of stored insulin from damaged beta cells. It eventually results in diabetes in some patients [16].

Quinine was first suspected as a cause of hypoglycemia in the 1920s and is now known to elevate insulin concentrations in patients being treated for malaria [20,21]. Those with cerebral malaria are most prone to hypoglycemia, possibly due to the high intake of glucose by malarial parasites, coupled with the increased insulin release. Quinine may rarely cause hypoglycemia in normal individuals [22]. Quinidine, an antiarrhythmic agent chemically related to quinine, can also enhance insulin secretion and produce hypoglycemia in ill, fasting patients [23].

Hypoglycemia has been reported in patients treated with disopyramide, an antiarrhythmic agent with pharmacologic properties similar to quinidine [24,25]. Ritodrine, a tocolytic agent that is usually infused for several days prior to delivery, can elevate plasma insulin and C-peptide levels and cause hypoglycemia in newborns and their mothers [26]. Rare cases of hypoglycemia associated with the angiotensin converting enzyme inhibitors enalapril and captopril have been reported; the mechanism is not known [27,28]. Hypoglycemia due to ethanol ingestion (alcoholic ketoacidosis) is a special case, discussed below.

HYPOGLYCEMIA ASSOCIATED WITH DEFICIENCIES IN COUNTERREGULATORY HORMONES. Glucocorticoid insufficiency, due either to primary adrenal disease or to panhypopituitarism, commonly causes hypoglycemia in children by decreasing glycogenolysis and gluconeogenesis in the liver [29]. In Addisonian adults, however, glucocorticoid deficiency is an uncommon cause of hypoglycemia [30]. Malnutrition may contribute to the development of hypoglycemia in these cases.

Table 116-2. Medication Errors That Can Result in Hypoglycemia

Prescribed	Dispensed
Acetazolamide (Diamox)	Acetohexamide (Dymelor)
Dyazide	Dymelor
Dialume	Diabinese
Tolectin	Tolinase
Diamox	Diabinese
Chlorpromazine	Chlorpropamide

Isolated growth hormone deficiency can be the result of congenital defects in pituitary development, vascular disease, therapeutic irradiation of the pituitary, and primary or metastatic neoplasia involving the pituitary. Patients with panhypopituitarism are prone to hypoglycemia because they lack adrenal glucocorticoids, are deficient in growth hormone, and are hypothyroid. There is increased sensitivity to insulin in these patients as well [30].

Although catecholamines play a significant role in preventing hypoglycemia, their absence does not predispose to hypoglycemia. Adrenalectomized patients with sympathetic denervation due to spinal cord transection maintain euglycemia. Glucagon deficiency is the rarest cause of hypoglycemia of endocrine origin.

Fasting Hypoglycemia Due to Inadequate Production of Endogenous Glucose

ORGAN DAMAGE

Liver. The critical role of the liver in maintaining normal blood glucose concentrations was first demonstrated in the 1920s when hypoglycemia was observed in hepatectomized dogs. In humans, hypoglycemia due to abnormal liver function does not occur until hepatic injury is severe. Only about 20 percent of normal liver biosynthetic capability is needed to maintain normal glucose homeostasis [31]. Hypoglycemia seldom occurs in the setting of isolated, limited hepatic failure and is not implicated in the pathogenesis of hepatic coma [32]. Standard tests of hepatocellular integrity (e.g., AST and ALT concentrations) or hepatic function (e.g., bilirubin concentration) do not correlate well with the liver's ability to maintain normoglycemia. The presence of structural damage to the liver (e.g., cirrhosis, chronic active hepatitis, metastatic liver disease) does not necessarily confer a risk of hypoglycemia.

Hypoglycemia due to toxic or infectious hepatitis is rare but does occur when the disorder is fulminant. Hepatotoxins that can impair gluconeogenesis and cause hypoglycemia include carbon tetrachloride, the *Amanita phalloides* mushroom toxin, and urethane. Drugs that cause hypoglycemia by inducing hepatocellular necrosis include acetaminophen, isoniazid, sodium valproate, methyldopa, tetracycline, and halothane [32].

Congestive heart failure (CHF) from any cause can lead to hepatic congestion and hypoglycemia in adults and children. Patients with this syndrome usually have severe CHF with cardiac cachexia, malnutrition, and muscle wasting. The mechanism by which CHF leads to hypoglycemia is not completely understood. There is no evidence of hepatocyte necrosis. It has been suggested that changes in hepatic blood flow alter the delivery of gluconeogenic precursors and that changes in intracellular redox state decrease the gluconeogenic capacity of the hepatocyte. Hypoglycemia in this setting resolves with successful treatment of the CHF [32].

Kidney. It has long been known that some patients with diabetes mellitus develop improved glucose tolerance with the onset of renal failure. A decrease in insulin requirements and more frequent episodes of hypoglycemia are also noted [33]. There is no correlation between degree of renal failure and severity of hypoglycemia in these patients. The mechanisms by which renal failure induce hypoglycemia are not completely understood. Some authorities suspect a decrease in the metabolic clearance rate of insulin in patients with renal failure. Deficiencies in the delivery of gluconeogenic substrates, specifically alanine, have been emphasized by some investigators [30]. Others have implicated hepatic insufficiency secondary to uremia [34].

Symptomatic hypoglycemia occurs in a significant fraction of diabetic patients receiving either chronic hemodialysis or chronic ambulatory peritoneal dialysis [35,36]. Any dialysis patient who experiences a change in mental status should be evaluated for hypoglycemia. The signs of neuroglycopenia are similar to those commonly induced by normal dialysis-induced fluid shifts, the "dialysis disequilibrium syndrome." The clinical picture includes fatigue, confusion, lethargy, and even coma. Hypoglycemia could cause the same signs and symptoms. Postdialysis hypoglycemia in diabetic patients, if prolonged, can be fatal [37]. The cause is not known but may involve increased glucose-stimulated insulin release due to the high glucose concentration in the dialysate and impaired clearance of insulin due to the underlying renal disease.

"Spontaneous" fasting hypoglycemia has also been reported to occur in nondiabetic patients with end-stage renal disease [38,39,40] It is not clear, however, whether these rare cases represent a distinct clinical entity [41] or instances of renal failure enhancing intercurrent disorders that predispose to hypoglycemia [42]. These might include drug ingestion, liver disease, and adrenal or pituitary insufficiency.

DRUGS AND POISONS THAT CAUSE NON-INSULIN-MEDIATED HYPOGLYCEMIA

Ethanol-Induced Hypoglycemia (Alcoholic Ketoacidosis). Individuals of all ages are susceptible to the hypoglycemic effects of ethanol, but foremost among them are children and chronic alcohol abusers. The most common history is ethanol consumption in the setting of poor dietary carbohydrate intake. Patients usually present to the emergency department in a stuporous or comatose state. There may be obvious signs of acute alcohol intoxication, but alcoholic hypoglycemia can occur up to 30 hours after the ingestion of ethanol-containing beverages. Blood glucose concentrations as low as 5 mg per deciliter have been recorded. Ketonuria and ketonemia are frequently present and reflect the appropriately low circulating insulin concentrations [32].

Ethanol causes hypoglycemia by suppressing hepatic gluconeogenesis. Glycogenolysis is not affected. When ethanol is oxidized to acetaldehyde and acetate, NAD^+ is reduced to NADH. The reduced NAD^+:NADH ratio produces an unfavorable intracellular environment for the oxidation of substrates of gluconeogenesis such as lactate and glutamate to pyruvate and alpha-ketoglutarate, respectively (Fig. 116-1). As a result, intracellular levels of pyruvate are below the Km (Michaels constant) of pyruvate carboxylase, one of the rate-limiting steps in glu-

coneogenesis. Ethanol also inhibits hepatic uptake of the gluconeogenic precursors glycerol, alanine, and lactate and inhibits the release of alanine from muscle [32].

Beta-Adrenergic Blockers. These agents prevent the normal glycogenolytic and gluconeogenic response to hypoglycemia. The nonselective beta-blockers propranolol, pindolol, and nadolol can reportedly predispose to hypoglycemia in diverse clinical settings. Both diabetics and nondiabetics being treated with hemodialysis are particularly susceptible. Neonates may also experience hypoglycemia during their first 24 hours life as a result of propranolol treatment of the mother for cardiac arrhythmias, hypertension, or thyrotoxicosis. Hypoglycemia in infants treated with propranolol for cyanotic heart disease or neonatal thyrotoxicosis has also been documented. Beta-blockers increase the risk of hypoglycemia in patients who are undernourished or who have liver disease [16,32].

Salicylates. Among children younger than 5 years of age salicylates are a major cause of fatal and nonfatal drug intoxication. Salicylate intoxication causes hypoglycemia commonly in children but only very rarely in adults [16,43]. The frequency of salicylate-induced hypoglycemia per se is difficult to ascertain due to the concomitant presence of acidosis and renal or hepatic impairment in many cases of intoxication.

The mechanism by which salicylates might induce hypoglycemia is unknown. Experimental evidence indicates that these drugs can uncouple oxidative phosphorylation, thereby impairing gluconeogenesis. They can also inhibit lipolysis, limiting the availability of free fatty acids for metabolism by muscle and as an energy source for hepatic gluconeogenesis.

Poisons. Several unusual substances can cause hypoglycemia. Hypoglycin is found in akee fruit, a staple of the Jamaican diet. The ripe fruit is edible, but immature fruit causes Jamaican vomiting sickness a few days after ingestion. This condition is most commonly observed in undernourished individuals. In addition to vomiting, affected patients have severe hypoglycemia due to inhibition of hepatic gluconeogenesis by hypoglycin.

Amanitatoxin is a cyclic polypeptide produced by the mushroom *A. phalloides*. It is the only toxic mushroom that affects the human liver. It causes hepatocellular necrosis, intralobular hemorrhage, and an acute inflammatory exudate that impairs hepatocellular function. Fatal hypoglycemia can result from the resulting complete depletion of hepatic glycogen and decreased capacity for gluconeogenesis [32].

SEPSIS. Sepsis has occasionally been implicated as a cause of hypoglycemia [44–47]. Shock and liver failure were intercurrent problems in some reported cases [45]. Under conditions of decreased hepatic reserve, the combination of circulatory failure and impairment of gluconeogenesis by endotoxin might be postulated to lead to hypoglycemia. Septic hypoglycemic patients are often acidotic, and the fatality rate is high [44,45]. In one study only 1 of 15 such patients survived 1 month after the onset of hypoglycemia and hypotension [45].

CONGENITAL ENZYME DEFICIENCIES. Congenital enzyme deficiencies and other abnormalities in the function of specific enzymes typically produce hypoglycemia in the context of glycogen storage disease or impaired hepatic gluconeogenesis. These uncommon conditions usually present as hypoglycemia in infancy and are reviewed extensively elsewhere [47].

Fasting Hypoglycemia Due to the Unavailability of Gluconeogenic Substrate

The prototypic disease in which substrate deficiency leads to hypoglycemia is nonketotic hypoglycemia of childhood. Patients with this disorder are usually diagnosed between 18 months and 5 years of age. The hallmark of the disease is a low basal blood concentration of the gluconeogenic precursor alanine. Hypoglycemia is corrected by infusion of alanine.

In adult populations, low levels of alanine are associated with chronic renal disease, and extrapolation from animal data suggests that glucocorticoid deficiency may result in the suboptimal release of alanine and other gluconeogenic precursors from muscle. Severe malnutrition from any cause diminishes the supply of gluconeogenic precursors and can lead to hypoglycemia. In severe malnutrition glycogen, fat, and lean body mass are reduced, adding to the propensity to develop hypoglycemia.

Laboratory Diagnosis of Fasting Hypoglycemia

Hypoglycemia is most readily diagnosed when the elements of Whipple's triad are satisfied. In critically ill patients, however, underlying medical and surgical problems may mimic fasting hypoglycemia and/or obscure the response to glucose administration. In these circumstances the diagnosis of hypoglycemia requires thoughtful assessment, particularly with respect to laboratory testing.

"NORMAL" BLOOD GLUCOSE CONCENTRATION. The laboratory diagnosis of hypoglycemia is generally straightforward, but even this simplest of diagnostic tests can be misleading if interpreted thoughtlessly. The normal plasma glucose concentration is 60 to 120 mg per deciliter (3.3–6.7 mM). Whole blood glucose concentrations are 15 to 20 percent lower. Fingerstick blood glucose determinations are performed on whole capillary blood and reflect this offset compared with plasma glucose determinations. Lack of awareness of this distinction may lead to inappropriate therapeutic decisions.

Symptoms of hypoglycemia generally occur when the plasma glucose concentration is less than 50 mg per deciliter (2.8 mM) or the whole blood glucose concentration is less than 40 mg per deciliter (2.2 mM). Fingerstick blood glucose determinations, even when made with a reflectance meter, can be less accurate at the lower end of their scale. Interpretation of fingerstick blood glucose determinations must account for the clinical context, accompanying symptoms, and subsequent response to glucose administration.

There are several physiologic exceptions to guideline values for diagnosing hypoglycemia in the ICU. After about 48 hours of starvation many individuals, particularly women, have a plasma glucose concentration less than 50 mg per deciliter (2.8 mM). After 72 hours of fasting the plasma glucose concentration

may approach 40 mg per deciliter (2.2 mM). These individuals are nonetheless asymptomatic; they do not fulfill Whipple's triad and are not physiologically or clinically hypoglycemic. The lack of symptoms is due to the ability to shift to utilization of ketones for maintenance of central nervous system function. Similarly "low" plasma glucose concentrations are also encountered in pregnancy, in which the normal fasting plasma glucose concentration is 60 mg per deciliter or less (3.3 mM). Again, there are no symptoms of hypoglycemia per se in these cases.

FACTITIOUS HYPOGLYCEMIA. Factitious "hypoglycemia" must always be considered when interpreting laboratory reports of low blood glucose concentrations. This term is applied to glucose concentrations that are reported to be low but come from a normoglycemic patient. This most commonly occurs as a result of storing blood samples at room temperature for long periods before laboratory analysis. As a result of anaerobic glycolysis by blood elements, the actual glucose concentration in the test tube may decline at a rate of about 7 percent per hour. The effect is enhanced if large numbers of white blood cells are present in the sample as the result of severe leukocytosis or leukemia. Analyzing specimens promptly, keeping them iced, or drawing them into tubes containing sodium fluoride will obviate this problem.

TESTING FOR KETONURIA. The differential diagnosis of fasting hypoglycemia is sometimes facilitated by testing the urine for ketones. Normally, the fasted state is associated with low circulating insulin levels that promote gluconeogenesis and lipolysis. When hypoglycemia is associated with ketonuria, the combination enhances the likelihood that the low glucose concentration is not due to overinsulinization.

OTHER STUDIES. The only essential test for the diagnosis of hypoglycemia per se is blood glucose. Urinary ketones are very useful in all but the most obvious cases of insulin overdosage. Additional tests should be ordered as appropriate to the patient's underlying medical condition and the differential diagnosis of hypoglycemia that is developed. In general, these should always include studies of hepatic and renal function. In addition, it is often desirable to obtain additional serum and plasma samples from any comatose, hypoglycemic patient *when they are first seen.* This allows appropriate assays for sulfonylureas or IRI/glucose ratios to be performed later, if indicated. A cosyntropin test may be performed if adrenal insufficiency is suspected as a cause of hypoglycemia.

Management of Hypoglycemia

When hypoglycemia is suspected, the principal diagnostic maneuver and the definitive treatment are the same: glucose administration. In the hospital setting, this normally takes the form of intravenous glucose, but if a patient is sufficiently alert and cooperative, oral carbohydrates (e.g., sucrose in orange juice or glucose tablets) are an acceptable alternative method of treatment. When there is any question that the patient might aspirate, the intravenous route is mandatory.

In general, all comatose patients, including trauma patients, should be given intravenous glucose. The treatment is lifesaving in the presence of hypoglycemic coma and harmless when given to patients with coma due to other causes. Traumatologists should always bear in mind that altered mental status due to hypoglycemia is sometimes the root cause of an accident. If possible, blood specimens for testing should be obtained before glucose is given, but glucose should never be withheld pending the results.

The initial treatment of hypoglycemia in the patient with stupor or coma consists of the intravenous injection of 50 ml of $D_{50}W$ over 3 to 5 minutes. Care must be taken to avoid subcutaneous extravasation; the solution is hypertonic and can cause local tissue damage and severe pain. If hypoglycemia is present, treatment with $D_{50}W$ usually leads to improved mental status within minutes, but elderly patients and patients with very prolonged hypoglycemia may have a delayed response.

This prompt improvement is gratifying but can be misleading. If the cause of the hypoglycemia was overinsulinization due to exogenous insulin in a known diabetic patient, no further treatment may be needed; however, there are many other causes of hypoglycemia. The initial bolus of glucose treats the symptoms of hypoglycemia but *not their cause*. The most common error in the management of the hypoglycemic patient is inadequate treatment leading to recurrence of symptoms.

After the first bolus of $D_{50}W$ glucose is given, an infusion of D_5W or $D_{10}W$ glucose should be started in any patient whose hypoglycemic episode is not due to exogenous short- or intermediate-acting insulin. The choice of D_5W or $D_{10}W$ glucose depends on the severity of the initial hypoglycemia. This infusion allows the critical care physician to evaluate the cause of the hypoglycemic episode while protecting the patient from recurrence.

If the history reveals that a long-acting insulin might have caused the hypoglycemic episode, continuation of the glucose infusion, fingerstick blood glucose testing, and periodic adjustment of the infusion rate may be required. The duration of therapy depends on the particular insulin preparation. It is obviously important to determine the underlying etiology of these cases of hypoglycemia. The most common problems are dietary errors (e.g., missing a snack or meal), heavy exercise undertaken without caloric supplementation, and inadvertent injection of short-acting in place of long-acting insulin. Other causes of hypoglycemia due to exogenous insulin include malingering and attempts at suicide and homicide.

When the cause of hypoglycemia is sulfonylurea ingestion, the patient should usually be admitted to the hospital because of the prolonged duration of action of most members of this class of drugs. Continuous intravenous glucose is mandatory. Oral carbohydrate should be provided if the patient can eat. It is particularly important that the glucose infusion be continued while the patient recovering from a sulfonylurea overdose is asleep. Cases of persistent sulfonylurea-induced hypoglycemia requiring up to 16 days of intravenous glucose have been reported. The typical patient with this condition requires 2 to 3 days of intravenous glucose therapy [16]. Recently the somatostatin analog octreotide was proposed as an adjunct to the treatment of severe oral agent overdosage [48]. Octreotide can inhibit sulfonylurea-induced insulin secretion, but there is as yet little clinical experience with its use.

If the history and physical examination do not immediately establish the underlying cause of hypoglycemia, continuation of the infusion and glycemia monitoring are required until it is established that these therapies are no longer needed. Severe unexplained cases of hypoglycemia require intensive care monitoring. Blood glucose should be monitored every 1 to 3 hours and the serum glucose concentration maintained at a target level of ≈100 mg per deciliter. The studies outlined in the section on differential diagnosis can be obtained as appropriate during continuous glucose infusion.

Intravenous glucose should continue either until a definitive diagnosis and treatment are established or until normoglycemia is demonstrated. To determine whether parenteral glucose is no longer needed, the infusion should be discontinued and blood glucose concentration measured every 15 minutes. If the patient is unable to maintain a blood glucose concentration greater than 50 mg per deciliter or if the patient becomes symptomatic, reinstitution of the glucose therapy is necessary. Depending on the etiology of the hypoglycemia (e.g., sulfonylurea overdosage, insulinoma) parenteral glucose infusion may be required for many days.

When hypoglycemia is due to an insulinoma or nesidioblastosis, it may rarely be necessary to supplement glucose infusion therapy with drugs that inhibit insulin secretion, pending definite surgical treatment. Diazoxide is a benzothiadiazine nondiuretic antihypertensive agent that blocks the secretion of insulin from both normal and neoplastic beta cells. To treat hypoglycemia, diazoxide can be given at a dose of 300 mg in D_5W infused at 100 ml per hour. Somatostatin is an inhibitor to insulin secretion produced in pancreatic islet delta cells. Experimental long-acting analogs have been used in the treatment of insulinoma, but results using one such analog have been disappointing [49]. These analogs may be more effective in cases of nesidioblastosis. The analog octreotide has been proposed as adjunctive therapy for oral agent-induced hypoglycemia [49] and quinine-induced hypoglycemia in malaria [21].

When hypoglycemia is due to impaired gluconeogenesis in the setting of liver disease, renal disease, or congestive heart failure, only treatment of the underlying condition will prevent recurrence.

When the etiology of severe, refractory hypoglycemia is obscure, one may attempt to increase gluconeogenic substrates and inhibit insulin action in the periphery by giving parenteral adrenocortical steroids. Hydrocortisone sodium succinate can be given at a dose of 100 mg per liter of glucose infused. This mode of therapy is most beneficial in patients whose hypoglycemia is due to adrenocortical insufficiency.

The primary action of exogenous glucagon in the treatment of hypoglycemia is the promotion of glycogenolysis. It is most effective in patients with ample liver glycogen stores. Glucagon can be a useful drug in out-of-hospital treatment of hypoglycemia due to overinsulinization in known diabetic patients. It is common practice to teach family members of "brittle" diabetic patients to administer parenteral glucagon. In the intensive care setting, however, there is seldom need to administer glucagon in lieu of, or in addition to, parenteral glucose.

Conclusion

The diagnosis of hypoglycemia must be considered in all cases of stupor and coma. Diagnosis is based on Whipple's triad. Evaluation of the triad requires appropriate initial therapy for true hypoglycemia and should take no more than a few minutes. After initial therapy for hypoglycemia has been given, it must be remembered that only the symptoms and not the cause have been treated. The most common cause of hypoglycemia is insulin overdosage in individuals with diabetes; these cases may require no further intervention. The most common error in the management of hypoglycemia is inadequate treatment of hypoglycemia due to other causes. Hypoglycemia due to intercurrent medical conditions often responds only to correction of the underlying disorder. Patients with sulfonylurea-

or insulinoma-induced hypoglycemia may require aggressive treatment of hypoglycemia with parenteral glucose for many days.

References

1. Whipple AO: The surgical therapy of hyperinsulinism. *J Int Chirurgie* 3:237, 1938.
2. Cahill GF Jr: Starvation in man. *N Engl J Med* 282:668, 1970.
3. Butler PC, Rizza RA: Regulation of carbohydrate metabolism and response to hypoglycemia. *Endocrinol Metab Clin North Am* 18:1, 1989.
4. Bauman WA, Yalow RS: Hyperinsulinemic hypoglycemia: Differential diagnosis by determination of the species of circulating insulin. *JAMA* 252:2730, 1984.
5. Albers N, Lohr M, Bogner U, et al: Nesidioblastosis of the pancreas in an adult with persistent hyperinsulinemic hypoglycemia. *Am J Clin Pathol* 91:336, 1989.
6. Fong TL, Warner NE, Kumar D: Pancreatic nesidioblastosis in adults. *Diabetes Care* 12:108, 1989.
7. Burch HB, Clement S, Sokol MS, et al: Reactive hypoglycemic coma due to insulin autoimmune syndrome: Case report and literature review. *Am J Med* 92:681, 1992.
8. Varga J, Lopatin M, Boden G: Hypoglycemia due to antiinsulin receptor antibodies in systemic lupus erythematosus. *J Rheumatol* 17:1226, 1990.
9. Uchigata Y, Takayama-Hasumi S, Kawanishi K, et al: Inducement of antibody that mimics insulin action on insulin receptor by insulin autoantibody directed at determinant on asparagine site on human insulin B chain. *Diabetes* 40:966, 1991.
10. Selinger S, Tsai J, Pulini M, et al: Autoimmune thrombocytopenia and primary biliary cirrhosis with hypoglycemia and insulin receptor autoantibodies: A case report. *Ann Intern Med* 107:686, 1987.
11. Redmon B, Pyzdrowski KL, Elson MK, et al: Hypoglycemia due to a monoclonal insulin-binding antibody in multiple myeloma. *N Engl J Med* 326:994, 1992.
12. Seino S, Fu ZZ, Marks W, et al: Characterization of circulating insulin in insulin autoimmune syndrome. *J Clin Endocrinol Metab* 62:64, 1986.
13. Daughaday WH, Trivedi B: Measurement of derivatives of proinsulin-like growth factor-II in serum by a radioimmunoassay directed against the E-domain in normal subjects and patients with nonislet cell tumor hypoglycemia. *J Clin Endocrinol Metab* 75:110, 1992.
14. Daughaday WH, Trivedi B, Baxter RC: Serum "big insulin-like growth factor II" from patients with tumor hypoglycemia lacks normal E-domain O-linked glycosylation, a possible determinant of normal propeptide processing. *Proc Natl Acad Sci USA* 90:5823, 1993.
15. Daughaday WH: Hypoglycemia in patients with non-islet cell tumors. *Endocrinol Metab Clin North Am* 18:91, 1989.
16. Seltzer HS: Drug-induced hypoglycemia: A review of 1418 cases. *Endocrinol Metab Clin North Am* 18:163, 1989.
17. Gerich JE: Oral hypoglycemic agents. *N Engl J Med* 321:1231, 1989.
18. Hargett NA, Ritch R, Mardirossian J, et al: Inadvertent substitution of acetohexamide for acetazolamide. *Am J Ophthalmol* 84:580, 1977.
19. Johnstone FD, Nasrat AA, Prescott RJ: The effect of established and gestational diabetes on pregnancy outcome. *Br J Obstet Gynaecol* 97:1009, 1990.
20. White NJ, Warrell DA, Chanthavanich P, et al: Severe hypoglycemia and hyperinsulinemia in falciparum malaria. *N Engl J Med* 309:61, 1983.
21. Phillips RE, Looareesuwan S, Molyneux ME, et al: Hypoglycaemia and counterregulatory hormone responses in severe falciparum malaria: Treatment with Sandostatin. *Q J Med* 86:233, 1993.
22. Limburg PJ, Katz H, Grant CS, et al: Quinine-induced hypoglycemia. *Ann Intern Med* 119:218, 1993.
23. Phillips RE, Looareesuwan S, White NJ, et al: Hypoglycaemia and antimalarial drugs: Quinidine and release of insulin. *Br Med J* 292:1319, 1986.
24. Goldberg IJ, Brown LK, Rayfield EJ: Disopyramide (Norpace)-induced hypoglycemia. *Am J Med* 69:463, 1980.
25. Nappi JM, Dhanani S, Lovejoy JR, et al: Severe hypoglycemia associated with disopyramide. *West J Med* 138:95, 1983.
26. Caldwell G, Scougall I, Boddy K, et al: Fasting hyperinsulinemic hypoglycemia after ritodrine therapy for premature labor. *Obstet Gynecol* 70:478, 1987.
27. Arauz-Pacheco C, Ramirez LC, Rios JM, et al: Hypoglycemia induced by angiotensin-converting enzyme inhibitors in patients with non-insulin-dependent diabetes receiving sulfonylurea therapy. *Am J Med* 89:811, 1990.
28. Buller GK, Perazella M: ACE inhibitor-induced hypoglycemia. *Am J Med* 91:104, 1991.
29. Fajans SS, Floyd JC Jr: Fasting hypoglycemia in adults. *N Engl J Med* 294:766, 1976.
30. Arky RA: Hypoglycemia, in DeGroot LJ, Cahill GF Jr, Martini L, et al. (eds): *Endocrinology*. New York, Grune & Stratton, 1979, pp 1099–1123.
31. Marks V: Hepatogenous and nephrogenic hypoglycemia, in Marks V, Rose FC (eds): *Hypoglycemia*. Oxford, Blackwell, 1981, pp 216–226.
32. Arky RA: Hypoglycemia associated with liver disease and ethanol. *Endocrinol Metab Clin North Am* 18:75, 1989.
33. Muhlhauser I, Toth G, Sawicki PT, et al: Severe hypoglycemia in type I diabetic patients with impaired kidney function. *Diabetes Care* 14:344, 1991.
34. Garber AJ, Bier DM, Cryer PE, et al: Hypoglycemia in compensated chronic renal insufficiency: Substrate limitation of gluconeogenesis. *Diabetes* 23:982, 1974.
35. Comty CM, Leonard A, Shapiro FL: Nutritional and metabolic problems in the dialyzed patient with diabetes mellitus. *Kidney Int* 1 (suppl):51, 1974.
36. Tzamaloukas AH, Murata GH, Eisenberg B, et al: Hypoglycemia in diabetics on dialysis with poor glycemic control: Hemodialysis versus continuous ambulatory peritoneal dialysis. *Int J Artif Organs* 15:390, 1992.
37. Greenblatt DJ: Insulin sensitivity in renal failure: Fatal hypoglycemia following dialysis. *N Y State J Med* 74:1040, 1974.
38. Rutsky EA, McDaniel HG, Tharpe DL, et al: Spontaneous hypoglycemia in chronic renal failure. *Arch Intern Med* 138:1364, 1978.
39. Avram MM, Wolf RE, Gan A, et al: Uremic hypoglycemia: A preventable life-threatening complication. *N Y State J Med* 84:593, 1984.
40. Bansal VK, Brooks MH, York JC, et al: Intractable hypoglycemia in a patient with renal failure. *Arch Intern Med* 139:101, 1979.
41. Pun KK: Hypoglycaemia and insulin resistance in uraemia associated with insulin fragments. *Med Hypotheses* 17:243, 1985.
42. Toth EL, Lee DW: "Spontaneous"/uremic hypoglycemia is not a distinct entity: Substantiation from a literature review. *Nephron* 58:325, 1991.
43. Miller SI, Wallace RJ Jr, Musher DM, et al: Hypoglycemia as a manifestation of sepsis. *Am J Med* 68:649, 1980.
44. Nouel O, Bernuau J, Rueff B, et al: Hypoglycemia: A common complication of septicemia in cirrhosis. *Arch Intern Med* 141:1477, 1981.
45. Scheetz A: Hypoglycemia and sepsis in two elderly diabetics. *J Am Geriatr Soc* 38:492, 1990.
46. Romijn JA, Godfried MH, Wortel C, et al: Hypoglycemia, hormones and cytokines in fatal meningococcal septicemia. *J Endocrinol Invest* 13:743, 1990.
47. Haymond MW: Hypoglycemia in infants and children. *Endocrinol Metab Clin North Am* 18:211, 1989.
48. Boyle PJ, Justice K, Krentz AJ, et al: Octreotide reverses hyperinsulinemia and prevents hypoglycemia induced by sulfonylurea overdoses. *J Clin Endocrinol Metab* 76:752, 1993.
49. Fajans SS, Vinik AI: Insulin-producing islet cell tumors. *Endocrinol Metab Clin North Am* 18:45, 1989.

117. Sick Euthyroid Syndrome in the Intensive Care Unit

Alan P. Farwell

Introduction

Critical illness causes multiple alterations in thyroid hormone concentrations in patients who have no intrinsic thyroid disease [1,2,3]. These effects are nonspecific and relate to the severity of the illness. Since a wide variety of illnesses tend to result in the same changes in serum thyroid hormones, such alterations in thyroid hormone indexes has been termed sick euthyroid syndrome [4,5]. These changes are rarely isolated and often are associated with alterations in other endocrine systems, such as reductions in serum gonadotropin and sex hormone concentrations [6,7] and increases in serum ACTH and cortisol levels [8]. Similar changes in endocrine function have been shown experimentally by the administration of cytokines from the interleukin and interferon families as well tumor necrosis factor α [9,10]. Thus, sick euthyroid syndrome should not be viewed as an isolated pathologic event but as part of a coordinated systemic reaction to illness that involves both the immune and endocrine systems.

The differentiation between sick euthyroid syndrome and intrinsic thyroid disease is a frequent diagnostic problem in the ICU. This chapter first reviews normal thyroid physiology and the changes in thyroid hormone metabolism seen with critical illness. Management of these patients and identification of those with intrinsic thyroid disease are then discussed.

Normal Thyroid Hormone Economy

REGULATION. Synthesis and secretion of thyroid hormone are under the control of the anterior pituitary hormone, thyrotropin (TSH). Secretion of TSH increases when serum thyroid hormone levels fall and decreases when they rise, in a classic negative feedback system (Fig. 117-1). Thyrotropin is also under the regulation of the hypothalamic hormone, thyrotropin-releasing hormone (TRH). The negative feedback of thyroid hormone is targeted mainly at the pituitary level but probably affects TRH release from the hypothalamus as well. In addition, input from higher cortical centers affects TRH secretion.

Under the influence of TSH, the thyroid gland synthesizes and releases thyroid hormone. Thyroxine (T_4) is the principal secretory product of the thyroid gland, comprising approximately 90 percent of the secreted hormone under normal conditions [11,12]. Thyroxine is also the most abundant thyroid hormone in serum, with a normal circulating level between 4.5 and 11.0 μg per deciliter. While some effects of thyroid hormone are attributed specifically to T_4, for the most part T_4 functions as a hormone precursor that is metabolized in peripheral tissues to a more active form.

METABOLIC PATHWAYS. The major pathway of T_4 metabolism is by sequential monodeiodination (Fig. 117-2) [13]. Removal of the 5'-, or outer ring, iodine by type I iodothyronine 5'deiodinase is the "activating" metabolic pathway, leading to the formation of the metabolically active form of thyroid hormone, 3,5,3'-triiodothyronine (T_3). Removal of the inner ring, or 5-, iodine by type III iodothyronine 5-deiodinase is an "inactivating" pathway, producing the metabolically inactive hormone, 3,3',5'-triiodothyronine (reverse T_3, rT_3). Under normal conditions, about 41 percent of T_4 is converted to T_3, about 38 percent is converted to rT_3, and about 21 percent is metabolized via other pathways, such as conjugation in the liver and excretion in the bile [14].

3,5,3'-triiodothyronine is the metabolically active thyroid hormone and exerts its actions via binding to chromatin-bound nuclear receptors and regulating gene transcription in responsive tissues [15]. Important in the understanding of the alterations in circulating thyroid hormone levels seen in critical illness is the fact that only about 10 percent of circulating T_3 is secreted directly by the thyroid gland, while more than 80 percent of T_3 is derived from conversion of T_4 in peripheral tissues. Thus, factors that affect peripheral T_4 to T_3 conversion have significant effects on circulating T_3 levels. Peripheral T_4 to T_3 conversion is catalyzed by type I 5'-deiodinase, found predominantly in the liver and kidney. Serum levels of T_3 are about 100-fold lower than those of T_4, with a normal circulating range between 60 and 180 ng per deciliter. Like T_4, T_3 is metabolized by deiodination, forming diiodothyronine (T_2), and by conjugation in the liver [14].

SERUM BINDING PROTEINS. Both T_4 and T_3 circulate in the serum bound to several proteins synthesized in the liver [1,16]. Thyronine-binding protein (TBG) is the major serum binding protein and binds approximately 80 percent of the serum thyroid hormones. The affinity of T_4 for TBG is about 10-fold greater than that of T_3; this is part of the reason circulating T_4 levels are higher than T_3 levels. Other serum binding proteins include transthyretin, which binds about 15 percent of T_4 but little, if any, T_3, and albumin, which has a low affinity but a very large capacity for binding T_4 and T_3. Overall, 99.97 percent of circulating T_4 and 99.7 percent of circulating T_3 is bound to plasma proteins.

FREE HORMONE CONCEPT. Essential to the understanding of the regulation of thyroid function and the alterations of circulating thyroid hormones seen in critical illness is the free hormone concept: only the unbound hormone has any metabolic activity. Laboratory measurements of serum total T_4 and T_3 measure both bound and unbound hormone. Because of the high degree of binding of T_4 and T_3 to the serum binding proteins, changes in either the concentrations of these proteins or the binding affinity of thyroid hormone to the serum binding proteins would have major effects on the total serum hormone levels. However, since the pituitary responds to and regulates the circulating free hormone levels, minimal changes in free

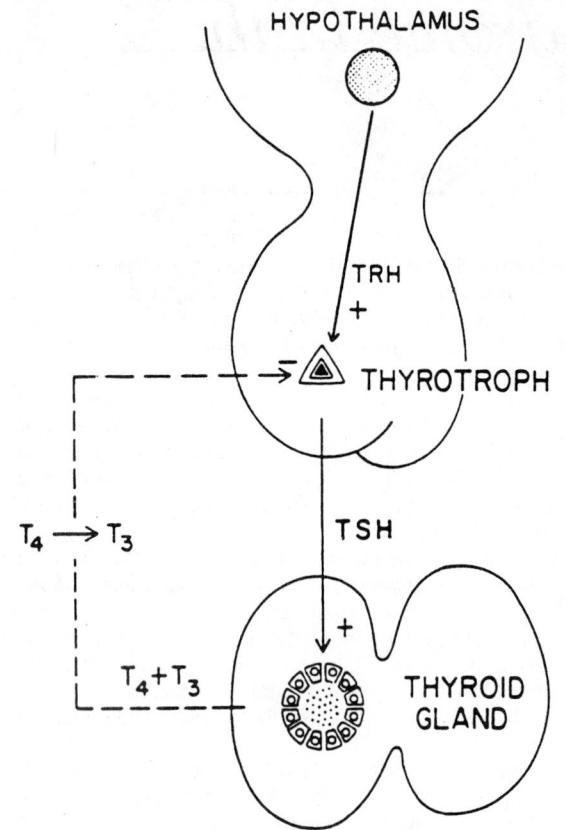

Fig. 117-1. The hypothalamic-pituitary-thyroid axis. The inhibitory effect of T_4 and T_3 on TSH secretion is shown by the dashed line and minus sign. The stimulatory effects of TRH on TSH secretion and TSH on thyroid secretion are shown by the solid lines and plus signs. T_4 and T_3 may also have an inhibitory effect on TRH secretion. TRH = thyrotropin-releasing hormone; TSH = thyrotropin; T_4 = thyroxine; T_3 = 3,5,3′-triiodothyronine. (From Toft AD: Thyrotropin: Assay, secretory physiology, and testing of regulation, in Braverman LE, Utiger RD (eds): *The Thyroid: A Fundamental and Clinical Text.* Philadelphia, JB Lippincott, 1991. With permission.)

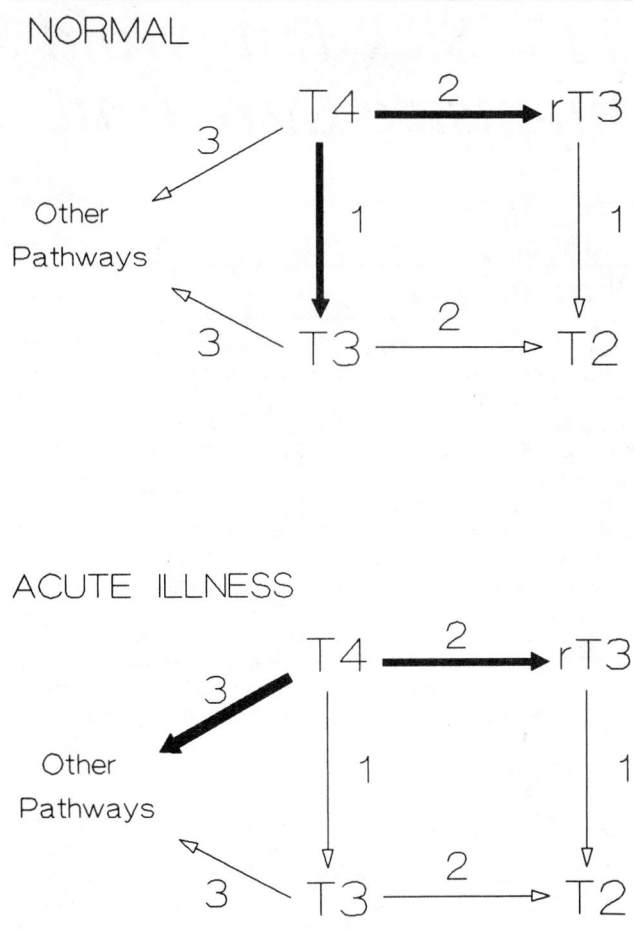

Fig. 117-2. Pathways of thyroid hormone metabolism. Thyroid hormones are metabolized by outer ring deiodination (1, type I 5′-deiodinase), inner ring deiodination (2, type III 5-deiodinase), or nondeiodinative pathways (3). Deiodination is the major route of T_4 metabolism in healthy individuals, while nondeiodinative pathways of metabolism assume a greater role in critically ill patients.

hormone concentrations, and thus overall thyroid function, would be seen.

Thyroid Hormone Economy in Critical Illness

The widespread changes in thyroid hormone economy in the critically ill patient occur as a result of (1) alterations in the peripheral metabolism of the thyroid hormones, (2) alterations in TSH regulation, and (3) alterations in the binding of thyroid hormone to TBG.

PERIPHERAL METABOLIC PATHWAYS. One of the first alterations in thyroid hormone metabolism in acute illness is impairment in T_4 to T_3 conversion in peripheral tissues by the acute inhibition of type I 5′deiodinase (Fig. 117-2) [1,2,3]. This enzyme is affected by a wide variety of factors (Table 117-1) [12,13,17]. Since deiodination of T_4 by type I 5′deiodinase is

the prime metabolic pathway for the generation of T_3 in peripheral tissues, T_3 production decreases markedly and T_3 levels fall soon after the onset of acute illness. In contrast, inner ring deiodination of T_4 to produce rT_3 is unaffected by acute illness. However, since rT_3 is subsequently deiodinated by type I 5′ deiodinase, degradation of rT_3 decreases and levels of this inactive hormone rise in proportion to the fall in T_3 levels. Thus, inhibition of type I 5′deiodinase decreases both T_3 production and T_4 and rT_3 degradation, leading to a decrease in serum T_3 levels and an increase in serum rT_3 and, to a lesser extent, serum T_4 levels [18]. However, as conversion of T_4 to T_3 decreases with acute illness and conversion of T_4 to rT_3 remains constant, other pathways of T_4 metabolism assume a more prominent role in thyroid hormone economy, so overall T_4 degradation remains relatively constant [14,19,20].

THYROTROPIN REGULATION. Serum TSH levels are usually normal early in acute illness [21,22]. However, TSH levels often fall as illness progresses, due to the effects of a variety of inhibitory factors that are common in the treatment of the critically ill patient (Table 117-2). Most common are the use of dopamine and increased levels of glucocorticoids, either en-

Table 117-1. Factors That Inhibit Type I 5'Deiodinase Activity

Acute and chronic illness
Caloric deprivation
Malnutrition
Glucocorticoids
Beta-adrenergic blocking drugs (e.g., propranolol)
Oral cholecystographic agents (e.g., iopanoic acid, sodium ipodate)
Amiodarone
Propylthiouracil
Fatty acids
Fetal/neonatal period

Table 117-2. Factors That Inhibit Thyroid-Stimulating Hormone Secretion

Acute and chronic illness
Caloric restriction
Glucocorticoids
Dopamine and dopamine agonists
Adrenergic agonists
Phenytoin
Carbamazepine
Somatostatin
IGF-1
Serotonin
Endogenous depression
Surgical stress
Thyroid hormone metabolites
Depressed thyroid-releasing hormone secretion

Table 117-3. Factors That Alter Binding of Thyroxine to Thyronine-Binding Protein

	Increase Binding	Decrease Binding
Drugs	Estrogens	Glucocorticoids
	Methadone	Androgens
	Clofibrate	L-asparaginase
	5-fluorouracil	Salicylates
	Heroin	Mefenic acid
	Tamoxifen	Antiseizure medications (phenytoin, tegretol), furosemide
Systemic factors	Liver disease	Inherited
	Porphyria	Acute illness
	HIV infection	Inherited

dogenous or exogenous, both of which have a direct inhibitory effect on TSH secretion. Indeed, pressor doses of dopamine may decrease TSH levels to normal in patients with preexisting primary hypothyroidism [23]. Decreased TRH secretion due to inhibitory signals from higher cortical centers also may play a role in decreasing TSH secretion [24]. Finally, certain thyroid hormone metabolites that are increased in nonthyroidal illness may play a role in the inhibition of TSH and TRH secretion [19,20].

SERUM BINDING PROTEINS. The binding of thyroid hormones to serum proteins is altered with acute illness (Table 117-3). Serum levels of transthyretin decrease rapidly after the onset of acute illness [25]. Serum albumin levels decrease, especially during prolonged illness, malnutrition, and high catabolic states. Thyronine-binding protein levels may be increased, as in liver dysfunction [16,26] and HIV infection [27], or decreased, as in severe or prolonged illness [28,29]. An acquired binding defect of T_4 to TBG is commonly seen in patients with critical illness [28] and is believed to result from the release of some as yet unidentified factor from injured tissues [30]. This factor has the characteristics of unsaturated fatty acids and also inhibits T_4 to T_3 conversion [17,31]. Many drugs, including high-dose furosemide [32] and antiseizure medications [33], also alter binding of T_4 to TBG. These alterations in serum binding proteins in critical illness make estimation of the free hormone concentrations difficult. Indirect measurements of free T_4 levels using T_3-resin uptake or TBG measurements often result in levels in the hypothyroid range, while measurements of free T_4 levels by equilibrium dialysis or ultrafiltration are normal or even elevated [34,35].

STAGES OF SICK EUTHYROID SYNDROME. The changes in serum concentrations of thyroid hormone that are observed in critically ill patients represent a continuum of changes that depends on the severity of the illness (Fig. 117-3). Thus, the wide spectrum of changes observed often results from the differing points in the course of the illness that the thyroid function tests were obtained.

Low T_3 State. Common to all of the abnormalities in thyroid hormone concentrations seen in critically ill patients is a substantial depression of serum T_3 levels, which can occur as early as 24 hours after the onset of illness [22,36]. In one study more than half of patients admitted to the medical service demonstrate depressed serum T_3 concentrations [37,38]. The development of low T_3 state can be explained solely by the impairment of peripheral T_4 to T_3 conversion through the inhibition of type I 5'deiodinase. As discussed above, this results in a marked reduction in T_3 production and rT_3 degradation, leading to reciprocal changes in serum T_3 and serum rT_3 concentrations. Clinically, these patients appear euthyroid, although mild prolongation in Achilles reflex time is found in some patients [1].

High T_4 State. Serum T_4 levels may be elevated early in acute illness due to either acute inhibition of type I 5'deiodinase or increased TBG levels. This is seen most often in the elderly [39] and patients with psychiatric disorders [40]. As the duration of illness increases, nondeiodinative pathways of T_4 degradation increase and return serum T_4 levels to the normal range.

Low T_4 State. As the severity and duration of the illness increase, serum total T_4 levels decrease into the subnormal range. Contributing to this decrease in serum T_4 levels are (1) a decrease in the binding of T_4 to serum carrier proteins, (2) a decrease in serum TSH levels, leading to decreased thyroidal production of T_4, and (3) an increase in nondeiodinative pathways of T_4 metabolism. The decline in serum T_4 levels correlates with prognosis in the ICU, with mortality increasing as serum T_4 levels drop below 4 μg pr deciliter and approaching 80 percent in patients with serum T_4 levels less than 2 μg per deciliter [22,41,42]. Despite marked decreases in serum total T_4 and T_3 levels in the critically ill patient, free hormone levels have been reported to be normal or even elevated [34,35,43,44]. If this is true, it would explain why most patients appear eumetabolic despite thyroid hormone levels in the hypothyroid range. Thus, the low T_4 state is unlikely to be a result of a hormone-deficient state and is probably more a marker of multisystem failure in these critically ill patients. In addition, administration of either T_4 or T_3 is ineffective in altering the grave prognosis of the low T_4 state [45,46].

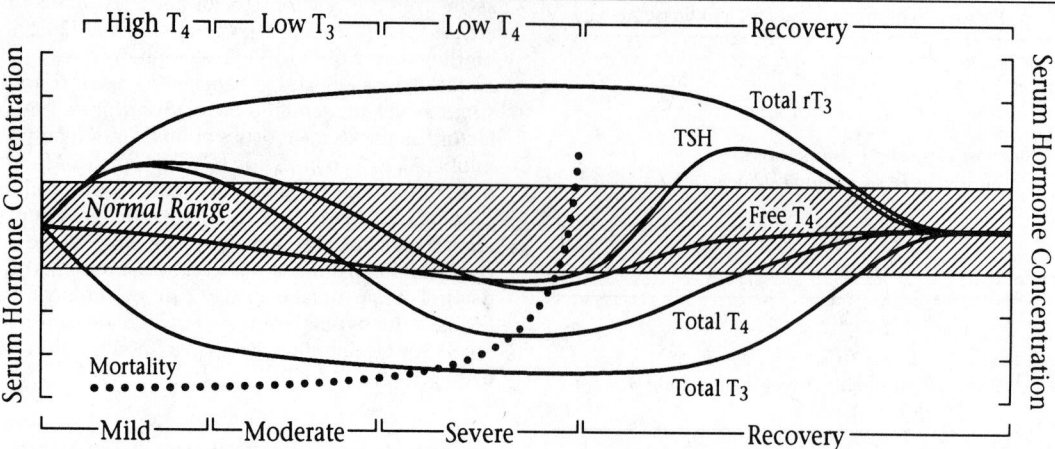

Fig. 117-3. Alterations in thyroid hormone concentrations with critical illness. Schematic representation of the continuum of changes in serum thyroid hormone levels in patients with nonthyroidal illness. These alterations become more pronounced with increasing severity of the illness and return to the normal range as the illness subsides and the patient recovers. A rapidly rising mortality accompanies the fall in total and free T_4 levels.

Recovery State. As acute illness resolves, so do the alterations in thyroid hormone concentrations. This stage may be prolonged and is characterized by modest increases in serum TSH levels [47]. Full recovery, with restoration of thyroid hormone levels to the normal range, may take up to several months after the patient is discharged from the hospital [38].

Alterations in Thyroid Function in Specific Critical Illnesses

CALORIC DEPRIVATION. Most, if not all, nonthyroidal illnesses in the ICU are associated with decreased caloric intake, catabolism, and/or malnutrition. Caloric deprivation is the most common inhibitory factor of type I 5'deiodinase [48,49,50]. Serum T_3 levels decrease and rT_3 levels increase within 24 hours of the onset of a fast. The decrease in serum T_3 levels may possibly be an adaptive response to preserve the total body protein stores. Indeed, restoring the serum T_3 to normal during starvation results in a marked increase in urinary nitrogen excretion [51]. Thus, the inhibition of T_4 to T_3 conversion in starvation can be viewed as a condition of adaptive hypothyroidism. Further support for the role of caloric deprivation in the development of euthyroid sick syndrome is the demonstration that serum thyroid hormone levels in critically ill patients receiving nutritional support return to normal levels [52].

HIV INFECTION. A unique pattern of changes in circulating thyroid hormone levels is seen in patients with HIV infection and those with AIDS [27]. A progressive increase in TBG levels is commonly observed and T_4 levels rarely decrease below the normal range. Serum rT_3 levels fail to rise with advancing infections and are only modestly increased in preterminal AIDS patients. Most striking is the observation that serum T_3 levels remain in the normal range despite progression of the HIV infection and are only mildly decreased in the critically ill AIDS

patient, suggesting that these "inappropriately normal" T_3 levels play a role in the wasting and weight loss seen in the terminal phases of this disease. In contrast to sick euthyroid syndrome, in AIDS patients admitted to the ICU with *Pneumocystis carinii* infections decreased serum T_3 levels correlate with increased mortality [53].

LIVER DISEASE. In contrast to the decrease in thyroid hormone levels seen in critically ill patients, individuals suffering from acute and chronic hepatocellular dysfunction often have marked elevations in total T_4 levels similar to those seen in patients with thyrotoxicosis [26,54]. The T_3 levels are also higher than expected with illness and tend to fall late in the course of terminal liver disease. The etiology of these increased thyroid hormone concentrations is the increased discharge of TBG following destruction of hepatocytes. Free hormone measurements remain in the normal range.

Management of the Critically Ill Patient with Abnormal Thyroid Function Tests

EVALUATION. Identification of the critically ill patient with intrinsic thyroid disease is often difficult and always a diagnostic challenge. Routine screening of an ICU population for the presence of thyroid dysfunction is not recommended due to the high prevalence of abnormal thyroid function tests and low prevalence of true thyroid dysfunction. Whenever possible, it is best to defer evaluation of the thyroid-pituitary axis until the patient has recovered from acute illness. In principle, when thyroid function tests are ordered in a hospitalized patient, it should be with a high clinical index of suspicion for the presence of thyroid dysfunction. For example, thyroid function should be evaluated in the patient admitted to the ICU with tachyarrhythmias when that patient also has a goiter, proptosis, and a tremor. Similarly, a large pericardial effusion, hypothermia, a goiter, and "hung-up" deep tendon reflexes suggests the diagnosis of hypothyroidism. In practice, however, thyroid function tests are ordered in the patient with less specific clinical findings and present a diagnostic dilemma. Because every test of thyroid hormone function can be altered in the critically

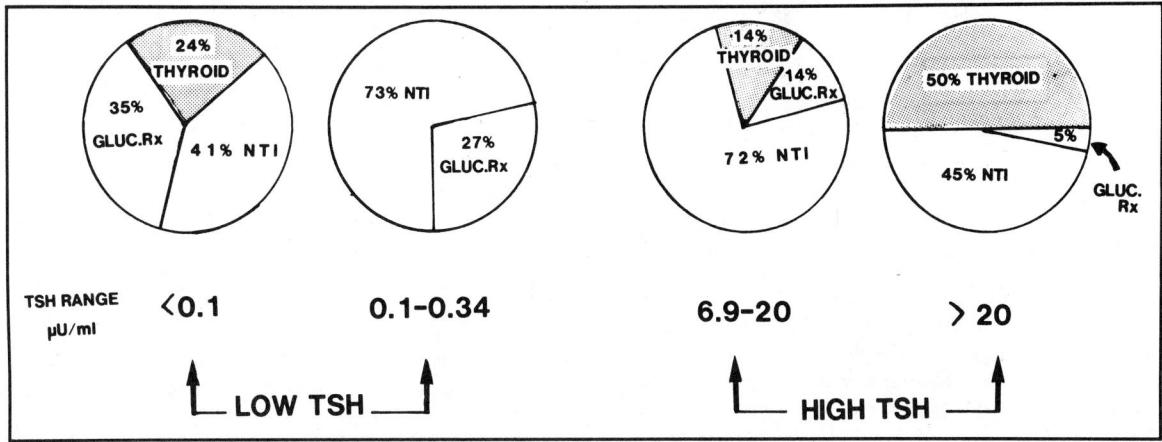

TSH RANGE
μU/ml

<0.1   0.1-0.34   6.9-20   >20

LOW TSH   HIGH TSH

Fig. 117-4. Clinical diagnostic classification of hospitalized patients with abnormal thyrotropin (TSH) values. The proportion of patients with thyroid disease (Thyroid), with nonthyroidal illness (NTI), and receiving glucocorticoid therapy (Gluc.Rx) among a large group of hospitalized patients, subdivided into four ranges of serum TSH concentrations. (From Spencer CA: Clinical utility and cost-effectiveness of sensitive thyrotropin assays in ambulatory and hospitalized patients. *Mayo Clin Proc* 63:1214, 1988. With permission.)

ill patient, no single test can definitively rule in or rule out the presence of intrinsic thyroid dysfunction.

Primary Test

SENSITIVE TSH ASSAYS. The development of the sensitive TSH assay has both helped and hindered the evaluation of thyroid function in the critically ill. These new assays have greatly expanded the lower range of the TSH assay, so the typical sensitive TSH assay has a lower limit of detection of 0.01 to 0.03 mU per liter, 20 to 30 times lower than the lower limit of the normal range [55,56]. With this improved sensitivity has come the recognition of an increased frequency of subnormal TSH values in hospitalized patients, indicating that transient abnormalities in TSH secretion are commonplace in acute illness. To what degree this TSH dysregulation represents clinically significant alterations in thyroid function is uncertain.

Abnormal TSH values have been reported in up to 20 percent of acutely ill patients [37,38,57]. In a study of 1580 hospitalized patients, abnormal TSH values were found in 17.2 percent, with more than 80 percent of these patients having no intrinsic thyroid dysfunction on follow-up testing when healthy [37,38]. Only 24 percent of patients with suppressed TSH values (TSH < assay limit of detection) and 50 percent of patients with TSH values greater than 20 mU per liter were found to have thyroid disease (Fig. 117-4). More important, none of the patients with subnormal but detectable TSH values and only 14 percent of patients with elevated TSH values less than 20 mU per liter were subsequently diagnosed with intrinsic thyroid dysfunction. Finally, the only patients found to have thyroid dysfunction with a normal TSH value were previously diagnosed patients on thyroid hormone replacement therapy. Thus, while a normal TSH level has a high predictive value of normal thyroid function, an abnormal TSH value alone is not helpful in the evaluation of thyroid function in the critically ill patient.

FREE T$_4$ INDEX. The free T$_4$ index (FTI) may be the most cost-effective screening test of thyroid disease [58,59,60] although many thyroidologists recommend serum TSH as the first test. The FTI is an estimate of the free T$_4$ concentration and is determined by multiplying total T$_4$ concentration by T$_3$- or T$_4$-

resin uptake, which is an inverse estimate of serum TBG concentrations and expressed as a percentage. Methods of direct measurement of free thyroid hormone levels are also available but may be no more accurate than the FTI [61,62,63]. In a healthy population, there is a close correlation between FTI and free T$_4$ levels measured directly. In the critically ill patient, this correlation breaks down, mainly due to difficulties in estimating TBG binding with the resin uptake tests. In spite of this, the sensitivity of the FTI in a recent large study of hospitalized patients was 92.3 percent, compared to 90.7 percent for the sensitive TSH test [38].

A possible limitation to the use of the FTI as a sole screening test for thyroid dysfunction is the recent recognition of "subclinical" thyroid disease as a distinct clinical entity [64]. By definition, patients with subclinical thyroid disease are those healthy individuals with an abnormal sensitive TSH value with an FTI in the normal range. As seen above, this pattern of TSH and FTI values is not uncommon in the critically ill patient and rarely indicates intrinsic thyroid disease on follow-up testing when the patient has recovered. In addition, there is no consensus on the indications for treatment in an individual healthy patient with subclinical thyroid disease. Finally, the "subclinical" aspects of this disorder make it less likely to have significant impact on the clinical course of the critically ill patient.

Secondary Tests

TOTAL T$_3$. As discussed above, serum T$_3$ concentrations are affected to the greatest degree by the alterations in thyroid hormone economy resulting from acute illness. Therefore, there is no indication for routine measurement of serum T$_3$ levels in the initial evaluation of thyroid function in the critically ill patient. This test should be obtained only if thyrotoxicosis is clinically suspected in the presence of a suppressed sensitive TSH value and an elevated or high normal FTI determination [65]. Thus, in patients with an elevated FTI and a suppressed TSH, the finding of an elevated serum T$_3$ concentration differentiates between thyrotoxicosis and the high T$_4$ state of sick euthyroid syndrome.

THYROID AUTOANTIBODIES. Autoantibodies to two intrinsic thyroid proteins, thyroglobulin and thyroid peroxidase (TPO), are commonly available. While significant titers of either or both of these antibodies indicate the presence of autoimmune thyroid disease, the presence of thyroid autoantibodies does not necessary indicate thyroid dysfunction. Thyroid autoantibodies do add to the sensitivity of abnormal TSH and FTI values in diagnosing intrinsic thyroid disease [37,38,66,67,68]. In one series, more than 60 percent of acutely ill patients with suppressed

TSH values and positive thyroid antibodies were subsequently diagnosed with thyroid disease, compared to less than 15 percent of patients with negative antibodies [37,38]. In patients with elevated TSH values less than 20 mU per liter, thyroid disease was present in 50 percent of those with positive antibodies, as opposed to less than 5 percent of those with negative antibodies.

DIAGNOSIS. As indicated above, the diagnostic significance of a single abnormal thyroid function test is low. The best single test to screen for thyroid dysfunction is the FTI, although subtle changes in thyroid function will be missed. A reasonable approach to the initial evaluation of thyroid function in the critically ill patient is to obtain both an FTI and TSH measurements in patients with a high clinical suspicion for intrinsic thyroid dysfunction. Assessment of these values in the context of the duration, severity, and stage of illness of the patient allows the correct diagnosis in most patients. For example, a mildly elevated TSH coupled with a low FTI is more likely to indicate primary hypothyroidism early in an acute illness as opposed to the same values obtained during the recovery phase of the illness. Similarly, the combination of an elevated TSH and low normal FTI is more likely to indicate thyroid dysfunction in the hypothermic, bradycardic patient than the tachycardic, normothermic individual. If both FTI and TSH are normal, thyroid dysfunction is effectively eliminated as a contributing factor to the clinical picture. If the diagnosis is still unclear, measurement of thyroid antibodies is helpful as a marker of intrinsic thyroid disease and increases the sensitivity of both the FTI and the TSH. Only in the case of a suppressed TSH and a mid- to high normal FTI is measurement of serum T_3 levels indicated.

TREATMENT WITH THYROID HORMONE. Whether sick euthyroid syndrome in critically ill patients represents an adaptive or a pathologic response to illness remains unclear. It is clear that supplemental thyroid hormone therapy, in the form of either L-T_4 or L-T_3, has no effect on outcome and is therefore not indicated [22,45,46]. One prospective study examined the effect of thyroid hormone therapy in ICU patients with serum T_4 levels less than 5 μg per deciliter but with no evidence of intrinsic thyroid dysfunction [45]. Either T_4 or placebo was given daily intravenously, with subsequent normalization of serum T_4 levels by day 5 in the T_4-treated group. There was no difference in mortality between the two groups and the elevation of TSH and serum T_3 concentrations seen in the recovery phase of acute illness was delayed in the T_4-treated group, suggesting that T_4 replacement was detrimental to the restoration of normal pituitary-thyroid regulation. Another study examined the effect of treatment with T_3 in patients with acute burn injuries and found no change in either mortality or basal metabolic rate [46].

Summary

The spectrum of alterations in thyroid hormone concentrations and regulation seen in the critically ill patient are the result of a coordinated systemic reaction to illness and most likely represent an adaptive response of the endocrine system to acute illness. Interpretation of thyroid function tests in the ICU patient and identification of patients with intrinsic thyroid dysfunction are often difficult and must take into consideration both the clinical assessment and the duration and severity of illness.

Whenever possible, it is best to defer the evaluation of thyroid function until the patient has recovered from the critical illness.

References

1. Chopra IJ, Hershman JH, Pardridge WM, Nicoloff JT: Thyroid function in nonthyroidal illness. *Ann Intern Med* 98:926, 1983.
2. Kaptein EM: Thyroid hormone metabolism in illness, in Hennemann G (ed): *Thyroid Hormone Metabolism.* New York, Marcel Dekker, 1986.
3. Nicoloff JT, Lopresti JS: Nonthyroidal illness, in Braverman LE, Utiger RD (eds): *The Thyroid.* 6th ed. Philadelphia, JB Lippincott, 1991.
4. Chopra IJ: Euthyroid sick syndrome: Abnormalities in circulating thyroid hormones and thyroid hormone physiology in nonthyroidal illness. *Med Grand Rounds* 1:201, 1982.
5. Morley JE, Slag MF, Elson MK, Shafer RB: The interpretation of thyroid function tests in hospitalized patients. *JAMA* 249:2377, 1983.
6. Quint AR, Kaiser FE: Gonadotropin determinations and thyrotropin-releasing hormone and luteinizing hormone-releasing hormone testing in critically ill postmenopausal women with hypothyroxinemia. *J Clin Endocrinol Metab* 60:464, 1985.
7. Woolf PD, Hamill RW, McDonald JV, et al: Transient hypogonadism caused by critical illness. *J Clin Endocrinol Metab* 60:444, 1985.
8. Parker LN, Levin ER, Lifrak ET: Evidence for adrenocortical adaptation to severe illness. *J Clin Endocrinol Metab* 60:947, 1985.
9. Fujii T, Sato K, Ozawa M, et al: Effect of interleukin-1 on thyroid hormone metabolism in mice: Stimulation by IL-1 of iodothyronine 5'-deiodinating activity (type I) in the liver. *J Clin Endocrinol Metab* 124:167, 1989.
10. Chopra IJ, Sakane S, Chua Teco GN: A study of the serum concentration of tumor necrosis factor-alpha in thyroidal and nonthyroidal illness. *J Clin Endocrinol Metab* 72:1113, 1991.
11. Larsen PR, Silva JE, Kaplan MM: Relationships between circulating and intracellular thyroid hormones: Physiological and clinical implications. *Endocr Rev* 2:87, 1981.
12. Koehrle J, Brabant G, Hesch RD: Metabolism of thyroid hormones. *Hormone Res* 26:58, 1987.
13. Leonard JL, Visser TJ: Biochemistry of deiodination, in Hennemann G (ed): *Thyroid Hormone Metabolism.* New York, Marcel Dekker, 1986.
14. Burger A: Nondeiodinative pathways of thyroid hormone metabolism, in Hennemann G (ed): *Thyroid Hormone Metabolism.* New York, Marcel Dekker, 1986.
15. Oppenheimer JH, Schwartz HL, Mariash CN, et al: Advances in our understanding of thyroid hormone action at the cellular level. *Endocr Rev* 8:288, 1987.
16. Robbins J: Thyroid hormone transport proteins and the physiology of hormone binding, in Braverman LE, Utiger RD (eds): *The Thyroid.* 6th ed. Philadelphia, JB Lippincott, 1991.
17. Chopra IJ, Huang T-S, Beredo A, et al: Evidence for an inhibitor of extrathyroidal conversion of thyroxine to 3,5,3'-triiodothyronine in sera of patients with nonthyroidal illness. *J Clin Endocrinol Metab* 60:666, 1985.
18. Chopra IJ, Chopra U, Smith SR, et al: Reciprocal changes in serum concentrations of 3,3',5'-triiodothyronine (reverse T3) and 3,3',5-triiodothyronine (T3) in systemic illnesses. *J Clin Endocrinol Metab* 41:1043, 1975.
19. Chopra IS, Santini F, Wu S, Hind RE: The role of sulfation and desulfation in thyroid hormone metabolism, in *Thyroid Hormone Metabolism,* Wu S, Visser TS (eds). Boca Raton, FL, CRC Press, 1994, pp. 119–138.
20. Nicoloff JP, LoPresti SS: Nonintegrated assessment of prereceptor regulation of thyroid hormone metabolism, in *Thyroid Hormone Metabolism,* Wu S, Visser TS (eds). Boca Raton, FL, CRC Press, 1994, pp. 75–84.
21. Faber J, Kirkegaard C, Rasmussen B, et al: Pituitary-thyroid axis in critical illness. *J Clin Endocrinol Metab* 65:315, 1987.
22. Kaptein EM, Weiner JM, Robinson WJ, et al: Relationship of altered

thyroid hormone indices to survival in nonthyroidal illness. *Clin Endocrinol (Oxf)* 16:565, 1982.

23. Kaptein EM, Spencer CA, Kamiel MB, Nicoloff JT: Prolonged dopamine administration and thyroid hormone economy in normal and critically ill subjects. *J Clin Endocrinol Metab* 51:387, 1980.

24. Jackson IM: Thyrotropin-releasing hormone. *N Engl J Med* 306:145, 1982.

25. Bellabarba D, Inada M, Varsano-Aharon N, Sterling K: Thyroxine transport and turnover in major nonthyroidal illness. *J Clin Endocrinol Metab* 28:1023, 1968.

26. Yamanaka T, Ido K, Kimura K, Saito T: Serum levels of thyroid hormones in liver diseases. *Clin Chim Acta* 101:45, 1980.

27. LoPresti JS, Fried JC, Spencer CA, Nicoloff JT: Unique alterations of thyroid hormone indices in the acquired immunodeficiency syndrome (AIDS). *Ann Intern Med* 110:970, 1989.

28. Kaptein EM, Grieb DA, Spencer CA, et al: Thyroxine metabolism in the low thyroxine state of critical nonthyroidal illness. *J Clin Endocrinol Metab* 53:764, 1981.

29. Chopra IJ, Solomon DH, Hepner GW, Morgenstein AA: Misleadingly low free thyroxine index and usefulness of reverse triiodothyronine measurement in nonthyroidal illness. *Ann Intern Med* 90:905, 1979.

30. Oppenheimer JH, Schwartz HL, Mariash CN, Kaiser FE: Evidence for a factor in the sera of patients with nonthyroidal disease which inhibits iodothyronine binding to solid matrices, serum proteins, and rat hepatocytes. *J Clin Endocrinol Metab* 54:757, 1982.

31. Chopra IJ, Huang T-S, Solomon DH, et al: The role of T4-binding serum proteins in oleic acid-induced increase in free T4 in nonthyroidal illnesses. *J Clin Endocrinol Metab* 63:776, 1986.

32. Stockigt JR, Lim CF, Barlow JW, et al: High concentrations of furosemide inhibit serum binding of thyroxine. *J Clin Endocrinol Metab* 59:62, 1984.

33. Burger AG: Effects of phamacological agents on thyroid hormone metabolism, in Braverman LE, Utiger RD (eds): *The Thyroid*. 6th ed. Philadelphia, JB Lippincott, 1991.

34. Surks MI, Chopra IJ, Mariash CN, et al: American Thyroid Association guidelines for the use of laboratory tests in thyroid disease. *JAMA* 263:1529, 1990.

35. Nelson JC, Weiss RM: The effect of serum dilution on free thyroxine concentration in the low T4 syndrome of nonthyroidal illness. *J Clin Endocrinol Metab* 61:239, 1985.

36. Bermudez F, Surks MI, Oppenheimer JH: High incidence of decreased serum triiodothyronine concentration in patients with nonthyroidal disease. *J Clin Endocrinol Metab* 41:27, 1975.

37. Spencer CA: Clinical utility and cost-effectiveness of sensitive thyrotropin assays in ambulatory and hospitalized patients. *Mayo Clin Proc* 63:1214, 1988.

38. Spencer C, Elgen A, Shen D, et al: Specificity of sensitive assays of thyrotropin (TSH) used to screen for thyroid disease in hospitalized patients. *Clin Chem* 33:1391, 1987.

39. Burrows AW, Shakespear RA, Hesch RD, et al: Thyroid hormones in the elderly sick: "T4 euthyroidism." *Br Med J* 4:437, 1975.

40. Spratt DI, Pont A, Miller MB, et al: Hyperthyroxinemia in patients with acute psychiatric disorders. *Am J Med* 73:41, 1982.

41. Slag MF, Morley JE, Elson MK, et al: Hypothyroxinemia in critically ill patients as a predictor of high mortality. *JAMA* 245:43, 1981.

42. Maldonado LS, Murata GH, Hershman JM, Braunstein GD: Do thyroid function tests independently predict survival in the critically ill? *Thyroid* 2:119, 1992.

43. Kaptein EM, Macintyre SS, Weiner JM, et al: Free thyroxine estimates in nonthyroidal illness: Comparison of eight methods. *J Clin Endocrinol Metab* 52:1073, 1981.

44. Slag MF, Morley JE, Elson MK, et al: Free thyroxine levels in critically ill patients: A comparison of currently available assays. *JAMA* 246:2702, 1981.

45. Brent GA, Hershman JM: Thyroxine therapy in patients with severe nonthyroidal illnesses and low thyroxine concentration. *J Clin Endocrinol Metab* 63:1, 1986.

46. Becker RA, Vaughan GM, Zeigler MG, et al: Hypermetabolic low triiodothyronine syndrome of burn injury. *Crit Care Med* 10:870, 1982.

47. Hamblin S, Dyer SA, Mohr VS, et al: Relationship between thyrotropin and thyroxine changes during recovery from severe hypothyroxinemia of critical illness. *J Clin Endocrinol Metab* 62:717, 1986.

48. Balsam A, Ingbar SH: Observations on the factors that control the generation of triiodothyronine from thyroxine in rat liver and the nature of the defect induced by fasting. *J Clin Invest* 63:1145, 1979.

49. Portnay GI, O'Brian JT, Bush J, et al: The effect of starvation on the concentration and binding of thyroxine and triiodothyronine in serum and on the response to TRH. *J Clin Endocrinol Metab* 39:199, 1974.

50. Visser TJ, Lamberts SWJ, Wilson JHP, et al: Serum thyroid hormone concentrations during prolonged reduction of dietary intake. *Metabolism* 27:405, 1978.

51. Gardner DF, Kaplan MM, Stanley CA, Utiger RD: Effect of tri-iodothyronine replacement on the metabolic and pituitary responses to starvation. *N Engl J Med* 300:579, 1979.

52. Richmand DA, Molitch ME, O'Donnell TF: Altered thyroid hormone levels in bacterial sepsis: The role of nutritional adequacy. *Metabolism* 29:936, 1980.

53. Fried JC, LoPresti JS, Micon M, et al: Serum triiodothyronine values: Prognostic indicators of acute mortality due to *Pneumocystis carinii* pneumonia associated with the acquired immunodeficiency syndrome. *Arch Intern Med* 150:406, 1990.

54. Chopra IJ, Solomon DH, Chopra U, et al: Alterations in circulating thyroid hormones and thyrotropin in hepatic cirrhosis: Evidence for euthyroidism despite subnormal serum triiodothyronine. *J Clin Endocrinol Metab* 39:501, 1974.

55. Nicoloff JT, Spencer CA: Clinical review 12: The use and misuse of the sensitive thyrotropin assays. *J Clin Endocrinol Metab* 71:553, 1990.

56. Spencer CA, LoPresti JS, Patel A, et al: Applications of a new chemiluminometric thyrotropin assay to subnormal measurement. *J Clin Endocrinol Metab* 70:453, 1990.

57. Szabolcs I, Ploenes C, Bernard W, Herrmann J: Screening of geriatric patients for thyroid dysfunction with thyrotropin-releasing-hormone test, sensitive thyrotropin and free thyroxine estimation. *Horm Metab Res* 22:298, 1990.

58. Kaplan MM, Larsen PR, Crantz FR, et al: Prevalence of abnormal thyroid function test results in patients with acute medical illnesses. *Am J Med* 72:9, 1982.

59. Helfand M, Crapo L: Screening for thyroid disease. *Ann Intern Med* 112:840, 1990.

60. DeGroot LJ, Mayor G: Admission screening by thyroid function tests in an acute general care teaching hospital. *Am J Med* 93:558, 1992.

61. Liewendahl K, Mahonen H, Tikanoja S, et al: Performance of direct equilibrium dialysis and analogue-type free thyroid hormone assays, and an immunoradiometric TSH method in patients with thyroid dysfunction. *Scand J Clin Lab Invest* 47:421, 1987.

62. Nuutila P, Irjala K, Viikari J, et al: Comparative evaluation of serum thyroxine, free thyroxine and thyrotropin determinations in screening of thyroid function. *Ann Clin Res* 20:158, 1988.

63. Tikanoja S: Ultrafiltration devices tested for use in a free thyroxine assay validated by comparison with equilibrium dialysis. *Scand J Clin Lab Invest* 50:663, 1990.

64. Cooper DS: Subclinical hypothyroidism. *Adv Endocrinol Metabol* 2:77–88, 1991.

65. Gavin LA, Rosenthal M, Cavalieri RR: The diagnostic dilemma of isolated hyperthyroxinemia in acute illness. *JAMA* 242:251, 1979.

66. Hawkins BR, Dawkins RL, Burger HG, et al: Diagnostic significance of thyroid microsomal antibodies in randomly selected population. *Lancet* 2:1057, 1980.

67. Rosenthal MJ, Hunt WC, Garry PJ, Goodwin JS: Thyroid failure in the elderly: Microsomal antibodies as discriminant for therapy. *JAMA* 258:209, 1987.

68. Sawin CT, Bigos ST, Land S, Bacharach P: The aging thyroid: Relationships between elevated serum thyrotropin level and thyroid antibodies in elderly patients. *Am J Med* 79:591, 1985.

IX. Hematologic Problems in the Intensive Care Unit

Section Editor
Jack E. Ansell

118. Acquired Bleeding Disorders

Jack E. Ansell

The critical care physician is often called on to manage patients with excessive posttraumatic or postsurgical bleeding or excessive hemorrhage during the course of a fulminant illness [1]. As such, a working knowledge of hemostatic reactions is an essential quality to possess. Table 118-1 briefly classifies hemorrhagic disorders that can be attributed to coagulation and platelet defects and indicates those entities that are likely to be seen in an intensive care setting. As the classification scheme indicates, coagulation and platelet disorders result from functional defects or quantitative deficiencies.

Although hemorrhage can also result from undue stress on a normal hemostatic system, this chapter focuses on pathologic bleeding, particularly the bleeding that results from acquired coagulation defects and acquired qualitative platelet defects. (See Chaps. 119 and 120 for discussions of hereditary coagulation disorders and quantitative platelet disorders.)

Platelet Physiology

Platelet reactions may be divided into three distinguishable events: adhesion, secretion, and aggregation [2]. Adhesion is the property of stickiness whereby platelets interact with certain surfaces, such as subendothelial collagen, and to a lesser extent, basement membrane and other subendothelial-supporting elements.

The platelet possesses a number of surface receptor molecules, many of which belong to the integrin family of adhesion receptors that serve as receptors for various ligands that participate in platelet adhesion. An essential non-integrin receptor that mediates adhesion, however, is the glycoprotein I_b-IX (GPI$_b$-IX) complex, which serves as a receptor for von Willebrand factor (vWF) [3]. Von Willebrand factor is a large multimeric plasma protein circulating in complex with factor VIII that links the platelet to subendotheial collagen. In the absence of von Willebrand factor (specifically, in von Willebrand's disease), or the absence of glycoprotein I_b (specifically, in Bernard-Soulier syndrome), platelet adhesion is abnormal while other platelet functions are generally maintained, including the release mechanism and aggregation [4].

After adherence to collagen, platelets are activated and undergo a release reaction and secrete a number of endogenous substances. Platelet activation requires an initiating event such as contact with collagen or exposure to thrombin. This leads to signal transduction mediated by effector molecules in the platelet membrane such as phospholipase C (PLC), phospholipase A_2(PLA$_2$), or adenyl cyclase (activation of the latter leads to platelet inhibition) [5]. Activation of these effector molecules is regulated by guanine nucleotide binding proteins (G proteins). Second messenger molecules are then generated, which in the the case of PLC leads to calcium release from the platelet-dense tubular system, and in the case of PLA$_2$ leads to arachidonic acid liberation and thromboxane A_2 (TxA$_2$) generation. TxA$_2$ diffuses across the platelet membrane, where it serves as a potent activator of nearby platelets. Although platelet activation, secretion, and aggregation can occur without TxA$_2$ formation, its relative importance is demonstrated by the mild

platelet disorder and potential bleeding that can occur with use of aspirin or nonsteroidal antiinflammatory drugs, agents that inhibit TxA$_2$ synthesis.

In the process of activation platelets change from a discoid structure to a spherical shape [3]. This process of change of shape involves pseudopod extension and internal contraction, and these events are energy dependent and intimately related to the platelet-contractile proteins, actin and myosin. As noted, the initiation and regulation of this process of shape change and secretion involves the liberation of calcium and generation of prostaglandins. Calcium activates phosphorylation enzymes that facilitate actin-myosin coupling. Levels of cyclic adenosine monophosphate (AMP) are also critical in regulating calcium levels in the platelet.

The release reaction involves the secretion of a number of endogenous platelet substances from platelet granules (Table 118-2). Many of these substances are agonists activating other

Table 118-1. Classification of Hemostatic Disorders and Sources of Pathologic Bleeding

I. Platelet disorders
  A. Quantitative platelet disorders (thrombocytopenia)
    1. Deficient or abnormal thrombopoiesis
      a. Stem cell defect: aplastic anemia
      b. Ineffective thrombopoiesis: B_{12} or folate deficiency
    2. Accelerated destruction, loss, or abnormal distribution
      a. Immunologic: Idiopathic thrombocytopenic purpura, drugs*
      b. Nonimmunologic: disseminated intravascular coagulation,* thrombotic thrombocytopenic purpura*
  B. Qualitative platelet disorders
    1. Congenital
      a. Adhesion defect: von Willebrand's disease
      b. Secretion defect: storage pool disease
      c. Aggregation defect: thrombasthenia
    2. Acquired
      a. Adhesion defect: uremia,* drugs*
      b. Secretion defect: drugs,* myeloproliferative disease
      c. Aggregation defect: drugs,* paraproteinemias, fibrin(ogen) degradation products*
II. Coagulation disorders
  A. Factor deficiencies
    1. Production defect
      a. Congenital: hemophilia
      b. Acquired: vitamin K deficiency,* liver disease,* drugs (coumarins)*
    2. Accelerated destruction
      a. Consumption: DIC,* fibrinolysis
      b. Loss: nephrotic syndrome
      c. Multifactorial: post–open heart surgery
    3. Dilutional: massive blood replacement*
  B. Inhibitors (anticoagulants)
    1. Antibodies to coagulation factors: factor VIII inhibitor
    2. Antibodies to phospholipid: lupuslike inhibitor
    3. Dysproteinemias
    4. Fibrin(ogen) degradation products*
    5. Heparin*

*Indicates those disorders likely to be seen in the intensive care unit DIC = disseminated intravascular coagulants.

Table 118-2. Substances Released by Platelets During Platelet Activation

δ-Granule (dense body)
  Agonists: ADP, ATP, serotonin, calcium
α-Granule
  Adhesive proteins: fibrinogen, fibronectin, vWF, thrombospondin, vitronectin
  Growth modulators: PDGF, CTAP III, TGF beta, platelet factor 4, thrombospondin
  Coagulation factors: factor V, HMWK, C1 INH, fibrinogen factor XI, protein S, PAI-1
Cytoplasmic factors
  Factor XIII, PDECGF
Lysosomes
  Lysosomal enzymes

PDGF = platelet-derived growth factor; CTAP III = connective tissue activating peptide; TGF beta = transforming growth factor; HMWK = high-molecular-weight kininogen; C1 INH = C1 inhibitor; PAI-1 = plasminogen activator inhibitor-1 (from reference 2).

platelets, chemicals influencing vascular tone, coagulation factors or phospholipid promoting thrombin formation, and factors promoting cellular growth [2]. Critical to this process is the exposure of another platelet receptor member of the integrin family of adhesive proteins, the glycoprotein II$_b$-III$_a$ complex, essential for the binding of fibrinogen [6]. These glycoproteins span the platelet membrane and are linked internally with the platelet-actin contractile protein. They bind fibrinogen at specific arginyl-glycyl-aspartic acid (RGD) recognition sites, a common mechanism of receptor recognition for adhesive proteins. Thus, fibrinogen serves as the bridge mediating platelet aggregation. As one might expect, platelet aggregation is defective if GP II$_b$-III$_a$ is absent (thrombasthenia, a rare congenital disorder) or if fibrinogen is absent (the rare congenital disorder of afibrinogenemia).

In summary, platelets are stimulated by adhesion to subendothelial elements. Calcium is liberated, and arachidonic acid is generated and channeled into thromboxane synthesis. Thromboxane A$_2$ mobilizes other platelets. Increases in cytosolic calcium regulate enzymes for actin-myosin coupling. The release reaction ensues, and platelets secrete their granular contents. These substances initiate similar reactions in nearby platelets. Fibrinogen receptors are exposed, and platelets begin to aggregate to form a platelet thrombus. This primary platelet plug must be stabilized by the deposition of fibrin, the end product of the coagulation cascade as described in the following discussion.

Coagulation Physiology

The coagulation phase of hemostasis involves a sequential series of chemical reactions in the blood between a number of proteins or coagulation factors that results in fibrin clot formation (Fig. 118-1) [7]. The participants in these reactions can be grouped into functional classes (Table 118-3): (1) the zymogens (proenzymes), or inactive precursors of factors XIII, XII, XI, X, IX, VII, II, and prekallikrein; (2) the cofactors (factors VIII, V, and high-molecular-weight kininogen), which accelerate the rate of zymogen activation; (3) fibrinogen, the final substrate from which a clot is formed; and (4) the inhibitors, which restrict or limit the degree of clot formation.

The zymogens XII, XI, X, IX, II, prekallikrein, and factor VII are serine proteases (having serine at the active center of the enzyme) that cleave specific peptide bonds in other zymogens, leading to their activation. Factor XIII is a transglutaminase that introduces covalent bonds between lysine and glutamine residues that lie between polymerized fibrin monomers. Many of the reactions in the coagulation cascade require divalent cations (Ca^{2+}) and occur much more rapidly on phospholipid surfaces (the platelet membrane or platelet factor 3).

All coagulation factors are synthesized in the liver, including factor VIII. Von Willebrand factor is synthesized by endothelial

Fig. 118-1. Coagulation cascade. HMW = high molecular weight; PL = phospholipid. (Adapted from Murano G: A basic outline of blood coagulation. *Semin Thromb Hemost* 6:140, 1980.)

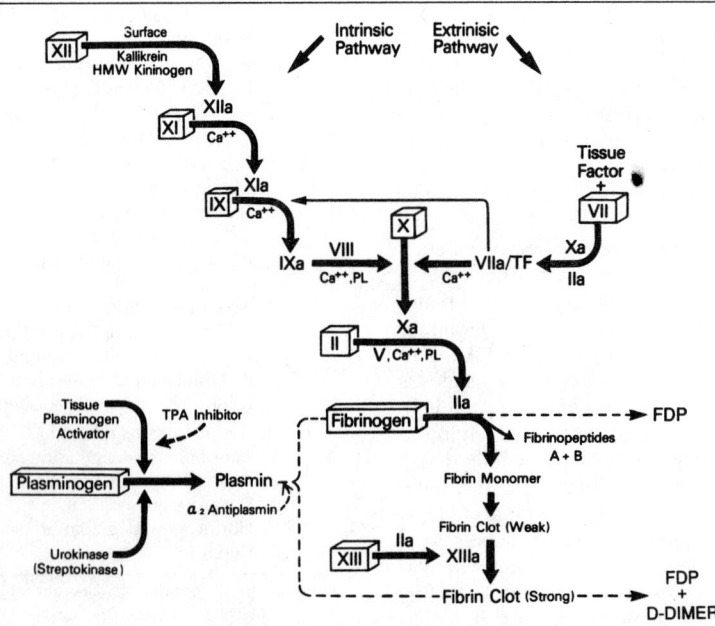

Table 118-3. Characteristics of Coagulation Factors

Factor	Descriptive name(s)	Source	Approximate half-life (hr)	Function
I	Fibrinogen	Liver	120	Substrate for fibrin clot (CP)
II	Prothrombin	Liver (VKD)	60	Serine protease (CP)
V	Proaccelerin; labile factor	Liver	12–36	Cofactor (CP)
VII	Serum prothrombin conversion accelerator; proconvertin	Liver (VKD)	6	Serine protease (EP)
VIII	Antihemophilic factor; globulin	Liver	12	Cofactor (IP)
IX	Plasma thromboplastin component; Christmas factor	Liver (VKD)	24	Serine protease (IP)
X	Stuart-Prower factor	Liver (VKD)	36	Serine protease (CP)
XI	Plasma thromboplastin antecedent	Liver	40–84	Serine protease (IP)
XII	Hageman factor	Liver	50	Serine protease, contact activation (IP)
XIII	Fibrin stabilizing factor	Liver	96–180	Transglutaminase (CP)
Prekallikrein	Fletcher factor	Liver	?	Serine protease, contact activation (IP)
High-molecular-weight kininogen	Fitzgerald factor; Flaujeac factor; or Williams factor	Liver	?	Cofactor, contact activation (IP)

VKD = vitamin K-dependent; CP = common pathway; EP = extrinsic pathway; IP = intrinsic pathway.

cells throughout the vascular system as well as by megakaryocytes. Factors II, VII, IX, and X require vitamin K for their normal synthesis. Vitamin K participates in a reaction that adds a carboxyl group to the gamma-carbon atom of glutamic acid residues in the precursors of these factors [8].

The gamma-carboxyglutamic acid residues are responsible for calcium and phospholipid binding. In their absence, the proteins circulate as nonfunctional precursors, because they cannot bind to phospholipid. As a result, measurement of the factors by functional assays, such as prothrombin time (PT) or partial thromboplastin time (PTT), shows very low levels. However, immunologic assays that use a precipitation reaction with heterologous antibodies show normal levels, because the nonfunctional proteins retain their antigenic characteristics.

COAGULATION REACTIONS. The sequence of coagulation reactions can be analyzed beginning with the last stage in the coagulation cascade, the formation of a fibrin clot (see Fig. 118-1). Fibrin formation can be divided into three steps: proteolysis and release of two small peptides, polymerization of the remaining fibrin monomers, and stabilization of the fibrin clot [9]. Thrombin, a serine protease, cleaves two small peptides (peptides A and B) from the amino terminal end of the alpha- and beta-chains of fibrinogen. The resulting fibrin monomers spontaneously polymerize to form a weak clot that is soluble in high-ionic-strength solutions. The fibrin monomers, held together by electrostatic forces, are then stabilized by the introduction of covalent disulfide bonds between the gamma- and alpha-chains by the action of factor XIII. Factor XIII must first be activated by exposure to thrombin.

Thrombin is derived from its inactive precursor, prothrombin or factor II [10], by a series of proteolytic steps initiated by activated factor X (X_a). X_a functions optimally in the presence of Ca^{2+}, factor V, and a phospholipid surface (the prothrombinase complex). Factor V is thought to maintain the integrity of the complex of X_a and II on the phospholipid surface, so that optimal concentration gradients can exist and allow the reaction to proceed at a maximal rate. In the process of throm-

bin formation, a prothrombin fragment (PTF1.2) is generated. Identification of this cleavage product in plasma has been used as a sign of hemostatic activation in settings of suspected hypercoagulability.

Factor X_a is derived from its inactive precursor, as are the other serine proteases. Two interrelated pathways of activation, termed the *extrinsic* and *intrinsic pathways,* are important. The rapidly acting extrinsic pathway is initiated by tissue factor, a transmembrane protein expressed in stimulated endothelial cells [11]. In the presence of calcium ions, tissue factor complexes with factor VII or VII_a, and it is thought that this complex activates small amounts of factor X. Activated factor X then feeds back to activate factor VII to VII_a in a cyclic fashion. The intrinsic pathway of factor X activation is mediated by a complex composed of activated factor IX, factor VIII, Ca^{2+}, and phospholipid. Factor VIII serves as a cofactor, and its activity is significantly enhanced by the feedback interaction with thrombin, which cleaves a number of sites to form an activated factor VIII light chain [12]. This cleavage of factor VIII also releases it from its binding to von Willebrand factor so that it can function in factor X activation. The phospholipid surface is provided by the platelet membrane (platelet factor 3), and IX_a is a serine protease that converts factor X to its active form.

Activated factor IX is derived from the proteolytic cleavage of its precursor in the presence of Ca^{2+} by activated factor XI. Recent studies have shown that factor IX can also be activated by the reaction product of tissue factor—factor VII (the extrinsic system)—and that this pathway has physiologic significance in vivo.

The initial steps of the intrinsic coagulation pathway are complex [13]. Factors XII, XI, prekallikrein, and high-molecular-weight kininogen (HMWK) are involved in the contact activation of the intrinsic system. Factor XII and prekallikrein reciprocally activate each other, and HMWK, a cofactor, participates in the binding of prekallikrein and factor XI to the surface where activation occurs. This sequence of reactions is initiated by the association of factor XII with a negatively charged surface. Many substances can serve this function in vitro, including glass, kaolin, celite, and endotoxin. Surfaces of physiologic importance in vivo appear to be collagen and subendothelial connective tissue that are exposed by injury, as well as platelet membrane phospholipid.

Factor XII undergoes a conformational change, leading to minimal activation, as well as making it highly susceptible to proteolytic cleavage by kallikrein. Activated factor XII (XII_a) then enzymatically converts prekallikrein to kallikrein, and the reciprocal nature of the interaction continues. XII_a is a pivotal factor with the ability to initiate several physiologic biochemical systems, including the kinin system, the fibrinolytic mechanism, the complement system, and factor XI in the coagulation cascade. Factor XI activation by XII_a occurs on a negatively charged surface where factor XI is bound by HMWK. The activation process continues with XI_a converting factor IX to its activated form.

INHIBITORY MECHANISMS. A number of inhibitory mechanisms limit the process of fibrin deposition, so that neither disseminated coagulation nor extensive local thrombosis occurs after injury. These mechanisms include "self-inhibitors," specific inhibitors, and compartmentalization of reactions (Fig. 118-2).

Activated procoagulants inhibit their own further generation (e.g., inhibitory activity of excess X_a on factor VII, and of excess thrombin on factors V and VIII). There are also specific inhibitors of coagulation factors. Antithrombin III is an important inhibitor of the activated serine proteases, including thrombin, X_a, IX_a, XI_a, XII_a and kallikrein [14], although its principal effect appears to be on factor X_a and thrombin. Heparin cofactor II, a recently recognized inhibitor, neutralizes the activity of thrombin (II_a) [15]. The inhibitory activity of both of these proteins is enhanced considerably by their association with heparin. Protein C is an inhibitor of activated factors V and VIII [16]. Protein C is a vitamin K–dependent serine protease that requires activation by thrombin in conjunction with an endothelial cell membrane–based protein (thrombomodulin). Protein S is a cofactor necessary for protein C function and serves to stabilize the inhibitor reaction on the platelet membrane [16]. Lastly, tissue factor pathway inhibitor is a very recently described inhibitor of the factor VII-X_a interaction, although its physiologic importance is still uncertain [17].

Another means of limiting the degree of coagulation is by compartmentalization of reactions. Most coagulation reactions have specific requirements for optimal activity, such as phospholipid surfaces. Compartmentalization, which limits interaction of all necessary factors, can limit these reactions.

Additional limiting factors include cellular clearance mechanisms and the fibrinolytic system. Activated coagulation factors are rapidly cleared from the blood by the reticuloendothelial cells, primarily those in the liver. The major component of the fibrinolytic system is plasminogen [18], a serine protease that must be activated to plasmin by specific activators, the major one being tissue plasminogen activator released from endothelial cells (see Fig. 118-1) [19]. Plasmin degrades fibrin clots as well as soluble fibrinogen to generate a number of fragments. These fibrin(ogen) degradation products (FDP) can inhibit additional fibrin monomer polymerization, and thus predispose to poor clot formation and bleeding. In addition to activators of plasminogen, there are also inhibitors of fibrinolysis, the major ones being alpha$_2$-antiplasmin and plasminogen activator inhibitor [20].

Laboratory Evaluation of Hemostasis

To understand the pathophysiology of hemostatic derangements and to arrive at definitive diagnoses, great reliance must be placed upon the laboratory evaluation of these disorders.

PLATELETS. The platelet component of hemostasis can be measured both quantitatively and qualitatively. Thrombocytopenia can be estimated from the blood smear (one platelet per oil-immersion field is equivalent to 15,000 platelets/μl). More accurate counts can be performed by microscopy or electronic particle counting equipment. A bone marrow examination can provide information as to the cause of thrombocytopenia by indicating increased or decreased platelet production by quantitation of megakaryocytes (increased megakaryocytes suggest platelet destruction). Platelet size on peripheral blood smear may similarly be helpful; large platelets suggest a shortened survival and rapid platelet turnover.

Platelet functional impairment can also be a cause for a platelet-related hemostatic defect. The bleeding time (BT) measures various aspects of platelet function as well as vascular competency [21]. The bleeding time is usually prolonged with any qualitative defect and thus has low specificity. Its value as a screening test to indicate the likelihood of bleeding as a result of a qualitative platelet disorder is quite low, and its use is not recommended for this purpose [22]. However, it may be useful in specific disorders known to predispose to a long BT such as von Willebrand disease or uremia.

Platelet aggregation studies further delineate platelet function abnormalities. A suspension of platelets in plasma transmits relatively little light when placed in a spectrophotometric light path. As platelets aggregate in response to the addition of specific aggregating reagents (e.g., epinephrine, ADP, collagen), more light is transmitted. This change in light transmittance is recorded on a chart recorder as a primary wave of aggregation

Fig. 118-2. The coagulation cascade indicating the site of action of inhibitors. AT III = antithrombin III; PC/PS = protein C/protein S; TFPI = tissue factor pathway inhibitor; HCoF II = heparin cofactor II; t-PA = tissue plasminogen activator; PAI = plasminogen activator inhibitor; FDP = fibrin(ogen) degradation products.

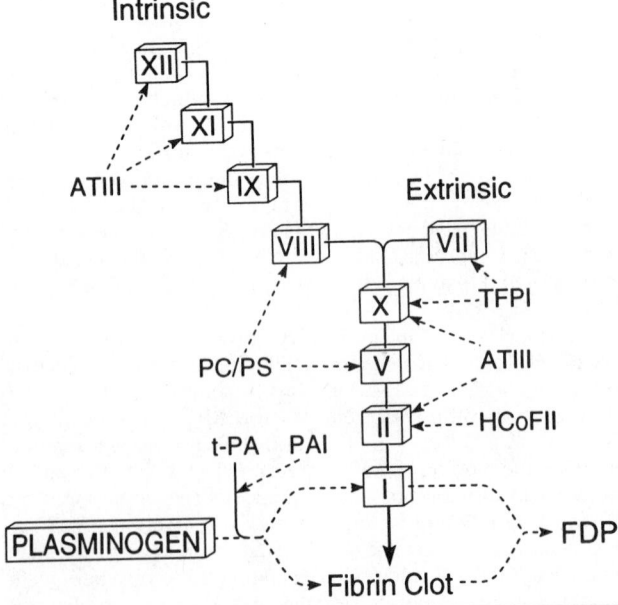

(response to the reagent added) and a secondary wave (response to the endogenous release of aggregating substances, such as adenosine diphosphate [ADP], after initial platelet activation).

Various disorders of platelet function have specific aggregation patterns. Other assays of platelet function include quantitation of the content of adenine nucleotides in platelet-dense bodies, measurement of the ability of platelets to take up and release serotonin, measurement of the availability of platelet factor 3, and assessment of the prostaglandin cascade, as well as others. Many of these assays are not routinely available in most hospitals and are of little value in the acute management of bleeding in the intensive care setting.

COAGULATION. The plasmatic or coagulation phase of hemostasis is readily accessible for evaluation (Fig. 118-3). The PT and PTT are two general screening tests of the extrinsic and intrinsic systems, respectively. The PT is initiated in the laboratory by the addition of tissue thromboplastin (tissue factor) and CaCl$_2$. A timer records the time it takes to form a fibrin clot, which is the end point of the PT. The activated PTT is initiated by the addition of a contact activator of factor XII, phospholipid, and CaCl$_2$. A fibrin clot is also the end point of this test.

The PT and PTT are prolonged in the presence of one or more factor deficiencies or in the presence of an acquired coagulation inhibitor. To determine whether a prolonged PT or PTT is attributable to a factor deficiency or an inhibitor, an "inhibitor screen" is performed. Although there are several methods of detecting an inhibitor, the basic concept is that the patient's plasma and pooled normal plasma are mixed in equal amounts, and the appropriate test (PT or PTT) is performed on the mixture. Complete to nearly complete correction of the abnormality after 60 minutes of incubation suggests a factor deficiency because the resulting mixture will have at least 50 percent of the deficient factor, which is adequate to produce a

normal clotting time. Little or no correction immediately or a loss of correction after incubation favors the presence of an inhibitor, because inhibitors neutralize the coagulation factors that are contributed by the normal plasma. The finding of an abnormal PT or PTT is not uncommon in seriously ill, hospitalized patients. Figure 118-4 outlines the approach to evaluation of a patient with a prolonged PT, PTT, or thrombin time (TT).

A TT is a measure of the time required to convert fibrinogen to a fibrin clot after the addition of purified thrombin to plasma. It is often a helpful assay because it is prolonged in only three circumstances: (1) the presence of deficient or functionally abnormal fibrinogen, (2) the presence of the anticoagulant heparin, and (3) the presence of a high titer of FDP.

FDP, which represents the proteolytic fragments of fibrinogen or fibrin produced by the effect of plasmin, can also be quantitated by a number of techniques. These include agglutination of latex beads coated with antisera to FDP or cross-linked fibrin fragments, agglutination of a specific strain of *Staphylococcus* that is sensitive to FDP, and by hemagglutination. Recently, antibodies specific for cross-linked fibrin fragments (d-dimer) have been developed [23]. Traditional assays detect proteolytic fragments of fibrinogen or fibrin, whereas the d-dimer test specifically detects fibrin fragments. When positive, this latter assay indirectly indicates that thrombin was initially generated, that it converted fibrinogen to fibrin, and that plasmin acted on fibrin; in other words, intravascular coagulation with secondary fibrinolysis or disseminated intravascular coagulation (DIC). A positive FDP does not discriminate between fibrinogen or fibrin proteolysis, and thus, between DIC and primary fibrinogenolysis.

Other important but less routine coagulation assays include biologic and immunologic measurements of specific coagulation factors, measurement of prothrombin consumption, measurement of the presence of fibrin monomers or fibrinopeptides A and B, various mixing experiments, plasminogen activity, and so on. A thorough description of these assays can be found in many textbooks of hemostasis, for example, Colman et al. [24].

Fig. 118-3. The plasmatic evaluation of hemostasis. A. Prothrombin time. B. Partial thromboplastin time. C. Thrombin time. HMW = high molecular weight; PL = phospholipid.

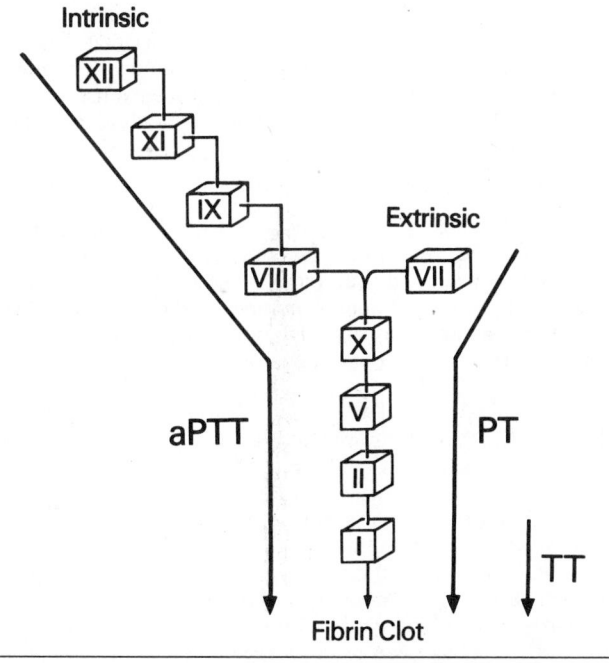

Acquired Qualitative Platelet Disorders

A reduction in the number of platelets is only one cause of a defective platelet phase of hemostasis. Poorly functioning platelets can also be responsible for a hemorrhagic tendency. Qualitative disorders of platelets may be acquired or congenital. The focus in this section is on acquired disorders, because they account for most qualitative platelet defects that are encountered in the intensive care unit. A discussion of thrombocytopenia can be found in Chapter 120.

Acquired disorders of platelet function affect the platelet reactions of adhesion, release, or aggregation [25]. Frequently, acquired disorders interfere with more than one of these reactions, whereas congenital defects are more restricted in this pathophysiology.

DRUGS. The most common cause of qualitative platelet disorders is drugs. The main offenders are aspirin and other nonsteroidal antiinflammatory medications [26] (see Chap. 154). Aspirin irreversibly acetylates and inactivates the enzyme cyclooxygenase, preventing the generation of prostaglandin intermediates and thromboxane A$_2$. The effect is permanent, rendering the platelet nonfunctional for its life span, and occurs

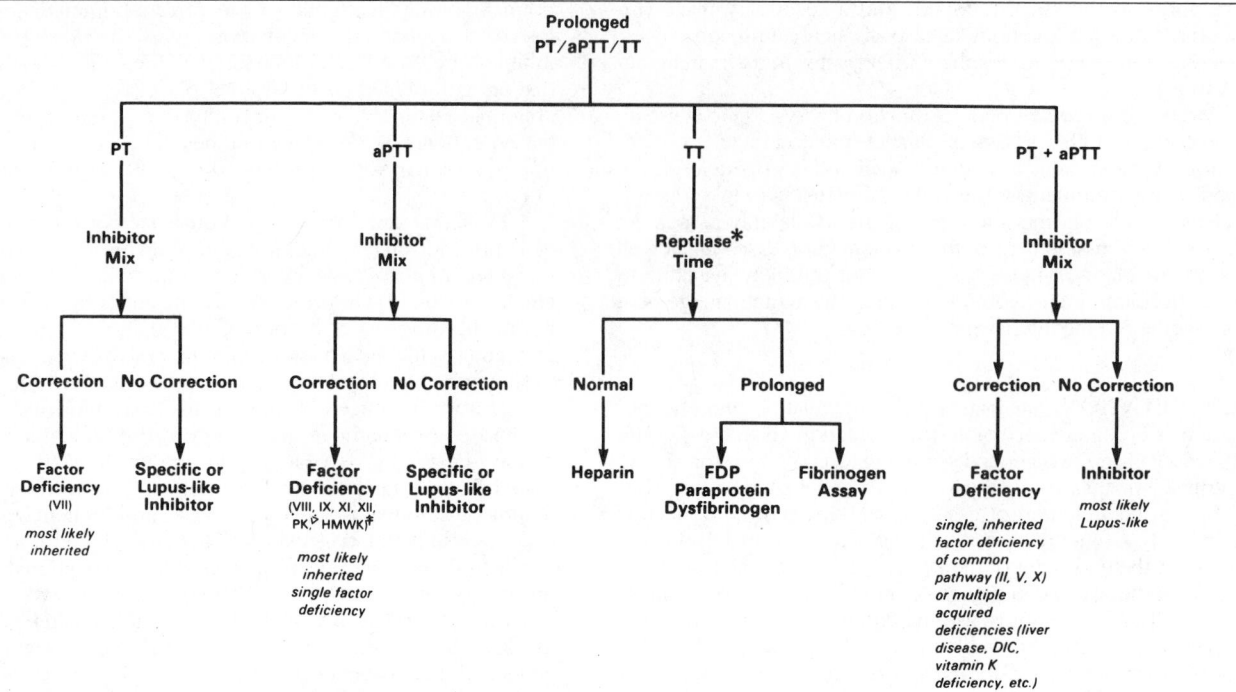

Fig. 118-4. Approach to the evaluation of a prolonged PT, aPTT, or TT.

only with acetylsalicylic acid and not with nonacetylated forms of aspirin. These platelets no longer undergo release, the bleeding time is prolonged, and secondary aggregation is poor or absent.

Aspirin is rapidly hydrolyzed to salicylate in the circulation (approximately 30 min) and affects only platelets, and perhaps, megakaryocytes, which are exposed during that time. One aspirin tablet (5 gr) is enough to prolong the bleeding time (usually 1½–2 times baseline) 2 hours later. The effect on these platelets, however, may be masked by new platelets entering the circulation over the next day or so, and hemostasis may return to normal within that time. However, in the patient who takes aspirin on a regular basis over several days, a period of 7 to 10 days is required for the production of adequate numbers of new platelets to normalize the bleeding time.

Because aspirin affects cyclooxygenase, it also interferes with prostacyclin production by endothelial cells, and thus removes an antiaggregatory substance from the circulation. There is good evidence, however, that this inhibitory effect requires higher doses of aspirin and is short acting because endothelial cells are able to generate new cyclooxygenase enzyme. Nonsteroidal antiinflammatory drugs other than aspirin cause a similar defect in cyclooxygenase activity, but the deficiency is reversible and lasts only as long as the drug is present in the circulation.

Two other medications used in the past to interfere with platelet function are dipyridamole (Persantine) and sulfinpyrazone, but their benefit is questionable, and their use as platelet function inhibitors is not recommended. Ticlopidine is a recently developed antiplatelet agent that does have clinical benefit and is used in some cases when aspirin is not effective (see Chap. 121).

A number of other drugs interfere with platelet function, many of which are commonly used in an intensive care setting. Table 118-4 lists the most likely offenders and their postulated mechanism of action. None of these drugs are known for their

tendency to induce spontaneous bleeding, but their use may exacerbate or enhance underlying hemostatic defects or worsen traumatic bleeding. Correction of a drug-induced platelet defect requires cessation of the medication.

Aspirin defects are not immediately reversible with the clearing of the drug from the bloodstream. If bleeding is serious, platelet transfusions can be administered, beginning with 6 to 8 units of random- or a single-donor pack of platelets. A baseline and posttransfusion bleeding time should be obtained to assess the response. The use of deamino-8-D-arginine vasopressin (DDAVP) has also been shown to improve the bleeding time in patients with some drug-induced qualitative platelet defects [27] (see the discussion under Uremia that follows). When drugs essential to the treatment of an individual cannot be easily discontinued, a risk-benefit assessment must be made carefully to determine whether to continue the drug in the face of bleeding.

UREMIA. Uremia is a common cause for a functional platelet defect [28]. The mechanism responsible for this qualitative defect is unknown, but it is probably related to the accumulation of an uncleared metabolite. A number of different substances have been incriminated, although none have been definitively shown to be the cause of platelet dysfunction in uremia. The bleeding time is often more than 15 or 20 minutes. Tests of adhesion and aggregation are often abnormal, and prostaglandin production may be impaired, as well as platelet factor 3 availability. Peritoneal dialysis and, to a lesser extent, hemodialysis have been shown to improve the bleeding time, but personal experience indicates that this is not always the case.

Studies that have used infusions of cryoprecipitate or DDAVP have been successful in correcting the bleeding time, suggesting that vWF may be important in this defect [29,30]. DDAVP is known to increase the synthesis and plasma levels of factor VIII and vWF and has been used therapeutically in hemophiliacs

Table 118-4. Drugs Associated With Platelet Dysfunction

Classification	Examples
Antibiotics	Penicillin and derivatives
	Nitrofurantoin
	Hydroxychloroquine
Antihistamines and antitussives	Diphenhydramine and others
	Glycerol guaiacolate
Antiinflammatory agents	Aspirin
	Other nonsteroidal antiinflam-
	matory agents
	Corticosteroids
Antithrombotic agents	Heparin
	Dextran
Calcium channel-blocking agents	Verapamil and others
Diuretics	Furosemide
Serotonin antagonists	Reserpine, cyproheptadine
Sympathetic blocking agents	Alpha-blockers (phentolamine)
	Beta-blockers (propranolol)
Tranquilizers and antipsychotic agents	Phenothiazines and derivatives
	Tricyclic antidepressants
Vasodilators	Sodium nitroprusside
	Nitroglycerin
Xanthine derivatives	Theophylline, caffeine
	Dipyridamole
Miscellaneous	Clofibrate
	Ethanol

[31]. Cryoprecipitate is a plasma fraction that is rich in factor VIII/vWF. Some studies suggest that these substances may increase the concentration of the large vWF multimers, which may enhance the aggregating ability of platelets. However, studies do not show abnormalities of vWF in patients with renal failure. Lastly, therapeutic improvement in the bleeding time has also been shown with the infusion of estrogens [32], but the mechanism of this effect remains unknown.

The infusion of donor platelets is not recommended in patients with uremia, because the platelet defect results from the plasma environment, and transfused platelets would be affected as much as endogenous platelets. When an invasive diagnostic procedure, such as a percutaneous biopsy, needs to be performed on a uremic individual, it may be safer to perform an open biopsy so that the surgeon has direct visualization and control of any sites of bleeding.

MYELOPROLIFERATIVE DISORDERS. Myeloproliferative disorders, such as essential thrombocythemia, chronic myelogenous leukemia, and myelofibrosis with myeloid metaplasia, are often associated with a qualitative platelet defect [33]. The defect arises from a stem cell abnormality, resulting in the production of abnormal platelets. Most often, the release reaction is defective and results in an aspirinlike defect in platelet aggregation studies. Bleeding as well as thrombosis may be a problem. The former should be amenable to platelet transfusions, although the bleeding time does not always return to normal as expected.

OTHER DISORDERS. Other conditions associated with functional platelet disorders include diseases associated with high plasma concentrations of FDP and paraproteinemias [25]. Both substances interfere with reactions on the platelet surface, lead-

ing to poor platelet plug formation. Platelet transfusions are not indicated, and correction of the defect depends on improvement of the underlying disease process and lowering the concentrations of FDP or paraproteins.

Acquired Coagulation Disorders

DEFICIENCY: ACQUIRED PRODUCTION DEFECT

Vitamin K Deficiency. Acquired coagulation factor deficiencies attributable to inadequate synthesis involve multiple factors, and can be attributed to either vitamin K deficiency, liver disease, or a combination of the two. The coumarin or indanedione anticoagulant drugs interfere with vitamin K metabolism and produce a deficiency of the vitamin K–dependent coagulation factors, thus producing a clinical state of apparent vitamin K deficiency and deficiencies of factors II, VII, IX, and X.

Vitamin K deficiency occurs predominantly in seriously and chronically ill patients [34], such as those seen in an intensive care unit. A lack of awareness on the part of the physician of the clinical setting and the pathophysiology of vitamin K deficiency is primarily responsible for the frequency of this easily preventable condition. Vitamin K is obtained not only from food (leafy colored vegetables, alfalfa) but also as a by-product of the metabolism of endogenous intestinal gram-positive bacteria. It is a fat-soluble vitamin that requires bile salts for normal absorption. It is rare to become deficient on the basis of poor intake alone, because the bacterial production of vitamin K is enough to maintain adequate factor production.

A clinical state of vitamin K deficiency occurs most commonly in patients with malabsorption caused by biliary disease, which leads to fat malabsorption, or in severely malnourished patients who are taking antibiotics that suppress the gram-positive flora of the gut. This condition is commonly seen in the postoperative patient on antibiotics who may have been malnourished preoperatively and is unable to eat postoperatively. Hematuria, melena, epistaxis, and ecchymoses are common manifestations of vitamin K deficiency. Severe gastrointestinal bleeding can occur as the deficiency persists; central nervous system bleeding can be fatal.

The characteristic laboratory findings in vitamin K deficiency include an initial prolongation of the PT caused by the rapid decline of factor VII, because it has the shortest half-life of the vitamin K–dependent coagulation factors (approximately 6 hr), and then a gradual prolongation of the PTT caused by depression of factor IX. A common clinical problem is the differentiation between liver impairment and vitamin K deficiency when both conditions may exist in a patient with a prolonged PT and PTT.

The diagnosis can be established by assaying the activity of two coagulation factors (e.g., factors VII and V); both are synthesized in the liver, but only one is vitamin K dependent. Another means of establishing the diagnosis is a therapeutic trial of parenteral vitamin K. Full correction of the coagulopathy should occur within 24 to 48 hours if the abnormality is caused by vitamin K deficiency and the liver is functioning normally.

Therapy depends on the degree of the hemostatic defect. Parenteral vitamin K (10 mg IM or 5 mg IV) corrects the PT in 12 to 24 hours. Fresh frozen plasma (initial dose 15–20 ml/kg followed by one-third this dose q8–12h) immediately replaces the vitamin K–dependent factors and corrects the PT. It should be used in a situation of abnormal coagulation studies with acute bleeding caused by vitamin K deficiency. When given intravenously, vitamin K must be administered slowly over several minutes, watching for untoward effects.

Liver Disease. Advanced liver disease is commonly associated with pathologic bleeding as a result of an accompanying coagulopathy. Altered coagulation occurs as a result of either decreased factor synthesis, production of an abnormal factor, increased factor consumption or, very rarely, primary fibrinolysis [35]. Because most of the coagulation factors are produced in the liver, the most common coagulopathy is attributable to impaired factor synthesis and results in multiple factor deficiencies. The vitamin K–dependent factors are particularly sensitive to liver impairment, especially factor VII. The contact activation factors (XII, XI, PK, HMWK) are less severely affected.

The liver has great potential to produce fibrinogen, and thus its concentration is not depressed until late-stage liver failure occurs. In certain states, dysfunctional fibrinogens may also be produced. This condition can be seen with hepatomas, cirrhosis, chronic active liver disease, and acute hepatic failure. Extensive studies have failed to show a consistent abnormality in the fibrinogen structure that is responsible for its reduced activity.

Many investigators have also shown that the coagulation mechanism can be activated in liver disease and results in disseminated intravascular coagulation. Activation is postulated to result from necrosis of hepatocytes and release of tissue thromboplastin, inadequate clearance of already activated factors by the liver's reticuloendothelial system, and depressed levels of naturally occurring inhibitors that are produced in the liver, such as antithrombin III. Intravascular coagulation results primarily in the consumption of factors II, V, VIII, XIII, and fibrinogen as well as the secondary activation of fibrinolysis and the generation of fibrin degradation products, which further impair clotting by inhibiting the polymerization of fibrin. There are usually multiple laboratory abnormalities, including a prolonged PT, PTT, TT, and a mildly elevated FDP and even D dimer. If portal hypertension exists, the spleen may be slightly enlarged and cause a mildly reduced platelet count because of hypersplenism. This constellation of abnormalities may be difficult to differentiate from DIC (see Table 118-6).

Treatment depends on the severity of the coagulopathy and the presence of bleeding and usually includes fresh frozen plasma. Treatment simply for the purpose of correcting an abnormal PT and PTT is not recommended. Because it takes a large volume of plasma to correct the abnormality, the correction is short lived, and the protein load contained in the plasma may be enough to induce hepatic encephalopathy in a patient who is predisposed. Factor IX concentrates should be avoided because of the risk of thrombosis.

DEFICIENCY: ACCELERATED DESTRUCTION OR LOSS

Consumption. Disseminated intravascular coagulation is conceptually a simple disorder, yet it is frustratingly complex in its diagnosis and treatment. It most often occurs in critically ill patients and is a common syndrome in the intensive care setting. DIC is a syndrome of accelerated destruction or consumption of certain coagulation factors [36,37]. It involves the pathologic activation of coagulation by an underlying disease process that leads to fibrin clot formation and secondary fibrinolysis, which then cause the consumption of coagulation factors, platelets, and red cells. It may not be apparent clinically, or it may be manifested by thrombosis, hemorrhage, or both, depending on the degree of activation and compensatory efforts of the body.

The fulminant syndrome is most often a life-threatening bleeding disorder. Bleeding results from the developing factor deficiency (primarily I, II, V, VIII, and XIII), thrombocytopenia, excessive fibrinolysis, and high levels of FDP and d-dimer superimposed on a vascular system already damaged by diffuse microvascular thrombi. Bleeding is typically manifested by diffuse superficial hemorrhage in the form of ecchymoses and petechiae, as well as oozing from the gingiva and other areas of the oral mucosa or from the gastrointestinal and urinary tracts.

Hemorrhage is classically from the microvasculature, but major vascular hemorrhage can occur as well, and central nervous system bleeding, which is not unusual, can be fatal. The most common causes of DIC include gram-negative septicemias [38], certain malignancies [39], surgery, trauma, and obstetric complications [40]. Table 118-5 lists several other potential causes of DIC as well.

PATHOPHYSIOLOGY. The pathophysiology of the consumption process depends on the underlying disease process or initiating event. The common, underlying mechanism is activation of the extrinsic, intrinsic, or common pathways of coagulation. In infections with gram-negative organisms, the lipopolysaccharide component of endotoxin can directly activate factor XII and the intrinsic pathway. More importantly, endotoxemia causes lysis and degranulation of granulocytes, releasing a substance with thromboplastic activity that initiates the extrinsic system of coagulation and is the major pathway of intravascular coagulation in these infections [36]. Acute promyelocytic leukemia is the neoplasm most commonly associated with DIC [41]. Lysis and release of a thromboplastic activity from promyelocytes is the cause of the intravascular coagulation. Adenocarcinomas similarly release a thromboplastic or procoagulant substance with the potential for activating the extrinsic system [42]. The pathophysiology of DIC in obstetric complications is variable. Puerperal sepsis with a gram-negative organism initiates coagulation through endotoxin. Abnormalities or complications that affect the placenta generally affect coagulation by releasing thromboplastic activity into the maternal circulation.

Table 118-5. Disorders Associated with Disseminated Intravascular Coagulation

1. Infection
   a. Gram-negative endotoxemia with hypotension or shock
   b. Severe gram-positive septicemia
   c. Rocky Mountain spotted fever
   d. Viral infection (herpes)
   e. Malaria (*Plasmodium falciparum*)
2. Complications of pregnancy and delivery
   a. Gram-negative sepsis
   b. Abruptio placentae
   c. Amniotic fluid embolism
   d. Retained dead fetus
   e. Toxemia
3. Pediatric disorders, especially in the newborn
4. Malignant diseases
   a. Metastatic carcinoma (prostate, pancreas, lung, stomach, colon, breast)
   b. Leukemia, especially acute promyelocytic leukemia
5. Liver diseases (cirrhosis)
6. Complications of surgery: extracorporeal circulation
7. Critical tissue damage
   a. Brain tissue destruction
   b. Massive trauma
   c. Heat stroke
   d. Extensive burns
8. Miscellaneous
   a. Hemolytic transfusion reactions
   b. Vasculitis
   c. Aneurysms
   d. Giant hemangioma
   e. Snake bites

Table 118-6. Laboratory Findings in Disseminated Intravascular Coagulation Compared with the Coagulopathy of Liver Disease

Test	Liver disease	DIC	
		Low grade	Fulminant
Prothrombin time*	Long	Normal, short	Long
Partial thromboplastin time*	Long	Normal, short	Long
Thrombin time*	Long	Normal, short, long	Long
Fibrinogen*	Low	High-normal-low	Low
Factor VIII	Normal-high	Normal-high	Low
Fibrin monomers	±	+	+ + + +
Fibrinopeptide A	±	+	+ + + +
Fibrin(ogen) degradation Products/d-dimer*	±	+ +	+ + + +
Euglobulin lysis time	Normal	Normal–short	Short
Antithrombin III	Low	Normal	Low
Platelet count*	Mildly low	Normal–mildly low	Low
Blood smear* *(Microangiopathic)*	No	±	+

*Indicates those tests easily obtained in a short period (e.g., 1–2 hr), which constitute a so-called DIC screen.
± (slightly positive) to + + + + (strongly positive).

In addition to direct effects on coagulation by the mechanisms described above, a number of cytokines or vascular factors may play an indirect role in coagulation activation. These include tumor necrosis factor-α, interleukin-1, and vascular factors [43].

DIAGNOSIS. The diagnosis of DIC is complicated by the fact that the clinical manifestations range from those of no findings to manifestations of an extensive thrombotic disease or a severe hemorrhagic disorder. Unless there are large vascular defects, bleeding is usually from the microvascular system and is generalized. The patient usually has evidence of an underlying disorder known to predispose to DIC. The definitive diagnosis is established in the laboratory (Table 118-6) by a constellation of abnormalities. Factor consumption and high titers of FDP, which inhibit fibrin monomer polymerization, produce prolongations of the PT, PTT, and TT. The fibrinogen concentration is reduced, and proteolytic fragments of fibrinogen and fibrin are elevated. The traditional FDP assay does not discriminate between fibrin and fibrinogen breakdown products and is less specific (but more sensitive) than the d-dimer assay, which is specific for fibrin proteolysis [44,45] (see discussion under Laboratory Evaluation of Hemostasis earlier in this chapter). The theoretical advantages, however, of the d-dimer assay over the standard FDP assay may not add much to the clinical diagnosis of DIC.

Thrombocytopenia occurs as a result of platelet consumption on microvascular clots and platelet activation by circulating thrombin. Red blood cells may be fragmented and lysed as a result of impact with intravascular fibrin strands, producing a microangiopathic hemolytic anemia with a low hemoglobin, high reticulocyte count, and signs of intravascular hemolysis (Fig. 118-5). More sophisticated tests can be performed, looking specifically for fibrin monomer formation, fibrinopeptides, or activation of fibrinolysis, but they are seldom necessary to confirm the diagnosis in clinically significant cases of DIC.

TREATMENT. The most important component in the treatment of DIC is correction of the underlying disease [46]. Supportive measures include plasma and platelet transfusions to replace the deficient factors, AT III and platelets. The often-cited danger of "feeding the fire" by replenishing these substances has never been clinically substantiated. The use of heparin remains controversial [47]. Theoretically, it has a role based on its ability to neutralize activated serine proteases (factors XII, PK, XI, IX, X, II) and interrupt the generation of thrombin, but clinical studies do not convincingly support its use.

In certain specific conditions such as purpura fulminans and acute promyelocytic leukemia heparin may be helpful and should be considered. Otherwise, patients must be considered on an individual basis. Table 118-7 provides general guidelines for treatment of DIC. If heparin is used, it should be started at low doses (5–10 units/kg/hr) and given by constant infusion without a loading dose. Some investigators recommend low-dose subcutaneous heparin [48], but the advantages of this over IV heparin are not substantiated.

Newer modes of therapy have been tested, but it is still too early to determine their efficacy or cost-effectiveness. These include concentrates of antithrombin III or protein C to neutralize activated coagulation factors [49,50], low-molecular-

Fig. 118-5. Microangiopathic blood smear showing fragmented red blood cells in DIC.

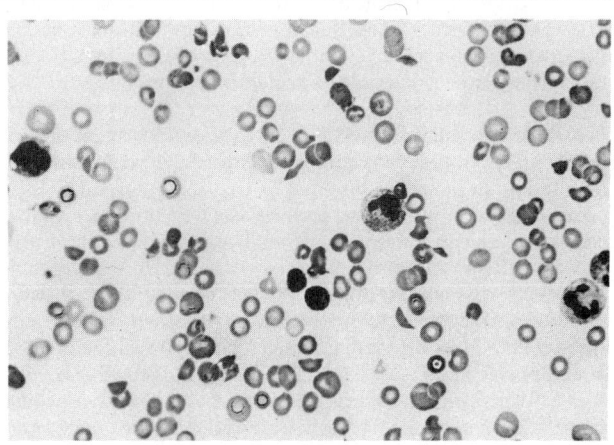

Table 118-7. Principles of Therapy for Disseminated Intravascular Coagulation (DIC)

1. Treat the underlying condition.
2. If the underlying condition is rapidly reversible, watch, wait, and support with fresh frozen plasma and platelets.
3. If the bone marrow is normal and the liver intact, fresh frozen plasma and/or platelets are less likely to be needed.
4. If there is actual or potentially serious bleeding or clotting, "consider" heparin therapy.
5. If the underlying disorder (and thus the DIC) is not rapidly reversible, "consider" heparin therapy.
6. If the patient has a surgically intact vascular system (i.e., no large holes in vessels), "consider" heparin therapy.
7. Depending on nos. 4, 5, and 6 above and a risk-vs.-benefit assessment, decide to treat or not to treat with heparin.
8. Remember, heparin may acutely worsen the hemorrhage, and evidence of its efficacy is available only in situations of more chronic forms of DIC, such as those seen with promyelocytic leukemia or prostatic carcinoma.

weight heparin [51], monoclonal antibodies to gram-negative endotoxin [52], or inhibitors of various modulators of coagulation [43].

Efficacy of therapy can be monitored by looking for a decrease in FDP or d-dimer, an increase in fibrinogen concentration, or the normalization of the PT and PTT. No single laboratory parameter is definitive, however, and the overall clinical status of the patient must be continually assessed.

Fibrinolysis. Fibrinolysis is often the result of the activation of the coagulation cascade, and in that sense, it is a secondary phenomenon. Whether conditions exist that will initiate fibrinolysis primarily is unclear, but there are conditions in which fibrinolysis is the major physiologic response. In this situation, plasminogen is activated by plasminogen activators, and plasmin enzymatically attacks fibrinogen, producing high levels of FDP. Low levels of fibrinogen and high titers of FDP cause a prolongation of the TT, PT, and PTT. Plasmin also destroys factors V and VIII, but other factors and the platelet count are normal, and fibrin monomers and cross-linked fibrin fragments (d-dimer) are not detectable. Conditions in which abnormalities of primary fibrinolysis are said to occur are in certain tumors, such as carcinoma of the prostate, and in extracorporeal open heart surgery [53].

The therapeutic approach to fibrinolysis usually involves the use of a combination of heparin and epsilon-aminocaproic acid (Amicar) as well as factor replacement with fresh frozen plasma. The combination is used because frequently there is a component of intravascular coagulation as well, and epsilon-aminocaproic acid alone could provoke thromboses.

Cardiopulmonary Bypass Surgery. With the advent of open heart surgery, a new and complex hemorrhagic syndrome seen in patients after cardiopulmonary bypass has emerged [54]. The cause of bleeding in these patients is often multifactorial, including inadequate heparin neutralization, postneutralization rebound effect of heparin, thrombocytopenia, functional platelet defects, disseminated intravascular coagulation, and excessive fibrinolysis [55]. Much research has focused on functional platelet defects as the major cause of postbypass bleeding [56], but extensive studies of DDAVP, a platelet function enhancing agent, to reduce postoperative hemorrhage have been unsuccessful [57]. Excessive fibrinolysis, however, is not uncommon in this setting and probably results from release of fibrinolytic

activator from damaged endothelium in the surgical field as well as from lysis of leukocytes during extracorporeal circulation. Recent studies of aprotinin, a serine protease inhibitor with a major inhibitory effect on plasmin, have shown efficacy in reducing blood loss in this setting [58]. In most cases of excessive postbypass bleeding it is often difficult to identify with certainty the abnormality that is predominantly responsible for the bleeding, so that hemorrhage is usually attacked on multiple fronts. Of course, surgical bleeding is always a consideration; the identification of such bleeding is essential because it may require surgical reexploration. For a further discussion of this subject the reader is referred to Chapter 162.

Massive Blood Replacement. Pathologic bleeding can occur in the setting of massive blood transfusions, particularly when the volume of blood received is given over a short interval and approximates the patient's normal blood volume. Labile coagulation factors (V and VIII) and platelets do not survive long in stored blood, and dilutional deficiencies of platelets and these labile coagulation factors may account for the hemorrhagic tendency [59]. Patients receiving such large amounts of blood, however, are often very ill, and it is difficult to attribute bleeding to one cause.

In patients who receive such large quantities of blood over short intervals, 1 unit of fresh frozen plasma should be given for every 5 units of blood transfused, although it is best to monitor hemostatic function and base replacement therapy on objective parameters. The platelet count should be monitored and platelet transfusions given only when serious thrombocytopenia attributable to dilution develops. A guideline to follow is 1 to 2 units of platelets for every 5 units of blood transfused. Although there is some controversy concerning the potential role of citrate-induced hypocalcemia in regard to the coagulopathy, there is little firm evidence that serious hypocalcemia does develop with massive transfusion or that it plays a role in the coagulopathy. Therefore, routine infusions with calcium gluconate or calcium chloride are not recommended.

INHIBITORS. Endogenous or spontaneously occurring pathologic inhibitors of coagulation may either be antibodies or soluble fragments of fibrinogen or fibrin that interfere with coagulation of blood and lead to a hemorrhagic disorder [60]. Inhibitor antibodies function by direct neutralization of a specific coagulation factor or by reacting with phospholipid and interfering with coagulation factor interaction. FDP interferes with the polymerization of fibrin monomer.

Antibodies to Specific Factors. Antibodies directed toward factor VIII are the most common neutralizing factor-specific antibodies [61]. They occur in 10 to 20 percent of patients with hemophilia but may be found in nonhemophilic individuals with autoimmune disorders (e.g., systemic lupus erythematosus and rheumatoid arthritis), during the postpartum period, and even in some elderly individuals without demonstrable underlying disease. Factor VIII antibodies in hemophiliacs generally first occur in patients younger than 20 years of age who have received multiple transfusions of products containing factor VIII; they usually have severe disease. The antibody is directed toward the coagulant moiety of the factor VIII complex, and its interaction is time and temperature dependent. The antibody is usually an IgG immunoglobulin.

Factor VIII antibodies often have a strong affinity, or neutralizing capacity, which produces a hemorrhagic state that is equivalent to severe hemophilia. Occasionally, weak antibodies are seen in hemophiliacs. Hemophiliacs with inhibitors typically respond to an infusion of factor VIII with a dramatic rise in inhibitor titer, which effectively neutralizes any further transfused factor VIII. These patients are notoriously difficult to treat when bleeding occurs because replacement therapy with factor VIII is ineffective. The diagnosis of factor VIII antibody can be presumed on the basis of a failure to respond to factor VIII infusions in a hemophiliac or by various mixing experiments. More specific quantitative assays are also available.

Treatment of hemophilia patients with factor VIII inhibitors is less than satisfactory (see Chap. 119 for details) [61]. In brief, prednisone and immunosuppressive agents have had little success. Intensive plasmapheresis can have a short-term effect. For active bleeding, patients have received factor IX and activated factor IX concentrates (which also contain activated factor X) in hopes of bypassing factor VIII. Alternatively, patients have been given high doses or constant infusions of factor VIII with some success. These patients should be treated in collaboration with a hematologist who is knowledgeable about coagulation and hemophilia. For patients without hemophilia who acquire a factor VIII antibody, prednisone or immunosuppressive agents are more effective and should be tried.

Factor IX inhibitors are relatively less common compared with factor XIII inhibitors and occur in approximately 5 percent of individuals with factor IX deficiency [62]. They have not been described in diseases other than hemophilia B. Much less frequently, inhibitors have been described against fibrinogen and factors V, VII, XI, XII, and XIII as well as vWF. Streptomycin and isoniazid have been incriminated in the causes of inhibitors to factors V and XIII, respectively.

Antibodies to Phospholipid. The other major variety of endogenous inhibitor is referred to as the *lupus inhibitor* and is present in as many as 10 percent of patients with systemic lupus erythematosus [63,64]. However, a similar inhibitor has now been demonstrated to occur in a number of other disease states, including other autoimmune disorders and various malignancies, HIV infection, as well as with certain drugs, particularly those known to produce a lupuslike syndrome (e.g., procainamide, hydralazine, chlorpromazine). The inhibitor is an immunoglobulin, most often of the IgG class, but occasionally IgM. Its interference with coagulation is instantaneous and not time dependent, as with factor VIII antibodies. Investigators have found it to interfere with, or to inhibit, various factors in the coagulation cascade, especially the intrinsic and common limbs.

Most consistent findings, however, favor the evidence that the antibody interacts with phospholipid and exerts its major influence on the reaction between activated factor X and factor II by interfering with their interaction with phospholipid. The in vivo significance of this inhibitor is minimal with regard to bleeding, because patients generally do not manifest a bleeding tendency unless coexistent defects, such as thrombocytopenia or other factor deficiencies, are also present. Paradoxically, however, there is a strong association between the presence of a lupus inhibitor and a thrombotic disorder [63]. This occurs more commonly in women, is associated with both venous and arterial thromboses, and is implicated as a cause of spontaneous abortions and intrauterine fetal death. Other manifestations include deep venous thromboses, pulmonary embolism, and strokes. The common underlying pathologic abnormality is the presence of antiphospholipid antibodies [65]. Some of these antibodies interfere with the coagulation cascade; others do not. However, thrombotic events can occur in either situation. Recent evidence has identified a cofactor for binding to phospholipid, specifically cardiolipin, called β_2-glycoprotein I (apolipoprotein H) [66], and this binding may be necessary for the development of thrombotic events.

The pathophysiology of thrombosis in this syndrome is un-defined, but some investigators have found evidence of deficient prostacyclin production in endothelial cells, inhibition of protein C activation, problems with fibrinolysis, and effects on platelets [67].

Patients with a lupus inhibitor commonly have a prolonged PTT or a measurable antiphospholipid antibody, but neither test is 100 percent sensitive, and both are much less specific for the clinical syndrome. A number of coagulation assays have been studied and recommended as screening and diagnostic tools for the identification of a lupus inhibitor [68]. When detected, treatment is long-term oral anticoagulant therapy in most cases and aspirin therapy in others. However, the presence of a lupus inhibitor alone without clinical problems is not an indication for therapy, which is usually not initiated unless a thrombotic epsiode develops.

References

1. Dyke C, Sobel M: The management of coagulation problems in the surgical patient. *Adv Surg* 24:229, 1991.
2. Plow EF, Ginsberg MH: The molecular basis of platelet function, in Hoffman R, Benz EJ Jr, Shattil SJ, et al (eds): *Hematology, Basic Principles and Practice*. New York, Churchill Livingstone, 1992, p 1165.
3. Fox JEB: The platelet cytoskeleton. *Thromb Haemost* 70:884, 1993.
4. Tschopp TB, Weiss HJ, Baumgartner HR: Decreased adhesion of platelets to subendothelium in von Willebrand's disease. *J Lab Clin Med* 83:296, 1971.
5. Brass LF: The biochemistry of platelet activation, in Hoffman R, Benz EJ Jr, Shattil SJ, et al (eds): *Hematology, Basic Principles and Practice*. New York, Churchill Livingstone, 1991, p 1176.
6. Plow EF, D'Souza SE, Ginsberg MH: Ligand binding to GPII$_b$-III$_a$: A status report. *Semin Thromb Hemost* 18:324, 1992.
7. Bloom AL: Physiology of blood coagulation. *Haemostasis* 20(suppl 1):14, 1990.
8. Bell RG: Metabolism of vitamin K and prothrombin synthesis: Anticoagulants and the vitamin K-epoxide cycle. *Fed Proc* 37:2599, 1978.
9. Mosesson MW: The roles of fibrinogen and fibrin in hemostasis and thrombosis. *Semin Hematol* 29:177, 1992.
10. Jackson CM: The biochemistry of prothrombin activation. *Br J Haematol* 39:1, 1978.
11. Rapaport SI: Regulation of the tissue factor pathway. *Ann NY Acad Sci* 614:51, 1991.
12. Hoyer LW: Hemophilia A. *N Engl J Med* 330:38, 1994
13. Griffin JH, Cochrane CG: Recent advances in the understanding of contact activation reactions. *Semin Thromb Hemost* 5:254, 1979.
14. Rosenberg RD: Actions and interactions of antithrombin and heparin. *N Engl J Med* 292:146, 1975.
15. Van Deerlin VMD, Tollefsen DM: Molecular interactions between heparin cofactor II and thrombin. *Semin Thromb Hemostas* 18:341, 1992.
16. Clouse LH, Comp PC: The regulation of hemostasis: The Protein C system. *N Engl J Med* 314:1298, 1986.
17. Broze GJ: The role of tissue factor pathway inhibitor in a revised coaglation cascade. *Semin Hematol* 29:159, 1992.
18. Lucas FV, Miller ML: The fibrinolytic system. *Cleve Clin J Med* 55:531, 1988.
19. Verstraete M, Collen D: Thrombolytic agents, in Fuster V, Verstraete M (eds): *Thrombosis in Cardiovascular Disorders*. Philadelphia, WB Saunders, 1992, p 175.
20. Krishnamurti C, Alving BM: Plasminogen activator inhibitor type 1: Biochemistry and evidence for modulation of fibrinolysis in vivo. *Semin Thromb Hemost* 18:67, 1992.
21. Rodgers RPC, Levin J: A critical reappraisal of the bleeding time. *Semin Thromb Hemost* 16:1, 1990.
22. Lind S: The bleeding time does not predict surgical bleeding. *Blood* 77:2547, 1991.
23. Greenberg CS, Devine DV, McCrae KM: Measurement of plasma

fibrin d-dimer levels with the use of a monoclonal antibody coupled to latex beads. *Am J Clin Pathol* 87:94, 1987.

24. Colman R, Hirsh J, Marder VJ, Salzman EW: *Hemostasis and Thrombosis*. Philadelphia, J.B. Lippincott, 1987.

25. Bick RL: Platelet function defects: A clinical review. *Semin Thromb Hemost* 18:167, 1992.

26. Stein B, Fuster V: Clinical pharmacology of platelet inhibitors, in Fuster V, Verstraete M (eds): *Thrombosis in Cardiovascular Disorders*. Philadelphia, 1992, W.B. Saunders, p 99.

27. Kobrinsky NL, Gerrard JM, Watson CM, et al: Shortening of bleeding time by 1-deamino-8-arginine vasopressin in various bleeding disorders. *Lancet* 1:1145, 1984.

28. Livio M, Benigni A, Remuzzi G: Coagulation abnormalities in uremia. *Semin Nephrol* 5:82, 1985.

29. Janson PA, Jubelirer SJ, Weinstein MJ, et al: Treatment of the bleeding tendency in uremia with cryoprecipitate. *N Engl J Med* 303:1318, 1980.

30. Mannucci PM, Remuzzi G, Pusineri F, et al: Deamino-8-D-arginine vasopressin shortens the bleeding time in uremia. *N Engl J Med* 308:8, 1983.

31. Mannucci PM: Desmopressin: A nontransfusional form of treatment for congenital and acquired bleeding disorders. *Blood* 72:1449, 1988.

32. Livio M, Mannucci PM, Vigano G, et al: Conjugated estrogens for the management of bleeding associated with renal failure. *N Engl J Med* 315:731, 1986.

33. Boneu B, Nouvel C, Sie P, et al: Platelets in myeloproliferative disorders. *Scand J Haematol* 25:214, 1980.

34. Ansell JE, Kumar R, Deykin D: The spectrum of vitamin K deficiency. *JAMA* 238:40, 1977.

35. Furie B: Coagulation disorders associated with liver disease, in Hoffman R, Benz EJ Jr, Shattil SJ, et al (eds): *Hematology, Basic Principles and Practice*. New York, Churchill Livingstone, 1992, p 1377.

36. Fruchtman S, Aledort LM: Disseminated intravascular coagulation. *J Am Coll Cardiol* 8:159B, 1986.

37. Berghaus GM: Pathophysiologic and biochemical events in disseminated intravascular coagulation: Dysregulation of procoagulant and anticoagulant pathways. *Semin Thromb Hemost* 15:58, 1989.

38. Philippe J, Offner F, Declerck PJ, et al: Fibrinolysis and coagulation in patients with infectious disease and sepsis. *Thromb Haemost* 65:291, 1991.

39. Bick RL: Coagulation abnormalities in malignancy: A review. *Semin Thromb Hemost* 18:353, 1992.

40. Finley BE: Acute coagulopathy in pregnancy. *Med Clin North Am* 73:723, 1989.

41. Kantarjian HM, Keating MJ, Walters RS, et al: Acute promyelocytic leukemia: MD Anderson Hospital experience. *Am J Med* 80:789, 1986.

42. Gordon SF: Cancer cell procoagulants and their role in malignant disease. *Semin Thromb Hemost* 18:424, 1992.

43. Bone RC: Modulators of coagulation: A critical appraisal of their role in sepsis. *Arch Intern Med* 152:1381, 1992.

44. Carr JM, McKinney M, McDonagh J: Diagnosis of disseminated intravascular coagulation. *Am J Clin Pathol* 91:280, 1989.

45. Boisclair MD, Lane DA, Wilde JT, et al: A comparative evaluation of assays for markers of activated coagulation and/or fibrinolysis: Thrombin-antithrombin complex, D-dimer and fibrinogen/fibrin fragment E antigen. *Br J Haematol* 74:471, 1990.

46. Schmaier AH: Disseminated intravascular coagulation: Pathogenesis and management. *J Intensive Care Med* 6:209, 1991.

47. Feinstein DI: Diagnosis and management of disseminated intravascular coagulation: The role of heparin therapy. *Blood* 60:284, 1982.

48. Bick RL, Scates S: Disseminated intravascular coagulation. *Lab Med* 23:161, 1992.

49. Blauhut B, Kramar H, Vinazzer H, et al: Substitution of antithrombin III in shock and DIC: A randomized study. *Thromb Res* 39:81, 1985.

50. Okajima K, Imamura H, Koga S, et al: Treatment of patients with disseminated intravascular coagulation by protein C. *Am J Hematol* 33:277, 1990.

51. Oguma Y, Sakuragawa N, Maki M, et al: Treatment of disseminated intravascular coagulation with low molecular weight heparin. *Semin Thromb Hemost* 16(suppl):34, 1990

52. Ziegler EJ, Fischer CJ, Sprung CL, et al: Treatment of gram negative bacteremia and septic shock with HA-1A human monoclonal antibody against endotoxin. *N Engl J Med* 324:429, 1991.

53. Stump DC, Taylor FB, Nesheim ME, et al: Pathologic fibrinolysis as a cause of clinical bleeding. *Semin Thromb Hemost* 16:260, 1990.

54. Mammen EF, Koets MH, Washington BC, et al: Hemostasis changes during cardiopulmonary bypass surgery. *Semin Thromb Hemost* 11:281, 1985.

55. Bick RL: Hemostasis defects associated with cardiac surgery, prosthetic devices, and other extracorporeal circuits. *Semin Thromb Hemostas* 11:249, 1985.

56. Michelson A: The platelet function defect of cardio-pulmonary bypass. *Blood* 82:107, 1993.

57. Ansell J, Klassen V, Lew R, et al: A randomized, double-blind study of the efficacy and safety of Desmopressin to reduce hemorrhage following cardiac surgery. *J Thorac Cardiovasc Surg* 98:237, 1992.

58. Bidstrup BP, Royston D, Sapsford RN, et al: Reduction in blood loss and blood use after cardiopulmonary bypass with high dose aprotinin (Trasylol). *J Thorac Cardiovasc Surg* 97:364, 1989.

59. Miller RD, Robbins TO, Tong MJ, et al: Coagulation defects associated with massive blood transfusion. *Ann Surg* 174:794, 1971.

60. Feinstein DI: Acquired inhibitors of blood coagulation, in Hoffman R, Benz EJ Jr, Shattil SJ, et al: (eds): *Hematology, Basic Principles and Practice*. New York, Churchill Livingstone, 1992, p 1380.

61. Kasper CK: Complications of Hemophilia A treatment: Factor VIII inhibitors. *Ann NY Acad Sci* 614:97, 1991.

62. Roberts HR, Lozier JN: Clinical aspects and therapy for hemophilia B, in Hoffman R, Benz EJ Jr, Shattil SJ, et al: (eds): *Hematology, Basic Principles and Practice*. New York, 1992, Churchill Livingstone, p 1325.

63. Gastineau DA, Kazmier FJ, Nichols WL, et al: Lupus anticoagulant: An analysis of the clinical and laboratory features of 219 cases. *Am J Hematol* 19:265, 1985.

64. Love PE, Santoro SA: Antiphospholipid antibodies: Anticardiolipin and the lupus anticoagulant in systemic lupus erythematosus and in non-SLE disorders. *Ann Intern Med* 112:682, 1990.

65. Lockshin MD: Antiphospholipid antibody syndrome. *JAMA* 268:1451, 1992.

66. McNeil HP, Simpson RJ, Chkesterman CN, et al: Anti-phospholipid antibodies are dirrected against a complex antigen that includes a lipid-binding inhibitor of coagulation: β_2-glycoprotein I. *Proc Natl Acad Sci* 87:4120, 1990.

67. Eisenberg GM: Antiphospholipid syndrome: The reality and implications. *Hosp Pract* 27:77, 1992.

68. Triplett DA: Laboratory diagnosis of lupus anticoagulants. *Semin Thromb Hemost* 16:182, 1990.

119. The Congenital Coagulopathies

Doreen B. Brettler and Peter H. Levine

The modern ability to diagnose and successfully treat most coagulation defects has changed the spectrum of clinical challenges for physicians who deal with such patients in the intensive care setting. This chapter emphasizes four disease states now increasingly seen in both medical and surgical units: (1) hemophilia A (classic hemophilia), (2) hemophilia A complicated by inhibitor antibody against factor VIII, (3) hemophilia B (Christmas disease), and (4) von Willebrand's disease.

The treatment for each of these coagulation disorders is unique to that disorder. Adequate treatment requires a precise diagnosis, including (1) identification of the deficient factor (or factors), (2) the precise quantitation of the factor level to allow an accurate prognosis and the calculation of replacement doses, and (3) determination of the presence or the absence of an inhibitor antibody against factors VIII or IX, a complication in 10 to 20 percent of persons with hemophilia A but very rare in those with hemophilia B.

Description of Hemophilia

Hemophilia A is an X-linked recessive bleeding disorder caused by decreased blood levels of properly functioning procoagulant factor VIII (also known as VIII:C, antihemophilic factor, or AHF). This disorder accounts for approximately 80 percent of the true hemophilias; thus the unqualified use of the term *hemophilia* is generally understood to refer to hemophilia A. Hemophilia B is also an X-linked recessive bleeding disorder and is indistinguishable from hemophilia A in its clinical manifestations. In hemophilia B, however, the defect is a decreased level of functional procoagulant factor IX (also known as IX:C, plasma thromboplastin component [PTC], or Christmas factor). The incidence of the hemophilias is in the range of 10 to 15 cases per 100,000 males.

Successful transfusion therapy for hemophilia was first reported in 1840 by Lane, using whole blood [1]. By 1923 Feissly reported the use of citrated plasma in hemophiliacs [2]. The therapy of hemophilia A, hampered by the volume restrictions imposed by whole blood or plasma transfusion, entered the modern era in 1964 with the description by Pool et al. [3] of the preparation of a crude AHF-rich plasma fraction through cryoprecipitation of fresh frozen plasma. More highly purified factor VIII fractions through glycine precipitation of fresh plasma [4] or through polyethylene glycol precipitation [5] were found therapeutically useful in 1964 and 1966, respectively. Prothrombin complex concentrates, rich in factors II, VII, IX, and X, and thus useful in hemophilia B, also appeared during this time [6].

It has long been known that hemophilia, with rare exception, is a disease of males. Hemophilia is an example of a typical X-linked recessive trait. Because the defective gene is located on the X chromosome, the male possesses no normal allele and manifests the clinical disorder. All of the sons of hemophilic males will be normal, but all of the daughters will be obligatory carriers of the trait [7]. Female carriers of hemophilia also may exhibit bleeding tendencies especially after trauma or surgery if their normal X chromosomes are randomly suppressed to a greater extent than normal (lyonization). Their factor levels may be less than 10 percent, making them similar to mild hemophiliacs.

The defect in hemophilia A is not a true absence of the factor VIII coagulant molecule, but rather a molecular defect in its procoagulant portion. Von Willebrand factor antigen (vWFAg), when measured by immunologic methods, is found to be present in normal amounts in all patients with hemophilia A [8]. In both hemophilia A and B, gene deletions, point mutations, and missense mutations have been found to account for the abnormal coagulation activity in individual families [9,10]. Whichever defect is present runs true in all family members.

Clinical Severity of Hemophilia

The frequency and severity of bleeding in hemophilia may be predicted from the factor VIII and IX procoagulant levels. Levels of factors VIII and IX are usually assayed in comparison with a reference standard that is prepared in each laboratory or obtained commercially and consists of pooled fresh frozen plasmas from many normal donors. Such standards are assumed to have factor VIII or IX levels of 100 percent, or in more recent terminology, they are said to contain 1 unit of factor VIII or IX activity per milliliter. The factor VIII or IX levels in a normal person on a given day may range typically between 50 and 200 percent (0.50–2 units/ml).

Individuals with factor VIII or IX levels that are equal to or less than 1 percent of normal (≤ 0.01 unit/ml) have spontaneous hemorrhages that require therapy two to four times per month on the average, although the amount of bleeding varies widely and the episodes are irregularly spaced [11]. Such patients are classified as severe hemophiliacs. Individuals with factor VIII or IX levels that are greater than 5 percent of normal (>0.05 unit/ml) are considered mild hemophiliacs and usually hemorrhage only with trauma or at surgery. Some mild cases of hemophilia are not diagnosed until adult life. Occasional "spontaneous" hemarthrosis may occur in such patients, especially in joints damaged by previously undertreated posttraumatic hemorrhage.

Patients whose factor VIII or IX levels fall between these two ranges are considered moderately severe, and their clinical pictures fall somewhere between the two extremes. If multiple untreated or suboptimally treated hemarthroses with subsequent joint damage have occurred in such a patient, the anatomic instability of these joints will cause frequent and severe bleeding, and the patient's condition will appear clinically more severe than the factor VIII or IX assay would suggest. This phenomenon probably explains the discrepancy between laboratory severity and clinical severity observed in some patients.

Within the kindred of a patient clinical and laboratory severity of the disorder is relatively constant; thus an individual with moderately severe hemophilia will have relatives with moderately severe hemophilia. The appearance of a more clinically severe course of the disease in a relative should raise the possibility in the patient either of established anatomic lesions that will predispose to frequent or severe hemorrhage or of the development of inhibitor antibody.

Clinical Manifestations of Hemophilia A and B

The clinical hallmarks of both hemophilia A and B are (1) a lack of excessive hemorrhage from minor cuts or abrasions because of the normalcy of platelet function in hemophilia, (2) joint and muscle hemorrhages, which lead to the most difficult and disabling long-term sequelae of this disorder, and (3) prolonged and potentially fatal postoperative hemorrhage. Infants and small children may have large ecchymoses from being carried or lifted and are occasionally mistaken for "battered" children in emergency departments.

The hemorrhagic lesions described below are found in both hemophilia A and B. Later in this chapter, those areas in which hemophilia B differs from classic hemophilia A will be emphasized.

HEMARTHROSIS. Hemarthrosis is most frequently involved, in descending order of frequency, with the knee, elbow, ankle, shoulder, hip, and wrist joints. Bleeding into the hand is rare and usually follows significant trauma, whereas the spine is rarely if ever involved.

The first episodes of acute hemarthrosis occur in childhood, but often not until the child begins to walk. Hemarthrosis is usually spontaneous or associated with imperceptible trauma. In a typical episode of hemarthrosis in an older child or adult, the onset of hemorrhage is signaled by an "aura," which consists of a vague warmth, a tingling sensation, or a sense of mild restlessness or anxiety. The aura may last up to 2 hours in some cases. A mild discomfort and a slight limitation of joint motion then occur, which are followed from 1 to several hours later by pain, joint swelling, cutaneous warmth, and an eventually severe limitation of motion, with the joint usually held in flexion. Once bleeding has stopped, the blood is reabsorbed, and the joint can return to normal over several weeks.

When pain, swelling, and severe limitation of motion are present, the hemorrhage is far advanced, and the process of synovitis begins. The synovitis may predispose the joint to further episodes of hemarthrosis and to the development of hemophilic arthropathy, the pathophysiology of which has recently been reviewed [11]. Unlike most conditions in medical practice, hemophilia should be treated as soon as symptoms suggestive of joint hemorrhage occur, long before the development of any physical findings. Only in this way can the long-term disabling sequelae be prevented.

The recognition of early acute hemarthrosis in the adult hemophiliac may be a more difficult problem. Such patients may (1) demonstrate periodic joint pain caused by established hemophilic arthropathy rather than bleeding, (2) have considerable fibrosis of the joint capsule, which prevents joint swelling, (3) develop chronic limitation of motion, which removes the value of this finding, and (4) often exhibit defense mechanisms that include repression or denial of the existence of hemorrhage. A short period of prophylactic correction of the hemostatic defect can help the patient to differentiate acute hemarthrosis from a background of chronic symptoms and signs.

Because severe hemophiliacs bleed spontaneously into muscles or joints approximately once weekly, a hemophiliac in an intensive care unit may well develop hemarthrosis during his or her stay in the unit unless already covered by factor VIII or IX infusion. The development of any joint or muscle pain should lead to immediate replacement therapy (see General Principles of Replacement Therapy, following). Additionally, nonsteroidal antiinflammatory agents are used successfully to control chronic joint paint secondary to arthropathy with no additional negative impact on the hemostatic system.

HEMATOMA. Small intramuscular hematomas are common and may sometimes resolve spontaneously, but large muscle hematomas may lead to severe sequelae through compression of vital structures. Large hematomas may produce fever, leukocytosis, severe pain, and low-grade hyperbilirubinemia caused by erythrocyte degradation. Large muscle hematomas that are not adequately treated may result in an eventual fibrous organization with contractures. Several important syndromes that may result from intramuscular hematomas in hemophiliacs are discussed below.

Psoas Hematoma. One of the most serious and potentially disabling lesions in hemophilia is hematoma of the psoas muscle or in the muscles of the retroperitoneum. Pain in the lower quadrant of the abdomen may mimic appendicitis, or the pain may be referred to the groin and may be mistaken for hemarthrosis of the hip joint. Because of distention of the body of the iliopsoas muscle, the leg is typically held in flexion at the hip, and the psoas sign is usually positive. Partial compression of the femoral nerve leads to the eventual development of pain on the anterior surface of the thigh. With further progression of the hematoma, increased pressure on the femoral nerve leads to paresthesia, hypesthesia, and eventual weakness of the quadriceps muscle. Permanent paralysis of the thigh flexors may be the end result.

Other Closed Space Hemorrhages. Bleeding into the muscles of the forearm may lead to median or ulnar nerve paralysis, or possibly to classic Volkmann's ischemic contracture of the hand. Calf lesions may lead to fixed equinovarus deformity at the ankle caused by muscle contractures or to peroneal or other nerve palsies [12]. Wrist bleeding, with nerve entrapment syndromes, is less common. Spontaneous or traumatic bleeding into the tongue or into the muscles or the soft tissues of the neck or throat may rapidly obstruct the airway and require prompt and vigorous therapy.

Hemophilic Cyst (Pseudotumor). Hemophilic cysts, or pseudotumors, begin as hematomas in muscle or subperiosteum. If inadequately treated, they will slowly organize, become highly vascular, grow by rebleeding, and cause pressure necrosis on surrounding muscle or bone. Such lesions may expand insidiously for several years, achieving huge dimensions, with a subsequent threat to life or limb [13]. The treatment is surgical excision, but an incomplete excision may lead to local recurrence. In younger patients, the small bones of the hand or the foot are the most common locations for pseudotumor, whereas in the adult, the pelvis and the femur provide the most usual locales.

INTRACRANIAL BLEEDING. Although relatively rare in hemophilia, intracranial bleeding remained the single major cause of death in hemophilia caused by hemorrhage, accounting for 25 percent or more of such deaths, before the occurrence of acquired immunodeficiency syndrome (AIDS) in persons with hemophilia. This lesion now accounts for many admissions to intensive care units. A history of antecedent trauma is obtained from approximately 50 percent of the patients. The advent of computed tomographic (CT) scanning and magnetic resonance (MRI) has led most experts to revise upwardly their index of suspicious bleeding after head trauma, because frequent examples of intracerebral bleeding have been seen in hemophiliacs after only "moderate" head injuries.

Bleeding may be subdural, epidural, subarachnoid, intracerebral, or, rarely, intraspinal. In one cooperative study of 2500 hemophiliacs studied over a 10-year period, 71 episodes of central nervous system bleeding were documented; there was a mortality rate of 34 percent, and 47 percent of the survivors were left with mental retardation, seizure disorders, or motor impairment [14]. In this study, survivors had been treated with sufficient clotting-factor concentrate to raise the factor VIII or IX level to 30 to 50 percent of normal for at least 10 to 14 days. Most centers would now treat more intensively than this. No recent studies have been done, but anecdotal data would suggest that the incidence of such severe sequelae has decreased markedly.

OTHER SITES OF HEMORRHAGE

Gastrointestinal Hemorrhage. Hematemesis, melena, and hematochezia are highly unusual in hemophilia. Their occurrence should raise the suspicion of an organic gastrointestinal lesion, and the appropriate diagnostic studies should be carried out.

Gingival Hemorrhage. Prolonged gingival oozing is common, especially with the shedding of deciduous teeth, the eruption of new teeth, or after instrumentation. If such oozing is sufficiently prolonged or severe enough to require therapy, several days of antifibrinolytic agent such as epsilon-aminocaproic acid (EACA, Amicar) or tranexamic acid usually suffice [15]. The infusion of coagulation factor is only occasionally needed.

Hematuria. Urinary bleeding is not rare and is usually painless unless a clot has formed in the ureter or the pelvis. Most hematuria subsides after several days without therapy. Inhibitors of fibrinolysis such as epsilon-aminocaproic acid should be avoided, because they may increase clot formation in the collecting system and lead to renal colic. If hematuria persists after several days, factor VIII or IX may be given for 2 to 4 days. Pyelography, ultrasound, or other studies are not carried out unless hematuria is chronic or recurrent.

Epistaxis. Nosebleeds are not unusual in the hemophiliac. If it is a prominent part of the hemorrhagic history in other than a severe hemophiliac, however, the possibility of either a local nasal lesion or a wrong diagnosis (von Willebrand's disease) should be considered. Nasal packing or cauterization may be required as well as factor concentrate infusion if the hemorrhage is severe enough (see Chap. 168).

Posttraumatic Hemorrhage. Delayed bleeding that follows trauma is well documented in hemophilia. The phenomenon of delayed bleeding may initially reassure (falsely) the patient or the physician after trauma. For this reason, treatment with factor concentrate should be given after significant trauma whether or not evidence of hemorrhage is apparent. Venipuncture (not arterial puncture) and the small subcutaneous or intradermal (not intramuscular) injections that are used in immunization are generally safe in hemophiliacs without factor concentrate infusion, but firm pressure must be maintained over the injection site.

The Patient and the Family

The extraordinary ramifications for individuals of this genetically transmitted, lifelong, painful, unpredictable, potentially crippling, extremely expensive, and much misunderstood illness are beyond the scope of this chapter. Yet without taking these ramifications into account, the efficacy of treatment will be impaired, and the outcomes will be poor. Lay organizations, such as the National Hemophilia Foundation, or local hemophilia societies are sources of materials and paramedical support.

The financial problems of hemophilia (estimated cost falls in the range of $40,000–$100,000 per patient per year) can ruin a family and must be addressed in advance. The vocational problems of adults with established arthropathy caused by prior years of suboptimal therapy are immense. There is reason to believe that the level of education of health care professionals about hemophilic health care is poor because of the relative rarity of the disease, the burst of recent therapeutic advances, and the general antipathy of most physicians toward working with the complex and confusing hemostatic mechanism.

General Principles of Replacement Therapy: Factor VIII

The hemostatically effective plasma level for each coagulation factor is different and depends in part on the nature, the extent, and the duration of the bleeding lesion. The dose of replacement factor is calculated in units: One unit is the activity of a given coagulation factor that is equivalent to that found in 1 milliliter of pooled, citrated, fresh frozen human plasma. The factor must be given in sufficient quantity to allow for the in vivo fall-off in plasma level, which will be determined by the metabolic half-life of the factor and its clearance. Further, each coagulation factor has a different apparent volume of distribution within the body.

Partly because of these complex factors, partly because of the variability of clotting factor assays, and partly because of the historical difficulty in obtaining reliable and stable sources of clotting factors for therapeutic use, there is no general agreement as to the optimum therapeutic program for the treatment of the hemophilias and few scientific data on the relative merits of various regimens. The program suggested here is in general agreement with those widely used in large U.S. hemophilia centers and has been successfully applied over the past 15 years in more than 400 hemophiliacs closely followed in our own region.

FACTOR VIII DOSE CALCULATION. The biologic half-life of factor VIII is between 8 and 12 hours, which includes an initial rapid decline in level caused by diffusion into extravascular pools. The minimum hemostatic level of factor VIII for most early and relatively mild hemorrhages is thought to be 30 percent (0.3 unit/ml plasma). Early bleeding into muscles or joints, for example, is permanently arrested by achieving this level in most episodes so treated [16]. Whether lesser amounts of concentrates could be used with equal outcomes is being studied.

In far-advanced joint or muscle bleeding or in other major hemorrhagic lesions (Table 119-1), a factor VIII level of 50 percent (0.5 unit/ml) should be achieved. For such advanced lesions to resolve, from one to several days of maintenance therapy are needed. The procedure consists of repeating the infusion at 24-hour intervals at approximately 75 percent of the original dose infused to compensate for the residual in vivo level that remains from the initial dose.

In the intensive care unit, for the treatment of life-threatening bleeding or for surgery (see Surgery in Hemophilia A and B, following), levels of 80 to 100 percent (0.8–1.0 unit/ml) should be achieved, and the factor VIII level kept above the 40 to 50

Table 119-1. Replacement Doses for Hemophilia A and B

Indication for therapeutic infusion*	Hemophilia A units VIII	Hemophilia B units IX
1. Life-threatening lesions	40–50 units/kg	80 units/kg
a. Suspected or established intracranial hemorrhage	yields 80–	yields 80%
b. Major trauma with bleeding	100% level	level in vivo
c. Gastrointestinal hemorrhage, severe	in vivo	
d. Surgery		
2. Major hemorrhage	40–50 units/kg	80 units/kg
a. Advanced joint or muscle bleeding	yields 80–	yields 80%
b. Neck, tongue, or pharyngeal hematoma	100% level	level in vivo
c. Head trauma without neurologic deficit	in vivo	
d. Severe physical trauma, no evidence of bleeding		
e. Severe abdominal pain		
f. Gastrointestinal hemorrhage		
3. Mild hemorrhage	15 units/kg	30 units/kg
a. Early joint or muscle bleeding	yields 30%	yields 30%
b. Severe epistaxis	level in vivo	level in vivo
c. Gingival or dental bleeding unresponsive to epsilon-aminocaproic acid		
d. Hematuria, if persistent		

*Typical initial doses of replacement products for hemophilia A and B. For category 2, subsequent doses are usually required; for category 1, several weeks' maintenance of minimal levels is mandatory. Factor VIII maintenance is generally by infusion at least every 12 hours, the half-life being 8 to 12 hours. For factor IX, maintenance infusions should be given at least every 24 hours, the half-life approximating 18 to 24 hours.

percent range by appropriate doses of factor VIII infused at intervals of 8 to 12 hours [17]. This more frequent infusion regimen decreases both the incidence of excessively low levels just before an infusion and the total amount of factor needed to maintain a given in vivo plasma level. Constant infusions of factor concentrate can also be given to keep a persistent level of greater than 30 percent, usually beginning with empiric dosing at 2 to 4 units/kg/hr after a bolus of 50 units per kilogram intravenously [18].

Dose calculation for factor VIII can be made by calculating the recipient's plasma volume in milliliters and then multiplying by the desired increment of factor VIII in units per milliliter. A simpler and reproducible dose calculation can be made from the following replacement formula: Each unit of factor VIII infused per kilogram body weight yields a 2-percent rise in plasma factor VIII level (i.e., 0.02 unit/ml). For example, to achieve an 80 percent level in vivo in a 70-kg individual with psoas hematoma or for whom surgery is planned would require 40×70 units/kg, or approximately 2800 units of factor VIII, assuming a starting point of essentially 0 percent factor VIII.

If a given minimal level is to be maintained over several days, this level can be achieved by (1) giving an initial infusion to twice the desired minimum, (2) giving one half this dose every 8 to 12 hours, assuming a half-life of 8 to 12 hours, and (3) performing factor VIII assays every several days for precise dose adjustments.

For example, a 50-kg individual with an extensive laceration should be maintained at above 30 percent factor VIII in vivo until healing is complete. An initial infusion is given to the 60 percent level, by 30×50 units/kg, or 1500 units of factor VIII. The patient then receives 750 units every 8 hours thereafter for 7 to 10 days. If on day 3, a factor VIII assay, which was drawn just before an infusion, returns at 20 percent, the dose infused can be adjusted upward on day 4.

For patients with major or life-threatening lesions, the measurement of in vivo factor VIII:C by standard laboratory assays is advisable because all of these calculations are only approximations, and the responses of individuals to variable sources of factor VIII vary in yield and stability. The substitution of the activated partial thromboplastin time or other screening test in place of a formal factor VIII assay should be avoided, because the results may be misleading in the extreme. It should be noted that if a person with congenital clotting disorder is in the intensive care unit, a hematologist with knowledge of hemophilia should be consulted and aid in following the patient. Also important is an active coagulation laboratory and a pharmacy or blood bank that can keep factor concentrate in adequate supply.

REPLACEMENT SOURCE. Wet frozen cryoprecipitate was the replacement source of choice years ago, but is rarely used as such at this time. The treatment for severe/moderate factor VIII deficiency is replacement with factor VIII concentrates that are lyophilized and treated with heat or solvent/detergents to inactivate viruses. There are now many different commercial factor VIII concentrates available, which are made from large pools of normal plasma and sold in lyophilized form. When reconstituted, one can administer 1000 units of factor VIII in a volume of 5 to 10 ml, depending on the product used. Each vial is labeled with the number of units contained, and such figures are reasonably accurate. These products not only allow accurate dose calculations but are convenient for home use. They are stable at home-refrigerator temperature for months to years and at room temperature for many months, and they can rapidly be prepared for self-administration. The major disadvantage is cost; current wholesale prices range from $.40 to $1.00 per factor VIII unit. The concentrates have made early and intensive home therapy possible, however, and thus overall costs of health care have greatly declined for patients treated with these materials [19]. The currently available concentrates are reviewed in Table 119-2.

Recombinant factor VIII has been available since December 1992. These concentrates are produced from mammalian cell lines, not from human plasma, and when compared with plasma-derived factor VIII are identical in function and similar in structure [20,21]. Safety and efficacy have been shown in more than 300 patients worldwide [21]. In hemophiliacs who have not been exposed to any human bloodborne viruses it should be considered as first-choice therapy.

Table 119-2. Current Factor Concentrates

Name (company)	Virus inactivated method	Comments
Factor VIII concentrates		
Monoclate P (Armour)	Pasteurized (60°, 10h)	Very high purity
Hemophil M (Baxter-Hyland)	Solvent/detergent	Very high purity
ARC—Method M (American Red Cross)	Solvent/detergent	Very high purity
Profilate OSD (Alpha)	Solvent/detergent	Intermediate purity
Koate HP (Bayer)	Solvent/detergent	High purity
Humate P (Behring/Armour)	Pasteurization	Intermediate purity
Melate SD (NY Blood Center)	Solvent/detergent	Intermediate purity
Kogenate (Bayer)	—	Recombinant
Recombinate (Hyland Baxter)	—	Recombinant
Helixate (Bayer/Armour)	—	Recombinant
Bioclate (Baxter Vyland/Armour)	—	Recombinant
Factor IX concentrates		
Alphanine SD (Alpha)	Solvent/detergent	Highly pure
Mononine (Armour)	Ultrafiltration	Highly pure
Factor IX complex concentrates		
Konyne 80 (Miles)	Dry heat	Contain factors II, VII, X
Proplex T (Hyland)	Dry heat	Contain factors II, VII, X
Profilnine SD (Alpha)	Solvent detergent	Contain factors II, VII, X
Bebulin (Immuno)	Vapor heated	Contain factors II, VII, X

In patients with mild hemophilia A, the use of DDAVP (desmopressin) should be considered first if the patient needs treatment. The general rule is that 0.3 μg/kg intravenously over 30 minutes will increase the factor VIII level threefold [22]. It should be given every 8 to 12 hours. Tachyphylaxis may occur after 3 to 4 days of use, and factor VIII levels should be checked periodically. Side effects include facial flushing, headache, and occasionally hyponatremia, especially in a patient not taking oral fluids who is on intravenous hydration. Serum sodium levels should be checked intermittently in these types of patients. If the patient develops tachyphylaxis or does not have an adequate rise in factor VIII levels with DDAVP, factor concentrate that is virally inactivated should be used. Because cryoprecipitate cannot be virally inactivated, and thus the risk of transmission of hepatitis C or HIV-1 exists (although it is very small), it should not be used.

SIDE EFFECTS OF REPLACEMENT THERAPY. Allergic reactions to factor VIII concentrates such as urticaria or fever are quite infrequent and very mild. Changing to a different product lot number for subsequent infusions is probably warranted, and subsequent reactions are rare. As with any plasma product,

reactions lasting more than a few minutes may be ameliorated with low-dose antihistamine therapy. It is important to note that patients who have had severe reactions to cryoprecipitate usually do not have reactions to factor VIII concentrate. Anaphylaxis to factor concentrate has been reported but is extremely rare.

With the infusion of large doses of factor VIII concentrate, usually in a surgical setting or for major trauma, recipients may develop hemolytic anemia. This infrequent side effect occurs only in recipients with type A or B erythrocytes, and is attributable to the presence of anti-A or anti-B antibodies in the concentrate. If red cell transfusion is necessary, type O cells should be given [23]. The process resolves as the dose of concentrate is decreased. This complication should not be seen with the more highly purified plasma-derived factor concentrates or recombinant factor concentrate.

The major side effect of replacement therapy has been human immunodeficiency virus (HIV) infection and AIDS (see following section). Another serious infectious complication is hepatitis, which may be of either A, B, or C types. In most series, the great majority of treated hemophiliacs have plasma levels of hepatitis B surface antibody, and a minority (2–10%) carry hepatitis-B surface antigen [24]. Presumably because of extensive plasma-product exposure early in life, the incidence of overt clinical hepatitis in moderately severe or severe hemophiliacs who received pooled commercial concentrate is surprisingly low. With the availability of the recombinant hepatitis B vaccine, all newly diagnosed persons with hemophilia should be vaccinated. Infants may start the three-injection series at birth. Thus hepatitis B is a problem that should be largely eliminated.

Most treated hemophiliacs have persistent mild elevations of serum transaminases. Although most such patients are asymptomatic, chronic active hepatitis and cirrhosis [25] have both been proved by biopsy in patients selected because of either symptoms or severely abnormal liver chemistries. When testing for hepatitis C became available it was found that approximately 80 to 85 percent of hemophiliacs transfused before concentrates were virally inactivated were hepatitis C antibody positive, signifying infection [26]. Whether hepatitis C infection will lead to a greater incidence of hepatocellular carcinoma, as suggested by some investigators [27], or increased death from liver failure remains to be elucidated.

The development of inhibitor antibody only occurs after exposure to factor VIII, tends to develop in patients with severe hemophilia younger than age 5 years, and occurs after a range of 5 to 30 treatments of factor concentrate. Recent data suggest that there may be a familial predisposition to the development of this complication. There does appear to be an increased incidence of factor VIII gene deletions in association with inhibitor development [28]. Treatment of patients with inhibitor antibodies is still problematic. (See section on treatment of inhibitor antibodies.)

HIV and Hemophilia

The problem regarding transmission of the human immunodeficiency virus (HIV) to patients with hemophilia is beyond the scope of this chapter. A few points, however, deserve emphasis here.

In retrospect, HIV was introduced into the U.S. blood supply, and thus into coagulation factor concentrates, in the late 1970s. By 1982, the year the first case of AIDS was reported in a hemophiliac, and 3 years before a test for HIV was widely available, more than half of U.S. hemophiliacs had been infected. Currently, approximately 40 to 50 percent of all U.S. hemophiliacs are HIV seropositive; among severe factor VIII–deficient patients, between 80 and 95 percent are seropositive. Once infected, the natural history is similar to that of patients in other risk groups [29]. If a hemophilia patient's HIV-1 serostatus is unknown, he should be assumed positive, especially if the patient is in the late adolescent or adult age-group. As with all patients, universal precautions should be practiced diligently.

In HIV-seronegative patients, every effort should be made to preserve seronegative status. This includes the use of the currently "safest" products (see Table 119-2), which now include recombinant factor VIII.

Inhibitor Antibody in Hemophilia

Between 15 and 30 percent of hemophiliacs develop an inhibitor antibody at some time in the course of their disease, usually during infancy or childhood and usually within the first 5 to 40 exposures to plasma products. The antibody results in the rapid clearance of infused factor VIII procoagulant activity from the plasma. Therefore, no significant increase in circulating factor VIII can usually be measured even after infusions of large doses. Because bleeding can no longer be reliably controlled, elective surgery should not be considered in such a patient.

Inhibitor antibodies in hemophiliacs have a highly unpredictable natural history. At times, very low titer and clinically weak antibodies, which are easily neutralized by factor VIII, are found to not have undergone anamnestic rises in titer after multiple challenges, only later to reach high titer unexpectedly. More common are the patients who develop rising antibody titers after each exposure to factor VIII. In rare cases, patients appear to have spontaneously lost their antibody despite multiple subsequent factor VIII challenges. The type of antibody response to factor VIII infusion and the patient's clinical response dictate therapy.

The therapy for patients with inhibitor antibody ranges from the total avoidance of all exposure to factor VIII in some centers to an aggressive megadose factor VIII replacement in others. Prothrombin complex concentrates (PCC), possibly because of its variable contamination with activated factor X, activated factor VII, phospholipid, or other procoagulant, is thought to be efficacious. It is usually given in large doses, 70 units of factor IX activity per kilogram of body weight. This regimen appears to control bleeding 50 percent of the time or somewhat less [30]. Activated prothrombin complex concentrates (aPCC, FEIBA, Autoplex) at doses of 70 units per kilogram have also been shown to be inconsistently efficacious. With both PCC and aPCC, no measurable factor VIII level is obtained, nor is shortening of the PTT seen, so their effectiveness can only be demonstrated empirically. Because of this, hemostasis cannot be guaranteed with their use. The use of immunosuppressive agents or corticosteroids has been abandoned in most centers because of their lack of efficacy and their serious side effects. (Such agents are efficacious in treating acquired circulating anticoagulants in nonhemophiliac patients).

In our experience, patients with low titer antibodies, which remain low in titer (e.g., <5 Bethesda units) after repeated therapy, often do well with increased doses of factor VIII concentrate. For those who fail to benefit or who have higher titers, PCC or aPCC is used. Both groups of patients are often on home therapy, and bleeding is more likely to be arrested when treatment is applied early rather than when the hemorrhage has progressed.

Porcine factor VIII in a purified form is available for treating patients with factor VIII inhibitor antibodies who are hospitalized with severe hemorrhages. Using empiric dosing of 100 to 300 units per kilogram of porcine factor VIII, measurable circulating factor VIII levels can be obtained. If the human inhibitor antibody titer is low (below 20 Bethesda units) the antibody often does not cross react with porcine factor VIII. However, If the patient has a very high titer antibody, porcine factor VIII will not likely be effective [31]. An alternative for the hemorrhaging inhibitor patient is plasmapheresis to remove the IgG antibody while giving very high doses of human factor VIII concentrates. Recently, columns that selectively remove IgG from plasma have become available and make the plasmapheresis more efficient. Recombinant factor VIIa is an experimental therapy for inhibitor patients that are bleeding. There have been case reports of surgery being done successfully with recombinant VIIa coverage as well as cessation of retropharyngeal hemorrhaging with this product [32,33]. Clinical trials are still ongoing to truly evaluate its efficacy. The summary of treatment for patients with inhibitor antibodies to factor VIII is seen in Table 119-3.

Because patients with inhibitor antibody depend on intensive and frequent use of all of a hemophilia center's comprehensive services (e.g., orthopedic, physiatric, psychiatric, social, financial) and because of their changing and complex replacement needs, all such patients should be followed, at a major hemophilia center. As indicated earlier, no invasive procedures, including central line placement, arterial catheters, or surgeries, should be done until consultation with a hematologist has been obtained.

Clinical Manifestations of Hemophilia B (Factor IX Deficiency)

The clinical manifestations of hemophilia B in general are identical to those of hemophilia A, although a few minor differences are noted. As is true for hemophilia A, this disease has an X-linked recessive mode of inheritance. The frequency of patients with hemophilia B who have severe degrees of deficiency of factor IX:C is somewhat less than is seen in hemophilia A. Thus the "average" hemophilia B patient may have somewhat milder manifestations than are seen in hemophilia A. Over the years, however, the chronic arthropathy of hemophilia B becomes indistinguishable from that of hemophilia A unless appropriate treatment programs are instituted.

FACTOR IX DOSE CALCULATION. The biologic half-life of factor IX is considerably longer than for factor VIII, and although estimates have varied considerably [34], a terminal half-

Table 119-3. Treatment of Inhibitors of Factor VIII

Concentrate	Dose	Comment
Porcine factor VIII	50–300 units/kg	Shortens PTT
Activated PCC (Feiba®, Autoplex®)	70 units/kg	Judge efficacy on clinical basis only
High-dose factor VIII with plasmapheresis	50–200 units/kg	Removes IgG antibody
Recombinant VIIa	—	Experimental

life (t½) of approximately 24 hours is generally accepted, with an initial rapid fall-off in plasma level that is attributable to diffusion into extravascular pools. The minimum hemostatic level for factor IX is in the range of 10 to 25 percent (0.10–0.25 unit/ml), a range significantly lower than the estimated 30 percent level needed for factor VIII. Although the longer half-life and lower minimum hemostatic level serve to ease the replacement of factor IX in a deficient patient, the low in vivo recovery of this factor, at 25 to 50 percent of the dose administered, works in the opposite direction and dictates larger starting doses.

The replacement dose for factor IX can be calculated from the estimated plasma volume and the level desired, correcting for the considerable extravascular diffusion of this small molecule. A simpler and reproducible dose calculation can be made from the following formula: Each unit of infused factor IX per kilogram of body weight yields a 1 percent rise in plasma IX level (i.e., 0.01 unit/ml). To achieve a 60 percent level in vivo in a 70-kg individual with major trauma would thus require 60 × 70 kg, or approximately 4200 units of factor IX, assuming a starting point of essentially 0 percent of factor IX. If a given minimal level is to be maintained over several days, this can be achieved by methods similar to those described for factor VIII, except that the half-life of 24 hours (as compared with approximately 12 hr for factor VIII) indicates the need for either lower or less frequent subsequent doses by a factor of 50 percent. For example, to maintain the above patient at a factor IX level of above 30 percent at all times, one could infuse 2100 units every 12 to 24 hours, after the initial loading dose of 4200 units. Factor IX assays should be monitored every few days for adequate control.

A minimal level of 20 percent (0.20 unit/ml) is generally targeted for most acute hemorrhages. Early bleeding into muscles or joints will be permanently arrested by a single infusion to this level in 95 percent of episodes. For more advanced joint or muscle bleeding or for other major episodes (see Table 119-1), a factor IX level of 40 percent should be achieved. For major trauma or surgery, initial levels of 60 to 80 percent may be required, maintaining the level at above 40 percent through repeated infusions for several days, and then at levels above 20 percent for a total of 7 to 10 days. For major orthopedic surgery, considerably longer treatment periods may be needed.

REPLACEMENT SOURCE. For patients with severe/moderate factor IX deficiency, prothrombin complex concentrates (PCC) are the major treatment source. Pooled plasma is absorbed with either tricalcium phosphate or dimethylaminoethyl (DEAE) cellulose, which binds factors II, VII, IX, and X [35]. After further fractionation steps, which generally include ethanol precipitation, heparin may be added in some methods to inhibit activation of these concentrated factors. A variety of studies have proved the efficacy of these concentrates in hemophilia B.

There are six commercial factor IX concentrates available in the United States, and others will soon be forthcoming. They are all currently virally inactivated. The cost of these materials is at least as high as that for factor VIII concentrate: current wholesale cost for factor IX concentrate is in the range of $0.30 to $0.95 per factor IX unit. As is true for factor VIII concentrates, the factor IX concentrates are accurate in their stated potency, stable at 4°C for many months, and can be rapidly prepared for intravenous infusion. High-purity factor IX concentrates (Alphanine®, Mononine®) have recently been introduced into the marketplace. They contain very little, if any, factor II, VII, X and thus may have decreased thrombotic side effects in ill, bedridden patients. They are the concentrates of choice in a patient who is in the intensive care unit or undergoing surgery. Recom-

binant factor IX is not yet available, but research on such a product is ongoing and clinical trials are in progress.

SIDE EFFECTS OF REPLACEMENT THERAPY. Possibly because of contamination by minute amounts of activated coagulation factors, the administration of large doses of PCC has been associated with the development of deep venous thrombosis or pulmonary embolus, especially in settings known to predispose to venous thrombosis, such as the postoperative state or in patients with liver disease [35]. Disseminated intravascular coagulation associated with the use of prothrombin complex concentrate in patients with severe liver disease has also been reported, as have myocardial infarctions in young patients [36].

In our experience, many major surgical procedures have been performed under simultaneous coverage with PCC and heparin (5000 units subcutaneously q8–12hr) without evidence of thrombotic complications. With the advent of the purer factor IX concentrates, the use of prophylactic heparin probably is unnecessary because the occurrence of thrombotic episodes appears significantly decreased.

Another major side effect has been the risk of both hepatitis B and C, which may be even more frequent than with the use of factor VIII concentrates because factor IX concentrates did not become virally inactivated as early as factor VIII concentrates. HIV infection and AIDS have become the major side effects of replacement therapy of factor IX deficiency. The reader is referred to the previous section on HIV infection and hemophilia. The development of inhibitor antibodies in patients with factor IX deficiency is rare, less common than in hemophilia A patients, but is more commonly associated with gene deletions. Treatment of patients with factor IX inhibitors is very problematic, with aPCCs (FEIBA, Autoplex) being the only treatment modality available. The efficacy, however, is inconsistent.

Surgery in Hemophilia A and B

Elective and emergency surgery in hemophilia can be safely carried out in patients without inhibitor antibodies, under adequate coverage with replacement coagulation factor. Surgery, however, should only be done in consultation with a hematologist knowledgeable in coagulation disorders.

As orthopedic, general, oral, and other types of surgery become increasingly commonplace in the hemophiliac, certain guidelines require reemphasis. Both physician and patient should consider the following points in an orderly and systematic manner before surgery is undertaken to minimize the chances of poor outcome.

One of the first concerns is whether the lesion will recur postoperatively. If the lesion developed because of suboptimal medical control of hemophilia, it may well recur. This principle is of special importance with respect to orthopedic surgery in hemophilia. Orthopedic surgery often fails when the patient has demonstrated unreliability in adhering to a conservative regimen. For this reason, elective orthopedic surgery should be preceded by a period of intense nonsurgical management that will emphasize to the patient the importance of basic medical principles (immediate infusion at the first sign of hemorrhage, appropriate physical therapy, and so forth). This also tests the patient's ability to adhere to the regimen.

The patient should be instructed to avoid antiplatelet medication before and after surgery. Aspirin, and aspirin-containing medications such as Darvon Compound, Empirin, and Percodan, can produce marked prolongation of the previously normal bleeding time in hemophiliacs [37].

Surgery should be scheduled for early in the week. Early scheduling assures the availability of laboratory services for factor assays as well as access to consultants during the first few days after surgery. The supply of replacement therapeutics must be secure. The expected dose of material needed for a period of at least 2 weeks should be available in the blood bank or pharmacy.

A preoperative conference between the patient, the patient's family, the surgeon, and the hematologist should occur just before admission to the hospital. The benefits of such planned communications are obvious. Many patients or family members may have an unstated fear of fatal bleeding and respond dramatically to reassurance on this issue. Admission orders should include the following: "Hemophiliac: IM medications contraindicated"; "Patient may not be given aspirin in any form, including Darvon Compound, Empirin, or Percodan"; and "Joint or muscle pain may indicate hemorrhage—notify M.D. at once for possible coagulation-factor infusion." These same instructions should be taped to the cover of the patient's chart holder to ensure their being seen by all house officers, nursing staff, medical students, anesthesiologists, and medical consultants. Pain can be managed with either a continuous intravenous morphine drip or patient-assisted narcotic delivery systems.

For major surgery, the factor VIII level should be brought to the range of 80 to 100 percent just before the surgery and then kept at more than 40 percent for 10 to 14 days. For extensive orthopedic surgery, 4 to 6 weeks of replacement may be required. For example, a 50-kg boy requires major surgery. To achieve a 100 percent factor VIII level, 50 units per kilogram are given, or 2500 factor VIII units. Within 8 to 12 hours, the child's VIII level will have fallen to approximately 50 percent. One could then give 1750 factor VIII units every 8 hours to keep him in the desired range. Because the biologic half-life of factor VIII is somewhat longer than 8 hours, however, smaller doses may be needed, and the program should be modified as needed according to periodic factor VIII assays.

For major surgery in hemophilia B, the factor IX level should be brought to 80 percent just before surgery and then kept at more than 30 percent for 10 to 14 days. For example, a 50-kg boy will require major surgery. To achieve a 80 percent factor IX level, give 80 units per kilogram, or 4000 factor IX units. Twenty-four hours later, his factor IX level will have fallen to approximately 40 percent; one could then give 2000 units of factor IX every 12 to 24 hours to keep him above the desired minimum. As previously noted, with major surgery the highly purified factor IX products should be used. With major surgery in both hemophilia A and B, constant infusion of concentrate with syringe pump devices should be considered. Factor levels are more consistent and fewer total units are used, decreasing expenses.

These theoretic calculations must be checked at least every third day (preferably daily for the first few days) by performing assays of factor VIII or IX on the patient's plasma. In the best of hands, there is considerable error in these estimates. Doses should be adjusted according to the actual levels observed in vivo. For very minor surgery, one-half as much therapy may suffice, but it will still need to be maintained for 7 to 10 days.

Von Willebrand's Disease

This is the most common congenital coagulopathy, occurring in approximately 1 of 200 in the general population. Most patients are asymptomatic and discovered only after routine screening for surgery or for other problems. The PTT is usually prolonged, as is the bleeding time, although the quantitative platelet count is normal. Type I von Willebrand's disease is the most common disorder. Factor VIII:C, von Willebrand factor antigen (VWF:Ag), and ristocetin cofactor (Ricof) activity are all usually mildly reduced. If these patients are symptomatic at all they may have increased bruising, epistaxis, menorrhagia, or gingival bleeding. Type III vWD patients are very rare. Their factor VIII:C, VWF, and RiCof levels are severely quantitatively depressed, and they may present with spontaneous hemorrhaging similar to that of a person with hemophilia. Type II vWD patients have quantitative defects in their VWF multimeric structure and tend mostly to present with mild clinical symptoms.

TREATMENT. The patient with classic type I vWD responds very well to DDAVP (desmopressin, Stimate) at doses similar to those used in mild hemophilia (0.3 μg/kg IV over 30–40 minutes) with excellent elevation in both the factor VIII:C level and vWF measurements [38]. DDAVP is now also available as an intranasal preparation. As with mild hemophilia, tachyphylaxis may occur after 3 to 4 days of use, and thus factor VIII levels should be checked periodically. DDAVP can be used also in type II VWD, except in patients who have type IIB disease, because in these cases DDAVP may cause transient but significant thrombocytopenia.

Type III vWD patients do not respond to DDAVP. For these patients and persons with type IIB vWD, treatment choices are controversial. Some hematologists use cryoprecipitate, which contains both factor VIII:C and VWF, calculating the doses on the increase of factor VIII:C desired and the units of factor VIII:C in each bag of cryoprecipitate (approximately 80 units). However, cryoprecipitate is not yet virally inactivated and holds some risks for transmission of blood-borne viruses. Thus, factor VIII concentrates have also been used to increase factor VIII:C levels. Some factor concentrates do contain VWF (Hemate P, Alphaeight) but the multimeric structure is abnormal. These concentrates will not predictably shorten the bleeding time, and thus efficacy of treatment should not be judged on this parameter alone [39].

However, for major bleeding resulting from surgery or severe trauma, correction of factor VIII:C levels is thought to be sufficient [40]. Dosing should be done every 24 hours as necessary to maintain the factor VIII:C level above 50% with dose calculations similar to those used to calculate doses in patients with hemophilia A. Because of sustained factor VIII level increases, less frequent concentrate doses may suffice, and thus those patients should have factor VIII levels checked repeatedly. Again, if a patient with Von Willebrand's disease, whether severe or mild, needs surgery or invasive intensive care unit monitoring, a hematologist skilled in coagulation problems must be consulted.

References

1. Lane S: Hemorrhagic diathesis: Successful transfusion of blood. *Lancet* 1:185, 1840.
2. Feisly R: Etudes sur l'hemophilie. *Bull Mem Soc Med Hosp Paris* 47:1778, 1923.
3. Pool JG, Hershgold EJ, Pappenhagen AR: High potency antihaemophilic factor concentrate prepared from cryoglobulin precipitate. *Nature* 203:312, 1964.
4. Wagner RH, Smith M, McLester WD: Precipitation of factor VIII with

aliphatic amino acids, in Brinkhous KM (ed): *The Hemophilias.* Chapel Hill, University of North Carolina Press, 1964, p 81.

5. Johnson AJ, Newman J, Howell MB, et al: Two large-scale procedures for purification of human anti-hemophilic factor (AHF). *Blood* 28:1011, 1966.

6. Tullis JL, Melin M, Jurigian P: Clinical use of prothrombin complexes. *N Engl J Med* 273:667, 1965.

7. Graham JB: Biochemical genetics of blood coagulation. *Am J Hum Genet* 8:63, 1956.

8. Hoyer LW, Rick ME: Implications of immunologic methods for measuring antihemophilic factor (factor VIII). *Ann NY Acad Sci* 240:97, 1975.

9. Gitschier J, Wood WI, Tuddenhan EG, et al: Detection and sequence of mutations in the factor VIII gene of hemophiliacs. *Nature* 315:427, 1985.

10. Montandon AJ, Green PM, Gianelli F, et al: Direct detection of point mutations by mismatch analysis: Application to hemophilia B. *Nucleic Acids Res* 17:3347, 1989.

11. Upchurch K, Brettler DB, Levine PH: Hemophilic arthropathy, in Kelley WN, Harris ED Jr, Ruddy S, et al (eds): *Textbook of Rheumatology.* 4th ed. Philadelphia, Saunders, 1993, p 1509.

12. Hoskinson J, Duthie RB: Management of musculoskeletal problems in the hemophilias. *Orthop Clin North Am* 9:455, 1978.

13. Gilbert MS: Characterizing the hemophilic pseudotumor. *Ann NY Acad Sci* 240:311, 1975.

14. Eyster ME, Gill FM, Blatt PM, et al: Central nervous system bleeding in hemophiliacs. *Blood* 51:1179, 1978.

15. Walsh PN, Rizza CR, Evans BE, et al: The therapeutic role of epsilon aminocaproic acid (EACA) for dental extractions in hemophiliacs. *Ann NY Acad Sci* 140:267, 1975.

16. Kasper CK: Hematologic care, in Boone DC (ed): *Comprehensive Management of Hemophilia.* Philadelphia, Davis, 1976, p 3.

17. Post M, Telfer MD: Surgery in hemophilic patients. *J Bone Joint Surg [Am]* 57:1136, 1975.

18. Bona RD, Weinstein RA, Weisman ST, et al: The use of continuous infusion of factor concentrates in the treatment of hemophilia. *Am J Hematol* 32:8, 1990.

19. Smith PS, Levine PH: The benefits of comprehensive care of hemophilia: A five year study of outcomes. *Am J Public Health* 74:616, 1984.

20. White G, MacMillan C, Kingdon H, et al: Recombinant factor VIII. *N Engl J Med* 320:166, 1989.

21. Schwartz RS, Abildgaard CF, Aledort LM, et al: Human recombinant DNA derived antihemophilic factor in the treatment of hemophilia A. *N Engl J Med* 323:1800, 1990.

22. Mariani G, Ciavarella N, Mazzuconi MG, et al: Evaluation of the effectiveness of DDAVP in surgery and bleeding episodes in hemophilia and Von Willebrand Disease. *Clin Lab Haematol* 6:229, 1984.

23. Seeler RA: Hemolysis due to anti-A and anti-B in factor VIII preparations. *Arch Intern Med* 130:101, 1972.

24. Allain JP: Transfusion support for hemophiliacs. *Clin Haematol* 3:99, 1984.

25. Aledort LM, Levine PH, Hilgartner M, et al: A study of liver biopsies and liver disease among hemophiliacs. Blood 66:367, 1985.

26. Brettler DB, Forsberg A, Dienstag JL, et al: The prevalence of antibody to HCV in a cohort of hemophilic patients. *Blood* 76:254, 1990.

27. Colombo M, Mannucci PM, Brettler DB, et al: Hepatocellular carcinoma in hemophilia. *Am J Hematol* 37:243, 1991.

28. Millar DS, Steinbrecher RA, Wieland K, et al: The molecular analysis of hemophilia A: Characterizations of six partial deletions in the factor VIII gene. *Hum Genet* 86:219, 1990.

29. Eyster ME, Ballard JO, Gail MH, et al: Predictive markers for the acquired immunodeficiency syndrome in hemophiliacs: Persistence of p24 antigen and low CD4 cell counter. *Ann Intern Med* 110:963, 1989.

30. Lusher JM, Shapiro SS, Palascek JE, et al: Efficacy of prothrombin complex concentrates in hemophiliacs with antibodies to factor VIII. *N Engl J Med* 303:421, 1980.

31. Kernoff PB, Thomas ND, Lilley PA, et al: Clinical experience with polyelectrolyte-fractionated porcine factor VIII concentrate in the treatment of hemophiliacs with antibodies to factor VIII. *Blood* 63:31, 1984.

32. Hedner U, Glazer S, Pingel K, et al: Successful of recombinant factor VIIa in a patient with severe hemophilia A during synovectomy. *Lancet* 2:1193, 1988.

33. Macik BG, Hohnekr J, Roberts HR, et al: Use of recombinant activated factor VII for treatment of a retropharyngeal hemorrhage in a hemophilic patient with high titer inhibitor. *Am J Hematol* 32:232, 1989.

34. Hermens WT: Dose calculation of human factor VIII and factor IX concentrates for infusion therapy, in Brinkhous KM, Hemker HC (eds): *Handbook of Hemophilia.* New York, American Elsevier, 1975, p 569.

35. Middleton SM, Bennett IH, Smith JK: A therapeutic concentrate of coagulation factors II, IX and X from citrated factor VIII-depleted plasma. *Vox Sang* 24:441, 1973.

36. Chavin SI, Siegel DM, Rocco TA Jr., et al: Acute myocardial infarction during treatment with an activated prothrombin complex concentrate in a patient with factor VIII deficiency and a factor VIII inhibitor. *Am J Med* 85:245, 1988.

37. Kaneshiro MM, Mielke CH, Kasper CK, et al: Bleeding time after aspirin in disorders of intrinsic clotting. *N Engl J Med* 281:1039, 1969.

38. Mannucci PM, Canciani MT, Rota L, et al: Response of factor VIII/ Von Willebrand factor to desmopressin in healthy subjects and patients with hemophilia A and von Willebrand disease. *Br J Haematol* 47:283, 1981.

39. Mannucci PM, Tenconi PM, Castanan G, et al: Comparison of four virus inactivated concentrates for treatment of severe von Willebrand Disease: A crossover randomized trial. *Blood* 79:3130, 1992.

40. White GC, Montgomery RR: Clinical aspects and therapy for von Willebrand disease, in Hoffman R, Benz EJ, Shattil SJ, et al (eds): *Hematology Basic Principles and Practice.* New York, Churchill Livingstone, 1991, p 1290.

120. Thrombocytopenia

Theodore E. Warkentin and
John G. Kelton

Thrombocytopenia is one of the most common laboratory abnormalities found in patients within an intensive care unit. Although most physicians fear the bleeding complications that can be secondary to the thrombocytopenia, life-threatening bleeding is distinctly uncommon in these patients. Rather, these patients are more likely to die of the underlying cause of the thrombocytopenia. Thrombocytopenia, like anemia, should not be considered as a diagnostic endpoint. It is the cause of the thrombocytopenia that poses the greatest risk for the thrombocytopenic patient. All too often, intensive care physicians treat thrombocytopenia with platelet transfusions. If platelet support is not accompanied by a more definitive treatment of the cause for the thrombocytopenia, then the thrombocytopenia usually recurs. Additionally, there are several important platelet-mediated thrombotic disorders (Table 120-1) in which platelet transfusions can worsen the disease course and potentially cause death. In this chapter, we present the approach we use in the investigation and management of thrombocytopenic patients in the intensive care unit setting.

Definition of Thrombocytopenia

Thrombocytopenia is defined as a platelet count below 150×10^9/L, which represents 2 standard deviations below the mean platelet count for a normal, healthy population. However, an alternate definition of thrombocytopenia may be appropriate for specific patient populations. For example, the "normal" platelet count range (mean ± 2 standard deviations) was approximately 275 to 900×10^9 per liter on the 12th postoperative day in one study of patients undergoing elective hip replacement surgery. An "abnormal" platelet count of 200×10^9 per liter in this study indicated a high probability that the patient had a cause for the lower than expected platelet count such as heparin-induced thrombocytopenia [1].

Although the normal platelet count range is relatively wide ($150–400 \times 10^9$/L), healthy individuals do not experience a marked day-to-day platelet count variability. Thus, an abrupt platelet count decline, even within the normal range, can signify a pathologic process (see platelet profile "E," Fig. 120-1).

Mechanism of Thrombocytopenia

There are four general explanations for thrombocytopenia: (1) increased platelet destruction (nonimmune or immune), (2) hemodilution, (3) platelet sequestration (virtually synonymous with hypersplenism), and (4) decreased platelet production. Usually, the mechanism of thrombocytopenia can be inferred from basic clinical and laboratory data, although in unusual situations a platelet survival study may be required. Determining the mechanism of thrombocytopenia is helpful in developing a differential diagnosis (Table 120-2).

History and Physical Examination

The explanation for thrombocytopenia can often be suspected by information obtained from the history and physical examination (Table 120-3). Often, the date of onset of the thrombocytopenia in relation to specific clinical factors (e.g., exposure to blood and heparin) provides important diagnostic clues (see Fig. 120-1).

The hallmark of severe thrombocytopenia is the presence of petechiae, which are pinpoint cutaneous hemorrhages usually found in dependent areas such as the back and posterior thighs in most intensive care unit patients. Ecchymoses are larger purpura (greater than 2 mm in diameter) and hematomas are large purpura that can be palpable. Although these larger purpura also can occur in thrombocytopenic patients, they are much less specific for thrombocytopenia and occur in patients with coagulation problems, corticosteroid-induced thinning of the skin, etc.

Laboratory Investigations

COMPLETE BLOOD COUNT (CBC) AND EXAMINATION OF THE BLOOD FILM. The most helpful laboratory test is the complete blood count and peripheral blood film. The results should be compared with previous blood counts whenever

Table 120-1. Thrombocytopenic Disorders Associated with Thrombosis

Diagnosis	Type of thrombotic complication	Possible relationship between platelet destruction and thrombosis
Heparin-induced thrombocytopenia	Macrovascular thrombosis (venous, arterial)	Causal
Thrombotic thrombocytopenic purpura/hemolytic uremic syndrome	Microvascular (arteriolar) thrombosis	Causal
Antiphospholipid antibody syndrome (lupus anticoagulant syndrome)	Macrovascular thrombosis; ?microvascular thrombosis	?Causal
Disseminated intravascular coagulation	Microvascular thrombosis	Collateral
Hemodilution	Macrovascular thrombosis (e.g., perioperative myocardial infarction)	Collateral

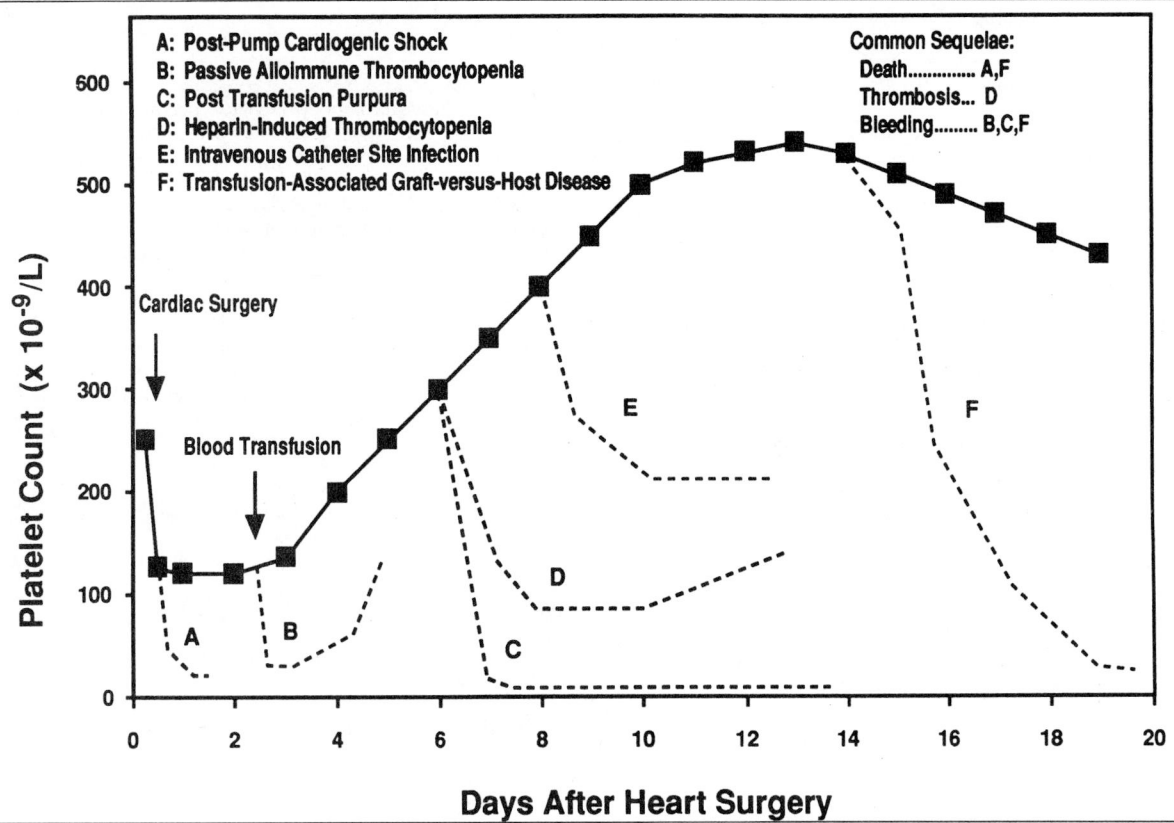

A: Post-Pump Cardiogenic Shock
B: Passive Alloimmune Thrombocytopenia
C: Post Transfusion Purpura
D: Heparin-Induced Thrombocytopenia
E: Intravenous Catheter Site Infection
F: Transfusion-Associated Graft-versus-Host Disease

Common Sequelae:
Death............. A,F
Thrombosis... D
Bleeding......... B,C,F

Fig. 120-1. Various platelet count profiles after heart surgery.

possible. Isolated thrombocytopenia is usually caused by increased platelet destruction, whereas thrombocytopenia accompanied by anemia and leukopenia is caused by decreased platelet production, hypersplenism, or hemodilution.

Evaluation of the mean platelet volume (MPV) may provide helpful diagnostic clues [2]. Normal megakaryocytes respond to thrombocytopenia by producing increased numbers of larger-sized platelets [3]. Hence, large platelets (increased MPV) are associated with destructive thrombocytopenic disorders, and a reduced MPV is often caused by decreased marrow production [2].

Inspection of the blood film can provide important diagnostic clues. One important reason to review the blood film is to exclude **pseudothrombocytopenia.** This is an ex vivo artifact usually caused by ethylenediaminetetra-acetic acid (EDTA)-dependent platelet agglutinins [4,5]. The platelet aggregates, which are not detected by the electronic particle counter, are readily observed microscopically. The correct platelet count can usually be determined by collecting the blood sample into alternate anticoagulants such as sodium citrate, or by counting platelets in a counting chamber using blood obtained by finger prick. Another pseudothrombocytopenic disorder known as "platelet satellitism" can be diagnosed by the characteristic rosetting of platelets around neutrophils or monocytes [6].

The blood film should be reviewed for several morphologic abnormalities that can indicate septicemia. These can include increased number, immaturity ("left shift"), or granularity ("toxic granularity") of the neutrophils. Pale blue cytoplasmic inclusions termed Döhle bodies, vacuoles, and protoplasmic extensions of neutrophils and monocytes can also indicate septicemia.

Less common morphologic abnormalities that suggest specific diagnoses include red cell fragments (thrombotic thrombocytopenic purpura, hemolytic-uremic syndrome, disseminated intravascular coagulation, preeclampsia), "tear drop" and nucleated red cells (infiltrative marrow disorders), "atypical" lymphocytes (viral infections, lymphoproliferative disorders), parasitic red cell inclusions (malaria), circulating myeloblasts or lymphoblasts (acute leukemia), or giant platelets (hereditary macrothrombocytopenia).

BONE MARROW ASPIRATE AND BIOPSY. Examination of the bone marrow is usually not helpful in evaluating thrombocytopenic patients in the intensive care unit. This is because the commonest cause for thrombocytopenia in this group of patients is increased platelet destruction. In these patients, the marrow typically is normal [7]. However, bone marrow examination is important in patients in whom the mechanism of thrombocytopenia is obscure, or in whom a disorder of decreased platelet production is suspected (pancytopenic patients without splenomegaly or hemodilution). The marrow can be virtually diagnostic in several important disorders, including megaloblastic anemia, hemophagocytosis, primary (e.g., acute leukemia, myelodysplasia) or secondary (e.g., metastatic carcinomatosis) neoplastic disorders, and aplastic anemia.

Assessment of Bleeding Risk

The physician should attempt to estimate the risk of bleeding when evaluating thrombocytopenic patients. Unfortunately, there are few data available to help the physician judge the risk

Table 120-2. Mechanism/Differential Diagnosis of Thrombocytopenia

Increased Platelet Destruction
  Septicemia
  Other disorders associated with systemic inflammatory response (acute pancreatitis, fat embolism syndrome, acute respiratory distress syndrome, severe allergic reactions)
  Extracorporeal circulation (note: predominantly hemodilution)
  Intravascular catheters and prostheses
  Cardiovascular, pulmonary hypertensive, and thrombotic disorders
  Glomerulonephritis, acute transplant rejection
  Disseminated intravascular coagulation
    Acute (trauma, shock, septicemia, intravascular hemolysis, snake bites, heat stroke, obstetric complications)
    Chronic (neoplasms, aortic aneurysms, hemangiomas)
  Drug-induced (immune) thrombocytopenia
    Heparin-induced thrombocytopenia
    Miscellaneous idiosyncratic drug-induced thrombocytopenia
  Autoimmune thrombocytopenia
    Idiopathic thrombocytopenic purpura (ITP)
    Secondary ITP (systemic lupus erythematosus and other rheumatic disorders, HIV infection, neoplastic lymphoproliferative disorders, solid tumors)
  Alloimmune thrombocytopenia
    Posttransfusion purpura, passive alloimmune thrombocytopenia
  Thrombotic microangiopathy
    Thrombotic thrombocytopenic purpura, hemolytic-uremic syndrome
Hemodilution
Platelet sequestration
  Hypersplenism
  Hypothermia
Decreased platelet production with isolated thrombocytopenia
  Alcohol-induced thrombocytopenia
  Congenital hypomegakaryocytic disorders (e.g., thrombocytopenia absent radii syndrome)
  Congenital (hereditary) thrombocytopenia with normal megakaryocyte numbers (e.g., hereditary macrothrombocytopenic disorders, Wiskott-Aldrich syndrome)
Decreased platelet production with pancytopenia
  Acute leukemia, myelodysplasia, primary myelofibrosis, aplastic anemia, paroxysmal nocturnal hemoglobinuria
  Megaloblastic anemia
  Antineoplastic chemotherapy or radiation
  Transfusion-associated graft-versus-host disease
  Hemophagocytosis
  Congenital marrow disorders (e.g., Fanconi anemia)

Table 120-3. Assessment of Thrombocytopenia in the Intensive Care Unit

Alcohol abuse
  Alcohol-induced thrombocytopenia, hypersplenism secondary to cirrhosis, septicemia, megaloblastic anemia secondary to folate deficiency
Numerous petechiae, mucosal blood blisters
  May indicate higher risk of life-threatening bleeding
Extremity swelling (venous thrombosis)
  Heparin-induced thrombocytopenia, chronic DIC (e.g., secondary to adenocarcinoma)
Pale, ischemic limb(s)
  Heparin-induced thrombocytopenia (large vessel arterial thrombosis), shock with DIC (microvascular ischemia)
Fever/chills
  Septicemia, acute heparin-induced thrombocytopenia following intravenous bolus heparin (rare)
Recent surgery
  Hemodilution
Conjunctival and upper body petechiae
  Bacterial endocarditis, fat emboli syndrome
Erythematous maculopapular rash
  Transfusion-associated graft-versus-host disease (rare, associated with pancytopenia)
Hypotension
  Septicemia, subacute retroperitoneal bleeding (hemodilution), adrenal insufficiency (septicemia, heparin-induced thrombocytopenia)
Drugs
  Heparin-induced thrombocytopenia (common); all other idiosyncratic drug-induced thrombocytopenic disorders are relatively uncommon
Intravascular catheters
  Heparin-induced thrombocytopenia, catheter-related septicemia
Recent blood transfusion
  Hemodilution (common), posttransfusion purpura (rare), passive alloimmune thrombocytopenia (rare), transfusion-associated graft-versus-host disease (rare, associated with pancytopenia), cytomegalovirus-associated immune thrombocytopenia (rare)
Remote blood transfusion
  Hypersplenism secondary to chronic hepatitis, human immunodeficiency virus-associated immune thrombocytopenia
Hepatomegaly or splenomegaly
  Hypersplenism (multiple causes), infiltrative marrow disorders (rare)
Lymphadenopathy
  Lymphoproliferative disorder (e.g., lymphoma, chronic lymphocytic leukemia)
Focal neurologic deficits
  Heparin-induced thrombocytopenia (thrombotic cerebrovascular accident), thrombotic thrombocytopenic purpura, hemolytic-uremic syndrome (rare), chronic disseminated intravascular coagulation secondary to adenocarcinoma
Renal failure
  Septicemia, thrombotic thrombocytopenic purpura/hemolytic-uremic syndrome, immediate or delayed severe hemolytic transfusion reaction (rare)
Very severe thrombocytopenia
  Autoimmune thrombocytopenia, drug-induced thrombocytopenia (note: heparin-induced thrombocytopenia more commonly >20 × 10⁹/L), posttransfusion purpura (rare)

of bleeding. Several clinical factors can impact on the bleeding risk, and are summarized here:

1. *Severity and cause of the thrombocytopenia.* In general, the risk of bleeding does not increase until the platelet count falls below 20×10^9 per liter and does not increase markedly until below 5×10^9 per liter. However, the risk appears to vary with the mechanism for the thrombocytopenia [8]. For example, most patients with immune thrombocytopenic disorders produce large, hyperfunctional platelets. At the same platelet count, the risk of bleeding is lower in these patients than in patients with decreased platelet production [8].

2. *Comorbid factors.* Many patients have one or more comorbid factors that influence risk of bleeding, including disruption of vascular integrity (recent surgery, trauma, intravascular catheters); coagulation disorders (liver dysfunction, vitamin K deficiency or pharmacologic antagonism, disseminated intravascular coagulation); platelet dysfunction (certain drugs,

uremia); and other poorly defined patient-dependent factors.

Prophylaxis of Thrombocytopenic Bleeding

Patients at increased risk for life-threatening hemorrhage (e.g., major head injury, recent neurosurgery, removal of pericardial drainage tubes after open heart surgery) should probably have the platelet count raised to above 50×10^9 per liter. Studies suggest that "blind" invasive procedures such as liver biopsy, paracentesis, and thoracentesis can be performed safely when the platelet count is greater than this level [9,10].

Prophylactic platelet transfusions are contraindicated in patients in patients with platelet-mediated thrombosis (heparin-induced thrombocytopenia, thrombotic thrombocytopenic purpura, hemolytic-uremic syndrome). This is because bleeding complications are relatively uncommon, and platelet transfusions may precipitate thrombotic complications.

Prophylactic use of desmopressin (DDAVP, 20 μg in 50 mL solution given over 20 minutes) has been shown to reduce the bleeding time in patients with certain platelet function disorders (e.g., uremia, cirrhosis) [11,12,13] and to reduce bleeding in some patients after open heart surgery [14,15]. Desmopressin is not effective in severely thrombocytopenic patients [11], but may be helpful in some patients with moderate thrombocytopenia (e.g., 20–100 × 10^9/L) [16]. Desmopressin releases large multimeric forms of von Willebrand factor from endothelial cells [17] and results in enhanced platelet-subendothelial interactions. However, increased von Willebrand factor synthesis and release typically occurs in certain postoperative [18] or traumatized patients, and may not be elevated further by desmopressin.

Treatment of Thrombocytopenic Bleeding

Platelet transfusions should be given to patients with life-threatening bleeding irrespective of the mechanism of thrombocytopenia. This approach is important even if the transfused platelets will be destroyed rapidly by the underlying disorder [19]. The reticuloendothelial system should be blocked using high-dose intravenous gammaglobulin in patients with immune thrombocytopenia [20]. The physician should simultaneously treat the underlying cause for the thrombocytopenia.

Causes of Thrombocytopenia in the Intensive Care Unit

Although there are a large number of potential causes of thrombocytopenia in an intensive care unit, several disorders are encountered relatively frequently, and may coexist (Fig. 120-2). However, certain rare thrombocytopenic disorders are important to recognize promptly (thrombotic thrombocytopenic purpura, intracranial hemorrhage in autoimmune thrombocytopenia, posttransfusion purpura), because rapid treatment can be life saving.

Thrombocytopenia Caused by Increased Platelet Destruction

Increased platelet destruction is the most important cause of thrombocytopenia in the intensive care unit. It is common and may be indicative of a potentially life-threatening disorder.

SEPTICEMIA. Sepsis is the most common cause of death in intensive care units [21] and also is a common cause of thrombocytopenia in these patients. Typically, thrombocytopenia is caused by increased platelet destruction, possibly by both immune and non-immune mechanisms. Occasionally, infection produces thrombocytopenia through other mechanisms, including decreased platelet production (e.g., marrow infiltration by *Mycobacterium avium-intracellulare* in acquired immune deficiency syndrome [AIDS] patients; hepatitis C–associated aplastic anemia), hypersplenism (malaria), or initiation of autoimmune platelet destruction (postviral or vaccination acute idiopathic thrombocytopenic purpura).

Thrombocytopenia typically occurs in patients with advanced infection caused by gram-positive bacteria, endotoxin-containing gram-negative bacteria, or fungi. In infected patients, the presence of thrombocytopenia is an important clue indicating a high probability of microbial invasion of the bloodstream (bacteremia). For example, approximately two-thirds of bacteremic patients develop thrombocytopenia [22,23,24], and thrombocytopenia occurs in more than 90% of patients with septic shock [25,26]. Blood cultures and careful clinical assessment of intravascular catheters should always be performed in hospitalized patients in whom unexplained thrombocytopenia occurs.

The pathophysiology of thrombocytopenia is debated. Occasionally, excess intravascular thrombin generation (DIC) can be demonstrated in these patients and could contribute to the thrombocytopenia. Investigators using dual radiolabels observed parallel increases in fibrinogen and platelet turnover in septic patients [27]. Other evidence implicating thrombin generation in septic patients includes elevated thrombin-antithrombin complexes and soluble fibrin monomer complexes [28], as well as elevated cross-linked D-dimer levels [29].

However, evidence for excess thrombin generation is usually not observed in patients with mild-to-moderate thrombocytopenia [23], suggesting that other mechanisms are responsible for the thrombocytopenia. Elevated platelet-associated IgG [30] and elevated circulating immune complexes [31] suggest that immune mechanisms could explain the thrombocytopenia in these patients. A humoral immune pathogenesis for malaria-associated thrombocytopenia was found by one group who observed that IgG localized to malarial antigens that became adsorbed to the platelet surface [32].

Platelet destruction in some instances could be related to direct effects of the infection. For example, certain bacterial toxins such as endotoxin [33,34] and *Staphylococcus aureus* α-toxin [35,36] directly activate platelets. Endogenous mediators of the sepsis syndrome such as platelet-activating factor [37] and tumor necrosis factor [38] could also be important in producing thrombocytopenia.

There is no evidence supporting the routine therapeutic role of anticoagulants or antiplatelet agents in improving outcomes in thrombocytopenic, septic patients. Some physicians use heparin in septic patients with DIC [25], but the efficacy of this approach remains unproven. We use heparin in patients with fulminant DIC, particularly when there is evidence of thrombotic complications (e.g., meningococcal septicemia in children

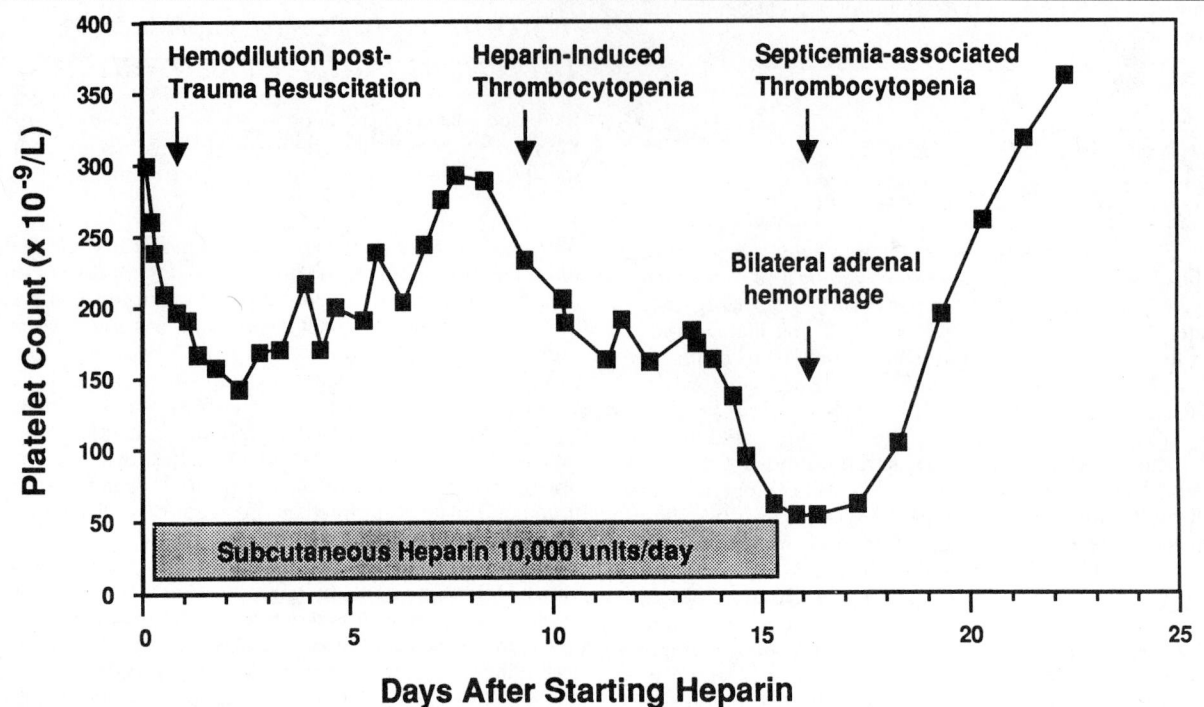

Fig. 120-2. Potential causes of thrombocytopenia in the intensive care unit.

resulting in necrosis of the extremities). The most important therapy remains the early introduction of appropriate antibiotic therapy [24], surgical drainage whenever appropriate, and aggressive hemodynamic support [39,40].

MISCELLANEOUS DESTRUCTIVE THROMBOCYTOPENIC DISORDERS. Thrombocytopenia is a common finding in patients with disorders associated with a *systemic inflammatory response,* such as acute pancreatitis, fat embolism syndrome [41], acute respiratory distress syndrome [42], and severe allergic reactions [43,44]. Although the mechanism for the increased platelet destruction in these syndromes is unknown, it may be mediated by endogenous inflammatory mediators. No specific therapeutic interventions for the thrombocytopenia have been described, and therapy is largely supportive.

Increased platelet destruction occurs in patients undergoing extracorporeal circulation (cardiopulmonary bypass surgery, hemodialysis, apheresis) [45,46]. However, significant thrombocytopenia is usually caused by other factors, such as hemodilution (approximately 50% in patients undergoing open heart surgery) [47].

Increased platelet turnover can be caused by indwelling intravascular prosthetic devices, including pulmonary artery (Swan-Ganz) catheters, prosthetic heart valves, dacron vascular grafts, intraaortic balloon pumps, arteriovenous Silastic cannulas, and ventriculojugular shunts [27,48,49]. Typically, the thrombocytopenia is mild because of compensatory increase in platelet production. The increased platelet turnover can normalize with progressive endothelialization of the implanted foreign material [49,50]. Thrombocytopenia in these patients should always prompt consideration of alternate diagnoses

such as catheter- or prosthesis-related infection, or heparin-induced thrombocytopenia [51].

Certain cardiovascular disease, including congenital or acquired valvular heart disease [52,53,54], cardiomyopathies [55], primary pulmonary hypertensive syndromes [56,57], or massive deep vein thrombosis or pulmonary embolism [58,59], has been associated with increased platelet consumption and thrombocytopenia. However, alternate explanations for the thrombocytopenia should be considered (e.g., heparin-induced thrombocytopenia or DIC secondary to adenocarcinoma in patients with thrombocytopenia complicating venous thromboembolic disease).

Thrombocytopenia can occur in some patients with immune-mediated glomerulonephritis, such as poststreptococcal glomerulonephritis [60]. Thrombocytopenia also can accompany acute renal transplant rejection [61].

DISSEMINATED INTRAVASCULAR COAGULATION. Disseminated intravascular coagulation (DIC) can be defined as a clinicopathologic spectrum of disorders characterized by excess thrombin generation within the circulation (see Chap. 118). Thrombocytopenia is a frequent finding in DIC and is believed to be related to thrombin-mediated platelet activation.

Patients can present with both acute and chronic DIC. Acute DIC is often seen in severe tissue injury [62], shock, septicemia [23], severe intravascular hemolysis, snakebites, heat stroke, and obstetric complications, such as placental abruption [63] and amniotic fluid embolism. Microvascular thrombotic complications can lead to severe acral tissue losses (e.g., symmetric gangrene of the hands and feet) [64,65,66]. This is classically observed in children with acute meningococcal septicemia or Rocky Mountain spotted fever.

Chronic DIC is usually seen in patients with adenocarcinoma, where it can result in a prothrombotic state, such as recurrent deep vein thromboses or nonbacterial marantic endocarditis with thromboembolic phenomena. This syndrome can cause life-threatening thromboembolic complications, including phlegmasia cerulea dolens, venous gangrene, and recurrent arterial thrombosis [67,68]. Less common age-specific explanations for a hemorrhagic syndrome accompanied by laboratory evidence for DIC include cavernous hemangiomas in neonates and young children [69,70], intrauterine deaths in pregnant women, and certain abdominal aortic aneurysms in elderly patients [71]. However, localized rather than disseminated intravascular thrombin generation occurs in these patients. Sometimes, adequate compensatory increase in coagulation factor synthesis occurs, and the laboratory abnormalities are limited to thrombocytopenia and elevated fibrin(ogen) degradation products.

There are no specific diagnostic tests for DIC. This is because laboratory tests cannot distinguish between physiologic thrombosis (normal postoperative hemostasis), localized pathologic thrombosis (deep vein thrombosis, particularly after treatment with lytic therapy), and generalized microvascular thrombosis (typical DIC). Thus, the results of hemostasis testing must be interpreted in the clinical context. DIC is discussed in more detail in Chapter 118.

HEPARIN-INDUCED THROMBOCYTOPENIA. Heparin-induced thrombocytopenia is an important cause of thrombocytopenia in hospitalized patients because of its high frequency and paradoxic risk of venous or arterial thrombosis [1,72,73,74]. In addition, there is evidence that certain patient populations [75,76] (including very ill patients in intensive care units) may be more likely to suffer adverse clinical sequelae from this drug reaction.

The incidence of heparin-induced thrombocytopenia varies widely in published studies [73]. The incidence is related to the type and dose of heparin used, as well as the definition of thrombocytopenia. At therapeutic doses of heparin, approximately 5 to 10 percent of patients treated with bovine lung heparin and 2 to 3 percent treated with porcine mucosal heparin develop a platelet count less than 100×10^9 per liter. In contrast, thrombocytopenia occurs in fewer than 1% of patients receiving low-dose heparin.

Mild-to-moderate thrombocytopenia is typical in heparin-induced thrombocytopenia. The mean platelet count reported in the literature is approximately 50×10^9 per liter [74,75]. It is rare for the platelet count to be below 20×10^9 per liter (contrast thrombocytopenia caused by quinine, quinidine, and sulfa drugs). Typically, the onset of thrombocytopenia is 6 to 10 days after initial heparin exposure. Although the frequency of heparin-induced thrombocytopenia is dose dependent, some patients develop thrombocytopenia and thrombotic sequelae even when receiving small amounts of heparin, including heparin given for line "flushes" or heparin that is bonded to pulmonary artery catheters [77,78,79].

Several clinical syndromes can occur with heparin-induced thrombocytopenia, including arterial thrombosis, venous thrombosis, DIC, hemorrhagic infarction (especially of the adrenal glands), and skin necrosis (especially at the sites of heparin injection). Arterial thrombosis most commonly affects the distal aorta and proximal lower limb arteries, but cerebrovascular and coronary artery thrombosis are described. Lower and upper limb venous thrombosis, which can progress to venous gangrene, have also been reported. Certain comorbid clinical factors such as vascular trauma resulting from placement of arterial or central venous catheters can localize thrombosis to the site of vascular injury [80]. Recently, patients have been reported to develop abrupt-onset thrombocytopenia and acute inflammatory reactions, termed "acute systemic reactions," after administration of intravenous bolus heparin [81]. Transient global amnesia has also been reported in heparin-induced thrombocytopenia patients after intravenous bolus heparin [82].

Bilateral adrenal hemorrhage merits special attention, as this complication has been reported in several patients in intensive care unit settings [79,83,84,85] (see Fig. 120-2). Patients sometimes present with unexplained abdominal pain and hypotension. Pathologic studies indicate adrenal vein thrombosis and hemorrhagic infarction, suggesting that the hemorrhage is secondary to prothrombotic effects of heparin-induced thrombocytopenia.

Heparin-induced thrombocytopenia is caused by heparin-dependent IgG that activates platelets through their Fc receptors [86] through an interaction with platelet factor 4 [87]. There is marked variability among normal individuals [88] and patients [76] in their Fc receptor numbers and platelet reactivity to Fc receptor stimuli, suggesting that this could be an important factor determining the differences in clinical sequelae. The high risk of thrombotic complications in patients with heparin-induced thrombocytopenia could be related to observations that heparin-dependent IgG causes platelets to produce platelet-derived microparticles that carry procoagulant activity [89].

Currently, optimal diagnostic testing for heparin-induced thrombocytopenia uses a platelet activation endpoint, such as platelet release [86,88,90], platelet microparticle formation [91], or aggregation of washed platelets [92]. Many centers use aggregation of platelets in citrated plasma, but the sensitivity may be as low as 50% [92,93].

The optimal treatment for heparin-induced thrombocytopenia remains unknown. For patients with thrombotic complications who require further anticoagulation, the options include warfarin (potential risk of warfarin-induced limb necrosis in this patient population) [93], ancrod (Arvin) [94] (potential risk of precipitating thrombosis in some patients with impaired fibrinolysis) [95], and the heparinoid danaparoid sodium (Orgaran) (possible risk of cross-reactivity with heparin-dependent IgG) [96]. We have some experience using two agents: ancrod and danaparoid. When ancrod is used as a defibrinogenating agent, it is important that warfarin not be started simultaneously with the ancrod, because a rapid decrease in the protein C levels (a natural anticoagulant) could worsen the thrombotic complications [93]. We give the ancrod for several days, then initiate warfarin when the thrombocytopenia has resolved. High-dose intravenous gammaglobulin [97], plasmapheresis [98], and thrombolytic therapy [99] may be beneficial in some patients. In our experience, use of vena caval filters may be associated with progression in limb-threatening thrombotic complications.

OTHER CAUSES OF DRUG-INDUCED THROMBOCYTOPENIA. Many antineoplastic drugs cause transient, sometimes severe, pancytopenia in a dose-dependent fashion. Admission to intensive care units is more often the result of life-threatening infections secondary to severe neutropenia rather than thrombocytopenic bleeding.

Many other drugs cause idiosyncratic thrombocytopenia [100,101,102] (Table 120-4). In some instances, immune mechanisms have been established. For example, drug-dependent IgG Fab binding to specific platelet glycoprotein complexes, such as GPIIb/IIIa (fibrinogen receptor) or GPIb/IX (von Willebrand factor receptor), has been implicated in the pathogenesis of quinine-, quinidine-, and vancomycin-induced thrombocytopenia. The platelet count is usually less than 20×10^9

Table 120-4. Drug-Induced Thrombocytopenia

Drug-dependent platelet-activating IgG (Fc receptor dependent)
   Standard (unfractionated) heparin, low-molecular-weight heparin, pentosan polysulfate, Arteparon (polysulfated chondroitin sulfate)

Drug-dependent increase in PAIgG (Fab-dependent, Fc-independent, binding to platelet GPIIb/IIIa or GPIb/IX or both)
   Quinine, quinidine, vancomycin

Drug-dependent increase in PAIgG (unknown GP localization)
   Ampicillin, cefotetan, cephamandole, cimetidine, diazepam, gold, ibuprofen, "sulfa" antibiotics, penicillin, piroxicam, ranitidine, rifampin

Probable drug-induced thrombocytopenia (established by drug rechallenge or drug-dependent non-PAIgG assays, e.g., complement fixation, platelet factor 3 assays)
   Acetaminophen, acetazolamide, actinomycin D, allyl-isopropyl-acetyl-carbamide, alprenolol, aminoglutethimide, amiodarone, antazoline, aspirin (acetylsalicylic acid), carbamazepine, cephalexin, cephalothin, chlorothiazide, chlorpheniramine, chlorthalidone, danazol, desferrioxamine, desipramine, diazoxide, diflunisal, difluoromethylornithine, digitoxin, digoxin, diphenylhydantoin, ethchlorvynol, furosemide, gentamicin, heroin, hydrochlorothiazide, imipramine, α-interferon, β-interferon, iodinated contrast agents (diatrizoate, iocetamic acid, iopanoic acid), isotretinoin, levamisole, lidocaine, meclofenamate, meprobamate, methicillin, methyldopa, mianserin, minoxidil, morphine, nalidixic acid, nomifensine, novobiocin, oxprenolol, paraaminosalicylic acid, phenylbutazone, piperacillin, pirenzepine, procainamide, spironolactone, stibogluconate, stibophen, sulfasalazine, tolmetin

Possible drug-induced thrombocytopenia (no rechallenge or in vitro testing)
   Amitriptyline, apalcillin, butobarbitone, captopril, chlordiazepoxide/clidinium bromide, chlorpropamide, clinoril, clonazepam, cocaine, etretinate, fenoprofen, glyburide [glibenclamide], indomethacin, isoniazid, levodopa, lincomycin, nitroprusside, oxyphenbutazone, oxytetracycline, pentamidine, primidone, sulindac, ticlopidine, tobramycin, tolbutamide, toluene

Drugs with high incidence of mild thrombocytopenia and positive direct PAIgG
   Valproic acid
   Amrinone ·

Drug-induced lupus anticoagulant syndrome and thromboembolism
   Procainamide

Drug-induced hemolytic-uremic syndrome
   Quinine

Drug-induced immune hemolytic anemia with thrombocytopenia
   Diclofenac, doxepin, glafenine, nomifensine

References for this table can be found elsewhere [100,101].

per liter in these patients (contrast heparin-induced thrombocytopenia), and mucocutaneous bleeding is frequent. Fatal intracranial hemorrhages have been reported. Patients in whom severe idiosyncratic drug-induced thrombocytopenia is suspected should have all potentially implicated drugs discontinued, with substitution (if necessary) using immunologically non–cross-reactive agents. High-dose intravenous gammaglobulin, with or without platelet transfusions, should be given to patients judged to be at high risk for serious hemorrhage. The benefit of corticosteroids is uncertain.

Rarely, drug-dependent immune mechanisms result in damage to the hemopoietic stem cell, resulting in life-threatening drug-induced aplastic anemia (e.g., gold, carbamazepine, chloramphenicol, sulfonamides, phenylbutazone).

AUTOIMMUNE THROMBOCYTOPENIA. Idiopathic thrombocytopenic purpura (ITP) is a relatively common autoimmune disorder caused by platelet-reactive IgG that results in premature destruction of the platelets by macrophages of the reticuloendothelial system (spleen, liver, marrow, lungs). In most patients, the antigenic targets are platelet GPIIb/IIIa and GPIb/IX [103]. Although an abrupt-onset (acute) thrombocytopenia can occur, for most adults, the thrombocytopenia is chronic, with intermittent exacerbations that can be severe. There is a 3:1 female predominance, and many patients are young adults or middle-aged.

Many patients with mild-to-moderate ITP are asymptomatic, and treatment is not required. However, severe thrombocytopenia (platelet count less than $20 \times 10^9/L$) and bleeding complications may necessitate urgent treatment. Platelet transfusions (10–20 random donor units) should be administered to any patient with life-threatening bleeding. Two approaches have been reported to raise the platelet count rapidly (within 24 hours) in the majority of ITP patients: high-dose intravenous gammaglobulin (1 g/kg given over 6–8 hours, for 2 consecutive days) [104,105] and high-dose intravenous methylprednisolone (1 g over 30 minutes for 3 consecutive days) [106]. Plasmapheresis has been used successfully in refractory patients [107].

Intravenous administration of Rh immune globulin (anti-D) to Rhesus-positive individuals will raise the platelet count to safe levels in approximately 75% of patients [108]. But because response is often not seen during the first 48 hours, this therapy is not recommended in urgent situations. However, Rh immune globulin is much less expensive than high-dose gammaglobulin treatment, and is preferred in appropriate situations (e.g., preparation for elective surgery).

Many treatments have been used for longer-term control of the thrombocytopenia [109,110]. The standard first-line agent is oral prednisone (0.25–1 mg/kg/day for 1–3 weeks, with subsequent tapering to zero or low maintenance doses). However, relapse during or after tapering of the prednisone is a common occurrence.

Splenectomy offers the best chance of cure (approximately 70%, with partial benefit in an additional 10–20% of patients). Prospective splenectomy candidates should receive pneumococcal, meningococcal, and, possibly, *Haemophilus influenzae* type b vaccination before planned splenectomy [111], to reduce the risk of postsplenectomy septicemia. Patients in whom splenectomy fails or who relapse after initial response should undergo investigations for a residual, "accessory" spleen.

Although many other medical treatments have been used to treat patients with refractory ITP (including danazol, α-interferon, dapsone, colchicine), consideration of cytotoxic agents alone (azathioprine, cyclophosphamide, or vinca alkaloids) or in combination [112] should be given for refractory ITP patients who continue to bleed.

SECONDARY AUTOIMMUNE THROMBOCYTOPENIA. Acute severe ITP can be triggered by viral infections (Epstein-Barr virus, cytomegalovirus, varicella, rubella), and in approximately 1 of 30,000 children receiving measles-mumps-rubella vaccination [113]. Symptomatic patients should receive high-dose intravenous gammaglobulin.

Chronic ITP can be associated with autoimmune (systemic lupus erythematosus, rheumatoid arthritis, "reactive" large granular lymphocytic disorders) and neoplastic (most commonly chronic lymphocytic leukemia and Hodgkin's/non-Hodgkin's lymphomas) disorders. Sometimes the thrombocytopenia responds to treatment of the underlying disorder, but usually one must treat the patient as though he or she had ITP.

Many patients who are infected with the human immunodeficiency virus (HIV) develop chronic thrombocytopenia, likely of humoral immune pathogenesis. HIV patients respond to conventional treatment for ITP, including corticosteroids, splenectomy, gammaglobulin, and Rh immune globulin. Many physicians prefer to give high-dose intravenous gammaglobulin because of the concern of exacerbating immunosuppression using prednisone or immunosuppressives. Splenectomy has been used successfully in these patients. The physician should always consider alternate explanations for thrombocytopenia in patients with chronic HIV infection, including effects of myelosuppressive anti-retroviral drugs, opportunistic infections involving marrow, marrow hypoplasia secondary to advanced retroviral burden, or neoplastic involvement of the marrow. The platelet count can rise with anti-retroviral treatment, e.g., zidovudine, but the rise is usually modest.

ALLOIMMUNE THROMBOCYTOPENIA. The alloimmune thrombocytopenic disorders are a rare but important cause of thrombocytopenia in adult patients. *Posttransfusion purpura* (PTP) is characterized by severe thrombocytopenia (platelet count usually less than 20×10^9/L) that begins 5 to 10 days after blood transfusion [114]. More than 95 percent of patients are women who are older than 40 years and who were presumably sensitized during previous pregnancies. The syndrome is caused by formation of high-titer platelet-specific alloantibodies (usually anti-Pl[A1]) that result in destruction of autologous platelets. Severe, life-threatening thrombocytopenia can persist for days to weeks. High-dose intravenous gammaglobulin is first-line treatment [115], although plasmapheresis appears to benefit some patients as well. *Passive alloimmune thrombocytopenia* (PAT) is a syndrome of abrupt thrombocytopenia that begins within hours of receiving a blood transfusion. It is caused by platelet-specific alloantibodies within the blood product [116,117].

THROMBOTIC MICROANGIOPATHIC DISORDERS. There are two major thrombotic microangiopathic disorders: thrombotic thrombocytopenic purpura (TTP) and hemolytic-uremic syndrome (HUS). Both of these disorders are characterized by thrombocytopenia, intravascular hemolysis (fragmented red cells known as schistocytes or "helmet" cells, elevated lactate dehydrogenase [LDH], elevated unconjugated bilirubin), and risk of organ dysfunction secondary to platelet-rich microvascular thrombosis. Particularly in HUS, the red cell fragmentation can be mild [118], and a markedly elevated LDH can be helpful as a rapid marker for intravascular hemolysis.

Thrombotic thrombocytopenic purpura (TTP) typically occurs in middle-aged adults, with a slight female preponderance (3:2) [119]. There is often a nonspecific flulike prodrome. Many patients develop multiorgan dysfunction, including the central nervous system (altered level of consciousness, focal deficits, seizures), kidneys (oliguric renal failure), heart (heart failure, dysrhythmias), lungs (respiratory distress syndrome), and pancreas (abdominal pain). Fever occurs in some patients.

The pathogenesis of TTP is unknown, although there is evidence for involvement of enzymic platelet-activating factors [120] and high multimeric forms of von Willebrand factor [121].

The treatment of choice for TTP is plasma, preferably given by apheresis [122]. The patient should receive fresh frozen plasma by infusion (75–100 ml/hr), pending the initiation of plasmapheresis. Some physicians use high-dose corticosteroids (prednisone 200 mg/day) as initial treatment for all patients with TTP, and reserve plasma exchange for those with renal or neurologic involvement or who failed to respond to prednisone [123]. Many physicians also routinely prescribe one or more antiplatelet agents, including aspirin, dipyridamole, dextran, ticlopidine, and prostacyclin [124]; however, the possible additional benefit of these therapies is not established.

The management of refractory TTP patients is uncertain. Some patients who respond incompletely, or who are refractory, to plasmapheresis may respond to more intensive plasma exchange or substitution of cryosupernatant (which lacks the large multimers of von Willebrand factor) for fresh frozen plasma [125]. Plasmapheresis should be continued even in patients who show no or minimal platelet count response, because microthrombotic complications could be prevented, and the prospect for eventual remission is high (>80%) [126,127]. Some physicians try adjunctive treatments such as splenectomy [126,127] or vincristine for refractory or relapsing TTP, but the efficacy remains unproven.

End-stage renal failure and persisting neurologic dysfunction are important long-term sequelae of TTP (approximately 10% each) [126]. Early or late relapse of the TTP occurs in approximately 25% of patients [126,127].

Hemolytic-uremic syndrome (HUS) can be considered a nephrotropic variant of TTP that typically occurs at the extremes of age, i.e., small children and the elderly. In many patients there is a bloody diarrheal prodrome, which in western societies is usually caused by verocytotoxin-producing *Escherichia coli* O157:H7 [128,129]. Shigatoxin-producing *Shigella dysenteriae* is a frequent trigger in nonwestern countries. Oliguric renal failure is the hallmark of HUS, with neurologic involvement less common than in TTP. Children without the diarrheal prodrome appear to be at increased risk for severe HUS and subsequent relapse [130].

HUS varies from a relatively mild illness that recovers with symptomatic treatment alone to a fulminant disorder resulting in fulminant renal failure and other life-threatening complications. A multicenter randomized controlled trial of plasma infusion did not show a patient or renal survival benefit, compared with supportive therapy [131]. However, the treated group demonstrated lower follow-up blood creatinine levels, less proteinuria, and less cortical necrosis. Based on the proven effectiveness of plasma treatment in TTP, we recommend plasmapheresis therapy for children with severe HUS.

Illnesses that resemble TTP or HUS have been reported in patients with various underlying conditions, including neoplasia, HIV infection, systemic lupus erythematosus, pregnancy and the postpartum period, bone marrow transplantation, and while receiving certain drugs (quinine, mitomycin C).

Hemodilution

Administration of large amounts of crystalloid, colloid, or red cell concentrates results in dilutional thrombocytopenia. In addition, administration of red cell concentrates can be associated with further thrombocytopenia, possibly related to transient splenic platelet sequestration initiated by the transfused leukocytes [132]. It is important to recognize that dilutional thrombocytopenia in the postoperative or posttrauma setting persists for 2 to 4 days, often followed by rebound thrombocytosis (see Fig. 120-1). The massive transfusion of trauma or surgical patients is a situation in which dilution can coexist with more dangerous causes for thrombocytopenia, such as DIC resulting from tissue injury or shock. Accordingly, platelet count and coagulation testing should be done frequently in these patients, because a disproportionate fall in the platelet count may indicate DIC rather than dilution [133]. Platelet transfusions should be given when diffuse microvascular bleeding occurs or is suspected, or if the platelet count falls to less than 50×10^9 per liter [133].

Platelet Sequestration (Hypersplenism and Hypothermia)

Hypersplenism is characterized by palpable splenomegaly and thrombocytopenia alone or with leukopenia and anemia. Hypersplenism is caused by a maldistribution of otherwise normal total platelet numbers. In hypersplenic patients, the splenic platelet pool is increased to as high as 60 to 90 percent of the total platelet mass (normal 30%) [134]. Because the platelet count in hypersplenism is usually 50 to 150 × 10^9 per liter, bleeding complications are unusual, and generally related to coexisting hemostatic problems, such as esophageal varices or coagulopathy secondary to cirrhosis. Only under very unusual circumstances is a splenectomy indicated to raise the platelet count. The postplatelet transfusion rise in the platelet count is suboptimal, because of splenic sequestration of the transfused platelets.

Thrombocytopenia is commonly observed in critically ill patients admitted to hospital with hypothermia [135]. Experimental studies in dogs indicate that transient hepatic sequestration of platelets is the cause [136].

Decreased Platelet Production and Isolated Thrombocytopenia

ALCOHOL-INDUCED THROMBOCYTOPENIA. Alcohol in large amounts can result in moderate to severe thrombocytopenia caused by marrow suppression that may take up to 2 weeks to recover. Megakaryocyte number is often normal, but reduced megakaryocyte number is associated with slower platelet count recovery [137]. Vacuolation of red and white cell precursors is typically observed. Alcohol reduces platelet production by impairing megakaryocyte maturation, rather than suppressing the progenitor megakaryocytic progenitor cells [137].

Decreased Platelet Production and Pancytopenia

ACUTE LEUKEMIA, MYELODYSPLASIA, APLASTIC ANEMIA. Severe thrombocytopenia is common in many patients with neoplastic and nonneoplastic stem cell disorders. Treatment is largely supportive, with prophylactic platelet transfusions indicated for severely thrombocytopenic patients. The threshold for platelet transfusions is controversial, and generally varies from 5 to 30 × 10^9 per liter depending on the center [138].

Aplastic anemia patients constitute a special patient group. The probability of successful marrow transplantation is reduced by blood transfusion [139,140]. Consequently, platelet transfusions should be avoided whenever possible. Ideally, leukodepleted, single-donor platelets obtained by pheresis should be used when necessary for these patients.

Immune mechanisms appear to exacerbate thrombocytopenia in some patients with myelodysplasia, and danazol may raise the platelet count [141].

MEGALOBLASTIC ANEMIA. The combination of decreased intake and increased tissue requirement for nutrients results in many critically ill patients being at increased risk for folic acid and, less often, vitamin B$_{12}$ deficiency. Particularly when red cell macrocytosis is evident, cytopenic patients should empirically be given folic acid (5 mg daily), and possibly vitamin B$_{12}$ (1000 μg once daily for 3 days). It can take 3 to 4 days for the peripheral blood counts to improve in severely megaloblastic patients.

TRANSFUSION-ASSOCIATED GRAFT-VERSUS-HOST DISEASE (GVHD). This very rare and usually fatal illness is characterized by an erythematous maculopapular rash, hepatitis, diarrhea, and pancytopenia secondary to severe marrow hypoplasia that follows a blood transfusion by several weeks [142,143]. Increased risk for transfusion-associated GVHD occurs in certain congenital and acquired immunodeficiency states, but rarely also in immunocompetent patients who share an HLA haplotype with HLA-homozygous blood donors (most likely in settings of directed donations among family members or in certain inbred populations). The syndrome is caused by engraftment of viable, alloreactive blood donor–derived T-lymphocytes, and can be prevented by irradiating the blood product before transfusion.

HEMOPHAGOCYTOSIS. The hallmark of the hemophagocytic syndromes is pancytopenia associated with engulfment of red cells, leukocytes, and platelets by macrophages on bone marrow examination. In some patients there is an associated T lymphocyte neoplasm that characteristically presents with fever, weight loss, lymphadenopathy, hepatomegaly, splenomegaly, and a fulminant progression terminating with septicemia [144]. In other patients, the trigger appears to be an infection, ranging from unusual to common organisms. There is no known specific therapy for these illnesses, and the prognosis is poor.

CONGENITAL THROMBOCYTOPENIC DISORDERS. There are several rare congenital disorders that can present with thrombocytopenia and absent or markedly reduced megakaryocytes. These include generalized stem cell disorders that typically cause pancytopenia (e.g., Fanconi anemia) and hypomegakaryocytic disorders that produce isolated thrombocytopenia (e.g., thrombocytopenia with absent radii syndrome, or TAR syndrome).

The most common congenital thrombocytopenic disorders, however, are characterized by generally mild to moderate thrombocytopenia, large platelet size, normal megakaryocyte numbers, normal platelet survival, autosomal dominant inheritance, and mild to moderate bleeding tendency. In some families, other abnormalities can be found, including leukocyte inclusions, sometimes accompanied by sensorineural deafness and nephritis [145]. Some patients are incorrectly diagnosed as having ITP, until awareness of the family history and lack of response to ITP treatment suggests the diagnosis. A rare X-linked disorder known as the Wiskott-Aldrich syndrome is characterized by very small platelets, immunodeficiency, and atopy.

References

1. Warkentin TE, Levine MN, Hirsh J, et al: Heparin-induced thrombocytopenia in patients treated with low-molecular-weight heparin or unfractionated heparin. *N Engl J Med* 332:1330, 1995.

2. Bessman JD: Platelets, in Bessman JD: Automated blood counts and differentials: A practical guide. Baltimore, Johns Hopkins University Press, 1986; p 57.

3. Corash L, Chen HY, Levin J, et al: Regulation of thrombopoiesis: Effects of the degree of thrombocytopenia on megakaryocyte ploidy and platelet volume. *Blood* 70:177, 1987.

4. Payne BA, Pierre RV. Pseudothrombocytopenia: A laboratory artifact with potentially serious complications consequences. *Mayo Clin Proc* 59:123, 1984.

5. Berkman N, Michaeli Y, Or R, et al: EDTA-dependent pseudothrombocytopenia: A clinical study of 18 patients and a review of the literature. *Am J Hematol* 36:195, 1991.

6. Bizzaro N: Platelet satellitosis to polymorphonuclears: Cytochemical, immunological, and ultrastructural characterization of eight cases. *Am J Hematol* 36:235, 1991.

7. Jones EC, Boyko WJ: Diagnostic value of bone marrow examination in isolated thrombocytopenia. *Am J Clin Pathol* 84:665, 1985.

8. Harker LA, Slichter SJ: The bleeding time as a screening test for evaluation of platelet function. *N Engl J Med* 287:155, 1972.

9. McVay PA, Toy PTCY: Lack of increased bleeding after liver biopsy in patients with mild hemostatic abnormalities. *Am J Clin Pathol* 94:747, 1990.

10. McVay PA, Toy PTCY: Lack of increased bleeding after paracentesis and thoracentesis in patients with mild coagulation abnormalities. *Transfusion* 31:164, 1991.

11. Mannucci PM, Vicente V, Vianello L, et al: Controlled trial of desmopressin in liver cirrhosis and other conditions associated with a prolonged bleeding time. *Blood* 67:1148, 1986.

12. Mannucci PM. Desmopressin: A nontransfusional form of treatment for congenital and acquired bleeding disorders. *Blood* 72:1449, 1988.

13. DiMichele DM, Hathaway WE: Use of DDVAP in inherited and acquired platelet dysfunction. *Am J Hematol* 33:39, 1990.

14. Salzman EW, Weinstein MJ, Weintraub RM, et al: Treatment with desmopressin acetate to reduce blood loss after cardiac surgery: A double-blind randomized trial. *N Engl J Med* 314:1402, 1986.

15. Czer LSC, Bateman TM, Gray RJ, et al: Treatment of severe platelet dysfunction and hemorrhage after cardiopulmonary bypass: Reduction in blood product usage with desmopressin. *J Am Coll Cardiol* 9:1139, 1987.

16. Kobrinsky NL, Tulloh H: Treatment of refractory thrombocytopenic bleeding with 1-desamino-8-D-arginine vasopressin (desmopressin). *J Pediatr* 112:993, 1988.

17. Ruggeri ZM, Mannucci PM, Lombardi R, et al: Multimeric composition of factor VIII/von Willebrand factor following administration of DDAVP: Implications for pathophysiology and therapy of von Willebrand's disease subtypes. *Blood* 59:1272, 1982.

18. Turner-Gomes SO, Andrew M, Coles J, et al: Abnormalities in von Willebrand factor and antithrombin III after cardiopulmonary bypass operations for congenital heart disease. *J Thorac Cardiovasc Surg* 103:87, 1992.

19. Carr JM, Kruskall MS, Kaye JA, et al: Efficacy of platelet transfusions in immune thrombocytopenia. *Am J Med* 80:1051, 1986.

20. Baumann MA, Menitove JE, Aster RH, et al: Urgent treatment of idiopathic thrombocytopenic purpura with single-dose gammaglobulin infusion followed by platelet transfusion. *Ann Intern Med* 104:808, 1986.

21. Parillo JE, moderator: Septic shock in humans: Advances in the understanding of pathogenesis, cardiovascular dysfunction, and therapy. *Ann Intern Med* 113:227, 1990.

22. Corrigan JJ Jr: Thrombocytopenia: A laboratory sign of septicemia in infants and children. *J Pediatr* 85:219, 1974.

23. Neame PB, Kelton JG, Walker IR, et al: Thrombocytopenia in septicemia: The role of disseminated intravascular coagulation. *Blood* 56:88, 1980.

24. Kreger BE, Craven DE, McCabe WR: Gram-negative bacteremia. IV. Re-evaluation of clinical features and treatment in 612 patients. *Am J Med* 68:344, 1980.

25. Corrigan JJ Jr, Jordan CM: Heparin therapy in septicemia with disseminated intravascular coagulation: Effect on mortality and on correction of hemostatic defects. *N Engl J Med* 283:778, 1970.

26. Milligan GF, MacDonald JAE, Mellon A, et al: Pulmonary and hematologic disturbances during septic shock. *Surg Gynecol Obstet* 138:43, 1974.

27. Harker LA, Slichter SJ: Platelet and fibrinogen consumption in man. *N Engl J Med* 287:999, 1972.

28. Okajima K, Yang WP, Okabe H, et al: Role of leukocytes in the activation of intravascular coagulation in patients with septicemia. *Am J Hematol* 36:265, 1991.

29. Voss R, Matthias FR, Borkowski G, et al: Activation and inhibition of fibrinolysis in septic patients in an internal intensive care unit. *Br J Haematol* 75:99, 1990.

30. Kelton JG, Neame PB, Gauldie J, et al: Elevated platelet-associated IgG in the thrombocytopenia of septicemia. *N Engl J Med* 300:760, 1979.

31. Poskitt TR, Poskitt PKF: Thrombocytopenia of sepsis: The role of circulating IgG-containing immune complexes. *Arch Intern Med* 145:891, 1985.

32. Kelton JG, Keystone J, Moore J, et al: Immune-mediated thrombocytopenia of malaria. *J Clin Invest* 71:832, 1983.

33. Csako G, Suba EA, Elin RJ: Endotoxin-induced platelet activation in human whole blood in vitro. *Thromb Haemost* 59:378, 1988.

34. Grabarek J, Timmons S, Hawiger J: Modulation of human platelet protein kinase C by endotoxic lipid A. *J Clin Invest* 82:964, 1988.

35. Arvand M, Bhakdi S, Dahlbäck B, et al: *Staphylococcus aureus* α-toxin attack on human platelets promotes assembly of the prothrombinase complex. *J Biol Chem* 265:14377, 1990.

36. Bhakdi S, Muhly M, Mannhardt U, et al: Staphylococcal α toxin promotes blood coagulation via attack on human platelets. *J Exp Med* 168:527, 1988.

37. Diez FL, Nieto ML, Fernandez-Gallardo S, et al: Occupancy of platelet receptors for platelet-activating factor in patients with septicemia. *J Clin Invest* 83:1733, 1989.

38. Van der Poll T, Büller HR, ten Cate H, et al: Activation of coagulation after administration of tumor necrosis factor to normal subjects. *N Engl J Med* 322:1622, 1990.

39. Li TCM, Phillips MC, Shaw L, et al: On-site physician staffing in a community hospital intensive care unit: Impact on test and procedure use and on patient outcome. *JAMA* 252:2023, 1984.

40. Reynolds HN, Haupt MT, Thill-Baharozian MC, et al: Impact of critical care physician staffing on patients with septic shock in a university hospital medical intensive care unit. *JAMA* 260:3446, 1988.

41. Gurd AR: Fat embolism: an aid to diagnosis. *J Bone Joint Surg* 52B:732, 1970.

42. Bone RC, Francis PB, Pierce AK: Intravascular coagulation associated with the adult respiratory distress syndrome. *Am J Med* 61:585, 1976.

43. Bousquet J, Huchard G, Michel FB: Toxic reactions induced by Hymenoptera venom. *Ann Allergy* 52:371, 1984.

44. Maestrelli P, Boschetto P, Zocca E, et al: Venous blood platelets decrease during allergen-induced asthmatic reactions. *Clin Exp Allergy* 20:367, 1990.

45. Hope AF, Heyns A du P, Lotter MG, et al: Kinetics and sites of sequestration of indium 111-labeled human platelets during cardiopulmonary bypass. *J Thorac Cardiovasc Surg* 81:880, 1981.

46. Hakim RM, Schafer AI: Hemodialysis-associated platelet activation and thrombocytopenia. *Am J Med* 78:575, 1985.

47. Harker L, Malpass TW, Branson HE, et al: Mechanism of abnormal bleeding in patients undergoing cardiopulmonary bypass: Acquired transient platelet dysfunction associated with selective α-granule release. *Blood* 56:824, 1980.

48. Harker LA, Slichter SJ: Studies of platelet and fibrinogen kinetics in patients with prosthetic heart valves. *N Engl J Med* 283:1302, 1970.

49. Harker LA, Slichter SJ, Sauvage LR: Platelet consumption by arterial prostheses: The effects of endothelialization and pharmacologic inhibition of platelet function. *Ann Surg* 186:594, 1977.

50. Stratton JR, Thiele BL, Ritchie JL: Natural history of platelet deposition on Dacron aortic bifurcation grafts in the first year after implantation. *Am J Cardiol* 52:371, 1983.

51. Walls JT, Boley TM, Curtis JJ, et al: Heparin induced thrombocytopenia in patients undergoing intra-aortic balloon pumping after open heart surgery. *ASAIO J* 38:M574, 1992.

52. Terai M, Nakazawa M, Takao A, et al: Thrombocytopenia in patients with aortopulmonary transposition and an intact ventricular septum. *Br Heart J* 57:371, 1987.

53. Jacobson RJ, Rath CE, Perloff JK: Intravascular hemolysis and

thrombocytopenia in left ventricular outflow obstruction. *Br Heart J* 35:849, 1973.

54. Steele PP, Weily HS, Davies H, et al: Platelet survival in patients with rheumatic heart disease. *N Engl J Med* 290:537, 1974.

55. Weidinger F, Glogar D, Sochor H, et al: Platelet survival in patients with dilated cardiomyopathy. *Thromb Haemost* 66:400, 1991.

56. Edwards BS, Weir EK, Edwards WD, et al: Coexistent pulmonary and portal hypertension: Morphologic and clinical features. *J Am Coll Cardiol* 10:1233, 1987.

57. Jubelirer SJ: Primary pulmonary hypertension: Its association with microangiopathic hemolytic anemia and thrombocytopenia. *Arch Intern Med* 151:1221, 1991.

58. Stahl RL, Javid JP, Lackner H: Unrecognized pulmonary embolism presenting as disseminated intravascular coagulation. *Am J Med* 76:772, 1984.

59. Mustafa MH, Mispireta LA, Pierce LE: Occult pulmonary embolism presenting with thrombocytopenia and elevated fibrin split products. *Am J Med* 86:490, 1989.

60. Kaplan BS, Esseltine D: Thrombocytopenia in patients with acute post-streptococcal glomerulonephritis. *J Pediatr* 93:974, 1978.

61. Bunting RW, Quay SC: Case records of the Massachusetts General Hospital. *N Engl J Med* 300:1262, 1979.

62. Kaufman HH, Hui KS, Mattson JC, et al: Clinicopathological correlations of disseminated intravascular coagulation in patients with head injury. *Neurosurgery* 15:34, 1984.

63. Coopland AT, Israels ED, Zipursky A, et al: The pathogenesis of defective hemostasis in abruptio placentae. *Am J Obstet Gynecol* 100:311, 1968.

64. Molos M, Hall J: Symmetrical peripheral gangrene and disseminated intravascular coagulation. *Arch Dermatol* 121:1057, 1985.

65. Hautekeete ML, Berneman ZN, Bieger R, et al: Purpura fulminans in pneumococcal sepsis. *Arch Intern Med* 146:497, 1986.

66. Kirkland KB, Marcom PK, Sexton DJ, et al: Rocky Mountain spotted fever complicated by gangrene: Report of six cases and review. *Clin Infect Dis* 16:629, 1993.

67. Sack G, Levin J, Bell W: Trousseau's syndrome and other manifestations of chronic disseminated coagulopathy in patients with neoplasms: Clinical, pathophysiologic, and therapeutic features. *Medicine (Baltimore)* 56:1, 1977.

68. Graus F, Rogers LR, Posner JB: Cerebrovascular complications in patients with cancer. *Medicine (Baltimore)* 64:16, 1985.

69. Kasabach HH, Merritt KK: Hemangioma with extensive purpura. *Am J Dis Child* 59:1063, 1940.

70. Shim WKT: Hemangiomas of infancy complicated by thrombocytopenia. *Am J Surg* 116:896, 1968.

71. Micallef-Eynaud PD, Ludlam CA: Aortic aneurysms and consumptive coagulopathy. *Blood Coagul Fibrinolysis* 2:477, 1991.

72. Warkentin TE, Kelton JG: Heparin and platelets. *Hematol Oncol Clin North Am* 4:243, 1990.

73. Warkentin TE, Kelton JG: Heparin-induced thrombocytopenia. *Progr Hemost Thromb* 10:1, 1991.

74. Warkentin TE, Kelton JG: Interaction of heparin with platelets, including heparin-induced thrombocytopenia, in Bounameaux H (ed): *Low-Molecular-Weight Heparins in Prophylaxis and Therapy of Thromboembolic Diseases.* Series: "Fundamental and Clinical Cardiology." New York, Marcel Dekker, 1994, p 75.

75. Boshkov LK, Warkentin TE, Hayward CPM, et al: Heparin-induced thrombocytopenia and thrombosis: Clinical and laboratory studies. *Br J Haematol* 84:322, 1993.

76. Chong BH, Pilgrim RL, Cooley MA, et al: Increased expression of platelet IgG Fc receptors in immune heparin-induced thrombocytopenia. *Blood* 81:988, 1993.

77. Laster J, Silver D: Heparin-coated catheters and heparin-induced thrombocytopenia. *J Vasc Surg* 7:667, 1988.

78. Moberg PO, Geary VM, Sheikh FM: Heparin-induced thrombocytopenia: A possible complication of heparin-coated pulmonary artery catheters. *J Cardiothorac Anesth* 4:226, 1990.

79. Homcy CJ, Southern JF: Case records of the Massachusetts General Hospital. *N Engl J Med* 321:1595, 1989.

80. Makhoul RG, Greenberg CS, McCann RL: Heparin-associated thrombocytopenia and thrombosis: A serious clinical problem and potential solution. *J Vasc Surg* 4:522, 1986.

81. Warkentin TE, Soutar RL, Panju A, et al: Acute systemic reactions to intravenous heparin bolus therapy: Relationship to heparin-induced thrombocytopenia [abstract]. *Blood* 80(suppl 1):160a, 1992.

82. Warkentin TE, Hirte HW, Anderson DR, et al: Transient global amnesia associated with heparin-induced thrombocytopenia. *Am J Med* 97:489, 1994.

83. Ernest D, Fisher MM: Heparin-induced thrombocytopaenia complicated by bilateral adrenal haemorrhage. *Intensive Care Med* 17:238, 1991.

84. Souid F, Pourria JL, Le Roux G, et al: Adrenal haemorrhagic necrosis related to heparin-associated thrombocytopenia. *Crit Care Med* 19:297, 1991.

85. Bleasel JF, Rasko JEJ, Rickard KA, et al: Acute adrenal insufficiency secondary to heparin-induced thrombocytopenia-thrombosis syndrome. *Med J Aust* 157:192, 1992.

86. Kelton JG, Sheridan D, Santos A, et al: Heparin-induced thrombocytopenia: Laboratory studies. *Blood* 72:925, 1988.

87. Kelton JG, Smith JW, Warkentin TE, et al: Immunoglobulin G from patients with heparin-induced thrombocytopenia binds to a complex of heparin and platelet factor 4. *Blood* 83:3232, 1994.

88. Warkentin TE, Hayward CPM, Smith CA, et al: Determinants of donor platelet variability when testing for heparin-induced thrombocytopenia. *J Lab Clin Med* 120:371, 1992.

89. Warkentin TE, Hayward CPM, Boshkov LK, et al: Sera from patients with heparin-induced thrombocytopenia generate platelet-derived microparticles with procoagulant activity: an explanation for the thrombotic complications of heparin-induced thrombocytopenia. *Blood* 84:3691, 1994.

90. Sheridan D, Carter C, Kelton JG: A diagnostic test for heparin-induced thrombocytopenia. *Blood* 67:27, 1986.

91. Warkentin TE, Santos AV, Hayward CPM, et al: Importance of platelet preparation in diagnostic testing for heparin-induced thrombocytopenia [abstract]. *Blood* 78(suppl 1):344a, 1991.

92. Greinacher A, Michels I, Kiefel V, et al: A rapid and sensitive test for diagnosing heparin-associated thrombocytopenia. *Thromb Haemost* 66:734, 1991.

93. Warkentin TE, Russett, JI, Johnston M, et al: Warfarin treatment of deep vein thrombosis complicating heparin-induced thrombocytopenia (HIT) is a risk factor for initiation of venous limb gangrene: report of nine patients implicating the interacting procoagulant effects of two anticoagulant agents [abstract]. *Thromb Haemost* 73:110, 1995.

94. Demers C, Ginsberg JS, Brill-Edwards P, et al: Rapid anticoagulation using ancrod for heparin-induced thrombocytopenia. *Blood* 78:2194, 1991.

95. Krishnamurti C, Bolan CD, Reid TJ III, et al: Pharmacology and mechanism of action of ancrod: Potential for inducing thrombosis [letter]. *Blood* 79:2492, 1992.

96. Magnani HN: Heparin-induced thrombocytopenia (HIT): an overview of 230 patients treated with orgaran (Org 10172). *Thromb Haemost* 70:554, 1993.

97. Frame JN, Mulvey KP, Phares JC, et al: Correction of severe heparin-associated thrombocytopenia with intravenous immunoglobulin. *Ann Intern Med* 111:946, 1989.

98. Bouvier JL, Lefebre P, Villain P, et al: Treatment of serious heparin-induced thrombocytopenia by plasma exchange: Report on 4 cases. *Thromb Res* 51:335, 1988.

99. Clifton GD, Smith MD: Thrombolytic therapy in heparin-associated thrombocytopenia with thrombosis. *Clin Pharm* 5:597, 1986.

100. Hackett T, Kelton JG, Powers P: Drug-induced platelet destruction. *Semin Thromb Hemost* 8:116, 1982.

101. Warkentin TE, Kelton JG: Acquired platelet defects. In: Bloom AL, Forbes CD, Thomas DP, et al (eds): *Haemostasis and Thrombosis.* 3rd ed. Edinburgh: Churchill Livingstone, 1994; p 767.

102. Kelton JG, Meltzer D, Moore J, et al: Drug-induced thrombocytopenia is associated with increased binding of IgG to platelets both in vivo and in vitro. *Blood* 58:524, 1981.

103. Kunicki TJ, Newman PJ. The molecular immunology of human platelet proteins. *Blood* 80:1386, 1992.

104. Bussel JB, Pham LC: Intravenous treatment with gammaglobulin in adults with immune thrombocytopenic purpura: Review of the literature. *Vox Sang* 52:206, 1987.

105. Boshkov LK, Kelton JG: Use of intravenous gammaglobulin as an immune replacement and an immune suppressant. *Transfus Med Rev* 3:82, 1989.

106. von dem Borne AEGK, Vos JJE, Pegels JG, et al: High dose intravenous methylprednisolone or high dose intravenous gammaglobulin for autoimmune thrombocytopenia. *Br Med J* 296:249, 1988.

107. Bussel JB, Saal S, Gordon B: Combined plasma exchange and intravenous gammaglobulin in the treatment of patients with refractory immune thrombocytopenic purpura. *Transfusion* 28:38, 1988.

108. Bussel JB, Graziano JN, Kimberly RP, et al: Intravenous anti-D treatment of immune thrombocytopenic purpura: Analysis of efficacy, toxicity, and mechanism of effect. *Blood* 77:1884, 1991.

109. Warkentin TE, Kelton JG: Current concepts in the management of immune thrombocytopenia. *Drugs* 40:531, 1990.

110. Berchtold P, McMillan R: Therapy of chronic idiopathic thrombocytopenic purpura in adults. *Blood* 74:2309, 1989.

111. Centers for Disease Control and Prevention: Recommendations of the Advisory Committee on Immunization Practices (ACIP): Use of vaccines and immune globulins in persons with altered immunocompetence. *MMWR* 42(No. RR-5):1, 1993.

112. Figueroa M, Gehlsen J, Hammond D, et al: Combination chemotherapy in refractory immune thrombocytopenic purpura. *N Engl J Med* 328:1226, 1993.

113. Nieminen U, Peltola H, Syrjälä MT, et al: Acute thrombocytopenic purpura following measles, mumps and rubella vaccination: A report on 23 patients. *Acta Paediatr* 82:267, 1993.

114. Kunicki TJ, Beardsley DS: The alloimmune thrombocytopenias: Neonatal alloimmune thrombocytopenic purpura and posttransfusion purpura. *Progr Hemost Thromb* 9:203, 1989.

115. Mueller-Eckhardt C, Küenzlen E, Thilo-Körner D, et al: High-dose intravenous immunoglobulin for post-transfusion purpura [letter]. *N Engl J Med* 308:287, 1983.

116. Nijjar TS, Bonacosa IA, Israels LG: Severe acute thrombocytopenia following infusion of plasma containing anti-Pl^A1. *Am J Hematol* 25:219, 1987.

117. Warkentin TE, Smith JW, Hayward CPM, et al: Thrombocytopenia caused by passive transfusion of anti-glycoprotein Ia/IIa alloantibody (anti-HPA-5b). *Blood* 79:2480, 1992.

118. Salant DJ, Colvin RB: Case records of the Massachusetts General Hospital. *N Engl J Med* 323:1050, 1990.

119. Kwaan HC: Clinicopathologic features of thrombotic thrombocytopenic purpura. *Semin Hematol* 24:71, 1987.

120. Murphy WG, Moore JC, Kelton JG: Calcium-dependent cysteine protease activity in the sera of patients with thrombotic thrombocytopenic purpura. *Blood* 70:1683, 1987.

121. Moake JL, Rudy CK, Troll JH, et al: Unusually large plasma factor VIII: von Willebrand factor multimers in chronic relapsing thrombotic thrombocytopenic purpura. *N Engl J Med* 307:1432, 1982.

122. Rock GA, Shumak KH, Buskard NA, et al: Comparison of plasma exchange with plasma infusion in the treatment of thrombotic thrombocytopenic purpura. *N Engl J Med* 325:393, 1991.

123. Bell WR, Braine HG, Ness PM, et al: Improved survival in thrombotic thrombocytopenic purpura-hemolytic uremic syndrome: Clinical experience in 108 patients. *N Engl J Med* 325:398, 1991.

124. del Zoppo GJ: Antiplatelet therapy in thrombotic thrombocytopenic purpura. *Semin Hematol* 24:130, 1987.

125. Byrnes JJ, Moake JL, Klug P, et al: Effectiveness of the cryosupernatant fraction of plasma in the treatment of refractory thrombotic thrombocytopenic purpura. *Am J Hematol* 34:169, 1990.

126. Hayward CPM, Sutton DMC, Carter WH Jr, et al: Treatment outcomes in patients with adult thrombotic thrombocytopenic purpura-hemolytic uremic syndrome. *Arch Intern Med* 154:982, 1994.

127. Onundarson PT, Rowe JM, Heal JM, et al: Response to plasma exchange and splenectomy in thrombotic thrombocytopenic purpura: A 10-year experience at a single institution. *Arch Intern Med* 152:791, 1992.

128. Karmali AM, Steele BT, Petric M, et al: Sporadic cases of haemolytic-uraemic syndrome associated with faecal cytotoxin and cytotoxin-producing Escherichia coli in stools. *Lancet* 1:619, 1983.

129. Chart H, Smith HR, Scotland SM, et al: Serological identification of *Escherichia coli* O157:H7 infection in haemolytic uraemic syndrome. *Lancet* 337:138, 1991.

130. Fitzpatrick MM, Walters MDS, Trompeter RS, et al: Atypical (non-diarrhea-associated) hemolytic-uremic syndrome in childhood. *J Pediatr* 122:532, 1993.

131. Loirat C, Sonsino E, Hinglais N, et al: Treatment of the childhood haemolytic uraemic syndrome with plasma: A multicentre randomized controlled trial. *Pediatr Nephrol* 2:279, 1988.

132. Bareford D, Chandler ST, Hawker RJ, et al: Splenic platelet-sequestration following routine blood transfusion is reduced by filtered/washed blood products. *Br J Haematol* 67:177, 1987.

133. Ciavarella D, Reed RL, Counts RB, et al: Clotting factor levels and the risk of diffuse microvascular bleeding in the massively transfused patient. *Br J Haematol* 67:365, 1987.

134. Aster RH: Pooling of platelets in the spleen: Role in the pathogenesis of "hypersplenic" thrombocytopenia. *J Clin Invest* 45:645, 1966.

135. Easterbrook PJ, Davis HP: Thrombocytopenia in hypothermia: A common but poorly recognized complication. *Br Med J* 291:23, 1985.

136. Pina-Cabral JM, Amaral I, Pinto MM, et al: Hepatic and splenic platelet sequestration during deep hypothermia in the dog. *Haemostasis* 2:235, 1974.

137. Gewirtz AM, Hoffman R: Transitory hypomegakaryocytic thrombocytopenia: Aetiological association with ethanol abuse and implications regarding regulation of human megakaryocytopoiesis. *Br J Haematol* 62:333, 1986.

138. Gmür J, Burger J, Schanz U, et al: Safety of stringent prophylactic platelet transfusion policy for patients with acute leukaemia. *Lancet* 338:1223, 1991.

139. Storb R, Prentice RL, Thomas ED: Marrow transplantation for treatment of aplastic anemia: An analysis of factors associated with graft rejection. *N Engl J Med* 296:61, 1977.

140. Storb R, Thomas ED, Buckner CD, et al: Marrow transplantation in thirty untransfused patients with severe aplastic anemia. *Ann Intern Med* 92:30, 1980.

141. Cines DB, Cassileth PA, Kiss JE: Danazol therapy in myelodysplasia. *Ann Intern Med* 103:58, 1985.

142. Anderson KC, Weinstein HJ: Transfusion-associated graft-versus-host disease. *N Engl J Med* 323:315, 1990.

143. Shivdasani RA, Haluska FG, Dock NL, et al: Brief report: Graft-versus-host disease associated with transfusion of blood from HLA-homozygous donors. *N Engl J Med* 328:766, 1993.

144. Falini B, Pileri S, De Solas I, et al: Peripheral T-cell lymphoma associated with hemophagocytic syndrome. *Blood* 75:434, 1990.

145. Greinacher A, Mueller-Eckhardt C: Hereditary types of thrombocytopenia with giant platelets and inclusion bodies in the leukocytes. *Blut* 60:53, 1990.

121. Antithrombotic Therapy

Jack E. Ansell

The intensive care physician must have a good understanding of antithrombotic therapy because intensive care patients either have or are at great risk of developing thromboemboli, and are candidates for antithrombotic therapy. This chapter focuses primarily on those drugs most likely to be used in an intensive care setting to treat or prevent thromboembolic disease.

There are three major classes of antithrombotic drugs currently in use: anticoagulants, antiplatelet agents, and thrombolytic or fibrinolytic agents. Thrombolytic agents have a direct therapeutic effect on thrombi in that they hasten their dissolution and clearance. Anticoagulants and platelet function inhibitors act indirectly and are always prophylactic because they prevent de novo initiation of thrombosis (primary prophylaxis) or they prevent extension of established thrombi (secondary prophylaxis). The agents that are discussed include heparin, low-molecular-weight heparin, warfarin, dextran, aspirin, ticlopidine, streptokinase, anisoylated streptokinase, urokinase, and tissue plasminogen activator. New antithrombotic agents are constantly being developed, such as new thrombin inhibitors, e.g., hirudin [1], or analogs of the fibrinolytic proteins, e.g., prourokinase [2]. Many of these agents are still under study and are not discussed here (see Chap. 43). However, much of what is covered can be applied to these newer agents because they share similar properties with currently used drugs.

Indications

Table 121-1 summarizes the major indications for antithrombotic therapy whether for primary or secondary prophylaxis. A more in-depth analysis of indications can be found in a recent consensus conference on antithrombotic therapy [3]. Based on the pathophysiology of thrombotic disease, certain agents are more effective in particular situations. Thus, anticoagulants are used primarily for venous disease, because coagulation and fibrin deposition play a major role in the pathogenesis of venous thromboemboli. Antiplatelet agents are commonly used for the treatment of arterial disease because platelets play a principal role in the pathogenesis of arterial thromboemboli. However, in the case of heparin, the most commonly used antithrombotic drug, there is much overlap in the situations in which it is used.

Contraindications

Table 121-2 summarizes the major contraindications for the use of these drugs. In general, all contraindications are relative, and a risk-benefit assessment must be made in each patient [4]. One must be particularly alert to the contraindications for thrombolytic therapy, particularly the warning to avoid invasive procedures because of the great potential for serious bleeding.

Pharmacologic Aspects of Antithrombotic Drugs

HEPARIN. Heparin is a glycosaminoglycan made up of repeating disaccharide units of D-glucosamine and uronic acid with a wide range in molecular weight from 5000 to 30,000 daltons [5]. Heparin is commercially derived from bovine lung or porcine intestinal mucosa. Heparin mediates its effect by binding to a plasma protein, antithrombin III (AT III), and altering its conformation and enabling AT III to bind more rapidly and neutralize the serine protease coagulation factors (II_a, IX_a, X_a, XI_a, and XII_a). Its predominant activity is directed toward factors X_a and II_a. Heparin contains a unique pentasaccharide essential for binding to AT III [6]. To neutralize thrombin, the serine protease must bind to both AT III and heparin, forming a ternary complex. This dual binding requires a minimal chain length of 18 monosaccharides. Factor X_a does not require simultaneous binding to heparin when bound to AT III and thus, smaller heparin chain lengths (including the critical pentasaccharide) can serve to neutralize X_a [7].

Another recently described antithrombin, heparin cofactor II, also mediates the effect of heparin, but its neutralizing activity is most active against thrombin [8].

Heparin's pharmacokinetic and pharmacodynamic behavior is complex [5]. Its biologic half-life varies with dose and the method of administration. For clinical purposes, an intravenous bolus should be considered to have a half-life of approximately 60 minutes. Heparin's pharmacodynamic behavior is influenced by the presence of heparin neutralizing proteins to which it binds (e.g., platelet factor 4, histidine-rich glycoprotein, factor VIII) and by its ability to bind to endothelial cells. Such binding properties account for poor bioavailability and recovery of heparin. Heparin-binding proteins may be increased in seriously ill patients and account for much of the heparin resistance seen in such patients. Reduced levels of AT III can also induce a

Table 121-1. General Indications for Antithrombotic Therapy for Primary and Secondary Prevention*

1. Venous thromboembolic disease
   a. Deep venous thrombosis (DVT)
   b. Pulmonary embolism (PE)
   c. Primary prophylaxis of DVT or PE
2. Arterial thromboembolic disease
   a. Prosthetic heart valves
   b. Mitral valve disease, especially with atrial fibrillation or a large heart
   c. Nonvalvular atrial fibrillation
   d. Unstable angina
   e. Mural cardiac thrombi
   f. Acute myocardial infarction
   g. Occlusive peripheral arterial disease
   h. Transient ischemic attacks
   i. Stroke
3. Disseminated intravascular coagulation
4. Maintenance of patency of vascular grafts, shunts, bypasses, and access catheters

**All indications must be judged in the context of the risks and benefits of antithrombotic therapy in the particular situation.

Table 121-2. Contraindications to Antithrombotic Therapy

1. General risk factors
   a. Preexisting coagulation or platelet defect, thrombocytopenia, or other bleeding abnormality
   b. Inaccessible ulcerative lesion (e.g., GI tract lesion)
   c. Central nervous system lesion (e.g., caused by stroke, surgery, trauma)
   d. Spinal anesthesia or lumbar puncture
   e. Malignant hypertension
   f. Bacterial endocarditis
   g. Advanced retinopathy
   h. Old age (>70 yr)
   i. Aspirin or other antiplatelet drug
   j. Neoplastic disease
2. Specific to warfarin (pertains to ambulatory patients)
   a. Early and late pregnancy
   b. Poor patient cooperation, understanding, or reliability
   c. Unsatisfactory laboratory or patient follow-up
   d. Occupational risk of trauma
3. Specific to thrombolytic agents
   a. Recent thoracic, abdominal (10 days), or CNS surgery (2 mo)
   b. Recent cerebrovascular accident (2 mo), trauma (10 days), neoplasm, or atrioventricular malformation
   c. Active internal bleeding
   d. Severe hypertension
   e. Known bleeding disorder
   f. Anticipated invasive procedures (e.g., arterial punctures, biopsies, central lines)

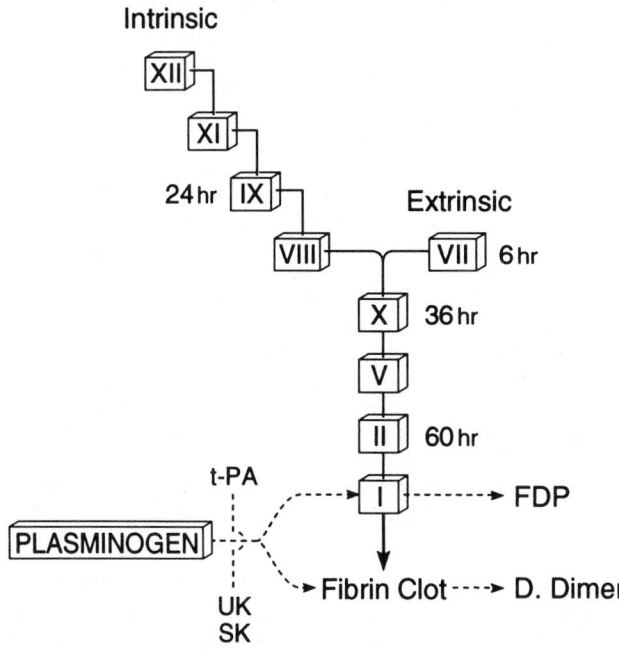

Fig. 121-1. Coagulation cascade. Numbers indicate the normal metabolic half-life in the absence of vitamin K of those factors that are vitamin K dependent.

state of heparin resistance, and low levels may occur in severe liver disease or situations where AT III is consumed (disseminated intravascular coagulation). Heparin's metabolic fate is not entirely clear. Most heparin is handled and excreted by the kidney, and approximately 25 percent is metabolized by the liver.

LOW-MOLECULAR-WEIGHT HEPARIN. Low-molecular-weight heparin (LMWH) is produced by chemical or enzymatic depolymerization of unfractionated heparin [9]. A number of different preparations are available that have an average molecular weight between 4000 and 6500 daltons. They contain a much higher proportion of the essential pentasaccharide for AT III binding, enabling the ATIII-LMWH complex to neutralize factor X_a, but they lack a substantial number of the larger monosaccharide chains (18 or more) required for binding to thrombin. Thus, the ratio of the relative neutralizing potency for X_a:II_a, which for unfractionated heparin is 1:1, is considerably higher for LMWH (approximately 3:1). Because of the average chain lengths of the LMWHs, they have significantly less ability to bind plasma proteins or to endothelial cells, or to interact with platelets. Consequently, they have a much greater bioavailability and predictability of response. They are also more uniformly absorbed from subcutaneous depots and have a longer plasma half-life, in the range of 2 to 4 hours. LMWHs are excreted almost entirely from the kidney.

WARFARIN. Warfarin, a synthetic derivative of the coumarin anticoagulants, is the most commonly used oral anticoagulant in the United States [10]. Warfarin interferes with the production of the vitamin K–dependent coagulation factors (Fig. 121-1) by interfering with the recycling of vitamin K. Recent evidence suggests that warfarin interferes with the reduction of vitamin K, which is oxidized during the gamma-carboxylation of glutamic acid residues in factors II, VII, IX, and X [11,12].

Warfarin affects only new factor synthesis, and the initial anticoagulant effect at the start of therapy is dependent on the normal survival (half-lives) of circulating factors II, VII, IX, and X. The 6-hour half-life of factor VII is the shortest, and its decline determines the rate of the initial prolongation of the prothrombin time. Factor IX has the next shortest half-life—24 hours—and its fall in concentration determines the rate of the initial prolongation of the partial thromboplastin time. Factors II and X have much longer half-lives of approximately 36 and 60 hours, respectively.

Warfarin is rapidly and almost completely absorbed after an oral dose and is highly protein bound in the serum. Peak anticoagulant effect occurs at 36 to 72 hours. Warfarin is a racemic mixture of stereoisomers; both the R and S isomers have different metabolic pathways and plasma half-lives [13]. The average circulating half-life of racemic warfarin is 36 hours, with a range of 15 hours to 60 hours. Changes in the metabolism and half-life of warfarin are primarily responsible for fluctuating prothrombin times and differing dose requirements. Rapid metabolizers require higher daily doses, and slow metabolizers require lower maintenance doses. Drug effects on warfarin metabolism may be stereoisomer specific.

DEXTRAN. Dextran is a polysaccharide derived from the action of bacteria on sucrose. High- and low-molecular-weight preparations (average polymer molecular weight of 70,000 and 40,000 daltons, respectively) are available, but the low-molecular-weight form is most commonly used. Primarily used as a plasma expander, dextran also has a mild effect on hemostasis [14]. Its mechanism of interference with hemostasis is unclear, but it appears to affect both platelet function and coagulation. Dextran enhances the susceptibility of fibrin clots to lysis by plasmin. In regard to platelet function, both adhesion and adenosine diphosphate (ADP)-induced aggregation are impaired.

ASPIRIN, TICLOPIDINE, AND OTHER PLATELET INHIBITORS. Aspirin, other nonsteroidal antiinflammatory agents, and other platelet inhibitors such as ticlopidine have a principal effect on platelet function, although aspirin in very high doses can also cause hypoprothrombinemia. Aspirin, in its acetylated form (acetylsalicylic acid), irreversibly acetylates cyclooxygenase, the key enzyme operating early in the prostaglandin cascade (see Fig. 118-1, Chapter 118), thus rendering exposed platelets impaired for the duration of their lifespan (7–10 days) [15]. Newly forming platelets from megakaryocytes in the bone marrow may also be affected if exposed to aspirin during their production. Nonsteroidal antiinflammatory agents may also affect cyclooxygenase, but in a reversible manner, such that their inhibiting effect dissipates as the drug is metabolized.

Ticlopidine is a new antiplatelet agent that mediates its effect by inhibiting platelet aggregation, possibly by interfering with the binding of von Willebrand factor and fibrinogen to the platelet membrane [16]. It is a thienopyridine derivative whose onset of action is delayed for up to 48 hours after beginning therapy, and its effect may persist for several days after cessation of therapy.

FIBRINOLYTIC AGENTS. Streptokinase and urokinase are plasminogen activators (see Fig. 121-1) [17,18]. Streptokinase is a bacterial protein produced by streptococci, and urokinase is a human protein produced in the kidney and excreted in the urine. Streptokinase binds to plasminogen in a 1:1 stoichiometric complex and alters the conformation of plasminogen so that this complex can then activate other plasminogen molecules by cleaving a specific peptide bond and forming plasmin. Urokinase directly cleaves a specific peptide bond in plasminogen, creating plasmin. Tissue plasminogen activator (t-PA) is the principal human plasminogen activator [19]. It is produced by various tissues, but vascular endothelium probably accounts for the major source of t-PA. Tissue plasminogen activator activates plasminogen directly, but is most active when both proteins are bound to fibrin. At physiologic or even therapeutic levels, t-PA has a low affinity for circulating plasminogen, and thus, systemic plasminemia and consequent hypofibrinogenemia are less likely to occur, unlike the case with streptokinase or urokinase. This fibrin (or thrombus) selectively confers great theoretical advantage to t-PA.

In an effort to impart greater fibrin specificity to streptokinase, plasminogen-streptokinase complexes have been synthesized with the plasminogen catalytic site blocked by various acyl derivatives [20]. Known as anisoylated plasminogen-streptokinase activator complex (APSAC, anistreplase), these complexes are protected from inactivation by alpha-2 antiplasmin and are not active against circulating plasminogen. However, because the fibrin binding site of plasminogen in the complex remains open, the complex can bind fibrin. The activity of the bound complex is dependent on the rate of hydrolysis of the acyl group. Thus, fibrin-bound APSAC is slowly deacylated and enzymatically active against fibrin.

Streptokinase and urokinase have a brief half-life in the body. Streptokinase has the additional problem of being neutralized by preformed streptococcal antibodies that reside in all individuals. Enough must be given to neutralize these antibodies before streptokinase has a measurable fibrinolytic effect. Being a foreign protein, streptokinase may induce hypersensitivity reactions in patients who receive it [21]. Urokinase is a human protein obtained commercially by purification from urine, by a technique of kidney cell cultures that synthesize the protein, or by recombinant DNA techniques [22]. Urokinase is not antigenic in humans and does not elicit hypersensitivity reactions. Clinically used, t-PA is obtained almost exclusively by recombinant

DNA techniques. Like urokinase, it is not antigenic in humans nor associated with hypersensitivity reactions. Tissue plasminogen activator has an extremely short half-life of approximately 5 minutes. The biologic half-life of APSAC is dependent primarily on the deacylation rate of plasminogen. This rate varies in different studies, but approximates 100 minutes for patients with acute myocardial infarction [23].

Clinical Use of Antithrombotic Drugs

HEPARIN. Full-dose heparin as it is used for the secondary prevention of thromboembolism is given by a continuous intravenous infusion, beginning with a loading dose to saturate protein and tissue-binding sites [5]. Heparin was traditionally given by intermittent IV boluses (e.g., q4h), but this mode of therapy, which produces "peaks and valleys" of plasma heparin concentrations, is associated with an increased risk of hemorrhage. Investigations have shown that a continuous infusion achieves a more constant therapeutic level of heparin, with a constant antithrombotic effect and a smaller risk of hemorrhage [24]. Full-dose heparin has also been administered by other routes, such as intermittent subcutaneous injections, but these modes of therapy are for special situations and not particularly relevant to the intensive care setting.

Heparin therapy is initiated with a loading dose of approximately 50 to 125 units per kilogram by IV bolus [25]. Larger doses are sometimes recommended for patients with extensive thromboembolic disease, especially with pulmonary embolism (see Chap. 60). The average loading dose is approximately 5000 to 7500 units for adults, but in patients with pulmonary embolism, a starting dose of 10,000 units may be advisable. This dose is immediately followed by a continuous infusion, starting at approximately 15 to 20 units/kg/hr. The average initial infusion dose is usually 1000 to 1200 units per hour. Clinical studies have shown that patients often fail to achieve a therapeutic degree of anticoagulation early in the course of therapy because of insufficient dosing. Nomograms for dose adjustment have been developed to assist physicians [25,26]. Clinical studies have shown that these are effective.

The effect of heparin is monitored most commonly by the activated partial thromboplastin time (aPTT). The aPTT should be assessed approximately 4 to 6 hours after beginning the infusion, with a goal of achieving a prolongation above control value of $1\frac{1}{2}$ to $2\frac{1}{2}$ times. The infusion should be altered by increments or decrements of 100 units per hour or multiples thereof for those aPTTs outside of therapeutic range, and the aPTT should be reassessed 2 to 4 hours later. Once a therapeutic level is established, the aPTT can be monitored once daily. It is important to understand that the aPTT response to heparin is highly reagent dependent. Studies have shown that a therapeutic heparin concentration ranges between 0.2 and 0.6 units per milliliter, but aPTT reagents may vary considerably in their response to heparin levels in this range [27]. It would be ideal to calibrate each new reagent lot against established heparin levels to determine a lot-specific therapeutic range, but this is seldom done. Continuous-infusion heparin generally requires an automated infusion device to control the rate of infusion. Depending on the patient's fluid volume requirements or limitations, heparin is diluted in the appropriate volume of IV solution.

Before the start of therapy, all patients should have a screening evaluation of their hemostatic system with prothrombin time, aPTT, and platelet count to exclude gross abnormalities of hemostasis.

Heparin is most often administered for a period of 5 to 7 days for patients with venous thromboembolic disease. The duration of therapy depends on the reasons for its use and the postheparin therapy plans. Experimental studies show that it takes 10 to 14 days for thrombi to adhere to venous endothelium, and thus, 10 days has traditionally been the suggested duration of heparin therapy. However, for most uncomplicated cases of deep venous thrombosis, 5 to 7 days of treatment have been shown to be just as appropriate, as long as the patient has achieved a therapeutic degree of anticoagulation with an oral anticoagulant before heparin is stopped [28,29]. Heparinized patients scheduled to undergo invasive procedures such as percutaneous biopsies or surgery should have heparin discontinued 4 to 6 hours before the procedure, unless a decision is made that the risk of recurrent thromboembolism is too great. In that case, surgery can be done while on heparin, keeping the aPTT as close to $1\frac{1}{2}$ times control value as possible, and understanding that surgical blood loss may be increased.

Early in the course of heparin therapy, it is not uncommon to experience difficulty in achieving or maintaining a therapeutic level of anticoagulation. Many patients initially require larger quantities of heparin, which decrease as the thrombotic process stabilizes. A relative degree of heparin resistance may be associated with more extensive thromboembolic disease, possibly because of low levels of antithrombin III from excessive consumption. However, heparin resistance is most likely attributable to the presence of heparin-binding proteins such as platelet factor 4, factor VIII, histidine-rich glycoprotein, and others, which prevent its binding to AT III [5]. These proteins are often increased in inflammatory conditions. Care must be taken to monitor the infusion rate, because heparin sensitivity is often reestablished after the first few days of therapy.

Complications. The intensive care physician must be aware of three potentially serious complications attributed to heparin. As one might expect, hemorrhage is the most common side effect and potentially the most serious. Bleeding has been reported in up to 30 percent of patients who have received heparin, with the occurrence of major bleeding episodes in up to 10 percent [30]. In general, one should expect at least a 5 to 10 percent incidence of bleeding, with half of these episodes being serious.

Reversal of the anticoagulant effect of heparin can be achieved by administration of protamine sulfate at a dose of 1 mg of protamine for every 100 units of heparin. The full neutralizing protamine dose can be given shortly after an IV bolus of heparin. Only 50 percent should be given at 1 hour and 25 percent at 2 hours. In patients receiving subcutaneous heparin, 50 percent neutralizing equivalency of the last heparin dose should be used; in patients receiving continuous intravenous infusions, 25 to 50 percent of the hourly total infusion can be used. In all cases, the neutralizing effect is monitored by the aPTT.

A second major side effect of heparin therapy, which has been widely recognized only within the last decade, is thrombocytopenia [31,32] (see Chap. 120). By a mechanism of peripheral consumption that is immunologic in nature, heparin causes an approximate 5 percent incidence of severe thrombocytopenia (platelet count <100,000/ml). Most investigators have found a higher incidence of severe heparin-induced thrombocytopenia with heparin derived from beef lung as opposed to porcine heparin. Thrombocytopenia generally occurs after 6 to 8 days of therapy (but it may occur sooner) and resolves within days of discontinuing therapy. The thrombocytopenia can be mild to severe and may be associated with

bleeding. A detailed discussion of heparin-induced thrombocytopenia can be found in Chapter 120.

A phenomenon associated with heparin-induced thrombocytopenia is recurrent or de novo thromboembolism, frequently involving the arterial circulation [31,33]. This condition may be induced by an effect of heparin on platelets, leading to spontaneous in vivo platelet aggregates and thromboemboli. In many patients with heparin-induced thrombocytopenia, a platelet-aggregating factor has been identified in the plasma and can be looked for by platelet aggregation or ^{14}C-serotonin release studies [34]. Therapy for heparin-induced thrombocytopenia may only require observation if the platelet reduction is mild. More serious reductions (<75,000/µl) require discontinuation of heparin and substitution of alternate therapy [35] (see Chap. 120). A risk-benefit assessment must be made in each situation.

One must be alert to the recurrence of thromboembolism during therapy. It may represent progression of the underlying thrombotic disorder or heparin-induced thromboembolism. The latter is associated with severe morbidity and mortality and requires the cessation of heparin and the use of an alternate anticoagulant [35]. Warfarin is often started immediately, but takes days to exert its full protective effect. More rapid-acting alternatives include low-molecular-weight dextran or antiplatelet therapy. Clinical reports have also shown that prostacyclin analogs and various low-molecular-weight heparin preparations may be effective. The new low-molecular-weight heparins have fewer platelet-associated effects, and in some cases do not cross-react with heparin-induced antibodies, but not in all cases. A new heparinoid (Orgaran), however, has little, if any, cross-reactivity and has been used effectively in this setting [36]. As of this writing, it is not available in North America.

The last potentially serious complication of heparin therapy is an uncommon syndrome of heparin-induced skin necrosis [37]. It is seen primarily with subcutaneous heparin therapy and produces a well-demarcated area of dermal necrosis similar to the findings in purpura fulminans. It may also be associated with thrombocytopenia and systemic thromboembolism. The cause is probably heparin-induced thrombosis of small capillaries. There is no specific therapy other than discontinuation of heparin and switching to an alternative anticoagulant.

LOW-MOLECULAR-WEIGHT HEPARIN. Currently, the low-molecular-heparins (LMWH) have their greatest applicability in the prevention of postoperative deep venous thrombosis (DVT) [38,39]. There are a number of commercial preparations of LMWH, each manufactured by different methodologies and each having different anti-factor X_a potencies. Thus, the dosing of LMWH is product specific, and one cannot simply substitute one preparation or brand for another as is done with unfractionated heparin. Low-molecular-weight heparin is given subcutaneously for the prophylaxis of deep venous thrombosis on a once- or twice-daily basis, depending on the product being used. Although several preparations are available in Europe and elsewhere, only one preparation is FDA approved for use in the United States at the time of this writing. Enoxaparin (Lovenox, Rhône-Poulenc Rorer) is approved for the prophylaxis of deep venous thrombosis in patients undergoing hip replacement surgery. It is given in a fixed dose of 30 mg twice daily, with the first dose given as soon as possible after surgery. LMWH has little effect on the aPTT, and monitoring of therapy is not necessary. It is given until the risk of postoperative DVT is significantly diminished. Other preparations for clinical use to prevent DVT will be approved for use in the United States. in the next few years. They will each have their specific dosage guidelines and frequency of administration.

Low-molecular-weight heparin has also been studied for its effectiveness in the treatment of established venous thrombosis, and early studies show favorable comparisons to standard heparin [9]. When used for established thrombosis LMWH has been given by subcutaneous or intravenous administration. There are still many unresolved issues pertaining to LMWH in its use for prophylaxis and especially treatment of DVT. These include questions of timing and frequency of administration, fixed or adjusted dosing, monitoring, neutralization with protamine, use in pregnancy, and others [9].

The side effects of low-molecular-weight heparin are similar to those of standard heparin but appear to be less frequent. In the prophylaxis studies, hemorrhage appears to be no more frequent and probably less frequent than with low-dose heparin. Thrombocytopenia has been reported as a complication of LMWH, but is significantly less likely to occur. In some cases of heparin-induced thrombocytopenia, LMWH has been successfully substituted as an alternative means of anticoagulation [35].

WARFARIN. Warfarin therapy is most often initiated during heparin therapy. Because it takes 3 to 5 days to achieve a satisfactory reduction of all of the vitamin K–dependent coagulation factors and to adequately interfere with both the intrinsic and extrinsic systems of coagulation, heparin is continued during this period after warfarin has been started. Studies have shown that heparin and warfarin can be started together, rather than delaying the start of warfarin for several days as had been the custom, without affecting the outcome [28,29]. The converse, treating patients with venous thromboembolic disease without an initial course of heparin, results in a worsening of the thrombotic condition [40].

Therapy is initiated by administering a fixed daily dose of warfarin for 3 days that is equal to or slightly higher than the anticipated maintenance dose (i.e., 5–10 mg) [10]. Warfarin is no longer started with a large loading dose. Such therapy causes a rapid and marked drop in factor VII levels that enhances the risk of bleeding. At the same time it does not adequately protect against clotting, because several days are required to interfere with the intrinsic cascade and to prolong the aPTT. The average maintenance dose is approximately 5 mg daily. Thus therapy is often started with 10 mg daily for 2 days. On the third day, the prothrombin time (PT) is assessed and the dose adjusted accordingly. Warfarin can also be given intravenously for patients who cannot take it orally. Intramuscular therapy should probably be avoided because of the risk of hemorrhage.

When the PT reaches the therapeutic level, heparin is discontinued. The PT is repeated approximately 4 hours later, at which time a drop of 2 to 3 seconds in the PT should be anticipated because of the absence of a heparin effect. When a maintenance dose is being determined, prothrombin times should be assessed daily or every other day. Once achieved, PTs can be assessed less frequently. However, intensive care patients, who are often seriously ill and receiving multiple and changing medications, may require daily assessment of the PT.

The monitoring of warfarin therapy has recently undergone a change because of the realization that prothrombin times performed with different thromboplastin reagents are not equivalent [41]. The concept of a safe and effective therapeutic range was established in the 1940s and 1950s using a human brain thromboplastin that is sensitive to a reduction in the vitamin K–dependent coagulation factors. Thromboplastin is a biologic reagent used to activate coagulation for the prothrombin time test and produces quite variable PT results, depending on its source of origin. In North America, manufacturers switched from human brain to rabbit brain thromboplastin in the 1950s and 1960s, the latter of which tends to be less sensitive to a reduction in the vitamin K–dependent coagulation factors. Thus, considerably more warfarin is required to achieve the same elevation of PT when using a rabbit brain or insensitive reagent versus a sensitive reagent. The consequences of this difference in reagents were clearly demonstrated by Hull et al [42] by showing a significantly higher rate of bleeding in patients monitored by an insensitive reagent versus a sensitive reagent without any difference in recurrent thromboembolism.

To avoid this problem it is best to compare all PT results with an international standard called the International Normalized Ratio (INR) [43]. The INR represents the PT ratio (PT divided by the mean of the normal range) one would obtain if an international reference thromboplastin had been used. Thus, manufacturers compare new thromboplastin preparations with an international standard and assign a sensitivity value called the International Sensitivity Index (ISI). The ISI can then be used to calculate an INR from the local PT by the formula:

$$[\text{PT Ratio}]^{\text{ISI}}$$

This calculation is done automatically by the hospital laboratory, and an INR is reported. According to the INR, the therapeutic range one should aim for is summarized in Table 121-3 [41]. Although monitoring therapy by use of an INR does not eliminate all variabilities, it is considerably better than using the raw PT in seconds, which can be quite variable depending on the sensitivity of the reagent used.

One of the major problems associated with warfarin therapy is maintenance of a therapeutic prothrombin time in the face of numerous factors that alter the body's response to warfarin. In the critically ill patient, the response to warfarin is even more variable. Complications can be avoided, however, because prothrombin times are readily available in the hospital, and a patient's response can be monitored daily. Nevertheless, physicians must be aware of the factors that affect the response to warfarin [10].

Table 121-4 lists the factors that determine the response to warfarin. The principal determinants are those conditions that influence the availability of either vitamin K or warfarin. Anything that makes vitamin K more or less available (e.g., the inadvertent administration of vitamin K in hyperalimentation fluids or the suppression of vitamin K–producing gut bacteria by antibiotics) will shorten or lengthen the PT. Factors that make warfarin more or less available (e.g., a decrease or increase in its rate of metabolism) will lengthen or shorten the PT. Particularly important are the effects on warfarin metabolism by other drugs. Table 121-5 lists the various mechanisms of drug-drug interaction and the common drugs that typify each mechanism [11].

Table 121-3. Therapeutic Range for Oral Anticoagulant Therapy Based on the International Normalized Ratio

Indication	Recommended INR
Prophylaxis of venous thrombosis	2.0–3.0
Treatment of venous thrombosis	
Treatment of pulmonary embolism	
Prevention of systemic embolism	
Tissue heart valves	
Acute myocardial infarction	
Valvular heart disease	
Atrial fibrillation	
Mechanical prosthetic valves	2.5–3.5
Recurrent systemic embolism	

Table 121-4. Factors That Determine Response to Warfarin Therapy

Too much or too little vitamin K	
Decrease in dietary vitamin K	Increase PT
Malabsorption of vitamin K	Increase PT
Suppression of gut bacteria	Increase PT
Increase in dietary vitamin K	Decrease PT
Too much or too little warfarin	
Decrease in absorption	Decrease PT
Changes in metabolism	Increase/decrease PT
Drug effects	Increase/decrease PT
Changes in factor production/metabolism	
Liver disease	Increase PT
Hypermetabolic states (fever)	Increase PT
Other illnesses	Increase PT
Technical/laboratory factors (problems with)	
Phlebotomy	Increase/decrease PT
Evacuated collection tubes	Increase/decrease PT
Handling specimens	Increase/decrease PT
Instrumentation	Increase/decrease PT
Different thromboplastin reagents	Increase/decrease PT

Complications. Complications of warfarin therapy are not uncommon [30]. The most frequent problem is hemorrhage, which usually develops as an extension of warfarin's physiologic effect. Minor hemorrhage has been reported in as many as 20 to 30 percent of patients on long-term therapy. Most cases involve minor bleeding, although serious morbidity and mortality may occur. Well-regulated patients probably experience no more than a 10 percent incidence of minor bleeding (e.g., hematuria or occult melena) and a less than 1 percent incidence of major hemorrhage during long-term follow-up. In an intensive care setting, the risks may well be higher. The most common sites of bleeding are the gastrointestinal tract, urinary tract, soft tissues, and the oropharynx. The risk of bleeding is positively influenced by the duration of therapy (with most bleeding occurring early on) and the intensity of treatment [44]. Comorbid conditions are the most important patient-specific factors associated with the risk of bleeding and include a history of GI bleeding, cerebrovascular disease, and renal disease as the most common. Concurrent use of aspirin or nonsteroidal antiinflammatory agents also enhances the risk of bleeding [45].

Reversal of the anticoagulant effect of warfarin is achieved by parenteral administration of vitamin K_1. Because vitamin K allows for only new-factor synthesis, full or nearly complete correction of the coagulopathy requires 24 to 36 hours in patients with normal liver function. In patients who require immediate correction of their warfarin-induced coagulopathy, replacement of the vitamin K–dependent coagulation factors by infusions of fresh frozen plasma (FFP) is necessary. Approximately 15 ml per kilogram of FFP should be given initially, and one-half this dose may be needed every 6 to 8 hours, because the half-life of infused factor VII is only 6 hours.

Plasma infusions should only be necessary until the liver is able to synthesize new factors in response to a dose of vitamin K. For complete correction without concern for future oral anticoagulation vitamin K can be given in a dose of 10 mg subcutaneously or 1 to 5 mg intravenously. Vitamin K should be held or used sparingly (1 mg) in patients who are expected to continued warfarin after control of their bleeding because reestablishing anticoagulant control can be very difficult after larger doses of vitamin K [46]. FFP can be relied on in this situation.

Hemorrhagic necrosis of the skin and subcutaneous fatty tissue is another well-known but uncommon complication of warfarin [47]. This complication is attributable in some cases to

Table 121-5. Drugs That Interact with Warfarin or Alter Its Effect on Hemostasis

Drug	Mechanism of interaction
Prolongs prothrombin time	
Amiodarone	Decreases clearance
Anabolic steroids	Unknown
Cephalosporins (2nd & 3rd generation)	Interferes with vitamin K recycling
Cimetidine	Decreases clearance
Clofibrate	Unknown
Disulfiram	Decreases clearance
Erythromycin	Unknown
Fluoroquinolones	Displaces binding to albumin
Glucagon	Unknown
Metronidazole	Decreases clearance
Miconazole	Decreases clearance
Omeprazole	Decreases clearance
Phenytoin	Unknown
Piroxicam	Unknown
Quinidine	Unknown
Phenylbutazone	Decreases clearance
Salicylates	Enhances hypoprothrombinemia
Sulfinpyrazone	Decreases clearance
Tamoxifen	Unknown
Trimethoprim/sulfamethoxazole	Decreases clearance
Vitamin E	Unknown
Reduces prothrombin time	
Alcohol	Increases clearance
Barbiturates	Increases clearance
Carbamazepine	Increases clearance
Cholestyramine	Decreases absorption
Griseofulvin	Increases clearance
Nafcillin	Increases clearance
Rifampin	Increases clearance
Sucralfate	Decreases absorption
Enhances risk of bleeding	
Aspirin	Inhibits platelet function
Heparin	Inhibits other coagulation factors
Penicillins	Inhibits platelet function

a deficiency of protein C, a vitamin K–dependent, naturally occurring inhibitor of activated factors V and VIII [48]. Because of protein C's short half-life of 6 hours, protein C concentration can be seriously reduced during the first few days of warfarin therapy before the coagulation factors are significantly reduced, thus leading to a hypercoagulable state. Patients at risk seem to be those who already have a heterozygous deficiency (approximately 50% of normal) of protein C. A similar deficiency of protein S, a cofactor for protein C, has also been implicated as a cause. This problem occurs more commonly in women and affects areas of abundant fatty tissue, such as the breasts, buttocks, or thighs. No specific therapy is available except for the discontinuation of warfarin, and in one case report, the early administration of vitamin K [49]. Other side effects of warfarin have been reported, including allergic phenomena and a peculiar discoloration of the toes called the purple toes syndrome, but these are rare and of lesser clinical significance.

Care must be taken in patients requiring surgery or invasive procedures while on warfarin [10]. Percutaneous closed biopsies or needle sticks, especially of noncompressible tissues, should be avoided. Open biopsies and even major surgery can be performed, but under close observation and with the prothrombin time kept below $1\frac{1}{2}$ times the control value. An assessment of the risk of recurrent thrombosis if anticoagulants are stopped versus the risk of excessive bleeding if they are not stopped must be made in each case. Generally, warfarin can be discontinued several days before a surgical procedure, allowing the PT to return to normal on its own, and then restarted postoperatively [10,50]. If anticoagulants must be maintained, then warfarin should be discontinued, and heparin should be started. Approximately 4 hours preoperatively, heparin can be discontinued; it can be restarted postoperatively if it is considered safe to do so.

Warfarin therapy during pregnancy should be avoided because it crosses the placenta and has been implicated in the genesis of fetal malformations [51]. Although warfarin is most dangerous during the first trimester because of the risk of causing fetal abnormalities and the last 3 weeks because of the risk of bleeding, it is advisable to avoid its use during the entire gestation period. Because heparin does not cross the placenta and its effect can be rapidly reversed, its use is indicated during pregnancy when needed.

DEXTRAN. The most common use for dextran as an antithrombotic agent is as an alternative agent for the primary prevention of deep venous thrombosis in patients at risk [52]. Its other major use is as an alternative antithrombotic medication for active thromboembolic disease in either the arterial or the venous circulation when heparin cannot be used. Dextran is not an overly effective antithrombotic agent but provides minimal efficacy in a number of conditions for prophylaxis or treatment. Its major use comes into play when heparin cannot be used and an alternative anticoagulant is sought.

Dextran carries the same risk of bleeding complications as oral anticoagulants in addition to occasional problems of allergic reactions, fluid overload, and renal failure. It is given by a loading dose of approximately 100 ml of a 10% solution by IV bolus that is followed by approximately 20 ml per hour or 500 ml daily. In most situations, whether for primary or secondary prophylaxis, dextran is infused for only a few days. For prophylaxis of postoperative thromboembolic complications, dextran must be started either before or during surgery to have a beneficial effect.

ASPIRIN. Aspirin and other nonsteroidal antiinflammatory drugs (NSAIDs) are used to interfere with platelet function, usually by inhibiting aggregation, in patients with arterial thromboembolic disease. Although aspirin has been studied in patients with venous thromboembolic disease, its effectiveness is well below that of anticoagulants, and it is generally not recommended in that situation.

NSAIDs other than aspirin generally interfere with platelet function only as long as the drug persists in the circulation. The half-life of aspirin in the acetylated form is approximately 30 to 60 minutes, but platelets exposed during that time are impaired for their lifespan. Thus a few days are required to recover from a single dose of aspirin and 1 week to 10 days are necessary to recover from chronic aspirin use.

Aspirin is currently recommended for primary and secondary prophylaxis in a number of cardiovascular and cerebrovascular thromboembolic disorders [53] (see Chap. 60). A controversy existed in the past concerning the optimal dose of aspirin necessary to impair platelet thromboxane synthesis without affecting endothelial cell prostacyclin synthesis. The latter substance is an antiaggregatory prostaglandin that is important in preventing platelet thrombi on vascular surfaces. Laboratory studies show that platelet cyclooxygenase is inhibited by a lower concentration of aspirin than is endothelial cell cyclooxygenase. Furthermore, endothelial cells can regenerate cyclooxygenase, whereas platelets cannot. Thus, even after a high dose of aspirin

or after prolonged use, prostacyclin synthesis is resumed, whereas platelet thromboxane synthesis is not.

Unfortunately, many of the early multicenter trials of platelet inhibition of aspirin employed excessive doses of aspirin that may have canceled out some of the potential beneficial effects. Currently, as little as 90 mg of aspirin ($\frac{1}{4}$ gr) is enough to produce a differential effect on thromboxane and prostacyclin synthesis. More recent studies, however, suggest that between 160 and 325 mg (one tablet) affords adequate protection in many cases [54], including a reduction in fatal and nonfatal myocardial infarction in males 50 years of age or older without previous known heart disease [55]; secondary prophylaxis in patients with known coronary artery disease who have stable or unstable angina [54]; after coronary angioplasty or coronary artery bypass grafting [56]; and in some patients with bioprosthetic valves who are not on anticoagulants [57] as well as patients with mechanical valves on oral anticoagulants [58]. For the secondary prevention of transient ischemic attacks (TIA), reversible ischemic neurologic deficits or stroke, low-dose acetylsalicylic acid appears to be as protective as higher dose therapy (1 g/day). Data do suggest, however, that aspirin is not beneficial for the primary prevention of TIA or stroke [55].

Ticlopidine is effective in a number of clinical conditions, but because of potentially serious side effects its use is recommended only for those individuals unable to take aspirin [16]. Side effects include diarrhea, skin rash, and a low incidence of neutropenia.

FIBRINOLYTIC AGENTS. Streptokinase, urokinase, tissue plasminogen activator (t-PA), and anisoylated plasminogen-streptokinase activator complex (APSAC or anistreplase) are used for a variety of thromboembolic conditions; their indications evolve according to new investigative studies. The major reason for reluctance in the use of thrombolytic agents has been the high rate of bleeding complications in the early therapeutic trials. However, with proper care and avoidance of invasive procedures, the rate of bleeding complications can be equivalent to the rate seen with heparin [59]. Table 121-6 summarizes the approved indications for thrombolytic therapy and the generally recommended therapeutic doses. Based on clinical investigations, streptokinase is approved for use in acute pulmonary embolism and deep venous thrombosis, arterial thrombosis, acute myocardial infarction, and occlusion of vascular access shunts. Urokinase is approved for pulmonary embolism, coronary artery thrombosis, and thrombotic occlusion of indwelling catheters. Tissue plasminogen activator is currently approved only for the treatment of acute myocardial infarction, although it is currently being used in a number of clinical thrombotic syndromes on an investigational basis, and indications are likely to expand in the future. Anistreplase is similarly approved for acute myocardial infarction alone.

The use of thrombolytic agents in myocardial infarction is discussed in great detail in Chapter 46. The discussion here briefly touches on their use in other thromboembolic conditions.

For the treatment of pulmonary embolism, urokinase and streptokinase were studied in two large clinical trials in the late 1960s [60,61]. Based on results from both studies, thrombolytic agents were beneficial primarily in regard to the more rapid dissolution of emboli and the improvement in hemodynamics and pulmonary vascular perfusion. There was no difference in overall mortality, but the trials were not expected to show this because of their limited size. Subsequent studies have since shown that some of these improvements are maintained for as long as 1 to 7 years after pulmonary embolism [62]. Recent

Table 121-6. Approved Indications and Suggested Doses for Thrombolytic Agents

Thrombolytic agent	Indication			
	Deep venous thrombosis	Pulmonary embolism	Acute myocardial infarction	Occluded caths/ art/veins
Streptokinase	250,000 IU × 30′ then 100,000 IU/hr × 24 hr	250,000 IU × 30′ then 100,000 IU/hr × 24 hr	1.5 × 10⁶ IU × 20′	250,000 IU × 60-120′
Urokinase	4400 IU/kg × 10′ then 4400 IU/hr × 24 hr	4400 IU/kg × 10′ then 4400 IU/hr × 24 hr	2 × 10⁶ IU bolus or 3 × 10⁶ IU over 90′	5000 IU
Alteplase (t-PA)	—	100 mg over 2 hr	60 mg × 1 hr (6–10 mg as bolus), 20 mg over 2nd hr, 20 mg over 3rd hr.	–
Anistreplase	—	—	30 U (1.25 × 10⁶ IU Streptokinase) bolus	—

investigations have studied the effectiveness of t-PA for the treatment of pulmonary embolism [63]. Although early and significant lysis of emboli was achieved (greater than that seen with urokinase or streptokinase), the long-term benefits of this therapy remain unclear, and no extensive head-to-head comparisons with heparin therapy have been conducted. In addition, hemorrhagic complications remain problematic, even with t-PA, which loses its clot selectivity at the doses used.

Although as many as 50% of patients with pulmonary embolism may be suitable candidates for thrombolysis [64], questions of long-term benefit and concerns about bleeding suggest that thrombolytic therapy is not recommended for the treatment of simple pulmonary embolism. However, in the setting of life-threatening embolism, particularly with hypotension or other serious hemodynamic changes, and without contraindications, thrombolytic therapy is an appropriate therapeutic option.

Similar results on a smaller basis have also been demonstrated for clot dissolution and preservation of venous function in patients with deep venous thrombosis [65,66]. Most studies, however, have been small, have not been rigorously randomized or blinded, and have focused more on short-term clot dissolution versus long-term outcomes, especially in regard to postphlebitic changes [67]. Accordingly, thrombolytic therapy cannot be recommended on a routine basis for patients with deep venous thrombosis.

Streptokinase and urokinase are both effective in restoring perfusion in patients with acute peripheral arterial occlusion, but not very effective in chronic arterial occlusion. Urokinase is frequently used to clear clotted indwelling catheters, particularly central venous catheters used in cancer patients.

The recommended doses for the various thrombolytic agents are outlined in Table 121-6. Large loading doses of streptokinase must be given to overcome antistreptococcal antibodies and hydrocortisone, 100 mg, should be given before, and every 12 to 24 hours during streptokinase therapy to prevent bothersome side effects. Anticoagulant therapy is initiated after thrombolytic therapy, usually in the form of heparin. It is started when the aPTT falls to approximately twice the control value as a result of cessation of thrombolytic drugs. A loading dose is not necessary unless the aPTT is well below therapeutic range. Therapy is then continued for a number of days, depending on the underlying condition.

Thrombolytic therapy does not require close monitoring of coagulation parameters, because a fixed dose is given in most situations. For short-term therapy, e.g., acute myocardial infarction, monitoring is probably even less essential. For longer duration therapy, however, monitoring may assume some im-

portance [68]. The major reason to monitor therapy is to ensure that at least a lytic state has been reached. For urokinase or streptokinase this can most conveniently be determined by a thrombin time that should be obtained before therapy and approximately 3 to 4 hours after initiation of treatment. The goal is to achieve a significant prolongation above the baseline value, which, for the thrombin time, is more than 3 seconds above the control value. If not achieved, a repeat loading dose should be given and its effect measured 3 hours later. Similar information can also be obtained by determining the fibrinogen concentration, which with streptokinase therapy should be reduced to the range of 1.5 g per liter. Patients who fail to achieve a fibrinolytic state with streptokinase should then be switched to urokinase, because antibody neutralization of streptokinase may be responsible.

Complications. Hemorrhage is the major complication of thrombolytic therapy, as it is with anticoagulants [69,70]. Of particular concern is the increased risk of cerebrovascular hemorrhage [71]. At a minimum, these agents are contraindicated in the setting of active internal bleeding, recent (within 2 months) cerebral vascular event or intracranial/intraspinal surgery, intracranial neoplasm, arteriovenous malformation or aneurysm, severe uncontrolled hypertension, or a known bleeding diathesis. Meticulous care must be exercised to exclude patients with recent surgery or recent invasive procedures and to avoid invasive procedures during therapy. Venous phlebotomy should be reduced to a minimum, and pressure dressings should be used over venipuncture sites. Contraindications to therapy must be closely observed to avoid treating patients at risk of bleeding.

Minor local bleeding can be controlled locally, but major bleeding requires discontinuation of therapy. Packed red cells can be given to replace blood loss, and FFP or cryoprecipitate can be given to correct the coagulopathy. The half-life of streptokinase and urokinase is very short (15 minutes) and of t-PA even shorter (5 minutes), and thus the lytic state resolves quickly. Rarely would one need to give aminocaproic acid to inhibit fibrinolysis.

Streptokinase is also associated with a high incidence of fever and allergic reactions [21], and some patients experience nausea, vomiting, and flushing with treatment. These reactions can be treated with antihistamines and antipyretics (acetaminophen). Some investigators recommend the regular use of hydrocortisone, 100 mg IV before starting therapy, and continuing it orally every 12 to 24 hours during treatment.

References

1. Markwardt F: Hirudin. *Semin Thromb Hemostas* 17:79, 1991.
2. Lijnen HR, Stump DC, Collen DC: Single-chain urokinase-type plasminogen activator: Mechanism of action and thrombolytic properties. *Semin Thromb Hemostas* 13:152, 1987.
3. Dalen JE, Hirsh JA: Third ACCP Consensus Conference on Antithrombotic Therapy. *Chest* 102(suppl):303S, 1992.
4. Harrington R, Ansell J: Risk benefit assessment of anticoagulant therapy. *Drug Safety* 6:54, 1991.
5. Hirsh J: Heparin. *N Engl J Med* 324:1565, 1991.
6. Lindahl U, Thunberg L, Backstrom G, et al: Extension and structural variability of the antithrombin-binding sequence in heparin. *J Biol Chem* 259:12368, 1984.
7. Hirsh J, Dalen J, Deykin D, Poller L: Heparin: Mechanism of action, pharmacokinetics, dosing considerations, monitoring, efficacy and safety. *Chest* 102(suppl):337S, 1992.
8. Tollefsen DM: Laboratory diagnosis of antithrombin and heparin cofactor II deficiency. *Semin Thromb Hemostas* 16:162, 1990.
9. Hirsh J, Levine MN: Low molecular weight heparin. *Blood* 79:1, 1992.
10. Ansell J: Oral anticoagulant therapy: Fifty years later. *Arch Intern Med* 153:586, 1993.
11. Hirsh J: Oral anticoagulant drugs. *N Engl J Med* 324:1865, 1991.
12. Bell RG: Metabolism of vitamin K and prothrombin synthesis: Anticoagulants and the vitamin K-epoxide cycle. *Fed Proc* 37:2599, 1978.
13. Porter RS, Sawyer WT, Lowenthal DT: Warfarin, in Evans WE, Schentag JJ, Jusko WJ (eds): *Applied Pharmacokinetics*. 2nd ed. Spokane, WA, Applied Therapeutics, 1986, pp 1057-1104.
14. Aberg M, Hedner U, Bergentz SE: The antithrombotic effect of dextran. *Scand J Haematol* 62:37 (suppl), 1977.
15. Stein B, Fuster V: Clinical pharmacology of platelet inhibitors, in Fuster V, Verstraete M (eds): *Thrombosis in Cardiovascular Disorders*. Philadelphia, W.B. Saunders, 1992, p 99.
16. Defreyn G, Bernat A, Delebassee D, et al: Pharmacology of ticlopidine: A review. *Semin Thromb Hemostas* 15:159, 1989.
17. Verstraete M: Biochemical and clinical aspects of thrombolysis. *Semin Hematol* 15:35, 1978.
18. Verstraete M, Collen D: Thrombolytic agents, in Fuster V, Verstraete M (eds): *Thrombosis in Cardiovascular Disorders*. Philadelphia, Saunders, p 175.
19. Loscalzo J, Brunwald E: Tissue plasminogen activator. *N Engl J Med* 319:925, 1988.
20. Smith RAG, Dupe RJ, English PD, et al: Fibrinolysis with acyl-enzymes: A new approach to thrombolytic therapy. *Nature* 290:505, 1981.
21. Dykewicz MS, McGrath KG, Davison R, et al: Identification of patients at risk for anaphylaxis due to streptokinase. *Arch Intern Med* 146:305, 1986.
22. Robbins KC, Barlow GH, Nguyen G, et al: Comparison of plasminogen activators. *Semin Thromb Hemostas* 13:131, 1987.
23. Nunn B, Esmail A, Fears R, et al: Pharmacokinetic properties of anisoylated plasminogen streptokinase activator complex and other thrombolytic agents in animals and in humans. *Drugs* 33:88, 1987.
24. Salzman EW, Deykin D, Shapiro RM, et al: Management of heparin therapy: Controlled prospective trial. *N Engl J Med* 292:1046, 1975.
25. Raschke RA, Reilly BM, Guidry JR, et al: The weight-based heparin dosing nomogram compared with a "standard care" nomogram. *Ann Intern Med* 119:874, 1993.
26. Hull RD, Raskob GE, Rosenbloom D, et al: Optimal therapeutic level of heparin therapy in patients with venous thrombosis. *Arch Intern Med* 152:1589, 1992.
27. Bain B, Forster T, Sleigh B: Heparin and the activated partial thromboplastin time: A difference between the in vitro and in vivo effects and implications for the therapeutic range. *Am J Clin Pathol* 74:668, 1980.
28. Hull RD, Raskob GE, Rosenbloom D, et al: Heparin for 5 days as compared with 10 days in the initial treatment of proximal venous thrombosis. *N Engl J Med* 322:1260, 1990.
29. Mohiuddin SM, Hillemen DE, Destache CJ, et al: Efficacy and safety of early versus late initiation of warfarin during heparin therapy in acute thromboembolism. *Am Heart J* 123:729, 1992.
30. Levine MN, Hirsh J: Hemorrhagic complications of anticoagulant therapy. *Semin Thromb Hemostas* 12:39, 1986.
31. Ansell J, Deykin D: Heparin-induced thrombocytopenia and recurrent thromboembolism. *Am J Hematol* 8:325, 1980.
32. Warkentin TE, Kelton JG: Heparin-induced thrombocytopenia. *Progr Hemost Thromb* 10:1, 1991.
33. Chang JC: White clot syndrome associated with heparin-induced thrombocytopenia: A review of 23 cases. *Heart Lung* 16:403, 1987.
34. Sheridan D, Carter C, Kelton JG: A diagnostic test for heparin-induced thrombocytopenia. *Blood* 67:27, 1986.
35. Cola C, Ansell J: Heparin-induced thrombocytopenia: Alternative therapies. *Am Heart J* 119:368, 1990.
36. Ortel TL, Gockerman JP, Califf RM, et al: Parenteral anticoagulation with the heparinoid Lomoparan (Org 10172) in patients with heparin-induced thrombocytopenia and thrombosis. *Thromb Hemost* 67:292, 1992.
37. White PW, Sadd JR, Nensel RE: Thrombotic complications of heparin therapy including six cases of heparin-induced skin necrosis. *Ann Surg* 190:595, 1979.
38. Nurmohamed MT, Rosendaal FR, Buller HR, et al: Low molecular weight heparin versus standard heparin in general and orthopaedic surgery: A meta-analysis. *Lancet* 340:152, 1992.
39. Mohr DN, Silverstein MD, Murtaugh PA, et al: Prophylactic agents for venous thrombosis in elective hip surgery. *Arch Intern Med* 153:2221, 1993.
40. Brandjes DPM, Heijboer H, Buller HR, et al: Acenocoumarol and heparin compared with acenocoumarol alone in the initial treatment of proximal-vein thrombosis. *N Engl J Med* 327:1485, 1992.
41. Hirsh J, Dalen J, Deykin D, et al: Oral anticoagulants: Mechanism of action, clinical effectiveness and optimal therapeutic range. *Chest* 102(Suppl):312S, 1992.
42. Hull R, Hirsh J, Jay R, et al: Different intensities of anticoagulation in the long-term treatment of proximal venous thrombosis. *N Engl J Med* 307:1676, 1982.
43. Kirkwood TBL: Calibration of reference thromboplastins and standardization of the prothrombin time ratio. *Thromb Haemost* 49:238, 1983.
44. Landefeld SC, Beyth RJ: Anticoagulant-related bleeding: Clinical epidemiology, prediction, and prevention. *Am J Med* 95:315, 1993.
45. Shorr RI, Ray WA, Daugherty JR, et al: Concurrent use of nonsteroidal anti-inflammatory drugs and oral anticoagulants places elderly persons at high risk for hemorrhagic peptic ulcer disease. *Arch Intern Med* 153:1665, 1993.
46. Shetty HG, Backhouse G, Bentley OP, et al: Effective reversal of warfarin-induced excessive anticoagulation with low dose vitamin K1. *Thromb Hemost* 67:13, 1992.
47. Faraci PA, Deterling RA, Stein A, et al: Warfarin induced necrosis of the skin. *Surg Obstet Gynecol* 146:695, 1978.
48. Clouse L, Comp PC: The regulation of hemostasis: The protein C system. *N Engl J Med* 314:1298, 1986.
49. van Amstel WJ, Boekhout-Mussert MJ, Loeliger EA: Successful prevention of coumarin-induced hemorrhagic skin necrosis by timely administration of vitamin K1. *Blut* 36:89, 1978.
50. Tinker JH, Tarhan S: Discontinuing anticoagulant therapy in surgical patients with cardiac valve prosthesis. *JAMA* 239:738, 1978.
51. Ginsberg JS, Hirsh J: Anticoagulants during pregnancy. *Annu Rev Med* 40:79, 1989.
52. Bergentz SE: Dextran in the prophylaxis of pulmonary embolism. *World J Surg* 2:19, 1978.
53. Hirsh J, Dalen JE, Fuster V, et al: Aspirin and other platelet-active drugs: The relationship between dose, effectiveness, and side effects. *Chest* 102(suppl):327S, 1992.
54. Cairns JA, Hirsh J, Lewis HD, et al: Antithrombotic agents in coronary artery disease. *Chest* 102(suppl):456S, 1992.
55. Physicians' Health Study Research Group: Final report on the aspirin component of the ongoing physicians' health study. *N Engl J Med* 321:129, 1989.
56. Stein PD, Dalen JE, Goldman S, et al: Antithrombotic therapy in patients with saphenous vein and internal mammary artery bypass grafts following percutaneous transluminal coronary angioplasty. *Chest* 102(Suppl):508S, 1992.
57. Stein PD, Alpert JS, Copeland J, et al: Antithrombotic therapy in patients with mechanical and biological prosthetic heart valves. *Chest* 102(Suppl):445S, 1992.

58. Turpie AGG, Gent M, Laupacis A, et al: A comparison of aspirin with placebo in patients treated with warfarin after heart-valve replacement. *N Engl J Med* 329:524, 1993.

59. Sharma GVRK, Cella G, Parisi AF, et al: Thrombolytic therapy. *N Engl J Med* 306:1268, 1982.

60. Sasahara AA, Hyers TM, Cole CM, et al (eds): The urokinase pulmonary embolism trial: A national cooperative study. *Circulation* 47(suppl 2:II):1, 1973.

61. Urokinase-streptokinase embolism trial: Phase 2 results: A cooperative study. *JAMA* 229:1606, 1974.

62. Goldhaber SZ: What role for thrombolysis in patients with pulmonary embolism? *J Crit Illness* 7:192, 1992.

63. Goldhaber SZ, Markis JE, Kessler CM, et al: Perspectives on treatment of acute pulmonary embolism with tissue plasminogen activator. *Semin Thromb Hemostas* 13:171, 1987.

64. Terrin M, Goldhaber SZ, Thompson B, et al: Selection of patients with acute pulmonary embolism for thrombolytic therapy: Thrombolysis in pulmonary embolism patient survey. *Chest* 95:279S, 1989.

65. Goldhaber SZ, Sors H: Treatment of venous thrombosis and pul-

66. monary embolism, in Fuster V, Verstraete M (eds): *Thrombosis in Cardiovascular Disorders*. Philadelphia, Saunders, 1992, p 465.

66. Rogers LQ, Lutcher CL: Streptokinase therapy for deep vein thrombosis: A comprehensive review of the English literature. *Am J Med* 88:389, 1990.

67. Sidorov J: Streptokinase vs heparin for deep venous thrombosis. *Arch Intern Med* 149:1841, 1989.

68. Conard J, Samama MM: Theoretic and practical considerations on laboratory monitoring of thrombolytic therapy. *Semin Thromb Hemost* 13:212, 1987.

69. Bovill EG, Terrin ML, Stump DC, et al: Hemorrhagic events during therapy with recombinant tissue-type plasminogen activator, heparin and aspirin for acute myocardial infarction. *Ann Intern Med* 115:256, 1991.

70. Sherry S: Bleeding complications in thrombolytic therapy. *Hosp Pract* 25(suppl 5):1, 1990.

71. Sloan MA: Stroke associated with thrombolytic therapy for acute myocardial infarction. *Heart Dis Stroke* 1:287, 1992.

122. Hypercoagulability and the Pathophysiology of Thrombosis in the Critically Ill Patient

Craig S. Kitchens

Although hypercoagulability has an ethereal definition, its consequence, thromboembolism, haunts intensive care units. Too frequently an otherwise good outcome of the disorder for which the patient was hospitalized is frustrated by thrombosis. Although studies have clarified pathophysiology, identified patients at risk, and verified effective and safe prophylaxis and treatment, it may be impossible to eliminate the occurrence of thromboembolism totally, but the risk of hypercoagulability can and should be minimized.

The final result of hypercoagulability, thrombosis, is usually caused by perversion of physiologic mechanisms (Fig. 122-1). Rather than bizarre or novel mediators, thrombosis results from a clot that occurs through physiologic pathways but at an unwanted time and place.

Hypercoagulability may be defined as any clinical condition in which a patient develops or is at risk of developing a thrombosis when an otherwise normal person would not [1,2]. Some refer to this situation as "prethrombotic" or "prothrombotic." Others [3] have developed more narrow definitions. In any event, thrombosis results from a pathologic increase in procoagulant forces, e.g., circulating tissue thromboplastin from tissue necrosis, or an absolute decrease in opposing forces, e.g., deficiency of antithrombin III.

A subset of hypercoagulability includes thrombophilic disorders [4], which for this discussion have the same relationship to thrombosis that hemophilic disorders have to hemorrhage. Inherited thrombophilic conditions are caused by specific disorders of regulatory coagulation proteins, the lack of which leads to a circumscribed but lifelong increased risk for thrombosis. Acquired thrombophilic conditions are disorders in which thrombosis is a primary aspect of a well-defined disease. Many other situations and states are referred to as hypercoag-

ulable in that they enhance coagulation but are not usually thought of as specific disease states. Examples include bed rest, prolonged automobile travel, or paralysis. Even as surgery, trauma, liver disease, or aspirin ingestion may precipitate bleeding in a person with hemophilia, any of several provocations such as heart failure, pregnancy, or trauma may precipitate thrombosis in a patient with thrombophilia. Many of these provocations are themselves considered risk factors for thromboembolism.

Risk Factors for Thrombosis

Table 122-1 lists many risk factors that may enhance the likelihood of thrombosis. A glance proves that most of these risks are pertinent in the intensive care unit (ICU) setting. Initially, these risk factors appear to be a miscellany of conditions. However, recalling Virchow's triad [1], one may sort most of these risks into at least one of Virchow's three categories to explain thrombosis: (1) *decreased flow,* thought to explain the hypercoagulability of congestive heart failure, bed rest, and dehydration; (2) *vessel wall changes,* explaining risks from varicosities and trauma from catheters or intraaortic balloon pumps; and (3) *intrinsic changes in blood* consistent with trauma, myocardial infarction, and congenital thrombophilia. Some risks are not yet well explained, such as the risk attributed to age, whereas other risks may fit several corners of the triad, for instance, the risk associated with malignancy.

The coagulation system may be viewed as the system that results in coagulation of blood. Limiting the extent of coagula-

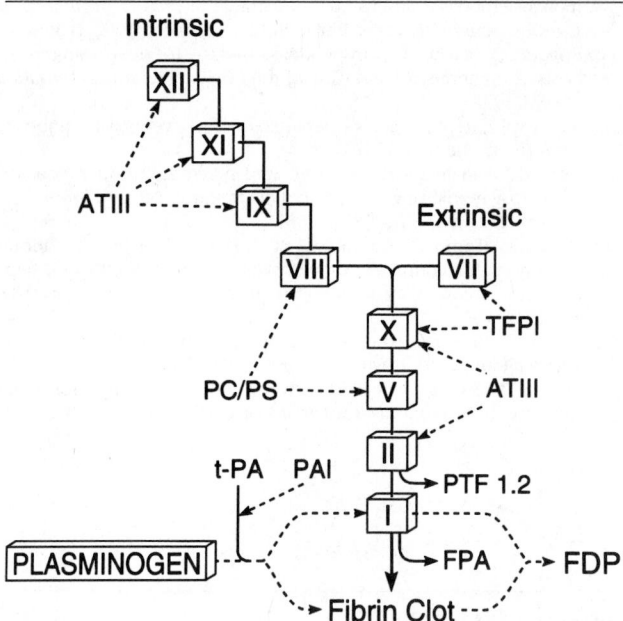

Fig. 122-1. Control points in coagulation. Dotted lines represent mechanisms of control to limit procoagulant forces. Antithrombin III (ATIII) complexes with activated serine proteases. Proteins C and S (PC/PS) limit activities of the cofactors (factors V and VIII) while tissue factor pathway inhibitor (TFPI) inhibits components of the extrinsic system. Plasminogen activator inhibitor-1 (PAI) modulates tissue plasminogen activator's activation of plasminogen into plasmin, which in turn cleaves the fibrin clot into fibrin degradation products (FDP). The activation of prothrombin (factor II) results in both the production of thrombin and prothrombin fragments 1 + 2 (F 1 + 2). Fibrinogen peptide A (FPA) is an activation product of thrombin cleavage of fibrinogen.

tion are the systems that regulate coagulation and lyse fibrin. These systems may be regarded as true agonists:antagonists. Coagulation is always occurring at a slow rate but can be accelerated by any number of physiologic and pathophysiologic activities. Whether systems can hold coagulation in check determines when, where, and to what extent blood coagulates.

In the traditional view, coagulation is initiated by either the intrinsic system or the extrinsic system, as discussed in Chapter 118. The intrinsic system activates factor XII by the so-called contact system, in which contact with activators alters this physicochemically sensitive factor. Activators include denuded en-

Table 122-1. Hypercoagulable Conditions

Inherited thrombophilia	Tissue damage
Acquired thrombophilia	▶Trauma
Massive obesity	▶Surgery
Puerperium	▶Acute myocardial infarction
Prior DVT	▶Malignancy
Prior PE	Sepsis
Congestive heart failure	High-dose estrogen therapy
Ascites	Paralysis
Varicosities	Immobilization
Dehydration	Bed rest
Age >40 years, especially >60 years	Pressor drug administration
	Endovascular devices
Vascular trauma	

dothelium, exposed collagen and other subendothelial materials, or certain negatively charged substances. Activated factor XII, in turn, activates in an accelerating manner the intrinsic chain, with the final product being the generation of thrombin.

In the extrinsic system, activation is initiated by the release of tissue factor (tissue thromboplastin), which is contained in virtually all mammalian cells. Disruption of the circulatory system results in tissue factor gaining entry into the circulatory system with subsequent activation of factor VII and ultimate production of thrombin.

It is believed that many of the hypercoagulable conditions enhance activation of coagulation through either the intrinsic system, the extrinsic system, or both.

Four mechanisms moderate procoagulant forces such that fibrin formation or thrombosis does not overwhelm physiology. These are (1) flow and dilution; (2) the clearance of activated coagulation factors by the reticuloendothelial system; (3) physiologic inhibitors of coagulation; and (4) the fibrinolytic system. Whereas each of these activities is closely interconnected and difficult to dissect from a physiologic point of view, such division enhances understanding.

That *flow and dilution* are important to check procoagulant forces is documented by several researchers' experience. Deykin [5] experimentally demonstrated that flow was important. Blood stagnated in a vein clots more rapidly or requires a weaker procoagulant stimulus than does flowing blood. With flow, one achieves dilution, which makes it more difficult for a critical mass of activated coagulants to accrue. Coagulation is thus retarded by way of dilution. Blood in a traumatized area is characterized by very slow or even interrupted flow by virtue of edema, disruption of blood vessels, and external pressure. As flow is impeded, coagulation is enhanced. Conversely, if blood undergoing activation escapes the bounds of local trauma and is diluted, propagation of coagulation outside the traumatized area is not permitted.

Clearance by the reticuloendothelial system is important in regulation of coagulation. Using an experimental model, Deykin [5] demonstrated that activated coagulation proteins are quickly cleared by passage through the liver. Hepatic insufficiency and slow hepatic blood flow impede the inhibitory forces of the liver.

The system of *natural inhibitors* is composed of antithrombin III, protein S, and protein C. These natural inhibitors neutralize procoagulants. Less is known about recently described inhibitors with regard to their physiologic importance. These include tissue factor pathway inhibitor (an inhibitor of factors VII and X) and heparin cofactor II, an antithrombinlike protein [4]. Antithrombin III neutralizes most activated serine proteases in a one-to-one stoichiometric manner. Antithrombin binds to thrombin, Xa, VIIa, and, to a lesser extent, IXa and XIa. Antithrombin III's activity is enhanced 1000- to 10,000-fold by heparin and is the mechanism of anticoagulant activity of heparin. Proteins C and S serve together, with protein C in its activated form neutralizing activated factors V and VIII. Protein S is a cofactor necessary for protein C activity.

The *fibrinolytic system* is composed of several proteins whose final expression is the production of plasmin that lyses fibrin and, to a lesser extent, fibrinogen and factors V and VIII. Plasmin is derived from plasminogen, which physiologically is activated by endogenous tissue plasminogen activator (tPA). Plasminogen activation is inhibited by plasminogen activator inhibitors, chief of which is plasminogen activator inhibitor-1 (PAI-1). Plasmin in turn is neutralized by its inhibitor, α_2 antiplasmin (α_2AP), alternatively known as α_2 plasmin inhibitor (α_2PI).

Although hypercoagulability can result from the overstimulation of physiologic coagulation by activation of either the intrinsic or extrinsic system, it can also occur from failure to neutralize physiologic activation. This failure may result from decreased flow and dilution, reticuloendothelial system insufficiency, decreased levels of inhibitors, or decreased fibrinolytic activity. These inadequacies may result in physiologic hemostasis becoming pathologic, resulting in thrombosis.

Repeated efforts have been made to monitor blood for evidence of hypercoagulability by laboratory methods. The notion that activation of coagulation factors consumes factors resulting in decreased levels of the native inactivated forms is not true. Coagulation factors are present in such excess molar amounts and the range of normal is so broad that it is impossible to detect accurately a decrease in inactivated coagulation factors as a result of activation. Conversely, efforts have been made to identify activated forms such as circulating thrombin. This is not possible because of the short half-life of thrombin attributable to rapid dilution, clearance, and neutralization by antithrombin III.

Thrombin has several activities once it is generated. Evidence that these activities have developed may lead one to deduce that thrombin has, in fact, been generated. Thrombin cleaves fibrinogen into not only insoluble fibrin, but small soluble activation peptides as well. These activation products include fibrinopeptide A (FPA) and fibrinopeptide B (FPB), the only known source of which is cleavage of fibrinogen by thrombin. Therefore detection of elevated levels of FPA or FPB indicates that thrombin has recently been generated. FPA has been proven to be beneficial in clinical studies in detecting recent thrombin generation.

When thrombin is released into the circulation it is quickly neutralized by antithrombin III, forming a thrombin:antithrombin III complex (TAT). Detection of the TAT complex using monoclonal antibodies allows one to conclude that thrombin has been generated. The monoclonal antibody does not recognize prothrombin, thrombin, or antithrombin III alone. This has also proven to be a useful marker in clinical studies for deducing the presence of thrombin.

One of the most promising markers for thrombin generation has been developed by Bauer and colleagues [6]. When thrombin is generated by the proteolytic action of factor Xa on prothrombin, activation peptides termed fragments $1 + 2$ ($F1 + 2$) are released from the amino terminal end of prothrombin. $F1 + 2$ has a short half-life; therefore its identification indicates that thrombin generation is quite recent. Assays for this activation product have been developed.

A similar story unfolds for the fibrinolytic system [6]. Whereas plasminogen may be reduced in extensive disseminated intravascular coagulation (DIC) or after activation with thrombolytic agents (e.g., therapeutic administration of tPA or streptokinase), in general, a reduction in plasminogen concentration is not a sensitive indicator that thrombosis has occurred. Plasmin also has a short half-life, being quickly neutralized by its inhibitor, α_2AP. Reduction of levels of α_2AP is occasionally useful in deducing the presence of plasmin. Alternatively, the plasmin:α_2AP complex (PAP) can be measured.

The best "footprint" of plasmin's existence, however, is detection of fibrin degradation products (FDP). Plasmin dissolves fibrin into many FDPs. Because FDPs are generated solely through plasmin digestion, one can deduce that plasmin has been generated by the detection of FDP.

Factor XIII is physiologically activated by thrombin. When fibrin monomers form, they are initially noncovalently cross-linked, but become cross-linked by the action of activated factor XIII. Cross-linked fibrin, when it is proteolyzed by plasmin, yields a unique FDP called D-dimer. This small fragment of fibrin, as it has been cross-linked by the action of factor XIII, implicates the production of thrombin. Because it is an FDP, it also implicates the circulation of plasmin. Accordingly, D-dimer assays are useful for deducing the generation of both thrombin and plasmin as might be found in DIC.

The detection of these footprints of plasmin and thrombin has only recently become possible by the use of modern technology to detect molecular species that exist in nanomolar concentrations [6,7]. The measurement of such fragments has been quite useful in experimental thrombosis and coagulation and is now on the verge of clinical use.

Inherited Thrombophilia

Five inherited thrombophilic conditions have been described. These disorders are congenital deficiencies of antithrombin III, protein C, protein S, or plasminogen, and so-called resistance to activated protein C [7a] (Table 122-2). These disorders have been recently thoroughly reviewed [4,8].

These deficiencies are transmitted in an autosomal dominant fashion, with affected persons having approximately one-half of the normal amount of the involved regulatory protein. Most likely, these persons manifest a heterozygous condition. A small number of patients have been described with homozygous deficiency of protein C or protein S, the presentation of which is neonatal purpura fulminans, a condition that is highly thrombotic and frequently lethal in the first few days of life. Homozygous deficiency of either antithrombin III or plasminogen has not been described.

Patients with heterozygous deficiency of these regulatory proteins frequently present with a thromboembolic event in the second or third decade of life, an important clinical clue to the diagnosis. Three other features of inherited thrombophilia are the recurrent nature of thrombosis, the presence of a family history consistent with an autosomal dominant pattern of inheritance, and the occurrence of thrombosis in unusual sites such as in the cerebral or splanchnic veins (Table 122-3). Only approximately 40 to 50 percent of patients fulfilling these criteria are shown to have an identifiable congenital thrombophilia. Clearly other, as yet poorly characterized or undescribed, regulatory proteins exist.

Persons with these inherited thrombophilic disorders have a

Table 122-2. Thrombophilic Disorders

Inherited Thrombophilias
   Antithrombin III deficiency
   Protein C deficiency
   Protein S deficiency
   Plasminogen deficiency
   Resistance to activated protein C
Acquired Thrombophilias
   Antiphospholipid syndrome
   Myeloproliferative syndrome
   Paroxysmal nocturnal hemoglobinuria
   Trousseau's syndrome

Table 122-3. Clinical Features of Congenital Thrombophilia

Initial thrombosis prior to age 40–45
Recurrent thrombotic episodes
Thrombosis in unusual sites
Positive family history

higher than normal plasma level of prothrombin fragment $F1+2$ even in the ambulatory setting, indicating an increased pace of ongoing coagulation. Administration of warfarin to an International Normalized Ratio (INR) of 2.5 to 3.5 reduces five-fold to 10-fold these patients' levels of $F1+2$ [9]. Whereas these patients are thrombophilic during their normal day-to-day activities, they become even more so when other provocative events (most commonly pregnancy, trauma, surgery, or infection) are additionally present, conditions that may very well result in an admission to an ICU. Patients with these deficiencies are at extreme risk for severe and fatal thromboembolic events during serious illness and must receive prophylactic anticoagulant therapy.

Acquired Thrombophilia

Numerous acquired disorders are alleged to be thrombophilic. These have been reviewed extensively elsewhere [4]. Some diseases, such as nephrotic syndrome and hepatic insufficiency, are characterized by acquired reductions of antithrombin III, protein C, or protein S. Four acquired conditions are notorious for thrombotic complications.

The *antiphospholipid syndrome* is a term used to define a broad spectrum of abnormalities, including the lupus anticoagulant, thrombocytopenia, hemolytic anemia, recurrent fetal wastage, leg ulcers, and the predilection for venous or arterial thrombosis [10,11]. This disorder is increasingly identified as an explanation for arterial thromboses, particularly in young persons for whom no other explanation is readily available. It can be detected by assessment of the presence of antiphospholipid antibodies, anticardiolipin antibodies, and lupus anticoagulant. Clinical features, laboratory assessment, pathophysiology, and treatment have been recently reviewed by experts in this condition [10,11]. The hypercoagulability accompanying this disorder usually responds well to anticoagulant prophylaxis or therapy.

The group of hematologic disorders known as the *myeloproliferative syndromes* (polycythemia vera, chronic myelogenous leukemia, essential thrombocythemia, and myelofibrosis) are often associated with deep venous thrombosis, pulmonary embolus, and thrombosis of the splanchnic veins, particularly the splenic vein. The hypercoagulability of polycythemia vera is well documented and is usually adequately treated by vigorous phlebotomy to bring hematocrits to the low-normal range. This is accompanied by prolonged survival of such patients [12]. Essential thrombocythemia is characterized by hyperproliferation of the megakaryocytic cell line. Platelet counts are often over a million and platelets frequently are large. Occasionally this disorder is accompanied by thrombosis. Should thrombotic manifestations become problematic, cytoreductive therapy aimed at reducing the platelet count, and antiplatelet agents inhibiting platelet function may be indicated [13,14].

Paroxysmal nocturnal hemoglobinuria (PNH) is a rare but extremely hypercoagulable disease. Indeed, the leading cause of death appears to be thrombosis, particularly thrombosis of the splanchnic vessels, with a peculiar predilection to hepatic vein thrombosis (Budd-Chiari syndrome). Thromboembolic manifestations are particularly present in the puerperium [15].

The fourth acquired thrombophilic disorder is *Trousseau's syndrome,* which refers to the hypercoagulability associated with adenocarcinoma. Although thromboembolic phenomena occur with many cancers, the features of Trousseau's syndrome are characteristic enough to warrant separate discussion. The clear association with mucinogenic adenocarcinoma casts fa-

vorable light on the notion that the hypercoagulability is caused, at least in part, by the excessive production and circulation of mucin with subsequent activation of the coagulation system. Tumors commonly associated with this syndrome include adenocarcinomas of the lung, pancreas, stomach, and colon. Characteristic features of this syndrome include recurrent migratory thrombosis resistant to warfarin therapy yet usually responsive to heparin, on which survival is dependent [16,17]. The tumor may be occult, being found only at autopsy.

Other Hypercoagulable States

A multitude of events in the ICU are associated with hypercoagulability (see Table 122-1). All patients in the ICU are on bed rest, which leads to decreased blood flow and stasis. Stasis itself enhances coagulation of blood, as proven in animal experiments [5,18]. Patients having strokes and not receiving prophylaxis frequently develop deep venous thrombosis. Nearly all the thrombosed extremities involve the paretic limb [19]. An older study [20] using sensitive methods showed that transmural myocardial infarction treated in the era of prolonged immobilization and before routine heparinization was clearly thrombogenic, with at least half the patients developing deep venous thrombosis. An even higher percentage developed thrombosis if their myocardial infarction was complicated by congestive heart failure. However, the incidence of deep venous thrombosis in both uncomplicated and complicated myocardial infarction was decreased fourfold to fivefold by early ambulation.

Multiple studies have shown that advancing age is associated with an increased risk of developing deep venous thrombosis. Although the mechanism(s) explaining this observation is not clear, aging itself in healthy persons is associated with increasing plasma levels of $F1+2$, FPA, and PAP, all of which triple from age 40 to 80 years [21].

Sepsis and inflammation are common in ICU patients. The boundaries between the coagulation system and the inflammatory system are now less distinct than ever. It is known that activation of the contact system also activates the complement system. Cytokines, such as tumor necrosis factor (TNF) [22,23], activate both the inflammatory and coagulation systems and may serve as mediators of hypercoagulability. Interleukins, to include therapeutic infusion of IL-2, affect the coagulation system [24,25]. White blood cells contain a variety of powerful enzymes, some of which are strongly proteolytic and may enhance coagulation through their involvement with inflammation and infection [26,27,28].

Tissue damage is characteristic of most patients in ICUs. This damage can result from surgery, trauma, burns, ischemia, necrosis, tumors that outgrow their vascular supply, tumors that die from chemotherapy, crush injuries, and sepsis, to mention but a few.

Trauma is associated with hypercoagulability [28a]. Using rabbits and escalating doses of tissue trauma, Borgstrom et al [29] demonstrated that as trauma increased, the propensity toward thrombosis increased. Serum from dogs with experimentally induced myocardial infarction causes thrombosis when infused into rabbits [30]. Before routine use of heparin for treatment of myocardial infarction, Murray et al [31] used radiofibrinogen studies to show that among patients admitted for unstable angina, the incidence of deep venous thrombosis was 34 percent in those patients who were subsequently proved to have had myocardial infarction yet only 7 percent for those who had not experienced infarction.

Several studies have shown that, among humans, increasing

levels of illness are associated with increasing changes in blood, which may explain, at least in part, the hypercoagulable nature of injured patients. As APACHE II scores increase among ICU patients, plasma levels of F1 + 2, D-dimer, and TAT increase [32]. Schmidt et al [33] showed that with increasing trauma, higher levels of circulating D-dimer were found. The longer this elevation persisted, the more likely a patient was to develop not only deep venous thrombosis and pulmonary embolus, but also acute respiratory distress syndrome. As trauma scores increase, others have found increasing plasma levels of D-dimer and falling levels of antithrombin III and protein S [34].

In an extensive review on the pathogenesis of venous thrombosis, Mammen [35] concluded that the hypercoagulability of surgery and trauma was attributable to three simultaneous events: (1) the increase in procoagulant activity caused by tissue damage and the escape of tissue factor into the circulation; (2) decreased flow caused by bed rest and the generally depressed circulation of the critically ill patient; and (3) "fibrinolytic shutdown" caused by increasing levels of PAI-1, which serves to impede generation of plasmin. PAI-1, as an acute phase reactant, increases in a variety of clinical situations, including trauma [34]. Increasing levels of PAI-1 were found in patients undergoing total hip replacement who are inadequately anticoagulated and subsequently develop thrombosis [36]. In general surgical patients, levels of PAI-1 increased with the extensiveness of the surgical procedure [37,38,39]. Modern experimental studies confirm older clinical observations made before routine prophylactic anticoagulation for surgical patients. Twenty years ago it was reported that among common gynecologic operations, the lowest rate of thromboembolism followed vaginal hysterectomies, a middle range followed abdominal hysterectomies, and the highest rate of thromboembolism complicated radical procedures such as the Wertheim operation [40].

Closed head injury is associated with hypercoagulability and disseminated intravascular coagulation [41]. In experimental head injury in rats, fixed amounts of head trauma result in reproducible amounts of fibrin deposition in the microcirculation [42]. The same investigators [43] found that in patients with head injury, there was a correlation between extent of head injury, hemostatic defects, and worsening clinical outcome. Olson et al [44] confirmed these findings in a large series of patients with head injuries. Head injuries not only lead to neurologic damage, paralysis, and venous stasis, but damaged brain tissue serves as a source of tissue thromboplastin released into the circulation, causing coagulation activation.

The hypercoagulability of cancer is related to cell death with the subsequent release of tissue factor into the circulation. Cell death can occur from either proliferation of defective cells incompatible with prolonged viability, tumors outgrowing their vascular supply, or effective therapy [45]. Additionally, cancer patients are frequently on bed rest. The placement of catheters and various other devices promotes coagulation. Nearly all patients having a variety of cancers have increased plasma markers indicative of a hypercoagulable state. Nearly half of all patients undergoing operation for cancer develop thromboembolism. Accordingly, prophylaxis should be strongly considered. There is increasing evidence that chemotherapy itself may be associated with thromboembolic events, because this complication peaks at the time of chemotherapy administration [46].

Intensivists frequently encounter female patients treated with hormonal therapy, either as contraceptives or for estrogen replacement. The role of estrogens in hypercoagulability has been debated vigorously for decades. In one early study using dosages of estrogen quite large by today's standard, 6 of 31 young women treated with birth control pills who underwent emergency abdominal operation developed deep venous thrombosis, whereas none of 19 similar patients not administered oral contraceptives developed deep venous thrombosis [47]. An exhaustive analysis of the literature in 1985 of oral contraceptives and cardiovascular disease concluded that there was a slight risk between the ongoing use of contraceptives and deep venous thrombosis in the high doses employed up to that time [48]. The bulk of patients having experienced thromboembolism and other cardiovascular events while on oral contraceptives were smokers and older than 35 years. Now that doses of estrogen in birth control pills are much lower, the risk appears to be attenuated. Lower doses of estrogens result in fewer changes in the hemostatic system that probably, although it is not proven, result in fewer thromboembolic catastrophes [49]. Using sensitive and modern markers for hemostatic activation, Saleh and associates [50] were unable to find increased levels of TAT or F1 + 2 in users of modern contraceptives. In a 1992 review of the modern era of oral contraceptives, it was concluded that there is no additional risk from estrogen use, with the caveats that patients are younger than 35 years of age, do not smoke, and do not have a personal history for previous thromboembolism [51]. Accordingly, such patients in an ICU are probably not at additional risk if they were taking oral contraceptives at admission. However, it would seem prudent to discontinue administration of such medications during admission to the ICU if only because of decreased indication.

Singh et al [52] analyzed blood samples from 97 nonsmoking women who received levonorgestrel (Norplant) subcutaneously for 5 years, finding that antithrombin III levels were slightly increased, vitamin K–dependent factors were slightly decreased, overall fibrinolytic activity was slightly decreased, and platelet aggregation was slightly increased compared with controls. They interpreted these changes as no net change in the coagulation system caused by this progestinol agent. Accordingly one may conclude that Norplant need not be removed in most patients for fear of thrombosis.

Women treated with estrogen replacement therapy do not appear to be at increased risk for thromboembolism. Changes in the hemostatic system do not clearly appear to favor coagulation [53]. However, using more sensitive markers, namely FPA and F1 + 2, Caine et al [54] found that women taking 0.625 mg daily of estrogen replacement had an increase in circulating levels of those markers, whereas those taking 1.25 mg daily had twice that increase. Accordingly, it seems that doses less than 1.25 mg cause less activation than higher doses. Clinical studies using modern doses of estrogen replacement have not shown an increased risk of thromboembolic disease [55]. One may conclude that estrogen replacement therapy in patients admitted to the ICU does not increase the risk for thromboembolic events above and beyond the risk expected from the age and condition for which they are admitted. By age criteria alone, most should receive prophylaxis, and it would seem reasonable to interrupt estrogen replacement therapy for the duration of the admission.

Men with prostate cancer are frequently treated with estrogens. Older studies documented an increased mortality in men taking 5 mg estrogen per day but not in those taking 1 mg estrogen per day [56]. Such patients, by age alone, qualify for prophylactic antithrombotic therapy. Whether to continue the estrogen treatment may depend on the clinical situation and the overall control of the disease by estrogen therapy.

Prophylaxis

Given the multitude of risk factors for thromboembolism that threaten the patient in the ICU and the frequency with which thromboembolism adversely affects outcome, it is natural to consider prophylaxis. The concept of prophylaxis against thromboembolic disease has grown enormously in the last two decades. When groups of patients who are clearly at high risk can be identified, the standard of care involves aggressive prophylaxis. Concerns of bleeding, although real, have dramatically decreased in the last several years as the use of commonly employed anticoagulant agents has evolved from a mysterious art-form to a clear science. De Takats [57], two decades ahead of his time, was one of the first to state clearly that lower doses of either parenteral or oral anticoagulant agents were required to confer prophylaxis against thromboembolic phenomena than the higher doses used to treat thromboembolism. The concept of prophylaxis against thrombosis matured during 1970 to 1980, coming to fruition with the NIH Consensus Conference of 1986 devoted to this topic [58]. That conference concluded that high-risk groups could be clearly identified, that a multitude of prophylactic measures were effective, and that prophylaxis needed to be used more aggressively and in more situations. Conversely, prophylaxis is grossly underused. Anderson et al [59] reported that as few as 25 percent of all patients qualifying for prophylactic anticoagulant therapy receive appropriate therapy. Kakkar and Stringer, early proponents of prophylactic anticoagulation, in a 1990 review concluded that heparin was unequivocally effective and needed to be more extensively employed [60]. Many physicians are still unduly overconcerned about bleeding, and some still doubt efficacy [61] despite the fact that prophylaxis has been proven to be effective in nearly every aspect of medicine.

The bulk of clinical evidence that has proved the efficacy of thrombosis prophylaxis has been generated by studies of surgical patients. Patients older than 40 years of age undergoing abdominal surgery have been the primary cohort for demonstrating the unequivocal efficacy of prophylactic anticoagulation in reducing deep venous thrombosis, pulmonary embolus, and fatal pulmonary embolus, as well as overall mortality. However, the use of prophylaxis should not be limited to this group. These surgical groups have served as ideal study groups, given the large number of candidates and operations performed. Such surgical patients are a more homogenous group than are the variety of patients and multitude of illnesses found in medical ICUs. Patients in intensive care settings are at least as likely to develop thrombosis. Double-blind, placebo-controlled studies, however, have not been published in sufficient number to prove with equal clarity the efficacy of anticoagulant prophylaxis in ICU patients, although some studies have strongly favored the efficacy of such treatment. Chalmers et al [62] performed a meta-analysis of 32 studies aimed at anticoagulating patients hospitalized for acute myocardial infarction. They noted that although the intent of these studies, namely, to reduce myocardial infarction, was not borne out, there was a 21 percent decrease in all-cause mortality. This highly statistically significant decrease in mortality was explained by deep venous thrombosis and pulmonary embolism in the treatment groups, occurring less than half as often as in the control groups. This analysis also showed a high hemorrhagic rate, namely, three times higher than control patients, but it must be recalled that these studies were completed using the inappropriately high intensity of oral anticoagulation that was the standard of care at that time.

Now nearly all patients sustaining myocardial infarction are treated with heparin for any of several reasons. Other ICU patients warrant prevention of fatal events by administration of anticoagulant drugs. In one randomized study involving critically ill patients, the incidence of deep venous thrombosis was decreased 50% (p < 0.05) by the administration of heparin, 5000 units subcutaneously twice daily from the time of admis-

sion [63]. In another randomized study, Halkin et al [64] studied acutely ill, immobilized patients. They used a similar dose of prophylactic heparin and found a 30 percent decrease in all-cause mortality. They noted a reduction in mortality in the treatment group from the time of admission, with the magnitude of protection becoming larger the longer the length of stay, which is compatible with our concept that deep venous thrombosis develops and propagates as a function of time in critically ill patients. Belch et al [65] prospectively studied a randomized group of 100 patients who were admitted for congestive heart failure, pneumonitis, or both. With low-dose heparin administration they found that 4 percent of their patients developed deep venous thrombosis, compared with 26 percent of the control group (p < 0.01). No patient in the treatment group but 4 percent of the patients in the control group sustained pulmonary embolism. In addition, patients receiving heparin prophylaxis had rates of bleeding similar to those who did not receive heparin. In a retrospective study of ICU patients, Pingleton et al [66] noted that the administration of heparin, 5000 units subcutaneously three times a day, eliminated pulmonary embolism from their intensive care patients. Their patients did not experience excessive bleeding with this dose of heparin.

Accordingly, most patients in an ICU should be offered thrombotic prophylaxis of some type. The most common prophylaxis employed is heparin, 5000 units subcutaneously either twice or thrice daily. Numerous studies, including those from ICUs, document no increase in bleeding [65,66]. It is possible that some patients, especially in the early stages of evaluation, may not be candidates for prophylaxis because of real concern for bleeding. In trauma patients where the total impact of injuries, to include hemorrhagic potential, is not known on admission, observation may be in order for 1 or 2 days. When analyzing prophylaxis in spinal cord injury patients, a recent consensus study [67] concluded that in the first 2 or 3 days, intermittent pneumatic compression devices are indicated until the risk of bleeding has been more thoroughly assessed. Conversely, this same consensus group concluded that one cannot continue without prophylaxis because of the unacceptably high rate (70%) of thromboembolic events in such patients. Indeed, this group of patients is at such high risk that low-dose heparin does not offer enough prophylaxis. Therefore, adjusted-dose heparin, at a dose sufficient to raise the partial thromboplastin time (PTT) to the very upper limits of normal, is recommended after the first few days of observation. Although not as effective for prophylaxis as adjusted-dose heparin, intermittent pneumatic compression devices are popular, acceptable, and effective in preventing thromboembolism in neurosurgical patients and cause no increase in bleeding.

The incidence of deep venous thrombosis and pulmonary embolism in stroke patients is very high, and the risk of recurrent stroke is especially high. Therefore, prophylaxis is required to prevent deep venous thrombosis and recurrent strokes, and there is also great concern about intracerebral bleeding. A recent consensus group [68] suggested that for patients with stroke-in-evolution, heparin at therapeutic doses was justified. For completed strokes, therapeutic levels of heparin appeared not to be justified, although low-dose heparin for prophylaxis against deep venous thrombosis is probably justified. For acute embolic strokes, heparin within the first 48 hours is not indicated because of fear of hemorrhagic transformation of the infarcted brain, particularly in hypertensive patients or in strokes that involve a large volume of tissue. If, after 48 hours, appropriate investigative imaging studies indicate that there has been no bleeding and the patient is not hypertensive, heparin should then be administered until concomitant initiation of warfarin therapy achieves an INR of 2.0 to 3.0.

Consensus was recently reached regarding the use of antithrombotic agents in coronary artery disease [69]. Patients with unstable angina qualify for aspirin therapy (160–325 mg) immediately and daily thereafter. Intravenous heparin in doses sufficient to raise the PTT to 1.5 to 2.0 times normal is also indicated. In acute myocardial infarction, those patients who are not undergoing thrombolytic therapy qualify for the aforementioned aspirin and heparin. Those with anterior Q-wave infarction are advised to receive anticoagulant therapy with warfarin to INRs of 2.0–3.0 for up to 3 years, which reduces the incidence of not only subsequent myocardial infarction but stroke, and all-cause mortality [70]. Patients who have atrial fibrillation, unless otherwise contraindicated, should be treated indefinitely with warfarin [71]. Patients who receive thrombolytic therapy [72] are discussed elsewhere in this text.

Intensive care patients with mechanical prosthetic heart valves who require invasive procedures represent special problems. There are few adequate studies to direct the practitioner scientifically, but a recent consensus group [73] recommended three possible courses. These are

1. To stop oral anticoagulant therapy, allowing the prothrombin time to achieve normal levels
2. To reduce warfarin dosage to provide "acceptable INR levels" such as from 1.3 to 1.8
3. To convert from warfarin to heparin therapy, stop the heparin immediately before an operation or procedure, only to restart it again, and then following heparinization, to restart warfarin.

Whereas all three of these recommendations seem adequate, there are certain advantages of option 2. The first option represents the least risk for bleeding but also the highest risk for thromboembolism. The third option has been strongly criticized because it requires much more time and expense and has no clear therapeutic advantage [74]. Additionally, by starting and stopping several medicines, chances of error increase.

The second option is recommended. Reducing warfarin therapy to an INR in the 1.3 to 1.8 range offers prophylaxis against thromboembolism, yet, in a double-blind trial involving total hip replacement, it is not associated with increased bleeding compared with controls [75]. More recently, two groups of investigators have shown that therapy to INRs in this range is associated with decreased levels of plasma F1 + 2 and therefore impacts on measurable products of coagulation, even at this low dosage [76,77].

A variety of other methods are available for prophylaxis, although their exact role has not been clearly established. Mechanical methods such as early ambulation [20], foot pedaling, calf stimulation, and elastic compression stockings have been shown to be effective [61]. Intermittent compression devices on the legs have been shown to be effective in a variety of models and are particularly acceptable to neurosurgeons and may be especially indicated when there are strong and reasonable concerns about the risk of bleeding [78].

Low-molecular-weight heparin has recently been approved for use [79]. Its role in ICU patients has yet to be proved, but the drug has potential, particularly if decreased bleeding and ease of monitoring prove to be as effective as indicated from multiple European studies [80]. Data exist supporting the efficacy and safety of low-molecular-weight heparin in the treatment and prophylaxis of thromboembolism. Whether one preparation of low-molecular-weight heparin can be substituted for another for various indications has not yet been established.

Use of filters placed in the inferior vena cava to prevent death from pulmonary embolism appears to do just that. However, these devices have side effects, such as obstruction with clots, filter migration, and perforation of the inferior vena cava [81].

Fifteen percent of patients in whom filters have been placed and adequately followed in a prospective manner develop obstruction of the inferior vena cava [82]. Being mechanical bioprosthetic devices, filters may also activate coagulation. With thrombophilic disorders, thrombotic events are hardly limited to deep venous thrombosis and pulmonary embolus. There may be an increase in activation of blood coagulation that presents itself by other thromboses such as in the visceral or cerebral veins [83]. In a critical review of inferior vena cava filters, Becker et al [84] pointed out that there were no controlled studies to properly address their precise role. Whereas there is a decrease in immediate death from pulmonary embolus, there is no evidence supporting an overall reduction in morbidity and mortality, especially when compared with no treatment, to anticoagulant administration, despite what is perceived by some to be contraindications for anticoagulants or thrombolytic therapy.

Laboratory Evaluation for Hypercoagulability

Because of the risk of thromboembolism in ICU patients, practitioners must be on constant alert for evidence of thromboembolism. Spiess and Davalle [85] concluded that the best monitor for thromboembolic events still is frequent examination of extremities for both venous and arterial insufficiency. Similarly, thromboembolism should always be kept in mind as a cause for changes in the patient's status. Physical examination should be enhanced by Doppler examinations and determinations of ankle-brachial indices (ABIs), particularly in patients who are unable to communicate their symptoms.

Laboratory monitoring of blood levels of F1 + 2, TAT, and D-dimer is still evolving. These markers have shown utility in developing the concept of hypercoagulability; yet their general use in the ICU has not arrived [7]. As these assays become commercially available and acceptable, this may change. Monitoring of FDP and D-dimer is available and frequently of use for the diagnosis of DIC.

The source of blood for any coagulation test has been a concern, and most coagulation experts insist that samples be drawn solely for coagulation purposes from a fresh venipuncture. Heparin contamination, even in extremely small concentrations, can obfuscate the results of the very tests for which the blood is drawn [86]. Czapek [87] concluded that the most common source of a prolonged PTT from patients in the ICU is blood samples drawn through a preexisting line. In her studies, the withdrawal of 10 cc through the line does not always prevent an artifactual elevation of the PTT, although this has not been universally agreed on [88].

Too frequently, practitioners attempt to use laboratory methods to screen for congenital thrombophilia in critically ill patients. This is not only inappropriate but actually serves as a frequent source of disinformation. Patients with congenital thrombophilia, like those with congenital hemophilia, are at risk because of the static congenital decrease in either antithrombin III, protein S, protein C, or plasminogen, all of which are affected by liver disease, DIC, ongoing thrombosis, and the therapy for ongoing thrombosis, namely, anticoagulants [89,90]. The least appropriate time to analyze for congenital thrombophilia is when patients are seriously ill. Levels of these four proteins are decreased in acutely ill patients. Accordingly, patients and their families may be inappropriately labeled as deficient in any of these regulatory proteins when such may not be the case. Because anticoagulant therapy for any of the hypercoagulable states including thrombophilia is the same, therapeutic decisions can be made independent of the levels of these proteins.

It is impossible to make the diagnosis of congenital thrombophilia definitively in intensely ill patients. If the family history indicates, blood from members of the patient's family may be assayed because these deficiencies are inherited in an autosomal dominant pattern. It is only when the patient is stable, with normal liver function, no longer treated with anticoagulant drugs, and has been returned to good health that such measurements are appropriate. Only patients having at least two of the four clinical features on Table 122-3 should undergo routine testing for antithrombin III, protein S, protein C, and plasminogen [4,8,91,92]. A low value for any of these proteins should be confirmed at least once at a separate time. Patients who have sustained thromboembolism but do not have these clinical features are more likely to have false-positive assays than true-positive diagnoses. The bulk of patients having had a thromboembolic event do not have an identifiable congenital thrombophilia [4,91].

References

1. Kitchens CS: Concept of hypercoagulability: A review of its development, clinical application, and recent progress. *Semin Thromb Hemost* 11:293, 1986.
2. Schafer AI: The hypercoagulable states. *Ann Intern Med* 102:814, 1985.
3. Joist JH: Hypercoagulability: Introduction and perspective. *Semin Thromb Hemost* 16:151, 1990.
4. Kitchens CS: Thrombophilia and thrombosis in unusual sites, Chap 64, in Colman RW, Hirsh J, Marder VS, et al (eds): *Hemostasis and Thrombosis: Basic Principles and Clinical Practice.* 3rd ed. Philadelphia, Lippincott, 1994, pp 1255–1273.
5. Deykin D: The role of the liver in serum-induced hypercoagulability. *J Clin Invest* 45:256, 1966.
6. Bauer KA: Laboratory markers of coagulation activation. *Arch Pathol Lab Med* 117:71, 1993.
7. Boisclair MD, Ireland H, Lane DA: Assessment of hypercoagulable states by measurement of activation fragments and peptides. *Blood Rev* 4:25, 1990.
7a. Sun X, Evatt B, Griffin JH: Blood coagulation factor Va abnormality associated with resistance to activated protein C in venous thrombophilia. *Blood* 83:3120, 1994.
8. Alving BM: The hypercoagulable states. *Hosp Pract (Off Ed)* 28(2):109, 1993.
9. Conway EM, Bauer KA, Barzegar S, et al: Suppression of hemostatic system activation by oral anticoagulants in the blood of patients with thrombotic diatheses. *J Clin Invest* 80:1535, 1987.
10. Lockshin MD: Antiphospholipid antibody syndrome. *JAMA* 268:1451, 1992.
11. Triplett DA: Antiphospholipid antibodies and thrombosis: A consequence, coincidence, or cause? *Arch Pathol Lab Med* 117:78, 1993.
12. Conley CL: Polycythemia vera. *JAMA* 263:2481, 1990.
13. Schafer AI: Essential thrombocythemia. *Prog Hemost Thromb* 11:69, 1991.
14. Kessler CM, Klein HB, Havlik RS: Uncontrolled thrombocytosis in chronic myeloproliferative disorders. *Br J Haematol* 50:157, 1982.
15. Greene MG, Frigoletto RD Jr, Claster S, et al: Pregnancy and paroxysmal nocturnal hemoglobinuria: Report of a case and review of the literature. *Obstet Gynecol Surv* 38:591, 1983.
16. Bell WR, Starksen FH, Ton S, et al: Trousseau's syndrome: Devastating coagulopathy in the absence of heparin. *Am J Med* 79:423, 1985.
17. Woerner EM, Rowe RL: Trousseau's syndrome. *Am Fam Physician* 38:195, 1988.
18. Wessler S: Studies in intravascular coagulation. III. The pathogenesis of serum-induced thrombosis. *J Clin Invest* 34:647, 1955.
19. Landi G, D'Angelo A, Boccardi E, et al: Venous thromboembolism in acute stroke: Prognostic importance of hypercoagulability. *Arch Neurol* 49:279, 1992.
20. Miller RR, Lies JE, Carretta RF, et al: Prevention of lower extremity venous thrombosis by early mobilization: Confirmation in patients with acute myocardial infarction by ^{125}I-fibrinogen uptake and venography. *Ann Intern Med* 84:700, 1976.
21. Bauer KA, Weiss LM, Sparrow D, et al: Aging-associated changes in indices of thrombin generation and protein C activation in humans: Normative aging study. *J Clin Invest* 80:1527, 1987.
22. Bauer KA, Ten Cate H, Barzegar S, et al: Tumor necrosis factor infusions have a procoagulant effect on the hemostatic mechanism in humans. *Blood* 74:165, 1989.
23. Schutze S, Machleidt T, Kronke M: Mechanisms of tumor necrosis factor action. *Semin Oncol* 19(Suppl 4):16, 1992.
24. Fleischmann JD, Shingleton WB, Gallagher C, et al: Fibrinolysis, thrombocytopenia, and coagulation abnormalities complicating high dose interleukin 2 immunotherapy. *J Lab Clin Med* 117:76, 1991.
25. Levi M, ten Cate H, vander Poll T, et al: Pathogenesis of disseminated intravascular coagulation in sepsis. *JAMA* 280:957, 1993.
26. Cohen JR, Sarfati I, Birnbaum E, et al: The inactivation of antithrombin III by serum elastase in patients with surgical infections. *Am Surg* 56:665, 1990.
27. Spillert CR, Lazaro EJ: Contribution of the monocyte to thrombotic potential. *Agents Actions* 34:28, 1991.
28. Colman RW: Platelet and neutrophil activation in cardiopulmonary bypass. *Ann Thorac Surg* 49:32, 1990.
28a. Geerts WH, Code KI, Jay RM, et al: A prospective study of venous thromboembolism after major trauma. *N Engl J Med* 331:1601, 1994.
29. Borgstrom S, Gelin LE, Zederfeldt B: The formation of vein thrombi following tissue injury: An experimental study in rabbits. *Acta Chir Scand* (Suppl) 247:1, 1951.
30. Moschos CB, Khan MI, Regan TJ: Thrombogenic properties of blood during early ischemic and nonischemic injury. *Am J Physiol* 220:1882, 1971.
31. Murray TS, Lorimer AR, Cox FC, et al: Leg-vein thrombosis following myocardial infarction. *Lancet* 2:792, 1970.
32. Bredbacka S, Blomback M, Wiman B, et al: Laboratory methods for detecting disseminated intravascular coagulation (DIC): new aspects. *Acta Anaesthesiol Scand* 37:125, 1993.
33. Schmidt U, Enderson BL, Chen JP, et al: D-dimer levels correlate with pathologic thrombosis in trauma patients. *J Trauma* 33:312, 1992.
34. Garcia Frade LJ, Landin L, Garcia Avello A, et al: PAI and D-D dimer levels are related to severity of injury in trauma patients. *Fibrinolysis* 5:253, 1991.
35. Mammen EF: Pathogenesis of venous thrombosis. *Chest* 102(Suppl 6):640S, 1992.
36. Rocha E, Alfaro MJ, Paramo JA, et al: Preoperative identification of patients at high risk of deep venous thrombosis despite prophylaxis in total hip replacement. *Thromb Haemost* 59:93, 1988.
37. D'Angelo A: Fibrinolytic shut-down after surgery: Impairment of the balance between tissue-type plasminogen activator and its specific inhibitor. *Eur J Clin Invest* 15:308, 1985.
38. Johnson EJ, Hariman H, Hampton KK, et al: Fibrinolysis during major abdominal surgery. *Fibrinolysis* 4:147, 1990.
39. Mellbring G, Dahlgren S, Wiman B: Plasma fibrinolytic activity in patients undergoing major abdominal surgery. *Acta Chir Scand* 151:109, 1985.
40. Walsh JJ, Bonnar J, Wright FW: A study of pulmonary embolism and deep leg vein thrombosis after major gynaecological surgery using labelled fibrinogen-phlebography and lung scanning. *J Obstet Gynaecol Br Commonw* 81:311, 1974.
41. Goodnight SH: Defibrination after brain-tissue destruction: A serious complication of head injury. *N Engl J Med* 290:1043, 1974.
42. van der Sande JJ, Emiss JJ, Lindeman J: Intravascular coagulation: A common phenomenon in minor experimental head injury. *J Neurosurg* 54:21, 1981.
43. van der sande JJ, Veltkamp JJ, Boekhout-Mussert RJ, et al: Hemostasis and computerized tomography in head injury: their relationship to clinical features. *J Neurosurg* 55:718, 1981.
44. Olson JD, Kaufman HH, Moake J, et al: The incidence and signifi-

cance of hemostatic abnormalities in patients with head injuries. *Neurosurgery* 24:825, 1989.

45. Luzzatto G, Schafer AI: The prethrombotic state in cancer. *Semin Oncol* 17:147, 1990.

46. Rickles RF, Levin M, Edwards RL: Hemostatic alterations in cancer patients. *Cancer Metastasis Rev* 11:237, 1992.

47. Sagar S, Stamatakis JD, Thomas DP, et al: Oral contraceptives, antithrombin III activity, and postoperative deep-vein thrombosis. *Lancet* 1:509, 1976.

48. Realini JP, Goldzieher JW: Oral contraceptives and cardiovascular diseases: A critique of the epidemiologic studies. *Am J Obstet Gynecol* 152:729, 1985.

49. Notelovitz M, Zauner C, McKenzie L, et al: The effect of low-dose oral contraceptives on cardiorespiratory function, coagulation, and lipids in exercising young women: A preliminary report. *Am J Obstet Gynecol* 156:591, 1987.

50. Saleh AA, Brockbank N, Dorey LG, et al: TAT complexes and prothrombin fragment 1 + 2 in oral contraceptive users. *Thromb Res* 73:137, 1994.

51. Mammen EF: Oral contraceptives and thrombotic risk: A critical overview. Chap 5, in Ramwell P, Rubanxi G, Schillinger E (eds): *Sex, Steroids and the Cardiovascular System.* Berlin, Springer, 1992, p 65.

52. Singh K, Viegas OA, Koh SC, et al: Effect of long-term use of Norplant implants on haemostatic function. *Contraception.* 45:203, 1992.

53. Notelovitz M, Kitchens C, Ware M, et al: Combination estrogen and progestogen replacement therapy does not adversely affect coagulation. *Obstet Gynecol* 62:596, 1983.

54. Caine YG, Bauer KA, Barzegar S, et al: Coagulation activation following estrogen administration to postmenopausal women. *Thromb Haemost* 68:392, 1992.

55. Devor M, Barrett-Connor E, Renvall M, et al: Estrogen replacement therapy and the risk of venous thrombosis. *Am J Med* 92:275, 1992.

56. Henriksson P: Estrogen in patients with prostatic cancer: An assessment of the risks and benefits. *Drug Saf* 6:47, 1991.

57. de Takats G: Anticaogulant therapy in surgery. *JAMA* 142:527, 1950.

58. NIH Consensus Conference Prevention of venous thrombosis and pulmonary embolism. *JAMA* 256:744, 1986.

59. Anderson FA Jr, Wheeler B, Goldberg RJ, et al: Physician practices in the prevention of venous thromboembolism. *Ann Intern Med* 115:591, 1991.

60. Kakkar VV, Stringer MD: Prophylaxis of venous thromboembolism. *World J Surg* 14:670, 1990.

61. Arcelus JI, Caprini JA, Traverso CI: International perspective on venous thromboembolism prophylaxis in surgery. *Semin Thromb Hemost* 17:322, 1991.

62. Chalmers TC, Matta RJ, Smith H Jr, et al: Evidence favoring the use of anticoagulants in the hospital phase of acute myocardial infarction. *N Engl J Med* 297:1091, 1977.

63. Cade JF: High risk of the critically ill for venous thromboembolism. *Crit Care Med* 10:448, 1982.

64. Halkin H, Goldberg J, Modan M, et al: Reduction of mortality in general medicine in-patients by low-dose heparin prophylaxis. *Ann Intern Med* 96:561, 1982.

65. Belch JJ, Lowe GDO, Ward AG, et al: Prevention of deep vein thrombosis in medical patients by low-dose heparin. *Scott Med J* 26:115, 1981.

66. Pingleton SK, Bone RC, Pingleton WW, et al: Prevention of pulmonary emboli in a respiratory intensive care unit: Efficacy of low-dose heparin. *Chest* 79:647, 1981.

67. Hull RD: Venous thromboembolism in spinal cord injury patients. *Chest* 102(Suppl 6):658S, 1992.

68. Sherman DG, Dyken JL Jr, Fisher M, et al: Antithrombotic therapy for cerebrovascular disorders. *Chest* 102(Suppl 4):529S, 1992.

69. Cairns JA, Hirsh J, Lewis HD Jr, et al: Antithrombotic agents in coronary artery disease. *Chest* 102(Suppl 4):456S, 1992.

70. Smith P, Arensen H, Holme I: The effect of warfarin on mortality and reinfarction after myocardial infarction. *N Engl J Med* 323:147, 1990

71. Laupacis A, Albers G, Dunn M, et al: Antithrombotic therapy in atrial fibrillation. *Chest* 102(Suppl 4):426S, 1992.

72. Cairns JA, Fuster V, Kennedy JW: Coronary thrombolysis. *Chest* 102(Suppl 4):482S, 1992.

73. Stein PD, Alpert JS, Copeland J, et al: Antithrombotic therapy in patients with mechanical and biological prosthetic heart valves. *Chest* 102(Suppl 4):445S, 1992.

74. Eckman MH, Beshansky JR, Durand-Zaleski I, et al: Anticoagulation for noncardiac procedures in patients with prosthetic heart valves: Does low risk mean high costs? *JAMA* 263:1513, 1990.

75. Francis DW, Marder VHJ, Evarts CMcC, et al: Two-step warfarin therapy: Prevention of postoperative venous thrombosis without excessive bleeding. *JAMA* 249:374, 1983.

76. Mannucci PM, Bottasso B, Tripodi A, et al: Prothrombin fragment 1+2 and intensity of treatment with oral anticoagulants. *Thromb Haemost* 66:741, 1991.

77. Millenson MM, Bauer KA, Kistler JP, et al: Monitoring "mini-intensity" anticoagulation with warfarin: Comparison of the prothrombin time using a sensitive thromboplastin with prothrombin fragment F_{1+2} levels. *Blood* 79:2034, 1992.

78. Caprini JA, Arcelus JI, Traverso CI, et al: Low molecular weight heparin and external pneumatic compression as options for venous thromboembolism prophylaxis: A surgeon's perspective. *Semin Thromb Hemost* 17:356, 1991.

79. Hirsh J, Dalen JE, Deykin D, et al: Heparin: Mechanism of action, pharmacokinetics, dosing considerations, monitoring, efficacy, and safety. *Chest* 102(Suppl 4):337S, 1992.

80. Hull RD, Pineo GF: Therapeutic use of low molecular weight heparins: The knowledge to date as applied to therapy. Semin Thromb Hemostas 19(Suppl 1):111, 1993.

81. Lofaso F, Messadi AA, Anglade MC, et al: Failure of the intracaval filter of Gunther to prevent recurrence of pulmonary embolism: Report of two cases. *Intensive Care Med* 16:457, 1990.

82. Kolachalam RB, Julian TB: Clinical presentation of thrombosed Greenfield filters. *Vasc Surg* 9:666, 1990.

83. Simon LS, Gorn AH: Case records of the Massachusetts General Hospital: A 38-year-old woman with fever, skin lesions, thrombocytopenia and venous thrombosis. *N Engl J Med* 322:754, 1990.

84. Becker DM, Philbrick JT, Selby JB: Inferior vena cava filters: Indications, safety, effectiveness. *Arch Intern Med* 152:1985, 1992.

85. Spiess BD, Davalle M: Coagulation monitoring in the surgical intensive care unit. *Crit Care Clin* 4:605, 1988.

86. Kitchens CS: Prolonged activated partial thromboplastin time of unknown etiology: A prospective study of 100 consecutive cases referred for consultation. *Am J Hematol* 27:38, 1988.

87. Czapek EE: Iatrogenic prolonged aPTT: A nondisease state. *JAMA* 227:1304, 1974.

88. Lew JKL, Hutchinson R, Lin ES: Intra-arterial blood sampling for clotting studies: Effects of heparin contamination. *Anaesthesia* 46:719, 1991.

89. Kitchens CS: Amelioration of antithrombin III deficiency by coumarin administration. *Am J Med Sci* 293:403, 1987.

90. Marciniak E, Gockerman JP: Heparin-induced decrease in circulating antithrombin III. *Lancet* 2:581, 1977.

91. Freed JA: Hypercoagulability: Should every patient with venous thrombosis be tested? *Postgrad Med* 90(6):157, 1991.

92. Genton E: Primary hypercoagulable state. *Cardiovasc Clin* 22:19, 1992.

123. The Hemolytic Anemias

Liberto Pechet

Hemolytic anemias are characterized by a shortened survival of red cells [1]. Clinically, one must distinguish a compensated hemolytic state in which the bone marrow capacity to increase its red cell production overcomes the deficit from an uncompensated state that results in anemia. Hemolytic anemias may also be classified by the site of the major hemolytic event. Intravascular hemolysis is said to occur when the red cells are both damaged and destroyed in the circulation. The most striking and life-threatening example is that of an incompatible ABO hemolytic-transfusion reaction. In extravascular hemolysis, although the initial damage to red cells usually occurs in the circulation, their actual destruction takes place in the reticuloendothelial system.

In most cases of extravascular hemolysis, a red cell membrane defect exists or develops, resulting in recognition and uptake by macrophages, primarily in the spleen and liver. Intravascular hemolysis is most often caused by traumatic events to the red blood cell membrane, resulting in its destruction.

Diagnosis

Many of the laboratory results from patients with hemolytic anemia may be better interpreted if they are based on a separation of intravascular from extravascular hemolytic states as described in Table 123-1. In brief, intravascular hemolysis is characterized by an acute anemia with increased plasma hemoglobin, hemoglobinuria (if the process is intense), and decreased or absent plasma haptoglobin. In extravascular hemolysis, the development of anemia is usually (but not universally) more insidious. Plasma hemoglobin is at most only mildly increased, but indirect (unconjugated) bilirubin is usually higher than 2 mg per deciliter, hemoglobinuria is absent, plasma haptoglobin is minimally decreased, and the peripheral blood smear shows spherocytes and polychromasia. Peripheral blood polychromasia, indicated by large bluish red cells on Wright-stained smears, is a marker of rapid hematopoiesis with an increased number of younger nonnucleated red cells, the reticulocytes.

In most cases of hemolysis, especially when the cause is known, bone marrow examination is not mandatory because the reticulocyte count is a good index of bone marrow activity. To quantitate reticulocytes, a special stain is necessary. When an underlying disease accompanies hemolysis, the bone marrow response may be suboptimal, resulting in an inadequate reticulocyte response. In such cases bone marrow examination may be necessary.

The Coombs test, using antiglobulin, separates immune from nonimmune hemolytic anemias. The direct Coombs test (direct antiglobulin test or DAT) is performed on the patient's red cells. The antiglobulin serum, containing anti-IgG or anticomplement antibodies, will agglutinate cells coated by either IgG antibodies or by components of the complement system. The presence of antibodies in the patient's serum is investigated by the indirect Coombs test (indirect antiglobulin test or IAT).

Clinical Manifestations

The clinical manifestations of hemolytic anemia depend on the severity of the anemia and the rapidity with which it has developed. In cases of chronic, mild, or moderate anemias and in the absence of heart disease, patients are usually asymptomatic. If the bone marrow's compensatory effort is handicapped (e.g., an intercurrent infection), an acute, severe exacerbation of anemia may ensue. Hypoplastic or aplastic crises may occur in any case of chronic hemolytic anemia, but are most common in patients with sickle cell anemia or hereditary spherocytosis.

Other clinical manifestations of hemolytic anemia are related to chronicity. They consist of signs and symptoms of folic acid deficiency if supplements are not given, chronic jaundice, and episodes of cholelithiasis. Patients with chronic hemolysis may present with acute, painful cholelithiasis, superimposed on chronic bilirubin gallbladder stones. Splenomegaly is found in most instances of significant chronic hemolysis, except for sickle cell anemia, where the initial splenomegaly of early childhood resolves because of repeated infarctions (autosplenectomy).

The presence of splenomegaly increases the risk of traumatic

Table 123-1. Laboratory Findings in Hemolytic States

Finding	Comment
Anemia	Present in acute or noncompensated chronic hemolysis
Spherocytes on blood smear	Present with extravascular hemolysis
Polychromasia and increased reticulocytes on blood smear	In all hemolysis with adequate bone marrow response
Bone marrow	Red cell hyperplasia in all cases of chronic hemolysis with intact bone marrow function
Red cell survival	Shortened in all hemolytic states
Red cell splenic uptake	Increased in extravascular hemolysis with intact splenic function
Red cell osmotic fragility	Characteristically increased in hereditary spherocytosis
Unconjugated (indirect) bilirubin	Increased, particularly in severe chronic extravascular hemolysis
G-6-PD	Decreased in G-6-PD deficiency, to be tested only after an interval from hemolytic episode when reticulocyte response has subsided
Plasma haptoglobin	Decreased, especially with intravascular hemolysis
Sugar-water test, Ham test	Positive in paroxysmal nocturnal hemoglobinuria (PNH)
Direct antiglobulin (Coombs test)	Positive in most immune hemolytic anemias
Indirect antiglobulin (Coombs test)	Positive in severe immune hemolytic anemia and with allosensitization
Hemoglobin electrophoresis	Abnormal in hemoglobinopathies with defect(s) in globin chains, such as S or C
Hemoglobin A$_2$	Increased in beta-thalassemias

or spontaneous rupture of the spleen, and has the potential of transforming a well-compensated patient into one with an acute abdominal emergency. Young patients with congenital hemolytic anemias may develop bone infarcts and, occasionally, pathologic fractures that result from an increase in hematopoiesis with encroachment on bone cortices. Because the courses of acquired hemolytic anemias and congenital hemolytic anemias are so different, the specific hemolytic syndromes of both groups will be discussed separately.

ACQUIRED HEMOLYTIC ANEMIAS

Drug-Induced Hemolytic Anemias. The drugs commonly involved in the development of immune hemolytic anemias, their mechanisms, and clinical manifestations are summarized in Table 123-2. A drug commonly implicated in the past, and best studied, is alpha-methyldopa [2]. Although approximately 15 percent of all patients receiving alpha-methyldopa develop a positive DAT, only 0.8 percent of those taking the drug for at least 3 months have clinically significant hemolysis. When hemolysis does develop, however, it may be quite severe, and the drug should be immediately discontinued. In most cases, transfusions are not necessary because the anemia develops slowly, and patients usually adjust to it.

When transfusion is necessary, packed red cells should usually be administered slowly, and use of a diuretic considered. Because of the presence of anti-Rh or other autoantibodies in the patients' serum, the blood bank may have difficulties in cross-matching these patients, which in turn may delay procurement of red cells. With replacement of the affected red cell population by newly formed unaffected red cells, the hemolysis slows down, and hematologic improvement is usually seen within 1 to 2 weeks. There is no evidence that corticosteroids are effective, but it has been suggested that they should be given if the hematologic condition deteriorates in spite of cessation of the drug.

Autoimmune Hemolytic Anemia. Autoimmune hemolytic anemia (AIHA) includes a group of immune disorders in which hemolysis is produced by autoantibodies directed against normal, unmodified erythrocyte surface antigens [3,4]. In most cases of AIHA, a positive DAT is present. Characterization of the antibody's specificity is mandatory, because it serves as a guide with respect to red cell transfusions. AIHA can be classified into two major categories: those caused by cold-reactive antibodies and those attributable to warm-reactive antibodies.

Cold-reactive AIHA, or *cold agglutinin syndrome,* is characterized by the presence of IgM antibodies, which react best at low temperatures. It is usually associated with complement activation and mostly intravascular hemolysis. Cold AIHA may occur de novo or may accompany infections or malignant diseases, the most common infections being *Mycoplasma pneumoniae* and infectious mononucleosis. The typical patient with cold agglutinin syndrome is an elderly individual (unless the disease is accompanying the two infections mentioned above) with cyanosis of the extremities when exposed to cold in association with severe anemia. When an underlying disease is found, its treatment usually results in improvement in hemolysis.

In the idiopathic type, however, no effective treatment is available. Corticosteroids are usually ineffective, nor is splenectomy always helpful. Immunosuppressive therapy has been tried with some benefit. It should be undertaken with great caution, preferably by someone experienced in the use of these agents. When transfusions are necessary, the red cells should be warmed to body temperature. Because exposure to cold triggers intravascular agglutination of erythrocytes and exacerbates the hemolysis, exposure to cold is to be avoided.

Warm-reactive AIHA, the more common of the two types of immune hemolysis, is usually induced by IgG autoantibodies that react best at body temperature. Hemolysis is mainly extravascular, splenic sequestration being the major site of red cell destruction. This type of AIHA may be idiopathic or secondary to an underlying disease. Diseases associated with warm AIHA are collagen vascular diseases, particularly lupus erythematosus; lymphoproliferative disorders, most commonly chronic lymphocytic leukemia; multiple myeloma, thymoma, and occasionally other malignancies; thyroid diseases; and viral infections, particularly in children. With treatment of the underlying disease, the hemolysis in warm-reactive AIHA usually abates.

The presenting symptoms are usually insidious but sometimes may develop acutely. Fever is reported quite frequently.

Table 123-2. Common Drug-Induced Immune Hemolytic Anemias (IHA)

Drugs	Type of IHA	Manifestation
Alpha-methyldopa L-Dopa Mefenamic acid	Antibodies directed against normal components of red cell membrane, usually Rh complex. Hemolysis may continue for weeks or months in the absence of the drug.	Chronic extravascular hemolysis, with positive direct and indirect antiglobulin test.
Sulfonamides Sulfonylureas Quinidine, quinine Phenacetin Isoniazid, rifampin Chlorpromazine P-amino-salicylic acid Insulin Stibophen	Immune complexes (antidrug antibody and drug) absorbed on the red cell membrane. Hemolysis abates when the drug is discontinued.	Acute intravascular hemolysis, with positive direct antiglobulin test.
Penicillin	The drug combines with red cell membrane and then is attacked by antipenicillin antibodies. Mild hemolysis may persist for weeks after the antibiotic is discontinued.	Extravascular hemolysis when >10 million units of penicillin are administered a day; positive direct antiglobulin test.
Cephalothin	Absorption on RBC, resulting in membrane modification that becomes immunogenic.	Hemolysis is rarely present and then very mild, Positivity of antiglobulin test creates difficulty for blood-banking procedures.

Physical examination shows moderate splenomegaly, mild to moderate nontender hepatomegaly, occasional lymphadenopathy, and frequently jaundice. In the warm type of AIHA, anti-IgG specificity can be demonstrated with the Coombs test. The indirect bilirubin is moderately increased. Urine as well as fecal urobilinogen are elevated. The peripheral blood smear shows many microspherocytes, polychromasia, and macrocytes.

In the idiopathic form, the administration of prednisone at 40 mg per square meter of body surface (60 mg/m² in children) per day results in a prompt and dramatic amelioration of anemia in approximately 80 percent of patients. A trial of high-dose intravenous gammaglobulin (1.0 gm/kg once, or 0.4 gm/kg daily for 3–5 days) may also be beneficial but is expensive. If no response is observed, splenectomy should be considered. Transfusions are sometimes necessary and may require the administration of red cells that are "incompatible" by usual blood bank techniques, because all cross-matches may yield a positive antiglobulin test. Some patients may present with an extremely severe clinical picture and may need exchange transfusions (particularly pediatric cases) or plasma exchange.

Once a patient has achieved remission on corticosteroids, a strategy has to be applied to taper therapy and to discontinue it if a complete remission is obtained. If a complete remission cannot be obtained, one must use the lowest dose that will result in compensated hemolysis, thus minimizing the many severe side effects of continuous corticosteroid administration.

Hemolytic Anemias Caused by Mechanical and Other Physical Damage to Red Cells.

Mechanical hemolysis develops when the red cells are traumatized in the circulation. When hemolysis takes place in small vessels, the term *microangiopathic hemolytic anemia* is used. It may develop with disseminated intravascular coagulation (DIC), severe peripheral vascular disease, malignant hypertension and eclampsia, disseminated cancer, thrombotic thrombocytopenic purpura (TTP), hemolytic uremic syndrome, and amyloidosis. Mechanical hemolysis may also be found with severely damaged cardiac valves, such as in severe atherosclerotic aortic valvular disease or after replacement of heart valves with a prosthesis, especially if there is a leak at the base of the valve. The term "Waring Blender syndrome" has been used for this syndrome. The hallmark of mechanical injury to red cells is the presence of schistocytes, which are fragmented, deformed, irregular, or helmet-shaped red cells seen in peripheral blood smears. Mechanical hemolytic anemia is generally not clinically serious, but its presence heralds an underlying abnormality of great importance. Because these anemias involve intravascular hemolysis with chronic hemoglobinemia, the patient excretes excess amounts of hemosiderin (iron) in urine and may need iron replacement.

Osmotic injury is seen after intravenous administration of hypotonic solutions, such as the inadvertent infusion of distilled water, perfusion of prostatic operative beds with water, or in freshwater drownings. Although it is a self-limited event, it may be life threatening if not detected and treated promptly with red cell transfusions. Severe thermal injury, such as third- or fourth-degree burns, may also result in acute hemolysis.

March hemoglobinuria is a rare condition that is seen after strenuous physical exercise (e.g., prolonged forced walking or running). It is caused by physical injury to erythrocytes in the vessels of the feet and is usually a benign condition.

Other causes of mechanical hemolysis include chemical injury, when agents directly injurious to erythrocytes, such as phenylhydrazine, benzene, or phenols are administered. Clostridial infections and malaria may be associated with acute intravascular hemolysis. Hemolysis associated with hypersplenism should also be mentioned, because an enlarged spleen may shorten the red cell life span by increasing sequestration and destruction of normal erythrocytes. This extravascular hemolysis may be accompanied by neutropenia and thrombocytopenia and can be corrected by splenectomy.

Paroxysmal Nocturnal Hemoglobinuria.

Paroxysmal nocturnal hemoglobinuria (PNH) is an acquired stem cell disorder manifested by severe intravascular hemolysis and thrombocytopenia with episodes of both abdominal and back pain and venous thrombotic events [5]. Increased hemolysis may be triggered by infections. The disease may evolve into acute myelocytic leukemia. A major complication of a hemolytic episode may be acute renal failure, probably related to severe hemoglobinuria and associated dehydration.

Treatment of this condition is directed at the anemia and loss of iron in the urine and at the acute complications, particularly thrombotic. Although iron deficiency requires iron therapy, hemolysis may be exacerbated after iron therapy, because this therapy increases the numbers of young red cells in the circulation that are more susceptible to the lytic action of complement. In most cases, however, iron may be given safely either orally or parenterally. Because these patients may require steroids for long periods, 15 to 40 mg alternate-day prednisone is recommended. When hemolysis is particularly severe or if an aplastic bone marrow develops, transfusions may be necessary.

Venous thrombosis, possibly related to abnormally sticky platelets (PNH affects not only red cells but platelets and white cells), may occur in hepatic, intraabdominal, and cerebral veins. One of the recently recognized complications of PNH is an insidious form of hepatic venous thrombosis (insidious Budd-Chiari syndrome). Fibrinolytic agents such as sreptokinase or tissue plasminogen activator may be effective if used during the acute episode [6]. Bone marrow transplantation may be considered early in the course of this disease [7]. Although oral anticoagulants are indicated whenever manifestations of venous thrombosis develop, heparin may result in hemolytic episodes.

Hemolytic Transfusion Reactions.

Hemolytic transfusion reactions are discussed in detail in Chapter 124.

Hemolytic Disease of the Newborn (Erythroblastosis Fetalis).

Hemolytic disease of the newborn (HDN) due to Rh incompatibility has become extremely rare with the administration of anti-Rh gamma globulins (Rhogam) at the time of delivery to Rh-negative mothers. Primary immunization occurs in approximately 15 percent of primigravid Rh-negative women who are carrying an Rh-positive fetus when numerous fetal cells enter the maternal circulation during labor and delivery. If an immunized woman becomes pregnant again with an Rh-positive fetus, the small number of fetal cells crossing the placenta during pregnancy may be sufficient to induce a profound secondary immune response with a rising anti-Rh maternal titer, which is manifested by a positive antiglobulin test. These IgG antibodies cross the placenta and attack fetal erythrocytes, resulting in development of intrauterine fetal hemolysis.

This can be avoided by the passive administration of anti-Rh gamma globulin immediately after the delivery of the first child and any subsequent children as well as after an abortion. However, women who have already been immunized to Rh antigens during previous pregnancies or by transfusions do not benefit from Rhogam administration.

In addition to the Rh system, other red cell antigens, particularly the AB group, may result in similar, albeit usually less severe, hemolytic disease of the newborn. All mothers at risk should be followed throughout each pregnancy by performing the indirect antiglobulin test and by following its titer when positive. If the titer increases, the fetus should be carefully monitored and amniocentesis performed between the 22nd and 27th weeks of pregnancy to examine for products of fetal red cell destruction. If there is evidence of HDN, induction of delivery between the 34th and 38th weeks may be indicated. If there is risk of severe HDN, such as hydrops fetalis or of stillbirth before 34 weeks, intrauterine transfusions to the fetus can be administered, followed by induction of labor at 34 weeks. Depending on the severity of HDN, exchange transfusion is instituted after delivery.

General Approach to the Patient with Severe Acquired Hemolytic Anemia. After an initial evaluation, the physician must decide whether the severity of the anemia compromises vital functions. If that is the case and the anemia appears to be treatable with corticosteroids, immediate treatment consists of administration of prednisone at 40 mg per meter square (60 mg/m^2 in children) per day. If heart failure is present, slow transfusion of red cells and diuretics should be added to steroids. This treatment may result in prompt and dramatic amelioration of the anemia. When red cell transfusions are necessary in life-threatening situations, they may pose a great challenge to the physician and the blood bank. In general, patients with immune forms of hemolytic anemia are serologically incompatible with their own and most donors' red cells by laboratory testing, resulting in great difficulties in cross-matching. After eliminating alloantibodies by absorption the blood bank will select the least incompatible donor out of a battery of many donors. The smallest quantity of red cells that provides benefit should be administered.

In severe cases and in emergency situations, one-half unit of packed (and preferably washed) red cells should initially be transfused slowly (1 cc/kg red cells in children). This red cell volume expansion may be sufficient to improve the cardiopulmonary distress caused by the severe anemia without provoking overt hemolytic reactions or pulmonary edema. Administration of a small volume of packed red cells may be periodically repeated under close observation and in association with diuretics when indicated, until the patient becomes stable. Finally, plasmapheresis may be tried to remove high titer antibodies.

After the patient has been stabilized, a thorough search for an underlying disease should be initiated. If discovered and treated successfully, the hemolytic anemia generally abates. The long-term outcome depends on eliminating an underlying agent or disease, or in idiopathic hemolytic anemias, inducing clinical remission by the use of immunosuppressive agents, particularly corticosteroids.

Congenital Hemolytic Anemias

HEMOGLOBINOPATHIES. The hemoglobinopathies are hereditary disorders related to structural defects in the composition or quantity of globin synthesis. Hemoglobin, the oxygen-carrying molecule of red cells, contains four iron-heme groups for each globin chain. Normal globin is a protein composed of four components: two alpha- and two beta-chains in approximately equal amounts for hemoglobin A, which forms 95 percent of the adult hemoglobin; two alpha- and two gamma-chains for hemoglobin F, fetal hemoglobin, which forms less than 2 percent of adult hemoglobin, and two alpha- and two delta-chains for hemoglobin A$_2$, which forms up to 3 percent of normal adult hemoglobin. The most prevalent hemoglobinopathies are sickle cell disease, hemoglobin C, and the thal-

assemia syndromes. In recent years the prenatal diagnosis of the hemoglobinopathies has become a practical reality [8].

Sickle Cell Disease. Among the most common inherited hemoglobinopathies, the sickle cell diseases include homozygous hemoglobin (Hb)S and doubly heterozygous HbS/C and HbS/thalassemia. The homozygous state (SS) results in sickle cell anemia, a severe disabling disease [9]. The defect consists of one amino acid substitution in the beta-globin chain. The abnormal gene is encountered primarily in the population of African ancestry and in certain Arabic groups. Deoxy Hb S (the hemoglobin in the deoxygenated state that is found in capillaries after having released oxygen) forms long, parallel, rodlike fibers that polymerize and form crescent-shaped (sickled) red cells. Sickling is a progressive process, which is preceded by repeated sickling-unsickling in response to various body oxygen tensions. It ultimately produces the irreversibly sickled cells that are both nonfunctional and have the propensity to occlude precapillary arterioles, resulting in infarction of surrounding tissues.

Sickle cell trait is generally an asymptomatic condition, except under situations of severe hypoxia. In some cases military recruits with sickle-cell trait have been found in basic training to have an increased risk of exercise-related sudden death [10]. Sickle-cell trait may also be associated with a renal tubular defect causing fixed urine specific gravity (inability to concentrate). Hemoglobin electrophoresis of individuals with the trait shows approximately equal amounts of both hemoglobin A and hemoglobin S, whereas in the homozygous state, hemoglobin S is found almost exclusively with or without elevation of fetal hemoglobin.

The clinical picture of sickle cell anemia is that of a relatively stable, severe hemolytic anemia that is interrupted by infections and by acute vasoocclusive or aplastic crises. Patients are repeatedly subject to vasoocclusive episodes leading to recurrent attacks of pain involving the chest, abdomen, and skeleton. These crises, secondary to red cell sequestration and infarction, must be differentiated from aplastic crises, usually occurring in relation to febrile illnesses and resulting in acute exacerbations of anemia that may be fatal if not promptly treated by transfusion. The loss of splenic function is partially responsible for the increased risk of death of overwhelming infection in childhood.

Growth and development are retarded from the second decade on, and bone disease develops with multiple infarctions. Osteomyelitis, particularly from salmonella infection, is common at all ages. Cardiomegaly from chronic anemia and, in some cases, chronic pulmonary disease secondary to repeated infections and infarctions, can develop. Hepatomegaly, hyposthenuria, hematuria, and occasionally nephrotic syndrome are encountered. Retinal detachment, blindness, and vitreous hemorrhages are the ocular complications.

Treatment of sickle cell anemia and its complications remains symptomatic despite efforts and various attempts at definitive therapy [11,12]. The approach to patients with sickle cell anemia depends on whether one is dealing with a painful vasoocclusive crisis or an aplastic crisis. The treatment of a vasoocclusive crisis relies on supportive measures: analgesics, intravenous fluids, and oxygen. Because of severe and prolonged pain, one should use narcotics for pain not responsive to acetaminophen or nonsteroidal antiinflammatory agents. Oxygen is commonly used to diminish hypoxia, but its benefits have not been substantiated unless the patient has a low PO$_2$. If acidosis is present, sodium bicarbonate is added, usually 1 ampule (44 mEq) to each liter of 1/4 normal saline in 5% glucose.

The acute chest syndrome is a complication characterized by fever, respiratory symptoms, pain in the thorax or abdomen, and lung infiltrates associated with hypoxemia. It is fatal in 2 to 14 percent of cases. The underlying pathology may involve pulmonary vasoocclusion. Antibiotics should be immediately instituted in the presence of fever, and arterial PO_2 should be monitored in an effort to bring it above 75 mm Hg with oxygen therapy (see Chap. 56). Exchange transfusions are indicated for those with evidence of diffuse pulmonary involvement [13].

Treatment is also supportive in the "right upper quadrant syndrome" manifested by pain, fever, and increased jaundice caused by acute cholecystitis, extrahepatic biliary tract obstruction, viral hepatitis, or infarction in the liver. Stroke may be another potential complication of sickle cell anemia. If CT scan or MRI examination is considered, one must be careful with the use of contrast dyes, even the newer non-ionic contrast agents, unless the hemoglobin is at least 5 gm/dl. In the presence of a confirmed stroke, exchange transfusions should be instituted promptly. Exchange, if well monitored, avoids hyperviscosity and blood volume perturbations. Priapism, another serious complication, should also be treated by exchange transfusion if only minimal response occurs after conservative therapy by 24 to 48 hours [13]. This same approach is recommended for most acute, severe sickle-related complications, high-risk pregnancies, or surgery. Deglycerolized or leukofiltered red cells are recommended for all patients with sickle cell disease. Because of frequent alloimmunization, all donor red cells should be checked for antigens in the Rh, K, MNS, and Fy blood groups, as well as for the sickle-cell trait. When emergency transfusion is required, O, Rh(C,D,E)-negative, K-negative red cells should be used [13].

Prevention of repeated infections, particularly by penicillin prophylaxis to at least age 5 and pneumococcal vaccine, should be routine. Prompt antibiotic treatment as soon as fever or infection develops is also indicated. To minimize problems throughout pregnancy, it is advisable to maintain a hematocrit of 25 percent because sickle cell blood is closest to normal viscosity at this level. At delivery, regional or spinal anesthesia should be used, and proper oxygenation should be ensured.

Certain agents that modify hemoglobin S, such as sodium cyanate, urea, zinc, and carbon monoxide, have been proposed as therapy, but so far they have been either impractical, too expensive, too toxic, or their efficacy not proved in controlled trials. More recently, efforts to optimize erythropoiesis by administering erythropoietin to increase fetal hemoglobin with hydroxyurea or butyrate have undergone initial trials [14,15].

Hemoglobin C Disease. Hemoglobin C disease is the next most common hemoglobinopathy in African-Americans. It is found in approximately 3 percent of this group. The defect also consists of one amino acid substitution on the beta-globin chain. The homozygous form, hemoglobin CC disease, is characterized by a mild anemia that results from a moderate hemolytic process and a suboptimal erythropoietic response by the bone marrow. The hematocrit is usually 32 to 34 percent, and the reticulocyte count is 3 to 6 percent. The association between S trait and C trait (SC) is quite common, occurring in 1 of every 833 African-Americans.

Although patients with hemoglobin SC disease tend to have a variable course with fewer total complications than in those with SS disease, they have been reported to develop thromboembolic complications, retinopathy, and renal papillary necrosis more frequently than patients with sickle cell anemia. Generally, because anemia and painful crises rarely need therapy in these patients, treatment is directed toward the complications. Meticulous prenatal care and hypertransfusions (or exchange transfusions) are recommended by some authorities during the third trimester of pregnancy.

Thalassemia Syndromes. Alpha- and beta-thalassemia, a heterogeneous group of inherited disorders, result from suboptimal synthesis of the alpha- or beta-globin chains. The remaining normal globin chains that are synthesized in normal amounts are unpaired and form intraerythrocytic inclusions that damage the red cell membrane and lead to hemolysis. Because generally alpha- and beta-thalassemia minor produce only minimal symptoms, therapeutic problems predominantly occur in beta-thalassemia major. (Deletion of all four alpha chains is usually fatal.)

Beta-thalassemia major (Cooley's anemia, Mediterranean anemia) and thalassemia intermedia [16] are severe diseases that were previously fatal in childhood or early adolescence if untreated. Thalassemia major is found in homozygotes, resulting in a transfusion-dependent anemia [17]. Repeated transfusions in turn lead to hemosiderosis and the complications of iron overload. The latter can, however, be reduced by chelation of iron with desferoxamine. The most common causes of death are cardiac arrhythmias and intractable congestive heart failure from iron overload or infections. Patients with thalassemia intermedia may require splenectomy, splenectomy and transfusions, or no treatment. Patients with thalassemia trait are asymptomatic; hence there is no need for specific treatment. Diagnosis is mandatory for genetic counseling and to avoid unnecessary iron therapy, which is potentially harmful. Bone marrow transplantation may be considered, to provide the patient with normal erythroid precursors to synthesize hemoglobin A [18].

OTHER INTRINSIC RED CELL DEFECTS

Primary Membrane Disorders. Any disorder affecting the membrane shape and the chemical composition of the red cells may result in a shortened red cell survival. The hemolysis that results from membrane defects is predominantly extravascular.

The prototype of these congenital diseases is hereditary spherocytosis (HS). It is transmitted as an autosomal dominant trait and is characterized by the presence of spherocytes on the peripheral blood smear, reticulocytosis, increased osmotic fragility, jaundice, splenomegaly, and a tendency to form gallstones. Although the anemia is usually mild, aplastic crisis may produce severe exacerbations. The antiglobulin test is negative in this disease, unless the patients have developed a superimposed immune disorder.

Depending on the degree of hemolysis and the size of the spleen, or if the spleen ruptures or infarcts, splenectomy may be indicated [19]. Even though spherocytes and abnormal osmotic fragility persist (the membrane defect remains), splenectomy results in a clinical cure. The anemia and signs of increased red cell production and destruction disappear as well as the tendency to cholelithiasis.

Another disorder of the red cell membrane is hereditary elliptocytosis (ovalocytosis). Demonstrable but usually mild hemolysis is found in only about 12 percent of these patients. Splenectomy is rarely indicated. Other rare conditions in this category include hereditary stomatocytosis and hereditary A-beta-lipoproteinemia (hereditary acanthocytosis).

Hereditary Hemolytic Anemias Due to Enzymatic Defects. The anemias caused by enzymatic defects result from abnormalities in red cell metabolism as a consequence of an enzyme deficiency. The most common defect is that found in patients with decreased *glucose-6-phosphate dehydrogenase* (G-6-PD) [20]. This enzyme is necessary for normal red cell metabolism because it catalyzes the first step in the hexose monophosphate shunt that counteracts oxidative processes.

The gene is carried on the X chromosome, being fully expressed in males and in females homozygous for the trait.

The abnormality is most prevalent in the Mediterranean countries as well as in Africa and China, apparently areas where malaria is, or was, prevalent. In the United States approximately 12 percent of the males of African ancestry are affected, and 25 percent of such females are heterozygous. The disease is not clinically manifested until, and unless, the affected person is exposed to an oxidizing drug, the effect of which cannot be counteracted in red cells deficient in the G-6-PD enzyme.

In Mediterraneans, a more severe type of G-6-PD deficiency is found, designated *G-6-PD Mediterranean*, in which the defect involves leukocytes as well as platelets. These patients present with chronic hemolysis that is exacerbated by the administration of oxidants. In all cases, drug-induced hemolysis is accompanied by the formation of Heinz bodies. These inclusions result from the oxidative denaturation of hemoglobin that precipitates and attaches to red cell membranes, rendering them susceptible to destruction in the spleen and liver.

In the African variety, where complete recovery occurs between hemolytic episodes, an improvement of anemia may occur even if the oxidant exposure is continued, because the newly generated red cells contain sufficient amounts of G-6-PD. In the Mediterranean form, no spontaneous improvement takes place as long as the oxidant is present, because the enzyme levels are very low even in young cells. In this type, exposure to fava beans may result in acute hemolysis that may occasionally be fatal.

The diagnosis of G-6-PD deficiency is established by quantitation of the enzyme in red cells. However, immediately after a hemolytic episode in the African variety, the enzyme level may be normal and thus mask a true deficiency. A definitive diagnosis of G-6-PD deficiency in the African variety cannot be established for 2 to 4 weeks after an acute hemolytic episode, at which time the red cells have sufficiently aged to have depleted their G-6-PD levels.

If hemolysis develops, precipitating agents should be withdrawn. Splenectomy is not indicated in the African variety, but occasionally may have a place in the chronic hemolysis of the Mediterranean variety. Red cell transfusion may be necessary in emergency situations associated with very severe hemolysis and anemia.

The next most common enzymatic deficiency is that of pyruvate kinase (PK), another enzyme important in the glycolytic pathway of red cells. Its absence is characterized by a chronic nonspherocytic anemia that varies in severity, ranging from severe neonatal jaundice that requires exchange transfusions to a chronic compensated hemolytic process in adults. Blood transfusions are required only during aplastic crises. Splenectomy in patients with severe PK deficiency may be occasionally beneficial.

GENERAL APPROACH TO THE PATIENT WITH CONGENITAL HEMOLYTIC ANEMIA. The clinician must first concentrate on counteracting the effects of severe anemia due either to excessive hemolysis or to aplastic crisis. There should be judicious use of packed red cells, or if frequent transfusions are necessary, filtered red cells, to eliminate antigens provided by plasma trapped with packed red cells as well as by leukocytes. In each case, the long-term effect of hemosiderosis must be weighed against the need for maintaining hematocrits compatible with growth and life. Chronic iron chelation therapy may be necessary to avoid hemosiderosis in transfusion-dependent patients. Because of the persistence of hemolysis with higher requirements for marrow response, a well-balanced diet should be ensured. In addition, oral supplements of 1 mg per day of folic acid should be administered throughout life. The need for splenectomy must be judged from case to case.

Whenever splenectomy is performed, penumococcal vaccine should be administered 2 to 3 weeks before the procedure. In addition, splenectomy should be deferred in children until they reach at least age 6 years; most clinicians prefer waiting until early adulthood. The presence of increased bilirubin metabolism, resulting in a high incidence of cholelithiasis in these patients, requires observation for any unexplained increase in their jaundice or for right upper quadrant symptoms. Cholecystectomy may be necessary at young ages. The avoidance of infections and their prompt treatment when present should reduce the incidence of aplastic crises.

References

1. Jandl JH: *Blood—Textbook of Hematology*. Boston, Little, Brown, 1987.
2. Petz LD: Drug-induced immune hemolysis. *N Engl J Med* 313:510, 1985.
3. Engelfriet CP, Overbeeke MAM, von dem Borne AE G Kr: Autoimmune hemolytic anemia. *Semin Hematol* 29:3, 1992.
4. Collins PW, Newland AC: Treatment modalities of autoimmune blood disorders. *Semin Hematol* 29:64, 1992.
5. Schreiber AD: Paraxysmal nocturnal hemoglobinuria revisited. *N Engl J Med* 309:723, 1983.
6. Sholar PW, Bell, WR: Thrombolytic therapy for inferior vena cava thrombosis in paroxysmal nocturnal hemoglobinuria. *Ann Intern Med* 103:539, 1985.
7. Antin JH, Ginsburg D, Smith RR, et al: Bone marrow transplantation for paroxysmal nocturnal hemoglobinuria: Eradication of the PNH clone and documentation of complete lymphohematopoietic engraftment. *Blood* 66:1247, 1985.
8. Kazazian HH, Boehm CD: Molecular basis and prenatal diagnosis of beta thalassemia. *Blood* 72:1107, 1988.
9. Johnson CS: Sickle cell anemia. *JAMA* 254:1958, 1985.
10. Kark JA, Posey DM, Schumacher HR, et al: Sickle-cell trait as a risk factor for sudden death in physical training. *N Engl J Med* 317:781, 1987.
11. Platt OS: Is there treatment for sickle cell anemia? *N Engl J Med* 319:1479, 1988.
12. Vichinsky EP: Comprehensive care in sickle cell disease: Its impact on morbidity and mortality. *Semin Hematol* 28:220, 1991.
13. Wayne AS, Kevy SV, Nathan DG: Transfusion management of sickle cell disease. *Blood* 81:1109, 1993.
14. Perrine SP, Ginder GD, Faller DW, et al: A short-term trial of butyrate to stimulate fetal-globin-gene expression in the B globin disorders. *N Engl J Med* 328:81, 1993.
15. Rodgers GP, Dover GJ, Uyesake N, et al: Augmentation by erythropoietin of the fetal-hemoglobin response to hydroxyurea in sickle cell disease. *N Engl J Med* 328:73, 1993
16. Nienhuis AW, et al: Thalassemia major: Molecular and clinical aspects. *Ann Intern Med* 91:883, 1979.
17. Fosburg MT, Nathan DG: Treatment of Cooley's anemia. *Blood* 76:435, 1990.
18. Weatherall D: Bone marrow transplantation for thalassemia and other inherited disorders of hemoglobin. *Blood* 80:1379, 1992.
19. Agre P, Asimos A, Casello JF, et al: Inheritance pattern and clinical response to splenectomy as a reflection of erythrocyte spectrin deficiency in hereditary spherocytosis. *N Engl J Med* 315:1579, 1986.
20. Beutler E: Glucose-6-phosphate dehydrogenase: New perspectives. *Blood* 73:1397, 1989.

124. Transfusion Therapy: Blood Components and Transfusion Complications

Richard S. Eisenstaedt

Blood components are often required in the care of critically ill patients, and, when used appropriately, may provide life-saving therapy without suitable alternatives. On occasion, components may be transfused without clear insight as to their expected value, in particular, whether those benefits exceed the potential risks that might be anticipated. In this chapter, the general indications for cellular and plasma components are reviewed, and the complications, both immediate and delayed, that arise from transfusion are discussed.

Blood Component Therapy

RED BLOOD CELLS. Most red cell transfusions are provided as citrate anticoagulated packed red blood cells (pRBC). Whole blood at donation is processed to remove platelets and plasma and then stored at 4°C as pRBC. During the period of storage, predictable changes occur (Table 124-1), including a leakage of intracellular potassium into the plasma space and depletion of intracellular 2-3 diphosphoglyceric acid (2-3 DPG). Hemoglobin displays increased oxygen affinity in the presence of lowered 2-3 DPG levels, although the clinical consequences of transfusing red cells that, in theory, may be less efficient in tissue oxygen delivery are not well documented [1]. Stored pRBC units have elevated plasma ammonia levels, elevated pCO_2, lowered pH, and increased amounts of microaggregate debris [2]. Platelet function deteriorates, and the clotting activity of the labile factors V and VIII falls.

The obvious indication for pRBC transfusion is inadequate oxygen-carrying capacity in patients who are bleeding acutely or chronically anemic. The exact level of anemia that warrants transfusion cannot be generalized. It is heavily dependent on additional considerations, such as (1) how rapidly the patient's anemia has evolved; (2) whether the patient has additional medical problems, especially preexisting myocardial or cerebral disorders that might make these organs especially vulnerable

to reduced oxygen delivery; and (3) whether the source of bleeding for patients with acute blood loss is identified and under control.

In making transfusion decisions physicians should focus not only on the reduction in blood oxygen content represented by the decreased hemoglobin concentration or hematocrit, but also on adaptive responses to anemia that may offset adverse sequelae. Such adaptations, including intravascular volume expansion and increased cardiac output, lowered blood viscosity, and decreased hemoglobin oxygen affinity, may provide adequate oxygen delivery to vital organs even in the face of decreased blood oxygen content and temper the need to augment such oxygen content through transfusion [3].

A recent Consensus Development Conference sponsored by the National Institutes of Health concluded that preoperative patients could often tolerate hemoglobin levels in the 7 to 8 gm per deciliter range without adverse sequelae, and that the traditional reliance on a hemoglobin of less than 10 gm per deciliter to trigger transfusion intervention was, for many, unnecessary [4]. Guidelines from this consensus report referred to stable operative patients and, clearly, may be inadequate to address the needs of critically ill patients in the intensive care setting, whose multisystem disease may impair their ability to adapt to and increase the risks of anemia.

A rational approach to red cell transfusion therapy avoids reliance on an arbitrary hemoglobin number and instead focuses on signs and symptoms reflecting inadequate oxygen-carrying capacity. Such parameters may include standard symptoms and physical findings reflecting myocardial or cerebral ischemia or may rely on more objective data such as mixed venous PO_2, oxygen consumption, or oxygen extraction.

Red cells may also be transfused in the form of whole blood or modified whole blood, wherein platelets are removed but plasma components spared. Whole blood may be the preferential form of red cell transfusion in two circumstances: (1) for patients who require intravascular volume expansion, usually because of acute blood loss, as well as augmentation of oxygen-carrying capacity; (2) for patients who require plasma components, usually because of coagulation factor depletion, as well as red cell replacement. In the former instance, decisions about the type of red cell component to transfuse should be mindful of the fact that pRBC plus crystalloid or colloid solutions may be perfectly adequate therapy for most patients who are acutely bleeding. In the latter instance, benefits in limiting donor exposure by providing plasma and red cells as one component are weighed against the predictable loss of factor V and factor VIII activity that occurs during whole blood storage [5]. Whole blood is often processed immediately after donation as a valuable source of platelets and a unique source of a variety of plasma proteins. Maintaining an adequate inventory of such specialized components inevitably limits the availability of whole blood.

Leukocyte-depleted packed red cells, which may be pre-

Table 124-1. Storage Lesions of Banked pRBC

Lesion	Theoretical consequences
Decreased RBC 2–3 DPG	Increased O_2 affinity
	Decreased tissue oxygenation
RBC potassium leak	Hyperkalemia
Increased plasma ammonia	Encephalopathy
Increased pCO_2, decreased pH	?
Increased microaggregate debris	Pulmonary injury
Decreased platelets, factors V, VIII	Coagulopathy

pRBC = packed red blood cells; 2-3 DPG = 2-3 disphosphoglyceric acid.

pared at donation or, using smaller pore-sized filters (20 to 40 μ), during transfusion, are indicated for patients who have immunologic reactions with leukocyte antigens suspected as the cause.

The leukocytes that contaminate red cell components have also been implicated in the transmission of cytomegalovirus (CMV), human T cell lymphotropic virus (HTLV) I and II, and other infections and will increase alloimmunization in patients receiving platelet transfusion. Newer filters may achieve even greater leukodepletion and have been recommended for immunosuppressed transfusion recipients such as premature neonates or recipients of allogeneic bone marrow transplantation [6].

The patient's own RBCs may be predonated some time in advance of anticipated need or may be salvaged perioperatively and, in either instance, used for autologous transfusion. By eliminating the threat of immune incompatibility as well as avoiding exposure to donor infections, autologous blood serves as the safest form of red cell transfusion [7].

Blood may also be donated by family and friends and designated for a specifically intended recipient. These designated donations lack the unique safety of autologous erythrocytes and may not be much different in overall benefit from homologous units donated anonymously by the community [8,9].

PLATELETS. Platelet transfusions are optimally indicated for patients who are thrombocytopenic, or, more rarely, who have qualitative defects of platelet function, who are bleeding as a direct consequence of the platelet defect, and for whom there are no more specific means of correcting the problem. Platelet therapy may also be appropriate for thrombocytopenic patients with an anticipated risk of bleeding by virtue of requiring surgery or an invasive procedure and may be given prophylactically to severely thrombocytopenic patients in the absence of bleeding or scheduled procedures. The platelet count that should prompt transfusion support is difficult to state in exact terms. In otherwise healthy individuals, platelet counts can fall to the 50,000 per microliter range before tests of platelet function, such as the bleeding time, become abnormal. Platelet transfusions have, therefore, been recommended for operative or otherwise bleeding patients when their platelet count falls to that range [10]. Delicate procedures involving the eye or central nervous system (CNS), in which even subtle increases in closed-space blood loss may cause catastrophic complications, often require more aggressive management to maintain platelet counts of 100,000 per microliter. In the absence of additional hemostatic threats, many patients will tolerate more severe thrombocytopenia, with platelet counts approximately 20,000 units per microliter, without clinically significant bleeding.

In addition to factors such as the magnitude of thrombocytopenia and the presence of anticipated bleeding, transfusion decisions should also be based on the mechanism, consumptive versus hypoproliferative, causing the lowered platelet count [11]. Platelet support is most ideally suited for circumstances in which inadequate marrow production is the principal cause of thrombocytopenia. In thrombocytopenic disorders such as immunologic thrombocytopenic purpura (ITP), the shortened survival of transfused platelets limits their therapeutic utility, although transfusions may be lifesaving in patients with ITP who are exsanguinating or bleeding into the CNS. Thrombocytopenia in critically ill patients is often related to sepsis, disseminated intravascular coagulation (DIC), or massive bleeding with both consumption and marrow suppression contributing. Platelet transfusions, their shortened survival notwithstanding, can be beneficial, along with simultaneous therapy specifically di-

rected toward eradicating or ameliorating those factors contributing to excessive platelet destruction.

Platelet transfusions should be used with great caution in patients with thrombotic thrombocytopenic purpura, because rapid agglutination of transfused platelets in the central nervous system and kidneys has led to acute renal failure and sudden death [12].

Decisions about platelet support should consider qualitative function as well as absolute numbers. Patients with hereditary defects of platelet function may require transfusion despite a perfectly normal platelet count. Acquired platelet function defects are far more common. Associated illness, such as liver disease or uremia, and a variety of drugs, including antiinflammatory agents and antibiotics, impair platelet function [13]. These acquired qualitative defects, encountered often in the critical care setting, contribute to the bleeding risk of thrombocytopenia when either defect alone might be adequately tolerated. Although knowledge of qualitative platelet injury might lower the threshold for platelet transfusion, the intensivist must also consider whether these newly transfused platelets will function adequately if the underlying cause of platelet function impairment has not been remedied.

Platelets are provided for transfusion in two forms: (1) separated from individual units of whole blood at the time of donation and pooled, from six to eight different donor units, to provide sufficient numbers of platelets and (2) harvested, using automated cell separators, from a single donor. Traditionally, most platelet transfusions have been provided as random pooled products, while the need for expensive hardware, dedicated technicians, and motivated donors limited the availability of single-donor products, often to alloimmunized recipients.

Although such alloimmunized recipients remain legitimate candidates for histocompatible single-donor products, one could argue that any patient would benefit by receiving a blood product from one donor versus six to eight, thus reducing the risk of transfusion-transmitted infections. Additional data suggest that patients with an anticipated long-term need for platelet support are less likely to become alloimmunized if antigen exposure is limited at the onset through single-donor platelet products [14].

The inability to meet the demand for platelet transfusions exclusively with single-donor products has created a logistical and ethical dilemma. In some regions, single-donor products are scarce and are limited exclusively for alloimmunized recipients who have become refractory to random pooled platelets. In other areas, blood procurement centers may harvest single-donor apheresis products in excess of the demand by alloimmunized recipients. There is no agreed-on method for rationing the excess. Some experts believe they should be used for patients, primarily with aplastic anemia or leukemia, who will need large numbers of platelets over long periods, as a means of decreasing or delaying alloimmunization. Others argue that patients with acute, transient needs for platelet support will benefit proportionately more from the reduced donor virus exposure that apheresis platelets offer.

A single unit of platelets raises the platelet count of a healthy recipient approximately 10,000 per microliter, and each single-donor apheresis product contains the equivalent of approximately 6 units of pooled platelet concentrate [10]. Although these figures offer a general framework for calculating the amount of platelet transfusion support required, it is understood that platelet transfusions are rarely given to healthy individuals but rather to patients who often have reasons for suboptimal response to therapy. Fever, sepsis, DIC, hypersplenism, and hemorrhage all shorten platelet survival [15]. Determining a posttransfusion platelet count, usually within 1 hour of the transfusion and 12 to 24 hours later, is essential to assess the adequacy of transfusion intervention.

GRANULOCYTES. Granulocyte transfusion would be logically indicated for neutropenic patients with infection. Problems harvesting an adequate number of properly functioning granulocytes, uncertainty regarding immunologic factors predicting granulocyte survival, and a high incidence of toxic reactions have dampened the initial enthusiasm toward this treatment. Although select patients with granulocytopenic infections may still benefit from a course of leukocyte transfusions, clinical trials demonstrate that most of these patients can be adequately supported with antimicrobials until the marrow recovers [16].

FRESH FROZEN PLASMA. Fresh frozen plasma (FFP) provides clotting factor replacement for individuals with severe deficiency of a single coagulation protein for which there is no more concentrated replacement source, as is the case for factor XI. More often, FFP is used for patients with multiple clotting factor deficiencies usually associated with massive bleeding, liver disease, vitamin K deficiency, or DIC. FFP should never be used as a volume expander in the absence of coagulopathy because colloid solutions such as albumin are equally effective and much safer [17].

The degree of coagulopathy that warrants FFP therapy is unclear. The prothrombin time (PT) has been the most relied on indicator to gauge coagulopathy, with a PT greater than 1.5 times control an often-quoted standard for FFP replacement. Whether treatment should be initiated for less severe PT abnormalities, or, conversely, whether FFP should be withheld unless the PT is more dramatically prolonged, remains unknown. Additional uncertainty in the use of FFP stems from the fact that the PT measures the interrelated activities of a number of coagulation factors, with a variety of patterns of factor deficiency yielding potentially identical PT values. Whether bleeding risk and, thus, FFP need is more related to the specific pattern of clotting factor deficiency or to the bottom-line PT prolongation is not known.

Most audits of FFP use show consistent patterns of overuse but, paradoxically, suggest that volumes transfused are often inadequate in situations in which need is documented. Four to 6 units of FFP are often needed per therapeutic intervention, considering that each unit contains less than one-tenth of the clotting factor activity found in a normal individual [5].

Decisions to transfuse FFP for patients with coagulopathy are clearly influenced by the presence of active bleeding or the threat of bleeding after a planned invasive procedure. Patients whose coagulopathy is not secondary to severe factor V or factor VIII depletion and who require erythrocytes as well as plasma replacement may be optimally treated with 1 unit of whole blood rather than pRBC and FFP from two different donors. Vitamin K replacement, rather than FFP, is indicated for patients with coagulopathy secondary to vitamin K deficiency unless the coagulopathy is life threatening.

Plasmapheresis at times requiring FFP replacement is used to treat a diverse group of disorders, including thrombotic thrombocytopenic purpura, hyperviscosity syndrome, myasthenia gravis, rapidly progressive glomerulonephritis, and a variety of rheumatic and neuromuscular diseases [18,19]. In critically ill patients, complications may arise from shifts in intravascular volume. Citrate reactions during rapid reinfusion of blood are not uncommon, and complications related to venous access or arising from rapid changes in drug levels may be encountered.

CRYOPRECIPITATE. Cryoprecipitate contains concentrated amounts of factor VIII, von Willebrand factor, and fibrinogen. Although it may be used to treat patients with hemophilia A and von Willebrand's disease, desmopressin [20], along with newer methods of producing factor VIII concentrate [21], offers safer alternatives. Hypofibrinogenemia (fibrinogen less than 100 mg per deciliter) secondary to DIC, especially in association with obstetrical complications, may require therapy with cryoprecipitate, 8 to 10 bags, often along with FFP.

ALBUMIN. Albumin is unique among blood components previously mentioned in that infectious contaminants are destroyed during manufacturing and purification, and immunologic reactions are rare. Albumin administration expands intravascular volume while simultaneously increasing plasma oncotic pressure. Despite theoretical benefits and a reassuringly low incidence of side effects, the clinical utility of albumin is debatable. Acute hypovolemia remains the most common indication for its use, although some critical care specialists argue that crystalloid solutions are equally effective and far less expensive [22]. Albumin is accepted as appropriate therapy for patients with extensive burns, but its efficacy in patients with hypoalbuminemia resulting from liver disease, nephrotic syndrome, or malnutrition is less well defined [23].

Complications of Transfusion

The complications associated with transfusions may be categorized by cause, i.e., infectious, immunologic, metabolic, or by time of occurrence, i.e., acute versus delayed (Table 124-2). To compare benefits and risks of transfusion properly, the clinician must be aware that most of the more ominous complications are totally inapparent at the time of transfusion and, indeed, may not become clinically manifest for years after the event. Similarly, demonstrable and clinically relevant acute reactions to blood products are not common. These facts explain the tendency to underestimate the magnitude of risk and a corresponding tendency toward overuse of blood products to the exclusion of safer alternatives. At the same time, transfusion risks should not be exaggerated and should never discourage transfusion therapy for critically ill patients in situations in which the expected benefits are quite tangible.

IMMUNOLOGIC COMPLICATIONS. Immunologic reactions may occur in response to antigens on red cells or on other cellular or plasma components and, with red cells, may be noted acutely or delayed for days or weeks after the transfusion.

Acute Hemolytic Transfusion Reactions. Acute hemolytic transfusion reactions (AHTR) are rare. When they occur, the cause is most likely careless clinical error leading to ABO mismatched transfusion and less often traced to recipient alloantibody, which, although difficult to detect, may still cause fulminant erythrocyte destruction [24].

The pathophysiologic consequences of AHTR are related to complement activation, initiation of an anaphylaxislike immune response, and the release of thromboplastic material from injured erythrocytes [25]. Vascular collapse, bronchospasm with impaired oxygenation, and bleeding manifestations of DIC are the major clinical manifestations. Gross hemoglobinuria and hemoglobinemia provide diagnostic clues, and a positive direct antiglobulin test may be noted. Because mortality is directly

Table 124-2. Acute Transfusion Reactions

Etiology	Signs	Diagnostic studies	Therapy
Acute hemolysis	Fever, back pain, hypotension, dyspnea, bleeding	Clerical review, urine, plasma hemoglobin, direct AGT	IV fluids Vasopressors, bronchodilators, O_2, corticosteroids, mannitol, furosemide, platelets, FFP, cryoprecipitates
Leukoagglutinin	Fever, dyspnea	Chest film Leukoagglutinating antibodies	Oxygen, ventilatory support
IgA anaphylaxis	Hypotension, dyspnea	Serum IgA level	Vasopressors, bronchodilators, oxygen
"Non-RBC" immune	Fever, urticaria, other skin rash	Rule out other etiologies	Acetaminophen, diphenhydramine
Bacterial contamination	Fever, septic shock	Blood cultures from patient and unit	Antibiotics
Volume overload	Dyspnea	Chest film	Diuretics

AGT = antiglobulin test; FFP = fresh frozen plasma.

related to the volume of incompatible blood administered [26], the transfusion should be stopped immediately if early signs of AHTR such as fever, backache, or flushing are noted while the cause is investigated. Therapy is largely supportive, with vasopressors, bronchodilators, and corticosteroids used for circulatory or respiratory distress. Renal injury in AHTR is probably more related to hypoperfusion and DIC-related cortical necrosis than to hemoglobin toxicity. Restoration of renal perfusion is the major goal. Furosemide or mannitol may be beneficial, along with adequate attention to maintaining intravascular volume. Platelet or clotting factor replacement may be required if consumptive coagulopathy is severe; heparin therapy has not been shown to be beneficial [27].

Delayed Hemolytic Transfusion Reactions. Delayed hemolytic transfusion reactions (DHTR) occur approximately once in several thousand transfusions [28]. Clinical signs, which are usually noted 1 to 3 weeks posttransfusion, include fever and findings related to hemolytic anemia [29]. The more severe sequelae of AHTR, including hypotension and renal failure, are rare. The diagnosis is easily overlooked in critically ill patients because the fever and anemia are incorrectly attributed to infection and bleeding. Classical serologic findings include a newly developing positive indirect antiglobulin test (AGT) and a weak, "mixed-field," positive direct AGT, although variations in the amount of alloantibody may lead to false negatives. Specific therapy, other than additional compatible red cell transfusion, is usually not needed.

Reactions to Leukocyte Antigens. Typical reactions to leukocyte antigens are clinically innocuous, with self-limited fever and urticaria, but these symptoms may be uncomfortable to the patient and interrupt transfusion therapy while more serious causes are excluded. They can be prevented by using a smaller pore-sized filter or by transfusing leukocyte-depleted red blood cells.

Patients may also develop far more alarming reactions characterized by fever, dyspnea, and hypotension, with chest radiographs showing infiltrates consistent with noncardiac pulmonary edema, the illness evolving as an acute respiratory distress syndrome (ARDS). Patients or donor units have been found to have leukoagglutinating antibodies [30]. Mechanical ventilation may be required, although respiratory function improves within 2 to 4 days in most instances. A small number of individuals with congenital IgA deficiency develop anaphylaxis after exposure to IgA in the plasma of donor units [31]. These patients should receive washed erythrocytes or red cells from IgA-deficient donors.

Graft-Versus-Host Disease. Graft-versus-host disease (GVHD), long recognized as a complication of bone marrow transplantation, has been increasingly noted after routine peripheral blood transfusion, especially in immunocompromised recipients such as premature newborn babies [32]. This problem has also been seen in recipients with normal immunity, such as those undergoing coronary bypass surgery after transfusion of blood recently donated by relatives [33]. The syndrome of GVHD includes dermatitis, hepatitis, gastroenteritis, and pancytopenia. Infectious complications are common and often lethal. Irradiation of the blood will prevent this complication.

Transfusion-Induced Immunosuppression. Transfusion-induced immunosuppression is suggested by a variety of in vitro tests, though the clinical consequences of such immunosuppression are arguable. Increased perioperative infection in trauma victims and decreased disease-free survival after curative colon cancer surgery have both been attributed, in part, to blood transfusion independent of other clinical variables [34].

INFECTIOUS COMPLICATIONS. The transmission of viruses carried by asymptomatic donors constitutes the major risk of blood transfusions.

Posttransfusion Hepatitis. Hepatitis C virus is the most common cause of posttransfusion hepatitis (PTH) and accounts for approximately 85 percent of cases previously called "non-A, non-B" hepatitis [35]. A small number of cases of PTH from hepatitis B continue to occur, despite rejection of all donors with hepatitis B surface antigen, and a small number of cases are caused by a hepatitis virus of unknown origin or by CMV or Epstein-Barr virus. Donor screening for hepatitis C antibody is the most recently implemented test to improve transfusion safety and, along with other measures, has lowered the overall risk of PTH to less than 1 percent of transfused patients [36].

Acute symptoms from PTH may be noted 1 to 3 months posttransfusion. They are characteristically mild and easily mistaken for a nondescript viral syndrome. Jaundice is unusual, and severe illness from overwhelming hepatic necrosis even less common. Indeed, unless one carefully screens transfusion recipients using serial blood tests of liver function, most cases will be missed, thus explaining the tendency of many physicians to underestimate this complication.

Although few transfusion recipients die of acute PTH, as many as one-half fail to recover entirely, going on to develop chronic liver disease [37]. The prognosis of chronic PTH is not known with certainty, but liver biopsy shows disturbing changes, such as chronic aggressive hepatitis with bridging necrosis or cirrhosis, in a significant percentage of patients [38]. More clear-cut delineation of the natural history of PTH, including therapy to improve the prognosis, promises to dramatically improve our understanding of this problem. Nonetheless, a complication affecting 1 percent of all transfusion recipients, that fails to resolve in half those affected, that may ultimately lead to cirrhosis with its attendant morbidity and mortality must be taken quite seriously. The long-term nature of the illness makes PTH an even more compelling risk when transfusing young patients or patients with reasonable life expectancy.

Human Immunodeficiency Virus. Human immunodeficiency virus (HIV) is efficiently transmitted by blood transfusion. An infected donor transmits virus to more than 90 percent of blood recipients, with both cellular and plasma components implicated [39]. The magnitude of the risk of transfusion-transmitted HIV (TT-HIV) infection has been lowered by rejecting from donation all individuals with behavioral risk for HIV exposure and by testing all donors for antibody to HIV (HIV-Ab), but neither mechanism has proved foolproof. Approximately 2 in 10,000 donors are found to be positive for HIV-Ab [40]. Curiously, half of these individuals report behavioral risk that should have prevented donation in the first place [41]. The enzyme-linked immunoassay (ELISA) for HIV-Ab has proved enormously useful as a screening test. However, donors who are recently infected may have HIV-viremia and transmit the virus to their blood recipients during the 4- to 12-week latent period before they produce detectable antibody [42].

Recognizing the inherent fallibility of the ELISA screening test for HIV, assessing its sensitivity at 95 to 99 percent, and using realistic estimates of the prevalence of virus among current blood donors, one can predict the current risk of TT-HIV at between 1:40,000 and 1:150,000 per unit of blood [43,44]. This risk may be viewed with reassurance by health care workers but still seems to conjure up fear out of proportion to its statistical likelihood among patients needing transfusion.

The prognosis of TT-HIV is analogous to that seen when HIV is transmitted by other routes. Exposed recipients may have a self-limited acute HIV illness but then become asymptomatic, with 5 to 10 percent per year converting from inapparent infection to reactivation of the virus and eventual immune destruction [45]. Premature newborn babies have a more accelerated illness with earlier progression to acquired immune deficiency syndrome (AIDS). New cases of TT-AIDS continue to occur both from individuals infected before screening was instituted in early 1985 and from recipients who continue to be exposed to HIV from donors falsely testing negative. Recipients exposed to TT-HIV can themselves transmit the virus to their sexual partners.

Whenever a blood donor is found to be HIV-Ab positive, prior blood recipients are traced, informed of the possibility that the blood they received could have been infected, and counseled about the benefits and risk of undergoing testing to determine exposure. Some individuals recommend that all patients who have received blood be informed of conceivable HIV exposure, whether or not an infected donor has been linked to their transfusion products. The magnitude of risk for any blood recipient is related to the time of transfusion (greatest risk being early 1985 before initiating routine donor HIV-Ab screening), to the location of donated blood (HIV prevalence

in the community related to HIV among donors), and to the number of donor exposures [46].

HTLV I and II. HTLV I and II are other retroviruses that may be transmitted by blood transfusion, although plasma components, such as FFP, cryoprecipitate, or factor VIII concentrate, are much less likely to be contaminated [47]. Individuals infected with HTLV-1 have an increased risk for T cell leukemia and lymphoma as well as for degenerative neurologic disease, all occurring years or decades after virus exposure. The natural history of HTLV-II, prevalent among intravenous drug users in the United States, is less understood.

A recent syndrome of CD4+ lymphocytopenia and immunodeficiency has been described in a small number of patients who are not infected with HIV. Although the cause and transmission of this syndrome are unknown, approximately 15 percent of cases had reported prior blood transfusion [48].

Cytomegalovirus. Cytomegalovirus (CMV) may be transmitted by cellular blood components, but it causes in most transfusion recipients an innocuous or inapparent illness. More serious problems from transfusion-CMV that may occur in immunosuppressed individuals, such as neonates or organ transplant recipients, can be avoided by using blood from CMV antibody–negative donors who have never been exposed to the virus [49].

Bacterial Infections. Bacterial infections may be transmitted by transfusion, usually from contamination of the unit during phlebotomy and storage. Platelets, which are stored at room temperature, offer more opportunity for bacterial growth than would be expected in refrigerated or frozen units [50]. Investigation of acute transfusion reactions should include blood cultures from the patient and cultures of the unit being transfused. Organisms contaminating blood components may be unusual; their growth in culture should not be dismissed as clinically irrelevant [51].

Other infectious agents that may persist in an individual's blood without causing symptoms overt enough to defer donation, such as might be seen with malaria, babesiosis, or *Yersinia enterocolitica* infection.

OTHER COMPLICATIONS

Volume Overload. Volume overload may be the most common metabolic complication of transfusion. Patients with chronic anemia often develop intravascular volume expansion as a physiologic adaptation to decreased oxygen-carrying capacity and are at particular risk, but even acutely bleeding patients may develop congestive problems if fluid management is imprecise. Underlying cardiac disease may contribute to the problem. Signs and symptoms are analogous to those seen in congestive heart failure. Acute infections or immunologic reactions to transfusion need to be considered in the differential diagnosis.

MASSIVE TRANSFUSION. Patients who are massively bleeding and require large amounts of blood are vulnerable to five additional complications associated with transfusion (Table 124-3) [52].

Hypocalcemia. Hypocalcemia occurs when citrate, which keeps banked blood anticoagulated, is administered in such large amounts that its metabolism is delayed and in vivo chelation occurs. Patients at risk often have liver disease that further impairs citrate detoxification. Although symptomatic hypocal-

Table 124-3. Complications Associated with Massive Transfusion

Hypocalcemia
Hyperkalemia
Coagulopathy
Respiratory distress
Hypothermia

cemia is a legitimate threat for transfused neonates, its incidence in adults has been overemphasized. The routine administration of additional calcium to asymptomatic adults who have received in excess of an arbitrarily defined number of units of blood in a 24-hour interval is usually not necessary.

Hyperkalemia. Hyperkalemia has also been associated with massive transfusion, invariably in the setting of renal failure and metabolic acidosis, which, independently, could cause this electrolyte disturbance. The role of transfusion in the pathogenesis of this problem is unclear. Plasma potassium concentrations in refrigerated blood are elevated, but these erythrocytes are able to reaccumulate leaked potassium as they warm to in vivo temperatures. The metabolic alkalosis that accompanies citrate metabolism may, in fact, facilitate hypokalemia.

Hypothermia. Hypothermia, with deleterious effects on cardiac function, may occur when large volumes of blood refrigerated at 4°C are transfused without equilibration to room temperature.

Acute Respiratory Distress Syndrome. Acute respiratory distress syndrome (ARDS), seen in the setting of massive bleeding, had been linked to transfused microaggregates occluding the pulmonary circulation. The pathogenesis is now believed to be related more to tissue trauma, hypotension, and other metabolic problems seen in critically ill patients, independent of their transfusion support, although the possibility that the blood products create additional injury cannot be excluded.

Coagulopathy. Coagulopathy frequently occurs in heavily bleeding patients. Again, this problem is not necessarily a complication of transfusion, but rather a result of the underlying injury causing platelet and clotting factor consumption that exceeds the patient's capacity to compensate. Replacement of lost erythrocytes alone eventually leads to recognizable deficiencies. The severity of coagulopathy from massive blood loss is hard to predict and should not be anticipated with a formula approach that mandates routine administration of FFP or platelets per arbitrary number of red cell units transfused. Anticipation of this complication should, instead, warrant careful monitoring of hemostasis with platelet counts, prothrombin time, and partial thromboplastin time determinations, with subsequent component support predicated on these values.

Hemochromatosis. Patients with chronic transfusion requirements from congenital hemolysis, thalassemia, or acquired aplastic anemia are at risk for transfusion-induced hemochromatosis. Transfusion of more than 100 units of red cells provides an additional 20 gm of iron that cannot be effectively metabolized or excreted and may be sufficient to cause parenchymal injury to the myocardium, liver, pancreas, and other organs. Phlebotomy, the therapy of choice for individuals with idiopathic hemochromatosis, is clearly contraindicated in patients who are transfusion dependent. Chelation therapy with deferoxamine is an acceptable alternative and should be insti-

tuted in patients at risk before symptoms of iron overload are manifest [53].

References

1. Collins JA: Massive blood transfusion. *Clin Haematol* 5:216, 1976.
2. Sohmer PR: Transfusion therapy in surgery, in Petz LD, Swisher SN (eds): *Clinical Practice of Transfusion Medicine.* New York, Churchill-Livingstone, 1989.
3. Welch HG, Meehan KR, Goodnough LT: Prudent strategies for elective red blood cell transfusion. *Ann Intern Med* 116:393, 1992.
4. Perioperative red blood cell transfusion. *JAMA* 260:2700, 1988.
5. Braunstein AH, Oberman HA: Transfusion of plasma components. *Transfusion* 24:281, 1984.
6. Rawal BD, David RE, Busch MP, et al: Dual reduction in the immunologic and infectious complication of transfusion by filtration/removal of leukocytes from donor blood soon after collection. *Trans Med Rev* 4 (suppl):36, 1990.
7. American Medical Association Council on Scientific Affairs: Autologous Blood Transfusion. *JAMA* 256:2378, 1986.
8. Page PL: Directed blood donations: Con. *Transfusion* 29:65, 1989.
9. Goldfinger D: Directed blood donations: Pro. *Transfusion* 26:70, 1989.
10. Eisenstaedt RS: Blood component therapy in platelet disorders, in Brain MD, Carbone PP (eds): *Current Therapy in Hematology-Oncology.* Toronto, BC Decker, 1988.
11. Tomasulo PA, Lenes BA: Platelet transfusion therapy, in Menitove JE, McCarthy LJ (eds): *Hemostatic Disorders and the Blood Bank.* Arlington, VA. American Association of Blood Banks, 1984.
12. Eisenstaedt RS, Colman RW, Marder VJ: Thrombotic thrombocytopenic purpura, in Colman RW, Hirsh J, Marder VJ, Salzman EW (eds): *Hemostasis and Thrombosis,* 2nd ed. Philadelphia, JB Lippincott, 1987.
13. Rao AK, Walsh PN: Acquired qualitative platelet disorders. *Clin Haematol* 12:201, 1983.
14. Sintnicolaas K, Vriesendorp HM, Sizoo W, et al: Delayed alloimmunization by random single donor platelet transfusion. *Lancet* 1:750, 1981.
15. Platelet transfusions. Primary hemostatic failure, in Beal, RW, Isbister JP (eds): *Blood Component Therapy in Clinical Practice.* Victoria, Australia, Blackwell Scientific Publications, 1985.
16. Clift RA, Buckner CD: Granulocyte transfusions. *Am J Med* 76:631, 1984.
17. Fresh Frozen Plasma: Indications and risks. Consensus Conference, NIH. *JAMA* 253:551, 1985.
18. Shumack KH, Rock GA: Therapeutic plasma exchange. *N Engl J Med* 310:762, 1984.
19. Consensus Conference: The utility of therapeutic plasmapheresis for neurological disorders. *JAMA* 256:1333, 1986.
20. Mannucci PM: Desmopressin: A nontransfusional form of treatment for congenital and acquired bleeding disorders. *Blood* 72:1449, 1988.
21. Mannucci PM, Colombo M: Virucidal treatment of clotting factor concentrates. *Lancet* 2:782, 1988.
22. Rackow EC, Falk JL, Fein IA, et al: Fluid resuscitation in circulatory shock: A comparison of the cardiorespiratory effects of albumin, hetastarch, and saline solutions in patients with hypovolemic and septic shock. *Crit Care Med* 11:839, 1983.
23. Alexander MR, Alexander B, Mustion AL, et al: Therapeutic use of albumin. *JAMA* 247:831, 1982.
24. Honig CL, Bove JR: Transfusion-associated fatalities: Review of bureau of biologics reports, 1976-1978. *Transfusion* 20:653, 1980.
25. Greenwalt T: Pathogenesis and management of hemolytic transfusion reactions. *Semin Hematol* 18:84, 1981.
26. Schmidt PJ: The mortality from incompatible transfusion, in Sandler SG, Nussbacher J, Schanfield MS (eds): *Immunobiology of the Erythrocyte.* New York, Alan R Liss, 1980.
27. Popovsky MA: Immune mediated transfusion reactions, in Nance SJ (ed): *Immune Destruction of Red Blood Cells.* Arlington, VA, American Association of Blood Banks, 1989.
28. Moore SB, Taswell HF, Pineda AA: Delayed hemolytic transfusion

reactions: Evidence of the need for an improved pre-transfusion compatibility test. *Am J Clin Pathol* 74:94, 1980.

29. Pineda AA, Taswell HF, Brzica SM Jr: Delayed hemolytic transfusion reaction: An immunological hazard of blood transfusion. *Transfusion* 18:1, 1978.

30. Popovsky MA, Moore SB: Diagnostic and pathogenetic considerations in transfusion-related acute lung injury. *Transfusion* 25:573, 1985.

31. Miller WV, Holland PV, Sugarbaker E, et al: Anaphylactic reaction to IgA, a difficult transfusion problem. *Am J Clin Pathol* 54:618, 1970.

32. Brubacker DB: Transfusion-associated graft versus host disease. *Hum Pathol* 17:1085, 1986.

33. Thaler M, Shamiss A, Orgard S, et al: The role of blood from HLA-homozygous donors in fatal transfusion-associated graft versus host disease after open-heart surgery. *N Engl J Med* 321:25, 1989.

34. Blumberg N, Triulzi DJ, Heal JM: Transfusion-induced immunomodulation and its clinical consequences. *Trans Med Rev* 4 (Suppl):24, 1990.

35. Aach RD, Stevens CE, Hollinger FB, et al: Hepatitis C virus infection in post transfusion hepatitis: An analysis with first and second generation assays. *N Engl J Med* 325:1325, 1991.

36. Donahue JG, Munoz A, Ness PA, et al: The declining risk of post-transfusion hepatitis C virus infection. *N Engl J Med* 327:369, 1992.

37. Dienstag JL: Non-A, non-B hepatitis: I. Recognition, epidemiology, and clinical features. *Gastroenterology* 85:439, 1983.

38. Lashner BA, Jonas KB, Tang HS, et al: Chronic hepatitis: Disease factors at diagnosis predictive of mortality. *Am J Med* 85:609, 1988.

39. Friedland GH, Klein RS: Transmission of human immunodeficiency virus. *N Engl J Med* 317:1125, 1987.

40. Cumming PD, Wallace EL, Schorr JB, et al: Exposure of patients to human immunodeficiency virus. *N Engl J Med* 321:941, 1989.

41. Ward JW, Kleinman SH, Douglas DK, et al: Epidemiologic characteristics of blood donors with antibody to human immunodeficiency virus. *Transfusion* 28:298, 1988.

42. Raevsky CA, Cohn DL, Wolf FC, et al: Transfusion associated human T-lymphotrophic virus type III lymphadenopathy associated virus infection from a seronegative donor—Colorado. *MMWR* 35:389, 1986.

43. Ward JW, Holmberg SD, Allen JR, et al: Transmission of human immunodeficiency virus (HIV) by blood transfusions screened as negative for HIV antibody. *N Engl J Med* 318:473, 1988.

44. Cohen MD, Munoz A, Reitz BA, et al: Transmission of retrovirus by transfusion of screened blood in patients undergoing cardiac surgery. *N Engl J Med* 320:1172, 1989.

45. Ward JW, Bush JJ, Perkin HA, et al: The natural history of transfusion-associated infection with human immunodeficiency virus. *N Engl J Med* 321:947, 1989.

46. Peterman TA, Lui KJ, Lawrence DN, et al: Estimating the risks of transfusion-associated acquired immunodeficiency syndrome and human immunodeficiency virus infection. *Transfusion* 27:371, 1987.

47. Guidelines for counseling persons infected with human T-lymphotropic virus type I (HTLV-1) and Type II (HTLV-II). *Ann Intern Med* 118:448, 1983.

48. Busch MP, Holland PV: Idiopathic CD4+ T-lymphocytopenia (ICL) and the safety of blood transfusions: What do we know and what should we do. *Transfusion* 32:794, 1992.

49. Adler SP: Transfusion associated cytomegalovirus infection. *Rev Infect Dis* 5:977, 1983.

50. Heal JM, Singal S, Sardisco E, et al: Bacterial proliferation in platelet concentrates. *Transfusion* 26:388, 1986.

51. Scott J, Boulton FE, Govan JRW, et al: A fatal transfusion reaction associated with blood contaminated with Pseudomonas fluorescens. *Vox Sanguinis* 54:201, 1988.

52. Holland PV: Transfusion reactions and other adverse effects, in Petz LD, Swisher SN (eds): *Clinical Practice of Transfusion Medicine.* New York, Churchill Livingstone, 1989.

53. Proper RD, Cooper B, Rufo BR, et al: Continuous subcutaneous administration of deferoxamine in patients with iron overload. *N Engl J Med* 297:418, 1977.

125. Granulocytopenia

F. Marc Stewart and Doreen B. Brettler

With the increased utilization of stem cell or bone marrow transplantation as well as cytotoxic chemotherapeutic and immunosuppressive drugs, granulocytopenia and its associated complications are more frequently encountered in intensive care unit settings. The isolation and purification of hemopoietic growth factors that directly stimulate granulocyte replication, differentiation, and function have opened *potential* therapeutic avenues for patients who are deficient in granulocyte numbers or those who require augmented phagocytic action.

Definitions

The term *granulocytes* refers to neutrophils, eosinophils, and basophils. Although *granulocytopenia* should therefore refer to absolute decreases in the number of all three of these cellular elements, in reality the terms *granulocytopenia* and *neutropenia* (an absolute decrease in neutrophils alone) are often used interchangeably [1]. In this chapter, *neutropenia* and *granulocytopenia* are used interchangeably unless otherwise noted. *Agranulocytosis* refers to a profound decrease in granulocytes; this term is most often used when the cause is secondary to a drug.

Normal total white counts and granulocyte counts are highly variable within the population. In a series of 291 normal adults, total white counts ranged from 4300 to 10,000 cells per cubic millimeter using 95-percent confidence levels, with neutrophil counts ranging from 1800 to 7200 cells per cubic millimeter [2]. In another series of 109 male students, the mean neutrophil count was found to be 4300 cells per cubic millimeter, with a range of 1800 to 6700 [3]. Black males may normally have slightly reduced neutrophil counts with a mean of 3700 ± 1400 cells per cubic millimeter versus 4400 ± 1400 for age-matched white males [4]. The definition of neutropenia is therefore not standardized, but an absolute neutrophil count below 1500 to 2000 cells per cubic millimeter is an accepted range. With neutrophil counts below 1000 per cubic millimeter, the incidence of infection begins to increase and below 500 cells per cubic millimeter, the chance of developing infection is high [5].

Neutrophil Precursors and Kinetics

Stem cells have the capacity for long-term reconstitution of the hemopoietic system. The earliest cell, a pluripotential stem cell, is generally dormant in the cell cycle, but when stimulated gives rise to progenitors that are restricted in their differentiation potential to a single lineage. As stem cells proliferate and become committed to a particular cell lineage and function, they gradually lose their capacity for self-renewal. The decision of a stem cell to self-renew or differentiate may be random (or stochastic), and further steps in the differentiation pathway may be regulated further by local factor concentrations or by contact with accessory cells present in the marrow microenvironment [6].

Isolation and identification of the "true" pluripotential stem cell has eluded investigators despite some claims of success [7]. Because stem cells are thought to resemble small lymphocytes, it is impossible to identify them with standard morphologic criteria. Early stem cells have specific surface antigen and staining characteristics, which distinguishes them from more committed progenitor cells.

Previously, with the perfection of techniques of culturing bone marrow cells in methylcellulose or semisolid agar, stem cells could be measured indirectly by counting the number of colonies formed on the culture plate. Because mature cells in a marrow specimen, i.e., granulocytes, cannot proliferate, each "colony" of cells is theoretically generated by a single stem cell. In the murine system, which closely mirrors human hemopoiesis, an early stem cell such as the high proliferative potential colony-forming unit, or HPP-CFC, eventually gives rise to multilineage progeny in vitro. The presence of murine colony-forming cells in vitro correlates with the marrow's in vivo capacity to rapidly repopulate the lethally irradiated animals after marrow transplantation [8].

A more committed stem cell, a colony-forming unit in culture (CFU-C) that differentiates only into myeloid cells, has been identified. CFU-Cs are assayed by placing bone marrow cells in semisolid agar with a growth stimulus, such as granulocyte-macrophage colony stimulating factors (GM-CSF)[9], and by counting granulocyte colonies of 50 to 2000 cells after a period of 7 days. CFU-Cs have now been measured in various neutropenic states, such as aplastic anemia and preleukemia, and have been found to be decreased [10,11]. Various combinations of growth factors in vitro preferentially stimulate the growth of different progenitor cells and have led to a wide variety of standardized clonogenic assays capable of assessing various lineage-specific stem cells.

With the advent of gene cloning techniques and recombinant technology, isolation and purification of numerous growth hormones governing granulocyte-macrophage production have been achieved [6]. Their relationships to progenitor cells in the differentiation sequence are illustrated in Figure 125-1. The myeloid specific factors, which include granulocyte-macrophage colony stimulating factor (GM-CSF), granulocyte stimulating factor (G-CSF), and macrophage colony stimulating factor (M-CSF) [12], prevent apoptotic cell death [13]. G-CSF or GM-CSF act in the granulocyte pool, whereas M-CSF affects primarily the macrophage pool. IL-5 has been found to stimulate eosinophilic precursors and B lymphocytes. IL-6 stimulates B-cell maturation and megakaryopoiesis. Early cycle dormant progenitors include IL-3, IL-6, IL-11, IL-12, leukemia inhibitory factor (LIF), stem cell factor (SCF), and IL-4. G-CSF, GM-CSF, and IL-6 also serve as synergistic factors for primitive dormant progenitor cells [6].

Fig. 125-1. Hemopoiesis and bone marrow kinetics

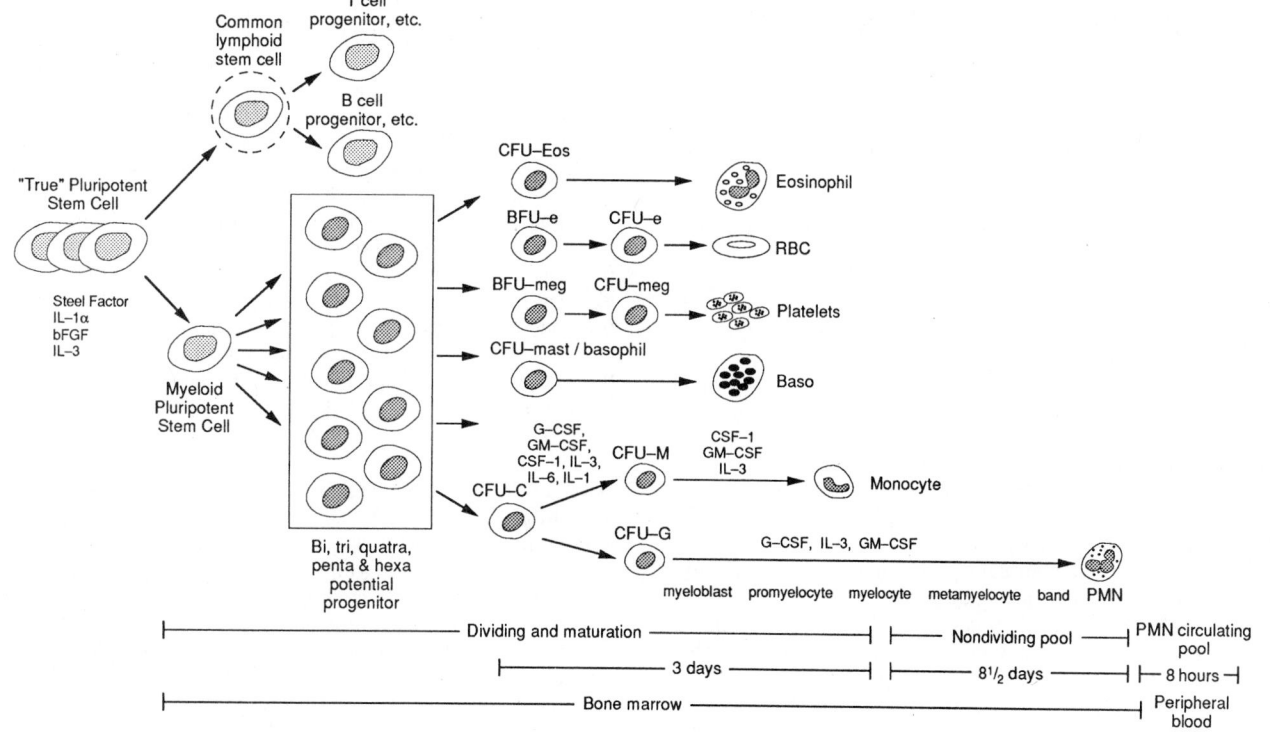

The granulocytes comprise a substantial amount of tissue. Although 60% are located in the marrow and 40% in other tissues, fewer than 1% of the total number of granulocytes are found in the blood [14]. Granulocytes are produced only in the marrow and move from there to the peripheral blood and into the tissues. The overall life span of the granulocyte is 10 to 14 days, including the time spent in the marrow of 6 to 9 days [15]. The committed stem cell pool (CFU-C) gives rise to the mitotic pool, which includes myeloblasts, promyelocytes, and myelocytes. The mitotic pool then gives rise to the nonmitotic pool, the metamyelocytes, the bands, and the polymorphonuclear cells (PMNs). In this pool there is no cell division, only maturation. Once mature cells are formed, they exit from the marrow and equilibrate between the circulating granulocyte pool and the marginal granulocyte pool, where they adhere to the postcapillary venules. Mature cells in the marginal pool are released into the circulation under conditions of stress, such as infection or hypoxia. The maturation scheme of the granulocyte is seen in Fig. 125-1.

The circulating granulocytes spend only 6 to 8 hours in the peripheral circulation and then migrate through endothelial cells to the tissues, where they survive another 2 to 4 days. The production rate of granulocytes is 1.6×10^9 cells/kg/day [15]. Because the terminal half-life ($t\frac{1}{2}$) of circulating granulocytes is very short, and current labeling techniques are problematic, routine measurements of white cell survival are not readily available [1].

Function of Granulocytes

The major function of the neutrophil is to protect the body against pyogenic infection. This function is accomplished through several mechanisms, beginning with movement of the neutrophil toward the site of infection or inflammation. This process of cell motility requires an adenosine triphosphate (ATP)-derived energy source and a functional intracellular contractile system composed of actin filaments that interact with myosin and other proteins to produce ameboid movement. Chemical signals from the environment stimulate and direct neutrophil movement or chemotaxis. After adhering to endothelial cells the neutrophil passes from the intravascular space through the vessel lumen and into the tissues to initiate phagocytosis. During phagocytosis the destruction of the organism is accomplished by metabolites of the respiratory burst and the myeloperoxidase system. The neutrophil recognizes and adheres to organisms that have undergone opsinization, or coating with specific plasma proteins such as IgG, C3b, and C3bi. The receptors for these proteins as well as chemotactic factors are found on the neutrophil surface membrane [16]. Once a neutrophil has adhered to an organism, cytoplasmic pseudopods surround it, and a portion of the neutrophil plasma membrane invaginates to encase the organism in a protected compartment termed a phagosome. Secondary granules and primary granules, which include enzymes such as lysozyme, collagenase, plasminogen activator, or myeloperoxidase, degranulate or release their contents into the phagosome and begin the process of lytic destruction of the microbe.

Phagocytosis causes membrane perturbation, which activates an oxidase enzyme that is located most probably in the plasma membrane. This enzyme then catalyzes the respiratory burst [16]. Oxygen accepts a single electron and is reduced to the superoxide anion O_2^- and then to hydrogen peroxide H_2O_2; both products are toxic to bacteria [16]. Singlet oxygen and hydroxyl radicals are also generated and may also participate in killing bacteria, although this has not been shown directly [17].

Perhaps more potent in bactericidal activity is the myeloperoxidase-halide system. Myeloperoxidase (MPO), which is present in azurophilic or primary granules, is released into phagosomes during degranulation. When this enzyme combines with hydrogen peroxide, it forms an enzyme-substrate complex that can generate a variety of compounds, including toxic halide oxidation products such as hypochlorous acid that can kill microorganisms [18].

Hemopoietic growth factors such as M-CSF, GM-CSF, or G-CSF have been shown to stimulate monocyte or neutrophil phagocytosis, antibody-dependent cell cytotoxicity, and superoxide generation. In contrast to G-CSF, GM-CSF inhibits neutrophil migration, perhaps accounting for some differences in their side effects when used therapeutically in vivo.

Patients with deficiencies of MPO are not troubled by major infections. Patients with chronic granulomatous disease (CGD), however, whose neutrophils cannot generate a respiratory burst, are subject to life-threatening, repeated infections, especially by catalase-producing organisms, such as *Staphylococcus aureus, Candida albicans,* and gram-negative bacteria [16]. Although a discussion of this and other qualitative neutrophil disorders is beyond the scope of this chapter, they should be considered in a patient who has a normal number of neutrophils but who has had repeated, overwhelming episodes of sepsis that began at an early age.

Differential Diagnosis

Granulocytopenia is usually associated with a deficiency of the total granulocyte pool (TGP). Occasionally the TGP is normal, and neutropenia is related to a shift of neutrophils out of the blood and into the tissues, e.g., in some cases of septicemia. The complex, severe clinical problems that occur in critically ill patients often confound the physician attempting to pinpoint a cause of neutropenia. In many patients multiple factors may contribute simultaneously to neutropenia. The most common causes in this setting include drugs such as antineoplastic agents, antibiotics, anticonvulsants, and antihistamines; sepsis or infection; alcohol; nutritional deficiencies (particularly folic acid); hemodialysis; and primary marrow disorders such as acute leukemia. The cause of neutropenia can most simply be divided into non–drug-induced and drug-induced neutropenia. In each category, the mechanism by which granulocytes are decreased may be one of (1) decreased production secondary to decreased marrow production or ineffective marrow production, (2) increased destruction secondary to immune or nonimmune etiologies, or (3) redistribution from the circulating to the marginal pool. A summary of the mechanisms of neutropenia is found in Table 125-1.

DRUG-INDUCED NEUTROPENIA. In the intensive care setting drugs are a frequent cause of neutropenia, and in any patient, a careful and detailed history of drug use is essential. The mechanisms of drug-induced neutropenia are varied and may be multiple for a single drug. Drugs such as cephalosporins have been shown to inhibit neutrophil production in some cases and in other cases may increase peripheral neutrophil destruction [19,20]. Because most critically ill patients receive multiple medications, the exact drug or mechanism producing neutropenia may be difficult to define.

Table 125-1. Mechanisms of Neutropenia

I. Drug-induced
  A. Decreased production
    1. Chemotherapy
    2. Alcohol
    3. Phenothiazines
    4. Radiation
  B. Increased destruction
    1. Penicillin
    2. Quinidine
    3. Procainamide
  C. Mechanism uncertain (many drugs)

II. Non–drug induced
  A. Decreased production
    1. Viral infections
    2. Replacement of marrow by tumor or leukemia
    3. Aplastic anemia
    4. Leukemia
    5. Human cyclic neutropenia
    6. Chronic benign neutropenia
    7. Congenital diseases (Kostmann's syndrome)
  B. Increased destruction
    1. Nonimmune mediated
      a Hypersplenism
      b. Renal dialysis
    2. Immune mediated
      a. Autoimmune neutropenia
      b. Felty's syndrome
      c. Systemic lupus erythematosus
      d. Paroxysmal nocturnal hemoglobinuria
    3. Ineffective granulopoiesis
      a. B_{12} deficiency
      b. Folate deficiency

Chemotherapeutic Agents. The cause of drug-induced neutropenia can be separated into decreased production and increased destruction. Chemotherapeutic drugs predictably will cause neutropenia in all persons who are given these drugs in high enough doses for a sufficient period [21]. Most chemotherapeutic agents interrupt deoxyribonucleic acid (DNA) synthesis (antimetabolites), block mitosis through disruption of the mitotic spindle (vinca alkaloids), or interfere with DNA *binding* (alkylating agents). Thus, it is the dividing pool, including the progenitor cells, that is affected. With most chemotherapeutic agents, the nadir of peripheral neutrophil counts occurs between 10 and 14 days after the onset of therapy. Earlier nadirs may occur when the marrow neutrophil reserves have been depleted from chronic illness, active infections, nutritional deficiency, or prior cytotoxic therapy. After treatment with aggressive multiagent chemotherapy regimens, absolute neutrophil counts often drop transiently to less than 500 to 1000 per cubic millimeter, and fever and infection may result in 5 to 40 percent of patients. Between day 21 and day 28, peripheral counts usually normalize and are heralded initially by a monocytosis and then perhaps by a rebound leukocytosis. In patients who undergo treatment for acute leukemia or patients who receive intensive therapy and bone marrow transplants, neutrophil counts fall precipitously over several days and must be monitored daily or twice daily. Neutropenia lasting from a week to several weeks is not uncommon. Fever indicative of infection occurs in almost every case.

A notable exception to the timetable outlined above for conventional chemotherapy is the granulocytopenia that is induced by *cis*-chloronitrosourea (CCNU and other stem cell toxic drugs, including melphalan, BCNU, and busulfan). Neutrophil counts reach their nadir at 30 to 36 days and may not recover until 6 weeks after administration. Inadvertent overdosages of these drugs may result in prolonged marrow aplasia and ultimately may be fatal.

When methotrexate clearance is prolonged, even low doses occasionally cause severe mucositis and neutropenia. After administration, diffusion of methotrexate from pleural effusions or ascitic fluid collections into the blood (the so-called "reservoir effect"), or underlying renal insufficiency may produce sustained, low levels of methotrexate and lead to toxicity. Leucovorin inhibits the cytotoxic effect of methotrexate [22].

Radiation in standard doses also can directly damage marrow stem cells when ports include marrow proliferative areas such as pelvis, skull, ribs, spine, and sternum. In general, radiation has a more permanent effect on marrow stem cell reserves than chemotherapy. Chronic exposure to low doses of radiation has no immediate adverse effect but may have delayed bone marrow effects. Even very small amounts of radiation targeted to painfully enlarged spleens seen in myeloproliferative disorders may produce profound myelosuppression, possibly because hemopoietic stem cells in these disorders circulate in high frequency through the spleen.

Alcohol. Alcohol in large doses can also directly suppress marrow precursor cells in culture and cause neutropenia. In neutropenia associated with chronic or acute alcoholism, other factors such as folate deficiency, congestive splenomegaly from cirrhosis, or other complicating medical problems may play a role.

Phenothiazines. There are a variety of drugs that will damage stem cell production that are idiosyncratically unrelated to dose or duration of the drug. A partial list is shown in Table 125-2. The term *agranulocytosis* refers to a syndrome of abrupt, profound neutropenia with nearly complete absence of circulating granulocytes. Fever and infection supervene and sepsis may be fatal. Drugs are a frequent cause. Phenothiazines, especially chlorpromazine, appear to cause an agranulocytosis that is dose related and serve as a model for idiosyncratic drug-induced suppression of granulopoiesis. It usually occurs in psychiatric patients who have been taking the drug for at least 2 to 15 weeks with a cumulative dose of 10 to 20 gm [23]. The drug inhibits both DNA and protein synthesis and thus is toxic to cycling progenitor cells [24].

In addition, cell culture studies have demonstrated the inhibition of CFU-C after the addition of phenothiazines. Agranulocytosis occurs in approximately 1 in 1300 patients treated, with granulocyte counts that are less than 500 cells per cubic millimeter. The syndrome is more common in females than in males (3:1), in whites, and in the elderly (70% patients >40 years of age) [23].

It is believed that a subset of patients are predisposed to the development of drug-induced agranulocytosis. The bone marrow of these patients is abnormal with an increased amount of precursor cells in the resting phases of G_0 and G_1. When exposed to phenothiazines, the limited amount of stem cells in cycle are destroyed, and because of their impaired proliferative capacity, granulocytopenia occurs. When agranulocytosis occurs, the drug must be stopped immediately. Recovery begins after the cessation of phenothiazine administration and should be complete within 2 weeks. Because of the severity of the neutropenia, however, the mortality rate secondary to sepsis is 30 to 40 percent, even with broad-spectrum antibiotics [24]. In 10 percent of patients on phenothiazines, a mild neutropenia occurs that will resolve spontaneously even if treatment is continued. Bone marrow studies show the persistence of granu-

Table 125-2. Drugs That Induce Neutropenia by Stem Cell Injury

1. Antibiotics
   a. Semisynthetic penicillins
   b. Penicillin
   c. Sulfonamides (Bactrim)
   d. Metronidazole
   e. Vancomycin
   f. INH
   g. Ciprofloxacin
   h. Beta-lactams
   i. Nitrofurantoin
   j. Metronidazole (Flagyl)
2. Antithyroid agents
   a. Propylthiouracil
   b. Methimazole
3. Cardiovascular agents
   a. Captopril
   b. Procainamide
   c. Quinidine
   d. Calcium channel blockers
4. Antiinflammatory agents
   a. Phenylbutazone
   b. Gold salts
   c. Nonsteroidal antiinflammatory agents
   d. Penicillamine
   e. Ibuprofen
5. Anticonvulsants
   a. Phenytoin (Dilantin)
   b. Carbamazepine (Tegretol)
6. Psychiatric drugs
   a. Phenothiazines
   b. Meprobamate
   c. Imipramine/desipramine
7. Gastrointestinal drugs
   a. Salicylazosulfapyridine (Azulfidine)
   b. Cimetidine
   c. Ranitidine
   d. Metoclopramide (Reglan)
8. Diuretics
   a. Chlorothiazide
   b. Hydrochlorothiazide
9. Antiviral agents
   a. Zidovudine
   b. Ganciclovir

locytic cells in contrast with their absence in granulocytosis. It appears that this syndrome and agranulocytosis are not related.

Other nonphenothiazine antipsychotic drugs such as clozapine, a tricyclic dibenzodiazepine, may cause agranulocytosis through an immune-mediated mechanism. Risk factors include increased age and female sex [25].

Antibiotics. Commonly used antibiotics that cause agranulocytosis or neutropenia include sulfonamides such as salicylazosulfapyridine (Azulfidine) [26] or trimethoprim-sulfamethoxazole [27], metronidazole (Flagyl), beta-lactams [19,20], vancomycin [28], isonicotinic acid hydrazide (INH), nitrofurantoin, levamisol, Augmentin, metronidazole, norfloxacin, oxacillin, methicillin, ampicillin, penicillin, ganciclovir, and ciprofloxacin. Bone marrow studies in patients with drug-induced agranulocytosis show a total lack of myeloid precursors or may show a predominance of myeloid cells that are in the early stage of differentiation. Any patient with drug-induced agranulocytosis must have the offending drug stopped immediately. Chloramphenicol classically causes aplastic anemia that is secondary to suppression of a pluripotent stem cell, but rare cases

of solitary neutropenia have been reported [29]. Neutropenia that rarely occurs with penicillin may be mediated by a drug-hapten mechanism and is usually seen when penicillin is administered in high doses.

Antiinflammatory/Analgesic Agents. Neutropenia caused by drugs can also occur secondary to peripheral destruction of mature neutrophils, which is often immune mediated. The classic description of this mechanism was with the analgesic aminopyrine, which caused precipitous episodes of agranulocytosis; it has subsequently been taken off the market [30]. Episodes occurred suddenly, after variable amounts of time on the drug. When 2 of the original 14 patients were rechallenged, an abrupt neutropenia was noted in approximately 12 hours. It has been thought that neutrophil lysis was caused by a drug-antibody immune complex, an "innocent bystander" type of reaction. Phenylbutazone has a chemical structure similar to aminopyrine. Other drugs such as ibuprofen and Tolmetin may cause neutropenia, but the mechanisms vary.

Gastrointestinal Agents. H_2 blockers such as cimetidine may cause neutropenia by receptor blockade. Ranitidine may act by a similar mechanism [31]. Sulfonamides such as salicylazosulfapyridine (Azulfidine) may cause neutropenia in patients with Crohn's disease [26]. Other drugs such as metoclopramide (Reglan) may suppress neutrophil production [32].

Anticonvulsants. Drugs such as diphenylhydantoin, carbamazepine [33], and trimethyloxazolidine may produce neutropenia after several weeks of use. Fever and a rash often herald the onset of neutropenia.

Cardiovascular Agents. Procainamide may cause peripheral destruction of neutrophils as well as agranulocytosis, and quinidine-induced neutropenia may be mediated in a similar manner [23]. Patients may present with acute fever and shock secondary to the lysis of cells. The bone marrow, in cases where there is peripheral destruction, will show the presence of the myeloid series as well as cells that are differentiating normally. White cell survival studies, which are carried out either by ^{51}Cr or DF ^{32}P labeling, will show a decreased half-life. However, survival studies are difficult to obtain routinely. Recently, captopril has been reported to cause neutropenia.

With each individual drug, the mechanism that causes neutropenia may be difficult to determine. A partial list of commonly used drugs is shown in Table 125-2; more detailed lists can be found in Finch [1] and in Young and Vincent [24]. The treatment of neutropenia when a drug cause is suspected is immediate withdrawal of the offending agent.

NON–DRUG-INDUCED NEUTROPENIA

Infections. Bacterial infections seldom cause neutropenia unless there is an overwhelming septicemia. Patients with septicemia-induced neutropenia often have deficient neutrophil reserves attributable to alcoholism, nutritional deficiency, prior chemotherapy, or radiation. Other rare bacterial infections that suppress neutrophil production include typhoid or paratyphoid [1,34].

Viral infections, such as infectious mononucleosis, infectious hepatitis, cytomegalovirus (CMV), measles, rubella, or chickenpox, may cause suppression of myeloid production. The cause is not clear, but at least in the case of hepatitis, it may represent a direct toxic effect of the virus on the bone marrow. The effect is usually transient and is reversed as the infection improves. Peripheral blood may show atypical lymphocytes.

Human immunodeficiency virus (HIV) may also cause leukopenia, and its presence should be ruled out in a person presenting with a low white count who is in a high-risk group for HIV infection. Leukopenia in asymptomatic HIV-infected individuals is related to lymphopenia. In AIDS patients, the frequency of leukopenia is between 40 and 65 percent and can be secondary to granulocytopenia as well [35]. The cause of neutropenia is multifactorial. Autoantibodies to granulocytes were found to be present in more than 50 percent of patients with AIDS or AIDS-related complex (ARC) in one study. Decreases in myeloid stem cells, perhaps secondary to a circulating inhibitory factor, have also been reported [36]. Because in vitro addition of GM-CSF or G-CSF in bone marrow cultures of AIDS patients may increase the amount of stem cells, AIDS patients may also have a deficiency of marrow stimulatory factors [37]. The cause of cytopenias in AIDS patients is complex and may also be caused by infiltration of marrow by other infectious agents (CMV, *Mycobacterium avium intracellulare*) or lymphoma, as well as by antiviral drugs such as zidovudine or ganciclovir. Human marrow growth factors have been used to improve the neutropenia in AIDS patients, as discussed in the Treatment section of this chapter.

CMV-associated neutropenia may be seen in organ and marrow transplant recipients or as a complication of anti-CMV therapy with ganciclovir. B19 parvoviral infections occasionally cause pure red cell aplasia and in a few cases, neutropenia [38]. The bone marrow contains abnormal erythroblasts, and the diagnosis is confirmed by isolation of the virus. The disorder may respond to intravenous immune globulin.

Hemodialysis. Hemodialysis leukopenia is a phenomenon of peripheral consumption of neutrophils that has recently been described [39]. A notable, although transient, granulocytopenia had been observed in patients with renal failure on hemodialysis. Leukocyte counts can drop as low as 1000 cells per cubic millimeter and can be associated with pulmonary infiltrates and shortness of breath. The mechanism has been shown to be secondary to the activation of complement, with the formation of C5a when the patient's plasma comes in contact with the cellophane membrane in the dialysis machine. C5a is a potent granulocyte-aggregating agent [40]. Thus in some patients on dialysis, aggregates of white cells are formed and sequestered in the lungs. The granulocytopenia resolves within 1 to 2 hours after dialysis is stopped. If granulocytopenia persists, other causes of neutropenia, especially drugs, should be sought [39].

Anaphylactic Shock. Allergic reactions to endotoxin or foreign proteins may cause the activation of complement, producing massive accumulations of neutrophils in the lung, leading to transient neutropenia. The mechanism is similar to that with hemodialysis.

Nutritional Deficiencies. In other disorders, production of stem cells and the mitotic pool may be quantitatively normal, but destruction of the cells may occur within the marrow, causing an ineffective granulopoiesis. It is rarely seen independently of other cellular elements in the marrow. Megaloblastic anemias, such as is seen with folate or vitamin B_{12} deficiency, are the common cause. Neutrophils are hypersegmented, and earlier forms are larger than normal. In the intensive care setting, these vitamins, particularly folate, should be supplied for patients who require total parenteral nutrition or those who fail to sustain adequate oral nutrition. Copper deficiency secondary to decreased intake or excessive zinc ingestion may produce neutropenia by several mechanisms [41,42].

Primary Hematologic Diseases. Neutropenia that is based on a direct bone marrow effect can also be the result of primary

hematologic disease. Acute leukemia may present as an isolated neutropenia, and a bone marrow differential cell count usually indicates more than 30% blasts. In acute leukemia, an inhibiting factor that suppresses the marrow has been found [43], contradicting the previous concept of a "packed marrow," physically impeding normal cell growth. In most cases, however, other cellular elements, such as platelets and erythrocytes, are suppressed; the diagnosis is easily confirmed by bone marrow aspirate or biopsy. Refractory anemia, preleukemia, and myelophthisic anemias with marrow infiltration by tumor may also cause a decrease in neutrophils and, again, are diagnosed by bone marrow.

The 5q- syndrome is associated with a deletion in a portion of chromosome 5, which contains the genes for GM-CSF, IL-3, IL-4, IL-5, M-CSF, and the M-CSF receptor. Inadequate production of these cytokines or a receptor abnormality may relate to the pathogenesis of this syndrome. Although the disorder usually presents as a macrocytic anemia with hypolobated megakaryocytes on marrow examination, neutropenia may occur in some cases.

Paroxysmal nocturnal hemoglobinuria (PNH) also represents a disease process in which complement plays a role in the neutropenia observed. However, the neutropenia is not isolated, and the characteristic finding is chronic hemolysis. The defect in erythrocytes has been shown to be caused by abnormal sensitivity to the lytic action of complement, perhaps secondary to an abnormal membrane component. The neutropenia may be secondary to the same defect, or it may be caused by a production defect [44]. Disorders of large granular lymphocytes (LGL), either clonal or nonclonal, produce cytopenias, particularly neutropenia. Other abnormalities associated with the clonal forms of this disease include a positive RF, positive ANA, polyclonal hypergammaglobulinemia, circulating immune complexes, and antineutrophil anitbodies [45].

Hypersplenism. Increased destruction of neutrophils may occur on a nonimmune or an immune basis. Nonimmune destruction or sequestration may be caused by hypersplenism, which can produce leukopenia or neutropenia. Liver disease, other causes of congestive splenomegaly, and storage diseases, such as Gaucher's, may produce splenomegaly and subsequent pooling of white cells in the spleen. Mild anemia and thrombocytopenia may be associated findings. The relative leukocyte differential usually remains normal.

Autoimmune Diseases. The diagnosis of immune destruction may be difficult to confirm. Unlike a Coombs test for erythrocytes, testing for antineutrophil antibodies is more difficult and lacks specificity. However, these tests are becoming more readily available [46].

Collagen vascular diseases, such as systemic lupus erythematosus (SLE), may cause neutropenia on an immune basis, although this has not been conclusively demonstrated. In one series, 50 percent of patients with SLE had neutropenia [47]. Felty's syndrome, the rheumatoid arthritis that is associated with splenomegaly and neutropenia, occurs in fewer than 1 percent of patients with rheumatoid arthritis. Of these patients, more than 90 percent have positive latex fixation titers [48]. Neutrophil counts are usually less than 2000 per cubic millimeter and may be severely depressed. Bone marrow shows an absence of mature myeloid cells, especially neutrophils. The mechanism may be multifactorial.

Some studies have shown increased IgG on the neutrophils of these patients or have demonstrated circulating antineutrophilic antibodies [49]. Others have shown a mononuclear suppressor cell that suppresses the growth of myeloid stem cells [50]. If patients are asymptomatic, no therapy is indicated. When recurrent severe infections occur, however, splenectomy may be indicated. Two-thirds of patients show a significant increase in neutrophil count with splenectomy, but in many patients this benefit is temporary [48]. Autoimmune neutropenia has been described in other disorders such as Crohn's disease [51].

OTHER UNCOMMON CAUSES OF NEUTROPENIA. There are several hereditary disorders that represent production defects that are only rarely encountered in the intensive care unit. *Kostmann's syndrome,* or infantile genetic agranulocytosis, is a disorder inherited as an autosomal recessive trait in which there is a profound peripheral neutropenia [52]. The bone marrow shows the presence of early myeloid precursors but an absence of myelocytes and more mature myeloid forms. Infants present with fever and multiple, serious infections, and most die within the first year of life. Although the neutropenia has been reversed by bone marrow transplantation [53], the chronic administration of G-CSF has led to normalization of neutrophil levels and elimination of infections. It is now the treatment of choice for this disease.

A group of patients may present later in life with occasional severely depressed neutrophil counts of 500 to 1000 per cubic meter but with a minimum of infectious complications. This condition is known as *chronic benign neutropenia*. It may be transmitted as a non–sex-linked autosomal dominant trait. The white count can be depressed for months to years. Kinetic studies show both decreased mitotic and reserve pools; agar culture studies show decreased CFU-C [54]. The diagnosis is often made inadvertently on a routine blood count. It is a diagnosis of exclusion after drug ingestion, collagen vascular disease, and malignancy have been ruled out. No treatment is required [55].

Human *cyclic neutropenia* is another uncommon disease. Patients complain of intermittent episodes of aphthous stomatitis, fever, malaise, and occasionally more severe infections. The diagnosis is made by demonstrating regularly occurring cycles of neutropenia, which may occur on the average of every 28 days. There may be cyclic variations of the platelets and of the reticulocyte count as well. Occasionally, it has been described in patients with Crohn's disease [56]. In canine studies, cyclic neutropenia has been shown to be a disorder of the pluripotent stem cells in the marrow, which is reversible by bone marrow transplantation [46]. The disease can be ameliorated by alternate-day corticosteroids. Recently, G-CSF has been used to treat this disorder successfully.

Evaluation

The diagnosis of the cause of neutropenia revolves around the history and the clinical setting. In the critically ill patient, it is extremely important to understand the relative factors that could influence neutrophil counts. It is helpful to construct a flow chart describing the time relation of neutropenia to the administration of drugs (including nonprescription drugs the patient may have taken prior to admission), the onset of infection, dialysis, etc. If no obvious precipitating factor is identified, the patient should be evaluated for occult infections or viral diseases. If neutropenia antedated admission to the intensive care unit, an attempt should be made to obtain previous blood counts to determine whether the patient has chronic neutropenia. The nutritional status of the patient should be assessed with regard to prior alcohol use and dietary factors or gastrointestinal factors that could lead to B_{12} or folate deficiency. A careful review of the vitamin supplements added to the par-

enteral nutritional infusions should be made. In an adult, physical findings of smooth tongue or cheilosis may suggest nutritional deficiencies. The presence of arthritis and splenomegaly should aid in making a diagnosis of an underlying collagen vascular disease such as SLE or Felty's syndrome. Splenomegaly alone may produce mild leukopenia, usually in association with other cytopenias secondary to sequestration. The differential count is usually normal in the leukopenia associated with splenomegaly. Massively enlarged spleens or enlarged spleens that are nontender and firm to palpation usually indicate a myeloproliferative process, lymphoma, or hairy cell leukemia. Underlying liver disease should be suspected in the absence of other causes of splenomegaly, and a careful assessment for spider angiomas, palmar erythema, gynecomastia, or ascites should be made. Rarely, hereditary factors must be considered. If a child receiving no medications presents with repeated infections, a congenital disorder must be entertained, such as Kostmann's syndrome.

The peripheral blood smear and possibly the bone marrow must be examined to rule out a primary hematologic problem such as acute leukemia or some form of myelophthisis. In severe neutropenia or agranulocytosis, where granulocytes are virtually absent on peripheral smear, the marrow is found likewise to be deficient in granulocytes, bands, and metamyelocytes, but often exhibits a predominance of promyelocytes. This presentation occasionally has been ascribed erroneously to acute promyelocytic leukemia, and careful review of the marrow is warranted. Promyelocytes with prominent Golgi apparatus typify the marrow cells observed in patients with agranulocytosis. The presence of blasts in the peripheral blood may be found in acute leukemia, but blasts are absent in classic agranulocytosis. Chromosomal abnormalities may be diagnostic in patients with acute promyelocytic leukemia (translocation of portions of chromosome 15 and 17) or other acute leukemias. Vacuolated bone marrow cells suggest a drug-induced idiosyncratic effect such as chloramphenicol. Patients with a history of poor nutrition or patients who are maintained on mechanical ventilators for prolonged periods without folate supplementation should have serum and erythrocyte folate levels measured. A history of alcohol abuse also should prompt an evaluation for folate deficiency. Folate should be routinely administered to these individuals. Although stores of vitamin B_{12} are not usually depleted by the short-term absence of the vitamin in the diet, levels should be obtained if there is unexplained macrocytosis, hypersegmentation of the neutrophils, a history of gastrointestinal tract surgery, or bacterial overgrowth that might have interfered with B_{12} absorption. Neutrophil survival times remain difficult to measure. Antinuclear antibodies or latex fixation studies may implicate collagen vascular diseases. Although the detection of antineutrophil antibodies is relatively nonspecific, a positive test and characteristic bone marrow may suggest an autoimmune process.

Treatment

Therapy for neutropenia depends on the cause and the degree of the neutropenia and whether a significant fever is present. Patients with acute granulocytopenia secondary either to an idiosyncratic response to a drug or to chemotherapy usually recover uneventfully after 10 to 14 days or less. However, mortality from severe drug-induced agranulocytosis is about 25 to 30 percent, and in leukemics undergoing induction chemotherapy, there is a mortality rate of 10 percent in centers with experience handling these patients.

In patients with drug-induced neutropenia any implicated

drug should be withdrawn if at all possible. Mild chronic leukopenia associated with drugs such as anticonvulsants may be tolerable if the patient's neutrophil count is above 500/mm^3 and no infection is present. If the patient is afebrile, contact with anyone with a known infection should be prevented. Reverse isolation (the patient in a private room, with entering visitors and personnel having to wear sterile gowns, masks, and gloves) is not necessary and is ineffective in preventing bacteremia in neutropenic patients or shortening the time the patient is hospitalized with fever [57]. Most infections are the result of endogenous microflora. A modified approach with careful attention to handwashing before entering the room and screening visitors for infection is recommended. In the intensive care unit, isolation from other patients who may harbor resistant organisms may be appropriate.

In the absence of fever, prophylactic antibiotics should not be started, because resistant organisms may then be selected out. However, in patients who undergo marrow transplantation where fever and neutropenia are expected in practically every patient, a number of infection prophylaxis protocols, often initiated before the transplant, have been employed with mixed success. These include agents given to prevent herpes simplex (acyclovir), *Pneumocystis carinii* pneumonia (Bactrim), and bacterial infections (bowel sterilizing antibiotics, systemic antibiotics [58], GM-CSF or G-CSF [59,60]), and in allograft recipients, CMV infections (ganciclovir [61], immune globulin [62], CMV seronegative [63,64]).

If a temperature of more than 38.3°C is present and the granulocyte count is less than 500 to 1000 per cubic millimeter (particularly if the neutrophil count is decreasing) even in the absence of localizing signs or symptoms, blood and urine cultures should be obtained and broad-spectrum antibiotics initiated immediately [65]. If CMV is suspected, "buffy coat" leukocyte cultures and urine cultures for CMV should be obtained periodically. Specimens from bone marrow aspirates and biopsies performed as part of the evaluation of neutropenia should be sent for acid-fast bacilli, mycobacteria, and fungal cultures, even though the yield from these cultures is low.

Infection with *S. aureus* or *S. epidermidis* or gram-negative bacteria, such as *Pseudomonas, Klebsiella,* or *Escherichia coli* [66,67], is not uncommon. In at least 20 to 50 percent of patients, however, a specific organism is not isolated nor a clear-cut source of infection identified [68]. Routine admitting chest radiographs do not appear to elucidate the cause or change the treatment approach in febrile, neutropenic patients, although follow-up films, particularly when fever does not respond to initial treatment, may be helpful [69]. Diagnosis with indium 111 IgG in febrile neutropenic patients may locate a source of infection in some. Its relevance with regard to treatment remains unknown [70], and it is not routinely recommended.

In an acute neutropenia secondary to chemotherapy or idiosyncratic drug reaction, antibiotic treatment for the febrile illness should be continued until bone marrow recovery occurs. In patients whose blood cultures show a pathogen, a full course of antibiotic therapy lasting 10 days to 2 weeks (or longer with fungal infections) is probably indicated. In patients whose neutropenia and infection clinically resolve, a brief course of antibiotics is probably sufficient. Earlier "discharge criteria" have been proposed in patients with no signs of active infection who have signs of early marrow recovery. A detailed algorithm as proposed by Pizzo is shown in Figure 125-2.

Antibiotic regimens used in neutropenic patients are varied but should include an antibiotic that acts against *Pseudomonas,* such as ceftazidime [71,72], aztreonam [73], or imipenem [74], often with an aminoglycoside such as gentamicin or tobramycin that is active against gram-negative organisms [75]. Monotherapy with imipenem alone may be equal to ceftazidime and

gentamicin [76]. Many centers also add vancomycin to this regimen if gram-positive organisms are strongly suspected, i.e., central catheter with exit site infection, inflamed skin wounds, or cellulitis. If an organism is isolated by culture and the patient remains neutropenic, the broad-spectrum antibiotic regimen should be continued rather than tailored more specifically. Antibiotic regimens for the neutropenic patient are discussed in more detail in Chapter 92 and in a recent review [77].

Since the early 1980s, indwelling catheters such as Portacaths, Hickman, Groshong, or Broviac catheters have been widely used in cancer patients receiving chemotherapy. Infections with gram-positive organisms such as *Staphylococcus epidermidis, Staphylococcus aureus,* or streptococci occur in these patients with or without neutropenia [78]. The change in incidence of these organisms is not caused by increased use of venous access devices but probably is related to shifts in the representative gastrointestinal microbial flora [79]. In most cases, the infections associated with indwelling catheters can be eradicated without removing the line [80]. However, if there is a subcutaneous "tunnel" infection, the catheter should be removed. Gram-negative catheter infections have a high recurrence rate after treatment, and fungemia in patients with catheters in place should prompt the removal of these devices.

In some centers, vancomycin is empirically added to the antibiotic regimen when a neutropenic febrile patient with an indwelling catheter begins antibiotic treatment. However, vancomycin is costly and is associated with synergistic ototoxicity in conjunction with aminoglycosides, Redman's syndrome, and occasionally cytopenias. Thus, a more common practice is to add vancomycin once a responsive bacteria is cultured or if a gram-positive infection is strongly suspected. In a series of 350 episodes of fever and neutropenia, the response to delaying initiation of vancomycin pending culture results was as good as when vancomycin was started immediately empirically [81]. Another unusual but important gram-positive infection includes those that produce the alpha-streptococcal shock syndrome, usually observed in neutropenic marrow transplant recipients and associated with shock and respiratory failure. Prophylaxis with the quinolones may predispose to this syndrome.

If fever persists even with broad-spectrum antibiotic therapy, especially if the patient is immunocompromised secondary to cancer or chemotherapy, fungal infection must be considered. In neutropenic patients with fever that persists beyond 5 days, empiric amphotericin-B should be added. However, this should be done in consultation with an infectious disease specialist. Itraconazole is being evaluated for treatment of patients with invasive *Aspergillus* disease. Surgery may be indicated as part of the treatment process for some forms of localized mycotic infections.

Other infections should be considered in patients with prolonged neutropenia. Pulmonary infiltrates are often categorized as diffuse or patchy. Bronchoalveolar lavage (BAL) may assist in the differential diagnosis of lung infiltrates and may identify pathogens such as *Pneumocystis carinii, Legionella,* and viral infections with cytomegalovirus (CMV), herpes simplex, or zoster. Diagnosis of a serious fungal infection is often difficult. The presence of fungal elements in the BAL specimen is not diagnostic for invasive fungal disease and may represent only colonization. Tissue biopsy confirmation remains the standard approach to confirm a diagnosis of invasive fungal disease in the lung. Transbronchial or open lung biopsy should be seriously considered if pulmonary infiltrates are present in the seriously ill patient. In patients with patchy infiltrates, care should be taken to perform a biopsy on the center of the lesion. However, in our experience in patients who have a nondiagnostic BAL, the use of empiric antibiotics is preferable to open lung biopsy because the results of the biopsy procedure very frequently do

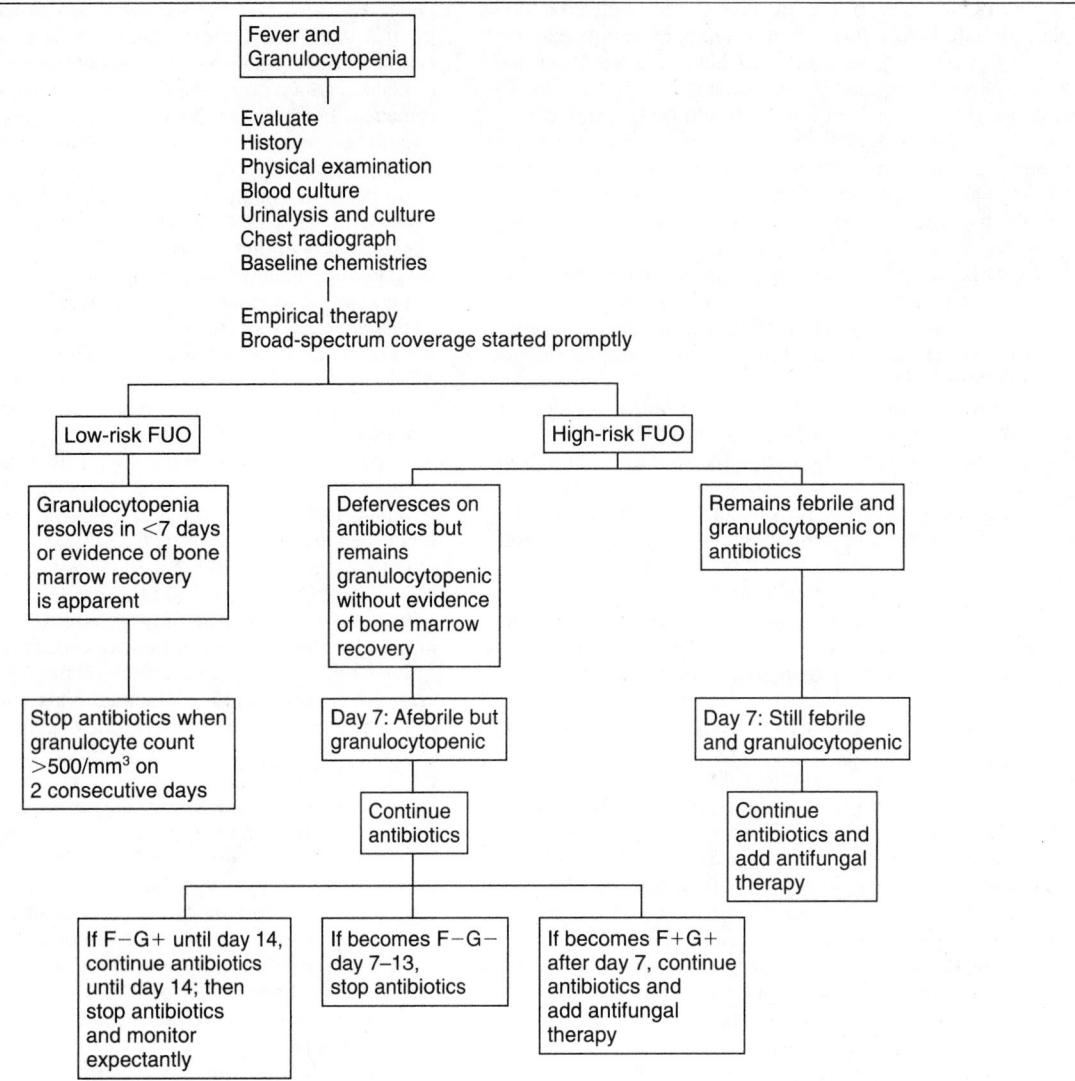

Fig. 125-2. Evaluation and management of fever and granulocytopenia. (Reproduced with permission from Pizzo PA, Meyers J, Freifeld AG, et al: Infections in the cancer patient, in DeVita VT, Hellman S, Rosenberg SA (eds): *Cancer Principles and Practice of Oncology.* 4th ed. Philadelphia, JB Lippincott, 1993, p. 2298.

not change therapy in a way that justifies its morbidity. In the situation where empiric antibiotics are causing serious complications, identification of a pathogen through an open biopsy procedure may be justified in spite of its marginal yield.

Daily examination of the skin, perianal area, mouth, sinuses, abdominal region, and central nervous system may show findings that direct diagnostic and therapeutic approaches. Rectal examinations should be performed very carefully if at all in neutropenic patients. Instrumentation procedures such as upper endoscopy have caused symptomatic bacteremia and fever in some. Severe neutropenia is not necessarily a contraindication to invasive procedures such as exploratory laparotomy in selected life-threatening situations [82,83]. Prophylactic antibiotics probably should be administered before invasive procedures that involve gastrointestinal or other bacteria-laden sites.

Some unique complications occur during the febrile neutropenic period of allogeneic bone marrow transplantation. In acute graft-versus-host disease (GVHD) alloreactive donor T lymphocytes may attack recipient tissues, including skin, liver, and gut. GVHD predisposes recipients to a variety of infections, including CMV, other viral infections, bacteremias, and fungal infections. CMV and other viruses cause neutropenia, although this occurs most frequently 40 to 80 days after transplant when the marrow has already regenerated. Ganciclovir possibly with immune globulin may result in some improvement, but overall the results of treatment are poor. Lymphopenia is a poor prognostic factor in CMV-infected marrow allograft recipients independent of their neutrophil levels.

WHITE CELL TRANSFUSIONS. In some studies, granulocyte transfusions have been found to be beneficial in certain clinical situations associated with prolonged neutropenia and resistant infections, although enthusiasm has waxed and waned over the years. Currently, granulocyte transfusions are administered rarely. Certain patient profiles may justify consideration of this modality. A febrile patient with granulocytopenia who is deteriorating with persistent growth of organisms from the blood unrelated to access devices continuing and in spite of appropriate broad-spectrum antibiotics might benefit from white cell transfusions. The decision to use transfusions should be made in conjunction with both a hematologist and an infectious disease consultant. The best responses have been seen in patients with a documented gram-negative bacteremia or a known source of infection [84,85].

In a review of multiple studies using white cell transfusions, Strauss concluded that in many the duration of transfusions was too short, and the amount of white cells collected was too low, making efficacy hard to assess [86]. With the advent of hemopoietic growth factors, such as G-CSF or GM-CSF, which mobilize leukocyte progenitors from the bone marrow to the peripheral blood and increase blood granulocyte numbers, large numbers of "functionally primed" leukocytes may be collected from normal donors by apheresis techniques [87]. In this context future studies may define a new role for granulocyte transfusions.

Currently, granulocyte transfusions are of questionable efficacy, may cause serious reactions in the patient, and their acquisition may place the donor at real, albeit minimal, risk. Therefore, for now they should be used in selected circumstances discussed above [88]. The incidence of granulocyte transfusion reactions is high, and even more problematic, an increased incidence of alloimmunization has been noted in which patients administered these transfusions no longer respond to transfused platelets [89].

HEMOPOIETIC GROWTH FACTORS (HGFs). The most recent approach to the problem of neutropenia has been the use of growth factors manufactured by recombinant technology.

Several prospective controlled trials have shown that G-CSF given prophylactically after moderately intense chemotherapy reduced the incidence of neutropenic fevers, decreased antibiotic use, and diminished the total number of hospitalizations and hospital days [90,91,92]. The results of these studies may only be applied to patients who receive a drug combination that is likely to have a 30 to 40 percent incidence of neutropenic fever or higher and likewise do not apply to patients with established fever and neutropenia. Studies addressing the latter question are in progress.

To reduce the duration of cytopenias and ultimately improve patient care, hemopoietic growth factors such as G-CSF or GM-CSF have been applied to (1) hasten marrow recovery or treat graft failure posttransplantation [59,60,93–98] and (2) mobilize peripheral blood progenitor cells for apheresis collection and cryopreservation [99,100]. The latter technique provides a source of autologous stem cells, i.e., committed progenitor cells that differentiate rapidly and reconstitute the hemopoietic system after ablative chemotherapy. With either autologous bone marrow or peripheral blood stem cells, GM-CSF reduced the number of neutropenic days. The number of hospital days, antibiotic days, and infections were variably affected. Overall, the use of cytokines in marrow transplantation is in its infancy. No definite advantages in terms of real patient benefit have been established consistently. Cost-effectiveness has also not been established consistently.

Anecdotal reports have suggested that drug-induced agranulocytosis responds to GM-CSF [101], but a more critical analysis of these cases raises the possibility that the same degree of recovery may have been achieved without GM-CSF. However, in patients with chronic neutropenia of various causes, a prospective controlled trial found that G-CSF significantly increased neutrophil levels and decreased infection and antibiotic use [102].

Recombinant human GM-CSF has been used to treat the neutropenia caused by HIV infection [103]. Increases in neutrophil counts and augmentation of neutrophil function were seen but were not sustained once the growth factor was withdrawn [104]. In vitro studies suggest that GM-CSF, M-CSF, and IL-3 stimulate HIV replication whereas G-CSF apparently does not [105]. Alternatively, in mononuclear cell systems the anti-HIV effect of zidovudine has been potentiated tenfold by GM-CSF [106]. GM-CSF has been shown to ameliorate the neutropenia caused by zidovudine, but in some cases has produced thrombocytopenia by unknown mechanisms. During treatment of CMV-infected AIDS patients, ganciclovir often has produced significant neutropenia. In a controlled trial in AIDS patients treated with ganciclovir for CMV retinitis [107], GM-CSF had a beneficial effect on neutrophil levels. Recombinant granulocyte stimulating factor has been used in neutropenic HIV-infected patients. Neutrophils, CD4 lymphocytes, and reticulocytes were increased [108].

Recombinant human G-CSF has also been used in primary marrow disorders such as myelodysplastic syndromes (MDS) and aplastic anemia, but its effects are transient and in MDS may increase the number of blasts in the marrow or peripheral blood.

Common side effects of GM-CSF or G-CSF include fever or mild bone pain. GM-CSF in high doses may result in edema, weight gain, or a flulike syndrome with fever and myalgias. In several patients, hypotension, pericardial effusions, and pleural effusions were noted. The dose schedules of the various growth factors and the indications for use are still under investigation. Current recommended dosages for G-CSF are 5 to 10 μg per kilogram given daily intravenously over 2 hours or subcutaneously. GM-CSF is administered at a dose of 250 μg per square meter daily intravenously over 2 hours or subcutaneously. Once the target neutrophil count has been surpassed after the nadir, the drug may be discontinued.

In vitro studies show that GM-CSF and other cytokines may stimulate leukemia cell growth [109] and the growth of small cell carcinoma cells and other neoplastic cells. Although there is no proof from controlled clinical trials that HGFs have caused increased recurrence rates in chemotherapy-treated leukemia or cancer patients, this remains an important concern for future analysis.

There are probably subsets of patients, presumably those without cytokine receptors on their tumors and those who experience minimal cytokine toxicity, who are benefited, whereas there may be subsets who are harmed. The challenge of the future is to define these subsets. However, it hoped that in certain primary bone marrow diseases and in the cytopenias induced by chemotherapy or bone marrow transplantation, use of these growth factors, singly or in combination, will be beneficial.

References

1. Finch S: Granulocytopenia, in William W (ed): *Hematology*. New York, McGraw-Hill, 1983.
2. Orfanakis NG, Ostlund RE, Bishop CR, et al: Normal blood leukocyte concentration values. *Am J Clin Pathol* 53:647, 1970.
3. Boggs DR: The kinetics of neutrophil leukocytes in health and disease. *Semin Hematol* 4:359, 1967.
4. Brown GO, Herbig FK, Hamilton JR: Leukopenia in negroes. *N Engl J Med* 175:1410, 1979.
5. Bodey GP, Buckley M, Sathe YS, et al: Quantitative relationships between circulating leukocytes and infection in patients with acute leukemia. *Ann Intern Med* 64:328, 1966.
6. Ogawa M: Differentiation and proliferation of hematopoietic stem cells. *Blood* 81:2844, 1993.

7. Spangrude GF, Heimfeld S, Weissman IL: Purification and characterization of mouse hematopoietic stem cells. *Science* 241:58, 1988.

8. Hodgson GS, Bradley TR: Properties of haematopoietic stem cells surviving 5-fluorouracil treatment: Evidence for a pre-CFU-S cell. *Nature* 281:381, 1979.

9. Quesenberry PJ, Levitt L: Hematopoietic stem cells. *N Engl J Med* 301:755, 1979.

10. Sullivan R, Quesenberry PJ, Parkman R, et al: Aplastic anemia: Lack of inhibitory effect of bone marrow lymphocytes on in vitro granulopoiesis. *Blood* 56:625, 1980.

11. Greenberg PL, Mara B: The preleukemic syndrome. *Am J Med* 66:951, 1979.

12. Nathan DG: Hope for hematopoietic hormones. *N Engl J Med* 317:626, 1987.

13. Williams GT, Smith CA, Spooncer E, et al: Haemopoietic colony stimulating factors promote cell survival by suppressing apoptosis. *Nature* 343:76, 1990.

14. Osgood EE: Hypoplastic anemias and related syndromes caused by drug idiosyncrasy. *JAMA* 152:816, 1953.

15. Robinson W, Mangalek K: Kinetics and regulation of granulopoiesis. *Semin Hematol* 12:7, 1975.

16. Tauber AI: Current views of neutrophil dysfunction. *Am J Med* 70:1237, 1981.

17. Tauber AI: The human neutrophil oxygen armory. *Biochem Sci* 7:411, 1982.

18. Klebanoff SJ: Oxygen metabolism and the toxic properties of phagocytes. *Ann Intern Med* 93:480, 1980.

19. Neftel KA, Hauser SP, Muller MR: Inhibition of granulopoiesis in vivo and in vitro by beta-lactam antibiotics. *J Infect Dis* 152:90, 1985.

20. Murphy MF, Metcalfe P, Grint PCA, et al: Cephalosporin-induced immune neutropenia. *Br J Haematol* 59:9, 1985.

21. Pennington JE: Fever, neutropenia and malignancy: A clinical syndrome in evolution. *Cancer* 39:1345, 1977.

22. Mayall B, Poggi G, Parkin JD: Neutropenia due to low-dose methotrexate therapy for psoriasis and rheumatoid arthritis may be fatal. *Med J Aust* 155:480, 1991.

23. Piscottia AJ: Immune and toxic mechanisms in drug induced agranulocytosis. *Semin Hematol* 10:279, 1973.

24. Young GA, Vincent PC: Drug induced agranulocytosis. *Clin Haematol* 9:483, 1980.

25. Alvir JMJ, Liberman JA, Safferman AZ, et al: Clozapine-induced agranulocytosis. *N Engl J Med* 329:162, 1993.

26. Jamshid K, Arlander T, Garcia M, et al: Azulfidine agranulocytosis with bone marrow toxicity. *Minn Med* 53:548, 1972.

27. De Manzini A, Peratoner L, Lepore L: Neutropenia caused by low-dose trimethoprim sulfamethoxazole in children with chronic pathology of the urinary tract. *Pediatr Med Chir* 12:49, 1990.

28. Morris A, Ward C: High incidence of vancomycin-associated leucopenia and neutropenia in a cardiothoracic surgical unit. *J Infect* 22:217, 1991.

29. Polak BP, Wesseling H, Schut D, et al: Blood dyscrasias attributed to chloramphenicol. *Acta Med Scand* 192:409, 1972.

30. Palva IP, Mustala OO: Drug induced agranulocytosis with special reference to aminophenazone. *Acta Med Scand* 187:109, 1970.

31. List AF, Beaird DH, Kummet T: Ranitidine-induced granulocytopenia: Recurrence with cimetidine administration. *Ann Intern Med* 108:566, 1988.

32. Harvey RL, Luzar MJ: Metoclopramide-induced agranulocytosis. *Ann Intern Med* 108:214, 1988.

33. Bertolino JG: Carbamazepine: What physicians should know about its hematologic effects. *Postgrad Med* 88:183, 1990.

34. Abdool Gaffar MS, Seedat YK, Coovadia YM, et al: The white cell count in typhoid fever. *Trop Geogr Med* 44:23, 1992.

35. Costello C: Hematologic abnormalities in human immunodeficiency virus (HIV) disease. *J Clin Pathol* 41:711, 1988.

36. Zon LI, Grossman JE: Hematologic manifestations of the human immune deficiency virus (HIV). *Semin Hematol* 25:208, 1988.

37. Stella CC, Ganser A, Hodzer D: Defective in vitro growth of hematopoietic progenitor cells in AIDS. *J Clin Invest* 80:286, 1987.

38. Elian JC, Frappaz D, Pozzeto B, et al: Transient erythroblastopenia and neutropenia revealing human parvovirus B19 infection. *Pediatrie* 673:675, 1991.

39. Craddock PR, Fehr J, Dalmasso AP, et al: Hemodialysis leukopenia. *J Clin Invest* 59:879, 1977.

40. Craddock PR, Hammerschmidt D, White JG, et al: Complement (C5a)-induced granulocyte aggregation in vitro. *J Clin Invest* 60:260, 1977.

41. Higuchi S, Higashi A, Nakamura T, et al: Anti-neutrophil antibodies in patients with nutritional copper deficiency. *Eur J Pediatr* 150:327, 1991.

42. Broun ER, Greist A, Tricot G, et al: Excessive zinc ingestion: A reversible cause of sideroblastic anemia and bone marrow depression. *JAMA* 264:1441, 1990.

43. Quesenberry PJ, Rappeport JM, Fountebuoni A, et al: Inhibition of normal murine hematopoiesis by leukemic cells. *N Engl J Med* 299:71, 1978.

44. Rosee WF: Paroxysmal nocturnal hemoglobinuria, in Williams W (ed): *Hematology.* New York, McGraw-Hill, 1983.

45. Loughran TP: Clonal diseases of large granular lymphocytes. *Blood* 82:1, 1993.

46. Weiden PL, Robinette P, Graham TC, et al: Canine cyclic neutropenia. *J Clin Invest* 53:950, 1974.

47. Logue GL, Schimm DS: Autoimmune granulocytopenia. *Annu Rev Med* 31:191, 1980.

48. Sienknecht CW, Urowitz MB, Pruzanski P, et al: Felty's syndrome: Clinical and serological analysis of 34 cases. *Ann Rheum Dis* 36:500, 1977.

49. Starkbaum G, Singer JW, Arend WP: Humoral and cellular immune mechanisms of neutropenia in patients with Felty's syndrome. *Clin Exp Immunol* 39:307, 1980.

50. Abdou NI, NaPombejara C, Balentine L, et al: Suppressor cell mediated neutropenia in Felty's syndrome. *J Clin Invest* 61:738, 1978.

51. Stevens C, Peppercorn MA, Grand RJ: Crohn's disease associated with autoimmune neutropenia. *J Clin Gastroenterol* 13:328, 1991.

52. Baehner RL, Boxer LA: Disorders of granulopoiesis and granulocyte function, in Nathan DG, Oski FA (eds): *Hematology of Infancy and Childhood.* Philadelphia, Saunders, 1981.

53. Rappeport JM, Parkman R, Newburger P, et al: Correction of infantile agranulocytosis by allogeneic bone marrow transplantation. *Am J Med* 68:605, 1980.

54. Dale DC, Guerry D, Wewerka JR, et al: Chronic neutropenia. *Medicine* 58:128, 1979.

55. Kyle RA: Natural history of chronic idiopathic neutropenia. *N Engl J Med* 302:908, 1980.

56. Lamport RD, Katz S, Eskreis D: Crohn's disease associated with cyclic neutropenia. *Am J Gastroenterol* 87:1638, 1992.

57. Nauseff W, Maki D: A study in the value of simple protective isolation in patients with granulocytopenia. *N Engl J Med* 34:448, 1981.

58. Attal M, Schlaifer D, Rubie H, et al: Prevention of gram-positive infections after bone marrow transplantation by systemic vancomycin: A prospective, randomized trial. *J Clin Oncol* 9:865, 1991.

59. Nemunaitis J, Rabinowe SN, Singer JW, et al: Recombinant granulocyte-macrophage colony-stimulating factor after autologous bone marrow transplantation for lymphoid cancer. *N Engl J Med* 324:1773, 1991.

60. Advani R, Chao NJ, Horning SJ, et al: Granulocyte-macrophage colony-stimulating factor (GM-CSF) as an adjunct to autologous hemopoietic stem cell transplantation of lymphoma. *Ann Intern Med* 116:183, 1992.

61. Laurence J, Coleman M, Allen SL, et al: Combination chemotherapy of advanced diffuse histiocytic lymphoma with the six-drug COP-BLAM regimen. *Ann Intern Med* 97:190, 1982.

62. Sullivan KM, Kopecky KJ, Jocom J, et al: Immunomodulatory and antimicrobial efficacy of intravenous immunoglobulin in bone marrow transplantation. *N Engl J Med* 323:705, 1990.

63. Bowden RA, Sayers M, Flournoy N, et al: Cytomegalovirus immune globulin and seronegative blood products to prevent primary cytomegalovirus infection after marrow transplantation. *N Engl J Med* 314:1006, 1986.

64. Appelbaum FR, Herzig GP, Ziegler JL, et al: Successful engraftment of cryopreserved autologous bone marrow in patients with malignant lymphoma. *Blood* 52:85, 1978.

65. Pizzo PA: Management of fever in patients with cancer and treatment-induced neutropenia. *N Engl J Med* 328:1323, 1993.

66. Levine AS, Graw RG, Young RC: Management of infections in patients with leukemia and lymphoma: Current concepts and experimental approaches. *Semin Hematol* 9:141, 1972.

67. Singer C, Kaplan M, Armstrong D: Bacteremia and fungemia complicating neoplastic disease. *Am J Med* 62:731, 1977.
68. Schimpf S: Intravenous sulfamethoxazole-trimethoprim plus ticarcillin as empiric antibiotic therapy for granulocytopenic patients. *Arch Intern Med* 141:844, 1981.
69. Donowitz GR, Harman C, Pope T, et al: The role of the chest roentgenogram in febrile neutropenic patients. *Arch Intern Med* 151:701, 1991.
70. Oyen WJG, Glaessens RAMJ, Raemaekers JMM, et al: Diagnosing infection in febrile granulocytopenic patients with indium-111-labeled human immunoglobulin G. *J Clin Oncol* 10:61, 1992.
71. Pizzo PA, Hathorn JW, Hiemenz J, et al: A randomized trial comparing ceftazidime along with combination antibiotic therapy in cancer patients with fever and neutropenia. *N Engl J Med* 315:552, 1986.
72. Sanders JW, Powe NR, Moore RD: Ceftazidime monotherapy for empiric treatment of febrile neutropenic patients: A meta-analysis. *J Infect Dis* 164:907, 1991.
73. Masur H: Aztreonam in the treatment of serious gram-negative infections in immunosuppressed patients. *Int Surg* 9:27, 1990.
74. Wade J, Bustamante C, Devlin A, et al: Imipenem vs piperacillin plus amilacin, empiric therapy for febrile neutropenic patients: A double-bind trial. *Programs and Abstracts of the 27th Interscience Conference on Antimicrobial Agents and Chemotherapy* 3315a, 1987.
75. Bodey GP, Bolivar R, Fainstein V: Infectious complications in leukemic patients. *Semin Hematol* 19:193, 1982.
76. Rolston KV, Berkey P, Bodey GP, et al: A comparison of imipenem to ceftazidime with or without amikacin as empiric therapy in febrile neutropenic patients. *Arch Intern Med* 152:283, 1992.
77. Armstrong D: Empiric therapy for the immunocompromised host. *Rev Infect Dis* 13:S763, 1991.
78. Gorelick MH, Owen WC, Seibel NL, et al: Lack of association between neutropenia and the incidence of bacteremia associated with indwelling central venous catheters in febrile pediatric cancer patients. *Pediatr Infect Dis J* 10:506, 1991.
79. Wade JC, Schimpff SC, Newman KA, et al: *Staphylococcus epidermidis:* An increasing cause of infection in patients with granulocytopenia. *Ann Intern Med* 97:503, 1982.
80. Pizzo PA: Diagnosis and management of infectious disease problems in the child with malignant disease, in Rubin RH, Young LS (eds): *Clinical Approach to Infection in the Compromised Host.* New York, Plenum Press, 1988.
81. Rubin M, Hathorn JW, Marshall D, et al: Gram positive infections and the use of vancomycin in 350 episodes of fever and neutropenia. *Ann Intern Med* 108:30, 1988.
82. Wade DS, Douglass H Jr, Nava HR, et al: Abdominal pain in neutropenic patients. *Arch Surg* 125:1119, 1990.
83. Rouquette-Gally AM, Boyeldieu D, Prost AC, et al: Autoimmunity after allogeneic bone marrow transplantation: A study of 53 long-term-surviving patients. *Transplantation* 46:238, 1988.
84. Higby D, Burnett D: Granulocyte transfusions: Current status. *Blood* 55:2, 1980.
85. Vogler W, Winton E: A controlled study of the efficacy of granulocyte transfusions in patients with neutropenia. *Am J Med* 63:548, 1977.
86. Strauss RG: Granulocyte transfusions: Uses, abuses and indications, in Kolins J, McCarthy LT (eds): *Contemporary Transfusion Practice.* Arlington, VA, American Association of Blood Banks, 1987.
87. Bensinger WJ, Price TH, Dale DC, et al: The effects of daily recombinant human granulocyte colony-stimulating factor administrations on normal granulocyte donors undergoing leukapheresis. *Blood* 81(7):1883, 1993.
88. Ford JM, Cullen MH, Roberts MM, et al: Prophylactic granulocyte transfusions. *Transfusion* 22:311, 1982.
89. Schiffer CA, Aisner J, Daly PA, et al: Alloimmunization following prophylactic transfusion. *Blood* 54:766, 1979.
90. Crawford J, Ozer H, Stoller R, et al: Reduction by granulocyte colony-stimulating factor of fever and neutropenia induced by chemotherapy in patients with small-cell lung cancer (r-metHuG-CSF). *N Engl J Med* 5:164, 1991.
91. Trillet-Lenoir V, Green JA, Manegold C, et al: Recombinant granulocyte colony-stimulating factor reduces the infectious complications of cytotoxic chemotherapy. *Eur J Cancer* 29A:319, 1993.
92. Pettengell R, Gurney H, Radford JA, et al: Granulocyte colony-stimulating factor to prevent dose-inhibiting neutropenia in non-Hodgkin's lymphoma: A randomized controlled trial. *Blood* 80:1430, 1992.
93. Link H, Boogaerts MA, Carella AM, et al: A controlled trial of recombinant human granulocyte-macrophage colony-stimulating factor after total body irradiation, high-dose chemotherapy, and autologous bone marrow transplantation for acute lymphoblastic leukemia or malignant lymphoma. *Blood* 80:2188, 1992.
94. Gorin NC, Coiffier B, Hayat, M, et al: Recombinant human granulocyte-macrophage colony-stimulating factor after high-dose chemotherapy and autologous bone marrow transplantation with unpurged and purged marrow in non-Hodgkin's lymphoma: A double-blind placebo-controlled trial. *Blood* 80:1149, 1992.
95. Khwaja A, Linch DC, Goldstone AH, et al: Recombinant human granulocyte-macrophage colony-stimulating factor after autologous bone marrow transplantation for malignant lymphoma: A British National Lymphoma Investigation double-blind, placebo-controlled trial. *Br J Haematol* 82:317, 1992.
96. Linch DC, Scarffe H, Proctor S, et al: Randomized vehicle-controlled dose-finding study of glycosylated recombinant human colony-stimulating factor after bone marrow transplantation. *Bone Marrow Transplant* 11:307, 1993.
97. Blaise D, Vernant JP, Fiere D, et al: A randomized, controlled multicenter trial of recombinant human granulocyte colony stimulating factor (Filgrastim) in patients treated by bone marrow transplantation (BMT) with total body irradiation (TBI) for acute lymphoblastic leukemia (ALL) or lymphoblastic lymphoma (LL). *Blood* 80:248a, 1992.
98. Powles R, Smith C, Milan S, et al: Human recombinant GM-CSF in allogeneic bone-marrow transplantation for leukaemia: Double-blind, placebo-controlled trial. *Lancet* 336:1417, 1990.
99. Crown J, Kritz A, Vahdat L, et al: Rapid administration of multiple cycles of high-dose myelosuppressive chemotherapy in patients with metastatic breast cancer. *J Clin Oncol* 11:1144, 1993.
100. Crump M, Ross M, Vredenburgh J, et al: Early toxicity after high-dose therapy and autologous bone marrow transplantation (ABMT) for breast cancer: Implications for outpatient management. *Blood* 80:70a, 1992.
101. Nand S, Bayer R, Prinz RA, et al: Granulocyte-macrophage colony stimulating factor for the treatment of drug induced agranulocytosis. *Am J Hematol* 37:267, 1991.
102. Dale DC, Bonilla MA, Davis MW, et al: A randomized controlled phase III trial of recombinant human granulocyte colony-stimulating factor (Filgrastim) for treatment of severe chronic neutropenia. *Blood* 81:2496, 1993.
103. Scadden DT, Bering HA, Levine JD, et al: Granulocyte-macrophage colony-stimulation factor mitigates the neutropenia of combined interferon alfa and zidovudine treatment of acquired immune deficiency syndrome-associated Kaposi's sarcoma. *J Clin Oncol* 9:802, 1991.
104. Groopman JE, Mitsuyasu RT, DeLeo MJ, et al: Effect of recombinant human granulocyte macrophage stimulating factor in myelopoiesis in the acquired human immunodeficiency syndrome. *N Engl J Med* 317:593, 1987.
105. Koyanagi Y, O'Brien WA, Zhao JQ: Cytokines alter production of HIV-1 from primary mononuclear phagocytes. *Science* 241:1733, 1988.
106. Perno CF, Yarchoan R, Cooney DA, et al: Replication of human immunodeficiency in monocytes. *J Exp Med* 169:933, 1989.
107. Hardy WD: Combined ganciclovir and recombinant granulocyte-macrophage colony-stimulating factor in the treatment of cytomegalovirus retinitis in AIDS patients. *J Acquir Immune Defic Syndr* 4:S22, 1991.
108. Miles SA, Mitsuyasu R, Fink N, et al: Recombinant granulocyte colony stimulating factor and recombinant erythropoietin may abrogate neutropenia and anemia of AIDS. *V International Conf AIDS* 550, 1989.
109. Young DC, Griffin JD: Autocrine secretion of GM-CSF in acute myeloblastic leukemia. *Blood* 68:1178, 1986.
110. Pizzo PA, Meyers J, Freifeld AG, et al: Infections in the cancer patient, in DeVita VT, Hellman S, Rosenberg SA (eds): *Cancer Principles and Practice of Oncology.* Philadelphia, JB Lippincott, 1993, pp 2292-2337.

126. The Acute Leukemias

Lawrence N. Shulman

With the advent of modern chemotherapy both acute myelogenous leukemia and acute lymphoblastic leukemia are now potentially curable. In the case of childhood acute lymphoblastic leukemia, approximately 60 to 70 percent of patients will be cured of disease [1]. In adults, the results in the treatment of acute myelogenous leukemia are more modest, but nevertheless, between 20 and 40 percent of patients will ultimately be cured of disease [2]. The treatment responsible for this success is highly toxic and causes many complications. Therefore, physicians caring for these patients must learn not only to manage the complications of the diseases, but also of the therapies employed. A basic understanding of leukemias is necessary for an understanding of their management, and therefore we begin with a brief description of each.

Acute Lymphoblastic Leukemia

Acute lymphoblastic leukemia (ALL) is a disease primarily of children, although it can occur at any age. The malignant cell is an immature lymphoid cell or lymphoblast that has a characteristic appearance in the blood or bone marrow, as shown in Figure 126-1. There is a fine, open nucleus, with rare indistinct nucleoli and scant cytoplasm. Although the morphology of these cells is relatively uniform from one patient to another, there are three distinct immunologic subtypes of ALL, all with different prognoses and complications, as shown in Table 126-1. The most common variety was previously known as "common" or "null cell" ALL. This accounts for approximately 70 percent of cases of ALL. These cells are now known to be pre-B cells and usually bear the common ALL antigen (CALLA or CD10) on their surface. This subtype has the best overall prognosis. The second variety is T cell ALL, accounting for approximately 25 percent of cases. The remainder of cases are truly B cell in type and have the worst prognosis, and this category is now considered by many to be a variant of small noncleaved cell lymphoma (Burkitt's lymphoma) rather than ALL. Though 60 to 70 percent of children presenting with ALL will be cured of their disease, only 20 to 40 percent of adults will. It is now known that a type of Philadelphia chromosome (t(9;22)), originally described as a marker for chronic myelogenous leukemia, is sometimes present in the leukemic blasts seen in the pre–B cell variety of ALL, and is associated with a very poor prognosis [3]. Whereas only 5 percent of children with ALL have blasts bearing the chromosomal marker, blasts from approximately 30 percent of adults with ALL express this translocation, and this in part accounts for the poor prognosis of ALL in adults.

All these diseases present with extensive infiltration of the bone marrow by leukemic cells, resulting in a displacement of the normal hematopoietic cells, leading to anemia, neutropenia, and thrombocytopenia. Some patients with ALL, particularly those with the T cell variety, also have a mediastinal mass, which, when large, can cause respiratory distress or embarrassment of the mediastinal vascular structures. All varieties of ALL are associated with a high incidence of leukemic meningitis. The frequency of this complication has been reduced, but not eliminated, by prophylactic treatment of the meninges with radiation and intrathecal chemotherapy.

Treatment of the patient with ALL is tailored depending on the immunologic type and the age of the patient, because both of these factors affect prognosis. Intensive induction chemotherapy followed by maintenance therapy for up to 2 years is a general treatment strategy. Induction therapy consists of vincristine and prednisone, sometimes with the addition of an anthracycline such as daunorubicin and L-asparaginase. Maintenance therapy usually includes methotrexate, 6-mercaptopurine, vincristine, and prednisone. Intrathecal methotrexate or cytosine arabinoside together with cranio-brainstem irradiation is a typical central nervous system (CNS) prophylaxis program. Newer, more intensive chemotherapy regimens are now in use for adult patients with ALL, and these appear to have improved the prognosis for these patients, but the intensity of the regimens has led to an increased incidence of therapy-related complications [4].

Acute Myelogenous Leukemia

Acute myelogenous leukemia (AML) is sometimes also referred to as acute nonlymphocytic leukemia or acute myeloblastic leukemia. The morphology of the leukemic blasts can be quite variable. Generally they are larger than lymphoblasts, contain more cytoplasm, and usually have large distinct nucleoli. Auer rods are sometimes present. An example is shown in Figure 126-2. There are seven subtypes included in the general category of AML as defined by the French-American-British (FAB) classification system and shown in Table 126-2 [5]. Though these different subtypes of AML are usually treated in a similar fashion, different manifestations of disease predictably occur with the different subtypes. The monocytic varieties, for instance, are more likely to demonstrate extramedullary tissue infiltration with leukemic cells with skin, gums, and meninges as common sites of involvement. Acute promyelocytic leukemia is often associated with disseminated intravascular coagulation (DIC), as is discussed later.

AML is a disease primarily of adults, although it sometimes occurs in children. Half of the patients are older than 50 years of age and often suffer from other comorbid diseases present in this age-group. Because of this, and because the disease in older patients may be inherently more resistant to chemotherapy than that seen in younger patients, the remission and cure rate in older patients is much lower than in younger patients. Initial induction therapy usually consists of a 7-day continuous infusion of cytosine arabinoside and 3 days of the anthracycline daunorubicin. With this regimen, approximately 60 to 70 percent of patients will enter a remission. Failure to enter a remission is caused by either resistant leukemic cells that persist after therapy or death of complications of the disease or therapy, usually infection or bleeding [6]. If patients enter a complete remission, they usually receive intensive consolidation therapy, or if they are an acceptable candidate, bone marrow transplantation. Bone marrow transplantation can be carried out either by using bone marrow from a human leukocyte antigen (HLA)-matched sibling or HLA-matched unrelated donor (allogeneic) or by using the patient's remission bone marrow, often treated in vitro by either chemotherapy or monoclonal antibodies (au-

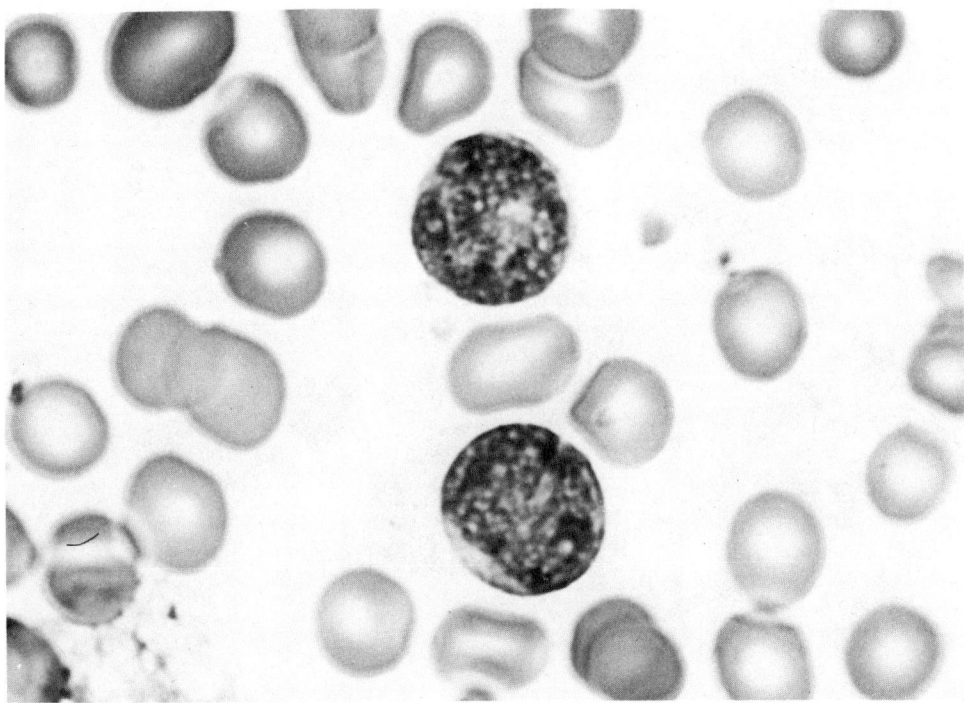

Fig. 126-1. Acute lymphoblastic leukemia. Note the scant cytoplasm and absence of granules.

tologous). The role of allogeneic and autologous transplantation in AML remains controversial, and its usage varies from one medical center to another [7].

Medical Complications of the Acute Leukemias

HYPERLEUKOCYTOSIS. In certain of the leukemias very high white blood cell counts can lead to leukostasis, resulting primarily in pulmonary or CNS compromise [8]. Patients presenting with hyperleukocytosis have a poorer prognosis and are less likely to attain a complete remission, usually because of fatal complications that can occur early in the course of treatment [9]. The likelihood of this complication arising is related to the type and size of the leukemic cell and the height of the white blood count. It occurs when the majority of cells are blasts. In addition, the hematocrit also plays a significant role in that a high hematocrit may add to whole blood viscosity.

Myeloblasts are significantly larger than lymphoblasts, and their nuclei are relatively rigid. This makes it relatively difficult for them to pass through small capillaries. This becomes much more significant when the white blood count is high, particularly over 100,000 per cubic millimeter. Therefore, in patients with AML or the myeloid blast crisis of chronic myelocytic leukemia, leukostasis must be considered a potential problem when the "blast count" (number of myeloblasts per cubic millimeter) approaches 100,000 per cubic millimeter.

Often at this level patients begin to develop respiratory compromise with pulmonary infiltrates and hypoxia. When pulmonary tissue is obtained from open lung biopsy or at autopsy, there are leukemic cell plugs in the arterioles and periarteriolar infiltrates with leukemic blasts. In any patient with leukemia and pulmonary infiltrates, infection is always a concern and must be ruled out. If the respiratory failure is attributable to leukostasis, the appropriate treatment is rapid institution of antileukemic chemotherapy.

More critical and frequent than pulmonary involvement is CNS involvement. Two major manifestations are usually seen. The first is impaired mental status due to leukostasis within the cerebral circulation. The patient typically has a blast count well in excess of 100,000 per cubic millimeter and is lethargic and disoriented but usually will not have focal neurologic signs. The treatment is reduction of the leukemic blast count with chemotherapy and, in severe cases, radiation therapy given to

Table 126-1. Classification of Acute Lymphoblastic Leukemia

Type	CALLA	Cytoplasmic Ig	T cell markers	% Pts
Pre-B Cell	Positive	Negative	Negative	70
T Cell	Negative (or Positive)	Negative	Positive	25
B Cell	Positive	Positive	Negative	<5

CALLA = common acute lymphoblastic leukemia antigen or CD10; Cytoplasmic Ig = cytoplasmic immunoglobulin.

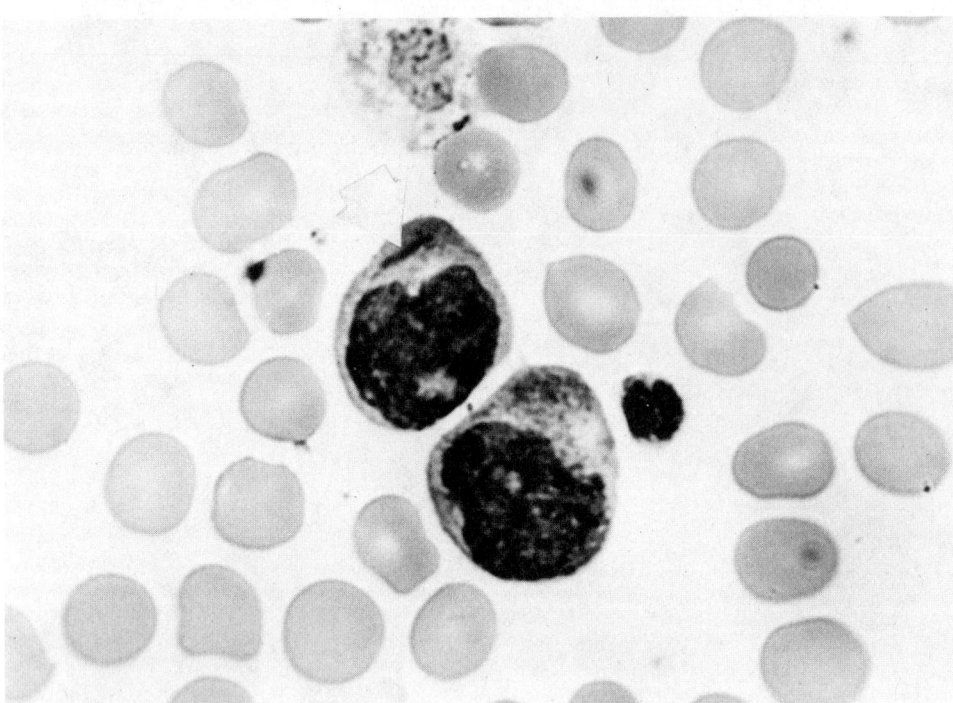

Fig. 126-2. Acute myeloblastic leukemia. An Auer rod present in the cytoplasm of the myeloblast at right is indicated by the arrow.

the brain and brainstem. With rapid institution of treatment, the neurologic signs will often disappear, and a full recovery can be seen. More devastating is CNS hemorrhage. The incidence of hemorrhage at the time of diagnosis and initiation of treatment is also closely related to the height of the blast count.

Patients with high blast counts are more likely to die early in induction therapy, and either pulmonary or CNS hemorrhage is usually the cause of death [10]. In the patient with hyperleukocytosis and evidence of leukostasis, prompt antileukemic therapy is indicated. Although some physicians use hydroxyurea as an initial means of lowering the blast count, most institute standard antileukemic therapy, which, in the previously untreated patient, usually lowers the blast count as rapidly. The role of leukopheresis is controversial. It can certainly lower the circulating leukemic cell concentration transiently and is used regularly in some institutions, but it has never been conclusively shown to diminish complications or improve survival when used in this circumstance.

Because leukostasis is dependent not only on the concentration of leukemic blasts in the blood but also on the whole blood

Table 126-2. Classification of Acute Myelocytic Leukemia

FAB Classification	Morphology	% Pts
M1	Myeloblastic without differentiation	29
M2	Myeloblastic with differentiation	30
M3	Promyelocytic	6
M4	Myelomonocytic	29
M5	Monocytic	6
M6	Erythroid	<1
M7	Megakaryocytic	<1

FAB = French-American-British Classification.

viscosity, there must be careful management of the hematocrit in these patients. Transfusion with red blood cells may cause a patient's condition to worsen acutely because of the increased viscosity caused by the increased hematocrit together with the high leukemic blast count. Therefore, if the patient can tolerate the degree of anemia present, red blood cell transfusions should be delayed until the blast count is reduced.

DISSEMINATED INTRAVASCULAR COAGULATION. Disseminated intravascular coagulation can be a serious complication in the patient with acute leukemia. Often this is a result of systemic bacterial or fungal infection. In these cases the DIC is usually mild to moderate, and the control of the DIC is dependent on the ability to control the underlying infection. As discussed later, prompt institution of antimicrobial therapy is essential to control serious infections in patients with acute leukemia of any variety.

Patients with acute promyelocytic leukemia (FAB classification M3) are particularly prone to develop DIC because of the release of a procoagulant from the primary azurophilic granules of leukemic promyeloblasts [11,12]. The prothrombin time (PT) and partial thromboplastin time (PTT) are often elevated, and there is usually thrombocytopenia and hypofibrinogenemia. Bleeding can be severe and occasionally is rapidly fatal. DIC often worsens as therapy is initiated because an increased amount of procoagulant is released when the leukemic blasts are lysed. When hypofibrinogenemia is present along with an elevated PT and PTT, the missing coagulation factors should be aggressively replaced with fresh frozen plasma, and if thrombocytopenia is present, then platelet transfusions should also be given. Prompt institution of antileukemic therapy is crucial because eradication of the leukemic blasts is the only means to stop DIC from continuing. The role of heparin in these patients is controversial. Although it counteracts the procoagulant activity present, there are no controlled studies to suggest that its use is beneficial in decreasing hemorrhage or improving survival.

NEUTROPENIA AND FEVER. Patients are often neutropenic at diagnosis because of involvement of the bone marrow with leukemic cells or during treatment because of the bone marrow suppressive effects of antileukemic therapy. Whatever the cause, neutropenia, as defined as an absolute granulocyte count of less than 500 per cubic millimeter, leaves the patient with poor defenses against bacterial or fungal infection. In the neutropenic patient, fever of greater than 100.5°F should be promptly evaluated with a physical examination, chest x-ray, and blood and urine cultures. It is important to remember that because the patient is neutropenic, there may not be an inflammatory response at a site of infection. Pyuria may not be present with a urinary tract infection, and so urine should be cultured even in the absence of white cells. After these tests are quickly performed, antibiotic therapy should be instituted. Many antibiotic regimens are now acceptable as first-line therapy, but these often include a synthetic penicillin such as ticarcillin or mezlocillin and an aminoglycoside such as gentamicin [13,14]. If a bacterial organism is subsequently identified, it is still preferable to use two antibiotic agents to which the organism is sensitive. Antibiotics must be continued until the granulocyte count is greater than 500 per cubic millimeter, even if fever resolves and there is no obvious site of infection [15].

In the patient who is persistently neutropenic and febrile and receiving multiple antibacterials, a repeat evaluation is necessary, including a careful physical examination looking for signs of soft tissue infection, particularly in the perirectal area, a chest x-ray, and repeat blood and urine cultures [16,17]. If no bacterial infection is found and neutropenia and fever persist, amphotericin may be added as an antifungal agent even in the absence of documented fungal infection. The timing of the addition of amphotericin in these patients is subject to judgment concerning the individual case.

Severe infection sometimes leads to septic shock, with hypotension, increased vascular permeability, third spacing of fluid in the lungs and other tissues, renal failure, and DIC. Administration of fluids, cardiotropic agents, and blood products may be necessary. Broad-spectrum antibiotic coverage should continue. Routine white blood cell transfusions are no longer considered appropriate in most patients. They are not clearly efficacious, are difficult to obtain, and can be hazardous to the recipient.

THROMBOCYTOPENIA. As with neutropenia, thrombocytopenia can be present either because of replacement of the bone marrow with leukemic blasts or because of suppressive effects of antileukemic therapy. When the platelet count falls below 20,000 per cubic millimeter, the incidence of serious spontaneous hemorrhage increases and platelet transfusions should be initiated. Single-donor platelets should be used when possible to minimize blood cell antigen exposure and, it is hoped, to delay or prevent alloimmunization. In the event of alloimmunization and a resultant poor response to platelet transfusion, platelets obtained from HLA-matched donors may improve the response as well as platelets obtained from family members. Family members should not be used as blood donors if the patient is being considered for allogeneic bone marrow transplantation because of a desire not to expose a patient to potential donor antigens.

TUMOR LYSIS SYNDROME. When patients with a high leukemic cell burden are treated with chemotherapy, large numbers of leukemic cells can be rapidly destroyed. This can result in a number of metabolic problems, including hyperuricemia, hypokalemia, hypocalcemia, and rarely, hyperkalemia [18,19]. These disorders are addressed individually.

Hyperuricemia. Patients often present with hyperuricemia because of the increased metabolic activity and large cellular burden of their leukemic blasts. In addition, with the initiation of antileukemic therapy and the destruction of the leukemic blasts, there is often a rapid increase in the serum uric acid level. Hyperuricemia can rapidly cause renal failure, leading to further elevation of the uric acid because of the renal failure. This can be prevented by the administration of allopurinol before the initiation of antileukemic therapy at a dose of 300 mg per day. This should be begun 24 hours before the initiation of chemotherapy when possible, and the patient should be well hydrated and the urine alkalinized if the uric acid level is high, because uric acid is more soluble in alkaline urine.

Hyponatremia. Hyponatremia is a common complication seen in patients with acute leukemia before and during treatment. There is a natriuresis suggestive of the syndrome of inappropriate secretion of antidiuretic hormone (SIADH). The mechanism for this is unclear, but the syndrome can often worsen after chemotherapy is initiated, suggesting that there may be a factor released from the leukemic cells that causes this to occur. The hyponatremia tends to be mild to moderate and resolves if the patient achieves a remission (see Chap. 79).

Hypokalemia. Hypokalemia develops in between 30 and 50 percent of patients being treated for acute leukemia (see Chap. 79). Potassium is lost in the urine, but the reason for this is not clear. It appears to happen more frequently with AML than ALL, particularly the M4 and M5 variety. This may be attributable to the release of lysozyme from the monoblasts present in these patients, but several studies have failed to show a correlation between lysozyme levels and the occurrence of hypokalemia. Aggressive replacement with potassium is essential. In addition, many of the antibiotics used today, particularly amphotericin, cause renal wasting of potassium.

Hyperkalemia. Hyperkalemia is a theoretical concern because potassium is a major intracellular constituent, which with leukemic cell lysis may be released into the blood, but clinically this does not often occur.

Hypocalcemia. Hypocalcemia is a relatively common finding in patients with high leukemic blast counts who have a rapid reduction in the leukemic cell burden from chemotherapy. The mechanism is not entirely clear but may relate to binding of calcium by phosphate that is lost by the degenerating leukemic cells and may also be due to renal loss (see Chap. 114). On occasion when large numbers of leukemic blasts are rapidly lysed, the calcium can fall to critical levels and even result in tetany. In spite of the high phosphate levels, calcium must be replaced, and patients need to be observed carefully for respiratory compromise secondary to tetany.

Hypercalcemia. On rare occasions hypercalcemia is present in acute leukemia. This is usually seen when the leukemic blast counts are high. Hypercalcemia is more often encountered in the blast crisis phase of chronic myelogenous leukemia. The treatment should focus both on control of the leukemia and on the usual treatments for hypercalcemia, including fluid administration, diuretics, diphosphonates, and calcitonin (see Chap. 114).

SIDE EFFECTS OF CHEMOTHERAPEUTIC AGENTS. Specific treatment programs for patients with acute leukemia are constantly changing. Not only are new drugs being used, but new dose schedules and combinations of old drugs are also being used. Because of this, toxic effects of these drugs are continually changing. In this section we list some of the more commonly used drugs and their major important side effects (Table 126-3). This is not meant to be an exhaustive list of the toxic effects of these drugs, but merely a highlighting of major toxic effects now known. In the case of the individual patient, it is always important to remember that these drugs are extremely potent, and expert consultation is indicated to attempt to identify the causes of toxic effects being seen.

Almost all the drugs used in the treatment of acute leukemias are bone marrow suppressants. Neutropenia and thrombocytopenia have been mentioned previously and are dealt with at greater length elsewhere in this text; therefore they are not included in the discussion of the individual medications.

Many of the medications listed are tissue vesicants and can result in severe soft tissue damage if extravasation occurs during administration [20]. These agents should be administered by persons experienced in their delivery, and if extravasation occurs, prompt consultation with the appropriate experts is indicated.

Cytosine Arabinoside (Cytarabine, Ara-C). This drug is a cycle active agent that inhibits DNA replication [21]. Cytosine arabinoside is used in many different dose schedules, resulting in different toxicities. Particularly when used in high-bolus dosage (so-called high-dose Ara-C or HiDAC), it can cause severe intestinal mucositis. In the worst cases there can be extensive denuding of the small and large intestine, resulting in ileus and gram-negative sepsis. Abdominal pain and diarrhea are usually present as well as fever. Unfortunately this usually occurs at the same time the patient becomes neutropenic, and the mortality rate is very high. High doses of this drug can also cause CNS toxicity, particularly cerebellar toxicity [22]. This is usually reversible but can be permanent. Patients older than 60 years are particularly prone to this complication. Hepatic toxicity is

also seen with an elevation of the transaminases and alkaline phosphatase, although this is usually mild and reversible. Some patients have a febrile reaction to this drug that in rare cases can be severe.

Anthracyclines and Anthraquinones (Doxorubicin, Daunorubicin, Mitoxantrone). These drugs bind to DNA and inhibit DNA replication, but the binding is not dependent on active DNA replication being present at the time of drug administration. All of these agents are cardiotoxic, and the likelihood of cardiotoxicity occurring increases with increasing total cumulative dose administered, though in the individual patient the dose causing cardiotoxicity is unpredictable [23]. Echocardiography, thallium scans, and other tests of cardiac function do not predict who will develop cardiac toxicity or when they will develop it. When it occurs, cardiomyopathy will often be sudden in onset with a rapid fall in the ejection fraction and cardiac output and is relatively resistant to the usual medications employed in the treatment of congestive heart failure, although they should be tried in any case. Cardiomyopathy is often rapidly fatal. Because these agents are metabolized to inactive by-products in the liver, they can be significantly more toxic when hepatic dysfunction is present. In patients with hepatic failure, bilirubin can be used to try to estimate an appropriate dose reduction, but these agents should be administered with extreme caution to anyone with liver failure.

Vincristine. This vinca alkaloid is an inhibitor of microtubular formation. It does not suppress the bone marrow in conventional doses. Vincristine is neurotoxic, causing peripheral neuropathy with decreased reflexes, impaired sensation, and pain. The occurrence of these findings is related to the height of individual doses, the frequency of administration, and the total cumulative dose. In most circumstances these findings resolve with time, although this may take months to years. An autonomic neuropathy can occur, sometimes leading to a profound intestinal ileus, functional small bowel obstruction, and, rarely, perforation.

Methotrexate. This drug is an inhibitor of dihydrofolate reductase. Toxicity includes mucositis, which can be severe, hepatitis, and less frequently pulmonary fibrosis. Increased toxicity can occur when it is administered to patients with pleural effusions, ascites, or other fluid collections. In these cases the methotrexate accumulates in these reservoirs and slowly reenters the circulation. This prolonged exposure is particularly toxic to the mucous membranes and bone marrow. Sometimes methotrexate is intentionally given in very high doses followed by administration of the antidote folinic acid (leucovorin), which bypasses the metabolic block. When given in high doses, it can cause renal failure, which further increases the toxicity of the drug because of decreased drug secretion in the urine. When used in this manner, the timely administration of folinic acid is essential, because a delay in its use can cause disastrous effects that cannot always be reversed by its subsequent administration. With serious methotrexate toxicity, intravenous folinic acid should be promptly administered and continued until methotrexate blood levels become undetectable.

Cyclophosphamide. This drug binds to DNA, inhibiting duplication at the time of cell replication. It is metabolized to its active form in the liver and excreted in the urine. It can be toxic to the bladder mucosa, and the likelihood of bladder toxicity occurring depends on the drug concentration in the urine and the length of time the urine remains in the bladder. When given in high doses, aggressive intravenous hydration is necessary to dilute the drug in the resulting urine. In the case of administra-

Table 126-3. Toxicities of Selected Chemotherapeutic Agents

Cytosine arabinoside	Bone marrow suppression
	Mucositis
	Neurotoxicity
	Hepatic toxicity
	Fever
Anthracyclines and anthraquinones	Bone marrow suppression
	Local tissue injury
	Mucositis
	Cardiomyopathy
Vincristine	Neurotoxicity
	Autonomic paralytic ileus
Methotrexate	Bone marrow suppression
	Mucositis
	Hepatitis
	Renal failure
Cyclophosphamide	Bone marrow suppression
	Hemorrhagic cystitis
	Cardiac toxicity
L-Asparaginase	Pancreatitis
	Hyperglycemia
	Coagulopathy
	Anaphylaxis
Etoposide	Bone marrow suppression
	Local tissue injury
	Cardiac arrhythmias
	Anaphylactic type 1 reaction

tion of very high doses, bladder catheterization may be indicated using a three-way Foley and continuous irrigation. At very high doses given over a short period, the drug can also be cardiotoxic [24].

L-Asparaginase. This bacterial by-product is frequently used in the treatment of ALL and less commonly in the treatment of AML. Because it is a foreign protein, anaphylaxis is always a risk, particularly when given intravenously. Appropriate resuscitative drugs and equipment should always be present during administration. The drug can also cause pancreatitis and hyperglycemia. Coagulation abnormalities can occur, and although they are often associated with mildly elevated PT and PTT, hypercoagulability is a greater concern [25].

Etoposide (VP-16). This agent can cause severe mucositis. Rapid administration can cause cardiac arrhythmias, probably secondary to other agents used in its preparation. Because of this the drug needs to be administered very slowly. Usually doses should be given over 45 to 60 minutes. Anaphylactic-like, type 1 reactions, consisting of urticaria, angioedema, flushing, rash, and hypotension, can occur to etoposide, even with the first dose administered [26]. These reactions tend not to be severe, are almost never fatal, and, when necessary, etoposide can usually be safely administered with steroid and diphenhydramine premedication in a patient with a previous allergic reaction.

References

1. Champlin R, Gale RP: Acute lymphoblastic leukemia: Recent advances in biology and therapy. *Blood* 73:2051, 1989.
2. Champlin R, Gale RP: Acute myelogenous leukemia: Recent advances in therapy. *Blood* 69:1551, 1987.
3. Fletcher A, Lynch E, Kimball V, et al: Translocation (9;22) is associated with extremely poor prognosis in intensively treated children with acute lymphoblastic leukemia. *Blood* 77:435, 1991.
4. Hoelzer D, Thiel E, Loffler H, et al: Intensified therapy in acute lymphoblastic and acute undifferentiated leukemia in adults. *Blood* 64:38, 1984.
5. Burns CP, Armitage JO, Frey AL, et al: Analysis of the presenting features of adult acute leukemia: The French-American-British classification. *Cancer* 47:2460, 1981.
6. Estey EH, Keating MJ, McCredie KB, et al: Causes of initial remission induction failure in acute myelogenous leukemia. *Blood* 60:309, 1982.
7. Santos GW: Marrow transplantation in acute nonlymphocytic leukemia. *Blood* 74:901, 1989.
8. Lichtman MA, Rowe JM: Hyperleukocytic leukemias: Rheological, clinical and therapeutic considerations. *Blood* 60:279, 1982.
9. Dutcher JP, Schiffer CA, Wiernik PH: Hyperleukocytosis in adult acute nonlymphocytic leukemia: Impact on remission rate and duration, and survival. *J Clin Oncol* 5:1364, 1987.
10. Creutzig U, Ritter J, Budde M, et al: Early deaths due to hemorrhage and leukostasis in childhood acute myelogenous leukemia. *Cancer* 60:3071, 1987.
11. Bauer KA, Rosenberg RD: Thrombin generation in acute promyelocytic leukemia. *Blood* 64:791, 1984.
12. Collins AJ, Bloomfield CD, Peterson BA, et al: Acute promyelocytic leukemia: Management of the coagulopathy during daunorubicin-prednisone remission induction. *Arch Intern Med* 138:1677, 1978.
13. Pizzo PA, Commers J, Cotton D, et al: Approaching the controversies in antibacterial management of cancer patients. *Am J Med* 76:436, 1984.
14. O'Hanley P, Easaw J, Rugo H, et al: Infectious disease management of adult leukemic patients undergoing chemotherapy: 1982–1986 experience at Stanford University Hospital. *Am J Med* 87:605, 1989.
15. Pizzo PA, Robichard KJ, Gill FA, et al: Duration of empiric antibiotic therapy in granulocytopenic patients with cancer. *Am J Med* 67:194, 1979.
16. Kramer BS, Pizzo PA, Robichaud KJ, et al: Role of serial microbiologic surveillance and clinical evaluation in the management of cancer patients with fever and granulocytopenia. *Am J Med* 72:561, 1982.
17. Barnes SG, Sattler FR, Ballard JO: Perirectal infections in acute leukemia: Improved survival after incision and debridement. *Ann Intern Med* 100:515, 1984.
18. Mir MA, Delamore IW: Metabolic disorders in acute myeloid leukaemia. *Br J Haematol* 40:79, 1978.
19. O'Regan S, Carson S, Chesney RW, et al: Electrolyte and acid-base disturbances in the management of leukemia. *Blood* 49:345, 1977.
20. Rudolph R, Larson DL: Etiology and treatment of chemotherapeutic agent extravasation injuries: A review. *J Clin Oncol* 5:1116, 1987.
21. Kremer WB: Cytarabine. *Ann Intern Med* 82:684, 1975.
22. Salinsky MC, Levine RL, Aubuchon JP, et al: Acute cerebellar dysfunction with high-dose Ara-C therapy. *Cancer* 51:426, 1983.
23. Schwartz RG, McKenzie WB, Alexander J, et al: Congestive heart failure and left ventricular dysfunction complicating doxorubicin therapy. *Am J Med* 82:1109, 1987.
24. Goldberg MA, Antin JH, Guinan EC, et al: Cyclophosphamide cardiotoxicity: An analysis of dosing as a risk factor. *Blood* 68:1114, 1986.
25. Homans AC, Rybak ME, Baglini RL, et al: Effect of L-asparaginase administration on coagulation and platelet function in children with leukemia. *J Clin Oncol* 5:811, 1987.
26. Kellie SJ, Crist WM, Pui CH, et al: Hypersensitivity reactions to epipodophyllotoxins in children with acute lymphoblastic leukemia. *Cancer* 67:1070, 1991.

127. Oncologic Emergencies

Harry L. Greene and Ana Maria Lopez

The concept of an *oncologic emergency* is one that has emerged over the past 30 years. At one time, it referred to either the mode of presentation or a preterminal occurrence in the natural history of a cancer. Recently, as cancers have become curable or successfully palliated with aggressive therapy, the term evolved to indicate events that are directly related to, or are complications of, this therapy. The oncologic emergencies to be discussed in this chapter are superior vena cava syndrome,

epidural spinal cord compression from metastatic tumors, hypercalcemia of malignancy, and malignant pericardial effusion.

The challenge to the intensive care physician faced with an oncologic emergency is to know when to apply the skill, technology, and aggressive measures available versus when to focus on measures of comfort. The decision is best made in collaboration with the primary care physician and an oncologist after the following questions have been answered: (1) What is the tumor type? (2) What is the extent of the disease? (3) Is curative or palliative therapy available? (4) Is cure or palliation a reasonable possibility in this patient? (5) What is the stage of the disease? (6) What are the patient's and family's wishes? (7) Are we simply trading modes of death? (8) Is this emergency cancer related?

Superior Vena Cava Syndrome

The superior vena cava (SVC) syndrome was first described by William Hunter in 1757 in a patient with obstructed venous return in the superior vena cava caused by a syphilitic aortic aneurysm. Any process that blocks the return of blood through the superior vena cava produces venous hypertension distal to the block and causes dilation of collateral vessels. This plethora of hypertensive, dilated, vessels, wending their way under the skin of the patient's body or through his or her vital structures, produces the signs and symptoms of SVC syndrome. The superior vena cava syndrome has gone from the category of an oncologic emergency to that of an oncologic urgency. Whether it is emergent or urgent is dependent on the rate of symptom development.

ETIOLOGY. The etiologies of the SVC syndrome have changed in frequency over time. In older series, fibrosing mediastinitis, aneurysm, pericarditis, infections, and tuberculosis were more prominent. In more recent series malignancy constitutes 78 percent of cases of SVC; other causes are mediastinal fibrosis (11%), thrombosis (7%), inflammatory lymph nodes (2%), radiation fibrosis (1%), and idiopathic (1%) [1].

Among the neoplasms (Table 127-1), bronchogenic cancer is

Table 127-1. Malignancies Causing Obstruction in the Superior Vena Cava Syndrome (67 cases)

Malignancy	No. patients
Lung (45 patients)	
Squamous cell carcinoma	12
Adenocarcinoma	11
Small cell carcinoma	12
Large cell carcinoma	8
Intermediate cell, undifferentiated cancer	2
Breast (7 patients)	
Adenocarcinoma	7
Lymphoma (8 patients)	
Lymphoblastic	4
Diffuse mixed	1
Histiocytic	1
Hodgkin's	1
Diffuse, well-differentiated lymphocytic	1
Thymus (2 patients)	
Malignant lymphocytic thymoma	1
Carcinoid	1
Testicular (3 patients)	
Embryonal cell carcinoma	1
Anaplastic seminoma	1
Spermatocytic seminoma	1
Unknown primary (2 patients)	
Adenocarcinoma	1
Anaplastic carcinoma	1

Source: Adapted from Paris JM, Marshke RF, Dines DL, et al: Etiologic considerations in superior vena cava syndrome. *Mayo Clin Proc* 56:407, 1981.

the most common cause of SVC syndrome (70%) with oat cell as the predominant cell type. Squamous cell, adenocarcinoma, and large cell neoplasms constitute, in decreasing frequency, the remaining lung cancer causes of superior vena cava syndrome. After lung cancer, lymphoma is next in frequency, followed in decreasing occurrence by breast cancer, thymic tumors, testicular cancer, and metastasis from an unknown primary. Of the benign causes of SVC syndrome, constituting less than 20 percent in most series, etiologies include dermoid, teratoma, thymoma, mediastinal fibrosis secondary to previous tuberculosis, actinomycosis, histoplasmosis, thyroiditis, thrombosis, sarcoidosis, inflammatory lymph nodes, sclerosing cholangitis, Peyronie's disease, and radiation fibrosis [2]. In the instances of SVC syndrome caused by thrombosis [3], an increasing number are caused by indwelling catheters for cardiac pacing, Swan-Ganz catheterization, peritoneal-venous shunts [4], central venous pressure lines, chemotherapy, or hyperalimentation cannulas. Other thrombotic causes include Behcet's, polycythemia vera, and paroxysmal noturnal hemoglobinuria.

PATHOPHYSIOLOGY. Any process that prevents blood from returning through the superior vena cava can produce SVC syndrome. These processes may be divided into intrinsic (e.g., thrombosis) or obstruction due to intraluminal catheters or direct tumor growth into, or along, the superior vena cava. Extrinsic processes that produce collapse of the SVC, such as trauma with hematoma, mediastinal or right hilar tumor growth, or lymph node enlargement, may also occlude the SVC.

The SVC is particularly subject to obstruction because of its thin walls, its low pressure, and the fact that it is surrounded by relatively firm nondistensible neighboring anatomic structures, such as the trachea, the sternum, the right mainstem bronchus, the ascending aorta, and the lymph nodes. The rate of development of the SVC syndrome depends on the rate of growth of the etiologic process. Those processes that are slow growing, such as benign tumors, often give adequate time for collateral compensation to develop. The malignant process usually occurs faster and may produce more dramatic symptoms.

An important concern in the pathophysiology of the syndrome is the location of the block with respect to the opening of the azygos system into the SVC (Fig. 127-1). If the block allows the azygos to function as a bypass system, most of the signs and symptoms are in the supraepigastric region. If, however, the azygos access to the SVC is impaired, the collaterals must flow inferiorly and find their way to the inferior vena cava and then back to the right atrium. Because of the circuitous nature of this flow, these patients are at greater risk than those in whom the azygos inlet is patent [5].

CLINICAL MANIFESTATIONS. The common symptoms of the SVC syndrome (Table 127-2) are related to poor venous return, increased intravenous pressure, collateral development, and a background of impaired pulmonary or cardiac function. Among the malignant etiology group, most admit to heavy smoking, with those who smoke two or more packs per day often presenting with oat cell carcinoma. Most patients are dyspneic. A change in cough or sputum production may suggest the lung as the etiology of the malignancy. Orthopnea is a common complaint in those with SVC syndrome, and the symptom may be increased in the prone position.

An astute patient will notice a collar that does not fit well or a necklace that begins to choke as the neck becomes engorged. If unilateral swelling takes place, one arm or hand may be difficult to get into a blouse or shirt sleeve or a glove may fit too tightly. Sometimes a spouse or friend may comment on the prominent venous pattern over the chest. As the cerebral ve-

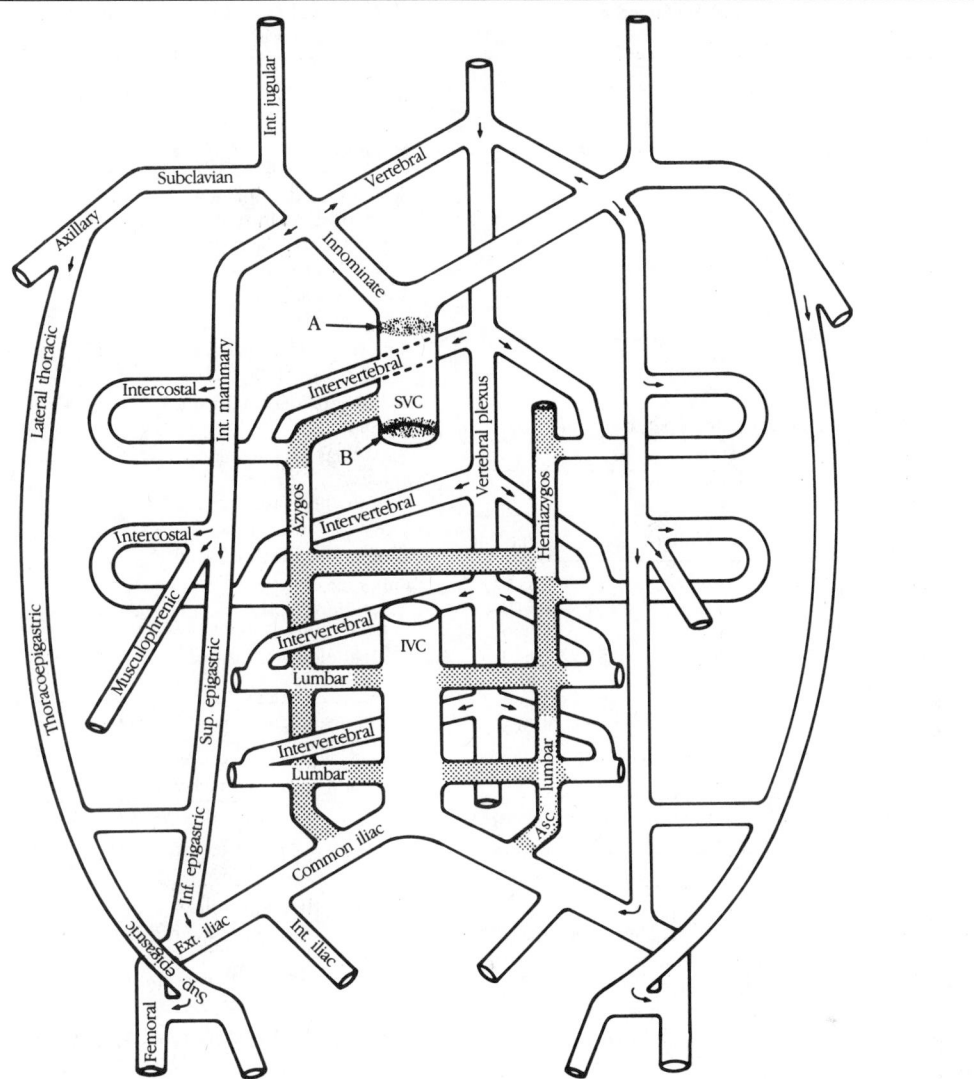

Fig. 127-1. Venous collateral system in superior vena cava (SVC) obstruction. Obstruction of the SVC at point A causes the blood to bypass the obstruction and return to the right atrium via the azygous system. Blockage at point B is much more severe because it causes the inferior vena cava (IVC) to become the only remaining major bypass route.

nous pressure begins to increase, headaches and nightmares may be noted, which are lessened when sleeping upright. A sense of vertigo, drowsiness, dry eyes, or teary eyes may be noted before lethargy is manifested. Chest pain is frequently mentioned.

Some patients with malignant etiologies will complain of back or rib pain, with the tumor tracking along the collateral veins of the lumbar or intercostal region to invade bone. Those with lymphomas may give a history of night sweats, fever, node swelling, weight loss, or pruritus. Those with benign etiologies may have had a goiter, previous tuberculosis, histoplasmosis, or an indwelling intravenous line (catheter or wire). For some, a previous history of chest trauma, thoracic surgery, or radiation therapy may help with the diagnosis. Patients may have noted a change in voice caused by laryngeal edema, or difficulty in swallowing caused by esophageal edema or invasion. Occasional patients will have had syncope.

Physical findings show increased respiratory rate and a mild tachycardia. Neck veins are prominent. Heart sounds are usually normal, but if diminished, coincident pericardial effusion must be considered.

The physical findings characteristic of the syndrome (Table 127-3) are edema of head, neck, arm(s), and trunk with dilated collateral vessels of the upper thorax if the lesion does not obstruct the azygous inlet [6]. The anterior abdominal vessels will be prominent if the azygos is obstructed with venous filling, which would flow from the thorax to the abdomen. The direction in which the abdominal vessels fill can be determined if the veins are flattened and allowed to refill. The supraclavicular fossae may be quite full, chemosis may be present, and facial plethora is common. Some patients appear cyanotic when desaturation of hemoglobin occurs because of slow flow. Some have a paralyzed vocal cord caused by impingement on the laryngeal or recurrent laryngeal nerve. A small percentage have Horner's syndrome.

DIAGNOSIS. The diagnosis of the SVC syndrome is strongly suggested by the characteristic signs and symptoms just described, and it is documented by demonstrating SVC obstruc-

Table 127-2. Common Symptoms of the Superior Vena Cava Syndrome

Symptom	Incidence (%)
Facial swelling	43
Trunk and/or extremity swelling	40
Dyspnea	20
Chest pain	20
Cough	20
Dysphagia	20
Dizziness	10
Syncope	10
Visual disturbance	10

Table 127-3. Physical Findings of the Superior Vena Cava Syndrome

Finding	Patients	
	Number	Percent
Thorax vein distention	56	67.0
Neck vein distention	49	59.0
Edema of face	47	56.0
Tachypnea	34	40.0
Plethora of face	16	19.0
Cyanosis	13	15.0
Edema of upper extremities	8	9.5
Paralyzed true vocal cord	3	3.5
Homer's syndrome	2	2.3

Source: Adapted from Perez CA, Presant CA, VanAmburg AL III: Management of superior vena cava syndrome. *Semin Oncol* 2:124, 1978.

Table 127-4. Chest X-ray Findings of the Superior Vena Cava Syndrome

Findings	No. patients		
	Bronchogenic carcinoma	Lymphoma	Total
Superior mediastinal mass (± pleural effusions or pulmonary lesions except right upper lobe)	10	12	32
Superior mediastinal and hilar mass	11	2	13
Superior mediastinal and right upper lobe mass	2		2
Superior mediastinal, right upper lobe, and hilar mass	2		2
Right hilar (or parahilar) mass			
With atelectasis	6		6
Without atelectasis	13		13
Bilateral hilar adenopathy	1		1
Other masses			
Left upper lobe	2		2
Right middle lobe	1		1
Right pleural effusion	1		1
Total	59*	14	73

* Pretreatment chest x-rays were not available for review on 11 patients with bronchogenic carcinoma.
Source: Adapted from Perez CA, Presant CA, VanAmburg AL III: Management of superior vena cava syndrome. *Semin Oncol* 2:124, 1978.

tion. A chest radiograph shows an abnormality more than 80 percent of the time (Table 127-4) [6]. A superior mediastinal mass can be seen in 70 percent of patients, with some also having a pleural effusion, hilar mass, or right upper lobe mass. A right hilar mass without a superior mediastinal mass is also seen about 10 percent of the time. Less frequent x-ray patterns are bilateral adenopathy, left upper lobe mass, right middle lobe masses, or isolated pleural effusion.

Lung tomography, radionuclide scans, and fluoroscopy have been used in the past but usually add little except expense to the patient's management. Superior vena cavagram can specifically localize the block, but it should be used only when doubt about treatment exists or the possibility of catheter-induced thrombosis is a consideration. The newest and probably most effective radiologic study is thoracic computed tomography (CT) with contrast. It allows visualization of the collateral system, localizes the mass, and gives clues to other possible impending complications (e.g., vertebral spread, internal jugular patency). Its major drawback is the need for the patient to be relatively immobile, and for those who are already dyspneic, any restraint may be frightening.

Plane film with coned-down views should be ordered for any symptomatic areas that do not evaluate well with CT (e.g., rib pain). Those with vertebral back pain should have myelography or magnetic resonance imaging (MRI), but if symptoms are minimal, this may be delayed until some relief of the intracerebral pressure has occurred with treatment to the thoracic mass. A delay of a few days is acceptable unless signs of the progression of back pain or neurologic symptoms develop, in which case radiation to the spine should begin as soon as possible. Other laboratory studies should include a complete blood count with differential. Some patients have myelophthisic

changes that will allow a tissue diagnosis to be made with a simple bone marrow biopsy (e.g., oat cell carcinoma, lymphoma).

DIFFERENTIAL DIAGNOSIS. After the syndrome has been diagnosed, the cause of the obstruction must be determined. Although thoracotomy will yield the etiology in virtually all patients, it is generally deferred pending other less invasive studies. In Perez' series, 63 percent of patients had positive sputum cytologies [6]. Palpable supraclavicular lymph nodes were positive on biopsy 84 percent of the time. Although palpable scalene node biopsies may be positive up to 85 percent of the time [1], in Perez' series, they were positive only 50 percent of the time [6].

Pleural effusion cytology is very helpful in those patients with effusion and has a yield up to 100 percent in some small series. One must be cautious when aspirating pleural fluid because of the frequently striking dilation of the intercostal vessels. Mediastinoscopy gives a tissue diagnosis up to 81 percent of the time. If the surgeon believes that the risks of bleeding are quite significant, however, one should proceed to limited thoracotomy rather than undertaking mediastinoscopy.

Bronchoscopy, using a flexible scope, seems to be one of the most practical approaches. It is well tolerated, affords an opportunity to view the vocal cords as well as the tracheobronchial tree, and allows for obtaining selected biopsy and cytology specimens (see Chap. 12). It gives a positive diagnosis 60 to 70 percent of the time with limited risk to the patient. As mentioned, suspicion of marrow involvement on peripheral smear should prompt a bone marrow biopsy. In the absence of myelophthisic changes or cytopenia, its yield will be low. Any suspicious skin nodules should be considered for biopsy because up to 10 percent of SVC syndrome may be caused by metastatic disease.

In summary, the histologic diagnosis should be made by the simplest, least invasive method available, beginning with sputum cytologies, pleural fluid analysis, skin or nodule biopsy, lymph node biopsy, and proceeding to bronchoscopy and finally to limited thoracotomy if necessary.

TREATMENT. Current practice dictates radiation and chemotherapy or radiation alone as a first approach to small cell carcinoma, lymphoma, and other lung neoplasms that cause severe SVC symptoms. Milder forms of SVC syndrome with chemotherapy-responsive tumors may be treated with chemotherapy first. After resolution of the obstruction, therapy reverts to that which is appropriate for the primary process. For those patients who have recurrence and for whom active agents or further radiation therapy is not a consideration, the focus should be on palliation and comfort.

The mainstay of therapy has been radiation, with daily fractions of 400 cGy for 3 or 4 days followed by decreasing doses of 150 cGy to 200 cGY per day until a total dose of 3000 cGy to 5000 cGy is achieved. The dose and rate are determined by the histology (e.g., small cell carcinoma and lymphoma often respond at lower doses than squamous cell carcinoma). Lower doses may be given that are dependent on other factors, such as prior chemotherapy, the patient's general condition, cytopenias, and tolerance for radiation therapy. The portals are constructed to encompass the tumor, the adjacent nodes, and any parenchymal lesions.

Treatments are usually given in five fractions per week, with the response observable in 3 to 5 days in the more radiosensitive histologies and by 7 days in the squamous histologies. Failure of response often suggests intravenous thrombosis as a complication of obstruction, a squamous histology, or prior treatment with recurrence. Table 127-5 shows the subjective and objective response rates in one series of 35 patients [7].

Chemotherapy has been used successfully without radiation therapy for the treatment of SVC syndrome caused by small cell carcinoma of the lung, but success is limited. Those patients who have responded in our own series have done so in 3 to 5 days. It remains to be seen whether this will be the treatment of choice for this type of cancer in the future.

Recent reports have called attention to the increasing incidence of SVC syndrome caused by thrombosis from indwelling catheters and wires [3,4]. For venous thrombosis, intravenous streptokinase has been given to produce fibrinolysis and resolution of the obstruction [3]. This enzyme has more theoretic appeal than the use of heparin, which prevents propagation of clot, but does little to resolve it.

The symptoms of SVC syndrome should be treated. Hypoxia is relieved with oxygen administration, and cerebral edema is treated with decadron, 4 to 8 mg orally or IV every 6 hours.

Table 127-5. Subjective and Objective Response of Superior Vena Cava Obstruction to Radiation Therapy

Type of response	Patients	Days to respond	Percent response
Subjective	27/35	3–4	77
	32/35	7	91
Objective	23/35	7	66
	31/35	14	89

Source: Adapted from Davenport D, Ferree C, Blake D, et al: Radiation therapy in the treatment of superior vena cava obstruction. *Cancer* 42:2600, 1978.

Decadron should be rapidly tapered with a usual course continuing for 3 days to a week. Steroids should not be used unless clearly indicated because of risks of fungal and *Pneumocystis carinii* infections. Some have advocated the use of diuretics, but there is little to be gained from their use because of the risk of depleting the intravascular volume and converting a partial SVC obstruction to a complete one. Attempts to reconstruct the SVC or to bypass it surgically usually are of short-lived efficacy and should be avoided except in highly selected situations [8]. Local relapse may occur in up to 20 percent of small cell lung cancer patients and 10 percent of those with other lung histologies. It is a rare occurrence in treated lymphoma patients.

The overall survival in most series is heavily related to the etiology. In the Mayo Clinic series of 86 patients, 55 died, and 50 patients had malignant diseases [1]. The average survival in this group was 7.7 months. In the Oncologic Mallinkrodt Institute series, 25 percent of patients survived to 1 year, and 10 percent were still alive at 30 months after therapy [4]. The histology was shown to be of importance, with 45 percent of lymphoma patients surviving to 30 months. Only 10 percent of bronchogenic lung cancer patients survived this long. Those with small cell carcinoma did better than those with other lung histologies [4]. The cause of death in those with recurrent or refractory SVC syndrome was cerebral anoxia, failure of the respiratory center with respiratory arrest, suffocation from laryngeal and tracheal edema, infection, or bleeding.

Epidural Spinal Cord Compression from Metastatic Tumors

As the survival of cancer patients has improved, metastatic epidural tumors that compress the spinal cord have emerged as an important cause of morbidity. Once suspected, their evaluation and management is a true oncologic emergency. The incidence of tumors that invade the epidural space in known cancer patients is estimated to be 5 percent at autopsy or 20,000 patients per year in the United States [9,10]. Although spinal metastases are rarely the cause of death in patients who are affected, the neurologic deficits and the pain that results from such metastases significantly diminish the functional quality of the patients' lives, especially because 30 percent of patients with documented spinal cord compression survive beyond 1 year. The interval between the diagnosis of cancer and the development of spinal cord compression varied from 0 to 19 years in one study of 130 patients.

ETIOLOGY AND PATHOPHYSIOLOGY. The lymphomas and multiple myeloma constitute most of the cases where spinal cord compression is the presenting sign of cancer in adults [11–14]. The most common tumors to cause spinal cord compression in children are lymphoma, sarcoma, and neuroblastoma [10]. Frequently, metastases originate in the vertebral body and extend posteriorly into the epidural space, the dura, and the spinal cord. Metastases directly to the dura and the spinal cord occur infrequently.

Primary tumors of the dura and the spinal cord are rare and represent only a small percentage of tumors that cause spinal cord compression [15]. Solid tumors produce the great majority of metastases to the spine [16]. In order of frequency, the lung, the breast, the prostate, and the kidney constitute the most common identified primary sites. Spinal cord lesions may also be the mode of presentation for cancer metastases from an unknown primary site. Overall, the thoracic vertebrae are involved in 70 percent of spinal cord compressions, whereas the lumbosacral and cervical vertebrae account for 20 percent and 10 percent, respectively. This distribution reflects the number of vertebrae, the size of the spinal canal at each level, and the nature of the primary tumors.

The vascularity and microanatomy of the bone marrow within the vertebrae provide an environment conducive to metastases [17]. Prostate and breast cancers frequently metastasize through Batson's plexus, a valveless network of vertebral veins that communicates with the intercostal and lumbar veins. Lung cancer most commonly metastasizes to the thoracic vertebrae; in small cell lung cancer, spinal cord compression occurs in 10 percent of the cases. Colorectal cancer metastasizes primarily to the lumbosacral spine in 6 to 14 percent of cases [15].

Hematologic malignancies once represented one of the leading causes of spinal cord compression. In one series, lymphoma accounted for 18 percent of the cases from 1964 to 1970, but dropped to 6 percent of the cases from 1974 to 1976 [11]. The drop in incidence of spinal cord compression in lymphomas probably reflects the use of total nodal radiation in recent years. Spinal cord compression currently occurs in approximately 5 percent of malignant lymphoma cases [13] and 10 percent of multiple myeloma cases [15]. Neurologic complications occur three times more frequently in non-Hodgkin's lymphoma compared with Hodgkin's lymphoma [14].

The mechanisms of cord compression include (1) pressure caused by enlarging vertebral body metastases, (2) pressure from enlarging retroperitoneal lymph nodes that extend through the foramina (most common in lymphomas), (3) pressure from a pathologic vertebral fracture and dislocation, (4) severe spinal angulation after vertebral collapse, (5) pressure caused by intradural metastases (rare), and (6) vascular compromise secondary to compression or thrombosis. This latter cause results in infarction of the spinal cord and very rapid irreversible loss of function. Animal models of cord compression have shown a pathophysiology proceeding from compression of the vertebral venous plexus causing cord edema, to venous hemorrhage, demyelination, and ischemia that, after a time, become irreversible [10,18].

CLINICAL PRESENTATION.

Four cardinal symptoms characterize the presentation of spinal cord compression: pain, weakness, autonomic dysfunction, and sensory loss. Pain is the initial symptom in 82 to 97 percent of patients [9,11]. In these cases, symptoms occur 5 days to 2 years before the diagnosis of cord compression by myelography.

The pain associated with spinal metastases consists of two types. The first presents as localized tenderness and pain over the involved vertebrae. Characteristically, it is constant, can awaken the patient from sleep, is worse in the supine position, and is exacerbated by movement. The second type of pain is radicular in nature, occurring most frequently in the lumbosacral spine (90%). Cervical spine (79%) and thoracic spine (55%) metastases exhibit radicular pain less frequently [11]. The pain may be unilateral or bilateral, but when the thoracic spine is involved, the pain is most frequently bilateral. The pain may be increased by neck motion, Valsalva, or straight leg raising.

Weakness as a symptom or physical finding exists at presentation 87 percent of the time [11]. One series showed weakness to be more frequent than pain at presentation [19]. The degree of weakness can vary from minimal to paralysis, with symptoms progressing to paraplegia in less than 48 hours in some instances.

Sensory deficits rarely present as the initial symptom, but usually develop during the clinical course of the disease in most patients. Sensory deficits to pinprick, position, and vibration are usually equally represented, although the patient may retain a sensation to gross touch.

Finally, autonomic dysfunction early on manifests as constipation or obstipation, and later as loss of bowel and bladder control. It represents a late and poor prognostic sign. Approximately two-thirds of those presenting with autonomic dysfunction ultimately develop paraplegia [11]. Additional autonomic findings may be a loss of perspiration below the level of the lesions. Other symptoms such as ataxia may occur, and herpes zoster infection may develop at the level of compression, especially in lymphomas [9].

Because ambulatory status commonly denotes the most obvious sign of compression, patients often are graded for prognostic purposes. The grades are as follows: (1) symptomatic but ambulatory, (2) retention of antigravity strength but loss of ambulation, and (3) paraplegia. Generally, fewer than 5 percent of paraplegics regain their ability to ambulate [11,19]. Reversal of symptoms usually occurs opposite to the order of occurrence [16,20].

DIAGNOSIS.

Multiple diagnostic modalities are available to aid in the diagnosis of spinal cord compression. Often, when pain is the only presenting symptom, the presence of spinal metastases is established first. Plain radiographs of the spine are the easiest, quickest, and least expensive initial evaluation available, providing useful information in 80 percent of cases. Abnormalities found on plain radiographs are loss of pedicles, vertebral compression fractures, and osteoblastic or osteolytic bone lesions [21,22]. Occasionally, breast cancer may present with a mixed osteoblastic-osteolytic picture. In one study, plain radiographs of the spine accurately predicted the presence or absence of spinal epidural metastases in 83 percent of cases with a sensitivity of 81 percent and a specificity of 86 percent. Rodichok et al. recommended proceeding to myelography in the presence of pain and abnormal plain radiographs whether or not the physical examination shows abnormal findings [21].

Bone scanning has been shown to be highly sensitive but not specific for malignant disease [23,24]. Overall accuracy in one study was only 63 percent [21]. The sensitivity in another study was demonstrated by a yield of 0.4 percent false-negative bone scans compared with 9.1 percent for plain radiographs [25]. Although bone scanning may frequently uncover spinal metastases when used as a screening procedure, it does not offer detailed information with regard to bone architecture and cord compression.

CT defines in detail the anatomy of vertebrae and the extent of metastases [26]. Therefore, if myelography cannot be performed or is contraindicated, CT can provide valuable information, especially to define the extent of disease before surgery [17]. It is good at evaluating the retroperitoneal region. Magnetic resonance imaging (MRI) has been shown to be useful for identifying central nervous system cancer, and when available, may have advantages over CT scanning when metastases are suggested. It can directly image the spinal cord without contrast or radiation exposure, and it provides the best resolution of cord metastasis. Unfortunately, those with metal implants, i.e., pacemakers or surgical clips, are not candidates for this procedure [27]. Many experts believe that MRI should be the primary radiologic procedure for diagnosing the location and extent of spinal cord compression [28]. The advantages of increased sensitivity for paraspinal masses, less invasiveness, and improved tolerance for patients are compelling, but are offset by the time required to image the entire cord. Studies comparing myelography with MRI suggest an advantage for MRI [29]. Contrast-enhanced MRI is especially helpful in identifying leptomeningeal and intramedullary lesions [30].

Myelography remains the diagnostic procedure of choice in many hospitals without MRI for delineating the presence and the extent of spinal cord compression. Myelography offers the advantage of being able to detect the upper and lower levels of a lesion and of detecting multiple lesions. Pantopaque, an oily nonabsorbable contrast material, or metrizamide, a water-soluble contrast material, are the two media most commonly used. Pantopaque has the advantage of providing follow-up noninvasive examinations if left in place. Metrizamide, because of its greater solubility and diffusibility, can better distinguish stenotic lesions from complete blocks. Generally, contrast is introduced through the lumbar spine until an obstruction is encountered. The anatomy above an obstruction is then defined by a cisterna magna or cervical spinal tap. It is crucial to see the upper and lower extent of the lesion. Myelography carries a risk of further neurologic deterioration (in the presence of complete block) and possible reaction to the contrast media.

Cerebral spinal fluid analysis is primarily helpful if an elevated protein level or positive cytologic studies are found, the latter of which may be positive in cases of concomitant meningeal carcinomatosis (see Chap. 24). Lumbar puncture (LP) should be combined with myelography because the spinal fluid that is removed below a complete block may not reaccumulate, thus making a repeat LP extremely difficult. It should be evaluated for protein, glucose, cytology, cell count, Gram stain, India ink preparation, and culture studies. Neurosurgical backup should be available, because up to 8 percent of patients develop paralysis within 48 hours of lumbar puncture.

DIFFERENTIAL DIAGNOSIS. The most common causes of back pain in oncology patients are lumbar sprain, strains, and disc disease. In those who have leukopenia, vertebral or epidural abscess are considerations. In those who are thrombocytopenic or receiving anticoagulants for clotting problems, epidural hematomas are a possibility. These are often rapidly progressive and may follow attempts at lumbar puncture in thrombocytopenic patients. Retroperitoneal metastasis, paraneoplastic neuropathy, or some neurolytic chemotherapy, such as vincristine or platinum, may produce pain or may cause severe neuropathy. Paraneoplastic neuropathy, transverse myelitis caused by radiation therapy, and Guillain-Barré syndrome may all mimic epidural cord compression.

TREATMENT. Treatment of spinal cord compression secondary to metastatic tumors has been controversial for years. Initially, surgical decompression was the treatment of choice. A variety of studies have shown satisfactory results (defined as the patient's ability to ambulate) in 21 to 46 percent of patients treated primarily with surgery [11,31–35]. Operative mortality ranged from 0 to 8.7 percent, depending on patient selection [32,34,35]. Radiation therapy emerged in the 1970s, not only as a valuable adjunct to surgery, but also in many instances as the therapeutic equivalent of surgery [11,36,37,38]. It is now considered the treatment of choice with exceptions as noted below.

Response rates for radiation therapy, defined as the ability to ambulate, range from 40 to 50 percent, depending on the status of the patient at presentation and the radiosensitivity of the tumor. Radioresponsive tumors respond at rates as high as 64 percent [11]. Radiation therapy ports are generally 8 cm wide and extend approximately two vertebrae above and two below the site of compression. The total dosage varies from 2000 to 4000 cGy delivered over 2 to 4 weeks. The initial three doses are 400 to 500 cGy followed by subsequent fractions of 200 cGy [15,19,33]. Radiation therapy alone appears to be of comparable benefit to laminectomy plus radiation and in some se-

ries is better than surgery alone [39]. Radiation doses exceeding 5000 cGy may be associated with the development of myelitis.

Surgery should be considered in the following settings: (1) if relapse occurs after radiation therapy, and radiation limits have been reached, (2) if the diagnosis of malignancy or the nature of the malignancy has not been previously established, and no more easily accessible site for biopsy is present, (3) if symptoms progress during radiation therapy, and the tumor is thought to be radioresistant, (4) when, in the opinion of the radiotherapist or oncologist, respiration may be compromised by radiation (i.e., severe cervical cord lesion where little room for swelling is present), (5) when spinal cord hematoma or abscess is suspected, and (6) when lesions rapidly progress. The surgical approach can be either posterior (laminectomy) or anterior (vertebral body resection and spine stabilization with methylmethacrylate and/or metal rods). Radiation therapy is frequently given postoperatively to those having residual spinal tumor.

Corticosteroids are uniformly recommended and should be started as soon as spinal cord compression is suspected. Steroids serve two purposes: to diminish edema secondary to the compression and to prevent edema formation during radiation therapy. The appropriate dose is not established, but most physicians recommend dexamethasone 16 to 24 mg IV bolus followed by 16 to 40 mg per day in divided doses every 6 hours [11,15,16,33]. Higher dosages of 100 mg per day for 3 days with rapid tapering have been used and may be more beneficial in relieving pain [40], but no differences in neurologic outcome have been noted. One recent review suggests an intravenous dose of 10 to 100 mg of dexamethasone followed by 4 to 24 mg orally every 6 hours. The authors suggest tapering the dose by one third every 3 to 4 days.

The type of tumor has a great influence on the successful treatment of spinal cord compression. In general, lymphomas and other radiosensitive tumors, such as breast cancer, show the best response rates, ranging from 52 to 64 percent [11,31]. Non–small cell lung cancer usually is least responsive to treatment and, in one series, showed a 17 percent response rate. The presence of paraplegia diminishes response rates to less than 10 percent [11,15,16,21,31]. As mentioned, the response of symptoms and deficits usually occurs in an order opposite to occurrence [20]. Prognosis is poor in those who develop paraplegia rapidly (e.g., over 1–2 days) or in those who have been paraplegic for an extended period before treatment.

Hypercalcemia of Malignancy

Hypercalcemia, a common metabolic disturbance in oncology patients, is a heterogeneous disorder (see Chap. 114). Serum calcium can be elevated by several mechanisms, and tumors show different propensities to produce hypercalcemia. It is a potentially life-threatening complication of those tumors that are not necessarily advanced enough to directly incapacitate the patient. Hypercalcemia is readily diagnosed as well as reversible in most acute situations. Treatment depends on several nonspecific approaches to lowering serum calcium and, of course, on the institution of effective therapy for the underlying malignancy. The appearance of hypercalcemia frquently occurs late in the course of oncologic illness and in 98 percent of patients the tumor has already been identified. The median survival for this group is from 1 to 3 months [41].

ETIOLOGY. It is possible to divide oncology patients with cancer-related hypercalcemia into three classes: bone metastases present, bone metastases absent, and hematologic malignancies [42,43]. The solid tumors most often responsible for hypercalcemia due to bone metastases are carcinomas of the breast, the lung (epidermoid and large cell types), and the kidney. Hypercalcemia has also been described in association with metastatic carcinomas of the ovary, the colon, and the thyroid as well as squamous carcinomas of the head and neck, the cervix, and the esophagus [43,44].

One study concluded that approximately 15 percent of cancer patients with hypercalcemia do not have evidence of bone metastases [44]. This fraction may actually be smaller, however, because this study used x-ray rather than radionuclide bone scans to survey for metastases. The most frequently mentioned tumors associated with hypercalcemia in the absence of bone metastases are squamous cell carcinomas of the lung and renal adenocarcinomas, but this "paraneoplastic" syndrome has also been described in a wide variety of tumors [45]. When present, the syndrome may include renal phosphate wasting, increased renal cyclic adenosine monophosphate (AMP), and a low 1,25-dihydroxy vitamin D.

Hypercalcemia in hematologic malignancies may be produced by direct bone invasion [46], production of humoral factors, or both [47]. Hypercalcemia is associated with multiple myeloma frequently enough to be an integral part of the clinical picture [46]; it is less frequently seen in lymphoma and HTLV1-associated T cell leukemia. In these situations, the elaboration of osteoclast activating factor by lymphocytes is believed to be etiologic [39]. Recent work has shown that the osteoclast-activating factor is really a collection of cytokines each of which is capable of causing bone resorbtion. Thus far, active cytokines include interleukin 1α (IL-α), interleukin 1β (IL-1β), tumor necrosis factor-α, tumor necrosis factor-β (lymphotoxin), and transforming growth factor α [48].

Because of the frequency with which hypercalcemia is observed in breast and lung cancers, it is worthwhile reviewing these in greater detail. Although ectopic parathyroid hormone (PTH) production has been reported in patients with breast cancer [49], the occurrence of hypercalcemia was thought to be primarily a result of bone metastasis. Recently developed more sensitive PTH assays, however, have identified a parathyroid hormone–related protein (PTHrP), resembling PTH at its amino terminus, in a broad array of solid tumors and in some breast cancers as well. Hypercalcemia has been estimated to occur in 7 to 25 percent of patients with disseminated breast cancer [50,51]. In approximately 25 percent of cases, hypercalcemia is precipitated by the institution of hormonal therapy with androgens, estrogens, antiestrogens, progestins, or by ablative surgery. No generally useful prognostic factors have been noted that help predict those patients who will show a hypercalcemic response to hormonal therapy. This response is probably a result of transient stimulation of tumor growth and may be predictive of a less aggressive tumor [52].

Lung cancer is frequently associated with hypercalcemia, but the pathogenesis of this effect is clearly different than in breast cancer. When patients with nonresectable lung cancer are grouped by histologic type and presence of bone metastases [53], hypercalcemia is seen in 23 percent of patients with epidermoid carcinoma, in 12.7 percent of patients with large cell anaplastic carcinoma, 2.5 percent of those with adenocarcinoma, and in none with small cell carcinoma. In this study, mechanisms of hypercalcemia other than bone metastases were shown to be important in that 44 percent of the hypercalcemic patients did not have detectable bone metastases, and adeno- and small cell carcinomas, with the highest rate of bone metastases, rarely produced hypercalcemia. It is now believed that hypercalcemia in patients with solid tumors (other than breast) is due to the PTHrP described above. Numerous investigations support this finding as described by Strewler [48].

It should also be mentioned that primary hyperparathyroidism, usually due to a parathyroid adenoma (much less frequently as a result of hyperplasia or a parathyroid carcinoma), may occur with increased frequency in patients with cancer, thus creating a difficult diagnostic problem. In two series of patients with primary hyperparathyroidism, 10 to 34 percent were found to have either antecedent, coexisting, or subsequent cancer, with only a few falling into the category of multiple endocrine adenomatosis [54]. (See references 55 and 56 and Chap. 114 for in-depth discussions on mineral metabolism.)

PATHOPHYSIOLOGY. Tumors may produce hypercalcemia as a result of direct bone lysis by metastatic lesions, the production of humoral substances (PTHrP), or the production, by bone metastases, of local factors that increase resorption of the surrounding bone (cytokines). In patients with bone metastases, there is no direct relation between the radiographic extent of metastatic disease and the levels of hypercalcemia. Other factors that affect serum calcium are the rate of bone destruction, the ability of a patient's kidneys to excrete an increased calcium load, and the relative equilibrium between bone resorption (both normal and tumor induced) and new bone formation. As an example of the latter, prostate or breast tumors with predominantly osteoblastic metastases may actually produce hypocalcemia.

Certain tumors (most frequently hypernephroma and squamous cell carcinoma of the lung) appear to produce hypercalcemia by secreting a PTHrP with similarities to native PTH [48,57]. Patients with these tumors have hypercalcemia and hypophosphatemia in the absence of bone metastases, and PTHrP can be measured by radioimmunoassay in their serum, in tumor tissue, and in the venous outflow from the tumor [42,48,57]. These patients have evidence of increased bone resorption and decreased phosphate reabsorption characteristic of native PTH activity, thus demonstrating similar action between PTH and PTHrP [48].

Although some features suggest the presence of ectopic PTH production (e.g., recent onset, higher calcium, lower levels of 1,25-dihydrocholecalciferol [57,58], a clinical picture consistent with malignancy, and less frequent nephrolithiasis and subperiosteal bone resorption), the distinction between PTHrP and concurrent primary hyperparathyroidism is now possible using newer assay methods [48].

Prostaglandins (PG) stimulate bone resorption in vitro, and their production appears to be associated with hypercalcemia in some patients who show improvement after treatment with inhibitors of PG synthesis [59]. However, the mechanism of PG-induced hypercalcemia in vivo and its importance in patients with hypercalcemia and malignancy are not clear at this time. The production of sterols similar to vitamin D, as observed in breast cancer patients [60], is not thought to have major clinical significance [40], but may be related to PTHrP effects [48].

Tumors present in bone may be capable of secreting locally diffusible substances that can produce bone resorption and hypercalcemia by the stimulation of endogenous osteoclasts. Although other tumors may be able to secrete substances (e.g., PG) that stimulate osteoclasts, a local tumor-host interaction has been most clearly documented in studies of the nonprostaglandin "osteoclast activating factor" (OAF) in multiple myeloma [61], which is the cytokine IL-1B [62,63] or tumor necrosis factor B [64].

CLINICAL MANIFESTATIONS. The protean clinical manifestations of hypercalcemia have been best described in patients with hyperparathyroidism. The effects of hypercalcemia depend on the degree of elevation of ionized serum calcium levels, the chronicity of this elevation, and the rate of rise of serum calcium. Therefore, the hypercalcemia of malignancy, which in general is more severe, of more recent onset, and rapidly progressive, will present a somewhat different clinical picture than primary hyperparathyroidism.

The neuromuscular sequelae of hypercalcemia are presumably mediated by the effects of calcium on excitable membranes. Changes in mental status, such as lethargy or depression, may be subtle early in the course of the disease, but psychotic behavior, obtundation, and finally coma can develop later [65]. The electroencephalogram (EEG) will typically show diffuse slowing and may show changes mimicking those seen with brain metastases [66]. Seizures can occur at very high calcium levels, and cerebrospinal fluid (CSF) protein may be significantly elevated [67]. Muscle weakness and myopathy can occur, and hyporeflexia is common.

Cardiovascular effects may be observed. Moderate hypertension can be produced by acute or chronic hypercalcemia [68], at least in part because of positive inotropism and vasoconstriction. However, because these patients are frequently volume depleted, blood pressure is frequently normal or low. It is well known that the spectrum of digitalis-toxic arrhythmias may develop more easily in a hypercalcemic patient. The most characteristic ECG changes of hypercalcemia are prolonged P-R interval (occasionally producing high-grade A-V block), shortened Q-T interval, and "coving" of the S-T segment [69]. The changes are not sufficiently sensitive or specific to be diagnostically reliable, but they may be useful in following the progression of serum calcium levels.

The earliest effect of hypercalcemia on the kidney is a decrease in concentrating ability. This can produce the typical symptoms of polyuria and polydipsia and result in dehydration and prerenal azotemia [70]. If a decrease in glomerular filtration rate (GFR) occurs by this mechanism, calcium excretion is impaired, and a vicious cycle develops. The acid-base effects of hypercalcemia may vary. A metabolic alkalosis can result from volume depletion and from the increased release of buffers from reabsorbed bone. In contrast, if nephrocalcinosis occurs, the tubular damage may produce a picture resembling proximal renal tubular acidosis with glycosuria, hypomagnesemia, and aminoaciduria. Calcium deposition, producing either nephrocalcinosis or nephrolithiasis with hydronephrosis, is uncommon in cancer patients because of the relatively short duration of hypercalcemia.

The gastrointestinal signs of hypercalcemia are seen early in the course of malignancy but are nonspecific. They include anorexia, nausea, vomiting, constipation, and abdominal pain. The pancreatitis and the peptic ulcer disease seen in association with hyperparathyroidism are rarely found with hypercalcemia in cancer patients.

Other problems that may occur are pruritus, bone pain, and soft tissue calcifications (if hypercalcemia is prolonged or after chronic phosphate therapy).

DIAGNOSIS. The diagnosis of hypercalcemia is simple to confirm once it is clinically suspected. There are several pitfalls, however, in the interpretation of serum calcium levels. Most laboratories report a total serum calcium level rather than the biologically active ionized calcium level. Ordinarily, approximately 40 percent of total serum calcium is bound to protein, primarily albumin. This percentage of calcium can be altered under different conditions, causing an increase or a decrease in the active calcium species for the same total calcium level. Thus a hypoalbuminemic patient may show more signs and

symptoms of hypercalcemia than would be expected from the total serum calcium.

Because 1 gm of albumin binds 0.8 mg of calcium, a decrease of 1 gm per deciliter in serum albumin concentration below the normal concentration of 4.0 can be corrected for by adding 0.8 mg per deciliter to the measured serum calcium, which produces a corrected serum value that is more indicative of the patient's clinical status. Changes in globulin concentration and pH also affect the percentage of bound calcium but to a much lesser extent [56]. One gram of globulin binds 0.16 mg of calcium so that the corrected calcium equals total serum calcium plus 0.6 mg per deciliter for each decrease or minus 0.6 mg per deciliter for each increase in globulin. A decrease in pH of 0.1 produces a corrected calcium equal to total serum calcium plus 0.12 mg per deciliter. A special case may occur with multiple myeloma [71] where the M-protein binds calcium so that total calcium levels are elevated, but ionized calcium may be normal.

In a hypercalcemic patient with cancer, the patient will be found in most cases to have bone metastases, which can be documented by radiographic or radionuclide studies. Patients who have resistant hypercalcemia with bone metastases or patients without bone metastases should have PTH and PTHrP levels measured to assess possible coincident hyperparathyroidism or tumor-related PTHrP production. Although certain features are more characteristic of primary hyperparathyroidism (higher PTH level relative to serum calcium, chloride-phosphate ratio >33, renal tubular acidosis-like syndrome, evidence of long-standing hypercalcemia), it is difficult to distinguish this endocrine disorder with certainty from ectopic secretion of PTH or PTHrP without performing an assay.

Venous effluent sampling from either the tumor bed or neck veins may be necessary to determine the source of PTH activity in rare cases. Other studies to determine the etiology of hypercalcemia in a patient without bone metastases, such as prostaglandin levels, nephrogenous cyclic AMP, urinary calcium, or 1,25-dihydroxycholecalciferol, are useful in the setting of a research protocol but have limited availability and would not significantly influence therapy.

The most common clinical setting in which hypercalcemia would be suspected is in a patient with a known malignancy whose mental status has changed. Although all of the benign causes of obtundation need to be considered in cancer patients, there are particular problems associated with malignancy that need to be given special attention (Table 127-6). Once the presence of hypercalcemia is established, the differential diagnosis is limited, and many potential causes can be eliminated by the patient's history (Table 127-7).

TREATMENT. A number of reviews on the treatment of hypercalcemia associated with malignancy have recently been published [39,72–75]. Although treatment of hypercalcemia may require immediate life-saving therapy, a plan for diagnosis, staging, and treatment directed at the underlying malignancy must be initiated at the same time the hypercalcemia is treated. A complete discussion of therapy appears in Chapter 114.

Several supportive measures deserve to be noted. When possible, ambulation should be encouraged to prevent the increased osteoclastic activity seen in immobilized patients either with or without underlying bone pathology, which might contribute to further increases in calcium levels. Although levels of 1,25-dihydroxycholecalciferol are markedly decreased [58] and intestinal calcium absorption is moderately decreased [76] in such patients, it would seem prudent to limit oral calcium intake (i.e., no more than 1 gm/day). If dietary supplements are provided, the calcium content must be checked. Commercially available preparations (e.g., Hepatic Aid, Amin Aid) with only

Table 127-6. Differential Diagnosis of Altered Mental Status with Particular Reference to the Oncology Patient

A. Nonfocal
　1. Toxic
　　a. Opiates
　　b. Barbiturates
　2. Metabolic
　　a. Hyperglycemia (hyperosmolar secondary steroid therapy or pancreatic disease)
　　b. Hypoglycemia (insulinoma, sarcoma)
　　c. Uremia (obstructive nephropathy)
　　d. Hypercalcemia
　　e. Hepatic coma
　　f. Hypoxia (lung metastasis, pulmonary emboli, pulmonary fibrosis)
　　g. Hypo- or hypernatremia (SIADH, DI)
　　h. Lactic acidosis
　　i. Cushing's syndrome (endogenous or iatrogenic)
　　j. Addison's disease (adrenal metastasis)
　　k. Hypopituitarism (brain tumor)
　3. Infectious: sepsis
　4. Circulatory collapse
　　a. Dehydration
　　b. Pericardial disease
　　c. Doxorubicin hydrochloride (Adriamycin) cardiomyopathy
　5. Postictal
B. Focal
　1. Brain metastasis
　　a. Mass effect
　　b. Obstructive hydrocephalus
　2. Intracerebral or subarachnoid hemorrhage
　　a. Thrombocytopenia
　　b. Thrombocytosis
　　c. Leukostasis
　3. CNS infection
　　a. Meningitis
　　b. Encephalitis
　4. Carcinomatous meningitis
　5. Subdural hematoma
　6. Vasculitis
　7. Cerebrovascular disease

SIADH = syndrome of inappropriate excretion of antidiuretic hormone; DI = diabetes insipidus.

Table 127-7. Differential Diagnosis of Hypercalcemia

1. Cancer
　a. With bone metastasis (solid tumor)
　b. Without bone metastasis (solid tumor)
　c. Hematologic (multiple myeloma, leukemia, lymphoma with bone involvement)
2. Primary hyperparathyroidism
3. Toxic
　a. Thiazides
　b. Milk-alkali
　c. Vitamin D or A toxicity
4. Endocrine
　a. Thyrotoxicosis
　b. Adrenal insufficiency
　c. Pheochromocytoma (usually in association with primary hyperparathyroidism)
5. Granulomatous disease
　a. Tuberculosis
　b. Sarcoidosis
6. Immobilization (especially with underlying bone disease)
7. Aritfactual
　a. Hyperalbuminemia or hypergammaglobulinemia
　b. Venous stasis (prolonged tourniquet application)

trace amounts of calcium can be obtained. Patients receiving parenteral nutrition should receive calcium-free hyperalimentation.

Because hypercalcemic patients are usually volume depleted, fluid replacement is necessary for supportive purposes [77]. Because of the large volumes involved and the frequent presence of nausea, hydration is best accomplished intravenously (see Chap. 114). If the patient is able to drink, oral hydration can be a valuable adjunct.

Oral and intravenous phosphate preparations have been used to treat hypercalcemia. These probably act by increasing the calcium-phosphorus solubility product, leading to increased calcium deposition in bone and other tissues [45]. Concern over inducing extraskeletal calcifications has limited the use of phosphate therapy. Phosphates should not be given to patients who have elevated phosphorus levels at the onset of therapy or who have significantly impaired renal function. Oral phosphates are most useful in chronic treatment of mild-moderate hypercalcemia, because the calcium-lowering effect takes several days to occur. Usual dosage is 2 gm of inorganic phosphorus per day in four divided doses. Two grams of phosphorus will be provided by 12.5 cc of Fleet Phospho-Soda or 8 caps of Neutra-Phos or Neutraphos-K. Diarrhea (particularly when concentrated solutions are used) may be a limiting side effect of oral phosphate therapy.

Oral phosphates may be particularly useful in multiple myeloma patients [78] and are associated with some relief of bone pain. These patients must be carefully chosen, however, because of the frequency of renal impairment in multiple myeloma. Intravenous phosphate therapy is effective in lowering markedly elevated calcium levels within several hours, and a single course of treatment lasts several days [79]. Although the frequency of complications can vary when a dose of phosphate of 1.5 to 3 gm (50–100 mM) is given slowly (6–8 hr), rapid IV infusions have resulted in severe hypotension and hypocalcemia. Because of these risks, IV phosphates should be reserved for use in acute situations where other measures have not been successful or where the patient is severely hypophosphatemic.

Mithramycin is a cytotoxic antibiotic that is virtually always effective in lowering calcium levels at doses much smaller than those used for the chemotherapy of tumors [80,81] (see Chap. 114). Although mithramycin has been used for chronic therapy [82], it is best reserved for treatment of acute episodes because of toxicities. It should be used earlier and more frequently in the course of therapy to shorten hospital stays and get the patient home sooner.

Diphosphonates have been shown to be effective in the acute treatment of the hypercalcemia of malignancy [72,83] (see Chap. 114).

Calcitonin causes hypocalcemia and hypophosphatemia by decreasing bone resorption and by increasing urinary calcium and phosphorus excretion [84,85,86] (see Chap. 114). Calcitonin is primarily of benefit in situations such as renal failure, where aggressive fluid therapy, mithramycin, and phosphates are dangerous.

Glucocorticoids are useful in the treatment of hypercalcemia associated with hematologic malignancies. The usefulness of glucocorticoids is possibly related to their in vitro inhibitory action on cytokines as well as a direct antitumor effect. They may also be effective in hypercalcemic patients with breast cancer, and are especially useful when the hypercalcemia has been induced by hormonal therapy. They are generally not effective in patients with other solid tumors, particularly when ectopic PTH activity is present [43]. Usual dosage is 40 to 60 mg prednisone (or equivalent) daily, and the effects are not seen for 3 to 4 days. If prolonged therapy is required, the complications of chronic steroid therapy, including further bone demineralization, must be considered. Large intravenous doses of 250 to 500 mg of hydrocortisone may be given every 8 hours with a taper to oral 10 to 30 mg per day when the calcium is controlled [87].

As previously mentioned, inhibitors of prostaglandin synthesis have been tried as calcium-lowering agents. However, they have been effective in only a small fraction of patients, and in the absence of a simple method of patient selection [88] the addition of these agents, which have numerous physiologic effects, would seem undesirable.

Gallium nitrate, initially developed as an anticancer drug, was noted to inhibit bone resorption by reducing the solubility of bone crystals that led to hypocalcemia [89] (see Chap. 114).

With this variety of causative factors and therapeutic options in the hypercalcemia of malignancy, it is useful to discuss treatment in several clinical situations. As previously mentioned, clinical findings do not always correlate with the degree of hypercalcemia, but calcium levels are useful guides in selecting approaches.

Mild Hypercalcemia. Patients with mild hypercalcemia (serum calcium 12–14 mg/dl) will often have some symptoms such as polyuria, constipation, nausea, and an altered level of consciousness. If patients are clinically dehydrated, they should receive at least 1 liter of intravenous or oral fluids before beginning furosemide. If it is anticipated that fluid management will not be a major problem, then infusion of normal saline can begin with 20 to 40 mEq KCl per liter at 300 cc per hour. This infusion may be supplemented by ad libitum oral fluid intake.

Furosemide should be given every 4 hours or more often to maintain urine output; dosage will vary, depending on the patient's previous experience with loop diuretics. In a patient without major cardiac or renal disease who has not previously received diuretics, furosemide doses of 10 to 20 mg IV every 4 hours are usually adequate. Magnesium supplementation should be given orally or IM. Total intake and output, weight, serum electrolytes, and urine electrolytes (at least within the first 12 hr) are parameters that should be monitored.

Although calcium levels should be decreased by 24 hours, symptoms of hypercalcemia (particularly mental status changes) may take several days to return to normal. For patients in whom fluid problems are expected, saline and furosemide therapy can still be attempted, but in a setting where hydration status can be closely followed by central venous or pulmonary artery pressure monitoring. If there is no response, and the patient's clinical picture is not deteriorating, saline and furosemide should be continued, and the patient should receive a single dose of 25 µg per kilogram of mithramycin, with consideration of the caveats for mithramycin therapy (see previous section and Chap. 114).

Severe Hypercalcemia. In patients who have severe hypercalcemia (levels >14), a dose of mithramycin should be given at the onset of therapy. For patients with coma where a more rapid effect is desired, intravenous phosphates may be added (2 gm elemental phosphorus over 6–8 hr). Two grams of phosphorus is provided by 80 cc of In-Phos (along with 130 mEq Na and 16 mEq K) or 30 cc Hyper-Phos-K (with 100 mEq K). Etidronate disodium (Didronel) may be used as well (7.5 mg/kg in 200 ml normal saline intravenously over 2 hours every 24 hours) [87,90,91].

Renal Failure. Patients with renal failure present an additional problem because of the risks involved in using saline infusion, mithramycin, and phosphate therapies. In severe renal failure where these treatments would pose major risks, two forms of therapy are available. The first is calcitonin, which probably

should be given in combination with prednisone for maximal effect [86]: 100 to 200 MRC units SC every 12 hours with prednisone 60 mg per day in 2 to 3 divided doses. The second form of therapy is dialysis. Both peritoneal dialysis and hemodialysis have been effective in treating hypercalcemia when a calcium-free dialysate is used [92,93] (see Chap. 81).

Long-Term Therapy. Long-term therapy for the hypercalcemia of malignancy becomes necessary in patients with slow-growing tumors or tumors that are at least partially sensitive to therapy. Close follow-up, adequate hydration, patient mobilization, and avoidance of high calcium intake provide the necessary support measures. Specific therapy that consists of either chronic phosphate therapy or intermittent treatment with mithramycin is not without problems. Chronic phosphate therapy is associated with the risk of producing extraskeletal calcification. Maintenance therapy with mithramycin is frequently found to be limited by drug toxicities.

Maintenance therapy consisting of calcitonin and glucocorticoids (to avoid "escape" from calcitonin) has not been studied in large groups, and the only currently available oral diphosphate preparation, Didronel, is not suitable for long-term therapy because of the occurrence of osteomalacia. Chronic therapy, then, depends primarily on control of tumor growth, adequate support measures, and acute treatment of symptomatic hypercalcemia.

Hypercalcemia and Breast Cancer. Because of the frequent occurrence of hypercalcemia in breast cancer, its management deserves special mention. These patients often respond to prednisone therapy, which should be tried in mild hypercalcemia before proceeding to more aggressive measures. In patients where the hypercalcemia has been produced by hormonal therapy, such therapy may be continued if the hypercalcemia is mild in the presence of support measures, on the assumption that hypercalcemia represents a "flare" of tumor stimulation before regression occurs. If the hypercalcemia is severe or persistent, the most prudent course is to acutely treat the hypercalcemia and substitute prednisone for the hormonal agent [50].

Malignant Pericardial Disease

Malignant pericardial disease represents a common cause of morbidity and mortality in patients with cancer [94,95,96]. Autopsy studies estimate the incidence of pericardial and cardiac metastases to be 2 to 20 percent [95–103]. In patients with metastases to the pericardium, approximately 36 percent die as a direct result of the pericardial involvement, while it plays a contributory role in the death of another 45 percent of patients [104]. Despite the morbidity of pericardial metastases, only 3 to 29 percent of these patients are diagnosed as having pericardial disease antemortem [99,104,105]. In a setting of extensive metastatic disease with its accompanying signs and symptoms as well as the absence of cardiac tamponade, the presence of pericardial metastases is often obscured. This situation undoubtedly contributes in part to the discrepancy between antemortem diagnosis and postmortem findings (see Chap. 34).

ETIOLOGY AND PATHOGENESIS. Malignant tumors of the pericardium may be primary or secondary. Primary tumors of the pericardium occur rarely and are usually sarcomas or mesotheliomas [106,107]. Secondary involvement of the pericardium constitutes the majority of instances of malignant disease of the pericardium and can occur as a result of direct invasion by adjacent tumors or by hematogenous or lymphatic metastasis from a distant primary tumor. Hematologic malignancies, breast cancer, and lung cancer account for 80 percent of all malignant pericardial disease, and in one autopsy series, the incidence for each disease was reported as 11 percent, 21 percent, and 10 percent, respectively [104]. Goudie reported pericardial disease in 31 percent of lung cancer patients [99]. Histologic subtypes of lung cancer were equally represented in another series [108]. As many as two-thirds of melanoma patients exhibit cardiac or pericardial metastases [108].

The nature of pericardial involvement varies widely and can dictate how the disease presents clinically. The possible mechanisms of involvement include tamponade secondary to effusion, impairment due to constriction, encroachment of the great vessels, impairment of coronary circulation, encasement of cardiac innervation, and combinations of the above.

DIFFERENTIAL DIAGNOSIS. Underlying malignancies are not the sole etiology of symptomatic pericardial disease in cancer patients. Posner reported on 31 patients with a variety of malignancies in whom pericardial disease was diagnosed antemortem. Malignant pericardial disease represented 58 percent of the cases, and 32 percent and 10 percent of the cases were attributed to idiopathic and radiation-induced pericarditis, respectively [97]. Other causes of pericardial disease in cancer patients are drug-induced pericarditis [109], purulent pericarditis [110], hypothyroidism, and autoimmune disorders.

Despite initial convictions that the heart and pericardium were radioinsensitive, widespread use of radiation in the treatment of mediastinal disease, especially in Hodgkin's disease, has resulted in extensive documentation of radiation-induced pericarditis [97,111–116]. Onset of symptoms varies from less than 1 month [114] to more than 17 years [115] after completion of radiation. Recent studies by radionuclide ventriculogram demonstrate decreased left ventricular ejection fractions at rest and during exercise in patients who received a single-port mediastinal radiation 5 to 15 years before examination [113]. Radiation, therefore, induces long-standing and late deficits in cardiac function as well as a constrictive pericarditis.

CLINICAL MANIFESTATIONS. Thurber, describing the signs and symptoms in 55 patients with malignant pericardial disease, reported the following clinical manifestations with their incidences: dyspnea (91%), cough (67%), pleural effusion (53%), hepatomegaly (50%), thoracic pain (48%), orthopnea (37%), venous distention (33%), leg edema (33%), cardiac enlargement (30%), rales (20%), dysphagia (18%), pulsus paradoxus (5%), and ascites (5%) [104].

Neoplasm constitutes the most frequent cause of cardiac tamponade in general medical practice [117]. As outlined in Chapter 21, patients with cardiac tamponade present with pulsus paradoxus, venous hypertension, narrow pulse pressure, tachycardia, and, if cardiac tamponade is severe, with shock. Symptoms include facial swelling, dyspnea, ill-defined chest discomfort, and at times, symptoms of pericarditis [118]. The symptoms and signs of malignant pericardial disease without tamponade differ little from nonmalignant pericarditis. Although facial swelling, arrhythmias, and tamponade occur frequently with malignant pericardial disease, idiopathic pericarditis more commonly presents with pain, fever, and a pericardial friction rub [97].

ECG abnormalities seen in pericardial disease include electrical alternans in cases of tamponade, and more commonly, tachycardia, diffuse S-T wave abnormalities, loss of voltage, premature ventricular contractions, or T-wave inversions [97,104,105,117,118,119]. Atrial arrhythmias may also occur [120], and, as reported by Biran, the ECG abnormalities listed above may commonly be the first indication of malignant pericardial involvement [121]. The chest x-ray is nonspecific, although enlargement of the cardiac silhouette is commonly present.

DIAGNOSIS. Beyond the clinical suspicion of pericardial disease based on signs and symptoms, echocardiography has become established as the procedure of choice in the diagnosis of pericardial effusions. Advantages of echocardiography are its noninvasiveness, accuracy, and ease of performance (see Chap. 7). Pericardial effusion is manifested first by the presence of an echo-free space between the left ventricular posterior wall and the pericardial lung interface. As effusions grow in size, the following findings are exhibited: (1) development of an echo-free space between the right ventricular wall and the chest wall, (2) swinging of the heart in the pericardial sac, (3) abnormal septal motion, and (4) late systolic mitral prolapse. Under optimal conditions, 15 to 20 cc effusions can be detected [122].

Unfortunately, serious problems exist with echocardiography in the diagnosis of pericardial disease. Technically, optimal studies may be impossible in as many as 10 percent of patients studied. Loculated effusions and pericardial masses may escape detection by M-mode echocardiography. Accuracy diminishes in the presence of constrictive pericardial disease, and pericardial neoplasms have been shown to constitute a basis for pseudopericardial effusion on M-mode examination [123].

CT provides a valuable diagnostic addition and alternative to echocardiography in patients in whom the latter is technically suboptimal. Although estimates of effusion size are comparable with both modalities, CT demonstrates superiority over M-mode echo in the evaluation of the degree of pericardial thickening, the presence of malignant nodules, and the extent of loculation [123]. Application of CT also provides the opportunity to search for clues to the neoplastic origin of the effusion. Cardiac catheterization may be used to confirm the diagnosis but is seldom needed.

Pericardiocentesis remains the initial invasive diagnostic procedure of choice in the work-up of pericardial effusion of possible malignant origin (see Chap. 8). It also represents the initial therapeutic measure performed in patients with tamponade. As a diagnostic procedure, pericardiocentesis yields information about an effusion with regards to its chemical nature (transudate vs. exudate), volume, cellularity (hemorrhagic, inflammatory, purulent), and whether it is infected or malignant. The procedure is not without risk. The most common complications cited are right ventricular puncture and hemopericardium and ventricular ectopy [108,121,124]. In one study of pericardiocentesis in 50 cancer patients, 4 patients developed hemopericardium (2 were thrombocytopenic) and in 3 patients, the procedure either directly or indirectly contributed to the patient's death [124]. Other complications include lacerations of the internal mammary and the coronary arteries, liver, lung or stomach [89].

Chemical and cellular analyses of pericardial fluid in 13 cancer patients showed the following mean values: glucose, 54 mg per deciliter; protein, 5.3 gm per deciliter; hematocrit, 12.9 percent; and white blood cells, 6000 per microliter with 46 percent neutrophils, 42 percent lymphocytes, and 12 percent monocytes [110]. None of these values are diagnostic of malignant effusions. In approximately 80 percent of effusions secondary to malignancies, cytological examination will be positive [124,125]. False-positive reports of malignant effusions are rare [126].

TREATMENT. Management of cardiac tamponade requires prompt treatment. Supportive measures, such as intravenous volume expansion and supplemental oxygen, should be provided as needed while preparing for definitive therapy. Because of the decrease in diastolic filling attributable to the increased cardiac rate and chamber compression, one should avoid medications that can lower blood pressure, reduce preload, or decrease heart rate, e.g., diuretics or beta-blockers. Pericardiocentesis provides the safest and most rapid mode of treatment available [108,109,124,127,128,129]. As time permits, ECG, chest x-ray, and echocardiography should be performed before pericardiocentesis.

Aspiration of pericardial fluid is indicated when the following are present: (1) dyspnea, shock, or impairment of consciousness, (2) peripheral venous pressure above 13 cm H_2O, (3) measured pulsus paradoxus less than 50 percent of the pulse pressure, or (4) a falling pulse pressure less than 20 mm Hg [130]. If tamponade is not present or has been relieved with pericardiocentesis and the effusion is not increasing in size, a trial of conservative therapy with antiinflammatory agents can be attempted. This approach is reasonable if the patient exhibits a pericardial friction rub and fever in the face of improving or stable malignant disease and the cytology is negative [97].

If the effusion increases in size, a diagnostic-therapeutic pericardiocentesis is indicated. Failure of fluid removal to relieve symptoms suggests possible constrictive-effusive pericarditis, particularly in the face of prior mediastinal irradiation [131]. Confirmation of constrictive-effusive pericarditis often necessitates the use of cardiac catheterization. Treatment then consists of pericardiectomy [131].

Cytologically verified malignant effusions should be treated after pericardiocentesis with chemotherapy or radiation (1500–3500 rads) [108,121,123]. Recurrent effusions may require sclerosis. Tetracycline had been the initial treatment of choice. It is no longer commercially available, but alternatives have been found. Doxycycline may be used (0.5–1 gm in 20 cc normal saline) [132,133]. In addition, chemotherapeutic agents and radioactive chromic phosphate and gold have been used in the past [108,119,122,134]. Other available sclerosing agents are nitrogen mustard 0.1 to 0.2 mg per kilogram, thiotepa 15 to 30 mg, fluorouracil 750 to 1000 mg, or bleomycin 15 to 30 units [135].

If sclerosis fails in the case of constrictive disease, pleuralpericardial window placement and pericardiectomy provide alternative modes of treatment in a patient with an expected reasonable survival [116,117,136]. Successful use of short-term, indwelling pericardial catheter drainage has been accomplished [134], although at least one episode of purulent pericarditis has been reported as a complication [124]. Flannery et al. suggested the following criteria in addition to hemodynamic compromise as indications for surgical intervention: (1) severe radiation-induced constrictive pericarditis, (2) fluid reaccumulation so rapid that pericardiocentesis is not a practical means of control, (3) prior radiation therapy that precludes the use of further radiation, or (4) uncertain cause of the effusion with negative cytologic findings [133].

The criteria that indicate the control of malignant pericardial effusion are: (1) a decrease in, or the disappearance of, pericardial effusion that lasts 30 days or more as assessed by radiography, echocardiography, and clinical examination, (2) the absence of symptoms of pericardial tamponade for more than 30 days, and (3) no requirement for pericardiocentesis 30 days after initiation of local or systemic therapy or both [129,137].

PROGNOSIS. The diagnosis of malignant pericardial disease has grave implications. Although the treatment of patients with lymphomas has resulted in prolonged disease-free survival for many patients [116–121], the treatment of pericardial disease secondary to nonhematologic tumors has met with limited success [97,108,134]. One series showed a mean survival of 15.6 months in patients with lung and breast cancer who responded to conservative treatment with pericardiocentesis and sclerosis [129]. In comparison, historical control groups survived a mean of 11.7 months when treated conservatively as opposed to 6.4 months when treated surgically with pericardial window placement.

Patients who present with tamponade have a poorer prognosis for survival, frequently only days in spite of treatment. Radiation-induced pericarditis has been associated with prolonged survival when successfully treated conservatively or with pericardiectomy [97,111]. Finally, although idiopathic pericarditis frequently responds to conservative management, survival is on the order of 9 months, with most patients dying of their underlying malignant disease [97].

References

1. Paris JM, Marschke RF, Dines DL, et al: Etiologic considerations in superior vena cava syndrome. *Mayo Clin Proc* 56:407, 1981.
2. McIntire FT, Sykes EM: Obstruction of the superior vena cava: A review of the literature and report of two personal cases. *Ann Intern Med* 30:925, 1949.
3. Katz PO, Hackshaw TT, Barish CF: Venous thrombosis as a cause of superior vena cava syndrome. *Arch Intern Med* 143:1050, 1983.
4. Gore JM, Matsumoto AH, Layden JJ: Superior vena cava syndrome, its association with indwelling balloon-tipped pulmonary artery catheters. *Arch Intern Med* 144:506, 1984.
5. Roswit B, Kaplan G, Jacobson HG: The superior vena cava obstruction syndrome in bronchogenic carcinoma. *Radiology* 61:722, 1953.
6. Perez CA, Presant CA, VanAmburg AL III: Management of superior vena cava syndrome. *Semin Oncol* 2:124, 1978.
7. Davenport D, Ferree C, Blake D, et al: Radiation therapy in the treatment of superior vena cava obstruction. *Cancer* 42:2600, 1978.
8. Lokich JJ, Goodman R: Superior vena cava syndrome. *JAMA* 231:58, 1975.
9. Barron KD, Hirand A, Araki S, et al: Experiences with metastatic neoplasms involving the spinal cord. *Neurology* 8:91, 1959.
10. Byrne TN: Spinal cord compression from epidural metastasis. *N Engl J Med* 327:614, 1992.
11. Gilbert RW, Kim JH, Posner JD: Epidural spinal cord compression from metastatic tumor: Diagnosis and treatment. *Ann Neurol* 3:40, 1978.
12. Mullins GM, Flynn JP, El-Mandi AM, et al: Malignant lymphomas of the epidural space. *Ann Intern Med* 74:416, 1971.
13. Friedman M, Kim TH, Pananon AM: Spinal cord compression in malignant lymphoma. *Cancer* 37:1485, 1976.
14. Haddad P, Thaell JF, Kiely JM, et al: Lymphoma of the spinal extradural space. *Cancer* 38:1862, 1976.
15. Garbell SC, Goodman RL: Spinal cord compression, in DeVita VT, Hellman S, Rosenberg SA (eds): *Cancer: Principles and Practice of Oncology*. Philadelphia, Lippincott, 1982, p 1589.
16. Brockman JE, Bloomer WD: Management of spinal cord compression. *Semin Oncol* 5:135, 1978.
17. Boland PJ, Lane JM, Sundaresan N: Metastatic disease of the spine. *Clin Orthop* 169:95, 1982.
18. Manabe S, Tanaka H, Higo Y, et al: Experimental analysis of the spinal cord compressed by spinal metastasis. *Spine* 14:1308, 1989.
19. Auld AW, Buerman A: Metastatic spinal epidural tumors. *Arch Neurol* 15:100, 1966.
20. Tarlov IM, Klinger H: Spinal cord compression studies: II. Time limits for recovery after acute compression in dogs. *Arch Neurol Psychol* 71:271, 1954.
21. Rodichok LD, Harper GR, Ruckdeschel JC, et al: Early diagnosis of spinal epidural metastases. *Am J Med* 70:1181, 1981.
22. Sellwood RB: The radiological approach to metastatic cancer of the brain and spine. *Br J Radiol* 45:647, 1972.

23. Lentle BC, Russell AS, Percy JS, et al: Bone joint scanning updated. *Ann Intern Med* 84:297, 1976.
24. O'Mara RE: Bone scanning in osseous metastatic disease. *JAMA* 229:1915, 1974.
25. Pistenma DA, McDougall R, Kriss JP: Screening for bone metastases. *JAMA* 231:46, 1975.
26. Lee BCP, Kazam E, Newman AD: Computed tomography of the spine and spinal cord. *Radiology* 128:95, 1978.
27. DiChiro G, Doppman JL, Dwyer AJ, et al: Tumors and arteriovenous malformations of the spinal cord: Assessment using MRI. *Radiology* 155:689, 1985.
28. Flynn DF, Shipley WU: Management of spinal cord compression secondary to metastatic prostatic carcinoma. *Urol Clin North Am* 18:145, 1991.
29. Carmody RF, Yang PJ, Seeley GW, et al: Spinal cord compression due to metastatic disease: Diagnosis with MR imaging versus myelography. *Radiology* 173:225, 1989.
30. Sze G, Krol G, Zimmerman RD, et al: Intramedullary disease of the spine: Diagnosis using gadolinium-DTPA-enhanced MR imaging *AJNR* 9:847, 1988.
31. Stark PJ, Henson RA, Evans SJW: Spinal metastases. A retrospective survey from a general hospital. *Brain* 105:189, 1982.
32. Nather A, Bose K: The results of decompression of cord or cauda equina compression from metastatic extradural tumors. *Clin Orthop* 169:103, 1982.
33. Hall AJ, MacKay NNS: The results of laminectomy for compression of the cord or cauda equina by extradural malignant tumor. *J Bone Joint Surg* 55B:497, 1973.
34. White WA, Patterson RH, Bergland RM: Role of surgery in the treatment of spinal cord compression by metastatic neoplasm. *Cancer* 27:558, 1971.
35. Brice J, McKissock W: Surgical treatment of malignant extradural spinal tumours. *Br Med J* 1:1339, 1965.
36. Kahn FR, Glicksman AS, Chu FCH, et al: Treatment by radiotherapy of spinal cord compression due to extradural metastases. *Radiology* 89:495, 1967.
37. Cobb CA, Leavens ME, Eckles N: Indications for nonoperative treatment of spinal cord compression due to breast cancer. *J Neurosurg* 47:653, 1977.
38. Milborn L, Hibbs GG, Hendrickson FR: Treatment of spinal cord compression from metastatic carcinoma. *Cancer* 21:447, 1968.
39. Karp DD, Kadish S, Kavanah M, et al: Oncologic emergencies, in Osteen R (ed): *Cancer Manual,* 8th ed. Boston, American Cancer Society, 1990, p 450.
40. Greenberg HS, Kim J, Posner JB: Epidural spinal cord compression from metastatic tumor: Results with a new treatment protocol. *Ann Neurol* 8:361, 1980.
41. Fisken RA, Heath DA, Bold AM: Hypercalcemia: A hospital survey. *Q J Med* 196:405, 1980.
42. Besarab A, Caro JF: Mechanisms of hypercalcemia in malignancy. *Cancer* 41:2276, 1978.
43. Fields ALA, Josse RG, Bergsagel DE: Metabolic emergencies: Hypercalcemia, in Devita VT, Hellman S, Rosenberg SA (eds): *Cancer: Principles and Practice of Oncology.* Philadelphia, Lippincott, 1982, p 1594.
44. Myers WPL: Hypercalcemia in neoplastic disease. *Arch Surg* 80:308, 1960.
45. Rodman JS, Sherwood LM: Disorders of mineral metabolism in malignancy, in Avioli LV, Krare SM (eds): *Metabolic Bone Disease.* New York, Academic, 1974, vol II, p 577.
46. Bergsagel DE: Plasma cell myeloma, in Williams WJ, Beutier E, Ersiev AJ, et al (eds): *Hematology.* 2nd ed. New York, McGraw-Hill, 1977.
47. O'Regan S, Carson S, Chesney RW, et al: Electrolyte and acid base disturbances in the management of leukemia. *Blood* 49:345, 1977.
48. Strewler GJ, Nissenson RA: Hypercalcemia in malignancy. *West J Med* 153:635, 1990.
49. Mauligit GM, Cohen JL, Sherwood LM: Ectopic production of parathyroid hormone by carcinoma of the breast. *N Engl J Med* 285:154, 1971.
50. Davis HL Jr, Wisely AN, Ramirez G, et al: Hypercalcemia complicating breast cancer. *Oncology* 28:126, 1973.
51. Jessiman AG, Emerson K Jr, Shah R, et al: Hypercalcemia in carcinoma of the breast. *Ann Surg* 157:377, 1963.
52. Mannheimer IH: Hypercalcemia of breast cancer. *Cancer* 18:679, 1965.
53. Bender RA, Hansen H: Hypercalcemia in bronchogenic carcinoma. *Ann Intern Med* 80:205, 1974.
54. Farr HW, Fahey TJ Jr, Nash AG, et al: Primary hyperparathyroidism and cancer. *Am J Surg* 126:539, 1973.
55. Agus ZS, Wasserstein A, Goldfarb S: Disorders of calcium and magnesium homeostasis. *Am J Med* 72:473, 1982.
56. Popovtzer MM, Knochel JP: Disorders of calcium, phosphorus, vitamin D, and parathyroid hormone activity, in Schorer RW (ed): *Renal and Electrolyte Disorders.* 2nd ed. Boston, Little, Brown, 1980.
57. Lafferty FW: Pseudohyperparathyroidism. *Medicine* 45:247, 1966.
58. Stewart AF, Horst R, Deftos LJ, et al: Biochemical evaluation of patients with cancer-associated hypercalcemia. *N Engl J Med* 303:1377, 1980.
59. Seyberth HW, Segre GV, Morgan JL, et al: Prostaglandins as mediators of hypercalcemia associated with certain types of cancer. *N Engl J Med* 293:1278, 1975.
60. Gordon GS, Cantino TJ, Erhardt L, et al: Osteolytic sterol in human breast cancer. *Science* 151:1226, 1966.
61. Mundy GR, Raisz LG, Cooper RA, et al: Evidence for the secretion of an osteoclast stimulating factor in myeloma. *N Engl J Med* 291:1041, 1974.
62. Kawano M, Yamamoto I, Iwato K, et al: Interleukin-IB rather than lymphotoxin as the major bone resorbing activity in human multiple myeloma. *Blood* 73:1646, 1989.
63. Yamamoto I, Kawano M, Sone T, et al: Production of interleukin potent bone resorbing cytokine by cultured human myeloma cells. *Cancer Res* 49:4242, 1989.
64. Garrett IR, Durie BGM, Nedwin GE, et al: Production of lymphotoxin bone-resorbing cytokine by cultured human myeloma cells. *N Engl J Med* 317:526, 1989.
65. Lehrer GM, Levitt MF: Neuropsychiatric presentation of hypercalcemia. *J Mt Sinai Hosp NY* 27:10, 1960.
66. Ailen EM, Singer FR: Electroencephalographic abnormalities in hypercalcemia. *Neurology* 20:15, 1970.
67. Krawitt EL, Bloomer HA: Increased cerebrospinal protein secondary to hypercalcemia of the milk-alkali syndrome. *N Engl J Med* 273:154, 1965.
68. Earll JM, Kurtzman NA, Moser RH: Hypercalcemia and hypertension. *Ann Intern Med* 64:378, 1966.
69. Bronsky D, Dubin A, Waldstein SS, et al: Calcium and the electrocardiogram: II. The electrocardiographic manifestations of hyperparathyroidism and marked hypercalcemia from various other etiologies. *Am J Cardiol* 7:833, 1961.
70. Epstein FH: Calcium and the kidney. *Am J Med* 45:700, 1968.
71. Lindegarde F, Zettervall O: Hypercalcemia and normal ionized serum calcium in a case of myelomatosis. *Ann Intern Med* 78:396, 1973.
72. Stewart AF: Therapy of malignancy-associated hypercalcemia: 1983. *Am J Med* 74:475, 1983.
73. Mazzaferri EL, O'Dorisio TM, LoBuglio AF: Treatment of hypercalcemia associated with malignancy. *Semin Oncol* 5:141, 1978.
74. Attie MF: Treatment of hypercalcemia. *Endocr Metab Clin North Am* 18:807, 1989.
75. List A: Malignant hypercalcemia: The choice of therapy. *Arch Intern Med* 151:437, 1991.
76. Coombs RC, Ward MK, Greenberg PB, et al: Calcium metabolism in cancer. *Cancer* 38:211, 1976.
77. Suki WN, Yium JJ, Von Minden M, et al: Acute treatment of hypercalcemia with furosemide. *N Engl J Med* 283:836, 1970.
78. Goldsmith RS, Bantos H, Hulley SB: Phosphate supplementation as an adjunct in the therapy of multiple myeloma. *Arch Intern Med* 122:128, 1968.
79. Goldsmith RS, Ingbar SH: Inorganic phosphate treatment of hypercalcemia of diverse etiologies. *N Engl J Med* 274:1, 1965.
80. Perlia CP, Gubisch NJ, Wolter J, et al: Mithramycin treatment of hypercalcemia. *Cancer* 25:389, 1970.
81. Kiang DT, Loken MK, Kennedy BJ: Mechanism of the hypocalcemic effect of mithramycin. *J Clin Endocrinol Metab* 48:341, 1979.
82. Lebbin D, Ryan WG, Schwartz TB: Outpatient treatment of Paget's disease of bone with mithramycin. *Ann Intern Med* 81:635, 1974.

83. Jung A: Comparison of two parenteral diphosphonates in hypercalcemia in patients with malignancy. *Am J Med* 72:221, 1982.

84. Vaughn CB, Vaitkevicius VK: The effects of calcitonin in hypercalcemia in patients with malignancy. *Cancer* 34:1268, 1974.

85. Hosking DJ: Treatment of severe hypercalcemia with calcitonin. *Metabol Bone Dis Relat Res* 2:207, 1980.

86. Sinstock ML, Mundy GR: Effect of calcitonin and glucocorticoids in combination on the hypercalcemia of malignancy. *Ann Intern Med* 93:269, 1980.

87. Skeel RT: *Handbook of Cancer Chemotherapy.* Boston, Little, Brown, 1991, p 395.

88. Brenner DE, Harvey HA, Lipton A, et al: A study of prostaglandin E2, parathormone, and response to indomethacin in patients with hypercalcemia of malignancy. *Cancer* 44:556, 1982.

89. Casciato DA, Lowitz BB: *Manual of Clinical Oncology.* Boston, Little, Brown, 1988, pp 448–450.

90. Dunagon WC, Ridner ML: *Manual of Medical Therapeutics.* Boston, Little, Brown, 1989, p 427.

91. Thieboud D, Jacquet AF, Burckhardt P: Dose response in the treatment of hypercalcemia of malignancy by a single dose infusion of the biphosphonate, AHPRBP. *J Clin Oncol* 6:762, 1988.

92. Miach PJ, Dearborn JK, Martin TJ, et al: Management of the hypercalcemia of malignancy by peritoneal dialysis. *Med J Aust* 1:782, 1975.

93. Eisenberg E, Gotch FA: Normocalcemic hyperparathyroidism culminating in hypercalcemic crisis: Treatment with hemodialysis. *Arch Intern Med* 122:258, 1968.

94. Mauch PM: Malignant pericardial effusions, in DeVita VT, Hellman S, Rosenberg SA (eds): *Cancer: Principles and Practice in Oncology.* Philadelphia, Lippincott, 1982, p 1571.

95. Guberman BA, Fowler NO, Engel PJ, et al: Cardiac tamponade in medical patients. *Circulation* 64:633, 1981.

96. Wilding G, Greene HL, Longo DL, Urba WJ: Tumors of the heart and pericardium. *Cancer Treat Rep* 15:165, 1988.

97. Posner MR, Cohen GI, Smarin AT: Pericardial disease in patients with cancer. *Am J Med* 71:407, 1981.

98. Hanfling SM: Metastatic cancer to the heart. *Circulation* 22:474, 1960.

99. Goudie RB: Secondary tumors of the heart and pericardium. *Br Heart J* 17:183, 1955.

100. Cohen G, Peery TM, Evans JM: Neoplastic invasion of the heart and pericardium. *Ann Intern Med* 42:1238, 1955.

101. DeLoach JF, Haynes JW: Secondary tumors of heart and pericardium. *Arch Intern Med* 91:224, 1953.

102. Gassman HS, Meadows R. Baker LA: Metastatic tumors of the heart. *Am J Med* 19:357, 1955.

103. Scott RW, Garvin CF: Tumors of the heart and pericardium. *Am Heart J* 17:431, 1938.

104. Thurber DL, Edwards JE, Achor RWP: Secondary malignant tumors of the pericardium. *Circulation* 26:228, 1961.

105. Bizan S, Hochman A, Levy TS, et al: Clinical diagnosis of secondary tumors of the heart and pericardium. *Chest* 55:202, 1969.

106. Poole-Wilson PA, Farnsworth A, Braimbridge MV, et al: Angiosarcoma of the pericardium. *Br Heart J* 38:240, 1976.

107. Sytman AL, MacAlpin RN: Primary pericardial mesothelioma: Report of two cases and review of the literature. *Am Heart J* 81:760, 1971.

108. Lokich JJ: The management of malignant pericardial effusions. *JAMA* 224:1401, 1973.

109. Ahmed M, Slayton RE: Report on drug-induced pericarditis. *Cancer Treat Rep* 64:353, 1981.

110. Agner RC, Gallis HA: Pericarditis: Differential diagnostic considerations. *Arch Intern Med* 139:407, 1979.

111. Brosios FC, Waller BF, Roberts WC: Radiation heart disease. *Am J Med* 70:519, 1981.

112. Applefield MM, Cole JF, Pollock SH, et al: The late appearance of chronic pericardial disease in patients treated by radiotherapy for Hodgkin's disease. *Ann Intern Med* 94:338, 1981.

113. Gottdiener JS, Katin MJ, Borer JS, et al: Late cardiac effects of the therapeutic mediastinal irradiation. *N Engl J Med* 308:569, 1983.

114. Martin RG, Ruckdeschel JC, Chang P, et al: Radiation related pericarditis. *Am J Cardiol* 35:216, 1975.

115. Scott DL, Thomas RD: Late onset constrictive pericarditis after thoracic radiotherapy. *Br Med J* 1:341, 1978.

116. Morton DL, Kagan AR, Roberts WC, et al: Pericardiectomy for radiation-induced pericarditis with effusion. *Ann Thorac Surg* 8:195, 1969.

117. Hancock EW: Cardiac tamponade. *Med Clin North Am* 63:223, 1979.

118. Spodick DH: Differential diagnosis of acute pericarditis. *Prog Cardiovasc Dis* 14:192, 1971.

119. Theologides A: Neoplastic cardiac tamponade. *Semin Oncol* 5:181, 1978.

120. Young JM, Goldman IR: Tumor metastasis to the heart. *Circulation* 9:220, 1961.

121. Biran S. Brufman G, Glein E, et al: The management of pericardial effusion in cancer patients. *Chest* 71:182, 1977.

122. Tajik AJ: Echocardiography in pericardial effusion. *Am J Med* 63:28, 1977.

123. Isner JM, Carter BL, Bankoff MS, et al: Computed tomography in the diagnosis of pericardial heart disease. *Ann Intern Med* 97:473, 1982.

124. Krikorian JG, Hancock EW: Pericardiocentesis. *Am J Med* 65:808, 1978.

125. King DT, Nieberg RK: The use of cytology to evaluate pericardial effusions. *Ann Clin Lab Sci* 9:18, 1979.

126. Zipf RE, Johnston WW: The role of cytology in the evaluation of pericardial effusions. *Chest* 62:593, 1972.

127. Cassell P, Cullum P: The management of cardiac tamponade. *Br J Surg* 54:620, 1967.

128. Smith FE, Lane M, Hodgins PT: Conservative management of malignant pericardial effusion. *Cancer* 33:47, 1974.

129. Spodick DH: Acute cardiac tamponade pathologic physiology, diagnosis and management. *Prog Cardiovasc Dis* 10:64, 1967.

130. Mann T, Brodie BR, Grossman W, et al: Effusive-constrictive hemodynamic pattern due to neoplastic involvement of the pericardium. *Am J Cardiol* 41:781, 1978.

131. Terry LN, Kligerman MM: Pericardial and myocardial involvement of lymphomas and leukemias. *Cancer* 25:1003, 1970.

132. Davis S, Sharma SM, Blumberg ED, et al: Intrapericardial tetracycline for the management of cardiac tamponade secondary to malignant pericardial effusions. *N Engl J Med* 299:1113, 1978.

133. Flannery EP, Gregoratos G, Corder MP: Pericardial effusions in patients with malignant diseases. *Arch Intern Med* 135:976, 1975.

134. O'Bryan RM, Tally RW, Brennan MJ, et al: Critical analysis of the control of malignant effusion with radioisotopes. *Henry Ford Hosp Med J* 16:3, 1968.

135. Casciato DA, Lowitz BB: *Manual of Clinical Oncology.* Boston, Little, Brown, 1988, p 444.

136. Hill GJ, Cohen BI: Pleural pericardial window for palliation of cardiac tamponade due to cancer. *Cancer* 26:81, 1970.

137. Matthews MJ: Problems in morphology and behavior of bronchopulmonary malignant disease, in Chahanian P (ed): *Lung Cancer: Natural History, Prognosis and Therapy.* New York, Academic, 1976, p 28.

138. Barek L, Lautin R, Ledor S, et al: Role of CT in the assessment of superior vena cava obstruction. *J Comput Tomogr* 6:121, 1982.

Index

Index